MATERNAL·FETAL MEDICINE

Principles and Practice

Third Edition

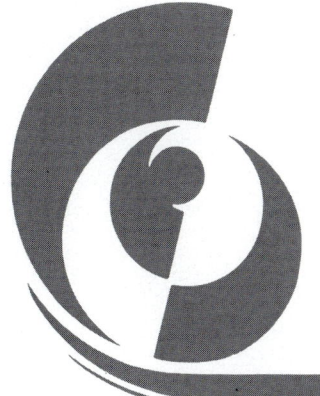

MATERNAL·FETAL MEDICINE

Principles and Practice

ROBERT K. CREASY, M.D.

Chairman and Emma Sue Hightower
Professor of Obstetrics, Gynecology,
and Reproductive Medicine
University of Texas
Houston, Texas

ROBERT RESNIK, M.D.

Professor and Chairman
Department of Reproductive Medicine
University of California, San Diego
San Diego, California

W.B. SAUNDERS COMPANY
A Division of Harcourt Brace & Company
Philadelphia, London, Toronto, Montreal, Sydney, Tokyo

W.B. SAUNDERS COMPANY
A Division of
Harcourt Brace & Company

The Curtis Center
Independence Square West
Philadelphia, Pennsylvania 19106

Library of Congress Cataloging-in-Publication Data

Maternal-fetal medicine : principles and practice / [edited by]
Robert K. Creasy, Robert Resnik.—3rd ed.

    p.   cm.

Includes bibliographical references and index.

ISBN 0–7216–6590–X

1. Obstetrics.   2. Perinatology.   I. Creasy, Robert K.   II. Resnik, Robert.
    [DNLM: 1. Embryology.   2. Fetal Diseases.   3. Pregnancy Complications.   4. Prenatal
    Diagnosis.   WQ 211 M425]

RG526.M34 1994   618.2—dc20

DNLM/DLC   92–48215

MATERNAL-FETAL MEDICINE   ISBN 0–7216–6590–X

Printed in the United States of America.

Last digit is the print number: 9   8   7   6   5   4   3

For
Judy and Lauren
and
Michelle, Bob, Andrew, and Jamie
with love and gratitude—for everything

CONTRIBUTORS

BARBARA ABRAMS, Dr.P.H., R.D.

Associate Professor, School of Public Health, University of California, Berkeley; Assistant Professor, Department of Obstetrics, Gynecology and Reproductive Sciences, University of California, San Francisco, San Francisco, California.

Maternal Nutrition

MICHAEL J. AMINOFF, M.D., FRCP

Professor of Neurology, School of Medicine, University of California, San Francisco School of Medicine; Attending Neurologist, University of California Medical Center, San Francisco, San Francisco, California.

Neurologic Disorders

ROBERT L. ANDRES, M.D.

Assistant Professor, Division of Maternal-Fetal Medicine, Department of Obstetrics, Gynecology and Reproductive Sciences, University of Texas Medical School at Houston; Attending Physician, Hermann Hospital and Lyndon Baines Johnson Hospital, Houston, Texas.

Social and Illicit Drug Use in Pregnancy

KURT BENIRSCHKE, M.D.

Professor of Pathology and Reproductive Medicine, University of California, San Diego; University of California Medical Center, San Diego, California.

Normal Development; Multiple Gestation: Incidence, Etiology, and Inheritance

RICHARD L. BERKOWITZ, M.D.

Professor and Chairman, Department of Obstetrics, Gynecology, and Reproductive Science, Mount Sinai School of Medicine; Chief of Obstetrics and Gynecology, The Mount Sinai Hospital, New York, New York.

Fetal Blood Sampling

MICHAEL L. BERMAN, M.D.

Professor, Department of Obstetrics and Gynecology, University of California, Irvine College of Medicine, Irvine, California.

Pelvic Malignancies, Gestational Trophoblastic Neoplasia, and Nonpelvic Malignancies

WATSON A. BOWES, Jr., M.D.

Professor, Department of Obstetrics and Gynecology, School of Medicine, University of North Carolina-Chapel Hill; Attending Staff, University of North Carolina Hospitals, Chapel Hill, North Carolina.

Clinical Aspects of Normal and Abnormal Labor

JOHN M. BOWMAN, O.C., M.D., CRCP, FRSC

Professor of Pediatrics and Child Health and Professor of Obstetrics, Gynecology, and Reproductive Sciences, Faculty of Medicine, University of Manitoba; Active Staff, Department of Pediatrics and Child Health, Children's Hospital and Women's Hospital; Director of the Rh Laboratory, Health Sciences Centre, Winnipeg, Manitoba, Canada.

Hemolytic Disease (Erythroblastosis Fetalis)

PETER C. BOYLAN, M.B., FRCOG

Master, National Maternity Hospital, Dublin, Ireland.

Fetal Acid-Base Balance

ROBERT A. BRACE, Ph.D.

Professor of Reproductive Medicine, University of California, San Diego School of Medicine, La Jolla, California.

Amniotic Fluid Dynamics

D. WARE BRANCH, M.D.

Associate Professor, University of Utah School of Medicine; Full-Time Staff, University of Utah Hospital, Salt Lake City, Utah.

The Immunology of Pregnancy; Immunologic Disorders

GERARD N. BURROW, M.D.

Dean and Professor of Internal Medicine, Yale University School of Medicine; Attending Staff, Yale–New Haven Hospital, New Haven, Connecticut.

Thyroid Disease and Pregnancy

TIMOTHY C. CAHILL, M.S.

Associate Specialist and Coordinator, Molecular Diagnostic Laboratory, Division of Medical Genetics, University of California, San Diego, School of Medicine, La Jolla, California.

Basic Genetics and Patterns of Inheritance

JOHN R. G. CHALLIS, Ph.D., D.Sc.

Professor, Departments of Obstetrics and Gynecology and Physiology, University of Western Ontario; Director, M.R.C. Group in Fetal and Neonatal Health and Development; Director, Lawson Research Institute; Vice-President, Research, St. Joseph's Health Centre, London, Ontario, Canada.

Characteristics of Parturition

JOSHUA A. COPEL, M.D.

Associate Professor of Obstetrics and Gynecology, Yale University School of Medicine; Director of Obstetrics and Chief of Maternal-Fetal Medicine, Yale-New Haven Hospital, New Haven, Connecticut.

Prenatal Diagnosis of Structural Heart Disease; Fetal Cardiac Arrhythmias: Diagnosis and Therapy

ROBERT K. CREASY, M.D.

Emma Sue Hightower Professor of Obstetrics, Gynecology, and Reproductive Sciences, University of Texas Medical School; Chairman, Department of Obstetrics, Gynecology and Reproductive Sciences, University of Texas Health Science Center at Houston; Chief, Obstetrics and Gynecology, Hermann Hospital; Physician-in-Chief, Obstetrics and Gynecology, Lyndon Baines Johnson Hospital, Houston, Texas.

Preterm Labor and Delivery; Intrauterine Growth Restriction; Cardiovascular and Renal Adaptation to Pregnancy

JOHN M. DAVISON, M.D., FRCOG

Professor of Obstetric Medicine and Consultant in Obstetrics and Gynaecology, Department of Obstetrics and Gynaecology, University of Newcastle upon Tyne, Newcastle upon Tyne, United Kingdom.

Renal Disorders

MICHAEL de SWIET, M.D., FRCP

Academic Sub Dean, Institute of Obstetrics, Royal Postgraduate Medical School, University of London; Consultant Physician at Queen Charlotte's and Chelsea Hospitals for Women, University College Hospital, Northwick Park Hospital, London, England.

Pulmonary Disorders; Rheumatologic and Connective Tissue Disorders

PHILIP J. DiSAIA, M.D.

Professor, Department of Obstetrics and Gynecology, University of California, Irvine College of Medicine; Attending Staff, University of California, Irvine Medical Center, Irvine, California.

Pelvic Malignancies, Gestational Trophoblastic Neoplasia, and Nonpelvic Malignancies

SHERMAN ELIAS, M.D.

Professor and Director, Division of Reproductive Genetics, Department of Obstetrics and Gynecology; Professor and Associate Chairman for Academic Affairs and Research, University of Tennessee, Memphis, Tennessee.

Prenatal Diagnosis of Genetic Disorders

ELIZABETH ANN FAGAN, M.Sc., M.D., MRCP

Honorary Senior Lecturer in Medicine, Royal Free Hospital and School of Medicine, London University; Wellcome Senior Graduate Research Fellow and Honorary Senior Lecturer in Medicine, Royal Free Hospital School of Medicine, London, England.

Diseases of Liver, Biliary System, and Pancreas

AVROY A. FANAROFF, M.B. (Rand), FRCPE

Professor of Pediatrics and Reproductive Biology, Case Western Reserve University; Director of Neonatology, Rainbow Babies and Childrens Hospital, University Hospital, Cleveland, Ohio.

Identification and Management of High-Risk Problems in the Neonate

ALAN W. FLAKE, M.D.

Assistant Professor of Surgery and Pediatrics, University of California, San Francisco School of Medicine; Active Staff, University of California, San Francisco Hospitals, San Francisco, California.

Fetal Therapy: Medical and Surgical Approaches

ROBERT GAGNON, M.D.

Associate Professor, Department of Obstetrics and Gynecology, University of Western Ontario; Active Teaching Staff, St. Joseph's Health Centre, London, Ontario, Canada.

Fetal Breathing and Body Movements

THOMAS J. GARITE, M.D.

Professor and Chairman, Department of Obstetrics and Gynecology, University of California, Irvine College of Medicine, Irvine, California.

Premature Rupture of the Membranes

RONALD S. GIBBS, M.D.

Professor and Chairman, Department of Obstetrics and Gynecology, University of Colorado School of Medicine, Denver, Colorado.

Maternal and Fetal Infections: Clinical Disorders

WILLIAM M. GILBERT, M.D.

Assistant Professor of Reproductive Medicine, Division of Perinatal Medicine, University of California, San Diego; Attending Staff, University of California, San Diego Medical Center, San Diego, California.

Disorders of Amniotic Fluid

J. CHRISTOPHER GLANTZ, M.D.

Assistant Professor of Obstetrics and Gynecology, Division of Maternal-Fetal Medicine, University of Rochester School of Medicine and Dentistry, Rochester, New York.

Significance of Amniotic Fluid Meconium

ROBERT H. GLASS, M.D.

Professor of Obstetrics, Gynecology and Reproductive Sciences, University of California, San Francisco School of Medicine; Attending Staff, University of California, San Francisco Hospitals and Clinics, San Francisco, California.

Gamete Transport, Fertilization, and Implantation; Recurrent Abortion

MITCHELL S. GOLBUS, M.D.

Professor of Obstetrics, Gynecology and Reproductive Sciences, University of California, San Francisco School of Medicine; Attending Staff, University of California, San Francisco Hospitals and Clinics, San Francisco, California.

Recurrent Abortion

BERNARD GONIK, M.D.

Associate Professor, Division of Maternal-Fetal Medicine, Department of Obstetrics, Gynecology and Reproductive Sciences, University of Texas Medical School at Houston; Active Staff, Hermann Hospital and Lyndon Baines Johnson General Hospital, Houston, Texas.

Intensive Care Monitoring of the Critically Ill Pregnant Patient

JAMES R. GREEN, M.D.*

Associate Clinical Professor, Obstetrics, Gynecology and Reproductive Sciences, University of California, San Francisco; Chief of Obstetrics, San Francisco General Hospital, San Francisco, California.

Placenta Previa and Abruptio Placentae

MICHAEL R. HARRISON, M.D.

Professor of Surgery and Pediatrics, Co-Director, Fetal Treatment Program, Chief, Division of Pediatric Surgery, University of California, San Francisco School of Medicine; Attending Staff, University of California, San Francisco Hospitals and Clinics, San Francisco, California.

Fetal Therapy: Medical and Surgical Approaches

MICHAEL A. HEYMANN, M.D.

Professor of Pediatrics and Obstetrics, Gynecology and Reproductive Sciences, Senior Staff Member, Cardiovascular Research Institute, University of California, San Francisco; Attending Physician, University of California Hospitals, San Francisco, California.

Fetal Cardiovascular Physiology

GABOR HUSZAR, M.D.

Senior Research Scientist, Department of Obstetrics and Gynecology, Yale University School of Medicine, New Haven, Connecticut.

Physiology of the Myometrium

ALAN H. JOBE, M.D., Ph.D.

Professor of Pediatrics, University of California, Los Angeles School of Medicine; Director of Perinatal Research, Harbor-UCLA Medical Center, Torrance, California.

Fetal Lung Development, Tests for Maturation, Induction of Maturation, and Treatment

KENNETH L. JONES, M.D.

Professor of Pediatrics, University of California, San Diego School of Medicine, La Jolla; Attending Physician, University of California, San Diego Medical Center, San Diego, California.

Effects of Therapeutic, Diagnostic, and Environmental Agents; Social and Illicit Drug Use in Pregnancy

OLIVER W. JONES, M.D.

Professor of Medicine/Pediatrics and Director, Division of Medical Genetics, University of California, San Diego (UCSD) School of Medicine; Attending Physician, UCSD Medical Center, La Jolla, California.

Basic Genetics and Patterns of Inheritance

ROBERT E. JORDON, M.D.

Professor and Chairman, Department of Dermatology, University of Texas Medical School at Houston; Active Staff, Hermann Hospital and Lyndon Baines Johnson General Hospital; Consultant, M.D. Anderson Cancer Center and St. Luke's Episcopal Hospital, Houston, Texas.

The Skin and Pregnancy

. . . .

*Dr. Green died in March 1993.

CHARLES S. KLEINMAN, M.D.

Professor of Pediatrics, Diagnostic Imaging, and Obstetrics and Gynecology, Yale University School of Medicine; Chief, Pediatric Cardiology, Yale-New Haven Hospital, New Haven, Connecticut.

Prenatal Diagnosis of Structural Heart Disease; Fetal Cardiac Arrhythmias: Diagnosis and Therapy

RUSSELL K. LAROS, Jr., M.D.

Professor, Department of Obstetrics, Gynecology and Reproductive Sciences, University of California, San Francisco; Chief of Obstetrics, Moffitt-Long Hospital, San Francisco, California.

Thromboembolic Disease; Maternal Hematologic Disorders

MARSHALL D. LINDHEIMER, M.D., FACP

Professor of Medicine and Obstetrics and Gynecology, University of Chicago's Pritzker School of Medicine; Director, Medical High-Risk Obstetrics Clinic, Chicago Lying-In Hospital; Attending Staff, University of Chicago Hospital and Clinics, Chicago, Illinois.

Renal Disorders

LAUREN LYNCH, M.D.

Associate Professor and Director of Maternal-Fetal Medicine Fellowship, Department of Obstetrics, Gynecology, and Reproductive Science, Mount Sinai School of Medicine; Assistant Attending, Obstetrics and Gynecology, The Mount Sinai Hospital, New York, New York.

Fetal Blood Sampling

ALASTAIR H. MacLENNAN, M.D., M.B.Ch.B., FRCOG, FRACOG

Associate Professor, Department of Obstetrics and Gynaecology, University of Adelaide; Senior Visiting Medical Specialist, Women and Children's Hospital, Adelaide, South Australia.

Multiple Gestation: Clinical Characteristics and Management

FRANK A. MANNING, M.D., M.Sc.(UXON), FRCS (Canada), FRCOG, FSOGC

Professor and Chairman, Department of Obstetrics and Gynecology, Faculty of Medicine, University of Manitoba; Head, Department of Obstetrics and Gynecology, Health Sciences Centre, Winnipeg, Manitoba, Canada.

General Principles and Applications of Ultrasonography; Fetal Biophysical Assessment by Ultrasound

RICHARD J. MARTIN, M.D.

Professor of Pediatrics and Reproductive Biology, Case Western Reserve University; Co-Director of Neonatology, Rainbow Babies and Childrens Hospital, Cleveland, Ohio.

Identification and Management of High-Risk Problems in the Neonate

GIACOMO MESCHIA, M.D.

Professor of Physiology, University of Colorado School of Medicine, Denver, Colorado.

Placental Respiratory Gas Exchange and Fetal Oxygenation

MARTHA J. MILLER, M.D., Ph.D.

Associate Professor, Department of Pediatrics, Division of Neonatology, Case Western Reserve University; Rainbow Babies and Childrens Hospital, Cleveland, Ohio.

Identification and Management of High-Risk Problems in the Neonate

HOWARD L. MINKOFF, M.D.

Professor of Obstetrics and Gynecology, SUNY Health Science Center at Brooklyn, Brooklyn, New York.

Human Immunodeficiency Virus

MANJU MONGA, M.D.

Assistant Professor, Department of Obstetrics, Gynecology, and Reproductive Sciences, University of Texas Medical School at Houston; Attending Staff, Hermann Hospital and Lyndon Baines Johnson General Hospital, Houston, Texas.

Cardiovascular and Renal Adaptation to Pregnancy

THOMAS R. MOORE, M.D.

Associate Professor, University of California, San Diego School of Medicine; Director, Division of Perinatal Medicine, University Medical Center, San Diego, California.

Diabetes in Pregnancy

SHAHLA NADER, M.D.

Associate Professor, Departments of Obstetrics, Gynecology and Reproductive Sciences, and Internal Medicine, University of Texas at Houston Medical School; Attending Physician, Hermann Hospital and Lyndon Baines Johnson General Hospital, Houston, Texas.

Other Endocrine Disorders of Pregnancy

KATHLEEN P. NICHOLS, M.D.

Assistant Clinical Professor of Anesthesiology, University of California, San Diego School of Medicine, Arizona Anesthesia and Analgesia, St. Mary's Hospital, Tucson, Arizona.

Anesthetic Considerations in the Complicated Obstetric Patient

JULIAN T. PARER, M.D., Ph.D.

Professor, Department of Obstetrics, Gynecology, and Reproductive Sciences, Associate Staff, Cardiovascular Research Institute, University of California, San Francisco; Director, Maternal-Fetal Medicine Fellowship Training Program, Attending Physician, University of California San Francisco Medical Center, San Francisco, California.

Fetal Heart Rate

VALERIE M. PARISI, M.D., M.P.H.

Associate Professor of Obstetrics and Gynecology and Director, Division of Maternal-Fetal Medicine, University of Texas Medical School at Houston; Attending Staff and Obstetrical Director, Labor and Delivery at Hermann Hospital; Attending Staff, Lyndon Baines Johnson General Hospital, Houston, Texas.

Fetal Acid-Base Balance; Cervical Incompetence

RONALD P. RAPINI, M.D.

Associate Professor of Dermatology and Pathology, University of Texas Medical School at Houston; Active Staff, Hermann Hospital and Lyndon Baines Johnson General Hospital; Consultant, M.D. Anderson Cancer Center, Houston, Texas.

The Skin and Pregnancy

ROBERT W. REBAR, M.D.

Professor and Director, Department of Obstetrics and Gynecology, University of Cincinnati College of Medicine; Attending Physician, University Hospital, Good Samaritan Hospital, Children's Hospital, Cincinnati, Ohio.

The Breast and the Physiology of Lactation

LAURENCE S. REISNER, M.D.

Professor and Vice Chairman, Department of Anesthesiology, Professor of Clinical Anesthesiology and Reproductive Medicine, University of California, San Diego School of Medicine; Director of Obstetric Anesthesia, University of California, San Diego Medical Center, San Diego, California.

Anesthetic Considerations in the Complicated Obstetric Patient

ROBERT RESNIK, M.D.

Professor and Chairman, Department of Reproductive Medicine, University of California, San Diego School of Medicine; Chief, Department of Obstetrics and Gynecology, University of California Medical Center, San Diego, California.

Anatomic Alterations in the Reproductive Tract; The Puerperium; Post-Term Pregnancy; Intrauterine Growth Restriction

BRYAN S. RICHARDSON, M.D.

Associate Professor, Department of Obstetrics and Gynecology and Department of Physiology, University of Western Ontario; Active Teaching Staff, St. Joseph's Health Centre; Consulting Staff, University Hospital, London, Ontario, Canada.

Fetal Breathing and Body Movements

JAMES M. ROBERTS, M.D.

Professor and Vice Chairman (Research), Department of Obstetrics, Gynecology and Reproductive Sciences, University of Pittsburgh; Director, Magee-Womens Research Institute, Pittsburgh, Pennsylvania.

Pregnancy-Related Hypertension

JAMES R. SCOTT, M.D.

Professor and Chairman, Department of Obstetrics and Gynecology, University of Utah School of Medicine; Chief, Obstetrics and Gynecology, University of Utah Hospital, Salt Lake City, Utah.

The Immunology of Pregnancy; Immunologic Disorders

LARRY D. SCOTT, M.D.

Professor of Medicine, Division of Gastroenterology, The University of Texas at Houston Medical School; Attending Staff, Hermann Hospital, Houston, Texas.

Gastrointestinal Disease in Pregnancy

B. LYNN SEELY, M.D.

Assistant Professor of Medicine, University of California, San Diego School of Medicine, La Jolla, California.

Thyroid Disease and Pregnancy

RALPH SHABETAI, M.D.

Professor of Medicine, University of California, San Diego School of Medicine; Chief, Cardiology Section, San Diego Veterans Administration Medical Center; Attending Cardiologist, University of California San Diego Medical Center, San Diego, California.

Cardiac Diseases

JOE LEIGH SIMPSON, M.D.

Faculty Professor and Chairman, Department of Obstetrics and Gynecology, University of Tennessee, Memphis, Memphis, Tennessee.

Prenatal Diagnosis of Genetic Disorders

RICHARD L. SWEET, M.D.

Professor and Chairman, Department of Obstetrics and Gynecology, University of Pittsburgh, Pittsburgh, Pennsylvania.

Maternal and Fetal Infections: Clinical Disorders

BRIAN TRUDINGER, M.D.

Associate Professor, University of Sydney at Westmead Hospital; Chairman, Department of Obstetrics and Gynaecology and Head, Maternal-Fetal Medicine, Westmead Hospital, Sydney, Australia.

Doppler Ultrasound Assessment of Blood Flow

ISABELLE WILKINS, M.D.

Assistant Professor, University of Texas Medical School at Houston and the Graduate School of Biomedical Sciences; Attending Staff, Hermann Hospital, Houston, Texas.

Nonimmune Hydrops

JAMES R. WOODS, Jr., M.D.

Professor of Obstetrics and Gynecology and Acting Chair, Department of Obstetrics and Gynecology, Director of Obstetrics and Maternal-Fetal Medicine, University of Rochester School of Medicine and Dentistry, Rochester, New York.

Significance of Amniotic Fluid Meconium

S. S. C. YEN, M.D., D.Sc.

Professor and W. R. Persons Chair, Department of Reproductive Medicine, University of California, San Diego, School of Medicine; Attending Physician, University of California, San Diego Medical Center, San Diego, California.

Endocrinology of Pregnancy

PREFACE

It is in many ways fulfilling to undertake the task of a third edition of this text. The need for another edition reflects the continuing progress of our knowledge base in the specialty, as well as the positive acceptance of the text by those for whom it is intended. We are indebted to the contributors of past editions both for their contributions to the progress within the field and for their role in having made the previous texts successful.

In keeping with the tradition, the goal of this edition is to delineate the basic foundation and principles upon which the practice of maternal and fetal medicine is performed. In the past four years, advances in both basic and clinical science have provided the necessity for some major revisions and for the addition of new chapters. Improved methods of investigation, enhancement in experimental design and implementation, along with improved methods of analyses, have led to a firmer foundation of our practice. Indeed, it has been a stimulating process for us to observe, examine, collate, and present the new information.

Major revisions have occurred throughout the text to provide current information and strategies. In reflection of the major changes in the field, it was thought necessary to devote separate new chapters to reproductive immunology, social and illicit drug use, percutaneous umbilical blood sampling, fetal therapy, disorders of amniotic fluid, premature rupture of membranes, human immunodeficiency virus, nonimmune hydrops, and anesthesia for high-risk pregnancy. We welcome and thank all of the new contributors and also give our thanks and appreciation to those who have contributed to the text again.

We mourn the passing of Jim Green, who contributed the chapter on placenta previa and abruption to this edition, as well as the first two editions. Jim was a clinician's clinician whose wisdom, compassion, and friendship will be missed.

The challenge of staying current and abreast of the marvelous advances in maternal and fetal medicine has been a worthy one. The stimulation of the students, residents, fellows, and practitioners makes the effort rewarding and we thank them all. We particularly wish to thank our secretaries, Onetia Materre and Jennifer White, for their extra hours and efforts in helping us to keep this third edition on track. We also wish to thank our editor, Lisette Bralow, and the W.B. Saunders staff for their assistance and cooperation in seeing the project to fruition. Finally, our special gratitude to our wives and children who by their understanding enabled us to have the time to bring this edition to reality.

ROBERT K. CREASY, M.D.
ROBERT RESNIK, M.D.

CONTENTS

PART III

Maternal and Fetal Pathophysiology

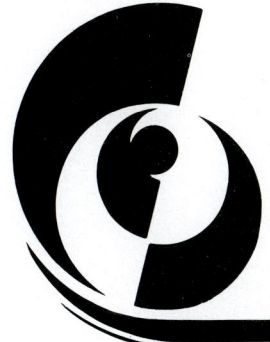

PART I

EARLY FETAL DEVELOPMENT AND THE ENVIRONMENT

REPRODUCTIVE GENETICS

CHAPTER

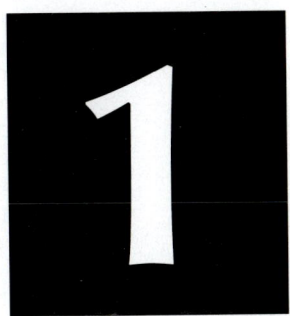

BASIC GENETICS AND PATTERNS OF INHERITANCE

OLIVER W. JONES, M.D., and TIMOTHY C. CAHILL, M.S.

GENE BIOCHEMISTRY, STRUCTURE, AND FUNCTION

Replication of Deoxyribonucleic Acid

Deoxyribonucleic acid (DNA) is the stuff of life, and after 4½ billion or so years, it is the best that processes of evolution could provide both to perpetuate and to diversify all living organisms. At some time during the evolutionary sequence, a major divergence in organic life occurred, resulting in the prokaryotes and the eukaryotes. Thus, all multicell animals, including humans, green plants, yeasts, fungi, molds, and some mammalian viruses, are composed of cells with membrane-covered central nuclei containing DNA, the genetic information. These are the eukaryotes. Prokaryotes, which include the bacterial viruses, bacteria, and the blue-green algae, have cell walls and cell membranes, but no central nucleus. The DNA molecules in these cells have no protective membrane. In general, eukaryotes contain considerably much more DNA per cell than prokaryotes. In addition, DNA in eukaryotes takes one of two forms: long, loosely coiled fibers termed *chromatin* or fibers tightly packed into rodlike structures called the *chromosomes*. In prokaryotes, DNA is constantly more chromatin-like, in that it takes the form of an extended loop within the cell. The prokaryotes, largely because of their relative simplicity and the ease in production of large quantities in short periods, have provided the research material for the remarkable amount of information biologists have learned during the past 25 years about genes and how they function. Somewhat more slowly,

knowledge about gene function in eukaryotes, especially humans, is emerging, and we are learning of the many remarkable and unique gene properties in these complex cells. In all likelihood, our knowledge of gene biology in both prokaryotes and eukaryotes will be required in order for us to understand the critical functions of each and to provide a better chance for the survival of any living organism.

With some rare exceptions, DNA in all living cells contains four chemical moieties: the nucleotides deoxyadenylic acid (dAMP), deoxythymidylic acid (dTMP), deoxycytidylic acid (dCMP), and deoxyguanylic acid (dGMP). In the DNA molecule, they are linked in linear sequence by phosphodiester bonds at the 3' or 5' position on a five-carbon sugar molecule (Fig. 1–1). This is the primary structure of DNA, a polynucleotide. All of the biological information characterizing the genetic uniqueness of the organism is determined by the sequence of nucleotides in the DNA molecule. The remarkable variability in genetic information can be exemplified by considering the number of different nucleotide sequences possible in the average mammalian gene, which is 1000 nucleotides in length. The variation in nucleotide sequences possible in a gene this size is 10^{600} (Szekely, 1980). Thus, the key to conservation of genetic information is precise replication of nucleotide sequences in DNA molecules. The catalyst for this type of reaction is called DNA polymerase. Kornberg and associates (1960) were the first to discover an enzyme that polymerized deoxyribonucleotides in a specific way in the bacterium *Escherichia coli* and that is capable *in vitro* of synthesizing a polynucleotide strand complementary to a DNA tem-

3

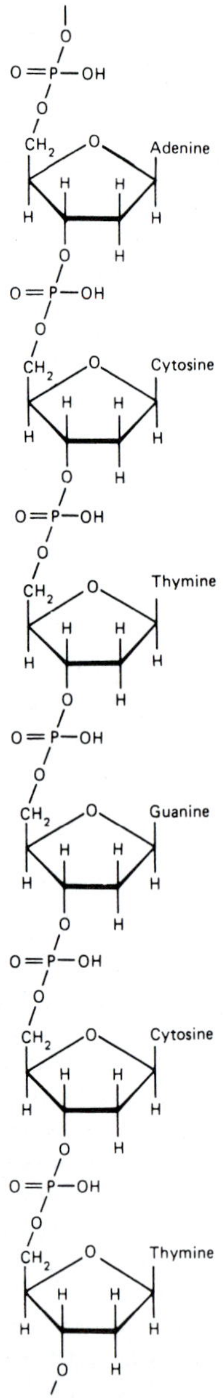

T or G—C) can occur. Thus, the number of A residues in DNA should equal the number of T residues, and the number of C residues should equal the number of G residues. This has proved to be the case, and as a result, the Watson and Crick double-helical structure of DNA can be considered diagrammatically as shown in Figure 1–2. This molecule is strictly complementary; the nucleotide sequence in one strand determines the sequence in the other. The implication is obvious: Each DNA strand serves as a template for a new complementary daughter strand, so that two new DNA molecules identical to the parent helical molecule are produced. This is a fundamental biological principle in molecular genetics. In the double helix, the two strands are parallel, but the direction is antiparallel (note that the 3' end of the molecule is complementary to the 5' end). The molecular structure of the gene is remarkable in its simplicity, but the mechanism for precise replication of the primary structure numerous times for generation after generation is quite complex and as yet not understood.

In order for replication to occur, the DNA complementary strands must separate to form replication forks. All available evidence to date suggests that for replication, DNA polymerase requires a small "primer" polynucleotide fragment. Using the chromosome of *E. coli* as a model for DNA replication shows the process to be complex and precise. Since

FIGURE 1–1. Chemical structure of a portion of a polydeoxyribonucleotide molecule (DNA) in single-strand form. Genetic information is determined by the sequence of bases, e.g., adenine, cytosine, thymine, guanine, in the polynucleotide strand. A single human gene has approximately 1000 bases in the polynucleotide. (From Szekely M: From DNA to Protein: Transfer of Genetic Information. Copyright © 1980, John Wiley & Sons, Inc. Reprinted by permission of John Wiley & Sons, Inc.)

plate. Single-strand DNA in circular form is a common chromosomal structure for many prokaryote cells, but in higher organisms, including humans, DNA molecules are double-stranded, and regions of the molecule may be circular. Two strands of DNA can be held together by hydrogen bonds, but among the nucleotides found in most DNA molecules, only complementary pairs adenine (A) and thymine (T) or guanine (G) and cytosine (C) form stable hydrogen bonds. Moreover, for the formation of a stable helical structure, only pairing between a purine and a pyrimidine (A—

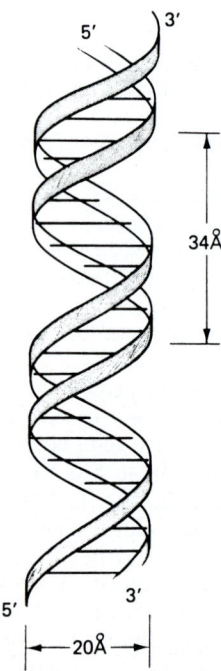

FIGURE 1–2. A diagrammatic presentation of the double-helical structure of a DNA molecule. One angstrom (Å) = 10^{-8} cm. The width of the double helix is 20 Å, and the length of one full turn is 34 Å. A sugar-phosphate linkage forms the backbone of the molecule and is aligned in an antiparallel direction. The base pairs (*horizontal lines*) hold the two strands together and are perpendicular to the axis of the double helix. (From Szekely M: From DNA to Protein: Transfer of Genetic Information. Copyright © 1980, John Wiley & Sons, Inc. Reprinted by permission of John Wiley & Sons, Inc.)

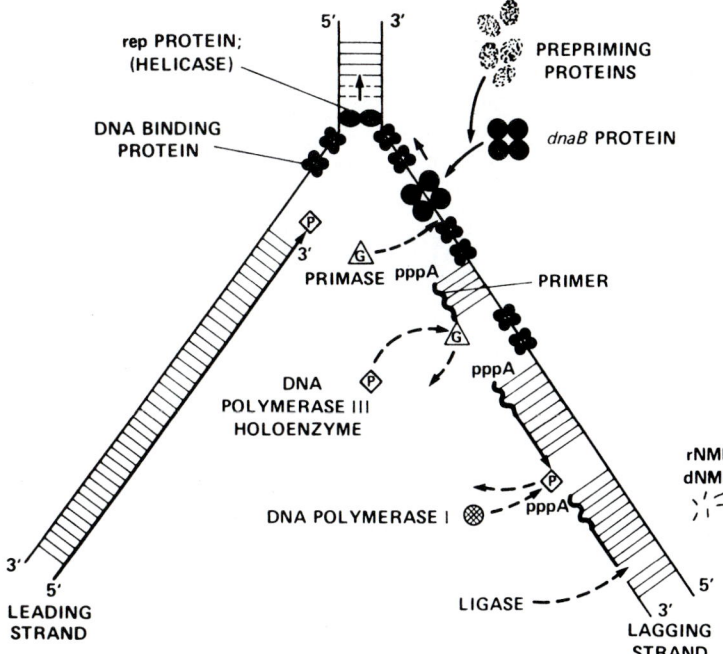

FIGURE 1–3. A model for the replication fork in the chromosome of *E. coli*. *rNMP* and *dNMP* represent ribonucleotide monophosphate and deoxyribonucleotide monophosphate molecules. *pppa* indicates the base adenine, linked to phosphate residues. (From Kornberg A: Aspects of DNA replication. Cold Spring Harbor Symposia on Quantitative Biology, **43**:1, 1978.)

Kornberg's discovery of DNA polymerase, now known as DNA polymerase I (DNA poly I), DNA polymerases II and III have been described. Currently, it is believed that the DNA poly III holoenzyme is mainly responsible for the polymerization process, and that poly I is involved in the DNA molecule maturation process as well as in DNA repair. The role of DNA poly II is poorly understood but may be related to alternative mechanisms for polymerization. As shown diagrammatically in Figure 1–3, the complementary strands of the chromosome (DNA molecule) separate under the influence of DNA binding proteins, which also stabilize the single-strand form of DNA for its template function (Kornberg, 1978). The enzyme helicase separates the strands and makes it possible for DNA poly III to catalyze continuous DNA replication of this single strand with growth in the 5'—3' direction. The opposite strand becomes a template for discontinuous DNA synthesis. Prepriming proteins become the dnaB protein, which binds to the single-strand DNA polynucleotide. The enzyme primase initiates synthesis of a very short segment of ribonucleotides or deoxyribonucleotides, the Okazaki fragments (Okazaki et al., 1969). These segments form a primer for extension of the polynucleotide by DNA poly III holoenzyme. The dnaB protein moves progressively in a 5'—3' direction, thus following the progress of the replication fork. Primase makes successive but discontinuous initiations of the lagging strand. The ribonucleic acid (RNA) and deoxyribonucleic acid (DNA) hybrid primers are removed, the gaps are filled by DNA poly I and 3'-hydroxyl, and 5'-phosphoryl ends are brought to closely adjacent positions. Another enzyme, DNA ligase, seals the ends, and a new progeny double helix is complete. This description, shown in Figure 1–3, suggests a replication fork starting at one end of the DNA duplex.

It is not an absolute requirement, for as shown in Figure 1–4, bidirectional replication of DNA can be initiated at any point on the molecule. Unwinding may start anywhere, but DNA synthesis will be both continuous and discontinuous, and to date it appears that DNA polymerase requires prior synthesis of small primer chains in order to initiate replication of the parent duplex. This is in contrast to the synthesis of messenger RNA, in which the enzyme RNA polymerase can scan the entire DNA molecule to transcribe selected segments into RNA without primers. The

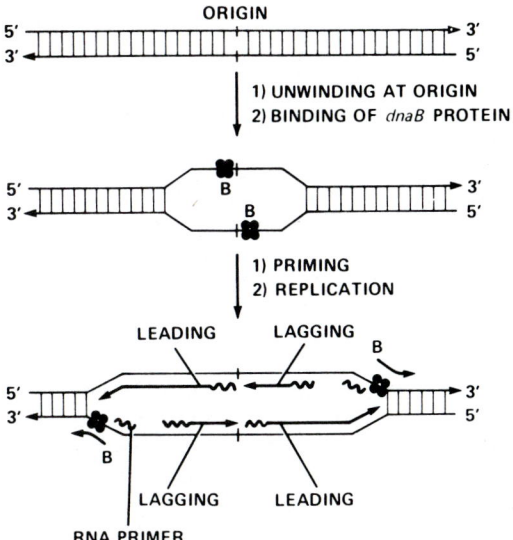

FIGURE 1–4. Model for role of dnaB protein in priming bidirectional DNA replication at chromosomal origin of replication. (From Kornberg A: Aspects of DNA replication. Cold Spring Harbor Symposia on Quantitative Biology, 1978.)

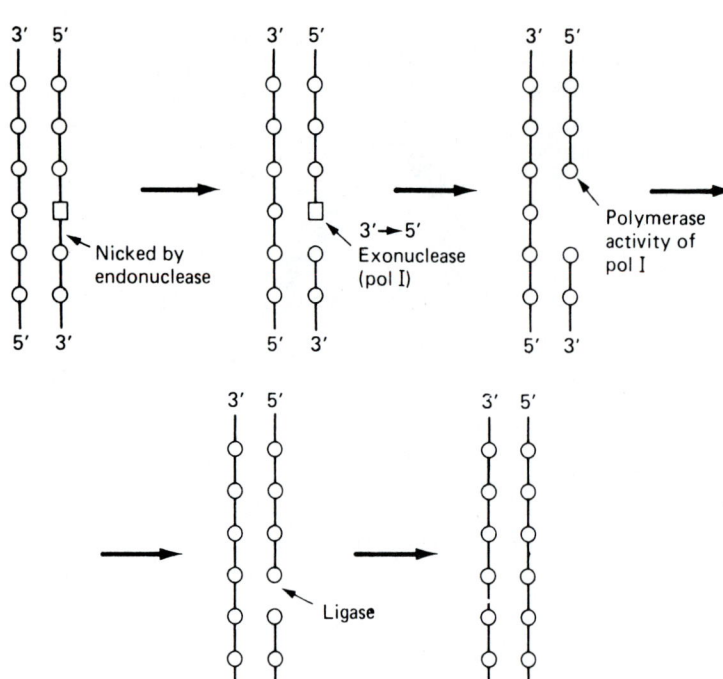

FIGURE 1–5. An illustrative model of DNA repair by DNA polymerase I and ligase. □ = site at which a mismatched nucleotide has been inserted into the polynucleotide strand. (From Szekely, M: From DNA to Protein: Transfer of Genetic Information. Copyright © 1980, John Wiley & Sons, Inc. Reprinted by permission of John Wiley & Sons, Inc.)

accuracy of replication is remarkable, but errors *in vivo* can occur. For example, hydrogen bonds can form between bases other than A—T and G—C, and so polymerases have some built-in mechanism to recognize only the properly matched bases. Nonetheless, the frequency of copying errors is estimated at approximately 10^{-8} to 10^{-9}. It is obviously to our advantage that evolution has provided a mechanism to ensure very high accuracy in replication of genetic material. In addition to the ability of the DNA polymerases to select only the proper nucleotides, there is a "proofreading" ability that can repair errors in replication. For example, when an incorrect nucleotide is inserted, an exonuclease function of DNA poly III can remove the nucleotide; then, functioning as a polymerase, DNA poly III can replace the improper base with the correct one. Other defects (mutations) can occur in the polynucleotide chain owing to chemicals or ultraviolet irradiation, i.e., thymine dimer (Fig. 1–5). When this error is noted, an endonuclease makes a "nick" in the double-strand molecule. The exonuclease property of DNA poly I removes a short sequence of nucleotides, including the damaged portion, and then its polymerase property inserts the proper nucleotides in the damaged region. Finally, polynucleotide ligase seals the "nick" by restoring the 3' and 5' phosphodiester linkage, and the repair is complete. Defects in the repair mechanism in humans may be found in genetic disorders, such as xeroderma pigmentosa, Fanconi's anemia, and ataxia and telangiectasia.

The Transcription Process

The Central Dogma, proposed by Crick in 1958, and modified in 1970 to account for the variable routes of

information transfer seen in certain viruses (Fig. 1–6), defines the fundamental transfer of biological information from a DNA polynucleotide molecule to its final product, a biologically functioning protein molecule. There is a mechanism whereby information in the DNA gene is transcribed into a variety of ribonucleotide (RNA) molecules, which perform important roles in the overall process of protein synthesis. One product of transcription is messenger RNA (mRNA). In one phase of this process, involving the enzyme RNA polymerase, mRNA is simply copied from a single strand of the DNA template. Thus, the ribonucleotides in mRNA are determined by the sequence and base-pairing with deoxyribonucleotides in the DNA strand. In addition, there must be a code system in this information transfer, so that genetic information determines the sequence of amino acids in the protein molecule through the mRNA intermediary.

This genetic code was "broken" after a period of intense research activity from several different labo-

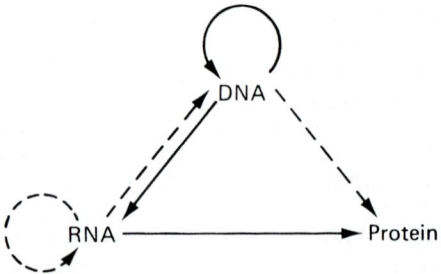

FIGURE 1–6. Routes of information transfer permitted by the Central Dogma. (From Szekely M: From DNA to Protein: Transfer of Genetic Information. Copyright © 1980, John Wiley & Sons, Inc. Reprinted by permission of John Wiley & Sons, Inc.)

Second letter

First letter	U	C	A	G	Third letter
U	UUU ⎫ phe UUC ⎭ UUA ⎫ leu UUG ⎭	UCU ⎫ UCC ⎬ ser UCA ⎪ UCG ⎭	UAU ⎫ tyr UAC ⎭ UAA ⎫ ter* UAG ⎭	UGU ⎫ cys UGC ⎭ UGA ter* UGG trp	U C A G
C	CUU ⎫ CUC ⎬ leu CUA ⎪ CUG ⎭	CCU ⎫ CCC ⎬ pro CCA ⎪ CCG ⎭	CAU ⎫ his CAC ⎭ CAA ⎫ gln CAG ⎭	CGU ⎫ CGC ⎬ arg CGA ⎪ CGG ⎭	U C A G
A	AUU ⎫ AUC ⎬ ile AUA ⎪ AUG met	ACU ⎫ ACC ⎬ thr ACA ⎪ ACG ⎭	AAU ⎫ asn AAC ⎭ AAA ⎫ lys AAG ⎭	AGU ⎫ ser AGC ⎭ AGA ⎫ arg AGG ⎭	U C A G
G	GUU ⎫ GUC ⎬ val GUA ⎪ GUG ⎭	GCU ⎫ GCC ⎬ ala GCA ⎪ GCG ⎭	GAU ⎫ asp GAC ⎭ GAA ⎫ glu GAG ⎭	GGU ⎫ GGC ⎬ gly GGA ⎪ GGG ⎭	U C A G

FIGURE 1–7. The genetic code. The letters *U, C, A,* and *G* correspond to the nucleotide bases in DNA. The three triplets *UAA, UAG,* and *UGA* with no amino acid allocated to them are nonsense codons providing termination of the polypeptide chain.

ratories in the 1960s (Fig. 1–7). Because DNA and mRNA contain only four different nucleotides each, and there are 20 or so known amino acids, some numerical combination of nucleotides should code for one amino acid. A triplet genetic codeword—a sequence of three nucleotides in DNA templating three complementary nucleotides in mRNA coding for a single amino acid—would provide more than 20 codewords. As seen in Figure 1–7, there are 64 codewords that thus far appear to be universal in all living organisms. This overabundance of triplet codewords (*codons*) suggested that the genetic code might be "degenerate," i.e., in which a given amino acid might have more than one codon. Alternatively, there could be several "nonsense" codons in the genetic dictionary that would not code for any amino acids. The latter possibility is less appealing, because the existence of a large number of nonsense codons would minimize flexibility in the primary structure of mRNA. We have been able to determine that the genetic code is largely degenerate, with only three nonsense codons that signal termination of protein synthesis. The initial discovery by Nirenberg and Matthaei (1961) opened the way for deciphering the genetic code; this finding was subsequently confirmed by several independent studies. There is little punctuation in the code; the reading begins with one codon and proceeds with each codon in succession. Thus, it has been shown in some instances that different "reading frames" can produce two different messages from the same nucleotide sequence (Fig. 1–8). Any mutation producing a "nonsense" codon will end protein synthesis at that point and yield incomplete proteins. Codons AUG and GUG define initiation sites for translation of mRNA. In addition, AUG codes for methionine and GUG codes for valine. These two codons represent the only "ambiguity" in the genetic code.

Protein Synthesis

Ribosomes are the sites for protein synthesis in all organisms. The early studies on protein synthesis gave a rather simplistic view of ribosomes and their precise function in protein synthesis. As expected, the more we have learned about these molecules, the more complex their function seems to be. A ribosome contains 50 to 70 proteins and three to four RNA molecules. The RNA molecules and protein are interwoven into a tightly knit structure that provides the site for polypeptide (protein) elongation. To do this, the ribosome must accommodate mRNA molecules, bind the peptidyl–transfer RNA (tRNA bound to the growing polypeptide chain at the position of insertion of the last amino acid), bind the aminoacyl–tRNA (tRNA carrying the next amino acid to be inserted), and bind to peptidyl transferase (the enzyme required for peptide bond formation between the last amino acid linked to the growing polypeptide chain and the next "incoming" amino acid). The ribosome must also recognize specific initiator sites on mRNA and "read" the message along its entire length, releasing a completed polypeptide molecule at the end of this process.

Transfer RNA (tRNA) is crucial in translation of the genetic message for protein synthesis. Transfer RNA molecules are relatively small, approximately 75 to 90 nucleotides in length. Within the molecular structure

AUGCGCGCUUCGAUAAAAAUGA

(a)	|met | arg | ala | ser | ile | lys | met |
(b)	| ala | arg | phe | asp | lys | asn |
(c)	| cys | ala | leu | arg |

FIGURE 1–8. Translation of a genetic message by three different "reading" frames. Amino acid sequences in (*a*) and (*b*) are sequences existing in proteins of bacteriophage IX 174. Different amino acid sequences in (*a*) and (*b*) are determined by the initial reading frame, AUG or GCG. In (*c*), the initial codon reading frame is UGC (cys). Thus, the fifth codon in this reading frame sequence will be UAA, which is a nonsense codon. Protein synthesis therefore will terminate at this point in (*c*). (From Szekely M: From DNA to Protein: Transfer of Genetic Information. Copyright © 1980, John Wiley & Sons, Inc. Reprinted by permission of John Wiley & Sons, Inc.)

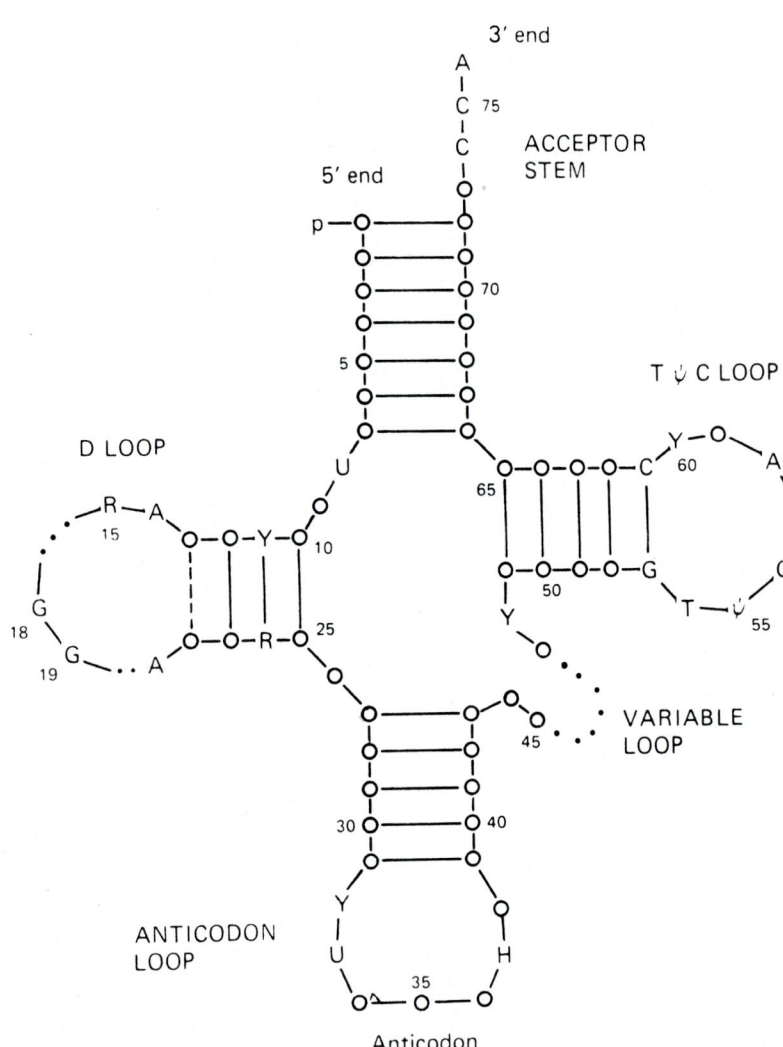

FIGURE 1–9. Generalized structure of transfer RNA (tRNA) showing invariant nucleotides. Y = pyrimidine; R = purine; H = modified purine. (Reproduced with permission from Rich A, RajBhandary UL: Transfer RNA: Molecular structure, sequence, and properties. Ann Rev Biochem **45**:805, 1976. © 1976 by Annual Reviews Inc.)

is a triplet nucleotide complementary to a codon on messenger RNA. This tRNA triplet is called the "anticodon." In addition, each tRNA molecule has a binding site specific for one amino acid; thus, each amino acid has at least one specific tRNA designed for it. There are 40 to 60 tRNA species per cell, so that, in fact, for almost every amino acid there is more than one tRNA molecule capable of binding and carrying that amino acid to its appointed destiny with the mRNA codon and the ribosome. On the other hand, the fact that there are still more triplet codewords than tRNA species suggests that some tRNA anticodons may recognize more than one codeword. An example of secondary structure of a tRNA molecule is shown in Figure 1–9, including the amino acceptor region and the anticodon site. These molecules are involved in initiation, elongation, termination, and release of the completed polypeptide chain. In particular, termination requires that a "nonsense" codon (UAA, UAG, or UGA) be "read" by the ribosome and tRNA in order for synthesis to cease. In addition, the nucleotide guanosine triphosphate (GTP) and magnesium ions are required throughout the translation process. Initiation and elongation of a polypeptide

chain are shown diagrammatically in Figure 1–10. AUG and GUG are the initiator codons on mRNA. The N-terminal is a formylated methionine residue (fMet), and the tRNA molecule, with the initiator anticodon plus the fMet molecule, constitutes a temporary peptidyl–tRNA and its binding site (P-site) on the ribosome. The A-site is the binding site for the next incoming aminoacyl–tRNA. As the next aminoacyl–tRNA (val) moves into position, elongation factors (EF–Tu) come into play, and GTP is involved in the reaction. Peptide bond formation takes place between fMet and valine. Aminoacyl–tRNA (val) now becomes the peptidyl–tRNA; the genetic message has moved along to the next codon (UUU), and the process continues. As already mentioned, termination occurs when any of the three "nonsense" codons, UAA, UAG, and UGA, is read. The final translocation from the aminoacyl to the peptidyl position must take place, and the "nonsense" codon must be read at the A-site in order for termination to occur. Release factors bind at the A-site, and hydrolysis of the bond between the polypeptide and the tRNA releases the protein molecule, which must still undergo some final post-translational changes in configuration.

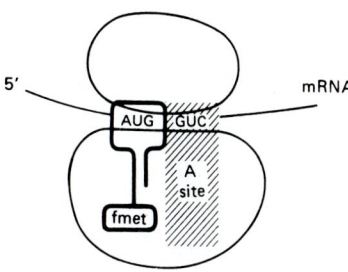

1. The A-site (shaded area) is free in the 70S initiation complex. GUC codon is present at this site

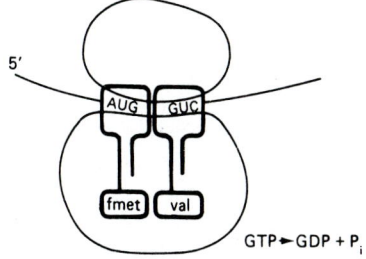

2. val–tRNA^{val} binds to A-site, by codon–anticodon annealing and interaction with ribosomal proteins. (EF–Tu involved)

GTP → GDP + P$_i$

FIGURE 1–10. Schematic representation of the events occurring in the ribosome in the process of elongation. Steps 1 to 4 lead to the incorporation of one amino acid into the peptide chain. (From Szekely M: From DNA to Protein: Transfer of Genetic Information. Copyright © 1980, John Wiley & Sons, Inc. Reprinted by permission of John Wiley & Sons, Inc.)

3. Peptide bond formation: peptidyl transferase produces fmet–val–tRNA^{val} (in A-site). Deacylated tRNA$_F^{met}$ remains in P-site

4. Translocation: deacylated initiator tRNA is replaced by peptidyl-tRNA in P-site. The A-site is free to accept the next aminoacyl–tRNA. Ribosome moved one codon further on mRNA. UUU codon is now exposed at the A-site.

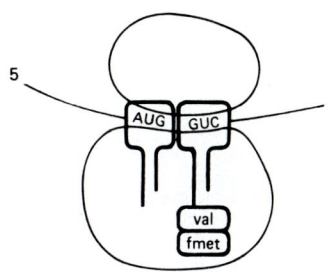

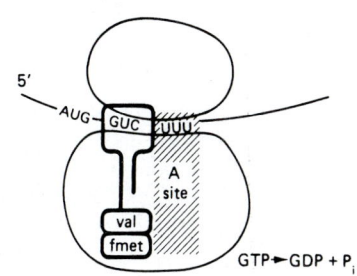

GTP → GDP + P$_i$

Organizational Structure of the Gene

Thus far, attention has been focused on the mechanisms leading to fidelity in replication of genetic information and the transfer of that information into functional proteins, most of which perform vital catalytic functions permitting not only the survival of the organism, but also growth and differentiation. Pure mature genes in humans are molecules of DNA in a double-helix form. In eukaryotes, these genes are packaged in structures called *chromosomes,* the dynamic unit of which is *chromatin,* a substance consisting of protein and DNA. The eukaryote chromosome contains a great deal of protein, which until recent years was considered a major determinant in the diversity of chromosome function. Moreover, it was anticipated that the protein constituency of the chromosome would also be quite diverse, reflecting the variable role assigned to it. Pure molecules of DNA are rather stiff structures, and so there was the added problem of how a relatively stiff linear molecule could be packaged in a membrane, the cell nucleus, which is often 200,000 times less in diameter than the length of the DNA molecule required to fit into it.

E. coli contains approximately four million base pairs of DNA. In contrast, a single mammalian somatic cell contains about five billion base pairs of DNA. An average protein consists of approximately 300 amino acids; on the basis of the triplet code, around 1000 DNA nucleotides must constitute the codon genetic information for the average protein. Accordingly, each mammalian somatic cell potentially contains information for five million different proteins, or five million genes. We know that in eukaryotes this formidable amount of genetic information is often packaged into more than one chromosome; in humans, the number is 46. In addition, it is fairly certain that for each chromosome, the genetic information is in the form of a continuous DNA molecule consisting of many functioning genes, between 1000 and 2000. Somehow, the basic genetic information embodied in DNA, together with the protein molecules cohabiting the chromosome, must solve the problem of fertilization and differentiation with absolute accuracy. To assure growth and continued development from a single fertilized egg and renewal of cells over a lifetime of many years, correct copying and expression must be accomplished billions of times. Then the process must continue repeatedly, generation after generation. During the past decade, the combined efforts of scientists in the fields of biochemistry, chemistry, and biophysics have brought about a clearer understanding of just how complex chromosomes are organized and how they function (Kornberg, 1974; Kornberg and Klug, 1981).

In mammals, chromosomes form a wide variety of shapes under specific functional conditions (Fig. 1–11). Earlier in the past decade it was known that the protein moiety of chromatin consists of a specific type of protein molecule called a *histone,* and that there are essentially five types of histones found in eukaryotic chromosomes. Approximately 20 per cent of the amino

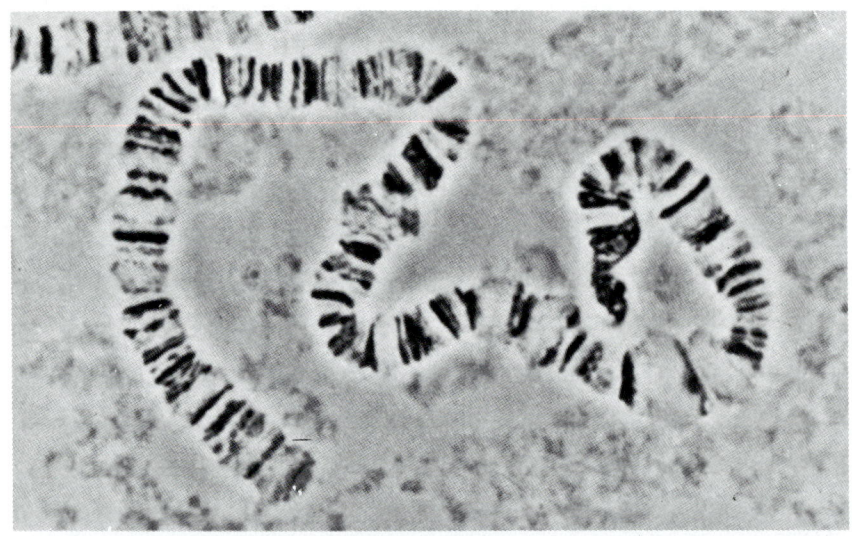

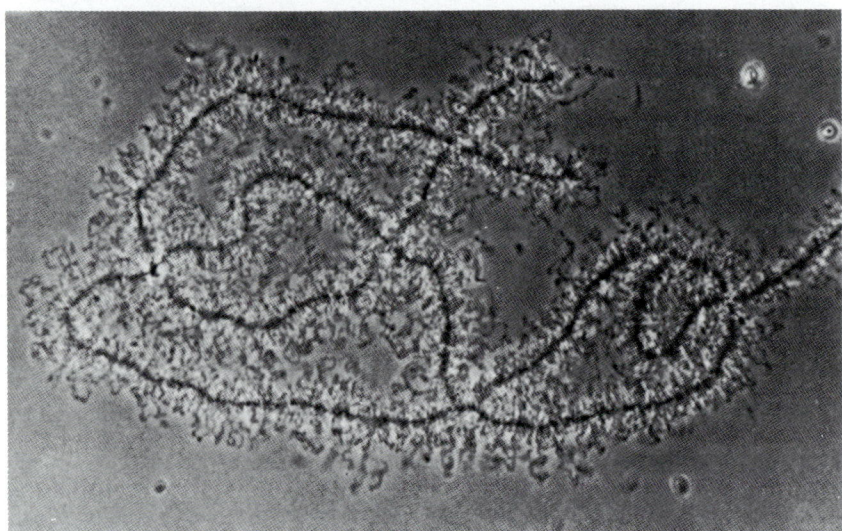

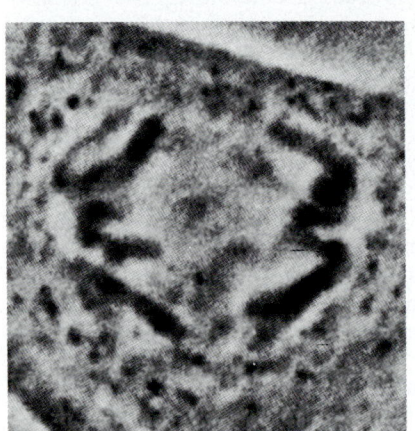
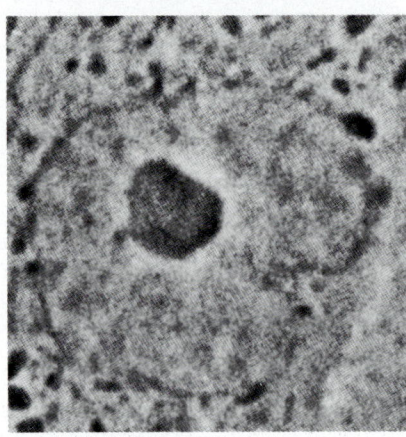

FIGURE 1–11. Various shapes of mammalian chromosomes under different functional conditions. (From Kornberg RD, Klug A: The nucleosome. Sci Am **244**:52, 1981. Copyright © 1981 by Scientific American, Inc. All rights reserved.)

acids in histones are positively charged and therefore develop an ionic interaction with negatively charged groups in DNA. X-ray diffraction studies suggested that chromatin contains a unit that regularly repeats every 100 ångströms (Å). DNA itself has no repeating units at regular 100-Å intervals, but when it combines with histones, repeating units appear. Biochemical experiments using enzymes that degrade DNA unless it is protected have led to the conclusion that chromatin consists of unprotected, bare DNA interspersed with protected regions bound to histones. Also, it has been shown that the protected regions occur at regular intervals along the DNA molecule and are approximately 200 DNA base-pairs in length. The studies of Kornberg and Klug (1981), among others, have demonstrated that the histone packages that bind to DNA at regular intervals consist of two identical tetramers (octamer), each of which can bind to about 25 nucleotide pairs of the DNA helix. These histone units have been designated H2A, H2B, H3, and H4. This putative octamer has subsequently been isolated from chromatin and has been confirmed to bind to a 200-nucleotide sequence of DNA (Kornberg and Klug, 1981). Moreover, it has been demonstrated that the DNA nucleotide strands bind on the outside of the octamer histone complex more like "strings on beads" than "beads on a string." As the 200-nucleotide sequence binds to the histone octamer, the double-helix DNA molecule forms a supercoil structure, ac-

counting for the chromatin packaging noted at regular 100-Å intervals. The fifth member of the chromatin histone family, histone 1 (H1), is located in juxtaposition to the supercoil and octamer. H1, in effect, seals off the complete structure of repeating units that have been collectively given the name *nucleosome* (Kornberg, 1974). The appearance of electron micrography of chromatin fibers in the chicken erythrocyte nucleus is demonstrated in Figure 1–12. Models of the nucleosome core and H1 function as proposed by Kornberg and Klug (1981) are shown in Figures 1–13 and 1–14. The nucleosome, the elementary subunit of the chromosome, is probably critical to the packing of DNA in the chromosome at various stages of the cell cycle. These proteins, as well as nonhistone proteins, may also be necessary in permitting uncoiling of the chromatin structure for gene replication and transcription during various stages of cell division, and perhaps differentiation. The histones may permit transcription of certain genes and not others at specific times in the life of the organism. Histones also influence sensitivity of DNA to nucleases, which may play an important role in viability of the organism, including aging.

The details remain shadowy and perplexing, but currently a perspective of the eukaryotic chromosome is emerging. Human chromosomes have the potential information for some five million genes, although most estimates of the actual number of functioning genes are closer to 100,000. The nucleosome is a

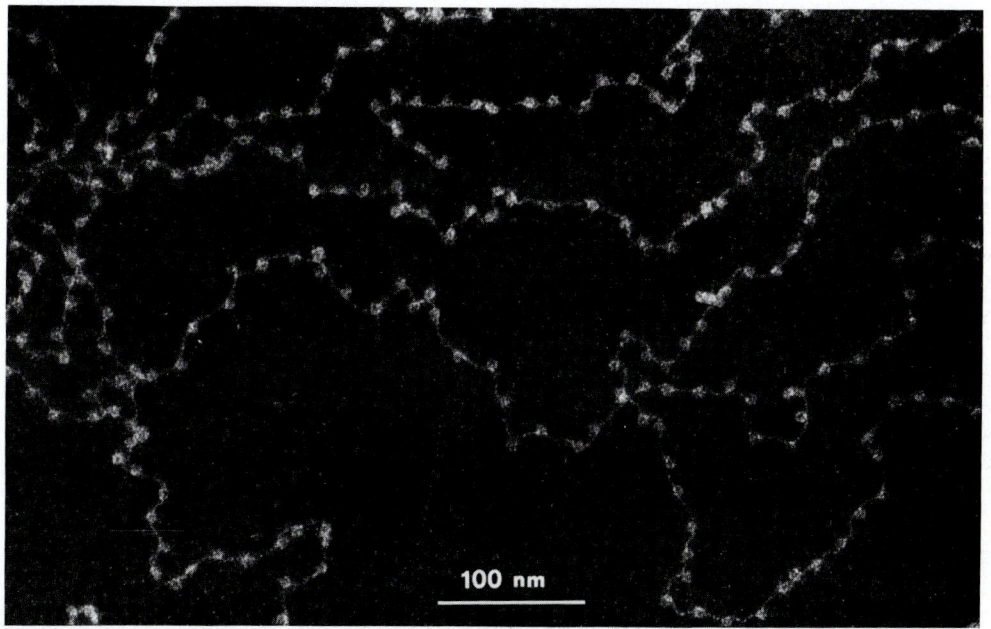

FIGURE 1–12. A darkfield electron micrograph of the edge of a chicken erythrocyte nucleus. The freshly isolated nuclei were gently suspended in 0.2 M KCl, then diluted 1:100 with 0.2 mM EDTA. After 10 minutes of swelling the solution was made 0.9% HCHO, and centrifuged through 10% HCHO pH 7 onto a glowed carbon-coated grid. The grid was washed in dilute Kodak Photo-flo, drained on the edge of bibulous paper, dried, stained for 30 seconds with 0.1% uranyl acetate, drained, and dried again (260,000X). (Courtesy of Dr. Ada L. Olins and Dr. Donald E. Olins.) (From Kornberg RD, Klug A: The nucleosome. Sci Am **244**:52, 1981. Copyright © 1981 by Scientific American, Inc. All rights reserved.)

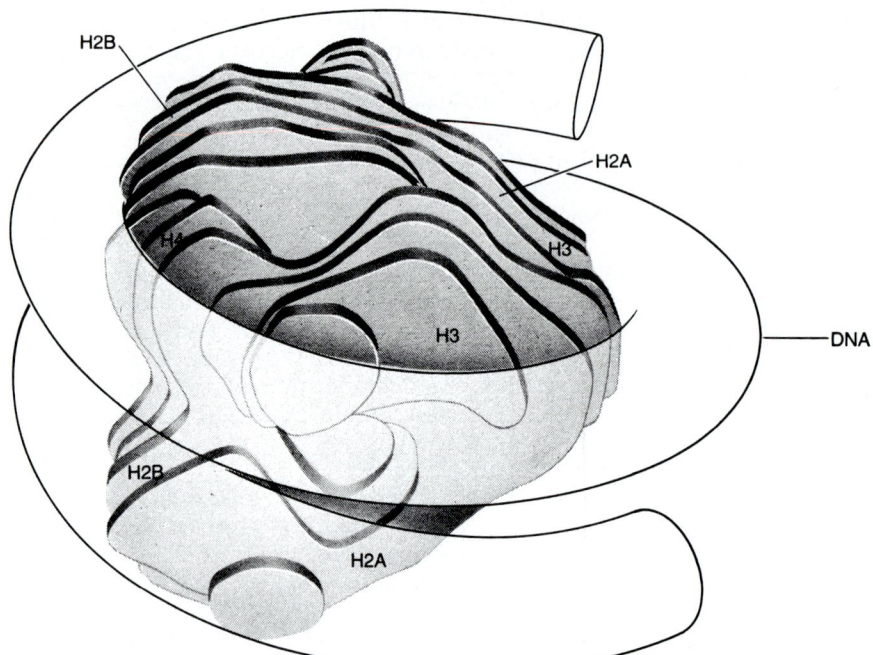

FIGURE 1–13. This model of nucleosome core was made by winding a tube simulating the DNA superhelix on a model of the histone octamer, which was built from a three-dimensional map derived from electron micrographs of the histone octamer. The ridges on the periphery of the octamer form a more or less continuous helical ramp on which a 146-nucleotide-pair length of DNA can be wound. The locations of the individual histone molecules (whose boundaries are not defined at this resolution) are proposed here on the basis of chemical crosslinking data. (From Kornberg RD, Klug A: The nucleosome. Sci Am **244**:52, 1981. Copyright © 1981 by Scientific American, Inc. All rights reserved.)

FIGURE 1–14. Role of the fifth histone, H1, is suggested by this model of the full nucleosome rather than the core particle. Two full turns (166 nucleotide pairs) of the DNA superhelix are wound on the histone octamer, represented schematically in this drawing as a drum-like object. The H1 molecule (whose actual shape is not yet known) is attached to sites on the particle at which DNA enters and leaves the nucleosome; in effect the H1 "seals off" the complete nucleosome. (From Kornberg RD, Klug A: The nucleosome. Sci Am **244**:52, 1981. Copyright © 1981 by Scientific American, Inc. All rights reserved.)

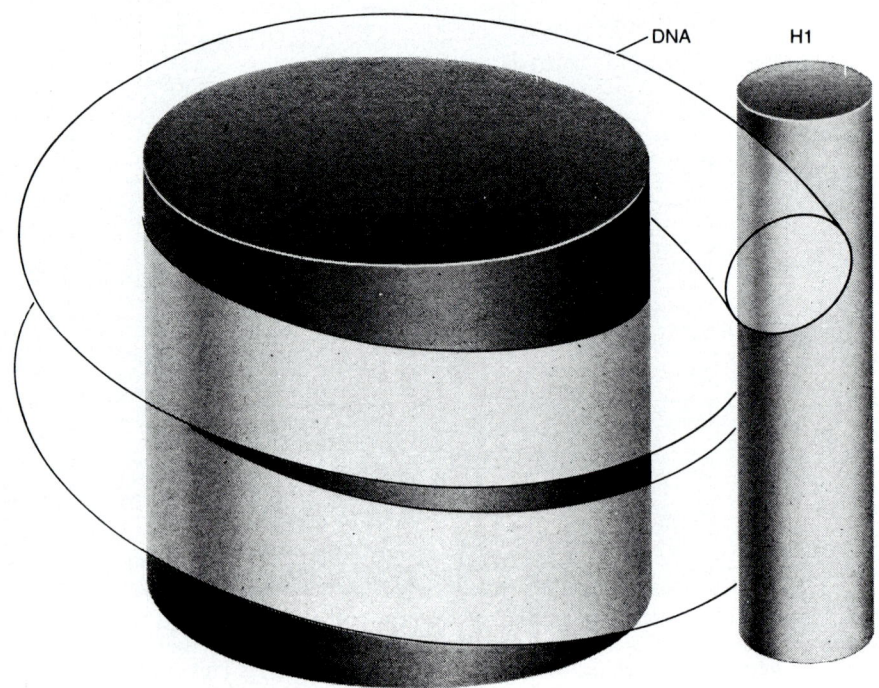

functional entity, but the role of the "linker" strand of unprotected DNA between nucleosomes and the degree of variability in "linker" length are unknown. In addition, the number of base pairs bound to the octamer histone core can vary, and its significance, too, is unknown. We do not know the mechanism for uncoiling the nucleosome for replication and transcription, nor whether some nucleosomes remain "silent" during the life of that particular organism. We also do not know the relationship of the nucleosome to regulatory regions on the gene. For some products, e.g., ribosomal RNA, there are literally hundreds of genes. Similar reiteration is seen in the multiple genes for transfer RNA. In contrast, many regions on the chromosome remain "silent"; the basis for and the control of the silent regions are unknown. Finally, the chromosomes of eukaryocytes possess DNA regions of relatively simple sequences. These regions may appear simply as alternating adenine and thymine (A—T) regions and are referred to as *satellite DNA* (not to be confused with metaphase chromosome satellites). They have also been related to constitutive heterochromatin, but certainly not all of these regions are heterochromatin. At first glance, their primary structure seems much too simple to serve as a functional gene, yet they appear too often and too consistently to be sporadic and functionless phenomena. The improving capability for DNA sequencing, and the growing use of eukaryotic cells for recombinant DNA research, increases the probability that a clear picture of the human chromosome, and its structure and function, will soon emerge.

CHROMOSOMES IN HUMANS

The Cell Cycle, Mitosis, and Meiosis

Cell Cycle

In normal mammalian somatic cells, the complete diploid set of chromosomes is duplicated, and the cell divides into two identical daughter cells approximately every 24 hours. A diagram of a characteristic cell cycle is depicted in Figure 1–15. During the G_1 phase, there is synthesis of RNA and proteins. In addition, the cell prepares for DNA replication. The S phase ushers in the period of DNA replication. Not all chromosomes are replicated at the same time, and as described previously, different segments of a given chromosome may be replicated at different intervals. During the G_2 phase, chromosome regions may be repaired, and the cell is made ready for mitosis. Both during and after replication, sister chromatid exchange may take place at regions on every chromosome. In this phenomenon, segments between two sister chromatids are exchanged repeatedly. As a result, the two chromatid arms of a mitotic chromosome have some parts of both chromatids. In the G_1 phase, as seen in Figure 1–15, DNA of every chromosome of the diploid set (2n) is present once. Between the S and G_2 phases, every chromosome doubles to become two identical polynucleotides, already referred to as sister chromatids. (One may also refer to the products of this doubling as sister chromosomes.) Thus, all DNA is now present twice ($2 \times 2n = 4n$).

Mitosis

Mitosis is shown diagrammatically in Figure 1–16. In *interphase* the somatic cell is resting. The beginning of mitosis is characterized by swelling of chromatin, which becomes visible under the light microscope by the end of *prophase*. Only two of the 46 chromosomes are shown in the schematic figure. In prophase, the two sister chromatids (chromosomes) lie closely adjacent. The nuclear membrane disappears, the nucleolus vanishes, and the spindle fibers begin to form. A protein called tubulin forms the microtubules of the spindle and connects with the centromeric region of each chromosome. After prophase, the cell is in *metaphase*; this is the important phase for cytogenetic technology, for it is in metaphase that virtually all clinical methods of examining chromosomes cause arrest of further steps in mitosis. Thus, we see all sister chromatids (4n) in a standard clinical karyotype. The centromeres of all chromosomes are located on an equatorial plane between the spindle poles. The two chromatids of each chromosome begin to separate and finally are connected only at the centromere region

FIGURE 1–15. Cell cycle of a dividing mammalian cell. In the G_1 phase, the diploid chromosome set (*2n*) is present once. After DNA synthesis (S phase), the diploid chromosome set is present in duplicate (*4n*). M = mitosis. (From Vogel F, Motulsky AG: Human Genetics: Problems and Approaches. New York, Springer-Verlag, 1979.)

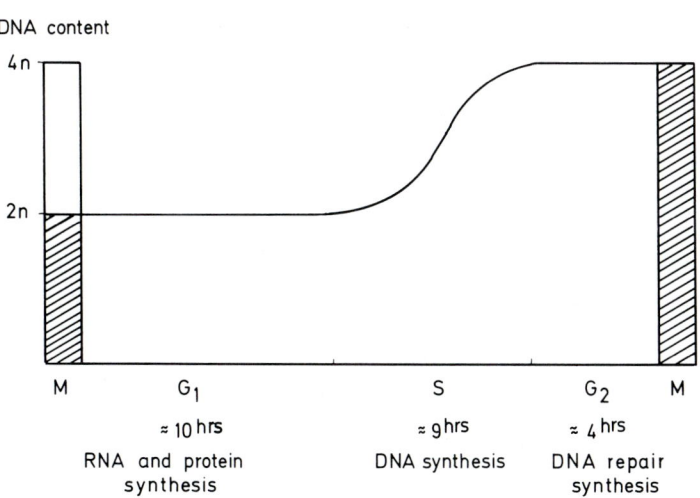

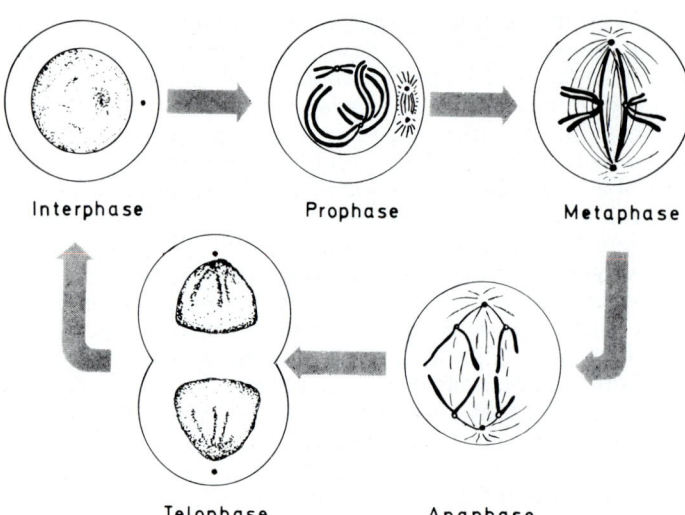

Interphase   Prophase   Metaphase

Telophase   Anaphase

FIGURE 1–16. Schematic representation of mitosis. Only two of the 46 chromosomes are present. (From Vogel F, Motulsky AG: Human Genetics: Problems and Approaches. New York, Springer-Verlag, 1979.)

(late metaphase to early *anaphase*). The centromeres then separate, and the half-chromosomes are drawn to the opposite poles by the spindle fibers. During *telophase*, chromosomes lose their visibility under the microscope, spindle fibers are degraded, tubulin is stored away for the next division, and a new nucleolus and nuclear membrane develop.

Meiosis

In mitotic cell division, the number of chromosomes remains constant for each daughter cell. In contrast,

one of the properties of meiotic cell division is the reduction in the number of chromosomes from the diploid number to the haploid number (from 46 to 23 in humans). The haploid number is found only in the germ cells; thus, following fertilization, the diploid chromosome number is restored. The selection of chromosomes from each homologous pair in the haploid cell is completely random, thereby ensuring genetic variability in each germ cell. Figure 1–17 depicts the stages of meiosis. DNA synthesis has already occurred before the first meiotic division and does not again occur during the two stages of meiotic division.

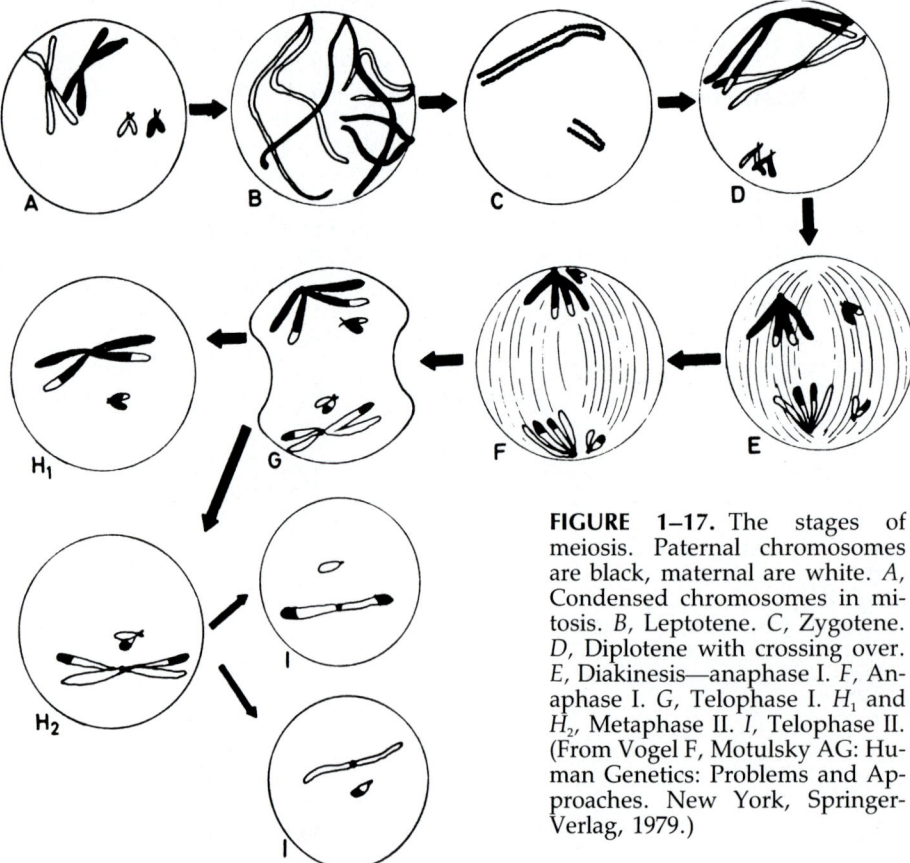

FIGURE 1–17. The stages of meiosis. Paternal chromosomes are black, maternal are white. *A*, Condensed chromosomes in mitosis. *B*, Leptotene. *C*, Zygotene. *D*, Diplotene with crossing over. *E*, Diakinesis—anaphase I. *F*, Anaphase I. *G*, Telophase I. *H₁* and *H₂*, Metaphase II. *I*, Telophase II. (From Vogel F, Motulsky AG: Human Genetics: Problems and Approaches. New York, Springer-Verlag, 1979.)

A major feature of meiotic division I is the pairing of homologous chromosomes at homologous regions, often at the chromosome ends (zygotene, Fig. 1–17C and D). The paired homologous chromosome regions are connected at a double-structured region, the synaptonemal complex. In the diplotene, four chromatids of each kind are seen in close approximation side by side (see Fig. 1–17D). Nonsister chromatids become separated, whereas the sister chromatids remain paired; the chromatid crossings (chiasmata) between nonsister chromatids can be seen (see Fig. 1–17D). The chromosomes now enter meiotic metaphase I, and during this division daughter nuclei also are formed (interkinesis; Fig. 1–17E and F). From each meiotic metaphase I, two daughter cells are formed (Fig. 1–17H_1 and H_2), and a random assortment of DNA along the chromosome has been accomplished. Meiotic division II is essentially a mitotic division of a fully copied set of haploid chromosomes. Through meiosis I, genetic information has become fourfold (2 × 2 homologous chromosomes), and after meiosis II, this genetic material is distributed to four cells as haploid chromosomes (23 in each cell). In addition to random crossing over, there also is random distribution of nonhomologous chromosomes to each of the final four haploid daughter cells. For these 23 chromosomes, the number of possible combinations in a single germ cell is 2^{23}, or 8,388,608. Thus $2^{23} \times 2^{23}$ equals the number of possible genotypes in the children of any particular combination of parents. This impressive number of variable genotypes is further enhanced by crossing

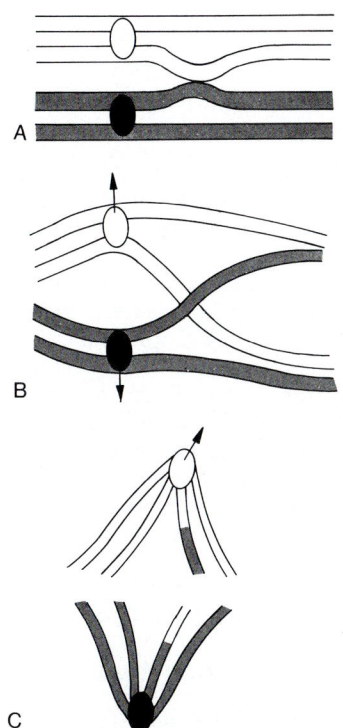

FIGURE 1–18. Crossing over and chiasma formation. *A*, Homologous chromatids are attached to each other. *B*, Crossing over with chiasma occurs. *C*, Chromatid separation occurs. (From Vogel F, Motulsky AG: Human Genetics: Problems and Approaches. New York, Springer-Verlag, 1979.)

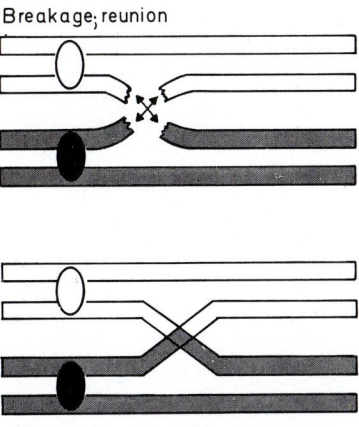

FIGURE 1–19. Breakage and reunion of nonsister chromatids in crossing over. (From Vogel F, Motulsky AG: Human Genetics: Problems and Approaches. New York, Springer-Verlag, 1979.)

over during the pairing of homologous chromosomes in meiosis I. Chiasma formation occurs as part of crossing over (Fig. 1–18). It reflects a crossing over between two nonsister chromatids and occurs through a phenomenon of breakage of nonsister chromatids at homologous points and reunion in a crosswise fashion (Fig. 1–19). Regular DNA replication is completed prior to meiosis I, but during meiotic prophase I, considerable "unscheduled" DNA replication can be detected, consistent with the repair at the breakage-reunion sites on the chromosome (Fig. 1–19).

There are crucial differences in meiosis between the two sexes. For example, in the male, meiosis is continuous in spermatocytes from puberty through adult life. After meiosis II, sperm cells acquire the ability to move effectively. The primordial fetal germ cells that produce oogonia in the female give rise to gonocytes at the same time in the male fetus. In these gonocytes, the tubules produce Ad (dark) spermatogonia as shown in Figure 1–20. During the middle of the second decade of life in males, spermatogenesis is fully established. At this point, the number of Ad spermatogonia is approximately 4.3×10^8 to 6.4×10^8 per testis, but herein lies a significant difference from cell division in oocytes. Ad spermatogonia undergo continuous divisions; during a given division one cell may produce two Ad cells, whereas another produces two Ap (pale) cells. These Ap cells develop into B spermatogonia and hence into spermatocytes that undergo meiosis (Fig. 1–20). Vogel and Rathenberg (1975) have calculated approximations of the number of cell divisions according to age. On the basis of these approximations, it can be estimated further that from embryonic age to 28 years, the number of cell divisions of human sperm is approximately 15 times greater than the number of cell divisions in the life history of an oocyte (Table 1–1).

In the primitive gonad destined to become female, the number of ovarian stem cells increases rapidly by mitotic cell division. Between the second and third months of fetal life, oocytes begin to enter meiosis (Fig. 1–21), and by the time of birth, mitosis in the female germ cells is finished, and only the two meiotic

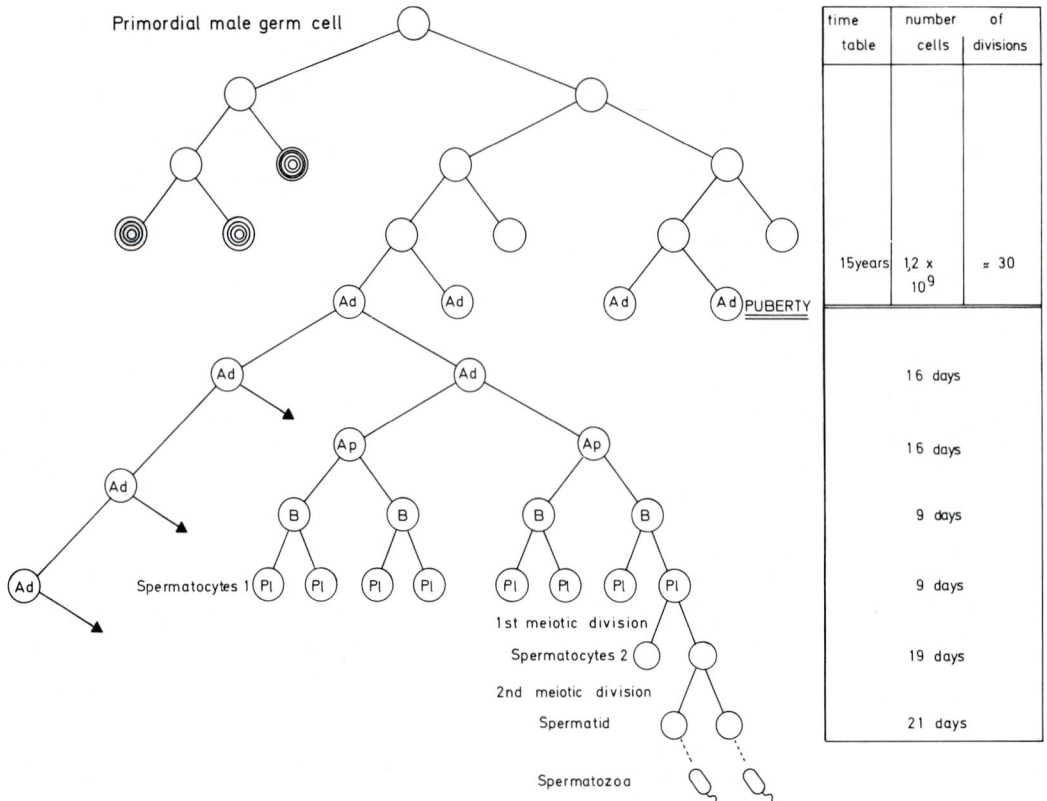

Primordial male germ cell

time table	number cells	of divisions
15years	1,2 × 10^9	≈ 30
	16 days	
	16 days	
	9 days	
	9 days	
	19 days	
	21 days	

FIGURE 1–20. Cell divisions during spermatogenesis. The overall number of cell divisions is much higher than in oogenesis. It increases with advancing age. Ad = dark spermatogonia; Ap = pale spermatogonia; B = spermatogonia; Pl = spermatocytes; concentric circles indicate cell atrophy. (From Vogel F, Motulsky AG: Human Genetics: Problems and Approaches. New York, Springer-Verlag, 1979.)

divisions remain to be fulfilled. After birth, virtually all stem cells are utilized; the oogonia either are transformed into oocytes or degenerate. Fetal germ cells increase from 6×10^5 at 2 months gestation to 6.8×10^6 during the fifth month. Decline begins at this time, to about 2×10^6 at birth. After birth in the female, meiosis remains arrested in the viable oocytes until puberty. At puberty, some oocytes start the division process again and complete meiotic metaphase II at the time of ovulation. If fertilization occurs, it does so at the time meiosis in the oocyte becomes complete. It is well known that in the female, only one of the four meiotic products develops into a mature oocyte, the other three becoming polar bodies that usually are not fertilized.

There are, then, two basic differences between meiosis in the male and meiosis in the female. They may be summarized as follows:

1. In females, one division product becomes a mature germ cell and three become polar bodies. In the male, all four meiotic products become mature germ cells.

2. In females, a low number of embryonic mitotic cell divisions occurs very early, followed by early embryonic meiotic cell division that continues to occur up to around the ninth month of gestation; division is then arrested for many years, commences again at puberty, and is completed only after fertilization. In the male, there is a much longer period of mitotic cell division, followed immediately by meiosis at puberty; meiosis is completed when spermatids develop into mature sperm.

Analysis of Human Chromosomes

Historical Aspects

The era of clinical human cytogenetics began just a little more than 30 years ago with the discovery that somatic cells in humans contain 46 chromosomes, not 48 as had previously been surmised. The utilization of a simple procedure, hypotonic treatment for spreading the chromosomes of individual cells, enabled medical scientists and physicians to study chromosomes in

TABLE 1–1.   Number of Cell Divisions in Spermatogenesis (From Embryonic Development to Meiosis)

From embryonic age to puberty	~30
Ad-type spermatogonia (one division/cycle is 16 days)	~23/year
Proliferation + maturation	4 + 2 = 6
Total	
At the age of 28	~380 divisions
At the age of 35	~540 divisions

(From Vogel F, Rathenberg R: Spontaneous mutation in man. Adv Hum Genet **5**:233, 1975.)

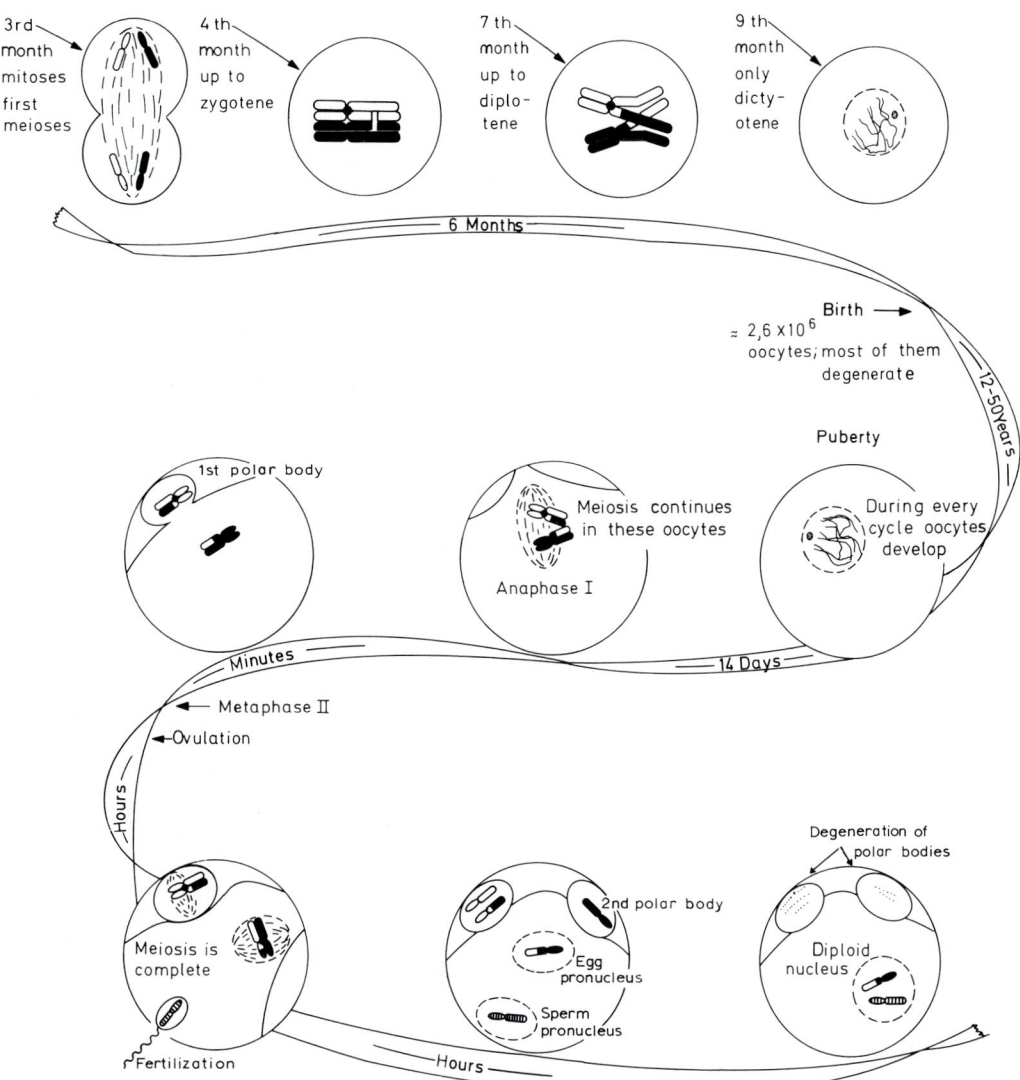

FIGURE 1–21. Meiosis in the human female. Meiosis starts after 3 months of development. During childhood, the cytoplasm of oocytes increases in volume but the nucleus remains unchanged. About 90 per cent of all oocytes degenerate at the onset of puberty. During the first half of every month the luteinizing hormone (LH) of the pituitary stimulates meiosis, which is now almost completed (end of the prophase that began during embryonic stage; metaphase I, anaphase I, telophase I, and—within a few minutes—prophase II and metaphase II). Then meiosis stops again. A few hours after metaphase I is reached, ovulation is induced by LH. Fertilization occurs in the fallopian tube. Then, the second meiotic division is complete. Nuclear membranes are formed around the maternal and paternal chromosomes. After some hours, the two "pronuclei" fuse, and the first cleavage division begins. (From Bresch C, Haussmann R: Klassiche und moleculare Genetik. 3rd ed. Berlin, Springer-Verlag, 1972.)

single cells rather than tissue sections. This new technical development ushered in the modern era of human cytogenetics. Between 1956 and 1959, new knowledge of clinical abnormalities in cytogenetics emerged at a rapid rate. In a short time, it was established that such birth defects as Down's syndrome, Turner's syndrome, Klinefelter's syndrome, Patau's syndrome, and cri du chat syndrome were in fact all abnormalities in chromosome number or structure. Many thought that this initial solution to the genetic aberration in these clinical entities would be followed for years to come by answers to many more baffling questions in clinical genetics. However, progress became frustratingly slow and uninformative. (Exceptions are investigations of other uncommon aneuploidies [variations in human metaphase chromosomes yielding more or less than the correct number of 46], the more obvious chromosome translocations, and rare genetic disorders involving increased chromosome instability.) Primarily, the problem lay in the inability to identify human metaphase chromosomes with precision. They could be spread and stained with ease, but except for size and location of the centromere relative to overall length, they all looked alike. Within major groups of chromosomes (e.g., chromosome pairs 6—12 and the X chromosomes), pairing was largely guesswork. Between 1968 and 1970, a significant technical breakthrough occurred when a group of investigators in

Denmark headed by Caspersson (1968) discovered a way to prepare metaphase chromosomes that removed virtually all ambiguity regarding the identification of each chromosome pair.

Constituency of DNA in the Human Chromosome

Characteristics of gene structure in the human chromosome are described earlier in this chapter, but additional characterization is useful to an understanding of the properties of the genetic material that give the characteristic staining patterns observed in procedures currently used in clinical and research studies.

The human genome is estimated to contain approximately 3.0×10^9 nucleotide pairs. (The *genome* is defined as the sum total of genes carried by all 46 chromosomes in the human.) Assuming that the average protein molecule contains around 300 amino acids, and recalling that the genetic code is triplet, we would expect the genome to contain five or six million genes. If all of these genes provided information for the synthesis of functional proteins, geneticists would be very nervous, because with the current mutation rate, new mutations might well accumulate in such numbers as to make normal chromosome function quite difficult. Thus, one expects to find a significant portion of the human genome remaining "silent," or in some other way nonfunctional during the lifetime of the organism, a phenomenon that occurs in humans. There are unique DNA sequences in the human genome that code for specific functional proteins; however, the genome also contains segments of highly repetitive nucleotide pairs, for example, sequences of alternating A—T regions. This material is located in the heterochromatic regions of the chromosome, largely around the centromere, and also on the long arm of the Y chromosome. In terms of length, it consists of two major sizes: short segments of 400 to 600 nucleotides alternating with unique nucleotide sequences about twice this length, and very short repetitive segments alternating with very long unique nucleotide sequences. Another subset of these repetitive sequences that have a bit more variation in their nucleotide content are classified as intermediary redundant DNA.

It has been estimated that in the human genome about 40 to 45 per cent of the DNA consists of repetitive DNA, most of which is in the intermediate redundant class, interdigitated with the unique sequences coding for functional proteins. Together, the intermediate redundant and unique nucleotide sequences compose about 80 per cent of all human DNA. The highly repetitive DNA sequences, about 6 to 10 per cent of the total genome, are relatively short, but are repeated many thousands of times.

The intermediate repetitive or redundant DNA sequences may be important in coding for ribosomal RNA. This genetic region is thought to be near the nucleolus organizer region on the short arms of the acrocentric chromosomes, numbers 13—15 and 21—22. This is a major piece of the genetic machinery in man, for it has been estimated that there are perhaps 400 to 450 genes in the human genome coding for

ribosomal RNA. Other studies have indicated that the intermediate repetitive DNA coordinates its function with the unique DNA sequences by providing the controlling mechanisms for functional protein synthesis.

In summary then, the human genome consists of 50,000 to 100,000 genes on 23 chromosome pairs. One of each pair of chromosomes is inherited from each parent. Each chromosome consists of a single DNA double helix combined with the histones into functional units, the nucleosomes, as described previously. For each chromosome, the whole DNA molecule consists of variable regions of unique nucleotide sequences coding for functional proteins, interspersed with highly repetitive and intermediate repetitive nucleotide sequences—the role of which is only partly understood at present. More often than not, these noncoding repetitive regions intervene in the coding sequence of the unique DNA. Special DNA sequences code for ribosomal and transfer RNA.

Preparation of Human Metaphase Chromosomes

Metaphase chromosomes can be prepared from any cell undergoing mitosis. During the day-to-day activity of almost any clinical or research cytogenetic laboratory, chromosome analysis will be obtained in cells derived from peripheral blood, bone marrow, amniotic fluid, skin, or other tissues in situ and in tissue cultures. For clinical cytogenetic diagnosis in living, nonleukemic individuals, metaphase cells from peripheral blood samples are the easiest to obtain. In order to obtain adequate numbers of metaphase cells from peripheral blood, mitosis must be induced artificially, and in most procedures, phytohemagglutinin, a mitogen, is used for this purpose. Specifically, T-cell lymphocytes are induced to undergo mitosis; thus, almost all chromosome analyses of human peripheral blood samples produce karyotypes of T lymphocytes. In general descriptive terms, a suspension of peripheral blood cells is incubated at 37°C in tissue culture media for 72 hours. Then the cells are incubated for 1 to 3 hours in a dilute solution of some spindle poison—colchicine or colchimid being most commonly used. Next, the chromosomes are spread in one dimension by a short treatment (10 to 30 minutes) in a hypotonic salt solution. The chromosomes are fixed in a mixture of alcohol and acetic acid, then gently spread on a glass slide for drying and staining.

Most cytogenetic laboratories currently use one or more of the staining procedures that stain each chromosome with variable intensity at specific regions, thereby providing "bands" along the chromosome; hence, the term *banding patterns*. All of the procedures are effective and provide different types of morphologic information about individual chromosomes. Most laboratories find a procedure or two that work well for them and use them for most of the routine work. For convenience in descriptive terminology, various banding patterns have been named for the methods by which they were revealed.

Some of the more commonly used methods are as follows: *G bands* are revealed by Giemsa staining in association with various other secondary steps—probably the most widely used banding technique. Quinacrine mustard and similar fluorochromes provide fluorescent staining for *Q bands*. The banding patterns are identical to those in G bands, but a fluorescence microscope is required. This was the technique used by Caspersson and colleagues (1968) to initiate the "banding era." In particular, Q banding is useful to identify the Y chromosomes in both metaphase and interphase cells. *R bands* are the result of "reverse" banding. They are produced by controlled denaturation, usually with heat. The pattern in R banding is opposite to that in G and Q banding: light bands produced on G and Q banding are dark on R banding, and dark bands on G and Q banding are light on R banding. *T bands* produce specific staining of the telomeric regions of the chromosome. *C bands* reflect constitutive heterochromatin and are located primarily on the pericentric regions of the chromosome.

Modifications and new procedures of band staining are constantly being developed. For example, a silver stain can be used to identify specifically the nucleolus organizer regions that were functionally active during the previous interphase. Other techniques enhance underlying chromosome instability and are useful in identifying certain aberrations associated with malignancies. Recent modifications of the basic culture-staining procedures have resulted in more elongated chromosomes, prophase-like in appearance, with more readily identifiable banding patterns.

The physiochemical basis for banding patterns is not fully understood, but probably involves both the protein and the nucleotide constituency of the chromosome. In terms of nucleotide composition, it has been suggested that Q bands and G bands indicate A—T–rich chromosome regions, whereas R bands indicate the G—C–rich regions. Figure 1–22 depicts the current designation for G banding on normal chromosomes. Starting from the centromeric region, each chromosome is organized into two regions: the P region (short arm) and the q region (long arm). Within each region, the area is further subdivided numerically. These numerical band designations greatly facilitate the descriptive identification of specific chromosomes. An ideogram of chromosomes 8 and 15 is shown on Figure 1–22.

Characteristics of the More Common Chromosome Aberrations in Humans

Aneuploidy

Aneuploidy is probably the chromosome abnormality most frequently seen in clinical cytogenetics. *Aneuploidy* refers to numeric abnormalities, which should be considered genome mutations. These numeric abnormalities can occur in three ways. The most significant is *nondisjunction*, which may occur in both mitosis and meiosis, but is observed more frequently in meiosis. It means simply that one pair of chromosomes fails to separate (disjoin) and is transferred in anaphase to one pole; thus, one cell will have both members of the pair, and one will have neither of that pair (Fig. 1–23). *Anaphase lag* is another event that can

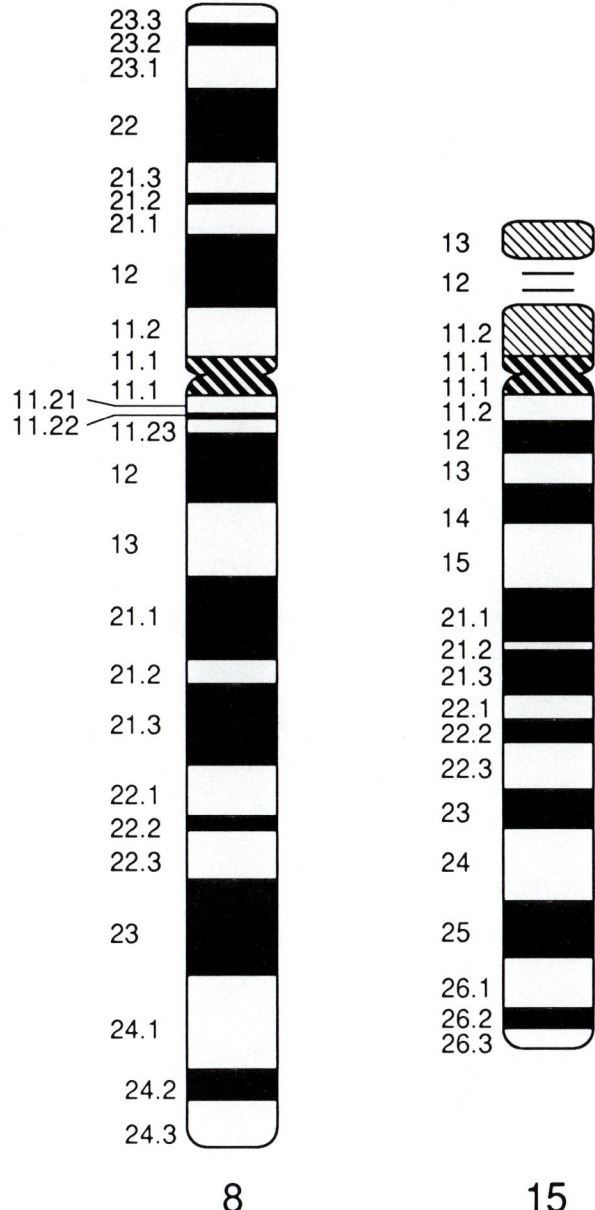

FIGURE 1–22. An ideogram of two representative chromosomes. Chromosome 8 and chromosome 15 represent arbitrary examples of schematic high-resolution, mid-metaphase Giemsa banding. At the level of resolution demonstrated in this figure, a haploid set of 23 chromosomes has a combined total of approximately 550 bands. Broad crosshatched areas represent the centromere, and the narrow crosshatched areas represent regions of variable size and staining intensity. A detailed ideogram of the entire human haploid set of chromosomes was published by the Standing Committee on Human Cytogenetic Nomenclature (1985).

lead to abnormalities in chromosome number; in this process, one chromosome of a pair does not move as rapidly during anaphase process as its sister chromosome and is lost. Often this loss leads to a mosaic cell population, one euploid and one monosomic (e.g., 45,XO/46,XX mosaicism). Finally, there is *polyploidization*. In affected fetuses, the whole genome is present

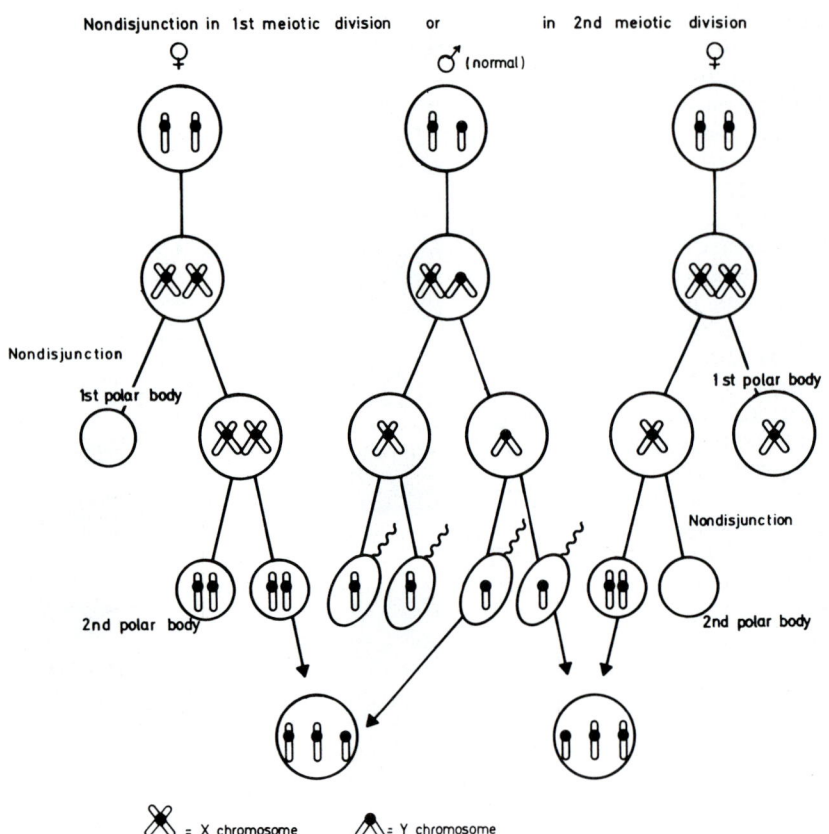

FIGURE 1–23. Nondisjunction of the X chromosome in the first and second meiotic divisions in a female. Fertilization is by a Y-bearing sperm. An XXY genotype/phenotype can result from both first and second meiotic division nondisjunction. (From Vogel F, Motulsky AG: Human Genetics: Problems and Approaches. New York, Springer-Verlag, 1979.)

more than once in every cell. When the increase is by a factor of one for each cell, the result is triploidy, with 69 chromosomes per cell.

Structural Alterations

Structural alterations in chromosomes constitute the other major group of cytogenetic abnormalities. *Deletion* may occur on the terminal segment of the short or long arm. Alternatively, a deletion may occur at some interstitial region anywhere on the chromosome. If the deleted fragment lacks a centromere, it will eventually be lost during subsequent cell division (Fig. 1–24). One example of a deletion mutation is seen in cri du chat syndrome, which results from deletion of part of the short arm of chromosome 5. A *ring chromosome* results from terminal deletions on both the short and long arms of the same chromosome (Fig. 1–25). In the process of *insertion*, an interstitial deleted segment is inserted into a nonhomologous chromosome (Fig. 1–26). A *duplication* represents an extra piece of chromosome material resulting from unequal crossing over. A deletion is the reciprocal of such an event. Duplications may be especially difficult to identify from banding patterns on metaphase chromosomes.

Inversions are another structural alteration in chromosomes. They more often involve the centromere (pericentric) rather than noncentromeric areas (paracentric). Figure 1–27 is a diagrammatic representation of a pericentric inversion. Inversions reduce pairing between homologous chromosomes. Thus, crossing over may be suppressed within inverted heterozygote

chromosomes. Because it may lead to retention within a species of multigene regions of the chromosome, this phenomenon has had some importance in genetic evolution. In order for homologous chromosomes to pair, one must form a loop in the region of the inversion (Fig. 1–28). If the inversion is pericentric, the centromere lies within the loop. When crossing over occurs, each of the two chromatids within the cross-over has both a duplication and a deletion. If gametes are formed with the abnormal chromosomes, the fetus will be monosomic for one portion of the chromosome and trisomic for another portion. One result of abnormal chromosome recombinants might be increased fetal wastage. When pericentric inversion occurs as a new mutation, usually the result is a phenotypically normal individual. However, when a carrier of a pericentric inversion reproduces, the pair-

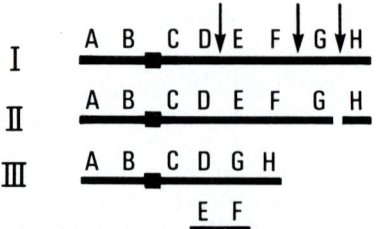

FIGURE 1–24. Diagrammatic examples of chromosome deletion; ■ indicates centromere. *I*, Arrows indicate break points. *II*, A single break at G–H produces an acentric fragment usually lost during subsequent division. *III*, Breaks at D–E and F–G produce an interstitial deletion, E–F, and reconstitution of the deleted chromosome.

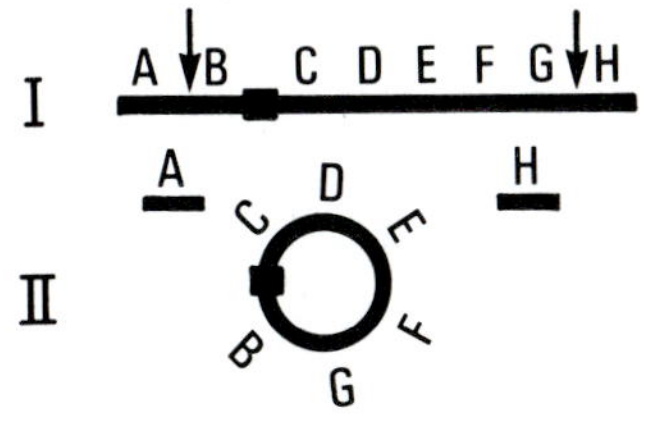

FIGURE 1–25. Diagrammatic example of a ring chromosome; ■ indicates centromere. In this example, terminal deletions A and H result in loss of these fragments and reunion of the broken chromosome ends to form a ring chromosome.

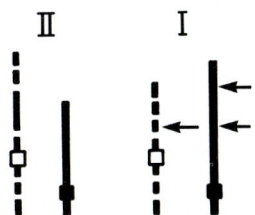

FIGURE 1–26. Diagrammatic example of an interstitial insertion. *I*, Arrows depict the break points. *II*, Deleted segment is inserted into a nonhomologous chromosome.

ing events just described may occur. If fertilization involves the abnormal gametes, there is a risk for abnormal progeny. When pericentric inversion is observed in a phenotypically abnormal child, parental karyotyping is indicated. An exception to this rule involves a pericentric inversion in chromosome 9, the most common inversion noted in humans. The author has observed an approximate 5 per cent frequency of this inversion in nearly 14,000 amniotic fluid cultures. In the 30 or so instances in which parental karyotyping was performed, invariably one or the other parent carried a pericentric inversion on one number 9 chromosome. One explanation for the apparently benign status of pericentric inversion in this chromosome could be that the pericentric region on chromosome 9 contains many highly repetitive or genetically "silent" regions in the nucleotide sequence, so that inversion in this region is of no clinical consequence. Alternatively, inversions involving relatively short DNA sequences may not be involved in crossing over.

Translocation is the most common form of chromosome structural rearrangement in humans. There are two types: reciprocal (Fig. 1–29) and Robertsonian (Fig. 1–30). If a translocation is balanced, phenotypic abnormalities are uncommon. Unbalanced translocations result in miscarriage, stillbirth or live birth with multiple malformations, developmental delay, and mental retardation. Reciprocal translocations nearly always involve nonhomologous chromosomes among any of the 23 chromosome pairs, including chromosomes X and Y. In contrast, Robertsonian translocations involve only acrocentric chromosome pairs 13, 14, 15 and 21, 22. They are joined end to end at the centromere and may be homologous, i.e., t21;21, or nonhomologous, i.e., t13;14.

Gametogenesis in heterozygous carriers of translocations is especially significant because of the increased risk for chromosome segregation which produces gametes with unbalanced chromosomes in the diploid set (Fig. 1–29). In a reciprocal translocation,

there will be four chromosomes with segments in common (Fig. 1–29). During meiosis homologous segments must match for crossing over so that in a translocation set of four a quadrivalent is formed. During meiosis I the four chromosomes may segregate randomly in two daughter cells with several results.

In 2:2 alternate segregation (Fig. 1–29), one centromere segregates to one daughter cell and the next centromere segregates to the other daughter cell. This is the only mode that leads to a normal or balanced normal karyotype. Adjacent segregation and 3:1 nondisjunction segregation all produce unbalanced gametes.

If a gamete is chromosomally unbalanced, the odds are probably increased for spontaneous abortion. In familial translocations, the risk of unbalanced progeny seems to depend on the method of ascertainment. For example, if a familial reciprocal translocation is ascertained by a chromosomally unbalanced live birth or stillbirth, the risk for subsequent chromosomally unbalanced children is approximately 15 per cent and the risk for spontaneous abortion or stillbirth is approximately 25 per cent. In contrast, if the ascertainment is unbiased, risk for chromosomally unbalanced live birth is 1 to 2 per cent, but the risk for miscarriage or stillbirth remains at 25 per cent.

There appears to be a parental sex influence on the risk for chromosomally unbalanced progeny associated with certain types of segregants. In general the risk for unbalanced progeny is higher if the female parent carries the translocation than it is with the paternal carrier. In addition, viable conceptuses are influenced by type of configuration produced during meiosis by the translocated chromosomes. In general, larger translocated fragments and more asymmetric pairing are associated with a greater likelihood for abnormal outcome of pregnancy.

Robertsonian translocation is named so in honor of an insect cytogeneticist, W. R. B. Robertson, who, in 1916, was the first to describe a translocation involving

FIGURE 1–27. An illustrative example of a possible mechanism for development of a pericentric inversion. *I*, Normal sequence of coded information on the chromosome. *II*, Formation of a loop involving a chromosome region. *III*, Breakage and reunion at the arrows, where the chromosome loop intersects itself. *IV*, Formation of the inverted information sequence after reunion.

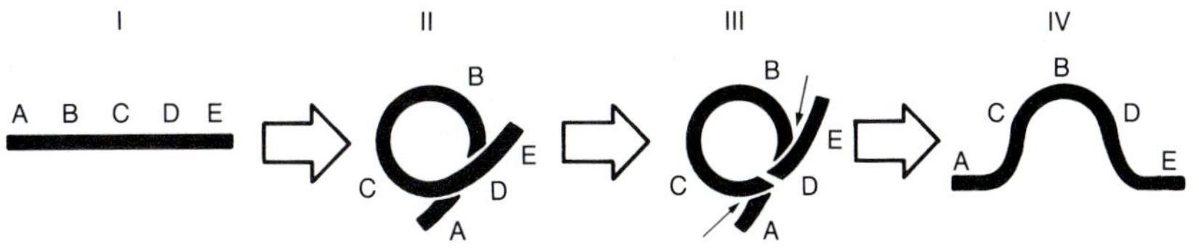

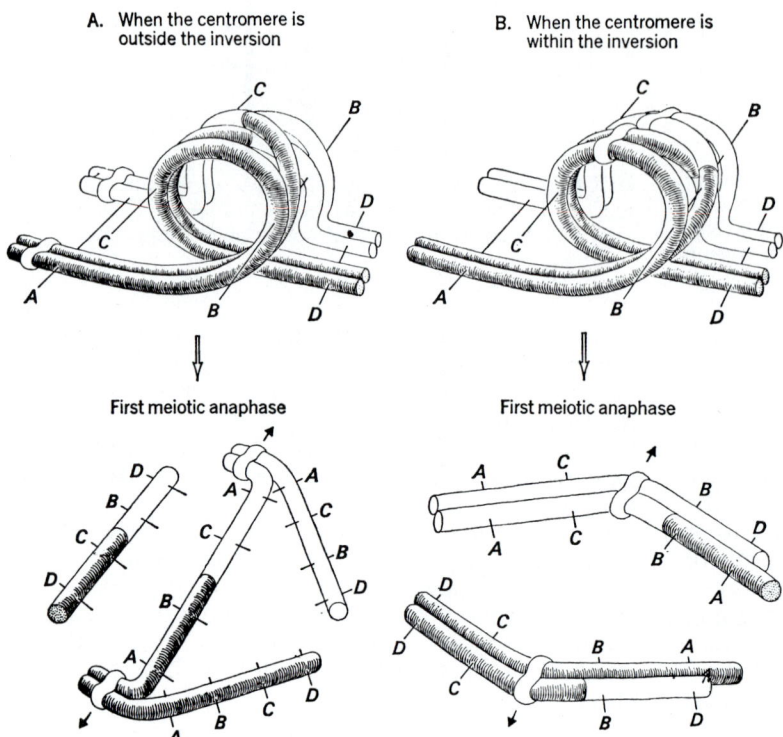

A. When the centromere is outside the inversion

B. When the centromere is within the inversion

First meiotic anaphase

First meiotic anaphase

FIGURE 1–28. Crossing over within the inversion loop of an inversion heterozygote results in aberrant chromatids with duplications or deficiencies. (From Srb AM, Owen RD, Edgar RS: General Genetics. 2nd ed. San Francisco, copyright © WH Freeman and Co, 1965. Reprinted by permission.)

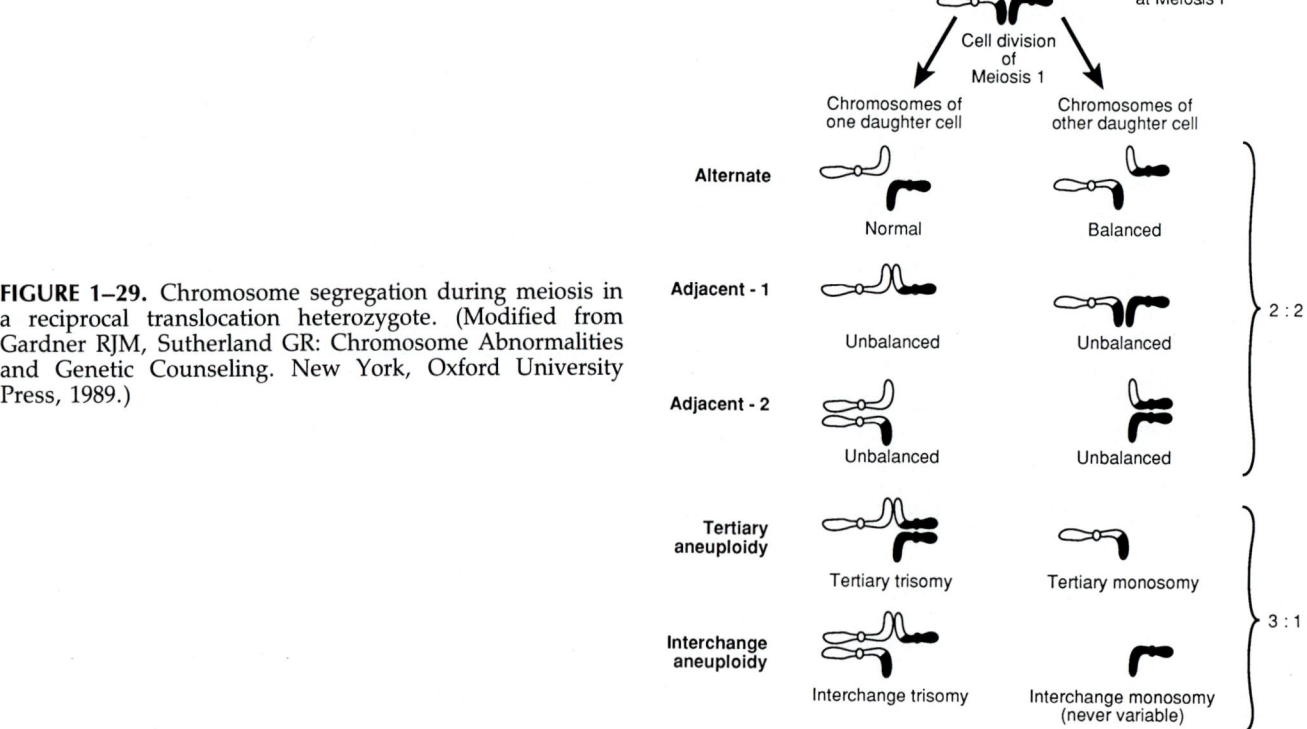

FIGURE 1–29. Chromosome segregation during meiosis in a reciprocal translocation heterozygote. (Modified from Gardner RJM, Sutherland GR: Chromosome Abnormalities and Genetic Counseling. New York, Oxford University Press, 1989.)

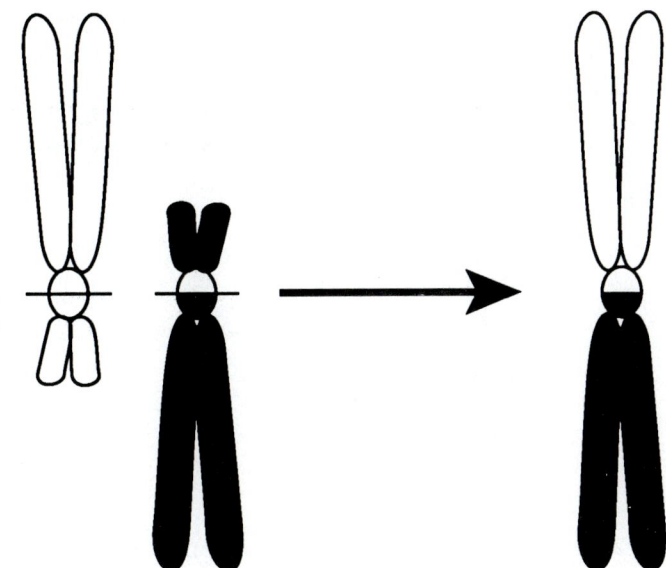

FIGURE 1–30. Formation of a centric fusion (monocentric) Robertsonian translocation. Robertsonian translocations involve only the acrocentric chromosomes.

two acrocentric chromosomes in insects. In the human karyotype, a Robertsonian translocation also involves only the acrocentric chromosomes. The Robertsonian translocation is also unique because the fusion of two acrocentric chromosomes usually involves the centromere (Fig. 1–30) or regions close to the centromere. However, reciprocal translocations may also include acrocentric chromosomes. Robertsonian translocations are nearly always nonhomologous. Most homologous Robertsonian translocations produce nonviable conceptuses. For example, translocation 14;14 would result in either trisomy 14 or monosomy 14, and both are nonviable.

The most common nonhomologous Robertsonian translocation in humans is 13;14. Approximately 80 per cent of all nonhomologous Robertsonian translocations involve chromosomes 13, 14, and 15. The next most common are translocations involving one chromosome from pairs 13, 14, and 15 and one chromosome from pairs 21 and 22.

Figure 1–31 illustrates gametogenesis in a nonho-mologous 14;21 Robertsonian translocation carrier. This illustration also represents the model for segregation during gametogenesis with any Robertsonian translocation. Translocation carriers theoretically produce six types of gametes in equal proportions. Monosomic gametes are generally nonviable as are many trisomies, for example trisomy 14 or 15. As illustrated in Figure 1–31, three gametes could result in viable conceptuses and one (B_1) could produce a liveborn, abnormal infant.

Robertsonian translocation 14;21 is the most medically significant in terms of incidence and genetic risk. In contrast, the most frequent Robertsonian translocation, 13;14, rarely produces chromosomally unbalanced progeny. Nonetheless, genetic counseling and at least consideration of prenatal diagnosis is recommended for all families with a chromosome Robertsonian or reciprocal translocation.

Isochromosome is a structural rearrangement often involving the X chromosome or, in certain forms of leukemia, chromosome 17. Abnormal division at the centromere has been offered as an explanation for the formation of an isochromosome. This explanation remains unproven. An alternative model is shown in Figure 1–32. In this model, a break occurs near the centromere in both ipsilateral short and long arms. Normal centromere division occurs in the derivative chromosome, and replication occurs as isochromosome for the short arm (p) and the long arm (q). Thus, the gametes will receive either isochromosome p or isochromosome q.

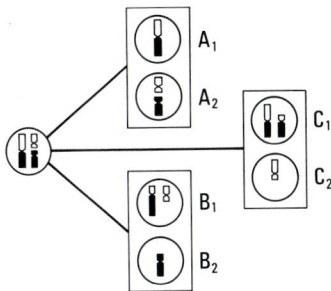

FIGURE 1–31. Gametogenesis for Robertsonian translocation. A_1 is balanced with 22 chromosomes including t(14q21q). A_2 is normal with 22 chromosomes. B_1 is abnormal with 23 chromosomes including t(14q21q) and 21. This gamete would produce an infant with Down's syndrome. B_2 is abnormal with 22 chromosomes and monosomy for chromosome 21. C_1 is abnormal with 23 chromosomes including t(14q21q) and 14. C_2 is abnormal with 22 chromosomes and no chromosome 14.

Prevalence of Chromosome Disorders in Humans

Genome mutations resulting in identifiable abnormalities in the human karyotype occur more frequently than mutations leading to mendelian hereditary disease. Tables 1–2, 1–3, and 1–4 summarize studies on incidence and mutation rates of genome

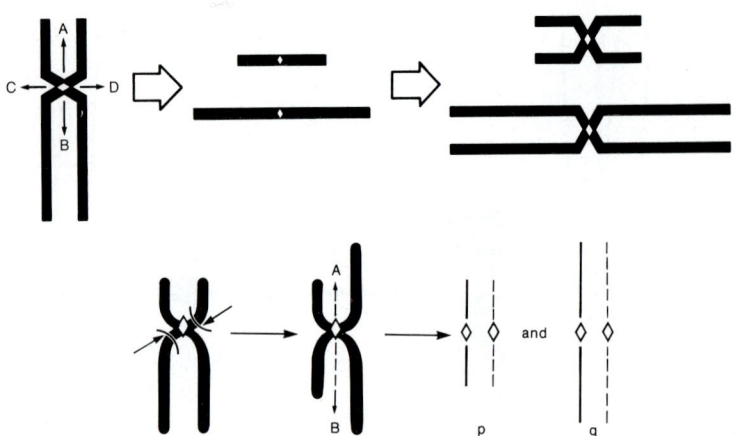

FIGURE 1–32. Alternative explanation for formation of isochromosome X. *Upper panel,* the centromere divides in plane C–D instead of normally in plane A–B. The products are metacentric chromosomes, and replication produces duplication of one arm and deficiency of the other arm of the original chromosome. *Lower panel,* two breaks, one in the short arm (p) and the other in the long arm (q), have occurred. A derivative chromosome is produced by ipsilateral chromatid exchange. The centromere divides in the normal plane. Replication produces gametes that contain isochromosome for the short arm (p) or long arm (q).

mutations (Nielsen and Silessen, 1975). Numerous studies have shown that trisomy 21 is the most common aneuploidy among liveborn humans. On the other hand, balanced reciprocal translocations occur almost as frequently. Trisomy 13 occurs at a much lower frequency than trisomy 18 or trisomy 21, owing possibly to increased fetal wastage with this mutation. Among sex chromosomes, aneuploidies 47,XYY and 47,XXY are seen in liveborn babies. Table 1–4 summarizes the mutation rate for several chromosome abnormalities. The mutation rate for most of the genome mutations, shown in Table 1–4, is nearly ten times greater than the mutation rate for genetic diseases such as achondroplasia, hemophilia A, and Duchenne muscular dystrophy. The cumulative data on genome mutations reveal an unanticipated finding. Chromosome analysis in newborns from several worldwide population samples shows the overall incidence of chromosome abnormalities to be 0.5 to 0.6 per cent. In a large study series of nearly 55,000

infants, more than two-thirds had no significant physical abnormality in association with genome mutations, and of the one-third with significant phenotype abnormalities, nearly 66 per cent had trisomy 21.

Phenotype-Genotype Correlations of Some Autosomal Abnormalities

Down's Syndrome

Down's syndrome (trisomy 21) is the most common numeric chromosome aberration in liveborn humans (Fig. 1–33). The overall incidence is one to two per 1000 live births. Physicians, nursing staff in newborn nurseries, and students nearly always make the diagnosis on the basis of physical aspects alone. The major features of the trisomy 21 phenotype and their incidence in infants are listed in Table 1–5. Hall (1966) noted at least four of these abnormalities in all of 48 newborns with Down's syndrome, and six or more in 89 per cent of them. Mental retardation is invariable. Overall the IQ ranges from 25 to 50, but the mean IQ for older patients is 24. The primary cause for early mortality is congenital heart disease, with a mortality rate of more than 40 per cent among the infants with

TABLE 1–2.   Incidence of Sex Chromosome Abnormalities in Seven Population Samples*

KARYOTYPE	TOTAL		RATE PER 1000	
47,XYY	28	} 35	0.81	} 1.02
47,XYY mosaics	7		0.20	
47,XXY	33	} 39	0.96	} 1.13
47,XXY mosaics	6		0.17	
46,XX (male)	2		0.06	
45,X/46,XY (male)	1		0.03	
			0.26	
46,X,inv(Y)	9			
45,X	2		0.10	} 0.39
45,X mosaics	6		0.29	
47,XXX	20	} 24	0.98	} 1.18
47,XXX mosaics	4		0.20	
Population samples	20,370 male 34,379 female	} 54,749		

*The samples came from Edinburgh, Ontario, Winnipeg, Boston, Moscow, and Århus, Denmark.
From Nielsen J, Silessen I: Incidence of chromosome aberrations among 11,148 newborn children. Hum Genet **30:**1, 1975.

TABLE 1–3.   Incidence of Autosomal Abnormalities (Genome and Chromosome Mutations) in 54,749 Newborns

KARYOTYPE	TOTAL	RATE PER 1000
47,+13	3	0.05
47,+18	8	0.15
47,+21	63	1.15
47,+marker chromosomes	12	0.22
47,+marker, mosaics	5	0.09
Deletions	5	0.09
Inversions	7	0.13
D/D translocations	43	0.79
D/G translocations	11	0.20
Reciprocal translocations	47	0.85
Unbalanced Y-autosomal translocations	2	0.04

Modified from Nielsen J, Silessen I: Incidence of chromosome aberrations among 11,148 newborn children. Hum Genet **30:**1, 1975.

Table 1–4. Mutation Rates for Genome Mutations Observed in Newborns

CONDITION	CALCULA-TION	MUTATION RATE
Sex chromosome trisomies		
XXY $\left.\begin{array}{c} \\ \text{including} \\ \end{array}\right\}$ XXX mosaics	$\dfrac{39}{2 \times 34{,}379}$	5.67×10^{-4}
	$\dfrac{24}{2 \times 20{,}370}$	5.89×10^{-4}
XXY and XXX together (X nondisjunction)		5.8×10^{-4}
XYY, including mosaics (Y nondisjunction)	$\dfrac{35}{2 \times 34{,}379}$	5.09×10^{-4}
Autosomal trisomies		
47, +21	$\dfrac{63}{2 \times 54{,}749}$	5.8×10^{-4}
47, +18	$\dfrac{8}{2 \times 54{,}749}$	7.3×10^{-5}
47, +13	$\dfrac{3}{2 \times 54{,}749}$	2.7×10^{-5}

Modified from Nielsen J, Silessen I: Incidence of chromosome aberrations among 11,148 newborn children. Hum Genet **30:**1, 1975.

Table 1–5. Trisomy 21: Major Phenotypic Features and Their Incidence

FEATURE	INCIDENCE (%)
Hypotonia	80
Poor Moro reflex	85
Hyperflexibility of joints	80
Excess skin on back of neck	80
Flat facial profile	90
Slant palpebral fissures	80
Anomalous auricles	60
Dysplasia of pelvis	70

cardiac lesions. Infectious disease poses a serious problem during infancy, and there is a 20-fold greater risk of developing acute leukemia during childhood. Under the best of circumstances, life expectancy is reduced. At least one large study reports a 31.1 per cent mortality rate in the first year of life, and 46 per cent by the end of the third year.

Trisomy 21 accounts for 94 per cent of all newborns with Down's syndrome. Between 1 and 2 percent have a mosaic trisomy 21/normal karyotype, and approximately 4 per cent of infants with Down's syndrome have translocations involving (1) chromosome 21 and chromosome 14 (most common), 15 (less common), or 13 (rare); (2) chromosome 21 and chromosome 22; or (3) the homologous chromosome 21. About 75 per cent of these translocations are new genome mutations and 25 per cent are familial. A rare mutation resulting in mild expression of the Down phenotype is an event producing a tandem duplication of the distal portion of the long arm of chromosome 21q21–22. Rare reciprocal translocations and tandem duplications suggest that the distal portions of the long arm on chromosome 21 are responsible for the Down phenotype. For example, when bands 21q21–22 are involved, variable expressions of the Down phenotype, including mental retardation, are observed. When band 21q21 but not q22 is involved, mental retardation is present, but most of the physical signs of Down's syndrome are absent.

Although clinical diagnosis of Down's syndrome is relatively simple, chromosomal confirmation is important, especially in mothers less than 35 years of age, because of the value of genotype confirmation to

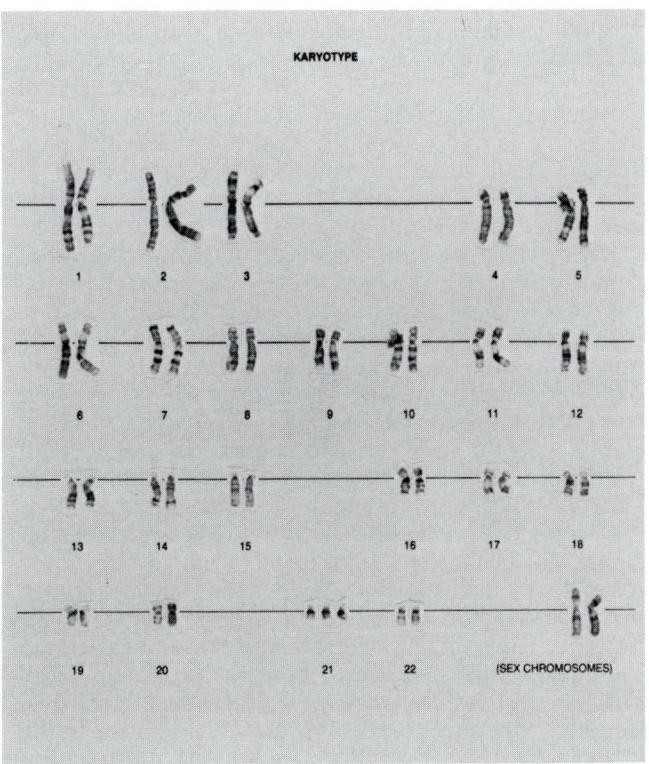

FIGURE 1–33. 47,XX, +21. A female with 47 chromosomes including trisomy 21.

Table 1–6. Frequency of Selected Chromosome Abnormalities in the Newborn

ABNORMALITY	FREQUENCY
Trisomy 21	1 in 800–1000 births
Trisomy 18	8000
Trisomy 13	20,000
XXY	1000 males
XYY	1000 males
XXX	950 females
XO	10,000 females

From Antenatal Diagnosis: Report of a Consensus Development Conference Sponsored by the National Institute of Child Health and Human Development. National Institutes of Health Publication No. 79–1973, April, 1979.

genetic counseling. An empiric recurrence risk for parents who have produced a child with trisomy 21 is estimated to be approximately 1 per cent. For parents of trisomy 21 infants, excluding the very rare parent who is mosaic at a low percentage for trisomy 21, this recurrence rate might be influenced only by increasing maternal age.

Maternal age seems to be of singular importance in relation to the incidence of Down's syndrome. Nonetheless, the source of the additional chromosome 21 in trisomy 21 is paternal approximately 25 per cent of the time. Moreover, it appears that paternal age may possibly become a significant factor by the fourth decade of life (Erickson, 1979; Steve et al., 1981). Table 1–6 summarizes the incidence of trisomy 21 in the newborn in comparison with other significant clinical aneuploidies, and Table 1–7 summarizes risks of producing liveborn trisomy 21 infants in relation to maternal age (Hook and Lindsje, 1978). As emphasized in the next section of this chapter, the incidence of all significant aneuploidies is greater when ascertained by amniocentesis at mid-trimester than by live births at term. A significant number of chromosomally abnormal fetuses identified during mid-trimester undergo spontaneous demise. For a relative comparison with the data in Table 1–7, the rate of detection of Down's syndrome fetuses at mid-trimester at a maternal age of 35 to 37 years is 0.9 per cent; 38 to 39 years, 2.7 per cent; 40 to 41 years, 3.2 per cent; 42 to 43 years, 5.6 per cent; and 44 years and older, 11 per cent (Vogel and Motulsky, 1979).

Irrespective of time of ascertainment, i.e., mid-trimester or birth, there is no question that maternal age is the most important associated factor. Age-related factors in Down's syndrome can be grouped broadly into two categories: maternal age–independent, and maternal age–dependent. The study and compilation of worldwide data by Lamson and Hook (1980) suggest one possible model consistent with incidence data. These investigators have proposed that Down's syndrome is a result of constantly accumulating biological processes. These processes continue at a constant background rate throughout the reproductive life of the female. At the time maternal age becomes a factor, the biological process is accumulating at a constant exponential rate superimposed on the background rate. Thus, both maternal age–independent and maternal age–dependent factors are continuously operative, with a progressive increase in the exponential incidence after age 30. Although experi-

mental studies of this situation are considerably fewer than those for trisomy 21, available evidence suggests that for other clinically significant trisomies—trisomy 13, trisomy 18, trisomy 9, and trisomy 8—maternal age is a significant factor. In contrast, the evidence of a higher risk for nondisjunction in very young mothers remains controversial and clearly needs more study.

The translocation form of Down's syndrome requires particular attention, although it represents just a small proportion of the total number of Down's syndrome infants born each year. Following ascertainment of a translocation form of Down's syndrome, parental chromosome analysis is imperative in order to differentiate between a familial translocation and a spontaneous genome mutation in the newborn. Obviously, the two alternatives imply different recommendations in genetic counseling. The estimate by Albright and Hook (1980), based on worldwide incidence data of Down's syndrome, is that the rate of familial translocation capable of producing Down's syndrome progeny is between 0.88 and 2.28 per cent in mothers under age 30, between 0.21 and 0.51 per cent in mothers over age 30, and between 0.47 and 1.22 per cent for all ages. The gametes that are theoretically possible when an individual carries the balanced translocation t(14;21) are summarized in Figure 1–31. The translocation t(21;22) produces a similar proportion of gametes, about one-third normal, one-third carrier, and one-third affected. If the translocation is t(21;21), progeny will be either trisomy 21 or monosomy 21 (nearly always nonviable). Numerous studies have confirmed a much lower actual number of affected liveborn than are estimated to be at risk because of a parental balanced translocation. Table 1–8 compares predicted (theoretic) outcomes with observed outcomes in progeny at risk for Down's syndrome because of parental translocation. It is pre-

Table 1–7. Risk of Giving Birth to a Down's Syndrome Infant in Relation to Maternal Age

MATERNAL AGE (YEARS)	FREQUENCY OF DOWN'S SYNDROME
30	1 in 885 births
31	826
32	725
33	592
34	465
35	365
36	287
37	225
38	176
39	139
40	109
41	85
42	67
43	53
44	41
45	32
46	25
47	20
48	16
49	12

From Hook EB, Lindsje A: Down syndrome in live births by single year maternal age interval in a Swedish study: Comparison with results from a New York State study. Am J Hum Genet **30**:19, 1978.

TABLE 1–8. Progeny of Translocation Carriers

	NORMAL	CARRIER	AFFECTED
Theoretic (if parent is a translocation carrier)	0.33	0.33	0.33
Observed			
Mother Dq Gq carrier	0.49	0.40	0.11
Father Dq Gq carrier	0.39	0.59	0.02
Mother Gq Gq carrier	0.46	0.52	0.01
Father Gq Gq carrier	0.34	0.66	—

From Thompson MW: Thompson and Thompson's Genetics in Medicine. 4th ed. Philadelphia, WB Saunders Company, 1986.

sumed that the difference between theoretic and observed rates is due to increased intrauterine loss of affected fetuses. Alternatively, there may be other prezygotic mechanisms operating that diminish the probability for fertilization or formation of an affected zygote. In any case, mid-trimester amniocentesis should be considered for pregnancies at risk for any type of parental translocation.

Trisomy 13

Figures 1–34 and 1–35 demonstrate the phenotype-genotype correlation for trisomy 13, a relatively uncommon genome mutation in humans. Approximately 50 per cent of liveborn babies with trisomy 13 will die within the first month. Nearly 20 per cent of all cases of trisomy 13 are caused by translocation, in contrast to trisomy 21. Like other autosomal trisomies, the incidence ascertained through mid-trimester amniocentesis is higher than that observed in liveborn babies. Central nervous system abnormalities are varied and severe in trisomy 13. Arhinencephaly or holoprosencephaly may be present. Usually there are severe intrauterine growth retardation and severe developmental delay. The head is sloping, with narrowness beginning at the forehead. There may be varied eye abnormalities, including hypertelorism, microphthalmia, anophthalmia, and coloboma of the iris. The ears are usually deformed, and there is nearly always severe bilateral cleft lip or palate. Postaxial polydactyly of the hands and feet is common. Internally there may be a wide variety of anomalies involving different organ systems. Less commonly, there are scalp defects at the vertex.

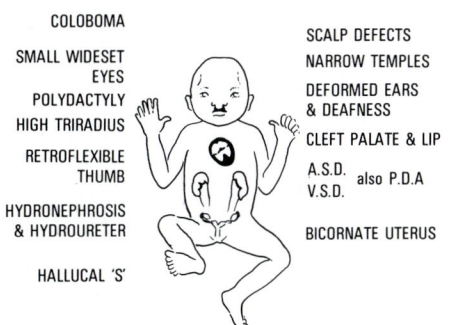

COLOBOMA
SMALL WIDESET EYES
POLYDACTYLY
HIGH TRIRADIUS
RETROFLEXIBLE THUMB
HYDRONEPHROSIS & HYDROURETER
HALLUCAL 'S'

SCALP DEFECTS
NARROW TEMPLES
DEFORMED EARS & DEAFNESS
CLEFT PALATE & LIP
A.S.D.   also P.D.A
V.S.D.
BICORNATE UTERUS

FIGURE 1–34. Various clinical manifestations of trisomy 13.

Trisomy 18

Figures 1–36 and 1–37 summarize diagrammatically the phenotype-genotype of trisomy 18. This mutation occurs in approximately one per 8000 newborns, but nearly 95 per cent of the mutations are aborted spontaneously. Even in 18 trisomic pregnancies carried to term, evidence for intrauterine growth retardation may be apparent by the third trimester. The mean survival time is in the range of 2 months, and only a small percentage survive up to 15 years. As noted earlier, this mutation is seen more frequently in babies of older mothers. Severe cardiac anomalies are common. In addition, 18 trisomics in particular seem to have an increased incidence of significant feeding problems, often requiring gavage for feeding and thereby increasing parental burden in infant care.

Triploidy

A rare numeric genome mutation is triploidy. Tetraploidy in liveborn humans is virtually nonexistent, but with the increasing utilization of mid-trimester amniocentesis and genetic analysis, diagnosis of triploidy during mid-trimester is occurring. A triploidy karyotype ascertained from mid-trimester genetic analysis is shown in Figure 1–38 (Porreco et al., 1980). The major phenotypic features of this abnormality are summarized in Table 1–9. The recurrence risk for triploidy is estimated to be exceedingly small.

Consideration of Abnormalities in Chromosome Structure

Mutations in genome structure are considerably more diverse in phenotype-genotype correlations, and so the sources of ascertainment for these types of mutations will be discussed primarily, with consideration of the wide variability of the genotype. The most common basis for parental karyotype assessment remains the abnormal newborn who reflects the phe-

TABLE 1–9. Phenotypic Features of the Triploidy Syndrome

FEATURE	APPROXIMATE PROPORTION IN REPORTED CASES (%)
Low birth weight	70
Cranial bone abnormalities	50
Ocular/ear anomalies	50
Micrognathia	20
Macroglossia	10
Cleft lip/palate	25
Syndactyly	70
Transverse palmar creases	50
Genital anomalies (XXY)	95
Omphalocele	10
Congenital heart defects	50
Kidney/adrenal anomalies	40
Hydatidiform changes in the placenta	66
Neural tube defects	20
Hydrocephalus	20

Reprinted with permission from Porreco RP, Matson MR, Young PE, et al: Diagnosis of a triploid fetus at genetic amniocentesis. Obstet Gynecol **56**:115. Copyright 1980 by American College of Obstetricians and Gynecologists.

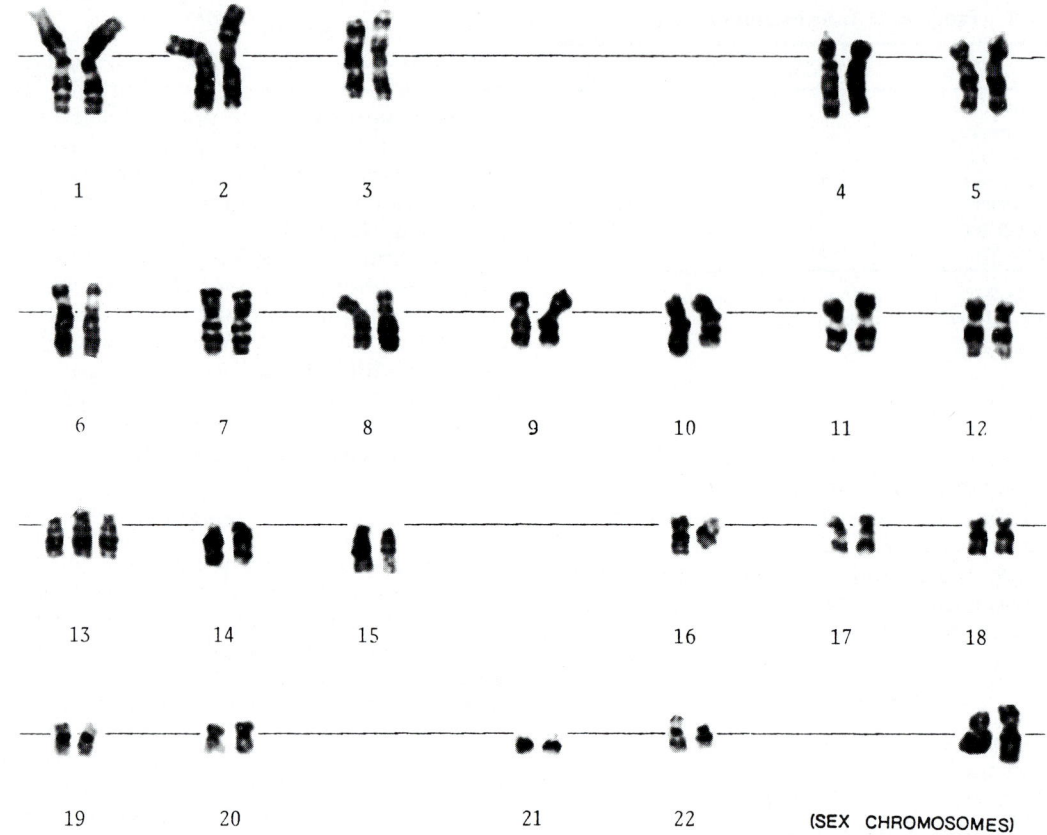

FIGURE 1–35. 47,XX, + 13. A female with 47 chromosomes including trisomy 13.

notypic expression of malsegregation of a balanced parental chromosome structural abnormality. Thus, ascertainment of abnormalities in chromosome structure includes: (1) chromosome screening studies in newborn infants (see Tables 1–2 and 1–3); (2) mid-trimester amniocentesis and genetic analysis because of other considerations (principally maternal age and the risk for chromosome nondisjunction); (3) a history of unexplained first-trimester spontaneous abortions; (4) a family history of stillborn or liveborn babies with unexplained anomalies and mental retardation; and (5) chromosome analysis performed because of multiple birth defects. When a mutation in chromosome structure is confirmed, consideration of additional family chromosome studies is indicated. When possi-

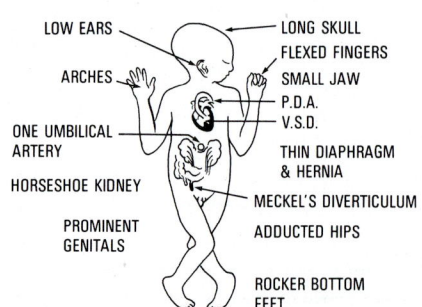

FIGURE 1–36. Various clinical manifestations of trisomy 18.

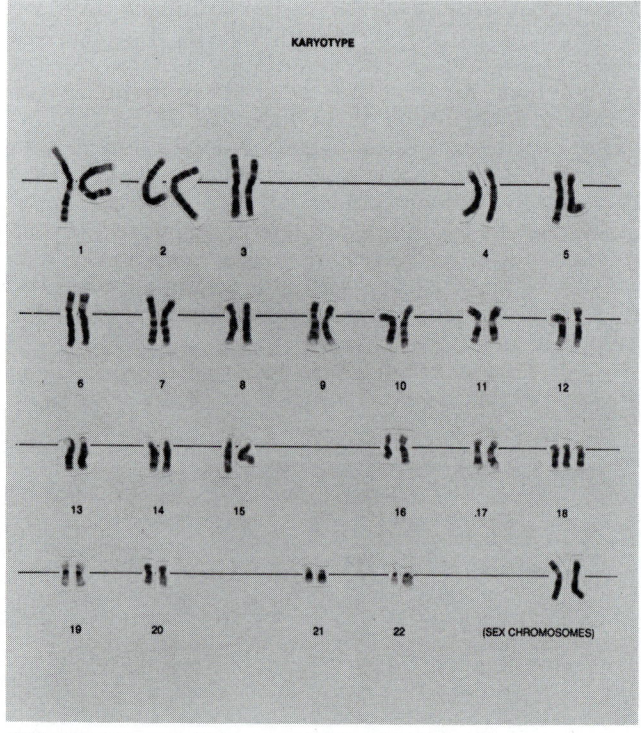

FIGURE 1–37. 47,XX, + 18. A female with 47 chromosomes including trisomy 18.

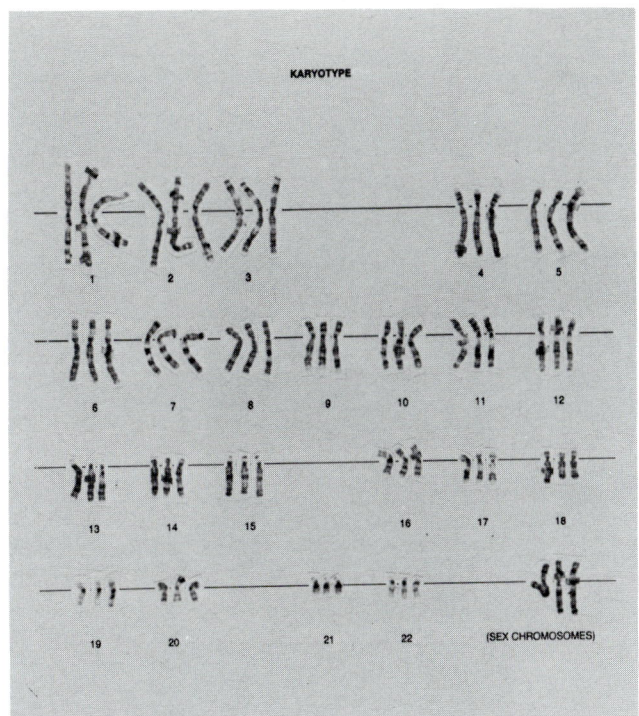

FIGURE 1–38. 69,XXX. There is an extra chromosome for every homologous pair in this genotype (triploidy).

ble, parental karyotyping should be performed first, in order to distinguish between familial transmission and new mutation for the chromosomal change under study. If the mutation proves to be familial, an extended family study is indicated.

Clinical and Biological Considerations of the Sex Chromosomes

Phenotypic sex in human beings is determined by the presence or absence of a Y chromosome. An increased number of either the X or the Y chromosome enhances the likelihood of mental retardation and other anatomic anomalies, irrespective of the sex phenotype. On the other hand, aneuploidy of the sex chromosome does not alter prenatal fetal development nearly as much as aneuploidy of an autosome. Numeric and structural sex chromosome aneuploidies are summarized in Table 1–10. Simpson (1976) provides an excellent reference for detailed clinical considerations of the varied abnormalities of the sex chromosomes. This discussion describes briefly only a few of the more common sex chromosome aberrations. Suffice it to say that abnormalities of the sex chromosomes or genes on the sex chromosomes may affect any of the stages of sexual and reproductive development.

Turner's Syndrome

Turner's syndrome occurs in only approximately one per 10,000 liveborn females, but is one of the chromosome abnormalities most commonly observed in studies of spontaneous abortuses. Although there is wide variability in the phenotypic expression of the Turner syndrome, it represents one sex chromosome abnormality that should be identifiable by physical examination of the newborn. Figures 1–39 and 1–40 demonstrate some of the variable physical characteristics in expression of Turner's syndrome as well as growth patterns for various individuals with the syndrome. Turner's syndrome is associated with a 45,XO genotype. Sex chromosome mosaics such as 46,XX/45,XO and structurally abnormal genotypes such as 46,X/delX and 46,X/isoX are all phenotypic females like those with 45,XO Turner's syndrome but have fewer of the typical manifestations associated with the 45,XO phenotype. Some of the common features of the 45,XO phenotype and the frequency with which they are seen are listed in Table 1–11. The paternally derived X chromosome is more often missing in the 45,XO genotype. Although there is inadequate information at present to permit assessment of longevity

TABLE 1–10.   Numeric and Structural X Chromosomal Aneuploidies in Humans

KARYOTYPE	PHENOTYPE	APPROXIMATE FREQUENCY
XXY	Klinefelter's syndrome	1 per 700 males
XXXY	Klinefelter variant	~1 per 2500 males
XXXXY	Low grade mental deficiency; severe sexual underdevelopment; radioulnar synostosis	Rare
XXX	Sometimes mild oligophrenia; occasionally disturbances of gonadal function	1 per 1000 females
XXXX	Physically normal; severe mental retardation	Rare
XXXXX		
XXY/XY and XXY/XX mosaics	Klinefelter-like, sometimes milder in symptomatology	~5–25% of all "Klinefelter-like" patients
XXX/XX mosaics	Like XXX	Rare
XO	Turner's syndrome	~1 per 2500 females at birth
XO/XX and XO/XXX mosaics	(Turner); very different degree of manifestation	Not uncommon
Various structural anomalies of X chromosomes		Not uncommon
XYY	Increased stature; occasional behavioral abnormalities	1 per 800 males
XXYY	Increased stature; otherwise resembling Klinefelter's syndrome	Rare

From Vogel F, Motulsky AG: Human Genetics: Problems and Approaches. New York, Springer-Verlag, 1979.

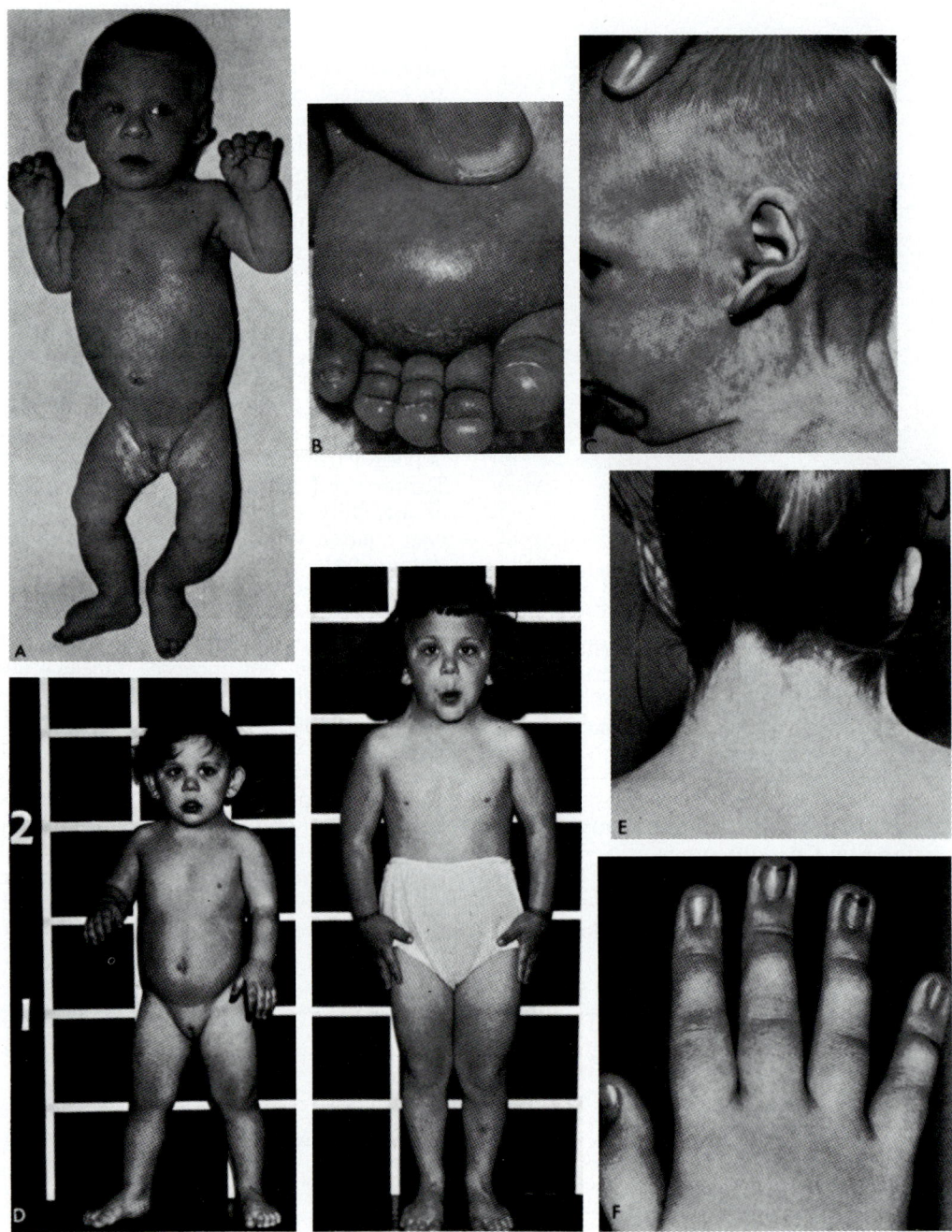

FIGURE 1–39. A female with Turner syndrome. *A* to *C*, At 1 month old. Note lymphedema, prominent ears, and loose folds of skin in posterior neck with low hair line. *D*, Same girl at 2 years (*left*) and 4 years (*right*), with height ages of 17 months and 3 years, respectively. *E*, Low posterior hair line and residual lateral neck web. *F*, Narrow, hyperconvex, deep-set fingernails; residual puffiness. (*A, B, C, E,* and *F* from Lemli L, Smith DW: The XO syndrome. A study of the differentiated phenotype in 25 patients. J Pediatr **63**:577, 1977. *D* from Smith DW: Recognizable Patterns of Human Malformation. 3rd ed. Philadelphia, WB Saunders Co, 1982.)

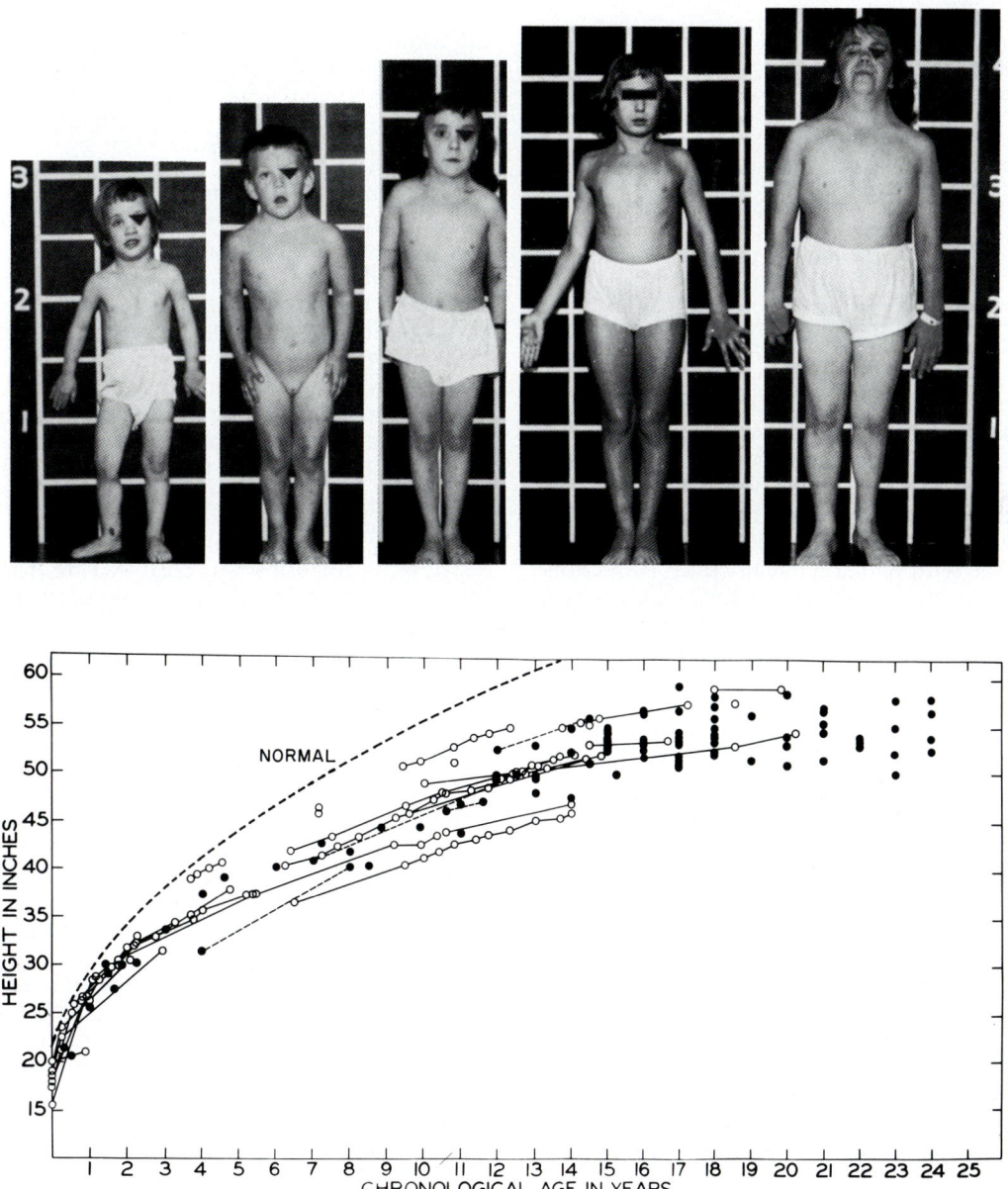

FIGURE 1–40. Turner's syndrome. *Top,* Five girls with the XO syndrome. Note the variability of features such as web neck and broad chest. *Bottom,* Linear growth of girls with the XO syndrome. *Open dots* represent patients evaluated at the University of Wisconsin; *closed dots* represent cases taken from the literature. (From Lemli L, Smith DW: The XO syndrome. A study of the differentiated phenotype in 25 patients. J Pediatr **63**:577, 1977.)

TABLE 1–11.   45,XO Phenotype: Major Features and Their Incidence

FEATURE	INCIDENCE (%)
Small stature, often noted at birth	100
Ovarian dysgenesis with variable degree of hypoplasia of germinal elements	90+
Transient congenital lymphedema, especially notable over the dorsum of the hands and feet	80+
Shield-like, broad chest with widely spaced, inverted, and/or hypoplastic nipples	80+
Prominent auricles	80+
Low posterior hairline, giving the appearance of a short neck	80+
Webbing of posterior neck	50
Anomalies of elbow, including cubitus valgus	70
Short metacarpal and/or metatarsal	50
Narrow, hyperconvex, and/or deepset nails	70
Renal anomalies	60+
Cardiac anomalies (coarctation of the aorta in 70% of cases)	20+
Perceptive hearing loss	50

and cause of death in adult life, the general health prognosis is good for childhood and young adult life in this phenotype. Renal anomalies, when present, rarely cause significant health problems, and in those cases in which congenital heart disease is part of the phenotype, surgery is generally effective.

The congenital lymphedema usually disappears during infancy, and when webbing of the neck poses a cosmetic problem, it may be corrected by plastic surgery. Short stature is a persistent problem. When the diagnosis of 45,XO genotype or a variant is missed during infancy or childhood, a complaint of persisting short stature or amenorrhea finally brings the patient to the physician. Often this delay precludes any specific therapy for the short stature. If a diagnosis is achieved early, however, height increase and external sexual development may be achieved, with the collaboration of a knowledgeable endocrinologist, by the appropriate use of androgen and estrogen replacement therapy. Affected patients are nearly always sterile, and the emotional adjustment to this issue should be part of any medical management of gonadal dysgenesis.

In rare variants of Turner's syndrome, some cells carry a Y chromosome. Occasionally, the Y chromosome line is found only in the germ cells, and the clinical manifestation in the individual may be virilization during adolescence or an unexplained growth spurt. In these cases, it is imperative to perform a gonadal biopsy for histologic and chromosome analysis. If a Y chromosome cell line is demonstrated in gonadal tissue, extirpation is indicated to prevent subsequent malignant transformation in gonadal cells.

Klinefelter's Syndrome

Klinefelter's syndrome, which occurs in approximately one per 700 to 1000 liveborn males, is associated with a 47,XXY genotype. In contrast to Turner's syndrome, there are relatively few so-called variants of Klinefelter's syndrome. The genotype 48,XXXY may be considered a variant, but as the number of X chromosomes increases, the greater the incidence of mental retardation, and the more the physical abnormalities appear to differ from those typical of Klinefelter's syndrome. Approximately 10 per cent of individuals with some of the Klinefelter's phenotype will be 47,XXY/46,XY mosaic, and they have a somewhat better prognosis for testicular function. In general, chromosome aneuploidies that include the Y chromosome are less likely to be diagnosed clinically during infancy or childhood. This is unfortunate, because testosterone replacement therapy is more effective if given prospectively when the patient is 11 to 12 years old. Major physical features of Klinefelter's syndrome are as follows (Fig. 1–41):

1. A tendency to long limbs with a low upper-to-lower segment ratio beginning in childhood; relatively tall, slim stature.

2. Small, soft testes and usually a small penis. Infertility is the rule. Gynecomastia is frequent, and cryptorchidism or hypospadias may be seen. Lack of virilization at puberty is common; indeed it is often the reason for the patient to seek medical attention.

3. There is a tendency toward mental dullness, with approximately 20 per cent of patients having an IQ below 80. Perhaps even more common is the incidence of behavioral and social problems often requiring professional help.

Therapy includes supportive care for the issues related to infertility, social and sexual immaturity, and androgen replacement. Prospective testosterone therapy has value in the medical management of Klinefelter's gonadal dysgenesis, and consultation with an endocrinologist should begin when the patient is about 11 years of age; a maximum therapeutic dose of testosterone should be achieved at 17 years of age and should be given monthly for the remainder of the patient's life.

XYY Syndrome

A great deal of medical, ethical, and sociolegal attention has been devoted to this particular aneuploidy. The incidence is approximately one per 800 to 1000 liveborn males, and it is clear that the genotype-phenotype is not often detected in childhood or, for that matter, during the lifetime of the affected individual. Certainly many males with a 47,XYY genotype have a normal phenotype and fall within societal norms for behavior. There is a pattern of variable abnormalities, however, that may be found more frequently in 47,XYY than in 46,XY males. These include a growth acceleration that appears in mid-childhood, sometimes mental dullness with volatile and antisocial behavior, some weakness in fine motor coordination, and an especially severe form of nodulocystic acne during adolescence. The tendency to tall stature is associated with the mid-childhood growth acceleration. The causal or even associated relationship between the 47,XYY genotype and, in particular, the more unacceptable forms of antisocial and illegal behavior remains a controversy. Currently the majority of observers believe that most people with 47,XYY syndrome function well in society.

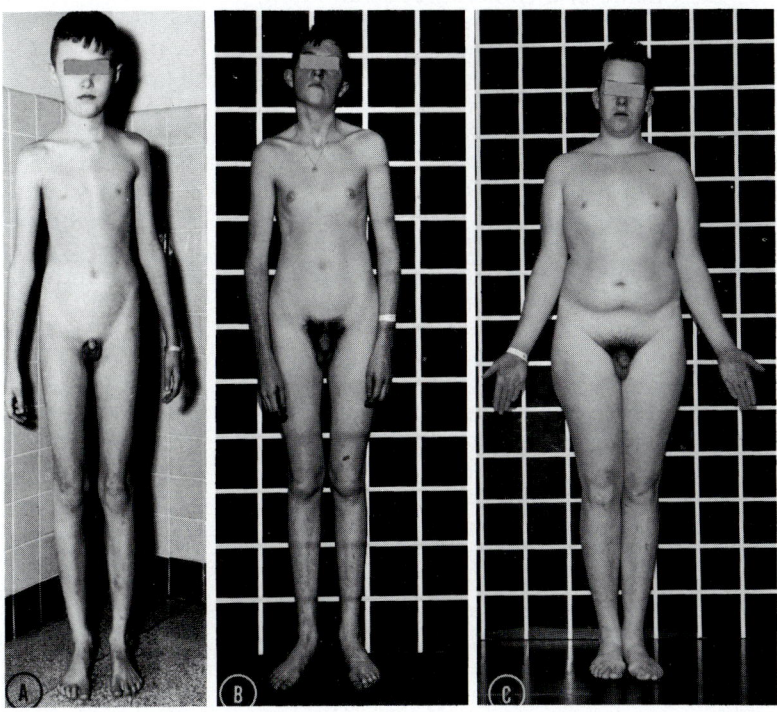

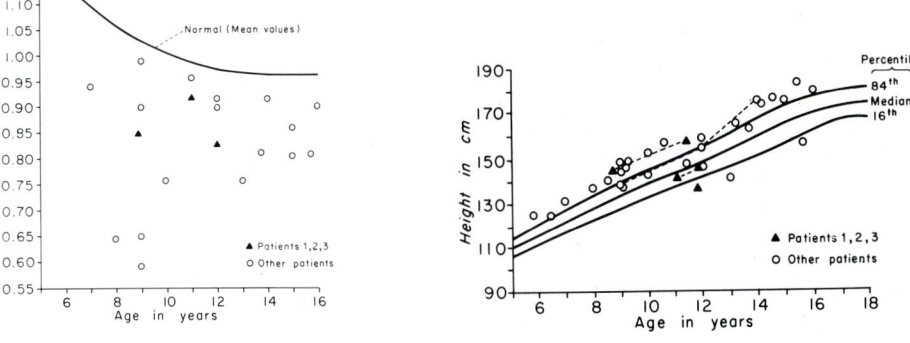

FIGURE 1–41. Klinefelter's syndrome. *A,* At 9 years; note the small penis and long legs. *B,* Untreated at 16 years; note the gynecomastia and scoliosis. *C,* Untreated at 21 years; note the obesity and hypovirilization. *D,* Various measurements in XXY patients and normals in childhood and adolescence. (From Caldwell PD, Smith DW: The XXY syndrome in childhood: Detection and treatment. J Pediatr **80**:250, 1972.)

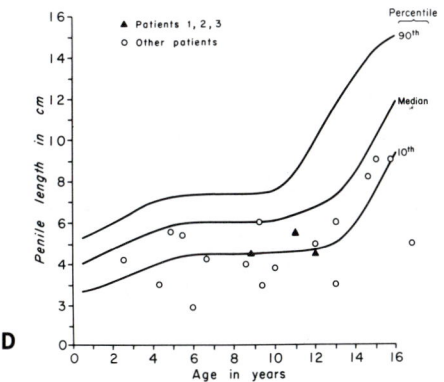

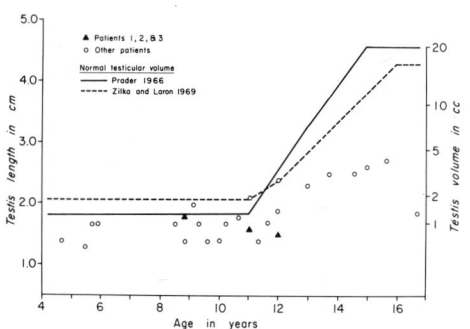

Unique Properties of the Sex Chromosomes

Dosage compensation is a genetic property thought to be unique to the X chromosome. Thus far, little mention has been made of a clinical assessment long used in the evaluation of individuals suspected of abnormalities of the sex chromosomes—in particular, the X chromosome. Barr and Bertram (1949) reported the observation of darkly staining masses called chromatin on the nuclear periphery of interphase nerve cells from female, but not male, cats. Subsequently, this phenomenon was observed in interphase cells from females of many species, including human females, and led to the simple test for the so-called *Barr body*, which numerically was always n-1, where *n* represents the total number of X chromosomes in the individual's genotype. Thus, normal females have one Barr body and normal males have none. This initial finding by Barr and Bertram was important in the development of human genetics, but with the increasing use of direct chromosome analysis and the ability to obtain necessary chromosomal diagnostic information within 24 hours, the utilization of Barr body analysis from interphase cells has diminished significantly. The legacy of the Barr body era relates more to what we know now about the phenomenon—namely that the Barr body represents one condensed and genetically inactive X chromosome during cell interphase. What Barr and Bertram had observed and reported for the first time was the phenomenon of dosage compensation for the X chromosome, although many years elapsed before the implications for mammalian genetics were clarified.

The problem is obvious; in humans and many mammals, the female has two X chromosomes and the male has one X and one Y chromosome. Why was it not also observed that gene products from the X chromosome in females were at least twice that of the gene products from the single X chromosome in males? The answer seems clear now, but it was a long time in coming; in the female, one X chromosome must be genetically inactive. Several investigative teams in the early 1960s provided an explanation. However, the dosage compensation mechanism is generally attributed to geneticist Mary Lyon, who based her hypothesis on experiments with X-linked coat color genes in the mouse. The *Lyon hypothesis* can be summarized as follows:

1. In the somatic cells of female mammals, only one X chromosome is genetically active. The genetically inactive X chromosome is condensed and appears in interphase cells as the sex chromatin (the Barr body).
2. Inactivation of the genetic functions of one X chromosome occurs early in embryonic life.
3. The genetically inactive X chromosome can be either paternal (X^P) or maternal (X^M) in different cells of the same organism. After the X chromosome that will be genetically inactive in a particular cell has been established (regulation), all the clonal descendants of that cell will follow the same regulation for that X chromosome, in that they will have the same genetically inactive X chromosome. Thus, inactivation of the X chromosome is random and then fixed.

Since this important milestone in 1961, considerable biochemical and genetic research has largely substantiated the Lyon hypothesis in humans, mice, and several other mammals. One of the more significant studies in humans utilized tissues from uterine leiomyomata and normal uterine tissue. One of the genes on the X chromosomes codes for an enzyme responsible for helping maintain the integrity of red blood cell membranes. This enzyme is glucose-6-phosphate-dehydrogenase, or G6PD. Two of the most common alleles for the enzyme are designated form A and form B. When uterine tumors from females heterozygous on the X chromosome for G6PD A and B were analyzed and compared with normal uterine tissue from the same individuals, it was noted that the tumor cells consistently showed only one of the allelic types (either A or B), whereas normal uterine tissue showed both A and B. The only acceptable conclusions from this research were (1) only one allele is active in the tumor cells; (2) the whole tumor was initiated by a single cell, thus it reflects a single cell clone; and (3) the specific X chromosome remains either active or inactive throughout the entire period of tumor growth.

The results of scientific research have supported in principle the Lyon hypothesis and its explanation of dosage compensation. As more has been learned about the X chromosome and embryogenesis, however, it appears that the X chromosome inactivation may not be operative in all cells. Furthermore, in certain instances inactivation is not random. Inactivation of the X chromosomes probably does not occur before the 16th day of the blastocyst stage. Moreover, there is evidence that inactivation does not occur at all in oocytes. In the mouse, there is evidence for genetic activity on both X chromosomes for specific enzymes. The blood group system Xg, the only blood group system with X-linked inheritance, does not appear to be under the same regulatory mechanism for dosage compensation that is predicted by the Lyon hypothesis.

Observations of structural abnormalities of the X chromosome have led to the conclusion that X chromosome inactivation is not always random. In general, when a structural abnormality involves only one X chromosome (i.e., deletion, isochromosome, ring chromosome), the abnormal X chromosome always appears to be the one inactivated. On the other hand, if the structural abnormality is a translocation between part of one X chromosome and an autosome, the "normal" X seems to be the one genetically inactive. Although this pattern is not proven, it is assumed that if the X chromosome translocated to an autosome is genetically inactivated, then part or all of that autosome might also become inactive, rendering that cell functionally monosomic for the autosome and thus nonviable. This phenomenon helps to explain why X-autosome translocation can produce the Turner phenotype in an individual and why some females heterozygous for X-linked recessive biochemical disorders, such as Duchenne muscular dystrophy, have phenotypic expression of that disorder. In this instance, if the mutant X chromosome is the one involved in the X-autosome translocation and the normal allele is inactive by virtue of being on the normal, inactive X chromosome, it is likely that the female will express the disease. Considerably more research is needed before all ramifications of X chromosome inactivation and dosage compensation are fully understood.

Chromosome Abnormalities in Abortuses and Stillbirths

It has been estimated that about 15 per cent of pregnancies terminate in spontaneous abortions, and that at least 80 per cent of those do so in the first trimester. The incidence of chromosome abnormalities in spontaneous abortuses during the first trimester has been reported to be as high as 61.5 per cent (Boué et al., 1975). In later spontaneous abortions, the incidence is reduced to around 5 per cent. Table 1–12 summarizes the genotype incidence in chromosomally abnormal abortuses. For comparison, note the incidence of chromosome abnormalities in liveborn babies (see Tables 1–2 and 1–3). At an incidence of 18 per cent, 45,XO is the most common chromosome abnormality found in first-trimester spontaneous abortions. Comparison with the relatively low incidence of 45,XO in liveborn babies suggests that most conceptuses with this genotype abort spontaneously. Trisomic embryos are seen for all autosomes except chromosomes 1, 5, 11, 12, 17, and 19. The studies of Creasy and colleagues (1976) offer comparison with the data in Table 1–12. Trisomy 16, the most common autosomal trisomy in spontaneous abortuses, is never seen in liveborn babies. Similarly, trisomy 22 is rare in liveborn babies, but is seen at virtually the same rate as trisomy 21 in abortuses. Comparison of the overall incidence of about one per 800 live births for trisomy 21 with the incidence in abortuses (Table 1–12) suggests that approximately three-fourths of trisomy 21 conceptuses abort spontaneously. Creasy and associates (1976) noted an incidence of 2.36 per cent for trisomy 13, 6.5 per cent for trisomy 14, and 10.04 per cent for trisomy 15 in spontaneous abortions, but in contrast, only

TABLE 1–12. Relative Frequency of Aberrations in Chromosomally Abnormal Abortuses

TYPE	INCIDENCE (%)
Trisomy	52
14	3.7
15	4.2
16	16.4
18	3.0
21	4.7
22	5.7
Other	14.3
45,X	18
Triploid	17
Tetraploid	6
Unbalanced translocation	3
Other	4
Total	*100*

Data from Carr DH, Gedeon M: Population cytogenetics of human abortuses. *In* Hook EB, Porter IH (eds): Population Cytogenetics: Studies in Humans. New York, Academic Press, 1977. Table from Thompson MW: Thompson and Thompson's Genetics in Medicine. 4th ed. Philadelphia, WB Saunders Co, 1986.

trisomy 13 is seen in liveborn babies, and at a very low frequency (see Table 1–3). Similarly, tetraploidies are seen in abortuses but not in liveborn babies.

Hassold (1980) has provided some additional insight into the issue of genome mutations in spontaneous abortuses. He was able to obtain karyotype analyses of at least two abortuses of each of a series of 40 women with recurrent spontaneous abortions. In 21 of these women, a normal karyotype in the first abortus was associated with a normal karyotype in the second abortus. The other 19 patients had abortuses with chromosome abnormalities. In this group, nine patients had chromosome abnormalities in two consecutive abortions, and in four of the nine, both spontaneous abortions were trisomic. This risk seems to be independent of maternal age. These results suggest that if a chromosome abnormality is identified in an abortus tissue, the probability is significant that a chromosome mutation will be seen in any subsequent abortus.

Information concerning the incidence of chromosome abnormalities in stillborn babies is much more limited, but it is estimated that about 5 per cent of stillborn infants have chromosome mutations. If the baby is small for gestational age and in addition has identifiable birth defects, the probability of a chromosome mutation increases to about 15 per cent. In the field of perinatal medicine, there will probably be more likelihood of obtaining diagnostic information from chromosome studies on stillborns than of karyotyping first-trimester spontaneous abortuses; however, each opportunity is too often missed.

At least 93 per cent of the chromosome aberrations in first-trimester abortuses reflect numeric abnormalities. Nonetheless, it seems reasonable, if chromosome data on a conceptus are unavailable, to karyotype both parents in an effort to ascertain a balanced chromosome structural abnormality. This would be of considerable importance to genetic counseling and to fetal monitoring during subsequent pregnancies. Various studies on parental karyotyping, using current spontaneous abortions as the selection factor, have suggested an incidence of translocation carriers that ranges from 3 to 31 per cent, with an average of 9.3 per cent. Ward and colleagues (1980) reported different results of chromosome studies in 100 couples who had experienced recurrent spontaneous abortions. In this study, couples who had already produced a congenitally abnormal liveborn child were specifically excluded from the study. No chromosome translocations were found in any of the individuals in this study. The authors routinely recommended analysis for couples when other causes of recurrent pregnancy wastage have been excluded, but they also suggest cytogenetic analysis as a first-order diagnostic study for these couples if they have already produced a congenitally defective liveborn child. Their reasoning is that in such a population subset, a chromosome translocation will be found in one parent about 36 per cent of the time. Chromosome analysis for couples might be indicated for evaluation of recurrent spontaneous abortions when other causes have been excluded. For patients who have already produced a child with multiple birth defects, and who in addition have recurrent first-trimester abortions, parental karyotyping should be done as part of the initial medical evaluation.

Summary of Indications for Chromosome Analysis

Of all the genetic aspects of maternal-fetal medicine, chromosome mutations constitute the category that most often requires the physician's attention. It is worthwhile, therefore, to review the indications for at least the consideration of chromosome analysis as part of the evaluation of fetus, infant, or parents. The following situations would justify chromosome analysis.

Unexplained First-Trimester Spontaneous Abortion

Every effort should be made to culture and karyotype fetal tissue from spontaneous abortions. Identification of a genomic mutation in the abortus provides a reason to concerned parents as well as useful information to a genetic counselor. Most abortuses represent sporadic mutations with little recurrence risk. On the other hand, when the mutation is a trisomy, the counselor may inform parents that a recurrence is possible.

Unexplained First-Trimester Spontaneous Abortion With No Fetal Karyotype

Usually, couples seek medical help because of recurrent first-trimester abortions, and there is no previous karyotype for aborted tissue. Many genetic centers currently recommend parental karyotyping after several (usually two or three) spontaneous abortions have occurred. The likelihood of a parental genome mutation is probably greatest if the couple has already produced a child with birth defects. When a parental chromosome structural abnormality is identified, genetic counseling and prenatal fetal monitoring in all subsequent pregnancies are advised.

Stillbirth

Unless an explanation is obvious, any evaluation of a stillborn infant should include chromosome analysis. Unless intrauterine demise occurred several days prior to delivery, tissue culture from a fascia lata biopsy after delivery is usually successful. The likelihood of finding a chromosome mutation is increased significantly if there is intrauterine growth retardation or phenotypic birth defects.

Abnormal Phenotype in a Newborn Infant

Most abnormal phenotypes in the newborn that are due to chromosome abnormalities will reflect abnormal autosomes. The important findings that should prompt karyotyping include low birth weight; early evidence of failure to thrive; any indication of developmental delay, in particular mental retardation; ab-

normal features of the head and face such as microcephaly, micrognathia, and abnormalities of eyes, ears, and mouth; abnormalities of the hands and feet; and congenital defects of various internal organs. A single isolated malformation or mental retardation without an associated physical malformation reduces significantly the likelihood of a chromosome abnormality. Disorders of the sex chromosomes are more apt to be associated with phenotypic ambiguity of the external genitalia and perhaps slight abnormality in growth pattern. Certainly any newborn manifesting sexual ambiguity should have a chromosome analysis. In addition to helping to exclude the possibility of a life-threatening genetic disorder, e.g., adrenogenital syndrome, the identification of sex genotype by chromosome analysis will assist attending physicians in their decisions about therapy and counseling for the parents. For the infant suspected of having autosome abnormalities, in whom the chromosomal genotype is urgently needed for making decisions about the infant's care, rapid chromosome analysis can be obtained by culture of bone marrow aspirate. When a familial chromosome mutation such as unbalanced translocation is detected in the infant, karyotyping of other kindred is indicated.

Diseases Associated With Increased Incidence of Malignancy

Although these disorders are relatively rare, for prognosis and genetic counseling, chromosome analysis should be part of the medical evaluation.

PATTERNS OF INHERITANCE

Two fundamental laws of genetics that are inviolate in diploid organisms were established by the experimental design, careful observation, and meticulous record-keeping of Gregor Mendel in 1857. These two laws are illustrated in Figure 1–42. Simply stated,

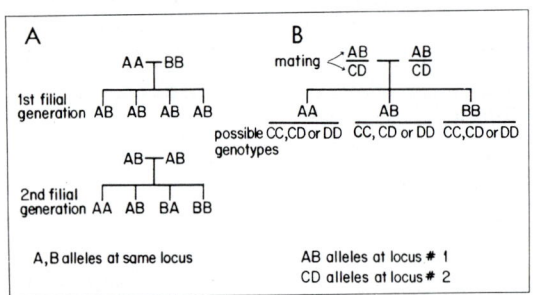

FIGURE 1–42. Mendel's first and second laws. *A*, With A and B representing alleles at the same locus, a mating of homozygous A and homozygous B individuals results in heterozygotes for A,B in each offspring. Mating of heterozygotes A,B results in the 1-2-1 segregation ratio in offspring. *B*, The segregation of genotypes for A and B at locus 1 is independent of the segregation of alleles C and D at locus 2. (Reproduced with permission from Kelly TE: Clinical Genetics and Genetic Counseling. Copyright © 1980 by Year Book Publishers, Inc., Chicago.)

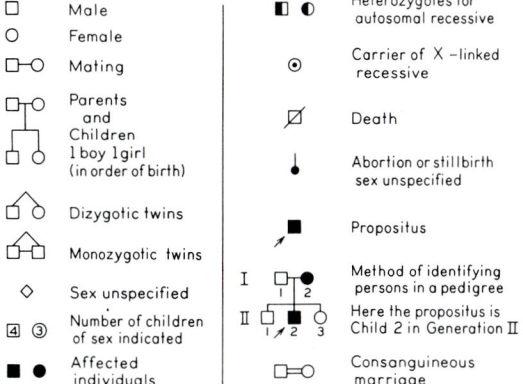

☐	Male
○	Female
☐—○	Mating
☐—○ (Parents and Children 1 boy 1 girl in order of birth)	Parents and Children 1 boy 1 girl (in order of birth)
	Dizygotic twins
	Monozygotic twins
◇	Sex unspecified
④ ③	Number of children of sex indicated
■ ●	Affected individuals
■ ◖	Heterozygotes for autosomal recessive
⊙	Carrier of X-linked recessive
⊘	Death
↓	Abortion or stillbirth sex unspecified
↗■	Propositus
I ☐—● 1 2	Method of identifying persons in a pedigree
II ☐—■—○ 1 2 3	Here the propositus is Child 2 in Generation II
☐═○	Consanguineous marriage

FIGURE 1–43. Symbols commonly used in pedigree charts. (From Thompson MW: Thompson and Thompson's Genetics in Medicine. 4th ed. Philadelphia, WB Saunders Co, 1986.)

Codominant Mode of Inheritance

Recessivity and dominance are relative concepts. For example, with the hemoglobinopathy sickle cell anemia (hemoglobin S), if one chooses anemia as the phenotypic expression of the gene function, the gene expression is consistent with autosomal recessive inheritance. If one considers the hemoglobin molecules, both hemoglobin S and hemoglobin A (normal) are expressed in individuals who are heterozygous (A/S). In terms of gene expression of the hemoglobin molecule, hemoglobin S and hemoglobin A are more correctly *codominant*. Another example of codominance are genes for the blood group antigens ABO. The individual with blood group AB has both A and B red cell surface antigens, and the allelic genes A and B are expressed codominantly.

Autosomal Dominant Mode of Inheritance

Figure 1–44 demonstrates the mode of inheritance for autosomal dominant disorders. McKusick's catalog of mendelian disorders describes 1864 autosomal dominant abnormalities (McKusick, 1990). In autosomal dominant inheritance, the disease is expressed in the heterozygote, and the probability of transmitting the gene to progeny is 50 per cent with each pregnancy. The pedigree in Figure 1–44 demonstrates what one would expect to see for any autosomal dominant disease: gene expression in each generation, approximately half of the offspring affected (both males and females), and father-to-son transmission. Although homozygotes for autosomal dominants have been described rarely in humans, it is generally conceded that in humans, the mutant autosomal dominant homozygous expression is lethal. A few autosomal disorders such as familial hypercholesterolemia have biochemical markers; however, the vast majority of the autosomal dominant diseases do not provide this laboratory advantage to the physician, who must rely on careful history-taking and physical examination for diagnosis and counseling.

The criteria for autosomal dominant inheritance may be summarized as follows:

1. Expression of the gene rarely skips a generation.
2. Affected individuals, if reproductively fit, transmit the gene expression to progeny with a probability of 50 per cent.
3. The sexes are affected equally, and there is father-to-son transmission.
4. A person in the kindred at risk who is not affected will not transmit the gene to progeny.

Mendel's first law is segregation, which occurs in the definite proportions of 1/4 + 1/2 + 1/4 (Fig. 1–42A). The second law describes independent assortment: when two or more pairs of different characters (alleles at different loci) are crossed, they segregate independently (Fig. 1–42B). In the jargon of medical genetics, *mendelian disorders* refer to single-gene phenotypes that segregate distinctly within families and generally occur in the proportions noted by Mendel in his experiments with garden peas.

In humans as well as many other mammalian species, kindred pedigrees reveal specific phenotypic or genotypic traits, depending on whether the responsible gene is on the X chromosome or an autosome. Because in diploid organisms all chromosomes (except sex chromosomes) are genetically paired, expression of a gene function or lack thereof depends on whether it (1) is expressed even when present on only one chromosome of a pair (dominant), or (2) is expressed only when present on both chromosomes (recessive). Therefore, both autosomal and sex-linked genes may be expressed as dominant or recessive.

Virtually any aspect of genetic evaluation requires development of a pedigree chart. Figure 1–43 illustrates some of the symbols useful in this process. This aspect of data gathering serves several functions. First, it assists the determination of transmission for the gene expression in question, i.e., recessive, dominant, sex-linked, or autosomal. Second, there is a greater likelihood that all possible genetic issues will be included in the data gathering when a formal pedigree chart is developed. Third, when consanguinity is present, the pedigree chart helps to relate the consanguinity to individuals in subsequent generations who are expressing the phenotype of a particular inheritable disorder.

FIGURE 1–44. Stereotype pedigree of autosomal dominant inheritance. Half the offspring of affected persons (7 out of 14) are affected. The condition is transmitted only by affected family members, never by unaffected ones. Equal numbers of males and females are affected. Male-to-male transmission is seen. (From Thompson MW: Thompson and Thompson's Genetics of Medicine. 4th ed. Philadelphia, WB Saunders Co, 1986.)

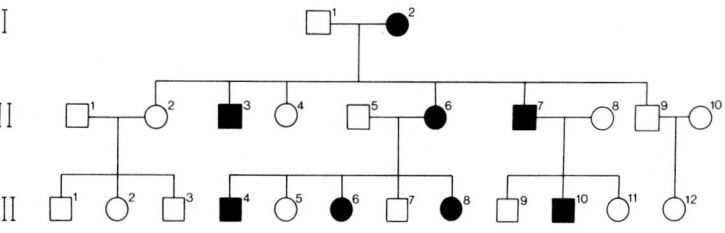

There are other characteristics that, although not exclusive properties of autosomal dominant disease, seem to be associated with this group of diseases more frequently. *Variable expressivity* is commonly seen in kindreds with autosomal dominant traits. In neurofibromatosis, for example, a kindred may have a range of phenotypic expression all the way from café au lait spots with a few tumors to extensive café au lait spots with massive neurofibromata. *Penetrance* is another term used to characterize autosomal dominant gene expression; it refers to whether or not there is any recognition of phenotypic expression of a particular mutant allele. If a gene is fully "penetrant," it is always expressed as part of the genome of that individual. On the other hand, in the autosomal dominant form of retinoblastoma, the gene expression is only 80 per cent penetrant. This means that a person who receives the gene for retinoblastoma from a parent has a 20 per cent chance that the gene will not be expressed by the usual identifiable means. In other words, the parent with bilateral retinoblastoma has a 40 per cent risk of having a child who develops the tumors. Penetrance may also be influenced by the means available to detect expression of the gene. For example, in autosomal dominant hypercholesterolemia, a myocardial infarct (a manifestation of gene expression and penetrance) may not appear until well into adult life. In this disorder there is a laboratory probe for gene expression, namely the serum cholesterol level, which becomes elevated quite early in life, well before the first chest pain of angina pectoris.

It is not uncommon for an autosomal dominant disorder to become manifest for the first time in a kindred as a new mutation. New mutations are also seen with sex-linked recessive disorders. For example, in achondroplastic dwarfism (autosomal dominant), nearly 80 per cent of parents represent new mutations. When this phenomenon can be identified with certainty, parents may be reassured that the recurrence risk is probably no greater than that for the general population. The recurrence risk for the affected "new mutant" is 50 per cent. In particular, new mutations for autosomal dominant diseases appear to be related to paternal age. Achondroplastic dwarfism, Apert's syndrome, Marfan's syndrome, and myositis ossificans all show an increasing rate of new mutations as paternal age exceeds 37 years. Other diseases such as hydrocephalus without spina bifida and microphthalmos or anophthalmia, basal cell nevus syndrome, Waardenberg's syndrome, Crouzon's disease, Treacher-Collins syndrome, and oculodentodigital syndrome may all prove to have increased mutation rates in association with higher paternal age.

Autosomal Recessive Mode of Inheritance

Currently, the number of identified autosomal recessive diseases is 631 (McKusick, 1990). Mutant genes are expressed only in homozygous individuals. Consanguinity often is a clue for autosomal inheritance when the specific gene mutation has not been identified. A stylized pedigree chart consistent with autosomal recessive inheritance is shown in Figure 1–45.

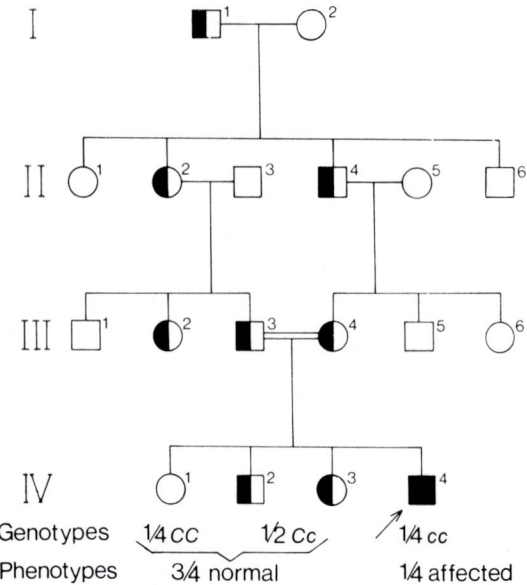

FIGURE 1–45. Stereotype pedigree of autosomal recessive inheritance, including a cousin marriage. A gene from a common ancestor I–1 has been transmitted down two lines of descent to "meet itself" in IV–4. (From Thompson MW: Thompson and Thompson's Genetics of Medicine. 4th ed. Philadelphia, WB Saunders Co, 1986.)

Primary features consistent with autosomal recessive inheritance may be summarized as follows:

1. Both males and females are affected.
2. Unless consanguinity or random selection of heterozygous matings in each generation occurs, mutant gene expression may appear to skip generations, in contrast to autosomal dominant inheritance, in which skipped generations are rarely seen.
3. Parents are usually unaffected, but sibs of affected homozygotes may be at risk. Affected individuals rarely have affected children.
4. Subsequent to identification of a propositus, the recurrence risk for homozygous affected progeny in each subsequent pregnancy is one chance in four.
5. Consanguineous parentage is often seen.

In virtually all autosomal disorders for which a specific defective gene product has been identified, the product has been found in some biochemical pathway reflecting a single gene mutation. In those disorders in which the biochemical and defective gene products are known, a biochemical laboratory test has provided confirmation for the autosomal recessive disease.

Sex-Linked Mode of Inheritance

In this instance, *sex-linked* refers to the X chromosome, and to date, at least 161 X-linked diseases are known (McKusick, 1990). For this group of genetic diseases, the male is considered to be hemizygous in relation to X-linked genes, whereas females can be homozygous or heterozygous. Hemophilia A and Duchenne muscular dystrophy are among the best-known X-linked recessive diseases. For illustrative

OVA

		X_H	X_H
	X_h	$X_H X_h$	$X_H X_h$
SPERM			
	Y	$X_H Y$	$X_H Y$

Daughters: 100 percent heterozygotes
Sons: 100 percent normal

FIGURE 1–46. Sex-linked recessive inheritance patterns. See text for explanation. (From Thompson JS, Thompson MW: Genetics in Medicine. 3rd ed. Philadelphia, WB Saunders Co, 1980.)

A

OVA

		X_H	X_h
	X_H	$X_H X_H$	$X_H X_h$
SPERM			
	Y	$X_H Y$	$X_h Y$

Daughters: 50 percent normal, 50 percent carriers
Sons: 50 percent normal, 50 percent affected

B

purposes, we shall use the symbol X_h to represent the recessive allele for hemophilia A on the X chromosome, and X_H to represent the normal or dominant allele. The diagrams in Figure 1–46 demonstrate progeny genotypes in matings between hemizygous affected males and homozygous normal females, as well as matings between hemizygous normal males and heterozygous, phenotypically normal females. When the father is affected, all sons will be hemizygous normal and all daughters will be heterozygous and phenotypically normal (Fig. 1–46A). In the other mating cross, each daughter will have a 50 per cent chance of being homozygous normal and a 50 per cent chance of being heterozygous but phenotypically normal (Fig. 1–46B). The son will have a 50 per cent chance of being hemizygous normal and a 50 per cent chance of being hemizygous affected. Males affected with Duchenne muscular dystrophy rarely reproduce, and so there is no increase in the gene pool through heterozygous females born to affected males. Characteristics of X-linked recessive inheritance may be summarized as follows:

1. A higher incidence of the disorder is noted in males than in females.
2. The mutant gene expression is never transmitted directly from father to son.
3. The mutant gene is transmitted from an affected male to all of his daughters.
4. The trait is transmitted through a series of carrier females, and affected males in a kindred are related to one another through the females.

An additional interesting aspect of X-linked recessive inheritance has been shown by observations for sporadic cases of hemophilia A and for another X-linked disorder, Lesch-Nyhan syndrome, a defect of the enzyme hypoxanthine guanine phosphoribosyltransferase, which is important in the "salvage" pathway biosynthesis of purine nucleotides. For the sporadic cases of these two disorders, there is an increase in the age of the maternal grandfather at which he

fathered the mother of an affected child—similar to the increase in paternal age for certain new dominant mutations.

In contrast to X-linked recessive inheritance, X-linked dominant diseases are nearly twice as common in females as in males (Fig. 1–47). For example, none of the sons of a male affected with vitamin D–resistant rickets is affected, but all of his daughters receive the mutant gene from him, and because the mutant is dominant, they all have the disease. A female with one X-linked mutant dominant allele will have the disease, and the transmission to her progeny, assuming a hemizygous normal mate, will be indistinguishable from that seen in autosomal dominant inheritance. As a group, the X-linked dominant disorders are relatively uncommon. Vitamin D–resistant rickets (hypophosphatemia) is one, and the X-linked blood group X is another. The distinguishing features of X-linked dominant inheritance are summarized as follows:

1. All daughters of affected males have the disorder, but no sons are affected.
2. Heterozygous affected females transmit the mutant allele at a rate of 50 per cent to progeny of both

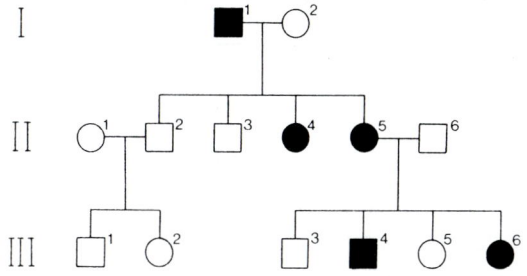

FIGURE 1–47. Stereotype pedigree of X-linked dominant inheritance. Affected males have no sons and no normal daughters. (From Thompson MW: Thompson and Thompson's Genetics of Medicine. 4th ed. Philadelphia, WB Saunders Co, 1986.)

sexes. If the affected female is homozygous, all her children will be affected.

3. The incidence of X-linked dominant disease may be twice as common in females as in males.

Multifactorial Inheritance

The class of multifactorially heritable disorders comprises the most frequently encountered genetic abnormalities in clinical medicine, and the least understood. Most of the genetically determined congenital disorders fall into this category. *Multifactorial inheritance* refers to determination by a combination of genetic and environmental factors. *Polygenic inheritance* is often used interchangeably, but this use is incorrect. *Polygenic inheritance* should be reserved for inheritance due to mutations in a large number of genes acting in an additive fashion.

In multifactorial inheritance, all relatives within the same degree (i.e., all first-degree relatives) may be considered collectively, and so it is important for purposes of counseling to characterize the closeness of relationship to the propositus, or proband. Table 1–13 summarizes for each degree of kindred relationship the relative number of genes in common with the new propositus.

There are at least three characteristics of particular importance in multifactorial inheritance. *Regression to the mean*, in practical terms, implies that parents who are particularly extreme in terms of their position on the normal curve for a given characteristic are more likely to have children who on the average are less extreme in position than the parents. For example, dull normal parents usually have children who on the average have intelligence that is higher than that of the parents, but still below the average of the general population. *Heritability* reflects the measure of the relative degree to which a given set of genes determines a given phenotype. *Threshold traits* depend on the developmental rate. The rate of development is determined by several factors, both genetic and environmental, and should be considered a continuous dynamic process. If a certain point in development is not reached at the appropriate time, a malformation may result; in such instances a continuous variable is established consisting of normal and abnormal groups separated by a threshold. In this method of analysis, information is collected on the incidence of the malformation in the general population and in different categories of relatives. From these data, an empiric risk for the malformation can be estimated on the basis of past experience, even without knowledge of the nature of the genetic and environmental factors in the etiology of the malformation.

Criteria for Multifactorial Inheritance

Carter (1976) and Thompson (1986) have described features of multifactorial inheritance in addition to those just discussed. The additional features are as follows:

1. The risks in relatives are greater than the risk in the general population, and the magnitude of the difference in the risks lessens as the general population incidence increases. There may be exceptions to this pattern if mating is nonrandom, if environmental variation is significant, or if dominant rather than additive genes are involved.

2. The recurrence risk for single-gene disorders after one or two affected children remains unchanged. In contrast, for multifactorial characteristics, the risk increases with each additional family member who is ascertained to be affected.

3. The more severe the malformation, the greater risk to relatives. For example, if a liveborn baby has unilateral cleft lip, the risk to future siblings is 2.5 per cent. If the liveborn baby has bilateral cleft lip and palate, the recurrence risk for future siblings is 6 per cent.

4. If there is a sex difference in the frequency of the trait, the risk to relatives is greater when the trait occurs in the less commonly affected sex. For example, the sex ratio for pyloric stenosis is 5:0; the difference in recurrence risk in relation to the sex of the propositus is shown in Table 1–14.

5. An increase in parental consanguinity is to be expected in multifactorial etiology, but the increase is less than that observed for rare autosomal recessive disorders.

Examples of disorders with multifactorial inheritance are numerous, and many can also be classified nosologically as *isolated malformations*. The following disorders are the most common.

TABLE 1–13.   Relationship to Genes in Common With Propositus

RELATIONSHIP TO PROPOSITUS	PROPORTION OF GENES IN COMMON WITH PROPOSITUS
Monozygotic twin	1
First-degree relative (parent; dizygotic twin or other sib; child)	1/2
Second-degree relative (grandparent; uncle or aunt; half-sib; nephew or niece; grandchild)	1/4
Third-degree relative (great-grandparent; great-grandchild; first cousin)	1/8

From Thompson MW: Thompson and Thompson's Genetics in Medicine. 4th ed. Philadelphia, WB Saunders Co, 1986.

TABLE 1–14.   Recurrence Risk of Pyloric Stenosis for First-Degree Relatives

	RISK (%)	GENERAL POPULATION RISK
Male relatives of male patients	4.6	× 10
Female relatives of male patients	2.6	× 25
Male relatives of female patients	18.2	× 35
Female relatives of female patients	8.1	× 80

From Kelly TE: Clinical Genetics and Genetic Counseling. Copyright © 1980 by Year Book Medical Publishers, Inc., Chicago. Reproduced with permission.

TABLE 1–15.   **Examples of Recurrence Risks for Cleft Lip With or Without Cleft Palate and Neural Tube Malformations**

FAMILY HISTORY	RISK FOR CLEFT LIP ± CLEFT PALATE (%)	RISK FOR ANENCEPHALY AND SPINA BIFIDA (%)
No sibs affected		
Neither parent affected	0.1	0.3
One parent affected	3	4.5
Both parents affected	34	30
One sib affected		
Neither parent affected	3	4
One parent affected	11	12
Both parents affected	40	38
Two sibs affected		
Neither parent affected	9	10
One parent affected	19	20
Both parents affected	45	43
One sib and one second-degree relative affected		
Neither parent affected	6	7
One parent affected	16	18
Both parents affected	43	42
One sib and one third-degree relative affected		
Neither parent affected	4	5.5
One parent affected	14	16
Both parents affected	44	42

Adapted from Thompson MW: Thompson and Thompson's Genetics in Medicine. 4th ed. Philadelphia, WB Saunders Company, 1986. Based on data from Bonaiti-Pellié C, Smith C: Risk tables for genetic counselling in some common congenital malformations. J Med Genet **11**:374, 1974.

Cleft Lip and Cleft Palate

The malformation cleft lip, with or without cleft palate, is etiologically distinct from cleft palate alone. In addition, cleft lip and/or palate may be part of a syndrome determined by a single mutant gene (approximately 30 are known), a syndrome related to a genome mutation (e.g., trisomy 13), or a syndrome related to a teratogenic agent (e.g., thalidomide). Cleft lip with or without cleft palate results from fusion failure of the frontal prominence with the maxillary process at about the seventh week of development. Sixty to 80 per cent of cases occur in males, and there is considerable variation in incidence among different ethnic groups: one per 1000 Caucasians, 1.7 per 1000 Japanese, and 0.4 per 1000 American Blacks. The recurrence risks are summarized in Table 1–15. The risk also varies with the severity of the defect, as noted by Fraser (1970). For bilateral cleft lip and palate, the risk is 5.6 per cent; for unilateral cleft lip and palate, the risk is 4.1 per cent; and for unilateral cleft lip without cleft palate, the risk is 2.6 per cent.

Cleft Palate

In this malformation, the secondary palate fails to fuse. The general incidence is approximately one per 2500. The disorder is more common in females. There is little ethnic variation in incidence, and the recurrence is about 2 per cent regardless of family history.

Pyloric Stenosis

Sex predilection and recurrence risks are shown in Table 1–14. Once the diagnosis has been made in the propositus, parents often make the diagnosis of subsequent affected siblings. It is of interest to note that clinical manifestations suggesting pyloric stenosis are often seen in newborns with single-gene metabolic disturbances. Protracted vomiting is one of the clinical manifestations.

Congenital Heart Disease

The overall incidence of congenital heart disease is five to seven per 1000 liveborn babies. Table 1–16, abstracted from Nora (1968), summarizes the recurrence risk for six common congenital heart defects.

Neural Tube Defects

This group of isolated malformations is of special importance because of the possibility of mid-trimester prenatal diagnosis as well as current considerations for prenatal screening of these disorders in all pregnancies. There is considerable variability in genetic expression of neural tube defects, ranging from an-

TABLE 1–16.   **Frequency of Six Common Congenital Heart Defects in Sibs of Probands**

ANOMALY	FREQUENCY IN SIBS (%)*	EXPECTED FREQUENCY (%)†
Ventricular septal defect	4.3	4.2
Patent ductus arteriosus	3.2	2.9
Tetralogy of Fallot	2.2	2.6
Atrial septal defect	3.2	2.6
Pulmonary stenosis	2.9	2.6
Aortic stenosis	2.6	2.1

*Data from Nora JJ: Multifactorial inheritance hypothesis for the etiology of congenital heart disease: The genetic-environmental interaction. Circulation **38**:604, 1968.
†$\sqrt{p}$, where p = population frequency of the specific defect. From Thompson MW: Thompson and Thompson's Genetics in Medicine, 4th ed. Philadelphia, WB Saunders Co, 1986.

encephaly to lumbar meningocele with little, if any, neurologic impairment. The defect results from failure of the neural tube to close within 28 days after conception (Fig. 1–48). The spectrum also includes encephalocele, iniencephaly, meningomyelocele, usually involving the lower thoracic and lumbar spine (often called spina bifida cystica), and spina bifida. The overall incidence in the British Isles is 4.5 to 5.0 per 1000 births, but in Ireland, Scotland, and Wales, 7.0 to 7.8 per 1000. The incidence in the United States is 1.5 to 2.0 per 1000 births, with a lower incidence in Blacks and Orientals. For anencephaly, any recurrence is apt to be the same malformation, but this may not be true for all types of neural tube defects. Table 1–15 shows the recurrence risk for both anencephaly and spina bifida.

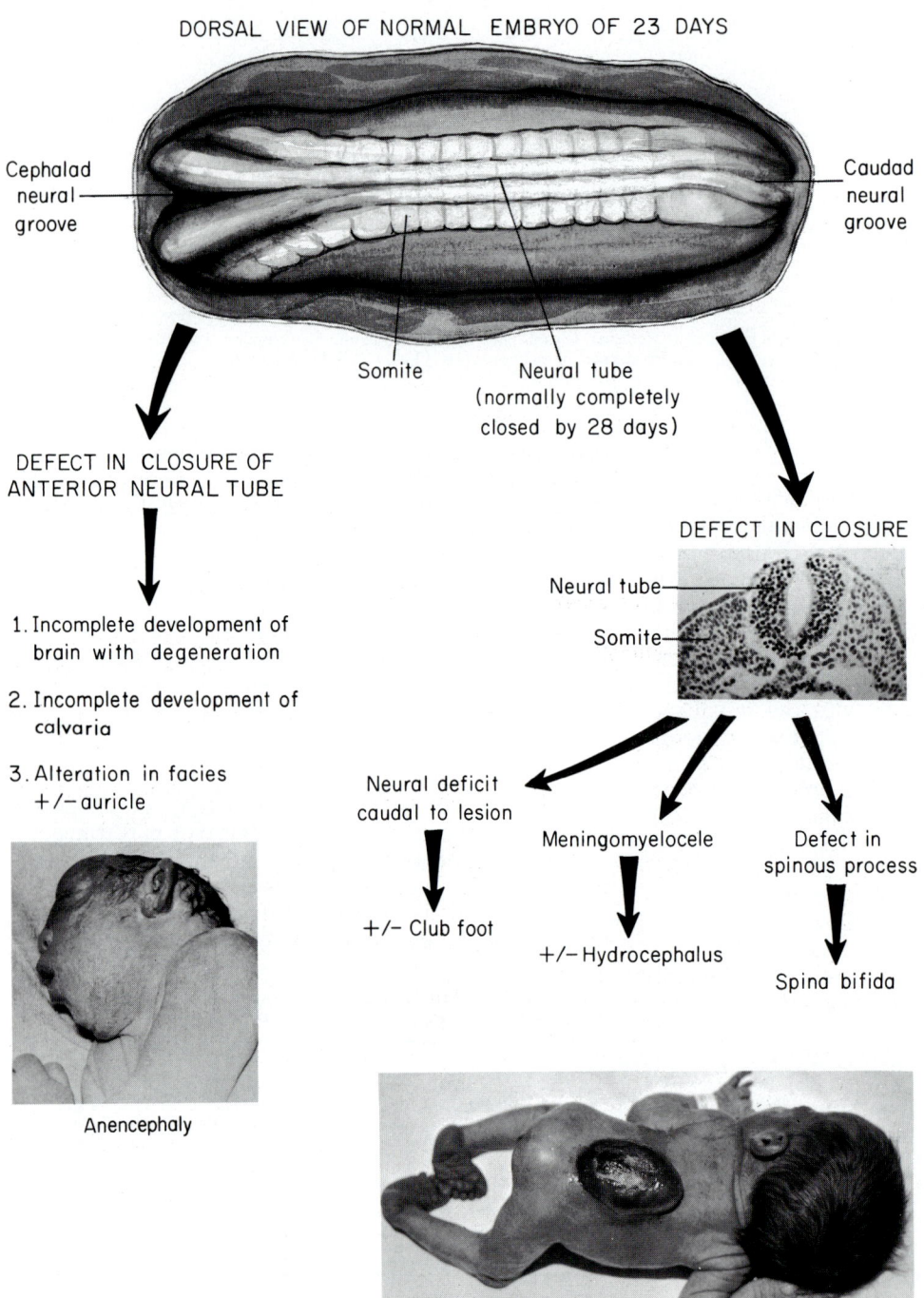

DORSAL VIEW OF NORMAL EMBRYO OF 23 DAYS

Cephalad neural groove

Caudad neural groove

Somite

Neural tube (normally completely closed by 28 days)

DEFECT IN CLOSURE OF ANTERIOR NEURAL TUBE

1. Incomplete development of brain with degeneration

2. Incomplete development of calvaria

3. Alteration in facies +/−auricle

Anencephaly

DEFECT IN CLOSURE

Neural tube

Somite

Neural deficit caudal to lesion

+/− Club foot

Meningomyelocele

+/−Hydrocephalus

Defect in spinous process

Spina bifida

FIGURE 1–48. Defects in closure of the neural tube. (From Smith DW: Recognizable Patterns of Human Malformation. 3rd ed. Philadelphia, WB Saunders Co, 1982.)

Meningomyelocele with partially epithelialized sac

TABLE 1–17. Metabolic Disorders and Their Estimated Frequency Among Newborn Infants in Massachusetts

DISORDER	TOTAL SCREENED	TOTAL DETECTED	FREQUENCY
Phenylketonuria*	981,361	67	1 in 15,000
Atypical phenylketonuria†	981,361	57	1 in 17,000
Iminoglycinuria	332,143	?34‡	? 1 in 10,000‡
Cystinuria†	332,143	21	1 in 16,000
Hartnup "disease"	332,143	18	1 in 18,000
Histidinemia	332,143	18	1 in 18,000
Galactosemia*	550,000	5	1 in 110,000
Maple syrup urine disease*	842,004	5	1 in 170,000
Argininosuccinic acidemia*	332,143	5	1 in 70,000
Cystathioninemia	332,143	3	1 in 110,000
Homocystinuria*	449,615	3	1 in 150,000
Hyperglycinemia (nonketotic)*	332,143	2	1 in 170,000
Propionic acidemia*	332,143	1	<1 in 300,000
Hyperlysinemia†	332,143	1	<1 in 300,000
Hyperornithinemia†	332,143	1	<1 in 300,000
Fanconi syndrome†	332,143	1	<1 in 300,000

*Disorders with definite clinical complications.

†Disorders that may or may not be associated with clinical disease.

‡Number of cases and frequency for iminoglycinuria may be falsely high because carriers for the disorder who have only hyperglycinemia later in life may have iminoglycinuria as young infants.

From Newborn screening for metabolic disorders. N Engl J Med **288**:1299, 1973. Reproduced with permission.

GENETIC ERRORS OF METABOLISM DETECTABLE AT OR SHORTLY AFTER BIRTH

Errors of metabolism are nearly always inherited as autosomal recessive disorders, are usually life-threatening, and are associated with major risks for permanent brain damage. Testing for many metabolic disorders, including athyrotic hypothyroidism, is done routinely in every newborn in many medical centers. Table 1–17 shows a screening summary published for Massachusetts in 1973, and a list of disorders for which screening in the newborn period is possible.

A *biochemical sequence* in living organisms is a stepwise series of reactions leading to production of a specific end-product important to the organism's metabolism. Each step is catalyzed by a specific enzyme, and succeeding reactions in the sequence may be blocked when there is a mutation involving the gene that directs synthesis of the enzyme normally catalyzing the reaction. These mutations nearly always involve substitution of a single amino acid in the wild-type enzyme polypeptide chain. A metabolic block may occur in either a biosynthetic or degradative pathway. The consequences of a metabolic block due to gene mutation may be one of two main types:

1. There is accumulation of all precursors prior to the block.
   a. Functional damage occurs to the organism as a result of the block.
   b. Overaccumulation of intermediate precursors may force biochemical activity into alternate pathways, creating disease from overproduction of toxic products.

2. There may be a deficiency of the normal end-product.

a. If the normal end-product itself is a substrate for a subsequent reaction, that reaction may be unable to proceed.
b. If the end-product is crucial to cell metabolism, the organism may be unable to survive.
c. Failure of end-product synthesis may also result in failure of normal control of the entire biochemical pathway due to lack of "feedback inhibition." Thus, intermediate products will continue to accumulate and become toxic to the cell.

The scheme shown in Figure 1–49 outlines a hypothetical sequence of biochemical reactions within a cell. In this outline, T_A is the membrane transport

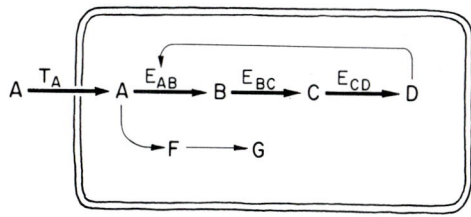

A, B, C, D — Substrate and Products of Major Pathway
F, G — Products of Minor Pathway
T_A — Transport System for A
E_{AB}, E_{BC}, E_{CD} — Enzymes Catalyzing Conversion of A to B, B to C, and C to D
— Cell Membrane

FIGURE 1–49. A hypothetical sequence of biochemical reactions. (From Rosenberg LE: Inborn errors of metabolism. *In* Bondy PK, Rosenberg LE (ed): Metabolic Control and Disease. 8th ed. Philadelphia, WB Saunders Co, 1980.)

system and catalyzes the transport of precursor A into the cell. In one aminoaciduria, Hartnup disease, there is defective transport of tryptophan, a precursor of nicotinamide biosynthesis. Thus, among other problems in these patients, a pellagra-like skin disorder appears. Gene mutations for any of the enzymes E_{AB}, E_{BC}, or E_{CD} would cause accumulation of the immediate precursor. In homocystinuria, for example, a lack of the enzyme cystathionine synthase causes accumulation of the immediate precursor, homocystine, as well as an earlier precursor, methionine. Forcing the alternative reaction, A→F→G, may produce quantities of these substances at concentrations that will be toxic to the cell. Deficiency of enzyme E_{CD} results in failure to produce end-product D and, as a consequence, failure of feedback to inhibit reaction E_{AB}, so that intermediates A, F, and G will accumulate.

Phenylketonuria (PKU) serves as a useful example of biochemical disorder in a metabolic pathway in which different gene mutations, each resulting in a different phenotype, have been identified. In addition to classic PKU, several genetic variants of PKU have been described (Schriver and Clow, 1980). Classic PKU is a result of a mutation in phenylalanine hydroxylase, the enzyme that normally converts phenylalanine to tyrosine (Fig. 1–50). As a result, there is enhancement of an alternate pathway, which increases cellular concentration of phenylpyruvic acid and its two derivative products. It is fortunate that, with the institution of newborn screening programs, untreated PKU is being seen less frequently, but patients with this disease who remain untreated suffer irreparable brain damage. As a secondary effect, due to the lack of tyrosine production in untreated patients, a mild expression of clinical albinism is seen. Mutation at another site in the pathway (reaction 3, Fig. 1–50) results in a deficiency of the enzyme tyrosinase, which blocks the conversion of tyrosine to melanin through DOPA, thus causing one form of albinism. Finally, a mutation that blocks the conversion of homogentisic acid to maleylacetoacetic acid produces the disorder *alkaptonuria*, a rare metabolic disease involving joints, cartilage, and skin.

Successful treatment of infants ascertained to have PKU has made it possible for affected individuals of both sexes to lead normal lives and successfully produce children. For the homozygous affected female who has been treated properly for PKU, has reached reproductive maturity, and is no longer receiving therapy (low phenylalanine diet), there is a special

prenatal consideration. In addition, during recent years there has been an ascertainment of PKU variants which, although not classic PKU, nonetheless involve hyperphenylalaninemia and elevated phenylpyruvic acid level (Schriver and Clow, 1980). Women with either of these abnormalities may produce infants who are mentally retarded and microcephalic and may have a greater than normal incidence of congenital heart disease. Lenke and Levy (1980) recently collected data on 524 pregnancies in 155 women with PKU. A low-phenylalanine diet was initiated in 34 cases after or shortly before pregnancy. Higher rates of mental retardation, microcephaly, and congenital heart disease were noted in the untreated pregnancies. Moreover, dietary treatment instituted during pregnancy was not universally successful in preventing congenital heart disease or mental retardation. Institution of treatment before pregnancy needs further evaluation but may be the means to successfully prevent the phenotypic damage to infants born to hyperphenylalaninemic mothers.

The metabolic disorders described thus far are not life-threatening to the newborn, but there are metabolic derangements that do pose a very real threat to survival unless recognized early in the neonatal period, for which even then appropriate therapy may not be successful. Table 1–18 summarizes metabolic diseases that may cause overwhelming illness in the neonate (Nyhan, 1977a). Many of these problems reflect disorders in the metabolism of branched-chain amino acids and result in neonatal acidosis. There are very sensitive laboratory techniques, e.g., amino acid analysis, gas chromatography, and enzyme analysis, that can establish the diagnosis for a specific metabolic derangement. The clinician must develop the skills to recognize early manifestations of these disorders in the neonate in order to initiate laboratory evaluation in the correct sequence for the appropriate diagnosis. Table 1–19 describes the primary manifestations of a metabolic disorder in the neonate; of particular interest is the observation of pyloric stenosis in this group. Table 1–20 describes the various metabolic diseases with protracted vomiting leading to pyloromyotomy. Nyhan (1977b) points out that in several instances the diagnosis was confirmed at surgery and notes further that in the case of a vomiting infant whom one suspects of having pyloric stenosis, but whose condition is acidotic rather than alkalotic, one is well advised to observe carefully for metabolic disease even when pyloric stenosis is confirmed.

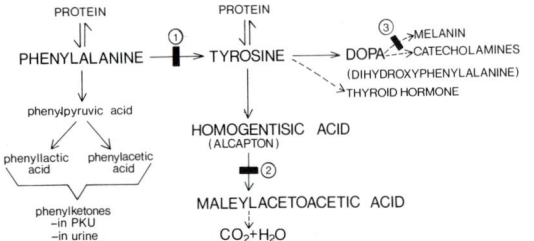

FIGURE 1–50. Scheme of pathways for phenylalanine and tyrosine metabolism. (From Thompson JS, Thompson MW: Genetics in Medicine. 3rd ed. Philadelphia, WB Saunders Co, 1980.)

GENETIC SCREENING FOR DONORS IN ARTIFICIAL INSEMINATION

As already noted, screening for specific genetic disease in newborns is an established procedure throughout much of the United States. Population screening for well-characterized genetic disorders such as Tay-Sachs disease and sickle cell anemia is also widely practiced. Recent reports of rare autosomal recessive diseases appearing in infants born to women made pregnant through artificial insemination by volunteer donors (Johnson et al., 1981; Shapiro and

TABLE 1–18.   Metabolic Disorders Occurring as Acute Overwhelming Disease in the Neonate

DISORDER	DETECTOR SUSPECT	DEFINITIVE DIAGNOSIS
Adrenogenital syndrome	17-ketosteroids	Urinary pregnanetriol; serum; α-OH progesterone; testosterone; DHA
Fructose intolerance	Fructosuria	Hepatic fructose-1-P-aldolase
Galactosemia	Urinary reducing substance	Gal-1-P-uridyl transferase
Hyperammonemia	Blood NH_3; orotic aciduria	Ornithine transcarbamylase; carbamyl phosphate synthetase
Argininosuccinic acidemia	Blood NH_3; urinary argininosuccinate	Argininosuccinate lyase
Citrullinemia	Blood NH_3; citrulline	Argininosuccinate synthetase
Hyperglycinemia, nonketotic	Glycinemia	Glycine-serine conversion
Hypervalinemia	Valinuria	Hypervalinemia; valine-α ketoglutarate transaminase
Isovaleric acidemia	Smell of sweaty feet; isovaleryglycinuria	Isovaleric acid in blood
Lactic acidemia	Attacks of acidosis and hyperventilation; growth retardation; ataxia; hypoglycemia	Lactic acid and alanine in blood and urine; hepatic fructose-1, 6-diphosphatase; pyruvate carboxylase; pyruvate decarboxylase
Lysosomal acid phosphate deficiency		Lysosomal acid phosphatase
Maple syrup urine disease	Urinary 2,4-DNP	Branched-chain amino acidemia; branched-chain ketoacid decarboxylase
Methylmalonic acidemia	Methylmalonic acid in urine	Methylmalonic acid in blood and urine; methylmalonyl CoA mutase
Propionic acidemia	Propionic acidemia; hyperglycinemia	Propionic acidemia; propionyl-CoA carboxylase
Pyroglutamic acidemia		Pyroglutamic acid in blood or urine

From Nyhan WL: An approach to the diagnosis of overwhelming metabolic disease in early infancy. Curr Prob Pediatr 7:3, 1977. Copyright © 1977 by Year Book Medical Publishers, Inc., Chicago. Reproduced with permission.

Hutchinson, 1981) poses the question of whether or not genetic screening should be developed for donors in artificial insemination programs and possibly for recipients as well. Although such screening is not likely to reduce the overall risk for birth defects in the progeny, there are several reasons why some type of genetic screening for both groups would be prudent.

The report by Timmons and associates (1981) from North Carolina is one of the few published studies thus far on this issue, although artificial insemination programs have some type of general donor screening questionnaire. In the Timmons study, 168 donor applicants and 89 recipients were screened. Nineteen of the 168 donors voluntarily withdrew. The study found that 52 (34.9 per cent) of the remaining 149 volunteers who were fully screened as potential donors had family histories warranting rejection or further investigation. Criteria for rejection, in addition to donor age over 36, included major malformations in donor or donor family, mendelian abnormalities, two or

more occurrences of fetal wastage or three or more first-trimester spontaneous abortions in a first-degree relative of either the donor or the recipient, families at high risk for common diseases, mental retardation, and geographic restrictions. The number of donors actually rejected was 17 (11.4 per cent), and an additional 16 (10.7 per cent) required matching with a recipient who did not have a family history for a similar multifactorial disorder. In the recipient group (89), 51 (57.3 per cent) had genetic disorders in their families. Perhaps of equal importance, the Timmons study points out that both donor and recipient often failed to perceive that certain disorders in the family were genetic. The question of whether or not there were hereditary problems in the family was ineffective, even when the donor or recipient had had formal medical training!

Both Timmons and associates (1981) and Johnson

TABLE 1–19.   Characteristics of Candidates for the Diagnosis of Metabolic Disease

Family history of sibling dying early
Overwhelming illness in the neonatal period
Vomiting, pyloric stenosis
Acute acidosis, anion gap
Massive ketosis
Deep coma
Seizures, especially myoclonic
Hiccups, chronic
Unusual odor

From Nyhan WL: Heritable metabolic disease in the differential diagnosis of asphyxia. In Gluck L (ed): Intrauterine Asphyxia and the Developing Fetal Brain. Copyright © 1977 by Year Book Medical Publishers, Inc, Chicago. Reproduced with permission.

TABLE 1–20.   Metabolic Diseases Manifesting as Vomiting Leading to Pyloromyotomy

DISORDER	NO. OF PATIENTS
Ketotic hyperglycinemia syndrome	1
Propionic acidemia	2
Defect in isoleucine metabolism	1
Methylmalonic acidemia	1
Phenylketonuria	3
Isovaleric acidemia	2*

*One patient was operated on at 4 days of age because of severe vomiting and a preoperative diagnosis of "intestinal obstruction." An "abnormal peritoneal band" was said partially to be obstructing the duodenum.

Data from Nyhan WL (ed): Heritable Disorders of Amino Acid Metabolism. New York, John Wiley, 1974. Table from Nyhan WL: Heritable metabolic disease in the differential diagnosis of asphyxia. In Gluck L (ed): Intrauterine Asphyxia and the Developing Fetal Brain. Copyright © 1977 by Year Book Medical Publishers, Inc., Chicago. Reproduced with permission.

and colleagues (1981) have made suggestions for systematic genetic evaluation of artificial insemination donors and recipients. These include (1) donor/recipient survey and family survey for genetic risk factors and genetic diseases; (2) Rh incompatibility testing; (3) sperm count and morphology studies; (4) carrier testing at least for Tay-Sachs disease, sickle cell anemia, and thalassemia; (5) banded chromosome analysis; and (6) genetic counseling. This type of survey needs to be developed in a practical way to give some assurance that at least for the screening provided, the future child will not be at increased risk for a genetic or chromosomal disorder transmitted by the biological father.

RECENT DEVELOPMENTS IN HUMAN GENETICS

Molecular Cytogenetics

The 1970s produced chromosome banding technology and unequivocal identification of each chromosome pair. The 1990s will witness molecular genetic technology dramatically change the speed of data collection, accuracy, and breadth of data derived from chromosome analysis. By the turn of the century, routine banded chromosome analysis may be as archaic as we now consider buccal smear and sex chromatin analysis to be.

High-resolution technology yields chromosome bands ranging in number from 500 to 2000 per 23 chromosomes. Under these conditions, the smallest chromosome deletion or duplication visible with a standard laboratory microscope would still be several million nucleotide pairs in length. Consistency in achieving 800 to 2000 bands per haploid chromosome set is difficult. This, plus added expense and time for routine analysis of such chromosomes, thwarted the use of 2000 band analysis. However, the combination of cytogenetic and molecular analysis has created an essentially new discipline of molecular cytogenetics which is likely to revolutionize chromosome analysis.

Several disorders, previously considered to be chromosomally normal by standard G-banded metaphase analysis, are now known to be associated with tiny deletions/duplications in chromosomes analyzed by high-resolution banding (Table 1–21).

Within this group, Prader-Willi syndrome and Angelman's syndrome have thus far been most informative. Approximately 60 per cent of all patients with phenotypic Prader-Willi syndrome have a detectable interstitial deletion at band q12 in chromosome 15 (Fig. 1–51). Deletions at precisely the same site are observed in approximately 50 per cent of patients with Angelman's syndrome. Molecular analysis at band q12, chromosome 15, has documented that the deleted 15q in patients with Prader-Willi syndrome is essentially always paternal in origin, whereas the deleted 15q in patients with Angelman's syndrome is maternal in origin. These observations suggest that maternal-derived chromosome 15 is necessary to prevent Angelman's syndrome and a paternal-derived chromo-

TABLE 1–21. Phenotype/Karyotype Correlations in Selected Microdeletion/Duplication Syndromes

DIAGNOSIS	PHENOTYPE
Langer-Giedion syndrome	Microcephaly, mental retardation, growth deficiency, lax skin, sparse hair, bulbous nose, multiple exostoses
Beckwith-Wiedemann syndrome	Gigantism, macroglossia, exomphalos, predisposition to certain embryonal tumors including Wilms' tumor
Aniridia with Wilms' tumor	Aniridia, Wilms' tumor, GU anomalies, mental retardation
Miller-Dieker syndrome	Mental retardation, cerebral agyria, cardiac defects, micrognathia
Prader-Willi syndrome	Hypotonia, hypogonadism, mental retardation, short stature, small hands and feet, obesity
Angelman's syndrome	Severe mental retardation, ataxia, speech almost absent, paroxysms of laughter, characteristic facies

some 15 is necessary to prevent expression of the Prader-Willi phenotype.

Recent molecular analysis in 20 to 30 per cent of patients with Prader-Willi syndrome who lack any recognizable deletion at band 15q12, demonstrated that in each instance, the patient had inherited both copies of the maternal chromosome 15 and no paternal 15. In fewer cases, some patients with Angelman's syndrome, but without deletion on chromosome 15, have inherited both paternal 15 chromosomes and none from the mother. The term for this phenomenon is uniparental disomy and raises the possibility of

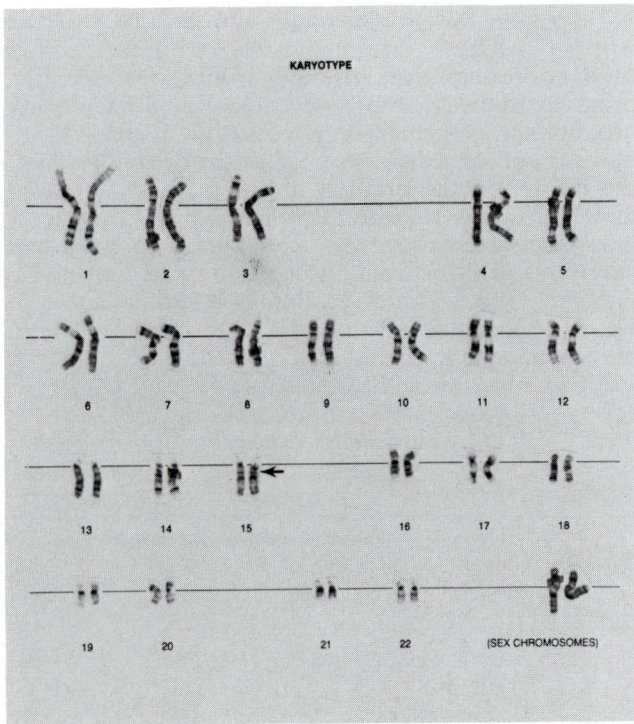

FIGURE 1–51. A karyotype demonstrating an interstitial deletion (*arrow*) at band q12 in chromosome 15.

imprinting as the pathogenesis for certain malformation/chromosomal syndromes.

In humans, triploidy (see Fig. 1–38) occurs when there is twice the normal chromosomal contribution from one parent. Fetal/placental phenotype appears to be influenced by parental source of the extra haploid (23) set of chromosomes. Triploidy, with two paternal sets and one maternal set of chromosomes, is usually associated with a large cystic placenta and frequent partial molar changes.

In contrast, if the parental chromosome contribution is two maternal sets and one paternal set, the placenta is usually small, underdeveloped, and noncystic. Correspondingly, the fetal phenotype is characterized by marked growth retardation in contrast to the android fetal phenotype (two paternal and one maternal complement) characterized by large head with CNS abnormalities, small body, syndactyly, and intrauterine growth retardation.

This is but one example of possible imprinting in humans (Hall, 1990). As will be noted in a subsequent section in this chapter, imprinting may be altered from one generation to another and, although not explicitly a mutation, may last the lifetime of that individual. The molecular basis for imprinting remains unresolved. However, it seems increasingly clear that normal human development requires both maternal and paternal genomes. We may soon discover that a surprising number of heretofore poorly understood abnormalities reflect defective genomic signals to the developing embryo.

Diagnostic Molecular Genetics

Advances in the field of molecular biology, collectively known as recombinant DNA technology, have revolutionized our understanding of the structure and function of the human genome. In 1982, McKusick noted that approximately 450 genes and other markers had been mapped on the human genome. By 1987, the number had increased to nearly 3500 (McAlpine et al., 1987), with greater than 1000 of these mapped genes being cloned (Schmidtke and Cooper, 1988). Proposals to begin sequencing the entire human genome began in the mid 1980s. These efforts culminated with the formation of the Human Genome Project, a multinational program dedicated to the construction of high-resolution genetic and physical maps as well as complete nucleotide sequencing of the entire human genome (National Research Council, 1988). With the Human Genome Project now under way, it is no longer unrealistic to predict that by the end of this century most if not all of the estimated 50,000 to 100,000 genes in the human genome will be mapped and the molecular defects that lead to disease phenotypes will be identified.

The application of recombinant DNA technology to the study of monogenic diseases has led to accurate carrier identification and prenatal diagnosis as well as a better understanding of the molecular basis for several of these disorders. Linkage analysis, using DNA sequence polymorphisms closely linked to a gene, is now commonly used for prenatal diagnosis for families at risk for disorders such as Huntington's disease and adult polycystic kidney disease, in which either the specific disease gene has not been cloned or the specific mutation in the gene has yet to be identified. Direct gene analysis is possible for disorders such as sickle cell anemia and cystic fibrosis, in which the specific gene has been cloned and the molecular defect is known.

What follows is a primer in recombinant DNA technology as well as a description of how the most recent technologic advances are currently being applied to the carrier identification and prenatal diagnosis of monogenic disorders.

The Human Genome

As stated previously, there are approximately 3 billion base pairs of DNA encoding for the estimated 50,000 to 100,000 genes in the human genome. Genes range in length from the hundreds to the millions of base pairs but compose only a small portion of the genome. The majority of DNA exists as intergenic sequences and serves little or no essential cellular function.

Structural genes are composed of an alternating series of exons and introns that vary widely in size and number. Exons compose the DNA coding region of a structural gene and are both transcribed into RNA and translated into protein without disturbing their original order. Introns, or intervening sequences, are not part of the coding region. These sequences are included in the primary RNA transcription product, but are subsequently spliced out before translation occurs (Fig. 1–52). As expected, it is within the exons that the majority of detectable mutations producing phenotypic change are found. Mutations detected in introns typically involve base changes at the exon-intron junction and therefore affect the RNA splicing process.

Recombinant DNA Technology

Restriction Endonucleases

Restriction endonucleases are a unique class of enzymes that recognize specific short nucleotide se-

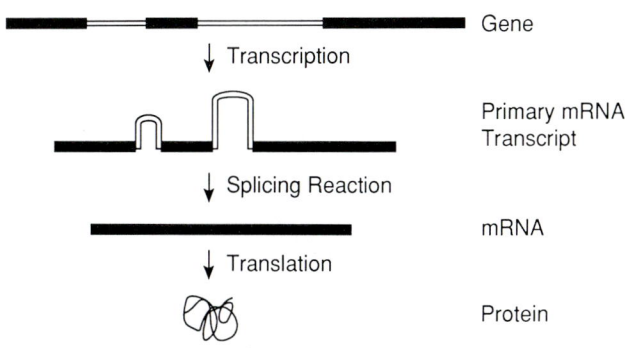

FIGURE 1–52. Transcription of DNA to RNA and translation of RNA to protein. Introns (□) are spliced out of the primary mRNA transcript and exons (■) are joined together to form mature mRNA.

quences in a double-stranded DNA molecule from any source and cleave both strands. In 1970, Smith and Wilcox made a chance discovery that the bacterium *Haemophilus influenzae* selectively degraded foreign bacterial virus DNA. This degradative activity was subsequently found to be due to the restriction endonuclease, HindII, which not only broke down foreign DNA but left its own DNA intact. Shortly thereafter, Kelly and Smith (1970) made the additional discovery that HindII was cleavage-specific. The enzyme recognized a specific nucleotide sequence and cleaved the foreign DNA only at that recognition site. Moreover, the enzyme cleaved all sites at which the recognition sequence occurred.

Since these initial discoveries, more than 100 restriction endonucleases that cleave DNA at sequence-specific sites from 4 to 8 base pairs have been isolated from various bacteria. Certain restriction endonucleases, for example, the enzyme EcoRI isolated from *Escherichia coli*, make staggered cuts at the recognition site, thus producing uneven or "sticky" ends:

$$\downarrow$$

$$5'\text{-G-A-A-T-T-C-}3'$$
$$3'\text{-C-T-T-A-A-G-}5'$$

$$\uparrow$$

$$\downarrow$$

$$5'\text{-G} \qquad + \qquad \text{A-A-T-T-C-}3'$$
$$3'\text{-C-T-T-A-A} \qquad\qquad \text{G-}5'$$

In this example, the enzyme cleaves between the G-A dinucleotide of both strands, yielding DNA fragments of varying lengths with frayed ends. Other restriction endonucleases, for example, the enzyme HaeIII isolated from *Haemophilus aegyptius*, make even cuts at the recognition site, thus producing blunt ends:

$$\downarrow$$

$$5'\text{pr-G-G-C-C-}3'$$
$$3'\text{-C-C-G-G-}5'$$

$$\uparrow$$

$$\downarrow$$

$$5'\text{-G-G} + \text{C-C-}3'$$
$$3'\text{-C-C} \qquad \text{G-G-}5'$$

In this example, the enzyme cleaves between the G-C dinucleotide of both strands (*arrows*), yielding DNA fragments of varying lengths that are fully base-paired.

The discovery of restriction endonucleases that are cleavage site–specific led directly to the development of cloning techniques. In 1973, Cohen and colleagues developed the first method of enzymatically combining DNA sequences from two different sources into a single DNA molecule. A *plasmid* is a circular piece of DNA transmitted genetically in the host cell, in this case a bacterium. By mixing EcoRI-digested *E. coli* plasmid pSC101 DNA with EcoRI-digested foreign DNA fragments and adding DNA ligase, Cohen and his collaborators could open the circular plasmid DNA, insert the foreign DNA, then close the circle, thus creating new hybrid plasmids containing one or more foreign DNA fragments inserted into the EcoRI rec-

ognition site of the pSC101 plasmid. This is illustrated in Figure 1–53. Later experiments found that if a foreign DNA fragment was inserted into autonomously replicating circular plasmid DNA, and if the recombinant molecule was used to infect a bacterial cell, the hybrid plasmid would replicate normally along with the host cell. Propagation of a DNA sequence by this method was termed *molecular cloning*. It was now possible to isolate a specific DNA sequence or gene in quantities large enough to permit the analysis of genome structure and function.

Genetic Probes

A human gene-specific probe is a recombinant DNA molecule used to detect the presence of a particular DNA sequence in the human genome. Probes can be prepared by various techniques. Examples include isolation of a portion of the gene, isolation of messenger RNA (mRNA), and synthesis of a single-stranded DNA fragment using specific mRNA as the template. A human gene-specific probe can be labeled with a radioisotope and, when mixed with denatured (single-stranded) human DNA, will hybridize only to its complementary sequence. As shall be seen later, the ability to detect specific sequences in the human genome allows for the study of DNA polymorphisms closely linked to disease genes. This in turn allows for carrier detection and prenatal diagnosis of monogenic disorders even without prior knowledge of the biochemical defect or of the nature of the mutation.

Typically, the use of a gene-specific probe requires the prior construction of a DNA sequence library from which the recombinant DNA molecule can be isolated and cloned. Once the recombinant molecule has been incorporated into a bacterial host and propagated, the DNA sequence of interest can be removed from the plasmid enzymatically and used as a probe. Two types of libraries will be described here. One can construct the genomic library by subjecting total human DNA to restriction endonuclease digestion, combining the fragments with an appropriate plasmid, introducing these recombinant DNA molecules into bacteria, and cloning each fragment. This type of library contains nontranscribed (intergenic) sequences as well as transcribed and translated sequences. One is therefore faced with the dilemma of isolating a particular clone of interest from millions of others. This can be overcome by construction of a complementary DNA library, which contains only transcribed and translated sequences. In 1970, two independent investigations (Baltimore, 1970; Temin and Mizutani, 1970) led to the discovery of the enzyme reverse transcriptase. This enzyme permits the synthesis of a double-stranded complementary DNA, or cDNA, using single-stranded mRNA as template. The cDNA library will therefore be representative of the mRNA expressed in the particular cell type from which it was derived and reduces the number of potential clones from the millions to the thousands. After the cDNA molecule is synthesized, it can be inserted into the appropriate plasmid and cloned. Once a cDNA molecule of interest has been cloned and isolated, it can be used as a probe

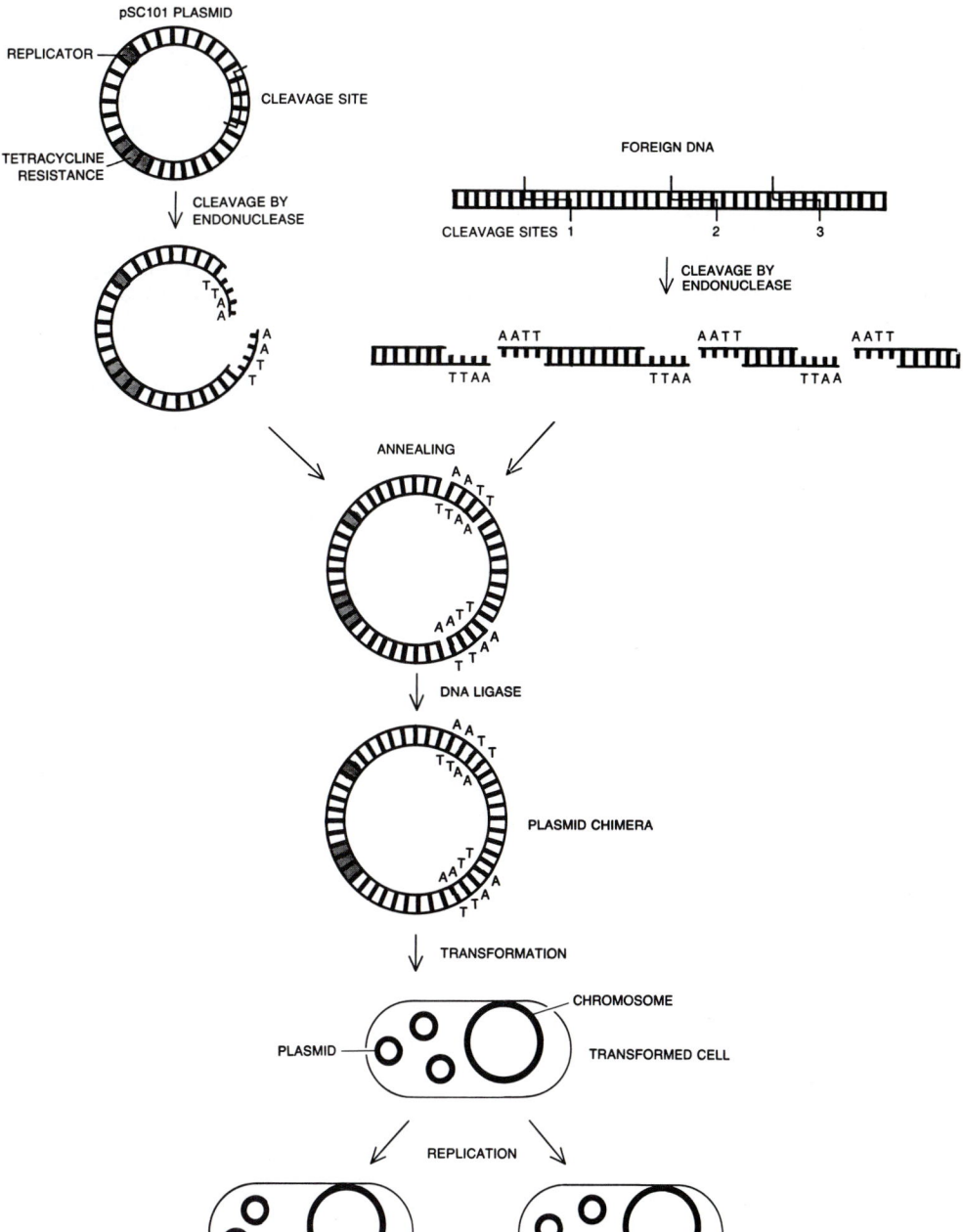

FIGURE 1–53. An illustrative scheme for insertion of a DNA probe into the chromosome of a bacterial plasmid. (From Cohen SN: The manipulation of genes. Sci Am **233**:24. Copyright © 1975 by Scientific American, Inc. All rights reserved.)

either to identify a particular gene or DNA sequence in the human genome or to pick out complementary clones from a genomic library.

A more simplified method of detecting changes in base sequence can be used if the mutation leading to an abnormal phenotype is known. Allele specific oligonucleotides (ASOs) of approximately 20 nucleotides, containing either the mutated or normal sequence, can be synthesized chemically and used as probes. Under the appropriate conditions, the ASOs bind only to their exact complementary sequences, thus making it possible to identify a specific molecular defect in an affected or carrier individual.

Southern Blotting

In 1975, Southern developed a technique which has proved to be an extremely powerful tool in analyzing the organization of the human genome as well as diagnosing monogenic disorders. The technique, known as *Southern blotting*, combines the abilities of restriction endonucleases to cleave DNA and of gene-specific probes to detect complementary sequences in the genome. The method consists of digesting genomic DNA with a site-specific restriction enzyme and separating the resultant fragments, according to size, by agarose gel electrophoresis (Fig. 1–54). Since a

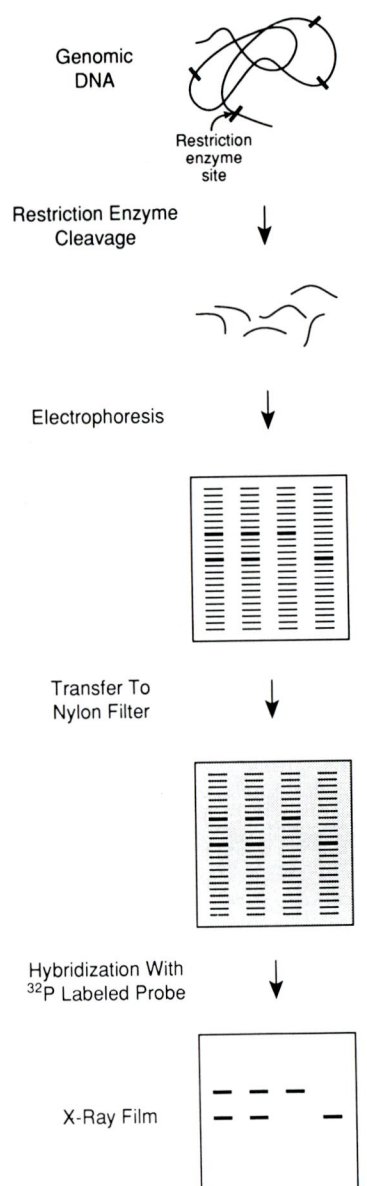

Genomic
DNA

Restriction
enzyme
site

Restriction Enzyme
Cleavage

Electrophoresis

Transfer To
Nylon Filter

Hybridization With
^{32}P Labeled Probe

X-Ray Film

FIGURE 1–54. Southern blotting. DNA is cleaved by a restriction enzyme, separated according to size by agarose gel electrophoresis, and transferred to a filter. After hybridization of the DNA to a labeled probe and exposure of the filter to X-ray film, complementary sequences can be identified.

restriction enzyme will cleave human genomic DNA into a continuum of fragments, the DNA appears as a "smear" in the agarose gel. The DNA fragments in the gel are then hydrolyzed with acid, denatured with an alkaline solution, and neutralized. A nitrocellulose or nylon filter is then placed on the gel, and the fragments are transferred onto the filter by a flow of salt solution through the gel perpendicular to the direction of electrophoresis. The DNA fragments are then immobilized on the filter either by being baked at 80°C or by a crosslinking of the fragments to the filter by exposure to ultraviolet light. This transfer of DNA fragments creates an exact copy of the electro-

phoretic separation pattern on the filter. A gene-specific probe, labeled with the radioisotope ^{32}P to a high specific activity, is then hybridized to the filter. After the filter is exposed to x-ray film, any fragments that are fully or partially complementary to the probe will be visible as distinct bands.

Identification, localization, and fine restriction mapping of a particular gene can be performed with the aid of Southern blotting. In addition, gene deletions and insertions, as well as single base substitutions within a restriction enzyme recognition site that alter fragment size, can be identified with this technique.

Polymerase Chain Reaction

The aforementioned technology has had a major impact on molecular genetics by allowing for the first time carrier detection and prenatal diagnosis of single gene disorders. Although the ability of recombinant DNA techniques to generate vital information concerning a particular disease in an at-risk family has never been questioned, adapting this technology for use in a clinical diagnostic laboratory environment has come under scrutiny. Linkage analysis typically requires the examination of multiple linked loci that are both proximal and distal to a gene. This is due to the risk of a meiotic recombination event occurring between a locus or loci and the gene of interest. Direct gene analysis may involve examination of multiple mutation sites, thus requiring the use of multiple probes or ASOs. It generally takes up to 2 weeks to culture enough cells from amniotic fluid or chorionic villi to obtain an adequate DNA sample (approximately 5/μg per restriction enzyme digest) for prenatal diagnosis, and an additional 1 to 2 weeks to perform Southern blotting with multiple probes. A further consideration involves the use of a radioisotope to label these probes, thus creating potential health hazards and disposal problems that need to be addressed. Because of the laboriousness of the technology and the requirement for special training in the handling of radioisotopes, molecular geneticists searched for ways to simplify existing techniques as well as more rapid alternative approaches to the diagnosis of inherited disorders.

The development of the polymerase chain reaction (PCR) (Saiki et al., 1985; Mullis and Faloona, 1987) and subsequent application to the area of molecular diagnosis has revolutionized the way DNA analysis is carried out in the clinical laboratory. The PCR not only simplifies the technology, thus allowing diagnosis to proceed with greater speed, but also provides the molecular geneticist with substantially more methodologies from which to choose when analyzing a particular gene or molecular defect. The PCR is an *in vitro* enzymatic synthesis technique that uses a DNA polymerase to amplify 10^6 to 10^7 copies of a targeted sequence of DNA. Minimal amounts of DNA isolated from cells present in a dried blood spot, a single hair root, or a single sperm can be used as template. The amplified target DNA can then be subjected to molecular analysis directly, thus eliminating the need for molecular cloning or for extraction of the microgram amounts of DNA required for Southern blotting.

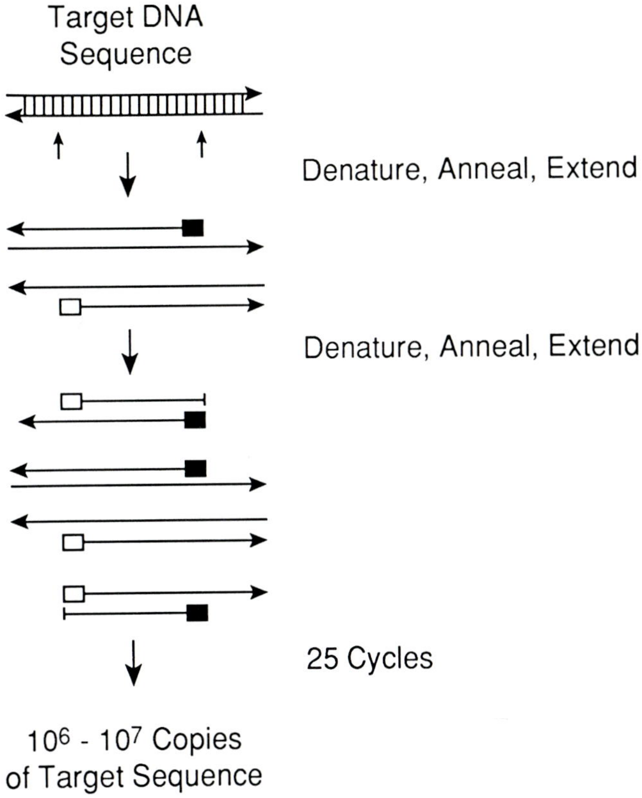

Target DNA
Sequence

Denature, Anneal, Extend

Denature, Anneal, Extend

25 Cycles

10^6 - 10^7 Copies
of Target Sequence

FIGURE 1–55. The polymerase chain reaction. Repeated synthesis of a specific target DNA sequence (*upper arrows*) results in exponential amplification. The reaction proceeds from the primers (□, ■) in the 3′ direction on both strands. The first two cycles of the PCR are shown.

To perform a PCR, the nucleotide sequences that flank the target DNA must be known. Two short chains of approximately 20 nucleotides (oligonucleotides) that complement opposite strands on either side of the target DNA are chemically synthesized and used as primers in the reaction (Fig. 1–55). A typical reaction consists of approximately 25 repeated cycles of three temperature-dependent steps. First, the DNA template is heat denatured at 94°C to form single strands. Second, the primers anneal to their complementary sequences; the orientation of the primers permits synthesis across the segment between them. The annealing temperature, normally between 35°C and 65°C, is dependent upon primer sequence and specificity. Third, a thermostable DNA polymerase initiates primer extension in both directions across the template. The primer extension products are then used as templates for subsequent cycles resulting in an exponential amplification of the original target sequence.

The molecular diagnostic applications of PCR technology became apparent immediately. Numerous PCR methodologies designed to detect polymorphic loci, point mutations, and deletions in single gene disorders soon followed. Working with the gene for hemophilia A, Kogan and colleagues (1987) demonstrated that a polymorphic locus or point mutation caused by an alteration in sequence that creates or destroys a restriction endonuclease cleavage site can be analyzed by enzyme digestion and gel electrophoresis of the amplified product. Saiki and colleagues (1986) developed a method by which amplified products containing the normal, hemoglobin S, or hemoglobin C alleles from the beta-globin locus were spot-ted onto a nitrocellulose or nylon filter (dot blot) and hybridized with radiolabeled ASOs to distinguish between the normal and mutant alleles. This method was subsequently found to be quite useful in the analyzing of mutations that do not involve a restriction enzyme site. A reverse dot blot method was also developed to analyze single gene disorders caused by a number of different mutations (Saiki et al., 1989). Here, the ASOs representing the normal and mutant alleles are fixed to a filter and hybridized to the labeled amplified product, thus eliminating the need for multiple hybridizations with multiple labeled probes. Wu and colleagues (1989) developed an allele-specific PCR (ASPCR) method for analyzing the hemoglobin S mutation that allows for direct detection of the normal or mutant allele without the need for restriction enzyme digestion or ASO hybridization. Two allele-specific primers, complementary to either the normal or mutant allele, are synthesized that differ only in the nucleotide at the 3′ terminus. Two separate PCR reactions under properly controlled conditions and containing one allele-specific primer plus an opposite strand primer will result in amplification only if there is complete homology between the allele-specific primer and the DNA template, thus identifying the presence of that particular allele. Haliassos and colleagues (1989) developed an additional method of detecting point mutations not involving a restriction site. Primer synthesis with a single base mismatch can create an artificial cleavage site. If an adjacent point mutation is contained within the recognition site, normal and mutant alleles can be distinguished by enzyme digestion and gel electrophoresis of the amplified product. Lastly, Chehab and colleagues (1987) demonstrated an extremely powerful method of detecting gene deletions in the alpha-globin loci by determining the presence or absence of more than one amplified product in a single PCR reaction. The method, known as multiplex PCR, has been further developed by Chamberlain and colleagues (1988, 1990) and involves the simultaneous amplification of numerous DNA sequences contained in a gene. If multiple primer sets are added to a single PCR and the amplified products are subjected to gel electrophoresis, an unknown gene deletion such as those found in the dystrophin gene of males with Duchenne muscular dystrophy or Becker's muscular dystrophy can be identified by the failure of a single primer set to amplify across its target sequence.

The development of PCR technology has greatly simplified molecular diagnosis of monogenic diseases. Southern analysis, a labor-intensive and costly technique, is no longer required for the diagnosis of an ever-increasing number of disorders. The PCR methodologies mentioned above can identify polymorphic loci, point mutations, and deletions with speed and accuracy and are readily adaptable to carrier identification and prenatal diagnosis.

DNA Sequencing

In-depth analysis of the structure and function of the human genome could not have proceeded without the development of techniques to determine the exact nucleotide sequence of DNA. Before the discovery of restriction endonucleases, it was not possible to determine the base sequence of a gene or DNA fragment because a method for cleaving DNA at specific sites, thus producing short fragments of defined length, did not exist. RNA molecules of approximately 80 nucleotides in length were the first nucleic acids to be sequenced in the mid-1960s. RNA sequencing proceeded with much success until the mid-1970s when, after the discovery of site-specific restriction enzymes, a number of methods appeared that permitted the sequencing of short fragments of DNA up to approximately 500 nucleotide pairs.

Foremost among these methodologies were the chemical cleavage method (Maxam and Gilbert, 1977) and the dideoxynucleotide chain termination method (Sanger et al., 1977) for sequencing DNA. Both of these methods have proved useful but extremely time consuming, requiring the molecular cloning of the DNA fragment of interest. After the development of PCR technology, DNA sequencing of the amplified product became possible. Initially, the PCR product was subcloned into a vector and subsequently sequenced with the dideoxynucleotide chain termination method. Direct sequence analysis was then developed, which utilized the amplified fragment as template for a sequencing reaction without subcloning, and has become the most powerful technique for detecting unknown or multiple mutations (Engelke et al., 1988, Gyllensten and Erlich, 1988). Direct sequencing has allowed for characterization of multiple mutations in hemophilia A (Higuchi et al., 1990), beta-thalassemia (Aulehla-Scholz et al., 1990), and Lesch-Nyhan disease (Sculley et al., 1991).

Linkage Analysis

Linkage analysis utilizes DNA polymorphisms to track the inheritance of a particular gene within a family. DNA polymorphisms exist throughout the human genome. A DNA polymorphism is simply an inheritable variation in base pair sequence. These variations in DNA sequence have been estimated to occur every 200 to 300 nucleotide pairs in the intergenic regions of the genome and have been identified within genes as well. These polymorphisms are transmitted by mendelian probabilities from one generation to the next. Intragenic polymorphisms and variations found to be closely linked to a disease gene can be used as genetic markers for molecular diagnosis. Theoretically, any single gene disorder should be amenable to carrier identification and prenatal diagnosis by linkage analysis without any previous understanding of the biochemical or molecular defect.

A polymorphism that results from a single nucleotide substitution which alters a restriction enzyme recognition site is called a restriction fragment length polymorphism (RFLP). Typically, two alleles are generated by a change in recognition site, which can be distinguished by size either on a Southern blot following restriction enzyme digestion of genomic DNA or on a gel following electrophoresis of restriction enzyme digested PCR products. The alleles behave codominantly and thus can be used for diagnosis in informative families by linking one of the alleles to the mutant gene of interest. Kan and Dozy (1978) first recognized the potential importance of RFLP analysis in molecular diagnosis when they performed a prenatal diagnosis of sickle cell anemia using an RFLP closely linked to the beta-globin locus. Provided a probe was available to detect an RFLP linked to a disease gene, linkage analysis quickly became accepted as a reliable method for prenatal diagnosis of a single gene disorder in which either the gene had not been cloned or the specific mutation had yet to be identified.

Variable number of tandem repeats (VNTR) is another type of polymorphism which results from a variation in the number of times a particular DNA sequence is tandemly repeated. VNTRs are highly polymorphic, possessing several alleles per locus, and like RFLPs can be distinguished by size using either Southern analysis or gel electrophoresis of PCR products. Short tandem repeats (STR) is another kind of polymorphism related to variation in number of tandem repeats. STRs differ from VNTRs in the size of their DNA repeat, which is typically 2 to 4 base pairs compared to 10 to 50 base pairs for VNTRs. An intragenic STR has recently proved useful for prenatal diagnosis of cystic fibrosis in families uninformative for the common mutation delta F508 (Mornet et al., 1992). Since more than two alleles are usually present at VNTR and STR loci, they have been found to be more informative and consequently more useful for prenatal diagnosis than RFLPs.

To perform linkage analysis within a family, DNA must be obtained from both parents and an affected offspring. The polymorphic locus or loci being analyzed must be fully informative, i.e., in the case of an

FIGURE 1–56. Schematic illustration of pedigree and prenatal diagnosis by DNA-probe analysis of restriction fragment length polymorphisms (RFLPs). On the left is the pedigree for two families. The darkened symbols represent heterozygosity or homozygosity for the disease gene. Members tested are listed numerically. Open triangles represent fetuses in putative pregnancies. (a) and (b) represent DNA restriction fragment lengths. The panels on the right represent gel electrophoresis patterns for RFLPs. (Modified from Emery AEH: An Introduction to Recombinant DNA. Copyright © 1984, John Wiley & Sons, Inc. Reprinted by permission of John Wiley & Sons, Inc.)

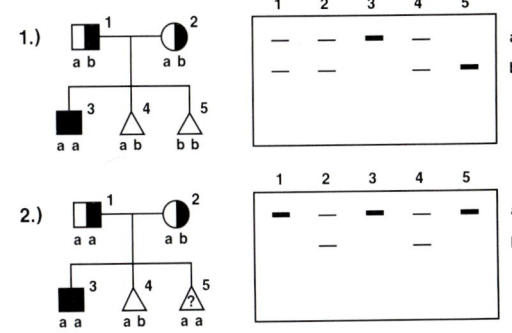

autosomal disorder, all four parental chromosomes must be distinguished. This is illustrated in Figure 1–56. In family 1, both parents are heterozygous for the RFLP alleles (a) and (b). The affected male is homozygous for allele (a), thus linking the mutant gene to this allele in both parents. This family is therefore fully informative at this RFLP locus. If prenatal diagnosis is performed, a genotype of (ab) would indicate a heterozygous carrier fetus (fetus 4), whereas a genotype of (bb) would indicate a homozygous normal fetus (fetus 5). In family 2, the mother is heterozygous for the RFLP alleles (a) and (b), but the father is homozygous for allele (a). The affected male is likewise homozygous for allele (a), thus linking the mutant gene to allele (a) in the mother, but failing to determine which paternal (a) allele is linked to the mutant gene. This family is therefore only partially informative at this RFLP locus. If prenatal diagnosis is performed, a genotype of (ab) would indicate either a heterozygous carrier or a homozygous normal fetus (fetus 4), whereas a genotype of (aa) would indicate either a heterozygous carrier or a homozygous affected fetus (fetus 5). In the case of fetus 5, the parents would face a 50 per cent risk of having an affected offspring. This risk can be altered by analyzing additional RFLP loci that are informative (heterozygous) for the father.

Meiotic recombination between an intergenic marker and the gene of interest should always be considered when performing prenatal diagnosis by linkage analysis. Approximately 30 to 40 recombinations occur per genome during meiosis I. A marker and a gene that are tightly linked have less of a risk of recombination and a greater likelihood of segregating together. To aid in identifying recombination events and to guard against possible misinterpretation of results, multiple closely linked markers located on either side of the gene are analyzed. It is usually preferable to use intragenic markers, if available, thereby reducing the risk of recombination in most genes to close to zero. Another consideration when performing linkage analysis for an X-linked disorder is the rate of new mutation. One-third of males affected with an X-linked disease are the result of new mutations, thus making it difficult to assign carrier status to mothers with only one affected son. For subsequent pregnancies it often becomes necessary to analyze siblings of the affected male or extended family members to more accurately determine carrier status in the mother.

Direct Gene Analysis

When a gene has been cloned and the mutation(s) responsible for the disease phenotype has been identified, carrier identification and prenatal diagnosis can be accomplished with direct detection methods. This increases the reliability of the analysis by eliminating the concern for meiotic recombination. Known point mutations, insertions, and deletions can be readily identified by Southern analysis or manipulation of PCR products by means of methods previously described. The application of this current technology to the diagnosis of specific single gene disorders will now be discussed.

Sickle Cell Disease

Sickle cell disease is an autosomal recessive disorder occurring most frequently among African nations. Approximately 1 in 12.5 American Blacks is heterozygous (carrier) for this disease, which results from a mutation in the beta-globin gene located on chromosome 11 and leads to the formation of abnormal sickle cell hemoglobin (Hb S). A newborn must be homozygous, i.e., inherit the sickle cell mutation from both parents, in order to be affected with this disorder. The characteristic clinical feature among patients with sickle cell disease is the abnormal or sickle appearance of red blood cells in the deoxygenated state. The phenotype consists of anemia, failure to thrive, repeated infections, and splenomegaly. Heterozygotes for this disorder have sickle cell trait. These individuals are asymptomatic, although sickling of red blood cells can occur when they are subjected to extremely low oxygen pressure. Carriers for sickle cell anemia are also immune to malarial infection. This heterozygote advantage has been used to explain the high mutant gene frequency in those regions of Africa where malaria is endemic.

Hb S was the first hemoglobin variant to be identified as well as the first point mutation to be detected directly. Consequently, Hb S has served as a molecular model for the development of much of the current DNA diagnostic technology. Hb S is due to a single nucleotide alteration (A→T) in the beta-globin gene which causes an amino acid substitution (glutamic acid → valine) at codon 6 of the beta-globin chain. This single point mutation, also called a missense mutation, is responsible for the development of the abnormal hemoglobin and, therefore, of the clinical manifestations of the disease. Hemoglobin C (Hb C) was the second abnormal hemoglobin to be detected and is likewise the result of a missense mutation: a single base change (G→A) in the beta-globin gene causing an amino acid substitution (glutamic acid → lysine) also at codon 6 of the beta-globin chain. About 1 in 100 American Blacks is a carrier for the Hb C mutation. Individuals who inherit the Hb S mutation from one parent and the Hb C mutation from the other parent (Hb SC disease) generally have a milder form of sickle cell disease.

Heterozygotes for the Hb S or Hb C mutation can be identified either by hemoglobin electrophoresis or DNA analysis. As stated previously, prenatal diagnosis of sickle cell disease using molecular diagnostic techniques was initially accomplished by RFLP analysis using a polymorphism adjacent to the beta-globin gene, which was generated by HpaI (isolated from *Haemophilus parainfluenzae*) digestion of genomic DNA (Kan and Dozy, 1978). Direct gene analysis by PCR is now used and greatly simplifies the diagnosis. The single nucleotide substitution found in Hb S destroys the CvnI (isolated from *Chromatium vinosum*) recognition site at codon 6 of the beta-globin gene. The Hb S mutation can be detected by altered fragment size after amplification of a 725 base pair (bp) fragment including this CvnI site followed by digestion of the PCR product and gel electrophoresis (Fig. 1–57). Amplified DNA from a homozygote for hemoglobin A (Hb A) has a normal CvnI recognition site in both beta-globin genes and shows bands at 201 bp and 180 bp after enzyme digestion. A homozygote for Hb S has an altered recognition site in both beta-globin genes and shows a single band at 381 bp. A hetero-

zygote (Hb AS) has an altered recognition site in one beta-globin gene and shows bands at 381 bp, 201 bp, and 180 bp. The digestion of the 725 bp fragment at two additional CvnI sites yields two constant bands at 256 bp and 88 bp, which serve as an internal control for the analysis. The Hb C mutation at codon 6 does not alter a known recognition site. Identification of this point mutation is therefore not amenable to restriction endonuclease digestion and gel electrophoresis of the amplified product. Prenatal diagnosis involving Hb S and Hb C carrier parents can be accomplished by hybridization of the PCR amplified product with A, S, and C ASOs as previously cited (Saiki et al., 1986).

Cystic Fibrosis

Cystic fibrosis (CF) is an autosomal recessive disorder most commonly found in Caucasian populations. The incidence of CF in North American Caucasians is approximately 1 in 2500, with a heterozygote frequency of 1 in 25. CF has an estimated frequency in American Blacks of 1 in 17,000, and is thought to be extremely rare among Asian populations. The CF gene has been cloned and its product, the cystic fibrosis transmembrane conductance regulator (CFTR), has been identified (Rommens et al., 1989; Riordan et al., 1989). The gene has 27 exons and is 250,000 bp in length, encoding a 1480 amino acid CFTR protein. A defective CFTR protein in CF patients results in the abnormal transport of chloride ions across epithelial cell membranes. The basic function of the CFTR protein has recently been identified as a chloride ion channel (Anderson et al., 1991).

The CF phenotype can be quite variable, but typically involves increased concentration of sweat chloride (>60 mEq/liter), chronic pulmonary disease with Pseudomonas colonization, and pancreatic insufficiency (see review by Boat et al., 1989). Meconium ileus is found in 5 to 10 per cent of newborns with CF. Two to 5 per cent of CF patients develop liver disease with a variable age of onset. About 98 per cent of CF males and less than 90 per cent of CF females are infertile. Although initial reports identified echogenic bowel in the second trimester as a marker for CF, this issue remains unresolved.

The CF gene was mapped to chromosome 7q3.1 by genetic linkage analysis. Tsui and colleagues (1985) first demonstrated linkage between the CF locus and a DNA polymorphism. Subsequently, numerous DNA markers more closely linked to the CF gene were identified, thus allowing for carrier detection and prenatal diagnosis in 1 in 4 risk pregnancies for couples with at least one living affected offspring. Certain alleles from some of these DNA polymorphisms yielded haplotypes that were found to be frequently associated with the CF gene. The tendency of specific alleles at two or more linked loci to occur together more often than by chance expectation is known as linkage disequilibrium. The linkage disequilibrium data generated from the analysis of these linked loci in large numbers of CF families enabled genetic counselors to provide risk probabilities to couples with 1 in 4 risk pregnancies when DNA from the affected

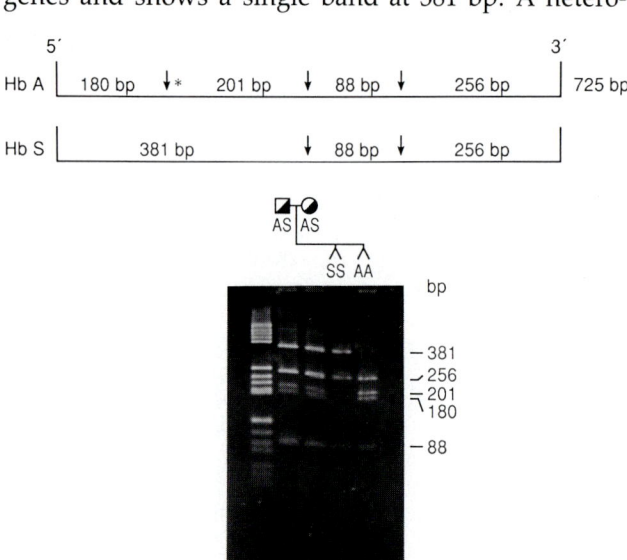

FIGURE 1–57. Direct gene analysis for sickle cell anemia. (*Top*) 725 bp amplified fragment from the *beta*-globin gene containing the Hb S mutation site. (↓) indicates CvnI recognition sites. (*) indicates the CvnI site altered by the Hb S mutation. (*Bottom*) Pedigree and agarose gel electrophoresis of CvnI digested amplified product. Lane 1: pBR322 HaeIII digested marker DNA. Lanes 2 and 3: father and mother with sickle cell trait. Lane 4: affected fetus (SS). Lane 5: normal fetus (AA).

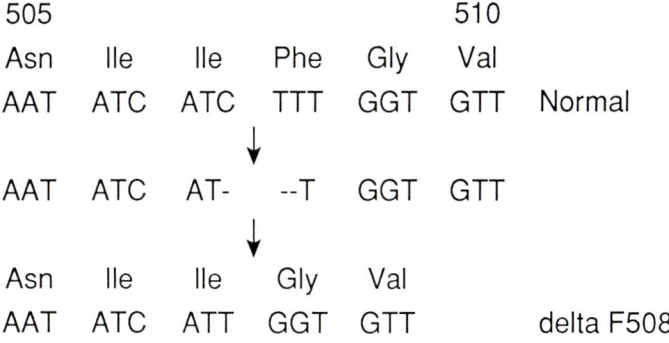

FIGURE 1–58. The delta F508 mutation. Positions 505 through 510 of the amino acid coding region are shown. A 3 base pair (CTT) deletion results in the loss of a phenylalanine residue at position 508. Asn = asparagine; Ile = isoleucine; Phe = phenylalanine; Gly = glycine; Val = valine.

offspring was not available, to couples with less than 1 in 4 risk pregnancies, and to relatives of CF families (Beaudet et al., 1989). In addition, because the majority of CF chromosomes were linked to a single haplotype, these data predicted that most CF cases are caused by a single mutation or a small number of mutations.

The cloning of the CF gene was followed immediately by the identification of a mutation found on the majority of Caucasian CF chromosomes. The mutation, designated delta F508, is a 3 bp deletion in exon 10 of the CF gene resulting in the loss of a phenylalanine residue at position 508 of the amino acid coding region (Fig. 1–58). This mutation accounts for approximately 70 per cent of CF chromosomes from North American Caucasians, is found in the homozygous or compound heterozygous state in the majority of CF patients with pancreatic insufficiency, and thus is associated with severe manifestation of the disease (Kerem et al., 1989). A gradient of distribution exists for the delta F508 mutation among CF chromosomes of European origin, ranging from approximately 70 per cent on CF chromosomes from Northern Europe to about 50 per cent on CF chromosomes from Southern Europe (European Working Group on CF Genetics, 1990). Indeed, other mutations with frequencies greater than 1 per cent have since been identified on CF chromosomes from Southern Europe, particularly of Spanish and Italian origin (Nunes et al., 1991). A worldwide survey of more than 13,000 CF chromosomes has established the overall frequency of the delta F508 mutation at 68 per cent of all CF mutations (Cystic Fibrosis Genetic Analysis Consortium, 1990). Direct analysis of the delta F508 mutation can be accomplished by manipulation of PCR products using a number of the methods previously described. In addition, the mutation may be easily detected by electrophoretic separation of normal and mutant amplified products on a polyacrylamide gel (Fig. 1–59). By amplifying across the deletion site using primers located in exon 10, one can identify the parents as heterozygotes for delta F508 since they show two bands at 98 bp and 95 bp. The band at 95 bp represents the CTT deletion that is representative of the mutation. Slowly migrating heteroduplexes, formed by the association of normal and mutant amplified sequences, are also visible. If prenatal diagnosis is performed, a single band at 98 bp would indicate a homozygous normal fetus (fetus 1), whereas a single band at 95 bp would indicate a homozygous affected fetus (fetus 2).

Since the cloning of the CF gene and the discovery of the delta F508 mutation, numerous additional mutations have been identified. Most of these mutations are either familial or found on CF chromosomes from Caucasian populations at frequencies less than 1 per cent. However, a small group of CF mutations has been identified in North American Caucasians at frequencies greater than 1 per cent, increasing the percentage of mutations detected by clinical diagnostic laboratories to as high as 85 per cent (Ng et al., 1991). Direct gene analysis of a relatively high percentage of CF mutations markedly improves the ability of the genetic counselor to provide risk probabilities to Caucasian couples seeking carrier detection and prenatal diagnosis because of family history. Using direct gene analysis, a relative of a CF patient can either be identified as a carrier or have his/her a priori risk reduced through Bayesian probabilities if no mutation is found. In addition, the low-risk spouse can also be tested and have his/her a priori risk modified (Table 1–22). For instance, if a mutation is identified in a high-risk individual and 80 per cent of CF mutations are ruled out in the low-risk spouse (carrier risk of 1 in 124), the probability of CF in an offspring would be 1 in 494. If the fetus inherits the mutation from the high-risk parent, the probability of CF becomes 1 in

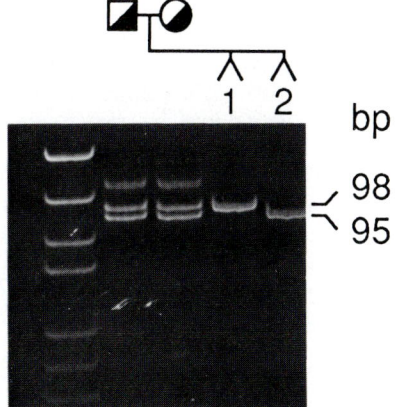

FIGURE 1–59. Direct gene analysis for the delta F508 mutation. Pedigree and polyacrylamide gel electrophoresis of the 98 bp and 95 bp amplified products. Lane 1: pBR322 HaeIII digested marker DNA. Lanes 2 and 3: delta F508 carrier father and mother. Slowly migrating heteroduplex bands are also seen. Lane 4: homozygous normal fetus (1). Lane 5: homozygous affected fetus (2).

TABLE 1–22. Individual Cystic Fibrosis Carrier Risk Probabilities After Mutation Analysis

PERCENTAGE OF DETECTABLE CYSTIC FIBROSIS MUTATIONS	CARRIER RISK FOR INDIVIDUAL WITH NEGATIVE TEST
0	1 in 25.5
70	1 in 82.7
75	1 in 99.0
80	1 in 124
85	1 in 165
90	1 in 246
95	1 in 491

Adapted from information appearing in Lemna WK, et al: Mutation analysis for heterozygote detection and the prenatal diagnosis of cystic fibrosis. N Engl J Med **322**:291, 1990.

248. Microvillar intestinal enzyme analysis could be pursued at this point, but should be approached with caution owing to the 2 per cent false-positive and the 8 per cent false-negative rates.

Duchenne Muscular Dystrophy and Becker's Muscular Dystrophy

Duchenne muscular dystrophy (DMD) is an X-linked recessive disorder affecting approximately 1 in 3500 males. Becker's muscular dystrophy (BMD) occurs less frequently than DMD and displays a similar but less severe phenotype. Both disorders have been shown to result from deletion mutations within the same gene. The clinical distinction between these two forms of muscular dystrophy is defined by severity and disease progression. DMD starts earlier in life and is more disabling, and affected males virtually never reproduce. BMD males may reproduce. Mental retardation is more frequent in DMD males, and although both DMD and BMD males may have cardiac complications, these complications are more severe in DMD males. Although not yet fully resolved, if mutation rates prove to be equivalent for both sexes, then approximately 30 per cent of DMD cases will represent new mutations. In contrast, approximately 10 per cent of BMD cases represent new mutations. This is a reflection of the higher reproductive fitness for BMD males. Carrier females for both DMD and BMD may occasionally demonstrate mild clinical features of muscular dystrophy (see review by Hyser and Mendell, 1988).

The gene for DMD/BMD has been mapped to the p21 region on the X chromosome by genetic linkage analysis and by studies involving DMD and BMD females, all of whom were found to have an X-autosome translocation disrupting the Xp21 region. Molecular cloning of the Xp21 region resulted in the isolation of intragenic DNA probes used for RFLP analysis as well as deletion analysis in a small number of cases (Kunkel et al., 1985; Ray et al., 1985). Carrier identification and prenatal diagnosis became highly accurate in families with more than one affected male. This proved to be more difficult in families with only one affected male due to the high rate of new mutation in the DMD/BMD gene and the possibility of intragenic recombination between the probe and the mutation site. These findings led directly to the discovery of the DMD/BMD gene and eventually to the cloning of a 14 kilobase (kb) cDNA representing the entire DMD/BMD mRNA transcript (Koenig et al., 1987). The DMD/BMD gene is approximately 2 million nucleotides (2000 kb) in length and is currently the largest gene identified in humans. At least 60 exons are present, with the majority of deletions occurring in a region corresponding to a 2000-nucleotide segment of the transcript. Hoffman and colleagues (1987) identified the DMD/BMD gene product, dystrophin, which was found to be deficient in muscle tissue from patients with DMD. In most DMD patients, dystrophin is decreased or absent, whereas most BMD patients have an abnormal dystrophin protein (Hoffman et al., 1988).

RFLP and deletion analysis for carrier identification and prenatal diagnosis can be performed by use of cDNA probes from the DMD/BMD gene (Darras and Francke, 1988, Darras et al., 1988). These probes permit detection of large deletions in the DMD/BMD gene in at least 50 per cent of carrier and affected individuals. RFLP analysis using the intragenic DNA probes already mentioned can be performed in cases that are uninformative with the cDNA probes. As previously cited, DMD/BMD gene deletions can also be detected by multiplex PCR (Chamberlain et al., 1988, 1990) (Fig. 1–60). Simultaneous amplification of nine separate regions of the DMD/BMD gene permits identification of at least 80 per cent of all deletions. PCR amplification of DNA from a male patient with DMD (lane 1) reveals a deletion in exon 48 of the DMD/BMD gene.

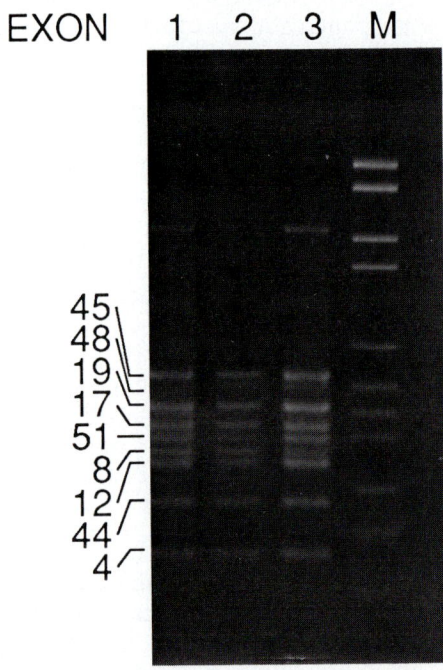

FIGURE 1–60. Direct gene analysis for mutations found in the dystrophin gene of patients with Duchenne or Becker's muscular dystrophy. Multiplex PCR of nine separate regions of the DMD/BMD gene was followed by electrophoresis of the amplified products. Exon locations are indicated at left. Lane 1: amplified DNA from a male DMD patient showing a deletion in exon 48. Lanes 2 and 3: amplified DNA from normal males. M: marker DNA. (Courtesy of Bradley W. Popovich, Ph.D., Oregon Health Sciences University, Portland.)

Amplification of DNA from two male controls (lanes 2 and 3) reveals a normal amplification pattern. Multiplex PCR has proved to be quite useful for prenatal diagnosis of a male fetus when the mother is a carrier of a known deletion. However, carrier identification in females is more difficult with this technique and usually requires confirmation with the cDNA probes.

The Fragile X Syndrome

The fragile X syndrome can best be described as an X-linked disorder with variable penetrance. Fragile X represents what is probably the most common cause of inheritable mental retardation in humans with an incidence of 1 in 1200 to 1500 males and 1 in 2000 to 2500 females. The fragile X phenotype is associated with a fragile site or constriction at band q27.3 on the X chromosome. The clinical picture in affected males is relatively nonspecific and variable but typically consists of mental retardation with particular speech impairment, prominent head, long face, large ears, and postpubescent macro-orchidism. Paternity is rare among affected males, suggesting a high frequency of new mutation. Retardation in affected females is less than in males, and there are no other distinguishing clinical features. Affected females may reproduce (see review by Brown, 1989).

The segregation pattern of the fragile X syndrome is peculiar. Sherman and colleagues (1984, 1985) studied the inheritance of the fragile X mutation in numerous families and determined that the risk of inheriting the fragile X phenotype depends on an individual's position in the pedigree (Sherman paradox). Approximately 30 per cent of carrier females are mildly mentally retarded, and 20 per cent of males who inherit a fragile X mutation are not clinically symptomatic. These carrier males are called normal transmitting males (NTM). Daughters of NTMs inherit the fragile X mutation, but are also clinically unaffected. However, grandsons of NTMs have a 40 per cent risk, and great-grandsons have a 50 per cent risk of displaying the fragile X phenotype.

The fragile X gene was mapped to Xq27.3 by genetic linkage analysis and subsequently cloned. A highly unstable region of DNA is located in the coding sequence of the fragile X gene, FMR-1 (Oberle et al., 1991; Verkerk et al., 1991; Yu et al., 1991). Mutations occurring in this region of instability during female meiosis and transmitted to offspring are the cause of the fragile X syndrome. The exact function of the FMR-1 gene is thus far unknown. It is not expressed in individuals with the fragile X phenotype (Pieretti et al., 1991). The unstable region of DNA in the FMR-1 gene is a $(CGG)_n$ trinucleotide repeat of variable length. The CGG repeat is highly polymorphic in normal noncarrier individuals. Carriers of a "premutation" exhibit an increase (amplification) in repeat number, which is further expanded in fragile X individuals. The mutation is unmethylated in NTMs, but is hypermethylated in affected males and in female symptomatic carriers. The significance of this observation remains unclear, but methylation in this region may suppress the FMR-1 gene, thus producing the clinical disorder.

After the isolation of FMR-1 and the discovery of its genetic instability, studies focused on the correlation between amplification of the CGG repeat and mutation status. Fu and colleagues (1991) determined the number of CGG repeats in normal individuals to range from 6 to 54. Amplification of repeats from 52 to greater than 200 were determined for carriers of premutations. Affected individuals had greater than 200 repeats. No distinct boundaries between normal and premutation, and between premutation and full mutation alleles, were seen. It was further observed that the risk of expansion of a premutation to a full mutation from a carrier female to offspring increased with the size of the premutation allele. These risk variations were in agreement with the observations of Sherman and colleagues (1984, 1985). There appears to be little or no change in the size of a premutation allele during male meiosis and subsequent transmission of the allele from NTM to female offspring. However, dramatic changes in size may occur during female meiosis and subsequent transmission of the premutation allele from female carrier to offspring. The risk of expansion of the premutation to a full mutation, and therefore of expression of the fragile X phenotype, increases with later generations.

DNA probes adjacent to the unstable region of the FMR-1 gene and capable of detecting variation in CGG repeats can be used for carrier identification and prenatal diagnosis of the fragile X syndrome and may soon replace chromosome analysis as the preferred method for genetic testing. This method is illustrated in Figure 1–61. The probe pE5.1 (Verkerk et al., 1991) is hybridized to PstI-digested DNA from normal, carrier, and affected individuals. Normal noncarrier males (lanes 1 and 7) and normal noncarrier females (lanes 3 and 6) show bands at approximately 1.0 kb. A carrier female (lane 2) shows a band at 1.0 kb indicating her normal X chromosome and an elevated band (greater than 52 repeats) indicating an unstable premutation on her other X chromosome. A normal transmitting male (lane 4) shows a single elevated band (greater than 52 repeats) indicating a premutation on his X chromosome. A female carrying a full mutation (lane 5) shows a band at approximately 1.0 kb and an elevated band (greater than 200 repeats), often seen as heterogeneous in length, indicating a full mutation. Affected males likewise show the elevated heterogeneous band, but not the band in the normal range.

Family screening for the CGG repeat offers a more sensitive basis for diagnosis and genetic counseling. With this technology, it may become possible to predict severity of the fragile X phenotype by analysis of asymptomatic first- and second-degree relatives. Ascertainment of progeny who do not have amplification of the CGG repeat is also possible. These individuals should not be at risk for the fragile X syndrome. It is anticipated that as more knowledge is gained concerning the CGG repeat, individuals with a fragile X phenotype who do not demonstrate amplification of the repeat sequence will be found. Other mutations that can produce the fragile X phenotype will then be discovered. Nonetheless, mutations involving triplet

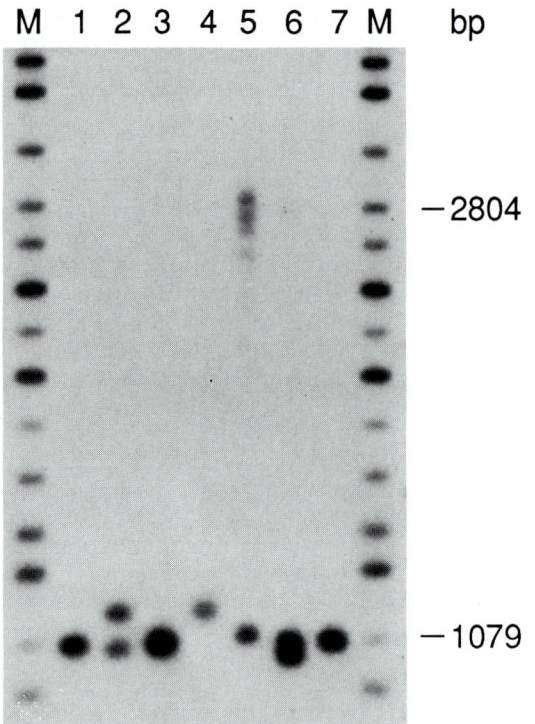

FIGURE 1–61. DNA-probe analysis for the fragile X syndrome by Southern blotting. The probe pE5.1 (Verkerk et al., 1991) is hybridized to PstI digested DNA. Normal bands are seen at approximately 1.0 kb. Premutation bands are elevated to greater than 52 triplet repeats. Full mutation bands of greater than 200 triplet repeats often appear as heterogeneous in length. Lanes 1 and 7: normal males. Lanes 3 and 6: normal females. Lane 2: carrier female. Lane 4: normal transmitting male. Lane 5: female carrying a full mutation. M-marker DNA. (Courtesy of Bradley W. Popovich, Ph.D., Oregon Health Sciences University, Portland.)

repeat sequences represent a new class of mutations that produce human disease.

Myotonic dystrophy (Brook et al., 1992; Fu et al., 1992; Mahadevan et al., 1992) and spinal and bulbar muscular atrophy (LaSpada et al., 1991) are other genetic disorders recently found to result from triplet repeat amplification. Triplet repeats are probably frequent in the human genome, but associations with other genetic disorders thus far have not been observed. Identification of premutation carriers based on triplet repeat number and development of risk probabilities for expansion to a full mutation in progeny represent a new dilemma for genetic counselors. The incidence of premutations in asymptomatic carriers as well as the range and associated risks for expansion of these alleles in progeny need to be determined in order to provide effective counseling for at-risk families.

CONCLUSION

The perinatologist will be involved with the practical issues of clinical genetics, which may provide favorable trends for the population at large in coming years. It can be anticipated that through prenatal diagnosis,

a decrease will be seen in incidence of chromosome abnormalities and genome mutations. Appropriate genetic counseling associated with DNA-probe analysis may lead to more informed reproductive decisions in kindreds with genetic disease, and new screening programs could reduce the incidence of a few single malformations, e.g., neural tube defects. Increasingly, clinical genetics will become one of the disciplines physicians will be expected to use for the care of their patients. The expanding knowledge gained through research in molecular biology and molecular genetics will provide the information necessary to physicians in formulating clinical approaches to genetic issues.

REFERENCES

Albright SG, Hook EB: Estimates of the likelihood that a Down's syndrome child of unknown genotype is a consequence of an inherited translocation. J Med Genet **17:**273, 1980.

Anderson MP, Gregory RJ, Thompson S, et al: Demonstration that CFTR is a chloride channel by alteration of its anion selectivity. Science **253:**202, 1991.

Aulehla-Scholz C, Basaran S, Agaoglu L, et al: Molecular basis of beta-thalassemia in Turkey: Detection of rare mutations by direct sequencing. Hum Genet **84:**195, 1990.

Baltimore D: RNA-dependent DNA polymerase in virions of RNA tumor viruses. Nature **226:**1209, 1970.

Barr ML, Bertram LF: A morphologic distinction between neurons of the male and the female and the behavior of the nucleolar satellite during accelerated nucleoprotein synthesis. Nature **163:**676, 1949.

Beaudet AL, Feldman GL, Fernbach SD, et al: Linkage disequilibrium, cystic fibrosis, and genetic counseling. Am J Hum Genet **44:**319, 1989.

Boat TF, Welsh MJ, Beaudet AL: Cystic fibrosis. In Scriver CL, Beaudet AL, Sly WS, Valle D (eds): The Metabolic Basis of Inherited Disease, 6th ed. New York, McGraw-Hill, 1989.

Bondy PK, Rosenberg LE (eds): Metabolic Control and Disease. 8th ed. Philadelphia, WB Saunders Company, 1980.

Boué J, Boué A, Lazar P: Retrospective and prospective epidemiological studies of 1500 karyotyped spontaneous human abortions. Teratology **12:**11, 1975.

Bresch C, Hausmann R: Klassiche und Moleculare Genetik. 3rd ed. Berlin, Springer-Verlag, 1972.

Brook JD, McCurrach ME, Harley HG, et al: Molecular basis of myotonic dystrophy: Expansion of a trinucleotide (CTG) repeat at the 3' end of a transcript encoding a protein kinase family member. Cell **68:**799, 1992.

Brown WT: The fragile X syndrome. Neuro Clinic **7:**107, 1989.

Caldwell PD, Smith DW: The XXY syndrome in childhood: Detection and treatment. J Pediatr **80:**250, 1972.

Carter CO: Genetics of common single malformations. Br Med Bull **32:**21, 1976.

Caspersson T, Foley GE, Kudynowski J, et al: Chemical differentiation along metaphase chromosomes. Exper Cell Res **49:**219, 1968.

Chamberlain JS, Gibbs RA, Ranier JE, et al: Deletion screening of the Duchenne muscular dystrophy locus via multiplex DNA amplification. Nucleic Acids Res **16:**11141, 1988.

Chamberlain JS, Gibbs RA, Ranier JE, Caskey CT: Multiplex PCR for the diagnosis of Duchenne muscular dystrophy. In Innis MA, Gelfand DH, Sninsky JJ, White TJ (eds): PCR protocols: A Guide to Methods and Applications. San Diego, Academic Press, Inc., 1990.

Chehab FF, Doherty M, Cai S, et al: Detection of sickle cell anemia and thalassaemias. Nature **329:**293, 1987.

Cohen SN: The manipulation of genes. Sci Am **233:**24, 1975.

Cohen SN, Chang ACY, Boyer HW, Helling RB: Construction of biologically functional bacterial plasmids in vitro. Proc Natl Acad Sci USA **70:**3240, 1973.

Creasy MR, Crolla JA, Alberman ED: A cytogenetic study of human spontaneous abortions using banding techniques. Hum Genet **31:**177, 1976.

Cystic Fibrosis Genetic Analysis Consortium: Worldwide survey of the delta F508 mutation—report from the Cystic Fibrosis Genetic Analysis Consortium. Am J Hum Genet **47:**354, 1990.

Darras BT, Blattner P, Harper JF, et al: Intragenic deletions in 21 Duchenne muscular dystrophy (DMD)/Becker muscular dystrophy (BMD) families studied with the dystrophin cDNA: Location of breakpoints on HindIII and BgIII exon-containing fragment maps, meiotic and mitotic origin of the mutations. Am J Hum Genet **43:**620, 1988.

Darras BT, Francke U: Normal human genomic restriction-fragment patterns and polymorphisms revealed by hybridization with the entire dystrophin cDNA. Am J Hum Genet **43:**612, 1988.

Engelke DR, Hoener PA, Collins FS: Direct sequencing of enzymatically amplified genomic DNA. Proc Natl Acad Sci USA **85:**544, 1988.

Erickson JD: Paternal age and Down syndrome. Am J Hum Genet **31:**489, 1979.

European Working Group on CF Genetics: Gradient of distribution in Europe of the major CF mutation and of its associated haplotype. Hum Genet **85:**436, 1990.

Fraser FC: The genetics of cleft lip and cleft palate. Am J Hum Genet **22:**336, 1970.

Fu Y-H, Kuhl DPA, Pizzuti A, et al: Variation of the CGG repeat at the fragile X site results in genetic instability: Resolution of the Sherman paradox. Cell **67:**1047, 1991.

Fu Y-H, Pizzuti A, Fenwick RG, et al: An unstable triplet repeat in a gene related to myotonic muscular dystrophy. Science **255:**1256, 1992.

Gardner RJM, Sutherland GR: Chromosome Abnormalities and Genetic Counseling. New York, Oxford University Press, 1989.

Gyllensten UB, Erlich HA: Generation of single-stranded DNA by the polymerase chain reaction and its application to direct sequencing of the HLA-DQA locus. Proc Natl Acad Sci USA **85:**7652, 1988.

Haliassos A, Chomel JC, Tesson L, et al: Modification of enzymatically amplified DNA for the detection of point mutations. Nucleic Acids Res **17:**3606, 1989.

Hall B: Mongolism in newborn infants. Clin Pediatr **5:**4, 1966.

Hall JG: Genomic imprinting: Review and relevance to human diseases. Am J Hum Genet **46:**857, 1990.

Hassold TJ: A cytogenetic study of repeated spontaneous abortions. Am J Hum Genet **32:**723, 1980.

Higuchi M, Wong C, Kochhan L, et al: Characterization of mutations in the factor VIII gene by direct sequencing of amplified genomic DNA. Genomics **6:**65, 1990.

Hoffman EP, Brown RH, Kunkel LM: Dystrophin: The protein product of the Duchenne muscular dystrophy locus. Cell **51:**919, 1987.

Hoffman EP, Fischbeck KH, Brown RH, et al: Characterization of dystrophin in muscle-biopsy specimens from patients with Duchenne's or Becker's muscular dystrophy. N Engl J Med **318:**1363, 1988.

Hook EB, Lindsje A: Down syndrome in live births by single year maternal age interval in a Swedish study: Comparison with results from a New York State study. Am J Hum Genet **30:**19, 1978.

Hyser CL, Mendell JR: Recent advances in Duchenne and Becker muscular dystrophy. Neuro Clinic **6:**429, 1988.

An international system for human cytogenetic nomenclature—high-resolution banding (1985). Report of the Standing Committee on Human Cytogenetic Nomenclature. Cytogenet Cell Genet (Karger, Bisel, 1985).

Jackman DA, Symons RH, Berg P: Biochemical method for inserting new genetic information into DNA of simian virus 40: circular SV40DNA molecules containing lambda phagegenes and the galactose operon of E. coli. Proc Natl Acad Sci USA **69:**2904, 1972.

Johnson WG, Schwartz RC, Chutorian AM: Artificial insemination by donors and the need for genetic screening. Late infantile GM₂-gangliosidosis resulting from this technique. N Engl J Med **304:**755, 1981.

Kan YW, Dozy AM: Antenatal diagnosis of sickle cell anemia by DNA analysis of amniotic fluid cells. Lancet **ii:**910, 1978.

Kelly TJ, Smith HO: A restriction enzyme from Haemophilus influenzae, II: Base sequence of the recognition site. J Mol Biol **51:**393, 1970.

Kerem B-S, Rommens JM, Buchanan JA, et al: Identification of the cystic fibrosis gene: Genetic analysis. Science **245:**1073, 1989.

Koenig M, Hoffman EP, Bertelson CJ, et al: Complete cloning of the Duchenne muscular dystrophy (DMD) cDNA and preliminary genomic organization of the DMD gene in normal and affected individuals. Cell **50:**509, 1987.

Kogan SC, Doherty M, Gitschier J: An improved method for prenatal diagnosis of genetic diseases by analysis of amplified DNA sequences. N Engl J Med **317:**985, 1987.

Kornberg A: Biological synthesis of deoxyribonucleic acid. Science **131:**1503, 1960.

Kornberg A: Aspects of DNA replication. Symp Quant Biol **43:**1, 1978.

Kornberg RD: Chromatin structure: A repeating unit of histones and DNA. Science **184:**868, 1974.

Kornberg RD, Klug A: The nucleosome. Sci Am **244:**52, 1981.

Kunkel LM, Monaco AP, Middlesworth W, et al: Specific cloning of DNA fragments absent from the DNA of a male patient with an X chromosome deletion. Proc Natl Acad Sci USA **82:**4778, 1985.

Lamson SH, Hook EB: A simple function for maternal-age-specific rates of Down syndrome in the 20-to-49 year age range and its biological implications. Am J Hum Genet **32:**743, 1980.

LaSpada AR, Wilson EM, Lubahn DB, et al: Androgen receptor gene mutations in X-linked spinal and bulbar muscular atrophy. Nature **352:**77, 1991.

Lemli L, Smith DW: The XO syndrome. A study of the differentiated phenotype in 25 patients. J Pediatr **63:**577, 1977.

Lemna WK, Feldman GL, Kerem B-S, et al: Mutation analysis for heterozygote detection and the prenatal diagnosis of cystic fibrosis. N Engl J Med **322:**291, 1990.

Lenke RR, Levy HL: Maternal phenylketonuria and hyperphenylalaninemia. N Engl J Med **305:**1202, 1980.

Mahadevan M, Tsilfidis C, Sabourin L, et al: Myotonic dystrophy mutation: An unstable CTG repeat in the 3' untranslated region of the gene. Science **255:**1253, 1992.

Maxam AM, Gilbert W: A new method of sequencing DNA. Proc Natl Acad Sci USA **74:**560, 1977.

McAlpine PJ, Van Cong N, Boucheix C, et al: The 1987 catalog of mapped genes and report of the nomenclature committee. Cytogenet Cell Genet **46:**29, 1987.

McKusick VA: The human genome through the eyes of a clinical geneticist. Cytogenet Cell Genet **32:**7, 1982.

McKusick VA: Mendelian Inheritance in Man. 9th ed. Baltimore, Johns Hopkins Press, 1990.

Mornet E, Chateau C, Simon-Bouy B, et al: Carrier detection and prenatal diagnosis of cystic fibrosis using an intragenic TA-repeat polymorphism. Hum Genet **88:**479, 1992.

Mullis KB, Faloona F: Specific synthesis of DNA in vitro via a polymerase-catalyzed chain reaction. Methods Enzymol **155:**335, 1987.

National Research Council: Mapping and Sequencing the Human Genome. Washington, D.C., National Academy Press, 1988.

Ng ISL, Pace R, Richard MV, et al: Methods for analysis of multiple cystic fibrosis mutations. Hum Genet **87:**613, 1991.

Nielsen J, Silessen I: Incidence of chromosome aberration among 11,148 newborn children. Hum Genet **30:**1, 1975.

Nirenberg NW, Matthaei JH: Characteristics and stabilization of DNAase-sensitive protein synthesis in E. coli extracts. Proc Natl Acad Sci USA **47:**1580, 1961.

Nora JJ: Multifactorial inheritance hypothesis for the etiology of congenital heart diseases: The genetic-environmental interaction. Circulation **38:**604, 1968.

Nunes V, Gasparini P, Novelli G, et al: Analysis of 14 cystic fibrosis mutations in five South European populations. Hum Genet **87:**737, 1991.

Nyhan WL: An approach to the diagnosis of overwhelming metabolic disease in early infancy. Curr Prob Pediatr **7:**1, 1977a.

Nyhan WL: Heritable metabolic disease in the differential diagnosis of asphyxia. In Gluck L (ed): Intrauterine Asphyxia and the Developing Fetal Brain. Chicago, Year Book Medical Publishers, 1977b.

Oberle I, Rousseau F, Heitz D, et al: Instability of a 550-base pair DNA segment and abnormal methylation in fragile X syndrome. Science **252:**1097, 1991.

Okazaki R, Okazaki T, Sakabe K, et al: In vivo mechanism of chain growth. Symp Quant Biol **33**:129, 1969.

Pieretti M, Zhang F, Fu Y-H, et al: Absence of expression of the FMR-1 gene in fragile X syndrome. Cell **66**:817, 1991.

Porreco RP, Matson MR, Young PE, et al: Diagnosis of a triploid fetus at genetic amniocentesis. Obstet Gynecol **56**:115, 1980.

Ray PN, Belfall B, Duff C, et al: Cloning of the breakpoint of an X;21 translocation associated with Duchenne muscular dystrophy. Nature **318**:672, 1985.

Rich A, RajBhandary UL: Transfer RNA: Molecular structure, sequence, and properties. Ann Rev Biochem **45**:805, 1976.

Riordan JR, Rommens JM, Kerem B-S, et al: Identification of the cystic fibrosis gene: Cloning and characterization of complementary DNA. Science **245**:1066, 1989.

Rommens JM, Iannuzzi MC, Kerem B-S, et al: Identification of the cystic fibrosis gene: chromosome walking and jumping. Science **245**:1059, 1989.

Saiki RK, Bugawan TL, Horn GT, et al: Analysis of enzymatically amplified β-globin and HLA-DQα DNA with allele-specific oligonucleotide probes. Nature **324**:163, 1986.

Saiki RK, Scharf S, Faloona F, et al: Enzymatic amplification of β-globin genomic sequences and restriction site analysis for diagnosis of sickle cell anemia. Science **230**:1350, 1985.

Saiki RK, Walsh PS, Levenson CH, Erlich HA: Genetic analysis of amplified DNA with immobilized sequence-specific oligonucleotide probes. Proc Natl Acad Sci USA **86**:6230, 1989.

Sanger F, Nicklen S, Coulson AR: DNA sequencing with chain-terminating inhibitors. Proc Natl Acad Sci USA **74**:5463, 1977.

Schmidtke J, Cooper DN: A comprehensive list of cloned human DNA sequences. Nucleic Acids Res **16**(Suppl):403, 1988.

Schriver CR, Clow CL: Phenylketonuria: Epitome of human biochemical genetics. N Engl J Med **303**:1336, 1980.

Sculley DG, Dawson PA, Beacham IR, et al: Hypoxanthine-guanine phosphoribosyltransferase deficiency: Analysis of HPRT mutations by direct sequencing and allele-specific amplification. Hum Genet **87**:688, 1991.

Shapiro DM, Hutchinson RJ: Familial histiocytosis in offspring of two pregnancies after artificial insemination. N Engl J Med **304**:757, 1981.

Sherman SL, Jacobs PA, Morton NE, et al: Further segregation analysis of the fragile X syndrome with special reference to transmitting males. Hum Genet **69**:289, 1985.

Sherman SL, Morton NE, Jacobs PA, Turner G: The marker (X) syndrome: A cytogenetic and genetic analysis. Ann Hum Genet **48**:21, 1984.

Simpson JL: Disorders of Sexual Differentiation: Etiology and Clinical Delineation. New York, Academic Press, 1976.

Smith DW: Recognizable Patterns of Human Malformation. 3rd ed. Philadelphia, WB Saunders Company, 1982.

Smith HO, Wilcox KW: A restriction enzyme from Haemophilus influenzae, I: Purification and general properties. J Mol Biol **51**:379, 1970.

Southern EM: Detection of specific sequences among DNA fragments separated by gel electrophoresis. J Mol Biol **98**:503, 1975.

Srb AM, Owen RD, Edgar RS: General Genetics. 2nd ed. San Francisco, WH Freeman and Co, 1965.

Steve J, Steve E, Stengel-Rutkowski S, Murken JD: Paternal age and Down's syndrome: Data from prenatal diagnoses (DFG). Hum Genet **59**:119, 1981.

Szekely M: From DNA to Protein: The Transfer of Genetic Information. New York, John Wiley & Sons, 1980.

Temin HM, Mizutani S: RNA-dependent DNA polymerase in virions of Rous sarcoma virus. Nature **226**:1211, 1970.

Thompson M: Thompson and Thompson Genetics in Medicine. 4th ed. Philadelphia, WB Saunders Company, 1986.

Timmons MC, Rao KW, Sloan CS, et al: Genetic screening of donors for artificial insemination. Fertil Steril **35**:451, 1981.

Tsui L-C, Buchwald M, Barker D, et al: Cystic fibrosis locus defined by a genetically linked polymorphic DNA marker. Science **230**:1054, 1985.

Verkerk AJMH, Pieretti M, Sutcliffe JS, et al: Identification of a gene (FMR-1) containing a CGG repeat coincident with a breakpoint cluster region exhibiting length variation in fragile X syndrome. Cell **65**:905, 1991.

Vogel F, Motulsky AG: Human Genetics: Problems and Approaches. New York, Springer-Verlag, 1979.

Vogel F, Rathenberg R: Spontaneous mutation in man. Adv Hum Genet **5**:223, 1975.

Ward BE, Henry GP, Robinson A: Cytogenetic studies in 100 couples with recurrent spontaneous abortions. Am J Hum Genet **32**:549, 1980.

Wu DY, Ugozzoli L, Pal BK, Wallace RB: Allele-specific enzymatic amplification of β-globin genomic DNA for diagnosis of sickle cell anemia. Proc Natl Acad Sci USA **86**:2757, 1989.

Yu S, Pritchard M, Kremer E, et al: Fragile X genotype characterized by an unstable region of DNA. Science **252**:1179, 1991.

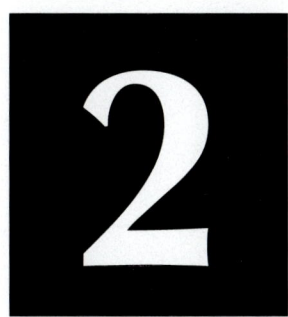

CHAPTER

2

PRENATAL DIAGNOSIS OF GENETIC DISORDERS

JOE LEIGH SIMPSON, M.D., and SHERMAN ELIAS, M.D.

Within recent years prenatal diagnosis has become possible for increasing numbers of genetic disorders by means of laboratory techniques surveyed in Chapter 1. Progress is as rapid as in any area of perinatology. Often the interval from research laboratory to clinical application is merely months or even weeks.

In this chapter we shall first review the principles of genetic counseling that must precede prenatal diagnosis. Then, we shall survey surgical techniques necessary for prenatal studies and consider current indications. The reader is also referred to several other publications for greater detail (Elias and Annas, 1987; Elias and Simpson, 1992; Simpson and Golbus, 1992; Simpson and Elias, 1992; Simpson 1991; Simpson, 1989, 1992).

PRINCIPLES OF GENETIC COUNSELING

Eliciting a Genetic History

Principles underlying counseling for genetic diseases are not dissimilar from those of counseling for other medical illnesses. Accurately eliciting information, communicating lucidly, sympathetically listening, and avoiding judgments are paramount.

For all pregnancies it is standard practice to determine whether the couple, or anyone in their families, has a disorder that might prove heritable. One inquires about the health status of first-degree relatives (sibs, parents, offspring), second-degree relatives (uncles, aunts, nephews, nieces, and grandparents), and third-degree relatives (first cousins). One should specifically record such abnormal reproductive outcomes as spontaneous abortions, stillborns, and anomalous liveborn infants. If one elicits a history of such a problem, counseling may either prove straightforward or it may be complex and require consultation with a geneticist. Drug exposure by the patient and her partner should be recorded, not merely those agents currently taken but to which exposure occurred prior to pregnancy.

In addition, noxious agents (e.g., cigarette smoking, work-related chemical exposures) should be noted.

Parental ages must be determined, for indeed the most common indication for prenatal diagnosis is advanced maternal age. A discussion is essential whenever a women is 35 years at estimated delivery date, regardless of a patient's difficulties in achieving pregnancy or a physician's personal opinions regarding pregnancy termination. Offspring of fathers in the fifth and sixth decade are at increased risk for new dominant mutations (e.g., achondroplasia). Unfortunately, the latter are not readily amenable to prenatal diagnosis, because many different genes could be involved.

Ethnic origin should be recorded. Ashkenazi Jews are at increased risk for offspring with Tay-Sachs disease and therefore should be screened to determine heterozygote status (frequency 1/27). Because in the United States some Jewish individuals are uncertain whether they are of Ashkenazic or Sephardic descent, we recommend offering screening to all Jewish couples. Although the frequency of Tay-Sachs carriers among non-Jewish individuals is lower (1 in 300) than among those of Jewish ancestry, we favor also offering screening to couples in which one partner is Jewish and the other is not. Increasing availability of prenatal diagnostic techniques also makes advisable routine heterozygote screening for β-thalassemia in Italians and Greeks, sickle cell anemia in African-Americans, and α-thalassemia in Southeast Asians and Filipinos. Cystic fibrosis will soon surely be added to this list, but as of the time of this writing it is not standard to screen for carriers of this disorder unless there is a positive family history.

Some obstetricians consider it useful to obtain genetic information through use of questionnaires or checklists, often constructed to require action only to positive responses. Table 2–1 reproduces a form recommended by the American College of Obstetricians and Gynecologists (ACOG, 1987).

61

TABLE 2–1. Prenatal Genetic Screen*

Name _____ Patient # _____ Date _____

1. Will you be 35 years or older when the baby is due? — Yes ___ No ___
2. Have you, the baby's father or anyone in either of your families ever had any of the following disorders?
   Down's Syndrome (mongolism) — Yes ___ No ___
   Other chromosomal abnormality — Yes ___ No ___
   Neural tube defect, i.e., spina bifida (meningomyelocele or open spine), anencephaly — Yes ___ No ___
   Hemophilia — Yes ___ No ___
   Muscular dystrophy — Yes ___ No ___
   Cystic fibrosis — Yes ___ No ___
   If yes, indicate the relationship of the affected person to you or to the baby's father: _____
3. Do you or the baby's father have a birth defect? — Yes ___ No ___
   If yes, who has the defect and what is it? _____
4. In any previous marriages, have you or the baby's father had a child born dead or alive, with a birth defect not listed in question 2 above? — Yes ___ No ___
5. Do you or the baby's father have any close relatives with mental retardation? — Yes ___ No ___
   If yes, indicate the relationship of the affected person to you or to the baby's father: _____
6. Do you, the baby's father, or a close relative in either of your families have a birth defect, any familial disorder, or a chromosomal abnormality not listed above? — Yes ___ No ___
   If yes, indicate the condition and the relationship of the affected person to you or to the baby's father. _____

   _____
7. In any previous marriage, have you or the baby's father had a stillborn child or three or more first-trimester spontaneous pregnancy losses? — Yes ___ No ___
   Have either of you had a chromosomal study? — Yes ___ No ___
8. If you or the baby's father are of Jewish ancestry, have either of you been screened for Tay-Sachs disease? — Yes ___ No ___
   If yes, indicate who and the results:_____
9. If you or the baby's father are black, have either of you been screened for sickle cell trait? — Yes ___ No ___
   If yes, indicate who and the results: _____
10. If you or the baby's father are of Italian, Greek or Mediterranean background, have either of you been tested for β-thalassemia? — Yes ___ No ___
    If yes, indicate who and the results: _____
11. If you or the baby's father are of Philippine or Southeast Asian ancestry, have either of you been tested for α-thalassemia? — Yes ___ No ___
    If yes, indicate who and the results:_____
12. Excluding iron and vitamins, have you taken any medications or recreational drugs since being pregnant or since your last menstrual period? (include non-prescription drugs) — Yes ___ No ___
    If yes, give name of medication and time taken during pregnancy: _____

*Any replying "YES" to questions should be offered appropriate counseling. If the patient declines further counseling or testing, this should be noted in the chart. Given that genetics is a field in a state of flux, alterations or updates to this form will be required periodically.

Questionnaire for identifying couples having increased risk for offspring with genetic disorders. (From American College of Obstetricians and Gynecologists: Antenatal Diagnosis of Genetic Disorders. ACOG Technical Bulletin No. 108, © September 1987. Washington, DC.)

Communication

In counseling, one should use terms that are readily understandable to patients, especially avoiding a patronizing attitude. It is useful to preface remarks with a few sentences recounting major causes of genetic abnormalities: cytogenetic, single gene (mendelian), polygenic/multifactorial (can be labeled "complex"), and environmental. It is helpful to write out unfamiliar words or use diagrams to reinforce important concepts. Repetition is essential. Allow time not only for couples to pose questions but to talk with each other to formulate their concerns and decisions. Although we find that most couples are able to make a decision of whether to proceed with prenatal diagnosis immediately after counseling, some require additional time and should be encouraged to reschedule so they have the opportunity to consider the issues further.

In complex cases, letters serve as a useful permanent record, allaying misunderstanding and helping to communicate with relatives. For more common problems—advanced maternal age, repetitive spontaneous abortions, previous offspring with neural tube defects, previous trisomic offspring—brochures and preprinted forms not only suffice, but have the advantage of emphasizing that a couple's problem is not unique.

Nondirective Counseling

Most geneticists subscribe to the thesis that a counselor should provide information but avoid dictating (directing) a particular course of action. Of course, completely nondirective counseling is probably a myth. For example, a counselor's unwitting facial expression invariably carries impact. Indeed, merely offering antenatal diagnostic services implies an element of approval. Nonetheless, one should attempt to provide objective information and to encourage couples to make their own decisions.

Confirmation of Diagnosis

Even if the diagnosis seems obvious, confirmation is always obligatory. One should not merely accept a patient's word or even a diagnosis made by a physician who lacks expertise about the condition. Of course, the anomalous individual should be examined, if possible. If the affected relative is alive but ill, cells should be cultured and frozen or immortalized (Epstein-Barr virus) for future DNA based diagnostic studies. Examining first-degree relatives may also be helpful if an autosomal dominant disorder like neurofibromatosis is suspected. Alternatively, one may have to rely upon medical records or laboratory tests.

Psychological Defenses

Psychological defenses underlie genetic counseling. If not appreciated, these defenses can impede the entire counseling process. Anxiety is usually low in couples requesting genetic counseling because of parental age or because of an abnormality in a distant relative. As long as the level of concern remains low, emotions are easily controlled and comprehension not impaired. However, couples who have had a stillborn infant, an anomalous offspring, or multiple repetitive abortions are inevitably more anxious. Their ability to retain information may be impaired.

Couples experiencing abnormal pregnancy outcomes show grief reactions similar to those that occur after the death of any loved one: denial, anger, guilt, bargaining, and resolution. In deference to these defenses, one should not attempt to offer definitive counseling immediately after the birth of an abnormal neonate or pregnancy loss. Usually, parents are best merely supported, the obstetrician avoiding specific discussion of risks in subsequent pregnancies, for fear of adding further to the immediate burden; nonetheless, any questions posed should be addressed. By 4 to 6 weeks couples are usually more receptive to counseling.

An additional psychological consideration is that of parental guilt or blame. It is natural to search for exogenous factors that might have caused an abnormal outcome. In the process of such a search, unjustifiable guilt often arises. The other spouse may be blamed subconsciously. Occasionally these emotions are understandable reactions—for example, in autosomal dominant or X-linked recessive traits. Fortunately, most couples can be assured that they could have done nothing to prevent the abnormal pregnancy.

Appreciating the psychological defenses just described helps one understand the failure of ostensibly intelligent couples to comprehend genetic information. One way to facilitate comprehension in anxious couples is for the physician personally to take the pedigree, despite the temptation to delegate this sometimes tedious responsibility. While the counselor is eliciting pedigree information, most couples visibly become more at ease. Interaction between the patient and her partner can also be observed. Thereafter, couples are more receptive to absorbing new and potentially troubling information. Communicating in easily comprehensible terms is essential, as alluded to previously. The ultimate principle is to allow couples to make their own decisions regarding pregnancy options.

TECHNICAL CONSIDERATIONS

Traditional Amniocentesis (≥15 weeks)

TECHNIQUE. Prenatal diagnosis often requires amniocentesis, the aspiration of amniotic fluid. This procedure is traditionally performed at 15 to 17 weeks gestation (menstrual weeks). At this stage of gestation, the amniotic fluid is sufficient (~200 ml) to allow removal of an adequate volume (20 to 30 cc) for testing. The ratio of viable to nonviable cells in the amniotic fluid is relatively high, and the time before fetal viability adequate to allow diagnostic studies so that pregnancy termination remains an option should a fetal abnormality be diagnosed.

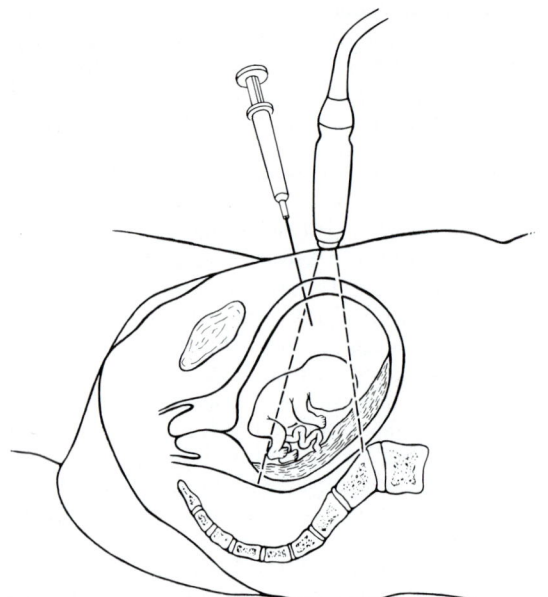

FIGURE 2–1. Amniocentesis performed concurrently with ultrasound.

An ultrasonographic examination with dynamic imaging should be performed immediately before amniocentesis in order to determine the fetal gestational age, placental location, optimal pockets of amniotic fluid, fetal cardiac movement to confirm viability, and number of fetuses. Although practiced routinely in most maternal-fetal medicine units, detailed anomaly assessment is not necessarily obligatory. However, consistency within a given center is essential; an institutional policy should be codified.

Concurrent use of ultrasound during amniocentesis is highly desirable (Fig. 2–1) to ensure proper needle placement. A 22-gauge spinal needle is preferred and nothing larger than a 20-gauge should be utilized. Rh immune globulin (RHIG), probably 300 μg, should be administered to the Rh-negative unsensitized patients at the time of amniocentesis, regardless of whether the placenta was traversed. In the United Kingdom and in some North American centers only 50 μg of Rh immunoglobin is administered.

Bloody amniotic fluid is aspirated in perhaps 1 to 2 per cent of amniocenteses. The blood is almost always maternal in origin, does not adversely affect amniotic cell growth, and usually does not presage subsequent pregnancy complications. Similarly, greenish amniotic fluid, which presumably is due to breakdown of hemoglobin within the amniotic sac, is also associated with no untoward pregnancy outcome (Karp and Schiller, 1977; Hess et al., 1986). By contrast, brown or dark red or wine-colored amniotic fluid is associated with an increased likelihood of poor pregnancy outcome. Pregnancy loss eventually occurs in about one-third of such cases (Milunsky, 1986). If the abnormally colored fluid is also characterized by elevated AFP, the outcome is especially unfavorable (fetal death, anencephaly, spontaneous abortion, or fetal abnormality). Brown amniotic fluid is also more likely to be associated with chromosomal abnormalities (7/56; 12.5

per cent) than is green fluid (1/35; 2.9 per cent) (Isada et al., 1990).

In multiple gestations, amniocentesis can usually be performed on all fetuses, provided that amniotic volume is adequate. Following aspiration of amniotic fluid from the first sac, 2 to 3 ml of indigo carmine, diluted 1:10 in bacteriostatic water, is injected before needle withdrawal. A second amniocentesis is then performed. The second needle is inserted in a site connoting the second fetus, preferably determined after visualizing the membranes separating the two sacs. Aspiration of clear fluid confirms that the second sac has been entered. In experienced hands, amniocentesis is performed successfully in well over 95 per cent of twin pregnancies, with ostensibly no increased risks over that of amniocentesis in singleton pregnancies (Elias et al., 1980; Anderson et al., 1991). Anderson and colleagues (1991) observed a post-procedure twin loss rate of 3.57 per cent up to 28 weeks that they interpreted as not increased over the sum of background twin loss rate plus the loss ratio associated with singleton amniocentesis.

Although other techniques for sampling multiple gestations are reported (Jeanty et al., 1990; Bahado-Singh et al., 1992), we still prefer the dye technique. In particular, there is the concern that single-puncture techniques could lead to contamination between sacs, resulting in diagnostic inaccuracies. Triplets and other multiple gestations can be managed similarly by sequentially injecting dye into successive sacs. So long as clear fluid is aspirated, one can rest assured that a new amniotic sac has been entered.

After amniocentesis, the patient may resume all normal activities. Common sense dictates that strenuous exercise such as jogging or aerobic exercise be deferred for a day or so. The patient should communicate to the obstetrician persistent uterine cramping, vaginal bleeding, leakage of amniotic fluid, or fever. There are no significant changes in fetal heart tracing following amniocentesis (Gianopoulos et al., 1986); accordingly, routine monitoring of women undergoing the procedure is not necessary.

SAFETY. Amniocentesis involves potential danger to both mother and fetus. Maternal risks are quite low, with symptomatic amnionitis occurring rarely. Such minor maternal complications as transient vaginal spotting and minimal amniotic fluid leakage occur in perhaps 1 per cent of cases, almost always being self-limited in nature.

The safety of traditional amniocentesis has been addressed by several large collaborative studies. In the United States, an NICHD-sponsored investigation revealed that 3.5 per cent of pregnant women who underwent amniocentesis during the years 1972 to 1975 experienced fetal loss after the procedure, compared with 3.2 per cent of concurrent controls (NICHD, 1976). This small difference was not statistically significant and, in fact, disappeared completely when corrected for maternal age. A later British collaborative study of the same period (1973 to 1976) found that the rate of fetal loss following amniocentesis was significantly greater than in controls (2.6 vs 1 per cent) (Working Party of Amniocentesis: 1978). However, in the British study a common indication for amniocentesis was elevated maternal serum alpha-fetoprotein (MSAFP), later recognized itself as a factor associated with fetal loss and adverse perinatal outcome. Analysis after excluding subjects undergoing amniocentesis for that indication lowered the differences between subject and control groups to less than 1 per cent, albeit still a significant difference (NICHD, 1979).

Neither the U.S. nor the U.K. collaborative study was conducted with high-quality ultrasonography and certainly not with concurrent ultrasound. Sometimes ultrasound was not employed at all. Moreover, some participating obstetricians were also relatively inexperienced in amniocentesis. For this reason there is an understandable temptation for obstetricians of this decade to assume that amniocentesis-related losses must be considerably less than the 0.5 per cent traditionally counseled. True, a procedure-related loss rate of this magnitude seems relatively high to these authors and perhaps to others. However, the one recent controlled study was a randomized one involving 30- to 34-year-old Danish women (Tabor et al., 1986). The loss rate was 1.7 per cent in the Danish amniocentesis group and only 0.7 per cent in the control group (p<0.05).

One possible explanation for the ostensible failure of quality ultrasonography to decrease loss rates is that loss rates in the original U.S. study—specifically in the control group—were spuriously high. Indeed, the reported loss rates after 16 weeks in controls (3.2 per cent) in the U.S. NICHD study was closer to that expected at only 8 to 9 weeks (Simpson et al., 1987; Simpson and Golbus, 1992), although confounding effects of maternal age and other variables make comparisons difficult. Perhaps some fetuses in the 1972–1975 U.S. NICHD control group (NICHD, 1976) were actually dead upon registration given that ultrasound was not routine. Nevertheless, it seems wise to continue to counsel that the risk of abortion secondary to amniocentesis is 0.5 per cent or only slightly less. It is prudent to tell patients that serious maternal complications and fetal injuries are "reported but very rare." However, very large surveys looking for rare anomalies have not been conducted. Observing a cluster of a specific anomaly in association with amniocentesis in a given center would produce the same dilemma as recently evoked by the issue of limb reduction defects and chorionic villus sampling.

Chorionic Villus Sampling

Although the most common diagnostic method, amniocentesis as currently commonly practiced has the disadvantage of being performed in the mid-second trimester (15 to 16 weeks). Even so-called early amniocentesis usually does not obviate this fundamental limitation, for only rarely is early amniocentesis performed before 13 weeks. A technique that could be performed during the first trimester is obviously highly desirable, not only to allow pregnancy termination early in gestation (a time associated with safer termination and substantial psychologic benefit) but also to maximize patient privacy. Early diagnosis is

also obligatory for treatment. One example is prevention of female pseudohermaphroditism in the treatment of 21-hydroxylase deficiency by administration of dexamethasone to the mother (Speiser et al., 1990). Chorionic villus sampling (CVS) makes possible first trimester diagnosis.

Techniques

TRANSCERVICAL APPROACH. The optimal time for transcervical sampling is 9 to 12 completed gestational weeks. In the U.S., CVS is now commonly performed with either the Portex catheter (Portex Limited, England) or a device of comparable diameter (1.5 mm). All these devices include a plastic cannula that encloses a metal obturator extending just distal to the catheter tip. In France, Dumez and others use a rigid biopsy instrument successfully (Dumez et al., 1985). Fetal viability must, of course, be confirmed before the procedure. Absolute contraindications to transcervical CVS include active cervical pathology (active herpes, gonorrhea, or chlamydia.) Relative contraindications include leiomyomata obstructing the cervical canal, multiple gestations, and markedly retroflexed retroverted uterus. If an Rh-negative patient is sensitized, it seems best to defer an invasive procedure as long as possible, specifically until amniocentesis at 16 to 18 weeks. The amount of fetal blood passing into the maternal circulation is not necessarily different between CVS and amniocentesis, but any exacerbation resulting from fetomaternal hemorrhage surely would be less deleterious the later the gestation.

For transcervical sampling the patient is placed in the lithotomy position, and the vagina cleaned with poviodone. The plastic catheter with its inner metal obturator is introduced transcervically into the placenta under concurrent ultrasonographic visualization. Optimal catheter placement is parallel to the long axis of the placenta and obviously away from either gestational sac or decidua (Fig. 2–2). The obturator is

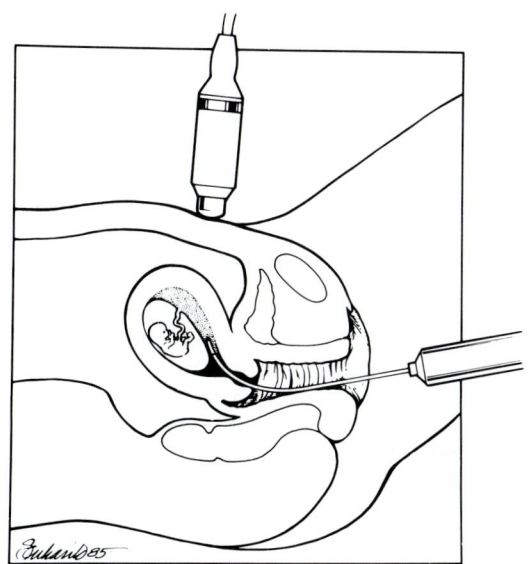

FIGURE 2–2. Diagram illustrating transcervical chorionic villus sampling.

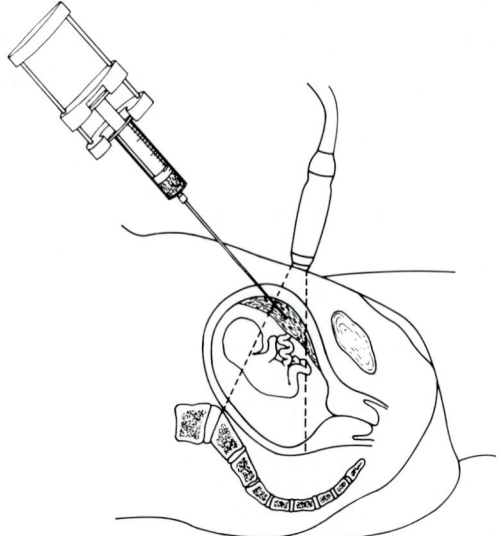

FIGURE 2–3. Diagram illustrating transabdominal chorionic villus sampling.

then removed and the catheter connected to a 20 or 30 cc syringe. By negative pressure, 10 to 25 mg of chorionic villi are aspirated. Adequacy of sample should be confirmed under a dissecting microscope. If another attempt is necessary, a new catheter should be employed.

TRANSABDOMINAL APPROACH. Transabdominal CVS is also most applicable at 9 to 12 weeks completed gestation; however, this procedure can be performed throughout the remainder of the pregnancy. Pioneered by Danish workers (Smidt-Jensen et al., 1985), the technique is now utilized in many U.S. centers. Using concurrent ultrasound, a 19- or 20-gauge spinal needle with stylet is passed into the placenta, with the device inserted lengthwise to the long axis of the placenta (Fig. 2–3). After stylet removal the spinal needle connects to a 20 or 30 cc syringe for aspiration.

Placentas especially amenable to the transabdominal approach include those located in the fundus or those located anterior in a slightly anteflexed uterus. Transabdominal chorionic villus sampling is often possible in certain circumstances when transcervical sampling is contraindicated (active herpes and cervical lesions). Women also potentially benefiting from transabdominal CVS include those with cervical leiomyomata or with a long, narrow, or an angulated endocervical canal. It may also prove particularly useful in late second and third trimesters in order to obtain rapid karyotypes (Holzgreve et al., 1987).

TRANSVAGINAL APPROACH. A final technique is transvaginal CVS, using a spinal needle as in transabdominal CVS. This technique may be preferable for a retroflexed uterus having a posterior placenta. Use of a needle attached to a transvaginal ultrasound probe may facilitate the procedure. Sidransky et al. (1990) reported 15 cases and our group has performed the procedure in about 20 cases (Shulman et al., 1992b).

Safety

Canadian and the United States NICHD collaborative studies initially reported the pregnancy loss rate in CVS patients to be 0.6 and 0.8 per cent, respectively, higher than in amniocentesis patients, neither figure statistically significant (Canadian Collaborative Trial, 1989; Rhoads et al., 1989). The Canadian study was randomized, whereas the U.S. study involved women who self-selected either amniocentesis or CVS. Remote obstetric complications (intrauterine growth retardation, abruptio placentae, premature delivery) also did not exceed those in women not undergoing CVS. Variables adversely influencing fetal loss rates are number of catheter passages, small sample size, and prior bleeding (Brambati et al., 1987; Rhoads et al., 1989). Fundal location is a risk factor (odds ratio 2.8) for transcervical CVS loss, relative to losses with posterior placentation (Golbus et al., 1992). All these factors invariably reflect technical difficulty.

Transabdominal and transcervical CVS appear equal in safety at 9 to 12 weeks. In a U.S. NICHD collaborative study, nearly 4000 subjects were randomized into transabdominal and transcervical groups. Loss rates of cytogenetically normal pregnancies were 2.5 per cent through 28 weeks following transcervical CVS and 2.3 per cent following transabdominal CVS (Jackson et al., 1992). Pursuant to assessing CVS-related risk, the absolute loss rate decreased by about 0.8 per cent during this randomized trial, in comparison with rates observed during the transcervical CVS versus amniocentesis self-selection study just cited. It is reasonable to conclude that this reflects both increasing operator experience and availability of both transcervical and transabdominal approaches. For example, with the availability of transabdominal CVS, some technically difficult transcervical CVS attempts (e.g., fundal placentation) could be eschewed in favor of a technically easier transabdominal approach. (Of course, the converse is also true.)

Brambati et al. (1990) also found no differences between transabdominal and transcervical CVS in an Italian randomized trial. Danish workers found transabdominal CVS to be associated with fewer losses than transcervical CVS; however, given the far greater Danish experience with transabdominal CVS, these results are not necessarily surprising. The clear consensus is that both TC and TA CVS are equal in safety.

The one major study at odds with U.S., Canadian, and Italian collaborative trials is that of the Medical Research Council (MRC, Working Party on the Evaluation of Chorionic Villus Sampling, 1991), predominantly involving United Kingdom and other European countries. Here the outcome measured was completed pregnancies following randomization to CVS or amniocentesis in the first trimester. The 4.4 per cent fewer completed pregnancies in the CVS cohort was both due to more unintended losses and to more intended terminations. The latter surely reflects some inexperience in cytogenetic interpretation because some terminations seem arguable in retrospect (i.e., confirmed placental mosaicism). The former is more difficult to assess, but it is clear that the experience of the MRC study operators was considerably less than that of those involved in the U.S. trial. For example, the only requirement for participation was 30 "practice" procedures. During the trial some centers contributed very few cases.

Few data exist for safety of CVS in multiple gestation. A U.S. study involving four centers showed a total loss rate of chromosomally normal fetuses (spontaneous abortions, stillborns, neonatal deaths) to be 5.0 per cent (Pergament et al., 1992), only slightly higher than the 4.0 per cent observed for singleton pregnancies (Rhoads et al., 1989).

A question has arisen concerning a possible association between limb defects and CVS. There have been no claims that other anomalies are increased. In 1991 Firth and co-workers reported five cases of limb reduction defects (LRD) among infants born to 539 mothers who had undergone transabdominal CVS. Oromandibular hypogenesis was present in four of the five; the fifth had a terminal transverse limb reduction alone. All cases occurred in a subset of 289 pregnancies in which the procedure was done at 56 to 66 menstrual days (8 to 9.5 gestational weeks or 6 to 7.5 embryonic weeks). In the U.S. NICHD trial only 10 per cent of cases were sampled this early.

In the United States, Burton and colleagues (1992) reported four cases of limb reduction defects among 260 pregnancies. All were transverse distal defects involving hypoplasia or absence of the fingers and toes; sampling had been performed at 9.5, 10, 10.5, and 11.5 weeks, respectively. Noteworthy is that three of these cases followed transcervical sampling with one particular device, which in that center was associated with a 11 per cent fetal loss rate (21 per cent with two passes). This catheter is slightly larger (1.4 vs 1.9 mm) and more rigid than the Portex catheter. Hsieh and colleagues in Taiwan (1991) reported severe limb abnormalities in fetuses following CVS at 8 to 9 weeks gestation: two of the pregnancies had been terminated following detection of the defect (at fetal anomaly screening by ultrasonography). However, the population from which the Taiwan cases were derived was not stated, nor were details available.

Are these reports of limb reduction anomalies due to a chance clustering of cases or do they actually reflect such malformations related to the CVS procedure? If the latter is true, several plausible mechanisms could be invoked.

1. Hypoperfusion due to fetomaternal hemorrhage or pressor substances released by perturbation of villi or the chorion. Indeed, limb malformations have been observed in hypoperfusion experiments in animals.
2. Embolization of chorionic villus material, or maternal clot, into the fetal circulation, again possibly leading to hypoperfusion. Direct observation of the fetus (embryoscopy) prior to abortion showed that ecchymoses appear if the placenta is agitated by a Hegar dilator, although this was not reported after CVS alone (Quintero et al., 1990).
3. Amniotic puncture and limb entrapment in exocoelomic gel (Shepard et al., 1991).

The potential association of limb reduction defects with CVS has been explored through various birth defects registries. The Italian Multicenter Birth Defects Registry (Mastroiacovo and Cavalcanti, 1991) reported that CVS has been performed in four of 118 cases with transverse limb reduction defects (3.4 per cent), compared with 15 of 6486 cases with other malformations

(0.2 per cent). Of note is that two of the four LRD cases were associated with 6- to 7-week CVS, a time at which CVS is no longer performed (WHO/EURO, 1992). Moreover, analysis of seven other EUROCRAT registries involving over 600,000 births showed that four of 336 cases (1.2 per cent) with limb reduction anomalies had been exposed to CVS, compared with 78 of 11,883 cases with other malformations (0.66 per cent) (Dolk et al., 1992). This difference was not statistically significant.

A major problem in assessing significance of LRD associated with CVS is that the background incidence of LRD is not precisely known. Perhaps the best data are incidence figures from British Columbia. Excluding LRD associated with chromosomal abnormalities and other known syndromes the incidence is 5:41/10,000 (one-third transverse defects; two-thirds longitudinal defects) (Froster-Iskenius and Baird, 1989). Unfortunately, determining the precise incidence beyond the general estimate stated will not be simple.

Despite considerable media attention, the reality is that few groups have shown increased LRD, especially when the CVS is performed at 9 to 12 gestational weeks. Certainly, the cluster reported by Burton et al. (1992) is not typical of the North American experience or that of experienced centers worldwide. For example, Table 2–2 compares the frequency of LRD among various centers worldwide as tabulated by the World Health Organization (WHO/EURO Meeting, 1992). Overall, worldwide experience shows no increased frequency for LRD above the observed background level, at least when sampling is performed by experienced centers during gestational weeks 9 to 12.

Of relevance is that the two reported clusters of infants with limb abnormalities were observed in centers with relatively limited experience. The high loss rates observed by the one U.S. center reporting a cluster has already been noted (Burton et al., 1992), and inexperience is expected to be associated with increased loss rates (WHO/EURO, 1992). Overall, observations suggest less than ideal surgical technique may be a correlate of any increased frequency of LRD that exists after CVS. Consistent with LRD being related to traumatic procedures are data of Brambati (WHO/EURO, 1992), whose highly experienced center reported a small cluster of LRD cases associated with very early CVS (7 to 8 weeks) but definitely not with traditional (9- to 12-week) CVS.

The WHO concluded that there is little evidence to suggest a substantive risk of congenital malformation

TABLE 2–2. Frequency of Reduction Defect (LRD) Following CVS Compared to Background Incidence Based on British Columbia Registry (WHO/EURO, 1992)

	TOTAL LIVE BIRTHS	TOTAL LRD	OVERALL INCIDENCE PER 10.00
CVS cases with known outcome	80,051	48	6.00
British Columbia Registry Data (1952–1984)	1,213,913	659	5.42

CVS cases derived from experienced centers. The 48 LRD cases include also the Oxford (N = 5) (Firth et al., 1991) and Chicago (N = 4) (Burton et al., 1992) clusters.

when CVS is performed after the eighth completed week of pregnancy in experienced centers. Still, patients must be informed of the controversy, and it is prudent to eschew CVS before 8 weeks. Even making worst-case estimates, the absolute risk would still be quite low. Because experience seems to be a more important factor in CVS safety than in amniocentesis, centers offering CVS should construct programs in such a way as to allow maintenance of skills and selection of the least traumatic approach (Boehm et al., 1993).

Safety of Early Amniocentesis

Limited experience is being reported on amniocentesis prior to 15 menstrual weeks. "Pilot" reports are promising in indicating that such a procedure would be beneficial for patients at increased risk for genetic disorders who otherwise must wait until 15 menstrual weeks for diagnosis. Some authorities perceived the need to provide prenatal diagnosis to women presenting immediately after the 12th week, the closing time for acceptance into most CVS programs; others believed that the initial reports of risks and complications following CVS were unacceptably high. Some centers reported moving toward earlier performance of amniocentesis almost inadvertently, when patients presented earlier than calendar dating anticipated. Reluctance to reschedule such patients resulted in attempting amniocentesis somewhat earlier than was standard practice (Hanson et al., 1987).

Initial reports of such experiences usually involved amniocentesis at 14 or 15 completed weeks (Henry et al., 1985; Luthard et al., 1985). Relatively few full reports are available, most remaining only in abstract form. However, Benacerraf et al. (1988) reported 100 consecutive patients undergoing amniocentesis between 11 and 14 weeks. Among 94 pregnancies allowed to continue, "all . . . were progressing normally at follow-up, which occurred at delivery or 1 month or more after the procedure." From the same institution, Penso et al. (1990) followed 407 women who underwent amniocentesis between 11 and 14 weeks, usually at 12 or 13 weeks. Loss rate within 4 weeks of the procedure was 2.3 per cent, with another 1.6 per cent loss thereafter. The neonatal care admission rate was 8.8 per cent; 6.6 per cent of neonates showed pulmonary complications, 1.6 per cent with respiratory distress syndrome. Nevin et al. (1990) reported 222 early amniocentesis; 60 per cent were performed at 14 weeks gestation, 27 per cent at 13 weeks, and 11 per cent at 12 weeks. The post-procedure spontaneous abortion rate was 1.4 per cent. No infant had respiratory stress syndrome (RDS). These authors concluded that although early amniocentesis appears to be safe and accurate for prenatal diagnosis, before (the procedure) becomes routine clinical practice, it requires appraisal by a randomized clinical trial.

In 1992 Hanson et al. updated their earlier work, their experience now encompassing 936 cases earlier than 13 weeks. About 75 per cent of procedures were performed in the 12th week and only 1.5 per cent at less than 11 weeks. They observed 0.7 per cent (7/936) losses within 2 weeks of amniocentesis, an additional 2.2 per cent (21/936) losses before 28 weeks and 0.4 per cent (4/936) stillbirths or neonatal deaths. The total losses (32/936 or 3.4 per cent) compared with 2.1 to 3.2 per cent in ultrasonographically normal pregnancies not undergoing a procedure.

Henry and Miller (1992) also reported favorable results in amniocentesis at 12, 13, and 14 weeks. Pregnancy losses prior to 28 weeks were 5/193 (2.6 per cent), 5/426 (1.2 per cent), and 18/1172 (1.5 per cent), respectively. These authors do not recommend amniocentesis before 12 weeks, although they have performed the procedure in selected cases at such early weeks gestation.

It would seem that amniocentesis at 12 to 14 weeks should be relatively safe, our own experience being favorable in singleton and in 6 twin gestations (Shulman et al., 1992a). However, reported data do not yet support the claim that early amniocentesis and traditional amniocentesis are equal in safety. The data base in no way even approaches that of CVS. These statements hold especially for amniocentesis at less than 12 weeks. *First*, most authors have described increased difficulty in obtaining the amniotic fluid sample at less than 13 weeks gestation. This presumably results from the tenting of the membranes by the needle, requiring a different needle insertion technique (Evans et al., 1989) and resulting in higher rates of failure (Hanson et al., 1987). *Second*, weeks 12 to 14 and especially earlier are among those most crucial for fetal lung development (Hislop and Fairweather, 1982). Given the documented increase in respiratory distress (2.1 relative risk) and neonatal pneumonia (2.5 relative risk) following even mid-trimester amniocentesis (Tabor et al., 1986), respiratory compromise following early amniocentesis is a clear concern. Indeed, Penso et al. (1990) found pulmonary complications in 6.6 per cent of early amniocentesis cases, 1.6 per cent having RDS.

Overall, it cannot yet be assumed that amniocentesis earlier than 14 weeks is as safe as traditional amniocentesis, although we and others are encouraged at 12 to 14 weeks. Earlier use should not be attempted routinely.

Fetal Blood Sampling

Prior to 1977, placentesis was used to sample fetal blood (Golbus et al., 1976b). Although this technique commonly produced mixed fetal/maternal blood samples, it was still satisfactory for the diagnosis of most hemoglobinopathies (Golbus, 1978; Ward et al., 1981; Cao et al., 1986). Later, fetoscopic visualization greatly improved fetal blood sampling, such that 100 per cent fetal blood was obtained more frequently. Thus, indications broadened to include hemophilia A and various immunologic diseases in which pure or nearly pure fetal blood was required. Still, fetoscopy usually resulted in fetal blood admixed with amniotic fluid. Additionally, fetoscopy was difficult if amniotic fluid was discolored. With the dramatic improvements in ultrasonographic technology occurring during the 1980s, percutaneous umbilical blood sampling (PUBS) gradually became possible, replacing fetoscopy and allowing nearly pure fetal blood to be obtained without amniotic fluid contamination in most cases.

During the fetoscopy era, absolute fetal loss rates appeared to be 4 to 7 per cent (Special Report, 1984; Alter, 1987), of which perhaps half were procedure-related. With PUBS, the corresponding fetal loss rate corrected for anomalous fetuses appears to be only 1 to 2 per cent (Daffos et al., 1985; Golbus et al., 1989). Preterm delivery occurs in 5 to 15 per cent of continuing pregnancies after fetoscopy (Ward et al., 1981; Alter, 1985; Golbus et al., 1989) but in only 5 per cent of pregnancies after PUBS, again corrected for anomalous fetuses (Daffos et al., 1985). It is unknown whether these results differ from those associated with late transabdominal CVS (Holzgreve et al., 1987), a procedure applicable for cytogenetic diagnosis but not fetal blood analysis.

Prior to sampling, the patient is usually premedicated with intravenous diazepam, and a local anesthetic is injected intra- and subdermally. Patients are typically given prophylactic intra-amniotic antibiotics after liver or skin biopsy, but not after blood sampling. If indicated, the patient is given Rh immunoglobin; the amount can be determined by performing a Kleihauer-Betke stain on maternal blood one hour after the procedure. The patient and fetus are observed for 4 to 6 hours before discharge.

Fetal Skin Sampling

Like fetal blood sampling, fetal skin sampling was also performed initially using fetoscopy. Using ultrasound guidance, the fetoscope was used first to visualize the fetal skin and then to be placed firmly on the appropriate fetal part. The trochar was withdrawn, a 20 cm biopsy forceps passed through the cannula, and skin specimens (2 mm) obtained. More recently, skin biopsies have been performed entirely under ultrasound guidance, again without direct visualization (Elias and Esterly, 1981; Elias, 1987; Gedde-Dahl and Weupper, 1987).

Biopsies of fetal skin still remain the only way to diagnose a few rare dermatologic disorders *in utero*. Epidermolysis bullosa (EB) and certain forms of ichthyosis are the major current indications. Analogous to the trend in genetic disorders once requiring fetal blood sampling, molecular elucidation of genodermatoses will doubtless further decrease indications of this already uncommon procedure. For example, one form of EB (albeit an autosomal dominant form for which skin biopsy is not appropriate) is potentially detectable by linkage to the keratin gene (McKenna et al., 1992).

Prior to fetal skin sampling the patient is usually premedicated with intravenous diazepam, and a local anesthetic injected intra- and subdermally. Patients are often given prophylactic intra-amniotic antibiotics after liver or skin biopsy but not after blood sampling. If indicated, the patient is given Rh immunoglobin. Patient and fetus are observed for 4 to 6 hours and then discharged. Procedure-related loss rates are assumed to be at least as high as for fetal blood sampling by fetoscopy, i.e., about 3 per cent.

Fetal Liver Sampling

Fetal liver sampling has also been reported with only a single institution, the University of California, San Francisco, currently providing this service in North America. With a 16.5 gauge thin-wall Lee biopsy needle (Becton-Dickinson, Rutherford, NJ), a single entry into the fetal liver is made immediately below the right costal margin. A 3 ml syringe is attached to the needle and negative pressure applied to bring liver tissue within the biopsy needle. After withdrawals, tissue is flushed from the needle with ice-cold 0.9 per cent saline. Approximately a dozen fetuses have been studied by liver biopsy by the San Francisco group and one other in London, with no fetal losses to date (Simpson and Golbus, 1992). Procedure-related loss rates of 2 to 3 per cent should be offered. Preparation of the patient prior to the procedure and management thereafter is nearly identical to that for fetal skin biopsy.

Fetal Muscle Biopsy

Almost all prenatal diagnoses of Becker-Duchenne muscular dystrophy (BDMD) can be accomplished by molecular genetic techniques (see Chapter 1). However, in a few families, meiotic recombination or homozygosity of multiple chromosomal RFLPs (see below per definition) preclude such a diagnosis. In these cases it may be possible to perform fetal muscle biopsy and to analyze the muscle fibers with a fluorescent anti-dystrophin antibody. Males with BDMD lack dystrophin, whereas unaffected male muscle cells contain this protein in abundance. The procedure is analogous to fetal skin or liver biopsy (Evans et al., 1991).

Analysis of Chorionic Villi or Amniotic Fluid Cells

The maternal-fetal medicine specialist must be well aware of the diagnostic pitfalls associated with analysis of chorionic villi or amniotic fluid cells. The most obvious problem is that cells may not grow, or growth may be insufficient for proper analysis. Fortunately, culture failures are relatively uncommon. Analysis of maternal rather than fetal cells is another theoretical possibility that could obviously result in an error in diagnosis. Fortunately, such maternal cell contamination has proved uncommon in experienced hands. In amniocentesis, maternal cell contamination can be minimized by discarding the first few drops of aspirated amniotic fluid. In chorionic villus sampling, examination of the specimen under a dissecting microscope allows one to distinguish villi from decidua.

CYTOGENIC ANALYSIS. Of more than theoretical concern is the possibility that chromosomal abnormalities in villi or amniotic fluid may fail to reflect fetal status. One reason is that chromosomal aberrations may arise in culture (*in vitro*). This possibility should be suspected whenever an abnormality is restricted to only one of the several culture flasks or clones from a single amniotic fluid or CVS specimen. In fact, cells containing at least one additional structurally normal chromosome are detected in 1 to 2 per cent of amniotic fluid or chorionic villus specimens (Simpson et al., 1982). If these abnormal cells are limited to a single culture or clone, the phenomenon is termed *pseudomosaicism*; no clinical significance is attached. Defined as presence of the same abnormality in more than one clone or culture flask, *true fetal mosaicism* occurs in about 0.1 to 0.3 per cent amniotic cultures (Hsu and Perlis, 1980; Worber and Stein, 1984) and in about 0.8 per cent of chorionic villi cultures (Ledbetter et al., 1990, 1992; Vejerslev and Mikkelsen, 1989). True mosaicism involving autosomes should probably be assumed to connote abnormal development, especially if ultrasound reveals any structural anomalies. Applicability of this principle is invariable if the mosaicism involves a common trisomy. Mosaicism involving sex chromosomes is less likely to be associated with fetal abnormalities. Of special note is that 45,X/46,XY mosaicism detected fortuitously at prenatal diagnosis is usually (90 to 95 per cent) associated with normal male development (Hsu, 1992).

Cell type is also important. Cytotrophoblasts derived from villi can be accumulated in metaphase within hours of sampling. Analysis of such cells can provide answers rapidly. However, discrepancies may arise between short-term cytotrophoblast cultures and long-term cultures initiated from the mesenchymal core of the villi (Ledbetter et al., 1990; 1992). Of the two techniques, long-term culturing is considered more definitive, but neither is categorically reliable. In direct cultures in particular, mosaicism and even nonmosaic aneuploidy involving monosomy X and lethal autosomal trisomies may not be definitive for fetal abnormalities.

The U.S. NICHD Collaborative studies involved 11,473 chorionic villus samples studied by direct method, long-term culture, or both. There were no incorrect sex predictions (Ledbetter et al., 1992). There were also no diagnostic errors involving 148 common autosomal trisomies (+13, +18, +21), 16 sex chromosomal aneuploidies, and 13 structural aberrations. In no case was a normal cytogenetic diagnosis with CVS followed by birth of a trisomic infant. Of 9 triploids all 3 studied were confirmed; no confirmation was possible in the single tetraploid case. Not confirmed were several rare trisomies (+16, +22, +7). Overall, accuracy is comparable with amniocentesis, but additional tests are necessary before definitive establishment of nonmosaic rare trisomies and, as in amniotic fluid analysis, polyploides. Of interest is that U.S. NICHD study also observed increased late loss rates (8.6 per cent) in pregnancies showing confirmed placental mosaicism, compared with 3.4 per cent in pregnancies without mosaicism (Wapner et al., 1992). However, there was no increased frequency of pregnancy complications.

A final caveat is that the neonatal phenotype cannot always be predicted on the basis of the chromosomal complement in amniotic fluid cells or chorionic villi. If a phenotypically normal parent carries the same balanced translocation as found in the fetus, reassurance is usually appropriate. On the other hand, if an ostensibly balanced translocation is detected in the fetus but in neither parent (a *de novo* translocation), the likelihood is clearly increased that the neonate will be phenotypically abnormal at birth. Presumably, the rearrangement is not always truly balanced. The risk for the fetus being abnormal has been calculated at 6.1 per cent for *de novo* reciprocal translocations, 3.7 per cent for *de novo* Robertsonian translocations, and 9.4 per cent for *de novo* inversion (Warburton, 1991). These risks are not chromosome specific but represent pooled data involving many chromosomes. These risks also refer only to structural abnormalities, not taking into account developmental delay (mental retardation), which of course is not evident at birth. The risk of phenotypic abnormalities associated with *de novo* marker chromosomes is 14.7 per cent if the marker lacks satellites and 10.9 per cent if satellites are present. With newer cytogenetic techniques (see later discussion) that enhance diagnosis, it is hoped that risks for marker chromosomes can be better defined based on determination of the specific chromosomes from which they are derived.

Diagnosis of Chromosomal Abnormalities by Fluorescent *In Situ* Hybridization (FISH)

This important new technique, which merges molecular genetics and cytogenetics, offers great diagnostic promise. Using DNA sequences present only on the chromosome in question, chromosome-specific probes (e.g., No. 21, the X, or the Y) can be created (Fig. 2–4). The probe is then labeled with a fluorochrome and used to challenge unknown DNA. Disomic cells (metaphase or interphase) will usually (80 to 90 per cent) show two separate signals; trisomic cells show three signals. (Because of geometric vicissitudes, not every trisomic cell will show three signals; however, the modal count readily indicates chromosomal complement.) Simultaneous use of different colored fluorochromes for different probes permits simultaneous assessment of multiple chromosomes. Computer-digitalized imaging is being used as an adjunct to assess the number of signals, particularly for multiple color probe analysis. Especially attractive is that FISH is applicable to interphase cells.

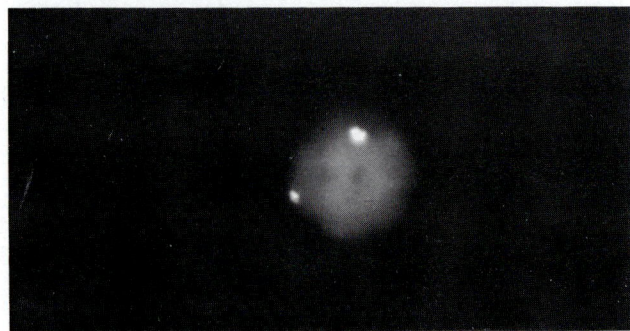

FIGURE 2–4. Fluorescent in situ hybridization (FISH) of interphase nucleus with a probe derived from the centromeric region of the X chromosome (alphoid repeats). Presence of two spots connotes two X chromosomes, thus in general derivation from a female (XX).

At present, sensitivity and specificity of FISH are still being assessed, and it would not yet be appropriate to consider FISH an alternative for metaphase analysis. However, FISH offers considerable advantage for rapid diagnosis and in circumstances in which metaphases cannot be obtained (e.g., fetal cells obtained from maternal blood) (Lebo et al., 1992). Analyzing amniotic fluid cells with five probes (21, 18, 13, X, and Y), Klinger et al. (1992) were able to diagnose corresponding trisomies. On a larger sample, the same group (Ward et al., 1992) reported a sensitivity of 88 per cent; analysis was sometimes uninformative. No false-positive trisomies were diagnosed, but a false-negative sex chromosome abnormality has been observed (Benn et al., 1992).

DNA AND ENZYME ANALYSES. In CVS, the accuracy of both molecular and biochemical (enzymatic) diagnoses for mendelian traits is nearly 100 per cent, comparable with amniotic fluid analysis. Such high accuracy could not have been assumed, for admixture of endometrial tissue could seriously compromise the diagnoses of enzyme errors. However, in the U.S. NICHD collaborative studies, there were no diagnostic errors in 283 mendelian disorders by enzymatic analysis (Desnick et al., 1992).

The most common biochemical disorders studied were lysosomal storage disease (81 per cent of all biochemical diagnoses), particularly Tay-Sachs disease. Diagnoses were also correctly made for amino acid and organic acid diseases, urea cycle defects, and various other diseases. However, in a few disorders (e.g., mucopolysaccharidosis type II, metachromatic leukodystrophy, Krabbe's disease), confirmatory analysis was necessary in amniotic fluid cells.

In the U.S. NICHD collaborative studies, many other cases (N = 318) were monitored for mendelian traits by molecular techniques. Disorders detectable by direct analysis were 100 per cent accurate, whereas those requiring RFLP analysis showed accuracy of the magnitude predicted on the basis of recombination. (See later discussion for pitfalls inherent in this approach.) That is, diagnosis was not 100 per cent accurate because of meiotic recombination, rather than diagnostic inaccuracy.

INDICATIONS FOR PRENATAL CYTOGENETIC STUDIES

All chromosomal disorders are detectable *in utero*. It is not appropriate, however, to study either by amniocentesis or CVS every pregnancy because for many couples the risks of such invasive procedures outweigh diagnostic benefits. Considered below are currently accepted indications.

Advanced Maternal Age

The most common indication for antenatal cytogenetic studies is advanced maternal age. The overall incidence of trisomy 21 is one per 800 liveborn births in the United States, but it is well known that the frequency increases with maternal age (Table 2–3). Tri-

TABLE 2–3. Maternal Age and Chromosomal Abnormalities (Live Births)

MATERNAL AGE	RISK FOR DOWN'S SYNDROME	TOTAL RISK FOR CHROMOSOME ABNORMALITIES*
20	1/1667	1/526*
21	1/1667	1/526*
22	1/1429	1/500*
23	1/1429	1/500*
24	1/1250	1/476*
25	1/1250	1/476*
26	1/1176	1/476*
27	1/1111	1/455*
28	1/1053	1/435*
29	1/1000	1/417*
30	1/952	1/384*
31	1/909	1/384*
32	1/769	1/322*
33	1/602	1/286
34	1/485	1/238
35	1/378	1/192
36	1/289	1/156
37	1/224	1/127
38	1/173	1/102
39	1/136	1/83
40	1/106	1/66
41	1/82	1/53
42	1/63	1/42
43	1/49	1/33
44	1/38	1/26
45	1/30	1/21
46	1/23	1/16
47	1/18	1/13
48	1/14	1/10
49	1/11	1/8

Data of Hook (1981) and Hook et al. (1983). Because sample size for some intervals is relatively small, confidence limits are sometimes relatively large. Nonetheless, these figures are suitable for genetic counseling.
*47,XXX excluded for ages 20–32 (data not available).

somy 21, trisomy 13, trisomy 18, 47,XXX, and 47,XXY all increase with advanced age, but 47,XYY, 45,X and *de novo* translocations do not.

It is now standard medical practice in the United States to offer prenatal chromosomal diagnosis to all women who at their expected delivery date will be 35 years or older. The choice of age 35 is largely arbitrary, however, having been chosen during an interval when risk figures were available only in 5-year intervals (i.e., 30 to 34 years, 35 to 39 years, 40 to 44 years). Flexibility is thus appropriate when answering inquiries from women younger than 35 years. Increasing numbers of women aged 33 or 34 years are now electing prenatal diagnosis.

The risk figures shown in Table 2–3 are applicable only for liveborns. The prevalence of abnormalities at the stage of gestation at which CVS or amniocentesis is performed is somewhat higher (Hook, 1981; Hook et al., 1983). For example, the risk for 35-year-old women is about 1/270 for Down's syndrome at the time of amniocentesis (mid-trimester); the risk is 1/385 at term. Risks of Down's syndrome reported in triple analyte screening or low MSAFP screening (see below) are, in fact, mid-trimester risks. That the frequency of chromosomal abnormalities is lower in liveborn infants than in first or second trimester fetuses reflects the disproportionate likelihood that fetuses lost sponta-neously between the time of prenatal testing (9 to 16 weeks) and term (40 weeks) will have chromosomal abnormalities (Hook, 1983; Hook et al., 1987). In fact, 5 per cent of stillborn infants show chromosomal abnormalities. It follows that some abnormal fetuses would have died *in utero* had iatrogenic intervention not occurred in the second trimester.

We shall discuss in detail the significance of low MSAFP with respect to autosomal trisomy. A logical corollary would be that normal or slightly elevated MSAFP (e.g., 1.0 to 2.4 multiples of the median [MOM]) decreases the risk of aneuploidy. For this reason, British workers in particular recommend against amniocentesis in older women (35 to 37 years) having normal or slightly increased MSAFP values ("screen negative"). This policy is especially recom-mended if hCG is not elevated and unconjugated estriol is not decreased. However, most U.S. authori-ties do not agree. Other chromosomal abnormalities that would otherwise have been detected by offering amniocentesis to all women age 35 years or older at estimated date of delivery, would be missed. More-over, in these pregnancies, potentially 100 per cent of Down's syndrome cases would be detected; combining age with MSAFP would by design lower the detection rate. In the U.S. there is no precedent for switching from a more sensitive screening test to a lesser sensi-tive one. The possible legal implications are self-evident.

Previous Child with Chromosomal Abnormality

After delivery of a child, or probably also of an abortus, with autosomal trisomy the likelihood that subsequent progeny will also have autosomal trisomy is increased. This holds even if parental chromosomal complements are normal. Although the risk is not so high as once believed, parental anxiety still dictates that antenatal chromosomal studies be discussed for all couples having a previous child with trisomy 21. Recurrence risks of perhaps 1 per cent are appropriate for genetic counseling (Stene and Mikkelsen, 1984).

Recurrence risk data following the birth of a liveborn infant trisomic for a chromosome other than No. 21 are limited. Risks of perhaps 1 per cent are appropriate either for the same or a different chromosomal abnor-mality. Thus, antenatal studies should be offered.

Parental Chromosomal Rearrangements

An important but uncommon indication for prenatal cytogenetic studies is the presence of a parental chro-mosomal abnormality. A balanced translocation is the usual indication, but inversions and other chromoso-mal abnormalities also arise. For either male or female heterozygotes having balanced reciprocal transloca-tions, pooled empiric risks approximate 12 per cent for unbalanced offspring (Boué and Gallano, 1984;

Daniel et al., 1989). For Robertsonian translocations, risks vary according to the chromosomes involved. For t(14q;21q), risks for unbalanced translocations are 10 per cent for offspring of heterozygous mothers and 2 per cent for offspring of heterozygous fathers (Boué and Gallano, 1984). For the other nonhomologous Robertsonian translocations, empiric risks for live-borns are less than 1 per cent. For homologous trans-locations 21q;21q, all liveborn offspring have Down's syndrome. For other homologous Robertsonian trans-locations (e.g., 13q;13q or 22q;22q), virtually all preg-nancies result in abortion.

Parental Inversions

The other parental chromosomal rearrangement of relevance to prenatal diagnosis is the inversion. Coun-seling is not dissimilar to that offered to individuals having a balanced translocation, although the cyto-logic mechanism responsible for abnormal offspring differs.

In chromosomal inversions, the normal sequence of genes is altered (Fig. 2–5). There are two types: para-centric and pericentric. In *paracentric* inversions, the rearrangement results from breakage, end-to-end re-versal, and reinsertion of a chromosomal segment in which break points occur on the same side of the centromere. In *pericentric* inversions, break points oc-cur on opposite sides of the centromere; reinsertion thus results in an altered arm ratio.

Individuals with inversions are phenotypically nor-mal; however, they may produce unbalanced gametes if during meiosis crossing-over (recombination) occurs within the inverted sequence. Crossing-over within a pericentric inversion gives rise to two duplication-deficiency products and two normal products (Fig. 2–5). Crossing-over within a paracentric inversion leads to one dicentric, one acentric, and two normal prod-ucts. Because acentric and dicentric products are usu-ally lost, all aberrant products of paracentric inversion are usually lethal. Abnormal liveborns will corre-spondingly be rare. However, individuals with a par-acentric inversion may experience repeated sponta-neous abortions and occasionally have had liveborn anomalous offspring.

Although empiric risk data for specific pericentric inversions are rarely available, pooled data indicate considerable risks to progeny. Females with an inver-sion are at greater risk (8 per cent) for abnormal unbalanced progeny than are males (4 per cent) (Boué and Gallano, 1984). Risk is also influenced by the length of chromosome involved in the inversion. In-dividuals with inversions involving relatively longer segments (30 to 60 per cent of the total chromosomal length) are, paradoxically, more likely to produce anomalous offspring than are those with pericentric inversion involving shorter or longer segments. A relatively short pericentric inversion segment is asso-ciated with decreased likelihood of recombination within the segment. Both relatively long and relatively short inversions yield large imbalances. If recombina-tion indeed occurs, such large imbalances are more likely to be lethal than small imbalances.

RECOMBINATION IN AN INV(18) HETEROZYGOTE

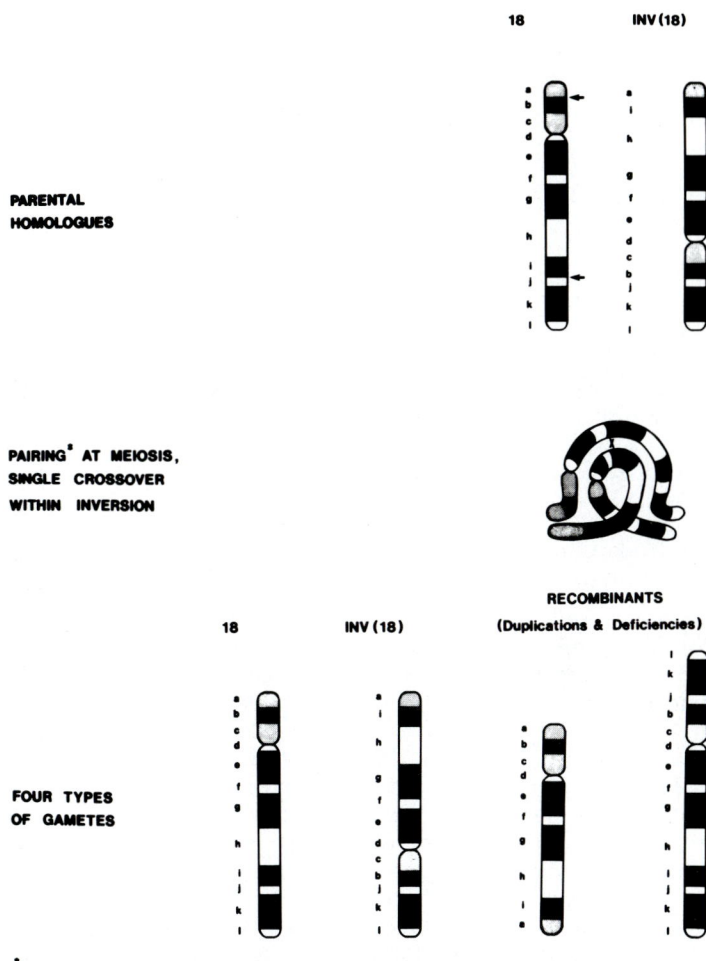

FIGURE 2–5. Diagram illustrating the breakpoints leading to an inversion in chromosome 18. The inversion loop resulting from pairing during meiosis is shown. As a result, crossing over at meiosis I would be expected to produce the four types of gametes shown. Two of the four would be genetically balanced, although one would show the inversion present in the parent. In addition, two types of gametes would be genetically unbalanced, showing complementary duplications and deficiencies. It is the chromosomal region outside the inverted segment that appears as a duplication or deletion. (Reproduced with permission from Martin AO, Simpson JL, Deddish DB, Elias S: Clinical implications of chromosomal inversions. A pericentric inversion in No. 18 segregating in a family ascertained through an abnormal proband. Am J Perinatol 1:81, 1983.)

Increased Risk of Aneuploidy due to Low MSAFP, Low Estriol, and Elevated HCG (Triple Analyte Screening)

Since at least 1987 maternal serum alpha-fetoprotein has been routinely employed in screening for neural tube defects, as will be discussed in greater detail later in this chapter. Elevated MSAFP can be indicative of an underlying fetal neural tube defect, whereas low MSAFP is associated with Down's syndrome (Merkatz, 1984; Cuckle et al., 1984). On the basis of low MSAFP women who would otherwise not have an invasive diagnostic procedure (i.e., <35 years of age at estimated delivery date) can thus be offered amniocentesis. In contrast to a single cut-off (e.g., 2.5 MOM) used to detect elevated MSAFP, a strict cut-off is not considered best for low MSAFP because the significance of a given value (e.g., 0.4 MOM) is greater for older than for younger women. Thus, a patient-specific risk using a likelihood ratio must be generated (see later).

Approximately 25 to 33 per cent of Down's syn-

drome infants can be detected on the basis of low MSAFP alone (DiMaio et al., 1987). As in evaluating elevated MSAFP, one must take into account maternal weight (Fig. 2–6) and gestational weight (Fig. 2–7). Overestimating gestational age can be associated with spurious "low" MSAFP value. Low unconjugated estriol (uE_3) (Canick, 1988; Wald et al., 1988) and elevated hCG (Bogart et al., 1987) are also associated with Down's syndrome. In pregnancies associated with fetal Down's syndrome the mean maternal serum values are 0.74 MOM for uE_3 and 2.03 MOM for hCG (Cuckle and Wald, 1992). An algorithm based on age, race, and analyte values for MSAFP, hCG, and estriol and maternal age has been devised to calculate a patient's specific risk for Down's syndrome. One uses individual MOM values to calculate likelihood ratios as illustrated in Figure 2–8 and Table 2–4. If the computer-generated algorithm risk is equal to or greater than that associated with a 35-year-old woman at mid-trimester having a fetus with Down's syndrome, i.e., 1/270, counseling and potential amniocentesis are usually appropriate. We recommend inform-

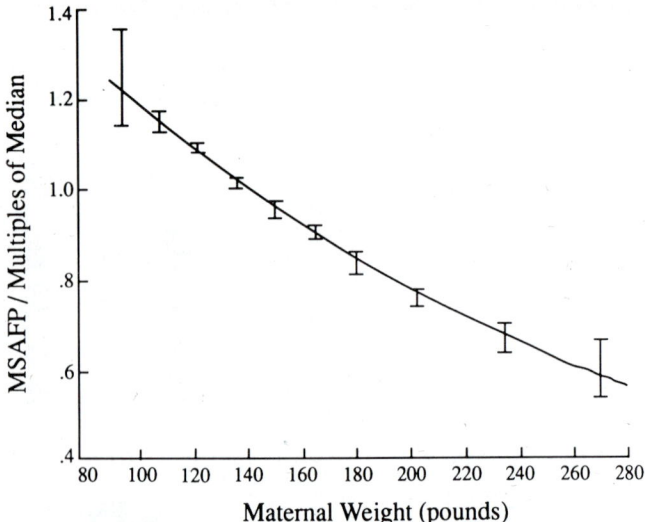

FIGURE 2–6. Maternal serum alpha-fetoprotein (MSAFP) v Maternal Weight. (From Gabbe SG, Niebyl JR, Simpson JL (eds): Obstetrics: Normal and Problem Pregnancies, 2nd ed. New York, Churchill Livingstone, 1991.)

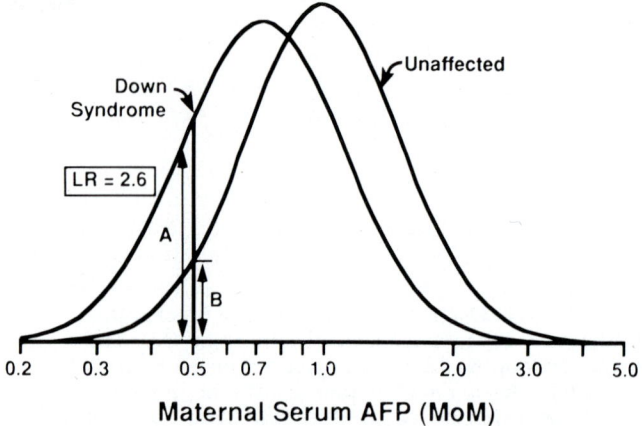

FIGURE 2–8. Schematic diagram illustrating likelihood ratio, which for Down's syndrome at MOM 0.5 is 2.6 (A/B = 2.6).

ing the patient only if her risk equals or exceeds 1/270. By taking into account age (≥35 years), AFP, uE_3, and hCG, approximately 60 to 70 per cent of Down's syndrome fetuses should theoretically be detected at an amniocentesis rate of 5 per cent. Indeed, cohort data involving 9530 cases (Phillips et al., 1992a) and by Haddow et al. (1992) involving over 25,207 cases confirm this sensitivity. Detection rate is relatively greater for older women (e.g., ages 30 to 34) and relatively lower for younger women. Nonetheless, even adolescent populations seem to benefit from triple analyte screening (Phillips et al., 1992b).

A problem with triple analyte screening as described is that trisomy 18 detection will decrease, given the fact that hCG in trisomy 18 is low rather than high as in Down's syndrome. In trisomy 18 pregnancies the median levels are 0.57 MOM for MSAFP, 0.49 for uE_3,

and 0.27 for hCG. Most cases (60 per cent) are detectable if amniocentesis is offered. This problem can be obviated by offering amniocentesis to couples in whom MSAFP is ≤0.75 MOM, uE_3 ≤0.60 MOM, and hCG ≤0.55 MOM (Canick et al., 1990).

A variation on the choice of analytes has been proposed by Macri et al. (1990), who advocate assaying free β-hCG rather than the traditional approach of assaying total hCG plus free β-hCG. However, comparison of multiple studies indicates that free β-hCG offers little or no advantage over traditional assays (Cuckle and Wald, 1992). Others measure only MSAFP and hCG, given that uE_3 adds only slightly to the sensitivity. However, use of uE_3 improves specificity, thus decreasing unnecessary amniocenteses. Many other analytes also show differences between pregnancies with Down's syndrome and pregnancies with normal fetuses. However, these analytes do not practically improve upon sensitivity and specificity of triple analyte screening (MSAFP, hCG, uE_3). The theoretical exception is neutrophil alkaline phosphatase (MOM); however, the assay for this analyte has not yet been

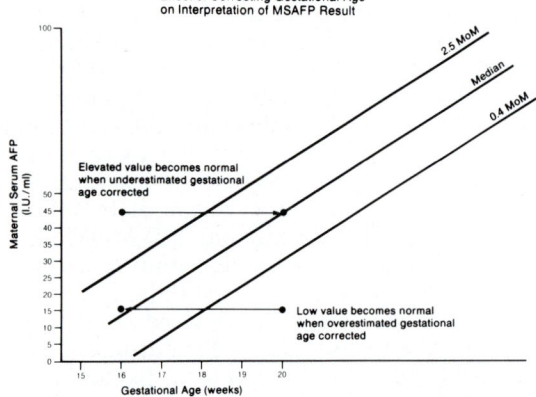

FIGURE 2–7. Median maternal serum α-fetoprotein (MSAFP) throughout gestation. Increasing values with increasing gestational age require accurate dating to interpret low or high MSAFP. (From Gabbe SG, Niebyl JR, Simpson JL (eds): Obstetrics: Normal and Problem Pregnancies, 2nd ed. New York, Churchill Livingstone, 1991.)

TABLE 2–4. Estimated Risk of a Down's Syndrome Term Pregnancy* for a 35-Year-Old Woman According to Various Serum AFP, uE_3, and hCG Levels (in MOMs)

CASE	AFP	uE3	hCG	RISK
1	ND	ND	ND	1:380
2	0.4	ND	ND	1:120
3	2.5	ND	ND	1:1800
4	0.4	0.5	ND	1:55
5	2.5	0.5	ND	1:170
6	0.4	2.0	ND	1:130
7	2.5	2.0	ND	1:3300
8	0.4	0.5	3.3	1:13
9	2.5	0.5	3.3	1:66
10	0.4	0.5	0.3	1:570
11	0.4	2.0	3.3	1:14
12	0.4	2.0	0.3	1:480
13	2.5	2.0	3.3	1:360
14	2.5	0.5	0.3	1:16000
15	2.5	2.0	0.3	1:65000

ND = test not done.
*Estimate using the algorithm described by Wald et al., 1992.

automated, the manual histochemical scoring of stained neutrophils now required being impractical for screening (Cuckle and Wald, 1992).

The possibility of first-trimester serum screening for aneuploidy is receiving increasing attention. It is appreciated that MSAFP is low in the first trimester in pregnancies with Down's syndrome (Milunsky et al., 1989; Spencer et al., 1992; Milunsky and Nebiolo, 1992); hCG is elevated in Down's syndrome but decreased in trisomies 21 and 18 (Kratzer et al., 1991). Usefulness of progesterone (P) and P:hCG ratios is less clear (Kratzer et al., 1991). However, for Down's syndrome the mean MOM hCG is 1.85 (Spencer et al., 1992), for SP1 0.40 to 0.90 and for PAPP-A only 0.23 (Brock et al., 1990; Brambati et al., 1991; Wald et al., 1992). In the first trimester MSAFP is also decreased in trisomy 18 (Milunsky et al., 1989) as is hCG (Spencer et al., 1992). Deriving a patient-specific risk based on the MSAFP, SP1, and PAPP-A could be envisioned, analogous to MSAFP, hCG, and uE_3 screening in the second trimester. Incorporating ultrasound data such as BPD/FL ratio (Platt et al., 1992b) could easily be incorporated as well into an algorithm.

Indication for Prenatal Diagnosis of Mendelian Disorders

Increasing numbers of mendelian disorders are now detectable *in utero* with high accuracy, both in chorionic villi as well as amniotic fluid cells. Initially only metabolic disorders could be detectable on the basis of enzyme analysis. Antenatal diagnosis of hemoglobinopathies and hemophilia later became possible through analysis of fetal blood, originally obtainable only by fetoscopy. DNA analysis now permits many other diagnoses. Any available nucleated cell will suffice (chorionic villi, amniotic fluid cells). The attractiveness of DNA analysis is that the nature of the mutant or absent gene product need not necessarily even be known. Given the rate of current advances, one might predict with confidence that in the foreseeable future all common mendelian disorders will be detectable. The rapid progress and increasing complexity required to diagnose mendelian traits dictate close liaison between obstetrician/gynecologist and geneticist.

Inborn Errors of Metabolism

Antenatal diagnosis is possible for approximately 100 inborn errors of metabolism, although increasingly DNA analysis is possible for some of these enzymopathies. Most are transmitted in an autosomal recessive manner, but a few display X-linked recessive or autosomal dominant inheritance. Couples at increased risk will usually be identified because they previously had an affected child. However, population screening identifies most Jewish couples who are at risk for Tay-Sachs disease. Nevertheless, metabolic disorders are so rare that it is unreasonable to expect obstetricians who are not geneticists to be fully cognizant of all of the diagnostic possibilities.

Detection of a metabolic error requires that the enzyme be expressed in amniotic fluid cells or chorionic villi. Although this requirement is fulfilled by most metabolic disorders, a prominent exception is phenylketonuria (PKU). (Fortunately, PKU can be detected by molecular techniques [Eisensmith and Woo, 1992].) All metabolic disorders detectable in amniotic fluid have proved detectable in chorionic villi. Cultured cells are usually necessary for diagnosis, although occasionally one can arrive at a diagnosis on the basis of a product in amniotic fluid. The most prominent example is 17α-hydroxyprogesterone, elevation of which indicates adrenal 21-hydroxylase deficiency (congenital adrenal hyperplasia) (Frasier et al., 1975). However, this disorder is perhaps best detected by analysis of linked HLA markers in nuclei obtained by CVS or amniocentesis (Speiser et al., 1990).

Disorders Detectable Solely by Tissue Sampling (Blood, Skin, Liver)

If a gene causing a given disorder is not expressed in amniotic fluid or chorionic villi, biochemical analysis of such tissues will provide no information concerning presence or absence of the disorder. However, the gene might still be expressed in other tissues—blood, skin, or liver. Techniques for obtaining samples have been discussed previously. Indications are rare.

Detection of Mendelian Disorders by Molecular Techniques

Molecular techniques were considered in Chapter 1. Increasing utilization and high accuracy have already been alluded to. Here we wish merely to note the two general approaches that must be applied clinically. It is convenient to divide mendelian disorders detectable by molecular techniques into those in which the molecular basis is known and those in which the precise molecular basis is unknown but in which the gene has been localized to a given chromosomal region.

Diagnosis When the Molecular Basis is Known

That the cause of a mendelian disorder is known usually implies perturbation of DNA (absence, point mutation, or duplication). This may involve a few or even one nucleotide in a coding region (exon). If a disorder is known to be characterized by *absence of DNA,* one can readily determine whether a probe does or does not recognize (hybridize) with the relevant sequence of DNA from an individual of unknown genotype. Failure of hybridization indicates that the individual lacks the DNA sequence in question; thus, the disorder can be deduced to be present. This approach is currently used to diagnose all forms of α-thalassemia, 80 per cent of Duchenne/Becker muscular dystrophy, a few forms of hemophilia, and about 20 per cent of β-thalassemia world-wide, but substantially higher in certain geographic regions.

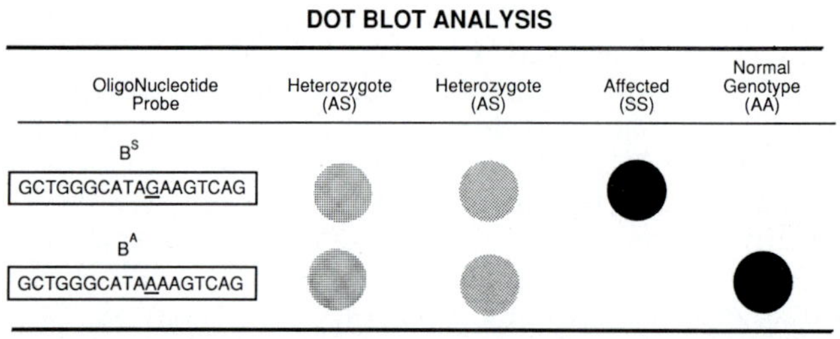

DOT BLOT ANALYSIS

FIGURE 2–9. Dot blot analysis. Oligonucleotides are constructed for sequences unique to normal DNa (B^A) and mutant DNA (B^s). DNA challenged by the oligonucleotide probe will be hybridized if and only if the DNA contains all nucleotides connoted by the probe. Thus, AS individuals will respond to both B^A and B^s probes, whereas AA or SS individuals will respond only to one of the two probes (B^A and B^s, respectively). Homozygous individuals respond with a stronger (darker) signal than heterozygous individuals. (From Simpson JL: Prenatal diagnosis and genetics. *In* Scott JR, et al (eds.): Danforth's Obstetrics and Gynecology, 4th ed. Philadelphia, JB Lippincott, 1989.)

A second approach becomes applicable if the etiology involves a *point mutation*. For example, in sickle cell anemia, the triplet (codon) designating the sixth amino acid has undergone a mutation from adenine to thymine. As a result, codon 6 connotes valine rather than glutamic acid, leading to the abnormal protein (β^s). Given that several restriction enzymes recognize the normal DNA sequence but not the mutant sequence at codons 5, 6, and 7, diagnosis becomes possible on the basis of length of DNA after exposure to the specific enzyme (Southern blotting).

A more straightforward approach becomes possible through construction of synthetic probes capable of hybridizing only to a specific sequence of approximately 15 nucleotides (oligonucleotides). Oligonucleotide probes can be designed to hybridize if and only if the (complementary) DNA of a given individual contains every single nucleotide in its correct sequence. Alteration of even a single nucleotide (e.g., in sickle cell anemia) will result in the oligonucleotide probe failing to hybridize. Sensitivity of oligonucleotide probes can also be enhanced by the use of polymerized chain reaction (PCR) to amplify the amount of DNA present in the unknown sample. Diagnoses can thus be made with small amounts of DNA, potentially even single cells. If the allele-specific oligonucleotide (ASO) hybridizes with DNA impregnated on a filter paper, it appears as a "dot blot" (Fig. 2–9). If hybridization does not occur, no such dot appears. Table 2–5 lists some common disorders for which a direct approach can be taken, allowing 100 per cent accuracy in diagnosis.

Diagnosis When the Molecular Basis is Not Known

The direct molecular approaches already described are applicable only when the precise molecular basis of a disorder is known. Actually, this requirement is fulfilled relatively infrequently. However, prenatal diagnosis is still often possible on the basis of linkage analysis, taking advantage of the ostensibly innocuous

differences in DNA that exist among individuals in the general population. These differences occur in the intervening sequences (introns) that are interspersed between coding sequences (exons).

Recall from Chapter 1 that clinically insignificant differences in DNA yield differences in DNA fragment lengths after exposure to a given restriction endonuclease. These differences are termed *restriction fragment length polymorphisms* (RFLPs). The principle underlying linkage analysis for prenatal diagnosis is that although diagnosis is not possible on the basis of analyzing the mutant gene *per se* (whose nature is unknown), a diagnosis still can be made on the basis of presence or absence of a nearby marker. Here the marker is a DNA variant capable of being recognized following exposure to a given restriction endonuclease (thus, RFLP).

To be diagnostically useful, a given RFLP must be near or preferably within the mutant gene of interest. One next needs to determine the relationship of the mutant to the status of the marker in a given family. Starting with an individual of known genotype, usually an affected child, one determines on which parental chromosome a given DNA fragment (RFLP marker) is located (*cis–trans* relationship). Is the marker located on the chromosome carrying the mutant gene, and is it located on the chromosome carrying the normal gene? For autosomal recessive traits the relationship must be deduced for both parents (heterozygotes). Figure 2–10 shows this approach.

Unfortunately, there are pitfalls in linkage analysis using RFLP. First, a RFLP may not be informative in a given family. If all family members show identical DNA fragment patterns, that particular RFLP is useless because affected and unaffected individuals cannot be distinguished from one another. If a given RFLP is uninformative, one searches for another RFLP that may prove informative. Second, the distance between the mutant gene and the RFLP is crucial because the likelihood of meiotic recombination is inversely related to this distance. During meiosis I, recombination can occur between homologous chromosomes. Genes are linked to one another if, after meiosis I, they remain together more often than expected by chance. Recombination can occur even between closely linked loci; thus, prenatal diagnosis based on linkage analysis is always less than 100 per cent accurate. Using polymorphic markers on both sides of the mutant can minimize but not exclude the likelihood of missing a recombination event.

Despite these caveats, RFLP analysis permits prenatal diagnosis of many disorders not heretofore de-

TABLE 2–5. Some Disorders Detectable by Direct DNA Analysis

Alpha-thalassemia
Beta-thalassemia (80 per cent worldwide; lower in the United States)
Duchenne-Becker muscular dystrophy (80 per cent)
Hemophilia A (rare)
Sickle cell anemia
Cystic fibrosis (50 per cent; 70 per cent in whites of northern European ancestry)

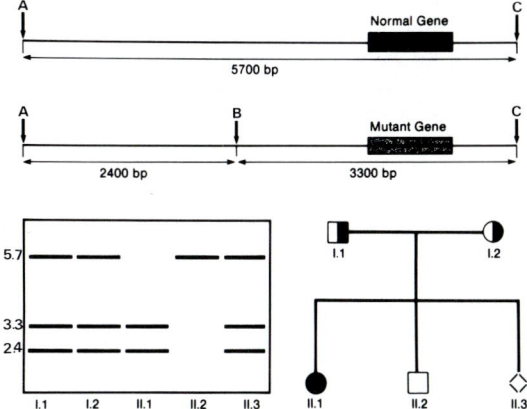

FIGURE 2–10. Restriction fragment length polymorphisms (RFLP), which are invaluable for certain prenatal diagnoses. Suppose a mutant gene is linked to another gene (B) that governs whether or not a restriction site (B) is present. If the repetitive segment is present, DNA is cut by a certain restriction enzyme (*arrow*) to produce 3300 and 2400-bp fragments long. If the segment is not present, the total fragment is 5700 long. The different lengths can function as markers to allow genotypes to be deduced. Suppose two obligate heterozygotes I.1 and I.2 have one affected child. Suppose further that a probe for the gene hybridizes to the region from A to C. The probe can thus identify three fragments (2400 bp, 3300 bp, 5700 bp). If the affected child shows only the 2400- and 3300-bp fragments, it can be deduced that the mutant allele is in association, i.e., on the same chromosome, as the gene conferring restriction site B and thus producing both 2400- and 3300-bp fragments. The normal allele must be in association with the allele not conferring restriction B and thus is designated by the 5700-bp fragment. Genotypes can thus be predicted from DNA analysis of chorionic villi or amniotic fluid cells. Fetus II.3 can be assumed to be heterozygous because all three fragments are present. (From Gabbe SG, Niebyl JR, Simpson JL (eds): Obstetrics: Normal and Problem Pregnancies, 2nd ed. New York, Churchill Livingstone, 1991.)

tectable. Because a potentially limitless number of RFLPs exist, virtually all single-gene (mendelian) disorders can be expected to become detectable eventually. This will especially become feasible as a more complete map of the human genome is developed. Table 2–6 lists some disorders already amenable to RFLP analysis. These include Huntington's disease, adult-onset polycystic kidney disease, and neufibromatosis. Cases of phenylketonuria, cystic fibrosis, forms of hemophilia A and B, Duchenne/Becker mus-

cular dystrophy, and β-thalassemia that are not amenable to direct analysis can usually be detected by RFLP analysis.

GENETIC HETEROGENEITY. Integral to prenatal diagnoses by molecular techniques is the concept of genetic heterogeneity. Clinically indistinguishable disorders may have different etiologies, particularly with respect to the abnormal nucleotide sequence. In this regard sickle cell anemia is atypical. A far more typical example of a mendelian disorder is cystic fibrosis.

Cystic fibrosis is the most common autosomal recessive trait in whites, 1 per 25 being a heterozygote. Approximately 75 per cent of individuals of north European extraction with cystic fibrosis show chromosomes No. 7 in which a deletion of three nucleotides (CTT) has occurred (Riordan et al., 1989). Deletion of these three nucleotides results in failure to code for phenylalanine at amino acid position 508 of the protein encoded by the gene, the cystic fibrosis transmembrane regulator (CFTR); hence the three nucleotide deletion is termed ΔF508, leading to an abnormality involving the CFTR. If both parents are heterozygotes, allele-specific oligonucleotide (ASO) probes readily permit prenatal diagnosis that is straightforward and that should be 100 per cent accurate. However, in some populations, the ΔF508 mutation is relatively rare, and in none is ΔF508 responsible for more than approximately 85 per cent of cystic fibrosis mutations. It is this genetic heterogeneity that makes arguable the initiation of cystic fibrosis carrier detection screening programs in all populations.

One would have hoped that the remaining CF mutations were relatively small in number, allowing screening programs to be initiated without great difficulty (multiplex PCR analyses). In fact, some 12 additional CF mutations in the North American Caucasian populations of the Northern European extraction only raise the number of recognizable CF mutations to 85 per cent. In the Ashkenazi Jewish population, one mutation (W1282X) in addition to ΔF508 allows 90 per cent of CF chromosomes to be detected. If only 75 per cent of CF mutations are detectable (as would be the case with Δ508 alone), one can detect 56 per cent of CF individuals in the general population (Table 2–7). With detection of the 85 per cent of CF chromosomes now possible, only 72 per cent of CF fetuses can be detected. If one partner is positive but the other is negative in a ΔF508 CF screening program, the latter still has a 1 in 100 risk

TABLE 2–6.   Examples of Disorders Detectable Through Linkage Analysis by Restriction Fragment Length Polymorphism (RFLP)

Adrenal 21-hydroxylase deficiency
Beta-thalassemia (20 per cent worldwide; higher in the United States)
Cystic fibrosis (50 per cent; 30 per cent in whites of northern European ancestry)
Duchenne muscular dystrophy (20 per cent)
Hemophilia A and B (most forms)
Neurofibromatosis (some forms)
Huntington's chorea
Adult-onset polycystic kidney disease

TABLE 2–7.   Likelihood of Detection of Cystic Fibrosis (CF) Given Various Frequencies of Detectable CF Mutations

DETECTABLE CF CHROMOSOMES (percentage)	DETECTION OF CARRIER STATUS (%)		
	BOTH PARENTS	**ONE PARENT**	**NEITHER PARENT**
70	49.0	42.0	9.0
75	56.3	37.5	6.2
80	64.0	32.0	4.0
85	72.3	25.5	2.2
90	81.0	18.0	1.0
95	90.3	9.5	0.2

Data of Lemna et al., 1990.

of being heterozygous at the CF locus at a position other than 508, i.e., three-fourths of CF mutations are excluded but one-fourth are not ($1/4 \times 1/25 = 1/100$).

The problem is that couples facing this dilemma (one member showing ΔF508 heterozygosity and the other showing no identifiable mutation) cannot be offered a definitive prenatal diagnosis. For these reasons population screening cannot yet be recommended (Elias et al., 1991). (See also Chapter 1.)

INDICATIONS FOR PRENATAL DIAGNOSIS AND GENETIC SCREENING IN POLYGENIC/MULTIFACTORIAL DISORDERS

Neural Tube Defects and Alpha-Fetoprotein

Failure of neural tube closure during embryogenesis leads to anencephaly, spina bifida (myelomeningocele or meningocele), encephalocele and other less common midline defects (e.g., lipomeningocele).

Anencephaly and spina bifida represent different manifestations of the same pathogenic process. Couples who have had a child with a neural tube defect (NTD) have approximately 1 per cent risk for any subsequent offspring having spina bifida and 1 per cent risk for subsequent offspring having anencephaly (2 per cent for any NTD) (Milunsky, 1992). This holds true regardless of the type of NTD present in the index case (proband). If a prospective parent has an NTD, the risk to the offspring is also about 2 per cent. Second-degree relatives (nieces, nephews, grandchildren) and third-degree relatives (first cousins) are less likely to be affected. A woman whose sister or brother had a child with NTD carries a lower (0.5 to 1.0 per cent) risk for offspring with NTD (Milunsky, 1992). For reasons that are unclear, risks are slightly lower if the father's sib had a child with NTD.

PREVENTION OF NEURAL TUBE DEFECTS

In 1991, the British Medical Research Council (MRC) Vitamin Study Group reported the results of a randomized trial demonstrating that oral supplementation of folic acid before conception and during early pregnancy reduced the recurrence risk of NTDs among women having a previously affected child by 70 per cent. These findings led to a recommendation from the United States Centers for Disease Control (1991) that all women who have had a pregnancy resulting in an infant or fetus with an NTD be treated with 4 mg daily of folic acid from at least 4 weeks before conception and through the first 3 months of pregnancy. More recently, based on an analysis of several studies in various centers throughout the world that have explored the potential protective benefit of folic acid in the general population, the CDC now recommends that all women of childbearing age "who are capable of becoming pregnant" should consume 0.4 mg of folic acid per day for the purpose of reducing the risk of having a pregnancy affected with spina bifida or other NTDs (1992). The expected risk decrease is approximately 50 per cent, and the rationale for the reduction in folic acid dosage is based on inadequate knowledge of the potential effects of high-dose folate as well as the possible confusion when diagnosing vitamin B_{12} deficiency.

Amniotic Fluid Alpha-Fetoprotein Analysis (AF-AFP)

Antenatal diagnosis of NTD can usually be accomplished by either high-quality ultrasonography or assay of amniotic fluid alpha-fetoprotein (AF-AFP). Through AF-AFP analysis, diagnosis of NTD is possible in all anencephaly cases and in all except the 5 to 10 per cent of spina bifida cases in which skin covers the lesion. Closed lesions are somewhat more common in encephalocele. Ultrasonography by experienced physicians should readily exclude anencephaly, and most cases of spina bifida can be detected by serial views of the vertebral column and third ventricle. Unfortunately, few ultrasonographers can state their own sensitivity or specificity for detecting NTD. Even in California prenatal diagnosis centers, Platt et al. (1992a) tabulated that only 92 per cent of open spina bifida was detected by ultrasonography. Until the situation can be shown to be different, AF-AFP analysis should remain the standard method for detecting NTD.

Amniotic fluid AFP may be spuriously elevated if the amniotic fluid is contaminated with fetal blood. This pitfall is eliminated by assaying amniotic fluid acetylcholinesterase (AChE) if the AFP is elevated. Acetylcholinesterase is present in the amniotic fluid of fetuses with open NTD but is absent, not simply decreased, in normal amniotic fluid. If AChE is absent but fetal hemoglobin is present, the elevated AFP can be assumed to be due to fetal blood.

Elevated AFP is also associated with certain other polygenic/multifactorial abnormalities (e.g., omphalocele, gastroschisis) and certain mendelian disorders (e.g., congenital nephrosis). In these conditions, AChE may or may not be elevated. Ultrasonographic studies should obviously be undertaken to determine the nature of any defect present. On the other hand, failure to detect an anomaly by ultrasound does not necessarily indicate that elevated amniotic fluid AFP was spurious or especially in presence of AChE. If amniotic fluid AFP is elevated and AChE is present, the fetus should be considered to be abnormal regardless of ultrasound findings.

Acetylcholinesterase in Early Amniocentesis

An unresolved issue in amniocentesis less than 13 to 14 weeks is interpreting the presence of AChE. Preliminary data on the predictive value for the presence of AChE are conflicting but encouraging. Accuracy is generally accepted at 13 weeks but not before. Crandall et al. (1989) tested AF-AFP and AChE in 360 samples obtained between 10 and 14 weeks gestation. All 11 open NTD cases had AF-AFP >3.0 MOM and showed the presence of AChE. Of the remaining 349, all were within normal AF-AFP range (>2.0 MOM).

A single normal case at 10 weeks gestation contained fetal blood and showed both elevated AF-AFP and a positive AChE. Overall, there was a false-positive AChE result in 17 per cent of samples less than 13 to 14 weeks gestation. In another report of women between 8 and 12 weeks gestation, AChE was present in 12 of 36 AF samples (Campbell et al., 1992). AChE measurement in amniotic fluid samples obtained by early amniocentesis before 13 weeks should not be relied on.

Maternal Serum Alpha-Fetoprotein (MSAFP) Screening

Because relatively few (5 per cent) NTDs occur in families who have had previously affected offspring, methods other than merely uncovering a positive family history are needed to identify couples in the general population at risk for NTD. Maternal serum AFP accomplishes this purpose, identifying couples with a negative family history who are at sufficient risk to justify amniocentesis.

Maternal serum alpha-fetoprotein (MSAFP) is greater than 2.5 multiples of the median (MOM) in 80 to 90 per cent of pregnancies characterized by a fetus with an NTD. Given overlap between MSAFP in normal pregnancies and MSAFP in pregnancies characterized by a fetus with an NTD, systematic approaches for evaluating elevated MSAFP values are necessary. In addition to NTD, elevated MSAFP occurs for the following reasons: (1) underestimation of gestational age, inasmuch as MSAFP increases as gestation progresses (see Fig. 2–7); (2) multiple gestation, 60 per cent of twins and almost all triplets having MSAFP values that would be elevated if judged on the basis of singleton values; (3) fetal demise, presumably due to fetal blood extravasating into the maternal circulation; (4) Rh disease, cystic hygroma, and other conditions associated with fetal edema and hence AFP transudation; (5) anomalies other than NTD, again generally characterized by edema or open skin defects.

For maximum accuracy the MSAFP assay should be performed at 16 to 18 weeks gestation. One must correct for certain other factors. MSAFP should be weight-adjusted because dilutional effects can result in heavier women having a spuriously low value (see Fig. 2–6). In addition, Blacks have higher mean levels than Caucasians. Obstetricians should also expect their referring laboratory to have generated their own normal values.

MSAFP values of 2.5 MOM or greater in the general population are usually considered elevated. Values above 2.0 MOM are considered by some authorities to be elevated in insulin-dependent diabetic women. In twin gestations MSAFP is generally considered abnormal only if 4.5 or 5.0 MOM or greater based on singleton pregnancy values. If elevated, a repeat MSAFP sample can substantially reduce the false-positive rate with little loss in the detection rate. We recommend repeating the MSAFP assay one week after the initial sample only if MSAFP is between 2.50 and 2.99 MOM and only if gestational age is 18 weeks or less. If not already performed before the initial

MSAFP assay, ultrasound is required before amniocentesis is offered. This will exclude erroneous gestational age, multiple gestations, or fetal demise. If there is no explanation for the elevated values, amniotic fluid should be obtained for AFP and acetylcholinesterase analysis. Amniotic fluid AFP is usually 5 SD above the mean in open NTD, whereas acetylcholinesterase is invariably present.

MSAFP screening identifies 90 per cent of anencephaly and 80 to 85 per cent of spina bifida, at the cost of 1 to 2 per cent of all pregnant women undergoing amniocentesis. If gestational age assessment is determined accurately before MSAFP sampling, the number of women having an initial elevated serum value will be reduced from about 5 per cent to about 3 percent. For every 15 women having unexplained elevated serum AFP, one will prove to have a fetus with NTD.

Unexplained Second Trimester MSAFP Elevations

In 1977, Wald et al. reported the mean birth weight to be 281 gm lower in pregnancies associated with unexplained elevated (>2.0 MOM) MSAFP than in pregnancies associated with normal second trimester MSAFP. MSAFP greater than 2.0 MOM was observed in 15.8 per cent of stillbirths, 14.8 per cent of neonatal deaths, and 16.3 per cent of infants less than 1500 gm. Only 5.8 per cent of normal singleton pregnancies showed MSAFP >2.0 MOM. In North Carolina, Burton and colleagues (1983) reported that patients with unexplained MSAFP elevations (>2.5 MOM) exhibited a significantly increased frequency of pregnancy complications. The frequency of fetal losses after 20 weeks was 4.0 per cent in women having unexplained MSAFP elevations, compared with 0.5 per cent in those with no elevation. Increases were observed for birth weight less than 2500 gm (15 vs 7.2 per cent), neonatal deaths (2.1 vs 0.5 per cent), and nonchromosomal congenital anomalies (6.2 vs 1.4 per cent). Similar claims concerning birthweight and other adverse conditions have been made by others (Brock et al., 1979; Crandall et al., 1983; Evans and Stokes, 1984).

Nelson et al. (1987) studied 166 patients with unusually high MSAFP levels (>5 MOM). Of these, 110 (66 per cent) had a subsequent pregnancy complication. The complication rate was 30 per cent if MSAFP was 4 to 4.9 MOM, 26 per cent if MSAFP was 3 to 3.9 MO, and 14 per cent if MSAFP was 2.5 to 2.9 MOM. This ostensible correlation between frequency of complications and degree of MSAFP elevation was partially confirmed by Robinson et al. (1989). From an initial sample of 35,787 women, 560 with unexplained MSAFP >2.5 MOM were identified. The frequency of stillbirths increased as MSAFP increased, although this relationship did not hold for intrauterine growth retardation.

With respect to pregnancy complications other than fetal demise or growth retardation, Clayton-Hopkins et al. (1982) reported that MSAFP values were elevated in pregnancies complicated by hypertension. This finding was also observed by Mizejewski and Risenberg (1985). In a case-control study by Milunsky and colleagues (1989), women whose pregnancies were characterized by obstetric complications were matched with women whose pregnancies had normal outcomes. Increased odds ratios were observed between elevated second trimester MSAFP and the following adverse perinatal outcomes and pregnancy complications: fetal death (8.1), low birth weight (4.0), "newborn complications" (3.6), oligohydramnios (3.4), placental abruption (3.0), preeclampsia (2.3), premature rupture membranes (2.0), and polyhydramnios (1.6). However, these complications are not independent of each other and corrections for multiple comparisons were apparently not made.

Although the aforementioned studies are intriguing, objections can be raised to the experimental designs of some. Biases of ascertainment probably exist in some studies. One obvious pitfall is ascertainment bias, which can arise if blood samples are preferentially submitted from women already suspected of having a complication. This pitfall was probably operative before MSAFP became routine, circa 1985. If some fetuses were moribund, if in fact not already dead, MSAFP might merely be secondarily elevated. Misclassification of a nonviable pregnancy as viable would contribute to an apparent association between MSAFP elevation and fetal demise and possibly other complications. If the purported association was applied clinically to women *known* to have viable pregnancies at the time of screening, risks would be overestimated.

Of great clinical significance is whether unexplained MSAFP elevation is predictive of complications in women not otherwise suspected of having obstetric problems. If unexplained MSAFP elevation merely identifies pregnancies already recognized clinically to be at increased risk as a result of pregnancy complications (i.e., preeclampsia, preexisting maternal conditions such as diabetes mellitus, bleeding), MSAFP measurements would add little to what the alert obstetrician already knows. Data are thus needed stating predictive value of elevated MSAFP in women known to have a viable pregnancy and manifesting no known risk factors.

Given that unexplained second trimester MSAFP elevations have been associated retrospectively with fetal losses and various pregnancy complications that adversely affect perinatal outcome, we are addressing whether the predictive value of this association could be enhanced by taking into account early third trimester MSAFP as well (Simpson et al., 1991). Although elevations of the latter are indeed correlated with certain pregnancy complications, cohort studies appear to show no advantage in adding third trimester MSAFP over that of second trimester measurement alone (Simpson et al., 1992a).

Polygenic/Multifactorial Disorders Detectable Only by Ultrasound

Anomalies inherited in a polygenic and multifactorial manner usually carry recurrence risks of 1 to 5 per cent for first-degree relatives (siblings, offspring, parent). This risk is sufficiently high to justify prenatal diagnosis for many couples. However, the number of genes responsible for these defects is unknown, albeit presumably more than one. Thus, diagnosis on the basis of a single enzyme assay or DNA analysis is not possible as of this writing. Diagnosis instead requires visualization of fetal anatomy, principally by ultrasound. Fetal visualization is also useful for certain mendelian disorders (e.g., autosomal recessive polycystic kidney disease, X-linked recessive aqueductal stenosis [hydrocephaly], and various skeletal dysplasias).

The typical couple is identified to be at risk on the basis of already having had a child with the anomaly in question, thus incurring a 1 to 5 per cent risk for another affected child. In order to allow maximum options in clinical management, an ultrasonographic diagnosis should ordinarily be made by 20 to 24 weeks gestation. This is sufficiently early to weigh the alternative options of pregnancy termination, fetal surgery, and delivery preterm or at term followed by neonatal surgery. Percutaneous uterine blood sampling and rapid karyotyping (Tipton et al., 1989) or second- or third-trimester transabdominal chorionic villus sampling (Holzgreve et al., 1987) are necessary to exclude chromosomal abnormalities if fetal or neonatal surgery is contemplated. A careful search for other defects is also necessary before this approach is pursued.

It cannot be overemphasized that antenatal ultrasonography for anomaly detection should be performed only by highly experienced physicians. Centers scanning patients only for fetal viability, multiple gestations, and placental location should explicitly inform their patients that anomaly assessment is not being attempted, especially if state-of-the-art equipment is not available. It should further be pointed out that almost no individual or center has experience of sufficient statistical power to allow definitive statement that a "normal" scan truly indicates absence of an anomaly.

PREIMPLANTATION PRENATAL DIAGNOSIS

Although CVS offers considerable advantages compared with amniocentesis with respect to time of diagnosis, it cannot be done until after organogenesis. This especially holds true now that it is recommended that CVS be avoided earlier than 9 weeks gestation because of the low but possibly finite risk of limb reduction defects. There are two disadvantages to delaying prenatal diagnosis until 9 weeks gestation (Simpson et al., 1990). *First*, earlier diagnosis may be necessary for certain treatment regimens. Successful metabolic treatment (i.e., dexamethasone) for fetal 21-hydroxylase deficiency, detectable at CVS, is possible; however, this is an especially propitious circumstance because the genital system is among the last of the organ systems to differentiate. *Second*, couples at exceptionally high risk for affected offspring may have repetitive abnormal fetuses at prenatal diagnosis and face multiple pregnancy terminations.

Preimplantation genetic diagnosis requires access to gametes (oocytes) or embryos before 6 days, the time at which implantation occurs. Potential approaches include (1) polar body biopsy, (2) aspiration of 1 to 2 cells from the 6 to 8 cell embryo at 2 to 3 days, and (3) trophectoderm biopsy of the 5- to 6-day blastocyst.

Polar Body Biopsy

In the absence of recombination (crossing-over), a polar body showing a mutant allele should be complementary to a primary oocyte carrying the normal allele. Thus, the normal oocyte could be allowed to fertilize *in vitro* and then be transferred for implantation and pregnancy. Conversely, if the polar body were normal, fertilization would not be permitted. Unfortunately, recombination can occur between homologous chromosomes. If crossing-over should occur, the single chromosome in the primary oocyte would be heterozygous for the two alleles. That is, the two chromatids of a single chromosome would differ in genotype. The genotype of the secondary oocyte then could not be predicted without further testing, i.e., biopsy of either the second polar body or the embryo *per se*. Recombination especially becomes a problem for genes located near the telomeres because such genes show recombination frequencies approximating 50 per cent. Nonetheless, this approach has been employed by Verlinsky et al. (1990, 1991) in pregnancies at risk for ZZ alpha-1-antitrypsin deficiency (N = 33), hemophilia A (N = 28), and ΔF508 cystic fibrosis (N = 22).

Polar body analysis and other forms of preimplantation genetic diagnosis would not be possible without polymerase chain reaction (PCR) to amplify DNA. One pitfall is that although a signal is theoretically possible with a single cell, a signal is not always observed after PCR even when DNA of a known type is present. This may be due either to loss of DNA or failure of amplification. In the hands of the one group that has attempted human polar body analysis (Verlinsky et al., 1990, 1991), PCR failed in 14 of 83 cases. Worse, PCR failure may be allele specific. A further problem is that pressing PCR to limits of its sensitivity greatly increases the risk of erroneous diagnosis due to contamination (e.g., from ambient normal cells).

Among 53 transfers by the same group, there were 4 pregnancies. Two resulted in biochemical pregnancies, one in a clinical spontaneous abortion, and one in a viable pregnancy. Unfortunately, the latter proved at CVS to be affected, thereby constituting an erroneous polar biopsy diagnosis.

Biopsy of the Eight-Cell Embryo

Biopsy at this stage requires obtaining cells contained within the zona pellucida. This can be obtained by direct aspiration with a pipette or by herniation following mechanical (razor) or chemical (pronase, EDTA) dissociation.

The sentinel work in this area has been conducted by Handyside and colleagues (1989, 1990, 1992) at Hammersmith Hospital (London). In the initial work on IVF human embryos, a single cell can be removed through a hole made in the zona pellucida by a drilling pipette (diameter 10–20 mm) containing acid Tyrode's solution. Embryonic sex was first determined in ongoing pregnancies at risk for X-linked recessive disorders, (e.g., adrenoleukodystrophy). After removal of the single cell, DNA was amplified by PCR and the product challenged with a probe for a repetitive Y chromosome sequence (Y long arm). In the initial work, embryos not showing a signal were assumed to be female and thus transferred. In 13 cycles, a mean of 5 embryos per cycle was available for biopsy. Predictably, half were female and hence transferred. Unfortunately, one diagnostic error occurred in the first 7 continuing pregnancies, presumably due to failed PCR (see later for comments on diagnostic problems): one embryo predicted to be 46,XX was shown at CVS to be 46,XY (Handyside et al., 1992). Griffin and colleagues (1992) now favor use of FISH (simultaneous X and Y probes) for determining embryonic sex.

More recently, ΔF508 cystic fibrosis has been diagnosed (Handyside et al., 1992). Here diagnosis required nested primer PCR to amplify DNA (Fig. 2–11). This technique proved successful in 12 of 16 single blastomeres from 13 embryos. Diagnosis was made by analyzing for presence or absence of the heteroduplex formation that occurs only if nonidentical single-stranded DNA reanneal together (Fig. 2–12). That is, mixing DNA from the biopsy that is presumptively normal with known mutant ΔF508 DNA would produce a heteroduplex that would confirm the diagnosis of normalcy. If a heteroduplex was not observed, the DNA in the biopsy would not be normal but rather ΔF508-like known mutant DNA. This approach was used in three couples, in which both parents were ΔF508 heterozygotes. In one of the three couples one homozygous normal and one heterozygous embryo were transferred, resulting in one homozygous normal liveborn.

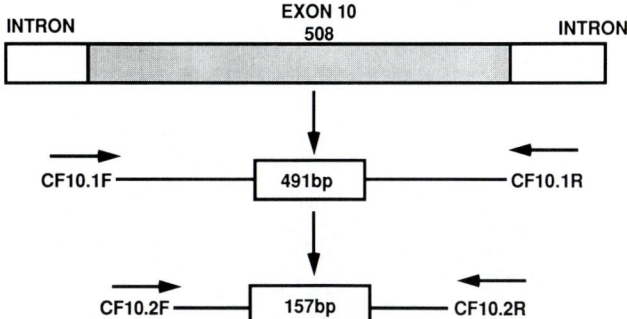

FIGURE 2–11. Diagram illustrating nested-primer polymerase chain reaction (PCR), specifically of a type enabling one to detect ΔF508 cystic fibrosis on the basis of analysis of a single cell. Polymerase chain reaction is first initiated for a 491-base pair fragment in exon 10, which contains the most common mutation in cystic fibrosis (ΔF508). After a given number of cycles (e.g., 30) with primers CF10.1F and CF10.1R, a 491-base pair sequence is generated. A second set of primers (CF10.2F and CF10.2R), internal to the first, is then constructed to generate a 157-base pair sequence. Nested-primer PCR allows far greater diagnostic sensitivity than possible on the basis of a traditional PCR.

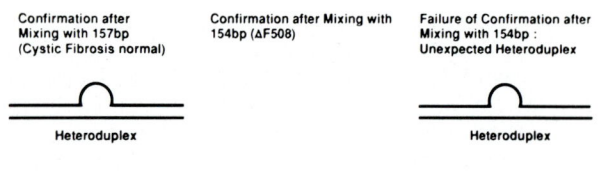

FIGURE 2–12. Heteroduplex analysis illustrating approach necessary to diagnose ΔF508 cystic fibrosis on the basis of analysis of a single cell, as would be accomplished for preimplantation genetics. Nested-primer PCR is first performed as shown in Figure 2–11. If the DNA fragment does not show ΔF508, a 157-base pair fragment (normal) is generated. If ΔF508 is present, the lack of three nucleotides results in a fragment that is only 154-base pairs in length. Although distinguishing between a 157-base pair and 154-base pair fragment is possible, this may be technically difficult. However, confirmation is easier after the unknown sample is denatured and mixed with either DNA from a normal individual (cystic fibrosis normal) or DNA from an individual known to show ΔF508. If DNA of the unknown individual (i.e., cell) is truly ΔF508, mixing with a 154-base pair fragment results in a homoduplex (middle diagram). Conversely, if the DNA from cell presumed to be ΔF508 is mixed with normal DNA (157-base pair fragment), one observes not only the 157- and 154-base pair fragments but also a heteroduplex resulting from incomplete reannealing when two dissimilar DNA fragments are placed together. The final figure (*right*) shows the presence of an unexpected heteroduplex, which would occur if the diagnosis of ΔF508 had been erroneous.

As discussed already with respect to polar body biopsy, the risk of contamination from ambient cells is a major diagnostic worry. Failed PCR is less catastrophic than contamination involving a normal cell, for only the latter would ordinarily lead to a false-negative diagnosis (Navidi et al., 1990). In autosomal recessive disorders in which the embryo was a heterozygote, PCR failure involving the normal allele would erroneously indicate the embryo to be affected and it would therefore not be transferred. The clinical consequence would be limited to a missed opportunity to achieve a pregnancy. Conversely, failing to amplify the abnormal allele would result in transfer of an embryo assumed erroneously to be homozygously normal but actually heterozygous. In either case allele-specific PCR failure would not result in a clinically significant error (i.e., false-negative diagnosis).

In the early experience of Handyside et al. (1992a), the pregnancy rate per embryo following blastomere aspiration was comparable with results obtained with in vitro fertilization without biopsy. These data reassure us that removing a single cell from the eight cell human embryo is not necessarily deleterious.

Blastocyst (Trophoectoderm) Biopsy

Diagnosis need not rely on PCR of a single cell if more cells are available. In fact, this could be accomplished by biopsying the 5- to 6-day blastocyst, an embryo with hundreds of cells rather than only 6 to 8 cells. In both murine and human models, the safest approach seems to involve slitting the zona and allowing 10 to 30 cells to extrude, followed by cutting off the herniated cells. This technique (Fig. 2–13) proved to be the least disruptive of four techniques evaluated by Carson et al. (1990) in the mouse and by Dokras et al. (1990) in the human. In the latter study, the frequency of hatching was not decreased after biopsy; however, biopsied human blastocysts have not yet been transferred.

Blastocysts can also be obtained by culture in vitro, but this process is relatively inefficient. After 3 to 4 days *in vitro*, embryonic development is not sustained efficiently to the blastocyst stage. An attractive yet still

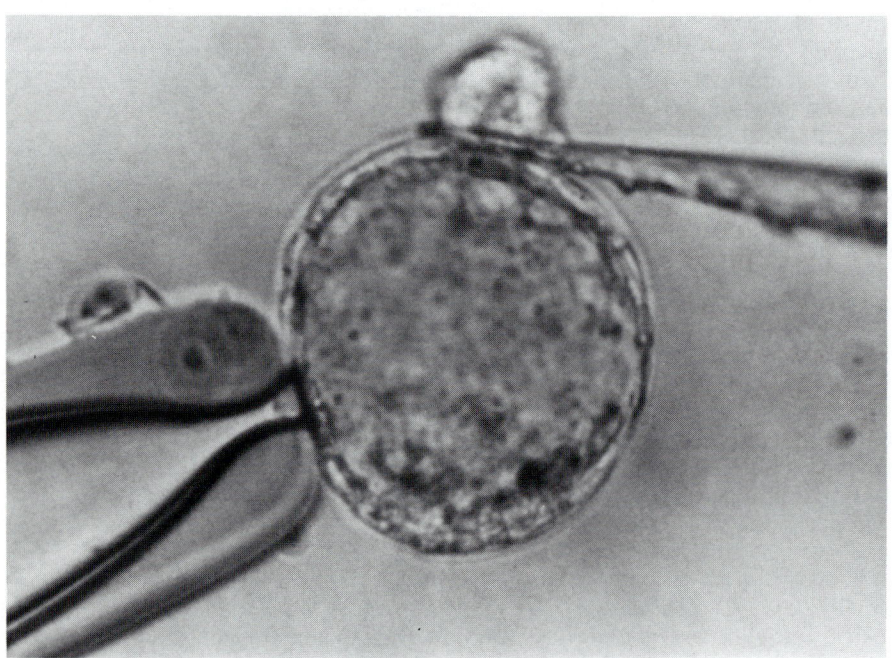

FIGURE 2–13. Trophoectoderm biopsy. (From Gabbe SG, Niebyl JR, Simpson JL (eds): Obstetrics: Normal and Problem Pregnancies. New York, Churchill Livingstone, 1991.)

unproved alternative involves uterine lavage, developed initially by Buster and colleagues (Buster et al., 1985; Bustillo et al., 1984) for use in infertile couples. Embryos recovered in this manner could be biopsied, with normal blastocysts being returned to the patient at risk for abnormal offspring.

In order to be practical, uterine lavage probably requires superovulation, as employed routinely by in vitro fertilization (IVF) programs to recover multiple embryos. Carson et al. (1991) superovulated 15 fertile women in 29 cycles, using 4 different ovulation induction regimens and using either natural intercourse or artificial intracervical donor insemination. Unfortunately, only 2 morulae, 1 blastocyst, and 4 unfertilized ova were recovered in 29 cycles. Formigli et al. (1990) had similarly disappointing results with superovulation. This discouraging experience in superovulated donors seems inexplicable. However, the potential dictates continued efforts.

ISOLATING AND ANALYZING FETAL CELLS IN MATERNAL BLOOD

The potential of recovering fetal cells from maternal blood for prenatal diagnosis was first raised by Walknowska et al, who in 1969 reported recovering "XY" metaphases in maternal blood of pregnant women carrying a male fetus. De Grouchy and Trubuchet (1971) also reported recovery of XY metaphases in pregnant women carrying a male fetus, and Y-chromatin positive cells in maternal blood were claimed by several groups (Siebers et al., 1975; Zilliacus et al., 1975). Herzenberg (1979) used flow-sorting techniques to recover lymphocytes on the basis of HLA-A2 antigen being present in the father but not in the mother; thus, sorted cells for HLA-A2 were presumably fetal in origin. However, skepticism persisted during the 1980s because confirmation of fetal origin was based solely on Y-chromatin analysis, a technique known to be characterized by less than 100 per cent specificity.

After nearly a decade of relative inactivity, various groups used polymerase chain reaction (PCR) to show that fetal cells actually exist in maternal blood. The first group to do so was Lo et al. (1989, 1990), who used the nested primer approach (see Fig. 2–11) to amplify for a Y sequence. This approach, also used in preimplantation genetics, greatly increased sensitivity (here manifested as ability to detect rare cells) over standard PCR. Women carrying a male fetus proved far more likely to show a Y-specific signal (hybridization) than those carrying a female fetus. Wachtel et al. (1991) and others (Bianchi et al., 1990; Mueller et al., 1990) later confirmed these results. The question then was identifying the particular cell type and analyzing it to determine fetal chromosomal status.

Trophoblasts

Trophoblasts are attractive candidate cells because of their intimate relationship with the uterus. Given the necessity of trophoblasts invading the uterus, it would not be surprising that some cells find their way into the maternal circulation. Indeed, in 1984 Covone et al. initially believed that trophoblasts could be isolated from peripheral blood of pregnant women at varying stages of gestation, beginning at 6 weeks. Separation was based on monoclonal antibody H315. This antibody reacts with a glycoprotein expressed on the surface of human syncytiotrophoblasts and other trophoblast cells, but not with peripheral blood cells. Unfortunately, Covone et al. (1988) later found that the H315-positive cells sorted from maternal blood were not fetal trophoblasts, but rather maternal cells that presumably had adsorbed H315 antigen *in vivo*.

Of 6000 monoclonal antibodies generated from placental tissue, Mueller et al. (1990) recovered 5 believed specific for fetal tissue. Maternal blood from pregnant women was then exposed to 2 of the 5 monoclonal antibodies and the presumptively isolated fetal cells subjected to PCR to detect Y sequences. Fetal sex was correctly identified in 7 of 7 males and 6 of 7 females. Bruch et al. (1991) used three monoclonal antibodies (GB17, GB21, GB25), which are directed against synctiotrophoblasts or (for GB72) also cytotrophoblasts. Flow-sorted cells subjected to PCR for Y-specific sequences yielded the predicted Y signal in 2 of the 3 samples tested.

Lymphocytes

Lymphocytes were actually the first fetal cells systematically sought in maternal blood, as we have already mentioned. The study already alluded to by Herzenberg and colleagues (Herzenberg et al., 1979; Iverson et al., 1981) involved couples in which the father but not the mother was HLA-A2 positive. Leukocytes from maternal blood were separated by Ficoll-Hypaque gradient and then subjected to fluorescence-activated cell sorting for HLA-A2-positive cells, which were assumed to be fetal. Fluorescein-stained cells were scored visually for presence or absence of Y-chromatin. Among 12 pregnancies resulting in male infants, 5 were positive for Y-chromatin (range 0.3 to 1.6 per cent of sorted cells). By contrast, seven mothers were delivered of infants whose lymphocytes failed to react with anti-HLA-A2 antiserum. No Y-chromatin cell was detected in these pregnancies.

Confirmation that lymphocytes were isolated was hindered by failure to document metaphases of fetal origin from lymphocytes flow-sorted on the basis of maternal-fetal HLA dissimilarities. In more recent studies, Tharapel et al. (1989; 1993), analyzed metaphases in 38 flow-sorted samples from pregnancies that usually involved male or aneuploid fetuses; all metaphases were 46,XX. These results could be explained by postulating these fetal lymphocytes are present but unresponsive to mitogens. That lymphocytes were present yet unresponsive to mitogens is consistent with the work of Yeoh and colleagues (1991). This group sorted on the basis of HLA dissimilarities and subjected these cells to PCR to confirm fetal origin.

Nucleated Red Cells (Erythroblasts)

The candidate cell being pursued at our institution is the nucleated fetal red cell (erythroblast) (Wachtel et al., 1991; Price et al., 1991; Elias et al., 1992; Simpson and Elias, 1992a and b). Bianchi et al. (1990) were the first to focus on this cell, sorting solely on the basis of transferrin receptor (CD71) positivity. PCR was then used to amplify for Y sequences. Of eight samples showing the Y sequence, six were derived from pregnancies in which women were carrying male fetuses.

In our experience, sorting on the basis of transferrin receptor (CD71) alone proved ineffective. Currently, sorting for fetal nucleated erythrocytes is on the basis of four criteria: cell size, cell granularity, transferrin receptor (CD71), and glycophorin-A, the major sialoglycoprotein of the erythroid cell membrane. Using the nested primers of Lo et al. (1990), male fetuses were correctly identified among flow-sorted samples in 12/12 (100 per cent) pregnancies; female fetuses were correctly identified in 5/6 (83 per cent) pregnancies (Wachtel et al., 1991). More recently, Bianchi and colleagues (1992) sorted not only on the basis of transferrin receptor positivity (CD71) but also on that of the presence of either glycophorin-A or the thrombospondin receptor (CD34). Ganshirt-Ahlert et al. (1992) sorted for erythroblasts, using magnetic-activated cell sorting. This group further believes that the basis of transferrin alone is not specific enough.

In Situ Hybridization for Diagnosis of Aneuploidy

In aggregate, several studies have amply verified the existence of fetal cells in maternal blood. However, PCR alone will rarely prove diagnostic, although there are exception cases. For example, if a mother is homozygous for an autosomal recessive disorder, a signal obtained after PCR amplification for the normal allele would connote a heterozygous fetus. Conversely, detection of a normal allele in cells obtained from a mother would connote a heterozygous fetus. By analogous reasoning, diagnosis of fetal hemoglobin Lepore-Boston inherited from the father was made following PCR amplification and hybridization of a sample of maternal blood (Camaschella et al., 1990).

Diagnosis of aneuploidy will almost certainly require technologies other than PCR alone. In fact, aneuploidy can be detected by FISH using chromosome-specific DNA probes. Success was first reported by Price et al. (1991), involving a blood sample taken prior to CVS; flow-sorting and FISH revealed trisomy 18 cells from the affected fetus. In the first case, 90 per cent of sorted cells showed a signal with the Y-probe, suggesting male origin; 9 per cent of sorted cells show three hybridization signals with the chromosome 18 specific DNA probe, suggesting trisomy 18. Overall, the data indicate a male fetus with trisomy 18, as shown in Figure 2–14. Since that time, several fetuses with trisomy 21 have been detected (Elias et al., 1992), and other groups have confirmed these findings.

As of this writing the sensitivity and specificity of FISH applied to flow-sorted fetal cells remain to be

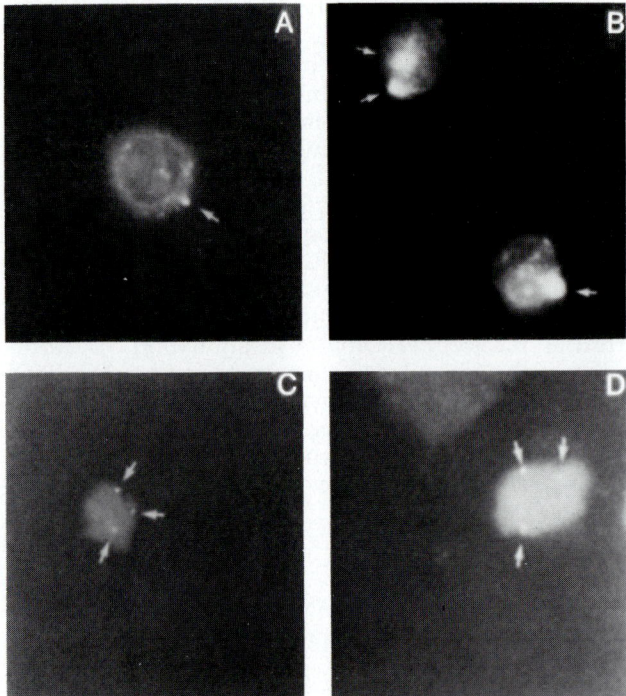

FIGURE 2–14. Flow sorted cells hybridized to various chromosome specific probes. The probes were labeled with biotin and visualized with fluorescent isothiocyanate (FITC)-streptaviden. All cells were from a single blood sample and analyzed in coded manner. *A,* Male cell of fetal origin. Fluorescent signal (*arrow*) in cell hybridized to PDP97 a probe, which identifies a repetitive sequence in the heterochromatic region on the long arm of the Y chromosome. *B,* Female cell of maternal origin (upper left) showing two signals (*arrows*) and male cell of fetal origin (lower right) showing a single signal (*arrow*). Cells are hybridized to an X chromosome-specific cosmid probe that identifies a pericentromeric repetitive sequence on the X chromosome. *C, D,* Trisomy 18 fetal cells sorted from maternal blood. Fluorescent signals (*arrows*) in cells hybridized to chromosome 18-specific cosmid contig probe, which identifies a single copy sequence on the distal long arm of chromosome 18. (From Price J et al: Prenatal diagnosis using fetal cells isolated from maternal blood by multiparameter flow cytometry. Am J Obstet Gynecol **165**:1737, 1991.)

determined. A major caveat is that FISH in flow-sorted cells is considerably more difficult than FISH in cells not subjected to flow sorting. In the initial clinical trials just under way, abnormal results will require confirmation by conventional invasive techniques such as CVS or amniocentesis. However, analysis of fetal cells isolated from maternal blood eventually could prove sufficiently accurate to allow definitive fetal diagnosis without an invasive diagnostic procedure.

REFERENCES

Alter BP: Antenatal diagnosis of thalassemia: A review. Ann NY Acad Sci **445**:393, 1985.
Alter BP: Prenatal diagnosis of hematologic diseases, 1986 update. Acta Haematol (Basel) **78**:137, 1987.
American College Obstetricians and Gynecologists: Technical Bul-

letin Number 108, September 1987: Antenatal Diagnosis of Genetic Disorders. ACOG, Washington, 1987.

Anderson RL, Goldberg JD, Golbus MS: Prenatal diagnosis in multiple gestation: 20 years experience with amniocentesis. Prenat Diagn **11**:263, 1991.

Bahado-Singh R, Schmitt R, Hobbins JC: New technique for genetic amniocentesis in twins. Obstet Gynecol **79**:304, 1992.

Benacerraf B, Green MF, Saltzman, DH, et al: Early amniocentesis for prenatal cytogenetic evaluation. Radiology **169**:709, 1988.

Benn P, Ciarleglio L, Lettieri L, et al: A rapid (but wrong) prenatal diagnosis. N Engl J Med **326**:1638, 1992.

Bianchi DW, Flint AF, Pizzimenti MF, et al: Isolation of fetal DNA from nucleated erythrocytes in maternal blood. Proc Natl Acad Sci USA **87**:3279, 1990.

Bianchi DW, Williams JM, Yih MC, et al: Fetal cells in maternal blood: prospects for non-invasive prenatal diagnosis. *Presented at the VIII International Congress of Human Genetics*, Washington, DC, 1991.

Bianchi DW, Zickwolf GK, Geifman OH, et al: Erythroid-specific antibodies enhance separation of fetal nucleated erythrocytes from maternal blood. Prenat Diagn **12**:52, 1992.

Boehm F, Salyer SL, Dev VG, et al: Chorionic villus sampling: Quality control—a continuous improvement model. Am J Obstet Gynecol. In Press.

Bogart MH, Pandian MR, Jones OW: Abnormal maternal chorionic gonadotropin levels in pregnancies with fetal chromosome abnormalities. Prenat Diagn **7**:623, 1987.

Boué A, Gallano PA: Collaborative study of segregation of inherited chromosome structural rearrangements in 1356 prenatal diagnoses. Prenat Diagn **4**:45, 1984.

Brambati B, Oldrini A, Ferrazzi E, et al: Chorionic villus sampling: An analysis of the obstetric experience of 1000 cases. Prenat Diagn **7**:157, 1987.

Brambati B, Lanzani A, Tului L: Transabdominal and transcervical chorionic villus sampling: Efficiency and risk evaluation of 2411 cases. Am J Med Genet **35**:160, 1990.

Brambati B, Lanzani A, Tului L: Ultrasound and biochemical assessment of first trimester pregnancy. *In* Chapman M, Grudzinskas G, Chard T (eds): The Embryo: Normal and Abnormal Development and Growth. New York, Springer-Verlag, 1991, p 181.

Brock DJH, Barron L, Duncan P, Scrimgeour JB, Watt M: Significance of elevated mid-trimester maternal plasma AFP values. Lancet **1**:1281, 1979.

Brock DJH, Barron L, Holloway S, et al: First trimester maternal serum biochemical indicators in Down syndrome. Prenat Diagn **10**:245, 1990.

Bruch JF, Metezeau D, Garcia-Fonknechten N et al: Trophoblast-like cells sorted from peripheral maternal blood using flow cytometry: A multiparametric study involving transmission electron microscopy and fetal amplification. Prenat Diagn **10**:787, 1991.

Burton BK, Sowers SG, Nelson LH: Maternal serum alpha-fetoprotein screening in North Carolina: Experience with more than 1200 pregnancies. Am J Obstet Gynecol **146**:439, 1983.

Burton BK, Pattanati MF: False positive acetycholinesterase (AChE) with early amniocentesis. Am J Hum Genet **43**:A227, 1988.

Burton BK, Schulz CJ, Burd LI: Limb anomalies associated with chorionic villus sampling. Obstet Gynecol **79**:726, 1992.

Buster JE, Bustillo M, Rodi IA, et al: Biologic and morphologic development of donated human ova recovered by non-surgical uterine lavage. Am J Obstet Gynecol **153**:211, 1985.

Bustillo M, Buster JE, Cohen SW, et al: Non-surgical ovum transfer as a treatment in infertile women. JAMA **251**:1171, 1984.

Camaschella C, Alfarno A, Gattardi E, et al: Prenatal diagnosis of fetal haemoglobin Lepore-Boston disease on maternal peripheral blood. Blood **75**:2101, 1990.

Campbell J, Cass P, Wathen N, et al: First trimester amniotic fluid and extraembryonic coelomic fluid acetylcholinesterase electrophoresis. Prenat Diagn **12**:609, 1992.

Canadian Collaborative CVS-Amniocentesis Clinical Trial Group: Multicenter randomized clinical trial of chorionic villus sampling and amniocentesis. Lancet **1**:1, 1989.

Canick JA, Palomaki GE, Osthanondh R: Prenatal screening for trisomy 18 in the second trimester. Prenat Diagn **10**:546, 1990.

Cao A, Falchi AM, Tuveri T, et al: Prenatal diagnosis of thalassemia major by fetal blood analysis: Experience with 1000 cases. Prenat Diagn **6**:159, 1986.

Carson SA, Smith AL, Scoggan JL, Buster JE: Superovulation fails to increase human blastocyst yield after uterine lavage. Prenat Diagn **8**:513, 1991.

Carson, SA, Gentry WL, Martin C, et al: Blastocyst microbiopsy in preimplantation diagnosis: Experience in mice. In Vitro Fertil Embryo Trans **7**:187, 1990.

Clayton-Hopkins JA, Olen PN, Blake AP: Maternal serum alpha-fetoprotein levels in pregnancy complicated by hypertension. Prenat Diagn **2**:47, 1982.

Covone AE, Kozma R, Johnson PM, et al: Analysis of peripheral maternal blood samples for the presence of placental-derived cells using Y-specific probes and McAb H315. Prenat Diagn **8**:591, 1988.

Covone AE, Johnson PM, Mutton, D, et al: Trophoblast cells in peripheral blood from pregnant women. Lancet **1**:841, 1984.

Crandall BK, Hanson FW, Tennant F: Acetylcholinesterase (AChE) electrophoresis and early amniocentesis. Am J Hum Genet **45**:A257, 1989.

Cuckle HS, Wald NJ, Lindenbaum RH: Maternal serum alpha-fetoprotein measurement: A screening test for Down syndrome. Lancet **1**:926, 1984.

Cuckle HS, Wald NJ: HCG, Estriol and Other Maternal Blood Markers of Fetal Aneuploidy. *In* Elias S, Simpson JL (eds.): Maternal Serum Screening for Fetal Genetic Disorders. New York, Churchill Livingstone, 1992, p 87.

Daffos F, Capella-Pavlovsky M, Forestier F: Fetal blood sampling during pregnancy with use of a needle guided by ultrasound: A study of 606 consecutive cases. Am J Obstet Gynecol **153**:655, 1985.

Daffos F, Forestier F, Capella-Pavlovsky M, et al: Prenatal management of 746 pregnancies at risk for congenital toxoplasmosis. N Engl J Med **318**:271, 1988.

Daniel A, Hook EB, Wulf G: Risks of unbalanced progeny at amniocentesis to carrier of chromosome rearrangements: data from US and Canadian laboratories. Am J Med Genet **33**:14, 1989.

Darras BT, Harper JF, Francke U: Prenatal diagnosis and detection of carriers with DNA probes in Duchenne's muscular dystrophy. N Engl J Med **316**:985, 1987.

de Grouchy J, Trubuchet C: Transfusion foeto-maternelle de lymphocytes sanguins et detection du sexe du foetus. Ann Genet **14**:133, 1971.

Desnick RJ, Schutte JL, Golbus MS et al: First trimester biochemical and molecular diagnosis using chorionic villus sampling: High accuracy in U.S. Collaborative Study. Prenat Diagn **12**:357, 1992.

DiMaio MS, Baumgarten A, Greenstein RM, et al: Screening for fetal Down's syndrome in pregnancy by measuring maternal serum alpha-fetoprotein levels. N Engl J Med **317**:342, 1987.

Dokras A, Sargent IL, Ross C, et al: Trophoectoderm biopsy in human blastocysts. Hum Reprod **5**:821, 1990.

Dolk H, Bertrand F, Lchat MF, for the EUROCAT Working Group: Chorionic villus sampling and limb abnormalities. Lancet **339**:876, 1992.

Dumez Y, Goossens B, Boue J, et al: Chorionic villi sampling using rigid forceps under ultrasound control. *In* Fraccaro M, Simoni G, Brambati B (eds.): First Trimester Fetal Diagnosis. New York, Springer-Verlag, 1985, p 38.

Eisensmith RC, Woo SLC: Molecular basis of phenylketonuria and related hyperphenylalaninemias: Mutations and polymorphisms in the human phenylaline hydroxylase gene. Hum Mutation **1**:13, 1992.

Elias S, Annas G: Reproductive Genetics and the Law. Chicago, Year Book Medical Publishers, 1987.

Elias S, Annas GJ, Simpson JL: Carrier screening for cystic fibrosis: Implications for obstetric and gynecologic practice. Am J Obstet Gynecol **164**:1077, 1991.

Elias S, Gerbie AB, Simpson JL, et al: Genetic amniocentesis in twin gestations. Am J Obstet Gynecol **138**:169, 1980.

Elias S, Esterly N: Prenatal diagnosis of hereditary skin disorders. Clin Obstet Gynecol **24**:1069, 1981.

Elias S: Use of fetoscopy for the prenatal diagnosis of hereditary skin disorders. Curr Probl Dermatol **16**:1, 1987.

Elias S, Price J, Klinger K, et al: Prenatal diagnosis of trisomy 18 using fetal cells isolated from maternal blood. Lancet. In Press.

Elias S, Simpson JL: Amniocentesis. *In* Milunsky A (ed): Genetic Disorders and the Fetus. Baltimore, Johns Hopkins University Press, 1992, p 33.

Evans J, Stokes IM: Outcome of pregnancies associated with raised serum and normal amniotic fluid alpha fetoprotein. Br Med J **288**:1494, 1984.

Evans MI, Drugan A, Koppitch FC, et al: Genetic diagnosis in the first trimester: the norm for the 1990's. Am J Obstet Gynecol **162**:1568, 1989.

Evans MI, Greb A, Kunkel LM, et al: In utero fetal muscle biopsy for the diagnosis of Duchenne muscular dystrophy. Am J Obstet Gynecol **165**:728, 1991.

Firth HV, Body PA, Chamberlain P, et al: Severe limb abnormalities after chorionic villus sampling at 56–66 days gestation. Lancet **337**:127, 1991.

Formigli L, Roccio C, Bellotti G, et al: Non-surgical flushing of the uterus for pre-embryo recovery: Possible clinical applications. Hum Reprod **58**:329, 1990.

Frasier SD, Thoneycroft IH, Weiss BA, et al: Elevated amniotic fluid concentration of 17alpha-hydroxyprogesterone in congenital adrenal hyperplasia. J Pediatr **86**:310, 1975.

Froster-Iskenius UG, Baird PA: Limb reduction defects in over one million consecutive live births. Teratology **39**:127, 1989.

Ganshirt-Ahlert D, Burschyk M, Garritsen HSP, et al: Magnetic cell sorting and the transferrin receptor as potential means of prenatal diagnosis from maternal blood. Am J Obstet Gynecol **166**:1350, 1992.

Gedde-Dahl Jr., Weupper KD (eds): Prenatal diagnosis of heritable skin diseases. Curr Probl Dermatol **16**:1, 1987.

Gianopoulous JG, Elias S, Simpson JL: Genetic amniocentesis: Ultrasonic monitoring of fetal activity and heart rate. Obstet Gynecol **67**:410, 1986.

Golbus MS, Kan YW, Naglich-Craig M: Fetal blood sampling in midtrimester pregnancies. Am J Obstet Gynecol **124**:653, 1976.

Golbus MS: The use of fetal blood for the prenatal diagnosis of genetic defects. Monogr Hum Genet **9**:222, 1978.

Golbus MS, McGonigle KF, Goldberg JD, et al: Fetal tissue sampling: The San Francisco experience with 190 pregnancies. West J Med **150**:423, 1989.

Golbus MS, Simpson JL, Fowler SE, et al: Risk factors associated with transcervical CVS losses. Prenat Diagn **12**:373, 1992.

Griffin DK, Wilton LJ, Handyside AH, et al: Dual fluorescent in situ hybridization for simultaneous detection of X and Y chromosome-specific probes for sexing of human preimplantation embryonic nuclei. Hum Genet **89**:18, 1992.

Haddow JE, Palomaki GE, Knight GJ, et al: Prenatal screening for Down's syndrome with use of maternal serum markers. N Engl J Med **327**:588, 1992.

Handyside AH, Pattinson JK, Penketh RJ, et al: Biopsy of human preimplantation embryos and sexing by DNA amplification. Lancet **1**:347, 1989.

Handyside AH, Kontogianni EH, Hardy K, et al: Pregnancies from biopsied human preimplantation embryo sexed by DNA amplification. Nature **344**:768, 1990.

Handyside AH, Delhanty JDA: Cleavage stage biopsy of human embryos and diagnosis of X-linked disease. *In* Edwards, R.G. (ed.): Preimplantation Diagnosis of Human Genetic Disease. London, Cambridge University Press, 1991, p 75.

Handyside AH, Lesko JG, Tarin JJ, et al: Birth of a normal girl after in vitro fertilization and preimplantation diagnostic testing for cystic fibrosis. N Engl J Med **327**:905, 1992.

Hanson FW, Zorn EM, Tennant FR, et al: Amniocentesis before 15 weeks' gestation: Outcome, risk and technical problems. Am J Obstet Gynecol **157**:217, 1987.

Hanson FW, Tennant F, Hune S, et al: Early amniocentesis: Outcome, risks and technical problems at ≤12.8 weeks. Am J Obstet Gynecol **166**:1707, 1992.

Henry G, Peakman D, Winkler W, et al: Amniocentesis before 15 weeks instead of chorionic villus sampling for earlier prenatal cytogenetic diagnosis. Am J Hum Genet **37**:A219, 1985.

Henry GP, Miller WA: Early amniocentesis. J Reprod Med **37**:396, 1992.

Herzenberg LA, Bianchi DW, Schroder J, et al: Fetal cells in the blood of pregnant women: Detection and enrichment by fluorescence-activated cell sorting. Proc Natl Acad Sci USA **76**:1453, 1979.

Hess LW, Anderson RL, Golbus MS: Significance of opaque amniotic fluid at second-trimester amniocentesis. Obstet Gynecol **67**:44, 1986.

Hislop A, Fairweather D: Amniocentesis and lung growth: An animal experiment with clinical implications. Lancet **2**:271, 1982.

Holzgreve W, Miny P, Basarans S, et al: Safety of placental biopsy in the second and third trimester. N Engl J Med **317**:1159, 1987.

Hook EB: Rates of chromosome abnormalities at different maternal ages. Obstet Gynecol **58**:282, 1981.

Hook EB: Chromosome abnormalities and spontaneous fetal death following amniocentesis: Further data and association with maternal age. Am J Hum Genet **35**:110, 1983.

Hook EB, Cross PK, Schreinemachers DM: Chromosomal abnormality rates at amniocentesis and in liveborn infants. JAMA **249**:2034, 1983.

Hook EB, Cross PK, Jackson LG, et al: Rates of 47, +21 and other cytogenetic abnormalities diagnosed in 1st trimester chorionic villus samples (CVS): Comparison with rates from 2nd trimester amniocentesis. Am J Hum Genet **41**:A276, 1987.

Hseih FJ, Chjen D, Tseng LH, et al: Limb-reduction defects and chorionic villus sampling. Lancet **337**:1091, 1991.

Hsu LYF, Perlis TE: United States survey on chromosome mosaicism and pseudomosaicism in prenatal diagnosis. Prenat Diagn **4**:97, 1980.

Hsu L: Prenatal diagnosis of chromosome abnormalities through amniocentesis. *In* Milunsky A (ed): Genetic Disorders and the Fetus, 3rd ed. Baltimore, Johns Hopkins Press, 1992, p 155.

Isada NB, Koppitch FC, Johnson MP, et al: Does the color of amniotic fluid still matter? Fetal Diagn Ther **5**:165, 1990.

Jackson LG, Fowler SE, Zachery JM, et al: A randomized comparison of transcervical and transabdominal chorionic villus sampling. N Engl J Med **327**:594, 1992.

Jeanty P, Shah D, Roussis P: Single needle insertion in twin amnio. J Ultrasound Med **9**:511, 1990.

Kan YW, Golbus MS, Dozy AM: Prenatal diagnosis of α-thalassemia: Clinical application of molecular hybridization. N Engl J Med **295**:1165, 1976.

Karp LE, Schiller HS: Meconium staining of amniotic fluid at midtrimester amniocentesis. Obstet Gynecol **50**:475, 1977.

Klinger K, Landes G, Shook D, et al: Rapid detection of chromosome aneuploides in uncultured amniocytes by using fluorescence in site hybridization (FISH). Am J Hum Genet **51**:55, 1992.

Kratzer PG, Golbus MS, Monroe SE, et al: First-trimester aneuploidy screening using serum human chorionic gonadotropin (hCG), free αhCG and progesterone. Prenat Diagn **11**:751, 1991.

Lebo RV, Lynch ED, Bird TD, et al: Multicolor in situ hybridization and linkage analysis order Charcot-Marie-Tooth type IA (CMTIA) gene region markers. Am J Hum Genet **50**:15, 1992.

Ledbetter DH, Martin AO, Verlinsky Y, et al: Cytogenetic results of chorionic villus sampling: High success rate and diagnostic accuracy in the U.S. Collaborative Study. Am J Obstet Gynecol **162**:495, 1990.

Ledbetter DH, Zachary JM, Simpson JL, et al: Cytogenetic results from the U.S. Collaborative Study on CVS: High diagnostic accuracy in over 11,000 cases. Prenat Diagn **12**:317, 1992.

Lemna WK, Feldman GL, Kerem BS, et al: Mutation analysis for heterozygote detection and the prenatal diagnosis of cystic fibrosis. N Engl J Med **323**:62, 1990.

Lo Y-MD, Wainscot JS, Gilmer MDG, et al: Prenatal sex determination by DNA amplification from maternal peripheral blood. Lancet **2**:1363, 1989.

Lo Y-MD, Patel P, Sampietro M, et al: Detection of single-copy fetal DNA sequence from maternal blood. Lancet **335**:1463, 1990.

Luthard FW, Luthy DA, Karp D, et al: Prospective evaluation of early amniocentesis for prenatal diagnosis. Am J Hum Genet **37**:A222, 1985.

Macri JN, Kasturi RV, Krantz DA, et al: Maternal serum Down syndrome screening: Free β-protein is more effective marker than human chorionic gonadotropin. Am J Obstet Gynecol **163**:1248, 1990.

Mastroiacovo P, Cavalcanti DP: Limb abnormalities and chorionic villus sampling. Lancet **337**:1091, 1991.

McKenna KE, Hughes AE, Bingham EA, Nevin NC: Linkage of

epidermolysis bullosa simplex to keratin gene loci. J Med Genet **29**:568, 1992.

Merkatz IR, Nitowsky HM, Macri JN, et al: An association between low maternal serum alpha-fetoprotein and fetal chromosomal abnormalities. Am J Obstet **148**:886, 1984.

Milunsky A: The prenatal diagnosis of neural tube and other congenital defects. In Milunsky A (ed): Genetic Disorders and the Fetus, 3rd ed. Baltimore, Johns Hopkins Press, 1992.

Milunsky A, Wands J, Brambati B, et al: First trimester maternal serum alpha-fetoprotein (MSAFP) screening for chromosome defects. Pediatr Res **21**:292A, 1988.

Milunsky A, Jick SS, Bruell CL, et al: Predictive values, relative risks and overall benefits of high and low maternal serum alpha-fetoprotein screening in singleton pregnancies: New epidemiologic data. Am J Obstet Gynecol **161**:291, 1989.

Milunsky A, Neliodo L: Screening for chromosome defects in the first and second trimesters of pregnancy. In Simpson JL, Elias S (eds): Maternal Serum Screening for Fetal Genetic Disorders. New York, Churchill Livingstone, 1992, p 75.

Mizejewski GJ, Risenberg HM: Alpha-fetoprotein: Use in predicting perinatal distress. In Mizejewski GJ, Porter IH (ed): Alpha-Fetoprotein and Congenital Disorders. Orlando, Academic Press, 1985, p 157.

MRC Vitamin Study Research Group, Prevention of neural tube defects: Results of the Medical Research Council vitamin study. Lancet **338**:131, 1991.

Mueller UW, Hawe, CS, Wright AE: Isolation of fetal trophoblast cells from peripheral blood of pregnant women. Lancet **336**:197, 1990.

Navidi W, Arnheim N: Using PCR in preimplantation genetic disease diagnosis. Hum Reprod **6**:836, 1991.

Nelson LM, Benson J, Burton BK: Outcomes in patients with unusually high maternal serum alpha-fetoprotein levels. Am J Obstet Gynecol **157**:572, 1987.

Nevin J, Nevin NC, Dornan JC, et al: Early amniocentesis: Experience of 222 consecutive patients, 1987–88. Prenat Diagn **10**:79, 1990.

NICHD Consensus Conference on Antenatal Diagnosis, NIH Publication No. 80-1973, December, 1979.

NICHD National Registry for Amniocentesis Study Group: Midtrimester amniocentesis for prenatal diagnosis: Safety and accuracy. JAMA **236**:1471, 1976.

Palomaki GE, Haddow JE: Maternal serum alpha-fetoprotein, age and Down syndrome risk. Am J Obstet Gynecol **156**:460, 1987.

Palomaki GE, Knight GJ, Kolza EM, et al: Maternal weight adjustment and low serum alpha-fetoprotein values. Lancet **1**:468, 1988.

Penso CA, Sanstrom MM, Garber MF, et al: Early amniocentesis: Report of 407 cases with neonatal follow-up. Obstet Gynecol **76**:1032, 1990.

Pergament E, Schulman JD, Copeland K, et al: The risk and efficacy of chorionic villus sampling in multiple gestations. Prenat Diagn **12**:377, 1992.

Phillips OP, Elias S, Shulman LP, et al: Maternal serum screening for fetal Down syndrome in women less than 35 years of age using alpha-fetoprotein, hCG and unconjugated estriol. A prospective 2 year study. Obstet Gynecol **80**:353, 1992a.

Phillips OP, Elias S, Shulman LP, et al: Maternal serum screening for fetal Down syndrome using alpha-fetoprotein (AFP), human chorionic gonadotrophin (hCG), and unconjugated estriol (uE3) in women less than 20 years of age. Pediatr Adol Gynecol, In Press.

Platt LD, Feuchtbaum L, Filly R, et al: The California Maternal Serum αfetoprotein Screening Program: The role of ultrasonography in the detection of spina bifida. Am J Obstet Gynecol **166**:1329, 1992a.

Platt LD, Medearis AL, Carlson DE, et al: Screening for Down syndrome with the femur length/biparietal diameter ratio: A new twist of the data. Am J Obstet Gynecol **167**:124, 1992b.

Price J, Elias S, Wachtel SS, et al: Prenatal diagnosis using fetal cells isolated from maternal blood by multiparameter flow cytometry. Am J Obstet Gynecol **165**:1737, 1991.

Quintero RA, Romero R, Mahoney MJ, et al: Fetal haemorrhagic lesions after chorionic villus sampling. Lancet **339**:193, 1990.

Recommendations for the use of folic acid to reduce the number of cases of spina bifida and other neural tube defects. MMWR **41**:1, 1992.

Rhoads GG, Jackson LG, Schlesselman SE, et al: The safety and efficacy of chorionic villus sampling. Initial findings from the U.S. Collaborative Study. N Engl J Med **320**:609, 1989.

Riordan JR, Rommens JM, Kerem BS, et al: Identification of the cystic fibrosis gene: Cloning and characterization of complementary DNA. Science **245**:1066, 1989.

Robinson L, Grau P, Crandall BF: Pregnancy outcomes after increasing maternal serum alpha-fetoprotein levels. Obstet Gynecol **74**:17, 1989.

Shepard T, Kapur RP, Fantel AG: Limb-reduction defects and chorion villus sampling. Lancet **337**:1092, 1991.

Shulman LP, Elias S, Phillips OP, et al: Early twin amniocentesis prior to 14 weeks' gestation. Prenat Diagn **12**:609, 1992a.

Shulman LP, Simpson, JL, Felken RE, et al: Transvaginal chorionic villus sampling using transabdominal ultrasound guidance. Prenat Diagn **12**:229, 1992b.

Sidransky E, Black SH, Soeken DM, et al: Transvaginal chorionic villus sampling. Prenat Diagn **10**:583, 1990.

Siebers JW, Knauf I, Hillemans HG: Antenatal sex determination in blood from pregnant women. Humangenetik **28**:273, 1975.

Simpson JL: Prenatal diagnosis and genetics. In Scott JR, DiSaia PJ, Hammond CB, Spellacy WN (eds): Danforth's Obstetrics and Gynecology, 6th ed. Philadelphia, JB Lippincott Co, pp 237, 1989.

Simpson JL: Genetic counseling and prenatal diagnosis. In Gabbe SG, Niebyl JF, Simpson JL (eds): Obstetrics: Normal and Problem Pregnancies, 2nd ed. New York, Churchill Livingstone, 1991, p 269.

Simpson JL: Advances in prenatal diagnosis: preimplantation genetics and recovery of fetal cells from maternal blood. Curr Opin **4**:295, 1992.

Simpson JL: Reproductive technologies and genetic advances in gynecology and obstetrics. Int J Gynecol Obstet **38**:261, 1992a.

Simpson JL, Martin AO, Verp MS, et al: Hypermodal cells in amniotic fluid cultures: Frequency interpretation and clinical significance. Am J Obstet Gynecol **143**:250, 1982.

Simpson JL, Mills JL, Holmes LB, et al: Low fetal loss rates after ultrasound-proved viability in early pregnancy. JAMA **258**:2555, 1987.

Simpson JL, Carson SA, Buster JE, Elias S: Future horizons in prenatal genetic diagnosis: preimplantation diagnosis and noninvasive screening. In Filkins K, Russo JF (eds): Human Prenatal Diagnosis. New York, Marcel Dekker, 1990, p 547.

Simpson JL, Elias S, Morgan CD, et al: Does unexplained second trimester (15 to 20 weeks gestation) maternal serum alpha-fetoprotein elevation presage adverse perinatal outcome? Am J Obstet Gynecol **164**:829, 1991.

Simpson JL, Elias S: Fetal cells in maternal blood: potential for noninvasive prenatal diagnosis. Proceedings of 13th World Congress of Obstetrics and Gynecology, Singapore, 1991. Lancaster, UK, Parthenon, 1992a, p 424.

Simpson JL, Elias S: Isolating and analyzing fetal cells in maternal blood: current status. Proceedings 5th International Congress on Early Fetal Diagnosis. Prague, Charles University Press, 1992b, p 424.

Simpson JL, Golbus MS: Genetics in Obstetrics and Gynecology. 2nd ed. Philadelphia, WB Saunders Co, 1992c.

Simpson JL, Palomaki GE, Elias S, et al: Elevated second trimester maternal serum alpha fetoprotein (MSAFP) is more predictive of certain pregnancy complications than elevated third trimester MSAFP: A cohort study. Am J Hum Genet **51**:A19, 1992d.

Smidt-Jensen N, Hahnemann N, Jensen PKA, et al: Transabdominal chorionic villi sampling for first trimester fetal diagnosis. In Fraccaro M, Simoni G, Brambati B (eds): First Trimester Fetal Diagnosis, New York, Springer-Verlag, 1985, p 51.

Special Report: The status of fetoscopy and fetal tissue sampling. Prenat Diagn **4**:79, 1984.

Speiser PW, Laforgia N, Kato K, et al: First trimester prenatal treatment and molecular genetic diagnosis of congenital adrenal hyperplasia (21-hydroxylase deficiency). J Clin Endocrinol Metab **70**:838, 1990.

Spencer K, Macri JN, Aitken DA, et al: Free β-hCG as first trimester marker for fetal trisomy. Lancet **339**:1480, 1992.

Stene J, Mikkelsen, M: Risk for chromosomal abnormality at amniocentesis following a child with a non-inherited chromosome aberration. Prenat Diagn 4:81, 1984.

Tabor A, Madsen M, Obel E, et al: Randomized controlled trial of genetic amniocentesis in 4606 low-risk women. Lancet 1:1287, 1986.

Tharapel AT, Jaswaney V, Dockter M, et al: Can fetal cells in maternal blood be selected through cytogenetic means? Am J Hum Genet 45(S):271, 1989.

Tharapel AT, Anderson KP, Simpson JL, et al: Are all terminal Xq deletions interstitial? Reevaluation of a deleted X-chromosome in a proband and her mother by southern blotting and by multiple FISH analyses. Fetal Diagn Ther 1993.

Tipton RE, Tharapel AT, Chang HT et al: Rapid chromosome analysis with the use of spontaneously dividing cells derived from umbilical cord blood (fetal and neonatal). Am J Obstet 161:1546, 1989.

Vejerslev LO, Mikkelsen M: The European collaborative study on mosaicism in chorionic villi sampling: Data from 1986 to 1987. Prenat Diagn 9:575, 1989.

Verlinsky Y, Ginsberg N, Lifchez A, et al: Analysis of the first polar body: Preconception genetic diagnosis. Hum Reprod 5:826, 1990.

Verlinsky Y: Biopsy of human gametes. In Verlinsky Y, Kuliev A (eds): Preimplantation Genetics. London, Plenum Press, 1991, p 39.

Wachtel SS, Elias S, Price J, et al: Fetal cells in the maternal circulation: Isolation by multiparameter flow cytometry and confirmation by PCR. Hum Reprod 6:1466, 1991.

Wald NJ, Cuckle HS, Stirrat GM, Bennett MJ, Turnbull ACI: Maternal serum alpha-fetoprotein and low birth-weight. Lancet 2:268, 1977.

Wald NJ, Cuckle HS, Densen JW, et al: Maternal serum unconjugated oestriol as an antenatal screening test for Down syndrome. Br J Obstet Gynaecol 95:334, 1988.

Wald NJ, Cuckle HS, Densen JW, et al: Maternal serum screening for Down syndrome: The effect of routine ultrasound scan determination of gestational age and adjustment for maternal weight. Br J Obstet Gynaecol 99:144, 1992.

Walknowska J, Conte FA, Grumbach MM: Practical and theoretical implications of fetal/maternal lymphocyte transfer. Lancet 1:1119, 1969.

Wapner RH, Simpson JL, Golbus MS, et al: Chorionic mosaicism: Association with fetal loss but not with adverse perinatal outcome. Prenat Diagn 12:347, 1992.

Warburton D: De novo balanced chromosome rearrangements and extra marker chromosome identified at prenatal diagnosis. Clinical significance and distribution of breakpoints. Am J Hum Genet 49:995, 1991.

Ward RH, Modell B, Fairweather DV, et al: Obstetric outcome and problems of a midtrimester fetal blood sampling for antenatal diagnosis. Br J Obstet Gynaecol 88:1073, 1981.

Working Party of Amniocentesis: An assessment of the hazards of amniocentesis. Br J Obstet Gynecol 85 (Suppl 2) 1, 1978.

Working Party in the Evaluation of Chorion Villus Sampling. Medical Research Council European Trial of Chorion Villus Sampling. Lancet 337:1491, 1991.

World Health Organization/European Regional Office (WHO/EURO): Risk evaluation of CVS. WHO/EURO, Copenhagen, Denmark, 1992. (Also summarized by Kuliev AM, Modell B, Jackson, L, et al: Chorionic villus sampling (CVS). World Health Organization/European Regional Office (WHO/EURO) Meeting Statement on the Use of CVS in Prenatal Diagnosis. J Assist Reproduc Genet 9:299, 1992.

Worber RG, Stern R: A Canadian collaborative study of mosaicism in amniotic fluid cell cultures. Prenat Diagn 4:131, 1984.

Yeoh SC, Sargent IL, Redman CWG, et al: Detection of fetal cells in maternal blood. Prenat Diagn 11:117, 1991.

Zilliacus R, de la Chapelle A, Schroder J: Transplacental passage of foetal blood cells. Scand J Haemetol 15:333, 1975.

THE PLACENTA

CHAPTER

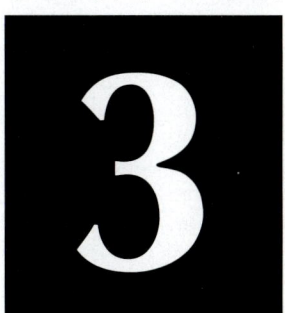

GAMETE TRANSPORT, FERTILIZATION, AND IMPLANTATION

ROBERT H. GLASS, M.D.

It is appropriate to consider the earliest stages of reproduction in a book devoted to perinatal medicine because many of the abnormalities of fetal development and well-being have their onset at gametogenesis, fertilization, or implantation. For example, failure of trophoblast to invade maternal blood vessels during implantation may increase the risk for subsequent development of pre-eclampsia (Brosens et al., 1972). This chapter examines how the sperm and egg arrive at the site of fertilization in the tube, how fertilization occurs, and how the embryo subsequently achieves its anchorage in the uterus.

SPERM TRANSPORT

Semen forms a gel almost immediately following ejaculation, but then is liquefied in 20 to 30 minutes by enzymes derived from the prostate gland. The alkaline pH of semen provides protection for the sperm from the acid environment of the vagina. This protection is transient, and most sperm left in the vagina are immobilized within 2 hours. The more fortunate sperm, by their own motility, gain entrance into the tongues of cervical mucus that layer over the ectocervix. It is only the sperm that enter the uterus; the seminal plasma is left behind in the vagina. This entry is rapid, and sperm have been found in mucus within 90 seconds of ejaculation (Sobrero and MacLeod, 1962). In the rabbit, inactivation of all sperm in the vagina 5 minutes after ejaculation does not interfere with fertilization, further attesting to the rapidity of transport. Uterine contractions propel the sperm

upward, and in the human they can be found in the tube 5 minutes after insemination (Settlage et al., 1973). It is possible that the first sperm to enter the tube are at a disadvantage. In the rabbit these early sperm have only poor motility, and disruption of the head membranes is common. The sperm in this vanguard are unlikely to achieve fertilization. Other sperm that have colonized the cervical mucus and the portion of the tubal isthmus nearest the uterus then make their way more slowly to the ampulla of the tube in order to meet the egg. Human sperm have been found in the fallopian tube as long as 85 hours after intercourse, but it is not known whether these sperm have retained their fertilizing ability (Ahlgren, 1975). In animals, the fertilizable life span is usually one-half the motile life span.

The attrition in sperm numbers from vagina to fallopian tube is substantial. Whereas an average of 200 million to 300 million sperm are deposited in the vagina, less than 100 achieve proximity to the egg. The major loss occurs in the vagina, with expulsion of semen from the introitus playing an important role. Other causes for loss are digestion of sperm by vaginal enzymes, phagocytosis of sperm all along the reproductive tract, and, to a limited extent, movement of sperm through the fallopian tube into the peritoneal cavity. There are also reports of sperm burrowing into or being engulfed by endometrial cells.

CAPACITATION

The discovery in 1951 that rat and rabbit spermatozoa must spend some hours in the female tract before acquiring the capacity to penetrate ova stimulated intensive research efforts to delineate the environmental conditions required for this change in the sperm to occur. The process by which the sperm are transformed is called *capacitation*. The most critical change in the sperm induced by capacitation is hyperactivated motility, which is vital for achieving zona penetration (Overstreet, 1983). Although capacitation classically has been defined as the change sperm undergo in the female reproductive tract, it is now apparent that sperm can acquire the ability to fertilize after a short incubation in defined media and without residence in the female reproductive tract. In addition to affecting sperm motility, capacitation changes the surface characteristics of sperm, causing removal of seminal plasma antigens, modification of their surface charge, and restriction of receptor mobility. These processes are associated with decreased stability of the plasma membrane and of the membrane lying immediately under it—the outer acrosomal membrane. This modification of the membranes cannot be demonstrated by routine electron microscopy, but changes in particle distribution within the membranes have been observed with freeze-fracture techniques. The membranes undergo further, more striking modifications when capacitated sperm reach the vicinity of an ovum or when they are incubated in follicular fluid. There is a breakdown and merging of the plasma membrane and the outer acrosomal membrane (acrosome reaction) (Bedford, 1970). The acrosome reaction (AR) is characterized by influx of Ca^{2+} and is dependent upon the calcium-binding protein calmodulin. The AR can be induced by a zona pellucida glycoprotein designated ZP_3, which also serves as a sperm receptor (Wassarman, 1987). The AR allows egress of the enzyme contents of the acrosome, the cap-like structure that covers the sperm nucleus. These enzymes, which include hyaluronidase, a neuraminidase-like factor, corona-dispersing enzyme, and a protease termed *acrosin*, are all thought to play roles in sperm penetration of the egg investments. Capacitation prepares sperm for the AR, which in turn prepares sperm for penetration of the zona pellucida.

EGG TRANSPORT

Egg transport encompasses the interval from ovulation to the entry of the egg into the uterus. The egg can be fertilized only during the early stages of its sojourn in the fallopian tube.

In rats and mice the ovary and the distal portion of the tube are covered by a common fluid-filled sac. Ovulated eggs are carried by fluid currents to the fimbriated end of the tube. By contrast, in primates, including women, the ovulated egg adheres, with its cumulus mass of follicular cells, to the surface of the ovary. The fimbriated end of the tube sweeps over the ovary in order to pick up the egg. Entry into the tube is facilitated by muscular movements that bring the fimbriae into contact with the surface of the ovary. Variations in this pattern surely exist, as evidenced by women who achieve pregnancy despite having only one ovary and a single tube located on the contralateral side.

Ciliary and Muscular Mechanisms

Although there can be a small negative pressure in the tube in association with muscle contractions, ovum pickup does not depend on a suction effect secondary to this negative pressure. In the rabbit, ligation of the tube just proximal to the fimbriae does not interfere with pickup. The cilia on the surface of the fimbriae have adhesive sites, which seem to have primary responsibility for the initial movement of the egg into the tube. This movement is dependent on the presence of follicular cells surrounding the egg, because removal of these cells prior to egg pickup prevents effective egg transport. In the ampulla of the tube the cilia beat in the direction of the uterus. In the human and the monkey this unidirectional beat is also found in the isthmus of the tube, whereas in the rabbit there are additional rows of cilia that beat in the direction of the ovary. The specific contribution of the cilia to egg transport in the ampulla and isthmus is an unresolved question. Most investigations have credited muscular contractions of the tubes as the primary force for moving the egg. Halbert and associates (1976) showed, however, that in the rabbit, interference with muscle contractility did not block egg transport. They concluded that cilia play a major role in this animal. Experimentally reversing a segment of the ampulla of the tube so that the cilia in this segment beat toward the ovary has the effect of interfering with pregnancy in the rabbit without blocking fertilization, the fertilized ova being arrested when they come in contact with the transposed area (Eddy et al., 1978). This finding also suggests that ciliary beat is crucial for egg transport, although in all likelihood cilia play a less important role in the human. Women who have Kartagener's syndrome, in which there is a congenital absence of dynein arms in the cilia that prevents them from beating, can nevertheless become pregnant. This deficiency in the cilia is found in the fallopian tubes as well as in the respiratory tract (Jean et al., 1979).

Muscular contractions of the tube are associated with a to-and-fro movement of the eggs rather than with a continuous forward progression. In most species, transport of the ovum through the tube requires approximately 3 days. The time it spends within the various parts of the tube varies from one species to another. Transport through the ampulla is rapid in the rabbit, but in women it requires 30 hours for the egg to reach the ampullary-isthmic junction. The egg remains at this point another 30 hours, at which time it begins rapid transport through the isthmus of the tube. The first cell division occurs approximately 24 hours following fertilization, and subsequent divisions are at 12-hour intervals. The embryo enters the uterus at the morula stage (16 to 32 compacted cells). Formation of the blastocyst with its differentiation into inner cell mass, which will give rise to the embryo, and trophectoderm cells, which are the precursors of the placenta, occurs in the uterus.

Hormonal and Other Influences

Modification of tubal function as a means of understanding its physiology has involved three major pharmacologic approaches: (1) altering levels of steroid hormones, (2) interference with or supplementation of adrenergic stimuli, and (3) treatment with prostaglandins. Although the literature on the effects of estrogen and progesterone on tubal function is abundant, it is clouded by the use of differing hormones, differing doses, and differing timing of injections. Because of these variations, it is difficult to obtain a coherent picture and to relate the experimental results to the *in vivo* situation. In general, pharmacologic doses of estrogen favor retention of eggs in the tube. This "tube locking" effect of estrogen can be partially reversed by treatment with progesterone.

The isthmus of the tube has an extensive adrenergic innervation. Surgical denervation of the tube, however, does not disrupt ovum transport. Prostaglandins of the E series relax tubal muscle, whereas those of the F series stimulate it. Although $PGF_{2\alpha}$ stimulates human oviductal motility *in vivo*, it does not cause acceleration of ovum transport.

The effect on fertility of removing different segments of the tube has been reviewed by Pauerstein and Eddy (1979), who noted that excision of the ampullary-isthmic junction in rabbits did not block fertility. There is also no block to fertility if small segments of the ampulla are removed, and pregnancy can occur even if the entire isthmus and uterotubal junction are excised. Although the fimbriae are thought to play a crucial role in fertility, spontaneous pregnancies have been reported following sterilization by fimbriectomy or following surgical repair of tubes whose fimbriated ends had been excised (Novy, 1980).

In most species a period of residence of the egg in the tube appears to be a prerequisite for full development. Rabbit eggs can be fertilized in the uterus, but they do not develop unless transferred to the tubes within 3 hours of fertilization (Glass, 1972). This and other work implies that there may be a component in uterine fluid during the first 48 hours following ovulation that is toxic to the egg (Adams, 1979). Indirect evidence of an inhospitable environment is also provided by studies indicating that there must be synchrony between development of the endometrium and development of the egg for successful pregnancy to occur. If the endometrium is in a more advanced stage of development than the egg, fertility is compromised. However, these studies were done in animals and may not be relevant to the human. Successful pregnancies have occurred in the human following the Estes procedure, in which the ovary is transposed to the uterine cornua and eggs are ovulated directly into the uterus, completely bypassing the tube, as well as when unfertilized human eggs and sperm have been placed directly into the uterus. This crucial difference between animal and human physiology is of more than academic importance. There has been considerable speculation concerning the use of drugs that could, by accelerating tubal transport, provide contraception by ensuring that the egg would reach the uterus when the uterus was in an unreceptive state.

Although this measure may work in animals, it would be of doubtful value in the human, because even the limited success with the Estes procedure indicates that perfect synchrony is not required.

Animal and human reproduction also differ in the occurrence of ectopic pregnancy. Ectopic pregnancies are rare in animals, and in rodents they are not induced even if the uterotubal junction is occluded immediately following fertilization; the embryos reach the blastocyst stage and then degenerate.

FERTILIZATION

Following ovulation, the fertilizable life span of the rabbit egg is between 6 and 8 hours. The fertilizable life span of human ova is unknown, but in the past estimates ranged between 12 and 24 hours. However, in human *in vitro* fertilization programs, immature oocytes can be cultured for as long as 36 hours and still be fertilizable (Dandekar et al., 1991). Equally uncertain is the fertilizable life span of human sperm, the most common estimate being 48 hours, although motility can be maintained after the sperm have lost the ability to fertilize.

Sperm Entry into the Egg

The acellular zona pellucida, which surrounds the egg at ovulation and remains in place until implantation, is made up of three glycoproteins designated ZP_1, ZP_2, and ZP_3. Acrosome intact sperm have specific binding proteins for ZP_3 (Bleil and Wassarman, 1990). Similarly, the zona pellucida contains receptors for sperm that are, with some exceptions, species-specific (Hartman and Gwatkin, 1971). The zona pellucida becomes impervious to other sperm once the fertilizing sperm penetrates, and thus it provides a bar to polyploidy. The initiation of the block to penetration of the zona (and the vitellus) by other sperm is mediated by release of materials from the cortical granules, organelles that are found just below the egg surface. A portion of these materials diffuse into the zona to make it impermeable to sperm while other portions coat the egg surface (Dandekar and Talbot, 1992). Penetration through the zona is rapid and may be mediated by the protease *acrosin*, which is bound to the inner acrosomal membrane of the sperm. The pivotal role assigned to acrosin has been disputed, however. For example, manipulations that increase the resistance of the zona to acrosin do not interfere with sperm penetration. Thus, sperm motility may be the most important factor in mediating zona penetration.

The postacrosomal region of the sperm head, which contains a specific binding and fusion protein (PH 30), makes initial contact with the vitelline membrane (Blobel et al., 1992). The egg membrane engulfs the sperm head, and subsequently there is fusion of egg and sperm membranes. The chromatin material of the sperm head decondenses and the male pronucleus is formed. The male and the female pronuclei migrate toward each other, and as they move into close proximity, the limiting membranes break down and a spindle is formed on which the chromosomes become arranged. Thus, the stage is set for the first cell division.

Preimplantation Loss

The clinician is interested not only in how normal fertilization takes place, but also in the occurrence of abnormal events that can interfere with pregnancy. It is worthwhile, therefore, to consider the failures that occur in association with *in vivo* fertilization. This information may bear on problems with *in vitro* fertilization. In one study a surgical method was used to flush the uteri of regularly cycling rhesus monkeys, and nine preimplantation embryos and two unfertilized eggs were recovered from 22 flushes. Two of the nine embryos were morphologically abnormal and probably would not have implanted (Hurst et al., 1976). Hendrickx and Kraemer (1968), using a similar technique in the baboon, found 10 of 23 recovered embryos to be morphologically abnormal; their results suggest that in nonhuman primates some ovulated eggs are not fertilized, and that many early embryos are abnormal and, in all likelihood, will be aborted. Similar findings have been reported in the human in the classic study of Hertig and colleagues (1959), who examined 34 early embryos recovered by flushing and pathologic examination of reproductive organs removed at surgery. Ten of these embryos were morphologically abnormal, including four of the eight preimplantation embryos. Because the four preimplantation losses would not have been recognized clinically, six losses would have been recovered in the remaining 30 pregnancies. Use of sensitive pregnancy tests suggests that approximately 25 to 40 per cent of conceptions may be lost before they are clinically perceived. Embryo survival during the *in vitro* fertilization process is even lower than that *in vivo*. Approximately 10 per cent of embryos will implant. Pregnancy rates are much higher because multiple embryos are usually transferred. This high rate of loss may be evidence for biologic selection against abnormal gametes and embryos throughout the reproductive process. For example, morphologically abnormal sperm are less successful than normal sperm in penetrating cervical mucus and in negotiating the uterotubal junction, although this selection does not seem to operate against chromosomally abnormal sperm that are morphologically normal. Another selective mechanism is the attrition of sperm numbers between the vagina and the area of the tube containing the egg, which decreases the chances for penetration of the egg by more than one sperm.

There is no direct information to indicate whether or not selection against chromosomally abnormal preimplantation embryos occurs. However, there is evidence that damaged preimplantation embryos are subject to selection. For example, brief treatment of preimplantation embryos *in vitro* with actinomycin D, a powerful teratogen when given to pregnant women after implantation, decreases the number of embryos that survive to term after reimplantation.

When only clinically diagnosed pregnancies are considered, the generally accepted figure for spontaneous abortion in the postimplantation period covering the first trimester is 15 per cent. Approximately 50 to 60 per cent of these abortions have chromosome abnormalities (Short, 1979), suggesting that a minimum of 7.5 per cent of all human conceptions are chromosomally abnormal. In contrast, only one in 200 newborns has a chromosome abnormality, attesting to the powerful selection mechanisms operating in early human gestation.

Loss of an Embryo Fertilized *In Vitro*

A number of the *in vivo* protective mechanisms are not present during *in vitro* fertilization. For example, the filtering effect of the cervical mucus and the uterotubal junction is not available *in vitro* to remove grossly abnormal sperm. Further, in most *in vitro* situations, relatively large numbers of sperm are placed in the vicinity of the egg, thus increasing the risk of penetration of the egg by more than one sperm. However, the sperm-blocking mechanism of the zona pellucida is so efficient that it prevents polyspermy from becoming a significant problem. Triploidy occurs in 1 to 3 per cent of recognized conceptions *in vivo* and in approximately 4 per cent of embryos following *in vitro* fertilization (Dandekar et al., 1990). These triploid embryos have only limited potential for development and in IVF programs are discarded.

IMPLANTATION

Implantation is the process by which an embryo attaches to the uterine wall and penetrates first the epithelium and then the circulatory system of the woman. The process is limited in both time and space. Implantation begins 2 to 3 days after the fertilized egg enters the uterus and is marked initially by apposition of the blastocyst to the uterine epithelium. A prerequisite for this contact is loss of the zona pellucida, which *in vitro* can be ruptured by contractions and expansions of the blastocyst. *In vivo* this activity is less critical, because the zona can be lysed by components of the uterine fluid. The exact nature and function of these components and of related proteins thought to mediate the implantation process—implantation-initiating factor, uteroglobin, and blastokinin—are uncertain. However, their production is known to depend on secretion of ovarian steroid hormones.

Trophoblast-Epithelium Interaction

Reports differ in their findings on changes in the surface charge of preimplantation embryos. There is evidence that blastocysts activated for implantation have a lower affinity for positively charged iron oxide than do inactive blastocysts, suggesting that a decrease in negative surface charge occurs just prior to implantation. There is also evidence, however, for an increase in negative charge at the blastocyst stage. In either case, it is unlikely that changes in surface charge are solely responsible for adherence of the embryo to the surface of epithelial cells. Binding of lectins to the embryo also changes during the preimplantation period, indicating that the surface glycoproteins of the embryo are in transition. It is reasonable to anticipate that these changes in configuration on the surface occur in order to enhance the ability of the embryo to adhere to the maternal surface. Antibodies against 140 kD adhesion glycoproteins can inhibit outgrowth of mouse blastocysts on extracellular matrices suggesting the importance of surface molecules in the implantation process (Sutherland et al., 1988).

As the embryo comes into close contact with the endometrium, the microvilli on the surface flatten and interdigitate with those on the luminal surface of the epithelial cells. A stage is reached at which the cell membranes are in very close contact and junctional complexes are formed. The embryo can no longer be dislodged from the surface of the epithelial cells by flushing of the uterus with physiologic solutions. Three types of subsequent interactions between the implanting trophoblast and the uterine epithelium have been described (Schlafke and Enders, 1975). In the first type, trophoblast cells intrude between uterine epithelial cells on their path to the basement membrane. Limited studies of embryos cultured on endometrial cells indicate that this is the pattern in the human (Lindenberg et al., 1989). In the second type, the epithelial cells lift off from the basement membrane, an action that allows the trophoblast to insinuate itself underneath the epithelium. In the third type, fusion of trophoblast with individual uterine epithelial cells occurs, as identified by electron microscopy in the rabbit (Larsen, 1961). This last process of gaining entry into the epithelial layer raises interesting questions concerning the immunologic consequences of mixing embryonic and maternal cytoplasm.

Trophoblast has the ability to phagocytose a variety of cells, but *in vivo* this process seems largely confined to removal of dead endometrial cells or cells sloughed from the uterine wall, and does not seem to play a major role in implantation. However, the embryo does secrete a variety of enzymes, which may be important for digesting the intercellular matrix that holds the epithelial cells together. Studies *in vitro* have demonstrated the presence of plasminogen activator in mouse embryos, and its activity is important in the attachment and early outgrowth stages of implantation. The embryo has been shown to be able, at a somewhat later stage of implantation, to digest *in vitro* a complex matrix composed of glycoproteins, elastin, and collagen, all of which are components of the normal intercellular matrix (Glass et al., 1983). Additional *in vitro* studies have shown that cells move away from trophoblast in a process called *contact inhibition* (Glass et al., 1979). Trophoblast then spreads to fill the spaces vacated by the co-cultured cells. Once the intercellular matrix has been lysed, this movement of epithelial cells away from trophoblast allows space for the implanting embryo to move through the epithelial layer. Trophoblast movement is aided by the fact that only parts of its surface are adhesive, the major portion being nonadhesive to other cells.

Embryonic Signals

Invasion by the trophoblast is limited by the formation of the decidual cell layer in the uterus, with fibroblast-like cells in the stroma being transformed into glycogen and lipoid-rich cells. In the human, decidual cells surround uterine blood vessels late in the menstrual cycle, but extensive decidualization does not occur until pregnancy is established. Ovarian steroids govern decidualization, and in the human a combination of estrogen and progesterone is critical. In animals, implantation is preceded by an increase in uterine stromal capillary permeability at the site where the blastocyst will attach. This localization and subsequent decidualization, as observed in rodents, raise the possibility that a signal from the embryo might be an important triggering stimulus. Thus, maternal recognition of pregnancy may depend on receiving signals released by the embryo. A number of stage-specific proteins have been found in association with the embryo. The presence of one of these proteins, embryo-derived platelet activating factor, has been correlated with pregnancy potential (O'Neill et al., 1989).

It has been suggested that the release of carbon dioxide by the embryo in the form of bicarbonate raises the pH of the embryo surface, which in turn increases its stickiness. Carbon dioxide also may act as a signal for decidual response in the mother (Boving, 1959).

Additional evidence that the embryo initiates implantation has been demonstrated in pigs (Heap et al., 1979). The pig blastocyst synthesizes estrogen starting on day 12 of pregnancy, which is 6 days before definitive attachment to the uterine wall. It is known that estrogen suppresses the release from the uterus of prostaglandins that ordinarily act as luteolytic agents, and that estrogen may also stimulate the pituitary to promote LH secretion, which is essential for maintenance of the corpus luteum. In rodents, however, even though the blastocyst has the enzyme capability for steroid metabolism, there is no proof that it also synthesizes steroids. Furthermore, implantation has been observed to occur in hamsters after ovariectomy, adrenalectomy, and treatment with inhibitors of steroidogenesis (Evans and Kennedy, 1980).

The human conceptus produces human chorionic gonadotropin (hCG) at about the time of implantation on day 6 of pregnancy. Human chorionic gonadotropin is luteotrophic and stimulates the corpus luteum to produce progesterone. Functioning of the corpus luteum is crucial during the first 7 to 9 weeks of pregnancy, and luteectomy early in human pregnancy can precipitate abortion (Csapo et al., 1973). Similarly, early pregnancy loss in primates can be induced by injections of anti-hCG serum.

In rodents, implantation can be interrupted by injection of prostaglandin inhibitors, such as indomethacin, which prevents the increase in endometrial vascular permeability normally seen just prior to implantation. Additional evidence for a role for prostaglandins in the earliest stages of implantation is the finding of increased concentrations of these substances at prospective implantation sites. The source of these prostaglandins is not known, but it is likely that the endometrial cells are one such source, and synthesis of prostaglandins may be stimulated by the tissue damage that accompanies implantation. It is known that the rabbit blastocyst contains prostaglandins, whereas there is no evidence of significant prostaglandin production by rat blastocysts *in vitro*.

Shelesnyak suggested that histamine may also initiate the decidual response (1952). He found that antihistamines administered directly into the uterus prevent the decidual response in rats. This report was disputed by other workers, who found systemic antihistamines ineffective in preventing the decidual response. However, it has been shown that there are two different receptors for histamines, H_1 and H_2, which are blocked by different agents. It is probable that early experiments demonstrating a lack of effect of systemic antihistamines may have utilized a block to only one of the receptors. When both receptors are blocked in rats, there is a decrease in the number of implantation sites. However, the histamine antagonists used to block the receptors may have an adverse effect on blastocysts, which could affect decidualization by blocking a signal from the embryo. Mast cells in the uterus are a major source of histamine, but it is possible that the embryo can also synthesize histamine, which would explain why the increase in capillary permeability and decidualization in the endometrium is localized to areas near the implanting embryo. For now the role of histamine in implantation is not established (Brandon, 1980).

One of the great mysteries associated with implantation is the mechanism by which a woman's body rejects a genetically abnormal embryo or fetus. One possibility is that the abnormal embryo is unable to produce a signal in early pregnancy that is recognizable by the woman's body. The embryonic signals are effective only in a proper hormonal milieu. Much of the knowledge concerning the hormone requirements for implantation in animals has been gained from studies in delayed implantation. In a number of species, preimplantation embryos normally lie dormant in the uterus for periods as long as 15 months before implantation is initiated. In other species, delayed implantation can be imposed by postpartum suckling or by performing ovariectomy on day 3 of pregnancy. This produces a marked decrease in synthesis of DNA and protein by the blastocyst. The embryo can be maintained at the blastocyst stage by injecting the female with progesterone. On the basis of these findings, hormonal requirements for implantation have been determined. In mice there is a requirement for estrogen and progesterone followed by estrogen to initiate implantation. In other species the nidatory stimulus of estrogen is not required, and progesterone alone is sufficient.

Although it is known that the hormone milieu of delayed implantation renders the embryo quiescent, it is not known whether the delay represents a direct effect on the embryo or whether there is a metabolic inhibitor in uterine secretions that acts on the embryo. Removal of the embryo in delay from the uterus to culture dishes allows rapid resumption of normal metabolism, suggesting that there has, in fact, been a release from the inhibitory effects of a uterine product.

CONCLUSIONS

There are many unanswered questions in the area of reproduction covered by this chapter. Some of the more intriguing are:

1. Why is gamete production so wasteful? Billions of sperm are produced, but only a few are ever successful in fertilizing an egg. Does this waste relate to early forms of reproduction—for example, those in fish, in which the sperm are released into the sea and large numbers are needed to guarantee that a few reach the egg? Does the overpopulation of sperm allow selection processes to take place, ensuring that the more abnormal sperm are filtered out before the tube is reached? Approximately 350 ova are ovulated during a woman's life, yet her ovaries contain over a million eggs at birth.

2. What is the purpose of capacitation? Is it needed to overcome the protective mechanisms that have been built into the sperm—specifically those that prevent premature release of sperm enzymes and premature invasion by sperm? Invasion of the egg is desirable, but invasion of other maternal cells might trigger immunologic reactions against sperm. Does capacitation free the sperm from some inhibitors, thus allowing hypermotility that may be needed for zona penetration?

3. Why are there so many abnormal embryos? Current estimates are that 50 per cent of embryos do not survive to term. Why is there a high rate of embryo loss, and specifically, why is there a high selection against abnormal embryos? Is it because of intrinsic programming defects within the embryo or an inability of the embryo to produce a signal recognizable by the woman's body, or does the maternal organism in some way recognize abnormality and react against it?

REFERENCES

Adams CE: Consequences of accelerated ovum transport, including a re-evaluation of Estes' operation. J Reprod Fertil 55:239, 1979.

Ahlgren M: Sperm transport to and survival in the human fallopian tube. Gynecol Invest 6:206, 1975.

Bedford JM: Sperm capacitation and fertilization in mammals. Biol Reprod 2(Suppl):128, 1970.

Bleil JD, Wassarman PM: Identification of a ZP3-binding protein on acrosome-intact mouse sperm by photo affinity crosslinking. Proc Natl Acad Sci USA 87(14):5563, 1990.

Blobel CP, Wolfsberg TG, Turck CW, Myles DG, Primakoff P, White JM: A potential fusion peptide and an integrin ligand domain in a protein active in sperm-egg fusion. Nature 356:248, 1992.

Boving BG: Implantation. Ann NY Acad Sci 75:700, 1959.

Brandon JM: Some recent work on the role of histamine in ovum implantation. Prog Reprod Biol 7:244, 1980.

Brosens I, Robertson WB, Dickson HG: The role of spiral arteries in the pathogenesis of pre-eclampsia. Obstet Gynecol Annual 1:177, 1972.

Csapo AI, Pulkkinen MO, Wiest WO: Effects of luteectomy and progesterone replacement therapy in early pregnant patients. Am J Obstet Gynecol 115:759, 1973.

Dandekar PV, Martin MC, Glass RH: Polypronuclear embryos after in vitro fertilization. Fertil Steril 53:510, 1990.

Dandekar PV, Martin MC, Glass RH: Maturation of immature oocytes by coculture with granulosa cells. Fertil Steril 55:95, 1991.

Dandekar PV, Talbot P: Perivitelline space of mammalian oocytes: Extracellular matrix of unfertilized oocytes and formation of a cortical granule envelope following fertilization. Mol Reprod Dev **31**:135, 1992.

Eddy CA, Flores JJ, Archer DR, Pauerstein CJ: The role of cilia in infertility: An evaluation by selective microsurgical modification of the rabbit oviduct. Am J Obstet Gynecol **132**:814, 1978.

Evans CA, Kennedy TG: Blastocyst implantation in ovariectomized, adrenalectomized hamsters treated with inhibitors of steroidogenesis during the pre-implantation period. Steroids **36**:41, 1980.

Glass RH: Fate of rabbit eggs fertilized in the uterus. J Reprod Fertil **31**:139, 1972.

Glass RH, Spindle AI, Pedersen RA: Mouse embryo attachment to substratum and the interaction of trophoblast with cultured cells. J Exp Zool **203**:327, 1979.

Glass RH, Aggeler J, Spindle AI, et al: Degradation of extracellular matrix by mouse trophoblast outgrowths: A model for implantation. J Cell Biol **96**:1108, 1983.

Halbert SA, Tam PY, Blandau RJ: Egg transport in the rabbit oviduct: The roles of cilia and muscle. Science **191**:1052, 1976.

Hartmann JF, Gwatkin RBL: Alteration of sites on the mammalian sperm surface following capacitation. Nature **234**:479, 1971.

Heap RB, Flint AP, Gadsby JE: Embryonic signals that establish pregnancy. Br Med Bull **35**:129, 1979.

Hendrickx AG, Kraemer DC: Preimplantation stages of baboon embryos. Anat Rec **162**:111, 1968.

Hertig AT, Rock J, Adams EC, Menkin MC: Thirty-four fertilized ova, good, bad and indifferent, from 210 women of known fertility. Pediatrics **23**:202, 1959.

Hurst PR, Jefferies K, Eckstein P, Wheeler AG: Recovery of uterine embryos in rhesus monkeys. Biol Reprod **15**:429, 1976.

Jean Y, Langlais J, Roberts KD, et al: Fertility of a woman with nonfunctional ciliated cells in the fallopian tubes. Fertil Steril **31**:349, 1979.

Larsen JF: Electron microscopy of the implantation site in the rabbit. Am J Anat **109**:319, 1961.

Lindenberg S, Hyttel P, Sjogren A, Greve T: A comparative study of attachment of human, bovine and mouse blastocysts to uterine epithelial monolayer. Hum Reprod **4**:446, 1989.

Novy MJ: Reversal of Kroener fimbriectomy sterilization. Am J Obstet Gynecol **137**:198, 1980.

O'Neill C, Collier M, Ryan JP, Spinks NR: Embryo-derived platelet-activating factor. J Reprod Fertil **37**(Suppl):19, 1989.

Overstreet J: Transport of gametes in the reproductive tract of the female mammal. In Hartmann JF (ed): Mechanism and Control of Animal Fertilization. New York, Academic Press, 1983.

Pauerstein CJ, Eddy CA: The role of the oviduct in reproduction. Our knowledge and our ignorance. J Reprod Fertil **55**:223, 1979.

Schlafke S, Enders AC: Cellular basis of interaction between trophoblast and uterus at implantation. Biol Reprod **12**:41, 1975.

Settlage DSF, Motoshima M, Tredway DR: Sperm transport from the external cervical os to the fallopian tubes in women: A time and quantitation study. Fertil Steril **24**:655, 1973.

Shelesnyak MC: Inhibition of decidual cell formation in the pseudopregnant rat by histamine antagonists. Am J Physiol **170**:522, 1952.

Short RV: When a conception fails to become a pregnancy. In Whelan J (ed): Maternal Recognition of Pregnancy. CIBA Fdn Symp 64 [NS], Amsterdam, Excerpta Medica, 1979.

Sobrero AJ, MacLeod J: The immediate postcoital test. Fertil Steril **13**:184, 1962.

Sutherland AE, Carlarco PG, Damsky CH: Expression and function of cell surface extracellular matrix receptors in mouse blastocyst attachment and outgrowth. J Cell Biol **106**:1331, 1988.

Wassarman PM: The biology and chemistry of fertilization. Science **235**:553, 1987.

CHAPTER

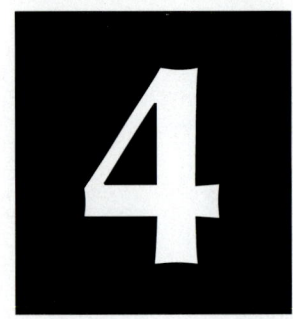

4

NORMAL DEVELOPMENT

KURT BENIRSCHKE, M.D.

The developing fertilized ovum enters the uterine cavity on about the fourth day after fertilization. The first differentiation of a human ovum into embryonic and future placental cells occurred in a 58-cell morula described by Hertig (1968). The specimen was 6 days old and had five embryonic cells, the "inner cell mass," and 53 trophoblastic cells constituted the wall of this uterine blastocyst. The polar bodies and an apparently degenerating zona pellucida were still present in the specimen, features destined to be lost shortly before implantation. Proliferation of the trophoblastic shell after this stage of development is rapid, and a segmentation cavity develops, with the more slowly reproducing embryonic cells assuming a marginal, "polar" position. The adjacent trophoblastic cells enlarge and secure implantation, which is assumed to take place on the sixth day after fertilization, although such a human specimen has not yet been described. With the very rapid enlargement occurring in the anchoring trophoblastic cells, the endometrial cells are dissociated by mechanisms discussed previously in this chapter. The entire blastocyst thus assumes an "interstitial" position, i.e., it sinks entirely into the endometrium at the site of attachment. The process may well be aided by the collapse of the blastocyst cavity that occurs at this time. Through this invasive activity, the blastocyst collapses, and through the deposition of fibrin or occasionally a coagulum at the site of penetration, the implanted trophoblastic shell comes to be surrounded by endometrium (decidua) on all sides. Perhaps some endometrial proliferation at the edges seals the defect. That portion of decidua lying between blastocyst and myometrium is the *decidua basalis*; that portion covering the defect is the *decidua capsularis*. Eventually, the latter comes to lie on the outside of the placental membranes. The decidua of the opposite side of the uterus is the *decidua vera*. At the time of implantation (day 6), the 0.1-mm morula can only be detected by a dissecting microscope. Within a few days, however, it will constitute a polypoid protrusion that can be detected readily by careful inspection of the endometrium. Thus, the approximately 14-day-old ovum shown in Figures 4–1

and 4–2 appeared to be a polyp. Occasionally, a small blood clot is attached to its surface, the *Schlusskoagulum*, whose presence may be detected clinically by spotting (Hartman's sign) and may lead to misinterpretation of the length of gestation. Decidual hemorrhages and small areas of necrosis at the site of trophoblastic penetration are common at this time and later.

MACROSCOPIC DEVELOPMENT

In the majority of recorded sites of early implantation, the ovum was found in the upper portion of the fundus. More recently it has been possible to follow the development of the placenta by ultrasonographic techniques. Thus, Rizos and colleagues (1979) found the 16-week placenta to be attached anteriorly in 37 per cent of patients, posteriorly in 24 per cent, in a fundal position in 34 per cent, and both anterior and posterior in 4 per cent. Others have employed sonography to measure placenta size and volume prenatally and have correlated their findings with fetal outcome (Hoogland et al., 1980). Of interest in this context is the finding from sonographic study that low implantation of the placenta in the uterus occurs frequently, with the formation of an apparent placenta previa. Moreover, it has been shown that such a low implantation may change through differential growth of the placenta and uterus and apparent marginal placental atrophy, so that at term the situation does not clinically resemble placenta previa (King, 1973). In the Rizos report, only five of 47 patients in whom placenta previa was diagnosed using ultrasound between 16 and 18 weeks were found actually to have this condition when delivered at term. These findings are of importance in our interpretation of the shape of the placenta at term and necessitate revision of former impressions.

Most commonly, the placenta develops at the uterine fundus. Through rapid expansion of the extraembryonic cavity (the exocoelom) and proliferation of the trophoblastic shell, the ovum bulges into the endo-

96

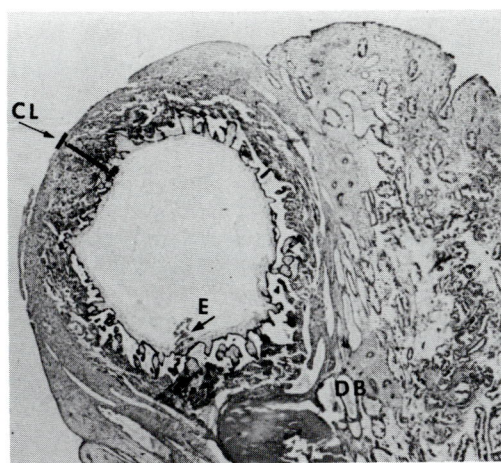

FIGURE 4–1. Implanted human embryo, of approximately 14 days gestational age. The implantation site projects into the endometrial cavity. Villi are just beginning to form. The secretory endometrium is undergoing decidualization. *CL* = chorion laeve; *E* = embryo; *DB* = decidua basalis. (H and E, × 16)

metrial cavity at the time of the first missed menstrual period. The surface is flecked by tiny hemorrhages and necrotic decidua. With continued expansion of the embryonic cavity, the surface bulges into the endometrial cavity and becomes attenuated. The peripheral villi atrophy and the future placental "membranes" form. They consist of decidua capsularis on the outside, hyalinized villi and trophoblast in the middle, and the membranous chorion laeve (and amnion) on the inside. The relationship of these membranes to the remainder of the uterus was sequentially traced in numerous pregnant uteri in a series collected by Boyd et al. (1970). Their observations suggested that the membranes truly fuse with the decidua vera of the side opposite to implantation in the fourth month of pregnancy, thereby obliterating the endometrial cavity. The decidua capsularis was seen to degenerate in their specimens prior to this time, and what is present on the outside of the term-delivered placenta they construed to be decidua vera attached to chorion. With the atrophy of peripheral villi and attachment of the membranes to the opposite side of the uterus, the macroscopic delineation of the placenta is essentially completed. We next turn our attention to the formation of amnion, yolk sac, and body stalk.

Figures 4–3 to 4–5 demonstrate the developing placenta and embryo at 7 weeks with an embryonic crown-rump length of 15 mm; the width of the entire specimen is approximately 25 mm. Through the "herniation" of the chorion laeve into the endometrial cavity, its surface has been smoothed and stretched. At the edge, the decidua is thrown into a fold and minute coagula are present (Fig. 4–3). When a tangential section is removed, the extension of the villous tissue for some distance onto the abembryonic pole of the cavity can be seen. The villi have already completely atrophied at the apex. The embryo is contained within the amnionic sac, which does not completely fill the chorionic cavity (Fig. 4–4). It is suspended within the cavity by a gel that liquefies upon touching,

the *magma reticulare.* When the sac is opened, the embryo and umbilical cord emerge (Fig. 4–5). An understanding of the morphogenesis of these structures is essential and can be gained from a study of Figure 4–2. In this histologic section the embryo is sectioned longitudinally. The ectoderm appears as a dark streak and is contiguous with the amnionic sac epithelium that lies below. On the other side of the embryo lie the endoderm and yolk sac. The mesoderm is seen to "flow" from the left caudal pole of the embryo onto the inner surface of the trophoblastic shell. This streak of mesoderm will ultimately become the substance of the umbilical cord. As the embryo grows and folds in such a manner as to enclose the endoderm, the amnion enlarges, and the embryo may be construed to herniate into this amnionic sac. A portion of the primitive yolk sac will be enclosed by the embryo to become its gut; another portion will be exteriorized (lying outside the amnionic sac) and will be connected by the omphalomesenteric (vitelline) vessels and duct. Most often these yolk structures disappear completely in later development; only in occasional term placentas can the calcified atrophic remnant of yolk sac be found at the periphery as a tiny (3 mm) yellow extra-amnionic disk. Once the amnionic sac has enclosed the entire embryo, it reflects on the umbilical cord, whose entire length it will eventually cover. At 8 weeks, the amnion is a thin, translucent membrane (Fig. 4–6). It does not fully expand to cover the inside of the entire sac until about 12 weeks. It never completely grows together with the chorion, however, so that in most term placentas the amnion may be dislodged from the chorion and the placental surface. The amnion does not have any blood vessels but is composed of a single layer of ectodermal epithelium, peripheral to which is a layer of delicate connective tissue with some macrophages (Bourne, 1962). Betraying the ectodermal origin of the amnion are small plaques of squamous metaplasia near the insertion of the term placenta's umbilical cord that must not be mistaken for amnion nodosum.

When the embryonic cells differentiate into meso-

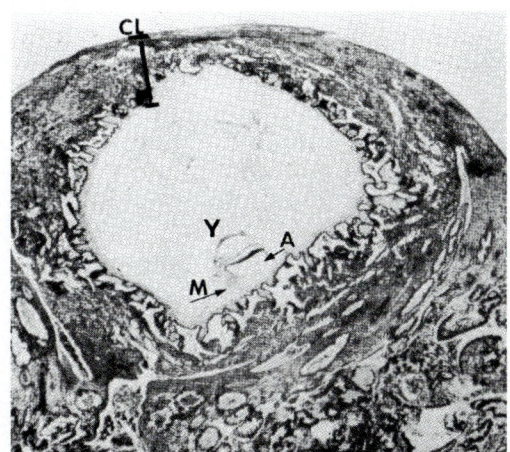

FIGURE 4–2. Same specimen as in Figure 4–1, with embryo sectioned longitudinally. *A* = amnion; *Y* = yolk sac (endoderm); *M* = mesoderm (developing cord); *CL* = chorion laeve (future membranes).

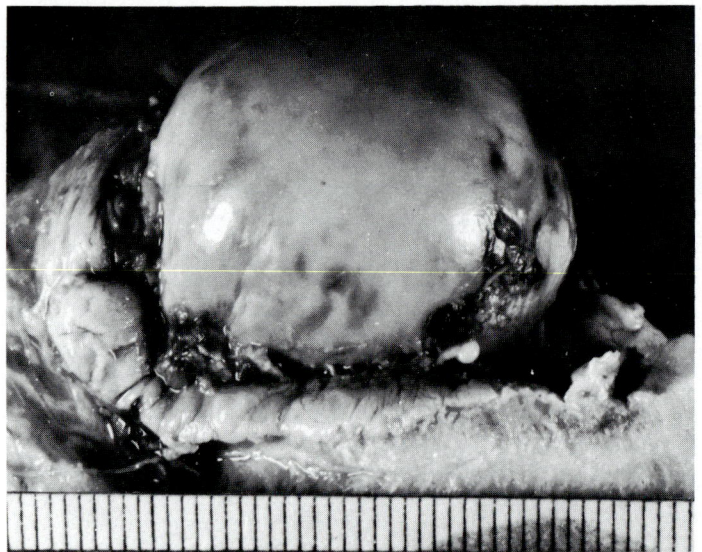

FIGURE 4–3. Endometrium with 7-week pregnancy. Note protuberance of flattened membrane projecting into endometrial cavity. (Courtesy of Dr. Jirasek, Praha.)

derm, endoderm, and ectoderm, the mesoderm is first clearly seen at the caudal pole of the embryonic disk (see Fig. 4–2). The mesodermal cells rapidly proliferate and send a column of cells streaming toward the inner surface of the trophoblastic cavity, which they then come to line. This column is ultimately destined to become the umbilical cord, and blood vessels as well as a rudimentary allantoic sac grow into this body stalk from the primitive yolk sac—hence the term *chorioallantoic vessels.* It is commonly thought that the *inner cell mass,* the future embryo, lies centrally in the early stages of implantation and that for this reason the umbilical cord comes to be attached to the center of the placenta. Aberrant attachment, such as at the margin or to the membranes (velamentous insertion), may be explained by one of two contradictory hypotheses. According to one hypothesis, the embryo had a less than perfect central position at the time of implantation and was perhaps even on the opposite side; thus, when the mesoderm proliferated the location of the cord was established on the surface of the endometrium, the area destined to become membranes. The other hypothesis suggests that normal, central implantation occurred, but that the area of implantation was less than optimal for placental development. Subsequently, the expansion of the placenta occurred to one side rather than in a uniform centrifugal manner. The already established location of the cord therefore changed from a central to a lateral position, a process called *trophotropism.*

This second hypothesis is supported by the much more common marginal or velamentous position of cords in multiple pregnancy, in which one can imagine there is competition for space by and collision of expanding placentas. Moreover, in term placentas marginal placental atrophy is often found, and the finding of succenturiate (accessory) lobes can best be explained by this mechanism. Also, the ultrasono-

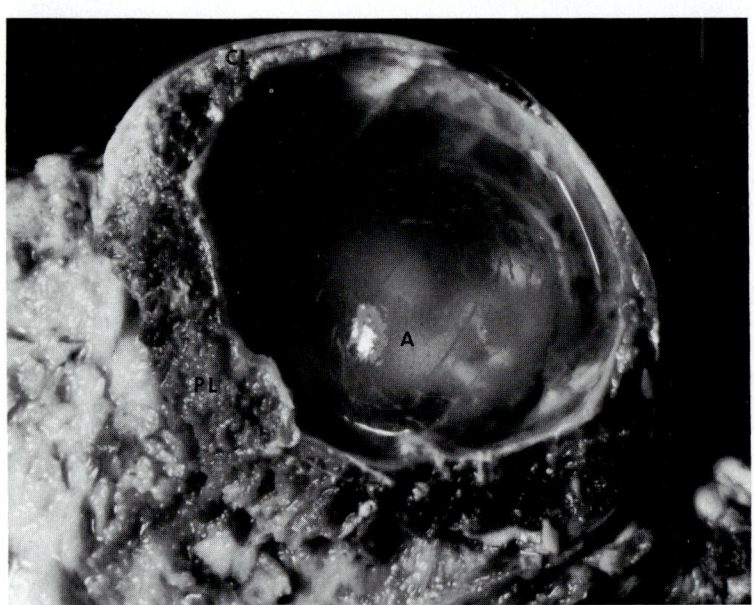

FIGURE 4–4. Same specimen as in Figure 4–3, with portion of chorion laeve (*CL*) removed to show partial atrophy of membranous villi, formation of definitive placenta (*PL*), and amnionic sac (*A*), which only partially fills chorionic cavity at this age. (Courtesy of Dr. Jirasek, Praha.)

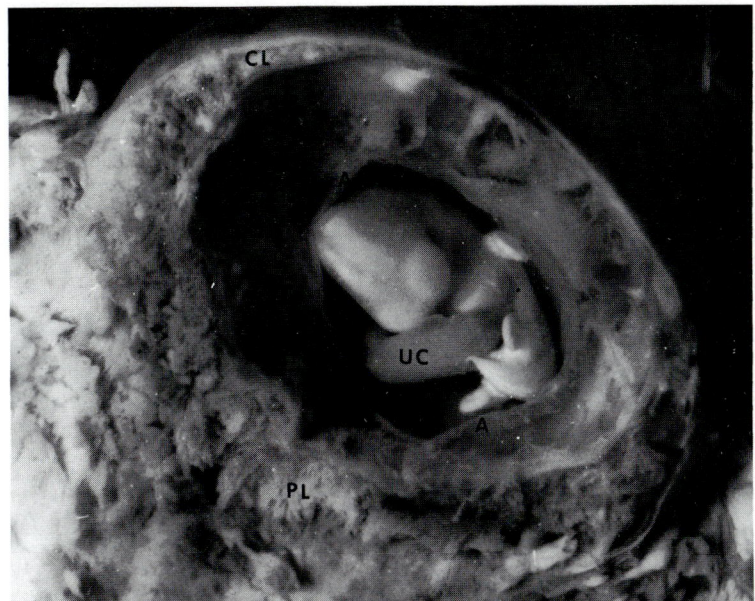

FIGURE 4–5. Same specimen as in Figure 4–3, with amnion (*A*) opened to disclose the 15-mm embryo and its umbilical cord (*UC*). (Courtesy of Dr. Jirasek, Praha.)

graphic finding of a "wandering" placenta favors this assumption, as does the fact that most of the few early embryos studied had a relatively central implantation. The first hypothesis is supported by the finding of a much higher frequency of velamentous insertion of the cord in aborted specimens than in term placentas (Monie, 1965).

The umbilical cord measures approximately 55 cm in length at term, but extreme variations occur for largely unknown reasons. Because a normal cord weighs as much as 100 gm and the segments of cord supplied with the placenta vary so much, the cord and membranes should be removed before the placental weight is ascertained. More often than not, the cord is spiraled, most commonly in a sinistral manner. Numerous theories have been presented to explain this helical arrangement, but the cause remains largely unknown. Because such twists do not exist in species with longitudinal orientation in bicornuate uteri, and because of the observed mobility of the primate fetus in its uterus simplex, it is most likely that fetal movements are the cause of the cord twisting (Benirschke, 1981; Lacro et al., 1987). The cord contains two umbilical arteries and one vein. A second rudimentary vein, the omphalomesenteric (vitelline) vessels, and the allantoic duct of early embryonic stages atrophy, and only on rare occasions are remnants of these structures found in the term cord. The two umbilical arteries anastomose through a variably constructed vessel within 2 cm of the insertion of the cord in almost all normal placentas. There are no nerves in the cord. True knots occur in a few umbilical cords, particularly very long ones, but much more common are so-called *false knots*. They represent redundancies (varicosities) of umbilical vessels that may protrude on the cord surface and have no clinical significance (Fig. 4–7).

The surface vessels of the placenta represent ramifications of the umbilical vessels and pursue a predictable course on the chorionic surface. In general, one arterial branch is accompanied by one branch of the vein, and each terminal pair of vessels supplies one fetal cotyledon. The arteries may be recognized by their superficial location, i.e., they cross over the veins. Anastomoses between superficial vessels do not occur; for that matter no such connections ever develop between villous vessels. Each district is isolated and distinct from the others (see Fig. 4–7). Two types of surface vascular arrangements have been observed, a very coarse and sparse vasculature and finely dispersed vessels. No significantly different fetal outcomes correlate with these features, however, and mixtures of the two types exist in single placentas. The number of terminal perforating vessels determines the number of fetal-placental cotyledons or districts. In most placentas this is around 20, somewhat more than the number of lobules that can be seen from the

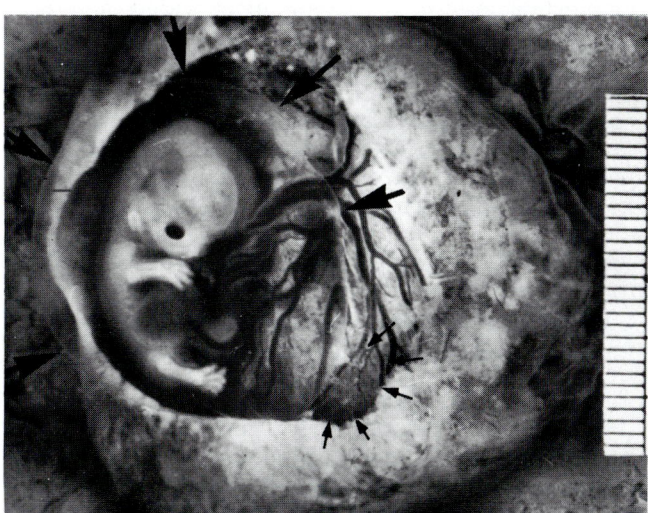

FIGURE 4–6. Pregnancy at 8 weeks with 20-mm embryo. The top portion of chorion laeve has been removed, thus disclosing amnion (*large arrows*) and extra-amnionic yolk sac (*small arrows*).

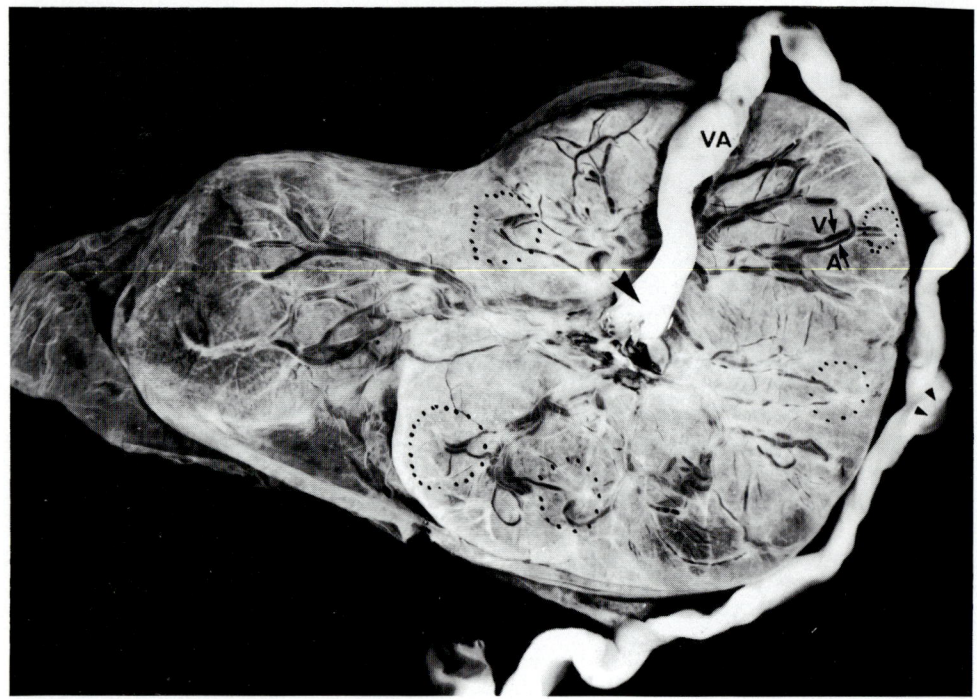

FIGURE 4–7. Term placenta, 530 gm, with lateral accessory (succenturiate) lobe to the left. The centrally inserted cord has a varicosity (*VA*) and a false knot (*small arrowheads*). At the base of the cord (*large arrowhead*) is the anastomosis between the two umbilical arteries. A surface artery (*A*) and vein (*V*) are labeled at top right, and several fetal cotyledons are indicated by dotted circles.

maternal side of mature placentas. In general there is correspondence of fetal lobules with maternal septal subdivisions when injection studies are performed of both circulations (Wigglesworth, 1967).

Authors who have performed such dual injections envisage that the intervillous circulation is achieved by the injection of blood from a decidual artery into the center of a fetal cotyledon, which there disperses from a central cavity in the villous tissue to the periphery of the cotyledon and to the undersurface of the chorion, whence it is drained by veins in the septa and decidual base (Ramsey, 1969). The loose central structure of cotyledons can be well demonstrated when a placenta is horizontally sectioned. This more conventional model of cotyledonary arrangement of villous structure and intervillous circulation has been challenged by Gruenwald (1975). He envisaged a different lobular architecture, with arterial openings occurring at the periphery of cotyledons, a concept that has not yet been unequivocally refuted. The former notion that all intervillous blood flows laterally to the *marginal sinus*, however, is no longer acceptable.

The normal term placenta from which membranes and cord have been trimmed weighs between 400 and 500 gm. There is an enormous amount of variability in placental size and shape, as there is in fetal weight. Some variations can be explained by racial differences, altitude, pathologic circumstances of implantation, diseases, or maternal habits such as smoking. However, in many cases the deviations from "normal" are as difficult to explain as the factors that ultimately determine fetal and placental growth in general. Systematic studies of placental structure have given some insight into the complexities; they are most recently summarized in the careful analysis by Teasdale (1980). Absolute growth as determined by DNA, RNA, and protein content occurs in the placenta to the 36th week

of gestation. Thereafter, proliferation of cells does not normally occur, and the placenta undergoes only further maturational changes. Previous studies have suggested an expansion of villous surface to between 11 and 13 sq m at term, whereas Teasdale's careful measurements suggest that the maximum is reached with 10.6 sq m at 36 weeks, decreasing to 9.4 sq m at term. The fetal-placental ratio is estimated to change from 5:1 in the third trimester to 7:1 at term, most rapidly increasing during the last month of gestation. Reasons for discrepancies of these measurements reported in the literature are partly explained by inconsistent handling of the organ at delivery. Thus, a variable amount of blood may be trapped, depending on the time of cord clamping. It is widely accepted now that the delivered placenta has a smaller volume, in particular is less thick, than before delivery, as ascertained by sonography (Bleker et al., 1977). Therefore, for quantitative assessment a histometric analysis must accompany such correlative study. Apparently, the slight increase in placental volume occurring in the last month of pregnancy results from an expansion of the "nonparenchymal" space—i.e., villous capillary size, decidua, septa, and fibrin. Thus, during the last month of gestation, fetal growth occurs without a commensurate increase in placental volume, indicating that changes must occur in perfusion or transport function of the placenta to ensure enhanced delivery of metabolic substrates to the fetus.

Macroscopically, a delivered, normal term placenta then can be described as a disk-shaped, round, or ovoid structure measuring 18 × 20 cm in diameter and having a thickness of approximately 2 cm. The cord is normally inserted near the center of the disk (marginal in 7 per cent and on the membranes in 1 per cent); it measures 40 to 60 cm in length and 1.5 cm in thickness, and has two arteries, one vein, and a number of helical spirals. The membranes are attached at the periphery and have some degenerated yellow decidua on their outer surface and a smooth, glistening inner amnionic surface. The amnion is only slightly adherent to the chorionic face of the placenta, from which it can be stripped by forceps, but it is firmly attached to the cord, upon which it reflects. The fetal surface of the placenta is blue because of the fetal villous blood content seen through the membranes. Irregular whitish plaques of subchorionic fibrin slightly project between fetal vessels and produce what has been referred to as a "bosselated" surface; it is indicative of a mature organ. The maternal surface usually has a film of loosely attached blood clot, which when removed discloses the thin, grayish layer of decidua basalis and fibrin that come away with delivery. In the fibrin, yellow granules and streaks of calcification characterize maturity. They are extremely variable in amount. The maternal surface is usually broken up into irregular lobules (cotyledons) by crevices that continue into partial or complete septa between fetal cotyledons. These septa are constructed of decidual cells and cellular trophoblast. On sectioning, the dark red villous tissue reflects the content of fetal blood. Loosely structured areas represent intervillous lakes, the presumed sites of first blood injections ("spurts") from decidual arteries.

MICROSCOPIC DEVELOPMENT

Complete interstitial implantation of the blastocyst is accomplished on the ninth day of gestation. The trophoblastic shell has proliferated appreciably, particularly at its basal portions, and most trophoblastic cells possess disproportionately large nuclei and form a syncytium. Within this mass of trophoblastic cells develop clefts (*lacunae*) that coalesce in order to form the most primitive type of the future intervillous space. At about this time or on the next day, the somewhat congested decidual vessels are tapped by the syncytium. The first maternal leukocytes have been observed on day 11 in this primitive intervillous space, soon to be followed by blood, thus establishing the primitive intervillous circulation (Hertig, 1968). At the same time the trophoblastic cells can be seen to differentiate into a central cellular type (*cytotrophoblast*, the future Langhans layer) and peripheral syncytiotrophoblast (Fig. 4–8). The syncytium never shows mitoses and grows by incorporation of cytotrophoblastic nuclei and cytoplasm, only the latter cells being capable of mitosis (Richart, 1961; Galton, 1962). On day 13 the first connective tissue may be observed in the central portion of the future villi. It will rapidly expand peripherally into the cell columns of trophoblast. Evidence suggests that this connective tissue core derives from the mesoderm of the body stalk (shown in Fig. 4–2) and not by central "delamination" from trophoblast. By the 30th day a truly villous ovum is formed, and the basic future development of the villous structure is delineated. Villi are found around the entire circumference at first, only to atrophy over the pole later. Commencing almost simultaneously, on the 14th day and subsequently, is the development of villous

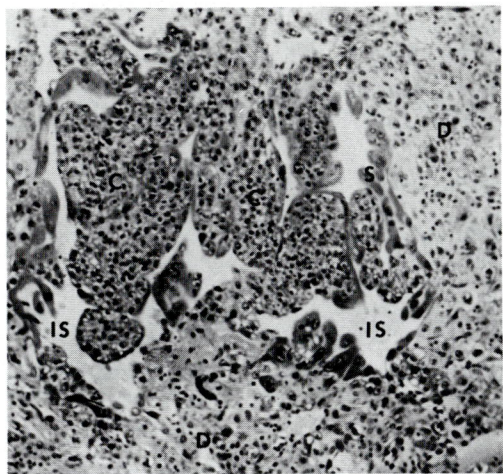

FIGURE 4–8. Trophoblastic shell of 13-day human ovum. Cell columns composed of solid cytotrophoblast (*C*) are covered by syncytiotrophoblast (*S*) lining the entire intervillous space (*IS*), which is still devoid of maternal blood. *D* = decidua. (H and E, × 300)

capillaries. Although Hertig (1968) has discussed in great detail how such a process also derives from delaminated trophoblastic cells by the internal detachment of angioblastic cells, more likely their origin is from fetal mesoderm or endoderm. These are not idle problems of the embryologist but pertain directly to an understanding of the genesis of hydatidiform moles. If villous connective tissue and vessels are definitely derived from the embryo (rather than the trophoblast), then hydatidiform moles must at one time have had an embryo. Occasional complete hydatidiform moles (CHM) have been shown to contain degenerated embryos, but in most CHM the embryo and its vessels have disappeared (Benirschke and Kaufmann, 1990). Villous vessels coalesce and connect to the omphalomesenteric and later allantoic vessels of the embryonic body stalk, and a true fetal circulation is active by 21 days (Moore, 1982). The initial fetal blood cells come from yolk sac, and only after the second month do they issue from fetal hematopoietic islands. With an established circulation the villi are now called tertiary villi.

The villous structure changes appreciably during further development, and gestational age can be crudely estimated from the histologic appearance of the villi. In young placentas the mesenchymal core of villi is extremely loosely structured, appearing almost edematous (Fig. 4–9). Capillaries are filled with nucleated cells and lie very close to the villous surface. This surface is uniformly covered by an inner cellular cytotrophoblast, which contains numerous mitoses and in turn is covered by a thick layer of syncytium that contains abundant organelles in its metabolically active cytoplasm. The syncytium is functionally the most important part of the placenta. With advancing age the villi elongate, lose their central edema, branch successively, and decrease in diameter. At term they contain little mesenchyma and are filled with distended capillaries. Cytotrophoblastic mitoses are rare after 36 weeks in normal placentas. The syncytium

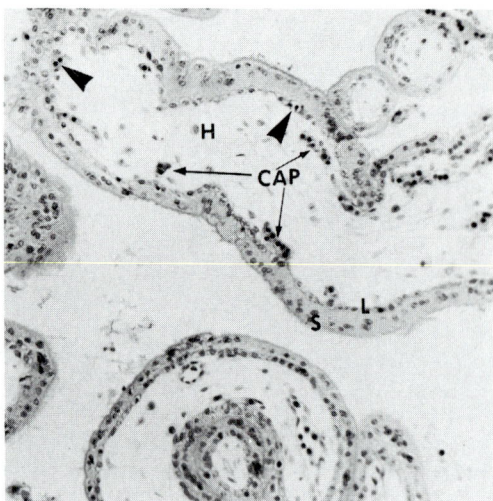

FIGURE 4–9. Villi of 30-day placenta. Note the very loosely structured mesenchymal core containing isolated macrophages, thin-walled fetal capillaries (*CAP*) filled with nucleated red blood cells, and the double-layered trophoblastic surface. *H* = Hofbauer cells; *L* = Langhans cells with mitoses at *heavy arrows* (cytotrophoblast); *S* = syncytium. (H and E, × 160)

tends to form buds and "knots," some of which break loose and are swept into the intervillous circulation, whence they reach the maternal lung. Fibrin is normally accumulated in ever-increasing quantities on the surface of villi, in the subchorionic area, and along the floor of the placenta, where Rohr and Nitabuch's fibrin layers mingle with decidua basalis. Near term, some of these fibrin deposits become calcified as a normal process that may become excessive in the postmature placenta. The amount of calcium varies greatly but has no deleterious influence on placental function. The placental septa, composed of cellular trophoblast ("X cells" or intermediate trophoblasts) and decidua, often undergo cystic change as a sign of maturity (Fig. 4–10). The X-cell has recently been the focus of attention. It is a separate lineage of trophoblast that is intimately related to fibrinoid deposition, the production of the "major basic protein" (MBP) and placental lactogen (hPL). Most so-called "placental site giant cells" are X-cells and are often confused with decidual stromal elements (Wasmoen et al, 1987; Benirschke and Kaufmann, 1990). These cells also infiltrate into the orifices of basal decidual spiral arterioles. Hustin and Schaaps (1987, 1988) have adduced evidence that they completely occlude these vessels in early pregnancy, thus allowing only a filtrate of maternal blood to enter the intervillous space. This hypothesis is one of the most interesting aspects of placental studies. The population of Hofbauer cells increases in the first 36 weeks and falls thereafter (Teasdale, 1980). Although their precise function is not well understood, recent immunohistochemical studies show that this large population of cells represents fully differentiated phagocytes (Wood, 1980). Following hemolysis they are seen to produce hemosiderin; in the chorionic surface they actively transport meconium after its discharge, and it is speculated that they remove antifetal antibodies.

At the site of implantation, trophoblastic cells intermingle extensively with decidua basalis; indeed, they penetrate into the superficial portions of myometrium. Frequently these areas are characterized by scattered lymphocyte infiltration as well as decidual necrosis (Pijnenborg et al., 1980). Cytotrophoblastic cells enter the opened mouths of maternal arterioles and penetrate deeply along their endothelial linings. Some trophoblastic cells infiltrate the decidua as well as myometrium, often fusing to form *placental giant cells* (Fig. 4–11), and others invade the spiral arterioles from the outside. They cause considerable local change, including fibrin deposition, and alter the normally contractile vessels to presumably rigid uteroplacental arteries. Thrombosis is not found normally but is a common finding when hypertensive changes are superimposed.

Electron-microscopic study of placental villi in general supports the findings made by light microscopy, but it adds significant new details. The arborization of villi and their complexity are best appreciated in scanning electron micrographs (Fig. 4–12). In the more peripheral areas of cotyledons, the villi appear histologically more mature, i.e., they are smaller and have more branches and less stroma. The syncytial surface is covered by numerous minute microvilli, and syncytial bridges are occasionally seen. In the central portion of the cotyledon the villi are plump and less

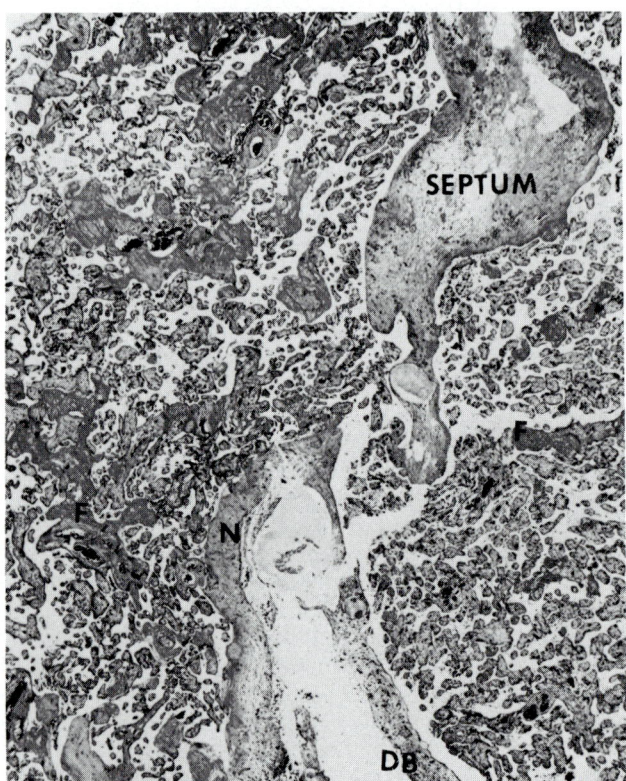

FIGURE 4–10. Term placenta; basal portion with septum constructed of decidua and trophoblast, forming small cysts. Villi are finely branched, and grayish masses of fibrin (*F*) are found throughout. At bottom is decidua basalis (*DB*), the only maternal tissue in a delivered placenta. Nitabuch's fibrin layer (*N*) is discontinuous. (H and E, × 64)

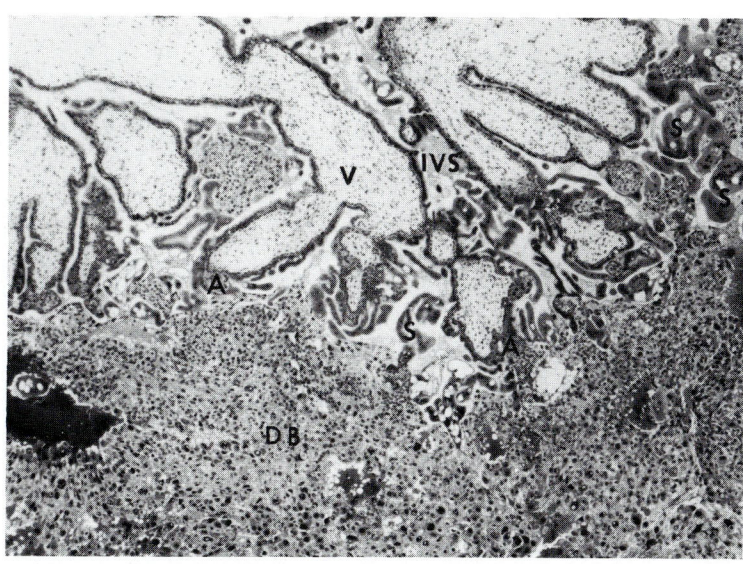

FIGURE 4–11. Implantation site of first trimester placenta. *IVS* = intervillous space; *A* = anchoring villi composed of cytotrophoblast; *S* = syncytial buds; *DB* = decidua basalis with maternal vessels and diffusely infiltrated placental giant cells; *V* = villi. (H and E, × 40) (From Benirschke K, Kaufmann P: The Pathology of the Human Placenta. New York, Springer-Verlag, 1990.)

branched. Freeze-fracture scanning electron microscopy discloses the proximity of fetal vessels to the basement membrane and the profuse microvillous surface of the syncytium (Fig. 4–13). With advancing maturity the Langhans cytotrophoblastic layer not only becomes less prominent but also is interrupted in many more places. Here, then, the fetal capillaries abut a thin layer of syncytium, presumably the most efficient site of transfer. These electron-micrographic features of maturity are also found more frequently in the periphery of cotyledons than in their more immature-appearing centers, but qualitative differences do not exist (Schuhmann and Wynn, 1980). The

slightly different electron-micrographic features of villi in part relate to the state of contraction of fetal capillaries (Fig. 4–14), and they may in part be the result of oxygen supply. Desmosomes have been identified by scanning and transmission electron microscopy in trophoblast (Reale et al., 1980). They interlock syncytium with cytotrophoblast, and when found with free membranes in the cytoplasm of the syncytium, they presumably represent the remnants of the fusion-incorporation process of cytotrophoblast into syncy-

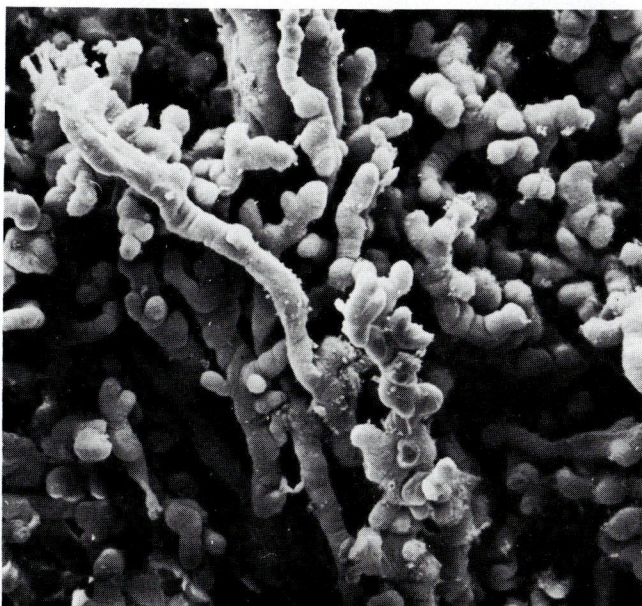

FIGURE 4–12. Scanning electron micrograph of mature villi at periphery of cotyledon. Note fine, uniform structure, rare adherence, and microvillous, velvety surface of terminal villi. (× 100) (From Sandstedt B: The placenta and low birth weight. Curr Top Pathol **66**:1, 1979.)

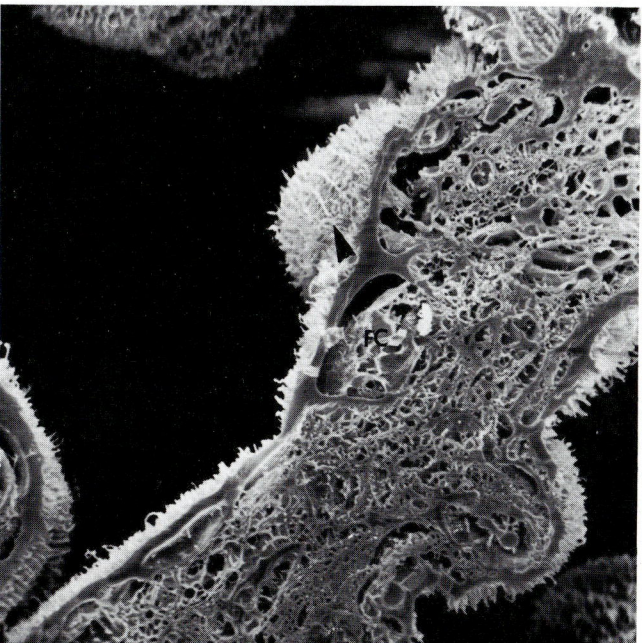

FIGURE 4–13. Freeze-fracture scanning electron microphotograph of term placental villus to show microvillous surface, often in rows (*arrow*), grayish trophoblast cytoplasm, and proximity of fetal capillary (*FC*) to black intervillous space. (× 250) (From Sandstedt B: The placenta and low birth weight. Curr Top Pathol **66**:1, 1979. Courtesy of Dr. B. Sandstedt.)

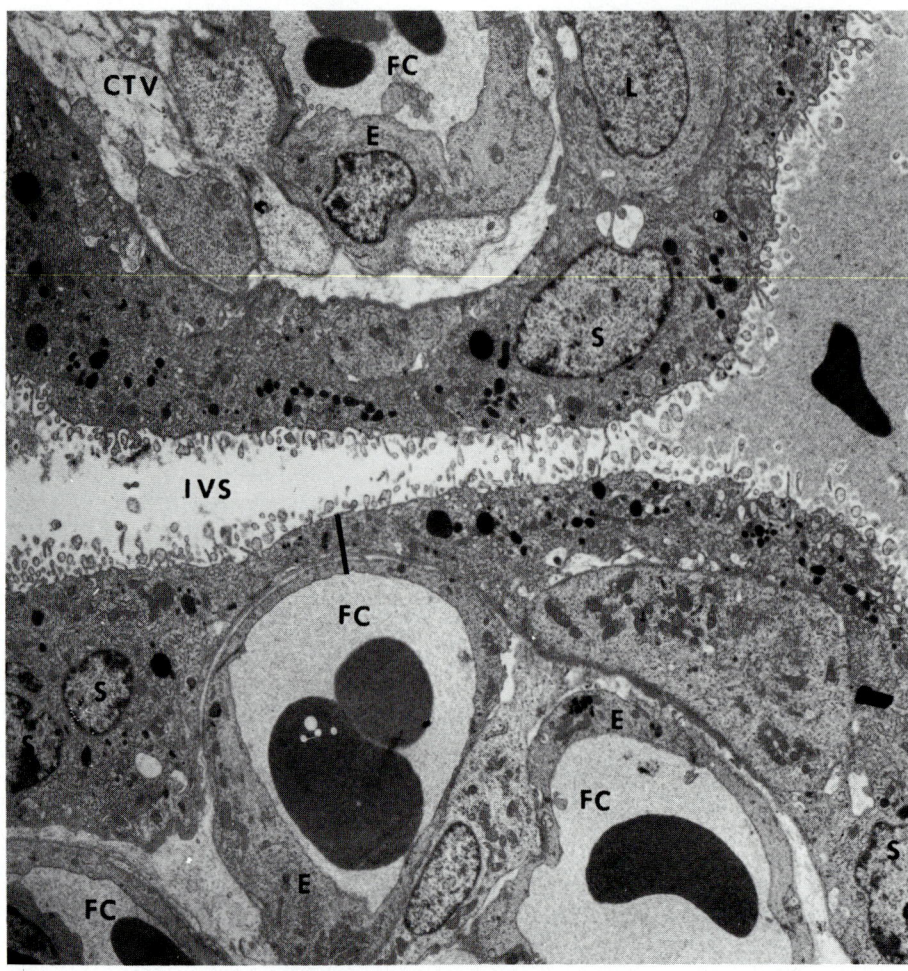

FIGURE 4–14. Transmission electron micrograph of two placental villi at 30 weeks gestation. At top the fetal capillary (*FC*) is contracted; at bottom, several capillaries are dilated. Note microvilli and shortest maternal-fetal exchange distance (indicated by *bar*). *S* = syncytial nuclei; *L* = Langhans cell nucleus; *IVS* = intervillous space; *E* = fetal capillary endothelium; *CVT* = connective tissue of villus. (× 5000) (Courtesy of Dr. R. M. Wynn.)

tium. The structure of the syncytiotrophoblastic cytoplasm is extremely complex. It is filled with minute vacuoles, ribosomes, mitochondria, and the other usual cytoplasmic components. Conversely, the cytotrophoblastic cytoplasm is relatively simple, reflecting its presumed primary function as precursor cells for syncytium.

REFERENCES

Benirschke K: Anatomy. *In* Berger GS, Brenner WE, Keith LG (eds): Second Trimester Abortion. Boston, John Wright, 1981.

Benirschke K, Kaufmann P: The Pathology of the Human Placenta. 2nd ed. New York, Springer-Verlag, 1990.

Bleker OP, Kloosterman GJ, Breur W, et al: The volumetric growth of the human placenta: A longitudinal ultrasonic study. Am J Obstet Gynecol **127**:657, 1977.

Bourne GL: The Human Amnion and Chorion. London, Lloyd-Luke, 1962.

Boyd JD, Hamilton WJ: The Human Placenta. Cambridge, Heffer and Sons, 1970.

Galton M: DNA content of placental nuclei. J Cell Biol **13**:183, 1962.

Gruenwald P: Lobular architecture of primate placentas. *In* Gruenwald P (ed): The Placenta and its Maternal Supply Line. Baltimore, University Park Press, 1975.

Hertig AT: Human Trophoblast. Springfield, IL, Charles C Thomas, 1968.

Hoogland HJ, deHaan J, Martin CB: Placental size during early

pregnancy and fetal outcome: A preliminary report of a sequential ultrasonographic study. Obstet Gynecol **138**:441, 1980.

Hustin J, Schaaps JP: Echocardiographic and anatomic studies of the maternotrophoblastic border during the first trimester of pregnancy. Am J Obstet Gynecol **157**:162, 1987.

Hustin J, Schaaps JP, Lambotte R: Anatomical studies of the uteroplacental vascularization in the first trimester of pregnancy. Trophoblast Res **3**:49, 1988.

King DL: Placental migration demonstrated by ultrasonography. Radiology **109**:167, 1973.

Lacro RV, Jones KL, Benirschke K: The umbilical cord twist: Origin, direction, and relevance. Am J Obstet Gynecol **157**:833, 1987.

Monie IW: Velamentous insertion of the cord in early pregnancy. Am J Obstet Gynecol **93**:276, 1965.

Moore KL: The Developing Human. 3rd ed. Philadelphia, WB Saunders Company, 1982.

Pijnenborg R, Dixon G, Robertson WB, Brosens I: Trophoblastic invasion of human decidua from 8 to 18 weeks by pregnancy. Placenta **1**:3, 1980.

Ramsey EM: New appraisal of an old organ: The placenta. Proc Am Philosph Soc **113**:296, 1969.

Reale E, Wang T, Zaccheo D, et al: Junctions on the maternal blood surface of the human placental syncytium. Placenta **1**:245, 1980.

Richart R: Studies of placental morphogenesis. I. Radioautographic studies of human placenta utilizing tritiated thymidine. Proc Soc Exp Biol **106**:829, 1961.

Rizos N, Doran TA, Miskin M, et al: Natural history of placenta previa ascertained by diagnostic ultrasound. Obstet Gynecol **133**:287, 1979.

Sandstedt B: The placenta and low birth weight. Curr Top Pathol **66**:1, 1979.

Schuhmann RA, Wynn RM: Regional ultrastructural differences in placental villi in cotyledons of a mature human placenta. Placenta **1**:345, 1980.

Teasdale F: Gestational changes in the functional structure of the human placenta in relation to fetal growth: A morphometric study. Am J Obstet Gynecol **137**:560, 1980.

Wasmoen TL, Benirschke K, Gleich GJ: Demonstration of immunoreactive eosinophil granule major basic protein in the plasma and placentae of non-human primates. Placenta **8**:283, 1987.

Wigglesworth JS: Vascular organization of the human placenta. Nature **216**:1120, 1967.

Wood GW: Mononuclear phagocytes in the human placenta. Placenta **1**:113, 1980.

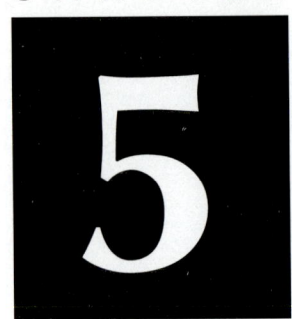

AMNIOTIC FLUID DYNAMICS

ROBERT A. BRACE, PH.D.

The purposes of this discussion are to supply quantitative information about amniotic fluid volume and to describe the current evidence regarding its formation and regulation. Aberrations of amniotic fluid accumulation in human disease states are discussed in greater depth in other sections of the text.

GESTATIONAL CHANGES

During late gestation in human pregnancy, intrauterine water content increases approximately 30 to 40 ml per day under normal circumstances. At term, total water accumulation is approximately 4000 ml, with 2800 ml in the fetus, 400 ml in the placenta, and 800 ml in the amniotic fluid. Volumes of amniotic fluid at various gestational ages have been studied by use of direct volumetric methods, indicator dilution techniques, and, more recently, quantitative ultrasonographic methods. In normal pregnancies, a wide range of volumes occurs, particularly during the latter half of gestation. Figure 5–1 demonstrates the progressive increase in amniotic fluid volume from 30 ml at 10 weeks to 190 ml at 16 weeks and to a mean of 900 ml at 32 to 35 weeks gestation, after which a decrease occurs. Figure 5–1 also provides a statistical definition of polyhydramnios and oligohydramnios as a function of gestational age. For example, 500 ml at 14 weeks is far in excess of normal, whereas 2000 ml at 33 weeks is not outside the 95 per cent confidence interval for normal pregnancies.

The gestational pattern of volume changes can vary considerably in individual women in that amniotic fluid volume may increase progressively until delivery or may begin to decrease as early as 24 weeks gestation. As seen in Figure 5–1, a decrease in mean volume begins to occur after 36 weeks and becomes more progressive, especially in post-term pregnancies. The rate of change in amniotic fluid volume is a strong function of gestational age. Figure 5–2 shows that fluid volume increases at a rate of 10 ml/week at the beginning of the fetal period. This increases to 50 to 60 ml/week at 19 to 25 weeks gestation and subsequently undergoes a gradual decrease until the rate of change equals zero (i.e., amniotic fluid volume is a

maximum) at 34 weeks. Thereafter amniotic fluid volume falls, with the decrease averaging 60 to 70 ml/week at 40 weeks. The decrease in post-term pregnancies has been found to be as high as 150 ml/week from 38 to 43 weeks gestation (Elliott and Inman, 1961). Although the basic mechanisms that produce these alterations in amniotic fluid volume throughout gestation are unclear, it is important to note that, when expressed as a percentage (Fig. 5–2), the rate of change in amniotic fluid volume decreases monotonically throughout the fetal period. Thus, the late decrease in amniotic volume represents a natural progression rather than an aberration.

The volume of amniotic fluid is important clinically because volumes in excess of 1.5 to 2 liters (polyhydramnios) or less than 0.5 liters (oligohydramnios) between 32 and 36 weeks gestation are often associated with fetal abnormalities and/or poor perinatal outcome (Chamberlain et al., 1984a,b). Polyhydramnios (also termed hydramnios) occurring during the second trimester spontaneously resolves in 40 to 50 per cent of the cases; the resolution is associated with a normal perinatal outcome (Zamah et al., 1982). Conversely, oligohydramnios in mid-pregnancy frequently is associated with poor pregnancy outcome (Mercer et al., 1984; Bastide et al., 1986).

BASIC MECHANISMS OF WATER TRANSPORT

An understanding of the mechanisms that regulate amniotic fluid dynamics requires knowledge of the biology of water transport. For a review of these principles as they apply to amniotic fluid accumulation, the reader is referred to a comprehensive review by Seeds (1980). Briefly, the active transport of water has not been demonstrated in biological tissues. Thus, net water accumulation occurs across body membranes only by passive mechanisms in response to hydrostatic and/or osmotic pressure gradients. If no such gradients exist, no net transfer of volume takes place. Seeds (1980) has reported that careful investigations to demonstrate the existence of transplacental chemical gradients that would be responsible for the

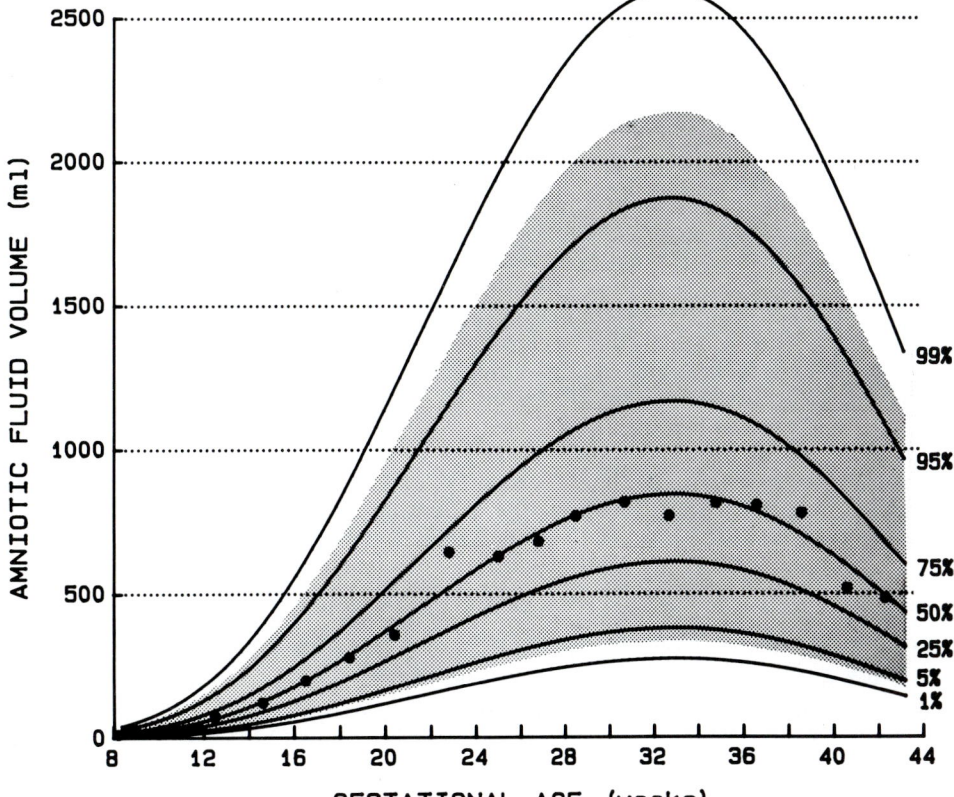

FIGURE 5–1. Amniotic fluid as a function of gestational age. Dots are means for 2 week intervals from 705 women. Shaded area is 95 per cent confidence interval. Percentiles calculated from polynomial regression. (From Brace RA, Wolf EJ: Normal amniotic fluid volume changes throughout pregnancy. Am J Obstet Gynecol **161:**382, 1989.)

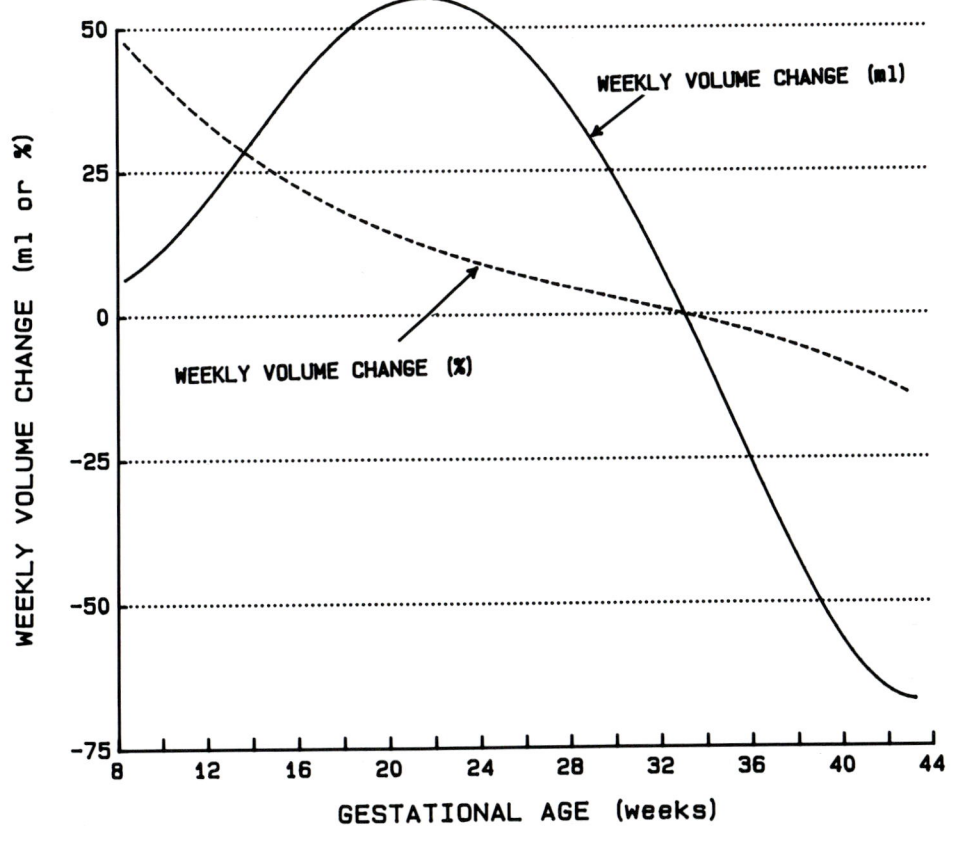

FIGURE 5–2. Weekly changes in mean amniotic volume. (From Brace RA, Wolf EJ: Normal amniotic fluid volume changes throughout pregnancy. Am J Obstet Gynecol **161:**382, 1989.)

net water transfer have been unsuccessful. However, since only exceedingly small chemical gradients would be necessary to explain the small daily net water transfer, it is entirely possible that current experimental techniques are not sufficiently sensitive to demonstrate their presence.

A second difficulty in understanding the factors involved in regulating water accumulation is that confusion has occurred over interpretation of studies that explored the movement of isotopically labeled water. As Seeds (1980) discussed in detail, data describing the diffusional movement of water molecules do not provide any information relevant to net volume changes, whereas only net volume changes affect amniotic fluid volume. This is illustrated by the fact that, as blood passes through a single capillary, each water molecule in the blood diffuses back and forth across the capillary wall 100 times in contrast to a net volume movement across the capillary membrane of less than 1 per cent (Landis and Pappenheimer, 1963). Because present techniques for measurement of the diffusional movement of water do not have a resolution anywhere near this ratio of one part in ten thousand, they cannot be used to study the factors that affect the net changes in amniotic fluid volume. Thus, in order for the regulatory mechanisms to be explored, net volume changes must be measured and related to the conditions being studied.

PATHWAYS FOR FLUID MOVEMENT

Amniotic fluid volume is the sum of the inflows and outflows of the amniotic space. Thus, a knowledge of the pathways for fluid movement is a prerequisite for understanding the volume regulatory mechanisms. Figure 5–3 summarizes these pathways. In the late gestation fetus, the excretion of urine and the swallowing of amniotic fluid are the two major pathways for

the formation and clearance of amniotic fluid. In early gestation, significant amounts of amniotic fluid are present before the establishment of fetal micturition or deglutition. Although the formation of amniotic fluid at this early stage is virtually unexplored, the most likely mechanism is an active transport of solute by the amnion into the amniotic space with water moving passively down the chemical potential gradient.

The amniotic fluid has been considered to be a stagnant pool of fluid. However, this view is far from accurate because, relative to amniotic fluid volume, large amounts of fluid enter and leave the amniotic space each day. Gitlin et al. (1972) injected several different proteins into the amniotic fluid of pregnant women and found that they were all cleared at essentially the same rate, which averaged 63 per cent per day. Because of the exponential nature of clearances, this corresponds to a net volume turnover in excess of 95 per cent of amniotic fluid volume per day. Thus, amniotic fluid circulates with a turnover time of approximately one day. This turnover rate of one volume per day is considerably less than that determined with isotopically labeled water (Liley, 1972; Lotgering and Wallenburg, 1986). However, as already discussed, the latter represents the diffusional exchange of water molecules rather than net volume movements.

Fetal Urine

It is clear that fetal urine is a major source of amniotic fluid in the latter half of pregnancy. Urine first enters the amniotic space at 8 to 11 weeks gestation (Abramovich and Page, 1973). As measured with real-time ultrasonographic techniques, there is a steady increase in the urine production rate throughout the latter half of gestation, as shown in Figure 5–4. Urine production per kilogram of body weight

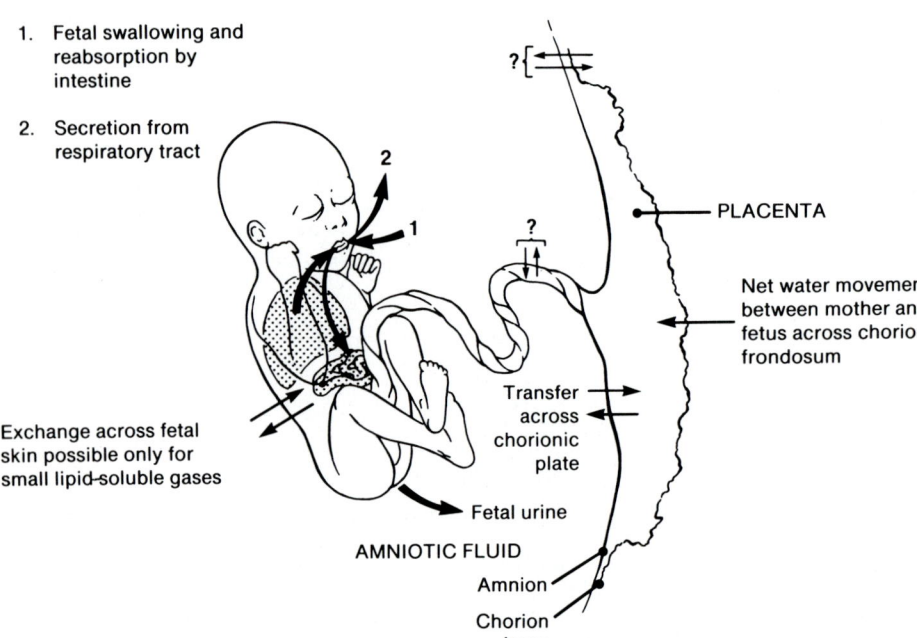

1. Fetal swallowing and reabsorption by intestine

2. Secretion from respiratory tract

PLACENTA

Net water movement between mother and fetus across chorion frondosum

Exchange across fetal skin possible only for small lipid-soluble gases

Transfer across chorionic plate

Fetal urine

AMNIOTIC FLUID

Amnion

Chorion laeve

FIGURE 5–3. Summary of the significant pathways of water and solute exchange between the amniotic fluid and fetus. (Modified from Seeds AE: Current concepts of amniotic fluid dynamics. Am J Obstet Gynecol **138:**575, 1980.)

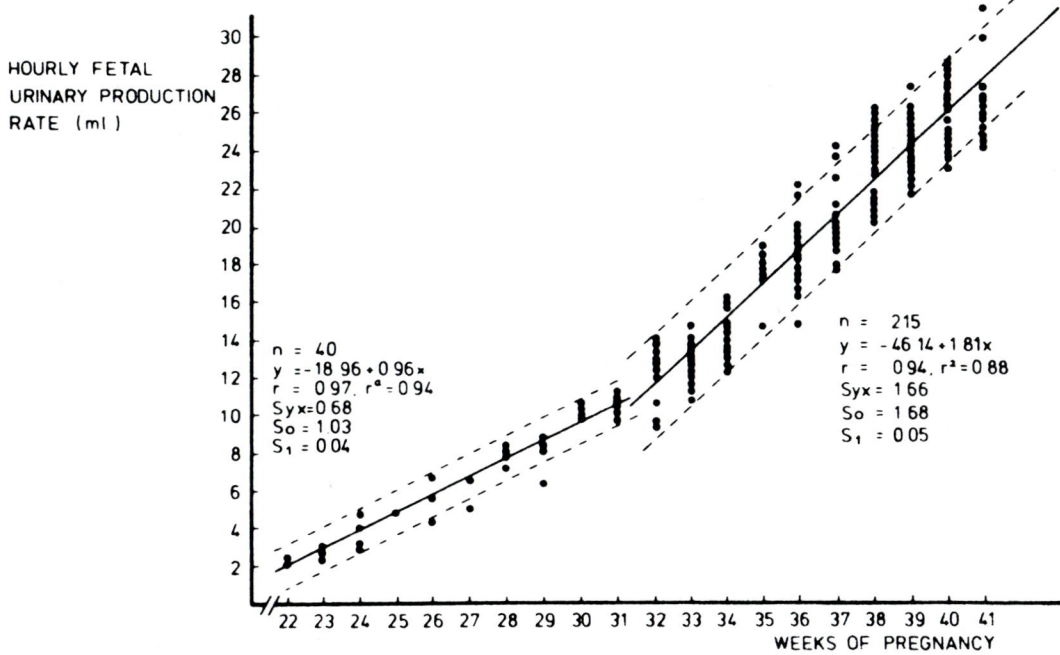

FIGURE 5–4. Increase in hourly fetal urinary production rates as determined by ultrasonographic techniques during human pregnancy. (From Kurjak A, Kirkinen P, Latin V, Ivankovic D: Ultrasonic assessment of fetal kidney functions in normal and complicated pregnancies. Am J Obstet Gynecol **141**:266, 1981.)

increases from approximately 110 ml/kg/24 hr at 25 weeks to approximately 190 ml/kg/24 hr at 39 weeks (Lotgering and Wallenberg, 1986). At term, fetal urine flow rate averages 500 to 600 ml per day. In near-term fetal sheep using direct methods for measuring urine production rates, similar values have been found (Gresham et al., 1972) although many find urine flow to average close to 1000 ml/day (Wlodek et al., 1988; Brace and Moore, 1991). Recently, Rabinowitz et al. (1989) found human fetal urine flow rates equal to twice those shown in Figure 5–4 when bladder volume measurements were made at 2- to 5-minute intervals rather than the 15- to 30-minute intervals used in previous studies. This difference is attributed to the fact that fetal micturition occurs at 20- to 25-minute intervals. As seen in Figure 5–4, there is a tendency for urine flow rate to decrease after 40 weeks gestation, but this may be better characterized as a failure to increase with advancing gestational age rather than as a decrease. Others found a clear reduction in human fetal urinary output in post-term pregnancies, particularly if oligohydramnios is present (Trimmer et al., 1990).

Any condition that prevents the formation of urine or prevents the entry of urine into the amniotic sac almost invariably results in oligohydramnios. Bain and Scott (1960) reviewed 50 cases of fetal urinary tract malformations, including 28 of renal agenesis, 17 of severe cystic dysplasia, and five of urethral atresia. In all but one case, oligohydramnios was observed. More recent reports fully support the concept that anuria or oliguria is a frequent cause of oligohydramnios (Chamberlain et al., 1984a). Even under less severe conditions, there is an association between a reduced fetal

urine production rate and amniotic volume. In growth-restricted fetuses, amniotic fluid volume is low, as is urine flow rate (VanOtterlo et al., 1977), although this is not found in all cases (Creasy, 1984). In addition, it has long been observed that fetal pulmonary hypoplasia is associated with reduced amniotic fluid in an entity known as Potter's syndrome. The oligohydramnios-associated pulmonary hypoplasia may be due to compression of the fetal chest by the uterine wall (Nakayama et al., 1983). Excess fluid loss from the lungs also contributes (Harding et al., 1990).

In contrast to the relationship between oligohydramnios and low urine flow rates, there is not a strong association between excess fetal urine production and hydramnios. Abramovich et al. (1979) reported that urine production in normal fetuses was not different from that in those with hydramnios. In diabetic pregnancy, it might be expected that fetal hyperglycemia would result in an increased solute load and urinary production rate. However, only 16 of 42 (32 per cent) diabetic patients, and only one of 10 hydramniotic patients, had fetal urinary production rates greater than the 95th percentile (Kurjak et al., 1981). Furthermore, VanOtterlo et al. (1977) found no increase in urinary output in diabetic pregnancies with hydramnios. However, an acute glucose load to pregnant sheep elevated fetal GFR as well as urinary output (Smith and Lumbers, 1989), again suggesting that alterations in fetal renal function may contribute to the association between polyhydramnios and diabetes.

Fetal Swallowing

The human fetus begins swallowing at roughly the same age at which urine first enters the amniotic space, that is, at 8 to 11 weeks gestation. Earlier studies suggested that the volume of amniotic fluid swallowed in late gestation averages 210 to 760 ml per day (Pritchard, 1965). Volumes in excess of 1000 ml per day have been measured in near-term fetal sheep when more detailed methods were used (Tomoda et al., 1985). Relative to fetal weight, swallowed volume increased from 100 ml/kg/day at the beginning of the third trimester to 500 ml/kg/day at term (Tomoda et al., 1985). These daily volumes do not include the amount of tracheal fluid from the lungs (see below) that is swallowed before it enters the amniotic space, and so the total swallowed volume may be considerably higher than these figures indicate. Recent studies have shown that the fetus swallows usually during episodes of fetal breathing activity (Harding et al., 1984) and that fetal breathing is suppressed before the onset of labor (Carmichael et al., 1984), so that the amount of amniotic fluid swallowed by the normal human fetus at or near term may have been underestimated.

It is clear that fetal swallowing plays an important role in determining amniotic fluid volume during the last half of gestation. In a review of 169 cases of hydramnios, Scott and Wilson (1957) were able to attribute the excess amniotic fluid volume to a disturbance in the fetal swallowing mechanism in 54 patients (32 per cent). Furthermore, all cases of esophageal atresia are associated with hydramnios unless there is a communication with the trachea that provides a route for swallowing. A large review of 1745 cases of hydramnios revealed esophageal abnormalities in 27 per cent and other conditions that interfered with fetal swallowing in 18 per cent (Moya et al., 1960). These suggestions that a lack of swallowing mediates the hydramnios is supported by the observation that, in fetal monkeys, esophageal ligation during the last trimester causes hydramnios (Minei and Suzuki, 1976). However, amniotic fluid volume returned to or was below normal with esophageal ligation prior to delivery.

Fetal Respiratory Tract

For many years there had been widespread acceptance of the idea that amniotic fluid entered the fetal lungs by way of the trachea and was absorbed by the capillaries lining the alveoli. Starting in the 1960s, considerable evidence began to accumulate which suggested that an outflow of lung fluid occurred through the trachea rather than an inflow of amniotic fluid. In 1972, Liley reviewed the topic and reported that, following intra-amniotic injection of contrast medium in over 800 patients, ". . . in only four instances, all highly pathological pregnancies, was any contrast medium detectable radiologically or histologically in the fetal or neonatal lung." This is supported by the observation that, although meconium staining of amniotic fluid is common, meconium aspiration is rare and occurs usually under conditions of severe fetal asphyxia. Studies in near-term fetal sheep have shown there is an outflow from the lungs of 200 to 400 ml per day (Adamson et al., 1973), and this is mediated

by an active transport of chloride ions across the epithelial lining of the developing lung. In addition, tracheal ligation in a number of species always leads to an abnormal distention of the fetal lungs. Thus, ample data support the concept that there is a relatively large volume of fluid flowing out of the lungs of the human fetus during normal pregnancy, although this has yet to be quantified.

Even though it is clear that an outflow of fetal lung fluid occurs, the relative contribution of lung fluid to amniotic fluid is unknown. Animal studies suggest that the lung fluid is usually swallowed before it enters the amniotic space (Brace, 1986). In humans, the phospholipids measured in amniotic fluid when L/S ratios are determined are of pulmonary origin and are not passed in significant quantities through the urine. Thus a significant fraction of the secreted lung fluid in human fetuses appears to enter the amniotic fluid.

Fetal Skin

It is possible that amniotic fluid may be derived from water transport across the highly permeable skin of the fetus during the first half of gestation. At 22 to 25 weeks, keratinization of the skin occurs, and it is generally accepted that significant amounts of water and solute are not transferred across this membrane after this time except for small lipid-soluble molecules such as carbon dioxide. However, as recently reviewed, there is ample evidence that the rate of water metabolism and transepidermal water loss is greater in premature newborns (32 to 37 weeks) than in full-term infants, and in very preterm infants (28 to 30 weeks), a further increase occurs (Brace, 1986).

Fetal Membranes

The amnion and chorion provide a large surface area for the potential transfer of both water and solute and hence may play an important role in the regulation of amniotic fluid balance. However, little is known about either net volume or solute movement across the membranes. As noted earlier, an inward transfer of solute across the amnion with water following passively is the most likely source of amniotic fluid very early in gestation. In the latter half of gestation, Liley (1972) and others have suggested that the net water transfer across the amnion is outward while the net electrolyte transfer is inward.

Although this may be correct, direct experimental evidence to support the idea is lacking even though there is indirect support for the concept. Following fetal death, amniotic fluid volume usually decreases, but this should be interpreted with caution because the membranes are undoubtedly changed with fetal death. By summing best estimates of inflows and outflows in the near term fetus (Fig. 5–5), it can be estimated that 200 to 500 ml/day may leave the amniotic space across the fetal membranes during late gestation. The driving force for this fluid movement is available because amniotic fluid has a lower osmolality than either maternal or fetal blood after the fetal

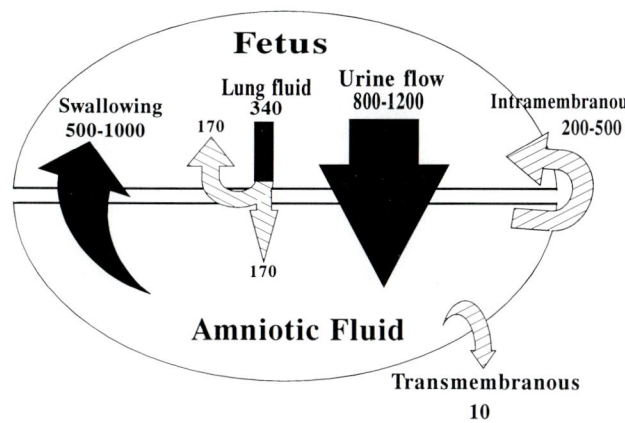

FIGURE 5–5. Estimates of inflows to and outflows from amniotic fluid in the near-term fetus. (From Gilbert WM, Moore TR, Brace RA: Amniotic fluid dynamics. Fetal Medicine Review **3**:89, 1991.)

skin keratinizes. However, quantitative estimates at normal amniotic osmolality suggest that only 10 ml/day may cross the transmembranous route and be absorbed by the uterus in sheep (Anderson et al., 1988). More recently (Gilbert and Brace, 1989), it has been estimated that 200 to 500 ml/day of ovine amniotic fluid are absorbed by the fetal blood, which perfuses the fetal surface of the placenta and perfuses the membranes (the amnion and chorion are vascularized in sheep, but not in humans). This has been referred to as "intramembranous" flow (Gilbert and Brace, 1989), and similar volumes may be absorbed across the fetal surface of the placenta in humans (Gilbert et al., 1991).

Recent studies indicate that the fetal membranes may be abnormal when amniotic fluid volume falls outside its normal range. The amniotic epithelial cell layer is one-half normal thickness in pregnancies complicated by oligohydramnios, whereas thicknesses greater than normal frequently occur with hydramnios (Hebertson et al., 1986). In addition, a chorionic lactogen receptor deficiency occurs in various forms of chronic hydramnios (Healy et al., 1985). Whether these produce or are caused by the aberrations in amniotic fluid volume has yet to be established. However, the observation that fetal prolactin levels are low in diabetic pregnancies (Saltzman et al., 1986) supports the possibility that altered membrane transport may play a role in the etiology of hydramnios.

Other Sources

It has been suggested that significant volumes of water are transferred between the amniotic fluid and the fetal vessels in the umbilical cord (Plentl, 1961). However, with the small surface area and a thickness that is thousands of times that of most membranes across which transfer occurs, it is unlikely that any significant volume exchanges occur across this surface. A more likely site of water and solute exchange is the fetal surface of the placenta in that the chorionic plate has a larger surface area and a rich supply of fetal blood just beneath its surface. Another relevant ob-

servation is that the density of sweat glands in the fetus is higher than in later life (Liley, 1972), but it is unknown whether the fetus sweats *in utero*. Finally, secretions from the nasal and buccal mucosa should be considered. The large amounts of saliva produced by the newborn suggest a similar production by the fetus, and experimental studies in late gestation sheep found that approximately 30 ml per day of fluid was secreted from the fetal head (Brace, 1986).

COMPOSITION OF AMNIOTIC FLUID

During the first third of gestation, amniotic fluid has an electrolyte composition and osmolality that are essentially the same as those of fetal and maternal blood (Fig. 5–6). When fetal urine begins to enter the amniotic sac, amniotic osmolality decreases slightly compared with fetal blood. After keratinization of the fetal skin, amniotic fluid osmolality decreases further with advancing gestational age, reaching values of 250 to 260 mOsm/kg water near term (Fig. 5–6). The amniotic fluid concentration of major solutes such as sodium and chloride ions parallels the changes in osmolality, and disease states involving major alterations in amniotic fluid electrolyte concentrations are virtually unknown. The low amniotic fluid osmolality, which is produced by the inflow of markedly hypotonic fetal urine (60 to 140 mOsm/kg water), provides a large potential osmotic force (19.3 mm Hg for each mOsm/kg gradient in osmolality for an ideal semipermeable membrane) for the flow of water outward across the fetal membranes as well as through the intramembranous pathway. In fetal monkeys, partial exchange of amniotic fluid with distilled water was followed by a restoration of solute concentrations within 24 hours while volume was reduced (Schruefer et al., 1972). In fetal sheep, infusion of one liter of an artificial amniotic saline was followed by a return to normal volume within 24 hours, whereas infusion of

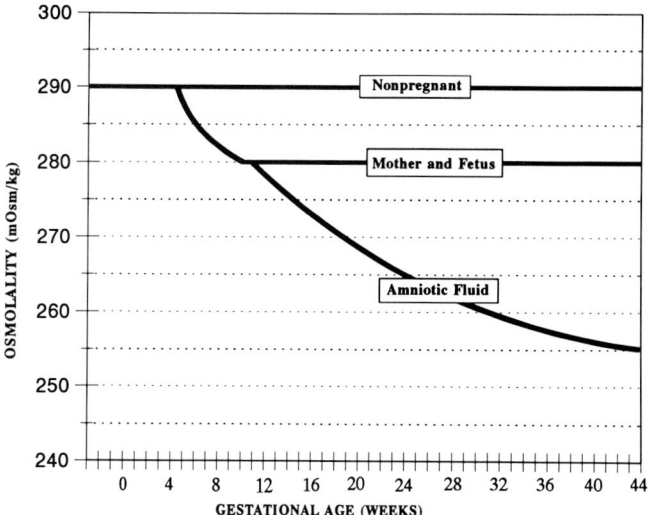

FIGURE 5–6. Gestation changes in osmolality of amniotic fluid and fetal and maternal blood. (From Gilbert WM, Moore TR, Brace RA: Amniotic fluid dynamics. Fetal Medicine Review **3**:98, 1991.)

one liter of isotonic mannitol reduced sodium concentration and elevated volume for more than 24 hours (Tomoda et al., 1987). These data show that both amniotic osmolality and composition play an important role in regulating amniotic fluid volume. This occurs primarily by altering the intramembranous movement of solutes and water, although transmembranous flow may change as well. From theory, the extent of intramembranous and transmembrane water and solute movement depends on the filtration and permeability characteristics of the fetal membranes, but these have yet to be determined *in vivo* in humans. In sheep, the filtration coefficient of the intramembranous pathway averages 5 per cent that of the placenta (Gilbert and Brace, 1990), whereas that of the transmembranous pathway is about 10-fold lower (Anderson et al., 1988).

Because of the large surface area of the chorioamnion, it has often been suggested there may be large amounts of water and solutes moving across the membranes. Thus, it is not surprising that membrane permeability frequently has been proposed to be an important regulator of amniotic fluid volume (Lingwood and Wintour, 1984). Although membrane permeability is critically important, little is known about the filtration and permeability characteristics of the membranes *in vivo* as they relate to amniotic fluid dynamics because of a sparsity of studies and sometimes conflicting interpretations. For example, the increase in amniotic fluid osmolality following the intravenous injection of hypertonic fluids into pregnant sheep was interpreted to be due to a net transmembranous movement of water (Ross et al., 1983). However, this was shown to be due to an increase in fetal urine osmolality (Woods, 1986). A great deal more information about intramembranous and transmembranous movements is needed in order to put in perspective the role of the membranes and fetal surface of the placenta in determining amniotic fluid volume.

REGULATION OF AMNIOTIC FLUID VOLUME

Although many theories have been advanced to explain the accumulation of amniotic fluid, there currently is little detailed knowledge of the determinants of amniotic fluid volume in the majority of circumstances. It is safe to state that, if amniotic fluid volume is regulated, then one or more of the inflows and/or outflows must be adjusted so as to maintain amniotic fluid volume at close to normal. However, it is not known whether amniotic fluid volume is, in fact, regulated. It has often been argued that amniotic fluid volume must be regulated because volume late in gestation falls within the range of 0.5 to 2 liters most of the time. This concept is supported by animal studies in which amniotic fluid volume returned toward normal following experimental increases or decreases in volume (Tomoda et al., 1987), but these observations do not prove that volume regulation exists.

Irrespective of the question of whether direct volume regulation occurs, it is clear that there are three main areas in which research is needed in order to provide a better understanding of the determinants of amniotic fluid volume. These are (1) water and solute transfer within and across the membranes including the fetal surface of the placenta, (2) regulation of inflows and outflows from the fetus, and (3) maternal effects on fetal fluid balance.

There are two approaches for understanding fluid movements between the fetus and the amniotic space. The first is to examine the regulation of the individual flows that enter and leave the amniotic space. A considerable amount is known about the regulation of fetal urine flow and composition. These are modulated by arginine vasopressin, aldosterone, angiotensin II, and atrial natriuretic peptide in ways that are qualitatively similar to regulation in the adult. The rate of production of fluid by the fetal lungs is affected by several hormones, including arginine vasopressin, and epinephrine (Brace, 1986), and the progressive decrease in flow that begins 3 days before delivery correlates inversely with plasma cortisol concentrations (Kitterman et al., 1979). In contrast, the factors that regulate fetal swallowing are poorly understood. In the human fetus, swallowing is reduced following intra-amniotic injection of an oil that tastes "vile," but injection of saccharin produced inconsistent results (Liley, 1972). Animal studies have shown that fetal swallowing of amniotic fluid per kilogram of body weight increases as gestation progresses, that neither the frequency nor the extent of swallowing depends on outflow from the trachea or the volume of the gastric compartment, that swallowing occurs only during episodes of fetal breathing activity, and that swallowing decreases to near zero prior to delivery or fetal demise (Brace, 1986). Recent data in humans indicate that fetal breathing activity may be absent before the onset of labor (Carmichael et al., 1984), suggesting that swallowing in human fetuses may also terminate prior to labor and delivery.

The second approach for understanding the regulation of inflows and outflows from the fetus is to consider the amniotic fluid as a reservoir for the fetus. Since all of the control mechanisms for fluid volume regulation within the fetus appear to be functional in the latter half of gestation, it is reasonable to assume that the fetus would maintain its fluid status at the expense of amniotic fluid volume. Thus, an overhydrated fetus would transfer its excess fluid into the amniotic space; conversely, a dehydrated fetus would restore its hydration by absorbing amniotic fluid.

Finally, the mother may affect amniotic fluid. Because fluid moves with relative ease between fetal and maternal blood across the placenta, the maternal effects on fetal hydration could be the ultimate controller of amniotic fluid volume. There are ample data showing that acute changes in maternal osmolality alter fetal hydration, but whether there are associated changes in amniotic fluid volume is less clear. In a study yet to be confirmed, Goodlin et al. (1983) reported that, if fetal anomalies and diabetes are excluded, there is a strong relationship between maternal plasma volume during pregnancy and amniotic fluid volume, so that subnormal plasma volume expansion is associated with oligohydramnios and elevated plasma volume with hydramnios. In addition, when the maternal plasma volume deficit was corrected with intravenous fluids, the oligohydramnios frequently was resolved. In contrast, studies in pregnant sheep have shown that severe sodium depletion over 6 days caused a large decrease in maternal plasma volume and sodium ion concentration with an increase in amniotic fluid volume (Phillips and Sundaram, 1966). Thus, the maternal effects on amniotic fluid have yet to be clearly delineated. Nonetheless, important studies are beginning to characterize the maternal effects on amniotic volume. For example, Kilpatrick et al. (1991) reported that ingestion of 2 liters of water in women with a low amniotic fluid index (AFI) resulted in a significant 31 per cent increase in AFI. More studies are needed in this area.

In summary, there is a wide range of amniotic fluid volumes during normal human pregnancy. Aberrations in volume outside the normal range are frequently associated with fetal anomalies or poor perinatal outcome or both (see Chapter 40). When fetal anomalies are excluded, there are three major determinants of amniotic fluid volume. These are the movements of water and solutes within and across the membranes, physiologic regulation by the fetus of flow rates such as urine production and swallowing, and maternal effects on transplacental fluid movement.

REFERENCES

Abramovich DR, Page KP: Pathways of water transfer between liquor amnii and the feto-placental unit at term. Eur J Obstet Gynaecol 3:155, 1973.

Abramovich DR, Garden A, Landial J, et al: Fetal swallowing and voiding in relation to hydramnios. Obstet Gynecol 54:15, 1979.

Adamson TM, Brodecky V, Lambert TF, et al: The production and composition of lung liquid in the in-utero foetal lamb. In Comline RS, et al (eds): Foetal and Neonatal Physiology. Cambridge, England, Cambridge University Press, 1973.

Anderson DF, Faber JJ, Parks CM: Extraplacental transfer of water in the sheep. J Physiol 406:75, 1988.

Bain AD, Scott JS: Renal agenesis and severe urinary tract dysplasia. A review of 50 cases with particular reference to the associated anomalies. Br Med J 1:841, 1960.

Bastide A, Manning F, Harmon C, et al: Ultrasound evaluation of amniotic fluid: Outcome of pregnancies with severe oligohydramnios. Am J Obstet Gynecol 154:895, 1986.

Brace RA: Amniotic fluid volume and its relationship to fetal fluid balance: Review of experimental data. Semin Perinatol 10:103, 1986.

Brace RA, Wolf EJ: Normal amniotic fluid volume changes throughout pregnancy. Am J Obstet Gynecol 161:382, 1989.

Brace RA, Moore TR: Diurnal rhythms in fetal urine flow, vascular pressures, and heart rate in sheep. Am J Physiol 261:R1015, 1991.

Carmichael L, Campbell K, Patrick J: Fetal breathing, gross fetal body movements, and maternal and fetal heart rates before spontaneous labor at term. Am J Obstet Gynecol 148:675, 1984.

Chamberlain PF, Manning FA, Morrison I, et al: Ultrasound evaluation of amniotic fluid volume. I. The relationship of marginal and decreased amniotic fluid volumes to perinatal outcome. Am J Obstet Gynecol 150:245, 1984a.

Chamberlain PF, Manning FA, Morrison I, et al: Ultrasound evaluation of amniotic fluid volume. II. The relationship of increased amniotic fluid volumes to perinatal outcome. Am J Obstet Gynecol 150:250, 1984b.

Creasy RK: Biophysical aspects of management of the growth retarded fetus. Semin Perinatol 8:56, 1984.

Elliott PM, Inman WHW: Volume of liquor amnii in normal and abnormal pregnancy. Lancet ii:836, 1961.

Gilbert WM, Brace RA: The missing link in amniotic fluid volume regulation: intramembranous absorption. Obstet Gynecol 74:748, 1989.

Gilbert WM, Brace RA: Novel determination of filtration coefficient of ovine placenta and intramembranous pathway. Am J Physiol. 259:R1281, 1990.

Gilbert WM, Moore TR, Brace RA: Amniotic fluid dynamics. Fetal Medicine Review 3:89, 1991.

Gitlin D, Dumate J, Morales C, et al: The turnover of amniotic fluid protein in the human conceptus. Am J Obstet Gynecol 113:632, 1972.

Goodlin RC, Anderson JC, Gallagher TF: Relationship between amniotic fluid volume and maternal plasma volume expansion. Am J Obstet Gynecol 146:505, 1983.

Gresham EL, Rankin JH, Makowski EL, et al: An evaluation of fetal renal function in a chronic sheep preparation. J Clin Invest 51:149, 1972.

Harding R, Bocking AD, Sigger JN, et al: Composition and volume of fluid swallowed by fetal sheep. Q J Exp Physiol 69:487, 1984.

Harding R, Hooper SB, Dickson KA: A mechanism leading to reduced lung expansion and lung hypoplasia in fetal sheep during oligohydramnios. Am J Ob Gyn 163:1904, 1990.

Healy DL, Herington AC, O'Herlihy C: Chronic polyhydramnios is a syndrome with a lactogen receptor defect in the chorion laeve. Br J Obstet Gynaecol 92:461, 1985.

Hebertson RM, Hammond ME, Bryson MJ: Amniotic epithelial ultrastructure in normal, polyhydramnic, and oligohydramnic pregnancies. Obstet Gynecol 68:74, 1986.

Kilpatrick SJ, Safford KL, Pomeroy T, et al: Maternal hydration increases amniotic fluid index. Obstet Gynecol 78:1098, 1991.

Kitterman JA, Ballard PL, Clements JA, et al: Tracheal fluid in fetal lambs: Spontaneous decrease prior to birth. J Appl Physiol 47:985, 1979.

Kurjak A, Kirkinen P, Latin V, et al: Ultrasonic assessment of fetal kidney function in normal and complicated pregnancies. Am J Obstet Gynecol 141:266, 1981.

Landis EM, Pappenheimer JR: Exchange of substances through capillary walls. In Handbook of Physiology, Circulation, Vol 2, Sec 2. Bethesda, American Physiological Society, 1963.

Liley AW: Disorders of amniotic fluid. In Assali NS (ed): Pathophysiology of Gestation. New York, Academic Press, 1972.

Lingwood BE, Wintour EM: Amniotic fluid volume and in vivo permeability of ovine fetal membranes. Obstet Gynecol 64:368, 1984.

Lotgering FK, Wallenburg HCS: Mechanisms of production and clearance of amniotic fluid. Semin Perinatol 10:94, 1986.

Mercer LJ, Brown LG, Petres RE, et al: A survey of pregnancies complicated by decreased amniotic fluid. Am J Obstet Gynecol 149:355, 1984.

Minei LJ, Suzuki K: Role of fetal deglutition and micturition in the production and turnover of amniotic fluid in the monkey. Obstet Gynecol 48:177, 1976.

Moya F, Apgar V, St James L, et al: Hydramnios and congenital anomalies. JAMA 173:1552, 1960.

Nakayama PD, Glick PL, Harrison MR, et al: Experimental pulmonary hypoplasia due to oligohydramnios and its reversal by relieving thoracic compression. J Pediatr Surg 18:347, 1983.

Phillips GD, Sundaram SK: Sodium depletion of pregnant ewes and its effects on foetuses and foetal fluids. J Physiol 184:889, 1966.

Plentl AA: Transfer of water across perfused umbilical cord. Proc Soc Exp Biol Med 107:622, 1961.

Pritchard JA: Deglutition by normal and anencephalic fetuses. Obstet Gynecol 25:289, 1965.

Rabinowitz R, Peters MT, Vyas S, et al: Measurement of fetal urine production in normal pregnancy by real-time ultrasonography. Am J Obstet Gynecol 161:1264, 1989.

Ross MG, Ervin MG, Leake RD, et al: Bulk flow of amniotic water in response to maternal osmotic challenge. Am J Obstet Gynecol 147:697, 1983.

Saltzman DH, Barbieri RL, Frigoletto FD: Decreased fetal cord prolactin concentration in diabetic pregnancies. Am J Obstet Gynecol 154:1035, 1986.

Schruefer JJ, Seeds AE, Behrman RE, et al: Changes in amniotic fluid volume and total solute concentration in the rhesus monkey following replacement with distilled water. Am J Obstet Gynecol **112**:807, 1972.

Scott JS, Wilson LK: Hydramnios as an early sign of oesophageal atresia. Lancet **ii**:569, 1957.

Seeds AE: Current concepts of amniotic fluid dynamics. Am J Obstet Gynecol **138**:575, 1980.

Smith FG, Lumbers E: Effects of maternal hyperglycemia on fetal renal function in sheep. Am J Physiol **255**:F11, 1989.

Tomoda S, Brace RA, Longo LD: Amniotic fluid volume and fetal swallowing rate in sheep. Am J Physiol **249**:R133, 1985.

Tomoda S, Brace RA, Longo LD: Amniotic fluid volume regulation: Basal values and responses to fluid infusion and withdrawal in sheep. Am J Physiol **252**:R380, 1987.

Trimmer KJ, Leveno KJ, Peters MT, et al: Observations on the cause of oligohydramnios in prolonged pregnancy. Am J Obstet Gynecol **163**:1900, 1990.

VanOtterlo LC, Wladimiroff JW, Wallenburg HCS: Relationship between fetal urine production and amniotic fluid volume in normal pregnancy and pregnancy complicated by diabetes. Br J Obstet Gynaecol **84**:205, 1977.

Wlodek ME, Challis JRG, Patrick J: Urethral and urachal urine output to the amniotic and allantoic sacs in fetal sheep. J Devel Physiol **10**:309, 1988.

Woods LL: Fetal renal contribution to amniotic fluid osmolality during maternal hypertonicity. Am J Physiol **250**:R235, 1986.

Zamah NM, Gillieson MS, Walters JH, Hall PF: Sonographic detection of polyhydramnios: A five-year experience. Am J Obstet Gynecol **143**:523, 1982.

CHAPTER

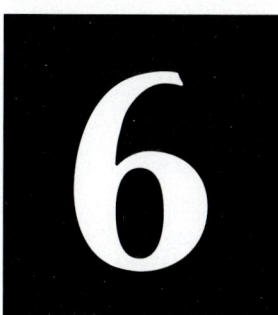

6

THE IMMUNOLOGY OF PREGNANCY

D. WARE BRANCH, M.D., and JAMES R. SCOTT, M.D.

Two unique and fascinating immunologic stories unfold during pregnancy. First, a fetus living in an isolated, sterile environment develops the essential framework of the immune system so that it can mount a respectable, albeit somewhat immature, immunologic response as a neonate and infant. The other story takes place at the maternal-fetal interface, where a combination of fetal and maternal immunologic factors conspire to allow, and perhaps encourage, the growth of the semi-allogeneic conceptus. To fully understand how these two stories evolve would be to completely understand immunology itself; as yet, only part of either story is revealed. This chapter will provide a review of the ontogeny of the fetal immune response and the immunologic relationship between the mother and conceptus. A basic understanding of these areas is not simply of academic interest; numerous diseases of the fetus or fetus and mother are due to aberrations in the normal immunology of pregnancy. Pathologic conditions now known or suspected to be due to immunologic mechanisms include certain neonatal and childhood illnesses, early pregnancy loss, fetal death, fetal growth impairment, preeclampsia, and preterm labor, as well as the obvious alloimmune hemolytic disease of the fetus and neonatal alloimmune thrombocytopenia.

FETAL AND NEONATAL IMMUNITY

Nature builds the structural framework of a normal immune system *in utero* and then completes immune development in the neonate and child. It is convenient to describe the immune system in terms of two interactive and complementary responses: *innate* and *adaptive*. In both systems, immune effector cells communicate with each other and with nonimmune cells via cytokines, small proteins secreted by the cells that have specific effects on other cells. A detailed discussion of the current understanding of cytokines and cytokine actions is beyond the scope of this chapter. For the purpose of brief description, the recognized cytokines can be categorized into *inflammatory, T cell derived lymphokines,* and *growth factors* (Table 6–1).

There is obviously a large overlap in terms of these somewhat arbitrarily assigned categories.

Innate immunity involves immune responses that depend only on the foreign nature of the inciting antigen; a specific antigen is not required for the immune response. The first line of defense in the innate immune system is comprised of physical and biochemical barriers to the entry of foreign material. In neonates, children, and adults, the most obvious physical barrier consists of the skin and mucosal surfaces, with the latter being further protected by substances in secretions such as lysozymes. Additionally, the fetus is even better protected by several layers of maternal tissue; even the amniotic fluid that surrounds the fetus has immunologic functions such as bacteriostasis.

The primary effector cells of innate immunity are phagocytes (monocytes or macrophages), granulocytes, and natural killer (NK) cells, all of which are derived from bone marrow stem cells. Both phagocytes and granulocytes destroy or remove foreign antigen by phagocytosis (Fig. 6–1). These cells are located throughout the body in areas where they are likely to encounter invading organisms. Consider, for example, the strategic location of alveolar macrophages and the tissue macrophages of the spleen and liver. NK cells are nonphagocytic lymphocytes that do not require specialized antigen presentation for the recognition of foreign antigen. They are particularly adept at recognizing the surface markers on virus-infected cells or tumor cells (Fig. 6–1). One of the primary cytokine groups of the innate immune system consists of the interferons, which are produced by virus-infected cells. Interferons activate NK cells and induce resistance to viral infection in neighboring host cells. Certain circulating factors, such as the acute phase proteins and complement, are also part of the innate immune system. C-reactive protein binds to the surface of certain types of bacteria and promotes phagocytosis. Complement is activated by the surface of some organisms via the alternative pathway. In turn, the complement system has the ability to lyse some bacteria without cellular help, and complement bound to the organism can facilitate phagocytosis.

115

Table 6–1. Cellular Sources, Target Cells, and Principal Activities of Cytokines

CYTOKINE	CELLULAR SOURCES	TARGET CELLS	PRINCIPAL ACTIVITIES
Inflammatory Cytokines			
Interleukin-1α	Macrophages	T and B cells	Lymphocyte activation, prostaglandin production
Interleukin-1β	Monocytes, LGLs, B cells, fibroblasts, endothelial cells	Macrophages, endothelial cells, fibroblasts	Macrophage stimulation, pyrexia, enhanced leukocyte-endothelial interaction, tissue regeneration, enhanced MHC expression
Tumor necrosis factor	Macrophages, cytotoxic T cells, NK cells	Macrophages, neutrophils, fibroblasts	Cachexia, enhanced leukocyte-endothelial interaction, macrophage activation, enhanced cytotoxicity
Interleukin-6	Macrophages, fibroblasts	Macrophages, endothelial cells, hepatocytes	Acute phase response, T cell activation, B cell antibody production, prostaglandin production
Interleukin-8	Macrophages, monocytes, endothelial cells, keratinocytes, fibroblasts	Neutrophils, T cells, basophils	Neutrophil activation and degranulation, chemotactic for neutrophils and T cells
T Cell Derived Lymphokines			
Interleukin-2	Activated CD4+ T cells, NK cells	CD4+ and CD8+ T cells	T cell growth and proliferation
Interleukin-3	Activated CD4+ T cells	Hematopoietic precursors, stem cells, mast cells	Promotes growth and differentiation of myeloid progenitor cells
Interleukin-4	Activated CD4+ T cells	B cells, eosinophils	B cell growth and differentiation, IgE production, eosinophilia
Interleukin-5	Activated CD4+ T cells	B cells	B cell differentiation, antibody isotype switching
Interleukin-6	Activated CD4+ T cells	B cells	B cell differentiation into plasma cells with high-rate antibody production
Interferon -γ	Activated CD4+ T cells, NK cells	CD4+ and CD8+ T cells, macrophages	Enhance MHC class II expression, macrophage activation, enhance endothelial-leukocyte interaction

Finally, some products of the activated complement cascade attract other phagocytes.

The adaptive immune system involves two types of antigen-specific immune responses: cellular and humoral (antibody). For many adaptive responses, the phagocytic cells, described above as part of the innate immune system, must first process ingested antigen and present it for recognition by the mature lymphocytes of the adaptive immune system (Fig. 6–2). Mature T cells recognize foreign antigen only when it is presented by a phagocytic antigen processing cell in the context of other self-antigens, specifically major histocompatibility complex (MHC) antigens. The T cells then develop surface receptors for the specific foreign antigen. When this antigen is again "seen" by the T cells, a complex arrangement of events results in proliferation of the T cells specific for the antigen ("clonal proliferation") (Fig. 6–2). The nature of the T cells involved strongly influences the immune response. So-called *cytotoxic* T cells kill target cells when they recognize and bind the specific antigen in the context of MHC antigens. T *helper* cells stimulate innate immune system responses and antibody production by B lymphocytes. Finally, T *suppressor* cells specifically suppress the activity of macrophages, B cells, and T helper cells.

The primary immune function of B lymphocytes is the production of immunoglobulins (antibodies) spe-

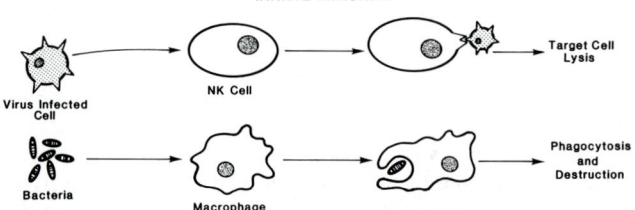

FIGURE 6–1. Summary of innate immunity. Surface antigens of viruses, bacteria, and tumors induce innate immune system function. In this system, natural killer (NK) cells and phagocytes, such as macrophages, can recognize certain antigens in a nonspecific fashion and either lyse the offending infected cells or tumor cells or ingest and destroy the offending organisms. Note that only the foreign nature of the antigen is required; antigen processing and major histocompatibility antigen participation are not necessary.

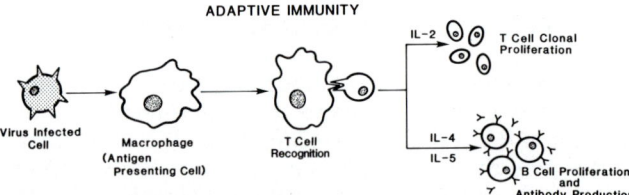

FIGURE 6–2. Summary of adaptive immunity. Adaptive immune responses initially require antigen processing and subsequent presentation to T cells. A T cell with a receptor specific for an inciting antigen will be activated and undergo clonal proliferation. In part, the type of cytokine produced by the activated T cell dictates the nature of the subsequent response. IL-2 is the primary growth factor required for clonal proliferation of T cells and stimulates the proliferation of cytotoxic and memory T cells. IL-4 and IL-5 stimulate B cell differentiation and proliferation for antibody production.

cific for a certain foreign antigen. The specificity of B cells is derived from a process known as gene rearrangement, which creates myriad possible immunoglobulin antigen-recognition sites and thus allows for a large immunoglobulin repertoire. Cells making antibodies that bind to the antigen are stimulated to undergo clonal proliferation and then differentiate into plasma cells, the mature antibody-secreting descendant of B lymphocytes. Antibodies facilitate the immune destruction of organisms or infected cells to which they are bound by promoting phagocytosis and membrane lysis.

In general terms, viruses and parasites tend to elicit the generation of T cell adaptive immune responses (cellular immune response), and bacteria tend to elicit B cell antibody responses (humoral immune response). The capacity of the adaptive immune system to respond to a new foreign antigen is virtually limitless. Throughout, the complex immune responses are modulated and regulated by cytokines. The final adaptive response is an impressive and changing array of immune stimulation and suppression.

Development of Fetal and Neonatal Innate Immunity

The immune effector cells of the innate immune system arise from hematopoietic progenitor cells first noted in the blood islands of the embryonic yolk sac. By 8 weeks gestation, the yolk sac is replaced by the fetal liver as the source of these cells, and by 20 weeks gestation, almost all of the hematopoietic progenitor cells are derived from the fetal bone marrow. These pluripotential hematopoietic cells respond to a variety of stimuli by differentiation and proliferation (Fauser and Messner, 1978, 1979; Messner and Fauser, 1980; Messner et al., 1981), giving rise to granulocytes and macrophages. In contrast to laboratory rodents, macrophage-like cells are found quite early in human gestation, appearing at the yolk sac stage of embryonic development (Beelen et al., 1990). Circulating monocytes, which differentiate into macrophages in the tissue, are present in the fetus by 16 weeks gestation (Steihm, 1975). The numbers of circulating monocytes in term neonates is similar to that in adults, but there are fewer tissue macrophages. This appears to be due to diminished monocyte infiltration into sites of inflammation in the neonate. The number of tissue macrophages does not reach adult levels until age 6 to 10 years (Klein et al., 1977). However, the phagocytic and antigen-processing capacities of neonatal macrophages are similar to those of adult cells.

Granulocytes appear in the fetal spleen and liver at 8 weeks gestation and in the fetal circulation by 12 to 14 weeks. In contrast to adults, no more than 10 per cent of the leukocytes in the fetal circulation are granulocytes, and a substantial number of these are functionally immature granulocyte precursors (Forestier et al., 1986). After delivery, the numbers of granulocytes increase dramatically, reaching or exceeding adult proportions by 48 to 72 hours. However, neonates are not so capable as adults of greatly increasing neutrophil production, a deficit that may contribute to the relatively high rate of neutropenia seen in severe neonatal infection. In addition, infiltration of inflammatory sites by neonatal neutrophils is diminished to about half that of adults and does not reach normal levels until age 2. Phagocytosis and bacterial killing by neonatal granulocytes are intact at levels comparable to those in adults (Gluck and Silverman, 1957; McCracken and Eichenwald, 1971).

NK cells are of uncertain lineage, but may be detected in the fetal liver after 8 weeks gestation (Uksila et al., 1983). By term, the proportion of NK cells in the circulation is similar to that of adults. However, neonatal NK cells have only 25 to 50 per cent of the cytolytic activity of adult cells (Lubens et al., 1982), and NK cytolytic activity does not reach adult levels until about the age of 5 years.

Many circulating protein components of the innate immune system appear by the middle of the second trimester. The fetal liver makes C4 and C2 as early as 8 weeks gestation (Colten, 1976; Colten and Goldberger, 1979). By 18 weeks gestation, C1, C3, C5, C7, and C9 are detectable in fetal serum, but the concentrations of these complement components remain low until the third trimester, when they begin to increase. By term, most complement proteins are found in levels approaching 50 per cent of adult levels (Ballow et al., 1974). Complement levels approach those of the normal adult by about one year of age. At term, the hemolytic activity of complement is about 40 per cent of adult levels for the classic pathway and 55 per cent of adult levels for the alternative pathway, but there is considerable individual variation (Johnston et al., 1979; Notarangelo et al., 1984).

Fetal and Neonatal Development of Adaptive Immunity

T cells also are derived from the pluripotential hematopoietic cells first seen in the yolk sac. In order to differentiate into T cells, these cells must first migrate to the thymus, an organ whose sole function appears to be T cell nurture and development. The fetal thymus is colonized by T cell precursors by 8 weeks gestation. Most are immature T cells, or stage I thymocytes, that express neither CD4 nor CD8 T cell surface adhesion molecules and are located in the cortical zone of the thymus. In the next stage of maturation, the thymocytes express both CD4 and CD8, but do not express the T cell receptor (TcR)-CD3 complex (TcR-CD3). After the final stage of maturation, the mature T cell expresses either the CD4 or CD8 molecule as well as the TcR-CD3 complex. By 12 to 16 weeks gestation, the fetal thymus contains T cells in each stage of development and in proportions similar to those found in the adult (Lobach et al., 1985). Compared to the adult, the mass of the thymus relative to the body weight is relatively large in late fetal life, infancy, and childhood, suggesting that the immune system is somehow triggered to greatly expand the T cell pool over this period. The gland begins to involute around the onset of puberty.

The sine qua non of the functional mature T cell is the TcR. This receptor is structurally similar to immunoglobulin, consisting of two disulfide-linked chains. Two TcR heterodimers have been described: one is the gamma/delta heterodimer and the other is the alpha/beta heterodimer. Cells bearing the gamma/delta TcR are the first to appear in the fetus, but their functional significance is unknown. They represent a small proportion of all T cells in postnatal life. The vast majority of mature circulating T cells express the alpha/beta heterodimer. To be functional, the TcR must be linked to the CD3 protein. This TcR-CD3 complex can bind specific antigen via TcR and subsequently initiate T cell activation and proliferation via transmembrane signalling by CD3. Some circulating T cells in the neonate do not express CD3 and are probably immature T cells. The proportion of these immature cells is greater in premature infants, probably contributing to the relative lack of T cell immunity in preterm infants.

Mature T cells recognize foreign antigen only when it is presented by antigen-presenting cells in the context of host (self) surface membrane antigens of the MHC system (Fig. 6–3). This absolute requirement for MHC antigen is known as "MHC restriction." Broadly speaking, there are two types of MHC antigens involved in this process. Class I MHC antigens (HLA-A, -B, and -C in humans) are present on most cells in the body. Antigen presented with class I MHC molecules is recognized by T cells with the CD8 surface adhesion molecule. CD8-positive T cells usually act as either cytotoxic or suppressor cells. Class II MHC molecules are expressed by far fewer cell types, including macrophages. Antigen presented with class II MHC molecules is recognized by T cells bearing the CD4 adhesion molecule. These T cells usually act as T helper cells, inducing other T cells to become active in the immune response. In the newborn, the proportion of CD4+ T cells and CD8+ T cells is similar to that of the adult (Griffiths-Chu et al., 1984; Solinger, 1985), and T helper cell function appears intact. However, several aspects of neonatal T cells are seemingly immature. For example, neonatal T cells make little interferon-γ in response to mitogen or antigen (Wilson et al., 1986). Furthermore, neonatal T cells have only about 50 per cent of the cytotoxic activity of adult cells after sensitization (Granberg and Hirvonen, 1980). Studies of perinatally acquired neonatal viral infections show that the specific T cell response is delayed compared to that of adults (Sullender et al., 1987) and is probably not normal until about 2 months of age.

Interestingly, neonatal T suppressor cells will suppress the proliferative response of adult T cells (e.g., maternal T cell proliferation), but not neonatal T cell proliferation (Olding et al., 1977; Oldstone et al., 1977). This paradoxical characteristic of fetal T suppressor cells is present by 8 weeks gestation (Unander and Olding, 1981) and may represent one way in which the conceptus protects itself from the maternal immune response. Stimulated neonatal T cells also suppress adult B cell immunoglobulin production (Oldstone et al., 1977).

The crucial role of the thymus and the development of a normal cellular immune system is evident in infants born with DiGeorge syndrome, a condition associated with aplasia or hypoplasia of the thymus. The embryologic lesion involves a failure of normal development of the thymus from the pharyngeal pouch. The condition is also associated with a failure of parathyroid gland development, also a pharyngeal pouch derivative, and with temporally related developmental abnormalities of the philtrum of the lip, ears, and aortic arch. Immunologically, the infants have moderate-to-severe T cell deficiency resulting in lymphopenia, susceptibility to viruses, and a propensity to graft-versus-host reactions following blood transfusions. The thymic development of T cells results in immune cells that can differentiate between self and non-self, and a failure of normal thymic development and function is implicated in the genesis of murine autoimmune disease (Theofilopoulos and Dixon, 1985).

Cells destined to become B cells differentiate from hematopoietic precursors in the fetal liver by 8 weeks gestation and the fetal bone marrow by 12 weeks. These pre-B cells do not have functional antigen receptors. The earliest B cells to appear bear surface IgM and are found in fetal liver at about 9 weeks gestation. B cells bearing IgG and IgA are present by 10 to 15 weeks gestation. Unlike adult B cells, fetal B cells that express IgG or IgA also express IgM. IgM-secreting plasma cells, which are the antibody-secreting cells derived from B lymphocytes, appear by 15 weeks gestation, while those that secrete IgG or IgA appear at 20 to 30 weeks gestation. However, significant production of IgM antibody does not occur until the early third trimester, and the levels of fetal IgM and IgA found in normal neonatal serum are 10 per cent and 1 per cent of adult levels, respectively. Neonatal levels of IgM are increased in infants suffering some intrauterine infections, indicating that the fetus can mount an antibody response. Total cord IgM concentrations >20 mg/dl suggest an intrauterine infection, and organism-specific IgM may be found. However, the ability of the neonate and, presumably, the fetus to respond to antigens is limited. For example, the

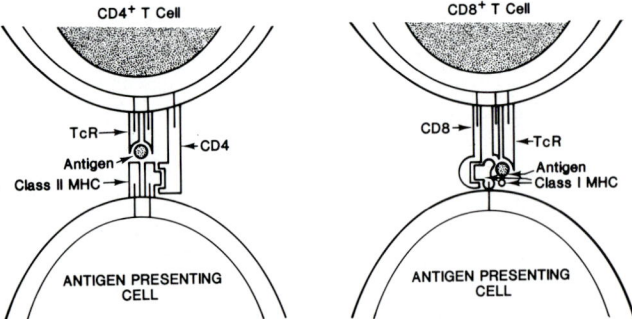

FIGURE 6–3. T cell receptor (TcR) and antigen recognition. T cells recognize foreign antigen in the context of self major histocompatibility antigen (MHC) when it is presented in this context by antigen presenting cells (e.g., macrophages). Antigen presented with class II MHC molecules (left side of figure) is recognized by T cells bearing the CD4 adhesion molecule. Such cells usually act as T "helper" cells. Antigen presented with class I MHC molecules (right side of figure) is recognized by T cells bearing the CD8 adhesion molecule. Such T cells usually act as cytotoxic T cells or T "suppressor" cells.

neonatal antibody response to bacterial polysaccharides is decreased, accounting in part for the neonate's susceptibility to certain bacterial infections (Baker et al., 1981).

Maternal IgG is transported across the placenta as early as the late first trimester, but the efficiency of transport is poor (Morell et al., 1986) so that total fetal IgG levels are low until the late second or early third trimester. For this reason, premature infants are not as well protected by maternal antibodies. The term neonate has IgG concentrations similar to or slightly greater than that of the adult, with virtually all the IgG being maternal in origin. Fetal and neonatal IgG production is limited, and IgG production similar to that of the adult is not reached until late childhood or early puberty.

Immunoglobulin proteins are composed of two identical heavy and two identical light amino acid chains (Fig. 6–4). The heavy and light chains are coded for by separate genes, and regions within each chain are coded for by corresponding gene segments. The antigen-binding portion of the molecule is made by the combination of highly variable regions within the heavy and light chains. An astonishingly wide diversity of immunoglobulin molecules can be generated by rearrangement of the gene segments responsible for the molecule in the developing B cells. Although a detailed description is beyond the scope of this review, the process of gene rearrangement allows a large number of different immunoglobulin molecules to be made from a relatively small number of somatic genes. Rearranged genes are present in pre-B cells and B cells, but each cell makes only one immunoglobulin, which is placed on its surface as an antigen receptor. When an antigen is recognized by the immunoglobulin expressed on the surface of the B cell, the B cell is stimulated to proliferate (clonal proliferation). Cells expressing antibody that binds the antigen more avidly are more strongly stimulated to proliferate. In this fashion, specific antibody-secreting cells are selected by antigen exposure.

Maturation of B lymphocytes into plasma cells is associated with the cell's acquiring the ability to secrete the antibody. This developmental process is regulated by the type of antigen, by local factors, and by the influences of other immune cells, including T cells and macrophages. For example, the production of antibodies to many protein antigens requires antigen processing by macrophages, antigen recognition by T helper cells, and eventual stimulation of B cells by T cell secreted cytokines such as interleukin-1 and interleukin-4. In contrast, plasma cells can develop independently of T cells in response to other antigens, particularly large compounds such as polysaccharides or lipopolysaccharides. This T cell independent B cell response is the last to appear in the human neonate, in part accounting for the poor neonatal antibody response to certain bacterial antigens such as the capsule of group B streptococci (Baker et al., 1981). The neonatal response to antigens requiring a T cell response appears to be normal (Van Tol et al., 1983).

The unfortunate consequences of poor antibody production are seen in X-linked hypogammaglobulinemia, a disease of males characterized by the absence of B cells in the peripheral circulation and markedly low levels of IgG as well as the absence of IgM and other classes of antibodies. Affected infants usually become ill with chronic bacterial infections as maternally acquired IgG gradually declines below significant levels starting at 4 to 6 months of age. The most severe of the congenital immunodeficiency syndromes is known as severe combined immunodeficiency syndrome. This disease occurs as an X-linked recessive, an autosomal recessive, or a sporadic form and is characterized by an absence of B and T cell immunity, probably due to a failure of the differentiation of hematopoietic stem cells. Individuals with this condition are susceptible to virtually any infection, viral or bacterial, and rarely live beyond the age of one year.

To summarize normal neonatal immunity, aspects of both the innate and adaptive immune responses are limited compared to that of the adult. In the adaptive system, both T cell and antibody responses are diminished. Neonatal protection by passively acquired maternal IgG is probably substantial, but is imperfect. As a consequence of these limitations, the neonate, and particularly the premature neonate, is relatively susceptible to systemic bacterial and viral infections.

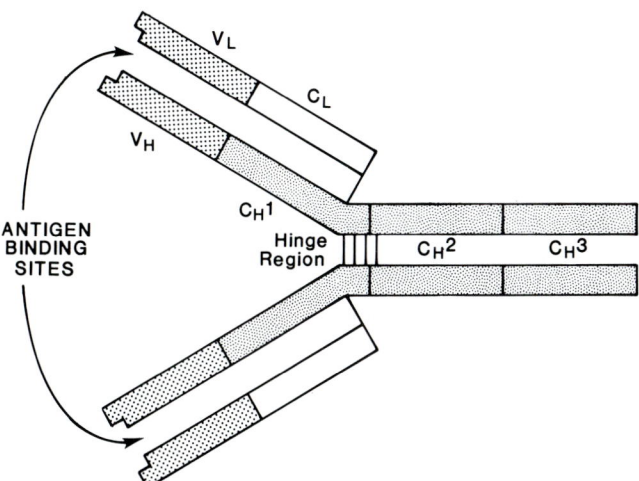

FIGURE 6–4. Basic IgG structure. The longer, inside chain is the "heavy" chain. It is structurally distinct for each class or subclass of antibody. The outside, shorter chain is the "light" chain. There is sequence variability at the amino-terminal end of both the heavy and light chains (V_H and V_L regions, respectively). The antigen binding sites are at the amino-terminal ends of these variable regions. The rest of the molecule has a relatively constant (C) structure, with three distinct domains (C_H1, C_H2, and C_H3, respectively). The hinge region between the C_H1 and C_H2 domains allows each binding site of antibody to operate independently.

MATERNAL-FETAL IMMUNOLOGY

Many reproductive immunologists consider the conceptus, with its tissues in intimate contact with maternal tissues, to be a "semi-allograft" since it bears antigens of paternal, as well as maternal, origin. Much of what is known about maternal-fetal immunology comes from investigations designed to explain how the fetal "semi-allograft" avoids immunologic attack by the mother. Such an approach is not surprising given medicine's tendency to focus on immunology primarily as it pertains to transplantation. As a result, reproductive immunologists have spent nearly two decades trying to make maternal-fetal immunology fit the immunologic concepts and assumptions derived from studies of allograft acceptance and rejection. There is a growing body of evidence that the immunologic relationship between the mother and conceptus does not strictly fit into the allograft model. Rather than being primarily destructive, and thus requiring abrogation, the normal immunologic interactions of mother and fetus may serve to promote the growth and development of the conceptus, a precept that makes good teleological sense. It seems unlikely that nature would engineer a complex alloimmune system primarily so that it would have to be overcome for the sake of reproduction (or manipulated when we learned to transplant tissues from one individual into the body of another). Yet pathologic alloimmune interactions between mother and conceptus occur, and at least part of normal maternal-fetal immunology involves avoiding these potentially harmful events.

Antigenic Status of the Trophoblast

Syncytiotrophoblast, which represents the vast majority of conceptus tissue in contact with maternal circulation, lacks both class I and class II MHC antigens (Faulk and Temple, 1976; Sunderland et al., 1981; Bulmer and Johnson, 1985a). Thus, the majority of the trophoblastic cells in contact with maternal tissues lack the determinants required for maternal T cell activation or for destruction by cytotoxic T cells. In contrast, some populations of extravillous cytotrophoblast express common framework determinants of class I MHC antigens, being recognized by monoclonal antibodies that recognize monomorphic determinants on class I antigens. These cells include cytotrophoblast of the anchoring columns, interstitial cytotrophoblast in the decidua and walls of the spiral arteries (Sunderland et al., 1981), and cytotrophoblast of the chorion laeve (Redman et al., 1984). However, these cells are unreactive to polyclonal antibodies that bind paternal MHC (HLA-A or -B) alloantigens (Redman et al., 1984), monoclonal antibodies to HLA-A or -B subclass specific determinants (Hunt et al., 1989), and to most monoclonal anti-MHC antibodies (Hsi, 1984). these findings indicate that the MHC antigens expressed by extravillous trophoblast are partial or muted in some way (Redman et al., 1984) and are qualitatively different from those expressed by other tissues. What is the class I MHC antigen expressed on by these cytotrophoblastic cells? It appears to be an unusual 40 kDa MHC class I chain associated with beta-2-microglobulin. Recent evidence suggests that the antigen may be HLA-G, a so-called nonclassic class I MHC antigen (Kovats et al., 1990; Ellis et al., 1990). HLA-G polymorphism is uncommon, perhaps allowing cytotrophoblast cells to express the gene product without engendering an immunologic response from the mother. HLA-G

mRNA has been identified in first trimester trophoblast (Kovats et al., 1990), as well as in term chorion (Hunt and Hsi, 1990). The role of HLA-G expression by early pregnancy trophoblast is uncertain, but it may function as an MHC antigen for the purpose of surveillance by cytotoxic cells that destroy infected cells without engendering a maternal anti-MHC response (Wei and Orr, 1990). Sanders and colleagues have shown that CD8 receptors can bind HLA-G in a fashion similar to that in which CD8 receptors bind to classic MHC class I antigens (Sanders et al., 1991). HLA-G expression may serve a protective role because it can reduce lytic activity by IL-2 activated NK cells (Sanders et al., 1991). Finally, some investigators feel that this fetal MHC antigen, or others like it, may be key to the normal development of the conceptus. According to this concept of "immunotropism" (Wegmann, 1987), the maternal recognition of fetal MHC antigen(s) or MHC-like antigen(s) prompts the local release of appropriate cytokines by maternal immune cells. Alternatively, it may be that fetal MHC antigen(s) play a role in the regulation of cell-cell interactions such as trophoblast invasion or the regulation of trophoblast binding of hormones or other molecules (Loke et al., 1991).

The strict regulation of class I antigen expression in the trophoblast probably occurs at the transcriptional or immediate post-transcriptional level. Hunt and colleagues have shown that syncytiotrophoblast contains no detectable class I MHC mRNA, while villous and extravillous cytotrophoblast has class I MHC mRNA (Hunt and Hsi, 1990). Yet little or none of the message is translated into class I surface antigens. The degree of suppression is substantial since neither exposure of human placental explants to interferon-γ nor systemic administration of interferon-γ to mice results in the expression of class I antigens (Hunt et al., 1987; Mattsson et al., 1989).

Class II MHC antigens also are not expressed by syncytiotrophoblast or cytotrophoblast, a fact that is not too surprising since these antigens are primarily expressed only by immunologic cells. The lack of classic class I MHC antigen and the absence of class II MHC antigen expression may well be a primary mechanism by which the conceptus maintains its immunologic inertness. A broader question is whether there are any alloantigens on trophoblast, MHC or otherwise, that might be recognized by the mother and induce an alloimmune response. One group has used an enzyme-linked immunoassay to detect anti-trophoblast antibodies in the sera of primiparas and multiparas (Davies and Browne, 1985). However, two other groups of investigators found no evidence of such antibodies. On the whole, trophoblast is remarkable for its lack of expression of antigens (either primary trophoblast antigens or paternal antigens) that result in a harmful maternal immune response.

In a different approach to the study of trophoblast antigenicity, investigators have found that trophoblast can induce a strong antigenic response in xenogeneic immunization. Most of the work has been done with membrane preparations of human syncytiotrophoblast. Numerous monoclonal and polyclonal antibodies to human trophoblast surface antigens have been generated, but none of the antigens thus identified appears to be entirely trophoblast specific. Perhaps the most interesting antigen system described by this approach is the trophoblast-lymphocyte cross-reactive (TLX) antigen system, described with polyclonal rabbit antisera raised against trophoblast membranes (Faulk and McIntyre, 1983; McIntyre and Faulk, 1982; McIntyre et al., 1983) The heteroantisera reacts with trophoblast and with several other cells, including maternal lymphocytes. Further work has shown that there are at least two antigens in the system. Antibody to one, designated TA1, blocks the maternal proliferative response to paternal cells in the mixed lymphocyte reaction. Some investigators hypothesize that the TLX antigens may be required for normal pregnancy in order to induce the production of protective blocking antibodies by the mother and to recruit suppressor lymphoid cells into the gestational tissues (Slapsys and Clark, 1982); however, this hypothesis remains unproven.

Maternal Immune Response in Pregnancy

GENERAL MATERNAL IMMUNITY. Working on the hypothesis that the mother's immune system must be suppressed in order for the semi-allogeneic conceptus to be tolerated, many investigators have attempted to show a relative suppression of the maternal systemic immune responses during pregnancy. For the most part, these studies have focused on maternal peripheral leukocytes and the potential immunosuppressive activity of pregnancy-associated proteins and hormones. Circulating leukocytes increase somewhat over the course of human pregnancy, rising to about 10,000 cells per mm^3 by the third trimester. This increase is primarily dependent upon an increase in the number of polymorphonuclear leukocytes. It also appears that the bactericidal activity of these leukocytes increases during pregnancy (Lawrence et al., 1980; Krause et al., 1987). Total circulating lymphocyte levels are unchanged during pregnancy (Sridama et al., 1982; Dodson et al., 1977; Glassman et al., 1985; Coulam et al., 1983; Gerhz et al., 1981). B cell function appears to be normal during pregnancy, and normal antibody responses to various vaccinations have been well documented (Brabin, 1985). Circulating levels of IgG, IgM, and IgA are essentially unchanged during uncomplicated pregnancy (Maroulis et al., 1971) and antibody-dependent cellular cytotoxicity is normal in pregnancy (Gonik et al., 1987). Total T cell numbers and T cell subpopulations are also unchanged during pregnancy (Glassman et al., 1985; Coulam et al., 1983). Although some investigators have found that lymphocyte responsiveness to various stimuli is decreased in pregnancy, the preponderance of evidence suggests that lymphocyte responsiveness is normal (Knoblach et al., 1976; Birkeland and Christoffersen, 1977; Poskitt et al., 1977) and overall cell-mediated cytotoxicity is maintained intact throughout pregnancy. Peripheral lymphocytes also appear to maintain their ability to produce lymphokines throughout gestation (Hauser et al., 1987; Feinberg and Gonik, 1991). Finally, the number of circulating NK cells is probably stable or only slightly decreased during pregnancy (Toder et al., 1984; Gregory et al., 1985). Although Gregory and colleagues reported that the cytotoxic activity of the NK cells was decreased during pregnancy (Gregory et al., 1985), the methodology of this work has been questioned (Feinberg and Gonik, 1991).

In spite of the overall normalcy of most immune function in pregnancy, an increased risk from certain infections has been suggested, perhaps because of decreased cellular immune responses to selected antigens (Gehrz et al., 1981; Weinberg, 1984). For example, there may be an increased incidence of poliomyelitis during pregnancy (Siegel and Greenberg, 1955; Weinstein et al., 1951), and the course of hepatitis A and B may be more severe in pregnant women than in nonpregnant women (Borhanmanesh et al., 1973; Morrow et al., 1968). An increased incidence and complication rate from malarial infection is also reasonably well documented during pregnancy (Diro and Beyboun, 1982). Most of the studies suggesting that pregnancy may lead to a higher incidence or worse course of certain infectious diseases are retrospective in nature and subject to bias. At this point, it is probably best to accept that maternal systemic immune function remains largely intact throughout pregnancy, even if certain infections might be more prevalent or virulent during gestation.

MATERNAL HUMORAL IMMUNE RECOGNITION OF THE CONCEPTUS. The maternal humoral recognition of fetal antigens is well established to occur in a limited proportion of pregnant women. Antipaternal (antifetal) leukocytotoxic antibodies are found in 35 to 65 per cent of multiparas and nearly 25 per cent of primiparas (Berke and Johansen, 1974; Beard et al., 1983; Ahrons, 1971). These antibodies are primarily of the IgG isotype and are directed against paternal MHC antigens. Less well-characterized, trophoblast antigens also may be involved in the maternal humoral alloimmune response. Billington and colleagues have demonstrated non-MHC antibodies that bind, but do not apparently damage, trophoblast in a majority of primiparous and multiparous women (Billington and Davies, 1987). In the mouse, the production of antipaternal (antifetal) antibodies occurs inconsistently and may be restricted to a few strains (Billington et al., 1983). As in the human, antipaternal (antifetal) antibodies were found most often among multiparas and are primarily of the IgG subclass (Bell and Billington, 1980).

It is one thing for the mother to produce antibodies against paternal (fetal) or trophoblast antigens, but it is quite another for these to actually damage the conceptus. At least some of the antipaternal (antifetal) antibodies will promote the lysis of paternal leukocytes in vitro (Van der Werf, 1971; Doughty and Gelsthorpe, 1974). Yet in spite of the presence of these alloantibodies in a modest proportion of pregnant women, there is no evidence of antibody-mediated damage to fetus or placenta. In part, this may be due to the elaboration of soluble HLA antigens by the fetus or suppression of the maternal alloantibodies by anti-idiotypic antibodies (Amsden et al., 1988; Reed et al., 1991). Finally, it may be that the placenta serves as an "antibody sponge," binding potentially damaging antibodies so that they cannot reach the fetus in sufficient concentration to be harmful.

MATERNAL CELLULAR IMMUNE RECOGNITION OF THE CONCEPTUS. One should keep in mind that the principal mediator of allograft rejection is the cellular immune system, and if the "semi-allogeneic" conceptus is to be rejected, this system would probably come into play. Thus, numerous studies have attempted to answer the question whether there are specific maternal cell-mediated responses against fetal alloantigens. At first glance, the data appear somewhat conflicting. Circulating maternal leukocytes with weak cytotoxic activity against fetal cells have been found by some investigators (Chardonnens and Jeannet, 1980). Two groups have found that maternal leukocytes are cytotoxic for trophoblastic cells isolated from their own placentae (Taylor and Hancock, 1975; Timonen and Saksela, 1976). Finally, incubation of neonatal or paternal cells with maternal lymphocytes has demonstrated sensitization to fetal (paternal) HLA antigens in several studies (Rocklin et al., 1973, 1982). But if cellular immunity to fetal (paternal) antigens were typical of pregnancy, one would expect a rapid secondary maternal lymphocyte reaction to paternal cells in mixed lymphocyte culture (as well as in subsequent pregnancies). A few investigators have reported such secondary maternal lymphocyte responses in mixed lymphocyte culture (Youtananukorn and Matangkasombut, 1973; Voisin, 1983; Chaouat and Voisin, 1979). However, a secondary immune response, indicative of prior sensitization, can be demonstrated only in time course studies. Such studies have failed to show a secondary maternal antifetal or antipaternal response (Car et al., 1974; Herva and Tiilikainen, 1977; Moen et al., 1980). In addition, Sargent and colleagues have investigated induction of chemotactic factor release and lymphocyte proliferation in primiparous and multiparous women. The kinetics of time course experiments were typical of primary immune responses rather than secondary immune responses (Sargent et al., 1982). In a follow-up study by the same group, pregnant women and their HLA-identical sisters were studied. The pregnant and nonpregnant sisters had identical primary immune responses to paternal cells (Moore et al., 1983). Taken together, the data show little or no evidence of a specific maternal cellular immune response to fetal (paternal) HLA antigens induced by pregnancy.

Some investigators have been able to demonstrate circulating maternal lymphocytes with weak cytotoxic activity against fetal cells (Wattanasak and Matangkasombut, 1983; Chardonnens and Jeannet, 1980). Redman et al. (1987) found maternal cytotoxic activity against paternal cells in 1 of 10 primiparas and a similar number of multiparas (Sargent et al., 1982). Another investigator found no evidence for maternal cell cytotoxic activity against fetal or paternal cells (Vanderbeeken et al., 1984), nor does cytotoxic T cell generation occur in the mouse (Billington et al., 1983). Thus, there appears to be a nearly virtual absence of antifetal cytotoxic T cells in normal pregnancy.

Even if cytotoxic T cells were present, it should be emphasized that *in vitro* trophoblast is resistant to cellular immune destruction (Zuckerman and Head, 1985, 1987; Clark and Chaouat, 1986). Experiments in rodents have shown that the induction of antipaternal

cytotoxic T lymphocytes has no effect on pregnancy outcome (Mitchison, 1953; Taylor, 1975). Interestingly, binding of trophoblastic cells by cytotoxic T cells may still occur, even though the trophoblastic cells are resistant to lysis (Johnson, 1989). It has also been shown that naive or interferon-activated NK cells do not kill trophoblastic cells (Johnson, 1989). However, interleukin-2 (IL-2) activated NK cells kill trophoblastic cells. This may be a potential mechanism for cell-mediated destruction of the conceptus in certain circumstances.

Immunology of the Maternal-Fetal Interface

IMMUNE CELLS AT THE MATERNAL-FETAL INTERFACE. There is an abundance of immunologically capable tissue in the luteal phase endometrium and decidua. Leukocytes are widely distributed throughout the upper level of the stroma of both the proliferative and luteal phase endometrium. Cells bearing B cell surface markers are distinctly rare, but T cells increase in number through the first half of the luteal phase (Bulmer and Johnson, 1985b; Bulmer et al., 1987). By the late luteal phase, many of these cells do not bear surface markers typical of mature T cells, but have markers suggesting that they are of T cell lineage. Bulmer and colleagues have found that most of these cells bear a surface antigen indicative of NK cells (Bulmer et al., 1987). These cells have the histologic appearance of large granular lymphocytes (LGLs), NK-like cells that are found in small numbers in the peripheral blood. LGLs function as effector cells of the innate immune system in that they do not require MHC for their cytotoxic activity and probably have undifferentiated or transformed cells as their primary targets. By early pregnancy, LGLs comprise the single largest population of immune cells in the decidua (Starkey et al., 1988), being especially prominent in the deeper decidua basalis and in the decidua parietalis. Redman and colleagues (1991) have shown that there are three subsets of LGLs in human decidua, each with a characteristic surface antigen expression. Taken together, decidual LGLs have weak cytotoxic activity against commonly used tumor targets; the LGLs of the largest of the three subsets are more cytotoxic than the others. However, decidual LGLs (as well as peripheral blood LGLs) do not lyse trophoblastic cells *in vitro* (King et al., 1989). The immunologic role, if any, of LGLs appears to be one of early and mid-pregnancy; by term, LGLs are relatively few in number.

The role of LGLs in early pregnancy is unknown. They are capable of secreting interleukin-1, interleukin-2, interferon, tumor necrosis factor-α, and colony stimulating factors. The relative abundance of LGLs and their ability to elaborate a variety of cytokines suggest that they may play a role in the regulation of trophoblastic cells or trophoblastic cell invasion. IL-2 induces the proliferation of decidual LGLs and enhances their cytotoxic activity against a standard tumor target (Redman et al., 1991). This feature of LGLs has led to speculation that IL-2 produced in decidual or trophoblastic tissues may result in trophoblastic cellular damage by activated LGLs.

Macrophages are present in substantial numbers in the luteal phase endometrium, but their numbers decline in the late secretory phase. However, during pregnancy, the majority of leukocytes in the portion of decidua underlying the point of trophoblastic invasion are macrophages. They remain the predominant leukocyte found close to the cytotrophoblast. In deeper areas of the decidua basalis and in other decidual tissues, 50 per cent or less of the leukocytes are macrophages. Unlike the LGLs, macrophages persist as pregnancy advances, especially in areas around interstitial trophoblast cells. They are also present in the decidua parietalis, where trophoblast does not occur. Interestingly, at term, some of the macrophages at the basal plate of the placenta are fetal in origin, possibly functioning as phagocytic cells for the processing and removal of debris at the maternal-fetal interface (Bulmer and Johnson, 1984).

MODULATION OF THE IMMUNE RESPONSE AT THE MATERNAL-FETAL INTERFACE. Several groups of investigators have focused attention on the role of immunosuppressive factors in implantation and early development of the conceptus. According to the generally held hypothesis, these factors play a role in abrogating the tendency for the maternal immune system to destroy the implanting conceptus by T cell or NK cell activity, or both. In the late 1970s, Clark and his co-workers reported the presence of suppressor cells in the murine decidua, which act to prevent the generation of cytotoxic lymphocytes (CTLs) *in vitro* (Clark and McDermott, 1978). A series of reports by the same group (Clark and McDermott, 1981; Slapsys and Clark, 1982, 1983; Slapsys et al., 1984; Clark et al., 1983; Daya et al., 1987) described a bimodal expression of suppressor cells in murine decidua, with the first appearing in the preimplantation period and the second in the postimplantation period. The first decidual suppressor cells to appear are large lymphocyte-like cells whose recruitment and activation are hormonally dependent (Clark and McDermott, 1981). The second are small granulated lymphocytic cells that lack T cell surface markers. Unfortunately, the relationship of these suppressor cells to LGLs or other immune cells identified by immunopathology is unknown. The recruitment or appearance of the small lymphocytic cells in the decidua seems to depend upon the presence of trophoblast cells. The small granulated lymphocytic cells, and perhaps the large cells, probably block the generation of CTLs by the elaboration of a soluble factor that blocks T cell responses to IL-2, thus suppressing the generation of CTLs. Investigations using human tissues indicate that small granular lymphocytes appear in human decidua (Daya et al., 1987), but these cells have not been as extensively studied as those in the mouse. According to Clark and colleagues, the immunosuppressive effect of the decidual suppressor cells is primarily due to the elaboration of a transforming growth factor-β_2-(TGF-β_2-)like molecule. This factor inhibits the generation of cytotoxic T cells and the activation of NK cells by blocking the action of IL-2 (Clark et al., 1985, 1986, 1988; Daya et al., 1987).

Working with both murine and human tissues, Chaouat and colleagues have found that trophoblastic cells elaborate an immunosuppressive factor(s) that inhibits the proliferative response of the mixed lymphocyte culture, the generation of cytotoxic T cells (Chaouat and Kolb, 1984; Chaouat et al., 1985; Menu et al., 1989), and the lytic activity of NK cells (Kolb et al., 1984). Supernatants from cultures of the human choriocarcinoma cell lines BeWo, JeG, and JAR appear to have similar activity by suppressing IL-2-dependent T cell proliferation (Chaouat et al., 1991). This soluble suppressor factor of trophoblast is inhibited by anti-TGF-β_2, and therefore may be a TGF-β_2-like molecule similar or identical to the one described by Clark et al.

Other suppressor factors have been described at the maternal-fetal interface, and there is currently no evidence that any one is more important than the other in achieving successful pregnancy. Parhar and Lala (1985a) found that dispersed human decidual cells suppressed NK cell lytic activity, the mixed lymphocyte culture proliferative response (Parhar and Lala, 1985b), and the generation of cytotoxic T cells (Lala et al., 1987). These investigators have identified the suppressor factor as prostaglandin E_2, which down-regulates IL-2 receptor expression and inhibits IL-2 production by T cells. Some investigators believe that the presence of PGE$_2$ is due to dispersion of the decidual cells (Wood et al., 1988) and that the relatively high concentrations of progesterone *in vivo* would suppress PGE$_2$ production (Clark et al., 1991).

Steroid hormones may also play a role in immunosuppression at the maternal-fetal interface, and their role in the regulation of the immune system in general is currently the subject of intense investigation. Maternal T cells bear progesterone receptors, and progesterone-treated T cells release an immunosuppressive factor (Szekeres-Bartho et al., 1985, 1986). This factor blocks NK-cell-mediated lysis of embryonic fibroblasts (Chaouat et al., 1991). Free cortisol levels are slightly elevated in pregnancy, and glucocorticoids inhibit IL-2 production and stimulate IL-4 production by T cells (Daynes et al., 1990). The steroid hormone 1,25 dihydroxyvitamin D_3, which is abundant in the placenta and decidua, has similar activities. Thus, both hormones tend to suppress T cell cytotoxic response and favor local antibody responses. In contrast, dehydroepiandrosterone (DHEA), but not DHEA-sulfate, enhances IL-2 production by activated T cells. According to the "microenvironment" theory of the regulation of the immune response proposed by Daynes and colleagues (Daynes et al., 1990), the local steroid hormone milieu profoundly affects the local immunologic response. Since the placenta and decidua are sites of considerable steroid hormone concentrations, normal pregnancy immunology may be primarily determined by the influences of the steroid milieu.

Finally, there may be an immunologic role for the numerous small proteins produced by the endometrium and early gestational tissues. The most notable of these is placental protein 14, also known as endometrial alpha-2-globulin. This protein is believed to exert an important local immunosuppressive effect (Van Cong et al., 1991). Its expression is under the influence of progesterone, again implicating this steroid hormone in an immunologic role.

IMMUNOTROPHIC FACTORS AT THE MATERNAL-FETAL INTERFACE. Some decidual or placental immunoregulatory factors may be immunotrophic, rather than immunosuppressive or immunologically damaging, in nature (Wegmann, 1984). Of the cytokines elaborated by LGL and macrophages, the colony stimulating factors are most likely to be relevant. For example, colony stimulating factor-1 (CSF-1), also known as macrophage CSF, is made by both LGLs and macrophages. It is present in murine gestational tissues and absent from nonpregnant endometrium (Pollard et al., 1987). In the mouse, trophoblastic cell receptors for CSF-1 have been identified (Muller et al., 1983; Hoshina et al., 1985), and CSF-1 induces at least one subset of murine placental cells to become adherent and phagocytic (Athanassakis et al., 1987). The responsive cells from murine placentae may be fetally derived macrophages or macrophage-like epithelial or trophoblastic cells (Guilbert et al., 1991). *In vitro* studies using human trophoblastic cells show that villous trophoblast have receptors for CSF-1 and that CSF-1 will increase hormone production in these cells (Pfeiffer-Ohlsson et al., 1984; Talamantes et al., 1980). Murine gestational tissue CSF-1 is induced by chorionic gonadotropin (Bartocci et al., 1986), and its production is abolished by ovariectomy or administration of antiprogestagen agents (Bartocci et al., 1986; Pollard et al., 1987). Administration of estradiol and progesterone sufficient to mimic pregnancy-like hormone levels induces uterine CSF-1 production in castrated mice (Pollard et al., 1987). Thus, the available data suggest that the appearance of CSF-1 in gestational tissues is related to the hormones of pregnancy and that CSF-1 has a trophic effect on trophoblastic cells in terms of steroid hormone and cellular growth and differentiation.

Granulocyte-macrophage colony stimulating factor (GM-CSF) is present in murine decidual cell culture supernatants and has been shown to have a trophic effect on preimplantation murine embryos (Robertson et al., 1991). GM-CSF also enhances trophoblast growth, as does interleukin-3 (Armstrong and Chaouat, 1989; Athanassakis et al., 1987). The administration of GM-CSF to a murine mating particularly prone to spontaneous resorption appears to decrease the number of resorptions (Chaouat et al., 1991). Other investigators have emphasized that GM-CSF, as well as other cytokines, are toxic to rapidly proliferating cells, and therefore may be toxic to trophoblast (Anderson et al., 1991). *In vitro* studies indicate that GM-CSF is toxic to 2-cell embryos as well as a choriocarcinoma line (Hill et al., 1987; Berkowitz et al., 1988).

The immunologic relationship between the mother and her fetus is certainly complex; much of it remains cloaked in mystery. It appears that mechanisms for protection of the conceptus from attack by the maternal immune system are part of normal early pregnancy. No doubt these mechanisms are multiple and complementary. In recent years, we have come to realize that the interplay between mother and fetus includes immunologic factors that are neither suppressive nor damaging in nature, but actually promote the growth and development of the gestational tissues.

REFERENCES

Ahrons S: Leukocyte antibodies: occurrence in primigravidae. Tissue Antigens 1:178, 1971.

Amsden AF, Smith RN, Chirakalwason N: The alloantibody response in the allogeneically pregnant rat. IV. Detection of maternal serum of specific antigen-antibody complexes. J Immunol 141:2295, 1988.

Anderson DJ, Hill JA, Haimovici F, Berkowitz RS: Adverse effects of immune cell products in pregnancy. *In* Wegmann TG, Gill TJ, Nisbet-Brown E (eds): Molecular and Cellular Immunobiology of the Maternal-Fetal Interface. New York, Oxford University Press, 1991.

Armstrong DT, Chaouat G: Effects of lymphokines and immune complexes on murine placental cell growth in vitro. Biol Reprod 40:466, 1989.

Athanassakis I, Bleackley PC, Paetkau V, et al: The immunostimulatory effect of T cells and T cell lymphokines on murine fetally derived placental cells. J Immunol 138:37, 1987.

Baker CJ, Edwards MS, Kasper DL: Role of antibody to native type III polysaccharide group B streptococcus in infant infection. Pediatrics 68:544, 1981.

Ballow M, Fung F, Good RA, et al: Developmental aspects of complement components in the newborn. Clin Exp Immunol 18:257, 1974.

Bartocci A, Pollard JW, Stanley ER: Regulation of colony-stimulating factor 1 during pregnancy. J Exp Med 164:956, 1986.

Beard RW, Braude P, Mowbray JF, et al: Protective antibodies and spontaneous abortion. Lancet ii: 1990, 1983.

Beelen RHJ, van Rees EP, Bos HJ, et al: Ontogeny of antigen-presenting cells. *In* Chaouat G (ed): The Immunology of the Fetus. Boca Raton, FL, CRC Press, 1990.

Bell SC, Billington WD: Major anti-paternal alloantibody induced by murine pregnancy is non-complement-fixing IgG1. Nature (London) 288:387, 1980.

Berke J, Johansen K: The formation of HLA antibodies in pregnancy. The antigenicity of aborted and term fetuses. J Obstet Gynaecol Br Commonwealth 81:222, 1974.

Berkowitz RS, Hill JA, Kurtz CB, et al: Effects of products of activated leukocytes (lymphokines and monokines) on the growth of malignant trophoblast cell in vitro. Am J Obstet Gynecol 158:199, 1988.

Billington WD, Davies M: Maternal antibody to placental syncytiotrophoblast during pregnancy. *In* Wegmann TG, Gill TJ (eds): Immunoregulation in Fetal Survival. New York, Oxford University Press, 1987.

Billington WD, Bell SC, Smith G: Histocompatibility antigens of mouse trophoblasts and their possible functional significance in maternal fetal immunological interactions. *In* Wegmann TG, Gill TJ (eds): Immunology of Reproduction. New York, Oxford University Press, 1983.

Birkeland SA, Christoffersen K: Cellular immunity in pregnancy: blast transformation and rosette formation of maternal T and B lymphocytes. Clin Exp Immunol 30:408, 1977.

Borhanmanesh F, Haghighi P, Hekmat K, et al: Viral hepatitis during pregnancy. Gastroenterology 64:304, 1973.

Brabin BJ: Epidemiology of infection in pregnancy. Rev Infect Dis 7:579, 1985.

Bulmer JN, Johnson PM: Macrophage populations in the human placenta and amniochorion. Clin Exp Immunol 57:393, 1984.

Bulmer JN, Johnson PM: Antigen expression by trophoblast populations in the human placenta and their possible immunobiological relevance. Placenta 6:127, 1985a.

Bulmer JN, Johnson PM, Bulmer D: Leukocyte populations in human decidua and endometrium. *In* Gill TJ, Wegmann TG, Nisbet-Brown E (eds): Immunoregulation and Fetal Survival. New York, Oxford University Press, 1987.

Bulmer JN, Johnson PM: Immunohistological characterisation of the decidual leukocytic infiltrate related to endometrial gland epithelium in early human pregnancy. J Reprod Immunol 7:364, 1985b.

Car MC, Stites DP, Fudenberg HH: Cellular immune aspects of the human fetal-maternal relationship. III. Mixed lymphocyte reactivity between related maternal and cord blood lymphocytes. Cell Immunol 11:332, 1974.

Chaouat G, Voisin GA: Regulatory T-cell subpopulations in pregnancy. I. Evidence for suppressive activity of the early phase of MLR. J Immunol **122**:1383, 1979.

Chaouat G, Kolb JP, Riviere M, et al: Local and systemic regulation of maternal antifetal cytotoxicity during murine pregnancy. Contrib Gynecol Obstet **14**:55, 1985.

Chaouat G, Kolb JP: Immunoactive products of murine placenta. II. Afferent suppression of maternal cell mediated immunity by supernatants from short term enriched cultures of murine trophoblast enriched maternal cell populations. Ann Immunol (*Inst Pasteur*) **135C**:205, 1984.

Chaouat G, Menu E, Szekeres-Bartho J, et al: Immunological and endocrinological factors that contribute to successful pregnancy. *In* Wegmann TG, Gill TJ, Nisbet-Brown E (eds): Molecular and Cellular Immunobiology of the Maternal-Fetal Interface. New York, Oxford University Press, 1991.

Chardonnens X, Jeannet M: Lymphocyte mediated cytotoxicity in humoral antibodies in pregnancy. Int Arch Allergy Appl Immunol **61**:467, 1980.

Clark DA, Chaput A, Walker C, et al: Active suppression of host-vs-graft reaction in pregnant mice. VI. Soluble suppressor activity obtained from decidua blocks the response to IL-2. J Immunol **134**:1659, 1985.

Clark DA, Chaouat G. Characterization of the cellular basis for the inhibition of cytotoxic effector cells by the murine placenta. Cell Immunol **102**:43, 1986.

Clark DA, Falbo M, Rowley RB, et al: Active suppression of host-versus-graft reaction in pregnant mice. IX. Soluble suppressor activity obtained from allopregnant mouse decidua that blocks the response to interleukin 2 is related to TGF-β. J Immunol **141**:3833, 1988.

Clark DA, Head JR, Drake BL, et al: Role of a factor related to transforming growth factor beta-2 in successful pregnancy. *In* Wegmann TG, Gill TJ, Nisbet-Brown E (eds): Molecular and Cellular Immunobiology of the Maternal-Fetal Interface. New York, Oxford University Press, 1991.

Clark DA, McDermott MR: Active suppression of host-versus-graft reaction in pregnant mice. III. Developmental kinetics, properties, and mechanism of induction of suppressor cells during first pregnancy. J Immunol **127**:1267, 1981.

Clark DA, McDermott MR: Impairment of host-vs-graft reaction in pregnant mice. I. Suppression of cytotoxic T cell generation in lymph nodes draining the uterus. J Immunol **121**:1389, 1978.

Clark DA, Slapsys RM, Chaput A, et al: Immunoregulatory molecules of trophoblast and decidual suppressor cell origin at the materno-fetal interface. Am J Reprod Immunol Microbiol **10**:100, 1986.

Clark DA, Slapsys RM, Croy BA, et al: Suppressor cell activity in uterine decidua correlates with success or failure of murine pregnancies. J Immunol **131**:540, 1983.

Colten HR: Biosynthesis of complement. Adv Immunol **22**:67, 1976.

Colten HR, Goldberger G: Ontogeny of serum complement proteins. Pediatrics **64**:775, 1979.

Coulam CB, Silverfield JC, Cazmar RE, et al: T lymphocyte subsets during pregnancy and the menstrual cycle. Am J Reprod Immunol **4**:88, 1983.

Davies M, Browne CM. Anti-trophoblast antibody responses during normal human pregnancy. J Reprod Immunol **7**:285, 1985.

Daya S, Rosenthal KL, Clark DA: Immunosuppressor factor(s) produced by decidua-associated suppressor cells: a proposed mechanism for fetal allograft survival. Am J Obstet Gynecol **156**:344, 1987.

Daynes RA, Araneo BA, Dowell TA, et al: Regulation of murine lymphokine production *in vivo*. III. The lymphoid tissue microenvironment exerts regulatory influences over T helper cell function. J Exp Med **171**:979, 1990.

Diro M, Beyboun SN: Malaria in pregnancy. South Med J **75**:959, 1982.

Dodson MG, Kerman RH, Lange CF, et al: T- and B-cells in pregnancy. Obstet Gynecol **49**:299, 1977.

Doughty RW, Gelsthorpe K: An initial investigation of lymphocyte antibody activity through pregnancy and in eluates prepared from placental material. Tissue Antigens **4**:291, 1974.

Ellis SA, Palmer MS, McMichael AJ: Human trophoblast and the choriocarcinoma cell line BeWo express a truncated HLA class I molecule. J Immunol **144**:731, 1990.

Faulk WP, McIntyre JA. Immunological studies of human trophoblast: markers, subsets and functions. Immunol Rev **75**:139, 1983.

Faulk WP, Temple A. Distribution of beta-2 microglobulin and HLA in chorionic villi of human placenta. Nature (London) **262**:799, 1976.

Fauser AA, Messner HA: Granuloerythropoietic colonies in human bone marrow, peripheral blood and cord blood. Blood **52**:1243, 1978.

Fauser AA, Messner HA: Identification of megakaryocytes, macrophages and eosinophils in colonies of human bone marrow containing neutrophilic granulocytes and erythroblasts. Blood **53**:1023, 1979.

Feinberg BB, Gonik B: General precepts of immunology. Clin Obstet Gynecol **34**:3, 1991.

Forestier F, Daffos F, Galacteros F, et al: Hematological values of 163 normal fetuses between 18 and 30 weeks of gestation. Pediatr Res **20**:342, 1986.

Gehrz RC, Christianson WR, Linner KM, et al: A longitudinal analysis of lymphocyte proliferative responses to mitogens and antigens during human pregnancy. Am J Obstet Gynecol **140**:665, 1981.

Glassman AB, Bennett CE, Christopher JB, et al: Immunity during pregnancy: lymphocyte subpopulation and mitogen responsiveness. Ann Clin Lab Sci **15**:357, 1985.

Gluck L, Silverman WA: Phagocytosis in premature infants. Pediatrics **20**:951, 1957.

Gonik B, Loo LS, West S, et al: Natural killer cytotoxicity and antibody-dependent cellular cytotoxicity to herpes simplex virus-infected cells in human pregnancy. Am J Reprod Immunol Microbiol **13**:23, 1987.

Granberg C, Hirvonen T: Cell-mediated lympholysis by fetal and neonatal lymphocytes in sheep and man. Cell Immunol **51**:13, 1980.

Gregory CD, Shah LP, Lee H, et al: Cytotoxic reactivity of human natural killer (NK) cells during normal pregnancy: a longitudinal study. J Clin Lab Immunol **18**:175, 1985.

Griffiths-Chu S, Patterson JAK, Berger CL, et al: Characterization of immature T cell subpopulations in neonatal blood. Blood **64**:296, 1984.

Guilbert LJ, Athanassakis I, Branch DR, et al: The placenta as an immune-endocrine interface: placental cells as targets for lymphohematopoietic cytokine stimulation. *In* Wegmann TG, Gill TJ, Nisbet-Brown E (eds): Molecular and Cellular Immunobiology of the Maternal-Fetal Interface. New York, Oxford University Press, 1991.

Hauser GJ, Lidor A, Zakuth V, et al: Immunocompetence in pregnancy: production of interleukin-2 by peripheral blood lymphocytes. Cancer Detect Prev **1**(Suppl):39, 1987.

Herva E, Tiilikainen A: Mixed lymphocyte culture reactions at delivery and in the puerperium: Effects of parity, HLA antigens, and maternal serum. Acta Pathol Microbiol Scand **85**:333, 1977.

Hill JA, Haimovici F, Anderson DJ: Products of activated lymphocytes and macrophages inhibit mouse embryo development in vitro. J Immunol **139**:2250, 1987.

Hoshina M, Nishio A, Bo M, et al: The expression of the oncogene *fms* in human chorionic tissue. Acta Obstet Gynecol Jpn **37**:2791, 1985.

Hsi BL, Yeh CJG, Faulk WP: Class I antigens of the major histocompatibility complex on cytotrophoblasts of human chorion laeve. Immunology **52**:621, 1984.

Hunt JS, Hsi BL: Evasive strategies of trophoblast cells: Selective expression of membrane antigens. Am J Reprod Immunol **23**:57, 1990.

Hunt JS, Andrews GK, Wood GW: Normal trophoblasts resist induction of class I HLA. J Immunol **138**:2481, 1987.

Hunt JS, Lessin D, King CR: Ontogeny and distribution of cells expressing HLA-B locus-specific determinants in the placenta and extra placental membranes. J Reprod Immunol **15**:21, 1989.

Johnson PM: Immunological intercourse at the feto-maternal interface. Immunol Today **10**:215, 1989.

Johnston RB, Altenburger KM, Atkinson AW, et al: Complement in the newborn infant. Pediatrics **645**:781, 1979.

King A, Birkby C, Loke TW: Early human decidual cells exhibit NK activity against K562 cell line but not against first trimester trophoblast. Cell Immunol **118**:337, 1989.

Klein RB, Fischer TJ, Gard SE, et al: Decreased mononuclear and polymorphonuclear chemotaxis in human newborns, infants and young children. Pediatrics **60**:467, 1977.

Knoblach V, Jouja V, Pospisil M: Feto-maternal relationships in normal pregnancy in mixed lymphocyte cultures. Arch Gynecol **220**:249, 1976.

Kolb JP, Chaouat G, Chassoux DJ: Immunoactive products of placenta. III. Suppression of natural killing activity. J Immunol **132**:2305, 1984.

Kovats S, Main EK, Librach C, et al: A class I antigen, HLA-G, expressed in human trophoblasts. Science **248**:220, 1990.

Krause PJ, Ingardie CJ, Pontius LT, et al: Post-defense during pregnancy: neutrophil chemotaxis and adherence. Am J Obstet Gynecol **157**:274, 1987.

Lala PK, Kearns M, Parhar RS: Immunology of the decidual tissue. In Gill TJ, Wegmann TG, Nisbet-Brown E (eds): Immunoregulation and Fetal Survival. New York, Oxford University Press, 1987.

Lawrence R, Murch J, Richards W, et al: Etiological mechanisms in the maintenance of pregnancy. Ann Allergy **44**:166, 1980.

Lobach DF, Hensley LL, Ho W, et al: Human T cell antigen expression during the early stages of fetal thymic maturation. J Immunol **135**:1752, 1985.

Loke YW, Grabowska A, King A: Human trophoblast-decidua interaction in vitro. In Wegmann TG, Gill TJ, Nisbet-Brown E (eds): Molecular and Cellular Immunobiology of the Maternal-Fetal Interface. New York, Oxford University Press, 1991.

Lubens RG, Gard SE, Soderberg-Warner M, et al: Lectin-dependent T-lymphocyte and natural killer cytotoxic deficiencies in human newborns. Cell Immunol **74**:40, 1982.

Maroulis GB, Buckley RH, Younger JB: Serum immunoglobulin concentrations during normal pregnancies. Am J Obstet Gynecol **109**:971, 1971.

Mattsson R, Holmdahl R, Schneynius A, et al: Allopregnancy in mice treated with recombinant rat interferon-gamma. (Abstract) J Reprod Immunol (Suppl):151, 1989.

McCracken GH, Eichenwald HF: Leukocyte function and the development of opsonic and complement activity in the neonate. Am J Dis Child **121**:120, 1971.

McIntyre JA, Faulk WP. Allotypic trophoblast-lymphocyte cross-reactive (TLX) cell surface antigen. Hum Immunol **4**:27, 1982.

McIntyre JA, Faulk WP, Verhulst SJ, et al: Human trophoblast lymphocyte cross-reactive (TLX) antigens define a new alloantigen system. Science **222**:1135, 1983.

Menu E, Kaplan L, Andreu G, et al: Immunoactive products of human placenta. I. An immunoregulatory factor obtained from explant cultures of human placenta inhibit CTL generation and cytotoxic effector cell generation. Cell Immunol **119**:341, 1989.

Messner HA, Fauser AA: Culture studies of human pluripotent hematopoietic progenitors. Blut **41**:327, 1980.

Messner HA, Izaquirre CA, Jamal N: Identification of T lymphocytes in human mixed hematopoietic colonies. Blood **58**:402, 1981.

Mitchison NA: The effect on the offspring of maternal immunization in mice. J Genet **51**:406, 1953.

Moen T, Moen M, Palbo V, et al: In vitro fetomaternal lymphocyte responses at delivery: No gross changes in MLC and PLT responsiveness. J Reprod Immunol **2**:213, 1980.

Moore MP, Sargent IL, Ting A, et al: Maternal cell-mediated immunity in pregnancy: Lymphocyte responses of mothers in their non-pregnant HLA-identical sisters to paternal HLA. Clin Exp Immunol **54**:91, 1983.

Morell A, Sidiropoulos D, Herrmann U, et al: IgG subclasses and antibodies to group B streptococci, pneumococci, and tetanus toxoid in preterm neonates after intravenous infusion of immunoglobulin to the mothers. Pediatr Res **20**:933, 1986.

Morrow RH, Smetana HF, Sai FT, et al: Unusual features of viral hepatitis in Accra, Ghana. Ann Intern Med **68**:1250, 1968.

Muller R, Verma IM, Adamson ED: Expression of c-onc genes: c-fos transcripts accumulate to high levels during development of mouse placenta, yolk sac and amnion. EMBO J **2**:679, 1983.

Notarangelo LD, Chirico G, Chiara A, et al: Activity of classical and alternative pathways of complement in preterm and small for gestational age infants. Pediatr Res **18**:281, 1984.

Olding LB, Murgita RA, Wigzell H: Mitogen-stimulated lymphoid cells from human newborns suppress the proliferation of maternal lymphocytes across a cell-impermeable membrane. J Immunol **119**:1109, 1977.

Oldstone MBA, Tishon A, Moretta L: Active thymus derived suppressor lymphocytes in human cord blood. Nature **269**:333, 1977.

Parhar RS, Lala PK: Changes in the host natural killer cell population in mice during tumor development. 2. The mechanism of suppression of NK activity. Cell Immunol **93**:265, 1985a.

Parhar RS, Lala PK: Local immunosuppression of lymphocyte alloreactivity by human decidual cells. Anat Rec **211**(3):147A, 1985b.

Pfeiffer-Ohlsson S, Goustin AS, Rydnert J, et al: Spatial and temporal pattern of cellular *myc* oncogene expression in developing human placenta: implications for embryonic cell proliferation. Cell **38**:585, 1984.

Pollard JW, Bartocci A, Arceci R, et al: Apparent role of the macrophage growth factor, CSF-1, in placental development. Nature **330**:484, 1987.

Poskitt PKF, Kurt EA, Paul BB, et al: Response to mitogen during pregnancy and the post-partum period. Obstet Gynecol **50**:319, 1977.

Redman CWG, McMichael AJ, Stirrat GM, et al: Class I MHC antigens on extravillus trophoblast. Immunology **52**:457, 1984.

Redman CWG, Arenas J, Mason DY, et al: Maternal alloimmune recognition of the fetus in human pregnancy. In Gill TJ, Wegmann TG, Nisbet-Brown E (eds): Immunoregulation and Fetal Survival. New York, Oxford University Press, 1987.

Redman CWG, Ferry BL, Jackson MC, et al: Immune cell populations in human early pregnancy decidua. In Wegmann TG, Gill TJ, Nisbet-Brown E (eds): Molecular and Cellular Immunobiology of the Maternal-Fetal Interface. New York, Oxford University Press, 1991.

Reed E, Beer AE, Hutcherson H, et al: The alloantibody response of pregnant women and its suppression by soluable HLA antigens and anti-idiotypic antibodies. J Reprod Immunol **20**:115, 1991.

Robertson SA, Lavranos T, Seamark RF: In vitro models of the maternal-fetal interface. In Wegmann TG, Gill TJ, Nisbet-Brown E (eds): Molecular and Cellular Immunobiology of the Maternal-Fetal Interface. New York, Oxford University Press, 1991.

Rocklin RE, Kitzmiller J, Garovoy MR: Maternofetal relation. II. Further characterization of an immunologic blocking factor that developed during pregnancy. Clin Immunol Immunopathol **22**:305, 1982.

Rocklin RE, Zuckerman JR, Alpert E, et al: Effective multiparity on human maternal hypersensitivity to fetal antigen. Nature **241**:130, 1973.

Sanders SK, Giblin PA, Kavathas P: Cell-cell adhesion mediated by CD8 and human histocompatibility leukocyte antigen G, a non-classical major histocompatibility complex class 1 molecule on cytotrophoblasts. J Exp Med **174**:737, 1991.

Sargent IL, Redman CWG, Stirrat GM: Maternal cell-mediated immunity in normal and preeclamptic pregnancies. Clin Exp Immunol **50**:601, 1982.

Siegel M, Greenberg M: Incidence of poliomyelitis in pregnancy. N Engl J Med **253**:841, 1955.

Slapsys RM, Clark DA: Active suppression of host-vs-graft reaction in pregnant mice. IV. Local suppressor cells in decidua and uterine blood. J Reprod Immunol **4**:354, 1982.

Slapsys RM, Beeson JH, Clark DA: The role of the trophoblast in the localization of decidua-associated suppressor cells. Am J Reprod Immunol **6**:66, 1984.

Slapsys RM, Clark DA: Active suppression of host-versus-graft reaction in pregnant mice. V. Kinetics, specificity, and in vivo activity of non-T suppressor cells localized to the genital tract of mice during first pregnancy. Am J Reprod Immunol **3**:65, 1983.

Solinger AM: Immature T lymphocytes in human neonatal blood. Cell Immunol **92**:115, 1985.

Sridama V, Pacini F, Yang SL, et al: Decreased levels of T helper cells: a possible cause of immunodeficiency in pregnancy. N Engl J Med **307**:352, 1982.

Starkey PM, Sargent IL, Redman CWG: Cell populations in human early pregnancy decidua: characterisation and isolation of large granular lymphocytes by flow cytometry. Immunology **65**:129, 1988.

Steihm ER: Fetal defense mechanisms. Am J Dis Child **129**:438, 1975.

Sullender WM, Miller JL, Yasukawa LL, et al: Humoral and cell-mediated immunity in neonates with herpes simplex virus infection. J Infect Dis **155**:28, 1987.

Sunderland CA, Redman CWG, Stirrat GM. HLA-A,B,C antigens are expressed on nonvillous trophoblasts of the early human placenta. J Immunol 127:2614, 1981.

Szekeres-Bartho J, Hadnagy J, Pacsa AS: The suppressive effect of progesterone during pregnancy: unique sensitivity of pregnancy lymphocytes. J Reprod Immunol 7:121, 1986.

Szekeres-Bartho J, Kilar F, Falkay G, et al: Progesterone-treated lymphocytes release a substance inhibiting cytotoxicity and prostaglandin synthesis. Am J Reprod Immunol 9:15, 1985.

Talamantes F, Ogren L, Markoff E, et al: Phylogenetic distribution, regulation of secretion, and prolactin-like effects of placental lactogens. Fed Proc 39:2582, 1980.

Taylor PV, Hancock KW: Antigenicity of trophoblast and possible antigen masking effects during pregnancy. Immunology 28:973, 1975.

Theofilopoulos AN, Dixon FJ: Murine models of systemic lupus erythematosus. Adv Immunol 37:269, 1985.

Timonen T, Saksela E: Cell-mediated anti-embryo cytotoxicity in human pregnancy. Clin Exp Immunol 23:462, 1976.

Toder V, Nebel L, Gleicher N: Studies of natural killer cells in pregnancy. I. Analysis at the single cell level. J Clin Lab Immunol 14:123, 1984.

Uksila J, Lassila O, Hirvonen T, et al: Development of natural killer cell function in the human fetus. J Immunol 130:153, 1983.

Unander AM, Olding LB: Ontogeny and postnatal persistence of a strong suppressor activity in man. J Immunol 127:1182, 1981.

Van der Werf AJM: Are lymphocytotoxic iso-antibodies induced by the early human trophoblast? Lancet i:595, 1971.

Van Tol MJD, Zijlstra J, Heijnen CJ, et al: Antigen-specific plaque-forming cell response of human cord blood lymphocytes after in vitro stimulation by T cell-dependent antigens. Eur J Immunol 13:390, 1983.

Van Cong N, Vaisse C, Gross M-S, et al: The human placental protein 14 (PP14) gene is localized on chromosome 9q34. Hum Genet 86:515, 1991.

Vanderbeeken Y, Vlieghe MP, Duchateau J, et al: Suppressor T-lymphocytes in pregnancy. Am J Reprod Immunol 5:20, 1984.

Voisin GA: Immunological interventions of the placenta in maternal immunological tolerance to the fetus. In Wegmann TG, Gill TJ (eds): Immunobiology and Reproduction. New York, Oxford University Press, 1983.

Wattanasak K, Matangkasombut P: Specific human maternal lymphocyte cytotoxic effects on cord blood lymphocytes. In Bratanov K (ed): Immunology of Reproduction. Sofia, Bulgaria, Bulgarian Academy of Science, 1983.

Wegmann TG: Fetal protection against abortion: is it immunosuppression or immunostimulation? Ann Immunol Instit Pasteur 135:309, 1984.

Wegmann TG: Placental immunotropism: maternal T cells enhance placental growth and function. Am J Reprod Immunol Microbiol 15:67, 1987.

Wei X, Orr HT: Different expression of HLA-E, HLA-F, and HLA-G transcripts in human tissue. Hum Immunol 29:131, 1990.

Weinberg ED: Pregnancy associated depression of cell mediated immunity. Rev Infect Dis 6:814, 1984.

Weinstein L, Aycock WL, Feemster RF: The relation of sex, pregnancy and menstruation to susceptibility in poliomyelitis. N Engl J Med 245:54, 1951.

Wilson CB, Westall J, Johnston L, et al: Decreased production of interferon-gamma by human neonatal cells. J Clin Invest 77:860, 1986.

Wood GW, Kamel S, Smith K: Immunoregulation and prostaglandin production by mechanically-derived and enzyme-derived murine decidual cells. J Reprod Immunol 13:235, 1988.

Youtananukorn V, Matangkasombut P: Specific plasma factors blocking human maternal cell-mediated immune reactivity to placental antigens. Nature 242:110, 1973.

Zuckerman F, Head JR: Possible mechanism of nonrejection of the feto-placental allograft: trophoblast resistance to lysis by cellular immune effectors. Transplant Proc 19:554, 1987.

Zuckerman F, Head JR: Susceptibility of mouse trophoblast to antibody and complement-mediated damage. Transplant Proc 17:925, 1985.

GESTATIONAL CHANGES OF THE REPRODUCTIVE TRACT AND BREASTS

CHAPTER

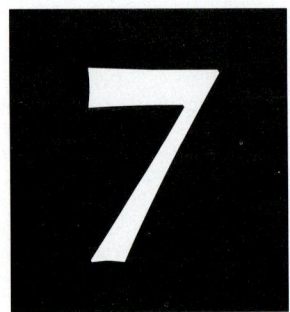

ANATOMIC ALTERATIONS IN THE REPRODUCTIVE TRACT

ROBERT RESNIK, M.D.

THE UTERUS

The uterus has the unique capacity to alter its shape and size dramatically to accommodate a rapidly growing fetus and placenta. Comparison of its dimensions in nonpregnant and pregnant states reveals a solid organ initially weighing 50 to 70 gm, reaching 800 to 1200 gm at term. It measures $7.5 \times 5.0 \times 2.5$ cm, with a capacity of 10 ml, before pregnancy, and $20 \times 25 \times 22.5$ cm with a 5-liter capacity prior to term delivery. Calculations obtained by ultrasound examination demonstrate a total intrauterine volume less than 300 cm³ at 6 weeks gestation, increasing to 4500 cm³ at 40 weeks (Gohari et al., 1977). These measurements are summarized in Table 7–1.

The mechanisms responsible for this growth are thought to be both hormonal and mechanical. During the first 6 weeks of pregnancy, uterine enlargement is due predominantly to hyperplasia and formation of new cells. Hypertrophy and stretching of muscle fibers account for the changes observed after the first trimester. The myometrium is known to be exquisitely sensitive to estrogens. Shortly following estrogen exposure, the uterus becomes hyperemic and edematous. Within 12 to 24 hours, marked increases in protein synthesis are observed, characterized by the appearance of RNA polymerase II and increases in the template capacity for RNA synthesis and, finally, net protein synthesis. These biochemical events following myometrial exposure to estrogen have been reviewed (Katzenellenbogen et al., 1979). Muscle fibers increase

in length from 50 to 500 μ, and in width from 5 to 15 μ, presumably owing to stretching caused by an expanding fetus and placenta.

The uterus assumes various shapes during the course of pregnancy. Prior to the sixth week, it retains a pyriform configuration. It becomes more globular by 12 weeks as it rises out of the maternal pelvis. At this point, the uterus becomes a sphere, ultimately assuming an ovoid appearance at term.

The distribution and direction of the muscle fibers are particularly well suited to the functions of coordinated contractile activity and postpartum hemostasis. The outermost layer consists of two thin longitudinal muscle bundles encompassing a transverse layer, which pass upward from the isthmus anteriorly, over the fundus, to the posterior uterine wall. The bulk of the organ is formed by the second, mid-layer component. This is a richly vascularized array of interlacing fibers that form "figures of eight" around blood vessels. The innermost layer, underlying the decidua, is circular, forming a triangular pattern, with more extensive development in the area of the isthmus and tubal insertions.

THE CERVIX AND ISTHMUS

Whereas the uterine corpus is made up primarily of smooth muscle, more than 85 per cent of the content of the cervix is fibrous connective tissue (Danforth,

TABLE 7–1. Dimensional Changes of Uterus During Pregnancy

	WEIGHT (gm)	LENGTH × WIDTH × DEPTH (cm)	CAPACITY (ml)	TOTAL INTRAUTERINE VOLUME (cm³)
Nonpregnant	50–70	7.5 × 5.0 × 2.5	10	<300 (early pregnancy)
Term	800–1200	20 × 25 × 22.5	5000	4500

1947). The cervix undergoes extensive change during pregnancy. It becomes soft, with a decrease in concentration of collagen as well as changes in the concentrations of various proteoglycans. The collagen fibers that remain are swollen and loosely associated. The endocervical cells demonstrate mitosis, and the squamocolumnar junction becomes visible during the process of "eversion." The extent of endocervical mucosal proliferation is such that it occupies about one-half of the entire cervical mass in late pregnancy, and the cells produce copious amounts of tenacious mucus. The cervix also changes its position, from an acute anteversion in early pregnancy to a more vertical configuration as the uterus rises out of the pelvis. The appearance and consistency of the external os undergo changes characterized by increased vascularity, softening, and dilation.

Functionally and anatomically, the cervix extends from the external to the histologic internal os and is lined by tall columnar epithelium. The area immediately above the cervix, extending from the histologic to the anatomic internal os for a distance of 5 to 10 mm in the nonpregnant state, is the isthmus or lowermost portion of the fundus (Aschoff, 1906). It is lined by a very thick layer of endometrial mucosa with a poorly developed stroma, no compacta, and a thin spongiosa layer. The importance of the isthmus is related to its presumed role in retention of the conceptus and to the likelihood that it is responsible for the formation of the lower uterine segment. Evidence in support of this likelihood is provided by the facts that the cavity of the isthmus increases in length to between 10 and 15 cm in late labor, and that the endometrium lining the lower segment, like that of the isthmus, does not become fully decidualized.

The factors that prepare the cervix for later pregnancy and labor, characterized by progressive softening and effacement with increasing development of the lower uterine segment, are under extensive investigation. The components of cervical tissue include collagen types I and III, proteoglycans (PGL), and elastin. Ripening of the uterine cervix in late pregnancy appears to be related to sharp decreases in collagen concentration and PGL, which influence the organization of collagen fibrils (Uldbjerg et al., 1983). It has been proposed that the simultaneous decrease in one PGL (decorin) and rise in two others (chondroitin sulfate PGL and biglycan) might be responsible for the cervical softening observed as term approaches (Uldbjerg et al., 1983; Norman et al., 1991). Recently it has been shown that large quantities of these two PGL accumulate in high concentrations in the cervical tissue taken from women who are immediately postpartum, compared to much lower concentrations in term women with unripe cervices (Norman et al.,

1993). These findings further support the role of PGL alterations in preparing the cervix before parturition.

It has also been suggested that human relaxin a polypeptide secreted by the corpus luteum, may also play a role in softening and effacement of the uterine cervix, but its precise contribution to this process has not been delineated. However, the application of porcine relaxin to the human cervix results in softening and effacement (Evans et al., 1983), and studies are currently under way to evaluate the effects of recombinant human relaxin on cervical ripening for the induction of labor.

THE VAGINA

Marked thickening of the vaginal mucosa occurs during pregnancy, with enlargement of the papillae, resulting in very prominent rugae. The cells contain increasing amounts of glycogen, and the rapid turnover results in sloughing of the surface layer and discharge of a whitish, acidic material. The increase in vascularity gives the vaginal tissues a bluish purple tint (Chadwick's sign). Other striking alterations in vaginal anatomy are hypertrophy of the musculature and a gradual softening of surrounding connective tissue, which permits the increased distensibility required for childbirth.

UTERINE BLOOD FLOW

Concomitant with the increase in uterine growth observed during pregnancy is a pronounced increase in uterine blood flow. Most of the data pertaining to the quantitative changes in flow occurring during pregnancy are obtained from laboratory animal models because there are obvious limitations to direct measurements in the human. From a nonpregnant baseline of between 30 and 40 ml/min, uterine blood flow increases to between 800 and 1200 ml/min in term pregnant sheep. Data obtained in humans suggest somewhat lower flows of approximately 500 ml/min, but measurements have been obtained under conditions of surgical intervention at the time of cesarean section, and the range of reported observations is wide (Metcalfe et al., 1955). During the last half of gestation, bulk uterine blood flow increases rapidly, although flow expressed per unit weight of the pregnant uterus and its contents is constant. Although the magnitude varies with the type of interspecies placental variation, in general the increasing oxygen demand of the growing fetus and placenta is satisfied by the increased uteroplacental blood flow and increasing oxygen extraction.

Despite the large increase in myometrial mass, studies utilizing radioactive microspheres in experimental animals demonstrate that myometrial and endometrial flows change little if at all during the second half of pregnancy, and that the increase in flow can be accounted for by the increase in placental circulation (Makowski et al., 1968). Specifically, at term less than 5 per cent of uterine blood flow is to the myometrium, 10 to 15 per cent is to the endometrium, and 80 to 85 per cent is to placental tissues. The pressure-flow relationship in the ovine uterus is such that blood flow is dependent on the pressure difference between the arterial and venous vasculature. Greiss et al. (1976) have shown that placental blood flow is not autoregulated, i.e., a decrease in arterial pressure does not result in a compensatory decrease in placental vascular resistance. However, it should be noted that within a human hemochorial placenta, the primary site of resistance to blood flow is in the distal uterine arteriolar bed. Consequently, the mechanisms of regulation are uncertain.

The mechanisms regulating changes in blood flow to the uterus are not thoroughly understood. There is, however, substantial evidence to suggest that blood flow to the nonpregnant uterus is, at least in part, under hormonal control. During the ovarian cycle of the sheep, uterine blood flow increases tenfold at the time of estrus coincidental with an increase in blood estradiol concentration, confirming previous observations that the uterine vasculature dilates in response to estrogen stimulation (Greiss and Anderson, 1969; Markee, 1932). These hormone-flow relationships are shown in Figure 7–1. The same phenomenon has been observed during the human menstrual cycle utilizing a thermal conductivity probe (Prill and Gotz, 1961). Additional evidence is provided by the observation that exogenous administration of estrogens to nonpregnant sheep induces increases in flow that approximate mid-pregnancy levels within 2 hours of exposure (Killam et al., 1973; Resnik et al., 1974). The striking response of the nonpregnant uterus to estrogens is shown in Figure 7–2. During the luteal phase of the cycle, blood flow decreases, possibly owing to the influence of progesterone, which has been shown to impede estrogen-induced increases in uterine blood flow (Resnik et al., 1977).

The fact that there is a 90-minute delay in uterine blood flow increase following estradiol injection directly into the uterine circulation, combined with the observation that the protein synthesis inhibitor cycloheximide inhibits the response, suggests that the estrogen action is mediated by another vasoactive chemical agent (Killam et al., 1973). Adenosine and the adenine nucleotides, histamine, acetylcholine, and bradykinin, as well as various prostaglandins including prostacyclin, have been shown to cause immediate increases in uterine blood flow, but their potential role as estrogen-induced mediators remains unclear (Resnik and Brink, 1978, 1980; Resnik et al., 1976).

Studies utilizing pregnant cows, which have a bicornuate uterus, reveal that uterine blood flow in early pregnancy is similar to that in nonpregnant cows until 13 days after mating. Blood flow to the gravid horn increases two- to threefold from day 14 to day 18, transiently decreases to flows observed in the ipsilateral nongravid horn from day 19 to day 25, and increases sharply at day 25 (Ford et al., 1979). Although no association between circulating estradiol levels and the abrupt increase in flow can be demonstrated, it is possible that sex steroids may have an influence on these early changes, either directly or by altering the ability of arterial smooth muscle to re-

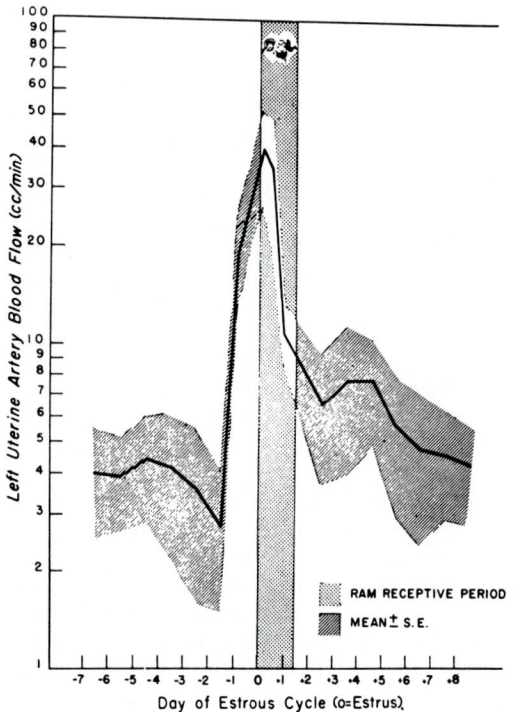

FIGURE 7–1. Graph of blood flow through one uterine artery during the estrous cycle of the nonpregnant ewe. Note the striking increase in flow at estrus. (From Greiss FC Jr, Anderson SG: Uterine vascular changes during the ovarian cycle. Am J Obstet Gynecol **103**:629, 1969.)

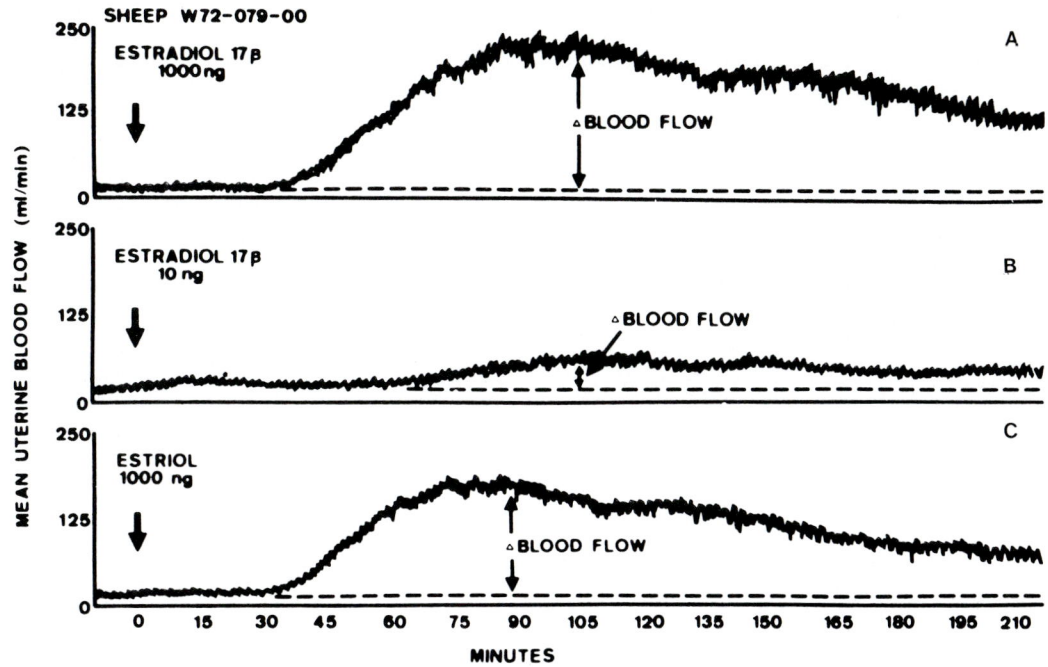

FIGURE 7–2. Graph of uterine blood flow response to 1000 ng of estradiol-17β (*A*), 10 ng of estradiol-17β (*B*), and 1000 ng of estriol (*C*) injected directly into the uterine artery of the nonpregnant sheep. (From Resnik R, Killam AP, Battaglia FC, et al: The stimulation of uterine blood flow by various estrogens. Endocrinology **94**:1192, 1974. © 1974, Baltimore, Williams & Wilkins.)

spond to norepinephrine (Pope and Stormshak, 1979). By 10 weeks gestation in the human, uterine blood flow approximates 50 ml/min, reaching 150 to 200 ml/min at 28 weeks. Again, the range of values is wide, and reported measurements have been obtained at the time of hysterotomy (Assali et al., 1960).

The progressive increase in uterine blood flow during gestation is totally derived from the increase in cardiac output and a ten- to 15-fold decrease in uterine vascular resistance (Dilts et al., 1969). Numerous biochemical factors have been implicated in the decrease in vascular resistance, including estrogen and progesterone levels, alterations in catecholamine metabolism and release, and the presence of vasodilator prostaglandins.

Administration of estrogen to the pregnant animal does not produce the dramatic increases in uterine blood flow observed in the nonpregnant animal, but does significantly augment flow nonetheless. Treatment of pregnant sheep with estradiol has been shown to increase uterine blood flow by 225 per cent in early pregnancy (38 days) and by 43 per cent near term. Flows specifically directed to placental tissues can be augmented by 25 per cent (Rosenfeld et al., 1976). These changes have been shown to parallel a decrease in uterine vascular resistance (Greiss and Marston, 1965). Although such experiments do not prove a cause-and-effect relationship between the sex steroids and the expansion of the uterine vasculature, they do demonstrate that the vasculature remains steroid sensitive during pregnancy and that it is not maximally vasodilated even during late gestation in sheep. Thus, it is clear that a number of anatomic, endocrinologic, and physiologic changes act in concert resulting in the

enormous increase in uterine blood flow observed during pregnancy. The precise regulating mechanisms are still not well understood.

REFERENCES

Aschoff L: Das untere Uterinsegment. Z Geburtschilfe Gyn **58**:328, 1906.

Assali NS, Rausamo L, Peltonen T: Measurement of uterine blood flow and uterine metabolism. Am J Obstet Gynecol **79**:86, 1960.

Danforth DN: The fibrous nature of the human cervix, and its relation to the isthmic segment in gravid and nongravid uteri. Am J Obstet Gynecol **53**:541, 1947.

Dilts PV Jr, Brinkman CR III, Kirschbaum TH, Assali NS: Uterine and systemic hemodynamic interrelationships and their response to hypoxia. Am J Obstet Gynecol **103**:138, 1969.

Evans MI, Dougan MB, Moawad AH, et al: Ripening of the human cervix with porcine ovarian relaxin. Am J Obstet Gynecol **147**:410, 1983.

Ford SP, Chenault JR, Echternkamp SE: Uterine blood flow of cows during the oestrous cycle and early pregnancy: Effect of the conceptus on the uterine blood supply. J Reprod Fertil **56**:53, 1979.

Gohari P, Berkowitz R, Hobbins JC: Prediction of intrauterine growth retardation by determination of total intrauterine volume. Am J Obstet Gynecol **127**:255, 1977.

Greiss FC Jr, Marston EL: The uterine vascular bed: Effect of estrogens during ovine pregnancy. Am J Obstet Gynecol **93**:720, 1965.

Greiss FC Jr, Anderson SG: Uterine vascular changes during the ovarian cycle. Am J Obstet Gynecol **103**:629, 1969.

Greiss FC Jr, Anderson SG, Still JG: Uterine pressure-flow relationships during early gestation. Am J Obstet Gynecol **126**:799, 1976.

Katzenellenbogen BS, Bhakoo HS, Ferguson ER, et al: Estrogen and anti-estrogen action in reproductive tissues and tumors. Recent Prog Horm Res **35**:259, 1979.

Killam AP, Rosenfeld CR, Battaglia FC, et al: Effect of estrogens on uterine blood flow of oophorectomized ewes. Am J Obstet Gynecol 115:1045, 1973.

Makowski EL, Meschia G, Droegemuller W, Battaglia FC: Distribution of uterine blood flow in pregnant sheep. Am J Obstet Gynecol 101:409, 1968.

Markee JE: Rhythmic uterine vascular changes. Am J Physiol 100:32, 1932.

Metcalfe J, Romney SL, Ramsey LH, Burwell CS: Estimation of uterine blood flow in women at term. J Clin Invest 34:1632, 1955.

Norman M, Ekman G, Ulmsten U et al. Proteoglycan metabolism in the connective tissue of pregnant and nonpregnant human cervix. An *in vitro* study. Biochemical J 275:515, 1991.

Norman M, Ekman G, Malmström A, et al. Changed proteoglycan metabolism in human cervix immediately after spontaneous vaginal delivery. Obstet Gynecol. In press.

Pope WF, Stormshak F: Effect of the ovine conceptus on in vitro responses of uterine arteries to prostaglandin E_2 and norepinephrine. Biol Reprod 20:847, 1979.

Prill HJ, Gotz F: Blood flow in the myometrium and endometrium of the uterus. Am J Obstet Gynecol 82:102, 1961.

Resnik R, Killam AP, Battaglia FC, et al: The stimulation of uterine blood flow by various estrogens. Endocrinology 94:1192, 1974.

Resnik R, Killam AP, Barton MD, et al: The effect of various vasoactive compounds upon the uterine vascular bed. Am J Obstet Gynecol 125:201, 1976.

Resnik R, Brink GW, Plumer MH: The effect of progesterone on estrogen-induced uterine blood flow. Am J Obstet Gynecol 128:251, 1977.

Resnik R, Brink GW: Effects of prostaglandins E_1, E_2, and $F_{2\alpha}$ on uterine blood flow in nonpregnant sheep. Am J Physiol 234:H557, 1978.

Resnik R, Brink GW: Uterine vascular response to prostacyclin in nonpregnant sheep. Am J Obstet Gynecol 137:267, 1980.

Rosenfeld CR, Morriss FH Jr, Battaglia FC, et al: Effect of estradiol-17β on blood flow to reproductive and nonreproductive tissues in pregnant ewes. Am J Obstet Gynecol 124:618, 1976.

Uldbjerg N, Ekman G, Malmström A, et al. Ripening of the human uterine cervix related to changes in collagen, glycosaminoglycans, and collagenolytic activity. Am J Obstet Gynecol 147:662, 1983.

CHAPTER

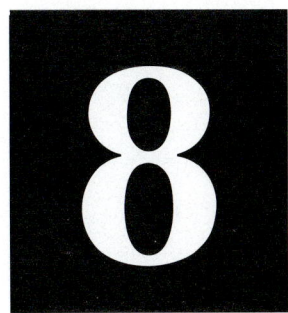

PHYSIOLOGY OF THE MYOMETRIUM

GABOR HUSZAR, M.D.

CELLULAR ASPECTS OF SMOOTH MUSCLE STRUCTURE

Unlike skeletal muscle, which is composed of continuous muscle fibers interrupted with Z-lines, the myometrial smooth muscle cells are dispersed within an extracellular matrix composed mainly of collagen fibers. The connective tissue integrates the myometrial contractile force that is generated within the individual muscle cells. The maximum force developed per cross-sectional area of smooth muscle often equals or exceeds that of striated muscle. This force-generating capacity is especially striking because the myosin content of smooth muscle is only about one-fourth that of skeletal muscle. Two other major properties distinguish smooth muscle from skeletal muscle: (1) the degree of shortening is about one order of magnitude greater in smooth muscle than in striated muscle and (2) smooth muscle can exert pulling force in any direction, whereas the contraction and force generation in skeletal muscle is always aligned with the axis of the muscle fibers. These characteristics of smooth muscles are caused by differences in the cellular organization of the contractile elements.

The myometrial cells communicate with one another through connections called *gap junctions* (Fig. 8–1). These cell-to-cell contacts are believed to facilitate the synchronization of myometrial function by conducting electrophysiologic stimuli. Although few gap junctions are seen in the myometria of nonpregnant women and women in early pregnancy, these structures become larger and more numerous close to term, at which point the frequency of Braxton Hicks contractions increases until the initiation of labor. It has been shown *in vitro* that an increase in the ratio of estrogen to progesterone favors the formation of gap junctions in uterine explants. The formation process is inhibited by indomethacin, an agent that inhibits prostaglandin synthesis. Subsequent administration of prostaglandins overcomes the indomethacin block. Oxytocin does not produce an effect, but isoxsuprine and isoproterenol decrease the number of gap junctions in *in vitro* systems. The process of gap junction formation may be viewed as an essential feature of the initiation of labor. Indeed, the area of myometrial gap junctions

in parturient rats was related to lower progesterone and higher estrogen concentrations. Furthermore, with respect to uterine activity, the area of gap junctions on the rat myometrium before, during, and after labor was directly proportional with the conduction velocity of the myometrial tissue and with the contractile properties, whether one considers the rate of rise in intrauterine pressure or the sum of intrauterine pressure during a contraction (Fig. 8–2).

The question of pacemaker activity in the myometrium is unresolved at present. Although the gap junctions help to integrate myometrial activity, no specific pacemaker cells have so far been identified in the uterus. It is not yet clear whether there is in fact an anatomic basis for pacemaker activity or whether pacing occurs as a consequence of the electrophysiologic and pharmacologic conditions.

ORGANIZATION OF THE MYOMETRIAL CELL

The structure of the smooth muscle cell can best be described by comparison with the well-known picture of striated muscle. A longitudinal section of rabbit psoas muscle is shown in Figure 8–3A in which the structural organization can be seen in two dimensions. In the longitudinal axis of the sarcomere (the contractile unit between two Z lines), repeating patterns of dense and light bands represent the filaments of myosin (thick filaments) and actin (thin filaments), respectively. The cross-sectional diagram shows the various phases of filament overlap. Each myosin filament is surrounded by thin actin filaments arranged in a hexagonal pattern; the sliding motion of these filaments against one another is the basis of the contraction-force generation process. Figure 8–3A is a schematic representation of the sarcomere in longitudinal section. The thick myosin filaments project the head part of the molecule, so-called subfragment-1, which contains adenosine triphosphatase (ATPase) and the actin combining active sites of myosin. These enzymatic sites interact with actin and ATP during the contraction and relaxation process.

The actin and myosin filaments of smooth muscle

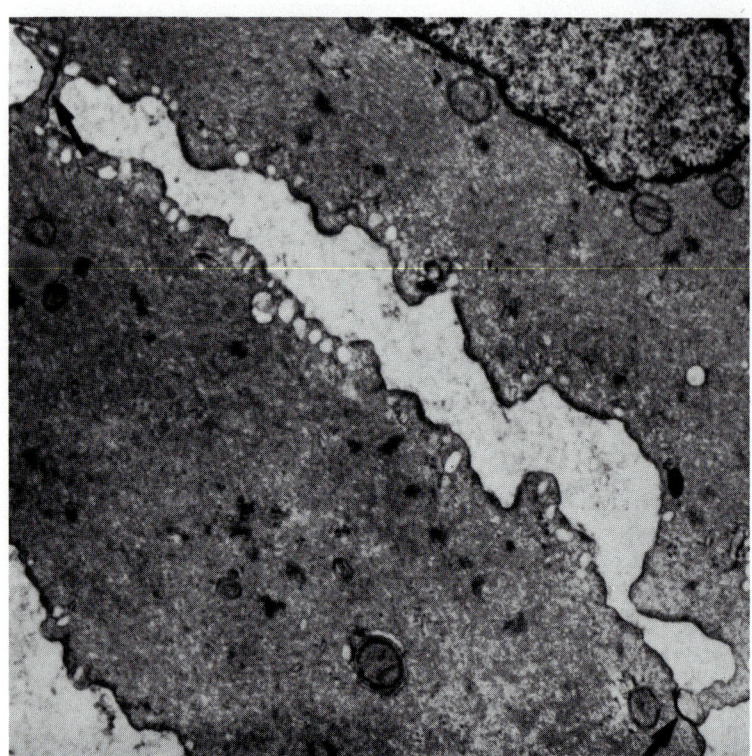

FIGURE 8–1. High magnification micrograph of rat myometrium during parturition. Arrow points to gap junction between two muscle cells. (Courtesy of Dr. R. Garfield, McMaster University, Hamilton, Canada.)

FIGURE 8–2. Relationship between percentage gap junction area, apparent conduction velocity of bursts of electrical activity, area of intrauterine pressure (IUP) cycles, and rate of rise of IUP cycles in sheep before, during, and after parturition. All values are mean ± S.E.M. Note the correspondence between changes in area gap junctions and changes in electrical conductance (conduction velocity) and mechanical activity (area and rate of rise of IUP cycles). (From Verhoeff A, Garfield RE: Ultrastructure of the myometrium and the role of gap junctions in myometrial function. *In* Huszar G (ed): The Physiology and Biochemistry of the Uterus in Pregnancy and Labor. Boca Raton, FL, CRC Press, 1986.)

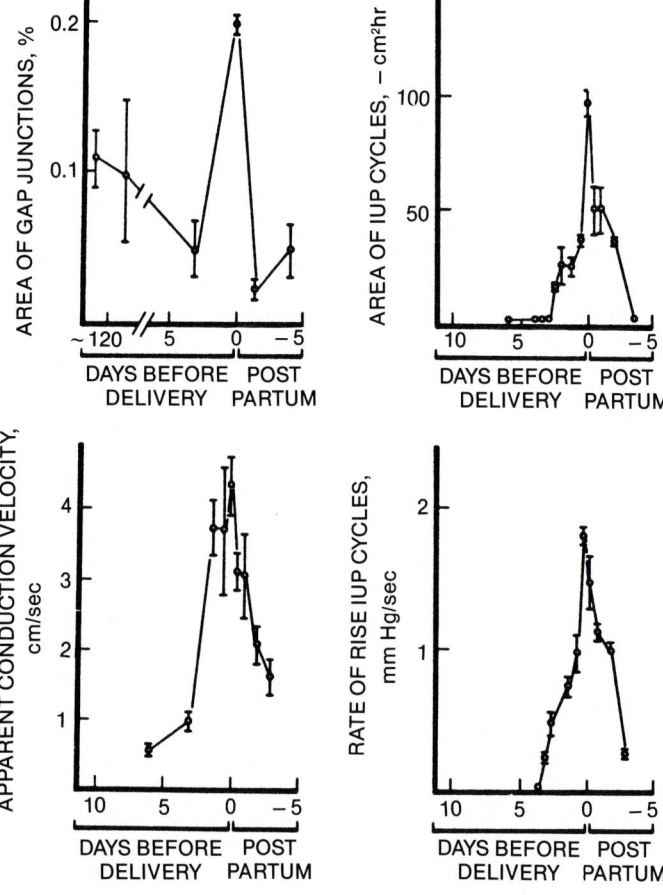

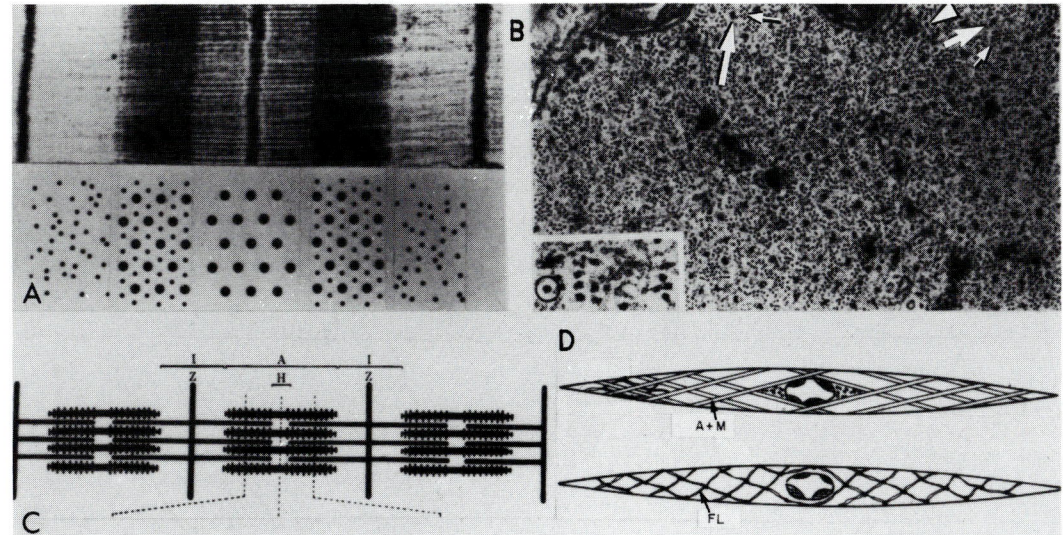

FIGURE 8–3. *A* and *C*, Electron microscopic and diagrammatic picture of longitudinal and cross sections of striated muscle, showing overlapping arrays of actin- and myosin-containing filaments, the latter with projecting crossbridges on them. *B*, Cross section of a smooth muscle cell. Thick filaments (*large arrows*) have a diameter of about 16 nM. Thin filaments (*small arrows*) have a mean diameter of about 7 nM. Intermediate filaments (*arrowhead*) are about 10 nM in diameter. *D*, Schematic diagram of the contractile apparatus: proposed arrangement of "contractile units." Each unit consists of a bundle of actin and myosin filaments (*A + M*) connecting opposite sites on the cell surface. The 10 nM filaments (*FL*) form a network between the actin-myosin filament groups. (*A* and *C* adapted from Huxley HE: The Croonian Lecture, 1970: The structural basis of muscular contraction. Proc R Soc Lond (Biol) **178**:131, 1971. *B* adapted from Somlyo AP, Somlyo AV: Ultrastructure of smooth muscle. *In* Daniels EE, Paton DM (ed): Methods in Pharmacology. New York, Plenum, 1974. *D* adapted from Stephens NL (ed): The Biochemistry of Smooth Muscle. Baltimore, University Park Press, 1977.)

are not organized into fibers and fibrils, as in striated muscle, but instead occur in random bundles throughout the muscle cells (Fig. 8–3*B*). In addition to the 15 to 18 nM thick (myosin) filaments and 6 nM thin (actin) filaments, which are known components of striated muscle, smooth muscle contains major filaments of a third type—the 10 nM intermediate filaments, which form a network linking protein structures known as *dense bodies*. The intermediate filaments and dense bodies do not play an active part in the contractile process. Rather, they are associated with the cell membrane and are distributed throughout the cytoplasm so as to form a network with attachment sites located over the entire cell (Fig. 8–3*D*). The 10 nM filaments link the individual actin and myosin filaments into integrated mechanical units. The intermediate filaments and dense bodies are analogous in function to the Z-lines of striated muscle. This organized yet highly flexible arrangement enables the uterus to adapt to virtually any shape and to generate the force necessary for labor even with fetuses of various positions and sizes.

The myosin filaments in striated muscle are bidirectional in each sarcomere, and the continuity of the filaments is interrupted by the Z lines. In smooth muscle, the myosin molecules are laid down in a unidirectional order, with the result that the myosin filaments are much longer than their counterparts in striated muscle (Fig. 8–4). Because of this uniform, uninterrupted polarity, the actin filaments are able to interact with myosin heads throughout the extended length of the thick filaments. This difference accounts for the fact that the maximal degree of shortening in smooth muscle is about 10 times greater than in striated muscle.

STRUCTURE OF CONTRACTILE PROTEINS

Myosin is the principal protein of muscle contraction. It is a structural protein laid down in thick myofilaments to optimize the actin-myosin interaction; it is also an enzyme that facilitates conversion of the chemical energy of ATP into motion and force generation during contraction. The myosin molecule is about 160 nM long and has a molecular weight of approximately 500,000 daltons (see Fig. 8–4). In smooth muscle it is composed of two heavy chains of 200,000 daltons and two light chains of about 20,000 and 15,000 daltons, respectively. The myosin molecule has two functional parts, the head and the tail. The globular head contains (1) the actin-combining site, where myosin and actin interact to generate force, (2) the ATPase site, where ATP is hydrolyzed and chemical energy is converted to mechanical force, and (3) the 20,000-dalton light chains that, when phosphorylated, constitute the key element of contractile regulation (the actin-myosin interaction) in smooth muscle. The tail of the myosin molecule is a helical rod that forms the "backbone" of the myofilaments and transmits the generated force.

An interesting aspect of the correlation between

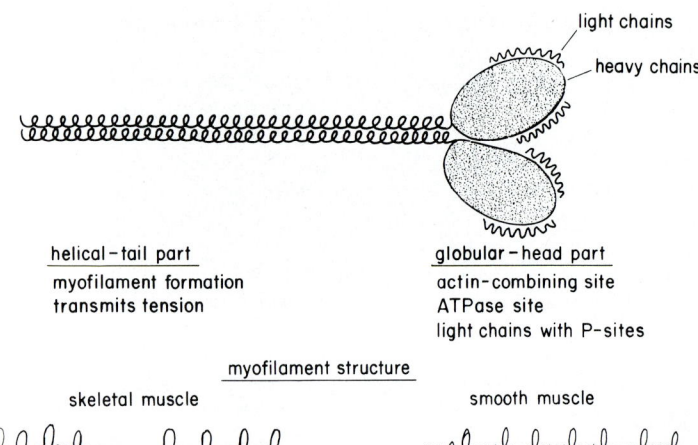

light chains

heavy chains

helical-tail part
myofilament formation
transmits tension

globular-head part
actin-combining site
ATPase site
light chains with P-sites

myofilament structure

skeletal muscle

smooth muscle

FIGURE 8–4. Schematic structure of myosin and myofilaments in skeletal and smooth muscle. Note that the myofilaments are bidirectional in the skeletal muscle but unidirectional in smooth muscle.

myosin structure and uterine contractility was recently recognized. Comparison of myosins isolated from nonpregnant and pregnant uteri of woman, rabbit, rat, and cow showed that the two types of myosins differed in enzymatic properties. Thus, as gestation brings about changes in myometrial function, new myosin isozymes specific to pregnancy are synthesized that apparently function more efficiently in pregnancy and labor.

The other major muscle protein is *actin*, a globular protein of 43,000 daltons. The actin monomers polymerize into long, thin filaments that originate in and are suspended between the dense bodies. When the actin and myosin filaments slide past one another during uterine contractions, the myosin heads and actin molecules form the so-called cross bridges that generate the contractile force of labor. Myometrial actin filaments also show isoformic changes related to pregnancy.

REGULATION OF MYOMETRIAL CONTRACTILITY

Calcium

The major role of calcium in contractile regulation is a factor common to both striated and smooth muscles (Fig. 8–5). In striated muscle, calcium effects the interaction of actin and myosin through *troponin*, a regulatory protein. In the absence of calcium, troponin blocks the interaction of these contractile proteins. When calcium is present, however, the actin-myosin interaction is promoted. These effects can be demonstrated both by contractility of isolated striated muscle strips and by *in vitro* measurements of actomyosin ATPase.

Several issues are currently under investigation with respect to the contractile state of the uterine muscle and the transport of calcium ions; these issues include the identification of the calcium pools that serve as the source of myoplasmic calcium; the sites of the cellular or extracellular compartments in which calcium can be sequestered at the time of relaxation; and characterization of the cellular processes that facilitate

the active transport of calcium across the cell membrane. The major sources of cytoplasmic calcium are the extracellular fluid (and the extracellular surface of the muscle cell membrane) and the intracellular calcium pool—essentially the sarcoplasmic reticulum. The sarcoplasmic reticulum sequesters calcium by active, ATP-fueled transport. The calcium concentration in smooth muscle cells is thus regulated by the cell membrane, the sarcoplasmic reticulum, and perhaps the mitochondria. The relative contributions of these three elements are the subjects of active research.

The mechanism by which calcium is transported through the cell membranes is at present not well understood. The main feature of this mechanism is a change in the action potential: that is, the cell membrane becomes permeable to calcium in response to neurotransmitters, hormones, or other physiologic stimulation. Parallel with the influx of calcium, cellular sodium and potassium ions move in the opposite direction. An interesting development in the understanding of transmembrane calcium transport (calcium gating) is the discovery of phospholipid effects. It appears that phosphatidic acid promotes the inward

REGULATION OF ACTIN-MYOSIN INTERACTION

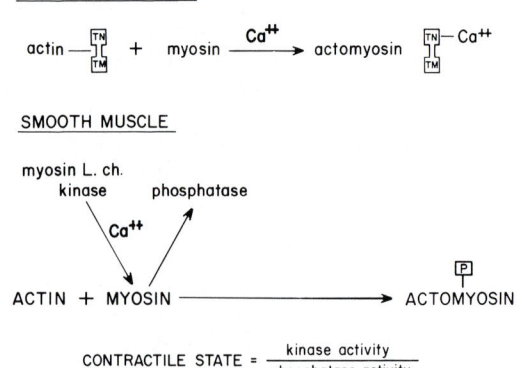

SKELETAL MUSCLE

SMOOTH MUSCLE

$$\text{CONTRACTILE STATE} = \frac{\text{kinase activity}}{\text{phosphatase activity}}$$

FIGURE 8–5. Calcium-mediated regulation of actin-myosin interaction in skeletal and smooth muscle. *TN* = troponin; *TM* = tropomyosin.

movement of calcium by increasing the permeability of the cell membrane. This phenomenon, together with increased turnover of phospholipids, takes place in response to the presence of cholinergic, alpha-adrenergic, and muscarinic drugs. The various agonists appear to stimulate activation of a phospholipase C, which subsequently hydrolyzes polyphospho-inositides in the cell membrane and releases inositol phosphates. Inositol 1,4,5-triphosphate (IP_3) appears to be the second messenger that stimulates the release of calcium from the sarcoplasmic reticulum. The calcium signal then initiates the influx of extracellular calcium.

The regulation of myoplasmic calcium concentration is in part based on the intracellular calcium stores for two reasons. First, it has been shown that the myometrium can contract in calcium-free media; thus the sarcoplasmic reticulum and mitochondria contain sufficient calcium in reserve for the initiation of contraction. Second, the biochemical and regulatory aspects of calcium transport by the sarcoplasmic reticulum and by the cell membrane are now well recognized. The known effects of various hormones and other agonists on the sarcoplasmic reticulum agree with our current concepts of myometrial contractility. An important possibility of oxytocin action is based on the inhibition of calcium-magnesium ATPase in the myometrial cell membrane. This enzyme is implicated in the transport of calcium from the intracellular to extracellular compartment. Oxytocin has been shown to inhibit the calcium-magnesium ATPase in membrane preparations of both the nonpregnant and pregnant uterus. The concentration of half maximum inhibitions was about 1 nM, which corresponds to the maximum of oxytocin binding to its myometrial receptors.

Myosin Light-Chain Phosphorylation

All evidence to date indicates that in smooth muscles the actin-myosin interaction is regulated through the enzymatic phosphorylation or dephosphorylation of the 20,000-dalton myosin light chains. Indeed, the actin-myosin interaction can take place only if the myosin light chain has been phosphorylated. Phosphorylation occurs through the action of myosin light-chain kinase, an enzyme that is activated by calcium. Relaxation of smooth muscle occurs when another enzyme, myosin light-chain phosphatase, removes the phosphate group from the myosin molecule. Actin does not "recognize" the dephosphorylated myosin; hence, no further actin-myosin interaction takes place.

The relationship between the actin-myosin interaction and myosin light-chain phosphorylation has been demonstrated *in vitro* in several actomyosin preparations. In studying smooth muscles from the human placenta at term, it was found that when the myosin light chains were phosphorylated, placental actomyosin ATPase activity simultaneously increased to about four times that of actin-unphosphorylated myosin. The relationship between myosin light-chain phosphorylation and the contractile state of muscle has also been confirmed in preparations that more clearly resemble *in vivo* conditions, such as in chicken gizzard fibers, porcine carotid arterial strips, and rat myometrium.

Myosin light-chain kinase has so far been shown to be influenced by three cellular regulatory systems. First, calcium in concentrations of about 10^{-6} molar is necessary for myosin light-chain kinase activity. Second, myosin light-chain kinase is active only if calmodulin is associated with the enzyme. This 16,500-dalton protein was isolated in uterine muscle and its amino acid sequence was determined. Finally, it has been shown that phosphorylation of the kinase by a cyclic adenosine monophosphate (cAMP)–dependent protein kinase inhibits myosin light-chain phosphorylation. The decrease in activity by phosphorylated myosin light-chain kinase is due to the enzyme's lower affinity for the calmodulin-calcium complex.

The phosphorylation and dephosphorylation of myosin light chains and myosin light-chain kinase offer an interesting regulatory system. First, when phosphorylation of the myosin light chain occurs, the actin-myosin interaction increases and the contractile state of the muscle is enhanced. When myosin light-chain kinase is phosphorylated and kinase activity decreases, less myosin light-chain phosphorylation occurs and the muscle relaxes. Second, the myometrium relaxes in response to dephosphorylation of the myosin light chains (although these two events do not show a close correlation because the smooth muscle cells can retain force without rephosphorylation of myosin light chains mimicking a catch-mechanism). This balance of kinase and phosphatase activities is presumably under common cellular control and, when fully elucidated, may prove to be very important in the regulation of myometrial contractility.

HORMONAL REGULATION OF MYOMETRIAL CONTRACTILITY

There is strong evidence that the three regulators of myosin light-chain kinase—calcium, calmodulin, and cAMP-mediated phosphorylation—are interrelated with the actions of hormones and pharmacologic agents in uterine contractility. As already discussed, the accumulation of calcium by the sarcoplasmic reticulum is an ATP-dependent enzymatic process mediated by various hormones and drugs. In *in vitro* sarcoplasmic reticulum preparations of bovine and human myometria, calcium uptake has been shown to be inhibited by prostaglandin $F_{2\alpha}$, oxytocin, and acetylcholine, hormones known to stimulate smooth muscle. Cyclic AMP, which promotes calcium uptake, depresses uterine contractility. The result of such postulated hormonal regulation is that prostaglandin $F_{2\alpha}$ and oxytocin would increase (whereas cAMP would decrease) not only the intracellular calcium levels, but also the rate of myosin light-chain phosphorylation and hence the contractile state of the uterus. These *in vitro* effects of hormones on the myometrial transport calcium agree with experimental findings. The intracellular calcium concentration increases during contraction and decreases when the uterine muscle is relaxed after administration of isoproterenol or other beta-adrenergic agents.

The inhibition of myosin light-chain kinase by cAMP offers an excellent model for the direct hormonal regulation of the actin-myosin interaction in the uterus. Cyclic AMP, or any agent that increases cellular levels of cAMP, promotes relaxation of smooth muscle. When cAMP-mediated myosin light-chain kinase phosphorylation diminishes activity, or when the action of cAMP reduces the intracellular levels of calcium in the uterine cytosol, the level of phosphorylated myosin light chains becomes lower.

In light of the interactions described so far, a number of drug and hormone effects that are familiar in everyday clinical practice can be explained in physiologic terms by the regulatory mechanisms of myosin light-chain kinase (Fig. 8–6). The main points are:

1. In smooth muscles enzymatic phosphorylation of the 20,000-mw light chain is necessary in order for actin-myosin interaction to occur.

2. Myosin light-chain kinase is the key enzyme for regulation of myometrial contractility.

3. Calcium is essential for myosin kinase light-chain activation; calcium binds to the kinase as a calmodulin-calcium complex. A second, as yet undefined, regulatory system causes a decline of the actin-myosin cross-bridge turnover during the contractile process. Thus, smooth muscles may retain tension even after the levels of cellular calcium and myosin light-chain phosphorylation become reduced.

4. Free calcium levels are regulated by the intracellular calcium pool, by the actions of the sarcoplasmic reticulum, and by the myometrial cell membrane. The membrane contains the calcium channels and the calcium-magnesium–stimulated ATPase system, both of which are important in the regulation of the transmembrane calcium transport.

5. The accumulation of calcium by the sarcoplasmic reticulum is an ATP-mediated enzymatic process that is modulated by various pharmacologic agents and hormones. Cyclic AMP promotes calcium sequestration in the myometrium; $PGF_{2\alpha}$ or oxytocin inhibits the process and thus causes higher free calcium levels in the cytoplasm.

6. Myosin light-chain kinase is inhibited by cAMP-mediated phosphorylation of the enzyme itself. Phosphorylation of the enzyme diminishes its affinity for the calcium-calmodulin complex.

7. Cellular cAMP levels depend on the relative activities of two enzymes, adenylate cyclase (cAMP synthesis) and phosphodiesterase (cAMP breakdown). Activation and inhibition of these enzymes determine myometrial cAMP levels. For example, smooth muscle relaxation may be caused by activation of adenylate cyclase with beta-adrenergic agonists or by inhibition of phosphodiesterase following the administration of theophylline or papaverine. The effects of the latter two agents recently have been demonstrated to cause myometrial relaxation *in vitro*.

8. Prostaglandins affect myometrial contractility. As of this writing, this can be best explained as caused by modulation of the calcium fluxes. Prostaglandins have been reported to change the calcium permeability of the membranes, thus influencing the levels of intracellular free calcium.

9. Various peptides and peptide hormones modulate myometrial function. For instance, oxytocin regulates intracellular calcium levels by inhibiting the calcium-magnesium ATPase of the myometrial cell membrane. Recent data suggest that *relaxin*, an insulin-like peptide hormone, causes an increase in cellular cAMP levels with simultaneous inhibition of myosin light-chain kinase phosphorylation and muscle relaxation. Also, there are peptides similar to the vasoactive intestinal peptide that have a powerful relaxing effect on the myometrium.

10. Finally, the muscle cells in the myometrium are not isolated; they are interconnected as a functional unit in the simultaneous labor action of the uterus. The essential parts of this functional and metabolic coordination are the gap junctions. Gap junction formation, along with other associated cellular events such as the levels of receptors for estrogen and oxytocin, are under the regulation of estrogen and progesterone.

For the purposes of tocolysis, it is important that

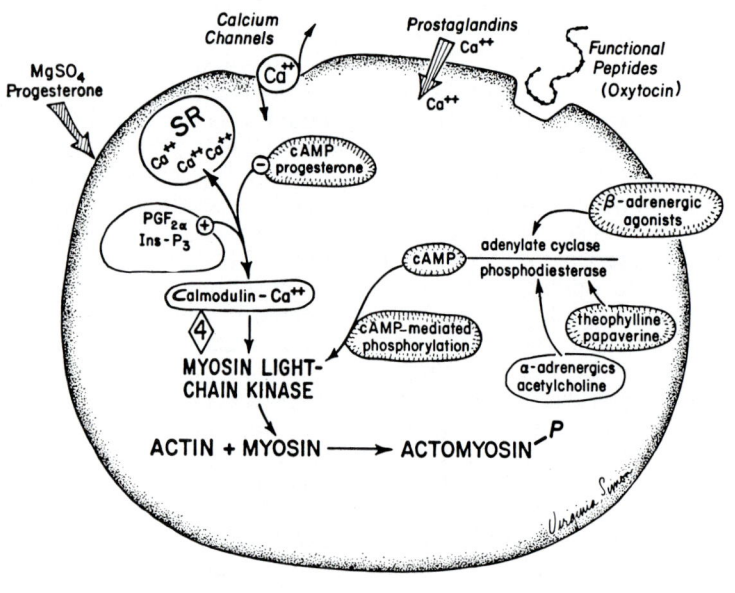

FIGURE 8–6. The contractile apparatus of the uterine smooth muscle cell: the MLCK is regulated through the calcium and cAMP pathways. Both calcium sequestration and cAMP levels in the cell are modulated by various drugs and hormones. Agonists circled with solid lines promote contractions: agonists in stippled areas promote relaxation. Specific sites that facilitate agonist interaction and have tocolytic potential include the adrenergic receptors, the calmodulin-MLCK interaction, the receptors for prostaglandins, the calcium channels, and the binding sites for functional peptides (OT, relaxin).

beta-adrenergic agonists activate adenylate cyclase, thus causing an increase in the cellular levels of cAMP. The increased cAMP concentration in turn diminishes myosin light-chain kinase activity through decreased binding of the calmodulin-calcium complex due to phosphorylation of the kinase and reduction of the cellular calcium levels. The latter effect is produced by the enhancement of calcium binding in the sarcoplasmic reticulum and by the cAMP effects on the ion transport across the cellular and mitochondrial membranes. (It modulates the sodium-potassium pump and sodium-calcium concentrations in the cytoplasm.) When myosin phosphorylation declines, the actin-myosin interaction diminishes and the myometrium relaxes. These events all contribute to the activities of myosin light-chain kinase and phosphatase and to the tocolytic effects of beta-adrenergic agents. The sequence and priority of the various myometrial regulatory processes are not yet known. The concept of cellular compartmentalization may eventually explain selected specific activation of one regulatory pathway in preference to another.

From the point of view of the clinician, the concept of the "tocolytic pathway" links the actin-myosin interaction, myosin phosphorylation, cAMP regulation of myosin light-chain kinase, the levels of cellular calcium, and the effects of beta-adrenergic agonists on adenylate cyclase activity. (A detailed discussion of the pharmacology of tocolytic therapy is presented in Chapter 33.)

The role of oxytocin in labor was quite puzzling until recently. It was apparent that oxytocin brought about uterine contractions, but no major increases in the circulating oxytocin levels were found during active labor. Fuchs and Soloff have successfully investigated the question of oxytocin action in rats and women. At the time of the initiation of labor, when the estrogen-progesterone ratio increases, there is an increase in myometrial estrogen receptors followed by an increase in oxytocin receptors. Thus, during labor the increased myometrial response to circulating oxytocin is due to greater numbers of oxytocin receptors in the myometrium. In keeping with this relationship between uterine function and oxytocin activities, the concentration of oxytocin receptors is much higher in the corpus than in the lower segment of the uterus or the cervix. When progesterone declines at the end of pregnancy and the influence of estrogen becomes predominant, the myometrium responds by synthesizing estrogen and oxytocin receptors. It is likely that a second messenger (e.g., inositol 1,4,5-triphosphate) is involved in the oxytocin-directed regulation.

SUMMARY

The main factor in the initiation of uterine contractions in labor is the rise in the estrogen-progesterone ratio. In women this increase may be perceived only on the cellular level, but not in measurable differences in plasma concentrations. The increased estrogen levels initiate the synthesis of estrogen receptors, with an increased myometrial response to estrogen. This is manifested in various effects, such as synthesis of oxytocin receptors, formation of myometrial gap junctions, changes in myometrial contractility, and increases in prostaglandin biosynthesis, in cellular inositol 1,4,5-triphosphate and calcium levels, and in myosin phosphorylation. Cervical collagen and glycosaminoglycan degradation and uterine catecholamine biosynthesis are also affected. The concomitant decrease in progesterone directly contributes to the initiation of labor by decreasing the stability of the uterine and membrane lysosomes that contain various enzymes. When these enzymes become available, various important functions are triggered (prostaglandin biosynthesis in the membranes, activation of cervical collagenase, and so on), and the complex cascade mechanism of labor proceeds. As of this writing, we have a general idea as to how the various hormones act on the surface receptors of the uterine muscle cells and a rough understanding of the components and regulation of myometrial contractility. However, there is a gap in our knowledge with respect to the exact mechanism(s) linking these extracellular and membrane-bound events of hormonal regulation to the intracellular processes of the myometrial muscle cell.

REFERENCES

Berridge MJ: Inositol triphosphate and diacylglycerol: two interacting second messengers. Annu Rev Biochem **56**:159, 1987.

Cooke R: The mechanism of muscle contraction. CRC Crit Rev Biochem **21**:53, 1986.

Fuchs A-R: The role of oxytocin in parturition. In Huszar G (ed): The Physiology and Biochemistry of the Uterus in Pregnancy and Labor. Boca Raton, FL, CRC Press, 1986.

Hartshorne DJ: Biochemistry of the contractile process in smooth muscle. In Johnson LR (ed): Physiology of the Gastrointestinal Tract. 2nd ed. New York, Raven Press, 1987, p. 423.

Huszar G: Cellular regulation of myometrial contractility and essentials of tocolytic therapy. In Huszar G (ed): The Physiology and Biochemistry of the Uterus in Pregnancy and Labor. Boca Raton, FL, CRC Press, 1986.

Huszar G, Roberts JR: Biochemistry and pharmacology of the myometrium and labor: Regulation at the cellular and molecular levels. Am J Obstet Gynecol **142**:225, 1981.

Verhoeff A, Garfield RE: Ultrastructure of the myometrium and the role of gap junctions in myometrial function. In Huszar G (ed): The Physiology and Biochemistry of the Uterus in Pregnancy and Labor. Boca Raton, FL, CRC Press, 1986.

CHAPTER

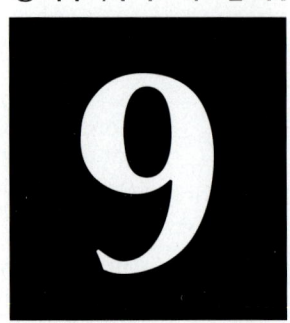

THE PUERPERIUM

ROBERT RESNIK, M.D.

THE REPRODUCTIVE ORGANS

The Uterus

The puerperium begins immediately after delivery of the placenta. Frequent, strong myometrial contractions rapidly induce a decrease in size, and within 24 hours the uterus becomes a globular hard mass approximately the size it was at 20 weeks gestation. The figure-of-eight interlaced muscle bundle of the middle uterine layer compresses blood vessels supplying the placental site, preventing hemorrhage. Within a week postpartum, the uterus has decreased in size by 50 per cent, to 500 gm. After 2 weeks, normal involution is such that the uterus cannot be felt by abdominal examination, and by 6 weeks it has returned almost to its nonpregnant dimensions.

Appropriate involution of the placental site is of great importance. After the placenta separates, only the basal portion of the decidua remains. Within 72 hours postpartum, two layers become apparent. The first layer is superficial and is sloughed with the lochia. The underlying layer contains residual endometrial glands and is a source of the new endometrium. By day 7, the surface epithelium and stroma begin to assume a nonpregnant appearance, and by the 16th day, complete restoration of proliferative endometrium has occurred. At this point, the endometrium is identical to that of the nonpregnant uterus in the proliferative phase of the cycle, except that remnants of hyalinized decidua remain and leukocytic infiltrates may be observed in the stroma (Sharman, 1953). The appearance of blood vessels underlying the placental site is shown in Figure 9–1.

The placental site itself takes longer to regenerate. Immediately following delivery, marked constriction of arterioles supplying the placental site occurs, and a fibrinoid endarteritis develops in a matter of hours. The area then undergoes hyalinization. Venous sites also become thrombotic and hyalinized (Anderson and Davis, 1968). The area then heals either by decidual sloughing produced by endometrial growth from areas adjacent to the placental site or by a process similar to that by which any denuded epithelial area regenerates. If this process does not proceed properly,

subinvolution is said to occur, which may result in significant late postpartum hemorrhage. The normal histologic appearance of the placental site 6 weeks postpartum is seen in Figure 9–2.

The Cervix

Following delivery of the placenta, the cervix has little tone and bears little resemblance to its nonpregnant state. Within 2 to 3 days, it resumes its customary appearance, but is still dilated to 2 or 3 cm. At 1 week postpartum, the gross appearance of the cervix is very like that in the nonpregnant state, although histologic examination shows regression of the endocervical hypertrophy (Glass and Rosenthal, 1950). As late as 6 weeks postpartum, involution is still occurring, with evidence of stromal edema and round cell infiltration, the latter persisting up to 3 or 4 months (McLaren, 1952). Thus, any evaluation of the cervix relative to repetitive mid-trimester loss should be delayed until at least 3 months after termination of pregnancy.

The Vagina

Immediately following delivery, the prominent vaginal rugae are not visible, and the vagina appears smooth and swollen. Within 3 weeks, the vascularity and edema regress, and rugae reappear. Histologically, the vaginal epithelium returns to its normal nonpregnant appearance in 6 to 10 weeks. At 6 weeks, it has completed involution, although varying degrees of mucosal and fascial relaxation may remain, manifested by a persistent cystocele and/or rectocele (Kistner, 1978).

RETURN OF OVULATION AND MENSTRUATION

Early studies demonstrate that the initial ovulation following delivery in nonlactating women occurs at a mean of 10 weeks, compared with 17 weeks for nursing women (Lyon and Stamm, 1946). With use of

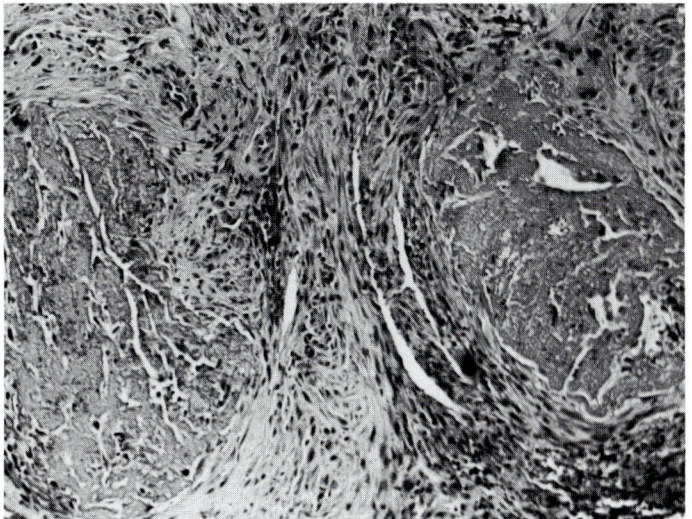

FIGURE 9–1. Maternal blood vessels of the placental site 2 weeks postpartum. Both vessels are filled with contracted thrombotic material, and early fibrocytic ingrowth is beginning at the periphery. ($\times$ 160)

sequential endometrial biopsies, a secretory pattern may be observed as early as day 44 (Sharman, 1951a). Other studies corroborate these earlier findings, but show that women who breast-feed for less than 28 days will ovulate at approximately the same time as women who do not breast-feed. Furthermore, ovulation can take place as early as 27 days after delivery (Cronin, 1968).

Return of menstruation in nonlactating women in-

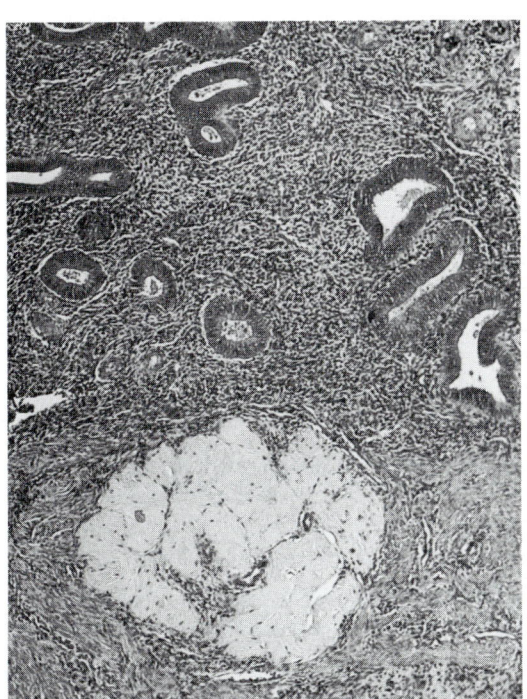

FIGURE 9–2. Normally involuted placental site blood vessels 6 weeks postpartum. Endometrium shows some inflammatory cell infiltration, irregular glandular lumen, and hemosiderin. Formerly thrombosed uteroplacental vessel is now completely "organized," and hyaline tissue has replaced thrombus. This vessel will now gradually become recanalized by new vascular growth. ($\times$ 64)

creases linearly up to 12 weeks postpartum, and 70 per cent will have menstruated by that time (Sharman, 1951b). The mean time to first menses is 7 to 9 weeks, but in lactating women, the longer the period of lactation, the longer the mean time to the first menstrual period. It is generally agreed that any menstrual period in the first 6 weeks is anovulatory, but once menstruation ensues, the percentage of subsequent menses that are ovulatory rises rapidly. The role of prolactin, as well as other polypeptide and steroid hormones, in ovarian function during the puerperium has been studied in detail (Rolland et al., 1975) and discussed in Chapter 10.

The physiologic basis for postpartum amenorrhea is not entirely clear, although it is known that gonadotropin activity is minimal for 2 to 3 weeks after delivery. It has been postulated that this may be due to a transient pituitary insensitivity to luteinizing hormone–releasing factor (LRF), and recent data suggest that normal postpartum women have a deficiency in endogenous LRF secretion (Sheehan and Yen, 1979; Liu and Park, 1988).

Disappearance of Chorionic Gonadotropin

Following normal term vaginal delivery, the disappearance of beta-human chorionic gonadotropin (β-hCG) from the maternal circulation follows a biexponential curve. The initial rapid half-life component averages 4.75 hours, and the slow component averages 32.2 hours. Total elimination from the circulation occurs at a median time of 14 days (Reyes et al., 1985). This is in contrast to that observed following first-trimester therapeutic abortions, following which the total elimination time is 37 days. Among pregnant women undergoing hysterectomy, β-hCG disappears from the maternal circulation in 12 days, similar to that observed following term delivery. These differences are presumably due to more definitive placental separation in term deliveries compared with therapeutic abortions (Marrs et al., 1975).

Table 9–1. **Cardiovascular Measurements Obtained Before Pregnancy and at Six and Twelve Weeks Postpartum**

	BEFORE PREGNANCY	6 WEEKS POSTPARTUM	12 WEEKS POSTPARTUM
Cardiac output (L/min)	4.3 ± 0.2	4.6 ± 2	4.9 ± 0.2*
Stroke volume (ml)	68 ± 3	81 ± 4*	79 ± 3*
End-diastolic volume (ml)	107 ± 6	124 ± 7*	119 ± 5*
Systemic vascular resistance	1349 ± 83	1277 ± 65	1154 ± 70*

*Statistically significant difference compared to before pregnancy values at $p = 0.025$ or less. Data from Capeless and Clapp (1991).

SYSTEMIC CHANGES IN THE PUERPERIUM

The changes that occur in other organ systems during the puerperium are of interest from a physiologic perspective and because the clinician often must distinguish between a normal postpartum finding and a pathophysiologic change. It is frequently stated that return to nonpregnant anatomy and function requires 6 to 8 weeks, implying a linear return to baseline. Inasmuch as this is not always the case, it is worthwhile to examine some of these changes in depth.

Cardiovascular System

Most of the major circulatory changes that occur during pregnancy return to basal, nonpregnant levels early in the puerperium. The changes of greatest hemodynamic significance observed in response to pregnancy include a dramatic augmentation of cardiac output and blood volume and a decrease in peripheral vascular resistance (see Chapters 46 and 47). Although these alterations do return to baseline within 6 weeks after delivery, less is known about the rate of return, which appears to be variable.

Data obtained in postpartum sheep demonstrate that much of the return to baseline nonpregnant physiology actually occurs within 2 weeks. In animals studied from day 8 to day 14 postpartum, cardiac output falls from 100 ml/kg/min in late pregnancy to 82 ml/kg/min during the second week. Nonpregnant values average 65 ml/kg/min, and it is therefore apparent that 50 per cent of the return to nonpregnant cardiac output is accomplished in the first 2 weeks. The same is true of systemic vascular resistance (Dilts et al., 1969).

Studies in humans utilizing a combination of Doppler ultrasonography and echocardiography reveal that cardiac output remains increased for at least 48 hours postpartum as a result of an increase in stroke volume, despite a decrease in heart rate. This is presumably a consequence of increased venous return secondary to the rapid decrease in uterine blood flow as well as mobilization of interstitial fluids. By 2 weeks postpartum, cardiac output had decreased by almost 30 per cent from the early puerperium, probably owing to decreased blood volume. Myocardial contractility is also reduced compared with that in late pregnancy; this may be due to a decrease in the end-diastolic volume or to an actual diminution in myocardial function (Robson et al., 1987).

More recent data obtained by M-mode electrocardiography would suggest that stroke volume, cardiac output, end-diastolic volume, and systemic vascular resistance remain strikingly elevated over the nonpregnant state as long as 12 weeks postpartum (Capeless and Clapp, 1991). The authors point out that the contribution of stroke volume to the total change in cardiac output has been underestimated in the past. Their data are summarized in Table 9–1.

Blood volume alterations also take place rapidly. A normal vaginal delivery is associated with a blood loss of approximately 500 ml, and losses may reach 1000 ml or more with cesarean section (Pritchard, 1965). By the third postpartum day, the blood volume increase observed during pregnancy has declined by 16 per cent of the predelivery peak (Ueland, 1976). There is additional evidence that other parameters such as heart rate, blood pressure, oxygen consumption, and total body water return to nonpregnant levels within a few days postpartum. Consequently, it appears that the rate of return of cardiovascular parameters to nonpregnant values is quite variable, with some functions returning in a matter of days, and others still elevated 12 weeks postpartum. It is no longer accurate to assume a linear return to the nonpregnant state in 6 weeks.

Urinary Tract

The functional changes that occur in the renal system during pregnancy appear to return to their nonpregnant baseline levels promptly postpartum. Renal plasma flow increases by about 200 to 250 ml/minute in late pregnancy, concomitant with inulin (glomerular filtration rate) and creatinine clearance. Studies of women throughout pregnancy and the postpartum period demonstrate that renal plasma flow, glomerular filtration rate, and serum creatinine clearance have returned to nonpregnant levels by 6 weeks (Sims and Krantz, 1958). Little information exists regarding very early changes, although renal plasma flow decreases substantially in the first 5 days.

In contrast to the physiologic dynamics, renal morphologic changes secondary to pregnancy may persist for several months. The classic changes in pregnancy include dilation of the calyces, renal pelvis, and ureters. By 5 days postpartum, intravenous pyelogram studies reveal the mean kidney length to be 1.5 cm greater than in nonpregnant women (Bailey and Rolleston, 1971). It has also been noted that 80 per cent of women demonstrate significant nonobstructive dilation of the lumbar aspect of at least one ureter, usually the right. Bladder function is altered, and 20 per cent of postpartum women have incomplete emptying, as demonstrated by residual contrast medium in the bladder after micturition. This generalized dilation may last 3 months or longer (Crabtree, 1942), and as many as 10 per cent of women have long-term, persistent changes in urinary tract anatomy (Spino and Fry, 1970).

The Liver

Many of the alterations observed in protein synthesis and serum levels are induced by increasing circulatory estrogen levels during pregnancy. These include alpha and beta globulins as well as fibrinogen and other clotting factors of liver origin, ceruloplasmin, and sex-steroid-, corticosteroid-, and thyroid-binding globulins. The return to normal levels usually occurs within 3 weeks postpartum. Serum albumin concentrations decrease in pregnancy owing to plasma volume increases as well as an accelerated catabolic degradation. Levels of free fatty acids, cholesterol, triglycerides, and lipoproteins are in the normal, nonpregnant range by 10 days, with a significant decrease noted within 24 hours (Fabian et al., 1968; Potter and Nestel, 1979).

It is also important to emphasize that enzymes such as SGOT and SGPT are not altered by pregnancy. Their elevation in the pregnant or puerperal period should be considered to represent a pathologic alteration. Alkaline phosphatase during pregnancy is derived from the placenta as well as liver and bone. The total serum alkaline phosphatase level, which is usually the only measurement made because most laboratories do not routinely measure and report the heat-labile and heat-stable fractions separately, does not return to nonpregnant baseline until 20 days postpartum (Zuckerman et al., 1965).

REFERENCES

Anderson WR, Davis J: Placental site involution. Am J Obstet Gynecol 102:23, 1968.
Bailey RR, Rolleston GL: Kidney length and ureteral dilatation in the puerperium. J Obstet Gynaecol Br Commonw 78:55, 1971.
Capeless EL, Clapp JF. When do cardiovascular parameters return to their preconception values? Am J Obstet Gynecol 165:883, 1991.
Crabtree EG: Anatomical and functional changes in the urinary tract. In Urologic Disease in Pregnancy. Boston, Little Brown, 1942.
Cronin TJ: Influence of lactation upon ovulation. Lancet 2:422, 1968.
Dilts PV Jr, Brinkman CR III, Kirschbaum TH, Assali NS: Uterine and systemic hemodynamic interrelationships and their response to hypoxia. Am J Obstet Gynecol 103:138, 1969.
Fabian E, Stark A, Kucerova L, Sponarova J: Plasma levels of free fatty acids, lipoprotein lipase, and post-heparin esterase in pregnancy. Am J Obstet Gynecol 100:904, 1968.
Glass M, Rosenthal AH: Cervical changes in pregnancy, labor and the puerperium. Am J Obstet Gynecol 60:353, 1950.
Kistner RW: Physiology of the vagina. In Havez ESE, Evans TN (eds): The Human Vagina. Amsterdam, North Holland, 1978.
Liu JH, Park KH: Gonadotropin and prolactin secretion increases during sleep during the puerperium in nonlactating women. J Clin Endocrinol Metab 66:839, 1988.
Lyon RA, Stamm MJ: The onset of ovulation during the puerperium. Cal Med 65:99, 1946.
Marrs RP, Kletzky OA, Howard WF, Mishell DR Jr: Disappearance of human chorionic gonadotropin and resumption of ovulation following abortion. Am J Obstet Gynecol 135:731, 1975.
McLaren HC: The involution of the cervix. Br Med J 1:347, 1952.
Potter JM, Nestel PJ: The hyperlipidemia of pregnancy in normal and complicated pregnancies. Am J Obstet Gynecol 133:165, 1979.
Pritchard JA: Changes in blood volume during pregnancy and delivery. Anesthesiology 26:393, 1965.
Reyes FI, Winter JSD, Faiman C: Postpartum disappearance of chorionic gonadotropin from the maternal and neonatal circulations. Am J Obstet Gynecol 153:486, 1985.
Robson SC, Dunlop W, Hunter S: Haemodynamic changes during the early puerperium. Br Med J 294:106, 1987.
Rolland R, Leguin RM, Schellekens LA, et al. The role of prolactin in the restoration of ovarian function during the early postpartum period in the human female. I. A study during physiological lactation. Clin Endocrinol 4:15, 1975.
Sharman A: Ovulation after pregnancy. Fertil Steril 2:371, 1951a.
Sharman A: Menstruation after childbirth. J Obstet Gynaecol Br Commonw 58:440, 1951b.
Sharman A: Postpartum regeneration of the human endometrium. J Anat 87:1, 1953.
Sheehan KL, Yen SSC: Activation of pituitary gonadotropic function by an agonist of luteinizing hormone-releasing factor in the puerperium. Am J Obstet Gynecol 135:755, 1979.
Sims EAH, Krantz KE: Serial studies of renal function during pregnancy and the puerperium in normal women. J Clin Invest 37:1764, 1958.
Spino FI, Fry IA: Ureteral dilatation in nonpregnant women. Proc R Soc Med 63:462, 1970.
Ueland K: Maternal cardiovascular dynamics. VII. Intrapartum blood volume changes. Am J Obstet Gynecol 126:671, 1976.
Zuckerman H, Sadovsky E, Kallner B: Serum alkaline phosphatase in pregnancy and puerperium. Obstet Gynecol 25:819, 1965.

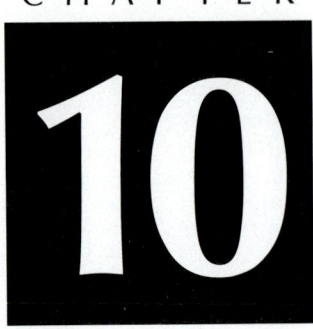

THE BREAST AND THE PHYSIOLOGY OF LACTATION

ROBERT W. REBAR, M.D.

DEVELOPMENT OF THE HUMAN BREAST

Embryonic and Prepubertal Development

The mammary gland is derived from ectoderm and is first anatomically apparent in the embryo 4 mm in length as a mammary band (Raynaud, 1961). By the time the embryo is 7 mm long, the mammary band and surrounding tissue have thickened to form a ridge (known as the *mammary crest* or *milk line*) extending along the ventrolateral body wall from the axillary to the inguinal region on each side. The epithelium along the caudal portions of this ridge regresses and the crest in the thoracic region further thickens to form a primordial mammary bud by the time the embryo measures 10 to 12 mm in length.

In different racial groups the breasts develop at slightly different heights, indicating utilization of slightly different levels of the ridge (Patten, 1953). Normally this variation occurs within rather narrow limits of the pectoral region, but not infrequently, supernumerary nipples may occur at other levels along the course of the milk line.

By the seventh week of development (17 mm), a lenticular mass of epithelial cells extends deep into the underlying mesenchyme. Although this mass of epithelial cells continues to increase in size, few outward changes can be detected in the fetal mammary bud until after the fifth month of intrauterine life. The primitive mammary bud then begins to form 15 to 25 secondary buds, which will provide the basis for the ductal system in the mature gland. These buds elongate into cylindrical cords that form the epithelial elements of the adult gland and develop lumina. With the development of a lumen, two concentric layers of cuboidal cells become evident: The inner layer of cells will form the secretory epithelium, and the outer layer will develop into the myoepithelium. By the time of birth, these epithelial ducts have undergone limited proliferation, presumably owing to stimulation by a number of hormones present in the fetal circulation in the last trimester of pregnancy. At birth the mammary structures are still rudimentary, but in some newborns secretion of "witch's milk" may be noted within the first few days after birth, no doubt as a result of the high prolactin levels present in every newborn (Friesen, 1973).

Recent investigations indicate that the human mammary gland does not involute rapidly after birth but remains active for a few months and often shows typical apocrine secretion (McKiernan et al., 1988). In general, the histologic appearance of the breast in early infancy is similar to the adult puerperal gland, but secretion of any milk in infancy seems to take place in dilated ducts, and definite alveoli at the ends of ducts are rarely seen. Myoepithelial cells are regularly present, and foci of extramedullary hematopoiesis may be found. No sex differences in breast development are apparent in infancy. It has been suggested that the infant's own gonadal secretions, which are increased for several months following birth, are responsible for the continued activity of the breast tissue for this brief interval after birth.

The gland then regresses, enters a quiescent stage, and grows proportionately with the remainder of the body until puberty. Some enlargement of the ducts does occur, but there is no lobuloalveolar development (Turner, 1952).

Pubertal and Postpubertal Development

With the onset of puberty in the girl, further growth of the breasts occurs, and the areolae enlarge and become more pigmented (Fig. 10–1). The growth involves an increase in connective tissue, adipose tissue, and vascular channels, but proliferation of the epithelial ducts and lobuloalveolar development are most prominent. Most of the molding of the breast, however, is due to accumulation of adipose tissue. Numerous studies have demonstrated that these changes are related to the increased secretion of estrogen and progesterone by the ovary (Mayer et al., 1961).

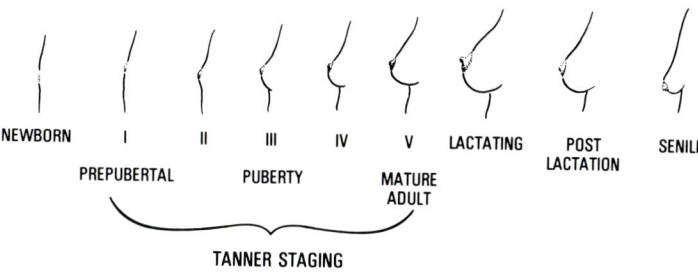

FIGURE 10–1. Profiles of the breast showing characteristic changes in configuration at different ages and with functional activity. (Adapted from Patten BM: Human Embryology. 2nd ed. New York, McGraw-Hill, 1953; and Marshall WA, Tanner JM: Variations in patterns of pubertal changes in girls. Arch Dis Child **44**:291, 1969.)

Breast Changes During the Menstrual Cycle

Cyclic changes, with proliferation and regression of ductal breast tissue, occur during each menstrual cycle (Aragona and Friesen, 1979). The proliferative changes reach a maximum late in each luteal phase. Histologic examination of normal breast tissue reveals that after puberty, mammary development consists of a slow, cyclic, progressive increase in glandular tissue with further division of the epithelial ducts to form rudimentary lobules and regression with each menses. No further growth occurs in nonpregnant women, and true alveoli are generally not present until the third month of pregnancy.

Breast Changes During Pregnancy and After Parturition

At the beginning of pregnancy, there is rapid growth and branching from terminal portions of the gland associated with some loss of interstitial adipose tissue (Cowie and Tindal, 1971). There is increased vascularity as well as infiltration of the interstitial tissue by lymphocytes, plasma cells, and eosinophils. Enlargement of the breasts is first noticeable after the second month. The nipples also increase in size, and the areolae become larger and more pigmented.

The greatest portion of the increase in the ductal system occurs during the first two trimesters. True glandular acini, necessary for milk secretion, appear early in the third month. During the last trimester the changes involve the differentiation of the acini in preparation for their secretory activity. In the final month of pregnancy, the enlargement of the breast results largely from hypertrophy of parenchymal cells of the alveoli with a hyaline, eosinophilic, proteinaceous secretion termed *colostrum*. Approximately 3 days postpartum the fat content of this secretion increases abruptly and it becomes typical milk.

The morphologic changes that occur postpartum have been summarized previously (Hollmann, 1974). The epithelial cells of the lumen increase in height, and the microvilli at the lumen become more numerous. The nuclei assume a more basal location in the cells and there is a marked increase in rough endoplasmic reticulum. The Golgi complex enlarges. Fat globules and granular protein vacuoles appear prominently.

The functional anatomy of the lactating breast is apparent upon gross inspection (Fig. 10–2). Because the nipple is supplied with smooth muscle fibers, it

projects as much as 2 cm beyond the areola in response to tactile or psychological stimuli. Beneath the areola are 15 to 20 sinuses that become engorged with milk when pressure is applied to the peripheral lactating glandular tissues. Milk is expressed by a relative compression of the subareolar sinuses by the lips and gums of the infant while suckling. Areolar expression of the milk results from compression of these sinuses. Many ductules connect the peripheral alveoli with the subareolar sinuses. These ductules have smooth muscle in their walls, and myofibrils also surround the individual alveoli. Surrounding the alveoli, which are lined with lactating cells, is a rich capillary bed and lymphatic supply. In fact, blood flow through the lactating mammary gland is 400 to 500 times the volume of milk secreted, with the blood flow influencing the volume of milk (Linzell, 1974).

Hormonal Effects on Mammary Development

The literature detailing hormonal control of mammary growth and development is vast (Topper and

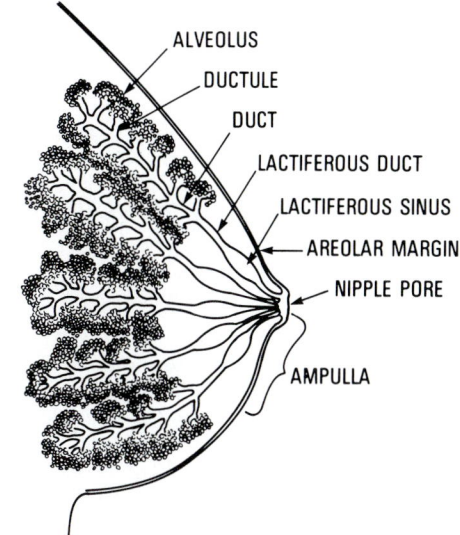

FIGURE 10–2. Detailed structural features of the lactating human mammary gland. The lactiferous sinuses rest beneath the areola and converge at the nipple pore. (Modified from Worthington BS: Lactation, human milk, and nutritional considerations. *In* Worthington BS, Vermeersch J, Williams SR (eds): Nutrition in Pregnancy and Lactation. St. Louis, CV Mosby, 1977.)

Freeman, 1980). Generally speaking, investigators have attempted to establish the simplest hormonal combinations necessary for ductal and lobuloalveolar development and have used hypophysectomized, adrenalectomized, and oophorectomized rats as models. Only limited studies have made use of human breast tissue, and results from animal experiments have generally been extrapolated to the human. That conclusions derived from such experiments also apply to women remains unsubstantiated in the majority of circumstances.

In their classic experiments, Lyons and co-workers (1958) demonstrated that a great many hormones were involved in mammary development, including prolactin, ACTH, growth hormone, TSH, LH, human placental lactogen, steroid hormones from the ovary and adrenal, thyroid hormones, and insulin (Fig. 10–3). Several of these hormones exert their influence only indirectly through effects on their respective target organs.

In vitro studies utilizing cultured mouse mammary tissue by Topper (1970) and Turkington (1972) have demonstrated that just three hormones, prolactin, insulin, and cortisol, are essential for mammary growth and function in this species. Insulin by itself induces mitosis of epithelial cells and lobuloalveolar formation in tissue culture. For complete differentiation of the secretory epithelial cells, however, all three hormones are required. Human placental lactogen can be substituted for prolactin in this experimental model.

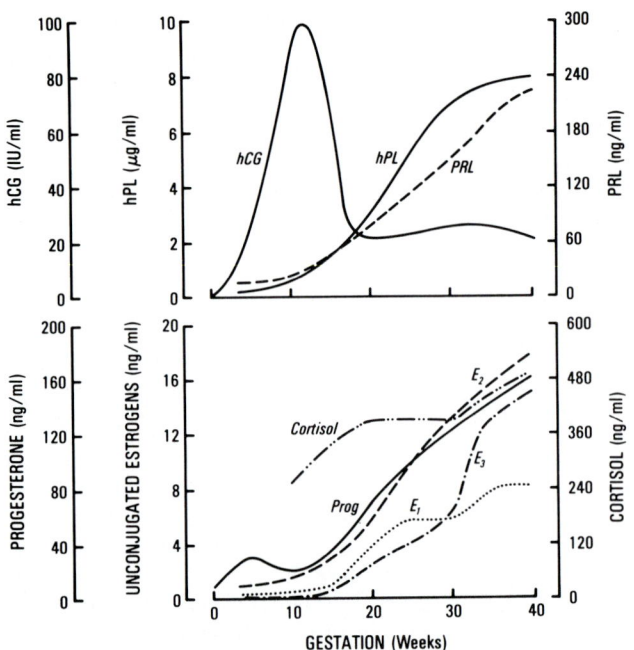

FIGURE 10–4. Serum concentrations of prolactin, hCG, hPL, cortisol, progesterone, and unconjugated estrogens during pregnancy. The values have been obtained from several sources in the literature. E_1 = estrone; E_2 = estradiol; E_3 = estriol.

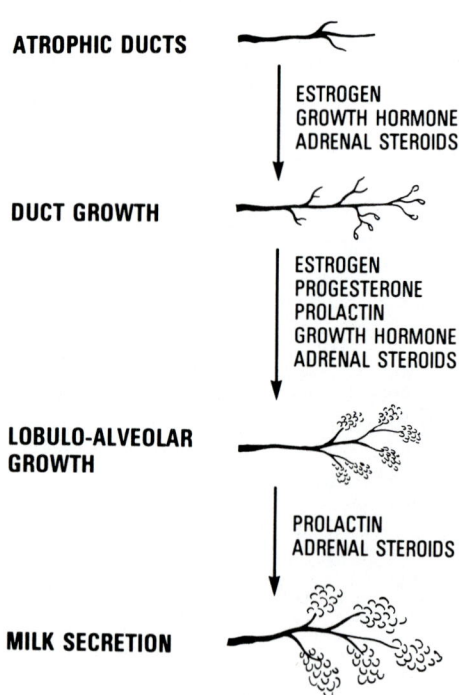

FIGURE 10–3. Multihormonal interaction in the development of the mammary gland and in the initiation of lactogenesis and lactation. Based on studies in the hypophysectomized, ovariectomized, adrenalectomized rat. (Adapted from Lyons WR, Li CH, Johnson RE: The hormonal control of mammary growth and lactation. Recent Prog Horm Res **14**:219, 1958.)

That the ovarian steroids estradiol-17β and progesterone are necessary for mammary development in women is based on clinical observations: No breast changes occur at puberty in girls with gonadal dysgenesis. Furthermore, enlargement of the breasts is frequently noted by women using oral contraceptive agents. Once breast development is complete, however, the effects of removal of the ovaries are less obvious. Numerous studies have established that estrogens generally stimulate growth of the duct system, whereas lobuloalveolar development depends on progesterone (Folley, 1948; Meites, 1965; Topper and Freeman, 1980).

During pregnancy, marked increases occur in a number of hormones now known to influence development of mammary tissue (Fig. 10–4). Progesterone and the estrogens estrone, estradiol, and estriol all increase dramatically in maternal blood as a result of synthesis by the maternal-fetal-placental unit (Jaffe, 1991). Both free and bound plasma cortisol levels increase as well. Levels of the placental hormones human chorionic gonadotropin (hCG) and human placental lactogen (hPL) are also increased, as is pituitary secretion of prolactin. No doubt these hormones act in concert to produce the mature gland present at parturition.

The placenta also secretes a number of other hormones that may play some role in the development of the breast during pregnancy. Those hormones produced by the placenta that have been identified thus far include thyrotropin-releasing hormone (TRH), gonadotropin-releasing hormone (GnRH), corticotropin-releasing hormone (CRH), growth hormone-releasing hormone (GHRH), corticotropin (ACTH), β-endorphin, β-lipotropin, α-melanocyte-stimulating hormone (MSH), oxytocin, relaxin, inhibin, placental TSH, a placental GH variant, and insulin-like growth factors I and II (Jeske et al., 1989).

ROLE OF HORMONES IN LACTATION

Current knowledge of the hormones involved in lactation is also derived from studies in species other than the human, and extrapolation to women may not be entirely justified. However, in humans as in other species it seems apparent that, as proposed by Lyons and co-workers (1958), the interaction of several hormones is required.

Pituitary and Placental Peptide Hormones

Prolactin

It is now evident that prolactin stimulates a number of intracellular biochemical events that are necessary for milk production. Experimental studies suggest that several of prolactin's effects require synergism with other hormones. Of all the hormones necessary for lactation, however, none is more important than prolactin.

CIRCULATING PROLACTIN CONCENTRATIONS. During pregnancy there is a progressive increase in prolactin concentrations in maternal serum, from a mean of less than 20 ng/ml in pre-pregnant women to an average of perhaps 200 to 300 ng/ml at term (see Fig. 10–4) (Fournier et al., 1974; Jaffe et al., 1973). After parturition, in women who are not breast-feeding, prolactin levels gradually fall to nonpregnant values in 4 to 6 weeks. In women who do breast-feed, basal prolactin levels remain elevated for the first 1 to 2 weeks. From about 2 weeks to 3 months postpartum, basal prolactin levels remain somewhat elevated, with an even more marked increase occurring with each episode of breast-feeding. Finally, approximately 3 months postpartum, basal concentrations are essentially normal and there are only slight if any increases in prolactin levels with breast-feeding (Tyson et al., 1972). As lactation continues, each suckling stimulus elicits progressively less prolactin release (Diaz et al., 1989).

As is true for almost all hormones, prolactin is secreted in a pulsatile manner. It appears that the number and duration of such secretory bursts of prolactin do not change as the hyperprolactinemia postpartum wanes (Nunley et al., 1991). Moreover, despite evidence that prolactin is found in plasma in a variety of molecular forms which change depending on the physiologic state (Larrea et al., 1989), the half-life of each secretory episode did not change relative to time after delivery (Nunley et al., 1991).

The pivotal role of prolactin in lactation in women was established with the use of the dopamine agonist 2-bromo-α-ergocryptine (bromocriptine) (Brun et al., 1973). When this agent is administered in the immediate postpartum period, prolactin levels fall to pre-pregnant values within hours, and breast engorge-

ment and lactation cease. Such observations demonstrate that prolactin is essential to the initiation of lactation. If estrogens are used to suppress lactation and breast engorgement, serum prolactin levels are actually somewhat higher than those seen in nursing women even though no milk is formed. Thus, it would seem that the action of prolactin at the breast is inhibited by high concentrations of estrogens. The high levels of estrogen present in a pregnant woman no doubt prevent milk formation. With the rapid fall in estrogens after delivery, the inhibitory effects of estrogens are removed, and prolactin is able to initiate lactation.

Administration of bromocriptine to women at any time postpartum will rapidly lower circulating prolactin levels and completely inhibit lactation. There is, however, considerable variation among species. Prolactin appears to play a role in the initiation of lactation in most species, but its role in maintaining lactation is more variable and less clearly understood. In women it appears that even late in the postpartum period low basal prolactin levels are necessary for the maintenance of lactation (Aragona and Friesen, 1979).

BINDING OF PROLACTIN TO ITS RECEPTORS. Mammary tissue is one of the targets of prolactin. Like other polypeptide hormones, prolactin appears to initiate its action by binding with specific receptors on the surface of mammary epithelial cells (Turkington, 1970; Kelly et al., 1991). Moreover, the extent of prolactin binding directly parallels milk synthesis (Hayden et al., 1979). Shiu and Friesen (1976) have shown that binding to receptors is necessary for prolactin hormone action by demonstrating that antibodies blocking the binding of prolactin to its receptors also block the stimulation of milk protein synthesis (casein) in explants of rabbit mammary glands in organ culture.

The numbers of receptors appear to differ in various physiologic states as well. Frantz and colleagues (1974) first demonstrated that prolactin binding activity in lactating rat mammary gland is three times that in pregnant tissue. It also appears that prolactin induces synthesis of its own receptor (Bohnet et al., 1977; Djiane et al., 1977; Posner et al., 1975), leading to a rapid increase in prolactin receptor numbers early in lactation. The induction of prolactin receptors can be blocked by progesterone (Djiane and Durand, 1977), suggesting that the inhibitory effect of progesterone on lactogenesis (discussed later) is at least in part at the level of the prolactin receptor. In male rats, treatment with estrogen leads to an induction of prolactin receptors in the liver (Waters et al., 1978). Immunocytochemical (Nolin and Witorsch, 1976) and autoradiographic (Aubert et al., 1978; Shiu and Friesen, 1980) studies suggest that prolactin may be internalized by mammary epithelial cells. Furthermore, the internalized prolactin may be either degraded in lysosomes or released intact by mammary cells, perhaps to act again (Shiu, 1979; Shiu and Friesen, 1980).

Prolactin receptors have now been characterized in microsomal membrane preparations from a number of tissues (Kelly et al., 1991). The physiologic function of prolactin in some of these tissues is not known, and many distinct and diverse effects have been ascribed to prolactin. Two forms of receptors have been identified, a short and a long form. The structure of the human prolactin receptor was identified by cDNA libraries prepared from human hepatoma (Hep G2) cells and a human breast cancer cell line (T-47D) (Boutin et al., 1989). The human prolactin receptor is a member of long form and contains 598 amino acids in its mature form. The receptor has an extracellular region of 210 amino acids, a single transmembrane region of about 24 amino acids, and then a lengthy cytoplasmic domain. The length of the cytoplasmic domain differs in short and long forms of the receptor. The extracellular region is glycosylated.

Action of Prolactin on Milk Protein Synthesis. Prolactin plays a key role in the induction of milk secretion by the differentiated mammary gland. Prolactin alone can stimulate the synthesis of milk proteins such as casein and alpha-lactalbumin in mammary tissue primed by insulin and cortisol (Juergens et al., 1965; Topper, 1970; Turkington et al., 1968, 1973). After binding of prolactin to its cell surface receptor, the molecular steps resulting in the synthesis of milk proteins have not been delineated (Kelly et al., 1991). Unlike with other polypeptide hormones, binding of prolactin to its receptor does not lead to activation of adenylate cyclase (Majumder and Turkington, 1971).

Data suggest that prolactin stimulates early RNA synthesis through the participation of membrane receptors and prostaglandins (Banerjee et al., 1978; Rillema and Wild, 1977; Turkington et al., 1973). Synthesis of polyamines may be stimulated as well (Shiu and Friesen, 1980). It is presumed that RNA initiates formation of protein kinases, which then "activate" functional proteins by phosphorylation. Additionally, gene expression further results in the activation of other "late" RNAs, which may include messenger RNAs for milk proteins.

Other Effects of Prolactin. Prolactin appears to have a number of other actions as well. *In vitro* studies with explants of rabbit mammary tissue have also established that prolactin, alone or in combination with insulin and hydrocortisone, stimulates the synthesis of milk fats in the mammary gland (Shiu and Friesen, 1980). Results of experiments in lower vertebrates have suggested that prolactin may play a role in maintaining the low sodium concentrations found in milk because it promotes sodium retention by the mammary gland (Bern and Nicoll, 1968). Other studies in rabbit mammary gland slices *in vitro* suggest that prolactin promotes the active transport of these ions out of the tissues (Falconer and Rowe, 1975, 1977). Finally, limited studies suggest that prolactin may play a role in the induction of the secretory immune system in the mammary gland as well (Shiu and Friesen, 1980). Prolactin appears to increase the number of IgA-bearing plasma cells in the mammary gland, although the mechanism is unknown (Weisz-Carrington et al., 1978).

In humans, although it is reasonable to assume that milk protein genes are regulated by prolactin, as in other species, the only gene that has been shown to be regulated by prolactin is a so-called prolactin-inducible protein (PIP). This protein was originally isolated from T-47D human breast cancer cells and is a secreted glycoprotein inducible by androgens and prolactin (Shiu and Iwasiow, 1985).

Human Growth Hormone and Placental Lactogen

Because both growth hormone (GH) and human placental lactogen (hPL) are structurally similar to prolactin (Niall et al., 1973), they have similar effects. However, the human prolactin gene is located on chromosome 6 while the genes for growth hormone and hPL are located on chromosome 17 (Truong et al., 1984). All three hormones are thought to be derived from a common ancestral gene that diverged about 4×10^8 years ago to give rise to separate prolactin and growth hormone lineages (Miller and Eberhardt, 1983; Walker et al., 1991). Human placental lactogen seems to have developed from one of the GH genes about 2×10^7 years ago. Although numerous investigators have demonstrated that these hormones, especially hPL, may be effectively substituted for prolactin in experimental animal models (Topper and Freeman, 1980), there are important differences among the three hormones.

Because pituitary GH is suppressed to very low levels in pregnancy (Yen et al., 1969), it probably does not play an important role in breast development and lactation in women. Furthermore, individuals with growth hormone deficiency often have normal breast development and lactate normally (Rimoin et al., 1968). In addition, GH is not released in response to suckling in women (Noel et al., 1974), although the responses vary among species (Cowie et al., 1980). Although GH is important for milk secretion in ruminants and is closely related to milk yield in cattle (Cowie et al., 1980), no such relationship has been established in humans.

These conclusions about the role of growth hormone have been complicated by the recent finding of a unique placental growth hormone variant, with concentrations increasing from mid-pregnancy until term (Frankenne et al., 1987, 1988). Although structurally distinct, the placental GH variant acts as a strong agonist to pituitary GH in binding to hepatic GH receptors. In contrast to the episodic, pulsatile secretion of pituitary GH, the placental GH variant appears to be secreted in a continuous manner, as evidenced by frequent measurements in women in the later half of pregnancy (Eriksson et al., 1989). The continuous secretion of placental GH, together with the suppression of pituitary GH, may indicate an important role for this GH variant as a regulator of maternal liver metabolism during pregnancy.

The role of hPL in mammary development and lactation is largely undefined. Concentrations of hPL increase progressively through pregnancy, with concentrations of perhaps 8 μg/ml present in maternal serum by the last few weeks of pregnancy (Grumbach et al., 1968). The plasma concentrations of hPL in the mother correlate positively with placental mass and are greater in multiple than in singleton gestations (Saxena et al., 1969). Throughout gestation, plasma concentrations of hPL exceed those of prolactin and both pituitary and placental GH. That the effects of hPL are distinct from those of prolactin and GH is supported by the recent identification of a distinct receptor for hPL in fetal and maternal liver (Freemark and Comer, 1989). Because of its short half-life (Kaplan et al., 1968), hPL disappears rapidly from maternal circulation following delivery and is generally undetectable 24 hours later. Thus, hPL is present in maternal serum in high concentrations when the lactogenic responsiveness of the breast is inhibited by the high concentrations of estrogens also present.

During pregnancy there is also a marked increase in maternal insulin-like growth factor I (IGF-I) concentrations (Furlanetto et al., 1978). Evidence suggests that this increase is due, at least in part, to hPL (Handwerger, 1991). Because plasma hPL concentrations increase markedly during gestation, Grumbach and co-workers (1968) have presented a cogent argument for a major role of hPL as a maternal "growth hormone" during the second half of pregnancy. They suggested that hPL acts as an antagonist of insulin action; by inducing glucose tolerance, lipolysis, and proteolysis in the mother, the transfer of glucose and amino acids to the fetus is promoted.

Oxytocin

The classic role of oxytocin in lactation is in the milk ejection reflex (discussed later). Evidence that oxytocin can exert galactopoietic actions in some species, such as goat, sheep, and rat, has long existed (Cowie et al., 1980). Several mechanisms to explain these galactopoietic effects have been suggested. Oxytocin may release hormones, such as growth hormone and prolactin, from the anterior pituitary (Benson and Folley, 1957). With the demonstration of retrograde blood flow in the pituitary stalk (Bergland and Page, 1978), the possibility that oxytocin may reach the adenohypophysis in very high concentrations makes this possibility attractive. Oxytocin may also increase membrane permeability, thereby increasing the supply of nutrients to the alveolar cells (Morag, 1968). By moving milk into the large ducts and cisterns, oxytocin may facilitate milk secretion by minimizing inhibitory pressures within the alveoli.

Steroid Hormones

Estrogens and Progestins

Estrogens appear to have a modulating influence on the responsiveness of the mammary gland to lactogenic hormones. Although they stimulate prolactin release in women (Yen et al., 1974), in large amounts estrogens inhibit lactation, apparently by a direct action on the mammary gland.

Specific binding sites for estradiol-17β have been detected in cytosol from the mammary glands of several species (Cowie et al., 1980) as well as human mammary tumors (McGuire et al., 1977). Most investigators have reported an increase in estrogen receptors on mammary tissue during lactation (Cowie et al., 1980; Hsueh et al., 1973), with a sharp decrease

on weaning (Leung et al., 1976). Furthermore, receptors appear to be modulated by prolactin (Leung and Sasaki, 1973). Since, as noted previously, estrogen can also increase prolactin receptors, there is a great deal of interaction between these two hormones.

Except for its role in mammary development, there is no evidence that progesterone plays a significant role in human lactation. High doses of progestin have little effect on the amount of milk or duration of lactation in some species (Karim et al., 1971). Progesterone can block induction of prolactin receptors in mammary tissue (Djiane and Durand, 1977), and so it may actually have an inhibitory effect in some circumstances. Progesterone receptors have been identified in human mammary tumors and normal mammary tissue from women with breast cancer (Cowie et al., 1980; Pollow et al., 1977).

Adrenal Steroids

Although studies in a number of animal species have demonstrated an effect of corticosteroids on milk secretion (Cowie et al., 1980), the role of adrenal steroids in human lactation is still unknown. Specific receptors for glucocorticoids have been detected in human mammary tumor tissue (Fazekas and MacFarlane, 1977). Furthermore, the greatest glucocorticoid binding in rat and mice mammary tissue has been observed in lactating animals (Cowie et al., 1980). In the rat, at least, evidence indicates that glucocorticoids play an important role in the regulation of several key mammary enzymes involved in milk synthesis (Cowie et al., 1980).

Other Hormones

Insulin and Serum Growth Factors

A number of *in vitro* and *in vivo* studies have demonstrated that insulin is necessary for the maintenance of normal lactation (Cowie et al., 1980). Because of the central anabolic role of this hormone in intermediary metabolism, it has sometimes been difficult to distinguish between actions of insulin directed at the mammary gland and effects mediated through its influence on overall metabolism in lactating animals. It has been suggested that during lactation insulin acts in two distinct ways (Baldwin and Louis, 1975). First, this hormone appears to be essential for maintenance or survival of alveolar cells in the mammary gland and at high concentrations is mitogenic to these cells. Second, insulin has direct effects on mammary epithelial cell metabolism, stimulating glucose entry into the cell and accelerating lipogenesis. Although large numbers of insulin-binding sites have been noted in mammary tissue from a variety of species, including humans (Aragona and Friesen, 1979; Topper and Freeman, 1980), the importance of insulin to lactation in humans remains to be defined.

Furthermore, a number of circulating growth factors with some properties of insulin have been identified in recent years. Epidermal growth factor (EGF), a potent mitogen and a polypeptide originally isolated from mouse submaxillary gland, has been reported in the serum of pregnant women (Ances, 1973). This factor causes proliferation of epithelial cells of mouse mammary glands and mammary carcinomas in organ culture (Aragona and Friesen, 1979). A possible role for IGF-I, discussed previously, also must be considered.

Thyroid and Parathyroid Hormones

Although thyroid hormone secretion appears to be important for adequate milk secretion, the evidence is confusing. Women with primary hypothyroidism also frequently have galactorrhea. Yet animals with deficient thyroid function have reduced milk secretion (Cowie et al., 1980). On the other hand, large doses of thyroid hormone also depress milk yield in both rats and rabbits (Cowie et al., 1980).

Removal of the parathyroid glands from lactating animals depresses lactation. Despite the large amounts of calcium secreted in milk, parathyroid activity in cows appears to be depressed during lactation (Cowie et al., 1980).

LACTATION

Initiation

There is considerable variation among different species as to when milk can first be detected in mammary alveoli during pregnancy. In humans, as noted earlier, the alveoli become distended with colostrum in the last trimester, but mammary secretion does not appear until approximately 3 days after delivery. Because maternal prolactin concentrations peak just before delivery, when no lactation occurs, and because estrogens inhibit puerperal lactation in the presence of elevated prolactin levels (Bruce and Ramirez, 1970; Brun et al., 1973), it is postulated that estrogens have a direct inhibitory effect on mammary epithelial cells. Following parturition, the rapid fall in estrogens allows the mammary gland to respond to lactogenic hormones. In addition, the high levels of progesterone in pregnancy inhibit the development of receptors for prolactin in mammary tissue until following delivery.

The Milk Ejection (Letdown) Reflex

In 1915 Gaines noted, "Milk secretion, in the sense of the formation of the milk constituents, is one thing; the ejection of milk from the gland after it is formed is quite another thing. The one is probably continuous, the other certainly discontinuous." He concluded that milk is actively ejected from the alveoli by a reflex contraction of the mammary gland musculature in response to the stimulus of milking, that the reflex has a latent period of 35 to 65 seconds, and that it can become conditioned. In 1930, Turner and Slaughter extended Gaine's observations by advancing the possibility "that one of the normal functions of the pituitary gland, which is so closely connected with the nervous system, is to regulate the discharging phase

of milk secretion. If this were the case, the nerve paths would lead to the pituitary gland causing the discharge of the hormone that would in turn bring about the well-known change in the (mammary) gland." Gunther (1942) noted that milk secretion in women is a continuous process and that an expulsive process actively assisted by contractile elements in the mammary gland occurs during suckling. She concluded that this expulsive process is regulated by a reflex arc, the stimulus being carried centrally by nerves and peripherally by humoral transmission by a hormone closely resembling posterior pituitary secretion. Thus, Gunther must be credited with introducing the concept of the neurohumoral nature of the milk ejection reflex in women.

In brief, impulses generated by suckling enter the spinal cord through the dorsal roots of the spinal nerves (Fig. 10–5). Neural pathways terminate in the magnocellular neurosecretory nuclei of the hypothalamus—the supraoptic and paraventricular nuclei. The precise mechanism by which the neurosecretory cells are activated is still unclear but may involve release of inhibin β from cells arising in the caudal nucleus of the solitary tract (Cunningham and Sawchenko, 1991). Oxytocin, a nonapeptide, is synthesized within neurons of both nuclei and is transported along the axons through the pituitary stalk to terminals in the posterior lobe of the pituitary gland in association with a cysteine-rich carrier protein, neurophysin I, also termed *estrogen-sensitive neurophysin* (ESN), at a rate of 1 to 4 mm/hour. Oxytocin and its neurophysin are formed from a common precursor known as proxyphysin (Russell et al., 1980). The rate of secretion of neurophysin I is influenced by estrogen (Legros et al., 1975). In the posterior pituitary the neurosecretory granules containing oxytocin are stored in nonterminal dilatations of the axon. The process by which oxytocin and its neurophysin are packaged in granules and transported down the axon has not been defined com-

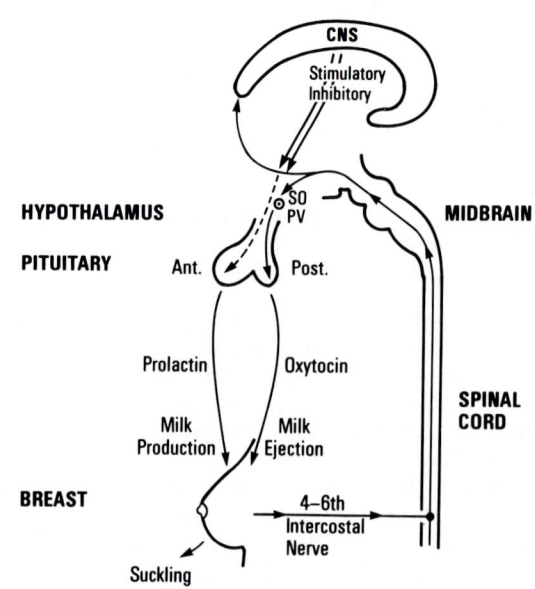

FIGURE 10–5. Neuroendocrine reflexes initiated by suckling. *PV* = paraventricular nucleus; *SO* = supraoptic nucleus; *Ant.* = anterior pituitary; *Post.* = posterior pituitary.

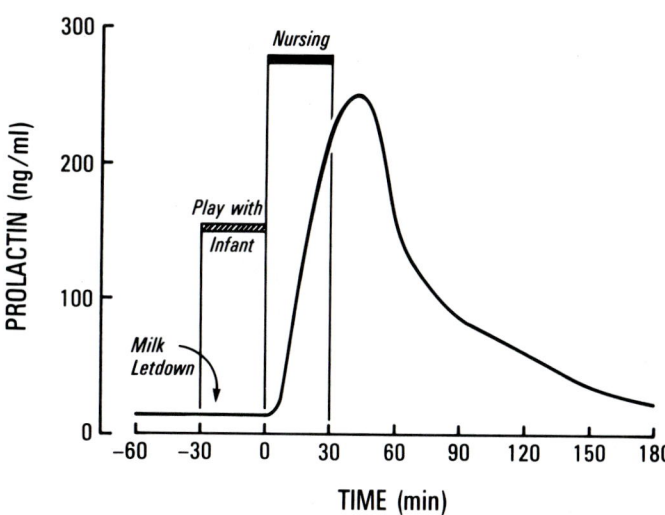

FIGURE 10–6. Schematic representation of serum prolactin concentrations during anticipation of nursing and during nursing in the first 40 days postpartum. The response decreases with time after delivery. No increase in growth hormone above basal levels was observed. (Adapted from Noel GL, Suh HK, Frantz AG: Prolactin release during nursing and breast stimulation in postpartum and nonpostpartum subjects. J Clin Endocrinol Metab **38**:413, © by The Endocrine Society, 1974.)

pletely. When the neurons are stimulated, the granules are conveyed to the terminal dilatations that end on capillary membranes and are probably released by calcium-dependent exocytosis. Because the rhythmic contraction of mammary tissue induced by suckling is closely mimicked by repeated intravenous injection of oxytocin at frequent intervals, oxytocin is apparently released in a pulsatile fashion (Cowie et al., 1980). Recordings from oxytocin neurons show a characteristic accelerated discharge followed by an arrest of firing before milk ejection (Cross et al., 1975). Furthermore, there is now clear evidence in all species studied that there is a rapid increase in circulating oxytocin levels in response to suckling (Cowie et al., 1980; Weitzman et al., 1980), and this release occurs without simultaneous release of vasopressin (Cobo, 1974).

It further appears that the myoepithelial cells are the effector cells for oxytocin. Richardson (1949) showed that myoepithelial cells surround each alveolus and that these cells contract in response to oxytocin, thus forcing milk out of the alveolar lumina. Hyperplasia of the myoepithelial cells occurs in the first half of pregnancy, and in late pregnancy the myoepithelial cells stretch to form thin, tenuous processes. Full development of these cells does not occur until lactation, when there is a great increase in the number of myofilaments in the cytoplasm. Specific, high-affinity binding of oxytocin to particulate constituents of mammary tissue also has been demonstrated (Soloff et al., 1977).

Although suckling is the primary stimulus for the milk ejection reflex, it has long been recognized that the reflex may be conditioned. The sight of the baby, the cry of the infant, and breast preparation may cause milk letdown, whereas pain, embarrassment, distraction, and anesthetics tend to inhibit the reflex.

A related reflex, termed the *draught reflex,* also contributes to the propulsion of milk through the duct system (Worthington, 1977). This reflex, noted by most lactating women as a prickly sensation in the breast, occurs several minutes after the onset of suckling. It serves to propel milk from the more distal ducts to the lactiferous sinuses. The reflex is important

in ensuring that the infant obtains sufficient milk at each feeding.

Effect of Suckling on Oxytocin and Prolactin

Noel and associates (1974) have demonstrated that both oxytocin and prolactin are released in response to suckling, but the patterns of release are clearly different (Fig. 10–6). When nursing women were allowed to hold their infants but not to breast-feed, serum prolactin concentrations did not increase despite the occurrence of the milk letdown reflex. Prolactin levels, however, did rise transiently with nursing. The increase in prolactin is apparently sufficient to maintain lactogenesis and an adequate milk supply for the next feeding. They concluded that neither psychic factors associated with the expectation of nursing nor the presumed release of oxytocin prior to milk letdown is effective in releasing prolactin. Also of note are the observations that ethanol is capable of inhibiting oxytocin as well as vasopressin release during lactation (Cobo, 1973) and that nicotine blocks the suckling-induced prolactin rise in lactating rats without affecting oxytocin release (Blake and Sawyer, 1972). It also appears that each episode of suckling is accompanied by an increase in skin conductance followed by an increase in both finger and breast temperature (Marshall et al., 1992), similar to the changes seen with menopausal hot flashes, and also suggesting hypothalamic activation.

The Mechanics of Suckling

A number of studies in animals and humans have demonstrated that the infant sucks the nipple to the back of its mouth, forming a "teat" from the nipple and stretched areola (Cowie et al., 1980). The base of this teat is compressed between the upper gum and the tip of the tongue, which is resting on the lower gum. The tongue is then applied to the lower surface of the teat from the front of the mouth to the back, pressing it against the hard palate. This action serves to strip the milk out from the milk cisterns. Thus, the mechanism of suckling is far different from the way in which one drinks from a straw.

Ovarian Function in the Puerperium

Following delivery, the hormones produced by the fetal-placental unit disappear rapidly. Whether the mother is nursing or not seems to be the major determinant of the timing of first ovulation (Fig. 10–7). Also important to the time of return of ovulation are the frequency of breast-feeding and the addition of solid food supplementation to the infant's diet (Stern et al., 1986). A study in Mexico indicated that in the absence of bleeding and supplementation, 100 per cent of breast-feeding mothers remained anovulatory for 3 months postpartum, and over 95 per cent

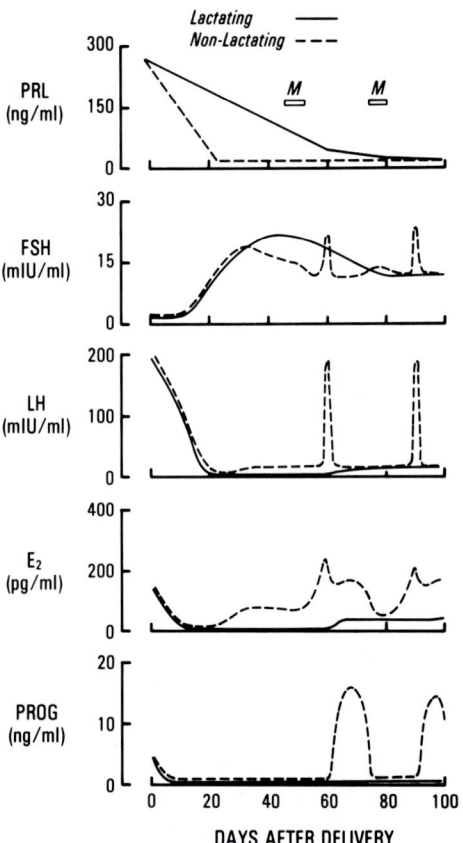

FIGURE 10–7. Schematic representation of serum concentrations of pituitary and gonadal hormones in lactating and nonlactating women in the puerperium. In the top graph, the *boxed M* refers to menses in the nonlactating woman. The lactating woman is still lactating at the end of the depicted period. Two LH surges are observed in the nonlactating woman. The elevated LH level immediately postpartum is no doubt due to cross reaction of assays with hCG, and the E_2 and progesterone *(Prog)* are of placental origin. (Based on Rolland R, Leguin RM, Schellekens LA, De Jong FH: The role of prolactin in the restoration of ovarian function during the early postpartum period in the human female. I. A study during physiological lactation. Clin Endocrinol 4:15, 1975.)

remained anovulatory for 6 months (Rivera et al., 1988). Postpartum women rarely ovulate before the 30th day after delivery (Vorherr, 1973). Furthermore, in most non-nursing mothers menstruation occurs by the third postpartum month, but both ovulation and menstruation are significantly delayed in nursing mothers.

On the basis of daily urinary pregnanediol glucuronide excretion, Gray and co-workers (1987) noted that the mean delay to first ovulation following delivery was 45.2 days in non-breast-feeding women and observed that no woman ovulated before 25 days after delivery. Over half of the women apparently ovulated prior to the first menses, but over 80 per cent of the first ovulatory cycles were abnormal based on pregnanediol excretion. It appears that the first menstrual period may occur following ovulation in breast-feeding women as well.

Rolland and co-workers (1975) have determined circulating hormone levels in normal breast-feeding women (see Fig. 10–7). Presumably as a result of pituitary suppression persisting from pregnancy, low levels of estradiol do not result in an increase in serum follicle-stimulating hormone (FSH) concentrations until approximately 2 weeks postpartum. Although immunoreactive luteinizing hormone (LH) levels are increased for perhaps 2 weeks postpartum, this is undoubtedly due to cross reaction of the antibodies with human chorionic gonadotropin (hCG). Human chorionic gonadotropin is detectable in the maternal circulation for as long as 14 days (Reyes et al., 1985), whereas measurements of the beta subunit of LH are extremely low during pregnancy (Hagen and McNeilly, 1975) and remain quite low until the tenth day postpartum (Miyake et al., 1978). In fact, the pituitary has been shown to be unresponsive to pituitary gonadotropin-releasing hormone (GnRH) in the early puerperium (Miyake et al., 1978). Subsequently, FSH but not LH rises above the normal range observed in eumenorrheic women. However, only after basal prolactin levels have fallen to normal does ovarian secretion of estradiol begin to rise. It appears that the hyperprolactinemia that is present postpartum is not due to an increase in the number of secretory pulses of prolactin per unit time, but rather to increased prolactin secretion during each pulse (Nunley et al., 1991).

Rolland and co-workers (1975) also noted that if prolactin is suppressed in the immediate postpartum period by bromocriptine, the levels of circulating estradiol fall below the normal range and FSH does not rise above normal. FSH and LH levels do increase during the second postpartum week with a high initial FSH/LH ratio (Kremer et al., 1989). An LH surge and ovulation then occur about 3 weeks postpartum, much earlier than ever observed in non-nursing mothers (Vorherr, 1973). Such data suggest that prolactin interferes either directly or indirectly with gonadal steroidogenesis.

The importance of prolactin and lactation to the return of gonadal function is perhaps even more dramatically demonstrated by studies of Kung hunter-gatherers in Africa (Konner and Worthman, 1980). Despite initiation of coitus soon after delivery and the lack of contraception, the average interval between births in this population is 44.1 months. It now appears that this long birth spacing is directly attributable to the pattern of nursing. Mothers nurse briefly and frequently (with a mean interval between nursing episodes of approximately 13 minutes), and infants are always in immediate physical proximity to their mothers until age 2 years or older. Infants even customarily sleep on the same skin mat with their mothers until weaned, and they are allowed to nurse at night as desired. Low levels of estradiol-17β and progesterone in the serum of the mothers correlated with the age of the infants and the intervals between nursing, but not with total nursing time. Because mean prolactin levels and frequent nursing are also correlated (Delvoye et al., 1977; Rolland et al., 1975), Konner and Worthman (1980) concluded that maternal ovarian function is apparently suppressed by a timing-dependent, prolactin-mediated effect of breast stimulation.

Recent data indicate that during the first 6 months postpartum, continued breast-feeding results in bone mineral loss from the lumbar spine (averaging 6.5 per cent), but not from the mid- or distal radius (Hayslip et al., 1989). At least one study has reported that lactating women regain bone mineral after cessation of lactation (Lamke et al., 1977). However, Wardlaw and Pike (1986) have noted that women aged 30 to 35 years who breast-fed for long periods (mean 10.7 months) had significantly lower bone densities of the ultra-distal forearm than women who breast-fed for a short term (mean 2.8 months). In addition, Goldsmith and Johnston (1975) found that women who had lactated tended to be poorly mineralized and had bone mineral deficits that were not fully recovered before menopause. It would be reasonable to conclude that bone mineral loss due to breast-feeding is most likely reversible in healthy postpartum women; however, breast-feeding may have adverse effects on the bone mineral of women with osteopenia from pre-existing disorders.

Composition of Colostrum and Milk

The composition of human milk has been extensively analyzed (Jenness, 1974, 1979; Howell et al., 1986). Milk is an emulsion of fat in water that is isotonic with plasma, with water being the major constituent. Mature human milk contains 3 to 5 per cent fat, 0.8 to 1.2 per cent protein, 6.8 to 7.2 per cent carbohydrate (calculated as lactose), and 0.2 per cent mineral constituents (Table 10–1). Human milk contains more than 100 known constituents, and additional components are continually being identified. Its energy content is 60 to 75 kcal/100 ml. The protein content is markedly higher and the carbohydrate content is lower in colostrum than in mature milk. In general, the fat content of milk does not vary consistently, but exhibits large diurnal variations, being highest in mid-morning and lowest during the night, and increasing during each nursing episode. Race, age, parity, and diet do not have much effect on milk composition, and there is no different in the composition of milk from each of the two breasts. Inadequate

TABLE 10–1. Approximate Composition of Human Colostrum, Mature Human Milk, and Cow's Milk (per 100 ml)

COMPONENTS	HUMAN COLOSTRUM	MATURE HUMAN MILK	COW'S MILK
Water (gm)	87	87	87
Total solids (gm)	13	13	13
Protein (gm)	7.9	1.1	3.5
Fat (gm)	1.3	4.5	3.7
Lactose (gm)	3.2	6.8	4.9
Ash (i.e., mineral content) (gm)	0.6	0.2	0.7
Proteins (% of total protein)			
Casein	—	40	82
Whey proteins	—	60	18
Major whey proteins (mg)			
α-Lactalbumin	333	263	40
Lactoferrin	384	168	—
Lysozyme	34	42	—
Albumin	36	52	23
IgA	364	142	40
Minerals (mg)			
Na	92	15	58
K	55	55	138
Cl	117	43	103
Ca	31	33	125
Mg	4	4	12
P	14	15	100
Fe	0.09	0.15	0.10
Vitamins (μg)			
A	89	53	34
C	4400	4300	1600
D		0.03	0.06
Riboflavin	30	43	157
Nicotinic acid	75	172	85
Thiamine	15	16	42

Based on data compiled by Jenness R: The composition of human milk. Semin Perinatol 3:225, 1979; and Worthington BS: Lactation, human milk, and nutritional considerations. *In* Worthington BS, Vermeersch J, Williams SR (eds): Nutrition in Pregnancy and Lactation. St. Louis, CV Mosby, 1977; and Casey CE, Hambidge KM: Nutritional aspects of human lactation. *In* Neville MC, Neifert MR (eds): Lactation. Physiology, Nutrition, and Breast-Feeding. New York, Plenum Press, 1983.

protein intake does not seem to affect the fat, protein, or lactose content of milk, but the volume of milk produced may be reduced.

The principal proteins in human milk are caseins, alpha-lactalbumin, lactoferrin, immunoglobulin A (IgA), lysozyme, and serum albumin (Bezkorovainy, 1977). Alpha-lactalbumin is a distinctive milk protein, being a component of the enzyme complex lactose synthetase, and its synthesis, as discussed earlier, is controlled by prolactin. Lactoferrin and IgA are found in greater quantities in colostrum than in later milk. Of note is the observation that the essential amino acid content of human milk appears to parallel what is optimal for human infants. A number of peptide hormones also are present in breast milk, and more are continually being identified. Epidermal growth factor and transforming growth factor-α are present and may play roles in the growth of newborn infants (Okada et al., 1991). Gonadotropin-releasing hormone, thyrotropin-releasing hormone, somatostatin, vasoactive intestinal polypeptide, growth hormone–

releasing hormone, and a gastrin-releasing peptide-like immunoreactive substance are all found in higher concentrations in milk than in maternal plasma (Takeyama et al., 1991). IGF-I and IGF-II and their binding proteins also are present and may contribute to the growth-promoting properties of human milk (Donovan et al., 1991). Prolactin is present and may play roles in lactation and in the intestinal absorptive function of the suckling newborn (Yuen, 1988). High levels of a parathyroid hormone–like protein may be important in extracellular calcium homeostasis in infants (Budayr et al., 1989; Bucht et al., 1992). Even naturally occurring benzodiazepines have been identified in human milk and may have sedative properties (Peña et al., 1991).

The major carbohydrate of human milk is lactose, but 30 or more oligosaccharides, all containing a reducing group and ranging from three to 14 saccharide units per molecule, are also present. These may comprise as much as 1 gm/100 ml in mature milk and 2.5 gm/100 ml in colostrum. Because many of these oligosaccharides are growth factors for certain strains of lactobacilli, they may have an effect on intestinal flora in infants. Some nucleotide sugars and lipid-bound and protein-bound carbohydrates are present as well.

The principal class of human milk lipids is triglycerides. The most common are palmitic and oleic acids. The fatty acid composition of milk fat is somewhat influenced by diet. When the diet is deficient in calories, the milk fat tends to resemble adipose tissue fat in fatty acid composition, no doubt as a result of lipolysis of maternal stores. When dietary intake is adequate, the main influence is the type of diet (Insull et al., 1959; Prentice et al., 1989).

The major mineral constituents of human milk are sodium, potassium, calcium, magnesium, phosphorus, and chloride. Iron, copper, and zinc contents of human milk vary considerably (Casey et al., 1989). Several other trace elements have been detected as well.

About 25 per cent, or 40 mg/100 ml, of the total nitrogen content of human milk represents nonprotein compounds, including urea, uric acid, creatine, creatinine, and free amino acids. The total nonprotein nitrogen content of colostrum is much higher than that of later milk. Of the free amino acids, glutamic acid and taurine are the most abundant. It has been suggested that taurine may be required for early stages of brain development in some species (Sturman et al., 1977). All of the vitamins, except for vitamin K, are found in human milk in nutritionally significant quantities.

At the end of the first postpartum week, a mother produces 550 ml of milk per day; by 2 to 3 weeks postpartum, her production has increased to approximately 800 ml per day, and it peaks at 1.5 to 2 liters per day.

Synthesis and Secretion of Milk

Carbohydrates and proteins in milk are synthesized within the rough endoplasmic reticulum, packaged within the Golgi apparatus, and released by merocrine secretion from Golgi vesicles (Hollmann, 1974). The specific site for triglyceride synthesis in the secretory cell is unclear but is also probably in the rough endoplasmic reticulum as a result of synthesis from glycerol and free fatty acids, which enter the cell by passive diffusion. Lipid droplets accumulate in the apical region of the cell and then empty into the lumen by attachment to the apical membrane, thus becoming part of the membrane (apocrine secretion). This process continues while the plasma membrane bulges into the lumen and envelops the apical fat droplet. The fat droplet does not fuse with the plasma membrane but remains separated from it by a thin layer of cytoplasmic origin. The fat droplet encased by this membrane is pinched off from the apical plasma membrane. The quantity of water in milk is regulated by the quantity of lactose, the principal osmotically active compound in milk. This is because the Golgi vesicles in which lactose is compartmentalized are permeable to water. A variable amount of cytoplasm is often released with the lipid droplets in *signet cells*. Occasionally, intact alveolar cells (the so-called Downey cells) are released into the lumen as well, and they are especially prominent in colostrum.

PRINCIPLES FOR NURSING

Maternal Nutritional Requirements

Obviously, the nutritional status of the mother during lactation is important (Filer, 1975). For each 20 calories of milk she produces, the nursing mother must consume an additional 30 calories. Under normal circumstances, a dietary caloric increase of approximately 500 to 1000 calories per day is observed in women who are maintaining body weight during lactation (Thomson et al., 1970; Whichelow, 1975). In most women the energy cost of lactation is met to a greater extent by fat loss than by increased energy intake, reduced expenditure of energy, or both (Schultz et al., 1980).

Unfortunately, no objective criteria exist for assessing the quantitative or qualitative adequacy of human milk. Recommendations for the dietary adequacy of the well-nourished lactating woman have not been determined. Diets recommended for lactating women include somewhat more of each nutrient, except vitamin D, than recommended for the nonpregnant female; they have been described elsewhere (Newman, 1981; Worthington, 1977; Casey and Hambidge, 1983). In general, recent studies indicate that human milk alone is adequate to meet the nutritional requirements of infants for at least the first 6 months of life.

Practical Aspects of Nursing

Ideally the decision whether to breast-feed her baby should be made by a mother in the prenatal period, after she has received instruction in its performance and the health benefits and practical advantages of nursing have been described to her (Berg, 1979; Riordan, 1983). No woman need be discouraged from breast-feeding because of small breast size. There is no correlation between the pre-pregnant size of the breast and the amount of milk produced postpartum. Milk production depends on the extent of mammary gland development during pregnancy and also seems to depend on proper antenatal and immediate postnatal breast stimulation. Problems resulting from inverted nipples or poor nipple protrusion usually resolve spontaneously during pregnancy. Prenatal rolling of the nipples to aid protractility may be of benefit.

After delivery, the timing of the first feeding may have significant effects on the success of nursing. Infants and mothers who initiate breast-feeding within the first hour after delivery have a higher success rate than those who delay nursing for several hours (Johnson, 1976). The frequency and duration of feedings are also important to successful nursing. In order to encourage optimal milk production, to condition the milk ejection reflex, and to avoid engorgement, a demand feeding schedule should be used. A schedule of at least 5 minutes at each breast at each feeding on the first postpartum day, gradually increasing over the next few days, will permit optimal milk letdown and generally not lead to sore nipples. Allowing less time at each breast at each feeding will result in a frustrated, hungry infant and a discouraged mother with engorged breasts.

Advantages of Nursing

From a nutritional point of view, human breast milk has not been improved on as a standard by which to evaluate any simulated formula (Committee on Nutrition, 1976). Compared with human milk, modified cow's milk formulas have a high solute load, may lack some beneficial and even essential components, and are not absorbed as easily or rapidly by the infants. Use of a mother's own colostrum and milk provides the nutritional advantages of an increased intake of minerals, vitamins, and protein as well as anti-infectious factors.

From an immunologic point of view, the most apparent role of human milk is to supply antibodies to the neonate (Butler, 1979). The IgA antibodies in milk probably protect the neonatal gastrointestinal tract from pathogens. IgG antibodies may provide some short-term systemic humoral immunity. Other nonantibody anti-infectious elements may also play important roles, but further studies are needed (Howell et al., 1986).

From a psychological point of view, the bonding established as a result of nursing leads to improved interactions between infant and mother that are measurable 2 years later (Lozoff et al., 1977). Other psychological advantages are more difficult to quantify (Oseid, 1979).

DISTURBANCES OF PUERPERAL LACTATION

Breast Engorgement and Nipple Tenderness

Engorgement, a common complication that typically affects both breasts, generally occurs between 2 and 4 days postpartum. It may occur in some women even when suggestions for nursing are properly followed or if the mother and infant must be separated. In this condition, edema of mammary tissues is associated with milk retention and vascular and lymphatic stasis. The breasts become swollen, firm, and tense, and there is therefore less nipple protrusion, making nursing more difficult. Except for possibly slight temperature elevation, systemic symptoms are uncommon, but the local discomfort is generally considerable. Treatment involves the use of warm moist compresses followed by hand or pump expression of milk and nursing.

Nipple tenderness is more difficult to treat than engorgement. The mother should know that some nipple tenderness is normal as the nipples become accustomed to nursing, but it will generally subside in a few days. The importance of proper technique in nursing to prevent or diminish nipple soreness and cracking should be emphasized (Berg, 1979). Appropriate treatment includes proper care of the nipples, beginning to nurse on the less sore breast to encourage milk letdown, changing nursing positions to rotate the major stress points on the nipples from the infant's mouth, and breaking the suction before removing the infant from the breast.

Declining Milk Production

Little is known about the causes of failing lactation in the human. A decline in milk production most frequently occurs in the first 3 months postpartum. In a 1943 study, Robinson reported that in 40 per cent of the 1100 women studied there was no recognized cause for failing lactation.

The regulation of lactation is complex, but basically it is a matter of the breast's producing the amount of milk for which there is a demand. In the early weeks of milk production many women over-produce, but if lactation continues, the supply and demand will gradually become equal. Obviously necessary to ensure adequate supply is to nurse on the demand of the infant. Supplemental feeding and the introduction of other foods should be delayed. Psychological stresses on the mother can reduce supply as well. As noted earlier, studies appear to show that milk yield among well-nourished women is higher than among malnourished women. In addition, lack of adequate rest and too much physical activity can interfere with milk letdown (Berg, 1979).

If lactation fails, formula feeding must be used. However, hormonal attempts to increase milk yield have been reported. Oral administration of thyroid-releasing hormone (TRH) has been observed to stimulate milk secretion without causing any endocrine dysfunction (Tyson et al., 1975).

Absence of Lactation

The complete absence of lactation, also known as agalactia, is rare. It is observed in persons with Sheehan's syndrome (postpartum pituitary necrosis) and may provide the first evidence of pituitary insufficiency (Sheehan, 1939). The disorder generally occurs as a result of postpartum hemorrhage and shock. The neurohypophysis is usually not involved, but can be in severe cases. Typically, fatigue and hypotension are also noted in the puerperium, and loss of pubic hair and other features common to hypopituitarism are observed thereafter. Partial or complete recovery with subsequent spontaneous pregnancies has been reported in some cases (Jackson et al., 1969).

Other Problems of and Contraindications to Nursing

Hyperbilirubinemia in the first 3 to 4 days of life, with its potential for kernicterus, is now often cited as a major problem for the breast-feeding infant even though kernicterus due to breast-feeding has not been reported in a healthy infant (Oseid, 1979). Human milk appears to contain an inhibitor, related to pregnanediol, that interferes with glucuronidation of fat-soluble bilirubin (Gartner and Lee, 1977). About 0.5 per cent of breast-fed infants develop unconjugated hyperbilirubinemia in the second week of life without showing any signs of illness. Other causes of hyperbilirubinemia should be sought. If the total bilirubin concentration increases to a high level, nursing can be transiently interrupted until it decreases. The mother can express milk manually during this interval. Infants with phenylketonuria and a few other rare amino acidurias should not be breast-fed even though human milk usually has less of the amino acid than cow's milk or standard formulas. Special low-level milk formulas must be given to affected children. Infants with galactosemia cannot nurse and need a formula containing sugars other than galactose. Primary lactose intolerance in infancy is rare, but acquired lactose or disaccharide intolerance may follow diarrhea. If this results, special formulas may be required.

Today infants with cleft palate may be fitted with dental prostheses to permit successful nursing. Premature and debilitated infants may be given manually expressed human milk by gavage.

A strong family history of breast cancer is not a contraindication to nursing. There is currently no evidence of any increased risk to the mother or infant (Vorherr, 1979).

Drugs and Nursing

A wide variety of agents may have effects on lactation and breast-feeding (Table 10–2). Drugs may affect lactation through a direct action on mammary tissue or by influencing prolactin secretion. Detailed discussion of such agents, which is beyond the scope of this chapter, has been published elsewhere (Dickey, 1979; Briggs et al., 1990). In general, gonadal and adrenal steroids can affect lactation through a direct effect on the breast. A wide variety of drugs, including phenothiazine derivatives, rauwolfia derivatives, substituted butyrophenones, tricyclic antidepressants, substituted thioxanthenes, α-methyldopa, opiates, and

thyroid-releasing hormone, act centrally to increase prolactin and cause lactation. Catecholamine precursors, monoamine oxidase inhibitors, ergot derivates, and barbiturates decrease secretion of prolactin and suppress lactation.

Many substances, including a wide variety of drugs, insecticides, and fungicides, may be transmitted to the neonate through human milk. Little is known about the effects of environmental pollutants on human development. For the present, women who breast-feed should be reassured that the risk of harm from the amounts of pollutants they encounter is negligible, unless they have been exposed to large quantities of known toxic substances during pregnancy or lactation.

Similarly, present data on drug excretion in human milk are limited in quality and amount. The available information has been exhaustively reviewed (Anderson, 1977, 1979, 1988). Only drugs that are necessary to the welfare of the mother should be prescribed. Lactating women should avoid drugs known to cross the placenta and to have harmful effects on the neonate. A current listing of agents contraindicated in nursing women (subject to change) may be found in Table 10–2, and additional information is published elsewhere (Briggs et al., 1990).

SUPPRESSION OF LACTATION

A variety of empiric measures to inhibit lactation have been used for several years and generally include mechanical compression of the breast, mild analgesics, and restriction of fluid intake. Because it is known that maternal fluid intake has no influence on lactogenesis (Duckman and Hubbard, 1950), only the first two measures are indicated (Harrison, 1979). Because such measures are frequently ineffective, estrogenic compounds began to be used for suppression of lactation in the late 1930s. A variety of estrogens have been tried, the best results being reported with long-acting preparations started as soon as possible after delivery (Morris et al., 1970; Vorherr, 1972; Schwartz et al., 1978). Still, the failure rate is typically 10 to 20 per cent. As noted previously, the inhibitory action of estrogen on lactation appears to be exerted at the mammary gland through blocking of the action of prolactin. Prolactin levels are not suppressed.

About half of all patients have continued or rebound breast engorgement after discontinuing the estrogen, indicating that the improvement in symptoms induced by such treatment is not sustained (Schwartz et al., 1978). Moreover, numerous clinicians have raised concerns about the possible association of estrogens with venous thrombosis and thromboembolism. Carcinoma of the breast, active hepatic disease, operative delivery, obesity, and age greater than 35 years are also regarded as contraindications.

Several studies have shown that bromocriptine prevents puerperal lactation and suppresses lactation once it has been established. It suppresses prolactin secretion through a direct effect on the pituitary and has been effective in all cases of increased prolactin secretion (Besser and Edwards, 1972). Bromocriptine, 5 mg twice a day, has been shown to be as effective

Table 10–2. Safety of Commonly Used Drugs for Lactating Women and Their Infants

CLASSIFICATION	AGENTS
Contraindicated (These drugs should not be used during lactation. If they are essential to the mother's health, breast-feeding should be discontinued at least temporarily.)	Amantadine* Amiodarone Antineoplastic agents Bromide Chloramphenicol Gold Iodide (including topical povidone-iodine in large amounts) Metronidazole Radiopharmaceuticals
Potentially Hazardous (Although not generally contraindicated these agents should be used with caution and should be avoided if possible.)	Acebutolol Alcohol (large amounts) Antihistamine/Decongestant combinations* Atenolol Benzodiazepines (lorazepam, oxazepam preferred)† Chlorthalidone* Contraceptives, estrogen-containing* Corticosteroids (high-dose, long-term; prednisolone preferred)† Estrogens* Lindane, topical Lithium Methimazole Narcotics (in addicts) Nitrofurantoin Quinolones (norfloxacin preferred)† Salicylates (high doses) Sulfonamides, long-acting Timolol
Probably Safe in Usual Doses (There are insufficient data to ensure that these agents have no effects in neonates, but if they occur they are probably infrequent and/or mild. The potential for rare allergic or idiosyncratic reactions should be kept in mind when prescribing these drugs to a lactating woman.)	ACE inhibitors Alcohol (occasional small amounts) Aminoglycosides Anticholinergics* Anticonvulsants Antihistamines* Barbiturates Butyrophenones Chloral hydrate Fluoxetine Histamine H_2-antagonists (famotidine preferred)† Isoniazid Nonsteroid anti-inflammatory agents (Ibuprofen preferred)† Phenothiazines Propylthiouracil Quinidine Salicylates (low doses) Spironolactone Tetracyclines Thiazides (short-acting) Tricyclic antidepressants (desipramine, nortriptyline preferred)† Verapamil

*Can potentially suppress lactation.
†Preferred agents distribute into milk less, have a shorter half-life, or both.

Table continued on following page

as diethylstilbestrol, 20 mg twice a day, and causes less rebound engorgement (Varga et al., 1972). In suppression of established lactation it is much more effective than diethylstilbestrol.

The recommended dosage of bromocriptine to prevent puerperal lactation is now 2.5 mg twice a day for 14 days, but therapy may be given for as long as 21 days if needed. From 2.5 to 7.5 mg may be given daily. Because about 30 per cent of women treated with bromocriptine develop significant lowered systolic and diastolic blood pressures, the first dose of bromocriptine should not be administered until after vital signs have stabilized and no earlier than 4 hours

after delivery. Blood pressure should be monitored during the first few hours of therapy. Other side effects, including dizziness, nausea, fainting, and syncope, have occurred in less than 10 per cent of treated patients. Rebound breast tenderness has been noted after therapy was discontinued in about 30 per cent of those treated; generally it is not severe and may be reduced if one tablet is given daily for a third week.

Although hypotension may occur with the start of therapy in some patients, several cases of hypertension now have been reported, sometimes with the initiation of therapy, but often during the second week of therapy (Watson et al., 1989). It appears that women

TABLE 10–2. Safety of Commonly Used Drugs for Lactating Women and Their Infants *Continued*

CLASSIFICATION	AGENTS
Safe in Usual Doses (The potential for rare allergic or idiosyncratic reactions should be kept in mind when prescribing these drugs to a lactating woman.)	Acetaminophen Antacids Aspirin (low doses) Caffeine Cephalosporins Corticosteroids (short courses) Digoxin Erythromycin Insulin Labetalol Lidocaine Magnesium sulfate Methyldopa Methylergonovine (short courses) Metoclopramide Metoprolol Oxymetazoline nasal spray Penicillins Progestins Propranolol Poliovirus vaccine Sulfisoxazole Theophylline Thyroid Vaccines Warfarin

Prepared by Philip O. Anderson, Pharm.D., Director, Drug Information Service, University of California, San Diego, Medical Center. Compiled from Anderson PO: Drugs and breast feeding. *In* Knoben JE, Anderson PO (eds): Handbook of Clinical Drug Data. 7th ed. Hamilton, IL, Drug Intelligence Publications, 1993, pp 106–128.

with antepartum pregnancy-induced hypertension are at increased risk for developing hypertension with therapy (Watson et al., 1989). Epilepsy, stroke, and myocardial infarction also have been reported (Iffy et al., 1986; Ruch and Duhring, 1989). Although there is no conclusive evidence documenting that ergot alkaloids are directly responsible, these potentially serious side effects should be considered whenever the postpartum use of bromocriptine is considered.

Recent studies have documented that another ergot derivative, cabergoline, given as a single dose of 1 mg, is at least as effective as bromocriptine given daily for 14 days in preventing puerperal lactation (Rolland et al., 1991; Melis et al., 1988). Because of a lower rate of rebound breast activity and a lower incidence of side effects, cabergoline may become the drug of choice for lactation inhibition.

In summary, an ergot derivative, estrogenic preparations, or breast binders and ice may be used to prevent immediate postpartum lactation and pain. Although the drugs are efficacious, their use has potential side effects that must be weighed against the transitory nature of the breast engorgement and discomfort.

REFERENCES

Ances IG: Serum concentrations of epidermal growth factor in human pregnancy. Am J Obstet Gynecol **115**:357, 1973.

Anderson PO: Drugs and breast feeding: A review. Drug Intell Clin Pharm **11**:208, 1977.

Anderson PO: Drugs and breast feeding. Semin Perinatol **3**:271, 1979.

Anderson PO: Drugs and breast feeding. *In* Knoben JE, Anderson PO (eds): Handbook of Clinical Drug Data. 6th ed. Hamilton, IL, Drug Intelligence Publications, 1988.

Aragona C, Friesen HG: Lactation and galactorrhea. *In* DeGroot LJ, Cahill GF Jr, Martini L, et al (eds): Endocrinology. Vol. III. New York, Grune & Stratton, 1979.

Aubert ML, Suard Y, Sizonenko PC, Krachenbuhl JP: Prolactin receptors: Study with dispersed cells from rabbit mammary gland. Abstract 19. 60th Annual Meeting, Endocrine Society, 1978.

Baldwin RL, Louis S: Hormonal actions on mammary metabolism. J Dairy Sci **58**:1033, 1975.

Banerjee MR, Terry PM, Sakai S, et al: Hormonal regulation of casein messenger RNA. In Vitro **14**:128, 1978.

Benson GK, Folley SJ: The effect of oxytocin on mammary gland involution in the rat. J Endocrinol **16**:189, 1957.

Berg RA: Nursing the newborn. Semin Perinatol **3**:241, 1979.

Bergland RM, Page RB: Can the pituitary secrete directly to the brain? (Affirmative anatomical evidence.) Endocrinology **102**:1325, 1978.

Bern HA, Nicoll CS: The comparative endocrinology of prolactin. Recent Prog Horm Res **24**:681, 1968.

Besser GM, Edwards CRW: Galactorrhoea. Br Med J **2**:280, 1972.

Bezkorovainy A: Human milk and colostrum proteins: A review. J Dairy Sci **60**:1023, 1977.

Blake CA, Sawyer CH: Nicotine blocks the suckling-induced rise in circulating prolactin in lactating rats. Science **177**:619, 1972.

Bohnet H, Gomez F, Friesen HG: Prolactin and estrogen binding sites in the mammary gland of the lactating and non-lactating rat. Endocrinology **101**:1111, 1977.

Boutin JM, Edery M, Shirota M, Jolicoeur C, Lesueur L, Ali S, Guld D, Djiane J, Kelly PA: Identification of a cDNA encoding a long form of PRL receptor in human hepatoma and breast cancer cells. Mol Endocrinol **3**:1455, 1989.

Briggs GG, Freeman RK, Yaffe SY: Drugs in Pregnancy and Lactation. 3rd ed. Baltimore, Williams & Wilkins, 1990.

Bruce JO, Ramirez VD: Site of action of the inhibitory effect of estrogen upon lactation. Neuroendocrinology **6**:19, 1970.

Brun F, Del Re R, del Pozo E, et al: Prolactin inhibition and suppression of puerperal lactation by Br-ergocryptine (CB-154): A comparison with estrogen. Obstet Gynecol **41**:884, 1973.

Bucht E, Carlqvist M, Hedlund B, Bremme K, Torring O: Parathyroid hormone-related peptide in human milk measured by a mid-molecule radioimmunoassay. Metabolism **41**:11, 1992.

Budayr AA, Halloran BP, King JC, Diep D, Nissenson RA, Strewler GA: High levels of a parathyroid hormone-like protein in milk. Proc Natl Acad Sci USA **86**:7183, 1989.

Butler JE: Immunologic aspects of breast feeding: Anti-infectious activity of breast milk. Semin Perinatol **3**:255, 1979.

Casey CE, Hambidge KM: Nutritional aspects of human lactation. *In* Neville MC, Neifert MR (eds): Lactation. Physiology, Nutrition, and Breast-Feeding. New York, Plenum Press, 1983.

Casey CE, Neville MC, Hambidge KM: Studies in human lactation: Secretion of zinc, copper and manganese in human milk. Am J Clin Nutr **49**:773, 1989.

Cobo E: Effect of different doses of ethanol on the milk-ejecting reflex in lactating women. Am J Obstet Gynecol **115**:817, 1973.

Cobo E: Neuroendocrine control of milk ejection in women. *In* Josimovich JB, Reynolds M, Cobo E (eds): Lactogenic Hormones, Fetal Nutrition, and Lactation. New York, John Wiley and Sons, 1974.

Committee on Nutrition, American Academy of Pediatrics: Commentary on breast-feeding and infant formulas including proposed standards for formulas. Pediatrics **57**:278, 1976.

Cowie AT, Tindal JS: The Physiology of Lactation. London, Edward Arnold, 1971.

Cowie AT, Forsyth IA, Hart IC: Hormonal Control of Lactation. New York, Springer-Verlag, 1980.

Cross BA, Dyball REJ, Dyer RG, et al: Endocrine neurons. Recent Prog Horm Res **31**:243, 1975.

Cunningham ET Jr, Sawchenko PE: Reflex control of magnocellular vasopressin and oxytocin secretion. TINS **14**:406, 1991.

Delvoye P, Demaegd M, Delogne-Desnoeck J, Robyn C: The influence of the frequency of nursing and of previous lactation experience on serum prolactin in lactating women. J Biosocial Sci **9**:447, 1977.

Diaz S, Seron-Ferre M, Cardenas H, Schiappacasse V, Brandeis A, Croxatto HB: Circadian variation of basal prolactin, prolactin response to suckling, and length of amenorrhea in nursing women. J Clin Endocrinol Metab **68**:946, 1989.

Dickey RP: Drugs affecting lactation. Semin Perinatol **3**:279, 1979.

Djiane J, Durand P: Prolactin-progesterone antagonism in self-regulation of prolactin receptors in the mammary gland. Nature **266**:614, 1977.

Djiane J, Durand P, Kelly PA: Evolution of prolactin receptors in rabbit mammary gland during pregnancy and lactation. Endocrinology **100**:1348, 1977.

Donovan SM, Hintz RL, Rosenfeld RG: Insulin-like growth factors I and II and their binding proteins in human milk: Effect of heat treatment on IGF and IGF binding protein stability. J Pediatr Gastroenterol Nutr **13**:242, 1991.

Duckman S, Hubbard JF: The role of fluid in relieving breast engorgement without the use of hormones. Am J Obstet Gynecol **60**:200, 1950.

Eriksson L, Frankenne F, Eden S, Hennen G, von Schoultz B: Growth hormone 24-h serum profiles during pregnancy—lack of pulsatility for the secretion of the placental variant. Br J Obstet Gynecol **96**:949, 1989.

Falconer IR, Rowe JM: Possible mechanism of action of prolactin on mammary cell sodium transport. Nature **256**:327, 1975.

Falconer IR, Rowe JM: Effect of prolactin on sodium and potassium concentrations in mammary alveolar tissue. Endocrinology **101**:181, 1977.

Fazekas AG, MacFarlane JK: Macromolecular binding of glucocorticoids in human mammary carcinoma. Cancer Res **37**:640, 1977.

Filer LJ: Maternal nutrition in lactation. Clin Perinatol **2**:353, 1975.

Folley SJ: Endocrine control of the mammary gland. II Lactation. Br Med Bull **5**:135, 1948.

Fournier PJR, Desjardins PD, Friesen HG: Current understanding of human prolactin physiology and its diagnostic and therapeutic applications. A review. Am J Obstet Gynecol **118**:337, 1974.

Frankenne F, Closset J, Gomez F, Scippo ML, Smal J, Hennen G: The physiology of growth hormones (GHs) in pregnant women and partial characterization of the placental GH variant. J Clin Endocrinol Metab **66**:1171, 1988.

Frankenne F, Rentier-Delrue FR, Scippo ML, Martial J, Hennen G:

Expression of the growth hormone variant gene in human placenta. J Clin Endocrinol Metab **64**:635, 1987.

Frantz WL, MacIndoe JH, Turkington RW: Prolactin receptors: Characteristics of the particulate fraction binding activity. J Endocrinol **60**:485, 1974.

Freemark M, Comer M: Purification of a distinct placental lactogen receptor, a new member of the growth hormone/prolactin receptor family. J Clin Invest **83**:883, 1989.

Friesen HG: Human prolactin in clinical endocrinology: The impact of radioimmunoassays. Metabolism **22**:1039, 1973.

Furlanetto RW, Underwood LE, Van Wyk JJ, Handwerger S: Immunoreactive somatomedin-C is elevated late in pregnancy. J Clin Endocrinol Metab **47**:695, 1978.

Gaines WL: A contribution to the physiology of lactation. Am J Physiol **38**:285, 1915.

Gartner LM, Lee K-S: Jaundice and liver disease. *In* Behrman RE (ed): Neonatal-Perinatal Medicine. Diseases of the Fetus and Infant. 2nd ed. St. Louis, CV Mosby, 1977.

Goldsmith NF, Johnston JO: Bone mineral: Effects of oral contraceptives, pregnancy, and lactation. J Bone Joint Surg **57(5)**:657, 1975.

Gray RH, Campbell OM, Zacur HA, Labbok MH, MacRae SL: Postpartum return of ovarian activity in nonbreastfeeding women monitored by urinary assays. J Clin Endocrinol Metab **64**:645, 1987.

Grumbach MM, Kaplan SL, Sciarra JJ, Burr IM: Chorionic growth-hormone prolactin (CGP): Secretion, disposition, biologic activity in man, and postulated function as the "growth hormone" of the second half of pregnancy. Ann NY Acad Sci **148**:501, 1968.

Gunther M: Lactation in women. Can Med Assoc J **47**:410, 1942.

Hagen C, McNeilly AS: The gonadotropic hormones and their subunits in human maternal and fetal circulation at delivery. Am J Obstet Gynecol **121**:926, 1975.

Handwerger S: Clinical counterpoint: The physiology of placental lactogen in human pregnancy. Endocr Rev **12**:329, 1991.

Harrison RG: Suppression of lactation. Semin Perinatol **3**:287, 1979.

Hayden TJ, Bonneg RC, Forsyth IA: Ontogeny and control of prolactin receptors in the mammary gland and liver of virgin pregnant and lactating rats. J Endocrinol **80**:259, 1979.

Hayslip CC, Klein TA, Wray HL, Duncan WE: The effects of lactation on bone mineral content in healthy postpartum women. Obstet Gynecol **73**:588, 1989.

Hollmann KH: Cytology and fine structure of the mammary gland. *In* Larson BL, Smith VR (eds): Lactation. A Comprehensive Treatise. Vol. I. New York, Academic Press, 1974.

Howell RR, Morriss FH Jr, Pickering LK (eds): Human Milk in Infant Nutrition and Health. Springfield, IL, Charles C Thomas, 1986.

Hsueh AJW, Peck EJ, Clark JH: Oestrogen receptors in the mammary gland of the lactating rat. J Endocrinol **58**:503, 1973.

Iffy L, TenHove W, Frisoli G: Acute myocardial infarction in the puerperium in patients receiving bromocriptine. Am J Obstet Gynecol **155**:371, 1986.

Insull WJ, Hirsch J, James T, Ahrens EH: The fatty acids of human milk. II. Alterations produced by manipulation of caloric balance and exchange of dietary fats. J Clin Invest **38**:443, 1959.

Jackson IMD, Whyte WG, Garrey MM: Pituitary function following uncomplicated pregnancy in Sheehan's syndrome. J Clin Endocrinol Metab **29**:315, 1969.

Jaffe RB, Yuen GH, Keye WR Jr, Midgley AR Jr: Physiologic and pathologic profiles of circulating human prolactin. Am J Obstet Gynecol **117**:757, 1973.

Jaffe RB: Endocrine physiology of the fetus and fetoplacental unit. *In* Yen SSC, Jaffe RB (eds): Reproductive Endocrinology. 3rd ed. Philadelphia, WB Saunders Company, 1991.

Jelliffe D, Jelliffe E: Human Milk in the Modern World. Oxford, Oxford University Press, 1978.

Jenness R: The composition of milk. *In* Larson BL, Smith VR (eds): Lactation. A Comprehensive Treatise. Vol. III. New York, Academic Press, 1974.

Jenness R: The composition of human milk. Semin Perinatol **3**:225, 1979.

Jeske W, Soszynski P, Rogozinski W, Lukaszewicz E, Latoszewska W, Snochowska H: Plasma GHRH, CRH, ACTH, β-endorphin, human placental lactogen, GH and cortisol concentrations at the third trimester of pregnancy. Acta Endocrinol **120**:785, 1989.

Johnson N: Breastfeeding at one hour of age. Am J Matern Child Nursing 1(1):12, 1976.

Juergens WG, Stockdale FE, Topper YJ, Elias JJ: Hormone-dependent differentiation of mammary gland in vitro. Proc Natl Acad Sci USA 54:629, 1965.

Kaplan SL, Gurpide E, Sciarra JJ, Grumbach MM: Metabolic clearance rate and production rate of chorionic growth hormone-prolactin in late pregnancy. J Clin Endocrinol Metab 28:1458, 1968.

Karim M, Ammar R, Elmahgoub S, et al: Injected progestogen and lactation. Br Med J 1:200, 1971.

Kelly PA, Djiane J, Postel-Vinay M-C, Edery M: The prolactin/growth hormone receptor family. Endocrinol Rev 12:235, 1991.

Konner M, Worthman C: Nursing frequency, gonadal function, and birth spacing among !Kung hunter-gatheres. Science 207:788, 1980.

Kremer JAM, Rolland R, Van der Heijden PFM, Thomas CMG, Lancranjan I: Return of gonadotropic function in postpartum women during bromocriptine treatment. Fertil Steril 51:622, 1989.

Lamke B, Brundin J, Moberg P: Changes of bone mineral content during pregnancy and lactation. Acta Obstet Gynecol Scand 56:217, 1977.

Larrea F, Escorza A, Valero A, Hernandez L, Cravioto MC, Diaz-Sanchez V: Heterogeneity of serum prolactin throughout the menstrual cycle and pregnancy in hyperprolactinemic women with normal ovarian function. J Clin Endocrinol Metab 68:982, 1989.

Legros JJ, Franchimont P, Burger H: Variation of neurohypophysial function in normally cycling women. J Clin Endocrinol Metab 41:54, 1975.

Leung BS, Sasaki GH: Prolactin and progesterone effect on specific estradiol binding in uterine and mammary tissues in vitro. Biochem Biophys Res Commun 55:1180, 1973.

Leung BS, Jack WM, Reiney CG: Estrogen receptor in mammary glands and uterus of rats during pregnancy, lactation and involution. J Steroid Biochem 7:89, 1976.

Linzell JL: Mammary blood flow and methods of identifying and measuring precursors of milk. In Larson BL, Smith VR (eds): Lactation. A Comprehensive Treatise. Vol I. New York, Academic Press, 1974.

Lozoff B, Brittenham GM, Truse MA, et al: The mother-newborn relationship: Limits of adaptability. J Pediatr 91:1, 1977.

Lyons WR, Li CH, Johnson RE: The hormonal control of mammary growth and lactation. Recent Prog Horm Res 14:219, 1958.

Majumder GC, Turkington RW: Adenosine 3′,5′-mono-phosphate-dependent and independent protein phosphokinase isoenzymes from mammary gland. J Biol Chem 246:2650, 1971.

Marshall WA, Tanner JM: Variations in patterns of pubertal changes in girls. Arch Dis Child 44:291, 1969.

Marshall WN, Cumming DC, Fitzsimmons GW: Hot flushes during breastfeeding? Fertil Steril 57:1349, 1992.

Mayer G, Klein M: Histology and cytology of the mammary gland. In Kon SK, Cowie AT (eds): Milk: The Mammary Gland and Its Secretion. Vol I. New York, Academic Press, 1961.

McGuire WL, Horwitz KB, Pearson OH, Segaloff A: Current status of estrogen and progesterone receptors in breast cancer. Cancer 39:2934, 1977.

McKiernan J, Coyne J, Cahalane S: Histology of breast development in early life. Arch Dis Child 63:136, 1988.

Meites J: Maintenance of the mammary lobulo-alveolar system in rats after adreno-orchidectomy by prolactin and growth hormone. Endocrinology 76:1220, 1965.

Melis GB, Mais V, Paoletti AM, Beneventi F, Gambacciani M, Fioretti P: Prevention of puerperal lactation by a single oral administration of the new prolactin-inhibiting drug, cabergoline. Obstet Gynecol 71:311, 1988.

Miller WL, Eberhardt NL: Structure and evolution of the growth hormone gene family. Endocrinol Rev 4:97, 1983.

Miyake A, Tanizawa O, Aono T, Kurachi K: Pituitary LH response to LHRH during puerperium. Obstet Gynecol 51:37, 1978.

Morag M: A galactopoietic effect from oxytocin administered between milkings in the cow. Ann Biol Anim Biochim Biophys 8:27, 1968.

Morris JA, Creasy RK, Hohe PT: Inhibition of puerperal lactation. Double-blind comparison of chlorotrianisene, testosterone enan-

thate with estradiol valerate and placebo. Obstet Gynecol 36:107, 1970.

Newman V: Nutrition in prevention. In Schneiderman LJ (ed): The Practice of Preventive Health Care. Menlo Park, CA, Addison-Wesley, 1981.

Niall HD, Hogan ML, Tregear GW, et al: The chemistry of growth hormone and the lactogenic hormone. Recent Prog Horm Res 29:387, 1973.

Noel GL, Suh HK, Frantz AG: Prolactin release during nursing and breast stimulation in postpartum and non-postpartum subjects. J Clin Endocrinol Metab 38:413, 1974.

Nolin JM, Witorsch RJ: Detection of endogenous immunoreactive prolactin in rat mammary epithelial cells during lactation. Endocrinology 99:949, 1976.

Nunley WC, Urban RJ, Kitchin JD, Bateman BG, Evans WS, Veldhuis JD: Dynamics of pulsatile prolactin release during the postpartum lactational period. J Clin Endocrinol Metab 71:287, 1991.

Okada M, Ohmura E, Kamiya Y, Murakami H, Onoda N, Iwashita M, Wakai K, Tsushima T, Shizume K: Transforming growth factor (TGF)-α in human milk. Life Sci 48:1151, 1991.

Oseid B: Breast-feeding and infant health. Semin Perinatol 3:249, 1979.

Patten BM: Human Embryology. 2nd ed. New York, McGraw-Hill, 1953.

Peña C, Medina JH, Piva M, Diaz LE, Danilowicz C, Paladini AC: Naturally occurring benzodiazepines in human milk. Biochem Biophys Res Commun 175:1042, 1991.

Pollow K, Sinnecker R, Schmidt-Gollwitzer M, et al: Binding of [³H] progesterone to normal and neoplastic tissue samples from tumor-bearing breasts. J Mol Med 2:69, 1977.

Posner BI, Kelly PA, Friesen HG: Prolactin receptors in rat liver: Possible induction by prolactin. Science 188:57, 1975.

Prentice A, Jarjou LMA, Drury PJ, Dewit O, Crawford MA: Breast milk fatty acids of rural Gambian mothers: effects of diet and maternal parity. J Pediatr Gastroenterol Nutr 8:486, 1989.

Raynaud A: Morphogenesis of the mammary gland. In Kon SK, Cowie AT (eds): Milk: The Mammary Gland and Its Secretion. Vol I. New York, Academic Press, 1961.

Reyes FI, Winter JSD, Faiman C: Postpartum disappearance of chorionic gonadotropin from the maternal and neonatal circulation. Am J Obstet Gynecol 153:486, 1985.

Richardson KC: Contractile tissues in the mammary gland with special reference to myoepithelium in the goat. Proc R Soc Lond (B) 136:30, 1949.

Rillema JA: Effect of prostaglandins on RNA and casein synthesis in mammary gland explants of mice. Endocrinology 99:490, 1976a.

Rillema JA: Action of prolactin on ornithine decarboxylase activity in mammary gland explants of mice. Endocrinol Res Commun 3:297, 1976b.

Rillema JA, Wild EA: Prolactin activation of phospholipase A activity in membrane preparations from mammary glands. Endocrinology 100:1219, 1977.

Rimoin DL, Holzman GB, Merimee TJ, et al: Lactation in the absence of human growth hormone. J Clin Endocrinol Metab 28:1183, 1968.

Riordan J: A Practical Guide to Breastfeeding. St. Louis, CV Mosby, 1983.

Rivera R, Kennedy KI, Ortiz E, Barrera M, Bhiwandiwala PP: Breastfeeding and the return to ovulation in Durango, Mexico. Fertil Steril 49:780, 1988.

Robinson M: Failing lactation. Lancet 1:66, 1943.

Rolland R, Lequin RM, Schellekens LA, De Jong FH: The role of prolactin in the restoration of ovarian function during the early postpartum period in the human female. I. A study during physiological lactation. Clin Endocrinol 4:15, 1975.

Rolland R, Piscitelli G, Ferrari C, Petroccione A, and The European Multicentre Study Group: Single dose cabergoline versus bromocriptine in inhibition of puerperal lactation: randomized, double blind, multicentre study. Br Med J 302:1367, 1991.

Ruch A, Duhring JL: Postpartum myocardial infarction in a patient receiving bromocriptine. Obstet Gynecol 74:448, 1989.

Russell JT, Brownstein MJ, Gainer H: Biosynthesis of vasopressin, oxytocin and neurophysins: isolation and characterization of two common precursors (propressophysin and prooxyphysin). Endocrinology 107:1880, 1980.

Saxena B, Emerson K, Selekow H: Serum placental lactogen levels as an index of placental function. N Engl J Med **281**:225, 1969.

Schwartz DJ, Evans PC, Garcia L-R: A clinical study of lactation suppression. Obstet Gynecol **42**:599, 1978.

Schutz Y, Lechtig A, Bradfeld RB: Energy expenditures and food intakes of lactating women in Guatemala. Am J Clin Nutr **38**:892, 1980.

Sheehan HL: Simmond's disease due to postpartum necrosis of the anterior pituitary. Q J Med **8**:277, 1939.

Shiu RPC, Friesen HG: Blockade of prolactin action by an antiserum to its receptors. Science **192**:259, 1976.

Shiu RPC: Prolactin receptors in human breast cancer cells in long term tissue culture. Cancer Res **39**:81, 1979.

Shiu RPC, Friesen HG: Mechanism of action of prolactin in the control of mammary gland function. Ann Rev Physiol **42**:83, 1980.

Shiu RPC, Iwasiow BM: Prolactin-inducible proteins in human breast cancer cells. J Biol Chem **260**(20):11307, 1985.

Soloff MS, Schroeder BT, Chakraborty J, Perlmutter AF: Characterization of oxytocin receptors in the uterus and mammary gland. Fed Proc **36**:1861, 1977.

Stern JM, Konner M, Herman TN, Reichlin S: Nursing behavior, prolactin and postpartum amenorrhea during prolonged lactation in American and !Kung mothers. Clin Endocrinol (Oxf) **25**:247, 1986.

Sturman JA, Rassin DK, Hayes KC, Gaull GE: Taurine in the developing kitten: Nutritional importance. Pediatr Res **11**:450, 1977.

Takeyama M, Kondo K, Takayama F, Kondo R, Murata H, Miyakawa I: High concentration of a gastrin-releasing peptide-like immunoreactive substance in pregnant human milk. Biochem Biophys Res Commun **176**:931, 1991.

Thomson AM, Hytten FE, Billewicz WZ: The energy cost of human lactation. Br J Nutr **24**:565, 1970.

Topper Y: Multiple hormone interactions in the development of mammary gland in vitro. Recent Prog Horm Res **26**:287, 1970.

Topper YJ, Freeman CS: Multiple hormone interactions in the developmental biology of the mammary gland. Physiol Rev **60**:1049, 1980.

Truong AT, Duez C, Belayew A, Renard A, Pictet R, Bell GI, Martial JA: Isolation and characterization of the human prolactin gene. EMBO J **3**:429, 1984.

Turkington RW, Brew K, Vanaman TC, Hill RL: The hormonal control of lactose synthetase in the developing mouse mammary gland. J Biol Chem **243**:3382, 1968.

Turkington RW: Stimulation of RNA synthesis in isolated mammary cells by insulin and prolactin bound to sepharose. Biochem Biophys Res Commun **41**:1362, 1970.

Turkington RW: Molecular biological aspects of prolactin. In Wolstenholme GEW, Knight J (eds): Lactogenic Hormones. Edinburgh, Livingstone, 1972.

Turkington RW, Majumder GC, Kadohama N, et al: Hormonal regulation of gene expression in mammary cells. Recent Prog Horm Res **29**:417, 1973.

Turner CW, Slaughter IS: The physiological effect of pituitary extract (posterior lobe) on the lactating mammary gland. J Dairy Sci **13**:8, 1930.

Turner CW: The Mammary Gland. Vol I. Columbia, MO, Lucus Brothers, 1952.

Tyson JE, Hwang P, Guyda H, Friesen HG: Studies of prolactin secretion in human pregnancy. Am J Obstet Gynecol **113**:14, 1972.

Tyson JE, Zanartu J, Perez A, Hacker R: Puerperal lactation in response to oral TRH. Clin Res **23**:243A, 1975.

Varga L, Lutterbeck PM, Pryor JS, et al: Suppression of puerperal lactation with an ergot alkaloid: A double-blind study. Br Med J **2**:743, 1972.

Vorherr H: Suppression of postpartum lactation. Postgrad Med J **52**:145, 1972.

Vorherr H: Contraception after abortion and postpartum. Am J Obstet Gynecol **117**:1002, 1973.

Vorherr H: Pregnancy and lactation in relation to breast cancer risk. Semin Perinatol **3**:299, 1979.

Walker WH, Fitzpatrick SL, Barrer HA, Saldan RP, Saunders GF: The human placental lactogen genes: Structure, function, evolution and transcriptional regulation. Endocr Rev **12**:316, 1991.

Wardlaw GM, Pike AM: The effect of lactation on peak adult shaft and ultradistal forearm bone mass in women. Am J Clin Nutr **44**:283, 1986.

Watson DL, Bhatia RK, Norman GS, Brindley BA, Sokol RJ: Bromocriptine mesylate for lactation suppression: A risk for postpartum hypertension? Obstet Gynecol **74**:573, 1989.

Waters MJ, Friesen HG, Bohnet HG: Regulation of prolactin receptors by steroid hormones and use of radioligand assays in endocrine research. In O'Malley BW, Birnbaumer L (eds): Receptors and Hormone Action III. New York, Academic Press, 1978.

Weisz-Carrington P, Roux ME, McWilliams M, et al: Hormonal induction of the secretory immune system in the mammary gland. Proc Natl Acad Sci USA **75**:2928, 1978.

Weitzman RE, Leake RD, Rubin RT, Fisher DA: The effect of nursing on neurohypophyseal hormone and prolactin secretion in human subjects. J Clin Endocrinol Metab **51**:836, 1980.

Whichelow MJ: Calorie requirements for successful breast feeding. Arch Dis Child **50**:669, 1975.

Worthington BS: Lactation, human milk, and nutritional considerations. In Worthington BS, Vermeersch J, Williams SR (eds): Nutrition in Pregnancy and Lactation. St. Louis, CV Mosby, 1977.

Yen SSC, Vela P, Tsai CC: Impairment of growth hormone secretion in response to hypoglycemia during early and late pregnancy. J Clin Endocrinol Metab **31**:29, 1969.

Yen SSC, Ehara Y, Siler TM: Augmentation of prolactin secretion by estrogen in hypogonadal women. J Clin Invest **53**:652, 1974.

Yuen BH: Prolactin in human milk: The influence of nursing and the duration of postpartum lactation. Am J Obstet Gynecol **158**:583, 1988.

ENVIRONMENTAL INFLUENCES ON FETAL DEVELOPMENT

CHAPTER

MATERNAL NUTRITION

BARBARA ABRAMS, Dr.P.H., R.D.

BACKGROUND

There have always been differing approaches and even controversies with regard to the role of food intake during pregnancy. Traditional beliefs from a wide variety of cultures present divergent approaches (Siefert, 1968). In some cultures, pregnant women are encouraged to eat an abundance of nutritious foods, such as leafy greens, soft fruits, and milk. In other cultures, foods that clearly make an important nutrient contribution to the diet, for example, eggs and milk, are forbidden during pregnancy. Such dietary prescriptions have not been limited to folk beliefs. The obstetric profession has changed its approach to nutritional management of pregnancy numerous times in the last century.

The first "scientific" scheme for dietary management of the pregnant woman was suggested by the physician Prowchownick in 1889. His diet, designed to stunt the growth of the fetus during the last weeks of gestation and hence facilitate vaginal delivery, was restricted in calories, fluid, and calcium and high in protein. This approach became popular in the United States and was used commonly until just after World War I, when it was suggested that the low level of preeclampsia seen in Germany during the war was the result of decreased meat intake. The dietary strategy that was developed in response to this observation limited weight gain and protein consumption. In the early 1940s, in another attempt to reduce the incidence of preeclampsia, sodium restriction was imposed in addition to the restriction of weight gain. As recently as the 1960s, medical textbooks recommended using strict dietary control to achieve weight gains of no

more than 20 to 25 pounds. At present, good nutritional care during pregnancy is based on the following general premises: women are encouraged to eat a variety of foods "to appetite," to achieve adequate weight gain as determined by their pre-pregnancy body mass index, and to breast-feed their infants after birth. This counsel is probably quite different from that given to their mothers and grandmothers.

CURRENT LIMITATIONS IN KNOWLEDGE

Nutrition and reproduction do not operate within a vacuum. Genetic, social, cultural, economic, and other factors inter-relate and make it extremely difficult to identify the independent influence of maternal nutritional status on pregnancy outcome. It is obvious that women cannot be experimentally starved to directly study the effect of poor nutrition on pregnancy outcome; thus, we must depend on data from epidemiology, food supplementation studies, and clinical observations. Difficulties in obtaining both accurate measures of nutritional status and reliable definitions of outcomes complicate the interpretation of research. The effect of a nutritional insult may depend on its timing during gestation, on its severity, or on both. Animal research is available, but applications of results are difficult owing to the great range of differences among the reproductive systems of mammalian species.

Despite these limitations, our understanding of the role of nutrition before and during pregnancy has increased substantially in the last two decades. The report *Nutrition During Pregnancy*, published by the

Institute of Medicine in 1990, reviewed the scientific evidence regarding weight gain, dietary intake, and nutrient supplementation during pregnancy and offered updated recommendations for nutritional care of the pregnant woman.

NUTRITIONAL INFLUENCES ON PREGNANCY OUTCOME

Maternal Body Size and Weight Gain During Pregnancy

It is now well established that both maternal pre-pregnancy body mass index and weight gain during pregnancy are determinants of fetal growth (IOM, 1990). Some, but not all, studies suggest an association between these factors and preterm delivery as well (Abrams et al., 1989; IOM, 1990). Underweight women or women with low pregnancy weight gains are at higher risk of delivering an infant weighing less than 2500 grams. Overweight women or those who gain a large amount of weight during pregnancy are more likely to deliver macrosomic babies. Figure 11–1 illustrates that the relationship between maternal weight gain and birth weight differs by pre-pregnancy weight for height: the impact of maternal weight gain on birth weight seems to decrease as pre-pregnancy weight for height increases. Thus, the Institute of Medicine recommends different amounts of weight gain at term based on a woman's pre-pregnancy weight for height or body mass index (Table 11–1). Additional factors may modify the weight gain goal as well. As their infants are at increased risk for low birth weight, young adolescents (less than 2 years postmenarche) and African-American women are advised to strive for weight gains at the upper end of their recommended ranges. Women less than 62 inches tall should aim for the lower ends of their target ranges. For twin gestations, weight gain in the range of 35 to 45 pounds is recommended; data are not yet available to support specific recommendations based upon maternal pre-pregnancy body mass.

Although the relationship between maternal weight

TABLE 11–1. Weight Gain Recommendations for Pregnancy

BMI* (WEIGHT FOR HEIGHT)	RECOMMENDED GAIN
Low (BMI <19.8 or <90% IBW†)	12.5–18 kg (28–40 lb)
Normal (BMI 19.8–26.0 or 90–120% IBW)	11.5–16 kg (25–35 lb)
High (BMI 26.0–29.0 or 120–135% IBW)	7–11.5 kg (15–25 lb)
Obese (BMI >29.0 or >135% IBW)	6 + kg (15 + lb)

*Body mass index = (weight in kg/height in m²). Tables for computing BMI are available (IOM, 1990).

$$or$$
$$= (weight\ in\ lb/height\ in\ in.^2) \times 700$$

†Ideal body weight, based on 1959 Metropolitan Life Insurance Company standards.

Reprinted with permission from Nutrition During Pregnancy. © 1990 by the National Academy of Sciences. Published by National Academy Press, Washington, DC.

gain and birth weight appears to be weak in very obese women, these pregnancies are at higher risk for both maternal complications (Abrams and Parker, 1988) and fetal mortality (NCHS, 1986). There are insufficient data to demonstrate exactly how much weight obese women should gain, therefore the Institute of Medicine recommended individual dietary assessment and counseling for each obese woman and a weight gain goal of at least 15 pounds (the estimated weight of the products of conception). They recognized that some obese women have healthy babies with lower gains. No evidence exists to suggest that it is safe or appropriate to impose a restrictive diet or encourage weight loss during pregnancy for any pregnant woman.

The weight gain recommendations just discussed concern *total* weight gain, which in reality is not known until delivery. Clinicians depend instead upon measurements of the rate and pattern of weight gain during the course of a pregnancy. Unfortunately, compared to the large literature on total weight gain during pregnancy, much less is known about the pattern of gestational weight gain (IOM, 1990). Weight gain grids commonly used during the last 30 years were based on two studies conducted in the 1950s, which described average weight change throughout pregnancy of women with reasonably good pregnancy outcomes. In addition to documenting the rapid increase of maternal weight related to preeclampsia, these investigators concluded that low gains during the second or third trimester increased the risk of low birth weight, and that even with an acceptable total gain, a low gain at one point was not completely compensated by a high gain at another (Thomson and Billewicz, 1957; Tompkins and Wiehl, 1951). Recently, results from a cohort of several thousand pregnant teenagers suggested that the pattern of maternal weight gain was predictive of both fetal size and preterm delivery (Hediger et al., 1989; Scholl et al., 1990). Limited additional data suggest an association between the pattern of weight gain and preterm delivery (IOM, 1990) and small-for-gestational-age deliveries (Abrams and Newman, 1991). Additional studies of the relationship between the pattern of gain and pregnancy outcome are needed.

For now, an example of a weight gain chart based on the new Institute of Medicine recommendations is

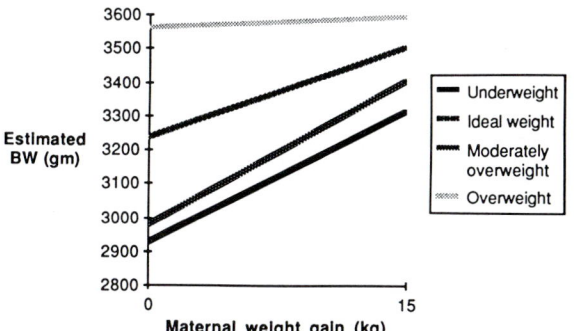

FIGURE 11–1. Birth weight of liveborn infants at term by pre-pregnancy body mass and weight gain adjusted for maternal age, race, parity, socioeconomic status, cigarette consumption, and gestational age (n = 2964). (From Abrams BF, Laros RK: Prepregnancy weight, weight gain, and birth weight. Am J Obstet Gynecol **154**:503, 1986.)

shown in Figure 11–2. This chart, with separate lines for women whose pre-pregnancy body mass indices are low, normal, and high, uses the recommended total target gain in Table 11–1 as the endpoints and a recommended rate of gain as the slope (IOM, 1990). Such charts are useful in allowing the clinician and the pregnant woman to visually track weight gain as pregnancy progresses. Despite the statistical associations described, it is important to remember that the pattern and the total amount of weight gain during pregnancy vary among individuals, and good pregnancy outcomes have occurred with gains much higher and lower than recommended.

Although the influence of weight gain during pregnancy on birth weight has been well documented, many pregnant women in the United States do not gain enough (NCHS, 1986), and results from the 1980 National Natality Study (Taffel and Keppel, 1986) indicated that the information a woman received from her physician or health care provider was related to her subsequent weight gain.

Thus, to promote adequate weight gain during pregnancy, guidelines on the importance of adequate nutrition and weight gain should be provided to all women. Recommendations for weight gain should be based on maternal pre-pregnancy body mass index, a goal should be formulated with the patient, and the pattern of gain should be plotted and monitored along with fetal growth. In cases in which weight gain deviates from expected, an assessment of dietary intake and activity patterns is needed either to allow appropriate intervention or to reassure the woman and her clinician that her weight gain is appropriate. Ideally, such an assessment should be done by a nutritionist or registered dietitian skilled in counseling perinatal patients.

Diet

The mother's diet must provide adequate nutrients to support the development of new maternal and fetal tissues, meet maternal maintenance costs, and provide for maternal activity. Additionally, fat deposits are laid down as energy reserves for lactation. Requirements vary by nutrient, stage of gestation, and number of fetuses, and may be further influenced by maternal body size and lifestyle factors (e.g., cigarette smoking). Increased requirements are met both through increased intake and through physiologic adjustments in absorption, excretion, and metabolism.

Evidence is increasing that diet *before* pregnancy may have an important influence on pregnancy outcome. Examples of this include the reduced risk of recurrence of neural tube defects with preconceptional folate supplementation (CDC, 1991; MRC Vitamin Study Research Group, 1991) and reduced risk of congenital anomalies through intensive preconceptional management of blood glucose (including dietary counseling) among women with diabetes (Kitzmiller et al., 1991). In one study, providing supplemental food to postpartum women significantly increased the birth weight of their subsequent infants (Caan et al., 1987).

Energy

Total caloric intake appears to be the most important nutritional factor relating to birth weight. It has been estimated that a typical pregnancy costs 80,000 additional calories over pre-pregnancy requirements or about 300 extra calories per day (NAS, 1989). This energy substrate intake will theoretically provide a weight gain of 10 to 12 kg at term. However, at least one recent study suggests that the actual requirements for energy may be lower. Using measurements of basal metabolic rate (BMR), body weight and fatness, physical activity, and mechanical efficiency of movement at 2- to 4-week intervals throughout the pregnancies of 162 well-nourished and healthy women in Scotland, the investigators determined the total energy requirement of pregnancy to be approximately 69,000

Prenatal Weight Gain Chart

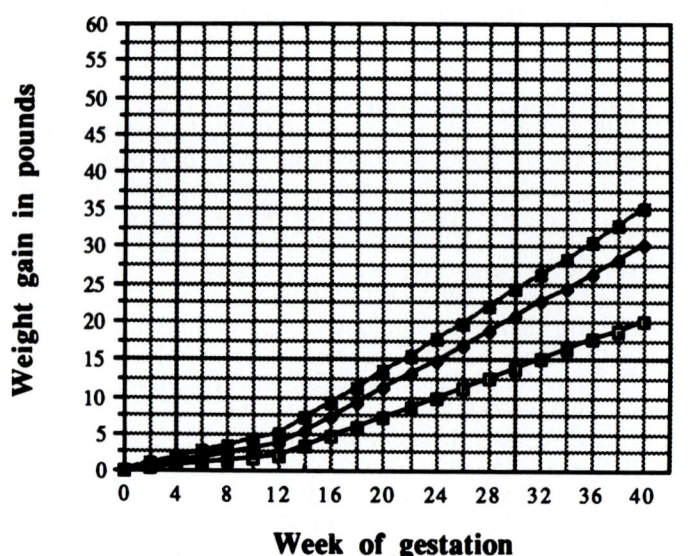

FIGURE 11–2. Prenatal weight gain chart. (Reprinted with permission from Nutrition During Pregnancy. © 1990 by the National Academy of Sciences. Published by National Academy Press, Washington, DC.)

calories. As discerned from weighed diet records, energy substrate intake increased by 22,000 calories, or approximately 100 to 150 calories per day during the second and third trimesters. The investigators believe that small reductions in physical activity, difficult to measure with any accuracy, may account for the difference between actual energy intakes and the energy cost of pregnancy (Durnin, 1991).

More research is clearly needed, especially in populations of women with poorer nutritional habits than this select sample, but these results do suggest that not all pregnant women need to increase their energy substrate intake during pregnancy as much as previously believed. Although energy substrate intake and maternal weight gain are important parameters of nutritional status, overall nutrition is more important than caloric intake alone. Nutrient density—the quantity of protein, vitamins, and minerals per 100 calories of food—is an important concept, because the current recommended increase for energy is only about 17 per cent, compared to increases of 20 to 100 per cent for vitamins and minerals. For example, a 300-calorie increase can be achieved by choosing one of several snacks: (1) a pint of low-fat milk, (2) a peanut butter sandwich on whole-grain bread, (3) six small cookies, or (4) a 12-oz can of soda and 10 slices of french-fried potatoes. The milk or sandwich has a superior nutrient-density profile, providing excellent amounts of additional nutrients besides calories; the cookies or soda and french fries are nutritionally empty. Since the pre-pregnancy diets of many American women are less than optimal in nutrient density, eating "to appetite" without additional education and guidance may result in dietary intake below standards in vital nutrients but excessive in calories, fat, and sodium.

Protein

Eating patterns in the United States tend toward diets that are adequate or even excessive in protein-rich foods. The estimated requirement for protein in pregnancy is 60 gm, about 15 gm over nonpregnant requirements (NAS, 1989). It is likely that a woman's pre-pregnant intake of protein already includes the recommended increase that is essential for fetal growth and development. Protein-containing foods can be excellent sources of vitamins and minerals such as iron, vitamin B_6, and zinc. However, animal proteins such as red meats and whole-fat milk and cheeses can provide excessive (and calorie-dense) fat if used in abundance. Consumption of lean animal foods (such as chicken and fish), low-fat or nonfat dairy products, and vegetable proteins (such as legumes) should be encouraged, especially in women with normal or high body mass indices.

Despite claims that pregnancy-induced hypertension can be prevented or treated with a high-protein diet, there is no evidence that a high protein intake during pregnancy is beneficial (Zlatnick and Burmeister, 1983). There is some evidence that "excessive amounts" of protein may be harmful (Rush, 1982).

Sodium

In the past, salt was forbidden to pregnant women, and diuretics were used at the first sign of edema. Because diuretics are now known to cause electrolyte imbalance, hyperglycemia, hyperuricemia, and other problems during pregnancy, they are rarely prescribed. Although sodium should not be restricted during pregnancy, excessive use should not be condoned, owing to its relationship to the development of hypertension in susceptible individuals. A diet of primarily natural foods can be safely salted "to taste." Processed foods are already high in sodium and should be consumed in moderation.

Iron

Hemodilution during pregnancy decreases hemoglobin concentration. Increasing iron intake through diet or supplements can limit the decrease. It is estimated that 500 mg of iron are needed for the increase in maternal red blood cell volume and 300 mg of iron for fetal erythropoiesis. Evidence exists that without supplemental iron, women can exhaust their iron stores by the end of pregnancy as measured by serum ferritin (Taylor et al., 1982). Therefore, daily supplementation of 30 mg of elemental iron during the second and third trimesters has been recommended for all women (IOM, 1990). Therapeutic iron in doses of 60 to 120 mg per day is prescribed for women who have diagnosed iron deficiency anemia. This is defined by a hemoglobin concentration of less than 11 gm/100 ml (hematocrit of less than 33 per cent) during the first and third trimesters, and a hemoglobin concentration of less than 10.5 gm/100 ml (hematocrit of less than 32 per cent) during the second trimester. Adjustments to these criteria accounting for altitude and maternal smoking are available (CDC, 1989). Women taking therapeutic doses of iron should also be supplemented with 15 mg of zinc and 2 mg of copper, as high doses of iron may interfere with the absorption and utilization of these nutrients. Additional guidelines for the diagnosis and management of anemia have been recently published (IOM, 1992).

To improve iron nutrition through diet, women should be aware of the best food sources of iron: meats, chicken, fish, legumes, leafy vegetables, and whole grain or enriched breads and cereals. Animal protein, "the meat factor," enhances iron absorption from the gut, as does ascorbic acid, and their effects are additive. Food cooked in cast-iron pans contains significant amounts of iron. Tea and coffee can bind iron in the gut and should be avoided at meals at which good sources of iron are eaten. Large doses of calcium or magnesium salts also decrease iron absorption. Since erythropoiesis depends on protein, vitamin B_{12}, and folate, dietary assessment and improvement of intake for those nutrients can provide therapeutic value in the treatment of anemia.

Calcium

The RDA for calcium is 1200 mg, which is sufficient to meet fetal needs and maintain maternal calcium balance. There is some evidence that calcium intake during pregnancy is inversely related to gestational hypertension, but not preeclampsia (Belizan et al., 1991; Marcoux et al., 1991). Further studies are needed. Low calcium intake has been defined as less than 600 mg per day (equivalent to a diet containing only one serving of a calcium-rich food in addition to nondairy foods). Women who are unable to increase their intake of calcium foods to achieve the RDA should be given a calcium supplement of 600 mg per day, especially if they are younger than 25 years and thus still increasing their bone density (IOM, 1990).

Cow's milk commonly fulfills a significant portion of the recommended calcium, vitamin D, and protein requirement but is not acceptable food for all pregnant women. Lactase deficiency is common among certain ethnic groups, including individuals of Asian, African, and Middle Eastern descent. Abdominal cramping, bloating, flatulence, and diarrhea associated with milk intake may be indicative of this disorder. Women who do not use milk because of personal preference or lactose intolerance should be counseled about culturally acceptable alternative food sources. Lower-lactose foods include cheese, yogurt, and special lactose-reduced milk. Canned fish with bones (such as salmon and sardines), fortified soy milk, tofu (soy bean curd) made with calcium sulfate, ground sesame seeds, and leafy green vegetables also provide calcium. Calcium and vitamin D supplements, accompanied by an increase in protein intake, may also be indicated.

Folate

Inadequate folate intake can lead to megaloblastic anemia. The recommended intake for folate is increased during pregnancy from 200 μg to 400 μg per day (NAS, 1989). Although it is possible to meet this requirement through a well-selected diet, some women, especially those in high-risk groups, may require daily supplementation of up to 300 μg folate (IOM, 1990). Dietary sources include eggs, leafy vegetables, oranges, legumes, and wheat germ. As mentioned previously, a recent randomized prevention trial in Great Britain reported that supplementation with folate before conception and during early pregnancy substantially reduced the risk of recurrent neural tube defects (MRC Vitamin Study Research Group, 1991). Subsequently, the Centers for Disease Control issued interim recommendations that women who have previously delivered infants with neural tube defects be given supplements containing 4 mg/day of folate, starting at least four weeks before conception and for the first three months of pregnancy (CDC, 1991). Multivitamins containing folate should not be used to achieve the desired level of supplementation, as potentially harmful quantities of other nutrients (such as preformed vitamin A) could be ingested. The Centers for Disease Control now also recommends that all women of childbearing age who are capable of becoming pregnant be advised to consume at least 400 μg of folate daily (CDC, 1992).

Other Nutrients

Processing of grains tends to remove zinc, pyridoxine (vitamin B_6), magnesium, and vitamin E. These nutrients are essential during pregnancy and are not replaced by enrichment. Encouraging the use of un-

refined whole grains can increase the intake of these vitamins and minerals. In addition, whole grains are excellent sources of dietary fiber. Other good food sources of zinc and pyridoxine include animal proteins and legumes. Magnesium is also found in legumes and vegetables, but not in animal proteins. Nuts and vegetable oils are excellent sources of vitamin E.

Supplements

Prenatal vitamin-mineral supplements are widely prescribed and can provide a false sense of security about a woman's diet. After examining all of the available evidence regarding the safety issues and justification for vitamin and mineral supplementation during pregnancy, the Institute of Medicine has concluded that routine supplementation of any nutrient, excepting iron, is unwarranted. A carefully chosen diet of unrefined grains, fruits, vegetables, lean meat or other protein sources, and dairy products or other calcium sources can provide adequate nutrition during pregnancy without supplementation. However, food habits of American women often differ from this pattern. Routine assessment of the dietary practices of every pregnant woman is necessary in order to determine the need for additional nutrient supplementation. Women who are unlikely to consume an adequate diet, even after counseling, and women who are in high-risk categories (Table 11–2) should take a daily multivitamin-mineral preparation beginning in the second trimester. Table 11–3 enumerates the recommended composition of this supplement, as well as additional guidelines for complete vegetarians and women with low calcium intake.

DIETARY GUIDANCE

Pregnancy creates a special demand for high-quality nutrients and also constitutes an excellent impetus for changing poor food habits. Recent studies have shown that providing nutritional counseling can improve both weight gain during pregnancy and birth weight (Orstead et al., 1985; Clements, 1988). Although preg-

TABLE 11–2. Nutritional Risk Factors in Pregnancy

Significant deviation of pregravid weight from ideal weight
Inadequate or excessive weight gain
Age less than 15 or more than 35 years
Psychological, social, cultural, religious, or economic factors that limit or affect adequacy of nutrition
History of obstetric problems, including previous low-birth-weight baby
Chronic illness, such as diabetes, thyroid, PKU, or sickle cell disease
Multiple gestation
Abnormal laboratory values, such as low hemoglobin level, glycosuria, abnormal blood glucose level, albuminuria, and ketonuria
Substance abuse
Eating disorders
Pica
Food allergies or intolerances
Bed rest

TABLE 11–3.   Recommended Levels of Vitamin and Mineral Supplementation

Multivitamin-mineral preparation for women with poor diets or high-risk categories:

Iron	30 mg	Vitamin B₆	2 mg
Zinc	15 mg	Folate	300 μg
Copper	2 mg	Vitamin C	50 mg
Calcium	250 mg	Vitamin D	5 μg (200 IU)

Supplementation for women in special circumstances:

Complete vegetarians (consume no animal products whatsoever):

10 μg (400 IU) Vitamin D

2 μ Vitamin B₁₂

Women under age 25 whose daily intake of calcium is less than 600 mg:

600 mg calcium

Women with low intake of vitamin D–fortified milk, especially those who have minimal exposure to sunlight:

10 μg (400 IU) Vitamin D

Reprinted with permission from Nutrition During Pregnancy. © 1990 by the National Academy of Sciences. Published by National Academy Press, Washington, DC.

nancy is considered a "teachable moment," dietary guidance will be effective only if the patient sees merit in the suggestions made and can apply the information to her own life experience.

Guides have been developed to translate nutritional recommendations into actual foods. A food guide for the reproductive years is found in Table 11–4. If a woman chooses daily the number of servings recommended from each group in the portion sizes defined, she will most likely be ingesting nutrients in adequate amounts, with the exception of iron and perhaps calories. As stated earlier, energy needs are highly individual; therefore, the need to add additional foods will be influenced by pre-pregnancy body mass index, weight gain during pregnancy, metabolic differences, number of fetuses, maternal activity, appetite, age, and other factors.

A low-fat diet including lean protein-rich foods, low-fat or nonfat dairy products, and limited amounts of added fat in food preparation is recommended for most women. However, women who are having difficulty achieving adequate weight gain may need to consume more fat in order to increase caloric intake. Items such as soft drinks, pastries, candy, fried foods, and salty snacks have poor nutrient density, and their consumption should be discouraged.

Nutrition education should be available to all women prior to or early in pregnancy, whether in a group or individually. Information regarding use of potentially hazardous substances, including cigarettes and alcohol, should be provided, as well as discussion of the average expected rate and amount of weight gain, the desirability of adequate exercise, and prenatal dietary recommendations. Later in pregnancy, information on infant feeding options and procedures—including encouragement to breast-feed—is part of the nutritional care plan. Individualized assessment of all patients includes a review of prepregnant weight, gestational weight gain, use of drugs, laboratory values (hemoglobin, hematocrit), medical and social problems, and dietary habits. Ask-

ing a woman what she usually eats and then recording an estimate of her intake during the previous 24 hours provides insight into her food patterns without a great investment of time and constitutes the basis for ongoing counseling. The presence of particular factors may indicate that a woman is at high risk for nutritional problems and needs in-depth nutrition assessment, counseling, and follow-up (see Table 11–2).

Basic nutritional assessment and guidance should be provided by the woman's primary health care provider before, during, and after pregnancy (Fig. 11–3). If problems are identified, intensive nutritional assessment and counseling are best performed by an experienced dietitian who understands the physiologic needs of pregnancy and the cultural food habits of the patients served and also is an effective communicator and counselor. Because nutrition is only one aspect of prenatal care, nutritional recommendations should support and complement the care given by other members of the medical team. A practical guide to the delivery of perinatal nutrition care is available from the Institute of Medicine (IOM, 1992). Table 11–5 outlines the basic recommendations for maternal nutrition care.

COMMON CLINICAL PROBLEMS

Clinicians are likely to encounter a number of nutrition problems in day-to-day prenatal care. Some of the issues frequently encountered are discussed.

ADOLESCENT PREGNANCY. Women under 17 years of age are at higher risk for short gestation, perinatal mortality, and low-birth-weight babies. Sociocultural factors heavily influence the outcome of these pregnancies. Physiologically, the young adolescent—within 2 years of menarche—is at highest risk, presumably because of the growth demands of her own body as well as of the fetus.

Diets chosen by female adolescents are notoriously variable and have been reported to be deficient in vitamin A, ascorbic acid, calcium, and iron both before and during pregnancy. Pica has been reported in as many as 20 per cent of adolescent pregnancies in some ethnic groups. Ingestion of vitamin supplements is erratic, and abuse of drugs, tobacco, and alcohol may be a problem. In addition, adolescent concern about body image may lead to dieting during pregnancy, resulting in inadequate energy and nutrient intake, small weight gain, and a low-birth-weight infant.

Assessment of each patient with regard to nutritional status, physical and emotional maturity, dietary habits, and educational needs, along with sensitive, on-going counseling can make an impact on poor dietary patterns. Women within 2 years of menarche may need additional energy substrates, protein, and calcium to meet growth needs (Story, 1990).

DIABETES. The diabetic pregnancy is discussed in Chapter 54.

NAUSEA AND VOMITING. Nausea and vomiting, which usually occur during the first trimester, can cause discomfort and anxiety as well as weight loss, ketosis, and dehydration in more severe cases. Management includes sympathetic reassurance that nausea

Table 11–4. **Food Guide for the Reproductive Years**

FOOD GROUP OR CATEGORY	FOOD	SERVING SIZE	NUMBER OF DAILY SERVINGS		MAJOR NUTRIENTS PROVIDED
			Nonpregnant	Pregnant/Lactating	
Protein sources	Meat	1 oz	5	7	Protein, iron, riboflavin, niacin, phosphorus, zinc, iodine, vitamins B₆ and B₁₂
	Fish	"			
	Cheese	"			
	Eggs	1			Emphasize those low in fat
	Beans, legumes	½ cup			Protein, iron, thiamine, phosphorus,
	Nuts, seeds	¼ cup			magnesium, zinc, vitamins B₆, E, and
	Nut butters	2 tbsp			folic acid
Calcium-rich foods*	Milk	1 cup	2	3	Calcium, phosphorus, riboflavin,
	Fortified soy milk	"			vitamins D, A, E, B₆, and B₁₂,
	Yogurt	"			magnesium, zinc, protein (not all of
	Tofu	9 oz			the foods listed provide all of these
	Cheese	1½ oz or ⅓ cup			nutrients)
	Dry milk	⅓ cup			Emphasize those low in fat
Grain products†	Whole-grain bread	1 slice	6+	6+	Thiamine, niacin, riboflavin, iron,
	Cereal, dry	1 oz or ¾ cup			phosphorus, zinc, fiber
	Wheat germ	4 tbsp			
	Pasta or rice	½ cup			
Vitamin C sources (fruits and vegetables)	Orange	1	2+	2+	Ascorbic acid, folate
	Grapefruit	½			
	Cantaloupe	¼			
	Strawberries	¾ cup			
	Tomatoes	1 cup			
	Greens	½			
	Peppers	"			
	Broccoli	"			
	Cabbage	"			
Leafy green vegetables	Broccoli	½ cup	1+	1+	Folate, vitamins A, E, B₆, riboflavin, iron, magnesium
	Brussels sprouts	"			
	Asparagus	"			
	Cabbage	"			
	Greens	"			
	Redleaf lettuce	1 cup			
	Romaine lettuce	"			
	Bok choy	"			
	Watercress	"			
Other fruits and vegetables		1 medium or ½ cup	2+	2+	Vitamins A, B complex, and E, magnesium, zinc, phosphorus

*Young women aged 11–24 years should consume 1 more serving of dairy products.
†Refined, enriched grain products in similar portions have significantly less fiber and smaller amounts of trace minerals than the grain products listed here.

Benefits of Maternal Nutrition Services

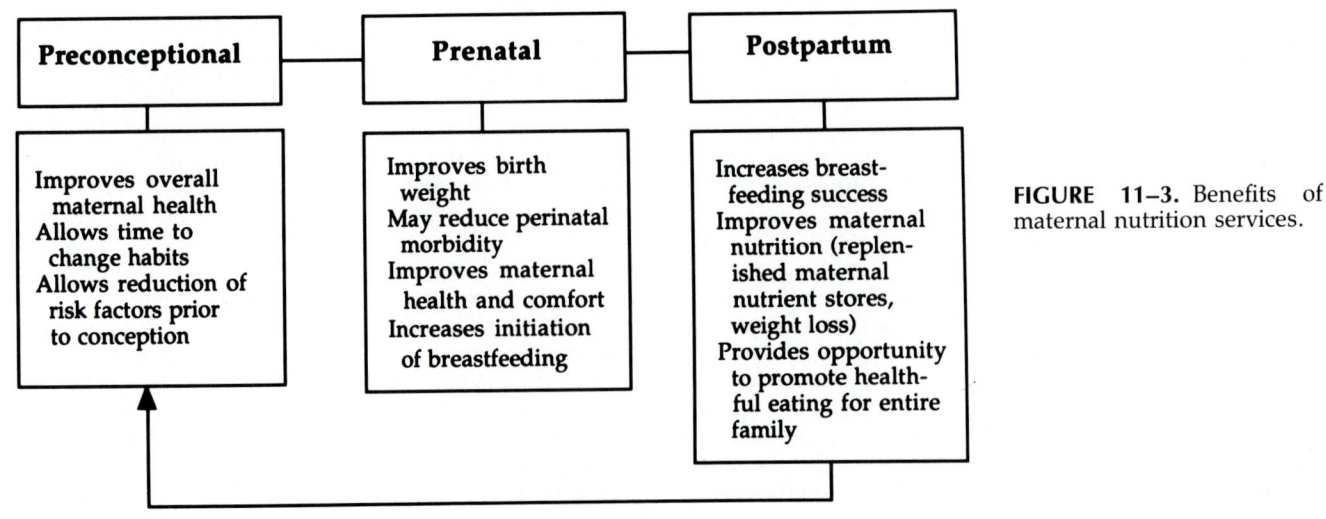

Preconceptional

Improves overall maternal health
Allows time to change habits
Allows reduction of risk factors prior to conception

Prenatal

Improves birth weight
May reduce perinatal morbidity
Improves maternal health and comfort
Increases initiation of breastfeeding

Postpartum

Increases breast-feeding success
Improves maternal nutrition (replenished maternal nutrient stores, weight loss)
Provides opportunity to promote healthful eating for entire family

FIGURE 11–3. Benefits of maternal nutrition services.

TABLE 11–5. General Guidelines for Maternal Nutrition Care

PRECONCEPTIONAL:
1. Assess weight status, hemoglobin or hematocrit, dietary intake, exercise habits, eating disorders, other parameters of nutritional status.
2. Offer basic guidance regarding healthful diet, exercise, and avoidance of harmful substances.
3. Provide individualized care to address risk factors such as obesity, anemia, phenylketonuria, or previous birth of infant with neural tube defect.

PREGNANCY:
1. Assess dietary intake; encourage a varied diet with good nutrient density.
2. Recommend and monitor weight gain based on pre-pregnancy weight for height.
3. Encourage moderate exercise as appropriate.
4. Counsel to avoid exposure to drugs and chemicals.
5. Supplement with prophylactic (30 mg elemental) iron; other nutrients based on assessments.
6. Provide education to all women on diet, weight gain, management of common pregnancy discomforts, and benefits of and preparation for breast-feeding.
7. Provide individual assessment and counseling by a perinatal nutritionist for women at risk for nutritional problems.

POSTPARTUM:
1. Provide assistance with initiation and maintenance of breast-feeding, including recommendations for nutritional needs of lactation.
2. Encourage varied diet with good nutrient density for all women.
3. Provide realistic, health-promoting advice regarding weight loss.
4. Counsel to avoid exposure to drugs and other harmful substances.

is common, is not harmful to the fetus, and will resolve. In addition, eating small, frequent meals consisting of dry, starchy foods and avoidance of strong odors can help. Results of a recent clinical trial indicate that vitamin B_6 supplementation (25 mg three times a day) may be helpful in the relief of vomiting and severe nausea during pregnancy (Sahakian et al., 1991). Psychological counseling and hospitalization may be necessary in severe cases (see also Chapter 57).

PICA. The craving and eating of nonfoods, such as laundry starch and clay, is known as pica and is common during pregnancy in certain ethnic groups. Cultural beliefs and iron deficiency anemia are both thought to contribute, although the etiology is unknown. Pica can replace the ingestion of nutritious foods and may bind dietary iron, leading to anemia. There is also the possibility that the substance ingested is toxic. Appropriate management includes detection of the practice, screening for and treating iron deficiency anemia, and counseling to discourage or at least minimize the ingestion of nonfoods.

HEARTBURN AND ACID INDIGESTION. Heartburn and acid indigestion are common complaints during pregnancy. Eating small, frequent, dry meals separately from fluid intake, avoiding greasy foods, and wearing loose-fitting clothing can provide some relief. Because antacids taken for symptomatic relief may bind iron in the gastrointestinal tract, excessive use should be

discouraged, especially if iron deficiency anemia is a problem.

CONSTIPATION. Constipation can be treated by increasing dietary fiber, fluid intake, and exercise. Good sources of dietary fiber include whole grains, bran, legumes, and fresh fruits and vegetables.

BED REST. Some women require bed rest during pregnancy due to hypertensive disorders, preterm labor, and other problems. Nutritional counseling can be especially important in these cases to help achieve (or control) weight gain, to help alleviate symptoms such as poor appetite or constipation secondary to medication or inactivity, and to assist the woman in creating a plan that allows access to foods that are both easy to prepare and nutritious (Herron and Dulock, 1987; IOM, 1992).

VEGETARIAN DIETS. Diets that exclude some or all animal products have become relatively popular in the last 20 years and can provide adequate nutrition during pregnancy if correctly balanced. Those that include dairy products are easily adapted to pregnancy. Vegetarian diets that exclude all animal products (vegan) can also be used successfully during pregnancy, but demand closer assessment and surveillance to ensure that the necessary nutrients are provided. Avoidance of all animal products can result in vitamin B_{12} deficiency. In addition, the vegan diet is often extremely low in fat and high in fiber; it is sometimes difficult to eat enough to satisfy caloric requirements. Calcium, riboflavin, and vitamin D intakes may be marginal if dairy products are not used, and iron and zinc intakes may be low as well. Dietary assessment indicates the potential difficulties that may exist, and counseling can dramatically upgrade the quality of the diet while the vegetarian pattern is maintained. Supplements may be indicated (see Table 11–3). The patient should also use iodized salt.

MATERNAL SOCIOECONOMIC CIRCUMSTANCES. A diet poor in quality and quantity may be the result of homelessness or an income too low to purchase enough nutritious food. Referral of the patient to local public or private agencies giving financial, housing, and food assistance is essential. WIC (the Women, Infants and Children Special Supplemental Food Program) is a valuable resource; knowledge of other community resources such as emergency food pantries or food banks is useful to the clinician as well. Counseling and education regarding low-cost, nutrient-dense foods, food budgeting, shopping, and preparation techniques can also help. Frequent follow-up is necessary.

REFERENCES

Abrams BF, Laros RK: Prepregnancy weight, weight gain, and birth weight. Am J Obstet Gynecol **154**:503, 1986.

Abrams B, Newman V: Small-for-gestational-age birth: Maternal predictors and comparison with risk factors of spontaneous preterm delivery in same cohort. Am J Obstet Gynecol **164**:785, 1991.

Abrams B, Newman V, Key T, Parker J: Maternal weight gain and preterm delivery. Obstet Gynecol **74**:577, 1989.

Abrams B, Parker J: Overweight and pregnancy complications. Int J Obes **12**:293, 1988.

Belizan JM, Villar J, Gonzalez L, Campodonico L, Bergel E: Calcium supplementation to prevent hypertensive disorders of pregnancy. N Engl J Med **325**:1399, 1991.

Caan B, Horgen DM, Margen S, et al: Benefits associated with WIC-supplemental feeding during the interpregnancy interval. Am J Clin Nutr **45**:29, 1987.

CDC (Centers for Disease Control): Recommendations for the use of folic acid to reduce the number of cases of spina bifida and other neural tube defects. MMWR **41**:1, 1992.

CDC (Centers for Disease Control): Use of folic acid for prevention of spina bifida and other neural tube defects—1983-1991. MMWR **40**:513, 1991.

CDC (Centers for Disease Control): CDC Criteria for anemia in children and childbearing-aged women. MMWR **38**:400, 1989.

Clements DF: The nutrition intervention project for underweight pregnant women. Clin Nutr **7**:205, 1988.

Durnin J: Energy requirements of pregnancy. Acta Paediatr Scand **373**(Suppl):33, 1991.

Hediger ML, Scholl TO, Salmon RW: Early weight gain in pregnant adolescents and fetal outcome. Am J Hum Biol **1**:665, 1989.

Herron M, Dulock H: Preterm Labor. 2nd ed. White Plains, NY, March of Dimes Foundation, 1987.

IOM (Institute of Medicine), Committee on Nutritional Status During Pregnancy and Lactation, National Academy of Sciences. Nutrition During Pregnancy. Washington, DC, National Academy Press, 1990.

IOM (Institute of Medicine), Subcommittee for a Clinical Application Guide, Committee on Nutritional Status During Pregnancy and Lactation, National Academy of Sciences. Nutrition During Pregnancy: An Implementation Guide. Washington, DC, National Academy Press, 1992.

Kitzmiller JL, Gavin LA, Gin GD, Jovanovic-Peterson L, Main EK, Zigrang WD: Preconception care of diabetes. Glycemic control prevents congenital anomalies. JAMA **265**:731, 1991.

Marcoux S, Brisson J, Fabia J: Calcium intake from dairy products and supplements and the risks of preeclampsia and gestational hypertension. Am J Epidemiol **133**:1266, 1991.

MRC Vitamin Study Research Group: Prevention of neural tube defects: Results of the Medical Research Council Vitamin Study. Lancet **338**:131, 1991.

NAS (National Academy of Sciences), National Research Council, Food and Nutrition Board: Recommended Dietary Allowances. 10th ed. Washington, DC, 1989.

NCHS (National Center for Health Statistics), Taffel SM: Maternal weight gain and the outcome of pregnancy: United States, 1980. Vital and Health Statistics, Series 21—No. 44. DHHS (PHS) 86—Public Health Service. Washington, DC, U.S. Government Printing Office, 1986.

Orstead C, Arrington D, Kamath SK, Olson R, Kohrs MD: Efficacy of prenatal nutrition counseling: Weight gain, infant birth weight, and cost-effectiveness. J Am Diet Assoc **85**:40, 1985.

Rush D: Effects of changes in protein and calorie intake during pregnancy on the growth of the human fetus. In Enken M, Chalmers I (eds): Effectiveness and Satisfaction in Antenatal Care. London, Spastics International Medical Publications, 1982.

Sahakian V, Rouse D, Sipes S, Rose N, Niebyl J: Vitamin B_6 is effective therapy for nausea and vomiting of pregnancy: a randomized, double-blind placebo-controlled study. Obstet Gynecol **78**:33, 1991.

Scholl TO, Hediger ML, Ances IG, Belsky DH, Salmon RW: Weight gain during pregnancy in adolescence: predictive ability of early weight gain. Obstet Gynecol **75**:948, 1990.

Siefert E: Changes in beliefs and practices in pregnancy. In Lydia J. Roberts Award Essays. Chicago, American Dietetic Association, 1968.

Story M: Nutrient needs during adolescence and pregnancy. In Nutrition Management of the Pregnant Adolescent: A Practical Reference Guide. Washington, DC, March of Dimes Birth Defects Foundation, US Department of Health and Human Services, and US Department of Agriculture, 1990.

Taffel SM, Keppel KG: Advice about weight gain during pregnancy and actual weight gain. Am J Public Health **76**:1396, 1986.

Taylor DJ, Mallen C, McDougall N, Lind T: Serum ferritin in women of reproductive age. Br J Obstet Gynecol **89**:1000, 1982.

Thomson AM, Billewicz WZ: Clinical significance of weight trends during pregnancy. Br Med J **1**:243, 1957.

Tompkins WT, Wiehl DG: Nutritional deficiencies as a causal factor in toxemia and premature labor. Am J Obstet Gynecol **62**:898, 1951.

Zlatnick FJ, Burmeister LF: Dietary protein and preeclampsia. Am J Obstet Gynecol **147**:354, 1983.

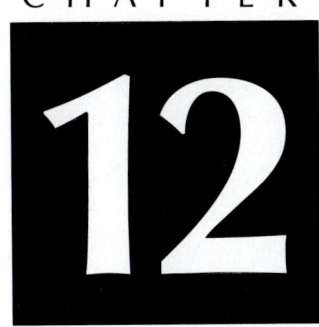

CHAPTER

12

EFFECTS OF THERAPEUTIC, DIAGNOSTIC, AND ENVIRONMENTAL AGENTS

KENNETH L. JONES, M.D.

Prior to 1960, the vast majority of birth defects were regarded as genetic in origin. The fetus was believed to occupy a privileged site within the uterus, protected from the effects of environmental agents to which the mother might be exposed.

Although the association between maternal rubella infection and abnormal fetal development was recognized in the early 1940s (Gregg, 1941), not until 20 years later did separate reports suggest that prenatal exposure to a drug, thalidomide, was the cause of serious defects in structural development (Lenz, 1961; McBride, 1961).

Since 1961, it has been demonstrated that a number of drugs and chemicals as well as certain byproducts of our contemporary technology can adversely affect fetal development. Nowhere has this latter issue been more dramatically illustrated than at Minimata Bay, Japan. There, between 1953 and 1965, the offspring of some women who ate shellfish contaminated with methyl mercury waste products released from large chemical plants on the bay developed symptoms of a generalized disorder of the central nervous system (Nishimura and Tanamura, 1976).

Recently, increased awareness of possible damage to the fetus by drugs given during pregnancy has led to a few well-controlled scientific studies as well as a vast array of anecdotal reports suggesting the teratogenic effect of various environmental agents. The pendulum has now swung in the opposite direction; virtually every drug is suspected of being a teratogen, and total pharmacologic prohibition throughout pregnancy has been proposed by many. Although few would argue the merits of that approach from a theoretic standpoint, practical considerations clearly dictate otherwise. Because of a number of circumstances, some medical and others related to employment, living conditions, or ignorance, the vast majority of pregnant women are exposed to a variety of agents. The purpose of this chapter is to outline what is known and what is not known about the most common pharmacologic agents with which women come into contact during pregnancy.

THERAPEUTIC AND DIAGNOSTIC AGENTS

Antipsychotic Drugs and Tranquilizers

Benzodiazepines

Three human studies of diazepam exposure during the first trimester of gestation have reported an increased relative risk of oral clefts. All the studies utilized retrospective data comparing diazepam use by mothers of children having oral clefts and mothers of children having no oral clefts. In two of the studies, however, the association was between first-trimester diazepam exposure and cleft lip with or without cleft palate, whereas in the third study the association was for cleft palate alone (Saxen and Saxen, 1975; Safra and Oakley, 1975; Saxen, 1975). As a result, a number of additional studies, none of which have confirmed this association, have been performed (Rosenberg et al., 1983; Shiono and Mills, 1984).

Regarding the other benzodiazepines, Czeizel documented the incidence of prenatal exposure to chlordiazepoxide, nitrazepam, or diazepam in children with isolated cleft lip with or without cleft palate, isolated posterior cleft palate, or multiple congenital anomalies including oral defects (Czeizel, 1988). In none of the three groups could an increased risk of drug exposure be documented.

None of the other benzodiazepines—including temazepam, prazepam, oxazepam, chlorazepate, lorazepam, midazolam, and alprazolam—have been studied with respect to teratogenicity.

In summary, no study has been performed from which it can be concluded that benzodiazepines are teratogenic in humans. However, it is important to realize that a study that would rule out the possibility that benzodiazepines are associated with a pattern of minor malformations, including developmental delay, has not been performed. In one study of 7 children prenatally exposed to benzodiazepines, prenatal and postnatal growth deficiency, craniofacial defects including telecanthus, epicanthal folds, upslanting palpebral fissures, a short nose with anteverted nares, dysplastic auricles and a high-arched palate, wide-spaced nipples, a webbed neck, and central nervous system abnormalities including mental retardation were noted (Laegreid et al., 1987). The findings in that study have not been confirmed.

Meprobamate and Chlordiazepoxide

Because meprobamate and chlordiazepoxide are minor tranquilizers and because a number of studies have evaluated pregnancy outcome in mothers exposed to both drugs, these two drugs are considered together.

In 1974, the outcome of 19,044 live births was evaluated in relation to the use of meprobamate and chlordiazepoxide (Milkovich and Van der Berg, 1974). A fourfold increase in the rate of defects was noted in offspring of mothers who took either agent during the first 42 days of gestation. No pattern of malformations was identified, although five of the 66 infants prenatally exposed to meprobamate had congenital heart defects. It is important to recognize, however, that the cardiac defects were not identical and that two of the children had defects in addition to the cardiac anomaly.

One other large study included 1870 children exposed *in utero* to meprobamate or chlordiazepoxide (Hartz et al., 1975). There was no increase in the incidence of structural defects in the prenatally exposed offspring. In addition, as judged according to mental and motor scores at 8 months and IQ scores at 4 years, there was no evidence that prenatal exposure to either drug caused mental deficiency.

These data suggest that neither meprobamate nor chlordiazepoxide is a human teratogen.

Phenothiazines

The most extensive study of phenothiazine use during pregnancy involved 12,764 pregnant Parisian women followed from 1963 to 1969 (Rumeau-Rouquette et al., 1977). Of the 315 women who took phenothiazines during the first trimester of pregnancy, 11 gave birth to children with malformations. It may be significant that eight of the 11 malformed children had been prenatally exposed to one of the phenothiazines with a 3-carbon aliphatic side chain, including acetylpromazine, trimeprazine, chlorpromazine, methotrimeprazine, methoxypromazine, and oxomemazine. Further breakdown of the data indicates that a total of 141 pregnant women in that study took a phenothiazine with a 3-carbon aliphatic side chain, eight of whose offspring (6 per cent) had malformations.

Therefore, the phenothiazines are probably not teratogenic in humans, although there remains some concern about the 3-carbon aliphatic side chain derivatives.

Tricyclic Antidepressants

Following an early report of three children with limb reduction abnormalities born to women who had taken imipramine or amitriptyline during pregnancy (McBride, 1972), further studies have indicated that these two drugs are not teratogenic in humans. The maternal drug histories of children with limb reduction defects from the birth defects surveillance programs in Atlanta and Los Angeles have been reviewed (Rachelefsky et al., 1972). Of the 43 children in Atlanta and five in Los Angeles with severe limb reduction defects, none had been prenatally exposed to either imipramine or amitriptyline. Other negative reports include studies of 20 normal neonates exposed to imipramine during the first trimester of pregnancy (Scanlon, 1969) and 81 offspring of women treated with 50 mg of imipramine three times a day for at least 2 months during pregnancy (Sim, 1972). In all instances, the children were judged to be normal, indicating that imipramine is not teratogenic in humans.

Lithium

A Register of Lithium Babies has been established to permit a prospective evaluation of the prenatal effects of lithium (Weinstein and Goldfield, 1975). As of 1975, 143 babies prenatally exposed to lithium had been reported to the Register. Thirteen had malformations, nine of which were defects in development of the heart and great vessels. Of particular significance, four of the nine defects were Ebstein's anomaly of the tricuspid valve, which occurs with a frequency of only one in 20,000 in the general population. As compelling as these data are, the methodology utilized in this study has been criticized by many because the study was retrospective and designed in such a way that pregnancy outcome (the presence of a normal or abnormal baby) was known by the reporting physician prior to the time the child was reported to the Register. Thus, the true incidence of Ebstein's anomaly and other cardiac defects in babies prenatally exposed to lithium is most likely far less than that reported to the Register. In order to more accurately determine that risk, a prospective study was designed in which pregnancy outcome was determined in 148 women ascertained because they contacted one of four Teratogen Information Services in North America because of their concern regarding the teratogenicity of lithium (Jacobson et al., 1992). In each case the contact was made early in pregnancy, long before pregnancy outcome was known. One of the women conceived a baby with Ebstein's anomaly, which was prenatally diagnosed at 16 weeks gestation and electively aborted. No other cardiac defect was noted.

Consistent with this much lower risk for Ebstein's anomaly, three case-control studies have been published. In none of the three could an association be documented between lithium and cardiac defects (Kallen, 1988; Zalystein et al., 1990; Edmonds and Oakley, 1990).

In summary, prenatal exposure to lithium is associated with an increased risk for Ebstein's anomaly. However, based on the one prospective cohort study as well as the three case-control studies, the risk is exceedingly small, clearly nowhere near the 500-fold increased risk suggested by data collected in the Register of Lithium Babies.

Hormones

Progestogens and Estrogen-Progestogen Combinations

Both progestogens and combinations of estrogens and progestogens (oral contraceptives) have been used therapeutically in early gestation for the management of threatened abortion and for a withdrawal pregnancy test. The most common reason for concern about these drugs, however, has been the continued use of birth control pills following conception by women unaware that they are pregnant.

A number of studies have been published regarding the teratogenic potential of these agents. Most of these have been retrospective in nature, and thus their results have been burdened with the well-known pitfalls of such studies. An early report found that six of 76 women studied because their children were noted to have transposition of the great vessels had taken sex steroids for threatened abortion during the first 6 weeks of gestation (Levy et al., 1973). Subsequently, a second study revealed that of 19 women who were identified by the fact that their children had a pattern of malformation referred to as the VACTERR (*v*ertebral, *a*nal, *c*ardiac, *t*racheo*e*sophageal, *r*enal, and *r*adial) association, 13 had taken a progestogen-estrogen compound or a progestogen alone during early pregnancy (Nora and Nora, 1975). In 1974, Janerich and associates investigated prenatal exposure to exogenous sex steroids in 108 children selected for study solely because they had a congenital limb defect. These patients, identified from their birth certificates as part of the Congenital Malformation Surveillance Program established by the New York State Department of Health in the early 1960s, were matched with normal controls. Fifteen of the 108 (14 per cent) had a history of exposure, as opposed to four (4 per cent) of the controls. In a second study by the same investigators, 104 children with congenital heart defects were identified from the same surveillance program (Janerich et al., 1977). Exposure to exogenous sex hormones was found to be 8.5 times more common among the infants with malformations than among controls. Of particular significance is a prospective cohort study in which data from the Collaboration Perinatal Project of the National Institute of Neurologic Disease and Stroke were analyzed (Heinonen et al., 1977). Of 1042 women identified as having received female sex hormones during early pregnancy, 19 gave birth to children with cardiovascular defects (18 per 1000). Only 385 of the 49,240 children not exposed *in utero* to these agents had cardiovascular malformations (7.8 per 1000). Based on these data, the authors suggested that prenatal exposure to female sex hormones was strongly associated with an increased risk for cardiovascular defects. However, re-evaluation of the same data base by Wiseman and Dodds-Smith (1984) led to a completely contradictory conclusion. Examination of the 19 cases described by Heinonen et al. (1977) as having a cardiovascular defect associated with prenatal exposure to a female sex hormone revealed that no sex hormone was administered in two cases, that the hormone was given after cardiac organogenesis had

occurred in five cases, that the hormone was given too early in gestation in two cases, and that two of the children had Down's syndrome. Thus, as opposed to 19, there were eight children prenatally exposed to sex hormones during the critical period of cardiac organogenesis whose cardiac defect potentially could have been related to prenatal sex hormone exposure.

Numerous reports suggesting that these sex hormones are not teratogenic add to the controversy. In interviews with 433 women selected because they gave birth to babies with one of eight major malformations, Down's syndrome, or multiple malformations, the proportion of women who had undergone a hormonal pregnancy test in each malformation group did not differ significantly from the proportion observed in the total (Oakley et al., 1973). In a second study, the prenatal exposure to sex hormones was evaluated in 88 children selected because they had conotruncal defects of the heart (Mulvihill et al., 1974). Four of the 88 had been exposed in the first trimester, whereas nine controls (patients with either a ventricular septal defect or a normal heart) had also been exposed prenatally to sex hormones.

The results of a prospective survey pertaining to progestins utilized for hormonal pregnancy tests were reported (Goujard and Rumeau-Rouquette, 1977). The drugs were classified according to whether they were testosterone or progesterone derivatives. Five (1.5 per cent) of the 355 women who received a testosterone derivative and 15 (1.8 per cent) of the 830 women who received a progesterone derivative gave birth to malformed babies. Neither of these figures represents a frequency significantly greater than that for women not receiving hormonal drugs.

The following four studies are particularly relevant because they permit conclusions regarding two of the most frequently used progesterone derivatives, medroxy-progesterone acetate and hydroxyprogesterone caproate, as well as progesterone itself.

Ressequie et al. (1985) reviewed medical records of 988 women who received progestins, primarily hydroxyprogesterone caproate (Delalutin), during pregnancy and documented through chart review any structural defects in their offspring. As compared with the incidence in a control group, no increased incidence of structural defects—including genitourinary, central nervous system, cardiovascular, and/or limb reduction defects—could be documented.

Rock et al. (1985) evaluated pregnancy outcome in 93 women who received progesterone either by suppository or intramuscularly in oil during the first trimester of pregnancy. Two of the 75 liveborn babies (2.6 per cent) were noted to have structural defects (one child with a meningomyelocele and one with an inguinal hernia).

Check et al. (1986) documented pregnancy outcome in 198 women treated with progesterone vaginal suppositories alone and 189 who had taken both progesterone suppositories and hydroxyprogesterone in the preimplantation period. Five of the 382 infants for whom information was available had structural defects (1.3 per cent).

Finally, the possible teratogenicity of progestogen (mostly medroxyprogesterone acetate) treatment for first-trimester vaginal bleeding has been studied prospectively. An increased incidence of structural defects could not be documented (Katz et al., 1985).

A comment is merited regarding the association of these agents with ambiguity of the external genitalia. For those progestins that are testosterone-derived, an increased risk exists for masculinization of the female genitalia (Schardein, 1980). These include ethinyl testosterone (ethisterone), 19-nor ethinyl testosterone (norethindrone), norgestrel, and norethynodiol—agents that have been used in the treatment of threatened or habitual miscarriage in addition to being used as the progestins in oral contraceptives.

Information regarding a potential lack of masculinization of the male genitalia in association with prenatal exposure to progestins is not available. However, Aarskog (1979) noted that 11 of 130 children selected because of hypospadias had been exposed to progestin or a progestin-estrogen combination during early gestation, as opposed to only 2 of 111 infants selected because of oral clefts. Although this study was retrospective, it seems significant, because a relationship was noted between the position of the urethral meatus and the week of gestation in which progestin treatment was begun; the more proximal openings were found in the offspring of mothers treated in the first month of pregnancy.

As conflicting as many of these results seem to be, the following practical conclusions are warranted.

1. If progestogens and/or progestogen-estrogen combinations are teratogenic in humans, the magnitude of the teratogenic risk is extremely small and is not biologically significant.
2. Progestin exposure during the vulnerable period may double the incidence of hypospadias in the offspring; however, it is important to recognize that the resulting risk, 140 per 10,000 male births, is extremely low.

Diethylstilbestrol (Stilbestrol)

In 1971, a new entity was observed when it was reported that the mothers of seven out of eight women between 15 and 22 years of age with vaginal adenocarcinoma had been treated with diethylstilbestrol (DES) beginning in the first trimester of pregnancy (Herbst et al., 1971). Subsequent studies indicate that the risk of vaginal cancer in prenatally exposed women is actually quite small. More than 2 million women have now been prenatally exposed to stilbestrol, of whom approximately 350 have been reported to have adenocarcinoma of the vagina. Recent studies have shown structural defects of the genital tract leading to reproductive problems in prenatally exposed females as well as genitourinary anomalies in prenatally exposed males (Kaufman et al., 1977; Gill et al., 1976). The frequency of these defects is unknown.

Clomiphene

There have been at least six separate, retrospectively ascertained case reports of babies with defects in neural tube closure (anencephaly and meningomyelocele) conceived after ovarian stimulation with clo-

miphene. However, only four infants with major malformations were observed in two surveys of a total of 321 pregnant women who received clomiphene to stimulate ovulation (Golbus, 1980). In a more recent prospective study of pregnancy outcome following clomiphene stimulation, a 2.3 per cent incidence of malformations was noted in 935 liveborn babies (Kurachi et al., 1983). This drug is not considered to be teratogenic in humans.

Adrenal Corticosteroids

Corticosteroids are potent teratogens in some rodents, but they are not considered to be teratogenic in humans.

Antihypertensive Agents

In that the use of antihypertensive agents is usually limited to the third trimester, effects on organogenesis have not, in most cases, been evaluated. Prenatal exposure to only the angiotensin-converting enzyme (ACE) inhibitors has clearly been associated with structural defects. A number of prenatally exposed children have been described with renal dysplasia leading to oligohydramnios and, subsequently, to consequent Potter sequence with joint contractures, loose skin, large ears, Potter facies, and death secondary to pulmonary hypoplasia (Brent and Beckman, 1991). Significantly, there is no evidence that the ACE inhibitors adversely affect organogenesis. Rather, they reduce uterine blood flow, leading to decreased placental perfusion and secondarily to severe fetal hypotension. In addition, since the ACE inhibitors cross the placenta, they block fetal ACE activity, thereby affecting systemic and renal hemodynamics in the fetus. Evidence to date suggests that the ACE inhibitors adversely affect fetal development only during the second and third trimesters of pregnancy. The incidence of adverse outcome in prenatally exposed infants is unknown.

Prenatal exposure to minoxidil has been associated in two of four cases reported with hypertrichosis, a known side effect of minoxidil treatment in both children and adults (Kahler et al., 1987; Rosa et al., 1987).

Antimicrobials

Penicillin has been widely used during pregnancy. Although no systematic, prospective evaluation of the prenatal effect of the drug has been undertaken, there is no evidence that it is teratogenic in humans.

A number of studies have indicated that *tetracycline* given beyond the fourth month of pregnancy results in deciduous teeth that appear yellow, fluoresce a bright yellow, are abnormally susceptible to caries, and display enamel hypoplasia (Baden, 1970). Tetracycline exposure *in utero* does not affect the permanent teeth.

Because of the well-known association between treatment of newborn infants with *sulfonamides* and the development of kernicterus, concern has been raised regarding maternal sulfonamide administration during the third trimester. However, in a study of 194 infants born to women who received sulfadiazine for rheumatic fever prophylaxis during pregnancy, no increase in incidence of kernicterus, hyperbilirubinemia, or prematurity was observed (Baskin et al., 1980).

A study of the prenatal effect of *sulfasalazine* and corticosteroids in pregnancy complicated by inflammatory bowel disease gave similar results (Mogadam et al., 1981). None of the 181 mothers receiving sulfasalazine, including 107 who received the drug throughout pregnancy, gave birth to a baby with jaundice. In addition, no increase in the incidence of structural defects was noted, suggesting that sulfasalazine and corticosteroids used in combination for inflammatory bowel disease are not human teratogens.

Because of the observed teratogenic effects of large doses of trimethoprim in rats, concern has been raised regarding prenatal exposure to *trimethoprim-sulfamethoxazole* combinations. The offspring of 120 women who received trimethoprim-sulfamethoxazole therapy for bacteriuria during pregnancy did not have a higher rate of structural defects (Williams et al., 1969).

Monnet and colleagues (1967) described five children with severe central nervous system abnormalities born to women treated with *isoniazid (INH)* during pregnancy. Since it is known that INH causes a deficiency of vitamin B_6, the authors suggested that treatment with this drug during pregnancy should be combined with administration of B_6. It should be emphasized, however, that no clear cause-and-effect relationship has been established between prenatal exposure to INH and central nervous system abnormalities.

A number of studies have shown that the incidence of eighth nerve damage is slightly increased in children prenatally exposed to *streptomycin*. The rate of affected offspring has been variable. In a report of 50 children whose mothers had received streptomycin and dihydrostreptomycin at various stages of pregnancy, two were mildly affected, one with a mild but perceptive hearing loss and the other with reduced reactivity to water at 30°C (Varpela et al., 1969). Ganguin and Rempt (1970) evaluated 44 children older than 4 years of age whose mothers had been treated during pregnancy with more than 10 gm of streptomycin. Five of the 44 (11 per cent) had perceptive hearing losses, with higher-frequency hearing most severely affected.

No increase in incidence of structural defects has been reported in the offspring of women treated with various combinations of antituberculosis drugs, including *rifampin* and *ethambutol*, during pregnancy (Jentgens, 1975). All of the offspring of 38 women who received ethambutol during pregnancy were followed for 1 to 9 years and were found to be normal (Bobrowitz, 1965).

The data for offspring of 206 pregnant women who received *metronidazole* treatment during pregnancy were reviewed by Peterson and associates (1966). Eight of the 207 viable infants had structural abnormalities (3.8 per cent), an incidence no different from that expected in the general population. This finding suggests that metronidazole is not teratogenic in humans.

In 1984, an Acyclovir in Pregnancy Registry was established in order to determine whether *acyclovir* is teratogenic in humans. As of 1990, 312 cases of oral or IV prenatal acyclovir exposure were prospectively ascertained during pregnancy; they were followed throughout the remainder of pregnancy, and the outcome was documented (Andrews et al., 1992). Among the 239 first-trimester exposures, there were 24 spontaneous abortions (10 per cent); 47 therapeutic abortions (19.6 per cent); 9 infants with structural abnormalities (3.8 per cent); and 159 liveborn infants without structural defects. No consistent defects were noted in the 9 affected infants. The 3.8 per cent incidence of structural defects is no greater than would be expected in the general population. These data should be helpful in counseling women who inadvertently become pregnant while taking the drug. However, based on the relatively small sample size, the following is recommended: "The safety of systemic acyclovir therapy among pregnant women has not been established. In the presence of life-threatening maternal HSV infections (e.g., disseminated infection that includes encephalitis, pneumonitis, and/or hepatitis), acyclovir administered IV is probably of value. Among pregnant women without life-threatening disease, systemic acyclovir treatment should not be used for recurrent genital herpes episodes or as suppressive therapy to prevent reactivation near term" (Andrews et al., 1992).

Because *ribavirin* is a potent teratogen in the offspring of all rodent species tested, and because it has not been evaluated in humans, the use of this agent has been contraindicated in human pregnancy by the FDA. Furthermore, because the agent is administered by aerosol, the Centers for Disease Control has indicated that "health-care workers who are pregnant or who may become pregnant and who are involved in direct patient care with patients who are receiving ribavirin through oxygen tent or mist mask should be counseled about risk-reduction strategies, including alternative job responsibilities" (Centers for Disease Control, 1988) It is important to emphasize, however, that no study has been performed to suggest that ribavirin is teratogenic in humans.

Anticonvulsants

Intrauterine *phenylhydantoin* exposure is associated with a wide spectrum of embryonic or fetal effects, manifested most severely as a specific pattern of malformation referred to as the *fetal hydantoin syndrome* (Hanson and Smith, 1975). The disorder consists of prenatal-onset growth deficiency, mental retardation, nail and digital hypoplasia, and craniofacial abnormalities consisting of a short nose with low nasal bridge, ocular hypertelorism, low-set or abnormal ears, and a wide mouth with prominent lips. The broad spectrum of severity of this disorder is illustrated by a group of 35 affected children subsequently evaluated (Hanson et al., 1976). Whereas four children had a pattern of malformation consistent with the fetal hydantoin syndrome, an additional 11 displayed several of the abnormalities seen in that disorder, but were much less severely affected. Of greatest significance, 38 per cent of the 35 children demonstrated developmental or mental deficiency. However, it is important to recognize that parental IQs were not documented in that study. Thus the extent to which the frequency of mental deficiency was determined by the prenatal hydantoin as opposed to other factors is unclear.

The possibility that prenatal exposure to *trimethadione* causes serious problems in the offspring was first suggested by German and co-workers (1970). Subsequently, a *fetal trimethadione syndrome* was detected, the principal features of which include prenatal-onset growth deficiency, mental deficiency, cardiac septal defects, and typical craniofacial abnormalities, consisting of a short upturned nose with a broad and low nasal bridge, prominent forehead, a very unusual upslant of the eyebrows, and a poorly developed overlapping helix of the external ear (Zackai et al., 1975). The incidence of this disorder in the offspring of women receiving trimethadione during pregnancy is unknown at this time.

Concern regarding the effects on the offspring of prenatal exposure to *valproic acid* was first suggested by Robert and Guiband (1982), who documented an increased incidence of meningomyelocele in prenatally exposed infants. Subsequently, Hanson et al. (1984) and DiLiberti et al. (1984) set forth a broader pattern of malformation, the principal features of which include a narrow bifrontal diameter, epicanthic folds connecting with an infraorbital crease, a broad nasal bridge with a short nose and anteverted nostrils, a long philtrum with a thin vermilion border, long thin fingers with hyperconvex nails, cardiovascular defects, and meningomyelocele. Although the incidence of this disorder in the offspring of women receiving valproic acid during pregnancy is unknown, the prevalence of meningomyelocele related to valproic acid monotherapy is estimated to be 2.5 per cent (Lindhout and Schmidt, 1986).

Until recently, *carbamazepine* was believed to be the drug of choice for women who require an anticonvulsant during pregnancy. However, Jones et al. (1989) described a pattern of malformation similar to that associated with prenatal exposure to hydantoin and valproic acid in offspring of women receiving carbamazepine during pregnancy. Thirty-five children, ascertained prospectively because their mothers took carbamazepine alone, were evaluated. Craniofacial defects including microcephaly with a narrow bifrontal diameter, upslanting palpebral fissures, and a short nose with a long philtrum were noted in 11 per cent, fingernail hypoplasia in 26 per cent, and developmental delay in 20 per cent. In that formal developmental testing was done in only 25 of the 35 prenatally exposed infants, the incidence of developmental delay may be less than the 20 per cent reported. Although no increased incidence of major malformations was documented in that study, Rosa subsequently documented a tenfold increase for meningomyelocele in babies born to women receiving carbamazepine without concurrent exposure to valproic acid during pregnancy (Rosa, 1991).

A pattern of anomalies similar to that observed in relation to hydantoin, valproic acid, and carbamazepine has been seen in infants exposed *in utero* to *barbiturates* such as phenobarbital and primidone (Berkowitz, 1979; Krauss et al., 1984; Myhree, 1981; Rudd 1979; Seip, 1976). At present, however, no study has been done to determine the incidence of problems in the offspring of women taking this class of anticonvulsants during pregnancy.

It is of particular interest that a similar phenotype exists for at least four of these agents. The reason for this similarity is possibly related to the fact that many of the anticonvulsants are metabolized through the same reactive oxidative metabolic system. Hydantoin and carbamazepine are metabolized to an epoxide intermediate, which is most likely the teratogenic agent as opposed to the specific anticonvulsant. The epoxide intermediate is then metabolized in a reaction catalyzed by the enzyme epoxide hydralase (Lindhout et al., 1984). Valproic acid inhibits production of the enzyme. Buehler et al. (1990) have presented data that suggest that the level of the epoxide hydralase is genetically determined and that susceptibility to teratogenesis in babies born to women who received hydantoin during pregnancy depends on the genetically determined level of the epoxide hydralase.

Relative to the usefulness of this observation in predicting the risk of the fetal hydantoin syndrome, 19 pregnant women with seizures who were treated with hydantoin had amniocentesis performed to determine the level of epoxide hydralase in amniocytes. In all four fetuses in which the epoxide hydralase activity was less than 30 per cent of the standard, the infants had clinical findings compatible with the fetal hydantoin syndrome, whereas the 15 fetuses with enzyme activity greater than 30 per cent lacked features of the fetal hydantoin syndrome. Although still preliminary, these data suggest that susceptibility to teratogenesis depends on the fetal level of the epoxide hydralase. This may well prove useful in determining which infants are at increased risk for structural defects induced by hydantoin. The same may well be true for the other anticonvulsants metabolized through the reactive oxidative metabolic system.

Miscellaneous Drugs

Warfarin and Its Derivatives

The major features of the warfarin embryopathy include prenatal-onset growth deficiency, mental deficiency, seizures, severe hypoplasia of the nose, and stippling in uncalcified epiphyseal regions, primarily the axial skeleton, proximal femur, and calcaneus (Shaul and Hall, 1977). Although the critical period for development of the facial abnormalities and epiphyseal stippling appears to be between the sixth and ninth weeks of gestation, controversy remains regarding the effect of these derivatives during the second and third trimesters. It had previously been suggested that the central nervous system abnormalities are secondary to exposure during the second and third trimesters. However, a recent report of a child with the Dandy-Walker deformity, agenesis of the corpus callosum, and Peters' anomaly of the right eye who was exposed to coumarin between the eighth and twelfth weeks of gestation indicates that central nervous system defects can occur following first-trimester exposure (Kaplan, 1985). Furthermore, none of 54 children exposed to acenocoumarol during the second and third trimesters had central nervous system defects. This suggests that the risk, if it exists, must be extremely small (Iturbe-Alessio et al., 1986). The incidence of problems in the offspring of women receiving warfarin is not clear at this time. In a review of 418 women taking warfarin derivatives during pregnancy, however, an adverse pregnancy outcome was judged to have occurred in one-third (Hall et al., 1980). In the same review, pregnancy outcome in 135 women on heparin treatment during pregnancy was examined. Although there were no malformations noted in the offspring, the overall frequency of fetal and neonatal death and morbidity was 36 per cent. It should be emphasized that many of the pregnant women selected for the review, particularly those treated with heparin, were seriously ill. Thus, the high incidence of adverse pregnancy outcome might well be due to the maternal illness rather than the drug therapy. In addition, in the majority of cases, the newborn infant was not adequately examined, so that subtle abnormalities such as those seen in warfarin embryopathy might not have been observed.

Aminopterin

When taken before 40 days gestation, aminopterin is always lethal to the embryo. Serious malformations as well as intrauterine growth deficiency have been reported in association with aminopterin ingestion later in the first trimester. Milunsky and associates (1968) reviewed and summarized the clinical data on eight fetuses or newborn infants whose mothers took folic acid antagonists during the first trimester of pregnancy. Aminopterin was the drug taken by the mother in seven cases; its methyl derivative, methotrexate, was taken in one case. Four of the pregnancies ended in abortions, two offspring died in the perinatal period, and two were living at the time of publication, one at 15 months of age. All had serious structural defects, including intrauterine growth deficiency, severe lack of ossification of the calvarium leading to a malformed head, prominent eyes secondary to hypoplastic orbital ridges, ocular hypertelorism, small low-set ears, severe micrognathia, and limb abnormalities, including missing bones and positional deformations.

Follow-up evaluations of three children so affected who survived the newborn period revealed postnatal growth deficiency in all cases and an IQ of 80 at 10 years in one, a developmental quotient of 75 at 18 months in a second, and normal development at 15 months of age in the third as defined by a Denver Developmental Assessment (Milunsky et al., 1968; Howard and Rudd, 1976; Shaw and Steinbach, 1968).

Bendectin and Debendox

Bendectin, an antiemetic formerly prescribed for morning sickness in early pregnancy, has been implicated as a potent human teratogen in two popular lay periodicals (Cathcart et al., 1979; Dowie and Marshall, 1980). The basis for this implication can be found in several case reports in which women who were prescribed or who took a preparation of doxylamine succinate, dicyclomine hydrochloride, and pyridoxine hydrochloride (the formulation of Bendectin in the United States until 1976 and the current formulation of Debendox in Britain) or doxylamine succinate and pyridoxine hydrochloride (the current formulation of Bendectin in the United States) had children with congenital malformations. The most common malformations cited have been limb reductions (Patterson, 1977; Dickson, 1977; Henderson, 1977; Donnai and Harris, 1978; Frith, 1978) and omphalocele and gastroschisis (Donnai and Harris, 1978; Menzies, 1978). In addition, epidemiologic studies have reported an association between cardiac defects (Rothman et al., 1979) and oral clefts (Golding and Baldwin, 1980) and maternal Bendectin use.

Determining the etiology of congenital malformations is always difficult, especially when the suspected agent is commonly used by pregnant women and the bulk of data is in the form of anecdotal case reports. Epidemiologic studies also have their shortcomings, particularly regarding the control of maternal recall bias and maternal exposure to other human teratogens. For example, in both epidemiologic studies just cited, the investigators used normal children as the control population, thereby falling into the trap of recall bias: mothers of malformed children are more likely to remember their drug exposures during pregnancy than are mothers of normal children.

Fortunately, there have been several other studies on the potential teratogenicity of Bendectin and Debendox that need to be considered. Milkovich and Van der Berg (1976) reported no association between severe congenital malformations and Bendectin in a prospective study of 628 women who took the drug in the first trimester. Using data from the Collaborative Perinatal Project, Shapiro and associates (1977) found no association between birth defects and either doxylamine or dicyclomine ingestion. Relying on Bendectin prescriptions to pregnant women for subject selection, Smithells and Sheppard (1978) demonstrated no higher incidence of birth defects in the offspring of 2298 women who were prescribed Bendectin. In a prospective study using Debendox prescriptions as a basis for maternal exposure, no increased rate of birth defects in the offspring of 620 women was observed following use in the first trimester (Fleming et al., 1981).

Of particular interest are three epidemiologic studies investigating the association between Bendectin (or Debendox) and limb reduction malformations, oral clefts, and cardiac defects. Most comprehensive was the study from the Centers for Disease Control Metropolitan Atlantic Congenital Defects Program, in which interviews with women having children with birth defects between 1968 and 1978 were reviewed for first-trimester exposure to either the two- or three-ingredient formulation of Bendectin (Cordero et al., 1981). Using offspring with congenital malformations other than those considered in the analysis as controls, the authors reported no association between first-trimester exposure to either formulation of Bendectin and limb reduction malformations or oral clefts (defined as cleft lip and/or cleft palate or isolated cleft palate). Also using children with congenital malformations other than those under consideration in the study as controls, Mitchell and associates (1981) observed no association between first-trimester use of Bendectin and oral clefts or cardiac defects. Finally, no association between Debendox use in pregnancy and limb reduction malformations has been recorded (Correy and Newman, 1981).

The bulk of available evidence suggests that Bendectin and Debendox are not human teratogens when taken in the first trimester of pregnancy, a conclusion also reached by the United States Food and Drug Administration Fertility and Maternal Health Drugs Advisory Committee (1980).

Isotretinoin

First licensed in the United States in 1982 with the brand name Accutane, isotretinoin (13-cis-retinoic acid) was recognized to be a human teratogen one year later (Rosa, 1983). A characteristic pattern of malformations has been delineated. Its principal features include severe defects of ear development; cardiovascular anomalies (conotruncal malformations including transposition of the great vessels, tetralogy of Fallot, double-outlet right ventricle, truncus arteriosus communis, aortic arch interruption, retroesophageal right subclavian artery, aortic arch hypoplasia); severe defects in central nervous system development; and thymic anomalies. As of 1987, the offspring of 57 women had been evaluated. There were nine spontaneous abortions, one malformed stillbirth, ten malformed live births, and 37 live births with no major malformations, leading to an absolute risk of 23 per cent for major malformations among fetuses that reach 20 weeks gestation.

It is important to recognize that all cases of the retinoic acid embryopathy have occurred in the offspring of women on isotretinoin at conception or during the first trimester of pregnancy. In a prospective study of pregnancy outcome in 88 women who completed or discontinued isotretinoin therapy prior to conception, neither an increased incidence of structural defects nor an increased rate of spontaneous abortions could be demonstrated (Dai et al., 1989). Furthermore, not a single case of the retinoic acid embryopathy occurred.

Penicillamine

Although the majority of pregnancies in which this drug has been used have resulted in normal outcome, five prenatally exposed infants, three of whom died in the neonatal period, have been born with cutis laxa (Rosa, 1986). It had previously been suggested that penicillamine could be safely used during pregnancy for the treatment of Wilson's disease. However, the mothers of two of the five children with cutis laxa were being treated for Wilson's disease.

Since the majority of pregnancies in which the fetus was exposed to penicillamine have normal outcomes, it is suggested that this drug should be continued during pregnancy for conditions such as Wilson's disease, in which alternative therapy is ineffective.

Diagnostic and Therapeutic Radiation

Prenatal exposure to ionizing radiation is associated with more emotion and less objectivity from the general public than virtually any other agent to which women are exposed during pregnancy. Brent and Gorson (1972) have set forth in detailed fashion the current knowledge regarding the effects of ionizing radiation on the developing embryo. More recently, the data pertinent to humans have been summarized together with some practical recommendations regarding prenatal exposure (Swartz and Reichling, 1978). From a clinical standpoint, diagnostic x-rays in the first trimester that deliver less than 5 rads to the fetus are not believed to be teratogenic. Concern about exposure to between 5 and 10 rads has been raised, but from a practical standpoint, serious risk to the fetus does not occur until the absorbed dose is 10 rads or more. Diagnostic x-rays deliver a relatively low dose to the female gonad. For example, a chest x-ray delivers 8 millirads, a cholecystogram 300 millirads, an upper GI series 558 millirads, an IVP 407 millirads, and a barium enema 805 millirads. On the other hand, the large doses of maternal radiation utilized in radiation therapy can lead to microcephaly and mental retardation in human offspring exposed *in utero*.

The question of radiation dose to the fetus often arises when pregnant women require radiologic examinations for diagnostic purposes or have inadvertently undergone x-ray examination during pregnancy. Table 12–1 illustrates the estimated radiation

Table 12–1. Estimated Ovarian Radiation Exposure from Common Radiologic Procedures*

PROCEDURE	ESTIMATED OVARIAN DOSE (millirads)	AVERAGE NUMBER OF FILMS PER EXAMINATION
Chest examination		
Radiography	8	1.4
Fluoroscopy	71	
Upper GI series		
Total	558	4.4
Radiography	360	
Fluoroscopy	198	
Barium enema		
Total	805	3.5
Radiography	439	
Fluoroscopy	366	
Intravenous or retrograde pyelography	407	5.0
Abdominal x-rays	289	1.7
Lumbar spine x-rays	275	2.5
Pelvic x-rays	41	1.5

*Ovarian dose approximates fetal exposure.
Adapted from Penfil RL, Brown ML: Genetically significant dose to the United States population from diagnostic medical roentgenology. Radiology **90**:209, 1968.

dose delivered to the ovaries during commonly used radiologic examinations. Ovarian dose is a reasonable approximation of fetal exposure.

ENVIRONMENTAL AGENTS

Occupational Chemicals

No adequate study has been done to evaluate the potential teratogenicity of the majority of occupational chemicals with which women come in contact during pregnancy. Based on animal experiments evaluating prenatal exposure to a variety of chemicals, as well as the frequency with which pregnant women come in contact with them, a number of compounds believed to be of concern in human pregnancy have been set forth by Koskineu and Hemminki (1985). However, it is important to note that the few studies that have been done in humans are either inconclusive or suggestive of a lack of teratogenicity. For example, Holmberg (1979) reported an increased incidence of prenatal exposure to a variety of organic solvents in children with congenital CNS defects entered in the Finnish Registry of Congenital Malformations. Unfortunately, that study was retrospective and involved only 14 children with central nervous system defects who were prenatally exposed to a variety of solvents, making definitive conclusions about any one of them impossible. Of some potential significance was the fact that eight of the offspring had defects in neural tube closure.

Exposure of a large number of individuals to chemicals at the Love Canal in Niagara Falls, New York in the mid-1970s provided an opportunity to study pregnancy outcome in a number of women exposed to benzene, dichloroethylene, lindane, chloroform, and toluene. Unfortunately, adequate pregnancy outcome studies were not performed. Although a preliminary survey revealed a pregnancy wastage 1.5 times higher than expected and structural defects in 6 of 57 births, the numbers were unsubstantiated and thus conclusions cannot be made (Schardein, 1985).

This complete lack of available data regarding the effects of occupational chemicals on human reproduction poses a significant frustration that will only become worse as more women enter the workplace and more chemicals that have not been adequately studied become available.

Pesticides

At present, no conclusive studies have been performed evaluating the potential teratogenic effect of pesticides. Given the large number of individuals who are in contact with these agents both at home and in the workplace, a prospective study regarding their embryonic-fetal effect is clearly necessary. The most commonly used pesticides both for agricultural purposes and for home use are the organophosphates and the carbamates. Both are acetylcholinesterase inhibitors, which act by binding to the acetylcholinesterase enzyme and thus allow acetylcholine to accumulate at the cholinergic neuroeffector junctions, at the skeletal muscle myoneural junctions, and in autonomic ganglia.

Contamination of the milk supply on the island of Oahu, Hawaii, between 1980 and 1982, by heptachlor provided the opportunity to investigate the teratogenicity of an organochlorine pesticide, an agent that also acts as a cholinesterase inhibitor (Marchand et al., 1986). Comparison of the incidence rates for 23 major malformations on Oahu from 1981 to 1983 with rates for the other Hawaiian islands, as well as the total United States, suggested that heptachlor is probably not a human teratogen. This negative study is particularly significant because organochlorine insecticides are lipid-soluble, remain in the environment for a long period of time, and are therefore potentially of greater concern. Since the organophosphates and carbamates do not persist in the environment, concern regarding their potential teratogenicity is less.

Hyperthermia

Retrospective studies have been reported suggesting that maternal hyperthermia is teratogenic in humans (Smith et al., 1978; Miller et al., 1978). Of greatest significance is a study of 23 retrospectively selected children who had been prenatally exposed to temperatures of 38.9°C or more between 4 and 14 weeks of gestation (Pleet et al., 1980). Similar patterns of malformations were noted that included (1) growth deficiency; (2) central nervous system defects including mental deficiency, microcephaly, hypotonia, and microphthalmia; and (3) variable dysmorphogenesis of the first and second branchial arches resulting in midface hypoplasia, micrognathia, cleft lip with or without cleft palate, and malformed ears. In six of the 23 cases, heat exposure was associated with sauna bathing or hot tub use, suggesting that hyperthermia, rather than an infectious agent, was the teratogenic agent.

A prospective study of 5566 women exposed to either hot tub, sauna, fever, or electric blanket during early pregnancy is particularly relevant (Milunsky et al., 1992). Exposure to heat in the form of hot tub, sauna, and/or fever was associated in all cases with an increased risk for neural tube closure defects. Of the three, the adjusted relative risk for hot tub use was the highest, 2.8 (95 per cent confidence limits, range 1.2 to 6.5). Exposure to electric blanket was not associated with an increased risk.

CONCLUSION

It is important to emphasize that the teratogenic potential of most agents is unknown at this time. Whereas only a few agents have been shown to be teratogenic in humans, the majority have not been adequately tested, creating an obvious dilemma for the physician attempting to provide optimum care for pregnant women. Although no easy answer seems forthcoming, it would seem prudent to provide all pregnant women with all the facts available regarding the teratogenic potential of any drug, chemical, or environmental agent to which they are exposed.

REFERENCES

Aarskog D: Association between maternal intake of diazepam and oral clefts. Lancet 2:921, 1975.

Aarskog D: Maternal progestins as a possible cause of hypospadias. N Engl J Med 300:75, 1979.

Andrews EB, Yankaskas BC, Cordero JF, et al: Acyclovir in pregnancy registry: Six years' experience. Obstet Gynecol 79:7, 1992.

Baden E: Environmental pathology of the teeth. In Gorlin RJ, Goldman HM (eds): Thomas' Oral Pathology. 6th ed. St. Louis, CV Mosby, 1970.

Baskin C, La S, Wenger NK: Sulfadiazine rheumatic fever prophylaxis during pregnancy: Does it increase the risk of kernicterus in the newborn? Cardiology 65:222, 1980.

Berkowitz FE: Fetal malformations due to phenobarbitone. A case report. S Afr Med J 500:100, 1979.

Bobrowitz ID: Ethambutol in pregnancy. Chest 66:20, 1965.

Brent R, Gorson RO: Radiation exposure in pregnancy. Curr Probl Radiol 2:3, 1972.

Brent RL, Beckman, DA: Angiotensin converting enzyme inhibitors, an embryopathic class of drugs with unique properties: Information for clinical teratology counselors. Teratology 43:543, 1991.

Buehler BA, Duane D, Van Waes M, et al: Prenatal prediction of risk of the fetal hydantoin syndrome. N Engl J Med 322:1567, 1990.

Cathcart J, Checkley J, Kelsey D: Common drug causing deformed babies. National Enquirer, Oct 1979, pp 20–21.

Centers for Disease Control: Assessing exposure of health care personnel to aerosols of ribavirin. MMWR 37:560, 1988.

Check JH, Rankin A, Teichman M: The risk of fetal anomalies as a result of progesterone therapy during pregnancy. Fertil Steril 45:575, 1986.

Cordero JF, Oakley GP, Greenberg F, James LM: Is Bendectin a teratogen? JAMA 245:2307, 1981.

Correy JF, Newman NM: Debendox and limb reduction deformities. Med J Aust 1:417, 1981.

Czeizel A: Lack of teratogenicity of benzodiazepine drugs in Hungary. Reproductive Tox 1:183, 1988.

Dai WS, Hsu M, Itri LM: Safety of pregnancy after discontinuation of isotretinoin. Arch Dermatol 125:362, 1989.

Dickson JH: Congenital deformities associated with Bendectin. Can Med Assoc J 117:121, 1977.

DiLiberti JH, Farndon PA, Dennis NR, Curry CJR: The fetal valproate syndrome. Am J Med Genet 19:473, 1984.

Donnai D, Harris R: Unusual fetal malformations after antiemetics in pregnancy. Br Med J 1:691, 1978.

Dowie M, Marshall C: The Bendectin cover-up. Mother Jones, Nov 1980, pp 43–56.

Edmonds LD, Oakley G: Ebstein's anomaly in maternal lithium exposure during pregnancy. Teratology 41:551, 1990.

Fleming DM, Knox JDE, Crombie DL: Debendox in early pregnancy and fetal malformations. Br Med J 283:99, 1981.

Frith K: Fetal malformation after Debendox treatment in early pregnancy. Br Med J 1:925, 1978.

Ganguin G, Rempt E: Streptomycinbehandlung in der Schwangerschaft und ihre Auswirkung auf das Gehor des Kindes. Z Laryngol Rhinol Otol 49:496, 1970.

German J, Kowal A, Ethlers KH: Trimethadione and human teratogenesis. Teratology 3:349, 1970.

Gill WB, Schumacher GFB, Bibbo M: Structural and functional abnormalities in the sex organs of male offspring of mothers treated with DES. J Reprod Med 16:147, 1976.

Golbus MS: Teratology for the obstetrician: Current status. Obstet Gynecol 55:269, 1980.

Golding J, Baldwin JA: Clefts of lip and palate and maternal drug consumption. I: Antinauseants. Read before Food and Drug Administration Fertility and Maternal Health Drug Advisory Committee, Washington, DC, Sept 15, 1980.

Goujard J, Rumeau-Rouquette C: First-trimester exposure to pro-

gestogen/oestrogen and congenital malformations (letter). Lancet 1:482, 1977.

Gregg NM: Congenital cataract following German measles in the mother. Trans Ophthalmol Soc Aust 3:35, 1941.

Hall JQ, Panti RM, Wilson KM: Maternal and fetal sequelae of anticoagulation during pregnancy. Am J Med 68:122, 1980.

Hanson JW, Smith DW: The fetal hydantoin syndrome. J Pediatr 87:285, 1975.

Hanson JW, Myrianthopoulos NC, Harvey MAS, et al: Risks to the offspring of women treated with hydantoin anti-convulsants with emphasis on the fetal hydantoin syndrome. J Pediatr 89:662, 1976.

Hanson JW, Ardinger HH, DiLiberti JH, et al: Effects of valproic acid on the fetus. Pediatr Res 18:306A, 1984.

Hartz SC, Heinonen OP, Shapiro S, et al: Antenatal exposure to meprobamate and chlordiazepoxide in relation to malformations, mental development and childhood mortality. N Engl J Med 29:726, 1975.

Heinonen OP, Sloan D, Monson RR, et al: Cardiovascular birth defects and antenatal exposure to female sex hormones. N Engl J Med 296:67, 1977.

Henderson IWD: Congenital deformities associated with Bendectin. Can Med Assoc J 117:721, 1977.

Herbst AL, Ulfelder H, Poskanzer DC: Adenocarcinoma of the vagina: Association of maternal stilbestrol therapy with tumor appearance in young women. N Engl J Med 284:878, 1971.

Holmberg PC: Central nervous system defects in children born to mothers exposed to organic solvents during pregnancy. Lancet 2:177, 1979.

Howard NJ, Rudd NL: The natural history of aminopterin-induced embryopathy. Presented at Birth Defects Conference, University of British Columbia, Vancouver, June 23–25, 1976.

Iturbe-Alessio I, del Carmen Fouseca M, Mutchinik O, et al: Risks of anticonvulsant therapy in pregnant women with artificial heart valves. N Engl J Med 315:1390, 1986.

Jacobson SJ, Jones K, Johnson K, et al: Prospective multicenter study of pregnancy outcome after lithium exposure during first trimester. Lancet 339:530, 1992.

Janerich DT, Piper JM, Glebatis DM: Oral contraceptives and congenital limb reduction defects. N Engl J Med 291:697, 1974.

Janerich DT, Dugan JM, Standfast SJ, Strite L: Congenital heart disease and prenatal exposure to exogenous sex hormones. Br Med J 1:1058, 1977.

Jentgens H: Antituberkulotische Therapie mit Ethambutol und Rifampicin in der Schwangerschaft. Prax Pneumol 30:42, 1975.

Jones KL, Lacro RV, Johnson KA, et al: Pattern of malformation in the children of women treated with carbamazepine during pregnancy. N Engl J Med 320:1661, 1989.

Kahler SG, Patrinos ME, Lambert GH, et al: Hypertrichosis and congenital anomalies associated with maternal use of minoxidil. Pediatrics 79:434, 1987.

Kallen B: Comments on teratogen update: Lithium. Teratology 38:597, 1988.

Kaplan LC: Congenital Dandy-Walker malformation associated with first-trimester warfarin. Teratology 32:333, 1985.

Katz Z, Lancet M, Skornik J, et al: Teratogenicity of progestogens given during the first trimester of pregnancy. Obstet Gynecol 65:775, 1985.

Kaufman RH, Binder GL, Gray PM, et al: Upper genital tract changes associated with exposure in utero to diethylstilbestrol. Am J Obstet Gynecol 128:51, 1977.

Koskineu K, Hemminki K: Environmental teratogenicity and embryotoxicity of occupational chemicals. In Hemminki K, Sorsa M, Vainio H (eds): Occupational Hazards and Reproduction. New York, Hemisphere Publishing Corp, 1985.

Krauss CM, Holmes LB, Van Lang QN, et al: Four siblings with similar malformations after exposure to phenytoin and primidone. J Pediatr 105:750, 1984.

Kurachi K, Aono T, Minagawa J, et al: Congenital malformations of newborn infants after clomiphene-induced ovulation. Fertil Steril 40:187, 1983.

Laegreid L, Olegard R, Wahlstrom J, et al: Abnormalities in children exposed to benzodiazepines in utero. Lancet 1:108, 1987.

Lammer EJ, Hayes AM, Schunior A, et al: Risk for major malformations among human fetuses exposed to isotretinoin (12-cis-retinoic acid). Teratology **35**:68A, 1987.

Lenz W: Kindliche Missbildungen nach Medikament-Einnahme wahrend der Graviditat? Dtsch Med Wochenschr **86**:2555, 1961.

Levy EP, Cohen A, Fraser FC: Hormone treatment during pregnancy and congenital heart disease. Lancet **1**:611, 1973.

Lindhout D, Hoppener RJ, Meinardi H: Teratogenicity of antiepileptic drug combinations with special emphasis on epoxidation (of carbamazepine). Epilepsia **25**:77, 1984.

Lindhout D, Schmidt D: *In utero* exposure to valproate and neural tube defects. Lancet **1**:1392, 1986.

Marchand LL, et al: Trends in birth defects for a Hawaiian population exposed to heptachlor and for the United States. Arch Environ Health **41**:145, 1986.

McBride WG: Thalidomide and congenital abnormalities. Lancet **2**:1358, 1961.

McBride WG: Limb deformities associated with iminodibenzyl hydrochloride. Med J Aust **1**:492, 1972.

Menzies CJG: Fetal malformation after Debendox treatment in early pregnancy. Br Med J **1**:925, 1978.

Milkovich L, Van der Berg BJ: Effects of antenatal expobamate and chlordiazepoxide hydrochloride on human embryonic and fetal development. N Engl J Med **291**:1268, 1974.

Milkovich L, Van der Berg BJ: An evaluation of the teratogenicity of certain anti-nauseant drugs. Am J Obstet Gynecol **125**:244, 1976.

Miller P, Smith DW, Shepard TH: Maternal hyperthermia as a possible cause of anencephaly. Lancet **1**:519, 1978.

Milunsky A, Graef JW, Gaynor MF: Methotrexate-induced congenital malformations with a review of the literature. J Pediatr **72**:790, 1968.

Milunsky A, Ulcickas M, Rothman KJ, et al: Maternal heat exposure and neural tube defects. JAMA **268**:882, 1992.

Mitchell AA, Rosenberg L, Shapiro S, Slone D: Birth defects related to Bendectin use in pregnancy. I. Oral clefts and cardiac defects. JAMA **245**:2311, 1981.

Mogadam M, Dobbins WO, Korelitz BI, Ahmed SW: Pregnancy in inflammatory bowel disease. Effect of sulfasalazine and corticosteroids on fetal outcome. Gastroenterology **80**:72, 1981.

Monnet P, Kalb JC, Pujol M: Doit-on craindre une influence teratogene eventuelle de l'isoniazide? Rev Tubercul (Paris) **31**:845, 1967.

Mulvihill JJ, Mulvihill CG, Neill CA: Prenatal sex-hormone exposure and cardiac defects in man. Teratology **9**:30A, 1974.

Myhree SA, Williams R: Teratogenic effects associated with maternal primidone therapy. J Pediatr **99**:160, 1981.

Nishimura H, Tanamura T: Clinical Aspects of the Teratogenicity of Drugs. New York, American Elsevier, 1976.

Nora AH, Nora JJ: A syndrome of multiple congenital anomalies associated with teratogenic exposure. Arch Environ Health **30**:17, 1975.

Oakley GP, Flynt JW, Falek A: Hormonal pregnancy tests and congenital malformations. Lancet **2**:256, 1973.

Patterson DC: Congenital deformities associated with Bendectin. Can Med Assoc J **116**:1348, 1977.

Peterson WF, Stauch JE, Ryder CO: Metronidazole in pregnancy. Am J Obstet Gynecol **94**:343, 1966.

Pleet HB, Graham JH, Harvey MA, Smith DW: Patterns of malformations resulting from the teratogenic effects of first trimester hyperthermia. Pediatr Res **14**:587, 1980.

Rachelefsky GS, Flynt JW, Ebbin AJ, Wilson MG: Possible teratogenicity of tricyclic antidepressants. Lancet **1**:838, 1972.

Ressequie LK, Hick JF, Bruen JA, et al: Congenital malformation among offspring exposed *in utero* to progestins. Olmstead County, Minnesota, 1936–1974. Fertil Steril **43**:514, 1985.

Robert E, Guiband P: Maternal valproic acid and congenital neural tube defects. Lancet **2**:934, 1982.

Rock JA, Wentz AC, Cole KA, et al: Fetal malformations following progesterone therapy during pregnancy: A preliminary report. Fertil Steril **44**:17, 1985.

Rosa FW: Teratogenicity of isotretinoin. Lancet **2**:513, 1983.

Rosa FW, Idanpaan-Heikkila J, Assauti R: Fetal minoxidil exposure. Pediatrics, **80**:120, 1987.

Rosa FW: Spina bifida in infants of women treated with carbamazepine during pregnancy. N Engl J Med **324**:674, 1991.

Rosa FW: Teratogenic update: Penicillamine. Teratology **33**:127, 1986.

Rosenberg L, Mitchell AA, Parsells JL, et al: Lack of relation of oral clefts to diazepam use during pregnancy. N Engl J Med **309**:1282, 1983.

Rothman KJ, Fyler DC, Goldblatt A, et al: Exogenous hormones and other drug exposures. Am J Epidemiol **109**:433, 1979.

Rudd NL, Freedom RM: A possible primidone embryopathy. J Pediatr **94**:835, 1979.

Rumeau-Rouquette C, Goujard J, Huel G: Possible teratogenic effects of phenothiazines in human beings. Teratology **15**:57, 1977.

Safra MJ, Oakley JP: Association between cleft lip with or without cleft palate and prenatal exposure to diazepam. Lancet **ii**:478, 1975.

Saxen I: Associations between oral cleft, and drugs taken during pregnancy. Int J Epidemiol **4**:37, 1975.

Saxen I, Saxen L: Association between maternal intake of diazepam and oral clefts. Lancet **2**:498, 1975.

Scanlon FJ: Use of antidepressant drugs during the first trimester. Med J Aust **2**:1077, 1969.

Schardein JL: Chemically Induced Birth Defects. New York, Marcel Dekker Inc, 1985.

Schardein JL: Congenital abnormalities and hormones during pregnancy: A clinical review. Teratology **22**:251, 1980.

Seip M: Growth retardation, dysmorphic facies and minor malformations following massive exposure to phenobarbitone in utero. Acta Paediatr Scand **65**:617, 1976.

Shapiro S, Heinonen OP, Suskind V, et al: Antenatal exposure to doxylamine succinate and dicyclomine hydrochloride (Bendectin) in relation to congenital malformation, perinatal mortality, birthweight and intelligence quotient score. Am J Obstet Gynecol **128**:480, 1977.

Shaul WL, Hall JF: Multiple congenital anomalies associated with oral anticoagulants. Am J Obstet Gynecol **127**:191, 1977.

Shaw EB, Steinbach HL: Aminopterin-induced fetal malformation. Survival of infant after attempted abortion. Am J Dis Child **115**:477, 1968.

Shiono PH, Mills JL: Oral clefts and diazepam use during pregnancy. N Engl J Med **311**:920, 1984.

Sim M: Imipramine and pregnancy. Br Med J **2**:45, 1972.

Smith DW, Clarren SK, Harvey MA: Hyperthermia as a possible teratogenic agent. J Pediatr **92**:878, 1978.

Smithells RW, Sheppard S: Teratology testing in humans: A method demonstrating safety of Bendectin. Teratology **17**:31, 1978.

Swartz HM, Reichling BA: Hazards of radiation exposure for pregnant women. JAMA **239**:1907, 1978.

United States Food and Drug Administration, Fertility and Maternal Health Drugs Advisory Committee: Draft guideline patient package insert; Bendectin and other combination drugs containing doxylamine and Vitamin B-6. Federal Register **45**:80740, 1980.

Varpela E, Hietalahti J, Aro MJT: Streptomycin and dihydrostreptomycin during pregnancy and their effect on the child's inner ear. Scand J Respir Dis **50**:101, 1969.

Weinstein MR, Goldfield MD: Cardiovascular malformations with lithium use during pregnancy. Am J Psychiatry **132**:529, 1975.

Williams JD, Condie AP, Brumfitt W, Reeves DS: The treatment of bacteriuria in pregnant women with sulpha-methoxazole and trimethoprim. Postgrad Med J **45**(Suppl):71, 1969.

Wiseman RA, Dodds-Smith IC: Cardiovascular birth defects and antenatal exposure to female sex hormones: A re-evaluation of some base data. Teratology **30**:359, 1984.

Zackai EH, Mellman WJ, Neiderer B, Hanson JW: The fetal trimethadione syndrome. J Pediatr **87**:280, 1975.

Zalystein E, Koren J, Einarson T, et al: A case-control study on the association between first-trimester exposure to lithium and Ebstein's anomaly. Am J Cardiol **65**:817, 1990.

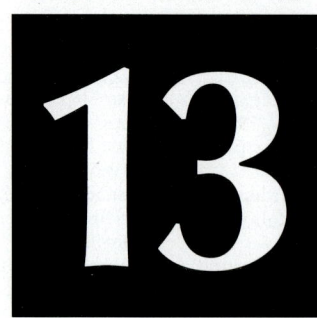

CHAPTER

13

SOCIAL AND ILLICIT DRUG USE IN PREGNANCY

ROBERT L. ANDRES, M.D., and KENNETH L. JONES, M.D.

The use of illicit drugs during pregnancy has received significant and widespread attention over the past decade. Although a great deal has been learned regarding the perinatal implications of drug use, many important questions remain unanswered. Furthermore, the use of alcohol and tobacco remains a significant factor contributing to perinatal morbidity.

Numerous issues complicate the interpretation of data collected from clinical research in this area. These include: (1) polydrug use (such as cigarettes and alcohol); (2) environmental effects (e.g., nutrition and the availability of prenatal care); (3) timing of exposure; (4) degree of exposure; and (5) appropriateness of control group. There is an increasing volume of basic research in the area of drug use in pregnancy, and this provides valuable data collected in a more controlled manner. This chapter will review the perinatal effects of social and illicit drug use in pregnancy, and offer recommendations concerning the management of these high-risk pregnancies.

PREVALENCE AND DRUG SCREENING

The National Institute of Drug Abuse Household Survey published in 1991 noted that 27 per cent of women between the ages of 18 and 25 and 14.7 per cent between the ages of 25 and 34 admitted to the use of an illicit drug within the preceding year. Alcohol use was reported by 80.1 per cent (18 to 25) and 77.3 per cent (25 to 34 years) and smoking in 40 per cent (18 to 25) and 35.6 per cent (25 to 34 years). It is not surprising that many women enter a pregnancy with a substance abuse problem. A universal intrapartum screening program conducted at the University of California, Davis showed that 20.5 per cent of patients were positive for cocaine (9.5 per cent), methamphetamine (7.5 per cent), or opiates (1.3 per cent) (Gillogley et al., 1990). A study involving 715 women enrolling in both public and private prenatal clinics concluded that 14.8 per cent had a positive urine toxicology screen for alcohol (1.0 per cent), marijuana (11.9 per

cent), cocaine (3.4 per cent), or opiates (0.3 per cent) (Chasnoff et al., 1990). Importantly, there was no significant difference in prevalence rates between patients seen at the public clinics (16.3 per cent) and the private clinics (13.1 per cent). Similarly, there was no significant difference between ethnic groups, with positive urine toxicologies noted in 14.1 per cent of black women and 15.4 per cent of white women. A recent survey of 36 hospitals demonstrated that the overall prevalence of substance abuse in pregnancy based on discharge diagnosis was 11 per cent, the range being 0.4 per cent to 27 per cent (Chasnoff, 1989a). The magnitude of this problem is illustrated by a recent report from the Institute of Medicine in which it is estimated that between 350,000 and 625,000 newborns are exposed to illict drugs each year (Institute of Medicine, 1990).

Alcohol use and smoking receive less attention in most prevalence studies. Zuckerman et al. (1989) showed that 41 per cent of the pregnant women in his series smoked cigarettes during the pregnancy and similar figures have been suggested by other authors (Gomby and Shiono, 1991). The prevalence of reported alcohol use in Zuckerman's investigation was 60 per cent, whereas a recent study of over 1700 women demonstrated that 25 per cent consumed alcohol while pregnant (Serdula et al., 1991).

Differences in reported prevalence rates (Table 13–1) are dependent upon the demographic characteristics of the population being studied and the methodology used for detection of the drugs (e.g., maternal urine, neonatal urine, neonatal meconium). Although meconium (Ostrea et al., 1989) and hair (Graham et al., 1989) have all been investigated as methods to detect drug exposure, urine testing remains the most frequently utilized screening tool. Meconium testing, which is currently available at relatively few centers, is a more sensitive screening test than urine and may eventually be the preferred method of detecting illicit drug use. A recent large-scale, prospective study of over 3000 neonates found that 44 per cent of the meconium samples collected were positive for cocaine, marijuana, or opiates. Among the women admitting

TABLE 13–1.   Prevalence of Illicit Drug Use in Pregnant Women

SUBSTANCE	OSTREA, 1992* (n = 3010) %	CHASNOFF, 1990 (n = 715) %	CENTERS FOR DISEASE CONTROL RHODE ISLAND, 1990 (n = 465) %	GILLOGLEY, 1990 (n = 1643) %
Cocaine	30.7	3.4	2.6	8.5
Opiates	20.5	0.3	1.7	1.2
Marijuana	11.5	11.9	3.0	—
Amphetamine	—	—	0.2	6.5
Any of above	44.3	14.8	7.5	20.5
Multiple	32	1.7	—	2.1

*Screening done on meconium; all others sampled maternal urine.

to illicit drug use (11 per cent), urine toxicology was positive in 52 per cent, whereas meconium testing identified 88 per cent as positive (Ostrea et al., 1992). The major disadvantage of urine drug screening is that it detects only relatively recent use rather than long-term or remote exposure. The metabolites of amphetamine are detectable for 24 to 72 hours following use, cocaine for 24 to 72 hours, opiates 24 to 48 hours, alcohol 8 hours, and LSD for 24 to 72 hours. Benzodiazepines can be detected for up to several weeks, and marijuana metabolites for 1 to 4 weeks (Hawks and Chiang, 1986). Selective urine drug screening appears to be a necessary adjunct to history taking in the detection of the drug-dependent pregnant woman. Several studies have pointed out the poor correlation between maternal self-report and urine toxicology (Gillogely et al., 1990; Zuckerman et al., 1989). Among the patients with positive urine drug screens in the intrapartum screening done by Gillogely et al. (1990), 48 per cent had denied drug use upon admission to the hospital. Numerous drug-screening criteria have been suggested, and a proposed set of indications is listed in Table 13–2. The design of any urine drug-screening program should include contributions from legal counsel and social service staff to address specific liability issues and local reporting laws.

ALCOHOL

The effects of alcohol on the fetus and newborn have been recognized for centuries. Aristotle noted that "foolish, drunk, or hare brained women for the most part bring forth children like unto themselves, difficult and listless" (Rosett and Weiner, 1984). In 1973, a pattern of anomalies was described in infants born to alcoholic women (Jones et al., 1973). In the years that followed, numerous studies reinforced the adverse fetal effects of maternal alcohol use (Hanson et al., 1978; Ouellette et al., 1977; Clarren and Smith, 1978; Olegard et al., 1979; Sokol et al., 1980). These data led to a report from the Surgeon General of the United States recommending that without an identifiable threshold, the safest course was abstinence (FDA Bulletin, 1981). Despite this recommendation and a report suggesting that the fetal alcohol syndrome is the leading recognized cause of mental retardation (Abel and Sokol, 1986), women have contin-

ued to drink alcohol while pregnant. The National Natality Survey demonstrated that 39 per cent of women admitted to alcohol use during their pregnancy (Prager et al., 1985), and a more recent publication showed that 25 per cent of the women questioned reported a continuation of drinking while pregnant. While it is encouraging to note that this figure decreased from 32 per cent in 1985 to 20 per cent in 1988, no such trend was apparent among the unmarried, those less than 24 years of age, smokers, and those with less formal education (Serdula et al., 1991). The prevalence of heavy or problem drinkers varies from 6 to 11 per cent, depending upon methodology and terminology (Abel and Sokol, 1989; Sokol et al., 1981), and these pregnancies are thought to be the most consistently and severely affected (Rosett et al., 1983).

TABLE 13–2.   Criteria for Urine Drug Screening

Physical appearance and demeanor
  Altered mental status
  Pupils extremely dilated or constricted
  Track marks/abscesses in extremities
  Inflamed or indurated nasal mucosa
Obstetric (past or present)
  Preterm labor/preterm delivery
  Low-birth-weight infant
  Intrauterine growth restriction
  Premature rupture of membranes
  Placental abruption
  Fetal death
  Unexplained congenital anomalies
  Suspected neonatal withdrawal symptoms
  Absent or erratic prenatal care
Medical
  AIDS/HIV infection
  Cellulitis
  Cirrhosis
  Endocarditis
  Hepatitis
  Pancreatitis
  Pneumonia
  Sexually transmitted diseases
Social
  Illicit drug use by partner
  Incarceration
  Prostitution
  Domestic violence

Modified from Chasnoff IJ: Perinatal effects of cocaine. Contemp Ob/Gyn **29**:164, 1987.

The pharmacokinetics of ethanol in the maternal-fetal unit have been studied extensively. There are data demonstrating an unimpeded and bidirectional movement of alcohol between the maternal and fetal compartments. Studies in human subjects (Idanpann-Heikkila et al., 1972), sheep (Brien et al., 1985, 1987; Clarke et al., 1988), guinea pigs (Clarke et al., 1986), and mice (Blakeley and Scott, 1984) demonstrate that maternal and fetal blood alcohol concentrations are equivalent. Investigations in the human (Brien et al., 1983) and in the pregnant ewe (Brien et al., 1987; Clarke et al., 1988) suggest that amniotic fluid levels rise more slowly than fetal blood levels, but remain detectable following the disappearance of ethanol from the fetal circulation. It is known that the activity of alcohol dehydrogenase in fetal liver is less than 10 per cent of that observed in the adult liver (Pikkarainen and Raiha, 1967; Clarke et al., 1989; Cumming et al., 1985). Therefore, the fetus is reliant upon maternal hepatic transformation of ingested ethanol and may be exposed to prolonged levels of ethanol in the amniotic fluid.

The mechanisms by which ethanol exerts its effects on the developing fetus are complex. Various animal models have been used to demonstrate that ethanol exposure interferes with protein synthesis (Dresoti et al., 1981; Henderson et al., 1980; Inselman et al., 1985) as well as the placental transfer of amino acids and glucose (Fisher et al., 1981; Gordon et al., 1985; Snyder et al., 1986; Marquis et al., 1984). Fetal hypoglycemia, hypoinsulinemia, and a decrease in fetal thyroid hormones and liver glycogen stores have also been demonstrated (Rose et al., 1981; Singh et al., 1984, 1986) and may contribute to abnormalities of fetal growth. Alterations in urinary metabolites of prostacyclin and thromboxane have been reported in neonates born to alcoholic women (Ylikorkala et al., 1988), suggesting that an alteration in the prostacyclin:thromboxane ratio and resultant vasoconstriction may explain in part the various fetal effects. Halmesmaki and co-workers (1990) have hypothesized that ethanol-exposed fetuses are subjected to chronic hypoxemia, reflected by elevated erythropoietin levels in cord blood samples.

The fetal alcohol syndrome (FAS) is a specific, recognizable pattern of malformations generally defined as (1) prenatal and postnatal growth deficiency; (2) central nervous system abnormalities; and (3) craniofacial abnormalities (Sokol and Clarren, 1989) (Fig. 13–1). Table 13–3 lists the specific criteria for FAS. The reported incidence of FAS varies widely from 1 in 2500 to 1 in 500 live births (Obe and Majewski, 1978; Olegard et al., 1979; Sokol et al., 1980; Clarren and Smith, 1978). A recent review of the available data concluded that the rate of FAS in the western world is 0.33 per 1000 live births (Abel and Sokol, 1991). The incidence of FAS among alcoholics is significantly greater and has been reported to be as high as 32 per cent (Jones et al., 1974). In addition to the craniofacial malformations, cardiovascular defects (Sandor et al., 1981) have been reported to occur with greater frequency in alcohol-exposed fetuses. It is important to note that the morphologic abnormalities characteristic of FAS have been observed in several animal models of chronic ethanol exposure (Clarren and Bowden,

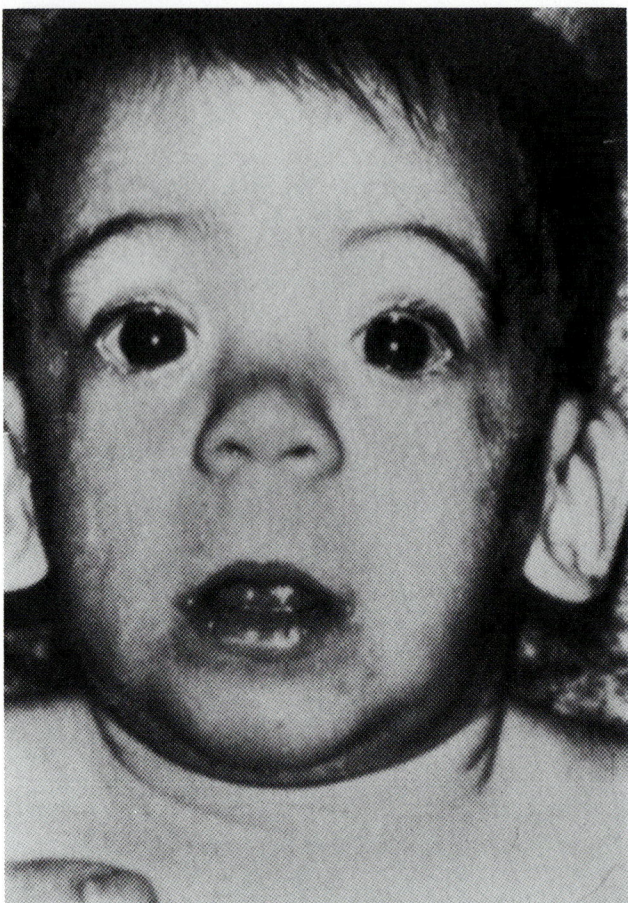

FIGURE 13–1. Nine-month-old infant with the fetal alcohol syndrome. (From Streissguth AP, Aase JM, Clarren SK, et al: Fetal alcohol syndrome in adolescents and adults. JAMA **265**:1961, 1991. Copyright 1991, The American Medical Association.)

1982; Ellis and Pick, 1980; Randall et al., 1977). Recent work (Streissguth et al., 1991) has shown that the effects of FAS persist into adolescence and adulthood. A mean IQ of 68 was noted among the 61 patients evaluated by this group of investigators.

Although a few reports have failed to show a significant effect of alcohol on birth weight (Tennes and Blackard, 1980; Marbury et al., 1983; Coles et al., 1985), the overwhelming majority of studies support the association (Hanson et al., 1978; Day et al., 1989; Kaminski et al., 1978; Ouellette et al., 1977; Rosett et

Table 13–3. Criteria for Fetal Alcohol Syndrome

Prenatal and/or growth restriction; failure to thrive (weight, length, and/or head circumference <10th percentile)
Central nervous system involvement including signs of neurologic abnormalities (irritability in infancy and hyperactivity during childhood), developmental delay, hypotonia, or intellectual impairment (mild-to-moderate mental retardation)
Characteristic facial dysmorphology (at least 2 of 3):
  Microcephaly (head circumference <3rd percentile)
  Microphthalmia and/or short palpebral fissures
  Poorly developed philtrum, thin upper lip (vermilion border), and flattening or absence of the maxilla

al., 1983; Halmesmaki, 1988; Little, 1977; Kaminski et al., 1981). Studies conducted in both cultured rat embryos (Brown et al., 1979) and C3H mice (Lochery et al., 1981) have shown a dose-dependent reduction in growth associated with ethanol exposure. Similarly, a decrease in mean fetal weight has been documented in the ovine fetus after chronic exposure to an intravenous ethanol infusion (Rose et al., 1981) and in beagles following chronic gastric lavage with ethanol (Ellis and Pick, 1980).

Mills et al. (1984) reported on over 30,000 pregnancies followed prospectively, noting a decrease in mean birth weight of 165 gm for babies born to patients reporting three to five drinks per day. Sokol et al. (1980) observed a similar decrease in birth weight (190 gm) when comparing nondrinkers to those using alcohol during their pregnancy. Data from the National Natality Survey conducted by the National Center for Health Statistics (Virji, 1991) demonstrated a significant difference in mean birth weight among those patients with moderate (1 to 13 drinks/week) alcohol use (3181.3 gm) and heavy (>2 drinks/day) alcohol use (2808.1 gm) compared to patients who were abstinent during pregnancy (3301.1 gm). Both Virji and Mills et al. demonstrated a dose-dependent increase in the incidence of low-birth-weight infant delivery. Among the "heavy" drinkers, 33 per cent (11/33) delivered a baby weighing <2500 gm (Virji, 1991). These differences remained significant after adjusting for smoking, maternal weight gain, parity, and level of education. Evidence also supports a decrease in mean birth length and in mean head circumference among infants with *in utero* exposure to ethanol (Ouellette et al., 1977; Smith et al., 1986; Day et al., 1989).

There are data from both animal models (Clarren and Astley, 1992) and human subjects (Kaminski et al., 1981; Kline et al., 1980; Harlap and Shiono, 1980) suggesting that the use of alcohol is associated with an increased risk of spontaneous abortion. However, there is little support for alcohol use as an independent risk factor for preterm delivery (Mills et al., 1984; Sokol et al., 1980; Kaminski et al., 1978; Day et al., 1989).

Counseling pregnant patients about a "safe" level of alcohol consumption is, to say the least, problematic. Although there is agreement that heavy alcohol use places the patient at a significant risk of delivering a low-birth-weight baby or an infant with FAS, a "safe" level of alcohol consumption has not been determined. At present there is no clear minimum threshold for the effects of alcohol on the fetus, and pregnant women should be counseled to abstain from its use. Obstetricians caring for patients with known alcohol abuse problems must be prepared to manage the multitude of medical problems encountered in this population (e.g., hepatic cirrhosis, esophageal varices, pancreatitis, delirium tremens). Patients contemplating breast feeding should be made aware of case reports linking alcohol in breast milk with pseudo-Cushing's syndrome (Binkiewicz et al., 1978) and hypoprothrombinemic bleeding (Hoh, 1969).

There is evidence that the risk of alterations in fetal growth (i.e., decreased head circumference and low birth weight) and of possibly the entire FAS can be significantly lowered by reducing alcohol intake dur-

TABLE 13–4. The T-ACE Questions Found to Be Significant Identifiers of Risk Drinking*

T	How many drinks does it take to make you feel high (TOLERANCE)?
A	Have people ANNOYED you by criticizing your drinking?
C	Have you felt you ought to CUT DOWN on your drinking?
E	Have you ever had a drink first thing in the morning to steady your nerves or get rid of a hangover (EYE-OPENER)?

*Alcohol intake sufficient to potentially damage the embryo or fetus.

ing the pregnancy (Rosett et al., 1983; Halmesmaki, 1988). Given this information it is clear that identifying the pregnant alcohol user is of critical importance. However, Sokol and Miller (1980) found that three of every four pregnant patients with alcohol abuse problems went undetected by the clinician. Several approaches to detecting alcohol use by way of patient interview have been studied (Ewing, 1984; Pokorny et al., 1972). Sokol et al. (1989) have reported on the T-ACE questionnaire (Table 13–4) in 971 pregnant patients. The probability of risk drinking increased from 1.5 per cent in those responding negatively to all four questions to 63 per cent for those answering positively to all four items. This brief screening tool for alcohol abuse should be included in every initial prenatal visit.

SMOKING

The deleterious effects of cigarette smoking on pregnancy outcome have been recognized for decades. A 1980 report from the Surgeon General stated that from 21 to 39 per cent of all low-birth-weight infants could be attributed to smoking (US Department of Health and Human Services, 1980), making this one of the most preventable causes of low birth weight (Institute of Medicine, 1985). Simpson (1957) is credited with reporting the relationship between cigarette smoking and an increase in the incidence of prematurity (birth weight <2500 gm). A dose-response effect of smoking on the incidence of low birth weight has been noted in several investigations (Meyer et al., 1976; Miller and Jekel, 1987; McDonald et al., 1992a). Data from the Ontario Perinatal Mortality Study demonstrated that women smoking >1 pack of cigarettes daily had a 130 per cent increase in their risk of delivering an infant weighing <2500 gm, while those smoking <1 pack per day increased their risk by 53 per cent (Meyer et al., 1976). The association with low birth weight is due primarily to intrauterine growth restriction and is observed across gestational ages (Davies et al., 1976; Hoff et al., 1986). A recent study by McDonald (1992a) concluded that the odds ratio for the delivery of a small-for-gestational-age infant (birth weight <5th percentile) was 3.19 (95 per cent CI 2.82–3.60) among women who smoke >20 cigarettes/day. For every 10 cigarettes smoked daily, the risk was shown to increase by a factor of 1.51.

Studies show that the average difference in birth weight between infants of smokers and those of nonsmokers ranges from 127 to 274 gm (Jeanty et al., 1987; Kline et al., 1987; Hebel et al., 1988; Pulkkinen, 1990).

As is true with the incidence of low birth weight, the effect of smoking on the difference in mean birth weight is thought to be dose-dependent (Hebel et al., 1988; Hoff et al., 1986; Beaulac-Baillargeon and Desrosiers, 1987; Haddow et al., 1987). A recent prospective cohort study of 772 mother-infant pairs found that women who were self-reported smokers delivered infants who were on the average 141.8 gm lighter than the infants born to nonsmokers (Abell et al., 1991). Differences in mean birth weight were observed in those smoking <10 cigarettes/day (–96 gm), 10 to 19 cigarettes/day (–183 gm) and >20 cigarettes/day (–200 gm), again suggesting a dose-dependent effect on birth weight.

The physiologic explanations for the adverse consequence of cigarette smoking during pregnancy center on the effects of carbon monoxide (CO) and nicotine. Carbon monoxide crosses the placenta (Longo and Ching, 1977) and binds to hemoglobin to form carboxyhemoglobin (HbCO), which has been shown to reduce the oxygen-carrying capacity of the blood (Astrup, 1972). Similarly, CO increases the affinity of hemoglobin for oxygen, which in turn interferes with oxygen delivery to the tissues (Longo, 1977). Studies in both the pregnant ewe (Longo and Hill, 1977) and in the human (Bureau et al., 1982) have shown that fetal HbCO levels exceed maternal HbCO levels, leading to a relatively prolonged fetal exposure to the effects of HbCO (Fig. 13–2).

Nicotine, a compound with a very basic character (pka = 7.8), readily crosses the placenta (Manning and Feyerabend, 1976) and reaches the fetal circulation. The concentration of nicotine in fetal serum has been shown to exceed maternal serum levels in the ewe (Monheit et al., 1983), in the rhesus monkey (Suzuki et al., 1974), and more recently in the human (Luck et al., 1985). Suzuki and colleagues (1980) have shown that uterine blood flow is reduced by as much as 38 per cent (Fig. 13–3) compared with control values

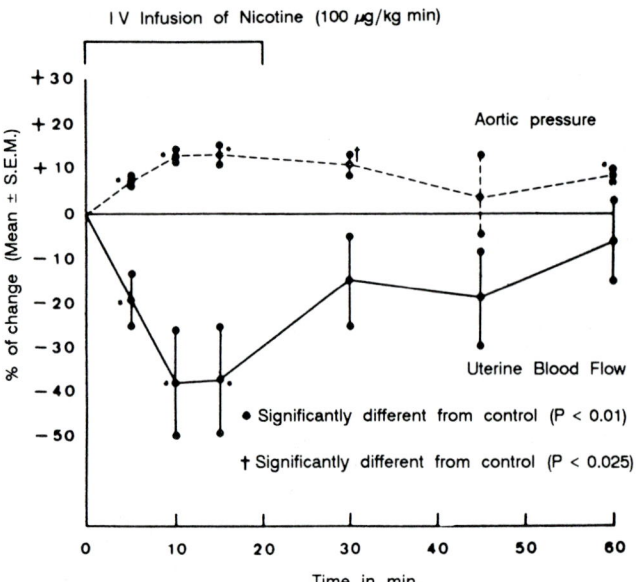

FIGURE 13–3. Changes in aortic pressure and uterine arterial blood flow in the pregnant rhesus monkey following intravenous infusion of nicotine. (From Suzuki K, Minei LJ, Johnson EE: Effect of nicotine upon uterine blood flow in the pregnant rhesus monkey. Am J Obstet Gynecol **136**:1009, 1980.)

following the intravascular infusion of nicotine to the pregnant rhesus monkey. Similar alterations in uterine blood flow have been reported by Monheit et al. (1983), who used the pregnant ewe. The effect of nicotine on fetal oxygenation and acid-base balance is controversial, with some studies showing a significant hypoxemia and acidemia (Suzuki et al., 1980; Manning et al., 1978) and others unable to demonstrate any changes in Pao$_2$ or pH (Monheit et al., 1983). The mechanism for uterine artery vasoconstriction is probably mediated through an increase in circulating catecholamines. Resnik et al. (1979) demonstrated a significant increase in both epinephrine (60.4 per cent) and norepinephrine (70.1 per cent) levels over control values following an infusion of nicotine to the pregnant ewe (Fig. 13–4). In addition, in the human, amniotic fluid catecholamine levels are significantly higher in smokers than in nonsmokers (Divers et al., 1981).

Smoking has emerged as an independent risk factor for preterm labor and delivery. Several studies have suggested an increase in the relative risk (range 1.4 to 1.8) of preterm delivery among smokers compared to women who do not smoke during their pregnancy (Guzick et al., 1984; Meyer et al., 1976; Mulcahy and Murphy, 1972). A recent prospective study from the National Institute of Child Health and Development showed that preterm birth (<37 weeks gestation) occurred in 6.8 per cent of nonsmokers compared to 8.1 per cent of women who smoked >1 pack of cigarettes daily. The adjusted odds ratio for preterm birth among the smokers was 1.2 (95 per cent CI = 1.1–1.4), with an attributable risk due to smoking of 4 per cent (Shiono et al., 1986). Also, a case-control study of 140 spontaneous preterm births and 280 term births found

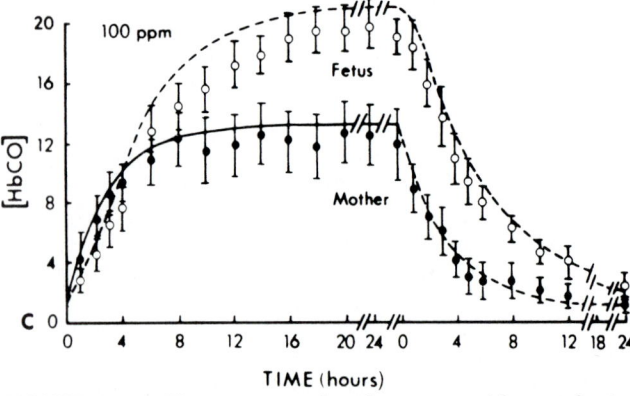

FIGURE 13–2. Time course of carbon monoxide uptake in maternal and fetal sheep exposed to carbon monoxide. The experimental results for the ewe (●) and fetal lamb (○) are the mean values (± S.E.M.). The theoretic predictions of the changes in maternal and fetal carboxyhemoglobin levels for the ewe and lamb are shown by the solid and interrupted lines, respectively. (From Longo LD: The biological effects of carbon monoxide on the pregnant woman, fetus, and newborn infant. Am J Obstet Gynecol **129**:69, 1977.)

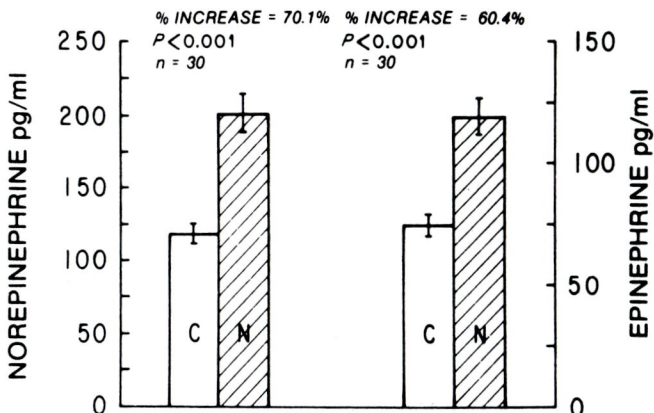

FIGURE 13–4. Plasma concentrations of norepinephrine and epinephrine in the control period (C) and during nicotine infusion (N). (Reproduced from Resnik R, Brink GW, Wilkes M: Catecholamine-mediated reduction in uterine blood flow after nicotine infusion in the pregnant ewe. J Clin Invest **63**:1133, 1979, by copyright permission of the American Society for Clinical Investigation.)

smoking to be an independent risk factor for preterm delivery (deHass et al., 1991). The relative risk for preterm birth among all smokers in this study was 1.6 (95 per cent CI = 0.9–2.9). Furthermore, the risk increased with increasing numbers of cigarettes smoked daily, so that in women smoking >10 cigarettes per day, the relative risk of preterm birth was 2.0 (95 per cent CI = 0.8–4.9).

Several authors (Williams et al., 1991; Meyer et al., 1976; Kramer et al., 1989) have noted an increase in the risk of placenta previa among smokers. In a case-control analysis, Williams et al. (1991) demonstrated the adjusted relative risk of placenta previa among smokers to be 2.6 compared to nonsmokers. It has been suggested that placental hypertrophy observed in women who smoke cigarettes increases the risk of implantation in the lower uterine segment over the cervical os. Placental abruption has also been reported to occur with greater frequency among smokers (Naeye, 1980; Meyer and Tonascia, 1977). Specific histologic changes found in the placentas of smokers include thickening of the villous membrane and the trophoblastic layer (Jauniaux and Burton, 1992; Van der Veen and Fox, 1982; Burton et al., 1989; Rush et al., 1986), changes that may affect the diffusional resistance for oxygen.

The risk of spontaneous abortion appears to be increased among smokers, with studies demonstrating a relative risk ranging from 1.1 to 1.8 (Armstrong et al., 1992; Kline et al., 1977; Himmelberger et al., 1978). There is no significant support for an association between smoking and congenital anomalies (McDonald et al., 1992b; Hemminki et al., 1983; Evans et al., 1979; Shiono et al., 1986).

There is evidence that reducing the number of cigarettes smoked per day has a positive impact on birth weight (McDonald et al., 1992a; Sexton and Hebel, 1984; MacArthur and Knox, 1988). Both McDonald and MacArthur have shown that if smoking is discontinued by the end of the first trimester, the patient is at no greater risk for fetal growth abnormalities than the nonsmoker. A prospective, randomized and controlled study of 935 smokers demonstrated a 92-gm increase in birth weight and a 0.6-cm increase in birth length in infants of a group of patients enrolled in a smoking intervention program. The patients in the smoking intervention program decreased their mean number of cigarettes from 10.7 to 6.4 daily while the other group continued at approximately 12 cigarettes per day. Given the evidence for various perinatal complications associated with cigarette smoking during pregnancy, clinicians should counsel women about the risks associated with smoking and encourage any attempts to stop or decrease the use of cigarettes during or before their pregnancy.

COFFEE

Caffeine-containing beverages, including coffee, are widely consumed by pregnant women. Concerns over the ingestion of caffeine during pregnancy extend back to a report linking the substance with skeletal malformations in mice (Nishimura and Nakai, 1960). Since that time, several other animal models have reinforced the potential for an association between caffeine use and birth defects (Nolen, 1988). These data led to a report from the United States Food and Drug Administration (1980) that recommended a limitation on caffeine intake during pregnancy. Although two studies have reported an association with ectrodactyly and cleft palate (Furuhashi et al., 1985; Borlee et al., 1978), clinical investigations offer little support for any causal link between caffeine and congenital anomalies. In fact, several authors (Rosenberg et al., 1982; McDonald et al., 1992b; Linn et al., 1982; Kurpa et al., 1983) have shown that there is no increase in the risk of fetal skeletal malformations, orofacial clefts, neural tube defects, or cardiac defects among coffee drinkers.

The association between spontaneous abortion and caffeine use is also controversial. Several authors have reported an increased risk of miscarriage (Weathersbee et al., 1977; Mau and Netter, 1974; Furuhashi et al., 1985), whereas others have failed to show any such increase in risk (Watkinson and Fried, 1985; Linn et al., 1982).

There is evidence supporting an increased risk of low-birth-weight infants among caffeine users. Martin and Bracken (1987) prospectively studied 3891 patients of whom 77 per cent consumed caffeine during their pregnancy. Those ingesting caffeine-containing products were divided into low (1 to 150 mg/day), moderate (151 to 300 mg/day), and heavy (>301 mg/day) use groups. The relative risks of delivering a low-birth-weight infant were 1.4, 2.3, and 4.6, respectively. The decreases in mean birth weight among low, moderate, and heavy users, compared with the control group, were 6, 31, and 105 gm, respectively. These differences persisted after controlling for numerous risk factors, including smoking. A similar decrease in mean birth weight (121 gm) was reported by Munoz et al. (1988) among a group of patients consuming >450 mg caffeine per day. In balance, the majority of published studies suggest an increased risk of delivering a low-birth-weight infant and/or a small decrease in mean birth weight (Watkinson and Fried, 1985; Furuhashi et al., 1985; Kuzma and Sokol, 1982; van der Berg, 1977; Mau and Netter, 1974). This effect was most prominent in those ingesting >300 mg/day (approximately 3 cups of coffee). It seems prudent to recommend that pregnant women who choose to consume coffee or other caffeine-containing substances limit their intake to 300 mg/day.

COCAINE

Cocaine is derived from the leaves of the *Erythroxylon coca* plant. It exerts its effect by interfering with the re-uptake of neutrotransmitter substances, such as dopamine and norepinephrine, at the presynaptic nerve terminals. This results in vasoconstriction, tachycardia, hypertension, and an increase in circulating catecholamines (Ritchie and Greene, 1985). The drug can be administered by intravenous injection or by "snorting" (intranasal) the powder form. The alkaloidal cocaine (free base), which is often referred to as "crack," is a heat-stable preparation that can be smoked as a cigarette, with absorption through the alveolar membranes (Medical Letter, 1986). The drug is metabolized by the action of plasma and hepatic cholinesterases (Stewart et al., 1979). Plasma cholinesterase activity may be diminished in pregnant women and in the fetus, leading to an accumulation of cocaine and an increase in the potential for toxicity (Hadeed and Siegel, 1989; Telsey et al., 1988). The major metabolites of cocaine are benzoylecognine and ecognine methyl ester, which are water soluble and excreted in the urine (Fish and Wilson, 1969). These metabolites are detectable in the maternal urine for 48 to 72 hours following the use of cocaine.

The medical complications of cocaine use in adults are well described (Cregler and Marx, 1986). Data support the hypothesis that the cardiovascular effects of cocaine are even more pronounced during pregnancy (Plessinger and Woods, 1990). This may be due to the effect of progesterone, which increases the metabolism of cocaine to norcocaine (a biologically active metabolite), or to the increasing sensitivity of alpha-adrenergic receptors associated with pregnancy (Woods and Plessinger, 1990).

The association between cocaine use during pregnancy and an increased risk of congenital anomalies is controversial. The hypothesized mechanism centers on the deformation/destruction of normally formed embryonic structures secondary to an interruption of blood supply. In general, the anomalies reported to occur more frequently among cocaine-exposed fetuses involve the extremities and the genitourinary, cardiovascular, and central nervous systems.

Basic science work offers support for the association. Webster and Brown-Woodman (1990) treated Sprague-Dawley rats with cocaine and noted the offspring to have hemorrhages involving the head, limbs, tail, and genital tubercle. They hypothesize that an interruption of blood flow led to necrosis and to disruption of both developing and normally formed structures. Several other investigators have reported an increase in anom-

alies related to *in utero* cocaine exposure (Finnell et al., 1990; Mahalik et al., 1980). Although negative studies have been published (Fantel and McPhail, 1982; Church et al., 1987), it is interesting to note that the specific anomalies demonstrated in animal models closely resemble the pattern of abnormalities observed clinically.

The possibility that cocaine may be associated with an increase in congenital anomalies was first suggested by Chasnoff et al. (1985). In this report, two cases of genitourinary tract abnormalities were discovered in 23 neonates. In a follow-up prospective study, 50 cocaine-exposed neonates underwent renal ultrasonography on days 2 to 3 of life and were compared to a group of 30 polydrug-exposed (non-cocaine) neonates. Among the cocaine group there were seven genitourinary tract malformations, but no genitourinary tract abnormalities were seen in the polydrug group (Chasnoff et al., 1988). However, a recently published prospective evaluation involving renal ultrasonography of 100 cocaine-exposed neonates failed to demonstrate a significant increase in the incidence of genitourinary tract anomalies (Rosenstein et al., 1990). Numerous clinical reports address the incidence of congenital anomalies among cocaine users. Retrospective (Madden et al., 1986; Gillogley et al., 1990; Cherukuri et al., 1988) and prospective (Hadeed and Siegel, 1989) investigations have been published suggesting that there is no significant increase in the risk of anomalies. Alternatively, there are reports, again retrospective (Chavez et al., 1989) as well as prospective (Bingol et al., 1987; Zuckerman et al., 1989), that demonstrate an increase in the incidence of congenital anomalies. A recent review of 119 cocaine-exposed neonates supports the association between cocaine use and congenital anomalies. When these infants were compared with 100 drug-free controls, the odds ratio for minor anomalies was 1.6, for major anomalies 4.99, and for genitourinary anomalies 6.5 (Little and Snell, 1991b). Congenital heart defects were also significantly more common in the cocaine-exposed group, a finding reinforced by a recent retrospective study of 114 cocaine-exposed neonates (Lipschultz et al., 1991).

In 1983 a report of two cases of placental abruption occurring in women admitting to cocaine use was published (Acker et al., 1983). This association between cocaine use and abruptio placentae seems plausible given the hypertensive effects of cocaine and the association between hypertension and placental abruption (Pritchard et al., 1970). Following this case report, Chasnoff and co-workers (1985) published their experience with a small group of cocaine-using women who were receiving prenatal care at their institution. Placental abruption was noted in 4 of 23 cocaine-using women, in contrast to 15 opiate-dependent women and 15 drug-free controls, in whom no cases of abruption were observed. Most investigations published since that time have been limited by a relatively small sample size, a lack of uniformity in diagnostic criteria for abruption, and inconsistent pathologic examinations of the placenta. The majority of studies support an increase in the relative risk of abruption among cocaine users, with several authors demonstrating a statistically significant increase in incidence (Chasnoff et al., 1989b; Hadeed and Siegel, 1989; Oro and Dixon, 1987; Chasnoff et al., 1987; Bingol et al., 1987; MacGregor et al., 1987; Neerhoff et al., 1989). A recent investigation retrospectively reviewed the records of 592 cocaine users and 4687 drug-free control patients. Placental abruption was diagnosed significantly more frequently among the cocaine users (11/592; 1.9 per cent) than among the controls (45/4677; 1.0 per cent) (Dombrowski et al., 1991).

A decrease in mean fetal weight has been demonstrated following administration of cocaine hydrochloride to pregnant rats (Fantel and McPhail, 1982; Church et al., 1987). The decrease in fetal weight was shown to develop independent of maternal weight changes, suggesting a direct effect of cocaine on fetal growth rather than simply the effect of maternal malnutrition. The impairment of fetal growth may be explained by the drug's vasoconstrictive effect on the uteroplacental circulation. Studies in both the pregnant ewe and the pregnant baboon have demonstrated a decrease in uterine blood flow following the intravenous administration of cocaine (Moore et al., 1986 [Fig. 13–5]; Woods et al., 1987; Morgan et al., 1991). Similarly, fetal hypertension, tachycardia, and hypoxemia have been demonstrated following maternal administration of the drug. Chronic fetal hypoxemia

(Soothill et al., 1986) and diminished uteroplacental blood flow (Creasy et al., 1972; Clapp et al., 1980) have been associated with suboptimal fetal growth.

Numerous studies have noted a decrease in mean birth weight associated with cocaine use during pregnancy (Kaye et al., 1989; Ryan et al., 1987; Zuckerman et al., 1989; MacGregor et al., 1989; Gillogley et al., 1990; Bingol et al., 1987; Chouteau et al., 1988; Chasnoff et al., 1989b; Hadeed and Siegel, 1989; Fulroth et al., 1989; Cherukuri et al., 1988; Oro and Dixon, 1987; Dixon and Bejar, 1989). Given the increase in morbidity and mortality associated with low-birth-weight infants (McCormick, 1985), the identification and elimination of any contributing factor are of utmost importance. A recent investigation demonstrated that the mean birth weight among 366 infants born to cocaine-using women (2663 gm) was 376 gm less than that for a control group that was well matched for factors associated with low birth weight (Kaye et al., 1989). The mean birth weight among infants born to 52 cocaine-using women receiving care at the Perinatal Center for Chemical Dependence at Northwestern University was 2829 gm, with 13 (25 per cent) weighing <2500 gm. The infants born to the drug-free control group were noted to have a mean birth weight of 3436 gm and 2 (5 per cent) weighed <2500 gm (Chasnoff et al., 1989b). The two groups were matched for maternal age, maternal weight gain, cigarette use, parity, and racial distribution.

The diagnosis of intrauterine growth restriction (IUGR) is often difficult in this population given the importance of an accurate evaluation of gestational age. However, numerous studies suggest a higher incidence of IUGR in women who use cocaine during pregnancy (Oro and Dixon, 1987; Hadeed and Siegel, 1989; Chasnoff et al., 1989b; Ryan et al., 1987; Cherukuri et al., 1988; MacGregor et al., 1987; Neerhoff et al., 1989; Fulroth et al., 1989; Keith et al., 1989). Keith and co-investigators noted a higher incidence of small-for-gestational-age neonates among 63 cocaine users (19 per cent) than among 123 drug-free control patients (6 per cent).

Several studies suggest that neonatal head circumference is significantly smaller than expected for gestational age (Little and Snell, 1991a; Chasnoff et al., 1989b; Fulroth et al., 1989; Gillogley et al., 1990; Bingol et al., 1987; Cherukuri et al., 1988; Ryan et al., 1987; Hadeed and Siegel, 1989; Oro and Dixon, 1987; Little et al., 1989). Whereas this finding is associated with the fetal alcohol syndrome (Smith et al., 1986; Day et al., 1989) and chromosomal abnormalities, it is not the typical pattern seen with "asymmetric intrauterine growth retardation." The significance of the diminished head circumference lies in its association with altered brain growth and with abnormal neurodevelopmental outcome (Ross and Frias, 1977). Postmortem examination of abortuses (Kapur et al., 1991) (Fig. 13–6) and computerized tomographic images of neonates (Chasnoff et al., 1986) support the occurrence of *in utero* cerebral hemorrhage. This may contribute to alterations in fetal brain growth and resultant microcephaly. A recent study observed that cocaine-exposed neonates have an increased cerebral blood flow velocity, a situation that predisposes to intracranial hemorrhage (van de Bor et al., 1990).

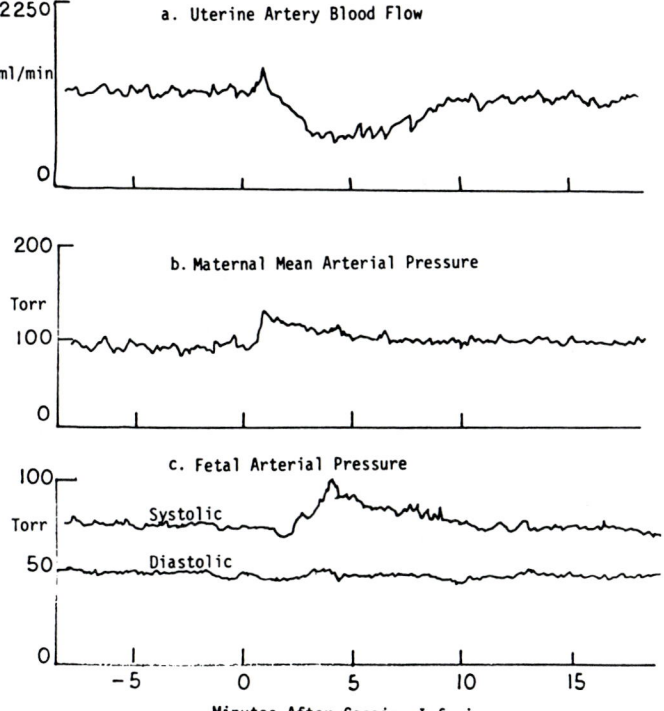

FIGURE 13–5. Maternal and fetal cardiovascular responses to cocaine infusion. *a,* Maternal uterine artery blood flow after infusion of 0.5 mg/kg of cocaine during 1 minute. *b,* Maternal mean arterial blood pressure response to cocaine infusion. *c,* Fetal arterial (systolic/diastolic) pressure response to infusion of 0.5 mg/kg of cocaine. (From Moore TR, Sorg J, Miller L, et al: Hemodynamic effects of intravenous cocaine on the pregnant ewe and fetus. Am J Obstet Gynecol **155**:883, 1986.)

The available data strongly support the association between cocaine use and preterm labor and delivery. Although the specific mechanism is not understood, studies utilizing both the pregnant rat (Daniel, 1964) and the pregnant rabbit (Hurd et al., 1991b) suggest that cocaine may have a stimulatory effect on myometrial contractility. Hurd and co-workers (1991a) have shown that cocaine blocks the extraneuronal re-uptake of catecholamines in the pregnant human uterus. They speculate that this may lead to an enhanced alpha-adrenergic-mediated contractile response in the myometrium and/or an increase in endometrial production of PGE_2 and $PGF_{2\alpha}$. Other investigators, utilizing human myometrial cell culture, have shown that cocaine has an inhibitory effect on adenylate cyclase and leads to intracellular mobilization of calcium (Molinar et al., 1992; Hertlendy et al., 1992). The administration of cocaine to the near-term pregnant ewe has not resulted in a significant increase in myometrial electromyographic activity or maternal plasma oxytocin concentrations (Owiny et al., 1992).

The overwhelming majority of data from clinical investigations support an increased incidence of preterm labor and delivery among cocaine-using women (Table 13–5) (Cherukuri et al., 1988; MacGregor et al., 1987; Keith et al., 1989; Chasnoff et al., 1989b; Hadeed and Siegel, 1989; Neerhoff et al., 1989; Little et al., 1989; Oro and Dixon, 1987; Gillogley et al., 1990). Ney and colleagues (1990) showed that among 141 patients with suspected preterm labor, 24 (17 per cent) had a positive urine toxicology screen, with 14 testing positive for cocaine. In contrast, of 108 control patients (no evidence of preterm labor), only 3 (2.8 per cent) had positive urine toxicology screens. A retrospective chart review of 55 "crack" cocaine users and a matched group of drug-free control patients showed a dramatic increase in preterm delivery (<37 weeks) among the cocaine group when compared to controls (50.9 per cent vs. 16.4 per cent) (Cherukuri et al., 1988). Among patients receiving their prenatal care in a specialized substance abuse clinic, the incidence of preterm delivery (defined as <38 weeks gestation) was 31 per cent (16/52) in contrast to a control group, in which 1 of 40 (3 per cent) delivered preterm (Chasnoff et al., 1989b).

Available data offer little support for an increase in depressed Apgar scores (Oro and Dixon, 1987; Keith et al., 1989; MacGregor et al., 1987; Kaye et al., 1989), premature rupture of the membranes (Mastrogiannis et al., 1990; Oro and Dixon, 1987; Keith et al., 1989), or spontaneous abortion (Ryan et al., 1987; Keith et al., 1989; Oro and Dixon, 1987) among cocaine-using women. Although precipitate delivery has been reported to occur more commonly among cocaine users (Chasnoff et al., 1987), a recent study suggests that cocaine has no effect on the duration of labor (Dombrowski et al., 1991).

Central nervous system abnormalities including periventricular/intraventricular hemorrhage (Dixon and Bejar, 1989; Kapur et al., 1991), cerebral infarction (Chasnoff et al., 1987, 1986; Tenorio et al., 1988), electroencephalographic changes, and seizure activity have been described (Doberczak et al., 1988; Kramer et al., 1990). Exposed neonates are thought to be at increased risk for the development of necrotizing enterocolitis (Porat and Brodsky, 1991; Telsey et al., 1988). This is supported by reports of intestinal ischemia in adults following cocaine ingestion (Nalbandian et al., 1985) and by cases of intestinal atresia-infarction that have been reported in exposed neonates (Hoyme et al., 1990).

Whether or not a true neonatal withdrawal follows *in utero* cocaine exposure is controversial (Doberczak et al., 1988; Fulroth et al., 1989; Oro and Dixon, 1987; Dixon and Bejar, 1989; Hadeed and Siegel, 1989; Ryan et al., 1987; Livesay et al., 1987). It would appear that neonatal withdrawal symptomatology is much less common after cocaine exposure than after opiate exposure (Ryan et al., 1987).

Although sudden infant death syndrome (SIDS) has been reported to occur more commonly among infants born to cocaine users (Chasnoff et al., 1989c), this

Table 13–5.   Incidence of Preterm Delivery*

AUTHOR	COCAINE USERS (%)		CONTROL (%)	
Keith et al., 1989	(17/63)	27	(9/123)	7
Chasnoff et al., 1989b	(16/52)	31	(1/40)	3
MacGregor et al., 1987	(6/24)	25	(2/70)	2.9
Gillogley et al., 1990	(44/139)	32	(48/299)	16
Oro and Dixon, 1987	(13/46)	28	(4/45)	9
Hadeed and Siegel, 1989	(13/32)	41	(8/29)	28
Neerhoff et al., 1989	(35/138)	25	(8/88)	9
Cherukuri et al., 1988	(28/55)	50.9	(9/55)	16.4
Little et al., 1989	(11/53)	21	(2/100)	2

*Preterm defined as <37 weeks except for studies by Chasnoff et al. (<38 weeks) and Hadeed and Siegel (<36 weeks).

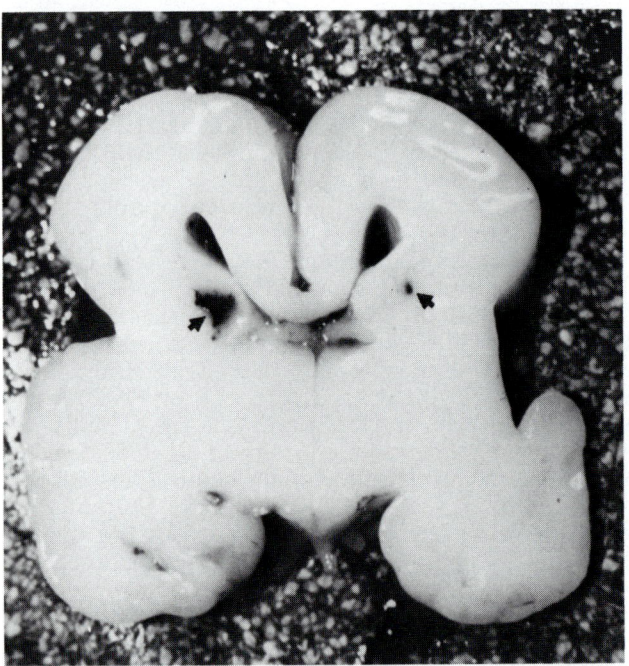

FIGURE 13–6. This coronal section of the fetal cerebrum shows bilateral hemorrhages (*arrows*) in the germinal matrices, left larger than right, found in fetus of mother using cocaine during the first trimester. (From Kapur RP, Shaw CM, Sheppard TH: Brain hemorrhages in cocaine-exposed human fetuses. Teratology **44**:11, Copyright © 1991. Reprinted by permission of Wiley-Liss, a Division of John Wiley and Sons, Inc.)

issue remains unsettled. A large-scale investigation has shown that the risk of SIDS in cocaine-exposed infants (5.6/1000 live births) is not significantly greater than that seen in a drug-free control group (4.0/1000) (Bauchner et al., 1988).

There is disagreement regarding the long-term consequences of *in utero* cocaine exposure. Several authors have observed a higher incidence of neurobehavioral abnormalities (e.g., sleeping patterns, feeding problems, hypertonia, tremors) in these infants (Oro and Dixon 1987; Chasnoff et al., 1989b). These infants appear to perform within the expected range on Bayley Scales and the Stanford Binet Test at age 2 to 3 years (Griffith et al., 1990; Chasnoff et al., 1992).

OPIATES

Opiates refer to naturally occurring substances, including morphine and codeine, that are recovered from the *Papaver somniferum* poppy. The term opioids refers to synthetic narcotics such as heroin, meperidine, fentanyl, propoxyphene, and methadone. Narcotics can be used orally, intranasally, intramuscularly, or intravenously. Most of the available data refer to the intravenous administration of heroin and, since its introduction in 1965 to treat opioid dependence, the oral administration of methadone (Dole and Nyswander, 1965).

No clear association has been established between opiate exposure and structural defects in the offspring. However, there is a well-defined neonatal withdrawal disorder called the neonatal abstinence syndrome (NAS). This disorder occurs in as many as two-thirds of exposed neonates (Stone et al., 1971; Wilson et al., 1973) and is generally clinically evident within 3 to 5 days. The clinical findings associated with neonatal withdrawal are listed in Table 13–6 (Stimmel and Jerez, 1985). The most common finding is central nervous system irritability, occurring in approximately 70 per cent of affected neonates (Cooper et al., 1983). Data exist to support a correlation between the severity of the neonatal withdrawal and both the daily metha-

done dose at delivery and the cumulative intake for the 3 months prior to delivery. A daily dose of less than 20 mg/day has been shown to be associated with a decrease in the incidence and the severity of neonatal withdrawal (Kandall et al., 1983; Madden, 1978; Ostrea et al., 1976). Long-term developmental sequelae have been reported and include an increased risk of behavioral and school-related problems. Interested readers are referred to an inclusive review by Wilson (1989).

Several perinatal complications have been reported to occur with greater frequency among opiate-dependent patients and their offspring. These include: (1) intrauterine growth restriction (Stone et al., 1971; Ostrea et al., 1976; Blinick et al., 1969; Fricker and Segal, 1978; Naeye et al., 1973a; Pellosi et al., 1975; Zelson et al., 1973; Kandall et al., 1977, 1976; Doberczak et al., 1987; Little et al., 1990; Chasnoff et al., 1982); (2) preterm delivery (Stone et al., 1971; Fricker and Segal, 1978; Pellosi et al., 1975; Little et al., 1990); (3) fetal death (Fricker and Segal, 1978; Zuspan et al., 1975; Rementeria and Nunag, 1973); (4) decreased head circumference (Doberczak et al., 1987; Chasnoff et al., 1982); (5) depressed Apgar scores (Ostrea et al., 1976); (6) meconium staining of the amniotic fluid (Ostrea et al., 1976; Blinick et al., 1969; Little et al., 1990); (7) premature rupture of the membranes (Ostrea et al., 1976); (8) multiple gestations (Ostrea et al., 1976); and (9) chorioamnionitis (Naeye et al., 1973a).

The association of maternal opiate use with altered fetal growth is supported by work in various animal models. Investigations in the pregnant rabbit (Taeusch et al., 1973; Roloff and Howalt, 1973; Raye et al., 1975) and in the pregnant mouse (Naeye et al., 1973b) have demonstrated delayed growth in the opiate-exposed offspring. Postmortem examination of 59 heroin-exposed newborns demonstrated a decrease in cell number in all organs studied (Naeye et al., 1973a). Other proposed mechanisms for altered fetal growth include decreased fetal growth hormone concentration (Cushman, 1972) and chronic fetal hypoxemia from cyclic opiate withdrawal (Cohen et al., 1980).

Clinical reports also support the association of opiate use with poor fetal growth. Chasnoff et al. (1982) compared 39 patients receiving low-dose methadone maintenance to 19 polydrug users and 27 drug-free women. A statistically significant decrease in mean birth weight was observed in the methadone group (2815 ± 613 gm) when compared to the drug-free control group (3492 ± 578 gm) and a significant decrease in head circumference was also noted in the methadone group (32.5 ± 1.9 cm) when compared to both the polydrug (33.8 ± 1.5 cm) and drug-free (34.6 ± 1.7 cm) groups. The decrease in head circumference has been reported by other authors (Doberczak et al., 1987). However, Lifschitz et al. (1983), reporting on 22 untreated heroin addicts, 21 polydrug users, and 28 drug-free patients, failed to demonstrate a difference in mean birth weight between groups that could not be explained by covariables such as smoking, prenatal care, maternal nutrition, race, or obstetrical risk.

The association of opiate use with preterm delivery is less clear than is the case with the use of other illicit drugs (e.g., cocaine). Although several studies have

TABLE 13–6. Neonatal Withdrawal Syndrome

Central nervous system symptoms	Respiratory system symptoms
Disturbance in sleep patterns	Nasal flaring
Hyperactivity	Nasal stuffiness
Hyperreflexia	Sneezing
Tremors	Tachypnea
Increased muscle tone	Yawning
Myoclonic jerks	Hiccups
Shrill cry	Gastrointestinal symptoms
Convulsions	Excessive sucking
Metabolic symptoms	Poor feeding
Fever	Vomiting
Hypoglycemia	Diarrhea
Mottling	
Sweating	
Yawning	
Vasomotor instability	

From Stimmel B, Jerez E: Alcohol and substance abuse during pregnancy. *In* Cherry SH, Berkowitz RL, Kase NG (eds): Medical, Surgical, and Gynecologic Complications of Pregnancy. Baltimore, Williams and Wilkins, © 1985, The Williams & Wilkins Company.

TABLE 13–7.   Signs of Opioid Intoxication in the Adult

Clouded mentation
Drowsiness
Analgesia
Euphoria
Decreased respirations
Diminished peristalsis with resultant constipation
Diminished drug seeking
Miosis

From Hoegerman G, Schnoll S: Narcotic use in pregnancy. Clin Perinatol 18:58, 1991.

suggested an increased rate of preterm delivery (Stone et al., 1971; Ostrea et al., 1976; Pellosi et al., 1975), others have failed to demonstrate such a relationship (Doberczak et al., 1987; Lifshitz et al., 1983). In balance, there is little support for an increase in the risk of preterm delivery among narcotic-dependent women.

The suggestion that methadone maintenance improves perinatal outcome and, more specifically, the incidence of fetal growth restriction is controversial. Several authors have observed an improvement in birth weight (Zelson et al., 1973; Kandall et al., 1976, 1977; Doberczak et al., 1987), whereas others have not demonstrated a significant difference (Rajegowda et al., 1972; Edelin et al., 1988). Regardless of the issue of fetal growth, the use of methadone in the pregnant narcotic user has several important advantages. The avoidance of intravenous drug use decreases the patient's risk of HIV infection and AIDS, hepatitis, and subacute bacterial endocarditis. In addition, the scheduled administration of methadone alleviates the pattern of recurrent withdrawal, which has been shown to result in significant fetal stress. Fetal hypoxemia, hypertension, bradycardia, and increased risk of intrauterine demise have been reported following drug withdrawal (Zuspan et al., 1975; Rementeria and Nunag, 1973; Cohen et al., 1980; Umans and Szeto, 1985). Drug-seeking behaviors, including prostitution, along with the increased risk of sexually transmitted diseases, may also be decreased by scheduled methadone administration.

Several issues specific to the antepartum and intrapartum management of the pregnant opiate user deserve mention. The clinician needs to be able to recognize the signs and symptoms of both narcotic intoxication and narcotic withdrawal (Tables 13–7 and 13–8) (Hoegerman and Schnoll, 1991). Given the risk of fetal withdrawal, narcotics with significant mixed agonist-antagonist properties (e.g., pentazocine) are contraindicated in opiate-dependent women. The American Academy of Pediatrics has suggested that, based on available data, women using heroin should not breast-feed their newborns, whereas women using appropriately prescribed narcotics for pain control (e.g., codeine), or 20 mg/day or less of methadone, can safely nurse their infants (Committee on Drugs, 1989).

MARIJUANA

The active ingredient in marijuana, tetrahydrocannabinol, causes a mild tachycardia, a slight increase in arterial pressure, and a generalized euphoria. The effects generally are evident within 30 to 60 minutes and last from 3 to 5 hours. Based on the National Institute on Drug Abuse Household Survey of 1990, it is estimated that 17.4 per cent of all women use marijuana during their pregnancy (Gomby and Shiono, 1991). Importantly, the concurrent use of other illicit drugs is common (Osterloh and Lee, 1989; Gibson et al., 1983; Linn et al., 1983), as is the use of tobacco and alcohol. Women who use marijuana tend to be younger, unmarried, less well-educated, and in a lower socioeconomic group than those who are not users (Fried et al., 1980).

The available data linking marijuana use to congenital anomalies are inconclusive. Early case reports associating its use with limb reduction defects (Hecht et al., 1968; Carakushansky et al., 1969) are difficult to interpret given the concurrent exposure to other illicit drugs. Numerous other authors have failed to observe an increase in the incidence of congenital anomalies in neonates with prenatal marijuana exposure (Tennes et al., 1985; Zuckerman et al., 1989; Linn et al., 1983; O'Connell and Fried, 1984). Reports of an increase in fetal alcohol syndrome–type features in exposed newborns (Qazi et al., 1985; Hingson et al., 1982) merit scrutiny and additional investigation.

Several studies have suggested an association between marijuana use and a decrease in birth weight and birth length. Zuckerman (1989) reported a 79-gm decrease in birth weight and a 0.5-cm decrease in birth length in babies born to women who used marijuana. Another investigation demonstrated a 105-gm difference in mean birth weight between users and nonusers (Hingson et al., 1982). Although a similar decrease in birth length (0.55 cm) was noted, Tennes and coworkers (1985) were not able to show a difference in mean birth weight among exposed neonates. Although other studies have suggested an impairment of fetal growth, they were not adequately controlled for confounding variables such as the use of additional illicit drugs or alcohol and tobacco (Gibson et al., 1983; Hatch and Bracken, 1986). Several investigations have shown that mean birth weight among marijuana-exposed newborns is no different from that among drug-free controls (Greenland et al., 1982; Fried and O'Connell, 1987; Fried et al., 1984).

There is little support for marijuana use as an independent risk factor for preterm delivery. A recent study reported a mean estimated gestational age at

TABLE 13–8.   Signs of Opioid Withdrawal in the Adult

Drug craving	Abdominal cramping
Lacrimation	Chills
Rhinorrhea	Flushing
Yawning	Muscle spasms and aches
Sweating	Tremors and irritability
Restless sleep	Hypertension
Mydriasis	Hyperventilation
Anorexia	Tachycardia
Vomiting	Piloerection
Diarrhea	

From Hoegerman G, Schnoll S: Narcotic use in pregnancy. Clin Perinatol 18:58, 1991.

delivery of 39.7 weeks for babies born to nonusers, compared with 40.2 weeks for babies of irregular and moderate users, whereas babies of heavy users were delivered at a mean gestational age of 38.8 weeks (Fried and O'Connell, 1987). The clinical significance of this difference in gestational age is unclear. Several studies have failed to show an increased incidence of preterm delivery in patients using marijuana (Tennes et al., 1985; Linn et al., 1983).

Although there is some evidence that newborns exposed prenatally to marijuana demonstrate changes in performance on the Brazelton Neonatal Behavioral Assessment Score (increased tremors and startles) (Fried and Makin, 1987), other investigators have shown no significant neonatal behavioral alterations (Tennes et al., 1985). There does not appear to be any effect of exposure on neurodevelopmental testing or on postnatal growth (Tennes et al., 1985; Fried and Watkinson, 1988).

AMPHETAMINE AND METHAMPHETAMINE

Amphetamine and methamphetamine belong to the general group of sympathomimetic amines. Their stimulatory effect on the sympathetic nervous system is mediated by an increase in the release of neurotransmitter substances from the presynaptic terminal. Amphetamine and methamphetamine can be taken orally or intravenously, or they can be smoked. The recent appearance of crystal methamphetamine ("ice"), a smokable form of the drug, has renewed concerns over the perinatal complications of amphetamine-like drugs (Cho, 1990).

Methamphetamine and amphetamine have been associated with delayed fetal growth and a significant decrease in mean birth weight and mean birth length (Oro and Dixon, 1987; Little et al., 1988; Naeye, 1983; Gillogley et al., 1990). Data collected from the University of California, Davis (Gillogley et al., 1990) show that the mean birth weight among the neonates of 106 amphetamine users (2947 gm) was significantly different from that of babies born to drug-free controls (3165 gm). However, the incidence of alcohol use in the amphetamine users was significantly greater than in the control group. Methamphetamine administered to the pregnant ewe has been shown to result in a decrease in uterine blood flow (Andres et al., 1992) and fetal hypoxemia (Burchfield et al., 1991).

Preterm birth is less clearly associated with amphetamine/methamphetamine than with cocaine. Although Oro and Dixon (1987) found a significant increase in the incidence of preterm birth among patients using cocaine and/or methamphetamine, other investigators have shown no difference in preterm birth or estimated gestational age at delivery (Little et al., 1988; Gillogley et al., 1990).

Studies in both animal models and humans suggest that amphetamine use may be associated with significant central nervous system effects. Rumbaugh and associates (1971) demonstrated areas of cerebral ischemia and infarction in rhesus monkeys given intravenous methamphetamine. Similarly, cerebral hemorrhage and ischemic stroke have been reported in adults using amphetamines (Delaney and Estes, 1980; Rothrock et al., 1988). Methamphetamine-exposed neonates have been shown to have a smaller mean head circumference compared to controls (Gillogley et al., 1990; Little et al., 1988; Oro and Dixon, 1987; Dixon and Bejar, 1989). Sonographic examination of term neonates exposed to methamphetamine suggests an increase in the incidence of intraventricular hemorrhage similar to that seen with preterm neonates at risk for hypoxemic encephalopathy (Dixon and Bejar, 1989). This difference was not noted in opiate-exposed neonates with similar demographic and life-style variables.

Although early investigations suggested an increased risk of congenital anomalies in amphetamine-exposed fetuses (Nelson and Forfar, 1971; Nora et al., 1970), the majority of data do not support the association of amphetamine/methamphetamine with congenital anomalies (Heinonen et al., 1977; Milkovich and van der Berg, 1977).

BENZODIAZEPINES

See discussion in Chapter 12.

SUMMARY

Providing obstetric care to women with illicit drug, alcohol, or smoking habits requires attention to several specific issues. Associations between illicit drug use and both human immunodeficiency virus and syphilis have been reported (Rolfs et al., 1990; Minkoff et al., 1990). Given the dramatic importance of these two conditions, appropriate screening is an absolute in this population. The risks of preterm labor and delivery, intrauterine growth restriction, and congenital anomalies are best addressed by frequent prenatal visits, appropriate use of sonographic examinations, and intensive patient counseling regarding the implications of their substance use.

Although not widely available, specialized multidisciplinary prenatal clinics designed for this population have been shown to improve outcome (MacGregor et al., 1989). This suggests that concerted efforts at rehabilitation and education along with intensive prenatal care can lead to an improved outcome for these patients and their newborns.

REFERENCES

Abel EL, Sokol RJ: Fetal alcohol syndrome is now leading cause of mental retardation. Lancet **1**:222, 1986.

Abel EL, Sokol RJ: Fetal diagnosis and therapy. Alcohol **2**:140, 1989.

Abel EL, Sokol RJ: A revised conservative estimate of the incidence of FAS and its economic impact. Alcohol Clin Exp Res **15**:514, 1991.

Abell TD, Baker LC, Ramsey CN: The effects of maternal smoking on infant birth weight. Family Medicine **23**:103, 1991.

Acker D, Sachs BP, Tracey KJ, et al: Abruptio placentae associated with cocaine use. Am J Obstet Gynecol **146**:220, 1983.

Andres RL, Dickinson JE, Deaver JE, et al: Ovine maternal and fetal vascular responses to acute methamphetamine administration. Abstract No. 563, Presented at the 39th Annual Meeting of the Society for Gynecologic Investigation, San Antonio, Texas, 1992.

Armstrong BG, McDonald AD, Sloan M: Cigarette, alcohol and coffee consumption and spontaneous abortion. Am J Public Health **82**:85, 1992.

Astrup P: Some physiological and pathological effects of moderate carbon monoxide exposure. Br Med J **4**:447, 1972.

Bauchner H, Zuckerman B, McClain M, et al: Risk of sudden infant death syndrome among infants with in utero exposure to cocaine. J Pediatr **113**:881, 1988.

Beaulac-Baillargeon L, Desrosires C: Caffeine-cigarette interaction on fetal growth. Am J Obstet Gynecol **157**:1236, 1987.

Bingol N, Fuchs M, Diaz V, et al: Teratogenicity of cocaine in humans. J Pediatr **110**:93, 1987.

Binkiewicz A, Robinson MJ, Senior B: Pseudo-Cushing's syndrome caused by alcohol in breast milk. J Pediatr Med **93**:965, 1978.

Blakeley PM, Scott WJ: Determination of the proximate teratogen of the mouse F.A.S.: 2. Pharmacokinetics of the placental transfer of ethanol and acetaldehyde. Toxicol Appl Pharmacol **72**:364, 1984.

Blinick G, Wallach RC, Jerez E: Pregnancy in narcotic addicts treated by medical withdrawal. Am J Obstet Gynecol **105**:997, 1969.

Borlee I, Lechat MF, Bouckaert P, et al: Le cafe facteur de risque pendant la grossesse? Louvain Med **97**:279, 1978.

Brien JF, Loomis CW, Tranmer J, et al: Disposition of ethanol in human maternal venous blood and amniotic fluid. Am J Obstet Gynecol **146**:181, 1983.

Brien JF, Clarke DW, Richardson B, et al: Disposition of ethanol in maternal blood, fetal blood and amniotic fluid of third-trimester pregnant ewes. Am J Obstet Gynecol **152**:583, 1985.

Brien J, Clark D, Smith G, et al: Disposition of acute, multiple dose ethanol in the near-term pregnant ewe. Am J Obstet Gynecol **157**:204, 1987.

Brown NA, Goulding EH, Fabro S: Ethanol embryotoxocity: Direct effects on mammalian embryos in vitro. Science **206**:573, 1979.

Burchfield DJ, Lucas VW, Abrams RM, et al: Disposition and pharmacodynamics of methamphetamine in pregnant sheep. JAMA **254**:1968, 1991.

Bureau MA, Monette J, Shapcott D, et al: Carboxyhemoglobin concentration in fetal cord blood and in blood of mothers who smoked in labor. Pediatrics **69**:371, 1982.

Burton GJ. Palmer ME, Dalton KJ: Morphometric differences between the placental vasculature of non-smokers, smokers and ex-smokers. Br J Obstet Gynecol **96**:907, 1989.

Carakushansky G, Neu RL, Gardner LI: Lysergide and cannabis as possible teratogens in man. Lancet **1**:150, 1969.

Centers for Disease Control, Atlanta, GA: Current trends: Statewide prevalence of illicit drug use by pregnant women—Rhode Island. MMWR **39**:225, 1990.

Chasnoff IJ, Hatcher R, Burns WJ: Polydrug and methadone-addicted newborns: A continuum of impairment? Pediatrics **70**:210, 1982.

Chasnoff IJ, Burns WJ, Schnoll SH, et al: Cocaine use in pregnancy. N Engl J Med **313**:666, 1985.

Chasnoff IJ, Bussey M, Savich R, et al: Perinatal cerebral infarction and maternal cocaine use. J Pediatr **108**:456, 1986.

Chasnoff IJ: Perinatal effects of cocaine. Contemp Ob/Gyn **29**:163, 1987.

Chasnoff IJ, Burns K, Burns W: Cocaine use in pregnancy: Perinatal morbidity and mortality. Neurotoxicol Teratol **9**:291, 1987.

Chasnoff IJ, Chisum GM, Kaplan WE: Maternal cocaine use and genitourinary tract malformations. Teratology **37**:201, 1988.

Chasnoff IJ: Drug use and women: Establishing a standard of care. Ann NY Acad Sci **562**:208, 1989a.

Chasnoff I, Griffith D, MacGregor S, et al: Temporal patterns of cocaine use in pregnancy. JAMA **261**:1741, 1989b.

Chasnoff IJ, Hunt C, Kletter R, et al: Prenatal cocaine exposure is associated with respiratory pattern abnormalities. Am J Dis Child **143**:583, 1989c.

Chasnoff IJ, Landress HJ, Barrett ME: The prevalence of illicit drug or alcohol use during pregnancy and discrepancies in mandatory reporting in Pinellas County Florida. N Engl J Med **322**:1202, 1990.

Chasnoff IJ, Griffith DR, Freier C, et al: Cocaine/polydrug use in pregnancy: Two-year follow-up. Pediatrics **89**:284, 1992.

Chavez GF, Mulinare J, Cordero JF: Maternal cocaine use during early pregnancy as a risk factor for congenital anomalies. JAMA **262**:795, 1989.

Cherukuri R, Minkoff H, Hansen RL, et al: A cohort study of alkaloidal cocaine ("crack") in pregnancy. Obstet Gynecol **72**:147, 1988.

Cho AK: Ice: A new dosage form of an old drug. Science **249**:631, 1990.

Chouteau M, Namerow PB, Leppert P: The effect of cocaine abuse on birth weight and gestational age. Obstet Gynecol **72**:351, 1988.

Church MW, Dintcheff BA, Gessner PK: Dose-dependent consequences of cocaine on pregnancy outcome in the Long-Evans rat. Neurotoxicol Teratol **10**:51, 1987.

Clapp JF, Szeto HH, Larro R, et al: Umbilical blood flow response to embolization of the uterine circulation. Am J Obstet Gynecol **138**:60, 1980.

Clarke DW, Steenhart NA, Brien JF: Disposition of ethanol and activity of hepatic and placental ADH and ALDH in the third-trimester pregnant guinea pig for single and short-term oral ethanol administration. Alcohol Clin Exp Res **10**:330, 1986.

Clarke DW, Smith GN, Patrick J, et al: Disposition of ethanol and its proximate metabolite, acetaldehyde, in the near-term pregnant ewe for short-term maternal administration of moderate-dose ethanol. Drug Metab Dispos **16**:464, 1988.

Clarke DW, Smith GN, Patrick J, et al: Activity of alcohol dehydrogenase and aldehyde dehydrogenase in maternal liver, fetal liver and placenta of the near-term pregnant ewe. Dev Pharmacol Ther **12**:35, 1989.

Clarren SK, Smith DW: The fetal alcohol syndrome. N Engl J Med **298**:1063, 1978.

Clarren SK, Bowden DM: The fetal alcohol syndrome: A new primate mode for binge drinking and its relevance to human ethanol teratogenesis. J Pediatr **101**:819, 1982.

Clarren SK, Astley SJ: Pregnancy outcome after weekly oral administration of ethanol during gestation in the pig-tailed macaque: Comparing early gestational exposure to full gestational exposure. Teratology **45**:1, 1992.

Cohen MS, Rudolph AM, Melmon KL: Antagonism of morphine by naloxone in pregnant ewes and fetal lambs. Dev Pharmacol Ther **1**:58, 1980.

Coles CD, Smith I, Fernhoff PM, et al: Neonatal neurobehavioral characteristics as correlates of maternal alcohol use during gestation. Alcohol Clin Exp Res **9**:454, 1985.

Committee on Drugs, American Academy of Pediatrics: Transfer of drugs and other chemicals into human milk. Pediatrics **84**:924, 1989.

Cooper JR, Altman F, Brown BS, et al: Research on the treatment of narcotic addiction—state of the art. Treatment Research Monograph Series NIDA. Rockville, MD, US Department of Health and Human Services, 1983.

Creasy RK, Barrett CT, de Sweit M, et al: Experimental intrauterine growth retardation in the sheep. Am J Obstet Gynecol **112**:566, 1972.

Cregler L, Marx H: Medical complications of cocaine abuse. N Engl J Med **315**:1495, 1986.

Cumming ME, Ong BY, Wade JG, et al: Ethanol disposition in newborn lambs and comparison of alcohol dehydrogenase activity in placenta and maternal sheep, fetal and neonatal lamb liver. Dev Pharmacol Ther **8**:338, 1985.

Cushman P: Growth hormone in narcotic addiction. J Clin Endocrinol Metab **35**:352, 1972.

Daniel EE: Effects of cocaine and adrenaline on contracture and downhill ion movements induced by inhibitors of membrane ATPase in rat uteri. Can J Physiol Pharmacol **42**:497, 1964.

Davies DP, Gray OP, Elwood PC, et al: Cigarette smoking in pregnancy: Associations with maternal weight gain and fetal growth. Lancet **1**:385, 1976.

Day NL, Jasperse D, Richardson G, et al: Prenatal exposure to alcohol: Effect on infant growth and morphologic characteristics. Pediatrics **84**:536, 1989.

deHass I, Harlow BL, Cramer DW, et al: Spontaneous preterm birth: A case-control study. Am J Obstet Gynecol **165**:1290, 1991.

Delaney P, Estes M: Intracranial hemorrhage associated with amphetamine abuse. Neurology **30**:1125, 1980.

Divers WA, Wilkes MM, Babakina A, et al: Maternal smoking and elevation of catecholamines and metabolites in the amniotic fluid. Am J Obstet Gynecol 141:265, 1981.

Dixon SD, Bejar R: Echoencephalographic findings in neonates associated with maternal cocaine and methamphetamine use: Incidence and clinical correlates. J Pediatr 115:770, 1989.

Doberczak TM, Thorton JC, Berstein J, et al: Impact of maternal drug dependency on birth weight and head circumference of offspring. Am J Dis Child 141:1163, 1987.

Doberczak TM, Shanzer S, Senie RT, et al: Neonatal neurologic and electroencephalographic effects of intrauterine cocaine exposure. J Pediatr 113:354, 1988.

Dole VP, Nyswander ME: A medical treatment for diacetylmorphine (heroin) addiction—a clinical trial with methadone hydrochloride. JAMA 193:646, 1965.

Dombrowski MP, Wolfe HM, Welch RA, et al: Cocaine abuse is associated with abruptio placentae and decreased birth weight, but not shorter labor. Obstet Gynecol 77:139, 1991.

Dresoti IE, Ballard J, Belling B, et al: The effects of ethanol and acetaldehyde on DNA sythesis in growing cells and on fetal development in the rat. Alcohol Clin Exp Res 5:357, 1981.

Edelin KC, Gurganious L, Golar K, et al: Methadone maintenance in pregnancy: Consequences to care and outcome. Obstet Gynecol 71:399, 1988.

Ellis FW, Pick JR: An animal model for the fetal alcohol syndrome in beagles. Clinical Exp Res 4:123, 1980.

Evans DR, Newcombe RG, Campbell H. Maternal smoking habits and congenital malformations: a population study. Br Med J 2:171, 1979.

Ewing JA: Detecting alcoholism: The CAGE questionnaire. JAMA 252:1905, 1984.

Fantel AG, McPhail BJ: The teratogenicity of cocaine. Teratology 26:179, 1982.

Finnell RH, Toloyan S, VanWaes M, et al: Preliminary evidence for a cocaine-induced embryopathy in mice. Toxicol Appl Pharmacol 103:228, 1990.

Fish F, Wilson WDC: Excretion of cocaine and its metabolites in man. J Pharm Pharmacol 21:1355, 1969.

Fisher SE, Atkinson M, Holzman I, et al: Effect of ethanol upon placental uptake of amino acids. Prog Biochem Pharmacol 18:216, 1981.

Food and Drug Administration: Surgeon General's advisory on alcohol and pregnancy. FDA Drug Bull 11:9, 1981.

Food and Drug Administration: Report on caffeine. Washington, DC, United States Government Printing Office, 1980.

Fricker HS, Segal S: Narcotic addiction, pregnancy and the newborn. Am J Dis Child 132:360, 1978.

Fried PA, Watkinson B, Grant A, et al: Changing patterns of soft drug use prior to and during pregnancy: A prospective study. Drug Alcohol Depend 6:323, 1980.

Fried PA, Watkinson B, Willan A: Marijuana use during pregnancy and decreased length of gestation. Am J Obstet Gynecol 150:23, 1984.

Fried PA, O'Connell CM: A comparison of the effects of prenatal exposure to tobacco, alcohol, cannabis and caffeine on birth size and subsequent growth. Neurotoxicol Teratol 9:79, 1987.

Fried PA, Makin JE: Neonatal behavioral correlates of prenatal exposure to marijuana in a low risk population. Neurotoxicol Teratol 9:1, 1987.

Fried PA, Watkinson B: Twelve and twenty-four month neurobehavioral followup of children prenatally exposed to marijuana cigarettes and alcohol. Neurobehav Toxicol Teratol 10:305, 1988.

Fulroth R, Phillips B, Durand DJ: Perinatal outcome of infants exposed to cocaine and/or heroin in utero. Am J Dis Child 143:905, 1989.

Furuhashi N, Sato S, Suzuki M, et al: Effects of caffeine ingestion during pregnancy. Gynecol Obstet Invest 19:187, 1985.

Gibson GT, Baghurst PA, Colley DP: Maternal alcohol, tobacco and cannabis consumption and the outcome of pregnancy. Aust N Z J Obstet Gynecol 23:15, 1983.

Gillogley KM, Evans AT, Hansen RL, et al: The perinatal impact of cocaine, amphetamine and opiate use detected by universal intrapartum screening. Am J Obstet Gynecol 163:1535, 1990.

Gomby DS, Shiono PH: Estimating the number of substance-exposed infants. In Behrman RE (ed.): The Future of Children. Los Altos, California, The Center for the Future of Children, The David and Lucille Packard Foundation, 1991, pp. 18–25.

Gordon BHJ, Streeter ML, Rosso P, et al: Prenatal alcohol exposure: Abnormalities in placental growth and fetal amino acid uptake in the rat. Biol Neonate 47:113, 1985.

Graham K, Karen G, Klein J, et al: Determination of gestational cocaine exposure by hair analysis. JAMA 262:3328, 1989.

Greenland S, Staisch KJ, Brown N, et al: The effects of marijuana use during pregnancy I. A preliminary epidemiologic study. Am J Obstet Gynecol 143:408, 1982.

Griffith DR, Chasnoff IJ, Freier MC: Developmental follow-up of cocaine exposed infants through three years. Infant Behav Dev 13:126, 1990.

Guzick DS, Daikoku NH, Kaltreider DF: Predictability of pregnancy outcome in preterm delivery. Obstet Gynecol 63:645, 1984.

Haddow JE, Knight GJ, Palomaki GE, et al: Cigarette consumption and serum cotinine in relation to birthweight. Br J Obstet Gynaecol 94:678, 1987.

Hadeed AJ, Siegel SR: Maternal cocaine use during pregnancy: Effect on the newborn infant. Pediatrics 84:205, 1989.

Halmesmaki E: Alcohol counselling of 85 pregnant problem drinkers: Effect on drinking and fetal outcome. Br J Obstet Gynaecol 95:243, 1988.

Halmesmaki E, Teramo AK, Widness AJ, et al: Maternal alcohol abuse is associated with elevated fetal erthropoietin levels. Obstet Gynecol 76:219, 1990.

Hanson JW, Streissguth AP, Smith DW: The effect of moderate alcohol consumption on fetal growth and morphogenesis. J Pediatr 92:947, 1978.

Harlap S, Shiono PH: Alcohol, smoking and the incidence of spontaneous abortions in the first and second trimester. Lancet 1:173, 1980.

Hatch EE, Bracken MB: Effect of marijuana use in pregnancy on fetal growth. Am J Epidemiol 124:986, 1986.

Hawks RL, Chiang CN (eds): Urine Testing for Drugs of Abuse. NIDA Research Monograph 73, 1986.

Hebel JR, Fox NL, Sexton M: Dose-response of birth weight to various measures of maternal smoking during pregnancy. J Clin Epidemiol 41:483, 1988.

Hecht F, Beals R, Lees MH, et al: Lysergic-acid-diethylamide and cannabis as possible teratogens in man. Lancet 2:1087, 1968.

Heinonen OP, Slone D, Shapiro S: Birth Defects and Drugs in Pregnancy. Littleton, MA, PSG, 1977.

Hemminki K, Mutanen P, Saloniemi I: Smoking and the occurrence of congenital malformations and spontaneous abortions: Multivariate analysis. Am J Obstet Gynecol 145:61, 1983.

Henderson GI, Hoyumpa AM, Rothschild MA, et al: Effect of ethanol and ethanol-induced hypothermia on protein synthesis in pregnant and fetal rats. Alcohol Clin Exp Res 4:165, 1980.

Hertlendy F, Molinar M: Cocaine directly affects signal transduction on human myometrial cells. (Abstract #44) Am J Obstet Gynecol 166:292, 1992.

Himmelberger DU, Brown BW, Cohen EN: Cigarette smoking during pregnancy and the occurrence of spontaneous abortion and congenital anomaly. Am J Epidemiol 108:470, 1978.

Hingson R, Alpert JJ, Day N, et al: Effects of maternal drinking and marijuana use on fetal growth and development. Pediatrics 70:539, 1982.

Hoegerman G, Schnoll S: Narcotic use in pregnancy. Semin Perinatol 18:58, 1991.

Hoh TK: Severe hypoprothrombinemic bleeding in the breast fed young infant. Singapore Med J 10:43, 1969.

Hoff C, Wetelecki W, Blackburn WR, et al: Trend associations of smoking with maternal, fetal, and neonatal morbidity. Obstet Gynecol 68:317, 1986.

Hoyme HE, Jones KL, Dixon SD, et al: Prenatal cocaine exposure and fetal vascular disruption. Pediatrics 85:742, 1990.

Hurd WW, Robertson PA, Riemer RK, et al: Cocaine directly augments the alpha-adrenergic contractile response of the pregnant rabbit uterus. Am J Obstet Gynecol 164:182, 1991b.

Hurd WW, Smith AJ, Gauvin JM, et al: Cocaine blocks extraneuronal reuptake of norepinephrine by the pregnant human uterus. Obstet Gynecol 78:249, 1991a.

Idanpann-Heikkila J, Jouppila P, Akerblom HK, et al: Elimination and metabolic effects of ethanol in mother, fetus and newborn infant. Am J Obstet Gynecol 112:387, 1972.

Inselman LS, Fisher SE, Spencer H, et al: Effects of intrauterine ethanol exposure on fetal lung growth. Pediatr Res 19:12, 1985.

Institute of Medicine: Treating Drug Problems. Gerstein DR, Harwood HJ (eds). Washington, DC, National Academy Press, 1990, p. 85.

Institute of Medicine: Preventing Low Birth Weight. Washington, DC, National Academy Press, 1985.

Jauniaux E, Burton GJ: The effect of smoking in pregnancy on early placental morphology. Obstet Gynecol 79:645, 1992.

Jeanty P, Cousaert E, deMaertalaer V, et al: Sonographic detection of smoking-related decreased fetal growth. J Ultrasound Med 6:13, 1987.

Jones KL, Smith DW, Ulleland CN, et al: Patterns of malformations in offspring of chronic alcoholic mothers. Lancet 1:1267, 1973.

Jones KL, Smith DW, Streissouth AP, et al: Outcome in offspring of chronic alcoholic women. Lancet 1:1076, 1974.

Kaminski M, Ruimeau-Roquette C, Schwartz D: Alcohol consumption in pregnant women and the outcome of pregnancy. Alcohol Clin Exp Res 1:155, 1978.

Kaminski M, Franc M, Lebouiver M, et al: Moderate alcohol use and pregnancy outcome. Neurobehav Toxicol Teratol 3:173, 1981.

Kandall SR, Albin S, Lowinson J, et al: Differential effects of maternal heroin and methadone use on birth weight. Pediatrics 58:681, 1976.

Kandall SR, Albin S, Gart LM, et al: The narcotic-dependent mother: Fetal and neonatal consequences. Early Hum Dev 1:161, 1977.

Kandall SR, Doberczak TM, Mauer KR, et al: Opiate vs. CNS depressant therapy in neonatal drug abstinence syndrome. Am J Dis Child 13:378, 1983.

Kapur RP, Shaw CM, Shepard TH: Brain hemorrhages in cocaine exposed human fetuses. Teratology 44:11, 1991.

Kaye K, Eklind L, Goldberg D, et al: Birth outcomes for infants of drug abusing mothers. NY State J Med 89:256, 1989.

Keith L, MacGregor S, Friedell S, et al: Substance abuse in pregnant women: Recent experience at the Perinatal Center for Chemical Dependence of Northwestern Memorial Hospital. Obstet Gynecol 73:715, 1989.

Kline J, Stein ZA, Susser M, et al: Smoking: A risk factor for spontaneous abortion. N Engl J Med 297:793, 1977.

Kline J, Shrout P, Stein Z, et al: Drinking during pregnancy and spontaneous abortion. Lancet 2:176, 1980.

Kline J, Stein Z, Hutzler M: Cigarettes, alcohol and marijuana: varying associations with birth weight. Int J Epidemiol 16:44, 1987.

Kramer LD, Locke GE, Ogunyemi A, et al: Neonatal cocaine related seizures. J Child Neurol 5:60, 1990.

Kramer MD, Taylor V, Hickok DE, et al: Smoking and placenta previa. Am J Epidemiol 130:804, 1989.

Kurpa K, Holmberg PC, Kuosma E, et al: Coffee consumption during pregnancy and selected congenital malformations: A nationwide case-control study. Am J Public Health 73:1397, 1983.

Kuzma JW, Sokol RJ: Maternal drinking behavior and decreased intrauterine growth. Alcohol Clin Exp Res 6:396, 1982.

Lifschitz MH, Wilson GS, Smith E, et al: Fetal and postnatal growth of children born to narcotic-dependent women. J Pediatr 102:686, 1983.

Linn S, Shoenbaum SC, Monson RR, et al: No association between coffee consumption and adverse outcomes of pregnancy. N Engl J Med 306:141, 1982.

Linn S, Schoenbaum SC, Monson RR, et al: The association of marijuana use with outcome of pregnancy. Am J Public Health 73:1161, 1983.

Lipschultz SE, Frassica JJ, Orav EJ: Cardiovascular abnormalities in infants prenatally exposed to cocaine. J Pediatrics 118:44, 1991.

Little BB, Snell LM, Gilstrap LC: Methamphetamine abuse during pregnancy: Outcome and fetal effects. Obstet Gynecol 72:541, 1988.

Little BB, Snell LM, Klein VR, et al: Cocaine abuse during pregnancy: Maternal and fetal implications. Obstet Gynecol 73:157, 1989.

Little BB, Snell LM, Klein VR, et al: Maternal and fetal effects of heroin addiction during pregnancy. J Reprod Med 35:159, 1990.

Little BB, Snell LM: Brain growth among fetuses exposed to cocaine in utero: Asymmetrical growth retardation. Obstet Gynecol 77:361, 1991a.

Little BB, Snell LM: Cocaine use during pregnancy and congenital anomalies: Further study. Am J Obstet Gynecol 164:350, 1991b.

Little RE: Moderate alcohol use during pregnancy and decreased infant birth weight. Am J Public Health 67:1154, 1977.

Livesay S, Ehrlich S, Finnegan LP: Cocaine and pregnancy: Maternal and infant outcome. Pediatr Res 21:238A, 1987.

Lochery EA, Randall CL, Goldsmith AA, et al: Effect of acute alcohol exposure during selected days of gestation in CH3 mice. Neurobehavior Toxicol Teratol 4:15, 1981.

Longo LD, Ching KS: Placental diffusing capacity for carbon monoxide and oxygen in unanesthetized sheep. J Appl Physiol 43:885, 1977.

Longo LD, Hill ED: Carbon monoxide uptake and elimination in fetal and maternal sheep. Am J Obstet Gynecol 232:324, 1977.

Longo LD: The biological effects of carbon monoxide on the pregnant woman, fetus and newborn. Am J Obstet Gynecol 129:69, 1977.

Luck W, Ngu H, Hansen R, et al: Extent of nicotine and cotinine transfer to the human fetus, placenta and amniotic fluid of smoking mothers. Dev Pharmacol Ther 8:384, 1985.

MacArthur C, Knox EG: Smoking and pregnancy: Effects of stopping at different stages. Br J Obstet Gynaecol 95:551, 1988.

MacGregor S, Keith L, Bachicha J, et al: Cocaine abuse during pregnancy: Correlation between prenatal care and perinatal outcome. Obstet Gynecol 74:882, 1989.

MacGregor S, Keith L, Chasnoff I, et al: Cocaine use during pregnancy: Adverse perinatal outcome. Am J Obstet Gynecol 157:686, 1987.

Madden JD: Problems pertaining to the care of newborn infants of drug addicted women. J Reprod Med 20:303, 1978.

Madden JD, Payne TE, Miller S: Maternal cocaine abuse and effect on the newborn. Pediatrics 77:209, 1986.

Mahalik MP, Gautieri RF, Mann DE: Teratogenic potential of cocaine hydrochloride in CF-a mice. J Pharm Sci 69:703, 1980.

Manning FA, Feyerabend C: Cigarette smoking and fetal breathing movements. Br J Obstet Gynaecol 83:262, 1976.

Manning F, Walker D, Feyerabend C: The effect of nicotine on fetal breathing movements in conscious pregnant ewes. Obstet Gynecol 52:563, 1978.

Marbury MC, Linn S, Monson R, et al: The association of alcohol consumption with outcome of pregnancy. Am J Public Health 73:1165, 1983.

Marquis S, Leichter J, Lee M: Plasma amino acids and glucose levels in the rat fetus and dam after chronic maternal alcohol consumption. Biol Neonate 46:36, 1984.

Martin TR, Bracken MB: The association between low birth weight and caffeine consumption during pregnancy. Am J Epidemiol 126:813, 1987.

Mastrogiannis D, Decavalas G, Verma U, et al: Perinatal outcome after recent cocaine usage. Obstet Gynecol 75:8, 1990.

Mau G, Netter P: Kaffee und alkoholkonsum. Ritikofaktoren in der Schwangerschaft. Geburtshilfe Frauenheilkd 34:1018, 1974.

McCormick M: The contribution of low birth weight to infant mortality and childhood morbidity. N Engl J Med 312:82, 1985.

McDonald AD, Armstrong BG, Sloan M: Cigarette, alcohol, and coffee consumption and prematurity. Am J Public Health 82:87, 1992a.

McDonald AD, Armstrong BG, Sloan M: Cigarette, alcohol, and coffee consumption and congenital defects. Am J Public Health 82:91, 1992b.

Medical Letter on Drugs and Therapeutics. "Crack." 28:69, 1986.

Meyer MB, Tonascia JA: Maternal smoking, pregnancy complications and perinatal mortality. Am J Obstet Gynecol 55:701, 1977.

Meyer MB, Jonas BS, Tonascia JA: Perinatal events associated with maternal smoking during pregnancy. Am J Epidemiol 103:464, 1976.

Milkovich L, van der Berg BJ: Effects of antenatal exposure to anorectic drugs. Am J Obstet Gynecol 129:637, 1977.

Miller HC, Jekel JF: Incidence of low-birth-weight infants born to mothers with multiple risk factors. Yale J Biol Med 60:397, 1987.

Mills J, Grabaed BI, Harley EE, et al: Maternal alcohol consumption and birth weight: How much drinking during pregnancy is safe. JAMA 252:1875, 1984.

Minkoff HL, McCall S, DeEhe I, et al: The relationship of cocaine use to syphilis and human immunodeficiency virus infections among inner city parturient women. Am J Obstet Gynecol 163:521, 1990.

Molinar M, Winn H, Hertelndy F: Cocaine activates the inositol cycle and potentiates the action of oxytocin in human myometrial cells. Abstract #231, p. 224, Society for Gynecologic Investigation, San Antonio, Texas, March, 1992.

Monheit AG, van Vunakis H, Key TC, et al: Maternal and fetal cardiovascular effects of nicotine infusion in pregnant sheep. Am J Obstet Gynecol 145:290, 1983.

Moore TR, Sorg J, Miller L, et al: Hemodynamic effects of intravenous cocaine on the pregnant ewe and fetus. Am J Obstet Gynecol 155:883, 1986.

Morgan MA, Silavin SL, Randolph M, et al: Effect of intravenous cocaine on uterine blood flow in the gravid baboon. Am J Obstet Gynecol 164:1021, 1991.

Mulcahy R, Murphy JF: Maternal smoking and the timing of delivery. J Irish Med Assoc 65:175, 1972.

Munoz L, Lonnerdal B, Keen CL, et al: Coffee consumption as a factor in iron deficiency anemia among pregnant women and their infants in Costa Rica. Am J Clin Nutr 48:645, 1988.

Naeye RL, Blanc W, Leblanc W, et al: Fetal complications of maternal heroin addiction: Abnormal growth, infections and episodes of stress. J Pediatr 83:1055, 1973a.

Naeye RL, Blanc WA, Leblanc W: Heroin and the fetus. Pediatr Res 7:321, 1973b.

Naeye RL: Abruptio placentae and placenta previa: Frequency, perinatal mortality and cigarette smoking. Obstet Gynecol 55:701, 1980.

Naeye RL: Maternal use of dextroamphetamine and growth of the fetus. Pharmacology 26:117, 1983.

Nalbandian H, Sheth N, Dietrich R, et al: Intestinal ischemia caused by cocaine ingestion: Report of two cases. Surgery 97:374, 1985.

National Institute on Drug Abuse: National household survey on drug abuse: Population estimates 1990. Washington DC, U.S. Government Printing Office, 1991, (DHHS Publication No. (ADM) 91–1732).

Neerhof MG, MacGregor SN, Retzky SS, et al: Cocaine abuse during pregnancy: Peripartum prevalence and perinatal outcome. Am J Obstet Gynecol 161:633, 1989.

Nelson MM, Forfar JO: Associations between drugs administered during pregnancy and congenital abnormalities of the fetus. Br Med J 1:523, 1971.

Ney JA, Dooley SL, Keith LG, et al: The prevalence of substance abuse in patients with suspected preterm labor. Am J Obstet Gynecol 162:1562, 1990.

Nishimura H, Nakai K: Congenital malformations in offspring of mice treated with caffeine. Proc Soc Exp Biol Med 104:140, 1960.

Nolen GA: The developmental toxicology of caffeine. Issues Rev Teratol 4:305, 1988.

Nora JL, Vargo TA, Nora AH, et al: Dexamphetamine: A possible environmental trigger in cardiovascular malformations. Lancet 1:1290, 1970.

Obe G, Majewski F: No elevation of exchange type aberrations in lymphocytes of children with alcohol embryopathy. Hum Genet 43:31, 1978.

O'Connell CM, Fried PA: An investigation of prenatal cannabis exposure and minor physical anomalies in a low risk population. Neurobehav Toxicol Teratol 6:345, 1984.

Olegard R, Sabel KG, Aronsson M, et al: Effects on the child of alcohol abuse during pregnancy: Retrospective and prospective studies. Acta Paediatr Scand 275:112, 1979.

Oro AS, Dixon SD: Perinatal cocaine and methamphetamine exposure: Maternal and neonatal correlates. J Pediatr 111:571, 1987.

Osterloh JD, Lee BL: Urine drug screening in mothers and newborns. Am J Dis Child 143:791, 1989.

Ostrea EM, Chavez CJ, Strauss ME: A study of factors that influence the severity of neonatal narcotic withdrawal. J Pediatr 88:642, 1976.

Ostrea EM, Parks P, Brady M: Rapid isolation and detection of drugs in meconium of infants of drug dependent mothers: An alternative to urine testing. J Pediatr 115:474, 1989.

Ostrea EM, Brady M, Gauge S, et al: Drug screening of newborns by meconium analysis: A large-scale, prospective, epidemiologic study. Pediatrics 89:107, 1992.

Ouellette EM, Rosett HL, Rosman NP, et al: Adverse effects on offspring of maternal alcohol abuse during pregnancy. N Engl J Med 297:528, 1977.

Owiny JR, Myers T, Massmann GA, et al: Lack of effect of maternal cocaine administration on myometrial electromyogram and maternal plasma oxytocin concentrations in pregnant sheep at 124–126 days' gestational age. Obstet Gynecol 79:82, 1992.

Pellosi MA, Fratarola M, Apuzzio J, et al: Pregnancy complicated by heroin addiction. Obstet Gynecol 45:512, 1975.

Pikkarainen PH, Raiha NC. Development of alcohol dehydrogenase activity in the human liver. Pediatr Res 1:165, 1967.

Plessinger MA, Woods JR: Progesterone increases cardiovascular toxicity to cocaine in nonpregnant ewes. Am J Obstet Gynecol 163:1659, 1990.

Pokorny AD, Miller BA, Kaplan HB: The MAST: A shortened version of the Michigan Alcoholism Screening Test. Am J Psychiatry 129:118, 1972.

Porat R, Brodsky N: Cocaine: A risk factor for necrotizing enterocolitis. J Perinatol 11:30, 1991.

Prager K, Malin H, Speigler D, et al: Smoking and drinking behavior before and during pregnancy of married mothers of liveborn infants and stillborn infants. Public Health Rep 99:117, 1985.

Pritchard JA, Mason R, Corle M, et al: Genesis of severe placental abruption. Am J Obstet Gynecol 108:22, 1970.

Pulkkinen P: Smoking in pregnancy, with special reference to fetal growth and certain trace element distribution between mother, placenta, and fetus. Acta Obstet Gynecol Scand 69:543, 1990.

Qazi QH, Mariano E, Milman DH, et al: Abnormalities in offspring associated with prenatal marijuana exposure. Dev Pharmacol Ther 8:141, 1985.

Rajegowda BK, Glass L, Evans HE, et al: Methadone withdrawal on newborn infants. J Pediatr 81:532, 1972.

Randall CL, Taylor WJ, Walker DW: Ethanol-induced malformations in mice. Alcohol Clin Exp Res 1:219, 1977.

Raye JR, Dubin JW, Blechner JN: Fetal growth restriction following maternal narcotic administration: Nutritional or drug effect. Pediatr Res 9:279, 1975.

Rementeria JL, Nunag NN: Narcotic withdrawal in pregnancy: Stillbirth incidence with a case report. Am J Obstet Gynecol 116:1152, 1973.

Resnik R, Brink GW, Wilkes M: Catecholamine-mediated reduction in uterine blood flow after nicotine infusion in the pregnant ewe. J Clin Invest 63:1133, 1979.

Ritchie J, Greene N: Local anesthetics. In Goodman A, Gillman L, Rall T, Murad F (eds): The Pharmacological Basis of Therapeutics. 7th ed. New York, Macmillan, 1985, pp. 309–10.

Rolfs RT, Goldberg M, Sharrar RG: Risk factors for syphilis: Cocaine use and prostitution. Am J Public Health 80:853, 1990.

Roloff DW, Howalt WF: The effect of chronic maternal morphine administration on lung development and growth of fetal rabbits. Pediatr Res 7:321, 1973.

Rose J, Strandhoy JW, Meis PJ: Acute and chronic effects of maternal ethanol administration on the ovine maternal-fetal unit. Prog Biochem Pharmacol 18:1, 1981.

Rosenberg L, Mitchell AA, Shapiro S, et al: Selected birth defects in relation to caffeine-containing beverages. JAMA 247:1249, 1982.

Rosenstein BJ, Wheeler JS, Heid PL: Congenital renal abnormalities in infants with in utero cocaine exposure. J Urol 144:110, 1990.

Rosett HL, Weiner L, Lee A, et al: Patterns of alcohol consumption and fetal development. Obstet Gynecol 61:539, 1983.

Rosett HL, Weiner L: Alcohol and the Fetus. New York, Oxford University Press, 1984.

Ross JJ, Frias JL: Microcephaly. In Vinken GW, Bruyn PW (eds): Handbook of Clinical Neurology. Amsterdam, Elsevier/North Holland Biomedical Press, 1977, pp. 507–524.

Rothrock JF, Rubenstein R, Lyden P: Ischemic stroke associated with methamphetamine inhalation. Neurology 38:589, 1988.

Rumbaugh CL, Bergeron RT, Scanlan RL, et al: Cerebral vascular changes secondary to amphetamine abuse in the experimental animal. Radiology 101:345, 1971.

Rush D, Kristal A, Blanc W, et al: The effects of maternal cigarette smoking on placental morphology, histomorphometry and biochemistry. Am J Perinatol 3:263, 1986.

Ryan L, Ehrlich S, Finnegan L: Cocaine abuse in pregnancy: Effects on the fetus and newborn. Neurotoxicol Teratol 9:295, 1987.

Sandor GG, Smith DF, MacLeod PM: Cardiac malformations in the fetal alcohol syndrome. J Pediatr 98:771, 1981.

Sexton M, Hebel JR: A clinical trial of change in maternal smoking and its effect on birth weight. JAMA 251:911, 1984.

Serdula M, Williamson DF, Kendrick JS, et al: Trends in alcohol consumption by pregnant women. 1985 through 1988. JAMA **265**:876, 1991.

Shiono PH, Klebanoff MA, Rhoads GG: Smoking and drinking during pregnancy. Their effects on preterm birth. JAMA **255**:82, 1986.

Shiono PH, Klebanoff MA, Berendes HW: Congenital malformations and maternal smoking during pregnancy. Teratology **34**:65, 1986.

Simpson WJ: A preliminary report on cigarette smoking and the incidence of prematurity. Am J Obstet Gynecol **73**:808, 1957.

Singh SP, Snyder AK, Singh SK: Effects of ethanol ingestion on maternal and fetal glucose homeostasis. J Lab Clin Med **104**:176, 1984.

Singh SP, Snyder AK, Pullen GL: Fetal alcohol syndrome: Glucose and liver metabolism in term rat fetus and neonate. Alcohol Clin Exp Res **10**:54, 1986.

Smith IE, Coles CD, Lancaster J, et al: The effect of volume and duration of prenatal ethanol exposure on neonatal physical and behavioral development. Neurobehav Toxicol Teratol **8**:375, 1986.

Snyder AK, Singh SP, Pullen GL: Ethanol-induced intrauterine growth retardation: Correlation with placental glucose transfer. Alcohol Clin Exp Res **10**:176, 1986.

Sokol RJ, Miller SI: Identifying the alcohol-abusing obstetric/gynecologic patient: A practical approach. Alcohol Health Res World **4**:36, 1980.

Sokol RJ, Miller SI, Reed G: Alcohol abuse during pregnancy: An epidemiologic study. Alcohol Clin Exp Res **4**:135, 1980.

Sokol RJ, Miller SI, Debanne S, et al: The Cleveland/NIAA prospective alcohol-in-pregnancy study: The first year. Neurobehav Toxicol Teratol **3**:203, 1981.

Sokol RJ, Clarren SK: Guidelines for use of terminology describing the impact of prenatal alcohol on the offspring. Alcoholism **13**:597, 1989.

Sokol RJ, Martier SS, Ager JW: The T-ACE questions: Practical prenatal detection of risk-drinking. Am J Obstet Gynecol **160**:863, 1989.

Soothill PW, Nicolaides KH, Bilardo K, et al: Uteroplacental blood velocity index and umbilical venous P_{O_2}, P_{CO_2}, pH, lactate, and erythroblast count in growth-retarded fetuses. Fetal Ther **1**:174, 1986.

Stewart DJ, Inaba T, Lucassen M, et al: Cocaine metabolism: Cocaine and norcocaine hydrolysis by liver and serum esterases. Clin Pharmacol Ther **252**:464, 1979.

Stimmel B, Jerez E: Alcohol and substance abuse during pregnancy. *In* Cherry SH, Berkowitz RL, Kase NG (eds): Medical, Surgical and Gynecologic Complications of Pregnancy. Baltimore, Williams and Wilkins, 1985.

Stone ML, Salerno LJ, Green M, et al: Narcotic addiction in pregnancy. Am J Obstet Gynecol **109**:717, 1971.

Streissguth AP, Aase JM, Clarren SK, et al: Fetal alcohol syndrome in adolescents and adults. JAMA **265**:1961, 1991.

Suzuki K, Horiguchi T, Comas-Urrutia AC, et al: Nicotine and cotinine in the amniotic fluid of smokers in the second trimester of pregnancy. Am J Obstet Gynecol **120**:64, 1974.

Suzuki K, Minei LJ, Johnson EE: Effect of nicotine upon uterine blood flow in the pregnant rhesus monkey. Am J Obstet Gynecol **136**:1009, 1980.

Taeusch HW, et al: Heroin induction of lung maturation and growth retardation in fetal rabbits. J Pediatr **82**:5, 1973.

Telsey A, Merrit A, Dixon S: Cocaine exposure in a term neonate: Necrotizing enterocolitis as a complication. Clin Pediatr **27**:547, 1988.

Tennes K, Avitable N, Blackard C, et al: Marijuana: Prenatal and postnatal exposure in the human. *In* Pinkert TM (ed): Consequences of Maternal Drug Abuse. Washington, DC, NIDA Research Monograph, No. 59, p. 48, 1985.

Tennes K, Blackard C: Maternal alcohol consumption, birth weight and minor physical anomalies. Am J Obstet Gynecol **138**:774, 1980.

Tenorio GM, Navzi M, Bickers GH, et al: Intrauterine stroke and maternal polydrug abuse. Clin Pediatr **27**:565, 1988.

U.S. Department of Health and Human Services: The Health Consequences of Smoking for Women; A Report of the Surgeon General. Washington, DC, U.S. Department of Health and Human Services, Public Health Service, Center for Disease Control. Center for Chronic Disease Prevention and Health Promotion, Office of Smoking and Health, 1980.

Umans JG, Szeto HH: Precipitated opiate abstinence in utero. Am J Obstet Gynecol **151**:441, 1985.

van de Bor M, Walther FJ, Sims ME: Increased cerebral blood flow velocity in infants of mothers who abuse cocaine. Pediatrics **85**:733, 1990.

Van der Berg, BJ: Epidemiological observations of prematurity: Effects of tobacco, coffee and alcohol. *In* Reed DN, Stanley FJ (eds): The Epidemiology of Prematurity. Baltimore, Urban and Schwarzenberg, 1977, pp 157–77.

Van der Veen F, Fox H. The effects of cigarette smoking on the human placenta: A light and electron microscopic study. Placenta **3**:243, 1982.

Virji SK: The relationship between alcohol consumption during pregnancy and infant birth weight. Acta Obstet Gynecol Scand **70**:303, 1991.

Watkinson B, Fried PA: Maternal caffeine use before, during and after pregnancy and effects upon offspring. Neurobehav Toxicol Teratol **7**:9, 1985.

Weathersbee PS, Olsen LK, Lodge JR: Caffeine and pregnancy: A retrospective survey. Postgrad Med **62**:64, 1977.

Webster WS, Brown-Woodman PDC: Cocaine as a cause of congenital malformation of vascular origin: Experimental evidence in the rat. Teratology **41**:689, 1990.

Williams MA, Mittendorf R, Lieberman E, et al: Cigarette smoking during pregnancy in relation to placenta previa. Am J Obstet Gynecol **165**:28, 1991.

Wilson GS, Desmond MM, Verniaud WM: Early development of infants of heroin-addicted mothers. Am J Dis Child **126**:457, 1973.

Wilson G: Clinical studies of infants and children exposed prenatally to heroin. Ann NY Acad Sci **562**:183, 1989.

Woods JR, Plessinger MA, Clark KE: Effect of cocaine on uterine blood flow and fetal oxygenation. JAMA **257**:957, 1987.

Woods JR, Plessinger MA: Pregnancy increases cardiovascular toxicity to cocaine. Am J Obstet Gynecol **162**:529, 1990.

Ylikorkala O, Halmesmaki E, Viinikka L: Urinary prostacyclin and thromboxane metabolites in drinking pregnant women and in their infants: Relation to the fetal alcohol effects. Obstet Gynecol **71**:61, 1988.

Zelson C, Lee SJ, Casalino M: Neonatal narcotic addiction: Comparative effects of maternal intake of heroin and methadone. N Engl J Med **289**:1216, 1973.

Zuckerman B, Frank DA, Hingson R, et al: Effects of maternal marijuana and cocaine use on fetal growth. N Engl J Med **320**:762, 1989.

Zuspan FP, Gumpel JA, Mejia-Zelaya A, et al: Fetal stress from methadone withdrawal. Am J Obstet Gynecol **122**:43, 1975.

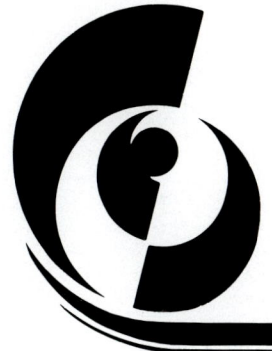

PART II

FETAL DIAGNOSTIC AND TREATMENT MODALITIES

ULTRASOUND IN PERINATAL MEDICINE

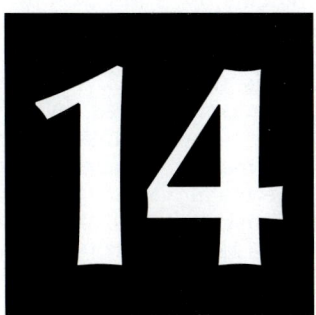

GENERAL PRINCIPLES AND APPLICATIONS OF ULTRASONOGRAPHY

FRANK A. MANNING, M.D., M.Sc. (OXON), FRCS (CANADA), FACOG, FSOGC

In the early 1960s a shift of major proportion occurred in the practice of obstetrics, and this shift was initiated by the pioneer work of the Scottish obstetrician the late Professor Ian Donald. Using a modification of wartime submarine detection devices (SONAR), Donald demonstrated that it was possible to create a fetal image based on the reflectance characteristics of its surface and internal structures (Donald and Brown, 1961). From these original observations flowed a series of technical advances that have continued to the present day. As a result of ultrasound imaging it is now possible to collect in considerable detail information pertaining to the morphometric, morphologic, and functional characteristics of the human fetus in health and disease. As a consequence, a balance has been introduced to the practice so that it is possible to have as much clinical detail regarding the fetus as is available concerning the mother. Paradoxically, it is now possible to gain as much or more information regarding structural and functional integrity of the fetus from prenatal ultrasound examination as is made available by direct examination of the newborn.

The fundamental and basic questions of fetal assessment are: What is the fetal age? How many fetuses are there? Are there structural/functional anomalies present? Is fetal growth appropriate? Is the fetus hypoxemic, and if so, how severe is the condition? Are the fetal environment and supporting structures normal?

Answers to these key clinical questions can be approximated by clinical methods, but can only be determined with certainty by the use of high-resolution dynamic ultrasound methods. The beneficial impact of ultrasound imaging in modern perinatal medicine has extended beyond the passive collection of fetal data. Now that accurate serial fetal observations are possible, it is also possible to better define the pathophysiology of common fetal diseases, the first step in the development of rational and tailored treatment modalities. Thus, for example, delivery solely on the basis of a clinical diagnosis of intrauterine growth restriction has been replaced by selective delivery of only those fetuses with evidence of placental dysfunction, whereas in the small but otherwise normal fetus and the fetus with growth failure secondary to lethal fetal anomaly, conservative management is usual. The dynamic aspect of the contemporary ultrasound image has made it possible to invade the fetus and its environment for diagnostic and therapeutic aims. The enhancement in the quality of perinatal care that may be achieved as a consequence of this advance has been considerable. Witness the dramatic improvement in the survival of the alloimmune anemic fetus secondary to ultrasound-guided intravascular transfusion (Harman and Manning, 1987) and the less dramatic, but nonetheless improved, outcome among selected fetuses with obstructive uropathy achieved by ultrasound-guided vesicoamniotic shunt placement (Harrison et al., 1982; Manning et al., 1983) (see also Chapter 25).

The impact of ultrasound on the practice of perinatal

medicine extends beyond direct clinical care. In days past, critical thought directed toward the understanding of fetal responses in health and disease was derived by extrapolation from observations and experiments in the nonhuman fetus. Today it is possible to examine the normal range of physiologic and pathophysiologic responses of the human fetus directly and without risk, thereby circumventing the problems of species variation inherent in all animal studies. Since human observation can occur without disturbing the fetal environment, the information recorded is not only specific to the human fetus, but also more accurate and reliable.

The application of dynamic ultrasound in its many modalities is now ubiquitous throughout perinatal medicine, and its clinical utility is under constant revision and expansion. Evidence to this effect is seen throughout this textbook: virtually all chapters dealing with aspects of fetal disease include a discussion of the application of ultrasound in its various guises. The intent of this chapter is to provide an overview of the many aspects of the application of ultrasound in the determination of fetal condition in health and disease and to present the contemporary concepts that govern its appropriate use.

ULTRASOUND IMAGING: TECHNICAL CONSIDERATIONS

The generation of an ultrasound pulse and the detection of echoes reflected from structures of varying density placed in the path of the ultrasound pulse is relatively simple. The ultrasound wave is produced by electrical excitation of artificial crystals (zirconium); exposure to high-energy electrons alters the lattice structure of the crystal, and the resulting brief deformation of the surface is propagated as a pressure wave. Conversely, external compression of the crystal by a pressure wave alters the lattice structure and results in the release of electrons (piezoelectric phenomenon). Altering the frequency of electrical pulses to the crystal determines the frequency of surface vibration; altering the power input determines the intensity of the pressure wave generated. Conversely, the strength of the signal produced within the crystal varies directly with the compression force applied to it, and the frequency varies directly with the rate at which compression occurs. These relationships are used to determine:

1. *The transducer frequency* (carrier frequency), which will vary from 2.25 MHz; (1 MHz = 1 million cycles per second) to 10 MHz. In fetal medicine, transducers with carrier frequencies of 3.5 to 5 MHz are the most practical.

2. *The transducer power,* typically measured as milliwatts per square centimeter. The upper limit of power considered to be safe for the fetus is 100 milliwatts per square centimeter (mW/cm^2); however, most dynamic B-mode ultrasound devices emit power far less than the maximum and operate in the range of 10 to 20 mW/cm^2. The power emitted by Doppler ultrasound devices is higher than with B-mode imaging, but

remains well within the recommended safety range. As signal processing improves, the amount of power output needed to maintain acceptable resolution has fallen. Most commercial equipment permits manipulation of power output, but governs the maximal output. As a general rule, one should use the minimal power necessary to ensure adequate image quality, but in some cases, as for example with the very obese patient, it will be necessary to use the maximal power available.

3. *The strength of the returning echo,* which is measured by the current it produces from within the transducer crystal. By this effect, echoes may be displayed according to brightness, hence the term *B-mode*. Modern equipment uses at least 64 and often 128 shades of gray to display echo strength, hence the term *gray scale*. The use of gray scale imaging greatly enhances the resolution of ultrasound images, permitting evaluation of target texture. The strength of the returning echo decreases exponentially with distance, and ultrasound devices use specialized (logarithmic) amplifiers to compensate for this effect. Sound wave reflections (echoes) occur at interfaces of varying density, the strength of the echo being directly proportional to difference in density; high-density structures (e.g., bone) are strong reflectors and low-density tissues (e.g., fat) are relatively weak reflectors. As in optics, the strength of a sound wave reflection is inversely related to angle of incidence between beam and target.

4. *The distance between the transducer and the reflective target,* which is determined by the time interval between pulse initiation and echo detection. This information is used to place the echoes in the appropriate position on the imaging screen, thereby generating complex target images. The speed at which the ultrasound signal traverses a structure varies directly with density (Table 14–1).

5. *The frequency of reflected echoes,* which is constant relative to the carrier frequency for a static target, but is altered by a moving target (the Doppler effect). The frequency of returning echoes is increased if the target is moving toward the transducer and decreased if the movement is away from the transducer. The frequency shifts are measured and (1) converted to either an audible sound, as with the simple ultrasound devices for detection of the fetal heart motion, or a trigger for the cardiotachometer used in continuous fetal heart rate recording devices (fetal monitors); or (2) displayed as a frequency/time plot and used to measure blood

TABLE 14–1.   Velocity of Sound Propagation in Biological and Nonbiological Media

MEDIUM	AVERAGE VELOCITY OF SOUND (m/sec)
Air	331
Water	1430
Fat	1450
Soft tissue (average)	1520
Brain	1540
Muscle	1580
Bone	4080

flow velocity waveforms in both maternal and fetal vessels; or (3) converted to colors based on the direction and magnitude of measured frequency shifts (color Doppler imaging).

The transducer functions in sequential fashion as the emitter and receiver of the ultrasound energy (the duty cycle) in a ratio of about 1:1000, respectively. The dynamic aspect of contemporary ultrasound imaging is created by the repetitive frequency of the duty cycle, set at or above the threshold of the human eye. This dynamic information may be displayed in B-mode or frequency spectrum (Doppler), or in both (color imaging), and, less commonly, may be displayed as a single B-mode line (time/motion display). Amplitude display of a single line (A-mode) is no longer used in obstetrics.

The shape of the dynamic ultrasound beam varies with the transducer construction and method of function. Transducers are generally classified as linear, annular, curvilinear, and sector; all but the mechanical sector scanners use sequential activation of the transducer crystals to produce and shape the ultrasound beam. Mechanical sector scanners are based on moving a single transducer through a prescribed arc. Transducer selection varies by availability and personal preference. Specialized transducers are available for transvaginal scanning.

Safety of Ultrasound Imaging

Because ultrasound information is created by spectral analysis of echoes produced when the target tissue is bombarded with sound energy, ultrasound imaging must be considered an invasive procedure carrying theoretical risks of tissue damage. Ultrasound energy is absorbed by tissues and transformed into other energy forms. Most sound energy is converted to heat, and the proportion of conversion increases directly with the emitting frequency. With low-level frequencies, a proportion of the energy is converted to movements within the target tissue, producing mechanical motion (vibration) called resonance. Low-frequency ultrasound can be used to create tissue disruption. This principle is applied therapeutically in physiotherapy. With diagnostic ultrasound, resonance does not occur, and most of the ultrasound energy is dissipated as heat. The amount of heat released per gram of tissue per unit of time varies directly with the intensity of the signal and inversely with the square of the distance from the emitting source. By convention, ultrasound energies are measured at the source and recorded as power per area, or watts per square centimeter. It is important to recognize that energy delivered to tissue varies inversely with the square of the distance. Thus, for example, if a target is 8 cm from an emitting source of 100 W/cm², the target will receive only 1/64, or 0.156 per cent, of the originally emitted energy. In special circumstances, with use of high-energy, low-frequency ultrasound, tissue disruption by cavitation can occur, but that effect does not occur with diagnostic ultrasound. For practical purposes a safe level of tissue ultrasound exposure has been arbitrarily defined as ≤100 mW/cm². Most commercial ultrasound instruments operate at ranges far lower than the maximal safe standard and produce energies of 10 to 20 mW/cm². Thus, a fetal target 8 cm from the course receives on average 0.01 to 0.03 mW/cm², or 0.01 to 0.03 per cent of the maximal safe levels. The total tissue energy is a function of exposure time. Diagnostic units employ pulsed ultrasound with a usual duty cycle of 1/1000, which, during 24 hours of continuous scanning, produces only 86 seconds of ultrasound exposure. Thus, ultrasound energy delivered to tissues varies with (1) frequency, (2) intensity (power), (3) exposure time, and (4) distance from emitting source.

At present there are no known examples of damage to target tissue from use of conventional diagnostic ultrasound imaging. Prospective studies of the biological effects of *in utero* exposure to ultrasound energies in the diagnostic range have failed to yield any differences in exposed offspring when compared to nonexposed sibling controls (Lyons and Coggrave-Toms, 1979). There is no doubt that exposure of tissue to high-energy (> 100 mW/cm²) continuous ultrasound in frequencies within the range used for diagnostic ultrasound can produce tissue damage (Edmonds, 1972). The relevance of this observation to current use of ultrasound in clinical obstetrics is questionable. It seems reasonable to state that diagnostic ultrasound in indicated circumstances carries no recognized inherent risk per se to the mother or her fetus and that it provides information that can produce major benefits in outcome of pregnancy.

CLINICAL APPLICATIONS OF ULTRASOUND: GUIDELINES FOR GENERAL APPLICATION (THE MINIMAL EXAMINATION)

Ultrasound imaging methods are employed widely in perinatal medicine, and their use continues to expand both in frequency and utility of application. Whereas it is generally held that this tool has been responsible for major advances in the practice of the specialty, there is not uniform agreement regarding its routine use. In most European countries, ultrasound assessment of pregnancy is done as a routine. In both the United States and Canada, universal ultrasound screening of all pregnancies has not been sanctioned, but rather the diagnostic procedure is recommended only for those pregnancies in which there are recognizable high-risk factors. The minimal criteria for conduct of an ultrasound examination in pregnancy have been developed and published by the Section of Obstetrics and Gynecology of the American Institute of Ultrasound in Medicine (AIUM) (Leopold, 1986) and are shown in Table 14–2. These criteria apply to the general examination and do not replace those for more detailed and specialized examinations in selected high-risk pregnancies. The guidelines assume that the operator has training in the use of ultrasound equipment and has at least a minimal understanding of the fetal anatomy and physiology and insight as to the relationship between the pregnancy risk factors and

Table 14–2. AIUM Guidelines (Minimal) for Obstetric Ultrasound Examination

First trimester
1. The location of the gestational sac should be documented; the embryo should be identified and the crown-rump length recorded.
2. Presence or absence of fetal life should be reported.
3. Fetal number should be documented.
4. Evaluation of the uterus (including cervix) and adnexal structures should be performed.

Second and third trimesters
1. Fetal life, number, and presentation should be documented.
2. An estimate of the amount of amniotic fluid (increased, decreased, normal) should be reported.
3. The placental location should be recorded and its relationship to the internal cervical os determined.
4. Assessment of gestational age should be accomplished by using a combination of biparietal diameter (or head circumference) and femur length. Fetal growth assessment (as opposed to age) requires the addition of abdominal circumference. If previous studies have been performed, an estimate of the appropriateness of interval change should be given.
5. Evaluation of the uterus and adnexal structures should be performed.
6. The study should include, but not necessarily be limited to, the following fetal anatomy: cerebral ventricles, spine, stomach, urinary bladder, umbilical cord insertion site on the anterior abdominal wall, and renal region.

the expected ultrasound findings. Only dynamic (real-time) ultrasound equipment should be used, and fetal examination with the older static ultrasound scanners is considered inappropriate and unsatisfactory. Adequate documentation of the results is considered to be essential for high-quality patient care. The AIUM recommendation is to maintain permanent records of the ultrasound images, appropriately labeled to identify the patient, the date of examination, and the scan orientation. Videotape records of the dynamic portion of the scan are not considered a requirement. The permanent record should also include a written interpretation of the observations, and a description of the examination should appear in the patient's medical record.

These AIUM-recommended minimal guidelines for ultrasound assessment vary according to gestational age.

In the *first trimester* the focus of the examination is directed primarily to determination of fetal age, number, and viability, and to detection of disease of contiguous structures. Crown-rump measurement is the recommended method for determining gestational age in the first trimester.

In the *second* and *third trimesters* the guidelines are more extensive and include assessment of fetal presentation, placental position (with particular reference to the relationship of the lower margin of the placenta to the lower uterine segment and the cervix), amniotic fluid volume, and a general survey of fetal anatomy which should include, but not necessarily be limited to, evaluation of the cerebral ventricles, spine, stomach, urinary bladder, kidney, and the region of insertion of the umbilical vessels into the fetal abdomen.

The required fetal morphometric measures are increased in number to include an estimate of head size, either by biparietal diameter or by head circumference, or both; determination of femur length; and measurement of the abdominal circumference in a plane at or near the intrahepatic junction of the umbilical vein and the portal sinus. When possible, a comparison of current with previous measurements should be evaluated and reported. The guidelines are summarized in Table 14–2.

PRINCIPLES AND GUIDELINES FOR ULTRASOUND ASSESSMENT OF THE FETUS AT RISK (THE EXTENDED EXAMINATION)

The AIUM guidelines need to be viewed in perspective; they describe the bare minimum of ultrasound information that should be obtained without reference to the expertise of the examiner and without reference to the presence of specific pregnancy risk factors. The principles of ultrasound fetal assessment for the perinatologist are different and may be summarized as follows:

1. The Criteria for Assessment of the Fetus at Risk Exceed the Minimal Criteria Described for the General Examination. In the specialized practice of maternal-fetal medicine, it is usual and recommended practice to collect considerably more information regarding the status of the fetus and its environment. The standard fetal ultrasound information regarding estimates of age, growth, structural integrity, and amniotic fluid volume should be supplemented with evaluation of fetal morphometric proportions, physiologic functions, umbilical cord structure and position, blood flow velocity waveform characteristics of the umbilical artery and intra-fetal vessels when indicated, and placental morphology.

2. The Criteria for the Assessment of The Fetus at Risk May Be Expected to Vary by Maternal and Fetal Risk Factors. The focus of ultrasound assessment may also be expected to vary according to the associated maternal risk factors and by the results of the current or preceding ultrasound examination. This concept, termed *disease-specific assessment*, has become a critical and necessary aspect of the complete ultrasound examination. As with most aspects of ultrasound assessment, disease-specific assessment is merely an intrauterine extension of a traditional and time-honored principle of extrauterine medicine: the search for the signs of a disease process will vary according to the understanding of the pathophysiology of the condition. Fetal medicine is replete with examples of application of this principle: (1) detection of a variance of fetal mass below the normal range for gestational age should trigger a detailed search for the underlying etiology; (2) in the diabetic pregnancy, the ultrasound examination is focused toward detection of macrosomia and of such anomalies as caudal regression syndrome and cardiac defects, which are common in this condition; (3) in alloimmune syndromes, fetal liver size and morphology are specifically assessed; (4) in multiple gestation, the ultrasound examination is extended so as to obtain information on the type of twinning present and the presence or absence of complications specific to the condition. When the principle of disease-specific assessment is considered in the light of the range and complexities of fetal disease, it is easy to see that annotation of appropriate universal criteria for ultrasound examination is neither simple nor direct, but rather must include both the basics and the focused examination.

3. **IN THE FETUS AT RISK, DYNAMIC ULTRASOUND ASSESSMENT IS USED BOTH AS A DIAGNOSTIC AND A MANAGEMENT TOOL.** The impact of this principle on the practice of fetal medicine is best viewed in a historical perspective. At its inception, ultrasound imaging in pregnancy was seen as a method for estimation of fetal viability, age, and number. As a diagnostic tool, it was confined to the domain of imaging specialists, usually radiologists, who were somewhat remote from direct clinical care and whose function was to provide a diagnosis but not a management plan. The concept of monitoring the pathophysiology of a given condition and the concept of integrating a wide spectrum of critical information into a rational management plan have now become integral aspects of ultrasound fetal assessment. The fetus is now viewed as a separate patient in whom the detection of a disease process, usually by ultrasound assessment, is the beginning step in formulating management. In this contemporary age, the collection of the needed uterine and fetal ultrasound information is done by the managing perinatologist. The information collected and considered includes (1) determination of the presence or absence of a given fetal risk condition, (2) monitoring the progression of such a condition, (3) estimating the probability that a given condition and/or an associated complication will cause serious or even lethal fetal or neonatal sequelae, (4) balancing the relative risks and benefits of continued intrauterine existence versus delivery and neonatal care, (5) consideration of the applicability and efficacy of the various forms of disease-specific intrauterine fetal therapy, (6) consideration of the potential value of ultrasound-guided invasive diagnostic procedures; and (7) integrating these data within the context of the maternal condition and the usual obstetric considerations. The relationship between the diagnostic and the management aspects of ultrasound fetal assessment is both intimate and dynamic. Once a diagnosis of a potentially serious fetal disorder has been established, the focus of ultrasound assessment is turned toward the balancing of fetal versus neonatal risks. In some clinical instances, the diagnosis per se dictates management: the ultrasound diagnosis of a lethal fetal anomaly, for example anencephaly, precludes the need for any further fetal assessment, and management departs from fetal considerations and is directed solely to avoidance of maternal morbidity. Similarly in the mature fetus, the diagnosis of severe dysmature intrauterine growth restriction obviates further assessment, and intervention is directed toward fetal indications. In most clinical instances, however, an ultrasound diagnosis is only the first albeit critical aspect

of ultrasound assessment, and subsequent evaluation is directed toward monitoring the progression of the fetal disease and in the balancing of relative fetal versus neonatal risks.

The ability to exclude fetal disease despite the presence of historical or maternal risk factors is an important aspect of ultrasound assessment. In the pre-ultrasound era, management protocols were empiric, based on the probability of existing fetal complications as derived from general experience. Thus, for example, for patients with diabetes, hypertension, suspected intrauterine growth restriction, and pregnancies that extended beyond 42 completed weeks, management by delivery at a predescribed fetal age was commonly recommended. In contemporary perinatal medicine, it has become possible to modify management of these high-risk circumstances according to the presence or absence of signs of fetal compromise as determined by direct ultrasound fetal assessment. The approach does not entirely obviate an aggressive obstetric approach to the management of many high-risk circumstances, but does permit many of these pregnancies to continue longer without undue fetal risk. Ultrasound-guided selective conservative management of the high-risk pregnancy can reduce the incidence of neonatal complications associated with immaturity and can be expected to reduce the incidence of induction and operative delivery in the mother, thereby reducing her risk of associated complications. A summary of the ultrasound evaluation of the high-risk fetus is shown in Table 14–3.

4. **ULTRASOUND DATA IN THE HIGH-RISK FETUS MUST BE INTERPRETED WITHIN THE OVERALL CLINICAL CONTEXT.** The highly reliable ultrasound information regarding the presence, progression, and risk associated with a fetal disease state cannot be interpreted in isolation, but rather needs to be considered in the light of maternal and obstetric factors. The integration of the maternal, fetal, and obstetric factors determines the need for, the frequency of, and the management plan that flows from any ultrasound examination. The fetal aspects of this equation have been discussed previously. The maternal aspects are of equal importance, and clearly fetal management decisions must be made in the light of the maternal condition. Serious and/or progressive pregnancy-related maternal disease is considered an indication for intervention and will override fetal considerations. Thus, for example, serial antepartum fetal assessment by ultrasound methods in the presence of severe progressive maternal hypertension is not warranted. Similarly, a diagnosis of a lethal fetal anomaly may not influence the mode of delivery in a patient with a history of a previous classic cesarean section. Assessment of the maternal condition will also influence the frequency of fetal ultrasound assessment. In the diabetic patient under poor control or in the patient with a medical condition that is associated with increased fetal risk (e.g., systemic lupus erythematosus), assessment of the fetus may be frequent. Interpretation of the fetal ultrasound findings are also influenced by obstetric factors. The favorability of the cervix for induction, fetal position, and a history of previous cesarean section may be expected to influence the management decisions that arise as a result of ultrasound fetal assessment.

TABLE 14–3. Ultrasound Assessment of the High-Risk Fetus: Extended Criteria

CRITERION	STANDARD METHOD/ PROCEDURES	ANCILLARY METHODS/ PROCEDURES	EXAMPLES OF CLINICAL APPLICATION
Fetal age determination	Parameter of head size (BPD, head circumference); femur length, abdominal circumference	Other long bone length (humerus, tibia, etc.); facial structures (mandible length, intraorbital diameter, pinna size); foot length	Differentiation of mistaken dates and IUGR; determination of risk to neonatal viability in threatened preterm labor
Fetal mass determination	Abdominal circumference alone; head circumference; femur length	Calculated fetal volume methods; total intrauterine volume	Detection of IUGR/macrosomia; determination of volume of blood for fetal transfusion
Determination of fetal number	General uterine survey; estimate of zygosity; assessment of membranes; determination of type of placentation; determination of fetal positions	US-guided invasive diagnostic/ therapeutic procedures (decompressing amniocentesis, selective fetal reduction)	Identification of twin-twin transfusion syndrome and identification and management of twin disparity growth syndrome
Fetal structural/functional integrity	Anatomic survey notation and assessment of dynamic physiologic variables	US-guided invasive diagnostic procedures (PUBS, CVS, amniocentesis, fetal biopsy)	Site selection for delivery of a fetus with treatable anomaly; avoidance of intervention for a lethal anomaly; specific intrauterine therapy
Environmental assessment	Assessment of position and morphology of the placenta and cord; amniotic fluid volume and its reflective characteristics; evaluation for the presence of abnormal structures within the uterine cavity (e.g., amniotic bands), uterine wall (fibroids); determination of fetal position	Doppler assessment of umbilical artery blood flow velocity waveform	Identification of placenta previa; identification of cord presentation; detection of intraplacental and intra-amniotic bleeding
Evaluation of immediate fetal risk	Amniotic fluid volume; fetal movement, breathing, and tone (modified biophysical profile score)	US-guided cordocentesis for fetal blood gas determination; blood flow velocity waveform assessment of intrafetal vessels	Balancing the risk of fetal versus neonatal morbidity and mortality

SPECIFIC APPLICATION OF ULTRASOUND IN PERINATAL MEDICINE

Determination of Fetal Age by Ultrasound

General Principles

Determination of gestational age and its correlate, the estimated date of confinement (EDC), is standard obstetric practice. They form the critical base from which pathologic deviations from the normal are recognized. The accuracy of the age estimate is not only critical in the planning of appropriate management, but may also alter profoundly the actual incidence of suspected high-risk factors in a population. For example, regarding the incidence of intrauterine growth restriction in a given population, the incidence of suspected disease is as high as 20 per cent when gestational age is based on menstrual history and as low as 5 per cent when based on ultrasound-derived dates. Similarly, the incidence of prolonged or post-term pregnancy (>294 completed days) is 9 per cent using menstrual dates, but only 3 per cent using ultrasound dates (Grennert et al., 1978). The importance of accurate gestational age estimates is now becoming more apparent earlier in pregnancy. Selection of appropriate transfusion volumes, either by intraperitoneal or intravascular routes, in alloimmunized fetuses depends upon accurate date estimates (Harman and Manning, 1987). Determination of accurate dates is now essential in plotting distribution

of maternal serum alpha-fetoprotein values. Selection of the appropriate temporal window for chorionic villus sampling depends upon such accurate estimates. Projecting toward the future, it is likely that new therapies such as stem cell transfusion and gene therapy will depend upon accurate dates.

Estimation of gestational age by ultrasound is based on the known relationship between fetal age and fetal size, in part and in whole. Since accurate measurement of a wide range of fetal physical parameters is feasible by contemporary ultrasound methods, it therefore becomes possible to construct distribution plots (nomograms) of given measurements against gestational age (Fig. 14–1). From such nomograms, mean fetal age and range of estimate can be calculated. Interestingly, virtually all such nomograms yield estimate accuracy at least comparable to that of data based on the last normal menstrual period (LNMP) and, importantly, the majority yield substantially better estimate accuracy.

The ultrasound method for fetal age determination has several other inherent advantages. Among these are the opportunity to select the most accurate variable for a given fetal age range (e.g., crown-rump as opposed to biparietal diameter [BPD]), to combine variables to refine predictive accuracy (e.g., BPD and femur length), and to measure variables sequentially.

The selection of the optimal method(s) and interpretation of predictive accuracy are dependent upon several basic principles. These are:

ACCURACY OF ULTRASOUND ESTIMATE OF FETAL AGE

NAME : _____

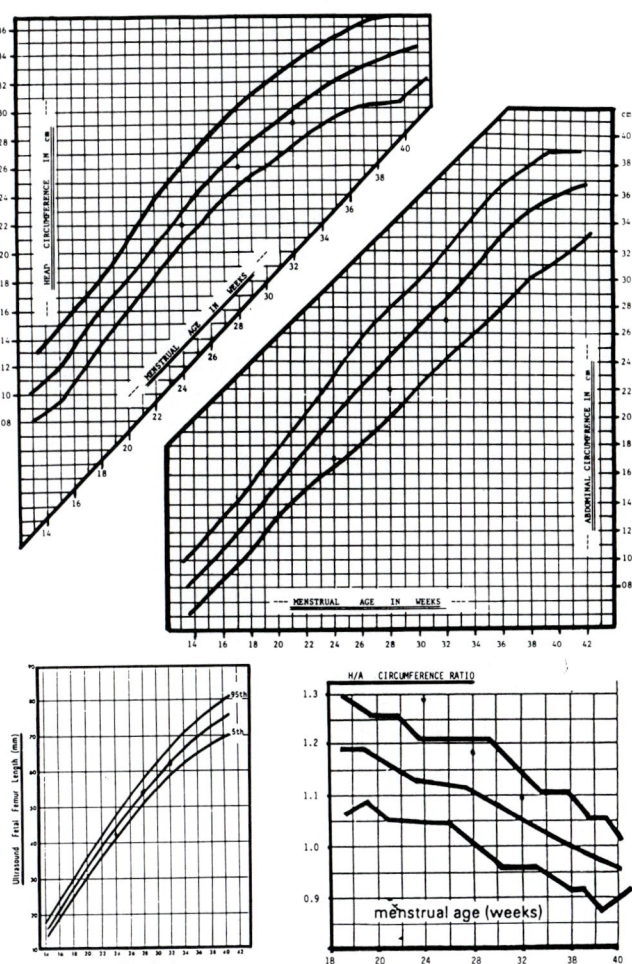

FIGURE 14–1. A typical fetal morphometric work sheet containing nomograms for head circumference, abdominal circumference, femur length, and intrafetal morphometric proportion (HC/AC ratio). Curves are constructed as the mean value ± 2 SD for gestational age as derived from a normal obstetric population. These composite graphs serve as a practical method for assessment of the rate of fetal growth. In this graph fetal morphometric parameters were determined at 24 weeks, then again at 28 and 32 weeks. Fetal head and abdominal circumferences are at about the 40th percentile for age, and these structures exhibit a normal growth rate. The femur length is near the mean for age, and growth rate is normal. Intrafetal morphometric proportions (HC/AC ratio) are normal.

IS INVERSELY RELATED TO FETAL AGE. The rate at which a fetus grows is not constant, but rather shows a progressive and sustained transition from the exponential rate evident at conception toward the linear rate evident in late pregnancy. The more rapid the growth rate, the more pronounced the incremental change in a given physical parameter per unit time. Further fetal growth is the net result of the interaction between intrinsic growth potential and environmental factors that may enhance or inhibit growth. The influence of environmental factors becomes progressively more apparent as gestational age advances. Hence, the distribution of physical measurements for a population of fetuses of the same age broadens as age advances (Fig. 14–2). Accordingly, the accuracy of a physical measurement parameter in predicting gestational age is inversely proportional to gestational age. This important clinical phenomenon has been observed for virtually every physical determinant of fetal age that can be measured by ultrasound.

THE OPTIMAL METHOD FOR ULTRASOUND DETERMINATION OF FETAL AGE VARIES WITH GESTATIONAL AGE. A gestational sac, signalling intrauterine pregnancy, has been identified from as early as the 25th day after the first day of the LNMP (conceptual age

11 days). The developing embryo has been visualized as early as the 34th day after LNMP (conceptual age 20 days), and fetal heart motion as early as the 38th day after LNMP (conceptual age 24 days). Whereas gestational sac volume can be used to estimate gestational age from as early as 4 weeks from LNMP, crown-rump length determination is the most practical early measure used. Crown-rump length can be determined from as early as 5 weeks to 12 weeks gestation and remains one of the most accurate methods of fetal age determination (Fig. 14–3). The range of error of estimate with crown-rump length is approximately 3 days (Robinson, 1973), and this index of age is substantially more accurate than estimates based upon menstrual history. From about the 12th week onward, crown-rump length determination becomes more difficult because of deflexion and variable position of the developing fetal head. At about the tenth or 12th week, the fetal head may be well visualized and intracranial anatomic landmarks identified. The BPD can be measured from about 12 weeks onward, and such measurements between the 12th and 20th weeks yield an estimate error of less than 7 days (Hadlock et al., 1982b). Although fetal long bone structures (humerus and femur) are seen as early as 10 weeks

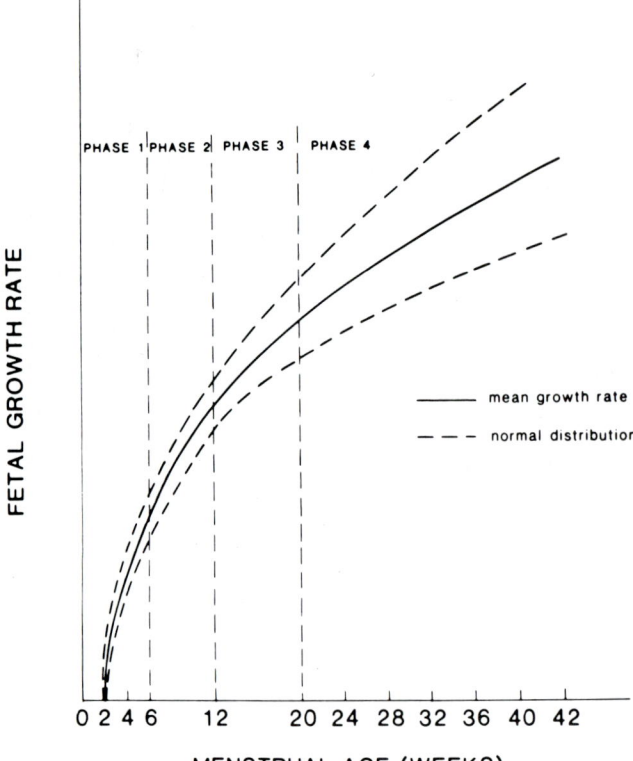

FIGURE 14–2. Theoretical plot of fetal growth rate against menstrual age.

Phase 1: 0–6 weeks

Conceptual growth is exponential at the onset with initial transition toward linear growth. Individual variability is minimal at this stage. Gestational sac volume can be measured by 4 weeks. The embryo is seen as early as 4.5 weeks (20 days conceptual age), and fetal heart activity is seen from as early as 5 weeks (24 days conceptual age).

Phase 2: 6–12 weeks

Growth rate is slowing, but individual variability still remains sharply restricted. Crown-rump measurement can be made from as early as 6 weeks and yields an estimated error of ± 3 days. At about 10 weeks the biparietal diameter (BPD) can be measured.

Phase 3: 12–20 weeks

Growth rate continues to slow and individual variability becomes more apparent. BPD can be measured from as early as 10 weeks; femur length and abdominal circumference are measured from as early as 14 weeks. Composite age estimates yield an error of estimate of about 1 week.

Phase 4: 20 weeks onward

Growth rate is slowing and individual variability becomes progressively more apparent as age advances. Composite age estimates yield an error of at least ± 1.5 weeks. Serial estimates of the growth rate derived from composite variables become the method of choice for age estimation. In late phase 4 (>32 weeks) the range of error of estimate (> ± 2.5 weeks) precludes accurate estimate of fetal age. Alternate clinical methods must be used.

gestation, accurate measurement of length is difficult before about 14 weeks gestation. Fetal long bone measurements are technically possible from about 14 to 16 weeks gestation onward.

THE TECHNICAL ERROR OF MEASUREMENT IS RELATIVELY CONSTANT. The axial resolution of a given ultrasound line is high, yielding discrimination to as high as 0.2 mm, and this axial resolution does not vary with absolute target size. Therefore, assuming that the target insonation angle is appropriate and the guiding landmarks are seen, the error of estimate due to axial resolution is constant and minimal. However, as ultrasound resolution has increased, selection of the start and end points for a given measurement have become more difficult. For example, BPD measurement by the older bistable B-mode methods was relatively simple because only the bony table of the calvarium produced a recognizable signal. With modern equipment, not only is the bone of the calvarium seen, but so are hair, skin, and subcutaneous tissue. It therefore becomes essential to assume that the beginning point of measurement is set at the calvarium surface and not the scalp surface.

ACCURACY OF GESTATIONAL AGE ESTIMATES BY ULTRASOUND INCREASES AS MORE VARIABLES ARE MEASURED. There is a clear relationship between a growing fetal physical parameter and gestational age. In the early days of ultrasound determination of fetal age the dimensions of the fetal head were the only fetal landmarks that could be measured in a reproducible and certain manner. Hence these dimensions, and in particular the BPD, became the mainstay of fetal age estimates. Now, using contemporary high-resolution ultrasound methods, we are presented with a large

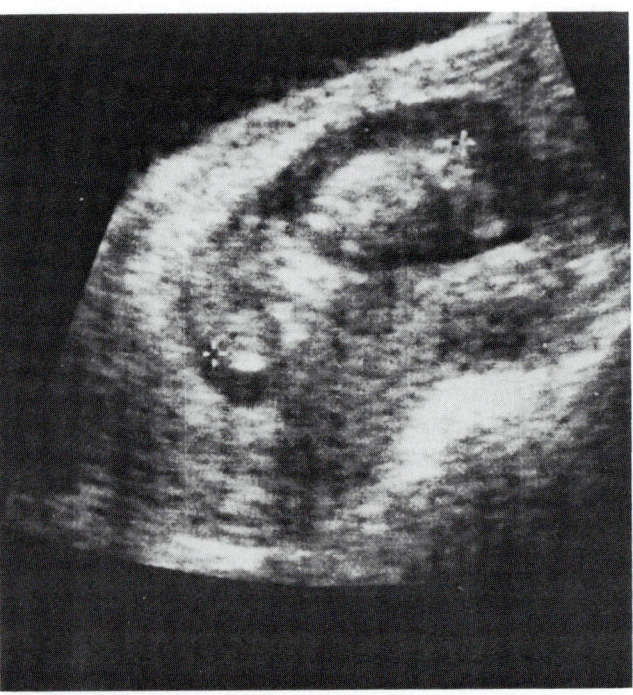

FIGURE 14–3. Crown-rump measurement in a 12-week fetus. Note that the fetal head at this age is very large relative to the thorax and abdomen.

spectrum of fetal physical parameters that may be measured simply and accurately. To date, all such parameters have been shown to be subject to the vicissitudes of the inherent population variability characteristic of later pregnancy, and no single variable shows an appreciable advantage in predictive accuracy.

The inherent variability in a fetal population of equal age is not constant across physical variables, but rather varies for each individual parameter. This principle is of some considerable clinical importance since it means that the error of estimate for the mean of composite variables will always be less than the error for any single variable. Thus, for example, Hadlock et al. (1983a), using a composite estimate of BPD, abdominal circumference, head circumference, and femur length, have shown improvement of predictive accuracy of 8 per cent in early pregnancy (12 to 18 weeks) and up to 28 per cent improvement in late pregnancy (36 to 42 weeks). It would seem reasonable therefore to conclude that all ultrasound estimates of fetal age beyond the crown-rump measurement stage should be based upon a range of variables. Which variables and how many variables should be included in the composite estimate are subjects undergoing active research. It seems obvious that there will be a point of ever-diminishing return by which the addition of further variables will no longer refine accuracy, but this point remains undefined at present. In our practice we use a composite of BPD, femur length, abdominal circumference, and foot length to estimate fetal age. Estimates of fetal age based upon only a single variable such as BPD should and will disappear from clinical practice.

IN LATER GESTATION THE ACCURACY OF FETAL AGE DETERMINATION IS ENHANCED BY SERIAL MEASUREMENTS. For reasons cited previously, determination of fetal age in later pregnancy (greater than 20 weeks) as based on a single ultrasound examination can be fraught with considerable error, the magnitude of which increases as gestational age advances (see Fig. 14–2). This clinical dilemma is common and usually occurs in the patient with an unknown or uncertain menstrual history who, for whatever reasons, enters for prenatal care at an advanced gestation. Since it is distinctly uncommon for dates to be underestimated by whatever menstrual data may be available, such patients are frequently considered to have possible intrauterine growth restriction. Determination of the rate of fetal growth by serial estimates of fetal physical parameters done at intervals spaced widely enough in time to account for the inherent measurement error (usually more than 2 weeks), is the method of choice for evaluation of such patients. The concept is based upon the curvilinear characteristics of the mean growth curve of the normal fetus (see Fig. 14–2) and requires a composite estimate rather than any single variable. Sabbagha et al. (1978) have described a method, termed *growth-adjusted sonographic age* (GASA), that was developed from this principle. This method uses estimates of BPD and abdominal circumference rate before 26 weeks and some 10 to 12 weeks later to calculate the slope of fetal growth (Tamura and Sabbagha, 1980). When applied correctly, the method yields an estimate error of 1 week more or less. The method, despite its theoretical appeal, is somewhat impractical since the first ultrasound scan must be done before 26 weeks. Accordingly, the method has not found widespread acceptance. An alternate method dependent upon the same principle involves serial composite measurements, usually two and preferably three such measurements, spaced at least 2 weeks apart, plotted against standard fetal growth curves. The method, when applied between 24 and 32 weeks gestation, yields an estimate error of 10 days more or less. Fetal age estimates beyond 32 weeks gestation are subject to major error and are not of real clinical value. In such cases management is best based upon assessment of fetal well-being and detection of ancillary signs of either excessive or reduced fetal growth.

Specific Fetal Measurements

Fetal Head Measurements

By convention the physical dimensions of the fetal head are measured in the plane of the BPD. This transverse plane transcribes the fetal head at an angle approximately 30 degrees to a line connecting the orbits and occiput and is just above the internal auditory meatus (Fig. 14–4). Within the plane lie the anterior falx, the cavum septum pellucidum, the anterior horn and lateral walls of the lateral ventricles, the choroid plexus, and the midbrain nucleus, the thalamus. Portions of the middle cerebral arteries and

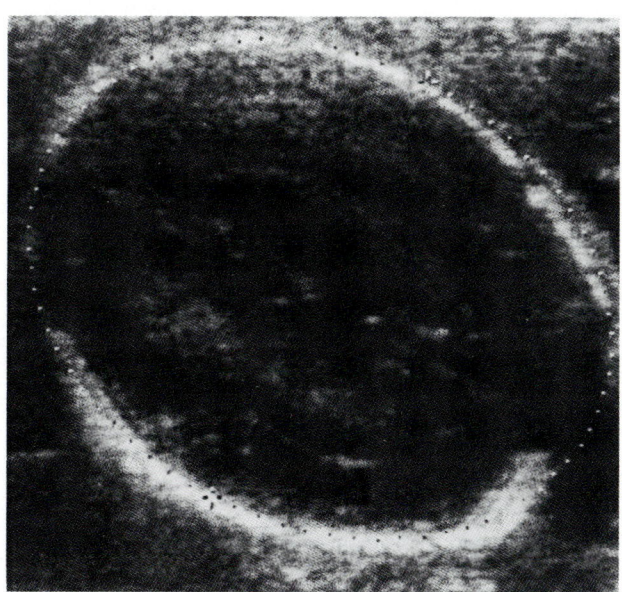

FIGURE 14–4. The fetal head in the plane of the biparietal diameter. Note the ovoid shape. The midline structure, the septum cavum pellucidum, is well visualized, as are the lateral walls of the lateral ventricle, the anterior horn, and the choroid plexus. Portions of the middle cerebral artery in the sylvian gyrus and branches of the circle of Willis are seen with dynamic mode imaging. In this fetus the BPD measures 71.3 mm, the head circumference is 258 mm, and the cephalic index is 77 per cent.

the vessels of the circle of Willis are usually seen in this plane. The definition of structure improves with advancing gestation, but accurate measurement depends upon recognition of most of these landmarks. Attention to detail is critical to measurement accuracy. Measurements at a plane above the true BPD will underestimate the true dimension, and tangential or oblique angulation may overestimate the true dimension.

Three fetal head dimensions are commonly measured. The BPD is measured as the distance between the outer surface of the proximal calvarium (outer skull table) to the inner surface of the distal calvarium (inner skull table) at the maximal width of the head in the previously described BPD plane. The long axis of the fetal head is measured from the outer surface of the front of the skull to the outer surface at the back of the skull. The head circumference (HC) is measured along the outer surface of the fetal skull in the plane of the BPD. With most modern equipment the measurements are obtained simultaneously using electronic planimetric calipers. For the most part, BPD and HC may be used interchangeably to estimate fetal age, with BPD being the most commonly used variable. The accuracy of estimate for either varies with gestational age, yielding an estimate error of $\pm$ 8 days before 20 weeks gestation, $\pm$ 12 days between 18 and 24 weeks, and $\pm$ 15 days after 24 weeks (Hadlock, 1985).

Because variation in fetal head shape is not uncommon and since BPD may vary with head shape, there are theoretical advantages to using head circumference as the method of choice. However, at the time of writing, BPD measurement is the most commonly reported parameter. Variation in head shape must be considered as well in interpretation of BPD measurements. Dolichocephaly, describing a fetal head shape in which the longitudinal axis is exaggerated and the transverse axis (BPD) is foreshortened, is commonly seen with breech presentation and with severe oligohydramnios. A BPD determination done in the dolichocephalic head will underestimate fetal age. In contrast, brachycephaly, in which the longitudinal axis is foreshortened and the transverse axis (BPD) exaggerated, while uncommon, may be observed. A BPD determination done in the brachycephalic head will overestimate fetal age.

The concept of cephalic index is designed to avoid these potential errors (Hohler, 1982). The predictive accuracy of the BPD is maintained provided the cephalic index, defined as the longitudinal length divided by BPD $\times$ 100, is within 78 $\pm$ 8 per cent. When the cephalic index falls outside this normal range, the use of head circumference rather than BPD is recommended.

The estimate of fetal age is determined from published nomograms. Many such nomograms exist as derived from study population that vary by ethnic and geographic factors. The selection of the appropriate nomogram will vary with the individual population characteristics.

Fetal Long Bone and Limb Measurements

Fetal limb anatomy, including the bony structures, may now be assessed easily by means of conventional high-resolution ultrasound equipment. The growth of the long bones (femur, tibia, fibula, humerus, radius, and ulna), all of which may be measured, as expected bear a direct relationship to fetal age (Jeanty et al., 1981b). By convention, femur length is the long bone measurement used most commonly as a fetal age determinant (O'Brien and Queenan, 1981). This measurement is made from the outer surface of the proximal end of the femur (greater trochanter) along the shaft of the femur to the distal end, not including the distal femoral epiphysis (Fig. 14–5). Such measurements become technically possible from about 14 weeks gestation onward. The range of error of estimate of fetal age by femur length varies with gestational age, ranging from as low as $\pm$ 7 days when done before 20 weeks to as high as $\pm$ 16 days when done beyond 36 weeks gestation (Hadlock, 1985).

The value of long bone assessment extends beyond determination of fetal age. Abnormalities of limb growth (e.g., short limb dystrophy) are detected by such assessment. Furthermore, long bone growth, in particular femur growth, bears a direct relationship to linear growth of the fetus. By this association fetal length may be determined according to the following formula (Fazekas and Kosa, 1978):

$$\text{Fetal length} = (\text{femur length (cm)} \times 6.44) + 4.51$$

The method yields an estimate of fetal length to within 1 cm when done after 36 weeks gestation (Manning et al., 1983a). Fetal length determination is a critical component of fetal mass-to-length ratios (ponderal

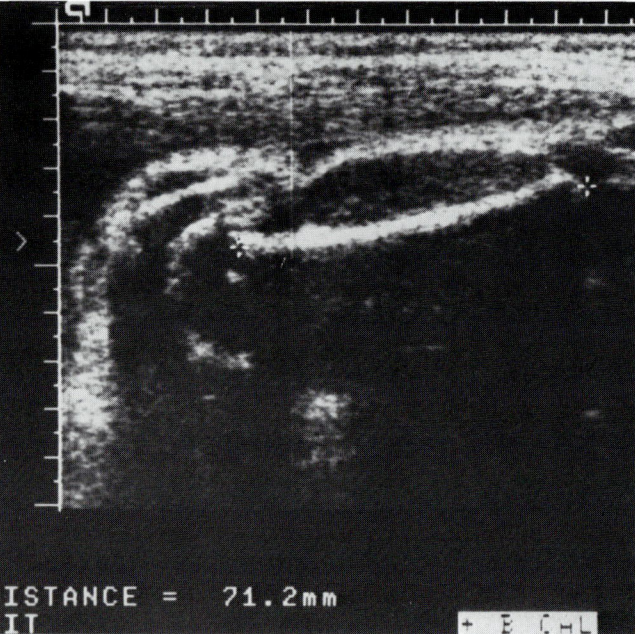

FIGURE 14–5. Ultrasound image of the femur in a fetus at term. The calipers are placed proximally on the greater trochanter and distally at the edge of the femur shaft. The slight curvature of the femur shaft is a usual and normal observation. Note the ossified distal femoral epiphysis appearing as an echogenic structure at the distal end of the femur. Bone shadowing is observed, and this is also a normal finding.

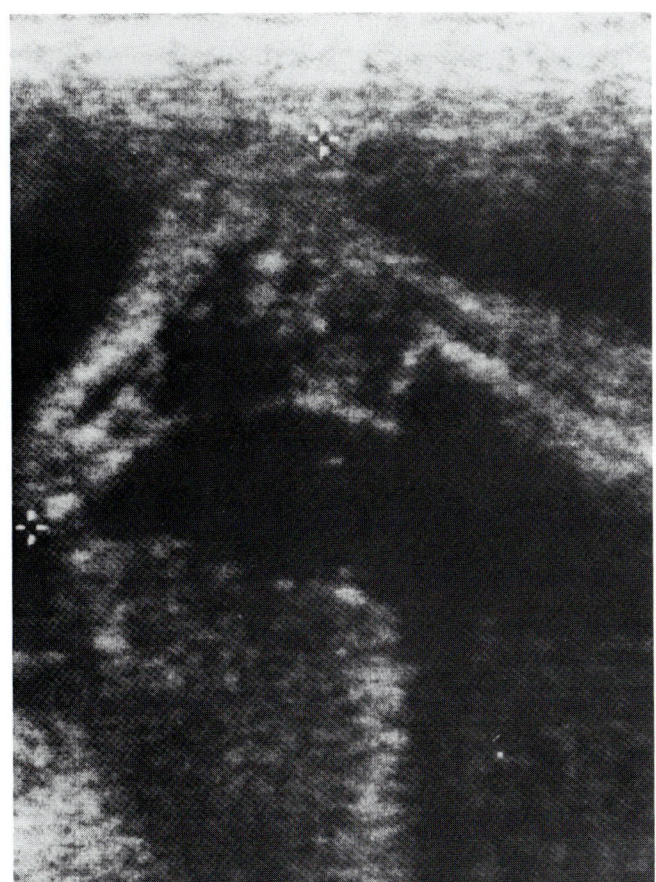

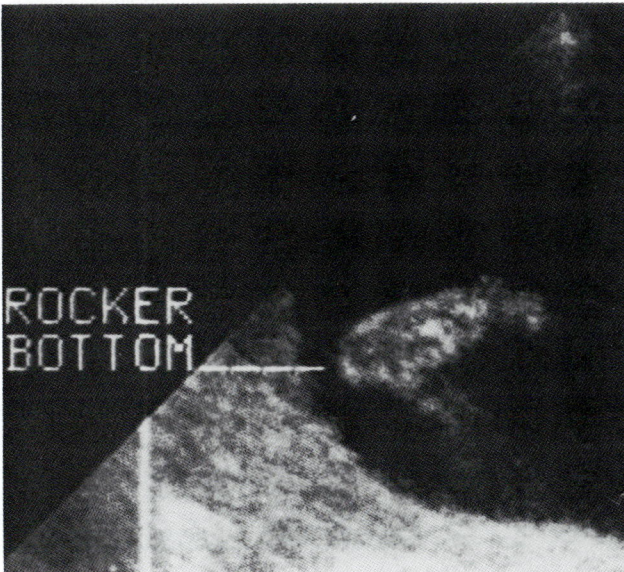

FIGURE 14–7. Fetal foot at 17 weeks gestation in a fetus with trisomy 13. The foot exhibits edema with loss of normal contour. This finding is not diagnostic of underlying karyotype abnormality but rather only an indication for further investigation.

FIGURE 14–6. Fetal foot in sagittal view. Foot length is 48.3 mm, consistent with a gestational age of 25.5 weeks. Fetal foot measurements are usually obtained without difficulty and are used in calculation of composite ultrasound fetal age estimates.

index) and may be used for recognition of abnormalities of fetal growth.

Assessment of anatomy and length of the fetal foot also holds promise as an ancillary method for determination of fetal age and condition (Fig. 14–6). The measurement is made from the outer surface of the heel to the distal end of the great toe. Fetal foot length yields an estimate of error comparable to femur length and BPD (Mercer et al., 1987). Fetal foot position may be used to detect contraction deformities; soft tissue defects may be seen with a variety of chromosomal abnormalities (Fig. 14–7).

Fetal Abdominal Circumference Determination

Measurement of fetal abdominal circumference at a plane just slightly superior to the umbilicus may be used to assess both fetal age and fetal mass (Campbell, 1977). Abdominal circumference (AC) is measured in the maximal transverse plane of the upper abdomen. Included within this plane are fetal liver, stomach, spleen, and a portion of the umbilical vein within the hepatic structure (Fig. 14–8). Measurement of the AC may be done directly by direct planimetric methods or calculated from the mean of two perpendicular

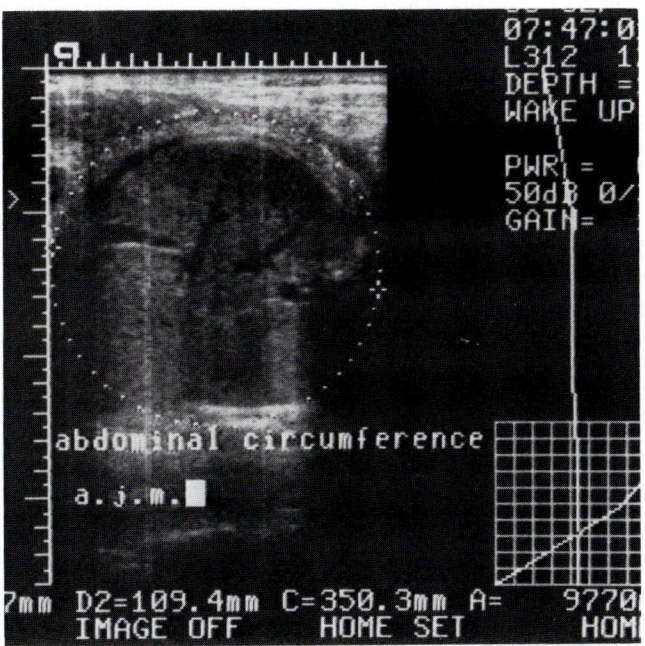

FIGURE 14–8. Transverse scan of the abdomen in a 36-week fetus. The fetal spine is at 3 o'clock. The echolucent intrahepatic portion of the umbilical vein is seen at 9 o'clock. Note the relatively homogeneous fetal liver and the echolucent branching of the hepatic vein. The inferior vena cava is seen as an echolucent circle just anterior and inferior to the fetal spine. This is the correct view from which to measure the fetal abdominal circumference. In this fetus, electronic calipers are used to record an abdominal circumference of 35.0 cm.

diameters. Because in the midline sagittal plane the fetal abdomen is ovoid, the accuracy of AC measurement depends critically on selection of the largest transverse plane. Fetal AC determination yields an estimate error of ± 12 days when done before 20 weeks gestation and an error of ± 21 days when done after 36 weeks (Hadlock et al., 1982a).

Ancillary Ultrasound Measures of Fetal Age

As stated previously, virtually any physical parameter of the growing, developing fetus may be expected to bear a direct relationship to fetal age. If one uses contemporary high-resolution dynamic ultrasound imaging, it is possible to measure a wide range of such fetal physical variables. Accordingly, the literature now contains many reports relating new parameters to fetal age. These variables include distal femoral epiphyseal size (Chinn et al., 1983), intraorbital diameter (Mayden et al., 1982), renal diameter (Jeanty et al., 1982), and gut structural characteristics (Goldstein et al., 1987). Even such variables as the morphology of the fetal external ear may be used to assess fetal age (Birnholz, 1983). By use of the dynamic mode, it has been possible to assess developmental movement patterns (Nijhuis et al., 1982) and gut peristalsis as markers of fetal age. What remains unclear at this writing is whether such ancillary measures, when considered alone or in combination, will be of any measurable value in refining the predictive accuracy of fetal age estimates as compared to estimates based on a composite assessment of head, long bone, and abdominal circumference measurements.

Estimation of Fetal Weight (Mass)

Fetal weight estimates, like fetal age estimates, commonly play a pivotal role in perinatal management decisions. Because perinatal weight correlates with neonatal survival, decisions regarding the appropriateness of intervention, observation, and management in the high-risk premature fetus may be strongly influenced by fetal weight estimates. As the field of fetal therapy continues to unfold, accurate fetal weight estimates have become even more important in calculating drug dosage and blood transfusion volumes (Harman and Manning, 1987). Most importantly, however, fetal weight estimates, when considered against age estimates, provide the basis for recognition of abnormal fetal growth patterns; the increased risk of perinatal death at the extremes of the normal growth curve has been well described (Lubchenco et al., 1972, Morrison and Olsen, 1985).

Because the recognition of fetal weight and age discrepancies is of such clinical importance, there is a great need for accurate methods to detect these aberrations of growth. Examination of the relationship between fetal physical dimension, as measured by ultrasound, and fetal mass presents an alternate and more direct method of calculating fetal weight. Such relationships have been explored extensively and a variety of formulas reported. Ultrasound estimates of fetal weight are subject to at least two critical sources of error. First, these measures assume a uniform relationship between linear measures of fetal structure and fetal volume. Although such relationships clearly exist, some variability is to be expected. Second, these estimates assume that in a given normal fetal population the relationship between volume and mass (density) is constant. Studies in normal neonates and in stillbirths indicate that perinatal density is not constant (Thompson et al., 1983). The average perinatal density is slightly less than water (mean 0.919 ± 0.7 gm/ml), but may range from 0.833 to 1.012 gm/ml. Thus, even in a population of normal fetuses in which volume is known with certainty, the average error of weight estimate will be about 8 per cent and may range as high as 21 per cent. Among fetuses with abnormal growth patterns, subcutaneous fat may be either reduced (IUGR) or increased (diabetic macrosomia), and therefore variation in fetal density may be even greater than in the normal population. Furthermore, within the individual fetus, the density of various structures differs; the mean density of the head is 0.571 gm/ml and of the body is 1.118 gm/ml. Therefore, variation in relative contribution to total mass, as may occur with asymmetric ("head-sparing") IUGR, may be expected to further compound the estimate error.

Since the fetus does not exhibit uniform density, it follows that estimates based upon the physical dimension of any given structure might vary in accuracy. Estimates of fetal weight, based upon head dimension alone, in which the fetal head contributes to only 20 per cent of total mass are so variable as to be of no clinical value. In contrast, estimates derived from body dimension (e.g., abdominal circumference) are considerably more accurate because the fetal body accounts for 80 per cent of total mass and the density of the trunk more closely approximates mean density. Following a principle that appears ingrained in all aspects of perinatal ultrasound, fetal weight estimates based upon a combination of fetal physical variables are substantially more accurate than most single variables. As would be predicted, the least error in estimate is achieved when true volume is known with certainty; true volume as measured by a water displacement method yields an estimate error of about 7.6 per cent (2 SD) (Thompson et al., 1983). Neonatal volume derived from direct measurement of physical dimensions yields an estimate error of about 8.2 per cent; the slight increase in estimate error is assumed to be due to the introduction of measurement error. The most exact estimate of fetal volume is based upon multiple serial ultrasound planes; this method, reported by McCallum and Brinkley (1979), is time-consuming and cumbersome, but yields an estimate error comparable to direct displacement methods (about 6.5 per cent; 2 SD). Composite measurement of head and abdominal and femur dimension, as described by Hadlock (1985), yields an estimate error of about 15 per cent. Fetal weight estimates based upon the summed volumes of fetal head, trunk, and limbs, as reported by Thompson et al. (1983), yield an estimate error of ± 16.2 per cent. Warsof et al. (1977), and more recently Shepard et al. (1982), have used head measurements (BPD) and trunk measurements (AC) to estimate fetal weight; despite the ease by which the method is used, it remains one of the least accurate, yielding a range of error of about 21.2 per cent (2 SD). Interestingly and inexplicably, estimates of fetal weight based upon abdominal circumference alone are reported to yield a range of estimate error of not greater than about 15 per cent (2 SD) (Campbell and Wilkin, 1975). The various ultrasonic methods for determining fetal weight are summarized in Table 14–4.

Because the error of estimate appears relatively constant for each method and because the normal fetus exhibits sustained growth, serial estimates made at intervals sufficiently spaced (usually more than 2 weeks) to account for estimate error permit detection of deviation from the expected normal growth rate. This method then is important in detecting growth rate abnormalities (Divon et al., 1986).

Evaluation of Fetal Growth

From conception to delivery and beyond, the developing infant exhibits circumferential and linear growth of a progressively slowing rate resulting in continuous incremental increases in volume and mass (see Fig. 14–2). Fetal growth may be viewed as the net integration of stimulatory and inhibitory influences arising intrinsically and environmentally. Accordingly and not surprisingly, fetal growth provides clear insight into a wide range of pathologic perinatal conditions. The complexities of fetal growth result in a wide spectrum of responses to abnormal growth-regulating factors. Consequently, there are no simple algorithms for ultrasound detection of growth abnormalities. Rather, the ultrasound detection of growth disturbances depends upon a consideration and evaluation of a number of morphologic and functional variables. Maximal discrimination of abnormal from normal fetal growth may be achieved only when such a wide range of variables is considered. Diagnosis of abnormality based upon assessment of any single set of variables, as for example fetal morphometrics, will be less accurate. This point merits added emphasis because it remains common practice for some ultrasound laboratories to report only fetal morphometrics (e.g., BPD, femur length, AC) in cases of suspected growth abnormality.

Reduced Fetal Growth

The ultrasound diagnosis of impaired or retarded fetal growth is of crucial interest to perinatologists because this is among the most frequent complications associated with death (Morrison and Olsen, 1985). A detailed discussion of the pathophysiology of fetal growth restriction is presented elsewhere in this text (see Chapter 36), but some additional comments are warranted here to underscore the basis for the diagnosis and management of this condition by ultrasound methods.

THE POPULATION OF FETUSES WITH GROWTH FAILURE IS HETEROGENEOUS BY ETIOLOGY AND PROGNOSIS. Growth failure or intrauterine growth restriction is defined by a birthweight at or below the 10th percentile for gestational age and sex. Assuming a normal (Gaussian) distribution, 10 per cent of the fetal population is classified as IUGR by this definition; in practice, the observed incidence of IUGR by this definition is 5 per cent. This population of small fetuses is heterogeneous by etiology and perinatal prognosis. Most IUGR fetuses (80 to 85 per cent) are categorized as "constitutionally small"; they are not at increased perinatal risk and do not require aggressive intervention. They comprise only a small proportion of the perinatal deaths associated with IUGR, and the fetal mortality rate of this group of IUGR fetuses is comparable to that of the appropriate-for-gestational-age nonanomalous fetuses (stillbirth rate 1.9 per 1000). From 10 to 15 per cent of IUGR fetuses exhibit true growth failure secondary to extrinsic factors commonly referred to as uteroplacental failure. These fetuses, described as having asymmetric IUGR, are at extreme perinatal risk and usually require early intervention to avoid mortality and major morbidity. The remaining 5 to 10 per cent of IUGR fetuses exhibit intrinsic growth failure secondary to one or more organ system anomalies (e.g., renal agenesis, short limb dystrophy), to chromosomal anomaly (e.g., trisomy 18) or to a combination of both. The prognosis for fetuses with intrinsic growth failure is variable, but is usually grim. Forewarning of the presence of lethal anomalies can prevent operative delivery and the attendant maternal risks. Assessment of fetal morphometric, morphologic, and functional data improves diagnostic accu-

TABLE 14–4. Estimation of Fetal Weight by Ultrasound Methods

METHOD	VARIABLES MEASURED	RANGE OF ESTIMATE ERROR ± 2 SD (PERCENTAGE)
Neonatal volume (Thompson et al., 1983)	Total volume by water displacement	7.6
Neonatal volume	Head, trunk, limb volume	8.2
Composite fetal volume (McCallum & Brinkley, 1979)	Serial ultrasound planes	6.5
Composite fetal volume (Hadlock, 1985)	HC, AC, femur	15
Composite fetal volume (Thompson et al., 1983)	Head, trunk, limb volume	16.2
Head/trunk volume (Shepard et al., 1982)	BPD and AC	21.2
Trunk volume only (Campbell and Wilkin, 1975)	AC	15

racy and the development of rational management strategies.

Ultrasound methods for detection of significant fetal growth failure are undergoing constant revision. Fetal morphometrics have been extremely useful in identifying the population of fetuses with IUGR. Diagnostic accuracy by ultrasound methods now exceeds 85 per cent compared to about 40 per cent detection by clinical means alone, and the clinical problem of "overdiagnosis" (false-positive) is also sharply reduced.

There are two major problems with basing diagnosis and management of IUGR solely on fetal morphometrics. First, morphometrics alone do not define the etiology or pathophysiology of the disease process. Second, the concept of growth failure "in evolution" must be considered. The ultimate disposition of extrinsic fetal growth failure will depend upon fetal age at onset, rate of progression, and the interval between disease onset and initial diagnostic observation. Consider, for example, the fetus with growth potential that falls in the 90th percentile of the normal population with late-onset extrinsic growth failure. Such a fetus may exhibit severe compromise and even death before the reduced growth rate propels it to less than the 10th percentile. Consideration of the wide spectrum of fetal information provided by dynamic ultrasound scanning can overcome these limitations. The additional information should include assessment of factors such as amniotic fluid volume. Recognition of a major organ or chromosomal anomaly will exclude most fetuses with IUGR due to intrinsic growth failure. Distinguishing the otherwise normal, small fetus from the asymmetric IUGR fetus, while more difficult, is essential since the management strategies are distinctly disparate. The asymmetric IUGR fetus often exhibits morphologic changes. Body proportion changes are characterized by a lesser effect on head growth and a more pronounced effect on trunk and limb growth (Hadlock et al., 1983b). A significant alteration in ratio of head circumference to abdominal circumference (more than 2 SD above the mean) yields a true-positive rate of diagnosis of 85 per cent (Campbell, 1977). An abnormal fetal ponderal index yields a true positive rate of 46.6 per cent (Hadlock et al., 1983b). Loss of subcutaneous fat, measured best in the region of the mid-thigh or paraspinal area, is strongly suggestive of asymmetric IUGR. Evaluation of the functional sequelae of growth failure provides insight to both the etiology and severity of disease. The volume of amniotic fluid can be assessed either subjectively or more objectively by measurement of the largest pocket of fluid or amniotic fluid index. The observation of oligohydramnios in fetuses known to have an intact genitourinary system and intact membranes is a powerful predictor of impending fetal jeopardy (Chamberlain et al., 1984b). Oligohydramnios in a fetus with morphometric evidence of IUGR virtually always indicates asymmetric severe (dysmature) IUGR and is considered by some to be an immediate indication for delivery (Bastide et al., 1986). The presence of normal amniotic fluid volume does not differentiate between the normal small fetus and the fetus with less severe dysmature IUGR (Hoddick et al., 1984; Manning et al., 1983b). Abnormalities in

Doppler flow velocity waveform in the umbilical artery and in select intrafetal vessels (middle cerebral artery, thoracic aorta) may be useful in defining the presumed etiology of IUGR, although its use is controversial (see Chapter 36). Assessment of acute fetal biophysical variables is also an important functional sign of IUGR. The presence of an abnormal biophysical profile score (less than 4) in the IUGR fetus is an indication for immediate delivery (Vintzileos et al., 1987a). Importantly, however, when these variables are normal it becomes reasonable and safe to extend the interval between observations, thereby permitting assessment of fetal growth rate.

Both Diagnostic Accuracy and Management Criteria Vary with the Certainty of Fetal Age Estimates. Virtually all ultrasound-derived fetal morphometric measures used to assess the adequacy of fetal growth and its pathologic deviation depend upon accuracy of the gestational age estimate. As described previously, estimates of fetal age from menstrual history carry considerable potential for error; as estimate error increases, the accuracy in calculation of growth parameter percentile ranking decreases. The important clinical corollary is that when fetal age is overestimated, the frequency of diagnosis of IUGR will increase. From a personal experience of more than 4000 patients referred with a clinical suspicion of IUGR, only about 25 per cent delivered a fetus with proven IUGR. In the vast majority of the remaining patients, the error in diagnosis could be attributed to uncertainty of dates. Campbell (1974) has similarly reported a high incidence of overdiagnosis of IUGR. When dates are known with certainty, as per known LNMP or early ultrasound measurements or both, the diagnosis of IUGR is achieved with some ease by confirmation of a major deviation of growth parameters below the lower distribution limit of the expected mean. With certain dates, the diagnosis of IUGR can usually be made from a single ultrasound examination. When dates are uncertain, a situation commonly encountered clinically, the diagnosis becomes more difficult, requiring serial assessment. By plotting the incremental change over time, one can determine the rate of growth. The interval between serial examinations varies directly with gestational age (see Fig. 14–1) and is usually at least 2 weeks. For each individual variable (BPD, HC, AC, femur, fetal weight estimate), the growth rate may be plotted against the normal curve. Assessment of fetal well-being is used adjunctively for each visit and offers considerable assurance that continued observation until the next scheduled visit is a safe and reasonable approach. A fetus exhibiting sustained growth in all variables may be safely categorized either as a normal small fetus or as of underestimated gestational age. Sharp differentiation of these two categories is inconsequential because obstetric intervention is unwarranted. Absence of or severe delay in fetal growth over serial examinations strongly suggests IUGR, and early intervention is warranted.

The management of the IUGR fetus varies not only with etiology but with gestational age at diagnosis. Intervention for the normal small fetus with a normal fetal biophysical profile score is not indicated, and the patient may be safely followed until the onset of spontaneous labor. Intervention for the IUGR fetus is frequently indicated, but the timing of intervention will vary with the severity of disease and gestational age. The major management dilemma arises when the fetus has an immature amniotic fluid phospholipid profile. In such cases expectant management up to probable or proven pulmonary maturity is recommended only when functional fetal assessment done at least twice weekly is normal. If the preterm dysmature IUGR fetus develops either oligohydramnios or sustained abnormalities by antepartum testing methods, immediate intervention is strongly warranted.

Fetal Macrosomia

The fetus with enhanced general growth or macrosomia is defined by a birth weight equal to or greater than the 90th percentile for gestational age and sex. The condition can usually be ascribed to one of three general causes. The most common reason is enhanced intrinsic growth potential, and the normal large fetus accounts for about 50 to 60 per cent of macrosomia. The condition is characterized by exaggerated, but proportionate, linear and circumferential growth. Such fetuses are not at risk for fetal asphyxia, but are at risk for birth trauma. Abnormal maternal glucose homeostasis accounts for about 35 to 40 per cent of macrosomic fetuses. While such fetuses may exhibit some enhancement of both linear and circumferential growth, they invariably exhibit abnormal fat deposition most evident in the malar cheek pad and the paraspinal area (Fig. 14–9). Fetuses with macrosomia due to maternal glucose intolerance are at increased risk of intrauterine death as well as birth trauma. Underestimation of fetal age is an unusual clinical error, accounting for only about 5 per cent of perinatal

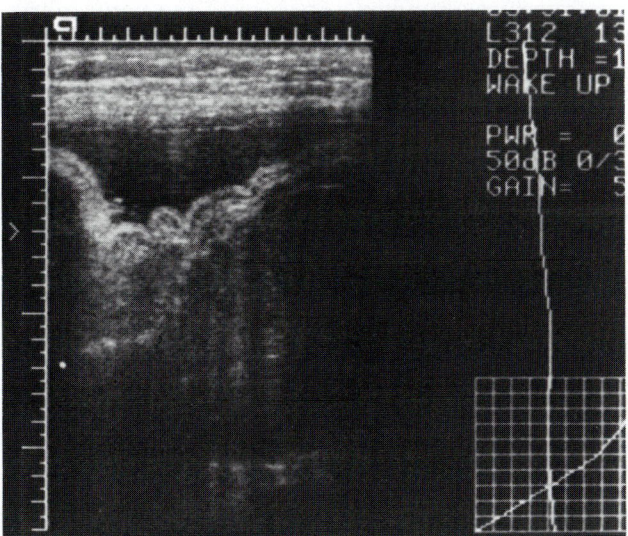

FIGURE 14–9. An ultrasound view of the occiput and posterior cervical region of a macrosomic fetus. The undulations of the skin are a typical feature in the fetus with increased subcutaneous fat.

macrosomia. Fetuses described as macrosomic on this basis are not at risk for fetal death or birth trauma.

Accurate detection of macrosomia beyond 36 weeks gestation would be of great value in avoiding the potential risk of birth trauma. Unfortunately, as of this writing there are no reliable methods for identifying the fetus weighing more than 4000 grams, a weight beyond which the risk of birth trauma rises sharply (Benedetti and Gabbe, 1978). Fetal weight estimates at this range yield significant error, and accordingly, the false-positive and false-negative rates of diagnosis of late macrosomia (more than 4000 grams) are high. Measurement of chest circumference or biacromial diameter as a predictor of shoulder dystocia has been studied (Elliott et al., 1982). The method, except in extreme cases, is relatively poor in predicting subsequent shoulder dystocia.

Fetal Developmental Anomalies: Detection and Assessment by Ultrasound

Principles

When discovery at delivery is used as the temporal reference, overt congenital anomalies occur at a frequency of about 1 to 3 per cent. The reported incidence of congenital anomaly at delivery must underestimate true incidence since lethal embryonic and early fetal anomalies will be excluded, as will anomalies not manifested until later life. Although congenital anomalies have always been a major prenatal problem and their rate of occurrence is constant, their relative clinical significance has increased dramatically since the introduction of dynamic ultrasound imaging. Among the unscreened population, anomalies account for about 15 to 20 per cent of perinatal mortality, whereas in the screened population in whom asphyxial death is reduced, anomalies now account for 65 to 70 per cent of all perinatal deaths. (A continuing fall in overall perinatal mortality, with a continuing rise in the proportion ascribed to anomaly, is the expected benefit of antenatal ultrasound fetal assessment.) The very definition of anomaly is under constant revision. On the basis of high-resolution dynamic ultrasound imaging methods, a spectrum of fetal anomalies is recognized ranging from primary *functional* defects (e.g., myotonic dystrophies and cardiac dysrhythmias without overt anatomic defect) to primary *structural defects* without overt functional fetal components (e.g., cleft palate) to the most common condition of *mixed functional and structural defects* (e.g., obstructive uropathy with renal dysgenesis and pulmonary hypoplasia). Anatomic derangements with functional defects may be primary (e.g., bradyarrhythmias with atrioventricular canal defects) or secondary (ascites with tachyarrhythmia) and may also be remote from the defective organ system (e.g., hydramnios with duodenal atresia, oligohydramnios with obstructive uropathy). In some conditions such as esophageal atresia and tracheal-esophageal fistula, alteration of amniotic fluid volume, a functional sequela, may be the only manifestation of the structural lesion.

Prenatal detection of congenital anomalies, while of

obvious clinical importance, is only the first step in unraveling this difficult and common clinical dilemma. The subsequent development of rational management strategies of the anomalous fetus must take into consideration both the fetus and the mother. Management depends upon consideration of such variables as expected prognosis for the lesion, demonstration of progressive pathophysiology, availability of treatment modalities if any, and the fetal age at the time of diagnosis. Consideration of these variables presents a wide range of management options. When fetal prognosis is hopeless, all efforts are directed toward minimizing maternal risk. When a structural lesion is identified and exhibits no progressive pathophysiology on serial evaluation (e.g., arrested hydrocephalus), conservative management may be indicated. In the mature fetus the presence of an anomaly amenable to neonatal therapy (e.g., omphalocele) should prompt appropriate referral and planning for postdelivery surgical repair.

In highly selected cases, *in utero* therapy may be indicated for a progressive, potentially lethal anomaly discovered in the grossly immature fetus. Such therapy may be either medical (e.g., chronotropic agents for fetal tachyarrhythmia with heart failure) or surgical (e.g., chronic diversion therapy for obstructive uropathy). A proposed clinical classification of fetal anomalies is shown in Table 14–5.

By conservative estimates there are at least 500 known developmental anomalies, the majority of which exhibit overt functional or structural characteristics or both. A detailed discussion of the ultrasound diagnosis of such anomalies falls beyond the scope of this chapter.

The detection rate of fetal anomalies by ultrasound is as difficult to define as is the actual incidence of anomalies, and is subject to the same compounding factors. Beyond 36 weeks of gestation, more than 85 per cent of all major anomalies can be detected by ultrasound assessment (Manning, 1983b). Chromosomal anomalies without overt structural or functional markers are not identified by ultrasound methods. The detection rate falls dramatically in earlier gestation since the anomalous condition may not yet be expressed (e.g., ureteropelvic obstruction) or the lesion

may be too small to be visualized (e.g., small myelomeningocele). As a general rule the earlier in gestation a lesion is detected, the worse the prognostic significance. Furthermore, the presence of an anomaly in one system should alert the clinician to the possibility of associated anomalies, not all of which may be detected by ultrasound. Thus, for example, the presence of obstructive uropathy is associated with karyotypic anomalies in about 8 per cent of cases (Manning et al., 1986). Almost all reports of anomaly detection by ultrasound emphasize the positive diagnostic accuracy, but there are few reports detailing negative predictive accuracy. Accordingly, the predictive accuracy parameters of ultrasound screening for anomalies, when applied to the population at large, remain essentially unexplored. The diagnostic acuity of ultrasound depends directly upon the intensity of examination. Whereas there are probably few, if any, structural abnormalities visible to the naked eye that cannot be detected by ultrasound imaging, the practicalities of the time constraints of examination introduce unavoidable error. A detection rate of 100 per cent, while a theoretic possibility, has not been achieved in the practical clinical setting. The reader is reminded that the probability of detection of a lesion is directly related to the index of suspicion. This factor accounts for the difficulties in achieving comparable diagnostic accuracy between the general population and that population referred with historical or other indicators of an increased risk of underlying anomaly.

Anomalies of the Head, Neck, and Face

The ultrasound assessment of the fetal head and facies may be divided into general assessment of shape and proportion and specific assessment of facial and intracranial architecture. The examination is done by sequential views rotating through the sagittal, parasagittal, coronal, and transverse planes.

In general assessment, the presence and shape of the calvarium are noted. Absence of the bony calvarium is the characteristic feature of the severe neural tube defect *anencephaly* (Fig. 14–10). This uniformly lethal anomaly may be detected from as early as 10 weeks gestation (menstrual age) and will always be

TABLE 14–5. A Clinical Classification of Fetal Anomalies

TYPE	PROGNOSIS	PROGRESSION*	PULMONARY MATURITY	MANAGEMENT	EXAMPLES†
I	Good	Nonprogressive	NA	Conservative	Intermittent fetal arrhythmia, unilateral multicystic renal disease, cystic hygroma, arrested hydrocephalus
II	Good	Progressive	Present	Delivery; give neonatal treatment	Chylothorax, ureteropelvic obstruction, arrhythmia with congestive heart failure
III	Good	Progressive	Absent	Intrauterine therapy or early delivery	Obstructive uropathy, arrhythmia with congestive heart failure, obstructive hydrocephalus
IV	Hopeless	NA		Conservative	Anencephaly, renal agenesis, holoprosencephaly, hypoplastic left ventricle

*As determined by serial ultrasound fetal assessment.
†For illustrative purposes only.
NA = nonapplicable.

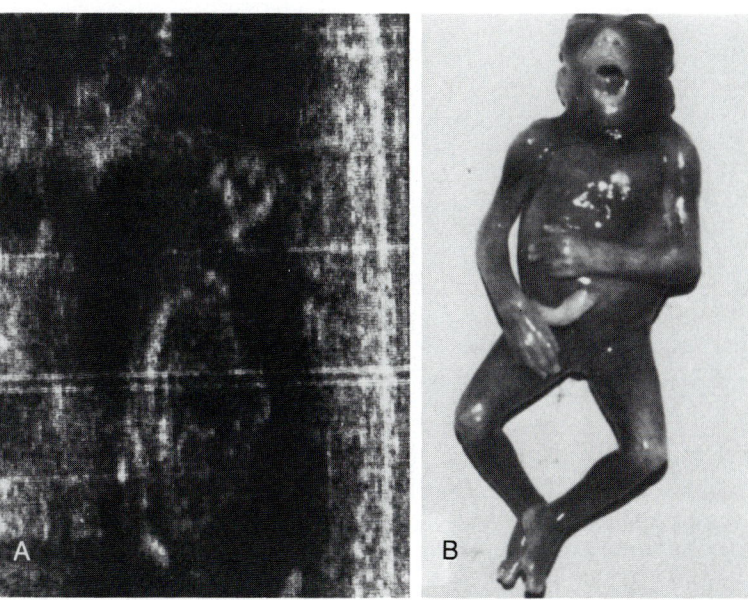

FIGURE 14–10. *A,* An ultrasound view in the sagittal plane of an anencephalic fetus. The fetal head is rotated to the right. The fetal eyes are visible and the complete absence of the calvarium is obvious. *B,* A photograph of the same anencephalic fetus. Note the prominence of the eyes and the complete absence of the calvarium.

overt by 16 weeks gestation. The lesion is associated with absence, to varying degrees, of cerebral tissue and gross distortion of intracranial architecture.

Herniation of meninges or cerebral tissue through a defect in the calvarium is the hallmark of *encephalocele.* A variant of neural tube defect, it is a midline lesion, and is usually posterior. Differentiation between large posterior encephalocele and cervical myelomeningocele can often be difficult. The prognosis varies with the size, location, and contents of the mass. Large defects and those containing neural elements carry the worst prognosis. Occasionally the encephalocele sac may contain almost all the cerebral cortex with resultant severe microcephaly; the prognosis in such cases is hopeless. In contrast, small encephaloceles composed of herniated meninges only have an excellent prognosis provided the intracranial architecture remains normal. Anterior encephalocele, more common in Asian populations, in general has a better prognosis than posterior encephalocele, although severe derangement of facial structure may be associated with anterior lesions.

Distortion and enlargement of the calvarium without herniation may be observed with thanatophoric dwarfism, the various cleidocranial dysplasias, and achondrospondylodysplasias. Marked cranial asymmetry may be observed with primary synostosis and with Apert's and Cruzon's syndromes.

Symmetric reduction in head size, termed *microcephaly,* is among the most difficult of fetal anomalies to classify. There is no clear relationship, except in the extreme, between head and brain size and the presence of normal brain function. Primary microcephaly may be due to either a nonpathologic normal distribution phenomenon or arrest of cerebral growth with resultant diminished head growth. Both conditions may be associated with reduced head dimensions, decrease in the ratio of head circumference to abdominal circumference, and reduced growth rate evident on serial measurement. Differentiation of normal from pathologic microcephaly can be extremely difficult.

Such differentiation is of major importance because the subsequent management strategies are widely divergent. Unequivocal diagnosis of pathologic microcephaly has a grim prognosis and should be reserved for those cases exhibiting extreme microcephaly (head circumference less than 4 SD below the mean for gestational age), absence or marked reduction in cerebral hemisphere volume, or extreme variance in head circumference to abdominal circumference ratio (less than 4 SD of the mean), or when environmental etiologic factors (e.g., high-dose radiation exposure, proven fetal cytomegalovirus infection) have been identified.

Soft tissue abnormalities of the fetal head and neck may be cystic or solid and often indicate underlying fetal functional or karyotypic abnormality. Generalized scalp edema is a characteristic feature of immune and nonimmune hydrops and of fetal congestive heart failure (Fig. 14–11). *Cystic hygroma* is manifested as multiple discrete cystic masses of varying size, primarily of the paraspinal cervical region, but occasionally involving the anterior neck. Cystic hygroma frequently is associated with the XO karyotype and variants (70 per cent of cases) and with trisomy 21 (20 per cent of cases), but also may be associated with a normal fetal karyotype (Phillips and McHahan, 1981). It is most commonly observed in the second trimester and usually decreases in size with advancing gestation. The neck webbing typical of Turner's syndrome is presumed to be a residual effect of cystic hygroma in early fetal life. Cystic hygroma must be differentiated from cavernous hemangioma. With Doppler flow ultrasound this differentiation is now simple since cystic hygroma never exhibits flow within the cystic mass, whereas venous flow is characteristic of cavernous hemangioma. Detection of cystic hygromas is an indication for fetal karyotype determination.

Localized nonedematous thickening (more than 5 mm) of the posterior nuchal subcutaneous tissue when observed before 20 weeks gestation has been reported as a sonographic sign of trisomy 21 (Benacerraf and

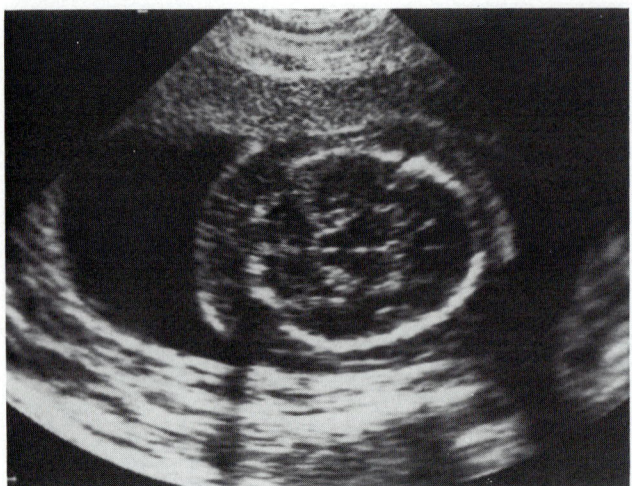

FIGURE 14–11. Ultrasound scan of the fetal head in the plane of the BPD demonstrating massive scalp edema secondary to immune (Rh) hydrops fetalis. The subcutaneous tissues of the scalp are grossly distended as a result of fluid accumulation. Scalp edema of this degree usually portends a very ominous prognosis.

Frigoletto, 1985). However, in the initial reports this finding was present in only 4 of 11 fetuses with Down's syndrome (36 per cent) and in one fetus with a normal karyotype. Furthermore, determination of subcutaneous thickness is angle-dependent, and false-positive results are reported (Toi et al., 1987). Nonetheless this finding should be considered as an indication for further karyotypic evaluation.

Evaluation of fetal facial structure, now possible with some considerable clarity, may offer insight into the presence of genetic and associated structural anomalies. The fetal face is visualized in the sagittal (profile), serial coronal (frontal view), and serial transverse views (Fig. 14–12). In the profile view, facial dimensions are assessed. Mandibular shortening and jaw retraction are suggestive of Pierre Robin and Treacher Collins syndromes and may also be seen with trisomy 13 and trisomy 18. Facial clefts ranging from cleft lip and palate to major facial cleft (bifid face) are best identified in the frontal and transverse scan planes (Fig. 14–12). The fetal lips and hard palate may be seen in great detail, and the diagnosis of cleft lip or palate or both is possible. However, the specificity and sensitivity of ultrasound diagnosis of these conditions remain undetermined. Observation of facial cleft should alert the clinician to the possibility of underlying karyotypic abnormality, especially trisomy 13 and trisomy 18.

Dynamic ultrasound imaging may permit visualization of the fetal tongue. Macroglossia may be seen in Beckwith's syndrome and with some forms of gangliosidosis. The fetal eye and orbits are well visualized, and nomograms for interorbital diameters have been published (Mayden et al., 1982). Both hypo- and hypertelorism may be identified and are suggestive but not diagnostic of associated anomalies. The exception is extreme hypotelorism, which is highly suggestive of holoprosencephaly. Examination of the fetal ear, while possible by ultrasound, has yet to be shown

to be of diagnostic value. Diminished pinna length is characteristic of trisomy 21, but a nomogram for fetal pinna length has not been reported. Determination of relative ear position is possible and may offer insight into the presence of associated anomalies. In the normal fetus a line extended from the midorbit will transect the pinna just above the external auditory meatus. In the fetus with low-set ears, the superior edge of the pinna falls below the extended midorbital line. Low-set ears are observed in a variety of conditions including Turner's syndrome, Potter's syndrome, trisomy 13, and trisomy 18. The clinical usefulness of ultrasound determination of ear level remains to be determined by prospective study.

Abnormalities of intracranial architecture are among the most common and most significant developmental anomalies. By means of contemporary high-resolution ultrasound methods, the fetal brain may be examined in remarkable detail.

Anomalies of the fetal brain can generally be assigned to two general categories: primary ventriculomegaly and primary brain tissue lesions.

Ventriculomegaly is defined as bilateral enlargement of the ventricular system beyond the upper limit (2 SD) of distribution for the normal population of equal age; in practice the ventricle-to-hemisphere ratio is used to determine ventriculomegaly (Jeanty et al., 1981a). In clinical practice the terms ventriculomegaly and hydrocephalus are used synonymously, although strictly speaking such interchange of terms is incorrect. Ventriculomegaly is of clinical significance only when shown to be progressive or associated with recognized underlying abnormalities. Pathologic ventriculomegaly is usually associated with one of four underlying conditions, and the prognosis varies substantially with these associations.

Holoprosencephaly results from disordered forebrain development and is characterized by the presence of a single ventricle (usually enlarged), absence of the corpus callosum, major forebrain dysgenesis, and facial abnormalities almost always involving the fetal eyes. In its most advanced form holoprosencephaly involves a markedly detailed single ventricle, absent forebrain, and cyclopia. The prognosis with holoprosencephaly is extremely poor, perinatal death is common, and severe mental retardation is uniform (Laurence and Coates, 1962; Chervenak et al., 1985). Accordingly, when the diagnosis of holoprosencephaly is made, heroic efforts for the fetus in the antepartum period (e.g., ventriculoamniotic shunt), intrapartum period (operative delivery for fetal indication), or neonatal period should be actively discouraged.

Ventriculomegaly due to *aqueductal stenosis* presents a major management dilemma. The condition is characterized by progressive dilatation of the lateral ventricle beginning initially in the anterior horn, then involving the entire lateral ventricle, with lateral displacement of the choroid plexus and of the middle cerebral artery and compression of the cerebral cortex (Fig. 14–13). Although proximal dilatation of the third ventricle may be observed, this sign is not uniform. The diagnosis of ventriculomegaly due to aqueduct stenosis is one of exclusion—that is, by ruling out posterior fossa lesion (e.g., Dandy-Walker cyst) and

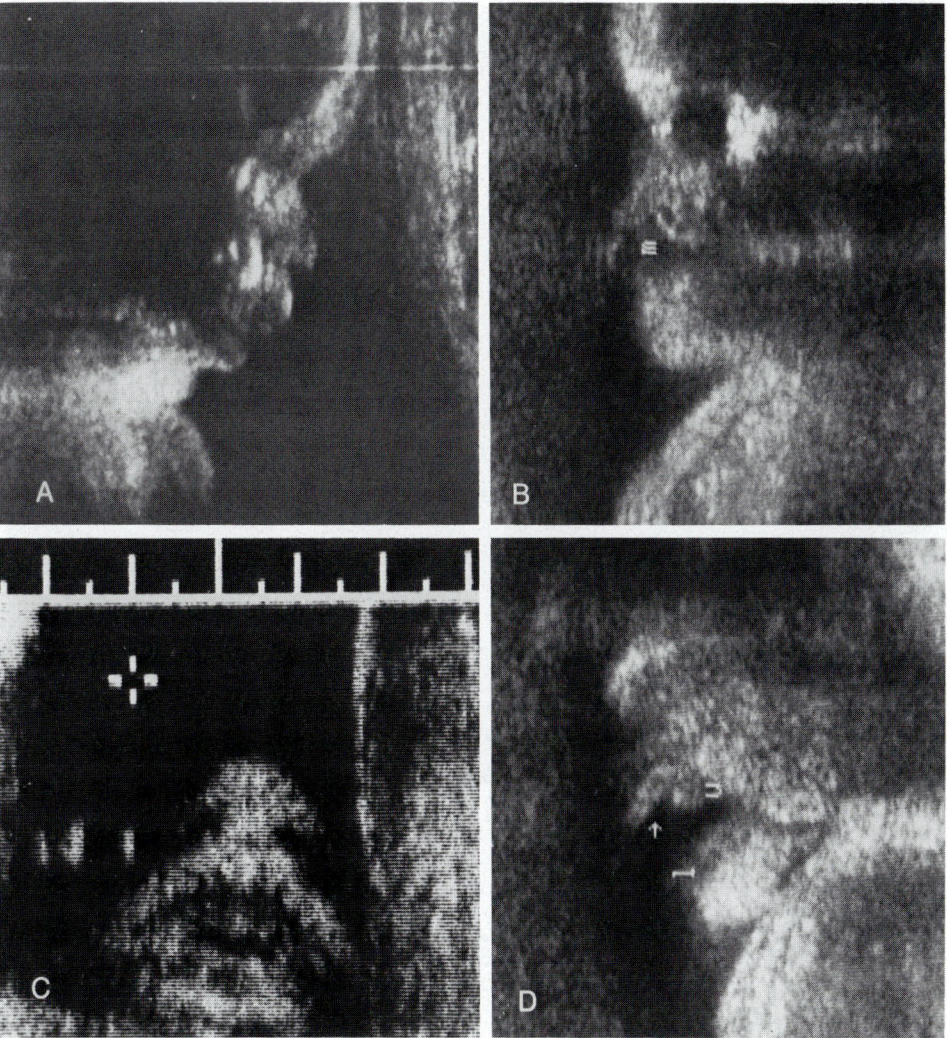

FIGURE 14–12. *A,* Fetal face in profile view at 24 weeks gestation. The medial aspects of the orbit, the nose, and the mouth are well visualized. *B,* A slightly rotated profile view of a 26-week fetus with a major cleft of the lip (marked by the letter m). *C,* A view of the fetal mouth and nose from an inferior angle. Note that the lips are well seen and are normal. The mouth is slightly open, permitting a view of the anterior gingiva. *D,* A slightly rotated inferior angle view of the mouth in a fetus with major clefting of the upper lip *(arrow);* "u" refers to upper lip and "l" to the lower lip.

associated neural tube defects. Characteristically the fetal calvarium is normal in shape and not enlarged with early disease; symmetric enlargement is observed with advanced disease.

The appropriate management of aqueductal stenosis is difficult to determine (Vintzileos et al., 1987b). Except in the extreme case, neither the extent of ventriculomegaly nor the degree of cortical tissue compression is a reliable prognostic indicator of adverse neurologic or intellectual sequelae. Perinatal outcome with ventriculomegaly due to aqueductal stenosis is usually, but not invariably, poor (Laurence and Coates, 1962; McCullough and Balzer-Martin, 1982). Spontaneous arrest of ventriculomegaly is reported (Laurence and Coates, 1967). Chronic ventricular decompression in the neonate is associated with high survival (>85 per cent), and may be associated with normal neurologic development and intellectual function in the majority of cases (65 per cent). However, it is invariably associated with major associated morbidity (infection, shunt revision, growth failure) (McCullough and Balzer-Martin, 1982). The value, if any, of fetal ventricular decompression remains unknown, although the procedure is technically possible and may be associated with intact outcome (Manning

et al., 1986). Although clear prognostic indicators are not available at present, it seems that the earlier the fetal age at diagnosis and the more progressive the ventriculomegaly, the worse the prognosis. Instability of the falx, termed the "wavering midline," is considered an indication of severe disease associated with a particularly poor outcome (Nelson et al., 1984).

Ventriculomegaly due to *major neural tube defect* is usually associated with definitive ultrasound signs and can be recognized with some certainty. The concordance of spinal neural tube defects and the Arnold-Chiari malformation is high (approximately 90 per cent). The Arnold-Chiari malformation, characterized by herniation of the cerebellar tonsils and midbrain structures into the foramen magnum, causes ventriculomegaly due to compression of the fourth and occasionally the third ventricle. Downward traction of the brain causes a reduction in the anterior calvarium, in turn producing a triangular head in the plane of the BPD, known as the lemon sign. The compression of the cerebellar hemisphere creates the so-called banana sign (Fig. 14–14). When these two signs are observed, the probability of a spinal defect approaches 100 per cent. Conversely, their absence conveys a high probability of a normal, intact spinal canal.

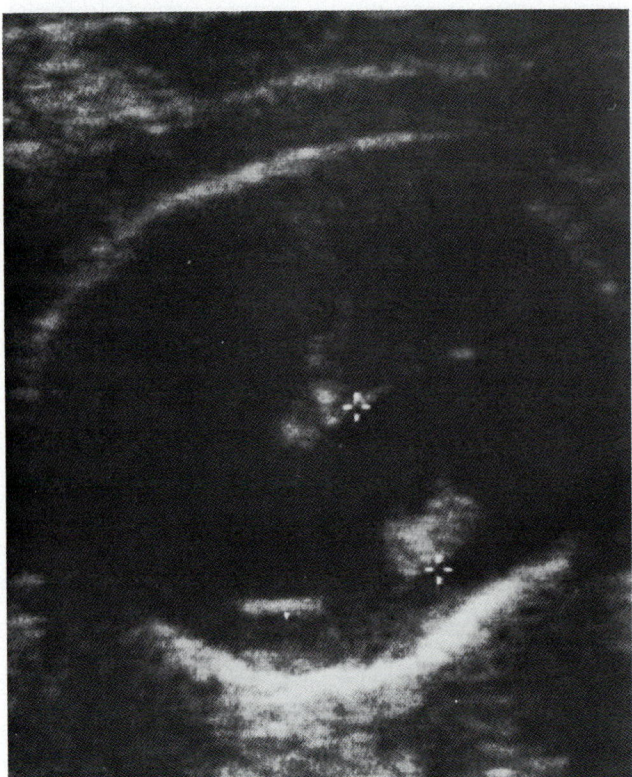

FIGURE 14–13. Fetal ventriculomegaly at 21 weeks secondary to aqueductal stenosis. Note that the fetal head is normal in shape and size. The key diagnostic features are the increase in ventricle size, as evidenced by an abnormal ventricle-to-hemisphere ratio (0.8125 in this case), and a prominent lateral shift of the choroid plexus. The midline structures were stable in this case and cortical mantle was seen. Disease was rapidly progressive; the fetus was delivered at 24 weeks and died.

Unilateral or occasionally bilateral *cystic cerebellar degeneration* (Dandy-Walker cysts) can cause ventriculomegaly due to compression of either the fourth or third ventricle. The prognosis with Dandy-Walker syndrome, while variable, is generally poor (Vintzileos et al., 1987b). Rarely, isolated saccular herniation of the ventricular wall, usually the posterior horn of the lateral ventricle, can cause extrinsic compression of the cerebrospinal fluid circulation (porencephalic cyst).

Abnormal closure of the neural tube is a relatively common lesion (incidence of approximately 1/1000 births) that produces a spectrum of anomalies ranging from absence of the dorsal laminae of the vertebral bodies (spina bifida), herniation of meninges (myelocele), herniation of meninges and neural elements (myelomeningocele) to absence of development of the forebrain and midbrain elements (anencephaly). The spinal lesion (excluding encephalocele and anencephaly) is most commonly located in the lumbar spine (approximately 70 per cent) or the sacral spine (approximately 20 per cent), and less commonly involves the thoracic or cervical spine. The prognosis varies with the location of the defect, being best with a low sacral lesion, and with the extent and nature of the defect. The smaller lesion without neural elements has

the most favorable prognosis. The lesion may involve a single or multiple vertebral bodies (Fig. 14–15).

Prenatal diagnosis of neural tube defects has improved dramatically in recent years because of the use of maternal serum alpha-fetoprotein screening and amniotic fluid alpha-fetoprotein and *N*-acetylcholinesterase determination as well as high-resolution dynamic ultrasound imaging (see Chapter 2).

Accuracy parameters of the ultrasound diagnosis or exclusion of neural tube defects is now of major importance, since subsequent clinical management depends upon the certainty of diagnosis. There is little doubt that the positive predictive accuracy of the

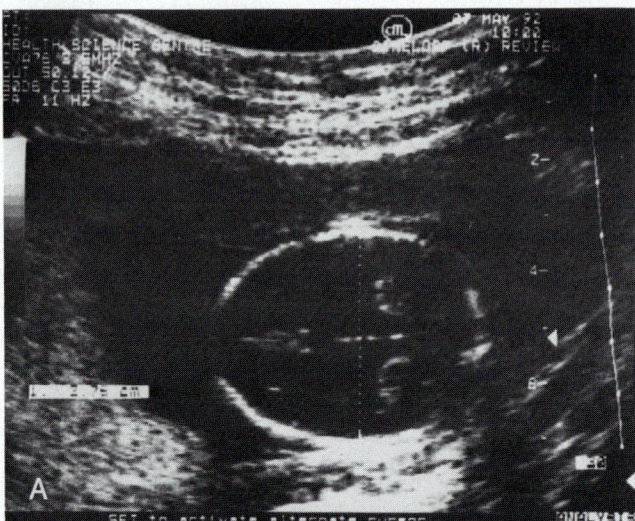

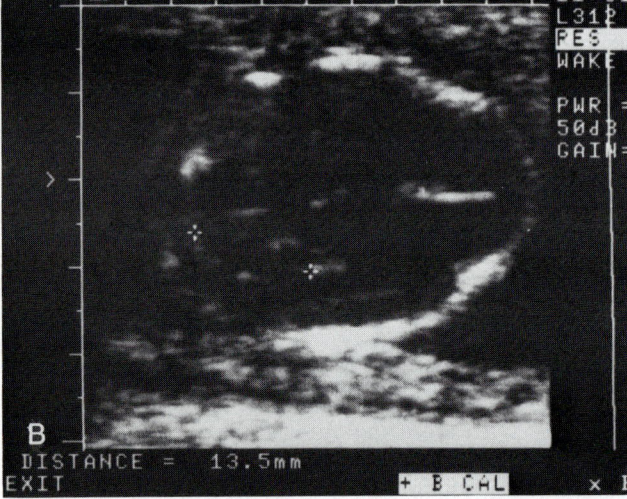

FIGURE 14–14. *A,* Normal fetal calvarium at 17 weeks gestation. This ultrasound image, in the BPD plane, demonstrates the normal symmetric shape of the calvarium and the normal cerebellar hemispheres (seen as faint circular echogenic structures in the posterior region of the image). *B,* The fetal calvarium at 18 weeks in a fetus with proven lumbosacral myelomeningocele. Note the collapse of the anterior calvarium disrupting the normal oval shape of the skull (lemon sign). The fetal cerebellar hemisphere (marked on the inferior side by the calipers) is elongated and flattened ("banana sign"). These are the typical cranial ultrasound signs of the Arnold-Chiari malformation seen in most fetuses with neural tube defect.

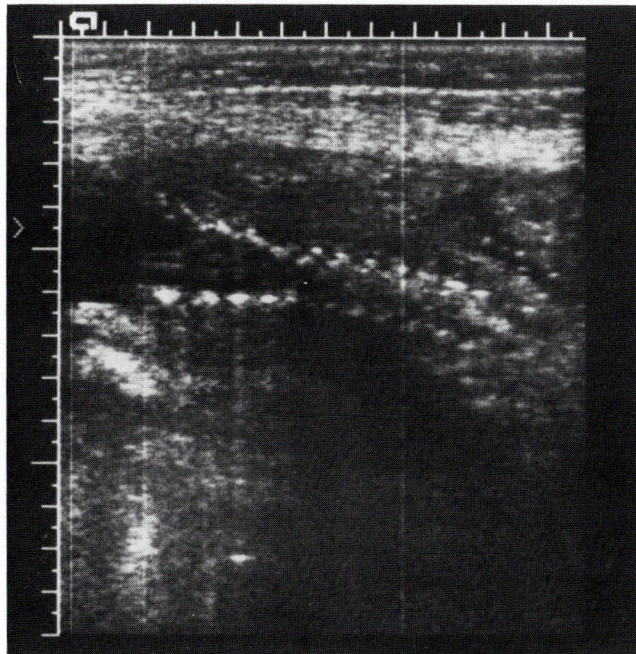

FIGURE 14–15. Longitudinal coronal scan of the fetal spine in a fetus with a large lumbosacral myelomeningocele. The splaying of the spinal process is a typical and diagnostic finding in this condition. The two echogenic parallel lines at the end of the splayed spine are a portion of the herniated spinal cord.

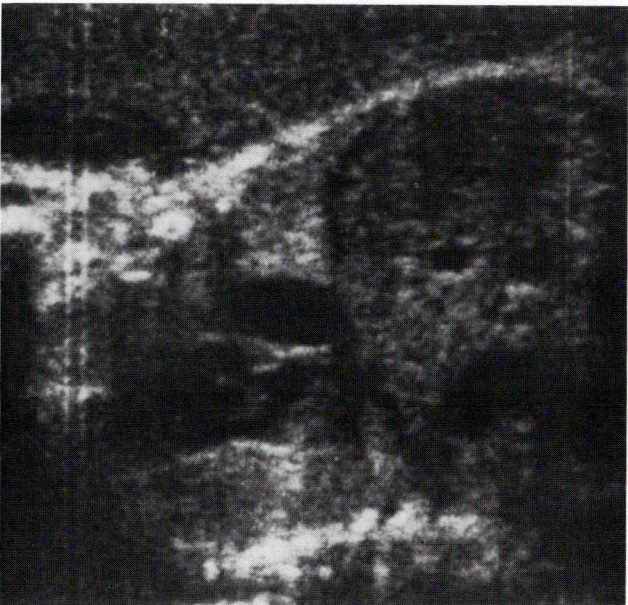

FIGURE 14–16. Coronal view (linear array) of fetal thorax and abdomen at 35 weeks gestation. Lung tissue and liver tissue vary in echodensity. The sonolucent diaphragm is well visualized bilaterally. The central echolucent structure in the thorax is the fetal heart.

ultrasound diagnosis of neural tube defect is high. The negative predictive accuracy, i.e., the certainty by which neural tube defect may be excluded, is not as reliable. The clinical significance of this uncertainty is accentuated by the now widespread use of maternal serum alpha-fetoprotein screening. Management of the patient with high alpha-fetoprotein and a normal ultrasound scan remains controversial. In many centers the presence of normal calvarium shape and normal cerebellar shape and the inability to detect any break in the continuity of the fetal spinal canal are taken as sufficiently strong evidence of the absence of a neural tube defect to preclude the use of invasive testing for this condition. In others, amniocentesis for amniotic fluid alpha-fetoprotein and acetylcholinesterase determination is recommended. The appropriate management course will vary with the expertise and experience of the ultrasonographer, the level of sophistication of the ultrasound equipment, and the patient's wishes.

Abnormalities of the Fetal Thorax and Heart

In the normal fetus the thoracic cavity is bell-shaped, with the inferior margin delineated by the markedly concave diaphragmatic leaves, which appear sonolucent (Fig. 14–16). Gross reduction in thoracic volume or distortion of shape is typical of a variety of disorders, including severe pulmonary hypoplasia associated with renal agenesis, asphyxiating thoracic dystrophy typical of thanatophoric dwarfism, and osteogenesis imperfecta and other skeletal dysplasias.

Diaphragmatic hernia is characterized by herniation of abdominal contents into the thoracic cavity (Fig. 14–17). The hernia, which may contain stomach, liver, spleen, and small bowel, causes displacement of the heart usually anterior and to the right. The defect in the diaphragm is usually not visible. Lethal pulmonary

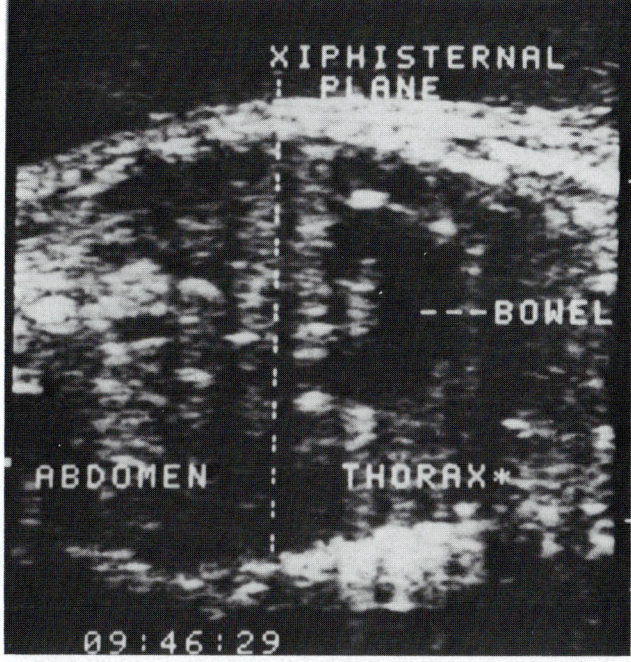

FIGURE 14–17. Sagittal scan of a fetus with a large diaphragmatic hernia. The echolucent mass in the fetal chest is a dilated loop of small bowel.

hypoplasia is a common result of diaphragmatic hernia presumed secondary to lung compression (Harrison et al., 1982, 1986).

Open fetal corrective surgery for this congenital lesion has been described (Longaker et al., 1991), but the advantages of this aggressive approach remain unproven. Interestingly, the mortality rate for diaphragmatic hernia varies directly with the age at diagnosis and with the presence or absence of hydramnios; the slope of the mortality curve reflects both the extent of the fetal lesion and the natural selection process occurring at the time of transition to pulmonary dependence. Antenatal diagnosis of diaphragmatic hernia confers a high probability of mortality (85 to 90 per cent), and when the lesion is associated with hydramnios, survival is unusual (Benacerraf and Adzick, 1987).

Pleural effusions are readily identified (Fig. 14–18) and may be secondary to anomalies of the thoracic duct (chylothorax), to generalized hypoproteinemia as seen with nonimmune hydrops, or to acquired immune hydrops. Forewarning of pleural effusion can be lifesaving for the newborn, although whether decompression should occur at or before delivery remains controversial (Lange and Manning, 1981; Benacerraf and Frigoletto, 1985). Recent clinical experience with chronic pleuro-amniotic shunt placement has been encouraging (Rodeck et al., 1988).

Lung tissue is well visualized, and specific malformations such as *cystic adenomatoid malformation* may be identified. The prenatal diagnosis of pulmonary hypoplasia by ultrasound has been reported, although the specificity and sensitivity of current techniques are not yet satisfactory (Nimrod et al., 1988; Sherer et al., 1990). Equating prenatal estimates of thoracic volume and lung volume to postnatal lung function falls outside the existing discrimination of contemporary ultrasound methods. Tracheoesophageal fistula may be suspected by ultrasound detection of hydramnios and the failure on repeated examination to visualize the fetal stomach. At present, however, a definitive ultrasound diagnosis of tracheoesophageal fistula is not possible.

A detailed description of the detection and management of *cardiac malformations* is outlined in Chapter 15.

Abnormalities of the GI Tract

The fetal stomach, small and large bowel, liver, pancreas, and spleen are usually easily visualized. Since the fetal GI tract normally contains fluid (swallowed amniotic fluid and local secretion), obstructive disorders are characterized by proximal dilatation creating echolucent masses. Persistent absence of stomach fluid, particularly when associated with hydramnios, is strongly suggestive of esophageal atresia. Occlusion of the pylorus of the stomach, which is rarely observed *in utero*, results in a distended stomach and associated hydramnios. Duodenal atresia is the most common congenital GI obstruction and results in the dilatation of the proximal duodenum and the antrum of the fetal stomach (prepyloric region); these areas of dilatation result in the classic "double bubble" sign of duodenal atresia (Fig. 14–19). Since duodenal atresia is frequently associated with trisomy 21, fetal karyotype determination is indicated when this lesion is detected. Jejunal or ileal atresia produces proximal dilatation, which appears as multiple echolucent areas. Using dynamic ultrasound imaging, one can observe marked preobstruction peristalsis. Large bowel obstruction rarely produces proximal dilatation, although occasionally this may be seen with anal atresia. Large bowel rupture due to meconium ileus is reported, producing complex echolucent abdominal mass with multiple scattered echogenic lesions (calcified meconium) (Brugman et al., 1979). Increased second-trimester bowel echogenicity has been associated with a significant risk of aneuploidy; the differential diagnosis should also include cystic fibrosis (Scioscia et al., 1992).

Anterior abdominal wall defects generally fall into one of two diagnostic categories. *Omphalocele* is an exaggerated umbilical hernia in which fetal liver and frequently fetal bowel extrude (Fig. 14–20). The omphalocele sac (peritoneum) is usually seen. Associated defects are common, and about 30 per cent of cases involve an abnormal karyotype, usually trisomy 13. Hence fetal karyotype determination is indicated. In contrast, *gastroschisis* is a rupture of the upper anterior abdominal wall, usually the left side, with extrusion of intestines but rarely fetal liver. Because the defect is not covered with peritoneum, the fetal intestine is free floating and may be scattered within the amniotic cavity (Fig. 14–21). Gastroschisis is not associated with an increased risk of karyotype anomaly.

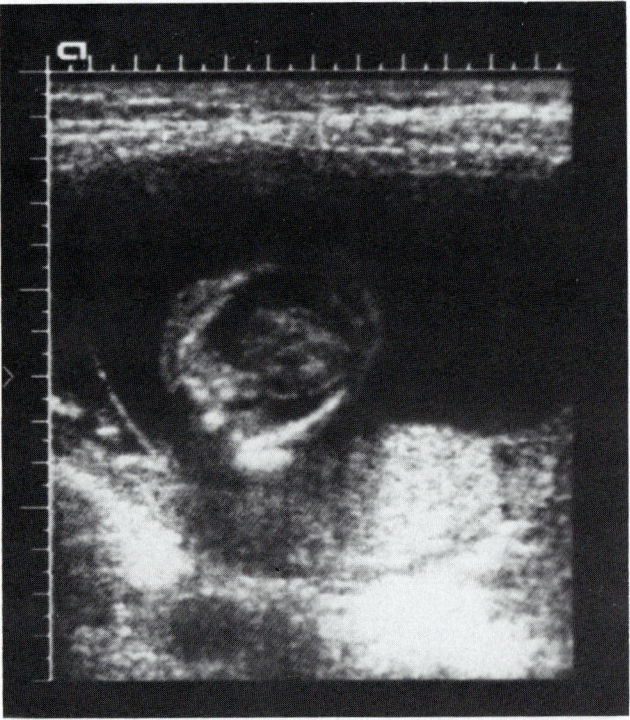

FIGURE 14–18. Transverse scan of the thorax at the level of the heart in a 16-week fetus with massive bilateral pleural effusion. The fetal heart is outlined by the echolucent fluid accumulation in the pleural space. A small pericardial effusion is also present.

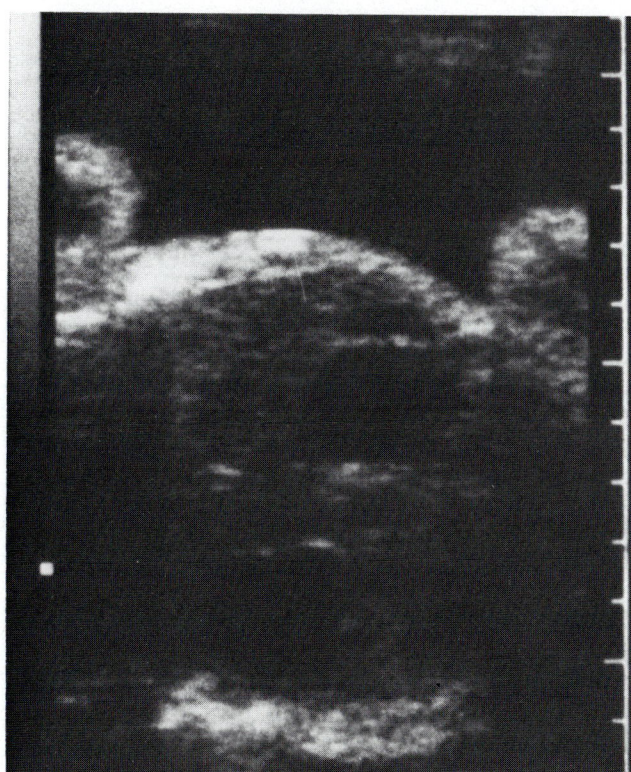

FIGURE 14–19. Longitudinal (sagittal) view of the fetal abdomen exhibiting the classic "double bubble" sign of proximal gut (duodenal) atresia. The two echolucent masses represent the dilated fluid-filled stomach and the dilated fluid-filled duodenum proximal to the atretic obstruction. Note the associated hydramnios, an almost uniform finding. Trisomy 21 is commonly associated with duodenal atresia.

Nonimmune hydrops is characterized by ascites, pleural and pericardial effusion, and generalized and often massive subcutaneous edema. Fetal prognosis varies with the underlying cause (Romero et al., 1986; Warsof et al., 1986). Nonimmune hydrops is always a diagnosis of exclusion and is considered after an immune etiology has been ruled out.

Abnormalities of the Genitourinary Tract

The genitourinary tract, including the fetal kidney, ureter, and bladder, is readily assessed by conventional ultrasound (Fig. 14–22). Abnormalities of the genitourinary tract may be broadly classified as *primary renal dysgenesis* of variable type and severity and as *obstructive disorders*. Ultrasound diagnosis of fetal renal disease is subject to error (Avni et al., 1985). Renal dysgenesis presents as a spectrum of disorders that may affect one or both kidneys. Renal agenesis, the most severe variant of dysgenesis, is usually bilateral, characterized by absence of recognizable renal tissue, absent fetal bladder, extreme oligohydramnios, and lethal pulmonary hypoplasia. Oligohydramnios is invariably present after 16 weeks gestation. The diagnosis of renal agenesis is usually problematic because oligohydramnios makes visualization of the renal fossa difficult, and adrenal tissue may be confused with

renal tissue. Serial evaluation over a 4- to 6-hour period to confirm absence of urine production, as evidenced by failure to visualize the fetal bladder, may be extremely useful in establishing the certainty of the diagnosis. Since fetal urine production is subject to diurnal variation, observation for less than 3 hours may produce false-positive results (Chamberlain et al., 1984a). In late gestation the differential diagnosis of severe oligohydramnios and reduced fetal size is either severe IUGR or renal agenesis. Since the perinatal prognosis and appropriate management are so radically different, considerable effort in establishing the correct diagnosis with certainty is required. Such determination may include ultrasound assessment by different examiners on different occasions. Less severe renal dysgenesis may present as unilateral (usual) or bilateral (uncommon) multicystic dysplasia (Fig. 14–23). Such lesions are characterized by increase in renal volume, distortion of renal architecture, multiple irregular-sized echolucent renal cysts, and areas of increased echogenicity and calcification. Bilateral disease may be associated with oligohydramnios and is invariably fatal. Unilateral disease is associated with normal amniotic fluid volume, evidence of contralateral renal function (bladder filling), and a favorable prognosis. Multicystic dysplastic disease must be differentiated from simple obstructive disorders. "Finnish" renal dysgenesis is characterized by massive enlargement of both kidneys and a general increase in echogenicity (Hobbins et al., 1979). Oligohydramnios is commonly but not invariably present. The condition is uniformly fatal.

Congenital urinary tract obstruction may occur at several sites. The most common site of obstruction is at the ureteropelvic junction, producing renal pelvis dilatation in milder cases and renal calyceal dilatation (hydronephrosis) with more severe obstruction (Fig.

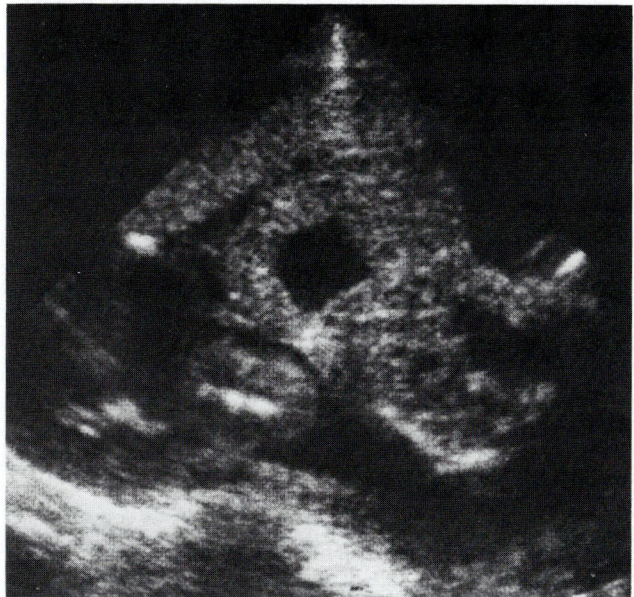

FIGURE 14–20. Transverse scan of the torso at the level just below the thoracoabdominal junction in a fetus with an omphalocele. The fetal abdominal cavity is seen to the right.

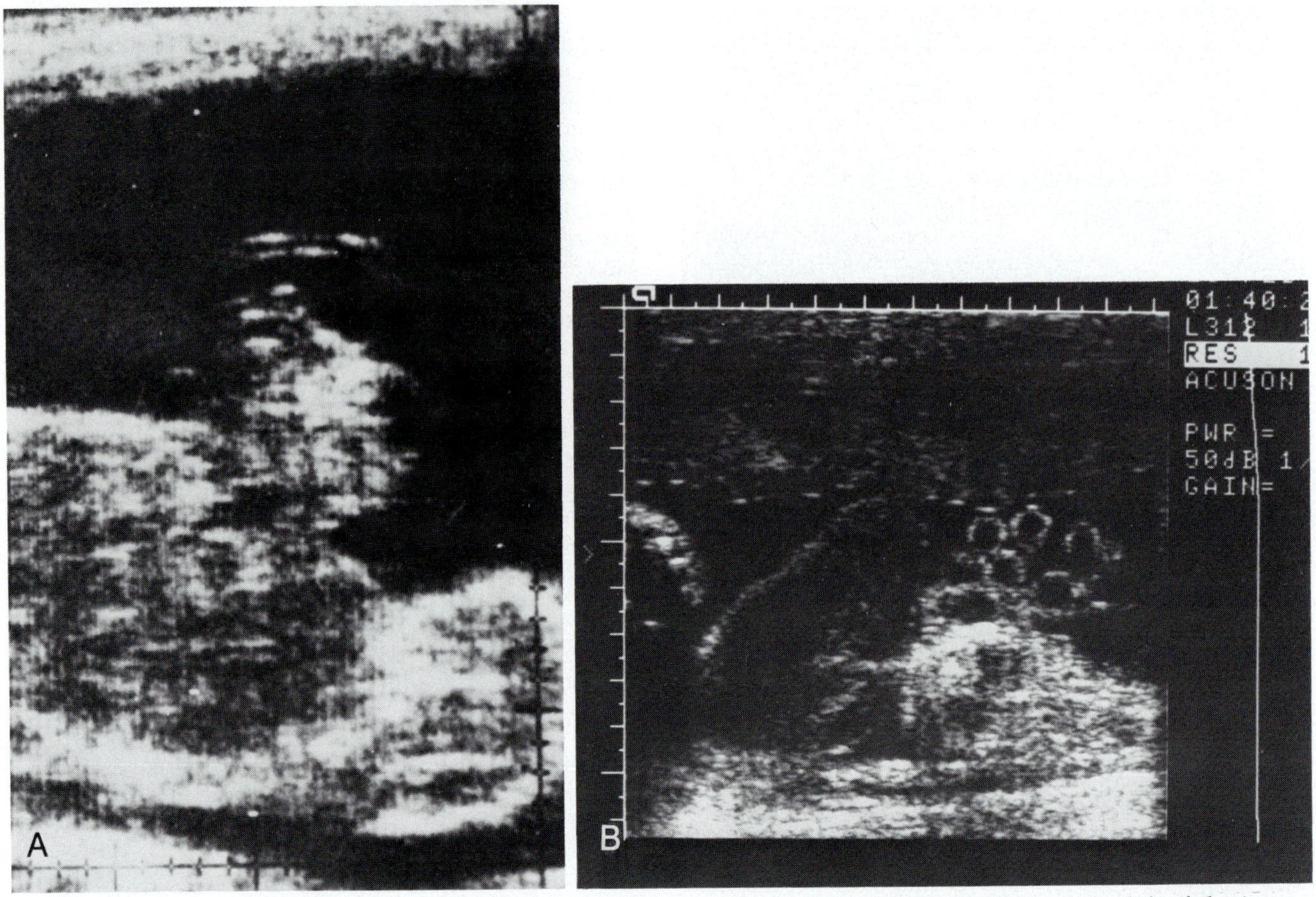

FIGURE 14–21. *A,* Longitudinal sagittal scan of a fetus with gastroschisis. The fetal head is toward the left of the image. Fetal small bowel is seen protruding from a defect in the fetal abdomen and floats freely in the amniotic cavity. *B,* A magnified view of the free loops of fetal bowel. The collection of echolucent circles is slightly dilated small bowel seen in transverse section.

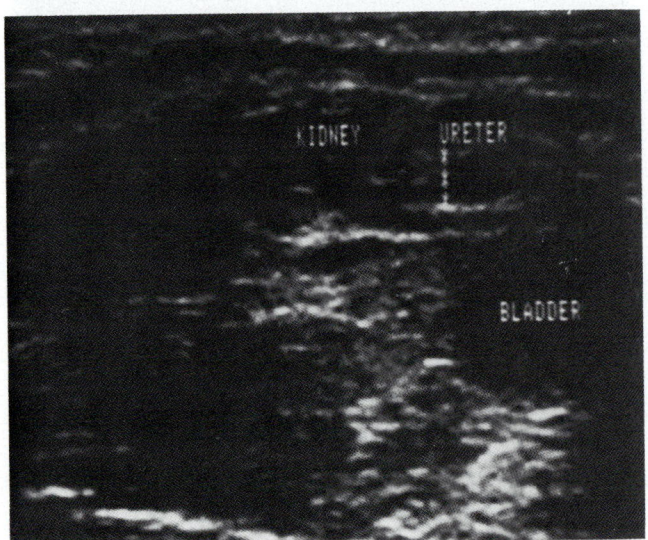

FIGURE 14–22. Coronal view of fetal abdomen demonstrating a normal left kidney and ureter and a normal bladder.

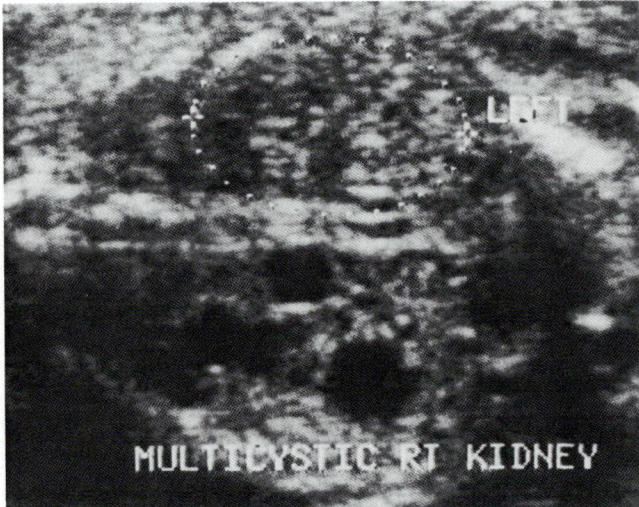

FIGURE 14–23. Coronal view of fetal abdomen demonstrating a normal left kidney and a markedly enlarged multicystic right kidney. Note the very irregular outline of the right kidney and the presence of coarse cysts and areas of increased echogenicity. At surgery (neonatal), the multicystic dysplastic right kidney was removed.

14–24). The lesion is usually but not invariably bilateral and is associated with normal fetal urine production and normal amniotic fluid volume. Most often the disease is slowly progressive, and early delivery usually is not indicated. Assessment of the newborn by a pediatric urologist is recommended. Outlet tract obstruction may be caused by posterior urethral valve syndrome (male fetus), urethral atresia, or persistent cloacal syndrome. Outlet production produces megalocystis, hydroureter, and hydronephrosis (Fig. 14–25). Oligohydramnios is common but not invariable. Pulmonary hypoplasia is a common associated finding. Posterior urethral valve syndrome may be recognized by observing dilatation of the proximal urethra. Persistent outlet obstruction, particularly when caused by posterior urethral valve syndrome, may be an indication for *in utero* diversion therapy (Manning et al.,

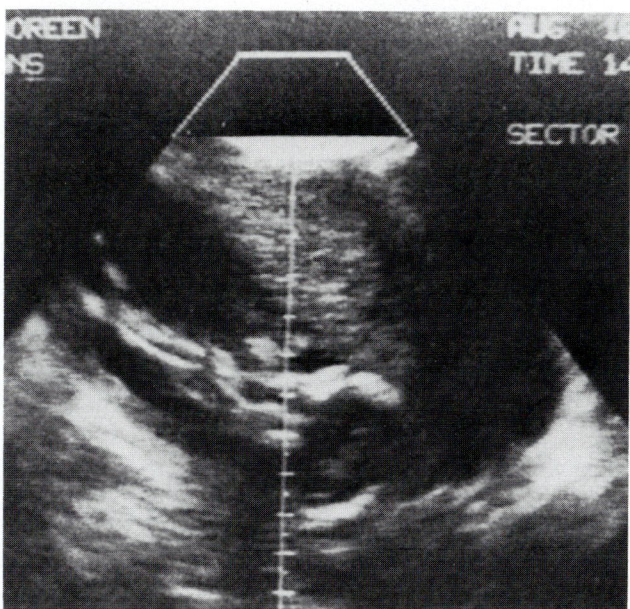

FIGURE 14–25. Longitudinal view of a fetus at 16 weeks gestation with bladder outlet obstruction. Note the extreme oligohydramnios, megacystis, and compression of the fetal thorax.

1986). The reader is referred to Chapter 25 for a detailed discussion of fetal therapy.

Anomalies of the Musculoskeletal System

As with all organ system anomalies, those of the musculoskeletal system are manifested as functional, structural, or combined lesions. Accordingly, a skeletal survey should include assessment of long bones, extremities, and digits, and determination of normal functional activities. Abnormalities of the calvarium, face, spine, and thoracic cage are frequently observed in conjunction with limb abnormalities.

Individual long bones are assessed for presence, length, proportion, shape, calcification, and epiphyseal and metaphyseal structure. As with most anomalies the detail of examination is a function of the index of suspicion (as when there has been a previously affected child).

The *skeletal dysplasias*, also termed *short-limb dystrophies*, are a complex group of anomalies with varying morphometric characteristics and prognosis. The diagnosis of skeletal dysplasia is based upon objective morphometric data pertaining to limb length and growth and subjective assessment of shape, density, and proportion. Nomograms for individual bone length and growth have been published (Jeanty et al., 1981b). *Thanatophoric dysplasia,* a uniformly fatal condition, presents as extreme shortening of limbs, thoracic cage deformity (with associated pulmonary hypoplasia), and relative cephalomegaly (Hobbins and Mahoney, 1985; McGuire et al., 1987). *Camptomelic dysplasia* is characterized by limb reduction and extreme bowing of the long bones. Although the prognosis is variable, perinatal death is usual. *Diastrophic dysplasia,* an autosomal recessive condition, involves

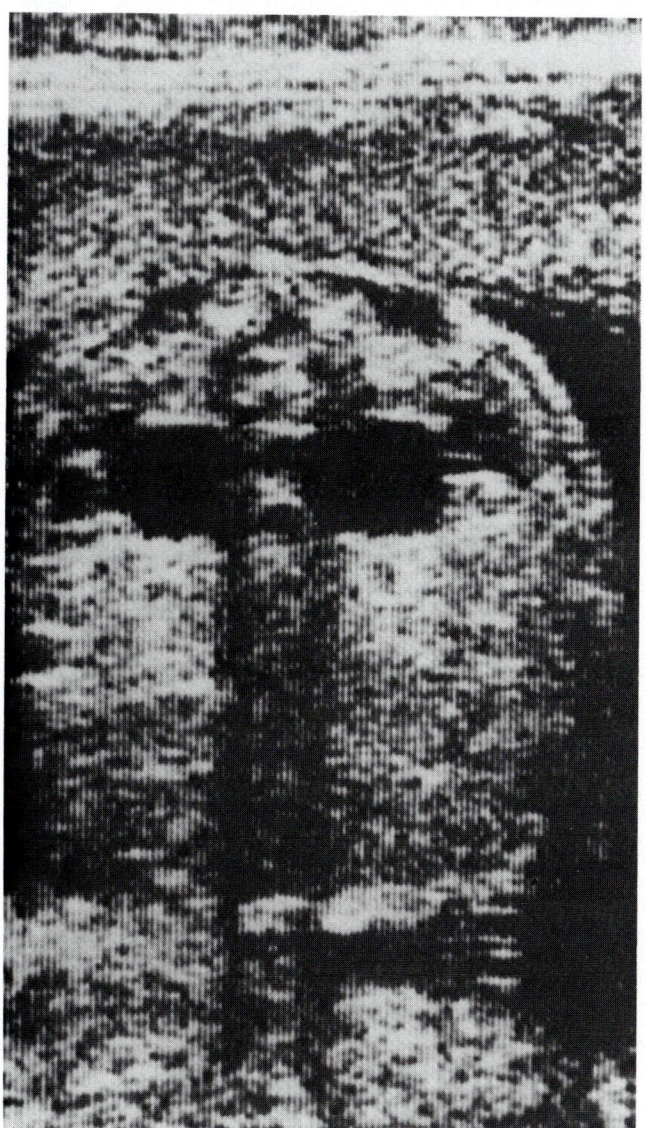

FIGURE 14–24. Severe bilateral ureteropelvic obstruction at 31 weeks gestation. Note the dilatation of renal pelvis bilaterally and the less pronounced dilatation of calyces. Amniotic fluid volume is normal.

severe limb shortening and frequently radical displacement of the thumbs (Hobbins and Mahoney, 1985). *Osteogenesis imperfecta* is seen as a spectrum of disease, ranging from mild camptomelia (bowing) to extreme demineralization, fracture, and short limbs (Chervenak et al., 1982). Spontaneous intrauterine fracture, indicated by displacement of bone elements and seen most often in the ribs, is diagnostic of a severe form of the disease. *Achondroplasia* presents as short limbs with marked flaring and enlargement of the metaphyses. *Chondroectodermal dysplasia* (Ellis–van Creveld syndrome) is part of an anomalad including cranial anomalies, limb shortening, chest deformity, and frequently polydactyly. *Hypophosphatasia* is characterized by short limb dystrophy and often extreme demineralization of the long bones. Absence of long bones is seen with the *TAR syndrome* (*t*hrombocytopenia and *a*bsent *r*adius) and with forms of syringomyelia and phocomelia.

The fetal extremities may be visualized with some clarity; such evaluation offers insight into the presence of both localized and generalized anomalies. Malrotation and malflexion of the feet (equinovalgus or equinovarus) may be diagnosed *in utero*. With subtle deformity, prolonged or repeated observation is necessary to avoid the false-positive result. Soft tissue edema of the feet may be recognized and is associated with a variety of chromosomal abnormalities including trisomy 13 and trisomy 18 and with Turner's syndrome and its variants (see Fig. 14–8). Multiple extreme flexion deformities typical of arthrogryposis multiplex congenita may be observed. In such cases the complete absence of normal flexion and extension motion of the limb is typical.

Functional abnormalities characterized by either excessive abnormal limb motion or absence of motion may be seen. Fetal tonic-clonic seizure disorders have been observed, associated with severe degenerative central nervous system disease, with spontaneous fetal intracerebral hemorrhage, and with opiate withdrawal. Hypomotility and hypotonia or paresis may be observed with primary anterior horn cell diseases such as Werdnig-Hoffmann syndrome and with severe myotonic dystrophy. Recognition of abnormal muscle group wasting or hypertrophy, both of which are typical of some muscular dystrophies and muscle glycogen storage disease, may theoretically be of clinical value.

Ultrasound Assessment of the Fetal Environment

Evaluation of the fetal environment—including amniotic fluid volume, umbilical cord structure, blood flow, fetal position, and placental morphology and site—is an integral part of ultrasound fetal assessment, providing insight into the presence of, or potential for, fetal disease.

Amniotic Fluid Volume

Clinicians have long recognized that abnormalities of amniotic fluid volume, either excessive or diminished, are associated with impending fetal disorders (see Tables 14–6 and 14–7). Amniotic fluid is readily seen with ultrasound, and therefore it is now possible to assess adequacy of volume. The volume of amniotic fluid may be judged by either subjective or objective methods; both methods in experienced hands yield comparable rates of predictive accuracy. By definition, the criteria for subjective assessment are difficult to categorize but include, in the case of oligohydramnios, the absence of fluid pockets throughout the uterine cavity and the impression of crowding of fetal small parts. In the case of hydramnios the criteria include multiple large pockets, the impression of the floating fetus, and free movement of the fetal limbs. Objective determination of amniotic fluid volume is based upon identification of the largest pocket of fluid and measurement of the vertical diameter. The objective method is subject to error due to variation in pocket size created by fetal movement. Accordingly, it is only of real value in detecting the extremes of fluid volume distribution and variation within the normal range.

There are two methods reported for determination of amniotic fluid volume. The first of these methods, measurement of the single largest pocket on a general scan of the uterus, is done initially to identify the presence and distribution of amniotic fluid, and then the largest pocket is identified and the vertical depth is measured. Amniotic fluid is described as decreased if the largest single pocket is less than 2 cm. Alternately used is the amniotic fluid index, in which the uterus is divided arbitrarily into four equal quadrants and the vertical depth of the largest pocket in each quadrant is measured; these results are summed and expressed in millimeters (Rutherford et al., 1987). By the amniotic fluid index method, amniotic fluid volume is described as normal if the summed value is greater than 80 mm and less than 180 mm. The predictive accuracy of the single pocket method and the amniotic fluid index is by and large comparable, and the method used in any given center is a matter of personal preference.

In using the objective method to determine oligohydramnios, one must avoid confusing approximated loops of cord with fluid pockets. Occasionally, amniotic fluid of extreme turbidity can suggest oligohydramnios (Fig. 14–26); the error is avoided by noting the characteristics of the umbilical cord and vessels. In day-to-day practice, subjective and objective methods of assessment of fluid volume may be used interchangeably. However, for reporting purposes, the

TABLE 14–6. **Causes of Polyhydramnios in 102 Pregnancies**

DIAGNOSIS	NO.	%
Idiopathic	68	67
Anomalies	13	13
Gestational and insulin-dependent diabetes	15	15
Twins	5	5

Adapted from Hill LM, Breckle R, Thomas ML, et al: Polyhydramnios: Ultrasonically detected prevalence and neonatal outcome. Obstet Gynecol **69:**21, 1987. Reprinted with permission from the American College of Obstetricians and Gynecologists.

TABLE 14–7. The Relationship of Amniotic Fluid Pocket to Perinatal Outcome*

LARGEST POCKET OF AMNIOTIC FLUID	NO. PATIENTS	% TOTAL	GROSS PNM	CORRECTED PNM	% MAJOR ANOMALY	% IUGR (<10th)	% MACROSOMIA (>90th)
>8 cm	243	3.2	32.9	4.12	4.3	3.8	33.3
2–8 cm	7096	93.8	4.65	1.97	0.54	4.9	8.7
1–2 cm	159	2.1	56.6	37.8	2.52	20.0	—
<1 cm	64	0.85	187.7	109.4	9.37	38.6	—

*From Chamberlain PF, Manning FA, Morrison I, et al: Ultrasound evaluation of amniotic fluid volume. I. The relationship of marginal and decreased amniotic fluid volumes to perinatal outcome. Am J Obstet Gynecol **150**:245, 1984b.

objective method is preferred because it is less subject to interobserver variability.

The risk of adverse perinatal outcome is increased in pregnancies associated with hydramnios and oligohydramnios (see Tables 14–6 and 14–7). Perinatal mortality shows a bimodal distribution, with values for the largest pocket of fluid (Fig. 14–27) increasing when the fluid pocket is greater than 8 cm or 2 cm or less. The selection of the end point for intervention for oligohydramnios in the structurally normal fetus should probably be set at less than 2 cm.

Oligohydramnios (fluid pocket less than 2 cm; AFI <80 mm) is in general related to one of three conditions: (1) rupture of membranes, (2) congenital absence of functioning renal tissue or obstructive uropathy, or (3) diminished renal perfusion with a resultant chronic reduction in fetal urine production, a consequence of hypoxemia-induced redistribution of fetal cardiac output. The presence of oligohydramnios in the fetus with intact membranes and a functional genitourinary tract usually signals significant fetal compromise and, in the fetus capable of extrauterine survival, an indication for prompt delivery. Aggressive management of oligohydramnios has been associated with a sharp fall in the corrected perinatal mortality rate (Bastide et al., 1986). The most common high-risk factors associated with oligohydramnios are post-term gestation (over 42 weeks) and IUGR (Manning et al., 1981; Chamberlain et al., 1984b). The management and outcome of post-term gestation are sharply altered by amniotic fluid volume monitoring (Johnson et al., 1986). The relationship between oligohydramnios and IUGR is less clear. However, the presence of oligohydramnios in a fetus with suspected growth failure is a powerful indicator of underlying asymmetric IUGR.

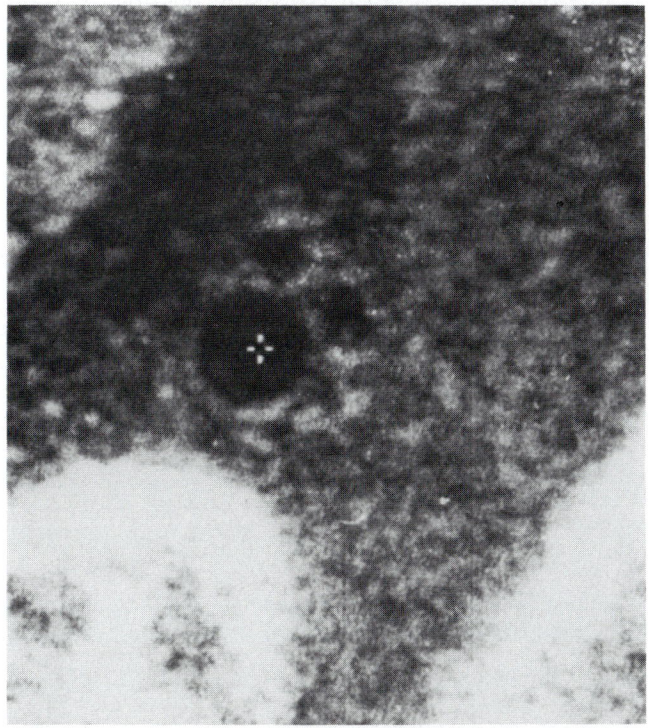

FIGURE 14–26. Close-up view of very echogenic amniotic fluid. The fetal umbilical cord and vessels (echolucent) are outlined. It is possible to confuse very echogenic amniotic fluid with oligohydramnios. With serial scan the echogenic amniotic fluid may suddenly become echolucent. The explanation for this phenomenon is unknown, but it may be caused by precipitation of amniotic fluid debris or blood.

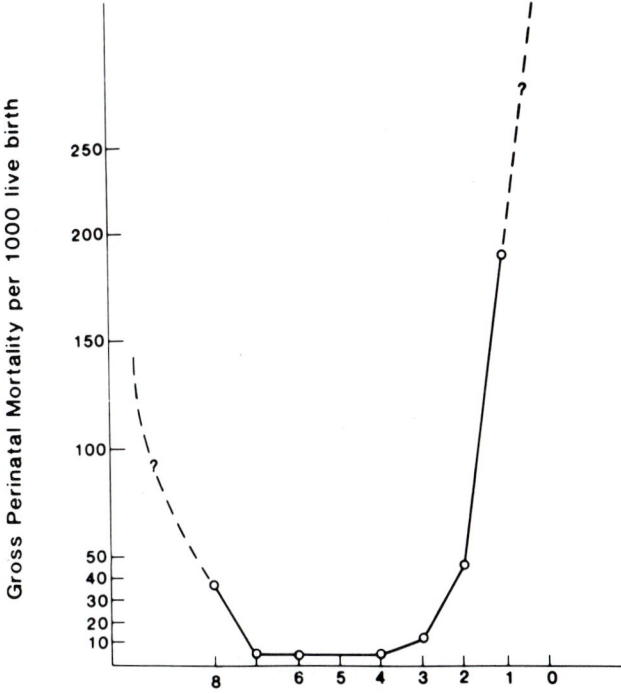

VERTICAL DIAMETER (CMS.) OF LARGEST POCKET OF AMNIOTIC FLUID

FIGURE 14–27. The relationship between perinatal mortality rate and the largest pocket of amniotic fluid as measured before delivery in 9760 high-risk patients.

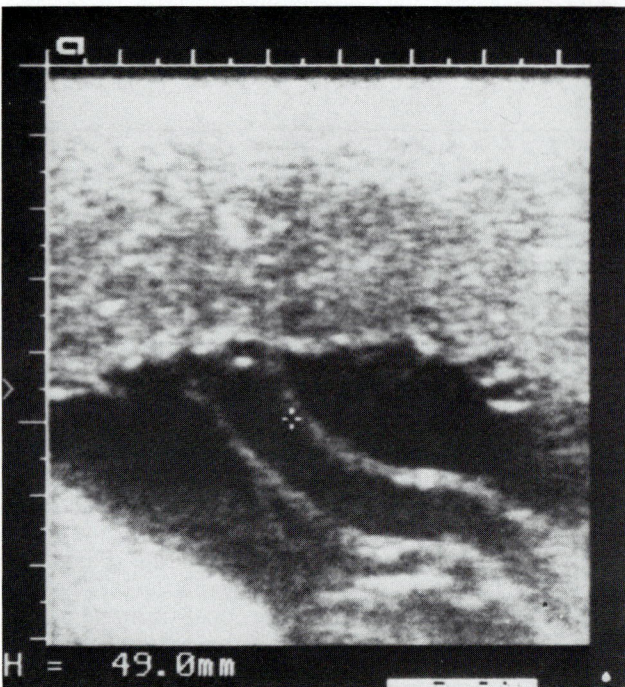

FIGURE 14–28. The fetal umbilical vein at its placental insertion. This is the usual and preferred site for ultrasound-guided fetal blood sampling and for intravascular transfusion.

The quality of amniotic fluid may be assessed by ultrasound. Turbidity created by vernix, debris, meconium, and intrauterine bleeding may be seen, and occasionally the fluid may appear opaque on ultrasound (Fig. 14–27). Meconium cannot be reliably identified by ultrasound assessment. In one study, amniotic fluid turbidity (free-floating particles) was noted to indicate a mature L/S ratio (Gross et al., 1985). This association cannot be reliable because debris may be seen as early as 14 weeks gestation. Prospective studies have also failed to confirm this association (Helewa et al., 1987). The reader is also referred to Chapters 5 and 40 for more detailed discussions of amniotic fluid physiology and abnormalities.

Assessment of the Umbilical Cord

The umbilical cord may be assessed in its entirety. The number of vessels may be determined, the presence of cord knotting (or entwining in monoamniotic twins) noted, and cystic and degenerative lesions identified (Hill et al., 1987b). Recognition of cord presentation is now possible, making prevention of cord prolapse a potential clinical reality (Lange et al., 1985).

Evaluation of the Placenta

The placenta can first be clearly recognized on ultrasonography between 14 and 16 weeks gestation. Prior to this time, it is usually possible to identify the site of placental implantation, which is characterized by a thickened portion of the intrauterine cavity.

However, clear discrimination of the placental edge from adjacent thickened decidua is difficult. Normally, the implantation site is in the region of the fundus, with an approximately equal anteroposterior distribution. In early gestation (less than 16 weeks), a low implantation site is associated with increased early fetal loss, although the association is by no means absolute. With advancing gestation, it becomes progressively easier to define the limits of the placenta and to evaluate its structural characteristics. Definition of the lower edge of the placenta in relation to the internal os is important in establishing the diagnosis of placenta previa. Evaluation of placental position and structural characteristics provides useful information in the management of the high-risk patient. The umbilical vein at its placental origin may be easily recognized by ultrasound (Fig. 14–28); this is the usual target site for cordocentesis (PUBS).

Developmental Anomalies of the Placenta

Occasionally, degenerative cystic spaces, termed *chorionic cysts* or *chorioangiomas,* develop within the placenta. They may be multiple or single and may reach a very large size. As a rule, this degenerative disorder is of no clinical significance. Large vascular channels are commonly seen within the normal placenta and may be confused with chorionic cysts. The vascular channel usually represents large fetal veins coursing over the fetal surface of the placenta, and with Doppler scanning it is usually possible to visualize a flow pattern within this vessel. Longitudinal scanning of the area confirms that the cystic areas represent vascular channels. Amniotic bands may also be identified (Fig. 14–29).

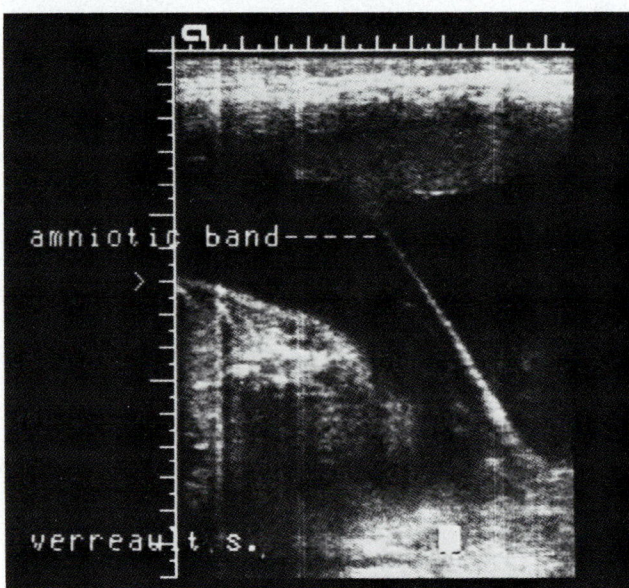

FIGURE 14–29. An amniotic band extending from the anterior uterine wall to its insertion in the posterior wall. The band is shiny and relatively fixed. Fetal limb amputation and facial malformation are complications that can result from this rare finding.

Grading of Placental Maturity

Grannum and colleagues (1979) reported a method of categorizing ultrasonographic characteristics of the maturing placenta. This method was based primarily on the identification and distribution of calcium deposits within the fetal component of placenta. In their preliminary report they noted a relationship between advancing placental grade and fetal pulmonary maturity, so that in the 23 patients with placental maturity grade III, the incidence of a mature lecithin to sphingomyelin (L/S) ratio (greater than 2.0) was 100 per cent. In 28 patients with grade II placental maturity, the incidence of mature L/S ratio was 87.5 per cent, and in 21 patients with grade I maturity, the incidence of L/S ratio was 67.7 per cent. They postulated that the observation of grade III placenta could lead to fewer amniocenteses and hence could reduce infant risk. In an expanded series of 314 patients, Harman and associates (1982) noted similar relationships, but also observed three of 84 (3.4 per cent) patients with grade III placenta to have immature phospholipid profiles (L/S less than 2, phosphatidyl glycerol absent). In these patients, addition of BPD was not useful in reducing false-positive results. These data suggest that placental grading alone may not be sufficiently accurate to predict pulmonary maturity and eliminate the need for amniocentesis.

Confirmation of Fetal Death

Dynamic ultrasound imaging methods can provide an absolute diagnosis of death *in utero*. Fetal heart motion can be identified routinely from 8 weeks gestation onward, and failure to observe fetal heart motion with adequate thoracic visualization indicates fetal demise. As gestation advances, the fetal cardiac motion becomes easier to detect. Dynamic ultrasound scanning is the primary method for establishing the diagnosis of fetal death, and ancillary methods (e.g., radiography for Spalding's sign and intravascular gas) are of less value. When the fetus has been dead for 2 or more days, fetal scalp edema (maceration) and overlap of cranial bones are seen. Some caution should be exercised by the inexperienced observer, however, because transmitted maternal pulsation can produce fetal heart structure motion, leading to an incorrect diagnosis of fetal bradycardia.

Determination of Fetal Lie, Position, and Attitude

Ultrasound imaging of the fetus allows the physician to determine fetal lie with certainty and to evaluate fetal position and attitude. Breech presentation is easily recognized, and with detailed scanning it is possible to identify the type of breech presentation.

Use of Ultrasound Scanning in Multiple Gestation

Multiple fetuses occur in up to 1 per cent of all pregnancies and are associated with a disproportionately high rate of perinatal morbidity. Ultrasound scanning is an extremely reliable method for detection of multiple pregnancies and should result in a false-negative rate approaching zero.

Although recognition of the presence of a multiple gestation is the first and key diagnostic step, it is also essential to attempt to define the type of multiple gestation. Whereas the risk of fetal and maternal complications is increased with all types of twinning, the fetal risks are greatest for monozygous twins. An estimate of the type of multiple gestation can be reached by assessment of placental number, fetal gender, and the presence or absence of a separating membrane as well as its thickness. The diagnosis of dizygotic twins can be made with almost complete certainty when the fetuses are of different sex. A certain diagnosis of monoamniotic twins can only be made by ultrasound, the typical findings being the inability to demonstrate a membrane on repeated scans and the observation of cord entanglement. Aggressive management of monoamniotic twins is strongly recommended since the mortality for this condition exceeds 50 per cent. Successful outcome with monoamniotic twinning diagnosed by antenatal ultrasound examination has been reported (Sutter et al., 1986).

Twin gestation may be detected by ultrasound as early as 6 to 8 weeks gestation and with reliability by 8 to 12 weeks. Detection is based on identification of two or more separate gestational sacs or fetuses. Interestingly, early detection of twins leads to a false-positive diagnostic rate of 60 to 70 per cent. In our experience, only one-third of patients in whom a diagnosis of multiple fetuses is made before 20 weeks gestation subsequently deliver more than one baby. This observation confirms the very high fetal wastage associated with multiple gestation. In early gestation (before 20 weeks), death of one twin is associated with gradual resorption of both twin and gestation sac. These changes can be monitored by ultrasound. Death of a twin fetus in late gestation is characterized by gradual decrease in fetal size and increasing echodensity; the latter phenomenon is likely due to loss of tissue fluid and to fetal compression.

From approximately 16 weeks onward, the fused amnions in diamniotic twins are clearly visible, particularly with a dynamic ultrasound method. Differentiation of the placentas in dichorionic twins is difficult except in late gestation. Early indices of gestational age (gestational sac volume, crown-rump length) are as accurate in multiple gestation as in singleton pregnancy. Similarly, in nondiscordant twins, biparietal diameter and abdominal circumference measurements are reliable indices of gestational age and weight. The BPD becomes less reliable after 28 to 30 weeks gestation in twin pregnancies.

Ultrasound monitoring of fetal growth and well-being is an important part of management of the twin gestation. Discordance of growth complicates up to 30 per cent of all twin gestations and is a major cause of fetal death and neonatal morbidity and mortality. Detection of discordant twins is relatively simple by ultrasound methods. At each visit fetal weight is calculated from abdominal circumference measurements, head growth is determined by BPD measure-

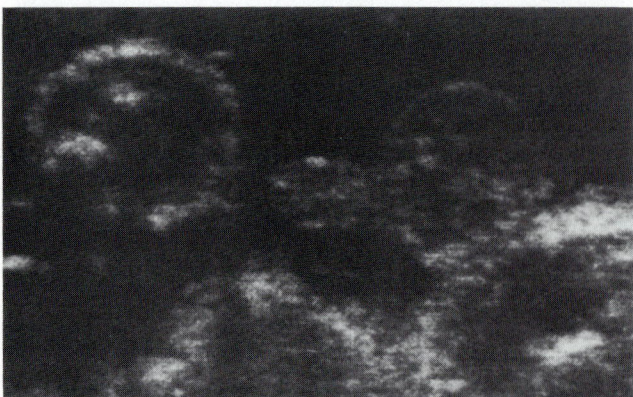

FIGURE 14–30. The penis and scrotum of a 32-week male fetus.

ment, and qualitative amniotic fluid volume determination is made for each twin. In addition, biophysical profile scoring is done for each twin. When discordance is defined as a birth weight difference of at least 30 per cent, this approach detects in excess of 95 per cent of all cases. When discordance is detected, amniocentesis of the larger twin is indicated and delivery may be considered if pulmonary maturity is present. See Chapters 37 and 38 for a detailed discussion of the multiple gestation.

Fetal Sex Determination

In the active fetus the perineum and external genitalia may be visualized and therefore fetal phenotypic sex assigned. External genitalia may be differentiated from as early as 16 weeks gestation and reliably from about 22 weeks onward. The diagnosis of the male fetus is direct, by notation of the penis and scrotum (Fig. 14–30). The characteristic undulating movement of the scrotum with fetal limb motion ("jello" sign) makes confusion with a loop of umbilical cord highly unlikely. The diagnosis of the female may be made either directly or by exclusion—that is, failure to identify the male genitalia. The latter method may lead to error if the male genitalia are flattened between the buttocks. Since misassignment of fetal sex may result in considerable consternation, the diagnosis should be withheld unless certain.

SUMMARY

It has been the intent of this discussion to provide a broad background on the use of ultrasound in clinical practice. More specific details with regard to its application in specific disorders may be found in those chapters dealing with clinical entities.

REFERENCES

Avni EF, Rodesch F, Schulman CC: Fetal uropathies: Diagnostic pitfalls and management. J Urol 134:921, 1985.

Baskett TF, Allen AC, Gray JH, et al: A fetal biophysical profile and perinatal death. Obstet Gynecol 70:375, 1987.

Bastide A, Manning FA, Harman CR, et al: Ultrasound evaluation of amniotic fluid: Outcome of pregnancies with severe oligohydramnios. Am J Obstet Gynecol 154:895, 1986.

Benacerraf BR, Barss VA, Laboda LA: A sonographic sign for the detection in the second trimester of the fetus with Down's syndrome. Am J Obstet Gynecol 151:1078, 1985a.

Benacerraf BR, Frigoletto FD: Mid-trimester fetal thoracentesis. J Clin Ultrasound 13:202, 1985.

Benacerraf BR, Frigoletto FD, Laboda LA: Sonographic diagnosis of Down's syndrome in the second trimester. Am J Obstet Gynecol 153:49, 1985b.

Benacerraf BR, Adzick NS: Fetal diaphragmatic hernia: Ultrasound diagnosis and clinical outcome in 19 cases. Am J Obstet Gynecol 156:573, 1987.

Benedetti TJ, Gabbe SG: Shoulder dystocia: A complication of fetal macrosomia and prolonged second stage of labour with midpelvic delivery. Obstet Gynecol 52:526, 1978.

Birnholz JC: The fetal external ear. Radiology 1417:819, 1983.

Boddy K, Dawes GS, Fisher R, et al: Foetal respiratory movements, electrocortical and cardiovascular responses to hypoxemia and hypercapnia in sheep. J Physiol (Lond) 243:599, 1974.

Brugman SM, Jjelland JJ, Thomasson JE, et al: Sonographic findings with radiologic correlation in meconium peritonitis. J Clin Ultrasound 7:306, 1979.

Campbell S: The assessment of fetal growth by diagnostic ultrasound. Clin Perinatol 1:507, 1974.

Campbell S: Ultrasound measurement of the fetal head to abdomen circumference ratio in assessment of growth retardation. Br J Obstet Gynecol 84:165, 1977.

Campbell S, Wilkin P: Ultrasonic measurement of fetal abdominal circumference in the estimation of fetal weight. Br J Obstet Gynecol 82:689, 1975.

Chamberlain PF, Manning FA, Morrison I, et al: Circadian rhythm in bladder volumes in the term human fetus. Obstet Gynecol 64(5):657, 1984a.

Chamberlain PF, Manning FA, Morrison I, et al: Ultrasound evaluation of amniotic fluid volume. I. The relationship of marginal and decreased amniotic fluid volumes to perinatal outcome. Am J Obstet Gynecol 150(3):245, 1984b.

Chamberlain PF, Manning FA, Morrison I, et al: Ultrasound evaluation of amniotic fluid volume. II. The relationship of increased amniotic fluid volume to perinatal outcome. Am J Obstet Gynecol 150(3):250, 1984c.

Chervenak FA, Berkowitz RL, Tontora M, et al: The management of fetal hydrocephalus. Am J Obstet Gynecol 155:933, 1985.

Chervenak FA, Romero RR, Berkowitz RL, et al: Antenatal sonographic findings of osteogenesis imperfecta. Am J Obstet Gynecol 143:228, 1982.

Chinn DH, Bolding DB, Callen PW, et al: Ultrasonographic identification of fetal lower extremity epiphyseal ossification centers. Radiology 147:815, 1983.

Divon MY, Chamberlain PF, Sipos L, et al: Identification of the small for gestational age fetus with the use of gestational age-independent indices of fetal growth. Am J Obstet Gynecol 155:1197, 1986.

Donald I, Brown TG: Demonstration of tissue interfaces within the body by ultrasound echo sounding. Br J Radiol 34:539, 1961.

Edmonds PD: Interactions of ultrasound and biological tissues. US DHEW Publications (FDA) 73-8008. Washington, DS, US Food and Drug Administration, 1972.

Elliott JP, Garite TJ, Freeman RJ, et al: Ultrasound prediction of fetal macrosomia in diabetic pregnancies. Obstet Gynecol 60:159, 1982.

Fazekas IG, Kosa F: Forensic fetal osteology. Budapest, Akademia Kiado, 1978, p.256.

Goldstein I, Lockwood C, Hobbins JC: Ultrasound assessment of fetal intestinal development in the evaluation of gestational age. Proceedings of the Society of Perinatologists and Obstetricians, Tampa, 1987.

Grannum PAT, Berkowitz RL, Hobbins JC: The ultrasonic changes in the maturing placenta and their relationship to fetal pulmonic maturity. Am J Obstet Gynecol 133:915, 1979.

Grennert L, Persson P, Gerrser G, et al: Benefits of ultrasound screening of a pregnant population. Acta Obstet Gynecol Scand 78 (Suppl):5, 1978.

Gross TL, Wolfson RN, Kuhnerol PM: Sonographically detected free floating particles in amniotic fluid predict a mature lethicin-sphingomyelin ratio. J Clin Ultrasound 13:405, 1985.

Hadlock FP: Determination of fetal age. In Athey PA, Hadlock FP (eds): Ultrasound in Obstetrics and Gynecology. St. Louis, CV Mosby Co, 1985.

Hadlock FP, Deter RL, Harrist RB, et al: Fetal abdominal circumference: Relation to menstrual age. Am J Radiol 139:367, 1982a.

Hadlock FP, Deter RL, Harrist RB, et al: Fetal biparietal diameter: A critical re-evaluation of the relation to menstrual age by means of realtime ultrasound. J Ultrasound Med 1:97, 1982b.

Hadlock FP, Deter RL, Harrist RB, et al: Computer assisted analysis of fetal age in the third trimester using multiple fetal growth parameters. J Clin Ultrasound 11:313, 1983a.

Hadlock FP, Deter RL, Harrist RB, et al: A date-independent predictor of intrauterine growth retardation: Femur length/abdominal circumference ratio. AJR 141:979, 1983b.

Harman CR: Evaluation of fetal lung morphology by ultrasound densitometry. Personal communication, 1986.

Harman CR, Manning FA: Alloimmune disease. In Pauerstein CJ (ed): Clinical Obstetrics. New York, John Wiley and Sons, 1987, pp 441–469.

Harman CR, Manning FA, Stearns E, et al: The correlation of ultrasonic placental grading and fetal pulmonic maturation in 563 pregnancies. Am J Obstet Gynecol 143:941, 1982.

Harman CR, Bowman JM, Manning FA, et al: Intrauterine transfusion—intraperitoneal versus intravascular approach: A case-control comparison. Am J Obstet Gynecol 162:1053, 1990.

Harrison MR, Golbus MS, Filly RA, et al: In utero treatment of urinary tract obstruction. Am J Obstet Gynecol 142:383, 1982.

Harrison MR, Adzick NS, Nakayama DK: Fetal diaphragmatic hernia: Pathophysiology, natural history and outcome. Clin Obstet Gynecol 29:490, 1986.

Helewa M, Manning FA, Harman CR, et al: Sonographic amniotic fluid free floating particles: Any relationship to fetal lung maturity. Obstet Gynecol 74:893, 1989.

Hill LM, Breckle R, Thomas ML, et al: Polyhydramnios: Ultrasonically detected prevalence and neonatal outcome. Obstet Gynecol 69:21, 1987a.

Hill LM, Kislak S, Runco P: An ultrasonic view of the umbilical cord. Obstet Gynecol Survey 42:82, 1987b.

Hobbins JC, Grannum PAT, Berkowitz RL, et al: Ultrasound in the diagnosis of congenital anomalies. Am J Obstet Gynecol 134:331, 1979.

Hobbins JC, Mahoney MJ: Skeletal dysplasias. In Sarden RC, James AM (eds): The Principles and Practice of Ultrasonography in Obstetrics and Gynecology. Norwalk, Conn., Appleton-Century-Crofts, 1985, p. 267ff.

Hoddick WK, Callen PW, Filly RA, et al: Ultrasonographic determination of qualitative amniotic fluid volume in intrauterine growth retardation: Reassessment of the 1 cm rule. Am J Obstet Gynecol 149:758, 1984.

Hohler CW: Cross-checking pregnancy landmarks by ultrasound. Contemp Obstet Gynecol 20:169, 1982.

Jeanty P, Dramaix-Wilmet M, Delbeke D, et al: Ultrasonic evaluation of fetal ventricular growth. Neuroradiology 21:127, 1981a.

Jeanty P, Kirkpatrick C, Dramaix-Wilmet M, et al: Ultrasound evaluation of fetal limb growth. Radiology 140:165, 1981b.

Jeanty P, Dramaix-Wilmet M, Elkhazen N, et al: Measurement of fetal kidney growth on ultrasound. Radiology 144:159, 1982.

Johnson JM, Harman CR, Lange IR, et al: Biophysical profile scoring in the management of the post-term pregnancy: An analysis of 307 patients. Am J Obstet Gynecol 154(2):269, 1986.

Lange IR, Manning FA: Antenatal diagnosis of congenital pleural effusions. Am J Obstet Gynecol 140(7):839, 1981.

Lange IR, Manning FA: Cord prolapse: Is antenatal diagnosis possible? Am J Obstet Gynecol 151(8):1083, 1985.

Laurence KM, Coates JS: Spontaneously arrested hydrocephalus: Results of the re-examination of 82 survivors from a series of 182 unoperated cases. Dev Med Child Neurol 13(Suppl):4, 1967.

Laurence KM, Coates JS: The natural history of hydrocephalus: Detailed analysis of 182 unoperated cases. Arch Dis Child 37:345, 1962.

Leopold GR: Antepartum obstetrical ultrasound examination guidelines. J Ultrasound Med Sci 5:244, 1986.

Longaker MT, Golbus MS, Filly RA, et al: Maternal outcome after open fetal surgery: A review of the first 17 human cases. JAMA 265:737, 1991.

Lubchenco LO, Searle DT, Brazie JV: Neonatal mortality rate: Relationship to birth weight of gestational age. J Pediatr 81:814, 1972.

Lyons EA, Dyke C, Cheang M: In utero exposure to diagnostic ultrasound: A six year follow-up. Radiology 166:687, 1988.

Manning FA, Harman CR, Lange IR, et al: Antepartum chronic vesicoamniotic shunts for obstructive uropathy. Am J Obstet Gynecol 145:819, 1983.

Manning FA, Hill LM, Platt LD: Qualitative amniotic fluid volume determination by ultrasound: Antepartum detection of intrauterine growth retardation. Am J Obstet Gynecol 139:254, 1981.

Manning FA, Lange IR, Morrison I, et al: Calculation of fetal length in utero: An ultrasound method. Proc SOGC, Vancouver, BC, June, 1983a. (abstract)

Manning FA, Lange IR, Morrison I, Harman CR: Determination of fetal health: Methods for antepartum and intrapartum fetal assessment. Curr Prob Obstet Gynecol 7(4):1, 1983b.

Manning FA, Harrison MR, Rodick C: Catheter shunts for fetal hydronephrosis and hydrocephalus: Report of the International Fetal Surgery Registry. N Engl J Med 315:336, 1986.

Mayden KL, Tortora M, Berkowitz RL: Orbital diameters: A new parameter for prenatal diagnosis and dating. Am J Obstet Gynecol 144(3):289, 1982.

McCallum WD, Brinkley TF: Estimation of fetal weight from ultrasound measurement. Am J Obstet Gynecol 133:195, 1979.

McCullough DC, Balzer-Martin LA: Current prognosis in overt neonatal hydrocephalus. J Neurosurg 57:378, 1982.

McGuire J, Manning FA, Lange IR, et al: Antenatal diagnosis of skeletal dysplasia using ultrasound. Birth Defects 23:367, 1987.

Mercer BM, Sklar S, Shariatnadar A, et al: Fetal foot length as a predictor of gestational age. Am J Obstet Gynecol 156:350, 1987.

Moessinger AC: Fetal lung growth in experimental utero-abdominal pregnancy. Obstet Gynecol 68:675, 1987.

Morrison I, Olsen J: Weight specific stillbirth and associated causes of death: An analysis of 765 stillbirths. Am J Obstet Gynecol 152:975, 1985.

Natale R, Clewlow F, Dawes GS: Measurement of fetal forelimb movements in the lamb in utero. Am J Obstet Gynecol 140:545, 1981.

Nelson LH, Anderson SG, Perry MF: The wavering midline: A diagnostic sign of fetal hydrocephalus. Am J Obstet Gynecol 149:662, 1984.

Nicolaides KH, Campbell S, Gabbe SG, et al: Ultrasound screening for spina bifida: Cranial and cerebellar signs. Lancet ii:72, 1986.

Nijhuis JG, Prechtl HFR, Martin CB Jr, et al: Are there behavioural states in the human fetus? Early Hum Dev 6:177, 1982.

Nimrod C, Nicholson S, Davies D, et al: Pulmonary hypoplasia testing in clinical obstetrics. Am J Obstet Gynecol 158:277, 1988.

O'Brien GD, Queenan JT: Growth of the ultrasound fetal femur during normal pregnancy. Am J Obstet Gynecol 141:833, 1981.

Phillips HE, McGahan PP: Intrauterine fetal cystic hygromas: Sonographic detection. AJR 136:799, 1981.

Platt LD, Eglington GS, Sipos L, et al: Further experience with the fetal biophysical profile score. Obstet Gynecol 61:480, 1983.

Robinson HP: Sonar measurement of fetal crown-rump length as a means of assessing maturity in the first trimester of pregnancy. Br Med J 4:28, 1973.

Rodeck CH, Fisk NM, Fraser DI, et al: Longterm in utero drainage of fetal hydrothorax. N Engl J Med 319:1135, 1988.

Romero R, Cullen M, Jeanty P: The diagnosis of congenital renal anomalies with ultrasound. II Infantile polycyctic kidney disease. Am J Obstet Gynecol 150:219, 1984.

Romero R, Copel J, Jeanty P, et al: Causes, diagnosis and management of non-immune hydrops. Clin Diagn Ultrasound 19:31, 1986.

Rutherford SE, Phelan JP, Smith CV, et al: The four-quadrant assessment of amniotic fluid volume: An adjunct to antepartum fetal heart rate testing. Obstet Gynecol 70:353, 1987.

Sabbagha RE, Hughey M, Depp R: The assignment of growth-adjusted sonographic age (GASA): A simplified method. Obstet Gynecol 51:383, 1978.

Schifrin BS, Guner V, Gergley RC, et al: The role of real time scanning in antenatal fetal surveillance. Am J Obstet Gynecol **140**:525, 1981.

Scioscia AL, Pretorius DH, Budorick NE: Second trimester echogenic bowel and chromosomal abnormalities. Am J Obstet Gynecol 1992, in press.

Sherer DM, Davis JM, Woods JR Jr: Hypoplasia: A review. Obstet Gynecol Surv **45**:792, 1990.

Shepard MJ, Richards VA, Berkowitz RL, et al: An evaluation of two equations for predicting fetal weight by ultrasound. Am J Obstet Gynecol **152**:47, 1982.

Socol ML, Manning FA, Murata Y, Druzin M: Maternal smoking causes fetal hypoxia: Experimental evidence. Am J Obstet Gynecol **142**(2):214, 1982.

Sutter JA, Arab H, Manning FA: Monoamniotic twins: Antenatal diagnosis and management. Am J Obstet Gynecol **155**:836, 1986.

Tamura RK, Sabbagha RE: Percentile ratios of sonar fetal abdominal circumference measurements. Am J Obstet Gynecol **138**:475, 1980.

Thompson TE, Manning FA, Morrison I: Determination of fetal volume in utero by an ultrasound method correlation with neonatal birth weight. J Ultrasound Med **2**:113, 1983.

Toi A, Simpson GF, Filly RA: Ultrasonically evident fetal nuchal skin thickening: Is it specific for Down's syndrome? Am J Obstet Gynecol **156**:150, 1987.

Vintzileos AM, Campbell WA, Nochimson DJ, et al: The use and misuse of the fetal biophysical profile. Am J Obstet Gynecol **156**:527, 1987a.

Vintzileos AM, Campbell WA, Weinbaum PJ, et al: Perinatal management and outcome of fetal ventriculomegaly. Obstet Gynecol **69**:5, 1987b.

Warsof SL, Gohari P, Berkowitz RL, et al: The estimation of fetal weight by computer assisted analysis. Am J Obstet Gynecol **128**:881, 1977.

Warsof SL, Nicholades KH, Rodeck C: Immune and non-immune hydrops. Clin Obstet Gynecol **29**:533, 1986.

Wenstrom KD, Weiner CP, Hanson TW: A five-year statewide experience with congenital diaphragmatic hernia. Am J Obstet Gynecol **165**:838, 1991.

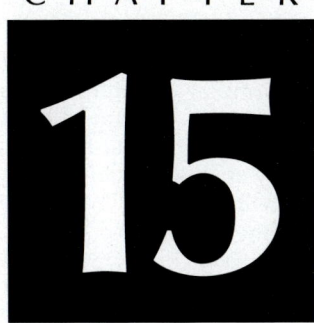

PRENATAL DIAGNOSIS OF STRUCTURAL HEART DISEASE

CHARLES S. KLEINMAN, M.D., and JOSHUA A. COPEL, M.D.

Despite the fact that congenital cardiac diseases constitute the most common lethal congenital malformations, carrying a tremendous burden of disability for the patients, their families, and society as a whole, the fetal cardiovascular system was the last of the major organ systems to be subjected to detailed examination during human pregnancy. During the last 10 to 15 years, however, fetal cardiac imaging has become almost commonplace and has led to the development of fetal cardiology as a new discipline within pediatric cardiology and perinatology.

The complex nature of congenital cardiac malformations, coupled with the dynamic nature of the tiny fetal heart, made complete examination virtually impossible prior to the development of ultrasound equipment with adequate resolution and the ability to examine a dynamic organ, which normally contracts between 110 and 160 times a minute. Because most early ultrasound scanners converted signals to composite images in the compound, or B-mode scan, only still pictures were available, and rapidly moving structures such as the heart were unaccessible.

In 1972, Winsberg used M-mode echocardiography to evaluate fetal cardiac motion against time. This first application of echocardiography for the examination of the human fetal heart attempted to estimate fetal cardiac output. It suggested that such technology could be used to evaluate fetal cardiac pump function, but that such examinations were unlikely to be of use in detecting abnormalities of fetal cardiac structure. In 1976, Morin speculated that the emerging technology in real-time sector scanning could offer the promise of simplifying techniques for the measurement of ventricular function in the fetus.

During the past 15 years, owing in large part to improvements in ultrasound technology, detailed evaluation of both normal and abnormal anatomy has become a reality (Kleinman et al., 1980; Allan et al., 1980; Sahn et al., 1980; Axel, 1983). The more recent application of pulsed and color flow Doppler techniques have made it possible to evaluate blood flow patterns within the central circulation of the human fetus throughout the second and third trimesters of pregnancy (Kleinman et al., 1986; Allan et al., 1987; Huhta et al., 1987; DeVore et al., 1987; Sharland et al., 1990; Copel et al., 1991).

The application of these techniques has made the prenatal diagnosis of complex structural heart disease a reality that is becoming commonplace in prenatal diagnostic centers. The information gleaned from these studies may have important practical implications for the management of pregnancy, delivery, and the neonatal period.

FETAL ECHOCARDIOGRAPHIC IMAGING TECHNIQUE

Although some authors have suggested that M-mode echocardiographic evaluation of cardiac chamber and blood vessel measurement should occupy a central position in the evaluation of fetal structural heart disease, we have relied primarily on two-dimensional imaging of the fetal heart to provide structural information. In so doing we apply the same sequential deductive imaging principle that provides the foundation for the echocardiographic analysis of cardiac structure in our postnatal echocardiographic program, reserving M-mode echocardiography for the analysis of cardiac arrhythmias, for analysis of ventricular function, and for the measurement of cardiac walls and septa in cases at risk for cardiomyopathies (Allan et al., 1982; Kleinman and Santulli, 1983; Kleinman and Donnerstein, 1985).

Two-dimensional echocardiography involves a tomographic analysis of fetal cardiac structure employing the same tomographic planes that are used in pediatric and adult echocardiography.

Examination can be performed with either a sector or linear array scanner. The higher frequency transducers (usually 5 mHz) provide better spatial resolution in the axial plane than do more powerful lower frequency transducers interfaced with the same scanner. We use a sector scanner with a transducer that has a focal point at the depth of the fetal heart from the maternal abdominal wall. The more sophisticated sector scanners, with dynamic focusing and annular phased array technology, provide high-resolution images that may be critical for the analysis of cardiac structure early in the second trimester, with very small fetal hearts. In general, newer linear or curvilinear array equipment provides adequate imaging for screening studies and, in some cases, detailed structural study of the fetal heart throughout the second and third trimesters.

More recently, dynamically focused high-frequency vaginal transducer probes have provided four-chamber imaging of the first-trimester fetal heart as early as the tenth week of gestation (Bronshtein et al., 1991).

The simplest and most important single view to obtain is the *four-chamber view* of fetal cardiac anatomy (Fig. 15–1). This view includes both atria and ventricles, with interposed interatrial and interventricular septa and atrioventricular valves. One can obtain this view by finding the cross-sectional image of the fetal abdomen at the level of the liver (used for the calculation of abdominal circumference) and angling the transducer slightly more cephalad on the fetus. This view is especially useful for assessing relative cardiac chamber sizes, for assessing the structure of the central portion of the fetal heart (involving the atrioventricular valves and the atrioventricular septum), and for detecting pericardial effusions.

In making the transition from cross-sectional imaging of the fetal abdomen to four-chamber imaging of the fetal heart, one should analyze the situs of the major abdominal organs and the fetal heart. Whereas the fetal liver is usually a midline organ that spans the entire fetal abdomen, it is usually a simple matter to lateralize the fetal stomach. The cardiac apex should normally be lateralized to the same side of the fetus

as the stomach. The inferior vena cava should be lateralized to the right side of the fetal abdomen, and should be traced into the morphologic right atrium of the fetal heart. When the fetal abdominal organs are oriented in situs inversus, the stomach bubble will be identified on the right side of the fetal abdomen and the inferior vena cava on the left. The latter blood vessel will be traced to its insertion into the morphologic fetal right atrium on the left side of the fetal chest. In such cases the "normal" position of the cardiac apex will be toward the right, that is, concordant with the position of the fetal stomach. In situations in which the fetal stomach and the fetal cardiac apex are not lateralized to the same side of the fetal body, there is a great likelihood of complex intracardiac malformations. Such fetuses often have *visceral heterotaxy* and may have critical forms of congenital heart disease, often involving abnormalities of the spleen (either *asplenia* or *polysplenia*) and malrotations of the gut. Most, but not all, such fetuses have defects of atrioventricular septation, anomalous pulmonary venous drainage, and possibly arterial transposition and associated pulmonary outflow tract obstruction. Such fetuses should be identified prior to birth, since sophisticated cardiac management may well be required in the immediate neonatal period. In our experience, an increasing number of fetuses have been identified to have congenital heart disease after initial level I scanning has identified abnormal viscero-atrial situs.

The identification of cardiac structures is facilitated by the recognition of some important landmarks. The more posterior atrial chamber, normally seen in a position closest to the fetal spine, contains the flap valve of the foramen ovale, which undulates within the *left atrial* cavity during real-time examination. This

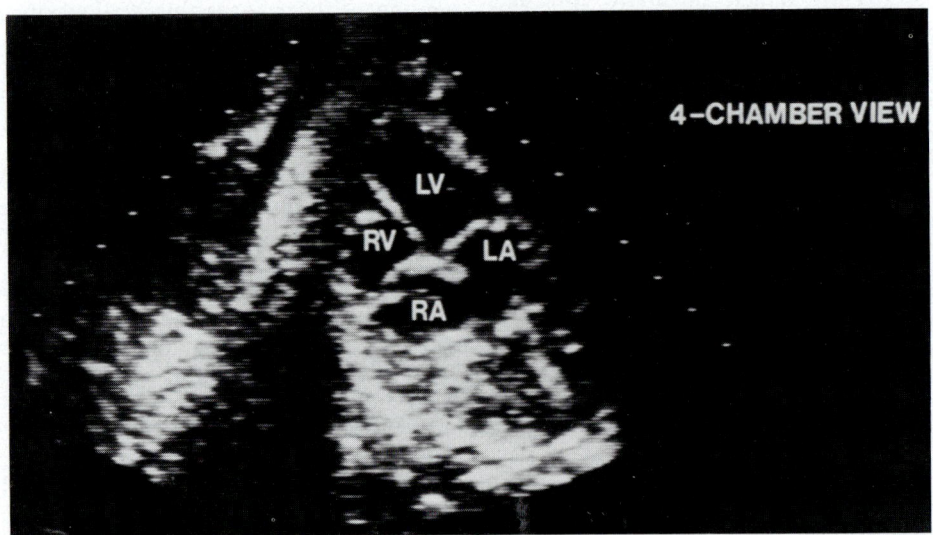

FIGURE 15–1. Four-chamber view of cardiac anatomy in a fetus at 36 weeks gestation. Echogenic structure at the apex of the right ventricle (RV) represents the moderator band. Interventricular septum separating RV and left ventricle (LV) is intact. Atrioventricular valves separate right and left atria (RA and LA) from their respective ventricles. The interatrial septum appears to have a large hole that represents the fetal foramen ovale. Note that at the center of the heart the atrioventricular valves insert into the junction of the atrial and ventricular septa with the tricuspid valve insertion slightly displaced toward the cardiac apex (apex is oriented toward the left upper aspect of the figure).

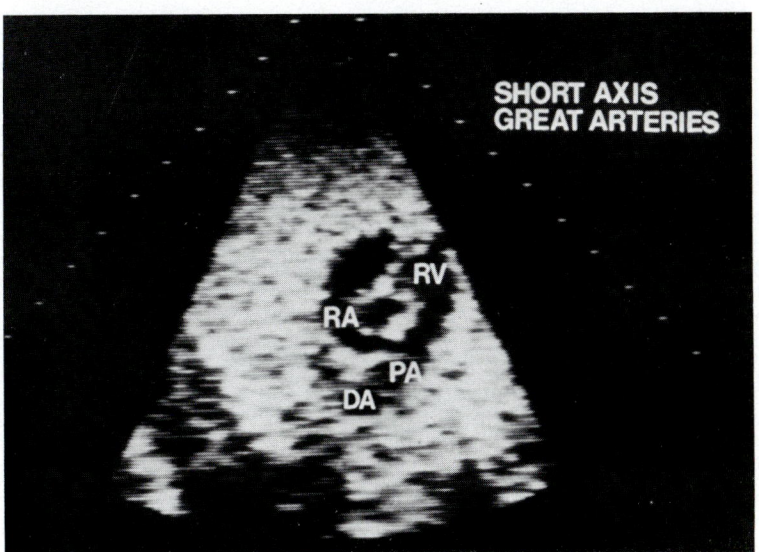

SHORT AXIS
GREAT ARTERIES

FIGURE 15–2. Short-axis view of the great arteries in a 38-week fetus. Aortic root appears as circular structure at the center. The aorta appears to be "wrapped" in the curvilinear right ventricular (RV) outflow tract leading to the pulmonary artery (PA), which in turn is continuous with the ductus arteriosus (DA).

undulation reflects unidirectional right-to-left shunting of blood across the foramen ovale. The more anterior ventricular chamber has a more coarsely trabeculated wall than does the posterior ventricle. A thick muscle bundle (moderator band) at the apex of the anterior ventricle and a papillary muscle inserting onto the interventricular septum identify this ventricle as the morphologic *right ventricle.* The two separate atrioventricular valves appear to insert close to the center of the heart, at the junction of the atrial and ventricular septa. However, the tricuspid valve (right atrioventricular valve) insertion is a few millimeters closer to the apex of the heart than the mitral valve (anatomic "marker" for identification of the morphologic *left ventricle*) insertion. In the vast majority of cases the entry of the inferior vena cava into the fetal *right atrium* can be appreciated, although it is also apparent that the inferior vena cava inserts close to the position of the foramen ovale, allowing much of the inferior vena caval (and thus umbilical venous) blood to gain preferential access to the fetal left atrium.

The sagittal or *long-axis view* of the fetal heart is obtained by orienting the tomographic imaging plane between the fetal left hip and right shoulder. This view provides demonstration of the origin of the aorta from the fetal left ventricle. In this view the anterior wall of the aorta appears to be continuous with the interventricular septum. The mitral valve is in continuity with the posterior wall of the aorta, and the aorta appears to arise completely from the left ventricular cavity. This view provides visualization of the anterior portion of the interventricular septum and is useful for the detection of "malalignment" defects within this septum, which lead to "over-riding" or "double-outlet" ventriculoarterial connections.

A subtle clockwise rotation of the transducer provides a *pulmonary artery/ductus view,* demonstrating the pulmonary artery to arise from the right ventricle. This artery appears to "dive" posteriorly to cross over the aorta and then "bifurcates" into the ductus arteriosus (which in turn continues into the descending aorta) and into the pulmonary artery. The latter divides into

smaller right and left pulmonary arteries. The crossing of the aortic and pulmonary arterial trunks is important to ascertain, since in "discordant" or "double-outlet" ventriculoarterial connections the two arteries are frequently parallel. The curvilinear "sweep" of ductus arteriosus into descending aorta can be confused with aortic arch if one is not careful to recognize that the aortic arch gives forth to the three great arterial branches (subclavian, left carotid, and left subclavian), which should be identified easily.

A further clockwise rotation of the transducer, into a position at right angles to the long axis view, provides the *short-axis view.* Slight caudad orientation will provide a short-axis cross-sectional view of the fetal ventricles, demonstrating the position of the interventricular septum between the two ventricles and often demonstrating the two small papillary muscles of the mitral valve. Slight cephalad orientation in the fetus demonstrates the great arteries in cross-section. In this view (Fig. 15–2), the aorta in cross-section appears as a small circular structure surrounded posteriorly by the left atrium and anteriorly by a curvilinear right ventricular outflow region leading into the pulmonary trunk.

FETAL CARDIAC FUNCTION

Echocardiographic studies of fetal cardiac structure have suggested that the fetal right ventricle is relatively volume-overloaded when compared with the fetal left ventricle. These conclusions were reached independently by several workers who observed that the fetal interventricular septum appears to "bow" into the left ventricular cavity during diastole (Sahn et al., 1980; Kleinman et al., 1980). More recently, several workers (Reed et al., 1986; De Smedt et al., 1987) have cited pulsed Doppler flow studies that show the human fetal right ventricle to have an output that exceeds the left ventricular output by a ratio of approximately 55/45. This contrasts with fetal lamb blood flow studies suggesting a 2/1 relationship (Rudolph and Heymann,

1970; Rudolph, 1985) between the outputs of these ventricles. Recent work in this same laboratory (Silverman et al., 1991) has demonstrated that the Doppler estimates of relative ventricular outputs correlate well with simultaneous measurements using the radionuclide microsphere and flow-probe techniques in the fetal lamb model. It is likely that the decreased ratio of right versus left ventricular output in the fetal human, compared with the fetal lamb, reflects the proportionately larger fetal brain, which imposes a larger requirement for left ventricular output on the human fetus.

Fetal echocardiographic studies are best interpreted in relation to the unique properties of the fetal circulatory system. These include the parallel circuitry in the fetal circulation, with communications between the atrial cavities at the level of the foramen ovale, and arterial communication across the ductus arteriosus. Perturbations in the fetal circulation are likely to have a structural impact on the fetal heart. An understanding of these alterations may provide added insights into the fetal adaptation to structural heart disease and may enable the pediatric cardiologist, neonatologist, and obstetrician to alter delivery plans and immediate neonatal management plans to allow a smoother transition to the postnatal circulatory pathway. For example, in situations in which prenatal evaluation has suggested that the neonate will be dependent upon persistent patency of the ductus arteriosus to provide adequate pulmonary or systemic blood flow, the fetus may receive prostaglandin E therapy to maintain ductal patency while plans for surgical therapy can be formulated, thereby avoiding severe hypoxemia or ischemia as the presenting sign of congenital cardiac disease (Neutze et al., 1977).

INDICATIONS FOR FETAL ECHOCARDIOGRAPHIC STUDY

Having demonstrated the feasibility of obtaining tomographic images of the structure of the fetal heart, we must now question whether it is feasible or cost-effective to attempt detailed echocardiographic studies on every pregnant woman. Despite the fact that universal screening could increase the number of cases of congenital heart disease diagnosed prenatally, this would require a prodigious commitment of human and financial resources that would be difficult to justify.

We have attempted to define, during the past 15 years, risk factors that place a given fetus at higher risk for significant congenital heart disease than the average pregnancy (0.4 to 0.8 per cent). We have defined a series of risk factors that constitute indications for echocardiographic studies in given pregnancies (Table 15–1). These risks have been grouped into fetal, maternal, and familial factors. During the 8-year period encompassing 1984 to 1991, 3513 fetuses underwent fetal echocardiographic examination at the Yale-New Haven Hospital. During this period, 213 cases of congenital cardiac disease were diagnosed (6.1 per cent). The most common indication for cardiac scan during this period was a familial or maternal history

TABLE 15–1. Indications for Detailed Fetal Echocardiographic Examination

Fetal risk factors
  Extracardiac anomalies
    Chromosomal
    Anatomic
  Fetal cardiac dysrhythmia
    Irregular rhythm
    Tachycardia (>200 beats/minute)
    Bradycardia (nonperiodic)
  Intrauterine growth retardation
  Nonimmune hydrops fetalis
  Suspected cardiac anomaly on level I scan
  Abnormal fetal situs

Maternal risk factors
  Congenital heart disease
  Cardiac teratogen exposure
    Lithium carbonate
    Progestins
    Amphetamines
    Alcohol
    Anticonvulsants
      Phenytoin
      Trimethadione
    Isoretinoin
  Maternal metabolic disorders
    Diabetes mellitus
    Phenylketonuria
  Polyhydramnios
  Maternal infections
    Rubella
    Toxoplasmosis
    Coxsackievirus
    Cytomegalovirus
    Mumps

Familial risk factors
  Congenital heart disease
    Previous sibling
    Paternal
  Syndromes
    Noonan
    Tuberous sclerosis

of congenital heart disease (Table 15–2), with a positive case finding rate of only slightly less than 2 per cent (17/1067 cases). It is our opinion that the small positive yield in this series does not detract from the cost-

TABLE 15–2. Positive Studies According to Referral Indications for Fetal Echocardiographic Examination

INDICATION	NO. OF PATIENTS STUDIED	NO. (%) POSITIVE STUDIES
Family history	310	3 (1%)
Previous child	215	3 (1.4%)
Maternal	49	0
Other	46	0
Dysrhythmias	182	3 (1.6%)
Extracardiac anomalies	117	21 (23.1%)
Cardiac teratogens	101	2 (2%)
Maternal diabetes	96	3 (3.1%)
Suspicious level I scan	40	20 (50%)
Aneuploidies	28	7 (25%)
Nonimmune hydrops	27	9 (33.3%)
Other	0	0
Total	1022	74 (7.2%)

effectiveness of performing fetal echocardiographic studies for this indication, in light of the important impact that negative studies may have on many families, especially when parental levels of anxiety regarding possible recurrent heart disease are high. Considerably higher positive yields were found in the groups of fetuses who were referred for specific fetal risk factors, including previous identification of extracardiac fetal malformations, fetal aneuploidies, nonimmune hydrops fetalis, and a suspicion of structural heart disease based on a level I ultrasound study (incidences in these groups varying from 25 to 50 per cent).

The association of structural heart disease with nonimmune hydrops fetalis in this study (14/65) is consistent with the concept that the fetal swelling associated with this condition represents congestive cardiac failure (Kleinman et al., 1982). It is interesting to note that since this concept was proposed, subsequent studies using Doppler flow techniques have demonstrated a high incidence of severe atrioventricular valve regurgitation in these fetuses (Silverman et al., 1985). Studies of the intrinsic properties of fetal myocardium (Friedman, 1973) have demonstrated that passive tension is higher in fetal than in adult ventricles, suggesting lower compliance of the myocardium of the fetus. In addition, at any given preload, fetal myocardium generates less active tension than adult myocardium. Such studies may explain the limited reserve that fetal hearts appear to demonstrate in the presence of severe ventricular outlet obstruction and the rapid development of fetal edema in the presence of ventricular diastolic volume loading, which may appear in the presence of atrioventricular valve regurgitation.

IMPORTANCE OF THE FOUR-CHAMBER VIEW

In a study that was carried out in our laboratory between January 1984 and December 1986, 1193 fetal echocardiograms were performed on 991 women carrying a total of 1022 fetuses (Copel et al., 1987). There were 31 sets of twins. Gestational ages at the time of examination varied from 18 weeks to term. Fetal echocardiographic studies involved the use of standard tomographic views. Seventy-four (7.2 per cent) of the fetuses had structurally abnormal hearts. In 71 (96 per cent), the four-chamber view of cardiac structure suggested that there was an abnormality of cardiac structure and/or flow. Examination of the four-chamber view had a sensitivity of 92 per cent and a 99.7 per cent specificity for predicting the existence of congenital heart disease. Positive predictive value was 95.8 per cent and negative predictive value was 99.4 per cent. On the basis of this study, it was concluded that a four-chamber screening view of the heart should be included as part of all routine obstetric ultrasound examinations. Such studies can be expected to detect over 95 per cent of the cases of congenital heart disease that exist in these fetuses. We emphasize that a four-chamber view of the heart cannot be considered to offer a comprehensive survey of cardiac structure that

rules out all forms of important fetal congenital heart disease, but rather offers an effective initial screening impression. In the ideal situation, once four-chamber screening of the heart becomes commonplace in all laboratories performing fetal ultrasound, one would hope that additional tomographic views of the heart and great arteries would become part of the ultrasound survey. Such examinations will improve case finding of previously unsuspected congenital heart disease and may offer more certain reassurances regarding normality as well. However, the fact that some congenital heart disease can be expected to be missed by four-chamber screening alone should not discourage the perinatal community from including such views in general fetal examinations. False-negative diagnoses during the 3-year period of study included transposition of the great arteries, aortic coarctation, and ventricular septal defect/pulmonic stenosis. False-positive studies included an incorrect identification of an overriding aorta, a case of suspected subaortic tunnel obstruction, and a case of aortic coarctation. It is important to recognize that even in a relatively experienced laboratory such as our own, where such studies have been ongoing since 1977, occasional errors have been made. These errors have been extremely rare in the past 5 years of our experience and have been limited primarily to missed cases of ventricular septal defect. We tend to avoid making a diagnosis of isolated ventricular septal defect, unless it is extremely large, involves great arterial malalignment, is in the atrioventricular septum, or has been visualized in multiple imaging planes at multiple examining sessions.

Review of the correct diagnoses established during this period (Table 15–3) demonstrates a relatively high incidence of "major" abnormalities that affect four-chamber anatomy, either due to direct identification of the structural abnormality (e.g., septal defects and atrioventricular valve abnormalities in atrioventricular

TABLE 15–3. Congenital Cardiac Malformations Identified in Decreasing Order of Frequency Encountered

INDICATION	NO. OF CASES	NO. ABNORMAL FOUR-CHAMBER VIEWS
Complete atrioventricular septal defect	16	16/16
Hypoplastic left heart syndrome	8	8/8
Ventricular septal defect	7	5/7
Pulmonic stenosis	6	6/6
Ebstein anomaly	5	5/5
Complex lesions	5	5/5
Tetralogy of Fallot	5	5/5
Ectopia cordis	4	4/4
Atrial isomerism	3	3/3
Double-outlet right ventricle	3	3/3
Pericardial effusion	2	2/2
Conjoined twins	2	2/2
Acardia	1	1/1
Isolated levocardia	1	1/1
Others	6	5/6
Total	74	71/74

septal defects [Fig. 15–3], ventricular hypoplasia in atrioventricular valve atresia, atrial and ventricular dilation in the Ebstein malformation of the tricuspid valve [Fig. 15–4]) or due to flow perturbations secondary to structural abnormalities that may exist outside the four-chamber tomographic view (e.g., right atrial dilation secondary to tricuspid valve, regurgitation in severe pulmonic stenosis [Figs. 15–5, 15–6], or right ventricular dilation in double-outlet right ventricle).

FETAL CONGENITAL HEART DISEASE: AN INDICATION FOR FETAL KARYOTYPING

Hook (1982) projected a 5 to 10 per cent frequency of chromosomal anomalies when congenital heart disease is identified in early infancy. We hypothesized that the association between congenital heart disease and chromosomal abnormalities would be even higher among fetuses diagnosed prenatally owing to the existence of lethal aneuploidy syndromes. During an 18-month period, between January 1985 and June 1986, 594 fetal echocardiographic studies were performed on 520 patients at the Yale Fetal Cardiovascular Center. Patients varied in age from 18 weeks gestation to term. Indications for scan were consistent with the criteria described above; 18 patients in the series were referred for scan after aneuploidy syndromes had already been diagnosed. Thirty-four of the 502 fetuses with previously unknown chromosomal status were found to have congenital cardiac malformations (6.8 per cent). Eleven of these 34 fetuses (32 per cent) had aneuploidy as well. This marked discrepancy from the data found in the pediatric literature may relate to nonviable fetuses identified *in utero* who escape pediatric case identification. On the basis of this study, we concluded that in all cases of prenatally diagnosed congenital heart disease, further evaluation should include amniocentesis, chorionic villus sampling, or fetal blood sampling for chromosome analysis. Subsequently, all cases of congenital heart disease diagnosed prenatally at Yale have been offered karyotyping since initiation of the study noted above. Through the end of 1990, 171 mothers were offered such testing, with 158 availing themselves of this study. Forty-five cases of aneuploidy were diagnosed (28.5 per cent). As one might expect, the incidence of aneuploidy was highest among fetuses noted to have multiple congenital anomalies (approximately 30 per cent), but the incidence of aneuploidy among fetuses with isolated congenital heart disease generally involving one or more ventricular septal defects (15 per cent) was also significant. Karyotyping should be performed regardless of the stage of pregnancy at which the congenital heart disease is detected. Abnormal results may suggest a management strategy involving much less aggressive neonatal resuscitation or may prevent the tragedy of a cesarean section for delivery of a nonviable infant.

IMPACT OF FETAL ECHOCARDIOGRAPHY ON OBSTETRIC MANAGEMENT

Despite the promise of four-chamber screening studies for the identification of fetal heart disease, there will still be a need for detailed fetal echocardiographic studies in a referral setting, involving a cooperative effort of experts in fetal ultrasound and congenital heart disease. Patients with specific risk factors for

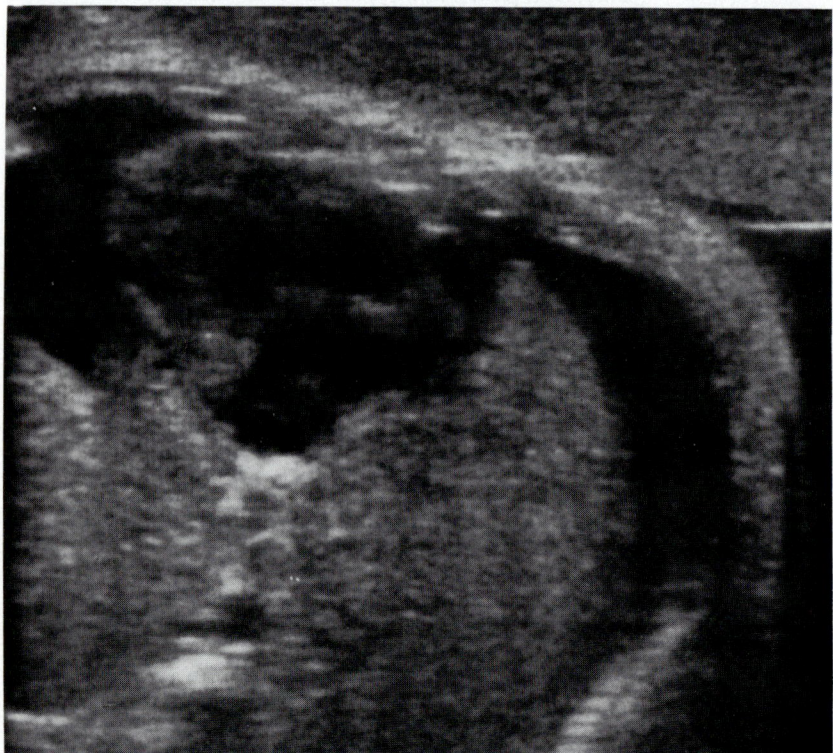

FIGURE 15–3. Four-chamber view of cardiac anatomy in a 32-week fetus with complete atrioventricular septal (canal) defect. Heart is oriented in same direction as the heart in Figure 15–1. Cardiac apex is at the upper left. Only one atrioventricular valve is seen. There is no interventricular septum in this view, and the interatrial septum is practically absent as well. In this view the heart appears to have two, rather than four, discrete cardiac chambers. This fetus also had pleural and pericardial fluid collections, representing fetal congestive heart failure. The four-chamber view of this fetal heart provided definitive diagnostic information.

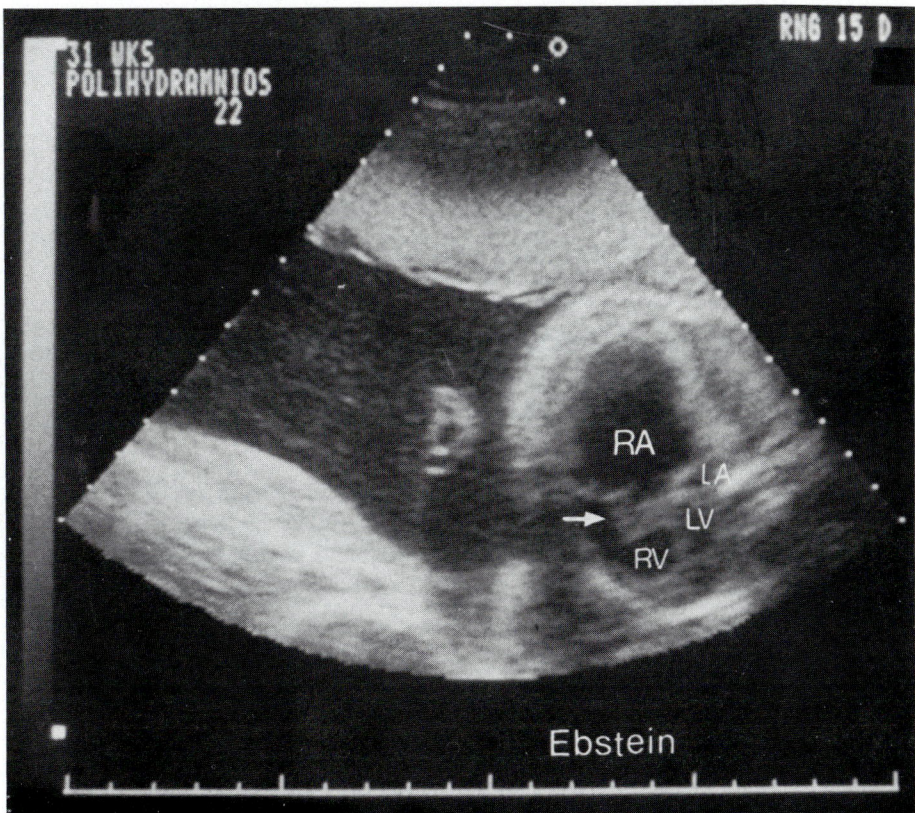

FIGURE 15–4. Four-chamber view of cardiac anatomy in a 31-week fetus with the Ebstein malformation of the tricuspid valve. The right atrial cavity (RA) is massively dilated and dwarfs the left atrial (LA) and ventricular (LV) cavities. The tricuspid valve (arrow) appears thickened and is displaced well into the right ventricular (RV) cavity.

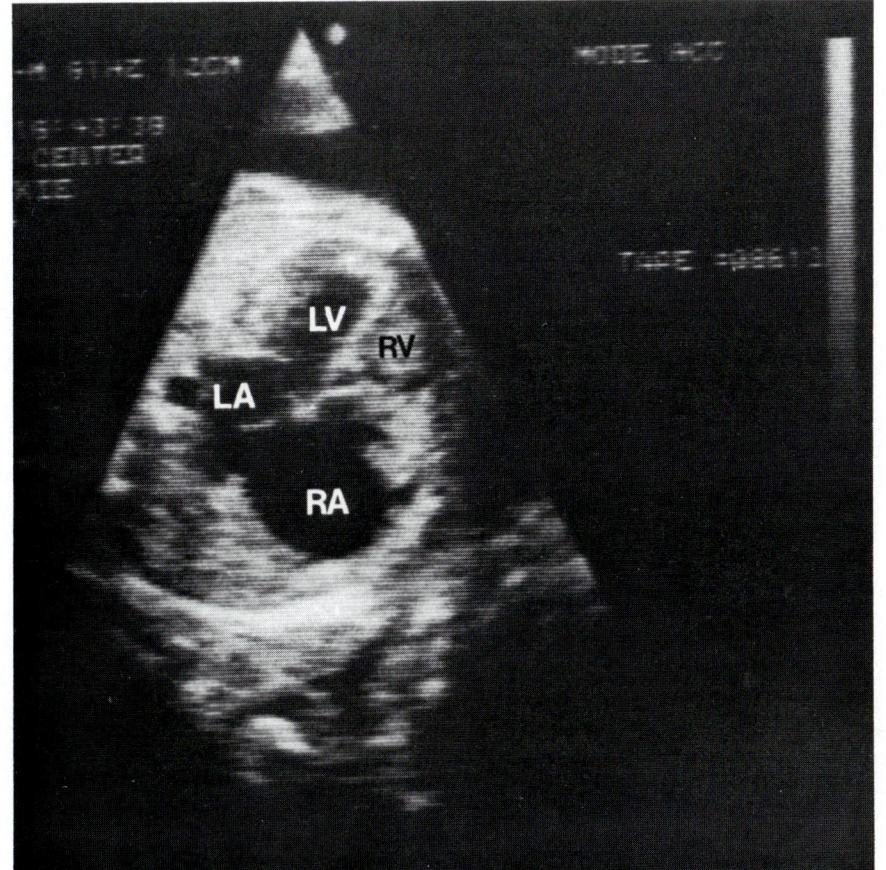

FIGURE 15–5. Four-chamber view of cardiac anatomy in a 27-week fetus who was twin A of a pregnancy in which twin B had a normal heart. This view suggested that cardiac flow patterns were disturbed. The right atrium (RA) is dilated and much larger than the left atrium (LA). The right ventricular cavity (RV) is much smaller than the left ventricular (LV) cavity, while the ventricular walls are extremely hypertrophic and impinge on the ventricular cavity volume. In this study the four-chamber view detected the presence of heart disease, although the cause of the flow disturbance in this view was not appreciated to be severe pulmonic stenosis with secondary tricuspid regurgitation.

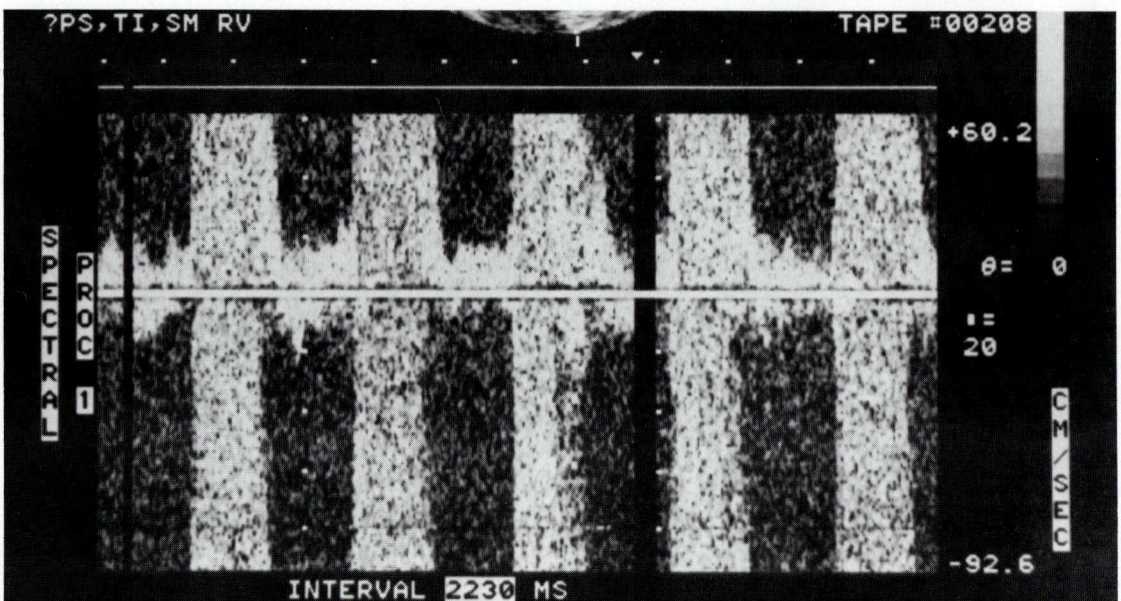

FIGURE 15–6. Pulsed Doppler echocardiographic study in a fetus who presented similarly to the patient whose four-chamber anatomy is seen in Figure 15–4. "Sample volume" of Doppler flow analyzer is positioned within the dilated right atrial cavity, using a "duplex" imager. The lower panel demonstrates holosystolic high-velocity tricuspid regurgitation. This was secondary to severe pulmonic stenosis. This infant underwent successful pulmonary balloon angioplasty shortly after birth, with resolution of tricuspid insufficiency.

fetal heart disease will continue to require such studies. Since the greatest number of fetal cardiac abnormalities still occur among fetuses who have not been identified to have well-defined risk factors, an increasing number of cardiac anomalies will be identified during obstetric scanning for other purposes, especially as fetal cardiac screening becomes a requisite part of the general fetal ultrasound scan. The total impact of these diagnoses is complex to evaluate.

Some anomalies will be incompatible with postnatal survival (e.g., structural heart disease associated with severe nonimmune hydrops fetalis). If these are found early in gestation, parents of such fetuses may choose to terminate the pregnancy. If diagnosis is beyond the time frame during which termination is an option, or if the parents are opposed to such a course, important benefits may be gleaned from the information obtained.

Many cardiac diagnoses are made later in pregnancy. This often reflects referrals because of suspicious-appearing hearts noted during obstetric sonography and the identification of extracardiac abnormalities with associated heart disease. In such cases, accurate prenatal diagnosis permits honest counseling for the parents and adequate medical planning for delivery and neonatal management (e.g., ensuring that prostaglandin E is prepared for administration after delivery of a fetus who is dependent upon persistent patency of the ductus arteriosus to provide adequate pulmonary or systemic blood flow). Delivery of such infants in an institution equipped to provide comprehensive neonatal, cardiac, and cardiac surgical therapy can be expected to improve outcome in many cases. Although survival statistics for the last 213 fetuses with congenital heart disease diagnosed at

the Yale-New Haven Hospital were not encouraging (51/213, 24 per cent), it is striking that 31 of the survivors (61 per cent) had malformations that rendered them dependent upon persistent patency of the ductus arteriosus to ensure continued pulmonary or systemic blood flow. A recent study completed at the Children's Hospital of Philadelphia (Chang et al., 1991) provides the first compelling evidence that prenatal identification of critical aortic outflow obstruction (in most cases hypoplastic left heart syndrome) had a statistically important effect on preoperative and postoperative morbidity, if not mortality, in a population of prenatally diagnosed patients compared with a matched population of patients diagnosed and transferred for therapy postnatally.

With continuing surgical advances, cardiac abnormalities that were considered hopeless only a few years ago are undergoing surgical correction today. For example, both neonatal cardiac transplantation and the Norwood procedure have been offered for neonates with the hypoplastic left heart syndrome (Norwood et al., 1981; Sade et al., 1986). The complexities of supporting such critically ill newborns until transport is arranged to one of the few centers offering these procedures argue for delivery to be accomplished at an institution capable of providing comprehensive maternal and neonatal care. It is also important to allow parents adequate time to consider their best options. "Informed consent" for surgery may be difficult in the best of circumstances, but with a critically ill neonate at issue, it may be an impossibility. Education of parents at one or more prenatal visits is essential for their active participation in deciding on expectant management versus transplantation or the Norwood procedure for their infant.

PRENATAL SURGICAL THERAPY

No discussion of prenatal diagnosis would be complete without some consideration of the potential for *in utero* therapy. In the case of congenital heart disease, this must include discussion of the potential for *in utero* cardiac surgery versus catheter therapies such as balloon angioplasty or valvuloplasty.

In consideration of such therapy, the work of Harrison and colleagues (1991) should serve as the paradigm. These workers have pioneered in the field of prenatal surgical therapy, including the development of protocols for fetal exteriorization and treatment of urinary tract obstruction and diaphragmatic hernia. In describing their innovative work, these investigators acknowledge the frustration that provided the initial impetus for this long-standing project. The frustration of dealing with infants who were already in an advanced state of deterioration at the time of birth from structural abnormalities that could have been mechanically corrected "if they had been operated on in time" provided some impetus, as did the identification of such abnormalities, often serendipitously, during "routine" ultrasound examinations of the fetus.

These workers emphasize the importance of refraining from potentially dangerous (to the mother and fetus) interventions until further information becomes available concerning the natural history of the untreated condition (usually employing serial ultrasound examinations) and until the pathophysiology of the natural and post-treatment condition is more fully understood. The latter information usually requires the development of an animal model.

Although the natural history of congenital heart disease in the fetus has been the subject of considerable investigation, animal models are only now being studied, with promising investigations taking place concerning techniques for surface cooling and rewarming of the exteriorized fetus undergoing cardiopulmonary bypass. Major problems still need to be addressed using this model of heart bypass (Verrier et al., 1991).

Recently, the Guy's Hospital group (Maxwell et al., 1991) reported their experience in attempting to perform balloon valvuloplasty on two fetuses identified to have critical aortic stenosis with associated left ventricular fibroelastosis. Neither procedure resulted in long-term survival, and these workers suggested that the presence of fibroelastosis had rendered the fetuses unsalvageable by the time of treatment. This same group recently reported two additional cases in which the valvuloplasty attempts proved to no avail when the aortic valve was unexpectedly found to be completely atretic rather than stenotic, and this condition prevented traversal of the valve by the catheter.

These cases underline the importance of having a scrupulously accurate diagnosis as well as knowledge of pathophysiology before counseling fetal invasion, regardless of how well-meaning the attempt at therapy is.

Considering the experience with postnatal valvuloplasty (surgical and/or transcatheter), in which valvular regurgitation may vary from mild to significant, and acknowledging the known limited diastolic reserve of the fetal heart, one is obliged to do some "groundwork" using an animal model for such therapy before attempting fetal invasion.

The potential for surgical or angioplasty intervention to dilate restrictive interatrial foramens has been postulated, since it has been suggested that such restriction, by decreasing atrial right-to-left shunting, could be a cause of left heart hypoplasia. Recently, Feit et al. (1991) demonstrated that the size of the fetal foramen ovale, indexed to the size of the interatrial septum, could be used to distinguish left heart obstructive lesions (in which the foramen ovale/atrial septal ratio was smaller than in normals) from right heart obstructive lesions (in which this ratio was larger than in normals). This study found, however, that this apparent difference could not be distinguished before the 19th week of gestation. In addition, several patients with left heart obstructive lesions were found to have predominantly left-to-right rather than right-to-left atrial level shunts, even in the absence of critical mitral or aortic obstruction. These findings suggest that, at least in some patients, the foramen ovale size, while reflecting transatrial flow volumes, may be a secondary phenomenon rather than causal in the pathophysiology of some cases of left heart hypoplasia.

The possibility of associated chromosomal abnormalities as well as extracardiac malformations in these patients must be appreciated and fully evaluated if the preoperative work-up of the patient is to be complete, since the question of "operability" of the patient is not solely dependent upon the potential existence of a technique for palliation of the cardiac structural disease, but rather involves evaluation of the fetus's potential to enjoy an independent existence postnatally.

As an important example, we review our experience with a subgroup of fetuses with severe cardiomegaly associated with right ventricular (and right atrial) dilation in whom the heart occupied more than 60 per cent of the thoracic cross-sectional area on ultrasound examination. All of these patients had significant pulmonary hypoplasia. The latter condition may well rule out the potential for survival, despite provision of aggressive cardiac surgical therapy.

Despite our seemingly pessimistic outlook toward fetal cardiac surgical therapy for congenital heart disease, we are actually cautiously optimistic that such therapy will ultimately become available and desirable in a limited number of fetuses. We believe, however, that considerably more groundwork must be laid before we can be confident that our diagnostic abilities, surgical skills, and knowledge of pathophysiology have reached the point where such treatments can be offered.

CONCLUSION

Prenatal diagnosis of structural heart disease is now widely available and, by identifying patients at risk, can reduce the frequency of unanticipated congenital heart disease. Further improvement in the rate of identification may be possible through routine screening of the four-chamber view of the heart. Any pregnancy with significant risk factors for fetal heart disease should be thoroughly evaluated with detailed fetal echocardiography rather than a simple screening four-chamber view.

Particular attention should be paid to performing fetal echocardiography in pregnancies found to have other structural anomalies, as coexistent heart disease may suggest the presence of a syndrome with specific inheritance patterns and may alter neonatal management plans. Similarly, any fetus with structural heart disease should undergo a thorough examination of all systems. If fetal heart disease is found, parental counseling should include a strong possibility of chromosomal abnormalities, and appropriate sampling for karyotyping should be offered.

Complete counseling is most easily accomplished with a team approach composed primarily of obstetricians and pediatric cardiologists, with further assistance from genetic counselors, pediatric cardiology nursing specialists, and willing parents in a similar situation to provide information to the parents regarding realistic expectations about the care their infants will require.

REFERENCES

Allan LD, Tynan MJ, Campbell S, et al: Echocardiographic and anatomical correlates in the fetus. Br Heart J 44:444, 1980.

Allan LD, Joseph MC, Boyd EGCA, Campbell S, Tynan M: M-mode echocardiography in the developing human fetus. Br Heart J 47:573, 1982.

Allan LD, Chita SK, Al-Ghazali W, Crawford DC, Tynan M: Doppler echocardiographic evaluation of the normal human fetal heart. Br Heart J 57:528, 1987.

Axel L: Real-time sonography of fetal cardiac anatomy. Am J Roentgenol 141:283, 1983.

Bronshtein M, Simmer EZ, Milo S, et al: Fetal cardiac abnormalities detected by transvaginal sonography at 12-16 weeks gestation. Obstet Gynecol 75:496, 1991.

Chang AC, Huhta JC, Yoon GY, et al: Diagnosis, transport, and outcome in fetuses with left ventricular outflow tract obstruction. J Thorac Cardiovasc Surg 102:841, 1991.

Copel JA, Pilu G, Green J, Hobbins JC, Kleinman CS: Fetal echocardiographic screening for congenital heart disease: The importance of the four-chamber view. Am J Obstet Gynecol 157:648, 1987.

Copel JA, Morotti R, Hobbins JC, et al: The antenatal diagnosis of congenital heart disease using fetal echocardiography: Is color flow mapping necessary? Obstet Gynecol 78:1, 1991.

De Smedt MCH, Visser GHA, Meijboom EJ: Fetal cardiac output estimated by Doppler echocardiography during mid- and late gestation. Am J Cardiol 60:338, 1987.

DeVore GR, Horenstein J, Siassi B, Platt LD: Fetal echocardiography. VII. Doppler color flow mapping. A new technique for the diagnosis of congenital heart disease. Am J Obstet Gynecol 156:1054, 1987.

Feit LR, Copel JA, Kleinman CS: Foramen ovale size in the normal and abnormal human fetal heart: An indicator of transatrial flow physiology. Ultrasound Obstet Gynecol 1:313, 1991.

Friedman WF: The intrinsic physiologic properties of the developing heart. In Friedman WF, Lesch M, Sonnenblick EH (eds): Neonatal Heart Disease. New York, Grune & Stratton, 1973.

Harrison MR, Golbus MS, Filly RA(eds): The Unborn Patient. 2nd ed. Philadelphia, W.B. Saunders Co., 1991.

Hook EB: Contribution of chromosome abnormalities to human morbidity and mortality. Cytogenet Cell Genet 33:101, 1982.

Huhta JC, Moise KJ, Fisher DJ, Sharif DS, Wasserstrum N, Martin C: Detection and quantitation of constriction of the fetal ductus arteriosus by Doppler echocardiography. Circulation 75:406, 1987.

Kleinman CS, Hobbins JC, Jaffe CC, Lynch DC, Talner NS: Echocardiographic studies of the human fetus: Prenatal diagnosis of congenital heart disease and cardiac dysrhythmias. Pediatrics 65:1059, 1980.

Kleinman CS, Donnerstein RL. Ultrasonic assessment of cardiac function in the intact human fetus. J Am Coll Cardiol 5:84S, 1985.

Kleinman CS, Donnerstein RL, DeVore GR, Jaffe CC, Lynch DC, Berkowitz RL, Talner NS, Hobbins JC: Fetal echocardiography in nonimmune fetal hydrops—A technique for evaluation of in utero heart failure. N Engl J Med 306:568, 1982.

Kleinman CS, Santulli TV Jr: Ultrasonic evaluation of the fetal human heart. Semin Perinatol 7:90, 1983.

Kleinman CS, Weinstein EM, Copel JA: Pulsed Doppler analysis of human fetal blood flow. In Kisslo J, Adams D, Mark DB (eds): Basic Doppler Echocardiography. New York, Churchill Livingstone, 1986, pp 173–185.

Maxwell D, Allan L, Tynan MJ: Balloon dilatation of the aortic valve in the fetus: A report of two cases. Br Heart J 65:256, 1991.

Morin FC III: Fetal Echocardiography. Doctoral Thesis for Doctor of Medicine Degree, Yale University School of Medicine, 1976.

Neutze JM, Starling MB, Elliot RB, Barratt-Boyes BG: Palliation of cyanotic congenital heart disease in infancy with type E prostaglandin. Circulation 55:238, 1977.

Norwood WI, Lang P, Castaneda AR, Campbell DN: Experience with operations for hypoplastic left heart syndrome. J Thorac Cardiovasc Surg 82:511, 1981.

Reed KL, Meijboom EJ, Sahn DJ, Scagnelli S, Valdes-Cruz LM, Shenker L: Cardiac Doppler flow velocities in human fetuses. Circulation 73:41, 1986.

Rudolph AM: Distribution and regulation of blood flow in the fetal and neonatal lamb. Circ Res 57:811, 1985.

Rudolph AM, Heymann MA: Circulatory changes during growth in the fetal lamb. Circ Res 26:289, 1970.

Sade R, Crawford F, Fyfe D: Symposium on hypoplastic left heart syndrome. J Thorac Cardiovasc Surg 91:937, 1986.

Sahn DJ, Lange LW, Allen HD, et al: Quantitative real-time cross-sectional echocardiography in the developing normal human fetus and newborn. Circulation 62:588, 1980.

Sharland GK, Chita SK, Allan LD: The use of color Doppler in fetal echocardiography. Int J Cardiol 28:229, 1990.

Silverman NS, Kleinman CS, Rudolph JA, et al: Fetal atrioventricular valve insufficiency associated with nonimmune hydrops: A two-dimensional echocardiographic and pulsed-Doppler ultrasound study. Circulation 72:825, 1985.

Silverman NH, Shiraishi H, Rudolph AM: Right ventricular output in the sheep fetus determined by pulsed Doppler sound. Circulation 84:(52):II-461, 1991.

Verrier ED, Vlahakes GJ, Hanley FL, et al: Experimental fetal cardiac surgery. In Harrison MR, Golbus MS, Filly RA (eds): The Unborn Patient: Prenatal Diagnosis and Treatment. Philadelphia, W.B. Saunders Co., 1991, pp 548–556.

Winsberg F: Echocardiography of the fetal and newborn heart. Invest Radiol 7:152, 1972.

CHAPTER

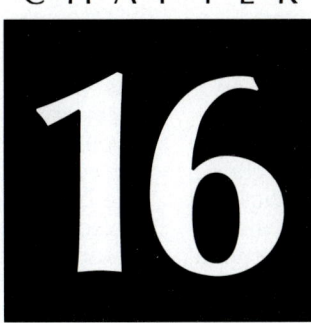

DOPPLER ULTRASOUND ASSESSMENT OF BLOOD FLOW

BRIAN TRUDINGER, M.D.

The ability to study blood flow noninvasively in the fetus, in the two placental circulations, and in the newborn is a major development in perinatal medicine. Clinical applications for this technology are still being established as the necessary evaluative studies and clinical trials are carried out.

Doppler ultrasound equipment has been used for many years to detect blood flow and heart motion. By selecting suitable signal parameters, especially frequency, it is possible to ensure that the frequency spectrum of the Doppler frequency shift falls within the audible range so that motion is heard. The development of real-time frequency spectrum analyzers has allowed a detailed visual display of the Doppler shift frequencies as a function of time. Duplex systems, which present B-mode image and allow a Doppler sample volume or range gate to be set to record from the vessel of interest, are widely available. Color coding of frequency shifts makes blood flow easily seen. Perinatal blood flow studies are now a potentially widely available clinical tool.

ULTRASOUND AND THE DOPPLER EFFECT

When an acoustic or ultrasound wave is backscattered from a target that is moving relative to the source of the wave, there is a change in frequency of the reflected wave relative to the transmitted wave. This is called the *Doppler effect* (for historical review see Eden, 1988). An ultrasound beam scattered by a moving column of red blood cells provides an example of this effect. The frequency of the returning or received echoes differs from the transmitted frequency, and this difference is the Doppler frequency shift (F_D). For blood cells moving with a velocity V, it is given by

$$F_D = F_1 - F_0 = \frac{2F_0 \, V_{\cos\theta}}{c}$$

where F_0 is the transmitted frequency, F_1 the received

frequency, c the velocity of sound in tissue, and θ the angle between the ultrasound beam and direction of flow. The important point in this equation is the proportionality of blood flow velocity to Doppler frequency shift. Using the Doppler equation, a frequency shift of close to 4000 (3896) Hz can be calculated for a 4-MHz beam interrogating an artery with blood flow velocity of 100 cm/sec in the direction of flow (angle θ close to zero). The velocity of sound in tissue is commonly assumed to be 1540 m/sec.

The choice of transmitting frequency (F_0) is influenced by a number of factors. Since the absorption of sound is proportional to frequency squared, better depth of penetration can be achieved with lower frequencies. Higher frequencies provide a greater frequency shift for the same velocity, and this has distinct advantages in recording. Scattering is proportional to the fourth power of frequency, and this also affects signal amplitude. The vessels to be studied in pregnancy are deep lying, and so it is necessary to use low frequencies. In practice, the highest frequency that can reach these vessels is chosen. For recording fetal umbilical and aortic and maternal uterine signals a 4-MHz transducer may be used, although some pulsed Doppler systems use a 1- or 2-MHz signal. Superficial vessels such as the neonatal cerebral circulation may be studied with an 8-MHz transducer.

The earliest display of the Doppler frequency shift signal was an audible sound because the Doppler frequency shift fell in the audible range. Frequency spectrum analyzers that operate in real time make possible a continuing visual display of the Doppler shift frequencies. Typically such machines have an analysis time of 5 to 12 msec. Frequency (Y axis) is displayed on a time base (X axis). The intensity or amplitude of the signal at each frequency level (bin) is displayed using a gray scale (Z axis). More recently, color Doppler systems allow colored display on the B-mode image of the sites (blood vessels) where movement of the echo reflector (blood flow), and hence a frequency shift, is occurring.

Across a vessel lumen blood flow may not always be forward or indeed in the same direction through the cardiac cycle. Adjacent vessels such as arteries and veins may have flow in opposite directions. It is necessary that the Doppler flow meter, or velocimeter, be directional; phase quadrature detection is now commonly used for this purpose. A nondirectional system assumes that all Doppler shift frequencies and therefore flow are in the same direction. To display forward and reverse flow simultaneously (directional separation), frequency-offset processing is used. This means that the zero Doppler frequency (no flow) is offset along the frequency axis (Y axis) with forward and reverse flow on different sides of this offset value.

Simple continuous-wave (CW) Doppler ultrasound systems can be used to display the flow velocity waveform Doppler frequency shift or sonogram as a function of time. These do not give range or positional information about the flow in the vessel under study. They do not allow spatial resolution. Very high velocities may be displayed, and the only limit to this is the spectrum analyzer analysis time. In order to obtain position and velocity information simultaneously, it is necessary to use a pulsed-wave (PW) Doppler ultrasound system. This allows for range gating. A velocity profile can be constructed by scanning across a vessel point by point. Mean velocity can be calculated. It is possible to determine volume flow if vessel area is also measured. However, pulsed-wave ultrasound introduces a limitation on maximal recordable velocity. The preceding pulse must travel to the vessel and return before the next is transmitted. Hence, the pulse repetition frequency (PRF) is related to vessel depth. The maximum Doppler frequency shift that can be accurately detected is one-half of the pulse repetition frequency. The *sample theorem* states that for accurate description, a signal must be sampled at a rate (F_s) at least as high as twice the highest frequency (F_h) in the spectrum. This sampling rate is sometimes referred to as the *folding frequency* or the *Nyquist frequency*. At lower sampling rates aliasing or foldover occurs. Considering the Doppler equation, it can be appreciated that increasing the angle θ or reducing the transmission frequency (F_0) will increase maximum recordable velocity and reduce the tendency toward aliasing. This same limitation applies to analysis by the frequency spectrum analyzer. Whereas a B-mode image is built up from the points of ultrasound waveform reflection of tissue interfaces (acoustic impedance mismatch), Doppler systems depend on detecting the change in frequency when the waveform strikes a moving target. Color Doppler systems overprint the two-dimensional B-mode image with color at the sites where a frequency shift (blood flow in a vessel) is detected with color coding of the frequency shift. Hard-to-identify vessels are readily located and jets of flow easily seen.

CIRCULATION HEMODYNAMICS RELEVANT TO DOPPLER STUDIES

Blood flow is influenced by all the components of the circulation categorized as pumps, pipes, resistances, and reservoirs. In addition, properties of blood itself are important. The pressure and flow waveforms are influenced by the cardiac contraction, physical properties of the arterial walls, the blood within, and the outflow impedance from the arterial tree. The *pressure pulse*, a time-varying pressure gradient between neighboring points in the artery, is generated by contraction of the heart. This gradient results in the blood flow, which is also pulsatile. The pressure pulse (wave) propagates down the aorta and its branches with an initial wave speed of 5 m/sec. The blood flow velocity (wave) travels more slowly, and it is this that is recorded by Doppler ultrasound systems (for review of circulation hemodynamics, see Caro et al., 1978).

In the ascending aorta there is forward flow (i.e., the instantaneous mean velocity in the vessel is away from the heart) for approximately one-fourth to one-third of the cardiac cycle. Flow begins at the time of opening of the aortic valve and rises rapidly to a peak. It then slowly falls until, at the time of closing of the aortic valve, there is a brief period of reverse flow. The blood is close to stationary for the remainder of the cardiac cycle. The pressure pulse and the velocity waveform both change in shape as they propagate down the aorta and its branches (Fig. 16–1).

The amplitude of the velocity waveform decreases progressively with distance from the heart, and the envelope changes as the sharp forward and reverse peaks are smoothed out. The pressure and velocity waveforms are also modified by the presence of reflected waves. Significant reflections occur at peripheral vascular beds, where a single artery branches into many small arteries or arterioles (e.g., the umbilical artery at the placenta), or at a single mismatched junction (e.g., the aortic bifurcation). In early systole, pressure and velocity waves are in phase. Later in systole this synchrony breaks down again due to the arrival of reflected waves.

The power of cardiac contraction that generates pressure (and flow) is almost entirely dissipated in the vascular tree. Resistance may be better thought of as the energy dissipated during the flow of blood through the vascular bed (Milnor, 1972). Arterioles contribute the major resistance to blood flow and have the greatest capacity for varying their resistance. Vascular distensibility, the creation of reflected waves, and the viscosity of blood also account for some energy loss. They all contribute to the changing form of the blood flow velocity waveform along the arterial tree.

Doppler Flow Studies

The information provided by Doppler ultrasound studies of blood flow consists of the blood flow velocity waveform and the volume blood flow.

Blood Flow Velocity Waveform

Real-time spectral analysis of the Doppler frequency shift signal yields the blood flow velocity waveform or sonogram. Simply observing these waveforms at various sites in the healthy body makes it clear that the shape of the waveform envelope can be considered a characteristic of the vascular site. Waveforms in arteries supplying low-impedance vascular beds (e.g.,

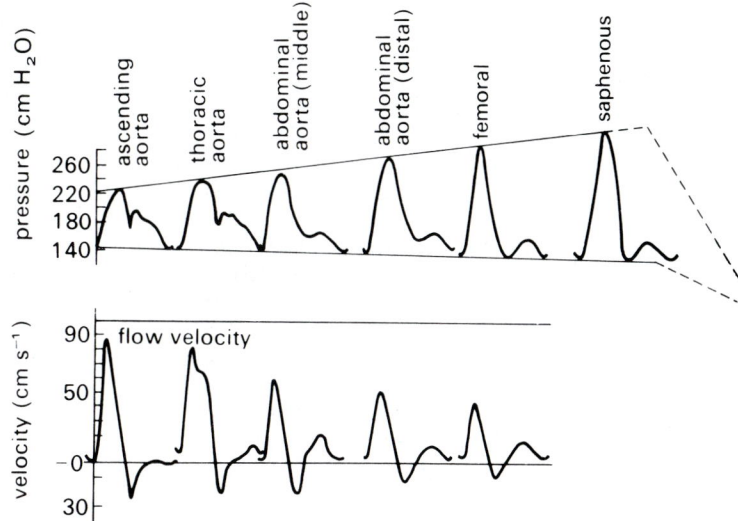

FIGURE 16–1. Matched records of pressure and flow velocity waveforms at different sites along the arterial tree of a dog. (From McDonald DA: Blood Flow in Arteries. London, Edward Arnold, 1974.)

internal carotid, umbilical, and uterine arteries in pregnancy) exhibit relatively high forward velocities throughout diastole. A triphasic waveform shape, in which there is a period of reverse flow in diastole, is characteristic of sites with high distal impedance, such as the external iliac artery. This is attributed to a large-amplitude reflected wave.

The development of methods of waveform analysis was initially directed toward the diagnosis of vessel stenosis as part of degenerative arterial disease. There was an attempt to define simple indices which relate waveform features to physiologic properties. The innate complexity of the Doppler data studied made this difficult. Peripheral impedance, vessel wall elasticity, degree and geometry of any proximal stenoses, and condition of the upstream pump all affect the waveform. Even in normal, presumably healthy subjects, blood flow patterns at a site such as the carotid birfurcation are complicated. However, the fetal circulation was far more suited to Doppler waveform analysis by simple empirical indices which might relate to physiologic parameters. This is because of the absence of degenerative arterial disease. Pathologic changes in the placental vasculature have been observed, but not at the level of the large arteries. Flow in the fetal aorta and umbilical artery is determined primarily by the placental impedance downstream and the cardiac contractility upstream. Insistence on recording only when the fetus is inactive and apneic eliminates the possibility of variability due to altered behavioral state, as well as the activity itself. In fetal compromise both placental resistance and cardiac activity may be changed, while a redistribution of cardiac output may also alter flow patterns to the various intrafetal vessel beds.

Volume Blood Flow

To measure volume blood flow, it is necessary to measure mean blood flow velocity (mean Doppler frequency shift). The cross-sectional area of the vessel must also be determined. To ensure uniform insona-

tion, the ultrasound beam must be wider than the vessel and homogeneous across its width (Gill, 1979). Good correlations between Doppler and electromagnetic flow probe measurements have been reported. In obstetric practice only two vessels, the umbilical vein and the descending aorta, are large enough to image and measure dimensions accurately. The system used most frequently for the measurement of human fetal volume blood flow has been a combined B-mode real-time and pulsed-wave Doppler duplex (Eik-Nes et al., 1980). The sources of error inherent in this methodology for quantitative assessment of volume blood flow are well known. They include (1) errors in measurement of the angle between the ultrasound beam and blood vessel, (2) errors in measurement of the vessel diameter (pulsations in arteries may produce changes in diameter that have been assessed in the fetal aorta to range to 19 per cent [Sindberg Eriksen et al., 1984]), (3) errors in positioning of the sample volume to ensure that the vessel is uniformly insonated but avoiding too large a sample volume, which might include extraneous signals, (4) errors in high-pass filtering of low-amplitude signals used to remove low-frequency vessel wall vibration signals (but that also remove low-flow velocities and so distort the calculation of the mean velocity). At the present time it is believed that these errors are too great for studies of volume blood flow to be performed in clinical practice. Other methods of measuring volume blood flow with ultrasound equipment are under study and may change this position.

RELEVANT PHYSIOLOGY OF THE FETAL CIRCULATION AND PLACENTAL BLOOD FLOW

The fetal circulation in comparison to that of the adult is characterized by a high heart rate and cardiac output and low blood pressure. This is accounted for by the low resistance of the umbilical placental circulation, which receives a large proportion of the cardiac output. Approximately 40 per cent of the combined ventricular output is destined for the umbilical placental circulation in the fetal lamb at term. Although umbilical placental blood flow increases throughout gestation, the proportion of cardiac output directed to this bed decreases. However, this circulation is relatively passive. Because resistance in this bed decreases with gestational age, a relatively greater decrease is necessary in peripheral resistance elsewhere in the fetus. This regulates the distribution of cardiac output (Rudolph and Heymann, 1970). Some 32 to 40 per cent of combined ventricular output is directed to the fetal carcass (nonvisceral flow). It has been suggested that this provides a reservoir so that vasomotor responses can effect a redistribution of the fetal circulation through a change in carcass flow. Changes in umbilical flow follow changes in fetal heart rate and arterial blood pressure (Rudolph, 1976). The possibility of changes in stroke volume and cardiac contractility also affecting this flow has also been shown (Kirkpatrick et al., 1976; Tonge et al., 1984). Growth of the placenta provides another mechanism for flow regulation. (See Chapter 18 for detailed discussion of fetal cardiovascular physiology.) Changes in ventricular output and its distribution can be expected to produce changes in the flow velocity waveforms.

Acute regulation of umbilical blood flow is not well understood. Acute changes in fetal arterial blood gas tensions produce a surprisingly slight effect on umbilical flow (Walker et al., 1976). Transient compression of the umbilical cord produces well-recognized changes in heart rate and blood pressure. Following the fall in umbilical blood flow, oxygen extraction can be increased to maintain oxygen consumption until the reduction in flow exceeds 50 per cent (Itskovitz et al., 1983). This fact would argue against the need for the fetus to finely regulate umbilical flow. A relatively stable umbilical flow waveform is therefore expected.

Uterine blood flow has two components, flow to the myometrium and flow to the placental implantation site. These components may be under entirely separate controls. In normal sheep pregnancy uterine flow increases, although the pressure gradient across the placental bed decreases (Clapp et al., 1982). This implies a greater decrease in resistance. This is attributed to placental growth, and it is the progressive increase in the number of vascular channels and cross-sectional area of the uteroplacental vascular bed that produces the fall in resistance and increase in flow. In human pregnancy uterine blood flow at term is estimated at 700 ml/min^{-1} (10 per cent cardiac output), of which 80 per cent is directed to the placental bed. Flow related to the weight of the uterus and its contents remains constant through pregnancy (for review, see Greiss, 1982) and has been related to oxygen consumption (Clapp, 1978) in experimental animal studies. Placentation brings into contact the maternal uteroplacental and fetal umbilical placental circulations. Uniform matching of perfusion optimizes exchange of oxygen (Longo, 1982) and nutrients between these two circulations and waste removal. If uteroplacental flow is reduced by microsphere embolization, a reduction occurs in umbilical flow (Clapp et al., 1982). In this circumstance the fetus redistributes

cardiac output to supply vital organs (Block et al., 1984). The fetal umbilical circulation can influence uteroplacental perfusion, as is seen after fetal death. The mediation of this perfusion balance between the two placental circulations is not clear; however, vasoactive prostaglandins and angiotensin have been implicated (Rankin and McLaughlin, 1979).

DOPPLER STUDIES OF THE UMBILICAL CIRCULATION

The umbilical arteries are ideal vessels from which to record blood flow velocity waveforms because they are of constant size, have no branches, and run the length of the cord in a pool of liquor. Upstream is the fetal heart and downstream the placenta. The effect of spiraling in the cord is unlikely to be important since the radius of curvature is many times greater than the vessel diameter (1 to 2 mm). Volume blood flow in

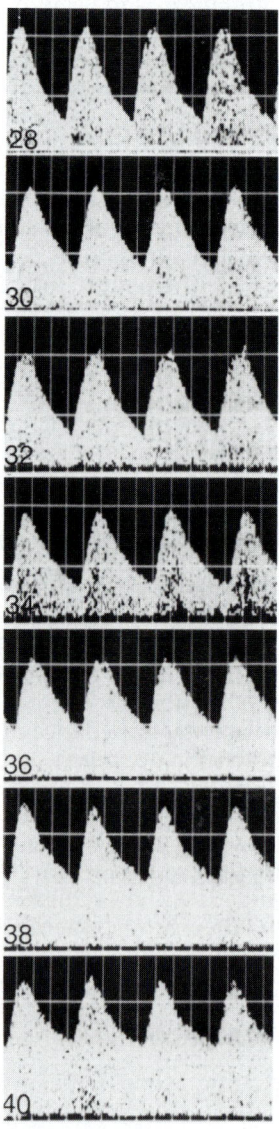

FIGURE 16–2. Sequential studies, from one normal pregnancy, of fetal umbilical artery flow velocity waveforms.

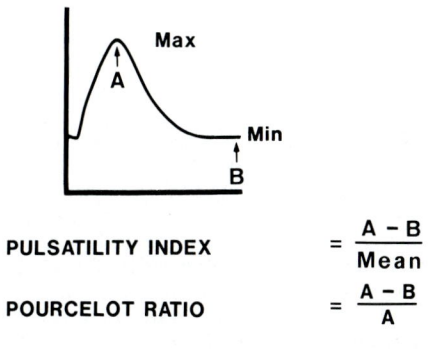

$$\text{PULSATILITY INDEX} = \frac{A - B}{\text{Mean}}$$

$$\text{POURCELOT RATIO} = \frac{A - B}{A}$$

$$\text{SYSTOLIC/DIASTOLIC RATIO} = A/B$$

FIGURE 16–3. The three commonly used indices of downstream impedance or resistance.

the umbilical circulation has been studied by measuring flow in the intrahepatic portion of the umbilical vein. These studies have not achieved the same place in perinatology as has the use of flow velocity waveforms.

Normal Pregnancy

The umbilical artery flow velocity waveform in normal pregnancy is characterized by an increase in end-diastolic flow velocity relative to peak systolic velocity with gestational age (Fig. 16–2). This has been ascribed to the decrease in umbilical placental resistance as the placenta and its vascular tree grow with advancing gestation. The umbilical artery runs unbranched to the small arteries and arterioles, the resistance vessels of its placental vascular bed. Here waveform reflection occurs. A number of indices have been used to quantitate flow velocity waveform patterns. The three main indices in use are the systolic/diastolic (A/B) ratio, the pulsatility index, and the resistance (Pourcelot) index (Fig. 16–3). The correlation between these indices in the umbilical circulation in late pregnancy is good (Table 16–1) (Thompson et al., 1986a). So close is the relationship between these indices that it is not possible for one index to provide more discriminatory information than does another. The ratio of systole to diastole has the advantage of being simplest to calculate and most descriptive of the visually recognized pattern changes in the waveform that all these indices quantitate. All indices contain the same intrinsic errors (Thompson et al., 1988a). The ratio of systole to diastole and the pulsatility index are not normally distributed. A normal range for the systolic/diastolic ratio for the second half of pregnancy is shown in Figure 16–4. After 28 weeks, the normal confidence interval can be approximated by straight lines, but during the second trimester the systolic/diastolic ratio falls exponentially. Care is necessary in the interpretation of results in the second trimester when very low diastolic flow velocities may be recorded in normal pregnancy. This difficulty is reduced if serial studies are carried out to demonstrate the normal increase in diastolic flow velocities as the placental vascular tree grows. When diastolic flow velocities are absent, the waveform has been quantitated by expressing the proportion of the cardiac period in which flow velocity is absent.

The study of the systolic/diastolic ratio (or indeed pulsatility index or resistance index) utilizes only the maximum flow velocity waveform. This is the waveform envelope produced by the fastest moving blood cells during the cardiac cycle. It is also possible to derive the velocity waveforms for the mean and first moment (for comparison see Thompson et al., 1986a, 1986b). The possible dependence of the various indices on fetal heart rate has been considered. All indices have been shown to demonstrate a significant but small correlation with this over the normal clinical range (120 to 160 beats/min). In clinical use this effect can be ignored. Outside the normal FHR range this effect is greater. The flow waveform varies along the umbilical cord. A higher value is observed close to the fetal abdominal wall and a lower value near the point of placental attachment. Again this effect is small in comparison to the difference between normal and complicated pregnancy. Recording in the mid-region away from the two ends is recommended.

Volume blood flow in the umbilical circulation has been assessed in normal pregnancy (Gill et al., 1981) by measuring flow in the intrahepatic portion of the common umbilical vein. Umbilical blood flow increases with gestation up to 35 weeks, although blood flow relative to fetal weight is constant at $120 \text{ ml} \cdot \text{min}^{-1} \cdot \text{kg fetus}^{-1}$. It decreases slightly after that time. This value agrees with values obtained by electromagnetic flow probe (Assali et al., 1960) and microsphere (Rudolph et al., 1971) techniques used in early pregnancy at the time of abortion. The average value obtained at 40 weeks is $90 \text{ ml} \cdot \text{min}^{-1} \cdot \text{kg fetus}^{-1}$.

Waveform Pattern Observed

Initial reports (Giles et al., 1982; Trudinger et al., 1985a) of the value of umbilical Doppler flow studies in recognition of fetal compromise have been confirmed by a number of groups (Erskine and Ritchie, 1985; Reuwer et al., 1984; Schulman et al., 1984). Fetal growth restriction is associated with an umbilical artery waveform pattern of low diastolic flow velocity (point B) relative to the high systolic peak velocity (point A), i.e., a high systolic/diastolic ratio. Furthermore, serial studies indicate that the systolic/diastolic ratio increases with deterioration of fetal condition (Fig. 16–5). In some cases the waveform pattern is so changed that diastolic flow is actually reversed (Fig. 16–6).

TABLE 16–1. Correlation Coefficient for the Three Waveform Indices Based on 133 Studies

	SYSTOLIC/DIASTOLIC RATIO	PULSATILITY INDEX
Pourcelot ratio	0.941	0.944
Pulsatility index	0.925	

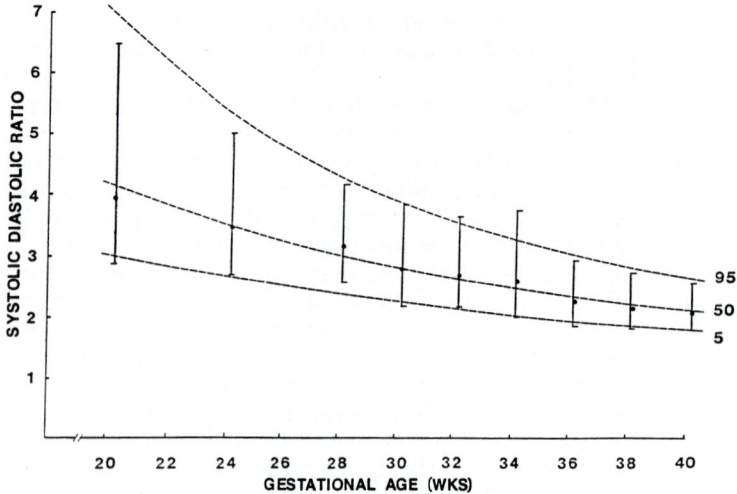

FIGURE 16–4. A normal range for the systolic/diastolic ratio from 20 weeks onward. At each gestation interval, the 90 per cent confidence interval is shown along with a smoothed curve. Each data point is based on studies from 35 normal pregnancies. (From Thompson RS, et al: Umbilical artery velocity waveforms: Normal reference values for AB ratio and Pourcelot ratio. Br J Obstet Gynaecol **95:**589, 1988a.)

Pathologic Correlations and Pathogenesis of Abnormal Waveform

Placental growth continues throughout pregnancy, as demonstrated by the increasing weight. The overall increase in placental size, with the resulting increase in numbers of tertiary stem villi and total numbers of small arterial channels, results in continuing expansion of the umbilical placental vascular tree and decreasing vascular resistance.

Giles et al. (1985a) carried out a study to correlate the umbilical artery flow velocity waveform pattern with the "resistance" vessels in the umbilical placental vascular tree. Since the major drop in arterial pressure across the umbilical placental vascular bed occurs in the small arteries and arterioles of the tertiary villi, these are the resistance vessels. Differences in these vessels were found on examination after delivery of pregnancies classified according to whether the antenatal umbilical Doppler studies were normal or abnormal. The modal tertiary villus small arterial vessel count was significantly less in the group with the abnormal umbilical artery blood flow velocity waveforms (FVW) (1 to 2 arteries/high power field) com-

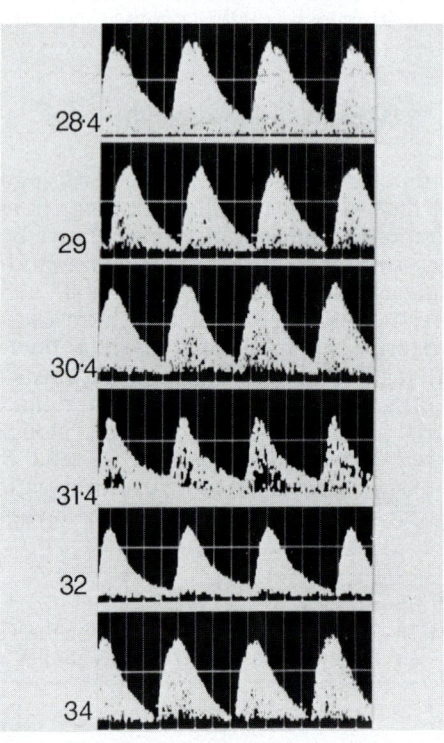

FIGURE 16–5. Sequential studies, from 28 to 34 weeks of gestation, of the umbilical artery flow velocity waveform in a woman with renal hypertension subsequently giving birth to a growth-restricted infant.

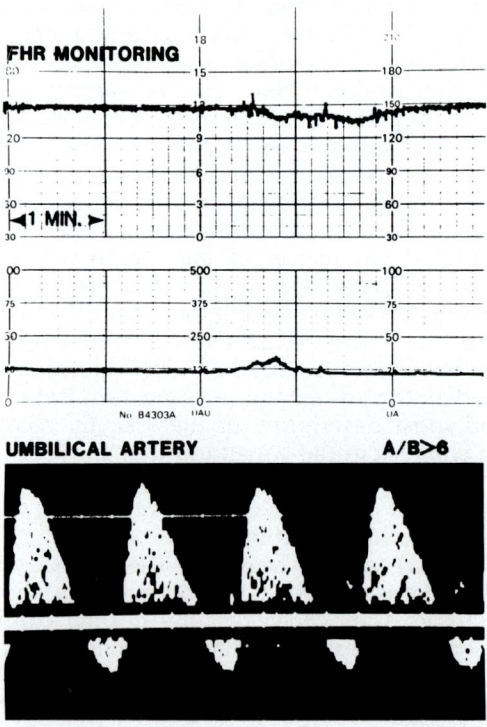

FIGURE 16–6. An umbilical artery flow velocity waveform in which umbilical placental impedance is so high that the diastolic component shows flow in a reverse direction. The non-stressed FHR tracing is nonreactive with a late deceleration evident. On the day following this study the patient gave birth to an infant of 1000 gm, at 33 weeks.

pared with the normal (7 to 8 arteries/field). This placental lesion of vascular sclerosis with obliteration of the small muscular arteries of the tertiary stem villi could be expected to cause an increase in flow resistance in the umbilical placenta. The author suggests that this lesion in the fetal placenta can best be described as "umbilical placental insufficiency." There has been discussion whether this lesion reflects a disappearance of vessels or whether these channels were never present in the villus tree. On serial studies of pregnancies with fetal compromise, an increase in the systolic/diastolic ratio may be seen, and this suggests vessel obliteration. A recently reported change in the walls of these resistance vessels (Fok et al., 1990) may be an earlier feature in the development of this vascular lesion.

In the past, a variety of histologic findings have been defined by investigators as possible indicators of placental insufficiency. These include the syncytial knot count, placental infarction, cytotrophoblast hypertrophy, deficiency of vasculoendothelial membranes, fibroid necrosis of villi, basement membrane thickening, stromal fibrosis, stromal edema, apparent placental hypovascularity, and villus maturation. These findings are extremely variable and are not consistently found in complicated pregnancies or those associated with fetal compromise. Fox (1978) stated that a pathologic basis for placental insufficiency cannot be defined. The author suggests that this failure to recognize this specific lesion in the past has been a consequence of patients being classified by maternal disease or fetal effect rather than by the disturbance in the arterial flow pattern. This is not to imply that the umbilical placental lesion is necessarily primary; it may be determined by factors of fetal or uterine origin.

The origins of the umbilical placental vascular obliteration are still to be determined. It is attractive to implicate the vasoactive prostaglandins, prostacyclin and thromboxane. Thromboxane is believed to be released by platelet aggregation, whereas prostacyclin is more a product of endothelial cells. They exhibit opposing actions. Vasoconstriction and, ultimately, vessel obliteration could well account for the increase in Doppler resistance index. Alterations in prostacyclin-to-thromboxane production ratios by placental tissue have been reported in pregnancy with hypertension (Walsh, 1985) and fetal growth restriction. Infusion of the stable thromboxane analogue U46619 caused a rise in systolic/diastolic ratio in fetal lambs (Trudinger et al., 1989), matching *in vitro* observations in perfused placentas (Mak et al., 1984). It is consistent with the local thromboxane release in the placenta producing the waveform changes seen in human pregnancy. To provide further support for this, it has been shown that fetuses in whom the umbilical Doppler study is abnormal have a significantly lower platelet count (Wilcox et al., 1990) than controls. This finding in the fetal circulation was independent of the maternal platelet count and whether or not pregnancy hypertension was present. Studies of platelet survival (Wilcox and Trudinger, 1991) confirm consumption in the fetal circulation in the presence of the placental vascular lesion defined by umbilical Doppler studies.

Experimental Models

To address the question of the meaning of the changing umbilical waveform pattern seen in fetal compromise, experimental models have been created in which the meaning of the waveform indices can be explained by manipulating a variety of governing parameters influencing blood flow. Physical and animal models have been used.

Physical modeling of the placental vasculature using a lumped electrical circuit equivalent with detailed attention to the branching of the umbilical arteries in the villus tree has been reported (Thompson and Trudinger, 1990). The validity of this approach was confirmed by demonstrating that the model predictions of volume flow were realistic for input parameters in the physiologic range and typical values for pressure and placental size. The great strength of this approach is that the effects of various parameters on the flow velocity waveforms can be examined individually. With this model, the pulsatility of the flow velocity waveform can be shown to be related to the pulsatility of the input pressure waveform. Another important observation is that the pulsatility index of the flow velocity waveform for a given placenta size (number of primary and secondary branches) will increase as the fraction of terminal vessels obliterated is increased, but it is not until 50 per cent or more of the terminal vessels are obliterated that the pulsatility index increases significantly (Fig. 16–7). This is a fundamental property of a vascular obliteration in the placental vascular tree. The Doppler umbilical flow waveforms are regarded as early predictors of vascular disease (relative to other clinical tests). However, the model results demonstrate that extensive disease is present before this detection and that the placenta has a large reserve capacity. Another prediction from such modeling relates to the altered capacitance of the umbilical placental vascular bed in association with arterial vessel obliteration. It is increased (reduced compliance). A consequence of this is the transmission of arterial pulses into the venous system so that they appear on the venous flow waveform (Fig. 16–8). This theoretical prediction has been observed clinically.

Animal studies have also been performed, most commonly in the fetal lamb. Calculated vascular resistance and umbilical artery velocity waveforms have been directly compared before and after microsphere embolization of the umbilical cotyledon vascular bed. This procedure caused a rise in both systolic/diastolic ratio and resistance (Trudinger et al., 1987a).

CLINICAL CORRELATIONS

Initial clinical studies with umbilical Doppler addressed the question of identification of the fetus subsequently born small for gestational age (SGA). Approximately two-thirds to three-quarters had a high-resistance umbilical Doppler result if studied close to the time of delivery. It was next appreciated that the small fetus with an abnormal umbilical study was at far greater risk of morbidity and mortality than those with a normal study. In a fetal study of 53 SGA

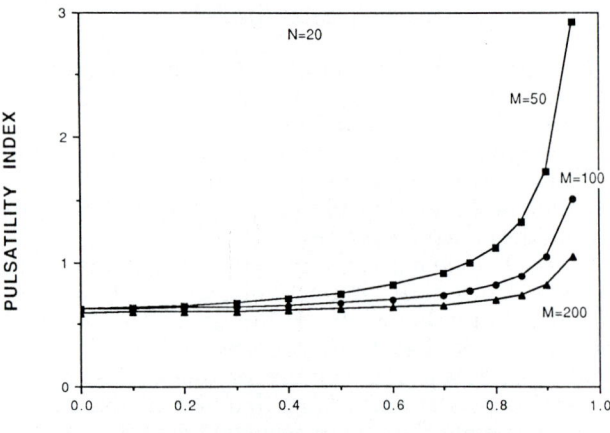

FIGURE 16–7. A mathematical model of the umbilical placental circulation was used to calculate the change in the umbilical artery pulsatility index in the presence of obliteration of an increasing fraction of the umbilical vascular bed. Three graphs are shown representing the circumstances of growth with increasing size and hence number of second-level (M) branches in the umbilical placental circulation. The number of primary branches (N) is held constant. As the placenta grows, the fraction of vessels needing to be obliterated to increase the pulsatility index beyond the normal range is increased. (Reprinted from Thompson RS and Trudinger BJ: Doppler waveform pulsatility index and resistance, pressure and flow in the umbilical placental circulation: An investigation using a mathematical model. Ultrasound Med Biol **16**:449, Copyright 1990, with permission from Pergamon Press Ltd., Oxford, UK.)

infants (birth weight less than the 10th percentile for gestational age), 34 exhibited a high systolic/diastolic ratio at the last study within a week of delivery (Trudinger et al., 1985b). Although these results were not available for clinical use, the mean gestational age at delivery was 37.3 weeks in the group with a normal study and 34.6 weeks (P<0.01) in the group with an abnormal study. Twenty-one of these infants were admitted to a tertiary-level neonatal nursery, and 19 had shown a high ratio antenatally (P<0.01). The six neonatal deaths in this series were all from the group with a high systolic/diastolic ratio on fetal study. This investigative approach has been followed throughout all at-risk pregnancies, regardless of whether birth weight was below the tenth percentile. The abnormal umbilical study predicts those at greatest risk of perinatal asphyxia and early neonatal morbidity.

I have reported on the outcome of 2178 high-risk singleton pregnancies studied over a 6-year period (Trudinger et al., 1991). Those with an abnormal result spent twice as long in the tertiary-level nursery. Conflicting results have been reported concerning fetal distress in labor. In most reported cases in which the umbilical study was done close to the time of delivery, a correlation has been demonstrated (for review see Low, 1991). Studies of fetal blood gases performed when there is reason to warrant cordocentesis demonstrate correlation between the degree of hypoxemia or acidemia and umbilical Doppler abnormality (Nicolaides et al., 1988). Whole population studies, unlike high-risk pregnancy studies, have not shown such

strong correlations, presumably because of the altered prevalence of an abnormal result.

The other common clinical situation in which abnormality of the fetal umbilical Doppler flow study is commonly evident is severe *preeclampsia*. Among a group of 21 mothers with severe preeclampsia (diastolic blood pressure greater than 110 mm Hg, proteinuria more than 1 gm/24 hrs), there were 18 fetuses with a high systolic/diastolic ratio (Trudinger et al., 1985b). This observation was independent of low birth weight. This observation implies that the umbilical flow study may be abnormal before fetal growth failure can be recognized. In severe pregnancy hypertension, abnormal umbilical Doppler has been correlated with adverse fetal outcome.

Doppler umbilical flow studies offer a convenient and easily applied method to monitor the effect of various obstetric therapies on placental blood flow. Following both fluid preload and lumbar epidural blockade there is an increase in diastolic flow velocities in the uteroplacental flow velocity waveform (Giles et al., 1987). This same change is also seen in the fetal umbilical waveform; this suggests dilatation of both placental circulations. The effect of various antihypertensive drugs used in pregnancy has been studied. There are reports of small increases of values of the index of resistance. Care is needed in interpreting such results, as changes in fetal blood pressure may produce this effect. The same explanation may account for reports of altered placental resistance in association with tocolysis. Maternal smoking has also been reported to increase the systolic/diastolic ratio.

The relationship between umbilical vein volume blood flow and the umbilical artery blood flow velocity waveform has been examined (Giles et al., 1986). Many fetuses subsequently born SGA maintain umbilical venous blood flow within the normal range even though the umbilical artery waveform exhibits a high resistance pattern with decreased diastolic velocity. When umbilical flow is expressed as a percentage of descending thoracic aorta flow, it is reduced (21 per cent) in the growth-restricted fetus in comparison with the normal fetus (40 per cent). This same observation has been made in growth-restricted fetal lambs following embolization of the maternal uterine circulation

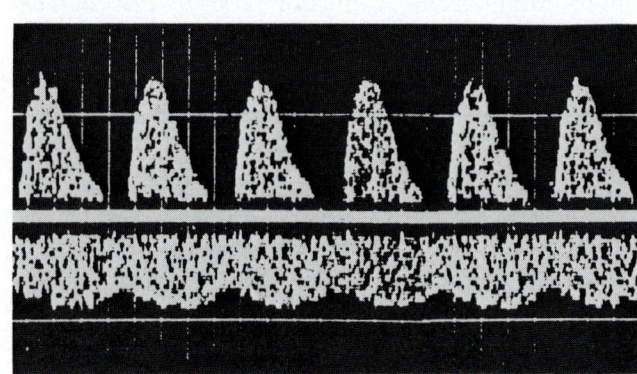

FIGURE 16–8. A recording of flow in the umbilical artery and vein. In the presence of high impedance in the umbilical placental vascular bed, venous pulsations in time with the cardiac impulse are noted. This is attributed to the decrease in capacitance.

(Block et al., 1984). It suggests an increase in cardiac output as the first response to maintain the umbilical circulation.

Doppler umbilical blood flow studies have been compared to other tests of fetal well-being. In the third trimester, they appear less efficient than ultrasound measurement of the abdominal circumference as an estimation of fetal weight and so recognition of the fetus subsequently born SGA (Chambers et al., 1989), but if the end point is changed to infant at risk of "fetal hypoxia" or operative delivery for fetal distress, they are more sensitive, with comparable positive predictive values (Newnham et al., 1990). These reports are in keeping with the notion of identification of fetus at risk of morbidity. In comparison to nonstressed fetal heart rate monitoring, umbilical Doppler was a more sensitive measure of both the SGA fetus and later asphyxia (Trudinger et al., 1986). This information is not surprising. Umbilical Doppler studies identify a vascular lesion in the fetal placenta. The lesion in the placenta may lead to fetal constraint and hypoxia. Failure of fetal growth and abnormal fetal heart rate tracings are consequences of the placental lesion, hence the suggested use of umbilical Doppler study to identify potential fetal compromise. It follows that the extent of fetal effect is better quantified by direct fetal testing (i.e., size–ultrasound measurement; behavior–biophysical profile; CNS function and heart rate control). Doppler umbilical blood flow studies by themselves should not provide an indication for delivery. They can be used to determine the need for an intensive fetal surveillance program. They are useful in detecting the false-positive nonreactive FHR due to pharmacologic depression or sleep. Acute events that may lead to fetal compromise, such as placental abruption, cord entanglement, or fetal maternal hemorrhage, are not predicted.

In the circumstance of ongoing pregnancy surveillance in a high fetal risk pregnancy, the value of serial studies is emphasized. Serial Doppler umbilical studies are useful to confirm continuing placental growth. A decreasing index of resistance indicates continuing expansion of the placental vascular bed. Even if the systolic/diastolic ratio is high, this decreasing or downward trend is associated with good fetal outcome (Trudinger et al., 1991). This trend on serial studies is particularly necessary in the second trimester, when the normal range for the systolic/diastolic ratio is wide. A decreasing trend on serial studies is of great value in confirming placental growth.

Umbilical Doppler studies have not emerged as useful in screening a total obstetric population. In the third trimester, they have been reported to be as efficient as a measurement of abdominal circumference at 34 weeks in predicting the SGA fetus at risk of asphyxia (Newnham et al., 1990). At 28 weeks they were a poor guide to later outcome (Beattie and Dornan, 1989).

Low-dose aspirin has been used as a therapy for the placental vascular pathology identified by an abnormally elevated index of resistance. The demonstrated placental vascular obliteration and fetal platelet consumption suggested the possibility of thromboxane release in the umbilical placental circulation. It was the rationale behind a controlled trial of low-dose aspirin therapy in the presence of an abnormal umbilical Doppler study (Trudinger et al., 1988) after 28 weeks. A dose of 150 mg soluble aspirin was used, but it is likely that lower doses will exert similar benefit and treatment might commence earlier in pregnancy. The treated pregnancies yielded infants with a 25 per cent increase in birth weight. Placental size was also greater, suggesting that placental growth and repair might be occurring. This improvement was not seen in pregnancies in which the Doppler studies were extremely abnormal with absent diastolic flow velocities. It was suggested that disease may be too advanced in these cases. Low-dose aspirin provides a means of treatment for placental insufficiency if the Doppler diagnosis is early and before marked fetal effect is established. It complements the use of low-dose aspirin to prevent proteinuria hypertension. The author has suggested that pregnancy hypertension may also be a consequence of the same placental pathology.

To date there have been four reports evaluating umbilical Doppler studies through the conduct of a randomized trial. It is important to understand that such a trial is specific to its design and clinical setting and the findings cannot be extrapolated without further test. In one study I conducted (Trudinger et al., 1987b), clinicians had access to all other fetal welfare assessments with umbilical Doppler availability randomized. Doppler availability was not associated with earlier delivery. Intervention rates in the two groups were similar. However, there was a significantly reduced incidence of fetal distress in labor and emergency cesarean section in the Doppler groups. Neonates spent less time in the tertiary-level nursery. A Dutch study (Omtzigt, 1990) was performed in which patients were randomized at the outset of pregnancy as to whether Doppler studies would be performed should an indication occur during the pregnancy. All other fetal welfare assessments were available. There was a significant reduction in fetal deaths in the group with access to umbilical Doppler studies. In a study (Newnham et al., 1991) of high-risk pregnancy using patients referred to an ultrasound department for fetal biometry, and deciding after this was known whether to include the patient, it was shown that umbilical Doppler studies were associated with no difference in outcome. These are interesting results and suggest that umbilical Doppler adds little to clinical management if the fetus is known to have a problem. Umbilical Doppler was compared to non-stressed fetal heart rate monitoring in a Swedish study (Almstrom et al., 1992) as a method of surveillance of fetuses identified as small by third-trimester biometry. The Doppler group had a lesser incidence of emergency cesarean section for fetal distress, and neonates required less tertiary-level care.

Changes in the umbilical artery waveform during contractions and in labor have been studied. The potential for clinical application of these studies during labor appears limited. During uterine activity, resistance indices may increase to peak at the height of each contraction. At the onset of labor, umbilical Doppler studies have been used as a screening mechanism to identify those at risk of fetal distress in labor (Fienkind et al., 1989).

Special Clinical Problems

MULTIPLE PREGNANCY. This presents major perinatal problems. Fetal and neonatal losses are high and prematurity is frequently seen. Fetal assessment is difficult; ultrasound imaging may be difficult with suboptimal measurements, and fetal heart rate monitoring may record the same fetus twice. Doppler umbilical studies provide an important new method of surveillance of the multiple gestation. To confirm identification of each fetus of a twin pair, it is imperative that the Doppler recording from the umbilical cord be carried out at the same time as the fetal heart movement is viewed on a real-time B-mode ultrasound image. Among twins with a birth weight appropriate for gestation based on singleton tables, the systolic/diastolic ratio falls within the normal singleton range (Giles et al., 1985b). When one or both fetuses were subsequently born SGA, the systolic/diastolic ratio was outside the normal range for at least one fetus in 78 per cent of cases. Management is difficult in the situation of discordancy in fetal well-being, when one fetus exhibits a high systolic/diastolic ratio and growth restriction, and the other normal studies. Early delivery implies a major penalty against the healthy fetus (Fig. 16–9) of the twin pair. It is difficult to justify this before 32 weeks. In my experience, the use of umbilical Doppler allows the recognition of this circumstance. Another important contributor to fetal loss in twin pregnancy is the *twin-twin transfusion syndrome*. In this case the systolic/diastolic ratio is similar and usually normal for both fetuses. The donor fetus is often small on ultrasound measurement with scant surrounding liquor, while the well-grown recipient exhibits polyhydramnios. The diagnosis of a twin-twin transfusion syndrome should be suspected when there is a discordancy in ultrasound size, or recent polyhydramnios, yet normal and similar umbilical flow studies. Some reports have suggested that discordant studies may also exist in this condition. This has not been so when rigid diagnostic criteria are used (Giles et al., 1990).

The high morbidity and mortality among twins justify intensive surveillance. It is my policy to perform Doppler studies on all multiple pregnancies at 28 and 34 weeks. In the absence of other complications, bed rest is advised only for patients with an abnormal result.

POST-DATE PREGNANCY. The use of umbilical Doppler studies at or beyond term has not been reported helpful. Poor discrimination of potential fetal compromise has been noted (Guidetti et al., 1987; Farmakides et al., 1988). It may be that the mature fetus is more susceptible to a degree of hypoxia. On the basis of observations made using models of the placenta, it has been reported that the larger the placenta (and so arterial branches), the greater is the fraction of vessels that need to be obliterated before the Doppler index of resistance becomes abnormal (Thompson and Trudinger, 1990). This would also explain the poor sensitivity of umbilical Doppler studies in this group.

RHESUS ISOIMMUNIZATION. This is becoming an uncommon problem in perinatal practice, but new techniques of fetal blood sampling and direct intravascular transfusion make salvage possible in most cases. The anemic fetus has a high cardiac output. Umbilical artery waveforms are normal in the presence of severe disease with high diastolic flow velocities. Within this normal range, such fetuses have been reported to exhibit an inverse correlation between the hematocrit and the blood flow waveform index of resistance (Rightmire et al., 1986). Volume blood flow in the umbilical vein has also been used to monitor these fetuses. A high blood flow has been reported in association with fetal anemia (Jouppila and Kirkinen, 1984), and this is correlated inversely with cord hemoglobin.

FETAL CARDIAC ARRHYTHMIAS. These can affect the flow velocity waveform in a manner depending upon the particular disturbance. (An example is shown in Figure 16–10.) By measuring volume blood flow in the umbilical vein and aorta in such cases it is possible to determine whether the fetus is maintaining adequate ventricular output (Tonge et al., 1984). Fetal therapy or delivery may be indicated if ventricular output is low.

DIABETES MELLITUS. In the mother this condition may be associated with either a large macrosomic fetus or a small growth-restricted fetus. The latter is more common in women with long-standing disease and vascular lesions. Those fetuses that exhibit abnormality in fetal welfare tests also show abnormality in umbilical blood flow studies (Fig. 16–11). In the case

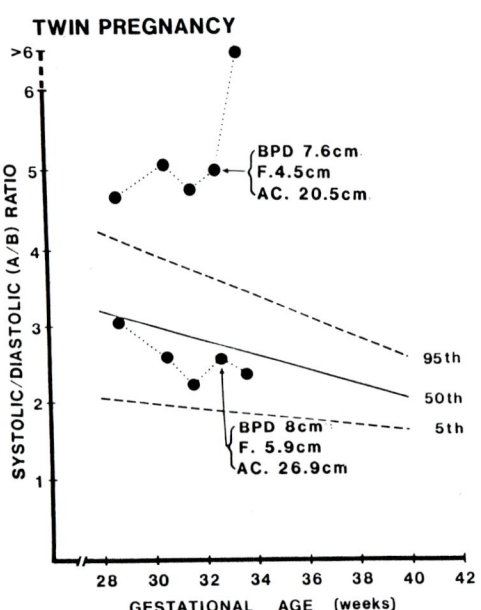

LSCS 33.5 wk
TWIN 1: BOY 1002gm
TWIN 2: GIRL 2065gm

FIGURE 16–9. Sequential systolic/diastolic ratio values in both fetuses of a twin pregnancy. The results of ultrasound measurement are also shown. Delivery was effected by elective cesarean because of concern for the smaller fetus.

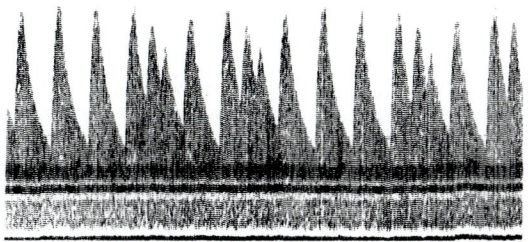

FIGURE 16–10. The umbilical artery flow velocity waveforms from a fetus with a variable heart block and ventricular extrasystoles associated with Gaucher's disease.

illustrated, deteriorating health of the macrosomic diabetic fetus was associated with an increasing umbilical blood flow resistance, yet earlier in pregnancy growth had been excessive. This serves to dissociate the metabolic drive to excess growth and the vascular insufficiency that deprives the fetus. The normal fetus of a well-controlled diabetic pregnancy exhibits normal umbilical flow studies.

THE LUPUS OBSTETRIC SYNDROME. This syndrome defines a group of mothers with high pregnancy wasting, both early and late, who have the lupus anticoagulant autoantibody in their blood and usually a positive anticardiolipin antibody (Lubbe and Liggins, 1985). Thrombosis dominates the clinical picture. It is believed that thrombosis occurs in the decidual and umbilical placental vessels and causes fetal death. Serial monitoring of umbilical flow studies in these patients allows recognition of a rise in umbilical placental resistance that is believed to precede fetal demise. This subject is discussed in greater detail in Chapter 31.

DOPPLER STUDIES OF INTRAFETAL VESSELS

Studies of the major arteries and veins within the fetus have been carried out. Most attention has been directed to the fetal aorta and cerebral arteries, although studies of renal, mesenteric, and femoral arteries have also been reported. Blood flow patterns in the fetal inferior vena cava and ductus venosus have also been recorded. Initial studies of these vessels used the same indices of resistance that had been applied to the umbilical circulation. The flow velocity waveform is influenced not only by the downstream resistance, but also by the upstream pump (heart). An approach in which attention is focused on the pump and possible circulation redistribution is emerging as more informative.

Fetal Aorta

Both blood volume and blood flow velocity waveforms may be measured in the fetal aorta. In the fetal descending thoracic aorta a flow of 191 ml $\cdot$ min^{-1} $\cdot$ kg fetus^{-1} has been measured (Eik-Nes et al., 1980). Volume flow studies have not been applied to clinical practice. The aortic flow velocity waveform has been recorded by pulsed Doppler. These waveforms have been analyzed by use of the same indices (systolic/diastolic ratio, resistance index, pulsatility index) as used for the umbilical circulation to assess downstream resistance. Because the placenta receives the largest fraction of aortic flow, the low resistance of this circulation has a dominant influence, but there

FIGURE 16–11. Sequential studies of the umbilical artery flow velocity waveform in a patient with poorly controlled diabetes mellitus. Delivery was effected at 34 weeks because of a persistent nonreactive FHR monitoring and the sequential studies of systolic/diastolic ratios. *A*, Plot of S/D sequential studies. *B*, Sequential Doppler studies.

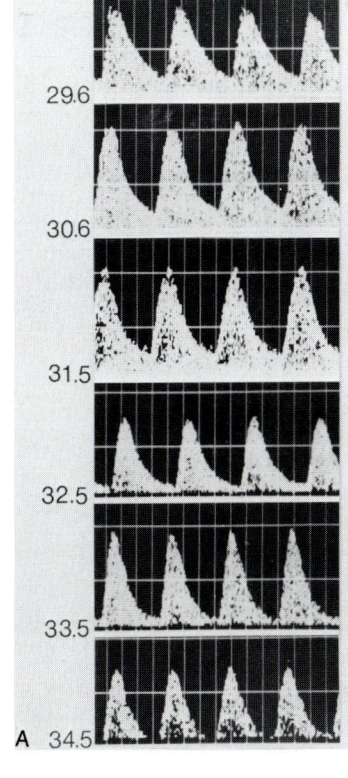

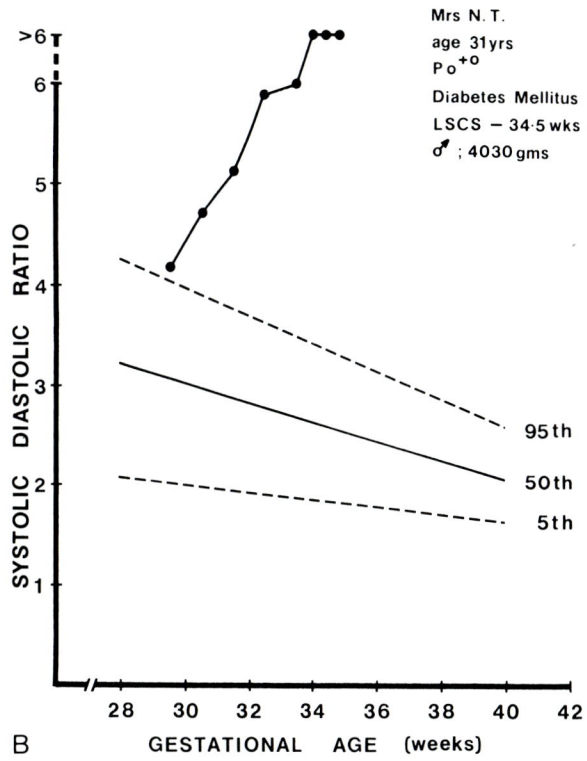

are other vascular beds that may influence this waveform.

The pulsatility index of the descending thoracic aorta changes little with gestation during the second half of pregnancy (Marsal et al., 1984). In fetal growth restriction, the pulsatility index is increased (Griffin et al., 1984; Jouppila and Kirkinen, 1986). This probably reflects the increase in placental flow resistance since the greatest part of flow is directed to that bed. There is no evidence that analysis of aortic FVW in this way provides superior or more discriminatory information in comparison to study of umbilical flow.

In experimental studies in fetal lambs (Trudinger, unpublished), the effect on the aortic flow waveform as a result of altering aortic blood flow through positive and negative inotropic stimulation was examined. Both peak and mean aortic flow velocity derived from the Doppler waveform envelope were strongly correlated with volume flow in the descending thoracic aorta. These parameters appeared as most useful in reflecting aortic flow and thus ventricular output. In human pregnancy, using principal component analysis, it has been shown that a reduction in peak mean aortic velocity (Soothill et al, 1986; Bilardo et al., 1990) correlated most strongly with fetal hypoxemia and hypercarbia in a group of fetuses in which umbilical blood sampling had been performed. Combining the animal and human data, it would appear that in the presence of marked fetal hypoxemia there is a reduction in blood flow in the aorta, the result of a reduced ventricular output. There is also evidence that indicates some circulatory redistribution with increased flow to cerebral vessels (see below). A reduction in combined ventricular output is also inferred from changes in the inferior vena cava flow pattern (see below). Direct measurement of cardiac chamber size in profoundly growth-retarded fetuses suggests dilatation (De Vore, 1988). These studies have not been evaluated in terms of clinical decision making. If umbilical Doppler studies are used to detect a placental lesion that might lead to fetal hypoxia, these studies would appear to offer the potential to determine whether that effect had yet occurred.

Fetal Cerebral Blood Flow

The internatal carotid and all the arteries of the circle of Willis can be imaged, and flow velocity waveforms from these vessels are available. In normal pregnancy these vessels show a low-resistance waveform pattern (Wladimiroff et al., 1987). There is a small change with gestation (van den Winjngaard et al., 1989). In fetal growth restriction it has been shown that this index is decreased (Arbeille et al., 1987). The separation is not as complete as one would like for a diagnostic test, and this has limited clinical application. It has been clearly shown that the more hypoxemic the fetus, the greater is the decrease in the indices of resistance (Vyas et al., 1990). The decrease in pulsatility index is presumed to be the result of cerebral vasodilation. It is popular to associate this with an increase in blood flow. The term "centralization of fetal flow" has been coined to describe the presumed redistribution of

cardiac output to maintain oxygen delivery to the fetal brain, although there are no actual human data on volume blood flow to this vascular bed.

Other Fetal Arteries

Studies of the fetal femoral artery flow velocity waveform have been carried out (Mari, 1991). A high-resistance waveform is seen and the pattern changes with gestation, reflecting increasing resistance. In fetal growth failure little change was seen.

Reports of recordings from fetal renal arteries have not provided a clear picture of change in fetal growth restriction (Vyas et al., 1989).

Inferior Vena Cava

Flow patterns in the fetal inferior vena cava have been recorded by means of duplex systems. Forward flow velocity to the atrium is greatest at the end of diastole and slows during systole until the atrioventricular valves reopen. It is a highly pulsatile waveform (Fig. 16–12). In profound fetal compromise with high umbilical Doppler resistance flow pattern, an entirely different waveform is seen (Fig. 16–13). This is clearly biphasic, with venous return to the atria augmented during the onset of diastole and after the atrioventricular valves reopen. Flow ceases or is reversed during the atrial contraction (Indik et al., 1991). Such a finding suggests a rise in venous pressure. Recently, flow in the ductus venosus has also been reported (Kiserud et al., 1991).

THE MATERNAL UTEROPLACENTAL CIRCULATION

Both pulsed (Campbell et al., 1983) and continuous-wave (Trudinger et al., 1985c; Schulman et al., 1986) Doppler have been used to study the uterine circulation. A low-resistance flow waveform pattern is recorded (Fig. 16–14), although in the first trimester high-resistance patterns are seen. The waveforms recorded from the main uterine artery trunk and its

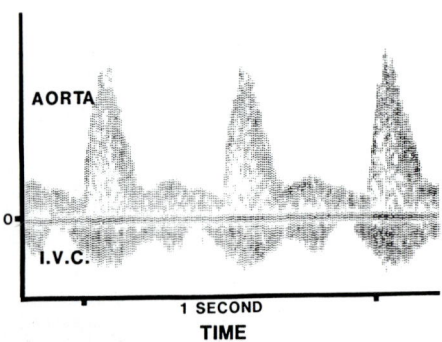

FIGURE 16–12. The flow velocity waveform from the fetal abdominal aorta and inferior vena cava at 34 weeks gestation in a normally grown fetus.

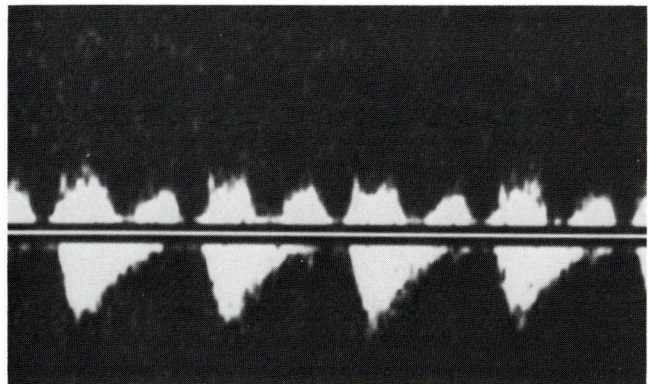

FIGURE 16–13. Waveforms from the fetal abdominal aorta and the inferior vena cava in profound fetal compromise at 32 weeks. The sample volume was positioned to include both vessels. Absent diastolic flow velocities are seen in the aortic waveform. The inferior vena cava shows high pulsatility with flow reversal at the time of the atrial contraction and isometric ventricular relaxation.

branches in the placental bed do differ (Chambers et al., 1988; Fleischer et al., 1986), so that the index of resistance used is lower in recordings from the placental bed. Recordings with continuous-wave ultrasound also lack certainty about recording site. Published studies associate adverse pregnancy outcome in terms of maternal hypertension or fetal growth restriction with a high-resistance waveform pattern. Others, however, have disputed this (Jacobsen et al., 1990; Newnham et al., 1990; Hanretty et al., 1988; Fleischer et al., 1986). There has been recent interest in the presence of a dicrotic notch in the waveform as a further marker of high resistance in the downstream bed.

It is presumed that the change in the uterine artery flow velocity waveform in pregnancy is due to an increase in flow and the associated trophoblast invasion of the spiral arteries. This has not been established. Based on this assumption, it was postulated that an increase in index of resistance of the uterine waveform might predict mothers who develop hypertension (Campbell et al., 1986). This finding has been

repeated (Steel et al., 1990). These authors reported that a uterine artery study at 18 and 24 weeks was reported to predict 63 per cent of mothers who will develop proteinuric hypertension and 33 per cent of fetuses born SGA. Recently, in a large screening study (Bewley et al., 1991), it was reported that an abnormal uterine study at 16 to 24 weeks increased the risk of adverse outcome by 9.8 times, but still the sensitivity for SGA detection was only 15 per cent and for proteinuric hypertension 24 per cent. Routine screening does not appear to be justified, although this is currently a field of active research.

REFERENCES

Almstrom H, Axelsson O, Cnattingius S, et al: Comparison of umbilical artery velocimetry and cardiotocography for surveillance of small for gestational age fetuses. Lancet **340**:936, 1992.

Arbeille PH, Roncin A, Berson M, et al: Exploration of the fetal cerebral blood flow by duplex doppler-linear array system in normal and pathological pregnancies. Ultrasound Med Biol **13**:329, 1987.

Assali NS, Rauromo L, Peltonen T: Measurement of uterine blood flow and uterine metabolism. VIII. Uterine and fetal blood flow and oxygen consumption in early human pregnancy. Am J Obstet Gynecol **79**:86, 1960.

Beattie RB, Dornan JC: Antenatal screening for intrauterine growth retardation with umbilical artery Doppler ultrasonography. Br Med J **298**:631, 1989.

Bewley S, Cooper D, Campbell S: Doppler investigation of uteroplacental blood flow resistance in the second trimester: A screening study for preeclampsia and retardation. Br J Obstet Gynaecol **98**:871, 1991.

Bilardo CM, Nicolaides KH, Campbell S: Doppler measurements of fetal and uteroplacental circulations: Relationship with umbilical venous blood gases measured at cordocentesis. Am J Obstet Gynecol **162**:115, 1990.

Block BSB, Llanos AJ, Creasy RK: Response of the growth retarded fetus to acute hypoxemia. Am J Obstet Gynecol **148**:879, 1984.

Campbell S, Griffin DR, Pearce JM: New Doppler technique for assessing uteroplacental blood flow. Lancet **1**:675, 1983.

Campbell S, Pearce KMF, Hackett G, et al: Qualitative assessment of uteroplacental blood flow: Early screening test for high-risk pregnancies. Obstet Gynecol **69**:649, 1986.

Caro CG, Pedley TJ, Schoter RC, et al: The Mechanics of the Circulation. Oxford, Oxford University Press, 1978.

Chambers SE, Hoskins PR, Haddad NG, et al: A comparison of fetal abdominal circumference measurements and Doppler ultrasound in the prediction of small-for-dates babies and fetal compromise. Br J Obstet Gynaecol **96**:803, 1989.

Chambers SE, Johnstone FD, Muir BB, et al: The effects of placental site on the arcuate artery flow velocity waveform. J Ultrasound Med **7**:671, 1988.

Clapp JF: The relationship between blood flow and oxygen uptake in the uterine and umbilical circulations. Am J Obstet Gynecol **132**:410, 1978.

Clapp JF, McLaughlin MK, Larrow R, et al: The uterine hemodynamic response to repetitive unilateral vascular embolization in the pregnant ewe. Am J Obstet Gynecol **144**:309, 1982.

De Vore GR: Examination of the fetal heart in the fetus with intrauterine growth retardation using M-Mode echocardiography. Semin Perinatol **12**:66, 1988.

Eden A: Christian Doppler, Thinker and Benefactor. Salzburg, The Christian Doppler Institute, 1988.

Eik-Nes SH, Brubakk AO, Ulstein MK: Measurement of human fetal blood flow. Br Med J **280**:283, 1980.

Erskine RLA, Ritchie JWK: Umbilical artery blood flow characteristics in normal growth-retarded fetuses. Br J Obstet Gynaecol **92**:605, 1985.

Farmakides G, Schulman H, Winter D, et al: Prenatal surveillance using non-stress testing and Doppler velocimetry. Obstet Gynecol **71**:184, 1988.

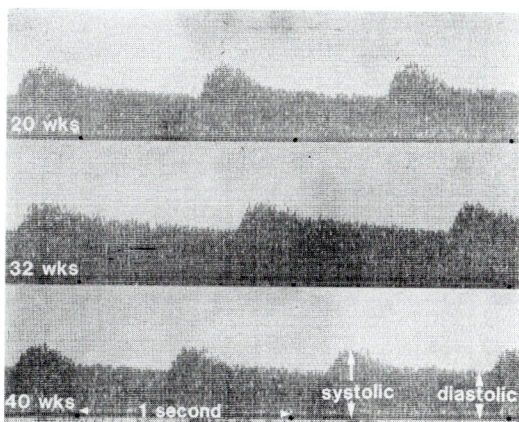

FIGURE 16–14. The normal flow velocity waveform from branches of the uterine artery in the placental bed.

Fienkind L, Abulafia O, Delke I, et al: Screening with Doppler velocimetry in labor. Am J Obstet Gynecol **161**:765, 1989.

Fleischer A, Schulman H, Farmakides G, et al: Uterine artery Doppler velocimetry in pregnant women with hypertension. Am J Obstet Gynecol **154**:807, 1986.

Fok R, Parlova Z, Benirschke K, Paul R: The correlation of arterial lesions with umbilical artery Doppler velocimetry in the placentas of small for date pregnancies. Obstet Gynecol **75**:578, 1990.

Fox H: Pathology of the placenta. In Bennington JL (Consulting Ed.): Major Problems in Pathology. Philadelphia, WB Saunders, Vol. VII in the series, 1978.

Giles WB, Trudinger BJ, Cook CM: Umbilical artery velocity time waveforms in pregnancy. J Ultrasound Med **1**(Suppl): 98, 1982.

Giles WB, Trudinger BJ, Baird PJ: Fetal umbilical artery flow velocity waveforms and placental resistance: Pathological correlation. Br J Obstet Gynaecol **92**:31, 1985a.

Giles WB, Trudinger BJ, Cook CM: Fetal umbilical artery flow velocity time waveforms in twin pregnancies. Br J Obstet Gynaecol **92**:490, 1985b.

Giles WB, Lingman G, Marsal K, Trudinger BJ: Fetal volume blood flow and umbilical artery flow velocity waveform analysis: A comparison. Br J Obstet Gynaecol **93**:46, 1986.

Giles WB, Lah FX, Trudinger BJ: The effect of epidural anaesthesia for caesarean section on maternal uterine and fetal umbilical artery blood flow velocity waveforms. Br J Obstet Gynaecol **94**:55, 1987.

Giles WB, Trudinger BJ, Cook CM, Connelly AJ: Doppler umbilical artery studies in the twin-twin transfusion syndrome. Obstet Gynecol **76**:1097, 1990.

Gill RW: Pulsed Doppler with B-mode imaging for quantitative blood flow measurement. Ultrasound Med Biol **5**:223, 1979.

Gill RW, Trudinger BJ, Garrett WJ, et al: Fetal umbilical venous flow measured in utero by pulsed Doppler and B-mode ultrasound. 1. Normal pregnancies. Am J Obstet Gynecol **139**:720, 1981.

Greiss FC: Uterine blood flow in pregnancy: An overview. In Moawad AH, Lindheimer MD (eds): Uterine and Placental Blood Flow. New York, Masson, 1982.

Griffin D, Bilardo K, Masin L, et al: Doppler blood flow waveforms in the descending thoracic aorta of the human fetus. Br J Obstet Gynaecol **91**:997, 1984.

Guidetti DA, Diven MY, Cavalieri RL, et al: Fetal umbilical artery flow velocimetry in postdate pregnancies. Am J Obstet Gynecol **1157**:1521, 1987.

Hanretty KP, Whittle M, Rubin PC: Doppler uteroplacental waveforms in pregnancy induced hypertension: A reappraisal. Lancet **1**:850, 1988.

Indik JH, Chau V, Reed KL: Association of umbilical venous with inferior vena cava blood flow velocities. Obstet Gynecol **77**:551, 1991.

Itskovitz J, LaGamma EF, Rudolph AM: The effect of reducing umbilical blood flow on fetal oxygenation. Am J Obstet Gynecol **145**:813, 1983.

Jacobson S-L, Imhof R, Manning N, et al: The value of Doppler assessment of the uteroplacental circulation in predicting preeclampsia or intrauterine growth retardation. Am J Obstet Gynecol **162**:110, 1990.

Jouppila P, Kirkinen P: Umbilical vein blood flow in the human fetus in cases of maternal and fetal anemia and uterine bleeding. Ultrasound Med Biol **10**:365, 1984.

Jouppila P, Kirkinen P: Blood velocity waveforms of the fetal aorta in normal and hypertensive pregnancies. Obstet Gynecol **67**:856, 1986.

Kirkpatrick SE, Pitlick PT, Nabiloff J, Friedman WF: The importance of the Frank-Starling relationship as a determinant of fetal cardiac output. Am J Physiol **231**:495, 1976.

Kiserud T, Eik-Nes S, Blaas H-GK, Hellevik LR: Ultrasonographic velocimetry of the fetal ductus venosus. Lancet **338**:1412, 1991.

Longo LD: Some physiological implications of altered uteroplacental blood flow. In Moawad AH, Lindheimer MD (eds): Uterine and Placental Blood Flow. New York, Masson, 1982.

Low JA: The current status of maternal and fetal blood flow velocimetry. Am J Obstet Gynecol **164**:1049, 1991.

Lubbe WF, Liggins GC: Lupus anticoagulant and pregnancy. Am J Obstet Gynecol **152**:322, 1985.

Mak KKW, Gude NM, Walters WAW, Boura ALA: Effects of vasoactive autocoids on the human umbilical-fetal placental vasculature. Br J Obstet Gynaecol **91**:99, 1984.

Mari G: Arterial blood flow velocity waveforms of the pelvis and lower extremities in the normal and growth-retarded fetuses. Am J Obstet Gynecol **165**:143, 1991.

Marsal K, Eik-Nes SH, Lindblad A, Lingman G: Blood flow in the fetal descending aorta. Intrinsic factors affecting fetal blood flow in fetal breathing movements and cardiac arrhythmia. Ultrasound Med Biol **10**:339, 1984.

Milnor WR: Pulsatile blood flow. N Engl J Med **187**:27, 1972.

Newnham JP, Paterson LL, James IR, et al: An evaluation of the efficacy of Doppler flow velocity waveform analysis as a screening test in pregnancy. Am J Obstset Gynecol **162**:403, 1990.

Newnham JP, O'Dea M, Reid K, et al: Doppler flow velocity waveform analysis in high-risk obstetric cases: A randomized controlled trial. Br J Obstet Gynaecol **98**:956, 1991.

Nicolaides KH, Bilardo CM, Soothill PW, Campbell S: Absence of end diastolic frequencies in umbilical artery: a sign of fetal hypoxia and acidosis. Br Med J **297**:1026, 1988.

Omtzigt AWJ: Clinical Value of Umbilical Doppler Velocimetry. PhD Thesis, University of Utrecht, 1990.

Rankin JHG, McLaughlin MK: The regulation of placental blood flows. J Devel Physiol **1**:30, 1979.

Reuwer PJ, Bruinse HW, Stoutenbeek P, Haspels AA: Doppler assessment of the fetoplacental circulation in normal and growth-retarded fetuses. Eur J Obstet Gynaecol Reprod Biol **18**:199, 1984.

Rightmire DA, Nicolaides KH, Rodeck C, Campbell S: Fetal blood velocities in rhesus isoimmunization: Relationship to gestational age and to fetal hematocrit. Obstet Gynecol **68**:233, 1986.

Rudolph AM: Factors affecting umbilical blood flow in the lamb in utero. In Rooth G, Brattenby LE (eds): Perinatal Medicine. Stockholm, Almquist and Wiksell International, 1976.

Rudolph AM, Heymann MA: Circulatory changes during growth in the fetal lamb. Circ Res **26**:289, 1970.

Rudolph AM, Heymann MA, Teramo KAW, et al: Studies on the circulation of the previable human fetus. Paediatr Res **5**:452, 1971.

Schulman H, Fleischer A, Stern W, et al: Umbilical velocity wave ratios in human pregnancy. Am J Obstet Gynecol **148**:986, 1984.

Schulman H, Fleischer A, Farmakides G, et al: Development of uterine artery compliance in pregnancy detected by Doppler ultrasound. Am J Obstet Gynecol **155**:1031, 1986.

Sindberg Eriksen P, Gennser G, Lindstrom K: Physiological characteristics of diameter pulses in the fetal descending aorta. Acta Obstet Gynecol Scand **63**:355, 1984.

Soothill PW, Nicolaidis KH, Bilardo CM, Campbell S: Relation of fetal hypoxia in growth retardation to mean blood velocity in the fetal aorta. Lancet **2**:1118, 1986.

Steel SA, Pearce JM, McParland P, Chamberlain GVP: Early Doppler ultrasound screening in prediction of hypertensive disorders of pregnancy. Lancet **225**:154, 1990.

Thompson RS, Trudinger BJ: Doppler waveform pulsatility index and resistance, pressure and flow in the umbilical placental circulation: An investigation using a mathematical model. Ultrasound Med Biol **16**:449, 1990.

Thompson RS, Trudinger BJ, Cook CM: A comparison of Doppler ultrasound waveform indices in the umbilical artery. I. Indices derived from the maximum velocity waveform. Ultrasound Med Biol **12**:835, 1986a.

Thompson RS, Trudinger BJ, Cook CM: A comparison of Doppler ultrasound waveform indices in the umbilical artery. II. Indices derived from the mean velocity and first moment waveforms. Ultrasound Med Biol **12**:845, 1986b.

Thompson RS, Trudinger BJ, Cook CM, Giles WB: Umbilical artery velocity waveforms: Normal reference values for AB ratio and Pourcelot ratio. Br J Obstet Gynaecol **95**:589, 1988a.

Thompson RS, Trudinger BJ, Cook CM: Doppler ultrasound waveform indices: AB ratio pulsatility index and Pourcelot ratio. Br J Obstet Gynaecol **95**:581, 1988b.

Tonge HM, Stewart PA, Waldimiroff JW: Fetal blood flow measurements during fetal cardiac arrhythmia. Early Human Dev **10**:23, 1984.

Trudinger BJ, Giles WB, Cook CM, et al: Fetal umbilical artery flow velocity waveforms and placental resistance: Clinical significance. Br J Obstet Gynaecol **92**:23, 1985a.

Trudinger BJ, Giles WB, Cook CM: Flow velocity waveforms in the maternal uteroplacental and fetal umbilical placental circulation. Am J Obstet Gynecol **152**:155, 1985b.

Trudinger BJ, Giles WB, Cook CM: Uteroplacental blood flow velocity time waveforms in normal and complicated pregnancy. Br J Obstet Gynaecol **92**:39, 1985c.

Trudinger BJ, Cook CM, Jones L, Giles WB: A comparison of fetal heart rate monitoring and umbilical artery waveforms in the recognition of fetal compromise. Br J Obstet Gynaecol **93**:171, 1986.

Trudinger BJ, Stevens D, Connelly A, et al: Umbilical artery flow velocity waveforms and placental resistance: The effects of embolization of the umbilical circulation. Am J Obstet Gynecol **157**:1443, 1987a.

Trudinger BJ, Cook CM, Giles WB, et al: Umbilical artery flow velocity waveform in high risk pregnancy: Randomized controlled trial. Lancet **1**:188, 1987b.

Trudinger BJ, Cook CM, Thompson RS, et al: Low dose aspirin therapy improves fetal weight in umbilical placental insufficiency. Am J Obstet Gynecol **159**:681, 1988.

Trudinger BJ, Connelly A, Hales JR, Wilcox G: The effects of prostacyclin and thromboxane analogue (U46619) on the fetal circulation and umbilical artery flow velocity waveforms. J Devel Physiol **11**:179, 1989.

Trudinger BJ, Cook CM, Giles WB, et al: Fetal umbilical artery velocity waveforms and subsequent neonatal outcome. Br J Obstet Gynaecol **98**:378, 1991.

Trudinger BJ, Stewart G, Cook CM, Connelly A, Exner T: Monitoring lupus anticoagulant positive pregnancies with umbilical artery flow velocity waveforms. Obstet Gynecol **72**:215, 1988.

van den Winjngaard JAGW, Groenenberg AIL, Wladimiroff JW, Hop WCJ: Cerebral Doppler ultrasound of the human fetus. Br J Obstet Gynaecol **96**:845, 1989.

Vyas S, Nicolaides KH, Campbell S: Renal artery flow velocity waveforms in normal and hypoxemic fetuses. Am J Obstet Gynecol **161**:168, 1989.

Vyas S, Nicolaides KH, Bowers S, Campbell S: Middle cerebral artery flow velocity waveforms in fetal hypoxemia. Br J Obstet Gynaecol **91**:797, 1990.

Walker AM, Oakes GK, Ehrenkranz R, et al: Effects of hypercapnia on uterine and umbilical circulations in conscious pregnant sheep. J Appl Physiol **41**:727, 1976.

Walsh SW: Pre-eclampsia—an imbalance in placental prostacyclin and thromboxane production. Am J Obstet Gynecol **152**:33, 1985.

Wilcox GR, Trudinger BJ, Cook CM, et al: Reduced fetal platelet counts in pregnancies with abnormal Doppler umbilical flow waveforms. Obstet Gynecol **75**:639, 1990.

Wilcox GR, Trudinger BJ: Fetal platelet consumption: A feature of placental insufficiency. Obstet Gynecol **77**:616, 1991.

Wladimiroff JW, Wijingaard JAGW, Degani S: Cerebral and umbilical arterial blood flow velocity waveform in normal and growth-retarded pregnancies. Obstet Gynecol **69**:705, 1987.

CHAPTER

17

FETAL BREATHING AND BODY MOVEMENTS

BRYAN S. RICHARDSON, M.D., and ROBERT GAGNON, M.D.

Pregnant women and the persons providing for their care have long recognized the importance of fetal movements as a measure of fetal health. During the last several years, fetal activity has been extensively studied with systematic investigation in animals, primarily the catheterized ovine fetus. In addition, the widespread use of real-time ultrasonic sector scanners has allowed for direct measurement of fetal movement in humans.

It has become evident that fetal breathing and body movements are important functions *in utero* and necessary for appropriate fetal growth and development. However, this activity contributes significantly to the fetal consumption of oxygen. Not surprisingly, experimental studies in unanesthetized animal preparations and clinical studies in high-risk pregnant patients indicate a decrease in such activity to be an adaptive mechanism whereby the fetus is able to decrease oxygen requirements when fetal oxygenation is compromised. Therefore, a decrease in fetal activity can be a marker of hypoxia, providing a basis for the use of activity parameters in the biophysical assessment of fetal health. However, physiologic as well as pathologic factors have been shown to affect fetal breathing and body movements, and an understanding of these is fundamental to the interpretation of fetal movement activity in the high-risk pregnant patient.

FETAL BREATHING MOVEMENTS: ANIMAL STUDIES

Physiology of Breathing Movements

Fetal breathing movements were initially characterized in the ovine fetus some 20 years ago by Dawes

et al. (1972), who used measurements from chronically implanted tracheal pressure catheters. Two types of breathing movements were distinguished. The first occurred relatively infrequently and consisted of single, brief, relatively deep inspiratory efforts recurring irregularly at a slow rate. The second, described as rapid irregular breathing, consisted of bursts of activity of much higher frequency (1 to 4 Hz) lasting from a few seconds to an hour; the inspiratory movements were irregular in both rate and depth. That fetal breathing movements are neurally generated was subsequently shown in acute animal preparations, as there is neural activity in the medulla during inspiration, and such activity in phrenic and external intercostal nerves coincides with respiratory movements and with deflections in the tracheal pressure trace (Bystrzycka et al., 1975). Diaphragmatic electromyographic (EMG) recordings as a further measurement of central respiratory drive demonstrate that after initiation of electrical activity in the diaphragm, tracheal pressure falls and tracheal flow begins and moves inward in the direction of the lungs at the rate of approximately 0.5 ml per breath (Maloney et al., 1975b). On completion of each fetal diaphragmatic EMG burst, tracheal pressure returns to normal; lung liquid flow is directed out of the lung and returns to zero between diaphragmatic EMG bursts. These observations confirm that the negative tracheal pressure measurements represent periods during which the fetal diaphragm descends into the abdomen, creating negative pressure in the chest and positive pressure in the fetal abdomen.

Although there is no evidence of a causal relationship between changes in arterial blood gas tension or pH and the onset of spontaneous fetal breathing movements, induced hypercapnia (Boddy et al., 1974) and metabolic acidosis (Hohimer and Bissonnette, 1981) have been found to affect the incidence and amplitude of respiratory movements in the ovine fetus, indicating the existence of functional chemoreceptors in the fetus. Further studies in the sheep fetus indicate that both central (Hohimer et al., 1983) and peripheral (Murai et al., 1985) chemoreceptor structures are active and capable of modulating the incidence of these movements.

There is also evidence from a number of species that normal lung growth is dependent upon the presence of fetal breathing movements of normal incidence and intensity, which may be important as a mechanical factor giving rise to intermittent pulmonary distention (Kitterman, 1984).

Biological Patterns of Breathing Movements

Episodes of rapid irregular fetal breathing movements occur up to 40 per cent of the time in chronically instrumented fetal sheep during the last third of pregnancy. As in postnatal life, these respiratory movements are affected by behavioral or sleep states and for the ovine fetus occur only during times of low-voltage electrocortical activity and electro-ocular activity characteristic of rapid eye movement (REM) sleep (Fig. 17–1) (Dawes et al., 1972). Although the to-and-fro movement of tracheal fluid is small for individual respiratory movements (<1 ml), there is an overall flow of fluid away from the lungs that is approximately five-fold greater during episodes of breathing movements than during apnea (Harding et al., 1984). A circadian rhythm in breathing activity has also been observed and is characterized by a two-fold increase in the incidence of rapid irregular breathing movements during the late evening over that measured during early morning hours (Boddy et al., 1973).

Fetal breathing movements in primates, although much less studied than in sheep, also are episodic,

with an incidence in the chronic rhesus monkey preparation noted to be approximately 50 per cent of the time near term (Martin et al., 1974). Recent studies in the baboon fetus report a similar overall incidence for breathing movements, which for this species are evident during times of electrocortical activity characteristic of both non-REM and REM sleep, albeit at an increased incidence and respiratory rate for the latter (Stark and Myers, 1992).

Developmental Changes

Developmental changes in fetal breathing activity are noted for the ovine species and are clearly dependent on the means by which this activity is measured. Whereas the incidence of fetal breathing movements as measured from tracheal pressure changes is lower in the younger gestational aged fetus (occurring approximately 20 per cent of the time at 90 days gestation; term 147 days), diaphragmatic EMG activity is almost continuous with increasing apneic modulation as gestation advances (Ioffe et al., 1987; Matsuda et al., 1992). However, the diaphragmatic EMG activity of the fetus of younger gestational age is primarily tonic in nature with a prolonged burst duration. With advancing gestation, phasic diaphragmatic activity becomes more pronounced in keeping with the increased incidence of fetal breathing movements as measured by tracheal pressure change in animals near term.

A developmental change in the pattern of breathing is also noted for the ovine fetus and appears to be related to the development of episodic variations in electrocortical activity characteristic of sleep states (Clewlow et al., 1983). Before 105 days gestation and with electrocortical activity still undifferentiated, breathing movements are nonepisodic and occur over short durations at frequent intervals. Thereafter, breathing movements become distinctly episodic and are associated with rapid eye movement as the elec-

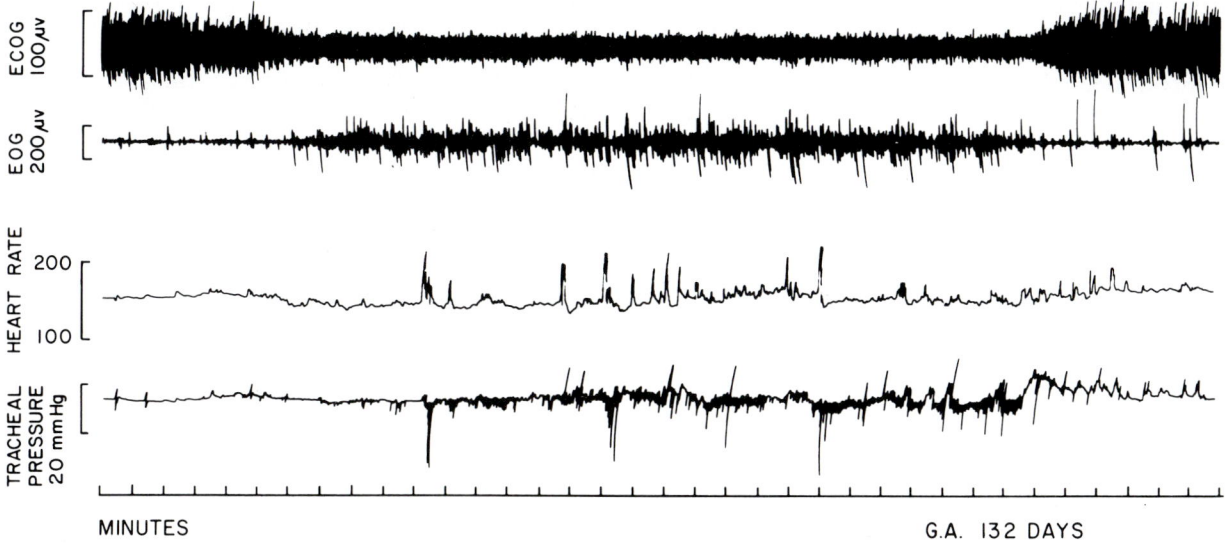

FIGURE 17–1. Chart recording demonstrating that electro-ocular activity (EOG) and fetal breathing movements normally occur during times of low-voltage electrocortical activity (ECOG).

trocorticogram begins to differentiate into high- and low-voltage patterns.

Parturition

The incidence of fetal lamb breathing movements decreases 2 or 3 days before the onset of labor and remains significantly reduced until delivery despite fetal blood gas and glucose concentrations within the normal range (Berger et al., 1986; Patrick et al., 1987b). The mechanism for this decrease in fetal breathing activity may relate to increasing concentrations of prostaglandin E_2, which is thought to play an important role in the onset of labor in sheep (Thorburn and Challis, 1979) and is known to diminish fetal breathing activity (Kitterman et al., 1983). Such a mechanism is further supported by the findings of Patrick et al. (1987b), during the last 12 hours before the onset of ACTH-induced labor in sheep, of a significant negative relationship between fetal arterial prostaglandin E_2 concentrations and the incidence of fetal breathing movements which fell to approximately 15 per cent of the time during early labor.

Hypoxia and Asphyxia

In the unanesthetized sheep fetus, moderate hypoxemia of short-term duration (reduction of arterial Po_2 from approximately 24 to 14 mm Hg for 1 to 2 hours) results in a decrease in fetal breathing movements to less than 10 per cent of the time (Boddy et al., 1974; Bocking and Harding, 1986). Similar responses to fetal hypoxemia are observed in chronic rhesus monkey preparations. It is noteworthy that fetal oxygen consumption increases some 30 per cent during periods of breathing activity when compared to apneic periods in the ovine fetus (Rurak and Gruber, 1983a), whereas neuromuscular blockade results in a 17 per cent decrease in oxygen consumption, presumably owing in part to a decrease in breathing activity and other gross body movements (Rurak and Gruber, 1983b). As such, the decrease in breathing activity when fetal oxygenation becomes compromised may serve as a protective mechanism whereby energy expenditure and thus oxygen requirements are also decreased. It should be noted that a maturational process is apparent for this fetal breathing response, with the preterm fetus showing less reduction in breathing activity at 0.7 to 0.8 of gestation (Clewlow et al., 1983; Bocking and Harding, 1986) and no reduction in breathing activity at 0.6 of gestation (Matsuda et al., 1992). Additionally, it has become apparent that the decrease in breathing activity in response to moderate hypoxemia reported for the ovine fetus near term shows adaptation over several hours with a return toward normoxic levels despite the persistence of the hypoxemic insult (Bocking et al., 1988; Koos et al., 1988).

Although the fetal breathing response to acutely induced hypoxemia has been well studied in the ovine fetus, information is limited on chronic reductions in fetal oxygenation. Worthington et al. (1981) have studied the effects of reduction of placental size in sheep

with resultant asymmetrical intrauterine growth restriction and chronic hypoxemia without acidemia. The incidence of fetal breathing movements was decreased to approximately 20 per cent. This finding was statistically significant, but involved 24-hour periods of observation, which would limit the effects of other influencing factors including the diurnal and periodic nature of breathing activity. A progression from decreased fetal breathing activity to prolonged apnea to abnormal breathing patterns has also been reported in both monkey (Manning et al., 1979) and sheep (Patrick et al., 1976; Chapman et al., 1978) fetuses prior to death *in utero*. Although abnormal breathing patterns, including gasping-type movements, were usually seen only with associated acidemia, decreased breathing activity and/or apnea were evident with hypoxemia alone, supporting hypoxemia as the stimulus for the alteration in behavioral activity rather than any associated acidotic change. However, in a recent study with prolonged and graded reductions in fetal arterial oxygen saturation over several days, a marked and significant decrease in fetal breathing activity was only noted as the degree of hypoxemia approached the level at which acidemia becomes apparent (Richardson et al., 1992). As such, fetal breathing assessment should be seen as a marker for moderate-to-severe hypoxemic changes, with heightened surveillance required for the extremely "high-risk" pregnancy as the time course for alteration prior to fetal demise may be relatively short.

Other Factors Affecting Breathing Movements

Numerous other factors alter breathing activity in chronic fetal animal preparations; these factors are outlined in Table 17–1.

FETAL BREATHING MOVEMENTS: HUMAN STUDIES

Physiology of Breathing Movements

Investigators in the late 19th century recognized and made kymographic recordings of rhythmic fetal movements transmitted to the surface of the maternal abdominal wall, which they described as fetal breathing movements (Wilds, 1978). However, it was not until the mid-1970s that it became possible to quantify fetal breathing and body movements by means of linear-array real-time imaging techniques. Thus began the systematic study of human fetal activity, with most investigators documenting visual interpretations of movement by means of an event marker from echoes displayed on a video screen (Patrick et al., 1978).

The accuracy of real-time scanning in the detection of fetal breathing movements was demonstrated by Fox and Hohler (1977). They measured fetal tracheal pressure in chronically catheterized fetal rhesus monkey preparations and simultaneously observed fetal breathing movements with a 3.5-MHz transducer. They observed fetal chest and abdominal wall move-

TABLE 17–1. Factors Affecting Fetal Breathing Movements in Sheep

Glucose concentration	
Hypoglycemia	Decreased FBM (Boddy and Dawes, 1975)
Glucose infusions	Increased FBM in fetuses with low blood glucose; no effect in normoglycemic fetuses (Richardson et al., 1982)
Temperature	
Increased core temperature	Increased FBM for 2–3 hours (Walker, 1988)
Barbiturates	
Phenobarbitone	Decreased FBM in mature fetuses (Boddy et al., 1976)
Caffeine	Increased FBM for 10–15 min (Piercy et al., 1977; Jansen et al., 1983)
Catecholamines	Increased FBM (Boddy and Dawes, 1975)
Diazepam	Decreased FBM (Piercy et al., 1977)
Doxapram	Increased FBM (Hogg et al., 1977; Jansen et al., 1983)
Ethanol	Variable effect on FBM depending on acute or chronic exposure (Patrick et al., 1985b; Smith et al., 1989)
General anesthesia	Total suppression of FBM (Maloney et al., 1975a)
Narcotics	
Methadone Morphine	Initial decrease followed by an increase in FBM with acute exposure (Szeto, 1983; Bennet et al., 1986; Hasan et al., 1988)
Prostaglandin E₂	Arrest of FBM (Kitterman et al., 1979)
Prostaglandin inhibitors	
Indomethacin Meclofenamate	Increased FBM for 12–18 hr (Kitterman et al., 1979; Patrick et al., 1987a)
Theophylline	Increased FBM (Bissonnette et al., 1990)

ments with the real-time scanner during the smallest tracheal pressure changes measured. The consistency of trained observers in the measurement of fetal breathing movements was subsequently demonstrated by Patrick et al. (1978). In this group, one-hour videotape recordings of fetal activity were independently analyzed by different observers. The correlation coefficient among observers who measured fetal breathing movements from the same recording was 0.94 while the average difference among observers was only 2.5 per cent.

Human fetal breathing movements are most readily visualized on longitudinal scanning, thus permitting visualization of both anterior fetal chest and abdominal wall echoes. During each fetal breathing movement, the anterior chest wall echoes move inward 0.5 to 5 mm and the anterior abdominal wall echoes move outward in the opposite direction about 3 to 8 mm. When posterior chest wall echoes are not over or near the fetal spine, both chest walls can be observed to move inward (toward each other) by 1 to 5 mm during breathing movements. Following each inspiratory movement, the chest walls move outward to the resting state and the anterior abdominal wall moves inward and returns to its resting state (Patrick et al., 1978). These paradoxic movements of the chest and abdominal wall echoes permit identification of each breath. As in the ovine fetus, the amplitude of chest

and abdominal wall movements during episodes of fetal breathing is variable. Likewise, the fetal diaphragm appears to be the primary muscular force generating these movements, as echoes that represent this structure descend into the fetal abdomen during, and return after, each fetal breath.

The incidence of human fetal breathing movements has been shown to correlate with induced changes in maternal end-tidal PCO_2, increasing with maternal breathing of 2 per cent and 4 per cent carbon dioxide and decreasing with maternal hyperventilation (Connors et al., 1988a). This would again suggest the existence of functional fetal chemoreceptors as previously noted for the ovine fetus. Increasing maternal arterial PO_2 with high concentrations (50 per cent) of inspired oxygen has no effect on fetal respiratory activity in normal fetuses (Devoe et al., 1984).

As seen with direct animal experimentation, circumstantial evidence from anomalous development of human fetuses supports the conclusion that loss of fetal breathing movements may play a role in abnormal lung growth with pulmonary hypoplasia, although loss of thoracic volume may be just as important if not more so (Liggins, 1984).

Biological Patterns of Breathing Movements

Breathing movements made by healthy human fetuses are episodic and separated by periods of apnea. Measurement of breath-to-breath intervals over the last 10 weeks of pregnancy reveals that only 3 per cent of these intervals are 6 seconds or longer (Patrick et al., 1980a). Therefore, in the absence of gross fetal body movements, it is reasonable to define fetal apnea as a period of 6 seconds or longer in humans.

Human fetal breathing movements are seen to occur approximately 30 per cent of the observed time over the last 10 weeks of pregnancy (Patrick et al., 1978; 1980b). Near term there is a clustering of fetal breathing and gross body movements into episodes lasting 20 to 60 minutes and recurring every 60 to 90 minutes, suggesting a relationship to behavioral state activity as previously noted for the animal studies (Fig. 17–2) (Patrick et al., 1978, 1980b). The use of mathematical time-domain and spectral methodology further demonstrates that these fetal movements are not random events (Campbell, 1980). This behavioral state relationship has been quantified by Junge and Walter (1980), with breathing movements reported to be present approximately 30 per cent of the time during fetal "active" periods (analogous to the rapid-eye-movement state) as determined by coincident recording of heart rate and body movements. Although breathing movements are decreased, they are still present approximately 14 per cent of the time during fetal "quiet" periods (analogous to the non-rapid-eye-movement state). The character of fetal breathing is also affected by sleep states, as Nijhuis et al. (1983) report fetal breathing rhythm to be more regular during "quiet" periods than during "active" periods.

As a result of the episodic nature of human fetal breathing movements, the percentage of time spent breathing can be substantially altered by the length of

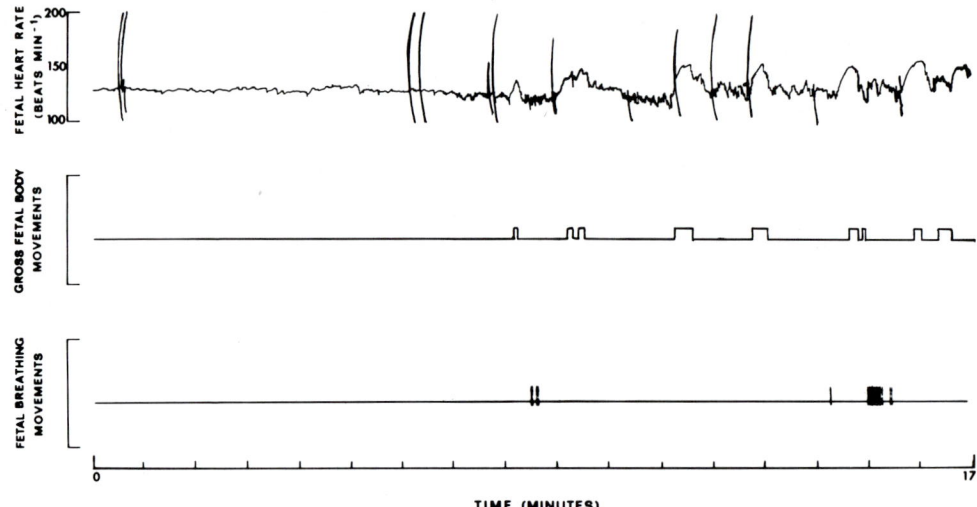

FIGURE 17–2. A chart recording of fetal heart rate, gross fetal body movements, and fetal breathing movements over a 17-minute observation period. For the first 8 minutes there were no gross fetal body movements and the fetal heart rate demonstrated no significant accelerations or decelerations. From 8 to 17 minutes a normal episode of gross fetal body movements accompanied by accelerations in the fetal heart rate occurred. (From Richardson B, Campbell K, Carmichael L, Patrick J: Effects of external physical stimulation on fetuses near term. Am J Obstet Gynecol **139**:344, 1981.)

recording time. It is thus necessary to record for a long enough period to be certain that the recording interval does not entirely consist of a normal period of fetal apnea. We have studied healthy patients over 24-hour observation intervals through the last 10 weeks of pregnancy (Patrick et al., 1978, 1980a, 1980b). Analysis of successive 5-minute intervals in each patient was performed to determine the percentage of intervals of 5 minutes and multiples of 5 minutes during which no fetal breathing movements were observed. This study demonstrated that approximately 25 per cent of 5-minute intervals, 15 per cent of 15-minute intervals, and 8 per cent of 30-minute intervals contained no fetal breathing movements (Fig. 17–3). It was also evident from this study that episodes of fetal apnea of up to 2 hours can occasionally occur in healthy human fetuses when recordings are made without attention to time of day or the relationship to maternal meals.

Throughout the last 10 weeks of pregnancy the

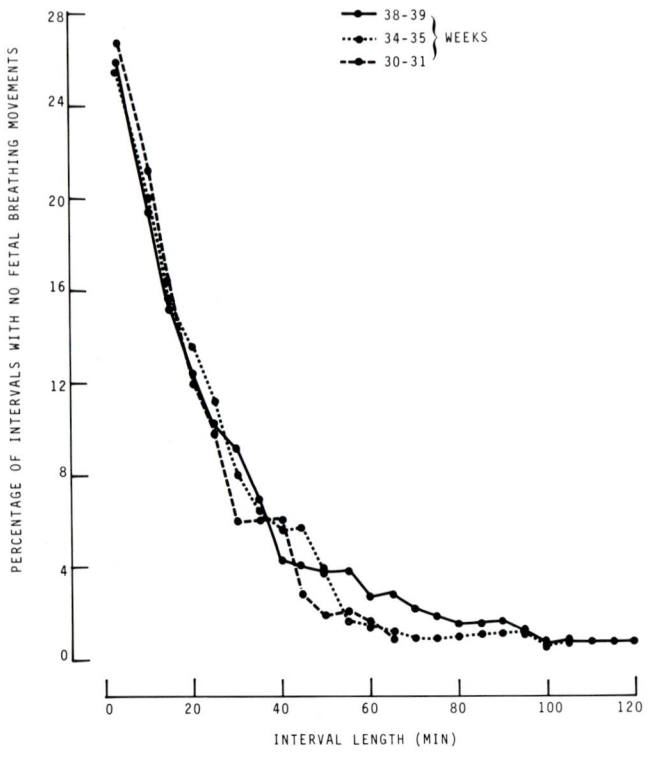

FIGURE 17–3. Composite plot of the percentage of intervals with no fetal breathing movements in nine fetuses at 30 to 31 weeks, 11 at 34 to 35 weeks, and 11 at 38 to 39 weeks, demonstrating a similar distribution at these different gestational ages. The longest apneic interval was 65 minutes at 30 to 31 weeks, 105 minutes at 34 to 35 weeks, and 120 minutes at 38 to 39 weeks. (From Patrick J, Campbell K, Carmichael L, et al: A definition of human fetal apnea and the distribution of fetal apneic intervals during the last ten weeks of pregnancy. Am J Obstet Gynecol **136**:471, 1980a.)

percentage of time a fetus spends breathing is increased significantly during the second and third hours following maternal meals, with the increase appearing to follow the normal postprandial increase in maternal blood glucose concentration (Fig. 17–4) (Patrick et al., 1978, 1980b). The observation that periods of fetal apnea are no longer than 45 minutes during the second and third hours after meals would indicate that this is an ideal time for clinical measurement of fetal breathing movements.

A prolonged significant increase in fetal breathing movements is also observed overnight while mothers are asleep (Fig. 17–4) (Patrick et al., 1978, 1980b; Natale et al., 1988). This may represent a circadian rhythm in fetal breathing activity, as previously described for the ovine fetus. There is also a circadian rhythm in maternal plasma estriol concentration, which is inversely related to the circadian rhythm in cortisol level at 30 to 35 weeks of pregnancy (Patrick et al., 1980c). This finding is consistent with the hypothesis that maternal cortisol or placental metabolites of cortisol might cross to the fetus and influence fetal hypothalamic pituitary and adrenal function. It is notable that the overnight increase in maternal cortisol level coincides with the overnight increase in fetal breathing movements. In women receiving exogenous glucocorticoids and with suppressed or absent circadian rhythms in cortisol concentration (Challis et al., 1981), this overnight increase in fetal breathing activity is not seen (Patrick et al., 1981). The data from these studies thus suggest that the overnight increase in fetal breathing normally seen in healthy fetuses during the last 10 weeks of pregnancy might be due to a circadian rhythm in fetal life that is modulated by a circadian rhythm in maternal glucocorticoids.

Developmental Changes

Rhythmic breathing movements can be observed from 10 weeks gestation onward, with a trend toward an increase in incidence thereafter, although they are still only evident 6 per cent of the recording time by 19 weeks gestation (de Vries et al., 1982, 1985). At this time breathing movements frequently occur alone, although they are sometimes seen in combination with other movement. Continuous 24-hour recordings of fetal breathing activity at 24 to 28 weeks gestation have been reported by Natale et al. (1988), with the mean incidence found to be 14 per cent. In this study no significant increase in fetal breathing activity occurred following maternal meals; however, a significant increase was noted overnight. Fetal breathing activity was now distinctly episodic and clustered with other behavioral variables, but the longest period of apnea was only 14 minutes, which is significantly less than that seen during the last 10 weeks of pregnancy. This would suggest that different normal values need to be used in the evaluation of fetal health at earlier gestations. It is of interest that there is a maturational change in the fetal respiratory response to carbon dioxide which parallels the change in the effect of gestational age on these movements, supporting this response as the possible mechanism whereby fetal breathing movements are decreased in the fetus of younger gestational age (Connors et al., 1989).

Although the overall percentage of time the fetus spends breathing remains little changed between 30 and 40 weeks of gestation, differences in patterns of breathing activity and in distributions of breath-to-breath intervals are evident (Patrick et al., 1980a). The mean rate of fetal breathing movements at 30 to 31

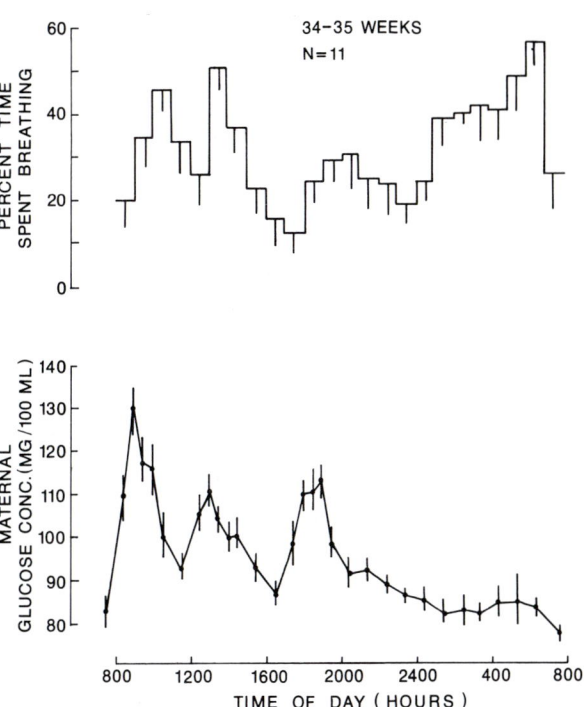

FIGURE 17–4. The percentage of time spent breathing by 11 fetuses at 34 to 35 weeks each hour of the day. Mothers were given meals at 0800, 1200, and 1700 hours. Fetuses made breathing movements a greater percentage of the time during the second and third hours following breakfast, lunch, and dinner. There was a prolonged significant increase in the percentage of time spent breathing between 0100 and 0700 hours. Peak glucose concentrations occurred at 0900, 1300, and 1800. (From Patrick J, Natale R, Richardson B: Patterns of human fetal breathing activity at 34 to 35 weeks gestational age. Am J Obstet Gynecol **132**:507, 1978.)

weeks is 58 and falls to 41 breaths per minute at 38 to 39 weeks. The distribution of breath-to-breath intervals is much broader at 30 to 31 weeks than at 38 to 39 weeks, when breath-to-breath intervals are more regular. These changes in respiratory rate and variability over this period suggest a maturation in the control of fetal breathing movements, which probably reflects the emergence of behavioral state influences.

Parturition

A number of reports suggest that patterns of human fetal breathing movements are changed in relation to human labor at term. We studied healthy women during electively induced labor at term and found that fetal breathing movements, although still present, were decreased to less than 10 per cent of the time during the latent phase of labor (Richardson et al., 1979). However, during the active phase of labor, breathing movements were virtually abolished and were present less than 1 per cent of the time. Similar findings have been reported by Wittman et al. (1979) and Boylan and Lewis (1980) in patients with both induced and spontaneous labor. Carmichael et al. (1984) demonstrated that there is a decrease in the incidence of fetal breathing movements at full term in fetuses within 3 days of spontaneous labor as compared with a similar group of term fetuses delivered more than 7 days following study. Their data also provided evidence that a significant decrease in breathing activity normally occurs in the days immediately preceding the onset of labor at term.

Assessment of Preterm Labor

Since fetal breathing activity is known to decrease during labor, its incidence has been proposed as a means of predicting fetuses at risk of preterm delivery in women who present in the hospital with signs of premature labor. Studies by Castle and Turnbull (1985) and subsequently Boylan et al. (1985) and Besinger et al. (1987) indicate that fetal apnea of 20 to 60 minutes' duration is a reliable indicator of true premature labor with subsequent premature delivery within 48 hours in almost all of these patients. However, Castle and Turnbull (1985) reported little benefit from tocolytic therapy in these patients, suggesting that they were in more advanced premature labor. This suggestion is further supported by our results (Richardson et al., 1979) for electively induced labor at term, when prolonged fetal apnea was only evident during active labor. In those same clinical studies of prematurely laboring patients, the presence of fetal breathing movements did not appear to be as reliable in predicting false premature labor, with a number of patients still delivering within the subsequent 48 hours. Our own experience supports this finding, for although the incidence of fetal breathing movements was decreased prior to preterm labor, breathing was not abolished and was still present about 15 per cent of the time over 2-hour observation intervals in women delivering prematurely within 12 hours of study (Pa-

trick and Richardson, 1985a). Given the wide range of variation in the incidence of fetal breathing movements when monitored over short time intervals, the observation of a decrease in this activity during early premature labor is not likely to be clinically useful in the predicting of outcome in these women.

Intrauterine Growth Restriction

In the assessment of fetal health, a decrease in breathing activity is presumed to reflect a decrease in oxygenation with resultant fetal hypoxemia and/or acidemia, although as noted in patients with impending labor, fetal breathing activity will also be decreased. It is therefore of interest that in patients with intrauterine growth restriction (IUGR) and presumed chronic fetal hypoxemia, the incidence of fetal breathing movements is reported to be variably decreased and appears dependent on the severity of IUGR (less than the tenth percentile versus less than the third percentile) and the conditions and duration of study (Luther et al., 1982; Dornan and Ritchie, 1983; van Vliet et al., 1985; Ruedrich et al., 1989; Gagnon et al., 1990; Bekedam et al., 1991). However there is considerable overlap with population norms, which would limit the usefulness of this parameter, at least as used clinically, as a marker of intrauterine growth restriction. Maternal hyperoxia (inspired oxygen concentration of 50 per cent) has been shown to increase the incidence of breathing movements in the IUGR fetus, with no such increases noted for the well-grown fetus (Dornan and Ritchie, 1983; Ruedrich et al., 1989; Gagnon et al., 1990; Bekedam et al., 1991). Although implicating fetal hypoxemia as the basis for the reduced incidence of breathing movements in the IUGR fetus, the induced increase in such activity is to a level similar to that of the well-grown fetus and, given the inherent periodicity of fetal breathing activity, is again unlikely to serve as a useful clinical marker.

Assessment of Fetal Health

The present use of fetal breathing movements in the assessment of fetal health is largely confined to its component part in biophysical profile scoring. Experience to date would suggest that the observation of the three dynamic biophysical variables—fetal breathing movements, gross body movements, and non-stress heart rate testing—do not improve the predictive value of a normal perinatal outcome compared to the observation of a single variable (Manning et al., 1980; Schifrin et al., 1981; Baskett et al., 1984). However, the predictive value for an abnormal perinatal outcome is improved and the false-positive rate decreased when test results are combined. For the dynamic fetal variables, the monitoring of body movements would appear to improve the positive predictive value of the biophysical profile more than the monitoring of breathing movements or non-stress testing (Platt et al., 1983; Vintzileos et al., 1983), although a recent report by Manning et al., (1990) would suggest the same for non-stress testing. However, as noted by

Devoe et al. (1988), such comparisons are without statistical relationship to physiologic incidence data, as the unweighted and somewhat arbitrary scoring system currently used does not provide for the quantification of the dynamic fetal variables and their normal population standards. Moreover, sequential rather than concurrent monitoring of these fetal activities, as used in biophysical profile scoring, does not respect the interdependence of these variables with behavioral state organization. It remains to be determined whether prolongation of the monitoring interval, as suggested for non-stress testing (Brown and Patrick, 1981), would be equally successful in improving the positive predictive value for poor perinatal outcome.

As presently scored within the biophysical profile, fetal breathing movements are more likely to be falsely abnormal at 26 to 33 weeks gestation when compared with 34 to 41 weeks (Baskett, 1988). This is not surprising, given the lower incidence of breathing activity in younger fetuses (Natale et al., 1988), and it emphasizes the need to establish population norms reflecting the biological patterns and known factors affecting this activity. It has also recently been stated that nonreactive non-stress testing and loss of fetal breathing are earlier signs of fetal acidosis and worsening hypoxemia as opposed to the loss of fetal movement and tone (Vintzileos et al., 1991). This would imply a hierarchy within the fetal brain for the control of these activities in response to onsetting hypoxemia and/or acidemia. Although this may be true, as suggested by studies in the ovine fetus (Richardson et al., 1992), the clinical evidence to date is again based on arbitrary standards without relation to normal values for a given population.

The predictive value for a normal perinatal outcome is high and similar among the dynamic fetal variables, and in the order of 95 per cent with little improvement when test results are combined (Manning et al., 1980; Schifrin et al., 1981; Baskett et al., 1984). Nonetheless, there continues to be a small number of patients with adverse perinatal outcome that was not predicted on the basis of dynamic fetal monitoring (Manning et al., 1987). This serves to emphasize that the monitoring of fetal breathing movements, as well as the other dynamic fetal variables, only allows for the assessment of fetal health at the time of testing, from which a probability of continued health may be formulated. An improvement in negative predictive value might occur with more frequent testing, but the time course over which these fetal variables become abnormal prior to fetal death is not known and may well change with the assorted disease processes and their severity. Anecdotal clinical reports indicate that in some instances deterioration in scoring profiles can occur over as short a time interval as 2 to 3 days (Baskett et al., 1984; Manning et al., 1987). It is not yet clear whether any one of the dynamic fetal variables is a more sensitive predictor of adverse perinatal outcome than the others, although the concurrent computer-assisted assessment with quantification of these variables, as proposed by Devoe et al. (1988), would again suggest a decrease in fetal breathing movements to be an earlier indicator of a deterioration in fetal health.

Other Factors Affecting Breathing Movements

Numerous other factors alter breathing activity in human fetuses; these factors are outlined in Table 17–2.

FETAL BODY MOVEMENTS: ANIMAL STUDIES

Physiology of Body Movements

There has been limited study of fetal body movements using fetal animal preparations; again most information has been obtained from the ovine fetus. Dawes et al. (1972) provided one of the first descriptions in sheep near term delivered into a warm saline bath with intact umbilical cords. Three different types of movement activity were observed. In the first, the lamb appeared awake, moved its limbs, raised its head, and opened its eyes. The second type involved only slow gentle extension of the limbs and seemed to correspond to non-REM sleep. The third type appeared to correspond to REM sleep since it entailed movements of the eyes and intermittent twitching of ears, lips, and limbs. Fetal movement activity has subsequently been characterized by use of EMG leads and/or transit time ultrasonography on different skeletal muscles including forelimb, neck (postural muscle activity), and trunk (Ruckebusch et al., 1977; Natale et al., 1981; Szeto et al., 1985). Simple fetal movements such as extension of the head and flexion or extension of the limbs have been identified, as have complex movements characterized by two to three repetitive elements involving combined movements of neck, limb, and trunk.

Biological Patterns of Body Movements

Ovine fetal movement activity is also affected by the behavioral state although the relationship is much

TABLE 17–2.   Factors Affecting Fetal Breathing Movements in Humans

Glucose concentration	
Glucose infusions	Increased FBM in patients who have fasted (Natale et al., 1978)
Cigarette smoking	Increased frequency of FBM although incidence unchanged (Fox et al., 1977; Thaler et al., 1980)
Caffeine	Increased FBM with chronic exposure; no effect with acute exposure (McGowan et al., 1987)
Ethanol	Dramatic decrease in FBM (Fox et al., 1978; McLeod et al., 1984)
Methadone	Decreased FBM with chronic exposure (Richardson et al., 1984)
Other drugs	Small-series reports have appeared on the effects of amylobarbital, diazepam, meperidine, methyldopa, salbutamol, and terbutaline (For a review see Lewis and Boylan, 1979)

less clear than that reported for breathing movements. Simple fetal movements, although episodic in nature, are seen during both high-voltage and low-voltage electrocortical activity characteristic of non-REM and REM sleep, respectively (Ruckebusch et al., 1977; Natale et al., 1981). Complex movements likewise usually occur in clusters and are particularly prevalent during the transition between electrocortical states, although this can also occur both in high-voltage and, to a lesser extent, during low-voltage electrocortical activity. Near term the ovine fetus also demonstrates short periods of wakefulness characterized by low-voltage electrocortical activity and nuchal muscle tone and a marked increase in gross movement activity (Ruckebusch et al., 1977; Szeto et al., 1985). As with breathing movements, a circadian rhythm in body movements has also been observed to be characterized by an increase in gross movement activity overnight, which becomes more pronounced near term with the establishment of the awake state (Ruckebusch et al., 1977).

Developmental Changes

A developmental change in the pattern of nuchal muscle activity is evident and appears to be related to behavioral state development (Clewlow et al., 1983). Prior to 105 days gestation and with electrocortical activity still undifferentiated, nuchal muscle activity is almost continuous and without obvious pattern or relationship to the other biophysical variables. Thereafter, nuchal muscle activity becomes episodic and, with the distinct differentiation of electrocortical activity after 120 days gestation, becomes clearly related to the high-voltage state. Gross body movement activity is also increased in the last few days prior to birth and probably relates to the appearance at this time of fetal wakefulness (Ruckebusch et al., 1977; Szeto et al., 1985).

Parturition

In the ovine fetus, forelimb movements, although decreased by approximately 50 per cent, continue to be evident throughout labor and linked to behavioral state activity (Natale et al., 1981). As labor becomes well established, movements are often associated with uterine contractions.

Hypoxia and Asphyxia

In the unanesthetized sheep fetus, moderate hypoxemia of short-term duration (reduction of arterial PO_2 from approximately 22 mm Hg to 14 mm Hg for 1 to 2 hours), induced either by reducing maternal inspired oxygen (Natale et al., 1981) or by reducing uterine blood flow (Bocking and Harding, 1986), results in a decrease in fetal forelimb and nuchal muscle activity to less than 30 per cent of control values. It should be noted that this degree of hypoxemia is sufficient to result in metabolic acidemia. With mild hypoxemia

(reduction of arterial PO_2 to approximately 16 mm Hg), nuchal muscle activity is decreased by only 10 to 15 per cent from control values (Woudstra et al., 1990). Although of probable biological significance and representing a protective adaptive mechanism, this small fall in fetal movement activity would be of little clinical use as an indicator of mild fetal hypoxemia. Fetal body movements should also be seen as a marker for moderate-to-severe hypoxemic change and, when markedly decreased, probably reflects a degree of hypoxemia close to that required for the onset of metabolic acidemia.

FETAL BODY MOVEMENTS: HUMAN STUDIES

Physiology of Body Movements

Human fetal body movements have been systematically studied over the last half of pregnancy by the use of linear-array real-time imaging techniques, as previously described for the study of human fetal breathing movements. The consistency of trained observers in the measurement of these movements has again been demonstrated by Patrick et al. (1982), who used 1-hour videotape recordings of fetal activity. When the percentage of time spent moving as detected by different observers was compared to the percentage of time spent moving as derived from the original chart recordings, the average variability among observers was only 4.6 per cent. The systematic study of fetal activity in healthy pregnancies by Patrick and colleagues has relied upon longitudinal scanning of the fetus, thus permitting the simultaneous measurement of fetal breathing activity. Although providing for the accurate measurement of fetal rolling and stretching movements, isolated movements of the fetal limbs are not as well visualized.

The neural activity of fetal motility and its motor effects may contribute to the development of muscles, joints, and even the fine structure of the central nervous system itself (Prechtl, 1987).

Biological Patterns of Body Movements

Human fetal gross body movements occur approximately 10 per cent of the time over the last 10 weeks of pregnancy with an average of 31 movements per hour over a 24-hour period (Patrick et al., 1982). As previously noted, near term there is a clustering of fetal breathing and gross body movements, suggesting a relationship to behavioral state activity (see Fig. 17–2) (Patrick et al., 1978, 1980b). Studies by Nijhuis et al. (1982) have now identified an inextricable linkage of gross body movement activity to other behavioral parameters, thus firmly establishing the existence of fetal behavioral states. Fetal body movements are frequent during state 2F (active periods analogous to the REM state), whereas they are much reduced or absent during state 1F (quiet periods analogous to the non-REM state). This gives rise to an "activity-quiescent" cycle with a duration of approximately 60 minutes by term, although with considerable variability. An additional "active" fetal period has been described, termed state 4F, which is characterized by frequent and vigorous gross body movements and, by inference from human neonatal studies, appears to represent periods of fetal wakefulness. These are usually seen no more than 10 per cent of the time and are of relatively short duration (5 to 10 minutes).

As a result of the episodic nature of human fetal gross body movements, it is again important to record for a long enough period to be certain that the recording interval does not entirely consist of a normal period of fetal quiescence. From our 24-hour observation studies on healthy pregnant patients through the last 10 weeks of pregnancy, we have determined that approximately 25 per cent of 5-minute intervals, 10 per cent of 15-minute intervals, and 5 per cent of 30-minute intervals contain no gross body movement activity (Fig. 17–5) (Patrick et al., 1982). It was also evident that episodes of fetal quiescence of up to 75 minutes can occasionally occur in healthy human fetuses when recordings are made without attention to time of day.

Near term there is an increase in the incidence and number of gross fetal body movements in the late evening, and this increase may correspond to increased periods of wakefulness (Fig. 17–6) (Patrick et al., 1982). Thus this time of day may be a useful period for women to record fetal activity as a screening test of fetal health. In contrast to fetal breathing movements, gross body movements are not influenced by maternal plasma glucose concentrations or maternal meals during the day (Fig. 17–6).

Relationship of Body Movements to Heart Rate Accelerations

The relationship of fetal body movements to heart rate accelerations is an important one and provides the basis for non-stress heart rate testing. Timor-Tritsch et al. (1978), using strain gauges placed on the maternal abdomen wall, reported that 99.8 per cent of all fetal movements of greater than 3 seconds duration are associated with fetal heart rate accelerations (>10 bpm). Patrick and co-workers (1984), using real-time ultrasound and abdominal EKG methods, reported that near term 92 per cent of all evident gross body movements were associated with fetal heart rate accelerations ($\geq$10 bpm and lasting $\geq$10 seconds), whereas 85 per cent of all accelerations occurred in association with body movements. Thus quantitative observations of fetal movements would appear to be interchangeable with fetal heart rate accelerations over the last few weeks of pregnancy. However, it remains to be determined whether the compromised fetus with a nonreactive non-stress test has a loss of fetal heart acceleration with body movement or rather becomes inactive and stops moving.

Developmental Changes

Longitudinal study of fetal movement activity over the first half of pregnancy reveals that movements even of the young fetus appear to be specific and with recognizable patterning (de Vries et al., 1982, 1985). Fetal movements can be observed from 8 weeks gestation onward with a developmental trend in the various movements evident including a gradual in-

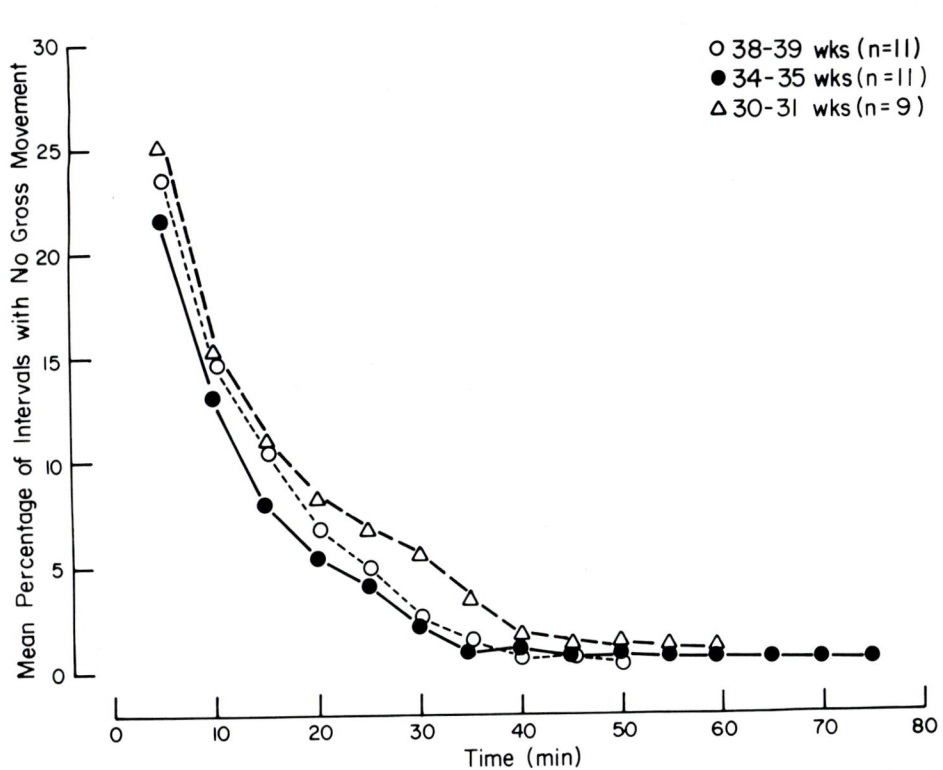

FIGURE 17–5. Composite plot of the percentage of intervals with no gross fetal body movements in nine fetuses at 30 to 31 weeks, 11 at 34 to 35 weeks, and 11 at 38 to 39 weeks, demonstrating a similar distribution at these different gestational ages. The longest period of fetal quiescence was 60 minutes at 30 to 31 weeks, 75 minutes at 34 to 35 weeks, and 50 minutes at 38 to 39 weeks. (From Patrick J, Campbell K, Carmichael L, et al: Patterns of gross fetal body movements over 24-hour observation intervals during the last 10 weeks of pregnancy. Am J Obstet Gynecol **142**:363, 1982.)

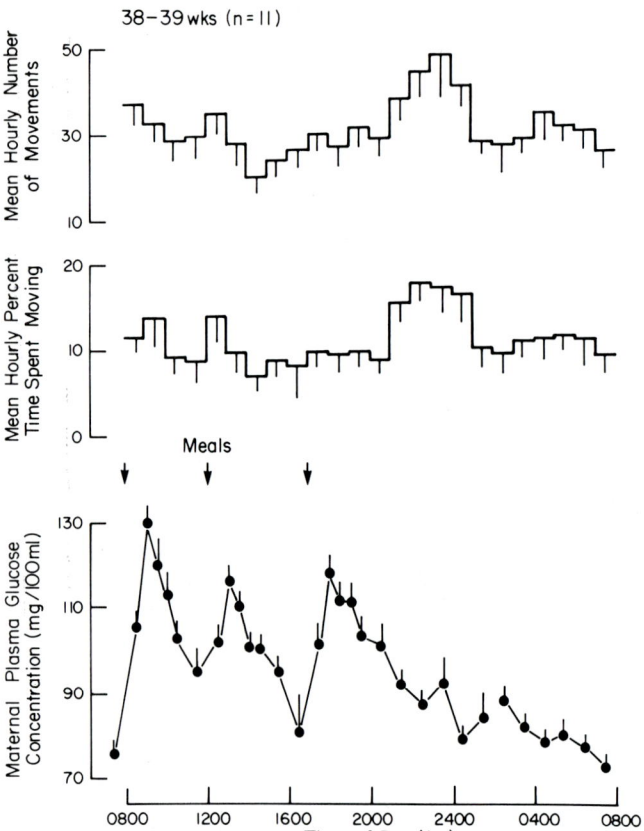

FIGURE 17–6. Maternal glucose concentrations, the average number of movements, and the percentage of time spent moving by fetuses plotted each hour of the day (± SEM) in 11 fetuses at 38 to 39 weeks gestational age. There was a peak in activity between 2100 and 0100 hours. (From Patrick J, Campbell K, Carmichael L, et al: Patterns of gross fetal body movements over 24-hour observation intervals during the last 10 weeks of pregnancy measured with a real-time scanner. Am J Obstet Gynecol **142**:363, 1982.)

crease in incidence (e.g., breathing movements and swallowing), an increase in incidence until a plateau is reached (e.g., general movements), or an increase in incidence followed by a decrease (e.g., startles). The majority of these movements, however, seem to occur at no regular interval with fetal quiescence usually no longer than 5 to 10 minutes (de Vries et al., 1985).

Continuous 24-hour recordings of gross fetal body movements at 24 to 28 weeks gestation have been reported by Nasello-Paterson et al. (1988) who found the mean incidence to be approximately 13 per cent, which is similar to the incidence reported over the last 10 weeks of pregnancy (Patrick et al., 1982). However, the total number of movements per hour shows a maturational decrease, suggesting that fetuses between 24 and 28 weeks gestation move significantly more often but with a shorter duration of movement than do fetuses between 30 and 39 weeks gestation. Although fetal movement activity is now becoming episodic and clustered with other behavioral variables, the longest period of quiescence was only 24 minutes, which is significantly less than observed during the

last 10 weeks of pregnancy, again suggesting that different norms need to be used in the evaluation of fetal health at earlier gestations. This group also noted a maturational change in the relationship of body movements to heart rate accelerations whereby the proportion of larger amplitudes of fetal heart rate accelerations (i.e., ≥15 bpm) increased with gestational age and the proportion of total heart rate accelerations associated with fetal body movements shifted from low amplitude types of accelerations (i.e., <15 bpm) to accelerations of higher amplitude (i.e., ≥15 bpm) as fetuses reached 32 weeks gestation (Fig. 17–7) (Natale et al., 1985). These maturational changes have obvious implications for non-stress test scoring in the fetus of younger gestational age.

Although the incidence of fetal body movements remains little changed over the last half of pregnancy, the emergence of behavioral states has a marked effect on the patterns of movement activity. As periods of coincidence of behavioral parameters give rise to clearly defined behavioral states, a maturational change in the duration of the so-called "activity-quiescent" cycle is seen with a progressive increase from approximately 20 minutes duration at 28 weeks of gestation to approximately 60 minutes by term, which is in fact similar in length to the sleep state cycling of the newborn infant (Nijhuis et al., 1982; Drogtrop et al., 1990).

Parturition

Gross fetal body movements, although somewhat reduced, continue to be evident throughout labor with a periodicity suggestive of "activity-quiescent" cycling (Richardson et al., 1979). Unlike fetal breathing movements, the incidence of gross body movements remains unchanged during the last 3 days prior to spontaneous labor at term (Carmichael et al., 1984).

Intrauterine Growth Restriction

The incidence and number of gross body movements is also variably decreased in patients with intrauterine growth restriction (Bekedam et al., 1985; Gagnon et al., 1988a; Ruedrich et al., 1989; Gagnon et al., 1990). Although of probable biological significance with a decrease in energy expenditure and thus oxygen requirements anticipated, considerable overlap with population norms is again evident, as previously discussed for fetal breathing movements. It is controversial whether maternal hyperoxia increases the incidence of these movements to a level similar to that of the well-grown fetus (Ruedrich et al., 1989; Gagnon et al., 1990). Given the inherent periodicity of fetal movement activity, this again is unlikely to serve as a useful clinical marker.

Assessment of Fetal Health

The potential usefulness of maternally perceived fetal movement activity as a measure of fetal health has long been recognized (Sadovsky and Polishuk, 1977). Recording of movement by the mother is simple, inexpensive, and readily available and does not require technical skill or sophisticated equipment. However, maternal perception of fetal activity can be

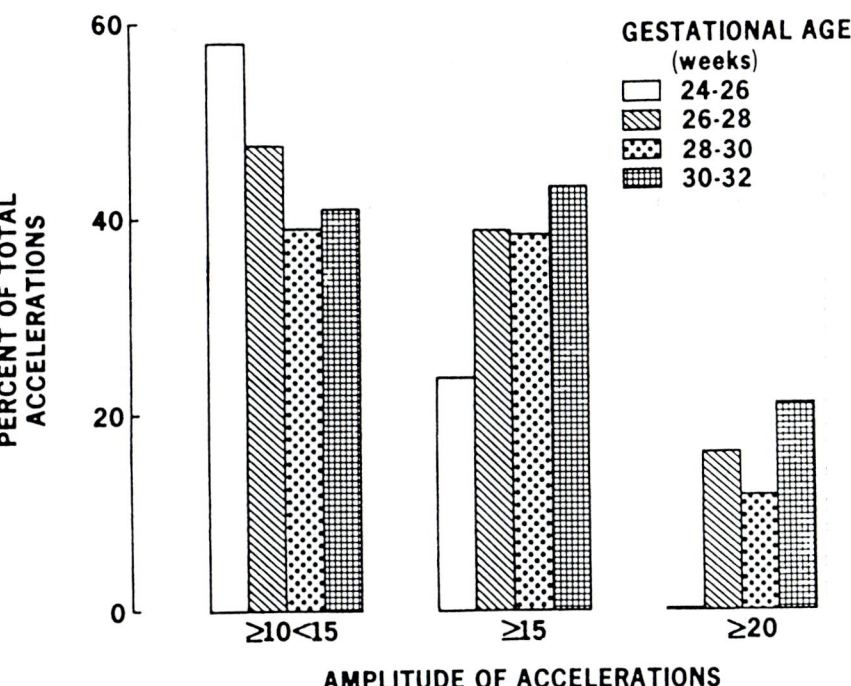

FIGURE 17–7. Frequency distribution of the amplitudes of fetal heart rate accelerations associated with fetal body movements. Significantly larger proportions of fetal heart rate accelerations ≥15 bpm and ≥20 bpm are associated with fetal body movements at 30 to 32 weeks gestation than at 24 to 26 weeks gestation (p <0.05). (From Natale R, Nasello C, Turliuk R: Longitudinal measurements of fetal breathing, body movements, heart rate, and heart rate accelerations and decelerations at 24 to 32 weeks of gestation. Am J Obstet Gynecol **151**:256, 1985.)

misleading, as some movements go undetected and others are wrongly recorded, instead representing Braxton Hicks contractions or maternal aortic pulsation and respiration. This contributes to the large intrapatient and interpatient variation in the monitoring of fetal movements and the difficulty in establishing population norms.

Connors et al. (1988b) have studied maternal perception of fetal activity from 24 weeks gestation until term. Although large interpatient variation in movement counts per hour was evident, only 2 per cent (28 to 40 weeks) to 4 per cent (24 to 27 weeks) of 1-hour observation periods were without perceived movement. When the observation period was extended to 2 consecutive hours, only five observations in one patient contained no movement. These findings correlate closely with the objective ultrasonography data reported by Patrick et al. (1982) and suggest that 2 hours is a sufficient period of time to allow for the normal periodicity of fetal movement activity.

The present use of fetal body movements in the assessment of fetal health is also dependent on its component part in biophysical profile scoring. Thus, much of the discussion on the predictive value of fetal breathing movements in the assessment of fetal health is also applicable to that for fetal gross body movements.

FETAL ACTIVITY AND VIBROACOUSTIC STIMULATION

Fetal Response to Stimulation

It is clinically important that periods of fetal quiescence combined with absence of heart rate accelerations may normally occur in human fetuses for up to 75 minutes, as described previously. As a result, there is some difficulty in separating healthy fetuses at rest from sick fetuses who are not moving because of hypoxemia and/or asphyxia. External physical manipulation of human fetuses does not change the overall pattern of gross fetal body movements (Richardson et al., 1981), nor does administration of glucose to women (Bocking et al., 1982). External vibroacoustic stimulation is the only stimulus that can reproducibly alter fetal heart rate and fetal movement patterns during the third trimester of human pregnancy (Gagnon et al., 1987b). This has led to substantial investigation into the safety and efficacy of the use of external vibroacoustic stimulation in assessing fetal health.

Structural Development of Fetal Sensory Receptors

The embryonic ear forms from an ectodermal thickening of the auditory placode, which is present in the 23-day-old human embryo (Altmann, 1950). As the placode invaginates into surrounding mesenchyme, a pit develops that assumes a vesicular shape and is termed the otocyst. In the 4- to 5-week embryo, the otocyst divides into two lobes; one lobe becomes the cochlea and the other the labyrinth (Ormerod, 1960). At 6 months, both the organ of Corti and the tunnel of Corti are present in all turns of the cochlea. Peripheral vibration-sensitive endings, including Meissner's and pacinian corpuscles which transmit vibrotactile stimuli, have been described in the hands of human fetuses at 24 weeks gestation. Therefore, by about the 24th week of intrauterine life, the cochlea and peripheral sensory end-organs have reached their normal development.

Functional Development of Fetal Sensory Receptors

In the adult, the ear responds to sound frequencies between approximately 20 and 20,000 Hz. Optimal response occurs at 2000 Hz (Schmidt, 1986). The nature of this frequency response is determined in large measure by the physical characteristics of the receiving organ, the nature of the external auditory canal, the tympanic membrane, and the ossicles that link the tympanic membrane through the middle ear to the fluids in the inner ear. Also, the ear is an impedance-matching device designed to receive sounds transmitted in air.

In utero the middle ear and external canals are filled with fluid, which would tend to dampen the frequency response of the tympanic membrane and ossicles and may prevent the middle ear from impedance matching. Therefore, fetuses probably require very high sound pressure levels to be able to detect sound.

Some evidence that human fetal auditory receptors are functional comes from records of evoked responses made from scalp electrodes during labor (Scibetta et al., 1971). Newborns exposed to sound stimuli have auditory brain responses (ABRs) that are neuroelectric signals recorded from EEG electrodes placed on the scalp. ABRs are now considered of value in evaluating newborn hearing function (Despland and Galambos, 1980). ABRs first appear between 26 and 28 weeks gestation in preterm human infants, and no ABRs can be detected before 26 weeks. The minimum stimulus intensity required to elicit evoked responses is 65 dB sound pressure level at 25 weeks (Starr et al., 1977); it decreases to 50 dB at 30 to 32 weeks (Uziel et al., 1980) and is adult-like at 35 weeks gestation (Uziel et al., 1980). More recently Blum et al. (1985) reported ABRs following external sound stimulation at 1000 Hz at 100 dB in a 35-week fetus with intact membranes, using magnetoencephalographic recordings of brain activity. The observation of ABRs as well as maturational changes have been confirmed in catheterized fetal lambs (Woods et al., 1984).

Fetal Sound Environment During Vibroacoustic Stimulation

In contrast to the neonate, the human fetus is surrounded by the fluid-filled amniotic cavity. Until recently it was not technically feasible to measure the fetal sound environment during the application of vibroacoustic stimulation (VAS) on the surface of the maternal abdomen using an electronic artificial larynx. Estimations of intrauterine sound pressure levels (SPLs) during VAS have varied from 90 to 111 dB (Smith et al., 1990), 95 dB (Birnholz and Benacerraf, 1983), 119 dB (Richards et al., 1991), and up to 139 dB (Gerhardt et al., 1988).

We measured the intrauterine background noise in ten women in active labor using a miniaturized hydrophone placed at the level of the fetal neck under ultrasonographic guidance (Benzaquen et al., 1990). In eight women no cardiovascular sound was audible, and the background intrauterine noise consisted pre-dominantly of low-frequency (i.e., less than 100 Hz) noise with maximum intensity of 85 dB at 12.5 Hz, which is the resonance frequency of the human body (Wasserman, 1990). Intermittent maternal bowel sounds and maternal vocalization featured well above the intrauterine background noise. During VAS, as used in clinical practice during active labor, the intra-uterine SPL increased to an average of 95 dB at frequencies between 87 and 20,000 Hz (Fig. 17–8) (Gagnon et al., 1992), which was similar to the overall SPL recently reported by Smith and associates (1990). In addition, our data indicated that a minimum thresh-old of 94 dB intrauterine SPL was necessary to elicit a reproducible fetal heart rate (FHR) response (Gagnon et al., 1992).

Gross Fetal Body Movements and Vibroacoustic Stimulation

Peiper (1925) reported that fetal movements occurred in response to the sound of an automobile horn within a few feet of the abdomen of near term pregnant women. The presence of a fetal "startle reflex" has been demonstrated during vibroacoustic stimulation (Leader et al., 1982). This "reflex" was defined as an immediate marked fetal response involving either trunk or limb movement that occurs during VAS and for about 2.5 seconds afterward.

Gelman and associates (1982) reported a significant increase in the number of fetal movements following a 2000-Hz, 110-dB stimulus applied on the maternal abdomen for one minute, but not after a 500 Hz stimulus. This increase in fetal activity persisted for 30 minutes after the stimulus. However, Schmidt and associates (1985), using sound stimulation without touching the maternal abdomen, were not able to observe any change in patterns of fetal activity or heart rate.

More recently, a prolonged increase in the incidence of fetal body movements has been reported following vibroacoustic stimulation with an electronic artificial larynx (Gagnon et al., 1986, 1987b; Yao et al., 1990). There was a significant but delayed increase in both number and incidence of gross fetal body movements between 10 and 30 minutes following a 5-second vibroacoustic stimulus. This delayed increase in body movements occurred in human fetuses only after 33 weeks gestation (Gagnon et al., 1986, 1987b). In fetuses between 26 and 32 weeks gestation, gross fetal body movements are not altered following VAS, demonstrating a maturational change in the fetal responses to VAS possibly related to the development of fetal behavioral states.

Fetal Breathing Movements and Vibroacoustic Stimulation

A significant decrease in fetal breathing movements has been reported only in term (>36 weeks) fetuses following vibroacoustic stimulation (Gagnon et al., 1987b). Figure 17–9 demonstrates a histogram plot of the mean percentage of total breath-to-breath intervals

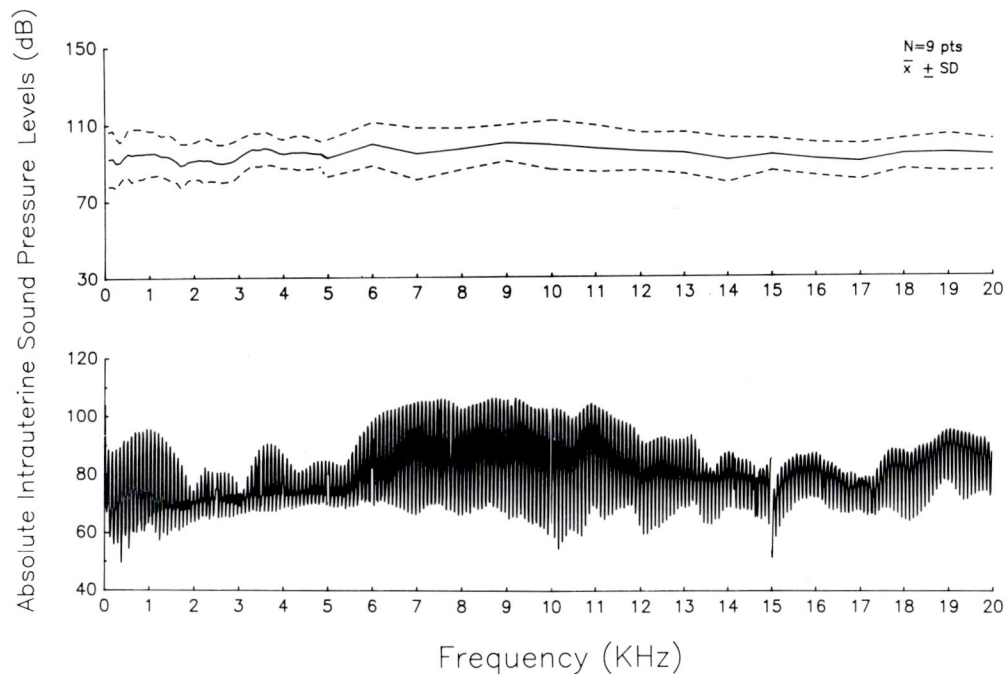

FIGURE 17–8. The mean (95 dB) ± 1 SD (15 dB) intrauterine sound pressure levels (re: 2×10^{-5} newtons/m²) during vibroacoustic stimulation at 0 cm from the surface of the maternal abdomen were plotted for frequencies between 87 and 20,000 Hz *(top)*. A typical example of intrauterine sound pressure levels recorded for frequencies between 87 and 20,000 Hz during vibroacoustic stimulation at 0 cm *(bottom)*. (From Gagnon R, Benzaquen S, Hunse C: The fetal sound environment during vibroacoustic stimulation in labor: Effect on fetal heart rate response. Obstet Gynecol **79**:950–955, 1992. Reprinted by permission from the American College of Obstetricians and Gynecologists.)

in successive 0.5-second increments in ten healthy term fetuses during the hour after control (N = 5) or vibroacoustic stimulation (N = 5). There is a skewed distribution of breath-to-breath intervals with a peak of 1.0 to 1.5 seconds after control, but during the hour after stimulus there is a broad distribution of breath-to-breath intervals at 1 to 2.5 seconds without a well-defined peak. This suggested that fetuses were breathing not only less frequently, but also more irregularly after stimulation, as is typical of a state of wakefulness (Nijhuis et al., 1982, 1983).

Fetal Heart Rate Response to Vibroacoustic Stimulation

In an attempt to detect deafness during the antenatal period, Johansson et al. (1964) found a significant increase in fetal heart rate for 5 seconds after application of a 3000-Hz stimulus at a sound pressure level of 110 dB for 1 second on the surface of the maternal abdomen. This effect on fetal heart rate has been noted by many authors (Davey et al., 1984; Grimwade et al., 1971; Jensen, 1984; Serafini et al., 1984) using different frequencies (range 500 to 3000 Hz) and sound pressure levels (range 70 to 130 dB). External stimulation with the electronic artificial larynx has produced the most reliable FHR response and is now widely used in clinical practice.

Using computerized fetal heart rate analysis, FHR responses to vibroacoustic stimulation in healthy human fetuses have been shown to be altered by

gestational age (Gagnon et al., 1987b). There is an immediate FHR response following stimulation characterized by an increase in duration of accelerations in fetuses from 26 weeks to term and an increase in basal fetal heart rate after 30 weeks gestation. There is also a delayed FHR response after 33 weeks gestation, which consists of an increase in the number of accelerations between 10 and 20 minutes following stimulus (Fig. 17–10) (Gagnon et al., 1987a, 1987b), and on occasion a persistent fetal tachycardia can last up to 1.5 hours following stimulation (Gagnon et al., 1987a, 1987b; Visser et al., 1989). The FHR response to VAS is believed to be due to a switch in fetal behavioral states from state 1F to state 4F, or due to a disruption of normal behavioral states. Numerous factors besides gestational age and unrelated to fetal hypoxemia and/or acidosis can alter fetal heart rate response to vibroacoustic stimulation; these factors are described in Table 17–3.

Clinical Significance

It is well documented that the presence of fetal body movements and FHR accelerations in response to VAS is associated with minimal risk (<1 per cent) of intrauterine death within a week (Smith et al., 1986). Although FHR accelerations induced by VAS may have the same predictive value for fetal outcome compared to currently used tests of antepartum fetal assessment, there are no randomized clinical trials that

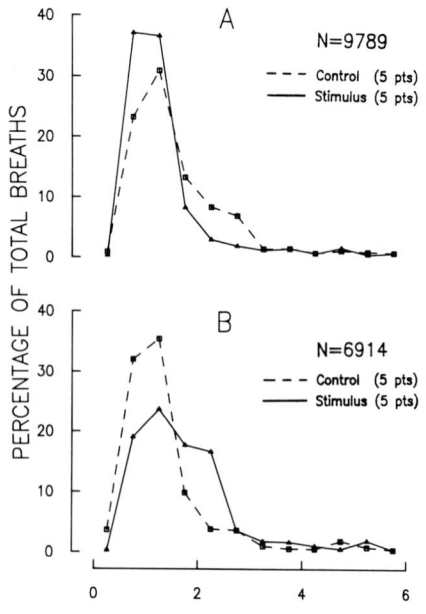

FETAL BREATH–TO–BREATH INTERVALS

(SECONDS)

FIGURE 17–9. Fetal breath-to-breath intervals were measured, and the histograms of the mean percentage of total breath-to-breath intervals in 0.5-second increments were plotted for 10 fetuses before stimulus (—) or control (---) *(A)*. The histograms of the mean percentage of total breath-to-breath intervals were also plotted for the same 10 fetuses after stimulus (—) or control (---) *(B)*. (From Gagnon R, Hunse C, Carmichael L, et al: Effects of vibratory acoustic stimulation on human fetal breathing and gross fetal body movements near term. Am J Obstet Gynecol **155**:1227, 1986.)

have shown that VAS can definitely replace biophysical profile testing (Richards, 1990).

Vibroacoustic stimulation has been shown to decrease testing time during antepartum fetal heart rate testing (Smith et al., 1986) and, in combination with assessment of amniotic fluid volume, might reduce the incidence of unexpected intrauterine fetal deaths (Clark et al., 1989).

Under certain conditions the FHR response to VAS

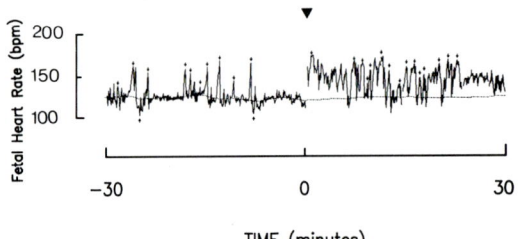

TIME (minutes)

FIGURE 17–10. A typical example of an increase in basal fetal heart rate and FHR accelerations following the application of a 5-second vibratory acoustic stimulus with an electronic artificial larynx. (From Gagnon R, Hunse C, Carmichael L, et al: External vibroacoustic stimulation near term: Fetal heart rate and heart rate variability responses. Am J Obstet Gynecol **156**:323, 1987a.)

TABLE 17–3.   Factors Affecting Fetal Heart Rate Response to Vibroacoustic Stimulation

Prestimulatory basal FHR	Inversely correlated with amplitude of first FHR acceleration (Gagnon et al., 1988b)
Prestimulus fetal behavioral state	FHR response more consistent during quiet (1F) sleep state (Devoe et al., 1990)
Intrauterine growth retardation	
≥32 weeks	Smaller amplitude and shorter duration of FHR response than normally grown fetus (Gagnon et al., 1988a)
<32 weeks	Rare FHR response (Gagnon et al., 1989)
Rupture of membranes	Decreased occurrence of FHR response (Richards et al., 1988)
Cervical dilatation	Inversely correlated with FHR response (Richards et al., 1988)
Intrauterine SPL reached during stimulus	Positively correlated with duration of first FHR acceleration (Gagnon et al., 1992)

may be difficult to interpret. The fetus may receive a subthreshold stimulus (Gagnon et al., 1992), have a high prestimulation baseline FHR (Gagnon et al., 1988b), or be immature (Gagnon et al., 1987b)—all factors that could lead to a falsely nonreactive test. Of more concern is the potentially reactive fetus following VAS in the presence of significant metabolic acidosis (Ingemarrsson et al., 1989), indicating that VAS may occasionally be a stimulus too strong to differentiate the healthy from the acidotic fetus. Therefore, if VAS is used to complement non-stress testing, these limitations should be taken into account when interpreting test results.

SUMMARY

The abundance of *in utero* movement activity and/or the resultant outcome from its limitation in either animal experimentation or human case reports would support an important role for such activity in fetal growth and development. With impairments in fetal oxygenation, a decrease in fetal neuromuscular activity may provide an adaptive mechanism whereby energy expenditure and thus oxygen requirements are decreased. Thus a lack of fetal activity, including both breathing and gross body movements, may serve as a marker for fetal hypoxemia and/or acidemia. However, a number of biological factors also affect these activities, the most important being the developmental aspects of the fetal behavioral state, which gives rise to the periodic nature of these movements. Gestational age, time of day, relationship to maternal meals, and maternal drug ingestion are also important considerations in the interpreting of fetal activity measurements. Additionally, it would appear that hypoxemia of a chronic nature must approach the level at which acidemia becomes apparent before a marked change in fetal behavioral activity is noted. Fetal biophysical assessment should be seen as a marker for moderate-to-severe hypoxemic change, with heightened surveillance required for the extremely "high-risk" pregnancy, as the time course for biophysical alteration before fetal demise may be relatively short.

REFERENCES

Altmann E: Normal development of the ear and its mechanics. Arch Otolaryngol 52:725, 1950.

Baskett TF, Gray JH, Prewett SJ, et al: Antepartum fetal assessment using a fetal biophysical profile score. Am J Obstet Gynecol 148:630, 1984.

Baskett TF: Gestational age and fetal biophysical assessment. Am J Obstet Gynecol 158:332, 1988.

Bekedam DJ, Visser GHA, de Vries JJ, Prechtl HFR: Motor behavior in the growth retarded fetus. Early Hum Dev 12:155, 1985.

Bekedam DJ, Mulder EJH, Snijders RJM, Visser GHA: The effects of maternal hyperoxia on fetal breathing movements, body movements and heart rate variation in growth retarded fetuses. Early Hum Dev 27:223, 1991.

Bennet L, Johnston BM, Gluckman PD: The central effects of morphine on fetal breathing movements in the fetal sheep. J Dev Physiol 8:297, 1986.

Benzaquen S, Gagnon R, Hunse C, et al: The intrauterine sound environment of the human fetus during labor. Am J Obstet Gynecol 163:484, 1990.

Berger PJ, Walker AM, Horne R, et al: Phasic respiratory activity in the fetal lamb during late gestation and labour. Respir Physiol 65:55, 1986.

Besinger RE, Compton AA, Hayashi RH: The presence or absence of fetal breathing movements as a predictor of outcome in preterm labor. Am J Obstet Gynecol 157:753, 1987.

Birnholz JC, Benacerraf BR: The development of human fetal hearing. Science 222:516, 1983.

Bissonnette JM, Hohimer AR, Conrad R, et al: Theophylline stimulates fetal breathing movements during hypoxia. Pediatr Res 28:83, 1990.

Blum T, Saling E, Bauer R: First magnetoencephalographic recordings of brain activity of a human fetus. Br J Obstet Gynaecol 92:1224, 1985.

Bocking A, Adamson L, Cousin A, et al: Effects of intravenous glucose injections on human fetal breathing movements and gross fetal body movements at 38 to 40 weeks gestational age. Am J Obstet Gynecol 142:606, 1982.

Bocking AD, Harding R: Effects of reduced uterine blood flow on electrocortical activity breathing and skeletal muscle activity in fetal sheep. Am J Obstet Gynecol 154:655, 1986.

Bocking AD, Gagnon R, Milne KM, White SE: Behavioral activity during prolonged hypoxemia in fetal sheep. J Appl Physiol 65:2420, 1988.

Boddy K, Dawes GS, Robinson JS: A 24-hour rhythm in the fetus. In Comline RS, Cross KW, Dawes GS, Nathanielsz PW (eds): Foetal and Neonatal Physiology. (Proceedings of the Sir Joseph Barcroft Centenary Symposium held at Cambridge, 25–27 July 1972). London, Cambridge University Press, 1973.

Boddy K, Dawes GS, Fisher R et al: Foetal respiratory movements, electrocortical and cardiovascular responses to hypoxaemia and hypercapnia in sheep. J Physiol (Lond) 243:500, 1974.

Boddy K, Dawes GS: Fetal breathing. Br Med Bull 32:1, 1975.

Boddy K, Dawes GS, Fisher RL, et al: The effects of pentobarbitone and pethidine on foetal breathing movements in sheep. Br J Pharmacol 57:311, 1976.

Boylan P, Lewis PJ: Fetal breathing in labor. Obstet Gynecol 56:35, 1980.

Boylan P, O'Donovan P, Owens OJ: Fetal breathing movements and the diagnosis of labor: A prospective analysis of 100 cases. Obstet Gynecol 66:517, 1985.

Brown R, Patrick J: The nonstress test: How long is enough? Am J Obstet Gynecol 141:646, 1981.

Bystrzycka EWA, Nail BS, Purves MJ: Central and peripheral neural respiratory activity in the mature sheep foetus and newborn lamb. Respir Physiol 25:199, 1975.

Campbell K: Ultradian rhythms in the human fetus during the last ten weeks of gestation: A review. Semin Perinatol 4(4):301, 1980.

Carmichael L, Campbell K, Patrick J: Fetal breathing, gross fetal body movements and maternal and fetal heart rates before spontaneous labor at term. Am J Obstet Gynecol 148:675, 1984.

Castle BM, Turnbull AC: The significance of preterm breathing. In Beard RW, Sharp F (eds): Preterm Labour and its Consequences. London, The Royal College of Obstetricians and Gynaecologists, 1985.

Challis J, Patrick J, Richardson B, Tevaarwerk G: Loss of diurnal rhythm in plasma estrone estradiol and estriol in women treated with synthetic glucocorticoids at 34 to 35 weeks gestation. Am J Obstet Gynecol 139:338, 1981.

Chapman RLK, Dawes GS, Rurak DW, Wilds PL: Intermittent breathing before death in fetal lambs. Am J Obstet Gynecol 131:894, 1978.

Clark SL, Sobey P, Jolley K: Nonstress testing with acoustic stimulation and amniotic fluid volume measurement: 5973 tests without unexpected fetal death. Am J Obstet Gynecol 160:694, 1989.

Clewlow F, Dawes GS, Johnston BM, Walker DW: Changes in breathing electrocortical and muscle activity in unanaesthetized fetal lambs with age. J Physiol 341:463, 1983.

Connors G, Hunse C, Carmichael L, et al: The role of carbon dioxide in the generation of human fetal breathing movements. Am J Obstet Gynecol 158:322, 1988a.

Connors G, Natale R, Nasello-Paterson C: Maternally perceived fetal activity from twenty-four weeks' gestation to term in normal and at risk pregnancies. Am J Obstet Gynecol 158:294, 1988b.

Connors G, Hunse C, Carmichael L, et al: Control of fetal breathing in the human fetus between 24 and 34 weeks' gestation. Am J Obstet Gynecol 160:932, 1989.

Davey DA, Dommisse J, Macnab M, Dacre D: The value of an auditory stimulatory test in antenatal fetal cardiotocography. Eur J Obstet Gynecol Reprod Biol 18:273, 1984.

Dawes GS, Fox HE, Leduc BM, et al: Respiratory movements and rapid eye movement sleep in the foetal lamb. J Physiol (Lond) 220:119, 1972.

de Vries JIP, Visser GHA, Prechtl HFR: The emergence of fetal behaviour. I. Qualitative aspects. Early Hum Dev 7:301, 1982.

de Vries JIP, Visser GHA, Prechtl HFR: The emergence of fetal behaviour. II. Quantitative aspects. Early Hum Dev 12:99, 1985.

Despland PA, Galambos R: The auditory brain stem response: A useful diagnostic tool in the intensive care nursery. Pediatr Res 14:154, 1980.

Devoe LD, Abduljabbar H, Carmichael L, et al: The effects of maternal hyperoxia on fetal breathing movements in third-trimester pregnancies. Am J Obstet Gynecol 148:790, 1984.

Devoe LD, Castillo RA, Searle N, Searle JS: Prognostic components of computerized fetal biophysical testing. Am J Obstet Gynecol 158:1144, 1988.

Devoe LD, Murray C, Faircloth D, et al: Vibroacoustic stimulation and fetal behavioural state in normal term human pregnancy. Am J Obstet Gynecol 163:1156, 1990.

Dornan JC, Ritchie JWK: Fetal breathing movements and maternal hyperoxia in the growth-retarded fetus. Br J Obstet Gynecol 90:210, 1983.

Drogtrop AP, Ubels R, Nijhuis JG: The association between fetal body movements, eye movements, and heart rate patterns in pregnancies between 25 and 30 weeks of gestation. Early Hum Dev 23:67, 1990.

Fox HE, Hohler CW: Fetal evaluation by real-time imaging. Clin Obstet Gynecol 20:339, 1977.

Fox HE, Steinbrecher M, Pessel D, et al: Maternal ethanol ingestion and the occurrence of human fetal breathing movements. Am J Obstet Gynecol 132:354, 1978.

Gagnon R, Benzaquen S, Hunse C: The fetal sound environment during vibroacoustic stimulation in labour: effect on fetal heart rate response. Obstet Gynecol 79:950, 1992.

Gagnon R, Hunse C, Carmichael L, Patrick J: Vibratory acoustic stimulation in 26- to 32-week small-for-gestational-age fetus. Am J Obstet Gynecol 160:160, 1989.

Gagnon R, Hunse C, Carmichael L, et al: Effects of vibratory acoustic stimulation on human fetal breathing and gross fetal body movements near term. Am J Obstet Gynecol 155:1227, 1986.

Gagnon R, Hunse C, Carmichael L, et al: External vibroacoustic stimulation near term: Fetal heart rate and heart rate variability responses. Am J Obstet Gynecol 156:323, 1987a.

Gagnon R, Hunse C, Carmichael L, Patrick J: Human fetal responses to vibratory acoustic stimulation from twenty-six weeks to term. Am J Obstet Gynecol **157**:1375, 1987b.

Gagnon R, Hunse C, Fellows F, et al: Fetal heart rate and activity patterns in growth-retarded fetuses: Changes after vibratory acoustic stimulation. Am J Obstet Gynecol **158**:265, 1988a.

Gagnon R, Hunse C, Patrick J: Fetal responses to vibratory acoustic stimulation: Influence of basal heart rate. Am J Obstet Gynecol **159**:835, 1988b.

Gagnon R, Hunse C, Vijan S: The effect of maternal hyperoxia on behavioral activity in growth-retarded human fetuses. Am J Obstet Gynecol **163**:1894, 1990.

Gelman SR, Wood S, Spellacy WN, Abrams RM: Fetal movements in response to sound stimulation. Am J Obstet Gynecol **143**:484, 1982.

Gerhardt KJ, Abrams RM, Kovaz B, et al: Intrauterine noise levels in pregnant ewes produced by sound applied to the abdomen. Am J Obstet Gynecol **159**:228, 1988.

Grimwade JG, Walker DW, Bartlett M, et al: Human fetal heart rate change and movement in response to sound and vibration. Am J Obstet Gynecol **109**:86, 1971.

Harding R, Sigger JN, Wickham PJD, Bocking AD: The regulation of flow of pulmonary fluid in fetal sheep. Respir Physiol **57**:47, 1984.

Hasan SU, Lee DS, Gibson DA, et al: Effect of morphine on breathing and behavior in fetal sheep. J Appl Physiol **64**:2058, 1988.

Hogg MIJ, Golding RH, Rosen M: The effect of doxapram on fetal breathing in the sheep. Br J Obstet Gynecol **84**:48, 1977.

Hohimer AR, Bissonnette JM: Effect of metabolic acidosis on fetal breathing movements in utero. Respir Physiol **43**:99, 1981.

Hohimer AR, Bissonnette JM, Richardson BS, Machida CM: Central chemical regulation of breathing movements in fetal lambs. Respir Physiol **51**:99, 1983.

Ingemarsson I, Alulkumaran S: Reactive fetal heart rate response to vibroacoustic stimulation in fetuses with low scalp blood pH. Br J Obstet Gynaecol **96**:562, 1989.

Ioffe S, Jansen AH, Chernick V: Maturation of spontaneous fetal diaphragmatic activity and fetal response to hypercapnia and hypoxemia. J Appl Physiol **63**:609, 1987.

Jansen AH, Ioffe S, Chernick V: Drug-induced changes in fetal breathing activity and sleep state. Can J Physiol Pharmacol **61**:315, 1983.

Jensen OH: Fetal heart rate response to a controlled sound stimulus as a measure of fetal well-being. Acta Obstet Gynaecol Scand **63**:97, 1984.

Johansson B, Wedenbergy E, Westen B: Measurement of tone response by the human fetus. A preliminary report. Acta Otolaryngol **57**:188, 1964.

Junge HD, Walter H: Behavioral states and breathing activity in the fetus near term. J Perinat Med **8**:150, 1980.

Kitterman JA: Fetal lung development. J Dev Physiol **6**:67, 1984.

Kitterman JA, Liggins GC, Clements JA, Tooley WH: Stimulation of breathing movements in fetal sheep by inhibitors of prostaglandin synthesis. J Dev Physiol **1**:453, 1979.

Kitterman JA, Liggins GC, Fewell JE, Tooley WH: Inhibition of breathing movements in fetal sheep by prostaglandins. J Appl Physiol **54**:687, 1983.

Koos BJ, Kitanaka T, Matsuda et al: Fetal breathing adaptation to prolonged hypoxaemia in sheep. J Dev Physiol **10**:161, 1988.

Leader LR, Baillie P, Martin B, Vermulen E: The assessment and significance of habituation to a repeated stimulus by human fetus. Early Hum Dev **7**:211, 1982.

Lewis P, Boylan P: Fetal breathing: A review. Am J Obstet Gynecol **134**:587, 1979.

Liggins GC: Growth of the fetal lung. J Dev Physiol **6**:237, 1984.

Luther ER, Gray JH, Scott K, et al: The effect of maternal glucose infusion on breathing movements in human fetuses with intrauterine growth retardation. Am J Obstet Gynecol **142**:600, 1982.

Maloney JE, Adamson TM, Brodecky V, et al: Modification of respiratory center output in the unanesthetized fetal sheep "in utero." J Appl Physiol **39**:552, 1975a.

Maloney JE, Adamson TM, Brodecky V, et al: Diaphragmatic activity and lung liquid flow in unanesthetized fetal sheep. J Appl Physiol **39**:587, 1975b.

Manning FA, Martin CB, Murata Y, et al: Breathing movements before death in the primate fetus (Macaca mulatta). Am J Obstet Gynecol **135**:71, 1979.

Manning FA, Morrison MB, Harman CR, Menticoglou SM: The abnormal fetal biophysical profile score. V. Predictive accuracy according to score composition. Am J Obstet Gynecol **162**:918, 1990.

Manning FA, Morrison I, Harman CR, et al: Fetal assessment based on fetal biophysical profile scoring: Experience in 19,221 referred high-risk pregnancies. Am J Obstet Gynecol **157**:880, 1987.

Manning FA, Platt LD, Sipos L: Antepartum fetal evaluation: development of a fetal biophysical profile. Am J Obstet Gynecol **136**:787, 1980.

Martin CB, Murata Y, Petrie RH, Parer JT: Respiratory movements in fetal rhesus monkeys. Am J Obstet Gynecol **119**:939, 1974.

Matsuda Y, Patrick J, Carmichael L, et al: Effects of sustained hypoxemia on the sheep fetus at mid-gestation: Endocrine cardiovascular and biophysical responses. Am J Obstet Gynecol **167**:531, 1992.

McGowan J, Devoe LD, Searle N, Altman R: The effects of long- and short-term maternal caffeine ingestion on human fetal breathing and body movements in term gestations. Am J Obstet Gynecol **157**:726, 1987.

McLeod W, Brien J, Carmichael L, et al: Maternal glucose injections do not alter the suppression of fetal breathing following maternal ethanol ingestion. Am J Obstet Gynecol **148**:634, 1984.

Murai DT, Lee C-CH, Wallen LD, Kitterman JA: Denervation of peripheral chemoreceptors decreases breathing movements in fetal sheep. J Appl Physiol **59**:575, 1985.

Nasello-Paterson C, Natale R, Connors G: Ultrasonic evaluation of fetal body movements over twenty-four hours in the human fetus at 24 to 28 weeks' gestation. Am J Obstet Gynecol **158**:312, 1988.

Natale R, Patrick J, Richardson B: Effects of maternal venous plasma glucose concentrations on fetal breathing movements. Am J Obstet Gynecol **132**:36, 1978.

Natale R, Clewlow F, Dawes GS: Measurement of fetal forelimb movements in lambs in utero. Am J Obstet Gynecol **158**:545, 1981.

Natale R, Nasello-Peterson C, Turliuk R: Longitudinal measurements of fetal breathing body movements, heart rate and heart rate accelerations and decelerations at 24 to 32 weeks of gestation. Am J Obstet Gynecol **151**:256, 1985.

Natale R, Nasello-Paterson C, Connors G: Patterns of fetal breathing activity in the human fetus at 24 to 28 weeks' gestation. Am J Obstet Gynecol **158**:317, 1988.

Nijhuis JG, Prechtl HFR, Martin CB, Botts RSGM: Are there behavioural states in the human fetus? Early Hum Dev **6**:177, 1982.

Nijhuis JG, Martin CB, Gommers S, et al: The rhythmicity of fetal breathing varies with behavioural state in the human fetus. Early Hum Dev **9**:1, 1983.

Ormerod FC: The pathology of congenital deafness in the child. *In* Ewing A (ed): The Modern Educational Treatment of Deafness. Manchester, Manchester University Press, 1960, p 811.

Patrick JE, Dalton KJ, Dawes GS: Breathing patterns before death in fetal lambs. Am J Obstet Gynecol **125**:73, 1976.

Patrick J, Natale R, Richardson B: Patterns of human fetal breathing activity at 34 to 35 weeks' gestational age. Am J Obstet Gynecol **132**:507, 1978.

Patrick J, Campbell K, Carmichael L, et al: A definition of human fetal apnea and the distribution of fetal apneic intervals during the last 10 weeks of pregnancy. Am J Obstet Gynecol **136**:471, 1980a.

Patrick J, Campbell K, Carmichael, L., et al: Patterns of human fetal breathing during the last 10 weeks of pregnancy. Obstet Gynecol **56**:24, 1980b.

Patrick J, Challis J, Campbell K, et al: Circadian rhythms in maternal plasma cortisol and estriol concentrations at 30 to 31, 34 to 35, and 38 to 39 weeks gestational age. Am J Obstet Gynecol **136**:325, 1980c.

Patrick J, Challis J, Campbell K, et al: Effects of synthetic glucocorticoid administration on human fetal breathing movements at 34 to 35 weeks' gestational age. Am J Obstet Gynecol **139**:324, 1981.

Patrick J, Campbell K, Carmichael L, et al: Patterns of gross fetal body movements over a 24-hour observation interval during the 1st 10 weeks of pregnancy measured with a real-time scanner. Am J Obstet Gynecol **142**:363, 1982.

Patrick J, Carmichael L, Chess L, Staples C: Accelerations of the human fetal heart rate at 38 to 40 weeks gestational age. Am J Obstet Gynecol **148**:35, 1984.

Patrick J, Richardson B: Clinical significance of fetal breathing and other movements. *In* Jones CT, Nathanielsz PW (eds): The Physiological Development of the Fetus and Newborn. London, Academic Press, 1985a.

Patrick J, Richardson B, Hasen G, et al: Effects of maternal ethanol infusion on fetal cardiovascular and brain activity in lambs. Am J Obstet Gynecol **151**:859, 1985b.

Patrick J, Challis JRG, Cross J: Effects of maternal indomethacin administration on fetal breathing movements in sheep. J Dev Physiol **9**:295, 1987a.

Patrick J, Challis JRG, Cross J, et al: The relationship between fetal breathing movements and prostaglandin E_2 during ACTH-induced labour in sheep. J Dev Physiol **9**:287, 1987b.

Peiper A: Sinnesempfindugen der kindes vor seiner geburt. Monalschr Kinderheilkd **29**:236, 1925.

Piercy WN, Day MA, Neims AH, Williams RL: Alteration of ovine fetal respiratory-like activity by diazepam, caffeine and doxapram. Am J Obstet Gynecol **127**:43, 1977.

Platt LD, Eglinton GS, Sipos L, et al: Further experience with the biophysical profile. Obstet Gynecol **61**:480, 1983.

Prechtl HFR: Prenatal development of postnatal behaviour. *In* Rauh H, Steinhausen H (eds): Psychobiology and Early Development. Elsevier Science Publishers, 1987.

Richards DS: The fetal vibroacoustic stimulation test: an update. Semin Perinatol **14**:305, 1990.

Richards DS, Abrams RM, Herhardt KJ, et al: Effects of vibration frequency and tissue thickness on intrauterine sound levels in sheep. Am J Obstet Gynecol **165**:438, 1991.

Richards DS, Cefalo RC, Thorpe JM, et al: Determinants of fetal heart rate response to vibroacoustic stimulation in labor. Obstet Gynecol **71**:535, 1988.

Richardson B, Natale R, Patrick J: Human fetal breathing activity during induced labor at term. Am J Obstet Gynecol **133**:147, 1979.

Richardson B, Campbell K, Carmichael L, Patrick J: Effects of external physical stimulation on fetuses near term. Am J Obstet Gynecol **139**:344, 1981.

Richardson B, Hohimer AR, Mueggler P, Bissonnette J: Effects of glucose concentration on fetal breathing movements and electrocortical activity in fetal lambs. Am J Obstet Gynecol **142**:678, 1982.

Richardson B, O'Grady JP, Olsen GD: Fetal breathing movements and the response to carbon dioxide in patients on methadone maintenance. Am J Obstet Gynecol **150**:400, 1984.

Richardson BS, Carmichael L, Homan J, Patrick JE: Electrocortical activity, electroocular activity and breathing movements in fetal sheep with prolonged and graded hypoxemia. Am J Obstet Gynecol **167**:553, 1992.

Ruckebusch Y, Gaujoux M, Eghbali B: Sleep cycles and kinesis in the foetal lamb. Electroencephalogr Clin Neurophysiol **42**:226, 1977.

Ruedrich DA, Devoe LD, Searle N: Effects of maternal hyperoxia on the biophysical assessment of fetuses with suspected intrauterine growth retardation. Am J Obstet Gynecol **161**:188, 1989.

Rurak DW, Gruber NC: Increased oxygen consumption associated with breathing activity in fetal lambs. J Appl Physiol **54**:701, 1983a.

Rurak DW, Gruber NC: The effect of neuromuscular blockade on oxygen consumption and blood gases in the fetal lamb. Am J Obstet Gynecol **145**:258, 1983b.

Sadovsky E, Polishuk WZ: Fetal movement in utero. Nature assessment, prognostic value, timing of delivery. Obstet Gynecol **50**:49, 1977.

Schifrin BS, Guntes V, Gergely RC, et al: The role of real-time scanning in antenatal fetal surveillance. Am J Obstet Gynecol **140**:525, 1981.

Schmidt W, Boos R, Gnirs LA, Schulze S: Fetal behavioural states and controlled sound stimulation. Early Hum Dev **12**:145, 1985.

Schmidt RF: Fundamentals of Sensory Physiology. 3rd ed. Berlin, Springer Verlag, 1986.

Scibetta JJ, Rosen MG, Hochburg CI, Chik L: Human fetal brain response to sound during labor. Am J Obstet Gynecol **109**:82, 1971.

Serafini P, Lindsay MJB, Nages DA, et al: Antepartum fetal heart rate response to sound stimulation: the acoustic stimulation test. Am J Obstet Gynecol **148**:41, 1984.

Smith GN, Brien JF, Carmichael L, et al: Development of tolerance to ethanol-induced suppression of breathing movements and brain activity in the near-term fetal sheep during short-term maternal administration of ethanol. J Dev Physiol **11**:189, 1989.

Smith CV, Phelan JP, Platt LD: Fetal acoustic stimulation testing (The Fas-test). II. A randomized clinical comparison with the nonstress test. Am J Obstet Gynecol **155**:131, 1986.

Smith CV, Satt B, Phelan JP, Paul RH: Intrauterine sound levels: Intrapartum assessment with an intrauterine microphone. Am J Perinatol **7**:312, 1990.

Stark RI, Myers MM: Effect of electroencephalographic state on fetal breathing activity in the baboon. Scientific abstract #264, Proceedings of the 39th Annual Meeting of the Society for Gynecologic Investigation, San Antonio, Texas, 1992.

Starr A, Amlie RN, Martin WH, et al: Development of auditory function in newborn infants revealed by auditory brainstem potentials. Pediatrics **60**:831, 1977.

Szeto HH, Hinman DJ: Prenatal development of sleep-wake patterns in sheep. Sleep **8**:347, 1985.

Szeto HH: Effects of narcotic drugs on fetal behavioral activity: Acute methadone exposure. Am J Obstet Gynecol **146**:211, 1983.

Thaler JS, Goodman JDS, Dawes GS: The effect of maternal smoking on fetal breathing rate and activity patterns. Am J Obstet Gynecol **138**:282, 1980.

Thorburn GD, Challis JRG: Control of parturition. Physiol Rev **59**:863, 1979.

Timor-Tritsch IE, Dierker LJ, Zador I, et al: Fetal movements associated with fetal heart rate accelerations and decelerations. Am J Obstet Gynecol **131**:276, 1978.

Uziel A, Marot M, Germain M: Les potentiels évoqué due nerf auditif et du tronc cérébral chez le nouveau-né et l'enfant. Rev Laryngol Otol Rhinol **101**:55, 1980.

van Vliet MAT, Martin CB, Nijhuis JG, Prechtl HFR: The relationship between fetal activity and behavioural states and fetal breathing movements in normal and growth-retarded fetuses. Am J Obstet Gynecol **153**:582, 1985.

Vintzileos AM, Campbell WA, Ingardia CJ, Nochimson DJ: The fetal biophysical profile and its predictive value. Obstet Gynecol **62**:271, 1983.

Vintzileos AM, Fleming AD, Scorza WE, et al: Relationship between fetal biophysical activities and umbilical cord blood gas values. Am J Obstet Gynecol **165**:707, 1991.

Visser GHA, Mulder HH, Wit HP, et al: Vibro-acoustic stimulation of the human fetus: Effects on behavioural state organization. Early Hum Dev **19**:285, 1989.

Walker DW: Effects of increased core temperature on breathing movements and electrocortical activity in fetal sheep. J Dev Physiol **10**:513, 1988.

Wasserman DE: Vibration: Principles, measurements and health standards. Semin Perinatol **14**:311, 1990.

Wilds PL: Observations of intrauterine fetal breathing movements—a review. Am J Obstet Gynecol **131**:315, 1978.

Wittman BK, Davison BM, Lyons E, et al: Real-time ultrasound observation of fetal activity in labour. Am J Obstet Gynecol **86**:178, 1979.

Woods JR, Plessinger M, Mack C: The fetal auditory brainstem response. Pediatr Res **18**:83, 1984.

Worthington D, Piercy WN, Smith BT: Effects of reduction of placental size in sheep. Obstet Gynecol **58**:215, 1981.

Woudstra BR, Aarnoudse JG, de Wolf THM, Zijlstra WG: Nuchal muscle activity at different levels of hypoxemia in fetal sheep. Am J Obstet Gynecol **162**:559, 1990.

Yao QW, Jakobsson J, Nymon M, et al: Fetal responses to different intensity levels of vibroacoustic stimulation. Obstet Gynecol **75**:206, 1990.

CHAPTER

FETAL CARDIOVASCULAR PHYSIOLOGY

MICHAEL A. HEYMANN, M.D.

BLOOD FLOW PATTERNS AND OXYGEN DELIVERY

In the mammalian adult, oxygenation occurs in the lungs, and oxygenated blood returns via the pulmonary veins to the left side of the heart to be ejected by the left ventricle into the systemic circulation. In the fetus, gas exchange occurs in the placenta, and the fetal lungs are nonfunctional as far as the transfer of oxygen and carbon dioxide is concerned. In order for oxygenated blood derived from the placenta to reach the systemic circulation, the fetal circulation is so arranged that several sites of intercommunication (shunts) are present. In addition, preferential flow and streaming occur to limit the disadvantages of intermixing of the oxygenated and deoxygenated blood returning to the heart. The patterns of blood flow to and from the fetal heart are shown diagrammatically in Figure 18–1. With fetal stress, these preferential streaming patterns may be modified even more to mitigate the adverse effects of disorders such as reduced umbilical blood flow and fetal hypoxemia. Little quantitative information regarding primate fetal circulation is available; the data presented here were obtained mainly from fetal lambs.

Venous Return to the Heart

About 40 per cent of total fetal cardiac output (about 200 ml per kg of fetal weight per min) is distributed to the placental circulation; a similar amount will return to the heart via the umbilical venous system. Because umbilical venous blood is the most highly saturated blood in the fetal circulation (Fig. 18–2), distribution of umbilical venous return is most impor-

tant in determining oxygen delivery to fetal tissues. After entering the intra-abdominal portion of the umbilical vein, a portion of umbilical venous blood flow supplies the liver; the remainder passes through the ductus venosus, which directly connects the umbilical vein–portal sinus confluence to the inferior vena cava (see Figs. 18–1 and 18–2). Unlike the umbilical and portal veins, the ductus venosus has no direct branches to the liver. Umbilical venous blood can enter the ductus venosus directly. Portal venous return, however, can reach the ductus venosus only through the portal sinus (Figs. 18–2 and 18–3) (Bristow et al., 1981). Approximately 50 per cent of umbilical blood flow passes through the ductus venosus; the remainder enters the hepatic–portal venous system and passes through the hepatic vasculature (Edelstone et al., 1978). The fetal liver receives its blood supply not only from the umbilical vein, but also from the portal vein and hepatic artery. In normal fetal lambs *in utero*, umbilical venous blood flow contributes approximately 75 to 80 per cent of total blood supply of the liver (Edelstone et al., 1978, 1980; Bristow et al., 1983). Portal venous blood flow accounts for about 15 per cent, and hepatic arterial blood flow from the aorta represents only 4 to 5 per cent. The distribution of blood flow from these sources to various parts of the liver is quite different. Hepatic arterial blood flow to the liver is equally distributed to the right and left lobes; however, the left lobe is supplied almost exclusively by umbilical venous blood (more than 95 per cent). In contrast, the right lobe receives both umbilical venous blood (about 60 per cent) and portal venous blood (about 30 per cent). Because umbilical venous blood supplies a major portion of flow to the right liver lobe by traversing the portal sinus, little if any portal venous blood reaches the ductus venosus. The

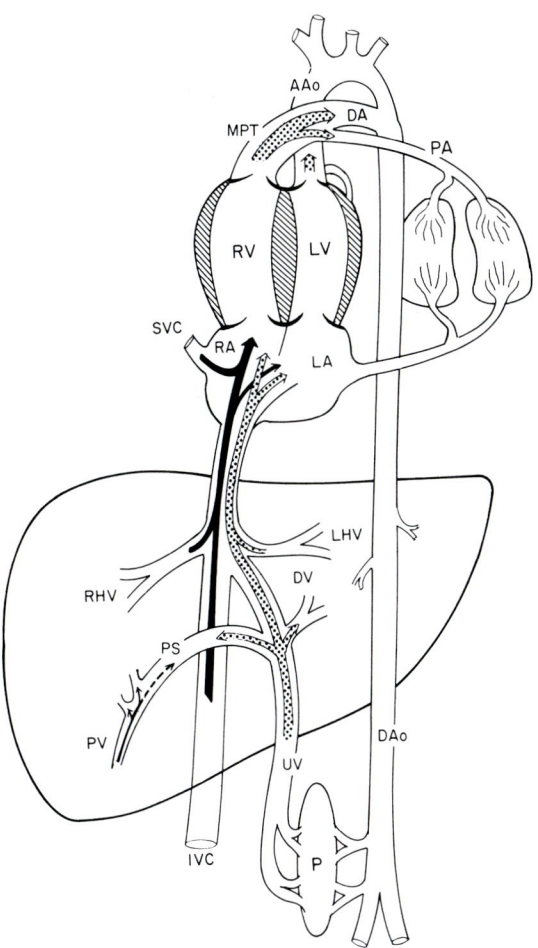

FIGURE 18–1. Diagrammatic representation of the normal fetal circulation and major fetal flow patterns. *IVC* = inferior vena cava; *P* = placenta; *UV* = umbilical vein; *PV* = portal vein; *PS* = portal sinus; *DV* = ductus venosus; *RHV* = right hepatic vein; *LHV* = left hepatic vein; *SVC* = superior vena cava; *RA* = right atrium; *LA* = left atrium; *RV* = right ventricle; *LV* = left ventricle; *MPT* = main pulmonary trunk; *AAo* = ascending aorta; *DA* = ductus arteriosus; *PA* = main branch pulmonary arteries; *DAo* = descending aorta.

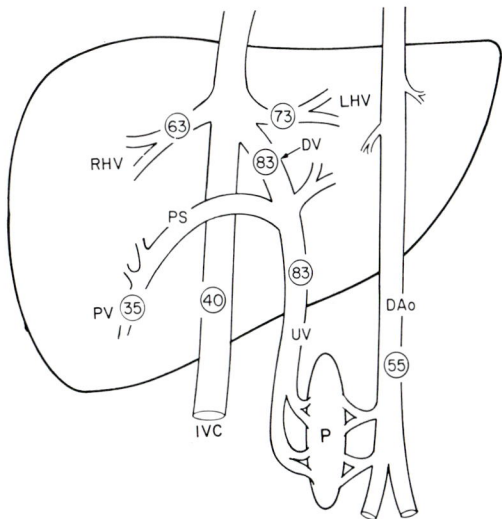

FIGURE 18–2. Representative normal hemoglobin oxygen saturation data (numbers indicate per cent saturation) in the umbilical, inferior vena caval, and hepatic venous drainage in fetal lambs. See Figure 18–1 for key to abbreviations.

desaturated inferior vena cava stream returning from the lower body produce preferential flow of umbilical venous return into the left atrium and thence the left ventricle and ascending aorta (Behrman et al., 1970; Edelstone and Rudolph, 1979; Reuss et al., 1981). Of particular importance is preferential streaming of umbilical venous blood to the brain and myocardium.

The preferential streaming of umbilical venous return to the left lobe of the liver and portal venous

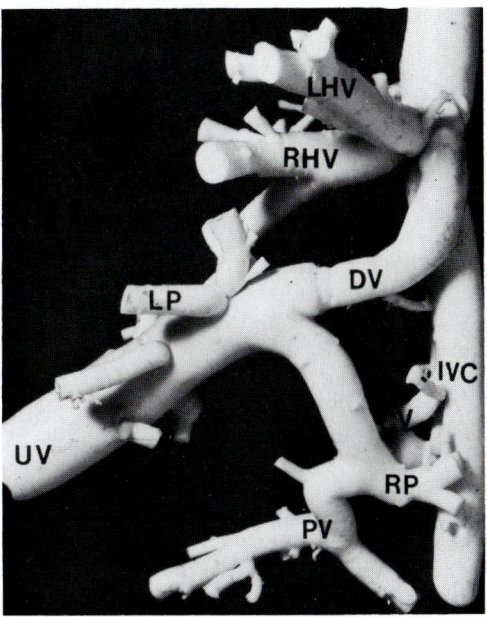

FIGURE 18–3. Silicone rubber cast of major vascular channels in the liver of a fetal lamb. *RP* and *LP* = right and left portal branches to liver parenchyma; *CV* = caudate lobe vein. See Figure 18–1 for key to other abbreviations. (From Bristow J, Rudolph AM, Itskovitz J: A preparation for studying liver blood flow, oxygen consumption, and metabolism in the fetal lamb *in utero.* J Dev Physiol **3**:255, 1981.)

blood in the ductus venosus, therefore, has pH, blood gas values, and hemoglobin oxygen saturation similar to those of umbilical venous blood. The portion of umbilical venous blood flow that passes via the ductus venosus directly into the inferior vena cava meets the systemic venous drainage from the lower body.

Blood flow through the thoracic inferior vena cava represents approximately 65 to 70 per cent of venous return to the heart; flow from the ductus venosus accounts for about one-third of this (Rudolph and Heymann, 1970; Edelstone et al., 1978). The two streams—one from the abdominal inferior vena cava and one from the ductus venosus—do not mix, and they demonstrate definite streaming within the thoracic inferior vena cava; the well-oxygenated blood derived from the ductus venosus occupies the dorsal and leftward portion of the inferior vena cava (Edelstone and Rudolph, 1979). This separation of the more highly saturated umbilical venous stream and the return to the right lobe also affects the distribution of oxygenated blood to the fetal body. The left hepatic lobe is perfused with umbilical venous blood, which has an oxygen saturation of 80 to 85 per cent, whereas the right lobe is perfused by a mixture of umbilical and portal venous blood, which has a much lower oxygen saturation (about 35 per cent) (see Fig. 18–2). The oxygen saturation of blood in the hepatic veins reflects this difference in perfusion saturation (Bristow et al., 1981, 1983). The oxygen saturation in left hepatic venous blood is about 10 per cent lower than umbilical venous blood, but about 10 per cent higher than right hepatic venous blood, in which the saturation more closely approximates that in the descending aorta. In fetal lambs, the ductus venosus and left hepatic vein drain into the inferior vena cava, essentially at a common point; partial valves are seen over the entrance of the hepatic vein and ductus venosus into the inferior vena cava (Bristow et al., 1981). Similarly, the entrance of the right hepatic vein into the inferior vena cava has a valve-like membrane overlying the ostium. This arrangement probably allows left hepatic venous blood to be distributed in a manner similar to that of ductus venosus blood, whereas right hepatic venous blood is distributed similarly to the abdominal inferior vena caval stream. This is particularly important because about half of umbilical venous return passes through the liver, thereby accounting for about 20 per cent of total venous return to the heart. In fetal lambs, left hepatic venous blood flow follows the same pattern as ductus venosus flow, with preferential streaming to the brain and heart (Bristow et al., 1983). Similarly, right hepatic blood flow follows the distribution pattern of abdominal inferior vena caval blood flow.

The inferior vena caval blood then enters the right atrium, and because of the position of the foramen ovale, more preferential streaming occurs. The foramen ovale is situated low in the interatrial septum, close to the inferior vena cava. The cephalad margin of the foramen, formed by the lower margin of the septum secundum, lies on the right side of the atrial septum; it is called the *crista dividens* and is positioned so that it overrides the orifice of the inferior vena cava. The crista dividens therefore splits the inferior vena caval blood stream into an anterior and rightward stream that enters the right atrium and a posterior and leftward stream that passes through the foramen ovale into the left atrium; it is this latter stream that has the more highly saturated blood returning from the umbilical circulation through the ductus venosus and left hepatic lobe. Despite this anatomic arrangement and the preferential streaming within the inferior vena cava, some mixing of blood does occur: a portion of the more highly saturated umbilical venous blood passes directly into the right atrium, and some desaturated abdominal inferior vena caval blood passes into the left atrium. The net result, however, is still a significantly higher saturation in the left atrium than in the right (Fig. 18–4).

Blood returning to the heart via the superior vena cava also streams preferentially once it reaches the right atrium. The crista interveniens, situated in the posterolateral aspect of the right atrial wall, effectively

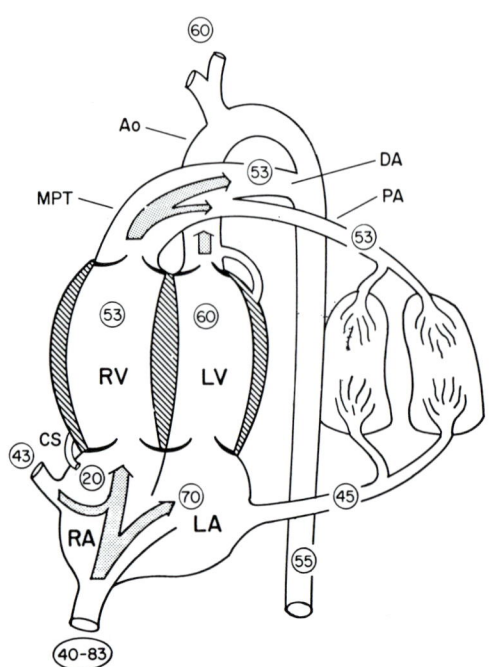

FIGURE 18–4. Representative normal hemoglobin oxygen saturation data (numbers indicate per cent saturation) in the heart and major vascular channels in fetal lambs. *CS* = coronary sinus. See Figure 18–1 for key to other abbreviations.

directs superior vena caval blood toward the tricuspid valve. The coronary sinus, which drains blood from the left ventricular myocardium, enters the right atrium between the crista dividens and the tricuspid valve; the very desaturated coronary venous return (saturation about 20 per cent), therefore, is also preferentially directed toward the tricuspid valve. This preferential streaming of superior vena caval and coronary sinus venous return to the right ventricle is also advantageous in the fetal circulation, because this very desaturated blood is preferentially directed toward the placenta for reoxygenation. Pulmonary venous return to the heart enters the left atrium, where it mixes with the portion of inferior vena caval blood that has crossed the foramen ovale to enter the left atrium.

Approximately 65 per cent of total cardiac output reaches the lower body and placenta and returns via the thoracic inferior vena cava to the heart (Fig. 18–5). Of this inferior vena caval return, approximately 40 per cent crosses the foramen ovale to the left atrium; the remaining 60 per cent enters the right ventricle across the tricuspid valve. The amount of inferior vena caval return crossing the foramen ovale therefore represents about 27 per cent of total fetal cardiac output. This blood then combines with pulmonary venous return (about 8 per cent of total fetal cardiac output) and represents the output of the left ventricle, or approximately 35 per cent of total fetal cardiac output. The venous return from the superior vena cava, the coronary sinus, and the remainder of the inferior vena caval return (about 40 per cent of total fetal cardiac output) enters the right ventricle and represents the portion of total fetal cardiac output ejected by the right

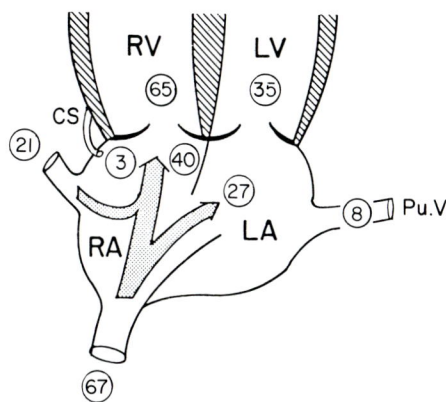

FIGURE 18–5. Representative values for percentages of fetal cardiac output (combined ventricular output) returning to the heart in fetal lambs. *Pu.V* = pulmonary vein; *CS* = coronary sinus. See Figure 18–1 for key to other abbreviations.

ventricle (about 65 per cent of total fetal cardiac output).

Cardiac Output and Its Distribution

In the fetus, because of the blood flow across the ductus arteriosus into the descending aorta, lower body organs are perfused by both the right and left ventricles (across the aortic isthmus). For this reason and also because of intracardiac shunting, it is customary to consider fetal cardiac output the total output of the heart, or combined ventricular output. In fetal lambs this is about 450 ml/kg/min. Unlike the adult, and because of the various sites of intracardiac and extracardiac shunting, the left and right ventricles in the fetus do not eject in series and therefore need not have the same stroke volume. In fact, as shown in Figure 18–6, the right ventricle ejects approximately two-thirds of total fetal cardiac output (about 300 ml/kg/min), whereas the left ventricle ejects only a little more than one-third (about 150 ml/kg/min) (Heymann et al., 1973a). Echocardiographic studies in human pregnancy have suggested that the right ventricle also dominates the left (Sahn et al., 1980; Reed et al., 1986; DeSmedt et al., 1987). Of the 65 per cent of cardiac output ejected by the right ventricle, only a small amount (8 per cent) flows through the pulmonary arteries to the lungs. The remainder (57 per cent) crosses the ductus arteriosus and enters the descending aorta. Since right ventricular output represents all superior vena caval and coronary sinus return, this allows unoxygenated venous blood to be preferentially returned to the placenta. Left ventricular output (about 35 per cent of cardiac output) enters the ascending aorta; in the fetal lamb, approximately 21 per cent reaches the brain, head, upper limbs, and upper thorax. About 10 per cent of cardiac output traverses the aortic isthmus and joins the blood flowing across the ductus arteriosus to perfuse the descending aorta. As shown in Figure 18–4, the level of hemoglobin oxygen saturation in the ventricles and great arteries is determined by the streaming patterns into, through,

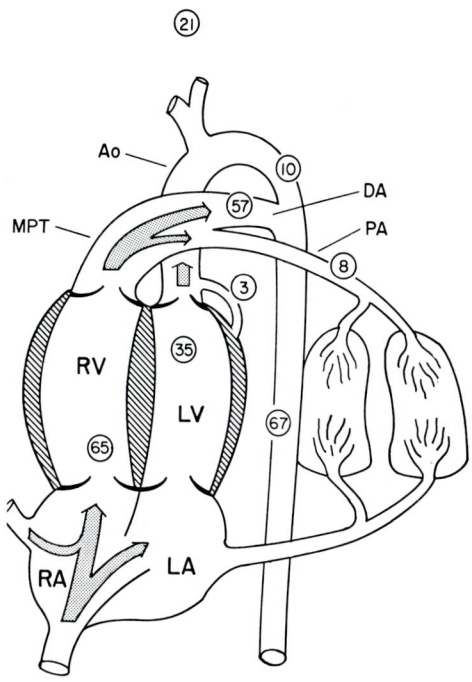

FIGURE 18–6. Representative normal values for percentages of total cardiac output (combined ventricular output) ejected by the heart and passing through the major arteries leaving the heart in fetal lambs. *Ao* = aorta. See Figure 18–1 for key to other abbreviations.

and out of the fetal heart. The highly saturated umbilical venous return streams preferentially across the foramen ovale into the left atrium, where it mixes with the relatively small amount of desaturated blood returning from the pulmonary veins. The net result is that blood ejected by the left ventricle to the ascending aorta is relatively well oxygenated (saturation about 60 per cent). On the other hand, the extremely desaturated coronary sinus venous return and the desaturated blood returning from the brain and upper body flow almost exclusively across the tricuspid valve into the right ventricle. This blood mixes with the inferior vena caval stream, which is primarily composed of desaturated blood returning from the lower body, but also contains some umbilical venous return. The net result is that the oxygen saturation of blood in the right ventricle is lower than that in the left. This blood perfuses the fetal lungs and also traverses the ductus arteriosus to the descending aorta, from which it perfuses lower body organs and also reaches the placenta for reoxygenation.

Blood gas and pH values in the fetus also reflect the preferential streaming patterns (Table 18–1). The data

TABLE 18–1. Normal Fetal pH and Blood Gas Data

	UMBILICAL VEIN	DESCENDING AORTA	ASCENDING AORTA
pH	7.40–7.43	7.36–7.39	7.37–7.40
Po₂(torr)	28–32	20–23	21–25
Pco₂(torr)	38–42	43–48	41–45

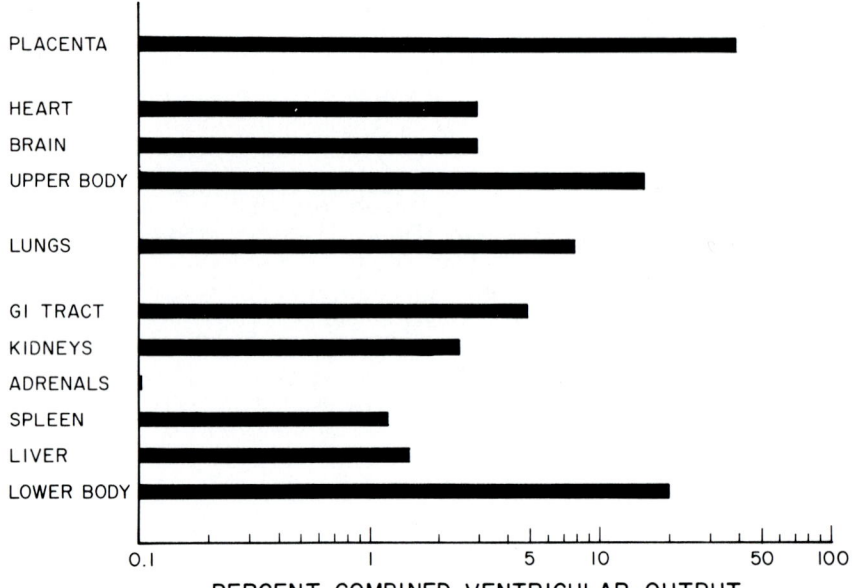

FIGURE 18–7. Representative normal values for the percentages of total cardiac output (combined ventricular output) distributed to different organs or parts in fetal lambs.

shown represent values usually found in healthy, catheterized fetal animals. There is interanimal as well as daily variability. During a normal uterine contraction, arterial blood has a lower partial pressure of oxygen (Po_2) than under truly resting conditions. In addition, over the last 7 to 10 days of gestation, Po_2 declines slightly and Pco_2 increases commensurately.

The distribution of blood flow to individual organs is shown in Figure 18–7. Because arterial blood supply to lower body organs is derived from both the left and right ventricles, it is customary to express organ flow as a percentage of the combined output of both ventricles, that is, of the combined ventricular output. Typical values are shown in Figure 18–7 (Rudolph and Heymann, 1970; Peeters et al., 1979). These values remain fairly constant throughout the latter third of gestation, the period in which such measurements have been made. There is, however, a slight increase in the percentage of combined ventricular output distributed to the heart, brain, and gastrointestinal tract in the 10 days prior to parturition. The flow distributed to the lungs increases from approximately 4 per cent to approximately 8 per cent of combined ventricular output between 125 and 130 days (0.85) of gestation. Organ blood flows are shown in Table 18–2. Umbilical placental blood flow is usually not considered in relationship to placental weight, which is quite variable, but rather is expressed in relationship to fetal weight, like combined ventricular output. Placental blood flow is approximately 200 ml/kg/min.

Intracardiac and Vascular Pressures

Vascular pressure in the fetus reflects the preferential streaming patterns described above. Although the ductus venosus is a fairly large, widely dilated structure, there is a high flow returning from the placenta through the umbilical veins and therefore resistance to flow; umbilical venous pressure is generally 3 to 5 mm Hg higher than that in the inferior vena cava (Fig. 18–8). Right atrial pressure is also higher than left atrial because of the greater volume of flow through the right atrium. Although the ductus arteriosus is widely patent, it too offers a small resistance to flow. Therefore, systolic pressures in the main pulmonary trunk and the right ventricle are slightly higher (1 to 2 mm Hg) than those in the aorta and left ventricle. The representative pressure data shown in Figure 18–8 would be expected in a fetus close to term. Arterial pressures increase slowly and progressively over the last third of gestation, reaching these values shortly before parturition. Measurement of intravascular pressures in the fetus reflects the additional amniotic pressure not found after birth. Because intra-amniotic pressure was used as the zero reference point, the values presented exclude this additional pressure and are therefore true vascular pressures.

MYOCARDIAL FUNCTION

Cardiac output is determined by the inter-relationships of preload, afterload, myocardial contractility,

TABLE 18–2. Organ Blood Flows in Normal Fetal Lambs Close to Term

ORGAN	BLOOD FLOW (ml/100 gm organ weight/ min)
Heart	180
Brain	125
Upper body	25
Lungs	100
GI tract	70
Kidneys	150
Adrenals	200
Spleen	200
Liver (hepatic arterial)	20
Lower body	25

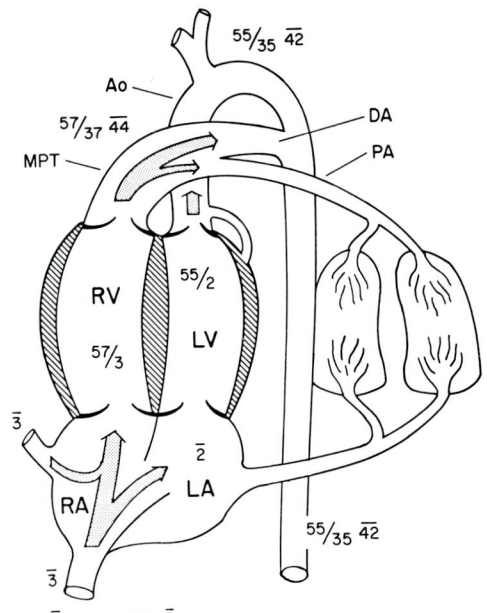

FIGURE 18–8. Representative normal pressures (mm Hg) in various vessels and cardiac chambers in fetal lambs. *Ao* = aorta. See Figure 18–1 for key to other abbreviations.

and heart rate. Preload or ventricular filling pressure reflects the initial muscle length, which by the Frank-Starling principle influences the development of myocardial force. Afterload, or the impedance to ejection from the ventricles, is reflected basically by arterial pressure. Contractility reflects the intrinsic inotropic capability of the myocardium. Studies of fetal myocardium show immaturity of structure, function, and sympathetic innervation relative to the adult (Friedman, 1973; Heymann and Rudolph, 1973b; Kirkpatrick et al., 1976; Gilbert, 1980, 1982). At all muscle lengths along the length-tension curve, the active tension generated by fetal myocardium is lower compared with adult myocardium (Friedman, 1973). In addition, resting, or passive, tension is higher in fetuses than in adults, suggesting lower compliance of fetal myo-

cardium. Studies in chronically instrumented, intact fetal lambs showed that after volume loading by the infusion of blood or saline, the right ventricle is unable to increase stroke work or output to the same extent as in the adult (Heymann and Rudolph, 1973b). This is particularly true in less mature fetuses, in whom right ventricular end-diastolic pressure is markedly elevated without any obvious change in right ventricular stroke work (Fig. 18–9). Other studies have demonstrated similar results for both the left and right ventricles, but with some ability to increase output or work at lower pressures, between 2 and 5 mm Hg (Kirkpatrick et al., 1976; Gilbert, 1980, 1982). More recently, the previously observed limitations in stroke work increase with increasing filling pressure has been shown to be afterload dependent and, for the left ventricle, also probably affected by right ventricular mechanical constraint (Hawkins et al., 1989; Teitel et al., 1991). Fetal and adult sarcomeres have equivalent lengths (Sheldon et al., 1976), but there are major ultrastructural differences between fetal myocardium and adult myocardium. The diameter of the fetal cells is smaller and, perhaps more importantly, the proportion of noncontractile mass (that is, of nuclei, mitochondria, and surface membranes) to the number of myofibrils is significantly greater than in the adult. In the fetal myocardium, only about 30 per cent of the muscle mass consists of contractile elements; in the adult the proportion is about 60 per cent. These ultrastructural differences are probably responsible for the age-dependent differences in performance (Friedman, 1973).

In newborn lambs, stroke volume is decreased at afterload levels considered low for adult animals (Downing et al., 1965). Gilbert (1982) has shown that in fetal animals, an increase in arterial pressure of about 15 mm Hg, produced by methoxamine infusion, depresses the cardiac function curve so that cardiac output averages 25 to 30 per cent less than normal. The extent of shortening is less in the fetus at any level of tension than in the adult, a potential explanation for the effects of afterload on stroke volume (Friedman, 1973).

In chronically instrumented fetal lambs, there is a

FIGURE 18–9. Right ventricular function curves in three fetal lambs of different gestational ages (term is about 145 days).

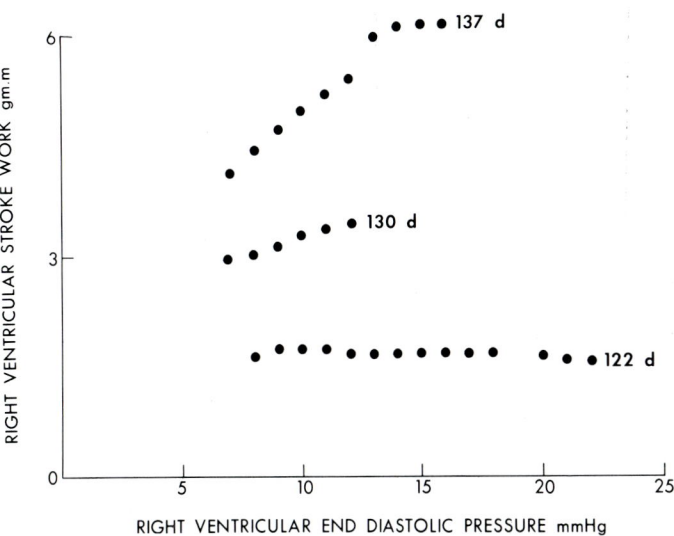

close relationship between cardiac output and heart rate. Spontaneous and induced changes in heart rate are associated with corresponding changes in left or right ventricular output. Increasing heart rate from the resting level of about 180 beats/min up to 250 to 300 beats/min increases cardiac output 15 to 20 per cent. Likewise, decreasing heart rate below the resting level significantly decreases ventricular output.

The fetal heart therefore appears to operate normally near the top of its cardiac function curve. An increase in heart rate can result in a modest increase in output. Above an atrial filling pressure of approximately 8 mm Hg, there is little or no increase in output because the length-tension relationship has reached a plateau. In addition, the fetal heart is sensitive to changes in afterload.

Sympathetic and Parasympathetic Innervation

Isolated fetal cardiac tissue has a lower threshold of response to the inotropic effects of norepinephrine than adult cardiac tissue and is also more sensitive to norepinephrine throughout dose-response curves (Friedman, 1973). Because isoproterenol, a direct beta-adrenergic agonist that is not taken up and stored in sympathetic nerves, has similar effects on fetal and adult myocardium, the supersensitivity of fetal myocardium to norepinephrine is probably due to incomplete development of sympathetic innervation in fetal myocardium. Myocardial concentrations of norepinephrine in the fetus within several weeks of term are significantly lower than in newborn animals, and activity of tyrosine hydroxylase, the intraneuronal enzyme responsible for the first transformation in catecholamine biosynthesis, is also reduced (Friedman, 1973). In contrast, adrenal gland tyrosine hydroxylase activity at the same gestational age is not suppressed, possibly because the decrease in myocardial activity is related to delayed sympathetic innervation rather than to a generalized immaturity. Monoamine oxidase, the enzyme responsible for oxidative deamination of norepinephrine, is also present in lower concentrations in the fetal heart than in the adult. Histochemical evaluation of the development of sympathetic innervation using the monoamine fluorescence technique has further substantiated the delayed development of sympathetic innervation of the fetal myocardium. At term, sympathetic innervation is incomplete. Patterns of staining indicate that there is a progression of innervation, starting at the area of the sinoatrial node and progressing toward the left ventricular apex (Friedman et al., 1968; Lebowitz et al., 1972).

Although sympathetic nervous innervation appears to begin developing in the fetal heart by about 0.55 gestation, beta-adrenergic receptors seem to be present much earlier and can be stimulated by appropriate agonists before 0.4 of gestation (Barrett et al., 1972). Prior to about 0.55 gestation (80 days gestation in the lamb), fetal myocardium may be affected by circulating catecholamines, but local reflex activity

through the sympathetic nervous system is not likely to play a major role in circulatory regulation.

Vagal stimulation at about 0.85 gestation produces bradycardia. Administering atropine at 0.55 gestation produces a modest increase in fetal heart rate (Vapaa-vuori et al., 1973), indicating that vagal innervation is present by this stage of development. Histochemical staining for acetylcholinesterase in close-to-term fetuses has shown that the concentrations of this enzyme, which is responsible for metabolism of acetylcholine, are similar to those found in adults.

Energy Metabolism

In the normal unstressed fetus, myocardial blood flow is about 180 ml/min/100 gm tissue, approximately 80 per cent more than in the adult. Fetal myocardial oxygen consumption, as measured in the left ventricular free wall, is about 400 μM/100 gm/min, similar to that in the adult. In adult sheep, free fatty acids provide the major source of energy for the myocardium, and carbohydrate accounts for only about 40 per cent of myocardial oxygen consumption (Fisher et al., 1980). In fetal sheep under normal conditions, however, free fatty acid concentrations are extremely low and almost all of the oxygen consumed can be accounted for by carbohydrate metabolism—glucose for 33 per cent, pyruvate for 6 per cent, and lactate for 58 per cent of the oxygen consumed by the left ventricular free wall.

ATPase activity in fetal myocardium is equal to that in adult myocardium, suggesting that energy utilization by the contractile apparatus is similar in fetal and adult myocardium (Friedman, 1973). Mitochondria from fetal myocardium demonstrate higher oxidative phosphorylation than those from adult myocardium. The higher oxygen consumption in fetal mitochondria uncoupled by DNP suggests that the augmented respiratory rate in mitochondria is a reflection of increased electron transport (Friedman, 1973). This is consistent with the greater cytochrome oxidase activity in fetal mitochondria.

CONTROL OF THE CARDIOVASCULAR SYSTEM

Maintenance of normal cardiovascular function, blood pressure, heart rate, and distribution of blood flow represents a complex inter-relationship between local vascular and reflex effects. These effects are initiated by the stimulation of various receptors and are mediated through the autonomic nervous system as well as through hormonal influences. Although some information is available about how these mechanisms affect the circulation after stress, little is known about their role in normal fetal cardiovascular homeostasis. To complicate the situation, other factors, such as sleep state, electrocortical activity, and uterine activity, transiently affect the circulation. As a result, this area of fetal physiology is difficult to study and the data are difficult to interpret.

Local Regulation

As the oxygen content of blood perfusing the fetus falls, blood flow to the brain, myocardium, and adrenal gland increases; conversely, pulmonary blood flow falls as oxygen content decreases. Local effects of changes in oxygen environment are less clearly established for other organs.

Many adult organs exhibit autoregulation, that is, the ability to maintain constant blood flow over a fairly wide range of perfusion pressures. In the fetus, the umbilical-placental circulation does not exhibit autoregulation and blood flow changes in relation to changes in arterial perfusion pressure (Berman et al., 1976). On the other hand, the cerebral circulation in fetal lambs does show autoregulatory capability (Papile et al., 1985).

Baroreflex Regulation

In chronically instrumented fetal lambs, the fetal heart rate slows after an acute increase in systemic arterial pressure (Shinebourne et al., 1972; Maloney et al., 1977). This baroreflex response, although present by 0.55 (80 days) gestation, is poorly developed early on, but the sensitivity of the reflex to induced changes in pressure increases with advancing gestation. Carotid denervation partially inhibits the response, and combined carotid and aortic denervation abolishes it. Parasympathetic blockade with atropine also abolishes the reflex. Although the existence of the arterial baroreflex is established, Dawes and associates (1980) have suggested that the threshold for fetal baroreflex activity is above the range of the normal fetal arterial blood pressure, and that this reflex is not important in controlling cardiovascular function *in utero.*

Carotid sinus and vagus nerve activity are synchronous with the arterial pulse, suggesting continuous baroreceptor activity (Biscoe et al., 1969; Ponte and Purves, 1973). Marked fluctuations in arterial blood pressure and heart rate are observed after sinoaortic denervation, although the average arterial blood pressure and heart rate are not different from control (Itskovitz et al., 1983).

The baroreflex in fetal animals is relatively insensitive and requires fairly marked changes in pressures to produce relatively minor responses. Sinoaortic denervation increases heart rate and blood pressure variability, however. Under normal circumstances, therefore, baroreceptor function acts to stabilize heart rate and blood pressure.

Chemoreflex Regulation

In general, chemoreceptor stimulation by sodium cyanide injection induces hypertension and bradycardia (Dawes et al., 1969; Goodlin and Rudolph, 1972). Central or carotid chemoreceptor stimulation causes hypertension and mild tachycardia with increased respiratory activity, whereas aortic chemoreceptor stimulation produces bradycardia with modest increases in arterial blood pressure. Because the carotid chemoreceptors are less sensitive than the aortic chemoreceptors, hypertension and bradycardia usually result. In chronically instrumented fetal lambs, sodium cyanide produces bradycardia with variable blood pressure changes, responses abolished by sinoaortic denervation (Itskovitz and Rudolph, 1982). Fetal hypoxia induced either by administration of low oxygen gas mixtures to, or by balloon occlusion of, the descending aorta in the ewe produces bradycardia and hypertension that are abolished by sinoaortic denervation of the fetus. Carotid sinus denervation alone does not have a major effect on the response. Aortic chemoreceptors therefore seem to play the major role in circulatory responses to hypoxia.

Autonomic Nervous System and Adrenal Medulla

As described earlier, sympathetic innervation of the heart is not complete until term or, in some species, until after delivery. On the other hand, cholinergic innervation as measured by the presence of acetylcholinesterase appears to be fully developed during fetal life. The innervation of other vascular beds also appears to proceed at different rates during gestation (Zink and Van Petten, 1981).

Adrenergic receptors are present in the fetus and have been demonstrated in myocardium (Cheng et al., 1980, 1981; Whitsett et al., 1982). Receptor populations that have been studied in the fetus exhibit characteristics similar to those in adults (Nuwayhid et al., 1975; Harris and Van Petten, 1979). The fetus possesses mature adrenergic receptors fairly early in gestation, but the concentration of receptors is different from that in adult organs (Cheng et al., 1980). The fetal concentration of receptors can be altered by administering thyroid hormone or isoxsuprine to the mother.

Injecting cholinergic or adrenergic agonists into fetal sheep produces responses as early as 0.4 (60 days) gestation (Barrett et al., 1972; Assali et al., 1977). Alpha-adrenergic stimulation with methoxamine produces an increase in arterial blood pressure, a small decrease in cardiac output, an increase in blood flow to the lungs, and a marked decrease in kidney and peripheral blood flow as early as 0.5 gestation. Beta-adrenergic stimulation by isoproterenol causes a response earlier in gestation and an increase in heart rate with little or no change in arterial blood pressure and cardiac output. Blood flow to both the myocardium and the lungs is increased. Administration of acetylcholine decreases blood pressure and heart rate and increases pulmonary blood flow markedly, particularly in fetuses close to term.

Although receptor affinity is well developed during fetal life, the response to a specific agonist is blunted relative to the adult. The maximal constrictor response to norepinephrine or nerve stimulation increases throughout the latter part of gestation and even more after birth (Wyse et al., 1977). The increase might result from gestational differences in neurotransmitter release in the fetus. During the last trimester of gestation, there is a progressive increase in maximal pressor response to ephedrine, which exerts its effect indirectly through neurotransmitter release; phenylephrine has a direct pressor effect (Harris and Van Petten, 1978). Also, neurotransmitter re-uptake in sympathetic nerve terminals is not fully mature in the fetus (Harris and Van Petten, 1979). Similarly, the differences between fetal and adult myocardium in respect to threshold and sensitivity to norepinephrine indicate an immature re-uptake mechanism for norepinephrine in the fetus (Friedman, 1973).

As gestation progresses, these variable rates of maturation of different components of the autonomic nervous system modify control mechanisms relating to the autonomic nervous system. The role of beta-adrenergic stimulation in resting circulatory regulation has been evaluated by pharmacologic blockade of beta-adrenergic receptors with propranolol. This component of the sympathetic nervous system exerts a positive influence over fetal heart rate that first appears at about 0.6 (80 to 90 days) gestation (Vapaavouri et al., 1973), but this influence is relatively small (Walker et al., 1978). During stress such as hypoxia or hemorrhage, however, beta-adrenergic activity does appear to be increased, because propranolol produces much greater changes in heart rate. Alpha-adrenergic control of the circulation has a somewhat clearer developmental pattern. Alpha-adrenergic blockade with phentolamine or phenoxybenzamine reduces arterial blood pressure very little, if at all, prior to 0.75 (100 to 110 days) gestation; thereafter there is a progressive increase in response, indicating a progressive increase in resting vascular tone attributed to alpha-adrenergic nervous activity. The parasympathetic nervous system exerts an inhibitory influence over fetal heart rate that is present by 0.55 (80 days) gestation (Vapaavouri et al., 1973; Walker et al., 1978). Parasympathetic blockade with atropine produces small changes at this age, with a progressive increase in parasympathetic control as gestation advances. After approximately 0.85 (120 to 130 days) gestation, no further increase is evident.

Hypoxemia or asphyxia increases circulating plasma catecholamine concentrations in fetal sheep (Comline et al., 1965; Jones and Robinson, 1975; Lewis et al., 1982). In fetuses younger than about 120 days gestation, when the adrenal gland becomes innervated, extremely low fetal blood oxygen concentrations are required to stimulate the adrenal gland; thereafter catecholamine secretion can be induced by more moderate hypoxemia (Comline et al., 1965). Infusing catecholamines to reach plasma concentrations that mimic those observed during hypoxemia produces circulatory changes similar to those seen during hypoxemia (Lorijn and Longo, 1980). Adrenal medullary responses to stress appear to play a role in circulatory adjustments; whether catecholamine secretion exerts a continuous regulatory function is not clear.

Hormonal Regulation of the Circulation

The Renin-Angiotensin System

The renin-angiotensin system is important in regulating the normal fetal circulation and its response to hemorrhage. The juxtaglomerular apparatus in the kidneys is well developed in fetuses and is present by 0.6 (90 days) gestation (Smith et al., 1974). Plasma renin activity, as well as circulating angiotensin II, is present in fetal plasma as early as about 0.6 (90 days) gestation (Broughton-Pipkin et al., 1974; Iwamoto and Rudolph, 1979a; Iwamoto et al., 1979b). The effects of fetal stress such as hemorrhage and hypoxia on the renin-angiotensin system are not absolutely clear. Small amounts of hemorrhage increase plasma renin activity (Broughton-Pipkin et al., 1974; Smith et al., 1974); other studies, however, have shown little effect (Robillard and Weitzman, 1980). Similarly, the effects of hypoxemia on the renin-angiotensin system in the fetus are controversial, but most likely hypoxemia is of little consequence.

When angiotensin II is infused to achieve plasma concentrations similar to those that occur after a moderate (15 to 20 per cent) hemorrhage, there are broad cardiovascular effects (Iwamoto and Rudolph, 1982). Arterial blood pressure increases markedly, and after an initial abrupt bradycardia, heart rate increases. Combined ventricular output increases as does blood flow to the lungs and myocardium. Renal blood flow decreases, but umbilical placental flow is unchanged; this latter phenomenon indicates vascular constriction in the umbilical-placental circulation because arterial blood pressure increases but flow does not. The increase in myocardial blood flow is probably caused by an increase in stroke work, and the large increase in pulmonary blood flow probably reflects the release of some other local pulmonary vasodilating substance such as one of the prostaglandins (Gryglewski, 1980).

Inhibiting the action of angiotensin II by specific inhibitors such as saralasin has somewhat variable effects. In unstressed fetal animals, however, there generally is a fall in mean arterial pressure and a slight decrease in heart rate (Iwamoto and Rudolph, 1979a). Combined ventricular output is unaltered, but umbilical-placental blood flow falls, probably in association with the fall in systemic arterial pressure. Blood flow to the peripheral tissues, adrenal glands, and myocardium increases. During hemorrhage, the effects of saralasin are markedly accentuated and result in profound hypotension and bradycardia.

Under normal resting conditions, endogenous angiotensin II appears to exert a tonic vasoconstriction on the peripheral vascular bed, thereby maintaining systemic arterial blood pressure and umbilical-placental blood flow. In response to hemorrhage, angiotensin II is released and produces more vasoconstriction in the periphery, as well as other cardiovascular effects, thereby maintaining systemic arterial blood pressure and umbilical blood flow.

Vasopressin

Arginine vasopressin (antidiuretic hormone) has been detected as early as 0.4 (60 days) gestation in fetal lambs (Drummond et al., 1980). Although hypoxia and hemorrhage, as well as many other stimuli such as hypotension and hypernatremia, induced a marked increase in plasma vasopressin concentrations (Rurak, 1978; Drummond et al., 1980), it is unlikely that vasopressin plays a major role in normal circulatory regulation. Maximal antidiuresis in adults occurs with vasopressin concentrations that have no discernible effects on systemic blood pressure. Fetal vasopressin concentrations are below this level.

Infusing vasopressin into fetal sheep to produce concentrations similar to those observed during fetal hypoxemia produces hypertension and bradycardia (Iwamoto et al., 1979b). Combined ventricular output decreases slightly, but the proportion distributed to the gastrointestinal tract and peripheral circulations falls, whereas that to the umbilical-placental, myocardial, and cerebral circulations increases. These findings indicate that vasopressin probably participates in fetal circulatory responses to stress not only directly but also by enhancing pressor responses to other vasoactive substances. Under resting conditions, however, vasopressin apparently has little regulatory function.

Atrial Natriuretic Factor

Atrial natriuretic factor, a potent volume-regulating family of peptides released from the atria and ventricles as well as other sites in response to stretch, also has vasoregulatory functions. It is present in fetal plasma, and concentrations are highest in blood leaving the right ventricle, indicating production in the right side of the heart (Hargrave et al., 1990). In the fetus, when infused to produce concentrations equivalent to those induced by stress, such as hypoxemia or volume loading, it produces pulmonary vasodilatation, suggesting a possible role in modulating right ventricular afterload.

Arachidonic Acid Metabolites

Although prostaglandins generally are locally active substances that do not normally circulate in adult blood, relatively high concentrations do normally circulate in the fetus (Challis and Patrick, 1980; Mitchell et al., 1978). It is likely that these prostaglandins are derived from the placenta. The fetal vasculature is also capable of producing prostaglandins, and the umbilical vessels, ductus arteriosus, and aorta produce significant amounts of prostaglandin E and prostacyclin (PGI_2).

Prostaglandins administered to the fetus have diverse and extensive cardiovascular effects. Prostaglandin E_1 (PGE_1) and prostaglandin E_2 (PGE_2) constrict the umbilical-placental circulation (Novy et al., 1974; Berman et al., 1978). Prostaglandin $F_2\alpha$ ($PGF_2\alpha$) and thromboxane also cause constriction, whereas PGI_2 dilates the umbilical-placental circulation. PGE_1, PGE_2, PGI_2, and PGD_2 produce pulmonary vasodilatation in the fetus, whereas $PGF_2\alpha$ produces constriction (Cassin, 1987). Infusing PGE_1 into fetal sheep has no effect on cardiac output or systemic pressure, but in addition to a reduction in umbilical-placental blood flow, there are increases in flow to the myocardium, adrenals, gastrointestinal tract, and peripheral tissues (Tripp et al., 1978). Of great interest is the role of prostaglandins in maintaining patency of the ductus arteriosus in the fetus. Although PGE_2 and PGI_2 are produced locally,

circulating prostaglandins most likely play the major role in actively relaxing the smooth muscle in the ductus arteriosus, thereby maintaining it in a dilated state *in utero* (Olley et al., 1975; Clyman, 1980, 1987).

The role of endogenous prostaglandin production in regulating the fetal circulation has been elucidated by administering inhibitors of prostaglandin synthesis to the fetus. Giving either indomethacin or salicylates markedly constricts the ductus arteriosus *in utero* (Sharpe et al., 1975; Heymann and Rudolph, 1976). Although PGE_2 produces umbilical-placental vasoconstriction, inhibition of prostaglandin synthesis has little effect on umbilical-placental vascular resistance, suggesting that prostaglandins do not normally regulate the umbilical-placental circulation. When prostaglandin synthesis is inhibited, the proportion of blood flow to the gastrointestinal tract, kidneys, and peripheral circulation decreases, indicating an increase in vascular resistance in these tissues. Vascular resistances to other tissues are essentially unchanged; perhaps prostaglandins play a role in regulating flow to the gastrointestinal tract and peripheral tissues only.

Although prostaglandins do not appear to be central to regulation of the resting fetal pulmonary circulation, PGI_2 may act to modulate tone and thereby maintain pulmonary vascular resistance relatively constant. However leukotrienes, also metabolites of arachidonic acid and potent smooth muscle constrictors, may play an active role in maintenance of the normally high fetal pulmonary vascular resistance. In newborns (Schreiber et al., 1985), leukotriene inhibition attenuates hypoxic pulmonary vasoconstriction. In fetal lambs, leukotriene receptor blockade (Soifer et al., 1985) or synthesis inhibition (LeBidois et al., 1987) increases pulmonary blood flow about eight-fold, suggesting a role for leukotrienes in maintenance of the normally high fetal pulmonary vascular resistance; the presence of leukotrienes in fetal tracheal fluid further supports this (Velvis et al., 1990).

Endothelial-Derived Factors

In addition to PGI_2, vascular endothelial cells can be stimulated to produce other vasoactive factors. These include potent vasoconstrictors, such as endothelin, and vasodilators, such as endothelium-derived relaxing factor (EDRF), as well as growth factors, such as platelet-derived growth factor, which not only is related to vascular growth but also has vasoactive properties. Little is known about the role of growth factors or of endothelin in the physiologic regulation of the fetal circulation, although endothelin is a potent umbilical-placental vasoconstrictor *in vitro*; substantially more is known about endothelium-derived vasodilators.

EDRF is now known to be nitric oxide (NO) and generally is called endothelium-derived nitric oxide (EDNO) (Ignarro, 1989). EDNO is produced by most endothelial cells in response to varied stimuli, generally involving specific receptors; smooth muscle relaxation is produced by a guanylate cyclase/cGMP mediated mechanism. In the fetus, EDNO is produced by umbilical vascular endothelium (Van de Voorde et al., 1987; Chaudhuri et al., 1991); nitroso compounds reduce umbilical vascular resistance *in vitro* (Myatt et al. 1991) and EDNO modulates resting umbilical vascular tone in fetal sheep *in utero* (Chang et al., 1992). Disturbances in normal EDNO production may also be involved in the genesis of preeclampsia (Pinto et al., 1991).

EDNO clearly is involved in regulation of vascular tone in the fetal pulmonary circulation, although it plays a far more important role in postnatal transition to air breathing. Superfused fetal sheep pulmonary arteries release EDRF when stimulated with bradykinin (Glasgow et al., 1990). In fetal lambs the vasodilating effects of bradykinin are attenuated by methylene blue and resting tone falls with N^w—nitro-L-arginine, an inhibitor of EDRF (EDNO) synthesis from precursor L-arginine (Moore et al., 1992), suggesting that a cGMP-dependent mechanism, such as EDNO production, continuously modulates or offsets the increased tone of the resting fetal pulmonary circulation. Inhibition of EDNO synthesis also blocks the pulmonary vasodilatation with oxygenation of fetal lungs *in utero* (Moore et al., 1992).

REFERENCES

Assali NS, Brinkman CR III, Woods JR Jr, et al: Development of neurohumoral control of fetal, neonatal, and adult cardiovascular functions. Am J Obstet Gynecol 129:748, 1977.

Barrett CT, Heymann MA, Rudolph AM: Alpha and beta adrenergic function in fetal sheep. Am J Obstet Gynecol 112:1114, 1972.

Behrman RE, Lees MH, Peterson EN, et al: Distribution of the circulation in the normal and asphyxiated fetal primate. Am J Obstet Gynecol 108:956, 1970.

Berman W Jr, Goodlin RC, Heymann MA, Rudolph AM: Pressure-flow relationships in the umbilical and uterine circulations of the sheep. Circ Res 38:262, 1976.

Berman W Jr, Goodlin RC, Heymann MA, Rudolph AM: Effects of pharmacologic agents on umbilical blood flow in fetal lambs in utero. Biol Neonate 33:225, 1978.

Biscoe TJ, Purves MJ, Sampson SR: Types of nervous activity which may be recorded from the carotid sinus nerve in the sheep foetus. J Physiol (Lond) 202:1, 1969.

Bristow J, Rudolph AM, Itskovitz J: A preparation for studying liver blood flow, oxygen consumption, and metabolism in the fetal lamb in utero. J Dev Physiol 3:255, 1981.

Bristow J, Rudolph AM, Itskovitz J, Barnes R: Hepatic oxygen and glucose metabolism in the fetal lamb. J Clin Invest 71:1, 1983.

Broughton-Pipkin F, Lumbers ER, Mott JC: Factors influencing plasma renin and angiotensin II in the conscious pregnant ewe and its foetus. J Physiol (Lond) 243,:619, 1974.

Cassin S: Role of prostaglandins, thromboxanes, and leukotrienes in the control of the pulmonary circulation in the fetus and newborn. Semin Perinatol 11:53, 1987.

Challis JRG, Patrick JE: The production of prostaglandins and thromboxanes in the feto-placental unit and their effects on the developing fetus. Semin Perinatol 4:23, 1980.

Chang J-K, Roman C, Heymann MA: Effect of endothelium—derived relaxing factor inhibition on the umbilical-placental circulation in fetal lambs in utero. Am J Obstet Gynecol 166:727, 1992.

Chaudhuri G, Buga GM, Gold ME, et al: Characterization and actions of human umbilical endothelium derived relaxing factor. Br J Pharmacol 102:331, 1991.

Cheng JB, Cornett LE, Goldfien A, Roberts JM: Decreased concentration of myocardial alpha-adrenoceptors with increasing age in foetal lambs. Br J Pharmacol 70:515, 1980.

Cheng JB, Goldfien A, Cornett LE, Roberts JM: Identification of beta-adrenergic receptors using (3H)dihydroalprenolol in fetal sheep heart: Direct evidence of qualitative similarity to the receptors in adult sheep heart. Pediatr Res 15:1083, 1981.

Clyman RI: Ontogeny of the ductus arteriosus response to prostaglandins and inhibitors of their synthesis. Semin Perinatol 4:115, 1980.

Clyman RI: Ductus arteriosus: Current theories of prenatal and postnatal regulation. Semin Perinatol 11:64, 1987.

Comline RS, Silver IA, Silver M: Factors responsible for the stimulation of the adrenal medulla during asphyxia in the foetal lamb. J Physiol (Lond) 178:211, 1965.

Dawes GS, Duncan LB, Lewis BV, et al: Cyanide stimulation of the systemic arterial chemoreceptors in foetal lambs. J Physiol (Lond) 201:117, 1969.

Dawes GS, Johnston BM, Walker DW: Relationship of arterial pressure and heart rate in fetal, newborn, and adult sheep. J Physiol 309:405, 1980.

DeSmedt MCH, Visser GHA, Meijboom EJ: Fetal cardiac output estimated by Doppler echocardiography during mid and late gestation. Am J Cardiol 60:338, 1987.

Downing SE, Talner NS, Gardner TM: Ventricular function in the newborn lamb. Am J Physiol 208:931, 1965.

Drummond WH, Rudolph AM, Keil LC, et al: Arginine vasopressin and prolactin after hemorrhage in the fetal lamb. Am J Physiol 238:E214, 1980.

Edelstone DI, Rudolph AM, Heymann MA: Liver and ductus venosus blood flows in fetal lambs in utero. Circ Res 42:426, 1978.

Edelstone DI, Rudolph AM: Preferential streaming of ductus venosus blood to the brain and heart in fetal lambs. Am J Physiol 237:H724, 1979.

Edelstone DI, Rudolph AM, Heymann MA: Effects of hypoxemia and decreasing umbilical flow on liver and ductus venosus blood flows in fetal lambs. Am J Physiol 238:H656, 1980.

Fisher DJ, Heymann MA, Rudolph AM: Myocardial oxygen and carbohydrate consumption in fetal lambs in utero and in adult sheep. Am J Physiol 238:H399, 1980.

Friedman WF, Pool PE, Jacobowitz D, et al: Sympathetic innervation of the developing rabbit heart. Circ Res 23:25, 1968.

Friedman WF: The intrinsic physiologic properties of the developing heart. In Friedman WF, Lesch M, Sonnenblick EH (eds): Neonatal Heart Disease. New York, Grune & Stratton, 1973.

Gilbert RD: Control of fetal cardiac output during changes in blood volume. Am J Physiol 238:H80, 1980.

Gilbert RD: Effects of afterload and baroreceptors on cardiac function in fetal sheep. J Dev Physiol 4:299, 1982.

Glasgow RE, Heymann MA: Endothelium-derived relaxing factor as a mediator of bradykinin-induced perinatal pulmonary vasodilatation. Clin Res 38:211A, 1990.

Goodlin RC, Rudolph AM: Factors associated with initiation of breathing. In Hodari AA, Mariona FG (eds): Proceedings of the International Symposium on Physiological Biochemistry of the Fetus. Springfield, IL, Charles C Thomas, 1972.

Gryglewski RJ: The lung as a generator of prostacyclin. Ciba Found Symp 78:147, 1980.

Hargrave B, Roman C, Morville P, Heymann M: Pulmonary vascular effects of exogenous atrial natriuretic peptide in sheep fetuses. Pediatr Res 27:140, 1990.

Harris WH, Van Petten GR: Development of cardiovascular responses to sympathomimetic amines and autonomic blockade in the unanesthetised fetus. Can J Physiol Pharmacol 56:400, 1978.

Harris WH, Van Petten GR: Development of cardiovascular responses to noradrenaline, normetanephrine and metanephrine in the unanesthetised fetus. Can J Physiol Pharmacol 57:242, 1979.

Hawkins J, Van Hare GF, Schmidt KG, et al: Effects of increasing afterload on left ventricular output in fetal lambs. Circ Res 65:127, 1989.

Heymann MA, Creasy RK, Rudolph AM: Quantitation of blood flow patterns in the foetal lamb in utero. In Proceedings of the Sir Joseph Barcroft Centenary Symposium: Foetal and Neonatal Physiology. Cambridge, Cambridge University Press, 1973a.

Heymann MA, Rudolph AM: Effects of increasing preload on right ventricular output in fetal lambs in utero. (Abstract) Circulation 48:IV–37, 1973b.

Heymann MA, Rudolph AM: Effects of acetylsalicylic acid on the ductus arteriosus and circulation in fetal lambs in utero. Circ Res 38:418, 1976.

Ignarro LJ: Biological actions and properties of endothelium-derived nitric oxide formed and released from artery and vein. Circ Res **65**:1, 1989.

Itskovitz J, Rudolph AM: Denervation of arterial chemoreceptors and baroreceptors in fetal lambs in utero. Am J Physiol **242**:H916, 1982.

Itskovitz, J, LaGamma EF, Rudolph AM: Baroreflex control of the circulation of chronically instrumented fetal lambs. Circ Res **52**:589, 1983.

Iwamoto HS, Rudolph AM: Effects of endogenous angiotensin II on the fetal circulation. J Dev Physiol **1**:283, 1979a.

Iwamoto HS, Rudolph AM, Keil LC, Heymann MA: Hemodynamic responses of the sheep fetus to vasopressin infusion. Circ Res **44**:430, 1979b.

Iwamoto HS, Rudolph AM: Effects of angiotensin II on the blood flow and its distribution in fetal lambs. Circ Res **48**:183, 1982.

Jones CT, Robinson RD: Plasma catecholamines in fetal and adult sheep. J Physiol (Lond) **248**:15, 1975.

Kirkpatrick SE, Pitlick PT, Naliboff JB, Friedman WF: Frank-Starling relationship as an important determinant of fetal cardiac output. Am J Physiol **231**:495, 1976.

LeBidois J, Soifer SJ, Clyman RI, Heymann MA: Piriprost: a putative leukotriene synthesis inhibitor increases pulmonary blood flow in fetal lambs. Pediatr Res **22**:350, 1987.

Lebowitz EA, Novick JS, Rudolph AM: Development of myocardial sympathetic innervation in the fetal lamb. Pediatr Res **6**:887, 1972.

Lewis AB, Evans WN, Sischo W: Plasma catecholamine responses to hypoxemia in fetal lambs. Biol Neonate **41**:115, 1982.

Lorijn RWH, Longo LD: Norepinephrine elevation in the fetal lamb: Oxygen consumption and cardiac output. Am J Physiol **239**:R115, 1980.

Maloney JE, Cannata JP, Dowling MH, Else W, Ritchie B: Baroreflex activity in conscious fetal and newborn lambs. Biol Neonate **31**:340, 1977.

Mitchell MD, Flint AP, Bibby J, et al: Plasma concentrations of prostaglandins during late human pregnancy: Influence of normal and preterm labor. J Clin Endocrinol Metab **46**:947, 1978.

Moore P, Velvis H, Fineman JR, et al: Endothelium derived relaxing factor inhibition attenuates the increase in pulmonary blood flow due to oxygen ventilation in fetal lambs. J Appl Physiol **73**:2151, 1992.

Myatt L, Brewer A, Brockman D: The action of nitric oxide in the perfused human fetal-placental circulation. Am J Obstet Gynecol **164**:687, 1991.

Novy MJ, Piasecki G, Jackson BT: Effect of prostaglandins E2 and F-2-alpha on umbilical blood flow and fetal hemodynamics. Prostaglandins **5**:543, 1974.

Nuwayhid B, Brinkman CR III, Su C, et al: Systemic and pulmonary hemodynamic responses to adrenergic and cholinergic agonists during fetal development. Biol Neonate **26**:301, 1975.

Olley PM, Bodach E, Heaton J, Coceani F: Further evidence implicating E-type prostaglandins in the patency of the lamb ductus arteriosus. Eur J Pharmacol **34**:247, 1975.

Papile L, Rudolph AM, Heymann MA: Autoregulation of cerebral blood flow in the preterm fetal lamb. Pediatr Res **19**:159, 1985.

Peeters LLH, Sheldon RE, Jones MD Jr, et al: Blood flow to fetal organs as a function of arterial oxygen content. Am J Obstet Gynecol **135**:637, 1979.

Pinto A, Sorrentino R, Sorrentino P, et al: Endothelial-derived relaxing factor released by endothelial cells of human umbilical vessels and its impairment in pregnancy-induced hypertension. Am J Obstet Gynecol **164**:507, 1991.

Ponte J, Purves MJ: Types of afferent nervous activity which may be measured in the vagus nerve of the sheep foetus. J Physiol **229**:51, 1973.

Reed KL, Meijboom EJ, Sahn DJ et al: Cardiac Doppler flow velocities in human fetuses. Circulation **73**:41, 1986.

Reuss ML, Rudolph AM, Heymann MA: Selective distribution of microspheres injected into the umbilical veins and inferior venae cavae of fetal sheep. Am J Obstet Gynecol **141**:427, 1981.

Robillard JE, Weitzman RE: Developmental aspects of the fetal renal response to exogenous arginine vasopressin. Am J Physiol **238**:F407, 1980.

Rudolph AM, Heymann MA: Circulatory changes during growth in the fetal lamb. Circ Res **26**:289, 1970.

Rurak DW: Plasma vasopressin levels during hypoxaemia and the cardiovascular effects of exogenous vasopressin in foetal and adult sheep. J Physiol (Lond) **277**:341, 1978.

Sahn DJ, Lange LW, Allen HD, et al: Quantitative real-time cross-sectional echocardiography in the developing normal human fetus and newborn. Circulation **62**:588, 1980.

Schreiber MD, Heymann MA, Soifer SJ: Leukotriene inhibition prevents and reverses hypoxic pulmonary vasoconstriction in newborn lambs. Pediatr Res **19**:437, 1985.

Sharpe GL, Larsson KS, Thalme B: Studies on closure of the ductus arteriosus. XII. In utero effects of indomethacin and sodium salicylate in rats and rabbits. Prostaglandins **9**:585, 1975.

Sheldon CA, Friedman WF, Sybers HD: Scanning electron microscopy of fetal and neonatal lamb cardiac cells. J Molec Cell Cardiol **8**:853, 1976.

Shinebourne EA, Vapaavuori EK, Williams RL, et al: Development of baroreflex activity in unanesthetized fetal and neonatal lambs. Circ Res **31**:710, 1972.

Smith FG Jr, Lupu AN, Barajas L, Bauer R, Bashore RA: The renin-angiotensin system in the fetal lamb. Pediatr Res **8**:611, 1974.

Soifer SJ, Loitz RD, Roman C, et al: Leukotriene end-organ antagonists increase pulmonary blood flow in fetal lambs. Am J Physiol **249**:H570, 1985.

Teitel DF, Dalinghaus M, Cassidy SC et al: In Utero ventilation augments the left ventricular response to isoproterenol and volume loading in fetal sheep. Pediatr Res **29**:466, 1991.

Tripp ME, Heymann MA, Rudolph AM: Hemodynamic effects of prostaglandin E_1 on lambs in utero. In Coceani F, Olley PM (eds): Prostaglandins and Perinatal Medicine. (Advances in Prostaglandin and Thromboxane Research Vol 4.) New York, Raven Press, 1978.

Van de Voorde J, Vanderstichele H, Leusen I: Release of endothelium-derived relaxing factor from human umbilical vessels. Circ Res **60**:517, 1987.

Vapaavuori EK, Shinebourne EA, Williams RL, et al: Development of cardiovascular responses to autonomic blockade in intact fetal and neonatal lambs. Biol Neonate **22**:177, 1973.

Velvis H, Krusell J, Roman C et al: Leukotrienes C_4, D_4, and E_4 in fetal lamb tracheal fluid. J Dev Physiol **14**:13, 1990.

Walker AM, Cannata J, Dowling MH, et al: Sympathetic and parasympathetic control of heart rate in unanesthetised fetal and newborn lambs. Biol Neonate **33**:135, 1978.

Whitsett JA, Pollinger J, Matz S: β-Adrenergic receptors and catecholamine-sensitive adenylate cyclase in developing rat ventricular myocardium: Effect of thyroid status. Pediatr Res **16**:463, 1982.

Wyse DG, Van Petten GR, Harris WH: Responses to electrical stimulation, noradrenaline, serotonin, and vasopressin in the isolated ear artery of the developing lamb and ewe. Can J Physiol Pharmacol **55**:1001, 1977.

Zink J, Van Petten GR: Noradrenergic control of blood vessels in the premature lamb fetus. Biol Neonate **39**:61, 1981.

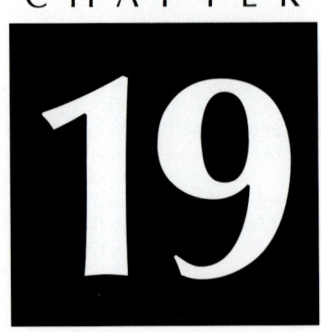

PLACENTAL RESPIRATORY GAS EXCHANGE AND FETAL OXYGENATION

GIACOMO MESCHIA, M.D.

Knowledge of respiratory gas exchange across the human placenta depends on the integrating of observations in pregnant patients with experimental findings in laboratory animals. This integration is necessary because data on the physiology of the human fetus are scant and could not be interpreted correctly in the absence of experimental evidence. The evidence in laboratory animals consists of a fairly comprehensive set of data in sheep with chronically implanted vascular catheters in the maternal and fetal circulation as well as a more limited but important set of data in nonhuman primates and other mammals.

TRANSPORT OF ATMOSPHERIC OXYGEN TO THE GRAVID UTERUS

The transport of oxygen from the atmosphere to the fetal tissues can be visualized as a sequence of six steps that alternate bulk transport with transport by diffusion (Fig. 19–1). The first three steps of this process are part of general physiologic knowledge and therefore are presented here briefly.

The first step—transport from the atmosphere to the alveoli—is by action of the respiratory muscles, which move air in and out of the lungs. This action maintains the oxygen pressure (P_{O_2}) in the alveoli at a level that is regulated by several physiologic mechanisms, some of which are driven by sensors of the P_{O_2}, P_{CO_2}, and pH of maternal blood. During pregnancy, the maternal organism is set to regulate arterial P_{CO_2} at a lower level than in the nonpregnant state (Gaensler, 1965).

In the second step, oxygen diffuses from the alveoli into the maternal red cells that circulate through the lungs. In the normal organism at sea level, the diffusion rate is so rapid that the P_{O_2} at the venous end of the pulmonary capillaries becomes virtually equal to the P_{O_2} in the adjacent alveoli. Nevertheless, the P_{O_2} of maternal arterial blood is somewhat less than the P_{O_2} in a sample of alveolar air, in part because some deoxygenated blood bypasses the lungs and in part because ventilation and perfusion of the alveoli are not matched evenly throughout the lungs. Under pathologic conditions that prevent the equilibration of P_{O_2} between alveoli and blood, increase the degree of uneven ventilation-perfusion, or shunt more deoxygenated blood directly into the arterial system, the P_{O_2} difference between alveolar air and arterial blood becomes larger.

In the third step, maternal blood—propelled by action of the maternal heart—transports oxygen from the lungs to the gravid uterus via the pulmonary veins, the left atrium, the left ventricle, the aorta, the uterine arteries, and branches of the ovarian and

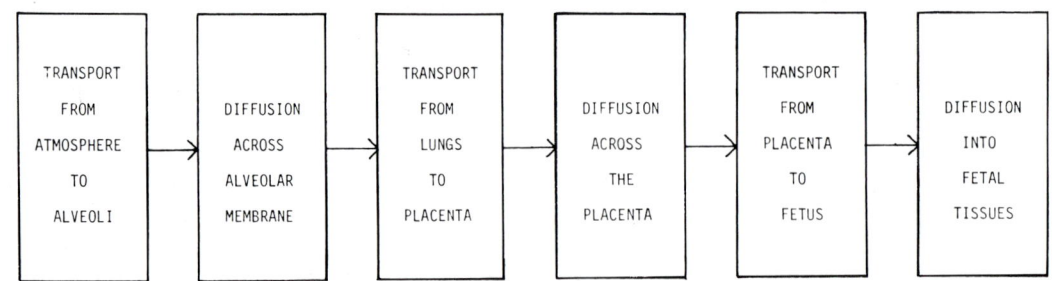

FIGURE 19–1. The transport of oxygen from the atmosphere to the fetal tissues in a sequence of steps that alternate bulk and diffusional transport. (From Meschia G: Supply of oxygen to the fetus. J Reprod Med **23**:160, 1979.)

TABLE 19–1.   Blood Oxygen Transport: Nomenclature, Symbols, Units, Methods of Measurement, and Interrelationships

NOMENCLATURE	SYMBOL	UNITS	METHODS OF MEASUREMENT
Free O_2	$[O_2]$	mM*	
O_2 bound to hemoglobin	$[HbO_2]$	mM*	
O_2 content	$[O_2\ Tot]$	mM*	e.g., Van Slyke apparatus
O_2 pressure	Po_2	mm Hg†	Po_2 electrode
Hemoglobin	$[Hb]$	mM*	Spectrophotometer
O_2 capacity	$[O_2\ CAP]$	mM*	
O_2 saturation	S	—	Spectrophotometer
O_2 saturation $\times$ 100	% S	—	

$[O_2\ Tot] = [HbO_2] + [O_2]$
$[O_2\ CAP] = 4\ [Hb]‡$
$S = [HbO_2] \div [O_2\ CAP]$
$[O_2] = \alpha_{O_2}\ Po_2$ (where $\alpha_{O_2} = O_2$ solubility coefficient)

*Another unit used often in reporting quantities of O_2 is ml_{STP} (one millimol = 22.4 ml_{STP}).
†The unit millimeters of mercury (mm Hg) is also called the torr.
‡Each hemoglobin molecule can combine with four molecules of oxygen.

vaginal arteries. Oxygen is transported by blood in two forms, free and bound to hemoglobin. In any blood samples, these two forms are in reversible equilibrium. The special nomenclature for the components of this equilibrium is summarized in Table 19–1.

OXYGEN UPTAKE BY THE UTERUS AND FETUS

The oxygen uptake by the uterus and the fetus can be calculated by measuring simultaneously uterine and umbilical blood flows and the oxygen content of blood samples drawn from four blood vessels: maternal artery, uterine vein, umbilical vein, and umbilical artery. A numerical example of these calculations is presented in Figure 19–2. The rationale, which is commonly known as the Fick principle, is as follows: Each milliliter of maternal blood in passing through

the pregnant uterus gives up a certain amount of oxygen, which one can calculate by measuring the difference in oxygen content between maternal arterial blood and uterine venous blood. The quantity of oxygen lost by each milliliter of blood is then multiplied by the milliliters of blood flowing through the pregnant uterus to obtain the uterine oxygen uptake. In the example shown in Figure 19–2, the uterine blood flow is 1412 ml/min, and the amount of oxygen lost by each milliliter of blood that passes through the uterus is 0.034 ml_{STP}/ml. Therefore, the oxygen uptake by the gravid uterus is $0.034 \times 1412 = 48$ ml_{STP}/min. Exactly the same reasoning is applied to the umbilical blood data in order to calculate the rate at which the fetus takes up oxygen from the placenta. Note that the oxygen uptake by the gravid uterus is greater than the oxygen uptake by the fetus. This is so because the placenta is metabolically active and consumes a relatively large fraction of the oxygen that the uterine circulation delivers to the gravid uterus.

Fetal growth is accompanied by an increase in fetal oxygen uptake. However, oxygen uptake and fetal weight do not grow proportionally. A 200-gm, mid-gestation fetal lamb has an average oxygen uptake of 0.460 $\mu M \cdot min^{-1}\ gm^{-1}$, whereas a 3000-gm near-term fetus has an average uptake of 0.340 $\mu M \cdot min^{-1}\ gm^{-1}$ (Bell et al., 1986). The difference in uptakes is much larger if the uptake is related to fetal dry weight, since fetal growth is accompanied by a decrease in fetal water content. Oxygen uptake expressed per unit fetal dry weight is about 2.5 times higher at mid-gestation. Given this complexity and the lack of comparable information for the human fetus, it is important to address the question whether fetal oxygen uptake measurements in experimental animals can be used to estimate human fetal oxygen uptake. If the aim is an accurate estimate the answer must be no, because there are several interspecies differences that are likely to affect oxygen demand. For example, in comparing near-term ovine and human fetuses of equal body weight, one must note that the human fetus has a much larger brain mass, has more adipose tissue, lives at a lower body temperature, and grows more slowly. It would be surprising if all these differences do not add up to a significant difference in oxygen uptake. It

---

Measured Quantities

Maternal arterial O_2 content (A): 0.143 ml_{STP}/ml of blood
Uterine venous O_2 content (V): 0.109 ml_{STP}/ml of blood
Umbilical arterial O_2 content (a): 0.078 ml_{STP}/ml of blood
Umbilical venous O_2 content (v): 0.115 ml_{STP}/ml of blood
Uterine blood flow (F): 1412 ml/min
Umbilical blood flow (f): 716 ml/min
Fetal body weight (BW): 4.0 kg
Uteroplacental unit weight (UPW): 1.0 kg

Calculations

O_2 uptake by the gravid uterus:	$(A - V) \times F = 48.0\ ml_{STP}$/min
O_2 uptake by the fetus:	$(v - a) \times f = 26.5\ ml_{STP}$/min
O_2 uptake per kg by fetus:	$(v - a) \times f \div BW =$ 6.6 ml_{STP}/min/kg
O_2 uptake per kg by fetus and uteroplacental unit:	$(A - V) \times F \div (BW + UPW)$ = 9.6 ml_{STP}/min/kg

FIGURE 19–2. Numerical example of the application of the Fick principle to a calculation of the oxygen uptake by the pregnant uterus and the fetus. Representative data from experiments in chronic sheep preparations during the last 2 weeks of pregnancy.

is interesting to note, however, that attempts to measure near-term fetal oxygen consumption rates in different species (i.e., horse, cattle, rhesus monkey, guinea pig) have yielded values of oxygen uptake per gram wet weight that are within ± 20 per cent of the fetal lamb value despite very large differences in body size, rate of growth, and body composition (Battaglia and Meschia, 1986). Therefore, it is fairly safe to assume that data in experimental animals provide an approximate estimate of human fetal oxygen demand.

Oxygen Pressures in Uterine and Umbilical Circulations

In chronic sheep preparations the PO_2 of umbilical venous blood, which is the most oxygenated blood of the fetal organism, is quite low in comparison to maternal arterial PO_2 (Table 19–2). The major reason for this large PO_2 difference is that the ovine placenta functions as a venous equilibration system. In order to understand how such a system works, one must consider its prototype, which is the concurrent exchanger presented in Figure 19–3. Two long, narrow channels are separated by a semipermeable membrane. Maternal blood is pumped through one channel and fetal blood is pumped through the other channel, in such a way that both streams run in the same direction. The arterial blood of the mother enters the exchanger with a PO_2 higher than that of fetal arterial blood. This establishes at the arterial end of the system a maternal-fetal PO_2 gradient that moves oxygen across the membrane. As the two bloodstreams proceed toward the venous end, there is a progressive decrease of PO_2 in the maternal blood and a progressive increase of PO_2 in the fetal blood. If the streams flow sufficiently slowly and/or the membrane is sufficiently permeable to oxygen, maternal and fetal blood can exit the exchanger with identical PO_2 values. Under no circumstances, as long as the mechanism of transfer is diffusion, can the recipient stream exit with a venous PO_2 higher than the venous PO_2 of the donor stream.

The structure of the ovine placenta is more complex than that of a concurrent exchanger. Some experimental evidence indicates that its flow pattern is crosscurrent. Nevertheless, it shares with the concurrent model a basic property, namely that the venous PO_2 of the umbilical circulation depends on, and cannot be higher than, the venous PO_2 of the uterine circulation (Rankin et al., 1971). An experimental demonstration of this fact is presented in Figure 19–4. Note that in every instance the umbilical venous PO_2 is less than the uterine venous PO_2. This means that the transfer of oxygen from the uterine to the umbilical circulation

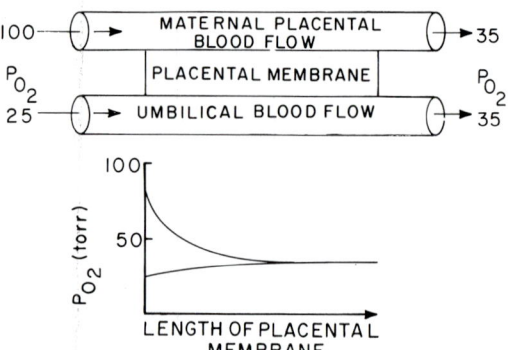

FIGURE 19–3. Concurrent model of transplacental oxygen diffusion.

does not attain the maximum level of performance of a venous equilibrator. In the attempt to explain this inefficiency, the following factors have been considered.

Shunts. Part of the uterine blood flow is shunted away from the area of exchange and perfuses the myometrium and the endometrial gland. A fraction of umbilical blood flow does not perfuse the placental cotyledons. In addition to anatomic shunts there are diffusional shunts within the maternal and fetal placental microcirculations (Fig. 19–5).

Uneven Perfusion. Both within and among the placental cotyledons there is a certain degree of uneven perfusion, i.e., the maternal/fetal blood flow ratio can be high in some parts of the placenta and low in others. This unevenness is a source of inefficiency. The greater the unevenness of perfusion ratios, the greater the PO_2 difference between the major placental veins of the mother and the fetus.

Oxygen-Diffusing Capacity. Placental oxygen-diffusing capacity is the rate of O_2 transport from placenta to fetus divided by the *mean* PO_2 difference between maternal and fetal red cells. Its value is a function of the surface and thickness of the placental barrier (the larger the surface and smaller the thickness the higher the diffusing capacity) and of the reaction rates of oxygen with hemoglobin (Longo et al., 1972). Placental oxygen-diffusing capacity has not been measured directly, but has been estimated from measurements of the diffusing capacity of the placenta for carbon monoxide (Bissonnette et al., 1979).

Some investigators believe that placental oxygen-diffusing capacity is a negligible hindrance to placental oxygen transport, but this belief depends on theoretical models that are not realistic. Experimental evidence in sheep indicates that most of the PO_2 difference between uterine and umbilical venous blood is due to a low oxygen-diffusing capacity that prevents the equilibration of maternal and fetal PO_2 across the placental barrier (Wilkening and Meschia, 1992). The role of placental oxygen-diffusing capacity in preventing the equilibration of maternal and fetal PO_2 becomes particularly important for an understanding of pathologic conditions. For example, in sheep severe fetal growth retardation is often associated with a low umbilical venous PO_2 (Bell et al., 1987). This low PO_2

TABLE 19–2. Representative PO_2 Values in Uterine and Umbilical Circulations of Sheep

LOCATION	PO_2 (mm Hg)
Uterine artery	72
Uterine vein	42
Umbilical vein	28
Umbilical artery	19

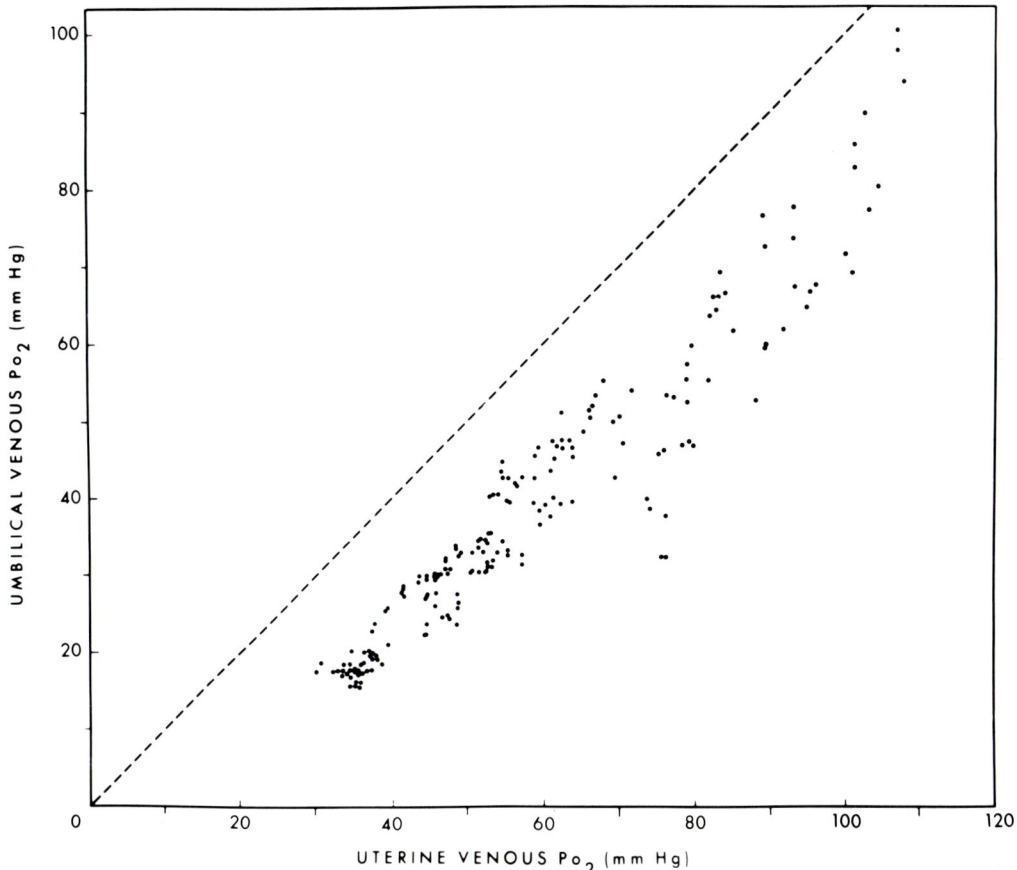

FIGURE 19–4. The relationship of umbilical venous P_{O_2} to uterine venous P_{O_2} in sheep. The *dashed line* is the line of identity. Uterine venous P_{O_2} was varied by administration of different gas mixtures to the mother and by displacing the oxyhemoglobin dissociation curve of maternal blood through changes of maternal blood pH. Note that each point is below the identity line. (From Rankin JHG, Meschia G, Makowski EL, Battaglia FC: Relationship between uterine and umbilical P_{O_2} in sheep. Am J Physiol **220**: 1688, 1971.)

is due to a small placental oxygen-diffusing capacity that requires the fetus to maintain a large transplacental P_{O_2} gradient in order to draw oxygen from the mother across the placenta.

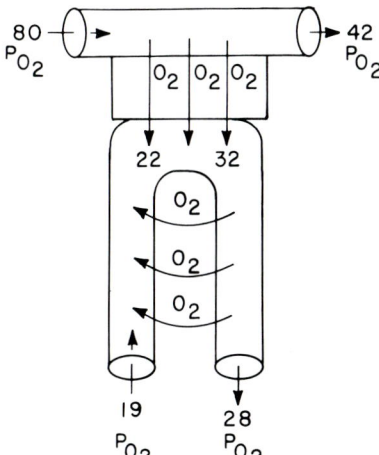

FIGURE 19–5. Example of a diffusional shunt. Fetal blood exiting the area of exchange decreases its P_{O_2} by donating oxygen to the incoming fetal arterial blood.

Is the Human Placenta a Venous Equilibrator?

In several species (e.g., guinea pig, rabbit) the placenta forms a countercurrent exchanger, which is more effective in transporting oxygen than a venous equilibrator. The effectiveness of the human placenta has been difficult to establish. One of the major problems has been variability in placental venous drainage. Experiments in the rhesus monkey, which has a placenta similar to the human placenta, were able to demonstrate that maternal placental venous drainage of fetally infused tritiated water was via either the left or right ovarian vein or via both (Wallenburg and vanKreel, 1977). Furthermore, in some cases drainage shifted from one vein to the other during the course of the experiment, showing that the position of the placenta in the uterus is not a reliable indicator of which vein draws the placenta preferentially (Battaglia et al., 1970). Thus, attempts to demonstrate the relation between maternal and fetal placental venous P_{O_2} in primates require a multiple venous sampling approach on the maternal side. By using this approach, a study of human placental venous drainage at elective cesarean section (Pardi et al., 1992) has found umbilical venous PO_2 to be lower than the PO_2 in the least oxygenated of the maternal veins (Fig. 19–6). This result agrees with previous findings in the rhesus monkey (Parer and Behrman 1967) and favors the concept that the human placenta is, like the ovine placenta, a venous equilibrator. More and diverse types of evidence are needed, however, for establishing this important concept on a firmer basis. It is interesting to note that in Figure 19–6 most of the points representing growth-retarded fetuses demonstrate a maternal-fetal venous PO_2 gradient that is greater than normal. This observation cautions against the commonly made assumption that the hypoxia of the growth-retarded human fetus is due to a low level of maternal placental perfusion. Other factors that influence the transplacental PO_2 gradient, e.g., the surface of the placental barrier, may play a more important role.

Factors That Determine Uterine Venous PO_2

The evidence in sheep, rhesus monkeys, and humans focuses attention on the uterine venous PO_2 as the primary determinant of the upper limit of umbilical venous blood PO_2 in these species. The factors that determine uterine venous PO_2 are shown in Figure 19–7. The immediately causative factors that determine uterine venous PO_2 are the oxygen saturation and the oxyhemoglobin dissociation curve of venous blood. The position of the oxyhemoglobin dissociation curve is shifted by pH, so that at any given saturation the PO_2 is inversely related to pH (Bohr effect). Because of the Bohr effect, maternal alkalosis can be detrimental to fetal oxygenation, via its effect on uterine venous PO_2 (Fig. 19–8).

The oxygen saturation of uterine venous blood, S_v,

is a function of four variables: the oxygen saturation of maternal arterial blood (S_A), the oxygen capacity of maternal blood (O_2 CAP), uterine blood flow (F), and the oxygen consumption rate of the gravid uterus ($\dot{V}O_2$):

$$S_v = S_A - \frac{\dot{V}O_2}{F \, [O_2 \, CAP]}$$

This equation is an application of the Fick principle.* It is an approximation that neglects the small contribution of free oxygen to the oxygen content of blood. Implicit in the equation are the three main types of hypoxia listed in textbooks of physiology, namely, low saturation of arterial blood (hypoxic hypoxia), reduced oxygen capacity (anemic hypoxia), and reduction in blood flow (circulatory hypoxia). These types of hypoxia, alone or in combination, decrease uterine venous saturation. A decrease in uterine venous oxygen saturation implies a decrease of uterine venous PO_2 and impairment of fetal oxygenation.

An important consequence of the inefficiency of a placenta which is a venous equilibrator and has a low oxygen-diffusing capacity is that it requires a relatively high uterine blood flow in order to provide a normal level of fetal oxygenation. For example, if we consider as valid the evidence that under normal physiologic conditions the umbilical venous PO_2 of a 35-week human fetus is about 30 torr (Bozzetti et al., 1987) and that uterine venous PO_2 must be at least 10 mm Hg higher than umbilical venous PO_2 (Pardi et al., 1992), then according to Figure 19–8, the uterine blood flow in late human pregnancy should be normally about one liter. Actual estimates tend to be lower (Thaler et al., 1990), suggesting that either the estimates have been biased toward small values by some measuring error, or the efficiency of the human placenta is greater than indicated by the uterine-umbilical venous PO_2 difference measured at cesarean section, or the oxygen demand of the human gravid uterus near term is even less than the conservative estimate of 30 ml$_{STP}$/min. The available data do not mesh easily together because

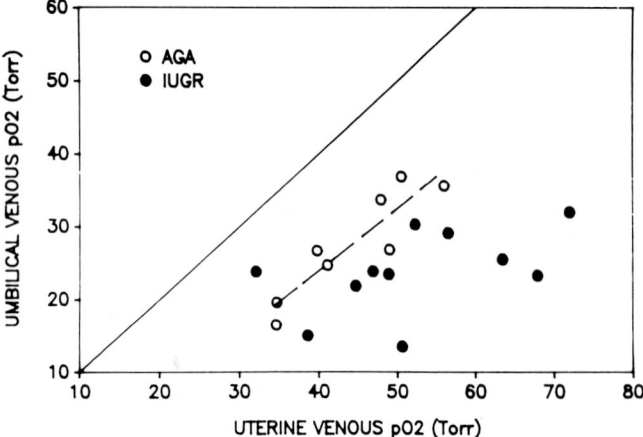

FIGURE 19–6. Relationship between uterine venous and umbilical venous PO_2 in normal (○) and IUGR (●) human pregnancies. (From Pardi et al.: Venous drainage of the human uterus: Respiratory gas studies in normal and fetal growth-retarded pregnancies. Am J Obstet Gynecol **166**:699, 1992).

....

*Derivation of equation for oxygen saturation of venous blood. Let $\dot{V}O_2$ = uterine oxygen consumption (mM/min); F = uterine blood flow (ml/min); A = arterial oxygen content (mM/ml); V = uterine venous oxygen content (mM/ml); [O_2 CAP] = oxygen capacity (mM/ml); S_A = oxygen saturation of arterial blood; and S_v = oxygen saturation of uterine venous blood.
According to the Fick principle:

$$\dot{V}O_2 = F(A - V)$$

Divide both sides of the equation by oxygen capacity:

$$\frac{\dot{V}O_2}{[O_2 \, CAP]} = F \frac{A}{[O_2 \, CAP]} - \frac{V}{[O_2 \, CAP]}$$

If we neglect the contribution of free oxygen to A and V:

$$\frac{A}{[O_2 \, CAP]} = S_A \text{ and } \frac{V}{[O_2 \, CAP]} = S_v$$

$$\therefore \frac{\dot{V}O_2}{[O_2 \, CAP]} = F \, (S_A - S_v)$$

$$\therefore S_v = S_A - \frac{\dot{V}O_2}{F \, [O_2 \, CAP]}$$

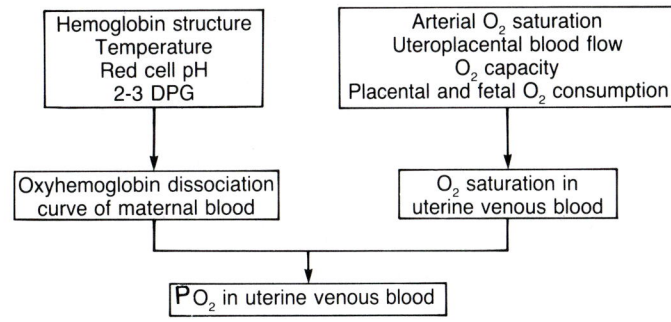

FIGURE 19–7. Factors that determine uterine venous P_{O_2}.

information about the human placenta and fetus depends on the effort of several independent research teams, each devoted to measuring only one or two of the many factors that contribute to fetal oxygen supply.

Figure 19–8 illustrates the effect of uterine blood flow variability on uterine venous P_{O_2} at three different pH values while the P_{O_2} of arterial blood, oxygen capacity, and uterine oxygen uptake are held constant.

TRANSPORT OF OXYGEN TO FETAL TISSUE

In recent years there has been considerable progress in the exploration of human fetal physiology by means of techniques for blood flow measurement and umbilical venous blood sampling *in utero.* The results of this effort, together with comparative data in sheep, allow us to construct a tentative picture of normal human fetal oxygenation and blood oxygen transport (Table 19–3).

In both the human and ovine fetus, arterial P_{O_2} is about one-fourth the maternal arterial P_{O_2} at sea level. This is a consequence partly of the structural and functional characteristics of the placenta, which require that the oxygenation of fetal blood take place at

a low P_{O_2}, and partly of the anatomy of the fetal circulation, which forms arterial blood by mixing the blood that returns from the placenta with deoxygenated blood returning from the fetal tissues.

Despite the very low P_{O_2} of its blood, the fetal lamb is capable of transporting large amounts of oxygen from the placenta to the sites of oxygen consumption within the fetal body. Three major adaptations make this possible. First, the hemoglobin of fetal red cells has a high affinity for oxygen (i.e., binds O_2 at low P_{O_2} values). This property enables the fetal red cells that circulate through the placenta to become highly saturated with oxygen. Second, the fetus has a very high cardiac output relative to its body size and metabolic rate. Third, the distribution of cardiac output between placenta and fetus and within the fetus creates a well-balanced oxygen uptake and delivery system (Battaglia and Meschia, 1986). The data that are available for the human fetus indicate the presence of a similar adaptive strategy with some intriguing quantitative differences from the ovine model.

At mid-gestation, the oxygen capacity of human fetal blood is approximately 6.5 mM, umbilical venous oxygen saturation and P_{O_2} are about 90 per cent and 50 torr, respectively (Bozzetti et al., 1987). The high P_{O_2} suggests that maternal placental blood flow is very high with respect to oxygen demand in early human gestation. By comparison, the mid-gestation ovine fetus has a somewhat lower oxygen capacity (5.7 ± 0.3 mM) and equally high umbilical venous oxygen saturation (89 ± 1 per cent). Note that a 90 per cent O_2 saturation is close to the highest value that one can reasonably expect for the oxygenation of blood by any respiratory organ. As gestation progresses toward

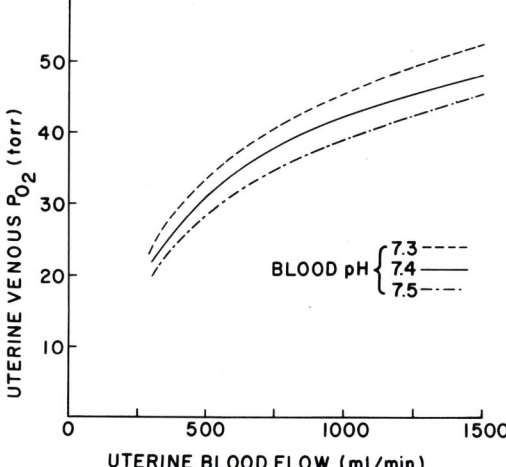

FIGURE 19–8. Uterine venous P_{O_2} as a function of uterine blood flow in a pregnant patient close to term. The figure was constructed on the assumption that the following values were constant: maternal arterial P_{O_2} 80 torr; maternal oxygen capacity 17.4 volumes per cent; oxygen consumption rate of the gravid uterus 30 ml_{STP}/minute.

TABLE 19–3. Representative Data for Blood O_2 Transport in a 35-Week Human Fetus and a Sheep Fetus at a Comparable Developmental Stage

	HUMAN FETUS (35-WEEK)	SHEEP FETUS (19-WEEK)
Blood O_2 capacity (mM)	9.4	6.7
Umbilical venous O_2 saturation (%)	70	81
Umbilical venous O_2 content (mM)	6.6	5.4
Umbilical venous P_{O_2} (torr)	28	28
Umbilical arterial O_2 saturation (%)	40	56
Umbilical arterial O_2 content (mM)	3.8	3.8
Umbilical arterial P_{O_2} (torr)	19	19
Cardiac output (ml · min^{-1} · kg^{-1})	500	500
Umbilical blood flow (ml · min^{-1} · kg^{-1})	120	216
Umbilical flow/cardiac output	0.24	0.43

term, umbilical venous oxygen saturation and P_{O_2} decline concomitantly with an increase in O_2 capacity. These changes occur in both species, but those described in humans are larger (Bozzetti et al., 1987; Soothill et al., 1986), so that in late gestation the human fetus has blood with substantially greater oxygen capacity and about 10 per cent lower umbilical venous oxygen saturation than the ovine fetus. Despite the difference in oxygen saturation, the two species have comparable umbilical venous P_{O_2} values because human fetal blood has slightly lower oxygen affinity than ovine fetal blood. Although the oxygen affinity of human fetal blood is not as high as in sheep, it still represents an important adaptation to the low P_{O_2} at which the human placenta oxygenates the fetus. Figure 19–9 compares the oxyhemoglobin dissociation curves of human adult and fetal blood and shows that at a P_{O_2} of 30 torr and blood pH 7.4, fetal blood is 73 per cent saturated with oxygen, whereas adult blood is only 60 per cent saturated.

In addition to umbilical venous P_{O_2} and oxygen saturation, we must consider oxygen content, which is the product of oxygen saturation and capacity. In this regard, the late-gestation human fetus has umbilical venous blood with higher oxygen content than the sheep fetus because the higher oxygen capacity more than compensates for the lower saturation. The next two important factors to be considered are umbilical blood flow and fetal cardiac output. The human umbilical blood flow is approximately 120 ml • min^{-1} (kg fetus)$^{-1}$ (Gill et al., 1984), which is about 40 per cent lower than umbilical blood flow measured in sheep (Battaglia and Meschia, 1986). Initial attempts to measure human fetal cardiac output suggested that it is also relatively small, but further investigations indicate that cardiac output is as high in the human as in the sheep fetus and approximately equal to 500 ml • min^{-1} (kg fetus)$^{-1}$ (Kenny et al., 1986, DeSmedt et al., 1987; Rizzo and Arduini, 1991). Therefore, there

seems to be a major difference between the two species in the distribution of fetal cardiac output. Whereas in fetal sheep umbilical blood flow represents approximately 40 per cent of cardiac output, in the late-gestation human fetus umbilical blood flow is less than 30 per cent of cardiac output (see Table 19–3). It is possible that this large difference results in part from errors of measurement. However, it seems clear that, in comparison to the ovine fetus, a high blood oxygen capacity (i.e., high hemoglobin content and hematocrit) and a low umbilical blood flow/cardiac output ratio are distinctive normal characteristics of the human fetus. Note that umbilical blood flow and oxygen capacity are interrelated. In anemic human fetuses, umbilical blood flow becomes greater than 120 ml • min^{-1} (kg fetus)$^{-1}$ and can be as high as in the sheep fetus (Jouppila and Kirkinen, 1984). To explore further the physiologic meaning of these data, it is important to realize that the function of the fetal circulation as an oxygen delivery system depends on an appropriate balance between umbilical blood flow and fetal somatic blood flow. It is intuitive that directing too much cardiac output into the somatic circulation would impair the umbilical uptake of oxygen and that directing too much cardiac output into the umbilical circulation would impair the supply of oxygen to fetal organs. It may seem that, theoretically, the optimum balance is to split the distribution of cardiac output evenly between the umbilical and somatic circulations, but in fact the optimum balance depends on a number of factors, among which oxygen capacity is quite important (Battaglia and Meschia, 1986). Everything else being equal, an increase in fetal oxygen capacity shifts the ideal balance in favor of the somatic circulation. Therefore, the high oxygen capacity of human fetal blood allows an increase of the somatic/umbilical blood flow ratio without compromising umbilical oxygen uptake. The enormous growth of the human fetal brain is probably responsible for creating the demand for a larger somatic blood flow. At term the human fetus and the ovine fetus weigh about the same, but the mass of the fetal human brain is about eight times greater. A larger cerebral mass implies greater oxygen demand and is likely to require a greater percentage of cardiac output directed to the fetal upper body at the expense of the fetal lower body and the umbilical circulation.

Because of its low blood P_{O_2}, the fetus is hypoxic in comparison to postnatal life. However, normally the fetus has access to all the oxygen that it needs and does not use anaerobic glycolysis as a terminal source of energy (Battaglia and Meschia, 1978). Furthermore, the low level of P_{O_2} in fetal arterial blood is physiologically useful because it is an essential component of the mechanisms that keep the ductus arteriosus open and the pulmonary vascular bed constricted. In order to counteract the pathologic connotation of the word "hypoxia," it is advisable to use the expression "physiologic hypoxia" to refer to the normal state of fetal oxygenation.

In the ordinary usage of the term *fetal hypoxia* means any decrease below normal in the level of fetal oxygenation. Such a decrease may come about in different ways, most commonly as a reduction in the P_{O_2} of

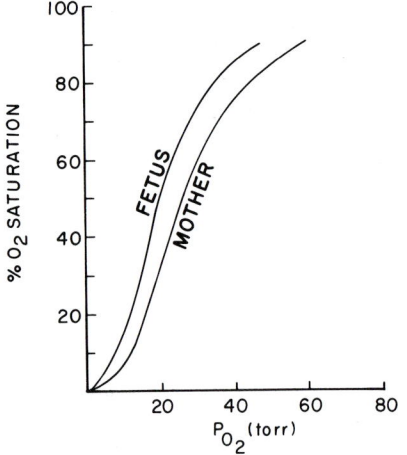

FIGURE 19–9. The oxyhemoglobin dissociation curves of maternal and fetal human blood at pH 7.4 and 37°C. (Adapted from Hellegers AE, Schruefer JJ: Nomograms and empirical equations relating oxygen tension, percentage saturation, and pH in maternal and fetal blood. Am J Obstet Gynecol 81:377, 1961.)

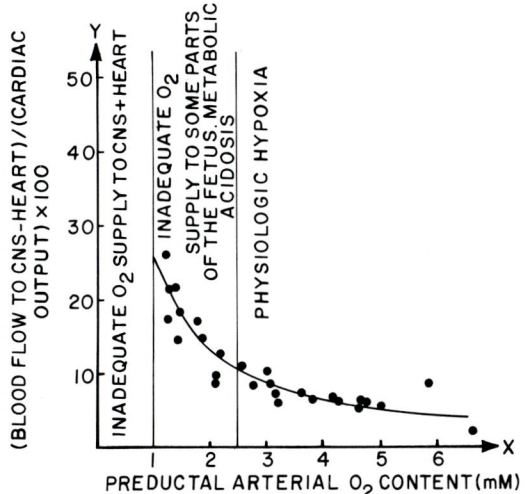

FIGURE 19–10. Hyperbolic relationship between the oxygen content in the preductal arteries of a fetal lamb and the percentage of cardiac output directed to the heart and the central nervous system. The curve was drawn according to the equation $y \cdot x = 0.26$. (Experimental data from Sheldon et al., 1979.)

umbilical venous blood (hypoxic hypoxia), in the oxygen capacity of fetal blood (anemic hypoxia, elevated levels of carbon monoxide), or in the perfusion rate of the umbilical circulation and the fetal body (circulatory hypoxia).

The circulation of a nonanesthetized, otherwise healthy sheep fetus reacts to an acute decrease in PO_2 in a predictable manner. As the PO_2 falls there is an increase of blood flow to the central nervous system (CNS) and the heart, although cardiac output and placental blood flow tend to remain constant. As a consequence, acute fetal hypoxia is characterized by a redistribution of cardiac output favoring CNS and heart at the expense of other parts of the fetal body.

The fraction of cardiac output directed to CNS and heart increases hyperbolically as the arterial oxygen content decreases (Fig. 19–10). The functional meaning of this relationship is that, in order to mount a successful defense against hypoxia, the fetus must keep constant (or nearly so) the flow of oxygen to CNS and heart, i.e., the product of blood flow times the oxygen content per milliliter of arterial blood. The limit of a successful circulatory defense against acute hypoxia is reached when the perfusion rate of the CNS and the heart has reached its maximum. In the fetal lamb this limit is in the vicinity of 1 mM oxygen content in the supraductal arteries. At this level, the flow of blood per gram of tissue is extremely high in the brain (approximately 4 ml/min/gm) and in the heart (approximately 7 ml/min/gm). Furthermore, the combined CNS and heart flow has become 26 per cent of fetal cardiac output (see Fig. 19–10). It is most likely that the circulation of the human fetus reacts similarly to acute hypoxia. However, under normal physiologic conditions the large O_2 demand of the human fetal brain requires a larger contribution of cardiac output to cerebral perfusion than in the fetal lamb. As a consequence, in response to acute hypoxia the human

fetus may not be able to produce a percentage increase in cerebral blood flow as dramatic as in a species with a small brain.

Between the region of oxygenation that defines physiologic hypoxia and the limit below which there is an insufficient oxygen supply to CNS and heart, there is a broad region (approximately between 2.5 and 1 mM arterial oxygen content in the fetal lamb) in which the supply of oxygen to parts of the fetal body other than CNS and heart becomes inadequate. In this region of oxygenation fetal blood accumulates lactic acid.

OXYGEN THERAPY

The inhalation of oxygen by a pregnant patient can increase dramatically the PO_2 of maternal arterial blood, but causes only a small increase in fetal arterial PO_2 (Table 19–4). This observation seems to contradict the empirical knowledge that oxygen therapy can be an effective measure for the temporary improvement of fetal oxygenation (oxygen toxicity in the mother is a major obstacle to the constant use of oxygen therapy). Indeed, some investigators have claimed that maternal oxygen inhalation cannot ameliorate fetal hypoxia because its effect on fetal PO_2 is "negligible." Others have claimed that the discrepancy of PO_2 changes in mother and fetus is the consequence of severe placental vasoconstriction in response to the high PO_2 of maternal blood. In order to dispel these misconceptions, it is necessary first to understand why fetal arterial PO_2 increases much less than maternal arterial PO_2 and then to focus attention on the effect that oxygen therapy has on the oxygen content of fetal blood.

The venous equilibration model of placental exchange and the characteristics of the maternal and fetal oxyhemoglobin dissociation curves readily explain the "small" effect of oxygen therapy on fetal PO_2. Consider the example shown in Figure 19–11, in which the oxygen contents of maternal and fetal blood are plotted against PO_2. The inhalation of 100 per cent oxygen by the mother causes the PO_2 of maternal arterial blood to increase from 90 to 500 torr (*step a*). This increase in PO_2 causes an increase of maternal arterial oxygen content equal to 1 mM (*step b*). These

TABLE 19–4. PO_2 of Maternal and Umbilical Blood at Different Levels of Maternal Oxygenation

	PO_2 (mm Hg)			
LOCATION	RHESUS MONKEY*		HUMAN†	
Maternal artery	108	257	91	583
Uterine vein	37	44	—	—
Umbilical vein	22	30	32	40
Umbilical artery	15	21	11	16

*Data from Behrman RE, Peterson EN, Delannoy CW: The supply of O_2 to the primate fetus with two different O_2 tensions and anesthetics. Respir Physiol 6:271, 1969.
†Data from Wulf KH, Künzel W, Lehmann V: Clinical aspects of placental gas exchange. *In* Longo LD, Bartels H (eds): Respiratory Gas Exchange and Blood Flow in the Placenta. Washington DC, DHEW Publication (NIH), 1972.

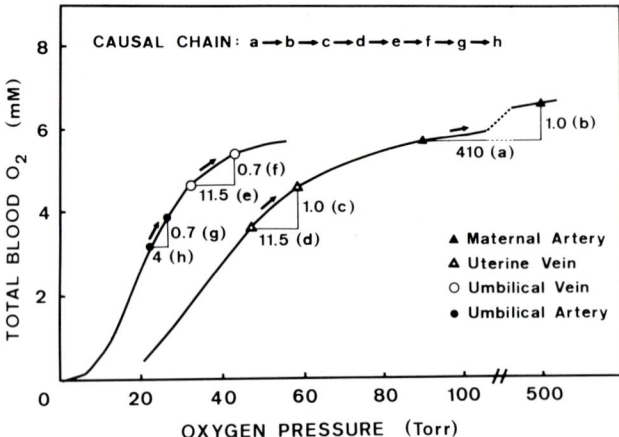

FIGURE 19–11. Example of the relationship between oxygen content and Po₂ in maternal and fetal blood before and after maternal inhalation of 100 per cent oxygen. (From Meschia G: Transfer of oxygen across the placenta. *In* Gluck L (ed): Intrauterine Asphyxia and the Developing Fetal Brain. Copyright © 1977 by Year Book Medical Publishers, Inc., Chicago. Reprinted by permission.)

changes in arterial Po_2 and oxygen content do not cause any appreciable change in the uterine blood flow. If we assume that they do not increase the uterine oxygen consumption rate—a correct assumption if fetal oxygen supply was already adequate prior to oxygen therapy—the law of conservation of matter requires that uterine venous oxygen content increase also 1 mM *(step c)*. The increase in uterine venous oxygen content causes the uterine venous Po_2 to increase 11.5 torr *(step d)*. Note that the "S" shape of the maternal oxyhemoglobin dissociation curve and the different positions of the arterial and venous points on this curve determine that an equal change of oxygen content is associated with a markedly smaller change of Po_2 in the uterine vein than in the maternal arteries. Note also that the assumption of a constant oxygen consumption rate maximizes the increase in venous Po_2. If the oxygen consumption of the gravid uterus were to increase in response to oxygen therapy, the increase of venous Po_2 would be less than indicated. Given an increase of 11.5 torr in the uterine venous Po_2, the umbilical venous Po_2 will increase by

an approximately equal value *(step e)*, as demonstrated by the experimental data shown in Figure 19–4. The increase in umbilical venous Po_2 is associated with an increase in umbilical venous oxygen content *(step f)*, whose magnitude is dictated by the slope of the oxyhemoglobin dissociation curve and by the position of the umbilical venous point on that curve. In this example, the oxygen content of umbilical venous blood increases 0.7 mM. If we assume no appreciable change in umbilical blood flow or oxygen uptake, it follows (again by application of the law of conservation of matter) that the oxygen content in the umbilical artery must increase also 0.7 mM *(step g)*. Since the arterial point is positioned on the steep part of the fetal oxyhemoglobin dissociation curve, an increase of 0.7 mM in oxygen content is associated with a Po_2 increase of only 4 torr *(step h)*. The end-result of this chain of events is that a Po_2 change of 410 torr in maternal arterial blood results in a Po_2 change of 4 torr in umbilical arterial blood.

If we were to focus our attention on fetal Po_2 changes by excluding other considerations, we might be tempted to conclude that maternal oxygen therapy has no appreciable effect on fetal oxygenation. To the contrary, what needs to be emphasized is that oxygen therapy can cause similar increments in the *oxygen content* of maternal and fetal blood. In the example under discussion, an increase of 1 mM in maternal blood was associated with an increase of 0.7 mM in fetal blood. Under somewhat different circumstances, the oxygen content of fetal blood can actually increase more than the oxygen content of maternal blood (Fig. 19–12).

PLACENTAL CARBON DIOXIDE TRANSFER

Carbon dioxide is an end product of fetal metabolism. In the fetal lamb the respiratory quotient (i.e., the moles of CO_2 produced per mole of oxygen consumed) is approximately 0.94.

The CO_2 produced by the fetus diffuses from the umbilical circulation into the placenta and from the placenta into the maternal blood, which brings it to the lungs for excretion. The diffusional transfer of CO_2 from fetus to mother requires that the Pco_2 of fetal

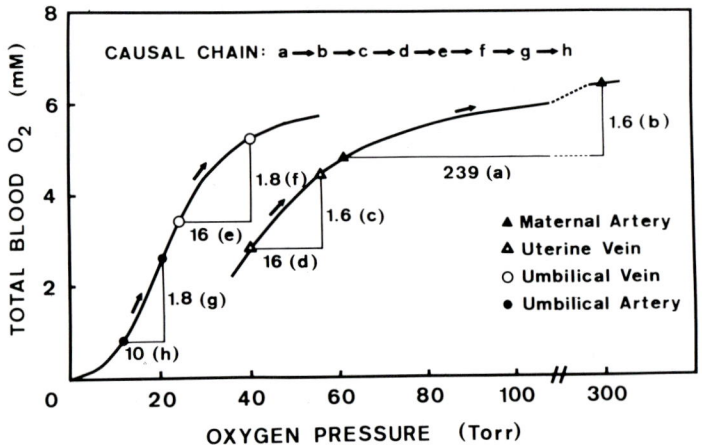

FIGURE 19–12. Example of the pronounced effect of oxygen therapy on fetal oxygen content in a case of fetal hypoxia secondary to maternal hypoxia. (From Meschia G: Transfer of oxygen across the placenta. *In* Gluck L (ed): Intrauterine Asphyxia and the Developing Fetal Brain. Copyright © 1977 by Year Book Medical Publishers, Inc., Chicago. Reprinted by permission.)

blood be higher than the P_{CO_2} of maternal blood. In chronic sheep preparations, umbilical venous P_{CO_2} is approximately 5 torr higher than uterine venous P_{CO_2}. The factors responsible for determining the magnitude of the P_{CO_2} gradient between fetal and maternal blood have not been analyzed in detail. A consequence of the high diffusibility of CO_2 across the placenta is that respiratory disturbances of acid-base balance in the mother cause—with a delay of a few minutes only—analogous disturbances in the fetus, as long as the two organisms are in communication via a well-perfused placenta. An abnormally low fetal P_{CO_2} (fetal respiratory alkalosis) is always secondary to a low maternal P_{CO_2}. To the contrary, an abnormally high fetal P_{CO_2} (fetal respiratory acidosis) can be due to a high maternal arterial P_{CO_2} or to inadequate gas exchange across the placenta, or to a combination of these two conditions.

There are probably substantial differences among mammals in the permeability of the placental barrier to bicarbonate ions. The epitheliochorial placenta of sheep has a very low permeability to bicarbonate as well as to other small anions such as chloride ions and ketoacids. If the mother develops metabolic acidosis or alkalosis, the bicarbonate concentration of fetal blood remains normal for several days. However, it is known that the hemochorial placenta of the rabbit or rhesus monkey is much more permeable to chloride ions than an epitheliochorial placenta. This suggests that the hemochorial placenta is permeable to bicarbonate and other ions, in which case metabolic disturbances of acid-base balance in the mother would cause analogous disturbances in the fetus. Unfortunately, there is no exact information, in the human or any other species with a hemochorial placenta, about the rate at which a metabolic disturbance of acid-base balance in the maternal compartment is transmitted to the fetal compartment.

REFERENCES

Battaglia FC, Meschia G: Principal substrates of fetal metabolism. Physiol Rev **58**:499, 1978.

Battaglia FC, Meschia G: An Introduction to Fetal Physiology. New York, Academic Press, 1986.

Battaglia FC, Makowski EL, Meschia G: Physiologic study of the uterine venous drainage of the pregnant Rhesus monkey. Yale J Biol Med **42**:218, 1970.

Behrman RE, Peterson EN, Delannoy CW: The supply of O_2 to the primate fetus with two different O_2 tensions and anesthetics. Respir Physiol **6**:271, 1969.

Bell AW, Kennaugh JM, Battaglia FC, et al: Metabolic and circulatory studies of fetal lamb at midgestation. Am J Physiol **250**:E538, 1986.

Bell AW, Wilkening RB, Meschia G: Some aspects of placental function in chronically heat-stressed ewes. J Devel Physiol **9**:17, 1987.

Bissonnette JM, Longo LD, Nevy MJ, et al: Placental diffusing capacity and its relation to fetal growth. J Dev Physiol **1**:351, 1979.

Bozzetti P, Buscaglia M, Cetin I, et al: Respiratory gases, acid-base balance and lactate concentrations of the midterm human fetus. Biol Neonate **51**:188, 1987.

DeSmedt MCH, Visser GHA, Meijboom EJ: Fetal cardiac output estimated by Doppler echocardiography during mid and late gestation. Am J Cardiol **60**:338, 1987.

Gaensler EA: Lung displacement: Abdominal enlargement, pleural space disorders, deformities of the thoracic cage. *In* Fenn WO, Rahn H (eds): Handbook of Physiology, Section 3: Respiration. Vol. II. Washington, DC, American Physiological Society, 1965.

Gill RW, Kossoff G, Warren PS, et al: Umbilical venous flow in normal and complicated pregnancy. Ultrasound Med Biol **10**:349, 1984.

Hellegers AE, Schruefer JJ: Nomograms and empirical equations relating oxygen tension, percentage saturation and pH in maternal and fetal blood. Am J Obstet Gynecol **81**:377, 1961.

Jouppila P, Kirkinen P: Umbilical vein blood flow in the human fetus in cases of maternal and fetal anemia and uterine bleeding. Ultrasound Med Biol **10**:365, 1984.

Kenny JF, Plappert T, Doubilet P, et al: Changes in intracardiac blood flow velocities and right and left ventricular stroke volumes in the gestational age in the normal human fetus: a prospective Doppler echocardiographic study. Circulation **74**:1208, 1986.

Longo LD, Hill EP, Power GG: Theoretical analysis of factors affecting placental O_2 transfer. Am J Physiol **222**:730, 1972.

Meschia G: Transfer of oxygen across the placenta. *In* Gluck L (ed): Intrauterine Asphyxia and the Developing Fetal Brain. Chicago, Year Book Medical Publishers, 1977.

Meschia G: Supply of oxygen to the fetus. J Reprod Med **23**:160, 1979.

Pardi G, Cetin I, Marconi AM, et al: Venous drainage of the human uterus: respiratory gas studies in normal and fetal growth retarded pregnancies. Am J Obstet Gynecol **166**:699, 1992.

Parer GT, Behrman RE: The oxygen consumption of the pregnant uterus and fetus of Macaca mulatta. Resp Physiol **3**:288, 1967.

Peeters LLH, Sheldon RE, Jones MD Jr, et al: Blood flow to fetal organs as a function of arterial oxygen content. Am J Obstet Gynecol **135**:637, 1979.

Rankin JHG, Meschia G, Makowski EL, et al: Relationship between uterine and umbilical venous P_{O_2} in sheep. Am J Physiol **220**:1688, 1971.

Rizzo G, Arduini D: Fetal cardiac function in intrauterine growth retardation. Am J Obstet Gynecol **165**:876, 1991.

Sheldon RE, Peeters LLH, Jones MD Jr, et al: Redistribution of cardiac output and oxygen delivery in the hypoxemic fetal lamb. Am J Obstet Gynecol **135**:1071, 1979.

Soothill P, Nicolaides KH, Rodeck CH, et al: Effect of gestational age on fetal and intervillous blood gas and acid base values in human pregnancy. Fetal Therapy **1**:168, 1986.

Thaler I, Manor D, Itskovitz G, et al: Changes in uterine blood flow during human pregnancy. Am J Obstet Gynecol **162**:121, 1990.

Wallenburg HCS, vanKreel BK: Placental and nonplacental drainage of the uterus in the pregnant rhesus monkey. Eur J Obstet Gynaecol Reprod Biol **7**:79, 1977.

Wilkening RB, Meschia G: Comparative physiology of placental oxygen transport. Placenta **13**:1, 1992.

Wulf KH, Künzel W, Lehmann V: Clinical aspects of placental gas exchange. *In* Longo LD, Bartels H (eds): Respiratory Gas Exchange and Blood Flow in the Placenta. Washington DC, DHEW Publications (NIH), 1972.

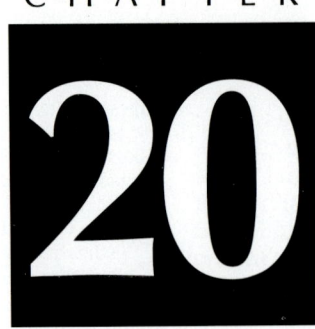

FETAL HEART RATE

....

JULIAN T. PARER, M.D., PH.D.

FACTORS CONTROLLING FETAL HEART RATE

Fetal heart rate analysis is the prime means by which a fetus is evaluated for adequacy of oxygenation, and so knowledge of its rate and regularity are of great importance to the obstetrician.

The average heart rate in the normal term fetus before labor is 140 beats/min. Earlier in pregnancy it is higher than this, although not substantially so. At 20 weeks the average fetal heart rate is 155 beats/min and at 30 weeks of pregnancy it is 144 beats/min. Variations of 20 beats/min above or below these values are seen in normal fetuses.

The fetal heart is similar to that of the adult in that it has its own intrinsic pacemaker activity that results in rhythmic contractions. The sinoatrial (SA) node, which is found in one wall of the right atrium, has the fastest rate of contraction and sets the rate in the normal heart (Fig. 20–1). The next fastest pacemaker rate is found in the atrium. Finally, the ventricle has a slower rate of beating than either the SA node or the atrium. In cases of complete or partial heart block in the fetus, variations in rate below normal can be seen. Typically a fetus with a complete heart block has a rate of about 50 to 60 beats/min.

Variability of the fetal heart rate from beat to beat, and longer-term trends in heart rate over periods of less than a minute, are important properties. Variability is of great prognostic importance clinically; valuable empiric interpretations can be made from its presence and also from its decrease or absence.

The mean fetal heart rate is the result of many physiologic factors that modulate the intrinsic rate of the heart, the most obvious being signals from the autonomic nervous system.

Parasympathetic Nervous System

The parasympathetic nervous system consists primarily of the vagus nerve (tenth cranial nerve), which originates in the medulla oblongata. Fibers from this nerve supply the SA node and also the atrioventricular (AV) node, the neuronal bridge between atrium and ventricle (see Fig. 20–1). Stimulation of the vagus nerve or injection of acetylcholine, the substance secreted at the nerve endings, results in a decrease in heart rate in the normal fetus owing to vagal influence on the SA node that decreases its rate of firing and the rate of transmission of impulses from atrium to ventricle. In a similar fashion, blocking of this nerve in a normal fetus by injecting a substance that blocks the effect of acetylcholine (e.g., atropine) causes an increase in the fetal heart rate of approximately 20 beats/min at term (Mendez-Bauer et al., 1963). This finding demonstrates that there is normally a constant vagal influence on the fetal heart rate tending to decrease it from its normal intrinsic rate.

The vagus nerve apparently also has another very important function: it is responsible for transmission of impulses causing beat-to-beat variability of fetal heart rate. Blocking the vagus nerve with atropine results in a disappearance of this variability. Hence, it has been postulated that there are two vagal influences on the heart—the first, a tonic influence tending to decrease its rate, and the second, an oscillatory influence that results in fetal heart rate variability (DeHaan et al., 1973). The vagal tone is not necessarily constant. Its influence increases with gestational age (Schifferli and Caldeyro-Barcia, 1973). In fetal sheep vagal activity increases as much as fourfold during acute hypoxia (Parer, 1983) or experimentally produced fetal growth retardation (Llanos et al., 1980).

Sympathetic Nervous System

Sympathetic nerves are widely distributed in the muscle of the heart at term. Stimulation of the sympathetic nerves will release norepinephrine and cause increases in fetal heart rate and the vigor of cardiac contractions, resulting in higher cardiac output. The sympathetic nerves are a reserve mechanism to improve the pumping activity of the heart during intermittent stressful situations. There is normally a tonic sympathetic influence on the heart. Propranolol, which blocks the action of these sympathetic nerves, causes a decrease in fetal heart rate of approximately 10 beats/min when administered to the normal sheep

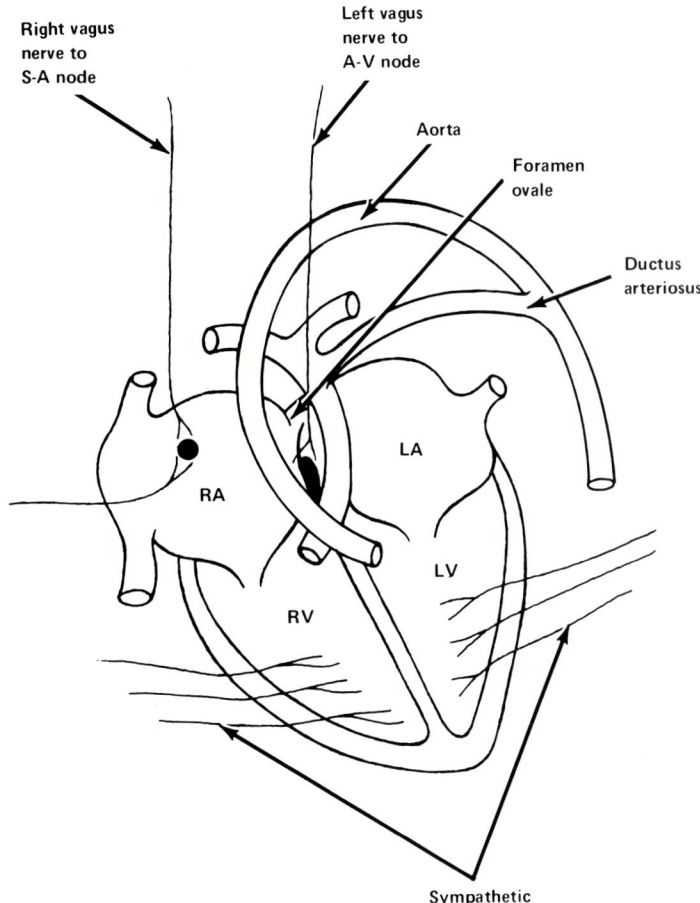

FIGURE 20–1. The fetal heart and its nervous connections. RA = right atrium; LA = left atrium; RV = right ventricle; LV = left ventricle. (From Parer JT: Physiological regulation of fetal heart rate. J Obstet Gynecol Nursing 5:265, 1976.)

fetus. As with the vagal tone, tonic influence increases as much as twofold during fetal hypoxia.

Fetal heart rate (FHR) variability decreases only slightly after blocking of the sympathetic nerves in primates. There is a commonly held theory that FHR variability is a result of the two neuronal inputs to the fetal heart, vagal and beta-adrenergic, each with a different time constant. Because atropine almost abolishes FHR variability, and propranolol decreases it only a little, it is unlikely that the theory is correct for the primate (Parer et al., 1981). However, there may be an important species difference in the transmission of FHR variability impulses. Both vagal and beta-adrenergic influences are probably important in the sheep (Dalton et al., 1983). One must keep this in mind, because sheep are used so frequently in fetal physiology studies.

Alpha-adrenergic activity is also important in altering the distribution of blood flow to specific organs during stress. Thus, during hypoxia there is vasoconstriction of certain vascular beds (e.g., gut, liver, lung) that allows preferential flow of blood with the available oxygen to vital organs (e.g., brain, heart, and adrenals), and blood flow to the placenta is maintained (see Chapter 18).

Several factors cause the parasympathetic and sympathetic nervous systems to increase their activity; they are discussed in the following pages.

Chemoreceptors

Chemoreceptors are found in both the peripheral and the central nervous systems. They have their most dramatic effects on the regulation of respiration, but they are still important in the control of the circulation. The peripheral chemoreceptors are in the carotid and aortic bodies, which are found in the arch of the aorta and the area of the carotid sinus (Fig. 20–2). The central chemoreceptors are in the medulla oblongata and respond to changes in the oxygen and carbon dioxide tensions in blood or cerebrospinal fluid perfusing this area.

In the adult, when oxygen in the arterial blood perfusing the central chemoreceptors is decreased or the carbon dioxide content is increased, a reflex tachycardia ordinarily develops. There is also a very substantial increase in arterial blood pressure, particularly with increases in carbon dioxide concentration; both of these effects are thought to be protective, in an attempt to circulate more blood through the affected areas in order to bring about a decrease in carbon dioxide tension or an increase in oxygen tension. Selective hypoxia or hypercapnia of the peripheral chemoreceptors alone in the adult produces a bradycardia, in contrast to the tachycardia and hypertension seen with central hypoxia or hypercapnia.

The interaction of the central and peripheral che-

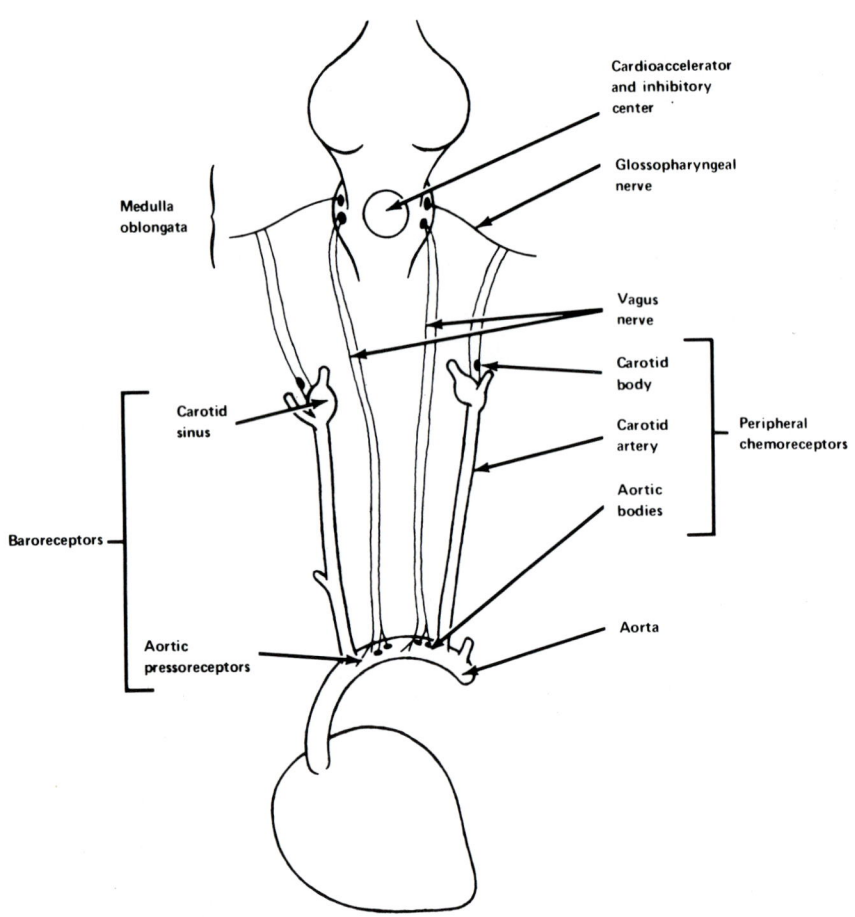

FIGURE 20–2. The peripheral chemoreceptors and baroreceptors and their input to the cardiac integrating center in the medulla oblongata. (From Parer JT: Physiological regulation of fetal heart rate. J Obstet Gynecol Nursing **5**:265, 1976.)

moreceptors in the fetus is poorly understood. It is known, however, that the net result of hypoxia or hypercapnia in the unanesthetized fetus is bradycardia with hypertension. During basal conditions, the chemoreceptors seem to contribute to the stabilization of the heart rate and blood pressure (Hanson, 1988).

Baroreceptors

In the arch of the aorta and in the carotid sinus at the junction of the internal and external carotid arteries are small stretch receptors in the vessel walls that are sensitive to increases in blood pressure (see Fig. 20–2). When pressure rises, impulses are sent from these receptors via the vagus or glossopharyngeal nerve to the mid-brain, resulting in further impulses via the vagus nerve to the heart, tending to slow it. This is an extremely rapid response, being seen with almost the first systolic rise of blood pressure. It is a protective, stabilizing attempt by the body to lower blood pressure by decreasing heart rate and cardiac output when blood pressure is increasing.

Central Nervous System

It has been established that in the adult the higher centers of the brain influence heart rate. Heart rate is increased by various emotional stimuli such as fear and sexual arousal. In fetal lambs and monkeys, the electroencephalogram or electro-oculogram shows increased activity at times in association with variability of the heart rate and body movements. At other times, apparently when the fetus is sleeping, body movement slows and the fetal heart rate variability decreases, suggesting an association between these two factors and central nervous system activity.

The hypothalamus is thought to be the area of dispatch of nerve impulses produced by physical expressions of emotion, including acceleration of the heart rate and elevation of the blood pressure. It has been shown in the fetal lamb that stimulating an electrode in the hypothalamus causes the fetal heart rate to increase, at least initially, followed by a decrease, probably because of the protective baroreflex mentioned earlier. The increases in blood pressure and heart rate appear to be mediated by the sympathetic nerves.

The medulla oblongata contains the vasomotor centers, integrative centers where the net result of all the inputs is either acceleration or deceleration of the heart rate. It is probably in these centers that the net result of numerous central and peripheral inputs is processed to generate irregular oscillatory vagal impulses, giving rise to fetal heart rate variability.

Hormonal Regulation

ADRENAL MEDULLA. The fetal adrenal medulla produces epinephrine and norepinephrine in response to stressful situations, e.g., asphyxia. Both of these substances act on the heart and cardiovascular system in a way similar to sympathetic stimulation; that is, they produce a faster heart rate, greater force of contraction of the heart, and higher arterial blood pressure. However, it is not clear whether catecholamines exert a regulatory function in the resting fetus, at least in sheep.

RENIN-ANGIOTENSIN SYSTEM. Angiotensin II seems to play a role in fetal circulatory regulation at rest, but its main activity is observed during hemorrhagic stress on a fetus.

VASOPRESSIN. Vasopressin has been shown to affect the distribution of blood flow in fetal sheep. However, this is probably operative only during hypoxia and possibly other stressful situations.

PROSTAGLANDINS. Arachidonic acid metabolites are found in high concentrations in the fetal circulation and in many tissues. Their main role seems to be in the regulation of umbilical blood flow as well as in maintaining the patency of the ductus arteriosus during fetal life.

OTHER HORMONES. Other hormones such as α-melanocyte-stimulating hormone (α-MSH), atrial natriuretic hormone, neuropeptide Y, thyrotropin-releasing hormone (TRH), and metabolites such as adenosine have also been described to be present in the fetus and to participate in the circulatory function regulation, but their importance is still not determined.

Blood Volume Control

CAPILLARY FLUID SHIFT. In the adult, when the blood pressure of the body is elevated by excessive blood volume, some fluid moves out of the capillaries into interstitial spaces, thereby decreasing the blood volume toward normal. Conversely, if the adult loses blood through hemorrhage, some fluid shifts out of the interstitial spaces into the circulation, thereby increasing the blood volume toward normal. There is normally a delicate balance between the pressures inside and outside the capillaries. This mechanism to regulate blood pressure is slower than the almost-instantaneous regulation found with the reflex mechanisms discussed previously. Its role in the fetus is imperfectly understood, although imbalances may be responsible for the hydrops seen in some cases of Rh isoimmunization and extreme fetal tachycardia. In addition, studies performed on sheep show that a fetus appears to be able to keep its blood volume closer to normal than an adult after reductions or expansions of volume (Brace and Gold, 1984).

INTRAPLACENTAL PRESSURES. Fluid moves down hydrostatic pressure gradients and also in response to osmotic pressure gradients. The actual value of these factors within the human placenta, where fetal and maternal blood closely approximate, is controversial. It seems likely, however, that there are some delicate balancing mechanisms within the placenta that prevent rapid fluid shifts between mother and fetus. The arterial blood pressure of the mother is much higher (approximately 100 mm Hg) than that of the fetus (approximately 55 mm Hg), and osmotic pressures are not substantially different. Hence, some compensatory mechanism must be present to equalize the effective pressures at the exchange points.

Frank-Starling Mechanism

The amount of blood pumped by the heart is determined by the amount of blood returning to the heart; that is, the heart pumps all of the blood that flows into it without excessive damming of blood in the veins. When the cardiac muscle is stretched prior to contraction by an increased inflow of blood, it contracts with a greater force than before and is able to pump out more blood. This mechanism has been studied in the unanesthetized fetal lamb and has been shown to be less well developed than in the adult sheep (Rudolph and Heymann, 1973), probably because the fetal heart muscle is not as well developed. It is likely that the same is true of the human fetus, which is generally more immature at birth than the lamb. As a consequence, increases in the filling pressure or preload produce minor if any changes in combined ventricular output, suggesting that the fetal heart normally operates near the top of its function curve.

The output of the fetal heart is also related to the heart rate. Some researchers have shown that spontaneous variations of heart rate relate directly to cardiac output, that is, as rate increases, output increases. However, different responses have been observed during right or left atrial pacing studies. No changes were observed in left ventricular output when the right atrium was paced, whereas the output decreased during left atrial pacing (Anderson et al., 1986). Clearly, additional factors are operating to explain such differences. This relationship between fetal heart rate and cardiac output has not been confirmed in human fetuses under physiologic conditions, because the spontaneous increase in heart rate has been found to be associated with a decrease in stroke volume, maintaining the cardiac output unchanged (Kenny et al., 1987).

In addition to heart rate and preload, cardiac output depends on afterload and intrinsic contractility. The fetal heart appears to be highly sensitive to changes in the afterload, represented by the fetal blood pressure. In this way, increases in afterload dramatically reduce the stroke volume or cardiac output. As has already been stated, the fetal heart is incompletely developed compared to that of adults. Many ultrastructural differences between the fetal and adult heart account for a lower intrinsic capacity of the fetal heart to contract. Each of these four determinants of cardiac output does not work separately, but rather they interact dynamically to modulate the fetal cardiac output during physiologic conditions. Cardiac output responses during hypoxic bradycardia are described later.

In clinical practice it is reasonable to assume that at modest variations of heart rate from the normal range, there are relatively small effects on the cardiac output. However, at extremes (for example, a tachycardia above 240 or a bradycardia below 60 beats/min), cardiac output and umbilical blood flow are likely to be hazardously decreased.

UMBILICAL BLOOD FLOW

Umbilical blood flow measured by ultrasonographic techniques is about 360 ml/min, or 120 ml/min/kg, in an undisturbed fetus at term. This figure is considerably less than that of a sheep, where it is approximately 200 ml/min/kg. The differences may be explained by the somewhat higher metabolic rate (body temperature 39°C) and lower hemoglobin concentration (10 gm/dl) in the fetal sheep. It is important to recognize this species difference because most of our information on fetal circulatory physiology comes from fetal sheep. The umbilical blood flow is approximately 40 per cent of the combined ventricular output, and about 20 per cent of this blood flow is shunted, that is, it does not exchange with maternal blood in sheep. Either it is carried through actual vascular shunts within the fetal side of the placenta or else it does not approach maternal blood closely enough to exchange with it.

Umbilical blood flow is unaffected by acute moderate hypoxia, but is decreased by severe hypoxia. There is no innervation of the umbilical cord, but umbilical blood flow decreases with the administration of catecholamines. It is also decreased by acute cord occlusion. There are no known means of increasing umbilical flow in cases in which it is thought to be decreased chronically. However, certain fetal heart rate patterns—namely, variable decelerations—have been ascribed to transient umbilical cord compression in the fetus during labor. Manipulation of maternal position either to the lateral or Trendelenburg's position can sometimes abolish these patterns; the implication is that cord compression has been relieved.

HYPOXIA/ASPHYXIA

Fetal Responses

Studies of chronically prepared animals have shown that a number of responses occur during acute hypoxia or asphyxia in the previously normoxemic fetus. There is little or no change in combined cardiac output and umbilical (placental) blood flow, but there is a redistribution of blood flow favoring certain vital organs—namely, heart, brain, and adrenal glands—and a decrease in the blood flow to the gut, spleen, kidneys, and carcass (Cohn et al., 1974). This initial response is presumed to be advantageous to a fetus in the same way as the diving reflex is in an adult seal, in that the blood containing the available oxygen and other nutrients is supplied preferentially to vital organs.

Fetal oxygen consumption decreased to values as low as 60 per cent of control (from approximately 8 to 5 ml/min/kg) during fetal hypoxia in the chronically instrumented fetus with arterial oxygen tension of 10 mm Hg (Parer, 1980). This decrease is rapidly instituted, stable for periods up to 45 minutes, proportional

to the degree of hypoxia, and rapidly reversible on cessation of maternal hypoxia. It is accompanied by a fetal bradycardia of about 30 beats/min below control (approximately 170 beats/min control to 140 beats/min hypoxia in fetal sheep) and an increase in fetal arterial blood pressure (approximately 54 mm Hg control to 61 mm Hg hypoxia mean pressure). There is also progressive fetal acidosis during fetal isocapnic hypoxia (fetal arterial pH 7.38 control to 7.33 after 25 minutes hypoxia). This is a metabolic acidosis due to lactic acid accumulation as a result of anaerobic metabolism primarily in those partially vasoconstricted beds where oxygenation is inadequate for normal basic needs (Mann, 1970). During fetal asphyxia, the increase in carbon dioxide tension superimposes a respiratory component on the acidosis.

The series of responses just described—that is, redistribution of blood flow favoring vital organs, decreased total oxygen consumption, and anaerobic glycolysis—may be thought of as temporary compensatory mechanisms that enable a fetus to survive moderately long periods (e.g., up to 30 minutes) of limited oxygen supply without decompensation of vital organs, particularly the brain and heart. The close matching of blood flow to oxygen availability to achieve a constancy of oxygen consumption has been demonstrated in the fetal cerebral circulation (Jones et al., 1977) and in the fetal myocardium (Fisher et al., 1982). In studies on hypoxic lamb fetuses, cerebral oxygen consumption was constant over a wide range of arterial oxygen contents because the decrease in arteriovenous oxygen content accompanying hypoxia was compensated for by an increase in cerebral blood flow.

However, during more severe asphyxia or sustained hypoxemia, these responses are no longer maintained, and a decrease in the cardiac output, arterial blood pressure, and blood flow to the brain and heart has been described (Fig. 20–3) (Yaffe et al., 1987). These changes may be considered to be a stage of decompensation, after which tissue damage and even fetal death may follow (Myers, 1972).

Metabolic Effects

It is known that the fetus depends partially on anaerobic metabolism for its energy needs during oxygen insufficiency (Low et al., 1975). It has also been shown in experimental animals that a newborn's ability to tolerate asphyxia depends on cardiac carbohydrate reserves. Whether this also applies to a human fetus is unknown, but clinical observations support the view that carbohydrate-depleted fetuses succumb more readily than those with normal reserves. A nutritionally growth-retarded fetus also is more susceptible to intrauterine asphyxia and depression than a normal fetus (Mann et al., 1974).

It has been stated that the prime aim of compensatory responses in hypoxia is maintenance of the circulation, and maintenance of the integrity of cardiac function is paramount in this regard. It is likely that carbohydrate availability is critical in supplying sub-

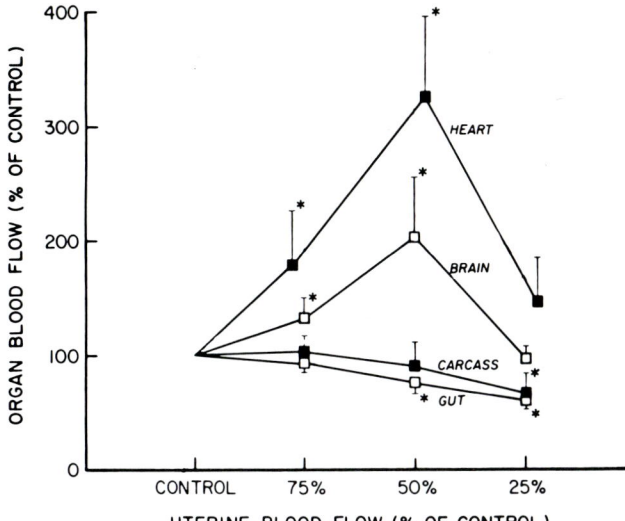

FIGURE 20–3. Changes of heart, brain, carcass, and gut blood flows during different degrees of fetal asphyxia produced by reduction of the uterine blood flow in sheep. The increase in heart and brain blood flow is reversed after more severe asphyxia. (Adapted from Yaffe H, et al: Cardiorespiratory responses to graded reductions of uterine blood flow in the sheep fetus. J Dev Physiol **9**:325, 1987 by permission of Oxford University Press.)

strates for glycolysis at more severe degrees of hypoxia.

Mechanisms of Responses

The cardiovascular responses to hypoxia are instituted rapidly and are mediated by neural and hormonal mechanisms (Fig. 20–4). As has been previously mentioned, the tonic influence of the autonomic nervous system on heart rate, blood pressure, and the umbilical circulation in a normoxemic fetus is quantitatively minor. This is in marked contrast to autonomic activity during hypoxia.

In studies using total pharmacologic blockade, it has been shown that parasympathetic activity is augmented three to five times and beta-adrenergic activity doubles when measured by heart rate response. The net result of these changes is a decrease in fetal heart rate during hypoxia. Augmented beta-adrenergic activity also may be important in maintaining cardiac output and umbilical blood flow during hypoxia, probably by increased inotropic effect on the heart.

Alpha-adrenergic activity is important in determining regional distribution of blood flow in hypoxic fetal sheep by selective vasoconstriction. As noted earlier, during hypoxia there is preferential blood flow to the brain, heart, and adrenals and decreased supply to the carcass, lungs, kidneys, and gut. Alpha-adrenergic blockade reversed the hypertension and increased peripheral resistance observed during fetal hypoxia. These changes are due to a decrease in the resistance in the gut, spleen, lungs, and probably carcass, indicating a participation of the alpha-adrenergic system in their vasoconstriction (Reuss et al., 1982).

Plasma concentrations of catecholamines, vasopressin, beta-endorphin, and atrial natriuretic factor increase during hypoxia in the fetus. The contributions of catecholamines to the circulatory responses to hypoxia were described earlier. Vasopressin contributes to the increase in blood pressure observed during hypoxia by decreasing umbilical and gut blood flows. Beta-endorphin and probably other endogenous opioids also participate in the response to hypoxia. The blockade of its receptors with naloxone further increases the hypertensive response by increasing the vasoconstriction in the kidneys and carcass. During hypoxia, a decrease in the fetal blood volume has been described. Atrial natriuretic factor may play a role in this response. Most of these results have been obtained from the chronically catheterized fetal sheep model. The relative contributions of these and other mediators to the cardiovascular response to hypoxia in a human fetus continue to be explored, because it is clear that the redistribution of blood flow is a powerful mechanism for protection of fetal organs from asphyxial damage during periods of oxygen insufficiency.

THE FETAL HEART RATE MONITOR

The fetal heart rate monitor is a device with two components, one to recognize and process heart rate and the other to recognize uterine contractions (Hon, 1968) (Fig. 20–5).

For recognition of fetal heart rate, the device uses the R wave of the fetal electrocardiogram complex, or

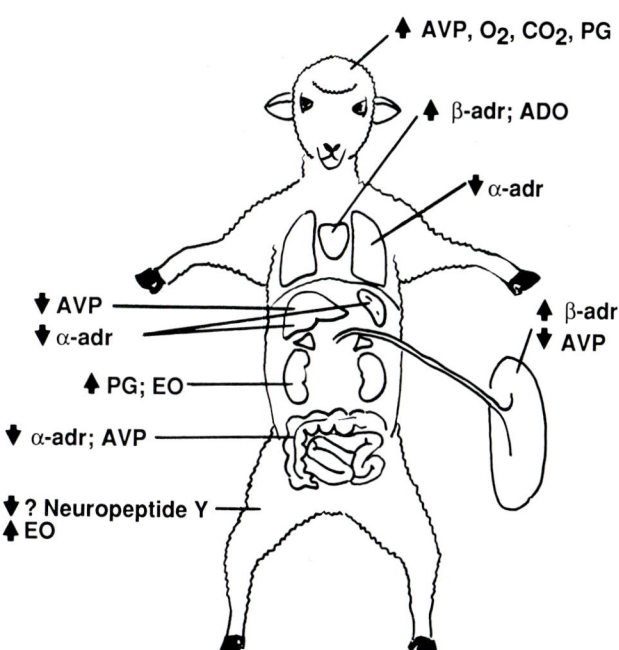

FIGURE 20–4. Summary of the mechanisms that are known to participate in the regulation of blood flow due to changes in vascular resistance in different organs and tissues during hypoxia in the fetal sheep. ↑ means increase in blood flow; ↓ means decrease in blood flow. ADO = adenosine; adr = adrenergic; AVP = arginine-vasopressin; EO = endogenous opioids; PG = prostaglandins.

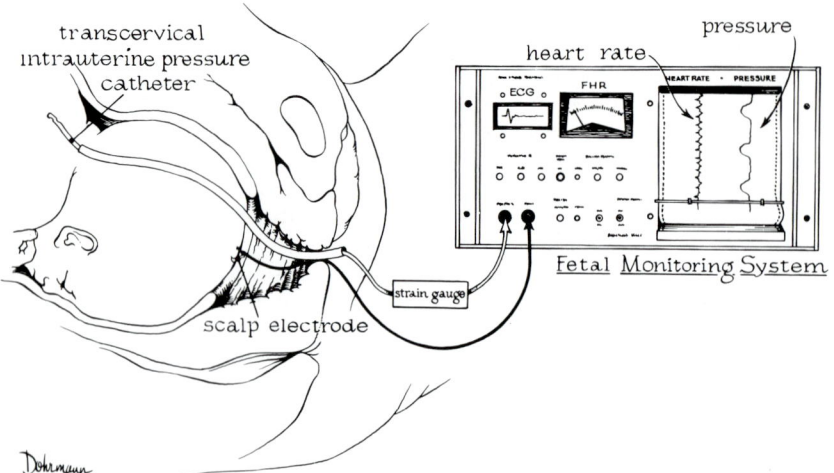

FIGURE 20–5. The fetal heart rate monitor, showing direct application, with fetal scalp electrode and intra-amniotic catheter.

a signal generated by the movement of a cardiovascular structure using ultrasound and the Doppler principle. Uterine contractions are detected either by an open-ended or balloon-tipped catheter inserted transcervically into the amniotic cavity and attached to a strain gauge transducer, or by an external device called a tokodynamometer, which is placed on the maternal abdomen and recognizes the tightening of the maternal abdomen during a contraction.

Monitoring with devices attached directly to the fetus or placed within the uterine cavity is called "direct," "internal," or "invasive." Devices that do not require direct connection with the fetus are called "noninvasive" or "external."

A critical component of the fetal monitor is the cardiotachometer. An understanding of its mode of action is essential for appreciating FHR variability. Within the monitor is a device for recognizing the cardiac event. Another device measures the interval between the events, and a third device rapidly divides the interval in seconds into 60 to give a rate for each interval between beats. These individual rates are then traced on a strip chart recorder moving at a specific speed. When the paper moves slowly, the recording appears as a "jiggly" line, representing the variability. If the intervals between heartbeats are identical, the line is straight, representing absence of variability or a flat or silent baseline.

Fetal Heart Rate Detection

FETAL ELECTRODE. The internal means of detecting FHR consists almost exclusively now of a small stainless steel spiral electrode attached to the fetal scalp. A second contact is bathed by the vaginal fluids. The wires traverse the vaginal canal and are connected to the machine. This mode gives the most accurate fetal heart rate tracing because of the discreteness of the signal, so that it accurately depicts beat-to-beat variability.

DOPPLER ULTRASOUND TRANSDUCER. The Doppler ultrasound transducer consists of a device affixed to the maternal abdominal wall that transmits a high-frequency sound of approximately 2.5 mHz. The signal is reflected from a moving structure, e.g., the ventricle wall, and the reflected beam is changed in frequency, depending on whether the wall moves away from or toward the source. The change in frequency with each systole is recognized as the cardiac event and is processed by the machine.

Although this device is simple to apply and can be used before rupture of membranes, it is sometimes unreliable during labor because of maternal and fetal movements. A greater disadvantage is that it may not give a valid indication of beat-to-beat variability, because the Doppler signal is broad and slurred and the machine is not always able to select accurately and consistently a point on this slurred curve representing the exact time of a cardiac event. Hence, an artificial short-term variability tends to be portrayed by this device, even up to variations of 5 beats/min. Long-term variability, however, may be accurately displayed.

Improvements in construction and logic have made the later-generation Doppler devices more accurate and easier to use. In particular, the technique of autocorrelation can be used to more accurately define the timing of the cardiac contraction by taking a number of points on the "curve" depicting the Doppler frequency shift. Earlier systems selected a threshold or peak of the curve, thereby making small errors in the timing of the contraction, which resulted in artifactual "variability."

SOURCES OF ARTIFACT AND ERROR. There are a number of opportunities for misinterpretation of FHR records (Klapholz et al., 1974). These can be due to electrical or signal defects, limitations of the machinery, or errors in interpretation of the records. These errors and their solutions are shown in Table 20–1.

Uterine Activity Detection

INTRA-AMNIOTIC CATHETER. The internal, invasive means of detecting uterine activity uses a soft plastic, open-ended or balloon-tipped catheter placed transcervically into the amniotic cavity (see Fig. 20–5). The open-ended catheter is filled with sterile water and transmits pressure changes caused by contractions to

TABLE 20–1.   Types of Errors in Fetal Heart Rate Monitoring and Their Solutions

TYPE OF ERROR	SOLUTION
Electrical or signal errors	
Faulty electrode material, legplate, or monitor	Replace defective parts
Intrinsic FEKG voltage too low	Use Doppler method
60-cycle interference	Ground the machine
Interference by maternal signal (maternal EKG or muscle movement, uterine contractions, equipment such as bedpans)	Recognize
Limitations of machinery	
Penlift (switch on back of certain machines that omits FHR more than 30 beats/min different from preceding beat, so it may omit arrhythmias)	Leave penlift out Record strip of fetal EKG directly
Averaging (may smooth variability)	Recognize that some ultrasound monitors take a running average of two or three beats
Halving or doubling (very slow rates may be doubled and very fast rates [>240 beats/min] may be halved by machine)	Auscultation
Short-term variability in Doppler signal due to indistinct FHR signal	Realize that short-term variability cannot always be reliably determined with a Doppler method
Interpretative errors	
Maternal signal being picked up because fetus is dead	Compare FHR pattern with maternal rate
Scaling error (using two speeds on some machines, which are capable of 1 and 3 cm/min)	Recognize that FHR pattern changes with recording rate, and use one rate all the time, preferably 3 cm/min
Nonrecognition of artifact ("good variability" may really be a noisy signal, especially with Doppler method)	Recognize
Arrhythmias (tend to be regular) confused with artifact (tend to be irregular)	Record fetal EKG directly

a strain gauge transducer. The pressure changes are translated to an electrical signal displayed and calibrated directly in mm Hg of pressure.

TOKODYNAMOMETER. An external device, the tokodynamometer is strapped to the maternal abdominal wall, generally over the uterine fundus. The tightening of the fundus with each contraction is detected by pressure on a small button in the center of the transducer, and uterine activity is displayed on the recorder. In a sense, it acts just like the hand placed on the abdomen to detect uterine activity. This simple device detects frequency and duration of uterine contractions, but cannot be calibrated for intensity as in direct pressure measurements. A modification of this device uses a circumferential ring that allows its attachment with a standard tension. This device can be at least partially calibrated.

A potential disadvantage is that the tokodynamometer works best with the mother in the supine position and moving as little as possible. This require-

ment may not be compatible with maternal comfort, fetal well-being, or progress of labor.

CHARACTERISTICS OF FETAL HEART RATE PATTERNS

Basic Patterns

The characteristics of the fetal heart rate pattern are classified as baseline or periodic (Hon and Quilligan, 1967). The baseline features, heart rate and variability, are those recorded between uterine contractions; periodic changes occur in association with uterine contractions.

Baseline Features

The baseline features of the heart rate are those predominant characteristics that can be recognized between uterine contractions. These consist of the following:

BASELINE RATE. The baseline fetal heart rate is conventionally considered to be between 120 and 160 beats/min. Values below 120 are termed bradycardia and those above 160, tachycardia.

FETAL HEART RATE VARIABILITY. In examining an FHR monitor tracing, in most cases one notes a "jiggly," irregular line. These jiggles demonstrate the FHR variability and represent a slight difference in interval, and therefore in calculated FHR, from beat to beat. If all intervals between heartbeats were identical, the line would be regular or smooth.

Two types of fetal heart rate variability are clinically recognized. First, *short-term variability* is considered to be the beat-to-beat fluctuation in heart rate that arises from the fact that there is a slightly different period between R waves of the electrocardiogram in the normal fetus. The second component is called *long-term variability*, and this can be described as either amplitude changes or frequency changes in the longer-term unidirectional changes of fetal heart rate, which occupy a cycle of less than one minute. The most commonly accepted quantitation of long-term variability in the United States is the approximate bandwidth of the amplitude fluctuations in long-term variability. Frequency changes in long-term variability have gained little popularity in clinical practice.

Periodic Patterns

Periodic patterns are the alterations in fetal heart rate that are associated with uterine contractions. These consist of (1) late decelerations, (2) variable decelerations, and (3) accelerations.

The Normal Pattern

The normal fetal heart rate pattern (Fig. 20–6) is accepted as that with a predominant heart rate of 120 to 160 beats/min. The beat-to-beat variability is present, and the long-term variability bandwidth is between 6 and 25 beats/min. There are no decelerative

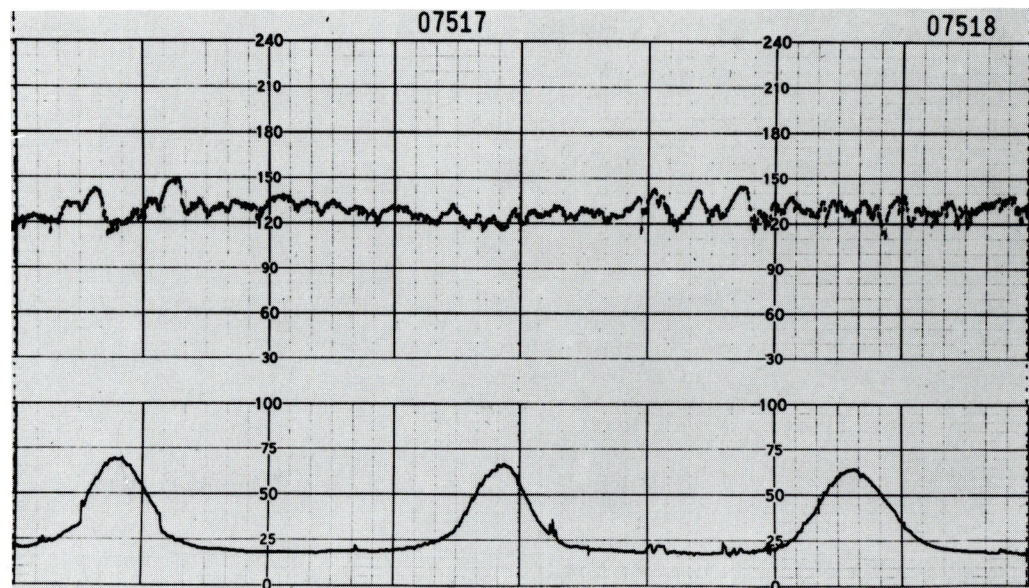

FIGURE 20–6. Normal FHR pattern with normal rate (about 130 beats/min) and normal short-term and long-term variability (amplitude range about 15 beats/min) and absence of periodic changes. This pattern represents a normally oxygenated fetus without evidence of asphyxial stress. Uterine contractions are 2 to 3 minutes apart, and about 60 mm Hg in intensity.

periodic changes, but there may be periodic accelerations (Table 20–2).

It is widely accepted in clinical practice that the fetus born with this normal heart rate pattern is virtually always vigorous and normally oxygenated if it is delivered at the time when the normal heart rate pattern is traced (Paul et al., 1975; Krebs et al., 1979; Parer, 1983). This will not hold, of course, should there be a subsequent traumatic delivery or a congenital anomaly inconsistent with extrauterine life.

In contrast to this high predictability of fetal normoxia and vigor in the presence of the normal pattern, there are a number of variant patterns that are not so accurately predictive of fetal asphyxia. However, when placed in the context of the clinical case, the progressive change in the patterns, and the duration of the variant patterns, reasonable judgments can be made about the likelihood of fetal asphyxial decompensation. Using this as a screening approach, impending intolerable fetal asphyxia can be presumed or, in certain cases, ruled out by the use of ancillary techniques such as the fetal stimulation test (Clark et al., 1984), vibroacoustic stimulation (Smith et al., 1986a), or fetal blood sampling (Wood et al., 1967; Beard et al., 1971; Tejani et al., 1976).

TABLE 20–2. Characteristics of Normal Fetal Heart Rate Patterns

Baseline rate	120 to 160 beats/min
Baseline variability (amplitude range)	>6 beats/min
Periodic patterns	None or accelerations
Fetal outcome	Vigorous; Apgar score >7 at 5 min

Variant Fetal Heart Rate Patterns

Baseline Rate

Bradycardia. The initial response of the normal fetus to acute hypoxia or asphyxia is bradycardia (Court and Parer, 1984). This statement is in contrast to some earlier beliefs whereby under acutely operated or anesthetized conditions a fetal tachycardia was sometimes noted in response to acutely imposed hypoxia. There is also a report of tachycardia occurring in experimental animals with very mild hypoxia, but clinically and experimentally the initial statement regarding bradycardia holds in the vast majority of cases because initially the vagal nerve activity is greater than the sympathetic activity.

There are a number of nonasphyxial causes of bradycardia. These include the bradyarrhythmias (for example, complete heart block), certain drugs (e.g., beta-adrenergic blockers or "caine" drugs), and hypothermia. There are other fetuses that have a heart rate below 120, but are otherwise totally normal and simply represent a normal variation outside our arbitrarily set limits of normal heart rate.

Bradycardia is arbitrarily distinguished from a deceleration, which is transient. A bradycardia is considered to represent a decrease in heart rate below 120 beats/min for 2 minutes or longer.

Prolonged bradycardia is considered to represent a prolonged stepwise decrease in fetal oxygenation (Fig. 20–7). This may be a consequence of fetal hypoxia due to vagal activity (and later hypoxic myocardial decompression), or the bradycardia may eventually result in fetal hypoxia because of the inability of the fetus to maintain a compensatory increase in stroke volume. As noted above, the hypoxic fetus has a

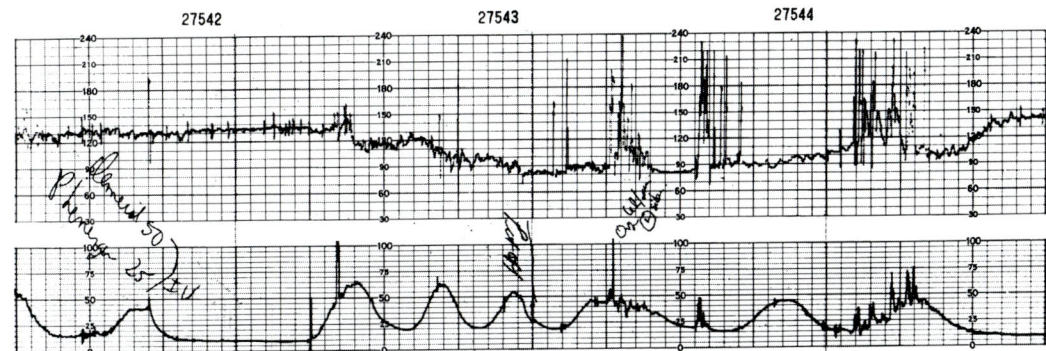

FIGURE 20–7. Prolonged fetal bradycardia due to excessive oxytocin-induced hyperstimulation of the uterus following intravenous infusion of Demerol and Phenergan into the same tubing. The heart rate is returning to normal at the end of the tracing, following appropriate treatment (signified by the notes "Pit off," "O₂ 61/min," and "side"). Note that FHR variability was maintained throughout this asphyxial stress, signifying adequate central oxygenation.

certain ability to increase stroke volume in response to bradycardia, but this breaks down at severe decreases in heart rate, probably below 60 beats/min. Under these conditions fetal cardiac output cannot be maintained, and therefore umbilical blood flow decreases. This results in insufficient oxygen transport from the fetal placenta to the fetal body and therefore results in eventual fetal hypoxic decompensation.

Reasons for the decreased heart rate may be a stepwise drop in oxygenation as occurs with maternal apnea or amniotic fluid embolus, a decrease in umbilical blood flow as occurs with a prolapsed cord, or a decrease in uterine blood flow as occurs with severe maternal hypotension.

A more complete discussion of bradycardias will appear later in this chapter.

TACHYCARDIA. Tachycardia is seen in some cases of fetal asphyxia, but never alone. That is, in the presence of normal fetal heart rate variability and absent periodic changes, the tachycardia must be assumed to be due to some other cause besides hypoxia. Tachycardia is sometimes seen on recovery from asphyxia and probably represents catecholamine activity following sympathetic nervous or adrenal medullary activity in response to this asphyxial stress, and withdrawal of vagal activity when the hypoxia is relieved.

There are a number of nonasphyxial causes of tachycardia. The most common of these is maternal or fetal infection, especially chorioamnionitis. Some drugs will cause tachycardia, for example, beta-mimetic agents or parasympathetic blockers such as atropine. Tachyarrhythmias occasionally occur, and at severe elevations of rate (e.g. above 240 beats/min), these may cause fetal cardiac failure with subsequent hydrops.

Baseline Variability

As noted above, normal FHR variability has two components, short-term (STV) and long-term variability (LTV). Usually they are both present, and the baseline has a jagged appearance, with unpredictable movements of heart rate upward or downward. The absence of either STV or LTV is a variant from normal.

There are four basic classes of heart rate variability:

(1) normal variability, in which the amplitude range of the variability is 6 beats/min or greater; (2) decreased variability, in which the amplitude range is less than 6 beats/min; (3) absence of variability, in which the amplitude range is less than 2 beats/min and the line looks "flat" or smooth; (4) saltatory pattern, or FHR variability of amplitude greater than 25 beats/min. Note that these classes are based primarily on the LTV. Superimposed on this classification is the visual estimate of "presence" or "absence" of STV. Generally, both types of variability exist together.

Although the physiologic origin and significance of FHR variability are not yet known for certain, there is a good deal of evidence to support the clinical belief that it represents an intact nervous pathway through cerebral cortex, mid-brain, vagus nerve, and cardiac conduction system. Thus, the integrity of this pathway is intact in the presence of normal FHR variability.

As described earlier, in the past FHR variability had been ascribed to an interaction between two branches of the autonomic nervous system—parasympathetic and beta-adrenergic—with different time constants. Because variability is primarily transmitted via the parasympathetic nerves in primates, this theory is unlikely to be true (Parer et al., 1981). It is more likely that variability is due to numerous sporadic inputs from various areas of the cerebral cortex and lower centers to the cardiac integratory centers in the medulla oblongata, which are then transmitted down the vagus nerve. Current theory suggests that these inputs decrease in the presence of cerebral asphyxia, and thus variability decreases after failure of the fetal hemodynamic compensatory mechanisms to maintain cerebral oxygenation.

The most important currently accepted aspect of these clinical correlates is the fact that, in the presence of normal FHR variability, no matter what other FHR patterns may be present, the fetus is not suffering cerebral tissue asphyxia because it has been able to successfully centralize the available oxygen and is thus physiologically compensated. In the presence of excessive asphyxial stress, however, as evidenced by severe periodic changes or prolonged bradycardia, this compensation may break down, and the fetus may have progressive central tissue asphyxia, i.e., asphyxia

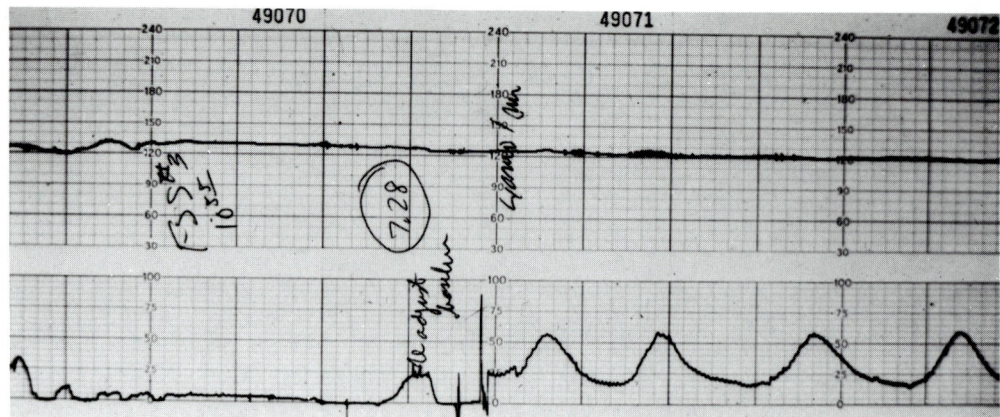

FIGURE 20–8. No variability of fetal heart rate. The patient was a severe preeclamptic receiving magnesium sulfate and narcotics. The normal scalp blood pH (7.28) assures one that the absence of variability is nonasphyxic in origin and that the fetus is not chronically asphyxiated and decompensating. The uterine activity channel has an inaccurate trace in the first half.

in cerebral and myocardial tissues. In this case, FHR variability decreases and eventually is lost.

There are several possible nonasphyxial causes of decreased or absent FHR variability: (1) absence of cortex (anencephaly); (2) narcotized or drugged higher centers (e.g., by morphine, meperidine, diazepam, magnesium sulfate) (Fig. 20–8); (3) vagal blockade (e.g., by atropine or scopolamine); and (4) defective cardiac conduction system (e.g., complete heart block) (Fig. 20–9).

The essence of the art of appropriate intrapartum FHR interpretation is noting a decrease or disappearance of FHRV in the presence of appropriate asphyxial stress patterns. Fortunately when labor begins most fetuses have normal STV and LTV, and so changes can be followed. Also, the ability of the clinician's eye to quantitate FHRV is excellent when compared to computer programs (Knopf et al., 1992).

Fetuses with unexplained virtual absence of FHRV and no periodic changes fall into three categories: (1) deep asphyxia with inability of the heart to manifest periodic changes, (2) congenital neurologic damage,

from either a developmental CNS defect or an *in utero* infection or asphyxial event (Kero et al., 1978), or (3) idiopathic reduced FHRV, with no obvious explanation, but no evidence of asphyxia or compromised CNS.

If the FHRV is reduced or absent on initial placement of the monitor, it becomes more difficult, or even impossible, for the clinician to determine whether progressive asphyxia is occurring and so ancillary testing will be necessary; if tests are not available, delivery may need to take place to "give the fetus the benefit of uncertainty."

Periodic Changes in Fetal Heart Rate

Late Decelerations. Late decelerations have the following characteristics (Hon and Quilligan, 1967). They are smooth and rounded in configuration and are the mirror image of the contraction; they are persistent, occurring with each contraction; their onset, nadir, and recovery are generally delayed 10 to 30 seconds after the onset, apex, and resolution of the

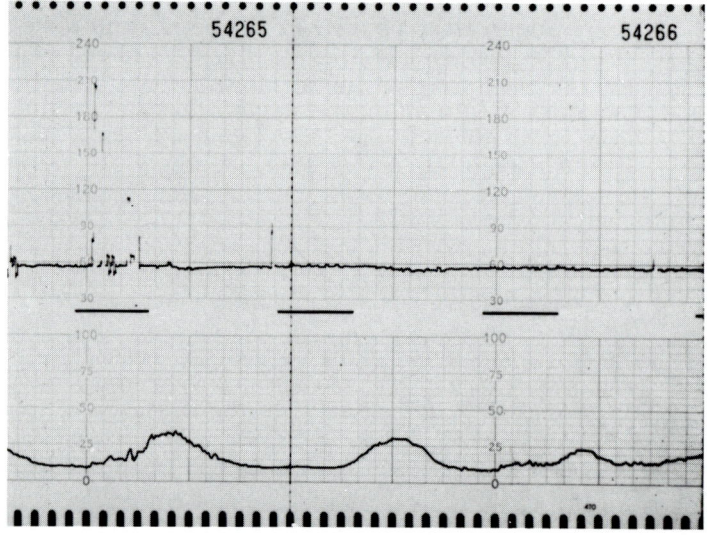

FIGURE 20–9. An unremitting fetal bradycardia. This does not signify asphyxia, because this fetus had complete heart block with ventricular rate of about 55 beats/min. Note the absence of fetal heart rate variability. There were serious cardiac structural defects, and the fetus died shortly after birth.

contraction; and the depth of the dip is related to the intensity of the contraction (Fig. 20–10).

Late decelerations are of two varieties (Martin et al., 1979; Parer et al., 1980; Harris et al., 1982; Parer, 1983):

1. The first type, *reflex late deceleration*, is seen when a sudden acute insult, e.g., reduced uterine blood flow due to maternal hypotension, is superimposed on a previously normally oxygenated fetus. These late decelerations are caused by a decrease in uterine blood flow (with the uterine contraction), beyond the capacity of the fetus to extract sufficient oxygen. The deoxygenated blood is carried from the fetal placenta through the umbilical vein to the heart and is distributed to the aorta, neck vessels, and head. Here, the low oxygen tension is sensed by chemoreceptors, and neuronal activity results in a vagal discharge, which causes the transient deceleration. The deceleration is presumed to be "late" because of the circulation time from the fetal placental site to the chemoreceptors and also because the progressively decreasing Po_2 must reach a certain threshold before vagal activity occurs. There may also be baroreceptor activity causing the vagal discharge (Martin et al., 1979). Between contractions, oxygen delivery is adequate and there is no additional vagal activity; thus the heart rate is normal. These late decelerations are accompanied by normal fetal heart rate variability and thus signify normal central nervous system integrity, i.e., the fetus is physiologically "compensated" in the vital organs (Fig. 20–11). The periodic change previously called "early deceleration" appears to simply be a variant of the reflex late deceleration (Fig. 20–12).

2. The second type of late deceleration, nonreflex late deceleration, is a result of the same initial mechanism, except that the deoxygenated bolus of blood from the placenta is presumed to be insufficient to support myocardial action, and so for the period of the contraction there is direct myocardial hypoxic depression (or failure) as well as vagal activity (Harris et al., 1982). This variety is seen without variability (Fig. 20–13), signifying fetal "decompensation," i.e., inadequate fetal cerebral and myocardial oxygenation.

It is seen most commonly in states of decreased placental reserve, e.g., with preeclampsia or intrauterine growth retardation or following prolonged asphyxial stresses, such as a long period of severe reflex late decelerations.

The distinguishing feature between reflex and nonreflex late decelerations is therefore the presence of FHR variability in the former. Each category has been shown to dichotomize into two groups based on pH, that of the reflex late deceleration group being in the normal range (Paul et al., 1975).

Severe late decelerations are those with a drop of more than 45 beats/min below the baseline and may be seen with reflex or nonreflex late decelerations (Kubli et al., 1969). There are heart rate and duration criteria for identifying mild and moderate late decelerations, but they are mainly of statistical rather than clinical importance.

When late decelerations are present, vigorous efforts should be made to eliminate them by optimizing placental blood flow and maternal hyperoxia. Vagal late decelerations, which in most cases are a result of an acute asphyxial episode, can generally be abolished. However, those caused by myocardial failure usually are seen when placental reserve is surpassed and the intermittent decreases in uterine blood flow with each contraction can no longer be tolerated (Fig. 20–14). The abolition of such late decelerations is unlikely.

VARIABLE DECELERATIONS. Variable decelerations (Fig. 20–15) have the following characteristics: (1) the appearance of the dip is variable in duration, depth, and shape from contraction to contraction; (2) variable decelerations are usually abrupt in onset and cessation, sometimes falling 60 beats/min in one or several beats, and are thus neurogenic (vagal) in origin; (3) they are described as severe when the decelerations are (a) below 60 beats/min, (b) 60 beats/min below baseline FHR, or (c) longer than 60 seconds in duration; and (4) variable decelerations without the criteria listed in (3) are classified as mild to moderate. Although other criteria have been proposed (Kubli et

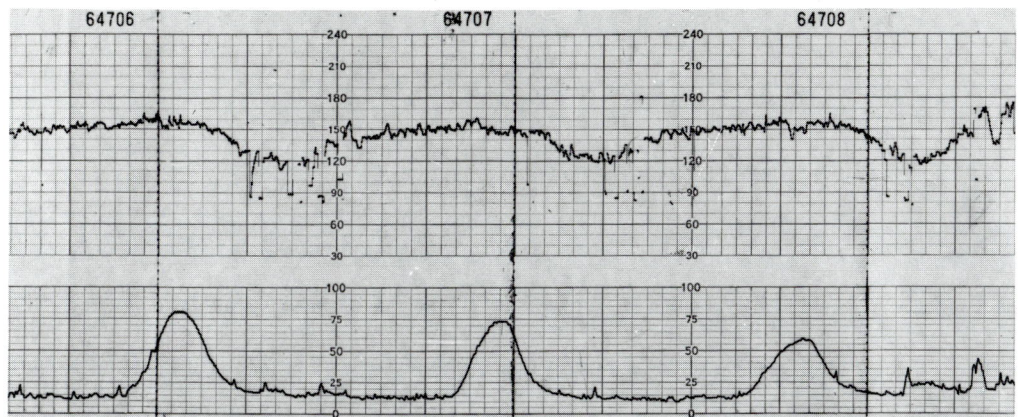

FIGURE 20–10. Late decelerations. These were recorded via Doppler ultrasound in the antepartum period in a severely growth-retarded (1700-gm) term baby born to a 32-year-old preeclamptic primipara. Delivery was by cesarean section because neither a direct fetal ECG nor fetal blood sample could be obtained owing to a firm, closed posterior cervix. The infant subsequently did well.

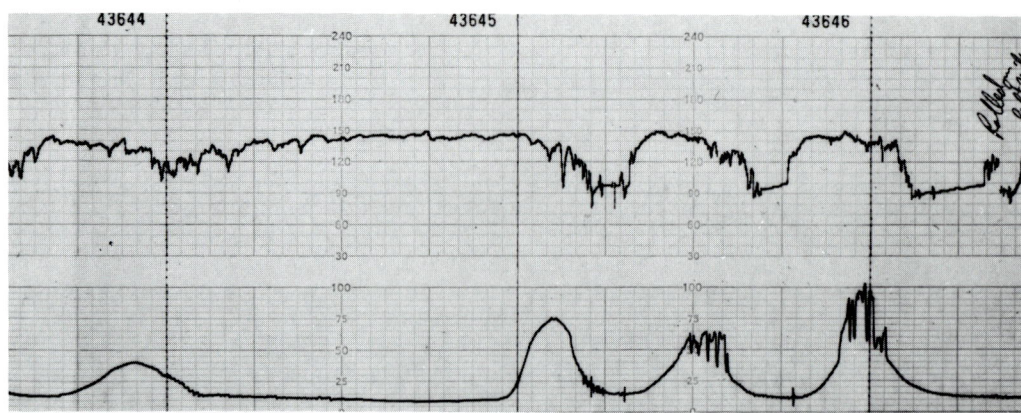

FIGURE 20–11. Reflex late decelerations. The FHR pattern was previously normal, but late decelerations appeared following severe maternal hypotension (70/30 mm Hg) after sympathetic blockade caused by a caudal anesthetic.

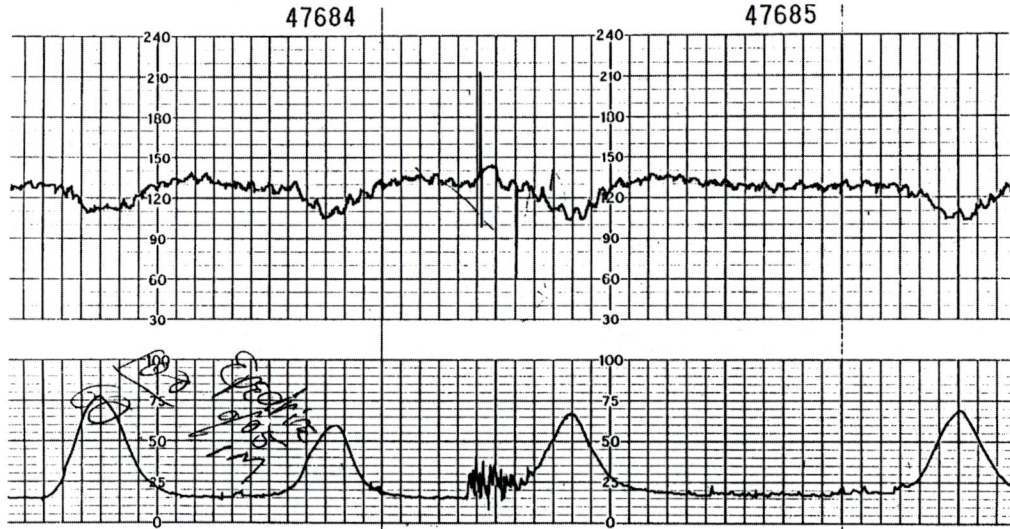

FIGURE 20–12. Early decelerations.

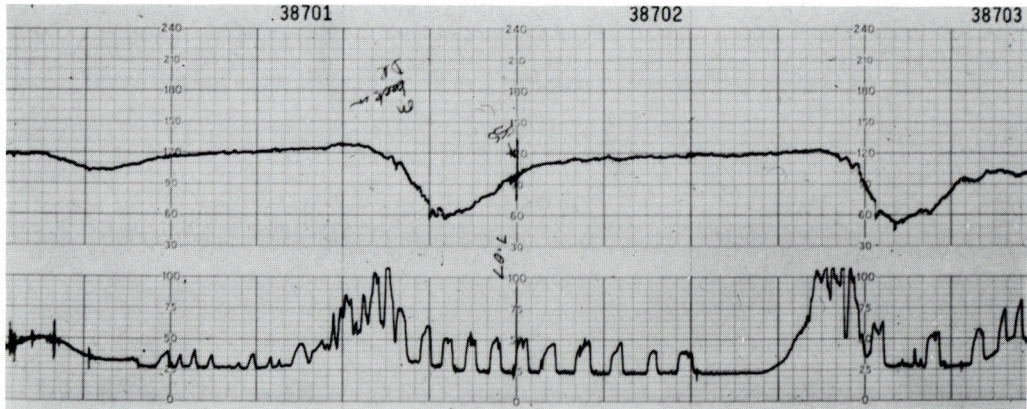

FIGURE 20–13. Nonreflex late decelerations with virtual absence of FHR variability. The decelerations represent transient asphyxic myocardial failure as well as intermittent vagal decreases in heart rate. The lack of FHR variability also signifies decreased cerebral oxygenation. Note the acidemia in fetal scalp blood (7.07). The baby, a 3340-gm female with Apgar scores of 3 (1 min) and 4 (5 min), was delivered soon after this tracing. Cesarean section was considered to be contraindicated owing to a severe preeclamptic coagulopathy.

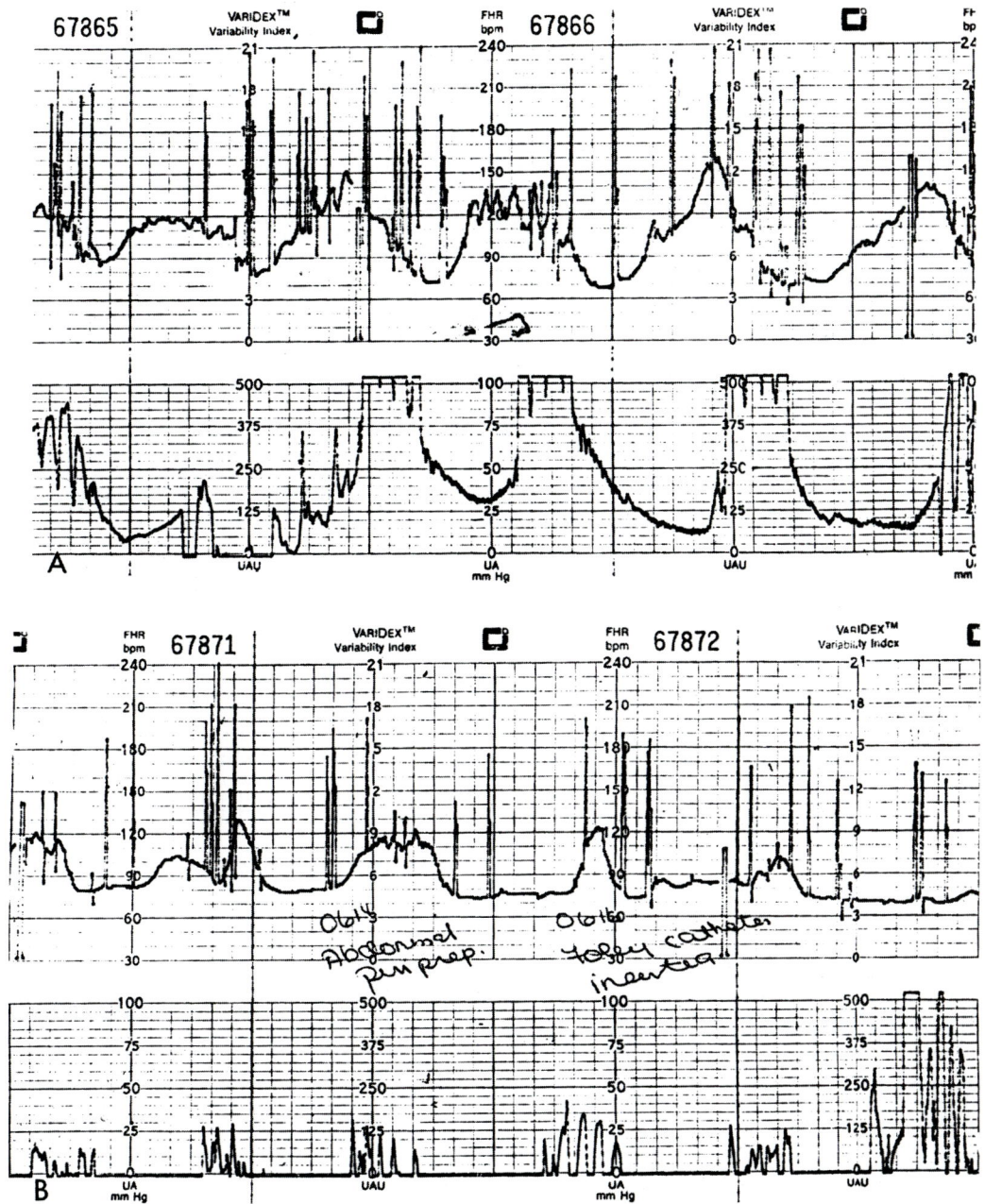

FIGURE 20–14. *A* and *B,* A case of fetal cardiorespiratory decompensation showing the evolution of the smooth baseline over 30 minutes. In this case the asphyxial stress is manifested as late decelerations. Death occurred *in utero* 30 minutes later.

al., 1969), Goodlin's "Rule of 60s" as presented here is the simplest and the most practical.

These abrupt decelerations in heart rate represent the firing of the vagus nerve in response to certain stimuli, either umbilical cord compression, generally in the first stage of labor, or substantial head compression, e.g., during pushing, late in the second stage of labor (Ball and Parer, 1992). Whether the fetus is still normoxemic in the central tissues (i.e., physiologically compensated) can be determined by observations of the maintenance of FHR variability. There are heart rate and duration criteria for mild and moderate variable decelerations, but these classifications

are of little importance. The major factor to observe is retention of baseline FHR variability.

The clinical significance of variable decelerations is that they represent insufficiency of umbilical blood flow. It is obvious why this is so if they are caused by compression of the umbilical cord. If they are caused by intense vagal activity, then the associated decrease in umbilical blood flow results from a drop in fetal cardiac output because of the relative inability of the fetus to maintain cardiac output at very low heart rates, e.g., below 60 beats/min.

When severe variable decelerations are present, vigorous efforts should be made to abolish them because

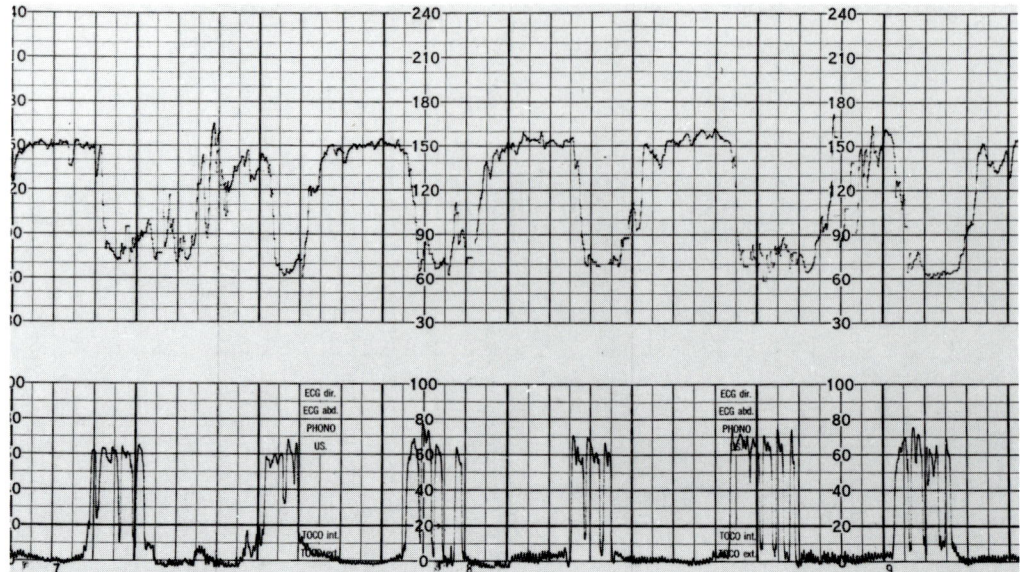

FIGURE 20–15. Variable decelerations. Intrapartum recording using fetal scalp electrode and tokodynamometer. The spikes in the uterine activity channel represent maternal pushing efforts in the second stage of labor. Note normal baseline variability between contractions, signifying normal central oxygenation despite the intermittent asphyxial stress represented by the severe variable decelerations.

it is likely that even the normally grown fetus with normal placental function eventually will decompensate, although usually not before 30 minutes (Fig. 20–16). The normal fetus, however, has a much greater ability to tolerate mild or moderate variable decelerations for a prolonged period.

Amnioinfusion. The theory of variable decelerations being caused by cord compression has given rise to the technique of amnioinfusion (Miyazaki and Nevarez, 1985). In this straightforward technique, sterile crystalloid is infused into the amniotic cavity through an intrauterine catheter, with an initial bolus of 250 to 1000 cc and a maintenance of about 2 to 3 cc/mm. This has been shown to result in a lowered incidence of severe variable decelerations and may allow a vaginal delivery instead of a cesarean section for presumed fetal asphyxia (Strong et al., 1990). It may also decrease the incidence of meconium aspiration when the meconium is thick (Wenstrom and Parsons, 1989). It appears to be more efficacious in premature fetuses than in term fetuses, and is not so effective in the second stage of labor, lending support to the theory that second-stage variable decelerations are due to head and not cord compression.

ACCELERATIONS WITH CONTRACTIONS. Accelerations sometimes occur with uterine contractions and have no adverse prognostic significance. They are probably similar to the accelerations that are seen with fetal movement in the antepartum period and thus are indicative of a reactive and healthy fetus. Accelerations with contractions probably represent the net result of greater sympathetic activity than parasympathetic activity during contractions in the case of a particular fetus.

"Shoulders" and the "overshoot" pattern probably represent a combination of sympathetic and vagal activity, with the sympathetic being predominant when the shoulders or overshoot occurs. There is no sound evidence that they have any prognostic significance as long as FHR variability is present.

The Influence of *In Utero* Treatment

It is now well recognized that fetal oxygenation can be improved, acidosis relieved, and abnormal FHR patterns abolished by certain modes of treatment. The events that result in fetal stress (recognized by FHR patterns) are presented in Table 20–3, together with the recommended treatment maneuvers and presumed mechanisms for improving fetal oxygenation. These should be the primary maneuvers carried out, and if the asphyxial insult is acute and the fetus was previously normoxemic, there is an excellent chance that the abnormal FHR pattern will be abolished. Late decelerations, if present, are most likely of the reflex type and not caused by myocardial failure.

During labor an FHR pattern with decreasing variability due to asphyxia is virtually always preceded by a heart rate pattern signifying asphyxial stress, e.g., late decelerations, variable decelerations (usually severe), or a prolonged bradycardia. In the antepartum period, however, before the onset of uterine contractions, this does not necessarily hold, and a fetus may develop decreasing or absent variability *without* periodic or base FHR changes. In addition, the normal evolution to decreased or absent variability sometimes occurs with relatively minor decelerations in cases of chorioamnionitis and dysmaturity.

If the FHR patterns cannot be improved, i.e., if the stress patterns indicative of peripheral tissue or central tissue asphyxia persist for a significant period, further diagnosis or delivery may be indicated.

Certain patterns are of such a severe character that

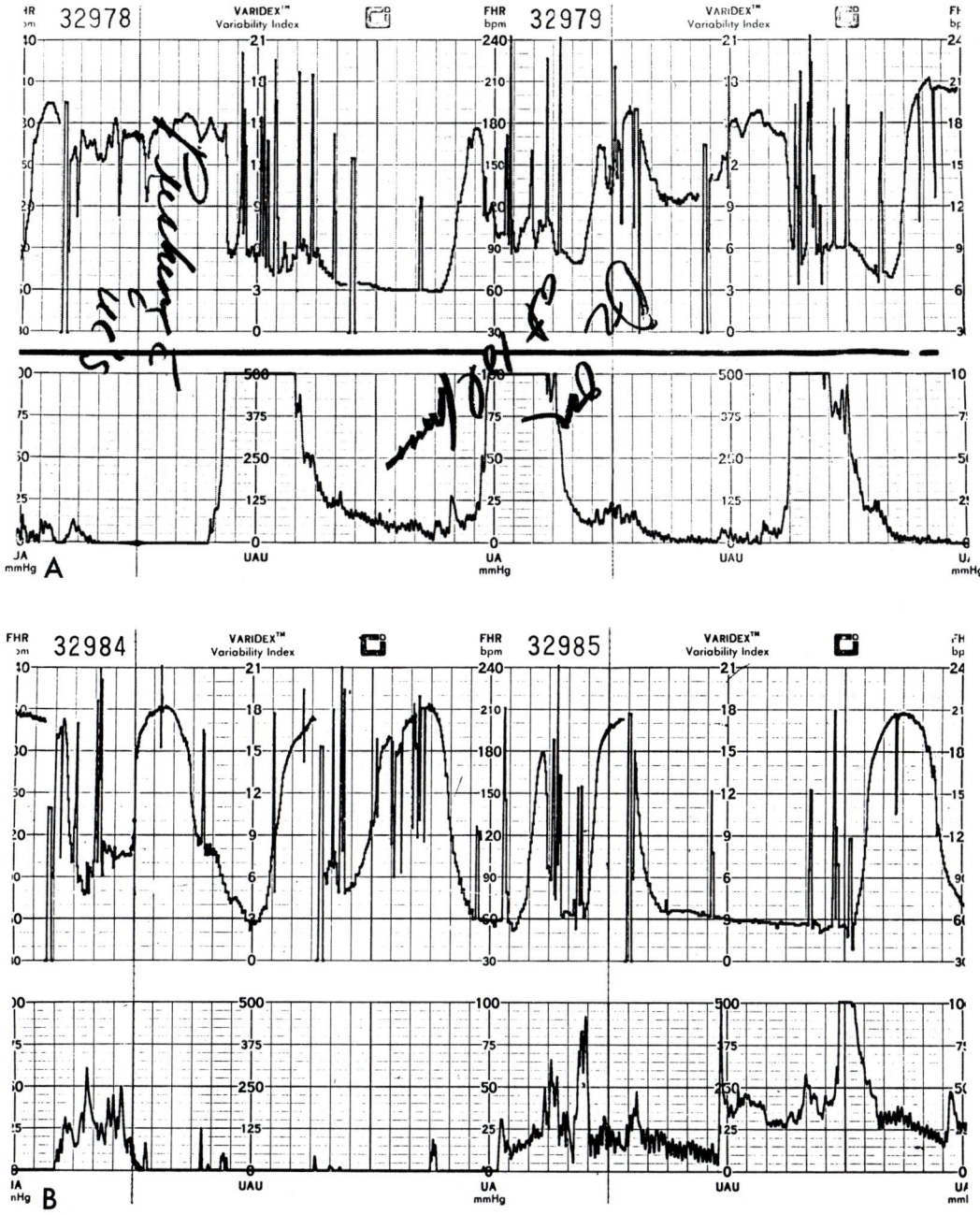

FIGURE 20–16. These tracings show a compensated fetus undergoing severe asphyxial stress (i.e., severe variable decelerations) (*A*), and its eventual decompensation 20 minutes later (*B*). Delivery was approximately 10 minutes after tracing *B*. Decompensation is signified by the virtual absence of FHR variability and the smoothness of the decelerations. Apgar scores 0, 0; neonatal death at 4 days of age.

TABLE 20–3.   Intrauterine Treatment for Variant FHR Patterns

CAUSES	POSSIBLE RESULTING FHR PATTERNS	CORRECTIVE MANEUVER	MECHANISM
Hypotension, e.g., supine hypotension, conduction anesthesia	Bradycardia, late decelerations	Intravenous fluids, position change, ephedrine	Return of uterine blood flow toward normal
Excessive uterine activity	Bradycardia, late decelerations	Decrease in oxytocin, lateral position	Same as above
Transient umbilical cord compression	Variable decelerations	Change in maternal position, e.g., left or right lateral, Trendelenburg	
		Amnioinfusion	"Pads" the cord, protecting it from compression
Head compression, usually second stage	Variable decelerations	Push only with alternate contractions	Same as above
Decreased uterine blood flow associated with uterine contraction below limits of fetal basal O_2 needs	Late decelerations	Change in maternal position, e.g., left lateral or Trendelenburg; establishment of maternal hyperoxia	Enhancement of uterine blood flow toward optimum; increase in maternal-fetal O_2 gradient
		Tocolytic agents, e.g., ritodrine or terbutaline	Decrease in contractions or uterine tonus, thus abolishing associated decrease in uterine blood flow
Prolonged asphyxia	Decreasing FHR variability*	Change in maternal position, e.g., left lateral or Trendelenburg; establishment of maternal hyperoxia	Enhancement of uterine blood flow to optimum; increase in maternal-fetal O_2 gradient

*NB: During labor this is virtually always preceded by a heart rate pattern signifying asphyxial stress, e.g., late decelerations (usually severe), severe variable decelerations, or a prolonged bradycardia. This is not necessarily so in the antepartum period, before the onset of uterine contractions.

immediate delivery without ancillary testing such as fetal scalp sampling is warranted if they cannot rapidly be relieved. They include patterns with a smooth baseline and severe, uncorrectable late or variable decelerations (Fig. 20–17) or a prolonged bradycardia below 60 beats/min with a smooth baseline. Such fetuses are either already asphyxiated or will soon become so.

Other Patterns

A number of patterns do not fit simply into the category of "basic patterns." They are less common, and their significance is generally more controversial.

Bradycardias

As noted previously, *bradycardia* is defined as a heart rate below 120 beats/min for 2 minutes or longer. This is to distinguish it from decelerations, which refers to a decrease in FHR below 120 beats/min for less than 2 minutes. These criteria are, of course, arbitrary; they have been developed primarily for communication and are not based strictly on a physiologic foundation.

A number of labels have been placed on various bradycardias, reflecting their appearance, occurrence, or presumed etiology; for example, prolonged bradycardia, prolonged end-stage bradycardia, and post—paracervical block bradycardia.

PROLONGED BRADYCARDIA. Moderate bradycardia,

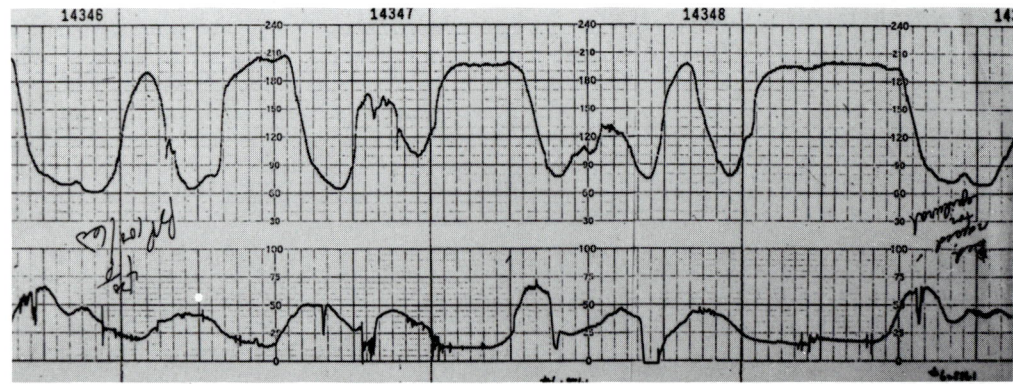

FIGURE 20–17. A sinister heart rate pattern in a 28-week fetus (gestational age determined after delivery) with baseline tachycardia, absence of heart rate variability, and severe periodic changes. The scalp blood pH was 7.0, and the fetus died shortly after this tracing. Cesarean section was not performed because the fetus was believed to be previable, although in fact it was 1100 gm. There is much artifact in the uterine activity channel.

i.e., not below 100 beats/min, may represent continuous head compression and therefore vagal activity. The reason for the vagal response to head compression is uncertain, but it may be caused by cerebral ischemia (Hon and Quilligan, 1967). It may also be caused by compression of the dura. Provided that FHR variability is maintained, prolonged moderate bradycardia is not associated with fetal acidosis. Some fetuses with moderate bradycardia may simply have rates below the arbitrary level of 120 beats/min; in fact, 110 beats/min has been proposed by some as the lower limit.

Prolonged bradycardia is generally applied to a sudden drop from a normal FHR to values below 120 beats/min, especially below 80 beats/min. As mentioned previously, bradycardia is the initial response of the fetus to acute asphyxia. It is probably a vagal response to peripheral or central chemoreceptor activity. The asphyxic stimulus may be caused by (1) a decrease in maternal oxygen tension, as during the apnea of a seizure; (2) a decrease in uterine blood flow, as during excessive uterine contractions or acute maternal hypotension; (3) a decrease in umbilical blood flow, as by cord compression (Fig. 20–18); or (4) loss of placental area, as in abruptio placentae. The extent of the bradycardia depends on the degree of fetal hypoxia. There may also be a baroreceptor influence causing the bradycardia with prolongation of asphyxia.

In rare cases, a prolonged bradycardia is the result of fetal hemorrhage, usually catastrophic, as occurs with tearing of vasa praevia or rupture of an anomalous fetal placental vessel. In such cases the fetus may be born not only asphyxiated, but in hemorrhagic shock.

Immediately upon recognition of a bradycardia, attempts should be made to optimize fetal oxygenation by maintenance of maternal blood pressure, avoidance of excessive uterine activity, position change, hydration, and possibly maternal hyperoxia (see Table 20–3). There is no need for grave concern if moderate bradycardia is not abolished. However, if the heart rate is below 100 beats/min, more vigorous efforts should be made to alleviate it, even in the presence of good FHR variability. An acute drop in heart rate to less than 60 beats/min usually results in fetal asphyxic decompensation, and it becomes an obstetric emergency to abolish it or deliver the baby before severe central asphyxia occurs (Fig. 20–19).

Fortunately, most sudden bradycardias resolve spontaneously or with various positional changes. However, they are of sufficient concern that many women whose babies exhibit several prolonged bradycardic episodes are brought to the delivery room for labor, in case the FHR does not recover after one of them. On rare occasions the bradycardia does not resolve, and the infants may be deeply depressed owing to asphyxia (see Fig. 20–19). Such cases are seen more commonly in post-date pregnancies and fortunately are rare. The etiology of the bradycardia is not always apparent, and some have ascribed it to excessive vagal activity.

PROLONGED END-STAGE BRADYCARDIA. This term refers to a sudden prolonged deceleration, generally late in the second stage of labor, in the presence of an otherwise normal FHR tracing (Fig. 20–20) (Herbert and Boehm, 1981). This pattern is not uncommon, and it will be seen much more frequently if one adopts the practice of taking the monitor to the delivery room and continuing to monitor FHR until the time of delivery.

Prolonged end-stage bradycardia is likely to be a vagal response to head compression as the head traverses the depths of the pelvis. Compression may cause a decrease in cerebral blood flow and brief local ischemia, which could produce a vagal output. Alternatively, the vagal discharge may be caused by compression of the dura.

The patterns were in the past generally managed by rapid termination of labor, either by forceps or encouragement to push. As with the spontaneous prolonged bradycardias, however, the results of expectant management have not been well tested. Position change (which is somewhat limited in the second stage) and discouragement from pushing sometimes

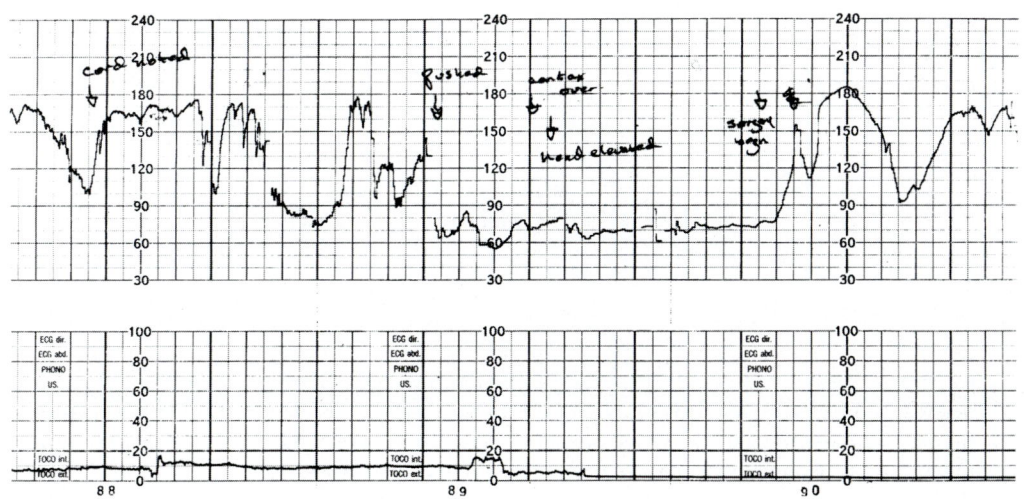

FIGURE 20–18. Bradycardia due to cord prolapse. The baby was delivered by cesarean section and did well.

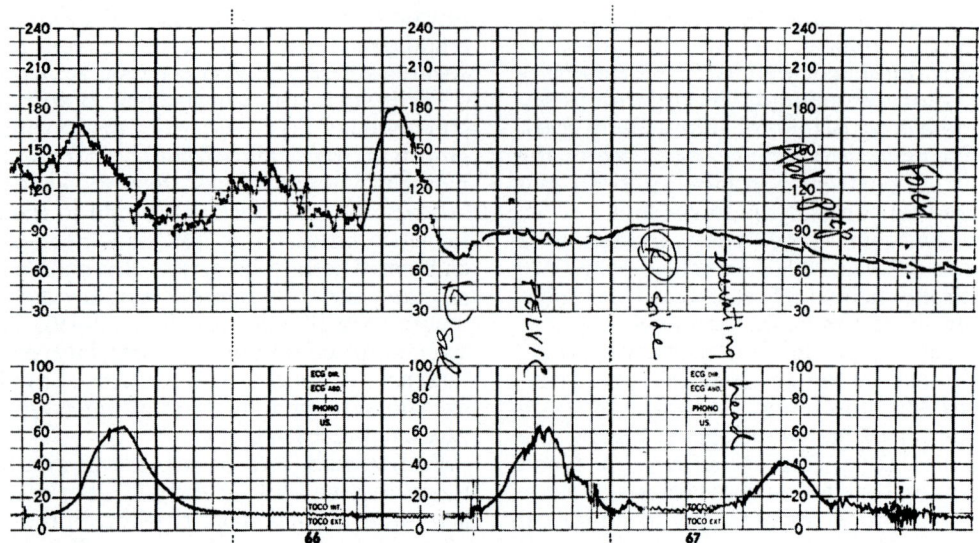

FIGURE 20–19. A sudden prolonged unremitting bradycardia, with lack of variability in a post-date (42 weeks) patient. The fetus was delivered by emergency cesarean section 9 min after the start of the deceleration, with Apgar scores of 2 (1 min) and 3 (5 min).

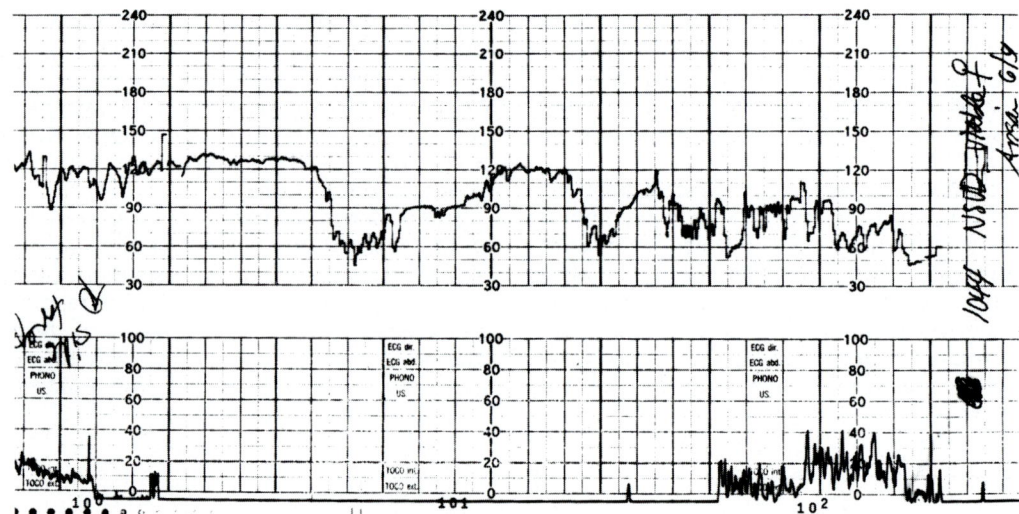

FIGURE 20–20. Prolonged end-stage bradycardia. This pattern is not uncommon in the final moments before delivery.

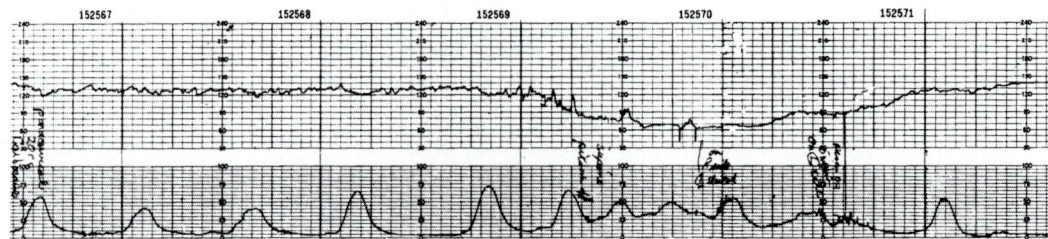

FIGURE 20–21. Bradycardia due to paracervical block anesthesia. Note the onset about 10 minutes after the administration of the anesthetic and its resolution about 5 minutes later.

appear to result in resolution of prolonged bradycardia. Elevation of the fetal head may also be efficacious, but studies purporting to demonstrate the benefit of the maneuver suffer from the defect of having no equivalent untreated group.

The current recommendation is that if the bradycardia is persistent and FHR variability decreases, the baby should be delivered as rapidly as possible. However, if variability is retained, efforts should be made to abolish the bradycardia or effect a spontaneous delivery. It is unusual for this pattern to result in absence of FHR variability and fetal decompensation in less than 10 minutes.

POST–PARACERVICAL BLOCK BRADYCARDIA. On the average, bradycardia occurs 7 minutes after paracervical block is administered and lasts 8 minutes (Fig. 20–21). The range in both of these values, the degree of bradycardia, and the associated FHR abnormalities are variable. Its incidence varies from 0 to 56 per cent, depending on drug, dosage, and definition. An average incidence is 15 per cent. Some fetal deaths have been associated with paracervical block bradycardia (Ralston and Shnider, 1978).

Although the etiology is controversial, the most likely cause of the bradycardia is a direct fetal toxic reaction to the local anesthetic drug, not necessarily because of direct fetal injection, but because of rapid uptake of the drug by the fetus, possibly via the uterine arteries. Fetal levels of such a drug can be high, though rarely higher than that of the mother. A further theory is that the local anesthetic agent causes spasm of the uterine arteries, resulting in decreased uterine blood flow and, hence, fetal asphyxia. Acidosis has been demonstrated by blood sampling in affected fetuses during the bradycardia (Ralston and Shnider, 1978).

One may minimize this undesirable side effect of paracervical block by using the lowest possible quantities of such drugs. Careful technique to ensure that the drug is placed just submucosally will avoid inadvertent fetal injection. Paracervical block is considered to be contraindicated if the fetus already has an abnormal heart rate pattern.

If bradycardia does develop, supportive management is recommended, i.e., position change and maternal hyperoxia, until it resolves. If the pattern does resolve and FHR returns to normal, no further evaluation is needed, but subsequent paracervical injection should be avoided.

Except in rare and profoundly abnormal cases, delivery should be avoided during the bradycardia, because the fetus is better able to get rid of the drug transplacentally than to detoxify it postnatally.

Arrhythmias

A complete discussion of fetal arrhythmias is presented in Chapter 21.

Sinusoidal Pattern

This is a regular, smooth sine wave-like baseline, with a frequency of approximately 3 to 6 per minute and an amplitude range of up to 30 beats/min. The regularity of the waves distinguishes it from long-term variability complexes, which are crudely shaped and irregular. Another distinguishing feature is the absence of FHR variability (Fig. 20–22).

The pattern was first described in a group of severely affected Rh-isoimmunized fetuses (Rochard et al., 1976), but has subsequently been noted in association with fetuses that are anemic for other reasons and in asphyxiated infants. It has also been described in cases of normal infants born without depression or acid-base abnormalities, although in these cases there is dispute about whether the patterns are truly sinusoidal or whether, because of the moderately irregular pattern, they are variants of long-term variability. Such patterns are also sometimes seen after administration of alphaprodine (Nisentil) to the mother. It is believed that an essential characteristic of the sinusoidal pattern is extreme regularity and smoothness.

If the sinusoidal pattern is seen in an Rh-sensitized patient with severe hemolysis, rapid intervention is needed. It may take the form of delivery or possibly intrauterine transfusion, depending on the gestational age and the preceding Rh data, treatment, and work-up (see Chapter 44).

Management in the absence of Rh disease is somewhat more difficult to recommend. If the pattern is persistent, monotonously regular, and unaccompanied by short-term variability and it cannot be abolished by the maneuvers just described, further evaluation of adequacy of fetal oxygenation, e.g., by fetal blood sampling, contraction stress test, fetal stimulation test, or a modified biophysical profile, is indicated. Non-alloimmune sinusoidal patterns have been associated with severe fetal asphyxia and fetal anemia due to fetal-maternal bleeding. However, if the pattern is irregularly sinusoidal or "pseudosinusoidal," intermittently present, and not associated with intervening periodic decelerations, it is unlikely to indicate fetal compromise. Hence, immediate delivery is not warranted. The aforementioned ancillary tests may assist in confirming normality in such cases.

Saltatory Pattern

This pattern consists of rapid variations in FHR with a frequency of 3 to 6 per minute and an amplitude range greater than 25 beats/min (Fig. 20–23). It is qualitatively described as excessive variability, and the variations have a strikingly bizarre appearance.

The saltatory pattern was associated with low Apgar scores in early discussions of FHR variability, but it was not possible to relate the time course of the pattern to the fetal depression (Hammacher et al., 1968). More specifically, fetuses with the pattern in the intrapartum period had a tendency toward low Apgar scores, but it was not clear whether the pattern was present immediately before delivery, or whether it preceded an evolution to a more serious FHR pattern.

The saltatory pattern is almost invariably seen during labor rather than antepartum. The etiology is uncertain. Clinical experience suggests, however, that it may be similar to that of the increased FHR variability seen in animal experiments with brief and acute hypoxia in the previously normoxemic fetus. This

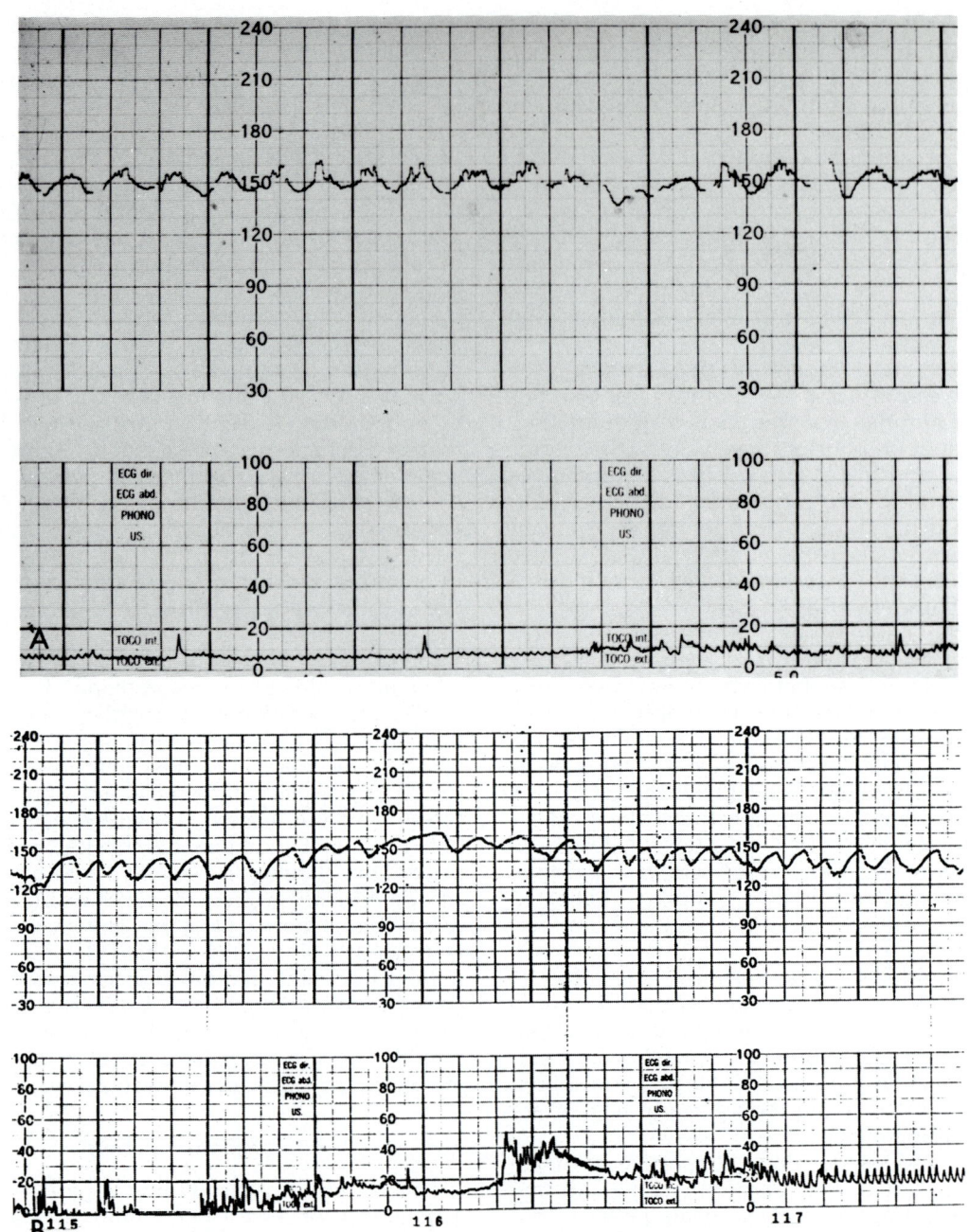

FIGURE 20–22. *A,* Sinusoidal pattern in a term fetus with severe hemolysis due to Rh disease. Cord hematocrit was 20 per cent, and the infant, delivered by cesarean section, was subsequently normal. This tracing was recorded by Doppler instrumentation, and the apparent short-term variability is artifactual. *B,* Recording by electrode in the same fetus a short time later.

increase is presumed to result from an increase in alpha-adrenergic activity, of which the primary function is to cause selective vasoconstriction of certain vascular beds. A secondary effect of this increased alpha-adrenergic activity may be excessive variability.

Because it is believed that the fetus with this pattern is hemodynamically compensated (although it may be moderately asphyxially stressed), we recommend that attempts be made to abolish it, by maneuvers such as the lateral position, avoidance of hypotension, avoidance of excessive uterine activity, and perhaps mater-

nal hyperoxia. We are not aware of any case of a saltatory pattern that has evolved directly into fetal decompensation; it probably is similar in significance to mild or moderate variable decelerations.

The Premature Fetus

Several investigators have examined both the antepartum and intrapartum FHR patterns of the premature and their relationship to fetal blood acid-base status (Zanini et al., 1980; Bowes et al., 1980). There

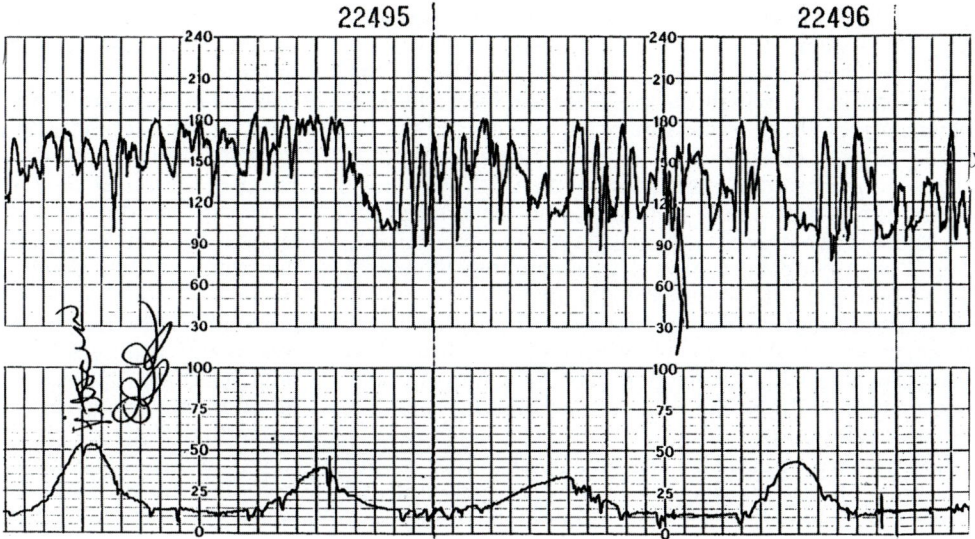

FIGURE 20–23. Saltatory pattern showing excessive FHR variability of up to 60 beats/min in brief intervals, probably representing mild asphyxial stress.

now seems little doubt that the same criteria used in the term fetus can be used for the premature. Important differences, however, are that prematures can quickly develop abnormal patterns and that these patterns tend to progress in severity much more rapidly than in the term fetus.

There are some commonly held and erroneous beliefs with regard to prematures. The first is that prematures normally have tachycardia. In fact, the average heart rate of the 28-week-old fetus is about 150 beats/min with a range of about 130 to 170 beats/min, i.e., only slightly above that of the term fetus. The second is that premature heart rates have "flat baselines." Most prematures have normal FHR variability, and its disappearance or absence should be managed as for a term fetus, even in the presence of a tachycardia. There is, however, a tendency for prematures to have a smaller amplitude of variability.

A further common misconception is that tachycardias result in decreased FHR variability. In our experience the large majority of fetuses with tachycardia have normal FHR variability, unless there is a component of decompensating asphyxia or drug effects.

Congenital Anomalies

Except as described for the dysrhythmias, the vast majority of fetuses with congenital anomalies have normal FHR patterns and a response to asphyxia similar to that of the normal fetus (Garite et al., 1979). There are several exceptions, e.g., complete heart block and anencephaly. Thus, aneuploid fetuses, such as those with Down's syndrome and trisomy 18, and fetuses with aplastic lungs, meningomyelocele, and hydrocephalus may give no FHR warning of defects. In one series it was noted that although there was no pathognomonic pattern in such fetuses, the rate of cesarean section for fetal distress was significantly increased (Garite et al., 1979).

An important exception is seen with Potter's syndrome. Affected fetuses are generally recognized as growth-retarded because of the oligohydramnios, and

they may have substantial variable decelerations, presumably for the same reason—that is, umbilical cord compression is more likely without the "padding" of adequate amniotic fluid. A number of such fetuses have been delivered by cesarean section for "fetal distress," with the tragic outcome being rapid neonatal death due to hypoplastic lungs.

There is no simple solution to the problem of heroic intervention (generally cesarean section) for the fetus who is destined to be severely defective or to die in the neonatal period. Genetic evaluation and high-resolution ultrasonography in certain high-risk groups may decrease the incidence of such problems, but in the case of a youthful primipara without significant family history of genetic disease, screening is not yet available, except possibly for open neural tube defects via alpha-fetoprotein measurements.

"Shoulders and Overshoot"

These terms are used to describe transient increases in FHR either preceding or immediately following a deceleration. They have an undeserved bad reputation. They probably represent the transient net result of dominance of sympathetic over parasympathetic activity. Some believe the "shoulders" may result from mild cord compression during which only the umbilical vein is compressed; this would produce a temporary fetal hypovolemia. However, there is little or no evidence to support this theory. It is unlikely that shoulders represent an asphyxial stress, and serious fetal compromise results from the associated decelerations. As with all patterns, the significance of the presence or absence of shoulders is secondary to the retention of FHR variability.

CURRENT INTRAPARTUM MANAGEMENT RECOMMENDATIONS

Fetal heart rate variability is thought to represent an intact neurologic pathway, which includes fetal cerebral cortex, mid-brain, vagus nerve, and cardiac conduction system. It is now well established that during asphyxia there is augmentation of blood flow to the brain and heart, which matches the degree of hypoxemia so that there is constancy of oxygen uptake by these organs. However, at severe degrees of hypoxia these compensatory mechanisms break down, augmentation of blood flow is limited, and oxygen uptake by these vital organs can no longer be maintained. This decompensation may occur as a consequence of acute profound stepwise asphyxia or may occur after the intermittent asphyxial stresses (during contractions) have occurred for a prolonged duration. This produces a cumulative oxygen debt, which eventually results in inability of the fetus to maintain oxygenation of the vital organs.

The clinical approach currently used is that in the presence of bradycardias, or of a prolonged series of late or variable decelerations, when fetal heart rate variability decreases or is intermittently lost, one must assume that the fetus is becoming severely centrally asphyxiated, unless one can demonstrate otherwise by other techniques.

It must be stressed that there are many other causes of decreased fetal heart rate variability besides asphyxia, and part of the art of clinical management is determining when asphyxia is the cause and when it is unlikely to be the cause.

The most important concept is that a decrease in fetal heart rate variability due to asphyxia during the intrapartum period almost invariably follows the asphyxial stress patterns: bradycardia, late decelerations, and variable decelerations. Exceptions to this evolution are rare, but it may be seen more often in acute infection, such as chorioamnionitis, in which reduced FHR variability may not be preceded by deep periodic changes. These three asphyxial stress patterns are not uncommon during labor, but only rarely result in fetal neurologic damage. There is a substantial fetal resistance due to the physiologic compensatory mechanisms noted above. The current clinical means by which we recognize asphyxial decompensation in the fetus is by noting the persistence and time course of changes in the fetal heart rate pattern. Experience suggests that a previously normoxemic baby can tolerate late decelerations or severe variable decelerations for at least 30 minutes before decompensating.

The evolution of intrapartum fetal heart rate patterns during asphyxia is established, and it is known that fetal heart rate variability decreases and then disappears before substantial fetal depression or fetal death *in utero*. This decrease in fetal heart rate variability is considered to correlate clinically with decreased CNS function, which is presumed to precede CNS damage.

From the point of view of clinical management, this is an important approach. It suggests that there is time for conservative management to alleviate the stress patterns before operative delivery is warranted. Thus with uncorrectable decreased fetal heart rate variability in the presence of persistent asphyxial stress patterns, delivery should be carried out immediately. In the presence of continued normal fetal heart rate variability with those stress patterns, one can conser-

vatively await a vaginal delivery in certain selected cases. Fetal blood sampling for acid-base measurement or fetal stimulation testing may be of value in uncertain cases. This approach does imply the ability to rapidly "rescue" the fetus if the need arises, and so decision-delivery times may need to be relatively short, of the order of 15 minutes or less.

Severe prolonged and sustained bradycardias are similar in some respects to the conditions already described. It has been noted that a bradycardia between 100 and 120 beats/min with normal fetal heart rate variability can be tolerated by most fetuses for essentially unlimited periods of time. In contrast, a fetal heart rate below 60 beats/min (in the absence of heart block) is an obstetric emergency that requires immediate delivery. There is some evidence that neurologic damage may begin at 10 minutes in such cases. It is our current belief that a sustained fetal heart rate below 80 beats/min should also be managed by immediate preparation for delivery, whereas rates of 80 to 100 can be handled more conservatively. In all of these cases the presence of fetal heart rate variability has persistently been the most important prognostic sign of continued fetal CNS integrity.

Recommendations for Usage of FHR Monitoring

Intrapartum fetal asphyxia appears to be infrequently associated with long-term neurologic morbidity. Subtle deleterious effects of intrapartum asphyxia may occur and not become manifest as cerebral palsy, but their incidence is not known. The incidence of cerebral palsy from all causes is 2 to 3 per 1000, but intrapartum asphyxia is only a relatively small part of this, possibly 10 per cent. Thus the number of fetuses that can benefit from electronic FHR monitoring, especially in the normal population, is probably less than 1 per cent, although in a high-risk group, such as premature or post-date fetuses, the proportion may well be higher.

In this section we will examine two areas: (1) the lack of substantial benefit in the various controlled trials of FHR monitoring, and (2) an effective and conservative approach that we have found clinically beneficial and without excessive detriment.

Controlled Trials of Electronic FHR Monitoring

The controlled trials of electronic FHR monitoring have shown little or no beneficial effect when compared with conventional management. This is not only puzzling, but of great concern to many clinicians who believe electronic FHR monitoring is effective because of numerous clinical observations and the physiologic basis of FHR patterns. Many obstetricians can show cases in which the use of electronic FHR monitoring undoubtedly led to early intervention and lessening of continued intrapartum asphyxia. Nonetheless, for several reasons the trials have not consistently shown a beneficial effect and in fact have shown the detrimental effect of increased cesarean section rates in the monitored group (Thacker, 1987).

One reason for this lack of consistent benefit is that, in earlier trials particularly, patient numbers were inadequate to show a difference in mortality rates when the intrinsic rate is so low. Also, criteria used for diagnosis of fetal asphyxia are generally dated and unsophisticated, bearing little relationship to modern criteria. In particular there has been little or no recognition of the importance of FHR variability in the determination of fetal status. The largest and most recent trial reports no description whatsoever of the FHR indices used to determine "abnormalities of fetal heart rate." A further effect of unsophisticated FHR interpretation is the tendency to diagnose fetal asphyxia too frequently, particularly in the presence of decelerations with normal FHR variability. This has the effect of elevating the cesarean section rate unnecessarily. Furthermore, response times are rarely noted in the trials. Clearly an asphyxiated fetus needs delivery and resuscitation before damage occurs, not according to some predetermined, arbitrary "standard" time, such as "cesarean section performed within 30 minutes." Brain damage apparently can occur in approximately 10 minutes in the case of total cessation of oxygen delivery; if our obstetric facilities cannot achieve delivery within this critical period, the fault does not rest with electronic FHR monitoring. Many of the intrapartum stillbirths in recent trials may well have been avoided with ideal response times, but such are either not discussed or are discussed in relation to a time frame that is more dependent on obstetric than on biologic (i.e., fetal) convenience.

A Conservative Approach

The almost dichotomous views of the proponents and opponents of electronic FHR monitoring can make it difficult for practicing obstetricians to take a stand in their practice. Physicians could opt for universal monitoring, or monitoring only high-risk patients, or not even use electronic monitoring at all. However, if they choose either of the last two courses, they must do so from a firm base of knowledge, based on intimacy with the literature on the subject. Few obstetricians opt for no electronic monitoring because they feel legally vulnerable. From the nursing care point of view, electronic monitoring is logistically easier than intermittent auscultation. Our current recommendations are as follows:

On admission to rule out labor, or in a patient in actual labor, an FHR record with either external or internal monitoring should be documented for approximately 20 minutes. In the case of an at-risk patient, the monitoring should continue throughout labor, although this need not be obsessively so in all cases. (There are difficulties with the definition of "high risk"; suffice it to say that such a patient is one who has a condition listed in publications on the subject.) Should the contractions be obvious and the FHR pattern be "normal" (normal rate, normal FHR variability, and absence of periodic changes except accelerations), the tokodynamometer need not be placed. The need for the tokodynamometer to measure contraction frequency, or for the intrauterine pressure catheter to measure intrauterine pressure, arises when cervical change is inadequate.

For a low-risk patient who continues to be low risk in that she does not develop any abnormality of labor or have risk factors appearing subsequently, electronic FHR monitoring may be intermittent. In such cases a short recorded strip of approximately 5 minutes every 30 minutes or in accordance with the hospital's policy or ACOG recommendation (ACOG Bulletin, 1989) for frequency of auscultation should be sufficient. Should equivocal changes in these short strips occur, continuous electronic FHR monitoring should be instituted until the condition of the fetus is resolved. During the second stage of labor, the frequency of recordings needs to be increased in accordance with the hospital's auscultation protocol. We believe, however, that when the second stage exceeds about 30 minutes, the institution of continuous monitoring is advisable.

Every effort should be made to minimize the intrusiveness of the monitor and associated activities because many couples find monitoring to be at variance with their wishes for a natural birth with minimal interference. Attendants should maintain an appropriate social interaction with the patient and make it obvious that she is more important than the machine, e.g., by making eye contact predominantly with her and not the record during examinations. Another way to minimize intrusiveness is to interpret knowledgeably, minimizing dramatic comments and activities.

Perhaps the most difficult aspect of monitoring is recognizing and predicting the fetus who is at risk of asphyxial damage without excessively overcalling the situation. The crucial step in this regard is in projecting the potential for asphyxial decompensation. This requires a dynamic approach to FHR interpretation, recognizing that oxygen levels in the fetus are continuously variable—from moment to moment, with contractions, and with longer cycles. It requires an understanding of the evolution of FHR patterns in relation to progressive decreases in oxygenation, for example, in the initially normoxemic fetus, the deepening of decelerations, the subsequent intermittent decrease or loss of variability, and finally the absence of variability as described above.

If, after 30 minutes, the decelerations (late or severe variable) become deeper despite attempts to abolish them, plans should be made for delivery. Should the projected time for a vaginal delivery be greater than the projected time for loss of FHR variability (i.e., asphyxial decompensation), then delivery should be carried out, generally by cesarean section. An alternative approach to noting retention of FHR variability in such cases of potential decompensation is to determine intermittently fetal acid-base status by fetal blood sampling or to confirm good fetal status by the fetal stimulation test.

With careful interpretation and conservative management, we believe that the rare cases of intrapartum asphyxia can be recognized, and in many cases, intervention can be carried out before asphyxial damage occurs. This goal need not be achieved at the expense of excessive cesarean section and other potential morbidity.

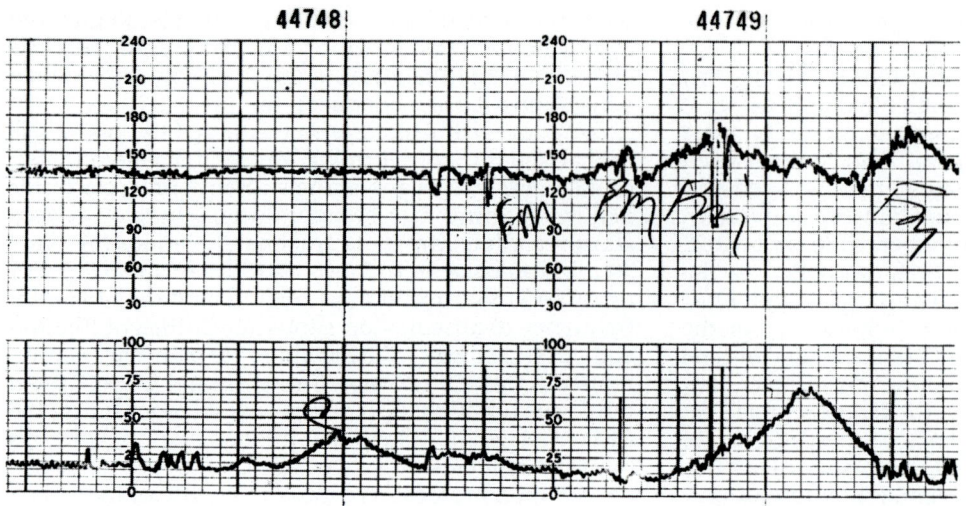

FIGURE 20-24. The reactive NST tracing also shows a transition from the nonreactive state (first half of trace), when there are no movements and poor fetal heart rate variability. Onset of activity (spikes on lower channel) is associated with a uterine contraction, accelerations of fetal heart rate, and increased fetal heart rate variability. The initial quiet state of this fetus does not signify fetal compromise.

ANTEPARTUM FETAL HEART RATE TESTING

The clinical methods available for detecting impending or actual fetal asphyxia are limited to beat-to-beat fetal heart rate measurement, quantitation of fetal movement, the biophysical profile (Manning et al., 1985; see Chapter 22), and fetal blood sampling. Only the first three can be used before rupture of membranes or with a closed cervix. The other tests of fetal surveillance, such as high-risk classification and ultrasound imaging, help us only to decide which fetuses require more definitive testing. These tests are relatively poor predictors of intrauterine asphyxia.

An approach to antepartum surveillance is evolving that includes the following:

1. Basic screening with fetal movement counting (Neldam, 1983; Grant and Elbourne, 1989).

2. Non-stress testing in cases of suspicious kick counts or in certain "high-risk" situations.

3. Contraction stress testing (CST) or biophysical profile (BPP) in the presence of nonreactive or suspicious non-stress testing.

4. In the case of a suspicious or positive CST, the biophysical profile may be done in an infant so premature that delivery seems unwarranted.

There is continued controversy regarding the relative merits (Freeman et al., 1982) and efficacy (Thacker and Berkelman, 1986) of these approaches.

Non-stress Testing

Non-stress testing consists of detecting the fetal heart rate, fetal movement, and uterine activity by external means, and noting accelerations of fetal heart rate with fetal movement and long-term variability. These parameters have been shown to be predictive of fetal outcome.

TECHNIQUE. Twenty minutes of good-quality fetal heart rate and tokodynamometer tracing are obtained with the patient in semi-Fowler's position or with a left lateral tilt. Blood pressure measurements are taken at frequent intervals. Fetal movements may be signified by maternal sensation, attendant's observation or palpation of maternal abdomen, and sharp upward marks on tokodynamometer tracing. Fetuses have been observed to have sleep or inactive cycles that often last 20 to 40 minutes and can last up to twice this time. If the fetus is initially inactive, it may be stimulated manually or the mother may be given appropriate liquid to ensure adequate glucose level. However, the utility of these maneuvers is in question.

The operator marks on the record any fetal movement and whether the fetal heart rate accelerates at least 15 beats/min with the movement. The baseline fetal heart rate is normal if within the range of 120 to 160 beats/min. The long-term amplitude variability, i.e., the irregular crude oscillations of three to six cycles per minute, should have an amplitude range of 10 beats/min on the external monitor. The beat-to-beat or short-term variability cannot reliably be read with the Doppler ultrasound device.

A variant of this test is the *fetal vibroacoustic stimulation test*. This test depends on the fetal response to an acoustic stimulation (generally produced by an artificial larynx) applied close to the maternal abdomen. This test has been validated and shortens the time required to produce a reactive test (Smith et al., 1986b).

INTERPRETATION. The following set of criteria for interpretation is one of several used successfully in various institutions (Schifrin, 1979; Keegan and Paul, 1980).

Reactive fetus: At least two fetal movements in 20 minutes with acceleration of fetal heart rate reaching a peak of a least 15 beats/min, long-term variability amplitude of at least 10 beats/min; baseline rate must be within normal range (Fig. 20–24).

Nonreactive fetus: No fetal movements or no acceleration of heart rate with movements; generally poor or no long-term variability; baseline rate may be outside (or within) normal range (Fig. 20–25).

Uncertain reactivity: Fewer than two fetal movements in 20 minutes or acceleration of less than 15 beats/min; long-term variability amplitude below 10 beats/min; abnormal baseline rate.

A "reactive test" is associated with survival of the

fetus for 1 week or more in more than 99 per cent of cases (Schifrin, 1979; Evertson et al., 1978).

A "nonreactive test" is associated with poor fetal outcome (i.e., perinatal death, low 5-minute Apgar score, late decelerations in labor) in approximately 20 per cent of cases. These prediction figures have been obtained from a summary of a large number of patients in reported clinical studies (Ott, 1978). In an earlier study in which the results of nonstress testing were "blinded" (not used in management), the ultimate stillbirth rate of nonreactive fetuses was 26 per cent.

Because of the high false-positive rate (80 per cent) in clinical application of this test, a nonreactive fetus requires further evaluation by means of the contraction stress test or the biophysical profile unless contraindicated. The false-positive rate of the contraction stress test is only about 50 per cent (Ott, 1978).

For the fetus with "uncertain reactivity," another non-stress test should be done within hours or days or should be followed by a CST or BPP, depending on the obstetrician's judgment. This decision is modified by the degree of abnormality and clinical conditions of each case.

The Contraction Stress Test (CST)

TECHNIQUE. The patient is placed in semi-Fowler's position or left lateral tilt to minimize supine hypotension. Blood pressure is recorded at frequent intervals. Baseline fetal heart rate and contraction pattern are determined for 10 minutes prior to any stimulation of contractions.

Common errors are that the tokodynamometer belt is too loose, giving poor contraction tracings, or that the ultrasonography transducer is not directed at the fetal heart, yielding a "noisy," poor-quality fetal heart rate tracing.

If there are three adequate contractions in a 10-minute period with a good tracing, the test is complete. The most common error in this period is accepting small, mild, irregular uterine activity for adequate contractions. If there are no uterine contractions or if there is inadequate frequency of contrac-

tions, they can be stimulated by either of two methods: nipple stimulation or oxytocin infusion. Nipple stimulation is carried out by manual nipple stimulation or application of warm packs to the breasts. Such stimulation should be limited to 2 minutes, with a 5-minute interval before restimulation, in order to avoid prolonged contractions and associated fetal bradycardia (Huddleston et al., 1984).

An alternative method of producing adequate uterine contractions is to begin oxytocin infusion via a small scalp vein needle in a hand vein at 1.0 mU/min. It is rarely necessary to exceed 10 mU/min. Oxytocin is increased every 15 minutes until the contraction rate is three in 10 minutes. If there are late decelerations with each contraction even at a lower frequency than this, the test is complete and the result is positive. It is important to have three recorded contractions in this 10-minute period, each with a duration of at least 1 minute. It is poor compromise to write "C," signifying a palpated contraction. If there is any doubt about the adequacy of the challenge, the oxytocin infusion should be continued or increased. After an interpretable test result, the oxytocin infusion is discontinued and the patient kept on the monitor until uterine activity has essentially ceased.

INTERPRETATION. The following are criteria used for interpretation of the CST:

Negative CST result: No late decelerations and normal baseline fetal heart rate.

Positive CST result: Persistent late decelerations with an adequate challenge; persistent late decelerations even with fewer than three uterine contractions per 10 minutes; possible absence of FHR variability (see Fig. 20–10).

Suspicious CST result: Intermittent late decelerations with an adequate challenge; variable decelerations (as occurs in the growth-retarded fetuses with oligohydramnios and may be due to the cord being compressed during contractions because it is unprotected by amniotic fluid); abnormal baseline fetal heart rate, i.e., less than 120 or more than 160 beats/min.

Unsatisfactory CST result: Poor-quality recording, perhaps due to maternal obesity or excessive fetal movement; inability to achieve three contractions in 10 minutes.

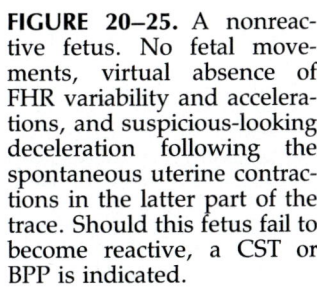 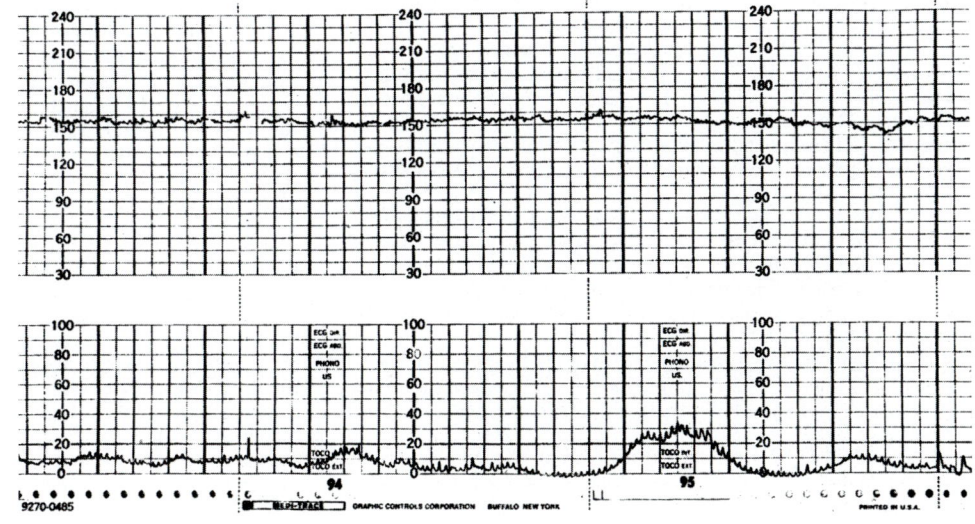

FIGURE 20–25. A nonreactive fetus. No fetal movements, virtual absence of FHR variability and accelerations, and suspicious-looking deceleration following the spontaneous uterine contractions in the latter part of the trace. Should this fetus fail to become reactive, a CST or BPP is indicated.

A fifth type of result, *hyperstimulation CST*, occurs when late decelerations or bradycardia occurs with excessive uterine activity, i.e., contractions closer than every 2 minutes or longer than 90 seconds in duration.

A negative CST result is associated with fetal survival for at least 1 week in more than 99 per cent of cases (Schifrin, 1979; Keegan and Paul, 1980).

A positive CST result has been associated with poor fetal outcome—perinatal death, low 5-minute Apgar score, or late decelerations in labor in approximately 50 per cent of cases, in a summary of numerous clinical surveys (Ott, 1978). In several early studies in which results of the testing were not used to determine management, the ultimate stillbirth rate of fetuses with a positive CST result was 22 per cent. However, because of the high false-positive rate, it is recommended that, if delivery is chosen, such patients be given a trial of labor with optimal fetal heart rate monitoring. A positive CST result is prognostically worse if it is accompanied by a nonreactive NST result with absence of FHR variability.

CONTRAINDICATIONS. There are certain contraindications to CST, including previous classic cesarean section; placenta previa; and presence of risk for preterm delivery—e.g., premature rupture of membranes, multiple gestation, incompetent cervix, and treatment for preterm labor.

THE BIOPHYSICAL PROFILE. This test is described in detail in Chapter 22. Some obstetricians use the test as the primary surveillance technique, whereas others use it to follow up on a nonreactive NST or to clarify the significance of a suspicious or positive CST. The biophysical profile has been reported to have a lower false abnormal rate than either the NST or CST (Manning et al., 1985).

REFERENCES

American College of Obstetricians and Gynecologists (ACOG) Technical Bulletin, Intrapartum Fetal Heart Monitoring, No. **132**, 1989.

Anderson PAW, Glick KL, Killam AP, et al: The effect of heart rate on *in utero* left ventricular output in the fetal sheep. J Physiol **372**:557, 1986.

Ball RH, Parer JT: The physiological mechanisms of variable decelerations. Am J Obstet Gynecol **166**:1683, 1992.

Beard RW, Filshie GM, Knight CA, Roberts GM: The significance of the changes in the continuous fetal heart rate in the first stage of labour. J Obstet Gynaecol Br Commwlth **78**:865, 1971.

Bowes WA, Gabbe SG, Bowes C: Fetal heart rate monitoring in premature infants weighing 1500 grams or less. Am J Obstet Gynecol **137**:791, 1980.

Brace RA, Gold PS: Fetal whole-body interstitial compliance, vascular compliance, and capillary filtration coefficient. Am J Physiol **247**:R800, 1984.

Clark SL, Gimovsky ML, Miller FC: The scalp stimulation test: A clinical alternative to fetal scalp blood sampling. Am J Obstet Gynecol **148**:274, 1984.

Cohn HE, Sacks EJ, Heymann MA, Rudolph AM: Cardiovascular responses to hypoxemia and acidemia in fetal lambs. Am J Obstet Gynecol **120**:817, 1974.

Court DJ, Parer JT: Experimental studies of fetal asphyxia and fetal heart rate interpretation. *In* Nathanielsz PW, Parer JT (eds): Research in Perinatal Medicine (I). New York, Perinatology Press, 1984, pp 113–169.

Dalton KJ, Phill D, Dawes GS, Patrick JE: The autonomic nervous system and fetal heart rate variability. Am J Obstet Gynecol **146**:456, 1983.

DeHaan J, Stolte LAM, Veth AFL, et al: The significance of short-term irregularity in the fetal heart rate pattern. *In* Dandenhausen JW, Saling E (eds): Perinatale Medezin. Vol 4. Stuttgart, Thieme Verlag, 1973.

Evertson LR, Gauthier RJ, Collea JV: Fetal demise following negative contraction stress test. Obstet Gynecol **51**:671, 1978.

Fisher DS, Heymann MA, Rudolph AM: Fetal myocardial oxygen and carbohydrate consumption during acutely induced hypoxemia. Am J Physiol **242**:H657, 1982.

Freeman RK, Anderson G, Dorchester W: A prospective multi-institutional study of antepartum fetal heart rate monitoring MI. Contraction stress test versus nonstress test for primary surveillance. Am J Obstet Gynecol **143**:778, 1982.

Garite TJ, Linzey EM, Freeman RK, Dorchester W: Fetal heart rate patterns and fetal distress in fetuses with congenital anomalies. Obstet Gynecol **53**:716, 1979.

Grant A, Elbourne D: Movement counting for assessment of fetal wellbeing. *In* Chalmers I, Enkin M, Keirse MJNC (eds): Effective Care in Pregnancy and Childbirth. Oxford, Oxford University Press, 1989, pp 440–454.

Hammacher K, Huter KA, Bokelmann J, Werners PH: Foetal heart rate frequency and perinatal condition of foetus and newborn. Gynaecologia (Basel) **166**:349, 1968.

Hanson MA: The importance of baro- and chemo-reflexes in the control of the fetal cardiovascular system. J Dev Physiol **10**:491, 1988.

Harris JL, Krueger TR, Parer JT: Mechanisms of late decelerations of the fetal heart rate during hypoxia. Am J Obstet Gynecol **144**:491, 1982.

Herbert CM, Boehm FM: Prolonged end-stage fetal heart rate deceleration: A reanalysis. Obstet Gynecol **57**:589, 1981.

Hon EH: An Atlas of Fetal Heart Rate Patterns. New Haven, CT, Harty Press, 1968.

Hon EH, Quilligan EJ: The classification of fetal heart rate. Conn Med **31**:779, 1967.

Huddleston JF, Sutliff G, Robinson D: Contraction stress test by intermittent nipple stimulation. Obstet Gynecol **63**:669, 1984.

Jones MD, Sheldon RE, Peeters LL, et al: Fetal cerebral oxygen consumption at different levels of oxygenation. J Appl Physiol **43**:1080, 1977.

Keegan KA, Paul RH: Antepartum fetal heart rate testing. IV. The nonstress test as a primary approach. Am J Obstet Gynecol **136**:75, 1980.

Kenny J, Plappert T, Doubilet P, et al: Effects of heart rate on ventricular size, stroke volume, and output in the normal human fetus: A prospective Doppler echocardiographic study. Circulation **76**:52, 1987.

Kero P, Antila K, Ylitalo V: Decreased heart rate variation in decerebration syndrome: Quantitative clinical criterion of brain death? Pediatrics **62**:307, 1978.

Klapholz H, Schifrin B, Myrick R: Role of maternal artifact in fetal heart rate pattern interpretation. Obstet Gynecol **44**:373, 1974.

Knopf K, Parer JT, Espinoza ME, et al: Comparison of mathematical indices of fetal heart rate variability with visual assessment in the human and sheep. J Dev Physiol **16**:367, 1992.

Krebs HB, Petres RE, Dunn LJ, et al: Intrapartum fetal heart rate monitoring. I. Classification and prognosis of fetal heart rate patterns. Am J Obstet Gynecol **133**:762, 1979.

Kubli FW, Hon EH, Khazin AF, Takemura H: Observations on heart rate and pH in the human fetus during labor. Am J Obstet Gynecol **104**:1190, 1969.

Llanos AJ, Green JR, Creasy RK, Rudolph AM: Increased heart rate response to parasympathetic and beta-adrenergic blockade in growth-retarded fetal lambs. Am J Obstet Gynecol **136**:808, 1980.

Low JA, Pancham SR, Worthington D, et al: The acid-base and biochemical characteristics of intrapartum fetal asphyxia. Am J Obstet Gynecol **121**:446, 1975.

Mann LI: Effects in sheep of hypoxia on levels of lactate, pyruvate, and glucose in blood of mothers and fetus. Pediatr Res **4**:46, 1970.

Mann LI, Tejani NA, Weiss RR: Antenatal diagnosis and management of the small-for-gestational-age fetus. Am J Obstet Gynecol **120**:995, 1974.

Manning FA, Morrison I, Lange IR, et al: Fetal assessment based on fetal biophysical profile scoring: Experience in 12,620 referred high-risk pregnancies. Am J Obstet Gynecol **151**:343, 1985.

Martin CB Jr, DeHann J, van der Wildt B, Jongsman HW, Dieleman A, Arts THM: Mechanisms of late decelerations in the fetal heart rate. A study with autonomic blocking agents in fetal lambs. Europ J Obstet Gynecol Repro Biol **9**:361, 1979.

Mendez-Bauer C, Poseirio JJ, Arellano-Hernandez G, et al: Effects of atropine on the heart rate of the human fetus during labor. Am J Obstet Gynecol **85**:1033, 1963.

Miyazaki FS, Nevarez F: Saline amnioinfusion for relief of repetitive variable decelerations: A prospective randomized study. Am J Obstet Gynecol **153**:301, 1985.

Myers RE: Two patterns of brain damage and their conditions of occurrence. Am J Obstet Gynecol **112**:246, 1972.

Neldam S: Fetal movements as an indicator of fetal well-being. Dan Med Bull **30**:274, 1983.

Ott WJ: Antepartum biophysical evaluation of the fetus. Perinatol Neonatol **2**:11, 1978.

Parer JT: The effect of acute maternal hypoxia on fetal oxygenation and the umbilical circulation in the sheep. Eur J Obstet Gynecol Reprod Biol **10**:125, 1980.

Parer JT: Handbook of Fetal Heart Rate Monitoring. Philadelphia, WB Saunders Company, 1983.

Parer JT, Krueger TR, Harris JL: Fetal oxygen consumption and mechanisms of heart rate response during artificially produced late decelerations of fetal heart rate in sheep. Am J Obstet Gynecol **136**:478, 1980.

Parer JT, Laros RK, Heilbron DC, Krueger TR: The roles of parasympathetic and beta-adrenergic activity in beat-to-beat fetal heart rate variability. *In* Kovach AGB, Monos E, Rubanyi G (eds): Cardiovascular Physiology—Heart, Peripheral Circulation and Methodology: Proceedings of the 28th International Congress of Physiological Sciences, Budapest, Hungary, 1980. (Advances in Physiological Science Vol 8, pp 327–329). New York, Pergamon, 1981.

Paul RH, Suidan AK, Yeh S, et al: Clinical fetal monitoring. VII. The evaluation and significance of intrapartum baseline FHR variability. Am J Obstet Gynecol **123**:206, 1975.

Ralston DH, Shnider SM: The fetal and neonatal effects of regional anesthesia in obstetrics. Anesthesiology **48**:34, 1978.

Reuss ML, Parer JT, Harris JL, Krueger TR: Hemodynamic effects of alpha-adrenergic blockade during hypoxia in fetal sheep. Am J Obstet Gynecol **142**:410, 1982.

Rochard F, Schifrin BS, Goupil F, et al: Nonstressed fetal heart rate monitoring in the antepartum period. Am J Obstet Gynecol **126**:699, 1976.

Rudolph AM, Heymann MA: Control of the foetal circulation. *In* Comline KS, Cross KW, Dawes GS, Nathanielsz PW (eds): Foetal and Neonatal Physiology. Proceedings of the Barcroft Centenary Symposium. Cambridge, Cambridge University Press, 1973.

Schifferli PY, Caldeyro-Barcia R: Effect of atropine and beta-adrenergic drugs on the heart rate of the human fetus. *In* Boreus L (ed): Fetal Pharmacology. New York, Raven Press, 1973.

Schifrin BS: The rationale for antepartum fetal heart rate monitoring. J Reprod Med **23**:213, 1979.

Schifrin BS, Dame L: Fetal heart rate patterns: Prediction of Apgar score. JAMA **219**:1322, 1972.

Smith CV, Nguyen HN, Phelan JP, Paul RH: Intrapartum assessment of fetal well-being: A comparison of fetal acoustic stimulation with acid-base determinations. Am J Obstet Gynecol **155**:726, 1986a.

Smith CV, Phelan JP, et al: Fetal acoustic stimulation testing II. A randomized clinical comparison with the non-stress test. Am J Obstet Gynecol **155**:131, 1986b.

Strong TH, Hetzler G, Sarno AP, Paul RH: Prophylactic intrapartum amnioinfusion: A randomized clinical trial. Am J Obstet Gynecol **162**:1370, 1990.

Tejani N, Mann LI, Bhakthavathsalan A: Correlation of fetal heart rate patterns and fetal pH with neonatal outcome. Obstet Gynecol **48**:460, 1976.

Thacker SD: The efficacy of intrapartum electronic fetal monitoring. Am J Obstet Gynecol **156**:25, 1987.

Thacker SD, Berkelman RL: Assessing the diagnostic accuracy and efficacy of selected antepartum fetal surveillance techniques. Obstet Gynecol **41**:121, 1986.

Wenstrom KD, Parsons MT: The prevention of meconium aspiration in labor using amnioinfusion. Obstet Gynecol **73**:647, 1989.

Wood C, Ferguson R, Leeton J, et al: Fetal heart rate and acid-base status in the assessment of fetal hypoxia. Am J Obstet Gynecol **98**:62, 1967.

Yaffe H, Parer JT, Block BS, et al: Cardiorespiratory responses to graded reductions of uterine blood flow in the sheep fetus. J Dev Physiol **9**:325, 1987.

Zanini B, Paul RH, Huey JR: Intrapartum fetal heart rate: Correlation with scalp pH in the preterm fetus. Am J Obstet Gynecol **136**:43, 1980.

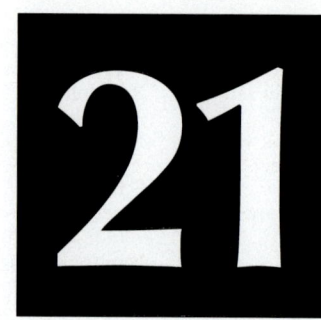

FETAL CARDIAC ARRHYTHMIAS: DIAGNOSIS AND THERAPY

CHARLES S. KLEINMAN, M.D., and JOSHUA A. COPEL, M.D.

Most disturbances of fetal cardiac rhythm represent isolated extrasystoles that are of little clinical importance to the human fetus. However, *sustained* arrhythmias may be associated with fetal heart failure, manifesting as nonimmune hydrops fetalis. Such fetuses may require antiarrhythmic therapy, which may be provided in a logical and well-planned fashion if the electrophysiologic mechanism of the arrhythmia is known and guides the selection of antiarrhythmic agents (Kleinman et al., 1980; Kleinman and Copel, 1991). Close monitoring of the maternal and fetal hemodynamic response to such therapy is essential.

In the following chapter, the application of fetal echocardiography for the analysis of fetal arrhythmias and for monitoring transplacental antiarrhythmic therapy will be discussed. The most commonly used antiarrhythmic agents will be discussed in the context of their use for fetal therapy, and a rationale will be proposed for the management of sustained fetal tachyarrhythmias.

For the purposes of this discussion, a "fetal arrhythmia" is defined as any irregularity of fetal cardiac rhythm not associated with uterine contraction or as a regular rhythm outside the range of 100 to 160 beats/minute.

THE YALE EXPERIENCE WITH FETAL ARRHYTHMIAS

During the past 14 years we have encountered 984 fetal patients with cardiac arrhythmias. In most cases, the reason for referral was an irregularity of fetal cardiac rhythm that was auscultated by the referring obstetrician. The most frequent finding on auscultation was the impression of a "skipping" of beats. In rare instances, patients were referred for evaluation of sustained tachy- or bradyarrhythmias.

Of these 989 fetuses, 878 were diagnosed as having isolated extrasystoles (Table 21–1). In most of these (806), the extrasystoles were judged to be supraventricular in origin, whereas 72 fetuses were thought to have ventricular or junctional or multifocal extrasystoles. The vast majority of these patients remained hemodynamically stable, with resolution of ectopic activity later in pregnancy or during the first several days of the neonatal period. Three patients who presented with isolated ectopy later presented with sustained supraventricular tachycardia and hydrops fetalis, and a fourth patient, who had blocked atrial bigeminy, developed sustained supraventricular tachycardia on the first day of life. On the basis of the small but finite (0.5 per cent) risk that a patient presenting with isolated extrasystoles will later develop sustained supraventricular tachycardia, we have recommended that such patients continue to have twice-weekly in-office checks of fetal heart rate until the time of delivery or until the arrhythmia resolves or deteriorates into sustained tachycardia.

One hundred and eleven fetuses presented with sustained arrhythmias (Table 21–1), including 47 with supraventricular tachycardia (SVT), 12 with atrial flutter, 2 with atrial fibrillation, 4 with ventricular tachycardia, 6 with sinus tachycardia, 1 with junctional tachycardia, 6 with sinus bradycardia, 7 with second-degree atrioventricular block, and 26 with complete heart block.

ECHOCARDIOGRAPHIC ANALYSIS OF FETAL CARDIAC RHYTHM

Although it would be preferable to utilize high-quality recordings of the fetal electrocardiographic

TABLE 21–1. Fetal Cardiac Arrhythmias (n = 984)

Isolated extrasystoles	878
Supraventricular tachycardia	47
Atrial flutter	12
Atrial fibrillation	2
Sinus tachycardia	6
Junctional tachycardia	1
Ventricular tachycardia	4
Second-degree AV block	7
Sinus bradycardia	1
Complete heart block	26

signal to analyze fetal cardiac rhythm, the technology required to obtain such signals against a background of sixty-cycle interference and interference from the maternal electrocardiographic signal is only now being developed, making echocardiographic recording of cardiac motion against time the cornerstone for the diagnosis of fetal cardiac arrhythmias.

M-mode Echocardiography

Using real-time techniques, an analysis of cardiac anatomy is performed. Two-dimensional imaging is used to analyze fetal cardiac anatomy. The two-dimensional image is then used to orient the position of the M-mode sampling line. M-mode echocardiographic recordings of cardiac motion against time are performed, with hard copy recordings made on a strip-chart recorder. These recordings, which are used to time electromechanical events in the fetal cardiac cycle, may be obtained by use of a single M-mode sampling line that intercepts both atrial and ventricular walls or the atrioventricular junction, including the atrioventricular valve mechanism. Such recordings may provide sufficient information to allow accurate timing of atrial and ventricular electrical events in the cardiac cycle. On occasion, however, the fetal heart may be oriented in a position that precludes one's obtaining a single M-mode line of information that intersects both atrial and ventricular structures. In such cases, use of the "dual M-mode" sampling capability of phased-array scanners allows simultaneous recording of atrial and ventricular wall motion. A "ladder-diagram" analysis of atrioventricular contraction sequence may then be constructed to provide accurate analysis of cardiac rhythm (Fig. 21–1) (Allan et al., 1983; Crowley et al., 1985; DeVore et al., 1983; Kleinman et al., 1983; Kleinman and Donnerstein, 1985; Kleinman and Copel, 1991).

Pulsed-Doppler Echocardiography

Using the two-dimensional image, the sample volume of a duplex pulsed-Doppler scanner may be placed within the cardiac chambers and great vessels to provide further information concerning the timing of mechanical events and their influence on ventricular filling and great arterial flow (Kleinman et al., 1984; Wladimiroff et al., 1983).

Color-Encoded M-mode Echocardiography

Doppler color flow mapping has added a new modality to the two-dimensional imaging of fetal cardiac structure by providing a cover overlay upon the two-dimensional gray-scale image of the fetal heart. This information may thus provide important physiologic flow information that may be considered when evaluating the gray-scale image of cardiac structure. This information, although rarely absolutely required to establish an anatomic diagnosis of congenital heart disease, may improve the accuracy of the prenatal structural diagnosis by imparting simultaneous flow information. The major shortcoming of color flow mapping is the lack of temporal resolution inherent in the color flow signal itself. Postnatally this is compensated for with the simultaneous inscription of an electrocardiogram, which is used to impart temporal resolution on the color flow information. With the lack of a fetal electrocardiographic signal, we have found that the use of color-encoded M-mode echocardiography may provide important insights into the analysis of fetal cardiac rhythm disturbances. By superimpos-

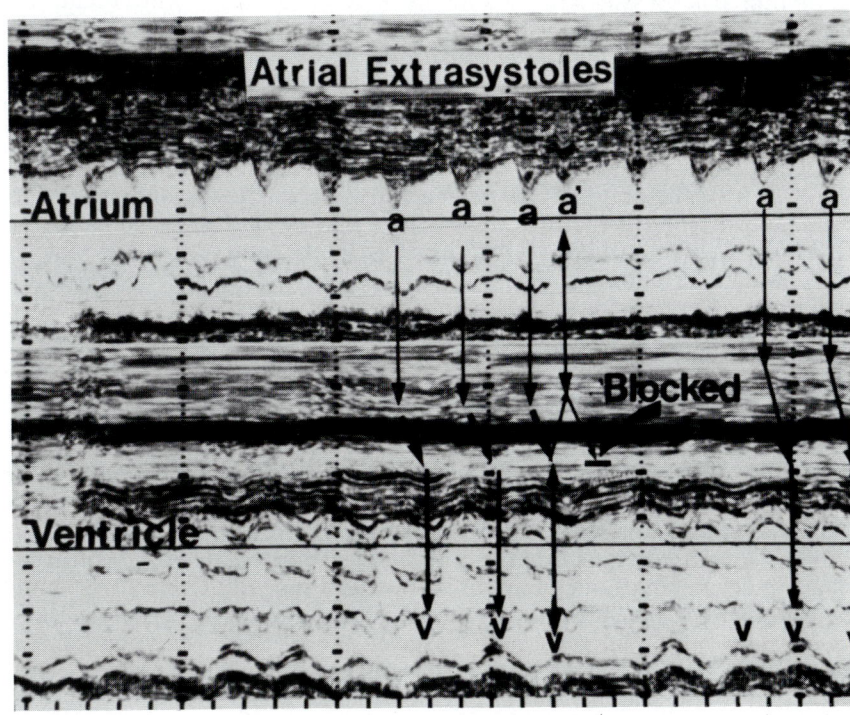

FIGURE 21–1. Ladder diagram analysis of fetal cardiac rhythm using dual M-mode echocardiographic recording of atrial and ventricular activity. Upper tracing represents atrial wall motion. Note that regular atrial rhythm, denoted by a, is interrupted by early contraction, a, which represents an atrial extrasystole. Simultaneously recorded ventricular wall echocardiogram shows regular undulations (v) following delay of conduction in the atrioventricular node. The atrial extrasystole has occurred too soon after the last normally conducted sinus beat and encounters the atrioventricular node while it is still refractory, resulting in block within this area and the absence of a ventricular response to the atrial beat.

ing the color flow information upon an M-mode echo-cardiogram, one may take advantage, simultaneously, of the cardiac-motion-against-time information that is inherent in the M-mode echocardiogram, which imparts temporal resolution upon the color flow data that is simultaneously inscribed. One can therefore use these hard-copy recordings of cardiac motion against time and cardiac flow against time to analyze the electromechanical characteristics of the fetal heart under study.

FETAL CARDIAC ARRHYTHMIAS: SHOULD THEY BE TREATED?

The existence of a technique for accurate diagnosis of fetal cardiac rhythm disturbances is necessary, but not sufficient to justify the administration of potent antiarrhythmic agents to pregnant women and their fetuses. The appropriate management of an arrhythmia requires an understanding of the natural history of the arrhythmia, a precise definition of the electrophysiologic mechanism of the arrhythmia, the pharmacology and pharmacokinetics of the antiarrhythmic agents in the maternal-fetal environment, and a detailed risk/benefit analysis.

The association of *hydrops fetalis* with sustained fetal supraventricular tachyarrhythmias is well described (Kleinman et al., 1982). It is also evident in studies from many centers that the mortality rate for severely hydropic neonates is prohibitively high, regardless of the underlying cause of the hydrops (Andersen et al., 1983). For this reason it seems reasonable that severely hydropic neonates with sustained supraventricular tachyarrhythmias are at extremely high risk, and that vigorous efforts at *in utero* therapy would be warranted if they could be applied with a reasonable expectation of success and at low risk to the mother. Even a moderate risk to the fetus would be acceptable, in light of the extremely poor prognosis for the neonate if the arrhythmia and hydrops remain untreated. The risk to the fetus increases proportionally with the degree of prematurity at the time of diagnosis.

The approach most reasonable for the fetus with sustained tachycardia without hydrops fetalis is dictated by an estimation of the risk/benefit ratio to the fetus and mother. If the diagnosis is made at a gestational age when pulmonary maturity is likely (and documented by amniocentesis) (Gluck, et al., 1974), delivery with provision of postnatal therapy is advisable. At increasing degrees of prematurity, immediate delivery is not a viable option. In this setting the decision regarding provision of therapy must depend upon considerations including (1) the potential risk of hydrops fetalis, (2) the potential risks of antiarrhythmic therapy, and (3) individual considerations, including the feasibility of providing medical follow-up to the mother and fetus. The risks of antiarrhythmic therapy are largely dependent upon the electrophysiologic mechanism of the arrhythmia, because this will determine which antiarrhythmic agents are to be used, and upon individual responses to each agent. The latter places a responsibility upon the treating physician to provide careful monitoring of the hemodynamic responses of both the mother and fetus under therapy. The decision to treat fetal arrhythmias must be based on an understanding of the natural history of the rhythm disturbance and cannot be predicated on the basis of subjective complaints of the patient or even, in most cases, on the frequency of the attacks.

Determining the likelihood of the development of hydrops fetalis in a given patient may be difficult or impossible. In our series, 28 of 47 fetal patients with supraventricular tachycardia were hydropic at the time of diagnosis and therefore warranted *in utero* therapy. Two additional patients, who presented with sustained tachycardia before the 34th week of gestation, were observed without therapy for 24 to 48 hours after presentation. Each fetus received antiarrhythmic therapy after pleural, pericardial, and/or ascitic effusions developed. Four additional patients received digoxin therapy of supraventricular tachycardia, despite the absence of fetal hydrops, after an exhaustive discussion of the pros and cons of such therapy was held with both parents.

The fact that not all fetuses with SVT develop hydrops fetalis is well known. It has been suggested that the "parallel" circuitry of the fetal cardiovascular system might impart some protection against the development of hydrops fetalis. However, the unique properties of the fetal cardiovascular system, including a physiologic "volume overload" on the right atrium and ventricle, as well as the intrinsic properties of the ventricular myocardium, make the fetus more, rather than less, susceptible to systemic edema in response to a variety of hemodynamic disturbances. It has been suggested (Kallfelz, 1979) that even a brief interlude of sinus rhythm interposed into an incessant tachycardia will provide the fetus with protection against the development of hydrops fetalis. That there is some "threshold" beyond which heart failure will develop seems likely, but this threshold is probably highly individual, making "blanket" recommendations regarding medical therapy unjustifiable.

Therapy for the hydropic fetus with sustained tachycardia is warranted. Furthermore, fetal SVT at virtually any gestational age is a potential medical emergency, especially when there is evidence of cardiovascular decompensation (hydrops fetalis). Unless there is no evidence of fetal hydrops and there is no doubt regarding pulmonary maturity, *in utero* therapy should be seriously considered in the management of this arrhythmia.

A rational approach to the treatment of a cardiac rhythm disturbance requires accurate identification of the electrophysiologic mechanism of the arrhythmia. As noted by Rae and Webb (1984) in their review of the management of SVT, "Certainly, the same therapy may be effective for many different types of SVT and an empiric approach may be successful, but logically directed therapy produces a greater chance of success in a shorter period of time and reduces the risk of causing acceleration, incessancy, or degeneration to life-threatening arrhythmias."

The pharmacologic treatment of *in utero* arrhythmias involves the administration of potent cardiac medications to the mother. The treatment of this "patient within a patient" therefore involves moral, ethical, and even legal considerations in compromising the autonomy of the mother's body and exposing her to the potential side effects that these agents may have.

Pulsed-Doppler analysis of ventricular diastolic filling characteristics has suggested that the normal fetal ventricle, like the ventricles of postnatal patients with restrictive cardiomyopathy, is dependent upon the active component of ventricular filling, following atrial systole. These findings are reminiscent of the studies of Friedman (1973), which suggested a relative "stiffness" of fetal lamb ventricular myocardium compared with the ventricular myocardium of later childhood and adulthood. We believe that the intrinsic "stiffness" of fetal myocardium makes the fetal heart more prone to the deleterious effects of excessive tachycardia, which foreshortens the diastolic filling period. The fetal heart therefore behaves as a heart with little "cardiac reserve" (Eik-Nes et al., 1984; Gill et al., 1984; Kleinman and Donnerstein, 1985). The intrinsic properties of the myocardium and the "parallel circuitry" of the fetal cardiovascular system and the paucity of pulmonary blood flow in the fetus explain why severe hemodynamic compromise leads to elevated right atrial pressure, and subsequently to systemic venous hypertension, and ultimately to systemic edema and third-spacing of fluid in the fetus.

ELECTROPHYSIOLOGY OF FETAL ARRHYTHMIAS

Tachyarrhythmias

Supraventricular Tachycardia

Sustained tachyarrhythmias have been the cardiac rhythm disturbances that carry the greatest clinical import for the involved fetus. Most of our tachycardic patients have been identified to have supraventricular tachycardia (SVT)(n = 47).

Supraventricular tachyarrhythmias may be reentrant (reciprocating) (related to a "circus movement" of electrical activity), automatic (arising in an "irritable" ectopic focus, above the bundle of His), or a manifestation of atrial flutter or fibrillation (Garson, 1990; Gillette, 1976; Reder and Rosen, 1981).

In the fetus and neonate the most common electrical mechanism underlying SVT involves an electrical impulse that reenters the atrium from the ventricle, resulting in a circular movement of repeated electrical stimulation that is faster than, and independent of, the normal sinus nodal pacemaker. Because the heart will beat at the rate of the fastest intrinsic pacemaker, this electrical stimulus drives the heart at a tachycardic rate. Such a circus movement may occur within the atrium or sinus nodal tissue (very rarely) or, much more frequently, within the atrioventricular (AV) node itself, due to a dissociation of conduction tissue within the AV node or due to a discrete accessory conduction pathway outside the AV node (e.g., the "Kent Bundle" in the Wolff-Parkinson-White [WPW] syndrome), which directly connects atrial and ventricular myocardium without interposing the delay to conduction that is inherent in AV nodal tissue.

AV nodal reentrant tachycardia (AVNRT) involves a "longitudinal dissociation" of conduction fibers within the AV node, resulting in two pathways with differing conduction velocities and refractory periods. The usual inciting mechanism is an extrasystole that is timed so that it encounters the fast conducting pathway (with longer refractory period) while it is still refractory following the preceding normal sinus beat. Atrioventricular conduction therefore occurs down the "slow" pathway. If conduction down this pathway is sufficiently slow to allow recovery of the fast pathway, "reciprocation" with ventriculoatrial conduction up the fast pathway to the atrium will occur, resulting in the establishment of a "circus movement" of electrical activity, which in turn results in the sudden initiation of tachycardia following the critically timed extrasystole.

Reentrant tachycardia is dependent upon the existence of an available pathway, with fibers that differ in conduction velocity and refractory periods, and appropriately timed extrasystoles. Reentrant tachycardias can be recognized by their tendency toward sudden onset and sudden termination (Figs. 21–2 through 21–5), with both events associated with pre-

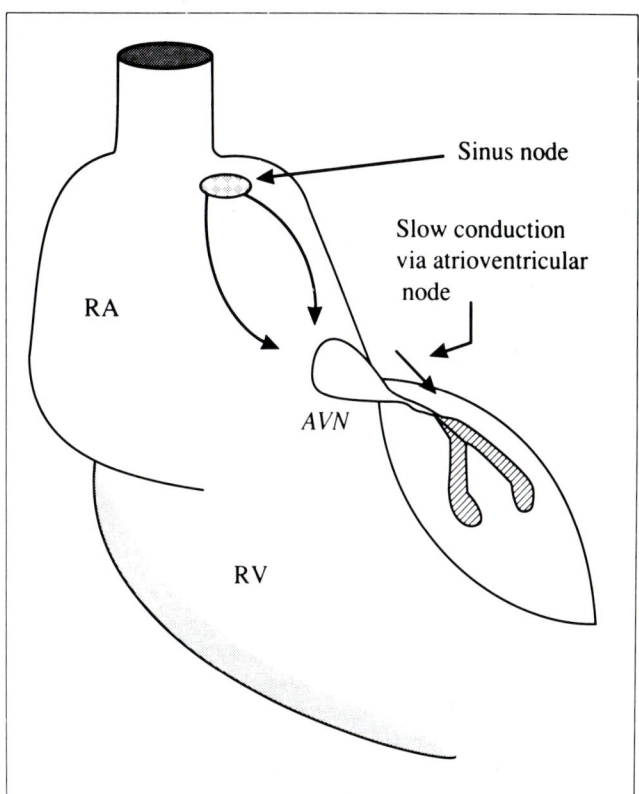

FIGURE 21–2. Schematic diagram of the cardiac conduction system during normal sinus rhythm. The sinus node is the primary pacemaker of cardiac rhythm. Cardiac impulses arising in the sinus node are conducted through atrial muscle until they reach the atrioventricular node (AVN). After slow conduction through the atrioventricular node, the impulse is conducted through the His-Purkinje system into the ventricular myocardium. (RA = right atrium; RV = right ventricle). (Reproduced with permission from Kleinman CS, Copel JC: Electrophysiologic principles and antiarrhythmic therapy. Ultrasound Obstet Gynecol 1:286, 1991.)

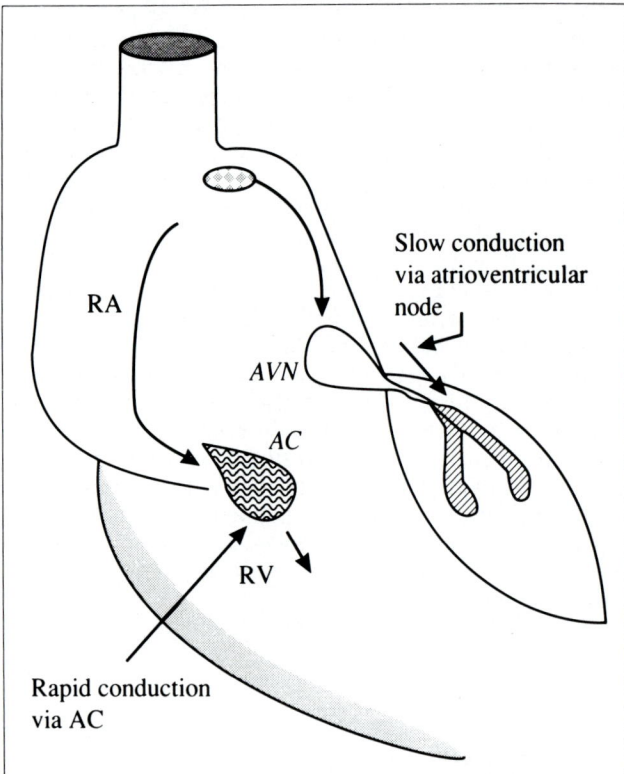

FIGURE 21–3. Schematic diagram of the cardiac conduction system in a patient with an accessory conduction pathway (AC) (Wolff-Parkinson-White syndrome). The accessory pathway conducts impulses into the ventricular muscle more rapidly than does the atrioventricular node, resulting in "preexcitation" of the ventricle. (Reproduced with permission from Kleinman CS, Copel JC: Electrophysiologic principles and antiarrhythmic therapy. Ultrasound Obstet Gynecol **1**:286, 1991.)

cipitating extrasystoles occurring at critical "coupling intervals" to the previous normal beats. These tachycardias usually have typical rates. For fetal SVT the typically encountered heart rate is in the 220 to 260 beat/minute range.

AV reentrant tachycardia (AVRT) is similar in many ways to AVNRT, in that both involve a reentrant circuit at the AV junction, requiring two electrical "limbs" with discrete electrical properties. Both AVRT and AVNRT may result in reentrant SVT of sudden onset (and cessation) following atrial or ventricular extrasystoles that occur at a critical "coupling interval" to the preceding sinus beat. In AVRT there is a discrete accessory conduction pathway that bypasses the usual delay within the AV node. This pathway directly connects atrial to ventricular muscle (in the WPW syndrome) and serves as the "fast" limb in the circus movement of electrical energy that results in SVT. This is the most common electrophysiologic mechanism underlying fetal supraventricular tachycardia.

Four of our 47 fetuses with reentrant SVT, four of our patients with atrial flutter, and one patient with atrial bigeminy *in utero* were diagnosed as having the WPW syndrome in the neonatal period. The first three

of these patients represented the only fetuses in our group who had protracted tachyarrhythmias postnatally, requiring multidrug therapy.

In both forms of reciprocating SVT, the arrhythmia is dependent upon a critical relationship between the conduction velocities and refractory periods within the two pathways for impulse conduction. Therapeutic interventions are logically aimed at perturbation of the delicate electrical balance between the two limbs of the electrical reentry circuit that are needed to support the tachycardia.

Postnatally, maneuvers that increase vagal tone, which in turn slow AV nodal conduction, may abruptly terminate reentrant tachycardia involving the AV node as part of the reentry circuit. Such maneuvers have been employed in the fetus, and several patients in our series who presented near term with SVT without hydrops have demonstrated that increased

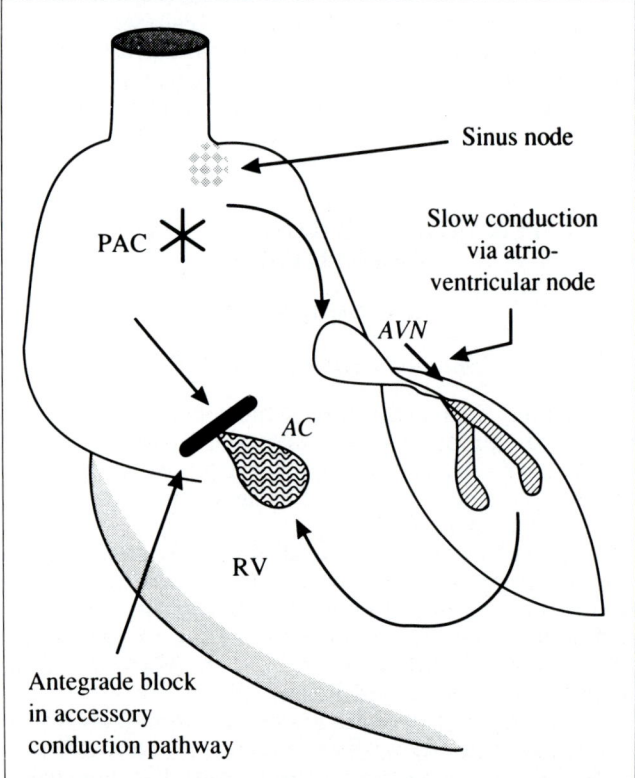

FIGURE 21–4. Schematic diagram of the cardiac conduction system in a patient with an accessory conduction pathway (AC). In order to establish orthodromic reciprocating supraventricular tachycardia, a premature atrial contraction (PAC) has occurred with a critical coupling interval that is shorter than the effective refractory period in the accessory conduction pathway. The impulse encounters the atrioventricular node (AVN) after its shorter refractory period. The impulse conducts slowly through the atrioventricular node and the ventricular muscle and then encounters the accessory conduction pathway in the retgrograde direction, after a significant time delay. (Reproduced with permission from Kleinman CS, Copel JC: Electrophysiologic principles and antiarrhythmic therapy. Ultrasound Obstet Gynecol **1**:286, 1991.)

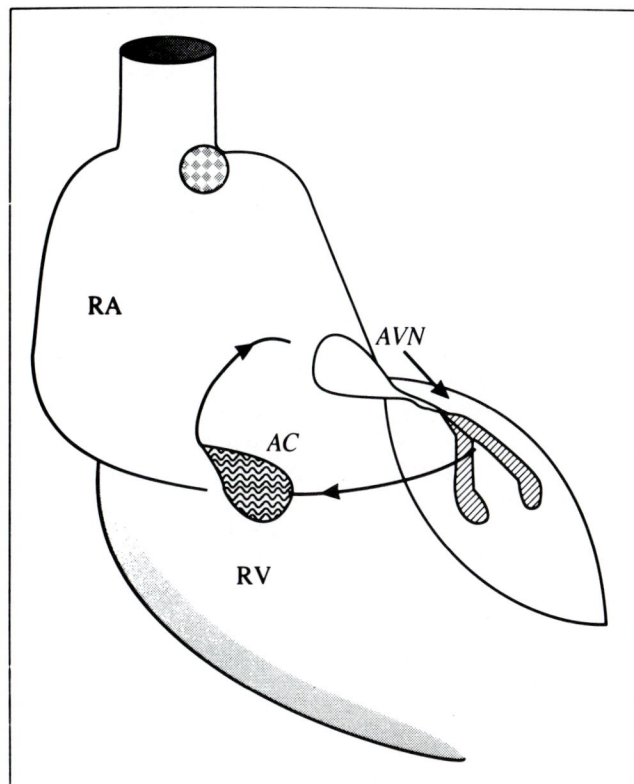

FIGURE 21–5. After retrograde reentry of the electrical impulse into the atrial muscle through the accessory pathway, a circular ("circus") movement of electrical energy is established. The wavefront in turn stimulates atrial and ventricular contraction at a rate governed by the properties of the electrical circuit, rather than by the sinus node. Each atrial stimulus is followed by a ventricular stimulus, and vice versa. (Reproduced with permission from Kleinman CS, Copel JC: Electrophysiologic principles and antiarrhythmic therapy. Ultrasound Obstet Gynecol **1**:286, 1991.)

vagal tone, caused by cord or head compression, will result in "breaks" in sustained episodes of SVT (Martin et al., 1984). Such maneuvers can hardly be recommended as a standard fetal therapy and provide no means of prophylaxis against repeated episodes of tachycardia.

Antiarrhythmic agents that depress conduction and prolong refractory periods in AV nodal or accessory conduction tissue can disturb the reentrant circuit and may be useful for the termination as well as prevention of AVNRT or AVRT. Such agents may include the cardiac glycosides (e.g., digoxin), beta-blockers (e.g., propranolol), calcium-channel blockers (e.g., verapamil), type Ia antiarrhythmics (e.g., quinidine and procainamide) type Ic antiarrhythmics (e.g., flecainide), and type III antiarrhythmics (e.g., amiodarone) (Antman et al., 1980; Lie et al., 1983; Rotmensch et al., 1982).

Ectopic or automatic tachycardias occur when there is spontaneous depolarization of a pacemaker focus within the atrium. These tachycardias, unlike the sudden-onset/sudden-cessation pattern of reentrant tachycardia, are usually incessant. Varying degrees of atrioventricular block may be seen in these patients

(Fig. 21–6). Whereas AV block will result in immediate termination of a tachycardia that is dependent upon reentry in either direction through the AV node, ectopic tachycardia is not dependent upon a circus movement of electrical energy and cannot logically be expected to respond to therapy aimed at AV reentry (Sapire et al., 1979).

Atrial Flutter/Fibrillation

The incidence of atrial flutter and fibrillation in our series (see Table 21–1) of patients suggests that these arrhythmias are rarer than SVT in fetal life. Our series also demonstrates that these patients may present with hydrops fetalis. The relatively high mortality rate in this subgroup of patients (Table 21–2) attests to the difficulties that we have encountered in controlling these arrhythmias *in utero*.

Atrial flutter appears to result from a circus movement of electrical energy within the body of the atrium itself (Fig. 21–7). The atrial rate in atrial flutter in the

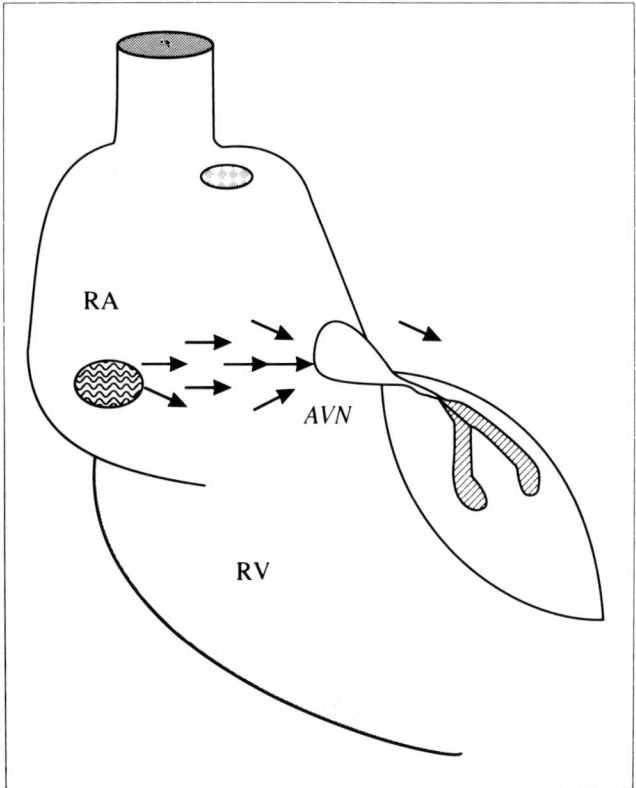

FIGURE 21–6. Schematic diagram of the cardiac conduction system in automatic atrial tachycardia. An ectopic focus within the atrial muscle has taken over pacemaker activity from the sinus node. Since the heart beats at the rate of the fastest intrinsic pacemaker, this ectopic focus "drives" the heart rate. Such tachycardia may, on occasion, be associated with varying degrees of atrioventricular block. (Reproduced with permission from Kleinman CS, Copel JC: Electrophysiologic principles and antiarrhythmic therapy. Ultrasound Obstet Gynecol **1**:286, 1991.)

TABLE 21–2. Fetal Supraventricular Tachyarrhythmias

SUPRAVENTRICULAR TACHYCARDIA	(n = 47)
Gestational age	19–39 weeks
Hydrops fetalis	30/47 cases
In utero control	31/34 cases
Postnatal control	3/34 cases
Congenital heart disease	1/47 cases
Deaths	2/47 cases
ATRIAL FLUTTER	(n = 12)
Gestational age	24–38 weeks
Hydrops fetalis	8/12 cases
In utero control	4/10 cases
Postnatal control	6/10 cases
Congenital heart disease	4/12 cases
Deaths	4/12 cases
ATRIAL FIBRILLATION	(n = 2)
Gestational age	19–38 weeks
Hydrops fetalis	0
In utero control	1/2 cases
Deaths	0

postnatal patient is typically 300 beats/minute, whereas in the fetus, monotonous atrial flutter rates of 400 to 460 are the rule rather than the exception (Fig. 21–8). Varying degrees of AV block may be seen in association with fetal atrial flutter, resulting in varying ventricular response rates, which may be fixed and unresponsive to fetal activity (in the case of fixed 2:1 AV block) or quite irregular (in cases with varying degrees of AV block). The almost invariable association of atrial flutter with some degree of AV block is important evidence that this arrhythmia does not involve atrioventricular reentry through the AV node as the underlying electrophysiologic mechanism.

Clinical experience has demonstrated that digoxin and/or verapamil may increase the degree of AV block, resulting in a slower ventricular response rate. Unlike the experience with postnatal therapy of atrial flutter, in which decreasing the ventricular response rate per se may lead to a decrease in the degree of heart failure, we have been disappointed to find that control of the ventricular response rate in fetuses with severe hydrops fetalis secondary to atrial flutter has not resulted in an improvement in the fetal hemodynamic status. This is probably attributable to the unique cardiovascular dynamics of the fetus, with relatively restrictive ventricular myocardium and a relatively volume-loaded right heart. From these observations in these fetuses, we have concluded that much of the fetal cardiovascular decompensation accompanying supraventricular tachyarrhythmias reflects diastolic rather than systolic dysfunction. Unless the atrial flutter is controlled, therefore, there will continue to be atrial contractions against a closed or partially closed atrioventricular valve, resulting in atrial pressure waves that will keep mean systolic venous pressure high, retarding the resolution of fetal edema and effusions. This makes it imperative that the therapeutic end point of antiarrhythmic therapy be restoration of normal sinus rhythm, with resumption of a 1:1 atrioventricular contraction sequence. This may well require incorporation of a type I antiarrhythmic agent such as quini-

dine, procainamide or flecainide in the antiarrhythmic protocol for atrial flutter, following control of ventricular response rate with digoxin and/or verapamil.

Atrial fibrillation appears to be even rarer in the fetus than is atrial flutter. Two of our patients responded to digoxin therapy alone, but if the arrhythmia had persisted despite control of the ventricular response rate, we would have opted for inclusion of a type I antiarrhythmic, for the same reasons that were outlined above in our discussion of atrial flutter.

The high (4/12 cases) mortality rate in our series of cases with atrial flutter/fibrillation reflects, in part, the difficulty that may be encountered in controlling this arrhythmia, but also reflects the association of congenital heart disease with this arrhythmia (4/12 cases). In all cases (2 with critical pulmonary outflow obstruction and tricuspid insufficiency, one with Ebstein malformation of the tricuspid valve with severe tricuspid insufficiency, and one with atrioventricular septal defect, AV valve insufficiency, and associated complete AV block), marked atrial dilation was associated with

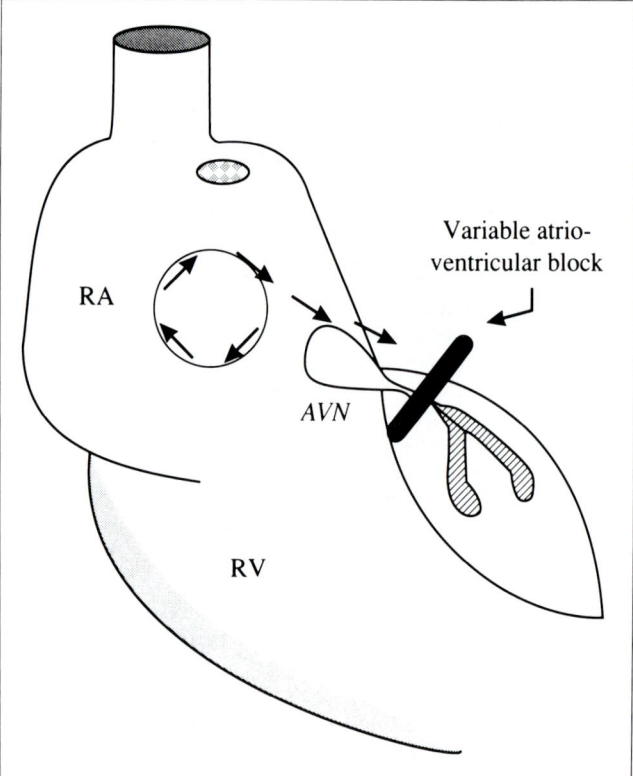

FIGURE 21–7. Schematic diagram of the cardiac conduction system in atrial flutter. In this situation the atrium flutters at a regular rate, governed by a circular movement of electrical energy. The wavefront of this "circus" movement is completely contained within the atrial muscle. The usual atrial rate in atrial flutter in the fetus is between 400 and 480 beats/minute. The ventricular rate is usually less than the atrial rate, owing to a variable degree of atrioventricular block at the level of the atrioventricular node. (Reproduced with permission from Kleinman CS, Copel JC: Electrophysiologic principles and antiarrhythmic therapy. Ultrasound Obstet Gynecol **1**:286, 1991.)

FIGURE 21–8. Dual M-mode echocardiographic recording of atrial (A) and ventricular (V) wall activity in a fetus with atrial flutter. Rapid and regular atrial wall undulations at a rate of 440 to 480 beats/minute are associated with a slower, irregular ventricular response rate. There is atrioventricular block of the atrial flutter, with persistence of the rapid atrial rhythm. Such findings rule out the possibility of atrioventricular reciprocation using the AV node as part of the reentry pathway. Hatched vertical lines are spaced at one-second intervals.

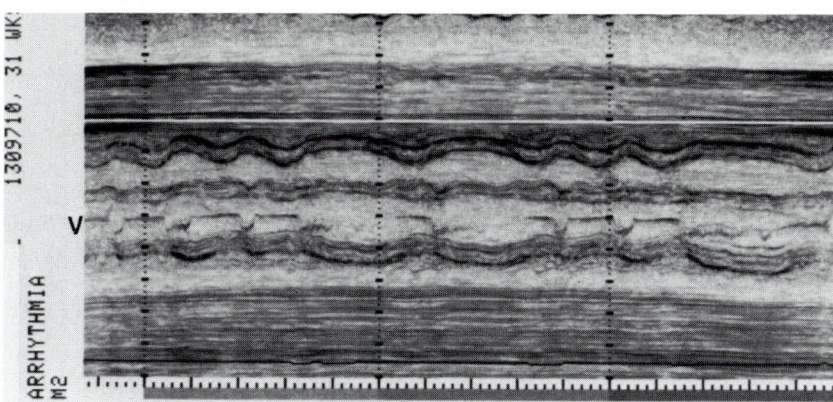

the development of atrial flutter. The four deaths in our series included three patients with associated congenital heart disease. Of interest is the fact that the only patient in our series of 47 cases of fetal reciprocating SVT with a congenital cardiac malformation had premature closure of the foramen ovale, and that fetus was one of the two who died, despite restoration of normal sinus rhythm for several days prior to its demise.

As we will reiterate below during our discussion of fetal complete heart block, the association of congenital heart disease with sustained fetal cardiac arrhythmias and hydrops fetalis is an ominous one that imparts an extremely poor prognosis for survival, with or without vigorous *in utero* and postnatal therapy.

Ventricular Tachycardia

We have encountered four patients with fetal ventricular tachycardia. In each case the heart rate during tachycardia did not fall into the "usual" range of 220 to 260 beats/minute that we have encountered in fetuses with AV recriprocating SVT. The common denominator in this group of patients with ventricular tachycardia was the finding of atrioventricular dissociation (the lack of a 1:1 relationship between atrial and ventricular contractions). AV dissociation may also be found in junctional tachycardia, but is not found in AV reciprocating supraventricular tachycardia. It is possible for fetuses with ventricular tachycardia to have a 1:1 relationship of retrograde atrial activity to each ventricular beat. This makes it impossible to rely solely upon atrioventricular dissociation as the means of diagnosing ventricular tachycardia in the fetus.

Not all neonates with ventricular tachycardia are ill, and not all require antiarrhythmic therapy. Three of our patients were free of hydrops fetalis, had normal cardiac structural scans, and were not treated *in utero*. None of these neonates received antiarrhythmic therapy, in light of the infrequency of episodes of tachycardia after birth, the lack of symptoms during tachycardia, and the lack of associated structural heart disease.

The fourth fetal patient developed tachycardia during labor, and this was associated with marked right ventricular and right atrial dilation. Therapy was not administered until after delivery. This patient had a

marked degree of right ventricular dilation and congestive heart failure associated with prolonged episodes of ventricular tachycardia. A diagnosis of arrhythmogenic right ventricular dysplasia was established, and the neonate was successfully treated with intravenous lidocaine, followed by chronic oral therapy with the lidocaine congener, mexiletine.

If a diagnosis of ventricular tachycardia is established in a previable fetus with evidence of congestive cardiac failure, antiarrhythmic therapy should be considered. In this setting digoxin should be avoided, and direct umbilical venous infusion of lidocaine, followed by oral maternal therapy with mexilitene, quinidine, procainamide, flecainide, propranolol, or phenytoin should be considered.

Sinus Tachycardia

We have encountered six fetuses with sinus tachycardia. These fetuses had baseline heart rates of approximately 180 to 190 beats/minute, with normal variations in rate around this baseline with associated fetal activity. In five fetuses no explanation for the tachycardia was found, even after the birth, despite careful monitoring and screening for abnormalities such as thyroid dysfunction. These fetuses remained well throughout the remainer of gestation and were well neonates, despite a baseline tachycardia, after birth, of approximately 155 to 165 beats/minute. Two of these fetuses were thought to have sinoatrial reentry tachycardia and progressively developed left ventricular dysfunction. One of the two responded well to digoxin therapy. The second developed progressive left ventricular dysfunction and continues to have marked left ventricular dysfunction, despite normalization of cardiac rhythm.

The sixth fetus with sinus tachycardia was the offspring of a mother with poorly controlled thyrotoxicosis and was found to have a large goiter and marked sinus tachycardia. Although the goiter resolved as maternal thyroid function was controlled better with propylthiouracil, the sinus tachycardia persisted. Hydrops fetalis did not develop. Administration of propranolol was considered, but was not given until the neonatal period, when the neonate was thought to be in impending thyroid storm. Beta blockade during the neonatal period was associated with the onset of severe congestive cardiac failure, despite the use of a rather low dose of propranolol. This neonate improved with a decrease in propranolol dose and administration of digoxin therapy.

Bradyarrhythmias

Sinus Bradycardia

Six fetuses with sinus bradycardia were seen at our institution during the past 14 years. Four of these fetuses were subsequently diagnosed to have left atrial isomerism with normal atrioventricular conduction. Postnatally they were diagnosed as having wandering supraventricular pacemakers, but none had associated hydrops fetalis. One of these patients required emergency systemic-to-pulmonary artery shunting in the neonatal period because of severe pulmonary outflow obstruction.

The two other patients with sinus bradycardia had baseline heart rates of 80 to 90 beats/minute, with normal heart rate variability on nonstress tests near term. Both fetuses tolerated labor and delivery well and remain normal infants.

In the presence of normal cardiac structure and normal heart rate responses to fetal activity, and in the absence of hydrops fetalis, moderate (heart rates between 80 and 100 beats/minute) sinus bradycardia does not appear to be an ominous fetal arrhythmia.

Blocked Atrial Bigeminy

Four fetuses in our series were found to have atrial bigeminy, with block of the extrasystolic beat, after referral for evaluation of severe (rates of 60 to 70 beats/minute) bradycardia. The referring obstetricians in each case had considered each fetus to have congenital complete heart block. In each case every second beat was a very "early" atrial extrasystole. It was so closely coupled to the previous sinus beat that either it encountered the AV node while it was still refractory (resulting in every second beat being blocked) or, if the AV node was no longer refractory, the ventricular contraction occurred before there was adequate filling of the ventricle. In the latter situation, while each extrasystolic beat resulted in a ventricular response, there was an inadequate stroke volume to create forward flow detectable with the usual continuous wave Doppler listening devices. One of these fetuses developed sustained SVT on the first day of life, and was diagnosed to have WPW syndrome following electrical cardioversion.

Second-Degree AV Block

Seven fetuses in our series had Mobitz type II atrioventricular block. These fetuses presented with irregular rhythms like those of our large series of patients with isolated ectopic beats, that is, on auscultation there was an irregular rhythm giving the impression of skipped beats. Unlike our large series of patients with extrasystoles, however, these fetuses were not found to have premature beats with varying postextrasystolic pauses, but rather were found, in-

deed, to have "skipped beats" (sinus beats that were not regularly conducted through the AV junction).

These fetuses had varying degrees of AV block prenatally. One of these fetuses remains in second-degree block. The others were born with varying degrees of Mobitz type I (Wenckebach) and Mobitz type II AV block, but had developed complete heart block by one month of age.

None of these had associated structural heart disease, and two mothers had a positive autoimmune antibody screen.

Complete Heart Block

Clinical experience with fetal complete heart block suggests that these fetuses may be divided into two discrete groups. Either these fetuses have complex congenital heart disease associated with heart block, or if cardiac structure is normal, the heart block appears to relate to immune complex-related damage to the fetal conduction tissue secondary to maternal autoantibodies (Litsey et al., 1985).

We have encountered 26 fetuses with complete heart block, and the reported experience is pooled with that of our colleagues from the University of California, San Francisco and the University of Heidelberg into a subgroup consisting of 55 patients. Of these 55 patients with congenital complete heart block (Table 21–3), 27 were found to have associated congenital heart disease, that is, abnormalities of atrioventricular connection such as ambiguous connections (in a setting of left atrial isomerism), discordant atrioventricular connection (corrected transposition of the great arteries), or atrioventricular septal defect in association with the Down syndrome.

The remaining 28 fetuses in the pooled series had no evidence of congenital heart disease. Twenty-one of the 28 mothers had positive autoantibody screens. Several mothers in this group had received medical attention for clinically diagnosable systemic lupus erythematosis. Several neonates required pacemaker insertion for a variety of clinical indications, including extreme bradycardia, ventricular arrhythmias, and/or congestive cardiac failure (Michaelsson and Engle, 1972).

The association between maternal autoimmune disease and fetal congenital heart block has been well established. Recent reports have shown immunofluorescent stains demonstrating selective binding of immune complexes to His-Purkinje tissue and fetal myocardium. This is associated with inflammatory

TABLE 21–3. Fetal Complete Heart Block (n = 55)

Congenital heart disease		29
Left atrial isomerism	17	
AV discordance	7	
Positive maternal antibody screen		19
Idiopathic		7
Hydrops fetalis		22
Mortality		29

From Schmidt KG, Ulmer HE, Silverman NH, et al: Perinatal outcome of fetal congenital complete atrioventricular block: a multicenter experience. J Am Coll Cardiol 17:1360, 1991.

infiltrates and fibrosis in the region of the AV node and Bundle of His. The immune complex binding and inflammatory infiltration of fetal ventricular myocardium may account for the clinical finding of congestive cardiomyopathy that has been reported by some groups (Litsey et al., 1985).

Maternal administration of beta agonists, such as ritodrine or terbutaline, may be associated with as much as a 50 per cent increase in fetal heart rate. This increase in ventricular rate has not been associated with diminution of fetal edema in our patients with heart block, hydrops fetalis, and structural heart disease, and has not improved the hemodynamic state of other investigators' patients with hydrops fetalis and congenital heart block in the absence of structural heart disease, probably because of the necessity of restoring a 1:1 atrioventricular contraction sequence in these fetuses. If systemic venous pressure is to be reduced sufficiently to allow resolution of hydrops fetalis, it is essential that "cannon a-waves" associated with atrial contraction against a closed atrioventricular valve be ameliorated.

The data from the combined series of cases suggest that fetuses with hydrops fetalis, associated congenital cardiac malformations, or ventricular escape rates of under 55 beats/minute have a particularly poor prognosis. While initial analysis of data suggested that slow atrial rate (<100/minute) also was a poor prognostic sign, this was true because all such fetuses had associated complex congenital heart disease (left atrial isomerism).

FETAL ANTIARRHYTHMIC AGENTS

Therapeutic Rationale

The treatment of arrhythmias remains one of the most specialized subdisciplines of cardiology, and the management of these patients, which is often difficult and frustrating, is associated with significant morbidity and mortality. The availability of "newer" antiarrhythmic agents offers the *promise* of more rapid and effective arrhythmia control, but only rarely have investigators demonstrated a significant improvement in mortality risks after inclusion of newer antiarrhythmic agents in the treatment of potentially life-threatening arrhythmias.

To complicate matters, virtually none of the available antiarrhythmic agents is without significant potential risk of undesired side effects, particularly the risk of "proarrhythmia." Proarrhythmia is the tendency of a particular antiarrhythmic agent, through its electrophysiologic activity, to cause rather than ameliorate arrhythmias (Morganroth, 1987). Such proarrhythmias may, in fact, be of equal or greater potential risk to the patient than the arrhythmia under therapy. Recently, for example, there have been reports of the utility of flecainide in the treatment of fetal supraventricular tachycardia (Allan et al., 1990). Nonetheless, the initial enthusiasm for the use of flecainide and encainide (related type IC antiarrhythmic agents) has been tempered by the ominous report from the CAST study involving double-blinded

placebo-controlled trials of prophylactic administration of these agents for suppression of cardiac arrhythmias following myocardial infarction (CAST Investigators, 1989). The initial and long-term results of this trial demonstrated a statistically significant increase in mortality rate from sudden arrhythmic death among post-myocardial infarction patients receiving flecainide and encainide. As a result, the FDA issued a strongly worded warning to physicians, suggesting that type IC antiarrhytmic agents be utilized only for the treatment of otherwise refractory life-threatening ventricular arrhythmias (encainide has recently been withdrawn by its manufacturer). Certainly, neither fetus nor mother fits into the mold of the patients who constituted the study population in the CAST study (older, male patients who had suffered myocardial infarctions). Nonetheless, the application of such medication for fetal therapy, which must be delivered by way of the mother, must be tempered by some degree of concern over the potential for causing potentially dangerous arrhythmias. The use of such an agent may, in fact, be considered if one postulates that the fetal arrhythmia is potentially life-threatening. On the other hand, one must also consider that in treating the fetus medically one is treating two patients, one within the other. Despite the mother's determination to do all that can be done for the fetus, which one often encounters when counseling mothers whose fetuses require medical therapy, the physician has a responsibility to keep in mind that the mother herself does not have a "life-threatening" condition, and in such a situation, it may be difficult to justify the use of agents with a significant intrinsic proarrhythmic potential.

The potential for interaction between potent antiarrhythmic agents must be considered as well. These medications exert their electrophysiologic effects by altering ion flux, and in some cases they interact at the level of the cell membrane. Efforts have been made to "classify" the electrophysiologic activity of these agents, and rational antiarrhythmic therapy must be based on a complete understanding of the underlying electrophysiologic mechanism and the electrophysiologic effect of the given antiarrhythmic agent. The wanton application of antiarrhythmic therapy with little consideration of the underlying electrophysiology and the potential hazards of additive therapy upon basic cellular electrophysiology and pharmacokinetics may well raise the risk of inadvertently precipitating a more dangerous situation such as proarrhythmia, impaired myocardial performance, impaired metabolism of concomitantly administered medications resulting in toxic accumulation of these agents, or, in some circumstances, changing an intermittent into an incessant arrhythmia (Blandon and Leandro, 1985).

Supraventricular Tachycardia

As previously discussed, the greatest initial success has been achieved in *in utero* treatment of fetal supraventricular tachyarrhythmias. Although there have been isolated reports involving the use of a number of antiarrhythmic agents in this setting (Allan et al.,

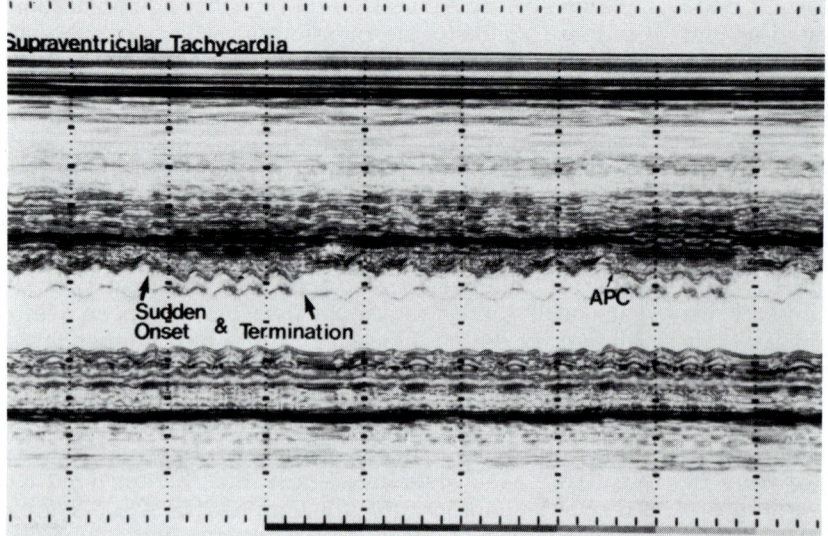

FIGURE 21–9. Single M-mode echocardiographic recording of ventricular wall motion in a fetus having short "runs" of supraventricular tachycardia. The ventricular wall undulations at a rate of 240 to 260 beats/minute (the hatched vertical lines are one second apart) occur in short paroxysms that are of sudden onset and sudden termination. In addition, the onset of these episodes follows an extrasystole. These characteristics suggest that this dysrhythmia is a "reentrant" tachycardia.

1990; Arnoux et al., 1987; Bergmans et al., 1985; Dumesic et al., 1982; Given et al., 1984; Golichowski et al., 1985; Hansmann et al., 1991; Johnson et al., 1987; Kerenyi et al., 1980; Lingman et al., 1980; Lusson et al., 1985; Spinnato et al., 1984; Teuscher et al., 1978; Wolff et al., 1980), there is little information available comparing these agents.

When M-mode or pulsed-Doppler echocardiography demonstrates sudden onset and termination of episodes of tachycardia, with induction of the arrhythmia by extrasystoles, this has been considered to be diagnostic of reentrant SVT. The onset and termination of the arrhythmia may not be observed until after a trial of antiarrhythmic therapy has begun. If therapy aimed at slowing conduction and increasing refractoriness in the slow AV conduction pathways results in AV nodal block without termination of the arrhythmia, one can rule out AVNRT or AVRT with the AV node

serving as one limb of the reentrant circuit as the mechanism of the arrhythmia. Further therapy should be directed by this information (Figs. 21–9, 21–10, 21–11).

Digoxin

Digoxin remains the drug of first choice in the treatment of *in utero* SVT. Our experience has suggested that maternal and fetal serum levels of this agent are usually similar, although the ratio of fetal to maternal level may vary from 0.6 to 1.0. It is well-known that pregnant women and neonates (and fetuses) may be demonstrated to have serum digoxin immunoreactivity, even in the absence of exogenous digoxin admininstration (Valdes, 1985). This finding may account for the suggestion that neonates may tolerate or even require higher serum levels of this

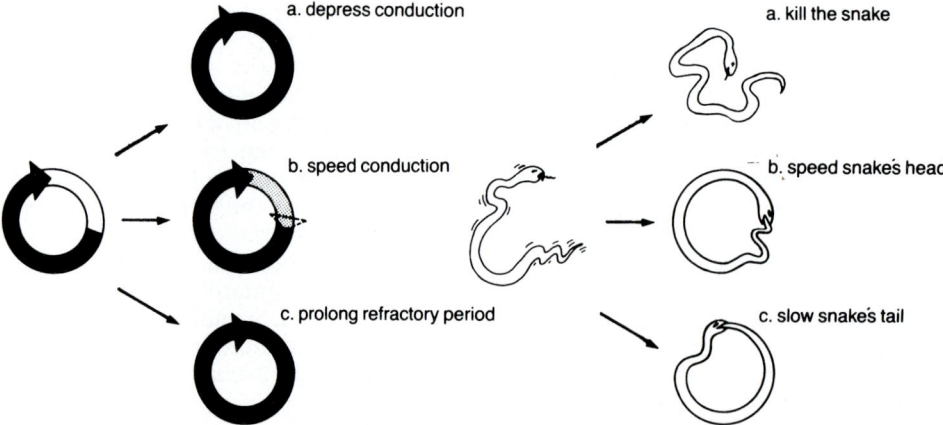

FIGURE 21–10. Three ways by which a circus movement can be terminated. *Left,* A circus movement can be stopped if conduction is completely blocked (a), if conduction is accelerated so that the front of the impulse reaches the previously depolarized tissue (b), or if the refractory period is prolonged so that the front of the impulse encounters tissue that can no longer be excited (c). *Right,* These three mechanisms can be viewed in terms of a snake traveling in a circle. The snake stops if it is killed (a), if it reaches ahead so as to bite its tail (b), or if its tail lags behind so as to be bitten by the advancing head (c). (Reproduced with permission from Katz, AM: Physiology of the Heart. 2nd ed. New York, Raven Press, 1992.)

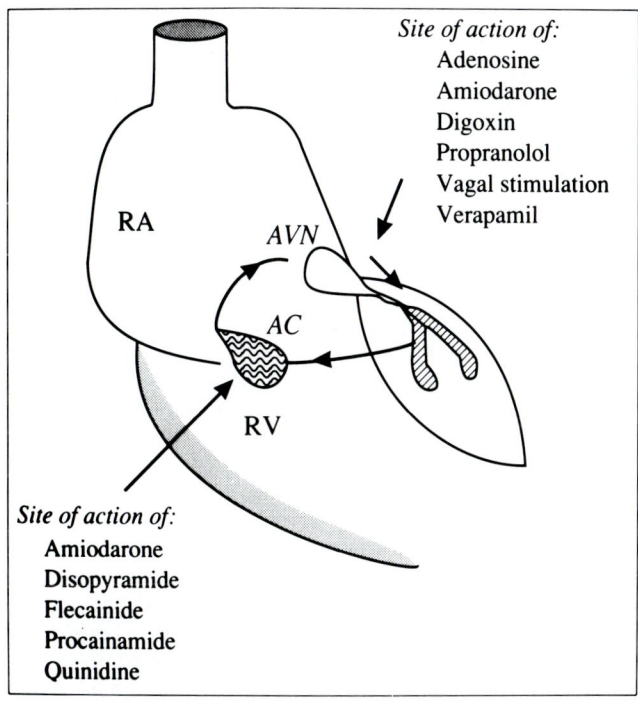

Site of action of:
Adenosine
Amiodarone
Digoxin
Propranolol
Vagal stimulation
Verapamil

RA

AVN

AC

RV

Site of action of:
Amiodarone
Disopyramide
Flecainide
Procainamide
Quinidine

FIGURE 21–11. Schematic diagram of the cardiac conduction system in a patient with an accessory conduction pathway and reciprocating orthodromic supraventricular tachycardia. This diagram demonstrates the site of action of the drugs that have been used to treat this arrhythmia. (Reproduced with permission from Kleinman CS, Copel JC: Electrophysiologic principles and antiarrhythmic therapy. Ultrasound Obstet Gynecol 1:286, 1991.)

agent than older children and adults, without developing clinical evidence of digoxin toxicity (Rogers et al., 1972). While exogenous digoxin and endogenous immunoreactive substance may be additive in serum assays for digoxin, there does not appear to be added risk of digoxin toxicity in fetuses and mothers receiving digoxin therapy (Ringel et al., 1987). This may well be due to recent findings that suggest that the immunoreactive substance does not appear to have significant Na^+-K^+ ATPase inhibition, thereby suggesting that the immunoreactive substance is not biologically active. While it may be of interest to monitor serum levels of digoxin, even prior to initiation of digoxin therapy, we have found this to be of no clinical value. We monitor both mother and fetus carefully for evidence of digoxin toxicity (which is a clinical rather than a laboratory diagnosis) while striving to attain maternal digoxin serum levels toward the "upper end" of the therapeutic range for our laboratory (2 ng/ml), in the absence of clinical evidence of digoxin toxicity. To attain these levels, in light of the limited oral absorption of digoxin during pregnancy, we have used the intravenous route for digoxin "loading" over the first 24 hours, followed by the use of rather large oral maintenance doses (0.50 to 0.75 mg/day). It has been suggested that little, if any, digoxin reaches the grossly hydropic fetus after maternal administration of this medication, and that this brings into question the use of this medication in the presence of hydrops fetalis.

Our clinical experience suggests that transplacental passage of this agent is impaired in the presence of hydrops fetalis, but some patients have resolved tachycardia and hydrops fetalis in the face of such therapy. It is certainly possible that these could have represented "spontaneous" resolution of tachycardia rather than a response to therapy, but we believe that the time course of these cases is strongly suggestive of a response to digoxin. This information has also led us to advocate the direct administration of digoxin, via umbilical venous puncture, if there has been no response to maternal administration of this medication. The fact that sustained tachycardia is likely to lead hydrops fetalis in a large (although we do not know how large) percentage of patients and that the latter condition is likely to reduce the effectiveness of digoxin therapy has led us to liberalize our use of this agent for the treatment of very premature fetuses with sustained or frequent prolonged episodes of reciprocating supraventricular tachycardia without hydrops fetalis.

The use of digoxin for the treatment of SVT in the setting of the WPW syndrome is undergoing reexamination in many centers because of the potential for a digoxin-induced shortening of the effective refractory period within the accessory conduction pathway. This may serve as the substrate for potentially fatal rapid conduction of atrial fibrillation, resulting in ventricular fibrillation (Wellens and Durer, 1973).

It is imperative to obtain informed consent from the parents of these fetuses before administering any antiarrhythmic medications. All parents who are being considered for transplacental therapy of SVT with digoxin should be informed about the risks associated with digoxin and the WPW syndrome and about our inability, to date, to diagnose the WPW syndrome from fetal echocardiographic tracings. It seems that the risk/benefit analysis is heavily weighted in favor of such therapy in previable fetuses with sustained SVT and severe hydrops fetalis. This analysis becomes somewhat less obvious with advancing fetal maturity and in the absence of florid hydrops fetalis.

Verapamil

As a blocker of slow inward calcium and sodium currents, verapamil is a potent agent for blocking AV nodal conduction and is therefore useful for the treatment and prophylaxis of reciprocating tachycardias involving AV nodal conduction as one limb of the reentry circuit.

Verapamil is a calcium channel blocking agent (type IV) and an extremely effective inhibitor of atrioventricular nodal conduction. This agent has multiple therapeutic uses and was originally introduced as an intravenous agent for the treatment of supraventricular tachycardia of the "reciprocating" type. When initially introduced to the therapeutic armamentarium, it quickly became the "drug of choice" for the treatment of neonates and infants with supraventricular tachycardia. It soon became apparent, however, that approximately 10 to 20 per cent of neonates with supraventricular tachycardia and associated congestive cardiac failure developed profound cardiac depression and cardiac arrest after intravenous administration of verapamil. Recent publications have stated that the use of this agent for the control of supraventricular tachycardia in an infant less than one year of age constitutes at best poor judgment and at worst medical malpractice (Garson, 1987). The rapid shift in the enthusiasm for this medication in this setting demonstrates a dramatic example of how even the best-intentioned of therapies may quickly prove to be a nightmare. It is believed that the immature myocardium, with its inherently limited systolic and diastolic "reserve," is extremely calcium channel dependent for contractile force. Administration of a profound calcium channel blocking agent, therefore, may well be expected to have an extremely negative effect on the myocardium of the already stressed immature heart. Addition of this agent to the therapy of a patient already receiving digoxin increases digoxin serum levels and bioavailability (Klein et al., 1980). Digoxin doses should be adjusted downward in order to avoid toxicity.

Quinidine

Quinidine is the oldest agent in the antiarrhythmic armamentarium (aside from the cardiac glycosides). It is a "type I" agent that blocks the sodium current responsible for the rapid phase O of the action potential and decreases conduction velocity in atrial, ventricular, His-Purkinje, and accessory conduction tissue. It also prolongs action potential duration and refractory periods of these tissues and may therefore be useful for therapy of reentrant tachycardias mediated by conduction through these tissues. Quinidine has not been particularly useful for the treatment of SVT owing to abnormal automaticity. It is one of the drugs of choice for control of rapid ventricular response to atrial fibrillation/flutter in the presence of an AV bypass tract and should be considered for early inclusion in the treatment protocol when M-mode echocardiography demonstrates atrial flutter or fibrillation. In this setting digoxin, verapamil, or propranolol should be administered first, in order to prevent the rapid ventricular response that may occur if the drugs' vagolytic action enhances AV nodal conduction at the outset of therapy or if the atrial refractory period is increased, thereby slowing the atrial flutter rate enough to allow for AV conduction of more of the atrial beats.

Quinidine undergoes extensive metabolism in the liver and is highly protein-bound in older children and adults, although it is less protein-bound in neonates (and presumably in fetuses) as well as in patients with cyanotic heart disease (and possibly in fetuses with a physiologically low PaO_2). These considerations may influence drug utilization by altering volume of distribution and plasma clearance of the agent.

Quinidine may prolong PR, QRS, and QT intervals postnatally and may precipitate ventricular tachycardia associated with excessive QT prolongation (which must be carefully sought in mothers taking the drug, but which cannot be monitored in utero). This effect on repolarization appears to be an idiosyncratic rather than a dose-related response. This "proarrhythmic"

potential (in as many as 2 to 5 per cent of adult patients taking this medication) of agents in this class (which includes procainamide and flecainide as well as quinidine) is cause for alarm and must be discussed with parents when informed consent is sought for inclusion of this agent in the treatment regimen.

Quinidine may result in noncardiac side effects, including gastrointestinal upset (7.8 per cent of cases), fever, skin rash, cinchonism, and autoimmune thrombocytopenia and hemolytic anemia.

The addition of quinidine to the treatment regimen of a patient receiving digoxin may lead to a twofold or greater increase in serum digoxin level. When this combination is used, therefore, digoxin serum levels should be monitored closely and the patients must be monitored closely for clinical evidence of digoxin toxicity.

Anecdotal reports of fetal thrombocytopenia, retinal damage, and intrauterine death associated with maternal quinidine administration have led us to use this agent sparingly (Hill and Malkasian, 1979). We have reserved its use for situations in which digoxin and adenosine have been unsuccessful in converting SVT in extremely immature fetuses with severe hydrops fetalis, or in fetuses who have atrial flutter and hydrops fetalis during early gestation, in which case we believe that risk/benefit analysis may warrant its use. Recent reports from other laboratories have documented the effective use of this agent, either alone or in combination with digoxin, for the therapy of fetal SVT and fetal atrial flutter. Transplacental passage of this agent appears to be highly variable (with cord levels varying from <25 per cent to as high as 94 per cent of the maternal serum level) (Rotmensch et al., 1983).

Quinidine cannot be administered intravenously because of its tendency to cause hemodynamic collapse when used by this route.

Procainamide

Procainamide is also a type I agent, with pharmacologic activity similar to that of quinidine. Our clinical experience with procainamide, which we have employed on two occasions when digoxin alone was unsuccessful in controlling in utero SVT, was disappointing. Our lack of success may have been related to the "low therapeutic" maternal serum levels of procainamide plus its active metabolite N-acetyl procainamide that were attained despite a high IV infusion rate.

Propranolol

Beta-blocking agents (type II antiarrhythmics) such as propranolol have been utilized on occasion for treatment of neonatal or fetal supraventricular tachycardia. These agents tend to slow atrioventricular conduction and may, on occasion, be useful in the postnatal period for therapy of reciprocating supraventricular tachycardia, especially for prophylaxis against recurrence of the arrhythmia.

We have had modest success with the combination of digoxin and the beta-blocking agent propranolol.

Transplacental transfer of propranolol has been demonstrated in the past, although the degree of transfer has been disputed. The broad therapeutic index of propranolol allows an increase in maternal dosage without untoward maternal effects, in efforts to attain "therapeutic" fetal drug levels. The risks of maternal propranolol therapy have been well described, and the potential for causing low birth weight, hypoglycemia, and sinus node depression must be weighed against the therapeutic goal of conversion of *in utero* tachycardia (Gladstone et al., 1975; Habib and McCarthy, 1977; Rubin, 1981; Wu et al., 1974).

Amiodarone

We mention amiodarone at this point only because it has been used by at least three groups for treatment of fetal supraventricular tachycardia. This class III antiarrhythmic agent has been released only recently in the United States for use as an antiarrhythmic agent for treatment of life-threatening arrhythmias. Prior to release in the United States this agent had been used extensively in Europe, Israel, and South America. It profoundly affects action potential duration and refractoriness within the atrium, AV node, accessory pathways, and ventricle and is useful for treatment of a variety of supraventricular and ventricular arrhythmias.

This agent has an unusual spectrum of toxicity, the most serious being pneumonitis, potentially leading to fatal pulmonary fibrosis. This complication has been reported to occur in 1 to 5 per cent of patients in some series and up to 10 per cent of patients in one series, although it does not appear to be a major risk in the pediatric age group (Garson, 1987). A proarrhythmic effect may result from QT prolongation. This agent also has a complex effect on the metabolism of thyroid hormones (it contains iodine in its molecule and has a molecular similarity to thyroxine). In 3 to 5 per cent of patients, hypothyroidism or hyperthyroidism may develop. A recent report from France demonstrated successful conversion of fetal SVT using amiodarone with resolution of hydrops fetalis (Arnoux et al., 1987; Lusson et al., 1985). However, this fetus was documented to have hypothyroidism in the neonatal period. Although the hypothyroidism resolved spontaneously, it is still cause for significant concern (Rovet et al., 1987). Hansmann and colleagues (1991) have advocated intravenous administration of this medication by direct umbilical venous route for treatment of refractory sustained fetal tachycardia. The intravenous form of this agent is currently unavailable in the United States.

The potentially severe side effects of this medication are compounded by the extraordinarily prolonged half-life (25 to 110 *days*). We have not included this agent in our therapeutic protocol and believe that only an extraordinary circumstance would warrant its inclusion in a rational treatment regimen.

Adenosine

Adenosine is an agent that has multiple effects, the most of important of which, for antiarrhythmic purposes, is inhibition of the sinus and atrioventricular nodes. It has become the drug of first choice for immediate intravenous therapy of reciprocating supraventricular tachycardia and may even be used with a reasonable degree of safety if ventricular tachycardia is incorrectly identified as supraventricular tachycardia. This is due to its extremely short half-life.

Adenosine has no effect on ectopic atrial focus tachycardia or atrial flutter. Its extremely short half-life of 10 to 30 seconds means that side effects are extremely transient. These may include dyspnea, flushing, and chest pain in the postnatal setting. The medication is generally administered as a rapid intravenous bolus at a dosage of 100 to 200 μg/kg of estimated dry body weight. Because of its extremely rapid protein binding, the medication must be administered by rapid intravenous push, and therefore it should be delivered directly to the fetal umbilical vein rather than via the maternal intravenous route.

This agent is extremely effective in "breaking" reciprocating supraventricular tachycardia that involves the atrioventricular node as part of the reentrant circuit (95 per cent of the clinically important supraventricular tachycardias of the fetus and neonate). It may result in a prolonged period of sinus rhythm, but owing to its extremely short half-life, it has no "prophylactic" effect to prevent recurrent episodes of tachycardia incited by atrial premature contractions. For this reason, although the medication may not provide long-term definitive therapy, it should at least be considered for inclusion early in the treatment protocol as a therapeutic/diagnostic trial. Should administration of this agent result in even a brief episode of sinus rhythm, one may then be reassured regarding the accuracy of the initial electrophysiologic diagnosis of the arrhythmia, and further therapy should be focused on the assumption that one is dealing with reciprocating supraventricular tachycardia. Further therapy should include medications that are likely to effect a "break" in the tachycardia and to prevent recurrent episodes of arrhythmia.

REFERENCES

Allan LD, Anderson RH, Sullivan ID, et al: Evaluation of fetal arrhythmias by echocardiography. Br. Heart J **50**:240, 1983.

Allan L, Chita S, Maxwell D, Priestley K: Use of flecainide in fetal atrial tachycardia. Br Heart J **64**:90, 1990.

Andersen HM, Hutchison AA, Fortune DW: Nonimmune hydrops fetalis: Changing contributions to perinatal mortality. Br J Obstet Gynaecol **90**:636, 1983.

Antman EM, Stone PH, Muller JE, Braunwald E: Calcium channel blocking agents in the treatment of cardiovascular disorders. Part I: Basic and clinical electrophysiologic effects. Ann Intern Med **93**:875, 1980.

Arnoux P, Seyral P, Llurens M, Djiane P, Potier A, Unal D, Cano JP, Serradimigni A, Rouault F: Amiodarone and digoxin for refractory fetal tachycardia. Am J Cardiol **59**:166, 1987.

Bergmans MGM, Jonker GJ, Kock HCLV: Fetal supraventricular tachycardia. Review of the literature. Obstet Gynecol Survey **40**:61, 1985.

Blandon R, Leandro I: Fetal heart arrhythmia: clinical experience with antiarrhythmic drugs. *In* Doyle EF, Engle MA, Gersony WM, Rashkind WJ, Talner NS (eds): New York, Springer-Verlag, 1985, p. 483.

The Cardiac Arrhythmia Suppression Trial (CAST) Investigators:

Preliminary report: effect of encainide and flecainide on mortality in a randomized trial of arrhythmia suppression after myocardial infarction. N Engl J Med 3:406, 1989.

Crowley DC, Dick M, Rayburn WF, Rosenthal A: Two-dimensional and M-mode echocardiographic evaluation of fetal arrhythmia. Clin Cardiol 8:1, 1985.

DeVore GR, Siassi B, Platt LD: Fetal echocardiography. III. The diagnosis of cardiac arrhythmias using real-time-directed M-mode ultrasound. Am J Obstet Gynecol 146:792, 1983.

Dumesic DA, Silverman NH, Tobias S, Golbus MS: Transplacental cardioversion of fetal supraventricular tachycardia with procainamide. N Engl J Med 307:1128, 1982.

Eik-Nes SH, Marsal K, Kristoffersen K: Methodology and basic problems related to blood flow studies in the human fetus. Ultrasound Med Biol 10:329, 1984.

Friedman WF: The intrinsic physiologic properties of the developing heart. In Friedman WF, Lesch M, Sonnenblick EH (eds): Neonatal Heart Disease. New York, Grune and Stratton, 1972, pp 87–111.

Garson A Jr: Supraventricular tachycardia. In Gillette PC, Garson A (eds): Pediatric Arrhythmias: Electrophysiology and Pacing. Philadelphia, W.B. Saunders, 1990.

Garson A Jr: Medicolegal problems in the management of cardiac arrhythmias in children. Pediatrics 79:84, 1987.

Gill RW, Kossoff G, Warren PS, Garrett WJ: Umbilical venous flow in normal and complicated pregnancy. Ultrasound Med Biol 10:349, 1984.

Gillette PC: The mechanisms of supraventricular tachycardia in children. Circulation 54:133, 1976.

Given BD, Phillippe M, Sanders SP, Dzau VJ: Procainamide cardioversion of fetal supraventricular tachyarrhythmia. Am J Cardiol 53:1460, 1984.

Gladstone GR, Hordof A, Gersony WM: Propranolol administration during pregnancy: Effects on the fetus. J Pediatr 86:9962, 1975.

Gluck L, Kulovich MV, Borer RC, Keidel WN: The interpretation and significance of the lecithin/sphingomyelin ratio in amniotic fluid. Am J Obstet Gynecol 120:142, 1974.

Golichowski AM, Caldwell R, Hartsough A, Peleg D: Pharmacologic cardioversion of intrauterine supraventricular tachycardia. A case report. J Reprod Med 30:139, 1985.

Habib A, McCarthy JS: Effects on the neonate of propranolol administered during pregnancy. J Pediatr 91:808, 1977.

Hansmann M, Gembruch U, Bald R, Manz M, Redel DA: Fetal tachyarrhythmias: Transplacental and direct treatment of the fetus. A report of 60 cases. Ultrasound Obstet Gynecol 1:162, 1991.

Harrison MR, Adzick NS, Longaker MT, Goldberg JD, Rosen MA, Filly RA, Evans MI, Golbus MS: Successful repair in utero of a fetal diaphragmatic hernia after removal of herniated viscera from the left thorax. N Engl J Med 32:1582, 1990.

Harrison MR, Golbus MS, Filly RA: The Unborn Patient: Prenatal Diagnosis and Treatment. Philadelphia, W.B. Saunders Co, 1990.

Hill LM, Malkasian GD Jr: The use of quinidine sulfate throughout pregnancy. Obstet Gynecol 54:366, 1979.

Johnson WH Jr, Dunnigan A, Fehr P, Benson DW Jr: Association of atrial flutter with orthodromic reciprocating fetal tachycardia. Am J Cardiol 59:374, 1987.

Kallfelz HC: Cardiac arrhythmias in the fetus diagnosis, significance and prognoses. In Godman MJ, Marquis RM (eds): Paediatric Cardiology. Vol. 2, New York, Churchill Livingstone, 1979.

Katz AM: Physiology of the Heart. 2nd ed. New York, Raven Press, 1992.

Kerenyi TD, Gleicher N, Meller J, et al: Transplacental cardioversion of intrauterine supraventricular tachycardia with digitalis. Lancet ii:393, 1980.

Klein GL, Bashore TM, Sellers TD, et al: Ventricular fibrillation in the Wolff-Parkinson-White syndrome. N Engl J Med 301:1080, 1979.

Klein HO, Lang R, Segni ED, Kaplinsky E: Verapamil-digoxin interaction. N Engl J Med 303:160, 1980.

Kleinman CS, Copel JC: Electrophysiologic principles and fetal antiarrhythmic therapy. Ultrasound Obstet Gynecol 1:286, 1991.

Kleinman CS, Donnerstein RL: Ultrasonic assessment of cardiac function in the intact human fetus. J Am Coll Cardiol 5:84S, 1985.

Kleinman CS, Donnerstein RL, DeVore GR, et al: Fetal echocardiography for evaluation of in utero congestive heart failure: A technique for study of nonimmune fetal hydrops. N Engl J Med 306:568, 1982.

Kleinman CS, Donnerstein RL, Jaffe CC, et al: Fetal echocardiography. A tool for evaluation of in utero cardiac arrhythmias and monitoring of in utero therapy: Analysis of 71 patients. Am J Cardiol 51:237, 1983.

Kleinman CS, Hobbins JC, Jaffe CC, et al: Echocardiographic studies of the human fetus: Prenatal diagnosis of congenital heart disease and cardiac dysrhythmias. Pediatrics 65:1059, 1980.

Kleinman CS, Valdes-Cruz LM, Weinstein EM, Sahn DJ: Two-dimensional Doppler echocardiographic analysis of fetal cardiac arrhythmias. Pediatr Res 18:124A, 1984.

Lie KI, Duren DR, Manger CV, et al: Long-term efficacy of verapamil in the treatment of paroxysmal supraventricular tachycardias. Am Heart J 105:688, 1983.

Lima JJ, Kuritzky PM, Schentag JJ, et al: Fetal uptake and neonatal disposition of procainamide and its acetylated metabolite: A case report. Pediatrics 61:491, 1978.

Lingman G, Ohrlander S, Ohlin P: Intrauterine digoxin treatment of fetal paroxysmal tachycardia. Br J Obstet Gynaecol 87:340, 1980.

Litsey SE, Noonon JA, O'Connor WN, et al: Maternal connective tissue disease in congenital heart block. Demonstration of immunoglobulin in cardiac tissue. N Engl J Med 312:98, 1985.

Lusson JR, Beytout M, Jacquetin B, Lamaison D, Cassagnes J: Traitment d'une tachycardie supraventriculaire foetale: association digoxine-amiodarone. Coeur 15:315, 1985.

Martin CB Jr, Nijhuis JG, Weijer AA: Correction of fetal supraventricular tachycardia by compression of the umbilical cord: report of a case. Am J Obstet Gynecol 150:324, 1984.

Michaelsson M, Engle MA: Congenital complete heart block: an international study of the natural history. Cardiovasc Clin 4:85, 1972.

Morganroth J: Risk factors for the development of proarrhythmic events. Am J Cardiol 59:32E, 1987.

Morganroth J, Anderson JL, Gentzkow GD: Classification by type of ventricular arrhythmia predicts frequency of adverse cardiac events from flecainide. J Am Coll Cardiol 8:607, 1986.

Nimrod C, Davies D, Harder J, et al: Ultrasound evaluation of tachycardia-induced hydrops in the fetal lamb. Am J Obstet Gynecol 157:655, 1987.

Parer JT: Handbook of Fetal Heart Rate Monitoring. Philadelphia, W.B. Saunders, 1983.

Rae AP, Webb CR: Management of supraventricular tachycardia. Cardiol in Prac 10:197, 1984.

Reder RF, Rosen MR: Basic electrophysiologic principles: application to treatment of dysrhythmias. In Gillette PC, Garson A Jr (eds): Pediatric Cardiac Dysrhythmias. New York, Grune & Stratton, 1981.

Ringel R, Hamyln J, Pinkas G: Is the plasma digoxin immunoreactivity of pregnancy associated with digitalis-like (Na + K-) ATPase inhibition? Pediatr Res 21:193A, 1987.

Rogers MC, Willerson JT, Goldblatt A, Smith TW: Serum digoxin concentrations in the human fetus, neonate and infant. N Engl J Med 287:1010, 1972.

Rotmensch HH, Belhassen B, Ferguson RK: Amiodarone: benefits and risks in perspective. Am Heart J 104:1117, 1982.

Rotmensch HH, Elkayem U, Frishman W: Antiarrhythmic drug therapy during pregnancy. Ann Intern Med 98:487, 1983.

Rovet J, Ehrlich R, Sorbac D: Intellectual outcome in children with fetal hypothyroidism. J Pediatr 110:700, 1987.

Rubin PC: Beta-blockers in pregnancy. N Engl J Med 305:1323, 1981.

Schmidt KG, Ulmer HE, Silverman NH, et al: Perinatal outcome of fetal congenital complete atrioventricular block: a multicenter experience. J Am Coll Cardiol 17:1360, 1991.

Spinnato JA, Shaver DC, Flinn GS, et al: Fetal supraventricular tachycardia: In utero therapy with digoxin and quinidine. Obstet Gynecol 64:730, 1984.

Stone PH, Antman EM, Muller JE, Braunwald E: Calcium channel blocking agents in the treatment of cardiovascular disorder. Part II: Hemodynamic effects and clinical applications. Ann Intern Med 93:886, 1980.

Strigl R, Pfeiffer U, Erhardt W, et al: Does the administration of the calcium antagonist verapamil in tocolysis with beta sympathomimetics still make sense? J Perinat Med 9:235, 1981.

Teuscher A, Bossi E, Imhof P, et al: Effect of propranolol on fetal tachycardia in diabetic pregnancy. Am J Cardiol **42**:304, 1978.

The Cardiac Arrhythmia Suppression Trial (CAST) Investigators: Preliminary report: effect of encainide and flecainide on mortality in a randomized trial of arrhythmia suppression after myocardial infarction. N Engl J Med **321**:386, 1989.

Valdes R Jr: Endogenous digoxin-immunoactive factor in human subjects. Fed Proc **44**:2800, 1985.

Wellens HJJ, Durrer D: Effect of digitalis on atrioventricular conduction and circus movement tachycardia in patients with the Wolff-Parkinson-White syndrome. Circulation **47**:1229, 1973.

Wolff F, Breuker KH, Schlensker KH, Bolte A: Prenatal diagnosis and therapy of fetal heart rate anomalies: with a contribution on the placental transfer of verapamil. J Perinat Med **8**:203, 1980.

Wladimiroff JW, Struyk P, Stewart PA, et al: Fetal cardiovascular dynamics during cardiac dysrhythmia. Case report. Br J Obstet Gynaecol **90**:573, 1983.

Wu D, Denes P, Dhingra R, et al: The effects of propranolol on induction of AV nodal reentrant paroxysmal tachycardia. Circulation **50**:665, 1974.

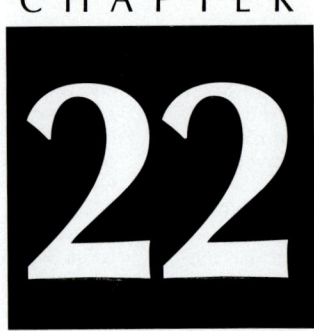

CHAPTER 22

FETAL BIOPHYSICAL ASSESSMENT BY ULTRASOUND

FRANK A. MANNING, M.D.

THE BIOPHYSICAL PROFILE

Monitoring of fetal biophysical activities plays a critical role in the identification of the asphyxiated fetus. Fetal asphyxial states define a spectrum of conditions ranging from transient episodes of hypoxemia without associated metabolic and/or respiratory acidosis to fixed severe acidosis. Asphyxia in the fetus, as is the case in every type of patient, produces effects on multiple organ systems, and therefore the signs of asphyxia are multiple and diverse. The degree of manifestation of these signs varies with the extent, duration, and chronicity of the asphyxial insult. Fetal hypoxemia and acidosis, either alone or in combination, produce reflex changes in distribution of cardiac output, the extent and duration of which vary with the nature of the insult.

The fetus retains a unique ability to redistribute its cardiac output away from organ systems not vital to fetal life (lung, kidney, gut) and toward vital organs (heart, brain, adrenals, placenta). This protective redistribution of cardiac output is reflex in origin, resulting from hypoxemic or acidemic stimulation of aortic body chemoreceptors (Cohn et al., 1974). With sustained or strong stimuli, the extent of this redistribution may be profound, resulting in near-total cessation of perfusion of the fetal lung and kidney, while flow to the brain and placenta increases substantially. Prolonged or repetitive stimuli initiating the redistribution reflex may result in diminished amniotic fluid production that is caused by decreased urine production and lung liquid flow. Asphyxia-induced oligohydramnios may further compound fetal asphyxia by rendering the umbilical cord more vulnerable to compression forces.

In the human fetus, asphyxia most commonly results from a chronic reduction in uteroplacental perfusion, aggravated by acute reduction in perfusion during uterine contractions including Braxton Hicks contractions. Human fetal asphyxia may then be best viewed as a chronic progressive disease, the extent and rate of progression being variable. In this context, the monkey model of partial prolonged asphyxia most

closely approximates the human condition (Myers, 1977). In the monkey fetus, partial prolonged asphyxia produced an initial increase in brain blood flow followed by a selective redistribution of cerebral flow so that cortical basal ganglia and thalamic blood flow decrease while brain stem perfusion remains unaltered or may increase. Presumably, cerebral edema develops as a result of translocation of brain fluid into the intracellular space. Biophysical functional correlates of these pathologic processes may be observed in the fetus. Central nervous system hypoxemia or asphyxia or both, even of a relatively minor degree, produces profound alteration in the frequency and patterning of biophysical activities and responses. Fetal hypoxemia in sheep, produced by administration of a hypoxic gas mixture to the ewe, consistently produces fetal apnea, which usually persists for some time after blood gas homeostasis of the fetus has been restored (Boddy and Dawes, 1975).

Human fetal correlates of the phenomenon have been observed. Maternal hypoxemia has been reported to be associated with prolonged fetal apnea (Manning and Platt, 1979). Under some experimental conditions maternal cigarette smoking has been shown to cause a fall in the incidence of fetal breathing movements (Manning et al., 1975; Manning et al., 1979), although this has not been confirmed in other studies (Thalar et al., 1980). In the chronically instrumented pregnant rhesus monkey model, cigarette smoke exposure produced a fall in fetal PO_2 (Socol et al., 1982). In fetal lambs, hypoxemia has been shown to produce a significant and sustained reduction in forelimb movement, and the effect exceeds the duration of the hypoxic insult.

These observations in animal and human fetuses suggest that asphyxia may result in significant alteration in central nervous system function and that this loss of function may lead to the absence of normal biophysical variables. Since central nervous system tissue is known to be among the tissues most sensitive to oxygen supply, it follows that observation of its function and output may be an important indirect indicator of fetal condition. The temporal and func-

TABLE 22–1. Relationship of Fetal Biophysical Profile Scoring to Perinatal Morbidity

AUTHOR*	TEST SCORE	FETAL DISTRESS %	LOW 5-MIN APGAR <7 %	IUGR (<3rd)	ADMISSION TO %	CORD pH (7.20) %	MECONIUM %	ANOMALY %
	Normal BPS (%)							
Baskett et al.	4079 (97.5)	8.2	0.9	4.9	—	—	—	—
Manning et al.	6500 (96.69)	12.8	3.7	3.4	4	2.2	8.7	3.7
	Equivocal BPS (%)							
Baskett et al.	66 (1.6)	27.8	7.6	30.3	—	—	—	—
Manning et al.	512 (1.99)	24.3	11.4	4.4	11.4	14.5	20.3	3.8
	Abnormal BPS (%)							
Baskett et al.	39 (0.9)	63	28.2	48.7	—	—	—	—
Manning et al.	373 (1.3)	60	23	34	28	28	22	5

*Data from Baskett TF, et al: Am J Obstet Gynecol **148**:630, 1984; and Manning FA, et al: Am J Obstet Gynecol, 1990a.
Abbreviations: BPS = biophysical profile score; IUGR = intrauterine growth retardation.

tional characteristics of fetal central nervous system function after recovery from asphyxia are not well studied. It does appear, however, that recovery of function may be delayed relative to restoration of normal blood gases.

In contrast, in animal models, return to normal biophysical activities after an asphyxial insult almost always indicates normal blood gas values. Variations in sensitivity to hypoxemia and asphyxia of specific areas of brain tissue responsible for initiation of biophysical activities are largely unexplored but are of major clinical interest. It is known, for example, that a fall in fetal PO_2 of as little as 6 torr can induce apnea in fetal lambs and monkeys (Boddy and Dawes, 1975; Martin et al., 1974). Whether the same degree of hypoxemia will alter other biophysical activities (for example, fetal tone or body movements), and to what extent, has not been studied. Therefore, it is uncertain whether increasing degrees of hypoxemia will result in progressive loss of given biophysical function or whether at a critical level of hypoxemia all such functions are lost at or near the same time. Clinical observation in the human fetus suggests that a gradient response exists, e.g., fetal breathing movements disappear early in the course of progressive hypoxemia and fetal movements disappear with more advanced disease. Interestingly, fetal breathing movements may reappear in the presence of extreme acidosis.

The biophysical signs of fetal asphyxia may be grouped into two main categories according to their temporal relationships to the asphyxial insult. Changes in biophysical activities occurring during the insult and for some variable time afterward may be termed "acute" or immediate effects and include such changes as loss of breathing movements, tone, movement, heart rate reactivity, and variability. The changes in amniotic fluid volume related to the asphyxial insult take some time to develop and therefore may be termed a "chronic" or "delayed" sign of fetal asphyxia.

The concept of multiple fetal biophysical variable monitoring to detect fetal asphyxia is based upon observation of these acute and chronic effects of asphyxia on organ function. By surveying the end result of specific organ function, one can estimate the presence, extent, and duration (chronicity) of the insult. Initially, asphyxia will cause a loss of acute variables (breathing, movement, tone, heart rate reactivity), while amniotic fluid volume may be normal. Recently the relationship between fetal blood gases, as determined in fetuses delivered by cesarean section before the onset of labor, and these acute biophysical variables has been assessed (Vintzileos et al., 1991). Fetal heart rate accelerations associated with fetal movement (nonstress test) and fetal breathing movements appear to be the most sensitive of these acute fetal biophysical variables, whereas fetal tone appears to be the least sensitive.

FETAL BIOPHYSICAL PROFILE SCORING AND PERINATAL MORBIDITY

To date there have been at least two large prospective clinical studies of the relationship between the fetal biophysical profile score and immediate neonatal morbidity (Baskett et al., 1984; Manning et al., 1990a); in both studies the incidence of perinatal morbidity, as measured by a variety of end points, rose progressively and significantly as the last test score fell (Table 22–1). The inverse linear correlation between last test and perinatal morbidity (Fig. 22–1) is in contradistinction to the inverse exponential relationship reported for perinatal mortality (Fig. 22–2). The explanation for these different distribution curves is based on the expected fetal adaptive compensatory responses to hypoxemia either alone or in combination with acidemia (asphyxia). The two major protective responses—the selective suppression of central nervous system regulatory centers and the reflex redistribution of cardiac output from nonessential to essential organs—are manifest directly as perinatal morbidity. Therefore, the correlation between a low fetal biophysical profile score and a low neonatal Apgar score is predicted and expected, since both tests measure the net output of oxygen-sensitive CNS system centers that generate acute biophysical activity. Similarly, the correlation of BPS with fetal distress as manifest by heart rate changes and the correlation of IUGR with the fetal biophysical profile score is expected; all are related to hypoxemia-induced (± acidosis) aortic arch chemoreceptor reflex redistribution of cardiac output. In contrast, the relationship between the fetal biophysical profile score and perinatal mortality reflects the *failure*

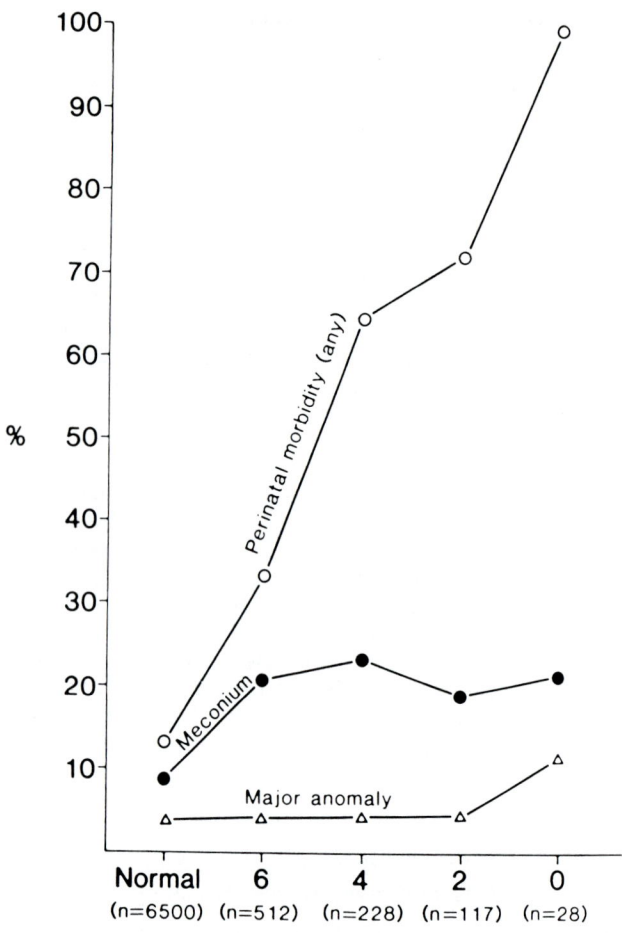

FIGURE 22–1. The relationship between any perinatal morbidity, as defined by the presence of fetal distress, admission to neonatal intensive care units, intrauterine growth retardation, 5-minute Apgar less than 7, and umbilical vein pH below 7.20—either alone or in any combination. A highly significant inverse linear correlation is observed. In contrast, no relationship between meconium staining of amniotic fluid and the presence of a major anomaly was observed. BPS = biophysical profile scoring. (From Manning FA, Harman CR, Morrison I, et al: Fetal assessment based on fetal biophysical profile scoring. IV. An analysis of perinatal morbidity and mortality. Am J Obstet Gynecol **162**:703, 1990a.)

were highly significant. Using fetal acidosis as the end point, the test accuracy parameters for the fetal biophysical profile score were a sensitivity of 90 per cent, a specificity of 96 per cent, a positive predictive accuracy of 82 per cent, and a negative predictive accuracy of 98 per cent. A similar relationship between cord pH at cesarean section before labor and the fetal biophysical profile score has been observed in our clinical unit. Among 557 high-risk fetuses, the umbilical venous pH in 495 fetuses with a normal score (BPS >8) was 7.35 + 0.13 (+2 SD); it was 7.21 + 0.23 in 39 fetuses with an equivocal score (BPS=6), and 7.13 + 0.16 in 23 fetuses with an abnormal score (BPS < 4) (Manning et al., unpublished data, 1992).

The relationship between umbilical blood gas values and the fetal biophysical profile score has also been examined in the antepartum period. Ribbert et al. (1990) studied the relationship in 14 severely growth-retarded fetuses in whom cordocentesis was done for karyotyping and noted a highly significant linear cor-

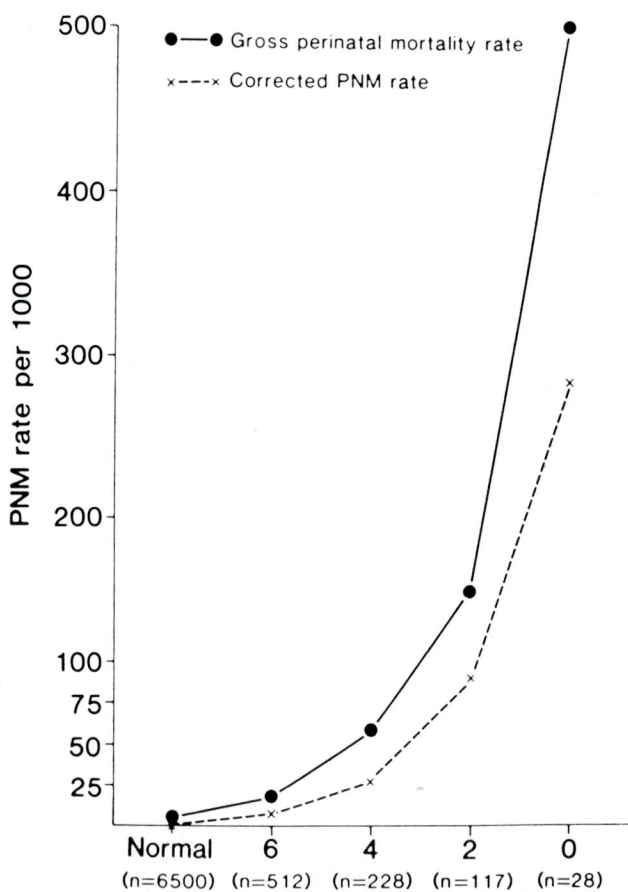

FIGURE 22–2. The relationship between perinatal mortality (PNM), either total or corrected for major anomaly, and the last biophysical profile scoring (BPS) result. This relationship is exponential, yielding a highly significant inverse correlation using log 10 conversion. (From Manning FA, Harman CR, Morrison I, et al: Fetal assessment based on fetal biophysical profile scoring. IV. An analysis of perinatal morbidity and mortality. Am J Obstet Gynecol **162**:703, 1990a.)

of the fetal adaptive responses. Thus, allowing for some clinical variation, the sharp rise in mortality may be expected to occur at the end of recruitment of all adaptive protective responses, an effect manifested clinically by a fetal biophysical profile score of 4 or less.

The relationship between the last fetal biophysical profile score and neonatal cord gases has been studied by Vintzileos et al. (1987) in 124 high-risk fetuses delivered by cesarean section before the onset of labor. A highly significant inverse linear correlation between last fetal biophysical profile score and cord pH was observed; mean venous pH in 102 fetuses with a normal score was 7.28, falling to a mean of 7.19 in the 13 fetuses with an equivocal score and to 6.99 in the 9 fetuses with an abnormal score. These differences

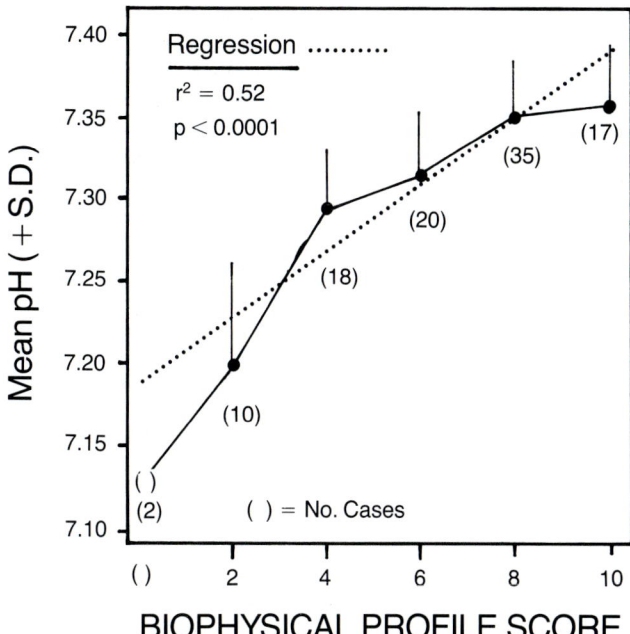

FIGURE 22–3. The relationship between fetal biophysical profile score and antenatal (cordocentesis) venous pH in 102 severely growth-restricted fetuses. Blood pH values are presented as the mean ± SD. (From Manning FA, Snijders R, Herman CR, et al: The relationship between fetal biophysical profile score and fetal pH. Am J Obstet Gynecol **168**:286, 1993.)

relation between venous pH and the biophysical profile score (r = 0.840, p <0.001), but did not find a similar significant correlation to umbilical venous P_{O_2} (r = 0.25) or P_{CO_2} (r = 0.25). These observations have now been expanded to include 102 severely growth retarded fetuses, again confirming the highly significant linear correlation between the fetal biophysical profile score and umbilical vein pH (r = 0.52, p = <0.0001) (Fig. 22–3) and demonstrating a weaker but significant linear correlation with umbilical vein P_{O_2} (r=0.42, p <0.01) (Manning et al., 1993).

Not all investigators have reported a correlation between test score and antepartum fetal blood gas values. Okamura et al. (1991) studied this relationship in 150 fetuses and noted no difference in mean pH or P_{O_2} among those fetuses with a normal, equivocal, or abnormal score. In this study, however, more than half the fetuses (53 per cent) had congenital malformations, a factor that may be expected to alter the fetal biophysical profile score results independent of blood gas values. Repeated episodes of hypoxemia with recovery between episodes may cause oligohydramnios, whereas acute variables may be normal. Progressive and severe asphyxia will produce both oligohydramnios and absent acute biophysical variables. Such a combined approach has both theoretical and proven advantages over any single variable assessment technique (Manning et al., 1985; Manning, 1985).

Central nervous system energy output and activity are not constant events but rather vary in nonrandom patterns. Fetal brain electrical activity as measured by

electrocortical leads exhibits rhythmic variations in both frequency and intensity. In general, an inverse relationship between the frequency and intensity of discharge is observed, resulting in two main patterns: low-frequency, high-voltage pattern (quiet sleep pattern) and high-frequency, low-voltage pattern (active sleep, REM sleep). In the fetus, an alternating pattern of these sleep states over a 20- to 40-minute period is usually observed. These patterns of sleep are coupled with alterations in biophysical activities. Thus, for example, in quiet sleep (low frequency, high voltage), fetal breathing movements tend to be absent or infrequent, isolated, and of large amplitude (fetal sighing), whereas during active sleep (high frequency, low voltage), bursts of fetal breathing movements of varying frequency and amplitude are observed. Similarly, rapid fetal eye movements are infrequent during quiet sleep and are usually observed only during active sleep (hence the designation rapid eye movement [REM] sleep).

The influence of sleep state on fetal biophysical activities is of major importance in the interpretation of fetal biophysical variable data. The observation of normal biophysical activities indicates a functional and therefore nonasphyxiated fetal central nervous sys-

TABLE 22–2. Biophysical Profile Scoring: Technique and Interpretation*

BIOPHYSICAL VARIABLE	NORMAL SCORE	ABNORMAL (Score = 0)
Fetal breathing movements	At least 1 episode of FBM of at least 30 sec duration in 30 min observation	Absent FBM or no episode of ≥30 sec in 30 minues
Gross body movement	At least 3 discrete body/limb movements in 30 min (episodes of active continuous movement considered as single movement)	2 or fewer episodes of body/limb movements in 30 min
Fetal tone	At least 1 episode of active extension with return to flexion of fetal limb(s) or trunk. Opening and closing of hand considered normal tone	Either slow extension with return to partial flexion or movement of limb in full extension or absent fetal movement with fetal hand held in complete or partial deflection
Reactive FHR	At least 2 episodes of FHR acceleration of ≥15 beat/min and of at least 15 sec duration associated with fetal movement in 30 min	Less than 2 episodes of acceleration of FHR or acceleration of <15 beats/min in 30 min
Qualitative AFV†	At least 1 pocket of AF that measures at least 2 cm in 2 perpendicular planes	Either no AF pockets or a pocket <2 cm in two perpendicular planes

*FBM = fetal breathing movement; FHR = fetal heart rate; AFV = amniotic fluid volume; AF = amniotic fluid.

†Modification of the criteria for reduced amniotic fluid from <1 cm to <2 cm would seem reasonable (see Chamberlain et al., 1984).

TABLE 22–3.   Biophysical Profile Scoring: Management Protocol

SCORE	INTERPRETATION	RECOMMENDED MANAGEMENT
10	Normal infant, low risk for chronic asphyxia	Repeat testing at weekly intervals; repeat twice weekly in diabetic patients and patients ≥42 wk gestation
8	Normal infant, low risk for chronic asphyxia	Repeat testing at weekly intervals; repeat twice weekly in diabetic patients and patients ≥42 wks; oligohydramnios indication for delivery
6	Suspected chronic asphyxia	Repeat testing in 4–6 hr; deliver if oligohydramnios present
4	Suspected chronic asphyxia	If ≥36 wk and favorable, then deliver; if ≥36 wk and L/S <2.0, repeat test in 24 hr; if repeat score <4, deliver
0–2	Strong suspicion of chronic asphyxia	Extend testing time to 120 min; if persistent score <4 deliver, provided gestational age is sufficiently advanced to permit possible neonatal survival

L/S, amniotic fluid lecithin: sphingomyelin

tem, rendering consideration of fetal sleep state unnecessary. In contrast, failure to recognize the presence of normal biophysical activities requires consideration of fetal sleep state. Both quiet sleep, a normal periodic fetal event, and fetal asphyxia, a pathologic fetal condition, can result in depression or absence of fetal biophysical activities, and the clinical significance of each cause is obviously different. Differentiation of these effects is achieved by extending the observation period beyond the minimal expected time for pattern shift (20 to 40 minutes) or repeating the observation at some later point. In either case, subsequent observation of normal activities confirms normality, whereas persistent absence of activities suggests an asphyxial etiology.

Fetal biophysical activities as a reflection of central nervous system activity and energy provide a direct window to brain function and an important indirect clinical indication of the state of fetal oxygenation. Detection of asphyxia is done for the most part by a method of exclusion, after ruling out absence of variables due to normal (intrinsic) central nervous system rhythms, the presence of circulating central nervous system depressant agents acquired from the mother (e.g., tranquilizers), or major fetal central nervous system trauma.

Fetal biophysical profile scoring is based on assessment of five discrete biophysical variables (Table 22–2); four of the variables (except for NST) are monitored simultaneously by dynamic ultrasound imaging method. Variables are coded as normal or abnormal according to fixed criteria and assigned a core of 2 if normal and 0 if abnormal. Thus, the score may range from 10 (all variables normal) to 0 (all variables abnormal) (Manning et al., 1980). The initial prospective open clinical study of the method, conducted in 1184 consecutive referred patients with high-risk pregnancies, yielded an overall perinatal mortality of 11.7 per 1000 (historical controls 65 per 1000) and a corrected perinatal mortality of 5 per 1000 (historical controls 40.6 per 1000) (Manning et al., 1981). Management was based on the BPS score according to fixed criteria (Table 22–3). An expanded study of 12,620 consecutive referred high-risk patients yielded a gross perinatal mortality rate of 7.35 per 1000 and a corrected PNM rate of 1.90 per 1000 (Manning et al., 1985). Experience with the method has accumulated in our own center and in other independent clinical laboratories; at least 57,255 tests in 24,699 high-risk patients have now been reported and are summarized in Table 22–4. This cumulative multi-center experience has yielded a gross perinatal mortality rate of 7.45 per 1000 and a corrected PNM rate of 2.12 per 1000.

Interestingly, the distribution of test results with this method is sharply dissimilar to that for single variable testing methods such as the NST alone or CST. In my experience (44,828 tests), a normal score is observed in 97.52 per cent of instances, an equivocal

TABLE 22–4.   Fetal Biophysical Profile Scoring and Perinatal Mortality

STUDY POPULATIONS	NO. PATIENTS	NO. TESTS	NO. PERINATAL DEATHS	CRUDE PNM RATE PER 1000	NO. CORRECTED* DEATHS	CORRECTED PNM RATE PER 1000	FALSE-NEGATIVE DEATHS†	FALSE-NEGATIVE RATE
Control population Manitoba low-risk untested population 1979–1982	65,979	—	943	14.1	586	8.81	—	—
Manitoba Prospective Study population-tested by BPS (Manning, 1987b)	19,221	44,828	141	7.35†	37	1.92‡	13	0.696
Baskett et al. (1987)	5034	11,075	32	7.60	13	3.10	2	0.5
Platt et al. (1983)	286	1112	4	14	2	7	2	7.4
Schifrin et al. (1981)	158	240	7	44	2	12.6	1	6.3
Total	24,699	57,255	184	7.45	54	2.12	18	0.748

*Corrected to exclude lethal anomaly and immune hydrops.
†Corrected stillbirth within 1 week of a last normal test.
‡Significantly less (p<0.01) than control population.

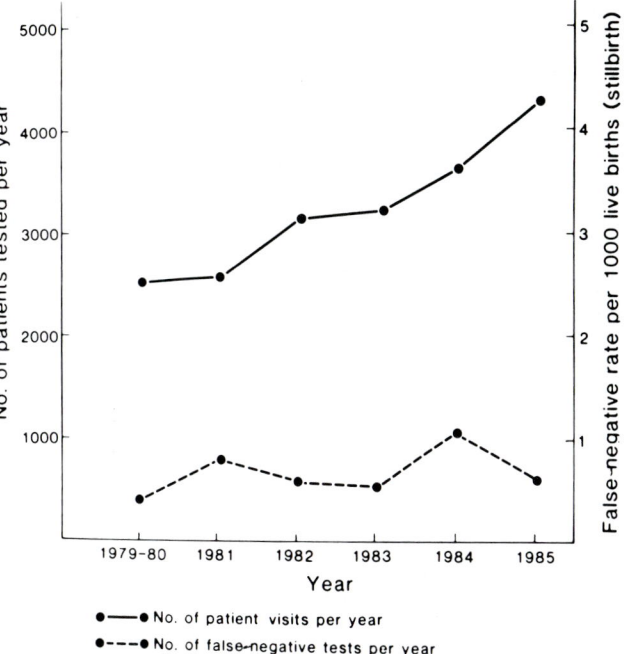

FIGURE 22–4. The false-negative rate, defined as stillbirth within 7 days of a normal fetal biophysical profile score (BPS >8), as described on an annual basis (1979 to 1984 inclusive). The false-negative rate has remained relatively constant despite a more than twofold increase in the number of high-risk patients studied annually.

score (BPS = 6) in 1.72 per cent, and an abnormal score (BPS<4) in 0.76 per cent. Accordingly, intervention based upon an equivocal score is not common. Therefore, PNM is sharply reduced without a significant increase in overall intervention rates. The selective nature of the testing method has been a distinct advantage. Further, despite the very high proportion of normal test results, the false-negative rate, defined as stillbirth occurring within a week of a last normal test result, remains low. I have observed the false-negative rate to range annually from as low as 0.411 to 1.01 per 1000, with a mean of 0.635 per 1000 (Fig. 22–4). Baskett et al. (1987), in a large study (5034 high-risk patients), report a false-negative rate of 0.5 per 1000.

The predictive accuracy of the abnormal test varies by end point used to measure outcome. In general there is a linear correlation between the degree of abnormality of the last test score and perinatal morbidity parameters, whereas an inverse exponential relationship is observed with perinatal mortality (Manning et al., 1990).

Recently this testing method has been modified to exclude the NST portion if the initial dynamic ultrasound monitored variables (fetal movement, breathing, tone, and amniotic fluid volume) are normal. The modification does not alter test accuracy, but does improve its efficiency (Manning et al., 1987a). Modification of the criteria for reduced amniotic fluid volume from the original definition (<1 cm) to a less severe criterion (<2 cm) would seem reasonable.

REFERENCES

Baskett TF, Gray JH, Prewett SJ, et al: Antepartum fetal assessment using a fetal biophysical profile score. Am J Obstet Gynecol **148**:630, 1984.

Baskett TF, Allen AC, Gray JH, et al: The biophysical profile score. Obstet Gynecol **70**:357, 1987.

Boddy K, Dawes GS: Fetal breathing. Br Med Bull **31**:1, 1975.

Chamberlain PF, Manning FA, Morrison I, et al: Ultrasound evaluation of amniotic fluid volume. I. The relationship of marginal and decreased amniotic fluid volume to perinatal outcome. Am J Obstet Gynecol **150**:245, 1984.

Cohn EH, Sacks EJ, Heyman MA, et al: Cardiovascular responses to hypoxemia and acidemia in fetal lambs. Am J Obstet Gynecol **120**:817, 1974.

Manning FA, Wyn Pugh E, Boddy K: Effect of cigarette smoking on fetal breathing movements in normal pregnancies. Br Med J **1**:552, 1975.

Manning FA, Feyerabend C: Cigarette smoking and fetal breathing movements. Br J Obstet Gynecol **83**:262, 1976.

Manning FA, Platt LD: Maternal hypoxemia and fetal breathing movements. Obstet Gynecol **53**:758, 1979.

Manning FA, Platt LD, Sipos L: Antepartum fetal evaluation: Development of a fetal biophysical profile. Am J Obstet Gynecol **136**:787, 1980.

Manning FA, Baskett TF, Morrison I, Lange IR: Fetal biophysical profile scoring: A prospective study in 1184 high-risk patients. Am J Obstet Gynecol **140**:289, 1981.

Manning FA, Morrison I, Lange IR, et al: Fetal assessment based on fetal biophysical profile scoring: Experience in 12,620 referred high-risk pregnancies. I. Perinatal mortality by frequency and etiology. Am J Obstet Gynecol **151**:343, 1985.

Manning, FA: Assessment of fetal condition and risk: Analysis of single and combined biophysical variable monitoring. Semin Perinatol **4**:168, 1985.

Manning FA, Morrison I, Lange IR, et al: Fetal biophysical profile scoring: Selective use of the non-stress test. Am J Obstet Gynecol **156**:709, 1987a.

Manning FA, Morrison I, Harman CR, et al: Fetal assessment by fetal BPS: Experience in 19,221 referred high-risk pregnancies. II. The false negative rate by frequency and etiology. Am J Obstet Gynecol **157**:880, 1987b.

Manning FA, Harman CR, Morrison I, et al: Fetal assessment based on fetal biophysical profile scoring. IV. An analysis of perinatal morbidity and mortality. Am J Obstet Gynecol **162**:703, 1990a.

Manning FA, Morrison I, Harman CR, et al: The abnormal fetal biophysical profile score. V. Predictive accuracy according to score composition. Am J Obstet Gynecol **162**:918, 1990b.

Manning FA, Snijders R, Harman CR, et al: The relationship

between fetal biophysical profile score and fetal pH. Am J Obstet Gynecol **168**:286, 1993.

Martin CB Jr, Murata Y, Petrie RH, et al: Respiratory movements in fetal rhesus monkeys. Am J Obstet Gynecol **119**:939, 1974.

Myers RE: Experimental models of perinatal brain damage: Relevance to human pathology. *In* Cluck L (ed): Intrauterine Asphyxia and the Developing Brain. Chicago, Year Book Medical Publishers, 1977.

Okamura K, Watanabe T, Endo H, et al: Biophysical profile and its relation to fetal blood gas level obtained by cordocentesis. Acta Obstet Gynecol Japonica **43**:1573, 1991.

Platt L, Eglinton G, Sipos L, et al: Further experience with the fetal biophysical profile. Obstet Gynecol **61**:480, 1983.

Ribbert LSM, Snijders RJM, Nicolaides KH, et al: Relationship of fetal biophysical profile and blood gas values at cordocentesis in severely growth-retarded fetuses. Am J Obstet Gynecol **163**:569, 1990.

Schifrin B, Guntes V, Gergely R: The role of real-time scanning in antenatal fetal surveillance. Am J Obstet Gynecol **140**:525, 1981.

Socol ML, Manning FA, Murata Y, Druzin M: Maternal smoking causes fetal hypoxia: Experimental evidence. Am J Obstet Gynecol **142**:214, 1982.

Thalar I, Goodman JD, Dawes GS: Effect of cigarette smoking on fetal breathing movements. Am J Obstet Gynecol **138**:292, 1980.

Vintzileos AM, Gaffrey SE, Salinger IM, et al: The relationship between fetal biophysical profile score and cord pH in patients undergoing Cesarean section before the onset of labour. Obstet Gynecol **70**:196, 1987.

Vintzileos AM, Fleming AD, Scorza WE, et al: Relationship between fetal biophysical activities and umbilical cord gas values. Am J Obstet Gynecol **165**:707, 1991.

CHAPTER

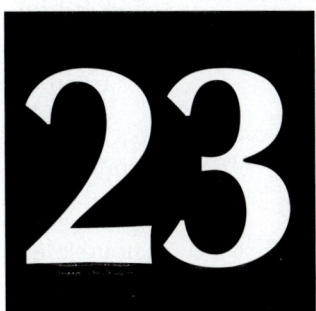

FETAL ACID-BASE BALANCE

PETER C. BOYLAN, M.B., F.C.C.O.G., and VALERIE M. PARISI, M.D., M.P.H.

ACID-BASE PHYSIOLOGY

General Considerations

Normal metabolism in both the fetus and adult results in a constant production of acids. These acids are buffered by various mechanisms that maintain extracellular fluid pH (the negative base 10 logarithm of hydrogen ion [H^+] concentration) within a narrow range. Although the concentration of hydrogen ions in extracellular fluid is very low, these protons are so reactive that even quite small changes can alter physiologic processes. Cardiac function, central nervous system function, and metabolic activity can be profoundly affected by changes in pH as small as 0.1 to 0.2 units, and an interval of 1 pH unit (6.8 to 7.8) is the widest range compatible with human life.

Calculation of pH by the Henderson-Hasselbalch Equation

The principal buffer of human extracellular fluid is the bicarbonate-carbonic acid system. The Henderson-Hasselbalch equation,

$$pH = pK + \log \frac{[HCO_3^-]}{[H_2CO_3]},$$

expresses the relationship between pH and the bicarbonate-carbonic acid concentrations in which pK is the carbonic acid dissociation constant (6.1) and [HCO_3^-] is the plasma bicarbonate concentration. The plasma carbonic acid concentration [H_2CO_3] is calculated from $PaCO_2$ and multiplied by the solubility factor for carbon dioxide in body fluids (0.031 mMol/liter/mm Hg PCO_2, or 1.2 mMol/liter at PCO_2 = 40).

Physiologic Principles of Acid-Base Balance

Arterial pH can provide only an estimate of total body acid-base balance because two-thirds of an acid or alkali load presented to the body will be buffered by intracellular fluid systems. This has led investigators to use the term "acidemia" instead of acidosis and "alkalemia" instead of alkalosis, thereby indicating that plasma pH measurements provide quantitative information about pH in the intravascular and interstitial compartments while providing only qualitative information about total body acid-base balance.

Proton shifts into the intracellular fluid in acidosis, and out of this fluid in alkalosis, are the body's first buffering response to a given acid or base load, and serve to maintain extracellular fluid pH in the appropriate physiologic range. The long-term maintenance of pH balance necessitates that input of acid (or base) to the body be matched by output of base (or acid) in order that the [HCO_3^-] to [H_2CO_3] ratio and the total bicarbonate content in the extracellular fluid remain constant. Regulation of pH in the adult is a function of the lungs (carbon dioxide balance) and the kidneys (bicarbonate balance). During fetal life, the placenta acts as the organ of respiration, allowing diffusion of oxygen from mother to fetus as well as diffusion of carbon dioxide produced by fetal metabolism across the intervillous space to be eliminated by maternal respiration. Additionally, the placenta assumes the fetal renal function of fixed acid elimination by allowing diffusion of fetal metabolic endproducts such as lactic, beta-hydroxybutyric, and uric acid across the intervillous space to be eliminated by the maternal kidney. These placental functions depend on normal umbilical blood flow from fetus to placenta as well as normal uterine blood flow from mother to placenta.

Fetal Acid-Base Physiology

Carbonic (Volatile) Acid

The major source of endogenous acid production is from combustion of glucose and fatty acids. During fetal oxidative metabolism, also called *aerobic glycolysis* or *cellular respiration*, the oxidation of glucose utilizes oxygen (O_2) and produces carbon dioxide (CO_2) according to the reaction:

$$C_6H_{12}O_6 + 6O_2 \rightleftarrows 6CO_2 + 6H_2O$$

Hydration of carbon dioxide is facilitated by erythrocyte carbonic anhydrase according to the reaction:

$$CO_2 + H_2O \rightleftarrows H_2CO_3 \rightleftarrows H^+ + HCO_3$$

Hemoglobin buffers the protons (hydrogen ions) formed by the dissociation of carbonic acid, while the bicarbonate generated leaves the erythrocyte in exchange for chloride. Simply stated, carbon dioxide generation is equivalent to carbonic acid formation, and most of the free hydrogen ion formed is buffered intracellularly. As blood passes through the organ of respiration (the lung in the adult and the placenta in the fetus), bicarbonate re-enters erythrocytes and combines with protons to form carbonic acid, which then dissociates to carbon dioxide and water. The carbon dioxide formed then diffuses across the placenta from the fetus and is excreted by the maternal lung. Carbon dioxide diffuses rapidly, in seconds, across the human placenta so that even large quantities produced by the fetus can be rapidly eliminated if maternal respiration, uteroplacental blood flow, and umbilical blood flow are normal.

The rate of fetal carbon dioxide production expressed on a molar basis is roughly equivalent to the fetal oxygen consumption rate (James et al., 1972). The PCO_2 of the veins draining the maternal uteroplacental bed reflects the contribution of carbon dioxide produced by fetal tissues as well as that produced by placental and uterine oxidative metabolism. In order for carbon dioxide to diffuse from fetus to mother, a PCO_2 gradient between fetal umbilical blood and maternal uteroplacental blood must be maintained, and adequate perfusion of both sides of the placenta must occur. Maternal PCO_2 is decreased during pregnancy to 34 mm Hg from the normal nonpregnant value of 40 mm Hg, thereby providing the necessary fetal-maternal gradient.

Noncarbonic (Nonvolatile) Acids

Fetal metabolism also results in the production of a number of noncarbonic (nonvolatile) acids. In the adult, dietary intake of the sulfur-containing amino acids cysteine and methionine is the major source of metabolism resulting in sulfuric acid formation. The fetus, however, produces noncarbonic acids primarily from two sources: (1) utilization of nonsulfur-containing amino acids resulting in uric acid formation and (2) incomplete combustion of carbohydrates and fatty acids resulting in production of lactic acid and the ketoacids (e.g., beta-hydroxybutyric acid). Fetal renal function is not sufficiently developed to handle excretion of these acids; therefore, they are transported via the umbilical circulation to the placenta, where they diffuse slowly (in contradistinction to carbon dioxide) across to the maternal circulation. The maternal kidney excretes noncarbonic acids produced by both maternal and fetal metabolism and in so doing also regenerates bicarbonate. Because the maternal glomerular filtration rate during normal pregnancy is increased by approximately 50 per cent, it should be noted that the maternal kidney filters and reabsorbs large quantities of bicarbonate daily.

While the fetus does have a limited ability to buffer an increase in acid production with bicarbonate stores and hemoglobin, the placental tissue bicarbonate pool may also play a role in buffering the fetus against changes in maternal pH or blood gas status. Aarnoudse et al. (1984) studied bicarbonate permeability in the perfused human placental cotyledon model and found that acidification of the maternal circulation to pH 7.06 for 30 minutes did not significantly alter fetal pH. Instead, there was an efflux of total carbon dioxide from the placenta into the maternal circulation in the form of bicarbonate, which was not matched by an influx of total carbon dioxide from the fetal circulation. By this mechanism, bicarbonate transfer could take place between the placental tissue pool and the maternal circulation while the transmission of maternal pH and blood gas changes to the fetal circulation would be minimized.

Alternatively, the fetus does have the ability to metabolize accumulated lactate in the presence of sufficient oxygen. However, this is also a slow process and for practical purposes is not thought to account for a large proportion of lactic acid elimination from the fetal compartment.

Factors Affecting Acid-Base Balance

Supply of oxygen and removal of carbon dioxide and acid metabolites by the placenta are, simply, what keep the fetal environment in a state of acid-base balance. The dependence of umbilical oxygen saturation and content, and fetal arterial base excess on uterine blood flow, is illustrated in Figure 23–1. Oxygen supply depends on adequate maternal oxygenation, blood flow to the placenta, transfer across the placenta, fetal oxygenation, and delivery to fetal tissues. Carbon dioxide removal is dependent on fetal blood flow to the placenta, transport across the placenta and pickup by maternal blood, and removal from the maternal circulation. Fixed acid equilibrium depends on a continued state of balance between production and removal.

Respiratory Factors in Fetal Acid-Base Balance

Respiratory acidosis is caused by those conditions resulting in increased carbon dioxide tension and subsequent decreased pH. In the fetus, this picture is usually associated with a decrease in PO_2 as well. The most common cause of acute respiratory acidosis in

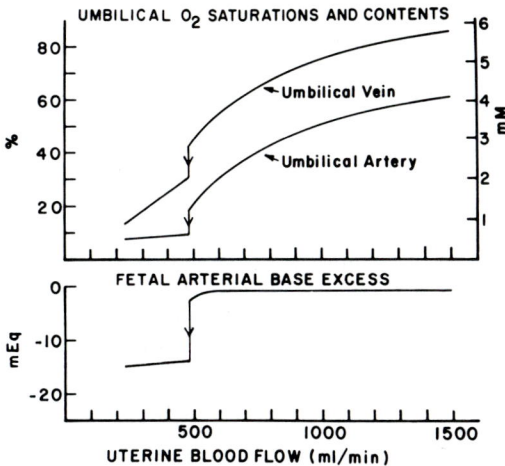

FIGURE 23–1. Effect of decreasing uterine blood flow on umbilical oxygen saturations and contents and the base excess of fetal blood in a 3-kg sheep fetus. (From Battaglia FC, Meschia G: An Introduction to Fetal Physiology. Orlando, Academic Press, Inc., 1986.)

the fetus is a sudden decrease in placental or umbilical perfusion. Cord compression, uterine hyperstimulation, and abruptio placentae are good examples because they cause a sudden inability of placental respiratory gas exchange secondary to decreased blood flow. If the etiologic factor(s) can be reversed, then the fetal respiratory acidosis can likely be reversed within a short time because transport of carbon dioxide (and oxygen) across the placenta is rapid under normal circumstances.

Factors that impair maternal alveolar ventilation by either decreasing minute ventilation or causing a ventilation-perfusion inequality will result in maternal respiratory acidosis. This will alter the transplacental carbon dioxide gradient so that the fetus will manifest a respiratory acidosis on the basis of the decreased carbon dioxide excretion capacity of the maternal lungs. Etiology of maternal hypoventilation is multifactorial. Induction of anesthesia or narcotic overdose may result in depression of the medullary respiratory center. Hypokalemia, neuromuscular disorders such as myasthenia gravis, and drugs that impair neuromuscular transmission such as magnesium sulfate in toxic doses may result in hypoventilation or even paralysis of the respiratory muscles. Finally, airway obstruction from foreign bodies or severe bronchospasm caused by an acute asthmatic attack may result in maternal respiratory acidosis. Again, restoration of normal fetal acid-base balance depends on the reversibility of the maternal etiologic factor(s).

Maternal respiratory alkalosis may occur when hyperventilation reduces the PCO_2 and subsequently increases pH. Severe anxiety, acute salicylate toxicity, fever, sepsis, pneumonia, pulmonary emboli, and acclimation to high altitudes are common etiologic factors. As in respiratory acidosis, restoration of maternal acid-base balance by appropriate treatment of the causative factor(s) will result in normalization of fetal blood gases.

Metabolic Factors in Fetal Acid-Base Balance

Fetal metabolic acidosis is characterized by loss of bicarbonate, high base excess, and a subsequent fall in pH. The etiology may be fetal or maternal and usually implies the existence of a chronic metabolic derangement. Intrauterine growth restriction and other conditions resulting from chronic uteroplacental hypoperfusion may result in fetal metabolic acidosis on the basis of decreased oxygen delivery and subsequent anaerobic metabolism and accumulation of noncarbonic acids.

Primary maternal metabolic acidosis can also cause fetal metabolic acidosis and is classified according to the status of the anion gap. In addition to bicarbonate and chloride, the remaining anions required to balance the plasma sodium concentration are referred to as "unmeasured anions" or the "anion gap." Reduced excretion of inorganic acids as in renal failure, or accumulation of organic acids as in alcoholic, diabetic, or starvation ketoacidosis, and lactic acidosis result in an increased anion gap metabolic acidosis. Bicarbonate loss seen in renal tubular acidosis, hyperparathyroidism and diarrheal states, and failure of bicarbonate regeneration will result in metabolic acidosis characterized by a normal anion gap. Fetal responses to these maternal conditions will be manifested by a pure metabolic acidosis with normal respiratory gas exchange as long as placental perfusion remains normal.

Prolonged fetal respiratory acidosis, as seen in cord compression and abruptio placentae, may also result in accumulation of noncarbonic acids from anaerobic metabolism characterized by blood gas measurements reflecting a mixed respiratory and metabolic acidosis.

ACID-BASE MONITORING IN LABOR

During labor the fetus is subjected continuously to intermittent episodes of relative hypoxia. With each contraction uterine blood flow diminishes, placental perfusion is reduced, and transplacental gaseous exchange is transiently impaired. The intermittent nature of uterine contractions appears teleologically designed to allow periods of recovery and resumption of normal oxygen supply. The vast majority of fetuses tolerate labor without incident or long-term damage because they enter labor with adequate reserve, although as labor progresses there is progressive reduction in fetal pH, PO_2, and bicarbonate level and increase in PCO_2 and base excess. Fetal scalp blood values during labor are summarized in Table 23–1.

The de novo development of asphyxia in a normal-sized term fetus who enters labor with good energy reserves and normal placental function, as evidenced by drainage of a normal volume of clear amniotic fluid, is unusual. When reserve is not adequate, for example in some cases of intrauterine growth restriction, uterine contractions may lead to a more rapid onset of fetal acidosis or may aggravate a pre-existing degree of acidosis. In most cases, there are premonitory signs that may be noted only for the first time in labor, such as drainage of meconium-stained fluid with thickness

Table 23–1. Fetal Scalp Blood Values in Labor*

	EARLY FIRST STAGE	LATE FIRST STAGE	SECOND STAGE
pH	7.33 ± 0.03	7.32 ± 0.02	7.29 ± 0.04
PCO_2 (mm Hg)	44 ± 4.05	42 ± 5.1	46.3 ± 4.2
PO_2 (mm Hg)	21.8 ± 2.6	21.3 ± 2.1	16.5 ± 1.4
Bicarbonate (mMol/liter)	20.1 ± 1.2	19.1 ± 2.1	17 ± 2
Base excess (mMol/liter)	3.9 ± 1.9	4.1 ± 2.5	6.4 ± 1.8

*Mean ± standard deviation.
(Abstracted from Huch R, Huch A: *In* Beard RW, Nathanielsz PW (ed): Fetal Physiology and Medicine. New York, Marcel Dekker Inc., 1984.)

of meconium related to the degree of associated oligohydramnios (Crowley et al., 1984) or ominous fetal heart rate patterns. Although preliminary efforts have been made to develop continuous tissue pH and PO_2 monitors for attachment to the fetal presenting part in labor, in practice fetal acid-base status assessment requires a fetal blood sample.

Fetal Blood Sampling

Saling and Schneider (1967) introduced the technique of obtaining a sample of blood from the fetal presenting part to evaluate fetal status during labor. A fetal blood sample may be obtained from the scalp or buttocks when indicated; it is the final determinant in making a firm diagnosis of fetal hypoxemia or acidosis. *Fetal distress* is a loose term often applied to abnormal fetal heart rate patterns, but there is poor correlation between abnormal patterns and abnormally low fetal blood sample values, although decreasing fetal blood pH is correlated with increasing severity of late decelerations (Paul et al., 1975) (Figure 23–2). A diagnosis of true fetal distress is best obtained by documentation of an abnormal fetal blood sample except in extreme, self-evident circumstances, such as cord prolapse or abrupt placental separation.

Indications for Fetal Blood Sampling

Clinical Suspicion of Fetal Hypoxia

If thick meconium drains at the time of rupture of membranes in labor, there may be underlying fetal hypoxia and it may be advisable to obtain a fetal blood sample, particularly if the fetal heart rate is not completely normal. Although thick meconium is not always associated with fetal acidosis, the development of meconium aspiration syndrome is linked to the presence of acidosis at birth (Mitchell et al., 1985). If no fluid drains at the time of rupture of membranes, continuous fetal heart rate monitoring may be indicated, although clinical experience suggests that clear fluid subsequently drains in the majority of cases. In institutions in which fetal heart rate monitoring by intermittent auscultation is the norm in low-risk cases, continuous fetal heart rate monitoring or a fetal blood

sample should be considered with any irregularity of the fetal heart, particularly bradycardia below 120 beats/min or tachycardia above 160 beats/min.

Abnormal Fetal Heart Rate Patterns

1. Absent short-term variability. In certain circumstances this pattern may be iatrogenic from central nervous system suppressants administered to the mother. However, a fetal blood sample may reveal evidence of fetal hypoxia in this situation.

2. Decreased short-term variability. In certain circumstances, such as at the onset of fetal monitoring, without maternal sedation or meconium-stained fluid, decreased variability may indicate fetal hypoxia.

3. Late decelerations that persist for more than 10 minutes and do not respond to conservative measures such as change of position.

4. Variable decelerations with reduced or absent short-term variability or persistent severe variable decelerations.

5. Patterns that are difficult to interpret or unusual (e.g., pseudosinusoidal).

Normal short-term variability is the most important element in determining whether or not a fetal blood sample should be obtained. Several investigators have demonstrated that normal variability is almost always associated with good fetal outcome (Boehm, 1977; Krebs et al., 1979; Parer, 1980). There is no doubt that with increasing experience in pattern interpretation, the need to obtain a fetal blood sample decreases. Clark and Paul (1985) have pointed out that at their institution only 2 per cent of patients undergo fetal blood sampling. While it may be said that a normal fetal heart rate pattern will almost always exclude fetal hypoxia, in the majority of abnormal patterns the fetus is not hypoxic, but without fetal blood sampling it is not possible to be sure, and the total clinical picture needs to be considered.

Interpretation of Results

There are five interdependent variables that may be taken into account when interpreting a fetal blood sample: pH, PCO_2, PO_2, HCO_3, and base excess. In the presence of a low pH, the most important decision is to distinguish between respiratory and metabolic acidosis because this may have a significant impact on patient management. Metabolic acidosis, associated with pH less than 7.20 and base excess greater than −6, requires consideration of delivery, while a fetus with respiratory acidosis may benefit from intrauterine resuscitation, and relatively immediate delivery may not be so crucial. Respiratory acidosis can occur with cord compression or uterine hyperstimulation, while metabolic acidosis more often represents a chronic condition in the fetus or may result from long-standing intrapartum hypoxia.

Maternal acid-base balance may influence fetal pH in exceptional circumstances, such as maternal acidosis due to renal tubular acidosis, and lower fetal pH. It is important to consider evaluation of maternal

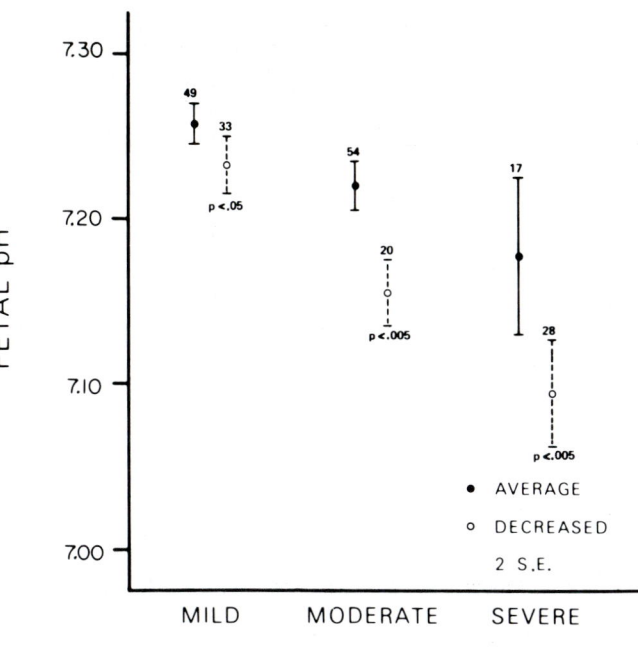

FIGURE 23–2. Relationship between fetal blood pH and severity of late decelerations at time of blood sampling. Each FHR classification is further divided into average (>5 beats per minute) or decreased (<5 beats per minute) FHR variability. (From Paul RH, Sudan AK, Yeh SY, et al: Clinical fetal monitoring: VII. The evaluation and significance of intrapartum baseline FHR variability. Am J Obstet Gynecol **123**:206, 1975.)

pH and blood gases when fetal values appear inappropriate.

Apart from distinguishing between respiratory and metabolic acidosis, it is important to interpret results in the light of clinical circumstances, taking into account stage of labor, color and volume of amniotic fluid, estimated fetal weight, gestational age, parity, and so on. It is particularly important to note that outcome in very low-birth-weight fetuses may be directly related to acid-base balance at birth (Westgren et al., 1984); these small fetuses may not tolerate even the most benign episodes of intrapartum hypoxia without becoming acidotic. However, low pH alone does not seem to predict subsequent development of cerebral palsy. (See section on acidosis in normal baby.)

Frequency of Fetal Blood Sampling

When should fetal blood sampling be repeated? There is no simple answer to this question because it depends entirely on the clinical circumstances, which may change with the progress of labor. This is only one aspect of care of the fetus during labor and must be viewed in context. As a general rule, a repeat sample should be obtained if the circumstances dictating the first sample do not resolve, or if delivery is not expected within 30 to 40 minutes. Persistence of an ominous pattern and an initial value of pH 7.22 and base excess of −2 in a primigravida at 3 cm with a fetus suspected of intrauterine growth restriction and no fluid drainage at rupture of membranes would dictate repetition within 30 minutes. On the other hand, a pH value of 7.30 and base excess of 0 in a similar primigravida draining a normal volume of clear amniotic fluid and whose heart rate pattern has improved would not require a second sample. Again,

experience of the clinician will often determine the necessity and frequency of resampling.

Contraindications

Fetal blood sampling should not be done when the fetus has a known or suspected blood dyscrasia (e.g., hemophilia or von Willebrand's disease). Fetal death due to excess blood loss has been reported in such cases (Ledger, 1978).

A potential disadvantage occurs with the use of the vacuum extractor after fetal blood sampling. Although this is not a contraindication to either procedure, one must be wary of using vacuum extraction on a fetus whose scalp has had numerous punctures for blood sampling. Amnionitis is considered a relative contraindication to FBS because of the possibility of increasing the risk of fetal scalp infection.

Fetal Complications

Fetal death due to exsanguination after blood sampling, caused by unsuspected fetal coagulopathy, has been reported (Mondanlou and Linzey, 1978). In addition, there have been isolated case reports of neonatal scalp bleeding after fetal blood sampling, possibly because scalp vasoconstriction resulting from fetal asphyxia, which had previously prevented bleeding, resolved after delivery.

The incidence of scalp infections has been cited as less than 1 per cent (Ledger, 1978), with the large majority requiring only local treatment (hair trimming, cleanliness). With the currently more common use of fetal heart rate monitoring via spiral electrodes, the incidence of fetal blood sampling complications is somewhat confused, because fetal heart rate monitoring almost always precedes fetal blood sampling.

Therefore, if the mortality rate resulting from coagulopathies is excluded, the infectious complications of fetal blood sampling are quantitatively minor and of less importance than the potentially irreversible problem of asphyxic brain damage that such sampling may help to avoid.

Effect on Incidence of Cesarean Section

Fetal blood sampling has the effect of limiting the increased incidence of cesarean section frequently seen in association with continuous electronic fetal monitoring. Chalmers (1978) showed that electronic fetal monitoring increased the incidence of cesarean section for dystocia as well as for fetal distress. Grant (1985) showed that fetal monitoring alone increased the incidence of cesarean sections by a factor of 2.7 (95 per cent confidence limits 1.9 to 3.8), while the addition of fetal blood sampling contained the increase to 1.9 (95 per cent confidence limits 1.6 to 2.2).

Only in exceptional circumstances should cesarean section be performed for fetal distress without first obtaining a fetal blood sample if it is available. In the majority of cases the result will be normal and labor may be allowed to continue. Exceptional circumstances would include the drainage of thick meconium in a primigravida at 1 cm dilation with either auscultated bradycardia or an ominous tracing on continuous electronic fetal monitoring. A policy of fetal blood sampling before cesarean section is undertaken for fetal distress will prevent many unnecessary cesarean sections and is compatible with excellent fetal outcome (O'Driscoll et al., 1977; MacDonald et al., 1985). Finally, improved perinatal outcome has been demonstrated only when fetal blood sampling has been considered an integral part of fetal monitoring in labor (Chalmers, 1978; MacDonald et al., 1985).

Umbilical Cord Acid-Base Measurement

Definition

There are cogent arguments, most of which revolve around the confirmation or exclusion of a diagnosis of birth asphyxia, to be made in favor of determining cord blood pH and gas measurements in every baby born. A long-accepted obstetric myth held that birth asphyxia was defined by low apgar scores. Even the ICD-CM 9 published by the U.S. Department of Health and Human Services defines severe birth asphyxia as "Apgar score of 0–3," and mild to moderate birth asphyxia as "Apgar score of 4–7." However, it has become increasingly clear from the literature (Sykes et al., 1982; Ruth and Raivio, 1988; Marrin and Bosco, 1988; American Academy of Pediatrics, 1986) that neonatal depression as determined by one and 5 minute Apgar scores alone is a poor reflection of birth asphyxia or predictor of long-term neurologic deficit.

Birth asphyxia remains a poorly defined term, although most obstetric and pediatric practitioners have come to accept a clinical definition that includes both neonatal depression and umbilical cord blood acidemia. A more rigorous definition would also include evidence of neonatal end-organ damage such as early seizures and cardiac or renal dysfunction. With the increasingly widespread use of umbilical cord blood gas determinations at delivery and the subsequent availability of good pediatric follow-up data, the American College of Obstetrics and Gynecology and the American Academy of Pediatrics are working toward a clinically meaningful and specific definition of birth asphyxia. Currently, however, umbilical cord blood pH at delivery provides the most sensitive reflection of birth asphyxia; the absence of acidemia excludes this diagnosis.

Normal Values

Umbilical cord blood gas values obtained at delivery from both artery and vein in a large series of consecutive term nulliparous women are presented in Table 23–2 (Thorp et al., 1989). These values are consistent with those reported by others (Yeomans et al., 1985; Nickelsen and Weber, 1987; Extermann et al., 1990). The definition of an abnormal cord arterial pH has in previous years been arbitrarily accepted as <7.20 without any support from the available data. In fact, when the definition of abnormal values as those more than 2 standard deviations below the mean is used, 7.20 falls well within the normal range for arterial pH in all the cited large studies. Review of the literature encompassing close to 19,000 deliveries sets the lower limit for normal arterial cord pH at 7.04 to 7.10. Although fewer data are available for venous cord blood pH values, the lower limit should be 7.14 to 7.20.

The next logical query regarding umbilical cord blood gases is: Does the statistical definition of an abnormal cord arterial pH have clinical significance as well? In their series of 1924 deliveries, Thorp et al. (1989) found that 2.1 per cent of newborns with normal Apgar scores (35/1690) had umbilical artery acidemia. Only three of these 35 acidemic babies had significant morbidity; one had transposition of the great vessels, one had meconium aspiration syndrome, and one developed early neonatal seizures with cerebral hemorrhage. Winkler et al. (1991) evaluated over 300 newborns with abnormal arterial pH and found that the only infants with neurologic deficit were those with arterial pH values <7.00. Gilstrap et al. (1989) also suggested that clinically significant acidemia at birth most likely does not occur until the arterial pH reaches 7.0.

TABLE 23–2.   Normal Umbilical Cord Blood Gas Values

	ARTERY	VEIN
pH	7.24 ± .07	7.32 ± .06
pO$_2$ (mm Hg)	17.9 ± 6.9	28.7 ± 7.3
pCO$_2$ (mm Hg)	56.3 ± 8.6	43.8 ± 6.7
Bicarbonate (mEq/L)	24.1 ± 2.2	22.6 ± 2.1
Base excess (mEq/L)	−3.6 ± 2.7	−2.9 ± 2.4

Data are expressed as mean ±1 S.D. (Thorp et al: Am J Obstet Gynecol **161**:600, 1989.)

Indications

Routine measurement of umbilical cord pH and gases at delivery is becoming increasingly common practice at institutions with large delivery services. Fortunately, the information gained from this data will frequently provide the means of understanding the physiologic events surrounding the birth of a baby with low Apgar scores, particularly if both venous and arterial samples are obtained. Additionally, the educational value for nurses, residents, pediatricians, and obstetricians is considerable.

While the authors advocate obtaining a full set of cord blood gases on all deliveries, this is currently not an American College of Obstetricians and Gynecologists (1991) standard of care, nor is it practical in all institutions. Strong consideration should be given to umbilical cord blood gas determinations in all high-risk deliveries and in all infants with unexpected delivery room complications. These indications include Apgar scores <7 at 1 or 5 minutes, meconium-stained amniotic fluid, known congenital anomalies, chorioamnionitis, prematurity, abnormal fetal heart rate tracings, and any other circumstance in which fetal condition may be in question. Two large studies have confirmed that while premature delivery results in significantly lower Apgar scores, those newborns have no significant differences in acid-base status when compared with term infants (Dickinson et al., 1992; Ramin et al., 1989). This is a particularly cogent finding as preterm infants with low Apgar scores may be assumed to have birth asphyxia unless this diagnosis is ruled out by cord blood gas analyses at delivery.

Technique

Immediately following delivery of the baby, a segment of cord approximately 20 to 30 cm in length is isolated by clamping, separated, and set aside for subsequent sampling (ACOG Committee Opinion, 1991). Arterial and venous samples are obtained in standard heparinized blood sampling syringes. At our institution a perinatal laboratory serves labor and delivery areas and the neonatal intensive care unit. Samples are delivered to the laboratory as quickly as is practical, so that results are available for pediatricians in cases of suspected birth asphyxia and for obstetricians to help in case review and for educational purposes. The result becomes a permanent part of the patient's record, just as the Apgar score does. After the cord has been doubly clamped, there are no significant changes in the blood gas values for 60 minutes with the specimens left at room temperature (Strickland et al., 1984). Once the specimens are placed on ice, the values are reliable for approximately 3 hours.

Acidosis in the Otherwise Normal Baby

The question arises as to whether the infant with an acidotic cord pH at birth but no other deviation from normal is at increased risk of developing neuro-logic abnormality. In normally grown infants, Dijxhoorn et al. (1985) found no evidence of a correlation between low umbilical pH values and abnormal neonatal neurologic evaluation. A low pH, by itself, does not predict abnormal behavior. Touwen et al. (1980, 1982), Jurgens-Van Der Zee et al. (1979), and Huisjes et al. (1980) followed a large group of infants for up to 6 years and found that unless there were other adverse perinatal influences at work, acidemia alone at birth did not predict adverse long-term developmental outcome.

Continuous Tissue Acid-Base Measurement in Labor

In current obstetric practice, continuous electronic fetal monitoring is the standard method of fetal monitoring in labor. For a variety of reasons, intermittent fetal blood sampling has not been as widely utilized. Stamm et al. (1976) described the use in newborns of an electrode that continuously measured subcutaneous pH. Others have adapted the electrode for use in the fetus.

Young (1981) has had extensive experience with continuous fetal tissue pH measurement in labor. He observed close correlation between tissue pH and scalp blood pH, and between final tissue pH and umbilical artery pH, although this has not been universal experience (Boos et al., 1978). Tissue pH values are generally agreed to be lower than arterial pH values by 0.026 to 0.06 pH units. There is a relationship between abnormal fetal heart rate patterns and reduced tissue pH and, as in the case of scalp pH measurements, the relationship is not constant. Young et al. (1979) found the lowest average tissue pH in association with late decelerations and tachycardia. Tissue pH changes appear to lag behind heart rate changes by approximately 3 minutes and recover approximately 5 minutes after heart rate recovery (Antoine et al., 1982).

Technical difficulties, mainly relating to attachment of the electrode to the fetal scalp, have inhibited the widespread acceptance of this method of fetal monitoring in labor, although with experience, satisfactory recording can be obtained in 60 to 90 per cent of cases (Antoine et al., 1982; Boos et al., 1978; Flynn and Kelly, 1980; Johnson et al., 1991).

Continuous Fetal Oxygen Monitoring

Although technically feasible (Aarnoudse et al., 1985), there are many limitations on the continuous measurement of fetal PO_2 in labor. It is likely that continuous PO_2 monitoring might contribute to an understanding of the etiology of fetal heart rate patterns in labor but will not enter routine clinical practice for the foreseeable future. Several investigators have recently reported on the use of a fetal oxygenation saturation monitor during labor (Dildy et al., 1993; Katz et al., 1993). This device is placed in contact with the fetal cheek after the membranes are ruptured and reads continuous O_2 saturation. Initial reports as to accuracy and feasibility have been promising. This type of technology has potential import in assessing the effects of labor on oxygen delivery to the fetus, and large trials are needed to determine its clinical usefulness.

Antepartum Fetal Acid-Base Assessment

Antepartum fetal blood samples may be obtained by inserting a needle, under ultrasound control, into the umbilical vein or artery (percutaneous umbilical blood sampling [see Chapter 24]) (Daffos et al., 1983), or directly into the fetal intrahepatic vein (Nicolini et al., 1990). Possible complications with cordocentesis include hematoma formation, spasm, infection, preterm labor, and fetal death. In practice the fetal loss rate in experienced hands is less than 1 per cent and is related to the number of attempts required to obtain a sample. Fetal blood sampling from the intrahepatic vein has the advantages of a larger target, no spasm, and no bleeding from the puncture site.

In the normal fetus it is apparent that both pH and PO_2 decrease significantly with advancing gestational age, while PCO_2 and base excess increase. Soothill et al. (1986a,b) and Nicolaides et al. (1989) obtained umbilical venous, arterial, and intervillous samples from over 200 fetuses between 16 and 38 weeks gestation and established normal ranges for pH, PO_2, PCO_2, bicarbonate, base excess, and lactate concentration. Samples were obtained both by fetoscopy and cordocentesis. Fetoscopically obtained umbilical venous samples had significantly higher PCO_2, lower pH, and more negative base excess values than blood obtained by percutaneous umbilical blood sampling. Other values did not differ by sampling method. The lower values obtained by fetoscopy were thought to be related to pre-sampling maternal fasting and sedation (Soothill et al., 1986a). Normal values in midtrimester and third trimester fetuses are given in Table 23–3 (Soothill et al., 1986b; Weiner, 1990). A fall in PO_2 is compensated for by a rise in fetal hemoglobin with advancing gestation, thus maintaining a constant fetal blood oxygen content throughout pregnancy. The progressive fall in fetal PO_2 with advancing gestation is probably due to increased oxygen consumption by the placenta. Lactate concentration has been reported to remain constant throughout gestation in umbilical arterial and intervillous samples, although Soothill et al. (1986a) found an increase in umbilical venous lactate concentration with advancing gestation. It is likely that lactate is a major component in supplying energy needs in human pregnancy, similar to that in the sheep (Burd et al., 1975).

Fetuses with intrauterine growth restriction (IUGR) have been reported to be more hypoxic, hypercapnic, acidotic, and to have higher lactate concentrations than normally grown controls (Nicolaides et al., 1989; Weiner and Williamson, 1989; Pardi et al., 1987; Soothill et al, 1987). The frequency of hypoxemia reported ranged from 28 to 36 per cent, depending on the gestational age and criteria for inclusion in the studies. Not surprisingly, the frequency of hypoxemia increased with additional abnormal indices such as reduced blood flow on Doppler studies (Weiner, 1990; Nicolini et al., 1990; Nicolaides et al., 1988) and abnormal fetal heart rate patterns (Visser et al., 1990).

There have been reports of emergency delivery undertaken as a result of abnormal results obtained at percutaneous umbilical blood sampling (Pearce and Chamberlain, 1987; Nicolaides et al., 1986) while others would suggest a much more cautious approach (Nicolini et al., 1990). The role of antepartum fetal blood sampling in determining management is not yet clear. Likewise, the exact role of antepartum fetal sampling for blood gas analysis in the management of intrauterine growth restriction remains unclear and further research is required. It is possible that it will join the fetal biophysical profile, Doppler analysis, and other indices in the total evaluation of complicated pregnancies.

Oxytocin and Fetal Acid-Base Balance

Infusion of oxytocin to a patient in labor can increase uterine activity and potentially accentuate the decrease in placental perfusion that is normally associated with contractions. However generated, contractions may provoke a hypoxic response in the fetus with inadequate respiratory and placental reserve. This is well illustrated by the inability of the fetus with severe intrauterine growth retardation to tolerate labor. In a comparative analysis of 54 cases of early neonatal seizures, which are frequently associated with birth asphyxia (Freeman, 1985), Minchom et al. (1987) noted an association between seizure occurrence and use of oxytocin to augment labor. However, they also cautioned that the association should not be used as evidence of cause and effect. MacDonald et al. (1985) found no evidence of an association between oxytocin use in labor and neonatal seizures but did observe an increase in seizure activity when labor lasted in excess of 5 hours. We and others have recently produced evidence that oxytocin does not cause fetal acidosis. A consecutive series of 1423 primigravidas at term, with singleton gestations and vertex presentation, was studied (Thorp et al., 1988). Oxytocin was infused in 43 per cent. The incidence of cord blood acidosis,

TABLE 23–3. Normal Umbilical Cord Blood Gas Values in Midtrimester Fetuses

	MIDTRIMESTER*		THIRD TRIMESTER†
	UMBILICAL ARTERY	UMBILICAL VEIN	UMBILICAL VEIN
pH	7.339 ± .03	7.358 ± .04	7.41 ± .02
pCO_2 (mm Hg)	42 ± 4	37 ± 4	36.1 ± 3
pO_2 (mm Hg)	34 ± 4	55 ± 7	34.6 ± 5
Bicarbonate (mMol/liter)	22 ± 1.5	20 ± 2	23.0 ± 1
Base excess (mMol/liter)	−3.5 ± 2.0	−4.2 ± 2.3	−0.6 ± 1
Lactate (mMol/liter)	1.10 ± .25	1.1 ± .25	—

Data are mean ± S.D. (From Soothill et al*: Obstet Gynecol **68**:173, 1986b and Weiner, CP†: Am J Obstet Gynecol **162**:1198, 1990.)

defined as venous pH less than 7.21, arterial pH less than 7.10, or venous pH less than 7.21 *and* arterial pH less than 7.10, was not influenced by oxytocin infusion (Table 23–4). There was no statistically significant difference in any of the arterial or venous cord blood gas parameters when oxytocin and no oxytocin groups were compared. Additionally, substratification to maximum oxytocin dose of less than or greater than 14 μ/min also failed to show a change in any blood gas parameters. Bidgood and Steer (1987) also found no evidence that oxytocin augmentation of spontaneous labor causes fetal acidosis. Several other studies have failed to document an adverse effect of oxytocin on perinatal outcome (Satin et al., 1992; Akoury et al., 1991; Cahill et al., 1992). However, if fetal distress is already proved, additional uterine activity, as produced by initiating oxytocin, is not desirable.

SUMMARY

Maintenance of acid-base balance is crucial to survival and normal development of the fetus and depends on a number of interrelated functions involving mother, placenta, and fetus. Until recently, direct measurement of fetal acid-base balance was confined to the most stressful period of fetal life, labor. The recent development of percutaneous umbilical blood sampling has allowed assessment of fetal acid-base balance before labor. Before percutaneous umbilical blood sampling for this purpose becomes established in clinical practice, it should be assessed critically and compared with existing methods of antepartum fetal assessment to see if it gives superior results without unacceptable side effects.

Our present state of knowledge allows a number of statements to be made: (1) Labor is characterized by a progressive tendency toward acidosis, which reflects the hypoxic stress of uterine contractions but which is rarely of clinical significance. (2) The ability to measure fetal scalp pH and blood gas composition should ideally be an integral part of intensive care of the fetus in labor so that the compromised fetus can be delivered expeditiously, and so that the mother will be protected from potential unwarranted operative intervention on the basis of an abnormal fetal heart rate pattern in the presence of normal fetal acid-base balance. (3) A true diagnosis of birth asphyxia depends on demonstration of cord artery pH and blood gas abnormalities in addition to other evidence of respiratory depression at birth. For this and other reasons, cord pH and blood gas measurement should be routine practice. (4) Chemical asphyxia, of itself, is not a good indicator of future neurologic abnormality.

Future developments in the investigation of acid-base balance in the fetus are likely to concentrate on two areas: (1) antepartum measurement and correlation with both existing methods of fetal assessment and with perinatal outcome and subsequent development, and (2) the influence of various aspects of the labor process on acid-base balance and what influence these changes have on long-term development.

REFERENCES

Aarnoudse JG, Deesley NP, Penfold P, et al: Permeability of the human placenta to bicarbonate: In vitro perfusion studies. Br J Obstet Gynaecol **91**:1096, 1984.

Aarnoudse JG, Huisjes HJ, Gordan H, et al: Fetal subcutaneous scalp PO_2 and abnormal heart rate during labor. Am J Obstet Gynecol **153**:565, 1985.

American College of Obstetricians and Gynecologists (ACOG) Committee Opinion. Committee on Obstetrics: Maternal and Fetal Medicine. Utility of umbilical cord blood acid-base assessment. Washington, DC, No. 91, February 1991.

Akoury HA, MacDonald FJ, Brodie G, et al: Oxytocin augmentation of labor and perinatal outcome in nulliparas. Obstet Gynecol **78**:227, 1991.

American Academy of Pediatrics: Committee on Fetus and Newborn: Use and abuse of the Apgar score. Pediatrics **78**:1148, 1986.

Antoine C, Silverman F, Young B: Current status of continuous fetal pH monitoring. Clin Perinatol **9**:409, 1982.

Battaglia FC, Meschia G: An introduction to fetal physiology. Orlando, Academic Press, 1986.

Bidgood KA, Steer PJ: A randomized control study of oxytocin augmentation of labour. 1. Obstetric outcome. Br J Obstet Gynaecol **94**:512, 1987.

Boehm FH: FHR variability: Key to fetal well-being. Contemp Obstet Gynecol **9**:57, 1977.

Boos R, Ruttgers H, Muliawan D, et al: Continuous measurement of tissue pH in the human fetus. Arch Gynecol **226**:183, 1978.

Burd LI, Jones MD, Simmons MA, et al: Placental production and foetal utilization of lactate and pyruvate. Nature **254**:710–711, 1975.

Cahill DJ, Boylan PC, O'Herlihy C: Does oxytocin augmentation increase perinatal risk in primigravid labor? Am J Obstet Gynecol **166**:847, 1992.

Chalmers I: Randomized controlled trials of intrapartum monitoring. *In* Thalhammer O, Baumgarten KV, Pollack (eds): Perinatal Medicine. Stuttgart, Georg Thieme, 1978.

Clark SL, Paul RH: Intrapartum fetal surveillance: The role of fetal scalp blood sampling. Am J Obstet Gynecol **153**:717, 1985.

Crowley P, O'Herlihy C, Boylan P: The value of ultrasound measurement of amniotic fluid volume in the management of prolonged pregnancies. Br J Obstet Gynaecol **91**:444, 1984.

Daffos F, Capolla-Pavlovsky M, Forestier F: Fetal blood sampling via the umbilical cord using a needle guided by ultrasound. A report of 66 cases. Prenatal Diag **3**:271, 1983.

Dickinson JE, Eriksen NL, Meyer BA, et al: The effect of preterm birth on umbilical cord blood gases. Obstet Gynecol **79**:575, 1992.

TABLE 23–4. The Effect of Oxytocin on Umbilical Cord Blood Gases

	OXYTOCIN	NO OXYTOCIN	P
VpH <7.21 (%)	6.5	5.3	NS
ApH <7.10 (%)	5.2	4.0	NS
ARTERIAL			
pH	7.23 ± .07	7.24 ± .07	NS
pCO_2 (torr)	56.8 ± 8.3	55.8 ± 9.0	NS
pO_2 (torr)	17.9 ± 7.3	17.9 ± 6.3	NS
Bicarbonate (mEq/liter)	23.9 ± 2.2	24.4 ± 2.2	NS
Base excess (mEq/liter)	−3.9 ± 2.7	−3.2 ± 2.6	NS
VENOUS			
pH	7.31 ± .06	7.32 ± .06	NS
pCO_2 (torr)	44.0 ± 6.3	43.5 ± 7.2	NS
pO_2 (torr)	28.5 ± 7.6	28.8 ± 6.9	NS
Bicarbonate (mEq/liter)	22.5 ± 2.0	22.8 ± 2.1	NS
Base excess (mEq/liter)	−3.1 ± 2.3	−2.6 ± 2.4	NS

Data are mean ± S.D. (Thorp et al: Am J Obstet Gynecol **159**:670, 1988.)

Dijxhoorn MJ, Visser GHA, Huisjes HJ, et al: The relation between umbilical pH values and neonatal neurological morbidity in full term appropriate-for-dates infants. Early Hum Dev 11:33, 1985.

Dildy GA, Clark SL, Loucks CA: Intrapartum fetal pulse oximetry: The effects of normal labor, variable deceleration and maternal oxygen administration on fetal arterial oxygen saturation. Am J Obstet Gynecol 168:341, 1993.

Extermann P, Irion O, Beguin F: Umbilical artery pH: Where does newborn acidemia begin? 10th Annual Meeting of the Society of Perinatal Obstetricians, Houston, Texas 1990.

Flynn AM, Kelly J: The continuous measurement of tissue pH in the human fetus during labour using a new application technique. Br J Obstet Gynaecol 87:666, 1980.

Freeman JM (ed): Prenatal and Perinatal Factors Associated with Brain Disorders. Bethesda, National Institutes of Health, 1985.

Gilstrap LC, Leveno KJ, Burris JB, et al: Diagnoses of birth asphyxia based on fetal pH, Apgar score and newborn cerebral dysfunction. Am J Obstet Gynecol 61:825, 1989.

Grant A: The Dublin randomized controlled trial of intrapartum fetal heart rate monitoring. D.M. Thesis, Oxford, England, University of Oxford, 1985.

Huch R, Huch A: In Beard RW, Nathanielsz PW (eds): Fetal Physiology and Medicine. New York, Marcel Dekker Inc., 1984.

Huisjes HJ, Touwen BCL, Hoekstra J, et al: Obstetrical-neonatal neurological relationship. A replication study. Eur J Obstet Gynecol Reprod Biol 10:247, 1980.

James EJ, Raye JR, Gresham EL, et al: Fetal oxygen consumption, carbon dioxide production and glucose uptake in a chronic sheep preparation. Pediatrics 50:361, 1972.

Johnson N, Johnson VA, Fisher J, et al: Fetal monitoring with pulse oximetry. Br J Obstet Gynaecol 98:36, 1991.

Jurgens-Van Der Zee AD, Bierman-Van Eendenburg MEC, Fidler VJ, et al: Preterm birth, growth retardation and acidemia in relation to neurological abnormality of the newborn. Early Hum Dev 3:141, 1979.

Katz M, Petrick T, Richichi K, et al: Oxygen saturation (SaO_2) monitoring in the presence of non-reassuring fetal heart rate (FHR) patterns. Am J Obstet Gynecol 168:341, 1993.

Krebs HB, Petres RE, Dunn LJ, et al: Intrapartum fetal heart rate monitoring. I. Classification and prognosis of fetal heart rate patterns. Am J Obstet Gynecol 133:762, 1979.

Ledger WJ: Complications associated with invasive monitoring. Semin Perinatol 2:187, 1978.

MacDonald D, Grant A, Sheridan-Pereira M, et al: The Dublin randomized controlled trial of intrapartum fetal heart rate monitoring. Am J Obstet Gynecol 152:425, 1985.

Marrin M and Bosco AP: Birth asphyxia: Does the Apgar score have diagnostic value? Obstet Gynecol 72:120, 1988.

Minchom P, Niswander K, Chalmers I, et al: Antecedents and outcome of very early neonatal seizures in infants born at or after term. Br J Obstet Gynaecol 94:431, 1987.

Mitchell J, Schulman H, Fleischer A, et al: Meconium aspiration and fetal acidosis. Obstet Gynecol 65:352, 1985.

Mondanlou HD, Linzey EM: An unusual complication of fetal blood sampling during labor. Obstet Gynecol 51:7s, 1978.

Nickelsen C, Weber T: Acid-base evaluation of umbilical cord blood: relation to delivery mode and apgar scores. Eur J Obstet Gynecol Reprod Biol 24:153, 1987.

Nicolaides KH, Soothill PW, Rodeck C, et al: Ultrasound-guided sampling of umbilical cord and placental blood to assess fetal wellbeing. Lancet 1:1065, 1986.

Nicolaides KH, Bilardo CM, Soothill PW, et al: Absence of end diastolic frequencies in umbilical artery: a sign of fetal hypoxia and acidosis. Br Med J 297:1026, 1988.

Nicolaides KH, Economides DL, Soothill PW: Blood gases, pH, and lactate in appropriate- and small-for-gestational-age fetuses. Am J Obstet Gynecol 161:996, 1989.

Nicolini U, Nicolaidis P, Fisk NM, et al: Limited role of fetal blood sampling in prediction of outcome in intrauterine growth retardation. Lancet 336:768, 1990.

O'Driscoll K, Coughlan M, Fenton V, Skelly M: Active management of labour: Care of the fetus. Br Med J 2:1451, 1977.

Pardi G, Buscaglia M, Ferrazzi E, et al: Cord sampling for the evaluation of oxygenation and acid-base balance in growth-retarded human fetuses. Am J Obstet Gynecol 157:1221, 1987.

Parer JT: The current role of intrapartum fetal blood sampling. Clin Obstet Gynecol 23:565, 1980.

Paul RH, Suidan AK, Yeh SY, et al: Clinical fetal monitoring. VII. The evaluation and significance of intrapartum baseline fetal heart rate variability. Am J Obstet Gynecol 123:206, 1975.

Pearce JM, Chamberlain GVP: Ultrasonically guided percutaneous umbilical blood sampling in the management of intrauterine growth retardation. Br J Obstet Gynaecol 94:318, 1987.

Ramin SM, Gilstrap LC, Leveno KJ, et al: Umbilical artery acid base status in the preterm infant. Obstet Gynecol 74:256, 1989.

Ruth JV and Raivio KO: Perinatal brain damage: predictive value of metabolic acidosis and the Apgar score. Br Med J 297:24, 1988.

Saling E, Schneider D: Biochemical supervision of the foetus during labour. J Obstet Gynaecol Br Commonw 74:799, 1967.

Satin AJ, Leveno KJ, Sherman ML, et al: High- versus low-dose oxytocin for labor stimulation. Obstet Gynecol 80:111, 1992.

Soothill PW, Nicolaides KH, Rodeck CH, et al: Effect of gestational age on fetal and intervillous blood gas and acid-base values in human pregnancy. Fetal Ther 1:168, 1986a.

Soothill PW, Nicolaides KH, Rodeck CH, et al: Blood gases and acid-base status of the human second trimester fetus. Obstet Gynecol 68:173, 1986b.

Soothill PW, Nicolaides KH, Campbell SP: Prenatal asphyxia, hyperlacticaemia, hypoglycaemia and erythroblastosis in growth-retarded fetuses. Br Med J 294:1051, 1987.

Stamm O, Latscha U, Janacek P, et al: Development of a special electrode for continuous subcutaneous pH measurement in the infant scalp. Am J Obstet Gynecol 124:193, 1976.

Strickland DM, Gilstrap LC, Hauth JC, et al: Umbilical cord pH and pCO_2: Effect of internal from delivery to determination. Am J Obstet Gynecol 148:191, 1984.

Sykes GS, Johnson P, Ashworth F, et al: Do Apgar scores indicate asphyxia? Lancet 1:494, 1982.

Thorp JA, Boylan PC, Parisi VM, et al: Effects of high-dose oxytocin augmentation on umbilical cord blood gas values in primigravid women. Am J Obstet Gynecol 159:670, 1988.

Thorp JA, Sampson JE, Parisi VM, et al: Routine umbilical cord blood gas determinations? Am J Obstet Gynecol 161:600, 1989.

Touwen BCL, Huisjes HJ, Jurgens-Van Der Zee AD, et al: Obstetrical condition and neonatal neurological morbidity. An analysis with the help of the optimality concept. Early Hum Dev 4:207, 1980.

Touwen BCL, Lok-Meijer TY, Huisjes HJ, et al: The recovery rate of neurologically deviant newborns. Early Hum Dev 7:131, 1982.

Visser GHA, Sadovsky G, Nicolaides KH: Antepartum heart rate patterns in small-for-gestational-age third-trimester fetuses: Correlations with blood gas values obtained at cordocentesis. Am J Obstet Gynecol 162:698, 1990.

Weiner CP, Williamson RA: Evaluation of severe growth retardation using cordocentesis—hematologic and metabolic alterations by etiology. Obstet Gynecol 73:225, 1989.

Weiner CP: The relationship between umbilical artery systolic/diastolic ration and umbilical blood gas measurements in specimens obtained by cordocentesis. Am J Obstet Gynecol 162:1198, 1990.

Westgren M, Holmqvist P, Ingemarsson I, et al: Intrapartum fetal acidosis in preterm infants: Fetal monitoring and long-term morbidity. Obstet Gynecol 63:355, 1984.

Winkler CL, Haugh JC, Tucker JM, et al: Neonatal complications at term as related to the degree of umbilical artery acidemia. Am J Obstet Gynecol 164(2):637, 1991.

Yeomans ER, Hauth JC, Gilstrap LC, et al: Umbilical cord pH, PCO_2 and bicarb following uncomplicated term vaginal deliveries. Am J Obstet Gynecol 151:798, 1985.

Young BK: Continuous fetal tissue pH monitoring in labor. J Perinat Med 9:189, 1981.

Young BK, Katz M, Klein SA: The relationship of heart rate patterns and tissue pH in the human fetus. Am J Obstet Gynecol 134:685, 1979.

CHAPTER

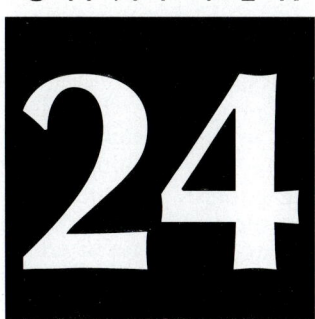

24

FETAL BLOOD SAMPLING

....

RICHARD L. BERKOWITZ, M.D., and LAUREN LYNCH, M.D.

INTRODUCTION

The use of ultrasonography to guide a needle into a portion of the fetal circulation has made fetal blood sampling a practical reality. This, in turn, has dramatically improved our ability to diagnose, and in some cases treat, a variety of disorders *in utero*. It was possible to obtain samples of fetal blood for diagnostic purposes in the '70s, but this required the use of a specially designed endoscope which permitted direct visualization of the cord root or a chorionic plate vessel (Hobbins and Mahoney, 1974; Rodeck and Campbell, 1979). The procedure, referred to as fetoscopy, was cumbersome and technically difficult to perform. As the trochar used to introduce a fetoscope into the uterine cavity had the equivalent size of a 14-gauge needle, and the procedure often took 30 minutes or longer to perform, it is not surprising that the pregnancy wastage rates were in the range of 5 to 7 per cent. Nevertheless, fetoscopic blood sampling procedures were performed in fetuses known to be at 25 per cent risk of having a recessive disorder that could not be diagnosed by amniocentesis, but could be detected by direct hematologic evaluation. These conditions included hemoglobinopathies such as sickle cell disease and thalassemia major, coagulopathies such as hemophilia A (factor VIII deficiency), and white blood cell disorders such as chronic granulomatous disease. Interestingly, many of these disorders can now be diagnosed by DNA analysis of material obtained by amniocentesis or chorionic villus sampling (CVS), and are rarely reasons for fetal blood sampling at the current time. However, the simplicity and relative safety of techniques utilizing ultrasonographic guidance have made fetal blood sampling available to a much larger population of patients, and the indications for performing this procedure have expanded considerably.

TECHNIQUE

In 1983, Daffos et al. described a method of obtaining fetal blood which involved the transabdominal introduction of a 20-gauge spinal needle under ultra-

sonographic guidance into a vessel within the root of the umbilical cord. Although many variations in technique have subsequently been described, they all utilize the same fundamental approach, and differ from fetoscopy in that visualization of the target vessel is obtained ultrasonographically, and only the sampling needle is introduced into the uterus. These techniques are collectively referred to as percutaneous umbilical blood sampling (PUBS), cordocentesis, or funipuncture.

The major differences in technique relate to the type of ultrasound transducer used and whether the operator works alone or in conjunction with a second individual who holds the transducer. If a linear array transducer is used, the operator may introduce the needle along its side and follow the progress of the tip by slightly rocking the transducer in the plane of its long axis. Only that portion of the shaft or tip traversing the sheet of ultrasound coming off the transducer face will be imaged with this approach, but with practice it is relatively easy to identify the tip at all times. The advantages of this approach are that the operator controls both the imaging and the movement of the needle. The disadvantages are that a sterile scanning gel and transducer sheath must be employed, and the operator has to learn to distinguish the needle tip from a cross-sectional cut through the shaft. A variation of this approach is to introduce the needle from the end, rather than the side, of a linear array transducer. This allows the entire shaft of the needle as well as the tip to be imaged if the needle is kept within the plane of the sound being transmitted from the transducer.

Another approach uses a sector or curved-array transducer placed fairly far from the needle entry site, but angled toward it. Again, the entire shaft of the needle can be visualized as long as it remains within the sheet of transmitted sound, and since the transducer is not adjacent to the needle entry site, it is not necessary to sterilize that portion of the abdomen which is used for imaging. This technique usually requires two individuals working as a team, although it is possible for the operator to hold the transducer in one hand and the needle in the other. In either case coordination is necessary in order to keep the shaft of the needle within the sheet of ultrasound. Finally, a variety of needle guides can be purchased which attach to the transducer and direct the needle along a predetermined course. The advantage to this approach is that the needle will go precisely to a specific target, but if the fetus moves or the patient develops a contraction with the needle in the uterus, redirection of the tip may be somewhat problematic.

Fetal vessels can be accessed within the cord or the fetus itself. It is easiest to enter the cord at either of its ends because it is anchored at these locations. Trying to place a needle into a floating loop of cord is difficult because of the target's potential for floating away. If the placenta is anterior, one can approach the cord root through the placental mass and never enter the amniotic fluid. Although this approach increases the potential for introducing fetal cells into the maternal circulation, it essentially protects the needle tip from being dislodged by movement of the fetus. If the placenta is posterior, however, it will be necessary to traverse the amniotic cavity in order to reach the target vessel and this, unfortunately, gives the fetus an opportunity to participate in the procedure. Obviously, this will also be true if the cord insertion site into the fetal abdominal wall is utilized. The hepatic vein is the most accessible vessel within the fetal body for blood sampling. Nicolini et al. (1990) have described their experience with 214 fetal blood sampling procedures performed at this location and report success rates of 91 per cent and 90 per cent for diagnostic and therapeutic procedures respectively. Furthermore, their fetal loss rates were comparable to those for blood sampling procedures done at the placental cord root. There have been reports of intrauterine transfusions done directly into the fetal heart (Bang, 1983), but this clearly has the potential to damage the cardiac valves or conduction system.

Once a sample of blood has been aspirated, it is essential to verify that it is fetal in origin. The most definitive way to do this is to compare the mean corpuscular volume (MCV) of the red cells with that of a sample of maternal blood. This is easily and quickly done on small aliquots of blood by a standard channelizing instrument. Since fetal red blood cells are considerably larger than those of an adult, the two samples will be readily identified as being from separate individuals or from the same one. In the absence of this capability, one can inject a small amount of sterile saline through the sampling needle under direct ultrasonic visualization. If the needle is in the umbilical vein, the microbubbles created by the injection will be seen to move toward the fetus within a cord vessel. If, however, the needle tip is in one of the umbilical arteries and is fairly close to the placental insertion site, it may not be possible to see movement of the microbubbles because they will flow toward the placenta and rapidly disappear into chorionic plate vessels. When it is necessary to verify that the sample is completely uncontaminated with either amniotic fluid or fetal blood, Forestier et al. (1988) recommend the performance of a battery of studies on the aspirated blood. These include a complete blood count with differential analysis and determination of anti-I and anti-i cold agglutinin, β-subunit of hCG, factors IX and VIIIC, and alpha-fetoprotein levels.

SUCCESS RATES AND SAFETY

The North American PUBS registry, which is maintained at Pennsylvania Hospital in Philadelphia, contains data collected from 16 centers in the United States and Canada. As of October 1991, 7462 diagnostic procedures performed on 6023 patients had been reported to this registry (Ludomirsky, 1991). The rate of failure to obtain a fetal blood sample was 5.7 per cent, with a range of 2 to 9.4 per cent. This figure diminished in proportion to the experience of the operators. There were 84 pregnancies that were felt to be lost as a direct consequence of the fetal blood sampling, for an incidence of 1.13 per cent per procedure and 1.39 per cent per patient. The range of losses for participating centers varied from 1 to 6.7 per cent, and this also was experience related. It should be noted that these figures reflect the operator's impression that a pregnancy loss was directly related to the procedure itself and not to the underlying fetal condition that necessitated the procedure. As many of these fetuses were quite sick at the time of the fetal blood sampling, it is certainly possible that a death *in utero* following the procedure might have been entirely unrelated to it. Nevertheless, the subjective nature of this assessment could be responsible for an underestimation of the true loss rates for percutaneous umbilical blood sampling.

The presumed causes of the fetal losses following PUBS procedures are listed in Table 24–1. The fact that chorioamnionitis was responsible for more than 25 per cent of these cases strongly suggests that strict attention should be paid to keeping the needle insertion site sterile during the procedure.

NORMATIVE FETAL VALUES

Before PUBS became available, normative fetal hematologic and biochemical values were obtained from abortuses or from a small number of fetuses undergoing fetoscopic blood sampling. The advent of a safer and easier technique, however, permitted sampling from a much larger number of fetuses at risk for conditions such as toxoplasmosis. Since most of these fetuses were not affected, their blood studies were used to establish normative values. In all of the published series, the normalcy of the sampled infants was confirmed at birth. It is important to remember that many fetal blood indices are gestational age–dependent, and it is imperative to take this into considera-

Table 24–1. Causes of 84 Fetal Losses Due to PUBS Procedures

1.	Chorioamnionitis	22
2.	PROM	16
3.	Exsanguination	12
4.	Severe bradycardia	13
5.	Thrombosis	5
6.	Unexplained	16
		Total 84

From North American PUBS Registry, Pennsylvania Hospital, Philadelphia, PA, October 1991.

TABLE 24–2. Hematologic Measurements According to Gestational Age in 2860 Normal Fetuses (Mean ± SD)

GESTATIONAL AGE (Weeks)	WBC ($\times 10^9$/L)	PLATELETS ($\times 10^9$/L)	RBC ($\times 10^{12}$/L)	HEMOGLOBIN (gm/100 ml)	HEMATOCRIT (%)	MCV (fl)
18–21 (n = 760)	4.68 ± 2.96	234 ± 57	2.85 ± 0.36	11.69 ± 1.27	37.3 ± 4.32	131.11 ± 10.97
22–25 (n = 1200)	4.72 ± 2.82	247 ± 59	3.09 ± 0.34	12.2 ± 1.6	38.59 ± 3.94	125.1 ± 7.84
26–29 (n = 460)	5.16 ± 2.53	242 ± 69	3.46 ± 0.41	12.91 ± 1.38	40.88 ± 4.4	118.5 ± 7.96
>30 (n = 440)	7.71 ± 4.99	232 ± 87	3.82 ± 0.64	13.64 ± 2.21	43.55 ± 7.2	114.38 ± 9.34

WBC = white blood cells; RBC = red blood cells; MCV = mean corpuscular volume.
From Forestier F: Principales normes biologiques chez le foetus. J Ped Puer **8:**436, 1991.

tion when prenatal studies are performed. Tables 24–2 through 24–5 contain normative data for the parameters most commonly used in prenatal assessment.

DIAGNOSTIC APPLICATIONS FOR FETAL BLOOD SAMPLING

Genetic Diseases

With the development of DNA technology, an expanding number of genetic diseases can be diagnosed in cells obtained from amniotic fluid or chorionic villi. Fetal blood sampling is now reserved for rapid karyotyping, diagnosing genetic hematologic disorders in families or diseases where DNA studies are not possible, and evaluating mosaicism which has been detected in studies of amniotic fluid or chorionic villi.

Karyotyping cultured amniocytes can take from 1 to 3 weeks. Sometimes, however, results must be obtained more rapidly. Karyotypes are usually available from fetal white blood cells within 48 to 72 hours and even more rapidly on direct preparations of material obtained by placental biopsy. The ultrasonographic detection of fetal morphologic malformations or severe intrauterine growth restriction is a common indication for rapid fetal karyotyping because management decisions may need to be made within a short period of time in these cases. If the need for karyotyping arises as the time limit approaches for a legal termination of pregnancy, or if delivery is imminent, fetal blood sampling may also be indicated.

Another indication for karyotyping fetal white blood cells is mosaicism detected in material obtained from amniotic fluid or chorionic villi. Depending on the chromosomal abnormality involved and the percentage of mosaicism found in the original sample, fetal blood sampling may either confirm or rule out the presence of an abnormal cell line. Approximately 1 per cent of chorionic villus samples reveal two popu-

lations of cells, but in 70 to 77 per cent of these cases the abnormal cell line is not present in the fetus (Ledbetter et al., 1990; Vejerslev and Mikkelsen, 1989). Although most cases of mosaicism found in chorionic villi can be effectively ruled out by amniocentesis, there have been a handful of cases of trisomy 21 mosaicism in which the chorionic villus culture revealed two cell lines, the amniotic fluid culture was entirely normal, yet true mosaicism was demonstrated in fetal blood (Ledbetter et al., 1990). Although this has only occurred in a small number of cases, it should be kept in mind in the counseling of patients with mosaicism detected on a CVS sample. Possible explanations for the discrepancies that may be found in studies of chorionic villi, amniotic fluid, and fetal blood include maternal cell contamination of the original sample, culture artifacts, mosaicism limited only to some fetal organs, and mosaicism confined to extraembryonic tissue.

Most common genetic blood disorders are now diagnosed by DNA analysis. However, sometimes the family is not informative by this type of study, or the location of the gene, for a particular disease, is not known. For example, a couple who has had a previous male child with severe combined immunodeficiency syndrome (SCIDS) without any other family history may have either an X-linked or autosomal recessive pattern of inheritance. If X-chromosome inactivation studies are inconclusive, fetal blood sampling to perform T cell analysis is the only diagnostic tool available for this family.

Hematologic Disorders

The majority of inherited hematologic disorders can now be diagnosed by the study of fetal DNA obtained from amniocytes or chorionic villi. Therefore, the antenatal detection of most congenital coagulopathies, hemoglobinopathies, white blood cell disorders, and

TABLE 24–3. Differential Cell Count According to Gestational Age in 732 Normal Fetuses (Mean ± SD)

GESTATIONAL AGE (Weeks)	LYMPHOCYTES (%)	NEUTROPHILS (%)	EOSINOPHILS (%)	BASOPHILS (%)	MONOCYTES (%)	ERYTHROBLASTS (% of RBCs)
18–21 (n = 186)	88 ± 7	6 ± 4	2 ± 3	0.5 ± 1	3.5 ± 2	45 ± 86
22–25 (n = 230)	87 ± 6	6.5 ± 3.5	3 ± 3	0.5 ± 1	3 ± 2.5	21 ± 23
26–29 (n = 144)	84 ± 6	8.5 ± 4	4 ± 3	0.5 ± 1	3 ± 2.5	21 ± 67
>30 (n = 172)	68.5 ± 15	23 ± 15	5 ± 3	0.5 ± 1	3 ± 2	17 ± 40

RBC = red blood cells.
From Forestier F: Principales normes biologiques chez le foetus. J Ped Puer **8:**436, 1991.

TABLE 24–4.   **Fetal Biochemical Assays According to Gestational Age**

	GESTATIONAL AGE (Weeks)	NUMBER OF FETUSES	MEAN	STANDARD DEVIATION
Alkaline phosphatase	<22	83	246.16	58.80
(U/liter)	22–25	114	251.42	55.38
	26–30	82	232.73	58.48
	>30	86	203.98	59.43
Gamma glutamyltransferase	<22	82	51.34	31.09
(U/liter)	22–25	119	70.09	43.08
	26–30	74	121.58	62.71
	>30	78	156.12	75.33
Cholesterol	<22	84	0.59	0.10
(gm/liter)	22–25	117	0.57	0.06
	26–30	84	0.58	0.11
	>30	99	0.61	0.11
Triglycerides	<22	85	0.62	0.19
(gm/liter)	22–25	119	0.41	0.06
	26–30	83	0.34	0.16
	>30	88	0.32	0.15
Total protein	<22	37	26.2	2.4
(gm/liter)	22–25	64	28.6	2.6
	26–30	39	32.4	3.7
	>30	44	39.9	5.2
Bilirubin	<22	83	15.48	2.80
(mg/liter)	22–25	117	16.52	2.62
	26–30	63	18.58	2.82
	>30	69	18.35	2.84

From Forestier F: Principales normes biologiques chez le foetus. J Ped Puer **8:**436, 1991.

immune disorders does not usually require direct analysis of fetal blood specimens. In some of these cases, family studies are noninformative and fetal blood sampling is necessary for diagnosis, but this is the exception rather than the rule. On the other hand, assessment of fetal anemia in cases of red blood cell isoimmunization or viral infection, and platelet counts in pregnancies affected by idiopathic thrombocytopenia (ITP) or alloimmune thrombocytopenia, require direct measurement of these parameters in fetal blood.

Since Liley's landmark study in 1961, the degree of fetal anemia in Rh isoimmunized pregnancies has usually been assessed by serial amniocenteses and studies of ΔOD 450 values as a function of gestational age. These values reflect the amount of bilirubin pigment in the amniotic fluid and, as such, are an indirect indicator of the degree of fetal hemolysis. All of the data in Liley's original paper, however, were collected at 28 weeks gestation or later, and extrapolation of the lines dividing the zones in the original graph to earlier gestational ages may not be appropriate. At least one recent study (Nicolaides et al., 1986) comparing amniotic fluid ΔOD 450 values with actual fetal hematocrits obtained concurrently found that the former values accurately reflected the degree of fetal anemia in the third trimester, but not in the second. Furthermore, there was no pattern to the inaccuracies; in some cases, high ΔOD 450 values inappropriately suggested the need for transfusion, and in other cases, low values were found in fetuses with significant anemia. These authors have argued, therefore, that in severely affected cases of Rh isoimmunization, determination of the fetal hemoglobin level is the most accurate way to determine the optimal timing of a transfusion prior to 27 weeks.

An additional reason for performing diagnostic fetal blood studies in cases of red blood cell isoimmunization is to determine the antigen status of the fetus when the father is a heterozygote for the offending antigen. There are many examples of women who have had a fetus requiring multiple transfusions *in utero* with one pregnancy, but delivered an antigen negative infant with absolutely no hematologic disorder in the next. In those cases, a single invasive

TABLE 24–5.   **Total IgM Antibody Levels According to Gestational Age in 1497 Normal Fetuses (mg/100 ml)**

GESTATIONAL AGE (Weeks)	NUMBER OF FETUSES	MEAN	STANDARD DEVIATION
18	20	1.18	0.57
19	21	1.52	0.70
20	88	1.86	0.98
21	220	2.18	1.08
22	270	2.53	1.32
23	230	2.95	1.46
24	140	3.21	1.43
25	120	3.92	1.95
26	90	4.58	2
27	62	4.90	2.8
28	61	5.08	2.10
29	47	5.92	2.32
30	25	6.26	2.79
31	13	6.56	1.79
32	19	5.65	1.89
33	18	7.17	2.64
34	9	9.53	3.58
35	10	9.47	2.91
36	4	7.72	4.52
37	6	10.36	5.91
38–40	5	11.82	5.51

From Forestier F: Principales normes biologiques chez le foetus. J Ped Puer **8:**436, 1991.

procedure can rule out the disease in an ongoing pregnancy, and no further diagnostic testing will be necessary.

Women with idiopathic thrombocytopenia have a 10 to 30 per cent chance of delivering a neonate with significant depression of its platelet count. Fortunately, spontaneous bleeding *in utero* rarely, if ever, occurs in this disorder. Nevertheless, most authorities advocate delivery by cesarean section if the fetal platelet count is less than 50,000/mm^3 in order to avoid the trauma that may result from labor. The fetal platelet count can be determined by scalp sampling during labor, but this predisposes the fetus to the potential for intracranial bleeding during the early first stage of labor, before its scalp is accessible for sampling. Furthermore, it may not be possible to have scalp sample platelet counts performed at inconvenient times in facilities where hematologists are not always available. An alternative approach is to perform fetal blood sampling in women with ITP at term, prior to the onset of labor. In this situation an elective cesarean section can be performed if severe fetal thrombocytopenia is discovered, or the patient can be offered a trial of labor if she is a candidate for a vaginal delivery. It should be noted, however, that fetal blood sampling may be technically difficult to perform in the late third trimester if the placental cord insertion site is in a location that can be obscured by the fetal body. Also, it should be remembered that the blood sampling procedure can cause hemorrhage or a vessel wall hematoma, which in turn can lead to acute fetal distress. This would lead to a cesarean section performed under emergency conditions, which is precisely what the operator has tried to avoid by doing the test in the first place. Obviously, the procedure should not be done for this indication unless the operator thinks that it will be technically easy. Furthermore, it would be wise to try to prospectively identify patients at greatest risk to have fetuses with thrombocytopenia. Two recent reports indicate that these women are likely to have had ITP before they became pregnant and have circulating antiplatelet antibodies (Samuels et al., 1990; Kaplan et al., 1990). It should be noted, however, that antiplatelet antibody testing is technically difficult to perform, and these studies should always be done in regional reference laboratories with demonstrated expertise in producing reliable results.

Alloimmune thrombocytopenia is the platelet equivalent of Rh disease. In this disorder the mother makes antibodies to antigens on the fetal platelets, and transplacental passage of these antibodies results in fetal thrombocytopenia. Unlike ITP this disorder is commonly associated with marked depression of the fetal platelet count, and this may result in intracranial hemorrhage occurring *in utero* long before the onset of labor. As severe thrombocytopenia and intracranial hemorrhage have been documented as early as 20 weeks gestation in this disorder, prolonged antenatal therapy is necessary to protect the fetus against the possibility of spontaneous bleeding. Since platelets have a life span of only 5 to 7 days, direct transfusions *in utero* would have to be done repeatedly if this were the therapeutic option chosen.

Fortunately, evidence exists which indicates that the majority of fetuses with alloimmune thrombocytopenia will respond to intravenous gammaglobulin at a dose of 1 gm/kg administered intravenously to the mother once a week (Bussel et al., 1988; Lynch et al., 1992). A randomized prospective study is currently being conducted to study the efficacy of this form of therapy alone, or in combination with low-dose dexamethasone, and to evaluate the use of high-dose prednisone "salvage therapy" for patients who fail to respond. This therapeutic approach requires fetal blood sampling to document the presence and degree of fetal thrombocytopenia, as well as to assess the response to treatment.

During the course of this investigation, and in a pilot study that preceded it, it was found that fetuses with platelet counts of less than 20,000/mm^3, and particularly those with counts of less than 10,000/mm^3, can exsanguinate from the cord puncture site after withdrawal of the needle in technically uncomplicated procedures. Therefore, patients with this disorder must be told that the risk of fetal blood sampling is higher in their case than for the population in general. We recommend that the blood sampling in these cases be done in a facility with access to rapid automated platelet counts at the time of the procedure, and a count should be determined before the sampling needle is withdrawn. A concentrate of washed maternal platelets should be prepared immediately prior to the procedure and be available when it is performed. If the fetal platelet count is found to be lower than 40 or 50,000/mm^3 a transfusion of maternal platelet concentrate can then be given to protect against excessive bleeding at the time of needle withdrawal from the vessel.

Infection

Isolated reports of the prenatal diagnosis of fetal infections by amniocentesis were published in the '60s and '70s. However, before fetal blood sampling became available, most patients exposed to teratogenic viruses or other microbes did not undergo diagnostic studies and were counseled about the risk of having an affected fetus based on published rates of neonatal infection. Many of these patients chose to terminate their pregnancies, but in the majority of cases their fetuses were actually not infected. The first infectious disease systematically studied *in utero* was toxoplasmosis. In 1988, Daffos and colleagues published their data on more than 700 pregnancies exposed to *Toxoplasma gondii* infection and demonstrated that 95 per cent were not infected. As a consequence, needless termination of pregnancy was avoided in these cases. Furthermore, by detecting those fetuses who were infected, they were able to selectively administer treatment *in utero*, which appeared to significantly reduce the incidence of severe sequelae of the disorder. Utilizing a combination of fetal blood sampling and amniocentesis, prenatal diagnoses of infections with cytomegalovirus (Lynch et al., 1991), parvovirus B19 (Gloning et al., 1990; Peters and Nicolaides, 1990; Nerlich et al., 1991; Naides and Weiner, 1989), rubella

(Daffos et al., 1984), and varicella-zoster virus (Cuthbertson et al., 1987) have been made.

Direct isolation of the organism from fetal blood or amniotic fluid is the most reliable evidence of fetal infection. However, this can be technically difficult and may take weeks. The fetus, like an adult, has both specific and nonspecific responses to any infection. The former may include production of specific IgM antibodies, but this is gestational age–dependent. Synthesis of specific IgM antibodies also appears to depend on the organism involved. For example, it has been found that almost 100 per cent of fetuses with congenital rubella infection produce specific IgM antibodies after 22 weeks (Daffos et al., 1984), whereas only 15 per cent of those infected with toxoplasma tested between 24 and 29 weeks produce specific IgM antibodies against the parasite (Daffos et al., 1988). Therefore, although detection of specific IgM antibodies in fetal blood is reliable evidence of fetal infection, their absence does not necessarily rule it out.

Nonspecific evidence of infection includes fetal thrombocytopenia, erythroblastosis, leukocytosis, eosinophilia, and elevated levels of gammaglutamyl transferase, lactic dehydrogenase, interferon (Raymond et al., 1990; Lebon et al., 1985), and total IgM antibodies. These findings are not all pathognomonic of fetal infection, and some of them can be seen in other conditions such as intrauterine growth restriction (Cox et al., 1988). Nevertheless, when fetal infection is of concern, positive nonspecific findings may be helpful in deciding whether to wait for culture studies to be completed or to inform the patient at that time that the chances of fetal infection are considerably higher than if these values were normal. Nonspecific findings may also reflect involvement of particular organs and be useful in determining the postnatal prognosis of the infant (Hohlfeld et al., 1991).

In the last several years, new technology has permitted direct identification of some of these teratogenic organisms without the need for repeated cultures. Lynch et al. (1991) reported the prenatal diagnosis of cytomegalovirus using fibroblast culture and indirect immunofluorescent staining with monoclonal antibodies. In those cases, the results were available in 48 hours. Polymerase chain reaction (PCR) studies were also successfully used in two cases in that series. In our experience, PCR analysis has been highly reliable in detecting cytomegalovirus in amniotic fluid.

In patients exposed to toxoplasmosis, the traditional method of parasite isolation has been mouse inoculation. Although fairly sensitive, this requires 3 to 6 weeks and is only done in a few laboratories in the United States. Fibroblast cell culture may provide a direct diagnosis in 4 days, but is only 50 per cent sensitive (Derouin et al., 1988). Preliminary data suggest that PCR analysis of amniotic fluid is both highly sensitive and specific for the toxoplasma organism, and a diagnosis can be made in only hours using this diagnostic modality (Grover et al., 1990).

Newer and faster methods for isolating the infecting organisms, plus safe access to the fetal circulation, have made the prenatal diagnosis of many fetal infections a reality. Fetal testing should be offered in pregnancies at risk for these infections, and automatic pregnancy termination should be considered a thing of the past. However, if the ultrasound examination of a fetus with hematologic or amniotic fluid evidence of infection is normal, it should be remembered that the infant may prove to be entirely asymptomatic at birth. At the present time it is extremely difficult to know how to counsel patients with these findings.

Drug Levels

Most of the existing data regarding transplacental passage of drugs has been derived from umbilical cord blood samples obtained at birth, often after administration of a single dose to the mother during labor. This approach has the obvious limitation of studying blood levels only after the baby has been delivered. In addition, labor or other conditions present at the time of delivery may affect fetal drug levels.

Pharmacologic studies under more physiologic conditions are now possible via fetal blood sampling. Several such studies have been reported for drugs such as aspirin, spiramycin, folic acid, fluorides, vitamin K, and low-molecular-weight heparins (Daffos, 1989; Mandelbrot et al., 1988; Forestier et al., 1987; Daffos and Forestier, 1988). In addition to determining drug levels, the effects of some of these drugs *in utero* can also be investigated. For example, Mandelbrot et al. (1988) reported that after maternal oral supplementation of vitamin K, fetal vitamin K levels were boosted 30-fold in the second trimester and 60-fold at term. However, despite elevated vitamin K concentrations, supplemented fetuses and neonates showed no increase in total or prothrombin coagulant activity, suggesting that the low prothrombin levels found during intrauterine life are not due to vitamin K deficiency. The same group also reported inhibition of fetal platelet aggregation after a single dose of 100 mg of aspirin was administered to the mother (Daffos and Forestier, 1988).

Fetal blood sampling can also be used to monitor the levels of drugs administered to the mother in order to treat the fetus. Some fetal disorders such as cardiac arrhythmias can be treated by administering drugs in this fashion. If the arrhythmia is not successfully abolished, fetal blood sampling can be performed to determine whether therapeutic levels have been achieved. Conversely, drugs given for maternal indications can have adverse effects on the fetus (e.g., chemotherapeutic agents). In this case, drug levels, as well as the impact on fetal hematologic parameters, can be studied by sampling fetal blood. The exact place for these potential uses of fetal blood sampling must be made on an individual basis at present, considering the benefits and risks of each situation.

Fetal Well-Being

Investigators have studied respiratory gases, acid-base balance, and lactate concentrations in fetal blood in an attempt to identify fetuses whose well-being was compromised *in utero*. It was hoped that this would prove to be useful when more conventional forms of fetal assessment were either equivocal or conflicting. Some case reports suggested that this might be the case, and a series by Nicolaides et al. (1989) found significantly more hypoxemia, hypercapnia, hyperlacticemia, and acidosis when 196 growth-restricted fetuses were compared with 208 who were appropriate in size for gestational age.

Nicolini and colleagues (1990), however, found that acid-base determination did not predict perinatal outcome in a group of growth-restricted fetuses. In their study 26 patients with structurally and karyotypically normal growth-restricted fetuses having absent end-diastolic flow on Doppler examination of the umbilical artery were compared to 20 patients with similar fetuses, but with end-diastolic flow evident on Doppler examination. The perinatal mortality was 65.4 per cent in the first group and 0 per cent in the latter. Significant differences in fetal blood values of P_{O_2}, P_{CO_2}, base equivalents, and nucleated red cell counts were demonstrable between the groups, but within the former these measurements did not discriminate between surviving fetuses and those who died perinatally. These authors therefore concluded that fetal blood sampling has a limited role in monitoring fetal well-being.

SUMMARY OF INDICATIONS REPORTED TO THE PUBS REGISTRY

As of October 1991, 63 per cent of the cases of diagnostic fetal blood sampling procedures reported to the PUBS registry were done either to determine a rapid karyotype or to evaluate hematologic status in pregnancies at risk for red blood cell isoimmunization (Ludomirsky, 1991) (Table 24–6). One-third of the procedures were performed to rule out fetal infection or to evaluate nonimmune hydrops, fetal acid-base status, twin-to-twin transfusion syndrome, or fetal platelet count. The remaining 4 per cent of procedures

TABLE 24–6. **Indications for Performing 7462 Diagnostic PUBS Procedures**

INDICATION	
1. Rapid karyotype	40%
2. Fetal red cell isoimmunization	23%
3. Fetal infection	8%
4. Nonimmune hydrops fetalis	7%
5. Fetal acid-base studies	6%
6. Twin-to-twin transfusion syndrome	5%
7. Alloimmune thrombocytopenia	4%
8. ITP	3%
9. Immunologic deficiencies	2%
10. Coagulation factor deficiencies	1%
11. Hemoglobinopathies	1%
12. Fetal drug levels (16)	
13. Fetal thyroid studies (5)	
14. R/O TAR syndrome (4)	
15. Paternity determination (1)	
16. R/O fetal phenytoin (Dilantin) toxicity (1)	

From North American PUBS Registry, Pennsylvania Hospital, Philadelphia, PA, October 1991.

were done for a variety of uncommon indications. Whereas the percentage of cases done to obtain a rapid karyotype was essentially the same as that reported to the registry in March 1989, the percentage of procedures performed to evaluate fetal red cell isoimmunization fell from 32 per cent to 23 per cent. Furthermore, the more recent data indicate an increase in the percentage of cases done for assessment of fetal infection, acid-base status, and twin-to-twin transfusion. Finally, while the overall percentage of procedures performed to determine the fetal platelet count remained constant, there was an increase in the percentage of cases of alloimmune thrombocytopenia and a concomitant decrease in the cases of ITP.

THERAPEUTIC APPLICATIONS OF THE TECHNIQUE

The value of fetal blood sampling is not limited to its use as a diagnostic modality. If access to the fetal circulation has been obtained, it is obvious that this can be used for the infusion of biologic or pharmacologic agents for therapeutic purposes. This technique has already been used to greatly improve our ability to effectively treat some conditions in utero, and holds the potential for even more exciting advances in the years to come (see also Chapter 25).

Transfusion of Blood Products

The greatest success achieved with intravascular therapy to date has been the treatment of fetal anemia. Although this condition is most commonly caused by red blood cell isoimmunization, severe fetal anemia can also be due to viral infections or large feto-maternal hemorrhages. As mentioned earlier, fetal blood sampling provides a more direct and objective measurement of fetal anemia than studies of amniotic fluid, and therefore more accurately indicates when transfusions should be performed in utero.

It has been known since the early 1960s that severely anemic erythroblastotic fetuses can respond to transfusions of packed red blood cells administered in utero (Liley, 1963). Until the early 1980s, however, the transfusions were performed intraperitoneally under fluoroscopic or ultrasonographic guidance. In 1981, Rodeck et al. demonstrated that intravascular transfusions could be performed in utero under fetoscopic visualization. One year later Bang and colleagues (1982) reported the successful transfusion of blood into the intrahepatic portion of the umbilical vein of a severely erythroblastotic fetus at 29 and again at 30 weeks. In these two procedures, a guide needle was introduced percutaneously under ultrasound guidance into the fetal abdomen near the umbilical vein, and through this a thin second needle was advanced into the lumen of the vein. Our group then described the successful transfusion of blood into an umbilical vessel at the cord root under ultrasonic visualization in a fetus at 31 weeks (Berkowitz et al., 1986). Since that time, several published series have attested to the feasibility and effectiveness of this approach to transfusing a fetus *in utero* (Grannum et al., 1986; Berkowitz et al., 1988; Poissonnier et al., 1989).

The major advantages to transfusing intravascularly, rather than into the peritoneal cavity, are that pre- and post-transfusion hematocrits can be measured, and the transfused cells are not dependent on lymphatic transport from the fetal peritoneal cavity for entry into the circulation. Hydropic fetuses in particular may be too sick to transport red blood cells via the lymphatic system and therefore might derive little or no benefit from a technically successful intraperitoneal transfusion. Furthermore, trauma associated with the introduction of the transfusion needle into the fetal abdomen has resulted in death *in utero*. On the other hand, intravascular transfusions can be technically difficult to perform in some cases and have also been associated with death *in utero*. In the absence of fetal hydrops, the intraperitoneal route may be preferable on some occasions for technical reasons.

In October 1991, the North American PUBS registry contained information regarding 2122 intravascular transfusions performed on 743 fetuses (Ludomirsky, 1991). Two hundred ninety two fetuses (39.3 per cent) in this group were hydropic before therapy was initiated. The perinatal survival rate was 74.6 per cent for the fetuses who were hydropic at the time of the first transfusion, and 91.1 per cent for those who were not, for an overall survival rate of 84.7 per cent. These are impressive results, especially for the hydropic group.

Concentrated platelet transfusions have been administered to severely thrombocytopenic fetuses *in utero*. This has been done as a single procedure immediately prior to delivery in order to avoid the necessity of performing an elective cesarean section, as well as on serial occasions for the management of alloimmune thrombocytopenia. As mentioned earlier, the relatively short half-life of platelets requires many repeated transfusions if maintenance of platelet counts at levels greater than 50,000/mm^3 is to be achieved over weeks or months of pregnancy. Nicolini et al. (1988) have described a patient who was given platelet transfusions *in utero* on seven separate occasions between 26 and 32 weeks gestation. We believe that this approach should be reserved for patients who have demonstrably failed to respond to medical therapy because of the morbidity and/or perinatal mortality that may be associated with multiple invasive procedures.

Drug Therapy

Most drugs cross the placenta to some degree, and several fetal conditions have been treated by administering therapeutic agents to the mother. Examples of this form of fetal therapy include: the treatment of fetal arrhythmias with various antiarrhythmic agents (Dumesic et al., 1982; Weiner and Thompson, 1988), prophylaxis and treatment of fetal toxoplasmosis with spiramycin and pyrimethamine/sulfadiazine, respectively (Daffos, et al., 1988), and treatment of neonatal alloimmune thrombocytopenia with intravenous gamma globulin (Bussel et al., 1988; Lynch et al., 1992). In some cases, however, the drugs must be

given directly into the fetal circulation because they cross the placenta poorly, if at all, or because the condition being treated requires bolus administration. For example, maternally administered digoxin is not always effective in treating supraventricular tachycardia in hydropic fetuses because transplacental passage of the drug is suboptimal in the presence of fetal congestive heart failure (Weiner and Thompson, 1988).

Another reason to inject a drug directly into the fetal circulation is that it would be dangerous if administered to the mother. An example of this is the use of muscle blocking agents to paralyze the fetus during invasive procedures such as intrauterine transfusions or prior to imaging with computed tomography or nuclear magnetic resonance (Daffos et al., 1988b).

Selective Termination

The first successful selective termination of an abnormal fetus in a twin pregnancy was reported by Aberg et al. in 1978. In that case cardiac puncture of a twin that had been diagnosed to have an inborn error of metabolism resulted in its death *in utero* at 24 weeks. The unaffected twin was delivered at 33 weeks and survived. Since that time a variety of methods of performing selective termination of an abnormal fetus in a multifetal pregnancy have been described. The method that is most widely accepted at the present time is the introduction of a cardiotoxic substance, such as potassium chloride, into the fetal circulation by direct cardiac puncture or injection into the umbilical vein.

Monochorionic placentas almost always have communications between the circulations of the two twins (see Chapter 37). If these communications exist, material injected into the vasculature of one fetus obviously has the potential to gain direct access to that of the other. Furthermore, published reports have described the death of the unaffected fetus within 24 hours of an apparently successful selective termination in twins with a monochorionic placenta (Donnenfeld et al., 1989; Golbus et al., 1988). This was thought to be due to exsanguination of the living fetus into the vasculature of the other one, presumably due to loss of the balanced pressure system in fetuses with a shared circulation. Finally, when significant communication exists between two placental circulations, death of one fetus *in utero* can result in embolization of thrombotic material into the living twin weeks after the death of the first (Enbom, 1985). Therefore, unless flow through all three vessels in the cord of the abnormal fetus can be occluded, selective termination of an abnormal twin having a monochorionic placenta is contraindicated.

In 1989, Chitkara et al. published the results of 17 selective termination procedures which had been performed at the Mount Sinai Medical Center in New York for a variety of fetal anomalies. That experience has now been expanded to include 42 patients. Except for one woman with triplets, all of the others presented with twins, and every patient appeared to have dichorionic membranes separating the sacs of each of the fetuses on ultrasonographic examination. All of the procedures were performed between 15.5 and 23.5 weeks gestation. The first six of these procedures were done over a 1½ year period from 1984 to 1986. Considerable technical difficulty was encountered in some of these early procedures, and a variety of different techniques were utilized. The latter included partial exsanguination, intracradiac injection of air, and intramyocardial or pericardial injection of saline, used independently or in combination. Two of these six patients delivered healthy normal infants at 38 and 31 weeks respectively, but the other four all lost the entire pregnancy within 3 days to 3.5 weeks following the procedure. The losses were due to either amnionitis or preterm labor in the absence of clinically evident infection.

From May 1986 through April 1992 an additional 36 procedures were performed. The first of the cases in this group was accomplished using a combination of partial exsanguination and the injection of intramyocardial normal saline, but all of the others were performed with the injection of KCl either directly into a cardiac chamber or into the umbilical vein at the cord root. As of May 1992, 34 of these patients had delivered viable infants who are all alive and well, two pregnancies were lost completely, and two were still ongoing. The two losses occurred 3 and 3.5 weeks following the procedure, and while the latter may have been directly related to the selective termination, the former seems to have been due to an incompetent cervix. Twenty-one of the women left with viable singletons delivered at 36 weeks or later, five delivered between 32 and 36 weeks, and the remaining seven delivered between 28 and 32 weeks. The woman who was reduced from triplets to twins delivered two healthy infants at 30½ weeks. All of the infants are alive, and 33 are developing normally. One child who delivered at 28 weeks has mild-to-moderate cerebral palsy at 3 years of age.

Aside from a single case of amnionitis associated with one of the losses in the first series of 6 patients, none of the mothers suffered any significant morbidity. Furthermore, there were no cases of clinically significant DIC caused by retention of the dead fetus following a selective termination procedure.

In the Mount Sinai series, the abnormal fetuses had a variety of anomalies, the most common being Down's syndrome. With the exception of a single case of acrania, however, none of the affected fetuses had an abnormality that was known to be lethal during the neonatal period. We feel that there is little justification in risking the life of a healthy twin by doing something that will occur naturally shortly after delivery. The only exception to this policy would be in cases where polyhydramnios in the sac of the anomalous twin threatens the well-being of the normal sibling because of its propensity to initate premature labor. That was the situation in the case where selective termination was performed because of acrania.

Twin-to-Twin Transfusion Syndrome

Although vascular communications are found in the placentas of almost all monochorionic twin pregnan-
cies, clinical signs of twin-to-twin transfusion syndrome occur in only 4 to 26 per cent of cases (Galea et al., 1982; Robertson and Neer, 1983). The pathophysiology of this condition is poorly understood. In general, however, the donor twin becomes anemic, growth restricted, and has associated oligohydramnios, while the recipient develops hydrops, cardiomegaly, and polyhydramnios.

The standard neonatal diagnostic criteria include differences in cord hemoglobin concentrations of 5 gm/dl or more, and in birth weights of 15 to 20 per cent or greater, although the latter is not necessarily present in the acute form of twin-to-twin transfusion syndrome (Rausen et al., 1965). Danskin and Neilson (1989), however, have found similar rates of these findings in twins with monochorionic and dichorionic placentas. Furthermore, there is evidence that the neonatal criteria used for diagnosing twin-to-twin transfusion may not apply to fetuses, especially during the second trimester. Fisk et al. (1990) reported sampling the blood of nine fetuses in six monochorionic pregnancies with typical ultrasonographic findings of twin-to-twin transfusion. In three of these cases both fetuses were tested, and only one pair had a hemoglobin discrepancy greater than 5 gm/dl. In this case and in one of the other two with concordant hemoglobin concentrations, placental vascular anastomoses were documented by injecting adult red blood cells into the donor's circulation and then recovering them from the recipient. Evidence of erythroblastosis was found in all of the fetuses sampled, but usually to a greater extent in the donor. Erythroblastemia in the recipient could result from either transfusion of donor erythroblasts or the action of donor erythropoietin on the recipient's marrow. In addition, erythroblastemia in the recipient may be secondary to hypoxia since four of the nine fetuses in this series were acidemic. Saunders and co-workers (1991) also described four cases of twin-to-twin transfusion syndrome studied by fetal blood sampling between 19 and 23 weeks gestation and found the mean hemoglobin difference to be only 1.7 gm/dl (range 1.2 to 2.7 gm/dl).

No form of therapy has consistently been successful in alleviating the twin-to-twin transfusion syndrome, although serial amniocentesis currently appears to be the best approach (Mahony et al., 1990; Urig et al., 1990; Elliott et al., 1991). Transfusion of the donor is unlikely to be useful since it would probably worsen the polycythemia in the recipient. Accidental bloodletting of the recipient was reportedly beneficial in two cases (Vetter and Scheider, 1988), but serial phlebotomy of the recipient may cause further blood loss from the already anemic donor.

None of the therapies mentioned above actually deals with the cause of the twin-to-twin transfusion syndrome. DeLia et al. (1990) have utilized a fetoscopically directed neodymium:YAG laser to ablate the vascular communications between the two placental circulations in three patients. Four of the six infants survived. Selective feticide has also been suggested as a mode of treatment. However, as mentioned earlier, terminating one member of a monochorionic pair by any means, without completely occluding the circulation of that fetus, could potentially lead to the death of the other or result in severe ischemic end-organ damage. Porreco et al. (1991) have reported successful occlusion of the single umbilical artery in an acardiac anencephalic twin by percutaneous placement of a thrombogenic coil.

Genetic Therapy

A variety of inherited disorders can now be successfully treated by bone marrow transplantation after birth. Although this approach is satisfactory in most cases, some potential advantages could accrue if bone marrow transplantation were performed *in utero*. Because the fetal immune system is immature, the chances of engraftment may be improved, and immunosuppression may not be necessary. Furthermore, if engraftment occurs *in utero*, subsequent fetal or neonatal damage may be avoided, such as congenital or neonatal infections in cases of severe combined immunodeficiency.

A possible disadvantage of attempting antenatal engraftment is potential inability to detect graft-versus-host disease prior to delivery. However, the use of HLA compatible grafts, or T cell depleted unmatched grafts, has significantly decreased the incidence of this complication (O'Reilly et al., 1989).

Animal data suggest that *in utero* stem cell transplantation is feasible provided it is done early in fetal life, but the chances of rejection increase as pregnancy progresses (Crombleholme et al., 1991). Chimeras have been successfully created *in utero* and maintained after birth in various species without immunosuppression (Flake et al., 1986). In the human, antenatal stem cell transplantation has thus far only been reported in two cases, and neither showed clear evidence of significant engraftment (Linch et al., 1986; Touraine et al., 1989).

Before *in utero* bone marrow transplantation is even considered, the genetic disorder must be diagnosable early in pregnancy, preferably in the first trimester. Furthermore, the condition must have been successfully treated by postnatal bone marrow transplantation. Finally, the family must understand that the risks and chances of success of this type of *in utero* therapy are unknown.

Some genetic disorders, such as Gaucher's disease, can now be treated by enzyme replacement because a mechanism has been found to transport the deficient enzyme into appropriate cells (Beutler, 1991). Although there is no need for *in utero* treatment of Gaucher's disease, it may serve as a model for the treatment of other enzymatic deficiencies. In the future, administration of the actual gene, instead of the missing enzyme, may be possible. If the normal gene becomes incorporated into the host's DNA, continuous enzyme replacement will be unnecessary. Access to the fetal circulation could potentially allow this type of therapeutic strategy to be attempted during fetal life.

CONCLUSION

Relatively safe and easy access to the fetal circulation has greatly increased diagnostic and therapeutic op-

tions for practicing perinatologists. As is true for any major new medical advance, it will take many years to properly define the optimal role for this invasive technology. There is no doubt, however, that this form of direct fetal access has enormously enhanced our ability to assess and treat our patients *in utero*.

REFERENCES

Aberg A, Mittelman F, Cantz M, Gehler J: Cardiac puncture of fetus with Hurler's disease avoiding abortion of unaffected co-twin. Lancet **2**:990, 1978.

Bang J: Clinical diagnostic techniques and laboratory method for congenital malformations and diseases: Ultrasound guided fetal blood sampling. International Symposium on Progress in Perinatal Medicine, Florence, Italy, May 1983.

Bang J, Bock JE, Trolle D: Ultrasound-guided fetal intravenous transfusion for severe rhesus haemolytic disease. Br Med J **284**:373, 1982.

Berkowitz RL, Chitkara U, Goldberg JD, et al: Intrauterine intravascular transfusions for severe red cell isoimmunization: Ultrasound guided percutaneous approach. Am J Obstet Gynecol **155**:574, 1986.

Berkowitz RL, Chitkara U, Wilkins IA, et al: Intravascular monitoring and management of erythroblastosis fetalis. Am J Obstet Gynecol **158**:783, 1988.

Beutler E: Gaucher's disease. N Engl J Med **325**:1354, 1991.

Bussel J, Berkowitz RL, McFarland JG, et al: Antenatal treatment of neonatal alloimmune thrombocytopenia. N Engl J Med **319**:1374, 1988.

Chitkara U, Berkowitz RL, Wilkins IA, et al: Selective second-trimester termination of the anomalous fetus in twin pregnancies. Obstet Gynecol **73**:690, 1989.

Cox WL, Daffos F, Forestier F, et al: Physiology and management of intrauterine growth retardation: A biologic approach with fetal blood sampling. Am J Obstet Gynecol **159**:36, 1988.

Crombleholme TM, Langer JC, Harrison MR, Zanjani ED: Transplantation of fetal cells. Am J Obstet Gynecol **164**:218, 1991.

Cuthbertson G, Weiner CP, Giller RH, Grose C: Prenatal diagnosis of second trimester congenital varicella syndrome by virus-specific immunoglobulin M. J Pediatr **111**:592, 1987.

Daffos F: Fetal blood sampling. Annu Rev Med **40**:319, 1989.

Daffos F, Capella-Pavlovsky M, Forestier F: Fetal blood sampling via the umbilical cord using a needle guided by ultrasound. Prenat Diagn **3**:271, 1983.

Daffos F, Forestier F: Pharmacologie antenatale. *In* Daffos F, Forestier F (eds): Medecine et biologie du foetus humain. Paris, Maloine, pp 431–432, 1988.

Daffos F, Forestier F, Capella-Pavlovksy M, et al: Prenatal management of 746 pregnancies at risk for congenital toxoplasmosis. N Engl J Med **318**:271, 1988a.

Daffos F, Forestier F, Grangeot-Keros L, et al: Prenatal diagnosis of congenital rubella. Lancet **2**:1, 1984.

Daffos F, Forestier F, Mac Aleese J, et al: Fetal curarization for prenatal magnetic resonance imaging. Prenat Diagn **8**:312, 1988b.

Danskin FH, Neilson JP: Twin-to twin transfusion syndrome: What are appropriate diagnostic criteria? Am J Obstet Gynecol **161**:365, 1989.

DeLia JE, Cruikshank DP, Keye WR: Fetoscopic neodymium: YAG laser occlusion of placental vessels in severe twin-twin transfusion syndrome. Obstet Gynecol **75**:1046, 1990.

Derouin F, Thulliez P, Confolfi E, et al: Early prenatal diagnosis of congenital toxoplasmosis using amniotic fluid samples and tissue culture. Eur J Clin Microbiol **7**:423, 1988.

Donnenfeld AE, Glazerman LR, Cutillo DM, et al: Fetal exsanguination following intrauterine angiographic assessment of selective termination of a hydrocephalic, monozygotic co-twin. Prenat Diagn **9**:301, 1989.

Dumesic DA, Silverman NH, Tobias S, Golbus MS: Transplacental cardioversion of fetal supraventricular tachycardia with procainamide. N Engl J Med **307**:1128, 1982.

Elliott JP, Urig MA, Clewell WH: Aggressive therapeutic amniocentesis for treatment of twin-twin transfusion syndrome. Obstet Gynecol 77:537, 1991.

Enbom JA: Twin pregnancy with intrauterine death of one twin. Am J Obstet Gynecol 152:424, 1985.

Fisk NM, Borrell A, Hubinont C, et al: Fetofetal transfusion syndrome: Do the neonatal criteria apply in utero? Arch Dis Child 65:657, 1990.

Flake AW, Harrison MR, Adzick NS, Zanjani ED: Transplantation of fetal hematopoietic stem cells in utero: The creation of hematopoietic chimeras. Science 233:776, 1986.

Forestier F, Cox WL, Daffos F, Rainaut M: The assessment of fetal blood samples. Am J Obstet Gynecol 158:1184, 1988.

Forestier F, Daffos F, Rainaut M, Toulemonde F: Low-molecular-weight heparin (CY 216) does not cross the placenta during the third trimester of pregnancy (letter). Thromb Haemost 7:57, 1987.

Galea B, Scott JM, Goel KM: Feto-fetal transfusion syndrome. Arch Dis Child 57:781, 1982.

Gloning KP, Schramm T, Brusis E, et al: Successful intrauterine treatment of fetal hydrops caused by parvovirus B19 infection. Behring Inst Mitt 85:79, 1990.

Golbus MS, Cunningham N, Goldberg JD, et al: Selective termination of multiple gestations. Am J Med Genet 31:339, 1988.

Grannum PA, Copel JA, Plaxe SC, et al: In utero exchange transfusion by direct intravascular injection in severe erythroblastosis fetalis. N Engl J Med 314:1431, 1986.

Grover CM, Thulliez P, Remington JS, Boothroyd JC: Rapid prenatal diagnosis of congenital toxoplasma infection by using polymerase chain reaction and amniotic fluid. J Clin Microbiol 28:2297, 1990.

Hobbins JC, Mahoney MJ: In utero diagnosis of hemoglobinopathies. Technique for obtaining fetal blood. N Engl J Med 290:1065, 1974.

Hohlfeld P, Vial Y, Maillard-Brignon C, et al: Cytomegalovirus fetal infection: Prenatal diagnosis. Obstet Gynecol 78:615, 1991.

Kaplan C, Daffos F, Forestier F, et al: Fetal platelet counts in thrombocytopenic pregnancy. Lancet 2:979, 1990.

Lebon P, Daffos F, Checoury A, et al: Presence of an acid-labile alpha-interferon in sera from fetuses and children with congenital rubella. J Clin Microbiol 21:775, 1985.

Ledbetter DH, Martin AO, Verlinsky Y, et al: Cytogenetic results of chorionic villus sampling: High success rate and diagnostic accuracy in the United States collaborative study. Am J Obstet Gynecol 162:495, 1990.

Liley AW: Liquor amnii analysis in the management of the pregnancy complicated by rhesus sensitization. Am J Obstet Gynecol 82:1359, 1961.

Liley AW: Intrauterine transfusion of foetus in haemolytic disease. Br Med J 2:1107, 1963.

Linch DC, Rodeck CH, Nicolaides K, et al: Attempted bone-marrow transplantation in a 17-week fetus. (Letter) Lancet 2:1453, 1986.

Lynch L, Bussel JB, McFarland JG, et al: Antenatal treatment of alloimmune thrombocytopenia. Obstet Gynecol 80:67, 1992.

Lynch L, Daffos F, Emanuel D, et al: Prenatal diagnosis of fetal cytomegalovirus infection. Am J Obstet Gynecol 165:714, 1991.

Ludomirsky A: Data presented at Sixth International Conference on Cordocentesis. Philadelphia, PA, October 21, 1991.

Mahony BS, Petty CN, Nyberg DA, et al: The "stuck twin" phenomenon: Ultrasonographic findings, pregnancy outcome, and management with serial amniocenteses. Am J Obstet Gynecol 163:1513, 1990.

Mandelbrot L, Guillaumont M, Leclercq M, et al: Placental transfer of vitamin K1 and its implications in fetal hemostasis. Thromb Haemost 30:60, 1988.

Naides SJ, Weiner CP: Antenatal diagnosis and palliative treatment of non-immune hydrops fetalis secondary to fetal parvovirus B19 infection. Prenat Diagn 9:105, 1989.

Nerlich A, Schwarz TF, Roggendorf M, et al: Parvovirus B19 infected erythroblasts in fetal cord blood. Lancet 1:310, 1991.

Nicolaides KH, Economides DL, Soothill PW: Blood gases, pH, and lactate in appropriate- and small-for-gestational-age fetuses. Am J Obstet Gynecol 161:996, 1989.

Nicolaides KH, Rodeck CH, Mibashan RS, et al: Have Liley charts outlived their usefulness? Am J Obstet Gynecol 155:90, 1986.

Nicolini U, Nicolaides P, Fisk NM, et al: Limited role of fetal blood sampling in prediction of outcome in intrauterine growth retardation. Lancet 2:768, 1990.

Nicolini U, Nicolaides P, Nicholas M, et al: Fetal blood sampling from the intrahepatic vein: Analysis of safety and clinical experience with 214 procedures. Obstet Gynecol 76:47, 1990.

Nicolini U, Rodeck CH, Kochenour NK, et al: In-utero platelet transfusion for alloimmune thrombocytopenia. Lancet 2:506, 1988.

O'Reilly RJ, Keever CA, Small TN, Brochstein J: The use of HLA-non-identical T-cell-depleted marrow transplants for correction of severe combined immunodeficiency disease. Immunodeficiency Rev 1:273, 1989.

Peters MT, Nicolaides KH: Cordocentesis for diagnosis and treatment of human fetal parvovirus infection. Obstet Gynecol 75:501, 1990.

Poissonnier MH, Brossard Y, Demedeiros N, et al: Two hundred intrauterine exchange transfusions in severe blood incompatibilities. Am J Obstet Gynecol 161:709, 1989.

Porreco RP, Barton SM, Haverkamp AD: Occlusion of umbilical artery in acardiac, acephalic twin. Lancet 1:326, 1991.

Rausen AR, Seki M, Strauss L: Twin transfusion syndrome. J Pediatr 66:613, 1965.

Raymond J, Poissonnier MH, Thulliez PH, et al: Presence of gamma interferon in human acute and congenital toxoplasmosis. J Clin Microbiol 28:1434, 1990.

Robertson EG, Neer KJ: Placental injection studies in twin gestation. Am J Obstet Gynecol 147:170, 1983.

Rodeck CH, Campbell S: Umbilical cord insertion as a source of pure fetal blood for prenatal diagnosis. Lancet 1:1244, 1979.

Rodeck CH, Holman CA, Karnicki J, et al: Direct intravascular fetal blood transfusion by fetoscopy in severe Rhesus isoimmunization. Lancet 1:625, 1981.

Samuels P, Bussel JB, Braitman LE, et al: Estimation of the risk of thrombocytopenia in the offspring of pregnant women with presumed immune thrombocytopenic purpura. N Engl J Med 323:229, 1990.

Saunders NJ, Snijders RJM, Nicolaides KH: Twin-twin transfusion syndrome during the 2nd trimester is associated with small intertwin hemoglobin differences. Fetal Diagn Ther 6:34, 1991.

Touraine JL, Raudrant D, Royo C, et al: In-utero transplantation of stem cells in bare lymphocyte syndrome. Lancet 1:1382, 1989.

Urig MA, Clewell WH, Elliott JP: Twin-twin transfusion syndrome. Am J Obstet Gynecol 163:1522, 1990.

Vejerslev LO, Mikkelsen M: The European collaborative study on mosaicism in chorionic villus sampling: Data from 1986 to 1987. Prenat Diagn 9:575, 1989.

Vetter K, Scheider KTM: Iatrogenous remission of twin transfusion syndrome. Am J Obstet Gynecol 158:221, 1988.

Weiner CP, Thompson MIB: Direct treatment of fetal supraventricular tachycardia after failed transplacental therapy. Am J Obstet Gynecol 158:570, 1988.

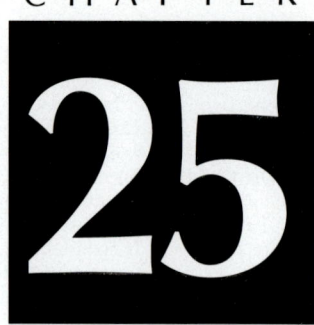

CHAPTER

25

FETAL THERAPY: MEDICAL AND SURGICAL APPROACHES

ALAN W. FLAKE, M.D., and MICHAEL R. HARRISON, M.D.

The impetus for *in utero* therapeutic intervention for fetal medical and surgical abnormalities arose from the clinical frustration of obstetricians, neonatologists, and pediatric surgeons involved in the treatment of certain abnormalities after birth. In many instances it was apparent that the damage had already been done. A simple anatomic defect, such as posterior urethral valves or a diaphragmatic defect, in an otherwise normal newborn, often led to devastating physiologic consequences *in utero,* which would result in death or nonviability after birth. Similarly, nonanatomic abnormalities such as erythroblastosis fetalis, which could be easily treated *ex utero,* could result in fetal death or nonviability *in utero.* In these cases, the rationale for prenatal intervention was compelling and obvious. Although less obvious, another category is fetuses with abnormalities which, although not lethal *in utero,* or in the neonate, might be better treated before birth. Treatment of the fetus, in many instances, offers a potential advantage over postnatal treatment because of the unique characteristics of fetal development. In this chapter we discuss specific medical and surgical interventions currently applicable to the fetus and briefly discuss some future possibilities for fetal intervention.

FETAL THERAPY FOR MEDICAL DISEASE

The concept of the fetus as a patient has evolved from our ability to make diagnoses and serial observations on the fetus, combined with increasing clinical experience and knowledge of the pathophysiology and natural history of fetal disease. Rh isoimmunization provided the first successful example of medical intervention in the developing fetus and provides a model for medical treatment of other fetal diseases (see Chapter 44). In the early 1960s, Sir William Liley, a pioneer in fetal treatment, performed the first successful prenatal transfusion of a hydropic fetus affected with Rh isoimmunization, and the field of fetal therapy was born (Liley et al., 1963). Since that time, a number of

other medical diseases have been successfully treated *in utero* either by direct treatment of the fetus, or transplacental treatment of the fetus via the mother.

Fetal disorders for which medical therapy may be appropriate are categorized in Table 25–1. Medical treatment of the fetus with cardiac dysrhythmias is addressed in detail in Chapter 21 and the prenatal induction of lung maturity is covered in detail in Chapter 28.

FUTURE DIRECTIONS IN PRENATAL MEDICAL THERAPY

Hematopoietic Stem Cell Transplantation

Although a large number of fetal diseases are potentially amenable to either surgical or medical prenatal treatment, the majority are relatively rare and, even in summation, fetal treatment would impact upon relatively few patients. In contrast, a relatively large number of patients are affected by hematopoietic derived diseases. These diseases, a large number of which can be diagnosed early in gestation, are listed in Table 25–2 and include the hemoglobinopathies, immunodeficiency diseases, and lysosomal storage diseases, to name a few.

Many of these diseases can be treated by conventional postnatal bone marrow transplantation (BMT). Unfortunately, application of conventional BMT has serious limitations (Sullivan, 1989; Clark, 1990). Only 35 per cent of candidates for BMT have an HLA identical donor available so that an optimal transplant can be performed. In addition, bone marrow conditioning (myeloablation) is usually required with its associated immunosuppression and risk of lethal infection. Rejection and graft-versus-host disease (GVHD) are constant threats, requiring further immunosuppressive therapy. By the time postnatal transplants are performed, most recipients have been ravaged by their underlying disease. Growth restriction, multiple transfusions, and recurrent infection

370

TABLE 25–1.   Nonanatomic Fetal Abnormalities Amenable to Prenatal Therapy

DISORDER	EXAMPLE	TREATMENT
Anemia	Rh isoimmunization	Transfusion: intraperitoneal or intravenous
	Other red blood cell antigens	Transfusion
Surfactant deficiency	Pulmonary immaturity	Glucocorticoids: transplacental
Biochemical defects	Multiple carboxylase deficiency	Biotin: transplacental
	Methylmalonic acidemia	Vitamin B_{12}: transplacental
	Menke's kinky-hair syndrome	Copper: transplacental
	Galactosemia	Galactose restriction during pregnancy
Cardiac arrhythmias	Supraventricular tachycardia	Digitalis: transplacental Propranolol: transplacental Procainamide: transplacental
	Heart block	Beta mimetics: transplacental
Endocrine deficiency	Congenital adrenal hyperplasia	Corticosteroids: transplacental
	Hypothyroidism and goiter	Thyroxin: transamniotic

result in a suboptimal clinical result. Finally, in many of the storage diseases, the neurologic damage begins early, perhaps *in utero,* and is not reversed by BMT (Parkman, 1986). In these fetuses, *in utero* treatment is not only advantageous, but necessary to cure the disease (Krivit et al., 1990). For all of these diseases the morbidity and mortality of the disease and its treatment remain significant and, in many cases, prohibitive for application of postnatal BMT. Therefore, although treatment is possible postnatally, many of these patients may be better served by fetal therapy. Transplantation of pluripotent hematopoietic stem cells (HSC) *in utero* may offer a number of advantages, which will reduce the morbidity and allow definitive treatment.

Rationale for Fetal HSC Transplantation

The rationale for prenatal HSC transplantation arises from aspects of immunologic (Soloman, 1971) and hematologic (Metcalf and Moore, 1971) ontogeny that are unique to fetal development. Early in gestation the fetus is tolerant of foreign antigen, recognizing foreign antigen as self, resulting in the induction of specific transplantation tolerance (Zanjani et al., 1992; Schwartz, 1989). Therefore, in contrast to postnatal BMT, the fetus will not reject the transplant, precluding the need for immunosuppression. If fetal liver is used as a source of donor cells, no mature T lymphocytes are present and GVHD does not occur (Touraine et al., 1987). In addition, during hematopoietic ontogeny, hematopoiesis migrates from the yolk sac to the fetal liver and finally to the bone marrow. Prenatal reconstitution would potentially allow normal post-

natal development, avoiding complications of the disease.

Longstanding hematopoietic chimerism in sheep and monkeys without GVHD has been created, without the need for immunosuppression, by early gestational fetal-to-fetal HSC transplantation (Flake et al., 1986; Harrison et al., 1989). Detailed analysis of the monkey chimeras confirms that these animals have normal immunologic response (Duncan et al., 1991) and that their donor hematopoietic compartment can respond normally to anemia-induced stress (Duncan et al., 1992).

Clinical Experience

Clinical experience has shown that current techniques of prenatal diagnosis and fetal transfusion make diagnosis and prenatal HSC transplantation feasible in humans well within the immunologic and hematopoietic window of opportunity. Mature T cells are not found in the fetal circulation until after 14 to 16 weeks gestation, and the bone marrow remains relatively empty until 18 to 20 weeks gestation. Clinical experience with HSC transplantation is limited in part because of the government moratorium on funding for use of fetal tissue for therapeutic purposes (Mason and Ryan, 1990) and the difficulty of obtaining intact fetal tissue. The reported clinical experience is summarized in Table 25–3. There have been a few promising successes, but in most cases no engraftment was

TABLE 25–2.   Congenital Hematopoietic Diseases Potentially Amenable to *In Utero* HSC

Disorders of erythropoiesis
  Thalassemia major
  Sickle cell anemia
  Diamond-Blackfan syndrome
  Fanconi anemia
Disorders of lymphopoiesis
  Severe combined immunodeficiency syndrome
  Bare lymphocyte syndrome
Disorders of myelopoiesis
  Chronic granulomatous disease
  Chediak-Higashi syndrome
  Wiskott-Aldrich syndrome
  Infantile agranulocytosis (Kostman's syndrome)
  Lazy leukocyte syndrome (neutrophil actin deficiency)
  Neutrophil membrane GP-180 deficiency
  Cartilage-hair syndrome
Metabolic errors of lysosomes of reticuloendothelial cells
  Mucopolysaccharidoses
    Hurler's disease (MSP I) (α-iduronidase deficiency)
    Hurler-Scheie syndrome
    Hunter disease (MSP II) (iduronate sulfatase deficiency)
    Sanfillippo B (MSP IIIB) (α-glycosaminidase deficiency)
    Morquio (MSP IV) (Hexosamine-6-sulfatase deficiency)
    Maroteaux-Lamy syndrome (MSP VI) (arylsulfatase B deficiency)
  Mucolipidoses
    Fabry disease (α-galactosidase A deficiency)
    Gaucher disease (glucocerebrosidase deficiency)
    Krabbe disease (galactosylceramidase deficiency)
    Metachromatic leukodystrophy (arylsulfatase A deficiency)
    Niemann-Pick disease (sphingomyelinase deficiency)
    Adrenal leukodystrophy
Disorder of osteoclast
  Infantile osteopetrosis

Table 25–3. Summary of Clinical Experience with Fetal Stem Cell Transplantation*

RECIPIENT AGE (wk)	DONOR CELL SOURCE	RECIPIENT DISEASE†	NO. PATIENTS	POSTNATAL FINDINGS AND CLINICAL OUTCOME	REFERENCE
17	T-cell-depleted auditory bone marrow	Rh disease	1	Survived with no evidence of engraftment	Linch et al., 1986
28	Fetal liver and fetal postnatal thymus	Bare lymphocyte syndrome	1	Clinically normal without infections. Lymphocytes have donor HLA expression	Touraine et al., 1989
26	Fetal liver and fetal thymus, 7–7.5 wk	SCID	1	Alive. Remains immunodeficient in protective isolation at <1 yr of age, plus evidence of donor cell engraftment	Touraine et al., 1989
12	Fetal liver, 7–10 wk	Thalassemia major	1	Engraftment, but remains anemic at <1 mo of age	Touraine et al., 1989
34, 23, 25	T-cell-depleted bone marrow	2, MCLD 1, thalassemia	3	No evidence of engraftment. Clinical status consistent with primary disease	Slavin et al., 1990

*A total of seven cases are described by three investigators. Engraftment was achieved in three fetuses given fetal cells early in gestation. Attempts to engraft T-depleted adult cells have been unsuccessful. Details of per cent and lineage of donor engraftment in chimeric recipients have not been published.
†SCID = severe combined immunodeficiency syndrome; MCLD = metachromatic leukodystrophy.

achieved. In many instances the indication, timing, dose, or donor source of cells has been suboptimal, providing an explanation for failure. It is necessary to pursue methods of improving engraftment in experimental models, but some of these questions can only be answered clinically.

Gene Therapy

Advances in molecular biology have made human gene therapy a clinical reality (Anderson, 1990), but many obstacles remain prior to general application (Anderson, 1984). Experimentally the challenge is to develop methods to efficiently introduce genetic material into an appropriate target cell, with minimal toxicity and in a manner in which expression of the gene product is normally regulated or, at least, within an appropriate range for therapeutic effect. The method that is closest to achieving this ideal is the use of retroviral vectors as gene delivery systems (Bernstein et al., 1985). Because of its immortality, multilineage expression, and ease of manipulation, and the frequency of hematopoietically based genetic disease, the HSC has been the most promising and most frequently studied target cell. However, postnatal studies, using bone marrow, particularly in large animals, have generally been disappointing (Kohn et al., 1987; Kantoff et al., 1987). Although gene expression can be achieved, the level of expression has been low and frequently transient. Improved efficiency in such systems will require improvement of vectors and potential techniques to cycle HSC so that maximal efficiency can be obtained.

As most genetic disease is progressive, particularly storage diseases with neurologic manifestations, it can be argued that the earlier therapy such as prenatal gene therapy is initiated, the better. There are also theoretical considerations and experimental data that support a physiologic advantage for prenatal gene therapy. Fetal liver, bone marrow, and peripheral blood contain a higher relative number of early progenitors than postnatal hematopoietic tissues, and a higher proportion of these cells may be cycling at any particular time. Studies in sheep and monkey *in utero* models show that the efficiency of transduction is higher with fetal derived HSC than with postnatal HSC and that persistence of durably transduced stem cells *in vivo* can be achieved (Kantoff et al., 1989). In addition, *in vitro* studies of human cord blood and premature blood support improved efficiency of transduction of fetal derived HSC (Ekhterae et al., 1988). Clinical application of prenatal gene therapy awaits further investigation. If methods of safely transducing vector into a large number of fetal cells are developed, there will undoubtedly be wide application.

Tolerance Induction for Organ Transplantation

Although now a routine procedure in older children and adults, organ transplantation remains a formidable challenge in the newborn (Najarian et al., 1990; Mavroudis et al., 1988). The long-term ramifications of neonatal and lifelong immunosuppression are unknown and disturbing (Tagge et al., 1987; Fricker et al., 1987; Krull et al., 1988). Tolerance induction for organ transplantation would reduce the need for lifelong immunosuppression. Successful induction and maintenance of tolerance are dependent upon early presentation of antigen and may require persistence of living cells (chimerism). Transplantation of "immortal" HSC *in utero* is a potential method of establishing tolerance.

Long-Term Catheterization of the Fetus

In many cases, medical therapy of the fetus would be greatly facilitated by long-term venous and arterial access to the fetus. Potential applications of such technology would include (1) multiple transfusions and exchange transfusions in Rh isoimmunization; (2) administration of short-acting medications as a continuous infusion, particularly for cardiac dysrhythmias; (3) *in utero* HSC transplantation for reconstitution, gene therapy, or tolerance induction; and (4) treatment of intrauterine growth restriction by the administration of vasoactive agents to improve placental blood flow or by providing intravenous nutrients to improve fetal nutrition and growth.

Direct placement of a catheter during open fetal surgery has a number of major drawbacks. We have developed experimental methods to laparoscopically place an extra-amniotic catheter into placental vessels. Experiments in the monkey model have resulted in successful, long-term catheterization of placental vessels with subsequent term delivery of normal monkey fetuses. If this approach can be safely translated to the clinical setting, it could introduce a number of new possibilities for fetal treatment.

FETAL THERAPY FOR SURGICAL DISEASE

The Fetus as a Surgical Patient

Correcting an anatomic malformation *in utero* with open fetal surgery jeopardizes the pregnancy and entails potential surgical risks to the mother as well as the fetus. Until risks of surgery, anesthesia, and preterm labor become relatively trivial, indications for open fetal surgery should remain limited to conditions which, if allowed to continue, will irreversibly interfere with fetal organ development, but if alleviated, would allow normal development to proceed. The minimum requirements for fetal intervention include the cooperative efforts of an obstetrician experienced in perinatal intervention, a sonographer experienced and skilled in fetal diagnosis, a surgeon experienced in operating on tiny preterm infants, and—in performing fetal procedures in the laboratory—a perinatologist working in a high-risk obstetric unit associated with a tertiary intensive care nursery, a geneticist experienced in syndromology and counseling, a reasonable and compassionate ethicist, and uninvolved professional colleagues who will monitor such innovative therapy (committee on human research). Malformations that qualify for consideration of fetal surgery should satisfy the following prerequisites:

1. Prenatal diagnostic techniques should identify the malformation and exclude other lethal malformations with a high degree of certainty.
2. The defect should have a defined natural history and cause progressive injury to the fetus which is irreversible after delivery.
3. Repair of the defect should be feasible and should reverse or prevent the injury process.
4. Surgical repair must not have excessive risk for the mother or her future fertility (Harrison et al., 1982b).

Table 25–4 lists the anatomic defects that theoretically may satisfy the requirements for open fetal sur-

TABLE 25–4. Anatomic Malformations That Interfere with Development and Theoretically May Benefit from Surgical Relief Before Birth

MALFORMATION	EFFECT ON DEVELOPMENT	
Urinary tract obstruction	→ Hydronephrosis/lung hypoplasia	→ Renal/respiratory failure
Diaphragmatic hernia	→ Lung hypoplasia	→ Respiratory failure
Cerebrospinal fluid obstruction	→ Hydrocephalus	→ Brain damage
Sacrococcygeal teratoma	→ High-output failure	→ Fetal hydrops/demise
Complete heart block	→ Low-output failure	→ Fetal hydrops/demise
Ventricular outflow obstruction	→ Pulmonary vascular hypoplasia	→ Pulmonary hypertension
Clefting/craniosynostosis	→ Craniofacial anomalies	→ Persistent deformity

gery. Our discussion will be limited to those defects that have actually satisfied our requirements and for which treatment *in utero* has been attempted.

The Fetus with Congenital Hydronephrosis

The approach to fetal hydronephrosis developed in the last decade is a paradigm for fetal treatment in general. A combination of clinical observation and experience, and simultaneous laboratory studies, defined the natural history and pathophysiology of the disease and allowed formulation of appropriate selection criteria for fetal treatment. From this large body of experimental and clinical work, for any individual case, the family can now be counseled about the prognosis and options in management ranging from termination of a hopeless pregnancy to prenatal intervention for a selected few fetuses.

Development of an Experimental Model

To study the pathophysiology of fetal urethral obstruction and the efficacy and feasibility of correction *in utero*, it was necessary to first develop an animal model before attempting a clinical approach. We created a model of severe bilateral hydronephrosis in the lamb by ligating the urachus and occluding the urethra with an ameroid constrictor or ligature at 95 to 105 days gestation (full term = 145 days) (Harrison et al., 1983). We then decompressed the obstruction by suprapubic vesicostomy at a second fetal operation 3 weeks later and compared obstructed, decompressed, and control lambs at birth (Harrison et al., 1982c). Uncorrected lambs did poorly with a high rate of stillbirth and hypoplastic lungs by weight. The renal pelvices, ureters, and bladder were markedly dilated mimicking the morphologic disease in human neonates. Seven of nine lambs corrected *in utero* were liveborn, with resolution of urinary tract dilatation and far less respiratory difficulty. However, this relatively late model of urinary obstruction did not reproduce

TABLE 25–5. Prognostic Criteria for the Fetus with Bilateral Obstructive Uropathy: Urine Composition and Volume

PREDICTED FUNCTION	SODIUM (mEq/ml)	CHLORIDE (mEq/ml)	OSMOLARITY (mOsmol)	OUTPUT (ml/hr)
Poor	>100	>90	>210	<2
Good	<100	<90	<210	>2

the typical cystic and dysplastic changes noted with severe human obstructive nephropathy.

To test whether earlier obstruction resulted in renal dysplasia, complete unilateral ureteral obstruction in fetal lambs was performed at the beginning of the second trimester (55 to 65 days gestation) (Glick et al., 1983). In this model the renal changes were both hydronephrotic, with ureteral and caliceal dilatation proximal to the obstruction, and dysplastic when examined at term. Twenty-five fetal lambs underwent early unilateral obstruction with subsequent decompression by end ureterostomy at predetermined time intervals (3, 6, and 9 weeks after obstruction) (Glick et al., 1984). Prenatal decompression prevented renal dysplasia, the degree of dysplasia and functional impairment being proportional to the length of time the kidney is obstructed. Other studies have shown that oligohydramnios-induced pulmonary hypoplasia associated with urinary obstruction is similar to that seen in human fetuses and that decompression of the obstructed urinary tract permits restoration of amniotic fluid volume and allows lung growth (Adzick et al., 1987; Docimo et al., 1989).

Natural History

Unrelieved urinary tract obstruction interferes with fetal development. The severity of damage at birth depends on the type, degree, and duration of obstruction (Harrison et al., 1981a). Although children born with partial bilateral obstruction at birth may have only mild hydronephrosis, which is easily treated, longstanding obstruction may result in advanced renal dysplasia incompatible with life. In addition, oligohydramnios secondary to decreased fetal urine output may produce pulmonary hypoplasia, which often is fatal at birth. Obviously, those with unilateral obstruction do not develop oligohydramnios and are not candidates for prenatal treatment. The presence of oligohydramnios requires bilateral obstruction and is a critical determinant of death (Harrison et al., 1982d). Fetuses identified with oligohydramnios at first examination in the early second trimester have a mortality rate of nearly 100 per cent. For those fetuses who develop oligohydramnios during serial ultrasonographic evaluations and prior to adequate pulmonary maturity for ex utero viability, morbidity and mortality are high. The major problem in management of these fetuses is determining which ones have severe enough obstruction to compromise renal and pulmonary function after birth, yet still have adequate renal function for salvage by prenatal decompression.

Based on a review with 20 fetuses with congenital bilateral hydronephrosis, prognostic criteria for "good" or "poor" fetal renal function were generated (Glick et al., 1985). The utility of these parameters has

been confirmed in recent prospective and retrospective studies as well as by our own clinical experience (Crombleholme et al., 1990). The prognostic criteria, normal renal echodensity and favorable urinary electrolytes (urine Na<100 mEq/L; Cl<90 mEq/L; Osm<210 mOsm) (Table 25–5) have proved reliable in the prediction of favorable neonatal and long-term outcome after in utero urinary tract decompression. The ultrasound appearance of the renal parenchyma provides valuable prognostic information if the renal parenchyma shows increased echogenicity or cystic changes, but is less predictive in their absence.

Management

From our cumulative clinical and laboratory experience, we use the following general guidelines for management of the fetus with hydronephrosis (Fig. 25–1). An initial ultrasonogram should be obtained to confirm the diagnosis, determine the anatomic level of obstruction, evaluate the volume of amniotic fluid, and rule out the presence of associated anomalies. If no associated anomalies are present and the amniotic fluid volume is adequate, the fetus should be followed by serial ultrasonography. If amniotic fluid volume remains adequate, the mother should receive routine obstetric care and the fetus can be treated after term delivery. If moderate-to-severe oligohydramnios develops, the fetus should undergo a complete prognostic evaluation to determine its potential for normal renal and pulmonary function after birth. For the fetus with predicted renal dysplasia, aggressive obstetric care or in utero decompression is not indicated. For the fetus with predicted good renal function, management options depend on fetal lung maturity. If the lungs are mature, immediate delivery and ex utero decompression is recommended. If the fetus's lungs are immature, in utero decompression is recommended. If the gestation is 28 weeks or later, but prior to adequate lung maturity, temporary decompression can be achieved with a percutaneously placed fetal vesicoamniotic shunt catheter. Before 28 weeks gestation, decompression by catheter placement has been unsuccessful largely due to frequent catheter obstruction and dislodgement (Crombleholme et al., 1988), and open fetal surgery is recommended.

We have performed open fetal surgery on eight fetuses with bilateral hydronephrosis selected from over 200 referrals over the past 11 years. In retrospect, our earliest attempts were on fetuses that would be excluded by our current selection criteria. One had a bilateral ureteropelvic junction obstruction with severe renal dysplasia; another had severe associated gastrointestinal anomalies which ultimately resulted in the child's death at 8 months of age, and another, a female, had a cloacal anomaly. One fetus was lost to

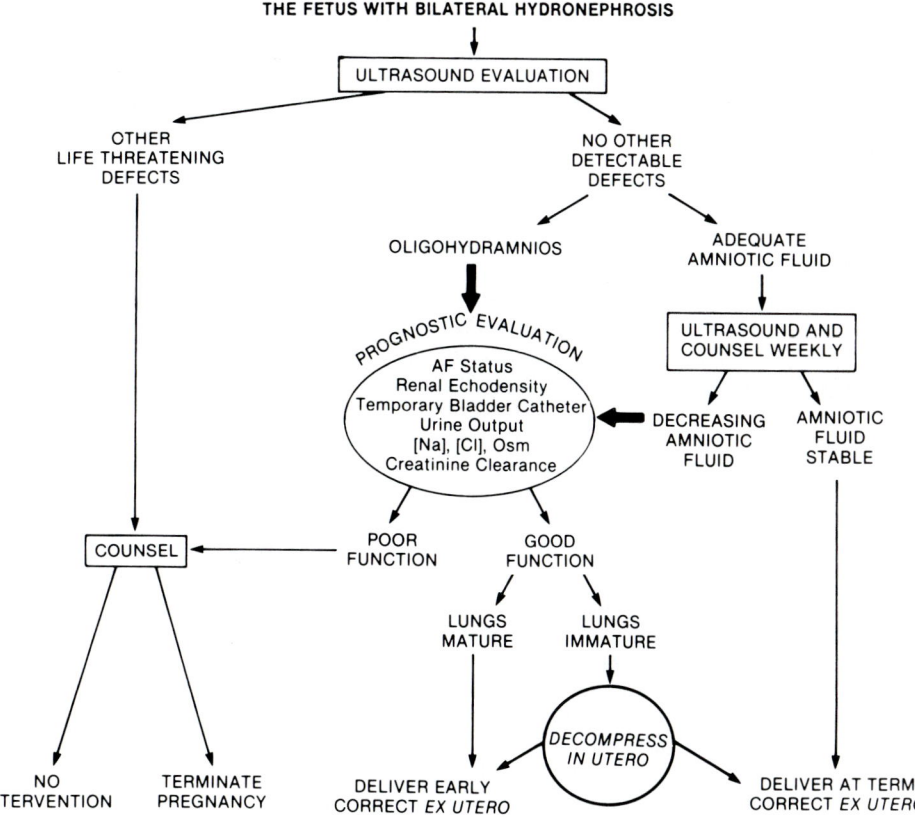

THE FETUS WITH BILATERAL HYDRONEPHROSIS

FIGURE 25–1. Management scheme for the fetus with bilateral hydronephrosis. Note that the development of prognostic criteria based on the assessment of fetal renal function allows improved counseling and management. (Reprinted with permission from Glick et al.: Management of fetus with congenital hydronephrosis. II. Prognostic criteria and selection for treatment. J Pediatr Surg **20:**376, 1985.)

preterm labor when the mother discontinued her oral tocolytic therapy. Of the remaining four patients, one died in the neonatal period of pulmonary and renal dysplasia, and the other three are alive and well. Two have normal renal function, and one required a renal transplant at 3 years of age. With our current selection criteria, we feel that an occasional, highly selected fetus with otherwise lethal obstructive uropathy will be salvaged by open fetal surgery.

The Fetus with Congenital Cystic Adenomatoid Malformation

Congenital cystic adenomatoid malformation (CCAM) represents a spectrum of disease characterized by cystic lesions of the lung. In the majority of cases, CCAM becomes manifest after birth and is easily treated *ex utero.* These cases present as pulmonary masses causing either respiratory difficulty or recurrent pulmonary infections in infancy or childhood. The more severe end of the spectrum has more recently been appreciated and is a lesion that results in fetal hydrops, pulmonary hypoplasia, and fetal demise.

Natural History

We have proposed a classification system of CCAM based on prenatal sonographic appearance, gross anatomy, and prognosis (Adzick et al., 1985a). CCAMs can be divided into macrocystic or microcystic types depending on the presence or absence of single or

multiple cysts greater than 5 mm in diameter respectively. The more favorable macrocystic lesion usually is not associated with hydrops and has a more favorable prognosis. The microcystic or solid lesion, however, frequently induces fetal hydrops and rapid fetal demise. The classification of micro- or macrocystic appearance remains somewhat predictive; however, we have had experience with macrocystic lesions that have resulted in fetal hydrops and, in a few cases, resolved before birth.

The invariably fatal outcome seen with large CCAMs is related to several factors, including development of hydrops, hypoplasia of the lung secondary to prolonged compression *in utero,* and in some cases, lack of early diagnosis and immediate postnatal surgery. The etiology for hydrops remains speculative, but the condition most likely results from vena caval obstruction or cardiac compression from extreme mediastinal shift caused by these lesions (Golladay and Mollitt, 1984). We therefore postulated that prenatal resection of the pulmonary mass might reverse the hydrops and allow sufficient lung growth to permit survival in these selected severe cases. We have demonstrated in the lamb model that *in utero* pulmonary resection is feasible and that compensatory growth of the opposite lung occurs (Adzick et al., 1986b).

Management

These patients should undergo ultrasonagraphy to confirm the diagnosis, evaluate for polyhydramnios or hydrops, determine the appearance of the lesion, and rule out other life-threatening anomalies. The majority of these patients have isolated small lesions, without hydrops, and are best treated by surgical resection after term delivery. In the early gestational fetus with a large CCAM, there is a much higher probability of trouble, and frequent serial sonography should be performed. Recommendations for management depend upon the presence or absence of associated hydrops and gestational age. If pulmonary maturity is established and hydrops evolves, the fetus should be emergently delivered and immediately resected *ex utero*. Fetuses that are between 28 weeks and lung maturity with evolving hydrops should undergo an attempt at steroid-induced lung maturation and immediate delivery with surfactant administration and emergent surgical resection if the hydrops is severe. The immature fetus (<28 weeks) with a large CCAM and evolution of hydrops should be immediately considered for *in utero* resection of the tumor.

In utero therapy has been attempted in selected cases of CCAM (Harrison et al., 1990a). Experience with attempted thoracentesis (four cases) or placement of thoracoamniotic shunts (three cases) in cases of macrocystic CCAM with associated hydrops resulted in rapid reaccumulation of cyst fluid or inadequate decompression to resolve the hydrops. A summary of six cases of open fetal surgery reveals that four out of six severely hydropic fetuses have been salvaged by open surgical resection of their CCAM and are currently doing well with a follow-up of 5 to 20 months, with two of the six cases being lost owing to preterm labor.

The Fetus with Congenital Diaphragmatic Hernia

Congenital diaphragmatic hernia (CDH) is perhaps the ultimate example of a simple anatomic defect that has devastating physiologic consequences during fetal development (Harrison et al., 1981b). The diaphragmatic defect is easily repaired after birth, but many patients with CDH will die with pulmonary insufficiency, despite optimal postnatal care, because their lungs are too hypoplastic to support extrauterine life. Pulmonary hypoplasia secondary to CDH appears to be secondary to compression of the developing fetal lungs by herniated abdominal viscera. The rationale for prenatal decompression of the fetal lungs is to allow lung development *in utero* and prevent pulmonary hypoplasia.

Development of an Experimental Model

A fetal lamb model was developed in which a balloon was progressively inflated in the left hemithorax of fetal lambs over the last trimester to simulate compression of the growing fetal lung by abdominal viscera (Harrison et al., 1980a). Lambs with inflated thoracic balloons deteriorated rapidly at term delivery and died of respiratory insufficiency despite maximal respiratory support, whereas deflation of the balloon (simulating *in utero* repair) midway through the third trimester resulted in sufficient lung growth to assure survival in all corrected lambs following delivery.

Simulated correction produced a significant increase in lung weight, air capacity, compliance, and area of the pulmonary vascular bed (Harrison, et al., 1980b).

Artificially created diaphragmatic defects in fetal lambs produce the same degree of pulmonary hypoplasia as the inflated balloon. Initial attempts at operative repair in the fetal lamb failed because increased intra-abdominal pressure secondary to replacement of herniated viscera into the abdomen caused umbilical venous compression and fetal demise. This problem was solved by placement of an abdominal Silastic patch to enlarge the abdomen and prevent increased intra-abdominal pressure after CDH repair. In contrast to unrepaired controls, repaired lambs survive at term and, at sacrifice, the lungs are well expanded as well as much larger and histologically mature (Harrison et al., 1981c; Soper et al., 1984). Fetal surgical repair ameliorates vascular changes and permits compensatory lung growth and development. The severity of pulmonary hypoplasia is determined by the timing, duration, and degree of visceral herniation.

Natural History

In general, the mortality rates associated with prenatally diagnosed CDH have been approximately 70 to 90 per cent (Adzick et al., 1985b; Benacerraf and Adzick, 1987; Sharland et al., 1992). After exclusion of cases with associated lethal anomalies or electively aborted, isolated CDH is associated with a mortality of 60 to 80 per cent, with few if any survivors if diagnosed prior to 24 weeks. Taken in combination, these studies show that the natural history of CDH is dismal in spite of optimal postnatal treatment. They also suggest that prenatally diagnosed CDH is not uniformly lethal and that better selection criteria for poor outcome are needed.

Defining prognostic criteria for individual cases of fetal CDH is difficult. Clearly there are prenatally diagnosed cases that do well with conventional therapy and therefore do not need fetal surgery, whereas others are beyond salvage by fetal surgery. Although not all agree, our experience suggests that the most important prognostic indicator is early gestational diagnosis. Unfortunately polyhydramnios, which is associated with poor outcome (Adzick et al., 1985b), usually occurs late in gestation and is therefore rarely useful in the selection for *in utero* repair. Early appearance of a large volume of visceral herniation, as suggested by the presence of herniated stomach and left lobe of the liver in the fetal chest and quantified by a decreased lung-to-thorax ratio at the level of a four-chamber view of the heart, appears to be associated with a poor prognosis. Although a fetus diagnosed prior to 24 weeks with a large volume of visceral herniation present has a dismal prognosis, there are exceptions who will survive with conventional management. Better selection criteria are therefore needed. With the current poor criteria, a minority of prenatal CDH fetuses actually undergo fetal surgery.

Management

All fetuses with CDH diagnosed prior to 28 weeks should undergo a detailed ultrasonography, amniocentesis or percutaneous umbilical blood sampling for karyotype determination, and a fetal cardiac echo to exclude other anomalies (Fig. 25–2). If an isolated CDH is present, detailed prognostic evaluation should be performed. The presence of early gestation (<24 weeks), stomach or liver in the chest, a low lung-to-thorax ratio, and/or the early appearance of polyhydramnios place the fetus in an early/severe category with a dismal prognosis. In these cases, fetal surgical repair is recommended in the context of a controlled/randomized trial (see below) to establish efficacy. When the fetus is equivocal by our prognostic criteria, appropriate parental counseling is provided, and the parents are allowed to choose fetal surgery or conventional management. Patients in the mild/late category are managed in a conventional fashion.

In the 3 years ending December 1991, 61 patients have been referred to our program for consideration of *in utero* repair, and fetal repair was attempted in 15 with severe isolated lesions diagnosed before 24 weeks gestation. Early experience was compromised by unexpected technical difficulties. Five fetuses died intraoperatively. With modifications in surgical technique, including combined thoracic and abdominal incisions and left lobar resection, these technical problems were overcome and the first survivals were achieved (Harrison et al., 1990b). Since that time, four of ten fetuses have survived and are now doing well at home. Further improvement in outcome will require improvement in the physiologic management of the maternal-fetal unit and improved methods of tocolysis. We are now initiating an evaluation of fetal surgery for treatment of CDH by means of a randomized controlled trial.

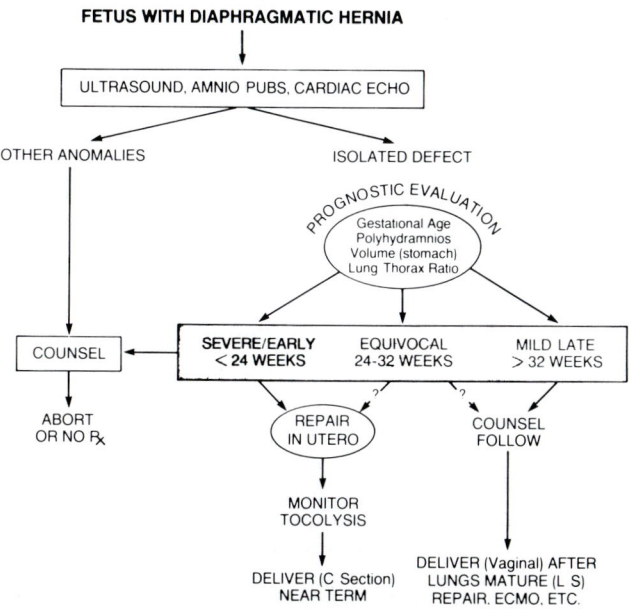

FIGURE 25–2. Management scheme for the fetus with CDH. (From Harrison MR: The fetus with a diaphragmatic hernia: Pathophysiology, natural history, and surgical management. *In* Harrison MR, Golbus MS, Filly RA (eds): The Unborn Patient. Philadelphia, WB Saunders Company, 1990, p 309.)

The Fetus with Sacrococcygeal Teratoma

Sacrococcygeal teratoma (SCT) is the most common tumor of the newborn, with an estimated incidence of 1 in 35,000 live births (Pantoja et al., 1976). The majority of cases remain asymptomatic *in utero* and are diagnosed after birth. Prenatal diagnosis is increasing, and this has allowed analysis of the natural history of SCT.

Natural History

A review of 27 cases of prenatally diagnosed SCT revealed that five cases were electively terminated, with 15 of the 22 remaining fetuses dying *in utero* or soon after birth (Flake et al., 1986). A more recent update confirmed the high mortality of fetal SCT, with 22 of 42 cases dying *in utero* or at birth (Bond et al., 1990). When placentomegaly or hydrops occurred, 15 of 15 fetuses died precipitously *in utero*. Presentation after 30 weeks was a relatively good prognostic sign, with six of eight fetuses surviving compared to one of 14 cases that presented prior to 30 weeks gestation (Flake et al., 1986). An additional prognostic indicator was that when a maternal indication for sonography was present 22 of 32 fetuses died, whereas nine of ten fetuses detected by routine screening sonography survived. Although diagnosis prior to 30 weeks gestation was associated with poor outcome, the incidental finding of SCT was favorable at any gestational age.

Death appears to result from secondary effects of the SCT rather than malignant invasion. Tumor mass and associated polyhydramnios frequently cause preterm labor and delivery, with fetal survival dependent upon fetal lung maturity. Massive hemorrhage into the tumor with secondary fetal exsanguination may occur spontaneously *in utero* or be precipitated by labor and delivery. Dystocia, secondary to tumor bulk, or tumor rupture may occur during vaginal delivery or cesarean section. In a few cases, placentomegaly and/or hydrops may occur, and high-output failure has been documented (Langer et al., 1989). The uniform association of precipitous death *in utero* after the appearance of placentomegaly/hydrops and confirmation of a vascular steal etiology of hydrops suggested our current belief that prenatal tumor resection might reverse hydrops and result in fetal salvage.

Management

All fetuses diagnosed with SCT undergo detailed sonographic evaluation to confirm the diagnosis and rule out associated anomalies (rare). An assessment of placental size, type of SCT, and the presence or absence of hydrops should be made. If diagnosis is serendipitous and the tumor small, an optimistic outlook can be given and the pregnancy followed with infrequent serial sonography to term vaginal delivery. If the tumor is large, or obstetric indications for sonography exist, a guarded prognosis should be given and the pregnancy followed by frequent sonography. If no placentomegaly or hydrops evolves, the fetus should be delivered by elective cesarean section to avoid dystocia or tumor rupture and hemorrhage. If placentomegaly/hydrops evolves after fetal pulmonary maturity is established, the fetus should be delivered by emergent cesarean section and treated *ex utero*. If placentomegaly/hydrops evolves prior to 28 weeks gestation and the tumor is anatomically amenable to easy resection (APSA type I SCT (Altman et al., 1974), we would recommend *in utero* tumor resection.

Clinical Experience

We have performed open surgery on only one fetus that presented with a large type I SCT, polyhydramnios, and placentomegaly at 21 weeks. Open fetal surgery was performed 3 weeks later owing to increasing fetal cardiac output (by echocardiography) and fetal hydrops, and the SCT was resected. The pregnancy ended 2 weeks later with preterm labor and neonatal demise due to prematurity, without evidence of residual SCT or hydrops.

This case was also complicated by signs of preeclampsia or the "mirror syndrome," a situation wherein the mother "mirrors" the fetal hydropic state with hypertension, edema, and gastrointestinal and renal dysfunction (Nicolay et al., 1964). We have observed massive placentomegaly in both cases wherein this syndrome complicated open fetal surgery of tumor masses, but have not seen the syndrome without placentomegaly in other fetal tumor resection cases.

The Fetus with Congenital Hydrocephalus

Although the rationale for prenatal decompression of congenital hydrocephalus remains compelling, there are a number of complicating factors that limit clinical application. First, fetuses with isolated high pressure hydrocephalus, which might benefit most from prenatal decompression, represent a minority of fetuses presenting with hydrocephalus. There is a high rate of associated CNS anomalies and secondary hydrocephalus which would not be expected to benefit from prenatal intervention. Frequently, diagnostic uncertainty exists making prediction of outcome difficult. In addition, the natural history of isolated congenital hydrocephalus has not been adequately defined in humans and experimental end points are difficult. Finally, results of 44 prenatal drainage procedures reported to the International Fetal Surgery Registry documented high procedure-related mortality (10.25 per cent), high residual neurologic morbidity (52.9 per cent), and a low rate of normal development in survivors (35.3 per cent) (Manning et al., 1986). We therefore currently advise against prenatal decompression pending improved accuracy of diagnosis, safety of intervention, and knowledge of the pathophysiology and natural history. The mature fetus with progressive hydrocephalus should be delivered early for *ex utero* decompression.

Future Directions in Prenatal Surgical Therapy

The remaining challenges in open fetal surgery involve primarily reduction of maternal and fetal risk.

It is unlikely that the list of anatomic diseases that are potentially amenable to fetal surgery (see Table 25–4) will expand significantly since the majority of anatomic abnormalities can be adequately treated after birth. However, the full potential of prenatal anatomic correction has not been realized because of prohibitive risk. For instance, cleft lip and palate could potentially be corrected *in utero* to take advantage of scarless fetal wound healing (Adzick and Longaker, 1992), or neural tube defects might best be closed *in utero*. These have not been attempted because of the prohibitive risk of fetal surgery for the treatment of nonlethal disease. If new surgical techniques, physiologic support systems, and tocolytic therapy can reduce the fetal and maternal risk to that of elective postnatal surgery, indications for fetal surgery could be liberalized.

Laparoscopic Approaches to Fetal Disease

The recent resurgence of interest in laparoscopic techniques has resulted in an explosion of new technology for laparoscopic procedures. However, the ability to perform major fetal surgery under direct vision through small puncture sites in the uterus has only recently become a realistic possibility. However, a number of modifications of current laparoscopic instrumentation and technique will be required to make fetal application possible. A large number of fetal procedures could possibly be done by laparoscopic technique (Table 25–6) reducing the maternal and fetal risk and the likelihood of preterm labor.

To determine feasibility of various procedures and to answer some of these questions, we have applied laparoscopic techniques experimentally in the sheep and monkey model. We have created and decompressed fetal obstructive uropathy in the fetal lamb and used an expandable wire stent to marsupialize the bladder. We have also created and repaired cleft lips in early gestational fetal lambs *in utero*, with subsequent documentation of scarless healing including regeneration of the muscle. Finally, we have placed long-term placental catheters in fetal monkeys by using laparoscopic technique without fetal or maternal compromise. Further developmental issues must be met before laparoscopic fetal surgery can be introduced clinically, but our experience has given us some cause for cautious optimism.

Maternal-Fetal Management and Risk

Fetal surgery is unique because of its inherent risk to both the mother and the fetus. Although maternal

TABLE 25–6. Endoscopic Fetal Surgery: Future Prospects

Catheters: vascular, bladder, chest
Vesicostomy
Cleft lip and palate
Amniotic bands
Parasitic twinning
Selective reduction pregnancy
Teratoma
Neural tube defects

safety is of overriding importance in any fetal surgical procedure, management of the maternal and fetal units are inseparable. Prior to human application, it was necessary to develop anesthetic, surgical, and tocolytic techniques, and to establish maternal safety by performing 102 fetal operations in 94 monkeys (Harrison et al., 1982a; Nakayama et al., 1984; Adzick et al., 1986a). Since that time, we have applied these techniques, and have continuously developed others, to improve maternal and fetal safety and to improve clinical outcome in approximately 40 fetal surgical cases.

Clinical Experience: Operative Technique

Maternal preparation begins with a 100-mg indomethacin suppository before operation and placement of arterial, central venous, and—if needed—Swan-Ganz catheters for intra- and postoperative maternal monitoring. We use postoperative indomethacin only as a last resort for control of intractable preterm labor because of its potential detremental effects on the fetus. Traditionally we have used halothane for uterine relaxation and for maternal and fetal anesthesia, but are now exploring other agents because of detrimental effects of halothane on placental perfusion. The current intra- and postoperative tocolytic regimen consists of a terbutaline drip, magnesium sulfate as required, and maintenance of optimal maternal volume status. The combination of gaseous anesthetic, tocolytic agents, and concern about maternal fluid-induced pulmonary edema have resulted in a number of cases of extreme maternal hypovolemia, which has been directly correlated with recalcitrant preterm labor. Our current approach uses a combination of invasive and noninvasive maternal-fetal monitoring techniques to maintain optimal volume status, optimal tocolysis, and optimal response to fetal physiologic compromise.

After induction of anesthesia, the mother is positioned supine with towels placed under her right side to avoid uterine caval compression. The uterus is exposed through a low transverse abdominal incision and delivered into the operative field. A large abdominal ring retractor serves a dual role (1) as fixed retraction to maintain exposure and (2) as an antenna for a fetal radiotelemeter. The position of the fetus and placenta are then determined by intraoperative ultrasonography and the hysterotomy planned to avoid the placenta and optimize fetal exposure. Excess amniotic fluid is aspirated through a trocar to allow uterine relaxation and uterine compression by the assistant's hand around the trocar. A small hysterotomy is performed with the electrocautery. After control of the membranes, the uterus can be opened hemostatically by use of a specially designed absorbable uterine stapler, which simultaneously compresses the myometrium and controls the membranes. The appropriate fetal part is then exteriorized for placement of fetal monitors; for obstructive uropathy, the lower extremities are brought out; for CDH, the left arm and thorax are exposed. Our current fetal monitoring consists of a pulse oximeter and a subcutaneously placed radiotelemeter. The radiotelemeter is left in the fetus until delivery and can continuously transmit fetal heart rate, temperature, and uterine amniotic fluid pressure to an external receiver. On completion of the fetal procedure, the fetus is returned to the uterine cavity and the amniotic fluid replaced with warm normal saline containing antibiotics. The uterine incision is meticulously closed, after removal of the staples, in three layers of absorbable sutures and fibrin glue to avoid postoperative amniotic fluid leak.

In the postoperative period the mother is intensively monitored in a fetal intensive care unit setting. Euvolemic status is maintained by clinical assessment, central pressure monitoring, and frequent correlation of clinical assessment with duplex scan examination of anatomy and flow of maternal and fetal vessels. This includes maternal uterine artery flow and caval filling, as well as fetal umbilical flow and waveform. The fetal heart is also examined at intervals to assess chamber size, contractility, and, when indomethacin is used, right-sided pressure (tricuspid regurgitation). Uterine contraction is monitored by tocodynamometry and, more recently, intrauterine pressure measurement. Tocolytic therapy with beta mimetics, magnesium sulfate, and as a last resort indomethacin is adjusted accordingly.

Maternal Outcome

There have been no maternal deaths and few major maternal complications in our entire series of nearly 40 patients. There was one case of mild pseudomembranous colitis secondary to antibiotics, which resolved with oral vancomycin. One patient developed an amniotic fluid leak from her hysterotomy site, presenting as abdominal pain several weeks after she returned home, and a second operation was required to close the leak. There have been three amniotic leaks, presenting as vaginal fluid leaks, which were presumably secondary to failure to control the membranes, with internal fluid dissection. These have not harmed the mother, but have resulted in oligohydramnios compromising the fetus. The maternal mirror syndrome has occurred in the two cases noted above, resulting in inability to control preterm labor and necessitating cesarean delivery of the fetus for maternal safety.

Effect on Reproductive Potential

A procedure to save a defective fetus which would render the mother incapable of having future normal children would be unacceptable in the majority of cases. Through retrospective analysis of detailed medical records maintained at the California Primate Research Center on 94 primates who had undergone fetal surgery, we found no reduction in fertility relative to colony controls (Adzick et al., 1986a; Adzick et al., 1985c). All of our patients who have attempted future pregnancies have been successful; thus far the count is nine normal pregnancies and normal children, all delivered by repeat cesarean section.

CONCLUSION

In summary, prenatal diagnosis has dramatically changed our perception of the fetus. The fetus is now appropriately considered a patient and fetal therapy for a wide variety of prenatally diagnosed abnormalities can be offered. Medical treatment of the fetus is currently the standard of care for a number of abnormalities and has potential for significant expansion. Its efficacy for many potential medical diseases, amenable to therapy, has yet to be established and further experimental work and clinical experience are required. More invasive therapeutic maneuvers involve significant risk for both fetus and mother, raising difficult questions about rights of the fetus and mother, risks and potential benefit. Because of the current high risk of open fetal surgery, it is imperative that efficacy be established by controlled clinical trials.

REFERENCES

Adzick NS, Harrison MR, Glick PL, et al: Fetal cystic adenomatoid malformation: Prenatal diagnosis and natural history. J Pediatr Surg 20:483, 1985a.

Adzick NS, Harrison MR, Glick PL, et al: Diaphragmatic hernia in the fetus: Prenatal diagnosis and outcome in 94 cases. J Pediatr Surg 20:357, 1985b.

Adzick NS, Harrison MR, Flake AW, et al: Automatic uterine stapling device in fetal surgery: Experience in a primate model. Surg Forum 36:479, 1985c.

Adzick NS, Harrison MR, Anderson JV, et al: Fetal surgery in the primate. III. Maternal outcome after fetal surgery. J Pediatr Surg 21:481, 1986a.

Adzick NS, Harrison MR, Hu LM, et al: Compensatory lung growth after pneumonectomy in fetal lambs: A morphometric study. Surg Forum 37:648, 1986b.

Adzick NS, Harrison MR, Hu L, et al: Pulmonary hypoplasia and renal dysplasia in a fetal lamb urinary tract obstruction model. Surg Forum 38:666, 1987.

Adzick NS, Longaker MT (eds): Fetal Wound Healing. New York, Elsevier Science Publishing, 1992.

Altman R, Randolf JG, Lilly JR. Sacrococcygeal teratoma. American Academy of Pediatrics Surgical Section Survey 1973. J Pediatr Surg 9:389, 1974.

Anderson WF: Prospects for human gene therapy. Science 226:401, 1984.

Anderson WF: News and comments. Clinical Protocols—The N2-TIL Human gene transfer clinical protocol. Hum Gene Ther 1:73, 1990.

Benacerraf B, Adzick NS. Fetal diaphragmatic hernia: Ultrasound diagnosis and clinical outcome in 19 cases. Am J Obstet Gynecol 156:573, 1987.

Bernstein A, Berger S, Huszar D, et al: Gene transfer with retrovirus vectors. In Setlow J, Hollaender A (eds): Genetic Engineering: Principles and Methods. New York, Plenum Press, 1985, 235 pp.

Bond SJ, Schmidt KG, Silverman NH, et al: Death due to high output cardiac failure in fetal sacrococcygeal teratoma. J Pediatr Surg 25:1287, 1990.

Clark J: The challenge of bone marrow transplantation. Mayo Clin Proc 65:111, 1990.

Crombleholme TM, Harrison MR, Langer JC, et al: Early experience with open fetal surgery for congenital hydronephrosis. J Pediatr Surg 23:1114, 1988.

Crombleholme TM, Harrison MR, Golbus, MS, et al: Fetal intervention in obstructive uropathy: Prognostic indicators and efficacy of intervention. Am J Obstet Gynecol 162:1239, 1990.

Docimo S, Luetic T, Crone RK, et al: Pulmonary development in the fetal lamb with severe bladder outlet obstruction and oligohydramnios: A morphometric study. J Urol 142:657, 1989.

Duncan BW, Harrison MR, Flake AW, et al: Immune response in hematopoietic chimeric rhesus monkeys. Surg Forum 42:373, 1991.

Duncan BW, Harrison MR, Crombleholme TM, et al: Effect of erythropoietic stress on donor hematopoietic cell expression in

chimeric rhesus monkeys transplanted in utero. Exp Hematol 20:350, 1992.

Ekhterae D, Crombleholme TM, Karson E, et al: Comparison of the efficiency of Neo® transfer into fetal and adult hematopoietic progenitors in vitro. Blood 72(Suppl 5):386a, 1988.

Flake AW, Harrison MR, Adzick NS, et al: Fetal sacrococcygeal teratoma. J Pediatr Surg 21:563, 1986a.

Flake AW, Harrison MR, Adzick NS, Zanjani ED: Transplantation of fetal hematopoietic stem cells in utero: The creation of hematopoietic chimeras. Science 233:776, 1986b.

Fricker F, Griffith BP, Hardesty RL, et al: Experience with heart transplantation in children. Pediatrics 79:138, 1987.

Glick PL, Harrison MR, Noall R, et al: Correction of congenital hydronephrosis in utero. III. Early mid-trimester urethral obstruction produces renal dysplasia. J Pediatr Surg 18:681, 1983.

Glick PL, Harrison MR, Adzick NS, et al: Correction of congenital hydronephrosis in utero. IV. In utero decompression prevents renal dysplasia. J Pediatr Surg 19:649, 1984.

Glick PL, Harrison MR, Adzick NS, et al: Management of the fetus with congenital hydronephrosis. II. Prognostic criteria and selection for treatment. J Pediatr Surg 20:376, 1985.

Golladay ES, Mollitt DL: Surgically correctable fetal hydrops. J Pediatr Surg 19:59, 1984.

Harrison MR, Jester JA, Ross NA: Correction of congenital diaphragmatic hernia in utero. I. The model: Intrathoracic balloon produces fatal pulmonary hypoplasia. Surgery 88:174, 1980a.

Harrison MR, Bressack MA, Churg AM: Correction of congenital diaphragmatic hernia in utero. II. Simulated correction permits fetal lung growth and survival at birth. Surgery 88:260, 1980b.

Harrison MR, Filly RA, Parer JRT, et al: Management of the fetus with a urinary tract malformation. JAMA 246:635, 1981a.

Harrison MR, deLorimier AA: Congenital diaphragmatic hernia. Surg Clin North Am 61:1023, 1981b.

Harrison MR, Ross NA, deLorimier AA, et al: Correction of congenital diaphragmatic hernia in utero. III. Development of a successful surgical technique using abdominoplasty to avoid compromise of umbilical blood flow. J Pediatr Surg 16:934, 1981c.

Harrison MR, Anderson J, Rosen MA, et al: Fetal surgery in the primate I. Anesthetic, surgical, and tocolytic management to maximize fetal-neonatal survival. J Pediatr Surg 17:115, 1982a.

Harrison MR, Golbus MS, Filly RA, et al: Fetal surgical treatment. Pediatr Ann 17:965, 1982b.

Harrison MR, Nakayama DK, Noall R, et al: Correction of hydronephrosis in utero. II. Decompression reverses the effects of obstrucution on the lamb lung and urinary tract. J Pediatr Surg 17:965, 1982c.

Harrison MR, Filly RA, Golbus MS, et al: Fetal treatment 1982. N Engl J Med 307:1651, 1982d.

Harrison MR, Ross NA, Noall R, et al: Correction of congenital hydronephrosis in utero. I. The model: Fetal urethral obstruction produces hydronephrosis and pulmonary hypoplasia in fetal lambs. J Pediatr Surg 18:247, 1983.

Harrison MR, Slotnick RN, Crombleholme TM, et al: In utero transplantation of fetal liver haematopoietic stem cells in monkeys. Lancet 2:1425, 1989.

Harrison MR, Adzick NS, Jennings RW, et al: Antenatal intervention for congenital cystic adenomatoid malformation. Lancet 336:965, 1990a.

Harrison MR, Adzick NS, Longaker MT, et al: Successful repair in utero of a fetal diaphragmatic hernia after removal of herniated viscera from the left thorax. N Engl J Med 322:1582, 1990b.

Kantoff PW, Gillio A, McLachlin J, et al: Expression of human adenosine deaminase in non-human primates after retroviral mediated gene transfer. J Exp Med 166:219, 1987.

Kantoff PW, Flake AW, Eglitis MA, et al: In utero gene transfer and expression: A sheep transplantation model. Blood 73:1066, 1989.

Kohn D, Kantoff PW, Eglitis MA, et al: Retroviral-mediated gene transfer into mammalian cells. Blood Cells 13:285, 1987.

Krivit K, Shapiro E, Kennedy W, et al: Treatment of late infantile metachromatic leukodystrophy by bone marrow transplantation. N Engl J Med 322:28, 1990.

Krull F, Hoyer PF, Offner G, et al: Renal handling of magnesium in transplanted children under cyclosporin A treatment. Eur J Pediatr 148:148, 1988.

Langer JC, Harrison MR, Schmidt KG, et al: Fetal hydrops and demise from sacrococcygeal teratoma: Rationale for fetal surgery. Am J Obstet Gynecol **160**:1145, 1989.

Liley AW: Intrauterine transfusion of the foetus in haemolytic disease. Br Med J **2**:1107, 1963.

Linch DC, Rodeck CH, Jones HM, Brent L: Attempted bone marrow transplantation in a 17-week fetus. Lancet **2**:1453, 1986.

Manning FA, Harrison MR, Rodeck C: Catheter shunts for fetal hydronephrosis and hydrocephalus. N Engl J Med **315**:336, 1986.

Mason J, Ryan KJ: Fetal tissue transplantation research. Fetal Diagn Ther **5**:2, 1990.

Mavroudis C, Harrison H, Klein JB, et al: Infant orthotopic cardiac transplantation. J Thorac Cardiovasc Surg **96**:912, 1988.

Metcalf D, Moore MAS: Embryonic aspects of hemopoiesis. *In* Neuberger A, Tatum EL (eds): Frontiers of Biology-Hematopoietic Cells. Amsterdam, North Holland Publishing, 172 pp, 1971.

Muller F, Dumez Y, Dommergues M, et al: Can fetal urinary biochemistry predict postnatal renal function? Fetal Ther. In press.

Najarian J, Frey DJ, Matas AJ, et al: Renal transplantation in infants. Ann Surg **212**:353, 1990.

Nakayama DK, Harrison MR, Seron-Ferre M, et al: Fetal surgery in the primate. II. Uterine electromyographic response to operative procedures and pharmacologic agents. J Pediatr Surg **19**:333, 1984.

Nicolay K, Gainey HL: Pseudotoxemic state associated with severe Rh immunization. Am J Obstet Gynecol **89**:41, 1964

Pantoja E, Llobet R, Gonzales-Flores B: Retroperitoneal teratoma: Historical review. J Urol **115**:520, 1976.

Parkman R: The application of bone marrow transplantation to the treatment of genetic diseases. Science **232**:1373, 1986.

Schwartz R: Acquisition of immunologic self-tolerance. Cell **57**:1073, 1989.

Sharland G, Lockhart SM, Heward AJ, Allan LD: Prognosis in fetal diaphragmatic hernia. Am J Obstet Gynecol **166**:9, 1992.

Slavin S, Neparstek E, Ziegler M, et al: Intrauterine bone marrow transplantation for correction of genetic disorders in man. (Abstract) Exp Hematol **18**:658, 1990.

Soloman J: Fetal and Neonatal Immunology. Amsterdam, North Holland Publishing, 1971.

Soper R, Pringle KC, Scofield JC: Creation and repair of congenital diaphragmatic hernia in the fetal lamb: Technique and survival. J Pediatr Surg **19**:33, 1984

Sullivan K: Current status of bone marrow transplantation. Transplant Proc **21**:41, 1989.

Tagge E, Campbell DA Jr, Dafoe DC, et al: Pediatric renal transplantation with an emphasis on the prognosis of patients with chronic renal insufficiency since infancy. Surgery **102**:692, 1987.

Touraine J, Roncarolo MG, Royo C, et al: Fetal tissue transplantation, bone marrow transplantation, and prospective gene therapy in severe immunodeficiencies and enzyme deficiencies. Thymus **10**:75, 1987.

Touraine JL, Raudrant D, Royo C, et al: *In utero* transplantation of stem cells in bare lymphocyte syndrome. (Letter). Lancet **1**:1382, 1989.

Zanjani ED, Ascensao JL, Flake AW, et al: The fetus as optimal donor and recipient of hemopoietic stem cells. Bone Marrow Transplant **10**(Suppl 1):107, 1992.

CHAPTER

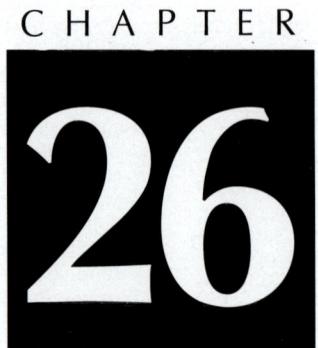

ENDOCRINOLOGY OF PREGNANCY

S. S. C. YEN, M.D., D.Sc.

The initiation, maintenance, and termination of pregnancy are dependent largely on the interaction of hormonal and neural factors. Proper timing of these neuroendocrine events within and between compartments (i.e., maternal, fetal-placental) is critical in directing the appropriate fetal growth and development and the timing of parturition.

Alterations of neuroendocrine-metabolic functions during pregnancy represent a most remarkable adaptive phenomenon in biological systems. Within the pregnant uterus, the fetal-placental-decidual unit produces extraordinary amounts of steroid and protein hormones, neuropeptides, and growth factors as well as cytokines. At present, there are more than 30 hormones identified, and their respective receptors have also been characterized. These substances appear to interact and to function in a manner resembling that of compressed hypothalamic-pituitary-target systems. It seems to be logical, and in some cases it has been proved, that these endocrine-paracrine-autocrine units conduct a unidirectional flow of nutrients from the mother to the fetus, to provide a favorable environment within the uterus for cellular growth and maturation, and to convey signals when the fetus is ready for extrauterine existence.

The fetus develops in an environment where respiration, alimentation, and excretory functions are provided by the placenta. Fetal tissue metabolism is directed largely to anabolism; body temperature is modulated by maternal metabolism, and fetal tissue thermogenesis is maintained at a basal level. Tissue and organ growth appear to be regulated by growth factors which function by autocrine or paracrine mechanisms during gestation (Fisher, 1986). In this milieu,

conventional endocrine control systems are largely modified, and newly added transient neuroendocrine systems appropriate to the intrauterine environment are evolved. Some insights into these remarkable adaptive systems are developed.

The production of steroid and peptide hormones and their relationship to placental neuropeptides and growth factors within the fetal-placental compartments are discussed. It is also our intent to provide an integrated functional perspective of the endocrine-metabolic adaptation during pregnancy.

ENDOCRINOLOGY OF IMPLANTATION

The sequence of morphologic and endocrinologic events that results in successful implantation of the blastocyst invokes both systemic and local mechanisms. The embryo initially depends on an inherent program of development, and the emergence of preimplantation signals soon follows. Nidation can be achieved only when the embryo and the endometrium reach a precise stage of synchronization. These processes in humans are prone to failure, as deduced from the high incidence of natural embryonic loss (50 per cent) and pregnancy loss after implantation (31 per cent) (Short, 1988; Wilcox et al., 1988).

Preimplantation Embryonal Signals

The human oocyte-corona-cumulus complex secretes relatively high levels of progesterone, estradiol, and prostaglandins (Shutt and Lopata, 1981). The corona cells may remain attached to the fertilized egg for 2 to 3 days both *in vitro* (Edwards et al., 1970) and *in vivo* (Ortiz and Croxatto, 1979), at which time the embryo is about to enter the uterine cavity. Preimplantation human embryos have the capacity to secrete hCG and to induce hCG and insulin-like growth factor (IGF-II) gene expressions (Fishel et al., 1984; Hug and Lopata, 1988; Öhlsson et al., 1989). The hormonal milieu for embryonic development within the oviducts may not be critical, since successful fertilization and early development can occur *in vitro* in the absence of oviductal factors (Edwards et al., 1980).

An embryo-derived platelet-activating factor (PAF) has been reported (O'Neill, 1985b). This factor appears to be responsible for the reduction of platelet count observed within 6 hours after fertilization and maintained for the first week of pregnancy in mice. This transient thrombocytopenia induced by an embryonic product also occurs in humans (O'Neill et al., 1985) and monkeys (Hearn, 1986). Although information is still limited, this phenomenon is speculated to be an embryonic signal for implantation since potent biologically active substances are released upon platelet activation, such as biogenic amines, histamines, serotonin, prostaglandins, and growth factors (O'Neill, 1985a; Rappolee et al., 1988).

Several growth factors—such as epidermal growth factor (EGF), transforming growth factor α (TGFα), TGF-β, and platelet-derived growth factor A (PDGF-A)—may also play a role as embryonic signals for implantation. Expressions of PDGF-A, TGFα, and TGF-β genes in preimplantation mouse embryos have been demonstrated (Nexo et al., 1980). Both EGF and TGFα and their common receptors have been mapped in human embryos (Hofmann et al., 1992). TGFα synthesized by the preimplanted embryos may stimulate angiogenesis and mitosis (Hofmann et al., 1992; Folkman and Klagsbrun, 1987). Since trophoblasts of preimplantation embryos grown in culture are shown to express TGFα/EGF receptors, TGFα may thus influence both embryonic and endometrial cells before implantation (Hofmann et al., 1992; Folkman and Klagsbrun, 1987). Experimental evidence also implicates insulin, IGF-II, and retinal binding protein (BP for vitamin A) in the development of preimplanted embryos (Öhlsson et al., 1989; Hemming et al., 1992; Liu et al., 1990). These growth factors are derived from embryos and demonstrate a paracrine/autocrine mode of action.

Embryonic-Maternal Interaction

Implantation is not a single event, but lasts for at least one week—from attachment and penetration of the blastocyst to the onset of decidua reaction in the endometrium. Although similar in the general pattern, there is considerable variation among species. In humans, the blastocyst is completely embedded into the endometrium—the interstitial implantation (Hearn, 1986). This process requires penetration of the firm basement membrane before the blastocyst enters the uterine decidua. The expression of type IV collagenase, a proteolytic enzyme, is increased at the time of implantation and may serve as a penetrating factor (Turpeenniemi-Hujanen et al., 1992).

Maternal recognition of the fetal semi-allograft invokes an immune response. Maternal decidua, which is in direct contact with fetal trophoblast, contains a relatively large number of macrophages and lymphocytes (Bulmer and Johnson, 1985), and decidua is a source of interleukin-1 (Romero et al., 1989). These cell types are capable of complex immunologic interactions, including allograft recognition, which is mediated in part by various cytokines and the major histocompatibility cell surface antigens (Unanue and Allen, 1987). Consequently, the regulation of cytokine production and major histocompatibility antigen expression at the maternal-fetal interface may play an important role in maternal immunologic recognition of the fetus and its subsequent survival.

Interleukin-1 (IL-1) is an immunoregulatory protein whose biological properties include stimulation of T-cell cytokine production, T- and B-cell proliferation, and foreign antigen recognition (Dinarello, 1988). There are two forms of IL-1, IL-1α and IL-1β, which have identical biological activities but are distinctly separate peptides encoded by separate genes (Dinarello, 1988).

HLA-DR is a major histocompatibility type II cell-surface antigen found mainly on activated lymphocytes and cells of monocyte-macrophage lineage. Antigen-presenting cells, many of which are tissue macrophages, couple foreign antigens to HLA-DR and then externalize the immune complex to the cytoplasmic membrane, where it is recognized by T and B lymphocytes (Unanue and Allen, 1987). The presence of HLA-DR-bearing cells in decidua has been demonstrated by immunohistochemistry (Bulmer and Johnson, 1985). Both HLA-DR and IL-1 expression are important for effective foreign antigen recognition and subsequent lymphocyte activation and proliferation (Kauma et al., 1990). The immunologic events during pregnancy are discussed in detail in Chapter 6.

Chorionic Gonadotropin (hCG)

The first decisive signal from the embryo to the maternal compartment is the secretion of hCG, and it appears in maternal circulation soon after implantation (9 days after ovulation) (Fig. 26–1). In fact, hCG is being secreted by the preimplantation embryos cultured *in vitro* (Fishel et al., 1984; Hug and Lopata, 1988). Incubation of hatched blastocysts with antiserum to β-hCG prevents embryonic attachment and causes embryo lysis, an observation that suggests that hCG may have a paracrine or autocrine function in the embryo in addition to its well-recognized role in sustaining corpus luteum function (Hearn, 1986).

CORPUS LUTEUM OF PREGNANCY

Following implantation, the hCG secreted by the trophoblast appears in the maternal circulation almost immediately and rescues corpus luteum function that otherwise would regress. A rise in circulating proges-

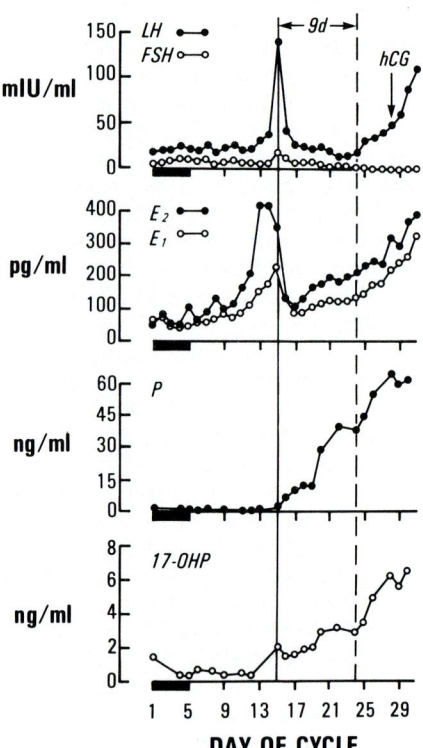

FIGURE 26–1. Hormonal patterns of a conception cycle in which hCG may be detectable in blood 9 days after LH peak. Note the rise of steroid hormones produced by the corpus luteum of early pregnancy.

amounts of *inhibin*. It has been demonstrated that pharmacologic rescue of the corpus luteum by hCG results in an increased inhibin production (Illingworth et al., 1990). As with relaxin, inhibin secretion by the corpus luteum of early pregnancy is limited in duration. As pregnancy advances, both inhibin and relaxin are produced by the decidual fetal membranes and placental tissue (McLachlan et al., 1987a, 1987b; Sakbun et al., 1990). The role of corpus luteum inhibin secretion is not entirely clear, but the suppression of pituitary FSH secretion to ensure the absence of folliculogenesis would be important.

Luteal-Placental Shift

Although the corpus luteum may continue to produce small amounts of progesterone for the duration of pregnancy, its functional capacity diminishes after the seventh week of gestation (Kemp and Niall, 1984; Johansson, 1969; Tulchinsky and Hobel, 1973). At this time, the luteal-placental shift occurs, by which the placental trophoblast and decidua assume the role of progesterone production and continue to be the principal source until parturition (Fig. 26–4). Thus, ovariectomy or corpus luteum removal before the eighth week of gestation invariably results in abortion (Csapo et al., 1973) but has no influence on the course of gestation if performed after the ninth week. The precise time course for these changes is given in Table 26–1.

terone, 17α-hydroxyprogesterone, and estradiol and estrone levels reflects the continued and augmented corpus luteum activity in response to hCG stimulation (Fig. 26–1). In addition, hCG appears to be responsible for the biosynthesis and secretion of relaxin and inhibin by the corpus luteum of early pregnancy.

Relaxin, a peptide hormone, is composed of A and B chains with a connecting peptide (C peptide). The structure of relaxin has remarkable similarities to insulin and insulin-like growth factors (Fig. 26–2) (Kemp and Niall, 1984). The human corpus luteum contains biologically active relaxin (Weiss et al., 1979). There are two genes (H1 and H2) for human relaxin, and both are located on chromosome 9. The transcription appears to be limited to the H2 gene in the corpus luteum of pregnancy (Kemp and Niall, 1984; Hudson et al., 1984). Serum relaxin concentration rises during the mid-luteal phase, reaching a maximal level of about 50 pg/ml 10 to 12 days after ovulation (Fig. 26–3) (Stewart et al., 1990). Thus, relaxin lags behind progesterone secretion by about 6 to 9 days. In a conception cycle, there is a rapid rise in relaxin parallel to that of hCG (Fig. 26–3). Exogenous hCG can induce relaxin secretion by the mature corpus luteum between days 8 and 10 after ovulation (Quagliarello et al., 1980). This early-appearing ovarian relaxin may function in conjunction with progesterone to reduce spontaneous uterine activity. Thus, relaxin plays a role in early pregnancy maintenance (Bigazzi and Nardi, 1981).

The corpus luteum of pregnancy secretes increasing

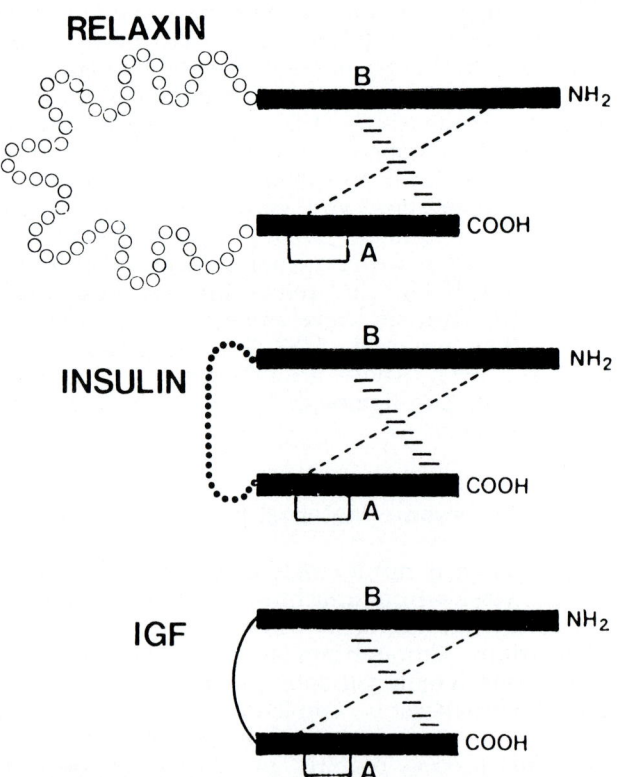

FIGURE 26–2. Diagrammatic depiction of the structure similarities among relaxin, insulin, and insulin-like growth factor.

FIGURE 26–3. Relaxin secretion by the early pregnancy corpus luteum and its relationship to the increments of hCG. *A,* Relaxin concentrations in a non-conceptive cycle followed by a conceptive cycle in the same subject. *B,* The relative changes in relaxin and hCG levels during a conceptive cycle; hCG values above 100 mIU/ml were off the scale. (Adapted from Stewart DR, Celniker AC, Taylor CA Jr, et al: Relaxin in the peri-implantation period. J Clin Endocrinol Metab **70:**1771, © by the Endocrine Society, 1990.)

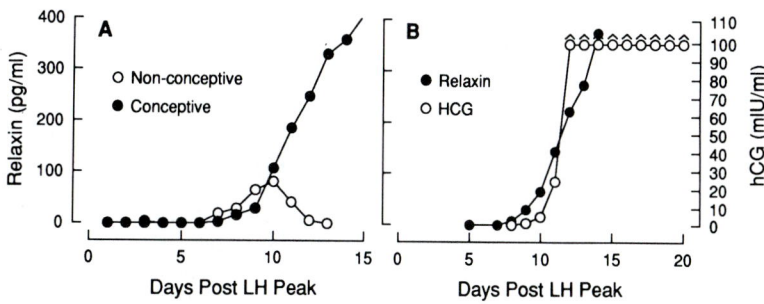

Effects of the Antiprogesterone (RU486)

The synthetic 19-nor steroid RU486 (mifepristone) (17β-hydroxy-11β-[4-dimethylaminophenyl]-17α[1-propynyl] estra-4, 9-dien-3-one) is a potent progesterone antagonist that inhibits the uterine actions of progesterone and has pronounced antifertility effects (Baulieu, 1989). In large doses, RU486 also has anti-glucocorticoid property. It acts by competitive antagonism of progesterone at the receptor level, with blockade of its biological effects in reproductive tissues including endometrium and cervix, and at the hypo-thalamic-pituitary level (Baulieu, 1989; Garzo et al., 1988). In normally cycling women at the mid-luteal phase, administration of RU486 induces premature menstruation (Garzo et al., 1988; Schaison et al., 1985; Shoupe et al., 1987). RU486 (600 mg), when administered to women during early pregnancy (49 days from last menstrual period) and followed 36 to 48 hours later by the administration of prostaglandin analogues, results in expulsion of the placenta within 4 to 19 hours and a fall in serum hCG with a 96 per cent overall success rate of pregnancy termination (Silvestre et al., 1990). The fall in hCG secretion caused by RU486 has been attributed to its inhibitory action on the decidualized endometrium and the detachment process that precedes expulsion of the placenta, but may also reflect an inhibitory effect exerted directly on the trophoblast as demonstrated *in vitro* (Das and Catt, 1987).

THE FETAL-PLACENTAL UNIT AS AN ENDOCRINE ORGAN

The placenta has evolved as an essential part of the reproductive organ in mammals and serves to transmit nutrients to the fetus, to excrete waste products into the maternal blood, and to modify maternal metabolism at various stages of pregnancy by means of its hormones. The human placenta achieves its mature architecture by the end of the first trimester of pregnancy. The functional unit is the *chorionic villus,* which consists of a central core of loose connective tissue and abundant capillaries connecting it with the fetal circulation. Around this core are two layers of trophoblast, an outer syncytium (*syncytiotrophoblast*) and an inner layer of discrete cells (*cytotrophoblast*), the latter becoming discontinuous as the placenta matures.

Cytotrophoblasts undergo morphologic and functional differentiation. Time-lapse cinematography reveals that after 24 to 48 hours in culture, cytotrophoblasts are transformed into multicellular aggregates (intermediate trophoblast), and at 72 hours these mononuclear cells fuse into multinuclear syncytiotrophoblasts (Kliman et al., 1986). The presence of syncytiotrophoblasts is associated with the appearance of immunocytochemical staining for hCG, chorionic somatomammotropin (hCS), and pregnancy-specific β₁-glycoprotein (SP₁). However, cytotrophoblasts also exhibit the capacity to produce hCG and hCS (Kliman et al., 1986; Kao et al., 1988).

The developing fetus and its placenta form an interdependent partnership in regulating the endocrine-metabolic processes during the course of pregnancy. This functional relationship, commonly known as the *fetal-placental unit,* is a unique endocrine system that produces a large number of hormones, including peptide, neuropeptides, steroid hormones, and peptide growth factors, many of which are identical with or at least mimic those produced by the hypothalamic-hypophyseal-target system.

Estrogens, androgens, and progestins are involved in pregnancy from implantation to parturition. They

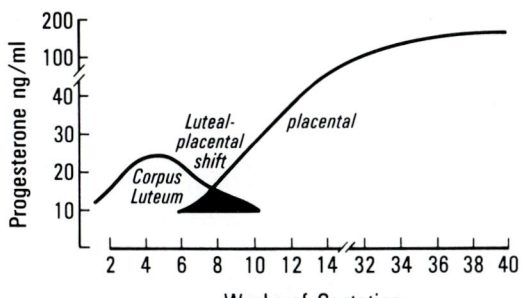

FIGURE 26–4. A shift of progesterone production from the corpus luteum to the placenta occurs at approximately the eighth to ninth week of gestation. The black area represents the estimated duration for this functional transition.

TABLE 26–1. Characteristics of Spontaneous Successful Human Pregnancies

Time of implantation relative to LH surge:	
Start (hCG = 0.5 μ/l)	8.4 ± 0.7 days
Finish (change of slope)	11.1 ± 0.7 days
Duration of active implantation	2.7 ± 0.3 days
hCG concentration doubling times:	
Peri-implantation	12.4 ± 2.4 h
After implantation	30.9 ± 3.7 h

Adapted from Lenton EA, Woodward AJ: The endocrinology of conception cycles and implantation in women. J Reprod Fertil **36**(Suppl):1, 1988.

are synthesized and metabolized in complex pathways involving the fetus, the placenta, and the mother.

FORMATION OF PROGESTERONE (MATERNAL-PLACENTAL UNIT)

Progesterone is synthesized by the placenta through hydroxylation from maternal cholesterol. This process is independent of fetal precursor and steroidogenesis, as evidenced by the unchanged plasma progesterone and urinary pregnanediol levels following fetal death *in utero* (Cassmer, 1959). Thus, the formation of progesterone by the placenta, with an almost unlimited amount of maternal substrate, represents an endocrine process that is exclusively a maternal-placental interaction.

Low-Density Lipoprotein (LDL) Pathway (Biosynthesis of Progesterone)

Cholesterol is carried in the maternal circulation by lipoproteins consisting of particles coated by proteins and is packaged within triglycerides and cholesterol esters. Specific high-affinity receptors for low-density lipoprotein (LDL) but not high-density lipoprotein (HDL) are present on the cell membrane of the trophoblast (Simpson and MacDonald, 1981; Cummings et al., 1982). After LDL is bound to surface receptors, it is internalized through the process of active endocytosis (Fig. 26–5). Within the trophoblast, LDL particles fuse with lysosomes where hydrolysis by lysosome enzyme occurs; the protein cast gives rise to amino acids. Hydrolysis of cholesterol esters gives rise to fatty acids and cholesterol (Winkel et al., 1980). The liberated cholesterol is then available to serve as precursor for C_{21} pregnenolone formation, the result of a

cytochrome P450 enzyme-dependent side-chain cleavage ($P450_{SCC}$) and hydroxylation by mitochondrial enzymes (Hall, 1986). Pregnenolone is readily converted to progesterone in a reaction catalyzed by 3β-hydroxysteroid dehydrogenase and Δ^5-Δ^4-isomerase enzymes (3β-HSD) (Ryan et al., 1966; Grimshaw et al., 1983).

Regulation

Progesterone formation appears to be modulated by β_2-adrenergic signal (stimulatory), hCG (stimulatory), and high concentrations of dehydroepiandrosterone and its sulfate (inhibitory). The enhancement of progesterone formation by β_2-adrenergic stimulation is mediated by intracellular Ca^{++} and cAMP (Kasugai et al., 1987). Accumulation of mRNAs encoding the hCG subunits and the $P450_{SCC}$ enzyme in response to cAMP accounts for the increase in hCG and progesterone biosynthesis (Branchaud et al., 1983). While the placental GnRH stimulates hCG secretion, it inhibits the production of progesterone by cultured trophoblasts (Branchaud et al., 1983; Ringler et al., 1989). Androgens attenuate progesterone production by the inhibitory effect on 3β-HSD enzyme, thereby reducing the formation of the progesterone from pregnenolone (Ryan et al., 1966; Grimshaw et al., 1983). In addition, estrogen may exert a tropic action on progesterone biosynthesis by regulating receptor-mediated LDL uptake (Albrecht and Pepe, 1990).

The human placenta is endowed with receptors for insulin-like growth factors IGF-I and IGF-II, and both IGF-I and IGF-II are produced in the placenta (Fant et al., 1986; Han et al., 1988; Marshall et al., 1974; Massague and Czech, 1982). The relative abundance of IGF-II mRNA is considerably greater than that of IGF-I (Han et al., 1988; Voutilainen and Miller, 1987). IGF-I stimulates $P450_{SCC}$ activity by about 20 per cent in cytotrophoblast in culture. In syncytiotrophoblast, IGF-I enhances the formation of progesterone twofold, an effect observed only in the presence of estrogen (Albrecht and Pepe, 1990). The potential effect of IGF-II on progesterone formation is unknown at present.

Progesterone Secretion

The maternal plasma progesterone concentration rises from 40 ng/ml in the first trimester to 160 ng/ml in the third trimester of pregnancy (Johansson, 1969) (Fig. 26–6). During the first trimester of pregnancy, serum progesterone levels exhibit episodic secretion and a remarkable postprandial decline with maximal nadir of 15 per cent and 13 per cent 1 hour after initiation of lunch and dinner meals (Nakajima, 1990). In contrast to the meal-related decline, there is a nocturnal rise in progesterone levels. The significance of these variations is unclear. The metabolic clearance rate of progesterone during pregnancy is unaltered from that of nonpregnant women (about 2000 liters per day) (Lin et al., 1972). At term, the placenta produces approximately 250 mg of progesterone per day and secretes mainly (90 per cent) into the maternal compartment and partially (10 per cent) into the fetal circulation. Because of the relative size of the compartments, the plasma concentration in the fetus is sevenfold higher than the maternal level (Tulchinsky and Okada, 1975). In plasma, most progesterone is

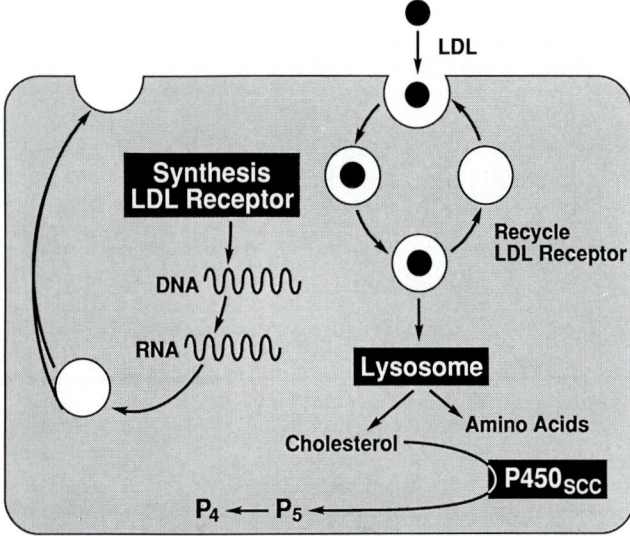

FIGURE 26–5. Pathways of LDL-cholesterol turnover and the biosynthesis of pregnenolone (P5) and progesterone (P4). The synthesis and recycling of LDL receptors are also depicted.

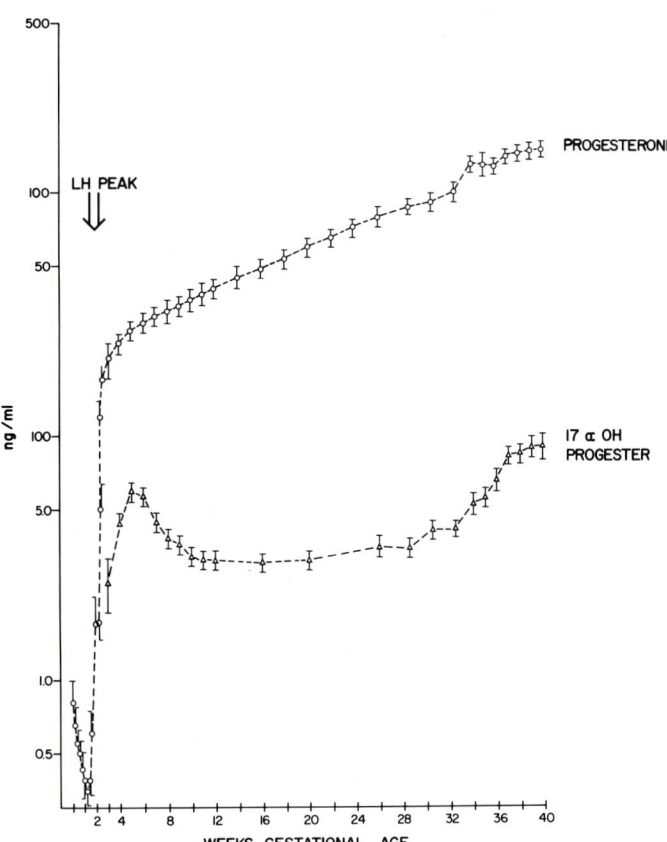

FIGURE 26–6. Relative circulating concentrations (mean ±SE) of progesterone and 17α-hydroxyprogesterone during the course of human pregnancy. (Courtesy of J. R. Marshall.)

bound to corticosteroid-binding globulin (CBG), and less than 10 per cent is in free form.

In contrast to serum progesterone levels, 17α-hydroxyprogesterone concentrations at mid-pregnancy are low and comparable to those observed during the luteal phase of the menstrual cycle (see Fig. 26–6). The placenta is unable to make 17-hydroxyprogesterone due to the *absence* of 17-hydroxylase activity. The substantial rise of 17α-hydroxyprogesterone after the 32nd week of gestation is largely due to the contribution by the fetal adrenal gland, which produces both 17α-hydroxyprogesterone and 17-hydroxypregnenolone (Tulchinsky et al., 1972). The latter compound can be converted by the placenta to 17α-hydroxyprogesterone. Thus, circulating levels of 17α-hydroxyprogesterone in late pregnancy reflect the functional activity of the fetal adrenal gland and the placenta transfer.

Function

The myometrium contains progesterone receptors, and progesterone is known to decrease uterine sensitivity to oxytocic stimulation. Thus, it works synergistically with relaxin (to be discussed) to reduce uterine motility and inhibit propagation of uterine contractions. This uterine quiescent effect of progesterone can be negated by the antiprogesterone RU486. Progesterone may also play a role in the coupling of bone resorption with bone formation by interaction with glucocorticoid receptors (Prior, 1990). In addition, progesterone may participate in the secretion of hCG and hCS, as well as progesterone itself; in cultured syncytiotrophoblasts, RU486 induces a dose-related inhibitory effect on the secretion of hCG, hCS, and progesterone. Its effects can be reversed by the addition of progesterone (Das and Catt, 1987).

FORMATION OF DEOXYCORTICOSTERONE IN PREGNANCY

Deoxycorticosterone (DOC), a potent mineralocorticosteroid, is elevated during pregnancy. Quantitative and time course studies reveal a two- to fivefold higher level of circulating DOC during the first trimester, followed by a progressive rise to levels of more than tenfold (1300 pg/ml) the nonpregnant value at term (Fig. 26–7) (Nolten et al., 1978; Parker et al., 1981). This marked elevation of circulating DOC during pregnancy is not derived from the adrenal secretion. It is produced by the kidney, where steroid 21-hydroxylase activity is present and converts plasma progesterone to DOC. The kidney 21-hydroxylase appears to be stimulated by estrogen (MacDonald et al., 1982). The rate of formation of DOC from plasma progesterone is proportional to the concentration of circulating progesterone in normal as well as in adrenalectomized

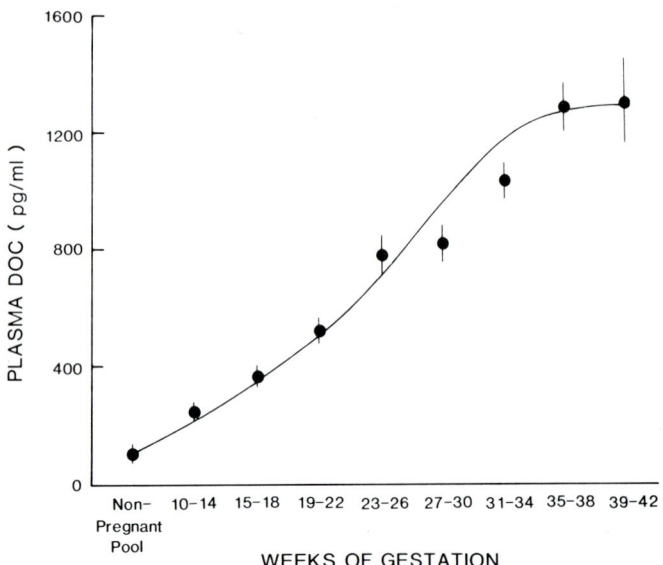

FIGURE 26–7. The progressive increase in plasma deoxycorticosterone (DOC) concentrations (mean ±SE) during the course of normal pregnancy. (Modified from Parker CR Jr, Everett RB, Whalley PJ, et al: Hormone production during pregnancy in the primigravid patient. II. Plasma levels of deoxycorticosterone throughout pregnancy of normal women and women who developed pregnancy-induced hypertension. Am J Obstet Gynecol **138**:626, 1980.)

subjects. This finding is consistent with the poor response of DOC to ACTH stimulation and dexamethasone suppression in late pregnancy. It should be noted, however, that there is marked individual variation in the rate of conversion of progesterone to DOC. Since DOC is a salt-retaining and hypertensive agent, it may play a role in the genesis of pregnancy-induced hypertension. However, DOC levels are not significantly elevated in women with this disorder (Parker et al., 1980).

FORMATION OF ESTROGENS (C_{18} STEROIDS)

The placenta represents the primary source of estrogen after 8 to 9 weeks of gestation. Four types of estrogens are produced by the placenta and the fetoplacental unit, and the formation of each follows unique pathways. Estradiol (E_2) and estrone (E_1) formations are dependent upon maternal and fetal contribution of androgens. The production of estriol (E_3) and estetrol (E_4) is governed exclusively by specific fetal androgenic precursors.

Estrone and Estradiol (E_1 and E_2)

The placenta lacks 17-hydroxylase and 17,20-desmolase activity (Diczfalusy, 1964) and therefore is unable to convert C_{21} compounds (progestins) to C_{19} steroids (androgens). Thus, the formation of E_1 and E_2 is dependent upon androgen precursors from the maternal and fetal adrenals. The placenta extracts dehydroepiandrosterone sulfate (DS) from the maternal and fetal circulations and, by hydrolyzing the sulfate (via sulfatase), converts it to free DHEA. The placenta is capable of converting DHEA to androstenedione (A) and testosterone (T), which are readily aromatized to form E_1 and E_2 (Fig. 26–8). E_1 and E_2, formed from circulating DS, are contributed to equally by the fetal and maternal adrenals and are released

mainly into the maternal circulation. Therefore, placental E_1 and E_2 production depends only partially on the availability of fetal precursors. Maternal serum T and A levels rise two- to threefold during pregnancy, and most of the serum T is bound to sex hormone–binding globulin (SHBG), the level of which is markedly elevated in the maternal compartment but very low in the fetal compartment regardless of the sex of the fetus (Fig. 26–9).

While maternal circulating levels of DS and DHEA do not change significantly during pregnancy, the production rates are increased. This paradox is due to the siphoning of circulating DHEA and DS by the placenta, resulting in a twice faster clearance in late pregnancy than in the nonpregnant state (Gant et al., 1971; Belisle et al., 1980). Thus, *the placenta functions as a sink for androgens which are irreversibly aromatized to estrogens*, a process of fundamental importance in pregnancy. The fetal adrenal produces DS in both the definitive and the fetal zones. This production is

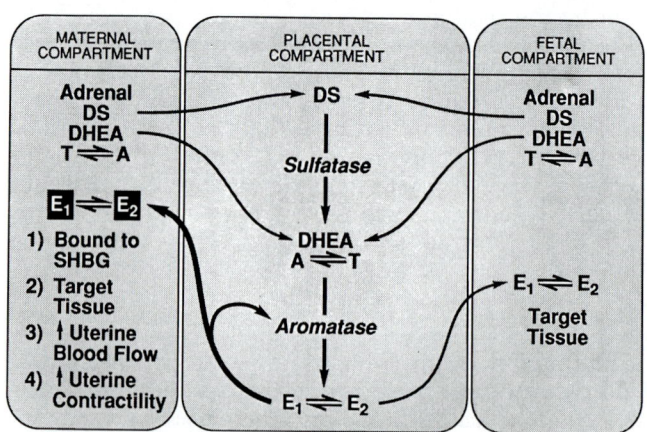

FIGURE 26–8. Diagrammatic illustration of the placental formation of estradiol (E_2) and estrone (E_1) from maternal and fetal androgen precursors—dehydroepiandrosterone (DHEA) and its sulfate (DS). T = testosterone; A = androstenedione.

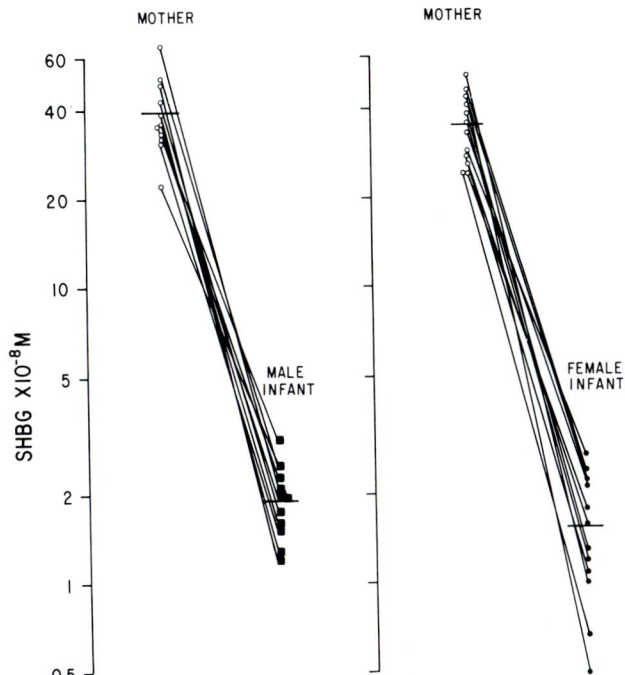

FIGURE 26–9. Sex hormone-binding globulin (SHBG) concentrations in paired samples from maternal and infant (cord blood) circulations. Note that there is no difference between male and female infants. (Courtesy of David Anderson.)

stimulated by hCG in early pregnancy, with a shift to ACTH stimulation after mid-gestation (Serón-Ferré et al., 1978).

This extensive extraction of androgens from maternal and fetal circulation provides a mechanism against excessive androgen action that otherwise might cause virilization of female fetuses. Thus, pregnancy in association with androgen-producing tumors, such as luteoma, does not usually cause virilization of the female fetus. However, the placenta is *not* capable of "aromatizing" synthetic 19-nor steroids, which are known to effect virilization *in utero*, causing female pseudohermaphroditism.

Because of the lack of 16-hydroxylase, the placenta cannot convert E_1 or E_2 to E_3 (Diczfalusy, 1964). Maternal serum E_2 levels rise throughout pregnancy until term, reaching 20 to 30 ng/ml (Tulchinsky et al., 1972). Sex hormone-binding globulin has a particularly high affinity for E_2, and hence total serum E_2 levels are higher than those of E_1 and E_3 (Fig. 26–10). However, the production of E_3 exceeds that of E_2 and E_1, as reflected by the urinary excretion rate of these three estrogens. Urinary excretion rates of E_1 and E_2 increase 100-fold from their preovulatory values to term. E_3, on the other hand, increases 1000-fold over the same period (Brown, 1956). The maternal liver metabolizes and conjugates E_1 and E_2, and only a small portion of each is converted to E_3.

Although the amount of placental secretion of E_1 and E_2 into the fetal circulation is small, the relative concentrations are high because of the smaller vascular compartment. To circumvent excessive estrogen effects, the fetus rapidly inactivates biologically active E_2 by hydroxylation and sulfurylation.

Estriol and Estetrol (E_3 and E_4)

The demonstration by Ryan in 1959 that the placenta contains an unlimited amount of aromatase enzyme has permitted a rapid advance in our understanding of estrogen formation by the placenta (Ryan, 1959). Because the placenta lacks 16-hydroxylase enzyme, it is essential that 16-hydroxylation of precursors be processed before reaching the placenta in order to achieve the formation of the 16-hydroxylated estrogen—E_3. The DS from the fetal adrenal is converted by the fetal liver to 16α-hydroxydehydroepiandrosterone sulfate (16α-OH-DS). This is the principal fetal contribution to E_3 biosynthesis (Magendantz and Ryan, 1964). In the placenta, 16α-OH-DS is cleaved by sulfatase to 16-OH-DHEA. The placenta converts 16-α-OH-DHEA initially to 16-OH-androstenedione and 16-OH-testosterone and then aromatizes these compounds to E_3 (Fig. 26–11). Thus, the fetus and placenta play a joint and obligatory role in the E_3 biosynthesis.

In the absence of fetal ACTH stimulation, there is little or no DS production by the fetal adrenal. This situation is found in congenital absence of the pituitary gland, in the anencephalic fetus, and when corticosteroids given to the mother cross the placenta and suppress fetal ACTH secretion. Levels of E_3 and E_4 are low or absent in cases of fetal death *in utero* and in placental sulfatase deficiency. In these instances, formation of E_1 and E_2 is in the lower range of normal, but E_3 is markedly reduced (Frandsen and Stakemann, 1961; Siiteri and MacDonald, 1963; Baulieu and Dray, 1963).

The placenta secretes E_3 mainly into the maternal circulation. In the mother, E_3 metabolism consists almost entirely of conjugation, and the steroid is then excreted in the urine as glucosiduronates. The urinary excretion rate of E_3 at term averages 30 mg/day.

The binding affinity of E_3 to estrogen receptors is similar to that of E_1 and E_2. However, the receptor retention time of E_3 is brief, and the biological activity is thus foreshortened. This reduced biological activity per molecule of E_3 is offset by the large quantity produced. Thus, E_3 is considered biologically important in estrogen-mediated events of pregnancy, i.e., increase in uterine blood flow (Resnik et al., 1974).

E_4 is 15α-hydroxyestriol, distinguished from E_3 by a fourth hydroxyl group on carbon atom 15. This fourth group is introduced predominantly in the fetal liver, catalyzed by the enzyme 15-hydroxylase, which is present only in fetal life (Bolte et al., 1964). E_4 secretion increases progressively only after mid-gestation. This uniquely fetal estrogen is capable of binding to estrogen receptors but is devoid of estrogenic activity (Gurpide et al., 1966; Martucci and Fishman, 1977). Thus, E_4 has been considered an endogenous antiestrogen, and it may have a "neutralizing" role, preventing the target cells, such as the fetal brain, from being exposed to massive amounts of free estrogen. In this context, the importance of endogenous antagonists as modulators of functional activity of target cells is viewed as a self-protective mechanism (Martucci and Fishman, 1977).

Because E_4 is entirely of fetal origin, it was hoped that its circulating level in the mother would accurately

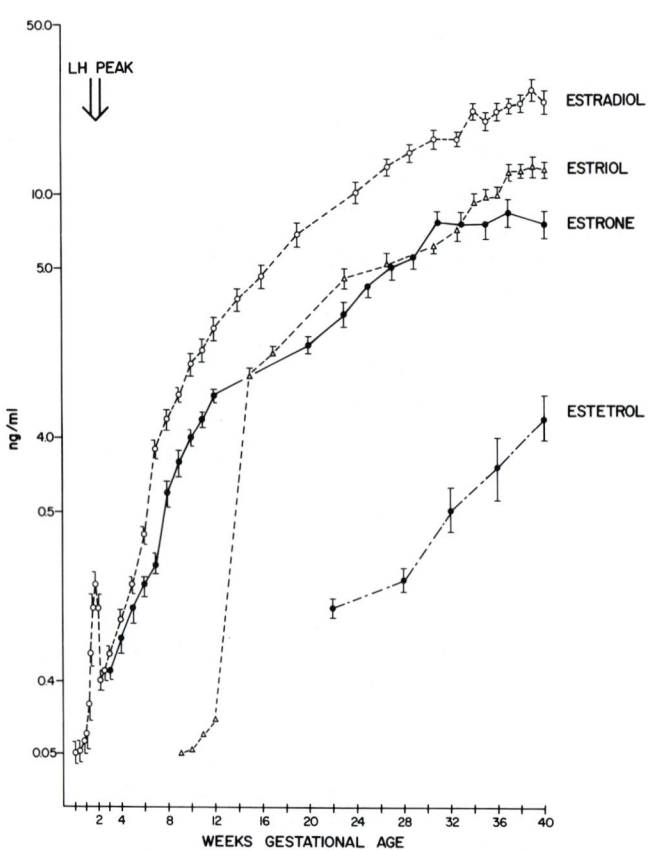

FIGURE 26–10. The relative concentrations (mean ±SE) and the incremental patterns of the four major estrogens plotted in the log scale during the course of pregnancy. (Courtesy of John Marshall.)

reflect fetal status; however, clinical experience has shown that plasma E_4 measurements are not useful for fetal monitoring (Tulchinsky et al., 1975).

Paracrine and Autocrine Functions of Estrogen

On the basis of experiments conducted *in vivo* in pregnant baboons and *in vitro* with human placental tissue, it appears that estrogen plays a positive role in the regulation of progesterone biosynthesis. This local control via autocrine or paracrine actions is accomplished by two interdependent mechanisms; estrogen induces an increased LDL receptor uptake for LDL and promotes the cytochrome $P450_{SCC}$ enzymatic activity. These effects of estrogens may thus accelerate the biosynthetic pathways for progesterone production (Albrecht and Pepe, 1990). Substantial reduction of progesterone secretion can be achieved by the administration of an antiestrogen (MER-25) during the second half of pregnancy in baboons (Castracane and Goldzieher, 1986).

In addition, estrogen has been shown to enhance the transplacental metabolism of *cortisol* to its biologically inactive metabolite *cortisone*. During early to midgestation, the placental 11β-hydroxysteroid dehydrogenase (11β-HSD) catalyzes interconversion of cortisol and cortisone and favors the formation of cortisol. The passage of cortisol to the fetus inhibits the ACTH release by the fetal hypothalamic-pituitary unit and thus reduces cortisol synthesis by the fetal adrenal. With increasing estrogen production in the second

half of gestation, an enhanced 11β-HSD oxidative activity occurs, resulting in an increased placental conversion of cortisol to cortisone (Baggia et al., 1990). As a consequence, the fetal hypothalamic-ACTH axis becomes disinhibited, and cortisol secretion by the fetal adrenals is activated (Pepe et al., 1990). These data obtained *in vivo* in baboons strongly suggest that placental estrogen plays a role in enhancing the fetal adrenal function by converting cortisol to biologically inactive cortisone with advancing gestation.

Enzymes for Estrogen Biosynthesis

As shown in Figure 26–11, the conversion of androgen precursors and the sulfurylated C_{19} steroids such as DS to estrogens in the placenta involves the action of four enzymatic systems: (1) sulfatase (sulfohydrolase), (2) 3β-hydroxysteroid dehydrogenase Δ^5, Δ^4-isomerase (3β-HSD), (3) aromatase, and (4) 17β-hydroxysteroid oxidoreductase.

SULFATASE. Sulfatase was originally found in the placenta; its presence in the chorion, amnion, and decidua has also been described (Warren and French, 1965; Mitchell et al., 1984). The relative abundance of sulfatase accounts for the large quantity of estrogen formation, particularly E_3. It converts DS to DHEA and 16-OH-DS to 16-OH-DHEA. In this process, free Δ^5 androgens are made available for biosynthesis of estrogens, and thus sulfatase is a rate-limiting enzyme in the formation of estrogens by the placenta. Sulfatase is also important in the conversion of estrone-sulfate to free estrone. Fetal membranes and decidua at term appear to have an increased ability to hydrolyze estrone sulfate and lead to a rise in free estrone which, in turn, may influence myometrial contractility (Mitchell et al., 1984). Both sulfatase mRNA and immunoreactivity are localized in the rough endoplasmic reticulum of the syncytial trophoblast, and immunoreactivity is more abundant during the transition between first and second trimesters than in term placenta (Salido et al., 1990). Although the syncytial trophoblast originates from the cytotrophoblast, neither sulfatase immunoreactivity nor its mRNA is detected in the cytotrophoblast at any stage of placental development (Salido et al., 1990). Prolactin and oxytocin have been shown to stimulate this enzymatic activity in decidual cells isolated before onset of labor (Braverman and Gurpide, 1986).

3β-Hydroxysteroid Dehydrogenase Δ^5, Δ^4-**Isomerase (3β-HSD).** This enzyme catalyzes the conversion of Δ^5 steroid to Δ^4 steroid—pregnenolone to progesterone and DHEA to androstenedione, and it is found in both mitochondrial and microsomal fractions. Both dehydrogenase/isomerase activities of 3β-HSD have been co-purified from human placenta as a monomer peptide of about 41,000 daltons, and the dehydrogenase and isomerase activities are inseparable (Thomas et al., 1989). Recent availability of cDNA for 3β-HSD has permitted studies of the expression of this enzyme; a single enzyme in human placenta is capable of the biosynthesis of both C_{19} and C_{21} Δ^4-3 ketosteroids from their corresponding Δ^5-3β-hydroxysteroids (Van Luu et al., 1989; Lorence et al., 1990). 3β-HSD is present in abundance in the placenta and hence it is not a rate-limiting enzyme.

Aromatase. Aromatase cytochrome P450 belongs to a functionally related multigene family. This enzyme binds C_{19} steroid substrate and catalyzes a series of reactions resulting in the formation of a phenolic A ring. Thompson and Siiteri (1974a, 1974b) demonstrated that the process of aromatization requires both P450 aromatase and a flavoprotein, NADPH-cytochrome P450 reductase. The latter is a ubiquitous protein present in most cells and serves to transfer NADPH to P450 aromatase. The aromatization of 1 mol C_{19} steroid requires 3 mol each of oxygen and NADPH, and this process is through the stereospecific 1β, 2β-hydrogen elimination mechanism (Osawa et al., 1987).

By means of immunohistochemistry, aromatase is localized exclusively in the endoplasmic reticulum of the syncytiotrophoblasts (Fournet-Dulguerov et al., 1987). Two aromatase P450 genes appear to exist, and both are located on chromosome 15 (Chen et al., 1988). It remains to be determined whether both of the genes are expressed. The NADPH cytochrome P450 reductase has also been purified, and mRNA encoding this enzyme has been isolated and cloned (Gonzalez and Kasper, 1982). These new advances will permit studies in the regulation of gene expression of the aromatase system.

17β-Hydroxysteroid Oxidoreductase (17β-HOR). The interconversion of estradiol and estrone and of testosterone and Δ^4 androstenedione is catalyzed by 17β-HOR. Two 17β-HOR activities are present in the human placenta; one localized in microsomes recognizes with equal affinity for estradiol, testosterone, and 20α-dihydroxyprogesterone, and the second has preferential high affinity for estradiol (Blomquist et al., 1985; Blomquist et al., 1987). The cDNA encode human placental 17β-HOR has been cloned, and the gene is localized on chromosome 17 (Van Luu et al., 1989a). These substrate-specific enzymatic activities have recently been confirmed by the demonstration of two distinct mRNA species in human placenta (Van Luu et al., 1989b).

REGULATORY PEPTIDES, NEUROPEPTIDES, AND GROWTH FACTORS

Human Chorionic Gonadotropin (hCG)

Heterogeneity of hCG Molecules

Human chorionic gonadotropin (hCG) is a glycoprotein hormone which consists of a 92-amino acid α-subunit noncovalently bonded to a 145-amino acid β-subunit. The single gene for the α-subunit is mapped to the long arm of chromosome 6 (6q), whereas the subunit for β-LH and β-hCG resides on the long arm of chromosome 19 (19q 13.3) in a complex cluster (Naylor et al., 1983). This cluster actually contains a total of 7 hCG-β-like genes: one gene for β-LH along with six genes for β-hCG arranged in tandem (Policastro et al., 1986; Jameson and Lindell, 1988). Only two of the β-hCG genes (hCG-β5 and hCG-β3) are expressed in human placental tissue (Jameson et al., 1986), leaving the remaining genes that are not transcribed—pseudogenes (Jameson and Lindell, 1988).

The hormone (holo hCG) and its uncombined subunits (free hCGα and free hCGβ) are secreted by the trophoblast throughout normal gestation as well as by benign and malignant trophoblastic tumors. In addition to free subunits, different molecular forms and fragments of hCG that vary in their carbohydrate and/or peptide structure are found in biological fluids (Amano et al., 1988; Wang et al., 1988). In particular, a carboxyl-terminal peptide spanning the C-terminal

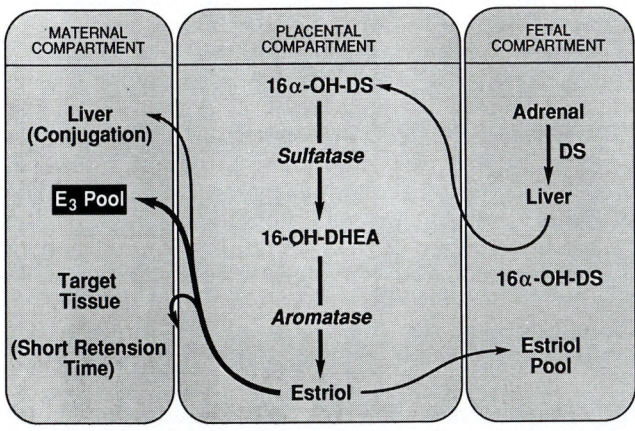

FIGURE 26–11. Diagrammatic illustration of placental formation of estriol (E_3) exclusively from the fetal precursor 16α-hydroxydehydroepiandrosterone sulfate (16α-OH DS).

portion of hCGβ (βCTP) and a low-molecular-weight form (M$_r$) of the β-subunit, called the β-*core fragment*, are present in the urine of pregnant women. The β-core fragment is composed of the β-6-40 disulfide linked to the 55-92 portion of hCGβ, and carbohydrate moieties are different from those of native hCGβ. It has no biological activity because it is unable to combine with the α-subunit (Kato and Braunstein, 1988; Berkin et al., 1988). The β-core fragment of β-subunit represents a major (70 to 90 per cent) form of immunoreactive hCG in urine during human pregnancy (Kato and Braunstein, 1988). In contrast, levels of both free hCGβ and β-core molecules in serum are very low (Blithe et al., 1988).

Although the precise origin of the β-core fragment is unclear, several studies indicate that it might be a degradation product of hCGβ in the kidney (Kato and Braunstein, 1988). In addition, there are other fragments of free and combined forms of the β-hCG. Thus, circulating β-subunit of hCG is modified by multiple fragmentations leading to microheterogeneity.

Human Chorionic Gonadotropin (hCG) Secretion

Human chorionic gonadotropin, produced by the syncytiotrophoblast, is secreted into the intervillous space. Serum hCG levels rise rapidly over the 10 days

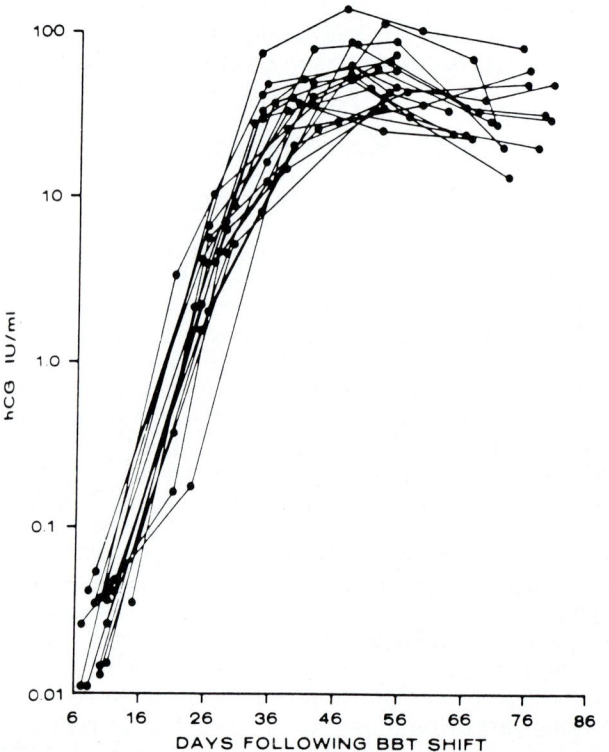

FIGURE 26–12. The exponential rise of circulating hCG following implantation and during first trimester of pregnancy. (From Braunstein GD, Kamdar V, Rasor J, et al: A chorionic gonadotropin-like substance in normal human tissues. J Clin Endocrinol Metab **49**:917, © by the Endocrine Society, 1979.)

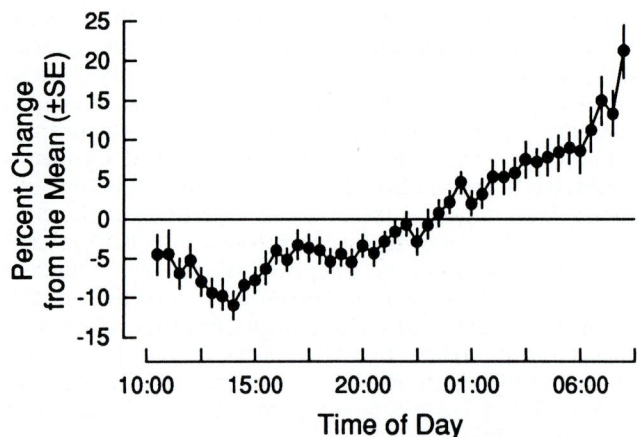

FIGURE 26–13. Diurnal pattern of hCG levels during first trimester of pregnancy. Data display per cent deviation from 24-hour mean. (From Nakajima ST, McAuliffe T, Gibson M: The 24-hour pattern of the levels of serum progesterone and immunoreactive human chorionic gonadotropin in normal early pregnancy. J Clin Endocrinol Metab **71**:345, © by the Endocrine Society, 1990.)

following implantation, with a mean doubling time of 30.9 hours (Pittaway et al., 1985; Lenton and Woodward, 1988; Braunstein et al., 1978). This exponential rise reaches a peak of about 100,000 IU/liter at the ninth week of gestation (Fig. 26–12) and is followed by a fall to 1000 IU/liter, where it remains until the end of pregnancy. In twin pregnancies, hCG levels 4 to 5 weeks after the last menstrual period are more than twofold higher than in singleton pregnancies (Jovanovic et al., 1977).

This pattern of secretion is a reflection of synthesis of subunits relative to holo hCG during the functional change of trophoblasts between early and late pregnancy placentas. Perfused placentas from early gestation released more hCG than α-subunit, whereas at 17 weeks, the amounts of α-subunit and hCG were equal. After 22 weeks of gestation, the placenta released more α-subunit than hCG, and at term the ratio of α-subunit to hCG release was 10:1 (Takemori et al., 1981). This changing ratio of subunits and hCG secretion between trophoblasts from early and late pregnancy was also demonstrated in culture and placental extracts (Kato and Braunstein, 1990).

Human chorionic gonadotropin (hCG) is secreted in episodic fashion and exhibits a 24-hour rhythm during the first trimester of pregnancy: a nadir at 1400 hours (12 per cent below the 24-hour mean), followed by a progressive rise in the evening, reaching a peak at 0700 hours (Fig. 26–13) (Nakajima et al., 1990). The regulatory mechanism for both the episodic and the 24-hour fluctuation of hCG secretion is unclear, and a host of factors may be involved such as alterations in metabolic clearance rate and/or volume of distribution of the hormone.

Human chorionic gonadotropin (hCG) is not unique during pregnancy. A remarkable characteristic of hCG (or hCG-like material) is its broad distribution. It is found in most, if not all, normal human tissues (Braunstein et al., 1979; Yoshimoto et al., 1979), in the urine and serum of normal men and women (Stenman et al.,

1987), and in many types of cancer cells (Vaitukaitis et al., 1976). Moreover, free α- and β-subunits as well as hCG have been found in the human pituitary gland (Hoerkmann et al., 1990). In nonpregnant women, the median level of hCG increases more than tenfold from reproductive age (median 0.05 IU/liter) to postmenopausal age (median 1.1 IU/liter). The findings that hCG levels follow a pulsatile pattern (Odell and Griffin, 1987) and that GnRH stimulates and ovarian steroids suppress serum hCG levels strongly suggest that pituitary hCG is under GnRH and sex steroid modulation (Stenman et al., 1987). The production of hCG-like material may represent incomplete regression of the fetal genome responsible for hCG biosynthesis (Hussa, 1980). Alternatively, the hCG may be produced by relatively undifferentiated stem cells which are responsible for cell renewal—i.e., not reaching the stage of repression of the hCG genome.

Human Chorionic Gonadotropin (hCG) Regulation

cAMP AND G PROTEINS. It has been demonstrated that hCG secretion by purified cytotrophoblasts in culture can be stimulated by 8-bromo-cAMP and is followed by increasing mRNA levels encoding the α- and β-subunits of the hormone (Ringler and Strauss, 1990). The demonstration that cytotrophoblast possesses functional adenylate cyclase activity establishes the adenylate cyclase-cAMP pathway in the activation of cellular responses to stimulatory agents *in vitro*. Factors that may trigger cytotrophoblast adenylate cyclase *in vivo* are not known.

The membrane-bound stimulatory and inhibitory quinine nucleotide regulatory proteins, G_s and G_i, are also present in the cytotrophoblast. Moreover, the coupling of G_s to adenylate cyclase in response to stimulation has also been demonstrated (Nielsen et al., 1988). Thus, the level of expression of adenylate cyclase activity is one determinant of the hCG synthesis and secretion of the differentiating trophoblast.

GnRH AND INHIBIN/ACTIVIN. It is now well established that the cytotrophoblast produces and secretes GnRH. The mechanisms regulating placental GnRH release are similar to those acting on hypothalamic GnRH (Petraglia et al., 1990a). Circulating GnRH levels are higher in pregnant women than in nonpregnant women. The time course and pattern of serum GnRH levels are parallel to those of hCG and are correlated with placental GnRH content, suggesting a placental origin of circulating GnRH and a regulating role of GnRH in hCG secretion within the placenta (Petraglia et al., 1990a; Siler-Khodr et al., 1984).

Evidence has accumulated that GnRH actively stimulates, in a dose-dependent manner, the release of hCG from the cultured trophoblasts (Khodr and Siler-Khodr, 1978; Siler-Khodr and Khodr 1981; Petraglia et al., 1987a). The presence of GnRH receptors on the placental cell membranes suggests that GnRH produced in situ is involved in the paracrine regulation of hormone secretion: the addition of a GnRH antagonist reduces hCG secretion in placental cells in culture and reverses the stimulatory effect of GnRH (Siler-Khodr et al., 1983). Trophoblasts from first-trimester

placenta in culture are more sensitive to GnRH stimulation of hCG secretion than those from late pregnancy placentas, an observation that confirms the secretory pattern of hCG (Siler-Khodr et al., 1986). While hCG stimulates progesterone production, GnRH inhibits the formation of progesterones and estrogens (Branchaud et al., 1983; Ringler et al., 1989). Collectively, these findings indicate a local regulatory loop between the secretion of GnRH, hCG, and placental steroids (Fig. 26–14).

Inhibin and activin synthesized in the cytotrophoblast may also partake in the regulation of hCG secretion, and they do so by way of modulating the GnRH activity (Fig. 26–14) (Petraglia et al., 1989b). The addition of inhibin antiserum to placental cell culture causes a significant increase in hCG secretion with a concomitant rise in GnRH release. This finding, together with the ability of a GnRH antagonist to reduce the inhibin antiserum effect on hCG secretion, suggests that the inhibitory action of inhibin on hCG secretion is a receptor-mediated event on placental GnRH. The suppressive effect of inhibin on hCG secretion is expressed only in the placenta of the later part of pregnancy and not in the first trimester (Mersol-Barg et al., 1990). Addition of purified inhibin has no effect on hCG or GnRH release, but it reverses the GnRH-induced hCG release from cultured placental cells (Petraglia et al., 1989b). Thus, placental inhibin may function as both an autocrine and paracrine factor in regulating hCG via GnRH.

Activin ($β_Aβ_A$), in contrast, has an opposite effect on hCG secretion. The addition of purified activin to placental culture augments the GnRH-induced release of hCG, and this effect can be significantly reduced by the addition of inhibin (Petraglia et al., 1989b).

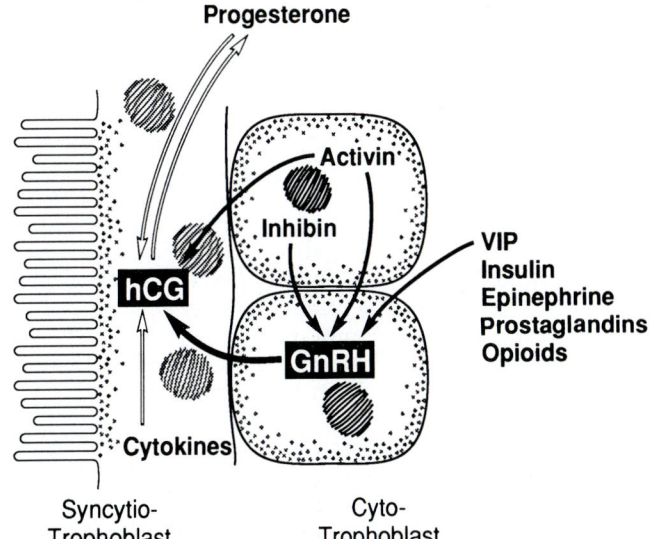

FIGURE 26–14. The regulatory system of GnRH and hCG between cytotrophoblasts and syncytiotrophoblasts. The autocrine and paracrine modes of regulation of GnRH by inhibin (inhibitory) and activin (stimulatory) as well as a host of modulating factors are depicted. The microvilli of the syncytiotrophoblast are depicted by the drawing of zigzag lines.

Thus, it would appear that placental GnRH plays a fundamental role in the regulation of hCG secretion, but its functional activity appears to be regulated by inhibin (inhibitory) and activin (stimulatory) in a receptor-mediated paracrine mode of action within the cytotrophoblast (Fig. 26–14).

Modulating Factors

This regulatory effect of inhibin/activin/GnRH on hCG production may be subject to modulation by other hormones, catecholamines and locally produced prostaglandins, growth factors, cytokines, and neuropeptides. Inhibin release is stimulated by both vasoactive intestinal peptides (VIP) and neuropeptide Y (NPY) (Petraglia et al., 1990a). Insulin and VIP are stimulatory on the release of placental GnRH in a dose-dependent fashion in cultured placental cells. Epinephrine and prostaglandins (PGE_2 and $PGF_{2\alpha}$) are also shown to increase GnRH release from the cultured placental cells. Since the trophoblast is endowed with β-adrenergic receptors and metabolizing enzymes for catecholamines, maternal and fetal sources of epinephrine may influence placental GnRH secretion (Petraglia et al., 1990a). Epidermal growth factor (EGF) has also been shown to stimulate hCG secretion in first-trimester placenta (Barnea et al., 1990).

Steroids and Opioid Peptides. Recent evidence provided by Petraglia et al. (1990a) suggests that placental steroid hormones and endogenous opioid peptides may also modulate the release of GnRH and thus hCG secretion. Estradiol and estriol potentiate while progesterone decreases the action of 8-bromo-cAMP on GnRH release from cultured placental cells. In addition, an augmenting effect of estriol and an inhibitory effect of progesterone on activin-stimulated GnRH are also observed. These observations are consonant with findings of a positive effect of estrogen and a negative effect of progesterone on basal and GnRH-stimulated hCG release, and hCG mRNA levels in human placenta (Ringler et al., 1989; Wilson et al., 1984; Maruo et al., 1986). It has been proposed that the decline of hCG secretion after 10 weeks of gestation may be causally related to the inhibitory effect of progesterone (Maruo et al., 1986; Wilson et al., 1980).

An inhibitory action of opioid peptides on placental GnRH release, similar to that found for hypothalamic GnRH neurons, has also been observed (Petraglia et al., 1990a). The presence of high-affinity opioid receptors in placental cell membranes (Belisle et al., 1988) would permit its modulation of GnRH release whether the source is placental, maternal, or fetal. Collectively, these findings suggest that the locally produced steroids and opioid peptides participate in the overall regulation of hCG secretion by the syncytiotrophoblast. The presence of receptors for estrogen, progesterone, and opioid peptides in human placenta (Younes et al., 1981) supports this formulation.

Cytokines. To date, two cytokines produced by the placenta, interleukin-1 (IL-1) and interleukin-6 (IL-6), have been shown to stimulate hCG secretion by the trophoblast.

IL-1, a critical mediator in immunologic responses, has a broad range of biological functions (Dinarello, 1988). The trophoblast and the macrophage are sources of IL-1 in the placenta (Main et al., 1987; Flynn et al., 1982). Using human recombinant IL-1 in concentrations of 10^{-11} to 10^{-9} mol/liter, Yagel (1989) has demonstrated IL-1 stimulated hCG release in trophoblasts from the first-trimester placenta. This effect of IL-1 is mediated by activating IL-6 and IL-6 receptor of the trophoblast.

Inhibin and Activin Secretion. Apart from its local regulatory effect on GnRH-hCG release, inhibin is secreted into the maternal circulation, and its concentrations are elevated to about three times the midluteal phase value during the course of pregnancy. Inhibin levels exhibit two peaks, the first occurring at 8 to 10 weeks gestation; thereafter, it declines and remains at relatively low levels during the second trimester. It rises to a second peak near term to a mean level higher than the first peak (Fig. 26–15) (Abe et al., 1990). The first peak of inhibin rise reflects corpus luteum secretion stimulated by hCG, and the inhibin levels after 10 weeks of gestation represent the placental source (McLachlan et al., 1987a, 1987b). Inhibin levels fall rapidly following delivery, as do levels of E_2 and P_4 (Kettel et al., 1991). Concentrations of inhibin in the cord blood are about half that in maternal serum, without significant differences between umbilical artery and umbilical vein (Abe et al., 1990; Kettel et al., 1991). The functional role of circulating inhibin during pregnancy other than the suppression of FSH secretion is unknown. Information regarding activin levels during pregnancy is not available at present. Since inhibin and activin are parts of the TGF-β family of peptides and they are potent growth and differentiation factors (Massague, 1986), the possibility that they may modulate placental and fetal cell growth and differentiation should be considered. In fact, expressions corresponding to TGF-β of inhibin and activin have already been demonstrated in multiple tissue sites during embryonic development in the rat (Roberts et al., 1991).

Functional Role of hCG

As depicted in Figure 26–16, hCG has multiple functions during the early stage of gestation. First, the

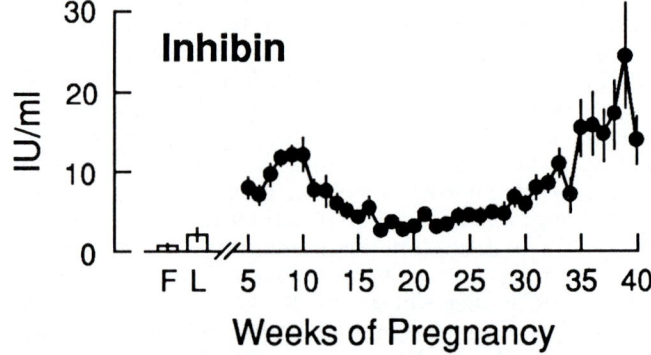

FIGURE 26–15. The mean (±SE) plasma inhibin concentrations in the midfollicular phase (F), in the midluteal phase (L), and during the course of normal pregnancy. (From Abe Y, Miyamoto HK, Yamaguchi M, et al: High concentrations of plasma immunoreactive inhibin during normal pregnancy in women. J Clin Endocrinol Metab **71**:133, © by the Endocrine Society, 1990.)

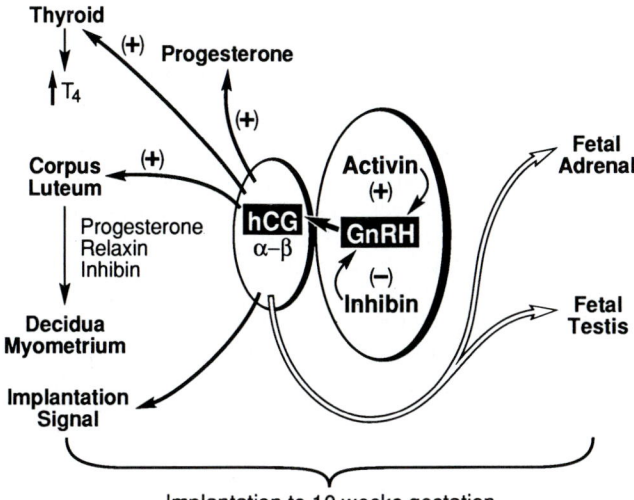

FIGURE 26–16. Diagrammatic representation of the functional role of hCG in the maternal and fetal compartments during the first 10 weeks of gestation. The GnRH/inhibin/activin system of the cytotrophoblast and the biosynthesis of hCG in the syncytiotrophoblast are depicted by ovals.

preimplantation embryo produces hCG and represents a signal of maternal-embryo dialogue at the time of implantation. Soon after, hCG provides luteotropic function for the corpus luteum rescue, resulting in enhanced production of progesterone and relaxin, which are essential for sustaining early pregnancy. Concomitantly, corpus luteum secretion of inhibin is heightened, thereby suppressing pituitary FSH secretion. Circulating hCG may also function to inhibit LH secretion by the maternal hypothalamic-pituitary unit. In addition to its luteotropic function, hCG has intrinsic thyrotropic activity, binding to the TSH receptor and stimulating iodide uptake and DNA synthesis in the thyroid gland (Hershman et al., 1988; Pekonen et al., 1988; Yoshikawa et al., 1989). The relative potency of hCG as a thyroid-stimulating factor is about 27,000 IU/liter hCG equivalent to 1 mIU of human TSH. As a consequence, serum T4 is modestly elevated and pituitary TSH secretion is suppressed—a state of mild thyroid hyperfunction in the early pregnancy (Hershman et al., 1988; Pekonen et al., 1988; Yoshikawa et al., 1989).

Human chorionic gonadotropin also exerts a stimulatory effect on placental progesterone biosynthesis and provides gonadotropic and adrenotropic input to the fetus during the first trimester of pregnancy (Serón-Ferré et al., 1978). Of special interest is the stimulation of Leydig cells in the male fetus during organogenesis to produce testosterone, which in turn is instrumental in the development of the internal genitalia. Conversion of testosterone to dihydrotestosterone by 5-α reductase in the external genital tissue determines the development of male genitalia.

METABOLIC HORMONES OF PREGNANCY
Human Chorionic Somatomammotropin

Human chorionic somatomammotropin (hCS), a single-chain 191-amino acid polypeptide hormone (mw

23,000) produced by the syncytiotrophoblast, is also known as chorionic growth hormone prolactin (CGP) and human placental lactogen (hPL). The 191-amino acid sequence has a remarkable similarity to human pituitary growth hormone (hGH) and prolactin (PRL), suggesting a common ancestral gene.

The regional organization of hCS and hGH gene cluster on the long arm of chromosome 17 has been described. Within this cluster, five related genes are aligned in the same transcriptional orientation in the order 5' to 3': hGN-N, hCS-L, hCS-A, hGH-V, hCS-B. Two genes, hCS-A and hCS-B, code for the same mature peptide and are responsible for hCS production by the trophoblast (Barsh, et al., 1983; Berrera-Saldana et al., 1983). Although hCS-L gene bears a high degree of sequence homology to hCS-A and hCS-B genes, it is not expressed in the placental tissue. The hGH-N gene codes for pituitary hGH, whereas the hGH-V gene codes for a peptide that differs from hGH in 13 of 191 amino acid residues, and it has been recently identified as human placental growth hormone (hPGH) (DeNoto et al., 1981; Seeburg, 1982). These findings provide the genetic basis for discerning the partial and complete hCS deficiency and the physiologic role of hPGH production during pregnancy.

Regulation

The ratio of cytotrophoblast to syncytiotrophoblast decreases progressively until the syncytial layer is the dominant trophoblastic component at term. This developmental change in trophoblast population is critical in the interpretation of gene expression and hormone production by the placenta, e.g., hCG versus hCS and neuropeptides versus protein hormones.

Using probes derived from clones bearing cDNAs corresponding to hCS and the α-subunit of hCG, Hoshina and associates (1982) have quantified their respective mRNA cytologically in sections of first-trimester and term human placentas. Whereas hCS mRNA is exclusively localized to the syncytial layer, hCGα mRNA is found in syncytial layer as well as in some differentiating cytotrophoblasts. Hybridization with the α-hCG probe is much greater in the first trimester than in term placenta sections. In contrast, hCS signals are comparable in both first-trimester and term placentas. These findings suggest that the transcription of hCG-α gene is initiated before the completion of syncytial formation, whereas hCS mRNA synthesis starts later in trophoblast differentiation, after syncytial formation. Furthermore, these data suggest that α-hCG mRNA synthesis becomes attenuated, but that hCS is transcribed at a constant rate during the course of placental development. The cellular hCS mRNA levels do not parallel the *in vivo* circulating levels of the hormone, which increase 20-fold from early gestation to term and parallel the growth of placental mass (syncytiotrophoblast). Thus, it is entirely consistent that *the content of hCS mRNA per unit of syncytial mass remains constant during gestation* (Hoshina et al., 1982).

Factors that regulate hCS synthesis and secretion are not fully understood. Indirect evidence suggests that an inhibitory action of somatostatin (SS) and a stimulatory role of growth hormone releasing factor (GRF) produced within the cytotrophoblast may function as regulators of hCS synthesis and secretion (Fig. 26–17). Expression of GRF mRNA in the cytotrophoblast of human placenta has been reported (Berry et al., 1992). The immunocytochemical staining of SS is most intense in early placentas, its intensity decreasing in placentas of advancing gestation (Watkins and Yen, 1980). This pattern of SS is opposite to that of hCS secretory activity and supports the notion that SS may play an inhibitory role. GRF (5×10^{-10}) stimulates (~ 30 per cent) hCS release in human trophoblast in culture (Hochberg et al., 1988), suggesting that GRF together with SS may function to modulate hCS secretion in the same way that the hypothalamus controls pituitary GH secretion. In addition, insulin stimulates hCS release in a dose-dependent manner (Hochberg et al., 1983) and dynorphin and angiotensin II produced locally (cytotrophoblast), acting via specific receptors, may also participate as regulators (Ahmed and Horst, 1986; Petit et al., 1989). The mechanism of action for these potential regulators of hCS secretion is mediated through cAMP and protein kinase C systems (Ringler and Strauss, 1990).

Human Placental Growth Hormone (hPGH)

Human placental growth hormone (hPGH) is composed of two forms—of 22 and 25 kilodaltons (K)

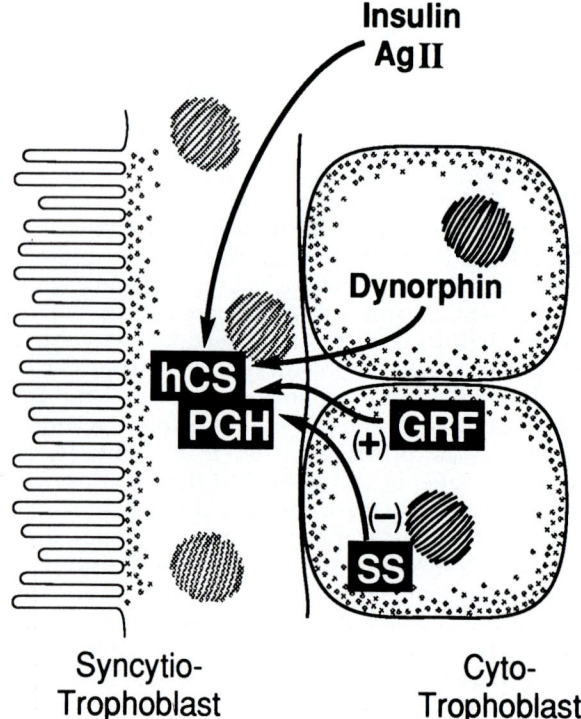

FIGURE 26–17. Diagrammatic depiction of a potential regulatory system of GRF/Somatostatin (SS) from cytotrophoblast in the release of hCS (possibly placental growth hormone) by the syncytiotrophoblast. The modulating role of dynorphin, insulin, and angiotensin II (Ag II) are also shown.

molecular weight—and the latter is probably glycosylated (Frankenne and Scippo, 1988). Both forms of hPGH are hGH-V gene products in distinction from pituitary hGH, which is encoded by hGH-N gene (Igout et al., 1988).

During the first trimester, pituitary GH is measurable in maternal serum and it is secreted in a highly pulsatile pattern (Eriksson et al., 1989). From 15 to 17 weeks gestation to term, serum pituitary GH is progressively replaced by increasing levels of hPGH, which displays a relatively constant, rather than episodic, 24-hour secretory profile (Eriksson et al., 1989). Simultaneously, the pituitary GH secretion is suppressed and unresponsive to secretagogues (Yen et al., 1970; Merimee et al., 1982). This suppression of pituitary GH secretion during the second half of pregnancy is probably due to the negative feedback action of elevated IGF-I levels during pregnancy (Daughaday et al., 1990). IGF-I levels are positively correlated with PGH (Wiedemann et al., 1976; Frankenne et al., 1988), suggesting that placental GH stimulates IGF-I production (Fig. 26–18).

The secretion of hPGH has been characterized. Using two distinct monoclonal antisera, one recognizes pituitary hGH and the other detects hPGH. Frankenne et al. (1988) developed specific RIAs for simultaneous measurements of hGH of pituitary and placental sources as well as hCS. The secretory pattern of pituitary hGH (22k) remains relatively constant between 4 and 6 µg/liter until 20 weeks, when a steady decline occurs, and becomes undetectable by the 35th week of gestation. The hPGH, in contrast, exhibits a progressive increase in mean concentration during the second half of pregnancy and becomes undetectable one hour after delivery, a pattern parallel to that of hCS (Fig. 26–19). These findings are complemented by the radioreceptor studies reported by Daughaday et al. (1990): levels are 2 to 3 times higher than values obtained by RIA, and the relative contribution of GH activities during late pregnancy are 85 per cent from PGH, 12 per cent from hCS, and less than 3 per cent from pituitary GH. Although much work remains to be done, hPGH may prove to be the major metabolic hormone of pregnancy, and hCG may further enhance, but is not essential for, the GH-like activity.

ENDOCRINE-METABOLIC ADJUSTMENTS IN PREGNANCY

Pregnancy in women is attended by pancreatic islet hypertrophy, hyperinsulinemia, and insulin resistance. Relative fasting hypoglycemia, elevations of plasma lipids, and hypoaminoacidemia are consistently observed, together with marked sensitivity to food deprivation (Table 26–2).

These changes are designed to serve a unique physiologic purpose of providing a preferential and uninterrupted supply of metabolic fuel from to mother to fetus, as dictated by the progressively increasing demand of the growing fetus. Accordingly, hormonal input from the fetoplacental unit in the regulation of such nutrient flow would be both economical and logical.

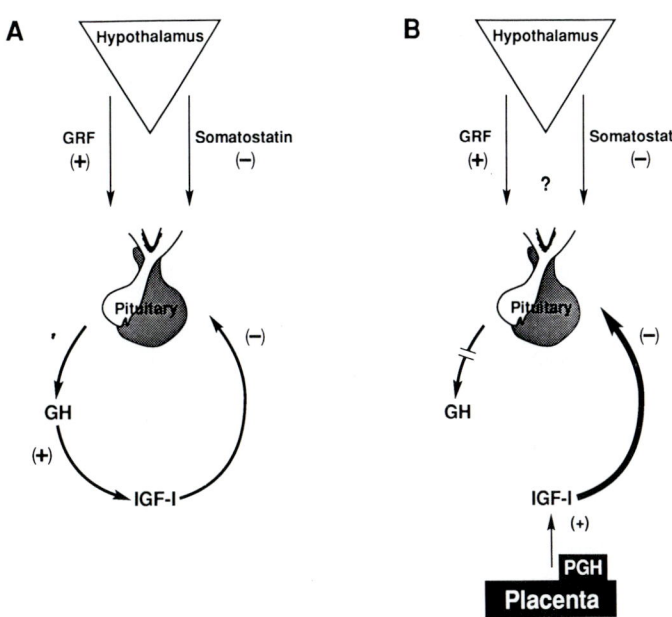

FIGURE 26–18. Diagrammatic depictions of hypothalamic-GH and IGF-I axis. *A,* In normal nonpregnant state, pituitary GH regulates the production of IGF-I, which in turn exerts a negative feedback action on GH release at the hypothalamic-pituitary level. *B,* During the second half of pregnancy, the GH-IGF axis is interrupted by progressive increase in placental GH (hPGH) and IGF-I production.

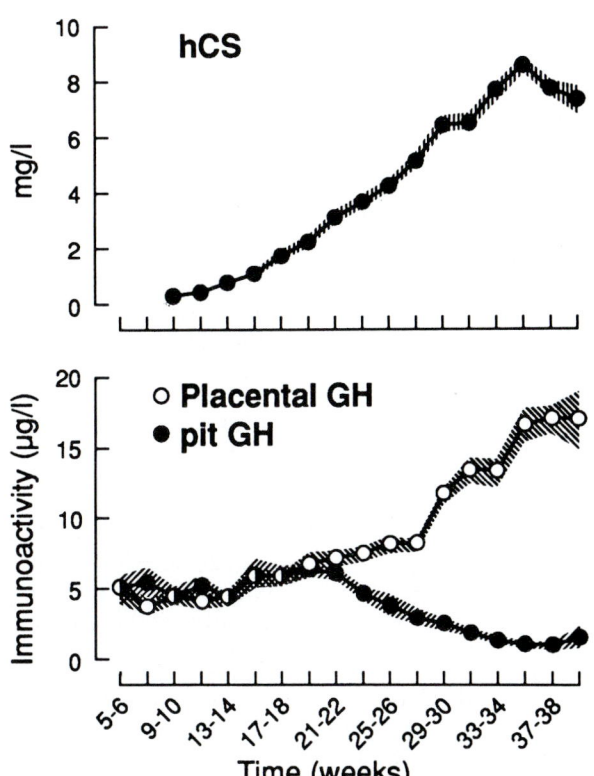

FIGURE 26–19. The time course of human placental growth hormone (hPGH) secretion and its parallelism to hCS and its divergence from that of pituitary growth hormone (PWGH) during pregnancy. (Modified from Frankenne F, Closset J, Gomez F, et al: The physiology of growth hormones (GHs) in pregnant women and partial characterization of the placental GH variant. J Clin Endocrinol Metab **66**:1171, © by the Endocrine Society, 1988.)

Modification of Metabolic Fuels

Peripheral Insulin Resistance and Hyperinsulinemia

It has long been established that pregnant women become progressively resistant to the hypoglycemic action of insulin. During the course of human gestation, an augmented plasma insulin response to a variety of insulinogenic stimuli occurs without affecting glucose levels (Fig. 26–20) (Spellacy and Goetz, 1963; Kalkhoff et al., 1964; Bleicher et al., 1964). The finding of maternal islet cell hyperplasia in all mammalian species examined to date supports the premise that pregnancy enhances insulin requirement. This phenomenon cannot be accounted for by a reduction of circulating insulin occasioned by an increased placental degradation (insulinase) since the disappearance rate of exogenous insulin in late pregnancy is identical to that in the nonpregnant state (Fig. 26–21) (Burt and Davidson, 1974). The lesser degree of glucose fall in response to exogenous insulin in late pregnancy thus reflects peripheral resistance to insulin.

A parallel increase in insulinogenic response to glucose and glucose disposition during the first trimester of pregnancy has been noted, suggesting that a more insulinotropic than anti-insulin effect is operating during early gestation. In contrast, a greater degree of hyperinsulinism in late pregnancy is unaccompanied by a parallel increase in glucose disposition, indicating the development of a greater anti-insulin effect concomitant with the enhanced insulinogenic activity (Yen et al., 1971; Yen, 1973; Buchanan et al., 1990). Despite the presence of peripheral resistance to insulin, the maternal circulating glucose pool appears

TABLE 26–2.   Basal Values for Insulin, Glucagon, and Plasma Metabolic Fuels in Young Women After Overnight Fast

MEASUREMENTS	NONGRAVID	LATE PREGNANCY
Glucose (mg/dl)	79 ± 2.4	68 ± 1.5*
Insulin (μU/ml)	9.8 ± 1.1	16.2 ± 2.0*
Glucagon (pg/ml)	126 ± 6.1	130 ± 5.2 (NS)
Amino acids		
(μ moles/L)	3.82 ± 0.13	3.18 ± 0.11*
(Alanine μ moles/L)	286 ± 15	225 ± 9*
FFA (μ moles/L)	626 ± 42	725 ± 21*
(mg/dl)	76.2 ± 7.0	181 ± 10*
Cholesterol (mg/dl)	163 ± 8.7	205 ± 5.7*

*Significant difference between nongravid and late pregnancy values.
NS = not significant.
Data from Freinkel N, Metzger BE, Nitzan M, et al: Facilitated anabolism in late pregnancy: some novel maternal compensations for accelerated starvation. *In* Malaisse WJ, Pirart J (eds): Diabetes. (International Series No. 312.) Amsterdam, Excerpta Medica, 1973, p 474.

to be diminished after intravenous glucose loading. The latter finding may reflect the progressive increase in maternal plasma volume and uteroplacental circulation, facilitating the uninterrupted extraction of maternal glucose by the fetoplacental unit.

The mechanism to account for the development of peripheral insulin resistance during the course of pregnancy is not entirely clear. It is likely that hPGH, hCS, and other diabetogenic hormones exert effects on insulin action by reducing the receptor binding sites and glucose transport in insulin-sensitive tissues (Ciaraldi et al., 1992). Nonetheless, more insulin is needed during pregnancy for maintenance of carbohydrate homeostasis. This homeostatic mechanism, however, may be interrupted by limited ability of the β cell to meet additional insulin requirements, such as that observed in diabetics.

In *gestational diabetes*, the development of hyperglycemia and retarded glucose utilization is associated with a significant increase in the circulating glucose pool. This event is related to an inability to release insulin acutely during the initial phase of a glucose challenge, followed by a delayed by sustained insulin secretion as demonstrated by two independent studies (Fig. 26–22) (Yen et al., 1971; Buchanan et al., 1990). After delivery, the rapid reversal of glucose intolerance

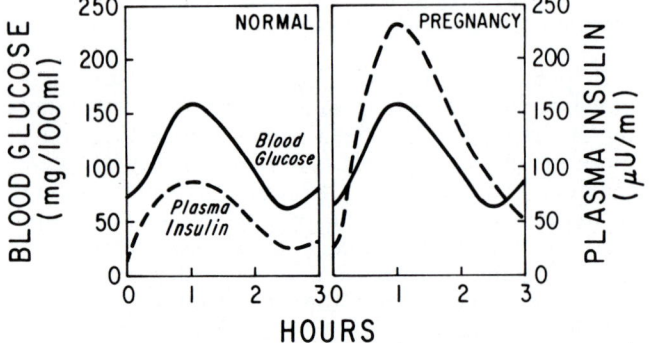

FIGURE 26–20. The augmentation of plasma insulin response to oral glucose load (100 gm) without modification of glucose levels in late pregnancy as compared to nonpregnant women (normal).

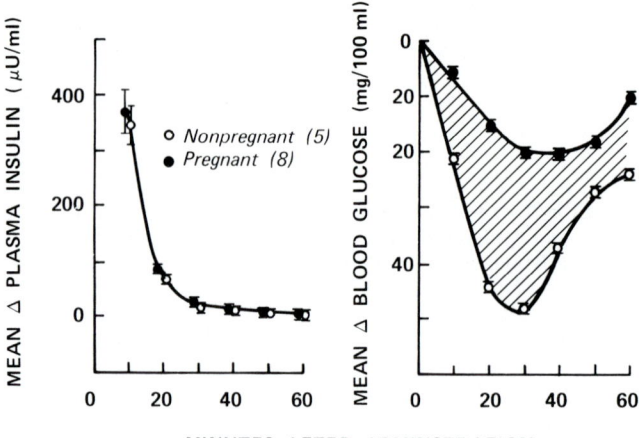

FIGURE 26–21. The identical disappearance curves of circulating insulin following IV insulin injection (0.1 U/kg) in pregnant and nonpregnant women (*left*). The marked reduction in blood glucose decline in response to exogenous insulin in pregnant women as compared to the nonpregnant women reflects peripheral insulin resistance (*right*). (From Burt RL, Davidson WF: Insulin half-life and utilization in normal pregnancy. Obstet Gynecol 4:161, 1974. Reprinted with permission from the American College of Obstetricians and Gynecologists.)

in gestational diabetes has been considered critical clinical evidence indicating that fetoplacental factors are diabetogenic and responsible for gestational diabetogenesis (Yen et al., 1971).

Interrelationship Among Glucose, Insulin, and Hyperlipemia in Pregnancy

Pregnancy is associated with hyperlipemia. Total plasma lipids increase significantly and progressively after 24 weeks of gestation. The rise of triglyceride, cholesterol, and free fatty acids (FFA) predominates (Freinkel et al., 1973). Pre-β-lipoprotein, a very-low-density lipoprotein (VLDL), which normally represents a very small percentage of total lipoprotein, is increased in pregnancy. Whereas LDL cholesterol increases toward late pregnancy, HDL cholesterol rises only during early pregnancy (Potter and Nestel, 1979).

The liver constitutes the first target for both absorbed glucose and endogenously secreted insulin. Thus, blood sugar levels reflect in part the glucose that has been spared by the insulin-mediated hepatic extraction and peripheral disposition. Following oral glucose (100 gm), despite a greater insulin output, the initial rate of decline of FFA is significantly lower in late pregnancy than at postpartum. It seems likely that the ongoing lipolytic activity characteristic of late pregnancy is disrupted less rapidly by both glucose and insulin, as suggested by Freinkel and co-workers (1973). In contrast, the acute increment in plasma triglyceride levels occurs more rapidly and in greater magnitude following oral glucose in late pregnancy than in nonpregnant women. This heightened triglyceride release in response to glucose is due principally to the increased formation and entry of VLDL, which may be causally related to: (1) estrogen-facilitated production of triglycerides by the liver and resulting

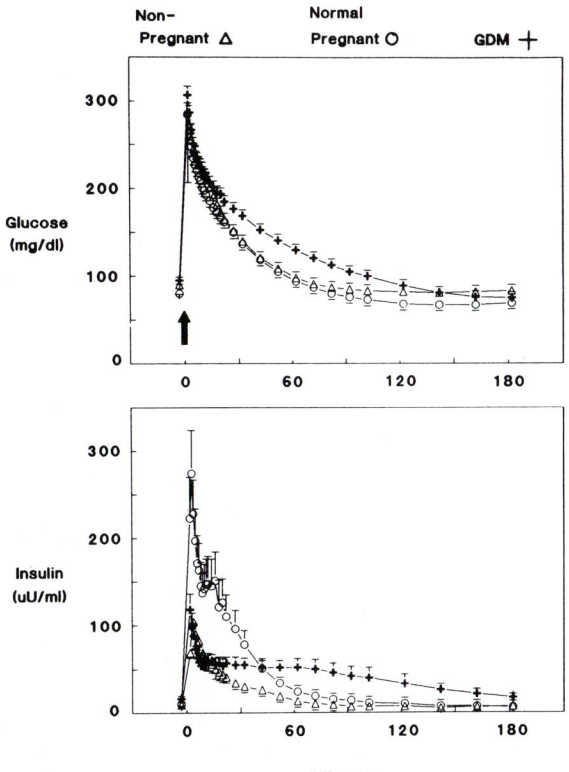

FIGURE 26–22. Comparisons of insulin and glucose responses to rapid IV glucose tolerance test (300 mg/kg) in normal nonpregnant and normal pregnant individuals, and in individuals with gestational diabetes (GDM). Note the elevated glucose values in GDM despite the sustained insulin secretion. (From Buchanan TA, Metzger BE, Freinkel N, Bergman RN: Insulin sensitivity and B-cell responsiveness to glucose during late pregnancy in lean and moderately obese women with normal glucose tolerance or mild gestational diabetes. Am J Obstet Gynecol **162**:1008, 1990.)

accumulation of hepatic triglyceride, or (2) increased availability of lipolytic hormones, such as hCS, hPGH, catecholamines, and cortisol (see below).

Regardless of the mechanism, an acute rise in triglycerides after oral glucose has certain unique implications for fuel economy during pregnancy. The placenta is poorly permeable to fat, whereas glucose and amino acids are readily transported by the placenta. Thus, the incorporation of an increased fraction of dietary glucose into VLDL provides a mechanism for minimizing the loss of excess glucose at a time of glucose surplus, retaining it for subsequent use as glycerol during fasting. In addition, fatty acids derived from VLDL may be subsequently mobilized to replenish fat stores in maternal adipose tissue. Thus, the important feature is the preservation of carbohydrate in the form of glycerol to be made available for fetal use when exogenous nutrients are insufficient (Freinkel et al., 1973).

The Role of Glucagon

In view of its known glycogenolytic, gluconeogenic, and lipolytic activities, glucagon dynamics in preg-

nancy have been investigated. Basal glucagon levels are unchanged during late pregnancy, but an unexplained decrease in basal glucagon concentrations occurs 6 to 8 weeks postpartum (Daniel et al., 1974; Leblanc et al., 1976). The suppression of glucagon by insulin-mediated glucose flux is maintained during pregnancy. The α cell response to amino acid stimulation is also preserved. However, the degree of glucagon suppression by 100 gm oral glucose appears to be greater in pregnant subjects than in postpartum subjects. Thus, glucagon cannot be implicated as a diabetogenic factor in normal pregnancy. Instead, the significantly greater decrement of glucagon at 120 and 180 minutes after glucose loading in pregnant women may actually facilitate anabolism (Freinkel et al., 1973).

Modification of Amino Acid Metabolism (Substrate Limitation of Gluconeogenesis)

Caloric deprivation in human pregnancy is accompanied by an exaggerated and accelerated hypoglycemia, hypoinsulinism, and hyperketonemia (Felig et al., 1972). During the course of a 3- to 4-day fast, maternal glucose levels fall markedly, while urea nitrogen excretion, reflecting hepatic gluconeogenesis, fails to increase above the levels observed in the nongravid state. This gestational exaggeration of fasting hypoglycemia occurs in the face of maternal hypoinsulinism and hyperketonemia, both of which would be expected to augment hepatic gluconeogenesis. This lack of appropriate gluconeogenesis during pregnancy is not due to altered hepatic processes; rather, it is related to the limited key substrate alanine, released by the muscle during starvation (Felig et al., 1972; Tyson et al., 1976). Although hyperaminoacidemia develops as a consequence of hypoinsulinism during starvation and is reflected by an increase in amino acids in the amniotic fluid compartment, alanine represents an exception in that it is selectively decreased (Felig et al., 1972). These findings indicate that the levels and kinds of amino acids in amniotic fluid, and probably the fetal compartment as well, may be profoundly influenced by maternal nutrition.

The significance of the altered gluconeogenesis in pregnancy is not entirely clear. The undeniable demands of the fetus during maternal fasting are met to some extent by accelerated muscle breakdown. However, even though fetal requirements are met during fasting, it is at the expense of the mother, whose homeostatic mechanism does not include sufficient gluconeogenesis to prevent maternal hypoglycemia. It is not clear whether normal muscle catabolism simply cannot keep up with the loss of glucose and amino acids to the fetus during fasting or whether there are additional restraints on muscle breakdown during pregnancy. The possibility of a continuous uptake of alanine by the placenta and preferential utilization by the fetus should also be considered.

Diabetogenic Hormones

Cortisol

Cortisol is a potent diabetogenic hormone. It exerts peripheral insulin antagonism and also promotes insulin secretion (Perley and Kipnis, 1966). Glucocorticoids are catabolic hormones that enhance protein breakdown in the muscle and increase circulating amino acids, particularly alanine. Indirectly, cortisol induces hyperglucagonemia due to increased alanine stimulation to α cells (Felig et al., 1976). Concomitantly with a reduction of glucose metabolism in the adipose tissue, it promotes lipolysis and elevates FFA (Perley and Kipnis, 1966). However, the effect of corticoids on lipolysis is operative only when insulin is absent or insufficient. In Cushing's disease or syndrome, with chronic glucocorticoid excess, continuous protein catabolism in the muscle is present (hence muscle wasting) and results in augmented hepatic gluconeogenesis (Doe et al., 1960). The development of hyperglycemia or diabetes in Cushing's disease or syndrome is related to both the decompensation of hyperinsulinism and chronic hyperglucagonemia.

Although serum cortisol is doubled during late pregnancy, much of the increase is attributable to biologically inactive hormones bound to transcortin or corticoid-binding globulin (CBG), which is in turn elevated under the influence of estrogen. However, a significant increase in plasma and urinary free cortisol levels with normal circadian rhythm occurs during late pregnancy (Fig. 26–23) (Cousins et al., 1983; Abou-Samra et al., 1984). The physiologic contribution of this elevated free cortisol to the diabetogenic potential of pregnancy is unclear, particularly since the biological half-life of cortisol during pregnancy has not been settled.

Pituitary GH

Pituitary GH, a potent diabetogenic factor, shares many similarities with metabolic change during pregnancy. It exerts an insulinotropic effect and peripheral resistance to insulin, increases lipolysis, and induces marked nitrogen retention (Yen, 1973). Most of the GH effects are mediated by the IGFs. Thus, growth hormone excess provides an excellent model to account for the metabolic changes during pregnancy. Acromegalic subjects, who have modest hyperglycemia, are associated with marked compensatory hyperinsulinism without affecting α cell function. The development of overt diabetes in approximately 25 per cent of acromegalics presumably is due to the decompensation of β cells to provide hyperinsulinism.

Pituitary hGH does not appear to play a role in the diabetogenic potential in pregnancy since its secretion in response to hypoglycemic and arginine stimuli is progressively diminished during pregnancy (Yen et al., 1970; Merimee et al., 1982). Furthermore, the observation of a GH-deficient dwarf due to deletion of hGH-N gene, in whom IGF-I levels increased from low to normal pregnant values and returned to low level after delivery (Merimee et al., 1982), strengthens the role of placental GH during pregnancy.

Placental Hormones

HUMAN CHORIONIC SOMATOMAMMOTROPIN (hCS). Human chorionic somatomammotropin (hCS) is immunochemically and biologically similar to pituitary

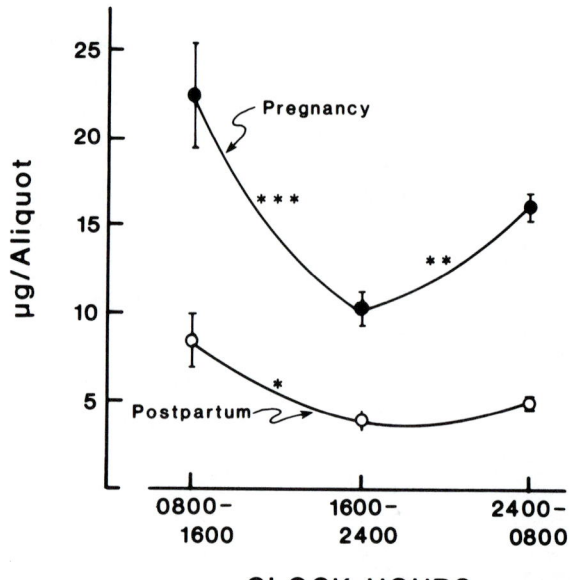

FIGURE 26–23. Mean (± SEM) urinary free corticoid levels during 8-hour intervals throughout the day in eight normal women studied during pregnancy (second and third trimesters) and postpartum. Asterisks indicate significant difference between levels: * =p<0.05; ** =p<0.01; *** =p<0.005. (From Cousins L, Rigg L, Hollingsworth D, et al: Qualitative and quantitative assessment of the circadian rhythm of cortisol in pregnancy. Am J Obstet Gynecol **145**:411, 1983.)

hGH. The rate of secretion is parallel to that of the fetal-placental growth curve, and it is independent of circulating metabolic fuel in normally fed pregnant women (Friesen et al., 1969). However, a transient decrease following acute hyperinsulinemia induced by exogenous glucose and an increase in response to exogenous insulin administration have been observed (Spellacy et al., 1971). Prolonged starvation in mid-pregnancy has been shown to induce a 30 per cent rise in hPL levels (Tyson et al., 1976). These findings, derived from highly unphysiologic circumstances, by themselves do not establish the regulation of hPL secretion by glucose or insulin. However, insulin at physiological concentrations does elicit a rapid increase in hCS release in placental cell culture (Hochberg et al., 1983). Nonetheless, one could argue that chronic hyperglycemia in diabetic pregnancies does not appear to suppress hCS secretion and, in fact, hCS concentration is higher than that in normal pregnancy, due to the larger placental mass. Moreover, during the 24-hour metabolic fluctuations in response to usual dietary intake and in the face of accelerated nocturnal hypoglycemia (Cousins et al., 1980), circulating hCS levels are maintained in a relatively constant range (Gillmer et al., 1977).

Although hCS has insulinotropic and anti-insulin properties and promotes lipolysis *in vitro* and *in vivo*, it has relatively weak anabolic activity (Friesen et al., 1969; Grumbach et al., 1968). In normal subjects, intravenous infusion and intramuscular injections of highly purified hCS promote a plasma insulin response to ingested glucose, with little effect on carbohydrate tolerance (Samaan et al., 1968; Beck and

Daughaday, 1967). In contrast, subclinical and overt diabetic subjects are much more sensitive to hCS, and a comparable blood level of hCS manifests a greater impairment of glucose tolerance in association with inadequate plasma insulin response (Samaan et al., 1968). Because of these biological properties, together with the large amounts secreted by the placenta, hCS is considered an important metabolic hormone of pregnancy.

FUNCTIONAL ROLE OF hCS VERSUS hPGH. The deficiency or absence of hCS secretion without accompanying abnormalities of the infant or mother has been observed (Wurzel et al., 1982; Parks et al., 1985). In these cases, the two genes, termed hCS-A and hCS-B, showed either heterozygous gene deletion or homozygous gene deletion to account for partial and total absence of hCS secretion, respectively (Parks et al., 1985). The recent demonstration that hPGH binds to human GH receptors (Daughaday et al., 1990) and possesses lactogenic and growth-promoting properties (Nickel et al., 1990) would indicate the importance of this placental hormone in the control of metabolic homeostasis of the maternal compartment in pregnancy.

Estrogen and progesterone may also participate in the regulation of glucose-insulin homeostasis during pregnancy. Inductions of hyperinsulinism and hypertrophy of islets following administration of estradiol and progesterone have been observed in humans and animals (Costrini and Kalkhoff, 1971; Kalkhoff et al., 1970). The accompanying glucose disposition, however, differs between progesterone and estradiol; exaggerated insulin response to glucose is associated with a significant lowering of the glucose level after estradiol treatment, whereas progesterone treatment induces a decreased sensitivity to the hypoglycemic action of insulin. In nonpregnant humans, despite a threefold increase in insulinogenic response induced by progesterone, there is no change in plasma glucose levels. These observations suggest that progesterone may exert a peripheral insulin antagonism as well. The possibility that the β-cytotropic effect of these steroids may be mediated through the paracrine action of IGF-I needs to be explored.

Summary

Maternal metabolic homeostasis appears to depend on the optimum balance between the insulinotropic effect and anti-insulin effect, which is regulated by a complex interaction of placental hormones, β cell activity, and peripheral tissue responsiveness. When compared with postpartum controls, normal glucose excursion (30 to 40 mg per 100 ml) in response to usual dietary intake appears to be maintained. This is accomplished by an increased insulin/glucagon ratio in the face of peripheral insulin resistance. However, during the sleeping hours (fasting phase of the day), an exaggerated hypoglycemia occurs which accounts for the progressive decrease in fasting plasma glucose levels. The continuous drain of circulating glucose by the fetal-placental compartment and the limitation of substrate (alanine) for gluconeogenesis are factors responsible for the accelerated nocturnal hypoglycemia characteristic of normal late pregnancy.

Maternal-fetal metabolic interactions must be viewed in terms of placental barriers to the exchange of substrate and hormones. Whereas the transplacental flux of free fatty acids is slow, glucose crosses the placenta freely, and amino acids are actively transported to the fetus against a concentration gradient. On the other hand, the placenta is relatively impermeable to insulin and other protein hormones. The regulation of maternal metabolism does appear to be directed by the fetus to ensure an appropriate and uninterrupted supply of fetal glucose and amino acid. Maximal conservation of maternal glucose and gluconeogenic precursors and heightened utilization of fat are operative (Fig. 26–24). The enhanced catabolism, particularly lipolysis, in the maternal compartment would constitute a unique system of sparing nonlipid fuel for the fetal compartment whenever food deprivation occurs. Thus, the increasing placental elaboration of protein and steroid hormones, with their anti-insulin and insulinogenic as well as lipolytic properties, represents an efficient means of providing a regulatory mechanism (Freinkel et al., 1973; Grumbach et al., 1968).

The clinical management of diabetes in pregnancy is discussed in Chapter 54.

CORTICOTROPIN-RELEASING FACTOR (CRF) AND PROOPIOMELANOCORTIN (POMC) SYSTEM

Proopiomelanocortin (POMC)

Recent studies have established a family of peptides originating from a common precursor, a glycosylated

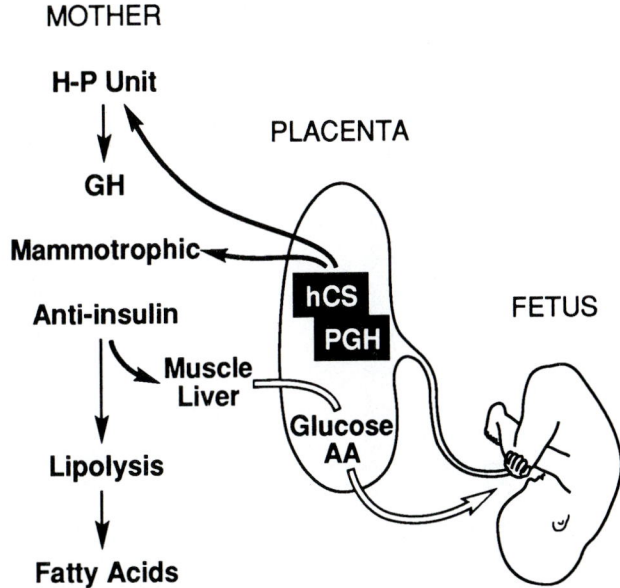

FIGURE 26–24. The proposed functional role of hCS and placental growth hormone (pGH) in the readjustment of maternal metabolic homeostasis with preferential transfer of amino acid and glucose to the fetus. GH = pituitary growth hormone.

protein with a molecular weight of 31,000. This large peptide, referred to as 31K ACTH-endorphin, or proopiomelanocortin (POMC), is enzymatically cleaved into several smaller component peptides, including β-lipotropic hormone (β-LPH), ACTH, α-melanocyte-stimulating hormone (α-MSH), and β-endorphin (Krieger and Liotta, 1979). It is now unequivocally established that these four peptides are present in the human brain, pituitary, and gonads as well as the placenta (Liotta et al., 1982).

Corticotropin-Releasing Factor (CRF)

The discovery, in 1982, that human placenta contains a corticotropin-releasing hormone (CRF) that induces the release of ACTH and β-endorphin from cultured rat anterior pituitary cells and human placental cells (Shibasaki et al., 1982; Sasaki et al., 1988; Petraglia et al., 1987b) has provided a clue to a CRH-POMC regulatory system of the placenta. Human placental CRF and its mRNA are identical to its hypothalamic counterpart. The CRF mRNA increases dramatically in late pregnancy placenta and is expressed in both cyto- and syncytiotrophoblasts (Fig. 26–25) (Frim et al., 1988), and immunocytochemical studies show a more intense staining with CRF antiserum in cytotrophoblast and intermediate trophoblast (Petraglia et al., 1990b). The CRF mRNA expression increases 20-fold from early to late pregnancy and parallels the rise in placental CRF content and maternal CRF concentration (Frim et al., 1988). CRF stimulates the secretion of ACTH, in a dose-related manner, by cultured placental cells.

Placental CRF-POMC System

The CRF-induced ACTH release is unaffected by glucocorticoids, whereas oxytocin and prostaglandins

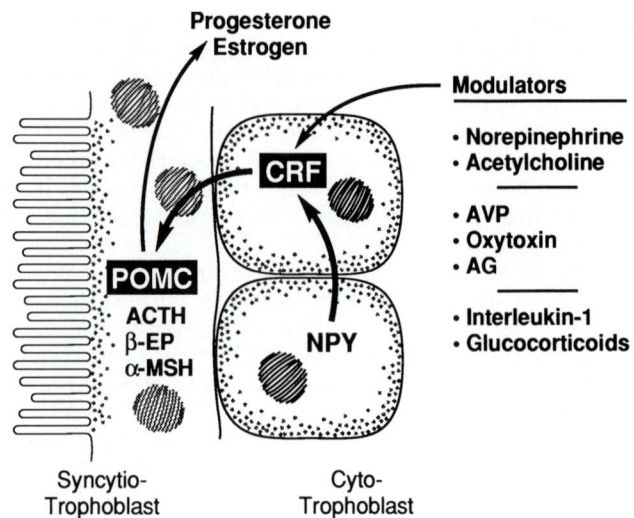

FIGURE 26–26. Diagrammatic depiction of the potential placental CRF-POMC system and its modulators.

stimulate the secretion of both CRF and ACTH. Thus, placental CRF may be involved in the processing of placental POMC peptides and ACTH and β-endorphin secretion (Fig. 26–26) (Petraglia et al., 1987b). Hypothalamic CRF, norepinephrine, acetylcholine, angiotensin II, vasopressin, oxytocin, and neuropeptide Y all have been shown to induce placental CRF release in culture (Petraglia et al., 1989b; Petraglia et al., 1989c). As in hypothalamic CRF counterpart, interleukin-1 (IL-1), but not IL-2, induces CRF release by the cultured placental cells (Petraglia et al., 1989b). While *in vivo* data are not available, the possibility that the neurotransmitters and neuropeptides may be involved in the stress-induced placental CRF responses has been proposed (Petraglia et al., 1990b; Plotsky, 1987).

Function

The functional role of placental CRF consists of an interdependent autocrine/paracrine control within the placenta and may also provide endocrine modes of regulation in the maternal and fetal compartments.

Autocrine/Paracrine Action

PROCESSING POMC. The formation of ACTH, β-LPH, β-EP and α-MSH from POMC is CRF-dependent and is dose-dependent. This effect of CRF is mediated through CRF receptors in the placenta and can be nullified by a synthetic antagonist to CRF (Petraglia et al., 1987b).

RESPONSE TO STRESS. The stressful event of labor may elevate CRF secretion. Under this circumstance both neurotransmitters (NE, Ach) and neuropeptides (AII, AVP, OT) are activated, and all are capable of inducing CRF release *in vitro* (Plotsky, 1987).

PARTURITION. Since both prostaglandins and glucocorticoids have the ability to stimulate CRF release (Robinson et al., 1988) and in view of their importance during labor and parturition, it is suggested that

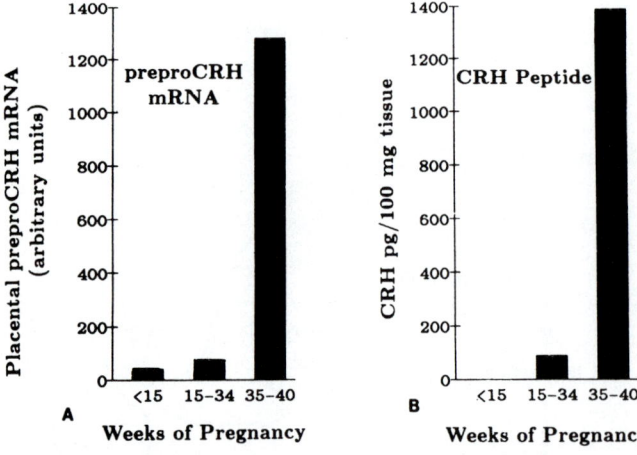

FIGURE 26–25. Changes in placental hCRH mRNA (*A*) and hCRH peptide (*B*) during gestation. (Reproduced from Frim DM, Emanuel RL, Robinson BG, et al: Characterization and gestational regulation of corticotropin-releasing hormone messenger RNA in human placenta. J Clin Invest **82**:287, 1988, by copyright permission of the American Society for Clinical Investigation.)

placental CRF is being activated at this time (Petraglia et al., 1990b).

IMMUNE FUNCTION. Interleukin-1, but not interleukin-2, stimulates the release of CRF from cultured trophoblasts, an effect similar to that of hypothalamic CRF secretion (Petraglia et al., 1989b). This regulatory function, if operative *in vivo*, would lead to a postulate of an interacting neuroendocrine-immune system in the human placenta.

Endocrine Role

CRF LEVELS IN MATERNAL COMPARTMENT. The placental source of elevated levels of CRF in the maternal circulation is well established (Petraglia et al., 1989b). The increased CRF levels during pregnancy occur mainly during the last trimester of pregnancy (approximately 600 pg/ml). These high levels of CRF are similar to the concentrations found in the rat hypothalamic portal blood and to those capable of stimulating ACTH release *in vitro* (Gibbs et al., 1982). Despite such high levels of CRF, maternal ACTH levels are elevated only slightly. This disparity can be explained by the presence of a CRF-binding protein (BP) which quenches circulating CRF and renders it unavailable for the corticotrope CRF receptors (Suda et al., 1989; Linton et al., 1990). The binding affinity of this BP for CRF is similar to that for the membrane-bound pituitary CRF receptors (Nishimura et al., 1988). This quenching effect of CRF-BP requires time (400 seconds), and thus the effectiveness of hypothalamic CRF on pituitary ACTH release in the maternal side should not be adversely affected by CRF-BP because the concentration of free CRF is high, the transient time is short, and the receptor number is high (Linton et al., 1990). The hypercortisolemia in late pregnancy cannot be fully attributed to placental ACTH or CRF release. Further studies are needed to improve our understanding of the placental-maternal regulations of the H-P-A axis during pregnancy.

β-ENDORPHIN (β-EP). As with ACTH, the relative contribution of placental β-EP to maternal and fetal compartment is also not fully understood. Plasma levels of β-endorphin immunoreactivity remain relatively low (mean 15 pg/ml) throughout pregnancy (Goland et al., 1981). With the onset of labor, there is a several-fold increase in β-endorphin with a further rise at delivery (Fig. 26–27). The molar ratio of β-endorphin to β-LPH does not alter during the course of pregnancy and labor—suggesting that the processing of the precursor molecule in pregnancy is similar to that in the nonpregnant state—or during the stress of delivery (Goland et al., 1981; Wardlaw et al., 1979). High levels of β-endorphin are also found in the cord plasma of the infant at term (mean 105 pg/ml). These levels are parallel to those of ACTH, indicating active secretion of both peptides by the fetal pituitary and/or by the placenta. There is evidence to suggest that hypoxia and acidosis may be major stimuli for the release of β-endorphin, β-LPH, and ACTH by the fetus (Wardlaw et al., 1979). Thus, elevation of β-endorphin level during labor and delivery and in fetal hypoxia-acidosis may reflect the expression of stress response. Nonetheless, the physiologic significance of

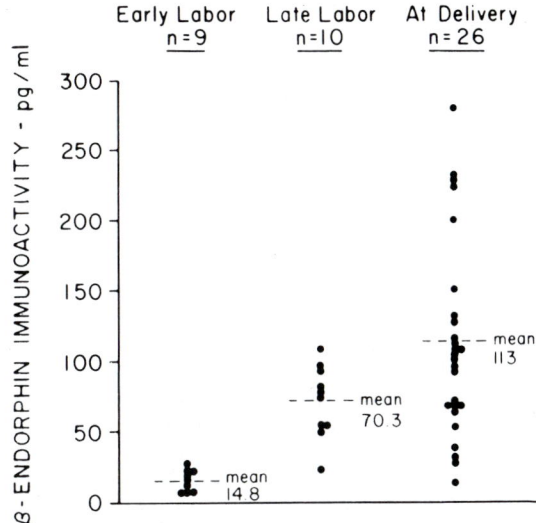

FIGURE 26–27. Concentrations of β-endorphin immunoreactivity in the plasma of women during early and late labor and at delivery. (From Goland RS, Wardlaw SL, Stark RI, Frantz AG: Human plasma β-endorphin during pregnancy, labor, and delivery. J Clin Endocrinol Metab **52**:74, © by the Endocrine Society, 1981.)

elevated β-endorphin levels in the maternal and fetal compartment remains to be elucidated.

CALCITROPIC HORMONES DURING PREGNANCY

It is estimated that 25 to 30 gm of calcium are deposited in the fetal skeleton during the second half of pregnancy, which is the only physiologic condition in which such massive shifts in calcium occur (Pitkin, 1985). Maternal calcium homeostasis is adjusted to include a positive calcium balance, an increased absorption of calcium by the small intestine, and alterations of calcitropic hormones, parathyroid (PTH), calcitonin, and 1,25-dihydroxyvitamin D_3 (1,25[OH]$_2$D$_3$).

Parathyroid Hormone

Parathyroid hormone (PTH) (84 amino acids, mw 9500) is synthesized in the parathyroid glands by sequential cleavage of pro-PTH. Circulating PTH is composed of at least three forms: (1) the intact hormone (1-84), which is biologically active with a half-life of 10 minutes and constitutes 10 per cent of the PTH pool; (2) the amino-terminal fragments, which are also biologically active, have a similar short half-life, and represent 10 per cent of the PTH pool; and (3) the carboxy-terminal fragments, which are biologically inactive and make up 80 per cent of the PTH pool. The heterogeneity of circulating forms of PTH represents a major problem in the understanding of the metabolism and inactivation of this hormone. Recently, however, the development of an immunoradiometric assay for the intact and biologically active forms of PTH has clarified this unsettled problem (Davis et al., 1988).

A *hypercalcemic hormone*, PTH is principally regulated by the calcium concentration in the extracellular fluid; a decrease in ionized calcium induces a prompt secretion of parathyroid hormone. In contrast to earlier studies, the serum PTH level is not found to be elevated. On the contrary, serum intact PTH declines during pregnancy while ionized calcium appears to be unaltered. Thus, the paradoxic hyperparathyroidism theory described previously is no longer held (Pitkin, 1985; Davis et al., 1988).

There is substantial evidence that the stimulatory effect of PTH on intestinal calcium transport reflects PTH-induced generation of 1,25(OH)D₃ by the kidney rather than a direct action of PTH on gut mucosa. PTH also enhances calcium reabsorption from the distal renal tubules. Finally, this hormone *promotes resorption of calcium from the bone.* Thus, all events of PTH action are directed at increasing serum calcium levels.

Calcitonin

Human calcitonin (CT) is secreted by the parafollicular or C cells of the thyroid gland. It is a 32-amino acid peptide hormone (mw 3200) with *hypocalcemic action.* CT secretion varies directly with changes in serum ionized calcium concentrations. The plasma half-life of this hormone is approximately 10 minutes. The calcium-lowering effect of CT is brought about through the reduction in bone resorption via a direct action on the bone. CT also inhibits parathyroid hormone–mediated bone resorption.

It appears that secretion of CT is elevated during pregnancy in both maternal and cord blood (Pitkin et al., 1979). Although several investigators have postulated a protective effect of CT on maternal skeleton, the roles of CT in the mother and the fetus are unclear at present (Pitkin et al., 1979).

Vitamin D and Metabolites

Vitamin D, like other steroid hormones, is derived from cholesterol. Vitamin D enters the circulation either from the skin, where it is formed by photosynthetic steps, or from the thoracic duct, which contains the absorbed dietary vitamin D. Vitamin D, as such, is a prohormone and is biologically inactive. During exposure to sunlight, the ultraviolet B portion of the solar spectrum produces the photochemical conversion of cutaneous 7-dehydrocholesterol to previtamin D₃ (Fig. 26–28). Immediately upon its formation, previtamin D₃ begins to isomerize by a temperature-dependent process to vitamin D₃. Following one exposure to sunlight, these processes continue for 3 days. Once vitamin D₃ is formed, the vitamin D–binding protein (owing to its high affinity to D₃) is translocated preferentially from the dermis to the circulation (Holick et al., 1980).

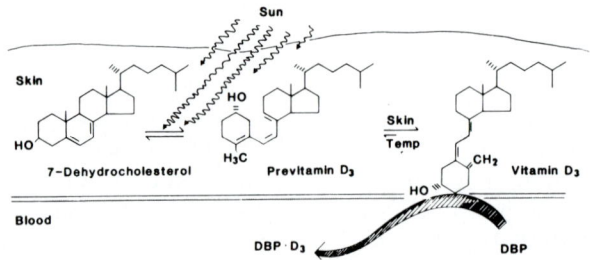

FIGURE 26–28. Diagrammatic representation of the formation of previtamin D₃ in the skin during exposure to the sun and its subsequent thermal conversion to vitamin D₃, which in turn is bound to vitamin D–binding protein (DBP) in plasma for transport into the circulation. (From Holick MF, MacLaughlin JA, Clark MB, et al: Photosynthesis of previtamin D₃ in human skin and the physiologic consequences. Science **210**:203, 1980. Copyright 1980 by the American Association for the Advancement of Science. Reprinted by permission.)

25-Hydroxyvitamin D₃

Transformation of circulating vitamin D₃ to biologically active D₃ requires several steps of hydroxylation. This process occurs first in the liver and gut, where 25-hydroxylation takes place with the formation of 25-hydroxyvitamin D₃ (25-OH D₃).

The concentration of 25-OH D₃ in maternal serum is higher than in cord serum, and there is a positive correlation between these levels (Cockburn et al., 1980). Because 25-OH D₃ crosses the placenta readily, this positive correlation has been interpreted as evidence for placental transport of 25-OH D₃. However, comparisons of serum concentrations of 25-OH D₃ are complicated by differences in the concentrations of vitamin D–binding protein (DBP) (Cooke et al., 1989). The maternal serum concentration of DBP increases 2.5-fold during pregnancy, and at term it is twice that of the cord serum (Bouillon et al., 1981). The lower levels of DBP and 25-OH D₃ in cord serum may reflect the immaturity of fetal liver function.

1,25-Dihydroxyvitamin D₃

The formation of 1,25-dihydroxyvitamin D₃ or, 1,25 (OH)₂D₃, the most potent vitamin D₃, occurs selectively in the kidney. This is because 1α-hydroxylase is found only in the kidney in the nonpregnant state. During pregnancy, however, additional synthetic sites for 1,25 (OH)₂D₃ are operational. These extrarenal sites of synthesis are the human placenta and decidua (Whitsett et al., 1981; Cockburn et al., 1980). Because the substrate, 25-OH D₃, is increased two- to threefold during pregnancy, and 1α-hydroxylase is present in the placenta and decidua, the synthesis of 1,25(OH)₂D₃ is also increased in pregnant women, resulting in an elevation of its circulating levels. Wilson and associates (1990) showed that 1,25(OH)₂D₃ levels rise during pregnancy in both free and total form as well as the DBP, but all concentrations fall dramatically during the first two weeks of lactation. This elevation probably explains how the mother increases intestinal absorption of calcium in anticipation of fetal and maternal needs for bone mineralization during pregnancy.

Osteocalcin

Osteocalcin (bone Gla-protein) is a bone-specific protein released into the circulation proportional to the rate of new bone formation (Brown et al., 1984). Serum osteocalcin measurement, as a clinical marker of bone turnover, is widely accepted. Studies in pregnant women have revealed a decreased level of osteocalcin in the second trimester, which returns to nonpregnant levels at term (Cole et al., 1987). Although this observation suggests the absence of accelerated bone turnover, the significance of this finding relative to calcium homeostasis during pregnancy remains to be examined.

PROLACTIN IN PREGNANCY

The Mother

In pregnancy, serum prolactin (PRL) concentration begins to rise in the first trimester and increases progressively to 10 times the nonpregnant concentration at term (Hwang et al., 1971; Tyson et al., 1972). When serum PRL concentrations are determined serially at weekly intervals in the same woman throughout pregnancy, an approximate linear pattern of rise is revealed (Rigg et al., 1977) (Fig. 26–29). The increase is probably related causally to supramaximal estrogen stimulation during the course of gestation and is a functional reflection of hypertrophy and hyperplasia of pituitary lactotropes.

The pulsatile nature of PRL release observed in nonpregnant women appears to be maintained during pregnancy. Sleep-induced PRL release also persists but with pulses of higher magnitude (Boyar et al., 1975). In pregnant women, as in nonpregnant women, an acute release of PRL occurs in synchrony with food ingestion (Quigley and Yen, 1979; Quigley et al., 1982). Thus, the food-entrained PRL release by the hypothalamic-pituitary system is also functionally unaltered (Fig. 26–30). The physiologic role of this food-entrained release during pregnancy is unclear. Infusion of PRL in humans induces glucose intolerance and increases plasma free fatty acid levels (McGarry and Beck, 1962). In hyperprolactinemic women, Gustafson

and colleagues (1980) have observed a reduced glucose tolerance in association with an exaggerated insulin response and a greater suppression of glucagon by glucose, a metabolic situation resembling that in normal pregnant women. Thus, hyperprolactinemia and the food-entrained PRL release may subserve endocrine-metabolic homeostasis in pregnancy.

In contrast to nonpregnant levels, prolactin levels in late pregnancy do not appear to be influenced by surgical stress or by anesthesia. This fact suggests that this aspect of neuroendocrine mechanisms is modified for the regulation of PRL secretion in late pregnancy (Rigg and Yen, 1977).

The Fetus

The pituitary gland of the human fetus is able to synthesize, store, and secrete prolactin early in gestation, with an accelerated increase in these functions during the last few weeks of intrauterine life (Aubert et al., 1975). At term, the mean umbilical vein concentration of PRL is higher than the mean maternal plasma level. The baby's PRL level returns progressively to the range usual in children by the end of the first week of postnatal life. Serum prolactin levels in *anencephalic infants* are essentially the same as those in normal infants (Fig. 26–31). Because lactotropes are anatomically isolated from the hypothalamus in the anencephalic fetus, this observation provides evidence that in the fetus, the principal hypothalamic control of PRL secretion by the pituitary, as in the adult, is through an inhibitory mechanism. The increase in fetal PRL secretion is probably due to a direct estrogenic stimulation of the fetal lactotropes. Although estriol production is markedly reduced in anencephalic infants, estrogen precursors of maternal adrenal origin are available, and indeed a low normal range of estradiol-17β and estrone levels has been found in their cord blood (Kenney et al., 1973). The physiologic role of fetal PRL is unknown. Experimental evidence indicates, however, that prolactin in the fetal compartment may participate in fetal lung maturation. Administration of PRL in pharmacologic amounts (1 mg) to the rabbit fetus leads to a rise in pulmonary lecithin levels, especially dipalmityllecithin, an active component of lung surfactant (Hamosh and Hamosh, 1977).

The Amniotic Fluid

The highest prolactin concentration is found in amniotic fluid, where it is five- to tenfold greater than in maternal serum (Hwang et al., 1971; Aubert et al., 1975). Of particular interest is the finding that this high concentration is present as early as the first trimester of pregnancy, when both fetal and maternal serum PRL concentrations are still relatively low (see Fig. 26–31). The human choriondecidua (but not the placenta) is capable of de novo biosynthesis of PRL that is immunologically and chemically identical to prolactin derived from the pituitary (Riddick and Kusmick, 1977; Golander et al., 1978; Bigazzi et al., 1979a).

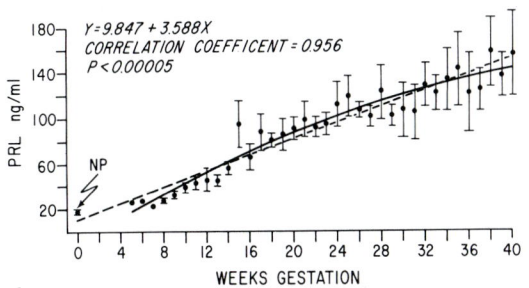

FIGURE 26–29. Serum prolactin concentration measured serially at weekly intervals as a function of duration of pregnancy. *Dashed line* = the linear regression; *solid line* = second order of regression; *NP* = nonpregnant value. (From Rigg LA, Yen SSC: Multiphasic prolactin [PRL] secretion during parturition in humans. Am J Obstet Gynecol **128**:215, 1977.)

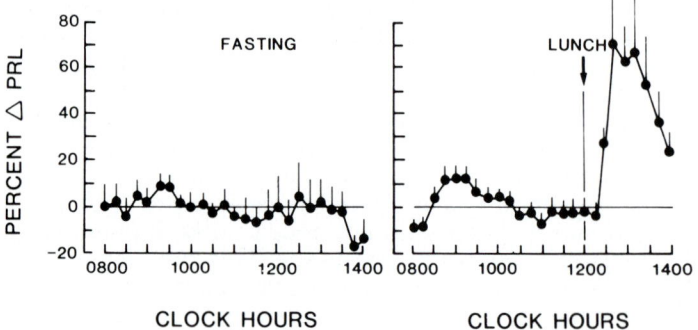

CLOCK HOURS   CLOCK HOURS

FIGURE 26–30. Mean (±SE) per cent change in serum prolactin levels in seven pregnant women during fasting and after ingestion of food at 1200 hours. (From Quigley ME, Ishizuka B, Ropert JF, Yen SSC: The food-entrained prolactin and cortisol release in late pregnancy and prolactinoma patients. J Clin Endocrinol Metab **54**:1109, © by The Endocrine Society, 1982.)

FIGURE 26–31. *Left,* Comparison of patterns of fetal and maternal plasma and amniotic fluid prolactin concentrations during pregnancy. *Right,* Plasma levels of normal and anencephalic newborns are compared with those of normal infants and adults. (Modified from Aubert ML, Grumbach MM, Kaplan SL: The ontogenesis of human fetal hormones. III. Prolactin. J Clin Endocrinol Metab **56**:155, © by The Endocrine Society, 1975.)

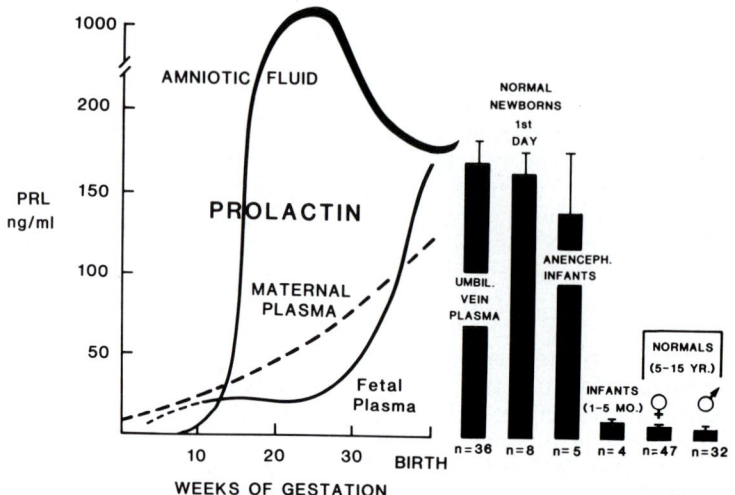

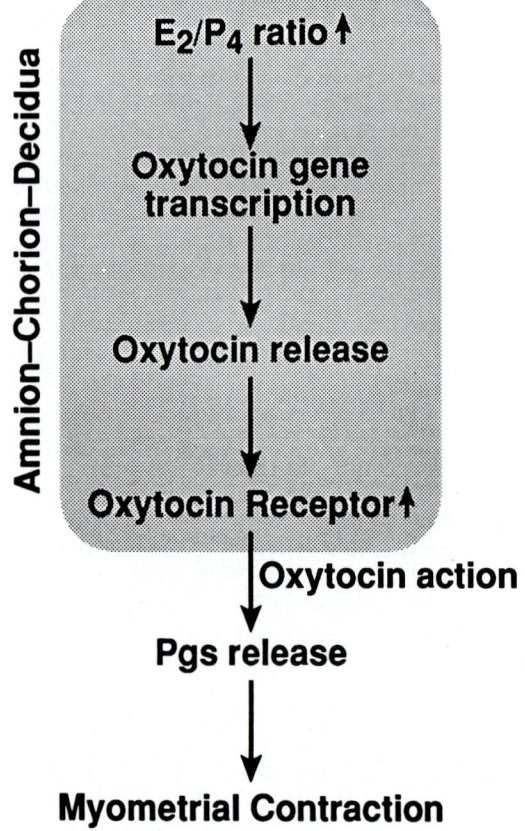

FIGURE 26–32. Diagrammatic illustration depicting the increase in oxytocin gene expression in the decidua-fetal membrane near term. It appears to be triggered by the increased E_2/P_4 ratio in these tissues. Together with increased oxytocin receptors, a paracrine action of oxytocin results in Pgs production and uterine contractions ensue.

The secretion of PRL by human decidual tissue *in vitro* (Bigazzi et al., 1979b) is not influenced by dopamine and dopamine agonists, which are known to modify pituitary PRL release. Prolactin binding has been demonstrated in amnion (McCoshen et al., 1982), and in fetal lung, adrenal, and liver of the rhesus monkey (Josimovich et al., 1977b). A 50 per cent decrease in amniotic fluid volume can be induced in rhesus monkeys by intra-amniotic injection of ovine prolactin, an effect that persists for about 24 hours (Josimovich et al., 1977a). Thus, locally produced PRL may participate in the regulation of osmotic exchange in the amniotic fluid compartment.

OXYTOCIN

Circulating oxytocin levels during pregnancy and labor have not been vigorously evaluated. Because of its short half-life (about 3 min) and the episodic nature of secretory events, frequent sampling is required to determine the relationship between changes in oxytocin levels and initiation of labor. In general, evidence suggests that oxytocin levels are very low and a clear increase occurs only during the second stage of labor.

Recent studies of human pregnant myometrium indicate that a 100- to 200-fold increase in oxytocin receptor concentration occurs during the course of gestation. More important, the levels of oxytocin receptors rise from late pregnancy values to a maximum during early labor (Fuchs and Fuchs, 1984). The rising receptor concentrations are paralleled by an increase in uterine oxytocin sensitivity during the second half of gestation. Circulating oxytocin is not essential for the initiation and maintenance of spontaneous labor; normal parturition can be achieved in the absence of endogenous oxytocin secretion by the neurohypophysis. The recent demonstrations, in both rat uterus and human fetal membranes and decidua, that oxytocin gene expression increases toward term have provided a new dimension for the role of oxytocin in the initiation of parturition. The signal for activating oxytocin gene expression in the fetal membrane and decidua remains to be determined, but the increased estradiol/progesterone ratio appears to play a significant role (Lefebvre et al., 1992; Chibbar et al., 1992). The current understanding of labor onset in pregnant women is depicted in Figure 26–32.

REFERENCES

Abe Y, Miyamoto HK, Yamaguchi M, Andoh A, Ibuki Y, Igarashi M: High concentrations of plasma immunoreactive inhibin during normal pregnancy in women. J Clin Endocrinol Metab **71**:133, 1990.

Abou-Samra AB, Pugeat M, Dechaud H, Nachury L, Bouchareb B, Ferre-Montagne M, Tournaire J: Increased plasma concentration of N-terminal lipotrophin and unbound cortisol during pregnancy. Clin Endocrinol **20**:221, 1984.

Ahmed MS, Horst MA: Opioid receptors of human placental villi modulate acetylcholine release. Life Sci **39**:535, 1986.

Albrecht ED, Pepe GJ: Placental steroid hormone biosynthesis in primate pregnancy. Endocr Rev **11**:124, 1990.

Amano J, Nishimura R, Mochizuki M, Kobata A: Comparative study of the mucin-type sugar chains of the human chorionic gonado-tropin present in the urine of patients with trophoblastic diseases and healthy pregnant women. J Biol Chem **263**:1157, 1988.

Aubert ML, Grumbach MM, Kaplan SL: The ontogenesis of human fetal hormones. III. Prolactin. J Clin Endocrinol Metab **56**:155, 1975.

Baggia S, Albrecht ED, Pepe GJ: Regulation of 11β-hydroxysteroid dehydrogenase activity in the baboon placenta by estrogen. Endocrinology **126**:2742, 1990.

Barnea ER, Feldman D, Kaplan M, Morrish DW: The dual effect of epidermal growth factor upon human chorionic gonadotropin secretion by the first trimester placenta in vitro. J Clin Endocrinol Metab **71**:923, 1990.

Barsh GS, Seeburg PH, Gelinas RE: The human growth hormone gene family: structure and evolution of the chromosomal locus. Nucleic Acids Res **11**:3939, 1983.

Baulieu EE: Contragestion and other clinical applications of RU486, an antiprogesterone at the receptor. Science **245**:13, 1989.

Baulieu EE, Dray FL: Conversion of ³H-dehydroisoandrosterone (3β-hydroxy-Δ⁵-androsten-17-one) sulfate to ³H-estrogens in normal pregnant women. J Clin Endocrinol Metab **23**:1298, 1963.

Beck P, Daughaday WH: Human placental lactogen: Studies of its acute metabolic effects and disposition in normal man. J Clin Invest **46**:103, 1967.

Belisle G, Schiff I, Tulchinsky D: The use of constant infusion of unlabeled dehydroepiandrosterone for the assessment of its metabolic clearance rate, its half-life, and its conversion into estrogens. J Clin Endocrinol Metab **50**:117, 1980.

Belisle S, Petit A, Gallo-Payet N, Bellabarba D, Lehoux JG, Lemaire S: Functional opioid receptor sites in human placenta. J Clin Endocrinol Metab **66**:283, 1988.

Berrera-Saldana HA, Seeburg PH, Saunders GF: Two structurally different genes produce the same human placental lactogen hormone. J Biol Chem **258**:3787, 1983.

Berry SA, Srivastava CH, Rubin LR, Phipps WR, Pescovitz OH: Growth hormone-releasing hormone-like messenger ribonucleic acid and immunoreactive peptide are present in human testis and placenta. J Clin Endocrinol Metab **75**:281, 1992.

Bigazzi M, Nardi E: Prolactin and relaxin: Antagonism on the spontaneous motility of the uterus. J Clin Endocrinol Metab **53**:665, 1981.

Bigazzi M, Pollicino G, Nardi E: Is human decidua a specialized endocrine organ? J Clin Endocrinol Metab **49**:847, 1979a.

Bigazzi M, Ronga R, Lancranjan I, et al: A pregnancy in an acromegalic woman during bromocriptive treatment: Effects on GH and PRL in the maternal, fetal and amniotic compartments. J Clin Endocrinol Metab **48**:9, 1979b.

Birker S, Armstrong EG, Gawinowicz-Kolks MA, Cole LA, Agosto GM, Krichevsky A, Vaitukaitis JL, Canfield RE: Structure of the human chorionic gonadotropin β-subunit fragment from pregnancy urine. Endocrinology **123**:572, 1988.

Bleicher SJ, O'Sullivan JB, Freinkel N: Carbohydrate metabolism in pregnancy. V. The interrelations of glucose, insulin and free fatty acids in late pregnancy and postpartum. N Engl J Med **271**:866, 1964.

Blithe DL, Akar AH, Wehmann RE, Nisula BC: Purification of β-core fragment from pregnancy urine and demonstration that its carbohydrate moieties differ from those of native human chorionic gonadotropin β. Endocrinology **122**:173, 1988.

Blomquist CH, Lindemann NJ, Hakanson EY: 17β-hydroxysteroid and 20α-hydroxysteroid dehydrogenase activities of human placental microsomes: kinetic evidence for two enzymes differing in substrate specificity. Arch Biochem Biophys **239**:206, 1985.

Blomquist CH, Lindemann NJ, Hakanson EY: Steroid modulation of 17β-hydroxysteroid oxidoreductase activities in human placental villi *in vitro*. J Clin Endocrinol Metab **65**:647, 1987.

Bolte E, Mancuso S, Eriksson G: Studies on the aromatization of neutral steroids in pregnant women. I. Aromatization of C-19 steroids by placentas perfused in situ. Acta Endocrinol **45**:535, 1964.

Bouillon R, VanAssche FA, VanBaelen H: Influence of the vitamin D binding protein on the serum concentration of 1,25-dihydroxy-vitamin D₃. J Clin Invest **67**:589, 1981.

Boyar RM, Finkelstein JW, Kapen S, Hellman L: Twenty-four hour prolactin secretory pattern during pregnancy. J Clin Endocrinol Metab **40**:1117, 1975.

Branchaud CL, Goodyer CG, Lipowski LS: Progesterone and estrogen production by placental monolayer cultures: effect of dehydroepiandrosterone and luteinizing hormone-releasing hormone. J Clin Endocrinol Metab **56**:761, 1983.

Braunstein GD, Kamdar V, Rasor J, Swaminathan N, Wade ME: Widespread distribution of a chorionic gonadotropin-like substance in normal human tissues. J Clin Endocrinol Metab **49**:917, 1979.

Braunstein GD, Karow WG, Gentry WC, Rasor J, Wade ME: First-trimester chorionic gonadotropin measurements as an aid in the diagnosis of early pregnancy disorders. Am J Obstet Gynecol **131**:25, 1978.

Braverman MB, Gurpide E: In vitro effects of human prolactin and oxytocin on sulfatase activity in isolated human decidual cells. J Clin Endocrinol Metab **63**:725, 1986.

Brown JB: Urinary excretion of oestrogen during pregnancy, lactation and the re-establishment of menstruation. Lancet **i**:704, 1956.

Brown JP, Delmar PD, Malaval L: Serum bone Gla-protein: A specific marker for bone formation in postmenopausal osteoporosis. Lancet **1**:1091, 1984.

Buchanan TA, Metzger BE, Freinkel N, Bergman RN: Insulin sensitivity and B-cell responsiveness to glucose during late pregnancy in lean and moderately obese women with normal glucose tolerance or mild gestational diabetes. Am J Obstet Gynecol **162**:1008, 1990.

Bulmer JN, Johnson PM: Immunohistological characterization of the decidual leucocytic infiltrate related to endometrial gland epithelium in early human pregnancy. Immunology **55**:35, 1985.

Burt RL, Davidson WF: Insulin half-life and utilization in normal pregnancy. Obstet Gynecol **43**:161, 1974.

Cassmer O: Hormone production of the isolated human placenta. Studies on the role of the foetus in the endocrine functions of the placenta. Acta Endocrinol **32**(Suppl 45):1, 1959.

Castracane VD, Goldzieher JW: The relationship of estrogen to placental steroidogenesis in the baboon. J Clin Endocrinol Metab **62**:1163, 1986.

Chen S, Besman MJ, Sparkes RS, Zollman S, Klisak I, Mohandas T, Hall PF, Shively JE: Human aromatase: cDNA cloning, Southern blot analysis, and assignment of the gene to chromosome 15. DNA **7**:27, 1988.

Chibbar R, Miller F, Mitchell BF: Regulation of oxytocin gene expression in human fetal membranes around the time of parturition. (Abstract 285) Proc Soc Gyn Invest, 1992.

Ciaraldi TP, Kettel LM, El-Roeiy A, Madar Z, Reichart D, Yen SSC, Olefsky J: Mechanisms of cellular insulin resistance in human pregnancy. J Clin Endocrinol Metab **75**:577, 1992.

Cockburn F, Belton NR, Purvis RJ: Maternal vitamin D intake and mineral metabolism in mothers and their newborn infants. Br Med J **281**:11, 1980.

Cole DEC, Gundberg CM, Stiek LJ: Changing osteocalcin concentrations during pregnancy and lactation: Implications for maternal mineral metabolism. J Clin Endocrinol Metab **65**:2, 1987.

Cooke NE, Haddad JG: Vitamin D protein (Gc-globulin). Endocr Rev **10**:294, 1989.

Costrini NV, Kalkhoff RK: Relative effects of pregnancy, estradiol and progesterone on plasma insulin and pancreatic islet insulin secretion. J Clin Invest **50**:992, 1971.

Cousins L, Rigg L, Hollingsworth D, Brink G, Aurand J, Yen SSC: The 24-hour excursion and diurnal rhythm of glucose insulin and C-peptide in normal pregnancy. Am J Obstet Gynecol **136**:483, 1980.

Cousins L, Rigg L, Hollingsworth D, Meis P, Halberg F, Brink G, Yen SSC: Qualitative and quantitative assessment of the circadian rhythm of cortisol in pregnancy. Am J Obstet Gynecol **145**:411, 1983.

Csapo AI, Pulkkinen MO, Wiest WG: Effects of luteoectomy and progesterone replacement in early pregnant patients. Am J Obstet Gynecol **115**:759, 1973.

Cummings SW, Hatley W, Simpson ER, Ohashi M: The binding of high- and low-density lipoproteins to human placental membrane fractions. J Clin Endocrinol Metab **54**:903, 1982.

Daniel RR, Metzger BE, Freinkel N, Faloona GR, Unger RH, Nitzan M: Carbohydrate metabolism in pregnancy. XI. Response of plasma glucagon to overnight fast and oral glucose during pregnancy and in gestational diabetes. Diabetes **23**:771, 1974.

Das C, Catt KJ: Antifertility actions of the progesterone antagonist RU486 include direct inhibition of placental hormone secretion. Lancet **2**:599, 1987.

Daughaday WH, Trivedi B, Winn HN, Yan H: Hypersomatotropism in pregnant women, as measured by a human liver radioreceptor assay. J Clin Endocrinol Metab **70**:215, 1990.

Davis OK, Hawkins DS, Rubin LP, Posillico JT, Brown EM, Schiff I: Serum parathyroid hormone (PTH) in pregnant women determined by an immunoradiometric assay for intact PTH. J Clin Endocrinol Metab **67**:850, 1988.

DeNoto FM, Moore DD, Goodman HM: Human growth hormone DNA sequence and mRNA structures: possible alternative splicing. Nucleic Acids Res **9**:3719, 1981.

Diczfalusy E: Endocrine functions of the human fetoplacental unit. Fed Proc **23**:791, 1964.

Dinarello CA: Biology of interleukin-1. FASEB J **2**:108, 1988.

Doe RP, Zinnerman HH, Flink EB, Ulstrom RA: Significance of the concentration of non-protein bound plasma cortisol in normal Cushing syndrome, pregnancy and during estrogen therapy. J Clin Endocrinol Metab **20**:1484, 1960.

Edwards RG, Steptoe PC, Purdy JM: Fertilization and cleavage in vitro of preovulatory human oocytes. Nature **227**:1307, 1970.

Edwards RG, Steptoe PC, Purdy JM: Establishing full-term human pregnancies using cleaving embryos grown in vitro. Br J Obstet Gynaecol **87**:737, 1980.

Eriksson L, Frankenne F, Eden S, Hennen G, von Schoultz B: Growth hormone 24-hour serum profiles during pregnancy—lack of pulsatility for the secretion of the placental variant. Br J Obstet Gynaecol **96**:949, 1989.

Fant M, Munro H, Moses AC: An autocrine/paracrine role for insulin-like growth factors in the regulation of human placental growth. J Clin Endocrinol Metab **63**:499, 1986.

Felig P, Kim YJ, Lynch V, Hendler R: Amino acid metabolism during starvation in human pregnancy. J Clin Invest **51**:1195, 1972.

Felig P, Wahren J, Sherwin R, Hendler R: Insulin, glucagon, and somatostatin in normal physiology and diabetes mellitus. Diabetes **25**:1091, 1976.

Fishel SB, Edwards RG, Evans C: Human chorionic gonadotrophin secreted by preimplantation embryos cultured in vitro. Science **223**:816, 1984.

Fisher DA: The unique endocrine milieu of the fetus. J Clin Invest **78**:603, 1986.

Flynn A, Finke JH, Hilfiker ML: Placental mononuclear phagocytes as a source of interleukin-1. Science **218**:475, 1982.

Folkman J, Klagsbrun M: Angiogenic factors. Science **235**:442, 1987.

Fournet-Dulguerov N, MacLusky NJ, Leranth CA, Todd R, Mendelson CR, Simpson ER, Naftolin F: Immunohistochemical localization of aromatase cytochrome P-450 and estradiol dehydrogenase in the syncytiotrophoblast of the human placenta. J Clin Endocrinol Metab **65**:757, 1987.

Frandsen VA, Stakemann G: The site of production of oestrogenic hormones in human pregnancy. Hormone excretion in pregnancy with anencephalic foetus. Acta Endocrinol (Kbh) **38**:383, 1961.

Frankenne F, Closset J, Gomez F, Scippo ML, Smal J, Hennen G: The physiology of growth hormones (GHs) in pregnant women and partial characterization of the placental GH variant. J Clin Endocrinol Metab **66**:1171, 1988.

Frankenne F, Scippo ML: Circulating forms and partial glycosylation of human placental growth hormone (hPGH). (Abstract 1129) Proceedings of the 70th Annual Meeting of The Endocrine Society, 1988.

Freinkel N, Metzger BE, Nitzan M, Daniel R, Surmacznsak BZ, Nagel TC: Facilitated anabolism in late pregnancy: Some novel maternal compensations for accelerated starvation. In Malaisse WJ, Pirart J (eds): Diabetes. (International Series No. 312.) Amsterdam, Excerpta Medica, 1973, p. 474.

Friesen HG, Suwa S, Pare P: Synthesis and secretion of placental lactogen and other proteins by the placenta. Rec Prog Horm Res **25**:161, 1969.

Frim DM, Emanuel RL, Robinson BG, Smas CM, Adler GK, Majzoub JA: Characterization and gestational regulation of corticotropin-releasing hormone messenger RNA in human placenta. J Clin Invest **82**:287, 1988.

Fuchs A-R, Fuchs F: Endocrinology of human parturition: a review. Br J Obstet Gynaecol **91**:948, 1984.

Gant NF, Hutchinson HT, Siiteri PK, MacDonald PC: Study of the metabolic clearance rate of dehydroepiandrosterone sulfate in pregnancy. Am J Obstet Gynecol 111:555, 1971.

Garzo G, Liu J, Ulmann A, Yen SSC: Effects of an antiprogesterone (RU486) on the hypothalamic-gonadotropin-ovarian-endometrial axis during the luteal phase of the menstrual cycle. J Clin Endocrinol Metab 66:508, 1988.

Gibbs DM, Stewart RD, Vale W, Rivier J, Yen SSC: Synthetic corticotropin-releasing factor stimulates secretion of immunoreactive β-endorphin/β-lipotropin and ACTH by human fetal pituitaries in vitro. Life Sci 32:547, 1982.

Gillmer MDG, Beard RW, Oakley NW, Brooke FM, Brudenell M, Chard T: Plasma human placental lactogen profiles over 24 hours in normal and diabetic pregnancy. Br J Obstet Gynaecol 84:197, 1977.

Goland RS, Wardlaw SL, Stark RI, Frantz AG: Human plasma β-endorphin during pregnancy, labor, and delivery. J Clin Endocrinol Metab 52:74, 1981.

Golander A, Hurley T, Barrett J, et al: Prolactin synthesis by human chorion-decidual tissue: A possible source of prolactin in the amniotic fluid. Science 202:311, 1978.

Gonzalez FJ, Kasper CB: Cloning of DNA complementary to rat liver NADPH-cytochrome c (P-450) oxidoreductase and cytochrome P-450b, mRNAs. Evidence that phenobarbital augments transcription of specific genes. J Biol Chem 257:5962, 1982.

Grimshaw RN, Mitchell BF, Challis JRG: Steroid modulation of pregnenolone to progesterone conversion by human placental cells in vitro. Am J Obstet Gynecol 145:234, 1983.

Grumbach MM, Kaplan SL, Sciarra JJ, Burr IM: Chorionic growth hormone-prolactin (CGP): Secretion, disposition, biologic activity in man, and postulated function as the "growth hormone of the second half of pregnancy." Ann NY Acad Sci 148:501, 1968.

Gurpide E, Schwers J, Welch MT, VandeWiele RL, Lieberman S: Fetal and maternal metabolism of estradiol during pregnancy. J Clin Endocrinol Metab 26:1355, 1966.

Gustafson AB, Banasiak MF, Kalkhoff RK, et al: Correlation of hyperprolactinemia with altered plasma insulin and glucagon: Similarity to effects of late human pregnancy. J Clin Endocrinol Metab 51:242, 1980.

Hall PF: Cytochromes P-450 and the regulation of steroid synthesis. Steroids 48:133, 1986.

Hamosh M, Hamosh P: The effect of prolactin on the lecithin content of fetal rabbit lung. J Clin Invest 59:1002, 1977.

Han VKM, Lund PK, Lee DC, E'Ercole AJ: Expression of somatomedin/insulin-like growth factor messenger ribonucleic acids in the human fetus: identification, characterization, and tissue distribution. J Clin Endocrinol Metab 66:422, 1988.

Hearn JP: The embryo-maternal dialogue during early pregnancy in primates. J Reprod Fertil 76:809, 1986.

Hemmings R, Langlais J, Falcone T, Granger L, Miron P, Guyda H: Human embryos produce transforming growth factors α activity and insulin-like growth factors II. Fertil Steril 58:101, 1992.

Hershman JM, Lee H-Y, Sugawara M, Mirell CJ, Pang X-P, Yanagisawa M, Pekary AE: Human chorionic gonadotropin stimulates iodide uptake, adenylate cyclase, and deoxyribonucleic acid synthesis in cultured rat thyroid cells. J Clin Endocrinol Metab 67:74, 1988.

Hochberg Z, Bick T, Perlman R: Two pathways of placental lactogen secretion by cultured human trophoblast. Biochem Med Metabol Biol 39:111, 1988.

Hochberg Z, Perlman R, Brandes JM, Benderly A: Insulin regulates placental lactogen and estradiol secretion by cultured human term trophoblast. J Clin Endocrinol Metab 57:1311, 1983.

Hoerkmann R, Spoettl G, Moncayo R, Mann K: Evidence for the presence of human chorionic gonadotropin (hCG) and free β-subunit of hCG in the human pituitary. J Clin Endocrinol Metab 71:179, 1990.

Hofmann GE, Drews MR, Scott Jr RT, Navot D, Heller D, Deligdisch L: Epidermal growth factor and its receptor in human implantation trophoblast: immunohistochemical evidence for autocrine/paracrine function. J Clin Endocrinol Metab 74:981, 1992.

Holick MF, MacLaughlin JA, Clark MB: Photosynthesis of previtamin D₃ in human skin and the physiologic consequences. Science 210:203, 1980.

Hoshina M, Boothby M, Boime I: Cytological localization of chorionic gonadotropin α and placental lactogen mRNAs during development of the human placenta. J Cell Biol 93:190, 1982.

Hudson P, John M, Crawford R, Haralambidis J, Scanlon D, Gorman J, Tregear G, Shine J, Niall H: Relaxin gene expression in human ovaries and the predicted structure of a human pre-prorelaxin by analysis of cDNA clones. EMBO J 3:2333, 1984.

Hug DL, Lopata A: Chorionic gonadotropin secretion by human embryos in vitro. J Clin Endocrinol Metab 67:1322, 1988.

Hussa RO: Biosynthesis of human chorionic gonadotropin. Endocr Rev 1:268, 1980.

Hwang P, Guyda H, Friesen H: A radioimmunoassay for human prolactin. Proc Natl Acad Sci 68:1902, 1971.

Igout A, Scippo ML, Frankenne F, Hennen G: Cloning and nucleotide sequence of placental hGH-V cDNA. Arch Int Physiol Biochim 96:63, 1988.

Illingworth PJ, Reddi K, Smith K, Baird DT: Pharmacological "rescue" of the corpus luteum results in increased inhibin production. Clin Endocrinol 33:323, 1990.

Jameson JL, Lindell CM: Isolation and characterization of the human chorionic gonadotropin β subunit (CGβ) gene cluster: regulation of a transcriptionally active CGβ gene by cyclic AMP. Mol Cell Biol 8:5100, 1988.

Jameson JL, Lindell CM, Habner JF. Gonadotropin and thyrotropin CG-α and β-subunit gene expression in normal and neoplastic tissues characterized using specific messenger ribonucleic hybridization probes. J Clin Endocrinol Metab 64:319, 1986.

Johansson EDB: Plasma levels of progesterone in pregnancy measured by a rapid competitive protein binding technique. Acta Endocrinol 61:607, 1969.

Josimovich JB, Merisko K, Boccella L: Amniotic prolactin control over amniotic and fetal extracellular fluid water and electrolytes in the rhesus monkey. Endocrinology 100:564, 1977a.

Josimovich JB, Merisko K, Boccella L, Tobon H: Binding of prolactin by fetal rhesus cell membrane fractions. Endocrinology 100:557, 1977b.

Jovanovic L, Landesman R, Saxena BB: Screening for twin pregnancy. Science 198:738, 1977.

Kalkhoff RK, Jacobson M, Lemper D: Progesterone, pregnancy and the augmented plasma insulin response. J Clin Endocrinol Metab 31:24, 1970.

Kalkhoff RK, Schalch DS, Walker JW, Beck P, Kipnis DM, Daughaday WH: Diabetogenic factors associated with pregnancy. Trans Assoc Am Physicians 77:270, 1964.

Kao LC, Caltabiano S, Wu S, Strauss III JF, Kliman HJ: The human villous cytotrophoblast: interactions with extracellular matrix proteins, endocrine function, and cytoplasmic differentiation in the absence of syncytium formation. Dev Biol 130:693, 1988.

Kasugai M, Kato H, Iriyama H, Kato M, Ninagawa T, Tomoda Y: The roles of Ca²⁺ and adenosine 3′,5′-monophosphate in the regulation of progesterone production by human placental tissue. J Clin Endocrinol Metab 65:122, 1987.

Kato Y, Braunstein GD: β-Core fragment is a major form of immunoreactive urinary chorionic gonadotropin in human pregnancy. J Clin Endocrinol Metab 66:1197, 1988.

Kato Y, Braunstein GD: Purified first and third trimester placental trophoblasts differ in in vitro hormone secretion. J Clin Endocrinol Metab 70:1187, 1990.

Kauma S, Matt D, Strom S, Eierman D, Turner T: Interleukin-1β, human leukocyte antigen HLA-DRα, and transforming growth factor-β expression in endometrium, placenta, and placental membranes. Am J Obstet Gynecol 163:1430, 1990.

Kemp BE, Niall HD: Relaxin. Vitamins and hormones. 41:79, 1984.

Kenny FM, Angsusingha K, Stinson D, Hotchkiss J: Unconjugated estrogens in the perinatal period. Pediatr Res 7:826, 1973.

Kettel LM, Roseff SJ, Bangah ML, Burger HG, Yen SSC: Circulating levels of inhibin in pregnant women at term: simultaneous disappearance with oestradiol and progesterone after delivery. Clin Endocrinol 34:19–23, 1991.

Khodr GS, Siler-Khodr TM: The effect of luteinizing hormone-releasing factor on human chorionic gonadotropin secretion. Fertil Steril 30:301, 1978.

Kliman HJ, Nestler JE, Sermasi E, Sanger JM, Strauss III JF: Purification, characterization, and in vitro differentiation of cytotrophoblasts from human term placentae. Endocrinology 118:1567, 1986.

Krieger DT, Liotta AS: Pituitary hormones in brain: where, how, and why? Science 205:366, 1979.

Leblanc H, Anderson JR, Yen SSC: Glucagon secretion in late pregnancy and the puerperium. Am J Obstet Gynecol **125**:708, 1976.

Lefebvre DL, Giaid A, Bennett H, Lariviére R, Zingg HH: Oxytocin gene expression in rat uterus. Science **256**:1553, 1992.

Lenton EA, Woodward AJ: The endocrinology of conception cycles and implantation in women. J Reprod Fertil **36**(Suppl):1, 1988.

Lin TJ, Lin SC, Erlenmeyer F, Kline IT, Underwood R, Billiar RB, Little B: Progesterone production rates during the third trimester of pregnancy in normal women, diabetic women, and women with abnormal glucose tolerance. J Clin Endocrinol Metab **34**:287, 1972.

Linton EA, Behan DP, Saphier PW, Lowry PJ: Corticotropin-releasing hormone (CRH)-binding protein: Reduction in the adrenocorticotropin-releasing activity of placental but not hypothalamic CRH. J Clin Endocrinol Metab **70**:1574, 1990.

Liotta AS, Houghten R, Krieger DT: Identification of a β-endorphin-like peptide in cultured human placental cells. Nature **295**:593, 1982.

Liu KH, Baumbach GA, Gillevet PM, Godkin JD: Purification and characterization of bovine placental retinol-binding protein. Endocrinology **127**:2696, 1990.

Lorence MC, Murry BA, Trant JM, Mason JI: Human 3β-hydroxysteroid dehydrogenase/$\Delta^5 \rightarrow^4$ isomerase from placenta: expression in nonsteroidogenic cells of a protein that catalyzes the dehydrogenation/isomerization of C21 and C19 steroids. Endocrinology **126**:2493, 1990.

MacDonald PC, Cutrer S, MacDonald SC, Casey ML, Parker CR Jr: Regulation of extra-adrenal steroid 21-hydroxylase activity: Increased conversion of plasma progesterone to deoxycorticosterone during estrogen treatment of women pregnant with a dead fetus. J Clin Invest **69**:469, 1982.

Magendantz HG, Ryan KJ: Isolation of an estriol precursor, 16α-hydroxydehydroepiandrosterone from human umbilical sera. J Clin Endocrinol Metab **24**:1155, 1964.

Main EK, Strizki J, Schochet P: Placental production of immunoregulatory factors: trophoblast is a source of interleukin-1. Trophoblast Res **2**:149, 1987.

Marshall RN, Underwood LE, Voina SJ, Foushee DB, Van Wyk JJ: Characterization of the insulin and somatomedin-C receptors in human placental cell membranes. J Clin Endocrinol Metab **39**:283, 1974.

Martucci C, Fishman J: Direction of estrogen metabolism as a control of its hormonal action—uterotropic activity of estradiol metabolites. Endocrinology **101**:1709, 1977.

Maruo T, Matsuo H, Ohtani T, Hoshina M, Mochizuchi M: Differential modulation of chorionic gonadotropin (CG) subunit messenger ribonucleic acid level and CG secretion by progesterone in normal placenta and choriocarcinoma cultured *in vitro*. Endocrinology **119**:858, 1986.

Massague J: The TGF-β family of growth and differentiation factors. Cell **49**:437, 1986.

Massague J, Czech MP: The subunit structures of two distinct receptors for insulin-like growth factors I and II and their relationship to the insulin receptor. J Biol Chem **257**:5038, 1982.

McCoshen JA, Tomita K, Fernandez C, Tyson JE: Specific cells of human amnion selectively localize prolactin. J Clin Endocrinol Metab **55**:166, 1982.

McGarry EE, Beck JC: Some metabolic effects of ovine prolactin in man. Lancet **ii**:915, 1962.

McLachlan RI, Burger HG, Healy DL, de Kretser DM, Robertson DM: Circulating immunoactive inhibin in the luteal phase and early gestation of women undergoing ovulation induction. Fertil Steril **48**:1001, 1987a.

McLachlan RI, Healy DL, Lutjen PJ, Findlay JK, de Kretser DM, Burger HG: The maternal ovary is not the source of circulating inhibin levels during human pregnancy. Clin Endocrinol (Oxf) **27**:663, 1987b.

Merimee TJ, Zapt J, Froesch ER: Insulin-like growth factor in pregnancy: studies in a growth hormone-deficient dwarf. J Clin Endocrinol Metab **54**:1101, 1982.

Mersol-Barg MS, Miller KF, Choi CM, Lee AC, Kim MH: Inhibin suppresses human chorionic gonadotropin secretion in term, but not first-trimester, placenta. J Clin Endocrinol Metab **71**:1294, 1990.

Mitchell BF, Cross J, Hobkirk R, Challis JRG: Formation of unconjugated estrogens from estrone sulfate by dispersed cells from human fetal membranes and decidua. J Clin Endocrinol Metab **58**:845, 1984.

Nakajima ST, McAuliffe T, Gibson M: The 24-hour pattern of the levels of serum progesterone and immunoreactive human chorionic gonadotropin in normal early pregnancy. J Clin Endocrinol Metab **71**:345, 1990.

Naylor SL, Chin WW, Goodman HM, Lalley PA, Grzeschik K, Sakaguchi AY: Chromosome assignment of genes encoding the alpha and beta subunits of glycoprotein hormones in man and mouse. Somatic Cell Mol Genet **9**:757, 1983.

Nexo E, Hollenberg MD, Figuerva A, Pratt RM: Detection of epidermal growth factor urogastrone and its receptor during fetal mouse development. Proc Natl Acad Sci USA **77**:2782, 1980.

Nickel BE, Kardami E, Cattini PA: The human placental growth hormone variant is mitogenic for rat lymphoma Nb2 cells. Endocrinology **126**:971, 1990.

Nishimura E, Bilezikjian L, Billestrup N, Perrin M, Vale W: Molecular characterization of bovine pituitary CRF receptors. (Abstract 01-18-06) Eighth International Congress of Endocrinology, 1988.

Nolten WE, Lindheimer MD, Oparil S, Ehrlich EN: Deoxycorticosterone in normal pregnancy. I. Sequential studies of the secretory patterns of deoxycorticosterone, aldosterone, and cortisol. Am J Obstet Gynecol **132**:414, 1978.

Nulsen JC, Woolkalis MJ, Kopf GS, Strauss JF III: Adenylate cyclase in human cytotrophoblasts: characterization and its role in modulating human chorionic gonadotropin secretion. J Clin Endocrinol Metab **66**:258, 1988.

Odell WD, Griffin J: Pulsatile secretion of human chorionic gonadotropin in normal adults. N Engl J Med **317**:1688, 1987.

Ohlsson R, Larsson E, Nilsson O, Wahlstrom T, Sundstrom P: Blastocyst implantation precedes induction of insulin-like growth factor II gene expression in human trophoblasts. Development **106**:555, 1989.

O'Neill C: Thrombocytopenia is an initial maternal response to fertilization in mice. J Reprod Fertil **73**:559, 1985a.

O'Neill C: Partial characterization of the embryo-derived platelet-activating factor in mice. J Reprod Fertil **75**:375, 1985b.

O'Neill C, Gidley-Baird AA, Pike IL, Porter RN, Sinosich MJ, Saunders DM: Maternal blood platelet physiology and luteal-phase endocrinology as a means of monitoring pre- and post-implantation embryo viability following in vitro fertilization. J In Vitro Fert Embryo Transfer **2**:87, 1985.

Ortiz ME, Croxatto HB: Observations on the transport, aging and development of ova in the human genital tract. *In* Talevar GP(ed): Recent Advances in Reproduction and Regulation of Fertility. Amsterdam, Elsevier/North-Holland, 1979, p 307.

Osawa Y, Higashiyama T, Fronckowiak M, Yoshida N, Yarborough C: Aromatase. J Steroid Biochem **27**:781, 1987.

Parker CR Jr, Everett RB, Whalley PJ, Quirk JG Jr, Gant NF, MacDonald PC: Hormone production during pregnancy in the primigravid patient. II. Plasma levels of deoxycorticosterone throughout pregnancy of normal women and women who developed pregnancy-induced hypertension. Am J Obstet Gynecol **138**:626, 1980.

Parker CR Jr, Winkel CA, Rush AJ Jr, Porter JC, MacDonald PC: Plasma concentration of 11-deoxycorticosterone in women during the menstrual cycle. Obstet Gynecol **58**:26, 1981.

Parks JS, Nielsen PV, Sexton LA, Jorgensen EH: An effect of gene dosage on production of human chorionic somatomammotropin. J Clin Endocrinol Metab **60**:994, 1985.

Pekonen F, Alfthan H, Stenman U-H, Ylikorkala O: Human chorionic gonadotropin (hCG) and thyroid function in early human pregnancy: circadian variation and evidence for intrinsic thyrotropic activity of hCG. J Clin Endocrinol Metab **66**:8, 1988.

Pepe GJ, Waddell BJ, Albrecht ED: Activation of the baboon fetal hypothalamic-pituitary-adrenocortical axis at midgestation by estrogen-induced changes in placental corticosteroid metabolism. Endocrinology **127**:3117, 1990.

Perley M, Kipnis DM: Effect of glucocorticoids on plasma insulin. N Engl J Med **274**:1237, 1966.

Petit A, Guillon G, Tence M, Jard S, Gallo-Payet N, Bellabarba D, Lehoux J-G, Belisle S: Angiotensin II stimulates both inositol phosphate production and human placental lactogen release from human trophoblastic cells. J Clin Endocrinol Metab **69**:280, 1989.

Petraglia F, Calza L, Giardino L, Sutton S, Marrkama P, Rivier J, Genazzani AR, Vale W: Identification of immunoreactive neuropeptide-t in human placenta: localization, secretion, and binding sites. Endocrinology 124:2016, 1989a.

Petraglia F, Lim ATW, Vale W: Adenosine 3', 5'-monophosphate, prostaglandins, and epinephrine stimulate the secretion of immunoreactive gonadotropin-releasing hormone from cultured human placental cells. Clin Endocrinol Metab 65:1020, 1987a.

Petraglia F, Sawchenko P, Rivier J, Vale W: Evidence for local stimulation of ACTH secretion by corticotropin-releasing factor in human placenta. Nature (Lond) 328:717, 1987b.

Petraglia F, Sutton S, Vale W: Neurotransmitters and peptides modulate the release of immunoreactive corticotropin-releasing factor from human cultured placental cells. Am J Obstet Gynecol 160:247, 1989b.

Petraglia F, Vaughan J, Vale W: Inhibin and activin modulate the release of GnRH, hCG and progesterone from cultured human placental cells. Proc Natl Acad Sci USA 86:5114, 1989c.

Petraglia F, Vaughan J, Vale W: Steroid hormones modulate the release of immunoreactive gonadotropin-releasing hormone from cultured human placental cells. J Clin Endocrinol Metab 70:1173, 1990a.

Petraglia F, Volpe A, Genazzani AR, Rivier J, Sawchenko PE, Vale W: Neuroendocrinology of the human placenta. Front Neuroendocrinol 11:6, 1990b.

Pitkin RM: Calcium metabolism in pregnancy and the perinatal period: a review. Am J Obstet Gynecol 151:99, 1985.

Pitkin RM, Reynolds WA, Williams GA, Hargis GKI: Calcium metabolism in normal pregnancy: a longitudinal study. Am J Obstet Gynecol 133:781, 1979.

Pittaway DE, Reish RL, Wentz AC: Doubling times of human chorionic gonadotropin increase in early viable intrauterine pregnancies. Am J Obstet Gynecol 152:299, 1985.

Plotsky PM: Regulation of hypophysiotropic factors mediating ACTH secretion. Ann NY Acad Sci 512:205, 1987.

Policastro PF, Daniels-McQueen S, Carle G, Boime I: A map of the hCBβ gene cluster. J Biol Chem 261:5907, 1986.

Potter JM, Nestel PJ: The hyperlipidemia of pregnancy in normal and complicated pregnancies. Am J Obstet Gynecol 133:165, 1979.

Prior JC: Progesterone as a bone-trophic hormone. Endocr Rev 11:386, 1990.

Quagliarello J, Goldsmith L, Steinetz B, Lustig DS: Induction of relaxin secretion in nonpregnant women by human chorionic gonadotropin. J Clin Endocrinol Metab 51:74, 1980.

Quigley ME, Ishizuka B, Ropert JF, Yen SSC: The food-entrained prolactin and cortisol release in late pregnancy and prolactinoma patients. J Clin Endocrinol Metab 54:1109, 1982.

Quigley ME, Yen SSC: A mid-day surge in cortisol levels. J Clin Endocrinol Metab 49:945, 1979.

Rappolee DA, Brenner CA, Schultz R, Mark D, Werb Z: Developmental expression of PDGF, TGF-α, and TGF-β genes in preimplantation mouse embryos. Science 241:1823, 1988.

Resnik R, Killam AP, Battaglia FC, et al: Stimulation of uterine blood flow by various estrogens. Endocrinology 94:1192, 1974.

Riddick DH, Kusmik WF: Decidua: A possible source of amniotic fluid PRL. Am J Obstet Gynecol 127:187, 1977.

Rigg LA, Lein A, Yen SSC: The pattern of increase in circulating prolactin levels during human gestation. Am J Obstet Gynecol 129:454, 1977.

Rigg LA, Yen SSC: Multiphasic prolactin (PRL) secretion during parturition in humans. Am J Obstet Gynecol 128:215, 1977.

Ringler GE, Kao L-C, Miller WL, Strauss JF III: Effects of 8-bromo-cAMP on expression of endocrine functions by cultured human trophoblast cells. Regulation of specific mRNAs. Mol Cell Endocrinol 61:13, 1989.

Ringler GE, Strauss JF III: In vitro systems for the study of human placental endocrine function. Endocr Rev 11:105, 1990.

Roberts VJ, Sawchenko PE, Vale W: Expression of inhibin/activin subunit mRNAs during rat embryogenesis. Endocrinology 128:3122, 1991.

Robinson BG, Emanuel RL, Frim DM, Majzoub JA: Glucocorticoid stimulates expression of corticotropin-releasing hormone gene in human placenta. Proc Natl Acad Sci USA 85:5244, 1988.

Romero R, Wu YK, Brody DT, Oyarzun E, Duff GW, Durum SK: Human decidua: a source of interleukin-1. Obstet Gynecol 73:31, 1989.

Ryan KJ: Biological aromatization of steroids. J Biol Chem 234:268, 1959.

Ryan KJ, Meigs R, Petro Z: The formation of progesterone by the human placenta. Am J Obstet Gynecol 96:676, 1966.

Sakbun V, Ali SM, Greenwood FC, Bryant-Greenwood GD: Human relaxin in the amnion, chorion, decidua parietalis, basal plate, and placental trophoblast by immunocytochemistry and Northern analysis. J Clin Endocrinol Metab 70:508, 1990.

Salido EC, Yen PH, Barajas L, Shapiro LJ: Steroid sulfatase expression in human placenta: immunocytochemistry and in situ hybridization study. J Clin Endocrinol Metab 70:1564, 1990.

Samaan N, Yen SSC, Gonzalez D, Pearson OH: Metabolic effects of placental lactogen (hPL) in man. J Clin Endocrinol Metab 28:485, 1968.

Sasaki A, Tampst P, Liotta AS, Margioris AN, Hood LE, Kent SBH, Krieger DT: Isolation and characterization of a corticotropin-releasing hormone–like peptide from human placenta. J Clin Endocrinol Metab 67:768, 1988.

Schaison G, George M, Lestrat N, Reinberg A, Baulieu EE: Effects of the antiprogesterone steroid RU486 during midluteal phase in normal women. J Clin Endocrinol Metab 61:484, 1985.

Seeburg PH: The human growth hormone gene family: nucleotide sequences show recent divergence and predict a new polypeptide hormone. DNA 1:239, 1982.

Serón-Ferré M, Lawrence CC, Jaffe RB: Role of hCG in regulation of the fetal zone of the human fetal adrenal gland. J Clin Endocrinol Metab 46:834, 1978.

Shibasaki T, Odagiri E, Shizume K, Ling N: Corticotropin-releasing factor–like activity in human placental extracts. J Clin Endocrinol Metab 55:384, 1982.

Short RV: When a conception fails to become a pregnancy. In Maternal Recognition of Pregnancy. Ciba Fdn Symp No. 64, Amsterdam, Excerpta Medica, 1988, pp 377–395.

Shoupe D, Mishell DR, Page MA, Madkour H, Spitz IM, Lobo RA: Effects of the antiprogesterone RU486 in normal women. II. Administration in the late follicular phase. Am J Obstet Gynecol 157:1421, 1987.

Shutt DA, Lopata A: The secretion of hormones during the culture of human preimplantation embryos with corona cells. Fertil Steril 35:413, 1981.

Siiteri PK, MacDonald PC: The utilization of circulating dehydro-isoandrosterone sulfate for estrogen synthesis during human pregnancy. Steroids 2:713, 1963.

Siler-Khodr TM, Khodr GS: Dose response analysis of Gn-RH stimulation of hCG release from human term placenta. Biol Reprod 25:353, 1981.

Siler-Khodr TM, Khodr GS, Valenzuela G: Immunoreactive GnRH levels in maternal circulation throughout pregnancy. Am J Obstet Gynecol 150:376, 1984.

Siler-Khodr TM, Khodr GS, Valenzuela G, Rhode J: GnRH effect on placental hormones during gestation. I. α-hCG, hCG and hCS. Biol Reprod 34:245, 1986.

Siler-Khodr TM, Khodr GS, Vockery BH, Nester JJ: Inhibition of hCG, α-hCG and progesterone release from human placenta tissue in vitro by a GnRH antagonist. Life Sci 32:2741, 1983.

Silvestre L, Dubois C, Renault M, Rezvani Y, Baulieu EE, Ulmann A: Voluntary interruption of pregnancy with mifepristone (RU486) and a prostaglandin analogue. N Engl J Med 322:645, 1990.

Simpson ER, MacDonald PC: Endocrine physiology of the placenta. Ann Rev Physiol 43:163, 1981.

Spellacy WN, Buchi WC, Schram JD, Birk SA, McCreary SA: Control of human chorionic somatomammotropin levels during pregnancy. Obstet Gynecol 37:567, 1971.

Spellacy WN, Goetz FE: Plasma insulin in normal late pregnancy. N Engl J Med 268:988, 1963.

Stenman U-H, Alfthan H, Ranta T, Vartiainen E, Jalkanen J, Seppala M: Serum levels of human chorionic gonadotropin in nonpregnant women and in men are modulated by gonadotropin-releasing hormone and sex steroids. J Clin Endocrinol Metab 64:730, 1987.

Stewart DR, Celniker AC, Taylor CA Jr, Cragun JR, Overstreet JW, Lasley BL: Relaxin in the peri-implantation period. J Clin Endocrinol Metab 70:1771, 1990.

Suda T, Iwashita M, Ushiyama T, Tozawa F, Sumitomo T, Nakagami Y, Demura H, Shizume K: Responses to corticotropin-releasing hormone and its bound and free forms in pregnant and nonpregnant women. J Clin Endocrinol Metab 69:38, 1989.

Takemori M, Nishimura R, Ashitaka Y, Tojo S: Release of human chorionic gonadotropin (hCG) and its alpha-subunit (hCGα) from perifused human placenta. Endocrinol Jpn **28**:757, 1981.

Thomas JL, Myers RP, Strickler RC: Human placental 3β-hydroxy-5-ene-steroid dehydrogenase and steroid 5-4-ene-isomerase: purification from mitochondria and kinetic profiles, biophysical characterization of the purified mitochondrial and microsomal enzymes. J Steroid Biochem **33**:209, 1989.

Thompson Jr EA, Siiteri PK: The involvement of human placental microsomal cytochrome P-450 in aromatization. J Biol Chem **249**:5373, 1974a.

Thompson Jr EA, Siiteri PK: Utilization of oxygen and reduced nicotinamide adenine dinucleotide phosphate by human placental microsomes during aromatization of androstenedione. J Biol Chem **249**:5364, 1974b.

Tulchinsky D, Frigoletto F, Ryan KJ, Fishman J: Plasma esterol as an index of fetal well-being. J Clin Endocrinol Metab **40**:560, 1975.

Tulchinsky D, Hobel CJ: Plasma human chorionic gonadotropin, estrone, estradiol, estriol, progesterone and 17α-hydroxyprogesterone in human pregnancy. III. Early normal pregnancy. Am J Obstet Gynecol **117**:884, 1973.

Tulchinsky D, Hobel CJ, Yeager E, Marshall JR: Plasma estrone, estradiol, estriol, progesterone and 17-hydroxyprogesterone in human pregnancy. I. Normal pregnancy. Am J Obstet Gynecol **112**:1095, 1972.

Tulchinsky D, Okada DM: Hormones in human pregnancy. IV. Plasma progesterone. Am J Obstet Gynecol **121**:293, 1975.

Turpeenniemi-Hujanen T, Rönnberg L, Kauppila A, Puistola U: Laminin in the human embryo implantation: analogy to the invasion by malignant cells. Fertil Steril **58**:105, 1992.

Tyson JE, Austin K, Farinholt J, Fiedler J: Endocrine-metabolic response to acute starvation in human gestation. Am J Obstet Gynecol **125**:1073, 1976.

Tyson JE, Hwang P, Guyda H, Friesen HG: Studies of prolactin secretion in human pregnancy. Am J Obstet Gynecol **113**:14, 1972.

Unanue E, Allen P: The basis for the immunoregulatory role of macrophages and other accessory cells. Science **236**:551, 1987.

Vaitukaitis JL, Boss GT, Braunstein GD, Rayford PL: Gonadotropins and their subunits: Basic and clinical studies. Rec Prog Horm Res **32**:289, 1976.

Van Luu T, Labrie C, Zhao HF, Couet J, Lanchance Y, Simard J, Leblanc G, Cote J, Berube D, Gagne R, Labrie F: Characterization of cDNAs for human estradiol 17β-dehydrogenase and assignment of the gene to chromosome 17: evidence of two mRNA species with distinct 5′-termini in human placenta. Mol Endocrinol **3**:1301, 1989a.

Van Luu T, Lachance Y, Labrie C, Leblanc G, Thomas JL, Strickler RC, Labrie F: Full length cDNA structure and deduced amino acid sequence of human 3β-hydroxy-5-ene steroid dehydrogenase. Mol Endocrinol **3**:1310, 1989b.

Voutilainen R, Miller WL: Coordinate tropic hormone regulation of mRNAs for insulin-like growth factor II and the cholesterol side-chain-cleavage enzyme, P-450scc, in human steroidogenic tissues. Proc Natl Acad Sci USA **84**:1590, 1987.

Wang H, Segal SJ, Koide SS: Purification and characterization of an incompletely glycosylated form of human chorionic gonadotropin from human placenta. Endocrinology **123**:795, 1988.

Wardlaw SL, Stark RI, Baxi L, Frantz AG: Plasma β-endorphin and β-lipotropin in the human fetus at delivery: Correlation with arterial pH and Po₂. J Clin Endocrinol Metab **79**:888, 1979.

Warren JC, French AP: Distribution of steroid sulfatase in human tissues. J Clin Endocrinol Metab **25**:278, 1965.

Watkins WB, Yen SSC: Somatostatin in cytotrophoblast of the immature human placenta: localization by immunoperoxidase cytochemistry. J Clin Endocrinol Metab **50**:969, 1980.

Weiss G, O'Byrne EM, Steinetz BG: Relaxin: A product of the human corpus luteum of pregnancy. Science **194**:948, 1979.

Whitsett JA, Yo M, Tsang RC: Synthesis of 1,25-dihydroxyvitamin D₃ by human placenta *in vitro*. J Clin Endocrinol Metab **53**:484, 1981.

Wiedemann E, Schwartz E, Frantz AG: Acute and chronic estrogen effects upon serum somatomedin activity, growth hormone, and prolactin in man. J Clin Endocrinol Metab **42**:942, 1976.

Wilcox AJ, Weinberg CR, O'Connor JF, Baird DD, Schlatterer JP, Canfield RE, Armstrong EG, Nisula BC: Incidence of early loss of pregnancy. N Engl J Med **319**:189, 1988.

Wilson EA, Jawad MJ, Dickson LR: Suppression of human chorionic gonadotropin by progestational steroids. Am J Obstet Gynecol **138**:708, 1980.

Wilson EA, Jawad MJ, Powell DE: Effect of estradiol and progesterone on human chorionic gonadotropin secretion *in vitro*. Am J Obstet Gynecol **149**:143, 1984.

Wilson SG, Retallack RW, Kent JC, Worth GK, Gutteridge DH: Serum free 1,25-dihydroxyvitamin D and the free 1,25-dihydroxyvitamin D index during a longitudinal study of human pregnancy and lactation. Clin Endocrinol **32**:613, 1990.

Winkel CA, Snyder JM, MacDonald PC, Simpson ER: Regulation of cholesterol and progesterone synthesis in human placental cells in culture by serum lipoproteins. Endocrinology **106**:1054, 1980.

Wurzel J, Parks JS, Herd HE, Nielsen PV: A gene deletion is responsible for absence of human chorionic somatomammotropin. DNA **1**:251, 1982.

Yagel S, Lala PK, Powell WA, Casper RF: Interleukin-1 stimulates human chorionic gonadotropin secretion by first trimester human trophoblast. J Clin Endocrinol Metab **68**:992, 1989.

Yen SSC: Endocrine regulation of metabolic homeostasis during pregnancy. Clin Obstet Gynecol **16**:130, 1973.

Yen SSC, Tsai CC, Vela P: Gestational diabetogenesis: Quantitative analyses of glucose-insulin interrelationship between normal pregnancy and pregnancy with gestational diabetes. Am J Obstet Gynecol **11**:792, 1971.

Yen SSC, Vela P, Tsai CC: Impairment of growth hormone secretion in response to hypoglycemia during early and late pregnancy. J Clin Endocrinol Metab **31**:29, 1970.

Yoshikawa N, Nishikawa M, Horimoto M, Yoshimura M, Sawaragi S, Horikoshi Y, Sawaragi I, Inada M: Thyroid-stimulating activity in sera of normal pregnant women. J Clin Endocrinol Metab **69**:891, 1989.

Yoshimoto Y, Wolfsen AR, Hirose F, Odell WD: Human chorionic gonadotropin-like material: Presence in normal human tissues. Am J Obstet Gynecol **134**:729, 1979.

Younes MA, Besch NF, Besch PK: Estradiol and progesterone binding in human term placental cytosol. Am J Obstet Gynecol **141**:1, 1981.

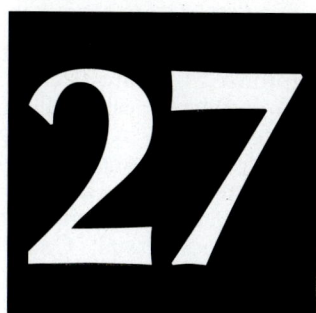

SIGNIFICANCE OF AMNIOTIC FLUID MECONIUM

JAMES R. WOODS, JR., M.D., and J. CHRISTOPHER GLANTZ, M.D.

Few topics in maternal and fetal medicine have attracted as diverse an interest or created as much controversy as meconium. Meconium-stained amniotic fluid has traditionally heralded imminent or existing fetal compromise, yet neonatal passage of the first meconium stool signals the onset of healthy gastrointestinal function. Meconium, if aspirated, complicates perinatal asphyxia. Its composition, however, represents a unique record of fetal swallowing, intestinal secretions, and intestinal absorption, and its presence in amniotic fluid may permit a better understanding of intestinal maturation and function under conditions of health and disease.

FORMATION AND COMPOSITION OF MECONIUM

Meconium forms relatively late in gastrointestinal development. The gastrointestinal tract originates from both early endoderm and splanchnic mesoderm by day 14 after fertilization and is lined by undifferentiated cuboidal cells by day 18 (Arey, 1974; Grand et al., 1976). Intestinal villi appear by 7 weeks, and active absorption of glucose and amino acids occurs at 10 and 12 weeks, respectively. By 12 weeks gestation, development of Meissner's and Auerbach's plexuses within the intestinal wall coincides with onset of peristalsis of the small intestine and colon. Meconium is first evident in the fetal intestine at approximately 70 to 85 days gestation (Smith, 1976).

The principal components of term fetal meconium are listed in Table 27–1. Large concentrations of bile pigments excreted by the biliary tract from the fourth month on give meconium its green color.

Meconium is composed primarily of water (72 to 80 per cent). At 16 to 17 weeks, the fetus swallows 2 to 7 ml/24 hr of amniotic fluid; at term it swallows up to 450 ml/24 hr (Pritchard, 1966). Amniotic fluid presumably accounts for most of the water in meconium, but our knowledge of the dynamics of water absorption in the fetal intestine is extremely limited.

The presence of low levels of primary and secondary bile acids in meconium reflects the immaturity of the fetal gastrointestinal system. In the adult, primary bile acids are synthesized and conjugated in the liver, secreted into the bile, released into the intestine, and then partially metabolized by intestinal bacteria to secondary bile acids. The fetus is capable of synthesizing both primary and secondary bile acids, but only negligible amounts of the latter, because it lacks intestinal bacteria (Sharp et al., 1971). Primary bile acids are present in the stool of neonates from birth. After the first meconium stool is passed, however, no secondary bile acids are detectable in the newborn stool or bile until about the fifth day. Presumably, then, secondary bile acids found in fetal meconium are acquired via transplacental passage. Maternal-to-fetal transfer of bile acids clearly occurs in intrahepatic cholestasis of pregnancy (Luukkainen et al., 1978). In this condition, bile acids are elevated in fetal serum and amniotic fluid, and they accumulate in meconium as a result of fetal swallowing.

Bile acids are normally absorbed in small amounts in the fetal jejunum and ileum, suggesting that the fetal carrier-mediated absorption mechanism in the ileum is incompletely developed (Lester et al., 1977). The neonate demonstrates increased ileal absorption of bile acids by 2 weeks and adult responses by 5 weeks. The bile salt pool and synthesis rate in the preterm fetus are low, which may account for the incomplete absorption of lipids at birth.

TABLE 27–1. **Composition of Term Fetal Meconium**

Water
Mucopolysaccharides
Cholesterol and sterol precursors
Protein
Lipid
Bile acids and salts
Enzymes
Blood group substances
Squamous cells
Vernix caseosa

The absence of bacteria in fetal meconium also explains why sterols in meconium differ from those in adult stool. Fetal swallowing accounts for similarities in meconium and amniotic fluid sterols (Miettinen and Luukkainen, 1968). Cholesterol is the predominant (99 per cent) sterol in fetal serum, whereas cholesterol precursors make up nearly 20 per cent of the total steroids in amniotic fluid and meconium. Noncholesterol sterols such as cholestanol and beta-cholestanol are higher in meconium than in amniotic fluid; this suggests that intestinal secretion of certain sterols may also occur.

Drug metabolites can accumulate in meconium. The mechanism may involve secretion into the bile with subsequent entry into the duodenal meconium, or alternatively, urinary metabolites may be ingested and directly incorporated into meconium. In rats, metabolites of morphine, cocaine, and cannabinoids can be found in meconium. These metabolites have also been detected in meconium of infants born to drug-abusing women (Ostrea et al., 1989).

In cystic fibrosis, a multisystem disease characterized by abnormal meconium, the duodenal fluid lacks the proteolytic enzymes needed to break down protein for absorption. As a consequence, protein, which contributes only 7 per cent of the dry weight of meconium in the healthy fetus, may exceed 80 per cent in the fetus with cystic fibrosis (Green et al., 1958). The viscous, rubbery consistency of meconium in cystic fibrosis patients appears to be a direct result of the elevated protein content.

PRESENCE OF MECONIUM IN AMNIOTIC FLUID

Physical Characteristics of Meconium

Meconium lacks intestinal bacteria, and it is this property that accounts for many of the differences in composition from adult stool. Once it has passed into amniotic fluid, however, meconium in concentrations exceeding 1 per cent enhances the ability of amniotic fluid to sustain bacterial growth (Florman and Tuebner, 1969).

The degree to which tissues stain when exposed to meconium depends on meconium concentration, length of exposure, and nature of the exposed tissue (Desmond et al., 1956; Miller et al., 1985). Vernix suspended in meconium stains yellow in 12 to 14 hours. Newborn fingernails stain yellow in 4 to 6 hours. The characteristics of the tissues may determine how much yellow or green pigment is absorbed (Bartman and Blanc, 1970).

Miller et al. exposed placentas in vitro to varying concentrations of and durations of exposure to meconium. Within 1 hour, surface staining was observed and was found to be proportional to length of exposure and concentration of meconium. Pigment accumulation in macrophages within the placenta depended upon length of exposure only, but it was observed in all placentas by 3 hours. Umbilical cord staining was noted at 1 hour with 5 per cent meconium and at 15 minutes with 10 per cent meconium. This

information can be important postpartum in determining the length of time meconium has been present, especially in cases of meconium aspiration. Meconium in pulmonary macrophages suggests antepartum *in utero* aspiration rather than birth asphyxia.

The influence of amniotic fluid meconium contamination upon fetal maturity testing remains controversial. Compounding the confusion are the multiple laboratory methodologies utilized to determine maturity, such as the lecithin-sphingomyelin (L/S) ratio and the phosphatidylglycerol (PG) level (Parker, 1981; Freer and Statland, 1981). The L/S ratio has been reported to increase (Wagstaff et al., 1974; Kulkarni et al., 1972) or decrease (Buhi and Spellacy, 1975) with addition of meconium to amniotic fluid samples. Hill and Ellefson (1983), using two-dimensional chromatograms, reported that meconium has a variable and unpredictable effect on L/S ratio. Tabsch et al. (1981) distinguished the effects of preterm meconium (passed before 35 weeks gestation) from term meconium on the L/S ratio. They concluded that an L/S ratio of less than 2.2 in the premature fetus with meconium-stained fluid may not be consistent with lung maturity, whereas a value less than 2.5 in the mature fetus with meconium-stained fluid should not be relied upon as an index of maturity. PG analysis using thin-layer chromatography can be difficult if not impossible with heavily stained amniotic fluid. However, the PG determination may be reliable in lightly stained amniotic fluids if the precipitated spot representing PG can be adequately discerned (Hill and Ellefson, 1983; Tsao and Zachman, 1982; Yambao et al., 1984; Schmidt-Sommerfeld et al., 1982). PG values determined by immunologic (agglutination) techniques may not be affected by meconium (Towers and Garite, 1989).

Such conflicting and variable results suggest that caution should be exercised in interpreting any tests for fetal lung maturity from meconium-contaminated amniotic fluid. In some cases, a reliable index of fetal maturity can be expected with current tests performed on meconium-stained amniotic fluid. However, the limits of current laboratory methods must be appreciated, and consultation with experienced laboratory personnel is recommended.

Ultrasonographic Detection of Meconium-Stained Amniotic Fluid

Amniotic fluid that appears echogenic or particulate on ultrasonography has been reported as consistent with *in utero* passage of meconium (Benacerraf et al., 1984). Unfortunately, vernix may also have this appearance (Hill and Breckle, 1986). In a small series, Sherer demonstrated that the positive predictive value of echogenic fluid on ultrasonography for the antenatal detection of meconium was only 10 per cent (Sherer et al., 1991). This is roughly equal to the frequency of meconium at delivery, and so is equal to chance. Since this ultrasonographic finding is not specific for meconium, it cannot be used with any certainty in making management decisions.

Ultrasonographic Diagnosis of Fetal Meconium Peritonitis

Neonatal intestinal disorders related to meconium have been recognized for decades. Only recently has real-time ultrasonography been used to detect *in utero* fetal abnormalities of intestinal function. Meconium peritonitis is a chemical inflammation of the peritoneum caused by the escape of sterile meconium through a perforation in the bowel. Significant morbidity and mortality can occur. The potential etiologies of fetal bowel perforation are diverse; they include intestinal atresias, congenital bowel and gut malrotation anomalies, volvulus, intussusception, and cystic fibrosis (Shalev et al., 1982; Narcarrow et al., 1985). *In utero* diagnosis of meconium peritonitis by ultrasonography has been reported (Shalev et al., 1982; Narcarrow et al., 1985; Williams et al., 1984; Curtis et al., 1983; Fleischer et al., 1983; Schwiner et al., 1984; Pan et al., 1983; Silverbach, 1983). A number of sonographic findings have been described: increased echogenicity of the bowel, acoustic shadowing suggesting calcifications, cystic abdominal masses consistent with granulation tissue from acute inflammation, polyhydramnios, ascites, and dilated intestinal loops filled with fluid. Serial ultrasonographic examinations should be performed in these fetuses to watch for worsening of the pathologic process. Amniocentesis should be considered to rule out chromosomal anomalies and to check for fetal maturity near term. Muller et al. (1985) have suggested that an echogenic fetal abdominal mass seen in patients presenting for prenatal diagnosis of cystic fibrosis may reflect meconium ileus. These masses can be observed at 16 to 20 weeks gestation and may correlate with decreased amniotic fluid intestinal enzyme levels assayed in affected fetuses.

The *in utero* diagnosis of fetal intestinal disorders demands careful managerial decisions based upon serial ultrasonographic examinations, amniotic fluid evaluation (when applicable), and fetal gestational age. Prenatal diagnosis of these abnormalities can alert the neonatal and pediatric surgical team to the need for immediate postnatal evaluation. *In utero* treatment of apparent meconium obstruction (meconium plug syndrome) has been reported by Samuel et al. (1986), in which amniography with Urografin was found to relieve meconium obstruction by stimulating the passage of copious watery meconium into the amniotic fluid. The potential risks inherent in this approach include meconium aspiration syndrome at delivery or *in utero* and the worsening of bowel distention in cases of fixed bowel obstruction (such as intestinal atresias). The recommendation of such therapy must await further reports of its efficacy and safety.

Theories of Meconium Passage

In Utero

The processes of intestinal peristalsis and defecation in the adult are a complex interaction of hormonal, myogenic, and neurogenic factors (for review see Davenport, 1971). Bowel activity in the adult is primarily controlled by local reflexes acting through intramural neural plexuses. Extrinsic innervation serves to modify this intrinsic reflex activity. Sympathetic innervation to the rectum, when stimulated, inhibits rectal activity while causing constriction of the internal anal sphincter. Parasympathetic activity increases motor activity in the rectum while it inhibits constriction of the internal anal sphincter. Unlike the internal sphincter, the external sphincter receives only somatic innervation. Since there is no direct inhibitory nerve activity, sphincter relaxation results from reduced neural stimulation.

The principal stimulus for peristalsis is increased intraluminal pressure and radial stretching of the bowel, which in turn activates two distinct neural pathways to produce contraction waves (Hirst, 1979). These descending contraction waves involving the longitudinal and circular muscles of the bowel act through cholinergic excitation (both may be blocked with atropine).

In the resting state, the external and internal rectal sphincters are constricted, with the latter retaining the higher resting tone. Sudden rectal distention produces relaxation of the internal sphincter and constriction of the external sphincter. Unless external sphincter constriction is voluntarily maintained, however, sphincter relaxation occurs and the rectal contents are discharged. In the adult, activity of the internal sphincter is independent of peristalsis, but responds primarily to rectal distention. The external sphincter responds to a number of stimuli, including rectal volume, abdominal pressure, dilatation, and anal stretch.

Our knowledge of the mechanisms of meconium passage and bowel peristalsis in the fetus is not nearly so substantive as in the adult.

Maturation Theory

Because meconium is seldom passed prior to 34 weeks, its presence in amniotic fluid may reflect gastrointestinal maturity in late gestation. Becker and co-workers (1940) first observed that meconium-stained amniotic fluid is a natural occurrence in certain species late in pregnancy. In these early experiments, radiopaque dye was injected into the amniotic cavity of pregnant guinea pigs in mid-gestation and sequential x-rays were taken until term. A progressive decrease occurred in the time the dye took to reach the small intestine. Many healthy fetuses routinely passed dye into the amniotic fluid in the last week of gestation. Moreover, some fetuses cleared the dye from the amniotic fluid by swallowing, an observation of clinical importance because we know very little about how meconium is cleared.

Clinical studies confirm that transit time to the fetal colon significantly decreases as gestation advances. In the 32-week fetus, transit time to the colon averages 9 hours, whereas the term fetus has a 4 1/2 hour transit time (McLain, 1963). The prolonged transit time in the preterm fetus has been attributed to poor gut musculature. Because peristalsis begins at 11 to 12 weeks in the human, and muscle development occurs even earlier, this explanation seems unlikely.

Immaturity of intrinsic and extrinsic innervation of the bowel may impair the ability of the premature fetus to pass meconium into the amniotic fluid. At autopsy, preterm (670 to 2000 gm) neonates demonstrate more unmyelinated nerve trunks and fewer ganglion cells in the distal 2.3 cm of the colon than are observed in older neonates and infants. Furthermore, as the fetus matures, its intestinal tract becomes more responsive to exogenous sympathomimetic agents (Grand et al., 1976). Although these maturational events do not explain why meconium is passed into the amniotic fluid, they must be considered an integral part of this process.

Theory of Fetal Distress

The relationship of fetal hypoxia, intestinal hyperperistalsis, and relaxation of the anal sphincter has been a consideration for many years. Meconium is a term derived from the Greek *mekonion*, a word for poppy juice or opium. Aristotle is credited with having drawn the analogy between the presence of this substance in the amniotic fluid and the "sleepy" newborn. Walker (1954) demonstrated that meconium was released more commonly when the oxygen saturation of the umbilical vein was below 30 per cent and that heavy meconium was more often associated with a lower oxygen saturation than was light meconium.

Our understanding of the relationship of meconium passage to fetal distress, however, is incomplete. In 12 to 25 per cent of deliveries complicated by fetal meconium passage, there is no demonstrable cause. Moreover, the fetal guinea pig, when exposed to maternal "anoxemia," swallows more rapidly, but manifests no significant increase in gastrointestinal motility (Becker et al., 1940). Hypoxia also fails to alter intestinal peristalsis in the monkey fetus. Saling (1968) suggested that meconium passage into amniotic fluid represents a compensatory redistribution of intestinal blood flow to more vital organs during hypoxia. In the adult, spinal shock, although it causes the external sphincter to become flaccid, produces constipation as a result of impaired defecation reflexes. If meconium is passed as a compensatory response to reduced intestinal blood flow, it must occur as an early event, while neurogenic reflexes are still intact.

Hon (1963) suggested that meconium is passed in response to parasympathetic stimulation during cord compression. That meconium is passed more commonly in the neurologically mature fetus and in the dysmature fetus supports this contention. However, meconium-stained amniotic fluid is not commonly associated with variable fetal heart rate deceleration unless other signs of fetal distress exist. Long-term single umbilical artery ligation causes the fetal lamb to pass meconium only after significant chronic fetal wasting has occurred (Emmanouilides et al., 1968). Signs of chronic intrauterine stress and meconium passage are frequently observed in the severely dysmature human fetus. Whether in these instances the fetus passes meconium in response to accelerated neurologic development or is at great risk of umbilical cord complications remains unclear.

Role of Intestinal Hormones

In 1971, Brown and colleagues successfully isolated an intestinal polypeptide from the upper small intestine, termed "motilin" for its stimulating action on motor function in the stomach. Motilin also produces muscle contractions in the esophagus, small intestine, and colon by acting directly on the smooth muscle. It elicits a myoelectric complex that slowly propagates along the smooth muscle of the small intestine and colon. Although this polypeptide is synthesized by cells distributed throughout the upper gastrointestinal tract, motilin-containing neurons have been identified in the submucosal and muscle layers of the stomach, small intestine, and colon and in the central nervous system (Chey and Lee, 1980).

Mean motilin levels in cord venous samples of healthy preterm (34 weeks) and term infants are 13 ± 4 pmol/liter and 32 ± 4 pmol/liter, respectively. Moreover, a fourfold increase in cord venous plasma motilin levels has been reported in eight term infants with abnormal fetal heart rate patterns, five of whom passed meconium *in utero* (Lucas et al., 1979). In another study using a different assay, umbilical cord blood motilin concentrations averaged 177 fmol/ml in 16 term neonates who passed antenatal meconium, compared to 111 fmol/ml in 22 term controls (Mahmoud, 1988). Fetal distress was not associated with elevated motilin levels in that study. Plasma motilin levels in preterm and term newborns increase rapidly after delivery. Because this rise is not observed in the preterm infant receiving intravenous fluids, this postdelivery response is attributed to enteral feedings (Lucas et al., 1980).

Although a possible relationship may exist between meconium passage and one or several of the intestinal polypeptides, little attention has been paid to this subject since the initial reports appeared. This relationship may help to explain the infrequent passage of meconium in the preterm fetus and the possible association of meconium-stained amniotic fluid with fetal distress. Unless additional studies are carried out, this assertion will remain intriguing, but poorly documented.

Incidence and Perinatal Outcome

Second-Trimester Passage of Meconium

The interpretation of meconium-stained amniotic fluid in the second trimester of pregnancy has become an issue as data emerge from large series of patients undergoing amniocentesis for genetic counseling. King and co-workers (1978) reported ten occurrences in 514 mothers. Seven of these ten patients subsequently delivered healthy infants, but the other three fetuses died *in utero* following the procedures. In another series, six of 234 mothers demonstrated amniotic meconium following genetic amniocentesis but encountered no problems and delivered healthy infants (Karp and Schiller, 1977). Allen (1985), reporting on a large series of 4709 consecutive mid-trimester genetic amniocenteses, found meconium-stained fluid in 79 cases (1.67 per cent). Only four of these 79 patients (5 per cent) sustained fetal death, all in the second trimester. There was no correlation between the degree of meconium-stained fluid and fetal outcome, as all cases of thick meconium were associated with a normal birth. Moreover, most patients with stained fluid in this study had clear fluid at the time of delivery, indicating the transient nature of midtrimester stained fluid. Svigos et al. (1981) found meconium on ten occasions in 520 consecutive midtrimester amniocenteses and concluded that second-trimester meconium usually does not indicate a poor fetal outcome. Only one fetus died, and the death was attributed to multiple skeletal anomalies.

A major problem with all studies in which meconium-stained amniotic fluid was encountered in the second trimester is the questionable ability of the clinician to distinguish meconium staining from blood pigment staining. Francoual et al. (1986) analyzed 78 amniotic samples in the third trimester by measuring both total hemoglobin and coproporphyrin concentrations, representing blood and meconium contamination, respectively. They found that simple visual observation by the obstetrician is not sufficient to distinguish meconium from old blood. Of 33 samples judged visually to be meconium stained, only five were solely contaminated with meconium. These investigators recommended biochemical testing of stained amniotic fluid to determine its composition. Legge (1981) similarly concluded that brown amniotic fluid from the second trimester was more often secondary to the presence of hemoglobin (both maternal and fetal) than of meconium. All green or brown fluids from genetic amniocentesis fluids tested by Hankins et al. (1984) using the Hemoccult slide test (guaiac reaction) were positive, suggesting intra-amniotic hemorrhage, not meconium. In this study of 83 discolored fluids out of 1227 amniocentesis samples, no differences were found in the incidence of spontaneous abortions, abnormal fetal karyotypes or anomalies, preterm labor, or the necessity for cesarean section when compared with case-matched control subjects.

Zorn et al. (1986) noted 110 discolored fluid samples out of 3349 midtrimester amniocentesis specimens. They examined 34 of these, utilizing spectrophotometry, electrophoresis, isoelectric focusing, and chromatography and concluded that 33 of the 34 specimens contained hemoglobin as the major discoloring agent. In this series, a 9 per cent spontaneous abortion rate was found in pregnancies complicated by stained fluid, as opposed to a 1.6 per cent miscarriage rate for the entire amniocentesis group. Sixty-two per cent of the women with discolored fluid gave a history of bleeding prior to their amniocentesis. Golbus and associates (1979) found that 36 of 3000 second-trimester amniocentesis specimens contained green-brown fluid that spectrophotometric analysis revealed to be aged blood pigments. Twenty-seven of these patients delivered healthy babies; in nine, the abnormal finding was associated with missed abortion.

The composite conclusions from these studies suggest that green- or brown-stained second-trimester amniotic fluid may contain not meconium, but rather degraded blood pigments. Biochemical testing (for hemoglobin or coproporphyrin) or the use of chromatography or electrophoresis rather than visual inspection is necessary to make this distinction accurately. Even this exercise may be academic, since ultimately many of these pregnancies involving discolored fluid continue to term without significant morbidity or mortality, and the amniotic fluid may be cleared of the abnormal pigment.

Third-Trimester Passage of Meconium

The incidence of antepartum meconium-stained amniotic fluid as taken from several studies varies from 6 to 11 per cent, reflecting the types of surveillance used and the nature of the study populations.

The use of amnioscopy for detection of meconium in amniotic fluid is largely of historic interest today. This technique is generally limited to those patients who are past the 37th week of gestation, so that sufficient cervical dilatation has occurred to permit visualization of the amniotic fluid through the amnioscope. Of 720 high-risk patients reported by Lee (1972), the initial examination was unsuccessful in 12.5 per cent. The presence of meconium was documented in 9.8 per cent of the patients and, not surprisingly, a higher incidence of meconium-stained amniotic fluid occurred in patients with postmaturity or toxemia. Although 1.4 per cent of the patients experienced artificial rupture of the membranes during the procedure and 15.7 per cent went into labor within 24 hours of the examination, active intervention in the presence of meconium-stained amniotic fluid produced a perinatal mortality rate of 4.1 per 1000. In another report of weekly amnioscopic examination of 508 patients, meconium was infrequently diagnosed (2.2 per cent) prior to labor and, by itself, was not associated with low Apgar scores or fetal acidosis at delivery (Saldana et al., 1976). Mandelbaum (1973), employing serial amniocentesis in 272 patients in the last 10 weeks of gestation, found 31 (11.3 per cent) to demonstrate antepartum meconium. Meconium was more often associated with hypertensive conditions and occurred less frequently in patients with diabetes mellitus or uncertain dates. Active intervention was recommended by the author, because 25.8 per cent of the babies in this high-risk group died *in utero* and 41.9 per cent had neonatal complications.

That disagreement exists as to proper management of the high-risk patient once antepartum meconium is detected reflects our inability to determine the duration of meconium staining and the factors involved in meconium passage. It is apparent, however, that the fetus should undergo additional antepartum evaluation if meconium is detected in the antepartum period and delivery is not imminent.

Intrapartum Passage of Meconium

The incidence of intrapartum meconium ranges from 1.5 to 18 per cent. More significantly, in patients in whom abnormal fetal heart rate patterns accompany the passage of meconium, there is a 3 to 22.2 per cent perinatal infant mortality rate and a 7 to 50 per cent neonatal morbidity rate (Abramovici et al., 1974; Fenton and Steer, 1962; Hobel, 1971; Krebs et al., 1980; Miller et al., 1975). However, the presence of intrapartum meconium and its association with low Apgar scores, acidosis, and abnormal fetal heart rate tracings remains controversial. A number of investigators have found lower Apgar scores following intrapartum observation of meconium-stained fluid (Miller and Read, 1981; Krebs et al., 1980; Starks, 1980; Cole et al., 1985; Steer et al., 1989). Although the 1- or 5-minute Apgar scores or both were statistically lower in the meconium than in the nonmeconium group, the absolute differences in Apgar scores differed between groups by only 1 or 2 points. Whether or not these differences in Apgar scores are clinically significant is unclear. These differences in Apgar scores may be attributed to vigorous endotracheal suctioning in the meconium babies, with neonatal depression on this basis alone, but this possibility has not been adequately addressed. Furthermore, a number of reports have found no difference in Apgar scores between meconium-stained and nonmeconium-stained fetuses (Meis et al., 1982; Mitchell et al., 1985; Dijxhoorn et al., 1986 and 1987). Dijxhoorn et al. (1986) could not correlate meconium in labor with neurologic status of the infants at 4 or 5 days of life. Even the presence of fetal acidosis (pH <7.25, as determined by scalp blood sampling during labor) and moderate-to-thick meconium was not sufficient to lower Apgar scores significantly in a study by Mitchell et al. (1985), although acidosis in this setting did correlate with an increased incidence of meconium aspiration syndrome. Yeomans et al. (1989) found that acidosis increased the incidence of meconium below the cords but *not* that of meconium aspiration syndrome.

A consistent association between meconium-stained fluid and fetal acidosis during labor or immediately postdelivery has not been demonstrated, although this issue remains controversial. Dooley et al. (1985) studied 58 infants with meconium below the vocal cords at delivery and compared their umbilical cord arterial blood gas values with those of 214 matched infants without meconium below the cords. No significant differences in mean pH, Pco_2, or base deficit were found between the two groups. Certain investigators (Krebs et al., 1980; Dijxhoorn et al., 1986) have made similar observations, whereas others (Starks, 1980; Miller and Read, 1981) suggest, on the basis of their data, that a relationship between amniotic fluid meconium and fetal blood gas values exists. Several studies have concluded that, in the absence of fetal heart rate abnormalities, meconium alone does not constitute fetal distress (Bochner et al, 1987; Miller et al., 1975).

If hypoxia during labor is associated with the presence of meconium, or in fact if it is the cause for passage of meconium intrapartum, it might be expected that ominous fetal heart rate tracings suggestive of hypoxia would frequently be found in association with discolored amniotic fluid. However, this relationship has not always been found. In certain studies, the occurrence of late decelerations is infrequently noted with meconium staining, and it is not necessarily found more often than in nonmeconium-stained groups (Miller and Read, 1981; Dooley et al.,

1985). Those studies that have correlated meconium with abnormal heart rate monitoring patterns have described repeated early and variable type decelerations, as well as decreased baseline variability and fewer accelerations of the fetal heart rate. These changes, however, have not been consistently related to low Apgar scores in the meconium-stained groups (Meis et al., 1982; Krebs et al., 1980). Dooley et al. (1985) noted that a rising FHT baseline and decreased variability were more common in infants who subsequently had meconium below the cords, although there was no increase in meconium aspiration syndrome. In labors complicated by thick meconium, Rossi found that the combination of fetal tachycardia and absent accelerations correlated with an increased risk of meconium aspiration syndrome (Rossi et al., 1989). Even so, these findings *plus* umbilical artery acidosis *and* a low 5-minute Apgar score predicted only 50 per cent of the infants with meconium aspiration syndrome.

The question whether the quality of meconium is "thin" or "thick" remains a clinical judgment. A number of investigators have tried to correlate thick meconium with a higher incidence of poor fetal outcome when compared with those associated with thinly stained fluid. Miller et al. (1975, 1981) could not conclusively demonstrate any difference in Apgar scores between fetuses exposed to thick or thin meconium-stained fluid. Krebs et al. (1980) concluded that both Apgar scores and fetal heart rate patterns were not different when comparing both groups. Abramovici et al. (1974) also documented that fetal scalp pH, Apgar scores, and ultimate fetal outcome could not be differentiated on the basis of "thin, watery meconium" versus "thick, firm, solid meconium." Conversely, Starks (1980) presented data that did demonstrate lower Apgar scores and fetal scalp blood pH values in the thick meconium group. Meis et al. (1978) showed that heavy meconium increased the risk of low Apgar scores, meconium aspiration syndrome, and death when compared to light meconium. In addition, "early" passage of meconium (meconium passed during or before the active phase of labor) carried a greater risk than "late" passage (meconium passed during the second stage, after clear fluid had been previously noted). The patients in the light meconium group were not at increased risk for adverse outcomes when compared to controls with clear fluid. Studies by Miller et al. (1975) and Bochner et al. (1987) came to the same conclusions. In a series of 238 pregnancies with meconium, Rossi et al. (1989) found that 19 per cent of infants with thick meconium had meconium aspiration syndrome, compared to 5 per cent of those with moderate and 3 per cent of those with thin meconium. Such contradictory views have not been completely resolved, although thick meconium in labor and at delivery is intuitively viewed by most obstetricians as a more ominous sign than is thin meconium.

Since meconium-stained fluid is a common finding intrapartum, with some reports quoting an incidence as high as 44 per cent in postdates pregnancies, any striking associations between meconium and the usual parameters signifying fetal distress should be readily apparent. However, despite continuing disagreement, investigators have failed to document consistently significant differences in Apgar scores, acidosis, and fetal heart rate patterns between meconium-stained infants and those with clear amniotic fluid. A quarter of a century ago, Fenton and Steer (1962) questioned the grave significance of meconium-stained fluid when ominous fetal heart rate patterns were not present. Current data appear to support this view, and meconium per se does *not* imply fetal distress during labor until other parameters support such a contention. Perhaps the most important clinical value of meconium-stained amniotic fluid is to alert the obstetrician to look further for signs of fetal compromise. When available, internal fetal heart rate monitoring should be considered with meconium-stained fluid. Finally, the necessity for careful suctioning of the nasopharynx of the infant at the time of delivery (see below) and the need to alert the pediatric staff should be anticipated.

MECONIUM ASPIRATION SYNDROME AND ITS PREVENTION

The meconium aspiration syndrome is characterized by mild-to-severe respiratory distress at birth. In its mildest form, the disease may present with neonatal tachypnea, associated with normal pH and lowered P_{CO_2}, which resolves within 2 to 3 days. In its more severe form, the syndrome can present as hypoxemia, acidosis, and respiratory failure a few hours after birth. The pathophysiology may involve a combination of mechanical obstruction of the small airways by particulate meconium, chemical pneumonitis, and the displacement of pulmonary surfactant by free fatty acids in meconium (Clark et al., 1987). Incidence is approximately 2 per cent in meconium-stained deliveries (Davis et al., 1985). Significant pulmonary vascular spasms can lead to right-to-left shunting through the patent foramen ovale or ductus arteriosus. Hypoxia may ultimately lead to convulsions, renal failure, disseminated intravascular coagulation, and heart failure (Brady and Goldman, 1986). Death can occur in up to 40 per cent of cases (Davis et al., 1985).

A major obligation of the obstetrician managing a patient with intrapartum meconium-stained fluid is to adequately suction the fetal oropharynx, ideally before the first breath is taken. Carson et al. (1976) demonstrated that suctioning of the fetus immediately after delivery of the head and before delivery of the thorax was effective in reducing the incidence and severity of meconium aspiration. Davis et al. (1985), Ting and Brady (1975), and Gregory et al. (1974) showed similar results of aggressive suctioning. These findings indicate that aspiration often occurs immediately following delivery. A plastic bulb or DeLee suction catheter has traditionally been used to clear the oropharynx, and the neonate often undergoes laryngoscopic visualization of the cords, with endotracheal suction if meconium is seen. These endotracheal procedures should be done on those infants with moderate or thick meconium. Since most studies have shown no increase in morbidity or mortality in otherwise normal newborns with only thin meconium, endotracheal procedures are not necessary for these infants.

Gage et al. (1981) studied the effectiveness of suction techniques in fetal kittens by injecting meconium labeled with radioactive technetium into the airway (trachea and oropharynx) via an endotracheal tube. Thirty seconds of bulb suctioning, followed by 30 seconds of DeLee suctioning, was performed before spontaneous breathing was permitted. In other trials of this study, the sequence of the two suction techniques was reversed. Subsequent scintigraphs of the fetal thorax with a gamma camera revealed that catheter suctioning consistently removed larger quantities of meconium as evidenced by decreasing radioactivity on sequential scintigraphs, whereas bulb suctioning removed significantly less meconium. These findings were confirmed by the differences in the amount of meconium suctioned by the two devices. The authors of this study concluded that catheter suction is more effective than bulb suction for removing meconium from the fetal oropharynx. Using a similar animal model, Pfenninger et al. (1984) demonstrated that oropharyngeal suction is superior to nasal suctioning, and although both methods should be used in succession, oropharyngeal suctioning should be carried out first. Unfortunately, even the most vigorous suctioning on the perineum will not remove meconium already aspirated into the lungs before birth, and thus will not eliminate the occurrence of meconium aspiration syndrome.

Amnioinfusion has been proposed as a way of diluting meconium and possibly decreasing the incidence of intrapartum meconium aspiration syndrome. In a randomized trial, Wenstrom and Parsons (1989) used intrauterine catheters to infuse 1000 cc saline into 36 laboring women with thick meconium and compared outcomes to those of 44 women with thick meconium who received routine care. Labor abnormalities, maternal and fetal electrolytes, 5-minute Apgar scores, and cord pH, were similar between groups. More patients in the control group had operative deliveries for fetal distress. There was a significant decrease in the incidence of meconium below the cords in the amnioinfusion group (2/36 vs 16/44). Although there were three cases of meconium aspiration syndrome in the control group and none in the amnioinfusion group, this difference was not statistically significant. Sadovsky et al. (1989) randomized 40 laboring women with more-than-trace meconium to either an amnioinfusion or control group. Meconium was analyzed spectrophotometrically. Of the amnioinfusion group, 79 per cent had thick meconium preinfusion; this decreased to 5 per cent postinfusion. The control group had 62 per cent thick meconium. There was a 29 per cent incidence of meconium below the cords in the control group, compared to zero per cent in the amnioinfusion group. There were no cases of meconium aspiration syndrome in either group. These studies suggest a potential benefit of amnioinfusion in decreasing the incidence of meconium below the cords, but further studies with larger numbers of patients are necessary to determine whether amnioinfusion can decrease the incidence of meconium aspiration syndrome.

In utero meconium aspiration has been suggested to occur by a number of investigators (Davis et al., 1985; Manning et al., 1978; Brown and Gleicher, 1981; Murphy et al., 1984; Turbeville et al., 1979). The evidence supporting this contention comes from autopsy studies showing meconium in the alveolar spaces both in stillborn infants and in newborns vigorously suctioned on the perineum before the first breath. Animal models have also been used to illustrate intrauterine meconium aspiration when the fetus is experimentally made hypoxic and acidotic (Block et al., 1981). Thus, in some cases meconium aspiration syndrome may not be preventable despite aggressive airway management at delivery.

MECONIUM AND DRUG TESTING

Meconium has been found to contain metabolites of various drugs for at least 3 days following administration. Assays of meconium passed in the first several days after birth may be a more sensitive method than urine screens for detecting recent maternal opiate, cocaine, and marijuana use. Whereas urine is rapidly excreted, meconium is usually not excreted prior to birth, and so potentially serves as a repository. In drug-abusing pregnant women, Ostrea et al. (1989) reported a 100 per cent detection rate using meconium, compared to a 37 per cent detection rate using urine. However, Maynard (1991) reported equal detection rates using urine and meconium in a group of women suspected of using drugs. Meconium may be easier to collect than urine for these purposes, and commercial assays are now available.

CONCLUSION

The significance and management of meconium passage *in utero* continues to be a challenge to the obstetrician. Although a sizable body of information exists concerning the pathophysiology of meconium-stained amniotic fluid, the practicing clinician must understand that these data are far from complete and often contradictory. From a practical standpoint, the discovery of meconium-stained fluid should alert the obstetrician to potential fetal and neonatal problems and encourage increased vigilance in managing such cases. However, the isolated presence of meconium-stained amniotic fluid must not compel the obstetrician to institute needless or harmful intervention. Future investigations are likely to clarify the meaning of *in utero* meconium passage and provide more definitive guidelines for optimal care.

REFERENCES

Gastrointestinal Physiology and Developmental Biology

Arey LB: Developmental Anatomy. Philadelphia, WB Saunders Company, 1974.
Becker RF, Windle WF, Barth EE, Schulz MD: Fetal swallowing, gastrointestinal activity and defecation *in utero*. Surg Gynecol Obstet 70:603, 1940.

Block JC, Kallenberger DA, Kern JD, Nepveux RD: *In utero* meconium aspiration by the baboon fetus. Obstet Gynecol 57:37, 1981.
Brown JC, Mutt V, Dryburgh JR: The further purification of motilin, a gastric motor activity stimulating polypeptide from the mucosa of the small intestine of hogs. Can J Physiol Pharmacol 49:399, 1971.
Chey WY, Lee KY: Motilin. Clin Gastroenterol 9:645, 1980.
Davenport HW (ed): Physiology of the Digestive Tract, 3rd ed. Chicago, Year Book Medical Publishers, Inc., 1971.
Emmanouilides GC, Townsend DE, Bauer RA: Effects of single umbilical artery ligation in the lamb fetus. Pediatrics 42:919, 1968.
Grand RJ, Watkins JB, Torti FM: Progress in Gastroenterology: Development of the human gastrointestinal tract. A review. Gastroenterology 70:790, 1976.
Hirst GDS: Mechanisms of peristalsis. Br Med Bull 35:263, 1979.
Lucas A, Christofides ND, Adrian TE, et al: Fetal distress, meconium and motilin. Lancet 1:718, 1979.
McLain CR: Amniography studies of the gastrointestinal motility of the human fetus. Am J Obstet Gynecol 86:1079, 1963.
Ostrea EM, Brady MJ, Parks PM, Asensio DC, Naluz A: Drug screening of meconium in infants of drug-dependent mothers: An alternative to urine testing. J Pediatr 115(3):474, 1989.
Pritchard JA: Fetal swallowing and amniotic fluid volume. Obstet Gynecol 28:606, 1966.
Smith CA: Physiology of the digestive tract. *In* Smith CA, Nelson NW (eds): The Physiology of the Newborn Infant. Springfield, Charles C Thomas, 1976.

Chemical and Physical Properties of Meconium

Bartman J, Blanc WA: Ultrastructure of human fetal placental membranes in chorioamnionitis and meconium exposure. Obstet Gynecol 35:554, 1970.
Benacerraf BR, Gatter MA, Ginsburgh F: Ultrasound diagnosis of meconium-stained amniotic fluid. Am J Obstet Gynecol 149:570, 1984.
Buhi WC, Spellacy WN: Effects of blood or meconium on the determination of the amniotic fluid lecithin/sphingomyelin ratio. Am J Obstet Gynecol 121:321, 1975.
Florman AL, Tuebner D: Enhancement of bacterial growth in amniotic fluid by meconium. J Pediatr 74:111, 1969.
Freer DE, Statland BE: Measurement of amniotic fluid surfactant. Clin Chem 27:1629, 1981.
Green MN, Clarke JT, Shwachman H: Studies in cystic fibrosis of the pancreas: Protein patterns in meconium. Pediatrics 21:635, 1958.
Hill LM, Breckle R: Vernix in amniotic fluid: Sonographic detection. Radiology 158:80, 1986.
Hill LM, Ellefson R: Variable interference of meconium in the determination of phosphatidylglycerol. Am J Obstet Gynecol 47:339, 1983.
Krebs HB, Petres RE, Dunn LJ, et al: Intrapartum fetal heart rate monitoring. III. Association of meconium with abnormal fetal heart rate patterns. Am J Obstet Gynecol 137:936, 1980.
Kulkarni BD, Bieniarz J, Burd L, Scommegna A: Determination of L/S ratio in amniotic fluid. Obstet Gynecol 40:173, 1972.
Lester R, Smallwood RA, Little JM, et al: Fetal bile salt metabolism: The intestinal absorption of bile salt. J Clin Invest 59:1009, 1977.
Lucas A, Adrian TE, Christofides ND, et al: Plasma motilin, gastrin and enteroglucagon and feeding in the human newborn. Arch Dis Child 55:673, 1980.
Luukkainen TJ, Lehtonen PJ, Hesso AE: Fetal sulfated and nonsulfated bile acids in intrahepatic cholestasis of pregnancy. J Lab Clin Med 92:185, 1978.
Mahmoud EJ, Benirschke K, Vaucher YE, Poitras P: Motilin levels in term neonates who have passed meconium prior to birth. J Pediatr Gastroenterol Nutr 7:95, 1988.
Miettinen TA, Luukkainen TJ: Gas liquid chromatographic and mass spectrometric studies on sterols in vernix caseosa, amniotic fluid and meconium. Acta Chem Scand 22:2603, 1968.
Parker SL: Laboratory variables in determining lecithin/sphingomyelin ratios. Am J Med Technol 47:901, 1981.
Saling E (ed): Fetal and Neonatal Hypoxia in Relation to Clinical Obstetric Practice. London, Edward Arnold, Ltd., 1968.
Schmidt-Sommerfeld E, Litmeyer H, Penn D: A rapid qualitative

method for detecting PG in amniotic fluid. Clin Chim Acta **119**:243, 1982.

Sharp HL, Peller J, Carey JB, Krivit W: Primary and secondary bile acids in meconium. Pediatr Res **5**:274, 1971.

Sherer DM, Abramowicz JS, Smith SA, Woods JR: Sonographically homogeneous echogenic amniotic fluid in detecting meconium-stained amniotic fluid. Obstet Gynecol **78**(5):819, 1991.

Tabsch KMA, Brinkman CR III, Bashore R: Effect of meconium contamination on amniotic fluid L/S ratio. Obstet Gynecol **58**:605, 1981.

Towers CV, Garite TJ: Evaluation of the new Amniostat-FLM test for the detection of phosphatidylglycerol in contaminated fluids. Am J Obstet Gynecol **160**:298, 1989.

Tsao FHC, Zachman RD: Determination of PG in amniotic fluid by a simple one-dimensional thin-layer chromatography method. Clin Chim Acta **118**:109, 1982.

Wagstaff TI, Whyley GA, Freedman G: Factors influencing the measurement of the L/S ratio in amniotic fluid. J Obstet Gynecol Br Commonw **81**:264, 1974.

Yambao TJ, Tawwater B, Chuachingco J, et al: Effect of meconium on the detection of phosphatidylglycerol. Am J Obstet Gynecol **150**:426, 1984.

Zorn EM, Hanson FW, Greve LC, et al: Analysis of the significance of discolored fluid detected at midtrimester amniocentesis. Am J Obstet Gynecol **154**:1234, 1986.

Clinical Relevance of Meconium-Stained Amniotic Fluid

Abramovici H, Brandes JM, Fuchs K, Timor-Tritsch I: Meconium during delivery: A sign of compensated fetal distress. Am J Obstet Gynecol **118**:251, 1974.

Allen R: The significance of meconium in midtrimester genetic amniocentesis. Am J Obstet Gynecol **152**:413, 1985.

Bochner CJ, Medearis AL, Ross MG, Oakes GK, Jones P, Hobel CJ, Wade ME: The role of antepartum testing in the management of postterm pregnancies with heavy meconium in early labor. Obstet Gynecol **96**(6):903, 1987.

Brady JP, Goldman SL: Management of meconium aspiration syndrome. *In* Thibeault DW, Gregory GA (eds): Neonatal Pulmonary Care. Norwalk, Appleton-Century-Crofts, 1986.

Brown BL, Gleicher N: Intrauterine meconium aspiration. Obstet Gynecol **57**:26, 1981.

Carson BJ, Cogey RW, Bowes WA, Simmons MA: Combined obstetric and pediatric approach to prevent meconium aspiration syndrome. Am J Obstet Gynecol **126**:712, 1976.

Clark DA, Nieman GF, Thompson JE, Paskanik AM, Rokhar JE, Bredenberg CE: Surfactant displacement by meconium free fatty acids: An alternative explanation for atelectasis in meconium aspiration syndrome. J Pediatr **110**(5):765, 1987.

Cole JW, Portman RJ, Lim Y, et al: Urinary beta-2-microglobulin in full-term newborns: Evidence for proximal tubular dysfunction in infants with meconium-stained amniotic fluid. Pediatrics **76**:958, 1985.

Curtis, MDe, Martinelli P, Saitta F, et al: Prenatal ultrasonic diagnosis of meconium peritonitis in a preterm infant. Eur J Pediatr **141**:51, 1983.

Davis RO, Philips JB III, Harris BA, et al: Fetal meconium aspiration syndrome occurring despite airway management considered appropriate. Am J Obstet Gynecol **151**:731, 1985.

Desmond MM, Lindley JE, Moore J, Brown CA: Meconium staining of newborn infants. J Pediatr **49**:540, 1956.

Dijxhoorn MJ, Visser GHA, Fidler VJ, et al: Apgar scores, meconium and acidaemia at birth in relation to neonatal neurological morbidity in term infants. Am J Obstet Gynecol **93**:217, 1986.

Dijxhoorn MJ, Visser GHA, Touwen BCL, Huisjes HJ: Apgar score, meconium and acidaemia at birth in small-for-gestational age infants born at term, and their relation to neonatal neurological morbidity. Br J Obstet Gynecol **94**:873, 1987.

Dooley SL, Pesavento DJ, Depp R, et al: Meconium below the vocal cords at delivery: Correlation with intrapartum events. Am J Obstet Gynecol **153**:767, 1985.

Fenton AN, Steer CM: Fetal distress. Am J Obstet Gynecol **83**:354, 1962.

Fleischer AC, Davis RJ, Campbell L: Sonographic detection of a meconium-containing mass in a fetus: A case report. J Clin Ultrasound **11**:103, 1983.

Francoual J, Lindenbaum A, Benattar C, et al: Importance of simultaneous determination of coproporphyrin and hemoglobin in contaminated amniotic fluid. Clin Chem **32**:877, 1986.

Gage JE, Taeusch HW, Treves S, Caldicott W: Suctioning of upper airway meconium in newborn infants. JAMA **246**:2590, 1981.

Golbus MS, Loughman WD, Epstein CJ, et al: Prenatal genetic diagnosis in 3000 amniocenteses. N Engl J Med **300**:157, 1979.

Gregory GA, Gooding CA, Phibbs RH, Tooley WH: Meconium aspiration in infants—a prospective study. J Pediatr **85**:848, 1974.

Hankins GDV, Rowe J, Quirk JG, et al: Significance of brown and/or green amniotic fluid at the time of second trimester genetic amniocentesis. Obstet Gynecol **64**:3, 1984.

Hobel CJ: Intrapartum clinical assessment of fetal distress. Am J Obstet Gynecol **110**:336, 1971.

Hon EH: Modern Trends in Human Reproductive Physiology. London, Butterworths, 1963.

Karp LE, Schiller HS: Meconium staining of amniotic fluid in midtrimester amniocentesis. Obstet Gynecol **50**(Suppl):47, 1977.

King CR, Prescott G, Pernoll M: Significance of meconium in midtrimester diagnostic amniocenteses. Am J Obstet Gynecol **132**:667, 1978.

Krebs HB, Peters RE, Dunn LJ, et al: Intrapartum fetal heart rate monitoring. III. Association of meconium with abnormal fetal heart rate patterns. Am J Obstet Gynecol **137**:936, 1980.

Lee KH: Supervision of high-risk cases by amnioscopy. Am J Obstet Gynecol **112**:46, 1972.

Legge M: Dark brown amniotic fluid—identification of contributing pigments. Br J Obstet Gynecol **88**:632, 1981.

Mandelbaum B: Gestational meconium in the high-risk pregnancy. Obstet Gynecol **42**:87, 1973.

Manning FA, Schreiber J, Turkel SB: Fatal newborn aspiration "*in utero*": A case report. Am J Obstet Gynecol **132**:111, 1978.

Maynard EC, Amoruso LP, Oh W: Meconium for drug testing. AJDC **145**:650, 1991.

Meis PJ, Hall M, Marshall JR, Hobel CJ: Meconium passage: A new classification for risk assessment during labor. Am J Obstet Gynecol **131**(5):509, 1978.

Meis PJ, Hobel CJ, Ureda JR: Late meconium passage in labor—A sign of fetal distress? Obstet Gynecol **59**:332, 1982.

Miller FC, Read JA: Intrapartum assessment of the postdates fetus. Am J Obstet Gynecol **141**:516, 1981.

Miller FC, Sacks DA, Yeh SY, et al: Significance of meconium during labor. Am J Obstet Gynecol **122**:573, 1975.

Miller PW, Coen RW, Benirschke K: Dating the time interval from meconium passage to birth. Obstet Gynecol **66**:459, 1985.

Mitchell J, Schulman H, Fleischer A, et al: Meconium aspiration and fetal acidosis. Obstet Gynecol **65**:352, 1985.

Muller F, Aubry MC, Gasser B, et al: Prenatal diagnosis of cystic fibrosis. II. Meconium ileus in affected fetuses. Prenat Diagn **5**:109, 1985.

Murphy JD, Vawter GF, Reid LM: Pulmonary vascular disease in fatal meconium aspiration. J Pediatr **104**:758, 1984.

Narcarrow P, Mattrey RF, Edwards DK, Skram C: Fibroadhesive meconium peritonitis: *In utero* sonographic diagnosis. J Ultrasound Med **4**:213, 1985.

Pan EY, Chen LY, Yang JZ, et al: Radiographic diagnosis of meconium peritonitis: A report of 200 cases including 6 fetal cases. Pediatr Radiol **13**:199, 1983.

Pfenninger E, Dick W, Brecht-Krauss D, et al: Investigation of intrapartum clearance of the upper airway in the presence of meconium-contaminated amniotic fluid using an animal model. J Perinat Med **12**:57, 1984.

Rossi EM, Philipson EH, Williams TG, Kalhan SC: Meconium aspiration syndrome: Intrapartum and neonatal attributes. Am J Obstet Gynecol **161**(5):1106, 1989.

Sadovsky Y, Amon E, Bade ME, Petrie RH: Prophylactic amnioinfusion during labor complicated by meconium: A preliminary report. Am J Obstet Gynecol **161**(3)613, 1989.

Saldana LR, Schulman H, Lin CC: Routine amnioscopy at term. Obstet Gynecol **47**:521, 1976.

Samuel N, Dicker D, Landman J, et al: Early diagnosis and intra-uterine therapy of meconium plug syndrome in the fetus: Risks and benefits. J Ultrasound Med **5**:425, 1986.

Schwiner SR, Vanley GT, Reinke RT: Prenatal diagnosis of cystic meconium peritonitis. J Clin Ultrasound **12**:37, 1984.

Shalev J, Paskel Y, Avigad I, Mashiach S: Spontaneous intestinal perforation *in utero*: Ultrasonic diagnostic criteria. Am J Obstet Gynecol **144**:855, 1982.

Silverbach S: Antenatal real-time identification of meconium cyst. JCU **11**:455, 1983.

Starks GC: Correlation of meconium-stained amniotic fluid, early intrapartum fetal pH and Apgar scores as predictors of perinatal outcome. Obstet Gynecol **56**:604, 1980.

Steer PJ, Eigbe F, Lissauer TJ, Beard RW: Interrelationships among abnormal cardiotocograms in labor, meconium staining of the amniotic fluid, arterial cord blood pH and Apgar scores. Obstet Gynecol **74**(5):715, 1989.

Svigos JM, Steward-Rattray SF, Pridmore BR: Meconium-stained liquor at second trimester amniocentesis: Is it significant? Aust NZ J Obstet Gynecol **21**:5, 1981.

Ting P, Brady J: Tracheal suction in meconium aspiration. Am J Obstet Gynecol **22**:767, 1975.

Turbeville DF, McCaffree MA, Bloch MF, Krous HF: *In utero* distal pulmonary meconium aspiration. South Med J **72**:535, 1979.

Walker J: Fetal anoxia. Obstet Gynecol Br Emp **61**:162, 1954.

Wenstrom KD, Parsons MT: The prevention of meconium aspiration in labor using amnioinfusion. Obstet Gynecol **73**(4):647, 1989.

Williams J III, Nathan RO, Worthen NJ: Sonographic demonstration of the progression of meconium peritonitis. Obstet Gynecol **64**:822, 1984.

Yeomans ER, Gilstrap LC, Leveno KJ, Burris JS: Meconium in the amniotic fluid and fetal acid-base status. Obstet Gynecol **73**(2):175, 1989.

CHAPTER

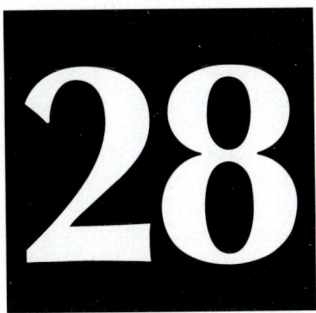

FETAL LUNG DEVELOPMENT, TESTS FOR MATURATION, INDUCTION OF MATURATION, AND TREATMENT

ALAN H. JOBE, M.D., PH.D.

AN OVERVIEW

Perinatal research and care have focused on the lung because successful lung function is so critical to newborn survival. In the recent past, lung immaturity in the preterm newborn uniformly resulted in rapid death. Modern obstetric management of the preterm pregnancy is oriented toward an optimal fetal outcome. Management includes attempts to delay delivery, the use of corticosteroids to mature the fetal lung, improvements in neonatal ventilatory techniques, and surfactant treatments. With intensive clinical management, lung function—in many cases—no longer limits survival of the preterm newborn. The complex process of lung maturation involves considerations of anatomy, physiology, and cell biology, all of which must be appreciated for a balanced understanding of lung functional development and maturation. Although the anatomy and physiology of lung development in the human and in experimental animals have been fairly well characterized, the cell biology, and thus the understanding of the mechanisms underlying the developmental changes, is in its infancy. Hyaline membranes were described in association with respiratory deaths early in this century, and von Neergaard (1929) reported the presence of air-fluid interfaces in lungs. However, there was no substantial increase in the understanding of lung immaturity until Pattle (1955) and Clements (1961) noted the presence of surfactant in pulmonary edema foam and lung extracts, and

Avery and Mead (1959) subsequently correlated respiratory failure with decreased surfactant levels in saline extracts of the lungs of infants with respiratory distress syndrome (RDS). Once the association between atelectasis with hyaline membranes and surfactant levels was appreciated, a massive research effort was focused on the development of the surfactant system. The first direct clinical benefit was the development by Gluck and colleagues (1971) of the lecithin/sphingomyelin (L/S) ratio using amniotic fluid to predict lung immaturity and the risk of RDS in preterm infants. The utility of phosphatidylglycerol measurements for lung maturity testing was recognized by 1976 (Hallman et al., 1976). The maturational effects of corticosteroids on developing systems were appreciated by the late 1960s, and Liggins and Howie first documented a decreased incidence in RDS with maternal corticosteroid treatments in 1972. Perhaps the greatest effect of lung research on infant care will result from the evolving surfactant treatment strategies for RDS and other neonatal lung diseases, a strategy that was developed in animal models in the 1970s primarily by Enhorning and Robertson and their colleagues (reviewed in Robertson and Lachman, 1988) and first demonstrated in humans by Fujiwara et al. in 1980. This progress in the application of research to the pulmonary care of the infant will continue as molecular and cell biologic observations improve the general understanding of lung development, injury, and repair.

LUNG STRUCTURAL DEVELOPMENT

Embryonic Development

Lung development is divided into the three periods of growth: embryonic, fetal, and postnatal (Boyden, 1977). The lung first appears as a ventral bud off the esophagus just caudal to the laryngotracheal sulcus. The grooves between the lung bud and the esophagus deepen, and the bud elongates within the surrounding mesenchyme and divides to form the future main-stem bronchus (Fig. 28–1). Subsequent dichotomous branching gives rise to the airway tree, which exactly develops into the conducting airways. The branching of the endodermal endothelium is under control of the underlying mesoderm because removal of the mesenchyme will stop branching, and transplantation of the mesenchyme from a branching airway to the more proximal airway structures will induce budding in the new location. Lobar airways are formed by about 37 days with progression to segmental airways by 42 days and subsegmental bronchi by 48 days. The pulmonary vasculature branches off the sixth aortic arch to form a vascular plexus in the mesenchyme of the lung bud. The pulmonary artery can be identified by about 37 days, and venous structures appear somewhat later. The 50 days of embryonic lung development have a direct impact on perinatal medicine because most major lung anomalies such as pulmonary agenesis, tracheoesophageal fistula, and bronchial anomalies occur during this period.

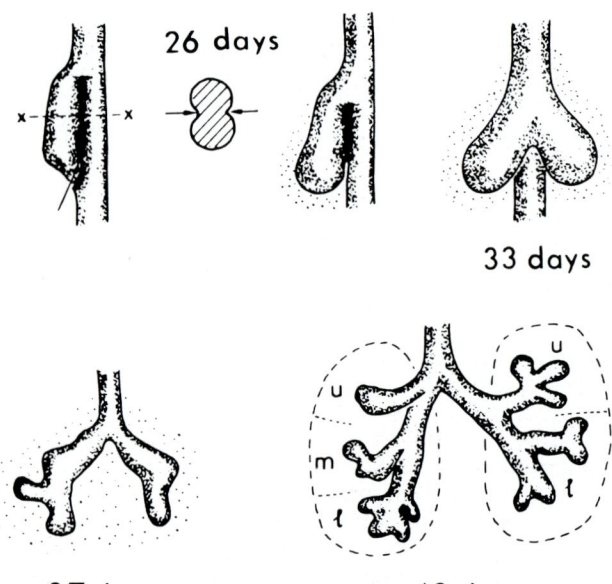

FIGURE 28–1. Embryonic lung development. At 26 days the lung first appears as a protrusion of the foregut. The lung bud becomes more prominent with deepening of the laryngotracheal grooves. By 33 days the lung bud has branched, and by 37 days the prospective main bronchi are penetrating the mesenchyme. Lobar and initial segmental bronchi have formed by 42 days. (Modified from Burri PW: *In* Fishman AP, Fisher AB (eds): Handbook of Physiology: The Respiratory System. Bethesda, MD, American Physiological Society, 1985.)

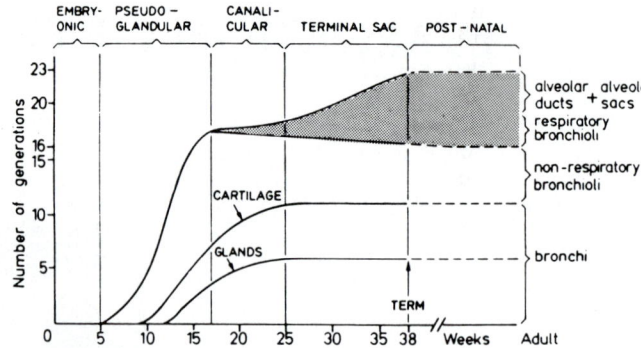

FIGURE 28–2. Timetable for the development of airways. Airway branching is indicated by generation number on the Y axis versus the fetal age. The times of appearance of glands and cartilage also are indicated. (Modified from Burri PW: *In* Fishman AP, Fisher AB (eds): Handbook of Physiology: The Respiratory System. Bethesda, MD, American Physiological Society, 1985.)

Fetal Lung Development

Pseudoglandular Stage

Fetal lung development is divided into the pseudoglandular, canalicular, and terminal sac stages based on the descriptive characteristics of airway development (Burri, 1985) (Fig. 28–2). The pseudoglandular period—from about the seventh to the 17th week—is characterized by the progressive division of the airways from the terminal bronchioles to the completion of respiratory bronchiolar appearance. By the end of the 16th week there are about 15 airway generations, depending somewhat on airway segment length, forming essentially all of the preacinar airways. The developing airways are lined with simple cuboidal cells that contain large amounts of glycogen. In general, epithelial differentiation is centrifugal in that the most distal tubules are lined with undifferentiated cells with progressive differentiation in the more proximal airways. Upper lobar development occurs earlier than lower lobe development in animals, and a similar pattern of development probably occurs in the human. Pulmonary arteries grow in conjunction with the airways, and the principal arterial pathways are present by 14 weeks. Pulmonary venous development occurs in parallel but with a different pattern that demarcates lung segments and subsegments. By the end of the pseudoglandular stage, airways, arteries, and veins have developed in the pattern corresponding to that found in the adult.

Canalicular Stage

The canalicular stage—between about 16 and 25 weeks gestation—represents the transformation of the previable lung to the potentially viable lung that can exchange gas. The three major events during this stage are the "birth" of the acinus, epithelial differentiation with the development of the potential air-blood barrier, and the start of surfactant synthesis within recognizable type II cells (Burri, 1985). The acinus is the tuft of airways and alveoli originating from a terminal bronchiole. The acinus includes two to four respiratory bronchioles with a terminal six to seven generations of branched buds. Its initial development is the critical first step for the development of the future gas exchange surface of the lung. As airway branching and canalization progress, the initially poorly vascularized mesenchyme surrounding the airways becomes more vascular and more closely associated with the airway epithelial cells. With subsequent fusion of the vascular and epithelial basement membranes, a structure comparable to the adult air-blood barrier is formed. Air-blood barriers of thickness comparable to the adult lung begin to appear by about 19 weeks. The total surface area occupied by the air-blood barrier increases exponentially through the canalicular stage with a resultant fall in the mean wall thickness and with an increased potential for gas exchange.

Epithelial differentiation is characterized by proximal-to-distal thinning of the epithelium by transformation of cuboidal cells into thin cells that line wide tubes. Thus the tubes grow both in length and in width with attenuation of the mesenchyme, which is simultaneously becoming vascularized. After about 20 weeks gestation in the human fetus, these cuboidal cells rich in glycogen begin to have more lamellar bodies in their cytoplasm, indicating the initiation of surfactant production. In the human there is a somewhat simultaneous development of acinar airway structures, epithelial differentiation, and surfactant synthesis, a pattern not necessarily seen in other mammalian species, where structural maturation may precede surfactant appearance or visa versa.

Terminal Sac Stage

The terminal sac stage encompasses the period of lung development from the potentially viable stages of prematurity at about 25 weeks to term. This stage is notable for the final branching of the air spaces. Nomenclature is confusing, as a terminal sac or saccule implies a wide, short, closed-end structure, but in fact the distal structures are elongating, branching, and widening until alveolarization is completed. Alveolarization is initiated from the terminal saccules by the appearance of septa in association with capillaries, elastin fibers, and collagen fibers. The definition of an alveolus in part depends on how much septation is required for its identification.

Alveolarization in the human was considered to be a postnatal event. However, recent morphometric studies using late-gestation human lungs have defined alveoli as shallow structures defined by crests (or septa) with elastin at the free margin of the primitive alveoli. Such structures have been identified by 28 weeks gestation with apparently continuous alveolar acquisition and maturation to term. The term human lung has been estimated as having between 10 and 150 million alveoli, indicating extensive alveolarization by term, as the adult lung contains about 300 million alveoli (Langston et al., 1984; Hislop et al., 1986). The major event of physiologic importance is the rapid increase in potential lung gas volumes and surface area after about 25 weeks gestational age (Fig. 28–3).

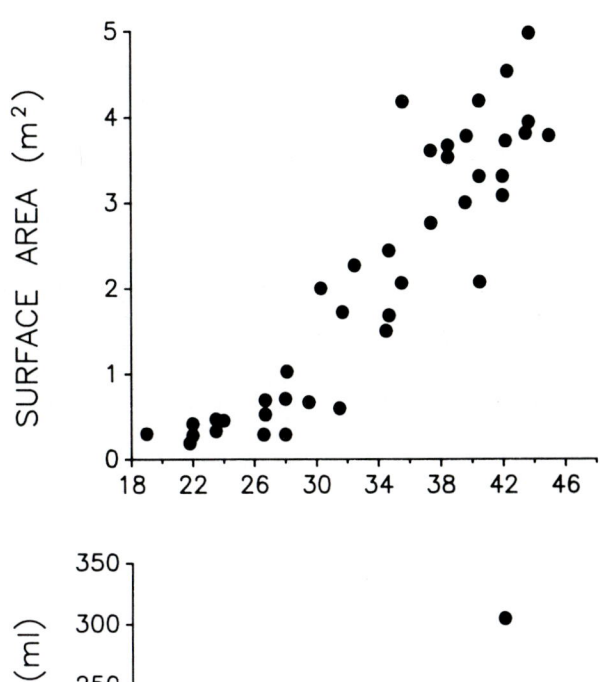

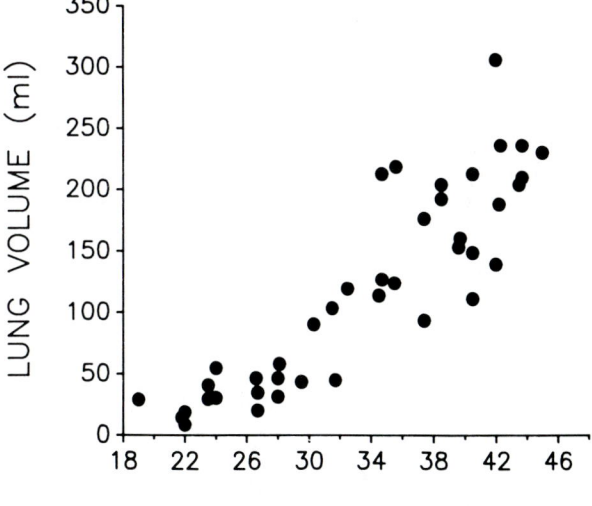

GESTATIONAL AGE

FIGURE 28–3. Changes in lung surface area and lung volume. Both potential air surface area and lung volume increase sharply after about 30 weeks gestational age. There can be large differences in these measurements between fetuses at comparable gestational ages. (Data from Langston C, et al: Am Rev Respir Dis **129**:607, 1984, as presented by Jobe A: The developmental biology of the lung. *In* Fanaroff AA, Martin RJ (eds): Neonatal-Perinatal Medicine. St. Louis, Mosby Year Book, 1992, p. 787.)

Pulmonary Hypoplasia

Although there are occasional embryonic developmental anomalies that result in unilateral pulmonary atresias and abnormal lung segmentation syndromes, diffuse pulmonary hypoplasia syndromes are much more common. Pulmonary hypoplasia diagnosed by low lung weight was found in 15 to 20 per cent of unselected autopsy series (Wigglesworth and Desai, 1982). The diagnosis of pulmonary hypoplasia by the anatomic criteria of airway number and radial alveolar counts is time consuming and not routinely undertaken. However, measurements of lung DNA content relative to body weight clearly separate infants with pulmonary hypoplasia from infants with normal lung development. The fetus must maintain the appropriate volume of fetal lung fluid in the airways and have the normal frequency and amplitude of fetal breathing movements for the lung to grow normally (Liggins, 1984). Fetal lung fluid volume can be decreased either by external chest compression (e.g., oligohydramnios) or by space occupation in the chest cavity (e.g., diaphragmatic hernia).

Somewhat arbitrary classifications of conditions associated with pulmonary hypoplasia are listed in Table 28–1. Thoracic compression syndromes probably are most destructive to lung growth during the canalicular period of human lung development from 16 to 24 weeks gestation. Simple oligohydramnios not associated with renal anomalies does not invariably result in pulmonary hypoplasia, but the earlier in gestation, the more severe it is, and the longer the duration, the more likely it is to become lethal (Thibeault et al., 1985). Pulmonary hypoplasia has been reported after only 6 days of ruptured membranes. Pulmonary hypoplasia secondary to decreased intrathoracic space may in some cases result from abnormal fetal breathing caused by diaphragm dysfunction as much as by the lack of thoracic space. Decreased fetal breathing despite maintenance of apparently normal fetal lung fluid and amniotic fluid volumes explains pulmonary hypoplasia in infants with severe central nervous system damage resulting in depressed fetal breathing and in infectious or developmental neuropathies and myopathies.

The causes of severe primary pulmonary hypoplasia are not known, but a number of infants with less severe degrees of pulmonary hypoplasia have been described. Some of these infants die after prolonged periods of ventilation or survive with residual lung disease. Infants with trisomy 21 or other syndromes may have anomalous lung development or may have abnormal fetal breathing patterns that can result in pulmonary hypoplasia. With improved treatments of severe RDS, preterm infants with variable degrees of pulmonary hypoplasia can be identified and the magnitude of the problem better recognized clinically.

TABLE 28–1. Clinical Syndromes Associated with Pulmonary Hypoplasia

Thoracic compression
  Renal agenesis (Potter's syndrome)
  Urinary tract outflow obstruction
  Oligohydramnios before 28 weeks gestational age
  Extra-amniotic fetal development
Decreased intrathoracic space
  Diaphragmatic hernia
  Pleural effusions
  Abdominal distention sufficient to limit chest volume
  Thoracic dystrophies
Decreased fetal breathing
  Intrauterine CNS damage
  Fetal Werdnig-Hoffmann syndrome
  Other neuropathies and myopathies
Other associations
  Primary pulmonary hypoplasia
  Trisomy 21
  Multiple congenital anomalies
  Erythroblastosis fetalis

Fetal Lung Fluid

The fetal airways are not collapsed, but filled with fluid from the canalicular period until delivery and the initiation of ventilation. Most information concerning quantitative aspects of fetal lung fluid is from the fetal lamb with sonographic and pathologic correlates available for the human. The fetal lung close to term contains enough fluid to maintain the airway volume approximately at the same volume as the functional residual capacity once air breathing is established (Strang, 1991). This volume is about 25 ml/kg body weight in the fetal lamb. The composition of fetal lung fluid is unique relative to other fetal fluids. The chloride content is high while the bicarbonate and protein contents are low (Adamson et al., 1969). Since the fetal lung fluid is in equilibrium with fetal P_{CO_2} values of about 45 mm Hg, the resulting pH of fetal lung fluid is low. This electrolyte composition is maintained by transepithelial ion secretion with bicarbonate reabsorption.

The fetal epithelium is essentially impermeable to protein. The resultant ion movements, together with possible effects of pulmonary microvascular pressures, cause a production rate for fetal lung fluid of 4 to 5 ml/kg/hr. Assuming a 3- to 5-kg fetus, the production of fetal lung fluid would be about 400 ml per day. In the human, some of this fluid is swallowed and some mixes with the amniotic fluid. The pressure in the fetal trachea exceeds that in the amniotic fluid by about 2 mm Hg; this indicates that an outflow resistance exists that maintains the fetal lung fluid volume in the fetal lung. The secretion of fetal lung fluid seems to be primarily an intrinsic metabolic function of the developing alveolar and airway epithelium because changes in vascular hydrostatic pressures, tracheal pressures, and fetal breathing movements do not greatly affect fetal lung fluid production.

While the presence of fetal lung fluid is essential for normal lung development, its clearance is equally essential for normal neonatal respiratory adaptation. Fetal lung fluid production can be completely stopped, and fluid adsorption occurs in near-term fetal sheep by vascular infusions of epinephrine at concentrations that approximate the levels of epinephrine present during labor (Brown et al., 1983). The epinephrine response switch of the air space epithelium from fluid secretion to absorption is absent in preterm fetal sheep and can be induced by short-term cortisol and T_3 infusions (Barker et al., 1990). In term guinea pigs, the Na^+ channel blocker amiloride mixed with fetal lung fluid will delay fluid clearance and cause respiratory distress (O'Brodovich et al., 1990).

Fetal lung fluid production decreases in the days just prior to the clinical detection of labor, and fetal lung fluid volume decreases to about 65 per cent of the maximal volumes present during fetal life (Bland, 1986) (Fig. 28–4). During active labor and delivery, a further 30 per cent of the fluid is cleared from the airways and alveoli, leaving only about 35 per cent of the fetal lung fluid to be adsorbed and cleared from the lungs with breathing. Most of the fluid moves rapidly into the interstitial spaces and subsequently directly into the pulmonary vasculature, with less than

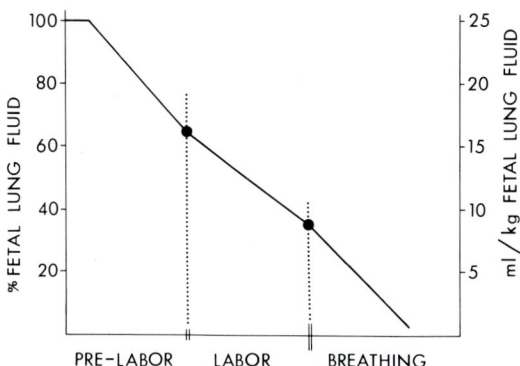

FIGURE 28–4. Loss of fetal lung fluid. The fetal lung fluid volume decreases before labor is clinically apparent. There is a further decrease in fluid volumes during labor, and the residual fluid rapidly moves from the airway and alveoli to the lung interstitium with breathing. The volume estimates are based on measurements in sheep and rabbits as reviewed by Bland (1986).

20 per cent of the fluid being cleared by pulmonary lymphatics. Clearance of the fluid from the interstitial spaces occurs over many hours.

The sequence of prelabor, labor, and delivery is an important regulator of the fetal lung fluid volume present at the initiation of air breathing (Strang, 1991). There are numerous reports of decreased lung compliance, increased incidence of early respiratory distress, and transient tachypnea of the newborn in infants delivered by cesarean section (Faxelius et al., 1982). The magnitude of the potential problem can be appreciated by the following estimates. In the apneic term unlabored newborn with a fetal lung fluid volume of 25 ml/kg, a normal blood volume of 80 ml/kg, and hematocrit of 50 per cent, the fetal lung fluid, which contains essentially no protein, would be equivalent to 62 per cent of the plasma volume. Cesarean section delivery, intubation, and ventilation could result in a crystalloid volume challenge of 25 ml/kg, which could destabilize cardiopulmonary function. Although this scenario is the extreme, many subtle abnormalities and a few severe difficulties of neonatal adaptation are likely to result from the presence of large amounts of alveolar and interstitial fluid in the lungs of infants. The ability of an infant to clear fetal lung fluid will be compromised by systemic hypoproteinemia and vascular volume overload.

SURFACTANT

Composition

Surfactant as recovered from lungs of all mammalian species contains 70 to 80 per cent phospholipids, about 10 per cent protein, and about 10 per cent neutral lipids, primarily cholesterol (Fig. 28–5). The phosphatidylcholine species of the phospholipids contribute about 60 per cent by weight to surfactant and are about 80 per cent of the phospholipids (King and Clements, 1972). The composition of the phospholipids in surfactant is unique relative to the lipid composition of the lung in general or other organs. About 60 per cent of the phosphatidylcholine species are saturated in that both fatty acids esterified to the glycerol-phosphorylcholine backbone are predominantly the 16 carbon saturated fatty acid, palmitic acid. Most other phosphatidylcholine species of surfactant have a fatty acid with one double bond in the 2 position of the molecule. Saturated phosphatidylcholine is the principal surface-active component of surfactant, and much less saturated phosphatidylcholine is present in lipid fractions of lung not associated with surfactant metabolism. Thus saturated phosphatidylcholine can be used as a relatively specific probe of surfactant metabolism. The acidic phospholipid, phosphatidylglycerol, is present in surfactant in small but relatively constant amounts that vary between 4 and 15 per cent of the phospholipids in different species (Van Golde et al., 1988). The composition of the phospholipids in the surfactant lipoprotein complex changes during late gestation. Surfactant phospholipids from the immature fetus or newborn contain relatively large amounts of phosphatidylinositol, which then decrease as phosphatidylglycerol appears with lung maturity (Kulovich et al., 1979). The switch from phosphatidylinositol to phosphatidylglycerol probably results from a fall in the circulating and lung tissue pools of free inositol in the fetus during late gestation (Hallman and Epstein, 1980). Although phosphatidylglycerol is a convenient marker for lung maturity, the presence of phosphatidylglycerol is not necessary for normal surfactant function.

Much of the protein found with surfactant isolated from alveolar lavages is serum protein that is not specific to surfactant. However, three surfactant-specific proteins have recently been characterized and their functions in part elucidated (Weaver and Whitsett, 1991). The gene for human SP-A is on chromosome 10. The primary translation product is about 24 kDa, which then is heavily glycosylated before secretion to yield a reduced protein of about 36 kDa. SP-A has a number of isoforms because of variable glycosylation. This protein has a collagen domain, and in its mature state, the protein is in the form of a collagen-

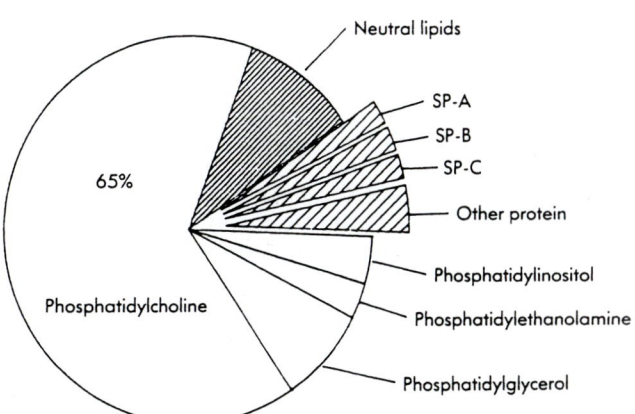

FIGURE 28–5. Composition of surfactant recovered by alveolar wash. The quantities of the different components are similar for surfactant from mature lungs of mammals.

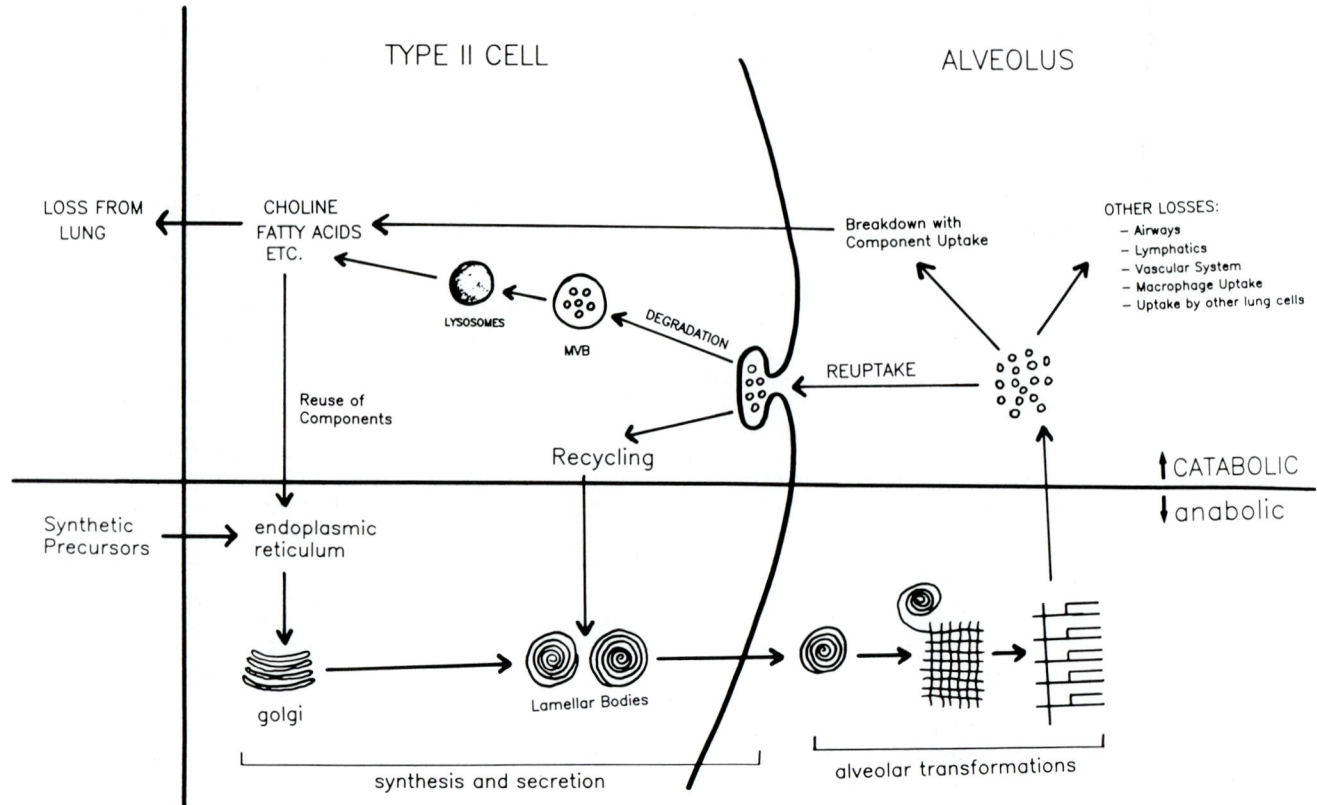

FIGURE 28–6. Sketch of the metabolic pathways of surfactant phosphatidylcholine from synthesis and secretion by the type II cell to alveolar transformations and re-uptake by the type II cell.

like triple helix and thus exists as a hexamer. Six of these hexamers then aggregate to form a final large protein shaped like a flower with a stem that has a molecular weight of 650 kDa. About 2 to 4 per cent of surfactant is SP-A. The protein is secreted with the surfactant lipids and is thought to be a lipid organizer as it may form the corner structures of tubular myelin. SP-A also may be a critical regulator of alveolar surfactant metabolism as this protein increases phospholipid uptake and inhibits surfactant secretion by type II cells *in vitro* via a receptor that recognizes the carbohydrate on SP-A (Possmayer, 1988). SP-A will influence the surface properties of phospholipids, but these effects are best demonstrated as a modest cooperative effect in the presence of the other surfactant proteins.

SP-B and SP-C are two hydrophobic proteins that are extracted with the lipids from surfactant by organic solvents and contribute 2 to 4 per cent to the surfactant mass. The SP-B gene is on human chromosome 2, and the primary translation product is 40 kDa. However, the primary secretion product is an 8-kDa hydrophobic protein. The SP-C gene is on chromosome 8, and its primary translation product is 22 kDa, which is reduced to an extremely hydrophobic 4 kDa protein when associated with alveolar surfactant. These two proteins are difficult to separate from the lipids of surfactant and from each other so that unambiguous functions for each of the proteins have not been established. However, the hydrophobic proteins per-

mit rapid adsorption and spreading of phospholipids on a surface and facilitate the development of low surface tensions on surface compression (Possmayer, 1990). Metabolic or regulatory functions of these proteins have not been identified. Surfactants prepared by organic solvent extraction of natural surfactants contain SP-B and SP-C, but lack SP-A. Such surfactants are virtually equivalent to natural surfactants when evaluated for *in vitro* surface properties or for function *in vivo*, suggesting that the hydrophobic proteins are more critical for the biophysical effects of surfactant than is SP-A (Yamada et al., 1990).

Surfactant Metabolism

The type II cell in the lung is the cell responsible for the major pathways involved in surfactant metabolism (Wright and Clements, 1987) (Fig. 28–6). The overall synthesis and secretion of surfactant should be viewed as a complex sequence of biochemical events, which result in the release by exocytosis of the lamellar bodies to the alveolus. The basic pathways for the synthesis of phospholipids are common to all mammalian cells. Specific enzymes within the endoplasmic reticulum utilize glucose, phosphate, and fatty acids as substrates for phospholipid synthesis (Rooney, 1985). The uniqueness of a phospholipid is determined by the character of the fatty acid side chains esterified to the glycerol carbon backbone and by the head group (choline, glycerol, inositol, and so on) linked to the phosphate. The interrelated pathways for the synthesis of lung phospholipids are outlined in Figure 28–7, and the enzymes referred to in the discussion below are identified by roman numerals on the figure. The 3-carbon backbone of each phospholipid is derived ultimately from glucose and enters the pathway as glycerol-3-phosphate. The de novo synthetic pathway then proceeds through two sequential acyltransferase reactions. A saturated fatty acyl-CoA (usually palmitic acid) is esterified to the 1-acyl position of glycerol-3-phosphate by glycerolphosphate acyltransferase (I). Then the 1-acyl-glycerol-phosphate phosphotransferase (II) esterifies either an unsaturated or saturated fatty acid to the 2-acyl position, generating diacylglycerophosphate (phosphatidic acid), which is the common precursor of the phospholipids. Phosphatidic acid is then either dephosphorylated to diacylglycerol by phosphatidic acid phosphatase (III) or converted to cytidine-5'-diphospho-diacyl-glycerol (CDP-diacylglycerol) by phosphatidate cytidyltransferase (VIII). CDP-diacylglycerol is the common precursor of phosphatidylglycerol and phosphatidylinositol. Phosphatidylglycerol is synthesized by a two-step pathway involving the enzymes glycerolphosphate phosphatidyltransferase (IX) and phosphatidylglycerolphosphatase (X). The diacylglycerol is the direct precursor of both phosphatidylethanolamine and phosphatidylcholine following the transfer of ethanolamine or choline from the CDP-ethanolamine or CDP-choline to the diacylglycerol by the appropriate phosphotransferase (IV, XII). However, the resulting phosphatidylcholines are in large part 1-acyl saturated, 2-acyl unsaturated.

A remolding of some of the 2-acyl-unsaturated phosphatidylcholines resulting from this de novo synthetic pathway occurs within the type II cell before packaging of the resulting saturated phosphatidylcholine into lamellar bodies for secretion. Two pathways for the synthesis of saturated phosphatidylcholine from unsaturated phosphatidylcholine have been proposed. Both initially involve the generation of 1-acyl, 2-lyso phosphatidylcholine by phospholipase A_2 (V). Lysophosphatidylcholine acyl transferase (VI) can make saturated phosphatidylcholine from lysophosphatidylcholine and a saturated acylcoenzyme A or saturated phosphatidylcholine can result from the transfer of a fatty acid from one lysophosphatidylcholine molecule to another as catalyzed by lysophosphatidylcholine-lysophosphatidylcholine acyl transferase (VII). Information derived from culture of type II pneumocytes indicates that the direct reacylation of lysophosphatidylcholine (enzyme VI) is the important pathway for saturated phosphatidylcholine synthesis (Van Golde et al., 1988).

Although the overall synthetic pathways are known, the details of how the components of surfactant con-

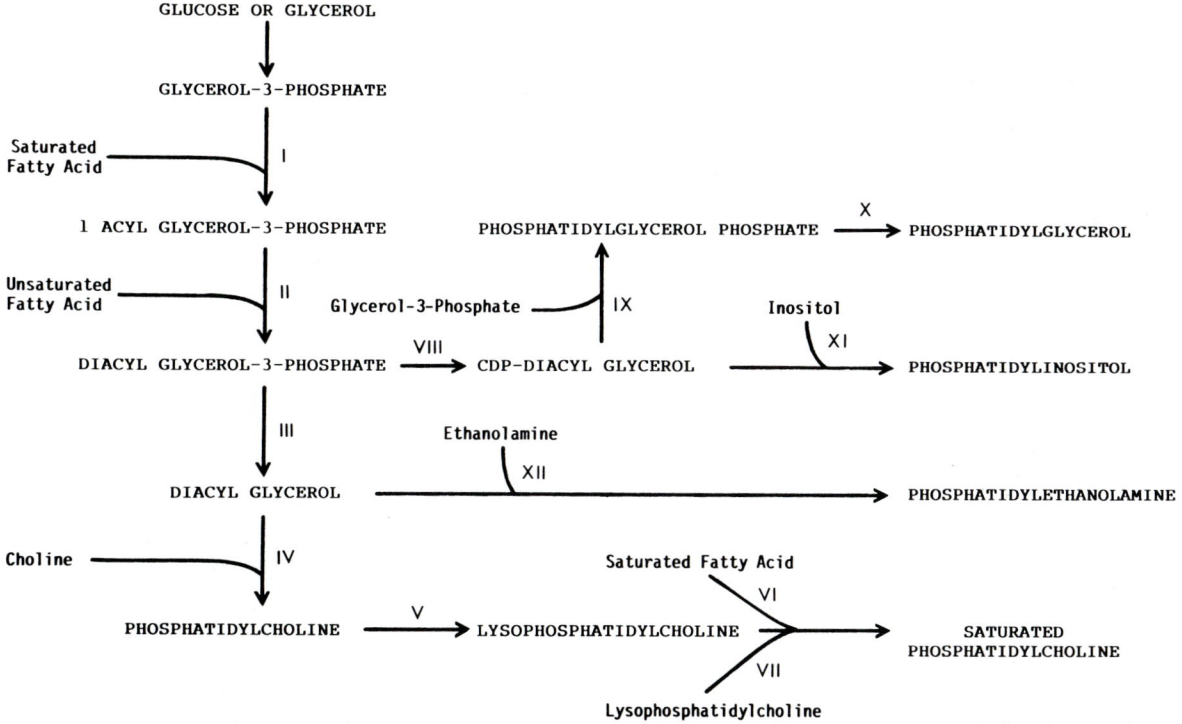

FIGURE 28–7. Biosynthesis of lung phospholipids. The figure outlines the major pathways and precursors for the synthesis of saturated phosphatidylcholine, phosphatidylethanolamine, phosphatidylinositol, and phosphatidylglycerol. The enzymes specific for each step are indicated by roman numerals: I = glycerophosphate acyltransferase; II = 1-acyl-glycerol-phosphate phosphotransferase; III = phosphatidic acid phosphatase; IV = CDP-choline diacylglycerol phosphotransferase; V = phospholipase A_2; VI = lysophosphatidylcholine acyl transferase; VII = lysophosphatidylcholine-lysophosphatidylcholine acyl transferase; VIII = phosphatidate cytidyltransferase; IX = glycerophosphate phosphatidyltransferase; X = phosphatidylglycerol phosphatase; XI = CDP-ethanolamine diacylglycerol phosphotransferase.

dense to form the surfactant lipoprotein complex within lamellar bodies remain obscure. The hydrophobic surfactant proteins may be integral to lamellar body formation. The development and maturation of the ability of the immature lung to process surfactant lipids from synthesis to secretion are essential if the fetus is to ventilate successfully after birth. Although the timing of appearance of synthetic enzymes has been documented, the development of secretion capability has not been defined. Once the type II cell has surfactant stores and can secrete surfactant, secretion can be stimulated by a number of mechanisms (Chander and Fisher, 1990). Type II cells have beta receptors and respond to beta agonists by increased surfactant secretion. Theoretically, if maternal administration of beta agonists to stop preterm labor caused the release of surfactant stores that were then lost into the amniotic fluid, the fetus could be made surfactant-deficient. However, the release of stored surfactant to the airways could facilitate the initiation of air breathing and be beneficial. No clinically important effects of beta agonists on surfactant metabolism in the human have been reported. Purines such as ATP are more potent stimulators of surfactant secretion than are beta agonists and may be important for surfactant secretion at birth. Surfactant secretion also occurs with mechanical stimuli such as lung distention and hyperventilation. The surfactant secretion that occurs with the initiation of ventilation following birth probably results from multiple stimuli such as the combined effects of elevated catecholamines and lung expansion.

After Avery and Mead (1959) observed that saline extracts of the lungs of infants with RDS had high minimum surface tensions, decreased alveolar and tissue surfactant pools were documented in animal models. In general, increasing surfactant pool sizes correlate with improving compliances during development, although other factors such as structural maturation also influence compliance measurements. The few measurements that exist indicate that infants with RDS have surfactant pool sizes on the order of 2 to 10 mg/kg body weight (Hallman et al., 1986). The quantity is similar to the amount of surfactant found in the alveoli of healthy adult animals, but much less than the amount of surfactant recovered from healthy term animals, which often have surfactant pool sizes of 100 mg/kg body weight. Although measurements have not been made for the term human, the large amounts of surfactant in amniotic fluid are consistent with large lung pool sizes. This pool size information, together with the clinical observations that preterm infants and animals respond remarkably to surfactant, indicates that in many infants surfactant deficiency is the primary problem (Jobe and Ikegami, 1987).

Synthetic and secretory pathways have been studied in the hope that stimulation would mitigate the surfactant deficiency. However, the kinetics of synthesis and secretion of surfactant indicate that short term stimulation will not likely have much acute effect on alveolar surfactant pools. There are long time delays between synthesis and the movement of surfactant components from the endoplasmic reticulum through the golgi apparatus to lamellar bodies for eventual secretion (Jobe, 1988). The net kinetics of that process

demonstrate maximal labeling of alveolar surfactant by about 15 hours in adult rabbits and 30 hours in adult sheep. The time delays are longer in the newborn—about 35 hours in newborn rabbits and 40 hours in newborn sheep. Similar time delays from synthesis to secretion of de novo synthesized surfactant phosphatidylcholine also were found in ventilated preterm lambs with RDS (Jobe et al., 1989) (Fig. 28–8). These characteristics of surfactant metabolism in the newborn indicate that the only effective way to quickly correct a surfactant deficiency is to treat with surfactant.

The other half of the metabolic equation from synthesis is catabolism, and catabolic and clearance characteristics of surfactant phospholipids also differ between adult and newborn animals. In adult rabbits, surfactant phosphatidylcholine is rapidly turned over so that secretion and clearance of surfactant from the alveoli are balanced with renewal of the total pool

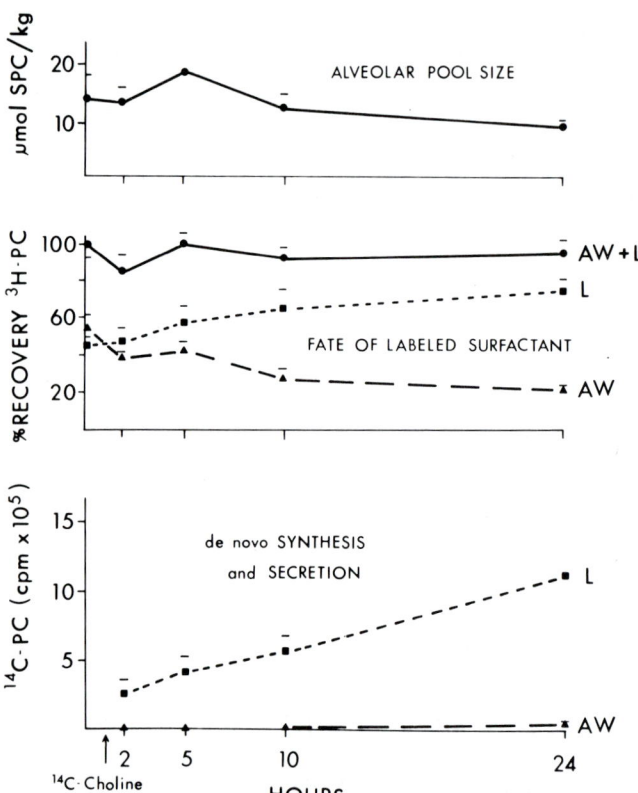

FIGURE 28–8. Labeling patterns of phosphatidylcholine in the lungs of preterm ventilated lambs. The figure is labeled to indicate the alveolar saturated phosphatidylcholine (SPC) pool size/kg, the per cent recovery of a trace dose of labeled phosphatidylcholine (PC) from labeled surfactant that had been mixed with the fetal lung fluid prior to birth, and the labeling of endogenously synthesized and secreted phosphatidylcholine following an intravascular injection of radiolabeled choline at 1 hr of age. The total lung recoveries were the sum of the alveolar wash (AW) plus lung tissue (L) recoveries (AW + L). The labeling patterns are consistent with recycling of surfactant phosphatidylcholine by the lungs. (Data from Jobe et al (1989) as presented in Jobe A: Phospholipid metabolism and turnover. In Polin RA, Fox WW (eds): Fetal and Neonatal Physiology. Philadelphia, WB Saunders Co., 1992, p 990.)

about every 5 hours. About 50 per cent of the surfactant that leaves the air spaces seems to be catabolized within the lung, primarily by type II cells and macrophages. The rest is taken back into type II cells and recycled for resecretion. This resecretion pathway is active for both the surfactant phospholipids and surfactant proteins SP-A and SP-B. The term newborn lung has very little catabolic potential for surfactant. Following the administration of either trace or treatment doses of surfactant to newborn animals, much of the surfactant becomes "lung tissue associated" in that it cannot be recovered by alveolar wash procedures. However, very little catabolism or clearance from the lung occurs. The half-life of lung phosphatidylcholine in the term lamb is on the order of 6 days (Glatz et al., 1982). As much as 95 per cent of the surfactant phosphatidylcholine that was secreted is taken back into type II cells and recycled into surfactant as intact lipids.

There is much less information available concerning the preterm human with RDS. Hallman and his colleagues (1986) measured the biological half-life of airway phosphatidylcholine and phosphatidylglycerol after surfactant treatment of infants with RDS. The half-life values for the surfactant phospholipid components were on the order of 30 hours. This time includes the combined effects of uptake of the lipids into lung tissue and dilution of the alveolar surfactant pool by secretion of endogenously produced surfactant and cannot be interpreted in terms of catabolic activity. Preterm ventilated lambs were found to have essentially no catabolism of endogenous surfactant, and a rough estimate of the turnover time for alveolar surfactant phosphatidylcholine was 13 hours, indicating very active movement of the surfactant through the metabolic pools (Jobe et al., 1989). Preterm lambs treated with 100 mg/kg surfactant did not catabolize the phosphatidylcholine from the treatment doses of surfactant over the first 24 hours of life. The preterm lambs seemed to integrate the exogenous surfactant into their metabolic pathways, presumably to reprocess the surfactants for the maintenance of surface properties (Ikegami et al., 1989). An important effect of surfactant treatments probably is to provide substrate for the metabolic pathways. The basic metabolic pathways for synthesis, secretion, and recycling are present in the preterm lung.

An understanding of the dynamics of surfactant metabolism is further complicated by form transitions within the alveolar space (see Fig. 28–6). Alveolar surfactant has a "life cycle" after secretion (Wright and Clements, 1987). The secreted surfactant phosphatidylcholine moves from secretion as lamellar bodies to a tubular myelin pool that is the reservoir in the hypophase from which the surface film is maintained. SP-A is thought to be critical for this transition. Area compression of the surface film is then thought to concentrate saturated phosphatidylcholine by squeezing out other lipids and surfactant proteins. New surfactant continually enters the surface film and "used" surfactant leaves in the form of small vesicles, which then are cleared from the air spaces. The major compositional difference between the large surface active aggregates of surfactant and the small vesicular

forms is that the small forms contain very little of the surfactant-specific proteins SP-A, SP-B, or SP-C (Magoon et al., 1983). These proteins may be critical for the regulation of the sequential transformations of the surfactant lipids within the air spaces. Just before and after birth, lamellar bodies are secreted to yield an alveolar pool that is essentially all in the large aggregate form (Bruni et al., 1988). This surfactant then begins to function with aeration of the lung. As the newborn goes through neonatal transition, the percentage of large aggregate forms falls and the small forms increase. The distribution of aggregate forms within a few hours of birth approximates that found in the adult animal. This transition after birth represents the establishment of the alveolar life cycle of surfactant.

Physiologic Effects of Surfactant on the Preterm Lung

The effect of surfactant on the preterm surfactant-deficient lung can be demonstrated by the pressure-volume relationships during quasi-static inflation and deflation (Fujiwara, 1984). Preterm surfactant-deficient rabbit lungs do not accumulate much gas on inflation until pressures exceed 25 cm H_2O (Fig. 28–9). The pressure needed to open a lung unit is related to the radius of curvature and surface tension of the meniscus of fluid at the mouth of each uninflated lung unit. In the uninflated lung there are many different units with different radii. The units with larger radii and lower surface tensions will "pop" open first since, with partial expansion, the radius increases and the forces needed to finish opening the unit fall. Surfactant treatment results in a striking decrease in the opening pressure to about 15 cm H_2O. Since the treatment

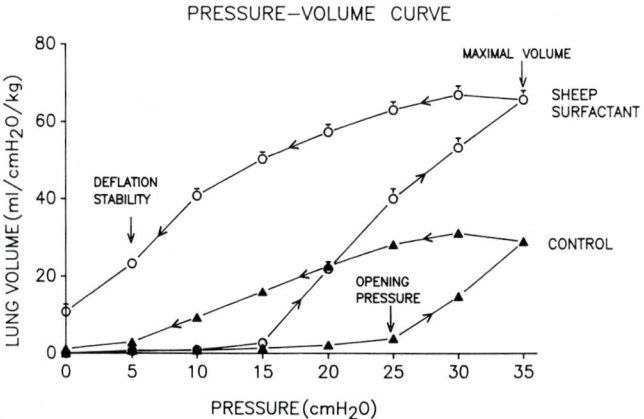

PRESSURE–VOLUME CURVE

FIGURE 28–9. Pressure-volume relationships for the inflation and deflation of surfactant-deficient and surfactant-treated preterm rabbit lungs. The arrowheads on the curves indicate the direction of the inflation-deflation sequence. The control lungs are from 27-day preterm rabbits. Surfactant deficiency is indicated by the high opening pressure, the low maximal volume at a distending pressure of 35 cm H_2O, and the lack of deflation stability at low pressures on deflation. In contrast, treatment of 27-day preterm rabbits with a natural surfactant strikingly alters the pressure-volume relationships.

does not alter the radii of the airways, the decreased opening pressure results from adsorption of the surfactant to the menisci. The subsequent inflation is more uniform as more units are opening at lower pressures so that there is less overdistention of the units that do open, as occurs in the surfactant-deficient lung.

A particularly interesting effect of surfactant on the surfactant-deficient lung is the increase in maximal volume at maximal pressure. In the example in Figure 28–9, maximal volume at 35 cm H_2O increased 2.5-fold with surfactant treatment to a volume that is similar to that achieved in a term newborn rabbit lung. Increased pressures above 35 cm H_2O in control lungs result in lung rupture with little further volume accumulation. This volume difference is potential gas exchange lung volume that can be realized only with the surfactant treatment. The opening pressures of many distal lung units in the surfactant-deficient lung exceed 35 cm H_2O and exceed the rupture pressure of the preterm lung. The traditionally described effect of surfactant is to stabilize the lung on deflation (Fujiwara, 1984). The surfactant-deficient lung completely collapses at low transpulmonary pressures, but the surfactant-treated lung retains about 40 per cent of the lung volume on deflation to 5 cm H_2O.

Dynamic lung mechanics also are altered by surfactant treatments. Time constants for inflation decrease, but time constants for deflation increase, resulting in less effective lung emptying (Noack et al., 1990). The clinical correlate is that a surfactant treatment increases the small functional residual capacity of infants with RDS. The most generally reported response of infants with RDS to surfactant treatments is a rapid improvement in oxygenation. Oxygenation can improve almost instantly, but improvements in Pco_2, compliances, and therefore ventilatory support variables change more gradually. There has been considerable discussion about why oxygenation improves without compliance changes. The explanation is the acute changes in lung volumes following surfactant treatments (Goldsmith et al., 1991). Large changes in gas-to-tissue space ratios are evident by histologic examination of surfactant-treated lungs or by simple gross inspection of excised lungs in animal models. These volume changes mean that all pressure-volume relationships for the lungs are altered. It is apparent by clinical observation that some infants have an acute increase in functional residual capacity after surfactant

Table 28–2. Pregnancy-Related Conditions Associated with Induced Lung Maturation

Accelerated maturation
Chronic maternal hypertension
Maternal cardiovascular disease
Placental infarction
Intrauterine growth retardation
Severe pregnancy-induced hypertension
Prolonged rupture of membranes
Hemoglobinopathies
Delayed maturation
Diabetes mellitus
RH isoimmunization with hydrops fetalis

Table 28–3. Effector Substances That Alter Lung Maturation in in Vitro Systems

Accelerate maturation
Corticosteroids
Thyrotropin releasing hormone (TRH)
T_3
Beta agonists
Prolactin
Epidermal growth factor (EGF)
Transforming growth factor α (TGF-α)
Estrogen
Delay maturation
Insulin
Androgens
Bombesin
Transforming growth factor-β

treatment. Therefore the rapid improvement in oxygenation results from reversal of the atelectasis and the stabilization of the lung to collapse at end expiration.

INDUCED LUNG MATURATION

After Liggins (1969) observed that fetal corticosteroid treatments resulted in early lung maturation in sheep, numerous clinical trials have documented that maternal corticosteroid treatments can decrease the incidence of RDS (Crowley et al., 1990). The decreased incidence of RDS needs to be interpreted within the context of maturational phenomena that occur spontaneously in the preterm infant. Most infants destined to deliver at term do not have mature lungs until about 36 weeks gestation. However, only about 50 per cent of infants born at 30 weeks gestational age have RDS. Although the incidence of RDS increases as gestational age decreases, occasional infants at 24 to 25 weeks gestational age have functional lung maturity. This spontaneous early lung maturation in the human fetus is thought to result from stress-induced maturation events that can be maternal, placental, or fetal in origin. Many specific abnormalities related to prematurity have been associated with early maturation (Table 28–2). However, each specific pregnancy-related condition is disputed because of inconsistent clinical findings. The inconsistences no doubt result in part because the comparison groups of preterm infants are not normal. Prematurity cannot be considered a normal condition. It is perhaps useful to think of the preterm infant with RDS as the normal unstressed preterm. In contrast, the preterm without RDS has experienced a stress sufficient to induce lung maturation.

The precise sequence of events resulting in spontaneous early lung maturation in the human has not been identified. There are pieces of information that can be combined to generate a working hypothesis. Explants of human lung at 14 to 20 weeks gestational age spontaneously differentiate in organ culture in the absence of hormonal stimuli, and agents such as corticosteroids and thyroid hormones accelerate this spontaneous maturation (Gross, 1990) (Table 28–3). Several agents such as insulin and transforming growth factor-beta tend to block lung maturation, and androgens delay maturation. Since at least half of the corticosteroid-treated fetuses do not seem to respond, it is reasonable to propose that fetal lung maturation normally is suppressed in favor of growth. If suppression is released by stress-related signals, then the lung is susceptible to either endogenously mediated maturational signals or to exogenous effectors. Corticosteroids are one class of agents that induce lung maturation, but many other agents also can influence lung maturation (Ballard, 1986).

The fetal lung responses to corticosteroids are multiple and affect many different systems that could influence a functional maturational response. The particular response depends on species, corticosteroid dose, and gestational age. In general, corticosteroids induce lung structural maturation by increasing gas exchange surface area as is reflected by lung volume measurements and influence lung structural proteins, such as collagen (Snyder et al., 1992). Type II cell maturation has been noted primarily in *in vitro* systems and less prominently following maternal corticosteroid treatments in animals. Biochemical markers of maturation include glycogen clearance from type II cells, increased fatty acid synthesis, increased beta receptors, and increased choline incorporation into surfactant phosphatidylcholine (Rooney, 1985). *In vivo*, animals demonstrate increased aeration and survival. Corticosteroid treatment of the fetal lung also decreases the tendency of that lung to develop pulmonary edema. Although it is generally considered that the primary effect of corticosteroids on the fetal lung is to induce surfactant synthesis, effects on enzymes in the synthetic pathway have not been consistently demonstrated across species, and surfactant pool sizes are not increased in some preterm lamb studies and in preterm ventilated rabbits (Ikegami et al., 1991).

The most reasonable synthesis of the available information is that corticosteroids affect many cell types in the fetal lung to stimulate maturation at the expense of growth. The integrated effects of multiple responses are reflected clinically by improved lung function. The magnitude of the effect of maternal corticosteroid clinically has been controversial, in part because of the large number of small studies, each emphasizing different outcomes. The randomized and controlled studies were recently analyzed using meta-analysis techniques to generate reasonable estimates and confidence intervals for outcomes following maternal corticosteroid treatments in studies that included over 3000 patients (Crowley et al., 1990). Maternal corticosteroid therapy decreased the incidence of respiratory distress by about 50 per cent, an effect noted at gestational ages less than 31 weeks in both male and female infants (Fig. 28–10). The treatment also decreased overall neonatal death by about 50 per cent and decreased other major morbidities such as intraventricular hemorrhage and necrotizing enterocolitis in the infants. Maternal corticosteroid treatments also have been reported to decrease the incidence of patent ductus arteriosus and to induce kidney tubular maturation (Clyman et al., 1981; NIH Publication 85-2695, 1985). Overall rates of maternal and neonatal infection as well as stillbirth were not changed. In an analysis

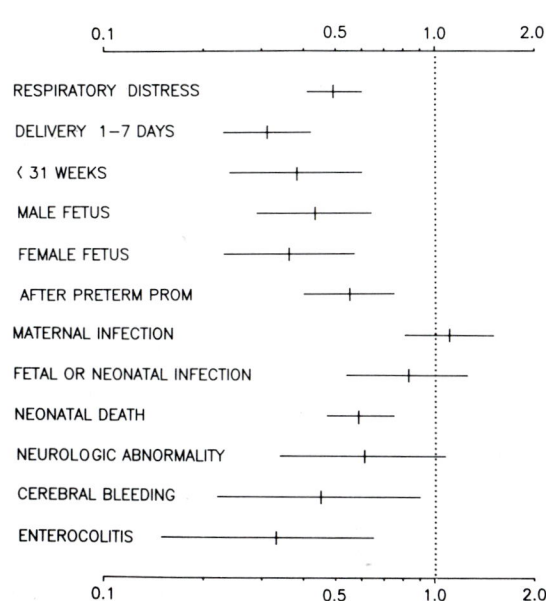

FIGURE 28–10. Meta-analysis of maternal corticosteroid treatments to prevent RDS. The odds ratio ± per cent confidence limits are shown for the indicated variables based on the results from 12 randomized controlled trials. The odds ratio gives the relationship between infants experiencing the event relative to the control infants. An odds ratio <1.0 with 95 per cent confidence limits <1 indicates a beneficial outcome while a ratio >1 indicates increased occurrence of the event relative to the control group. (Graph drawn from the data of Crowley, Chalmers and Keirse: The effects of corticosteroids administration before preterm delivery: an overview of the evidence from controlled trials. Br J Obstet Gynecol **97**:11, 1990.)

of seven studies, maternal corticosteroids decreased respiratory distress without increasing neonatal infection in pregnancies with prelabor rupture of membranes. These beneficial effects on the newborn tended to persist since neurologic abnormalities were numerically fewer in the corticosteroid exposed infants and overall long-term outcomes were good.

The published clinical research record for maternal corticosteroids contrasts with the lack of wide acceptance of this treatment. When surveyed, only about 50 per cent of perinatologists and obstetricians in the United States say that they frequently use corticosteroids (Taslimi et al., 1989), and this usage may be an overestimate based on the data for 1765 infants weighing less than 1500 gm tracked by the National Institute of Child Health Neonatal Network (Hack et al., 1991). An average of just 16 per cent of the infants had been exposed to maternal corticosteroid with a center range of 1 to 33 per cent. Perinatologists have given a number of reasons for not using maternal corticosteroids. Based on the United States collaborative trial, the treatment was influenced by race and fetal sex, although no such relationships were found in other studies or were present in the extensive meta-analysis. Similarly, there is conflicting information about whether maternal corticosteroid treatments work at very early gestational ages in the human (Papageorgiou et al., 1989; Garite et al., 1992). The treatment requires efforts to delay the preterm delivery for 24 to

TABLE 28–4. Component Elements of the Developing Lung That Contribute to Respiratory Failure in the Preterm Infant

ELEMENT	CLINICAL CONSEQUENCES IF IMMATURE
Surfactant	Atelectasis/respiratory distress syndrome
Airways	Pulmonary interstitial emphysema
Alveoli	Inadequate gas exchange
Airway fluid clearance	Pulmonary edema/transient tachypnea
Endothelial and epithelial barriers	Interstitial and alveolar edema

72 hours for the therapy to be effective. However, delayed delivery, if not contraindicated, is potentially beneficial independent of corticosteroid use. Maternal corticosteroids do not suppress maternal immunity, and other harmful effects have not been reported with any consistency (Cunningham and Evans, 1991). Corticosteroid treatments alone decrease RDS and mortality by 50 per cent, a very good result, but a result that indicates that the treatment is not universally effective. Also, depending on the patient mix, perhaps only 50 per cent of women who will deliver prematurely will be candidates for corticosteroid treatments. In the others, delivery will be imminent or there will be a contraindication to corticosteroid use. With an increased focus on the early diagnosis of preterm labor, more women should be eligible for treatment.

Nevertheless, treatments that would be more rapid in effect, without contraindications, and more potent would be helpful. Increased potency could mean a larger and more rapid maturational effect and/or more infants responding. The only lung maturational agent other than corticosteroids that has been systematically evaluated in the human is thyrotropin releasing hormone (TRH). The rationale for the use of TRH is that thyroid hormones induce lung maturation when given to the fetus, and the combined use of thyroid hormones and corticosteroids stimulate surfactant synthesis *in vitro* in human lung explants and lung tissues from other animals more rapidly and to a greater extent than either agent alone (Gross, 1990). Thyroid hormones are not a reasonable choice for maternal treatments since high and toxic maternal doses would be required to get enough placental transfer to mature the fetus. TRH does cross the placenta, and its use will elevate fetal T_3, T_4, and prolactin levels (Moya et al., 1986). In one trial, Morales et al. (1989) found a nonsignificant decrease in the incidence of RDS with the combined use of corticosteroids and TRH to 28 versus 44 per cent with steroids alone. However, time on mechanical ventilation and bronchopulmonary dysplasia were decreased significantly. In a large four-center trial comparing the efficacy of corticosteroids versus corticosteroids plus TRH for the prevention of RDS, there was no effect on incidence of RDS, but time in oxygen and the requirements for mechanical ventilation were decreased, indicating a decrease in bronchopulmonary dysplasia (Ballard et al., 1992). Thus the additive effect of TRH is on the late-outcome variable—bronchopulmonary dysplasia. The mechanisms by which this occurs are unknown at present.

INTEGRATED LUNG MATURATION

Many of the severe difficulties experienced by preterm infants do not result from RDS caused by surfactant deficiency alone. Bronchopulmonary dysplasia can result from prolonged ventilation of the preterm lung that initially functions relatively normally as a gas exchange organ (O'Brodovich and Mellins, 1985). The transition from the immature to the mature lung involves multiple alterations in the lungs (Table 28–4). The air leak syndrome of pulmonary interstitial emphysema is usually associated with RDS and the use of high ventilatory pressures. The pathophysiology of pulmonary interstitial emphysema is the development of multiple air leaks in distal bronchi with the appearance of parenchymal pockets and bronchial cuffs of air that disrupt gas exchange. This sequence of events indicates inadequate development of the structural support elements for the airways. Pulmonary edema syndromes are common in the preterm infant. The tendency of the preterm lung to develop proteinaceous pulmonary edema seems to result from ventilation, since the fetal lung epithelium is quite impermeable to protein. In experimental animals the tendency to pulmonary edema increases as gestational age decreases and can be decreased by fetal treatment with corticosteroids before birth (Ikegami, 1991). The proteinaceous pulmonary edema can inactivate surfactant and aggravate the surfactant deficiency and thus increase the severity of RDS.

Bronchopulmonary dysplasia, pulmonary interstitial emphysema, and pulmonary edema are common clinical problems that illustrate the need for integrated pulmonary development. Such maturity includes not only the synthesis and secretion of adequate amounts of surfactant, but also development of sufficient gas exchange surface to support life, formation of an adequate structural matrix for airway and alveolar function, development of endothelial and epithelial barriers and lymphatic function sufficient to control fluid and protein fluxes in and out of the lungs, and maturation of metabolic properties of the lung such as antioxidant systems and vasoactive substance clearance pathways on the pulmonary vascular epithelium. Even if the lung were sufficiently mature to sustain life, other organ systems must function in concert to permit gas exchange. Respiratory drive and the control of respiration are poorly developed in the tiny infant. The problem of apnea results from the immature central nervous system—pulmonary control mechanisms that often result in prolonged ventilation and bronchopulmonary dysplasia. Immaturity of the muscles of breathing, which results in fatigue and apnea, may also contribute to respiratory failure. The preterm infant's inadequate control of head position and pharyngeal musculature can result in airway obstruction and acute respiratory failure. Adequate postnatal lung function requires the integrated maturation of many aspects of lung development as well as maturation of other organ systems.

EVALUATION OF FETAL LUNG MATURITY

Tests of fetal lung maturation depend upon amniotic fluid composition reflecting the status of the fetal lung.

The lung secretes fetal lung fluid and any surfactant released into that lung fluid throughout late gestation. The flow of fluid out of the lung is episodic and the swallowing or release of this fluid to the amniotic cavity is controlled by the larynx (Bland, 1986). Clements and Tooley (1977) aptly described the amniotic fluid as the fetal cesspool, containing all fetal excretions as well as desquamated cells and other biological matter of variable volume and composition.

Early amniotic fluid tests were nonspecific tests of general fetal maturation that correlated with gestational age. For example, the staining patterns of amniotic fluid cells evaluated skin maturation. Tests such as amniotic fluid creatinine and osmolarity probably evaluate the maturation of the fetal kidneys, whereas optical density measurements such as ΔOD-450 and OD-650 probably are nonspecific measurements of fetal maturity (Nelson et al., 1985). In normal pregnancies, any test of gestational age or general fetal maturation state—independent of which organ is targeted by the test—will correlate well with the degree of fetal lung maturity because maturational events are normally linked closely with gestational age. A remarkable aspect of maturation in the human fetus is the extraordinary inducibility of lung maturation at gestational ages as early as 25 weeks (Gluck et al., 1974). Thus a test of lung maturation in the abnormal pregnancy is *not* a test of gestational age. Other evaluations are necessary to coordinate interpret gestational age and the status of fetal lung maturity if appropriate clinical decisions are to be made.

Lecithin-Sphingomyelin Ratio

The L/S ratio was introduced by Gluck et al (1971). This test remains the most used and the standard against which other tests are compared. The test depends upon the flow of fetal lung fluid into the amniotic fluid being sufficient to change amniotic fluid phospholipid composition in a timely manner relative to changes in fetal lung maturation. The results are expressed as the ratio of a lecithin (phosphatidylcholine) fraction enriched by cold acetone precipitation for saturated phosphatidylcholine to sphingomyelin. Sphingomyelin is a general membrane lipid and is a nonspecific component of amniotic fluid not related to lung maturational events. The sphingomyelin content per milliliter of amniotic fluid tends to fall from about 32 weeks gestational age to term while the more saturated lecithin concentration, a large part of which is from the fetal lung, increases. The L/S ratio for normal pregnancies is less than 0.5 at 20 weeks gestational age and gradually increases to a value of 1.0 at 32 weeks gestational age. A value of 2.0 is achieved by 35 weeks gestational age, and empirically RDS is unlikely if the L/S ratio is more than 2.0 (Gluck et al., 1974) (Fig. 28–11).

Because amniotic fluid volumes change during gestation and cannot be accurately measured clinically, the use of the lecithin measurement standardized against an internal control, sphingomyelin, is thought to correct for changes in amniotic fluid volume and to yield a number that should be more accurate than an

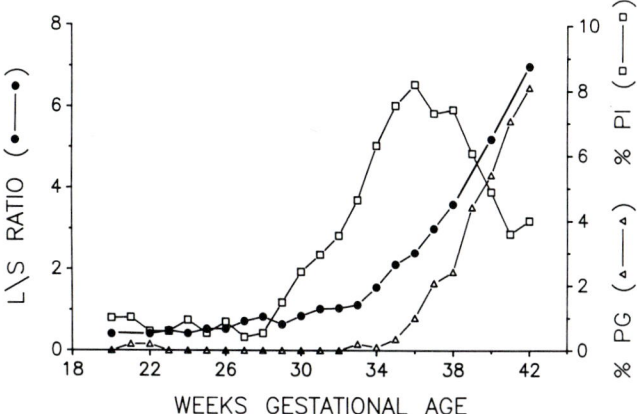

FIGURE 28–11. Lecithin/sphingomyelin (L/S) ratio, percentage phosphatidylglycerol (PG), and percentage phosphatidylinositol (PI) in amniotic fluid from normal pregnancies as a function of gestational age. Each measurement has a distinct profile versus gestational age. (Data from Gluck L et al: Am J Obstet Gynecol **120**:142, 1974, and Hallman et al: Am J Obstet Gynecol **125**:613, 1976, as shown in Jobe A: The developmental biology of the lung. *In* Fanaroff AA, Martin RJ (eds): Neonatal-Perinatal Medicine. St. Louis, Mosby Year Book, 1992, p 792.)

absolute measurement of surfactant phospholipids in the amniotic fluid. Assuming equal losses of the phosphatidylcholines and sphingomyelin during the L/S ratio procedure, the use of a ratio also avoids technical difficulties related to extraction efficiencies and quantification. The value of 2.0 indicates a low risk for RDS at any point in gestation prior to 35 weeks, and L/S ratios can increase rapidly in complicated pregnancies associated with induced lung maturation (Gluck et al., 1974). Values of less than 1.0 are associated with a very high incidence of RDS, while less RDS will be observed in infants who have values of 1.0 to 1.5, and values of 1.5 to 2.0 indicate a modest risk of RDS. The test is not very good at predicting who will not develop RDS. In general, the lower the L/S ratio, the more severe the RDS is likely to be.

The basic test has been modified by numerous investigators. Physicians using this and other tests of lung maturity need to be aware of some of the details and pitfalls of amniotic fluid analysis (Frier and Statland, 1981). Each hospital should establish its own standards and evaluate the predictability of the test for the occurrence of RDS. However, this is seldom done despite the introduction of changes in procedure. Many inaccurate predictions probably result from technical errors or inappropriate numeric criteria for a given procedure. Ideally, amniotic fluid should be sent to the laboratory immediately after collection. However, it can be stored for as long as 24 hours at room temperature and for 10 days at 4° C without significant changes in the L/S ratio (Schwartz et al., 1981). Amniotic fluid can be frozen indefinitely.

A major variable that will change the L/S ratio is the initial centrifugation of the amniotic fluid. Although Gluck et al. (1974) did not give specific average gravitational force recommendations for the centrifugation, very low forces on the order of 300 to 500 × gravity for 10 minutes should be used to remove cellular debris while leaving the surfactant aggregates in suspension. Most of the surfactant in amniotic fluid is present as a suspension of large lamellar body forms that will be removed at higher centrifuged forces resulting in a low L/S ratio. Following phospholipid extraction of the amniotic fluid with chloroform and methanol, the lipid extract is dried and exposed to ice-cold acetone to solubilize the unsaturated phosphatidylcholines away from the saturated phosphatidylcholines that are from the fetal lung. This is a qualitative step that can yield variable results (Hobson et al., 1986). The nonsolubilized phospholipids are then separated by thin layer chromatography. The next difficulty is the quantification of the L/S ratio from the thin layer plates. A clinically useful measurement needs to be rapid, and different spray reagents have been used to detect the phosphatidylcholine and sphingomyelin spots. Different ratios result from the different reagents because the staining characteristics of the phospholipids are not linearly related with molar amounts of the phospholipids on the thin-layer plate (Moore, 1982). Once the spots are identified, they are quantified by planimetry or by reflectance densitometry. It should be recognized that neither measurement technique is very accurate. The L/S ratio will not be reliable if amniotic fluid is heavily contaminated with blood or meconium, because the cold acetone precipitation step does not separate small amounts of saturated phosphatidylcholines from large amounts of contaminating unsaturated phosphatidylcholines and because the contaminants contain sphingomyelin, which will lower the ratio.

Lung Profile

Surfactant from the mature lung contains not only saturated phosphatidylcholine, but also another unique lipid, phosphatidylglycerol, which is about 10 per cent of the surfactant lipids by weight. Phosphatidylglycerol is absent from fetal lung fluid early in gestation and only appears at the time of normal lung maturity at about 35 weeks gestational age (Hallman et al., 1976) (see Fig. 28–11). Phosphatidylglycerol also is absent from the amniotic fluid or tracheal aspirates of infants with RDS, and it appears in the lungs as the disease resolves (Hallman et al., 1977). Phosphatidylglycerol is inducible and can be detected before 30 weeks gestational age in infants with early lung maturation. The presence of phosphatidylglycerol, as opposed to its absence, can be used as a yes or no answer about the risk of RDS. Phosphatidylglycerol is present in appreciable amounts only in lung tissue and surfactant; in other organs, trace amounts of phosphatidylglycerol are present as a precursor of cardiolipin. Thus amniotic fluid contaminated with blood or meconium can be analyzed for phosphatidylglycerol (Strassner et al., 1980).

Phosphatidylglycerol and phosphatidylinositol share a common precursor, CDP-diacylglycerol. Prior to lung maturation, the high levels of inositol in the fetus result in a characteristic increase in amniotic fluid phosphatidylinositol from about 26 weeks gestational age to 35 weeks gestational age. Phosphatidylglycerol appears in amniotic fluid as the percentage of phosphatidylinositol falls (Hallman et al., 1976). Phosphatidylglycerol and phosphatidylinositol thus have developmental profiles that are different from each other and different from the L/S ratio. The lung profile is a test that combines the L/S ratio with measurements of the percentage of phosphatidylglycerol and phosphatidylinositol and the amount of phosphatidylcholine that was cold-acetone precipitable relative to the total amount of phosphatidylcholine extracted from the amniotic fluid (Kulovich et al., 1979). The test is based on sound information about changes in surfactant phospholipids with development and has the advantage of providing enough information to stage lung maturation and thus to better predict infants at risk of RDS. The increased information provided by the lung profile is at the expense of increased difficulty in making the measurements. The test is performed by two-dimensional thin-layer chromatography of the lipid extracts of amniotic fluid, a demanding technique that is not easy for the clinical laboratory. The thin-layer plates yield somewhat variable separations of the phospholipids, and experience in interpretation is necessary.

Other Tests for Phospholipids

Numerous other tests for lung maturity have been reported (Nelson et al., 1985). The number of proposed tests in part reflects the dissatisfaction of both investigators and clinical laboratories in the L/S ratio. The investigators have sought tests that would be more quantitative and would better predict which infant is not at risk for RDS. Clinical laboratories do not like to perform the L/S ratio because it is labor intensive, time consuming, and requires the use of organic solvents and thin-layer chromatography. Also, the interpretation of the chromatogram is somewhat subjective and requires considerable experience. In the other biochemical tests of amniotic fluid phospholipids a ratio is not used, and thus there is no attempt to control for amniotic fluid volume. Although theoretically desirable, the use of a ratio probably makes little difference in most clinical situations (Nelson et al., 1985).

Various investigators have measured total phospholipids, total phosphatidylcholine, saturated phosphatidylcholine, and palmitic acid content of amniotic fluid with success (Frier and Statland, 1981). The phospholipids can be quantified chemically, by enzyme assay, by high-performance liquid chromatography, or by using the amniotic fluid phospholipids as a thromboplastin in clotting assays. If these tests are carefully performed, all are probably comparable to the L/S ratio under most circumstances, but in most reports the values that distinguish infants destined to develop RDS have not been carefully defined.

The presence of phosphatidylglycerol in amniotic fluid seems to predict accurately the absence of RDS. Therefore, a number of tests less complicated than the lung profile have been proposed. Several solvent systems for the one-dimensional separation of phospha-

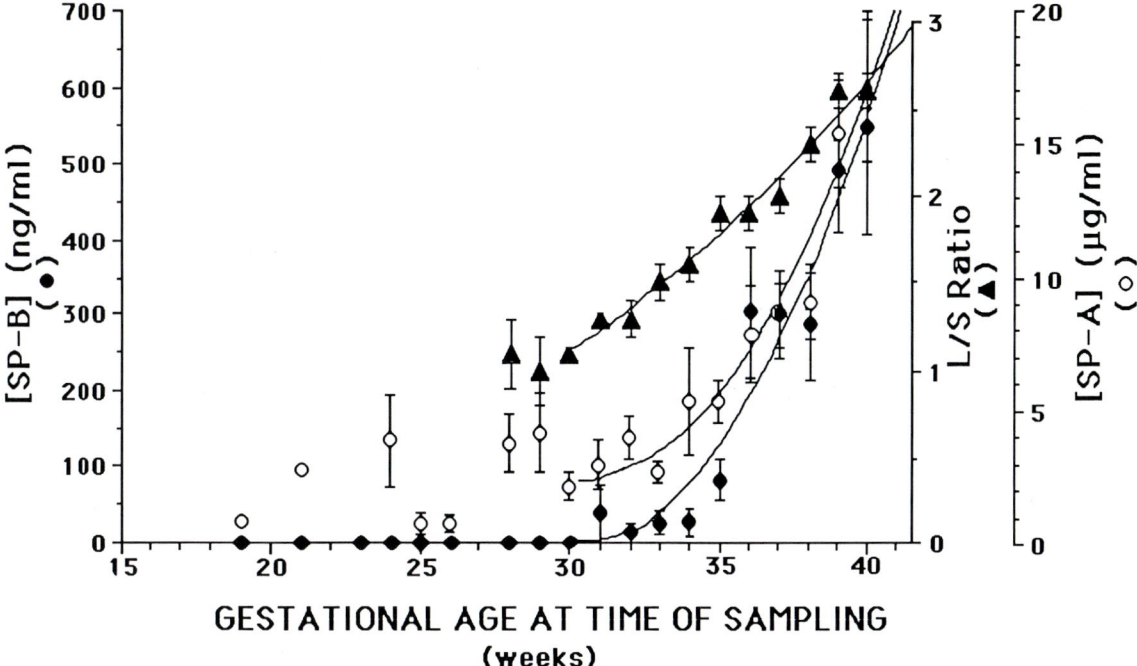

FIGURE 28–12. Mean human amniotic fluid L/S ratios (SP-A) and (SP-B) concentrations at various gestational ages. The values are expressed as mean ± SD. SP-A (open circle) and SP-B (closed circle) were measured by ELISA; L/S (closed triangle) was determined by thin-layer chromatography. Best fit second order polynomial regression lines are given for amniotic fluid samples from 30- to 40-wk gestations. (Reprinted from Pryhuber GS et al: Ontogeny of surfactant proteins A and B in human amniotic fluid as indices of fetal lung maturation. Pediatr Res **30**:597, 1991.)

tidylglycerol from the other phospholipids in amniotic fluid have been described, but they must be used with caution because other phospholipids tend to contaminate the phosphatidylglycerol spot (Gross et al., 1981). An agglutination test using antibodies specific for phosphatidylglycerol is now available as a commercial kit. This can be used as a rapid, semiquantitative measurement of phosphatidylglycerol in amniotic fluid (Lockitch et al., 1984).

Biophysical Tests for Surfactant

Since surfactant has unique surface properties, these properties can be used to detect surfactant in amniotic fluid. Surface properties are concentration dependent and sensitive to interfering substances and thus tend to be qualitative. Although elaborate measurements of surface tension, adsorption of surfactant to a surface, and other surface properties can be done with surfactant isolated from amniotic fluid using a surface balance, such measurements are extremely tedious and exacting and not practical for clinical use. Clements et al. (1972) proposed a simple bedside test that is commonly called the *shake test, bubble stability test,* or *foam test.* Serial dilutions of amniotic fluid are mixed with ethanol and the tubes shaken. The amount of bubbles at the surface at 15 minutes at the different dilutions are interpreted as a positive, intermediate, or negative test for lung maturity. A positive test virtually excludes the presence of RDS, whereas a negative test often occurs in the presence of normal lungs. A similar

bedside bubble test called the *tap test* uses a mixture of amniotic fluid, 6 N HCl, and diethyl ether and may give more reliable results than the shake test (Guidozzi and Gobetz, 1991). Surface properties also can be tested by measurements of surface tension on the basis of the size of drops from a capillary tube or by the movement of amniotic fluid in a capillary tube (Sing, 1980). The changes of phospholipid composition in amniotic fluid can be monitored by fluorescent probes that associate with the lipid micelles (Ashwood et al., 1986). The molecular rotation of probes such as diphenyl-hexatriene can be monitored by a fluorescent polarization assay as an indirect measurement of phospholipid composition and thus used to test for lung maturity. The test is rapid, sensitive, and probably as predictive as the L/S ratio; however, special instrumentation is required.

Other Tests of Maturation

Surfactant contains not only phospholipids, but also the surfactant-associated proteins, other proteins, and enzymes that could be used to evaluate lung maturity. The 35,000 molecular weight surfactant-associated protein SP-A increases in amniotic fluid in parallel with the phospholipids (Fig. 28–12). Polyclonal and monoclonal antibodies to the protein are now available, and enzyme-linked immunoassays have been developed (Kuroki et al., 1985), and analysis of SP-A content can be used to predict RDS (Hallman et al., 1988). Measurement of SP-A is not more predictive of RDS than

MAJOR STEPS IN PATHWAY   EFFECTORS OF PATHWAY

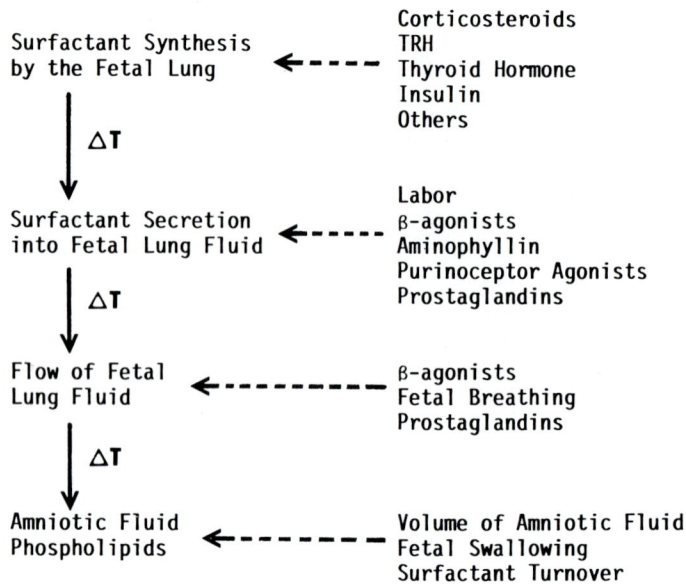

FIGURE 28–13. Fetal lung-amniotic fluid relationships. The time relationship between increased surfactant synthesis and secretion as a manifestation of lung maturity and the reflection of those events in the amniotic fluid are not known even for the normal fetus. The multiple complications that occur with preterm delivery may influence this rather distant relationship between surfactant metabolism within the type II cell and the amniotic fluid. The figure indicates some of the factors that probably modulate this relationship.

the L/S ratio and may give false-positive results in preeclampsia (Hallman et al., 1989). The lipophilic surfactant protein SP-B also has a maturational profile in amniotic fluid, but is less reliable as an indicator of lung maturation (Pryhuber et al., 1991). In the near future assays of surfactant-associated proteins may replace other procedures for lung maturity testing because the test is easy to perform.

Reasons for Incorrect Assessment of Lung Maturity

The L/S ratio and other currently used tests of lung maturation are based on the premise that the amniotic fluid accurately reflects the degree of differentiation of the type II cell population in the developing alveoli of the fetal lung. When complexities of the pathway from fetal surfactant synthesis to its arrival in the amniotic fluid are considered together with the multiple known effectors of the steps on this pathway, it is surprising that these tests of lung maturation work for the evaluation of complicated pregnancies (Jobe, 1986) (Fig. 28–13). Amniotic fluid phospholipids are very far downstream in both distance and time from the type II cell. Although the path length is known, the time delays are unknown in the human. The effectors of the pathways are the same effectors that occur in preterm labor and pregnancy-associated abnormalities. As an indication that the delays between a maturational event and a change in amniotic fluid phospholipids may be long, maternal corticosteroids do not consistently alter amniotic fluid maturation indices.

SURFACTANT FOR RDS

The possibility that surfactant could be used to treat RDS was suggested by the observations of Avery and

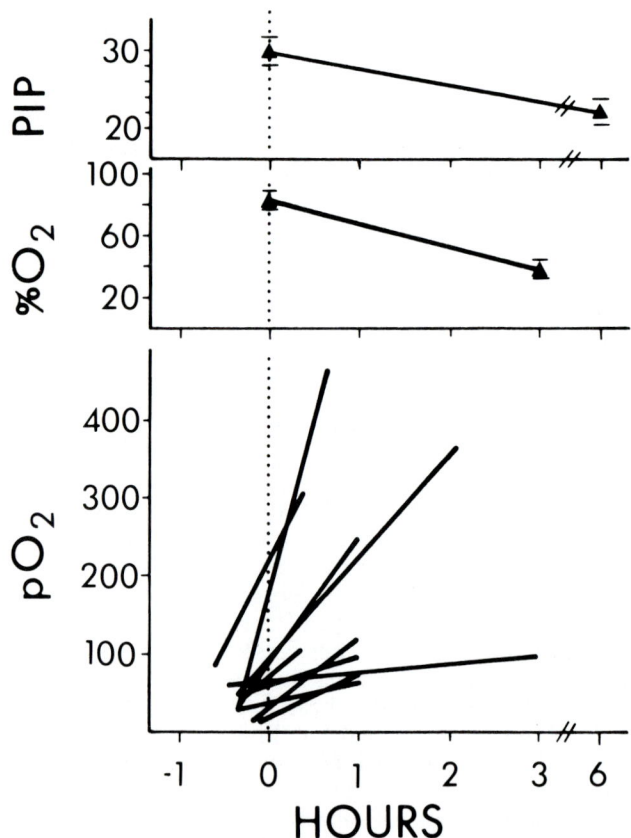

FIGURE 28–14. Response of first 10 infants treated with surfactant. The infants had improved oxygenation and improved ventilation within a short time after receiving the bovine lung derived surfactant. (Redrawn from Fujiwara T et al: Artificial surfactant therapy in hyaline membrane disease. Lancet **1**:55, 1980.)

Mead in 1959. Fujiwara et al. (1980) first reported clinical responses in infants with RDS treated with a bovine lung source surfactant (Fig. 28–14). The infants with severe RDS all had an improvement in oxygenation with several remarkable rapid increases in Po_2. The inspired oxygen concentration and ventilatory pressures could be lowered shortly after the surfactant treatment. Surfactant for RDS became a generally available clinical reality with the licensure of surfactant in 1990 following a number of years of careful clinical trials (Enhorning et al., 1985). Two surfactant preparations are currently in use in the United States: (1) a surfactant composed only of synthetic lipids and an emulsifying agent—Exosurf, and (2) a surfactant made from bovine lung that contains lipids and the two lipophilic surfactant proteins, SP-B and SP-C—Survanta.

Each of these surfactants has been evaluated for two indications—for the treatment of tiny preterm infants at risk for RDS immediately following birth and for the treatment of infants with RDS. Either treatment strategy is effective in decreasing the severity of respiratory symptoms and infant mortality (Long et al., 1991; Hoekstra et al., 1991). The choice of treatment strategy probably does not influence complications or outcomes for larger infants with RDS, but early treatment may benefit the very immature infant weighing less than 1 kg at birth (Kendig et al., 1991). In the early trials, delivery room treatment was contrasted with treatments many hours after birth; in present-day clinical practice, however, there is a tendency to merge the two treatment strategies so that treatment is given as soon after birth as is practical and when some respiratory distress is apparent. A surfactant treatment should not interfere with neonatal resuscitation and initial stabilization.

The multiple clinical trials have consistently shown that mortality from RDS and overall infant mortality are decreased by about 30 per cent (Soll, 1991) (Fig. 28–15). These remarkable effects are reflected by large decreases in the incidence of pneumothorax, oxygen requirements, and ventilatory requirements over the first several days of life. A disappointment has been the lack of consistent decrease in the incidence of bronchopulmonary dysplasia in surfactant-treated survivors of RDS. Presumably, those infants whose lives are saved by surfactant treatment are the infants most likely to develop bronchopulmonary dysplasia, in part explaining the lack of decrease of this chronic lung disease. Although isolated trials report either increases or decreases in the occurrences of common neonatal problems such as patent ductus arteriosus and intraventricular hemorrhage, surfactant treatments do not seem to affect the nonpulmonary complications of prematurity. In an effort to further improve outcomes and better maintain lung function, most surfactants are now being used in multiple-dose strategies.

Although surfactant treatments are effective, infants still die of both RDS and other complications of prematurity. The preterm infant with induced or spontaneous early maturation should have a less complicated clinical course than the infant at the equivalent gestational age with RDS and an increased likelihood of other problems of prematurity. Therefore, obstetric management should not be altered because RDS can be treated with surfactant. The most effective way to prevent RDS is to prevent preterm delivery. If preterm delivery is inevitable, then attempts to mature the fetus are reasonable. Infants that received maternal corticosteroids seemed to respond better to surfactant than untreated infants (Farrell et al., 1989). This clinical observation is supported by experimental demonstrations that both preterm lambs and rabbits have augmented postnatal surfactant treatment responses following fetal exposure to corticosteroids (Ikegami et al., 1987, 1991).

REFERENCES

Adamson TM, Boyd RDH, Platt HS, Strang LB: Composition of alveolar liquid in the foetal lamb. J Physiol (Lond) **204**:159, 1969.

Ashwood ER, Tait JF, Foerder CA, et al: Improved fluorescence polarization assay for use in evaluating fetal lung injury. III. Retrospective clinical evaluation and comparison with the lecithin/sphingomyelin ratio. Clin Chem **32**:260, 1986.

Avery ME, Mead J: Surface properties in relation to atelectasis and hyaline membrane disease. Am J Dis Child **97**:517, 1959.

Ballard PL: Hormones and Lung Maturation. New York, Springer Verlag, 1986.

Ballard RA, Ballard PL, Creasy RD, et al: Respiratory disease in very low birth weight infants after prenatal thyrotropin-releasing hormone and glucocorticoid. Lancet **339**:510, 1992.

Barker PM, Markiewicz M, Walters DV, et al: Synergistic action of T_3 and hydrocortisone on epinephrine-induced readsorption of lung liquid in the fetal sheep. Pediatr Res **27**:588, 1990.

Bland RD: Lung fluid balance before and after birth. *In* Johnston BM, Gluckman PD (eds): Respiratory Control of Lung Development in the Fetus and Newborn, Ithaca, NY, Perinatology Press, 1986, pp 162–208.

Boyden EA: Development and growth of the airways. *In* Hodson WA (ed): Development of the Lung. New York, Marcel Dekker, 1977, pp 3–35.

Brown MJ, Oliver RE, Ramoden CA, et al: Effects of adrenaline and of spontaneous labor on the secretion and adsorption of lung liquid in the fetal lamb. J Physiol (Lond) **344**:137, 1983.

Bruni R, Baritussio A, Quaglino D, et al: Postnatal transformations of alveolar surfactant in the rabbit: Changes in pool size, pool

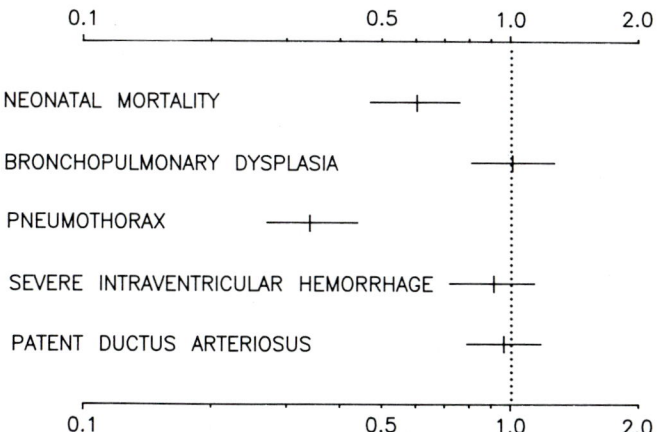

FIGURE 28–15. Meta-analysis of results of 12 randomized controlled trials using natural source surfactants to treat infants with respiratory distress syndrome. Results are shown as odds ratios ± 95 per cent confidence limits. (Data from Soll, 1991.)

morphology and isoforms of the 32–38 kD apolipoprotein. Biochim Biophys Acta **958**:255, 1988.

Burri PW: Development and growth of the human lung. *In* Fishman AP, Fisher AB (eds): Handbook of Physiology: The Respiratory System. Bethesda, MD, American Physiologic Society, 1985, pp 1–46.

Chander A, Fisher AB: Regulation of lung surfactant secretion. Am J Physiol **258**:241, 1990.

Clements JA: Surface tension of lung extracts. Proc Soc Exp Biol Med **95**:170, 1961.

Clements JA, Platzker ACG, Tierney DF, et al: Assessment of the risk of respiratory distress syndrome by a rapid test for surfactant in amniotic fluid. N Engl J Med **268**:1077, 1972.

Clements JA, Tooley WH: Kinetics of surface active material in fetal lung. *In* Hodson WA (ed): Development of the Lung. New York, Marcel-Dekker, 1977, pp 349–366.

Clyman RI, Ballard PL, Snideman S, et al: Prenatal administration of betamethasone for prevention of patent ductus arteriosus. J Pediatr **98**:123, 1981.

Crowley P, Chalmers I, Keirse MJN: The effects of corticosteroid administration before preterm delivery: An overview of the evidence from controlled trials. Br J Obstet Gynaecol **97**:11, 1990.

Cunningham D, Evans E: The effects of betamethasone on maternal cellular resistance to infection. Am J Obstet Gynecol **165**:610, 1991.

Enhorning G, Sherman A, Possmayer F, et al: Prevention of neonatal respiratory distress syndrome by tracheal instillation of surfactant: A randomized trial. Pediatrics **76**:145, 1985.

Farrell EE, Silver RK, Kimberlin LV, et al: Impact of antenatal dexamethasone administration on respiratory distress syndrome in surfactant-treated infants. Am J Obstet Gynecol **161**:628, 1989.

Faxelius G, Bremme K, Lagercrantz H: An old problem revisited—hyaline membrane disease and cesarean section. Eur J Pediatr **189**:121, 1982.

Frier DE, Statland BE: Measurement of amniotic fluid surfactant. Clin Chem **27**:1629, 1981.

Fujiwara T: Surfactant replacement in neonatal RDS. *In* Robertson B, Van Golde LMG, Batenburg JJ (eds): Pulmonary Surfactant. New York, Elsevier, 1984, pp 479–503.

Fujiwara T, Maeta H, Chida S, et al: Artificial surfactant therapy in hyaline membrane disease. Lancet 55, 1980.

Garite TJ, Rummey PJ, Briggs GG, et al: A randomized, placebo-controlled trial of betamethasone for the prevention of corticosteroid distress syndrome at 24 to 28 weeks gestation. Am J Obstet Gynecol **166**:646, 1992.

Glatz T, Ikegami M, Jobe A: Metabolism of exogenously administered natural surfactant in the newborn lamb. Pediatr Res **16**:711, 1982.

Gluck L, Kulovich MV, Boerer RC Jr, et al: Diagnosis of the respiratory distress syndrome by amniocentesis. Am J Obstet Gynecol **109**:440, 1971.

Gluck L, Kulovich MV, Borer RC, et al: The interpretation and significance of the lecithin/sphingomyelin ratio in amniotic fluid. Am J Obstet Gynecol **120**:142, 1974.

Goldsmith LG, Greenspan JS, Rubenstein SD, et al: Immediate improvement in lung volume after exogenous surfactant: alveolar recruitment versus increased distention. J Pediatr **119**:424, 1991.

Gross I: Regulation of fetal lung maturation. Am J Physiol **259**:L337, 1990.

Gross TL, Wilson MV, Kuhnert PM, Sokol RJ: Clinical laboratory determination of phosphatidylglycerol: One- and two-dimensional chromatography compared. Clin Chem **27**:486, 1981.

Guidozzi F, Gobetz L: The tap test—a rapid bedside indicator of fetal lung maturation. Br J Obstet Gynaecol **98**:479, 1991.

Hack M, Hobar JD, Malloy MH, et al: Very low birthweight outcomes of the NIH-CHD Neonatal Network. Pediatrics **87**:587, 1991.

Hallman M, Kulovich M, Kirkpatrick E, et al: Phosphatidylinositol and phosphatidylglycerol in amniotic fluid: Indices of lung maturity. Am J Obstet Gynecol **125**:613, 1976.

Hallman M, Feldman BH, Kirkpatrick E, et al: Absence of phosphatidylglycerol in respiratory distress syndrome in the newborn. Pediatr Res **11**:714, 1977.

Hallman M, Epstein BL: Role of myo-inositol in the synthesis of phosphatidylglycerol and phosphatidylinositol in the lung. Biochem Biophys Res Commun **92**:1151, 1980.

Hallman M, Merritt TA, Pohjavuori M, et al: Effect of surfactant substitution on lung effluent phospholipids in respiratory distress syndrome: Evaluation of surfactant phospholipid turnover, pool size, and the relationship to severity of respiratory failure. Pediatr Res **20**:1228, 1986.

Hallman M, Arjomaa P, Mizumoto et al: Surfactant proteins in the diagnosis of fetal lung maturity I. Predictive accuracy of the 35 kD protein, the lecithin/sphingomyelin ratio, and phosphatidylglycerol. Am J Obstet Gynecol **158**:531, 1988.

Hallman M, Arjomaa P, Hoppu K, et al: Surfactant proteins in the diagnosis of fetal lung maturity. II. The 35 kd protein and phospholipids in complicated pregnancy. Am J Obstet Gynecol **161**:965, 1989.

Hislop AA, Wigglesworth JS, Desai R: Alveolar development in the human fetus and infant. Early Hum Devel **13**:1, 1986.

Hobson DW, Spillman T, Cotton DB: Effect of acetone precipitation on the clinical prediction of respiratory distress syndrome when utilizing amniotic fluid lecithin/sphingomyelin ratios. Am J Obstet Gynecol **154**:1023, 1986.

Hoekstra RE, Jackson JC, Myers TF, et al: Improved neonatal survival following multiple doses of bovine surfactant in very premature neonates at risk for respiratory distress syndrome. Pediatrics **88**:10, 1991.

Ikegami M, Berry D, El Kady T, et al: Corticosteroids and surfactant change lung function and protein leaks in the lungs of ventilated premature rabbits. J Clin Invest **79**:1371, 1987.

Ikegami M, Jobe A, Yamada T, et al: Surfactant metabolism in surfactant-treated preterm ventilated lambs. J Appl Physiol **67**:429, 1989.

Ikegami M, Polk D, Tabor B, Lewis J, et al: Corticosteroid and thyrotropin-releasing hormone effects on preterm sheep lung function. J Appl Physiol **70**:2268, 1991.

Jobe A: Surfactant and the developing lung. *In* Thibeault D, Gregory GA (eds): Neonatal Pulmonary Care. New York, Appleton-Century-Crofts, 1986, pp 75–100.

Jobe A: Metabolism of endogenous surfactant and exogenous surfactants for replacement therapy. Semin Perinatol **12**:231, 1988.

Jobe A: The developmental biology of the lung. *In* Fanaroff AA, Martin RJ (eds): Neonatal-Perinatal Medicine. St. Louis, Mosby-Year Book, 1992, pp 783–801.

Jobe A, Ikegami M: Surfactant for the treatment of respiratory distress syndrome. Am Rev Respir Dis **136**:1256, 1987.

Jobe A, Ikegami M, Seidner S, et al: Surfactant phosphatidylcholine metabolism and surfactant function in preterm, ventilated lambs. Am Rev Respir Dis **139**:352, 1989.

Kendig JW, Notter RH, Cox C, et al: A comparison of surfactant as immediate prophylaxis and as rescue therapy in newborns of less than 30 weeks gestation. N Engl J Med **324**:865, 1991.

King RJ, Clements JA: Surface active materials from dog lung. II. Composition and physiological correlations. Am J Physiol **223**:715, 1972.

Kulovich MV, Hallman MB, Gluck L: The lung profile. I. Normal pregnancy. Am J Obstet Gynecol **135**:57, 1979.

Kuroki Y, Takahashi H, Fukuda Y, et al: Two-site "simultaneous" immunoassay with monoclonal antibodies for the determination of surfactant apoproteins in human amniotic fluid. Pediatr Res **19**:1017, 1985.

Langston C, Kida K, Reed M, et al: Human lung growth in late gestation and in the neonate. Am Rev Respir Dis **129**:607, 1984.

Liggins GC, Howie RN: A controlled trial of antepartum glucocorticoid treatment for prevention of the corticosteroid distress syndrome in premature infants. Pediatrics **50**:515, 1972.

Liggins GC: Growth of the fetal lung. J Dev Physiol **6**:237, 1984.

Liggins GC: Premature delivery of foetal lambs infused with glucocorticoid. J Endocrinol **45**:515, 1969.

Lockitch G, Wittman BK, Mura SM, et al: Evaluation of the amniostat-FLM assay for assessment of fetal lung maturity. Clin Chem **30**:1233, 1984.

Long W, Thompson T, Sundell H, et al: Effects of two rescue doses of a synthetic surfactant on mortality rate and survival without bronchopulmonary dysplasia in 700- to 1350-gram infants with respiratory distress syndrome. J Pediatr **118**:595, 1991.

Magoon MW, Wright JR, Baritussai A, et al: Subfractionation of lung surfactant. Implications for metabolism and surface activity. Biochim Biophys Acta **750**:18, 1983.

Moore P: The lecithin-sphingomyelin ratio in amniotic fluid by thin layer chromatography: three areas of difficulty. Med Lab Sci **39**:237, 1982.

Morales WJ, Obrien WF, Angel JL, et al: Fetal lung maturation: The combined use of corticosteroids and thyrotropin-releasing hormone. Obstet Gynecol **73**:111, 1989.

Moya F, Mena P, Heusser F, et al: Response of the maternal, fetal and neonatal pituitary-thyroid axis of thyrotropin-releasing hormone. Pediatr Res **20**:982, 1986.

Nelson GH, Nelson SJ: Theoretical effects of amniotic fluid volume changes on surfactant concentration measurements. Am J Obstet Gynecol **152**:870, 1985.

NIH Publication 85-2695. Prevention of RDS: Effects of antenatal dexamethasone administration. Washington, DC, 1985.

Noack G, Curstedt T, Grossman G, et al: Passive expiratory flow-volume recordings in immature newborn rabbits. Respiration **57**:1, 1990.

O'Brodovich HM, Mellins RB: Bronchopulmonary dysplasia. Unresolved neonatal acute lung injury. Am Rev Respir Dis **132**:694, 1985.

O'Brodovich H, Hannam V, Seear M, et al: Amiloride impairs lung water clearance in newborn guinea pigs. J Appl Physiol **68**:1758, 1990.

Papageorgiou AN, Doray J-L, Ardila R, et al: Reduction of mortality, morbidity, and respiratory distress syndrome in infants weighing less than 1000 grams by treatment with betamethasone and ritodrine. Pediatrics **83**:493, 1989.

Pattle RE: Properties, function and origin of the alveolar lining layer. Nature **175**:1125, 1955.

Possmayer F: A proposed nomenclature for pulmonary surfactant-associated proteins. Am Rev Respir Dis **138**:990, 1988.

Possmayer F: The role of surfactant associated proteins. Am Rev Respir Dis **142**:749, 1990.

Pryhuber GS, Hull WM, Fink I, et al: Ontogeny of surfactant proteins A and B in human amniotic fluid as indices of fetal lung maturity. Pediatr Res **30**:597, 1991.

Robertson B, Lachman B: Experimental evaluation of surfactants for replacement therapy. Exp Lung Res **14**:279, 1988.

Rooney SA: The surfactant system and lung phospholipid biochemistry. Am Rev Respir Dis **131**:439, 1985.

Schwartz DB, Engle MJ, Brown DJ, et al: The stability of phospholipids in amniotic fluid. Am J Obstet Gynecol **141**:294, 1981.

Sing EJ: Capillary method for assessment of pulmonary maturity in utero with the use of amniotic fluid. Am J Obstet Gynecol **136**:228, 1980.

Snyder JM, Rodgers HF, O'Brien JA, et al: Glucocorticoid effects on rabbit fetal lung maturation in vivo: an ultrastructural morphometric study. Anat Rec **232**:133, 1992.

Soll RF: Natural surfactant extract treatment of RDS. *In* Chalmers I (ed): Oxford Database of Perinatal Trials Version 1.2, Disk issue 6. Autumn, 1991.

Strang LB: Fetal lung liquid: secretion and readsorption. Physiol Rev **71**:991, 1991.

Strassner HT Jr, Golde SH, Mosley GH, et al: Effect of blood in amniotic fluid on the detection of phosphatidylglycerol. Am J Obstet Gynecol **138**:697, 1980.

Taslimi MM, Sibai BM, Amon E, et al: A national survey on preterm labor. Am J Obstet Gynecol **160**:1352, 1989.

Thibeault DW, Beatty EC Jr, Hall RT, et al: Neonatal pulmonary hypoplasia with premature rupture of fetal membranes and oligohydramnios. J Pediatr **107**:273, 1985.

Van Golde LMG, Batenburg JJ, Robertson B: The pulmonary surfactant system: Biochemical aspects and functional significance. Physiol Rev **68**:374, 1988.

Von Neergaard: Neue Auffassungen uber einen Grundbegriff der atemmechanik. Z Ges Exp Med **66**:373, 1929.

Weaver T, Whitsett JA: Function and regulation of expression of pulmonary surfactant-associated proteins. Biochem J **273**:249, 1991.

Wigglesworth JS, Desai R: Is fetal respiratory function a major determinant of perinatal survival? Lancet **1**:264, 1982.

Wright JR, Clements JA: Metabolism and turnover of lung surfactant. Am Rev Respir Dis **135**:426, 1987.

Yamada T, Ikegami M, Jobe A: Effects of surfactant subfractions on preterm lung function. Pediatr Res **27**:592, 1990.

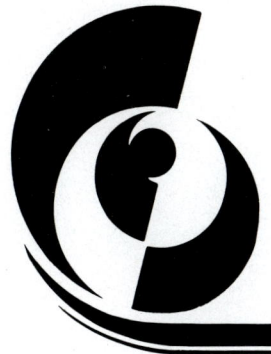

PART III

MATERNAL AND FETAL PATHOPHYSIOLOGY

PREGNANCY WASTAGE

CHAPTER

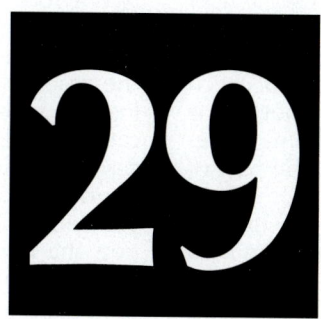

RECURRENT ABORTION

ROBERT H. GLASS, M.D., and MITCHELL S. GOLBUS, M.D.

Approximately 15 per cent of recognized pregnancies end in a first-trimester spontaneous abortion. For most women such an abortion is a random event, but an estimated 0.4 per cent of women have three consecutive spontaneous abortions, and they are categorized as having *recurrent abortion*. This chapter is concerned with abortion probability and the possible causes for recurrent abortion.

A distinction should be made between the rate of abortion in clinically apparent pregnancies (15 per cent) and the much higher rate found when very early pregnancies are surveyed. A study of 34 early embryos, which were recovered by flushing and pathologic examination of reproductive organs removed at surgery, revealed that 10 of these embryos were morphologically abnormal, including four of the eight preimplantation embryos (Hertig et al., 1959). The abnormal embryos would, in all likelihood, have been aborted. On the basis of this information and other data, Leridon (1977) concluded that only one-third of ova exposed to sperm survive to birth. The results of sensitive pregnancy tests also indicate that there is an early pregnancy loss of more than 40 per cent (Miller et al., 1980). Three-quarters of the losses are not evident clinically and can be diagnosed only by a pregnancy test. If all women were monitored in each cycle by pregnancy testing, it is likely that many would be found to have repetitive abortions. However, we will concentrate our discussion on those women who have had three *clinically evident* first-trimester spontaneous abortions.

In discussing the recurrence rates of spontaneous abortions, most authors use the clinically evident abortion rate of approximately 15 per cent as a figure for comparison. Malpas (1938), using theoretical calculations, stated that a woman with a history of three

consecutive abortions had a 73 per cent chance of aborting in the next pregnancy. In 1946 Eastman presented statistical calculations indicating that after three abortions the risk was 83.6 per cent. These early papers established the concept that the probability for a subsequent abortion increases dramatically with each successive abortion and that after three abortions the chances for successful pregnancy are very low. In subsequent studies on the efficacy of many types of treatment, the researchers used these pessimistic figures for comparison rather than establishing their own control figures. If a particular treatment increased the salvage rate to 70 per cent, it was considered curative. However, later studies indicate that the risk of abortion after three consecutive abortions is, in fact, only 20 to 55 per cent (Warburton and Fraser, 1964; James, 1963b; MacNaughton, 1964; Poland et al., 1977; Vlaanderen and Treffers, 1987). It is not surprising, therefore, that treatment with a wide range of approaches was followed by successful pregnancies in a reasonable percentage of women with recurrent abortion. These cures were not due to the therapy; rather, the claims for success were based on a comparison to the now discredited figures of Malpas (1938) and Eastman (1946).

More than one-half of spontaneous first-trimester abortion specimens that undergo karyotyping are found to have a chromosomal abnormality, which is the major cause for spontaneous abortion. Trisomy is the most common finding (52 per cent), with triploidy (20 per cent) and monosomy X (15 per cent) the next most common (Boue et al., 1975). The lack of autosomal monosomy and the low frequency of certain types of trisomy suggest that these abnormalities lead to very early developmental arrest. In addition to the high percentage of chromosomal abnormalities in aborted specimens, another 20 per cent of specimens are morphologically abnormal (Boue et al., 1975). Single-gene defects that are not diagnosed by chromosomal analysis could account for other early pregnancy losses. Just as there are inherited gene defects, such as Tay-Sachs disease or tuberous sclerosis, that cause early childhood deaths, and other gene defects such as α-thalassemia that cause late *in utero* demise, single-gene defects that cause early embryonic death and spontaneous abortion probably occur. It is unlikely that we will ever have an impressive list of such disorders because the product of an early abortion is rarely subjected to biochemical studies, which, moreover, would represent blind guesswork on the part of the investigators.

Whereas a minimum of 7.5 per cent of human embryos are chromosomally abnormal (based on a 15 per cent spontaneous abortion rate and a 50 per cent incidence of chromosomal abnormalities in aborted specimens), only one in 200 infants has a chromosomal abnormality, indicating that there is selection against abnormal embryos and fetuses. There also may be selection even earlier against abnormal gametes. Percentages of morphologically abnormal sperm are lower in the cervix and tube than in the ejaculate, suggesting that the cervical mucus and the uterotubal junction act as filters (Krzanowska, 1974). However, these filters probably are not effective against genetically abnormal sperm that are morphologically normal. The manner in which abnormal embryos and fetuses are lost is unknown. In some species the embryo transmits a signal that is recognized by the mother, and that triggers maternal mechanisms necessary for embryo survival (Heap et al., 1979). Pig blastocysts secrete estrogen on day 12 of pregnancy, 6 days before definitive attachment of the embryo to the uterus. The estrogens decrease prostaglandin secretion into the maternal circulation and thereby prevent the luteolytic effect of prostaglandins. Estrogen also increases the secretion of luteinizing hormone. Both of these effects result in maintenance or enhancement of function of the corpus luteum. In the human, chorionic gonadotropin (hCG) is secreted at the time of implantation, and this, too, stimulates the corpus luteum. Perhaps genetically abnormal embryos cannot produce a normal signal.

Genetic abnormalities may affect the cell surface of the embryo, resulting in abnormal arrangements of surface glycoproteins and interfering with attachment of the embryo to the uterine epithelium. Alternately, the genetic abnormality may cause a programmed cell death of the embryo, as demonstrated in chromosomally abnormal mice (Wudl et al., 1977). Although it is common to speak in terms of maternal selection against abnormal embryos, this notion is, in our view, an unproven cause of failure of pregnancies involving genetically abnormal embryos.

CAUSES OF RECURRENT ABORTION

Genetic Factors

A few of the chromosome abnormalities that result in spontaneous abortion arise from transmission of structurally aberrant chromosomes from the parents. *Translocation* describes the situation in which a fragment of one chromosome becomes attached to the broken end of another. A *reciprocal* translocation involves two chromosomes in a mutual exchange of broken-off fragments. A *Robertsonian* translocation is a special category of reciprocal translocation involving two acrocentric chromosomes, in which breakage occurs close to the centromere in the short arm of one chromosome and in the long arm of the other. One of the resulting chromosomes is extremely small and is lost in subsequent mitotic divisions. An individual carrying a balanced reciprocal translocation in which essentially no genetic material has been lost will be phenotypically normal, but may have reproductive problems. Depending on the type of meiotic segregation the involved chromosomes undergo, the zygote may be (1) normal, (2) a balanced translocation carrier like the parent, (3) trisomic for part of a chromosome, or (4) monosomic for part of a chromosome. These last two conditions will almost always lead to spontaneous abortion.

Karyotypic examinations of couples with two or more spontaneous abortions reveal that 2.78 per cent (43/1544) are balanced reciprocal translocation carriers (Rott et al., 1972; de la Chapelle et al., 1973; Papp et al., 1974; Byrd et al., 1977; Khudr, 1974). This 5 per cent rate of "positive" results for a given couple can be increased by altering the indication for karyotyping. Byrd and associates (1977) found a 3.4 per cent incidence of translocation carriers among mothers and fathers with two or more spontaneous abortions, but a 13.6 per cent translocation rate in couples with a history of abortion plus fetal malformation.

The introduction of chromosome banding techniques has allowed recognition of smaller, more subtle translocations. Using these methods, a slightly higher incidence (4.76 per cent, or 4 of 84) of balanced translocation carriers is detected in couples with two spontaneous abortions. Some reports have quoted higher rates of "positive" results by including chromosomal variations such as pericentric inversions, large satellites on acrocentric chromosomes, and long Y chromosomes (Khudr, 1974; Rott et al., 1972). These are normal variants found in the general population and should not be implicated in recurrent abortions unless detailed population studies are done. In view of the preceding data on balanced translocation carriers, a chromosome study, including banding, is appropriate for a couple with three or more spontaneous abortions. It is reassuring if both the husband and wife have normal karyotypes, but this is not absolute proof that the abortions are not caused by chromosomal abnormalities inherited from the parents. Jagiello (1981) reported that testicular biopsy showed the male partner of a woman who had six spontaneous abortions to have abnormalities of meiosis, even though his blood karyotype was normal.

In considering patients with recurrent abortion, the question arises as to whether having one chromosomally abnormal spontaneous abortion increases the risk of a chromosome abnormality and, therefore, of abortion in the next pregnancy. When karyotypes of two consecutive abortuses are performed, there is a correlation between the normal or abnormal characters of the two specimens (Golbus, 1981). If the first abortus is chromosomally normal, then the second abortus has a 66 per cent chance of being chromosomally normal. If the first abortus is chromosomally abnormal, there is a 75 per cent chance that the second abortus is also chromosomally abnormal. This means that some couples who have recurrent chromosomally abnormal conceptions (almost all of which result in spontaneous abortions) present with a complaint of recurrent abortions. This condition has no treatment, but if it is diagnosed by karyotyping of successive abortuses and the woman then becomes pregnant, chorionic villus sampling or amniocentesis for prenatal diagnosis should be performed. Moreover, any treatment to prevent abortion will be futile, and inclusion of this group in evaluating the efficacy of a therapy will create a negative bias. Amniocentesis or chorionic villus sampling should also be offered if either parent is a translocation carrier (see also Chapter 2).

Anomalies of the Reproductive Tract

Midline fusion and canalization of the müllerian ducts are requisites for normal uterine and vaginal development. Failure of one of these processes, either total or partial, is thought to occur in one of every 700 women. The double uterus and its variants, reflecting failure of midline fusion or resorption of septa, have long been recognized as factors in pregnancy wastage. However, the association is not clear-cut. Many women with recognized anomalies of the uterus have successful pregnancies. In addition, there are many women with unrecognized anomalies who do not undergo medical scrutiny because they do not have problems referable to the abnormalities. Even those who have pregnancy wastage can at times achieve subsequent success without surgical intervention. Although malformations of the uterus can be consistent with satisfactory reproductive performance, it is also true that reproductive failure may be caused by uterine malformations. A hysterosalpingogram should be obtained if a woman has two or more consecutive abortions or has repeated premature births. A bicornuate uterus, a septate uterus, or a single uterine horn can contribute to early pregnancy wastage. Significant improvements in pregnancy salvage have been reported in uncontrolled series following use of the Strassman (1966) metroplasty and a variety of techniques for removal of a uterine septum, including resection by means of hysteroscopy. March and Israel (1987) reported that 87 per cent of pregnancies following hysteroscopic incision of septate uteri either resulted in a term birth or were beyond 20 weeks of gestation at the time of their report. One-half of the women had had three or more pregnancy losses, whereas the other half had had only one or two losses. The authors stress the need for laparoscopic monitoring of the hysteroscopic procedures.

It is important to emphasize the need for investigation of renal anomalies in all women found to have genital malformations. In the series reported by Jones (1957), 5.3 per cent of patients with genital anomalies also had abnormal renal structures. In the subgroup of patients with vaginal agenesis, the renal anomaly rate is close to 50 per cent (Capraro and Gallego, 1976); an equally high rate is seen with uteri derived from single müllerian ducts.

Both uterine myomas and intrauterine adhesions have been implicated in recurrent abortion (Siegler, 1967), myomas being found in 18 per cent of women with two or more abortions in one report (Robins, 1972). Whereas DES exposure in utero may increase the risk for spontaneous abortion, the long-term outlook is good.

Inadequate Luteal Phase

Inadequate luteal phase is due to a relatively deficient secretion of progesterone by the corpus luteum. The progesterone levels are insufficient to properly stimulate the endometrium. A related but rare condition is the absence of progesterone receptors in the endometrium. Approximately 3 to 4 per cent of infertile women are diagnosed as having an inadequate luteal phase. The incidence may be 25 to 30 per cent in women with recurrent abortion (Balasch et al., 1986).

An inadequate luteal phase also may be more common in women who have elevated levels of prolactin, those who are perimenopausal, and those taking clomiphene citrate. Whereas the hallmark is a deficient secretion of progesterone from the corpus luteum, the etiology in some cases may reside in abnormal follicle-stimulating hormone secretion in the follicular phase or abnormal gonadotropin-releasing hormone pulses.

The diagnosis of an inadequate luteal phase has been made on the basis of serum progesterone levels or by the histologic examination of tissue obtained by endometrial biopsy. Because of the pulsatile nature of progesterone secretion, a single value may not be representative even of the values for that day. Despite this reservation, a progesterone level of 15 ng/ml at the midpoint between the luteinizing hormone surge and the onset of menses is reassuring. Values below 10 ng/ml at the same time in the cycle are strongly suggestive of a luteal phase deficiency, with values between 10 and 15 ng/ml subject to varying interpretations. One can obtain correct timing for the progesterone assay by using urinary LH kits to determine the day of ovulation and measuring the progesterone level 6 to 7 days later. The endometrial biopsy can be painful, expensive, and subject to variation in interpretation by different observers. Moreover, an isolated biopsy showing evidence of an inadequate luteal phase (a lag of more than 2 days in endometrial development) is found in approximately 30 per cent of cycles. Only if it is found in two cycles is the diagnosis established (Murthy et al., 1970). Despite these drawbacks to the endometrial biopsy, it remains the classic method for diagnosing an inadequate luteal phase.

Two principal approaches have been taken in the investigation of the role of progesterone deficiency in recurrent abortion. The first, which has not proved useful, was implication of low pregnanediol levels in pregnancy as a cause for abortion and, as a corollary, treatment with exogenous progesterone or progestins. The second approach has been to diagnose the insufficient effect of progesterone on the endometrium during the luteal phase of the menstrual cycle (inadequate luteal phase) and to initiate treatment with exogenous hormone a few days after ovulation. Both approaches are described in detail.

Shearman and Garrett (1963), in a study of women with two or more consecutive abortions, found no increase in salvage rate when the 17-hydroxyprogestrone caproate was used in women whose pregnanediol levels were below normal or whose pregnanediol excretion rate decreased more than 2.5 ng/24 hr from one week to the next before the 12th week of pregnancy. A double-blind study of the effects of oral medroxyprogesterone acetate on pregnancy salvage using similar consecutive abortion criteria found no advantage of active drug over the placebo (Goldzieher, 1964). These last two studies indicated that recurrent aborters with low pregnanediol excretion rates have a spontaneous salvage rate approximating 80 per cent. In another report, dydrogesterone or a placebo was given to pregnant women who had ferning of the cervical mucus in early pregnancy, with no observed difference between the hormone and the placebo groups and an overall salvage rate of 85 per cent (MacDonald et al., 1972). An argument in favor of hormone treatment was advanced by Hensleigh and Fainstat (1979) who, in an uncontrolled study, used progesterone to treat 11 patients who presented in early pregnancy with cramping and/or vaginal bleeding and serum progesterone levels below 15 ng/ml. In nine of the 11, the response to treatment was elevated serum progesterone levels, and eight delivered at term. The ninth woman delivered an anencephalic infant at 30 weeks. Two patients continued to have progesterone levels below 15 ng/ml; one aborted and the other delivered at term. However, in a similar study, treatment of high-risk women with 17-hydroxyprogesterone caproate starting at 6 weeks of a viable pregnancy did not increase fetal survival (Reijnders et al., 1988).

Harrison (1985) reported that women with a history of three consecutive abortions had a higher salvage rate (10 of 10 births) when given injections of human chorionic gonadotropin than women given placebo injections (3 of 10 births). Treatment was initiated before the 8th week of gestation and after fetal heart activity was seen on ultrasonography. The low number of subjects limits the impact of this finding.

These studies on the use of hormonal agents were restricted to pregnancies that were well established. It is possible that those patients at greatest risk may lose pregnancies earlier. An argument has been advanced, therefore, that hormone deficiency, specifically progesterone deficiency (inadequate luteal phase), must be corrected prior to implantation to prevent recurrent abortion. Jones (1968) stated that of 120 women with pregnancy wastage, 34 (28 per cent) had inadequate luteal phases and, with treatment, 31 of 34 (91 per cent) had liveborn children. An endometrial biopsy was used to make the diagnosis of inadequate luteal phase. Treatment consists of progesterone via vaginal suppositories or daily intramuscular injection. Syn-

thetic progestins should not be used because of questions regarding teratogenicity and high doses may be luteocytic. Because hormone abnormalities in the follicular phase may be a cause for an inadequate luteal phase, clomiphene citrate has been used as an alternative to treatment with progesterone.

Despite the abundance of clinical information, there are, unfortunately, no well-controlled studies of treatment of the inadequate luteal phase that provide convincing information on pregnancy outcome. For that reason, the theory that inadequate luteal phase is a cause of recurrent abortion remains unproven. However, in clinical practice the combination of recurrent pregnancy loss and a diagnosis of an inadequate luteal phase warrants the use of progesterone vaginal suppositories (25 or 50 mg twice a day) starting 2 to 3 days postovulation and continuing until menses. Progesterone is also available by injection or by micronized pills. The woman should be warned that the period may be delayed a few days by use of progesterone. If pregnancy occurs, the medication is continued until 8 weeks of gestation, at which time there should be ample progesterone production by the placenta. Another therapy is the use of clomiphene citrate, 50 mg daily for 5 days starting between days 3 and 5 of the menstrual cycle. With either therapy, a biopsy should be repeated during a treatment cycle to confirm therapeutic efficacy of the medications. Biopsy provides only a very slight risk of precipitating abortion even if it is done in a pregnancy cycle.

Immunologic Factors

The fetus contains paternal antigens that are foreign to the mother, and classic immunologic theory would suggest that the fetus should be rejected much as a skin graft from a donor is rejected. However, circumstances exist in which there is a positive effect for the target of an immunologic reaction. Thus, immunologic diversity may be beneficial. For example, breeding of genetically dissimilar mice results in higher fetal weights compared with those of fetuses derived from mating of inbred strains.

Conversely, a number of studies have implicated genetic similarity (increased sharing of human leukocyte antigens [HLA]) as a cause of recurrent abortion (Beer et al., 1983; McIntyre et al., 1984). A theory has been advanced that, because of this sharing, the woman's immunologic system does not receive the usual stimulation by paternal antigens carried by the fetus. Without this stimulation, blocking antibodies that could cover the antigenic sites on the trophoblast or interfere with immune cell function are not produced, and the trophoblast is vulnerable to either damaging antibodies or maternal immune cells (Rocklin et al., 1976). However, not all studies have found increased sharing of HLA to be more prevalent in recurrent aborters, and indeed not all women with successful pregnancies have blocking antibodies.

Despite this ambiguity, women with recurrent abortion have been transfused or injected subcutaneously with white blood cells obtained either from their partners or from third parties to stimulate production of antibodies. In a controlled trial, Mowbray et al. (1985) compared this treatment to the injection of the woman's own white blood cells. The experimental group had 22 women, of whom 17 had live births after injection of the husband's cells. In comparison, the 27 women treated with their own cells had 10 live births. This difference is statistically significant. More recent studies have been unable to confirm an advantage for allogeneic leukocyte immunization (Cauchi et al., 1991). A recent Workshop on Unification of Immunotherapy Protocols (Coulam, 1991) concluded that proof of efficacious treatment for recurrent spontaneous abortion does not exist and that immunotherapy should be performed only at centers that are undertaking studies of the process. An attempt to initiate a multi-center study with a standardized protocol to conclusively evaluate immunotherapy failed when only one center showed an interest in participating. Transfusion of foreign leukocytes is not without hazards, including the risk of hepatitis and AIDS. A few pregnancies, subsequent to the injections of paternal white cells, have been complicated by intrauterine growth restriction and preeclampsia.

McIntyre et al. (1984) divide recurrent aborters into primary (no children) or secondary (children or still-birth) and suggest different causes for the abortions in each group. They claim that primary aborters lack a blocking antibody to an antigen that is shared by both trophoblast and lymphocytes and is located in proximity to the HLA locus. These patients benefit from paternal leukocyte transfusions. The secondary aborters, who have an immunologic cause for pregnancy loss, have an abnormal antibody response to trophoblast; McIntyre et al. (1984) found that the latter group does not benefit from transfusions. However, Mowbray et al. (1985) found no difference in the response between primary and secondary aborters.

We recommend caution until further controlled studies are available to provide guidance for the usefulness of white blood cell transfusions in the treatment of recurrent abortion. The limited hazards of the treatment must be clearly understood by physicians and patients. Currently, treatment should be offered only as part of well-controlled research studies approved by institutional human experimentation committees. The reader is referred to Chapters 6 and 31 for a more detailed discussion of the sharing of leukocyte antigens as a cause of recurrent abortion.

Systemic Lupus Erythematosus

Systemic lupus erythematosus (SLE) commonly has been implicated as a causal factor in abortion, but the clinical data are not convincing (del Junco, 1986). Despite the ambiguity, a number of mechanisms for SLE-induced abortions have been suggested. One involves transplacental passage of antinuclear antibodies (ANA) including anti-Ro/SSA. The latter also has been incriminated as a cause of congenital complete heart block. Cowchock et al. (1984) found ANA in four of 14 (28 per cent) women who had unexplained recurrent abortion, whereas the antibody was present in only one of six women who had repetitive abortions

that could be ascribed to a specific cause. None of the women in these groups had clinical SLE. Harger et al. (1989) used a titer cut-off of 1:80 and found a positive result in 6.9 per cent of women with recurrent abortion compared to less than 1 per cent in controls. However, pregnancy outcomes in women with titers of 1:80 or higher and a history of three or more pregnancy losses did not differ significantly from that of controls. Thus routine testing for ANA in women with recurrent abortion is of questionable value.

Recent attention has focused on the role of antibodies to phospholipids (lupus anticoagulant, anticardiolipin) in pregnancy loss (Lubbe et al., 1984; Unander et al., 1987). These antibodies could cause damage by reacting against phospholipids on platelet cell membranes and vascular endothelial cells. Despite its name, lupus anticoagulant can be found in the absence of SLE. Whereas *in vitro* it is associated with elevated activated partial thromboplastin times, *in vivo* it is associated with thrombosis. Although lupus anticoagulant and anticardiolipin antibodies have been implicated mostly in mid- and third-trimester pregnancy loss, they also can be found in association with early pregnancy loss. Treatment with prednisone, aspirin, heparin, or immunoglobulins can lead to successful pregnancies, although these are often complicated by growth retardation and preeclampsia. The role of antiphospholipid antibodies in abnormal reproduction is discussed in detail in Chapter 31.

Diabetes Mellitus and Other Diseases

It is almost a reflex for the physician to order a glucose tolerance test when faced with the problem of recurrent abortion. Despite an occasional case report (Pedowitz and Shlevin, 1957), however, there seems to be no conclusive evidence that unsuspected diabetes or even overt diabetes that is adequately controlled is a cause of recurrent abortion (Kalter, 1987). For that reason, the authors see no value in the routine ordering of a glucose tolerance test. Similarly, syphilis has not been implicated in recurrent first-trimester abortion, and a serologic study need not be routine in the diagnosis of this problem. Bacteriuria is often sought, but its connection with abortion has not been established.

Infection

Toxoplasma gondii can invade the placenta and be transmitted to the fetus. Although some authors have implicated this parasite as a cause of recurrent abortion, most work suggests that it is not a significant factor. Kimball and associates (1971) found the dye test for Toxoplasma antibodies to be positive in 31.0 per cent of women with no history of abortion, in 38.5 per cent of women with sporadic abortion, and in 32.9 per cent of women with recurrent abortion.

Listeria monocytogenes can cause abortion in animals. However, in one study of abortions in 554 women (including 74 with recurrent abortion), there was no bacteriologic or serologic evidence of Listeria infection (Rabau and David, 1963).

Herpesvirus infection in the first 20 weeks of pregnancy was found to be associated with a 34 per cent abortion rate, compared with a 10.6 per cent abortion rate in the controls (Nahmias et al., 1971). The role of this virus, if any, in recurrent abortion has not been established.

Approximately 3 per cent of pregnant women shed cytomegaloviruses. These agents can cause a variety of congenital anomalies, but it is not known whether they cause recurrent abortion.

Chlamydia trachomatis is one of the most common sexually transmitted pathogens, and there is evidence that implicates the organism in salpingitis. Studies have shown that Chlamydia can also infect the mouse trophoblast *in vitro* (Banks et al., 1982). However, there is only an isolated report indicating that Chlamydia can be cultured from human abortuses (Schachter, 1967). One of the strains of Chlamydia cultured from human abortuses has been shown to cause abortion in cattle (Page and Smith, 1974), but Chlamydia is so commonly found in the cervix that it is doubtful whether the culture of this organism from the cervix of women with recurrent abortion will prove useful in providing evidence of an etiologic role for this organism. It has been suggested that antichlamydial antibodies are more common in women with recurrent abortion, but further evidence is needed.

Mycoplasma is commonly found in the vagina and cervix. Caspi and co-workers (1972) cultured mycoplasma from the products of conception of 31 per cent of spontaneous abortions, but only 5 per cent of specimens from therapeutic abortions were culture-positive. Stray-Pedersen and colleagues (1978) have reported significantly higher colonization of the endometrium with T mycoplasma in women with a history of recurrent abortion than in normal fertile women. This finding could be interpreted as implicating mycoplasma as a cause of abortion. An alternative explanation is that women who have had abortions have undergone repeated instrumentation of the uterus, which could transfer mycoplasma from the cervix into the uterus. Moreover, Harger et al. (1983) reported that 13 of 19 women (68 per cent) successfully treated for *Ureaplasma urealyticum* had successful pregnancies, but that six of seven women who were treatment failures also had normal pregnancies. At this time the relationship of mycoplasma to recurrent abortion remains to be determined; because mycoplasma is so commonly found in the vagina and cervix, it may be difficult to prove a causal relationship.

Psychological Factors

The effect of psychological treatment of recurrent abortion was reported by Tupper and Weil (1962) and by James (1963a). The study group consisted of 38 women (24 of whom had borne children) who had had three consecutive abortions and were again pregnant. Treatment consisted largely of a weekly interview with a psychiatrist and access to the psychiatrist by telephone at other times. In addition, sexual rela-tions were prohibited during the first 3 to 4 months of pregnancy, although no rationale for the proscription was given. There were also rare prescriptions of small doses of pentobarbital or meprobamate. Hormones were never given. Nineteen of the women received only an initial evaluation and then returned, because of geographic or other unspecified conditions, to their own family physicians for prenatal care. Of the women in this group, 13 had spontaneous abortions, compared with only two of 19 in the group receiving psychotherapy (a statistically significant difference). The two groups seemed comparable in terms of number of previous abortions, age, education, length of marriage, and occupation. Similarly, Stray-Pedersen and Stray-Pedersen (1984) found that counseling and psychological support for women with a history of unexplained recurrent abortion was associated with a successful pregnancy rate of 86 per cent, whereas women who had no such care had only a 33 per cent successful pregnancy rate.

Male Factor

Sperm are filtered at the level of the cervix, which provides a barrier to the entry of morphologically abnormal sperm into the uterus. Therefore, the evaluation of sperm in cases of recurrent abortion, from the standpoint of shape and form, would seem to be an unproductive procedure. It has been suggested, however, that recurrent abortion may be secondary to a decreased DNA content of sperm, although this concept has received little support (Joel, 1966). Recurrent abortion also may be associated with very high sperm counts (Joel, 1966; MacLeod and Gold, 1957). In summary, the role, if any, of the male in recurrent abortion is at present unknown.

Miscellaneous Factors

Both cigarette smoking and alcohol ingestion have been implicated as factors in spontaneous abortion (Kline et al., 1980). There is a higher rate of abortion in women who smoke a half pack a day than in nonsmokers. In addition, there is a statistically significant higher number of heavy smokers (14 to 80 cigarettes each day) among women with euploid abortions compared with controls.

In the same study, 17 per cent of women who aborted reported drinking two times per week, whereas only 8.1 per cent of women whose pregnancies went beyond 28 weeks reported similar alcohol intake. The data suggest that a mean of one ounce of absolute alcohol twice a week is the minimum threshold dose for increasing the risk of an abortion.

The association of maternal age with the incidence of trisomy is well known. There is also an increase in euploid spontaneous abortions in association with increasing maternal age, the increase in risk being notable at age 36.

Ecker and co-workers (1992) have described a factor, possibly gamma interferon, in the sera of women with unexplained recurrent abortion. The presence of this factor in early pregnancy is associated with a high risk of subsequent abortion. The authors suggest that postovulatory use of progesterone for its immune suppressive effect may be of value.

DIAGNOSTIC PROTOCOL

Given the many uncertainties raised in this chapter, what is a rational approach to the investigation of spontaneous abortion? If a woman has had only one abortion, reassurance is in order, with some discussion of the protective effects of abortion against the birth of chromosomally abnormal children. Improvement of general health by eliminating tobacco or alcohol may be helpful. After two consecutive abortions, most couples want some investigation of the problem. Currently, only chromosomal abnormalities and uterine malformations can be definitely implicated in the etiology of recurrent abortion. It would be reasonable to obtain a hysterogram in a woman who has two consecutive abortions. Because of the expense and the probability that there is at least a 60 per cent rate of spontaneous cure after two abortions, we usually obtain karyotypes only after a couple has had three or more consecutive abortions. Karyotypes are also done if, in addition to one or two abortions, the couple has had a child or fetus with congenital malformations. Moreover, if at any time karyotypic analysis of a fetus or abortus shows it to have a translocation, parental karyotypes should be obtained. If either parent has a translocation, chorionic villus sampling or amniocentesis should be offered in every subsequent pregnancy. There is some indication that future pregnancies of a woman who has a trisomic abortus are at increased risk of also being trisomic and she should be offered prenatal diagnosis (Jacobs, 1977).

Most physicians would feel uncomfortable with such a minimal investigation. Further studies may be justified by the realization that information is not available to prove or to disprove other factors as causes of recurrent abortion. Therefore, it is reasonable to perform serum progesterone determinations or endometrial biopsies, as well as tests for lupus anticoagulant and anticardiolipin antibodies.

The case for treating couples who have recurrent abortion and positive cultures for Ureaplasma is not proved. Despite this lack of proof, the authors have elected to treat couples with positive cultures for Ureaplasma with doxycycline, 100 mg daily for the first 10 days of each menstrual cycle, until negative cultures are obtained. Treatment early in the cycle minimizes the risk of exposing a fetus to the antibiotic.

Immunologic studies are available only in limited areas. Further controlled studies are needed to prove the value of white blood cell injections to stimulate the maternal immune system.

Finally, psychological support in the form of frequent visits, sympathetic counseling, and ready access to the physician should be part of the care of every couple with recurrent abortion.

REFERENCES

Balasch J, Creus M, Márquez M, et al: The significance of luteal phase deficiency on fertility: A diagnostic and therapeutic approach. Hum Reprod **1**:145, 1986.

Banks J, Glass RH, Spindle A, et al: *Chlamydia trachomatis* infection of mouse trophoblast. Infect Immunol **38**:368, 1982.

Beer AE, Quebbeman JF, Semprini AE, et al: Recurrent abortion: Analysis of the roles of parental sharing of histocompatibility antigens and maternal immunological responses to paternal antigens. *In* Isojima S, Billington WE (eds): Reproduction and Immunology. Amsterdam, Elsevier, 1983.

Boue J, Boue A, Lazar P: Retrospective and prospective epidemiological studies of 1500 karyotyped spontaneous human abortions. Teratology **12**:11, 1975.

Byrd JR, Askew DE, McDonough PG: Cytogenetic findings in fifty-five couples with recurrent fetal wastage. Fertil Steril **28**:246, 1977.

Capraro VJ, Gallego MB: Vaginal agenesis. Am J Obstet Gynecol **124**:98, 1976.

Caspi E, Solomon F, Sompolinsky D: Early abortion and mycoplasma infection. Isr J Med Sci **8**:123, 1972.

Cauchi MN, Lim D, Young DE, et al: Treatment of recurrent aborters by immunization with paternal cells—controlled trial. Am J Reprod Immunol **25**:16, 1991.

Coulam CB: Workshop A: Unification of immunotherapy protocols. Am J Reprod Immunol **25**:1, 1991.

Cowchock S, Dehoratius RD, Wapner RJ, et al: Subclinical autoimmune disease and unexplained abortion. Am J Obstet Gynecol **150**:367, 1984.

de la Chapelle A, Schroder J, Kokkonen J: Cytogenetics of recurrent abortion or unsuccessful pregnancy. Int J Fertil **18**:215, 1973.

del Junco DJ: Association of autoimmune conditions with recurrent intrauterine death. Clin Obstet Gynecol **29**:959, 1986.

Eastman NJ: Habitual abortion. *In* Meigs JV, Sturgis S (eds): Progress in Gynecology. Vol I. New York, Grune & Stratton, 1946.

Ecker J, Laufer M, Hill JA: Measurement of embryotoxic factors is predictive of pregnancy outcome in women with a history of recurrent abortions. The Pacific Coast Fertility Society 40th Annual Meeting, Indian Wells, California, April 8–12, 1992, Abst 0–011.

Golbus MJ: Chromosome aberrations and mammalian reproduction. *In* Mastroianni L, Biggers J, Sadler W (eds): Fertilization and Embryonic Development *in Vitro*. New York, Plenum Press, 1981.

Goldzieher JW: Double blind trial for a progestin in habitual abortion. JAMA **188**:651, 1964.

Harger JH, Archer DF, Marchese SG, et al: Etiology of recurrent pregnancy losses and outcome of subsequent pregnancies. Obstet Gynecol **62**:575, 1983.

Harger, JH, Rabin BS, Marchese SG: The prognostic value of antinuclear antibodies in women with recurrent pregnancy losses: A prospective controlled study. Obstet Gynecol **73**:419, 1989.

Harrison RF: Treatment of habitual abortion with human chorionic gonadotropin: Results of open and placebo-controlled studies. Eur J Obstet Reprod Biol **20**:159, 1985.

Heap RB, Flint AP, Gadsby JE: Embryonic signals that establish pregnancy. Br Med Bull **35**:129, 1979.

Hensleigh PA, Fainstat T: Corpus luteum dysfunction: Serum progesterone levels in diagnosis and assessment of therapy for recurrent and threatened abortion. Fertil Steril **32**:396, 1979.

Hertig AT, Rock J, Adams EC, et al: Thirty-four fertilized ova, good, bad and indifferent from 210 women of known fertility. Pediatrics **23**:202, 1959.

Jacobs PA: Epidemiology of chromosome abnormalities in man. Am J Epidemiol **105**:180, 1977.

Jagiello G: Pinpointing male reproductive dysfunction. Contemp Ob/Gyn **17**:65, 1981.

James WH: The problem of spontaneous abortion. X. The efficacy of psychotherapy. Am J Obstet Gynecol **85**:38, 1963a.

James WH: Notes toward an epidemiology of spontaneous abortion. Am J Hum Genet **15**:223, 1963b.

Joel CA: New etiologic aspects of habitual abortion and infertility with special reference to the male factor. Fertil Steril **17**:374, 1966.

Jones G: Luteal phase defects. *In* Behrman SJ, Kistner RW (eds): Progress in Infertility. Boston, Little, Brown, 1968.

Jones WS: Obstetric significance of female genital anomalies. Obstet Gynecol **10**:113, 1957.

Kalter H: Diabetes and spontaneous abortion: A historical review. Am J Obstet Gynecol **156**:1243, 1987.

Khudr G: Cytogenetics of habitual abortion. Obstet Gynecol Surv **29**:299, 1974.

Kimball AC, Kean BH, Fuchs F: The role of toxoplasmosis in abortion. Am J Obstet Gynecol **111**:219, 1971.

Kline J, Stein Z, Susser M, et al: Environmental influences on early reproductive loss in a current New York City study. *In* Porter IH, Hook EB (eds): Human Embryonic and Fetal Death. New York, Academic Press, 1980.

Krzanowska H: The passage of abnormal spermatozoa through the uterotubal junction of the mouse. J Reprod Fertil 38:81, 1974.

Leridon H: Human Fertility: The Basic Components. Chicago, University of Chicago Press, 1977.

Lubbe WF, Butler WS, Palmer SJ, et al: Lupus anticoagulant in pregnancy. Br J Obstet Gynaecol 91:357, 1984.

MacDonald RR, Goulden R, Oakey RE: Cervical mucus, vaginal cytology and steroid excretion in recurrent abortion. Obstet Gynecol 40:394, 1972.

MacLeod J, Gold RZ: The male factor in fertility and sterility. Fertil Steril 8:36, 1957.

MacNaughton MC: The probability of recurrent abortion. J Obstet Gynaecol Br Commonw 71:784, 1964.

Malpas P: A study of abortion sequences. J Obstet Gynaecol Br Emp 45:932, 1938.

March CM, Israel R: Hysteroscopic management of recurrent abortions caused by septate uterus. Am J Obstet Gynecol 156:834, 1987.

McIntyre JA, McConnachie PR, Taylor CG, et al: Clinical immunologic and genetic definitions of primary and secondary recurrent spontaneous abortions. Fertil Steril 42:849, 1984.

Miller JF, Williamson E, Glue J, et al: Fetal loss after implantation. Lancet 2:554, 1980.

Mowbray JF, Liddell H, Underwood JL, et al: Controlled trial of treatment of recurrent spontaneous abortion by immunisation with paternal cells. Lancet 1:941, 1985.

Murthy YS, Arronet GH, Parekh MC: Luteal phase inadequacy. Obstet Gynecol 36:758, 1970.

Nahmias AJ, Josey WE, Naib ZM, et al: Perinatal risk associated with maternal genital herpes simplex virus infection. Am J Obstet Gynecol 110:825, 1971.

Page LA, Smith PC: Placentitis and abortion in cattle inoculated with chlamydiae isolated from aborted human placental tissue. Proc Soc Exp Biol Med 146:264, 1974.

Papp Z, Gardo S, Dolhay B: Chromosome study of couples with repeated spontaneous abortions. Fertil Steril 25:713, 1974.

Pedowitz P, Shlevin EL: Perinatal mortality in the unsuspected diabetic. Obstet Gynecol 9:524, 1957.

Poland BJ, Miller JR, Jones DC, et al: Reproductive counseling in patients who have had a spontaneous abortion. Am J Obstet Gynecol 127:685, 1977.

Rabau E, David A: *Listeria monocytogenes* in abortion. J Obstet Gynaecol Br Commonw 70:481, 1963.

Reijnders FJL, Thomas CMG, Doesburg WH, et al: Endocrine effects of 17α-hydroxyprogesterone caproate during early pregnancy: A double blind clinical trial. Br J Obstet Gynaecol 95:462, 1988.

Robins SA: Uterotubography. *In* Robbins LL (ed): Golden's Diagnostic Roentgenology. Vol 4. Baltimore, Williams & Wilkins Co, 1972.

Rocklin RE, Kitzmiller JL, Carpenter CB, et al: Maternal fetal relation. N Engl J Med 295:1209, 1976.

Rott HD, Richter E, Rummel WD, et al: Chromosomenbefunde bei ehepaaren mit gehauften aborten. Arch Gynaekol 213:110, 1972.

Schachter J: Isolation of Bedsoniae from human arthritis and abortion tissues. Am J Ophthalmol 63(Suppl):1082, 1967.

Shearman RP, Garrett WJ: Double blind study of effect of 17-hydroxyprogesterone caproate on abortion rate. Br Med J 1:292, 1963.

Siegler AM: Hysterosalpingography. New York, Hoeber, 1967.

Strassman EO: Fertility and unification of double uterus. Fertil Steril 17:165, 1966.

Stray-Pedersen B, Eng J, Reikvam TM: Uterine T-mycoplasma colonization in reproductive failure. Am J Obstet Gynecol 130:307, 1978.

Stray-Pedersen B, Stray-Pedersen S: Etiologic factors and subsequent reproductive performance in 195 couples with a prior history of habitual abortion. Am J Obstet Gynecol 148:140, 1984.

Tupper C, Weil RJ: The problem of spontaneous abortion. IX. The treatment of habitual aborters by psychotherapy. Am J Obstet Gynecol 83:421, 1962.

Unander AM, Norberg R, Hahn L, et al: Anticardiolipin antibodies and complement in ninety-nine women with habitual abortion. Am J Obstet Gynecol 156:114, 1987.

Vlaanderen W, Treffers PE: Prognosis of subsequent pregnancies after recurrent spontaneous abortion in first trimester. Br Med J 295:92, 1987.

Warburton D, Fraser FC: Spontaneous abortion risks in man: Data from reproductive histories collected in a medical genetics unit. Am J Hum Genet 16:1, 1964.

Wudl LR, Sherman MI, Hillman N: Nature of lethality of t mutations in embryos. Nature 270:137, 1977.

C H A P T E R

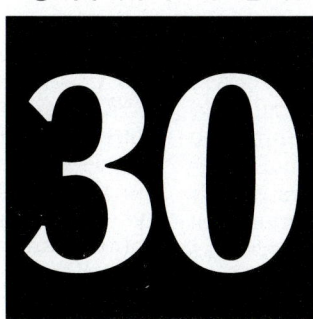

30

CERVICAL INCOMPETENCE

VALERIE M. PARISI, M.D., M.P.H.

HISTORICAL PERSPECTIVES

Although the term *cervical incompetence* was first popularized in the 1940s and 1950s to describe recurrent mid-trimester pregnancy loss heralded by painless dilatation of the cervix, recognition of this clinical entity dates back to the 17th century. In the *Practice of Physick*, written in 1658, Cole and Culpepper describe cervical incompetence and its possible etiologies:

. . . the second fault in women which hindered conception is when the seed is not retained or the orifice of the womb is so slack that it cannot rightly contract itself to keep in the seed; which is chiefly caused by abortion, or hard labor and childbirth, whereby the fibers of the womb are broken in pieces one from another and they, and the inner orifice of the womb, overmuch slackened.

Initial use of the term cervical incompetence has been attributed to Gream in an 1865 issue of the Lancet. The early 1900s saw the advent of operative procedures on the cervix for the prevention of recurrent pregnancy loss. Herman (1902) performed the Emmet trachelorrhaphy on three women with recurrent pregnancy loss, two of whom later had successful pregnancies. Child (1922) described an operative procedure to restore functional integrity of the internal cervical os.

In the 1940s, both Palmer and LaComme (1948) and Lash and Lash (1950) reported surgical operations to repair anatomic defects in the nonpregnant cervix. Shirodkar (1955) and McDonald (1957) introduced methods of transvaginal cervicoisthmic cerclage that remain the most commonly used procedures for the treatment of cervical incompetence. Benson and Durfee (1965) advocated a transabdominal approach for the placement of a cerclage in those few patients in whom the transvaginal approach had failed, or in whom cervical scarring or congenital abnormality was so severe as to make the transvaginal approach technically impossible. Various minor modifications of these procedures have been added over the last three decades with respect to choice of suture material and perioperative adjunctive antimicrobial and tocolytic therapy, but the basic techniques of cervical cerclage have remained unchanged.

Crucial to the management of patients with incompetent cervix is the accuracy of diagnosis. This disorder has remained largely a diagnosis of exclusion, as there is no single pathognomonic clinical or laboratory feature. It is therefore extremely important that an exhaustive search be made for other common causes of recurrent pregnancy loss before operative therapy for cervical incompetence is undertaken (Table 30–1). Recent advances in diagnostic modalities such as hysteroscopy, ultrasonography, and the prediction and early diagnosis of preterm labor by risk assessment and home uterine activity monitoring have added considerably to our ability to distinguish women with cervical incompetence from those with other causes of recurrent pregnancy loss.

ANATOMIC CONSIDERATIONS

The uterine cervix and corpus are derived from fusion of the distal müllerian ducts and subsequent central atrophy (Crosby and Hill, 1962). The cervix consists primarily of fibrous tissue with only 10 to 15 per cent smooth muscle (Danforth, 1947). The cervicoisthmic histologic transition from fibrous to muscular tissue varies from a narrow 1- to 2-mm zone to a relatively wide 5- to 10-mm zone (Danforth, 1947), while the proportion of cervical smooth muscle varies from 29 per cent in the upper third to 6.4 per cent in the lower third (Rorie and Newton, 1967). During pregnancy, the muscular uterine isthmus distends and

TABLE 30–1. Etiologies of Second-Trimester Pregnancy Loss

1. Chromosomal abnormalities
2. Uterine factors
   a. Congenital anomalies
   b. Intrauterine synechiae
   c. Leiomyomata
3. Immunologic factors
4. Infectious factors
   a. Cervicitis (cervical and lower genital tract infection)
   b. Systemic infection
5. Idiopathic preterm labor
6. Incompetent cervix

elongates between the 12th and 20th weeks of gestation, making its inferior border with the fibrous cervix the functional internal os. It is this anatomic and histologic junction that is responsible for retaining the products of conception *in utero* during normal pregnancy. It would seem that primary disorders of this sphincteric mechanism could result from abnormalities in both the muscular isthmus and the upper cervix as well as derangement of the cervical fibrous tissue, resulting in decreased cervical resistance.

Cervical biopsies obtained just before and after parturition by Danforth et al. (1960) revealed fewer crosslinks and greater dissociation and disorganization of the collagen bundles. Additionally, during normal pregnancy at term, an increased proportion of soluble collagen fragments was demonstrated in the cervix (Kleissl et al., 1978; von Maillot and Zimmermann, 1976). Decreased amounts of hydroxyproline, a major component of mature collagen, were also found. This suggests that cervical effacement may indeed reflect a true change in the biochemical and, subsequently, the biophysical structure of cervical connective tissue at term.

The role of elastin in the function of the cervicoisthmic sphincter is still under question. In the 1960s, Danforth et al. (1960) and Pinto et al. (1965) reported finding relatively few fibers of elastin in the cervical stroma and subsequently believed them to be of little or no clinical significance. More recently, however, Leppert et al. (1982) assayed the amino acids desmosine and isodesmosine in cervical tissue obtained from pregnant women and monkeys. These amino acids are found only in elastin and comprise 1.54 to 1.57 per cent of the cervical tissue studied, an amount thought to be clinically significant by this group of investigators. This group also reported (1987) that women with incompetent cervix had a decrease in cervical elastic fibers compared to normal pregnant and nonpregnant women. These differences were based on both light microscopy and biochemical findings.

Structural changes in the cervix have also been attributed to estrogen and progesterone administration (Asplund, 1952) and have been postulated to occur in multiple gestations with an increased production of relaxin from the corpus luteum (Haning et al., 1985).

ETIOLOGIC FACTORS

Although undocumented by experimental evidence, the currently accepted etiology of cervical incompetence is classified into three major categories: congenital factors, spontaneous or iatrogenic cervical trauma, and hormonal influences.

Congenital Factors

In utero exposure to diethylstilbestrol (DES) is the most commonly mentioned of these factors. The National Institutes of Health estimates that up to 6 million people may have been exposed to diethylstilbestrol *in utero* before the Food and Drug Administration banned its use for recurrent pregnancy loss (Robboy et al., 1983). In the late 1970s, reports of poor pregnancy outcome and structural genital tract abnormalities in those women exposed to DES *in utero* began to appear in the literature (Kaufman et al. 1977, 1980; Cousins et al., 1980b; Mangan et al., 1982; Stillman, 1982). Singer and Hochman (1978), Goldstein (1978), and Ben-Baruch et al. (1981) specifically reported cervical incompetence attributed to DES exposure, while Nunley and Kitchin (1979) reported successful treatment of DES-related incompetent cervix by cervical cerclage.

Both upper and lower genital tract structural abnormalities have been reported to occur with a frequency of 33 to 66 per cent in women exposed to DES *in utero* (Kaufman and Adam, 1978; Sandberg, 1976). Readily visible cervicovaginal structural abnormalities are present in approximately one-quarter to one-half of these women (Scully et al., 1978; Herbst and Cole, 1978). Upper genital tract abnormalities documented by hysterosalpingography and hysteroscopy include the well-described T-shaped uterus, various other abnormalities of uterine cavity shape, intrauterine defects such as synechiae and diverticula, and structural alterations of the fallopian tube (Kaufman et al., 1984). Cervical changes such as growth resembling collars, hoods, septa, and cockscombs, and abnormal mucus and incompetence have been reported with DES exposure (Stillman, 1982).

It is well established that DES-exposed women have an increased incidence of preterm labor and delivery as well as an increased perinatal mortality rate when compared with controls (Cousins, 1980a). Within this population, it seems to be the group of DES-exposed women with gross cervicovaginal abnormalities that accounts for the poor reproductive outcomes (Berger and Goldstein, 1980; Sandberg et al., 1981; Cousins, 1984). More recently, however, Ludmir and associates (1987) have reported that of 36 DES-exposed women with normal cervicovaginal anatomy and no prior pregnancy losses, 16 (44 per cent) required emergency cerclage. Of the remaining 20 women who did not require cerclage, five (25 per cent) delivered prior to 30 weeks compared with one of 16 in the emergency cerclage group. There were five perinatal deaths (5 per cent), with an average gestational age of 24 weeks in the no-cerclage group as compared with none in the emergency cerclage group. Ludmir concluded that normal cervicovaginal anatomy in the DES-exposed woman does not accurately rule out the development of incompetent cervix and subsequent perinatal loss.

Spontaneously occurring congenital structural uterine abnormalities have also been associated with an increased incidence of reproductive loss that is usually attributed to both incompetent cervix and preterm labor (Heinonen et al., 1982; Rock and Murphy, 1986). It is difficult, however, to distinguish true structural cervical incompetence from progressive cervical effacement and dilatation secondary to increased uterine activity. It is entirely possible that these are not distinct entities but rather opposite ends of a spectrum.

Cervical Trauma

Cervical incompetence attributed to trauma may be iatrogenically induced during obstetric or gynecologic operative procedures or may be the result of a spontaneous obstetric laceration caused by precipitous labor. Overzealous mechanical dilatation of the cervix prior to curettage for either diagnosis or therapeutic termination of pregnancy has been blamed for cervical incompetence and subsequent pregnancy loss (Hulka and Higgins, 1961; Johnstone et al., 1976), as has cervical conization performed for the diagnosis and treatment of intraepithelial neoplasia (Jones et al., 1979). Information suggests that first-trimester termination of pregnancy is no longer a risk factor for cervical incompetence if performed after 1973 by an experienced operator with the use of laminaria (Schuly et al., 1983). Similarly, a review of the literature on pregnancy outcome after cervical conization indicates a minimal role for this procedure in the etiology of cervical incompetence, the major risk factor being the extent of the cone biopsy (Harger et al., 1983; Novy, 1985).

Hormonal Factors

Serum relaxin levels in multiple gestations resulting from menotropin treatment are 2.6 times normal (Haning et al., 1985). It is postulated that hyperrelaxinemia might be a factor in premature births associated with multiple gestations after menotropin treatment and that hyperrelaxinemia may also be an endocrine-determined cause of cervical incompetence. The clinical utility of serum relaxin levels as predictors of cervical incompetence in these pregnancies remains to be determined by further investigation. The relative overdistention caused by multiple gestations and polyhydramnios may also affect the competence of the cervicoisthmic junction and play a role in the increased incidence of second-trimester pregnancy loss in these patients. It is not yet clear whether these circumstances warrant a diagnosis of true cervical incompetence or preterm labor. Cervical cerclage in multiple gestations does not improve outcome (Dor et al., 1982; Weekes et al., 1977).

DIAGNOSIS

Unfortunately, despite the exponential growth of medical diagnostic technology in recent years, there remains no *specific* test or criterion for the accurate diagnosis of cervical incompetence. Perhaps true cervical incompetence is not a specific anatomic entity but rather a functional one with multifactorial causes that make definitive diagnosis difficult. A history of second-trimester pregnancy loss has long been regarded as the cornerstone in the diagnosis of cervical incompetence. However, as Harger (1983) points out in his comprehensive review of cervical cerclage, "Regardless of the cause of the pregnancy loss, the cervix always dilates before the conceptus emerges from the uterus. Cervical dilatation is, then, merely a final common pathway for many causes of pregnancy loss." It is imperative, therefore, that before the diagnosis of cervical incompetence is made in the woman with a history of second-trimester pregnancy loss, or in the

nulliparous woman with significant risk factors, an exhaustive search be made for other possible causes. Investigation of uterine activity, whether idiopathic or secondary to other factors such as infection, should be high on this list. It is not unreasonable to assume that the cause for recurrent pregnancy loss may be found and appropriately treated, thereby obviating surgical intervention and cerclage placement.

A variety of methods for the diagnosis of cervical incompetence have been developed over the years and can be classified by their application in the pregnant or nonpregnant state. First is the carefully taken history of rapid, relatively painless cervical effacement and dilatation resulting in second-trimester pregnancy loss, usually with the delivery of a live fetus, and sometimes a completely intact gestational sac. These women may complain of increasing vaginal discharge, spotting, and/or a feeling of pelvic pressure, menstrual-like cramping, or "heaviness." Some uterine activity may be present but is usually less intense than what would be expected to result in delivery. The nulliparous patient who is at risk for mid-trimester pregnancy loss also needs careful symptomatic evaluation.

Several techniques for the diagnosis of cervical incompetence have been suggested for use in the nonpregnant woman: passage of a No. 8 Hegar dilator with ease through the internal cervical os (Lash and Lash, 1950; Jennings, 1972), the traction test measuring the pressure necessary to pull a Foley catheter inflated with 1 ml of water through the internal cervical os (Bergman and Svennerud, 1957; Peterson and Keifer, 1973), abnormal cervical canal and isthmic funnel angle by hysterogram (Lash and Lash, 1950; Lash, 1960), and a two-stage uterine balloon to detect differential pressure gradients (Mann et al., 1961). It must be remembered, however, that despite the changing hormonal influences of the menstrual cycle, neither cervical anatomy nor cervical function is the same in the pregnant state as in the nonpregnant state. This observation reduces the value of these tests to being suggestive rather than diagnostic.

The current standard in the diagnosis of cervical incompetence during pregnancy is the documentation of cervical effacement, shortening, or dilatation in the absence of premature labor. Frequent serial cervical examination by the same person combined with careful patient education as to the warning signs and symptoms of cervical change are utilized for women at high risk of cervical incompetence. Unfortunately, these practices depend on subjective evaluations by both patient and physician, and on the "normal" values for cervical status at any given gestational age. At least three studies (Parikh and Mehta 1961; Floyd 1961; and Schaffner and Schanzer 1966) have demonstrated that a significant percentage of both primigravidas (15 to 16 per cent) and multigravidas (17 to 35 per cent) had cervical dilatation of 1 to 2 cm in the mid to late second trimester of pregnancy. None of these authors observed a significant difference in the incidence of preterm delivery in these patients when compared to similar groups with a closed cervix. These studies indicate the importance of caution in making the diagnosis of cervical incompetence on the basis of cervical examination *alone,* particularly late in the second trimester when this may be a "normal" finding or the result of unrecognized uterine activity rather than the more classic presentation of cervical incompetence.

There has been much recent interest in the ability of early serial ultrasound examinations of the cervix to aid in the diagnosis of incompetence during pregnancy. The recent advent of transvaginal ultrasound transducers has added significantly to our diagnostic abilities in this area. Ayers et al. (1988) prospectively evaluated cervical length in 142 normal term pregnancies by serial ultrasonography every 4 to 6 weeks from 12 weeks to 36 weeks of gestation. Cervical length was fairly constant at 52 ± 12 mm until 34 weeks, at which time gradual cervical shortening was observed. There was no difference in cervical length between multiparas and nulliparas, nor was there much interobserver difference in cervical length measurements (3 to 5 per cent).

Several investigators (Sarti et al., 1979; Jackson et al., 1984; Costantini et al., 1986; Laing, 1985) have reported the use of ultrasonographic visualization of both cervical shortening and canal dilatation as helpful in the diagnosis of incompetence in those women at risk. Three more recent studies (Michaels et al., 1986; Varma et al., 1987; and Ayers et al., 1988) prospectively evaluated a total of 365 women at risk for cervical incompetence because of previous obstetric history by serial cervical ultrasonography. Thirty-seven per cent of these patients never showed incompetent cervix on ultrasonography and went on to deliver at term. Importantly, these women were spared an unnecessary cerclage procedure. Additionally, all three authors concluded that early diagnosis of cervical shortening and dilatation by ultrasonography assists in the diagnosis of both silent preterm labor and cervical incompetence. The early diagnosis of these entities before the onset of clinical symptoms allows a better opportunity for prompt and effective therapeutic interventions.

Ultrasonographic assessment of the cervix has also been reported to be of use in the accurate placement of a cerclage at the level of the internal os (Wheelock et al., 1984), and in the postoperative assessment of suture location (Parulekar and Kiwi, 1982), as well as pregnancy management and outcome (Rana et al., 1990). Both the No. 2 nylon suture commonly used in the McDonald procedure and the 5-mm Mersilene tape used in the Shirodkar procedure can be visualized ultrasonographically, and the length of the cervix from the suture to the external os can be measured serially.

It is my routine practice to follow women at risk or with a history suggestive of cervical incompetence by weekly cervical examination and serial ultrasonographic assessment of cervical length and dilatation. Figures 30–1A and B and 30–2A and B show the ultrasonograms of cervical configuration and length obtained pre- and postoperatively in a patient with cervical incompetence. Cervical "beaking" (widening of the proximal portion of the cervix by amniotic fluid) is noted preoperatively, and the sutures are seen postoperatively as the hyperechoic areas in the anterior portion of the cervix.

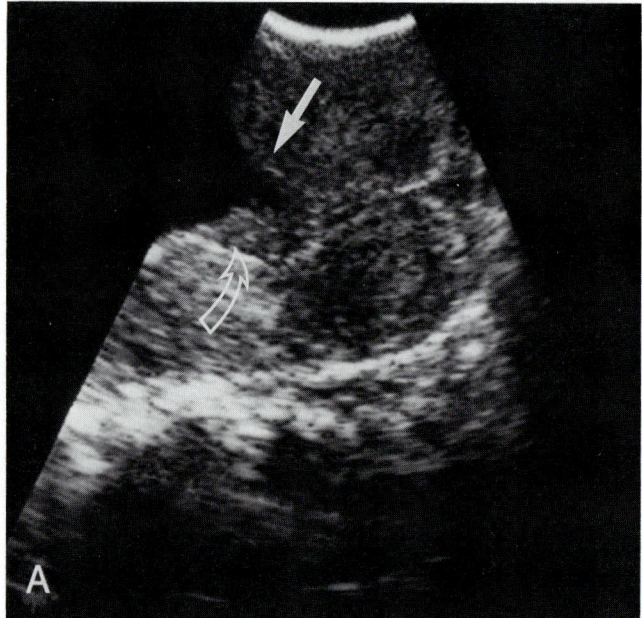

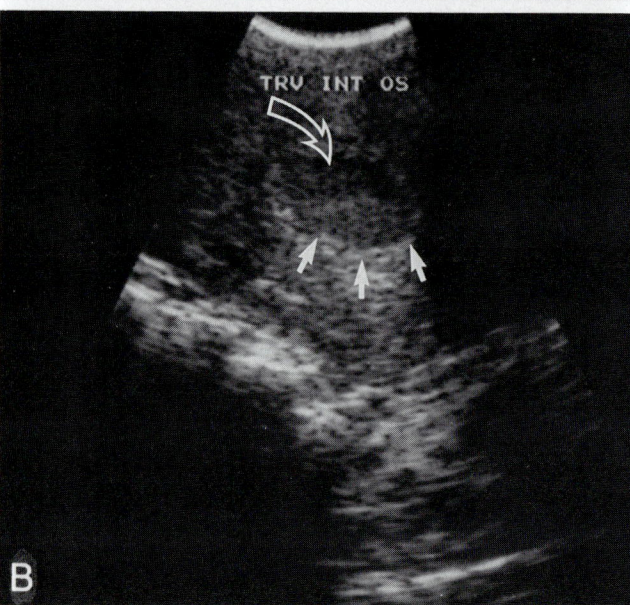

FIGURE 30–1. *A,* Transvaginal ultrasound in the sagittal view through the cervix at 16 weeks gestation. Cervical length is 2.0 cm. Note the funneling/beaking present at the level of the internal os (*solid arrow*) with debris (probably a blood clot) at the internal os (*open arrow*). *B,* Transvaginal ultrasound in the coronal (transverse) view of the cervix (posterior aspect shown by *closed arrows*) at the internal os in the same patient, showing dilatation of the cervix and debris (probably a blood clot) in the os (*open arrow*).

TREATMENT

Despite the lack of objective scientific or experimental evidence for its efficacy, cervical cerclage has become the standard treatment for cervical incompetence. Other noninvasive modalities such as treatment with progesterone or beta-agonists, pessary insertion, and prolonged bed rest have been advocated by var-

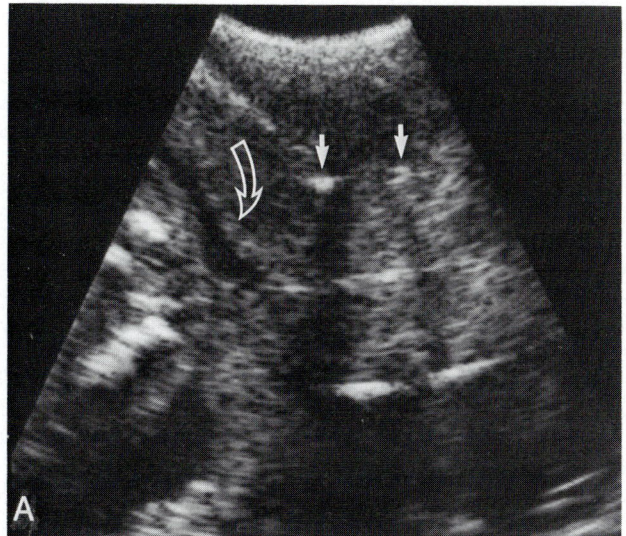

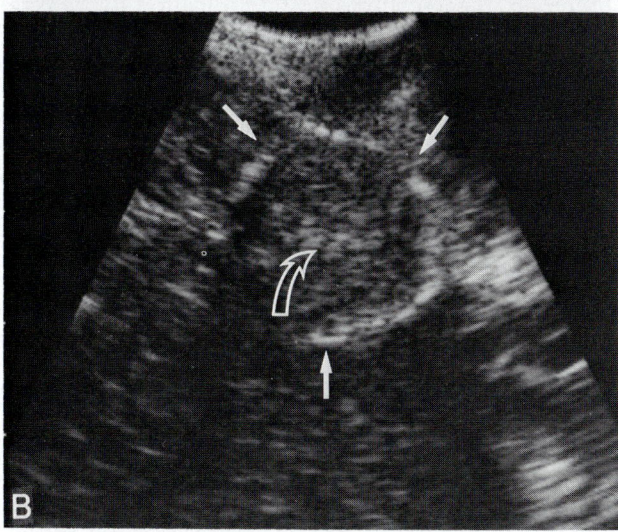

FIGURE 30–2. Postoperative ultrasound images of the same patient as in Figure 30–1 after McDonald cerclage placement. *A,* Transvaginal, sagittal view of the cervix. Note the two sutures (*closed arrows*) placed anteriorly with shadowing through the body of the cervix. Also note the resolution of funneling at the internal os (*open arrow*). *B,* Transvaginal, coronal (transverse) view of the cervix at the level of one of the sutures seen as a hyperechoic ring (*closed arrows*). Note the central cervical canal shadow indicating no dilatation and no debris (*open arrow*). (Images in Figure 30–1 and 30–2 are courtesy of Dr. Jude Crino, University of Texas Medical School at Houston.)

ious investigators, but have never gained widespread acceptance.

Data on the outcome of pregnancies treated by cervical cerclage are most often presented as reports of case series (Barter et al., 1958; Seppala and Vara, 1970; Lauersen and Fuchs, 1973; Toaff et al., 1977; Harger, 1980). These data boast success rates of 75 to 90 per cent; however, they are seriously flawed by the practice of comparing pregnancy outcome with that of previous pregnancies in the same woman. The inappropriateness of this type of comparison and the serious biases thus created have been reviewed by Chalmers (1984). Furthermore, good evidence exists to support the fact that repeated mid-trimester pregnancy loss does not preclude subsequent *spontaneous,* successful pregnancy outcome. One hundred couples with a history of three consecutive pregnancy losses had a 71 per cent chance of successful outcome if they had a normal karyotype and hysterosalpingogram (Tho et al., 1979). Harger et al. (1983) reported a pregnancy success rate of 73 per cent after recurrent pregnancy loss in 155 couples studied. In a review of the Norwegian experience, Bakketeig et al. (1979) reported that, although the risk of delivery between 16 and 36 weeks increases nearly four times after one preterm delivery, the next pregnancy has an 85 per cent probability of going to term. This number decreases to 70 per cent after two preterm deliveries, but both percentages remain within the range reported as "successes" with cervical cerclage.

In an effort to focus on a more homogeneous group of patients at risk for incompetent cervix, Keirse et al. (1978) and Rush (1979) retrospectively reviewed pregnancy outcome in patients with similar obstetric histories of mid-trimester abortion or preterm delivery. They compared women treated with cerclage with those women with similar histories managed without a cerclage during the same chronologic interval. Both studies suggested no significant benefit from cervical cerclage, although such observational studies are tainted by bias in the selection of patients for cerclage.

It seems clear from these data that well-designed, randomized controlled trials would be the method of choice for resolving the issue of efficacy of cerclage. To date, the results of four such trials have been published. Dor et al. (1982) randomly allocated 50 patients with twin gestations resulting from ovulation induction into a group managed with double silk McDonald cerclage at 13 to 14 weeks and a control group without cerclage. There was no statistically significant difference in preterm premature rupture of membranes, gestational age at delivery (<33 weeks and <37 weeks), or perinatal mortality. Although fetal and neonatal losses in both groups occurred at similar gestational ages, three women in the cerclage group had spontaneous loss between 14 and 17 weeks compared to two losses in the control group at 15 and 16 weeks. It seems that the extra miscarriage in the cerclage group is responsible for the small difference in mortality (28 per cent as opposed to 22 per cent) and illustrates the difficulty in assigning blame for pregnancy loss to the procedure of cerclage itself.

Rush et al. (1984) randomly allocated 194 "high-risk" women with singleton pregnancies to have a nylon McDonald cerclage or to be managed without cerclage. The risk of mid-trimester loss or preterm delivery in these patients was calculated to be 30 per cent. There was a statistically significant increase in hospital admission and tocolytic therapy for preterm labor in the cerclage group. These women also had an increased incidence of preterm premature rupture of membranes. Unfortunately, there was no difference in gestational age at delivery (<33 weeks and <37 weeks) or perinatal mortality between the groups.

Lazar and Gueguen (1984) used a weighted scoring system to assess patient eligibility for their trial. This approach excluded both women at high risk who should be managed with cerclage and those at low risk who should be managed without cerclage; these investigators hoped to identify a group at "moderate" risk. Unfortunately, the study group of 506 women turned out to be at low risk with a preterm delivery rate of 6 per cent. The study was conducted at four clinical centers with random allocation of patients to a McDonald cerclage group or a control group managed without cerclage. In reality, 90 per cent of the cerclage group had the suture placed and 11 per cent of the control group also had a cerclage placed. Randomization was violated in one of the centers, with cerclages being placed more frequently in women perceived to be at greater risk. These data are included in the publication because statistical analysis of the results was unchanged after their exclusion. As observed by Rush et al. (1984), hospitalization and treatment with tocolytics were significantly more frequent in the cerclage group. These women also reported a perceived increase in uterine activity. There was no evidence from this trial to suggest that cerclage prolonged gestation or decreased perinatal mortality.

It is interesting to note that in all three trials fewer pregnancies in the cerclage groups reached 33 weeks, although the difference is not statistically significant at the $p < 0.05$ level. One cannot help but be alarmed by the increased incidence of hospitalization and treatment for preterm labor in the cerclage groups, suggesting a role for cerclage placement itself in the etiology of preterm labor. These epidemiologic data are supported by a retrospective analysis of uterine activity in 96 patients with cervical cerclage (Robichaux et al., 1990). These women had daily home uterine activity monitoring from 20 weeks of gestation onward. Preterm labor developed in 23 per cent and 12 per cent had preterm delivery secondary to failed tocolysis or preterm premature rupture of membranes. Uterine activity in those women who developed preterm labor was significantly greater than in those women who delivered at term. Although randomization has eliminated bias from these trials, their treatment effects were not large enough to allow confident separation from chance effects. Statistically, precision depends on the number of cases with adverse outcome in a trial, which in turn is maximized by increasing the degree of risk in the population studied as well as by increasing the number of patients studied. Grant's (1986) review of the cerclage trials includes statistics on the pooled data from all three trials. This analysis *suggests* that the risk of preterm delivery is in fact increased by cerclage. This drastic statement must be tempered with the knowledge that even the pooled data reveal confidence limits that do not provide evidence of statistical significance and may still be compatible with a beneficial effect of cerclage on prolongation of pregnancy.

Most recently, the Medical Research Council/Royal College of Obstetricians and Gynaecologists reported results of a large, multicenter, randomized trial of cervical cerclage which included 905 women (1988). Previous second-trimester loss or preterm delivery accounted for 74 per cent of the patients and previous cervical surgery for an additional 11 per cent. Women were enrolled in the study because their obstetricians were "uncertain" as to the advisability of cerclage. After randomization to either cerclage or no surgery, 92 per cent were actually treated as allocated. The cerclage group had statistically fewer deliveries at less than 33 weeks (13 per cent vs. 18 per cent $p = .03$), fewer infants less than 1500 gm (11 per cent vs. 16 per cent $p = .01$), and fewer pregnancy losses including miscarriage, stillbirth, and neonatal death (8 per cent vs. 12 per cent $p = 0.06$). The percentage of deliveries occurring between 33 and 36 weeks was similar. The authors concluded that while there was statistically significant benefit in the cerclage group, the differences were not large and would require 20 to 25 cerclage procedures to prevent one preterm delivery. As none of the other randomized trials has reported significant benefit of cerclage, they feel that it is uncertain as to how much of this apparent benefit is real. Unfortunately, there were not sufficient numbers of women in each subgroup by indication for cerclage to make stratification analyses reliable. However, it would seem from the raw data that the benefit of cerclage is concentrated in the groups of women with one or more previous pregnancy losses or preterm deliveries. As an example, in the cerclage group only 2 of 40 women with the poorest obstetric history delivered before 33 weeks (5 per cent) compared with 41 of 285 women with a relatively good history (14 per cent).

After careful examination of all the available data on the diagnosis of cervical incompetence and the efficacy of cerclage as a therapeutic modality, the clinician is not left with a clear mandate. The decision to place a cerclage should not be made lightly, as there are significant risks to the continuation of the pregnancy, yet the efficacy of cerclage appears to be related to the severity of the criteria for the diagnosis of incompetence. This continues to be a clinical problem requiring intensive observation of the patient at risk, and a significant degree of sound clinical judgment in the choice of patients for cerclage placement.

Surgery in Nonpregnant State

These techniques are uncommon in clinical practice today, as the diagnosis of cervical incompetence is usually confirmed during pregnancy. The major disadvantage of preconceptual cerclage placement is that it does not allow for the relatively high rate of spontaneous first-trimester loss or the possibility of a genetically abnormal fetus. Nonetheless, there is the occasional well-selected patient who may benefit from these procedures.

Lash Procedure

Named for the investigators who pioneered it (Lash and Lash, 1950), this procedure was intended to correct a structural defect within the body of the cervix that was thought to result from poor healing of an obstetric laceration or vigorous dilatation of the cervix prior to curettage. A transverse incision in the anterior cervical mucosa is made approximately 2 cm above the external os and the bladder reflected as necessary.

The observed defect is then plicated with interrupted sutures of 2–0 chromic catgut. It is suggested that larger lesions be excised in an elliptical fashion prior to suture plication. Lash (1960) reported a 78 per cent fetal survival rate after surgery in 79 women compared with 11 per cent preoperatively. These data, however, are based on previous reproductive history in the same women and must be viewed with that criticism in mind. Lees and Sutherst (1974) suggested that these women suffered from a 50 per cent infertility rate postoperatively, although Lash's original report (1960) reported a 16 per cent infertility rate.

Mann Isthmic Cerclage

Mann et al. (1961) described a transvaginal cervicoisthmic cerclage that was undertaken preconceptually in order to facilitate dissection of an abnormally shortened or scarred cervix and to enable placement of the suture at the level of the internal os. The original description of the technique suggests dissection of the cervix both anteriorly and posteriorly to the level of the peritoneal reflection. A nonabsorbable suture is placed circumferentially at the level of the internal os as in the Shirodkar procedure, except that the uterosacral ligaments and a small amount of cervical tissue both anteriorly and posteriorly are incorporated in the suture with a curved Mayo needle. The suture is tied anteriorly over a No. 4 Hegar dilator and a second suture placed 1 to 2 cm distal to the first. The cervicovaginal incisions are closed with interrupted absorbable sutures. Mann et al. (1961) reported an 85 per cent success rate with his procedure, again compared with previous reproductive history in the same women . Although this operation is uncommon today, it may yet be appropriate as an alternative to postconceptual placement of a transabdominal cervicoisthmic cerclage in the patient with a markedly foreshortened or severely scarred cervix.

Surgery During Pregnancy

Perioperative Considerations

Once the diagnosis of cervical incompetence is made and the decision to place a cerclage is reached, timing is of great importance. It is generally agreed that elective cerclage placement has a significantly higher success rate than those procedures performed after cervical effacement and dilatation have occurred (Kuhn and Pepperell, 1977; Harger, 1980; Rock and Murphy, 1986; Branch, 1986). Waiting until the early second trimester (13 to 16 weeks) provides the following advantages: (1) sonographic confirmation of fetal viability by cardiac activity at 10 to 12 weeks essentially reduces to a minimum the opportunity of spontaneous miscarriage (Christiaens and Stoutenbeek, 1984); (2) significant anatomic fetal abnormalities as well as the presence of a partial molar pregnancy can usually be detected by diagnostic ultrasonographic evaluation by 14 to 16 weeks; (3) early amniocentesis (13 to 15 weeks) or chorion villus sampling (9 to 12 weeks) can be done preoperatively to diagnose chromosomal, DNA, or metabolic abnormalities in those pregnancies at risk.

While early second trimester seems the optimal time for elective cerclage placement, this does not preclude surgery if the diagnosis is made at a later gestational age, although there is no consensus with regard to an upper limit for surgery. As neonatal intensive care technology continues to improve and mortality statistics for very-low-birth-weight babies continue to fall, it seems reasonable to withhold cerclage placement at that gestational age when there is significant opportunity for fetal survival.

Efforts at constructing a scoring system to predict efficacy of cerclage in patients with cervical incompetence have been made by Ger et al. (1991) and Block and Rahhal (1976). Although the numbers of patients are relatively small (47), Ger and colleagues conclude that cerclage is most efficacious in preventing preterm delivery and fetal loss in patients with three or more of five criteria for the diagnosis of cervical incompetence: (1) previous premature delivery or mid-trimester abortion without cause, (2) visual evidence of surgical or obstetric trauma to the cervix, (3) history of painless premature labor or rapid delivery, (4) progressive dilatation or dilatation greater than 2 cm on initial examination during mid-trimester, and (5) previous diagnosis of cervical incompetence with previous cerclage.

Contraindications to cerclage placement during pregnancy include rupture of membranes, evidence of cervical or intrauterine infection, major congenital anomalies of the fetus, vaginal bleeding of undetermined cause, and active labor irrespective of etiology. Careful monitoring often reveals some degree of uterine activity when it is performed in those women undergoing emergency cerclage for significant cervical effacement or dilatation. Although there is disagreement in the literature concerning the appropriateness of perioperative tocolytic therapy for these patients (Novy et al., 1987; Novy, 1982; Repke and Niebyl, 1985), the approach has been to achieve uterine quiescence in these women for 6 to 12 hours preoperatively by treatment with indomethacin, 25 mg orally every 6 hours, and to continue that therapy for 24 hours postoperatively.

Several studies have documented an increase in maternal plasma concentration of the prostaglandin $F_2\alpha$ metabolite PGFM after transvaginal McDonald cerclage (Bibby et al., 1979; Toplis et al., 1980; Novy et al., 1987). An in-depth study of maternal plasma prostaglandin E and F concentrations after both transabdominal and transvaginal cerclage placement was undertaken by Novy et al. (1987). Their data confirm earlier observations that PGFM increases rapidly (by the end of the operative procedure) and returns to preoperative values within 6 to 8 hours. Additionally, the PGE_2 metabolite (PGEM-II) increases and returns to normal levels in a fashion similar to that of PGFM. There was no significant difference in plasma levels of either metabolite when timing of the procedure (first trimester as opposed to second trimester) or type of procedure (McDonald as opposed to Shirodkar cerclage) was evaluated. Transabdominal cervicoisthmic cerclage did not result in a further increased plasma concentration of prostaglandin metabolites as compared with the transvaginal approach, but did result in prolongation of the duration of the rise in plasma concentration by 6 to 8 hours. These data give support to the clinical tenet that the cerclage procedure itself is not responsible for a sustained outpouring of prostaglandins that might be likely to initiate labor, and that those women who do manifest significant uterine activity more than 12 to 24 hours after cerclage are likely to have infection, idiopathic preterm labor, or some other underlying cause for their contractions.

A recent report by Arias (1988) advocates the use of cervical cerclage in patients with complete placenta previa and vaginal bleeding prior to 30 weeks of gestation. In a randomized trial, 12 patients underwent cerclage and 11 patients were managed with bed rest in the hospital, tocolytics, and steroids. The cerclage group had a significant improvement in pregnancy prolongation (7.9 as opposed to 2.7 weeks), gestational age at delivery (35.1 as opposed to 31.6 weeks), and birth weight (2723 gm as opposed to 1817 gm). However, there was no statistically significant difference in perinatal mortality or morbidity or in the total number of units of blood transfused to the mothers. Delivery was undertaken if bleeding recurred or if fetal pulmonary maturity was reached. While this is indeed a novel approach to the treatment of placenta previa, the technical difficulties and risks of cerclage placement in these patients at such an advanced gestational age warrant further carefully undertaken trials before acceptance into clinical practice.

Morbidity associated with cervical cerclage of all types includes both complications related to the procedure itself (anesthetic risks, bleeding, maternal soft tissue injury, spontaneous suture displacement, rupture of membranes, and infection) and those associated with subsequent delivery (cervical laceration, increased incidence of cesarean section). Bleeding that requires transfusion is a rare complication of cerclage. In a report of 202 elective transvaginal procedures, Harger (1980) noted no blood loss greater than 150 ml. Benson and Durfee (1965) transfused two of 13 patients undergoing transabdominal cerclage, while Novy (1982) reported one transfusion in 16 transabdominal procedures and an average blood loss of less than 150 ml.

Perioperative rupture of membranes is a common complication of emergency cerclage when the cervix is substantially effaced, dilated, or both and the membranes either at or prolapsed past the external os. When the process of cervical incompetency is far advanced, Olatunbosun and Dyck (1981) reported a 17 per cent incidence of intraoperative rupture of membranes compared with 30 per cent in Harger's (1980) series. The incidence of perioperative rupture of membranes in elective cerclage procedures is much lower, but the association with risk of amniorrhexis still exists, as several studies (Harger, 1980; Hofmeister et al., 1968; Jennings, 1972; Lauersen and Fuchs, 1973; Peters et al., 1979) report incidences of 1.1 per cent to 9 per cent in the perioperative period.

Chorioamnionitis, accompanied by significant maternal morbidity and even mortality (Dunn et al., 1959), and resulting from cervical cerclage placement, has been reported with varying frequency from 1 per cent (Harger, 1980; Kuhn and Pepperell, 1977) to 6 to 8 per cent (Peters et al., 1979; Aarnoudse and Huisjes, 1979). After studying 115 pregnant women undergoing cerclage, Charles and Edwards (1981) suggested that the incidence of postoperative chorioamnionitis was related to the timing of surgery; they reported that the incidence of chorioamnionitis was increased 2.6 times and the incidence of premature rupture of membranes before 32 weeks was increased three times if cerclage was performed after the 20th week of gestation. They also suggested that prophylactic antibiotics be used when surgery is done after 18 weeks. Other maternal morbidity associated with cerclage placement includes vesicovaginal and urethrovaginal fistulas (Bates and Cropley, 1977; Ulmsten, 1977), as well as ulceration of the trigone of the bladder from erosion of the knot of the cerclage (Hortenstine and Witherington, 1987).

Displacement of the cervical suture has been reported by Toaff et al. (1977) and by Harger (1980) to occur in approximately 3 per cent of cases, although Aarnoudse and Huisjes (1979) and Cushner (1963) have reported incidences of 12 to 13 per cent. It is generally agreed that when the initial cerclage becomes displaced, subsequent attempts have a very low success rate in prolonging pregnancy to viability (none of six in Harger's series, and two of seven in Aarnoudse's group).

The long-range sequelae of cervical cerclage procedures include events that occur with the onset of labor and the delivery process. Lindberg (1979) and Thurston (1963) have reported uterine rupture in women whose labors began before the suture could be removed. It has also been postulated that the cervix may not dilate normally in response to labor after a cerclage has been in place, despite its removal at the appropriate time. This is thought to be a result of fibrous scar tissue formation in the cervix as a reaction to the foreign body (Harger, 1980; Hofmeister et al., 1968; Kuhn and Pepperell, 1977). Fibrous cervical tissue would neither efface properly before the onset of labor nor dilate gradually in response to uterine contractions. The reported incidence of cervical lacerations at delivery thought to be related to cerclage placement ranges from less than 1 per cent (Lauersen and Fuchs, 1973) to approximately 13 per cent (Harger, 1980; Smith and Scragg, 1969). A desire to avoid both this potential morbidity and the need for suture removal and subsequent placement during future pregnancies has led some authors to advocate routine cesarean section as the delivery method of choice for patients with a cervical cerclage. While this seems justified in the patient who requires transabdominal cervicoisthmic cerclage in order to avoid the additional laparotomies involved in suture removal and replacement, it seems unwise to add the additional morbidity of cesarean delivery to those patients with sutures that can be easily removed transvaginally.

Ultimately, the decision for cerclage placement should be made on an individual basis after weighing the relative risks and benefits of the procedure, the strength of the diagnosis of cervical incompetence, and the certainty with which other conditions in the differential diagnosis have been ruled out.

Shirodkar Cerclage

In a 1955 report, Shirodkar first described his cerclage procedure utilizing maternal fascia lata as the "suture" material (Shirodkar, 1955). He used aneurysm needles to thread the fascia lata strip submucosally after first incising the vaginal epithelium both anteriorly and posteriorly in a transverse fashion and reflecting the vesicovaginal and rectovaginal fascia to the level of the internal os. Shirodkar tied the suture anteriorly, cut the ends short, and then closed both anterior and posterior incisions with fine, absorbable material. In the last 30 years, many modifications of the original procedure have evolved, including tying the knot posteriorly, leaving the ends of the knot exposed for easier removal, and replacing fascia lata with either No. 2 Mersilene or nylon or a 5-mm Mersilene band mounted on its own atraumatic needles. Instead of tunneling the suture submucosally, some obstetricians, including the author, advocate inserting a curved, long Allis clamp into the incisions both anteriorly and posteriorly and placing lateral traction on the submucosal tissue in order to place the cerclage next to the body of the cervix and medial to the uterine vessels. Caspi et al. (1990) randomized 90 women to Shirodkar cerclage or a new technique using anterior colpotomy only, and tying a 0.6-mm nylon suture posteriorly. Pregnancy outcomes were similar, and the authors felt the technique was simpler and suture removal easier.

Some advocate that the Shirodkar type of cerclage should be anchored to the cervix both anteriorly and posteriorly to avoid the complication of suture displacement. If the 5-mm Mersilene tape is used, this can be done by means of a fine silk suture placed to anchor the tape to the cervical tissue, whereas if a No. 2 Mersilene thread suture is used, the cerclage may be anchored directly if an extra bite of cervical tissue is taken both anteriorly and posteriorly. Further technical details can be found in reviews by Branch (1986) and by Rock and Murphy (1986).

McDonald Cerclage

A simpler procedure requiring no submucosal dissection was described in 1957 by McDonald and has gained widespread popularity because of its simplicity and its application to the emergency situation. The original series reported by McDonald (1957) included 70 patients in whom cerclage was performed with No. 4 silk suture on a Mayo needle. The purse-string suture is begun anteriorly at the junction of the ectocervix and rugated vagina, and five or six bites of cervix are taken in a circumferential fashion deep into the body of the cervix, but avoiding entry into the endocervical canal. McDonald cautioned that the suture must be placed deeply in the posterior aspect of the cervix as this was the most likely site for the suture to become displaced postoperatively. The suture is tied anteriorly, and the ends left long enough to facilitate removal at term or at the onset of labor. Variations of McDonald's original technique have also developed over the years and include the use of braided nylon, Mersilene thread and Mersilene bands,

reentering the cervix at the previous point of exit with successive bites to place the suture entirely submucosally, and placing two sutures approximately 1 cm apart to prevent the posterior suture from tearing and to add substance and length to the cervix (Hofmeister et al., 1968). See reviews by Branch (1986) and by Rock and Murphy (1986).

Transabdominal Cervicoisthmic Cerclage

Although first described by Benson and Durfee (1965), the transabdominal approach to cerclage placement has been extensively studied and continually updated by Novy (1977, 1982, 1985; Novy et al., 1987) and others (Wallenburg and Lotgering, 1987; Herron and Parer, 1988). The criteria used by Benson and Durfee included congenitally short or amputated cervix; previously unsuccessful cerclage with cervical scarring; deeply notched, multiple cervical defects; and unhealed forniceal lacerations or subacute cervicitis. Suggested timing of cerclage is between 10 and 14 weeks of gestation so that uterine manipulation for visualization of both anterior and posterior leaves of the broad ligament can be easily accomplished. Novy (1982) has modified the selection criteria by eliminating those patients with cervical infection and adding the patient who is a candidate for emergency cerclage with marked cervical effacement, dilatation less than 4 cm, and membranes intact in whom a transvaginal approach would be thought unfeasible. In his series of 16 procedures, all cerclages were placed in the second trimester of pregnancy in order that fetal structural, metabolic, and chromosomal abnormalities could be ruled out by the appropriate diagnostic means and that the time in which first-trimester spontaneous miscarriage could occur had passed.

All authors describe essentially the same surgical technique. The peritoneal cavity is entered via either the Pfannenstiel or the vertical incision, the peritoneal reflections divided transversely and bladder advanced carefully, avoiding wide lateral dissection that might injure the massive vascular plexus present during pregnancy. At the level of the uterine isthmus, the space between the ascending and descending branches of the uterine artery is identified and developed by blunt dissection medial to the uterine arteries and veins, and lateral to the connective tissue of the uterine isthmus. Upward traction on the uterine fundus by an assistant exposes the region of the internal os, and the vessels are placed on traction. After the tunnel has been developed in the vascular space bilaterally, the posterior leaf of the broad ligament is punctured bilaterally and a 5-mm Mersilene tape is passed under direct vision to lie over the posterior peritoneum at the level of the insertions of the uterosacral ligaments. The Mersilene band is tied snugly anteriorly with a single square knot, and the cut ends are sutured to the band with fine nonabsorbable sutures. The peritoneum and abdomen are then closed in routine fashion. See reviews by Novy (1982, 1985) and by Branch (1986).

There are additional risks associated with the transabdominal procedure. Two laparotomies are required, one for cerclage placement and one for subsequent cesarean section. Emergency removal of the suture can sometimes be accomplished by posterior colpotomy but may be accompanied by substantial hemorrhage from tearing of the intensely vascular parametrial venous plexus. It is therefore prudent to leave the cerclage in place and perform elective cesarean section, and to leave the cerclage in place interconceptually if the decision for future childbearing is made. In summary, transabdominal cervicoisthmic cerclage seems to have a definite place in management of cervical incompetence in a very small and well-defined population.

Emergency Cerclage

The diagnosis of cervical incompetence occasionally will not be made until the patient presents with advanced effacement and dilatation of the cervix and the membranes located at the level of the external os or bulging into the vagina. Under these emergency circumstances the prognosis for fetal survival decreases significantly, but a cerclage may still be placed if appropriate conditions are met. The patient should be placed at bed rest in Trendelenberg position, and uterine activity should be monitored. Ultrasonographic examination should be performed to ensure fetal viability and to rule out major congenital anomalies. If a diagnosis of abruptio placentae or chorioamnionitis is suspected, cerclage placement is contraindicated. Tocolytic therapy may be warranted in the presence of mild uterine activity without evidence of infection, abruption, or progressive cervical change.

Placement of a cervical cerclage of any type under these circumstances is difficult at best. Bulging or prolapsed membranes are prone to rupture intraoperatively at the slightest provocation; however, several authors have reported techniques by which this risk may be reduced.

Olatunbosun and Dyck (1981) described placing six to ten stay sutures of No. 0 silk or Mersilene at the edges of the cervix, which when placed on traction tend to move the protruding membranes back into the uterine cavity, thus facilitating cerclage placement. Novy (1985) has suggested gently replacing the membranes by using gauze on a ring forceps covered by either a condom or finger cot so as to avoid trauma to the amniotic sac. Several authors (Orr, 1973; Holman, 1973; Didolkar, 1986) have described using a No. 16 French Foley catheter with a 30-cc balloon to avoid inadvertent perforation of the membranes during cerclage. The tip of the catheter is cut off and the catheter inserted through the external os. The balloon is inflated slowly and acts to keep the membranes from prolapsing through the cervix (Fig. 30–3A). Either a McDonald or a Shirodkar cerclage may then be placed and tied with the catheter in place. The balloon is then deflated and the catheter withdrawn (Fig. 30–3B). If the membranes are particularly tense and no other maneuvers are helpful, Goodlin (1979) has advocated transabdominal amniocentesis to temporarily reduce amniotic fluid volume and assist in spontaneous replacement of the membranes within the uterus.

Sheerer et al. (1987) have reported a noninvasive

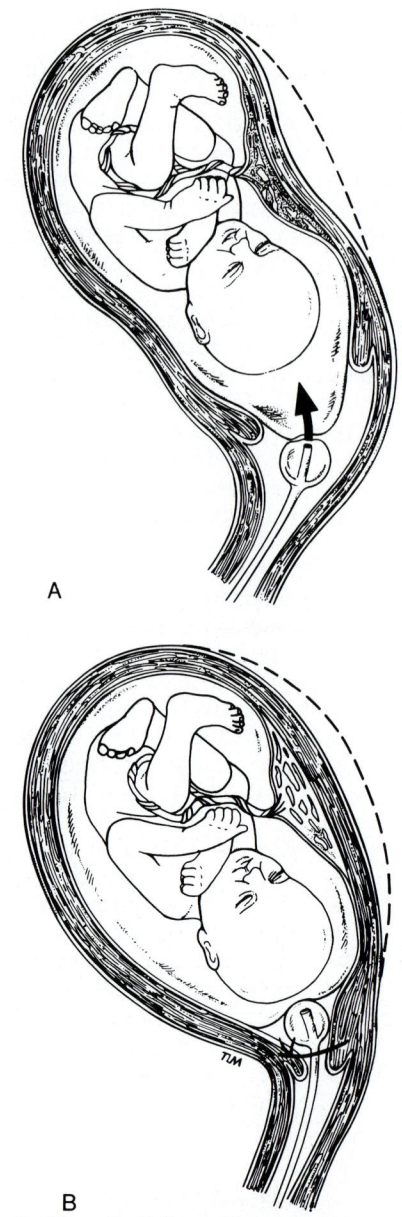

A

B

FIGURE 30–3. Use of a Foley catheter in emergency cerclage placement with bulging membranes. *A*, The tip of the catheter is cut off and the balloon inflated. The balloon is then placed against the membranes to displace them upward into the cervical canal. *B*, A cerclage is placed with the balloon and membranes well advanced inside the uterus. The balloon is then deflated and the Foley catheter removed.

technique for the replacement of prolapsed membranes without direct contact. Four patients underwent emergency cerclage between 21 and 23 weeks gestation and had cervical dilatation of at least 3 cm and membranes prolapsed 3 to 7 cm below the external os by visualization and ultrasound confirmation. All patients were placed in Trendelenburg position with shoulder supports and received general anesthesia. The urinary bladder was then filled with up to 1000 cc of 0.45 per cent saline. This was carried out under direct visualization of the cervix by speculum examination, and the bladder infusion was stopped when the membranes were seen to recede into the cervical canal. After sonographic documentation, a cerclage of either the McDonald or Shirodkar type was placed, and the bladder was emptied (Fig. 30–4). There were no reported postoperative complications, and the mean delivery time was 31 ± 6.8 weeks; all four infants were doing well at the time of the initial report.

A Cervical Incompetence Scale (CIS) was devised by Kokia et al. (1991) in order to evaluate the appropriateness of emergency cerclage placement and to predict outcome. Cervical effacement, dilatation, and protrusion of fetal membranes through the cervix were each scored as 0 to 3 points. Twenty-four women presenting in the second trimester underwent emergency McDonald cerclage. Women with CIS of 0 to 3 points had fewer postoperative complications (33 per cent vs. 87.5 per cent), fewer pregnancy losses (22.2 per cent vs. 75 per cent), and significantly longer gestation (33.2 weeks vs. 24.4 weeks), when compared to those women with CIS scores of 5 to 8. Corroboration of these data by other investigators will potentially help the clinician to counsel and manage patients who require emergency cerclage procedures.

Recent reviews of experience with emergency cerclage offer more hope than the original 10 per cent success rates of the earlier literature (Harger, 1980). Chryssikopoulos et al. (1988) reviewed 40 emergency cerclage placements and reported a perinatal mortality rate of 42.3 per cent, a preterm delivery rate of 53 per cent, but a 20 per cent rate of infants with birth weights >2500 gm. In a review of 20 patients presenting for emergency cerclage, Kelly et al. (1992) found that cervical dilatation of >3.5 cm was predictive of poor outcome (0 per cent survival), whereas dilatation <3.5 cm correlated with 83 per cent survival. Neither effacement nor protrusion of membranes was predictive of outcome, and perioperative tocolysis did not affect outcome.

SUCCESS OF CERCLAGE PROCEDURES

As previously mentioned, success rates for cerclage procedures have been uniformly reported using the patients' previous reproductive performance as controls to establish the efficacy of the procedure. The simple statistical truth is that this is not a valid approach for the proof of efficacy of an intervention. Keeping this in mind, the "success" rates (fetal survival) for Shirodkar cerclage vary only minimally from approximately 75 per cent (Stromme et al., 1960; Barter et al., 1958; Robboy, 1973) to 85 per cent (Shirodkar, 1967; Lauersen and Fuchs, 1973; Harger, 1980; Charles and Edwards, 1981), as compared with fetal survival rates of 10 to 30 per cent in those same series before cerclage. Similar data have been collected after McDonald cerclage with fetal survival ranging from 73 per cent (Harger, 1980; McDonald, 1980) to 89 per cent (Jennings, 1972; Toaff et al., 1977) after cerclage, as compared to 7 to 50 per cent before cerclage in those same women. Three series combining a total of 35 pregnancies treated with transabdominal cervicoisthmic cerclage report fetal survival rates of 82 to 100 per cent as compared with 11 to 44 per cent before treatment in those same women (Benson and Durfee, 1965; Watkins, 1972; Novy, 1982).

As in most other areas of medicine, practicing obstetricians tend to have strong feelings as to which type of cerclage is more effective, despite the fact that data from four studies in which a comparison was made have shown no significant difference in the fetal survival rate (Harger, 1980; Kuhn and Pepperell, 1977; Robboy, 1973; Peters et al., 1979). Conceptually, the Shirodkar procedure would seem to provide stronger circumferential support as it is placed high enough to be at the level of the internal os, whereas the McDonald procedure may be easier to accomplish under emergency circumstances. Frieden et al. (1990) report

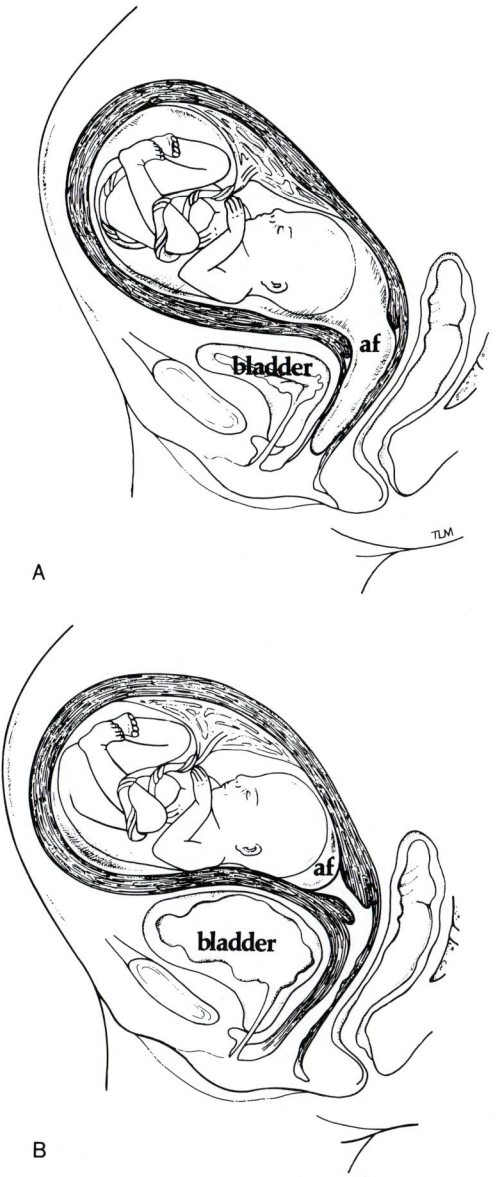

FIGURE 30–4. *A,* Incompetent cervix with membranes bulging into the vagina. *B,* Note that distention of the bladder with 0.45 per cent saline results in displacement of the membranes back inside the uterus and allows for cerclage placement without direct manipulation of the membranes.

the experience of one surgeon with 66 Shirodkar procedures. Mean operative blood loss was 25 ml, term delivery rate was 88 per cent, and corrected perinatal survival (after exclusion of cases unrelated to the diagnosis of cervical incompetence or the placement of cerclage) was 100 per cent. This was compared to a pre-cerclage survival rate of 35 per cent in this same group of women. Irrespective of personal preference and retrospective analyses, the questions of true efficacy of cervical cerclage in preventing second-trimester pregnancy loss and increasing fetal survival, and the superiority of one technique over the others, remain to be answered by an appropriately controlled, randomized, prospective clinical trial.

CONSERVATIVE THERAPY

Through the years there have been a number of nonsurgical approaches to the management of patients with supposed cervical incompetence, although none of these techniques has gained widespread acceptance or been proved efficacious in a controlled trial. The administration of hydroxyprogesterone caproate intramuscularly along with a program of bed rest was suggested by Sherman (1966). Various types of vaginal pessaries were also used in an attempt to change the axis of the cervical canal and prevent alleged gravitational forces from causing cervical dilatation and subsequent delivery (Vitsky, 1963; Oster and Javert, 1966). Yosowitz et al. (1972) described an inflatable plastic cuff for the treatment of incompetent cervix. The device was constructed of two fluid inflatable plastic balloons that could be applied over the internal cervical os transvaginally. This could be accomplished at an office visit without anesthesia. If labor ensues or term is reached, the device can be removed by cutting and emptying the balloons.

Bed rest and tocolysis with beta-adrenoceptor agents has been advocated as an alternative to cerclage in patients with supposed cervical incompetence (Rivera-Alsina et al., 1983). It is likely, however, that those patients successfully treated by this regimen had true premature labor as a cause of early cervical change; in fact, on careful review of the patient population in this study, 40 per cent of the group had premature labor listed as a criterion for cervical incompetence.

SUMMARY

The diagnosis of cervical incompetence remains one of exclusion, made on the basis of careful history and physical examination and possibly with the aid of transvaginal ultrasonography. The decision to place a cerclage in women so diagnosed requires careful clinical judgment and a weighing of the risks and benefits attendant to the procedure. The last decade has seen some progress in the early diagnosis of cervical incompetence in women at risk, as well as a higher success rate for emergency cerclage procedures. However, our ability to develop specific diagnostic criteria for cervical incompetence and to successfully diagnose the disorder in women at risk in time to intervene effectively awaits a better understanding of the biochemistry of the cervix and the physiology of the interaction between uterine activity and cervical compliance.

REFERENCES

Aarnoudse JG, Huisjes HJ: Complications of cerclage. Acta Obstet Gynaecol Scand **58**:255, 1979.

Arias F: Cervical cerclage for the temporary treatment of patients with placenta previa. Obstet Gynecol **71**:545, 1988.

Asplund J: The uterine cervix and isthmus under normal and pathological conditions. A clinical and roentgenological study. Acta Radiol **91**(Suppl):3, 1952.

Ayers JWT, DeGrood RM, Compton AA, et al: Sonographic evaluation of cervical length in pregnancy: Diagnosis and management of preterm cervical effacement in patients at risk for premature delivery. Obstet Gynecol **71**:939, 1988.

Bakketeig LS, Hoffman HJ, Harley EE: The tendency to repeat gestational age and birthweight in successive births. Am J Obstet Gynecol **135**:1086, 1979.

Barter RH, Dusbabek JA, Riva HL, et al: Surgical closure of the incompetent cervix during pregnancy. Am J Obstet Gynecol **75**:511, 1958.

Bates JL, Cropley T: Complications of cervical cerclage. Lancet **2**:1035, 1977.

Ben-Baruch G, Menczer J, Mashiach S, Serr DM: Uterine anomalies in diethylstilbestrol-exposed women with fertility disorders. Acta Obstet Gyneacol Scand **60**:395, 1981.

Benson RC, Durfee RB: Transabdominal cervicouterine cerclage during pregnancy for the treatment of cervical incompetency. Obstet Gynecol **25**:145, 1965.

Berger MJ, Goldstein DP: Impaired reproductive performance in DES-exposed women. Obstet Gynecol **55**:25, 1980.

Bergman R, Svennerud S: Traction test of demonstrating incompetence of the internal os of the cervix. Int J Fertil **2**:163, 1957.

Bibby JG, Brunt J, Mitchell MD, Turnbull AC: The effect of cervical encerclage on plasma prostaglandin levels during early human pregnancy. Br J Obstet Gynaecol **86**:19, 1979.

Block MF, Rahhal DK: Cervical incompetence: A diagnostic and prognostic scoring system. Obstet Gynecol **47**:279, 1976.

Branch W: Operations for cervical incompetence. Clin Obstet Gynecol **29**:240, 1986.

Caspi E, Schneider DF, Mor Z, Langer R, Weinraub Z, Bukovksy I: Cervical internal os cerclage: Description of a new technique and comparison with Skirodkar operation. Am J Perinatol **7**:347, 1990.

Chalmers I: Confronting Cochrane's challenge to obstetrics. Br J Obstet Gynaecol **91**:721, 1984.

Charles D, Edwards WR: Infectious complications of cervical cerclage. Am J Obstet Gynecol **141**:1065, 1981.

Child CG: Sterility and Conception. New York, Appleton-Century-Crofts, 1922.

Christiaens GCML, Stoutenbeek P: Spontaneous abortion in proven intact pregnancies. Lancet **2**:571, 1984.

Chryssikopoulos A, Botsis D, Vitoratos N, et al: Cervical incompetence: A 24-year review. Int J Gynecol Obstet **26**:245, 1988.

Costantini S, Valenzano M, Venturini PL, et al: Ultrasonic evaluation of cervical incompetence. Biol Res Pregnancy Perinatol **7**:11, 1986.

Cousins L: Cervical incompetence, 1980: A time for reappraisal. Clin Obstet Gynecol **23**:467, 1980a.

Cousins L, Karp W, Lacey C, et al: Reproductive outcome of women exposed to diethylstilbestrol in utero. Obstet Gynecol **56**:70, 1980b.

Cousins L: Cervical Incompetence. In Creasy RK, Resnik R (eds): Maternal-Fetal Medicine. Philadelphia, W. B. Saunders Company, 1984.

Crosby WM, Hill EC: Embryology of the müllerian duct system. Obstet Gynecol **20**:507, 1962.

Cushner IM: The management of cervical incompetence by pursestring suture. Am J Obstet Gynecol **87**:882, 1963.

Danforth DN: The fibrous nature of the human cervix and its relation to the isthmic segment in gravid and nongravid uteri. Am J Obstet Gynecol **53**:541, 1947.

Danforth DN, Buckingham JC, Roddick JW: Connective tissue changes incident to cervical effacement. Am J Obstet Gynecol 80:939, 1960.

Didolkar SM: Foley catheter and cervical cerclage. Miss Med J 35:846, 1986.

Dor J, Shaley J, Mashiach S, et al: Elective cervical suture of twin pregnancies diagnosed ultrasonically in the first trimester following induced ovulation. Gynecol Obstet Invest 13:55, 1982.

Dunn LJ, Robinson JC, Steer CM: Maternal death following suture of incompetent cervix during pregnancy. Am J Obstet Gynecol 78:335, 1959.

Floyd WS: Cervical dilatation in the midtrimester of pregnancy. Obstet Gynecol 18:380, 1961.

Frieden FJ, Ordorica SA, Hoskins IA, et al: The Shirodkar operation: A reappraisal. Am J Obstet Gynecol 163:830, 1990.

Ger JO, Rogo KO, Sinei SK: Cervical incompetence: assessment of a scoring system for patient selection of cervical cerclage. Int J Gynecol Obstet 34:325, 1991.

Goldstein DP: Incompetent cervix in offspring exposed to diethylstilbestrol in utero. Obstet Gynecol (Suppl) 52:735, 1978.

Goodlin RC: Cervical incompetence, hourglass membranes and amniocentesis. Obstet Gynecol 54:748, 1979.

Grant A: Cervical cerclage: Evaluation studies. In Proceedings of a Workshop on Prevention of Preterm Birth. Paris, INSERM, 1986.

Haning RV Jr, Steinetz B, Weiss G: Elevated serum relaxin levels in multiple pregnancy after menotropin treatment. Obstet Gynecol 66:42, 1985.

Harger JH: Comparison of success and morbidity in cervical cerclage procedures. Obstet Gynecol 56:543, 1980.

Harger JH: Cervical cerclage: Patient selection, morbidity and success rates. Clin Perinatol 10:321, 1983.

Harger JH, Archer DF, Marchese SM, et al: Etiology of recurrent pregnancy losses and outcome of subsequent pregnancies. Obstet Gynecol 62:574, 1983.

Heinonen PK, Saarikoski S, Pystynen P: Reproductive performance of women with uterine anomalies. Acta Obstet Gynecol Scand 61:157, 1982.

Herbst AL, Cole P: Epidemiologic and clinical aspects of clear cell adenocarcinoma in young women. In Herbst AL (ed): Intrauterine Exposure to Diethylstilbestrol in the Human. American College of Obstetricians and Gynecologists, Proceedings of Symposium on DES, 1978.

Herman GE: Notes on Emmet operation as a prevention of abortion. J Obstet Gynaecol Br Commonw 2:256, 1902.

Herron MA, Parer JT: Transabdominal cerclage for fetal wastage due to cervical incompetence. Obstet Gynecol 71:865, 1988.

Hofmeister FJ, Schwartz WR, Vondrak BF, et al: Suture reinforcement of the incompetent cervix. Am J Obstet Gynecol 101:58, 1968.

Holman MR: An aid for cervical cerclage. Obstet Gynecol 42:478, 1973.

Hortenstine JS, Witherington R: Ulcer of the trigone: A late complication of cervical cerclage. J Urol 137:109, 1987.

Hulka JF, Higgins G: Trauma to the internal cervical os during dilatation for diagnostic curettage. Am J Obstet Gynecol 82:913, 1961.

Jackson G, Pendleton HJ, Nichol B, Wittmann BK: Diagnostic ultrasound in the assessment of patients with incompetent cervix. Br J Obstet Gynaecol 91:232, 1984.

Jennings CL: Temporary submucosal cerclage for cervical incompetence. Report of 48 cases. Am J Obstet Gynecol 113:1097, 1972.

Johnstone FD, Beard RJ, Boyd JE, et al: Cervical diameter after suction termination of pregnancy. Br Med J 1:68, 1976.

Jones JM, Sweetnam P, Hibbard BM: The outcome of pregnancy after cone biopsy of the cervix: A case control study. Br J Obstet Gynaecol 86:913, 1979.

Kaufman RH, Adam E: Genital tract anomalies associated with in utero exposure to diethylstilbestrol. Isr J Med Sci 14:347, 1978.

Kaufman RH, Binder GL, Gray PM, et al: Upper genital tract changes associated with exposure in utero to diethylstilbestrol. Am J Obstet Gynecol 128:51, 1977.

Kaufman RH, Adam E, Binder GL, et al: Upper genital tract changes and pregnancy outcome in offspring exposed in utero to diethylstilbestrol. Am J Obstet Gynecol 137:299, 1980.

Kaufman RH, Noller K, Adam E, et al: Upper genital tract abnormalities and pregnancy outcome in diethylstilbestrol-exposed progeny. Am J Obstet Gynecol 148:973, 1984.

Keirse MJN, Rush RH, Anderson ABM, Turnbull AC: Risk of preterm delivery in patients with previous preterm delivery and/ or abortion. Br J Obstet Gynaecol 85:81, 1978.

Kelly TF, Troyer LR, Piacquadio KM, et al: Predictors of success in the emergent cerclage. Am J Obstet Gynecol 166:398, 1992.

Kleissl HP, Van der Rest M, Naftolin F, et al: Collagen changes in the human uterine cervix at parturition. Am J Obstet Gynecol 130:748, 1978.

Kokia E, Dor J, Blankenstein J, et al.: A simple scoring system for the treatment of cervical incompetence diagnosed during the second trimester. Gynecol Obstet Invest 31:12, 1991.

Kuhn RJP, Pepperell RJ: Cervical ligation: A review of 242 pregnancies. Aust N Z J Obstet Gynaecol 17:79, 1977.

Laing FC: Ultrasound Evaluation of Obstetric Problems Relating to the Lower Uterine Segment and Cervix. In Sanders PC, James AE (eds): The Principles and Practice of Ultrasonography in Obstetrics and Gynecology. Norwalk, CT, Appleton Century-Crofts, 1985.

Lash AF: Fertility and reproduction following repair of the incompetent internal os of the cervix. Fertil Steril 11:531, 1960.

Lash AF, Lash SR: Habitual abortion: The competent internal os of the cervix. Am J Obstet Gynecol 59:68, 1950.

Lauersen NH, Fuchs F: Experience with Shirodkar's operation and postoperative alcohol treatment. Acta Obstet Gynaecol Scand 52:77, 1973.

Lazar P, Gueguen S: Multicentred controlled trial of cervical cerclage in women at moderate risk of preterm delivery. Br J Obstet Gynaecol 91:731, 1984.

Lees DH, Sutherst JR: The sequelae of cervical trauma. Am J Obstet Gynecol 120:1050, 1974.

Leppert PC, Keller S, Cerreta J, et al: Conclusive evidence for the presence of elastin in human and monkey cervix. Am J Obstet Gynecol 142:179, 1982.

Leppert PC, Yu SY, Keller S, et al: Decreased elastic fibers and desmosine content in incompetent cervix. Am J Obstet Gynecol 157:1134, 1987.

Lindberg BS: Maternal sepsis, uterine rupture, and coagulopathy complicating cervical cerclage. Acta Obstet Gynaecol Scand 58:317, 1979.

Ludmir J, Landon MB, Gabbe SG, Mennuti MT: A prospective study of cerclage in the DES-exposed pregnant patient. Am J Obstet Gynecol 157:665, 1987.

Mangan CE, Borow L, Burtnett-Rubin MM, et al: Pregnancy outcome in 98 women exposed to diethylstilbestrol in utero, their mothers, and unexposed siblings. Obstet Gynecol 59:315, 1982.

Mann EC, McLaren WD, Hoyt OB: The physiology and clinical significance of the uterine isthmus. Am J Obstet Gynecol 81:209, 1961.

McDonald IA: Suture of the cervix for inevitable miscarriage. J Obstet Gynaecol Br Commonw 64:346, 1957.

McDonald IA: Cervical cerclage. Clin Obstet Gynaecol 7:461, 1980.

Michaels WH, Montgomery C, Karo J, et al: Ultrasound differentiation of the competent from the incompetent cervix: Prevention of preterm delivery. Am J Obstet Gynecol 154:537, 1986.

MRC/RCOG Working Party on Cervical Cerclage. Interim report of the Medical Research Council/Royal College of Obstetricians and Gynaecologists multicentre randomized trial of cervical cerclage. Br J Obstet Gynaecol 95:437, 1988.

Novy MJ: Managing reproductive failure by transabdominal isthmic cerclage. Contemp Obstet Gynecol 10:17, 1977.

Novy MJ: Transabdominal cervicoisthmic cerclage for the management of repetitive abortion and premature delivery. Am J Obstet Gynecol 143:44, 1982.

Novy MJ: Combating recurrent abortion and premature delivery with cervical cerclage. Contemp Obstet Gynecol Special Issue, 1985, p. 113.

Novy MJ, Ducsay CA, Stanczyk FZ: Plasma concentrations of prostaglandin F_{2a} and prostaglandin E_2 metabolites after transabdominal and transvaginal cervical cerclage. Am J Obstet Gynecol 156:1543, 1987.

Nunley WC, Kitchin JD: Successful management of incompetent cervix in a primigravida exposed to diethylstilbestrol in utero. Fertil Steril 31:217, 1979.

Olatunbosun OA, Dyck F: Cervical cerclage operation for a dilated cervix. Obstet Gynecol 57:166, 1981.

Orr C: An aid to cervical cerclage. Aust NZ J Obstet Gynaecol **13**:114, 1973.

Oster S, Javert CT: Treatment of the incompetent cervix with the Hodge pessary. Obstet Gynecol **28**:206, 1966.

Palmer R, LaComme JL: La béance de l'orifice interne, cause d'avortment a repetition une observation de dechirure cervico-isthmique repare chirugicalement, avec gestation a term consec-utive. Gynecol Obstet (Paris) **47**:905, 1948.

Parikh MN, Mehta AC: Internal cervical os during the second half of pregnancy. J Obstet Gynaecol Br Commonw **68**:818, 1961.

Parulekar SG, Kiwi R: Ultrasound evaluation of sutures following cervical cerclage for incompetent cervix uteri. J Ultrasound Med **1**:223, 1982.

Peters WA, Thiagarajah S, Harbert GM: Cervical cerclage: Twenty years experience. South Med J **72**:933, 1979.

Peterson PG, Keifer WS: Diagnosis of an incompetent internal cervical os. Am J Obstet Gynecol **116**:498, 1973.

Pinto RM, Rabow W, Votta RA: Uterine cervix ripening in term pregnancy due to the action of estradiol 17B. Am J Obstet Gynecol **92**:319, 1965.

Rana J, Davis SE, Harrington JT: Improving the outcome of cervical cerclage by sonographic follow-up. J Ultrasound Med **9**:275, 1990.

Repke JT, Niebyl JR: Role of prostaglandin synthetase inhibitors in the treatment of preterm labor. Semin Reprod Endocrinol **3**:259, 1985.

Rivera-Alsina ME, Saldana LR, Arias JW: Nonsurgical treatment of cervical incompetence. Texas Med **79**:40, 1983.

Robboy MS: The management of cervical incompetence. Obstet Gynecol **41**:108, 1973.

Robboy SJ, Noller KJ, Kaufman RT, et al: An Atlas of Findings in the Human Female After Intrauterine Exposure to Diethylstilbes-trol. Washington, DC, US Department of Health and Human Services, National Institutes of Health, 1983.

Robichaux III AG, Stedman CM, Hamer C: Uterine activity in patients with cervical cerclage. Obstet Gynecol **76**:63S, 1990.

Rock JA, Murphy AA: Anatomic abnormalities. Clin Obstet Gynecol **29**:886, 1986.

Rorie DK, Newton M: Histological and chemical studies of the smooth muscle in human cervix and uterus. Am J Obstet Gynecol **99**:466, 1967.

Rush RW: Incidence of preterm delivery in patients with previous preterm delivery and/or abortion. South Afr Med J **56**:1085, 1979.

Rush RW, Issacs S, McPherson K, et al: A randomized controlled trial of cervical cerclage in women at high risk of spontaneous delivery. Br J Obstet Gynaecol **91**:724, 1984.

Sandberg EC: Benign cervical and vaginal changes associated with exposure to stilbestrol in utero. Am J Obstet Gynecol **125**:777, 1976.

Sandberg EC, Riffle NL, Higdon JV, et al: Pregnancy outcome in women exposed to diethylstilbestrol *in utero.* Am J Obstet Gynecol **140**:194, 1981.

Sarti DA, Sample WF, Hobel CJ, Staisch KJ: Ultrasonic visualization of a dilated cervix during pregnancy. Radiology **130**:417, 1979.

Schaffner F, Schanzer SN: Cervical dilatation in the early third trimester. Obstet Gynecol **27**:130, 1966.

Schuly KF, Grimes DA, Cates W Jr: Measures to prevent cervical injury during suction curettage abortion. Lancet **1**:1182, 1983.

Scully RE, Robboy SJ, Welch WR: Pathology and pathogenesis of diethylstilbestrol. Related disorders of the female genital tract. *In* Herbst AL (ed): Intrauterine Exposure to Diethylstilbestrol in the Human. American College of Obstetricians and Gynecologists, Proceedings of a Symposium on DES, Chicago, 1978.

Seppala M, Vara P: Cervical cerclage in the treatment of incompetent cervix. Acta Obstet Gynaecol Scand **49**:343, 1970.

Sheerer LJ, Lam L, Katz M: A new technique for cervical cerclage in the presence of prolapsed fetal membranes. Orlando, Society for Perinatal Obstetricians, 1987.

Sherman AI: Hormonal therapy for control of the incompetent os of pregnancy. Obstet Gynecol **28**:198, 1966.

Shirodkar VN: A new method of operative treatment for habitual abortions in the second trimester of pregnancy. Antiseptic **52**:299, 1955.

Shirodkar VN: Long-term results with the operative treatment of habitual abortion. Triangle **8**:123, 1967.

Singer MS, Hochman M: Incompetent cervix in a hormone-exposed offspring. Obstet Gynecol **51**:625, 1978.

Smith SC, Scragg WH: Premature cervical dilatation and the Mc-Donald cerclage. Obstet Gynecol **33**:533, 1969.

Stillman RJ: In utero exposure to diethylstilbestrol: Adverse effects on the reproductive tract and reproductive performance in male and female offspring. Am J Obstet Gynecol **142**:905, 1982.

Stromme WB, Wagner RM, Reed SC: Surgical management of the incompetent cervix. Obstet Gynecol **15**:635, 1960.

Tho PT, Byrd JR, McDonough PG: Etiologies and subsequent reproductive performance in 100 couples with recurrent abortion. Fertil Steril **32**:389, 1979.

Thurston JC: Rupture of uterus following Shirodkar suture. Br Med J **2**:1293, 1963.

Toaff R, Toaff ME, Ballas S, et al: Cervical incompetence: Diagnostic and therapeutic aspects. Isr J Med Sci **13**:39, 1977.

Toplis PJ, Shephard JH, Youssefniejadian E, et al: Plasma prosta-glandin concentrations after cerclage in early pregnancy. Br J Obstet Gynaecol **87**:669, 1980.

Ulmsten U: Complication of cervical cerclage. Lancet **2**:1350, 1977.

Varma TR, Patel RH, Pillai U: Ultrasonic assessment of cervix in "at risk" patients. Int J Gynaecol Obstet **25**:25, 1987.

Vitsky M: The incompetent cervical os and the pessary. Am J Obstet Gynecol **87**:144, 1963.

Von Maillot KV, Zimmermann BK: The solubility of collagen of the uterine cervix during pregnancy and labour. Arch Gynaekol **220**:275, 1976.

Wallenburg HCS, Lotgering FK: Transabdominal cerclage for closure of the incompetent cervix. Eur J Obstet Reprod Biol **25**:121, 1987.

Watkins RA: Transabdominal cervico-uterine suture. Aust NZ J Obstet Gynaecol **12**:62, 1972.

Weekes ARL, Menzies DN, de Boer CH: The relative efficacy of bed rest, cervical suture, and no treatment in the management of twin pregnancy. Br J Obstet Gynaecol **84**:61, 1977.

Wheelock JB, Johnson TRB, Graham D, et al: Ultrasound-assisted cervical cerclage. J Clin Ultrasound **12**:307, 1984.

Yosowitz EE, Haufrect F, Kaufman RH, et al: Silicone-plastic cuff for the treatment of the incompetent cervix in pregnancy. Am J Obstet Gynecol **113**:233, 1972.

CHAPTER

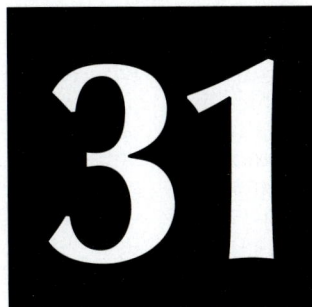

IMMUNOLOGIC DISORDERS

．．．．．．．．．．．．．．．．．．．．．．．．

JAMES R. SCOTT, M.D., and D. WARE BRANCH, M.D.

Research advances in reproductive immunology now being applied clinically represent new and rapidly changing areas in the modern practice of maternal-fetal medicine. The purpose of this chapter is to incorporate scientifically sound guidelines into a practical clinical approach to perinatal problems of alloimmune and autoimmune etiology.

ALLOIMMUNE PREGNANCY LOSS

Clinical spontaneous abortion is the most common complication of human pregnancy, with approximately 2 to 5 per cent of couples suffering recurrent early losses. Because the majority of patients have no demonstrable reason for their repetitive miscarriages, it has long been suspected that alloimmune factors may be responsible. Since the conceptus is immunogenetically foreign, one might intuitively predict that the early fetoplacental unit would routinely be rejected from its implantation site in the immunologically dynamic female reproductive tract. Predominant theories hold that rejection does not occur because the semi-allogeneic conceptus evokes an immunotolerant response from the mother that results in successful implantation and growth (Wegmann, 1984; Athanassakis et al., 1987; Clark and Chaouat, 1989) (see Chapter 6). Conversely, a defective maternal immune response leads to spontaneous abortion.

Over the past decade, reproductive immunologists have interpreted data from a variety of studies as evidence for alloimmune causes of recurrent miscarriage. Parental sharing of human leukocyte antigens (HLA) or trophoblast-lymphocyte cross-reacting (TLX) antigens were originally linked to habitual abortion (Beer et al., 1981; McIntyre et al., 1983). It was proposed that the mechanisms normally leading to successful pregnancy were not triggered because the pregnant woman failed to immunologically recognize the implanting fetoplacental unit. Therefore, the maternal alloimmune system rejected the conceptus much in the same manner as any allograft rejection. There are inconsistencies with this once popular concept since histocompatibility between donor and host is usually associated with a decreased risk of immu-

nologic rejection of transplanted organs. Some have suggested that antipaternal leukocytotoxic antibodies must be present for the success of early pregnancy (Mowbray et al., 1985), but this assertion has not been confirmed by other investigators. In reality, most couples with recurrent pregnancy loss (RPL) are histoincompatible, and only a small percentage of pregnant women make antibodies directed against paternal HLA. It is doubtful, therefore, that either HLA typing or tests for maternal antipaternal cytotoxic antibodies are useful markers in the clinical management of RPL (Scott, 1989; Ho et al., 1991).

Current hypotheses to explain alloimmune causes of pregnancy loss now center on two general categories: (1) abnormalities in molecular events at the maternal-fetal interface, or (2) a lack of necessary peripheral immunosuppressive factors in the maternal circulation.

Local Events

Transformation of endometrial stromal cells into decidual cells, as well as the invading trophoblast at the fetomaternal junction, seems to play a key role in the successful implantation and subsequent development of the embryo (Clark et al., 1991; Mori et al., 1992). Throughout the menstrual cycle and pregnancy, variable numbers of macrophages and lymphocytes are present in the endometrium and decidua (Daya et al., 1985). Also present are a heterologous group of larger, granular, non-T-cell lymphocytes that express *in vitro* natural killer, natural suppressor, and antibody-dependent and -independent allogeneic cytotoxicity (Redman et al., 1991).

Cytokines appear to be the principal language of the trophoblast/decidua system, but other bioactive substances produced by the endometrium (e.g., hormones, enzymes, growth factors, and endometrial proteins) may be important. Certain products of activated lymphocytes and macrophages appear to be immunosuppressive; some are probably important for implantation, growth, and development of the early placenta and embryo (immunotropic) (Wegmann, 1984); and others may cause abortion when expressed

467

(immunodystrophic) (Clark et al., 1986; Toder et al., 1990; Anderson et al., 1991). Supernatants from decidual cell suspensions contain factors capable of blocking the action of Il-2, which is the primary mediator of cytotoxic lymphocytes. This activity at the maternal-fetal interface is believed to direct an immunosuppressive response, thereby safeguarding the conceptus from immune attack (Daya et al., 1987). Conditioned media from decidual biopsies from missed abortions in humans have been reported to be deficient in suppressor cell activity as compared with biopsies from presumably normal pregnancies (Daya et al., 1985). However, the lack of class I major histocompatability complex (MHC) antigens on syncytiotrophoblast, together with the atypical nature of HLA antigen expression on extravillous cytotrophoblast and the complete absence of class II MHC determinants on either trophoblast layer, seems to preclude trophoblast involvement, either as a classic immunogen for maternal sensitization or as a target for MHC-directed cytotoxic T cells. Nevertheless, certain products of immune cells have adverse effects on fetal tissues if present during specific intervals of development. For example, class I MHC antigen expression may be induced by gamma interferon (γ-INF). Theoretically, secretion of γ-INF by lymphocytes in the endometrium of some women could induce class I MHC antigen expression, providing a mechanism for cytotoxic lymphocyte attack that culminates in abortion (Feinman et al., 1987). Granulocyte-macrophage colony-stimulating factor (GM-CSF), which is present in decidual cell supernatants, enhances trophoblast growth and prevents spontaneous fetal resorption (Chaouat et al., 1990), whereas injections of tumor necrosis factor (TNF) dramatically increase the per cent of fetal resorptions in animal models (Berkowitz et al., 1988). The interrelationship of these molecular changes in the pre-implantation endometrium and decidua has not been thoroughly studied in the human. Consequently, this is a rapidly developing area of research, but there are currently no practical clinical tests available for these factors.

Circulating Suppressive Factors

One popular concept to explain maternal immunotolerance of the fetus proposes that maternal serum factors inhibit cell-mediated immune function. The basis for this hypothesis centers on three important suppositions: (1) there is a maternal cellular immune response to the conceptus in all pregnancies that must be blocked, (2) circulating blocking antibodies develop in all successful pregnancies, and (3) the absence of blocking antibodies is associated with spontaneous abortion. Although blocking antibodies and other pregnancy-maintaining factors in maternal peripheral blood have been widely accepted as necessary for normal pregnancy, they have never been well characterized biochemically or immunologically. Although the antigens against which they are directed remain unclear, these antibodies or factors could theoretically function in one of several ways to prevent rejection of the fetus. The antibodies could be directed against maternal lymphocytes to prevent them from reacting with receptors on fetoplacental tissues, or they could react with antigen-specific receptors on the fetoplacental semi-allograft and block recognition of the foreign antigens by maternal lymphocytes. Another possibility is that blocking factors are anti-idiotypic antibodies directed against the antigen-specific combining sites (idiotypes) on other antibodies (Burlingham, 1988). Similar idiotypes function as antigen receptors on the surface of T lymphocytes. Therefore, anti-idiotypic antibodies would bind to antigen receptors and prevent maternal lymphocytes from interacting with the target cells of the conceptus.

Blocking factors are usually identified by *in vitro* tests such as the mixed lymphocyte reaction (MLR). However, the clinician should be aware of several pitfalls with these assays: (1) a wide variability in the proliferative response has been found among different patients and between the same couples tested at different times, (2) no uniform method exists for reporting the results, and (3) the presence of blocking factors is dependent on the equation used for calculation of MLR data (Park et al., 1990).

A number of studies have reported the presence of blocking antibodies in women with successful pregnancies and their absence in women with recurrent pregnancy loss (RPL) (Rocklin et al., 1976; Stimson et al., 1979). Investigators have also found that sera from women with RPL inhibit the development of *in vitro* mouse preimplantation embryos (Abir et al., 1990; Hill et al., 1992) and that a lymphocyte-derived, progesterone-induced blocking factor has an antiabortive effect (Szekeres-Bartho and Chaouat, 1990). However, others have cast doubt on the importance of this information because (1) blocking antibodies frequently do not appear until late in the first or second trimester of the first pregnancy (Rocklin et al., 1982), (2) agammaglobulinemic women have normal pregnancies (Zak and Good, 1959; Holland and Holland, 1966; Kobayashi et al., 1980), and (3) animals rendered incapable of producing immunoglobulins or mounting a humoral immune response also have successful pregnancies (Rodger, 1985).

In summary, there is currently no consensus on which tests that have been advocated to detect immunologic abnormalities in couples with recurrent miscarriages are clinically important or how they should be used to determine which patients will benefit from immunologic treatment.

Immunotherapy

Even though no immunologic mechanism has yet been unequivocally proved to cause RPL in humans, a number of "immunotherapy" treatments have been advocated. There are many medical centers around the world that now offer immunization with paternal or donor leukocytes or with other fractions containing trophoblast antigens.

The rationale for immunotherapy is borrowed from transplantation medicine, where studies in animals and humans suggest that such immunizations may induce a beneficial immunosuppression. Prior to the

TABLE 31–1. Results of Immunotherapy in Recurrent Abortion Patients

INVESTIGATOR	CELL SOURCE	ROUTE	PATIENTS	LIVE BIRTHS
Beer, 1988	Paternal	ID	121	100 (83%)
Mowbray et al., 1987	Paternal	ID, SC, IV	244	181 (74%)
Takakuwa et al., 1990	Paternal	ID	42	33 (78%)
Smith and Cowchock, 1988	Paternal	ID, SC, IV	58	29 (50%)
Carp et al., 1990	Paternal	ID, SC, IV	81	61 (75%)
Alexander et al., 1988	Paternal	ID, SC, IV	30	24 (80%)
Reznikof-Etievant, 1988	Paternal	ID, SC, IV	35	30 (80%)
McIntyre et al., 1986	Third party	IV	23	20 (87%)
Unander and Lindholm, 1986	Third party	IV	105	100 (95%)
Beer, 1988	Third party	ID	21	15 (71%)
Johnson et al., 1988	Trophoblast	IV	21	16 (76%)
Peters and Coulam, 1990	IVIgG	IV	4	3 (75%)
Mueller-Echardt et al., 1991	IVIgG	IV	38	27 (71%)
Totals			843	639 (76%)

ID = intradermal; SC = subcutaneous; IV = intravenous.

introduction of modern immunosuppressives, pretransplant blood transfusions in allograft recipients were used to decrease the risk of immunologic rejection (Opelz and Terasaki, 1980). Long-term survival of kidney grafts is reportedly increased with either donor-specific or third-party blood; the buffy coat appears to be responsible for this beneficial effect (Norman et al., 1986). Although the exact mechanism of immunosuppression in transplant patients is unknown, several possibilities exist (Sollinger et al., 1984). Leukocyte immunizations induce MLR-blocking antibodies (Nagarkatti et al., 1983; Singal et al., 1983), which some have found to be anti-idiotypic in nature (Takeuchi et al., 1985; Singal et al., 1983). Immunizations may also generate peripheral suppressor T cells (Takeuchi et al., 1985; Leivestad and Thorsby, 1984). In animal models, the rate of fetal resorptions or abortions is decreased by prior immunization with spleen cells or blood from a paternally related strain (Chaouat et al., 1988; Antezak and Allen, 1988). The immunizations correlate with the formation of anti-MHC antibodies (Chaouat et al., 1985), the recruitment of decidual suppressor cells (Clark, 1984; Clark et al., 1987), and the induction of MLR suppressor activity by decidual cell supernatants (Chaouat et al., 1985). This background information has led to similar clinical therapeutic approaches to improve the maternal immune response and to prevent rejection of the fetus in recurrent aborters.

A variety of immunization regimens have been utilized in the treatment of RPL patients for whom all nonimmunologic causes have been ruled out (Table 31–1) (Alexander et al., 1988; Beer, 1988; Carp et al., 1990; Johnson et al., 1988; McIntyre et al., 1986; Mowbray et al., 1985; Reznikoff-Etievant et al., 1988; Smith and Cowchock, 1988; Takakuwa et al., 1990; Unander and Lindholm, 1986), but only three have been prospective, randomized trials (Table 31–2) (Cauchi et al., 1991; Ho et al., 1991; Mowbray et al., 1985). Immunization with paternal lymphocytes has resulted in live birth rates of 50 to 83 per cent, whereas random donor leukocyte injections have produced successful pregnancy rates of 71 to 95 per cent. Whether these treatments result in higher live birth rates than in untreated pregnancies is still uncertain (Scott et al., 1987; Roman, 1984; Alberman, 1988). It must be remembered that there is a reasonable chance of a successful pregnancy (40 to 60 per cent) in unexplained recurrent aborters even without treatment. The conflicting results from prospectively randomized trials emphasize the need for further properly designed studies with larger numbers to confirm the value of immunotherapy in these patients. Moreover, similar rates of successful pregnancies have been achieved with other methods of treatment such as intravenous immune globulin (Mueller-Echardt et al., 1991, Peters and Coulam, 1990) and trophoblast membrane fractions (Johnson et al., 1988).

Although potential maternal and fetal risks are associated with immunization using any type of cells or blood products, remarkably few complications have been reported in hundreds of treated mothers or their offspring who have now been observed through childhood (Reginald et al., 1987). No one has reported

TABLE 31–2. Published, Prospective, Randomized Trials of Immunotherapy in Recurrent Abortion Patients

INVESTIGATOR	CELL SOURCE	ROUTE	PATIENTS	LIVE BIRTHS
Mowbray et al., 1985	Paternal	ID, SC, IV	22	17 (77%)
	Maternal	ID, SC, IV	27	10 (37%)
Ho et al., 1991	Paternal	ID	20	13 (65%)
	Third Party	ID	6	5 (83%)
	Maternal	ID	28	14 (50%)
Cauchi et al., 1991	Paternal	ID, SC, IV	21	13 (62%)
	Saline	ID, SC, IV	25	19 (76%)

ID = intradermal; SC = subcutaneous; IV = intravenous.

transfusion reactions, anaphylaxis, or viral infection in treated mothers, but one case each of maternal platelet alloimmunization, blood group sensitization, and cutaneous graft-versus-host-like reaction (Katz et al., 1992) have occurred. At the Third International Congress of Reproductive Immunology held in Toronto in 1986, investigators from around the world summarized the information available on the infants of immunized mothers. Adverse outcomes were rare but included placental abruption, placenta accreta, oligohydramnios, preeclampsia, fetal growth retardation, preterm delivery, renal anomalies, and trisomy 21 and 13, as well as an unusual case of an undefined neonatal immunodeficiency disease. Overall, the prevalence of fetal or neonatal problems has not been higher than one would expect compared to the general population of untreated recurrent miscarriage patients matched for age.

Immunotherapy for potential alloimmune causes of RPL justifiably remains controversial, and cautious interpretation of the results is warranted at this time. Currently, the diagnosis of alloimmune-mediated RPL is one of exclusion. There is no agreement among investigators regarding which patients should receive immunotherapy or how they might be identified, and there is also confusion as to what constitutes an appropriate response to immunotherapy. The major questions that remain are: (1) What is the actual success rate with and without immunotherapy? (2) Exactly which patients should be offered immunotherapy? (3) If effective, what is the optimal source of white cells and what is the best regimen? and (4) Are there any unanticipated long-term risks? Because of these questions, immunotherapy remains experimental at this time.

AUTOIMMUNE PREGNANCY LOSS

Antiphospholipid Antibodies and Antiphospholipid Syndrome

Antiphospholipid antibodies have become of great interest to obstetricians because they are now known to be associated with fetal loss. They are acquired autoantibodies, induced by an unknown process, which are directed against negatively charged phospholipids abundantly distributed in cell membranes.

Originally, a peculiar circulating anticoagulant was described in two patients which prolonged the prothrombin time and did not correct in a mixture with normal plasma (Conley and Hartmann, 1952). Since no bleeding tendency was found, the phenomenon was long considered to be a laboratory nuisance with no clinical implications. It was erroneously termed the lupus anticoagulant (LA) because it was encountered predominantly in patients with systemic lupus erythematosus (SLE) (Feinstein and Rapaport, 1972). The paradoxical thrombotic tendency associated with the circulating anticoagulant was recognized later. *In vitro* studies showed that LA was caused by antibodies reactive with phospholipids needed for the formation of the prothrombin-activator complex during the coagulation process and was also associated with false-positive biologic reactions for syphilis (Triplett, 1989). In tests for syphilis (e.g., VDRL), cardiolipin, a phospholipid derived from bovine hearts, is the main antigen. Subsequently, highly sensitive immunoassays for cardiolipin were developed, which demonstrated that LA and anticardiolipin antibodies (aCL) are closely related (McNeil et al., 1989). Therefore, the term "antiphospholipid antibodies" (aPL) is now used as the most appropriate nomenclature for this heterogeneous group of antibodies.

A tremendous number of papers on aPL have appeared in the literature during the past decade, and this continues to be one of the most significant new areas of research in reproductive immunology. Clinical correlations with thrombosis, fetal loss, thrombocytopenia, ischemic brain disease, valvular heart disease, and livedo reticularis have been found for both LA and aCL, not only in SLE patients but also in patients with no apparent underlying disease. This heterogenous clinical picture combined with the presence of antiphospholipid antibodies is now known as the antiphospholipid syndrome (APS), and this is what is encountered most frequently in obstetric patients. To be classified as having APS, a patient must fulfill the clinical and laboratory criteria outlined in Table 31–3.

Laboratory Determination and Interpretation

Antibodies designated aPL can be regarded as a family of related autoantibodies that have different specificities and are defined by different laboratory tests.

Unfortunately, there is no international agreement on the determination of LA. Three major criteria are necessary for the diagnosis: (1) an abnormal phospholipid-dependent coagulation reaction, (2) proof that this abnormality is due to an inhibitor of clotting rather than a factor deficiency, and (3) evidence that the inhibitor activity is directed at phospholipids and not to specific coagulation proteins (Triplett, 1989). Phospholipid-dependent coagulation tests include the activated partial thromboplastin time (APTT), kaolin clotting time (KCT), and dilute Russell viper venom time (dRVVT) (Brandt et al., 1987; Margolis, 1958; Thiagarajan et al., 1986). Prolongation of the clotting

TABLE 31–3. Clinical and Laboratory Criteria for the Antiphospholipid Syndrome (APS)

CLINICAL FEATURES	LABORATORY FEATURES
Pregnancy loss	Lupus anticoagulant (LA)
Fetal death	
Recurrent pregnancy loss	
Thrombosis	Anticardiolipin antibodies
Venous	IgG, medium- or high-positive
Arterial, including stroke	
Autoimmune thrombocytopenia	
Other	Anticardiolipin antibodies
Coombs' positive hemolytic	IgM, medium- or high-positive
anemia	and LA
Livedo reticularis	

Patients with APS should have at least one clinical and one laboratory feature at some time in the course of their disease. Laboratory tests should be positive on at least two occasions more than 8 weeks apart.

time of these tests must persist after addition of an equal volume of normal plasma in order to exclude factor deficiencies. Phospholipid specificity is proved by a progressive increase in partial thromboplastin time upon dilution of thromboplastin or by a decrease in the test system (platelet neutralization procedure) (Triplett et al., 1983). Although there is a great deal of controversy over which test to use, the advantages of the APTT are its availability and the fact that most physicians are familiar with its interpretation (Triplett, 1989).

The immunoassay for aCL is a standardized test using sera from the Antiphospholipid Standardization Laboratory in Louisville, Kentucky. Results are calibrated against these standards and determined as GPL (IgG aCL) or MPL (IgM aCL) units, which should be reported in semiquantitative terms as either negative, low-positive, medium-positive, or high-positive (Harris, 1990). Most low-positive IgG and isolated IgM results in the absence of LA are considered analogous to a low false-positive antinuclear antibody titer (ANA) and are of questionable clinical significance (Harris et al., 1986; Branch, 1991). Recent work suggests that all binding may depend on a serum cofactor (Galli et al., 1990; McNeil et al., 1990; Matsuura et al., 1990).

Although the majority of patients have LA and aCL, they are not always concordant in a given patient. At least 79 per cent of patients with LA have aCL (Branch et al., 1987; Triplett, 1989); fewer patients with aCL have LA, although the overlap increases at progressively higher levels of aCL. Therefore, when considering the diagnosis of APS, the physician should obtain both a coagulation assay sensitive for the detection of LA and an immunoassay for aCL performed in a reliable laboratory.

Prevalence

During pregnancy, aPL antibody levels are not significantly different from nonpregnant levels (Sammaritano et al., 1990); less than 2 per cent of normal pregnant females have IgG aCL and less than 4 per cent have IgM aCL (Harris and Spinnato, 1991). In this population, over 80 per cent of the positive results were in the low-positive range, with only 0.2 per cent of IgG and 0.7 per cent of IgM results in the clinically significant medium- or high-positive range. Other studies have also confirmed the relatively small proportion of positive results in unselected obstetric patients (Branch and Scott, 1992a; Lockwood et al., 1989). For this reason, aPL testing in the general population as a screening test for pregnancy complications seems unwarranted. In contrast, testing for aPL in patients with recurrent pregnancy loss or fetal deaths is more productive since the prevalence of positive results is approximately 10 per cent (Petri et al., 1987; Parke et al., 1991; Out et al., 1991a; Branch and Scott, 1991). Indications for testing in the obstetric population are shown in Table 31–4.

The prevalence of aPL antibodies in patients with SLE is approximately 30 to 40 per cent (Feinstein, 1985; Harris et al., 1985; Triplett et al., 1985). The fetal loss rate in patients with SLE and aPL is 73 per cent, compared to 19 per cent in SLE patients without aPL.

TABLE 31–4. Indications for Anticardiolipin and Lupus Anticoagulant Test in Obstetric Population*

1. SLE or other autoimmune disease
2. Unexplained second- or third-trimester pregnancy losses
3. Recurrent first-trimester fetal losses
4. Presence or history of unexplained thrombocytopenia
5. History of unexplained venous thrombosis or pulmonary embolus
6. History of unexplained stroke, transient ischemic attacks, myocardial infarction, or other arterial occlusion
7. False-positive VDRL test
8. Abnormal PTT or PT test
9. Severe or early-onset atypical preeclampsia

*Diagnosis of antiphospholipid syndrome relies on criteria suggested in Table 31–3 and on the clinician's judgment.

However, well over half the women with APS who present with obstetric problems have no underlying autoimmune disease (Branch, 1991). The risk of fetal loss in patients without SLE but with LA or aCL is also high, with a wide variation in the reported prevalence (Petri et al., 1987; Edelman et al., 1986; Unander et al., 1985; Harris et al., 1986; Lockshin et al., 1989; Lubbe and Liggins, 1988; Triplett, 1989; Branch et al., 1992b). Differences in the methodology and sensitivity of LA and aCL assays between laboratories probably explain these divergent prevalences. In SLE patients, it has also been shown that fluctuations of aPL may occur during the course of the disease and influence prevalence rates in cross-sectional studies. Furthermore, patient selection accounts for some discrepancies. When studies on the prevalence of aPL in the absence of SLE include patients with thrombosis, recurrent fetal losses, or other clinical autoimmune stigmata, the prevalence increases. In other words, the firm relationship between fetal loss and aPL is only apparent in patients with a prior history of thrombosis, fetal loss, SLE, or other autoimmune manifestations.

Clinical Manifestations

It is now generally accepted that a small subset (5 to 10 per cent) of patients with pregnancy loss has significantly positive tests for aPL as the only recognizable explanation (or marker) for their problem. A history of mid-trimester fetal death (loss of pregnancy after the detection of fetal heart tones) appears to be a specific clue for APS. Ninety per cent of patients with aPL as the "cause" of their pregnancy loss experience at least one mid-trimester fetal death. The more consecutive pregnancy losses, the worse the prognosis is for future pregnancies.

It is again important to emphasize that many patients with APS do not have other diagnosed autoimmune diseases. However, aPL antibodies are associated with a variety of serious medical problems, including thromboembolic disease, stroke, and thrombocytopenia. Thirty to 50 per cent of women with APS have a history of thrombotic episodes, and over 80 per cent of the thrombotic events occur while the patient is pregnant or taking oral contraceptives (Branch et al., 1992b).

TABLE 31–5.   Summary of APS Pregnancies Treated with Prednisone and Low-Dose Aspirin

AUTHOR AND YEAR	NUMBER OF PREGNANCIES	SPONTANEOUS ABORTIONS	FETAL DEATHS*	LIVE BIRTHS
Lubbe and Liggins, 1988	18	NA	NA	15 (78%)
Gatenby et al., 1989	27	NA	NA	17 (63%)
Ordi et al., 1989	9	0	2 (22%)	7 (78%)
Lockshin et al., 1989	11	3 (27%)	6 (55%)	2 (18%)
Cowchock, 1991	19	NA	NA	13 (68%)
Reece et al., 1990	18	3 (17%)	1 (5%)	14 (78%)
Branch, 1992b	39	8 (21%)	8 (21%)	23 (59%)†

*Fetal deaths defined as intrauterine death of a fetus proven to be alive after 10 weeks' gestation.
†Includes two neonates that subsequently succumbed to complications of prematurity.

Pathogenesis

The mechanism of aPL, pregnancy loss, and thrombotic events has not been resolved. Placental thrombosis is a prominent feature in patients with APS, and decidual vessel thromboses, small placentas, and placental infarctions have all been reported (Nilsson et al., 1975; DeWolf et al., 1982; Out et al., 1991b). However, these lesions are nonspecific, and the degree of placental pathology is not always sufficient to explain the fetal death. The original hypothesis proposed an imbalance of local prostacyclin and thromboxane production, leading to vasoconstriction, platelet aggregation, and intravascular thrombosis (Carreras et al., 1981). Subsequent studies have not confirmed the original work (Haaselaar et al., 1988; Dudley et al., 1990). Other proposals for the thrombotic tendency include decreased activation of protein C (Cariou et al., 1986; Freyssinet and Cazenave, 1987), inhibition of fibrinolysis (Tsakiris et al., 1989), platelet activation (Weiner et al., 1991a), and decreased functional antithrombin III. Although animal studies strongly suggest a pathogenic role for aPL (Branch et al., 1990; Blank et al., 1991), it is still not certain whether these antibodies are the cause of fetal loss or simply represent epiphenomena reflecting other mechanisms of thrombosis.

Pregnancy Management

The presence of a positive test for aPL does not invariably indicate a poor prognosis, and some patients with APS have achieved successful pregnancies without specific medical therapy. Consequently, the physician should establish a well-documented history of previous unexplained fetal deaths or the presence of underlying autoimmune disease (SLE, APS) before considering therapy. However, many reports suggest that women with APS and previous pregnancy loss can be treated during the next pregnancy to improve the chance of delivering a live infant.

Prednisone (40 to 60 mg per day) and low-dose aspirin (80 mg per day), or in other doses or combinations, were initially used in pregnant patients with LA and eventually in patients with aCL; these results are summarized in Table 31–5. Direct comparison of these studies is virtually impossible because of the nature of the patients (e.g., SLE versus no SLE and numbers of previous fetal deaths) and their diagnoses (LA and aCL versus LA alone or aCL alone). Although no prospective randomized trials have been published, the pregnancy outcome was improved in all series but one.

Treatment with corticosteroids is potentially complicated by numerous minor side effects and by several serious adverse effects. Maternal side effects reported in the treatment of these pregnancies include gestational diabetes, hypertension, oropharyngeal candidiasis, facial acne, facial abscess, postpartum adrenal insufficiency, pneumonia, mycobacterial infection, osteoporosis leading to vertebral collapse, and osteonecrosis of the hip (Branch and Scott, 1991, Lubbe and Liggins, 1988).

The most attractive alternative to corticosteroids and low-dose aspirin treatment is subcutaneous heparin treatment, with or without low-dose aspirin. The results seem comparable to those achieved with corticosteroids (Table 31–6). The treatment regimen at the University of Utah includes one low-dose aspirin taken daily throughout pregnancy in an attempt to prevent or ameliorate preeclampsia. Treatment with subcutaneous heparin, 15,000 units daily, is begun after first-trimester documentation of a live fetus, and the dose is adjusted upward in the second trimester to achieve anticoagulation. The most significant risks are bleeding from trauma, heparin-induced osteoporosis, and idiosyncratic thrombocytopenia (Branch and Scott, 1991). Fortunately, the latter is uncommon in preg-

TABLE 31–6.   Summary of APS Pregnancies Treated with Heparin or Heparin and Low-Dose Aspirin

AUTHOR AND YEAR	NUMBER OF PREGNANCIES	SPONTANEOUS ABORTIONS	FETAL DEATHS*	LIVE BIRTHS
Rosove et al., 1987	15	NA	NA	14 (93%)
Cowchock, 1991	8	NA	NA	6 (75%)
Branch, 1992b	19	1 (5%)	2 (11%)	16 (84%)†

*Fetal deaths defined as intrauterine death of a fetus proven to be alive after 10 weeks' gestation.
†Includes two neonates that subsequently succumbed to complications of prematurity.

nancy (Kelton et al., 1988). To avoid osteoporosis, it may be helpful for women treated with either corticosteroids or heparin to take at least 1 gm of calcium daily and to exercise regularly. The concomitant use of corticosteroids and heparin should be avoided because this combination has not been shown to be better than either alone in achieving a live birth. Moreover, several cases of severe osteoporosis with fractures have occurred in women with APS treated with a combination regimen (Branch and Scott, 1991).

The use of low-dose aspirin (80 mg per day) alone has also been suggested, and preliminary results are promising (Tchobroutsky et al., 1988; Lockshin et al., 1989). These reports support the use of aspirin alone, particularly for women who are pregnant for the first time or are considered to be at low risk for fetal loss. Other therapeutic approaches that have been tried include intravenous immunoglobulin (Scott et al., 1988; Carreras et al., 1988; Parke et al., 1989; Wapner et al., 1989), plasma exchange (Frampton et al., 1987), and azathioprine (Gregorini et al., 1986), but none appear to be superior to the usual regimens.

Even with treatment, patients with APS frequently have complicated pregnancies. Therefore, careful antepartum management including serial monitoring for fetal growth and well-being are essential. Fetal loss may occur despite treatment, and complications include maternal thrombocytopenia, chorea gravidarum, severe early-onset preeclampsia, fetal growth retardation, fetal distress, and thrombotic episodes. The rather high rate of preeclampsia in patients with APS has prompted a search to determine whether APS may present or manifest itself as preeclampsia. In a series of patients with severe early-onset preeclampsia, 16 per cent were found to have significant levels of aPL (Branch et al., 1989). Three of these women suffered serious peripartum or postpartum sequelae including cerebral infarction, amaurosis fugax, transient global amnesia, deep venous thrombosis, pulmonary embolus, and autoimmune flare. Moreover, treatment of APS patients during pregnancy does not appear to markedly diminish the risk or severity of preeclampsia, which is often an important contributor to preterm delivery (Branch et al., 1992b). The typical sequence of fetal compromise develops as limitation of fetal growth, followed by abnormalities of the fetal heart rate tracing indicative of hypoxemia and decreased amniotic fluid volume (Druzin et al., 1987). With any of these findings, twice-weekly fetal cardiotocography and once-weekly ultrasonographic measurements of the amniotic fluid volume have been recommended as soon as delivery for fetal distress would be considered. The pregnancies of six untreated women with APS have also been successfully managed under close fetal surveillance with Doppler velocimetry (Trudinger et al., 1988), but this method of fetal surveillance remains controversial.

While close fetal monitoring is a key to successful pregnancy, the relative contribution of fetal surveillance versus pharmacologic treatment is yet to be determined. Even careful fetal surveillance cannot prevent fetal or neonatal death before 22 to 24 weeks gestation. Although preterm delivery is a common result of obstetric complications, children born to women treated for APS during pregnancy follow a course similar to that of infants born at the same gestational age (Pollard et al., 1992).

Several women with APS have developed similar features of an autoimmune flare in the postpartum period consisting of unexplained fever, pleurisy, pulmonary infiltrates, pleural effusion, thromboses, and cardiomyopathy (Kochenour et al., 1987). Perhaps the most dangerous feature is thrombosis, but the pleural-pulmonary disease is potentially life-threatening. After infection is thoroughly excluded, women with unexplained fever and pleural-pulmonary disease are treated with corticosteroids and supportive care. Finally, the role of long-term prophylactic aspirin or anticoagulation in nonpregnant patients with APS is unresolved. Certainly, this therapy should be considered in all patients who have already suffered a life-threatening thrombotic episode.

Subclinical Autoimmunity

Although other autoantibodies have also been suggested as the etiology of reproductive disorders, this is a less well-defined and more controversial entity. The idea that a "subclinical" autoimmune condition or polyclonal B lymphocyte abnormality may in some way cause other reproductive problems arose primarily from the observation that patients with RPL often have detectable levels of other autoantibodies in infertility (Gleicher, 1991). This has stimulated further interest in the role of these autoantibodies in infertility (Gleicher et al., 1989), endometriosis (Kennedy et al., 1989), preeclampsia, and fetal death. However, the literature in this area is marked by differences in autoantibody measurements, types of assays, and a variety of conclusions (Gleicher et al., 1987). Most published reports have focused on ANA, but other autoantibodies or autoimmune aberrations have also been implicated (Gleicher, 1991). Given the currently available data, it is difficult to support the routine performance of autoantibody "profiles" in the evaluation of patients with these disorders. The statistical chance of obtaining false-positive tests in normal patients increases with the number of tests performed, and no reasonable recommendation is currently available regarding the management of patients with positive tests (Branch, 1989).

IMMUNE THROMBOCYTOPENIA IN PREGNANCY

Immunologic thrombocytopenia can be broadly classified as two diseases with similar fetal but different maternal consequences: (1) autoimmune (formerly termed idiopathic) thrombocytopenic purpura (ATP), and (2) alloimmune (formerly termed isoimmune) thrombocytopenic purpura. An increased perinatal morbidity and mortality are associated with both disorders; however, maternal and neonatal thrombocytopenia can also be asymptomatic or result from other complications of pregnancy.

Thrombocytopenia in women is now frequently first

noted by the obstetrician on a complete blood count as part of routine automated prenatal screening tests. Despite conflicting reports, the normal values for platelet counts do not usually change significantly during pregnancy (Romero and Duffy, 1980; Sejeny et al., 1975). The mean antepartum platelet count for healthy pregnant women is 246,000/mm³; approximately 7.6 per cent will have a platelet count below 150,000/mm³, and fewer than 1 per cent will have a count below 100,000/mm³. The most common condition confused with autoimmune thrombocytopenic purpura during the last half of pregnancy is atypical preeclampsia or the HELLP syndrome. Since the thrombocytopenia often occurs first, this diagnosis should always be considered even with very subtle signs of preeclampsia. Thrombocytopenia may also signal the presence of AIDS, SLE, APS, sepsis, cocaine abuse, thrombotic thrombocytopenic purpura, transfusion reaction, or blood dyscrasias, or it may be drug-induced. In the neonate, thrombocytopenia is sometimes present in prematurity, in infection, and in infants born to women who are Rh immunized or are preeclamptic.

What constitutes a platelet count in an asymptomatic pregnant woman that is low enough for concern is a matter of controversy, but specific evaluation is usually not necessary unless the count is below 100,000/mm³. "Incidental" mild thrombocytopenia during pregnancy is fairly common, and the risk of severe neonatal thrombocytopenia in the offspring of women with no history of immune thrombocytopenia before pregnancy is minimal (Burrows et al., 1988a; Burrows and Kelton 1990; Samuels et al., 1990). The thrombocytopenia in these patients is often secondary to a laboratory artifact (pseudothrombocytopenia) such as platelet clumping induced by EDTA in the collection tube, clotting of blood samples because of improper techniques of blood withdrawal, or an inadequate amount of anticoagulant (Solanki and Blackburn, 1985; Payne and Pierre, 1984). Pseudothrombocytopenia due to EDTA-induced clumping, large platelets, or platelet cold agglutinins can be confirmed by examination of a stained peripheral blood smear. One method is to collect a finger-stick blood sample by using an ammonium oxalate Unopette (Bectin-Dickinson, Rutherford, New Jersey) and to count the blood cells by phase microscopy. The second method involves collection of an additional venous blood sample and anticoagulation of one test tube of blood with EDTA and another with 3.8 per cent sodium citrate. Smears are prepared from both vials, and platelet counts are determined on both test tubes. Once the diagnosis of pseudothrombocytopenia is established, no further treatment is needed for either mother or infant.

Autoimmune Thrombocytopenic Purpura

ATP is the most common autoimmune bleeding disorder encountered during pregnancy. The coexistence of ATP and pregnancy is fairly common since the disease usually presents in the second to third decade of life and has a female preponderance of 3:1.

It is characterized by the production of IgG antibodies directed against both maternal and fetal platelets. The spleen is a major site of antiplatelet antibody production (McMillan et al., 1972; Karpatkin, 1980), and the thrombocytopenia occurs as a result of increased platelet destruction. IgG antibody binds to the platelets and renders them more susceptible to sequestration and premature destruction in the reticuloendothelial system, and the rate of destruction exceeds the compensatory ability of the bone marrow to produce new platelets.

Both direct and indirect assays of antiplatelet antibodies have been developed. Approximately 90 per cent of patients with ATP have increased levels of bound immunoglobulins, primarily IgG, on the platelet surfaces. This platelet-associated IgG (PAIgG) correlates directly with the severity of thrombocytopenia in the mother but not in the fetus (Karpatkin, 1980; Kelton et al., 1982). Increased levels of unbound circulating antiplatelet antibody also may be present, but unbound antibody is less reliable as a predictor of thrombocytopenia in the mother or fetus (Karpatkin, 1980; Scott et al., 1980).

The overall course of ATP is not influenced significantly by pregnancy. However, pregnancy may be adversely affected by ATP, and the primary risk is hemorrhage in the peripartum period. Because the placenta selectively transports maternal IgG antiplatelet antibodies into the fetal circulation, fetal thrombocytopenia may also occur and result in hemorrhagic consequences.

Diagnosis

Most women with ATP have a history of easy bruising, petechiae, ecchymoses, or other bleeding manifestations (Fig. 31–1). The diagnosis is based on four findings: (1) a maternal platelet count repeatedly less than 100,000/mm³, with or without megathrombocytes on the peripheral smear; (2) bone marrow aspirate with normal or increased numbers of megakaryocytes; (3) exclusion of other diseases or drugs associated with thrombocytopenia; and (4) the absence of splenomegaly (Karpatkin, 1980; Kelton et al., 1982). The presence of antiplatelet antibodies is not strictly required for the diagnosis, but is confirmatory. The prothrombin time, partial thromboplastin time, and bleeding time are generally within normal limits.

Treatment

The goal of treatment in pregnancy is to minimize the risk of hemorrhage in both the mother and the fetus. Therapy should not necessarily focus on restoration of a normal platelet count.

CORTICOSTEROIDS. Glucocorticoid drugs are the cornerstone of therapy in pregnancy. Prednisone, 1 to 2 mg/kg per day, is given in divided doses for 2 to 3 weeks. A rise in platelet count to more than 50,000/mm³, accompanied by a decrease in clinical bleeding, is usually achieved within 21 days (Martin et al., 1984). Platelet response of some degree will be seen in more than 70 per cent of patients, with a complete remission achieved in up to 25 per cent

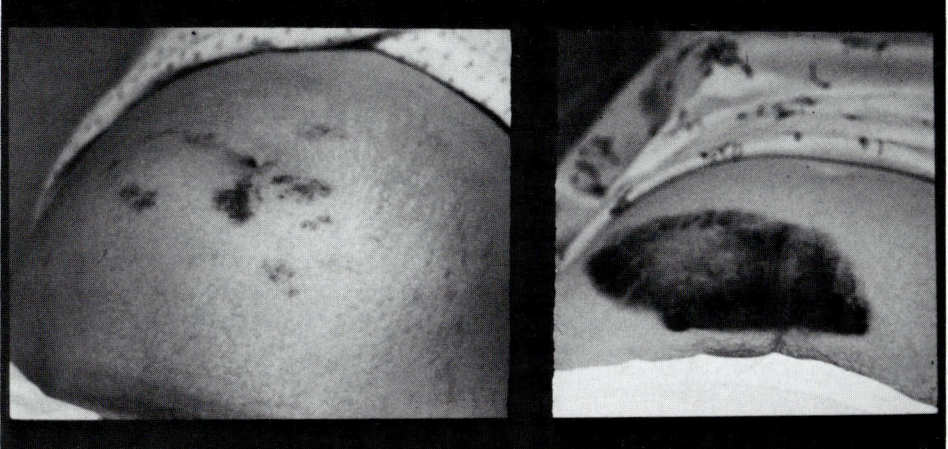

Figure 31–1. Two pregnant patients with ATP who sustained skin ecchymoses for minor trauma to the abdomen.

(Karpatkin, 1971). The corticosteroid dose is usually tapered by 10 to 20 per cent decrements at 2-week intervals, until the lowest dosage to maintain the platelet count above 50,000/mm³ is reached. Corticosteroids function therapeutically in four ways: (1) they decrease antiplatelet antibody production by the reticuloendothelial system; (2) they interfere with the interaction of antiplatelet antibody at the platelet surface and lead to a decrease in PAIgG; (3) they decrease the clearance of antibody-coated platelets by macrophages in the spleen and liver, effecting an increase in platelet survival; and (4) they improve abnormal capillary fragility (Martin et al., 1984). Dexamethasone and betamethasone, which easily cross the placenta, do not insure a normal fetal platelet count (Yin and Scott, 1985; Christiaens et al., 1990). The side effects of corticosteroids in pregnancy include steroid-induced moon facies, diabetes mellitus, psychosis, adrenocortical insufficiency, and osteoporosis.

SPLENECTOMY. This operation, which removes the site of destruction of damaged platelets as well as the major source of antibody production, is indicated in patients with ATP who are refractory to or unable to tolerate corticosteroids. A complete remission is obtained in 80 per cent of patients. The postsplenectomy platelet count increases rapidly and is often normal within 1 to 2 weeks (Karpatkin, 1971; Schwartz et al., 1980). In pregnant patients, the surgery is associated with a risk of spontaneous abortion or preterm labor and is technically difficult late in pregnancy. If splenectomy is unavoidable, surgery is best performed in the second trimester; however, it has also been combined safely with cesarean section at term. With careful preoperative preparation and surgical technique, operative morbidity and mortality are uncommon. Corticosteroids should be continued preoperatively and tapered postoperatively in splenectomy patients (McMillan, 1981). It is important to recognize that splenectomy does not always protect the fetus from thrombocytopenia because antibodies to platelets also are produced in other lymphoid tissues (Scott et al., 1983).

IMMUNOGLOBULIN. Immune globulin is a pooled concentrate of immunoglobulins collected from many donors. High doses of immune globulin (400 mg/kg

per day for 5 days) given intravenously (IVIgG) usually induce a peak platelet count within 7 to 9 days. More than 80 per cent of patients treated with this regimen will have a peak platelet count greater than 50,000/mm³; in 30 per cent of patients, the duration of the response lasts for more than 30 days (Imbach and Jungi, 1983; Bussel and Pham, 1987). While the mechanism of action is not clear, it seems to involve depression of antiplatelet antibody production, interference with antibody attachment to platelets, inhibition of macrophage receptor-mediated immune complex clearance, and interference with platelet receptor mechanisms in the reticuloendothelial system (Bussel and Pham, 1987; Barton and Saleh, 1987; Fehr et al., 1982). In responders, only 2 or 3 days of IVIgG therapy may be needed, and higher doses of 800 mg or 1 gm/kg may suffice as a single or double infusion (Newland, 1989). Although expensive, IVIgG therapy initiated 1 to 2 weeks prior to delivery or surgery is useful in obstetric patients who must undergo operative procedures or who develop bleeding problems and require emergency treatment. IgG is selectively transported across the placenta, and the amount transferred increases with gestational age and dose. Thus, maternally infused IgG may also have a beneficial fetal effect after 32 weeks of gestation (Sidiropoulous et al., 1986). However, it does not guarantee a normal platelet count in the fetus, as verified by the birth of thrombocytopenic infants following IgG administration to the mother. There have been no reports of HIV transmission with IVIgG, but adverse effects include thrombosis, alopecia, liver function disturbances, transient neutropenia, chills, nausea, flushing, tightness of the chest, wheezing, anaphylactic reactions in patients with IgA antibodies (Ben-Chetrit and Putterman, 1992), and occasional reports of non-A, non-B hepatitis from specific batches (Kurtzberg et al., 1987; Gutteridge et al., 1988). Therefore, the use of IVIgG should be carefully monitored and offered only for specific indications.

OTHER THERAPIES. The use of other agents has been reserved for patients who are refractory to corticosteroids and splenectomy. Those most commonly used—such as azathioprine, cyclophosphamide, vinca alkaloids, and danazol—are to be avoided in pregnancy because of their toxicity and potential adverse effects on the fetus (Warkentin and Kelton, 1990; Smollen and Scott, 1992). Plasmapheresis has also been tried, but the results of this treatment are variable (Branda et al., 1978; Weir et al., 1980).

PLATELET TRANSFUSIONS. Platelet transfusions should be considered only as a temporary measure to control life-threatening hemorrhage or to prepare a patient for splenectomy or cesarean section. Survival of transfused platelets is decreased in patients with ATP since antiplatelet antibodies also bind to donor platelets; thus, the usual elevation in platelets of approximately 10,000/mm³ per unit of platelet concentrate is not achieved in ATP patients. Nevertheless, 6 to 10 U can be used during the perioperative period to temporarily control hemostasis (Martin et al., 1984; Cruikshank, 1982).

Obstetric Management

Maternal mortality from ATP in pregnancy is low; no deaths have been reported in the past 10 years. The major maternal risk is peripartum bleeding associated with vaginal or cesarean delivery.

Since the placenta is permeable to circulating maternal antiplatelet antibody, the fetal thrombocytopenia that frequently occurs may result in clinical bleeding such as purpura, ecchymoses, hematuria, melena, or intracranial hemorrhage (which is also the most common cause of perinatal death). These hemorrhagic complications are extremely rare if the infant's platelet count remains above 50,000/mm³ (Scott et al., 1980), which is in close agreement with a platelet count of 50,000 to 70,000/mm³ generally considered necessary to avoid excessive bleeding at surgery (Rote and Lau, 1985). Most cases of intracranial hemorrhage have been reported in infants born vaginally (Jones et al., 1977, Samuels et al., 1990). Although it is not clear that vaginal delivery per se is the causative factor in intracranial bleeding, it seems prudent to avoid labor and vaginal delivery in any instance in which the fetus is markedly thrombocytopenic. However, it is difficult to predict during the antepartum period which baby will be thrombocytopenic.

The obstetric management of ATP patients remains controversial. If, as some authors have proposed, universal cesarean section is used, the operation will be performed unnecessarily in over 75 per cent of cases in which the fetal platelet count is greater than 50,000/mm³ (Scott et al., 1980). If, as others have suggested, the decision for cesarean section is based on a maternal platelet count less than 100,000/mm³ (Territo et al., 1973), a significant number of infants delivered abdominally will have normal platelet counts (Scott et al., 1980). Despite reports to the contrary (Clark et al., 1987), the fetal platelet count does not correlate closely enough with maternal PAIgG, circulating antiplatelet antibody levels, or previous treatment regimens to determine the safest route of delivery for an individual ATP patient (Scott et al., 1983; Colvin, 1985; Burrows and Kelton, 1990). The futility of using any maternal factor as a predictor of fetal involvement is illustrated by patients with twins, one of which has a normal platelet count and the other

thrombocytopenia (Scott et al., 1983). Unless there is a definite benefit to the infant in each case, cesarean section cannot be advised lightly in patients with ATP because of the risk of maternal bleeding at surgery.

Because of these difficulties, the use of fetal scalp blood sampling for platelet determinations in early labor or at the time of elective induction has been suggested as one way for obstetricians to determine the safety of vaginal delivery (Ayromlooi, 1978; Scott et al., 1980). This method, which utilizes a pediatric Unopette system (Bectin-Dickinson, Rutherford, New Jersey), is widely available and allows at least 80 per cent of infants of ATP mothers to undergo safe vaginal delivery. As with scalp blood sampling performed for any reason, technical problems can occur with limited cervical dilatation, a high presenting part, or a falsely low platelet count if blood clots are present in the sample.

Recently, percutaneous umbilical cord sampling (PUBS) has been proposed to determine the fetal platelet count (Daffos et al., 1983; Moise et al., 1988; Daffos et al., 1985; Forestier et al., 1988; Hobbins et al., 1985; Scioscia et al., 1988). This procedure requires expertise available in a tertiary care setting, but provides a more accurate platelet count than fetal scalp sampling. The true risk of PUBS in ATP is not well established, since only a small number of actual thrombocytopenic fetuses have undergone this procedure. Because of reports of occasional cord hematomas or other mishaps (Chenard et al., 1990; Daffos et al., 1985; Weiner et al., 1991b), PUBS is generally not recommended until pulmonary maturity is present (i.e., 36 to 37 weeks) in the event that complication from the sampling procedure necessitates emergency cesarean section.

The risk of fetal thrombocytopenia and bleeding has recently been shown to be lower than previously reported (Samuels et al., 1990; Burrows and Kelton, 1988b; Matthews et al., 1990; Cook et al., 1991). Morbidity is uncommon even in thrombocytopenic infants. Therefore, the emphasis should be placed on vaginal delivery unless a markedly thrombocytopenic infant is identified. External fetal monitoring rather than scalp electrodes should be used in any patient in early labor until the fetal platelet count is known. Injectable anesthetics and forceps manipulations should be avoided, and careful attention should be given to the repair of lacerations or the episiotomy.

Delivery should be accomplished in a setting where platelets, fresh frozen plasma, and immune globulin are available for the mother; and a neonatologist or pediatrician familiar with the disorder should be present to promptly treat any hemorrhagic complications in the neonate. It is important to recognize that the platelet count of the affected newborn infant will usually fall after delivery and that the lowest platelet count is not reached for several days. Although most infants are asymptomatic and the thrombocytopenia is self-limited, daily platelet counts should be obtained. For the infant who develops serious thrombocytopenia, treatment with high-dose immune globulin, sometimes combined with corticosteroids or platelet or exchange transfusions, is effective in raising the platelet count (Pearson and McIntosh, 1978; Ballin et al., 1988; Wenske and Gaedicke, 1984). Early in the puerperium, breast-feeding may theoretically induce neonatal thrombocytopenia due to the passage of antiplatelet antibodies in the colostrum.

Alloimmune Thrombocytopenia

Alloimmune thrombocytopenic purpura should be suspected when a thrombocytopenic infant is delivered from a mother with a normal platelet count. The disorder is the result of maternal alloimmunization by platelet antigens that are lacking on her own platelets, similar to neonatal hemolytic anemia caused by fetomaternal blood incompatibility. Fetomaternal incompatibility for the platelet-specific antigen PLA1 (Zwa) is responsible for most of the serologically proven cases of neonatal alloimmune thrombocytopenia. The antigen is inherited as a codominant trait; 69 per cent of women are homozygous PLA1-positive and 28 per cent are heterozygous (Shulman and Jordan, 1982). Several other antigens including PL^{A2}, Br, KO, Bak, Yuk, and class I HLA antigens may also be involved. In contrast to Rh immunization, many cases of alloimmune thrombocytopenia occur in infants of primiparas not previously exposed to the sensitizing stimulus or blood transfusions, and the diagnosis is not usually made until after delivery. Although 98 per cent of mothers are PLA1-negative, alloimmune thrombocytopenia occurs in only 1 to 2 per 10,000 newborns, indicating that unknown factors prevent sensitization from occurring more frequently (Smollen and Scott, 1992). It is possible that in some cases the disorder remains subclinical because the maternal anti-PLA1 antibodies are not strong enough to induce thrombocytopenia in the infant (Tanning and Skibsted, 1990). The more frequent development of PLA1 antibodies in association with a certain maternal HLA phenotype seems to be another reason. A woman possessing the DR3 antigen is 76.5 times more likely to form anti-PLA1 antibodies than a woman who is DR3-negative (Muller, 1987). Future siblings of an infant with alloimmune thrombocytopenia have approximately a 75 per cent chance of also having the disorder (Shulman and Jordan, 1982).

When PLA1-negative persons are transfused with any blood product containing platelets or possibly even soluble platelet antigen (particularly if they have been previously immunized by virtue of pregnancy or transfusion), they occasionally develop a potent complement-fixing antibody to PLA1 (Shulman and Jordan, 1982). This may result in a profound thrombocytopenia 5 to 8 days following the transfusion. Thus the transfused PLA1 platelets and the patient's own platelets are destroyed. This process may continue for several weeks. Some investigators have hypothesized that concurrent with the development of alloantibody to PLA1, an autoantibody also emerges that accounts for the destruction of the patient's own platelets. Others believe that soluble PLA1 antigen settles on the patient's own platelets, which are then destroyed by the alloantibody. Plasmapheresis, with or without immunosuppressive therapy with prednisone, appears to be the treatment of choice.

Obstetric Management

Although less common than autoimmune thrombocytopenia, alloimmune thrombocytopenia appears to have more serious consequences for the infant. Neurologic abnormalities occur in about 25 per cent of infants (Muller, 1987; Reznikoff-Etievant et al., 1988), and neonatal mortality rates of 10 to 15 per cent have been reported (McIntosh et al., 1973). Intracranial hemorrhages, which occur in 15 to 30 per cent (Burrows et al., 1988b), have been detected in about 10 per cent of affected infants by sonography in utero (Reznikoff-Etievant et al., 1988; Deaver et al., 1986). Therefore, serial ultrasonographic examinations to detect this complication may be useful. Although antepartum maternal administration of corticosteroids and IVIgG have been reported to elevate the fetal platelet count (Bussel et al., 1988; Bussel et al., 1990), others have disputed this (Mir et al., 1988; Nicolini et al., 1990, Marzusch et al., 1992). In one case, even direct intravascular fetal transfusions of IV IgG were unsuccessful in raising the fetal platelet count (Scott and Branch, 1992). Although serial fetal transfusion of PLA1-negative platelets has been recommended (Kaplan et al., 1988; Murphy et al., 1990), this treatment is not universally accepted because of the potential risks involved with repeated cordocenteses. Intracranial hemorrhage has also occurred as early as the end of the first trimester when intrauterine platelet transfusion is not yet possible (Giovangrandi et al., 1990). However, fetal platelet transfusions may have merit in severely thrombocytopenic fetuses during the third trimester to minimize the risk of fetal intracranial bleeding and in preparation for delivery. An adverse outcome in one infant was reported after *in utero* platelet transfusion (Kay et al., 1992). This may have resulted from generalized systemic fetal vascular endothelial damage because several cell types, including umbilical endothelial cells, contain surface molecules similar to the receptor containing the PLA1 antigen.

The obstetric management of alloimmune thrombocytopenia is similar to that for ATP, but a stronger case can be made for antepartum fetal blood sampling and delivery by cesarean section near term for significant fetal thrombocytopenia. PLA1-negative platelet concentrates should be available for immediate transfusion of the thrombocytopenic neonate (McIntosh et al., 1973). These can be obtained by plasmapheresis from the mother or from known PLA1-negative donors and can be stored for up to 5 days. Prior to infusion, the platelets must be washed to remove maternal antibody. Once the maternal antiplatelet antibody has been cleared from the infant's circulation, the disorder is self-limiting.

REFERENCES

Abir R, Zusman I, Ben Hur H, et al: The effects of serum from women with miscarriages on the *in vitro* development of mouse pre-implantation embryos. Acta Obstet Gynecol Scand **69**:27, 1990.

Alberman E: The epidemiology of repeated abortion. *In* Beard RW, Sharp F (eds): Early Pregnancy Loss. London, Springer-Verlag, 1988, pp 9–17.

Alexander SA, Latinne D, Debruyere M, et al: Belgian experience with repeat immunization in recurrent spontaneous abortions. *In* Beard RW, Sharp F (eds): Early Pregnancy Loss. London, Springer-Verlag, 1988, pp 355–365.

Anderson DJ, Hill JA, Haimovici F, et al: Adverse effects of immune cell products in pregnancy. *In* Wegmann TG, Gill TJ, Nisbet-Brown E (eds): Molecular and Cellular Immunobiology of the Maternal Fetal Interface. New York, Oxford University Press, 1991, pp 207–218.

Antezak DF, Allen WR: A non-genetic development defect in trophoblast formation in the horse: Immunological aspects of a model of early abortion. *In* Beard RW, Sharp F (eds): Early Pregnancy Loss. London, Springer-Verlag, 1988, pp 123–140.

Athanassakis I, Bleackley RC, Paetkau V, et al: The immunostimulatory effect of T cells and T cell lymphokines on murine fetally derived placental cells. J Immunol 18:37, 1987.

Ayromlooi J: A new approach to management of immunologic thrombocytopenia in pregnancy. Am J Obstet Gynecol 130:235, 1978.

Ballin A, Andrew M, Ling E, et al: High-dose intravenous gamma globulin therapy for neonatal autoimmune thrombocytopenia. J Pediatr 112:789, 1988.

Barton JC, Saleh MN: Case report: Immune thrombocytopenia: Effects of maternal gammaglobulin infusion in maternal and fetal serum, platelet, and monocyte IgG. Am J Med Sci 293:112, 1987.

Beer AE: Pregnancy outcome in couples with recurrent abortions following immunologic evaluation and therapy. *In* Beard RW, Sharp F (eds): Early Pregnancy Loss. London, Springer-Verlag, 1988, pp 337–349.

Beer AE, Queebeman JF, Ayers JW, et al: Minor histocompatibility complex antigens, maternal and paternal immune responses and chronic habitual abortions in humans. Am J Obstet Gynecol 141:987, 1981.

Ben-Chetrit E, Putterman C: Transient neutropenia induced by intravenous immune globulin. N Engl J Med 326:270, 1992.

Berkowitz RS, Hill JA, Kurtz CB, et al: Effects of products of activated leukocytes (lymphokines and monokines) on the growth of malignant trophoblast cells in vitro. Am J Obstet Gynecol 158:199, 1988.

Blank M, Cohen J, Toder V, Shoenfeld Y: Induction of anti-phospholipid syndrome in naive mice with mouse lupus monoclonal and human polyclonal anticardiolipin antibodies. Proc Natl Acad Sci USA 88:3069, 1991.

Branch DW, Andres R, Digre KB, Rote NS, Scott JS: The association of antiphospholipid antibodies with severe preeclampsia. Obstet Gynecol 73:541, 1989.

Branch DW: Antiphospholipid syndrome: Laboratory concerns, fetal loss, and pregnancy management. Sem Perinatol 15:230, 1991.

Branch DW: Critique of Gleicher N, El-Roeiey A, Confino E, Friberg J: Reproductive failure because of autoantibodies: Unexplained infertility and pregnancy wastage. Am J Obstet Gynecol 160:1381, 1989.

Branch DW, Dudley DJ, Mitchell MD, et al: Immunoglobulin G fractions from patients with antiphospholipid antibodies cause fetal death in Balb C mice: A model for autoimmune fetal loss. Am J Obstet Gynecol 163:210, 1990.

Branch DW, Rote NS, Dostal DA, et al: Association of lupus anticoagulant with antibody against phosphatidylserine. Clin Immunol Immunopathol 42:63, 1987.

Branch DW, Scott JR: Clinical implications of anti-phospholipid antibodies: The Utah experience. *In* Harris EN, Exner T, Hughes GRV, Asherson RA (eds): Phospholipid-Binding Antibodies. Boca Raton, CRC Press, 1991, pp 355–346.

Branch DW, Scott JR: Immunological aspects of pregnancy loss: Alloimmune and autoimmune considerations. *In* Reece EA, Hobbins JC, Mahoney MJ, et al (eds): Medicine of the Fetus and Its Mother. Philadelphia, JB Lippincott, 1992a, pp 217–233.

Branch DW, Silver RM, Blackwell JL, et al: Outcome of pregnancies in women with antiphospholipid syndrome: An update of the Utah experience. Obstet Gynecol 80:615, 1992b.

Branda RF, Tate DY, McCullough JJ, et al: Plasma exchange in the treatment of fulminant idiopathic thrombocytopenic purpura. Lancet i:688, 1978.

Brandt JT, Triplett DA, Musgrave K: The sensitivity of different coagulation reagents to the presence of lupus anticoagulants. Arch Pathol Lab Med 111:120, 1987.

Burlingham WJ: What is known about blocking factors in renal allograft recipients? Am J Reprod Immunol Microbiol 16:15, 1988.

Burrows RF, Caco CC, Kelton JG: Neonatal alloimmune thrombocytopenia: Spontaneous in utero intracranial hemorrhage. Am J Hematol 28:98, 1988a.

Burrows RF, Kelton JG: Incidentally detected thrombocytopenia in healthy mothers and their infants. N Engl J Med 319:142, 1988b.

Burrows RF, Kelton JG: Low fetal risks in pregnancies associated with idiopathic thrombocytopenic purpura. Am J Obstet Gynecol 163:1147, 1990.

Bussel JB, Berkowitz RL, McFarland JG, et al: Antenatal treatment of neonatal alloimmune thrombocytopenia. N Engl J Med 319:1374, 1988.

Bussel JB, McFarland JG, Berkowitz RL: Antenatal management of fetal alloimmune and autoimmune thrombocytopenia. Transfusion Medicine Reviews 4:149, 1990.

Bussel JB, Pham LC: Intravenous treatment with gamma globulin in adults with immune thrombocytopenia purpura: Review of the literature. Vox Sang 52:206, 1987.

Cariou R, Tobelem G, Soria C, et al: Inhibition of protein C activation by endothelial cells in the presence of lupus anticoagulant. N Engl J Med 314:1193, 1986.

Carp HJA, Toder V, Mashiach S, et al: Recurrent miscarriage: A review of current concepts, immune mechanisms, and results of treatment. Obstet Gynecol Surv 45(10):657, 1990.

Carreras LO, Defreyn G, Machin SJ, et al: Arterial thrombosis, intrauterine death and "lupus" anticoagulant: Detection of immunoglobulin interfering with prostacyclin formation. Lancet i:244, 1981.

Carreras LO, Perez GN, Vega HR, et al: Lupus anticoagulant and recurrent fetal loss: Successful treatment with gammaglobulin. Lancet ii:393, 1988.

Cauchi MN, Lim D, Young DE, et al: Treatment of recurrent aborters by immunization with paternal cells—controlled trial. Am J Reprod Immunol 25:16, 1991.

Chaouat G, Clark DA, Wegmann TG: Genetic aspects of the CBA × DBA/2 and B10 × B10. A model of murine pregnancy failure and its prevention by lymphocyte immunization. *In* Beard RW, Sharp F (eds): Early Pregnancy Loss. London, Springer-Verlag, 1988, pp 89–102.

Chaouat G, Kolb JP, Riviere M, et al: Local and systemic regulation of maternal antifetal cytotoxicity during murine pregnancy. Contrib Gynecol Obstet 14:54, 1985.

Chaouat G, Menu E, Clark DA, et al: Control of fetal survival in CBA × DBA/2 mice by lymphokine therapy. J Reprod Fertil 89:447, 1990.

Chenard E, Bastide A, Fraser WD: Umbilical cord hematoma following diagnostic funipuncture. Obstet Gynecol 76:994, 1990.

Christiaens GCML, Niewenhuis HK, Von Dem Borne AEGK, et al: Idiopathic thrombocytopenic purpura in pregnancy: A randomized trial on the effect of antenatal low dose corticosteroids on neonatal platelet count. Br J Obstet Gynaecol 97:893, 1990.

Clark DA, Chaouat G, Guennet JL, et al: Local active suppression and successful vaccination against spontaneous abortion in CBA/J mice. J Reprod Immunol 10:79, 1987.

Clark DA, Chaouat G: What do we know about spontaneous abortion mechanisms? Am J Reprod Immunol Microbiol 19:28, 1989.

Clark DA, Chaput A, Tutton D: Active suppression of host-versus-graft reaction in pregnant mice. VII. Spontaneous abortion of allogeneic CBA/J × DBA/2 fetuses in the uterus of CBA/J mice correlates with deficient non-T suppressor cell activity. J Immunol 136(5):1668, 1986.

Clark DA, Lea RG, Podor T, et al: Cytokines determining the success or failure of pregnancy. Ann NY Acad Sci 626:524, 1991.

Clark DA: Local suppressor cells and the success or failure of the foetal allograft. Ann Inst Pasteur Immunol 135:321, 1984.

Colvin BT: Thrombocytopenia. Clin Haematol 14:661, 1985.

Conley CL, Hartmann RC: A hemorrhagic disorder caused by circulating anticoagulant in patients with disseminated lupus erythematosus. J Clin Invest 31:621, 1952.

Cook RL, Miller RC, Katz VL, et al: Immune thrombocytopenic purpura in pregnancy: A Reappraisal of Management. Obstet Gynecol 78:578, 1991.

Coulam CB: Unification of immunotherapy protocols. Am J Reprod Immunol 25:1, 1991.

Cowchock FS: Alternative approaches to treatment of women with antiphospholipid antibodies and fetal loss. *In* Harris EN, Exner T, Hughes GRV, Asherson RA: Phospholipid-Binding Antibodies. Boca Raton, CRC Press, 1991, pp 347–354.

Cruikshank DP: Idiopathic thrombocytopenic purpura. *In* Queenan JT, Hobbins JC (eds): Protocols for High-Risk Pregnancies. Oradell, Medical Economics Books, 1982, pp 89–92.

Daffos F, Capella-Pavlovsky M, Forestier F: A new procedure for fetal blood sampling in utero: Preliminary results of 53 cases. Am J Obstet Gynecol 146:985, 1983.

Daffos F, Capella-Pavlovsky M, Forestier F: Fetal blood sampling during pregnancy with the use of a needle guided by ultrasound: A study of 606 consecutive cases. Am J Obstet Gynecol 153:655, 1985.

Daya S, Clark DA, Devlin MC, et al: Preliminary characterization of two types of suppressor cells in the human uterus. Fertil Steril 44:778, 1985.

Daya S, Rosenthal KL, Clark DA: Immunosuppressor factor(s) produced by decidua-associated suppressor cells: A proposed mechanism for fetal allograft survival. Am J Obstet Gynecol 56:344, 1987.

Deaver JE, Leppert PC, Zaroulis CG: Neonatal alloimmune thrombocytopenic purpura. Am J Perinatol 3:127, 1986.

DeWolf F, Carreras LO, Moerman P, et al: Decidual vasculopathy and extensive placental infarction in a patient with repeated thromboembolic accidents, recurrent fetal loss, and a lupus anticoagulant. Am J Obstet Gynecol 142:829, 1982.

Druzin ML, Lockshin MD, Edersheim TG, et al: Second trimester fetal monitoring and preterm delivery in pregnancies with systemic lupus and/or circulating anticoagulant. Am J Obstet Gynecol 157:1503, 1987.

Dudley DJ, Mitchell MD, Branch DW: Pathophysiology of antiphospholipid antibodies: Absence of prostaglandin-mediated effects on cultured endothelium. Am J Obstet Gynecol 162:953, 1990.

Edelman PH, Rouquette AM, Verdy E, et al: Autoimmunity, fetal losses, lupus anticoagulant: Beginning of systemic lupus erythematosus or new autoimmune entity with gynaeco-obstetrical expression? Hum Reprod 1:295, 1986.

Fehr J, Hofmann V, Kappeler U: Transient reversal of thrombocytopenia in idiopathic thrombocytopenic purpura by high-dose intravenous gamma globulin. N Engl J Med 306:1254, 1982.

Feinman MA, Kliman HJ, Main EK: HLA antigen expression and induction by interferon in cultured human trophoblasts. Am J Obstet Gynecol 157:1429, 1987.

Feinstein DI: Lupus anticoagulant, thrombosis and fetal loss. N Engl J Med 313:1348, 1985.

Feinstein DI, Rapaport SI: Acquired inhibitors of blood coagulation. *In* Spaet TN (ed): Progress in Hemostasis and Thrombosis. New York, Grune & Stratton, 1972, pp 75–95.

Forestier F, Cox WL, Daffos F, et al: The assessment of fetal blood samples. Am J Obstet Gynecol 158:1184, 1988.

Frampton G, Cameron JS, Thom M, et al: Successful removal of antiphospholipid antibody during pregnancy using plasma exchange and low dose prednisone. Lancet 2:1023, 1987.

Freyssinet JM, Cazenave JP: Lupus like anticoagulants modulation of the protein C pathway and thrombosis. Thromb Haemost 58:679, 1987.

Galli M, Comfurius P, Maassen C, Hemker HC, et al: Anticardiolipin antibodies (ACA) directed not to cardiolipin but to a plasma protein cofactor. Lancet 335:1544, 1990.

Gatenby PA, Cameron K, Shearman RP: Pregnancy loss with antiphospholipid antibodies: Improved outcome with aspirin containing treatment. Aust NZ J Obstet Gynaecol 29:294, 1989.

Giovangrandi Y, Daffos E, Kaplan C, et al: Very early intracranial hemorrhage in alloimmune thrombocytopenia. Lancet 2:310, 1990.

Gleicher N: Autoimmunity and reproductive failure. Ann NY Acad Sci 623:537, 1991.

Gleicher N, El-Roeiy A, Confino E, et al: Is endometriosis an autoimmune disease? Obstet Gynecol 70:114, 1987.

Gleicher N, El-Roeiy A, Confino E, et al: Reproductive failure because of autoantibodies: Unexplained infertility and pregnancy wastage. Am J Obstet Gynecol 160:1376, 1989.

Gregorini G, Setti G, Remuzzi G: Recurrent abortion with lupus anticoagulant and preeclampsia: A common final pathway for two different diseases? Case Report. Br J Obstet Gynaecol 93:194, 196, 1986.

Gutteridge CN, Veys P, Newland AC: Safety of intravenous immunoglobulin for treatment of autoimmune thrombocytopenia. Acta Hematol 79:88, 1988.

Harris EN, Chan JKH, Asherson RA, et al: Thrombosis, recurrent fetal loss, and thrombocytopenia, predictive value of the anticardiolipin antibody test. Arch Intern Med 146:2153, 1986.

Harris EN, Gharavi AE, Hughes GRV: Anti-phospholipid antibodies. Clin Rheum Dis 11:591, 1985.

Harris EN, Spinnato JA: Should anticardiolipin tests be performed in otherwise healthy pregnant women? Am J Obstet Gynecol 165:1272, 1991.

Harris EN: The second international anti-cardiolipin standardization workshop/the Kingston anti-phospholipid antibody study (KAPS) group. Am J Clin Pathol 4:476, 1990.

Hasselaar P, Derksen RHWM, Blokzijl L, et al: Thrombosis associated with antiphospholipid antibodies cannot be explained by effects on endothelial and platelet prostanoid synthesis. Thromb Haemost 59:80, 1988.

Hill JA, Polgar K, Harlow BL, et al: Evidence of embryo- and trophoblast-toxic cellular immune response(s) in women with recurrent spontaneous abortion. Am J Obstet Gynecol 166:1044, 1992.

Ho HN, Gill TJ, Hsieh HJ, et al: Immunotherapy for recurrent spontaneous abortions in a Chinese population. Am J Reprod Immunol 25:10, 1991.

Hobbins JC, Grannum PA, Romero R, et al: Percutaneous umbilical blood sampling. Am J Obstet Gynecol 152:1, 1985.

Holland NH, Holland P: Immunologic maturation in an infant of an agammaglobulinemic mother. Lancet 2:1152, 1966.

Imbach P, Jungi TW: Possible mechanisms of intravenous immunoglobulin treatment in childhood idiopathic thrombocytopenic purpura. Blut 46:117, 1983.

Johnson PM, Chia KV, Hart CA, et al: Trophoblast membrane infusion for unexplained recurrent miscarriage. Br J Obstet Gynecol 95:342, 1988.

Jones RW, Asher MI, Rutherford CJ, et al: Autoimmune (idiopathic) thrombocytopenic purpura in pregnancy and the newborn. Br J Obstet Gynaecol 84:679, 1977.

Kaplan C, Daffos F, Forestier F, et al: Management of alloimmune thrombocytopenia: Antenatal diagnosis and in utero transfusion of maternal platelets. Blood 72:340, 1988.

Karpatkin S: Autoimmune thrombocytopenic purpura. Am J Med Sci 261:127, 1971.

Karpatkin S: Autoimmune thrombocytopenic purpura. Blood 56:329, 1980.

Katz I, Fisch B, Amit S, et al: Cutaneous graft-versus-host-like reaction after paternal lymphocyte immunization for prevention of recurrent abortion. Fertil Steril 57:927, 1992.

Kay HH, Hage ML, Kurtzberg J, et al: Alloimmune thrombocytopenia may be associated with systemic disease. Am J Obstet Gynecol 166:110, 1992.

Kelton JG, Inwood MJ, Barr RM, et al: The prenatal prediction of thrombocytopenia in infants of mothers with clinically diagnosed immune thrombocytopenia. Am J Obstet Gynecol 144:449, 1982.

Kelton JG, Sheridan D, Santos A, et al: Heparin-induced thrombocytopenia: Laboratory studies. Blood 72:925, 1988.

Kennedy SH, Nunn B, Cederholm-Williams SA: Cardiolipin antibody levels in endometriosis and systemic lupus erythematosus. Fertil Steril 52:1061, 1989.

Kobayashi RH, Hyman CJ, Steihm ER: Immunologic maturation in an infant born to a mother with agammaglobulinemia. Am J Dis Child 134:942, 1980.

Kochenour NK, Branch DW, Rote NS, et al: A new postpartum syndrome associated with anti-phospholipid antibodies. Obstet Gynecol 69:460, 1987.

Kurtzberg J, Friedman HS, Kinney TR, et al: Management of human immunodeficiency virus-associated thrombocytopenia with intravenous gammaglobulin. Am J Pediatr Hematol Oncol 9:299, 1987.

Leivestad T, Thorsby E: Effects of HLA-haploid identical blood transfusions on donor-specific immune responsiveness. Transplantation 37:175, 1984.

Lockshin MD, Druzin ML, Qamar T: Prednisone does not prevent recurrent pregnancy fetal death in women with antiphospholipid antibody. Am J Obstet Gynecol 160:439, 1989.

Lockwood CJ, Romero R, Feinburg RF, et al: The prevalence and biologic significance of lupus anticoagulant and anticardiolipin antibodies in a general obstetric population. Am J Obstet Gynecol **161**:369, 1989.

Lubbe WF, Liggins GC: Role of lupus anticoagulant and autoimmunity in recurrent pregnancy loss. Sem Reprod Endocrinol **6**:181, 1988.

Margolis J: The kaolin clotting time. A rapid one stage method for diagnosis of coagulation defects. J Clin Pathol **11**:406, 1958.

Martin JN, Morrison JC, Files JC: Autoimmune thrombocytopenic purpura: Current concepts and recommended practices. Am J Obstet Gynecol **150**:86, 1984.

Marzusch K, Schnaidt M, Dietl J, et al: High-dose immunoglobulin in the antenatal treatment of neonatal alloimmune thrombocytopenia: Case report and review. Br J Obstet Gynaecol **99**:260, 1992.

Matsuura E, Igarashi Y, Fujimoto M, Ichikawa K, et al: Anticardiolipin cofactor(s) and differential diagnosis of autoimmune disease. (Letter) Lancet **336**:177, 1990.

Matthews JH, Benjamin S, Gill DS, et al: Pregnancy-associated thrombocytopenia: Definition, incidence and natural history. Acta Haematol **84**:24, 1990.

McIntosh S, O'Brien RT, Schwartz AD, et al: Neonatal isoimmune purpura: Response to platelet infusions. J Pediatr **82**:1020, 1973.

McIntyre JA, Faulk WP, Nichols-Johnson VR, et al: Immunologic testing and immunotherapy in recurrent spontaneous abortion. Obstet Gynecol **67**:169, 1986.

McIntyre JA, Faulk WP, Verhulst SJ, et al: Human trophoblast-lymphocyte cross-reactive (TLX) antigens define a new alloantigen system. Science **222**:1135, 1983.

McMillan R: Chronic idiopathic thrombocytopenic purpura. N Engl J Med **304**:1135, 1981.

McMillan R, Longmire RL, Yelenosky R, et al: Immunologic synthesis *in vitro* by splenic tissue in idiopathic thrombocytopenic purpura. N Engl J Med **286**:681, 1972.

McNeil HP, Chesterman CN, Krilis SA: Anticardiolipin antibodies and lupus anticoagulants comprise separate antibody subgroups with different phospholipid binding characteristics. Br J Haematol **73**:506, 1989.

McNeil HP, Simpson RJ, Chesterman CN, Krilis SA: Antiphospholipid antibodies are directed against a complex antigen that includes a lipid-binding inhibitor of coagulation: B2 glycoprotein I (apolipoprotein H). Proc Natl Acad Sci USA **87**:4120, 1990.

Mir N, Samson D, House MJ, et al: Failure of antenatal high-dose immunoglobulin to improve fetal platelet count in neonatal alloimmune thrombocytopenia. Vox Sang **55**:188, 1988.

Moise KJ, Carpenter RJ, Cotton DB, et al: Percutaneous umbilical cord blood sampling in the evaluation of fetal platelet counts in pregnant patients with autoimmune thrombocytopenic purpura. Obstet Gynecol **72**:346, 1988.

Mori T, Takakura K, Narimoto K, et al: Endocrine and immune implications of human endometrial decidualization in implantation. Ann NY Acad Sci **626**:321, 1992.

Mowbray JF, Gibbins C, Liddell H, et al: Controlled trial of treatment of recurrent spontaneous abortion by immunization with paternal cells. Lancet **1**:941, 1985.

Mowbray JF, Underwood JL, Michel M, et al: Immunization with paternal lymphocytes in women with recurrent miscarriage. Lancet **2**:679, 1987.

Mueller-Echardt G, Heine O, Polten B: IVIF to prevent recurrent spontaneous abortion. Lancet **337**:728, 1991.

Muller JY: Neonatal alloimmune thrombocytopenia: Clinical immunology and allergy. *In* Engelfriet CP, Borne AE (eds): Alloimmune and Autoimmune Cytopenias. Philadelphia, Balliere Tindal, 1987, pp 427–442.

Murphy MF, Pullon HWH, Metcalfe P, et al: Management of fetal alloimmune thrombocytopenia by weekly *in utero* platelet transfusions. Vox Sang **58**:45, 1990.

Nagarkatti PS, Joseph S, Singal DP: Induction of antibodies by blood transfusions capable of inhibiting responses in MLC. Transplantation **37**:695, 1983.

Newland AC: The use and mechanisms of action of intravenous immunoglobulin: An update. Br J Haematol **72**:301, 1989.

Nicolini U, Tannirandorn Y, Gonzalez P, et al: Continuing controversy in alloimmune thrombocytopenia: Fetal hyperimmunoglobulinemia fails to prevent thrombocytopenia. Am J Obstet Gynecol **163**:1144, 1990.

Nilsson IM, Astedt B, Hedner U, et al: Intrauterine death and circulating anticoagulant, "antithromboplastin." Acta Med Scand **197**:153, 1975.

Norman DJ, Barry JM, Fischer S: The beneficial effect of pretransplant third-party blood transfusions on allograft rejection in HLA identical sibling kidney transplants. Transplantation **41**:125, 1986.

Opelz G, Terasaki PI: Dominant effect of transfusions on kidney graft survival. Transplantation **29**:153, 1980.

Ordi J, Barquinero J, Vilardelli, et al: Fetal loss treatment in patients with antiphospholipid antibodies. Ann Rheum Dis **48**:798, 1989.

Out HJ, Bruinse HW, Christiaens GCML, et al: Prevalence of antiphospholipid antibodies in patients with fetal loss. Ann Rheum Dis **50**:553, 1991a.

Out HJ, Kooijman CD, Bruinse HW, Derksen RHWM: Histophysiological findings in placentae from patients with intra-uterine fetal death and antiphospholipid antibodies. Europ J Obstet Gynecol Reprod Biol **41**:179, 1991b.

Park MI, Edwin SS, Scott JR, et al: Interpretation of blocking activity in maternal serum depends on the equation used for calculation of mixed lymphocyte culture results. Clin Exp Immunol **82**:363, 1990.

Parke A, Maier D, Wilson D, et al: Intravenous gammaglobulin and antiphospholipid antibodies and pregnancy. Ann Intern Med **110**:495, 1989.

Parke AL, Wilson D, Maier D: The prevalence of antiphospholipid antibodies in women with recurrent spontaneous abortion, women with successful pregnancies, and women who have never been pregnant. Arthritis Rheum **34**:1231, 1991.

Payne BA, Pierre RV: Pseudothrombocytopenia: A laboratory artifact with potentially serious consequences. Mayo Clin Proc **59**:123, 1984.

Pearson HA, McIntosh S: Neonatal thrombocytopenia. Clin Lab Haematol **7**:111, 1978.

Peters AJ, Coulam CB: Pregnancy outcome after the use of intravenous immunoglobulin for the treatment of recurrent spontaneous abortion. (Abstract) Fertil Steril Program Suppl, 1990, p 821.

Petri M, Golbus M, Anderson R, et al: Antinuclear antibody, lupus anticoagulant, and anticardiolipin antibody in women with idiopathic habitual abortion. A controlled, prospective study of 44 women. Arthritis Rheum **30**:601, 1987.

Pollard JK, Scott JR, Branch DW: Growth and development of children from women treated during pregnancy for the antiphospholipid syndrome. Obstet Gynecol **80**:365, 1992.

Redman CWG, Ferry BL, Jackson MC, et al: Immune cell populations in human early pregnancy decidua. *In* Wegmann TG, Gill TJ, Nisbet-Brown E (eds): Molecular and Cellular Immunobiology of the Maternal Fetal Interface. New York, Oxford University Press, 1991, pp 110–128.

Reece EA, Gabrielli S, Cullen MT, et al: Recurrent adverse pregnancy outcome and antiphospholipid antibodies. Am J Obstet Gynecol **163**:162, 1990.

Reginald PW, Beard RW, Chapple J, et al: Outcome of pregnancies progressing beyond 28 weeks gestation in women with a history of recurrent miscarriage. Br J Obstet Gynaecol **94**:643, 1987.

Reznikoff-Etievant MF, Durieux I, Huchet J, et al: Human MHC antigens and paternal leucocyte injection in recurrent spontaneous abortions. *In* Beard RW, Sharp F (eds): Early Pregnancy Loss. New York, Springer-Verlag, 1988, pp 375–384.

Reznikoff-Etievant MF: Management of alloimmune neonatal and antenatal thrombocytopenia. Vox Sang **55**:192, 1988.

Rocklin RE, Kitzmiller JL, Carpenter CG, et al: Maternal-fetal relation: Absence of an immunologic blocking factor from the serum of women with chronic abortions. N Engl J Med **295**:1209, 1976.

Rocklin RE, Kitzmiller JL, Garvoy MR: Further characterization of an immunologic blocking factor that develops during pregnancy. Clin Immunol Immunopathol **22**:305, 1982.

Rodger JC: Lack of a requirement for a maternal humoral immune response to establish or maintain successful allogeneic pregnancy. Transplantation **40**:372, 1985.

Roman E: Fetal loss rates and their relation to pregnancy order. J Epidemiol Commun Health **38**:29, 1984.

Romero R, Duffy T: Platelet disorders in pregnancy. Clin Perinatol **7**:327, 1980.

Rosove MH, Tabsh K, Wassertrum N, et al: Heparin therapy for pregnant women with lupus anticoagulant or anticardiolipin antibodies. Obstet Gynecol **75**:630, 1987.

Rote NS, Lau JL: Immunologic thrombocytopenic purpura. Clin Obstet Gynecol **28**:84, 1985.

Sammaritano LR, Gharavi AE, Lockshin MD: Antiphospholipid antibody syndrome: Immunologic and clinical aspects. Semin Arthritis Rheum **20**:81, 1990.

Samuels P, Bussel JB, Braitman LE, et al: Estimation of the risk of thrombocytopenia in the offspring of pregnant women with presumed immune thrombocytopenic purpura. N Engl J Med **323**:229, 1990.

Schwartz SI, Hoepp IM, Sachs S: Splenectomy for thrombocytopenia. Surgery **88**:497, 1980.

Scioscia AL, Grannum PAT, Copel JA, et al: The use of percutaneous blood sampling in immune thrombocytopenic purpura. Am J Obstet Gynecol **159**:1066, 1988.

Scott JR, Branch DW, Kochenour NK, et al: Intravenous globulin treatment of pregnant patients with recurrent pregnancy loss due to antiphospholipid antibodies and Rh immunization. Am J Obstet Gynecol **159**:1055, 1988.

Scott JR, Branch DW: Unpublished data. 1992.

Scott JR, Cruikshank DP, Kochenour NK: Fetal platelet counts in the obstetric management of immunologic thrombocytopenic purpura. Am J Obstet Gynecol **136**:495, 1980.

Scott JR: Habitual abortion—Recommendations for a reasonable approach to an enigmatic problem. *In* Soules MR (ed): Controversies in Reproductive Endocrinology and Infertility. New York, Elsevier Co, 1989, pp 95–106.

Scott JR, Rote NS, Branch DW: Immunologic aspects of spontaneous abortion and fetal death. Obstet Gynecol **70**:645–656, 1987.

Scott JR, Rote NS, Cruikshank DP, et al: Antiplatelet antibodies and platelet counts in pregnancies complicated by autoimmune thrombocytopenic purpura. Am J Obstet Gynecol **145**:932, 1983.

Sejeny SA, Eastham RD, Baker SR: Platelet counts during normal pregnancy. J Clin Pathol **28**:812, 1975.

Shulman NR, Jordan JV: Platelet immunology. *In* Colman RW, Hirsh J, Marder VJ, Salzman EW (eds): Hemostasis and Thrombosis: Basic Principles and Clinical Practice. Philadelphia, JB Lippincott, 1982, pp 274–342.

Sidiropoulous D, Herrman U Jr, Morell A, et al: Transplacental passage of intravenous immunoglobulin in the last trimester of pregnancy. J Pediatr **109**:505, 1986.

Singal DP, Fagnilli L, Joseph S: Blood transfusions induce anti-idiotypic antibodies in renal transplant patients. Transplant Proc **15**:1005, 1983.

Smith JB, Cowchock S: Immunologic studies in recurrent spontaneous abortion: Effects of immunization of women with paternal mononuclear cells on lymphocytotoxic and mixed lymphocyte reaction blocking antibodies and correlation with sharing of HLA and pregnancy outcome. J Reprod Immunol **14**:99, 1988.

Smollen MA, Scott JR: Immunologic thrombocytopenic purpura. *In* Coulam CB, Faulk WP, McIntyre JA (eds): Immunology and Obstetrics. New York, WW Norton, 1992, pp 632–639 .

Solanki DL, Blackburn BC: Spurious thrombocytopenia during pregnancy. Obstet Gynecol **65**:14S, 1985.

Sollinger HW, Burlingham WJ, Sparks EMF, et al: Donor-specific transfusions in unrelated and related HLA mismatched donor recipient combinations. Transplantation **38**:612, 1984.

Stimson WH, Strachman AF, Shepherd A: Studies on the maternal immune response to placental antigens: Absence of a blocking factor from the blood of abortion-prone women. Br J Obstet Gynaecol **86**:41, 1979.

Szekeres-Bartho J, Chaouat G: Lymphocyte-derived progesterone-induced blocking factor corrects resorption in a murine abortion system. Am J Reprod Immunol **23**:26, 1990.

Takakuwa K, Goto S, Hasegawa I, et al: Result of immunotherapy on patients with unexplained recurrent abortion: A beneficial

treatment for patients with negative blocking antibodies. Am J Reprod Immunol **23**:37, 1990.

Takeuchi H, Sakagami K, Seki Y, et al: Anti-idiotypic antibodies and suppressor cells induced by DST in potential kidney transplant recipient. Transplant Proc **17**:1059, 1985.

Tanning E, Skibsted L: The frequency of platelet alloantibodies in pregnant women and the occurrence and management of neonatal alloimmune thrombocytopenic purpura. Obstet Gynecol Surv **45**:521, 1990.

Tchobroutsky C, Clauvel JP, Sutan Y, et al: Successful pregnancies in antiphospholipid syndrome without prednisone. Clin Exp Rheumatol **6**:213, 1988.

Territo M, Finklestein J, Oh W, et al: Management of autoimmune thrombocytopenia in pregnancy and the neonate. Obstet Gynecol **41**:579, 1973.

Thiagarajan P, Pengo V, Shapiro SS: The use of the dilute Russell viper venom time for the diagnosis of lupus anticoagulants. Blood **68**:869, 1986.

Toder V, Strassburger D, Irlin Y, et al: Nonspecific immunopotentiators and pregnancy loss: Complete Freund adjuvant reverses high fetal resorption rate in CBA × DBA12 mouse combination. Am J Reprod Immunol **24**:63, 1990.

Triplett DA: Antiphospholipid antibodies and recurrent pregnancy loss. Am J Reprod Immunol **20**:52, 1989.

Triplett DA, Brandt JT, Kaczor D, Schaeffer J: Laboratory diagnosis of lupus inhibitors: A comparison of the tissue thromboplastin inhibition procedure with a new platelet neutralization procedure. Am J Clin Pathol **79**:678, 1983.

Triplett DA, Brandt JT, Maas RL: The laboratory heterogeneity of lupus anticoagulants. Arch Pathol Lab Med **109**:946, 1985.

Trudinger BH, Stewart GJ, Cook CM, et al: Monitoring lupus anticoagulant-positive pregnancies with umbilical flow velocity waveforms. Obstet Gynecol **72**:215, 1988.

Tsakiris DA, Marbet GA, Matnis DE, et al: Impaired fibrinolysis as an essential contribution to thrombosis in patients with lupus anticoagulant. Thromb Haemost **61**:175, 1989.

Unander AM, Lindholm A: Transfusions of leukocyte-rich concentrates: A successful treatment in selected cases of habitual abortion. Am J Obstet Gynecol **154**:516, 1986.

Unander AM, Norberg R, Hahn L, Arfora L: Anticardiolipin antibodies and complement in 99 women with habitual abortion. Am J Obstet Gynecol **156**:114, 1987.

Wapner RJ, Cowchock FS, Shapiro SS: Successful treatment in two women with antiphospholipid antibodies and refractory pregnancy losses with intravenous immunoglobulin infusions. Am J Obstet Gynecol **161**:1271, 1989.

Warkentin TE, Kelton JG: Current concepts in the treatment of immune thrombocytopenia. Drugs **40**(4):531, 1990.

Wegmann TG: Fetal protection against abortion: Is it immunosuppression or immunostimulation? Ann Immunol Instit Pasteur **135**:309, 1984.

Weiner HM, Vardinon N, Yust I: Platelet antibody binding and spontaneous aggregation in 21 lupus anticoagulant patients. Vox Sang **62**:111, 1991a.

Weiner CP, Wenstrom KD, Sipes SL, et al: Risk factors for cordocentesis and fetal intravascular transfusion. Am J Obstet Gynecol **165**:1020, 1991b.

Weir AB, Poon M, McGowan EI: Plasma exchange in idiopathic thrombocytopenic purpura. Arch Intern Med **140**:1101, 1980.

Wenske G, Gaedicke G: ITP in pregnancy and the neonatal period. Blut **48**:377, 1984.

Yin CS, Scott JR: Failure of maternal dexamethasone treatment to prevent immunologic thrombocytopenia in the infant. Obstet Gynecol **152**:316, 1985.

Zak SJ, Good RA: Immunological studies of human sera gamma globulins. J Clin Invest **38**:579, 1959.

DISORDERS OF PARTURITION

C H A P T E R

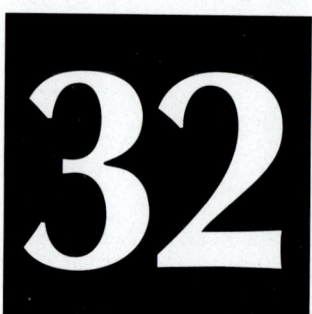

CHARACTERISTICS OF PARTURITION

JOHN R. G. CHALLIS, Ph.D., D.Sc.

The incidence of preterm labor, accounting for 7 to 10 per cent of all deliveries, has remained relatively unchanged for several years. This condition accounts for a substantial proportion of the perinatal mortality and morbidity statistics. It is now clear that about one-third of preterm deliveries are associated with infection, but whether they are driven by an infective process remains an area of active investigation. Other predisposing factors may include socioeconomics, lifestyle, and work habits. Medical variables including history, multiple gestations, and a previous preterm labor are recognized as risk factors (Creasy, 1980, 1991). A further proportion (up to 50 per cent) of patients present in idiopathic preterm labor, supporting the suggestion that this is a syndrome rather than a specific disease process (Romero et al., 1991) and that it will be difficult to evaluate a single diagnostic marker or mode of management. In this chapter we shall discuss controls of normal labor and examine potential mechanisms that may lead to preterm parturition.

LESSONS FROM THE SHEEP MODEL OF PARTURITION

In species such as the sheep, labor results from a complex interplay of fetal and maternal endocrine factors and can be viewed as the outcome of an integrated sequential maturation of a series of endocrine organ communication systems (Fig. 32–1). The sequence begins at the level of the fetal brain or hypothalamus and is transmitted through the pituitary to the fetal adrenal gland, where increased cortisol output provides the stimulus to the subsequent maternal endocrine changes (Thorburn and Challis, 1979;

Challis and Olson, 1988). Altered placental steroidogenesis results in a decrease in progesterone secretion into the maternal circulation and a later increase in plasma concentrations of unconjugated estrogens. These changes are followed by an increase in prostaglandin $F_{2\alpha}$ ($PGF_{2\alpha}$) levels in maternal utero-ovarian venous plasma, resulting from an increase in placental prostaglandin H synthase activity (see below) and an altered cellular pattern of expression of this enzyme in the placenta (Boshier et al., 1991). $PGF_{2\alpha}$, also produced in the fetal membranes and endometrium, activates uterine contractility after the myometrium has undergone preparedness for labor. Cervical biochemical changes accompany the pattern of myometrial contractility that leads to birth.

The classic experiments of Liggins, Thorburn, and associates in the sheep and goat emphasized the role of the fetus in the triggering of labor. Their studies dictated much of the thinking and research thrusts of the 1970s. It is well established that the sheep fetus, through increased activity of its pituitary-adrenal axis and increased cortisol output from the fetal adrenal gland during late gestation, provides the signal for the onset of birth (Liggins et al., 1973). Hypophysectomy of the fetal lamb *in utero* obliterates the normal prepartum increase in fetal adrenal weight and rise in plasma cortisol concentrations and prolongs gestation. On the other hand, infusion of adrenocorticotropic hormone (ACTH) to fetal sheep *in utero* results in a precocious increase in fetal adrenal weight, rise in plasma cortisol concentrations, and premature delivery that, endocrinologically, may resemble the sequence of events seen at full term (Liggins et al., 1973; Thorburn and Challis, 1979).

In the sheep fetus there is an increase in the ability of the fetal pituitary gland to secrete ACTH in re-

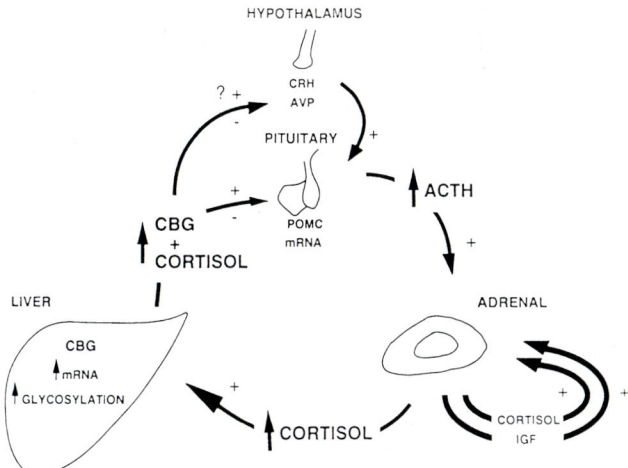

FIGURE 32—1. Working model for activation of the hypothalamic-pituitary-adrenal axis in the fetal sheep. Hypothalamic neuropeptides stimulate an increase in pituitary pro-opiomelanocortin (POMC), mRNA abundance, and ACTH release. Fetal ACTH activates fetal adrenal function; in part this action is mediated by cortisol. We suggest that ACTH also stimulates insulin-like growth factor (IGF) expression in the fetal adrenal and that IGFs influence fetal adrenal growth and differentiated function. Fetal cortisol stimulates an increase in corticosteroid-binding globulin (CBG) mRNA in the fetal liver and a rise in plasma CBG. In turn this binds cortisol and maintains a low free cortisol concentration in plasma and a low negative feedback effect of cortisol at the hypothalamic and pituitary level. Cortisol may influence post-translational processing of POMC so that more $ACTH_{1-39}$ is secreted. Thus, birth results from a positive feed-forward cascade involving the entire hypothalamic-pituitary-adrenal axis, with cortisol occupying a central role.

sponse to stimulation by corticotropin-releasing hormone (CRH) during late gestation (Norman and Challis, 1987). This change is followed by an increase in responsiveness of the fetal adrenal gland to secrete cortisol in response to ACTH stimulation. ACTH increases the steroidogenic machinery of the adrenal gland, including effects on adenylate cyclase activity and on gene expression for key enzymes in the pathway to cortisol production (Challis and Olson, 1988). Cortisol may itself modulate the mechanism by which ACTH activates fetal adrenal function (Challis et al., 1985). It also alters the pattern of fetal pituitary ACTH secretion to increase levels of the bioactive forms of this peptide in plasma. Cortisol actually preserves low levels of glucocorticoid negative feedback at the hypothalamus and pituitary by stimulating production of its own circulating binding protein, corticosteroid-binding globulin (CBG), from the fetal liver. It thereby perpetuates a positive pituitary-adrenal cascade in the fetus leading to birth (Challis and Brooks, 1989).

The role of the human fetus in initiating labor is less well defined. In anencephaly, after exclusion of patients with polyhydramnios, the mean length of gestation is similar to that of a control population, although there is a marked increase in the incidence of both premature and postmature births. The distribution is similar to that reported subsequently for rhesus monkeys after experimental fetal exencephaly (Thorburn and Challis, 1979). The output of fetal

corticosteroids increases during late pregnancy (Fencl et al., 1980); however, until recently (see below) there was little evidence to suggest that cortisol produced by the human fetus had a role analogous to that in the sheep. For example, in both monkeys and women, exogenous glucocorticoids failed to induce parturition, except in some patients already classified as post-term (Liggins et al., 1977).

One reason for the differences between the sheep model and the primate lies in the specialized nature of the fetal adrenal cortex. In primates the fetal zone of the fetal adrenal secretes substantial amounts of C_{19} estrogen precursor steroids, whereas in the sheep these are produced mainly in the placenta under the influence of fetal adrenal cortisol at term. In human pregnancy the maternal adrenal secretes about 50 per cent of the C_{19} precursors utilized for placental estradiol production, and this may mask further a fetal contribution to the initiation of parturition. It will be argued later that C_{19} steroids from the fetal adrenal may provide part of the fetal signal to birth in primates. It is possible that one steroid (cortisol) from the adult zone of the fetal adrenal may facilitate fetal organ maturation while a second steroid (dehydroepiandrosterone sulfate, DHAS) from the fetal zone may contribute to estrogen production and delivery through intrauterine mechanisms (see below). Recent studies have suggested that cortisol of fetal origin stimulates output from the placenta of peptides such as CRH (Robinson et al., 1988). CRH concentrations are elevated in the maternal plasma of patients in preterm labor, without infection (Warren et al., 1992), raising the possibility of using plasma CRH in the diagnosis of this condition.

It is also possible that in human pregnancy other triggers of fetal origin are transported through the amniotic fluid to influence steroid or prostaglandin production in the fetal membranes or decidua. It is likely that the key to human labor lies within trophoblast-derived structures, the amnion and chorion and the adjacent decidua. For these reasons, a number of investigators have sought changes in the production of steroid hormones and prostaglandins that may occur locally within the human decidua and fetal membranes. Such changes might provide a signal to the onset of birth without being reflected in maternal peripheral plasma hormone concentrations.

ROLE OF PROSTAGLANDINS IN HUMAN PARTURITION

A commonly held view is that prostaglandins (PGs), produced within the intrauterine tissues, play a central role in the stimulus to myometrial contractility in different species, including humans (Novy and Liggins, 1980; Okazaki et al., 1981; Bleasdale and Johnston, 1984; Challis and Olson, 1988). Three major lines of evidence support a role for prostaglandins in the onset of labor. During parturition there is an increase in the concentration of prostaglandin E_2 (PGE_2) and prostaglandin $F_{2\alpha}$ ($PGF_{2\alpha}$) in amniotic fluid, and of their metabolites in maternal plasma and urine. Administration of drugs such as aspirin and indomethacin, which are prostaglandin synthase inhibitors, suppresses uterine activity and prolongs the length of pregnancy. Further, the primate myometrium is exquisitely sensitive to the stimulatory effects of exogenously administered prostaglandins (Novy and Liggins, 1980; Bleasdale and Johnston, 1984; Challis and Lye, 1986).

There is substantial evidence of changes in prostaglandin production during labor in animals and in humans, but it should be noted that most investigators have failed to demonstrate large increases in prostaglandin synthesis prior to the onset of human parturition. Concentrations of PGE and PGF in amniotic fluid increase with progressive dilation of the cervix (Keirse and Turnbull, 1973), and these changes are accompanied by a rise in the concentration of unesterified arachidonic acid, the obligate precursor of PGE_2 and $PGF_{2\alpha}$ (MacDonald et al., 1974; Keirse and Turnbull, 1976). The concentration of PGE in amniotic fluid exceeds that of PGF before the onset of active labor (Dray and Frydman, 1976), but the relative increase in PGF is greater than PGE during labor. In amniotic fluid the concentration of 6-keto $PGF_{1\alpha}$, the hydrolytic breakdown product of prostacyclin (PGI_2), does not change with labor (Mitchell, 1986). This is of interest because PGI_2 inhibits contractility of human and sheep myometrium (Omini et al., 1978; Lye and Challis, 1982; Lumsden and Baird, 1986). Thus not only is there an increase in the concentration of stimulatory PGs, but their formation is favored over that of inhibitory eicosanoids. This pattern of PG output, increased PGE_2 and PGF_2 relative to 6-keto $PGF_{1\alpha}$, can be reproduced in vitro by treating decidual tissue with estrogen (Olson et al., 1983b).

BIOSYNTHESIS AND METABOLISM OF PROSTAGLANDINS (PGs)

To understand factors responsible for changes in production of PGs, it is necessary to review key steps in their biosynthetic and metabolic pathways. PGs are formed from unesterified arachidonic acid released from membrane phospholipids such as phosphatidylinositol and phosphatidylethanolamine. Key enzymes in this initial step are phospholipase C (PLC), which catalyzes formation of diacylglycerol from phosphatidylinositol, and phospholipase A_2 (PLA_2). Free arachidonate is converted to prostaglandins through activity of prostaglandin H synthase (PGHS). This enzyme contains cyclooxygenase activity, which is responsible for conversion of arachidonic acid to the unstable endoperoxide PGG_2, and peroxidase activity, through which PGG_2 is converted to PGH_2 (DeWitt, 1991). PGH_2 is substrate for different synthases and isomerases leading to formation of primary prostaglandins. In turn, metabolism of PGs proceeds, initially, through the action of an NAD^+ type I 15-hydroxyprostaglandin dehydrogenase (PGDH) to form 15-keto compounds, which are essentially inactive biologically. These are rapidly converted through $\Delta^{13,14}$ reductase to 13,14 dihydro 15-keto derivatives, the major circulating PG metabolites. In turn these undergo beta oxidation and

omega oxidation to form a variety of metabolites that are excreted in urine (Mitchell, 1990).

Arachidonic acid can also be metabolized through 5-, 12-, or 15-lipoxygenase and epoxygenase pathways to form leukotrienes, hydroxyeicosatetraenoic acids (HETE), and epoxides (Fig. 32–2). These compounds may have direct stimulatory actions on the myometrium. They are elevated in amniotic fluid at the time of labor (Romero et al., 1989a), even in the absence of significant changes in cyclooxygenase products (Walsh, 1991). It has been reported that arachidonate metabolism proceeds preferentially through the lipoxygenase pathways during the latter part of human pregnancy, but that nearer to labor there is a progressive switch to cyclooxygenase products (Rose et al., 1990). This change in metabolism may thereby lead to production of more potent agonists to the myometrium. A direct role of lipoxygenase products in uterine preparedness for labor is unexplored.

Major sites of PG synthesis and metabolism have been evaluated by in vitro incubation techniques, by studies with dispersed cells or with mixed cells in short-term tissue culture, and by immunohistochemistry. Results from different laboratories are generally confirmative, although interpretation of the in vivo situation from the in vitro measurements can be made only with caution, and the relative quantitative significance of different sites of production remains unresolved.

Amnion contains predominantly phospholipase and PGHS activity with little PGDH. It produces primarily PGE_2 and probably accounts for much of the increase in amniotic fluid PGE_2 concentrations with labor (Lundin-Schiller and Mitchell, 1990; Challis and Olson, 1988). Immunoreactive (IR-) PGHS was localized to amniotic epithelial cells by immunohistochemistry (Price et al., 1989). These studies will need repeating with recognition of separate constitutive and inducible forms of PGHS (PGHS-I and PGHS-II), which are products of different genes. Chorion contains PGHS activity, but is the major site of PGDH activity in the human fetal membranes. PGDH is localized to the chorionic trophoblast cells; its distribution and activity do not change significantly with labor. However, we have recently found that PGDH immunostaining is weak or undetectable in some, but not all, patients in preterm labor without infection at <31 weeks and at 31 to 36 weeks gestation. Further, undetectable IR-PGDH was correlated with undetectable PGDH mRNA transcripts by northern blot analysis. This raises the possibility that a deficiency or reduced expression of this gene in the membranes of some patients may lead to diminished metabolism and consequent availability of primary PGs in intrauterine tissues, thereby predisposing to preterm delivery.

Decidua is a mixture of decidualized stromal cells, bone marrow–derived macrophages, and other cell types including, at its interface with chorion, occasional invasive trophoblasts. It contains PG synthetic and metabolic activities (Casey and MacDonald, 1988), although the latter could be derived in part from contaminating trophoblasts. "Decidual cells" obtained at spontaneous labor produced increased amounts of PGE_2 and PGF_2 in vitro, compared to cesarean section

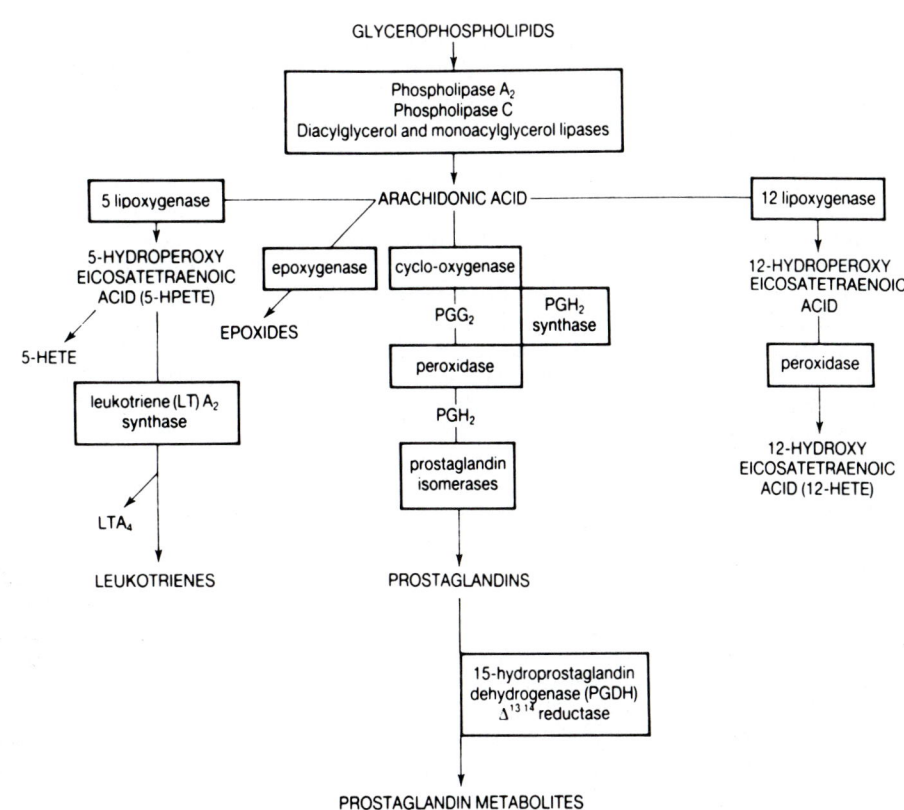

FIGURE 32—2. Pathways of arachidonic acid metabolism.

tissue (Skinner and Challis, 1985). Since there is some transmembrane transfer of PGs, albeit low (Nakla et al., 1986), $PGF_{2\alpha}$ produced de novo as a result of decidual activation could pass back into the amniotic fluid in increasing amounts at the time of labor. A current view is that decidual $PGF_{2\alpha}$ is the major stimulus to the myometrium in labor. However, this is based on *in vitro* evidence, and most investigations have ignored any contribution of the myometrium itself to eicosanoid generation. Decidua, like chorion, contains 9-ketoreductase activity and has the ability to interconvert PGE_2 to $PGF_{2\alpha}$. The source of this PGE_2 could be de novo production or the amnion after limited transmembrane transfer. However, the K_m for decidual 9-ketoreductase is such that it is unlikely to be important at physiologic concentrations of PGE_2 *in vivo*.

Bleasdale et al. (1983) demonstrated the substrate specificity of PLA_2 in human chorioamnion. They showed that the specific activity of this enzyme increased in the amnion but not in chorion or decidua, between 13 and 17 weeks of gestation and at term (38 to 41 weeks). There was no further change with labor. The specific activity of PLC increased in a similar manner during pregnancy. However, no change was detected in diacylglycerol lipase activity in either the decidual tissue or the fetal membranes. Conversely, PGHS activity in amnion, but not in decidua or chorion, was greater in tissue collected after labor of spontaneous onset than in tissue collected at elective cesarean section at term (Okazaki et al., 1981). Aitken et al. (1990, 1992) have shown recently that the abundance of nonpancreatic PLA_2 mRNA in amnion and

chorion is much less than in the placenta. In the latter tissue, PLA_2 mRNA did not change during late pregnancy, but increased with labor. Further studies of PLA_2 and PLC gene expression and localization are required for different isozymes. Similar measurements are required for the type I and type II forms of PGHS.

STIMULATORS OF PROSTAGLANDIN SYNTHESIS

Over the past five years an impressive list of stimulants to PG synthesis by intrauterine tissues has emerged. Some of these agents affect PGHS expression and/or activity; others appear to act through PLA_2 or PLC. The list includes steroids, growth factors, cytokines, and placental peptides. Again, interpretation of these data is made with the caution that studies are conducted on cells or tissue explants *in vitro*, and often effects of individual agents have been examined independently of other stimulants or inhibitors.

The availability of free calcium is a major factor influencing prostaglandin output by fetal membranes (Bleasdale et al., 1983; Bleasdale and Johnston, 1984). It has been suggested that the probable site of calcium action is through stimulation of PLA_2 and PLC, and through inhibition of the enzyme diacylglycerol kinase, thereby preventing the resynthesis of phosphatidylinositol. However, others have argued that the changes in calcium that may occur *in vivo* are unlikely to be great enough to influence phospholipase activity. The importance of Ca^{2+} for prostaglandin synthesis was demonstrated by the use of intact dispersed cells *in vitro*. Removal of extracellular calcium from the incubation medium bathing amnion cells or blocking calcium entry into the cells with D-600 (verapamil) attenuated PGE_2 output (Olson et al., 1983a). Conversely, if the intracellular calcium concentration was increased by addition of the calcium ionophore A23187 to the extracellular medium, there was a two- to threefold increase in prostaglandin output. It is possible that the effects of calcium on PG production may be mediated by intracellular calcium-binding proteins. For example, the stimulatory effect of A23187 on PG output by amnion and decidual tissue is inhibited, in a dose-dependent manner, by the calmodulin antagonist trifluoperazine (Warrick et al., 1985).

Several years ago it was recognized that samples of newborn (fetal) urine contained a moiety that exhibited a tissue-specific stimulation of PGE_2 output from human amnion cells maintained in monolayer tissue culture (Casey et al., 1983). This activity is also present in amniotic fluid in late gestation (Mitchell et al., 1984). The effects of human fetal urine on the output of PGE_2 by amnion cells are similar to those obtained during incubation with epidermal growth factor (EGF). EGF is present in human amniotic fluid and stimulates PGE_2 output from amnion cells. Amnion cells contain EGF receptors, and it is now known that EGF increases the rate of synthesis of PGHS (Casey et al., 1987). Thus, there is potentiation of arachidonic acid–stimulated PGE_2 output from amnion by the further addition of EGF. In Swiss 3T3 cells, others have shown that human platelet-derived growth factor (PDGF) stimulates prostaglandin synthesis in two distinct time phases. The first phase, which occurs within 60 minutes, is directly on prostaglandin synthesis from exogenous arachidonic acid, and is independent of protein synthesis. The second phase, occurring at 2 to 4 hours after addition of PDGF, requires rapid translation of PGHS and is blocked by cycloheximide (Habenicht et al., 1985).

Platelet-activating factor (PAF, acetyl glycerol ether phosphoryl choline) is present in amniotic fluid at term and in term fetal membranes. Amnion possesses the enzymes responsible for its synthesis and metabolism (Billah and Johnston, 1983; Bleasdale and Johnston, 1984; Ban et al., 1986). Addition of PAF to amnion cells in culture or in incubation provokes a two- to threefold increase in the output of PGE_2 by these cells, the effect resembling that seen with the stimulating calcium ionophore A23187. In platelets, PAF stimulates inositol phospholipid turnover and increases the availability of diacylglycerol. This compound is rich in arachidonic acid, and its transient formation is associated with activation of protein kinase C. In addition, inositol triphosphate (IP3) formed from phosphatidylinositol-4-phosphate or phosphatidylinositol-4, 5-biphosphate releases calcium from intracellular stores. Okazaki et al. (1984) have shown that protein kinase C activity is present in human fetal membranes. It seems likely that PAF, derived from amniotic fluid and perhaps from the fetal lung or kidney (Ban et al., 1986) or synthesized within amnion, activates PLC with resultant PG generation through the protein kinase C pathway. More recently,

several groups have shown that activation of protein kinase C by addition of phorbol esters or diacylglycerol to amnion cells stimulates PGE_2 output by increasing de novo synthesis of PGHS. The effect on PGE_2 is potentiated by addition of the calcium ionophore A23187 (Zakar and Olson, 1988).

Prostaglandin output is also influenced by modulators of cyclic AMP (cAMP)-dependent protein kinase. Amnion tissue possesses beta-receptors, classified as belonging to the β_2 subtype. The possibility has been raised that catecholamines, present in amniotic fluid in increasing concentration during late pregnancy as a result of fetal adrenal medullary maturation (Divers et al., 1981), might stimulate adenylate cyclase and influence PG production through such receptors (DiRenzo et al., 1984). Both amnion and decidua contain active adenylate cyclase systems, which can be stimulated with beta-agonists such as isoproterenol and with PGE_1, forskolin, and cholera toxin (DiRenzo et al., 1984; Warrick et al., 1985). The effects of forskolin and cholera toxin on cAMP output by amnion and decidual cells are associated temporally with an increase in the output of PG by these tissues. The effects of activators of adenylate cyclase on prostaglandin biosynthesis can be mimicked by addition of dibutyryl cAMP (dbcAMP) or phosphodiesterase inhibitors such as methylxanthine (MIX) to the cells in incubation (Warrick et al., 1985). Interestingly, the effects of MIX and of the calcium ionophore A23187 in stimulating prostaglandin output by amnion cells are partially additive. These studies help explain the disappointing lack of efficacy of β_2-sympathomimetic drugs in sustaining uterine quiescence in the treatment of preterm labor. Although these compounds are effective in the short term, their continuous administration may be associated with a return of uterine contractility. In part this is clearly attributable to down-regulation of the beta-receptor, reduced ability to generate cAMP, and reduced responsiveness of the tissues. If β-mimetics also provoke output of stimulatory PGs, they are acting in a milieu where their effectiveness is counteracted by enhanced production of the compounds that their usage is intended to antagonize. Administration of these compounds as pulses or short infusions may prove to circumvent this problem and to improve their long-term usefulness (Casper and Lye, 1986).

Infection and Preterm Labor

As noted earlier, approximately 30 to 40 per cent of preterm labors are associated with degrees of chorioamnionitis and low-grade infection (Romero et al., 1991). Romero and colleagues (Romero et al., 1987, 1989b) have shown that the concentrations of products of both PGHS and lipoxygenase pathways of arachidonic acid metabolism are elevated in the amniotic fluid of these patients. In contrast, there was no elevation in amniotic fluid eicosanoid concentrations of patients in defined preterm labor that was responsive to tocolytic management. The site of increased eicosanoid production is probably the intrauterine tissues. Lopez-Bernal et al. (1989) showed that the output of PGE_2 by amnion and choriodecidua obtained at preterm labor at which there was evidence of infection was significantly greater than that from tissues of patients in preterm labor without infection, or at term elective cesarean section, or at preterm cesarean section for severe preeclampsia. The output of PGE_2 from tissues during preterm labor without infection was not different from that of tissues obtained at elective preterm cesarean section. Both of these groups had lower outputs of PGE_2 from amnion and choriodecidua than from tissues at term cesarean section or spontaneous labor. Thus, infection-associated preterm labor may show increases in PG output. In the absence of infection, PG output does not appear to be causally activated (see below).

Several mechanisms have been suggested to explain the increased output of PGs at the time of infection and preterm labor. Bacterial phospholipases may directly release arachidonic acid from intrauterine (amnion, decidua) phospholipid stores (Bennett et al., 1987; Lamont et al., 1990). Alternatively, bacterial endotoxins, including lipopolysaccharide (LPS) and lipoteichoic acid (LTA), may stimulate PGs directly or may stimulate increased output of cytokines such as interleukin-1 (IL-1) and tumor necrosis factor (TNF) from amnion and decidual cells. These cytokines are elevated in amniotic fluid from patients with preterm labor and infection. Their addition to amnion or decidual cells *in vitro* provokes PG output. Further IL-1 stimulates output from decidua of other cytokines including IL-6 and IL-8, a chemotactic peptide for neutrophils and T cells, thereby setting up a positive cytokine-PG cascade. This is particularly likely since macrophages and bone marrow—derived cells are major constituents of decidua. Endotoxins will provoke release of cytokines from these cells. In turn, cytokines will stimulate PG output from decidualized stromal cells or amniotic epithelial cells. In addition cytokines may cause release of other uterotonins, including oxytocin and CRH, from decidua, membranes, and/or placenta. These compounds may affect the myometrium directly or indirectly (see below). LPS and LTA also inhibit replication of amnion cells and presumably contribute to premature rupture of the membranes (Casey et al., 1990).

The paradigm of infection-driven preterm labor has been suggested as a way of understanding controls of PG production and labor at term. However, as indicated above, preterm labor in the absence of infection can occur without the demonstrable changes in amniotic fluid PG concentrations, and without enhanced PG biosynthetic activity in the fetal membranes. Furthermore, MacDonald et al. (1991) have argued that changes in PG and cytokine concentrations in the amniotic fluid of women in preterm labor with infection are not consistent. In that case, the events discussed above may describe an association rather than a cause of preterm labor. It remains possible that other uterotonins are produced which affect the myometrium. For example, preproendothelin mRNA is present in amnion (Sunnergren et al., 1990). Endothelin-1 (ET-1) stimulates smooth muscle contractility. Its expression in decidua is decreased by progesterone and increased by transforming growth factor beta-1 (TGFβ-1) (Casey and MacDonald, 1992). Progesterone

also increases the activity of the enkephalinase enzyme that metabolizes ET-1 (Casey et al., 1991). This action is blocked by TGFβ (Casey and MacDonald, 1992). Further work is required to characterize fully these relationships in tissues from patients at term and preterm labor. During *in vitro* culture of amnion cells, ET-1 output was stimulated by IL-1 and by epidermal growth factor, and the effects of these compounds were inhibited by cycloheximide (Sunnergren et al., 1990). At present, however, there is insufficient evidence to conclude that ET-1 causes myometrial activation, either term or preterm.

Placental CRH and Parturition

It is now well recognized that certain peptides, hitherto described as being of pituitary or hypothalamic origin, are also produced by the placenta and fetal membranes, and may affect myometrial activity at term and in pathologic pregnancies. Corticotropin-releasing hormone (CRH) is one such peptide. PreproCRH mRNA is present in placental tissue; the concentration of translated peptide and its mRNA abundance increases in the placenta during gestation; and secretion occurs into both maternal and fetal compartments (Goland et al., 1986; Sasaki et al., 1987; Frim et al., 1988; Robinson et al., 1988; Riley and Challis, 1991). Maternal plasma CRH concentrations rise at full term and are increased in preterm labor in the absence of infection (Campbell et al., 1987; Warren et al., 1992). These results do not establish a cause and effect relationship, but do establish an association between CRH and labor that warrants further study.

By immunohistochemical methods, CRH was localized to syncytiotrophoblasts and intermediate trophoblasts in the placenta, to chorionic trophoblasts, and to invasive trophoblast cells in the decidua (Riley et al., 1991). In culture, CRH output from placenta, membranes, and decidua can be stimulated by glucocorticoids and attenuated by progesterone (Jones et al., 1989). In placental cells, this action appears to be exerted through an increased rate of transcription, as judged by the significant increase in preproCRH mRNA after dexamethasone treatment (Robinson et al., 1988). CRH output from placental tissue is also increased by prostaglandins, cytokines, and vasopressin (Riley and Challis, 1991). It has been suggested that CRH output may be stimulated by glucocorticoids of fetal adrenal origin. In turn, placental CRH stimulates output from the placenta of POMC-derived peptides including ACTH and β-endorphin (Petraglia et al., 1987; Margioris et al., 1988). Secretion of these peptides into the maternal or fetal circulation is nonsuppressible and potentially stimulated by glucocorticoids. Placental CRH and ACTH would therefore drive fetal pituitary-adrenal activation as a positive, feed-forward loop (Challis and Brooks, 1989; Fig. 32–3).

The importance of the placental CRH-ACTH axis in the process of parturition may be that both peptides stimulate prostaglandin output from cultures of placental, decidual, and chorionic cells (Jones and Challis, 1989). Presumably this effect is mediated through cAMP-dependent protein kinases. Futhermore, Quar-

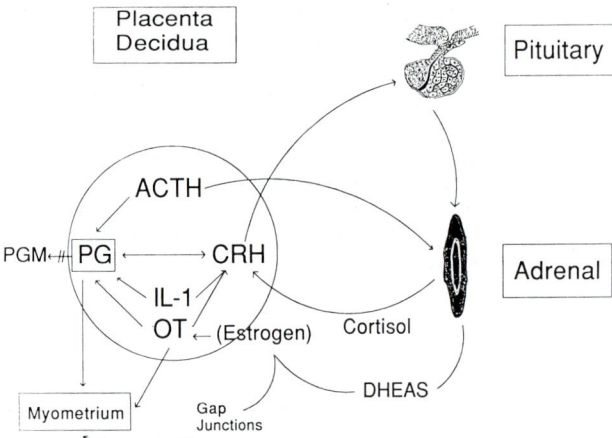

FIGURE 32–3. Diagrammatic representation of the interrelationships among the placenta decidua, pituitary, and adrenal in human pregnancy. CRH, ACTH, prostaglandins, IL-1, and oxytocin are made within the placenta and fetal membranes. The paracrine and autocrine interrelationships between them result in increased prostaglandin production. Placental CRH is secreted into the fetal compartment where it may stimulate the fetal pituitary. Placental ACTH may stimulate adrenal output of cortisol and the estrogen precursor dehydroepiandrosterone sulfate (DHEAS). Endogenous fetal pituitary ACTH also drives these pathways. Cortisol (secreted from the fetal adrenal as cortisol sulfate) is hydrolyzed in the placenta, stimulates CRH mRNA, and perpetuates the cascade. It is proposed that the major effects of estrogen are on myometrial protein and gap junction formation. Myometrial contractility is increased in response to prostaglandins and oxytocin, perhaps acting in conjunction with CRH.

tero and Fry (1989) have shown that CRH directly stimulated contractility of human myometrial strips. CRH potentiated oxytocin-induced contractions. Its action was inhibited by indomethacin, suggesting that this effect might be mediated, at least in part, by prostaglandins. These studies collectively raise the issue of whether placental CRH secretion increases in response to fetal compromise, for example, in hypoxemia, with or without reduced uteroplacental blood flow, leading to preterm labor in the absence of infection.

INHIBITORS OF PROSTAGLANDIN SYNTHESIS

Human amniotic fluid contains both stimulatory and inhibitory activities toward prostaglandin generation in a microsome-enriched preparation of bovine seminal vesicles (Cohen et al., 1985). Since these assays were carried out in the presence of excess arachidonic acid, the effects are presumably exerted through changing PGHS activities rather than on PLA$_2$ or PLC. Cohen et al. (1985) reported that the activity of the stimulatory fraction increased, while that of the inhibitory fraction decreased, with gestational age. Previous work had identified an endogenous inhibitor of prostaglandin synthesis (EIPS) in the blood and amniotic fluid of pregnant women. There was a significant

decrease in EIPS activity in amniotic fluid between early pregnancy (15 to 17 weeks) and term, with a further fall at the time of labor (Saeed et al., 1982; Mitchell et al., 1983), although there was no change in EIPS activity in maternal plasma during gestation.

Wilson et al. (1985) have reported the presence of two components from amniotic fluid that specifically inhibited PLA$_2$ activity in an endometrial cell assay system. These components did not affect PGHS. The protein(s) isolated by Wilson et al. (1985) had molecular weights of 150,000 to 260,000 and 70,000 to 80,000 daltons and were specific for PLA$_2$. It is likely that these molecules belong to the annexin family of proteins. The annexins are substrates for tyrosine kinases and influence PLA$_2$ mobilization and Ca^{2+} mobilization. It is believed that they bind to phospholipids, thereby preventing PLA$_2$ from gaining access to its substrate(s). Recently Myatt, Everson, and colleagues (personal communication) have used immunohistochemistry to localize annexin I to the apical surface of the syncytiotrophoblast. They have shown that the amounts of annexin I measured by western blot analysis and of annexin I mRNA determined by northern blotting decrease with labor. The factors regulating these changes are unknown at the present time. However, these studies indicate that PG output may be affected by modulation of PLA$_2$ activity through members of the annexin family.

STEROID PRODUCTION BY INTRAUTERINE TISSUES

In sheep and many other animal species, birth is preceded by a decrease in the maternal peripheral plasma concentration of progesterone and by a coincident increase in estrogen concentrations, the so-called withdrawal of the progesterone block to the myometrium, and change in the progesterone/estrogen ratio (Thorburn and Challis, 1979). It is clear now that human parturition is not preceded by dramatic changes in progesterone or estrogen concentrations in maternal peripheral plasma either at term or in association with preterm labor (Block et al., 1984; Smit et al., 1984). Similarly, there are no significant changes in the bound or free fractions of estrogen or progesterone nor in the ratios between them in maternal plasma, with the approach of labor (Anderson et al., 1985).

For these reasons various investigators have examined the possibility that changes in steroid production may occur within the intrauterine tissues in late pregnancy, and that the products of such activities would be effective in a paracrine or autocrine fashion and would not be recognized in the peripheral circulation (Challis, 1985; Challis and Mitchell, 1988). Substrate for steroid biosynthesis in the membranes could be derived from fetal plasma, maternal plasma, or amniotic fluid. In amniotic fluid, concentrations of dehydroepiandrosterone sulfate (DHAS) and estrone sulfate (E$_1$S) rise during late pregnancy, and these precursors are converted to estrogen in the membranes. Chorion and decidua have estrone sulfate sulfohydrolase activities. The B$_{max}$ of this enzyme is significantly higher in tissue collected from patients in spontaneous labor, compared to samples obtained at elective cesarean section, while the K_d is unchanged (Chibbar et al., 1986). Activity of 3β-hydroxysteroid dehydrogenase (3βHSD) (pregnenolone to progesterone conversion) was greater in decidua from patients at elective cesarean section than from those in spontaneous labor, although activity in chorion did not differ between these groups. The fetal membranes also contain 17, 20α-hydroxysteroid dehydrogenase activity capable of interconverting estrone and estradiol and progesterone and 20α-dihydroprogesterone. Alterations of this enzyme could influence the local bioactive concentration of progesterone and estrone.

In the placenta, 3βHSD and aromatase activities have been localized by immunohistochemistry to the syncytiotrophoblast. Type I 3βHSD is present in some cells of the amniotic epithelium, weakly in decidual stromal cells, but intensely in the trophoblast layer of the chorion and in intermediate trophoblasts that have invaded decidua (Riley et al., 1992). This localization of 3βHSD is similar to that of CRH (see above), suggesting the possibility of local production of progesterone and autocrine and/or paracrine regulation of CRH expression in the fetal membranes.

OXYTOCIN

Oxytocin is present in maternal and fetal blood during late gestation, and secretion within the two vascular compartments is relatively independent (Forsling, 1979). In women, there is high-amplitude "spurt" release of oxytocin in maternal blood during labor. Umbilical arterial concentrations of oxytocin and vasopressin are higher than those in the umbilical vein, thereby implying fetal secretion. Mean concentrations increase progressively through the first and second stages of labor to reach a peak at delivery (Chard et al., 1971). It is likely that the changing endocrine milieu of late pregnancy may facilitate the release and action of oxytocin. In sheep, Roberts and Share (1969) showed that more oxytocin was released in response to vaginal distention in an estrogen-dominated animal and that progesterone dominance reduced oxytocin output.

Interest in the role of oxytocin in the processes of labor has been renewed with the demonstration of oxytocin gene expression in the placenta and decidua and with the finding that oxytocin antagonists inhibit uterine activity in animals and in women. Lefebvre et al. (1992) reported a dramatic 150-fold increase in the abundance of oxytocin mRNA in rat uterine tissue on days 18 and 21 of pregnancy. At term, uterine oxytocin mRNA exceeded hypothalamic oxytocin mRNA by 70-fold. Immunoreactive oxytocin in uterine tissue showed a corresponding rise at term. This material eluted as two peaks with high-performance liquid chromatography; one peak corresponded with the oxytocin nonapeptide, the second with oxytocin non-covalently associated with neurophysin. In situ hybridization demonstrated that most of the oxytocin mRNA was present in the epithelial cell layer of the endometrium. These observations may have direct relevance to human pregnancy. Chibbar et al. (1992) have shown that the oxytocin gene is expressed in human chorion and decidua, and that oxytocin mRNA abundance is significantly greater in tissues from laboring women than in tissues collected at term elective cesarean section, in the absence of labor. The levels of oxytocin mRNA in amnion and placenta were much less than in chorion and decidua. In preliminary studies Chibbar et al. (1992) suggested that chorio-decidual oxytocin gene expression was increased by estrogen. Thus, oxytocin may be increased by estrogen in a manner that could effect paracrine regulation of myometrial contractility at term or preterm labor. These observations may obviate efforts to explain oxytocin effects on the uterus as resulting from differences in the amplitude or frequency of oxytocin pulses in maternal peripheral plasma.

Estrogen also modulates uterine responsiveness to oxytocin and has a central role in the increasing capacity of oxytocin to stimulate myometrial contractility during late pregnancy. Estrogen increases the number of myometrial oxytocin receptors (Fuchs et al., 1983; Alexandrova and Soloff, 1980). Local estrogen production in chorio-decidua or systemic estrogen could account for the 12-fold increase in the myometrial oxytocin receptor number and enhanced uterine responsiveness to exogenous oxytocin that occur between 13 and 17 weeks of pregnancy and term (Fuchs et al., 1984). After the onset of labor, either preterm or at term, oxytocin receptor levels were maximal and significantly higher than at term but without labor. Oxytocin receptors are also present in decidual tissue. Oxytocin stimulates the output of PGE and PGF by decidua and myometrial tissue *in vitro* (Fuchs et al., 1981, 1982), an action that may lead to enhanced myometrial stimulation. The number of oxytocin receptors in amnion and in chorio-decidua increases with labor, suggesting that these are target tissues for oxytocin, and that local oxytocin may contribute to the overall stimulus to PG generation at parturition.

RELAXIN

Experiments in animals have suggested that relaxin may exert inhibitory effects on myometrial activity, which can be distinguished easily from those of progesterone. The inhibitory effect of relaxin is more rapid in onset than is that of progesterone, and it is primarily one of frequency modulation. Although spontaneous myometrial contractility is suppressed, sensitivity to oxytocin, but not to exogenous prostaglandins, is maintained (Porter, 1979; Schwabe et al., 1978). Also, relaxin elevates uterine cAMP concentrations, in common with some other uterine relaxants (Sanborn et al., 1980). Whether this effect is causally related to the action of relaxin in suppressing myometrial activity has not been established. Alternatively, it has been reported that relaxin stimulates production of PGI_2 by the myometrium (Richardson et al., 1984). It may therefore suppress uterine contractility by both direct and indirect actions.

The highest concentrations of relaxin in maternal plasma are found during the first trimester of human pregnancy, with lower but stable concentrations being present during the rest of gestation (Quagliarello et al., 1979). The concentration of relaxin in cord blood is low, and the corpus luteum was formerly regarded as the major site of production. However, Sakbun et al. (1990) showed recently that relaxin mRNA was present in human fetal membranes. The greatest abundance of message was in decidua, followed by placental trophoblast and chorion. By immunohistochemistry the protein was localized to chorionic trophoblasts and to extravillous (intermediate) trophoblasts. These studies suggest that relaxin could function as a locally produced myometrial relaxant of late pregnancy. This would allow oxytocin sensitivity to develop in a uterus in which spontaneous contractility was suppressed.

DEVELOPMENT OF MYOMETRIAL ACTIVITY

If prostaglandins and oxytocin are among the uterotonins that lead to increased myometrial activation, they can only do so if the uterus has developed the capacity to respond in a synchronous fashion (Lye and Challis, 1989). Thus, the appearance of oxytocin and PG receptors and the development of gap junctions between myometrial cells are considered as necessary prerequisites of labor. There is now abundant electron-microscopic evidence showing that the number of gap junctions in the myometrium increases at term parturition and in preterm labor (Garfield, 1988). Work from Garfield's laboratory in particular has shown that the appearance of gap junctions is influenced by steroid hormones. Withdrawal of progesterone, as after ovariectomy of the rat, or withdrawal of progesterone action, as after administration of the antagonist RU486, increases the number of gap junctions in the myometrium (Garfield, 1988). Exogenous estrogen increases the number of gap junctions and the levels of mRNA for connexin-43, the major gap junction protein (Petrocelli and Lye, 1992). Other work has suggested that the increased appearance of gap junctions at term is due to altered transport and processing of these proteins. These steps also appear to be mediated by steroid hormones.

The control of myometrial activity per se has been described in several reviews (Huszar and Naftolin, 1984; Roberts, 1984). Briefly, it depends upon the enzymatic phosphorylation of the myosin light chains to allow interaction with actin to form actomyosin. Myosin light chain kinase (MLCK) is a key enzyme in effecting this phosphorylation. Calcium, after binding to calmodulin, is essential for the activation of MLCK. Thus, agents that influence the availability of calcium affect MLCK activity and myometrial contractility. Within the myometrial cell, calcium levels are regulated by the intracellular calcium pool, through sequestration within storage vesicles (sarcoplasmic reticulum) and by fluxes of calcium across the cell membrane. These fluxes may be effected through calcium channels or through the calcium-magnesium–dependent ATPase system. Oxytocin appears to stimulate myometrial activity by preventing extrusion of calcium through this latter system. Agents such as

prostaglandins cause release of calcium from intracellular pools or prevent uptake of calcium into those pools.

Progesterone and beta-agonists acting through cyclic AMP-dependent protein kinases promote sequestration of calcium within the sarcoplasmic reticular pools. MLCK activity is also influenced directly through phosphorylation by cAMP-dependent kinases and thus by the intracellular cAMP concentration. In turn, the levels of cAMP within the cell reflect the balance between adenylate cyclase and phosphodiesterase activity. Beta-adrenergic stimulation or beta-sympathomimetic drugs such as terbutaline and isoproterenol, which stimulate adenylate cyclase, thus inhibit MLCK activity. Drugs such as theophylline and alpha-adrenergic effectors, which inhibit phosphodiesterase activity and prevent cAMP breakdown, also elevate intracellular cAMP levels with resultant activation of cAMP-dependent kinases.

These observations provide a rationale for methods currently used to stop labor and for the development of new methods to suppress myometrial contractility. Beta-mimetics act through cyclic AMP-dependent protein kinases to affect MLCK activity and Ca^{2+} availability. Drugs that block prostaglandin production or analogues of prostacyclin that may inhibit uterine activity will be of continued interest. Calcium channel blockers exert their action directly on the myometrium to reduce the availability of calcium necessary for MLCK activation. These drugs may also exert indirect effects on prostaglandin generation. In this chapter we have focussed on prostaglandins. However, we have indicated the need to remain open to the possibility that other agents, separately or synergistically, participate in stimulating myometrial contractility. We have seen that the underlying etiology of preterm labor may be varied and that this syndrome is unlikely to be diagnosed through any one single factor or measurement. Recognition of different precipitating events to preterm labor should allow the rational development and use of different and appropriate management strategies.

REFERENCES

Aitken MA, Rice GE, Brennecke SP: Gestational tissue phospholipase A₂ messenger RNA content and the onset of spontaneous labour in the human. Reprod Fertil Dev 2:575, 1990.

Aitken MA, Rice G, Brennecke SP: Relative abundance of human placental phospholipase A₂ messenger RNA in late pregnancy. Prostaglandins 43:361, 1992.

Alexandrova M, Soloff MS: Oxytocin receptors and parturition: 1. Control of oxytocin receptor concentrations in the rat myometrium at term. Endocrinology 106:730, 1980.

Anderson PJB, Hancock KW, Oakey RE: Non-protein-bound estradiol and progesterone in human peripheral plasma before labor and delivery. J Endocrinol 104:7, 1985.

Ban C, Billah MM, Truong ET, Johnston JM: Metabolism of platelet-activating factor (1-0-alkyl-2-acetyl-sn-glycero-3-phosphocholine) in human fetal membranes and decidua vera. Arch Biochem Biophys 246:9, 1986.

Bennett PR, Rose MP, Myatt L, Elder MG: Preterm labor: Stimulation of arachidonic acid metabolism in human amnion cells by bacterial products. Am J Obstet Gynecol 156:649, 1987.

Billah MM, Johnston JM: Identification of phospholipid platelet-activating factor (1-0-alkyl-2-acetyl-sn-glycero-3-phosphocholine) in human amniotic fluid and urine. Biochem Biophys Res Commun **113**:51, 1983.

Bleasdale JE, Okazaki T, Sagawa N, et al: The mobilization of arachidonic acid for prostaglandin production during parturition. *In* MacDonald PC, Porter J (eds): Fourth Ross Conference on Obstetric Research: Initiation of Parturition. Prevention of Prematurity. Columbus, OH, Ross Laboratories, 1983.

Bleasdale JE, Johnston JM: Prostaglandins and human parturition: Regulation of arachidonic acid mobilization. Rev Perinat Med **5**:151, 1984.

Block BSB, Liggins GC, Creasy RK: Preterm delivery is not predicted by serial plasma estradiol or progesterone concentration measurements. Am J Obstet Gynecol **150**:716, 1984.

Boshier DP, Jacobs RA, Han VKM, et al: Immunohistochemical localization of prostaglandin H synthase in the sheep placenta from early pregnancy to term. Biol Reprod **45**:322, 1991.

Campbell EA, Linton EA, Wolfe CDA, et al: Plasma corticotropin-releasing hormone concentrations during pregnancy and parturition. J Clin Endocrinol Metab **64**:1054, 1987.

Casey ML, MacDonald PC, Mitchell MD: Stimulation of prostaglandin E2 production in amnion cells in culture by a substance(s) in human fetal and adult urine. Biochem Biophys Res Commun **114**:1056, 1983.

Casey ML, Mitchell MD, MacDonald PC: Epidermal growth factor-stimulated prostaglandin E2 production in human amnion cells:specificity and nonesterified arachidonic acid dependency. Mol Cell Endocrinol **53**:169, 1987.

Casey ML, MacDonald PC: Decidual activation: The role of prostaglandins in labor. *In* MacDonald PC, Challis JRG, Roberts JM, Nathanielz PW, et al (eds): NIH Workshop on Initiation of Labor. Ithaca, Perinatology Press, 1988, p 141.

Casey ML, Cox SM, Ward RA, et al: Cytokines and infection-induced preterm labor. Reprod Fertil Dev **2**:499, 1990.

Casey ML, Smith JW, Nagai K, et al: Progesterone regulated cyclic modulation of enkephalinase in human endometrium. J Biol Chem **266**:23041, 1991.

Casey ML, MacDonald PC: The endothelium-enkephalinase system: women, men and babies. Proc Endocr Soc, San Antonio, 1992.

Casper RF, Lye SJ: Myometrial desensitization to continuous but not to intermittent beta-adrenergic agonist infusion in the sheep. Am J Obstet Gynecol **154**:301, 1986.

Challis JRG: Factors responsible for parturition. *In* Beard RW, Sharp F (eds): Preterm Labour and Its Consequences. 13th Study Group of Royal College Obstetrics and Gynaecology, 1985.

Challis JRG, Huhtanen D, Sprague C, et al: Modulation by cortisol of adrenocorticotropin-induced activation of adrenal function in fetal sheep. Endocrinology **116**:2267, 1985.

Challis JRG, Lye SJ: Parturition. *In* Clarke JR (ed): Oxford Review of Reproductive Biology. Vol. 8. Oxford, Clarendon Press, 1986.

Challis JRG, Mitchell BF: Steroid production by the fetal membranes in relation to the onset of parturition. *In* McNellis D, Challis J, MacDonald P, Nathanielz P, Roberts J (eds): The Onset of Labor: Cellular and Integrative Mechanisms. Ithaca, NY, Perinatology Press, 1988, p 233.

Challis JRG, Olson DM: Parturition. *In* Knobil E, Neill J (eds): The Physiology of Reproduction. New York, Raven Press, 1988, p 2177.

Challis JRG, Brooks AN: Maturation and activation of hypothalamic-pituitary-adrenal function in fetal sheep. Endocrine Rev **10**:182, 1989.

Chard T, Hudson CN, Edwards CRW, Boyd NRH: Release of oxytocin and vasopressin by the human fetus during labor. Nature **243**:352, 1971.

Chibbar R, Hobkirk R, Mitchell B: Sulfohydrolase activity for estrone sulfate and dehydroepiandrosterone sulfate in human fetal membranes and decidua around the time of parturition. J Clin Endocrinol Metab **62**:90, 1986.

Chibbar R, Miller, Mitchell BF: Regulation of oxytocin gene expression in human fetal membranes around the time of parturition. Proc Soc Gynecol Invest, San Antonio, abstr 285, 1992.

Cohen DK, Craig DA, Strickland DM, et al: Prostaglandin biosynthesis stimulatory and inhibitory substances in human amniotic fluid during pregnancy and labor. Prostaglandins **30**:13, 1985.

Creasy RK: Prevention of preterm labor. *In* Mead Johnson Symposium on Perinatal and Developmental Medicine **15**:37, 1980.

Creasy RK: Preventing preterm birth. N Engl J Med **235**:727, 1991.

DeWitt DL: Prostaglandin endoperoxide synthase: regulation of enzyme expression. Biochem Biophys Acta **1083**:121, 1991.

DiRenzo GC, Venincasa MD, Bleasdale JE: The identification and characterization of beta-adrenergic receptors in human amnion tissue. Am J Obstet Gynecol **148**:398, 1984.

Divers WA, Wilkes MM, Babknia A, Yen SSC: An increase in catecholamines and metabolites in the amniotic fluid compartment from middle to late gestation. Am J Obstet Gynecol **139**:483, 1981.

Dray F, Frydman R: Primary prostaglandins in amniotic fluid in pregnancy and spontaneous labor. Am J Obstet Gynecol **126**:13, 1976.

Fencl M, Stillman RJ, Cohen J, Tulchinsky D: Direct evidence of sudden rise in fetal corticoids late in human gestation. Nature **287**:225, 1980.

Forsling M: The neurohypophyseal hormones. *In* Ellendorf F (ed): Physiology and Control of Parturition in Domestic Animals. Amsterdam, Elsevier, 1979.

Frim DM, Emanuel RL, Robinson BG, et al: Characterization and gestational regulation of corticotropin-releasing hormone messenger RNA in human placenta. J Clin Invest **82**:287, 1988.

Fuchs A-R, Husslein P, Fuchs F: Oxytocin and the initiation of human parturition. II. Stimulation of prostaglandin production in human decidua by oxytocin. Am J Obstet Gynecol **141**:694, 1981.

Fuchs A-R, Fuchs F, Husslein P, et al: Oxytocin receptors and human parturition; a dual role for oxytocin and the initiation of labor. Science **215**:1396, 1982.

Fuchs A-R, Periyasamy S, Alexandrova M, et al: Correlation between oxytocin receptor concentration and responsiveness to oxytocin in pregnant rat myometrium: Effects of ovarian steroids. Endocrinology **113**:742, 1983.

Fuchs A-R, Fuchs F, Husslein P, Soloff MS: Oxytocin receptors in the human uterus during pregnancy and parturition. Am J Obstet Gynecol **150**:734, 1984.

Garfield RE: Structural and functional studies of the control of myometrial activity and labor. *In* McNellis D, Challis J, MacDonald P, Nathanielsz P, Roberts J (eds): The Onset of Labor: Cellular and Integrative Mechanisms. Ithaca, NY, Perinatology Press, 1988, p 55.

Goland RS, Wardlaw SL, Stark RI, et al: High levels of corticotropin-releasing hormone immunoactivity in maternal and fetal plasma during pregnancy. J Clin Endocrinol Metab **63**:1199, 1986.

Habenicht AJR, Goerig M, Grulich J, et al: Human platelet-derived growth factor stimulates prostaglandin synthesis by activation and by rapid de novo synthesis of cyclooxygenase. J Clin Invest **75**:1381, 1985.

Huszar G, Naftolin F: The myometrium and uterine cervix in normal and preterm labor. N Engl J Med **311**:571, 1984.

Jones SA, Brooks AN, Challis JRG: Steroids modulate corticotrophin-releasing factor production in human fetal membranes and placenta. J Clin Endocrinol Metab **68**:825, 1989.

Jones SA, Challis JRG: Local stimulation of prostaglandin production by corticotropin-releasing hormone in human fetal membranes and placenta. Biochem Biophys Res Commun **159**:192, 1989.

Keirse MJNC, Turnbull AC: E prostaglandins in amniotic fluid during late pregnancy and labour. J Obstet Gynaecol Br Commonw **80**:970, 1973.

Keirse MJNC, Turnbull AC: The foetal membranes as a possible source of amniotic fluid prostaglandins. Br J Obstet Gynaecol **83**:146, 1976.

Lamont RF, Anthony F, Myatt L, et al: Production of prostaglandin E2 by human amnion *in vitro* in response to addition of media conditioned by microorganisms associated with chorioamnionitis and preterm labor. Am J Obstet Gynecol **162**:819, 1990.

Lefebvre DL, Giaid A, Bennett H, et al: Oxytocin gene expression in rat uterus. Science **256**:1553, 1992.

Liggins GC, Fairclough RJ, Grieves SA, et al: The mechanism of initiation of parturition in the ewe. Recent Progr Horm Res **29**:111, 1973.

Liggins GC, Forster CS, Grieves SA, Schwartz AL: Control of parturition in man. Biol Reprod **16**:39, 1977.

Lopez-Bernal A, Hansell DJ, Khong TY, et al: Prostaglandin E production by the fetal membranes in unexplained preterm labour and preterm labour associated with chorioamnionitis. Br J Obstet Gynaecol **96**:1133, 1989.

Lumsden MA, Baird DT: The effect of intrauterine administration of prostacyclin on the contractility of the nonpregnant uterus. Prostaglandins 31:1011, 1986.

Lundin-Schiller S, Mitchell MD: Review: The role of prostaglandins in human parturition. Prostagl Leukotr and Essential Fatty Acids 39:1, 1990.

Lye SJ, Challis JRG: Inhibition by PGI–2 of myometrial activity in non-pregnant ovariectomized sheep. J Reprod Fertil 66:311, 1982.

Lye SJ, Challis JRG: Paracrine and endocrine control of myometrial activity. In Gluckman PD, Nathanielsz PW (eds): The Liggins Symposium. Ithaca, NY, Perinatology Press, 1989.

MacDonald PC, Schultz FM, Duenhoelter JH, et al: Initiation of human parturition. 1. Mechanism of action of arachidonic acid. Obstet Gynecol 44:629, 1974.

MacDonald PC, Koga S, Casey ML: Decidual activation in parturition:examination of amniotic fluid for mediators of the inflammatory response. Ann NY Acad Sci 622:315, 1991.

Margioris AN, Grino M, Protos P, et al: Corticotropin-releasing hormones and oxytocin stimulate the release of placental pro-opiomelanocortin peptides. J Clin Endocr Metab 66:922, 1988.

Mitchell MD: Pathways of arachidonic acid metabolism with specific application to the fetus and mother. Semin Perinatol 10:242, 1986.

Mitchell MD: Pathways of arachidonic acid metabolism. In Mitchell MD (ed): Eicosanoids in Reproduction. Boca Raton, FL, CRC Press, 1990.

Mitchell MD, Strickland DM, Brennecke SP, Saeed SA: New aspects of arachidonic acid metabolism and human parturition. In MacDonald PC, Porter J (ed): Fourth Ross Conference on Obstetric Research: Initiation of Parturition. Prevention of Prematurity. Columbus, OH, Ross Laboratories, 1983.

Mitchell MD, MacDonald PC, Casey ML: Stimulation of prostaglandin E_2 synthesis in human amnion cells maintained in monolayer culture by substance(s) in amniotic fluid. Prostagl Leukotr Med 15:399, 1984.

Nakla S, Skinner K, Mitchell BF, Challis JRG: Changes in prostaglandin transfer across human fetal membranes obtained after spontaneous labor. Am J Obstet Gynecol 155:1337, 1986.

Norman LJ, Challis JRG: Synergism between systemic CRF and AVP on ACTH release in vivo varies as a function of gestational age in the ovine fetus. Endocrinology 120:1052, 1987.

Novy MJ, Liggins GC: Role of prostaglandins, prostacyclin and thromboxanes in the physiologic control of the uterus and in parturition. Semin Perinatol 4:45, 1980.

Okazaki T, Casey ML, Okita JR, et al: Initiation of human parturition. XII. Biosynthesis and metabolism of prostaglandins in human fetal membranes and uterine decidua. Am J Obstet Gynecol 139:373, 1981.

Okazaki T, Ban C, Johnston JML: The identification and characterization of protein kinase C activity in fetal membranes. Arch Biochem Biophys 229:27, 1984.

Olson DM, Opavsky MA, Challis JRG: Prostaglandin synthesis by human amnion is dependent upon extracellular calcium. Can J Physiol Pharmacol 61:1089, 1983a.

Olson DM, Skinner K, Challis JRG: Estradiol-17β and 2-hydroxyestradiol-17β-induced differential production of prostaglandins by cells dispersed from human intrauterine tissues at parturition. Prostaglandins 25:639, 1983b.

Omini C, Pasargiklian R, Folco GC, et al: Pharmacological activity of PGI_2 and its metabolite 6-oxy-$PGF_2\alpha$ on human uterus and fallopian tubes. Prostaglandins 15:1045, 1978.

Petraglia F, Sawchenko PE, Rivier J, Vale W: Evidence for local stimulation of ACTH secretion by corticotropin-releasing factor in human placenta. Nature 328:717, 1987.

Petrocelli T, Lye SJ: Regulation of the level of the gap junction protein, connexin-43, in the rat myometrium. Proc Soc Gynecol Invest, abstr 233, 1992.

Porter DG: The myometrium and the relaxin enigma. Anim Reprod Sci 2:77, 1979.

Price TM, Kauma SW, Curry TE, Clark MR: Immunohistochemical localization of prostaglandin endoperoxide synthase in human fetal membranes and decidua. Biol Reprod 41:701, 1989.

Quagliarello J, Szlachter N, Steinetz BG, et al: Serial relaxin concentrations in human pregnancy. Am J Obstet Gynecol 135:43, 1979.

Quartero HWP, Fry CH: Placental corticotropin-releasing factor may modulate human parturition. Placenta 10:439, 1989.

Richardson M, Mitchell MD, MacDonald PC, Casey ML: Effect of relaxin on prostacyclin production by human myometrial cells in monolayer culture. (Abstract 402) Society for Gynecologic Investigation, San Francisco, 1984.

Riley SC, Challis JRG: Corticotropin-releasing hormone production by the placenta and fetal membranes. Placenta 12:105, 1991.

Riley SC, Walton JC, Herlick JM, Challis JRG: The localization and distribution of corticotropin-releasing hormone in the human placenta and fetal membranes throughout gestation. J Clin Endocrinol Metab 72:1001, 1991.

Riley SC, Walton JC, Luu-The V, Labrie F, Challis JRG. Immunohistochemical localization of 3β-hydroxy-5-ene-steroid dehydrogenase/$\Delta^5 \rightarrow \Delta^4$ isomerase in human placenta and fetal membranes throughout gestation. J Clin Endocrinol Metab 75:956, 1992.

Roberts JM: Current understanding of pharmacologic mechanisms in the prevention of preterm birth. Clin Obstet Gynecol 27:592, 1984.

Roberts JS, Share L: Effects of progesterone and estrogen on blood levels of oxytocin during vaginal distention. Endocrinology 84:1076, 1969.

Robinson BG, Emanuel RL, Frim DM, Majzoub JA: Glucocorticoid stimulates expression of corticotropin-releasing hormone gene in human placenta. Proc Natl Acad Sci USA 85:5244, 1988.

Romero R, Quintero R, Emamian M, et al: Arachidonate lipoxygenase metabolites in amniotic fluid of women with intra-amniotic infection and preterm labor. Am J Obstet Gynecol 157:1454, 1987.

Romero R, Wu YK, Mazor M, et al: Amniotic fluid concentration of 5-hydroxy-eicosatetraenoic acid is increased in human parturition at term. Prostaglandins Leukotr Essent Fatty Acids 35:81, 1989a.

Romero R, Wu YK, Sirtori M, et al: Amniotic fluid concentrations of prostaglandin $F_{2\alpha}$, 13,14-dihydro-15-keto-prostaglandin $F_{2\alpha}$ (PGFM) and 11-deoxy-13,14-dihydro-15-keto-11,16-cyclo-prostaglandin E_2 (PGEM-II) in preterm labor. Prostaglandins 37:149, 1989b.

Romero R, Avila C, Brekus CA, Morotti R: The role of systemic and intrauterine infection in preterm parturition. Ann NY Acad Sci 622:355, 1991.

Rose MP, Myatt L, Elder MG: Pathways of arachidonic acid metabolism in human amnion cells at term. Prostaglandins Leukotr Essent Fatty Acids 39:303, 1990.

Saeed SA, Strickland DM, Young DC, et al: Inhibition of prostaglandin synthesis by human amniotic fluid: Acute reduction in inhibitory activity of amniotic fluid obtained during labor. J Clin Endocrinol Metab 55:801, 1982.

Sakbun V, Ali SM, Greenwood FC, et al: Human relaxin in the amnion, chorion, decidua parietalis, basal plate, and placental trophoblast by immunocytochemistry and northern analysis. J Clin Endocrinol Metab 70:508, 1990.

Sanborn BM, Kuo HS, Weisbrodt NW, Sherwood OD: The interaction of relaxin with the rat uterus. 1. Effect on cyclic nucleotide levels and spontaneous contractile activity. Endocrinology 106:1210, 1980.

Sasaki A, Shinkawa O, Margioris AN, et al: Immunoreactive corticotropin-releasing hormone in human plasma during pregnancy, labor, and delivery. J Clin Endocrinol Metab 64:224, 1987.

Schwabe C, Steinetz B, Weiss G, et al: Relaxin. Recent Progr Horm Res 34:123, 1978.

Skinner KA, Challis JRG: Changes in the synthesis and metabolism of prostaglandins by human fetal membranes and decidua at labor. Am J Obstet Gynecol 151:519, 1985.

Smit DA, Essed GGM, de Haan J: Predictive value of uterine contractility and the serum levels of progesterone and oestrogens with regard to preterm labour. Gynecol Obstet Invest 18:252, 1984.

Sunnergren KP, Word RA, Sambrooke JF, et al: Expression and regulation of endothelin precursor mRNA in avascular human amnion. Mol Cell Endocrinol 68:R7, 1990.

Thorburn GD, Challis JRG: Endocrine control of parturition. Physiol Rev 59:863, 1979.

Walsh SW: Evidence for 5-hydroxyeicosatetraenoic acid (5-HETE) and leukotriene C_4 (LTC_4) in the onset of labor. Ann NY Acad Sci 622:341, 1991.

Warren WB, Patrick SL, Goland RS: Elevated maternal plasma corticotropin-releasing hormone levels in pregnancies complicated by preterm labor. Am J Obstet Gynecol 166:1198, 1992.

Warrick C, Skinner K, Mitchell BF, Challis JRG: Relation between cyclic AMP and prostaglandin output by dispersed cells from human amnion and decidua. Am J Obstet Gynecol **153**:66, 1985.

Wilson T, Liggins GC, Aimer GP, Skinner SJM: Partial purification and characterization of two compounds from amniotic fluid which inhibit phospholipase activity in human endometrial cells. Biochem Biophys Res Commun **131**:22, 1985.

Zakar T, Olson OM: Stimulation of human amnion prostaglandin E₂ production with activators of protein kinase C. J Clin Endocr Metab **67**:915, 1988.

CHAPTER

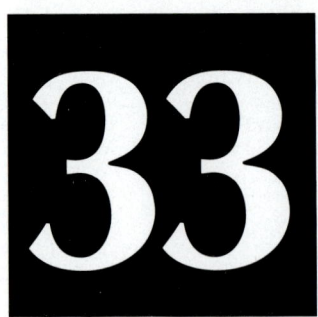

PRETERM LABOR AND DELIVERY

ROBERT K. CREASY, M.D.

Preterm labor and delivery have been a significant cause of perinatal morbidity and mortality for centuries. Although the introduction of refinements in neonatal care has improved outcome for small neonates, there has been no consistent documented decrease in the incidence of low-birth-weight, preterm newborns for many decades. The problem of preterm birth has actually been magnified as the other causes of perinatal morbidity and mortality have decreased, so that preterm delivery is now the single most important problem to overcome in improving the outcome of the gestation with a nonanomalous fetus.

DEFINITION

Traditionally, all newborns weighing less than 2500 gm were classified as premature, but it is now known that as many as one-third of such neonates are born near term but restricted in growth (see Chapter 36). A *preterm birth* is any delivery, regardless of birth weight, that occurs before 37 completed weeks from the first day of the last menstrual period (American Academy of Pediatrics, 1967; World Health Organization, 1969). However, the lower limits of gestational age at which the phrase *preterm labor and delivery* can be used have never been well defined. Pregnancies ending before 20 completed weeks gestation are termed *abortions;* therefore, it seems reasonable to define preterm labor and delivery as occurring between 20 and 37 completed weeks (140 and 259 days) of gestation.

INCIDENCE AND PERINATAL MORTALITY AND MORBIDITY

The true incidence of preterm delivery is not as well documented as might be expected, owing in part to lack of differentiation of growth-restricted from preterm infants. The British Perinatal Mortality Survey, excluding 8 per cent of births because of uncertain gestational age, found that 3.4 per cent of births occurred before 251 days and another 6.1 per cent between 252 and 265 days gestation (Butler and Bonham, 1963). In the United States, data from a study of

birth certificates for most of the country revealed the incidence of preterm birth to be 9.4 per cent in 1981 which rose to 10.7 per cent in 1989 (Monthly Vital Statistics 1991). Significant racial differences exist with 8.8 per cent of white births and 18.9 per cent of black births having occurred preterm. A large multicenter trial in which gestational age was carefully assessed revealed an incidence of delivery before 36 weeks of 9.6 per cent, adding credence to the birth certificate—derived data (Cooper et al., 1993). Thus, the overall preterm birth rate is approximately 10 per cent and will probably vary among different populations depending upon risk factors present.

Preterm births account for the majority of perinatal deaths in nonanomalous newborns. In England, 62 per cent of perinatal deaths and 85 per cent of neonatal deaths unrelated to anomalies were noted in births occurring between 22 and 37 weeks of gestation (Rush et al., 1976). More recently, in a study of 33,401 pregnancies, 83 per cent of neonatal mortality occurred in births of less than 37 completed weeks, and 66 per cent of the neonatal losses occurred with birth before 29 weeks (Cooper et al., 1993). Gestational age is a better predictor of survival before 29 weeks, but birth weight appears to be a better predictor after that gestational age. In addition, prior to 29 weeks, mortality rate in male infants was approximately double that of females, and twin infants had a 3 to 4 times increase in mortality in comparison to singleton infants. Gender, plurality, and ethnicity show minimal differences after this gestational age. A major improvement in survival occurs between 25 and 26 weeks of gestation (Table 33–1). These survival rates from special centers are likely to be higher than the survival rates reached under all circumstances. Although survival following delivery before 26 weeks does occur, the possibility of survival without serious long-term impairment is relatively low (Yu et al., 1986; Nwaesei et al., 1987).

Since survival exceeds 90 per cent by 30 completed weeks of gestation, and approximately 80 to 90 per cent of otherwise uncomplicated preterm birth occurs after this gestational age, neonatal morbidity problems become of paramount importance between 30 and 36 weeks. Data from the large multicenter trial cited

TABLE 33–1. Predicted Survival by Gestational Age and Weekly Improvement in Neonatal Survival

GESTATIONAL AGE (Weeks)	SURVIVAL BY GESTATIONAL AGE (%)	WEEKLY IMPROVEMENT IN SURVIVAL (%)
22	0.0	0.0
23	1.8	1.8
24	9.9	8.1
25	15.5	5.6
26	54.7	39.2
27	67.0	12.3
28	77.4	10.4
29	85.2	7.8
30	90.6	5.4
31	94.2	3.6
32	96.5	2.3
33	97.9	1.4

Adapted from Cooper RL, Goldenberg RL, Creasy RK, et al: A multicenter study of preterm birth weight and gestational age specific mortality. Am J Obstet Gynecol **168**:78, 1993.

above are summarized in Table 33–2 (Robertson et al., 1992). Extension of the otherwise uncomplicated pregnancy past 36 weeks gestation results in a decrease in neonatal respiratory distress syndrome (3.3 to 0.4 per cent, at 36 and 37 weeks), and past 32 weeks, a decrease in patent ductus arteriosus (9.3 to 1.8 per cent, at 32 and 33 weeks) and necrotizing enterocolitis (5.6 to 1.8 per cent, at 32 and 33 weeks). Grades 3 and 4 intraventricular hemorrhage decrease rapidly after 27 weeks and are usually absent after 32 completed weeks. Survival of small neonates has continued to improve. The number of major handicaps has not risen but has remained static or has improved (Jones and Davies, 1981; Nwaesei et al., 1987).

EPIDEMIOLOGY OF PRETERM LABOR

Socioeconomic Status

Numerous reports show a strong correlation between preterm births and low socioeconomic status, the latter being defined on the basis of educational level or of occupation and income (Illsley and Thompson, 1976; Fedrick and Anderson, 1976; Papiernik and Kaminski, 1974). Although Black women are reported to have an incidence of preterm birth that is approximately double that of Caucasian women at all educational levels, Black women who have more than 16 years of education have approximately two-thirds the preterm rate of those with less than 8 years of education (U. S. Department of Health and Human Services, Public Health Service, 1984). Longitudinal studies of more than 30,000 births over 10 years show that there is a higher incidence of preterm delivery at both low and high maternal age (Bakketeig and Hoffman, 1981). The incidence is higher for women less than 20 years of age, not only for the first pregnancy but also for the second or third. Mothers 35 years or older at first delivery are at the highest risk. However, maternal age exceeding 35 years is not associated with an increased incidence of preterm births unless childbearing begins after 35 years.

Socioeconomic status also may have an impact on the nutritional status of a patient. The nutritional level at the time of conception affects the incidence of preterm delivery; the rate in women weighing less than 50 kg at the start of pregnancy is three times the rate in women weighing 57 kg or more (Fedrick and Anderson, 1976). Several recent studies also demonstrate that inadequate weight gain during pregnancy is associated with an increased risk of preterm delivery of perhaps 50 to 60 per cent (Abrams et al., 1989; Hediger et al., 1989; Scholl et al., 1989).

Medical History

The incidence of preterm labor and birth correlates with previous reproductive performance in all reports. A history of one previous preterm birth is associated with a risk of recurrent preterm labor that varies between 17 and 47 per cent, the incidence rising with two or more previous preterm births (Keirse et al., 1978; Bakketeig and Hoffman, 1981; Roberts et al., 1990). With each birth that is not preterm, the risk of a subsequent preterm birth decreases (Table 33–3). Although some reports suggest an increased incidence of subsequent preterm labor following one first abortion, properly controlled reports show no risk (Keirse et al., 1978; Linn et al., 1983). Most but not all reports show an increased risk of preterm delivery after multiple first-trimester abortions (Papaevangelou et al., 1973). However, there appears to be little question that second-trimester abortions are associated with subsequent increased risk.

Incompetence of the cervix (see Chapter 30) due to an inherent defect, which can lead to preterm delivery, is relatively rare. The rate of preterm birth following cerclage approximates 30 per cent (Medical Research Council, 1988; Rush et al., 1984). Cervical incompetence may occur because of dilation of the cervix beyond 8 mm at induced abortion or cone biopsy, but its incidence and its effect on preterm labor and delivery are poorly delineated. Preterm delivery rates ranging from 0 to 33 per cent have been reported to follow cone biopsy (see review by Weber and Obel, 1979).

Approximately 3 to 16 per cent of all preterm births have proved to be associated with uterine anomalies. The risk of preterm labor with a specific uterine anomaly is not known, however, because the incidence of uterine anomalies is not established. In one series of 265 pregnancies occurring in 126 patients with proven uterine anomalies, 29 per cent ended in abortion. The incidence of preterm labor varies from 4 to 17 per cent in patients with a septate uterus to between 20 and 80 per cent in those with other proven anomalies (Heinonen et al., 1982) (Table 33–4). In addition, the T-shaped uterus that may be present in women exposed *in utero* to diethylstilbestrol is often associated with preterm labor and birth (Herbst et al., 1980). Preterm birth rates of approximately 15 to 30 per cent have been reported in these patients. The incidence is greatest in those patients with associated demonstrated malformations of the genital tract. Multiple large leiomyomata may also increase the risk.

TABLE 33–2.   Neonatal Morbidity Rates by Gestational Age at Birth

GESTATIONAL AGE	24	25	26	27	28	29	30	31	32	33	34	35	36	37–38
Respiratory distress syndrome	66.7	87.0	92.6	83.9	64.3	52.8	54.7	37.3	28.0	33.9	13.5	6.4	3.3	4
Intraventricular hemorrhage grades III & IV	25.0	30.4	29.6	16.1	3.6	2.8	1.9	2.0	.9	.0	.0	.0	.0	.0
Sepsis	25.0	8.7	33.3	35.5	25.0	25.0	11.3	13.7	2.8	5.4	3.5	2.3	1.3	.3
Necrotizing enterocolitis	8.3	17.4	11.1	9.7	25.0	13.9	15.1	7.8	5.6	1.8	3.1	.3	.9	.0
Patent ductus arteriosus	33.3	60.9	48.1	38.7	42.9	44.4	22.6	15.7	9.3	1.8	1.7	1.3	.4	.3
Phototherapy for hyperbilirubinemia	66.7	43.5	9.26	80.6	67.9	75.0	73.6	58.8	63.6	43.8	29.3	16.4	9.0	3.5
Exchange transfusion for hyperbilirubinemia	.0	4.3	3.7	6.5	.0	2.8	.0	.0	.9	.0	.9	.3	.4	.2
Hypoglycemia	8.3	17.4	14.8	9.7	7.1	8.3	5.7	3.9	4.7	3.6	4.4	4.4	1.1	.9
None of the above	16.7	4.3	.0	.0	7.1	5.6	9.4	21.6	28.0	40.2	58.5	74.8	86.6	94.8
Admission to NICU or intensive care unit	100.0	100.0	100.0	100.0	100.0	100.0	94.3	96.1	98.1	83.9	70.3	41.6	24.1	10.2
N	12	23	27	31	28	36	53	51	107	112	229	298	544	4803

From Robertson PA, Sniderman SH, Laros RK Jr, et al: Neonatal morbidity according to gestational age and birth weight from five tertiary centers in the United States, 1983 through 1986. Am J Obstet Gynecol **166**:1629, 1992.

Habits During Pregnancy

A number of publications indicate that there is a relationship between strenuous and physically demanding employment and preterm labor (Mamelle et al., 1984; McDonald et al., 1988; Luke et al., 1992), whereas other reports show no deleterious effects (Berkowitz et al., 1983; Hartikainen-Sorri and Sorri, 1989). In one prospective study preterm delivery was highest in women with standing occupations and lowest in those with active jobs, such as nurses, physicians, and athletes (Teitelman et al., 1990). The reported increased incidence of low-birth-weight newborns delivered of female physicians during residency training has been shown to be due to an increase in fetal growth retardation and not to preterm delivery in one report (Grunebaum et al., 1987), but others indicate that the spontaneous preterm birth rate is also increased (Schwartz, 1985; Miller et al., 1989).

Maternal smoking not only decreases birth weight but also increases the incidence of preterm birth, the risk increasing with the number of cigarettes a day smoked (Meyer and Tonascia, 1977; Fedrick and Anderson, 1976; Wen et al., 1990). Parous smokers may be at especially high risk (Cnattingius et al., 1993). It is not known whether the association between alcohol or narcotic addiction and low birth weight produces its affect on fetal growth or gestational age.

The frequently reported anecdotal association of preterm labor and psychological trauma has received further support from studies demonstrating an association between adverse life events and preterm labor and delivery (Newton and Hunt, 1984; Lobel et al., 1992).

Pregnancy Complications

Asymptomatic bacteriuria is associated with a higher rate of preterm labor if there is underlying renal disease or if acute pyelonephritis develops (Kincaid-Smith, 1968). Any systemic infection, such as bacterial pneumonia or acute appendicitis with sepsis, increases uterine activity, and endotoxins have been shown to stimulate myometrial activity in experimental studies. Chronic hypertension may necessitate preterm induction but has not been clearly shown to cause spontaneous preterm birth, even though preeclampsia may lead to a slightly increased risk of preterm labor

TABLE 33–3.   Risk of Preterm Birth in Subsequent Births

FIRST BIRTH	SECOND BIRTH	SUBSEQUENT PRETERM BIRTH (%)
Not preterm		4.4
Preterm		17.2
Not preterm	Not preterm	2.6
Preterm	Not preterm	5.7
Not preterm	Preterm	11.1
Preterm	Preterm	28.4

From Bakketeig LS, Hoffman HJ: Epidemiology of preterm birth: Results from a longitudinal study of births in Norway. *In* Preterm Labor. Elder MG, Hendricks CH (eds). London, Butterworths, 1981, p. 17.

TABLE 33–4.   Incidence of Preterm Labor According to Uterine Anomaly

ANOMALY	NO. OF PATIENTS	PATIENTS WITH PRETERM LABOR NO.	PATIENTS WITH PRETERM LABOR %
Unicornuate	8	3	37
Didelphic	17	6	37
Bicornuate			
Bicollis	5	4	80
Unicollis	66	18	27
Arcuate	33	6	18
Septate			
Complete	24	1	4
Incomplete	36	6	17

Adapted from Heinonen PK, Saarikoski S, Pystynen P: Reproductive performance of women with uterine anomalies. Acta Obstet Gynecol Scand **61**:157, 1982.

(Bakketeig and Hoffman, 1981). Diabetes is not a risk factor unless complications such as polyhydramnios develop. Women who have been treated for pituitary adenomas may be at higher risk (Magyar and Marshall, 1978), but treatment with bromocriptine does not increase the risk (Singer et al., 1977). Patients with hyperthyroidism, heart disease, obstetric cholestasis, hepatitis, and anemia are also at increased risk, but the exact risk is not clear (Klebanoff et al., 1991). Abdominal surgery during the last two trimesters is usually associated with excessive uterine activity that may progress to preterm labor (Holbrook et al., 1989).

Assisted reproductive technologies (ART) are associated with a preterm birth incidence of approximately 27 per cent (Australian Institute of Health and Welfare, 1992). In part this is due to an incidence of multiple pregnancies of approximately 20 per cent, and the associated increased preterm delivery rate, but the incidence in singleton ART pregnancies is also quite high being approximately 15 per cent.

Approximately 30 to 50 per cent of multiple gestations end spontaneously before 37 completed weeks (Neilson et al., 1988; Gummerus and Halonen, 1987). This occurrence may be related to overdistention of the uterus, since preterm labor and delivery also occur in 30 to 40 per cent of pregnancies complicated by polyhydramnios (Kirbinen and Jouppila, 1978). Fetal anomalies, such as anencephaly associated with polyhydramnios or renal agenesis associated with oligohydramnios, are likely to be associated with preterm labor (Honnebier and Swaab, 1973; Ratten et al., 1973). Multiple congenital anomalies and central nervous system anomalies also carry higher risk. Unexplained elevation of maternal serum alpha-fetoprotein is associated with an increased incidence of preterm birth, the incidence increasing as the multiple of the median increases (Wenstrom et al., 1992).

Antepartum hemorrhage, from placenta previa, abruption of the placenta, or normally implanted placenta, is commonly associated with preterm birth (Roberts, 1970). Indeed, it is the highest risk factor in some reports (Bakketeig and Hoffman, 1981). First-trimester bleeding in one report also doubled the risk of subsequent preterm labor in the index pregnancy (Williams et al., 1991).

Some cases of preterm labor with intact membranes are caused by systemic or intrauterine infection, but as of this writing the exact incidence, specific organisms, and pathogenesis are poorly understood (for review see Gibbs et al., 1992). Such intrauterine infection may even be present without clinical signs of maternal infection, and in as many as 15 to 25 per cent of preterm deliveries, intrauterine infection has been implicated (Naeye, 1979; Romero and Mazor, 1988). Colonization of the lower genital tract with various bacteria such as Chlamydia trachomatis, Ureaplasma urealyticum, group B streptococci, Gardnerella vaginalis, Trichomonas vaginalis, and various anaerobes has been implicated in some but not all reports in causing preterm births (Minkoff et al., 1984; Gravett et al., 1986; Sweet et al., 1987; McDonald et al., 1992). In two reports demonstrating no relationship between lower genital tract chlamydial infection and preterm labor, there was an increase of preterm delivery in a subset of patients with proven IgM antibody against C. trachomatis (Sweet et al., 1987). Phospholipase A_2 activity has been detected in the lower genital track of pregnant women and is independently associated in increasing amounts in the presence of bacterial vaginosis, Trichomonas vaginalis and Chlamydia trachomatis (McGregor et al., 1992).

Infectious organisms may also reach the intrauterine milieu by transplacental passage from the maternal circulation and may cause preterm labor, examples being Listeria monocytogenes, Treponema pallidum, and mycobacteria. Other implicated organisms are viruses such as cytomegalovirus, herpes, rubella, hepatitis, smallpox, and chickenpox, and protozoans such as Toxoplasma gondii and Plasmodium falciparum (Remington and Klein, 1983; Polk, 1984).

Illicit drug use in pregnancy is associated with preterm birth: cocaine use in pregnancy has an attendant incidence of preterm birth of 20 to over 50 per cent in matched studies (Chasnoff et al., 1989; Cherukuri et al., 1988). Iatrogenic preterm delivery may also occur, a situation that should be avoidable.

PREDICTION OF PRETERM LABOR

The early symptoms of preterm labor are so subtle as to be frequently overlooked by the patient, nurse, and physician, with the result that as few as 10 to 20 per cent of patients who have received routine antenatal care, and present in preterm labor, are candidates for long-term therapy to prevent preterm birth (Zlatnick, 1972; Stubblefield, 1984). Contraindications to such treatment are rupture of the fetal membranes (30 to 40 per cent), advanced cervical dilation, maternal hemorrhage, fetal anomalies, and evidence of severe fetal compromise. Achieving a reduction in the number of preterm births is therefore dependent not only upon development of effective therapeutic drugs, but also upon the ability to identify patients in the early stages of preterm labor. The patient group to monitor closely would be those at increased risk of developing preterm labor, but ideally all patients should be screened. Ideally, an accurate means of predicting preterm labor should enable not only early treatment of the patient in preterm labor, but also its actual prevention through modification of lifestyle or selective use of prophylactic tocolytic agents.

Risk-Scoring Indices

Several systems based on epidemiologic information described previously have been proposed for the specific purpose of predicting spontaneous preterm labor. (Papiernik, 1969; Creasy et al., 1980b). Scoring evaluation is usually performed at the initial visit, with emphasis placed upon rescoring later in gestation and the value of observing cervical changes. Prospective studies of these risk-scoring systems in general reveal sensitivities of 40 to 60 per cent and positive predictive values of only 15 to 30 per cent (Creasy et al., 1980b; Main et al., 1987a). A simple method, based upon a retrospective analysis of over 7000 patients, is shown

TABLE 33–5. **Major and Minor Risk Factors in Prediction of Spontaneous Preterm Labor**

MAJOR RISK FACTORS
Multiple gestation
DES exposure
Hydramnios
Uterine anomaly
Cervix dilated >1 cm at 32 weeks
Second trimester abortion × 2
Previous preterm delivery
Previous preterm labor term delivery
Abdominal surgery during pregnancy
History of cone biopsy
Cervical shortening <1 cm at 32 weeks
Uterine irritability
Cocaine abuse

MINOR RISK FACTORS
Febrile illness
Bleeding after 12 weeks
History of pyelonephritis
Cigarettes—more than 10/day
Second trimester abortion × 1
More than 2 first-trimester abortions

Presence of one or more major factors and/or two or more minor factors places patient in risk group.
Adapted from Holbrook RH Jr, Laros RK Jr, Creasy RK: Evaluation of a risk-scoring system for prediction of preterm labor. Am J Perinat **6**:62, 1989.

in Table 33–5 (Holbrook et al., 1989). It is unlikely that further refinements in the use of epidemiologic data will be able to improve prediction to the degree that would warrant intervention or treatment to prevent preterm labor. At present these systems are mainly used to identify patients who are at greater risk, but only deserve enhanced surveillance. Other biochemical or biophysical measurements are needed to improve prediction of preterm labor.

Biochemical Prediction Indices

The study of the mechanisms of parturition has led to the finding that steroid hormones play an important role in certain animal species and may be involved in human parturition (see Chapter 32). Serum estradiol and progesterone concentrations in peripheral blood have been assessed in patients developing preterm labor, but results have been inconsistent, with low and normal progesterone and low-normal and high estradiol levels reported in patients who develop preterm labor (Csapo et al., 1974; TambyRaja et al., 1974). Weekly serum progesterone and estradiol measurements collected prospectively in 17 patients who developed spontaneous preterm labor were not found to be significantly different from measurements in 42 patients who delivered at term, in part owing to wide variability of values, and there was no change in estradiol or progesterone level before preterm or term parturition (Block et al., 1984). Measurement of serum progesterone and estradiol on a weekly basis does not improve prediction of preterm labor.

Plasma levels of prostaglandin or its metabolites have also been measured prior to the onset of preterm labor, without any evidence of elevation in most cases. Further evaluation of this potential biochemical pre-

dictor is necessary. The suggestion that elevated levels of major basic protein might identify patients destined to develop preterm labor (Coulam et al., 1987) appears to be negated by normal variability.

Fetal fibronectin, a component of the extracellular matrix, has been shown in cross-sectional studies to be present in cervicovaginal secretions in only 3 to 4 per cent of patients between 21 and 37 weeks (Lockwood et al., 1991). Longitudinal studies of women at high risk of preterm labor have revealed a positive test to have a positive predictive value of preterm delivery of 46 per cent, a sensitivity of 93 per cent, a specificity of 52 per cent, and a negative predictive value of 94 per cent (Nageotte et al., 1993). These encouraging studies will need further confirmation, in low-risk as well as high-risk patients.

Biophysical Prediction Indices

Approximately 25 per cent of patients with cervical effacement before 34 weeks deliver before term, with early engagement being an ominous sign (Leveno et al., 1986; Stubbs et al., 1986). A positive predictive value of only 25 per cent does not warrant active treatment. Use of the cervical score, defined as cervical length in centimeters minus cervical dilatation in centimeters, may prove to be superior. Although the cervical score has only been evaluated in multiple pregnancies, in two studies in which 154 of 294 pregnancies ended preterm, a score of ≤0 had a positive predictive value of between 66 and 75 per cent for all patients, and only 2/154 preterm births occurred within one week of a score of one or more (Neilson et al., 1988; Newman et al., 1991) (Table 33–6). The positive predictive value increased the earlier in gestation that a score of ≤0 was obtained. It is necessary to evaluate this approach in singleton pregnancies. Cross-sectional data of endovaginal ultrasound evaluation of the cervix reveal a risk of preterm delivery of 35 per cent if the cervical length is less than 3.4 cm (Anderson et al., 1990).

Uterine activity may be an important marker for identifying patients who are destined to experience preterm labor. Discontinuous studies reveal that there are two types of uterine contractile activity reported, high-frequency, low-amplitude contractile waves and a higher-amplitude wave form (Braxton Hicks) occurring at much longer intervals. The latter type increases in frequency as gestation advances, with the onset of active labor at term being gradual (Caldeyro-Barcia

TABLE 33–6. **Prediction of Preterm Delivery by use of the Cervical Score in Multiple Gestations**

PRETERM DELIVERY	PPV*
110/223†	66%
44/71‡	75%

*PPV = Positive predictive value.
†Data from Neilson JP, Verbuyl DA, Crowther CA, et al: Preterm labor in twins: Prediction by cervical assessment. Obstet Gynecol **72**:719, 1988.
‡Data from Newmann RB, Godsey RK, Ellings JM, et al: Quantification of cervical change: Relationship to preterm delivery in multifetal gestation. Am J Obstet Gynecol **165**:264, 1991.

and Poseiro, 1960). Longitudinal studies in 109 normal pregnant women, monitored for 24 hours twice a week for the last half of pregnancy and delivering at term, revealed that hourly contraction frequency increases throughout gestation (Moore, Iams, Creasy et al., 1993). There is a marked diurnal rhythm with peak uterine activity occurring at night during sleep (see Fig. 33–1). The 95th percentile of uterine activity rises to four contractions per hour at 36 weeks during daylight hours, but may be as high as seven or eight contractions per hour at night (Fig. 33–2). Significant individual variability can also occur.

An increase in baseline uterine activity days to weeks before the establishment of clinical preterm labor has been described (Bell, 1983; Katz et al., 1986a). The frequency of uterine contractions, measured by use of a portable tocodynamometer at home, was significantly greater in women at high risk of preterm labor who subsequently developed it than in those high-risk women who did not (Katz et al., 1986a). This difference in baseline activity could be seen in many patients several weeks before preterm labor. Main and colleagues (1988) randomly monitored a group of indigent patients without other preterm labor risk factors during their antenatal outpatient visits at 28 to 32 weeks of gestation. If the highest number of uterine contractions noted during these random samplings was less than six, the preterm labor rate was 4 per cent; with six or more, the preterm labor rate was 27 per cent with a sensitivity of 71 per cent. Patients with multiple gestations delivering at term also have significantly more uterine activity than those with term singleton gestations, the difference becoming more pronounced as term approaches (Newman et al., 1986a). At present it would appear that the positive predictive values of uterine activity monitoring are not

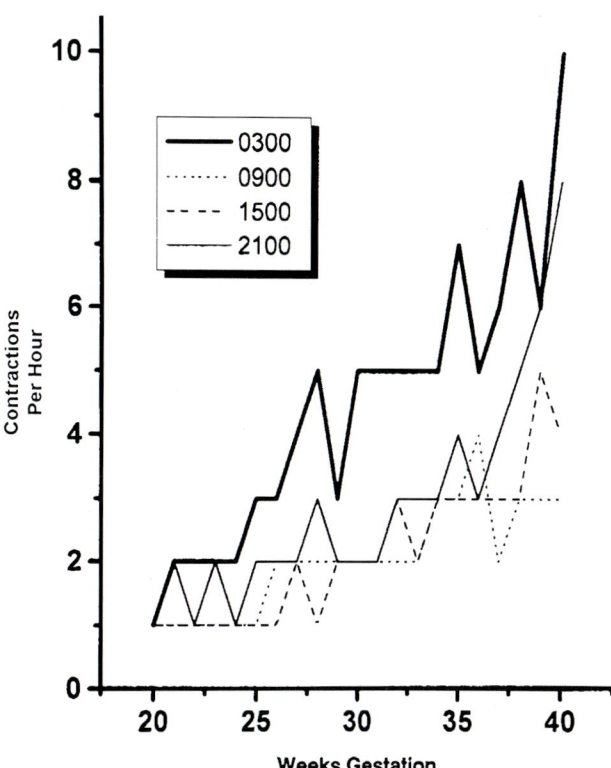

FIGURE 33–2. The 95th percentile of uterine contractions per hour as a function of four different times of day in normal singleton pregnancy. (From Moore TR, Iams, JD, Creasy RK, et al: Diurnal and gestational patterns of uterine activity in normal human pregnancy. Presented to Society of Perinatal Obstetricians, San Francisco, 1993.)

adequate to warrant treatment to prevent preterm labor, but merely to select out a high-risk group for further evaluation and surveillance.

It has also been suggested that the response of the uterus to mammary stimulation may help to predict preterm labor. In a prospective study of 94 high-risk patients, a positive response (seen in 50 per cent of patients) had a positive predictive value of 34 per cent and a sensitivity of 84 per cent and no patient delivered preterm within 1 month of a negative test (Eden et al., 1991).

PREVENTION OF PRETERM LABOR

As is evident from the foregoing discussion, the systems currently available to predict preterm labor are not discriminating enough to serve as a reliable basis for easy evaluation of ways to prevent preterm labor. Prophylactic approaches may be assessed in multiple gestations, wherein the incidence of preterm labor approaches 50 per cent, but the additional fetus and uterine overdistention make interpretation of information gained from such studies difficult to apply to the singleton gestation.

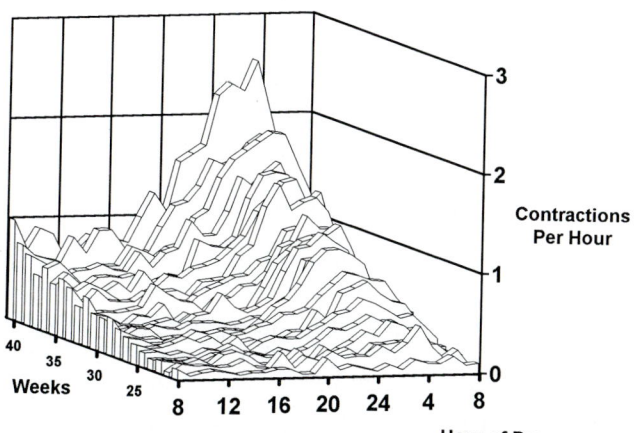

FIGURE 33–1. Contractions per hour (CPH) as a function of gestational age (weeks) and time of day in normal singleton pregnancy. (From Moore TR, Iams, JD, Creasy RK, et al: Diurnal and gestational patterns of uterine activity in normal human pregnancy. Presented to Society of Perinatal Obstetricians, San Francisco, 1993.)

Because there is epidemiologic information indicating a relationship between poor nutritional status and adverse outcome of pregnancy, including preterm birth, appropriate dietary advice should be given to all pregnant women. There are suggestions that hypovolemia, or a lack of the volume expansion that normally occurs in pregnancy, may be associated with preterm delivery (Rahia et al., 1956; Goodlin et al., 1981), but whether dietary approaches can alter this problem remains to be shown. It is prudent, however, to offer proper dietary counseling to any pregnant patient (see Chapter 11). It is also suitable to encourage reduction, preferably cessation, of maternal cigarette smoking and use of any unnecessary drugs. In addition, there are numerous suggestions that acute psychosocial trauma may precipitate preterm labor, but few controlled trials are available; however, affected patients should be observed closely for preterm labor and given psychological support as appropriate.

Bed Rest

Several observational reports have suggested that bed rest may be useful in preventing preterm births in multiple gestations, but no studies have been reported in singleton gestations. Four controlled trials have assessed the role of in-hospital bed rest in twin pregnancies, and none has shown any benefit (Table 33–7). If bed rest is to help decrease mortality, it should be instituted before 25 weeks. The issue of reduced activity in the home setting in either singleton or twin gestations remains to be addressed prospectively. Uterine activity does decrease following a rest period in normal singleton pregnancies (Moore et al., 1993).

Infection and Antibiotic Usage

As indicated earlier, preterm labor has been associated with occult amnionitis. Many bacterial species that may be present in the lower genital tract can theoretically initiate preterm labor through their high phospholipase A_2 activity leading to prostaglandin synthesis (Bejar et al., 1981; McGregor et al., 1992). Random treatment of nonbacteriuric pregnant patients with daily tetracycline therapy, as part of a study of bacteriuria in pregnancy, resulted in fewer preterm births (Elder et al., 1971). Although retrospective nonrandomized trials have indicated some benefit of treatment, three prospective trials using erythromycin or clindamycin have shown no decrease in preterm births

(For reviews see Gibbs et al., 1992; Kirschbaum, 1993). Other large prospective trials are ongoing.

Coitus

An association between coitus and preterm labor has been theorized (Goodlin et al., 1971; Wagner et al., 1976). Coitus may also contribute to the pathogenesis of intrauterine infection (Naeye, 1979). It is also known that the uterus contracts with orgasmic activity and that semen contains prostaglandins; the suggestion has been made that either of these mechanisms could trigger preterm labor. However, most pregnant women continue to have coitus, and the spontaneous preterm labor rate is only 5 to 10 per cent. Thus, routine recommendations against coitus cannot be advised. The use of condoms may be suggested in certain patients, and cessation of coitus between 20 and 36 weeks in very high-risk patients, such as those with two or three previous preterm deliveries, may be considered. Another approach is to have patients monitor themselves for uterine contractions two to three hours after coitus, when coitus-related increases in uterine activity should have returned to normal (Brustman et al., 1989; Moore et al., 1993). If regular painless contractions are noted at this time these patients should seek medical advice.

Surgery

Cervical cerclage appears to be effective treatment of incompetent cervix (see Chapter 30). Although there are suggestions that it may be a valuable procedure for preventing preterm labor, there is currently no evidence to support this view. Indeed, it is possible that placement of a cerclage after 20 weeks may actually promote uterine contractions, because plasma concentrations of prostaglandins are elevated shortly after the procedure (Bibby et al., 1979). If cervical incompetence is a factor in preterm labor, it might be particularly evident in the overdistended uterus associated with multiple gestations, in which cerclage has not been shown to be effective. Controlled trials in singleton gestations show an increased incidence of subsequent painful contractions leading to rehospitalization, the need for tocolytics, and a trend toward more preterm births in those patients having a cervical suture placed (Lazar et al., 1984; Rush et al., 1984). The rate of preterm birth following cerclage is approximately 30 per cent (Medical Research Council, 1988).

Table 33–7. **Four Randomized Studies of Bed Rest in Hospital in Twin Gestation to Prevent Preterm Delivery (PTD)**

AUTHOR / YEAR / NO. OF PATIENTS	TIME OF HOSPITALIZATION	OUTCOME
Hartikainen-Sorri et al. 1984 **N = 146**	30 weeks	No change
Saunders et al. 1985 **N = 212**	32 weeks	30% PTD in Rx vs 19% in controls (p <0.05)
Crowther et al. 1989 **N = 139**	34 weeks	No change
MacLennan et al. 1990 **N = 141**	26–30 weeks	PTD before 32 weeks 16% in Rx vs 8% in controls

Pharmacologic Therapy

The hypothesis that preterm labor may be initiated by a decrease in progesterone has led to studies testing the possibility that administration of progesterone or a similar compound might prevent preterm labor and delivery. Although, progesterone or 6α-methyl-17α-hydroxyprogesterone (medroxyprogesterone) has no beneficial effect on inhibiting preterm labor (Fuchs and Stakeman, 1960; Ovlisen and Iversen, 1960), a recent meta-analysis of five randomized controlled trials of injections of 17α-hydroxy-progesterone caproate to prevent preterm labor and delivery has revealed a significant decrease in preterm birth (odds ratio 0.50; 95 per cent confidence limits 0.30 to 0.85) (Keirse et al., 1989). These positive effects were not associated with a decrease in perinatal mortality or with neonatal respiratory distress. Further evaluation of this preventive modality is needed, perhaps using oral medication.

Prospective studies with low-dose beta-adrenergic agents have not demonstrated any beneficial effects in six twin trials and five singleton trials when assessed by meta-analysis (Keirse et al., 1989). However, terbutaline and ritodrine have been shown to decrease the recurrence rate of preterm labor (Brown and Tejani, 1980; Creasy et al., 1980a). Thus, the usefulness of prophylactic beta-adrenergic treatment remains to be clarified. As indicated later in this chapter, there is a close correlation between uterine-inhibiting effects and maternal pulse rate elevation when beta-adrenergic drugs are used. If these agents are to be beneficial in preventing preterm labor, it is likely that they will need to be used in doses causing a mild maternal tachycardia. Prostaglandin synthetase inhibitors and calcium antagonists have not been evaluated for safety or efficacy in preventing preterm labor.

In summary, there is at present no proven method for preventing the initiation of preterm labor.

EARLY DETECTION OF PRETERM LABOR

At present our ability to predict preterm labor is not discriminatory enough to warrant routine prophylactic treatment, which in itself is not well-established. Therefore, attention must be directed to preventing preterm birth by inhibition of preterm labor, once it has been diagnosed, through use of tocolytic drugs. However, the efficacy of tocolytic agents decreases markedly if the cervix is more than 80 per cent effaced or more than 3 to 4 cm dilated, or if the membranes are ruptured when therapy is instituted (Renaud et al., 1974). In addition, any significant reduction in the overall preterm birth rate is unlikely if, as indicated earlier, only 10 to 20 per cent of patients receiving routine obstetric care are candidates for treatment. Thus, every attempt should be made to detect preterm labor early in its evolution.

Symptoms

Unfortunately, the symptoms of preterm labor are frequently so subtle and insidious that they are not recognized until labor and cervical dilation are far advanced or the membranes rupture. The early symptoms and signs of preterm labor are listed in Table 33–8. The uterine contractions are frequently painless and often described as menstrual-like cramps or vague tightenings. In a study of 100 women in established preterm labor and having uterine contractions at least every 4 to 5 minutes, it was found that only 45 women recognized that they were having contractions every 10 minutes, and only half of these women described them as painful (Katz et al., 1990). Backache or pelvic pressure was described as constant. A sudden increase in vaginal discharge or a pink-stained discharge was reported by 30 to 50 per cent of patients. Similar findings have been reported by Iams et al. (1990), who also found that patients with preterm rupture of the membranes had many similar symptoms, but these occurred less frequently. These symptoms and signs may be seen in approximately 5 to 20 per cent of patients not in preterm labor, depending on the factor. The presence of these warning symptoms and signs indicates a need for further evaluation and/or observation of the patient. They have not been shown to be of value in predicting the subsequent development of preterm labor.

Preterm Birth Prevention Programs

A number of preterm birth prevention programs have been developed (Herron et al., 1982; Creasy, 1983; Papiernik, 1985; Mahan, 1983; Main et al., 1985a; Meis et al., 1987). These programs have varied somewhat in design, but in general include (1) special education and close observation of patients thought to be at increased risk of preterm labor, (2) education of health care providers of the importance of preterm delivery as a reproductive problem and the subtle symptoms of early preterm labor, (3) patient detection of painless contractions or the sampling of uterine activity by a home ambulatory monitor, and (4) prompt treatment with a tocolytic agent once a diagnosis is made. In addition, some programs have utilized a weekly evaluation of the cervix. The emphasis of most of these programs has been on the early detection of preterm labor rather than the prevention of preterm labor. More recent use of these approaches has focused on low-risk as well as high-risk patients (Yawn and Yawn, 1989).

The results of these programs have varied from no demonstrable effect in an inner-city population (Main et al., 1985a) to a 50 per cent reduction in preterm births and an approximately 70 per cent reduction in perinatal mortality and morbidity in a higher-income well-educated population based upon a historical con-

TABLE 33–8. Symptoms of Early Preterm Labor

Uterine contractions—frequently painless
Menstrual cramps
Constant backache
Pelvic pressure
Increased vaginal discharge
Blood-stained vaginal discharge

trol (Herron et al., 1982; Creasy, 1983). In general, positive results have been more difficult to demonstrate in patients of lower socioeconomic status than in those of higher socioeconomic status in the United States (Meis et al., 1987). A randomized control trial of inner-city patients revealed no difference in outcome between the intervention and control groups, but a greater than 30 per cent decrease in preterm birth in both groups over the study period (Mueller-Heubach et al., 1989). A large multi-center study in low-income patients in the United States revealed marked heterogeneity of program effects between centers, the differences in intervention effects not being readily explainable (Collaborative Group on Preterm Birth Prevention, 1993). This large study indicated that positive results of lower preterm birth rates cannot be reliably attained in patients of lower socioeconomic status with this approach. Overall results have been better in well-educated and motivated populations.

In France, a positive impact has been more pronounced in patients with less education, in whom the preterm labor rate is higher (Papiernik et al., 1985). French social support programs, including financial incentives for first-trimester perinatal care and more liberal maternity leave, are thought to be part of the basis of the differences in results in the two countries. In addition, emphasis was placed on educating patients to recognize uterine activity and changing their work or daily habits to reduce uterine activity. Thus this approach was aimed more at the prevention of preterm labor in all patients. Papiernik has also pointed out that a lag time of up to 4 years may occur from the institution of intervention policies to the time when positive results may be seen, in part as a result of patients' evolving acceptance of the new program (Papiernik et al., 1986). National surveys in France revealed a decrease in preterm birth (36 weeks and less) from 8.2 to 5.6 per cent. Unfortunately, hospital surveys have since revealed an increase in preterm births from 6.6 per cent in 1984 to 7.7 per cent in 1986, raising doubt as to the basis of the original improvement (Breart, 1991).

Weekly evaluation of the cervix to detect rather than predict preterm labor has been proposed (Herron et al., 1982). Preterm labor was initially diagnosed in 18.2 per cent of asymptomatic patients when the weekly cervical examination revealed changes (Holbrook et al., 1987). Although the study pointed out the value of such examinations, a cost-to-benefit analysis has not been done. The exact role of cervical examination in preterm birth prevention has not been established. A baseline examination in high-risk patients and a re-evaluation of the cervix when there is a possibility of preterm labor appears appropriate. Potential adverse effects of frequent cervical examinations (increased infectious morbidity, rupture of the membranes, and stimulation of preterm labor) were not reported in this study or in others (Bouyer et al., 1986; Mueller-Heubach et al., 1988).

Ambulatory Uterine Monitoring

It has been suggested that the use of daily sampling may help with the early detection of uterine activity.

Due to the observation that patients accurately perceive only approximately 15 per cent of uterine contractions (Newman et al., 1986b), portable tocodynamometers have been developed and assessed, using the guard-ring principle suggested by Smyth (1957). Patients can wear the sensor at home, record for periods of up to 3 hours, and transmit the recordings by telephone. In general, advice has been to sample uterine activity twice a day for one hour. Katz and colleagues (1986a) demonstrated that the home monitor could accurately detect uterine activity and reported that there was a sudden and significant increase in frequency of uterine contractions in the 24 hours prior to a clinical diagnosis of preterm labor. Once this change from baseline uterine activity is seen, the patient is immediately re-monitored for one hour at home or seen by the physician.

In the first reported observational trial, using matched controls, all monitored patients were candidates for tocolysis versus only one-third of control patients (Katz et al., 1986b). The overall preterm birth rate was 12 per cent in the monitored versus 41 per cent in controls.

The first randomized trial in patients at very high risk also revealed more patients to be candidates for tocolysis (92 per cent versus 45 per cent) and lower preterm birth rates (15 versus 45 per cent) in the monitored patients (Morrison et al., 1987). Since then a number of various trials have been reported (Iams et al., 1988; Hill et al., 1990; Mou et al., 1991; Dyson et al., 1991; Blondel et al., 1992). As a result of the various reports, there is controversy over the relative contributions of the daily nursing contact versus the uterine activity information. Only one trial (Mou et al., 1991) has addressed the issue of whether monitoring by itself, and without nursing support, is capable of improving early detection of preterm labor. In this trial, in which preterm labor was diagnosed with equal frequency in monitored and control patients, the mean cervical dilatation was significantly less at the time preterm labor was diagnosed in the monitored group (1.4 vs 2.4 cm p <0.001), and there were significantly more patients in the monitored group at each dilatation from less than 1 through less than 4 cm.

Various reviews of the subject have been reported, the reviews also demonstrating methodologic deficiencies in the reported studies (Grimes and Schulz, 1992). All of the reviews conclude that daily contact of high-risk patients and home monitoring of uterine activity appear to decrease preterm births, but that the contribution of the uterine activity data by itself is unproven (DATTA, 1989; Rhoads et al., 1991; Sacks et al., 1991; Grimes and Schulz, 1992).

Of particular note in these trials of home uterine activity is the increased number of control patients, approximately 40 per cent, who are candidates for tocolysis at the time of diagnosis of preterm labor. This is double the incidence previously observed and suggests that attention, education, and focus on the possibility of a preterm labor is of benefit. The presence of preterm premature rupture of the membrane is also decreased in the control patients. This also suggests that many cases of preterm premature rupture of the membranes are due to unrecognized preterm labor.

DIAGNOSIS OF PRETERM LABOR

The diagnosis of preterm labor is frequently difficult to make. Meta-analysis of 12 randomized and controlled trials of beta-adrenergic tocolysis has revealed a placebo effect, or misdiagnosis in many patients. In patients receiving a placebo, 27 to 89 per cent had delivery delayed for 48 hours, and 37 per cent delivered at term (King et al., 1988). Although bed rest and hydration may not be placebo treatment, it is unlikely that such measures will stop true preterm labor in half the cases, and the use of hydration and sedation to differentiate true from false preterm labor has not proved useful (Pircon et al., 1989). In most trials, the admission criteria include the presence of regular activity, but it is obvious that not all patients with regular uterine contractions proceed to preterm birth. If the membranes are ruptured and uterine contractions are present, the diagnosis is established. The diagnosis becomes more difficult if the membranes are intact. Preterm labor is diagnosed with intact membranes if cervical change is documented or the cervix is already 2 cm dilated or 80 per cent effaced. The success rate of bed rest and hydration in these conditions drops to less than 20 per cent (Ingemarsson, 1976). Current criteria for diagnosis of preterm labor are summarized in Table 33–9. Importantly, awaiting cervical change in order to diagnose preterm labor does not compromise efficacy of tocolysis (Utter et al., 1990).

Inhibition or cessation of fetal breathing movements is a physiologic event of term labor, thought to be mediated by elevated fetal prostaglandin concentrations (Dawes, 1984). In three reports of ultrasonic evaluation of fetal breathing movements in patients being observed for preterm labor, the absence of fetal breathing movements correlated well (38/43) with delivery within 48 hours, but the presence of the respiratory activity did not rule out preterm delivery (Castle and Turnbull, 1983; Boylan et al., 1985; Besinger et al., 1987). Fetal breathing movements are still present in approximately 10 to 15 per cent of patients delivering preterm within 12 hours of study (Patrick and Richardson, 1985). The concentration of prostaglandin F metabolite in maternal serum of patients being observed for preterm labor who actually delivered preterm has been reported to be double that in those who did not, and was decreased by beta-agonist agents only in patients successfully treated (Weitz et al., 1986).

TABLE 33–9. Criteria for Diagnosis of Preterm Labor

	Gestation 20–37 weeks	
	and	
	Documented uterine contractions	
	(4/20 min, 8/60 min)	
	and	
Ruptured membranes	*or*	Intact membranes
		and
		Documented cervical change
		or
		Cervical effacement of 80%
		or
		Cervical dilatation 2 cm

In patients presenting preterm with regular uterine contractions and intact membranes, the presence of fetal fibronectin in the cervicovaginal secretions had a positive predictive value of preterm delivery of 83 per cent and a sensitivity of 82 per cent (Lockwood et al., 1991).

Thus the utilization of contractions and cervical status, or the absence of fetal breathing movements, or the presence of fetal fibronectin in cervicovaginal secretions all have a false-positive predictive value of 10 to 20 per cent.

MANAGEMENT

Initial Patient Assessment

Before considering the use of a tocolytic agent, one must establish the diagnosis, search for treatable conditions that may be triggering preterm labor, and consider whether there are any maternal or fetal contraindications to attempting labor inhibition.

The patient with suspected preterm labor should initially be placed at bed rest in the lateral decubitus position, and external tocographic and fetal heart rate recording should be instituted. If the membranes are intact, a careful evaluation of the cervix is then performed. If it is decided to withhold drug therapy and await confirmation of the diagnosis in the form of progressive cervical change, frequent digital examination may be required so that the patient does not pass unidentified to an advanced stage of cervical dilatation. A diagnosis of preterm labor is established if the criteria outlined in the preceding section are met.

Owing to the frequent association of preterm labor and urinary tract infections, a urinary microscopic examination and culture should be performed, and antibiotic and antipyretic treatment should be instituted as appropriate. There is currently no information available to prove that cultures of the cervix are useful in regard to treatment of preterm labor (Gibbs et al., 1992; Kirschbaum, 1993). However, if the labor is progressive or the membranes rupture, culture evidence of herpes, Chlamydia, or hemolytic Streptococcus may alter subsequent perinatal management. The cost-effectiveness of routine cervical cultures remains to be determined. A more worrisome infection causing preterm labor is chorioamnionitis. If fever is present and its source obscure, amniocentesis to search for bacteria is indicated. Chorioamnionitis may also be present without maternal signs or symptoms in the presence of intact membranes, except for the preterm labor. Amniotic fluid cultures will be positive in 0 to 24 per cent of patients (Gibbs et al., 1992). A large study of 264 women in preterm labor with intact membranes revealed positive amniotic fluid cultures in 9.1 per cent, but 22 per cent in those going on to preterm delivery (Romero et al., 1989). However, routine amniocentesis to rule out an infectious cause of preterm labor in an otherwise asymptomatic patient has yet to be proved effective. The role of subclinical infection as a cause of preterm labor has also been studied using serum C-reactive protein (Potkul et al.,

1985; Handwerker et al., 1984; Dodds and Iams, 1987). When C-reactive protein was elevated in these three reports, tocolysis failed in 63 to 85 per cent of patients versus 6 to 29 per cent when measurement was less than 0.8 mg/dl. It has been suggested that amniotic fluid cultures be obtained if the C-reactive protein is elevated. It may also be of value in refractory preterm labor, although not all investigators have found infection to be a significant cause of persistent preterm labor (Duff and Kopelman, 1987). As culture results are not immediately available, if amniocentesis is performed, glucose concentrations in the amniotic fluid may provide further insight. Amniotic fluid glucose concentrations below 14 mg/dl have a sensitivity of 87 per cent, a positive predictive value of 63 per cent, and a negative predictive value of 98 per cent in the detection of a positive culture (Romero et al., 1990).

Tocolytic treatment is contraindicated for a variety of obstetric medical reasons (Table 33–10). Many conditions are relative contraindications, wherein tocolysis can be attempted if the risk of preterm birth and associated morbidity and mortality is high, but intensive monitoring of mother and fetus is necessary. Maternal medical conditions such as diabetes mellitus may be adversely affected by some tocolytic agents, such as beta-adrenergic drugs. Such agents can be used if there are resources for close glycemic observation and control. Minor degrees of vaginal bleeding or spotting are often seen in association with preterm labor owing to cervical change, but may also represent a minor abruption. In such cases, if the fetus is not in distress and uterine tonus is normal, tocolytic treatment can be used with continued close observation.

If the cervix is dilated more than 4 to 5 cm when tocolytic treatment is begun, there is only a minimal chance of prolonging the gestation for a significant period (Renaud et al., 1974). Occasionally, however, such a patient is observed whose uterine activity is highly sensitive to initial treatment. If the gestation is between 25 and 27 weeks, delay of delivery for 1 to 2 weeks may significantly alter perinatal outcome, and use of tocolysis can be considered, particularly in twin

TABLE 33–10. Contraindications to Tocolytic Inhibition of Preterm Labor

Absolute contraindications	Severe pregnancy-induced hypertension
	Severe abruptio placentae
	Severe bleeding from any cause
	Chorioamnionitis
	Fetal death
	Fetal anomaly incompatible with life
	Severe fetal growth retardation
Relative contraindications	Mild chronic hypertension
	Mild abruptio placentae
	Stable placenta previa
	Maternal cardiac disease
	Hyperthyroidism
	Uncontrolled diabetes mellitus
	Fetal distress
	Fetal anomaly
	Mild fetal growth retardation
	Cervix more than 5 cm dilated

gestations. Thus, the severity of any associated disease, individualization of patient care, and the tocolytic agent available must all be considered when the decision is made whether or not to inhibit the preterm labor process.

Preterm labor and rupture of the membranes are discussed in Chapter 41.

Pharmacologic Treatment

There is little evidence to support the use of sedatives or narcotics as tocolytic agents. However, the use of mild sedation may be beneficial, in order to allay the significant anxiety and fear so frequently seen in the patient in preterm labor. These agents ideally should not be used if delivery is likely to occur in the next few hours, because of the potential for neonatal depression.

A few trials have been reported on the combined use of antibiotics and tocolytic agents. Two limited trials using adjunctive erythromycin for 7 days showed significantly better prolongation of pregnancy in the groups receiving antibiotics (McGregor et al., 1986; Winkler et al., 1988). One larger study of 95 patients using intravenous ampicillin followed by erythromycin showed no benefit from the adjunctive antibiotic (Newton et al., 1989). Another study of 150 patients, using adjunctive ampicillin or erythromycin orally, demonstrated improved prolongation of pregnancy with either antibiotic (approximately 30 days versus 17 days for tocolytics alone) and fewer preterm births (55 per cent versus 85 per cent) in the group receiving ampicillin plus tocolytics (Morales et al., 1988). Thus when antibiotics have been used, the results are inconsistent; nor has there been consistent improvement in perinatal mortality with their use.

The mechanism of smooth muscle contractility is discussed in detail in Chapter 8. The pharmacologic agents currently in use in various hospitals and countries for preterm labor tocolysis include beta-adrenergic agonists, magnesium sulfate, prostaglandin inhibitors, and calcium antagonists. Ethanol, previously used extensively, has fallen from favor owing to the necessity to cause maternal inebriation. When compared with ritodrine, it also produced a higher incidence of adverse neonatal outcomes (Zervoudakis et al., 1980). The efficacy of tocolytic agents in delaying delivery for 1 to 3 days seems to have been proved, but their ability to cause a decrease in preterm births and their attendant morbidity are still controversial (Hemminki and Starfield, 1978; King et al., 1988; Larsen et al., 1986; Canadian Preterm Labor Investigation Group, 1992).

Beta-Adrenergic Agonists

The beta-adrenergic agonists, currently the most widely used tocolytic agents, include isoxsuprine, hexoprenaline, fenoterol, orciprenaline, ritodrine, salbutamol, and terbutaline.

MECHANISM OF ACTION. The beta-adrenergic agents that are used clinically are derivatives of epinephrine that have been formulated to maximize the beta$_2$-adrenergic effects on the uterus, although all have some beta$_1$-adrenergic activity. The responses of various tissues to beta-adrenergic stimulation are summarized in Table 33–11.

PHARMACOLOGY. The metabolism of the beta-adrenergic tocolytics is different from that of endogenous catecholamines, as the former are not substrates for catecholamine-o-methyl transferase. Information indicates that most of the clinically utilized beta-adrenergic agonists are excreted unaltered, or as conjugates, by the kidney. Minimal information is available on placental transfer except that some agents such as ritodrine and terbutaline cross into the fetus, whereas others such as fenoterol and hexoprenaline probably cross to a lesser degree.

Intravenous administration provides greater bioavailability than do other routes. The concentration of ritodrine in maternal serum increases with increasing infusion rates, and the concentrations can vary by more than 100 per cent from patient to patient at low infusion rates (Carritas et al., 1990a). The therapeutic blood concentration is not established, in part due to the degree of uterine activity and cervical change that may be present as well as differences in plasma clearance. This may explain some of the negative efficacy reports of studies wherein a rigid protocol is observed rather than individualization of treatment. After cessation of infusions, there is an initial rapid half-life of approximately 6 minutes followed by a second disposition half-life of approximately 2½ hours. Intramuscular administration achieves peak plasma concentrations within 10 minutes, with the concentrations being one-half to one-third within 2 hours (Gonik et al., 1988; Carritas et al., 1990b). Oral administration of ritodrine results in peak concentrations at approximately 1 hour, with plasma concentrations being one-fourth of peak concentrations within 4 hours (Carritas et al., 1989).

There is a reduction in myometrial beta-adrenergic receptors in pregnant women treated with a beta-agonist (Berg et al., 1985). In pregnant sheep, beta-adrenergic intravenous treatment for 24 hours leads to a loss of myometrial beta-adrenergic receptors and

a decrease in adenyl cyclase activity (Carritas et al., 1987), and increases uterine prostaglandins (Casper and Lye, 1987). The continuous exposure to beta-adrenergic stimulation led to a reduction of inhibition of oxytocin stimulated contractility in sheep. Intermittent administration of ritodrine revealed no change in the myometrial beta-adrenergic receptors or adenyl cyclase activity and maintenance of inhibition of oxytocin-induced contractility (Carritas et al., 1991). In this latter report, although adrenergic receptor loss was again observed with continuous infusion, the loss of contractility inhibition was not observed, possibly owing to lower plasma levels of ritodrine.

CLINICAL EFFICACY. The effectiveness of the different beta-adrenergic drugs used clinically for tocolysis is comparable. There is little consistent evidence that supports the superiority of one agent over another. There is evidence that beta-adrenergic therapy can delay delivery for 3 days, but its impact on preterm birth remains controversial (Larsen et al., 1986; King et al., 1988; Creasy and Katz, 1984; Leveno et al., 1990; Canadian Preterm Labor Investigators Group, 1992; Higby et al., 1993). The large Canadian study, although complicated by including patients with ruptured membranes (27 per cent), revealed fewer patients in the ritodrine group delivering within 7 days (-9.0; 95 per cent confidence interval -14.8 to -3.2), and a nonsignificant difference, in favor of ritodrine, of delivery occurring at less than 32 weeks (-9.2; 95 per cent confidence interval -18.6 to 0.2). There was also a nonsignificant trend of fewer neonatal deaths at 24 to 27 weeks (-7.2; 95 per cent confidence interval of -19.1 to 4.7). There was one case of pulmonary edema in the treatment group (0.3 per cent).

DOSAGE AND ADMINISTRATION. The beta-adrenergic agents may be administered intravenously, intramuscularly, subcutaneously, or orally. (The subcutaneous route has not been widely assessed for all the drugs.) It is usually recommended that treatment be initiated by intravenous infusion using a calibrated infusion pump. Before initiation of treatment, the patient is placed in the lateral tilt or decubitus position so that supine hypotension can be avoided. An intravenous infusion is established, and continuous external recording is made of fetal heart rate and uterine activity. Prior to initiating tocolytic therapy, baseline information is obtained (Gonik and Creasy, 1986). This can include maternal weight, blood tests such as serum potassium and glucose, complete blood count and colloid osmotic pressure, and urinalysis. The blood tests are repeated at 6- to 12-hour intervals. Intake and output are recorded, the total recommended intake being between 1500 and 2500 ml. The lungs should be auscultated every 6 to 12 hours for evidence of early pulmonary edema. The drug should be infused by means of an infusion pump. The incidence of pulmonary edema may be lower if 5 per cent dextrose in water is used as maintenance fluid rather than isotonic saline (Philipsen et al., 1981). The initial dose is the lowest recommended by the manufacturer of the particular agent. The dose is then usually increased at 10- to 30-minute intervals, the infusion rate adjusted according to uterine activity, or until adverse maternal effects are noted. The infusion rate

TABLE 33–11. Response of Various Tissues to Beta-Adrenergic Receptor Activity

Beta$_1$-adrenergic responses	Cardiac ↑ Heart stroke ↑ Stroke volume Bowel ↓ Motility Metabolic ↑ Lipolysis ↑ Intracellular K$^+$
Beta$_2$-adrenergic responses	Smooth muscle ↓ Vascular tone ↓ Uterine activity ↓ Bronchiolar tone Kidney ↑ Renin ↓ Urinary output Metabolic ↑ Glycogenolysis ↑ Insulin release

probably should not be increased further if maternal pulse rate reaches 130 beats/min or if systolic pressure falls below 80 to 90 torr. Once tocolysis is achieved, some physicians continue the infusion for another 6 to 24 hours. On the other hand, Carritas et al. (Carritas et al., 1983; Carritas, 1988) have recommended that once labor is halted, the infusion rate should be slowly reduced until the lowest inhibitory rate is established, and the maintenance rate should be continued for 12 hours.

Intramuscular or subcutaneous treatment is then given, followed by oral therapy, or oral medication is begun directly. The new route of administration should be started approximately 30 minutes before cessation of intravenous treatment. Intramuscular or subcutaneous injections may be given every 2 to 4 hours for 24 hours prior to initiation of oral medication. Oral doses are administered every 2 to 4 hours. It has been shown that oral terbutaline and ritodrine decrease the recurrence rate of preterm labor (Brown and Tejani, 1980; Creasy et al., 1980a). After 24 hours of oral therapy, the patient can ambulate, with a modified bed rest routine. If the contractions do not resume, the patient may be sent home to continue oral therapy until 36 or 37 weeks gestation.

Owing to the recognition of potential desensitization, there has been increasing interest in intermittent bolus administration of beta-adrenergic drugs. The use of a pump to administer a very low dose of terbutaline (0.3 to 0.5 mg/hr) with intermittent boluses of approximately 0.250 mg at times of peak activity has been recommended (Lam et al., 1988). This approach appears to be associated with the need for less agonist, fewer side effects, and less recurrent preterm labor, but confirmatory data are needed.

Although set doses of oral medication are frequently recommended by a manufacturer, it is often difficult to ascertain the proper dosage if contractions are not present at the initiation of oral treatment. In this situation, one may utilize the maternal pulse rate response. There is a close correlation between the maternal pulse rate and serum levels of ritodrine. In addition, Lipshitz (1977) has demonstrated a close correlation between the time of onset of uterine inhibitory effects and the time of increase in maternal pulse rate following the administration of oral fenoterol. A sustained mild tachycardia indicates the probability of a uterine effect.

The dose, frequency, and routes of administration for two drugs currently used in the United States by many centers, terbutaline and ritodrine, are listed in Table 33–12. The two agents listed are used as examples and not to indicate their superiority, in efficacy or safety, over other agents approved or in use in other countries.

Maternal Effects. Although formulated so as to maximize their uterine effects and minimize extrauterine effects, the beta-adrenergic drugs can significantly influence maternal cardiovascular and metabolic physiology.

Maternal Cardiovascular Effects. As indicated earlier, the beta-adrenergic tocolytic drugs do stimulate both beta$_1$ and beta$_2$ receptors of the maternal cardiovascular system. The more serious side effects include hypotension, cardiac arrhythmias, myocardial ischemia, and pulmonary edema. The reported incidences of these serious complications vary between 0.3 and 5 per cent. In addition, intravenous administration of the drug can be associated with mild palpitations in at least one-third of patients and flushing in 10 to 15 per cent (Merkatz et al., 1980), and with chest pain in 8 per cent (Canadian Preterm Labor Investigators Group, 1992). These effects may necessitate discontinuing treatment in as many as 10 per cent of patients (Robertson et al., 1981).

The altered cardiovascular physiology of pregnancy and labor (see Chapter 46) probably predisposes patients to some of the potentially adverse effects of beta-adrenergic treatment. There is a significant increase in plasma volume, which is more pronounced in twin gestations, and hyperdynamic cardiac function. These features may become more pronounced with beta-adrenergic treatment.

Stimulation of the arteriolar beta$_2$ receptors results in peripheral vasodilatation and potential hypotension. However, the increase in pulse rate and the increase in cardiac output up to 50 per cent over the already increased cardiac output of normal pregnancy (Bieniarz et al., 1974; Wagner et al., 1981; Finley et al., 1984) tend to compensate for the arteriolar dilatation. Among 343 patients treated parenterally with either isoxsuprine or terbutaline, treatment had to be discontinued in only three patients because of hypotension (Robertson et al., 1981). Most reports indicate that diastolic pressure tends to fall and systolic pressure to rise, resulting in a widening of pulse pressure.

Cardiac arrhythmias observed are usually asymptomatic and include premature nodal and ventricular contractions that commonly respond quickly to cessation of treatment (Benedetti, 1983). Myocardial ischemia has been reported by several authors (Benedetti, 1983; Katz et al., 1981; Ying and Tejani, 1982) and has been seen with several different agents. The occurrence or severity of the myocardial ischemia seems to occur mainly at high heart rates (over 120 to 130 beats/min). Measurement of the creatine kinase isoenzyme MB (Meinen, 1981; Steyer et al., 1979; Ying and Tejani, 1982) during beta-adrenergic tocolysis has not revealed any evidence of subclinical myocardial damage. Maternal deaths have also been reported in association with beta-adrenergic therapy, frequently in patients with unrecognized cardiac disease or myocarditis (Kubli, 1977; Barden et al., 1980). The presence of known cardiac disease is a contraindication to beta-adrenergic tocolysis.

Pulmonary edema has been the most common serious adverse side effect, and usually responds to

Table 33–12. Dosages of Ritodrine and Terbutaline for Tocolytic Treatment Used at the University of California, San Francisco

	IV	IM	PO
Ritodrine	0.050–0.350 mg/min	5–10 mg q2–4h	20 mg q2–4h
Terbutaline	0.010–0.080 mg/min	0.250–0.500 mg q3–4h	2.5–5 mg q2–4h

cessation of the beta-adrenergic infusion and institution of appropriate treatment (Katz et al., 1981; Wagner et al., 1981). However, if it is not recognized and acted upon quickly, it can lead to adult respiratory distress syndrome. Predisposing factors are twin gestations (approximately half of reported cases) in which mean plasma volume expansion is greater than in singletons, persistent heart rate over 130 beats/min, anemia below 9 gm per cent, and iatrogenic fluid overload. The beta-adrenergic drugs stimulate the renin-aldosterone system, decrease urinary output, and also decrease colloid osmotic pressure by approximately 20 per cent after 24 hours of infusion (Lammintausta and Erkkola, 1979; Gonik et al., 1985; Armson et al., 1992) (see Chapter 51). Experimental studies in the baboon over 24 hours have revealed that these agents cause an increase in extracellular fluid, retention of sodium, and a slow progressive rise in pulmonary capillary wedge pressure (Hauth et al., 1983). Sodium retention is probably the primary cause of fluid retention and volume expansion (Armson et al., 1992). Pulmonary edema during tocolysis is also increased in the presence of maternal infection (Hatjis and Swain, 1988). All these factors predispose the patient to volume overload over time, particularly if the colloid osmotic pressure drops below 15 mm Hg. The majority of reported cases mention pulmonary edema occurring 30 to 60 hours after initiation of treatment, whether or not intravenous treatment is continuing. The concomitant use of corticosteroids to induce fetal lung maturity and beta-adrenergic tocolytics in patients developing pulmonary edema has led to the suggestion that corticosteroids may be a predisposing factor. However, the incidence of corticosteroid therapy in patients who develop pulmonary edema is similar to that in the overall preterm labor population which receives tocolytics, indicating that corticosteroids are not a factor in the pathogenesis of the beta-adrenergic—associated pulmonary edema (Robertson et al., 1981). With the recognition of fluid dynamics, and recognition of the importance of close observation of intake and output and observance of fluid restriction, the incidence of the side effect of pulmonary edema appears to be decreasing, being only 0.3 per cent in the recent large Canadian trial.

Maternal Metabolic Effects. The increase in cyclic AMP production that occurs secondary to beta-adrenergic stimulation leads to an increase in hepatic glycogenolysis and maternal hyperglycemia, the increase in glucose levels being very rapid. The elevation in maternal glucose begins to decrease after the peak, which occurs within 3 hours of initiation of intravenous treatment (Young et al., 1983), but the concentration is still elevated at 24 hours. It is unclear how long the modest hyperglycemia persists. Chronic treatment with oral terbutaline, but not oral ritodrine, has been reported to be associated with maternal glucose intolerance (Main et al., 1985b, 1987b). Insulin secretion is apparently increased secondary to the hyperglycemia and to direct stimulation of the $beta_2$ receptors of the pancreatic islet cells, as the increase in insulin and glucagon occurs before the peak in glucose and free fatty acids (Lipshitz and Vinik, 1978). The acute alterations in carbohydrate metabolism are usually not of consequence in the normal patient but may be associated with ketoacidosis in the insulin-dependent diabetic (Thomas et al., 1977; Steel and Parboosingh, 1977; Miodovnik et al., 1985) and even, though rarely, in nondiabetics (Leopold and McEvoy, 1977). These potential effects on carbohydrate metabolism make other tocolytics, such as magnesium sulfate, the first-line choice in patients with diabetes mellitus in whom preterm labor is diagnosed. However, concomitant intravenous insulin and beta-adrenergic tocolysis can be used successfully if necessary.

$Beta_1$ stimulation leads to mobilization of free fatty acids and glycerol and an increase in production of beta-hydroxybutyrate and acetoacetate (Lunell et al., 1977). This increase in fixed fatty acids is accompanied by a rise in lactate as a result of increased muscle glycogenolysis, but only rarely has maternal acidosis of a significant degree been observed, perhaps because of the underlying state of mild respiratory alkalosis that exists in pregnancy (Richards et al., 1983).

Concomitant with the hyperglycemia is the development of hypokalemia (Young et al., 1983; Smith and Thompson, 1977). Although plasma potassium concentrations are reduced at first, they return to near normal by 24 hours and do not decrease during oral treatment. Urinary excretion of potassium is not increased. There is no evidence at present to support the need for exogenous potassium treatment during the acute hypokalemia, although some advocate its use, particularly if the serum potassium level falls below 3 mEq/liter. No changes are known to occur in serum magnesium, calcium, or phosphate concentration. Decreased serum iron transferring level and iron binding capacity have been observed (Kauppila et al., 1978), suggesting activation of hematopoiesis.

Other Maternal Effects. It is not rare for patients to experience some nausea and occasional emesis, in addition to some restlessness and general agitation with beta-adrenergic tocolysis. Paralytic ileus also occurs rarely as does dermatitis (Robertson et al., 1981; Horowitz and Creasy, 1978).

FETAL AND NEONATAL EFFECTS. The majority of the beta-adrenergic drugs, except perhaps hexoprenaline, cross the placenta, although little is known about the kinetics of transfer in human pregnancy. Studies using the experimental chorionic sheep preparation with short-term infusions of ritodrine into the fetus reveal increases in fetal heart rate, cardiac output, and blood flow to the adrenals, heart, and brain (Siimes et al., 1978). Similar effects on regional blood flow were seen when ritodrine was infused into the maternal sheep at rates that did not cause an increase in fetal heart rate. Prolonged infusions of ritodrine into the fetal lamb have shown resultant hypoxemia, lactacidemia without pH changes, and hyperglycemia (Bassett et al., 1989). These alterations returned to normal ranges within 72 hours, indicating that tachyphylaxis also occurs in the fetus. In the human, there are no changes in fetal heart rate at low infusion rates, but mild tachycardias occur, and there may be an increase in beat-to-beat variability with higher infusion rates (Unbehaun, 1974). One echocardiographic study on neonates exposed to beta-adrenergic drugs reported interventricular septal thickening, an effect correlating with duration of exposure, and an effect absent at follow-up (Nuchpuckdee et al., 1986). Focal myocardial necrosis and nuclear cell enlargement, mainly of the right ventricle, have been described in fetuses and newborns dying of noncardiac diseases associated with prematurity (Bohm and Adler, 1986). Isolated cases of abnormal fetal rhythms, abnormal electrocardiograms, congestive failure, and hydrops have been reported (Katz and Seeds, 1989).

Suggestions that prolonged treatment of the mother may be associated with increased fetal weight are yet to be proved. In addition, although beta-adrenergic treatment has been observed to accelerate lung maturity in experimental animals, this effect has not been well documented in human pregnancy.

Neonatal hypoglycemia, hypocalcemia, ileus, and hypotension have been reported to be more common in a retrospective review of mothers treated with isoxsuprine and delivered within 48 hours of treatment (Brazy and Pupkin, 1979). Similar retrospective findings were reported by Epstein and colleagues (1979) with use of terbutaline, isoxsuprine, and fenoterol in a small series. In numerous other trials these problems have not been noted in prospective studies. If these adverse neonatal effects are a problem, the incidence is unlikely to be high, particularly if the interval from the last maternal drug administration to delivery exceeds 24 hours.

The incidence of periventricular-intraventricular hemorrhage in preterm neonates exposed to beta-adrenergic agents has been reported to be increased (Groome et al., 1992; Dolfin et al., 1984) but this finding has not been observed by others (Levene et al., 1982; van de Bor et al., 1986; Laros et al., 1991).

Follow-up studies by Freysz and associates (1977) of children exposed *in utero* to beta-adrenergics show normal growth and development at 2 years of age. Studies of children 6 years after exposure could find no significant alterations in anthropometric measurement, neurologic tests, or general behavior, but decreased school performance as evaluated by teachers (Hadders-Algra et al., 1986).

Magnesium Sulfate

Although magnesium sulfate has been used extensively in obstetrics for the treatment of preeclampsia, it has been used to any degree as a tocolytic only for the past two decades. In many centers in Europe and the United States there has been an increasing interest in magnesium sulfate for tocolysis.

MECHANISM OF ACTION. Although it has been known for many years that magnesium has a depressant effect on myometrial contractility, the precise mechanism of action remains unknown. Elevated concentrations of magnesium have a central depressant effect, altering nerve transmission by affecting acetylcholine release and sensitivity at the motor end-plate. However, magnesium also suppresses contractility of isolated myometrial strips *in vitro* in a dose-dependent manner, suggesting a direct cellular action (Harbert et al., 1969). It is theorized that magnesium has a competitive antagonist role with calcium, decreasing the intracellular free calcium that is necessary for the actin-

myosin interaction of smooth muscle contractility (see Chapter 8).

PHARMACOLOGY. Myometrial contractility is inhibited when maternal serum levels of magnesium are 5 to 8 mg/100 ml (Harbert et al., 1969; Petrie, 1981). Deep tendon reflexes may be lost when concentrations reach 9 to 13 mg/100 ml, and respiratory depression defects occur at 14 mg/100 ml or higher. Magnesium is excreted almost entirely by the kidney, with at least 75 per cent of the infused dose of magnesium (for the treatment of preeclampsia) excreted during the infusion and at least 90 per cent excreted by 24 hours (Cruikshank et al., 1981; Pritchard, 1955). As magnesium is reabsorbed by a transport-limited mechanism, the glomerular filtration rate significantly affects excretion. Increases in maternal serum magnesium result in maternal hypocalcemia, the total calcium level falling by approximately 25 per cent (Cruikshank et al., 1981; Green et al., 1983), and an increase in parathyroid hormone, but no change in maternal phosphate or calcitonin level (Cruikshank et al., 1979). Hypocalcemia results from increased urinary excretion. In most cases it is asymptomatic, although symptoms have been reported (Savory and Monif, 1971). Magnesium ions cross the placenta rapidly, with fetal and newborn levels generally increasing proportionately with maternal levels (Cruikshank et al., 1979). Total calcium levels in the fetus or newborn are unchanged or minimally reduced (Savory and Monif, 1971; Cruikshank et al., 1979). The mean half-life of neonatal hypermagnesemia secondary to maternal therapy is reported to be over 40 hours (Dangman and Rosen, 1977).

Magnesium sulfate effects on the cardiovascular system have been studied in patients with severe pregnancy-induced hypertension (Cotton et al., 1984). Under these circumstances, a 4-gm intravenous bolus over 15 minutes resulted in a mild lowering of mean arterial blood pressure, no depression of myocardial work, and no effect on oxygen consumption or transport, or on pulmonary capillary wedge pressure.

CLINICAL EFFICACY. The reports concerning tocolytic efficacy have been observational or have mainly been comparisons with various beta-adrenergic agents. Success of tocolytic agents in delaying delivery is, in general, comparable to that of the beta-adrenergic agents (Elliott, 1984; Beall et al., 1985; Hollander et al., 1987; Spisso et al., 1982). A randomized investigation of magnesium sulfate tocolysis, in which mean maximum serum concentration in the treatment group was 6.6 mg/dl, showed no difference between treatment and controls in outcomes, except for decreased births between 33 and 35 weeks of gestation (Cox et al., 1990). Thirty-nine per cent of the treatment group reached term versus 26 per cent of controls, a nonsignificant difference statistically.

DOSAGE AND ADMINISTRATION. Before therapy is begun, the patient should be evaluated as already outlined. In addition, serum magnesium concentrations may be obtained and repeated every 6 to 8 hours. An initial loading dose of 4 to 6 gm administered intravenously over 20 minutes has been recommended (Petrie, 1981; Spisso et al., 1982), followed by a maintenance dose of 1 to 3 gm/hr. The relation between serum magnesium concentration and tocolysis success is poorly established (Madden et al., 1990). Individual titration is strongly recommended, based upon response and side effects up to 8 mg/dl. Intravenous therapy is continued for approximately 24 hours; some physicians then give oral beta-adrenergic treatment. Because pulmonary edema has been observed with magnesium sulfate treatment (Elliott et al., 1979), it is prudent to maintain careful observation of intake and output, and perhaps to restrict total fluid intake as with beta-adrenergic treatment. Constant monitoring of deep tendon reflexes and serum magnesium and calcium levels is appropriate. Calcium gluconate should be readily available to reverse any untoward toxic effects of magnesium.

It had previously been suggested that continuing oral magnesium, given as a gluconate (or oxide), may be effective in doses of 500 mg to 2 gm every 2 to 4 hours, even though serum levels of magnesium are only in the 2.5 mg per cent range with 1 gm every 4 hours (Martin et al., 1987). This regimen is not of value in preventing the initiation of preterm labor in high risk patients (Martin et al., 1992). A comparison of oral magnesium with oral ritodrine for continuing treatment showed comparable efficacy in inhibiting recurrent preterm labor and a similar incidence of side effects (Ricci et al., 1991).

MATERNAL EFFECTS. Flushing, a sense of warmth, headache, nystagmus, nausea, dizziness, dryness of the mouth, and lethargy in up to 45 per cent of patients may be observed, particularly during the intravenous loading dose (Hollander et al., 1987; Cox et al., 1990). Blurred vision or diplopia occurs in over three-fourths of patients (Dirge et al., 1990). Transient ischemia (Sherer et al., 1992) urticarial eruption (Thorp et al., 1989), maternal hypothermia (Rodis et al., 1987), and neuromuscular blockade in conjunction with nifedipine tocolysis (Snyder and Cardwell, 1989) have been the subject of isolated reports. If renal function is impaired, and thus magnesium excretion reduced, hypermagnesemia leading to respiratory and cardiac impairment is possible. High serum magnesium concentrations may theoretically alter the amount of muscle relaxant needed during general anesthesia. As indicated earlier, pulmonary edema has also been reported in patients receiving both magnesium and corticosteroid therapy.

Serum concentrations of both ionized and non-ionized calcium decrease during magnesium infusions with urinary output of calcium significantly elevated (Smith et al., 1992). Serum phosphorous and parathyroid hormone increase. These changes can lead to decreased bone density at 1 to 11 weeks postpartum if magnesium treatment is prolonged.

FETAL AND NEONATAL EFFECTS. Maternal magnesium sulfate treatment is frequently used in the presence of maternal hypertensive disease, which by itself may increase the risks of neonatal depression. In addition, many different regimens of maternal magnesium treatment using varying periods of treatment make interpretation of reports difficult. Green and associates (1983) found no significant alterations in neurologic state or Apgar scores with mean umbilical cord magnesium concentrations of 3.6 mg/100 ml.

Stone and Pritchard (1970) observed no correlation between cord magnesium levels, Apgar scores, and depression in newborns whose mothers had received intramuscular magnesium therapy for preeclampsia. However, respiratory and motor depression has been observed in infants with umbilical cord magnesium concentrations between 4 and 11 mg/100 ml (Lipshitz and English, 1967; Savory and Monif, 1971). Petrie (1981) reports that it is not unusual to have decreased muscle tone and drowsiness in newborns whose mothers were given magnesium for tocolysis (with maternal serum levels of 4 to 7 mg/100 ml). Fetal heart rate variability has been reported to be unchanged, increased or decreased. At plasma concentrations of 6 to 8 mg/dl for 24 hours, 50 per cent of fetuses have a nonreactive non-stress test and only 20 per cent have sustained respiratory movements affecting the biophysical profile interpretation (Peaceman et al., 1989).

Magnesium therapy for more than 7 days can result in demineralization of long bones in more than 50 per cent of fetuses (Holcomb et al., 1991), and congenital rickets have been reported (Lamm et al., 1988).

BETA-ADRENERGIC AGONISTS AND MAGNESIUM SULFATE. If either beta-adrenergic treatment or magnesium sulfate treatment fails as an initial tocolytic, it has been reported that a combination of the two may be more effective (Hatjis et al., 1987). Few reports are available at present, and some investigators have urged caution (Ogburn et al., 1985) regarding the potential for cumulative side effects.

Prostaglandin Synthesis Inhibitors

Since prostaglandins have a significant stimulatory role in established labor, there has naturally been an assessment of the role of prostaglandin synthesis inhibitors in the treatment of preterm labor.

MECHANISM OF ACTION. There is evidence that prostaglandins mediate the processes of uterine contractions and labor. Aspirin and other nonsteroidal compounds such as indomethacin, naproxen, or fenoprofen have been shown to depress synthesis of prostaglandins by inhibiting the cyclooxygenase enzyme necessary for the conversion of arachidonic acid to the various prostaglandins (Vane, 1971). Prostaglandins promote uterine activity by increasing myometrial gap junctions, and by stimulating an increase in intracellular calcium. In isolated human myometrial strips that contract with the addition of oxytocin or prostaglandin $F_{2\alpha}$, spontaneous contractions are abolished by the addition of indomethacin, but the strips remain responsive to exogenous prostaglandin $F_{2\alpha}$ (Garrioch, 1978).

PHARMACOLOGY. Indomethacin is absorbed after oral and rectal administration, plasma concentrations peaking 1 to 2 hours after oral administration and somewhat sooner than with the rectal route (Alvan et al., 1976). The drug is extensively protein-bound and is eliminated unchanged in pregnant women (Trager et al., 1973). Indomethacin readily passes across the placenta, and umbilical artery serum concentrations equilibrate with maternal concentrations by 5 hours after oral administration. The half-life in the full-term neonate is approximately 15 hours; it is almost half again longer in preterm neonates (Bhat et al., 1979). More than 90 per cent of the drug is protein-bound in the neonate.

CLINICAL EFFICACY. Zuckerman and colleagues (1974) reported, in an observation trial of indomethacin, that tocolysis was achieved in 40 of 50 patients. In a small prospective, randomized, controlled trial, it was found that preterm delivery occurred within 24 hours in one of 15 patients treated with indomethacin versus nine of 15 controls (Niebyl et al., 1980). Dudley and Hardie (1985) reported their observations of 167 patients treated with indomethacin for tocolysis, usually for only 24 to 48 hours. Delivery was delayed for more than 72 hours in 79 per cent of patients. Comparison trials with beta-adrenergics reveal at least comparable tocolytic effectiveness (Morales et al., 1989; Besinger et al., 1991).

DOSAGE AND ADMINISTRATION. Most reports have used a 100-mg rectal suppository of indomethacin as a loading dose followed by 25 mg orally every 6 hours. To avert the possible development of oligohydramnios, most treat for only 48 hours (see below).

MATERNAL EFFECTS. Although indomethacin has a reversible effect on cyclooxygenase (the effect is gone as soon as blood levels are normal), it has been associated with postpartum hemorrhage (Reiss et al., 1976). Gastrointestinal side effects may also be seen, but they may be kept to a minimum if the drug is taken with meals. Prolonged administration may be associated with headaches, dizziness, depression, and psychosis (Tepperman et al., 1977), but these latter effects have not been reported during brief tocolytic treatment. The incidence of these side effects is not well defined. In general, this agent should not be used in patients with drug-induced asthma, coagulation disorders, hepatic or renal insufficiency, or peptic ulcer disease.

FETAL AND NEONATAL EFFECTS. A number of reports have raised the concern that prostaglandin synthetase inhibitors may cause constriction of the ductus arteriosus in utero and perhaps pulmonary hypertension in neonates. Administration of acetylsalicylic acid to intact fetal lambs results in a constriction of the ductus arteriosus in the last 0.2 per cent of gestation, an effect not seen earlier in gestation (Heymann and Rudolph, 1978; Rudolph and Heymann, 1978). Indomethacin has been used clinically to effect pharmacologic closure of the patent ductus in preterm infants (Heymann et al., 1976). Fetal echocardiographic studies during maternal indomethacin therapy are limited. In one report, partial fetal ductal constriction was noted in seven of 14 fetuses, the cardiovascular effects resolving within 23 hours of treatment cessation at 26 to 31 weeks of gestation (Moise et al., 1988). In a randomized double blind study of indomethacin versus nylidrin tocolysis, ductal constriction was observed in 9 of 14 indomethacin patients (at 26-34 weeks) versus none of 13 nylidrin patients (Eronen et al., 1991). In a study of 53 fetuses during indomethacin tocolysis, ductal constriction was observed in 61 per cent at 31 to 34 weeks, 43 per cent between 27 and 30 weeks, and none under 27 weeks (Tulzer et al., 1992). Isolated cases of primary pulmonary hypertension, in association with maternal

indomethacin therapy for preterm labor, have also been reported (Manchester et al., 1967; Goudie and Dossetor, 1979). Csaba and associates (1978) reported abnormal cardiopulmonary adaptation in five of ten newborns exposed in utero to indomethacin. Besinger et al. (1991) reported three of 25 neonates with primary pulmonary hypertension after prolonged indomethacin tocolysis. Although indomethacin is suspect as the etiologic factor in these cases, pulmonary hypertension may occur in preterm neonates for other reasons, such as sepsis and asphyxia.

Accumulating clinical evidence indicates that the incidence of fetal death and perinatal morbidity may be no higher in those patients treated for 24 to 72 hours before 34 weeks than in those treated with placebo or beta-adrenergics or not treated at all (Zuckerman et al., 1984; Amy and Thiery, 1985; Niebyl and Witter, 1986; Dudley and Hardie, 1985; Morales et al., 1989). However, although the normal fetus may tolerate transient partial ductal narrowing if it occurs, in a growth-restricted fetus, with decreased umbilical blood flow and attendant increased dependence on ductal flow, partial constriction of the ductus could be more problematic.

Prolonged administration of indomethacin to rhesus monkeys results in the development of oligohydramnios and small kidneys in the fetus (Novy, 1978). Oligohydramnios has also been observed in human pregnancies in which indomethacin has been given for a number of days (Cantor et al., 1980; Itskovitz et al., 1980). The development of oligohydramnios is thought to be secondary to a decrease in fetal urine excretion. However, 5-hour infusions of indomethacin in the term lamb fetus actually leads to an increase in urinary flow (Walker et al., 1992). Indomethacin therapy in preterm neonates may also be complicated by oliguria and decreases in glomerular filtration, urinary sodium excretion, and free water clearance, all of which return to normal after cessation of treatment (Cifuentes et al., 1979). In addition, these renal effects may be transient, providing a possible explanation for the reports of oligohydramnios developing in some but not all pregnancies (Seyberth et al., 1983). Symptomatic polyhydramnios has also been successfully treated with indomethacin (Cabrol et al., 1987; Kirshon et al., 1990). In summary, it would appear that indomethacin can lead to oligohydramnios, particularly after long-term use, but that its onset is not predictable.

Aspirin affects platelet aggregation in the neonate as well as the mother, even if aspirin treatment has been discontinued a week before delivery (Bleyer and Breckenridge, 1970; Corby and Schulman, 1971). However, there has been no evidence to indicate that the incidence of intraventricular hemorrhage or other major bleeding problems is higher in the observational trials. The combination of cocaine and indomethacin has been reported to cause fever, anuria, neonatal edema, and gastrointestinal bleeding (Carlan et al., 1991). The inhibition of prostaglandin synthesis during induced fetal hypoxemia in the lamb adversely affects metabolism, leading to severe acidosis (Hooper et al., 1992).

Calcium Antagonists

Owing to the central role that cytoplasmic free calcium has in smooth muscle contractility, interest has arisen in the use of the newer calcium antagonists as tocolytic drugs.

MECHANISM OF ACTION. Agents such as nifedipine are believed to inhibit the influx of calcium ions through the cell membrane, primarily by affecting the calcium channels (Fleckenstein, 1977).

PHARMACOLOGY. Plasma concentrations of nifedipine peak in 30 to 60 minutes after oral administration, but sublingual administration can result in more rapid increases in the blood (Forman et al., 1981; Ferguson et al., 1989). The half-life is reported to be 1 to 2 hours, with elimination through the kidney and gut.

DOSAGE AND ADMINISTRATION. A loading dose of 10 mg of nifedipine by sublingual administration (after breaking the capsule) is usually used, to be repeated after 20 minutes if contractions persist and perhaps repeated in another 20 minutes. Oral therapy is then begun with 10 to 20 mg every 4 to 6 hours. The duration of treatment has not been established.

CLINICAL EFFICACY. In a small observational trial, nifedipine abolished uterine activity and prevented delivery for 3 days in all of 10 patients treated (Ulmsten et al., 1980). Moderate flushing was observed along with a transient increase in heart rate, without hypotension. Use of nifedipine has been compared with that of ritodrine in a control population using 20 patients in each group (Read and Wellby, 1986). Nifedipine was significantly more successful in delaying delivery and in causing additional days to be gained than either no treatment or ritodrine. Flushing was a bothersome side effect of nifedipine. A most recent randomized trial of nifedipine or ritodrine in 66 patients showed nonsignificant differences in successful tocolysis, but more side effects occurred with ritodrine (Ferguson et al., 1990).

MATERNAL EFFECTS. These agents cause vasodilatation and flushing is frequent, possibly accompanied by headache or nausea, which is usually transient. Hepatotoxicity has been observed during tocolysis (Sawaya and Robertson, 1992), and adjunctive treatment with magnesium can result in neuromuscular blockade (Snyder and Caldwell, 1989).

FETAL EFFECTS. Clinical studies are limited in number and the interpretation is frequently complicated by use of other tocolytic beta-adrenergic drugs. The worrisome feature at the present time derives from observations in animals. Significant decreases in fetal arterial PO_2 and pH have been observed following maternal administration of nicardipine in the rhesus monkey, probably due to decreased uterine blood flow (Ducsay et al., 1987). Similar fetal acidemic responses, including fetal demise, have been seen with maternal administration of nicardipine or nifedipine in sheep (Harake et al., 1987; Parisi et al., 1989).

Miscellaneous Tocolytic Drugs

Oxytocin-antagonists have been proposed as tocolytic agents, potentially being of value by blockade of oxytocin receptors. Their potential appeal, if efficacious, would be lack of significant side effects. Two uncontrolled studies of short-term infusions of one analogue resulted in inhibition of premature labor in all 13 patients in one study and in 9 of 12 patients in the other (Åkerlund et al., 1987; Andersen et al., 1989). A recent report of 2-hour infusions of an oxytocin antagonist, in a randomized, blind, placebo controlled trial resulted in more significant inhibition of preterm contractions in the treated group than in the control group (Goodwin et al., 1993). Further trials of this approach are needed.

Diazoxide, which is used as an antihypertensive, also has an inhibitory effect on smooth muscle contractility (Landesman et al., 1969). However, the drug has diabetogenic effects and can cause significant hypotension.

Aminophylline, a phosphodiesterase inhibitor, has also been suggested as a tocolytic drug, but only minimal information on its use is available.

Summary

A number of agents can suppress smooth muscle contractility. At present, all of these tocolytic drugs appear to have certain drawbacks and potential adverse side effects. In addition, their use necessitates close observation of the patient under controlled circumstances. Their success depends on use early in the course of preterm labor, but they should not be given until the diagnosis of preterm labor is relatively secure. That they can delay delivery for a few days appears to be well established, but their ability to decrease the incidence of preterm birth remains to be proved.

As of this writing, the beta-adrenergic drugs and magnesium sulfate are the most widely used drugs in the United States for tocolysis. The prostaglandin inhibitors—and possibly the calcium antagonists—may be considered as third choices if used under close supervision before 30 weeks. Further controlled trials of these latter two agents are not only warranted on the basis of current clinical information but are indicated and needed. The oxytocin antagonists also await further testing.

MANAGEMENT OF PROGRESSIVE PRETERM LABOR

There are numerous situations in which attempts to inhibit preterm labor are not indicated, in which tocolytic therapy is unlikely to succeed for many days, or indeed in which tocolytic therapy is failing. The decision must be made whether any other therapy is indicated, how the labor and delivery should be managed, and where the patient should be delivered. There is ample evidence that the delivery of small preterm newborns is best accomplished in a specialized perinatal center. Preterm infants delivered in an intensive care setting have a greater chance for survival and less short- and long-term morbidity than those who are transferred following birth for specialized neonatal care (Usher, 1977). Short-term tocolytic therapy can frequently delay delivery sufficiently to permit transfer of the mother and fetus to a center with specialized neonatal facilities and trained nurse and physician specialists. The regionalization of perinatal care can make available the appropriate level of care through cost-effective utilization of resources (Scott et al., 1984). Survival and morbidity have been addressed earlier in this chapter, but it should be recalled that most neonatal survival information is derived from specialized centers.

Fetal Age and Size

As neonatal survival is based upon both gestational age and birth weight, some information is needed on both of these issues for clinical management. Accurate determination of fetal age frequently is impossible. The use of ultrasound to estimate fetal weight has a considerable error, but this error is minimized as the fetal size decreases toward 500 gm. Errors in the range of 50 to 75 gm have now been reported for fetuses between 500 and 900 gm (Key et al., 1983). Therefore, if accurate measurements of the fetus are attainable by ultrasound, this may aid in the difficult decision-making process. It should also be remembered that there is a clinical tendency to underestimate fetal weight, and this can result in no intervention with poorer final neonatal outcome (Paul et al., 1979).

Fetal Lung Maturation

Two decades ago, on the basis of the observation in sheep that glucocorticoid administration to the fetus resulted in accelerated fetal lung maturation, the results of the first trial of antenatal glucocorticoid therapy in humans was reported by Liggins and Howie (Liggins and Howie, 1972; Liggins, 1977). They reported that antenatal glucocorticoid administration of 12 mg of betamethasone to mothers, on two occasions 24 hours apart, resulted in a significant decrease in the incidence of respiratory distress syndrome and an associated decrease in perinatal mortality in newborns delivered before 34 weeks. This effect was noted only if delivery occurred after more than 24 hours had elapsed from the first dose and before 7 days. The positive effect on lowering the incidence of respiratory distress syndrome in newborns delivered at less than 30 weeks, although present, was not as marked. Since that time there have been at least 12 more controlled trials demonstrating a decrease in respiratory distress syndrome if mothers are given either betamethasone or dexamethasone (usually 6 mg in four doses). A meta-analysis of 12 randomized controlled trials (Crowley, 1989) has shown that antenatal glucocorticoid therapy decreased respiratory distress syndrome, an effect more marked if delivery occurred more than 24 hours after starting treatment but within 7 days (odds ratio .31, 95 per cent confidence limits 0.23 to 0.42) (Fig. 33–3). Neonatal mortality was also significantly reduced. Data available in four trials revealed a decrease in periventricular hemorrhage, and from three trials, a decrease in necrotizing enterocolitis. No effect of gender was seen. It would appear that efficacy

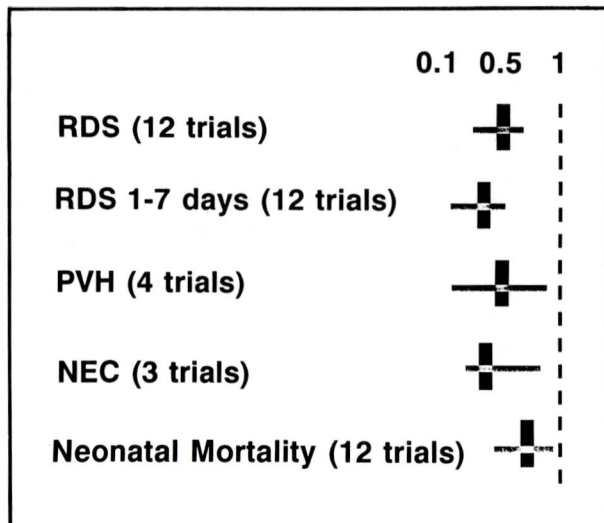

FIGURE 33–3. Meta-analysis of prenatal glucocorticoid randomized trials. Odds ratio and confidence intervals of effects. RDS = respiratory distress syndrome; RDS 1-7 days = respiratory distress syndrome in infants born preterm 1-7 days after starting treatment; PVH = periventricular hemorrhage; NEC = necrotizing enterocolitis. (Adapted from Crowley P: Promoting pulmonary maturity. *In* Chalmers I, Enkin M, Keirse MJNC (eds): Effective Care in Pregnancy and Childbirth. New York, Oxford University Press, 1989.)

of antenatal glucocorticoid therapy has been well established in patients who have intact membranes when treatment is begun and deliver between 30 and 34 weeks of gestation, with a probable but decreased effect before 30 weeks. However, there is still debate as to whether there is lack of benefit in specific situations, whether the treatment has value in multiple gestations in which numbers studied have been few and confounding variables more pronounced, whether a second course of therapy should be used if the pregnancy is extended more than 7 days, and whether there is any value in using corticosteroids if the membranes are ruptured (see Chapter 41). These analyses revealed no consistent effect on the incidence of maternal or neonatal infection with intact membranes.

Long-term follow-up of infants exposed *in utero* to antenatal corticosteroid therapy at 3 and 6 years has not demonstrated any adverse effect upon growth, physical development, motor or cognitive skills, or school progress (Collaborative Group, 1984; MacArthur et al., 1982).

Owing to the persistent presence of respiratory distress syndrome and chronic lung disease (defined as need for additional oxygenation at 28 days of life) in newborns with weights less than 1500 grams, other approaches have been evaluated. The administration of prenatal thyrotropin-releasing hormone, which crosses the placenta barrier to the fetus, increases tri-iodothyronine, and prolactin. Increases in fetal glucocorticoid, tri-iodothyronine, and prolactin are more effective than glucocorticoid alone in accelerating lung compliance and surfactant production in the lamb (Schellenberg et al., 1988). A randomized controlled trial of TRH and glucocorticoid versus glucocorticoid alone in gestations of less than 32 weeks has recently been reported (Ballard et al., 1992). When one full course of treatment was given and delivery occurred within 10 days, there was no difference in the incidence of respiratory distress syndrome in newborns under 1500 grams. However, the incidence of chronic lung disease was 18 per cent in the combined therapy group versus 44 per cent with glucocorticoids alone (p<0.01), and fewer cases of chronic lung disease or death (19 per cent versus 38 per cent, p<0.01) occurred with combined treatment. No short-term adverse effects were noted. A large study in Australia is currently being performed to see if these beneficial results can be duplicated.

Fetal Heart Rate Monitoring

Perinatal asphyxia is a risk factor for short- and long-term sequelae in the preterm infant as well as the term infant. In a study of 30 preterm newborns with metabolic acidosis at delivery matched with 60 preterm infants for birth weight, but without acidosis, neonatal mortality was higher in the acidotic newborns (23 per cent versus 3 per cent), and the incidence of major neurologic deficits at 12 months was also higher (8 of 30 versus 8 of 60) (Low et al., 1992). Apgar scores also reflect gestational age, and thus umbilical cord blood analysis is important to determine the presence of newborn acidosis (see Chapter 23).

Although there is controversy over the value of continuous fetal heart rate monitoring in normal term infants (see Chapter 20), it is indicated in the preterm infant during labor. A reduction in neonatal mortality and morbidity rates has been observed in fetuses under 1500 gm when continuous monitoring is used (Paul and Hon, 1974; Neutra et al., 1978). When fetal heart rate recordings are normal, there are few neonatal deaths, whereas severe variable or late decelerations and decreased baseline variability are associated with increased neonatal morbidity and mortality; also, ominous periodic patterns with normal baseline variability, or decreased variability without ominous patterns, is not associated with neonatal mortality or acidosis (Zanini et al., 1980; Bowes et al., 1980). If there is prompt response to ominous patterns, the preterm neonate may still evidence perinatal asphyxia but need not have increased morbidity and mortality (Bowes et al., 1979).

Delivery

Analgesia and *anesthesia* of choice for labor and delivery of the preterm infant are not well established. Epidural anesthesia, by relaxation of the pelvic floor, should offer less soft tissue impact on the presenting part and therefore presumably may result in less trauma. However, it must be remembered that epidural anesthesia can cause maternal hypotension leading to potential fetal distress. Central nervous system depressant drugs are usually avoided, but if they are needed and there is available neonatal resuscitation, the depression can be dealt with as if the newborn had been given these drugs for a surgical procedure.

Episiotomy is usually advised for vaginal deliveries to help effect controlled delivery, reduce resistance, and reduce the length of the second stage, but there is minimal significant information on the benefit of routine episiotomy to the preterm neonate.

Low forceps deliveries have been encouraged with the idea of protection of the head of the premature fetus. However, once again, data to support this potential benefit have not been established (Barrett et al., 1983; Schwartz et al., 1983; Tejani et al., 1987).

Route of delivery remains a controversial issue for the very small preterm infant, particularly if the fetus is presenting as a breech. As of this writing, there is no convincing evidence to support the concept that vaginal delivery should not be the mode of delivery when (1) the presentation is cephalic, (2) labor is progressing normally, and (3) the fetal heart rate is within normal limits. This approach assumes the capability to respond quickly to an ominous event by immediate cesarean section and available neonatal intensive care.

The effect of labor and route of delivery on periventricular-intraventricular hemorrhage has been particularly difficult to evaluate. A prospective study of 230 newborns weighing less than 1750 grams has been reported wherein sonographic examinations of the head were performed within 30 minutes of birth and serially until 7 days of life (Shaver et al., 1992). The overall incidence of hemorrhage was similar in newborns delivered by the vaginal and abdominal routes. Early hemorrhage (detected in the first hour after birth) was less frequent after cesarean birth than after vaginal delivery but no less frequent than after vaginal delivery with forceps. Late hemorrhage was more common in abdominal deliveries regardless of duration of labor. Grades 3 and 4 hemorrhages were highest in vaginal deliveries without forceps or abdominal deliveries after the active phase of labor. Cord blood acid-base status was similar in those with no hemorrhage or with early or late hemorrhage.

Retrospective studies strongly support the abdominal delivery approach as the method of delivery of the preterm breech (less than 1750 gm, less than 34 weeks) (Duenhoelter et al., 1979; Main et al., 1983). Prospective randomized trials have not been done to confirm this concept. It has been reported that a trial of labor can be undertaken if the presentation is a complete or frank breech (Karp et al., 1979). However, if the preterm breech presents as a footling, with the associated increase in cord prolapse and entrapment of the aftercoming head, cesarean section is indicated. The incidence of incomplete breech presentation is higher in small preterm fetuses than at term. In addition, the incidence of congenital anomalies is higher, nearly 20 per cent in some reports, when the preterm fetus is in breech presentation (Karp et al., 1979; De Crespigny and Pepperell, 1979). Thus, there is a need for careful ultrasound evaluation of the preterm breech to attempt to rule out lethal congenital anomalies. Experience with external cephalic version in early labor is too minimal to judge its potential role.

REFERENCES

Abrams B, Newman V, Key T, et al: Maternal weight gain and preterm delivery. Obstet Gynecol **74**:577, 1989.

Åkerlund M, Strömberg P, Hauksson A, et al: Inhibition of uterine contractions of premature labour with an oxytocin analogue. Results from a pilot study. Br J Obstet Gynecol **94**:1040, 1987.

Alvan G, Orne M, Bertilsson L, et al: Pharmacokinetics of indomethacin. Clin Pharmacol Ther **18**:364, 1976.

American Academy of Pediatrics, Committee on Fetus and Newborn: Nomenclature for duration of gestation, birthweight, and intrauterine growth. Pediatrics **39**:935, 1967.

Amy JJ, Thiery M: The prevention of preterm labour. Prostaglandin Perspectives **1**:9, 1985.

Anderson HF, Nugent CE, Wanty SD, et al: Prediction of risk of preterm delivery by ultrasonographic measurement of cervical length. Am J Obstet Gynecol **163**:859, 1990.

Anderson LF, Lyndrup J, Akerlund M, et al: Oxytocin receptor blockade: A new principle in the treatment of preterm labor? Am J Perinatol **6**:196, 1989.

Armson BA, Samuels P, Miller F, et al: Evaluation of maternal fluid dynamics during tocolytic therapy with ritodrine hydrochloride and magnesium sulfate. Am J Obstet Gynecol **167**:758, 1992.

Australian Institute of Health and Welfare National Perinatal Statistics Unit. Assisted conception in Australia and New Zealand 1990. Sydney, ISSN 1038 – 7234, 1992.

Bakketeig LS, Hoffman HJ: Epidemiology of preterm birth: Results from a longitudinal study of births in Norway. In Elder MG, Hendricks CH (eds): Preterm Labor. London, Butterworths, 1981.

Ballard RA, Ballard PL, Creasy RK, et al: Respiratory disease in very-low-birthweight infants after prenatal thyrotropin-releasing hormone and glucocorticoid. Lancet **339**:510, 1992.

Barden TP, Peter JB, Merkatz IR: Ritodrine hydrochloride: A beta – mimetic agent for use in preterm labor. Obstet Gynecol **56**:1, 1980.

Barrett J, Boehm F, Vaughn W: The effect of type of delivery on neonatal outcome in singleton infants of birth weight of 1000 grams or less. JAMA **250**:625, 1983.

Bassett JM, Hanson C, Weeding CM: Metabolic and cardiovascular changes during prolonged ritodrine infusion in fetal lambs. Obstet Gynecol **73**:117, 1989.

Beall MH, Edgar BW, Paul RH, et al: A comparison of ritodrine, terbutaline and magnesium sulfate for the suppression of preterm labor. Am J Obstet Gynecol **153**:854, 1985.

Bejar R, Curbello V, Davis C, Gluck L: Premature labor. II. Bacterial sources of phospholipase. Obstet Gynecol **57**:479, 1981.

Bell R: The prediction of preterm labour by recording spontaneous antenatal uterine activity. Br J Obstet Gynaecol **90**:884, 1983.

Benedetti TJ: Maternal complications of parenteral betasympathomimetic therapy for premature labor. Am J Obstet Gynecol **145**:1, 1983.

Berg G, Anderson R, Ryder G: β-adrenergic receptors in human myometrium during pregnancy: Changes in the number of receptors after β-mimetic treatment. Am J Obstet Gynecol **151**:392, 1985.

Berkowitz GS, Kelsey JL, Holford, et al: Physical activity and the risk of spontaneous delivery. J Reprod Med **28**:581, 1983.

Besinger RE, Compton AA, Hayashi RH: The presence or absence of fetal breathing movements as a predictor of outcome in preterm labor. Am J Obstet Gynecol **157**:753, 1987.

Besinger R, Niebyl J, Keyes WG, et al: Randomized comparative trial of indomethacin and ritodrine for the long-term treatment of preterm labor. Am J Obstet Gynecol **164**:981, 1991.

Bhat R, Vidyasager D, Vadapalli MO, et al: Disposition of indomethacin in preterm infants. J Pediatr **95**:313, 1979.

Bibby JG, Brunt J, Mitchell MV: The effect of cervical encerclage on plasma prostaglandin concentrations during early human pregnancy. Br J Obstet Gynaecol **86**:19, 1979.

Bieniarz J, Ibankovich A, Scommegna A: Cardiac output during ritodrine treatment in premature labor. Am J Obstet Gynecol **118**:910, 1974.

Bleyer WA, Breckenridge RJ: Studies on the detection of adverse drug reactions in the newborn. II. The effects of prenatal aspirin on newborn hemostasis. JAMA **213**:2049, 1970.

Block BSB, Liggins GC, Creasy RK: Preterm delivery is not predicted by serial plasma estradiol or progesterone concentration measurements. Am J Obstet Gynecol **150**:716, 1984.

Blondel B, Breart G, Berthoux Y, et al: Home uterine activity monitoring in France. A randomized controlled trial. Am J Obstet Gynecol **167**:424, 1992.

Bohm N, Adler CP: Focal necrosis, fatty degeneration and subendocardial nuclear polyploidization in the myocardium in newborns. Eur J Pediatr **136**:149, 1986.

Bouyer J, Papiernik E, Dreyfus J, et al: Maturation signs of the cervix and prediction of preterm birth. Obstet Gynecol **68**:209, 1986.

Bowes WA, Gabbe SG, Bowes C: Fetal heart rate monitoring in premature infants weighing 1500 grams or less. Am J Obstet Gynecol **137**:791, 1980.

Bowes WA, Halgrimson M, Simmons MA: Results of intensive perinatal management of very low birth weight infants (501 to 1500 gm). J Reprod Med **23**:245, 1979.

Boylan P, O'Donovan P, Owen OJ: Fetal breathing movements and the diagnosis of labor: A prospective analysis of 100 cases. Obstet Gynecol **66**:517, 1985.

Brazy JE, Pupkin MJ: Effects of maternal isoxsuprine administration on preterm infants. J Pediatr **94**:444, 1979.

Breart G: Evaluation of the preterm birth rate in France. In Berendes H, Kessel S, Jaffe S (eds). Advances in the Prevention of Low Birth Weight: An International Symposium. Washington, DC National Center for Education in Maternal and Child Health, 1991, p 13.

Brown SM, Tejani N: Terbutaline sulphate in the prevention of recurrence of premature labor. Obstet Gynecol **57**:22, 1980.

Brustman L, Raptoulis M, Langer O, et al: Changes in the pattern of uterine contractility in relationship to coitus during pregnanies at low and high risk for preterm labor. Obstet Gynecol **73**:166, 1989.

Butler NR, Bonham DG (eds): Perinatal Mortality. The First Report of the British Perinatal Mortality Survey. Edinburgh, Churchill Livingstone, 1963, pp. 115–145.

Cabrol D, Landersman R, Mueller J, et al: Treatment of polyhydramnios with prostaglandin synthetase inhibitor (indomethacin). Am J Obstet Gynecol **157**:422, 1987.

Caldeyro-Barcia R, Poseiro J: Physiology of uterine contraction. Clin Obstet Gynecol **3**:386, 1960.

Canadian Preterm Labor Investigators Group: The treatment of preterm labor with beta-adrenergic agonist ritodrine. N Engl J Med **327**:308, 1992.

Cantor B, Tyler T, Nelson RM, et al: Oligohydramnios and transient neonatal anuria. A possible association with the maternal use of prostaglandin synthetase inhibitors. J Reprod Med **24**:220, 1980.

Carlan SJ, Stromquist C, Angel JL, et al: Cocaine and indomethacin: Fetal anuria, neonatal edema, and gastrointestinal bleeding. Obstet Gynecol **78**:501, 1991.

Carritas SN: A pharmacologic approach to the infusion of ritodrine. Am J Obstet Gynecol **158**:380, 1988.

Carritas SN, Chiao JP, Kridgen P: Comparison of pulsatile and continuous ritodrine administration: Effects on uterine contractility and β-adrenergic receptor cascade. Am J Obstet Gynecol **164**:1005, 1991.

Carritas SN, Chiao JP, Moore JJ, et al: Myometrial desensitization after ritodrine infusion. Am J Physiol **253**:E410, 1987.

Carritas SN, Lin LS, Toig G, et al: Pharmacodynamics of ritodrine in pregnant women during preterm labor. Am J Obstet Gynecol **147**:752, 1983.

Carritas SN, Venkataramanan R, Cotroneo M, et al: Pharmacokinetics of orally administered ritodrine. Am J Obstet Gynecol **161**:32, 1989.

Carritas SN, Venkataramanan R, Darby MJ, et al: Pharmacokinetics of ritodrine administered intravenously. Recommendations for changes in the current regimen. Am J Obstet Gynecol **162**:429, 1990a.

Carritas SN, Venkataramanan R, Cotroneo M, et al: Pharmacokinetics and pharmacodynamics of ritodrine after intramuscular administration to pregnant women. Am J Obstet Gynecol **162**:1215, 1990b.

Casper RF, Lye SJ: β-Adrenergic receptor agonist infusion increases plasma prostaglandin F levels in sheep. Am J Obstet Gynecol **157**:998, 1987.

Castle BM, Turnbull AC: The presence or absence of fetal breathing movements predict the outcome of premature labor. Lancet **ii**:471, 1983.

Chasnoff IJ, Griffith DR, MacGregor SN, et al: Temporal patterns of cocaine use in pregnancy. JAMA **261**:1714, 1989.

Cherukuri R, Minkoff H, Hansen RL, et al: A cohort study of alkaloidal cocaine ("crack") in pregnancy. Obstet Gynecol **72**:147, 1988.

Cifuentes RF, Olley PM, Balie JW: Indomethacin and renal function in premature infants with persistent patent ductus arteriosus. J Pediatr **95**:583, 1979.

Cnattingius S, Forman MR, Berendes HW, et al: Effect of age, parity, and smoking on pregnancy outcome: A population-based study. Am J Obstet Gynecol **168**:16, 1993.

Collaborative Group on Antenatal Steroid Therapy: Effects of antenatal dexamethasone administration in the infant. Long-term follow up. J Pediatr **104**:259, 1984.

Collaborative Group on Preterm Birth Prevention: Multicenter randomized controlled trial of a preterm birth prevention program. Am J Obstet Gynecol. In Press.

Cooper RL, Goldenberg RL, Creasy RK, et al: A multicenter study of preterm birth weight and gestational age specific mortality. Am J Obstet Gynecol **168**:78, 1993.

Corby DG, Schulman I: The effects of antenatal drug administration on aggregation of platelets of newborn infants. J Pediatr **79**:307, 1971.

Cotton DB, Gonik B, Dorman KF: Cardiovascular alterations in severe pregnancy-induced hypertension: Acute effects of intravenous magnesium sulfate. Am J Obstet Gynecol **148**:162, 1984.

Coulam CB, Wasmoen I, Creasy RK, et al: Major basic protein as a prediction of preterm labor: A preliminary report. Am J Obstet Gynecol **156**:790, 1987.

Cox SM, Sherman LM, Leveno KY. Randomized investigation of magnesium sulfate for prevention of preterm birth. Am J Obstet Gynecol **163**:767, 1990.

Creasy RK: Prevention of preterm birth. Birth Defects **19**(5):97, 1983.

Creasy RK, Golbus MS, Laros RK, et al: Oral ritodrine maintenance in the treatment of preterm labor. Am J Obstet Gynecol **137**:212, 1980a.

Creasy RK, Gummer BA, Liggins GC: A system for predicting spontaneous preterm birth. Obstet Gynecol **55**:692, 1980b.

Creasy RK, Katz M: Beta-adrenergic tocolytics: Basic research and clinical experience in the United States. *In* Fuchs F, Stubblefield PG (eds): Preterm Birth: Causes, Prevention and Management. New York, Macmillan, 1984.

Crowley P: Promoting pulmonary maturity. *In* Chalmers I, Enkin M, Keirse MJNC (eds): Effective Care in Pregnancy at Childbirth. Oxford University Press, New York, 1989, Chapter 45.

Crowther CA, Neilson JP, Verkuyl DAA, et al: Preterm labour in twin pregnancies: Can it be prevented by hospital admission? Br J Obstet Gynaecol **96**:850, 1989.

Cruikshank DP, Pitkin RM, Donnelly E, et al: Urinary magnesium, calcium and phosphate excretion during magnesium sulphate infusion. Obstet Gynecol **58**:430, 1981.

Cruikshank DP, Pitkin RM, Reynolds WA, et al: Effects of magnesium sulphate treatment on perinatal calcium metabolism. I. Maternal and fetal responses. Am J Obstet Gynecol **134**:243, 1979.

Csaba IF, Sulyok E, Ertl T: Clinical note: Relationship of maternal treatment with indomethacin to persistence of fetal circulation syndrome. J Pediatr **92**:484, 1978.

Csapo A, Pohanka O, Kaihola HL: Progesterone deficiency and premature labour. Br Med J **I**:137, 1974.

Dangman BC, Rosen TS: Magnesium levels in infants of mothers treated with magnesium sulfate. Pediatr Res **11**:415, 1977.

Dawes GS: The central control of fetal breathing and skeletal muscle movements. J Physiol **346**:1, 1984.

De Crespigny LJC, Pepperell RJ: Perinatal mortality and morbidity in breech population. Obstet Gynecol **53**:141, 1979.

Diagnostic and Therapeutic Technology Assessment (DATTA): Home monitoring of uterine activity. JAMA **261**:3027, 1989.

Dirge KB, Varner MW, Schiffman JS: Neuroophthalmologic effects of intravenous sulfate. Am J Obstet Gynecol **163**:1848, 1990.

Dodds WG, Iams JD: Maternal C-reactive protein and preterm labor. J Reprod Med **32**:527, 1987.

Dolfin T, Skidmore MB, Fong KW, et al: Perinatal factors that influence the incidence of subependymal and intraventricular hemorrhage in low-birth-weight infants. Am J Perinatol **1**:107, 1984.

Ducsay CA, Thompson JS, Wu AT, et al: Effects of calcium entry blocker (nicardipine) tocolysis in rhesus macaques: Fetal plasma concentrations and cardiorespiratory changes. Am J Obstet Gynecol **157**:1482, 1987.

Dudley DKL, Hardie MJ: Fetal and neonatal effects of indomethacin used as a tocolytic agent. Am J Obstet Gynecol **151**:181, 1985.

Duenhoelter JH, Wells CE, Reisch JS, et al: A paired controlled study of vaginal and abdominal delivery of the low-birth-weight breech fetus. Obstet Gynecol **54**:310, 1979.

Duff P, Kopelman JN: Subclinical intra-amniotic infection in asymptomatic patients with refractory preterm labor. Obstet Gynecol **69**:756, 1987.

Dyson DC, Crites YM, Ray DA, et al: Prevention of preterm birth in high-risk patients: The role of education and provider contact versus home uterine monitoring. Am J Obstet Gynecol **154**:756, 1991.

Eden RK, Sokol RJ, Sorokin Y, et al: The mammary stimulation test: A predictor of preterm delivery. Am J Obstet Gynecol **164**:1409, 1991.

Elder HA, Santamarina BAG, Smith S, et al: The natural history of asymptomatic bacteriuria during pregnancy: The effect of tetracycline on the clinical course and outcome of pregnancy. Am J Obstet Gynecol **111**:441, 1971.

Elliott JP: Magnesium sulfate as a tocolytic agent. Am J Obstet Gynecol **147**:277, 1984.

Elliott JP, O'Keeffe DF, Greenberg P, et al: Pulmonary edema associated with magnesium sulfate and betamethasone administration. Am J Obstet Gynecol **134**:717, 1979.

Epstein MF, Nichols E, Stubblefield PG: Neonatal hypoglycemia after beta-sympathomimetic tocolytic therapy. J Pediatr **94**:440, 1979.

Eronen M, Pesonen E, Kurki T, et al: The effects of indomethacin and a β-sympathomimetic agent on the fetal ductus during treatment of premature labor. A randomized double-blind study. Am J Obstet Gynecol **164**:141, 1991.

Fedrick J, Anderson ABM: Factors associated with spontaneous preterm birth. Br J Obstet Gynaecol **83**:342, 1976.

Ferguson JE, Dyson DC, Schutz T, et al: A comparison of tocolysis with nifedipine or ritodrine: Analysis of efficacy and maternal, fetal and neonatal outcome. Am J Obstet Gynecol **163**:105, 1990.

Ferguson JE, Schutz T, Perske R, et al: Nifedipine pharmacokinetics during preterm labor tocolysis. Am J Obstet Gynecol **161**:1485, 1989.

Finley J, Katz M, Rojas-Perez M, et al: Cardiovascular consequences of β-agonist tocolysis: An echocardiographic study. Obstet Gynecol **64**:787, 1984.

Fleckenstein A: Specific pharmacology of calcium in myocardium, cardiac pacemakers, and vascular smooth muscle. Ann Rev Pharmacol Toxicol **17**:149, 1977.

Forman A, Andersson K-E, Ulmsten U: Inhibition of myometrial activity by calcium antagonists. Semin Perinatol **5**:288, 1981.

Freysz H, Willard D, Lehr A, Misser J: A long-term evaluation of infants who receive a beta-mimetic drug while in utero. J Perinat Med **5**:94, 1977.

Fuchs F, Stakeman G: Treatment of threatened premature labor with large doses of progesterone. Am J Obstet Gynecol **79**:172, 1960.

Garrioch DB: The effect of indomethacin on spontaneous activity in the isolated human myometrium and on the response to oxytocin and prostaglandin. Br J Obstet Gynaecol **85**:47, 1978.

Gibbs RS, Romero R, Hillier SL, et al: A review of premature birth and subclinical infection. Am J Obstet Gynecol **166**:1515, 1992.

Gonik B, Benedetti T, Creasy RK, et al: Intramuscular versus intravenous ritodrine hydrochloride for preterm labor management. Am J Obstet Gynecol **159**:323, 1988.

Gonik B, Creasy RK: Preterm labor—its diagnosis and management. Am J Obstet Gynecol **154**:3, 1986.

Gonik B, Creasy RK, Chambers SL: Colloid osmotic pressure alterations with ritodrine hydrochloride therapy. (Abstract) Eighth Annual Midwestern Conference on Perinatal Research, 1985.

Goodlin RC, Keller DW, Raffin M: Orgasm during late pregnancy and possible deleterious effects. Obstet Gynecol **38**:916, 1971.

Goodlin RC, Quaife MA, Dirksen JW: The significance, diagnosis, and treatment of maternal hypovolemia as associated with fetal/maternal illness. Semin Perinatol **5**:163, 1981.

Goodwin TM, Paul R, Silver H, et al: The effect of the oxytocin antagonist atosiban on preterm uterine activity in the human. Am J Obstet Gynecol. In Press.

Goudie BM, Dossetor JFB: Effect on the fetus of indomethacin given to suppress labor. Lancet **2**:1187, 1979.

Gravett MG, Nelson HP, DeRouen T, et al: Independent associations of bacterial vaginosis and *Chlamydia trachomatis* infection with adverse pregnancy outcome. JAMA **256**:1899, 1986.

Green KW, Key TC, Coen R, Resnik RK: The effects of maternally administered magnesium sulfate on the neonate. Am J Obstet Gynecol **146**:29, 1983.

Grimes DA, Schulz KF: Randomized controlled trials of home uterine activity monitoring: A review and critique. Obstet Gynecol **79**:137, 1992.

Groome LJ, Goldenberg RL, Cliver SP, et al: Neonatal periventricular-intraventricular hemorrhage after maternal β-sympathomimetic tocolysis. Am J Obstet Gynecol **167**:873, 1992.

Grunebaum A, Minkoff H, Blake D: Pregnancy among obstetricians: A comparison of births before, during and after residency. Am J Obstet Gynecol **157**:79, 1987.

Gummerus M, Halonen C: Prophylactic long-term oral tocolysis of multiple pregnancies. Br J Obstet Gynaecol **94**:249, 1987.

Hadders-Algra M, Touwen BCL, Huisjes HJ: Long-term follow-up of children prenatally exposed to ritodrine. Br J Obstet Gynaecol **93**:156, 1986.

Handwerker SM, Tejani NA, Verma UL, et al: Correlation of maternal C-reactive protein with outcome of tocolysis. Obstet Gynecol **63**:220, 1984.

Harake B, Gilbert RD, Ashwal S, et al: Nifedipine: Effects on fetal and maternal hemodynamics in pregnant sheep. Am J Obstet Gynecol **157**:1003, 1987.

Harbert GM, Cornell GW, Thornton WN: Effect of toxemia therapy on uterine dynamics. Am J Obstet Gynecol **105**:94, 1969.

Hartikainen-Sorri AL, Jouppila P: Is routine hospitalization needed in antenatal care of twin pregnancy? J Perinat Med **12**:31, 1984.

Hartikainen-Sorri AL, Sorri M: Occupational and socio-medical factors in preterm birth. Obstet Gynecol **74**:13, 1989.

Hatjis CG, Swain M: Systemic tocolysis for premature labor is associated with an increased incidence of pulmonary edema in the presence of maternal infection. Am J Obstet Gynecol **159**:723, 1988.

Hatjis CG, Swain M, Nelson LH, et al: Efficacy of combined administration of magnesium sulfate and ritodrine in the treatment of preterm labor. Obstet Gynecol **69**:317, 1987.

Hauth JC, Hankins GD, Kuell TJ, Pierson WP: Ritodrine hydrochloride infusion in pregnant baboons. I. Biophysical effects. Am J Obstet Gynecol **146**:916 1983.

Hediger ML, Scholl TO, Belsky DH, et al: Patterns of weight gain in adolescent pregnancy: effects on birth weight and preterm delivery. Obstet Gynecol **74**:6, 1989.

Heinonen PK, Saarikoski S, Pystynen P: Reproductive performance of women with uterine anomalies. Acta Obstet Gynecol Scand **61**:157, 1982.

Hemminki E, Starfield B: Prevention and treatment of premature labour by drugs: Review of controlled clinical trials. Br J Obstet Gynaecol **85**:411, 1978.

Herbst AL, Hubby MM, Blough RR, et al: A comparison of pregnancy experience in DES-exposed and DES-unexposed daughters. J Reprod Med **24**:62, 1980.

Herron M, Katz M, Creasy RK: Evaluation of a preterm birth prevention program: Preliminary report. Obstet Gynecol **59**:452, 1982.

Heymann MA, Rudolph AM: Effects of acetylsalicylic acid on the ductus arteriosus and circulation in fetal lambs in utero. Circ Res **38**:418, 1978.

Heymann MA, Rudolph AM, Silverman NH: Closure of the ductus arteriosus in premature infants by inhibition of prostaglandin synthesis. N Engl J Med **295**:530, 1976.

Higby K, Xenakis EM-J, Pauerstein CJ: Do tocolytic agents stop preterm labor? A critical and comprehensive review of efficacy and safety. Am J Obstet Gynecol. In Press.

Hill WC, Fleming AD, Martin RW, et al: Home uterine activity monitoring is associated with a reduction in preterm birth. Obstet Gynecol **76**:13S, 1990.

Holbrook RH Jr, Falcon J, Herron M, et al: Evaluation of the weekly cervical examination in a preterm birth prevention program. Am J Perinatol **4**:240, 1987.

Holbrook RH Jr, Laros RK Jr, Creasy RK: Evaluation of a risk-scoring system for prediction of preterm labor. Am J Perinat **6**:62, 1989.

Holcomb WL Jr, Shackelford GD, Petrie RH: Magnesium tocolysis and neonatal bone abnormalities: A controlled study. Obstet Gynecol **78**:611, 1991.

Hollander DI, Nagey DA, Pupkin MJ: Magnesium sulfate and ritodrine hydrochloride: A randomized comparison. Am J Obstet Gynecol **156**:631, 1987.

Honnebier WJ, Swaab DF: The influence of anencephaly upon intrauterine growth of fetus and placenta and upon gestational length. J Obstet Gynaecol Br Commonw **80**:577, 1973.

Hooper SB, Harding R, Deayton J, et al: Role of prostaglandins in the metabolic responses of the fetus to hypoxia. Am J Obstet Gynecol **166**:1568, 1992.

Horowitz J, Creasy RK: Allergic dermatitis associated with administration of isoxsuprine. Am J Obstet Gynecol **131**:225, 1978.

Iams JD, Johnson F, O'Shaughnessy R, et al: A prospective random trial of home uterine contraction monitoring in pregnancies at risk of preterm birth. Am J Obstet Gynecol **159**:595, 1988.

Iams JD, Stilson R, Johnson F, et al: Symptoms preceding preterm labor and preterm ruptured membranes. Am J Obstet Gynecol **162**:486, 1990.

Illsley R, Thompson B: Social characteristics identifying women at risk for premature delivery. *In* Turnbull AC, Woodward FP (eds): Prevention of Handicap through Antenatal Care. Amsterdam, Associated Scientific Publishers, 1976.

Ingemarsson J: Effect of terbutaline on premature labor. A double-blind placebo-controlled study. Am J Obstet Gynecol **125**:520, 1976.

Itskovitz J, Abramovici H, Brandes JM: Oligohydramnios, meconium and perinatal death concurrent with indomethacin treatment in human pregnancy. J Reprod Med **24**:137, 1980.

Jones RA, Davies PA: The outcome for preterm infants. *In* Elder MG, Hendricks CH (eds): Preterm Labor. London, Butterworths, 1981.

Karp LE, Doney JR, McCarthy T, et al: The premature breech. Trial of labor or cesarean section? Obstet Gynecol **53**:89, 1979.

Katz M, Gill PJ, Newman RB: Detection of preterm labor by ambulatory monitoring of uterine activity: A preliminary report. Obstet Gynecol **68**:773, 1986b.

Katz M, Goodyear K, Creasy RK: Early signs and symptoms of preterm labor. Am J Obstet Gynecol **162**:1150, 1990.

Katz M, Newman RB, Gill PJ: Assessment of uterine activity in ambulatory patients at high risk of preterm labor. Am J Obstet Gynecol **154**:44, 1986a.

Katz M, Robertson PA, Creasy RK: Cardiovascular complications associated with terbutaline treatment for preterm labor. Am J Obstet Gynecol **139**:605, 1981.

Katz VL, Seeds JW: Fetal and neonatal cardiovascular complications from β-sympathomimetic therapy for tocolysis. Am J Obstet Gynecol **161**:1, 1989.

Kauppila A, Tuimala R, Likorkala O, et al: Effects of ritodrine and isoxsuprine with and without dexamethasone during late pregnancy. Obstet Gynecol **51**:288, 1978.

Keirse MJNC, Grant A, King JF: Preterm labour. *In* Chalmers I, Enkin M, Keirse MJNC (eds): Effective Care in Pregnancy and Childbirth. New York, Oxford University Press, 1989, pp 694–745.

Keirse MJNC, Rush RW, Anderson AB, Turnbull AC: Risk of preterm delivery or abortion. Br J Obstet Gynaecol **85**:81, 1978.

Key TC, Dattel BJ, Resnik R: The ultrasonographic estimation of fetal weight in the very low-birth-weight infant. Am J Obstet Gynecol **145**:574, 1983.

Kincaid-Smith P: Bacteriuria and urinary infection in pregnancy. Clin Obstet Gynecol **11**:533, 1968.

King JF, Grant A, Keirse MJNC: Beta-mimetics in preterm labour: An overview of the randomized controlled trials. Br J Obstet Gynaecol **95**:211, 1988.

Kirbinen P, Jouppila P: Polyhydramnion. A clinical study. Ann Chir Gynaecol Fen **67**:117, 1978.

Kirschbaum T: Antibiotics in the treatment of preterm labor. Am J Obstet Gynecol. In Press.

Kirshon B, Mari G, Moise KJ Jr: Indomethacin therapy in the treatment of symptomatic polyhydramnios. Obstet Gynecol 75:202, 1990.

Klebanoff MA, Shiono PH, Selby JV, et al: Anemia and spontaneous preterm birth. Am J Obstet Gynecol 164:59, 1991.

Kubli F. In Anderson A, Beard R, Brudenell JM, Dunn PM (eds): Preterm Labor. Proceedings of the Fifth Study Group of the Royal College of Obstetricians and Gynecologists, London, 1977.

Lam F, Gill P, Smith M, et al: Use of the subcutaneous terbutaline pump for long-term tocolysis. Obstet Gynecol 72:810, 1988.

Lamm CI, Norton KI, Murphy RJC, et al: Congenital rickets associated with magnesium sulfate infusion for tocolysis. J Pediatr 113:1078, 1988.

Lammintausta R, Erkkola R: Effect of long-term salbutamol treatment on renin-aldosterone system in twin pregnancy. Acta Obstet Gynecol Scand 58:447, 1979.

Landesman R, DeSouza JA, Coutinko EM, et al: The inhibiting effect of diazoxide in normal term labor. Am J Obstet Gynecol 103:430, 1969.

Laros RK Jr, Kitterman JA, Heilbron D, et al: Outcome of very low birth weight infants exposed to β-sympathomimetics in utero. Am J Obstet Gynecol 164:1657, 1991.

Larsen JF, Eldon K, Lange AP, et al: Ritodrine in the treatment of preterm labor: Second Danish Multicenter study. Obstet Gynecol 67:607, 1986.

Lazar P, Gueguen S, Dreyfus F, et al: Multicentered controlled trial of cervical cerclage in women at moderate risk of preterm delivery. Br J Obstet Gynaecol 91:731, 1984.

Leopold D, McEvoy A: Salbutamol-induced ketoacidosis. Br Med J 2:1152, 1977.

Levene MI, Fawer CL, Lamont RF: Risk factors in the development of intraventricular hemorrhage in the preterm neonate. Arch Dis Child 57:410, 1982.

Leveno KJ, Cox K, Roark ML: Cervical dilatation and prematurity revisited. Obstet Gynecol 68:434, 1986.

Leveno KJ, Little BB, Cunningham FG: The national impact of ritodrine hydrochloride for inhibition of preterm labour. Obstet Gynecol 76:12, 1990.

Liggins GC: Prenatal glucocorticoid treatment: Prevention of respiratory distress syndrome. In Moore TD (ed): Report of the 70th Ross Conference on Pediatric Research. Columbus, OH, Ross Laboratories, 1977.

Liggins GC, Howie RN: A controlled trial of antepartum glucocorticoid treatment of the respiratory distress syndrome in premature infants. Pediatrics 50:515, 1972.

Linn S, Schoenbaum S, Monson R, et al: The relationship between induced abortion and outcome of subsequent pregnancies. Am J Obstet Gynecol 146:136, 1983.

Lipshitz J: The uterine and cardiovascular effects of oral fenoterol bromide. Br J Obstet Gynaecol 84:737, 1977.

Lipshitz J, English IC: Hypermagnesemia in the newborn infant. Pediatrics 40:856, 1967.

Lipshitz J, Vinik AI: The effects of hexoprenaline, a beta$_2$-sympathomimetic drug, on maternal glucose, insulin, glucagon, and free fatty acid levels. Am J Obstet Gynecol 135:761, 1978.

Lobel M, Dunkel-Schetter C, Scrimshaw PC: Prenatal maternal stress and prematurity. A prospective study of socioeconomically disadvantaged women. Health Psychol 11:32, 1992.

Lockwood CJ, Senjei AE, Dische MR, et al: Fetal fibronectin in cervical and vaginal secretions as a predictor of preterm delivery. N Engl J Med 325:669, 1991.

Low JA, Galbraith RS, Muir DW, et al: Mortality and morbidity after intrapartum asphyxia in the preterm fetus. Obstet Gynecol 80:57, 1992.

Luke B, Keith L, Minogue J, et al: Work during pregnancy: the association between occupational fatigue, obstetric history and preterm delivery. (Abstract) American College of Obstetricians and Gynecologists Annual Clinical Meeting, Las Vegas, 1992, p 22.

Lunell NO, Joelsson I, Larsson A, Persson B: The immediate effect of a beta-adrenergic agonist (salbutamol) on carbohydrate and lipid metabolism during the third trimester of pregnancy. Acta Obstet Gynecol Scand 56:475, 1977.

MacArthur BA, Howie R, Dezoete JA, et al: School progress and cognitive development of 6-year-old children whose mothers were treated with betamethasone. Pediatrics 70:99, 1982.

MacLennan AH, Green RC, O'Shea R, et al: Routine hospital admission in twin pregnancy between 26 and 30 weeks gestation. Lancet 335:267, 1990.

Madden C, Owen J, Hauth JC: Magnesium tocolysis: Serum levels versus success. Am J Obstet Gynecol 162:1177, 1990.

Magyar DM, Marshall JR: Pituitary tumors and pregnancy. Am J Obstet Gynecol 32:739, 1978.

Mahan C: New strategies for preventing an old problem: Low birthweight. J Fla Med Assoc 70:722, 1983.

Main D, Katz M, Chiu G, et al: Intermittent weekly contraction monitoring to predict preterm labor in low risk women: a blinded study. Obstet Gynecol 72:757,1988.

Main D, Main E, Maurer M: Cesarean section versus vaginal delivery for the breech fetus weighing less than 1500 grams. Am J Obstet Gynecol 146:580, 1983.

Main D, Richardson D, Gabbe S, et al: Prospective evaluation of a risk scoring system for predicting preterm births in indigent inner city women. Obstet Gynecol 69:61, 1987a

Main DM, Gabbe SG, Richardson D, et al: Can preterm births be prevented? Am J Obstet Gynecol 151:892, 1985a.

Main DM, Main EK, Strong SE, et al: The effects of oral ritodrine therapy on glucose tolerance in pregnancy. Am J Obstet Gynecol 152:1031, 1985b.

Main EK, Main DM, Gabbe SG: Chronic oral terbutaline therapy is associated with maternal glucose intolerance. Am J Obstet Gynecol 157:644, 1987b.

Mamelle N, Laumon B, Lazar P: Prematurity and occupational activity during pregnancy. Am J Epidemiol 119:309, 1984.

Manchester D, Margolis HS, Sheldon RE: Possible association between maternal indomethacin therapy and primary pulmonary hypertension of the newborn. Am J Obstet Gynecol 126:467, 1967.

Martin RW, Gaddy DK, Martin JN, et al: Tocolysis with oral magnesium. Am J Obstet Gynecol 156:433, 1987.

Martin RW, Perry KG, Hess LW, et al: Oral magnesium and the prevention of preterm labor in a high-risk group of patients. Am J Obstet Gynecol 166:144, 1992.

McDonald AD, McDonald JC, Armstrong B, et al: Prematurity and work in pregnancy. Br J Indust Med 45:56, 1988.

McDonald HM, O'Loughlin JA, Jolley P, et al: Prenatal microbiological risk factors associated with preterm birth. Br J Obstet Gynaecol 99:190, 1992.

McGregor JA, French JI, Jones W, et al: Association of cervicovaginal infections with increased vaginal fluid phospholipase A$_2$ activity. Am J Obstet Gynecol 167:1588, 1992.

McGregor JA, French JI, Reller LB, et al: Adjunctive erythromycin treatment for idiopathic preterm labor: Results of a randomized, double-blinded, placebo-controlled trial. Am J Obstet Gynecol 154:98, 1986.

Medical Research Council Royal College of Obstetricians and Gynaecologists Working Party on Cervical Cerclage: Interim report of the Medical Research Council Royal College of Obstetricians and Gynaecologists multicenter randomized trial of cervical cerclage. Br J Obstet Gynaecol 95:437, 1988.

Meinen K: Radioimmunoassay procedure of serum myoglobin in case of a long term tocolysis with beta-sympathomimetics. Gynecol Obstet Invest 12:37, 1981.

Meis PJ, Ernest JM, Moore ML, et al: Regional program for prevention of premature birth in northwestern North Carolina. Am J Obstet Gynecol 157:550, 1987.

Merkatz IR, Peter JB, Borden TP: Ritodrine hydrochloride: A betamimetic agent for use in preterm labor. II: Evidence of efficacy. Obstet Gynecol 56:7, 1980.

Meyer MB, Tonascia JA: Maternal smoking, pregnancy complications and perinatal mortality. Am J Obstet Gynecol 128:494, 1977.

Miller NH, Katz VL, Cefalo RC: Pregnancies among physicians. J Reprod Med 34:790, 1989.

Minkoff H, Grunebaum AN, Schwarz RH, et al: Risk factors for prematurity and premature rupture of membranes: A prospective study of the vaginal flora in pregnancy. Am J Obstet Gynecol 150:965, 1984.

Miodovnik M, Peros N, Holroyde JC, et al: Treatment of premature labor in insulin-dependent diabetic women. Obstet Gynecol 65:621, 1985.

Moise KJ, Huhta JC, Dawood S, et al: Indomethacin in the treatment of preterm labor: Effects on the human fetal ductus arteriosus. N Engl J Med **319**:327, 1988.

Monthly Vital Statistics Report. Advance Report on Final Natality Studies. **40**(Suppl):8, 1991.

Moore TM, Iams JD, Creasy RK, et al: Diurnal and gestational patterns of uterine activity in normal human pregnancy. Presented to Society of Perinatal Obstetricians, San Francisco, California, 1993.

Morales WJ, Angel JL, O'Brien WF, et al: A randomized study of antibiotic therapy in idiopathic preterm labor. Obstet Gynecol **72**:829, 1988.

Morales WJ, Smith SG, Angel JL, et al: Efficacy and safety of indomethacin versus ritodrine in the managment of preterm labor: a randomized study. Obstet Gynecol **74**:67, 1989.

Morrison JC, Martin JN, Martin RW, et al: Prevention of preterm birth by ambulatory assessment of uterine activity: A randomized study. Am J Obstet Gynecol **156**:536, 1987.

Mou SM, Sunderji SG, Gall S, et al: Multicenter randomized clinical trial of home uterine activity monitoring for detection of preterm labor. Am J Obstet Gynecol **165**:858, 1991.

Mueller-Heubach E, Barnett B, Reddick D, et al: Does weekly cervical examination increase the risk of premature rupture of membranes and chorioamnionitis? (Abstract 36) Presented at the Society of Perinatal Obstetricians, Las Vegas, Nevada, 1988.

Mueller-Heubach E, Reddick D, Barnett B, et al: Preterm birth prevention: Evaluation of a prospective controlled randomized trial. Am J Obstet Gynecol **160**:1172, 1989.

Naeye RL: Coitus and associated amniotic fluid infections. N Engl J Med **301**:1198, 1979.

Nageotte MP, Casal D, Senjei AE: Fetal fibronectin in patients at increased risk of a premature birth. Am J Obstet Gynecol. In Press.

Neilson JP, Verkuyl DAA, Crowther CA, et al: Preterm labor in twin pregnancies: Prediction by cervical assessment. Obstet Gynecol **72**:719, 1988.

Neutra R, Feinberg S, Greenland S, et al: Effect of fetal monitoring on neonatal death rates. N Engl J Med **299**:324, 1978.

Newman RB, Gill PJ, Katz M: Uterine activity during pregnancy in ambulatory patients. Comparison of singleton and twin gestations. Am J Obstet Gynecol **154**:530, 1986a.

Newman RB, Gill PJ, Wittreich P, Katz M: Maternal preception of prelabor uterine activity. Obstet Gynecol **68**:765, 1986b.

Newman RB, Godsey RK, Ellings JM, et al: Quantification of cervical change: Relationship to preterm delivery in multifetal gestation. Am J Obstet Gynecol **165**:264, 1991.

Newton ER, Dinsmor MJ, Gibbs RS: A randomized, blinded placebo-controlled trial of antibiotics in idiopathic preterm labor. Obstet Gynecol **74**:562, 1989.

Newton R, Hunt L: Psychosocial stress in pregnancy. Br Med J **288**:1191, 1984.

Niebyl JR, Witter FR: Neonatal outcome after indomethacin treatment for preterm labor. Am J Obstet Gynecol **155**:747, 1986.

Niebyl JR, Blake DA, White RD, et al: The inhibition of premature labor with indomethacin. Am J Obstet Gynecol **136**:1014, 1980.

Novy MJ: Effects of indomethacin on labor, fetal oxygenation and fetal development in Rhesus monkeys. Adv Prostaglandin Thromboxanc Rcs **4**:285, 1978.

Nuckpuckdee P, Brodskyr N, Porat R, et al: Ventricular septal thickness and cardiac function in neonates after in utero ritodrine exposure. J Pediatr **109**:687, 1986.

Nwaesei CG, Young DC, Byrne JM, et al: Preterm birth at 23 to 26 weeks gestation: Is active management justified? Am J Obstet Gynecol **157**:890, 1987.

Ogburn PL, Hansen CA, Williams PP, et al: Magnesium sulfate and β-mimetic dual-agent tocolysis in preterm labor after single-agent failure. J Reprod Med **30**:53, 1985.

Ovlisen G, Iverson J: Treatment of threatened premature labor with 6 α-methyl-17 α-acetoxyprogesterone. Am J Obstet Gynecol **79**:172, 1960.

Papaevangelou G, Vrettos AS, Papadratos C, Alexiou D: The effect of spontaneous and induced abortion on prematurity and birth weight. J Obstet Gynaecol Br Commonw **80**:418, 1973.

Papiernik E: Le coéfficient de risque d'accouchement prématuré. Presse Med **77**:793, 1969.

Papiernik E, Bouyer J, Dreyfus J, et al: Prevention of preterm birth: A perinatal study in Haguenau, France. Pediatrics **76**:154, 1985.

Papiernik E, Bouyer J, Yaffe K, et al: Women's acceptance of a preterm birth prevention program. Am J Obstet Gynecol **155**:939, 1986.

Papiernik E, Kaminski M: Multifactorial study of the risk of prematurity at 32 weeks of gestation. J Perinat Med **2**:30, 1974.

Parisi VM, Salinas J, Stockan EJ: Fetal vascular responses to maternal nicardipine administration in the hypertensive ewe. Am J Obstet Gynecol **161**:1035, 1989.

Patrick J, Richardson B: Clinical significance of fetal breathing and other movements. In Jones CT, Nathanielz PW (eds): The Physiological Development of the Fetus and Newborn. London, Academic Press, 1985.

Paul RH, Hon EH: Clinical fetal monitoring. V. Effect on perinatal outcome. Am J Obstet Gynecol **118**:529, 1974.

Paul RH, Kohn KS, Monfared AH: Obstetric factors influencing outcome in infants weighing from 1001 to 1500 grams. Am J Obstet Gynecol **133**:503, 1979.

Peaceman AM, Meyer BA, Thorp JA, et al: The effect of magnesium sulfate tocolysis on the fetal biophysical profile. Am J Obstet Gynecol **161**:771, 1989.

Petrie RH: Tocolysis using magnesium sulfate. Semin Perinatol **5**:266, 1981.

Philipsen T, Eriksen PS, Lynggard F: Pulmonary edema following ritodrine-saline infusion in premature labor. Obstet Gynecol **58**:304, 1981.

Pircon RA, Strassner HT, Kirz DS, et al: Controlled trial of hydration and bed rest alone in the evaluation of preterm uterine contractions. Am J Obstet Gynecol **161**:775, 1989.

Polk BF: Infectious processes and preterm labor. In Fuchs F, Stubblefield PG (eds): Preterm Birth: Causes, Prevention and Management. New York, Macmillan, 1984, p 86.

Potkul RK, Moawad AH, Ponto KL: The association of subclinical infection with preterm labor: The role of C-reactive protein. Am J Obstet Gynecol **153**:642, 1985.

Pritchard JA: The use of the magnesium ion in the management of eclamptogenic toxemias. Surg Gynecol Obstet **100**:131, 1955.

Rahia CE, Lind J, Johanson C, et al: Relationship of premature birth to heart volume and hemoglobin per cent in pregnant women. Ann Pediatr Finn **2**:69, 1956.

Ratten GJ, Beischer NA, Fortune DW: Obstetric complications when the fetus has Potter's syndrome. Am J Obstet Gynecol **115**:890, 1973.

Read MD, Wellby DE: The use of a calcium antagonist (nifedipine) to suppress preterm labour. Br J Gynaecol **93**:933, 1986.

Reiss U, Atad J, Reuinstein I, et al: The effect of indomethacin in labour at term. Int J Gynaecol Obstet **14**:369, 1976.

Remington JT, Klein JO: Infectious Diseases of the Fetus and Newborn Infant. 2nd ed. Philadelphia, WB Saunders Company, 1983.

Renaud R, Irrmann M, Gandar R, Flynn MG: The use of ritodrine in the treatment of premature labour. J Obstet Gynaecol Br Commonw **81**:182, 1974.

Rhoads GG, McNellis DC, Kessel SS: Home monitoring of uterine contractility. Am J Obstet Gynecol **165**:2, 1991.

Ricci JM, Hariharan S, Helfgott A, et al: Oral tocolysis with magnesium chloride: A randomized controlled prospective clinical trial. Am J Obstet Gynecol **165**:603, 1991.

Richards SR, Chang FE, Stempel LE: Hyperlactacidemia associated with acute ritodrine infusion. Am J Obstet Gynecol **146**:1, 1983.

Roberts G: Unclassified antepartum haemorrhage incidence and perinatal mortality in a community. J Obstet Gynaecol Br Commonw **77**:492, 1970.

Roberts WE, Morrison JC, Hamer C, et al: The incidence of preterm labor and specific risk factors. Obstet Gynecol **76**:85S, 1990.

Robertson PA, Herron M, Katz M, Creasy RK: Maternal morbidity associated with isoxsuprine and terbutaline tocolysis. Eur J Obstet Gynecol Reprod Biol **11**:317, 1981.

Robertson PA, Sniderman SH, Laros RK Jr, et al: Neonatal morbidity according to gestational age and birth weight from five tertiary centers in the United States, 1983 through 1986. Am J Obstet Gynecol **166**:1629, 1992.

Rodis JF, Vintzileos AM, Campbell WA, et al: Maternal hypothermia: An unusual complication of magnesium sulfate therapy. Am J Obstet Gynecol **156**:435, 1987.

Romero R, Kimenez C, Lokda AK, et al: Amniotic fluid glucose concentration: A rapid and simple method for the detection of intraamniotic infection in preterm labor. Am J Obstet Gynecol 163:968, 1990.

Romero R, Mazor M: Infection and preterm labor. Clin Obstet Gynecol 31:553, 1988.

Romero R, Sirtori M, Oyarzun E, et al: Infection and labor. V. Prevalence, microbiology, and clinical significance of intraamniotic infection in women with preterm labor and intact membranes. Am J Obstet Gynecol 16:817, 1989.

Rudolph AM, Heymann MA: Hemodynamic changes induced by blockers of prostaglandin synthesis in the fetal lamb in utero. Adv Prostaglandin Thromboxane Res 4:231, 1978.

Rush RW, Issacs S, McPherson K, et al: A randomized controlled trial of cervical cerclage in women at high risk of spontaneous preterm delivery. Br J Obstet Gynaecol 91:724, 1984.

Rush RW, Keirse MJNC, Howat P, et al: Contribution of preterm delivery to perinatal mortality. Br Med J 2:965, 1976.

Sacks BP, Hellerstein S, Freeman R, et al: Home monitoring of uterine activity. Does it prevent prematurity? N Engl J Med 325:1374, 1991.

Saunders MC, Dick JS, Brown IM, et al: The effects of hospital admission for bed rest on the duration of twin pregnancy: A randomized trial. Lancet 2:793, 1985.

Savory J, Monif G: Serum calcium levels in cord sera of the progeny treated with magnesium sulfate for toxemia of pregnancy. Am J Obstet Gynecol 110:556, 1971.

Sawaya GF, Robertson PA: Hepatotoxicity with the administration of nifedipine for treatment of preterm labor. Am J Obstet Gynecol 167:512, 1992.

Schellenberg JC, Liggins GC, Manzoi MK, et al: Synergistic hormonal effects on lung maturation in the sheep. Am J Physiol 65:94, 1988.

Scholl TO, Hediger ML, Salman RW, et al: Influence of prepregnant body mass and weight gain for gestation on spontaneous preterm delivery and duration of gestation during adolescent pregnancy. Am J Hum Biol 1:657, 1989.

Schwartz D, Miodovnik M, Lavin J: Neonatal outcome among low birth weight infants delivered spontaneously or by low forceps. Obstet Gynecol 62:283, 1983.

Schwartz RW: Pregnancy in physicians: Characteristics and complications. Obstet Gynecol 66:672, 1985.

Scott KE, Peddle LJ, Rees EP: Impact of regional organization and planned services to reduce perinatal mortality. In Fuchs F, Stubblefield PG (eds): Preterm Birth: Causes, Prevention and Management. New York, Macmillan, 1984.

Seyberth HW, Rascher W, Hackenthal R, et al: Effect of prolonged indomethacin therapy on renal function and selected vasoactive hormones in very low-birth-weight infants with symptomatic patent ductus arteriosus. Pediatrics 103:979, 1983.

Shaver DC, Bada HS, Korones SB, et al: Early and late intraventricular hemorrhage: The role of obstetric factors. Obstet Gynecol 80:831, 1992.

Sherer DM, Cialone PR, Abramowicz JS, et al: Transient symptomatic subendocardial ischemia during intravenous magnesium sulfate tocolytic therapy. Am J Obstet Gynecol 166:33, 1992.

Siimes ASI, Creasy RK, Heymann MA, Rudolph AM: Cardiac output and its distribution and organ blood flow in the fetal lamb during ritodrine administration. Am J Obstet Gynecol 132:42, 1978.

Singer A, Cooke ID, Tachman E: Cervical incompetence and premature delivery after bromocriptine therapy for infertility. Lancet 2:503, 1977.

Smith LG Jr, Burns PA, Schanler RJ: Calcium homeostasis in pregnant women receiving long-term magnesium sulfate therapy for preterm labor. Am J Obstet Gynecol 167:45, 1992.

Smith SK, Thompson D: The effects of intravenous salbutamol upon plasma and urinary potassium during premature labour. Br J Obstet Gynaecol 84:344, 1977.

Smyth CN: The guard-ring tocodynamometer: Absolute measurement of intra-amniotic pressure by a new instrument. J Obstet Gynaecol Br Commonw 64:59, 1957.

Snyder SW, Cardwell MS: Neuromuscular blockade with magnesium and nifedipine. Am J Obstet Gynecol 161:35, 1989.

Spisso KR, Harbert GM, Thiagoriajah S: The use of magnesium sulfate as the primary tocolytic agent to prevent delivery. Am J Obstet Gynecol 142:840, 1982.

Steel JM, Parboosingh J: Insulin requirements in pregnant diabetics with premature labor controlled by ritodrine. Br Med J 1:880, 1977.

Steyer M, Rink K, Schlesing H: Serum creatine-kinase MB during fenoterol tocolysis. Z Geburtshilfe Perinatol 183:339, 1979.

Stone SR, Pritchard JA: Effect of maternally administered magnesium sulfate on the neonate. Obstet Gynecol 35:574, 1970.

Stubblefield PG: Causes and prevention of preterm birth. An overview. In Fuchs F, Stubblefield PG (eds): Preterm Birth: Causes, Prevention and Management. New York, Macmillan, 1984.

Stubbs TM, Van Dorsten P, Miller MC: The preterm cervix and preterm labor: Relative risks, predictive values, and change over time. Am J Obstet Gynecol 155:829, 1986.

Sweet RL, Landers DV, Walker C, Schacter J: Chlamydia trachomatis infection and pregnancy outcome. Am J Obstet Gynecol 156:824, 1987.

TambyRaja RL, Anderson ABM, Turnbull AC: Endocrine changes in premature labour. Br Med J 2:67, 1974.

Teitelman AM, Welch LS, Hellenbrand G, et al: Effect of maternal work activity on preterm birth and low birth weight. Am J Epidemol 131:104, 1990.

Tejani N, Verma U, Hameed C, et al: Method and route of delivery in the low birth weight vertex presentation correlated with early periventricular intraventricular hemorrhage. Obstet Gynecol 69:1, 1987.

Tepperman HM, Beydoun SN, Abdul-Karim RW: Drugs affecting myometrial contractility in pregnancy. Clin Obstet Gynecol 20:423, 1977.

Thomas DJB, Gill B, Brown P, Subbs WA: Salbutamol-induced diabetic keto-acidosis. Br Med J 2:1152, 1977.

Thorp JM Jr, Katz VL, Campbell D, et al: Hypersensitivity to magnesium sulfate. Am J Obstet Gynecol 161:889, 1989.

Trager A, Naschel H, Zaumseil J: The pharmacokinetics of indomethacin in pregnant and parturient women and in their newborn infants. Zentralbl Gynaekol 95:635, 1973.

Tulzer G, Gudmundsson S, Tews G, et al: Incidence of indomethacin-induced fetal ductal constriction. J Maternal-Fetal Invest 1:267, 1992.

Ulmsten U, Anderson K-E, Wingerup L: Treatment of premature labor with the calcium antagonist nifedipine. Arch Gynecol 229:1, 1980.

Unbehaun V: Effects of sympathomimetic tocolytic agents on the fetus. J Perinat Med 2:17, 1974.

US Department of Health and Human Services, Public Health Service, National Center for Health Statistics: Vital Statistics of the United States, 1980. Vol 1, Natality. Hyattsville, 1984.

Usher R: Changing mortality rates with perinatal intensive care and regionalization. Semin Perinatol 1:309, 1977.

Utter GO, Dooley SL, Tamura RK, et al: Awaiting cervical change for the diagnosis of preterm labor does not compromise the efficacy of ritodrine tocolysis. Am J Obstet Gynecol 163:882, 1990.

Van de Bor M, van Bel F, Lineman R, et al: Perinatal factors of periventricular – intraventricular hemorrhage in preterm infants. Am J Dis Child 140:1125, 1986.

Vane JR: Inhibition of prostaglandin synthesis as a mechanism of action for aspirin-like drugs. Nature New Biol 231:232, 1971.

Wagner JM, Morton MJ, Johnson KA, et al: Terbutaline and maternal cardiac function. JAMA 246:2697, 1981.

Wagner NN, Butler JC, Sanders JP: Prematurity and orgasmic coitus during pregnancy: Data on a small sample. Fertil Steril 27:911, 1976.

Walker MPR, Moore TM, Brace RA: Urinary and cardiovascular responses to indomethacin infusion in the ovine fetus. Am J Obstet Gynecol 167:834, 1992.

Weber T, Obel E: Pregnancy complications following conization of the uterine cervix. Acta Obstet Gynecol Scand 58:259, 1979.

Weitz CM, Ghodgaonkar RB, Dubin NH, Niebyl JR: Prostaglandin F metabolite concentration as a prognostic value in preterm labor. Obstet Gynecol 67:496, 1986.

Wen SW, Goldenberg RL, Cutter GR, et al: Smoking, maternal age, fetal growth and gestational age at delivery. Am J Obstet Gynecol 162:53, 1990.

Wenstrom KD, Sipes SL, Williamson RA, et al: Prediction of pregnancy outcome with single versus serial maternal serum α-fetoprotein tests. Am J Obstet Gynecol **167**:1529, 1992.

Williams MA, Mittendorf R, Lieberman E, et al: Adverse infant outcomes associated with first trimester vaginal bleeding. Obstet Gynecol **78**:14, 1991.

Winkler M, Baumann L, Ruckhaberle KE, et al: Erythromycin therapy in threatened preterm delivery. A preliminary report. J Perinat Med **16**:253, 1988.

World Health Organization: Prevention of perinatal morbidity and mortality, Public Health Papers **42**, Geneva, WHO, 1969.

Yawn BP, Yawn RA: Preterm birth prevention in a rural practice. JAMA **262**:230, 1989.

Ying YK, Tejani NA: Angina pectoris as a complication of ritodrine hydrochloride therapy in premature labor. Obstet Gynecol **60**:385, 1982.

Young DC, Toofanian A, Leveno KJ: Potassium and glucose con-centrations without treatment during ritodrine tocolysis. Am J Obstet Gynecol **145**:105, 1983.

Yu VYH, Loke HL, Szymonowicz W, et al: Prognosis for infants born at 23–28 weeks gestation. Br Med J **293**:1200, 1986.

Zanini B, Paul R, Huey J: Intrapartum fetal heart rate. Correlation with scalp pH in the preterm fetus. Am J Obstet Gynecol **136**:43, 1980.

Zervoudakis IA, Krauss A, Fuchs F: Infants of mothers treated with ethanol for premature labor. Obstet Gynecol **137**:713, 1980.

Zlatnick FJ: The applicability of labor inhibition to the problem of prematurity. Am J Obstet Gynecol **113**:704, 1972.

Zuckerman H, Reiss U, Rubinstein I: Inhibition of human premature labor by indomethacin. Obstet Gynecol **44**:787, 1974.

Zuckerman H, Shalev E, Gilad G, et al: Further study of the inhibition of premature labor by indomethacin. Part I. J Perinat Med **12**:19, 1984.

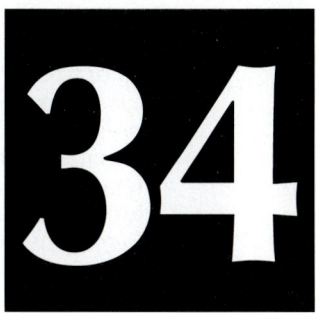

POST-TERM PREGNANCY

ROBERT RESNIK, M.D.

In 1902, Ballantyne described the problem of the post-term pregnancy for the first time in modern obstetric terms. Although the language used to describe the entity in early 20th century Scotland was different from that of today, Ballantyne's words clearly reflected current thinking when he said, "The post-mature infant . . . has stayed too long in intrauterine surroundings; he has remained so long *in utero* that his difficulty is to be born with safety to himself and his mother. The problem of the . . . postmature infant is intranatal."

During the ensuing years, the issue of post-term pregnancy, its risk, and its management have generated great controversy. However, an abundance of older as well as more recent data has firmly established that although the fetal risk of a prolonged pregnancy is small, it is real. Consequently, the pregnancy that continues beyond 42 weeks requires careful surveillance.

EPIDEMIOLOGY

By definition, a *term gestation* is one completed in 38 to 42 weeks. Pregnancy is considered prolonged, or post-term, when it exceeds 294 days or 42 weeks. The frequency of this occurrence has been reported to range from 7 to 12 per cent. The chances that parturition will occur precisely at 280 days after the first day of the last menstrual period (40 weeks) is 5 per cent. Approximately 4 per cent of all pregnancies proceed beyond 43 weeks.

One of the major problems in delineating the extent of risk beyond term is related to the limited reliability of the last menstrual period (LMP) as a basis for accurately predicting gestational age. It should be noted that, until recently, almost all epidemiologic studies pertaining to fetal and neonatal risks of delayed parturition were based upon the LMP. Only recently has the more precise technology of ultrasound biometry been applied to the issue of pregnancy dating for the post-term gestation, and the data confirm that the LMP is a relatively poor predictor of true gestational age. For example, the incidence of post-term gestation fell from 7.5 per cent by menstrual dating to

2.6 per cent when based upon early ultrasound examination, and to 1.1 per cent when the diagnosis required menstrual and ultrasound dates to reach 294 days or more (Boyd et al., 1988). Furthermore, Kramer et al. (1988), in a study of pregnancies believed to be post-term on the basis of their LMP, found that ultrasound criteria confirmed the post-term gestation in only 86 of 725 women studied. Consequently, the true incidence of post-term gestation is not known but seems very likely to be lower than previously thought.

Nevertheless, virtually all reports up to the present time, even given their inherent limitations, suggest a small increase in perinatal morbidity and mortality when pregnancy goes beyond 42 weeks gestation. One of the earliest and most frequently cited studies was provided by the National Birthday Trust of Britain in 1958, when a detailed study was undertaken to examine over 17,000 births in the United Kingdom from March 3 to 9 of that year (Butler and Alberman, 1969). Figure 34–1 demonstrates that the perinatal mortality rate begins to increase after 42 weeks gestation, doubling at about 43 weeks, and is four to six times higher at 44 weeks than at term. It should be emphasized that although this increase is striking, 95 per cent of babies delivered at 44 weeks survive the perinatal period. Numerous other reports since that time confirm this increase in risk (Nakano, 1972; Sachs and Friedman, 1986; Eden et al., 1987).

Another source of controversy resulted from a widely quoted publication by Clifford (1954). In his classic description of the undernourished postmature infant, Clifford suggested that the risk of postmaturity was limited to the primigravid pregnancy. It has now been clearly established that although the perinatal mortality rate in the multigravid pregnancy after 42 weeks is lower, some degree of risk remains.

ETIOLOGY

Our knowledge of the mechanism of parturition is increasing rapidly, and the pertinent physiologic and biochemical findings have been reviewed in Chapter 32. Despite the advances, we do not have a clear understanding about why some pregnancies are ab-

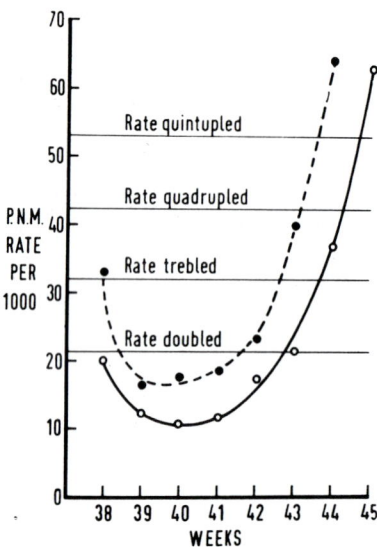

FIGURE 34–1. Perinatal mortality rate for all prolonged pregnancies (*solid line*), which increases markedly after 42 weeks gestation, and for prolonged pregnancies with superimposed toxemia (*hatched line*). (From McClure-Browne JC: Post-maturity. Am J Obstet Gynecol 85:573, 1963.)

normally prolonged. Observations in human pregnancies provide intriguing clues, however, that an anatomic or biochemical abnormality in the fetus or amnion may predispose to failure of normal timing of parturition. For example, it is known that anencephalic fetuses without pituitary glands frequently have prolonged gestation, in contrast to those in which pituitary glands have developed normally. The potential role of the pituitary-adrenal axis in human pregnancy is further suggested by the findings of Naeye (1978), who noted that 10 of 19 post-term fetuses whose deaths were attributed to congenital malformations had marked adrenal gland hypoplasia and that three did not have anencephaly. This evidence is consistent with the clinical studies in which injections of glucocorticoids into the amniotic cavity of post-term women resulted in the onset of labor (Nwosu et al., 1976).

In sheep, the surge in cortisol level is preceded by an increase in the production and plasma concentration of conjugated estrogens and a decrease in progesterone. With the exception of one study (Turnbull et al., 1974), this finding has not been confirmed in human parturition. It is of interest, however, that the rare human pregnancy with a placental sulfatase deficiency, resulting in low estriol levels, is often associated with prolongation of gestation.

It is clear that until the complex mechanism of normal parturition in humans has been clarified, the etiology of prolonged gestation as well as of preterm labor will remain obscure.

DIAGNOSIS

When one considers the rapidly accelerating risk of fetal morbidity and mortality between 42 and 43 weeks gestation and again at 43 to 44 weeks (see Fig. 34–1),

it becomes apparent that no historically derived or laboratory measurement of fetal age provides the precision required in the management of the post-term pregnancy. Traditional landmarks such as last menstrual period, uterine size, and first auscultation of fetal heart tones may be off by 2 weeks or more in terms of accurate determination of gestational age. Even sensitive sonographic determinations such as the crown-rump length in the first trimester have a range of several days. In fact, in any given gestation, the actual fetal age is known only when the time of ovulation and conception have been studied, as in the infertile couple who undergo ovulation induction or other assisted reproductive procedures (e.g., IVF).

In many cases, the obstetrician is faced late in pregnancy with the management of a potentially post-term patient without adequate early pregnancy data to accurately make the diagnosis. However, it is known that amniotic fluid volume tends to decrease in the post-term gestation, and that the risks to the fetus may well be related to the degree of oligohydramnios. Diminished amniotic fluid volume is associated with higher rates of intrapartum fetal distress and cesarean section (Leveno et al., 1984), and Bochner et al. (1987) observed almost a 24-fold increase in cesarean section for the indication of fetal distress among women whose largest amniotic fluid pocket was less than 3 cm. The incidence of meconium-stained amniotic fluid in the post-term gestation was reported to be 37 per cent in those women with adequate amniotic fluid volume but increased to 71 per cent when the amniotic fluid volume was decreased (Phelan et al., 1984). Consequently, if there is a question of the accuracy of dates, the finding of normal amniotic fluid volume is very reassuring. The amniotic fluid index shown in Figure 34–2 is a useful clinical tool in defining the adequacy of amniotic fluid volume. When the volume decreases sharply over time, or falls below 60 to 70 mm, oligohydramnios becomes a concern. However, it should be emphasized that there is little agreement among investigators regarding how oligohydramnios should be defined or the degree of risk its finding imposes.

FETAL COMPLICATIONS

Aberrations in Fetal Growth

Since the report of Clifford (1954) and his description of the postmature-dysmature neonate with wasting of subcutaneous tissue, meconium staining, and peeling of skin, many have focused their attention on the problems of the undernourished post-term fetus. In fact, only 10 to 20 per cent of true post-term fetuses exhibit any of the findings described by Clifford. Indeed, *macrosomia* is a far more common complication because, under most circumstances, the fetus continues to grow *in utero*. Twice as many post-term fetuses weigh > 4000 grams compared to term infants (Zwerdling, 1967; Eden et al., 1987), and birth injuries due to difficult forceps deliveries and shoulder girdle dystocia—including cephalohematomas, fractures, and brachial plexus palsy—are more common (Usher et

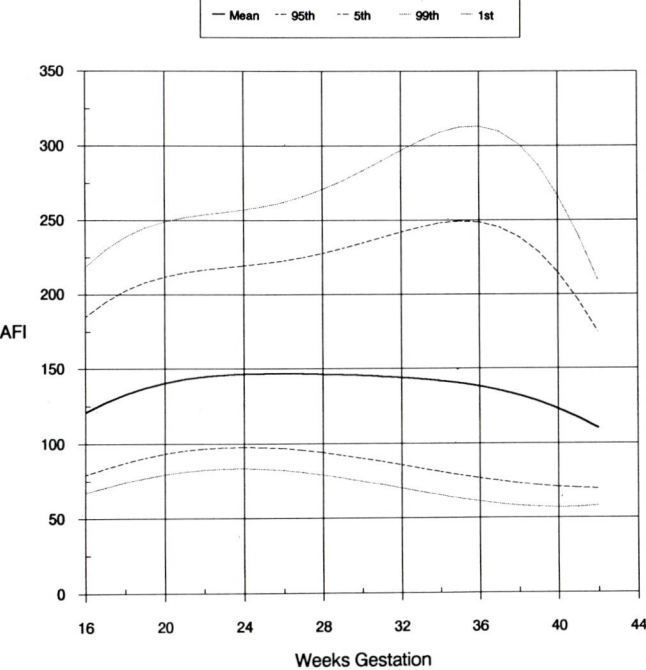

AMNIOTIC FLUID INDEX

FIGURE 34–2. The mean and various percentiles for amniotic fluid index. Data obtained from 768 patients. (Adapted from Moore TR, Cayle JE: Amniotic fluid index in normal human pregnancy. Am J Obstet Gynecol **162**:1168, 1990.)

al., 1988). A recent study of fetal growth characterization in 7000 post-term infants confirms a gradual shift toward higher birth weights and head circumference between 273 and 300 days of gestational age (McLean et al., 1991). These findings are further reinforced by a study of 519 pregnancies beyond 41 weeks in which 23 per cent of the newborns weighed >4000 grams and 4 per cent >4500 grams (Pollack et al., 1992).

Meconium Staining and Pulmonary Aspiration

Virtually all studies of post-term gestation report a markedly higher incidence of meconium-stained amniotic fluid, and the greater risk of meconium aspiration syndrome in these infants is well recognized (Eden et al., 1987). The presence of oligohydramnios further complicates the risks of meconium staining due to the lack of fluid to dilute the meconium, resulting in thicker, more tenacious material in the oropharynx and lower in the respiratory tract.

FETAL EVALUATION AND MANAGEMENT

It is generally accepted that careful ante- and intrapartum fetal monitoring can reduce perinatal mortality in the post-term gestation virtually to that of the term fetus (Eden et al., 1982; Freeman et al., 1981; Hauth et al., 1980; Phelan et al., 1985; Johnson et al., 1986).

Furthermore, there is little controversy regarding the management of the post-term patient in the presence of a cervix suitable for easy induction of labor (Bishop score 5 or greater). What remains controversial are two key clinical issues: (1) which fetal testing modality provides the greatest prognostic accuracy, and (2) whether patients who reach 41 to 42 weeks gestational age with an unripe cervix are better served by cervical ripening and induction or by continuous antenatal monitoring.

Non-stress Test

There is consensus that the non-stress test is a simple test to perform and that the combined findings of adequate baseline beat-to-beat variability and accelerations of the fetal heart rate with fetal movement are reassuring. Fleischer et al. (1985) reported a series of 228 women whose pregnancies proceeded beyond 42 weeks gestation and who were followed with weekly non-stress tests beginning at 41 weeks gestation. They were able to reduce the fetal and neonatal morbidity well below that in unmonitored patients but still had two stillbirths, three neonatal deaths, and a cesarean section rate substantially higher than in those born at term. It has also been noted that when an otherwise reactive non-stress test is associated with fetal heart rate decelerations, perinatal morbidity is similar to that of patients with a nonreactive test (Phelan et al., 1984). Finally, and of particular concern, is the finding of poor outcome in 10 pregnancies following a reactive non-stress test, including one neonatal and four antepartum deaths, four cases of fetal distress upon admission in labor, and one brain-damaged child (Miyazaki and Miyazaki, 1981). Similar findings have been reported by Barss et al. (1985). If fetal heart rate decelerations are observed during monitoring of the post-term gestation, there is a higher perinatal morbidity and mortality (Benedetti and Easterling, 1988; Small et al., 1987). Because of these disturbing reports, the use of the non-stress test as a single technique to evaluate the post-term gestation is not recommended.

Contraction Stress Test

In contrast, the contraction stress test, although more time consuming, appears to be an earlier and more sensitive indicator of fetal hypoxia. In a study of 679 post-term patients followed with weekly CSTs, no perinatal deaths occurred in the study group (Freeman et al., 1981). However, the post-term group did have a higher incidence of meconium-stained amniotic fluid, macrosomia, fetal distress in labor, and cesarean section.

Doppler Flow Velocity Wave Form

Most studies reported to date suggest that there are no significant changes in the systolic/diastolic ratio in the umbilical artery in fetuses who have gone well beyond term. There does not appear to be a relationship between Doppler flow velocity findings and outcome (Farmakides et al., 1988; Guidetti et al., 1987; Stokes et al., 1991).

Biophysical Profile

More recently, the role of amniotic fluid volume has been shown to be crucial in the assessment of the post-term gestation. Frequently, the evaluation includes all components of the biophysical profile test, including the non-stress test, fetal body and respiratory movements, and flexion, as well as amniotic fluid volume determination. Phelan and associates (1985) have shown that post-term pregnancy outcome was significantly improved if an adequate volume of amniotic fluid was present. "Adequate" was defined as a pocket greater than 1 cm in vertical dimension as well as fluid being present throughout the uterine cavity. The incidence of cesarean section for fetal distress was 2 per cent in those patients with adequate fluid volume compared with 16 per cent when fluid was considered to be adequate but decreased. Further, the incidence of abnormal antepartum fetal heart rate tests, associated with decelerations and/or bradycardia, was inversely related to amniotic fluid volume.

Johnson et al. (1986) utilized the biophysical profile for evaluation of 307 patients whose pregnancies had gone beyond 294 days. In twice-weekly testing, those with normal tests (including normal amniotic fluid volume) had no perinatal mortality, and morbidity was equal to a comparison group undergoing elective induction of labor with a favorable cervix. This study also showed a clear relationship between morbidity and inadequate amniotic fluid volume (defined as a pocket less than 2 cm in vertical dimension).

Finally, based upon their experience with 19,221 high-risk pregnancies followed with the biophysical profile alone, Manning et al. (1987) recommend twice-weekly profile testing with delivery if oligohydramnios develops.

Given these findings in the aggregate, the most effective antenatal monitoring approach associated with the lowest perinatal mortality would appear to be the biophysical profile used twice weekly beginning at 41 to 42 weeks gestational age. There remains disagreement regarding the definition of oligohydramnios, which probably accounts for some minor differences in outcome (Crowley et al., 1984; Phelan et al., 1985; Manning et al., 1981, 1987). It is for these reasons that we prefer the use of the amniotic fluid index (see Fig. 34–2).

Fetal Monitoring versus Induction of Labor

Despite the fact that antenatal monitoring can virtually eliminate perinatal mortality in the post-term gestation, the morbidities of meconium staining, increased cesarean section for a diagnosis of fetal distress, and macrosomia with its associated complications still exist. The continuing concern regarding morbidity has been addressed by an alternative approach, that of cervical ripening with prostaglandin gel followed by induction at 41 weeks gestation. Dyson et al. (1987) evaluated such an approach in a study of 302 patients who were at a minimum of 287 days gestation and who had no other risk factors. The control group of 150 patients received twice-weekly non-stress testing and amniotic fluid volume determinations. They underwent induction of labor only if the cervix ripened spontaneously or if antepartum fetal tests were abnormal. The induction group of 152 patients underwent cervical ripening with prostaglandin gel followed by labor induction utilizing oxytocin and amniotomy. The induction group had a significantly lower incidence of fetal distress, meconium aspiration, and cesarean section. In fact, the cesarean section rate among patients with induction was 14.5 per cent compared with 27 per cent in those followed with conventional management.

Dyson's data were not confirmed by a multi-institutional trial (Medearis, 1990). However, a more recent report from Canada (Hannah et al., 1992) demonstrated that among 1701 women induced with intracervical prostaglandin E_2 gel, the cesarean section rate was 21.2 per cent compared to 24.5 per cent (p = 0.03) in patients followed by fetal monitoring. This difference was due to a lower cesarean section rate for a diagnosis of fetal distress. Excluding congenital malformations, there were no perinatal deaths in the induction group, two stillbirths in the monitoring group, and no differences in neonatal morbidity. Although there is no significant difference in the perinatal mortality rate in the two groups, the authors point out that a sample of 30,000 women would have been required to show a difference. It is noteworthy that 0.5 mg prostaglandin E_2 cervical gel is now FDA-approved for use (Prepidil), and studies are under way to evaluate other dose-administration regimens.

It seems appropriate to recommend the following steps to evaluate and manage the post-term gestation:

1. Weekly cervical examinations should be performed starting at 41 to 42 weeks gestation, with induction in the presence of a readily inducible cervix (Bishop score 5 or greater).

2. If the cervix is unfavorable for induction, twice-weekly fetal testing should be done utilizing the biophysical profile.

3. In the presence of an abnormal fetal test, or with oligohydramnios as the only finding, delivery should be accomplished by the safest route for the fetus.

4. During the intrapartum period, careful fetal heart rate evaluation should be performed, with fetal scalp blood pH sampling if indicated and available. Since the presence of meconium in the amniotic fluid is associated with a lower umbilical arterial pH, particular attention should be given to this finding (Miller and Read, 1981). Consideration should also be given to the use of *saline amnioinfusion*. Two separate studies report a decrease in the cesarean section rate for fetal distress (Miyazaki and Taylor, 1983) and a decrease in meconium aspiration (Wenstrom and Parsons, 1989) utilizing this technique.

The data from studies utilizing routine induction at 41 to 42 weeks gestational age rather than antenatal monitoring remain somewhat controversial, although there may be some benefit in decreasing the cesarean section rate. It is prudent to recognize that this issue remains unresolved and that neither approach can, at this time, be considered superior to the other.

DEVELOPMENTAL EFFECTS OF POST-TERM GESTATION

Studies on subsequent development of children from prolonged pregnancies are difficult to evaluate, because investigators have not separated those neonates asphyxiated *in utero* and growth-retarded (dysmature) post-term neonates from otherwise normally born neonates. A study of neonatal behavior among 106 postmature infants revealed an increased number of illnesses and sleep disorders during the first year of life as well as diminished social competence (Vineland Social Maturity Scale) at 1 year of age. Also, and not unexpectedly, the incidence of fetal distress was high, and those babies asphyxiated *in utero* had a higher incidence of abnormal neurologic signs in the neonatal period (Lovell, 1973). All infants had signs of desquamation of skin and wasting of subcutaneous tissue, however, and the group of children studied was not compared with any children born post-term who did not have these physical findings at birth.

Field and co-workers (1977) have reported outcome in a group of 40 postmature offspring all of whom had parchment-like skin and long, thin bodies. At birth their Brazelton interaction and motor scores were lower than term controls, and at 4 months they scored lower on the Denver Developmental Scale. By 8 months, the Bayley motor scores of the post-term subjects were equivalent to those of control infants, but the mental scores were slightly lower. This study differs in at least one significant way from that of Lovell (1973): the Apgar scores at 5 minutes in the two groups were identical, thus partially correcting for *in utero* asphyxia.

In a large retrospective review, Zwerdling (1967) observed that post-term infants weighing less than 2500 gm had a neonatal mortality rate seven times that for post-term infants as a whole, confirming the additional risk of the occasionally observed abnormal growth pattern (dysmaturity) in some post-term infants. This increase in mortality rate was observed up to 2 years of age. Data on growth and intelligence revealed no differences between prolonged-gestation and normal-gestation children at age 5, however. These findings are confirmed in a more recent prospective study in which 129 children born of prolonged pregnancy were compared with 184 term controls (Shime et al., 1986). At 1 year, and again at 2 years of age, there were no differences between the two groups with respect to IQ, physical milestones, and intercurrent illnesses.

It is clear that the child of a post-term gestation must be evaluated in follow-up studies in relation to the presence or absence of antepartum or intrapartum asphyxia and of the dysmaturity syndrome (long fingernails, skin desquamation, and decreased subcutaneous tissue). It is entirely possible that later development is normal in the absence of these factors.

REFERENCES

Ballantyne JW: The problem of the postmature infant. J Obstet Gynaecol Br Emp **2**:36, 1902.
Barss VA, Frigoletto FD, Diamond F: Stillbirth after nonstress testing. Obstet Gynecol **65**:541, 1985.
Benedetti TJ, Easterling T: Antepartum testing in post-term pregnancy. J Reprod Med **33**:252, 1988.
Bochner CJ, Medearis Al, Davis J, et al: Antepartum predictors of fetal distress in post-term pregnancy. Am J Obstet Gynecol **157**:353, 1987.
Boyd ME, Usher RH, McLean FH, et al: Obstetric consequences of post-maturity. Am J Obstet Gynecol **158**:334, 1988.
Butler NR, Alberman ED: The second report of the 1958 British Perinatal Mortality Survey. Edinburgh, E & S Livingston, Ltd., 1969, p 327.
Clifford SH: Postmaturity—with placental dysfunction. J Pediatr **44**:1, 1954.
Crowley P, O'Herlihy C, Boylan P: The value of ultrasound measurement of amniotic fluid volume in the management of prolonged pregnancies. Br J Obstet Gynaecol **91**:444, 1984.
Dyson DC, Miller PD, Armstrong MA: Management of prolonged pregnancy: Induction of labor versus antepartum fetal testing. Am J Obstet Gynecol **156**:928, 1987.
Eden R, Gergely RZ, Schifrin BS, Wade ME: Comparison of antepartum testing schemes for the management of the postdate pregnancy. Am J Obstet Gynecol **144**:683, 1982.
Eden R, Seifert L, Winegar A, Spellacy WN: Perinatal characteristics of uncomplicated post-date pregnancies. Obstet Gynecol **69**:296, 1987.
Farmakides G, Schulman H, Ducey J et al. Uterine and umbilical artery Doppler velocimetry in post-term pregnancy. J Repro Med **33**:259, 1988.
Field TM, Dabiri C, Hallock N, Schuman HH: Developmental effects of prolonged pregnancy in the postmaturity syndrome. J Pediatr **90**:836, 1977.
Fleischer A, Schulman H, Farmakides G, et al: Antepartum nonstress test and the postmature pregnancy. Obstet Gynecol **66**:80, 1985.
Freeman RK, Garite TJ, Modanlou H, et al: Postdate pregnancy: Utilization of contraction stress testing for primary fetal surveillance. Am J Obstet Gynecol **140**:128, 1981.
Guidetti DA, Divon MY, Cavalieri RL et al: Fetal umbilical artery flow velocimetry in post-date pregnancies. Am J Obstet Gynecol **157**:1521, 1987.
Hannah ME, Hannah WJ, Hellmann J, et al: Induction of labor as compared with serial antenatal monitoring in post-term pregnancy. N Engl J Med **326**:1587, 1992.
Hauth JC, Goodman MT, Gilstrap LC III, Gilstrap JER: Post-term pregnancy. J Obstet Gynecol **56**:467, 1980.
Johnson JM, Harman CR, Lange IR, Manning FA: Biophysical profile scoring in the management of the post-term pregnancy. Am J Obstet Gynecol **154**:269, 1986.
Kramer MS, McLean FH, Boyd ME, et al: The validity of gestational age estimation by menstrual dating in term, preterm and post-term gestations. JAMA **260**:3306, 1988.
Leveno KJ, Quirk JG, Cunningham FG et al: Prolonged pregnancy: I. Observations concerning the causes of fetal distress. Am J Obstet Gynecol **150**:465, 1984.
Lovell KE: The effect of postmaturity on the developing child. Med J Austr **1**:13, 1973.
Manning FA, Baskett TF, Morrison I, Lange I: Fetal biophysical profile scoring: A prospective study in 1184 high risk patients. Am J Obstet Gynecol **140**:289, 1981.
Manning FA, Morrison I, Harman CR, et al: Fetal assessment based on fetal biophysical profile scoring: Experience in 19,221 referred high risk pregnancies: II. An analysis of false negative deaths. Am J Obstet Gynecol **157**:880, 1987.
McClure-Browne JC: Postmaturity. Am J Obstet Gynecol **85**:573, 1963.

McLean FH, Boyd ME, Usher RH: Post-term infants: Too big or too small? Am J Obstet Gynecol **164**:619, 1991.

Medearis AL: Post-term pregnancy: Active labor induction (PGE₂ gel) not associated with improved outcomes compared to expected management: A preliminary report. *In* Proceedings of the 10th Annual Meeting of the Society of Perinatal Obstetricians. January 23–27, 1990. Washington D.C., Society of Perinatal Obstetricians, 1990, p 17.

Miller FC, Read JA: Intrapartum assessment of the postdate fetus. Am J Obstet Gynecol **141**:516, 1981.

Miyazaki FS, Miyazaki BA: False reactive nonstress tests in postterm pregnancies. Am J Obstet Gynecol **140**:269, 1981.

Miyazaki FS, Taylor NA: Saline amnioinfusion for relief of variable or prolonged decelerations. A preliminary report. Am J Obstet Gynecol **146**:670, 1983.

Moore TR, Cayle JE: Amniotic fluid index in normal human pregnancy. Am J Obstet Gynecol **162**:1168, 1990.

Naeye RL: Causes of perinatal mortality. Excess in prolonged gestations. Am J Epidemiol **108**:429, 1978.

Nakano R: Post-term pregnancy: A five year review from Osaka National Hospital. Acta Obstet Gynecol Scand **51**:217, 1972.

Nwosu VC, Wallach EE, Bolognese RJ: Initiation of labor by intra-amniotic cortisol instillation in prolonged human pregnancy. Obstet Gynecol **47**:137, 1976.

Phelan JP, Platt LD, Yeh S-Y, et al: Continuing role of the nonstress test in the management of post-dates pregnancy. Obstet Gynecol **64**:624, 1984.

Phelan JP, Platt LP, Yeh S-Y, et al: The role of ultrasound assessment of amniotic fluid volume in the management of the post-date pregnancy. Am J Obstet Gynecol **151**:304, 1985.

Pollack RN, Hauer-Pollack G, Divon MY: Macrosomia in post-dates pregnancy: The accuracy of routine ultrasonographic screening. Am J Obstet Gynecol **167**:7, 1992.

Sachs BP, Friedman EA: Results of an epidemiological study of post-date pregnancy. J Reprod Med **31**:162, 1986.

Shime J, Librach CL, Gare DJ, Cook C-J: The influence of prolonged pregnancy on infant development at one and two years of age: A prospective controlled study. Am J Obstet Gynecol **154**:341, 1986.

Small JL, Phelan JP, Smith SV, et al: An active management approach to the post-date fetus with a reactive nonstress test in fetal heart rate decelerations. Obstet Gynecol **70**:636, 1987.

Stokes HJ, Roberts RV, Newnham JP. Doppler flow velocity wave form analysis in post-date pregnancies. Aust N Z J Obstet Gynecol **31**:27, 1991.

Turnbull AC, Patten PT, Flint APF, et al: Significant fall in progesterone and rise in estradiol levels in human peripheral plasma before the onset of labor. Lancet i:101, 1974.

Usher RH, Boyd ME, McLean FH et al: Assessment of fetal risk in post-date pregnancies. Am J Obstet Gynecol **158**:259, 1988.

Wenstrom KD, Parsons MT: The prevention of meconium aspiration in labor using amnioinfusion. Obstet Gynecol **73**:647, 1989.

Zwerdling MA: Factors pertaining to prolonged pregnancy and its outcome. Pediatrics **40**:202, 1967.

NORMAL AND ABNORMAL LABOR

C H A P T E R

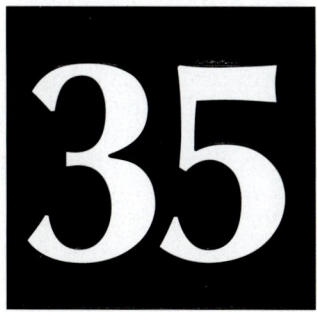

CLINICAL ASPECTS OF NORMAL AND ABNORMAL LABOR

WATSON A. BOWES, Jr., M.D.

NORMAL LABOR AND ITS LIMITS

The proper management of labor and delivery depends on a thorough understanding of the anatomy and physiology of normal labor. Moreover, the recognition and management of labor abnormalities require a knowledge of the limits of labor and of the physiologic response of both the mother and the fetus to the stress of labor and delivery.

The uterus contracts throughout normal pregnancy. These contractions are irregular in timing and intensity, discoordinate in distribution, and, for the most part, entirely painless. Such uterine activity continues in normal pregnancy until late in the third trimester, when the contractions become more frequent, of greater and more consistent intensity, and more coordinated. Also, during the latter part of the third trimester, effacement (shortening) and dilation of the cervix begins. The beginning of clinical labor has been described as the onset of painful uterine contractions associated with effacement and dilation of the cervix. The precise onset of this combination of events frequently cannot be ascertained, and for practical purposes clinicians must rely on the patient's best estimate of when her contractions began or when they became regular in consistency and intensity. The specific onset of cervical effacement and dilation can rarely be documented in cases of spontaneous onset of labor, and not uncommonly both effacement and dilation occur late in the third trimester, prior to the onset of regular or noticeable uterine contractions. The precise onset of labor is difficult to determine, and much of what is written about false labor, prodromal labor,

and the latent phase of labor is influenced by this uncertainty.

These prelabor changes of the cervix were studied by Hendricks and colleagues (1970), who reported the findings of serial cervical examinations of 303 patients in the third trimester. Cervical dilation began earlier and was of greater magnitude in multiparas than in primiparas. Cervical effacement, on the other hand, began earlier and was of greater magnitude in primiparas than in multiparas. These authors introduced the concept of the "cervical coefficient," which is the product of cervical dilation (in centimeters) times the percentage of effacement. They found that at any point in prelabor the cervical coefficient is relatively the same for all patients regardless of parity. The mean cervical dilation during the last 3 days prior to the onset of labor is 1.8 cm for nulliparas and 2.2 cm for multiparas. Their study stressed the importance of the prelabor preparation of the cervix and its influence on the duration of labor. It also pointed out the difficulty of using a specific time for onset of labor if it is defined as the beginning of cervical dilation.

It has been the convention to regard labor as divided into three stages:

First stage: from onset of labor to full dilation of the cervix.

Second stage: from full dilation of the cervix to delivery of the infant.

Third stage: from delivery of the infant to delivery of the placenta.

Pritchard and MacDonald (1980) have described a fourth stage of labor as the hour following the delivery of the placenta.

One of the most thorough evaluations of the first

stage of labor is that by Friedman (1978), conveniently summarized in a monograph. He divides the first stage of labor into two major phases, described as follows:

Latent phase: from the onset of regular uterine contractions to the beginning of the active phase.

Active phase: from the time the rate of cervical dilation begins to change rapidly to full dilation. (The active phase usually begins at about 3 to 4 cm of dilation.)

Data from several thousand patients, in whom cervical dilation and the station of the presenting fetal part were documented throughout labor, were used to establish normal limits of labor for nulliparous and multiparous patients. A group of nulliparas and a group of multiparas were selected in whom there were no apparent complications of labor and who delivered normal infants. From these cases the norms for ideal labor were determined (Table 35–1). Descent of the fetal head in relationship to the ischial spines was found to begin well before the second stage. The rate of descent increased late in the first stage and continued in a linear manner into the second stage of labor until the perineal floor was reached. Data for the maximum rate of descent and the length of the second stage of labor in all patients are given in Table 35–1.

The intelligent management of labor depends on an understanding of its mechanism as well as the norms and limits of its progress. One of the most important and helpful studies for understanding the mechanism of labor was that of Caldwell and associates (1935). This report was the culmination of a study of over 1000 roentgenologic examinations of the pelvis and fetal head, performed before, during, or after labor, in relation to the known details of delivery and the facts ascertained by vaginal examination. Many of the findings of this and later studies by the same authors (Caldwell et al., 1940) are incorporated in a monograph by Steer (1959). A complete review of these important works is beyond the scope of this text. However, a study of these contributions will substantially increase one's understanding of the influence of the pelvic architecture on normal and abnormal labor. Several of the important findings of these studies are worth reemphasizing.

With a gynecoid or android type of pelvis, the fetal head will engage in the transverse position 60 to 70 per cent of the time. The anthropoid pelvis predisposes to engagement in the occiput anterior or posterior position. After the fetal head enters the pelvis in the transverse position, it is carried downward and backward until it impinges on the sacrum low in the midpelvis. It is at this point that internal rotation begins.

Internal rotation usually occurs in the midpelvis. Anterior rotation of the fetal head is practically complete when the head makes contact with the lower aspects of the pubic rami.

The common occurrence of engagement and descent predominantly in the posterior pelvis is usually associated with a normal progress of labor and spontaneous delivery. However, when engagement and descent occur predominantly in the forepelvis, there is a higher incidence of abnormal progress of labor and a higher rate of operative delivery. If the fetal head is descending in the posterior pelvis, the cervix will usually be felt posteriorly in the vagina, while engagement and descent in the forepelvis must be suspected if the cervix is palpated in a forward position, closer to the symphysis than to the sacrum.

The increasing use of the vacuum extractor and the cesarean operation for delivery of second-stage arrest of labor has also contributed to the lessening of emphasis on knowledge about pelvic types and their influence on descent and rotation of the fetal head. However, the relationship between pelvic architecture and the position of the fetal head will often allow useful prediction or explanation of abnormal labor, especially in the descent phase.

A careful clinical examination frequently discloses the essential dimensions and shape of the pelvis. In general the characteristics of the anterior segment of the inlet will correspond to the anterior portion of the lower pelvis. A subpubic arch with a well-rounded apex and ample space between the ischial tuberosities is associated with a gynecoid anterior segment at the inlet. A subpubic arch with a narrow angle and straight rami, convergent side walls, and prominent spines is associated with a narrowed, android anterior segment at the inlet. A narrow subpubic arch with straight side walls is characteristic of an anthropoid anterior segment at the inlet. Finally, a wide subpubic arch with straight or divergent side walls and a wide interspinous diameter will be associated with a flat anterior segment at the inlet.

The posterior segment can best be characterized by palpation of the sacrospinous ligament and the sacrosciatic notch. A narrow notch (associated with a short sacrosciatic ligament—less than two finger breadths) suggests an android posterior segment. A

TABLE 35–1. **Characteristics of Labor in Nulliparas and Multiparas***

CHARACTERISTIC	NULLIPARAS		MULTIPARAS	
	ALL PATIENTS	**IDEAL LABOR**	**ALL PATIENTS**	**IDEAL LABOR**
Duration of first stage (hr)				
Latent phase	6.4 (±5.1)	6.1 (±4.0)	4.8 (±4.9)	4.5 (±4.2)
Active phase	4.6 (±3.6)	3.4 (±1.5)	2.4 (±2.2)	2.1 (±2.0)
Total	11.0 (±8.7)	9.5 (±5.5)	7.2 (±7.1)	6.6 (±6.2)
Maximum rate of descent (cm/hr)	3.3 (±2.3)	3.6 (±1.9)	6.6 (±4.0)	7.0 (±3.2)
Duration of second stage (hr)	1.1 (±0.8)	0.76 (±0.5)	0.39 (±0.3)	0.32 (±0.3)

*All values given are ± 1 SD.

Data from Friedman EA: Labor: Clinical Evaluation and Management. 2nd ed. New York, Appleton-Century-Crofts, 1978.

sacrosciatic ligament length of two to three finger breadths is suggestive of a gynecoid posterior segment. If the ligament is directed backward and the spines are close together, the posterior segment of the inlet is probably anthropoid. If the ligament is directed laterally and the spines are far apart, the posterior segment of the inlet is likely to be flat.

These assessments of pelvic configuration can be made at the time of a pelvic examination when the patient is admitted to the labor unit or can be part of the initial examination when the patient registers for prenatal care. The advantages of performing the assessment when the patient is hospitalized in labor are the increased relevance of the information at that time and the probability that the individual performing the examination will be incorporating the results into a comprehensive assessment of the patient's labor.

One of the most important aspects of the management of labor is accurate and thorough documentation of the progress of labor or the lack of it. Most authorities agree that a graphic display of intrapartum data that allows a prompt visualization of the status and progress of cervical dilation and, in some cases, descent of the presenting part is an essential adjunct to intrapartum patient monitoring. This may be accomplished with a simple record of cervical dilation plotted against time on ruled graph paper, or by a more comprehensive recording of all intrapartum data related in graphic form to the progress of cervical dilation. If the data about effacement and dilation of the cervix and station and position of the presenting part are recorded only in narrative form, early and significant abnormalities of labor may not be recognized as soon as if a more visual display of labor progress is available. This is especially important if more than one attendant follows the patient, as frequently occurs in a labor that is longer than normal or a labor that overlaps a change of shift in the hospital. A tabular and graphic display of intrapartum data is entirely in keeping with the concept that labor and delivery are worthy of intensive surveillance and also affords a convenient method of reviewing labor events in situations of an untoward fetal or maternal outcome. The compulsiveness, form, and orderliness of documenting labor events need not interfere with compassionate, family-centered care of a woman in labor. In fact, the challenge of modern obstetrics is to manage a pregnancy with the least interference and yet with the capability of recognizing and correcting at the earliest possible moment incipient complications.

MANAGEMENT OF LABOR ABNORMALITIES

Abnormalities of the First Stage

Abnormalities of the first stage of labor occur in 8 per cent of patients, according to Friedman (1978), with a much higher incidence among primiparas than among multiparas. Philpott and Castle (1972a) found that 11 per cent of primiparas had abnormal progress of the first stage of labor requiring oxytocin augmentation.

By defining the limits of cervical dilation and descent of the fetus with regard to time in normal labor, Friedman (1978) described abnormalities of labor, identified associated problems, detailed the prognosis for mother and fetus, and recommended a course of management for each abnormality.

Prolonged Latent Phase

On the basis of the 95th percentile limit of the distribution of latent phase durations in the primiparous population, 20 hours is considered the definition of an abnormal latent phase. For multiparas, 14 hours is the corresponding definition of prolonged latent phase. On some occasions it is difficult to ascertain the difference between a prolonged latent phase and so-called false labor. Friedman (1978) found that prolongation of the latent phase was associated with excessive sedation, prematurely administered epidural anesthesia, unfavorable cervical status, or myometrial dysfunction. Latent phase prolongation, however, is not predictive of other more ominous labor abnormalities, is not caused by cephalopelvic disproportion (CPD), should not result in a higher than expected number of cesarean births, and is not associated with an increased risk of depression or asphyxia of the newborn. The management of this abnormality of the first stage of labor includes deep sedation designed to fully relax the mother or oxytocin augmentation to improve uterine contractions. Friedman (1978) prefers the former, but his data suggest that either approach is effective in most cases. He also states that amniotomy is not effective therapy for this abnormality.

One of the major problems with the evaluation and management of the latent phase of labor is knowing at what hour labor began. For this reason, some authorities have used the time of admission to the hospital as a convenient starting point for judging when to intervene in the progress of labor (Philpott and Castle, 1972a; Beazley and Kurjak, 1972; O'Driscoll and Meagher, 1980). Friedman (1978), on the other hand, regards the onset of regular contractions as the beginning of labor and recommends intervention when the duration of the latent phase of labor reaches 20 hours in the primipara. He has found that either adequate sedation ("therapeutic narcosis") or oxytocin augmentation will result in the resumption of normal cervical dilation. Because most patients are exhausted after 20 hours of labor, Friedman prefers therapeutic narcosis over oxytocin augmentation. For narcosis, he recommends morphine sulfate, 15 to 20 mg, with 10 to 15 mg more if the first dose has not made the patient somnolent and therefore inhibited uterine contractions. The obvious advantage of this therapy is that the patient awakens rested and refreshed and prepared for the active phase of labor.

Critics of this approach, especially O'Driscoll and Meagher (1980), argue that awaiting 20 hours of latent phase before considering the labor abnormal only promotes exhaustion and discourages the patient. They advocate an *active management of labor*, which has been practiced and evaluated for two decades at the National Maternity Hospital in Dublin. This involves several important features as follows:

1. Admission to the labor unit only when patients are having painful uterine contractions as well as complete effacement of the cervix, ruptured membranes, or passage of blood-stained mucus.

2. Amniotomy soon after admission for those patients who have intact membranes.

3. The use of oxytocin augmentation of labor if there is less than 1 cm per hour progress of labor. Oxytocin infusion is begun at 4 mU/minute and increased by 6 mU/minute every 15 minutes until there are seven contractions per 15 minutes. The oxytocin infusion rate does not exceed 40 mU/minute.

4. Continuous electronic fetal heart rate monitoring is used only if there is meconium-stained amniotic fluid and after fetal scalp pH has been performed to rule out fetal acidosis.

5. A nurse-midwife is in constant attendance with the patient throughout labor.

6. The patient is assured that if her labor exceeds 12 hours, cesarean delivery will be performed.

7. The progress of labor is documented on a simple graphic form, and all cases are reviewed daily by the senior obstetrician in charge of the unit.

8. This approach to the management of labor is confined to nulliparas.

The active management protocol, with minor modifications, has now been evaluated on several obstetric services in the United States as well as other countries and has consistently resulted in a decrease in the incidence of cesarean delivery for dystocia in nulliparas without increasing maternal or neonatal morbidity (Lopez-Zeno et al., 1992; Turner et al., 1988; Boylan et al., 1991; Akoury et al., 1988).

Protraction Disorders

Protraction disorders are those in which progress of cervical dilation and descent of the fetal head occur at a slower than normal rate in the active phase of labor. The rate of cervical dilation for nulliparas should be 1.2 cm or more per hour, and for multiparas, 1.5 cm or more. For descent of the fetal head, the rate for nulliparas should be 1.0 cm or more per hour, and for multiparas, 2.0 cm per hour.

Beazley and Kurjak (1972) analyzed the labor records of 460 nulliparas and 276 multiparas giving birth in London. Philpott and Castle (1972b), in a similar study of 625 Rhodesian African primiparas, developed norms for labor, departures from which constitute indications for therapeutic intervention. Hendricks and colleagues (1970) studied 303 patients delivered at University Hospital in Cleveland, Ohio. Serial cervical examinations were performed prior to and during labor, and a curve for mean cervical dilation in active labor was developed. Although derived by somewhat different analytic methods and from different populations, the "active phase" of Friedman (1978), the "partograph" of Beazley and Kurjak (1972), the "action line" of Philpott and Castle (1972b), and the "cervical dilation vs. time after admission" of Hendricks and colleagues (1970) result in remarkably similar descriptions of the active phase of labor (Fig. 35–1). The patient whose cervical dilation versus time curve

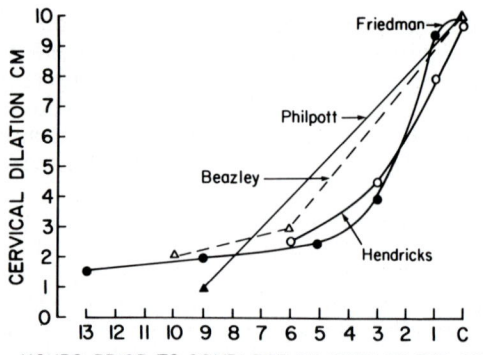

FIGURE 35–1. Labor curves as defined by cervical dilation versus time in several study populations (Beazley and Kurjak, 1972; Friedman, 1978; Hendricks et al., 1970; Philpott and Castle, 1972). Because "onset of labor" is defined somewhat differently by the various authors, the labor curves were superimposed by using complete cervical dilation as the common end point. The similarity of the "active phases" of labor among the various populations studied is illustrated.

crosses to the right of any these so-called norms is in the population deserving of attention. Of course, the precise time when that cross-over occurs depends on when the beginning of labor is established for purposes of clinical evaluation. As long as it is taken into account that most primiparas reach the hospital several hours after contractions have begun and with the cervix dilated 2 cm or more, the concept of using time of admission or alleged time of onset of contractions as time zero for management purposes will not make a great deal of difference, particularly when those labors beyond the latent or prelabor phase are considered.

Friedman (1978) found protraction disorders in primiparas to be frequently associated with CPD, use of conduction anesthesia, and fetal malposition. Whether these factors are related in a cause-and-effect manner is not known. Moreover, he found oxytocin augmentation and therapeutic narcosis of little value in these cases. He also noted unusually high neonatal mortality and morbidity rates when this labor abnormality was terminated by mid-forceps delivery. However, the diagnosis of a primary dysfunctional labor, i.e., the labor that persists at a cervical dilation rate of less than 1.2 cm/hr, is usually made in retrospect after oxytocin augmentation has been used and found not to increase the dilation rate. The experiences of Beazley and Kurjak (1972) and O'Driscoll and Meagher (1980) suggest that an early, more active use of oxytocin, as described in the active management of labor, will effectively correct most protraction disorders, although these authors do not specifically separate the protraction disorders from the arrest disorders. Those who advocate the active management of labor point out that the use of x-ray pelvimetry is unnecessary in the nulliparous patient because rupture of the uterus will not occur with the recommended oxytocin augmentation. Therefore, in nulliparous patients with suboptimal progress of labor of any source, it is safe to use a trial of oxytocin to determine if labor will progress to completion.

Ganström et al. (1991) have demonstrated significant differences in the collagen content and collagen remodelling in the cervix and lower uterine segment in patients with protracted labors as compared to those with normal labors. This may explain why some patients with protracted labor do not respond to oxytocin augmentation.

Arrest Disorders

Arrest disorder is defined by Friedman (1978) as the cessation of cervical dilation or of the descent of the fetal head in the active phase of labor for more than 2 hours. In their pure form, arrest disorders differ from protraction abnormalities in that prior to the arrest of progress, the rate of cervical dilation or descent of the fetal head is normal. The arrest of progress might also complicate a protraction disorder. In either situation, Friedman (1978) found that approximately one-half of the cases of arrest disorder were associated with cephalopelvic disproportion. Philpott and Castle (1972b) also found that patients whose labor progress crossed the "action line" (i.e., those with protraction or arrest disorders) had smaller pelvic measurements and more often required cesarean delivery for CPD.

Because of the frequent association between arrest disorders and cephalopelvic disproportion, Friedman (1978) recommends radiographic cephalopelvimetry followed by cesarean delivery for those who have CPD and oxytocin augmentation for the remainder. He has shown that 80 per cent of women with arrest disorders who do not have CPD will deliver following oxytocin augmentation. Philpott and Castle (1972b) and O'Driscoll and Meagher (1980) hold that radiographic studies are not required, especially in primiparas, and that a trial of oxytocin augmentation is indicated in all protraction and arrest disorders. If mother and fetus are carefully monitored and if the augmentation is discontinued when there is no progress in 4 to 6 hours, there is no danger to the patients. This approach is, in fact, followed on most United States obstetric services, where radiographic cephalopelvimetry is seldom used in the management of abnormal labor in vertex presentations (O'Brien and Cefalo, 1982; Parsons and Spellacy, 1985; Floberg et al., 1987). A notable exception is the use of the fetal-pelvic index by Thurnau et al. (1988). This technique combines ultrasound measurement of the fetal head and abdominal circumferences (HC and AC, respectively) and the radiographic measurement of the maternal pelvic inlet and mid-pelvic circumferences (IC and MC, respectively). The fetal-pelvic index is the sum of the two greatest positive circumference differences (HC − IC, HC − MC, AC − IC, AC − MC, respectively). A positive fetal-pelvic index value indicates the presence of fetal-pelvic disproportion, and a negative fetal-pelvic index value indicates the absence of fetal-pelvic disproportion. The fetal-pelvic index was found to have a 94 per cent positive predictive value for cesarean delivery of patients with abnormal labor patterns. Thurnau and Morgan (1988a) have had similar success in using the fetal-pelvic index obtained prior to indicated induction of labor to predict the need for operative delivery. Enthusiasm for the fetal-pelvic index in the management of labor awaits the success of this technique, as confirmed by others, and the performance of radiographic measurements by computed tomography, which exposes the mother and fetus to substantially less radiation than conventional x-ray pelvimetry (Federle et al., 1982).

Several authors have evaluated the effect of ambulation on the progress of labor. Flynn and co-workers (1978) found that patients who ambulated had more rapid labor with fewer instances of fetal distress than a similar number of patients who labored in bed. Williams and associates (1980), studying 48 ambulated patients, could find no differences in duration of labor or frequency of fetal distress compared with control patients. Read and colleagues (1981) studied 14 patients whose labors were regarded as requiring augmentation because of lack of progress attributed to inadequate contractions. In eight patients who were randomized to an ambulation study protocol, there was as rapid progress of labor as in six control patients whose labors were augmented with oxytocin. These studies suggest that ambulation is not detrimental to the progress of labor or the well-being of the fetus, although it has not been established whether ambulation is clearly beneficial or is a substitute for pharmacologic augmentation of labor in cases of abnormal progress.

Abnormalities of the Second Stage

Abnormalities of Rotation and Descent

Textbooks of obstetrics have traditionally discussed the first and second stages of labor as if they were separate clinical and biologic entities, which, in fact, they are not. Descent and rotation of the fetal head frequently occur prior to complete dilation of the cervix, a phenomenon that is clear to most clinicians and is confirmed by the studies of Friedman (1978). Arrest of descent and rotation, whether it occurs before or after complete dilation of the cervix, is a matter of concern and requires evaluation. Arbitrary limits on the duration of the second stage of labor probably resulted from the misinterpretation of the data presented by Hellman and Prystowsky (1952). In that study, it was shown that patients in whom the second stage of labor was longer than 2 hours were at increased risk for perinatal and maternal morbidity. This observation was interpreted by many clinicians to mean that delivery of the fetus should be accomplished, by whatever means, before 2 hours of the second stage had elapsed. This interpretation occasionally resulted in traumatic mid-forceps operations or unnecessary cesarean deliveries, not to mention the overzealous use of the vacuum extractor.

Cohen (1977) demonstrated that if patients with fetal distress or traumatic delivery are excluded, the duration of the second stage bears no relationship to perinatal outcome. If there are no serious fetal heart rate abnormalities, if the mother is well hydrated and reasonably comfortable, and if there is some progress of descent or rotation of the fetal head, regardless of how slow, there is no need for operative delivery.

TABLE 35–2.   Perinatal Morbidity in Shoulder Dystocia

STUDY	NO. OF CASES	INCIDENCE (%)	DEATHS RELATED TO SHOULDER DYSTOCIA	BRACHIAL PLEXUS INJURY	FRACTURE OF CLAVICLE OR HUMERUS
Swartz (1960)	31	15	5	15	3
McCall (1962)	105	63	2	3	4
Seigworth (1966)	51	38	5	8	2
Kahn (1966)	24	?	8	2	2
Benedetti and Gabbe (1978)	33	37	0	3	5
Total	244		20	31	16

Rather, uterine contractions should be assessed and, if inadequate, should be augmented with oxytocin. Posterior presentations, brow presentation, marked degrees of asynclitism, and very large infants will be associated with longer labors even with adequate contractions.

Shoulder Dystocia

Shoulder dystocia is the problem encountered when, following the delivery of the head, the anterior shoulder does not deliver either spontaneously or with gentle traction by the accoucheur. This complication, which was reviewed by Resnik (1980), occurs with the frequency of 0.15 to 0.63 per cent, or about one in 300 deliveries (Table 35–2). The specific etiology of this complication is not known, although it most frequently occurs in association with a large infant (more than 4000 gm) whose bisacromial diameter fails to engage in the pelvis in the usual oblique dimension. This results in the anterior shoulder being caught immediately above the symphysis. Other features of the maternal history that predispose to shoulder dystocia are a previous large infant, obesity, diabetes, and multiparity. Prolonged second stage of labor is a warning sign of fetal-maternal dystocia whether it be cephalopelvic disproportion or shoulder dystocia. Also, mid-pelvic delivery with forceps or vacuum extractor has been associated with shoulder dystocia. Benedetti and Gabbe (1978) demonstrated the cumulative effect of some of these features on the occurrence of difficult shoulder delivery. The incidence of shoulder dystocia in labors with infants weighing more than 4000 gm and in which there was a prolonged second stage and a mid-pelvic delivery was 23 per cent, in contrast to labors with none of these features, in which the incidence of shoulder dystocia was 0.07 per cent.

Maternal morbidity includes frequent fourth-degree perineal lacerations, cervical lacerations, postpartum hemorrhage, and endometritis. Perinatal morbidity and mortality are extensive (see Table 35–2). The perinatal mortality rate directly related to the complications ranges from zero to 33 per cent. Deaths are usually due to prolonged asphyxia associated with a delay in delivery of the infant.

The prolonged sequelae of asphyxia from shoulder dystocia have not been well studied. In 5- to 10-year follow-ups of 46 of 97 infants who survived deliveries complicated by shoulder dystocia, McCall (1962) found 13 (28 per cent) children with neuropsychiatric dysfunction (Table 35–3).

These data suggest that there may be permanent damage in some children as a result of shoulder dystocia, but the specific risk is difficult to ascertain. Brachial plexus injuries result from extensive lateral traction on the head of the infant during the delivery process. Many affected infants recover with time, but some have permanent neuromuscular disability. Fractures of the clavicle and humerus, which occur to the posterior shoulder and arm as a result of posterior shoulder delivery, heal without permanent residua.

Management of this complication of the second stage of labor includes assessment of each patient in labor for risk factors for shoulder girdle dystocia. The weight of large infants is notoriously underestimated prior to birth. The use of real-time ultrasonography in laboring patients for detection of the large infant has not been particularly helpful. The lack of amniotic fluid, the engaged vertex, and maternal obesity all interfere with the gathering of accurate sonographic measurements of the fetus during labor. In the patient suspected of having a large infant (>4000 gm), mid-pelvic deliveries with forceps or a vacuum extractor should be used with caution, especially if there is arrest of descent or rotation in the second stage of labor. The more liberal use of cesarean section is advised for patients with a number of risk factors for shoulder dystocia, but the relative maternal-fetal risks of such a policy have not yet been assessed in a prospective study. The studies of Morgan and Thurnau (1988b) in predicting delivery outcome for infants weighing 4000 grams or greater are promising and may provide a more effective means of selecting patients for elective cesarean delivery to prevent serious neonatal injuries from shoulder dystocia.

Shoulder dystocia may occur in the absence of any of the predisposing factors mentioned; therefore, all

TABLE 35–3.   Neuropsychiatric Dysfunction in 13 Children Surviving Shoulder Dystocia

DYSFUNCTION	OCCURRENCE IN SURVIVORS		INCIDENCE IN GENERAL POPULATION (%)
	No.	%	
Mental retardation	2	4.3	3
School grades below those expected	5	11.0	10
Speech dysfunction	7	15.0	6–13

Data from McCall JO Jr: Shoulder dystocia: A study of aftereffects. Am J Obstet Gynecol 83:1486, 1962.

physicians and nurse-midwives delivering infants should be familiar with the procedures for the management of shoulder girdle dystocia. The first sign of shoulder dystocia is recoil of the fetal chin into the perineum immediately following delivery of the head. This has been called by some the "turtle sign." When it is seen, or when the anterior shoulder does not appear beneath the symphysis pubis with the gentlest traction, shoulder dystocia must be suspected, and further attempts to deliver the anterior shoulder by lateral traction of the fetal vertex should be avoided

Exaggerated flexion of the mother's legs, i.e., knees to chest, known as the McRobert's maneuver, will often result in delivery of the shoulder (Gonik et al., 1983). If this simple and painless procedure does not promptly allow delivery, an assistant should apply downward pressure with the closed fist immediately above the symphysis pubis. This maneuver frequently will push the anterior shoulder to an oblique angle under the symphysis pubis. The maneuver may be combined with the insertion of the operator's second and third fingers against the anterior shoulder to rotate it to an oblique angle. Fundal pressure is not useful in the management of shoulder dystocia and may be counterproductive.

If these measures have not promptly resulted in delivery of the infant, this author recommends that the posterior shoulder should be delivered by the following method (Barnum, 1945). The operator inserts a hand in the vagina along the sacrum until the posterior forearm is encountered. It is then firmly grasped and drawn across the chest of the fetus into the vagina. This maneuver may cause a fracture of the humerus or clavicle, which is a remedial skeletal injury without the potential long-term sequelae of a brachial plexus injury. Once the posterior arm is delivered, rotation of the fetus and delivery of the opposite arm can usually be accomplished without difficulty.

Abnormalities of the Third Stage

Placental Separation and Control of Uterine Bleeding

The third stage of labor is defined as the time from delivery of the infant to delivery of the placenta. For all practical purposes, one should include the hour after the delivery of the placenta in the third stage of labor because it is during this time that the patient is at greatest risk for postpartum hemorrhage.

Following the delivery of the infant, the uterus contracts and placental separation occurs by cleavage along the plane of the decidua basalis. Placental separation is usually complete by the time two contractions have occurred, although several additional contractions may be necessary to accomplish expulsion of the placenta from the uterus. Large venous sinuses are exposed following separation of the placenta, and control of bleeding from these sinuses depends primarily on contraction of uterine muscle and only secondarily on coagulation and thrombus formation in the placental site. The average blood loss at the time of a normal vaginal delivery is about 600 ml

(Pritchard, 1965). In the young healthy parturient, acute blood loss is well tolerated because of the increased blood volume of pregnancy and the decrease in vascular volume that occurs with the reduction of the uteroplacental circulation at the time of birth.

Management of the placenta in the third stage is a matter of debate among qualified obstetricians. Manual removal of the placenta, if performed promptly, has been shown to be associated with no increase in puerperal morbidity and has the advantages of immediately identifying retained placental fragments and intrauterine extensions of cervical lacerations and shortening the time of placental removal (Thomas, 1963; Blanchette, 1977). However, this is not a painless procedure in the unanesthetized patient and is unnecessarily invasive in most cases. Gentle massage of the uterine fundus will encourage uterine contractions and help one to detect changes in the shape of the uterus that signal placental separation. Vigorous fundal massage accomplishes nothing, is painful, and, when combined with excessive traction on the umbilical cord of a placenta implanted in the fundus of the uterus, may promote uterine inversion. In cases in which the placenta has not delivered with gentle cord traction and uterine massage after 30 minutes, manual removal of the placenta should be accomplished either under general anesthesia or after a tocolytic drug has been given intravenously in combination with sufficient parenteral analgesia.

Rarely, placental retention will be due to placenta accreta, which is the result of defective decidua basalis and is characterized by the attachment and growth of chorionic villi directly into the myometrium. If the placenta cannot be removed manually and placenta accreta is suspected, hysterectomy is usually required to avoid catastrophic hemorrhage. The etiology of placenta accreta is not known, but there is a strong association with implantation of the placenta in the lower uterine segment, placenta previa, and prior cesarean delivery. A report of 22 cases of placenta accreta by Read and co-workers (1980) suggests that in cases of focal or partial placenta accreta without excessive blood loss, conservative management may be successful. The conservative approach includes curettage of the retained placenta or suturing of the bleeding site (in cases of cesarean delivery) and should be considered only when the preservation of fertility is of utmost importance and with the awareness that hysterectomy will be necessary if the conservative approach does not promptly control the blood loss.

The episiotomy and vaginal or cervical lacerations are also sources of blood loss in the third stage of labor. Careful inspection of the vagina and cervix immediately after delivery will identify lacerations of these structures so that they can be repaired promptly. Prompt repair also facilitates the management of an unexpected hemorrhage in the immediate recovery period by allowing attention to be directed immediately to uterine atony.

In the event of an immediate postpartum hemorrhage, the patient's vital signs should be monitored frequently, adequate intravenous lines established promptly, adequate fluid replacement started with lactated Ringer's infusion, and preparations made for blood transfusion. Thereafter, a very prompt review of possible sources of hemorrhage should be accomplished, including (1) uterine atony, (2) cervical, vaginal, or uterine lacerations, (3) coagulopathies (spontaneous or iatrogenic), (4) adherent placenta (accreta), and (5) uterine inversion. A real-time ultrasound scanner can be helpful in identifying retained portions of placenta or residual blood clots within the uterus.

As the usual source of hemorrhage is uterine atony, intravenous oxytocin should be given in amounts adequate to compensate for the decreased sensitivity of the postpartum uterus to this drug (Hendricks, 1962). Usually, 20 to 30 units of oxytocin in 1000 ml of fluid given at an infusion rate not to exceed 100 mU/min will suffice. Because this amount of oxytocin will far exceed the threshold for its maximum antidiuretic effect (Munsick, 1970), it must be recognized that fluid overloading is a potential danger in these patients. Bolus injections of oxytocin may cause hypotension and should be avoided, especially in patients who are at risk of volume depletion from hemorrhage (Hendricks and Brenner, 1970). Methylergonovine or ergonovine maleate, given in doses of 0.2 mg IM, is often effective in maintaining uterine tonus, but such drugs should not be given intravenously because of the danger of hypertension, central nervous system vasospasm, and hemorrhage (Browning, 1974).

Increasingly, the 15-methyl analogue of prostaglandin $F_{2\alpha}$ (carboprost tromethamine) is being used to treat uterine atony if oxytocin infusion is not successful (Buttino and Garite, 1986). The recommended dose is 250 μg IM, which can be repeated within a few minutes if the first injection does not suffice. Prostaglandin, particularly $PGF_{2\alpha}$, should be used with great caution, if at all, in patients with cardiovascular disease or obstructive lung disease (asthma).

In some cases, uterine atony and uterine hemorrhage persist in spite of all measures taken to enhance uterine contractions and after other possible sources of vaginal or cervical hemorrhage have been excluded. In these situations, exploratory laparotomy is often necessary (see also Chapter 51).

During preparation for laparotomy, several measures can be employed that may adequately control the hemorrhage and avoid an operative procedure. One is the use of a large Foley catheter balloon as a tamponade to halt bleeding from a low placental implantation site (Bowen and Beeson, 1985). Another is packing of the uterine cavity with sterile gauze. Although no well-designed study has been made to prove that this measure is effective, there is retrospective evidence that uterine packing is successful in controlling hemorrhage due to atony in some cases (Hester, 1975). Finally, in hospitals where the necessary facilities and personnel are available, selective embolization of pelvic vessels adequately controls hemorrhage in some patients (Alvarez et al., 1992).

In those situations in which all of the procedures have been tried in vain, laparotomy is performed to identify any sources of occult intra-abdominal bleeding such as unexpected uterine laceration, and to control the bleeding by appropriate arterial ligations or, in the most extreme and refractory cases, to perform hyster-

ectomy. When laparotomy is performed for postpartum hemorrhage, the patient should be placed in semi-lithotomy position and the sterile drapes should be applied in such a way that one observer can, with a sterile speculum, examine the vagina and cervix to determine when the bleeding has ceased. If major uterine lacerations are not found, the uterine arteries should be ligated by the method described by O'Leary and O'Leary (1974). If this measure does not control uterine bleeding, the hypogastric arteries should be ligated. Burchell (1968) has described the pelvic vascular supply and has demonstrated that the transient decreases in blood pressure and blood flow through regional vessels that occur at the time of internal iliac artery ligation are responsible for the control of hemorrhage. Because of the ample collateral circulation, there appear to be no long-term consequences of hypogastric artery ligation, and women have delivered normal infants in pregnancies following bilateral hypogastric artery ligation. Occasionally, a patient complains of mild bladder dysfunction and buttocks pain in the immediate postoperative period, but these symptoms are transient.

In cases of extensive postpartum hemorrhage, the use of a central venous pressure line or a Swan-Ganz catheter facilitates more accurate monitoring of the cardiovascular status of the patient and avoids serious errors of hydration and pulmonary edema (Swan, 1975; Berkowitz and Rafferty, 1980). Watson (1980) has written an excellent summary of the management of postpartum hemorrhage, including the indications and rationale for central cardiovascular monitoring (see Chapter 51).

Inversion of the Uterus

Inversion of the uterus is a rare but dramatic complication of the third stage of labor and the immediate puerperium that must be recognized and corrected promptly to avoid serious long-term morbidity (Watson et al., 1980). Uterine inversion is probably related to fundal implantation of the placenta, which results in thinning of the uterine wall in the area of implantation. Fundal implantation occurs in only 10 per cent of all pregnancies, but has been found in virtually all reported cases of acute puerperal uterine inversion in which the site of placental implantation has been recorded (McCullagh, 1925; Watson et al., 1980). The thin fundal area of the myometrium invaginates as the placenta separates, whereupon the inversion proceeds, with the uterus virtually delivering itself inside out. With this scenario in mind, one can easily imagine that vigorous fundal pressure or excessive cord traction may contribute to the tendency to inversion in the uterus predisposed by fundal implantation of the placenta. Complete uterine inversion occurs when the inverted fundus extends beyond the cervix, usually looking like a beefy red mass at the vaginal introitus. Incomplete inversions are those in which the inverted fundus has not extended beyond the external cervical os. These cases will not be so obvious and may be detected only when bimanual or visual examination of the cervix is performed. In cases of postpartum hemorrhage in which the uterine fundus cannot be palpated abdominally, incomplete uterine inversion should be suspected.

Tocolytic drugs including magnesium sulfate (Grossman, 1981) and beta-mimetic compounds (Catanzarite et al., 1986) have been used to assist in the reinversion of the uterus. However, because of the extensive blood loss and shock that often are associated with uterine inversion, an anesthesiologist should be summoned as soon as the diagnosis is recognized so that general anesthesia will be available if reinversion using tocolysis fails.

The technique of reinversion is the same whether accomplished with intravenous tocolysis or under general anesthesia. The uterus is reinverted with gentle but firm and persistent pressure applied on the fundus to elevate it into the vagina (Johnson, 1949). This technique, which presumably results in reinversion by indirect traction on the round ligaments when the uterus is elevated into the abdomen, is successful in most cases. Authorities disagree about whether the placenta, which is often attached to the inverted fundus, should be removed prior to attempts to reinvert the fundus. The practical matter is that the Johnson technique for reinversion is accomplished more easily if the placenta is not in place. If the diagnosis is made and reinversion is accomplished promptly, there are no long-term sequelae. However, if the complication is unrecognized and reinversion is delayed, tissue edema will magnify the constriction of the cervix around the inverted fundus, making reinversion difficult. Tissue necrosis and damage to the bladder or urethra may ensue.

If the Johnson method of reinversion is not successful, laparotomy should be performed. The first step is to grasp the round ligaments about 1 inch into the inverted uterus and to exert traction while an assistant elevates the uterus with a hand in the vagina. This procedure, described by Huntington (1921), may fail because the inverted fundus is too tightly trapped below the cervical ring, in which case the Haultain (1901) procedure may be performed. In this latter procedure, a longitudinal incision is made posteriorly through the inverted fundus that allows ample room to reinvert the fundus. The incision is then closed, leaving the equivalent of a classic cesarean incision on the posterior surface of the uterus. If uterine inversion is recognized and treated promptly, an operative procedure is rarely necessary to accomplish reinversion.

The third stage of labor and the immediate puerperal recovery period are a crucial time for the parturient. Occasionally, uterine hemorrhage goes undetected or, when recognized, is treated inadequately. Acute tubular necrosis, pituitary necrosis, and adult respiratory distress syndrome—all recognized complications of puerperal shock and hypoxia—can be avoided by careful observation of all patients during this time and by deliberate and aggressive management of hemorrhage if it occurs.

INDUCTION OF LABOR

Induction of labor is *elective* (i.e., performed for the convenience of the patient or professional staff) or is *indicated* for medical, obstetric, or fetal complications of pregnancy.

Elective Induction

Elective induction of labor is usually justified on one or more of the following grounds: to assure the patient that the physician with whom she has good rapport will be present during delivery, to ensure that labor will occur when maximum physician, nursing, and support personnel coverage is available in case of labor complications, and to enable the patient to plan for care of her home and other children and allow her husband to make suitable arrangements to be with her during labor and delivery.

In 1968, Keettel reported a series of elective inductions of labor at the University of Iowa from 1957 to 1966. There were 738 elective inductions at term, representing only 3.8 per cent of the total number of patients delivered (19,183 patients). During this period, there was strict adherence to the criteria for term induction, and oxytocin was not used until a latent period of 6 to 8 hours had elapsed after rupture of the membranes. In the second series, there was a remarkable reduction of complications, including one-half the incidence of low-birth-weight infants. In this group of 738 patients, there was only one perinatal death—a 2800-gm infant who died of hyaline membrane disease. A neonatal mortality rate of 0.1 per cent is certainly no greater than would be expected in any group of term infants. Criteria for elective induction of labor at the University of Iowa were as follows: single fetus at term with an estimated weight in excess of 2800 gm; engaged vertex presentation; and cervix partially effaced, dilated at least 2 cm, and not posterior. With these criteria, 89 per cent of patients were in labor within 4 hours and only 3.4 per cent required oxytocin infusions.

More recently, there have been several reports supporting the concept of the safety and convenience of the elective induction of labor at term (Cole et al., 1975; Tylleskär et al., 1979). Unfortunately these studies, although prospective and well controlled, report too few patients to be completely reassuring. Any series of healthy pregnant women at term will have a very low incidence of complications regardless of how labor is managed. Series of fewer than 200 patients do not suffice to establish the safety of elective induction. Two long-term studies, one of which entailed follow-up of the children until they reached 8 years of age, have shown no higher frequency of neurologic or developmental abnormalities in infants born following elective induction of labor (Black and McBride, 1979; Friedman et al., 1979).

There are reports of an increased rate of neonatal hyperbilirubinemia with use of oxytocin to augment or induce labor. The first of these reports was by Chalmers and colleagues (1975). The specific cause for the hyperbilirubinemia has not been proved. Sims and Neligan (1975) and Lange and co-workers (1982) published evidence that the hyperbilirubinemia associated with induced labor is related to a slight overall decrease in maturity of infants born of induced labor.

Friedman and Sachtleben (1976) relate the increase in hyperbilirubinemia to fetal trauma as a result of the higher number of forceps deliveries among patients with induced labor. Other investigators believe that red cell trauma occurs from the more intense uterine contractions that result from oxytocin induction or augmentation (D'Souza et al., 1979). Buchan (1979) demonstrated a direct effect of oxytocin on red cell deformability that may be partly responsible for the higher rate of neonatal hyperbilirubinemia encountered with oxytocin induction.

Whether carefully monitored oxytocin-induced contractions are of greater intensity and frequency than those observed in spontaneous labor is a controversial issue. Johnson and co-workers (1970) found that in 26 patients with oxytocin-stimulated labor the uterine contractions were of greater amplitude and greater frequency than in 26 control patients in spontaneous labor. Conversely, Anderson and Schooley (1975) could find no difference in uterine activity in a comparison of 20 patients in oxytocin-induced labor with 20 patients in spontaneous labor. Nevertheless, uterine hyperactivity is undoubtedly more common when oxytocin induction of labor is being performed on a clinical service, simply because there is always the possibility of infusion errors when oxytocin is being given. Liston and Campbell (1974) have demonstrated that fetal distress occurs with greater frequency when oxytocin is required for labor induction than when only amniotomy is required. Moreover, the same study showed that an increase in oxytocin requirement was accompanied by an increase in rate of fetal distress. On the other hand, Thorp et al. (1988), comparing 704 patients who had received no oxytocin with 556 whose labors had been augmented with oxytocin, could find no difference in umbilical arterial pH (7.24 +/− 0.07 vs. 7.23 +/− 0.07, respectively). In smaller numbers of patients in whom umbilical arterial base excess was also measured, there was no difference between those patients who had received oxytocin and those who had not. If there is proper intrapartum monitoring and prompt response to signs of fetal distress, the use of oxytocin does not cause fetal asphyxia.

Increasingly, it has been recognized that the cascade of physiologic events that precede and result in labor are largely mediated in and by the fetus and are, in most cases, signals of fetal maturity. This evidence of fetal readiness for the transition to extrauterine life is one of the most reassuring aspects of spontaneous labor. Furthermore, in the absence of spontaneous labor one must always be aware, in undertaking elective induction, that fetal preparation for extrauterine life may not be complete. Moreover, it has been shown that elective induction of labor is associated with a higher rate of cesarean delivery than spontaneous onset of labor, especially in nulliparous patients (Yudkin et al., 1979). Parents involved in an elective induction of labor must be made fully to understand the risk of the rare complication of functional fetal immaturity and the increased chance of operative delivery even when the closest attention has been paid to proper timing and appropriate intrapartum monitoring. Given this respective awareness and acquiescence

by physician and parents, there are, indeed, some situations in which elective induction of labor is appropriate for personal, geographic, or emotional reasons.

It is suggested that if an obstetrics service concludes that elective induction of labor is permissible, the professional staff, including physicians and nurses from labor and delivery and the nursery and the appropriate hospital administrators, should collectively agree on criteria for patient selection, draw up a protocol for the labor induction procedure, including lines of authority and areas of professional responsibility, and determine charges for the procedure. After establishing such standards of care, there should be periodic review of patients whose pregnancies have been terminated by elective induction. Such a review will determine whether the criteria for patient selection are being neglected, whether the protocol for safe labor induction is being violated, and whether unexpected or preventable maternal or neonatal morbidity is occurring as a result of the induction procedure. It is clear that careful professional supervision of all patients in labor and delivery is necessary to maintain a low morbidity rate. This is especially true for labor induction. Indeed, one of the most attractive arguments for elective induction is that it ensures adequate coverage of the labor and delivery unit while the patient is in labor (Pinkerton et al., 1975; Cole et al., 1975).

An objective classification for selection of patients who are "favorable" for induction of labor was described by Bishop (1964) and is shown in Table 35–4. Bishop stated that a pelvic score of 9 or more, in the term multipara, was associated with no failed inductions of labor in his series and that the average duration of labor was 4 hours. It is important to point out that this scoring system has not assessed the induction of the nulliparous patient or the preterm patient.

One of the most obvious dangers of elective labor induction is the unexpected delivery of a premature infant. Consequently, scrupulous attention to confirmation of gestational age is necessary. It is suggested that the following criteria be fulfilled before a patient is considered a candidate for induction:

1. A well-established ovulation date, which can be determined by one of the following:
   a. A regular menstrual history prior to the last menstrual period. The last menstrual period

TABLE 35–4.   Pelvic Scoring Table for Selection of Patients For Elective Induction*

FACTOR	POINTS ASSIGNED			
	0	1	2	3
Dilation (cm)	0	1–2	3–4	5–6
Effacement (%)	0–30	40–50	60–70	80
Station	−3	−2	−1 or 0	+1 or +2
Consistency	Firm	Medium	Soft	
Position	Posterior	Mid	Anterior	

*Total pelvic score is obtained by adding the points for each factor.
Adapted from Bishop EH: Pelvic scoring for elective induction. Obstet Gynecol **24**:266, 1964.

should not be considered normal if it occurred following cessation of oral contraceptive use.
  b. Basal body temperature chart demonstrating a biphasic rise.
  c. Clomiphene induction of ovulation followed by early confirmation of ovulation in pregnancy.
  d. Artificial insemination.
2. Examination of the patient by the 14th week of pregnancy in which the uterine size was consistent with estimated gestational dates.
3. Fetal heart tones heard with a fetoscope (not a Doppler instrument) by the 20th week of pregnancy.
4. Fetal weight estimated as 6 lb (2700 gm) or more.
5. A pelvic score of 9 or more in the multiparous patient (Bishop, 1964). With these criteria, the patient should be considered for elective induction of labor 40 weeks (280 days ± 3 days) after the last menstrual period (if menstrual interval is 28 days), or 266 days ± 3 days after the suspected ovulation date.

The study of Keettel (1968) demonstrates the effective use of amniotomy in the induction of labor in patients at term with favorable cervical status. Only 3.4 per cent of his patients required a subsequent oxytocin infusion. The mechanism by which amniotomy induces labor is not entirely clear, but Mitchell and associates (1977) have shown that artificial rupture of the membranes is followed by a substantial increase in plasma prostaglandins. In a small proportion of patients, an oxytocic agent is necessary. In such cases oxytocin should be given by intravenous infusion, preferably by constant infusion pump, with adequate monitoring of fetal heart rate, uterine contractions, and maternal vital signs. Intravenous infusion avoids the unpredictable and uncontrollable absorption of the drug that may occur when an oxytocic agent is administered by another route (buccal, vaginal, or intramuscular). To date there is no evidence that prostaglandins or other agents are safer or more effective than oxytocin for augmentation of uterine contractions after amniotomy (Ounsted et al., 1978).

Indicated Induction

Indications for induction of labor constitute those situations in which the prolongation of the pregnancy is dangerous for either the mother or the fetus and in which there are no contraindications to amniotomy or the augmentation of uterine contractions. Maternal indications include severe pregnancy-induced hypertension, fetal death, and chorioamnionitis. Fetal indications for pregnancy termination include any condition in which a variety of fetal tests demonstrate significant fetal jeopardy in any of the following complications of pregnancy: diabetes mellitus, post-term pregnancy, hypertensive complications of pregnancy, intrauterine growth restriction, isoimmunization, chorioamnionitis, and premature rupture of the membranes with established fetal maturity.

Contraindications to induction of labor in these situations include any condition in which spontaneous labor and delivery would be more dangerous for the mother or fetus than abdominal delivery, such as fetal distress, shoulder presentation, unengaged fetal presenting part, uncontrolled hemorrhage, placenta previa, and previous uterine incision that would preclude a trial of labor.

The following are *relative* contraindications to induction of labor: grand multiparity (five or more previous pregnancies beyond 20 weeks gestation), multiple pregnancy, suspected cephalopelvic disproportion, breech presentation, inability to adequately monitor the fetal heart rate throughout labor, and previous low transverse cesarean delivery. These situations are all controversial, and there are mitigating circumstances under which induction of labor might be attempted in any of them.

If the cervical status is favorable and the vertex is well engaged (pelvic score 9 or more), the preferred method of labor induction is amniotomy followed, when necessary, by a closely monitored oxytocin infusion. If the cervical status is not favorable, as is common when delivery is indicated for maternal or fetal complications, there are several methods for improving it; they are discussed in the next section.

Cervical Ripening

The anatomy, histology, and physiology of cervical ripening have been reviewed by Huszar and Walsh (1991). It is clear that the softening, shortening, and eventual dilation of the cervix, which are manifestations of cervical ripening, may occur independent of uterine contractions. Histochemical studies have shown that cervical ripening is due to the gradual dissociation and scattering of the previously densely packed, orderly collagen bundles characteristic of the nonpregnant cervix. Liggins (1978) suggests that cervical ripening is analogous to the remodelling of connective tissue that follows tissue injury. Glycosamine glycan protein and glycoprotein complexes control the arrangement and density of collagen fibers within the cervix, and it has been shown that both the content and the type of glycosamine glycan change in the cervix as term approaches.

A number of mechanical and pharmacologic methods for inducing changes in the cervix ("ripening") have been studied.

OXYTOCIN. A summary of five trials of oxytocin used to effect cervical ripening, although including only 90 oxytocin-treated patients, demonstrated that oxytocin is an ineffective cervical ripening agent (Keirse and van Oppen, 1989). The past approach of serial repetitive oxytocin inductions of labor, in the face of an unprepared cervix, which is tedious and exhaustive to the patient, should probably be abandoned.

HYDROPHILIC CERVICAL INSERTS. There are several types of hydrophylic cervical inserts that have been shown to be effective in ripening the cervix for induction of labor. These include *Laminaria digitata* (kelp); Dilapan, a copolymer of polyacrylonitrile; and Lamicel, a polyvinyl alcohol polymer sponge impregnated with 450 mg of magnesium sulfate. Laminaria insertion has been shown to effectively ripen the cervix (Cross and Pitkin, 1978; Rosenberg et al., 1980); but a retrospective study by Kazzi et al. (1982) suggests that maternal and neonatal infectious morbidity is increased by preinduction insertion of Laminaria, although other reports do not confirm an increase in infection or premature rupture of the membranes. Johnson and co-workers (1985) reported a series of patients having preinduction cervical ripening in whom a single 5-mm Lamicel was as effective as 4 mg of PGE_2 gel in the upper vagina. Also, Lamicel caused less uterine activity and fetal distress than prostaglandin gel.

FOLEY CATHETER. Following antiseptic preparation of the cervix, a Foley catheter (size 18 to 26) with a 30-ml balloon is inserted through the cervix 12 to 24 hours prior to induction of labor (Embry and Mollison, 1967; Leiberman et al., 1977). The specific method of action of the Foley catheter in improving cervical effacement and dilation is not known, although it may be through local release of tissue prostaglandins in the cervix or lower uterine segment. Studies comparing the Foley catheter to prostaglandin application for ripening of the cervix have been contradictory. Tromans et al. (1981) found the Foley catheter to be less effective than pharmacologic agents, whereas Schreyer et al. (1989) found the Foley catheter as effective as PGE_2 vaginal tablets for cervical ripening.

LOCAL PHARMACOLOGIC APPLICATIONS. Prostaglandin E_2 (PGE_2) suspended in a cellulose gel and administered through a catheter in the extraovular space or inserted as a tablet or gel in the vagina has been evaluated in a number of studies and found to be effective for preinduction ripening of the cervix (Shepherd and Knuppel, 1981). Labor induced solely by the use of PGE_2 appears physiologically more similar to spontaneous labor than is labor induced by either amniotomy or oxytocin infusion (Lamont et al., 1991). The major side effects of prostaglandin are nausea, pyrexia, and uterine contractions, although these are not common when use is confined to the low doses recommended for cervical ripening. However, uterine rupture in a multiparous patient has been reported in association with intracervical prostaglandin E_2 gel for induction of labor (Maymon et al., 1991). Intrauterine deaths in association with preinduction cervical ripening using local PGE_2 have been reported; it is presumed that such deaths are related to increased uterine tone and decreased uteroplacental perfusion (Quinn and Murphy, 1981). The amount of PGE_2 suspended in the gel medium for vaginal or extraovular application has varied from 0.25 to 5 mg, with lower doses resulting in fewer uterine contractions but less cervical ripening. A controlled trial including 226 patients randomized to either prostaglandin E_2 given by intracervical gel (0.5 mg) or vaginal pessary (2.5 mg) found no difference in efficacy or safety (Poulsen et al., 1991). The method of action of PGE_2 in ripening the cervix is probably a direct chemical action on the cervical collagen, resulting in an increase in the ground substance and separation of the tightly woven collagen bundles (Uldbjerg et al., 1981). Also, PGE_2 in amounts as low as 0.25 mg, when applied through the cervix into the extra-ovular space, has been reported to cause uterine contractions (Laube et al., 1986). Consequently, if PGE_2 is used for preinduction cervical ripening, the fetal heart rate should be monitored as if the patient were in early labor.

Gels containing 150 mg of *estradiol valerate* have also been inserted in either the extra-amniotic space or the posterior fornix of the vagina on the evening before induction of labor (Gordon and Calder, 1977). The improvement in cervical ripening appears to be equivalent to that induced by PGE_2, with less uterine activity (Tromans et al., 1981). Presumably, the mechanism of action is an alteration of cervical collagen.

Purified porcine *relaxin*, a polypeptide hormone, suspended in a gel and applied in the vagina, was shown by MacLennan and co-workers (1986) to ripen the cervix. In their randomized, controlled study there were no untoward effects in the 71 patients treated with the drug. Recombinant human relaxin is currently being investigated as an agent for cervical ripening.

ABNORMAL PRESENTATIONS

Breech Presentation

Breech presentation occurs in approximately 3 to 4 per cent of all deliveries. Its incidence decreases with advancing gestation. Weisman (1944), using periodic radiographic examination throughout pregnancy, found that at 18 to 22 weeks gestation 24 per cent of fetuses were in breech presentation, at 28 to 30 weeks 8 per cent, at 34 weeks 7 per cent, and at 38 to 40 weeks 2.8 per cent. It is generally agreed that higher rates of neonatal morbidity and mortality are associated with breech presentation than with cephalic presentation at all gestational ages and birth weights (Brenner et al., 1974). There is less agreement as to what can be done to eliminate the risk for the infant in breech presentation at the time of delivery.

Part of the problem may be inherent in the etiology of breech presentation itself. Term breech presentation is associated with fundal-cornual implantation of the placenta, which occurs in only 7 per cent of all pregnancies (Stevenson, 1950). This association suggests that breech presentation in many cases is related to a space problem in the uterus, and that given the fundal-placental implantation, an otherwise normal fetus finds it more comfortable to assume a breech position. Other studies have suggested that breech presentation may result from abnormal motor ability or diminished muscle tone in the fetus. Braun and colleagues (1975), reporting from a dysmorphology clinic, have shown that there is a higher than expected incidence of breech presentation (corrected for gestational age) in a variety of congenital disorders. Specifically, among infants with neuromuscular disorders there is an inordinately high rate of breech presentation at delivery (Axelrod et al., 1974; Ralis, 1975). Furthermore, McBride and associates (1979) found that 100 children delivered at term in breech and studied at 5 years of age scored less well on motor skills than children delivered in cephalic presentations regardless of the method by which the breech delivery was accomplished. These studies suggest that, at least in some cases, the fetus remains in a breech position because it is less capable of movement within the uterus. If these concepts are accurate, the outcome for the fetus in a breech presentation might depend to a great extent on the reason it is in the breech position rather than on the actual mode of delivery.

Speculation aside, there are some inherent risks to the fetus in a breech presentation during labor and delivery: prolapse of the umbilical cord (especially in the footling breech); trapping of the after-coming head by the incompletely dilated cervix (in the low-birth-weight, preterm fetus weighing less than 2000 gm); cephalopelvic disproportion; and trauma resulting from an extension of the head or nuchal position of the arms. Because of these risks, there has been an increase in the use of cesarean delivery for the pregnancy complicated by breech presentation. A policy of cesarean delivery for all term pregnancies in labor with a breech presentation might result in the lowest possible perinatal morbidity and mortality rates (Wright, 1959). However, such a policy would result in a substantial increase in maternal morbidity. Consequently, there has been an effort to establish the proper role of cesarean delivery in maintaining the lowest morbidity for both mother and infant in pregnancies complicated by breech presentation. One approach is to correct some breech presentations by an external version maneuver. A second approach is to identify those patients at highest risk for complications of vaginal breech delivery and deliver them by cesarean. The remainder are allowed a trial of labor with constant fetal monitoring and availability of the skillful assistance needed in breech delivery.

External version has been shown to reduce substantially the incidence of breech presentation. Studies in Europe and the United States including more than 680 patients have confirmed the relative safety and effectiveness of external version and have demonstrated a significant reduction in cesarean deliveries for the breech presentation (Brocks et al., 1984; Dyson et al., 1986; Morrison et al., 1986; Stine et al., 1985).

The use of tocolysis has improved the success of external version performed after 36 weeks gestation. Performing the procedure at this time in pregnancy allows prompt intervention by cesarean delivery if unrelenting fetal distress occurs. The recent prospective controlled studies of external version have demonstrated that after 36 weeks gestation there was an 18 per cent incidence of spontaneous version of breech to vertex presentation. External version was successful in 70 per cent of cases. The incidence of cesarean delivery in all patients undergoing a trial of version was 31 per cent, whereas the incidence of cesarean delivery in patients with a breech presentation not managed with a trial of labor was 63 per cent. Consequently, the net benefit to the women was a 50 per cent reduction in cesarean births.

There are no particular benefits for the fetus. The risks for the fetus, however, appear to be justifiably low. In the 684 cases of external version included in the recent published reports, there was one case of acute fetal distress in which emergency cesarean delivery was required (Dyson et al., 1986). There was

also one fetal death, which occurred 3 weeks after external version, and one maternal death due to an amniotic fluid embolus 4 days after an external version (Stine et al., 1985). It is not known whether either of these deaths was due to the external versions.

Contraindications to external version include uterine anomalies, third-trimester bleeding, multiple gestation, oligohydramnios, evidence of uteroplacental insufficiency, a nuchal cord as identified by ultrasonography, previous cesarean delivery or other significant uterine surgery, obvious cephalopelvic disproportion, or any maternal condition precluding the use of tocolytic drugs.

Primiparity, maternal obesity, advanced gestation, anterior implantation of the placenta, and excessive fetal weight have been associated with decreased success of version, but are not in themselves contraindications.

The procedure should be preferably performed in the hospital in which cesarean delivery can be accomplished if unrelenting fetal distress occurs. A real-time ultrasonographic scan is performed to confirm the breech presentation, to detect multiple gestation, oligohydramnios, or fetal abnormalities, and to measure fetal dimensions.

Following a reactive non-stress test, a tocolytic drug is administered (terbutaline sulfate, 250 μg SQ or 5 μg/min IV, or ritodrine hydrochloride 100 μg/min IV). (Some obstetricians may first prefer to make an attempt at version without tocolysis, and if this is unsuccessful, then proceed with external version under tocolysis.) When uterine relaxation occurs, the version is attempted. One person may elevate and laterally displace the breech while a second person manipulates the fetal head in the opposite direction. Mineral oil on the abdomen facilitates movement of the hands during the procedure. A forward roll is attempted, and if this is unsuccessful, a backward roll is tried. The fetal heart rate should be monitored intermittently with Doppler or with real-time scanning. Fetal bradycardia will occur in about 20 per cent of cases, but almost always subsides when the manipulation ceases. External fetal heart rate monitoring is continued for one hour, after which the patient is discharged.

Patients who are Rh negative and who have a negative antibody titer should be given one unit (300 μg) of Rh immune globulin, because of the risk of fetal-maternal transfusion associated with version (6 to 28 per cent) (Gjode et al., 1980; Marcus et al., 1975).

If version is not attempted or if it has been unsuccessful and the patient is in labor with a breech presentation, vaginal delivery may be chosen if three criteria are met. These are: the fetus is in frank (complete) breech position; the estimated fetal weight is 2000 to 3800 gm; and the patient has a normal gynecoid pelvis, as confirmed by radiographic pelvimetry, with the following measurements: inlet transverse 12 cm or greater, inlet AP 11 cm or greater, bispinous diameter 9.5 cm or greater. Using criteria similar to these, Collea and associates (1980) performed a prospective, randomized study of 208 patients with term frank breech presentations. Half the patients were delivered by cesarean section soon after admission to the hospital in labor. The other half were evaluated for vaginal delivery. Sixty patients were found to be candidates for vaginal delivery, 49 of whom delivered without a perinatal death. The remaining 11 patients had cesarean deliveries because of complications that occurred during labor. Transient brachial plexus injury occurred in two of the infants who were delivered vaginally. Of the 148 women who delivered by cesarean section, 73 (49 per cent) had significant puerperal morbidity, while only 7 per cent of the women who delivered vaginally had postpartum complications.

These observations emphasize the recurrent dilemma for the obstetrician, i.e., the balancing of morbidity risks for two patients (mother and fetus) who must be cared for simultaneously. This study, the only randomized prospective evaluation of term breech delivery, suggests that with careful selection of patients, vaginal delivery of certain fetuses in breech presentation can be accomplished without serious neonatal morbidity. Bowes and co-workers (1979) studied 460 singleton breech infants delivered on a service that incorporated criteria for selection of patients for vaginal delivery similar to those previously listed. Among infants weighing over 2500 gm, there were several cases of neonatal morbidity and one neonatal death that might have been avoided by a policy of prompt cesarean delivery of all patients with breech presentation. Green and co-workers (1982) reviewed 770 term breech deliveries at the Royal Victoria Hospital in Montreal. They concluded that the increase in cesarean births for breech presentation from 22 per cent to 94 per cent over the duration of the study had not reduced unfavorable perinatal outcomes significantly.

Using the criteria previously listed, one would deliver by cesarean section about 65 to 70 per cent of patients with breech presentation at the onset of labor.

The method of pain control for a vaginal breech delivery is another controversial issue. Conduction anesthesia has been used with good results (Crawford, 1974), and a case can be made for its preventing the mother from pushing uncontrollably in the second stage and allowing for an easier and more comfortable application of the Piper forceps to the after-coming head. However, in a recent study of 643 single term breech presentations, epidural analgesia was associated with longer duration of labor, increased need for augmentation of labor with oxytocin, and a significantly higher cesarean delivery rate in the second stage of labor (Chadha et al., 1992). Moreover, vaginal breech delivery should probably be attempted with a competent anesthetist or anesthesiologist who can administer a prompt general anesthetic in the event that there is difficulty delivering the after-coming head or arms in the nuchal position.

Fetal monitoring is essential during labor with a breech presentation. Because the fetal abdomen and the insertion of the umbilical cord will be in the lower uterine segment during the late first stage and the second stage of labor, significant variable decelerations are more likely to be encountered than with cephalic presentation. For this reason, membranes should be left intact as long as possible to provide some hydraulic

protection against umbilical cord compression. Vaginal breech deliveries are more often associated with significant fetal acidosis than are cephalic presentations (Hill et al., 1976). Therefore, one must exercise careful judgment as to when to intervene for "fetal distress." Fetal blood samples can be obtained from the buttock when there is a suspicious or ominous fetal heart rate pattern, and if the pH obtained between contractions is below 7.25 early in the second stage, abdominal delivery should be considered.

The use of oxytocin for induction of labor or augmentation of abnormal labor is not contraindicated (Collea et al., 1978), but its use must be monitored with extraordinary caution.

Finally, it must be stated that the technique of breech vaginal delivery is not so frequently or skillfully taught as in the past because there are fewer opportunities for such teaching. Consequently, if the physician is unsure about his or her skills for vaginal delivery of a breech presentation, a cesarean section is the safest method.

Careful selection of patients for either cesarean or vaginal delivery does not necessarily ensure a birth free from asphyxia or trauma. Calvert (1980) has shown that infants born by cesarean delivery for breech presentation have a higher incidence of birth asphyxia than a comparable group of infants in cephalic presentation who were born by cesarean delivery. He points out that even through a uterine incision there may be some difficulties in delivering an infant in breech presentation. His recommendation for more liberal use of the classic uterine incision for breech presentation would, however, substantially increase maternal morbidity.

Skillful, atraumatic delivery of the infant regardless of the route of birth is essential in keeping infant morbidity at a minimum. Milner (1975) has shown that application of forceps to the after-coming head is associated with a reduction in the rate of neonatal mortality from breech delivery. The well-illustrated publication by Piper and Bachman (1929), describing the use of the forceps designed by Piper and presenting in detail the method of breech delivery, should be standard reading for all physicians planning to assist in the vaginal delivery of a breech presentation. Even when delivery is performed by cesarean section, forceps should be available (use of Piper forceps is not necessary) and should be applied through the uterine incision to the after-coming head if there is any difficulty with its extraction.

The experience, judgment, and skill of the obstetrician are perhaps the most important ingredients in protecting both mother and infant from the risks of breech presentation, and these are the most difficult factors to study. The role of physician experience in outcome of breech presentation is illustrated by the report of Alexopoulos (1973) of 476 cases of breech delivery of infants with birth weights of 1500 gm or more who were managed in 1963 and 1964 by physicians in training. Twenty-two (5 per cent) of the infants were stillborn or died within one week of the delivery, most as a result of trauma. Of the survivors, 70 (16 per cent) had significant morbidity related to birth asphyxia or trauma, including 12 children who at 8

TABLE 35–5. **Prognostic Index for Vaginal Breech Delivery***

FACTOR	POINTS ASSIGNED		
	0	1	2
Parity	0	>1	—
Gestational age (weeks)	39	38	37
Estimated fetal weight	>8 lb	7 lb 1 oz to 7 lb 15 oz	<7 lb
	(3630 gm)	(3176–3629 gm)	(3175 gm)
Previous breech deliveries (birth weight >2500 gm)	0	1	2
Dilation (cm)	2	3	4
Station	−3 or higher	−2	−1 or lower

*Index is obtained by adding the points for each factor.
Adapted from Zatuchni GI, Andros GJ: Prognostic index for vaginal delivery in breech presentation at term. Prospective study. Am J Obstet Gynecol **98**:854, 1967.

years of age were mentally retarded, or were having seizures, or had cerebral palsy. This is in contrast to the report by Graves (1980) of 141 singleton breech deliveries from 1957 through 1976 managed by four fully trained obstetricians in a single private practice. Three infants with birth weight of 1500 gm died, all of whom had severe congenital anomalies. Two infants had significant trauma related to the delivery process, one a mild subdural hematoma and the other a fractured clavicle; both infants recovered without sequelae. Of interest is that the cesarean delivery rate for breech presentation in this series increased from 5 per cent between 1957 and 1966 to 12 per cent between 1966 and 1971, and to 71 per cent between 1971 and 1976.

The role of radiographic pelvimetry in the selection of patients for cesarean delivery is controversial. Apart from prolapse of the umbilical cord, which is far more common in footling than in frank breech presentation, the major risk to the fetus in breech presentation from labor and delivery is trapping of the fetal head by the pelvis. Unlike the head in cephalic presentation, the after-coming head in breech presentation enters the pelvis without benefit of molding, as well as with the ever-present danger that flexion of the head on the thorax will be incomplete. Because it has not undergone molding, the fetal head has a substantially larger cephalic diameter in breech than it would in a vertex presentation even if the fetus were larger, and its passage through the pelvis is much more difficult. Excluding major congenital anomalies, the most common cause of death in term infants who do not survive breech delivery is intracranial hemorrhage associated with lacerations of the tentorium cerebelli. Potter and co-workers (1960) studied 13 term infants without congenital defects who died of intracranial injury as a result of vaginal breech delivery. In seven of the 13 mothers, pelvic radiographs (five of which were obtained in the puerperium) revealed diminished pelvic capacity. In the remaining six patients, radiographs were not obtained. Beischer (1966) reviewed the outcome of term breech presentation in 64 patients who had pelvic contraction as documented by radiographs. Thirteen patients were delivered by cesarean; all infants survived. In the 51 infants vaginally delivered there were four deaths, three of which were due to tentorial tears. That study, together with the report of

Todd and Steer (1963) of 1006 term breech deliveries, suggests that the radiographic pelvic measurements below which vaginal delivery of a breech is not safe are (1) anteroposterior diameter of the inlet 11 cm, (2) widest transverse of the inlet 12 cm, and (3) interspinous diameter 9 cm. Any other encroachment on the space below the inlet also contraindicates vaginal delivery. Pelvimetry performed with computed tomography (CT) exposes the fetus to substantially less radiation and is performed with greater facility in most hospitals than conventional x-ray pelvimetry (Kopelman et al., 1986). Also, pelvimetry by magnetic resonance imaging has been used for breech presentation, but the cost and the greater time required for this procedure make it less practical than pelvimetry by CT scanning (Van Loon et al., 1990).

The study by Zatuchni and Andros (1967) suggests that careful clinical screening of patients with breech presentations at term will identify those who can safely accomplish a vaginal delivery. Their screening criteria did not include radiographic pelvimetry. Upon admission to the hospital in labor, their patients were evaluated according to their "prognostic index," as shown in Table 35–5. In a prospective study of 139 term breeches—exclusive of cases with prolapsed cord, severe congenital anomalies, and uterine bleeding—Zatuchni and Andros (1967) found that all perinatal mortality and morbidity occurred in patients with an index of 3 or less, and that cesarean delivery of all patients with such an index would have resulted in an abdominal delivery rate of 21.5 per cent.

Collea and associates (1980), using radiographic pelvimetry as one criterion for selecting patients, found that of 115 patients selected for vaginal delivery by randomization, 52 (45 per cent) had "below-normal" pelvic measurements and were delivered by cesarean section.

Most authorities agree that radiographic pelvimetry has a place in determining the safest method of delivery for a patient in labor at term with a breech presentation.

Transverse Lie (Shoulder Presentation)

Transverse lie occurs in approximately one in 300 deliveries (Seeds and Cefalo, 1982). Cruikshank and

White (1973), reporting on 118 shoulder presentations, found that prematurity (38 per cent) and high parity (87 per cent had already borne three or more infants) were the two most frequently associated conditions. Premature rupture of membranes (30 per cent) and placenta previa (10 per cent) are also seen more commonly in transverse lie than in longitudinal presentation. The high perinatal mortality rates of 3.9 to 24 per cent associated with transverse lie (Seeds and Cefalo, 1982) are almost surely due to the high prevalence of low-birth-weight infants in shoulder presentations, although prolapse of the umbilical cord occasionally results in perinatal death of a term infant in transverse lie. These accidents usually happen most unexpectedly, when spontaneous rupture of the membranes occurs outside the hospital setting. In such cases the patient is usually admitted to the hospital with a severely asphyxiated or dead fetus.

Diagnosis of transverse lie can usually be suspected upon palpation of the abdomen. Not infrequently, the patient notes that the fetus is in an unusual position and draws this fact to the attention of the physician. Confirmation of the fetal position can be accomplished by either real-time ultrasonography or a single AP radiograph. The former is preferred because it provides additional information about location of the placenta, fetal maturity, and fetal weight.

Management of the patient in whom the diagnosis of transverse lie has been confirmed depends on the length of gestation, the size of the fetus, the position of the placenta, and whether the membranes have ruptured. If the patient is in labor with a transverse lie and the expected fetal weight and gestational age are below those compatible with a reasonable (10 per cent) chance for survival, no intervention is necessary beyond attempts to stop labor in the interest of gaining fetal weight and maturity. A fetus of this size (usually less than 600 gm) eventually is delivered vaginally in shoulder presentation (*conduplicato corpore*) without undue trauma to the mother. However, if the gestational age or expected fetal weight is such that the chance for neonatal survival, in the absence of severe asphyxia or trauma, is greater than 10 per cent, cesarean delivery is usually necessary, especially if the membranes are ruptured or placenta previa is present.

The role of external version in the management of transverse lie is highly controversial. Prior to 37 weeks gestation in patients who are not in labor, external version should not be attempted because of the danger of cord entanglement or placental trauma and the difficulty of maintaining the normal axial lie following version. Moreover, there is the possibility that spontaneous version to a longitudinal lie will occur with additional growth and maturity of the fetus or with the onset of contractions. When a transverse lie is identified at or beyond 37 weeks gestation with intact membranes, however, and cephalopelvic disproportion and placenta previa are not present, external version often results in a longitudinal lie and a normal vaginal delivery.

Edwards and Nicholson (1969) demonstrated the benefits of a policy of admitting to the hospital all patients beyond 37 weeks gestation in whom a diagnosis of "unstable lie" is made. Their protocol in such patients was to search for etiologic factors and, in those in whom cephalopelvic disproportion and placenta previa were excluded, to perform external version followed by induction of labor after 38 weeks gestation. In 102 patients so managed, 86 delivered vaginally with only one case of cord prolapse and no perinatal deaths. In 50 cases of unstable lie at or beyond 37 weeks gestation in which the onset of spontaneous labor was awaited, there were 10 cases of prolapsed cord and four perinatal deaths. Their experience suggests that when a transverse or oblique lie is identified at or beyond 37 weeks gestation, thorough etiologic evaluation and admission to the hospital should be considered.

Patients in early labor with intact membranes and a transverse lie might also be candidates for external version provided cephalopelvic disproportion and placenta previa are excluded (Flowers, 1966). The use of tocolytic drugs to facilitate external version of a transverse lie is also reasonable when combined with all the precautions already mentioned as well as continuous fetal monitoring, with standby preparations for abdominal delivery if fetal distress or prolapse of the fetal arm should occur.

If fetal mobility is restricted by well-advanced labor or the absence of amniotic fluid, or if placenta previa or cephalopelvic disproportion is detected, abdominal delivery of transverse lie is mandatory. Most authorities advise a low vertical or classic uterine incision in such cases, although Cruikshank and White (1973) found an extraordinarily high maternal morbidity rate (21 per cent severe intraperitoneal infection and 8.3 per cent maternal death) to be associated with classic incisions for delivery of patients with shoulder presentations. The low transverse incision often suffices in cases of a back-up transverse lie, and the high transverse incision described by Durfee (1972) can be used in cases of a back-down shoulder presentation. Finally, a technique of intra-abdominal version to allow use of a low transverse incision has been described (Pelosi et al., 1979). Using the transverse rather than a vertical incision decreases the overall maternal morbidity of cesarean delivery by reducing acute puerperal complications associated with vertical incisions and by allowing the option of subsequent pregnancies to be managed with a trial of labor and vaginal delivery. However, the choice of uterine incision should always be made with the primary purpose of abdominal delivery in mind, i.e., to avoid fetal trauma and asphyxia.

Deflection Abnormalities

Brow and face presentations are manifestations of different degrees of deflection of a cephalic presentation and therefore can be considered together. The current literature regarding brow and face presentations has been reviewed by Seeds and Cefalo (1982). Brow and face presentations each occur with a frequency of about one in 500 deliveries, although it is likely that the incidences would be higher if careful assessment of all fetal presentations were made early in labor. About 50 per cent of such diagnoses are not made until the second stage of labor; many of the deflection problems diagnosed early in labor correct themselves spontaneously as labor progresses. With the exception of anencephaly, which almost always results in a face presentation, fetal anomalies do not seem to account for deflection problems in labor. Cephalopelvic disproportion, increased parity, prematurity, and premature rupture of membranes are commonly reported as etiologic factors in brow and face presentations. Apart from prematurity and anencephaly, the major problem associated with deflection presentations is dysfunctional labor in brow presentation. Friedman (1978) found that face presentation, contrary to generally held clinical impressions, did not appear to affect the course of labor to any significant degree in either nulliparas or multiparas. Brow presentation, on the other hand, was associated with abnormalities of descent and longer second stage of labor compared with vertex presentation in matched controls. This is not surprising in light of the fact that with brow presentation the largest dimension of the head, the mento-occipital diameter, must negotiate the inlet of the pelvis. Consequently, successful descent, rotation, and delivery of a brow presentation in the term infant depend on conversion to either a face or a vertex presentation. Moreover, it is often the delay in labor associated with this conversion that results in a more careful assessment of fetal position and the recognition of a brow presentation. Perinatal mortality rates for brow and face presentations are higher than for vertex presentations, but the increase can be accounted for by fetal anomalies (anencephaly), prematurity, and asphyxia and trauma associated with manipulation during vaginal delivery.

Management of deflection presentations begins with recognition of the abnormality. An emphasis on careful vaginal examination and a description of the position and characteristics of the presenting fetal part as an essential element in labor monitoring will enhance the awareness and diagnosis of deflection problems. If on vaginal examination the lambdoid sutures and the posterior fontanelle cannot be easily identified as occupying a central position in the pelvis, an abnormal presentation or deflection of a cephalic presentation must be suspected. Palpation of the anterior fontanelle or one of the orbits clearly identifies a deflection problem. Furthermore, in cases of abnormal descent or prolonged second stage of labor, deflection of the fetal head should be considered one of the possible causes and the patient should be re-evaluated with this in mind. When deflection of the fetal head is identified in association with abnormal progression of labor, cephalopelvic disproportion must be suspected. Friedman (1978) found that 10.9 per cent of patients with brow presentation had clinical and radiographic evidence of cephalopelvic disproportion, compared with 2.7 per cent of controls with vertex presentations. If progress of labor is arrested and cephalopelvic disproportion is suspected, cesarean delivery is indicated. If labor progresses and there is evidence of resolution of a brow presentation to either a face or vertex presentation, labor should be managed with the expectation of vaginal delivery. If labor is arrested and there are poor uterine contractions in the absence

of cephalopelvic disproportion, the use of a carefully monitored course of oxytocin augmentation may be warranted. Seeds and Cefalo (1982) suggest that radiographic pelvimetry be considered in these situations to exclude cephalopelvic disproportion.

The majority of brow presentations convert spontaneously to either face or vertex presentations, and 70 to 90 per cent of face presentations result in spontaneous delivery. If the brow presentation fails to convert or the face presentation rotates to a persistent mentum posterior, cesarean delivery is required. If uncorrectable fetal distress occurs, labor should be terminated by abdominal delivery. It is generally agreed that to rotate the fetal head or to convert its deflection position either manually or with forceps is excessively dangerous to fetus and mother.

Compound Presentation

A compound presentation exists if an extremity is adjacent to the presenting part. This complication of labor occurs in approximately one in 1000 deliveries and is associated with high rates of prematurity (31 to 61 per cent) and fetal mortality (16 to 22 per cent) (Breen and Wiesmeier, 1968; Weissberg and O'Leary, 1973; Cruikshank and White, 1973). Cord prolapse, which occurs in 11 to 20 per cent of cases, is the most common intrapartum complication (Seeds and Cefalo, 1982). The vertex-arm combination is the most common among the compound presentations and has the best prognosis.

Management includes early diagnosis and careful fetal monitoring, with retraction of the presenting extremity and normal vaginal delivery occurring in the majority of patients. If fetal distress or cord prolapse occurs or labor progress ceases, abdominal delivery should be accomplished promptly. Stimulation or manipulation of the presenting extremity to encourage retraction within the uterus is a controversial issue. Cruikshank and White (1973) found that in 16 of 32 compound presentations the presenting extremity could be manually replaced, 15 of which resulted in uneventful vaginal deliveries. However, Seeds and Cefalo (1982), in their review of the literature regarding compound presentation, advise against manipulation of the prolapsed part. Indeed, spontaneous retraction of the extremity occurs so frequently that attempts to re-place it may not be necessary and, in certain cases, may encourage prolapse of the umbilical cord.

OPERATIVE DELIVERY

Cesarean Delivery

The evolution of cesarean delivery as a safe procedure with extraordinarily low maternal and fetal mortality rates is one of the most important developments in modern perinatal medicine. Maternal mortality rates from cesarean operations in the 19th century were 85 per cent or greater, with the operation being performed only in the most extraordinary circumstances to save the life of the mother (Eastman, 1932). By the early decades of the 20th century, several important innovations in surgical care had occurred—including aseptic technique, reliable anesthesia, and the control of hemorrhage by proper suturing of tissue planes as well as ligation of severed blood vessels. Specifically for the cesarean operation, introduction of the low-segment incision, allowing exclusion of the uterine wound from the peritoneal cavity, dramatically decreased the risk of postoperative peritonitis as a complication of puerperal endometritis (Frank, 1907). The later additions of blood transfusion and antibiotic therapy further reduced the morbidity and mortality of cesarean delivery to the extent that, in 1950, D'Esopo published a remarkable study reporting 1000 consecutive cesarean deliveries without a single maternal death. The decrease in maternal morbidity of cesarean delivery made the operation a reasonable alternative for delivery of the fetus at increased risk of asphyxia or trauma from labor and vaginal delivery. This decrease, together with more sophisticated methods of detecting chronic and acute fetal distress, including ultrasonography, continuous fetal heart monitoring, and fetal scalp blood sampling, changed the indications for and frequency of cesarean section for delivery. Prior to 1960, cesarean deliveries generally constituted less than 5 per cent of births and were done primarily for maternal indications such as placenta previa, radiographically documented cephalopelvic disproportion, and failure of induction in severe preeclampsia. After 1960, more cesarean deliveries were performed primarily for fetal indications, the proportion of abdominal deliveries on some obstetric services being as high as 20 to 25 per cent. In September, 1980, a Consensus Development Conference sponsored by The National Institute of Child Health and Human Development in conjunction with The National Center for Health Care Technology addressed the issue of the rising rate of cesarean childbirth (Rosen, 1981). Four indications were found to account for 90 per cent of the increase—dystocia (30 per cent), repeat cesarean delivery (25 to 30 per cent), breech presentation (10 to 15 per cent), and fetal distress (10 to 15 per cent). The cesarean section rate in the United States reached a plateau in 1988, and by 1989 there were encouraging signs that it was beginning to decline (Taffel et al., 1991). The decline is largely the result of an increase in vaginal birth after cesarean delivery. It is likely that the cesarean delivery rate will decline even further as the active management of labor reduces the incidence of primary cesarean delivery for dystocia.

Complications

Although cesarean delivery can be regarded as a reasonably safe surgical procedure, it is associated with higher risks of morbidity and mortality than vaginal delivery. The mortality rate of cesarean delivery varies greatly depending on the source of the data. Evrard and Gold (1977), reporting on deliveries in Rhode Island from 1965 to 1975, found the mortality rate of cesarean delivery to be 26 times higher than that of vaginal delivery. On the other hand, Frigoletto and co-workers (1980) reported on 10,231 consecutive cesarean deliveries at Boston Hospital for Women between 1968 and 1978 without a single maternal death.

It is apparent that the mortality risk in cesarean delivery depends on the associated medical complications in the patient requiring abdominal delivery and the skill of the medical team performing the procedure. Data from the Professional Activities Survey of the Commission of Professional and Hospital Activities for the year 1978, which include about 1 million births and 100,000 cesarean deliveries, showed the rates of maternal death per 100,000 births to be 9.8 for vaginal deliveries, 40.0 for all cesarean deliveries (Rosen, 1981), and 18.4 for repeat cesarean deliveries. Acute maternal complications of cesarean delivery include anesthesia accidents (e.g., problems with intubation, drug reactions, aspiration pneumonitis), blood loss, bowel or bladder injury, and, on rare occasions, amniotic fluid or air embolism. Frequently, cesarean delivery must be performed under emergency conditions soon after the patient is admitted to the hospital. Patient anxiety, obesity, an incompletely emptied stomach, acute hemorrhage from a placental accident, a low blood volume and constricted vascular space in association with pregnancy-induced hypertension, and hypotension secondary to vena caval and aortic compression by the pregnant uterus are just a few of the problems frequently encountered in patients requiring emergency cesarean delivery. These problems challenge even the most skilled anesthesiologist.

Febrile puerperal complications occur in 20 to 30 per cent of patients undergoing cesarean delivery. These include atelectasis, pneumonia, endomyometritis, urinary tract infection, wound infections, ileus, sepsis from indwelling venous catheters, and thromboembolic disease. Green and Sarubbi (1977) used a computer-designed discriminant analysis program to evaluate 15 risk factors related to morbidity following cesarean delivery. They found general anesthesia, obesity, hematocrit of 30 per cent or less, and labor prior to delivery to be the four statistically significant factors. More than 80 per cent of patients with two or more of these risk factors developed postoperative febrile disease requiring antibiotic therapy.

It would appear that the safest, most atraumatic method of delivery for an infant is by cesarean section, and the recent increase in cesarean delivery rates undoubtedly is due in great measure to the concern about the dangers to the fetus of labor and vaginal delivery. Nevertheless, abdominal delivery is also associated with uncommon but significant dangers to the infant, including fetal asphyxia due to uteroplacental hypoperfusion induced by conduction anesthesia or maternal position, neonatal respiratory morbidity, and scalpel lacerations. Maternal hypotension and its deleterious effect on uteroplacental perfusion are well-known dangers of the supine position. Conduction anesthesia, by blocking vasoconstriction in the lower extremities through the sympathetic nervous system, can further reduce cardiac output and further compromise uterine blood flow. Corke and associates (1982) have demonstrated that even brief episodes of hypotension (<2 minutes) will be reflected in cord blood gases as a metabolic acidosis suggestive of neonatal asphyxia.

Cesarean delivery has long been recognized to be associated with an increase in neonatal respiratory morbidity at all gestational ages (Clifford, 1934; Usher et al., 1964; Bryan et al., 1990). The frequency of this complication, its specific etiology and pathophysiology, and the mortality rate associated with it are all matters of dispute. However, every intensive care nursery staff is all too familiar with the otherwise normal, term, full-sized infants who are admitted with severe respiratory illness following elective cesarean delivery, a number of whom do not survive (Maisels et al., 1977; Flaksman et al., 1978). This syndrome may be due to a number of problems, without a clearcut and similar pathophysiology in each case, but the common denominator is cesarean delivery; moreover, the syndrome is most often seen when the operative delivery was performed in the absence of labor. Some cases of respiratory morbidity following cesarean delivery are due to true iatrogenic prematurity, in which inaccurate gestational dates result unexpectedly in a premature infant. Even careful attention to the duration of pregnancy and the use of amniotic fluid tests of fetal lung maturity have not completely eliminated the problem, however. Schreiner and colleagues (1979) and Heritage and Cunningham (1985) suggest that neonatal respiratory disease following elective repeat cesarean delivery, which is usually manifested as mild transient tachypnea of the newborn (wet lung syndrome), is in its most severe form persistence of the fetal circulation. These observations, together with the studies of Boon and associates (1981) demonstrating the reduced air volume in the lungs of infants delivered by cesarean compared with those delivered vaginally, suggest that the neonatal respiratory disease following cesarean delivery is due to incomplete adaptation of the fetal lung to extrauterine respiration. The specific sequence and timing for this adaptation to extrauterine cardiorespiratory status are still unknown. Nor is it known if the physiologic and mechanical events of labor and delivery are necessary to complete pulmonary adaptation. Studies such as those by Bowers and co-workers (1982) and Cohen and Carson (1985), showing a higher incidence of neonatal respiratory morbidity following repeat cesarean delivery performed in patients not in labor than in those in whom labor had ensued prior to the procedure, suggest, at least, that labor is the signal that crucial physiologic changes have occurred to prepare a fetus for extrauterine life.

Accidental lacerations of the fetus during cesarean delivery have been reported (Gerber, 1974), although the incidence is unknown. The frequency of these accidents appears to be related to the experience of the surgeon, the most common situation being a well-thinned-out lower uterine segment in a patient who has ruptured membranes; in these cases the uterus at the incision site may be only 2 or 3 mm thick. Usually these inadvertent scalpel lacerations of the fetus are of only cosmetic importance, but the author knows of one infant who died as a result of a thrombosis of the sagittal sinus secondary to a scalpel incision incurred during cesarean delivery.

Long-term maternal complications of cesarean delivery include hemorrhage from delayed necrosis of the uterine wound (Madsen and Olsen, 1977), bowel obstruction due to intra-abdominal adhesions, endometriosis in the uterine incision, placenta accreta, and cesarean delivery in subsequent pregnancies. Cesarean delivery also accounts for added risks to infants of future pregnancies; these dangers include a higher than usual incidence of placenta previa (Singh et al., 1981), fetal death due to antepartum rupture of vertical uterine incisions, and the neonatal respiratory disease associated with subsequent elective cesarean delivery.

Indications

Reducing the frequency of maternal and neonatal complications of cesarean delivery begins with a proper respect for the dangers of the procedure and careful selection of patients to be delivered in this manner. In general, the indication for cesarean delivery is any situation in which delivery of the fetus must be accomplished and in which induction of labor, a trial of labor, additional labor, or vaginal delivery of the fetus is deemed to be of greater risk to the mother or the fetus than abdominal delivery. This straightforward generalization, although constituting a more rational approach than a simple list of absolute indications for the operation, does not do justice to the complexities of the decision in each case. As the fetal indications for cesarean delivery have multiplied, so have the dilemmas of balancing the benefits and risks of operation for the two patients involved. For example, in placenta previa, vaginal delivery subjects both mother and fetus to unacceptable risks of exsanguination, and cesarean delivery is clearly in the best interests of both patients. In the case of a difficult mid-forceps delivery for fetal distress or failure of progress in the second stage of labor, however, the fetus will most certainly benefit from an expeditious abdominal delivery, and the mother's risks from the two procedures are a matter of serious debate. At the other end of the spectrum is the case of a footling breech presentation or genital herpes simplex infection, in which the operation is done entirely for the benefit of the fetus with no advantages to the mother apart from the statistical reassurance that it may help her infant. Countless other situations could be used as examples of the difficult decision that faces both physician and mother when evaluating the proper method of delivery.

The Consensus Development Statement on Cesarean Childbirth (Rosen, 1981) has done much to clarify the indications for cesarean delivery and to draw attention to specific situations in which the need for cesarean section can be reduced by thorough evaluation of patient and facility.

The problem of dystocia, which includes both proven cephalopelvic disproportion and the less well-defined problem of "failure of labor to progress," was found by the Consensus Development Conference to account for 30 per cent of the increase in cesarean delivery rates in the United States. Studies by Silbar (1986), and Seitchik and colleagues (1986), suggest that the increase in cesarean birth rate for dystocia is due, in part, to an increased incidence of large infants causing an absolute increase in fetal-pelvic disproportion. To what degree the use of the electronic cardiotocograph has contributed to the increasingly frequent diagnosis of CPD or "failure of labor to progress" is not known. Haverkamp and associates (1979), however, in a prospective controlled study of fetal heart rate monitoring, found that cesarean delivery was more often performed for CPD in the group of patients for whom the continuous labor-fetal monitoring data were available to the physicians than in the group of patients in whom a nurse at the bedside was documenting uterine contractions and fetal heart rate data by palpation and auscultation. It is tempting to speculate that in the absence of data about absolute intrauterine pressure values and subtle fetal heart rate decelerations, there is longer and more vigorous oxytocin augmentation of desultory labors before cesarean section is considered. Or does the nurse at the bedside allay anxiety and thereby contribute to a normal labor pattern and less fetal distress?

The diagnosis of fetal distress, which accounted for 10 to 15 per cent of the increase in cesarean delivery rate, is often made in the context of a labor that is not progressing normally. Zalar and Quilligan (1979) have shown that the use of fetal scalp blood sampling substantially reduces the number of cesarean deliveries performed for presumed fetal distress. Moreover, as further experience is gained with reading fetal monitoring tracings, one is less likely to perform operative deliveries for abnormal but not necessarily ominous fetal heart rate changes. Consequently, judicious interpretation of continuous fetal heart rate monitoring data and persistent attention to factors that will improve the fetal environment often allow the additional time needed for successful labor and vaginal delivery.

The waning enthusiasm for mid-pelvic forceps deliveries has also contributed to the increased number of cesarean deliveries in the "dystocia" category.

Repeat cesarean delivery accounted for 25 to 30 per cent of the increase in cesarean delivery rate (Rosen, 1981). However, previous cesarean delivery that was performed through a low transverse uterine incision for a nonrecurring indication (presumed cephalopelvic disproportion not included) need not be an indication for repeat cesarean delivery. In hospitals with appropriate facilities, i.e., services and staff for prompt emergency cesarean birth, a patient with a previous cesarean delivery can be allowed a trial of labor. Rosen et al. (1991), in a meta-analysis of 31 studies which included 11,417 trials of labor, found that the maternal morbidity was significantly lower after a trial of labor than after an elective repeat cesarean. The intended route of delivery, the presence of an unknown type of scar, and the use of oxytocin made no difference in the rate of uterine wound dehiscence. Small series of patients have addressed the question of safety of vaginal birth after cesarean (VBAC) in patients with breech presentation (Sarno et al., 1989), twin gestation (Strong et al., 1989), and post-term pregnancy (Yeh et al., 1984). Although each of these reports has noted no greater incidence of complications as compared to VBAC with a vertex, term, singleton pregnancy, the small number of patients in each series demands continued caution in recommending VBAC for such patients.

Intrapartum rupture of a low transverse uterine scar, which occurs in 0.5 to 1 per cent of women who undertake a trial of labor after a cesarean delivery, is a serious emergency and can result in a perinatal death (Scott, 1991). Furthermore, puerperal morbidity is more common in women who have a cesarean after a trial of labor than for those having a repeat elective abdominal delivery. After being fully informed about the risks and benefits of trial of labor and vaginal birth after cesarean delivery, women are not universally enthusiastic. More than 25 per cent will choose to have a repeat elective cesarean if given the chance (Joseph et al., 1991). Thurnau et al. (1991) have found that the fetal-pelvic index using a combination of radiologic and ultrasonographic determinations of the pelvic and fetal dimensions will predict the outcome in over 90 per cent of women attempting a trial of labor after cesarean delivery. There are good reasons to encourage vaginal birth after cesarean, and such a policy will continue to reduce the cesarean delivery rate. Nevertheless, some patients, after being well informed, may select an elective, repeat cesarean delivery.

Breech presentation as an indication for cesarean delivery has already been discussed. With the current criteria for the management of breech presentation, it is unlikely that the incidence of abdominal delivery will fall much below 60 per cent even when these criteria are applied rather liberally by obstetric personnel with an enthusiasm for vaginal delivery of breech presentation.

Reducing Morbidity of Cesarean Delivery

When cesarean delivery must be done, the following measures will ensure the lowest morbidity and mortality risks for mother and infant: anesthesia administered by a skilled anesthesiologist; attention to maternal position and blood volume in the peripartum period; prophylactic antibiotics; use of a transverse uterine incision whenever possible; awaiting the onset of labor whenever possible in cases of repeat cesarean delivery; and the presence of an individual skilled in newborn resuscitation.

There is endless debate about the preferred method of anesthesia for cesarean delivery. The reviews of this subject by Datta and Alper (1980) and by Reisner (1980) demonstrate that equally good neonatal and maternal outcomes can be obtained with local infiltration, spinal, epidural, or general anesthesia, provided it is administered by skilled individuals fully aware of the unique physiologic problems of the pregnant patient and her fetus. Each form of anesthesia may be associated with complications.

Spinal anesthesia is associated with the highest incidence of hypotension and should always be accompanied by uterine displacement, maternal prehydration, and (more controversial) prophylactic ephedrine administration. It should also be recognized that operative levels of anesthesia are achieved with doses of local anesthetic agents well below those required in the nonpregnant patient. Most important for the obstetrician is the awareness that with spinal anesthesia the time from onset of anesthesia to delivery of the infant is directly related to the degree of fetal metabolic acidosis resulting from uteroplacental hypoperfusion (Crawford, 1965). Simply because the patient is alert is no reason to procrastinate in delivering the infant. There is perhaps as much, if not more, need for prompt delivery of the infant following spinal anesthesia as there is with general anesthesia.

Epidural anesthesia is associated with maternal hypotension less commonly than spinal anesthesia. However, Jouppila and colleagues (1978) have shown that epidural anesthesia is associated with a decreased clearance of xenon-133, especially when hypotension occurs. These authors presume that xenon-133 clearance reflects uteroplacental perfusion. One of the major disadvantages of epidural block for cesarean delivery is the time required for the onset of operative anesthesia, which may preclude its use in many emergency situations.

General anesthesia, which has the advantage of rapid onset, is also associated with decreased uteroplacental perfusion during induction of the anesthesia (Jouppila et al., 1979). Pulmonary aspiration of gastric contents (Mendelson's syndrome) is always a major threat with general anesthesia, and this risk is accentuated by the delayed gastric emptying in patients in labor; this subject has been reviewed by Cohen (1982). There is evidence that the particulate antacids, which are commonly used preoperatively to neutralize gastric acidity, may themselves cause pulmonary damage if aspirated, and their use has not eliminated Mendelson's syndrome. A nonparticulate antacid such as sodium citrate given 10 to 45 minutes before anesthesia should significantly decrease the risk from aspiration without contributing added hazard. Perhaps the most important safeguard against the aspiration syndrome is skillful intubation while cricoid pressure is applied.

In cases managed with general anesthesia as well as those with conduction anesthesia, prompt delivery of the infant is important, the crucial time being that from the incision of the uterus to delivery (Crawford et al., 1973). To avoid hypoxia from altered uteroplacental and umbilical blood flow, this time should be not more than 90 seconds.

Adequate volume replacement is important in preventing hypotension when regional anesthesia is used. Prehydration with 1000 ml of saline or lactated Ringer's injection frequently compensates for vasodilation following onset of anesthesia. The supine position is a well-known but frequently neglected danger in all pregnant women in the third trimester (Marx and Bassell, 1982). Often during the preparation for surgery and administration of the anesthetic the patient is left flat on her back. Appropriate wedges, left lateral tilt of the table, and even operating with the patient in the lateral position have been shown to avoid supine hypotension and to reduce fetal asphyxia.

The use of prophylactic antibiotics for cesarean delivery was reviewed by Swartz and Grolle (1981). Twenty-six studies reporting on the use of various prophylactic antibiotic regimens all demonstrated a

reduction in the incidence of febrile morbidity and endomyometritis. A reduction in wound infection and urinary tract infection rates was a less consistent finding. It is not clear that prophylactic antibiotics reduce the incidence of the uncommon complications of septic thrombophlebitis and pelvic abscess. The impact of antibiotic therapy in preventing puerperal morbidity is greatest in patients who have been in labor prior to cesarean delivery. Single-drug regimens are as effective as those using two or more drugs, and short regimens (less than 12 hours) are as effective as more prolonged courses of therapy. Moreover, administering the antibiotic immediately after cord clamping is as effective as starting prior to the operation and avoids unnecessary therapy of the infant. These findings suggest that a three-dose course of a single antibiotic (such as mefoxin or ampicillin) administered over an 8-hour period with the first dose being given immediately after the cord is clamped to every patient in whom a cesarean is performed (with the exception of a purely elective procedure) will, at minimal expense and risk, result in a substantial reduction in puerperal morbidity and hospitalization. Gonik (1985) has demonstrated that a single dose of cefotaxime given immediately after the cord was clamped was as effective as three doses of the same medication over a 12-hour period.

Several studies, including those by Saravolatz et al. (1985) and Leveno et al. (1984), have demonstrated that irrigation with an antibiotic solution during a cesarean birth is as effective as parenteral antibiotics in reducing puerperal infection. In addition to equal prophylaxis, irrigation techniques are more cost-effective than parenteral antibiotics.

Because prophylactic antibiotic therapy has not reduced the rate of serious post–cesarean section morbidity resulting in prolonged hospitalization, Ledger (1980) has emphasized the proper selection of antibiotic therapy for patients who become symptomatic with endomyometritis. He has demonstrated a substantially better outcome when the initial drug regimen contains an antimicrobial agent effective against anaerobes. Specifically, he found that 100 women with symptoms of post–cesarean delivery endomyometritis who were treated with clindamycin-gentamicin had no serious sequelae and only five required addition of a third antibiotic, compared with 100 similar patients treated with penicillin-gentamicin, four of whom required prolonged hospitalizations owing to serious infections and 25 of whom required a third antibiotic.

In cases in which chorioamnionitis is suspected, therapeutic rather than prophylactic antibiotic regimens should be used. This may mean adding specific coverage for anaerobic organisms with drugs such as clindamycin, as just described. It is for these situations that there has been a renewed interest in the use of extraperitoneal cesarean operations (Perkins, 1980). This technique, which was popular in some centers prior to the introduction of antibiotics, is considered by many to be overly complicated, time-consuming, and dangerous as well as unnecessary. Perkins (1980) and Hanson (1978) have demonstrated that the operation can be performed without additional hazard to the mother or infant, does not require substantially more time, and may, when chorioamnionitis is present, provide the advantage of less contamination of the peritoneal cavity with infected secretions. The risks and benefits of the extraperitoneal operation vis-à-vis those of the standard intraperitoneal approach will have to be tested in a prospective controlled study before definitive statements can be made about the role of the former approach in modern operative obstetrics.

The advantages of the transverse uterine incision over the vertical uterine incision for cesarean delivery were first recognized by Kerr (1926), who pointed out that low vertical incisions almost always extend into the thicker muscle layers of the fundus and are more frequently complicated by improper healing and subsequent rupture. Also, when the entire uterine incision can be covered by the bladder peritoneum, there is less risk of postoperative ileus, peritonitis, and subsequent adhesions and bowel obstruction.

The advantages of awaiting the onset of labor before performing repeat cesarean delivery are to eliminate iatrogenic prematurity and to reduce the risk of neonatal respiratory illness due simply to the lack of the late alterations in neonatal pulmonary physiology that normally allow the transition to extrauterine life. Awaiting the onset of labor also results in thinning of the lower uterine segment, which decreases blood loss and facilitates development of the bladder flap during the procedure.

Finally, the presence of an individual skilled in neonatal resuscitation is essential, especially when cesarean delivery is performed for fetal distress. It is not only courteous, but often *vitally important*, to inform the pediatrician or nursery personnel as early as possible of an impending cesarean delivery. Special equipment, drugs, and blood products may need to be assembled for a sick neonate. It is a disservice to a mother to perform a major operation on her in the interest of her fetus and not to follow up with the most expert care of the newborn.

Cesarean hysterectomy is occasionally lifesaving, especially in cases of uncontrolled hemorrhage from the site of a placenta previa, placenta accreta, or a ruptured uterus. Also, cesarean hysterectomy may be the treatment of choice in women with chorioamnionitis who desire sterilization and in whom there is an indication for cesarean delivery. However, for other indications such as cervical intraepithelial neoplasia and a request for sterilization with a repeat cesarean delivery, the operation is associated with sufficient morbidity to make its usefulness in these situations doubtful. Park and Duff (1980), in a review of cesarean hysterectomy including 3913 operations, found the following complication rates: 0.71 per cent maternal mortality, 3 per cent bladder injury, 0.4 per cent vesicovaginal fistula, 0.25 per cent ureteral injury, and 0.97 per cent intraperitoneal bleeding requiring reoperation. Supracervical cesarean hysterectomy is justified in cases of life-threatening hemorrhage when the patient's vital signs are unstable. Complete removal of the cervix is one of the most difficult and time-consuming aspects of the cesarean hysterectomy procedure, especially when there has been substantial effacement and dilation of the cervix.

Summary

Cesarean delivery, which is performed in approximately 20 per cent of parturients, is associated with significant mortality and morbidity rates for mother and infant. The procedure should be used only when it will substantially reduce the risks of mortality and morbidity to both patients, and it should be performed with careful attention to all of the details that minimize the dangers of the operative procedure for both patients.

Obstetric Forceps Delivery

In 1988 the American College of Obstetricians and Gynecolgists issued a Committee Opinion establishing new definitions for obstetric forceps. These definitions, which were incorporated in the ACOG Technical Bulletin entitled Operative Vaginal Delivery (1991), are as follows:

Outlet forceps
1. Scalp is visible at the introitus without separating labia
2. Fetal skull has reached pelvic floor
3. Sagittal suture is in anteroposterior diameter or right or left occiput anterior or posterior position
4. Fetal head is at or on perineum
5. Rotation does not exceed 45 degrees

Low forceps
Leading point of fetal skull is at station $>/= +2$ cm, and not on the pelvic floor
   a. Rotation $</= 45$ degrees (left or right occiput anterior to occiput anterior, or left or right occiput posterior to occiput posterior)
   b. Rotation >45 degrees

Mid-forceps
Station above $+2$ cm but head engaged

The new classification reflects what has been widely recognized among practicing obstetricians, that there are two types of forceps deliveries—low-forceps deliveries which are usually quite simple and uncomplicated for both mother and infant, and mid-forceps deliveries, which in some cases may be quite difficult and may cause substantial trauma to either patient.

Obstetric forceps were first used by members of the Chamberlen family in the 17th century, but were not widely accepted until 100 years later (Castiglioni, 1947). William Smellie was the first to systematically teach the principles of forceps deliveries. It is clear that he also was fully aware of the potential dangers of the instruments; he wrote, in the introduction to Volume II of *Treatise on the Theory and Practice of Midwifery* (Johnstone, 1952), ''If these expedients (forceps) are used prematurely when the nature of the case does not absolutely require such assistance, the mischief that may ensue will often over balance the service for which they were intended and this consideration is one of my principal motives for publishing this second volume.''

Prior to the publication of the 1988 ACOG definition of obstetric forceps, several studies compared the outcome of mid-forceps deliveries with cesarean deliveries performed in relatively similar circumstances. These studies, using previous definitions of mid-forceps, included a substantial number of patients whose deliveries would now be classified as low forceps. Cardozo et al. (1983) compared mid-pelvic forceps delivery (Kielland forceps) with cesarean delivery. There was a greater incidence of low 5-minute Apgar scores, need for intubation, and admission to the neonatal intensive care unit among infants delivered by cesarean. Traub et al. (1984) found no difference in the rates of neonatal depression between infants delivered by mid-forceps and those delivered by cesarean. Dierker et al. (1985) found no difference in short-term neonatal outcome when 176 mid-forceps deliveries were compared with a similar number of cesarean deliveries, with the exception that cephalhematomas occurred more frequently in the infants delivered by forceps. Gilstrap et al. (1984) compared 234 indicated mid-forceps deliveries with 111 cesarean deliveries. Using cord blood data, Apgar score, and the incidence of seizures in the neonates, they found no difference in the frequency of neonatal asphyxia.

Recently, Hagadorn-Freathy et al. (1991) prospectively evaluated forceps deliveries comparing outcomes as designated by the old (ACOG, 1965) and the new (ACOG, 1988) classifications. When the 1965 classification was used, there was no difference in outcome comparing outlet forceps to mid-forceps deliveries. When the deliveries were reclassified according to the 1988 criteria, mid-forceps deliveries had lower cord pH values and a higher incidence of fetal injury as compared to outlet or low forceps deliveries. Friedman (1973) showed that the highest perinatal mortality rate associated with mid-forceps operations occurred when protraction or arrest disorders or combinations of these abnormalities preceded the forceps operation. Davidson and co-workers (1976) found that if the time required for the cervix to dilate in the first stage of labor from 7 cm to 10 cm exceeded 2 hours, forceps deliveries were consistently difficult, whereas if the dilation time was less than 2 hours, an easy forceps delivery could be expected. Hughey and colleagues (1978), reviewing 458 mid-forceps rotations performed between 1967 and 1976, found several high-risk features that were predictive of complications in such operations, among which were first stage of labor longer than 8 hours, second stage of labor longer than 1 hour, maternal age less than 21 years or more than 35 years, first pregnancy, parity six or more, gestational age less than 37 weeks or greater than 43 weeks, fetal weight less than 2500 gm or more than 4500 gm, the occiput transverse position, and persistent back pain. If three or more of these factors were present, there was a 50 per cent or greater chance of an unfavorable newborn outcome if mid-forceps rotation was performed.

There are few studies of long-term follow-up of infants delivered with forceps. Friedman and colleagues (1984) published results from a collaborative perinatal project in which children delivered by mid-forceps demonstrated lower IQ scores and a higher prevalence of suspected speech, language, and hearing abnormalities than children born spontaneously. McBride and co-workers (1979) studied 700 5-year-old children, all of whom were born at term, 175 by mid-forceps delivery. Using a variety of neurologic, hearing, visual acuity, and development tests, these authors found no differences related to the method of delivery among the children who had been born in cephalic presentation. Dierker et al. (1986) compared 110 children 2 years of age or older who had been delivered by mid-forceps to a similar number of children of the same age delivered by cesarean. They found five cases of abnormal development in the children delivered by mid-forceps and seven cases among those delivered by cesarean. Seidman et al. (1991) related obstetric interventions to medical examinations and intelligence tests performed on more than 32,000 17-year-old men and women inducted into the Israeli Defense Forces. The mean intelligence scores for those who had been delivered by forceps and vacuum extractor were not statistically different from those who were delivered spontaneously or by cesarean. The studies that demonstrated no untoward long-term effect of operative vaginal delivery are those in which the infants were born after 1970. A more conservative attitude about obstetric force, which has characterized the past two decades, may have been responsible for the salutary outcomes noted in recent studies of both short-term and long-term effects of operative vaginal delivery.

Mid-forceps deliveries, as defined by the 1991 ACOG criteria, should be undertaken with caution and with a willingness to abandon the procedure in favor of cesarean delivery if there is difficulty with proper application of the instrument or if the head does not easily descend or rotate.

Vacuum Extraction

The vacuum extractor was introduced into modern obstetrics by Malmström in 1954. Since that time it has largely replaced the use of obstetric forceps in Scandinavia and continental Europe, but has had only sporadic and isolated popularity in the United States. The use of the vacuum extractor for obstetric delivery, including a detailed account of the technique of application and use of the Malmström instrument, was reviewed by Halme and Ekbladh (1982).

The indications for delivery with the vacuum extractor are virtually the same as those for the use of forceps: arrest of labor in the second stage, a maternal indication for shortening of the second stage of labor (e.g., cardiovascular or cerebrovascular disease, maternal exhaustion), fetal distress, and elective low pelvic delivery.

Contraindications to vacuum extraction include cephalopelvic disproportion, face or brow presentation, breech presentation, unengaged fetal head, premature infant, and incompletely dilated cervix.

Maternal complications of vacuum extractor delivery, including cervical and vaginal trauma, are generally agreed to be less frequent and less severe than those of forceps delivery; this is one of the major advantages of the instrument. Minor fetal complications include cephalohematomas and retinal hemorrhages, which are usually benign and self-limited.

More serious complications, such as subgaleal hemorrhage (4 per cent) and intracranial hemorrhage (2.5 per cent), are usually associated with prolonged labor and fetal asphyxia, but are probably less common than in forceps deliveries performed under the same circumstances.

Vaca and Keirse (1989) summarized a number of prospective controlled trials of vacuum extractor versus forceps deliveries. In this meta-analysis, as well as in the randomized controlled trial reported by Johanson et al. (1989), failure to deliver with the chosen instrument occurred more often with the vacuum extractor, significant maternal trauma (third- and fourth-degree perineal and extensive vaginal lacerations) occurred more commonly with forceps, and scalp injury (exclusive of cephalhematomas) occurred more commonly with the vacuum extractor. At present, the selection of one or another means of midpelvic delivery depends on the obstetrician's experience with each procedure and the availability of personnel and facilities for performing a cesarean delivery.

Two major advantages of the vacuum extractor are the ease with which it can be applied and the need for less anesthesia than is required for either forceps or cesarean delivery. Moreover, it is far easier to teach and to learn the appropriate skill required to safely use the extractor than to acquire a similar level of skill with either forceps or cesarean delivery. The Silastic cup, a recent modification of the vacuum extractor, further simplifies the application of the instrument. Studies by Maryniak and Frank (1984) and by Berkus and co-workers (1985) support the safety of the Silastic vacuum extractor and the ease with which it can be applied. It has replaced the Malmström vacuum extractor on many obstetric services in the United States.

ANALGESIA AND ANESTHESIA FOR LOW-RISK LABOR AND VAGINAL DELIVERY

A review by Myers and Williams (1982) brings a much-needed perspective to the role of analgesia and anesthesia in the management of labor. These authors review the data about the effect of anxiety on uteroplacental circulation and its relation to fetal asphyxia. Experiments on animals and humans suggest that the appropriate use of analgesia and anesthesia often improves the status of the fetus by reducing the catecholamine release that results from maternal pain and anxiety. In the past, there has often been a categorical rejection and fear of analgesic and anesthetic medications on the grounds that they cross the placenta and sedate the fetus. Although it is true that most of the agents used are rapidly transported to the fetus, the drug levels in the fetus are usually relatively low and the effect of such drugs is reasonably transient. Moreover, as Myers and Williams (1982) have pointed out, pharmacologic depression of the central nervous system may be beneficial to the fetus for whom there is risk of hypoxia. The decrease in central nervous system metabolism resulting from the drug therapy reduces oxygen requirements, lactate formation, edema, and tissue damage.

Barrier and Sureau (1982), in a review of the effect on the fetus and neonate of drugs used in labor and delivery, concluded that in the absence of complicated labor or fetal asphyxia, no long-term effects of obstetric anesthesia or analgesia can be demonstrated. Brackbill (1979), a psychologist, in a similarly exhaustive review of the literature, comes to a different conclusion, that analgesic and anesthetic medications have demonstrable effects on the neonate that may last for months. The difficulties of performing accurate and meaningful short-term evaluation to demonstrate the effect of obstetric medication on neonates is discussed by Amiel-Tyson and colleagues (1982) in their presentation of a new neurologic and adaptive capacity score (NACS) for just such a purpose. The problems involved in the short-term evaluation of the neonate are multiplied many times by the variety of compounding variables in long-term follow-up studies. In the midst of this dilemma, the practicing obstetrician and anesthesiologist can best serve the mother and her infant by using those drugs and procedures that provide sufficient analgesia and anesthesia to relieve anxiety, promote a normal labor, prevent fetal asphyxia, and accomplish delivery with as little trauma as possible.

One of the most important assets of a modern facility offering a full range of services is the presence of a qualified obstetric anesthesiologist. The physiologic changes that characterize pregnancy result in metabolic, respiratory, and cardiovascular phenomena not encountered in the nonpregnant state. These changes, together with the presence of the fetus *in utero*, are a challenge for the anesthesiologist. Furthermore, high-risk obstetric patients frequently have fetal or maternal problems that further complicate the already difficult task of administering anesthesia to two patients simultaneously (see Chapter 64).

The number of maternal and fetal-neonatal complications that are attributed to improperly administered anesthetic and analgesic drugs is evidence of the complexity of the anesthesiologist's task. It is no surprise that the studies by Williams and Hawes (1979) and Paneth and co-workers (1982) have shown that the survival rate of infants, corrected for birth weight and other risk factors, is highest in facilities with the greatest degree of perinatal sophistication. This is due, in part, to the capability of rapid response to fetal and maternal emergencies, a capability that requires an anesthesiologist. It is unfortunate that the number and distribution of trained obstetric anesthesiologists are not sufficient to make such perinatal services available to all women in labor.

The choice of drug and anesthetic technique for labor and delivery depends on the skill and experience of the individual who performs the procedure, the progress of labor, other complications of pregnancy or labor, and the desires of the patient. With proper antenatal psychological preparation, many patients require minimal, if any, analgesia or anesthesia throughout labor, and uncompromised, healthy infants are born in most of these cases. Nothing should be done to discourage such a practice. Furthermore, everything should be done to facilitate birthing in quiet, pleasant, and friendly surroundings in which the parturient is accompanied by a friend or family.

There is considerable evidence that a supportive birth attendant (doula) reduces the need for analgesia and anesthesia and, in some populations, reduces the incidence of dystocia (Sosa et al., 1980; Kennell et al., 1991).

Analgesia

Sedatives and narcotic analgesics are frequently administered alone or in combination in the first stage of labor. All drugs of this type rapidly appear in the fetal circulation when administered to the mother. Predictably, there will be some sedation of the infant, depending on the specific drug given, the amount, the time, and the route of administration. The drug most commonly used for pain is meperidine in doses of 50 to 100 mg IM or 25 to 50 mg IV. To enhance its effect, provide some sedation, and prevent nausea, a phenothiazine such as promethazine, 25 mg, is often given as well. The half-life of meperidine is increased and is more variable in pregnant women than in nonpregnant subjects. Furthermore, with evidence of fetal hypoxia, higher levels of meperidine will be found in umbilical blood samples after the same maternal dose (Barrier and Sureau, 1982). If the neonate appears depressed as the result of the recent maternal administration of meperidine, injection of the narcotic antagonist naloxone may be indicated (0.04 mg IV or 0.2 mg IM).

The use of patient-controlled infusion pumps for administering analgesic medications in labor has been shown to increase effectiveness of pain control while decreasing the amounts of drug that are administered (McIntosh and Rayburn, 1991).

The use of epidural and intrathecal injections of narcotic analgesics is a promising means of providing analgesia of relatively long duration with relatively smaller doses of drugs (Scott et al., 1980; Booker et al., 1980). Early studies suggest that the intrathecal administration of morphine requires lower doses of medication and is more reliable in relieving the pain of labor than injection of the drug into the epidural space (Baraka et al., 1981; Crawford, 1981).

Paracervical Block

Paracervical block was a popular form of anesthesia for the first stage of labor until it was implicated in several fetal deaths and was shown to be associated with fetal bradycardia in 25 to 35 per cent of cases (Rosefsky and Petersiel, 1968; Goddard, 1971; Freeman et al., 1972). Death in some cases was related to direct injection of large doses of local anesthetic agents into the fetus, whereas the fetal bradycardia was probably a response to rapid uptake of the drug from the highly vascular paracervical space. This form of anesthesia is still used, especially in hospitals in which epidural anesthesia is not available, and if used wisely in low-risk patients, it is safe and effective for the first stage of labor (Paul and Freeman, 1972). The anesthetic should be administered with great care to avoid direct fetal injection, using the smallest amount of drug possible. Chloroprocaine (1 to 2 per cent) should be used rather than lidocaine or mepivacaine if repeated doses will be required (Freeman and Arnold, 1975). Any physician using regional anesthesia techniques must be aware of the maternal and fetal effects of the drugs used. This topic was reviewed by Ralston and Shnider (1978).

Pudendal Block

Pudendal block is perhaps the most common form of anesthesia used for vaginal delivery. When successful it provides adequate pain relief for episiotomy, spontaneous delivery, forceps or vacuum extraction delivery from a low pelvic station, and repair of perineal, vaginal, or cervical lacerations. Because the local anesthetic agent is injected well away from the parauterine vasculature, uteroplacental blood flow and fetal heart rate are not affected to the same degree as in paracervical block. Occasionally, vaginal hematomas may be caused by pudendal nerve block, but the most dreaded complication is a retropsoas or pelvic abscess (Wenger and Gitchell, 1973; Svancarik et al., 1977). It is surprising that this complication does not occur more frequently, inasmuch as the injection is made through a nonsterile field inhabited by numerous potential pathogens. The infrequency of infections in Alcock's canal is probably due to the prolonged compression of the paravaginal tissues by the fetal head, which prevents hematoma formation. The success of pudendal nerve block depends on a clear understanding of the anatomy of the pudendal nerve and surrounding structures. The anatomic study by Klink (1953) clarifies the course of the pudendal nerve, describes the variations of the nerve and its branches, and discusses the anatomy in relation to the performance of successful regional anesthesia; this article, with its valuable illustrations, is an excellent resource.

Spinal Anesthesia

Low spinal anesthesia, often referred to as saddle block, is an effective means of anesthesia. It is relatively simple to perform and provides prompt, reliable pain relief that is adequate for spontaneous delivery or instrument delivery from the low pelvic or mid-pelvic station. It usually consists of 4 mg of tetracaine administered in a hyperbaric solution at the L4–L5 interspace with the patient sitting. Although this technique is intended to anesthetize only the "saddle region," the level of anesthesia sometimes is as high as T10. Because of the ease of administration and the reliability of this form of anesthesia, it has been a favorite of obstetricians practicing in hospitals in which anesthesiologists are available only for cesarean delivery or other emergencies. Because of the profound sympathetic block that occurs with spinal anesthesia, however, saddle block may be associated with profound hypotension and a decrease in uteroplacental perfusion. Furthermore, it may interfere with voluntary abdominal pushing effort far more than epidural anesthesia, frequently resulting in delivery of the infant by forceps. The popularity of this form of obstetric anesthesia is waning because it is being replaced by epidural anesthesia and because many patients insist on unmedicated, natural delivery.

Epidural Anesthesia

Epidural anesthesia is being used with increasing frequency, especially in hospitals in which anesthesiologists are available to patients in labor 24 hours a day. In experienced hands, epidural anesthesia has an excellent safety record (Crawford, 1985). Though it is the most difficult form of anesthesia to administer, it has the advantage of providing excellent pain relief for the first and second stages of labor and for delivery without altering the consciousness of the mother. Lumbar epidural block has replaced the caudal epidural technique because less drug is required to achieve satisfactory analgesia. Bupivacaine and chloroprocaine are the drugs most commonly used, the former providing more prolonged anesthesia but a greater delay in onset. The use of combinations of local anesthetics and narcotics also has been shown to provide excellent analgesia with less motor blockade (Lysak et al., 1990)

Continuous lumbar epidural anesthesia has been associated with late decelerations in fetal heart rate suggestive of decreased uteroplacental perfusion in as many as 20 per cent of cases. This is more common with bupivacaine than with chloroprocaine or lidocaine (Abboud et al., 1982). Also, the use of oxytocin to augment labor in cases in which continuous epidural anesthesia is used has been reported to increase the frequency of late decelerations noted on fetal monitoring (McDonald et al., 1974). When uterine hypertonus or maternal hypotension is associated with the augmentation of contractions in patients with epidural anesthesia, fetal heart rate patterns indicating uteroplacental insufficiency are seen in as many as 70 per cent of cases (Schifrin, 1972). The incidence of uteroplacental insufficiency with epidural anesthesia can be reduced by prehydration of the mother and avoidance of the supine position (Collins et al., 1978).

The effect of epidural anesthesia on the duration of labor is not entirely clear. Epidural anesthesia appears to lengthen the second stage of labor and is associated with an increased need for oxytocin augmentation and instrument delivery (Willdeck-Lund et al., 1979). This potential problem may be offset by the benefits of epidural anesthesia in reducing the maternal acidosis caused by excessive bearing-down efforts and in decreasing catecholamine release in the mother by effective anesthesia in the second stage (Pearson and Davies, 1973). One thing is perfectly clear: When epidural anesthesia is used, the obstetrician must be constantly aware of the dangers of uteroplacental hypoperfusion.

An additional benefit of epidural anesthesia for patients having a cesarean delivery is that opioids can be injected into the epidural space to provide prolonged postoperative analgesia (Cousins and Mather, 1984). The rare occurrence of serious respiratory depression (1/1200) appears to be the only major complication. Transient nausea, urinary retention, and pruritus have also been reported in patients treated with epidural opioids.

A serious question in many hospitals is, Who should be allowed to administer epidural anesthesia to women in labor? A number of residency training programs in obstetrics and gynecology include a rotation on obstetric anesthesia, during which the obstetric resident learns to perform epidural anesthesia under the direction of a qualified obstetric anesthesiologist. Is that resident then capable of administering epidural anesthesia in the management of labor in a hospital that does not have 24-hour in-house coverage by an anesthesiologist (Romine et al., 1970)? If an anesthesiologist places the epidural catheter and administers the initial dose, are nurses or nurse-midwives qualified to give additional doses (Scott and Sinclair, 1982; Crawford, 1985)? Should nurse anesthetists be trained to provide continuous lumbar epidural anesthesia? Because of the paucity of anesthesiologists either trained or willing to provide continuous epidural anesthesia for women in labor, these issues have practical, fiscal, and medicolegal implications and need to be addressed.

LABOR MONITORING

The term fetal monitoring has become almost synonymous with continuous electronic fetal monitoring. The latter subject is discussed in detail in Chapter 20. The more comprehensive term *labor monitoring* means the conduct and management of the labor event from its onset to its completion. The primary goal of labor monitoring is to achieve delivery of a healthy infant from a healthy mother with as little trauma as possible. A secondary goal is to accomplish this delivery in a manner that is not degrading to the mother and enhances and strengthens family relationships in a way that is consistent with the cultural and personal expectations of the patient. In a narrower context this latter goal has been defined as "reducing bonding failure" (Ounsted et al., 1982). Certainly a healthy and supportive family unit will augment the growth and development of the newborn. To accomplish these goals requires attention to all the details of the labor and delivery process as they relate to a specific patient's medical, obstetric, and psychosocial situation. One of the paradoxes of modern obstetric care is that the increase in technology that has contributed substantially to the identification and correction of the pathophysiologic abnormalities of labor may depersonalize the labor event and may even introduce phenomena that alter maternal and fetal physiology and create substantial maternal and family anxiety. The outcry against such depersonalization has come from many quarters and has resulted in the re-examination of the management of labor and delivery. Indeed, it has been found that many of the traditional hospital obstetric practices, such as the perineal shave, enemas, and isolation of the patient from her family and friends, are not beneficial. More liberal use of ambulation and positions of comfort in labor and delivery have been found to be physiologically beneficial. Furthermore, the presence of family members or supportive friends may decrease anxiety, shorten the duration of labor, and reduce the need for medications.

Perhaps the most important figure in this entire scenario is the bedside nurse in the labor and delivery unit. It is the role of the nurse to bridge the gap between the most sophisticated obstetric technology and the expectations and needs of the patient and her family. The nurse must have a thorough understanding of the physiology and pathophysiology of labor, must be able to collect, record, and interpret the data throughout the labor, and must anticipate both maternal and fetal problems. Furthermore, the nurse must provide timely communications to the physicians responsible for the patient's care and frequently must help to interpret in an intelligible and compassionate manner the course of labor to the patient and her family. This implies a one-to-one nurse/patient ratio for patients in active labor. All of these goals should be accomplished in a facility in which there can be an immediate response to a fetal or maternal emergency in the form of prompt delivery or resuscitation when necessary.

REFERENCES

Abboud TK, Khoo SS, Miller F, et al: Maternal, fetal, and neonatal responses after epidural anesthesia with bupivacaine, 2-chloroprocaine, or lidocaine. Anesth Analg **61**:638, 1982.

Akoury HA, Brodie G, Caddick R, et al: Active management of labor and operative delivery in nulliparous women. Am J Obstet Gynecol **158**:255, 1988.

Alexopoulos KA: The importance of breech delivery in the pathogenesis of brain damage. End results of a long-term follow-up. Clin Pediatr **12**:248, 1973.

Alvarez M, Lockwood CJ, Ghidini A, et al: Prophylactic and emergent arterial catheterization for selective embolization in obstetric hemorrhage. Am J Perinatol **9**:441, 1992.

American College of Obstetricians and Gynecologists. Obstetrics forceps. ACOG Committee Opinion 59. Washington, DC, ACOG, 1988.

American College of Obstetricians and Gynecologists. Operative vaginal delivery. ACOG Technical Bulletin 152. Washington, DC, ACOG, 1991.

Amiel-Tyson CL, Barrier G, Shnider SM, et al: A new neurologic and adaptive capacity scoring system for evaluating obstetric medications in full-term newborns. Anesthesiology **56**:340, 1982.

Anderson GC, Schooley GL: Comparison of uterine contractions in spontaneous and oxytocin- or $PGF_{2\alpha}$ induced labors. Obstet Gynecol **45**:284, 1975.

Axelrod FB, Leistner HL, Porges RF: Breech presentation among infants with familial dysautonomia. J Pediatr **84**:107, 1974.

Baraka A, Noueihid R, Hajj S: Intrathecal injection of morphine for obstetric analgesia. Anesthesiology **54**:136, 1981.

Barnum CG: Dystocia due to the shoulders. Am J Obstet Gynecol **50**:439, 1945.

Barrier G, Sureau C: Effects of anaesthetic and analgesic drugs on labour, fetus, and neonate. Clin Obstet Gynaecol **9**:351, 1982.

Beazley JM, Kurjak A: The influence of a partograph on the active management of labour. Lancet **2**:348, 1972.

Beischer NA: Pelvic contraction in breech presentation. J Obstet Gynaecol Br Commonw **73**:421, 1966.

Benedetti TJ, Gabbe SG: Shoulder dystocia. A complication of fetal macrosomia and prolonged second stage of labor with midpelvic delivery. Obstet Gynecol **52**:526, 1978.

Berkowitz RL, Rafferty TD: Pulmonary artery flow-directed catheter use in the obstetric patient. Obstet Gynecol **55**:507, 1980.

Berkus MD, Ramamurthy RS, O'Connor PS, et al: Cohort study of

Silastic obstetric vacuum cup deliveries. I. Safety of the instrument. Obstet Gynecol **66**:503, 1985.

Bishop EH: Pelvic scoring for elective induction. Obstet Gynecol **24**:266, 1964.

Black BP, McBride WG: Children born after elective induction of labour. Med J Aust **2**:362, 1979.

Blanchette H: Elective manual exploration of the uterus after delivery: A study and review. J Reprod Med **19**:13, 1977.

Booker PD, Wilkes RG, Beddard J: Obstetric pain relief using epidural morphine. Anaesthesia **35**:377, 1980.

Boon AW, Milner AD, Hopkin IE: Lung volumes and lung mechanics in babies born vaginally and by elective and emergency lower segmental cesarean section. J Pediatr **98**:812, 1981.

Bowen LW, Beeson JH: Use of a large Foley catheter balloon to control postpartum hemorrhage resulting from a low placental implantation. A report of two cases. J Reprod Med **30**:623, 1985.

Bowers SK, MacDonald HM, Shapiro ED: Prevention of iatrogenic neonatal respiratory distress syndrome: Elective repeat cesarean section and spontaneous labor. Am J Obstet Gynecol **143**:186, 1982.

Bowes WA Jr, Taylor ES, O'Brien M, Bowes C: Breech delivery: Evaluation of the method of delivery on perinatal results and maternal mortality. Am J Obstet Gynecol **135**:965, 1979.

Boylan P, Frankowski R, Rountree R, et al: The effect of active management of labor on the incidence of caesarean section for dystocia in nulliparae. Am J Perinatol **8**:373, 1991.

Brackbill Y: Obstetrical medication and infant behavior. In Osofsky JD (ed): Handbook of Infant Development. New York, John Wiley & Sons, 1979.

Braun FHT, Jones KL, Smith DW: Breech presentation as an indicator of fetal abnormality. J Pediatr **86**:419, 1975.

Breen JL, Wiesmeier E: Compound presentations: A survey of 131 patients. Obstet Gynecol **32**:419, 1968.

Brenner WE, Bruce RD, Hendricks CH: The characteristics and perils of breech presentation. Am J Obstet Gynecol **118**:700, 1974.

Brocks V, Philipsen T, Secher NJ: A randomized trial of external cephalic version with tocolysis in late pregnancy. Br J Obstet Gynaecol **91**:653, 1984.

Browning DJ: Serious side effects of ergometrine and its use in routine obstetric practice. Med J Aust **1**:957, 1974.

Bryan H, Hawrylyshyn P, Hogg-Johnson S, et al: Perinatal factors associated with the respiratory distress syndrome. Am J Obstet Gynecol **162**:476, 1990.

Buchan PC: Pathogenesis of neonatal hyperbilirubinaemia after induction of labour with oxytocin. Br Med J **2**:1255, 1979.

Burchell RC: Physiology of internal iliac artery ligation. J Obstet Gynaecol Br Commonw **75**:642, 1968.

Buttino L Jr, Garite TJ: The use of 15 methyl F2 alpha Prostaglandin (Prostin 15M) for the control of postpartum hemorrhage. Am J Perinatol **3**:241, 1986.

Caldwell WE, Moloy HC, D'Esopo DA: Further studies on the mechanism of labor. Am J Obstet Gynecol **30**:763, 1935.

Caldwell WE, Moloy HC, D'Esopo DA: The more recent conceptions of the pelvic architecture. Am J Obstet Gynecol **40**:558, 1940.

Calvert JP: Intrinsic hazard of breech presentation. Br Med J **281**:1319, 1980.

Cardozo LD, Gibb DM, Studd JWW, Cooper DJ: Should we abandon Kielland's forceps? Br Med J **287**:315, 1983.

Castiglioni A: A History of Medicine. New York, Alfred A. Knopf, 1947.

Catanzarite VA, Moffitt KD, Baker ML, et al: New approaches to the management of acute uterine inversion. Obstet Gynecol **68**:78, 1986.

Chadha YC, Mahmood TA, Dick MJ, et al: Breech delivery and epidural analgesia. Br J Obstet Gynecol **99**:96, 1992.

Chalmers I, Campbell H, Turnbull AC: Use of oxytocin and incidence of neonatal jaundice. Br Med J **2**:116, 1975.

Clifford SH: A consideration of the obstetrical management of premature labor. N Engl J Med **210**:570, 1934.

Cohen M, Carson BS: Respiratory morbidity benefit of awaiting onset of labor after elective cesarean section. Obstet Gynecol **65**:818, 1985.

Cohen S: The aspiration syndrome. Clin Obstet Gynaecol **9**:235, 1982.

Cohen WR: Influence of the duration of second stage of labor on perinatal outcome and puerperal morbidity. Obstet Gynecol **49**:266, 1977.

Cole RA, Howie PW, MacNaughton MC: Elective induction of labour. A randomized prospective trial. Lancet **1**:767, 1975.

Collea JV, Chein C, Quilligan EJ: The randomized management of term frank breech presentation. A study of 208 cases. Am J Obstet Gynecol **137**:235, 1980.

Collea JV, Robin SC, Weghorst GR, Quilligan EJ: The randomized management of term frank breech presentation: Vaginal delivery vs. cesarean section. Am J Obstet Gynecol **131**:186, 1978.

Collins KM, Bevan DR, Beard RW: Fluid loading to reduce abnormalities of fetal heart rate and maternal hypotension during epidural analgesia in labour. Br Med J **2**:1460, 1978.

Corke BC, Datta S, Ostheimer GW, et al: Spinal anesthesia for Cesarean section: The influence of hypotension on neonatal outcome. Anaesthesia **37**:658, 1982.

Cousins ML, Mather LE: Intrathecal and epidural administration of opioids. Anesthesiology **61**:276, 1984.

Crawford JS: Maternal and cord blood at delivery. II. Parameters of respiratory exchange: Elective cesarean section. Am J Obstet Gynecol **93**:37, 1965.

Crawford JS: Appraisal of lumbar epidural blockade in patients with singleton fetus presenting by breech. J Obstet Gynaecol Br Commonw **81**:867, 1974.

Crawford JS: Experiences with epidural morphine in obstetrics. Anaesthesia **36**:207, 1981.

Crawford JS: Some maternal complications of epidural analgesia for labour. Anaesthesia **40**:1219, 1985.

Crawford JS, Burton M, Davies P: Anaesthesia for section: Further refinements of a technique. Br J Anaesth **45**:726, 1973.

Cross WG, Pitkin RM: Laminaria as adjunct in induction of labor. Obstet Gynecol **51**:606, 1978.

Cruikshank DP, White CA: Obstetric malpresentations: Twenty years' experience. Am J Obstet Gynecol **116**:1097, 1973.

Datta S, Alper MH: Anesthesia for cesarean section. Anesthesiology **53**:142, 1980.

Davidson AC, Weaver JB, Davies P, Pearson JF: Relation between ease of forceps delivery and speed of cervical dilation. Br J Obstet Gynaecol **83**:279, 1976.

D'Esopo DA: A review of cesarean section at Sloan Hospital for Women 1942–1947. Am J Obstet Gynecol **59**:77, 1950.

Dierker LJ Jr, Rosen MG, Thompson K, et al: The midforceps: Maternal and neonatal outcomes. Am J Obstet Gynecol **152**:176, 1985.

Dierker LJ Jr, Rosen MG, Thompson K, Lynn P: Midforceps deliveries: Long-term outcome of infants. Am J Obstet Gynecol **154**:764, 1986.

D'Souza SW, Black P, Macfarlane T, Richards B: The effect of oxytocin in induced labour on neonatal jaundice. Br J Obstet Gynaecol **86**:133, 1979.

Durfee RB: Low classical cesarean section. Postgrad Med **51**:219, 1972.

Dyson DC, Ferguson JE II, Hensleigh P: Antepartum external cephalic version under tocolysis. Obstet Gynecol **67**:63, 1986.

Eastman NJ: The role of Frontier America in the development of cesarean section. Am J Obstet Gynecol **24**:919, 1932.

Edwards RL, Nicholson HO: The management of the unstable lie in late pregnancy. J Obstet Gynaecol Br Commonw **76**:713, 1969.

Embry MP, Mollison BG: The unfavorable cervix and induction of labor using a cervical balloon. J Obstet Gynaecol Br Commonw **74**:44, 1967.

Evrard JR, Gold EM: Cesarean section and maternal mortality in Rhode Island: Incidence and risk factors 1965–1975. Obstet Gynecol **50**:594, 1977.

Federle MP, Cohen EA, Rosenwein MF, et al: Pelvimetry by digital radiography: a low-dose examination. Radiology **143**:733, 1982.

Flaksman RJ, Vollman JH, Benfield DG: Iatrogenic prematurity due to elective termination of the uncomplicated pregnancy: A major perinatal health care problem. Am J Obstet Gynecol **132**:885, 1978.

Floberg J, Belfrage P, Ohlsen H: Influence of pelvic outlet capacity on labor. A prospective pelvimetry study of 1429 unselected primiparas. Acta Obstet Gynecol Scand **66**:121, 1987.

Flowers CE: Shoulder presentation. Am J Obstet Gynecol **96**:145, 1966.

Flynn AM, Kelly J, Hollins G, Lynch PF: Ambulation in labor. Br Med J **2**:591, 1978.

Frank F: Suprasymphyseal delivery and its relation to other operations in the presence of contracted pelvis. Arch Gynaecol **81**:46, 1907.

Freeman DW, Arnold NI: Paracervical block with low doses of chloroprocaine. Fetal and maternal effects. JAMA **231**:56, 1975.

Freeman RK, Gutierrez NA, Ray ML, et al: Fetal cardiac response to paracervical block anesthesia. Part I. Obstet Gynecol **113**:583, 1972.

Friedman EA: Patterns of labor as indicators of risk. Clin Obstet Gynecol **16**:172, 1973.

Friedman EA: Labor: Clinical Evaluation and Management. 2nd ed. New York, Appleton-Century-Crofts, 1978.

Friedman EA, Sachtleben MR: Neonatal jaundice in association with oxytocin stimulation of labour and operative delivery. Br Med J **1**:198, 1976.

Friedman EA, Sachtleben MR, Wallace BA: Infant outcome following labor induction. Am J Obstet Gynecol **133**:718, 1979.

Friedman EA, Sachtleben-Murray MR, Dahrouge D: Long-term effects of labor and delivery on offspring: A match-pair analysis. Am J Obstet Gynecol **150**:941, 1984.

Frigoletto FD Jr, Ryan KJ, Phillippe M: Maternal mortality rate associated with cesarean section: An appraisal. Am J Obstet Gynecol **136**:969, 1980.

Ganstrom L, Ekman G, Malmstron A.: Insufficient remodelling of the uterine connective tissue in women with protracted labour. Br J Obstet Gynaecol **98**:1212, 1991.

Gerber AH: Accidental incision of the fetus during cesarean delivery. Int J Gynaecol Obstet **12**:46, 1974.

Gilstrap LC III, Hauth JC, Schiano S, Connor KD: Neonatal acidosis and method of delivery. Obstet Gynecol **63**:681, 1984.

Gjode P, Rasmussen TB, Jorgenson J: Feto-maternal bleeding during attempts at external version. Br J Obstet Gynaecol **87**:571, 1980.

Goddard WB: Fetal monitoring in a private hospital. Observations of fetal bradycardia following paracervical block anesthesia. Am J Obstet Gynecol **109**:1145, 1971.

Gonik B: Single- versus three-dose cefotaxime prophylaxis for cesarean section. Obstet Gynecol **65**:189, 1985.

Gonik B, Stringer CA, Held B: An alternate maneuver for management of shoulder dystocia. Am J Obstet Gynecol **145**:882, 1983.

Gordon AJ, Calder AA: Estradiol applied locally to ripen unfavorable cervix. Lancet **ii**:1319, 1977.

Graves WK: Breech delivery in twenty years of practice. Am J Obstet Gynecol **137**:229, 1980.

Green JE, McLedan F, Smith LP, Usher R: Has an increased cesarean section rate for term breech delivery reduced the incidence of birth asphyxia, trauma, and death? Am J Obstet Gynecol **142**:643, 1982.

Green SL, Sarubbi EA Jr: Risk factors associated with post cesarean section febrile morbidity. Obstet Gynecol **49**:686, 1977.

Grossman RA: Magnesium sulfate for uterine inversion. J Reprod Med **26**:261, 1981.

Hagadorn-Freathy AS, Yeomans ER, Hankins GDV: Validation of the 1988 ACOG forceps classification system. Obstet Gynecol **77**:356, 1991.

Halme J, Ekbladh L: The vacuum extractor for obstetric delivery. Clin Obstet Gynecol **25**:167, 1982.

Hanson H: Revival of the extraperitoneal cesarean section. Am J Obstet Gynecol **130**:102, 1978.

Haultain FWN: The treatment of chronic uterine inversion by abdominal hysterotomy with a successful case. Br Med J **2**:974, 1901.

Haverkamp AD, Orleans M, Langendoerfer S, et al: A controlled trial of the differential effects of intrapartum fetal monitoring. Am J Obstet Gynecol **134**:399, 1979.

Hellman LM, Prystowsky H: Duration of the second stage of labor. Am J Obstet Gynecol **63**:1223, 1952.

Hendricks CH: Uterine contractility at delivery and in the puerperium. Am J Obstet Gynecol **83**:890, 1962.

Hendricks CH, Brenner WE: Cardiovascular effects of oxytocic drugs used postpartum. Am J Obstet Gynecol **108**:751, 1970.

Hendricks CH, Brenner WE, Kraus G: The normal cervical dilatation pattern in late pregnancy and labor. Am J Obstet Gynecol **106**:1065, 1970.

Heritage CK, Cunningham MD: Association of elective repeat cesarean delivery and persistent pulmonary hypertension of the newborn. Am J Obstet Gynecol **152**:627, 1985.

Hester JD: Postpartum hemorrhage and re-evaluation of uterine packing. Obstet Gynecol **45**:501, 1975.

Hill JG, Eliot BW, Campbell AJ, Pickett-Heaps AA: Intensive care of the fetus in breech labor. Br J Obstet Gynaecol **83**:271, 1976.

Hughey MJ, McElin TW, Lussky R: Forceps operations in perspective. I. Midforceps rotation operations. J Reprod Med **20**:253, 1978.

Huntington JL: Acute inversion of the uterus. Boston Med Surg J **15**:376, 1921.

Huszar GM, Walsh MP: Relationship between myometrial and cervical functions in pregnancy and labor. Semin Perinatol **15**:97, 1991.

Johanson R, Pusey J, Livera N, et al: North Staffordshire/Wigan assisted delivery trial. Br J Obstet Gynaecol **96**:537, 1989.

Johnson AB: A new concept in the replacement of the inverted uterus and a report of nine cases. Am J Obstet Gynecol **57**:557, 1949.

Johnson IR, Macpherson MBA, Welch CC, Filstie GIM: A comparison of Lamicel and prostaglandin E2 vaginal gel for cervical ripening before induction of labor. Am J Obstet Gynecol **151**:604, 1985.

Johnson WL, Depp R, Hunter CA Jr: Comparison of spontaneous, oxytocin-stimulated and hypertonic saline-induced labor by different methods of record analysis. Am J Obstet Gynecol **107**:268, 1970.

Johnstone RW: William Smellie, The Master of British Midwifery. London, E & S Livingstone, 1952.

Joseph GF Jr, Steman CM, Robichaux AG: Vaginal birth after cesarean section: The impact of patient resistance to a trial of labor. Am J Obstet Gynecol **164**:1441, 1991.

Jouppila P, Kuikka J, Jouppila R, Hollmen A: Effect of induction of general anesthesia for cesarean section on intervillous blood flow. Acta Obstet Gynecol Scand **58**:249, 1979.

Jouppila R, Jouppila P, Kuikka J, Hollmen A: Placental blood flow during cesarean section under lumbar extradural anesthesia. Br J Anaesth **50**:275, 1978.

Kahn PK: Dystocia of the fetal shoulder. Intern Surg **45**:137, 1966.

Kazzi GM, Bottoms SF, Rosen MG: Efficacy and safety of laminaria digitata for preinduction cervical ripening of the cervix. Obstet Gynecol **60**:440, 1982.

Keettel WC: Inducing labor by rupturing membranes. Postgrad Med **44**:199, 1968.

Keirse JNC, van Oppen ACC: Preparing the cervix for induction of labour. *In* Chalmers I, Enkin M, Keirse MJNC (eds): Effective Care in Pregnancy and Childbirth. New York, Oxford University Press, 1989, p 988.

Kennell J, Klaus M, McGrath S, et al: Continuous emotional support during labor in a US Hospital. JAMA **265**:2197, 1991.

Kerr JMM: The technic of cesarean section with special reference to the lower uterine segment incision. Am J Obstet Gynecol **12**:729, 1926.

Klink EW: Perineal nerve block. An anatomic and clinical study in the female. Obstet Gynecol **1**:137, 1953.

Kopelman JN, Duff P, Karl RT, et al: Computed tomographic pelvimetry in the evaluation of breech presentation. Obstet Gynecol **68**:455, 1986.

Lamont RF, Neave S, Baker AC, Steer PJ: Intrauterine pressures in labours by amniotomy and oxytocin or vaginal prostaglandin gel compared with spontaneous labour. Br J Obstet Gynaecol **98**:441, 1991.

Lange AP, Westergaard JG, Secher NJ, Skovgard I: Neonatal jaundice after labor induced or stimulated by prostaglandin E2 or oxytocin. Lancet **1**:991, 1982.

Laube DW, Zlatnik FJ, Pitkin RM: Preinduction cervical ripening with prostglandin E2 intracervical gel. Obstet Gynecol **68**:54, 1986.

Ledger WJ: Management of postpartum cesarean section morbidity. Clin Obstet Gynecol **23**:621, 1980.

Leiberman JR, Piura B, Chaim W, Cohen A: The cervical balloon method for induction of labor. Acta Obstet Gynecol Scand **56**:499, 1977.

Leveno KJ, Quirk JG Jr, Cunningham FG, et al: Perioperative antimicrobials at cesarean section: Lavage versus three intravenous doses. Am J Obstet Gynecol **149**:463, 1984.

Liggins GC: Ripening of the cervix. Semin Perinatol **2**:261, 1978.

Liston WA, Campbell AJ: Dangers of oxytocin induced labor to fetuses. Br Med J **3**:606, 1974.

Lopez-Zeno JA, Peaceman AM, Adashek JA, et al: A controlled trial of a program for the active management of labor. N Engl J Med **326**:450, 1992.

Lysak SZ, Eisenach JC, Dobson CE II: Patient-controlled epidural analgesia during labor: a comparison of three solutiions with a continuous infusion control. Anesthesiology **72**:44, 1990.

McBride WG, Black BP, Brown CJ, et al: Method of delivery and developmental outcome at five years of age. Med J Aust **1**:301, 1979.

McCall JO Jr: Shoulder dystocia: A study of aftereffects. Am J Obstet Gynecol **83**:1486, 1962.

McCullagh WM III: Inversion of the uterus: A report of three cases and an analysis of 223 recently recorded cases. J Obstet Gynaecol Br Emp **32**:280, 1925.

McDonald JS, Bjorkman LL, Reed EC: Epidural analgesia for obstetrics: A maternal, fetal, and neonatal study. Am J Obstet Gynecol **120**:1055, 1974.

McIntosh DG, Rayburn WF: Patient-controlled analgesia in obstetrics and gynecology. Obstet Gynecol **78**:1129, 1991.

MacLennan AH, Green RC, Grant P, et al: Ripening of the human cervix and induction of labor with intracervical purified porcine relaxin. Obstet Gynecol **68**:598, 1986.

Madsen P, Olsen CE: Severe haemorrhage from the non-pregnant uterus as a result of cicatricial necrosis after cervical caesarian section. Acta Obstet Gynecol Scand **56**:535, 1977.

Maisels MJ, Rees R, Marks K, Friedman Z: Elective delivery of the term fetus: An obstetrical hazard. JAMA **238**:2036, 1977.

Malmström T: Vacuum extractor: An obstetrical instrument. Acta Obstet Gynecol Scand **33**(Suppl 4):1, 1954.

Marcus RG, Crewe-Brown H, Krawitz S, Katz J: Fetomaternal hemorrhage following successful and unsuccessful attempts at external version. Br J Obstet Gynaecol **82**:578, 1975.

Marx GF, Bassell GM: Hazards of the supine position in pregnancy. Clin Obstet Gynecol **9**:255, 1982.

Maryniak GM, Frank JB: Clinical assessment of the Kobayashi Vacuum extractor. Obstet Gynecol **64**:431, 1984.

Maymon R, Shulman A, Pomeranz M, et al: Uterine rupture at term pregnancy with the use of intracervical prostaglandin E2 gel for induction of labor. Am J Obstet Gynecol **165**:368, 1991.

Milner RDG: Neonatal mortality of breech deliveries with and without forceps to the aftercoming head. Br J Obstet Gynaecol **82**:783, 1975.

Mitchell MD, Flint APF, Bibby J, et al: Rapid increases in plasma prostaglandin concentrations after the vaginal examination and amniotomy. Br Med J **2**:1183, 1977.

Morgan MA, Thurnau GR: Efficacy of the fetal-pelvic index in patients requiring labor inductions. Am J Obstet Gynecol **159**:621, 1988a.

Morgan MA, Thurnau GR: Efficacy of the fetal-pelvic index for delivery of neonates weighing 4000 grams or greater: a preliminary report. Am J Obstet Gynecol **158**:1133, 1988b.

Morrison JC, Myatt RE, Martin JN Jr: External cephalic version of the breech presentation under tocolysis. Am J Obstet Gynecol **154**:900, 1986.

Munsick RA: Renal hemodynamic effects of oxytocin in antepartal and postpartal women. Am J Obstet Gynecol **108**:729, 1970.

Myers RE, Williams MV: Lost opportunities for the prevention of fetal asphyxia: Sedation, analgesia, and general anesthesia. Clin Obstet Gynaecol **9**:369, 1982.

O'Brien WF, Cefalo RC: Evaluation of x-ray pelvimetry and abnormal labor. Clin Obstet Gynecol **25**:157, 1982.

O'Driscoll K, Coughlan M, Fenton V, Skelly M: Active management of labor: Care of the fetus. Br Med J **2**:1451, 1977.

O'Driscoll K, Meagher D: Active Management of Labour. Philadelphia, WB Saunders Company, 1980.

O'Leary JL, O'Leary JA: Uterine artery ligation for control of postcesarean section hemorrhage. Obstet Gynecol **43**:849, 1974.

Ounsted C, Roberts JS, Gordon M, Milligan B: Fourth goal of perinatal medicine. Br Med J **284**:879, 1982.

Ounsted MK, Hendrick AM, Mutch LMM, et al: Induction of labour by different methods in primiparous women: Some perinatal and postnatal problems. Early Hum Dev **2**:227, 1978.

Paneth N, Kiely JL, Wallenstein S, et al: Newborn intensive care and neonatal mortality in low-birth-weight infants. A population study. N Engl J Med **307**:149, 1982.

Park RC, Duff WP: Role of cesarean hysterectomy in modern obstetric practice. Clin Obstet Gynecol 23:601, 1980.

Parsons MT, Spellacy WN: Prospective randomized study of x-ray pelvimetry in the primigravida. Obstet Gynecol 66:76, 1985.

Paul RH, Freeman RK: Fetal cardiac response to paracervical block anesthesia. Part II. Obstetric Gynecol 113:592, 1972.

Pearson JF, Davies P: The effect of continuous lumbar epidural analgesia on maternal acid-base balance and arterial lactate concentration during the second stage of labour. J Obstet Gynaecol Br Commonw 80:225, 1973.

Pelosi MA, Apuzzio J, Fricchione D, Gowda VV: The intra-abdominal version technique for delivery of transverse lie by low segment cesarean section. Am J Obstet Gynecol 136:1009, 1979.

Perkins RP: Role of extraperitoneal cesarean section. Clin Obstet Gynecol 23:583, 1980.

Philpott RH, Castle WM: Cervicographs in the management of labour in primigravidae. I. The alert line for detecting abnormal labor. J Obstet Gynaecol Br Commonw 79:592, 1972a.

Philpott RH, Castle WM: Cervicographs in the management of labour in primigravidae. II. The action line and treatment of abnormal labor. J Obstet Gynaecol Br Commonw 79:599, 1972b.

Pinkerton JHM, Martin DH, Thompson W: Selective planned induction in conditions of civil strife. Lancet I:197, 1975.

Piper EB, Bachman C: The prevention of fetal injuries in breech delivery. JAMA 92:217, 1929.

Potter MG, Heaton CH, Douglas GW: Intrinsic fetal risk in breech delivery. Obstet Gynecol 15:158, 1960.

Poulsen HK, Moller LK, Westergaard JG, et al: Open randomized comparison of prostaglandin E2 given by intracervical gel or vagitory for preinduction cervical ripening and induction of labor. Acta Obstet Gynecol Scand 70:549, 1991.

Pritchard JA: Changes in the blood volume during pregnancy and delivery. Anesthesiology 26:393, 1965.

Pritchard JA, MacDonald PC (eds): Williams' Obstetrics. 16th ed. New York, Appleton-Century-Crofts, 1980, p. 426.

Quinn MA, Murphy AJ: Fetal death following extraamniotic prostaglandin gel: Report of two cases. Br J Obstet Gynaecol 88:650, 1981.

Ralis ZA: Traumatizing effect of breech delivery on infants with spina bifida. J Pediatr 87:613, 1975.

Ralston DH, Shnider SM: The fetal and neonatal effects of regional anesthesia in obstetrics. Anesthesiology 48:34, 1978.

Read JA, Cotton DB, Miller FC: Placenta accreta: Changing clinical aspects and outcome. Obstet Gynecol 56:31, 1980.

Read JA, Miller FC, Paul RH: Randomized trial of ambulation versus oxytocin for labor enhancement: A preliminary report. Am J Obstet Gynecol 139:669, 1981.

Reisner LS: Anesthesia for cesarean section. Clin Obstet Gynecol 23:517, 1980.

Resnik R: Management of shoulder girdle dystocia. Clin Obstet Gynecol 23:559, 1980.

Romine JC, Clark RB, Brown WE: Lumbar epidural anaesthesia in labour and delivery: One year's experience. J Obstet Gynaecol Br Commonw 77:722, 1970.

Rosefsky JB, Petersiel ME: Perinatal deaths associated with mepivacaine paracervical-block anesthesia in labor. N Engl J Med 278:530, 1968.

Rosen MG (Chairman): Consensus Task Force on Cesarean Childbirth. NIH Publication No. 82–2067, 1981.

Rosen MG, Dickinson JC, Westhoff CL: Vaginal birth after cesarean: A meta-analysis of morbidity and mortality. Obstet Gynecol 77:465, 1991.

Rosenberg LS, Tejani NA, Varanasi M, et al: Preinduction ripening of the cervix with laminaria in the nulliparous patient. J Reprod Med 25:60, 1980.

Saravolatz LD, Lee C, Drukker B: Comparison of intravenous administration with intrauterine irrigation with ceforanide for nonelective cesarean section. Obstet Gynecol 66:513, 1985.

Sarno AP, Phelan JP, Ahn MO, et al: Vaginal birth after cesarean delivery. Trial of labor in women with breech presentation. J Reprod Med 34:831, 1989.

Schifrin BS: Fetal heartrate patterns following epidural anaesthesia and oxytocin infusion during labour. J Obstet Gynaecol Br Commonw 79:332, 1972.

Schreiner RL, Stevens DC, Smith WL, et al: Etiology of the respiratory distress following elective cesarean section. (Abstract #107) Pediatr Res 13:505, 1979.

Schreyer P, Sherman DJ, Ariely S, et al: Ripening the highly unfavorable cervix with extra-amniotic saline instillation or vaginal prostaglandin E2 application. Obstet Gynecol 73:938, 1989.

Scott DB, Sinclair CJ: Advances in regional anaesthesia and analgesia. Clin Obstet Gynaecol 9:273, 1982.

Scott JR: Mandatory trial of labor after cesarean delivery: an alternative viewpoint. Obstet Gynecol 77:881, 1991.

Scott PV, Bowen FE, Cartwright P, et al: Intrathecal morphine as sole analgesic during labour. Br Med J 2:351, 1980.

Seeds JW, Cefalo RC: Malpresentations. Clin Obstet Gynecol 25:145, 1982.

Seidman DS, Laor A, Gale R, et al: Long-term effects of vacuum and forceps deliveries. Lancet 337:1583, 1991.

Seigworth GR: Shoulder dystocia. Review of 5-year experience. Obstet Gynecol 28:764, 1966.

Seitchik J, Holden AEC, Castillo M: Amniotomy and oxytocin treatment of functional dystocia and route of delivery. Am J Obstet Gynecol 155:585, 1986.

Shepherd JH, Knuppel RA: The role of prostaglandins in ripening the cervix and inducing labor. Clin Perinatol 8:49, 1981.

Silbar EL: Factors related to the increasing cesarean section rates for cephalopelvic disproportion. Am J Obstet Gynecol 154:1095, 1986.

Sims DG, Neligan GA: Factors affecting the increasing incidence of severe nonhaemolytic neonatal jaundice. Br J Obstet Gynaecol 82:863, 1975.

Singh PM, Rodrigues C, Gupta AN: Placenta previa and previous cesarean section. Acta Obstet Gynecol 60:367, 1981.

Sosa R, Kennell J, Klaus M, et al: The effect of a supportive companion on perinatal problems, length of labor, and mother-infant interaction. N Engl J Med 303:597, 1980.

Steer CM (ed): Moloy's Evaluation of the Pelvis in Obstetrics. Philadelphia, WB Saunders Company, 1959.

Stevenson CS: The principal cause of breech presentation in single term pregnancies. Am J Obstet Gynecol 60:41, 1950.

Stine LC, Phelan JP, Wallace R, et al: Update on external cephalic version performed at term. Obstet Gynecol 65:642, 1985.

Strong TH, Phelan JP, Ahn MO, et al: Vaginal birth after cesarean delivery in twin gestation. Am J Obstet Gynecol 161:29, 1989.

Svancarik W, Chirino O, Schaefer G Jr, Blythe JG: Retropsoas and subgluteal abcesses following paracervical and pudendal anesthesia. JAMA 237:892, 1977.

Swan HJC: Balloon flotation catheters: Their use in hemodynamic monitoring in clinical practice. JAMA 233:865, 1975.

Swartz DP: Shoulder girdle dystocia in vertex delivery. Clinical study and review. Obstet Gynecol 15:194, 1960.

Swartz WH, Grolle K: The use of prophylactic antibiotics in cesarean section. A review of the literature. J Reprod Med 26:595, 1981.

Taffel SM, Placek PJ, Moien M, et al: 1989 U.S. cesarean section rate steadies—VBAC rate rises to nearly one in five. Birth 18:2, 1991.

Thomas WO: Manual removal of the placenta. Am J Obstet Gynecol 86:600, 1963.

Thorp JA, Boylan PC, Parisi VM, Hesline EP: Effects of high-dose oxytocin augmentation on umbilical cord blood gas values in primigravid women. Am J Obstet Gynecol 159:670, 1988.

Thurnau GR, Morgan MA: Efficacy of the fetal-pelvic index as a predictor of fetal-pelvic disproportion in women with abnormal labor patterns that require labor augmentation. Am J Obstet Gynecol 159:1168, 1988.

Thurnau GR, Scates DH, Morgan MA: The fetal-pelvic index: a method of identifying fetal-pelvic disproportion in women attempting vaginal birth after cesarean delivery. Am J Obstet Gynecol 165:353, 1991.

Todd WD, Steer CM: Term breech: Review of 1006 term breech deliveries. Obstet Gynecol 22:583, 1963.

Traub AI, Morrow RJ, Ritchie JWK, Dornan KJ: A continuing use of Kielland's forceps. Br J Obstet Gynaecol 91:894, 1984.

Tromans PM, Beazley JM, Shenouda PI: Comparative study of estradiol and prostaglandin E2 vaginal gel for ripening the unfavorable cervix before induction of labor. Br Med J 282:679, 1981.

Turner MJ, Brassil M, Gordon H: Active management of labor associated with a decrease in the cesarean section rate in nulliparas. Obstet Gynecol 71:150, 1988.

Tylleskär J, Finnstrom O, Leijon I, et al: Spontaneous labor and elective induction—a prospective randomized study. I. Effects on mother and fetus. Acta Obstet Gynecol Scand **58**:513, 1979.

Uldbjerg N, Ekman G, Malstrm A, et al: Biochemical and morphological changes in human cervix after local application of prostaglandin E2 in pregnancy. Lancet **1**:267, 1981.

Usher R, McLean F, Maughan GB: Respiratory distress syndrome in infants delivered by cesarean section. Am J Obstet Gynecol **88**:806, 1964.

Vaca A, Keirse MJNC: Instrumental vaginal delivery. *In* Chalmers I, Enkin M, Kierse MJNC (eds): Effective Care in Pregnancy and Childbirth. Oxford, Oxford University Press, 1989, pp 1216–1233.

Van Loon AJ, Mantinoh A, Thiun CJ, Mooyaart EL: Pelvimetry by magnetic resonance imaging in breech presentation. Am J Obstet Gynecol **163**:1256, 1990.

Watson P: Postpartum hemorrhage and shock. Clin Obstet Gynecol **23**:985, 1980.

Watson P, Besch N, Bowes WA Jr: Management of acute and subacute puerperal inversion of the uterus. Obstet Gynecol **55**:12, 1980.

Weisman AI: An antepartum study of fetal polarity and rotation. Am J Obstet Gynecol **48**:550, 1944.

Weissberg SM, O'Leary JA: Compound presentation of the fetus. Obstet Gynecol **41**:60, 1973.

Wenger DR, Gitchell RG: Severe infections following pudendal block anesthesia: Need for orthopedic awareness. J Bone Joint Surg **55**:202, 1973.

Willdeck-Lund G, Lindmark G, Nilsson BA: Effect of segmental epidural block on the course of labour and the condition of the infant during the neonatal period. Acta Anesthesiol Scand **23**:301, 1979.

Williams RL, Hawes WE: Cesarean section, fetal monitoring, and perinatal mortality in California. Am J Public Health **69**:864, 1979.

Williams RM, Thom MH, Studd JW: A study of the benefits and acceptability of ambulation in spontaneous labor. Br J Obstet Gynaecol **87**:122, 1980.

Wright RC: Reduction of perinatal mortality and morbidity in breech delivery through routine use of cesarean delivery. Obstet Gynecol **14**:758, 1959.

Yeh S, Huang X, Phelan JP: Postterm pregnancy after previous cesarean section. J Reprod Med **29**:41, 1984.

Yudkin P, Frumar AM, Anderson ABM, Turnbill AC: A retrospective study of induction of labour. Br J Obstet Gynaecol **86**:257, 1979.

Zalar RW, Quilligan EJ: The influence of scalp sampling on the cesarean section rate for fetal distress. Am J Obstet Gynecol **135**:239, 1979.

Zatuchni GI, Andros GJ: Prognostic index for vaginal delivery in breech presentation at term. Prospective study. Am J Obstet Gynecol **98**:854, 1967.

CHAPTER

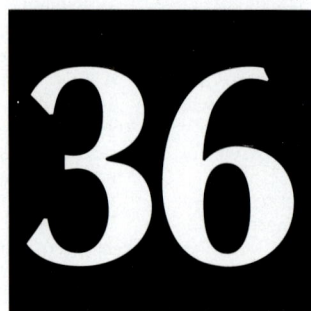

INTRAUTERINE GROWTH RESTRICTION

ROBERT K. CREASY, M.D., and ROBERT RESNIK, M.D.

Human pregnancy, similar to pregnancy in other polytocous animal species, may be affected by conditions that restrict the normal growth of the fetus. The growth-restricted fetus is at higher risk for perinatal morbidity and mortality, the risk rising with the severity of the growth restriction. This chapter reviews the various etiologies of fetal growth restriction and considers the methods of antepartum recognition and diagnosis along with clinical management. The term intrauterine growth restriction is preferred over intrauterine growth retardation, which frequently connotes mental retardation to the patient.

DEFINITIONS

The World Health Organization (1969) classifies all newborns weighing less than 2500 gm as having low birth weight. In the past, these infants were classified as premature, but it is now recognized that all low-birth-weight babies are not necessarily born before 37 completed weeks, or preterm. Many low-birth-weight babies are born near term, having sustained intrauterine growth restriction (IUGR). Low-birth-weight infants have traditionally been placed in one of the following three classifications (Battaglia, 1970; Yerushalmy, 1970):

1. Newborns delivered before 37 completed weeks gestation who are appropriate size for gestational age (AGA): preterm neonate.

2. Newborns delivered before 37 completed weeks gestation who are small for gestational age (SGA): preterm and growth-restricted neonate.

3. Newborns delivered after 37 completed weeks gestation who are small for gestational age (SGA): term growth-restricted neonate.

The combined use of gestational age and birth size assists in differentiating the specific problems of preterm birth and fetal growth restriction. Another clinical classification, that of asymmetric or symmetric growth restriction, is discussed later in this section.

The diagnosis of IUGR is in part dependent upon an accurate evaluation of gestational age. The last menstrual period is a reliable index of gestational age if the mother is seen early in gestation, unless there is a history of irregular menstrual cycles or conception occurred soon after discontinuation of oral contraceptives. As IUGR, particularly asymmetric IUGR, is rarely detected clinically prior to 22 to 24 weeks, uterine size should equate with gestational age up to that time (Murphy, 1969). Ultrasonographic evaluation is particularly useful in dating pregnancies if performed before biologic variation begins to have a significant impact, i.e., before 22 weeks gestation (see Chapter 14). Methods are also available to date the gestation retrospectively by physical and neurologic examination of the newborn (Dubowitz et al., 1970). Such methods rely on the development of various physical characteristics and responses throughout the latter part of gestation. Unfortunately, the usefulness of these characteristics for growth-restricted fetuses has not yet been verified. It is possible that the appearance of these various milestones of growth and maturation can be delayed or accelerated with different types of IUGR. For instance, skeletal maturation is also delayed with severe growth restriction (Roord et al., 1978). In a small series, fetal cerebellar growth has been reported to be unaffected by fetal growth restriction (Reece et al., 1987).

Different standards for fetal growth throughout gestation have been reported. These standards set the normal range, on the basis of statistical considerations, between two standard deviations of the mean (2.5th to 97.5th percentile) or between the tenth and 90th percentiles for fixed gestational ages. The standards most widely used in the United States in the 1960s and 1970s were those developed in Denver, Colorado (Lubchenco et al., 1966; Battaglia and Lubchenco, 1967). The Denver standards do not, however, reflect the increase in median birth weights that has occurred over the last two decades or the birth weight standards for babies born at sea level. More contemporary standards are available from large geographic regions such as the State of California, based on data from over 2 million singleton births between 1970 and 1976 (Williams et al., 1982), and from Canada, based upon over one million singleton births and over 10,000 twin gestations between 1986 and 1988 (Arbuckle et al., 1993) (Fig. 36–1). Comparison of the 1986–1988 Canadian data with data from births in Canada in 1970–1972 reveals less than 100 gm difference at the 10th percentile prior to 36 weeks, but approximately 150 to 200 gm greater weights at the 10th percentile from the latter time period (Fig 36–1). Comparison of the recent Canadian data and the California data at the 10th percentile reveals approximately 150 gm greater weights in Canada prior to 34 weeks and only 100 gm greater weights after that time. The California data are within 100 gm of recent data from Alabama in 1984–1986 at the 10th percentile (Goldenberg et al., 1989).

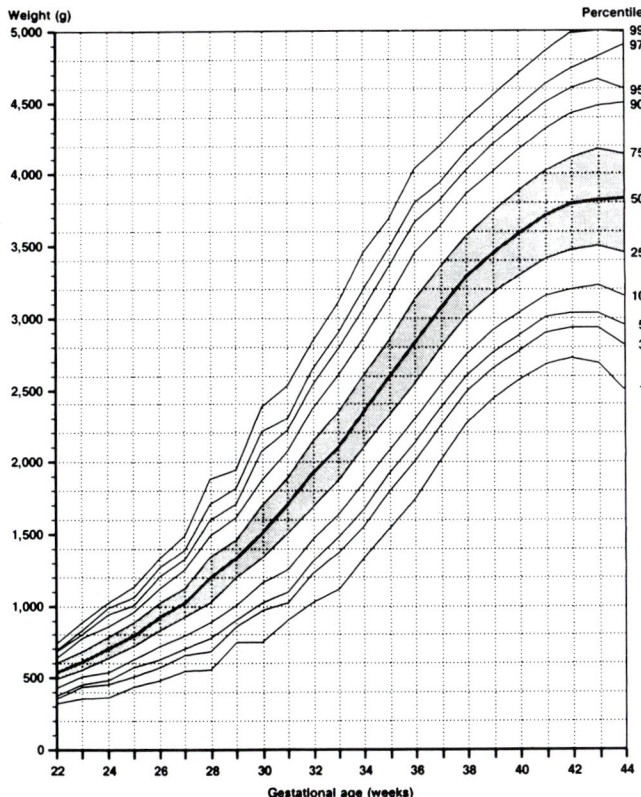

FIGURE 36–1. Birth weight percentiles for male singleton live births, Canada 1986–1988. (From Arbuckle TE, Wilkins R, Sherman GT: Birth weight percentiles by gestational age in Canada. Obstet Gynecol **81**:39, 1993. Reprinted with permission from the American College of Obstetricians and Gynecologists.)

The tenth percentile for the data from Denver approximates that from other sites up to 30 to 32 weeks. It would seem that different population standards are in close proximity prior to 30 to 32 weeks of pregnancy, but after that time fetal environmental issues affect these standards. In addition, there appears to have been a probable small but definite increase in birth weights at the 10th percentile over the last two decades.

The reliance on only gestational age and birth weight neglects the issue of body size and length and the clinical observations that there are two main clinical types of IUGR infants: the infant who is of normal length for gestational age but whose weight is below normal (asymmetrically small), and the infant whose length and weight are both below normal (symmetrically small). One method used to evaluate this issue is the ponderal index, calculated by the formula:

$$\frac{birth\ weight\ (gm)}{crown\text{-}heel\ length\ (cm)^3} \times 100$$

(Miller and Hassanein, 1971; Daikoku et al., 1979). Infants with a ponderal index of less than the tenth percentile for gestational age or a crown-rump length less than the third percentile are defined as growth-restricted. This index in term infants is not affected significantly by differences in race or sex. The disadvantage of this index is the potential error introduced by cubing the length. At present, it is not clear whether the asymmetric IUGR and symmetric IUGR are two distinct entities or are merely reflections of the severity of the growth restriction process (chromosomal aberrations and infectious disease being excluded).

It is also important to recognize that there is currently no acceptable means, except perhaps by the ponderal index, to classify a newborn as having IUGR whose weight is more than 2500 gm. The newborn who weighs 2800 gm at birth may be growth restricted if the mother has had three previous infants weighing greater than 3700 gm, but the classification systems would place such an infant in the normal growth category (see review, Brar and Rutherford, 1988).

RATE OF FETAL GROWTH

Data obtained from study of induced abortions and spontaneous deliveries indicate that the rate of fetal growth increases from 5 gm a day at 14 to 15 weeks gestation to 10 gm a day at 20 weeks, and to 30 to 35 gm a day at 32 to 34 weeks. Thus, the substrate needs of the fetus are relatively small in the first half of pregnancy, after which the rate of weight gain rises precipitously. The mean rate peaks at approximately 230 gm/week at 33 to 36 weeks gestation, after which it decreases, reaching zero weight gain, or even weight loss, at 41 to 42 weeks gestation (Fig. 36–2) (Williams et al., 1982). However, if growth rate is expressed as the percentage of increase in weight over the previous week, the maximum percentage of increase occurs in the first trimester and steadily decreases thereafter.

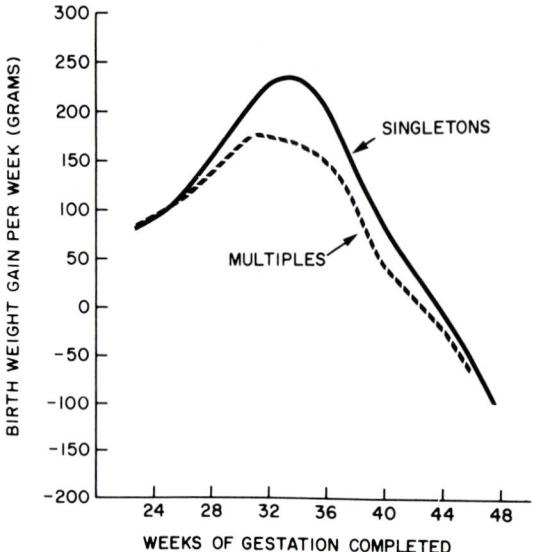

FIGURE 36–2. Median growth rate curves for single and multiple births in California, 1970–1976. (From Williams RL, Creasy RK, Cunningham GC, et al: Fetal growth and perinatal viability in California. Obstet Gynecol **59**:624, 1982. Reprinted with permission from the American College of Obstetricians and Gynecologists.)

INCIDENCE OF INTRAUTERINE GROWTH RESTRICTION

The incidence of IUGR varies depending on the population under examination, the geographic location, and the standard growth curves used as reference. In general, approximately one-third of all infants weighing less than 2500 gm at birth have sustained IUGR, and approximately 4 to 8 per cent of all infants born in developed countries, and 6 to 30 per cent in developing countries, are classified as growth-restricted (Gruenwald, 1963; Scott and Usher, 1966; Lugo and Cassady, 1971; Galbraith et al., 1979; Kramer, 1987).

PERINATAL MORTALITY AND MORBIDITY OF IUGR

IUGR is associated with an increase in fetal and neonatal mortality and morbidity rates. Reports from the mid-1960s revealed the stillbirth rate to be doubled in those fetuses 15 to 25 per cent under mean birth weight for gestational age and to have increased eightfold in those 25 per cent or more underweight (below the 2.5th percentile); in those fetuses 40 per cent or more underweight, there was only a 50 per cent chance of survival (Scott and Usher, 1966). The neonatal mortality rate was increased tenfold in neonates who were below the 2.5th percentile, but only minimally increased in those between the 2.5th and tenth percentiles. Reports in the early 1980s indicated that despite overall advances in the preceding decade in perinatal medicine, the perinatal mortality rate was still higher when IUGR was present. Infants weighing between 1500 and 2500 gm near term (38 to 42 weeks) had a perinatal mortality rate five to 30 times that of

infants between the tenth and 50th percentiles, and in infants weighing less than 1500 gm near term, the perinatal mortality rate was increased 70 to 100 times (Williams et al., 1982). With birth weights below the tenth percentile, the fetal mortality rate increases as gestation advances if the birth weight does not increase. For instance, the fetal mortality rate for an infant weighing 1250 gm born at 38 weeks is greater than that of an infant of the same weight born at 32 weeks. In general, fetal mortality rates are 50 per cent again higher than neonatal rates, and male fetuses with IUGR have a higher mortality rate than female fetuses. The 10 to 30 per cent increase in incidence of minor and major congenital anomalies associated with IUGR accounts for 30 to 60 per cent of the IUGR perinatal deaths (50 per cent of stillbirths and 20 per cent of neonatal deaths) (Scott and Usher, 1966; Ounsted et al., 1981). Infants with symmetric IUGR are more likely to die in association with anomalous development or infection. The incidence of mortality in the preterm newborn is higher if IUGR is also present (Teberg et al., 1988). The incidence of intrapartum fetal distress approximates 40 to 50 per cent (Low et al., 1972; Lin et al., 1991), with morbidity events tending to be higher in the symmetrically growth restricted fetus. Specific morbidities are discussed later and in Chapter 63.

ETIOLOGY OF INTRAUTERINE GROWTH RESTRICTION

Genetic Factors

There has been a great deal of interest in determining the relative contribution of factors that produce birth weight variation, namely the maternal and fetal genetic factors and the environment of the fetus. It is estimated that approximately 40 per cent of total birth weight variation is due to the genetic contributions from mother and fetus, approximately half in each, and the remaining 60 per cent from the fetal environment (Penrose, 1961; Polani, 1974).

Although both parents' genes affect childhood growth and final adult size, the maternal genes have the main influence on birth weight. The classic horse-pony crossbreeding experiments demonstrated the important role of the mother (Walton and Hammond, 1938). Foals of the maternal horse and paternal pony are significantly larger than foals of the maternal pony and paternal horse, and foals of each cross are comparable in size to foals of the pure maternal breed. These results clearly demonstrate the maternally related constraint on fetal growth. Similar conclusions are reached from family studies in humans. Low and high birth weights recur in families with seemingly normal pregnancies. Sisters of women with IUGR babies tend to have IUGR babies, a trend that is not seen in their brothers' babies (Johnstone and Inglis, 1974). There is also a greater similarity in birth weights of infants of maternal half siblings and full siblings than of paternal half siblings and full siblings (Morton, 1955). It has also been observed that mothers of IUGR infants frequently were growth-restricted at birth themselves (Ounsted and Ounsted, 1966). Although there is some evidence that the maternal phenotypic expression is a factor affecting fetal growth, in particular maternal height, the evidence for such an influence is not convincing.

The one definite paternal influence on fetal growth and size at birth is through the contribution of a Y chromosome rather than an X chromosome. The male fetus grows faster than the female fetus and weighs approximately 150 to 200 gm more than the female at birth (Karn and Penrose, 1951; Thomson et al., 1968). It has also been demonstrated that the greater the antigenic dissimilarity between parents, the larger the fetus.

Specific maternal genotypic disorders can cause IUGR, an example of which is phenylketonuria (Saugstad, 1972). Infants born to homozygously affected mothers almost always have IUGR, but whether the reason is an abnormal amount of metabolite crossing from mother to fetus or an inherent problem in the fetus is unknown.

There is a significant association between IUGR and congenital malformations. Such abnormalities may be due to established chromosomal disorders or to various dysmorphic syndromes, such as various forms of dwarfism. Some of these are the expression of a specific gene abnormality with a known inheritance pattern, and others are only presumed to be the result of a gene mutation or an adverse environmental influence.

Birth weights and lengths in 21-trisomic infants are below normal (Chen et al., 1972; Peuschel et al., 1976). The frequency distribution of birth weights in 21-trisomic infants is shifted to the left of the normal curve after 34 weeks gestation, resulting in gestational ages 1 to 1.5 weeks less than normal, and birth weights and lengths are less than controls from 34 weeks until term. This effect is more marked after 37 weeks gestation, but birth weights are still only approximately one standard deviation from mean weight. Birth weights in translocation trisomy 21 are comparable to those in primary trisomy 21. Birth weights of newborns who are mosaic for normal and 21-trisomic cells are lower than normal but higher than those of 21-trisomic infants (Polani, 1974). Newborns with trisomy 13 and trisomy 18 also have below-normal birth weights, the 18-trisomics frequently having IUGR and associated mental retardation (Chen et al., 1972). Although only 2 to 5 per cent of IUGR infants have a chromosomal abnormality, the incidence rises to 20 per cent if IUGR and mental retardation are both present (Chen et al., 1970; Anderson, 1976). Placental weights of 21-trisomic infants are similar to those of a control group, but those of 13- and 18-trisomics are reduced. Newborns with other autosomal abnormalities such as deletions (numbers 4, 5, 13, and 18) and ring chromosome structure alterations also have impaired fetal growth.

Although abnormalities of the female (X) and male (Y) sex chromosomes are frequently lethal—80 to 95 per cent result in first-trimester spontaneous abortions—they may be the cause of IUGR in a newborn (Polani, 1974). Infants with XO sex chromosomes have a lower mean birth weight than control infants (approximately 85 per cent of normal for gestational age) and are approximately 1.5 cm shorter at birth. Mosaics of 45,X and 46,XX cells are affected to a lesser degree. Although a paucity of reports prevents definite conclusions at present, it would appear that the repressive effect on fetal growth is increased with the addition of X chromosomes, each of which results in a 200- to 300-gm lowering of birth weight (Barlow, 1973).

There are numerous other dysmorphic syndromes, particularly those causing abnormal brain development, with which intrauterine growth restriction is associated (see Chapter 1).

The overall contribution that chromosomal and other genetic disorders make to human IUGR is estimated to be 5 to 15 per cent. Approximately 25 per cent of fetuses with early-onset fetal growth restriction, or symmetric IUGR may have chromosomal abnormalities, and karyotyping via cordocentesis may be considered (Weiner and Williamson, 1989). A genetic basis should be strongly considered when IUGR is encountered with associated neurologic impairment (Hill, 1978).

Infection

Infectious disease is known to cause IUGR, but the number of organisms with this effect is poorly defined. There is sufficient evidence for a causal relationship between IUGR and infectious disease for only two viruses, rubella and cytomegalovirus, and for a possible relationship with varicella-zoster and human immunodeficiency virus (Klein and Remington, 1990) (see Chapters 42 and 43). With rubella infection, the infected cells usually remain viable for many months. IUGR is thought to arise as a result of capillary endothelial damage during organogenesis, resulting in a decreased number of cells that have a cytoplasmic mass that is within normal range (Alford, 1976). In rubella-infected newborns, growth of the adrenals and thymus is particularly limited, and brain growth tends to be more restricted than in IUGR associated with poor uteroplacental perfusion. Cytomegalovirus infection results in cytolysis and localized necrosis within the fetus. Affected newborns have various organs of subnormal size, owing mainly to a decrease in cell number, unlike those with IUGR resulting from maternal vascular disease (Naeye, 1967). The growth rate of various individual fetal organs is altered in an unpredictable fashion by cytomegalovirus.

As of this writing, there are no bacteria known to cause IUGR. Protozoan infections due to *Toxoplasma gondii*, *Plasmodium*, or *Trypanosoma cruzi* can also cause IUGR (Klein and Remington, 1990).

Although the incidence of maternal infections with various organisms may be as high as 15 per cent, the incidence of congenital infections is estimated to be no more than 5 per cent. It is currently believed that infectious disease can account for no more than 5 to 10 per cent of human IUGR.

Fetal Cardiovascular Anomalies

Newborns with cardiac malformations are frequently of low birth weight and length for gestation, with the possible exception of those with tetralogy of Fallot and transposition of the great vessels (Richards et al., 1955). The subnormal size of many infants with cardiac anomalies (as low as 50 to 80 per cent of normal weight with septal defects) is associated with a subnormal number of parenchymal cells in organs such as the spleen, liver, kidneys, adrenals, and pancreas (Naeye, 1965a). The thymus is minimally affected, except in IUGR secondary to altered uteroplacental perfusion. The basis of IUGR in congenital cardiac malformations would appear to be abnormal hemodynamics. This explanation is not completely satisfactory, however, because anomalies that appear to be compatible with a normal fetal circulation, such as atrial septal defects, are more likely to be associated with low birth weight than are anomalies that usually alter the systemic fetal circulation, such as transposition of the great vessels.

Approximately 25 per cent of newborns with a single umbilical artery weigh less than 2500 gm at birth and some of these are born preterm (Froehlich and Fujikura, 1966). Twin-twin transfusion secondary to vascular anastomoses in monochorionic-monozygotic twins frequently results in IUGR of one twin, usually the donor (see Chapters 37 and 38). Abnormal umbilical cord insertions into the placenta are also occasionally associated with poor fetal growth (Shanklin, 1970).

Congenital heart disease, single umbilical artery, and monozygotic twins are relatively rare and probably account for no more than 1 to 2 per cent of all human IUGR.

Multiple Gestation

Multiple pregnancies are associated with a high progressive decrease in fetal and placental weight as the number of offspring increases in humans and various animal species (Barcroft and Kennedy, 1939; McKeown and Record, 1952). In both singleton and twin gestations there is a relationship between total fetal mass and maternal mass. The increase in fetal weight in singleton gestations is linear from approximately 22 to 24 weeks until approximately 34 to 38 weeks (Gruenwald, 1966; Williams et al., 1982). During the last weeks of pregnancy, the increase in fetal weight declines, actually becoming negative after 42 weeks in some pregnancies. If nutrition is adequate in the neonatal period, the slope of the increase in neonatal weight parallels the increase in fetal weight seen before 34 to 38 weeks. The decline in fetal weight increase has been reported to occur when the total fetal mass approximates 3000 to 3500 gm for either singleton or twin gestations. When growth rate is expressed incrementally, it is evident that the weekly gain in singletons peaks at approximately 220 to 240 gm/week at 34 weeks of gestation (see Fig. 36–2). In individual twin fetuses, the incremental weekly gain peaks at 160 to 170 gm/week at 28 to 32 weeks gestation (Williams et al., 1982).

More recent studies in triplets indicate that growth of individual triplets may continue in a linear fashion well beyond a total combined weight of 3500 gm (Jones et al., 1991). However, others have reported that prior to 35 weeks triplets grow at about the 30th percentile for singletons, and by 38 weeks the average weight of each triplet is at the tenth percentile (Elster et al., 1991).

The decrease in weight of twin fetuses, frequently with mild IUGR, is usually due to decreased cell size, the exception being severe IUGR associated with monozygocity and vascular anastomoses, wherein cell number may also be decreased (Naeye, 1965b; Naeye et al., 1966). These changes in twins are similar to those seen in IUGR secondary to poor uterine perfusion or maternal malnutrition. Twins with mild IUGR have an acceleration of growth after birth, so that their weight equals the median weight of singletons by one year of age. This observation supports the thesis that the etiology of poor fetal growth in twin gestations is an inability of the environment to meet fetal needs, rather than an inherent diminished growth capacity of the twin fetus. The example of twin fetuses supports the thesis derived from normal singleton pregnancies that the human fetus seldom is able to express its full potential for growth. Any one of the components of the environment may limit fetal growth, as described in the following sections. The incidence of IUGR in twins is 15 to 25 per cent (Houlton et al., 1981; Secher et al., 1985; Arbuckle et al., 1993), and as the incidence of multiple gestations is less than 1 per cent, these pregnancies probably account for less than 3 per cent of all human IUGR.

Inadequate Maternal Nutrition

Numerous animal studies have demonstrated that undernutrition of the mother due to protein or caloric restriction can adversely affect fetal growth (Brasel and Winick, 1972; Dobbing, 1970). Direct extrapolation of information from experiments using small animals, in which the fetal-to-maternal mass is much greater than in human pregnancy and the fetal/neonatal growth rate reaches its maximum after birth, must be done with caution. Such animal studies, however, have engendered important concepts. Winick (1971) has reported that there are three phases of fetal growth: cellular hyperplasia, followed by both hyperplasia and hypertrophy, and then predominantly hypertrophy. Thus, if there is a decrease in available substrate, the timing of the decrease will be reflected in the type of IUGR that is observed. If the insult occurs early in pregnancy, the fetus is likely to be born with a decrease in cell number and cell size, such as might be observed with severe chronic maternal undernutrition or an inability to increase uteroplacental blood flow during gestation. However, if the insult occurs late in gestation, such as with twin gestation, the fetus is likely to have a normal cell number but a restriction of cell size, which can be returned to normal with adequate postnatal nutrition.

The importance that maternal nutrition has in fetal growth and birth weight has been demonstrated by studies in Russia and Holland, where women, unfortunately, suffered inadequate nutrition during World War II. The population in Leningrad underwent a prolonged period of poor nutrition, and so preconceptual nutritional status as well as gestational nutrition was poor, and birth weights were reduced by 400 to 600 gm (Antonov, 1947). In Holland, there was a famine for approximately 6 months, thus permitting an evaluation of the effect of malnutrition during each of the trimesters of pregnancy in a group of women previously well nourished (Stein and Susser, 1975a). Birth weights declined approximately 10 per cent, and placental weights 15 per cent, only when undernutrition occurred in the third trimester with caloric intake below 1500 gm. The difference in severity of the IUGR in these two populations suggests the importance of pre-pregnancy nutritional status, an idea that has been substantiated (Love and Kinch, 1965; Kramer, 1987; Abrams and Newman, 1991). The more recent studies clearly show that inadequate weight gain in pregnancy (defined as less than 0.27 kg/week, or less than 10 kg at 40 weeks, or based upon suggested weight gain for body mass indices [see Chapter 11]) is associated with an increased risk of IUGR.

At present, it is still unclear whether generalized caloric intake reduction or specific substrate limitation such as protein or key mineral restriction, or both, are important in producing IUGR (see Chapter 11). Decreases in zinc content of peripheral blood leukocytes have been reported to correlate positively with IUGR (Meadows et al., 1981; Wells et al., 1987), and serum zinc concentrations of less than 60 μg/dl in the third trimester are associated with a fivefold increase in low-birth-weight newborns (Neggers et al., 1991). Similarly, an association between low serum folate levels and IUGR has been reported (Goldenberg et al., 1992a). Although there is no convincing evidence that high-protein supplementation is beneficial (Stein et al., 1978; Rush et al., 1980), caloric supplementation can improve birth weights by 50 to 225 gm, the largest increase being demonstrated when the net energy increment exceeds 430 kcal/day in an otherwise poorly nourished population (Prentice et al., 1983). However, Warshaw (1985) has pointed out that, in a fetus receiving decreased oxygen delivery due to decreased uteroplacental perfusion and which has adapted by slowing metabolism and growth, it may not be advisable to increase substrate delivery. This important question remains open.

As maternal body mass and plasma volume are correlated, it has been shown that reduced plasma volume or prevention of plasma volume expansion may lead to decreased cardiac output and uterine perfusion and a resultant decrease in fetal growth (Daniel et al., 1989; Rosso et al., 1992).

Another maternal nutrient that may be important to fetal growth is oxygen. The median birth weight of infants of women living more than 10,000 feet above sea level is approximately 250 gm less than that of infants of women living at sea level (Lichty et al., 1957). This difference may not be simply an effect of maternal hypoxemia, however, because women living at high altitudes usually have greater oxygen-carrying capacity. Also, placental weight is higher in relation to birth weight at high altitudes than at sea level (Kruger and Arias-Stella, 1970). Pregnancies complicated by maternal cyanotic heart disease usually result in IUGR, but it is unclear whether abnormal maternal hemodynamics or the reduction in oxygen saturation, by approximately 40 per cent in the umbilical vein, may account for poor fetal growth (Novy et al., 1968). The association between hemoglobinopathies and IUGR may be due to a decrease in either blood viscosity or fetal oxygenation (Pritchard et al., 1973). Patients with chronic pulmonary disease, such as poorly controlled asthma, cystic fibrosis, or bronchiectasis, or those with severe kyphoscoliosis may be at increased risk (Palmer et al., 1983; Kopenhager, 1977; Thaler et al., 1986).

Placental Factors

Although size of the placenta does not of necessity equate with function, our inability to evaluate human placental function properly has resulted in studies of the interrelationships of size, morphometry, and clinical outcome. In general, the birth weight increases with increasing placental weight in both animals and humans (Dawes, 1968; Aherne, 1966). IUGR without other anomalies is usually associated with a small placenta. A small placenta is not always associated with an IUGR newborn, but the large infant from an otherwise normal pregnancy does not have a small placenta. Placental weight increases throughout normal gestation, whereas in IUGR pregnancy, the placental weight plateaus after 36 weeks or earlier, and the placenta (after being trimmed of the membranes and cord) weighs less than 350 gm (Molteni et al., 1978). As normal gestation advances, there is a greater increase in fetal weight than in placental weight. Thus, there is an increase in the fetal-placental weight ratio in large-for-gestational-age (LGA), appropriate-for-gestational-age (AGA), and small-for-gestational-age (SGA) infants in the last half of gestation. In all three categories, when the ratio is greater than 10, there is an increased incidence of depressed newborns, suggesting that it is not only the IUGR fetus that may outgrow the capacity of the placenta to effect adequate transfer of necessary nutrients.

The villous surface area and the capillary surface area increase as normal gestation advances (Aherne and Dunnill, 1966). It is not known whether the relative villous surface area available for exchange can keep up with the metabolic needs of the enlarging fetus (Baur, 1977), but because the capillary vessels are closer to the periphery of the villi, the efficiency per unit may be improved as gestation progresses (Aherne, 1975). In placentas of IUGR babies, the mean surface area and the capillary surface area are reduced, implying a diminished diffusing capacity (Aherne and Dunnill, 1966). Cytotrophoblastic hyperplasia, thickening of the basement membrane, placental infarction, and chorionic villitis are commonly present in placentas from pregnancies complicated by maternal vascular disease and IUGR (Fox, 1964, 1967; Salafia et al., 1992).

Although it is reasonable to infer functional capacity from morphometry studies, and perhaps from ultrasound investigations (see Chapter 14), one must remember that relative physiologic investigations have not been performed in human gestations. It is useful to an understanding of basic mechanisms to know that urea permeability is proportional to placental size in sheep (Kulhanek et al., 1974), but we do not know how this finding relates to human placental function in the normal or IUGR-associated placenta. Recent information from cordocentesis studies reveals a decrease in α-aminonitrogen, particularly branched-chain amino acids, in plasma of the IUGR fetus, but it is not known whether this is causally related or consequent to the IUGR (Cetin et al., 1990).

Placental hemangiomas of the circumvallate placental anomaly may also reduce the area for nutrient transfer, but this disorder accounts for less than 1 per cent of IUGR (Shanklin, 1970). As the placenta has its own metabolic needs and is interposed between fetus and mother, a large placenta could theoretically cause IUGR. With severe maternal undernutrition, placental weight is reduced more than fetal weight, and when normal maternal nutrition resumes, placental weight recovers before fetal weight (Stein and Susser, 1975b). However, most evidence indicates that the larger the placenta, the larger the fetus.

Uterine-Placental Perfusion

Substantial evidence from experimental animal studies suggests that alterations in uteroplacental perfusion affect both the growth and the status of the placenta as well as the fetus. Ligation of the uterine artery of one horn of the pregnant rat results in IUGR of those fetuses nearest the constriction (Wigglesworth, 1964). Fetal and placental weights in guinea pigs, mice, and rabbits are lowest in the middle of each uterine horn, where arterial perfusion is lowest (Dawes, 1968; Duncan, 1969). Repetitive embolization of the uterine vascular bed during the last one-fourth of gestation in the sheep gives rise to localized hyalinization and fibrinoid changes in the placenta (Creasy et al., 1972) and results in a 40 per cent reduction in placental weight and alterations in organ growth patterns similar to those observed in IUGR fetuses from pregnancies complicated by maternal hypertensive disease. In addition, umbilical blood flow is reduced, and fetal oxidative metabolism is decreased (Creasy et al., 1972; Clapp et al., 1980, 1981). Doppler umbilical artery flow-velocity wave-form studies also indicate a reduction of umbilical blood flow in some human IUGR (Trudinger, 1987) (see Chapter 16).

That uteroplacental blood flow is decreased in pregnancies complicated by maternal hypertensive disease has been strongly suggested by results of various studies. The clearance of radioactive sodium, or xenon, from the intervillous space is reduced in preeclamptic patients (Browne and Veall, 1953; Dixon et al., 1963; Kaar et al., 1980). Obstructive arterionecrosis, which can result in local ischemia of villi, is frequently seen in histologic examination of the implantation site in pregnancies complicated by preeclampsia and IUGR (Dixon and Robertson, 1961; Brosens et al., 1977). Similar obstructive lesions are not present in normotensive IUGR pregnancies, although there is frequently a reduction of the normal endovascular migration of trophoblast in such pregnancies, suggesting that even without hypertension the vascular response

at the implantation site is altered in some cases of IUGR (Robertson et al., 1976). The etiology of the cytotrophoblastic proliferation and placental infarction described is not known, but these changes are generally related to ischemia and vascular disease. Uteroplacental flow-velocity wave-form studies using Doppler methods, in pregnancies complicated by hypertension, have shown a higher incidence of IUGR in those pregnancies in which abnormal wave-forms were recorded. These are thought to reflect abnormally increased resistance to blood flow (Campbell et al., 1987; Fleischer et al., 1986). High-resistance hypertension is associated with a marked decrease in fetal weight in comparison to low-resistance hypertension (Easterling et al., 1991). Increasing uteroplacental resistance, recorded with this methodology, has been positively correlated with fetal hypoxemia as determined by cordocentesis in IUGR fetuses (Soothill et al., 1986).

There are only fragmentary suggestions relating abnormal maternal vascular anatomy and IUGR. Intrauterine growth restriction may occur at a higher frequency when the pregnancy is in a unicornuate uterus, in which vascular abnormalities are likely but unproven (Andrews and Jones, 1982). Patients with two (rather than the usual one) ascending uterine arteries on each side of the uterus have a higher rate of IUGR (Burchell et al., 1978). However, pregnancy after bilateral ligation of the internal iliac and ovarian arteries is not associated with IUGR (Mengert et al., 1969; Shinagawa et al., 1981).

As exercise might affect uterine perfusion, this has been extensively studied, and the effect has been quite variable (Hall and Kaufman, 1987; Clapp and Capeless, 1990; Clapp et al., 1992). If there is an adverse effect it would appear to occur at high levels of exercise (more than 50 per cent of pre-pregnancy levels) and mainly result in a decrease in neonatal fat mass.

Recurrent antepartum hemorrhage from either premature separation of the placenta or placenta previa is associated with an increased incidence of IUGR (Hibbard and Jeffcoate, 1966; Varma, 1973) (see Chapter 39).

Clinical maternal vascular disease and the presumed decrease in uteroplacental perfusion can account for 25 to 30 per cent of IUGR infants. Undiagnosed decreased perfusion may be the cause of IUGR in an otherwise normal pregnancy, such as with recurrent idiopathic fetal growth restriction. Galbraith et al. (1979) reported that a prior IUGR infant was the factor most often associated with a subsequent IUGR birth. A previous low-birth-weight infant is significantly associated with a subsequent birth of decreased weight, decreased ponderal index, and decreased head circumference (Goldenberg et al., 1992b). This finding of symmetric growth restriction is in contrast to the asymmetric IUGR usually seen with maternal vascular disease. However, low-dose aspirin therapy directed against vascular disease has been used successfully to prevent recurrent idiopathic IUGR (Wallenberg and Rotmans, 1987) and to improve fetal weight in patients with abnormal umbilical artery wave-forms (Trudinger et al., 1988).

Severe IUGR, in addition to a very high fetal loss

rate, may be found in women who have antiphospholipid antibodies such as lupus anticoagulant antibodies, many of whom do not have a diagnosis of systemic lupus erythematosus (Carreras et al., 1981; Branch et al., 1985). Paradoxically, this "anticoagulant" is associated with decidual vasculopathy and placental infarction and probably decreased uteroplacental perfusion. Anti-cardiolipin antibodies may also play a role in IUGR. In a group of 37 pregnancies diagnosed by ultrasound as being complicated by IUGR, which was confirmed at birth, 24 per cent were positive for anticardiolipin antibodies, but negative for lupus anticoagulant factor (Polzin et al., 1991). IUGR not attributable to maternal or fetal disease states can also be associated with decreased platelet life span and enhanced platelet thromboxane production (Wallenberg and Rotmans, 1982; Wilcox and Trudinger, 1991). This can lead to increased platelet aggregation and a resultant decreased uteroplacental perfusion.

Vascular disease becomes more prevalent with advancing age. In a recent large study, controlled for confounding variables, the incidence of small-for-gestational-age births was increased more in nulliparous patients than in multiparous above the age 30 (Cnattingius et al., 1993).

Environmental Toxins

Maternal cigarette smoking decreases birth weight approximately 135 to 300 gm, the fetus being symmetrically smaller (Miller and Hassanein, 1974; Haworth et al., 1980; Wen et al., 1990). If smoking is stopped prior to the third trimester, its adverse effect on birth weight is reduced (Rantakallo, 1978). The mechanism whereby cigarette smoking decreases fetal growth is not well established, but most interest centers on the increased carboxyhemoglobin concentrations in maternal and fetal blood and relative fetal hypoxemia (Longo, 1977). Reduction in birth weight is also effected by maternal alcohol ingestion of one to two drinks per day (Mills et al., 1984). Cocaine use in pregnancy decreases birth weight, but the reduction of head circumference is more pronounced than the reduction in birth weight, which is similar to that caused by maternal alcohol ingestion (Little and Snell, 1991). Prolonged use of other drugs such as steroids, dilantin, Coumadin, and heroin has been implicated in IUGR (see Chapter 13).

Maternal and Fetal Hormones

In general, there is limited transfer of the various circulating maternal hormones into the fetal compartments (see Chapters 54 to 56).

Although the effects of hypothyroidism or hyperthyroidism on fetal size are not striking, studies in the subhuman primate indicate that when the mother and fetus are athyroid, there is retarded osseous development and reduced protein synthesis in the fetal brain (Thorburn, 1974; Holt et al., 1973).

Maternal diabetes without vascular disease is frequently associated with excessive fetal size (see Chapter 54). Although insulin does not cross the placenta, fetal hyperinsulinemia is frequently seen with maternal diabetes, as well as hyperplasia of the pancreatic islet cells. These changes are thought to occur as a result of maternal hyperglycemia, which leads to fetal hyperglycemia and an increased response of the fetal pancreas.

Fetal hypoinsulinemia produced experimentally in the rhesus monkey results in IUGR (Hill et al., 1972), and infants have been born, although rarely, with severe IUGR and requiring insulin treatment at birth, suggesting hypoinsulinemia *in utero* (Sherwood et al., 1974; Liggins, 1974). If nutrient transfer becomes limited owing to placental disease secondary to maternal vascular disease, the fetus of the diabetic mother can sustain IUGR.

Even though human growth hormone is present early in gestation, there is minimal evidence that it regulates fetal weight, although a deficiency may retard skeletal growth (Liggins, 1974). Convincing evidence is also lacking that adrenal hormones have a role in producing IUGR in humans.

A number of small polypeptides with *in vitro* growth-promoting activity have been purified. There is a correlation between birth weight and cord blood levels of insulin-like growth factor I, but not insulin-like growth factor II (Gluckman et al., 1983; Ashton et al., 1985). The exact role of these peptides as fetal growth factors and their relationship to IUGR are currently not known.

DIAGNOSIS OF INTRAUTERINE GROWTH RESTRICTION

Determination of Cause

An attempt should be made to determine the cause of fetal aberrant growth prior to delivery, in order to provide appropriate counseling, perform ultrasonographic evaluation for both growth and delineation of anatomy, and obtain neonatal consultation.

Frequently, the cause will be readily apparent. Among patients with significant chronic hypertensive disease, those who take prescribed medications known to be associated with prenatal growth deficiency, and those fetuses with congenital and/or chromosomal abnormalities, the diagnosis is easily established and management plans can be made. However, at times the causal factors may be more elusive. For example, growth restriction associated with preeclampsia may antedate the appearance of hypertension and/or proteinuria by several weeks (Nova et al., 1992). In many instances, a careful history, maternal examination, and ultrasound evaluation will reveal the etiology.

History and Physical Examination

Clinical diagnosis of IUGR by physical examination alone is inaccurate, and frequently the diagnosis is not made until after delivery. In a 5-year review reported by Cetrulo and Freeman (1977), the diagnostic accuracy by clinical assessment alone in 148 patients identified as being at risk for fetal growth restriction was 37 per cent, and the diagnosis was missed in 55 per cent of another at-risk population.

Techniques such as tape measurement of the uterine fundus are helpful in documenting continued growth if performed repeatedly by the same observer, but are not sensitive enough to detect accurately the majority of infants with IUGR (Beazley and Underhill, 1970). It has been shown that experienced obstetricians attempting to estimate fetal size are accurate to within 450 gm in 80 per cent of cases, but their accuracy drops to only 40 per cent for infants weighing less than 2270 gm (Loeffler, 1967).

In spite of the inaccuracy of such indicators, fetal assessment and specific aspects of the patient's history increase the clinician's index of suspicion about suboptimal fetal growth, without which more definitive laboratory investigation might not be considered. As discussed earlier, maternal disease entities such as hypertension (in particular, severe preeclampsia and chronic hypertension with superimposed preeclampsia), chronic antepartum hemorrhage, cyanotic congenital heart disease, and insulin-dependent diabetes with vascular disease carry a high incidence of IUGR. The diagnosis of a multiple gestation suggests the likelihood of diminished fetal growth relative to gestational age as well as preterm birth. Additional maternal risk factors include documented rubella and cytomegalovirus infections, heavy smoking, heroin and cocaine addiction, alcoholism, and poor nutritional status both before conception and during pregnancy. Previous obstetric history is also pertinent, inasmuch as correlation between weights of siblings is high (Billewicz and Thomson, 1973). The history may be significant if one considers a hypothetical situation in which a third-born infant weighs 2800 gm and the two preceding siblings had birth weights exceeding 3700 gm. Although the youngest may not meet strict weight criteria for the diagnosis of IUGR, it is likely that fetal growth did not reach full potential.

Endocrine Testing

The use of *estriol* as measured in either maternal urine or blood to diagnose or monitor the growth-restricted pregnancy is now of only historical interest due to the greater diagnostic accuracy of fetal antepartum heart-rate testing and ultrasound. Most studies show that estriol values are in the low to low-normal range, and the endocrine abnormalities in these fetuses have been extensively reviewed (Tulchinsky, 1977).

Human placental lactogen (hPL), a polypeptide of placental origin, has also been utilized to diagnose IUGR. However, hPL correlates better with placental size than with fetal weight (Spellacy et al., 1976), and there is considerable overlap between normal and abnormal values in growth-restricted pregnancies. Consequently, this hormone is rarely utilized for clinical evaluation.

Ultrasonography

Currently, ultrasonographic evaluation of the fetus is the preferred and accepted modality for the diagnosis of inadequate fetal growth. It offers the advantages of reasonably precise estimation of fetal weight, determination of interval fetal growth, and measurement of several fetal dimensions in order to describe the pattern of growth abnormality. The use of these measurements requires accurate knowledge of gestational age. Accordingly, if a patient is known to be at risk for a fetal growth abnormality, it is recommended that the crown-rump length be determined in the first trimester (Robinson, 1973; Robinson and Fleming, 1975). The application of ultrasound technology to fetal growth is reviewed extensively in Chapter 14, and only a few additional comments will be made here.

Measurement of the head and abdominal circumferences, the ratio of the two, and femur length allows the clinician to utilize accepted formulas to estimate fetal weight, and to determine whether a fetal growth aberration represents an asymmetric, symmetric, or mixed pattern (Fig. 36–3). Insults occurring early in pregnancy, such as infection, exposure to certain drugs or other chemical agents, and chromosomal abnormalities and other congenital malformations, are likely to affect fetal growth at a time of development when cell division is the predominant mechanism of growth. Consequently, musculoskeletal dimensions may be adversely affected as well as organ size, and *symmetric* growth restriction is observed. Given this set of circumstances, one might expect to find that femur length and head circumference are low for a given gestational age, as are abdominal circumference and overall fetal weight.

At the other end of the spectrum, an insult occurring later in pregnancy, usually characterized by inadequate fetal nutrition, is more likely to result in *asymmetric* growth restriction. In this type, femur length and head circumference are within normal limits, but abdominal circumference is decreased because of subnormal liver growth, and there is a paucity of subcutaneous fat. The most common disorders that limit fetal substrates for metabolism are the hypertensive complications of pregnancy, which are associated with decreased uteroplacental perfusion, and placental infarcts, which limit trophoblastic surface area for substrate transfer. In fact, a fall-off in the interval growth of the abdominal circumference is one of the earliest findings in late onset or asymmetric IUGR.

Frequently, these patterns of growth abnormality merge, particularly after long-standing fetal nutritional deprivation. An example of this mixed pattern is seen in Figure 36–4, which demonstrates fetal growth in a patient with severe ulcerative colitis, in whom uteroplacental blood flow and placental function were presumably normal, but maternal caloric intake was profoundly decreased.

Most estimates of fetal weight are derived from measurements of the biparietal diameter, abdominal circumference, and femur length (Hadlock et al., 1984; Woo and Wan, 1986). The ratio of femur length to abdominal circumference has also been reported to be

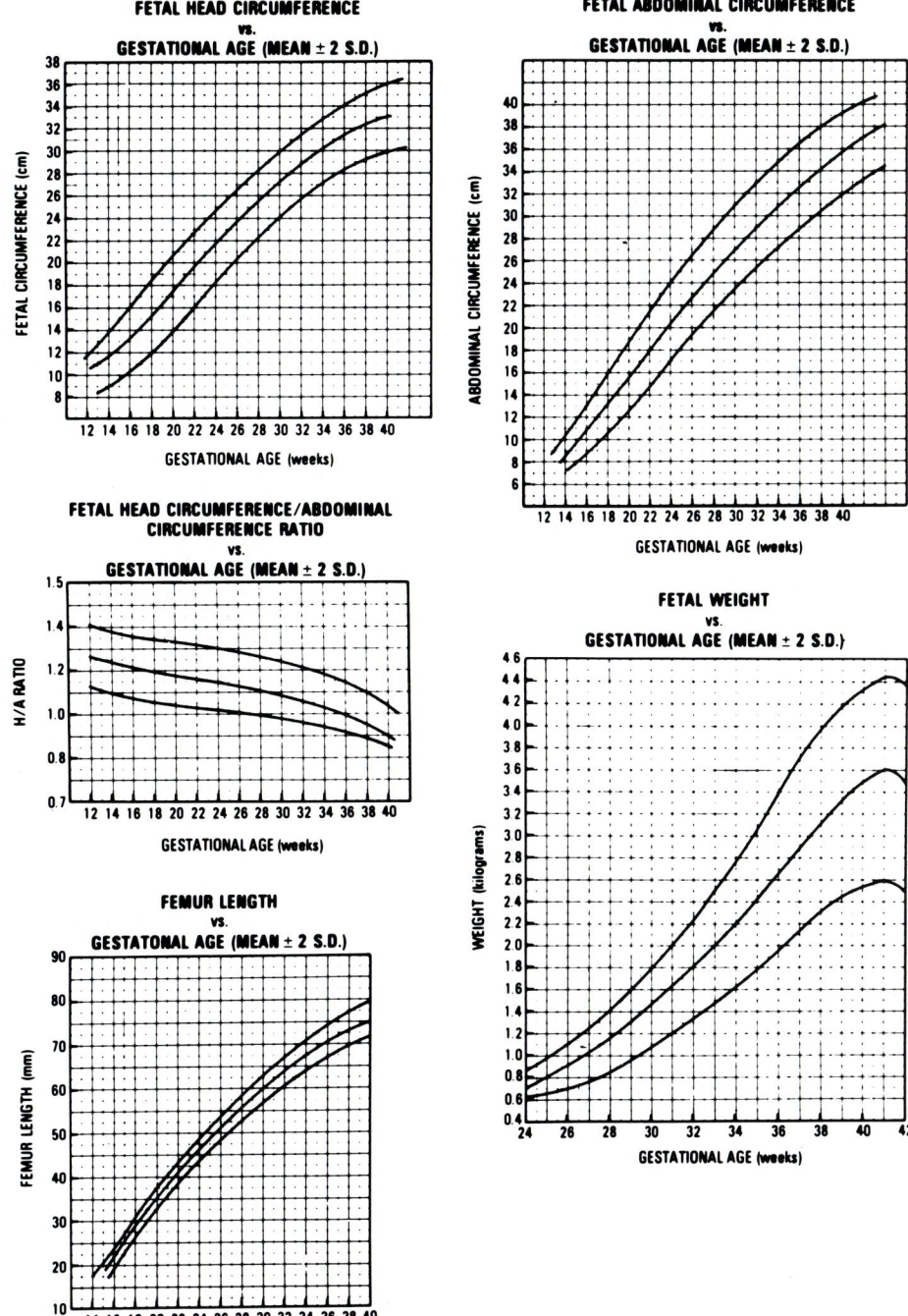

FIGURE 36–3. Composite of fetal body measurements used for serial evaluations of fetal growth.

of value in improved diagnostic accuracy in the asymmetrically growth-restricted fetus (Hadlock et al., 1983).

MANAGEMENT OF THE IUGR PREGNANCY

The prohibitive perinatal morbidity and mortality rates among IUGR infants have been discussed previously. A major current controversy involves the timing of delivery for such infants in order to ensure that intrauterine demise will not occur because of

chronic oxygen deprivation. This problem is underscored by the fact that if deaths among congenitally infected and anomalous infants are excluded, the perinatal risk is still higher for growth-restricted babies than for AGA newborns. Although opinions vary regarding the role of preterm versus term delivery of the SGA infant, it is generally prudent to deliver the growth-restricted infant prior to term in the presence of maternal hypertensive disease, as soon as fetal lung maturity has been achieved.

In an attempt to assess the role of preterm delivery in the presence of suboptimal growth, Perry and

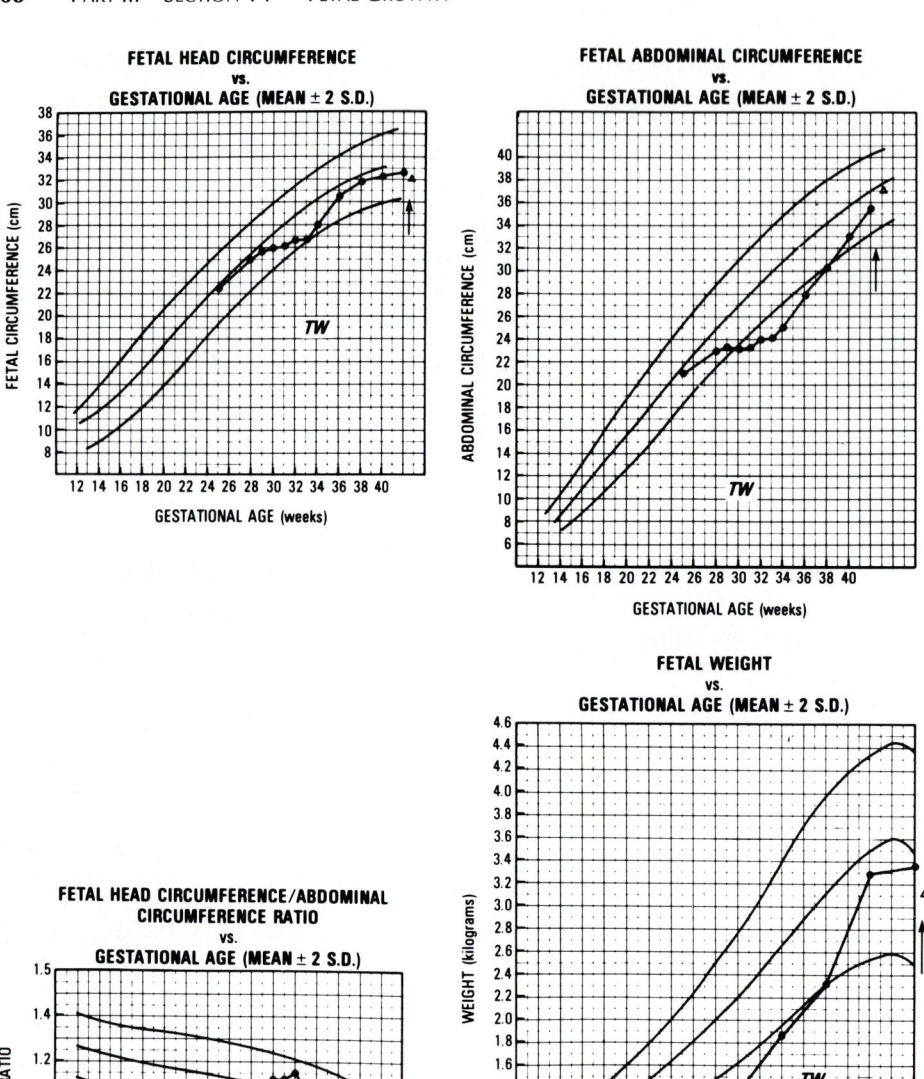

FIGURE 36–4. Serial fetal body measurements in a mother with severe ulcerative colitis. Note that fetal growth begins to decrease markedly in mid-gestation but returns to normal following the initiation of central hyperalimentation at approximately 28 to 30 weeks.

associates (1976) retrospectively reviewed initial neonatal outcome in 58 growth-restricted infants. Those delivered between 38 and 42 weeks gestation appeared to have a better prognosis—higher Apgar scores at birth and a lower incidence of neonatal asphyxia—than those born between 28 and 37 weeks. Furthermore, all perinatal deaths were in the preterm group. The value of this study is somewhat limited due to its retrospective nature and because only 13 of 58 fetuses were accurately diagnosed antepartum as having IUGR and no specific management protocol was in use at the time. However, the study does suggest some differences between preterm and term births and emphasizes the continued risk of respiratory distress syndrome associated with spontaneous or induced preterm delivery. Preterm delivery is indicated in the IUGR fetus demonstrating abnormal fetal function tests and perhaps in the absence of demonstrable

fetal growth. However, the risks of prematurity as well as neonatal complications unique to the IUGR infant must be considered.

In a study designed to reduce or prevent the risk of fetal growth restriction, Wallenburg and Rotmans (1987) demonstrated that low-dose aspirin and dipyridamole may be of value in preventing recurrent idiopathic fetal growth restriction. In a controlled trial of these agents in 24 multigravid women with a history of two or more pregnancies complicated by idiopathic IUGR, the incidence in the treated group was reduced to 13 per cent compared to 61 per cent in controls. Theoretically, low-dose aspirin (1 mg/kg/day) and dipyridamole (225 mg) decrease thromboxane A_2 synthesis, thus increasing the ratio of prostacyclin to thromboxane, with improvement of the uteroplacental circulation. As indicated earlier in this chapter, low-dose aspirin therapy, in a randomized placebo-controlled double blind trial of 46 patients with abnormal umbilical artery Doppler studies, revealed an increased birth weight of approximately 500 gm in the treatment group if the systolic-diastolic ratio was between the 95th and 99.5th percentile (Trudinger et al., 1988). These interesting studies will need confirmation.

ANTEPARTUM FETAL TESTING

At the current time, when a pregnancy is complicated by abnormal fetal growth, most perinatal centers utilize the *biophysical profile* (BPP) and/or *umbilical flow velocimetry* to evaluate fetal condition. These diagnostic modalities are discussed in depth in Chapters 22 and 16 respectively, but some additional comments are pertinent here and worthy of reemphasis.

Biophysical Profile

This technique is theoretically appealing inasmuch as it provides a multi-dimensional survey of fetal physiologic parameters. In particular, amniotic fluid volume assessment is a uniquely important aspect of the profile because oligohydramnios is such a frequent finding in the IUGR pregnancy. This is presumably due to diminished fetal blood volume, renal blood flow and urinary output. Human fetal urinary production rates may be measured with considerable accuracy (Rabinowitz et al., 1989), and three separate studies have shown decreased urinary production rates in the presence of fetal growth restriction (Wladimiroff and Campbell, 1974; Kurjak et al., 1981; Nicolaides et al., 1990). The significance of amniotic fluid volume (AFV) with respect to fetal outcome has been well documented during the last few years. Manning et al. (1981) reported the diagnostic value of AFV measurement in discriminating normal from aberrant fetal growth. Among 91 patients with normal AFV, 86 had infants whose birth weights were appropriate for gestational age. In contrast, 26 of 29 with decreased AFV had growth-restricted infants. The outcome of pregnancies with oligohydramnios is associated with severe fetal compromise (Chamberlain et al., 1984; Bastide et al., 1986).

It is likely that the chronic hypoxic state frequently observed in the IUGR fetus is responsible for diverting blood flow from the kidney to other organs more critical during fetal life (see Chapter 19). Nicolaides et al. (1990) have observed reduced fetal urinary flow rates in the IUGR fetus, and the degree of reduction is well correlated with the degree of fetal hypoxemia as reflected by fetal blood PO_2 measured following cordocentesis.

The predictive accuracy of the biophysical profile has been validated by recent reports. In a study of 19,221 high-risk pregnancies, Manning et al. (1987) observed that the fetal death rate following a normal biophysical profile (score 8 or higher) was 0.726/1000 births; only 14 fetuses died. Of the total patient population, approximately 4380 were pregnancies complicated by IUGR, and only four died following a normal test, yielding a false-negative test rate of less than 1/1000.

More recently, in an analysis of perinatal morbidity and mortality among patients followed with the BPP, a highly significant inverse correlation was observed for IUGR and last test score. When the last test score was 8 or higher, only 3.4 per cent of 6500 high-risk patients had infants with IUGR. Conversely, when the last test score was 4 or 2, the incidence of IUGR increased to 29 per cent and 41 per cent respectively (Manning et al., 1990).

Doppler Ultrasound Assessment of Fetal Blood Flow

There has been great interest during the last few years in the role of maternal and fetal blood flow velocity to predict and evaluate fetal growth restriction, as well as other fetal complications (see Chapter 16 for a detailed discussion). Whether the technique is of clinical value is dependent upon two issues: (1) Does abnormal uteroplacental or fetal vascular flow, as determined by Doppler technology, accurately predict the presence of IUGR? (2) Does reduced or absent end-diastolic flow aid in clinical management decisions—specifically, timing of delivery?

Current data would suggest that the sensitivity and positive predictive value of both uteroplacental and fetal blood flow velocity are too low to be of clinical value in the prediction of IUGR. Although it is beyond the scope of this chapter to review all the recent studies that address this technology, a few are noteworthy. In a study of 145 pregnant women of whom 85 ultimately delivered growth-restricted infants, the investigators found no difference in the mean resistance index of uteroplacental flow for growth-restricted compared to normal infants. The sensitivity of a single observation was only 29 per cent and the positive predictive value 66 per cent (Chambers et al., 1989). Jacobson et al. (1990) examined uteroplacental flow at 20 and 24 weeks in 93 pregnancies and found a positive predictive value of only 33 per cent. More recently, Bewley et al. (1991) showed that the sensitivity and predictive value of this measurement was so low that one could not justify its use as a routine test.

Some investigators have observed a better correlation between fetal blood flow and IUGR (Giles et al., 1986; Fleischer et al., 1985). However, Divon and co-workers (1989) found that traditional ultrasound-derived estimation of fetal weight was a better predictor of IUGR than was the S/D ratio. Others have reported a poor correlation between umbilical artery velocimetry and the ultimate diagnosis of IUGR (Dempster et al., 1989; Sijmons et al., 1989; Beattie and Dornan, 1989).

Some studies have suggested a role for umbilical velocimetry in the prediction of fetal distress in the IUGR fetus. Rochelson et al. (1987) observed fetal distress in 20 of 38 infants who had abnormal S/D ratios, but the sensitivity and positive predictive values were only 57 per cent and 24 per cent respectively. Brar and Platt (1988) observed fetal distress in 6 of 8 growth-restricted infants in whom reversal of end-diastolic flow had occurred.

There is little question that diminished fetal blood flow velocity is associated with fetal hypoxemia and acidosis. Nicolaides et al. (1988) reported hypoxemia in 80 per cent and acidosis in 46 per cent of 59 growth-restricted fetuses with absent end-diastolic blood flow and in whom fetal blood was sampled by cordocentesis. This correlation has been confirmed by some (Ferrazzi et al., 1988) but not all studies (Laurin et al., 1987; Divon et al., 1989).

Review of currently available data clearly demonstrates that although abnormal uteroplacental and umbilical velocity wave-forms are frequently observed in growth-restricted infants, the low sensitivity and positive predictive values preclude their routine use as screening tools for the presence of IUGR or as predictors of fetal distress. This subject has been extensively reviewed by Low (1991).

Cordocentesis

Fetal blood gases and other metabolic parameters measured from umbilical blood samples obtained by cordocentesis have also been utilized to aid in determining fetal condition in the growth-restricted fetus. Normative values have been reported at various gestational ages, and it is clear that, compared to the AGA fetus, the SGA fetus is more frequently hypoxemic, hypercapneic, hyperlacticacidemic, and acidotic (Nicolaides et al., 1989; Pardi et al., 1987; Marconi et al., 1990). Furthermore, abnormal fetal heart rate patterns are more commonly observed when fetal hypoxemia or acidosis is present (Visser et al., 1990). However, among 32 fetuses with absent umbilical end-diastolic flow, umbilical blood gases failed to discriminate between fetuses that would survive and those that would die (Nicolini et al., 1990).

Antepartum Therapy

Maternal hyperoxia has been shown to increase umbilical PO_2 and pH in the hypoxemic, acidotic growth-restricted fetus (Nicolaides et al., 1987). Among surviving fetuses, there was also an improvement in mean velocity of blood flow through the thoracic aorta. More recently, Battaglia and co-workers (1992) treated 17 of 36 women with pregnancies complicated by IUGR with maternal hyperoxia, and confirmed improvement in both blood gases and Doppler flow. They also observed a significant improvement in perinatal mortality in the oxygen-treated patients. Although the numbers of patients studied at the current time are too few to draw definitive conclusions, it is possible that this type of therapy may be of value in prolonging pregnancy in the very premature, growth-restricted and hypoxemic fetus.

Results of studies, considered in the aggregate, would suggest that traditional ultrasound-derived estimates of fetal weight remain the most accurate means of detecting inadequate fetal growth, as well as defining the pattern and rate of growth as gestation progresses. Furthermore, since striking abnormalities in fetal vascular flow velocity may be observed much earlier than changes in the BPP, and have only a low-to-moderate sensitivity and positive predictive value, the BPP remains the most effective method of evaluating fetal condition in the growth-restricted fetus. Amniotic fluid volume estimates are an integral and prognostically helpful component of the BPP evaluation. Antepartum evaluation should be undertaken at least twice weekly, and the timing of delivery influenced by the presence or absence of maternal vascular disease, fetal growth, and the BPP score. Doppler velocimetry is still considered a research tool and should be used only as an additional laboratory finding, rarely altering management decisions.

Intrapartum Management

That the growth-restricted infant is at risk of intrapartum asphyxia has been well documented by the second British Perinatal Mortality Survey, which demonstrated a fivefold increase in SGA infants over the intrapartum stillbirth rate in normally grown infants at a comparable gestational age (Butler and Alberman, 1969). It has long been recognized that lower Apgar scores and meconium aspiration, as well as other manifestations of poor oxygenation during labor, occur with greater frequency among SGA infants. The problem of intrapartum asphyxia has been further elucidated by studies demonstrating the acid-base status of growth-restricted infants at the time of delivery. If moderate-to-severe metabolic acidosis is defined as an umbilical artery buffer base value of less than 37 mEq/liter (normal is >40 mEq/liter), almost one-half of IUGR neonates show signs of acidosis at the time of delivery (Low et al., 1972). These findings document the problems of oxygenation during labor in such infants and emphasize that intensive fetal observation is required during this critical period.

Cesarean delivery of the IUGR infant should be seriously considered when antepartum tests indicate deteriorating fetal status and the uterine cervix is unfavorable for induction. During labor, continuous electronic fetal heart rate monitoring with a scalp electrode should be employed. At the time of delivery, a combined obstetric-pediatric approach is necessary to decrease the possibility of meconium aspiration, because approximately one-half of all neonates born through meconium will have meconium in the trachea (Gregory et al., 1974; Carson et al., 1976).

NEONATAL COMPLICATIONS AND LONG-TERM SEQUELAE

The growth-restricted fetus may have numerous complications in the neonatal period, complications related to the etiology of the growth insult as well as antepartum and intrapartum factors. These include neonatal asphyxia, meconium aspiration, hypoglycemia and other metabolic abnormalities, and polycythemia. These are discussed in greater detail in Chapter 63. Recent data by Low and colleagues (1992) show that fetal growth restriction has a deleterious effect on cognitive function, independent of other variables. Utilizing numerous standardized tests to evaluate learning ability, and excluding those children with genetic or major organ system malformations, almost 50 per cent (37 of 77) of children born small for gestational age had learning deficits at ages 9 to 11 years. Blair and Stanley (1990) also reported a strong association between IUGR and spastic cerebral palsy in newborns delivered after 33 weeks. This association was highest in IUGR infants who were short, thin and of small head size (Blair and Stanley, 1992). Newborns at or above the tenth percentile for weight, but with abnormal ponderal indices, were also at risk for spastic cerebral palsy.

REFERENCES

Abrams B, Newman V: Small-for-gestational-age birth: Maternal predictors and comparison with risk factors of spontaneous preterm delivery in the same cohort. Am J Obstet Gynecol **164**:785, 1991.

Aherne, W: A weight relationship between the human foetus and placenta. Biol Neonate **10**:113, 1966.

Aherne, W: Morphometry. In Gruenwald P (ed): The Placenta and Its Maternal Supply Line. Baltimore, University Park Press, 1975.

Aherne W, Dunnill MS: Quantitative aspects of placental structure. J Pathol Bacteriol **91**:123, 1966.

Alford CA Jr: Rubella. In Remington JS, Klein JO (eds): Infectious Diseases of the Fetus and Newborn Infant. Philadelphia, WB Saunders Co., 1976.

Anderson NG: A five-year study of small for dates infants for chromosomal abnormalities. Aust Paediatr J **12**:19, 1976.

Andrews MC, Jones HW Jr: Impaired reproductive performance of the unicornuate uterus: Intrauterine growth retardation, infertility, and recurrent abortion in five cases. Am J Obstet Gynecol **144**:173, 1982.

Antonov AN: Children born during siege of Leningrad in 1942. J Pediatr **30**:250, 1947.

Arbuckle TE, Wilkins R, Sherman GJ: Birth weight percentiles by gestational age in Canada. Obstet Gynecol **81**:39, 1993.

Ashton IK, Zapf J, Einschenk I, et al: Insulin-like growth factors (IGF) I and II in human foetal plasma and relationships to gestational age and fetal size during mid pregnancy. Acta Endocrinol **10**:558, 1985.

Barcroft J, Kennedy JA: The distribution of blood between the fetus and placenta in sheep. J Physiol **95**:173, 1939.

Barlow P: The influence of inactive chromosomes on human development: Anomalous sex chromosome complements and the phenotype. Hum Genet **17**:105, 1973.

Bastide A, Manning FA, Harman C, et al: Ultrasound evaluation of amniotic fluid: Outcome of pregnancies with severe oligohydramnios. Am J Obstet Gynecol **154**:895, 1986.

Battaglia FC: Intrauterine growth retardation. Am J Obstet Gynecol **106**:1103, 1970.

Battaglia C, Artini PG, d'Ambrogio G, et al: Maternal hyperoxygenation in the treatment of intrauterine growth retardation. Am J Obstet Gynecol **167**:430, 1992.

Battaglia FC, Lubchenco LO: A practical classification of newborn infants by weight and gestational age. J Pediatr **71**:159, 1967.

Baur R: Morphometry of the placental exchange area. Adv Anat Embryol Cell Biol **53**:3, 1977.

Beattie RB, Dornan JC: Antenatal screening for intrauterine growth retardation with umbilical artery Doppler ultrasonography. Br Med J **298**:631, 1989.

Beazley JA, Underhill RA: Fallacy of the fundal height. Br J Med **4**:404, 1970.

Bewley S, Cooper D, Campbell S: Doppler investigation of uteroplacental blood flow resistance in the second trimester: A screening study for preeclampsia and intrauterine growth retardation. Br J Obstet Gynaecol **98**:871, 1991.

Billewicz WZ, Thomson AM: Birth weights in consecutive pregnancies. Br J Obstet Gynaecol **80**:491, 1973.

Blair E, Stanley F: Intrauterine growth and spastic cerebral palsy. I. Association with birth weight for gestational age. Am J Obstet Gynecol **162**:229, 1990.

Blair E, Stanley F: Intrauterine growth and spastic cerebral palsy. II. The association with morphology at birth. Early Hum Dev **28**:91, 1992.

Branch DW, Scott JR, Kochenour NK, et al: Obstetric complications associated with the lupus anticoagulant. N Engl J Med **313**:1322, 1985.

Brar HS, Platt LD: Reverse end-diastolic flow velocity on umbilical artery velocimetry in high risk pregnancies: An ominous finding with adverse pregnancy outcome. Am J Obstet Gynecol **159**:559, 1988.

Brar HS, Rutherford SP: Classification of intrauterine growth retardation. Semin Perinatol **12**:2, 1988.

Brasel JA, Winick M: Maternal nutrition and prenatal growth. Experimental studies of effects of maternal undernutrition on fetal and placental growth. Arch Dis Child **47**:479, 1972.

Brosens I, Dixon HG, Robertson WB: Fetal growth retardation and the arteries of the placental bed. Br J Obstet Gynaecol **84**:656, 1977.

Browne JCM, Veall N: The maternal placental blood flow in normotensive and hypertensive women. J Obstet Gynaecol Br Emp **60**:141, 1953.

Burchell RC, Creed F, Rasoulpour M, Whitcomb M: Vascular anatomy of the human uterus and pregnancy wastage. Br J Obstet Gynaecol **85**:698, 1978.

Butler NR, Alberman ED: In Butler NR (ed): Perinatal Problems: The Second Report of the British Perinatal Mortality Survey. Edinburgh, Churchill Livingstone, 1969.

Campbell S, Bewley S, Cohen-Overbeek T: Investigation of the uteroplacental circulation by Doppler ultrasound. Semin Perinatol **11**:362, 1987.

Carreras LO, Vermylen J, Spitz B, et al: "Lupus" anticoagulation and inhibition of prostacyclin formation in patients with repeated abortion, intrauterine growth retardation, and intrauterine death. Br J Obstet Gynaecol **88**:890, 1981.

Carson BS, Losey RW, Bowes WA Jr, Simmons MA: Combined obstetric and pediatric approach to prevent meconium aspiration syndrome. Am J Obstet Gynecol **126**:712, 1976.

Cetin I, Corbetta C, Sereni LP, et al: Umbilical amino acid concentrations in normal and growth-retarded fetuses sampled in utero by cordocentesis. Am J Obstet Gynecol **162**:253, 1990.

Cetrulo CL, Freeman RF: Bioelectric evaluation in intrauterine growth retardation. Clin Obstet Gynecol **20**:979, 1977.

Chamberlain PF, Manning FA, Morrison I, et al: Ultrasound evaluation of amniotic fluid. I. The relationship of marginal and decreased amniotic fluid volume to perinatal outcome. Am J Obstet Gynecol **150**:245, 1984.

Chambers E, Hoskins PR, Haddad NG, et al: A comparison of fetal abdominal circumference measurements and Doppler ultrasound in the prediction of small-for-dates babies and fetal compromise. Br J Obstet Gynaecol **96**:803, 1989.

Chen ATL, Chan Y-K, Falek A: The effects of chromosome abnormalities on birth weight in man. II. Autosomal defects. Hum Hered **22**:209, 1972.

Chen ATL, Sergovich FR, McKim JS, et al: Chromosome studies on full term, low birth weight mentally retarded patients. J Pediatr **76**:393, 1970.

Clapp JF, Capeless EL: Neonatal morphometrics after endurance exercise during pregnancy. Am J Obstet Gynecol **163**:1805, 1990.

Clapp JF, Rokey R, Treadway JL, et al: Exercise in pregnancy. Med Sci Sports Exerc **24**(suppl):S294, 1992.

Clapp JF 3d, Szeto HH, Larrow R, et al: Umbilical blood flow response to embolization of the uterine circulation. Am J Obstet Gynecol **138**:60, 1980.

Clapp JF 3d, Szeto HH, Larrow R, et al: Fetal metabolic response to experimental placental vascular damage. Am J Obstet Gynecol **140**:446, 1981.

Cnattingius S, Forman MR, Poerendes HW, et al: Effect of age, parity and smoking on pregnancy outcome: A population based study. Am J Obstet Gynecol **168**:16, 1993.

Creasy RK, Barrett CT, de Swiet M, et al: Experimental intrauterine growth retardation in the sheep. Am J Obstet Gynecol **112**:566, 1972.

Daikoku NH, Johnson JWC, Graf C, et al: Patterns of intrauterine growth retardation. Obstet Gynecol **54**:211, 1979.

Daniel SS, James LS, Stark RI, et al: Prevention of the normal expansion of maternal plasma volume: A model for chronic fetal hypoxaemia. J Dev Physiol **11**:225, 1989.

Dawes GS: The placenta and foetal growth. *In* Dawes GS (ed): Foetal and Neonatal Physiology. Chicago, Year Book Medical Publishers, 1968.

Dempster J, Mires GJ, Patel N, Taylor TJ: Umbilical artery velocity wave forms: Poor association with small-for-gestational age babies. Br J Obstet Gynaecol **96**:692, 1989.

Divon MY, Girz BA, Lieblich R, Langer O: Clinical management of the fetus with markedly diminished umbilical artery end-diastolic flow. Am J Obstet Gynecol **161**:1523, 1989.

Dixon GH, Browne JCM, Davey DA: Choriodecidual and myometrial blood flow. Lancet **2**:369, 1963.

Dixon HG, Robertson WB: Vascular changes in the placental bed. Pathol Microbiol **23**:262, 1961.

Dobbing J: Undernutrition and the developing brain. Am J Dis Child **120**:411, 1970.

Dubowitz LMS, Dubowitz V, Goldberg CG: Clinical assessment of gestational age of the newborn infant. J Pediatr **77**:1, 1970.

Duncan SLB: The partition of uterine blood flow in the pregnant rabbit. J Physiol **204**:421, 1969.

Easterling TR, Benedetti TJ, Carlson KC, et al: The effect of maternal hemodynamics on fetal growth in hypertensive pregnancies. Am J Obstet Gynecol **165**:902, 1991.

Elster AD, Bleyl JL, Craven TE: Birth weight standards for triplets under modern obstetric care in the United States 1984–1989. Obstet Gynecol **77**:387, 1991.

Ferrazzi E, Pardi G, Bauscaglia M, et al: The correlation of biochemical monitoring versus umbilical flow velocity measurements of the human fetus. Am J Obstet Gynecol **159**:1081, 1988.

Fleischer A, Schulman H, Farmakides G, et al: Umbilical artery velocity wave forms and intrauterine growth retardation. Am J Obstet Gynecol **151**:502, 1985.

Fleischer A, Schulman H, Farmakides G, et al: Uterine artery Doppler velocimetry in pregnant women with hypertension. Am J Obstet Gynecol **154**:806, 1986.

Fox H: The villous cytophoblast as an index of placental ischemia. J Obstet Gynaecol Br Commonw **71**:885, 1964.

Fox H: The significance of placental infarction in perinatal morbidity and mortality. Biol Neonate **11**:87, 1967.

Froehlich LA, Fujikura R: Significance of a single umbilical artery. Am J Obstet Gynecol **94**:174, 1966.

Galbraith RS, Karchmar EJ, Piercy WM, Low JA: The clinical prediction of intrauterine growth retardation. Am J Obstet Gynecol **133**:281, 1979.

Gluckman PD, Barrett-Johnson JJ, Butler JH, et al: Studies of insulin like growth factor I and II by specific radioligand assays in umbilical cord blood. Clin Endocrinol **19**:405, 1983.

Goldenberg RL, Cutter GR, Hoffman HJ, et al: Intrauterine growth retardation: Standards for diagnosis. Am J Obstet Gynecol **161**:271, 1989.

Goldenberg RL, Hoffman HJ, Cliver SP, et al: The influence of previous low birth weight or birth weight, gestational age, and anthropometric measurement in the current pregnancy. Obstet Gynecol **79**:276, 1992b.

Goldenberg RL, Tamura T, Cliver SP, et al: Serum folate and fetal growth retardation: A matter of compliance? Obstet Gynecol **79**:71, 1992a.

Gregory GA, Gooding CA, Phibbs RH, Tooley WH: Meconium aspiration in infants a prospective study. J Pediatr **85**:848, 1974.

Gruenwald P: Chronic fetal distress and placental insufficiency. Biol Neonate **5**:215, 1963.

Gruenwald P: Growth of the human fetus. I: Normal growth and its variation. Am J Obstet Gynecol **94**:1112, 1966.

Hadlock FP, Deter RL, Harrist RB: A date-independent predictor of intrauterine growth retardation: Femur length/abdominal circumference ratio. Am J Radiol **141**:979, 1983.

Hadlock FP, Harrist RB, Carpenter RD, et al: Sonographic estimation of fetal weight. Radiology **150**:535, 1984.

Hall DC, Kaufman DA: Effects of aerobic and strength conditioning on pregnancy outcomes. Am J Obstet Gynecol **157**:1199, 1987.

Haworth JC, Ellestad-Sayed JJ, King J, et al: Fetal growth retardation in cigarette smoking mothers is not due to decreased maternal food intake. Obstet Gynecol **137**:719, 1980.

Hibbard BM, Jeffcoate TNA: Abruptio placentae. Obstet Gynecol **27**:155, 1966.

Hill DE: Physical growth and development after intrauterine growth retardation. J Reprod Med **21**:335, 1978.

Hill DE, Holt AB, Reba R, Cheek DB: Alterations in the growth pattern of fetal rhesus monkeys following the *in utero* injection of streptozotocin. Pediatr Res **6**:336, 1972.

Holt AB, Cheek DB, Kerr GR: Prenatal hypothyroidism and brain composition in a primate. Nature (London) **243**:413, 1973.

Houlton MCC, Marivate M, Philpott RH: The prediction of fetal growth retardation in twin pregnancy. Br J Obstet Gynaecol **88**:264, 1981.

Jacobson SL, Imhof R, Manning N, et al: The value of Doppler assessment of the uteroplacental circulation in predicting preeclampsia or intrauterine growth retardation. Am J Obstet Gynecol **162**:110, 1990.

Johnstone F, Inglis L: Familial trends in low birth weight. Br Med J **3**:659, 1974.

Jones JS, Newman RB, Miller MC: Cross-sectional analysis of triplet birth weight. Am J Obstet Gynecol **164**:135, 1991.

Kaar K, Joupilla P, Kuikka J, et al: Intervillous blood flow in normal and complicated late pregnancy measured by means of an intravenous Xe^{133} method. Acta Obstet Gynecol Scand **59**:7, 1980.

Karn MN, Penrose LS: Birth weight and gestation time in relation to maternal age, parity and infant survival. Ann Eugen **16**:147, 1951.

Klein JO, Remington JS: Current concepts of infections of the fetus and newborn infant. *In* Remington JS, Klein JO (eds): Infectious Diseases of the Fetus and Newborn Infant. 3rd ed. Philadelphia, WB Saunders Co., 1990, Chapter 1.

Kopenhager T: A review of 50 pregnant patients with kyphoscoliosis. Br J Obstet Gynaecol **84**:585, 1977.

Kramer MS: Determinants of low birth weight: methodological assessment and meta-analysis. Bull WHO **65**:663, 1987.

Kruger H, Arias-Stella J: The placenta and the newborn infant at high altitudes. Am J Obstet Gynecol **106**:586, 1970.

Kulhanek JF, Meschia G, Makowski EL, Battaglia FC: Changes in DNA content and urea permeability of the sheep placenta. Am J Physiol **26**:1257, 1974.

Kurjak A, Kirkinen P, Latin V, Ivankovic D: Ultrasonic assessment of fetal kidney function in normal and complicated pregnancies. Am J Obstet Gynecol **141**:266, 1981.

Laurin J, Marsal K, Persson PH, Lingman G: Ultrasound measurement of fetal blood flow in predicting fetal outcome. Br J Obstet Gynaecol **94**:940, 1987.

Lichty JA, Ting RY, Bruns PD, Dyar E: Studies of babies born at high altitude. Am J Dis Child **93**:666, 1957.

Liggins GC: The influence of the fetal hypothalamus and pituitary on growth. *In* Elliot K, Knight J (eds): Size and Birth. Amsterdam, Associated Scientific Publishers, 1974.

Lin C-C, Su S-J, River LP: Comparison of associated high-risk factors and perinatal outcome between symmetric and asymmetric fetal intrauterine growth retardation. Am J Obstet Gynecol **164**:1535, 1991.

Little BB, Snell LM: Brain growth among fetuses exposed to cocaine in utero: asymmetrical growth retardation. Obstet Gynecol **77**:361, 1991.

Loeffler FE: Clinical fetal weight prediction. J Obstet Gynaecol Br Commonw **74**:675, 1967.

Longo LD: The biological effects of carbon monoxide on the pregnant woman, fetus and newborn infant. Am J Obstet Gynecol **129**:69, 1977.

Love EJ, Kinch RAH: Factors influencing the birth weight in normal pregnancy. Am J Obstet Gynecol **91**:342, 1965.

Low JA: The current status of maternal and fetal blood flow velocimetry. Am J Obstet Gynecol **164**:1049, 1991.

Low JA, Boston RW, Pancham SR: Fetal asphyxia during the antepartum period in intrauterine growth retarded infants. Am J Obstet Gynecol **113**:351, 1972.

Low JA, Handley-Derry MH, Burke SO, et al: Association of intrauterine fetal growth retardation and learning deficits at age 9 to 11 years. Am J Obstet Gynecol **167**:1499, 1992.

Lubchenco LO, Hansman C, Boyd E: Intrauterine growth in length and head circumference as estimated from live births at gestational ages from 26 to 42 weeks. Pediatrics 37:403, 1966.

Lugo G, Cassady G: Intrauterine growth retardation: Clinicopathologic findings in 233 consecutive infants. Am J Obstet Gynecol **109**:615, 1971.

Manning FA, Harman CR, Morrison I, et al: Fetal assessment based on fetal biophysical profile scoring. Am J Obstet Gynecol **162**:703, 1990.

Manning FA, Hill LM, Platt LD: Qualitative amniotic fluid volume determination by ultrasound: Antepartum detection of intrauterine growth retardation. Am J Obstet Gynecol **139**:254, 1981.

Manning FA, Morrison I, Harman CR et al: Fetal assessment based on fetal biophysical profile scoring: Experience in 19,221 high-risk pregnancies. Am J Obstet Gynecol **157**:880, 1987.

Marconi AM, Cetin I, Ferrazzi E, et al: Lactate metabolism in normal and growth-retarded human fetuses. Pediatr Res **28**:652, 1990.

McKeown T, Record RG: Observations on foetal growth in multiple pregnancy in man. J Endocrinol 8:386, 1952.

Meadows NJ, Ruse W, Smith MF, et al: Zinc and small babies. Lancet **2**:1135, 1981.

Mengert WF, Burchell RC, Blumstein RW, Daskal JL: Pregnancy after bilateral ligation of the internal iliac and ovarian arteries. Obstet Gynecol **34**:664, 1969.

Miller HC, Hassanein K: Diagnosis of impaired fetal growth in newborn infants. Pediatrics **48**:511, 1971.

Miller HC, Hassanein K: Maternal smoking and fetal growth of full-term infants. Pediatr Res **8**:960, 1974.

Mills JL, Graubard BI, Harley EE, et al: Maternal alcohol consumption and birthweight. How much drinking during pregnancy is safe? JAMA **252**:1875, 1984.

Molteni RA, Stys SJ, Battaglia FC: Relationship of fetal and placental weight in human beings: Fetal/placental weight ratios at various gestational ages and birth weight distributions. J Reprod Med **21**:327, 1978.

Morton NE: The inheritance of human birth weight. Ann Hum Genet **20**:125, 1955.

Murphy PJ: The estimation of fetal maturity with retarded fetal growth. J Obstet Gynecol Br Commonw **76**:1070, 1969.

Naeye RL: Unsuspected organ abnormalities associated with congenital heart disease. Am J Pathol **47**:905, 1965a.

Naeye RL: Organ abnormalities in a human parabiotic syndrome. Am J Pathol **46**:892, 1965b.

Naeye RL: Cytomegalovirus disease: The fetal disorder. Am J Clin Pathol **47**:738, 1967.

Naeye RL, Benirschke K, Hagstrom JWC, Marcus CC: Intrauterine growth of twins as estimated from liveborn birth weight data. Pediatrics **37**:409, 1966.

Neggers YH, Cutter GR, Alvarez JO, et al: The relationship between maternal serum zinc levels during pregnancy and birthweight. Early Hum Develop **25**:75, 1991.

Nicolaides KH, Bilardo CM, Soothill PW, Campbell S: Absence of end-diastolic frequencies in umbilical artery: A sign of fetal hypoxia and acidosis. Br Med J **297**:1026, 1988.

Nicolaides KH, Bradley RJ, Soothill PW, et al: Maternal oxygen therapy for intrauterine growth retardation. Lancet **i**:942, 1987.

Nicolaides KH, Economides DL, Soothill PW: Blood gases, pH, and lactate in appropriate and small-for-gestational age fetuses. Am J Obstet Gynecol **161**:996, 1989.

Nicolaides KH, Peters MT, Vyas S: Relation of rate of urine production to oxygen tension in small-for-gestational age fetuses. Am J Obstet Gynecol **162**:387, 1990.

Nicolini U, Nicolaidis P, Fisk NM, et al: Limited role of fetal blood sampling in prediction of outcome in intrauterine growth retardation. Lancet **336**:768, 1990.

Nova A, Sibai B, Barton J, et al: Severe fetal IUGR may antedate clinical evidence of preeclampsia by several weeks. Abst. 48, Society of Perinatal Obstetricians, Orlando, 1992. Am J Obstet Gynecol **166**:294, 1992.

Novy MJ, Peterson EN, Metcalfe J: Respiratory characteristics of maternal and fetal blood in cyanotic congenital heart disease. Am J Obstet Gynecol **100**:821, 1968.

Ounsted M, Moar V, Scott WA: Perinatal morbidity and mortality in small-for-dates babies: The relative importance of some maternal factors. Early Hum Dev 5:367, 1981.

Ounsted M, Ounsted C: Maternal regulations of intrauterine growth. Nature **187**:777, 1966.

Palmer J, Dillon-Baker C, Tecklin JS, et al: Pregnancy in patients with cystic fibrosis. Am Intern Med **99**:596, 1983.

Pardi G, Buscaglia M, Ferrazzi E, et al: Cord sampling for the evaluation of oxygenation and acid-base balance in growth-retarded human fetuses. Am J Obstet Gynecol **157**:1221, 1987.

Penrose LS, Penrose LS (eds): Recent Advances in Human Genetics. London, Churchill Livingstone, 1961, p 55.

Perry CP, Harris RE, DeLemons RA, Null DM: IUGR infants: Correlation of gestational with maternal factors, mode of delivery and perinatal survival. Obstet Gynecol **48**:182, 1976.

Peuschel SM, Rothman KJ, Ogilvy JD: Birth weight of children with Down's syndrome. Am J Ment Defic **80**:442, 1976.

Polani PE: Chromosomal and other genetic influences on birth weight variation. In Elliot K, Knight J (eds): Size at Birth. Amsterdam, Associated Scientific Publishers, 1974.

Polzin WJ, Koppelman JN, Robinson RD, et al: The association of antiphospholipid antibodies with pregnancies complicated by fetal growth restriction. Obstet Gynecol **78**:1108, 1991.

Prentice AM, Watkinson M, Whitehead RG, et al: Prenatal dietary supplementation of African women and birth weight. Lancet **i**:489, 1983.

Pritchard JA, Scott DE, Whalley PJ, et al: The effects of maternal sickle cell hemoglobinopathies and sickle cell trait on reproductive performance. Am J Obstet Gynecol **117**:662, 1973.

Rabinowitz R, Peters MT, Sanjay V, et al: Measurement of fetal urine production in normal pregnancy by real time ultrasonography. Am J Obstet Gynecol **161**:1264, 1989.

Rantakallo P: The effect of maternal smoking on birth weight and the subsequent health of the child. Early Hum Dev **2**:371, 1978.

Reece EA, Goldstein I, Gianluigi G, et al: Fetal cerebellar growth unaffected by intrauterine growth retardation. A new parameter for prenatal diagnosis. Am J Obstet Gynecol **157**:632, 1987.

Richards MR, Merrit KK, Samuels JH, Langman A: Congenital malformations of the cardiovascular system in a series of 6053 infants. Pediatrics **15**:12, 1955.

Robertson WB, Brosens I, Dixon G: Maternal uterine vascular lesions in the hypertensive complications of pregnancy. In Lindheimer MD, Katz AL, Zuspan FP (eds): Hypertension in Pregnancy. New York, John Wiley & Sons, 1976.

Robinson HP: Sonar measurements of fetal crown-rump length as a means of assessing maturity in the first trimester of pregnancy. Br Med J **4**:28, 1973.

Robinson HP, Fleming JEE: A critical evaluation of sonar crown-rump length measurements. Br J Obstet Gynaecol **82**:701, 1975.

Rochelson BL, Schulman H, Fleischer A, et al: The clinical significance of Doppler umbilical velocimetry in the small for gestational age fetus. Am J Obstet Gynecol **156**:1223, 1987.

Roord JJ, Ramekers LHF, van Engelshoven JMA: Intrauterine malnutrition and skeletal retardation. Biol Neonate **34**:167, 1978.

Rosso P, Donoso E, Braun S, et al: Hemodynamic changes in underweight pregnant women. Obstet Gynecol **79**:908, 1992.

Rush D, Stein Z, Susser M: A randomized controlled trial of prenatal supplementation in New York City. Pediatrics **65**:683, 1980.

Salafia CM, Vintzileos AM, Silberman L, et al: Placental pathology of idiopathic growth retardation at term. Am J Perinatol **9**:179, 1992.

Saugstad LF: Birth weights in children with phenylketonuria and in their siblings. Lancet **1**:809, 1972.

Scott KE, Usher R: Fetal malnutrition: Its incidence, causes and effects. Am J Obstet Gynecol **94**:951, 1966.

Secher NJ, Kaern J, Hansen PK: Intrauterine growth in twin pregnancies: prediction of fetal growth retardation. Obstet Gynecol **66**:63, 1985.

Shanklin DR: The influence of placental lesions and the newborn infant. Pediatr Clin North Am **17**:25, 1970.

Sherwood WG, Chance GW, Hill DE: A new syndrome of pancreatic agenesis. Pediatr Res **8**:360, 1974.

Shinagawa S, Nomura Y, Kudoh S: Full-term deliveries after ligation of bilateral internal iliac arteries and infundibulopelvic ligaments. Acta Obstet Gynecol Scand **60**:439, 1981.

Sijmons EA, Reuwer PJ, van Beek E, Bruinse HW: The validity of screening for small-for-gestational age and low-weight-for-length infants by Doppler ultrasound. Br J Obstet Gynaecol **96**:557, 1989.

Soothill PW, Nicolaides KH, Bilardo K, et al: Uteroplacental blood velocity index and umbilical venous pO_2, pCO_2, pH, lactate and erythroblast count in growth retarded fetuses. Fetal Ther **1**:174, 1986.

Spellacy WN, Usategui-Gomez M, Fernandez-Decastro A: Plasma human placental lactogen, oxytocinase, and placental phosphatase in normal and toxemic pregnancies. Am J Obstet Gynecol **127**:10, 1976.

Stein Z, Susser M: The Dutch famine, 1944–1945, and the reproductive process. I. Effects on six indices at birth. Pediatr Res **9**:70, 1975a.

Stein Z, Susser M: The Dutch famine, 1944–1945, and the reproductive process. II. Interrelations of caloric rations and six indices at birth. Pediatr Res **9**:76, 1975b.

Stein Z, Susser M, Rush D: Prenatal nutrition and birth weight: Experiments and quasi-experiments in the past decade. J Reprod Med **21**:287, 1978.

Teberg AJ, Walther FJ, Pena IC: Mortality, morbidity and outcome of the small-for-gestational age infant. Semin Perinatol **11**:84, 1988.

Thaler I, Bronstein M, Rubin AE: The course and outcome of pregnancy associated with bronchiectasis. Br J Obstet Gynaecol **93**:1006, 1986.

Thomson AM, Billewicz WZ, Hytten FE: The assessment of fetal growth. J Obstet Gynaecol Br Commonw **75**:906, 1968.

Thorburn GD: The role of the thyroid gland and kidneys in fetal growth. *In* Elliot K, Knight J (eds): Size at Birth. Amsterdam, Associated Scientific Publishers, 1974.

Trudinger BJ: The umbilical circulation. Semin Perinatol **11**:311, 1987.

Trudinger BJ, Cook CM, Thompson RS, et al: Low-dose aspirin therapy improves fetal weight in umbilical placental insufficiency. Am J Obstet Gynecol **159**:681, 1988.

Tulchinsky D: Endocrine evaluation and diagnosis of IUGR. Clin Obstet Gynecol **20**:969, 1977.

Varma TR: Fetal growth. J Obstet Gynaecol Br Commonw **80**:311, 1973.

Visser GHA, Sadovsky G, Nicolaides KH: Antepartum heart rate patterns in small-for-gestational age third trimester fetuses: Correlations with blood gas values obtained at cordocentesis. Am J Obstet Gynecol **162**:698, 1990.

Wallenberg HCS, Rotmans N: Enhanced reactivity of the platelet thromboxane pathway in normotensive and hypertensive pregnancies with insufficient fetal growth. Am J Obstet Gynecol **144**:523, 1982.

Wallenberg HCS, Rotmans N: Prevention of recurrent fetal growth retardation by low-dose aspirin and dipyridamole. Am J Obstet Gynecol **157**:1230, 1987.

Walton A, Hammond J: The maternal effects on growth and conformation in the Shire horse–Shetland pony crosses. Proc R Soc Biol **125**:311, 1938.

Warshaw JB: Intrauterine growth retardation: Adaptation or pathology? Pediatrics **76**:998, 1985.

Weiner CP, Williamson RA: Evaluation of severe growth retardation using cordocentesis—hematologic and metabolic alterations by etiology. Obstet Gynecol **73**:225, 1989.

Wells JL, James DK, Luxton R, et al: Maternal leucocyte zinc deficiency at start of third trimester as a predictor of fetal growth retardation. Br Med J **294**:1054, 1987.

Wen SW, Goldenberg RL, Cutter GR, et al: Smoking, maternal age, fetal growth and gestational age at delivery. Am J Obstet Gynecol **162**:53, 1990.

Wigglesworth JS: Experimental growth retardation in the foetal rat. J Pathol Bacteriol **88**:1, 1964.

Wilcox GR, Trudinger BJ: Fetal platelet consumption: A feature of placental insufficiency. Obstet Gynecol **77**:616, 1991.

Williams RL, Creasy RK, Cunningham GC, et al: Fetal growth and perinatal viability in California. Obstet Gynecol **59**:624, 1982.

Winick M: Cellular changes during placental and fetal growth. Am J Obstet Gynecol **109**:166, 1971.

Wladimiroff JW, Campbell S: Fetal urine production rates in normal and complicated pregnancies. Lancet **ii**:151, 1974.

Woo JS, Wan MC: An elevation of fetal weight prediction using simple equation containing the fetal femur length. J Ultrasound Med **5**:453, 1986.

World Health Organization: Prevention of perinatal morbidity and mortality. *In* Public Health Papers, 1969, p 42.

Yerushalmy J: Relation of birth weight, gestational age, and the rate of intrauterine growth to perinatal mortality. Clin Obstet Gynecol **13**:107, 1970.

MULTIPLE GESTATION

CHAPTER

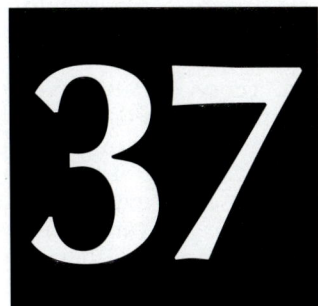

37

INCIDENCE, ETIOLOGY, AND INHERITANCE

KURT BENIRSCHKE, M.D.

INCIDENCE

The incidence of twinning is surely underestimated. Figures usually given derive from national or regional birth statistics and rely on the reporting by physicians or other personnel attending births. They do not accurately reflect the occurrence of twins at conception because the much higher prenatal mortality of twins (as abortion or fetus papyraceus) is not taken into account.

Guttmacher (1953) suggested that 1.05 to 1.35 per cent of pregnancies were twins, the reason for such wide variation of incidence being that the frequency of the twinning process varies widely in different populations. Data collated from various countries reveal that the variability relates largely to the ethnic stock of the population under consideration. Moreover, although the dizygotic twinning rate varies widely under different circumstances, the monozygotic twinning rate is "remarkably constant," usually between 3.5 and four per 1,000 (Bulmer, 1970).

When the twinning rate of a population is known, the frequencies of triplets, quadruplets, and so on can be calculated roughly by employing Hellin's hypothesis. It states that when the frequency of twinning is n, that of triplets is n^2, of quadruplets n^3, and so on. The highest number recorded so far is nine offspring (Benirschke and Kim, 1973). For many reasons on which we are not fully agreed, the overall incidence of twinning has been decreasing slightly during the last two decades owing to a decline in the incidence of dizygotic twins.

TYPES OF TWINS

Twins who possess characteristics that make them virtually indistinguishable are referred to as "identi-cal," whereas others who are very unlike are considered "fraternal." The former always have the same gender, but the latter may be of different gender. The terms identical and fraternal, although popular, are scientifically less useful and are best replaced by the terms monozygotic and dizygotic, to indicate the mechanism of origin of the two types of twins. An important reason for this preference is that monozygotic twins with discordant phenotypes, e.g., cleft lip, would be misclassified as fraternal.

In order to assess the frequency of monozygotic (MZ) and dizygotic (DZ) twins, Weinberg's differential method is commonly used. This suggests that the frequency of MZ twins can be deduced from a twin sample when the sex of the twin pairs is known. Thus, if male and female conceptuses were approximately equal and all twins were fraternal (DZ), then there would be 50 male-female pairs, 25 male-male pairs, and 25 female-female pairs in every 100 pairs of twins. Any excess of like-sex twins is assumed to be the population of MZ twins. This number then can be calculated by employing the following formula:

$$\text{MZ twins} = \frac{\text{like-sex pairs} - \text{unlike-sex pairs}}{\text{number of pregnancies}}$$

When this formula is applied to national birth statistics, it is seen that approximately one-third of twins in the United States are monozygotic. Moreover, the very high twinning rate of the Yoruba tribe in Nigeria results from a higher frequency of double ovulation, whereas the low twinning rate in Japan is the result of a lower frequency of double ovulation. Also, this formula supports the notion that MZ twinning occurs

575

with a relatively uniform incidence in different populations and rises only slightly with advancing maternal age (Bulmer, 1970). In contrast, DZ twinning increases with maternal age to about 35 years and then falls abruptly. It also increases with parity, is higher in conceptions that occur in the first 3 months of marriage, and decreases in periods of malnutrition, such as during World War II. James (1981) has deduced that DZ twinning also increases with coital frequency, and numerous studies indicate that DZ twins occur in certain families presumably because of the presence of genetic factors leading to double ovulation. These are expressed in the mother but may be transmitted through males. Only very few pedigrees suggest that MZ twinning is inherited, and most authorities conclude that it is a random event.

Much has been written about the possible occurrence of "third twins," i.e., twins that may arise from possibly irregular ovulation events such as polar body fertilization. Bulmer (1970) concluded that such an event is unlikely to have been described. More recently, however, Bieber and colleagues (1981) have suggested that the development of an acardiac triploid twin represents such an example. As will be seen, the topic is important because the evidence that DZ twins come from two ovulations does not rest on very firm knowledge. Goldgar and Kimberling (1981) have developed a genetic model to discriminate between dizygotic and polar body twins. They find that only near-centromeric genetic loci can confidently be used to make such a crucial distinction.

Twins may also derive from fertilization by sperm of two fathers, and the suggestion by James (1981) that DZ twinning is influenced by coital rates relates to this phenomenon of superfecundation. Few cases have been verified. In the ninth reported case, one white twin male and one black twin male were presumably conceived by two documented events one week apart (Harris, 1982).

CAUSES OF TWINNING

The causes of both types of twinning are poorly understood. It is commonly assumed that dizygotic twinning occurs because of double ovulation, and occasional cases support this assumption. Meyer and Meyer (1981) describe two 14-day implantation sites with two corpora lutea of similar age in contralateral ovaries. Moreover, multiple pregnancy can be induced by induction of ovulation, and the polyovulation can be followed via ultrasonography (Schenker et al., 1981; Martin et al., 1991). Serum gonadotropin levels in twin-prone Nigerian women are higher than in controls (Nylander, 1981), and lower levels are found in Japanese women, who are less likely to produce fraternal twins (Soma et al., 1975). For these and other reasons, we assume that DZ twinning is the result of somewhat elevated serum gonadotropin levels leading to double ovulation. Moreover, it is assumed that gonadotropin levels are influenced by maternal age, nutrition, parity, and, among other factors, maternal genotype.

Although these assumptions may be correct, they are not proven, and the existence of two corpora lutea

is rarely ascertained. In addition, the occurrence of two ova in one follicle is well documented, as are many abnormal fertilization events. More important questions about the validity of this concept of DZ twinning are statistical, however, and as yet unanswered. Excess nonrighthandedness is found not only in MZ and DZ twins but also in their close relatives (Boklage, 1981). The same observations have been made with respect to certain forms of schizophrenia, suggesting that the traditional MZ and DZ divisions may be incorrect, that perhaps there is a full spectrum between the two classes, and that the MZ twinning process relates to a factor interfering with the brain symmetry development of the embryo.

The mechanism leading to monozygotic twinning is even more obscure. That such twins exist can be verified not only by their physical similarity but also by their identity in genetic characters. Exhaustive blood group analysis, finding no differences in the face of different parental markers, was formerly employed to verify identity. Chromosomal markers have been employed for the diagnosis of MZ twins with apparently greater assurance (McCracken et al., 1978; Morton et al., 1981), but most recently direct comparison of DNA variations is being used for zygosity diagnosis. The determination of restriction fragment lengths polymorphism (RFLP) compares fragments of DNA and is decisive. Moreover, it can employ a variety of tissues, including blood and placenta (Derom et al., 1985; Hill and Jeffreys, 1985). The facts that MZ twins occur slightly more frequently with advancing maternal age (Bulmer, 1970), that malformations often occur, that conjoined twins develop, and that MZ twinning can be induced by teratogens (Kaufman and O'Shea, 1978) have led to the hypothesis that MZ twins result from a teratologic event. Boklage (1981) suggests it to be a disturbance in the process of symmetry development in the embryo. It has been possible to produce monozygotic twins by the separation of early blastomeres in several animal species (Triturus, Ovis, Bos, Mus, and perhaps others), but such physical events do not occur in early embryonic stages. Because of these uncertainties, it has been convenient to speak of the "twinning impetus," an external and perhaps teratogenic agency, that is randomly distributed and that may lead to twins only up to a certain stage, before the embryonic axis is established. Experiments in mice with vincristine support this hypothesis (Kaufman and O'Shea, 1978). If teratogens were to have their effect later, twins would not be seen but anomalies in the singleton would develop. It is further assumed that this twinning impetus may lead to separation of embryonic cells but that it will not lead to a splitting of already formed cavities. Therefore, when the embryonic events are plotted against embryonic age, one may deduce from the placental configuration the approximate timing of the twinning process (Fig. 37–1).

PLACENTATION IN TWINNING

There are two principally different placental types, monochorionic and dichorionic (Fig. 37–2), and it is essential that they be so identified at birth. Indeed, it

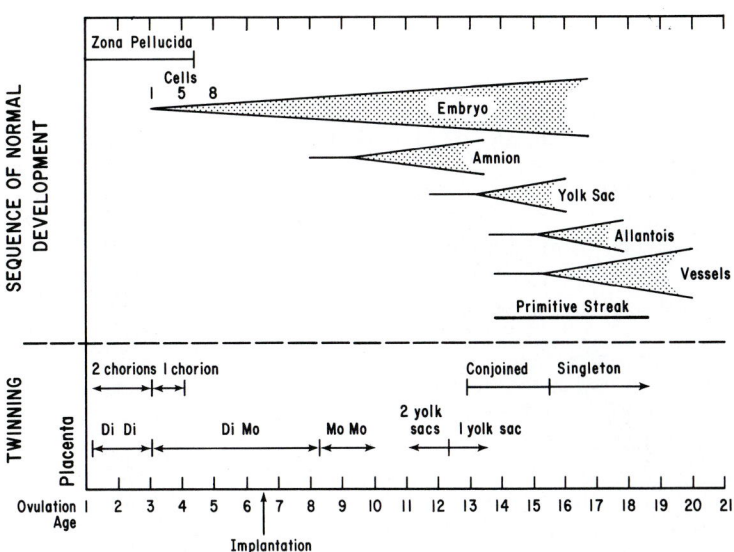

FIGURE 37–1. Schematic representation of monozygotic twinning event superimposed on temporal events of embryogenesis. The embryonic events in the upper portion are sketched according to the publications of early human embryos by Hertig (1968). The twinning event is depicted in the lower portion with resulting placental types indicated (DiDi = diamnionic, dichorionic; DiMo = diamnionic monochorionic; MoMo = monoamnionic, monochorionic). (From Benirschke K, Kim CK: Multiple pregnancy. N Engl J Med **288**:1276, 1973. Reprinted by permission from The New England Journal of Medicine.)

is also desirable to differentiate these prenatally by ascertaining the thickness of the "dividing membranes" sonographically. Winn et al. (1989) established criteria for this measurement and suggested, with an 82 per cent accuracy, that a thickness of maximally 2 mm is diagnostic of monochorionicity. Numerous surveys of placental types of twins have shown that heterosexual (assuredly DZ) twins always have a dichorionic placenta and that monochorionic twins have always been of the same sex. These are the basic facts that lead us to assume that all monochorionic twins are monozygotic.

Some MZ twins may be endowed with dichorionic placentas, i.e., twins that separated in the first 2 days after fertilization (see Fig. 37–1). The majority of MZ twins, however, have a placenta with diamnionic and monochorionic membranes. Monoamnionic twins, which are by necessity also monochorionic, occur least commonly (incidence about 1 per cent). Conjoined twins are monoamnionic and less common still, because it becomes increasingly difficult for a rapidly growing embryo to submit to the twinning impetus.

Dizygotic twins always have dichorionic placentation. Their placentas may be separated or intimately fused (Fig. 37–3). If they are fused, a ridge develops in the central fusion plane that allows easy distinction from the monochorionic placenta. Blood vessels never cross from one side to the other, and when the

dividing membranes (that portion separating the two sacs) are carefully dissected, four separate layers can be identified, one amnion on either side and two chorions in the middle. Between the two chorions one finds degenerated trophoblast and atrophied villi, features that render the dividing membranes of a diamnionic dichorionic twin pair opaque. Differential expansion of the fetal sacs often causes the membranes of one placenta to push away those of the other (Fig. 37–4), a feature that must not be confused with monochorionic placentation.

Twenty to 30 per cent of MZ twins have dichorionic placentation. Most commonly their placentation is diamnionic monochorionic. The latter type is invariably fused, and the dividing membranes consist of two translucent amnions only. When they are separated from each other, the single chorion on the placental surface is evident. It carries the fetal blood vessels and various types of interfetal vascular communications that occur regularly in monochorionic twins. The two principal types of membrane relationships are shown in Figures 37–5 and 37–6. Monoamnionic twins are least common and carry a mortality rate of approximately 50 to 60 per cent because frequent encircling of the cords and knotting lead to cessation of umbilical blood flow. The perinatal mortality rate of diamnionic monochorionic twins is next highest (about 25 per cent) because of the high frequency of the interfetal

FIGURE 37–2. The two principal types of twin placentation. *Left,* diamnionic monochorionic placenta, always monozygotic. *Right,* diamnionic dichorionic placenta, which may or may not be fused.

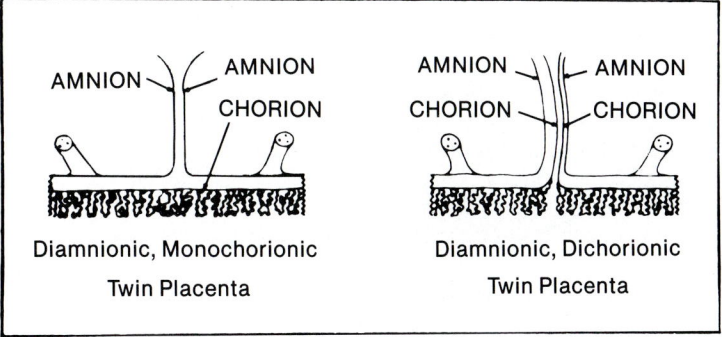

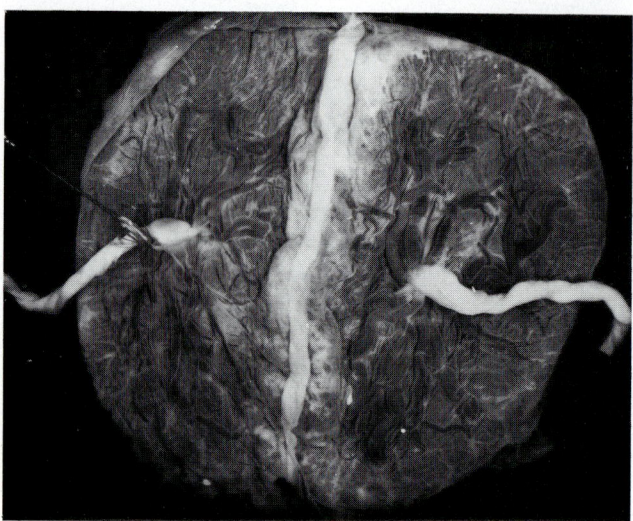

FIGURE 37–3. Diamnionic dichorionic twin placenta, fused. The cord on the left had a single umbilical artery. Note the close approximation of two placental disks with ridge formed by membranes in center.

FIGURE 37–4. Diamnionic dichorionic (separate) twin placenta in which the membranous sac of the right twin has pushed away the left membranes so that fusion of dividing membranes occurs over the left placenta ("irregular chorionic fusion").

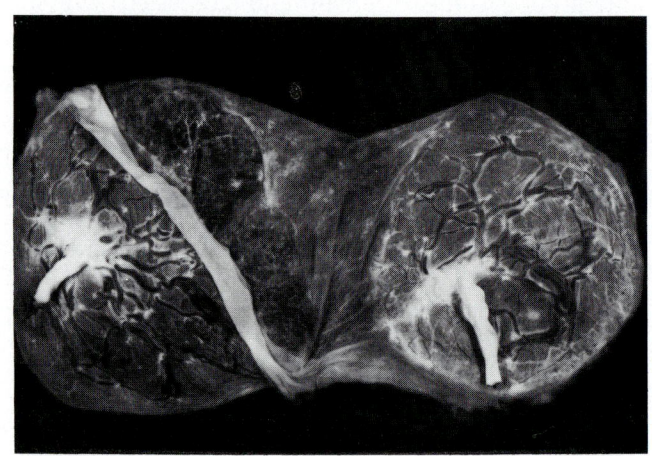

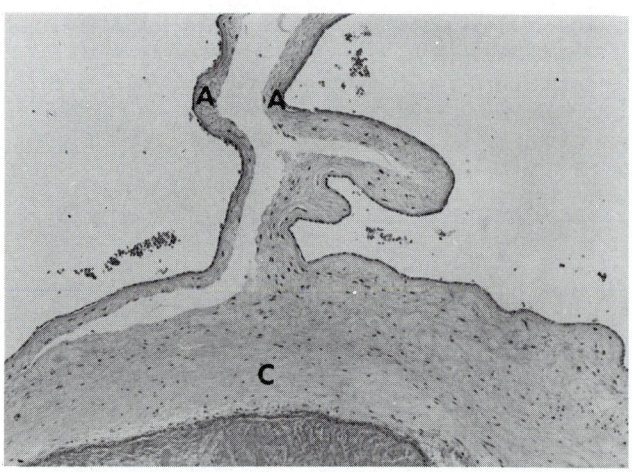

FIGURE 37–5. T section at the point of dividing membranes in diamnionic *(A)* monochorionic *(C)* twin placenta.

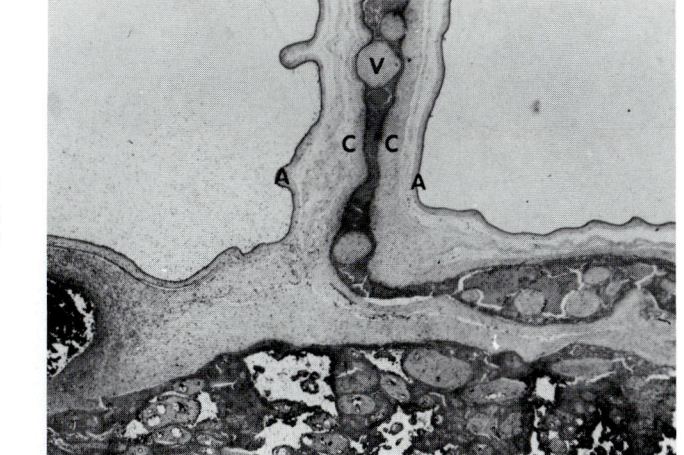

FIGURE 37–6. T section at point of dividing membranes in diamnionic *(A)* dichorionic *(C)* fused twin placenta showing degenerated villi *(v)* and trophoblast *(dark area)* between the membranes. Note inflammation of chorial vessel at left.

transfusion syndrome. Dichorionic twins have the lowest mortality rate (8.9 per cent).

The relationship of placentas among triplets, quadruplets, and higher orders of multiple birth generally follows the same principles, except that monochorionic and dichorionic placentations may coexist (Fig. 37–7). With these higher numbers, there is more frequent association of placental anomalies, particularly marginal and velamentous insertions of the cord (Figs. 37–7 and 37–8) and single umbilical artery (see Fig. 37–3). The etiology of these anomalies may be related to the crowding of placentas and competition for space or to primary disturbances of nidation of the blastocysts.

VELAMENTOUS INSERTION OF CORD AND VASA PREVIA

With the six to nine times higher incidence of velamentous cord insertion in twin placentas and an even higher incidence in higher-order multiple births, the presence of vasa previa in multiple pregnancy must be anticipated. It is a serious complication, often lethal because of exsanguination during delivery. Membranous vessels originating from a cord with velamentous insertion radiate toward the placental surface and are not protected by Wharton's jelly. Therefore, they may thrombose or may be compressed during labor. Sinusoidal fetal heart patterns may indicate this complication (Antoine et al., 1982). When the membranes are ruptured during delivery and these vessels accidentally have a transcervical position (vasa previa), the rupture may lead to exsanguinating hemorrhage. Not only may the first twin exsanguinate, but as has been repeatedly described, the second twin may exsanguinate through interfetal placental anastomoses if the placentation is monochorionic. Vasa previa may exist not only over the cervical os, but also over the dividing membrane when the second twin's cord has a velamentous insertion on the dividing

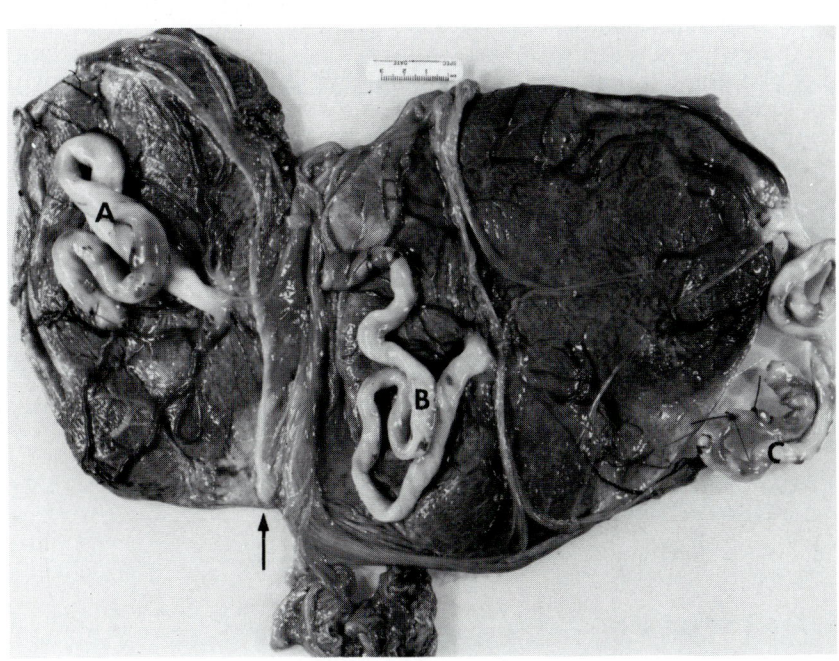

FIGURE 37–7. Placenta of male triplets at 36 weeks. Triplet A has a separate chorion (ridge indicated by *arrow*) from diamnionic monochorionic pair B and C *(right)*. Note marginal cord insertion of C. Anastomoses existed between B and C, but A was isolated.

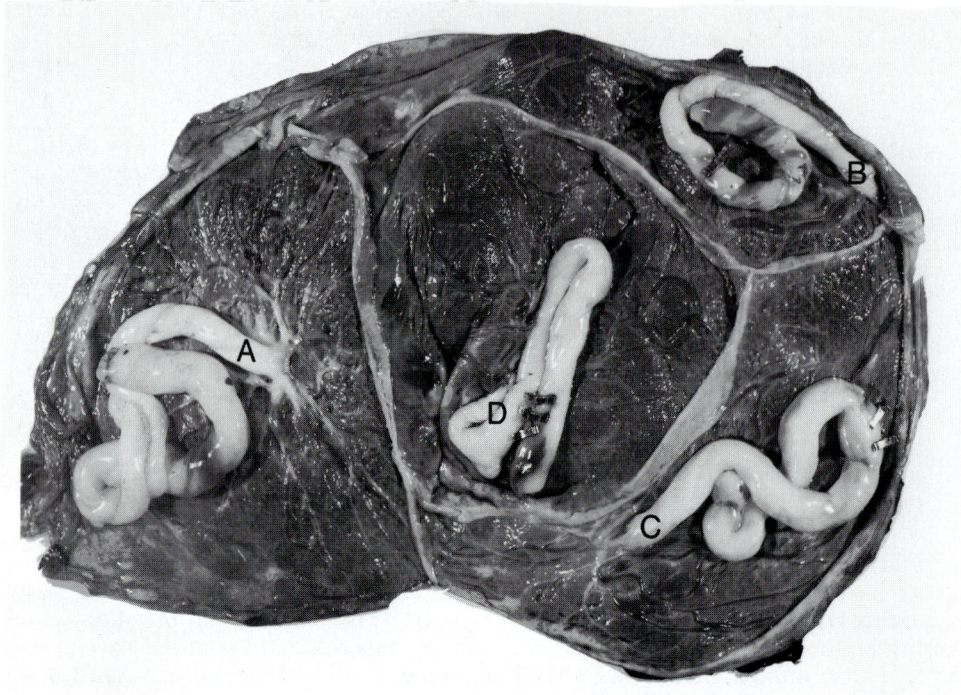

FIGURE 37–8. Placenta of quadruplets at 28½ weeks. A, C, and D are female; B is male. Placenta is tetrachorionic and intimately fused. Birth order is indicated by letters. Cord B is marginally inserted. Despite intimate fusion, there are no anastomoses.

membranes. Fetal hemorrhage leading to death within 3 minutes has been observed when the diamnionic dichorionic membranes of the second twin were ruptured (Benirschke and Driscoll, 1967). In nine cases collected by Antoine and colleagues (1982), no first twin survived and 62.5 per cent of the second twins eventually succumbed as the result of this hemorrhage.

The gloom with which this entity has formerly been discussed is no longer warranted (Van Drie and Kammeraad, 1981). When vaginal bleeding is not judged with certainty to be the result of a placenta previa, the use of 1-hour hemoglobin electrophoresis is helpful for the detection of fetal blood, as is the Kleihauer-Betke technique, particularly because it can be done more quickly and in the delivery suite at any time. It must be pointed out, however, that massive external hemorrhage may not always occur to alert the obstetrician to the presence of vasa previa (Fig. 37–9). Anticipation of the possible existence of vasa previa in multiple births is therefore necessary.

MONOAMNIONIC TWINS

Monoamnionic twins are all monozygotic because all must have also a single chorion. Monoamnionic twins are the least common, their occurrence variably recorded as from one in 33 to one in 661 twin births. In the series reported by Benirschke and Driscoll, (1967), three of 250 pairs had this type of placenta, and three of the six fetuses died from various complications. The most common complication is encircling and knotting of cords with cessation of umbilical blood flow. Indeed, double survival of monoamnionic twins is so uncommon that such cases were deemed worthy

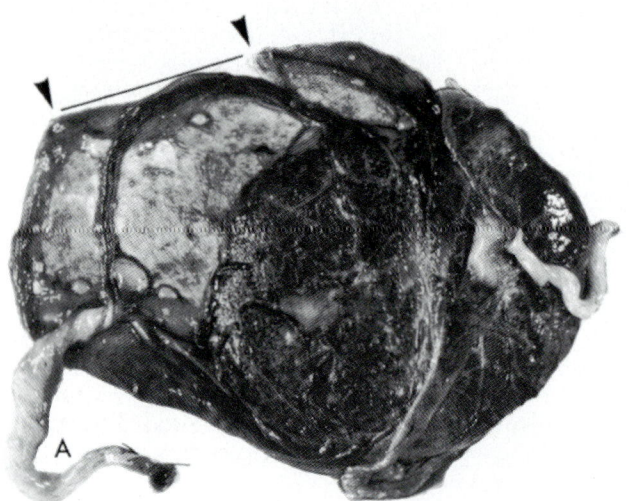

FIGURE 37–9. Fatal vasa previa in twin A of an intimately fused diamnionic dichorionic twin placenta. The disrupted vessel is indicated by *arrows*. Mother admitted 4 hours after rupture of membranes with no history of significant bleeding. Twin A had Apgar score of 1 and could not be resuscitated. Twin B lived. Left half of placenta had marked pallor (on maternal surface) because of fetal hemorrhage.

of report (Colburn and Pasquale, 1982). The extent of the knotting of cords is at times astonishing and testimony to the degree of fetal movements. Care must be exercised when the cord of the first-delivered twin is clamped because the cord of the second twin may be inadvertently severed before its birth (McLeod and McCoy, 1981). Locking is another but less common complication of monoamnionic twins. Although most monochorionic twins have interfetal placental anastomoses, such vessel communications are not invariably found. Through these anastomoses blood is exchanged between the twins, and if one succumbs before birth, thromboplastin, presumably originating in the macerating fetus, may lead to disseminated intravascular coagulation in the other twin. Although this phenomenon is restricted to monochorionic placentation, it occurs in monoamnionic as well as diamnionic twin placentas and can occur in triplets as well (Thomas, 1974). An alternative view for demise of the second twin has now assumed greater likelihood: that severe and acute hypotension develops through exsanguination into an already dead twin via large anastomoses (Yoshioka et al., 1979).

Because of the high mortality rate—the double survival is currently only 40 per cent (Colburn and Pasquale, 1982)—antenatal diagnosis is desirable. This has been achieved by amniography and, more recently, by ultrasonography (see Chapters 14 and 38). With such a diagnosis, however, a clear course of action must await accumulation of adequate statistics that delineate exactly when in the course of pregnancy one or both twins are likely to succumb from cord encircling. This information is currently not available.

The cords of monoamnionic twins most commonly arise near each other on the placenta, and in rare circumstances they are partially fused; less commonly they are velamentous (McLeod and McCoy, 1981). The fusion of cords, of course, represents a gradual transition to the invariably monoamnionic conjoined twins that are thought to form only slightly later, at the end of the twinning spectrum shown in Figure 37–1. Conjoined twins may have two cords with three vessels each, forked cords, anomalous vessels, or, at the other end of the spectrum, one cord with only one artery and one vein. Congenital anomalies, although more common among twins in general, are particularly common in monoamnionic and conjoined twins. The more frequent occurrence of *sirenomelia*—100 to 150 times more common in twins than in singletons (Wright and Christopher, 1982)—has led to insight into the relationship of this anomaly with pulmonary hypoplasia, a regular finding in sirens owing to a deficient urinary tract. When one monoamnionic twin is a siren and the other is normal, the amniotic fluid produced by the second twin apparently protects the siren from developing pulmonary hypoplasia. When the placenta is diamnionic, this protection does not occur (Wright and Christopher, 1982).

DIAMNIONIC MONOCHORIONIC TWINS

Diamnionic monochorionic (DiMo) twins are monozygotic, the placenta is fused, and the cords often have a marginal or velamentous insertion. The diagnosis is readily apparent from the absence of a ridge at the base of the dividing membranes (see Figs. 37–3, 37–7, and 37–9) and the translucency of the dividing membranes. When the membranes are dissected, one amnion can be readily stripped from the other, leaving a single (placental) chorionic plate that carries the fetal blood vessels. The amnions do not necessarily meet at the vascular equator of the two placental beds, but may shift irregularly from one side to the other, presumably because of fetal movements and the relative fluid contents of the two sacs. The diamnionic monochorionic placenta is the most common type seen in MZ twins; approximately 70 per cent have this conformation (see Fig. 37–1).

The DiMo placenta, and less commonly the monoamnionic twin placenta, nearly always possesses interfetal blood vessel communications. The anastomosis is more often an artery-to-artery (arterioarterial) than a vein-to-vein communication, and sometimes both types are present and multiple. These vessels allow blood to shift readily from one side to the other, equalizing volumes and pressures. They are most readily demonstrated, after the amnion has been removed, by careful inspection, by stroking blood from one side to the other, or by injection. It is generally impractical to inject the entire placenta from the cord, as rather large volumes are needed and the blood must not be clotted. One can verify the existence of anastomoses more readily by first cutting off the cords and then injecting water or milk into those vessels that are thought to be anastomotic. The large anastomoses have important practical clinical implications. Through these communications, the second twin may exsanguinate if vasa previa of the first twin are ruptured or, of course, if the cord of the first twin is not clamped. Indeed, because twins are sometimes not detected before delivery, the occasional practice of permitting placental transfusion to occur should be done only when twins assuredly do not exist. Otherwise the second twin may rapidly exsanguinate through these commonly large-caliber vessels.

It must also be realized that the interfetal anastomoses of larger caliber may lead to significant shifts of blood between fetuses. This is particularly important when one dies. The vascular bed of the dead twin will relax and a substantial amount of blood from the survivor may enter the dead twin, causing anemia in the survivor, possibly with destructive consequences. It now appears likely that the appreciable frequency of cerebral palsy of a surviving monochorionic twin results from acute hypotension after one twin dies because of major blood shifts between the twins through placental anastomoses (Yoshioka et al., 1979; Liu et al., 1992). This feature is then grossly similar to the appearance of the twins shown in Figure 37–12, who died from the transfusion syndrome, here with an arteriovenous anastomosis. One twin has much more blood than the other, and when this is due to large blood vessel anastomoses rather than the arteriovenous shunt to be described next, such twins have been erroneously diagnosed as having the *classic transfusion syndrome*. Twins with such marked differences in blood content near term are never the result of this syndrome.

The most important anastomosis, the arteriovenous shunt, is also the most difficult to diagnose. It is not a direct communication, but occurs when one cotyledon is fed by an artery from one twin and is drained by a vein into the other twin. It is diagrammatically shown in Figure 37–10; the common vascular relationships at a twin vascular equator are seen in Figure 37–11. In order to recognize such a shared cotyledon, one must follow all terminal arterial branches (arteries cross over veins) and ascertain whether there is a vein returning to the same twin, as is normal (seen on the left of Fig. 37—11), or whether the cotyledon is drained to the other twin (seen on the right of Fig. 37–11). To verify the existence of a common or shared cotyledon, one may inject the artery with water; the shared cotyledon will rise and blanch and then the water will drain from the vein of the other twin. Arteriovenous shunts may exist singly or in multiple, and they may be in opposing directions. When they are not accompanied by artery-to-artery or vein-to-vein anastomoses, one fetus continuously donates blood into the recipient (Fig. 37–10), which is the basis of the twin transfusion syndrome. This syndrome leads to plethora and hypervolemia (hypertension) of the recipient and anemia (hypotension) of the donor. Cardiac compensation (hypertrophy in the recipient) ensues first, followed by a wide spectrum of bodily growth differences (Figs. 37–12 and 37–13). A common symptom is rapid uterine growth due to hydramnios of the recipient; it is thought to be secondary to excessive fetal urination. The hydramnios usually manifests between 20 and 30 weeks of pregnancy, may reach enormous quantities, and is frequently the cause of premature delivery. The amnionic sac of the donor may be dry and may develop amnion nodosum. The severity and time of noted growth discrepancy probably depend on the size and the number as well as the direction of arteriovenous shunts. At times one twin dies *in utero*, the hydramnios disappears, and the pregnancy goes to term with one twin normal and the other a fetus

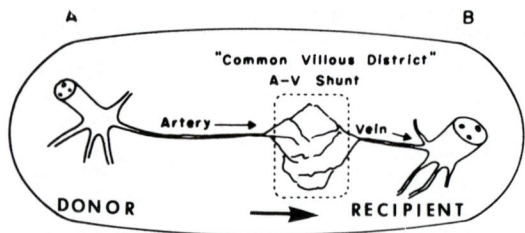

FIGURE 37–10. Monochorionic placenta with shared cotyledon, the basis for the twin transfusion syndrome.

papyraceus (Benirschke and Driscoll, 1967). When the twins are born, usually prematurely, they may differ remarkably in size; indeed, they may be so discordant that they seem to be DZ twins. Catch-up growth occurs postnatally but often is incomplete, and the twins remain discordant even though they are monozygotic. This is one more reason not to speak of "identical" twins.

The prenatal diagnosis of the transfusion syndrome can usually be made when mid-trimester hydramnios complicates a twin pregnancy. Wittmann and co-workers (1981) have differentiated the condition from other discrepancies of twin growth by the use of ultrasonography. The recipient is more active, and the hydramnios can be associated with the larger twin. These authors advocate the use of tocolytic agents and report that amniocentesis is rapidly followed by reaccumulation of hydramnios. Digoxin therapy and other means of prenatal treatment have been attempted, generally with mediocre success (De Lia et al., 1985a). More incisive is the laser obliteration of interfetal placental anastomoses at the height of hydramnios by fetoscopy (De Lia et al., 1985b). Although this therapy is currently only possible when the placenta has a posterior location, it is definitive and has greatly prolonged pregnancies that were formerly doomed (see also Chapter 38).

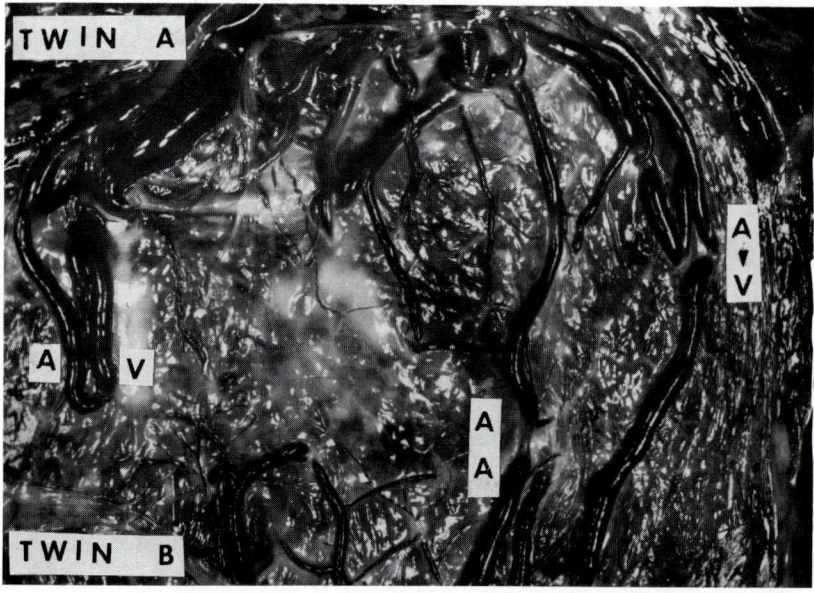

FIGURE 37–11. Diamnionic monochorionic placenta showing a portion of the "vascular equator." The amnions have been stripped off; only the chorionic surface is seen. Twin A has a normal cotyledonary supply at left with an artery (above veins) feeding a cotyledon that is drained back into Twin A. In the middle, an interfetal arterioarterial anastomosis is seen. At the right an arteriovenous shunt (A to B) is demonstrated. These twins came to term because the arterioarterial anastomosis immediately compensated for any inequality of blood volume arising from the arteriovenous shunt.

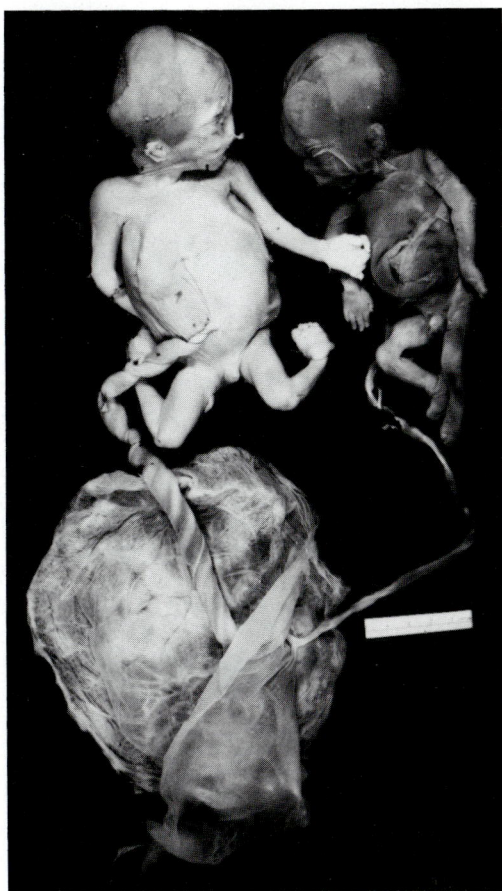

FIGURE 37–12. Diamnionic monochorionic twin abortus secondary to the twin transfusion syndrome. The "donor" *(right)* appears plethoric because he died *in utero* (maceration) and blood returned to him through the arteriovenous shunt. Note discrepancy in size, thick cord of recipient, and hydramneic (large) sac.

ABNORMALITIES OF TWIN GESTATION

Fetus Papyraceus

When one of the fetuses in a multiple gestation dies before birth and the pregnancy continues, the fluid of the dead twin's tissues is gradually absorbed, the amniotic fluid disappears, and the fetus is compressed and becomes incorporated into the membranes. Hence, it is called a fetus compressus, fetus papyraceus, or membranous twin. The condition occurs in both dizygotic and monozygotic twins.

The fetus papyraceus has important practical and theoretical implications. First, a birth with such an association is not usually entered into statistics as a twin gestation, and hence the frequency of twinning is underestimated. Fetus papyraceus is also often not recognized at birth. Figure 37–14 shows a twin placenta from what was thought to be an abruptio placentae of a singleton birth. One placenta was normal, the other a shriveled, diminutive, and separate organ of a dizygotic fetus papyraceus. The small embryo must have died early, but the preservation of the cord is remarkable. It is possible that this fetus papyraceus

was a chromosomally abnormal conceptus that would ordinarily have been aborted had it not been for the normal twin. This would support one hypothesis for the rapid fall in rate of twin gestation in women over 35 years. Another, less well understood hypothesis purports ovarian failure in older women to be the cause of the decline (Bulmer, 1970).

Fetus papyraceus in DiMo twins is also often overlooked. The example illustrated in Figure 37–15 was so small and compressed that its formerly presumably normal structure could be deduced only from radiographs (Fig. 37–16) in order for it to be differentiated from an acardiac twin. This fetus papyraceus is particularly interesting because it was associated with aplasia cutis of the surviving twin. The diffuse form of this unusual skin condition has always been associated with MZ twins, one a fetus papyraceus, in cases in which the placenta has been examined (Mannino et al., 1977). The inference is that diffuse, patchy aplasia cutis (in contrast to that in scalp midline) is the result of a prenatal insult associated with the death of one monozygotic twin.

Another insight into prenatal life afforded by the fetus papyraceus relates to the mechanism that leads to amnion nodosum. When one twin dies, so does the amnion of its sac. This occurs earliest on the diamnionic dividing membranes (Fig. 37–17). Because the amnion does not possess blood vessels, its growth and maintenance must be supported by nutrients and oxygen from adjacent tissues. The large area of dividing membranes, which are in contact only with amnionic fluid, must be maintained by this fluid. The amnion dies because of the disappearance of fluid or deficiency of its oxygen content. Amnion nodosum, or impaction of vernix, occurs secondarily after epithelial death.

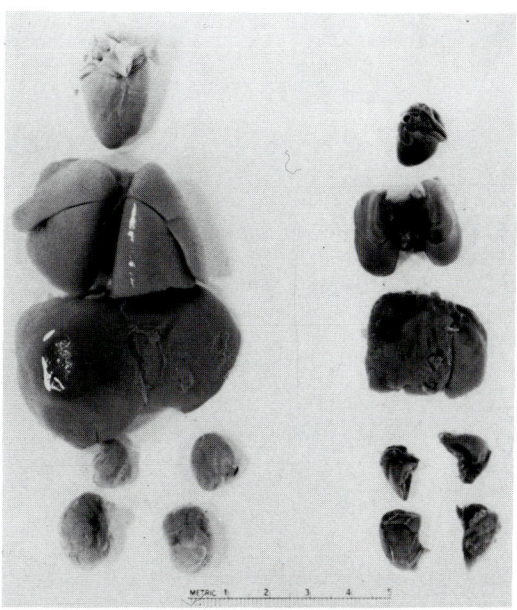

FIGURE 37–13. Hearts, lungs, livers, adrenals, and kidneys of monozygotic twins with transfusion syndrome shown in Figure 37–12. Most marked discrepancies of size exist in hearts, lungs, and livers.

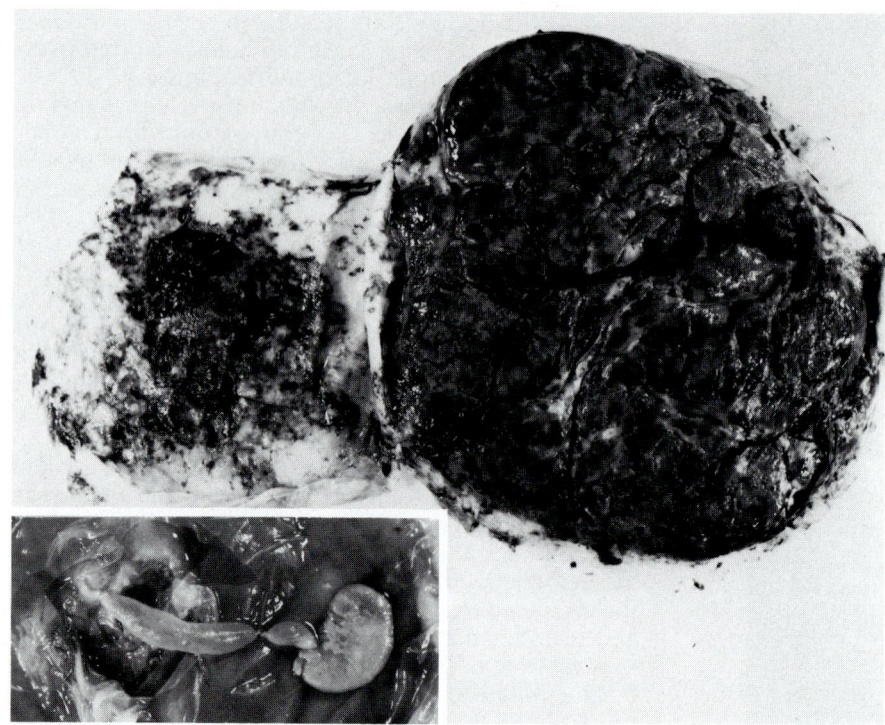

FIGURE 37–14. Placenta of 35-year-old woman thought to have abruptio placentae. Diamnionic dichorionic separate twin placentas, maternal surface. Normal twin from right. Degenerated twin placenta left. Inset shows fetus papyraceus, attached to cord. Embryo was golden-yellow, about 1 cm.

FIGURE 37–15. Diamnionic monochorionic twin placenta with small, round fetus papyraceus (see Fig. 37–16) compressed in the thickened membranes at left. Surviving twin from right had aplasia cutis.

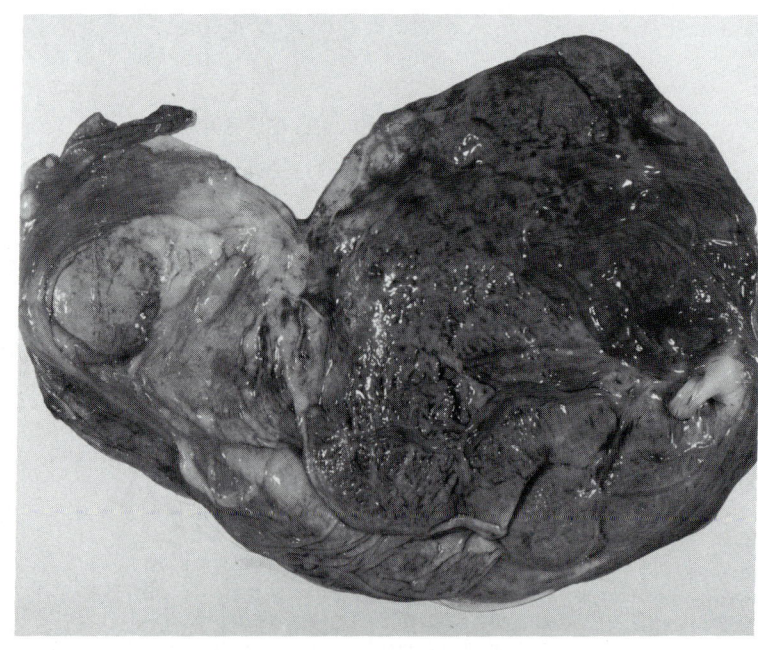

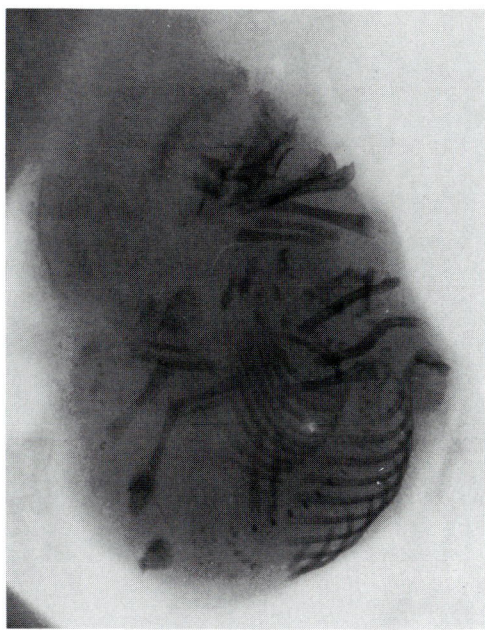

FIGURE 37–16. Radiograph of fetus papyraceus shown in Figure 37–15. Note the complete presence of skeleton, including skull *(top left)* of fetus, ruling out acardiac twin.

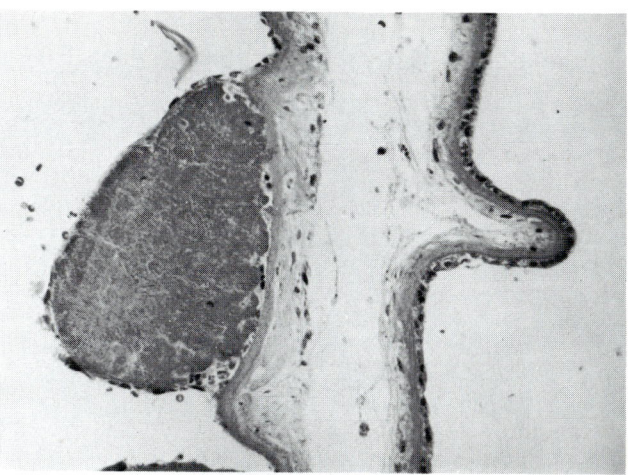

FIGURE 37–17. Amnion of dividing membranes in diamniotic monochorionic twin placenta. Twin and amnion at right were living. Twin at left had died, and nodule of impacted vernix is present on degenerated amnionic surface.

Acardiac Twin

The most bizarre malformation recorded, acardiac twin, occurs only in one of monozygotic twins. The normal twin maintains the acardiac by perfusion through two anastomoses, one artery-to-artery and one vein-to-vein. The circulation of the acardiac is therefore reversed, and most authors have assumed that this reversal of circulation may also be the cause of the malformation (Benirschke and Harper, 1977). This concept is challenged by the occasional observation of an acardiac with different chromosomal constitution from that of the always diploid normal twin. Two trisomic acardiac fetuses and one triploid acardiac have been described, findings that suggest major errors in fertilization (Bieber et al., 1981; Moore et al., 1990). Genetic study in Bieber's case indicated the likelihood of origin by fertilization of a polar body for the triploid embryo. It is then remarkable that for every acardiac for which adequate placental examination has been made, a monochorionic (usually monoamnionic) placenta has been found, thought to be diagnostic of monozygosity. Occasionally, an acardiac fetus is also a fetus papyraceus (Fig. 37–18), and only radiographs show its identity. Acardiacs usually have no heart, as the name implies. Occasionally, however, a misshapen heart is found, commonly two-chambered. The wide range of sizes and shapes among acardiacs has led to a complex taxonomy. Most often, acardiacs possess legs but lack arms and often have no head or one that is markedly abnormal. An acardiac may look like an inside-out teratomatous mass (Fig. 37–19), although it can be distinguished from a teratoma by the presence of an umbilical cord. The cord is invariably short, betraying the immobility of the acardiac, and usually it possesses only one artery. Of course, acardiacs do not survive and have occasionally been removed before term (Robie et al., 1989).

Other Anomalies

It has long been known that malformations occur more commonly in twins than in singletons; this increase is due to the higher incidence of structural defects in monozygotic twins (Schinzel et al., 1979). These anomalies may be concordant, but more frequently they are discordant, even in MZ twins. The reasons for the genesis of some anomalies are more readily comprehended than for others, such as the discordant development of conjoined twins and perhaps acardiac anomaly and aplasia cutis. Perhaps some other disruptions occur as a result of interfetal vascular embolization or coagulation, such as poren-

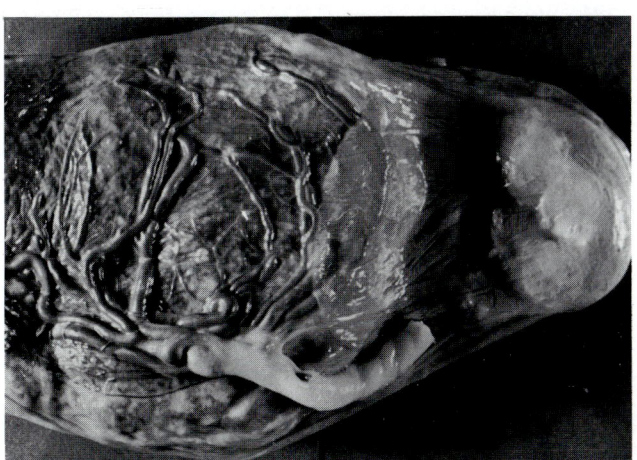

FIGURE 37–18. Diamnionic monochorionic twin placenta with acardiac fetus papyraceus in separate amnion at right. Diagnosis of acardiac nature was accomplished only by roentgenography.

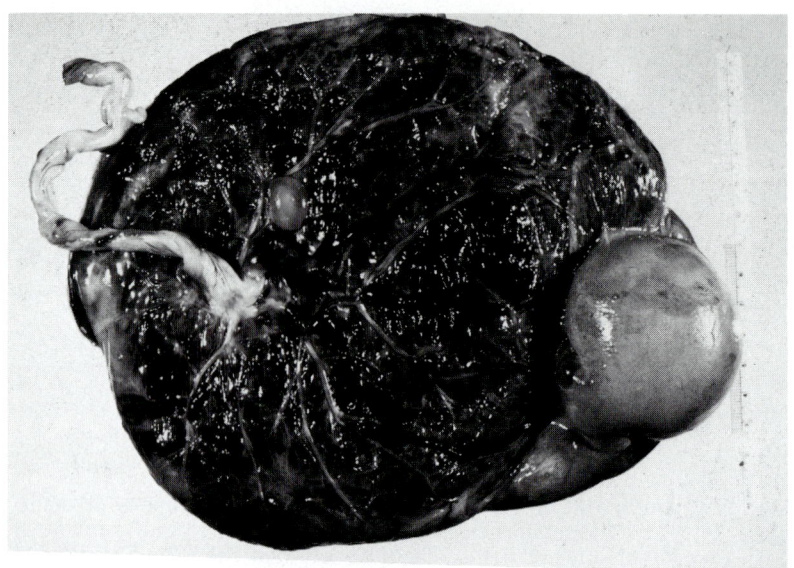

FIGURE 37–19. Diamnionic monochorionic term twin placenta with acardiac amorphus at right. It was a skin-covered ball of fat with few bones and had a very short umbilical cord. (Courtesy of the late N. Eastman.)

cephaly, and deformations due to crowding are explicable. There are a large number of structural defects, however, whose pathogenesis appears to be linked in some way to the twinning process itself. Thus, anencephaly and sirenomelia occur inexplicably commonly as discordant anomalies in MZ twins. These and other considerations, detailed by Schinzel and colleagues (1979), suggest that further studies may provide significant insight into not only the poorly understood twinning process but also the pathogenesis of many congenital anomalies.

Perhaps the most perplexing discordance occurs in the so-called heterokaryotic monozygotic twins, i.e., MZ twins with different karyotypes and phenotypes. On first impression, the idea of MZ twins with different karyotypes would appear to be contradictory. If, however, chromosomal nondisjunction of cells occurs just before or at the time of twinning, then the process that causes mosaicism in a singleton could lead to MZ twins with different chromosome sets. Most often this has been described for the sex chromosomes, and XO/XXX, XO/XX, and even XO/XY twins have been reported with appropriate divergence of phenotypes. Sixteen such cases of divergence in gonadal dysgenesis have been described (Pedersen et al., 1980), to which cases of discordance for trisomy 21 and some cases of acardiac twin must be added. These are the exceptional events, but they indicate how complex the twinning process is.

"Disappearance" of a Twin

A word may be said about the apparent frequency of twins diagnosed in early pregnancy by ultrasonography and their "disappearance" in later development. Figure 37–14 clearly indicates that even early embryonic death can be recognized in term placentas. The author has critically examined a number of term placentas from pregnancies in which twins had been ultrasonographically diagnosed in early stages, but no

fetus papyraceus or other structure resembling a twin was found. The conclusion is that great care must be exercised when diagnosing twin pregnancy by ultrasonography merely from the presence of two apparent cavities.

The Chimeras

On rare occasions, blood grouping or lymphocyte karyotype examination of fraternal twins has shown the coexistence of two genetically dissimilar cell types. This state is referred to as *blood chimerism*, because the solid tissues do not participate in the admixture. Blood chimerism is best explained by the existence of transplacental anastomoses in fraternal twins that allow the bone marrow–like blood cell precursors circulating in one embryo to settle in the other twin. Because it happens so early in embryonic life this graft is tolerated as "self" and settles permanently without any ill effect. Although this occurs with regularity in marmosets and frequently in twin cattle, it must be very uncommon in humans, in whom such anastomoses between the presumably dichorionic twins only rarely have been identified (Lage et al., 1989). The very tight junction between intimately fused placentas in DZ twins and tetrachorionic quadruplets has never been associated with such chimerism.

IDENTIFICATION OF TWIN ZYGOSITY

The zygosity of twins is of interest to the twins, their parents, and physicians who may treat the children in the future, as well as to scientists. An attempt should be made to establish the zygosity at birth and to register the objective findings in the chart. This time is particularly valuable because of the availability of the placenta, examination of which can aid materially in the process.

The most efficient way to identify zygosity is as

follows: Gender examination allows the classification of male-female pairs as fraternal or dizygotic. They should also have a dichorionic placenta that may be separated or fused. Next, the placenta is studied in detail, and twins with a monochorionic placenta (monoamnionic or diamnionic) can be set aside as being of monozygotic ("identical") origin, irrespective of whether they have dissimilar phenotypes. If doubt exists upon gross examination of the dividing membranes, then a transverse section (see Figs. 37–5 and 37–6) should be studied histologically. There then remain the like-sex twins with dichorionic placental membranes whose zygosity cannot instantly be known. They must be studied genetically, and several means of discriminating study exist. One may study a variety of enzyme markers (complex) or, more conventionally, the blood groups. If parents have dissimilar blood groups, DZ twins are more likely to have dissimilar blood groups. The larger the dissimilarity of parents, the more likely that DZ twins will differ in one marker or another. The difficulty occurs when parents have similar antigenic distribution and also when the blood bank undertaking these studies does not possess all antibodies needed to completely type the blood. Moreover, it is impossible to ascertain monozygosity with this method, although one can approach high probabilities. For these reasons, chromosome markers have been employed; they are considered by some to be more discriminating and easier to use (McCracken et al., 1978; Morton et al., 1981). Different banding patterns (Q and C bands) can be identified readily on at least five pairs of human chromosomes, and most individuals are polymorphic at several of these markers. Monozygotic twins always have an identical pattern, and dizygotic twins do not. The only reservation about this method is that the twin pairs who have been studied for chromosomal polymorphism were not newborns and their chorionic status was unknown; most of them must have been monochorionic (see Fig. 37–1). In each case, the placental anastomoses of the monochorionic placenta, by necessity, would have led to admixtures of would-be different cells. It is mandatory, therefore, to conduct such studies only in dichorionic twins in the future. The study of DNA polymorphism is currently the best way to approach these difficult problems (Derom et al., 1985; Hill and Jeffreys, 1985).

Cameron (1968), who examined gender, placentas, and genotypes of 668 consecutive twin pairs in Birmingham, England, found the following distribution: 35 per cent were DZ, because they were male and female; 20 per cent were MZ, because they were monochorionic (and had the same gender); 45 per cent had the same gender but dichorionic membranes; when these last were genotyped, 37 per cent were found to be DZ because of genetic differences, and 8 per cent to be MZ because of genetic identity.

REFERENCES

Antoine C, Young BK, Silverman F, et al: Sinusoidal fetal heart rate pattern with vasa previa in twin pregnancy. Obstet Gynecol **27**:295, 1982.

Benirschke K, Driscoll SG: The Pathology of the Human Placenta. New York, Springer-Verlag, 1967.

Benirschke K, Harper V: The acardiac anomaly. Teratology **15**:311, 1977.

Benirschke K, Kim CK: Multiple pregnancy. N Engl J Med **288**:1276, 1973.

Bieber FR, Nance WE, Morton CC, et al.: Genetic studies of an acardiac monster: Evidence of polar body twinning in man. Science **213**:775, 1981.

Boklage CE: On the distribution of nonrighthandedness among twins and their families. Acta Genet Med Gemellol (Roma) **30**:775, 1981.

Bulmer MG: The Biology of Twinning in Man. Oxford, Clarendon Press, 1970.

Cameron AH: The Birmingham twin survey. Proc Soc Med **61**:229, 1968.

Colburn DW, Pasquale SA: Monoamniotic twin pregnancy. J Reprod Med **27**:165, 1982.

De Lia JE, Emery MG, Sheafor SA, et al: Twin transfusion syndrome: successful in utero treatment with digoxin. Int J Gynaecol Obstet **23**:197, 1985a.

De Lia JE, Rogers JG, Dixon JA: Treatment of placental vasculature with a neodymium-yttrium-aluminum-garnet laser via fetoscopy. Am J Obstet Gynecol **151**:1126, 1985b.

Derom C, Bakker E, Vlietnnck R, et al.: Zygosity determination in newborn twins using DNA variants. J Med Genet **22**:279, 1985.

Goldgar DE, Kimberling WJ: Genetic expectations of polar body twinning. Acta Genet Med Gemellol (Roma) **30**:257, 1981.

Guttmacher AF: The incidence of multiple births in man and some other uniparae. Obstet Gynecol **2**:22, 1953.

Harris DW: Letter to the editor. J Reprod Med **27**:39, 1982.

Hertig AT: Human Trophoblast. Springfield, Ill, Charles C Thomas, 1968.

Hill AVS, Jeffreys AJ: Use of minisatellite DNA probes for determination of twin zygosity at birth. Lancet **2**:1394, 1985.

James WH: Dizygotic twinning, marital stage and status and coital rates. Ann Hum Biol **8**:371, 1981.

Kaufman MH, O'Shea KS: Induction of monozygotic twinning in the mouse. Nature **276**:707, 1978.

Lage JM, VanMarter LJ, Mikhail E: Vascular anastomoses in fused, dichorionic twin placentas resulting in twin transfusion syndrome. Placenta **10**:55, 1989.

Liu S, Benirschke K, Scioscia AL, et al.: Intrauterine death in multiple gestation. Acta Genet Med Gemellol (Roma) **41**:5, 1992.

Mannino, FL, Jones KL, Benirschke K: Congenital skin defects and fetus papyraceus. J Pediatr **91**:559, 1977.

Martin NG, Shanley S, Butt K, et al: Excessive follicular recruitment and growth in mothers of spontaneous dizygotic twins. Acta Genet Med Gemellol (Roma) **40**:291, 1991

McCracken AA, Daly PA, Zolnick MR, et al.: Twins and Q-banded chromosome polymorphisms. Hum Genet **45**:253, 1978.

McLeod FN, McCoy DR: Monoamniotic twins with an unusual cord complication. Case report. Br J Obstet Gynaecol **88**:774, 1981.

Meyer WR, Meyer WW: Report on a very young dizygotic human twin pregnancy. Arch Gynecol **231**:51, 1981.

Moore TR, Gale S, Benirschke K: Perinatal outcome of forty-nine pregnancies complicated by acardiac twinning. Am J Obstet Gynecol **163**:907, 1990.

Morton CC, Covey LA, Nance WE, et al.: Quinacrine mustard and nucleolar organizer region heteromorphisms in twins. Acta Genet Med Gemellol (Roma) **30**:39, 1981.

Nylander PPS: The factors that influence twinning rates. Acta Genet Med Gemellol (Roma) **30**:189, 1981.

Pedersen IK, Philip J, Sele V, et al.: Monozygotic twins with dissimilar phenotypes and chromosome complements. Acta Obstet Gynecol Scand **59**:459, 1980.

Robie GF, Payne GG, Morgan MA: Selective delivery of an acardiac, acephalic twin. N Engl J Med **320**:512, 1989.

Schenker JG, Yarkoni S, Granat M: Multiple pregnancies following induction of ovulation. Fertil Steril **35**:105, 1981.

Schinzel AAGL, Smith DW, Miller JR: Monozygotic twinning and structural defects. J Pediatr **95**:921, 1979.

Soma H, Takayama M, Kiyokawa T, et al.: Serum gonadotropin levels in Japanese women. Obstet Gynecol **46**:311, 1975.

Thomas DB: Intrauterine intraventricular haemorrhage and disseminated intravascular coagulation in a triplet pregnancy. Aust Paediatr J **10**:25, 1974.

Van Drie DM, Kammeraad LA: Vasa previa. Case report, review and presentation of a new diagnostic method. J Reprod Med **26**:577, 1981.

Winn HN, Gabrielli S, Reece EA et al.: Ultrasonographic criteria for the prenatal diagnosis of placental chorionicity in twin gestations. Am J Obstet Gynecol **161**:1540, 1989.

Wittmann BK, Baldwin, VJ, Nichol B: Antenatal diagnosis of twin transfusion syndrome by ultrasound. Obstet Gynecol **58**:123, 1981.

Wright JCY, Christopher CR: Sirenomelia, Potter's syndrome and their relationship to monozygotic twinning. A case report and discussion. J Reprod Med **27**:291, 1982.

Yoshioka H, Kadomoto Y, Mino M et al.: Multicystic encephalomalacia in liveborn twin with a stillborn macerated co-twin. J Pediatr **95**:798, 1979.

CHAPTER

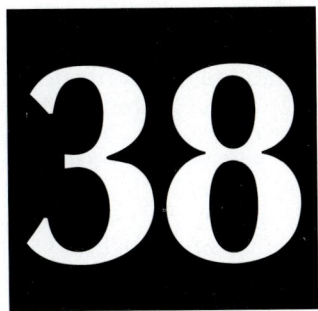

38

MULTIPLE GESTATION: CLINICAL
CHARACTERISTICS AND MANAGEMENT

ALASTAIR H. MacLENNAN, M.D.

CLINICAL CHARACTERISTICS OF MULTIPLE GESTATION

Mortality and Morbidity

Multiple pregnancy remains a high-risk situation, with published perinatal mortality rates in developed countries ranging between 47 and 120 per 1000 births for twins and between 93 and 203 per 1000 births for triplets (Lipitz et al., 1989). The increased risk of perinatal death in a twin pregnancy compared with a singleton pregnancy is now approximately fivefold higher, the risk being slightly higher for the second twin (Botting et al., 1987). The increased risk of death in twins persists during the first year of life, and it is not until the second year that mortality rates for twins are the same as for singletons (MacGillivray, 1978).

Approximately 10 per cent of preterm deliveries are twin gestations, and they account for 25 per cent of the perinatal deaths in preterm deliveries (Rush et al., 1976). The large majority of the deaths in preterm multiple deliveries occur with gestations less than 32 weeks and birth weights under 1500 gm (Fowler et al., 1991). Intrauterine growth restriction is also common in multiple gestation and makes an important contribution to the high incidence of low-birth-weight and stillborn babies. In general, the greater the number of fetuses in a gestation, the smaller their weight for gestational age (Fig. 38–1). Most studies of twin pregnancies show that more than 50 per cent of twins are born weighing less than 2500 gm. In the United States, the average birth weight of the first twin is 2390 gm and of the second twin 2310 gm (Keith et al., 1980).

The high rates of prematurity and intrauterine growth restriction in multiple gestation are also associated with a significant incidence of neonatal morbidity. The cost of a twin pregnancy to the parents and the community is much more than double that of a singleton pregnancy, as demonstrated by the fact that currently approximately every sixth baby receiving neonatal intensive care at Queen Victoria Hospital in Adelaide, Australia, is the product of a multiple gestation.

Two-thirds of twins at birth show some signs of growth restriction (Miller and Merritt, 1979). Follow-up studies of growth-restricted twins show a tendency for persistence of short stature and lower weight percentiles; at 6 years of age the mean weight and height for such twins are between the 10th and 25th percentiles. Ten to 13 years after birth, twins with more than a 36 per cent discrepancy in birth weight will still have, in general, a significant disparity in size.

Intelligence quotient (IQ) tests show a slight reduction in the mean IQ of twins and a further reduction in the mean IQ of triplets, but IQ measurements do not fully reveal the subsequent developmental handicaps of children born of multiple gestations. More sophisticated developmental tests of these children's learning ability and motor skills, e.g., hand-eye coordination, suggest that twins who have evidence of growth restriction at birth are significantly disadvantaged compared with their more fully grown singleton counterparts.

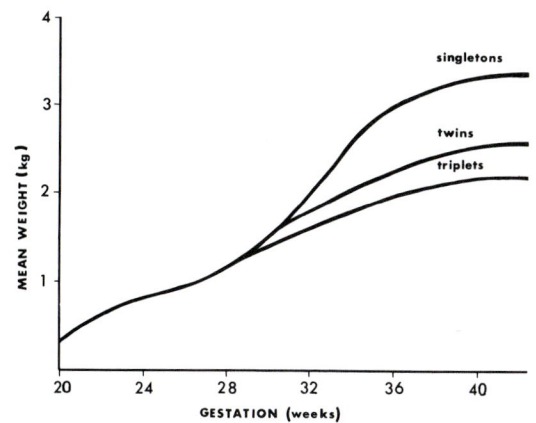

FIGURE 38–1. Mean fetal growth rates in singleton and multiple pregnancies.

In a developmental study of small-for-gestational-age (SGA) infants from both singleton and multiple pregnancies, Fitzhardinge and Steven (1972) found little in the way of major neurologic problems such as cerebral palsy, seizures, and hearing or visual defects in these infants. However, in later childhood 36 per cent of SGA infants were failing at school, 25 per cent had minimal brain dysfunction, 60 per cent had electroencephalographic abnormalities (without seizures), and 30 per cent had speech deficits. Of course, not all infants born of a multiple pregnancy show signs of intrauterine growth restriction, and if they do not suffer any of the complications of prematurity, their normal development seems more assured. Nevertheless, the majority of infants born of a multiple gestation will be of low birth weight (less than 2500 gm) and are at risk of significant short-term and long-term handicaps.

Maternal Mortality and Morbidity. Maternal mortality and morbidity rates are increased in multiple pregnancy. The maternal complications are numerous and are discussed later. Together they contribute to the high incidence of physical discomfort, prolonged hospitalization, surgical delivery, and social inconvenience associated with multiple pregnancy. The high risks of multiple pregnancy are generally underestimated by the lay public, who often simply view the pregnancy as twice as interesting and exciting with twice the expected happy result. The inexperienced obstetrician should not be so mistaken and would do well to refer the patient to a high-risk perinatal unit early in her pregnancy, where an experienced perinatal team can try to anticipate and cope with the many problems of multiple gestation.

Risk Factors

The antenatal risk factors in multiple gestation that correlate with higher perinatal mortality and morbidity rates are shown in Table 38–1. Clearly, the risks increase enormously with triplets, quadruplets, and so on. Late detection or nonrecognition of multiple pregnancy until delivery also correlates with a poor outcome and is an important argument in favor of routine, early ultrasound screening in all pregnancies. Other than ultrasonography, the only early prognostic sign of poor fetal outcome in twin pregnancy is the serum alpha-fetoprotein level, which is normally raised twofold in twin pregnancy. Levels more than

Table 38–1. Antenatal Risk Factors in Multiple Gestation

More than two fetuses	Premature rupture of membranes
Discordancy of fetal size	
Low maternal age	Preterm labor
Low maternal parity	Antepartum hemorrhage
Serum alpha-fetoprotein more than 4 × median	Pregnancy-induced hypertension
Late detection	Polyhydramnios
Monozygosity	Single fetal death
Black ethnicity	Malpresentation or labor outside a major center

four multiples of the median for singleton pregnancy correlate with an increased incidence of twins with birth weights less than 2500 gm (Wald et al., 1978).

Monozygosity may be suspected antenatally when ultrasonographic examination shows a single placenta, like sex, and a monochorionic septum (Barss et al., 1985). The perinatal mortality rate among monozygotic twins is approximately twice that of dizygotic twins. Monoamnionic twins have an even higher mortality rate, approaching 50 to 60 per cent. Intrapartum risk factors are malpresentation in labor, delay of more than 30 minutes between delivery of the first and second babies, premature separation of the placenta, increasing morbidity in relation to the birth order, and nonrecognition of the second or third fetus until birth. Postnatal risk factors are related to prematurity, the degree of intrauterine growth restriction, and the presence or absence of neonatal intensive care at delivery, with outcome being improved if tertiary care is available at delivery.

Complications

Abortion. Inevitable abortion is at least twice as common in multiple pregnancy as in singleton pregnancy, and a continuing pregnancy with resorption of one or more of the embryos may be even more common. Less than half the twin pregnancies diagnosed via ultrasound during the first trimester are finally delivered as twins (Varma, 1979). A vanishing twin can be an explanation for discordance between chorionic villus karyotype and fetal karyotype (Reddy et al., 1991). Some twins may be silently absorbed, whereas the demise of others is associated with bleeding and uterine activity. Only occasionally can a fetus papyraceus or remnants of the second placenta be found at delivery of the live twin, but as discussed in Chapter 37, many such occurrences may be missed. Obstetricians should exert great caution about informing the patient of the presence of a multiple pregnancy solely on the basis of ultrasound examination in the first trimester. Unless there are early pregnancy complications, the need for such early routine ultrasound examinations is debatable.

Congenital Anomalies. Malformations are approximately twice as common in twin infants as in singleton infants and four times as common in triplets. Kohl and Casey (1975) reported that in twin infants the incidence of major malformations was 2.12 per cent and of minor malformations 4.13 per cent. No particular malformation predominates in twin gestations, although cardiac anomalies are reported as not being involved in the overall increase. Monozygotic twins have twice the incidence of fetal abnormalities compared with dizygotic twins (Cameron et al., 1983). Conjoined twins are a rare complication of monozygotic twinning, occurring about once in every 1500 twin pregnancies. Rodis et al (1990) calculate that the risk of a woman aged 33 having a twin pregnancy with at least one fetus with Down's syndrome is the same as that of a woman aged 35 with a singleton pregnancy. Thus, prenatal testing should be considered at an earlier age. Prenatal testing presents problems, which are discussed later in this chapter.

HYPEREMESIS GRAVIDARUM. Excess nausea and vomiting should always alert the physician to the possibility of multiple pregnancy and the need for ultrasonographic screening. An increase in nausea or vomiting is common in multiple pregnancy and may be associated with the increased hormonal levels in such pregnancies. Other differential diagnoses must be excluded, such as urinary tract infection, hydatidiform mole, and psychosocial problems. The treatment for hyperemesis associated with multiple pregnancy is the same as for singleton pregnancy.

PREGNANCY ANEMIA. Maternal blood volume in twin pregnancy is approximately 500 ml greater than in singleton pregnancy, and, of course, the fetal demands are proportionately greater. Thus, iron and folate deficiency anemias are more common, the incidence varying with the nutritional status of the local population. Iron supplementation of 60 to 80 mg and folic acid supplementation of 1 mg per day are recommended in multiple pregnancy, along with a varied high-protein diet.

PREGNANCY-INDUCED HYPERTENSION. In multiple pregnancy, hypertension is more common, occurs earlier, and is more severe than in singleton pregnancy. Approximately 40 per cent of twin pregnancies and 60 per cent of triplet pregnancies will be complicated by hypertension. The exact incidence is hard to determine, perhaps because many multiple pregnancies terminate before the peak period at which symptoms are manifested. Most studies suggest, however, that in multiple pregnancy there is at least a threefold increase in the incidence of pregnancy-induced hypertension and also an increase in the severity of the disease, even in patients who have had previously uncomplicated singleton pregnancies.

POLYHYDRAMNIOS. The uterus and its twin contents often reach a volume of 10 liters or more and weigh in excess of 10 kg. Approximately one-third of this volume is amniotic fluid. Acute polyhydramnios does occur, particularly with monoamnionic twins. It has been reported as occurring in 5 to 8 per cent of multiple pregnancies and is another factor contributing to the high incidence of preterm labor in such gestations. Acute polyhydramnios before 28 weeks gestation has been reported as occurring in 1.7 per cent of all twin pregnancies (Steinberg et al., 1990). The perinatal mortality in such cases reaches 90 per cent but as will be discussed later, serial amniocentesis may significantly improve the fetal survival rate (Mahony et al., 1990).

PRETERM DELIVERY. The incidence of preterm delivery (before 37 weeks) in twin gestations approaches 50 per cent (Rush et al., 1976). This incidence is 12 times higher than that seen in singleton pregnancy, and the average length of gestation decreases inversely with the number of fetuses present (Table 38–2). Most neonatal deaths in multiple premature births are associated with gestations of less than 32 weeks and birth weights under 1500 gm. As one would expect, prolonged rupture of the membranes is also associated with a high mortality rate. The critical period, on the basis of current perinatal mortality figures, would

TABLE 38–2. Average Length of Gestation in Relation to Number of Fetuses*

NO. FETUSES	NO. PREGNANCIES	WEEKS COMPLETED
Singleton	82	39
Twins	21	35
Triplets	5	33
Quadruplets	3	29

*For pregnancies beyond 20 weeks with known ovulation date; length of gestation calculated from 2 weeks before ovulation.

From Caspi E, Ronen J, Schreyer P, et al: The outcome of pregnancy after gonadotrophin therapy. Br J Obstet Gynaecol 83:967, 1976.

appear to be between *26 and 32 weeks* gestation. The 1990 data from the Neonatal Intensive Care Unit of the Queen Victoria Hospital, Adelaide, Australia, for all low-birth-weight infants show that the mortality rate for babies less than 600 gm at birth is more than 80 per cent, and yet the mortality rate for babies over 1000 gm is less than 10 per cent. Thus, the period of growth between 600 and 1000 gm would certainly appear to be critical, and it corresponds in singleton pregnancies to between 26 and 29 weeks gestation. Mindful of such statistics, Lukacs and colleagues (1984), and others, have found antenatal sonographic fetal weight estimation to be a relatively accurate predictor of birth weight at these limits of viability. Birth weights of infants weighing between 500 and 1500 gm were accurately predicted to within 10 per cent in 92 per cent of pregnancies studied by Key et al. (1983). Thus, with regard to the mode of delivery, should termination of the pregnancy in these circumstances be necessary or inevitable, cesarean section may compromise the mother unnecessarily if the estimated fetal weight is less than 600 gm but may be warranted if the estimated weight is higher.

In view of the high incidences of preterm labor and perinatal mortality between 26 and 32 weeks gestation, many obstetricians used to admit patients with multiple pregnancies to the hospital around this time. Bed rest, cervical sutures, steroids, and prophylactic tocolytic agents have not been shown to prevent or ameliorate the effects of preterm delivery. A randomized controlled trial of routine hospitalization between 26 and 30 weeks gestation failed to show any benefit from such a policy, and indeed there was a trend toward a greater morbidity and mortality in the group randomly allocated to inpatient care (MacLennan et al., 1990). Several small trials have studied the use of prophylactic beta-sympathomimetic drugs, e.g., ritodrine (O'Connor et al., 1979), terbutaline (Skjaerris and Aberg, 1982), and oral salbutamol (Ashworth et al., 1990), and have failed to demonstrate a significant improvement in gestational age or birth weight in treated twin pregnancies. (The doses used in some of these trials may have been too small to achieve the optimal tocolytic effect.) Beta-mimetics have a smaller margin of safety in multiple pregnancy, in which there is a greater increase in blood volume and cardiac output with an increased risk of pulmonary edema than in singleton pregnancy (see Chapter 33). The prevention of preterm delivery in multiple pregnancy is discussed under Management of Multiple Gestation.

INTRAUTERINE GROWTH RESTRICTION. Two-thirds of twin infants show clinical and objective signs (neonatal body water turnover) of intrauterine growth restriction (Miller and Merritt, 1979; MacLennan et al., 1981). Approximately 70 per cent of the infants born of multiple gestation are significantly growth-restricted, and the incidence and degree of growth restriction in multiple pregnancy increase toward term. Disparity in growth rates between twins *in utero* can often be great, especially with twin transfusion syndrome.

TWIN TRANSFUSION SYNDROME. Approximately 15 per cent of monochorionic twin pregnancies show clinical evidence of twin-to-twin transfusion, and in these cases the perinatal mortality for both twins is high. The pathology of such vascular anastomoses is described in Chapter 37 (see Fig. 37–10). The recognition and treatment of this important complication are discussed later in this chapter.

HEMORRHAGE. Surprisingly, most studies of multiple gestation show only a small increase in the incidence of antepartum hemorrhage, despite the larger area of placentation and the expected increase in rates of placenta previa, accidental hemorrhage, and vasa previa. However, the risk of uterine atony and of postpartum hemorrhage is significantly increased, presumably owing to overdistention of the uterus during multiple pregnancy.

NEUROLOGIC DAMAGE. Cerebral palsy, microcephaly, porencephaly, and multiple encephalomalacia occur more frequently in multiple gestations than in singleton pregnancies and more frequently when delivery is preterm (Bejar et al., 1990). Monochorionic infants have a significantly higher incidence of antenatal necrosis of the cerebral white matter than dichorionic infants or singletons. Ischemic necrosis and cavitary brain lesions have been described many times after the fetal demise of one co-twin. This risk appears higher if death occurs in later gestation, but has been described in cases where death of the co-twin has occurred early in the second trimester (Anderson et al., 1990). This risk should be discussed with the patient if selective termination is considered at midgestation for fetal anomaly. There is evidence to suggest that emboli of thromboplastic material from the dead fetus are transported via vascular placental shunts to the brain, bowel, kidneys, and lungs.

The diagnosis of white matter necrosis in surviving infants is made after delivery by echoencephalography. Serial studies show that cavitary lesions and cerebral atrophy develop two or more weeks after the acute stage of necrosis in the white matter (Bejar et al., 1988). The demonstration of cavitary lesions and cerebral atrophy in the first few days after birth would indicate that these lesions occurred antenatally and not during the intrapartum period.

The incidence of necrosis of the cerebral white matter in twins is not accurately known, but has been reported as approximately 14 per cent in multiple gestations delivered at less than 36 weeks gestation (Bejar et al., 1990). This necrosis occurs not only in the presence of the demise of a co-twin, but also—and significantly more often—with monochorionic pregnancies, polyhydramnios, hydrops, and placental vascular connections, particularly vein-to-vein anastomoses.

INTRAPARTUM COMPLICATIONS. Malpresentation, cord prolapse, cord entanglement (particularly in monoamnionic twins), incoordinate uterine action, fetal distress, and surgical intervention are all more common during labor in multiple gestation than in singleton gestation. Locking or collision of twins is extremely rare, despite the disproportionate amount of attention given to this occurrence.

MANAGEMENT OF MULTIPLE GESTATION

If the outcome of multiple pregnancy is to improve, the prime objectives must be the prevention of preterm delivery and the recognition and effective management of intrauterine growth restriction, twin-twin transfusion syndrome, and evidence of a risk of antenatal neurologic damage. There seems little doubt, on review of the perinatal mortality and morbidity statistics, that all multiple pregnancies should be managed in high-risk perinatal units with neonatal intensive care facilities. General practitioners and obstetricians with access to only primary care facilities should at least request shared-care facilities at a unit specializing in perinatal medicine. Contact with such a unit should ideally occur from the time a multiple pregnancy is diagnosed. Such a recommendation will obviously meet with practical problems in some areas of the world, but all patients with multiple gestation should have antenatal access to tertiary-care perinatal facilities.

Early Diagnosis

The merits of routine ultrasonographic screening of all pregnancies before 20 weeks gestation are still debated. However, early detection of multiple pregnancy has many advantages with regard to its management, and routine ultrasonographic screening of all pregnancies may be justified solely on the basis of the high morbidity and mortality rates of multiple gestation. Studies show that prior to the routine use of ultrasonography, less than 50 per cent of twin pregnancies were diagnosed before the end of the critical period (32 weeks). Diagnosis of multiple gestation late in pregnancy or at delivery correlates with a high risk for a poor perinatal outcome. Some reports of twin pregnancies show that routine early ultrasonographic screening for multiple pregnancy is effective, both for detecting nearly all such pregnancies and for instituting therapy, which may significantly improve the perinatal outcome (Persson et al., 1979). As mentioned earlier, a very early ultrasonographic diagnosis of multiple pregnancy must be made with caution, because one or more of the fetuses may be absorbed. It should also be remembered that ultrasonography gives only a two-dimensional image, and an extra sac or fetus may occasionally be missed, particularly if hydramnios is present.

For detection of multiple pregnancy, some authors have suggested the routine assay of one of several hormones that are generally raised in the presence of more than one fetus. Placental lactogen, chorionic

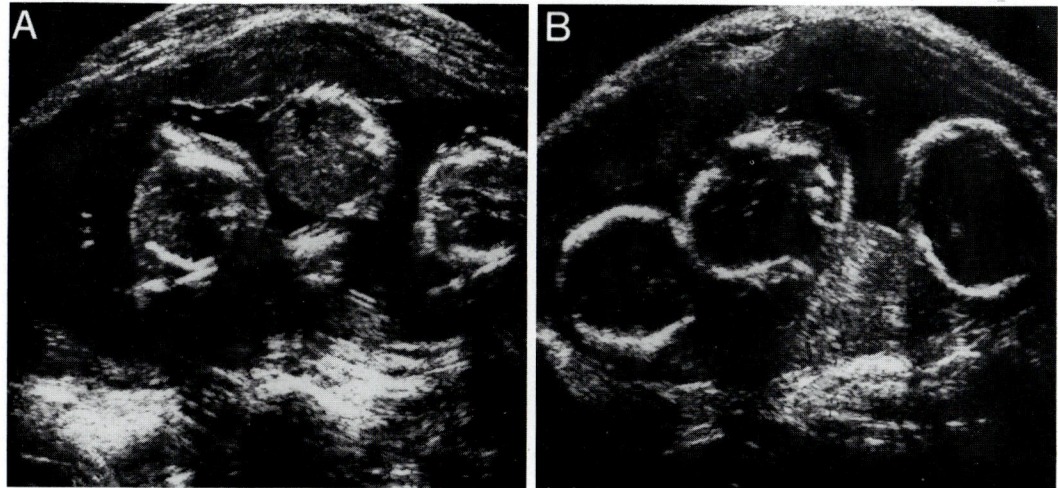

FIGURE 38–2. Ultrasonogram of triplets at 18 weeks gestation, showing trunk areas *(A)* and cross sections of the three heads *(B)*.

gonadotrophin, alpha-fetoprotein, estriol, and pregnanediol have all been reported as elevated in multiple pregnancy, but owing to variability in results there is still no biochemical test that will clearly differentiate multiple from singleton pregnancy, and ultrasonography remains the best screening test to date (Fig. 38–2).

Antenatal Care

Early diagnosis of multiple pregnancy is helpful because it gives time for the patient to be educated about the many ways in which her pregnancy will differ from a singleton pregnancy and for the patient and her family to be motivated to cooperate in the extra antenatal care and potential hospitalization associated with multiple pregnancy. There is merit in running special antenatal classes for such patients and their husbands. These classes can explain the need for increased nutrition, rest, and antenatal fetal monitoring, include tours of the neonatal intensive care unit, and give details of the special sources of postnatal support for parents after multiple births.

Early referral to a specialized perinatal unit allows time for the patient to gain confidence in her new attendants and for baseline values of fetal growth to be established, such as dating of the pregnancy by ultrasonography. When levels of alpha-fetoprotein are raised more than four multiples of the median, there is a high risk of a poor outcome, even when neural tube defects are not present. As multiple pregnancy is more common in older women, amniocentesis or chorionic villus biopsy may be indicated to rule out chromosomal anomalies; these procedures are not contraindicated in twin gestation, but introduce potential medical and ethical dilemmas.

Patients considering genetic testing in twin pregnancy must be carefully counseled beforehand about the dilemma they will face if one twin is found to have a severe abnormality and the other is thought to be normal. One possibility is selective abortion. The

risk of such a procedure cannot be accurately assessed yet. A review of 12 published case reports (Redwine and Hays, 1986) noted that cardiac puncture with fetal exsanguination or air embolization of the abnormal twin resulted in successful delivery of the healthy twin in nine of these cases without maternal morbidity in any instance. However, as discussed earlier, neurologic damage in the surviving twin is a potential risk, although in this circumstance the twins are likely to be dichorionic with less chance of vascular anastomoses. If selective abortion is an option, careful identification of each twin is necessary at the initial amniocentesis. A small amount of indigo-carmine dye can be inserted into the first sac after initial aspiration of the amniotic fluid to ensure that the second sample is indeed from the second sac. Careful sonographic mapping of both fetuses, with any differences recorded on video, is also helpful. A small amount of radiopaque dye may be added to the second sac, so that if there is any doubt 3 weeks later as to which sac is which, a single x-ray can be performed to identify the second twin.

Several other controversies about the management of multiple pregnancy persist, mainly because there is a lack of properly controlled prospective clinical trials. Most management approaches aim at the prevention of preterm delivery and the recognition and treatment of intrauterine growth restriction. The principal controversial aspects of such management are dealt with in this discussion. Whatever doubts there are as to their precise effectiveness, however, the perinatal statistics for multiple pregnancies managed in specialized units remain better than for those managed elsewhere (O'Connor et al., 1981), and referral of patients with multiple pregnancies to tertiary-care perinatal units is strongly recommended. A summary of the suggested intrapartum management of multiple pregnancy is shown in Figure 38–3.

Policies of Unproven Value

BED REST. Hospitalization and/or prolonged bed rest has previously been advocated in twin pregnancy

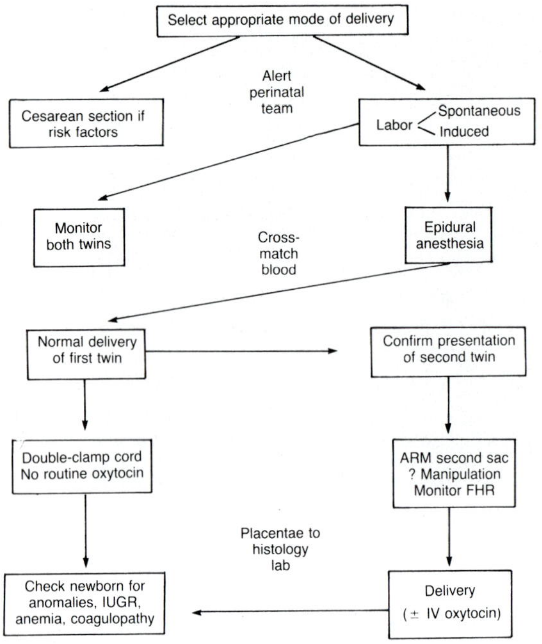

FIGURE 38–3. Flow chart for the management of multiple birth.

to improve perinatal outcome. Nonrandomized retrospective studies of this practice gave conflicting results. Recently, however, several prospective randomized controlled trials have been published, and all four studies give similar results and come to the same conclusion that routine hospitalization of women with twin gestations is not worthwhile (Crowther, 1991). An overview of the trials is shown in Table 38–3. There is even a trend to suggest that hospitalization might be disadvantageous with regard to gestational age at delivery and early neonatal death, although maternal hypertension may be reduced with rest. Hospital admission was both costly and socially inconvenient to the women and their families. The earliest admission in the trials was at 26 weeks gestation (MacLennan et al., 1990), and rest before this gestation has not been studied.

There seems to be no merit in routinely admitting women to the hospital for rest unless they have other major risk factors. There may be some logic in advo-

cating decreased work and exercise during multiple pregnancy, but even this advice has not been tested.

Cervical Cerclage. There may occasionally be an indication to insert a cervical suture, but this procedure should be considered only when there are definite signs of cervical incompetence during the second trimester (see Chapter 30). The routine use of cervical cerclage has not been found to prolong multiple pregnancy, and there may actually be a greater risk of premature labor after insertion of a cervical suture (Sinka et al., 1979; Grant, 1989). Although there may be merit in frequent, gentle assessment of the cervix to detect true cervical incompetence or early evidence of preterm labor, generally a conservative approach to cervical cerclage seems appropriate.

Beta-Adrenergic Agents. Meta-analysis of the published randomized trials to date suggests that the use of low-dosage beta-adrenergic drugs in twin pregnancy does not appear to influence the incidence of preterm labor (Kierse et al., 1989). The use of these agents is still open to question (Prescott, 1980), however, and when higher dosages are used, the mean gestational age at delivery may be higher, as may the mean birth weight (TambyRaja and Ratnam, 1979). The efficacy of prophylactic administration of tocolytic agents in multiple pregnancy remains to be determined, but if they are used, doses may be required that result in an increase in maternal heart rate (TambyRaja and Ratnam, 1979; Lipshitz, 1977). The use of these agents to inhibit established preterm labor is discussed in Chapter 33.

Cervical Assessment. Weekly digital cervical examinations (Newman et al., 1991) or a single examination at 32 weeks gestation (Neilson et al., 1988) has been found to better predict the risk of preterm labor in multiple pregnancy. However, the sensitivity and specificity of such a test are not high. Patients found to have a ripe cervix are eligible for more intensive monitoring and early tocolysis but the only randomized controlled trial yet published of hospitalization for increased rest and monitoring in twin pregnancies, where cervical dilatation has been found, showed no improvement in the perinatal outcome in the hospitalized group (Crowther et al., 1989). The policy of routine cervical examination remains an unproven intervention.

Uterine Activity Monitoring. The value of home uterine activity monitoring remains controversial in

TABLE 38–3. Overview of Randomized Controlled Trials of Hospitalization in Twin Pregnancy

OUTCOME	ODDS RATIO	95% C.I.	0.1	0.5	1	2	10
Low birth weight	0.83	0.65–1.06					
Preterm delivery	1.35	1.02–1.78					
Stillbirth	0.82	0.38–1.77					
Neonatal death	2.84	1.02–7.87					
Perinatal death	1.31	0.70–2.43					
Admission to level 3	1.12	0.76–1.66					
Hypertension	0.55	0.32–0.97					

Data from Crowther CA: Hospitalization for bed rest in multiple pregnancy. *In* Chalmers I (ed): Oxford Database of Perinatal Trials, Version 1.2, Disc Issue 6, Record 3375, Autumn 1991.

singleton pregnancy and is discussed in Chapter 33. The technology and related services are not available in many countries. In multiple gestations, uterine activity is significantly increased during the 24 hours before the diagnosis of labor (Garite et al., 1990). In a small randomized controlled trial, Knuppel et al. (1990) allocated 45 twin pregnancies either to daily home uterine activity monitoring and perinatal nursing or to an education group. Preterm labor was diagnosed at an earlier stage in the monitored group, and with tocolysis this led to significantly fewer preterm births. A recent prospective trial of 189 twin gestations revealed that patient education and self-palpation decreased the incidence of preterm birth in comparison to standard obstetric care; the addition of home uterine activity monitoring markedly decreased the incidence of preterm birth and further improved neonatal outcome in comparison to both standard care and education and palpation (Dyson et al., 1991). Further trials of this expensive service are required before its widespread use can be advocated.

AVOIDANCE OF COITUS. There is no evidence that coitus should be avoided in multiple pregnancies with intact membranes. In a study of 126 twin pregnancies, Neilson and Mutambira (1989) could find no correlation between coitus and the onset of preterm or term labor.

Fetal Monitoring in Multiple Pregnancy

This aspect of the management of multiple pregnancy presents several problems. Clinical estimation of uterine size or the interpretation of fetal movement patterns may not be helpful when only one of the twin fetuses is in jeopardy. In particular, the value of fetoplacental hormone assays is questionable. Although estriol and human placental lactogen levels are generally raised in multiple pregnancy, unless both fetuses are significantly growth-restricted, levels of these hormones may not be low. In a study of the value of hormone assays in twin pregnancy, Duncan and co-workers (1979) concluded that the analysis of hormone levels can be expected to contribute to the prevention of only a small proportion of perinatal deaths in such pregnancies. Although actual hormone levels per se are poor predictors of twin growth restriction, falling levels may predict some cases of growth restriction, if such observations are incorporated in a scoring system that includes clinical and ultrasonographic measurements (Houlton et al., 1981). At present, ultrasonography and antenatal cardiotocography appear to be the best predictors of intrauterine growth restriction in multiple gestation.

ULTRASONOGRAPHY. Serial ultrasound examinations, particularly if fetal weight or trunk area can be estimated, appear to be the optimal method of detecting intrauterine growth restriction in multiple pregnancy. Serial cephalometry in twin pregnancy can detect about 50 per cent of small-for-dates fetuses, but few studies claim greater success because of the technical and interpretive problems associated with the measurement of biparietal diameter (BPD) in multiple pregnancy. The product of crown-rump length × trunk area may provide a sensitive index of growth

restriction in twin pregnancy and prevents an error in BPD measurement (Neilson, 1981). However, the BPD can still be a useful measurement, especially if the BPD of either twin is more than 3 weeks behind the normal rate of growth as calculated from a singleton growth chart, or if there is discordance between the twin BPD measurements of more than 0.6 mm. Leveno and colleagues (1980) reported a 2.7 per cent mortality when the difference in the twin BPD was 0 to 6 mm and a 20 per cent mortality rate with a difference of 7 mm or more. Obviously, the value of the ultrasonographic information partly depends on the experience of the ultrasonographer and the sophistication of the equipment used. Ideally, however, all measurements of twin size (BPD, crown-rump length, trunk area) should be made, with notice taken of any discordance, either between the growth rates of the twins or between their growth and normal singleton growth. Lukacs and associates (1984) have found the estimation of fetal weight from these measurements in multiple pregnancy to be useful and relatively accurate. Measurements of umbilical artery flow velocity (Giles et al., 1988) appear to be another useful and additional biophysical predictor of twin growth, and randomized studies in this developing area of fetal monitoring are awaited (see Chapter 16). Ultrasonographic examinations should be conducted every 3 to 4 weeks from 23 weeks gestation on, to monitor the growth of each fetus.

ANTENATAL FETAL HEART RATE MONITORING. Non-stress cardiotocography to assess fetal well-being in patients with multiple pregnancy is feasible and of clinical value (Blake et al., 1984). Bailey and co-workers (1980) found it to be a better predictor of perinatal mortality and morbidity than serial estriol or serial BPD measurements. However, non-stress cardiotocography requires the simultaneous presence of a monitor and an operator for each fetus and perhaps real-time ultrasonography for accurate localization of each fetus. Therefore, performance of non-stress cardiotocography before 34 weeks gestation is not indicated unless clinical or ultrasonographic measurements suggest the presence of intrauterine growth restriction prior to that date. Although routine cardiotocography after 34 weeks gestation is debatable from a cost-efficiency point of view, it certainly should be considered if any other risk factors are present. There is at least a theoretical concern that the use of a contraction stress test in multiple frequency might precipitate preterm delivery, and thus this test may be inappropriate.

ASSESSMENT OF PULMONARY MATURITY. Amniocentesis to determine amniotic fluid surfactant levels is not necessary unless there is a strong indication for preterm delivery, in which case the fetuses should be delivered regardless of pulmonary maturity. Nevertheless, there are still occasions when a knowledge of fetal pulmonary maturity may help the timing of delivery in a multiple pregnancy. In such cases, amniocentesis of one sac is usually sufficient to obtain information regarding the risk of future hyaline membrane disease in each infant. Most studies suggest that there is a close correlation between the lecithin-sphyngomyelin (L/S) ratios in both sacs, and an L/S ratio of 2.5 or more in any sample should safely allow for most intersac variations. However, one report has stated that there may be marked differences between twin pairs (Obladen and Gluck, 1977), and therefore an effort should be made to obtain fluid from both sacs before elective induction.

Twin-Twin Transfusion

This syndrome is a complication of monozygotic-monochorionic twinning and is associated with a poor perinatal outcome. Clinical suspicion of the antenatal presence of a twin transfusion syndrome should be aroused when ultrasonographic examination suggests single placentation and a single chorion, disparity in fetal size, and polyhydramnios in the sac of the larger twin. There may be little or no liquor around the smaller fetus ("stuck twin sign"). Fetal hydrops suggesting congestive cardiac failure is usually a terminal sign. There may be a difference in Doppler velocimetry umbilical artery systolic/diastolic rates between the twins. Such signs may occur between 20 and 30 weeks gestation, and the option of immediate delivery (by cesarean section) will depend on the chances of viability, potential morbidity in the surviving twin, and related ethical issues.

Fetal blood sampling by cordocentesis is an option that may have several advantages. Similar blood groups help to establish monozygosity, and an inter-twin hemoglobin of >5 g/dl confirms the diagnosis. The degree of anemia in the smaller twin may help to determine the need for urgent intervention.

If extreme prematurity prevents delivery, several radical interventions can be considered in view of the high mortality associated with expectant management. Repeated decompression amniocentesis has been reported as being successful (Urig et al., 1990), but in a review of treatment modalities for this syndrome, Blickstein (1990) concludes that although it may sometimes be performed for maternal reasons, the efficacy from the fetal point of view is poor. Selective fetocide of the donor has been an option, but risks the outcome of the other twin. Intrauterine transfusion of the anemic twin risks congestive cardiac failure in the donor twin, and although maternal digoxin can be given, when signs of fetal congestive cardiac failure appear, this is a late sign. The surgical removal of one twin by hysterotomy at 21 weeks gestation has also been described (Urig et al., 1988).

Fetoscopically directed occlusion of the placental vascular anomaly seems possible as a major option for the future as this management addresses the cause of the syndrome. After developing the technique in an animal model, DeLia et al. (1990) have used the neodymium:YAG laser via the fetoscope to successfully occlude placental vessels in severe twin transfusion syndrome. In the first three human pregnancies reported to have been treated by this technique, four fetuses survived. Additional applications of this technique include ablating the blood supply to an acardiac twin and ablating the blood supply to placental chorioangiomas causing significant preterm polyhydramnios. However, this technique is only possible in a few centers with special expertise and special equipment, and experience of large numbers treated has

yet to be reported. Until laser ablation of placental vessel anastomoses is an established and proven technique, repeated amniocentesis may be the best of the difficult options until delivery is possible.

Polyhydramnios

This is common in late pregnancy and may contribute to the high incidence of preterm labor. However, when it occurs in the mid-trimester of pregnancy, the perinatal mortality is more than 70 per cent. Although early polyhydramnios in one sac is often associated with twin-twin transfusion syndrome or fetal anomaly, it can also occur for unknown reasons in any diamniotic pregnancy. One sac may be severely polyhydramniotic and the other sac oligohydramniotic, and as a result the fetus in the latter sac is squashed against the uterine wall—the "stuck twin" phenomenon. The extremely high mortality rates for these fetuses merits radical intervention, and if delivery of viable babies is not possible, serial amniocentesis is currently the preferred option. Using this technique, Mahoney et al. (1990) reported survival of 11 of 16 fetuses. Two of these survivors had severe handicap. When the gestational age is borderline for viability, rest and fetal monitoring until delivery is necessary as the only other option for the stuck twin.

When polyhydramnios occurs in both sacs before 32 weeks gestation, one useful option is indomethacin therapy (Lange et al., 1989). This drug should be used only with monitoring of the amniotic fluid volume lest oligohydramnios occur and for as short a time as clinically relevant.

Monoamniotic Twins

A relatively small number of cases of monoamniotic twins have been reported in the English literature. The perinatal mortality is around 50 per cent, but most of this occurs before 32 weeks gestation. Although prophylactic preterm delivery and cesarean section have been advocated to reduce the chance of cord entanglement, the reported data do not support very early delivery or the avoidance of vaginal delivery (Tessen and Zlatnik, 1991).

Acardiac Twinning

This abnormality occurs in 1 in 100 monozygotic twin pregnancies (see Chapter 37). The acardiac fetus may be mistaken for a twin who has died or an anencephalic fetus. The ultrasonographic features of absent head and trunk regions but increased body soft tissue facilitate the diagnosis. There is a 50 per cent mortality reported for the pump twin (Moore et al., 1990), with a worse prognosis in the presence of polyhydramnios, preterm labor, and pump-twin cardiac decompensation. When the acardiac size-to-pump weight is less than 25 per cent, mortality is less, and this finding may encourage conservative management. More recent interventions for high-risk cases include acardiac umbilical ligation or selective hysterotomy.

Single Fetal Death

When death of one fetus occurs in early pregnancy, absorption of the missed abortion usually occurs without major complications. However, later in pregnancy, morbidity and mortality in the remaining fetus are high. In reviewing the literature, Embom (1985) estimated that 46 per cent of the remaining twins will suffer major morbidity or death. The prognosis for the remaining twin depends on the cause of death of the first twin, the degree of shared fetal circulation, the gestational age, and the time between death of the first twin and delivery of the second. Clearly, the pathology that caused the first twin's demise may also affect the second. As discussed earlier, hypotension, hypoxia, and thromboembolism may lead to multicystic encephalomalacia in the surviving twin (Bejar et al., 1988). Similar lesions have been described in the renal cortex. Disseminated intravascular coagulation can occur in rare instances in both the surviving fetus (Moore et al., 1969) and the mother (Skelly et al., 1982). There is no policy that can avoid the risk of these complications. Management depends on the viability of the live fetus. A non-stress test and a biophysical profile score should be performed and, if fetal distress is found, delivery of the viable fetus should be considered. Expectant management of a closely monitored fetus until 34 weeks is usually adopted for the remainder of patients without fetal distress who do not go into labor. Early delivery after 34 weeks gestation, pulmonary maturity having been demonstrated, may be appropriate. Staff must not forget the sensitive and confused feelings of the parents of a live and a dead twin. Mourning of the lost twin should not be impeded, and every effort should be made to give the parents and the siblings an experience of the dead baby and to offer long-term counseling and support.

Intrapartum Management

The optimal route of delivery of twin gestations remains controversial, and although there has been an increased emphasis on the use of cesarean section, there are no prospective studies that apply in all situations. The method of delivery must be assessed individually and must take into account the presentation of the twins, the gestational age, the presence of maternal or fetal complications, the experience of the obstetrician, and the availability of anesthesia and neonatal care. A flow chart of intrapartum management is shown in Figure 38–3.

The management is in part determined by the presentation of the twins (Table 38–4). In general, considerations regarding breech presentation for singleton gestations (see Chapter 35) also apply to twin gestations, with the additional rare possibility of locked twins. Very-low-birth-weight fetuses (750 to 1500 gm) appear to have a better outcome when delivered by cesarean section, although this issue has not been tested prospectively. Bell et al. (1986) noted that there has been a marked increase in the cesarean section rate in uncomplicated twin pregnancies over the last

TABLE 38–4. Incidence of Presentations in Twin Deliveries

PRESENTATION	INCIDENCE (%)
Vertex-vertex	40
Vertex-breech	26
Breech-vertex	10
Breech-breech	10
Vertex-transverse	8
Miscellaneous	6

20 years; however, review of 1168 cases during that period did not show an improvement in the condition of the infants at birth.

Although in general cesarean section should be used with liberal indications, it would seem appropriate to permit a vaginal delivery with vertex-vertex twin presentations if there are no abnormalities. If one of the twins is in breech position, vaginal delivery may be appropriate if one has excluded fetal head deflexion, cephalopelvic disproportion, and significant fetal compromise.

Although many patients enter into labor spontaneously, it may be necessary to induce labor owing to the high incidence of maternal and fetal complications. In general, the uterus containing a multiple pregnancy is easy to stimulate. However, because of overdistention of the uterus and possible uteroplacental insufficiency, any induction must be performed carefully and with monitoring of both fetuses. Amniotomy of the first sac with or without oxytocin augmentation is currently the accepted practice. In my experience, low doses of prostaglandins E_2 and $F_{2\alpha}$ can also be successfully and safely used to induce labor (MacLennan, 1990). It is rare to find unfavorable cervical status in late multiple pregnancy. If any cervical ripening agent is used, both fetuses must be monitored continuously from the beginning of the ripening process, because the fetal distress that sometimes develops secondary to mild contractions induced by the ripening agent may otherwise not be detected. Thus, unfavorable cervical status can be an indication for cesarean section.

Both twins should be continuously monitored by abdominal ultrasonography, which is possible even with triplets. As labor becomes established, the use of two ultrasound devices to monitor both twins becomes more difficult; therefore, after abnormal fetal presentation that would preclude artificial rupture of the membranes has been excluded, amniotomy should be considered in order to attach a fetal skin electrode to monitor the first twin. The second twin can then continue to be monitored with ultrasonography in an easier manner.

Controversy persists regarding appropriate analgesia and anesthesia for labor in twin gestations. Because all types of regional anesthesia may conceivably alter the progress of labor, some authors believe that small amounts of intramuscular medication with pudendal block are the best combination. However, there are two advantages to regional analgesia with epidural or caudal block. First, the patient is unlikely to involuntarily push a small first twin through an incompletely dilated cervix. Second, adequate regional analgesia facilitates delivery of the second twin without delay if internal manipulation is necessary. A pudendal block is inadequate for the latter procedure. If regional anesthesia is employed, it is important to prevent inferior vena caval compression due to the excessively enlarged uterus. Labor should be conducted with the patient in the lateral decubitus position, and cesarean section, if necessary, should be performed with adequate lateral tilting of the patient.

Delivery of the First Twin

The crux of a safe twin vaginal delivery is preparation. When possible, the obstetrician in charge should have at hand (1) recent measurements of fetal size and position, (2) cross-matched blood, (3) effective epidural anesthesia, (4) dual fetal monitoring, (5) intravenous fluids (including oxytocin if necessary), and (6) an anesthetist, another obstetrician, and a neonatal team with two resuscitative facilities. Maternal expulsive efforts should not be encouraged until there is both full dilation of the cervix and a visible presenting part. Delivery of the first twin can be conducted as for a singleton. Epidural anesthesia makes both forceps delivery and occiput posterior position more common (Hoult et al., 1977), and spontaneous rotation is less likely to occur in twin pregnancy. Under these conditions, however, forceps delivery should present no problem to the experienced obstetrician. If it has been considered safe to conduct a breech delivery of the first twin, then an assisted breech delivery is appropriate, rather than a breech extraction. Obviously, routine oxytocic augmentation should be delayed until the birth of the second twin. It is useful to double-clamp the first umbilical cord, so that blood lost from the first cord does not compromise the hemodynamics of the second twin through anastomoses between the placental circulations.

Delivery of the Second Twin

Following delivery of the first twin, the well-being and the presentation of the second twin should be ascertained immediately.

Potential problems facing the second twin include delayed delivery, prolonged anesthesia, cord prolapse, placental separation, malpresentation, and operative delivery. Although there is no need dramatically to expedite delivery of the second twin when the fetal heart rate is normal, there is no hemorrhage, and the second cord does not present, morbidity is increased if delivery of the second twin is delayed. Thus, delivery before 30 minutes has elapsed after the delivery of the first twin is frequently recommended.

The presenting part of the second twin should be identified soon after delivery of the first twin. Internal version should rarely be necessary, except in the case of a transverse lie. External version of a breech presentation to a cephalic presentation before rupture of the second sac is another option. Access to real-time ultrasonography in the delivery room may aid this maneuver. External version of the second twin from the breech or transverse lie can usually be successfully achieved without hazard (Chervenak et al., 1983), and once the presentation is cephalic, the membranes are ruptured and the fetal heart monitored until delivery. However, the second twin can be delivered in a breech or cephalic presentation. To avoid breech extraction or a high-forceps delivery of the second twin, it is advisable to have an oxytocic infusion ready for administration should spontaneous uterine activity be incoordinate. In most cases, delivery of the second twin in these circumstances will be simple and can be conducted normally. Cord prolapse or fetal distress may occasionally require rapid delivery of the second twin. With epidural analgesia further manipulation, such as breech extraction, is possible, although it should be performed as gently as possible. Although version and extraction can be dangerous, Adam et al. (1991) could not demonstrate an increase in perinatal mortality or morbidity when the non-vertex second twin weighing >1500 gm was delivered either vaginally or by cesarean section. Delivery of the second twin by cesarean section should rarely be necessary if all the appropriate preparations for a twin delivery, as just outlined, have been made. However, a retrospective survey of 2364 twin births by Kelsick and Minkoff (1982) showed that vaginal delivery of the breech second twin was associated with a higher perinatal mortality (corrected for death before labor and congenital malformations) when the baby weighed less than 2 kg compared with those delivered by cesarean section. In infants over this weight, cesarean section held no such advantage.

An oxytocin infusion is kept running for 2 to 3 hours after delivery to reduce the chances of postpartum hemorrhage. The placenta and membranes can be inspected and sent for histologic examination to help determine zygosity. Infants of multiple births require special neonatal care, being at greater risk of fetal anomalies and intrauterine growth restriction. Blood samples should be taken to detect twin transfusion syndrome, hypoglycemia, and coagulopathy.

Locked Twins

It is important to emphasize that this condition is rare, occurring in approximately one in every 817 twin gestations (Cohen et al., 1965). Hypertonicity, monoamnionic twinning, or a reduced amount of amniotic fluid may contribute to interlocking of the fetal heads. The most common form, interlocking of the fetal chins, should be suspected if there is a delay during labor in which the first twin is in breech and the second twin is in a cephalic presentation. Currently, delay in the descent of any breech presentation should be an indication for cesarean section. A breech-cephalic twin presentation merits a radiograph or ultrasonogram at the beginning of labor, and cesarean section can be chosen if the twins are interlocked.

Higher Order Births

Three, four, and more fetuses are associated with increasing maternal and perinatal mortality and morbidity. They stretch the mother, the family, and the community resources because of the many complications associated with their pregnancy, birth, and future development. The incidence of higher order births was fairly constant at around one per 10,000 births until the 1980s, when a tripling in such births occurred (Fig. 38–4). This increase is most probably due to the direct influence of fertility programs. Fertility drugs have induced multiple ovulation, and *in vitro* fertilization programs and associated procedures have transferred three or more eggs or embryos per cycle.

In Australia, where there is a high ratio of fertility programs per head of population, the current incidence of higher order births is four per 10,000. Thus, a major preventative measure is the recommendation that GIFT and IVF procedures only transfer a maximum of 2 to 3 eggs or embryos. Gonadotrophins to induce ovulation should only be used by specialists monitoring follicular development with ultrasonography and hormonal assays. Greater control of these modern techniques should see a reduction in higher order births.

MULTIFETAL PREGNANCY REDUCTION. Although there are moral, ethical, and psychological concerns about reducing the number of fetuses in early pregnancy, this is now an option for the woman found to have a higher order multiple pregnancy. The term *multifetal pregnancy reduction* is used rather than *selective reduction* as in the latter a specific fetus with an abnormality is selectively terminated. Multifetal pregnancy reduction is usually performed transabdominally between 10 and 12 weeks of pregnancy by means of potassium chloride injection into the pericardium of the most accessible fetuses. Usually, a twin pregnancy is left to progress. Composite data from centers with the most experience suggest an ultimate live birth rate of 75 to 80 per cent (Evans et al., 1993). Fetal reduction before 12 weeks and dizygosity should reduce the risk of neurologic damage in the surviving fetuses.

MANAGEMENT OF HIGHER ORDER PREGNANCIES. Antenatal care should be given at a major perinatal center. Recent improvement in the perinatal mortality and morbidity for triplets appears to be due to improved neonatal care as the high rate of prematurity has not changed (Creinin et al., 1991). All the antenatal complications discussed earlier in this chapter occur more commonly in higher order pregnancy. There is a need for a multicenter randomized controlled trial on the value of routine hospitalization and rest for triplet pregnancies. However, many higher order pregnancies require admission for complications such as pregnancy hypertension, polyhydramnios, intrauterine growth restriction, antepartum hemorrhage, and maternal discomfort. Tocolysis, cervical cerclage, and progesterone have all been advocated for higher order pregnancies without supportive control data. In view of their lack of effectiveness in twin pregnancy, these prophylactic interventions should only be used selectively when the clinical situation suggests their therapeutic need. The published experience of the management of quadruplets, quintuplets, and the like is relatively sparse (Petrikovsky and Vintzileos, 1989). There may be merit in the use of corticosteroids to accelerate fetal lung maturation. It would be hard to justify very premature delivery of the other fetuses for the sake of one very small fetus, but serial amniocentesis is an option when polyhydramnios in one or more sacs is compromising another fetus or the mother.

MODE OF DELIVERY. There are no randomized controlled studies to support a preference of either abdominal or vaginal delivery. Precipitate premature vaginal delivery may not allow the option of cesarean section. However, most authors on this subject tend to advocate cesarean section as the preferred route of delivery. There is usually a reduction in the Apgar score and cord gas values by birth order regardless of the route of delivery chosen, but recent reviews suggest that this trend is less for the abdominal route (Petrikovsky and Vintzileos, 1989). Controversy exists also for the optimal uterine incision in multifetal pregnancy. Some authors suggest that a low vertical incision should be performed as it can be easily extended. Malpresentations of the fetuses will be likely, and the chosen incision should allow speed of delivery with the least trauma to the infants. The logistics of a high-order birth put a strain on any major perinatal center as there should be a full neonatal team for each infant, and in view of the likely prematurity, these infants will occupy much of the neonatal intensive care team's time for many weeks thereafter. The parents have been and will be under enormous stress and require long-term support in view of the likely medical and social complications of multiple birth. It behooves us as perinatologists to remind our colleagues specializing in the managment of infertility that many of the enormous problems created by higher order births are preventable.

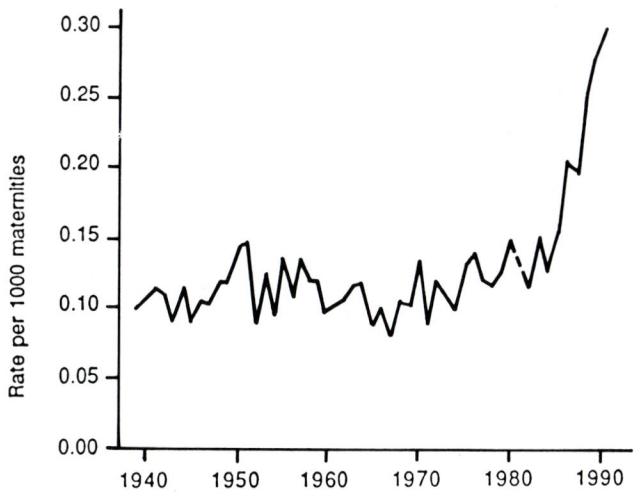

Triplet and higher order births
England and Wales 1939 - 1990

FIGURE 38–4. Triplet and higher order births in England and Wales, 1939 to 1990.

REFERENCES

Adam C, Allen AC, Baskett TF: Twin delivery: Influence of the presentation and method of delivery on the second twin. Am J Obstet Gynecol **165**:23, 1991.

Anderson RL, Golbus MS, Curry CJR et al: Central nervous system damage and other anomalies in surviving fetus following second trimester antenatal death of co-twin. Prenatal Diag **10**:513, 1990.

Ashworth MF, Spooner SF, Verkuyl DAA et al: Failure to prevent preterm labour and delivery in twin pregnancy using prophylactic oral salbutamol. Br J Obstet Gynaecol **97**:878, 1990.

Bailey D, Flynn AM, Kelly J, O'Connor M: Antepartum fetal heart rate monitoring in multiple pregnancy. Br J Obstet Gynaecol **87**:561, 1980.

Barss VA, Benacerraf BR, Frigoletto FD: Ultrasonographic determination of chorion type in twin gestation. Obstet Gynecol **66**:779, 1985.

Bejar R, Vigliocco G, Gramajo H, et al: Antenatal orgin of neurologic damage in newborn infants. Part II. Multiple gestations. Am J Obstet Gynecol **162**:1230, 1990.

Bejar R, Wozniak P, Allard M, et al: Antenatal origin of neurologic damage in newborn infants. Part I. Preterm infants. Am J Obstet Gynecol **159**:357, 1988.

Bell D, Johansson D, McLean FH, Usher RH: Birth asphyxia, trauma and mortality in twins: Has cesarean section improved outcome? Am J Obstet Gynecol **154**:235, 1986.

Blake GD, Knuppel RA, Ingardia CJ, et al: Evaluation of non-stress fetal heart rate testing in multiple pregnancy. Obstet Gynecol **63**:528, 1984.

Blickstein I: The twin-twin transfusion syndrome. Obstet Gynecol **76**:714, 1990.

Botting BJ, MacDonald-Davies I, MacIarlane AJ: Recent trends in the incidence of multiple births and associated mortality. Arch Dis Child **62**:941, 1987.

Cameron AH, Edwards JH, Derom R, et al: The value of twin surveys in the study of malformation. Europ J Obstet Gynecol Reprod Biol **14**:347, 1983.

Chervenak FA, Johnson RE, Berkowitz RL, et al: Intrapartum external version of the second twin. Obstet Gynecol **62**:160, 1983.

Cohen M, Kohl SG, Rosenthal AH: Fetal interlocking complicating twin gestation. Am J Obstet Gynecol **91**:407, 1965.

Creinin M, Katz M, Laros R: Triplet pregnancy: Changes in morbidity and mortality. J Perinatol **11**:207, 1991.

Crowther CA: Hospitalization for bed rest in multiple pregnancy. In Chalmers I (ed): Oxford Database of Perinatal Trials, Version 1.2, Disc Issue 6, Record 3375, Autumn 1991.

Crowther CA, Neilson JP, Verkuyl DAA, et al: Preterm labour in twin pregnancies: Can it be prevented by hospital admission? Br J Obstet Gynaecol **96**:850, 1989.

DeLia JE, Cruikshank DP, Keye WR: Fetoscopic neodymium: YAG laser occlusion of placental vessels in severe twin-twin transfusion syndrome. Obstet Gynecol **75**:1046, 1990.

Duncan SLB, Ginz B, Wahab H: Use of ultrasound and hormone assays in the diagnosis, management and outcome of twin pregnancy. Obstet Gynecol **53**:367, 1979.

Dyson DC, Crites YM, Ray DA, et al: Prevention of preterm birth in high-risk patients: The role of education and provider contact versus home uterine monitoring. Am J Obstet Gynecol **164**:756, 1991.

Embom JA: Twin pregnancy with intrauterine death of one twin. Am J Obstet Gynecol **152**:424, 1985.

Evans MI, Littmann L, King M, et al: Multiple gestation: The role for multifetal pregnancy reduction and selective termination. In Phelan J (ed): Multiple Gestation Clinics In Perinatology (in press).

Fitzhardinge PM, Steven EM: The small-for-date infant. II. Neurological and intellectual sequelae. Paediatrics **50**:50, 1972.

Fowler MG, Kleinman JC, Kiely JL et al: Double jeopardy: Twin infant mortality in the United States, 1983 and 1984. Am J Obstet Gynecol **165**:15, 1991.

Garite TJ, Bentley DL, Hamer CA et al: Uterine activity characteristics in multiple gestations. Obstet Gynecol **76**:56S, 1990.

Giles WB, Trudinger BJ, Cook CM: Umbilical artery flow velocity waveforms and twin pregnancy outcome. Br J Obstet Gynaecol **72**:894, 1988.

Grant A: Cervical cerclage to prolong pregnancy. In Chalmers I, Enkin M, Keirse MJNC (eds): Effective Care in Pregnancy and Childbirth. Oxford University Press, 1989, pp 644–646.

Hoult IJ, MacLennan AH, Carrie LES: Lumbar epidural in labour: Relation to fetal malposition and instrumental delivery. Br Med J **1**:14, 1977.

Houlton MCC, Marivate M, Philpott RH: The prediction of fetal growth retardation in twin pregnancy. Br J Obstet Gynaecol **88**:264, 1981.

Jeffrey RL, Bowes WA Jr, Delaney JJ: Role of bed rest in twin gestation. Obstet Gynecol **43**:822, 1974.

Keith L, Ellis R, Berger GS, et al: The Northwestern University multihospital twin study. Am J Obstet Gynecol **138**:781, 1980.

Kelsick F, Minkoff H: Management of the breech second twin. Am J Obstet Gynecol **144**:783, 1982.

Key TC, Dattel BJ, Resnik R: The ultrasonic estimation of fetal weight in the very low-birth-weight infant. Am J Obstet Gynecol **145**:574, 1983.

Keirse MJNC, Grant A, King JF: Preterm labour. In Chalmers I, Enkin M, Keirse MJNC (eds): Effective Care in Pregnancy and Childbirth. Oxford University Press, 1989, pp 694–745.

Knuppel RA, Lake MF, Watson DL et al: Preventing preterm birth in twin gestation: Home uterine activity monitoring and perinatal nursing support. Obstet Gynecol **76**:24S, 1990.

Kohl SG, Casey G: Twin gestation. Mt Sinai J Med **42**:523, 1975.

Komromy B, Lamp L: Value of bed rest in twin pregnancies. Int J Gynecol Obstet **14**:262, 1977.

Lange IR, Harman MD, Ash KM et al: Twin with hydramnios: Treating premature labour at source. Am J Obstet Gynecol **160**:552, 1989.

Leveno KJ, Santos-Ramos R, Duenhoelter JH, et al: Sonar cephalometry in twin pregnancy: Discordancy of the biparietal diameter after 28 weeks' gestation. Am J Obstet Gynecol **138**:615, 1980.

Lipitz S, Reichman B, Paret G, et al: The improving outcome of triplet pregnancies. Am J Obstet Gynecol **161**:1279, 1989.

Lipshitz J: The uterine and cardiovascular effects of oral fenoterol hydrobromide. Br J Obstet Gynaecol **84**:737, 1977.

Lukacs HA, MacLennan AH, Verco PW: Ultrasonic fetal weight estimation in multiple and singleton pregnancy. Aust Paediatr J **20**:59, 1984.

MacGillivray I: Twin Pregnancies. In Wynn RM (ed): Obstetrics and Gynaecology Annual. New York, Appleton-Century-Crofts, 1978.

MacLennan AH: Australian clinical trials with prostaglandins E_2 and $F_{2\alpha}$ to induce labour. Reprod Fertil Dev **2**:557, 1990.

MacLennan AH, Green RC, O'Shea R et al: Routine hospital admission in twin pregnancy between 26 and 30 weeks gestation. Lancet **335**:267, 1990.

MacLennan AH, Millington G, Grieve A, et al: Neonatal body water turnover: A putative index of perinatal morbidity. Am J Obstet Gynecol **139**:948, 1981.

Mahony BS, Petty CN, Nyberg DA, et al: The "stuck twin" phenomenon: Ultrasonographic findings, frequency outcome and management with serial amniocentesis. Am J Obstet Gynecol **163**:1513, 1990.

Miller HC, Merritt TA: Fetal Growth in Humans. Chicago, Year Book Medical Publishers, 1979.

Moore CM, McAdams AJ, Sutherland J: Intrauterine disseminated intravascular coagulation: A syndrome of multiple pregnancy with a dead fetus. J Pediatr **74**:523, 1969.

Moore TR, Gales S, Benirshke K: Perinatal outcome of forty-nine pregnancies complicated by acardiac twinning. Am J Obstet Gynecol **163**:907, 1990.

Neilson JP: Detection of the small-for-dates twin fetus by ultrasound. Br J Obstet Gynaecol **88**:27, 1981.

Neilson JP, Mutambira M: Coitus, twin pregnancy and preterm labour. Am J Obstet Gynecol **160**:416, 1989.

Neilson JP, Yerkuyl DAA, Crowther CA, et al: Preterm labor in twin pregnancies: Prediction by cervical assessment. Obstet Gynecol **72**:719, 1988.

Newman RB, Godsey RK, Ellings JM, et al: Quantification of cervical change: Relationship to preterm delivery in the multifetal gestation. Am J Obstet Gynecol **165**:264, 1991.

Newton ER: Antepartum care in multiple gestation. Semin Perinatol **10**:19, 1986.

Obladen M, Gluck L: RDS and tracheal phospholipid composition in twins: Independent of gestational age. J Pediatr **90**:799, 1977.

O'Connor MC, Arias E, Royston JP, Dalrymple IK: The merits of special antenatal care for twin pregnancies. Br J Obstet Gynaecol **88**:222, 1981.

O'Connor MC, Murphy D, Dalrymple IK: Double blind trial of ritodrine and placebo in twin pregnancy. Br J Obstet Gynaecol **86**:707, 1979.

Persson PH, Grennert L, Gennser G, et al: On improved outcome of twin pregnancies. Acta Obstet Gynecol Scand **58:**3, 1979.

Petrikovsky BM, Vintzileos AM: Management and outcome of multiple pregnancy of high fetal order: Literature review. Obstet Gynecol Surv **44:**578, 1989.

Powers FW, Miller TC: Bed rest in twin pregnancy: Identification of a critical period and its cost implications. Am J Obstet Gynecol **134:**23, 1979.

Prescott P: Sensitivity of a double blind trial of ritodrine and placebo in twin pregnancy. Br J Obstet Gynaecol **87:**393, 1980.

Reddy KS, Petersen MB, Antonarakis SE, et al: The vanishing twin: An explanation of discordance between chorionic villus karyotype and fetal karyotype. Prenatal Diag **11:**679, 1991.

Redwine FO, Hays PM: Selective birth. Semin Perinatol **10:**73, 1986.

Rodis JF, Egan JFX, Craffey A, et al: Calculated risk of chromosomal abnormalities in twin gestations. Obstet Gynecol **76:**1037, 1990.

Rush RW, Keirse MJNC, Howat P, et al: Contribution of preterm delivery to perinatal mortality. Br Med J **2:**965, 1976.

Saunders MC, Dick JS, Brown IM, et al: The effects of hospital admission for bed rest on the duration of twin pregnancy: A randomized trial. Lancet **2:**793, 1985.

Sinka DP, Nandakumar VC, Brough AK: Relative cervical incompetence in twin pregnancy. Acta Genet Med Gemellol (Roma) **28:**327, 1979.

Skelly H, Marivale M, Norman R, et al: Consumptive coagulopathy following fetal death in a triplet pregnancy. Am J Obstet Gynecol **142:**595, 1982.

Skjaerris J, Aberg A: Prevention of prematurity in twin pregnancy by orally administered terbutaline. Acta Obstet Gynecol Scand (Suppl) **108:**39, 1982.

Steinberg LH, Hurley VA, Desmedt E, et al: Acute polyhydramnios in twin pregnancies. Aust NZ J Obstet Gynaecol **30:**196, 1990.

TambyRaja RL, Ratnam SS: Endocrine changes during salbutamol therapy for the prevention of prematurity in twins. Singapore J Obstet Gynaecol **10:**58, 1979.

Tessen JA, Zlatnik FJ: Monoamniotic Twins: A retrospective controlled study. Obstet Gynecol **77:**832, 1991.

Urig MA, Clewell WH, Elliot JP: Twin-twin transfusion syndrome. Am J Obstet Gynecol **163:**1522, 1990.

Urig MA, Simpson GE, Elliot JP, et al: Twin-twin transfusion syndrome: The surgical removal of one twin as a treatment option. Fetal Ther **3:**185, 1988.

Varma TR: Ultrasound evidence of early pregnancy failure in patients with multiple conceptions. Br J Obstet Gynaecol **86:**290, 1979.

Wald NJ, Cuckle H, Stirrat GM, et al: Maternal serum α-fetoprotein and birth weight in twin pregnancies. Br J Obstet Gynaecol **88:**592, 1978.

PLACENTAL ABNORMALITIES

CHAPTER

PLACENTA PREVIA AND ABRUPTIO PLACENTAE

JAMES R. GREEN, M.D.

Third-trimester bleeding complicates about 3.8 per cent of all pregnancies. Placenta previa is documented by vaginal examination or at cesarean section in 22 per cent of cases, and strong evidence of abruptio placentae is found in 31 per cent (Hibbard and Jeffcoate, 1966). In the remaining 47 per cent of cases, the bleeding can be ascribed either to early labor (so-called marginal separation) or local lesions of the lower genital tract, or no source can be identified. Therefore, third-trimester bleeding ultimately proves to be of little consequence in about half the cases, but in the other half it is potentially life-threatening.

Vaginal bleeding in the third trimester is alarming to the pregnant woman and usually prompts immediate consultation with her physician. It is the responsibility of the physician to decide without delay whether the cause is benign or potentially life-threatening to the mother, fetus, or both. The potential harm from either procrastination or unnecessary intervention may be extreme.

PLACENTA PREVIA

Definition and Classification

Placenta previa is defined as implantation of the placenta in the lower uterine segment in advance of the fetal presenting part. Various degrees of placenta previa have been described, but the terminology is confusing. The major difficulty with classification systems is accounting for the potentially changing relationship between the placenta and the cervix during the third trimester and especially as labor progresses. Degrees of placenta previa are usually described with reference to the internal cervical os prior to the onset of labor. The following classification is commonly accepted in the United States:

1. *Total (complete) placenta previa:* The placenta covers the internal cervical os entirely. When the placenta is concentrically implanted about the cervical os, *central placenta previa* is the term often used.
2. *Partial placenta previa:* The placenta covers part of the internal cervical os.
3. *Marginal placenta previa:* The placental edge just reaches the internal cervical os. If the placental edge is within a short distance of the internal os (on the order of 2 cm), the designation of marginal placenta previa is probably still appropriate.
4. *Low-lying placenta:* The placental edge is implanted in the lower uterine segment but does not encroach on the internal cervical os. Once known as a "lateral placenta previa," the low-lying placenta is not generally considered a true placenta previa for the purpose of management. Nevertheless, the distinction between a low-lying placenta and a marginal placenta previa can be difficult.

Although some distinctions in outcome may be made among the different degrees of true placenta previa, all are potentially associated with life-threatening hemorrhage during labor. The degree of placenta previa cannot alone predict the clinical course accurately, nor can it serve as the sole guide for management decisions. Thus, the importance of such classifications has diminished.

Incidence and Etiology

The incidence of placenta previa at the time of delivery varies widely in published series, but averages approximately one in 200 to 250 births. The observed variability in incidence is explained in part by the definitions employed. Of greater importance is the ratio of nulliparas to multiparas in a population, because placenta previa is largely a problem of parous women. Its incidence is only one in 1500 nulliparas, compared with one in 20 grand multiparas (Hibbard, 1981).

It is important to recognize that these statistics relate to *symptomatic* placenta previa and the few asymptomatic cases discovered incidentally late in pregnancy by pelvic examination. There is evidence that low implantations are much more common early in pregnancy, but that the great majority of these "resolve" and never become symptomatic. A low-lying placenta may be diagnosed by ultrasonography in up to 45 per cent of women in the second trimester (Wexler and Gottesfeld, 1977). Approximately 5 per cent of women having second-trimester sonograms prior to genetic amniocentesis have total placenta previa, but in 90 per cent of these the condition "resolves" as pregnancy progresses, without becoming symptomatic (Wexler and Gottesfeld, 1979).

Resolution may not be an entirely appropriate term, since a high rate of other complications has been observed in women with early placenta previa, despite apparent "resolution" in 97 per cent (Newton et al., 1984). Forty-five per cent of these women had significant antenatal complications, including antepartum hemorrhage, abruptio placentae, and suspected intrauterine growth restriction. Statistically significant increases in prematurity and perinatal mortality were seen in this group. Placenta previa diagnosed in early pregnancy should possibly place the woman in a high-risk category.

The strong association between placenta previa and parity has suggested that "endometrial damage" is an etiologic factor. Presumably, each pregnancy "damages" the endometrium underlying the implantation site, rendering the area unsuitable for implantation. Subsequent pregnancies are more likely to become implanted in the lower uterine segment by a process of elimination. This effect is most clearly seen with prior term pregnancies, but multiple early pregnancy terminations may also be related to an increased incidence of placenta previa.

The women at highest risk are those with prior placenta previa or multiple prior cesarean sections. The risk of recurrent placenta previa is as high as 4 to 8 per cent (Kelly and Iffy, 1981). The risk of placenta previa increases with the number of prior cesarean sections, rising to 10 per cent with four or more (Clark et al., 1985).

Subsequent growth of the placenta after low implantation is either centripetal (resulting in central placenta previa) or unidirectional toward the more richly vascularized fundus. The latter mechanism is common, as demonstrated by the finding of an eccentric, marginal, or even velamentous insertion of the cord. The association of velamentous cord insertions with placenta previa and the pathologic entity of vasa previa are both consistent with a dynamic process sometimes called "placental migration." Unidirectional growth of the placenta coupled with disappearance of the early placenta at the original implantation site results in a placenta that appears to have moved away from its original location. The insertion point of the cord on the membranes marks the original location of the definitive placenta. The primary implantation site is probably low in the great majority of cases. An alternative mechanism involving fundal implantation with unidirectional growth toward the cervix has been suggested, but this mechanism has been observed only rarely with serial sonograms. Therefore, a fundal placenta in the second trimester is reassuring evidence that a placenta previa will not exist in the third trimester.

Diagnosis

The hallmark of placenta previa is the sudden onset of painless bleeding in the second or third trimester of pregnancy. The absence of abdominal pain and uterine contractions is often stated to be an important distinguishing feature between placenta previa and abruptio placentae. This distinction is sometimes incorrect; in up to 10 per cent of cases of placenta previa there is coexisting abruption of the normally implanted portion of the placenta with resulting signs and symptoms of abruption. In nearly one in four cases, there are signs of labor with or without rupture of the membranes (Hibbard, 1981).

The initial episode of bleeding has a peak incidence at about the 34th week of pregnancy, although one-third of cases become symptomatic before the 30th week and one-third after the 36th week (Crenshaw et al., 1973). Bleeding may begin without an obvious inciting cause, such as a pelvic examination, intercourse, or onset of labor. The patient may awake in the night to find herself lying in a pool of blood. In these cases the bleeding may be precipitated by formation of the lower uterine segment with consequent detachment of a portion of the placenta. The earlier the presentation, the more likely intercourse will be found to be the proximate inciting factor and the more likely the placenta previa is complete.

Absence of bleeding prior to term does not rule out placenta previa. In approximately 10 per cent of cases, bleeding begins only with the onset of labor, and in these situations one is more likely to find a partial or marginal placenta previa, or a low-lying placenta.

A careful abdominal examination can help to raise or lower the suspicion of placenta previa. Usually the uterus will be soft. The absence of contractions in 75 per cent of previa cases makes abruption less likely. The lie of the fetus is especially important. In 35 per cent of cases the fetus is either in a breech or transverse lie (Cotton et al., 1980). If the vertex is presenting, it is often high above the pelvic brim and may be difficult to palpate if the placenta is anterior. Any of these findings makes placenta previa more likely. Conversely, if the presenting part is the vertex and it is deeply engaged, placenta previa is less likely than other causes of bleeding such as a heavy show and placental abruption. Hearing the placental souffle via stethoscope or Doppler device just above the pelvic brim may be helpful, but is an inconsistent finding.

Some authors advocate a speculum examination of the vagina and cervix as the first step to rule out a lower genital source of the bleeding. Two points should be considered before it is decided to proceed in this fashion. First, the bivalve speculum can be easily as traumatic as a finger, especially if the placenta is located behind the anterior vaginal fornix, and heavy bleeding may be precipitated. Second, extrauterine sources of bleeding are much more likely to be benign, and immediate diagnosis of such causes is not mandatory. It has therefore been our practice to defer the speculum examination in most cases until we obtain sonographic evidence that placenta previa does not exist.

Ultrasonographic localization of the placenta has been available for some time and is now considered a necessary step in the evaluation of the patient with bleeding, except when the bleeding is heavy enough to mandate immediate surgical intervention irrespective of the source. Ultrasonographic diagnosis is discussed in detail in Chapter 14, but some comments are pertinent to this discussion. Accurate communication between the ultrasonographer and the obstetrician is critical and depends on common definitions; terms such as *marginal placenta previa* and *low-lying placenta* must mean the same thing to both. It is highly desirable that the obstetrician personally review the sonogram with the ultrasonographer. This will allow a mapping of the placenta and selection of the uterine incision that best avoids it should cesarean section be necessary.

Transabdominal sonography is highly accurate but not infallible. There are no markers to locate the internal cervical os precisely. As a consequence, both false-positive and false-negative results have been reported. The latter are particularly worrisome because they can lead to a potentially catastrophic management plan. The rate of false-negative results has been reported to be as high as 7 per cent (Cotton et al., 1980). The most common reasons for missing placenta previa are positions of the fetal head that obscure the region of the cervix and failure to scan the *lateral* uterine walls (Laing, 1981). In addition, the presence of blood in the area of the cervix can create the illusion that amniotic fluid is present, falsely ruling out placenta previa. False-positive results are harder to define, unless the absence of placenta previa is confirmed immediately by digital examination or at the time of cesarean section. More often, there is a variable interval between the sonogram and the event that confirms or rules out the diagnosis. It is well known that overfilling of the bladder can result in a false-positive diagnosis because of compression of the lower uterine segment. The diagnosis should be reported only if the condition appears to persist after stepwise emptying of the bladder.

In the past several years, transvaginal sonography has been used for placental localization. Despite the potential for probe-induced trauma to the placenta, this approach has been demonstrably safe in experienced hands. The transvaginal approach is considered by many ultrasonographers to offer superior definition of the spatial relationship of the placental margin to the internal cervical os. In one recent series, transvaginal sonography was 100 per cent sensitive in the diagnosis of placenta previa (Farine et al., 1990). Nevertheless, both false-positive and false-negative results have been reported (Leerentveld et al., 1990). The two approaches should be considered complementary. Generally, a transabdominal scan is performed first. If the placenta is clearly fundal in location, or if a complete placenta previa is seen, the transvaginal examination is unnecessary, however small the attendant risk. When a partial or marginal placenta previa or a low-lying placenta is seen, a transvaginal scan may provide useful information. This is especially true when technical difficulties (such as an over- or underfilled bladder, a low presenting part or posterior placental location) prevent optimal transabdominal examination.

Magnetic resonance imaging (MRI) has also been used to confirm the diagnosis in small series of patients with placenta previa diagnosed by ultrasonography (Powell et al., 1986). Preliminary results suggest that MRI may eventually replace ultrasonography as the diagnostic method of choice. The major advantages are better imaging of soft tissue structures, better definition of the cervix, and less potential error due to overfilling of the bladder. To date, however, there have been no series directly comparing the two modalities.

A rate of spontaneous resolution of approximately 90 per cent can be anticipated in asymptomatic women with ultrasonographically detected placenta previa in the second trimester (Wexler and Gottesfeld, 1979). For those women who remain asymptomatic, no special measures or restriction of activity (including intercourse) seems indicated until 26 to 28 weeks gestation, at which time another sonogram should be obtained. If the condition persists at this examination, it is more likely that it will be present at the time of delivery and will cause symptoms, either before or at delivery. The patient should subsequently be managed expectantly, like the symptomatic patient. Nevertheless, even when present into the mid-third trimester, asymptomatic placenta previa has approximately a 75 per cent chance of resolution by the time of delivery (Comeau et al., 1983).

The probability of resolution has not been established for women with symptomatic placenta previa, but it is certainly a good deal lower. Despite this, periodic ultrasonographic examinations should be performed in women being managed expectantly, and a final diagnostic ultrasonogram should be obtained shortly before elective delivery by cesarean section.

The Double Set-Up Examination

In the past, the double set-up examination has been considered the final diagnostic step in the management of placenta previa, given the acknowledged inaccuracies of earlier noninvasive diagnostic procedures. With the improved accuracy of diagnostic ultrasound, the indications for performing a double set-up examination are limited.

In the face of active hemorrhage mandating immediate delivery, fetal malposition precluding vaginal delivery, or clear ultrasonographic evidence of com-

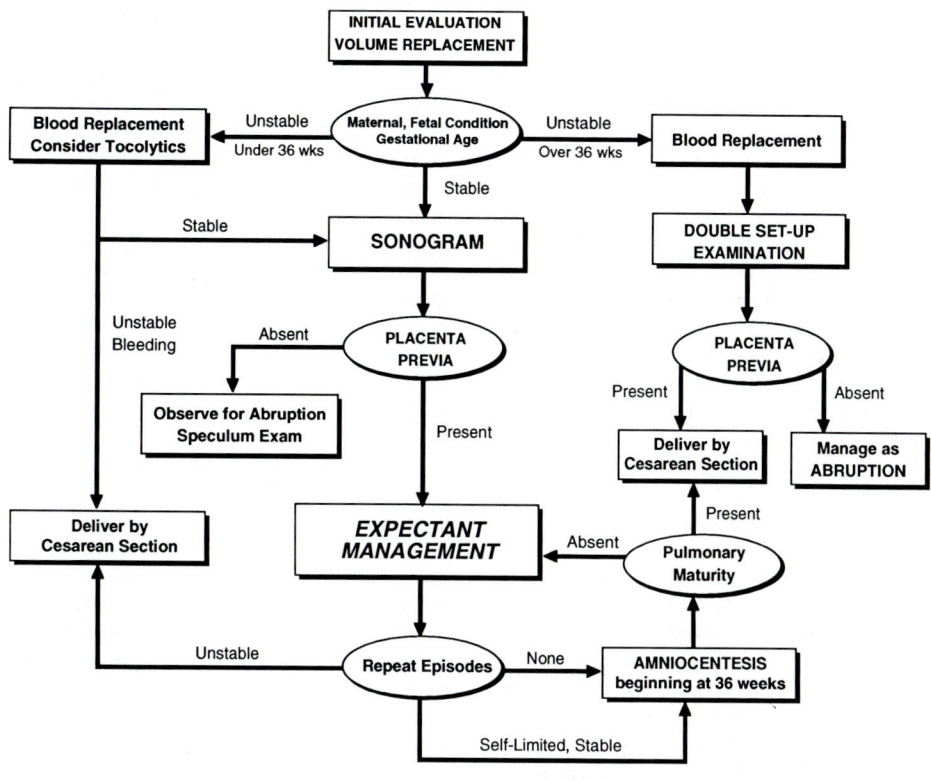

FIGURE 39–1. Outline of the initial stabilization, diagnostic procedures, and plan of management for patients presenting with bleeding in the latter half of pregnancy.

plete placenta previa, little is to be gained from the double set-up examination. The examination is indicated when the ultrasonographic evidence is inconclusive or when the patient presents with ongoing, but not life-threatening, uterine bleeding in labor. Under these conditions, a digital vaginal examination may be performed with certain precautions. At least four units of crossmatched blood should be available for the mother. The examination should be carried out in the operating room, allowing for immediate delivery in case of severe hemorrhage. A qualified anesthesiologist, instruments, a scrub nurse, and an experienced operating team in addition to the examining physician should be present. The patient should be prepared in the same manner as for elective surgery under general anesthesia, including abdominal preparation, insertion of a bladder catheter, and use of oral antacids, if indicated.

With the current accuracy of ultrasonographic placental localization, the digital examination is now more often undertaken to rule out marginal placenta previa than to confirm central implantation sites. Thus, the best procedure to follow (and the safest) is to sweep the vaginal fornices gently, using prior sonographic information to direct attention to the most critical quadrant. If the fetal presenting part is clearly felt through a thin lower uterine segment in all quadrants, vaginal delivery is probably feasible. In this event, the membranes can be ruptured and induction of labor begun. A boggy sensation, particularly in the same quadrant as might be expected from the sonogram, is

not diagnostic of placenta previa. Distinguishing placenta from clot or amniotic fluid can be difficult. Nevertheless, such a finding is usually sufficient reason to terminate the procedure and proceed to cesarean section. Digital probing of the cervical canal carries the danger of severe hemorrhage and rarely yields the information necessary to pursue the vaginal approach with confidence. In the absence of convincing evidence that a placenta previa does not exist, cesarean section is indicated.

Management

Two major factors have been responsible for the dramatic reduction in both maternal and perinatal mortality rates over the past 40 years: the expectant management approach and the liberal use of cesarean section rather than vaginal delivery. As a result, the maternal mortality rate has fallen from between 25 and 30 per cent to less than 1 per cent. The total perinatal mortality rate has fallen from between 60 and 70 per cent to under 10 per cent in the past 5 years. The major features of my approach to the management of placenta previa are illustrated in Figure 39–1.

General Measures

Any woman with bleeding in the late second trimester or the third trimester should be evaluated immediately in the hospital. Even in the absence of signs of maternal hypovolemia, it is wise to establish a large-bore intravenous line and to obtain a blood count and cross-matched blood. If the mother's condition is unstable from a cardiovascular standpoint, adequate fluid and blood replacement is the first priority. Simultaneously, the condition of the fetus can be determined by at least a 15-minute electronic monitor strip, during which time evidence of uterine activity is also sought. Only when the conditions of both the mother and fetus are stable and ongoing hemorrhage is not worrisome should attention be directed to establishing the diagnosis by ultrasonography. If the diagnosis of placenta previa is confirmed, a plan for the timing and method of delivery is outlined with the patient.

Timing of Delivery

The goal of management for placenta previa is to obtain the maximum fetal maturation possible while minimizing the risk to both the fetus and the mother. Since the 1940s, an expectant approach has been increasingly advocated as one that optimizes this goal. The basis for this approach is that episodes of bleeding are usually self-limited and not fatal to either the fetus or the mother in the absence of inciting trauma (e.g., intercourse, pelvic examination) or labor. Under carefully controlled conditions, delivery of the fetus may be safely delayed to a more advanced stage of maturity in a significant proportion of cases. An additional advantage to this approach is that a small proportion of cases, particularly those discovered early with lesser degrees of placenta previa, will resolve to an extent permitting vaginal delivery at term.

Once the diagnosis is established, the clinician must decide whether the patient is a suitable candidate for expectant management. If the pregnancy has reached 36 weeks or more at the time of initial presentation, the chance that the fetus is already mature favors delivery or, preferably, documentation of lung maturity via amniocentesis. One should be wary of relying on the menstrual history for dating these pregnancies. Bleeding in the first trimester of pregnancy occurs in up to one-third of cases and is often mistaken for a menstrual period. As a result, the length of gestation may be underestimated and delivery may be inappropriately delayed.

Evidence of concomitant abruption or fetal distress is a clear contraindication to expectant management, unless the fetus is grossly immature and the mother's condition is good. Heavy vaginal bleeding to the point of maternal hypovolemia or the presence of labor represent relative contraindications that must be weighed carefully. In the past, these conditions have been considered absolute contraindications, but some physicians have pursued an alternative approach with considerable success. In a study by Cotton and associates (1980), approximately 20 per cent of the patients lost in excess of 500 ml of blood at the initial episode, and yet half of these women were managed expectantly with a mean gain of 16.8 days. A total of 14 patients in labor at the time of the initial episode, including five with initial blood loss estimated in excess of 1000 ml, were treated with tocolytics. In this

group there was a mean gain of 3.4 weeks with no perinatal deaths. Such an aggressively expectant approach allows approximately 66 per cent of women to be managed expectantly (Cotton et al., 1980), as opposed to only 43 to 46 per cent in earlier series (Hibbard, 1969; Crenshaw et al., 1973). Blood loss that continues in excess of the volume being replaced, however, represents a contraindication to expectant management.

The expectation for success, i.e., delivery of a live, mature baby, depends to some extent on the length of gestation at first presentation and the degree of placenta previa. These factors are interdependent: The greater the degree of placenta previa, the earlier the bleeding is noted in pregnancy. About 50 per cent of patients with complete placenta previa are first noted to have bleeding at less than 30 weeks, compared with only 18 per cent of patients with marginal placenta previa (Crenshaw et al., 1973). Forty-eight per cent of patients with complete placenta previa are ultimately delivered after 36 weeks, and 76 per cent of patients with marginal placenta previa achieve that gestational length. The association between the degree of placenta previa and the length of time gained by expectant management has not been a uniform finding, and there is enough variation to preclude accurate prediction of the time of delivery in the individual case.

Placenta previa is characterized by repetitive hemorrhage. The majority of investigators find that the number of bleeding episodes is not related to the degree of placenta previa or to the prognosis for perinatal survival. Therefore, no specific cutoff in terms of number of episodes can be rationally established.

In contrast, the total amount of blood lost antenatally appears to relate directly to perinatal mortality (Hibbard, 1969). This effect may be nullified by the aggressive use of transfusions in the presence of maternal hypovolemia or anemia. Cotton and associates (1980) reported that no perinatal losses occurred in the 25 per cent of their expectantly managed patients who required transfusion for these indications. It is generally recommended that sufficient blood be transfused to maintain the maternal hematocrit at 30 per cent or greater, both to optimize oxygen supply to the fetus and to protect the mother against potential future loss. No rational limit in number of units transfused can be set. Rather, one has to question at each episode whether the risks to the mother and fetus outweigh the potential benefits of continued expectant management.

Improvements in neonatal intensive care over the past two decades have changed the outlook for the fetus considerably and have rendered outcome statistics from older series inappropriately discouraging. Nevertheless, in the most recent series, perinatal survival is still critically dependent on the gestational age at delivery. This relationship, shown in Table 39—1, clearly illustrates the negative impact of shortened gestation. Despite an aggressively expectant approach, including selected use of tocolytics, 20 per cent of women are still delivered earlier than 32 weeks, and these cases account for 73 per cent of all perinatal deaths (Cotton et al., 1980). They certainly remain the

**TABLE 39–1. Perinatal Mortality Rate
by Gestational Age**

	GESTATIONAL AGE (weeks)*			
	<27	27–32	33–36	>36
Births	8	27	63	76
Survivors	0 (0)	19 (70.3)	59 (93.6)	74 (97.4)
Deaths	8 (100)	8 (19.7)	4 (6.4)	2 (2.6)
Fetal	6 (75)	0 (0)	4 (6.4)	1 (1.3)
Neonatal	2 (25)	8 (19.7)	0 (0)	1 (1.3)

*The numbers in parentheses are percentages.
From Cotton DB, Read JA, Paul RH, Quilligan EJ: The conservative aggressive management of placenta previa. Am J Obstet Gynecol 137:687, 1980.

most difficult group to manage. The use of cervical cerclage (see Chapter 30) has been proposed to prevent further placental detachment, but there is still too little information available to recommend this approach except in unusual circumstances.

With expectant management, there is no sharp peak in the incidence of deliveries at any given week of gestation, but rather a steady rise as the pregnancy advances (Fig. 39–2A) (Brenner et al., 1978). The cumulative delivery rate, illustrated in Figure 39–2B, demonstrates the distressingly high rate of preterm deliveries. The probability that the pregnancy will be maintained for 1, 2, or 4 more weeks is a function of the gestational age already attained (Fig. 39–3). It can be seen, for example, that the fetus at 32 weeks has an 80 per cent probability of achieving 36 weeks *in utero* with potentially significant gains in maturity. Conversely, the fetus at 36 weeks has only a slightly better than 50–50 chance of gaining an additional 2 weeks *in utero*, with considerably less significant gain in maturity.

In the past, expectant management was believed to mandate continuous hospitalization until delivery. The current costs of hospitalization, as well as its psychological toll, make management in the home an option worth considering under carefully controlled circumstances. A minimum of 72 hours of hospitalization is advised, because nearly one-third of women initially selected for expectant management require delivery within this time (Cotton et al., 1980). Outpatient management should be considered if the patient is highly motivated, clearly understands the necessity of severe restriction of activity (and is able to comply), is constantly attended by a responsible adult, and has ready transportation to the hospital within 15 minutes at all times. In the absence of atypical maternal serum antibodies, the requirement that fully crossmatched blood be available at all times is not justifiable. The majority of our patients in recent years have been successfully managed at home.

The ideal method of terminating the expectant period is cesarean section under elective, rather than emergent, circumstances. Although it is not clear that emergent delivery influences perinatal survival independent of shortened gestation, significantly more newborns born under emergent conditions are anemic (27.7 per cent) than those born electively (2.9 per cent) (Cotton et al., 1980). If one selects 37 to 38 weeks as

the time for elective termination, only 24 to 30 per cent of patients remain undelivered (Brenner et al., 1978; Cotton et al., 1980). By choosing 36 weeks as the cutoff, the potential pool of candidates for elective termination constitutes approximately 50 per cent of the entire group. For this reason, we favor initiating weekly assessment of lung maturity by amniocentesis at 36 weeks, so that *elective* delivery may be performed as soon as lung maturity is documented. Waiting beyond 36 weeks in the hope of resolution of the placenta previa is probably justifiable only in the asymptomatic woman with a marginal previa or low-lying placenta.

Method of Delivery

Cesarean section has replaced attempts at vaginal delivery for all but a small minority of patients with placenta previa. The only circumstances under which the vaginal approach might be considered are the following: (1) a dead fetus, (2) major fetal malformation, (3) a clearly previable fetus, (4) advanced labor

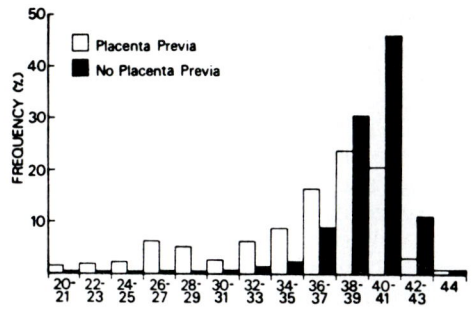

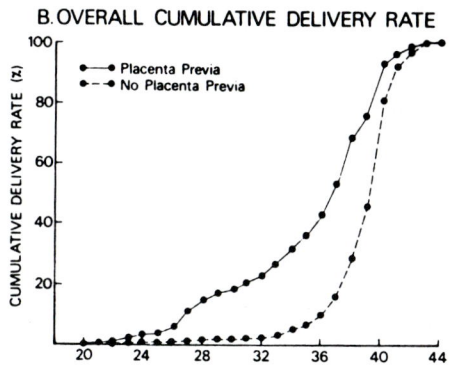

Gestational Age (Weeks)

FIGURE 39–2. Time of delivery in patients with and without placenta previa. *A,* The proportion (percentage) of patients delivered in each 2-week interval is shown. Despite the clear association of placenta previa with preterm delivery, the most common time for delivery is between 38 and 39 weeks. *B,* The cumulative delivery rate in percentages is shown; 25 per cent of patients with placenta previa are delivered at or before 32 weeks, and 50 per cent are delivered before 37 weeks. (From Brenner WE, Edelman DA, Hendricks CH: Characteristics of patients with placenta previa and results of "expectant management." Am J Obstet Gynecol **132**:180, 1978.)

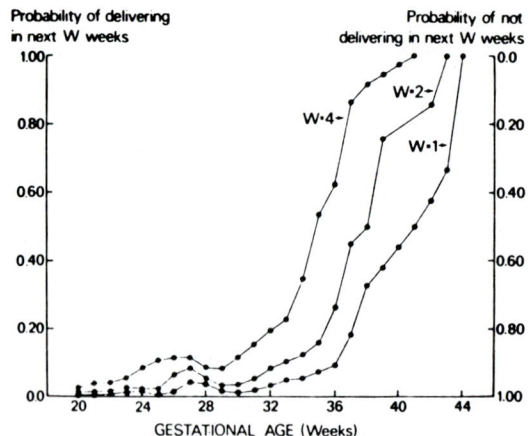

FIGURE 39–3. Graph showing the probability that pregnancy in a patient with placenta previa can be maintained for some time longer (1, 2, or 4 weeks). The fetus at 32 weeks has an 80 per cent chance of remaining *in utero* for 4 weeks; the fetus at 36 weeks, however, has only a 50 per cent chance of gaining 2 additional weeks of gestation. (From Brenner WE, Edelman DA, Hendricks CH: Characteristics of patients with placenta previa and results of "expectant management." Am J Obstet Gynecol **132**:180, 1978.)

with engagement of the fetal head. A posterior placenta previa is likely to obstruct engagement of the presenting part and represents a relative contraindication to attempts at vaginal delivery even in these circumstances. Prolonged attempts are unwise from the standpoint of both accumulated blood loss and increased risk of uterine rupture with placenta previa.

In the presence of a living, viable fetus, cesarean section is the delivery method of choice. The advantage in terms of perinatal survival is striking, and it is especially important to recognize that this advantage applies as much, if not more, to marginal and partial placenta previa as to total placenta previa. The benefits of the abdominal route (Table 39–2) should invalidate attempts at vaginal delivery, especially with marginal placenta previa (Crenshaw et al., 1973). If a sonogram made within several days of the delivery date is inconclusive, the option of performing a double set-up examination should be considered. As stated before, if placenta previa cannot be ruled out on this examination, the wisest course in the majority of circumstances is to proceed with cesarean section. Although a low-lying placenta does not contraindicate

TABLE 39–2. Perinatal Mortality Rate at Various Gestational Ages as a Function of the Route of Delivery

GESTATIONAL AGE (WEEKS)	VAGINAL DELIVERY		CESAREAN SECTION	
	NUMBER	MORTALITY RATE (%)	NUMBER	MORTALITY RATE (%)
Less than 32	21	81	8	63
32 to 35	14	43	7	14
36 or more	28	36	30	3

Adapted from Crenshaw C, Jones DED, Parker RT: Placenta previa: A survey of twenty years experience with improved perinatal survival by expectant therapy and cesarean delivery. Obstet Gynecol Survey **28**:461, © by Williams and Wilkins, 1973.

labor, the potential for placental abruption mandates close monitoring during labor.

The final choice of uterine incision can be made only after the abdomen is opened. If the fetal lie is longitudinal and ultrasonography does not show the placenta to be implanted on the anterior surface of the uterus above the bladder reflection, a low transverse uterine incision may be selected as long as the lower segment appears to be reasonably well formed. In all other circumstances a vertical incision is preferred, either in the lower segment or in the contractile segment (classic incision), the exact placement being the one that best avoids the placenta and affords easy, atraumatic extraction of the fetus. If the placenta cannot be avoided, it is generally best to seek its edge quickly, gaining access to the amniotic sac and the fetus through the membranes, rather than to cut or tear through the placenta itself. The procedure can be associated with extensive maternal blood loss, 1500 ml or more being common. It is prudent to have four units of crossmatched blood available in the operating room, perhaps more if the placenta is known to be anterior. Especially in this latter circumstance, a unit of low-titer O-negative blood should be available for the infant because trauma to the placenta can cause fetal blood loss.

Blood loss may also continue after delivery of the placenta. Normally the blood vessels supplying the intervillous space are occluded by myometrial contractions. The lower uterine segment is only weakly contractile, and may be ineffective in occluding vessels. Major bleeding vessels can be controlled by suturing, but the use of multiple sutures to control generalized bleeding is usually futile. We have had some success with direct injections of pitocin (10 units diluted in approximately 30 ml of saline), methergine, or 15-methyl $PGF_{2\alpha}$ into the area. Packing of the area and manual compression of the ascending branches of the uterine arteries may be useful as temporizing measures, but are rarely sufficient in themselves. Ultimately, bilateral uterine artery or bilateral hypogastric artery ligation or total abdominal hysterectomy may be necessary.

Complications

Placenta Accreta

Placenta accreta is strongly associated with placenta previa, occurring in as many as 15 per cent of cases (Breen et al., 1977). This association is due to the thin, poorly formed decidua of the lower segment, which offers little resistance to deeper invasion by the trophoblast. The incidence of placenta accreta is as high as 67 per cent in the woman with placenta previa and multiple prior cesarean sections (Clark et al., 1985). Placenta accreta and its more advanced forms (increta and percreta) are justifiably feared as the most serious maternal complications. Five out of six maternal deaths in Hibbard's (1969) series were directly attributed to this condition. In almost all cases, nothing short of total abdominal hysterectomy is lifesaving, and if contiguous organs are involved, even this may not suffice.

Vasa Previa

Vasa previa is uncommon, occurring in about one in 3000 deliveries, but is among the most lethal fetal conditions. It is defined as a velamentous insertion of the cord in the lower uterine segment so that the cord vessels course unsupported through the membranes in advance of the fetal presenting part and often across the cervical os. The unsupported fetal vessels are prone to tearing, especially at the time of spontaneous or artificial rupture of the membranes, with resultant fetal exsanguination leading to death in at least 75 per cent of cases. Membrane rupture is not invariably the proximate cause of tearing of the vessels (Pent, 1979). Furthermore, the perinatal loss even in the absence of bleeding from torn fetal vessels approaches 50 to 60 per cent owing to compression of the vessels by the presenting part and extreme compromise of the placental circulation. Making the diagnosis in time to save the fetus requires a high index of suspicion. Direct palpation of the vessels or visualization by amnioscopy is sometimes possible, but a negative result of either procedure in the face of severe variable decelerations of the fetal heart rate does not exclude the diagnosis. The onset of vaginal bleeding coincident with membrane rupture should prompt testing for fetal blood content. Immediate delivery by cesarean section is the only way to save the fetus in vasa previa.

Intrauterine Growth Restriction and Congenital Abnormalities

Varma (1973) has reported a 16 per cent rate of fetal growth restriction in association with placenta previa. He also found a good correlation between the occurrence of such restriction and multiple episodes of antepartum bleeding. These findings should serve as a reason for caution in expectant management, even though other researchers have found the rate of fetal growth to be normal in expectantly managed patients (Brenner et al., 1978). Nearly all reports confirm an approximate doubling of the rate of serious congenital malformations in cases of placenta previa, the most common being major anomalies of the central nervous system, cardiovascular system, respiratory tract, and gastrointestinal tract. A detailed fetal anatomic survey at initial sonographic diagnosis and serial sonographic evaluation of fetal growth should be performed in all cases.

Fetal Anemia and Rh Isoimmunization

Cesarean section itself is a risk factor for large fetal-maternal hemorrhage, and it is highly likely, although unproved, that placenta previa is an additional risk factor. For the Rh-negative woman who is identified as a candidate for immune prophylaxis, attempts to detect excessive fetal-maternal hemorrhage are clearly indicated (see Chapter 44). If excessive hemorrhage is detected, the appropriate dose of immune globulin is given and its sufficiency is documented by a positive indirect Coombs' test 48 hours after treatment. It should also be remembered that fetal-maternal transfusion can occur during antepartum bleeding episodes and perhaps should prompt testing after each episode in the Rh-negative woman unless the father is known to be Rh-negative. Even in the absence of documented fetal-maternal hemorrhage, antenatal Rh immune globulin prophylaxis is desirable.

ABRUPTIO PLACENTAE

Definition

The term abruptio placentae denotes separation of a normally implanted placenta prior to the birth of the fetus. The diagnosis is most commonly made in the third trimester, but the term may be used after the 20th week of pregnancy when the clinical and pathologic criteria are met. This is a uniquely dangerous condition to both the mother and the fetus because of its pathologic sequelae.

Pathophysiology

Abruptio placentae is initiated by bleeding into the decidua basalis. In most cases the source of the bleeding is small arterial vessels in the basal layer of the decidua that are pathologically altered and prone to rupture. In some cases the bleeding may be initiated from fetal-placental vessels. The resultant hemorrhage splits the decidua, leaving a thin layer attached to the placenta. As the decidual hematoma grows there is further separation. Compression by the expanding hematoma leads to obliteration of the overlying intervillous space. Ultimately there is destruction of the placental tissue in the involved area. This area may often be identified on gross inspection of the placenta by an organized clot lying within a cup-shaped depression on the maternal surface. From the standpoint of the fetus, this occurrence represents a loss of surface area for exchange of respiratory gases and nutrients.

In a small proportion of cases, the process may be self-limited and of no further consequence to the pregnancy. More often, bleeding continues, and the blood under pressure will seek the path of least resistance. If the initial point of separation is toward the center of the placenta there may be continued dissection and separation in the decidua as well as extravasation into the myometrium and through to the peritoneal surface. This results in the so-called *Couvelaire uterus*. Once the blood reaches the edge of the placenta it may continue to dissect between the decidua and the fetal membranes and gain access to the vagina through the cervix. It may pass through the membranes into the amniotic sac, causing the port wine discoloration that is almost pathognomonic of abruption. The amount of blood that eventually finds its way through the cervix is often only a small portion of that lost from the circulation, and in no way is it a reliable indication of the severity of the condition.

Classification

The severity of abruptio placentae may be classified according to clinical criteria, anatomic criteria, or both.

In the United States, a system of clinical classification first proposed by Page and colleagues (1954) is usually followed (Table 39–3). A rough correlation with the anatomic extent of placental separation may be made. Cases are assigned to grade 0 only in retrospect by the finding of a small area of adherent clot at the periphery of the placenta. This entity used to be called "marginal sinus rupture." It cannot be distinguished prospectively with any certainty from an early stage of abruption destined to become more severe. The proportions of mild, moderate, and severe cases are 48 per cent, 27 per cent, and 24 per cent, respectively (Bernstein, 1981). This classification is entirely retrospective, being assigned after delivery. A prospective classification, offering guidance for management, remains to be defined.

Incidence and Etiology

The reported incidence of abruptio placentae varies widely in published series according to the population studied and the diagnostic criteria applied. Knab (1978) found a range from 0.49 to 1.29 per cent in the series he reviewed, with a mean incidence of 0.83 per cent, or one per 120 deliveries. Abruption severe enough to kill the fetus is less common, being found only once in each 420 deliveries (Pritchard et al., 1970). It is not clear whether the overall incidence of abruption is stable or has declined over the past 2 or 3 decades.

Numerous factors have been suggested to play a causal role in abruptio placentae, but a unifying etiologic concept is still lacking. Underlying disease of the decidua and uterine blood vessels seems to explain best the diversity of associated factors that have been described. Women who suffer abruption have a remarkably poor reproductive history and future reproductive potential. For pregnancies culminating in abruption, there is evidence of long-standing pathologic fetal-maternal relationship, in that 81 per cent of infants born at less than 36 weeks gestation are below the mean birth weight for gestational age (Hibbard and Jeffcoate, 1966). Thus, abruptio placentae may be viewed as the final, dramatic expression of long-standing pregnancy disorder.

A detailed discussion of potential etiologic factors may be found elsewhere (Preucel et al., 1981). Some factors that have been suggested to play an etiologic role in the development of abruptio placentae are as follows:

TRAUMA. Although it has been anecdotally related to severe abruption, trauma accounts for only a small minority of cases. Nevertheless, a high index of suspicion should be maintained. Most cases associated with trauma will evolve within 24 hours of the precipitating event. Even in the absence of vaginal bleeding, close observation and continuous monitoring of the fetus is warranted after significant abdominal trauma in late pregnancy.

SHORT UMBILICAL CORD OR UTERINE ANOMALY. Extreme shortening of the umbilical cord, sudden decompression of the uterus (at the time of membrane rupture or after delivery of a first twin), and the presence of a uterine anomaly or myoma at the implantation site may be implicated only infrequently in abruptio placentae.

INFERIOR VENA CAVAL COMPRESSION. In theory, compression of the inferior vena cava can raise pressure in the intervillous space and promote forceful detachment of the placenta, but this occurrence has not been proved in human pregnancy and fails to account for the pathologic findings, which are predominantly found in the decidua.

MATERNAL HYPERTENSION. Mild abruption is not associated with clinically apparent hypertension. However, nearly 50 per cent of cases of severe abruption with a dead fetus are associated with maternal hypertension, about half chronic and half pregnancy-related (Pritchard et al., 1970); this rate represents a five-fold increase over the rate of hypertension in patients without abruption. Golditch and Boyce (1970) found the incidence of toxemia with abruption to be 13.9 per cent in mild abruption, 25.7 per cent in moderate abruption, and 52.1 per cent in severe abruption. These observations are consistent with the hypothesis that underlying maternal vascular disease is etiologic in both the hypertension and the abruption, and that abruption may be an even more sensitive indicator of vascular pathology than hypertension.

FOLIC ACID DEFICIENCY. Hibbard and Jeffcoate (1966) argued persuasively that dietary deficiency, in particular folic acid deficiency, may cause abruption by altering trophoblastic growth in the critical period during which the interface between the mother and the fetus is established. They estimated the risk of abruptio placentae in folic acid–deficient women to be

TABLE 39–3. Classification of Abruptio Placentae According to Major Maternal and Fetal Signs

GRADE	CONCEALED HEMORRHAGE	UTERINE TENDERNESS	MATERNAL SHOCK	COAGULOPATHY (OVERT)	FETAL DISTRESS	COMMENTS
0	No	No	Absent	No	No	A retrospective diagnosis by examination of the placenta. No symptoms.
1	No	No	Absent	No	No	Includes the diagnosis of "marginal sinus rupture." Blood loss variable.
2	Yes	Yes	Absent	Rare	Yes	Will usually progress to grade 3 unless delivery is effected promptly.
3	Extensive	Yes	Present	Common	Fetal death	Major maternal complication (e.g., renal cortical necrosis).

about 10 per cent. Numerous subsequent studies, however, have failed to substantiate this observation. Folic acid supplementation has no apparent effect if begun after the sixth week of pregnancy.

CIGARETTE SMOKING. Maternal cigarette smoking is associated with the finding of decidual necrosis on pathologic examination. It is not surprising, therefore, that both an increased incidence of abruption and an increase in fetal deaths due to abruption are seen among women who smoke more than 10 cigarettes per day (Naeye et al., 1977). This is one potential etiologic factor that is an appropriate target for preventive measures.

MATERNAL AGE AND PARITY. Abruptio placentae has long been known to occur more frequently in older women, but this increase merely reflects the effect of increased parity (Hibbard and Jeffcoate, 1966). The incidence is less than 1 per cent among primigravidas and rises to about 2.5 per cent among grand multiparas. At least part of the increase may be ascribed to shortened time between pregnancies with resultant chronic malnutrition. Alternatively, it may reflect permanent damage to the endometrium, as with the association between placenta previa and parity. The incidence of abruptio placentae has been found to have declined in some studies, perhaps reflecting the effects of widely available family planning and limitation of family size.

COCAINE ABUSE. Case reports of abruption with maternal cocaine use have appeared with increasing frequency over the past several years. The reason for this association may relate to the vasoactive properties of cocaine. The risk of cocaine use is not known but may be substantial, particularly with heavy use of free-base, or "crack," cocaine. Approximately 5 per cent of women with documented cocaine use in late pregnancy at our institution have pregnancies that terminate with abruptions (see Chapter 13).

Recurrence

Abruptio placentae is clearly not an "accident" in the great majority of cases, but rather an expression of a pathologic process of long duration. No better evidence exists than the risk of recurrent abruption in subsequent pregnancies. The risk of recurrence has been reported to be 5.5 to 16.6 per cent, as much as 30 times the incidence in the general population. Pritchard and colleagues (1970) noted that 7 per cent of women with abruption severe enough to kill the fetus will have the same outcome in a subsequent pregnancy. After two consecutive abruptions, the risk of a third rises to 25 per cent. About 30 per cent of all subsequent pregnancies of women who have experienced an abruption fail to produce a healthy child (Hibbard and Jeffcoate, 1966).

Clearly, these are high-risk pregnancies. However, a management plan proven to prevent recurrent morbid outcomes remains to be defined. Although there may be ongoing evidence of an abnormal fetal-maternal relationship, such as suspected intrauterine growth restriction, the timing of the final event is unpredictable. The prenatal course in many women

with abruption is completely normal. In fact, many women have had normal biophysical tests within 24 hours of an abruption. In the absence of a reliable method for predicting when abruption will occur, a program of planned preterm delivery is not justified in most cases.

Perinatal Mortality Rate

The overall perinatal mortality rate attributable to abruptio placentae has been nearly four per 1000 (Naeye et al., 1977). This figure represented 15 per cent of all perinatal deaths in the series. All sizable series reported to date have involved cases occurring before the widespread application of electronic fetal monitoring, and it is likely that the case fatality rate of 25 to 50 per cent for the fetus has been significantly reduced. Nevertheless, important limitations still exist in our ability to minimize the impact of this condition. The three major causes of perinatal death in abruption are fetal anoxia, prematurity, and fetal exsanguination. In most large series nearly half the fetuses who ultimately are stillborn have already died at the time of admission to the hospital. Effective intervention in this subgroup may prove to be impossible. The impact of prematurity has been lessened, but by no means eliminated, by improvements in neonatal intensive care. More than 20 per cent of abruption cases become manifested between 28 and 32 weeks; a similar proportion occur before 28 weeks with poor chance for intact survival (Blair, 1973).

Diagnosis

The classic symptoms and signs of abruptio placentae are vaginal bleeding, abdominal pain, uterine contractions, and uterine tenderness. The clinician must be aware that all of these are not invariably present and that the absence of one or more does not exclude the diagnosis or necessarily suggest a mild form.

Although vaginal bleeding is the hallmark of abruptio placentae, about 10 per cent of affected women present with only concealed hemorrhage; this may be particularly dangerous for both the fetus and the mother. When the initial point of separation is in the center of the implantation site, a large portion of the placenta separates before retroplacental blood gains access to the space between the membranes and the decidua and ultimately to the vagina. When external bleeding is noted, it is characteristically dark and nonclotting. In some cases it is serosanguineous, having been extruded from a retroplacental clot. The observed amount of bleeding gives little or no indication of the total loss from the maternal circulation and cannot be used to gauge the severity of the problem or to guide replacement therapy. Serial measurements of fundal height and abdominal girth are useful to detect large retroplacental blood collections, but stable measurements do not exclude the diagnosis or reliably predict a benign course for the mother and fetus.

Abdominal pain is a less constant presenting symptom than vaginal bleeding, being found in some series in only slightly over half of cases at admission. Its presence probably indicates extravasation of blood into the myometrium. In mild cases, the pain may be intermittent and difficult to distinguish from the pain of labor. In severe cases the pain is characteristically sharp, sudden in onset, and severe. The initial episode may subside, only to be followed by an intermittent crampy pain or a persistent dull pain in the lower abdomen or back. There may be associated nausea and vomiting and a feeling of faintness even in the absence of objective signs of hypovolemia.

Uterine contractions are present in the majority of cases but may be difficult to appreciate clinically. They are characteristically of high frequency but low amplitude, and if the baseline uterine tonus is elevated, they may not be palpable and may not register reliably on an external tocodynamometer. A case of total placental abruption that clearly demonstrates this point is illustrated in Figure 39–4. In severe cases the uterus may become so rigid that outlining the fetus is difficult or impossible. Uterine tenderness may be generalized or localized to the site of placental detachment. When it is localized, the point of maximal tenderness often corresponds to the area in which the patient's pain is perceived. Especially in cases in which the placenta is implanted posteriorly, uterine tenderness may be absent and the pain is often in the lower back.

Additional findings may help to make the correct diagnosis. Evidence of maternal hypovolemia beyond that expected on the basis of *observed* blood loss is highly suggestive. Evidence of fetal distress or fetal death suggests the loss of a large portion of villous exchange area.

Ultrasonography, although useful to exclude placenta previa, is not sensitive enough to exclude abruptio placentae reliably. Nevertheless, a spectrum of findings can be used to support the diagnosis. Acute hemorrhage is characteristically hyperechoic or isoechoic compared with the placenta and may therefore be misinterpreted as an abnormally thick placenta (Nyberg et al., 1987). Resolving hematomas become hypoechoic within one week, and sonolucent within 2 weeks. Prospective use of ultrasonography to guide the decision for expectant management as opposed to delivery has been suggested (Rivera-Alxina et al., 1983), but firm criteria have not been established. The size of the hematoma, its location (retroplacental, marginal, intra-amniotic), and change in size over time are all factors to consider. It must be emphasized, however, that valuable time should not be lost performing a sonogram in the presence of obvious fetal distress or an unstable maternal condition.

The differential diagnosis includes all other potential causes of third-trimester bleeding. When pain is the predominant presenting complaint (especially if bleeding is absent or minimal), several other diagnoses may be entertained. If there is maternal shock, diffuse abdominal pain, and tenderness, a uterine rupture is possible. Most such cases mandate prompt laparotomy for maternal indications, and the true diagnosis becomes readily apparent. Abdominal pain and tenderness and uterine contractions may also be seen with chorioamnionitis; in most instances, severe presenting symptoms will argue for uterine evacuation, but, if the diagnosis is in doubt, an amniocentesis and examination of the fluid for bacteria or blood may be helpful. Finally, appendicitis and pyelonephritis may occasionally be difficult to distinguish from abruption.

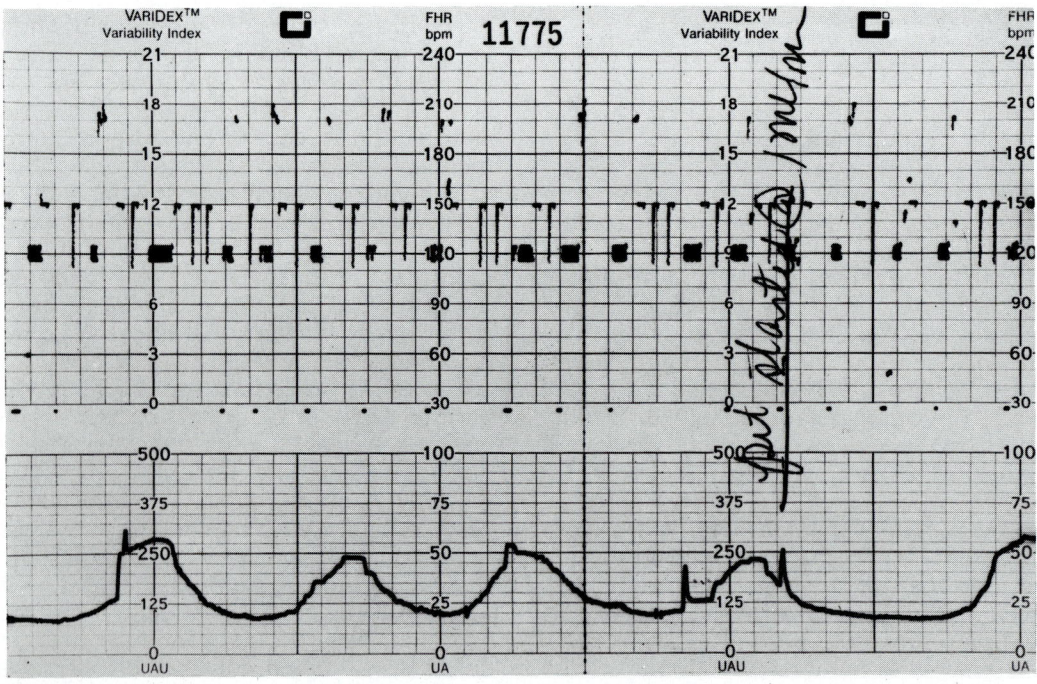

FIGURE 39–4. Internal monitor tracing from a case of severe abruption. The upper panel shows artifact only; the fetus is dead. The lower panel is derived from a calibrated internal pressure transducer and shows modest elevation of the baseline tonus and uterine tachysystole. Five contractions occur in a 7-minute period.

Management

General Measures

Any patient with suspected abruptio placentae should be hospitalized immediately. If the fetus is alive on admission, delay in instituting an effective plan for delivery may have dire consequences. In Knab's (1978) series, 22 per cent of all perinatal deaths occurred after hospitalization but before delivery, 30 per cent of these within 2 hours of admission.

A rapid evaluation of the mother's condition is made, including postural vital signs and abdominal examination. A blood pressure reading in the normal range may be misleading, because an underlying hypertensive condition may be revealed only after intravascular volume is restored. Postural changes may be absent until a large portion of intravascular volume is lost. The vital signs are repeated at least every 15 minutes thereafter. If the fetus is alive (as determined by auscultation), an external fetal monitor is placed and evidence of fetal distress is sought. If the diagnosis of abruptio placentae is clinically favored over that of placenta previa, it is highly desirable to perform ultrasonographic examination in the labor and delivery suite with portable equipment.

A large-bore intravenous line is placed, and through it the initial blood samples for the laboratory may be drawn. The initial infusate may be normal saline, lactated Ringer's solution, or Plasmalyte. If there is evidence of maternal hypovolemia, at least two such lines should be placed and secured well, because subsequent attempts at intravenous placement may become progressively more difficult. Serious consideration should be given at this time to the placement of a central vascular catheter. A Swan-Ganz catheter is ideal for monitoring blood and fluid replacement, but the potential for coagulopathy in severe abruption makes placement via the internal jugular or subclavian vein potentially hazardous (see Chapter 51). A central venous catheter placed via an antecubital vein is frequently a wise compromise. A bladder catheter should be placed in all but the mildest cases to monitor urine output. Finally, oxygen should be administered at 8 liters/minute via nasal prongs.

The initial hemoglobin and hematocrit readings may be falsely reassuring, especially if the patient's symptoms are of recent onset. However, if these values are lower than the last recorded prenatal values, the clinician should anticipate the need for additional crossmatched blood. Baseline electrolyte and renal function studies are useful for later comparison when massive transfusion is required as well as for later detection of renal complications. (Coagulation studies are discussed under "Complications.")

It cannot be emphasized strongly enough that loss of blood from the intravascular compartment is usually underestimated and that the more severe the loss the more gross the underestimate becomes. Crossmatched blood must be available to replace the loss already incurred and potential further loss. It is a good practice to have four units available for future needs.

Method and Timing of Delivery

Once the diagnosis is established and cardiovascular resuscitation is well under way, a rational plan for effecting delivery of the fetus must be established. This is the single most important therapeutic goal. The method and timing of delivery depend on the condition and gestational age of the fetus, the condition of the mother, and the status of the cervix.

If the fetus is immature and the abruption is judged to be mild, an expectant approach may be followed. Indeed, it is impossible in some cases to distinguish between idiopathic preterm labor and mild abruptio placentae. In the absence of fetal distress or maternal complications, a trial of tocolytic treatment may be undertaken. There is evidence that such pregnancies may be successfully prolonged without increased jeopardy to the mother or fetus (Sholl, 1987). Delivery should be effected, however, if the abruption is moderate or severe. If the fetal heart rate tracing is normal and the uterus relaxes well between contractions, an attempt at vaginal delivery may be considered. Even prior to the introduction of electronic fetal monitoring, there was no increase in perinatal mortality rate with mild abruption, irrespective of the interval from diagnosis to delivery, as long as the auscultated heart rate was normal (Golditch and Boyce, 1970). In some cases the use of intravenous oxytocin is required to augment uterine activity. Caution must be exercised because the uterine response may be erratic and the risk of uterine rupture is increased, especially in multiparas. No specific time limit may be rationally applied as long as intensive fetal and maternal surveillance reveals no advancement in abruption severity and the labor is progressing.

Amniotomy is advantageous in nearly all cases. It probably reduces extravasation of blood into the myometrium and entry of thromboplastic substances into the maternal circulation, and it may stimulate labor. A major advantage is that amniotomy allows placement of a fetal scalp electrode for heart rate monitoring and an intra-amniotic catheter. (The former gives assurance of fetal well-being or demonstrates evidence of fetal distress, which is usually manifested by late decelerations or loss of variability.) Careful calibration of the pressure transducer gives a reliable measure of resting baseline tonus and the contraction pattern. A resting tonus higher than 15 mm Hg is associated with deficits of uterine blood flow, compounding the deleterious effects of the reduced exchange area and frequent contractions. In such cases the prospect for vaginal delivery of a healthy infant is small unless the labor is far advanced, and early resort to cesarean section may be necessary.

Numerous studies of abruption over the past 25 years have demonstrated improved perinatal survival with increased and early use of cesarean section for delivery. The advantage seems to be limited to those cases classified as moderate (Knab, 1978). Overall in collected series the perinatal mortality rate with cesarean section is 16.7 per cent, and that with vaginal delivery is 31.5 per cent. Unfortunately, in none of these series was the question examined prospectively, and all were conducted prior to the availability of electronic fetal monitoring. Therefore, the clinician must still consider each case as unique in deciding the appropriate method of delivery. If the fetus is dead, vaginal delivery should be attempted in order to minimize maternal morbidity. If the fetus is alive but shows definite evidence of distress, immediate abdominal delivery should be effected unless contraindicated by the mother's condition. In this regard, it should be noted that clinically evident disseminated intravascular coagulation is uncommon in the presence of a living fetus, and an unsubstantiated fear of coagulopathy should not be regarded as a contraindication to abdominal delivery. Gross prematurity has a tremendously negative impact on perinatal survival, and the question has been raised whether there is a definable gestational age below which death *in utero* is merely traded for neonatal death if delivery is carried out. Unfortunately, the compounding effects of prematurity and abruptio placentae have not been sufficiently studied to define this theoretic limit. At present it is best for the physician to act in the interest of any fetus considered "viable"; the quality of neonatal care in a given institution is critically important in defining this term with any comfort.

Meticulous attention to correct surgical technique is more important than "shotgun" prophylactic therapy for coagulopathy in avoiding major intraoperative and postoperative complications. Particular emphasis should be placed on ligation or cautery of small bleeding points that might be overlooked in the routine case.

Complications

Hemorrhagic Shock

Obstetric shock was often used in the past to describe cases of abruption. The term implies that the degree of shock is out of proportion to the blood lost. This is now generally held to be incorrect, because the observed blood loss in abruption grossly under-represents the actual loss of circulating volume, particularly in severe cases. A median volume of 2500 ml of blood contained within the uterus at the time of delivery has been found in severe abruption, and even this fails to account for additional losses into the myometrium (Pritchard and Brekken, 1967). Both the magnitude and the frequency of undertransfusion increase with increasing severity of abruption when the volume of transfusion is based on observed antepartum blood loss.

Shock is characterized by tissue hypoperfusion. Rational therapy should be aimed at restoring effective perfusion by restoring effective circulating blood volume. This restoration is necessary to avoid major complications such as ischemic necrosis of the kidneys and often requires massive amounts of blood product replacement. Replacement can be effectively monitored only if there is objective evidence that perfusion to critical organs is adequate. The most accessible organ for monitoring is the kidney. A urine output of 30 ml/hr (preferably 60 ml/hr) affords excellent evidence that perfusion is adequate. If oliguria persists after volume expansion, however, other methods for monitoring effective circulating volume are necessary. The use of central monitoring techniques is more commonly required when severe preeclampsia com-

plicates replacement therapy, because there is no definable "end point" for blood pressure and because intrinsic renal disease may render urine output a false indicator of effective circulating volume. If a central venous pressure (CVP) catheter is employed, a value of 12 to 15 cm H_2O is usually associated with adequate circulating blood volume in the absence of cardiac decompensation. Pulmonary capillary wedge pressure (PCWP) via a Swan-Ganz catheter is currently believed to better reflect circulatory adequacy than the CVP. In pregnancy, the normal PCWP is 10 to 15 mm Hg. A PCWP below 10 mm Hg is associated with clinically evident shock. (See Chapter 51 for further discussion of maternal shock.)

Balanced salt solution can be infused until cross-matched blood is available. If there is clear evidence of massive hemorrhage on admission, the initial use of type-specific blood may be necessary. Initial fluid therapy must be vigorous, often with volumes well in excess of the actual hemorrhage, because moderate-to-severe shock is associated with significant fluid shifts from the intravascular to the extravascular compartment. Subsequent fluid therapy is aimed at maintaining an adequate circulating blood volume and a hematocrit of 30 per cent or greater. Such a hematocrit level helps to avoid cellular anoxia and damage, and it becomes especially important in massive transfusion situations in which banked blood essentially replaces the patient's own blood. Banked blood older than 7 days is characterized by significant decreases in erythrocyte 2,3-diphosphoglycerate concentration and a consequent increase in oxygen affinity. As a result of its use, release of oxygen to the tissues may be significantly impaired.

Massive transfusion may be defined as transfusion in excess of one to one-and-one half times the patient's estimated circulating blood volume, but defining it as administration of 10 or more units makes more sense in the clinical situation. Several problems may be encountered in this situation. The first is a coagulation disorder that may confuse the diagnosis of disseminated intravascular coagulation in abruptio placentae. Banked blood is generally fractionated into packed red blood cells and plasma; administration of the former effectively precludes replacement of the procoagulants lost with the patient's own blood. In the absence of overt coagulopathy, the prophylactic replacement of platelets and other procoagulants is usually unnecessary and wasteful. As an alternative, blood samples may be taken for coagulation analysis after each four to six units administered. A platelet count less than 50,000/mm^3 indicates the need for platelet transfusion. Each bag of platelet concentrate administered can be expected to raise the count by 7000 to 10,000/mm^3 ml. Similarly, a fibrinogen level less than 100 mg/100 ml may indicate the need for replacement. It is important, however, as will be discussed, to seek further evidence for disseminated intravascular coagulation before undertaking therapy with fresh-frozen plasma or cryoprecipitate. (See Chapters 51 and 53 for further discussion of hematologic disorders.) Banked blood is also characterized by loss of potassium from red blood cells and can raise the serum potassium to dangerous levels in the massively transfused patient. The serum potassium level should be checked after each four to six units infused, and continuous monitoring by electrocardiogram is highly desirable.

Disseminated Intravascular Coagulation

Disorders of coagulation are discussed comprehensively in Chapters 51 and 53, but it is pertinent to review here the pathophysiology and management of disseminated intravascular coagulation (DIC) with abruptio placentae. Clinically significant coagulopathy is encountered in only about 10 per cent of cases of abruption, but it is much more common in severe abruption marked by death of the fetus or massive hemorrhage. Proper management of this disorder demands an understanding of its pathophysiology as well as correct interpretation of various laboratory tests of hemostasis and blood coagulation.

A general outline of the clotting and fibrinolytic systems is shown in Figure 39–5. Thrombus formation is initiated by platelets, which adhere to the site of blood vessel injury. The process makes available platelet factor 3, which interacts with factors XI, XII, and XIII to form the intrinsic activator complex. Alternately, the extrinsic pathway involves the interaction of tissue thromboplastins released at the site of injury and factor VII, leading to the formation of the extrinsic activator complex. Either the intrinsic or the extrinsic activator complex can interact with factors X and V in the common pathway, resulting in the generation of thrombin. A proteolytic enzyme, thrombin acts on fibrinogen to cause the formation of fibrin monomer, which spontaneously polymerizes to form fibrin polymer. This unstable product is stabilized in the presence of factor XIII, resulting in the formation of the fibrin clot.

The extraordinary potency of the clotting mechanism is illustrated by the fact that sufficient potential thrombin exists in 10 ml of blood to clot 2500 ml of plasma. The unimpeded action of thrombin could result in total coagulation of the blood in the absence of equally potent counterbalancing factors, the most important of which is the *fibrinolytic system*. Circulating plasminogen (profibrinolysin) is converted to plasmin (fibrinolysin) by a variety of plasminogen activators. Plasmin is a proteolytic enzyme that can cleave a variety of substrates. When plasmin acts on fibrinogen and fibrin, fragments are produced that are collectively termed *fibrin degradation products* (FDP). Certain of these fragments serve as antithrombins, both by competing with fibrinogen for available thrombin and by forming nonclottable complexes with fibrin monomer. Thus, the fibrinolytic system is a potent anticoagulation mechanism. Normal hemostatic function depends on the critical balance between the coagulation and fibrinolytic systems in order to maintain the fluid state of the vascular system while allowing the local formation of clots at various sites of injury. This balance is clearly disturbed in a number of cases of abruptio placentae.

The nature of the coagulopathy in abruption has been a subject of frequent debate. One early theory held that the inability to clot was a direct result of consumption of procoagulants in the retroplacental clot. Measurement of the fibrin contained within the retroplacental clot shows it to be present in the same concentrations as in whole blood, however, making simple consumption alone an unlikely explanation for the coagulopathy. Alternatively, it has been suggested that primary activation of the fibrinolytic system causes digestion of circulating fibrinogen with resultant hypofibrinogenemia. This mechanism is also unlikely because only a minority of patients with severe hypofibrinogenemia secondary to abruption show abnormal clot lysis.

By far the most popular and cogent hypothesis is illustrated in Figure 39–6. Entry of thromboplastins into the circulation from the site of placental injury is the inciting event and continues to feed the process as long as the placenta remains undelivered. The thromboplastins initiate widespread intravascular activation of the clotting cascade. Clotting factors are

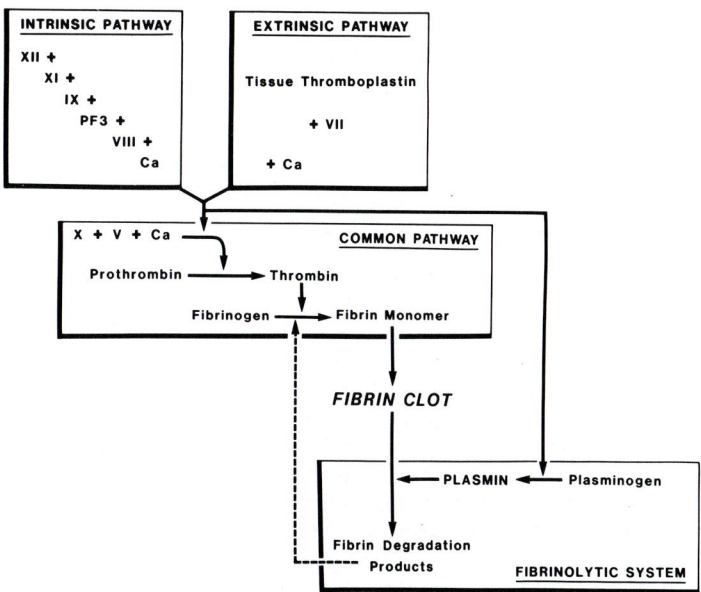

FIGURE 39–5. General outline of coagulation and fibrinolytic systems. *Solid lines* indicate stimulation; *broken lines* indicate inhibition.

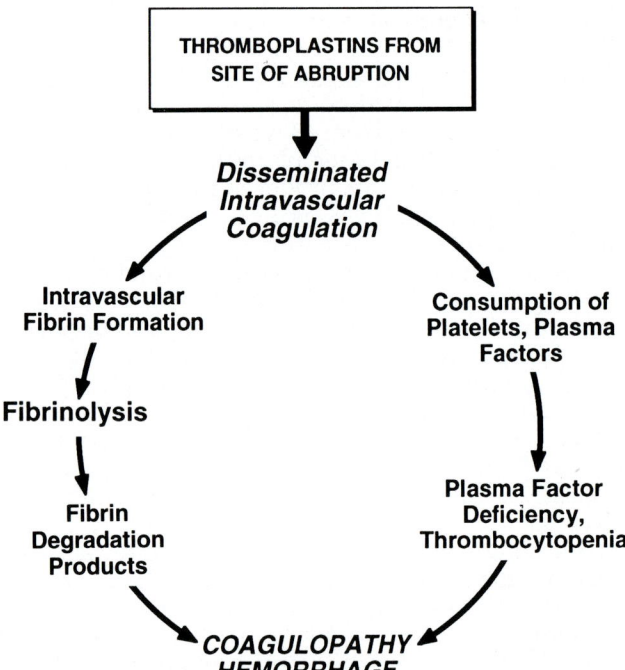

```
┌─────────────────────────┐
│  THROMBOPLASTINS FROM   │
│    SITE OF ABRUPTION    │
└─────────────────────────┘
```

Disseminated Intravascular Coagulation

Intravascular Fibrin Formation

Consumption of Platelets, Plasma Factors

Fibrinolysis

Fibrin Degradation Products

Plasma Factor Deficiency, Thrombocytopenia

COAGULOPATHY HEMORRHAGE

FIGURE 39–6. Pathogenesis of the coagulation disorder in abruptio placentae. The entry of thromboplastic materials from the site of placental injury causes a widespread intravascular initiation of the clotting cascade. It is rare to observe evidence of intravascular thrombus formation because the fibrinolytic system rapidly dissolves the clot. Activation of the fibrinolytic system, in concert with consumption of procoagulants (especially fibrinogen), is responsible for the coagulopathy seen with severe abruption.

consumed in the process. It is unusual, in the absence of severe shock, to see clinical evidence of this disseminated intravascular coagulation, such as plugging of vascular beds with end-organ infarction. Lack of such evidence is testimony to the secondary activation of the fibrinolytic system, which may be viewed as a protective mechanism in this clinical setting. The costs of maintaining the fluid state of the blood are the further depletion of fibrinogen (through the proteolytic action of fibrinolysin) and the production of fibrin (and fibrinogen) split products (FSP), which are potent thrombin inhibitors. The end result of this process is a coagulation disorder characterized by severe hypofibrinogenemia, moderate-to-severe depletion of other procoagulants and platelets, and the presence of circulating anticoagulants. Although this disorder is potentially a life-threatening complication of abruption, milder degrees of the coagulopathy should perhaps best be viewed as a protection against the potentially greater devastation of widespread clotting.

Diagnosis. The diagnosis of disseminated intravascular coagulation is sometimes obvious, with bleeding from needle puncture sites or uncontrollable hemorrhage at surgery. Nevertheless, a significant coagulation disorder can exist without obvious clinical signs as long as the physical integrity of the vascular system is maintained. The advantage in earlier diagnosis is that the need for blood component therapy may be anticipated. The tests that are most helpful in

establishing the diagnosis are listed in Table 39–4. (The ranges for normal values should be modified according to local laboratory standards.) In the absence of markedly abnormal values, a trend toward the abnormal range on serial testing can be helpful in establishing the presence of significant coagulopathy. The whole blood clotting time is insensitive because it will remain essentially normal even with a moderate coagulation disorder. Nevertheless, it is a valuable bedside test if performed serially. If blood fails to clot within 8 minutes or if the clot fails to retract and lyses within 2 hours, a marked coagulopathy is present, and ordering appropriate replacement products need not await confirmatory tests. The fibrinogen level is a sensitive indicator of the process on serial testing, but an initially normal result does not rule out DIC. In many hospital laboratories it is more convenient to perform serial thrombin times, which are mainly influenced by fibrinogen levels. The platelet count will usually fall in concert with fibrinogen levels, but there are sometimes striking differences in magnitude; in almost all such cases, the degree of fall in the fibrinogen level exceeds that in the platelet count. Presumably this difference reflects the fact that platelets are being consumed, while fibrinogen is being both consumed and digested.

The most sensitive laboratory test for diagnosing abruption-related coagulopathy is the determination of fibrin-fibrinogen degradation products by one of a variety of techniques, including assays for D-dimer. The absence of these in the circulation makes the diagnosis of abruption highly suspect. Their presence at abnormal levels confirms the presence of a coagulopathy, but gives only qualitative information as to severity of the process.

Serial testing of coagulation function should be done at least every 4 hours until delivery; more frequent testing is indicated by worsening of the patient's condition or the need for massive transfusion. Serial determination of fibrin split products is rarely helpful in guiding therapy once an abnormal result is found. More useful information is obtained from serial fibrinogen determinations (or thrombin times) and platelet counts.

Both the prothrombin time and the partial thromboplastin time are variably affected by the DIC associated with abruption. A normal result in either or both does not rule out the condition, but abnormal results are almost invariably accompanied by abnormalities in fibrinogen levels. Therefore, we do not rely on these two tests.

Treatment. Delivery of the fetus and placenta is the ultimate treatment of DIC with abruptio placentae, because it removes the source of thromboplastin that is feeding the process. Clear evidence of spontaneous resolution after delivery has been presented by Pritchard and Brekken (1967). With removal of the placenta, fibrinogen levels rise by an average of 9 mg/100 ml/hour. Even in the most severe cases, it is uncommon for clinically evident coagulopathy to persist beyond 12 hours after delivery. The postpartum rise in the platelet count is delayed because of the time required for maturation and release of new platelets by the bone marrow. Therefore, the platelet count may not fully normalize until several days postpartum.

TABLE 39–4. Coagulation Tests in Diagnosis of Abruptio Placentae

TEST	WHAT IT MEASURES	NORMAL VALUE	VALUE IN ABRUPTION
Bleeding time	Vascular integrity and platelet function	1–5 min	Usually normal; test of little clinical use in diagnosing abruption.
Whole blood clotting time	Intrinsic pathway Common pathway Platelet function Fibrinolytic activity	Clot formation: 4–8 min Clot retraction: <1 hr Clot lysis: none in 24 hr	Clot formation abnormality indicates severe deficiency. Abnormal retraction with thrombocytopenia.
Fibrinogen	Fibrinogen level	400–650 mg/100 ml	Usually decreased (see text).
Platelet count	Number of platelets	>140,000/mm³	Usually decreased (see text).
Fibrin degradation products	Fibrin and fibrinogen degradation products	<10 μg/ml	Nearly always elevated; most sensitive test.
Euglobulin clot lysis time	Fibrinolytic activity	None in 2 hr	Difficult to interpret with low fibrinogen levels.
Prothrombin time	Factors II, V, VII, X (extrinsic and common pathways)	10–12 sec	Normal to prolonged.
Partial thrombo-plastin time	Factors II, V, XIII, IX, X, XI (intrinsic and common pathways)	24–38 sec	Normal to prolonged.
Thrombin time	Factors I, II Circulating split products Heparin effect	16–20 sec	Parallels fall in fibrinogen; good marker of abruption severity.
RBC morphology	Microangiopathic hemolysis	Absence of RBC distortion or fragmentation	Presence of distortion or fragmentation is uncommon but indicates risk of renal cortical necrosis.

Specific therapy aimed at DIC in the antepartum and intrapartum periods is palliative and may be counterproductive in most cases. Administered procoagulants, including platelets, will suffer the same fate as the patient's own; they will be consumed and destroyed. Their indiscriminate use merely "fuels the fire" and results in production of increased amounts of fibrin split products. Except in specific circumstances, it has not been demonstrated that procoagulant administration favorably alters the course for either the fetus or the mother. In the series reported by Pritchard and Brekken (1967), fibrinogen replacement was employed in less than 10 per cent of patients, despite the presence of severe coagulopathy in nearly four times that number. Vigorous blood and volume replacement using packed red blood cells and crystalloid is usually all that is necessary.

The only clear indication for procoagulant replacement is severe coagulopathy (fibrinogen level less than 100 mg/100 ml, platelet count less than 50,000 cells/mm³) in a patient who requires cesarean section. In such a patient, perioperative administration of fibrinogen and other procoagulants may be necessary.

The various blood replacement products commonly employed are shown in Table 39–5. Fresh whole blood is rarely available and should not be viewed as offering any advantage over component therapy in the great majority of cases. Fibrinogen is the specific procoagulant most often needed. Approximately 4 gm are necessary to raise the concentration by 100 mg/100 ml. It may be administered as fresh-frozen plasma if there is a concurrent need for volume expansion. A minimum of 4 units is necessary. Alternatively, fibrinogen may be administered as cryoprecipitate, which contains three to ten times the fibrinogen per unit volume as plasma. The fibrinogen content of a bag of cryoprecipitate is variable but averages 0.25 gm. Therefore,

15 to 20 bags will usually be needed for initial treatment. Fibrinogen concentrates are no longer available in the United States, because these pooled products carried an inordinate risk of hepatitis. Platelet concentrates are indicated when the platelet count is less than 50,000 cells/mm³ in a patient undergoing surgery. Each bag can be expected to raise the platelet count by 7000 to 10,000 cells/mm³. The need for subsequent replacement is guided by serial coagulation tests. Once delivery is accomplished, further replacement is often unnecessary because the process usually resolves fairly rapidly. Formation of a normal clot signals that frequent coagulation tests are no longer required.

The use of heparin in the DIC associated with abruption has been controversial. It is now nearly universally condemned, except in the rare circumstance in which there is evidence of microvascular plugging (manifested by progressive renal dysfunction or gangrene of the digits) without evidence of abnormal bleeding.

Similarly, the use of epsilon-aminocaproic acid (EACA), a potent inhibitor of the fibrinolytic system, is indicated under only extraordinary circumstances. Use of this agent carries the danger of unchecked intravascular coagulation with subsequent infarction. It should be utilized only by those completely familiar with the management of coagulation disorders, and even then only with the concomitant use of heparin.

Ischemic Necrosis of Distant Organs

Ischemic damage to the kidneys is among the most severe maternal complications of abruptio placentae. The damage takes the form of either acute tubular necrosis or bilateral cortical necrosis and is caused by anoxia due to hemorrhagic shock or microvascular obstruction by fibrin deposition. Both forms are char-

TABLE 39–5. **Blood Replacement Products**

COMPONENT	VOLUME/ UNIT*	FACTORS PRESENT	COMMENTS
Fresh whole blood	500	RBC All procoagulants	Rarely indicated, as it is difficult to obtain.
Packed RBC	200	RBC only	
Fresh-frozen plasma	200–400	All procoagulants; no platelets	Contains approximately 1 gm fibrinogen per unit.
Cryoprecipitate	20–50	Fibrinogen; factors VIII, XIII	Variable fibrinogen content (averages about 0.25 gm per bag).
Fibrinogen	—	—	No longer available in United States.
Platelet concentrate	35–60	Platelets; small amounts of fibrinogen; factors V, VIII	Each unit raises the platelet count by about 8000/mm^3.

*Volume depends on individual blood bank.

acterized in the early phase by oliguria or anuria, and they may be impossible to distinguish. Acute tubular necrosis tends to appear somewhat late in the clinical course and is reversible in the majority of cases with time. Renal cortical necrosis tends to occur early in the course of abruption and leads to death from uremia within 1 to 2 weeks unless chronic dialysis is initiated. The key to prevention of either of these complications is vigorous blood and fluid therapy to combat hypovolemic shock. Renal cortical necrosis has not been observed in more than 300 consecutive cases of severe abruption treated with this approach (Pritchard et al., 1970).

In addition to the kidneys, hypoxic damage has been observed in the liver, adrenal glands, and pituitary gland. Anterior pituitary necrosis (Sheehan's syndrome) may lead to later symptoms of hypopituitarism.

Fetal Complications

Because abruptio placentae is probably the end result of a long-standing pathologic process, it is not surprising that there is a high incidence of growth restriction and congenital abnormalities. Birth weight in about 80 per cent of infants born before 36 weeks gestation is below the mean for gestational length (Hibbard and Jeffcoate, 1966). In addition, there is a three-fold increase in the rate of major malformations, mostly involving the central nervous system. There may be significant fetal bleeding in some cases of abruption, with a resultant neonatal anemia (Golditch and Boyce, 1970). I have also seen a transient coagulopathy in some newborns, the etiology of which remains unknown.

OTHER PLACENTAL ABNORMALITIES

CHORIOANGIOMA. Placental chorioangiomas (hemangiomas) are the most common benign tumors of the placenta. Although small chorioangiomas are relatively common, they are of little consequence. Multiple and/or large tumors (over 5 cm) are associated with a variety of complications, including polyhydramnios, hydrops fetalis, preeclampsia, preterm labor, fetomaternal transfusion, abruptio placentae, ab-

normal presentation, and elevated amniotic fluid alpha-fetoprotein.

The diagnosis should be entertained in the investigation of all cases of polyhydramnios. In many cases, however, the diagnosis will be made as an incidental finding on ultrasonographic examination. Chorioangiomas characteristically appear as complex masses on the fetal surface of the placenta, and their vascular nature can be demonstrated with Doppler studies (Grundy et al., 1986). In some cases, however, they may be multiple and distributed throughout the placental substance (O'Malley et al., 1981). In these cases, they may be difficult to differentiate from other causes of placental thickening.

A high incidence of fetal death (up to 30 per cent) has been reported with large tumors that are associated with polyhydramnios or, occasionally, with oligohydramnios (Engel et al., 1981). Frequent antenatal surveillance should be carried out in these cases. Both positive oxytocin challenge tests and sinusoidal heart rates have been reported in association with chorioangiomata (Hurwitz et al., 1983).

REFERENCES

Blair RG: Abruption of placenta: A review of 189 cases occurring between 1965 and 1969. J Obstet Gynaecol Br Commonw 80:242, 1973.

Breen JL, Neubecker R, Gregori CA, Franklin JE: Placenta accreta, increta and percreta: Survey of 40 cases. Obstet Gynecol 49:43, 1977.

Brenner WE, Edelman DA, Hendricks CH: Characteristics of patients with placenta previa and results of "expectant management." Am J Obstet Gynecol 132:180, 1978.

Clark SL, Koonings PP, Phelan JP: Placenta previa/accreta and prior cesarean section. Obstet Gynecol 66:89, 1985.

Comeau J, Shaw L, Marcell CC, Lavery JP: Early placenta previa and delivery outcome. Obstet Gynecol 61:577, 1983.

Cotton DB, Read JA, Paul RH, Quilligan EJ: The conservative aggressive management of placenta previa. Am J Obstet Gynecol 137:687, 1980.

Crenshaw C, Jones DED, Parker RT: Placenta previa: A survey of twenty years experience with improved perinatal survival by expectant therapy and cesarean delivery. Obstet Gynecol Survey 28:461, 1973.

Engel K, Haln T, Karschnia R: Sonographic diagnosis of a placental tumour with high-grade intrauterine foetal development deficiency, increasing anhydramnia and subsequent foetal death. Geburtshilfe Fraunheilkd 41:570, 1981.

Farine D, Peisner DB, Timor-Tritsch IE: Placenta previa—is the traditional diagnostic approach satisfactory? J Clin Ultrasound **18**:328, 1990.

Golditch IM, Boyce NE: Management of abruptio placentae. JAMA **212**:288, 1970.

Grundy HU, Byersa L, Walton S, et al: Antepartum ultrasonographic evaluation and management of placental chorioangioma. A case report. J Reprod Med **31**:520, 1986.

Hibbard BM, Jeffcoate TNA: Abruptio placentae. Obstet Gynecol **27**:155, 1966.

Hibbard LT: Placenta previa. Am J Obstet Gynecol **104**:172, 1969.

Hibbard LT: Placenta previa. *In* Sciarra JJ (ed): Gynecology and Obstetrics. Vol. 2. New York, Harper & Row, 1981.

Hurwitz A, Milwidsky A, Yarkoni S, Palti Z: Severe fetal distress with hydramnios due to chorioangioma. Acta Obstet Gynecol Scand **62**:633, 1983.

Kelly JV, Iffy L: Placenta previa. *In* Iffy L, Kaminetzky HA (eds): Principles and Practice of Obstetrics and Perinatology. Vol. 2. New York, John Wiley & Sons, 1981.

Knab DR: Abruptio placentae: An assessment of the time and method of delivery. Obstet Gynecol **52**:625, 1978.

Laing FC: Placenta previa: Avoiding false-negative diagnoses. J Clin Ultrasound **9**:109, 1981.

Leerentveld RA, Gilberts EC, Arnold MJ, Wladimiroff JW: Accuracy and safety of transvaginal placental localization. Obstet Gynecol **76**:759, 1990.

Naeye RL, Harkness WL, Utts J: Abruptio placentae and perinatal death: A prospective study. Am J Obstet Gynecol **128**:740, 1977.

Newton ER, Barss V, Cetrulo CL: The epidemiology and clinical history of asymptomatic midtrimester placenta previa. Am J Obstet Gynecol **148**:743, 1984.

Nyberg DA, Cyr DR, Mack LA, et al: Sonographic spectrum of placental abruption. AJR **148**:161, 1987.

O'Malley BP, Toi A, deSa DJ, Williams GL: Ultrasound appearances of placental chorioangioma. Radiology **138**:159, 1981.

Page EW, King EB, Merrill JA: Abruptio placentae; dangers of delay in delivery. Obstet Gynecol **3**:385, 1954.

Pent D: Vasa previa. Am J Obstet Gynecol **134**:151, 1979.

Powell MC, Buckley J, Price H, et al: Magnetic resonance imaging and placenta previa. Am J Obstet Gynecol **154**:565, 1986.

Preucel RW, Lavin JP, Colman RW: Placental abruption and premature separation. *In* Sciarra JJ (ed): Gynecology and Obstetrics. Vol. 2. New York, Harper & Row, 1981.

Pritchard JA, Brekken AL: Clinical and laboratory studies on severe abruption placenta. Am J Obstet Gynecol **97**:681, 1967.

Pritchard J, Mason R, Corley M, Pritchard S: Genesis of severe placental abruption. Am J Obstet Gynecol **108**:22, 1970.

Rivera-Alxina ME, Saldana LR, Maklad N, Korp S: the use of ultrasound in the expectant management of abruptio placentae. Am J Obstet Gynecol **146**:924, 1983.

Sholl JS: Abruptio placentae: Clinical management in nonacute cases. Am J Obstet Gynecol **156**:40, 1987.

Varma TR: Fetal growth and placental function in patients with placenta praevia. J Obstet Gynaecol Br Commonw **80**:311, 1973.

Wexler P, Gottesfeld KR: Second trimester placenta previa: An apparently normal placentation. Obstet Gynecol **50**:706, 1977.

Wexler P, Gottesfeld KR: Early diagnosis of placenta previa. Obstet Gynecol **54**:231, 1979.

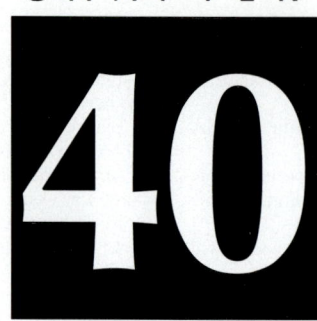

DISORDERS OF AMNIOTIC FLUID

WILLIAM M. GILBERT, M.D.

The mechanisms regulating amniotic fluid production and removal have been discussed in detail in Chapter 5. It is clear that any disease state that affects the normal balance, even slightly, will result in an aberration of amniotic fluid volume. A normal volume of amniotic fluid is frequently an indicator of fetal health, although exceptions may occur. Conversely, a paucity or excess of fluid, oligohydramnios and polyhydramnios respectively, is often an indicator of a significant fetal disorder.

The diagnosis of abnormal amniotic fluid volume requires that the clinician immediately initiate a logical and detailed study into possible etiologies. Whereas the cause of oligohydramnios is usually readily apparent, polyhydramnios is more frequently idiopathic. This section will provide a brief overview of the general approach to disorders of amniotic fluid volume. The reader will find more detail regarding specific fetal entities in their respective chapters.

OLIGOHYDRAMNIOS

Early definitions of oligohydramnios included the subjective impression of decreased amniotic fluid volume as determined by uterine size. With the advent and refinement of ultrasound imaging, a more accurate modality for estimation of amniotic fluid volume became available (see Chapter 22). In spite of this technology, estimations of amniotic fluid volume are frequently nonquantitative, with volumes recorded as "low, normal, or high." Early attempts to quantify amniotic fluid volume were based upon measurements of the largest single vertical pocket of fluid. As part of an overall evaluation of fetal status, the biophysical profile was developed utilizing five physiologic variables (Manning et al., 1980). One of the most important of these variables is that of amniotic fluid volume, and initial reports suggested that a single vertical pocket measuring at least 1 cm in two perpendicular planes was "normal." More recent data demonstrate that the 1-cm vertical pocket guideline is too low and that perinatal mortality rates are lowest when a single vertical pocket is between 2 and 8 cm, rising rapidly

as measurements decrease below 2 cm (Chamberlain et al., 1984).

The amniotic fluid index (AFI) has been utilized to sum the largest vertical fluid pockets in each of the four quadrants of the uterus (Phelan et al., 1987). The technique is shown in Figure 40–1. Pockets of amniotic fluid that contain multiple loops of umbilical cord are avoided. In addition, an effort is made to maintain the ultrasound transducer perpendicular to the plane formed by the floor. It has been shown that the AFI is a highly sensitive means of predicting poor pregnancy outcomes (Phelan et al., 1987).

The gestational age changes in the AFI have been studied, and the normal range is demonstrated in Figure 40–2 (Moore and Cayle, 1990). The establishment of these normal values allows for an accurate determination of amniotic fluid volume for a given gestational age, as well as for following trends over time. For example, marked changes observed over time in the amniotic fluid volume of a patient with diabetes mellitus may indicate adequacy of maternal glycemic control as well as fetal well-being. Additionally, a gravida with dehydration may be observed to have oligohydramnios, which responds favorably to maternal hydration. Quantitatively, oligohydramnios is defined as an AFI less than the fifth percentile for gestational age.

Oligohydramnios is associated with an increase in perinatal morbidity and mortality at any gestational age, but especially in the second trimester of pregnancy, when the risk of perinatal loss reaches 80 to 90 per cent (Barss et al., 1984; Mercer and Brown, 1986). Renal agenesis or urinary tract obstruction often presents during this period, at a time when fetal urine flow begins to contribute significantly to the formation of amniotic fluid. When amniotic fluid appears to be virtually absent, perinatal mortality rates approach 90 per cent (Moore et al., 1989). The major cause of fetal/neonatal demise is pulmonary hypoplasia and abnormal or absent renal function. Normal amniotic fluid volume is required for the normal development of the fetal lungs, and second-trimester oligohydramnios of any etiology may result in pulmonary hypoplasia, although the precise mechanism for aberrant development is not known.

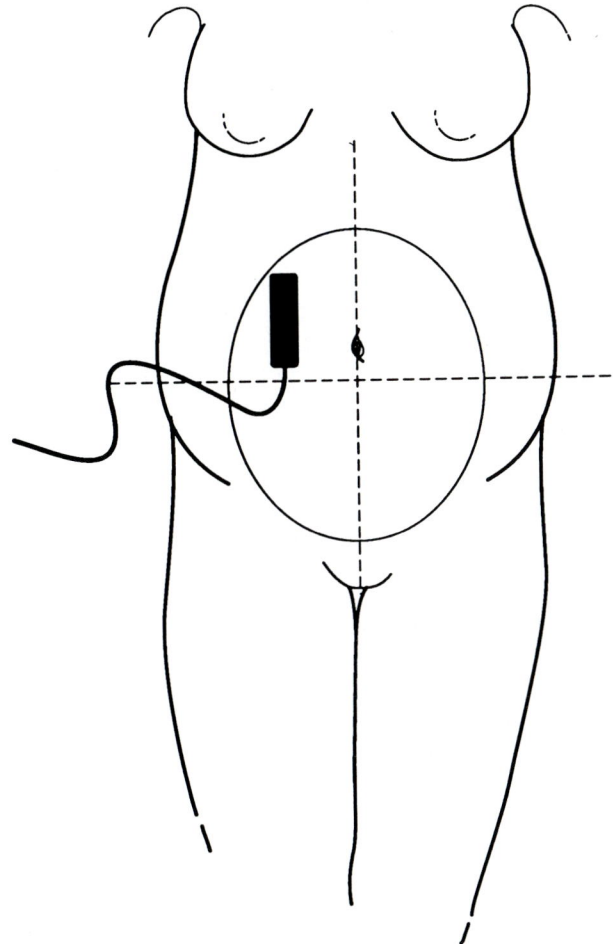

FIGURE 40–1. Schematic diagram of technique for measuring the four-quadrant amniotic fluid index (AFI). The uterus is divided into four quadrants (dotted lines), the ultrasound transducer is held perpendicular to the floor, and the largest vertical pocket of amniotic fluid is measured in each quadrant and summed.

Second-trimester oligohydramnios may also be the result of premature rupture of the membranes with loss of amniotic fluid. These fetuses have a much better prognosis than those with renal abnormalities, most likely due to the fact that amniotic fluid volume was normal prior to the rupture of the membranes and because the extent of volume loss is variable. Furthermore, the outcome is related to the gestational age at which the rupture of membranes occurs. The earlier and more complete the fluid loss, especially prior to 24 to 25 weeks gestation, the greater is the chance of pulmonary underdevelopment incompatible with life. The reader is referred to Chapter 41 for a more detailed discussion of these issues.

The amniotic fluid should be considered an extension of the fetal vascular compartment. When the fetus is well hydrated and has a normal plasma volume, urine output and amniotic fluid volume are normal. Conversely, if the fetus has a depleted vascular volume, urine output decreases and oligohydramnios will result. Intrauterine growth retardation from many causes, particularly severe preeclampsia,

is often associated with oligohydramnios. The mechanism involves fetal vascular volume deficit, leading to a decrease in glomerular filtration and urinary flow rates. In addition, the chronic hypoxic state resulting from preeclampsia leads to shunting of fetal blood flow away from the kidneys (Peeters et al., 1979). Indeed, fetuses with growth retardation have been observed to have abnormal urine flow rates (Kurjak et al., 1981). Conversely, the growth-retarded fetus with an early and severe symmetrical growth aberration may have normal or increased amniotic fluid volume. This should alert the observer to consider fetal aneuploidy as the cause (Schneider et al., 1981; Barkin et al., 1987).

Amniotic fluid volume also decreases in the postterm fetus, although the mechanism is unclear. It has been suggested that deterioration in placental function causes a less efficient transfer of water from the mother to the fetus in the post-date gestation, although there are no data to support this hypothesis. Nevertheless, the observation of oligohydramnios in this clinical situation is of considerable significance because it is associated with a marked increase in the incidence of meconium aspiration syndrome and perinatal asphyxia (Miyazaki et al., 1981; Leveno et al., 1984) and is often used as the basis for the decision to deliver the fetus (Rutherford et al., 1987). The evaluation of the post-date fetus should include the measurement of the AFI, and the relative importance of the AFI in the management scheme is discussed in detail in Chapter 34.

Therapeutic approaches for the patient with oligohy-

Amniotic Fluid Index

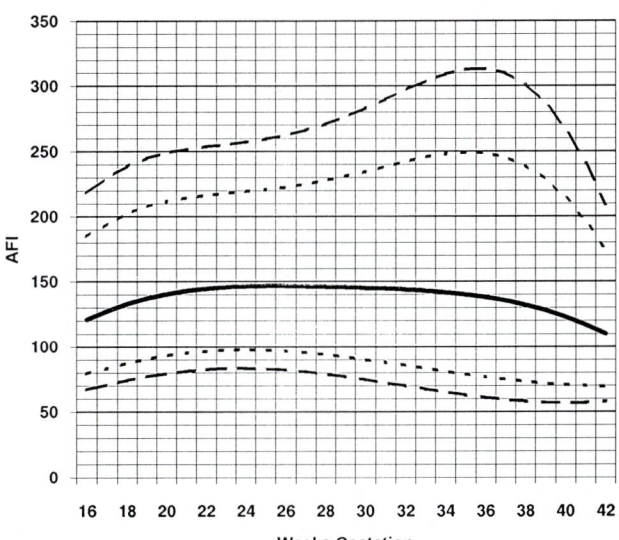

FIGURE 40–2. Normal values for the amniotic fluid index (AFI in mm). The graphs represent the distribution of 709 normal pregnancies. Outer lines indicate the 1 per cent and 99 per cent curves. Inner dashed lines indicate the fifth and 95th confidence limits. The center line is the mean value. (From Moore TK and Cayle JE: The amniotic fluid index in normal pregnancy. Am J Obstet Gynecol **162**:1168, 1990.)

dramnios are limited. When oligohydramnios is the result of a structural defect, e.g., urinary tract obstruction, *in utero* surgical diversion of urine flow has had some promising results (see Chapter 25). Crombleholme et al. (1990) found an improvement in outcome when either vesico-amniotic catheters or open drainage procedures were performed. When amniotic fluid volume was restored to normal, either because of the procedure or on its own, the perinatal survival was 94 per cent. However, when oligohydramnios persisted, the outcome was poor. It should also be emphasized that, in order to have optimal benefit, urinary diversion must be accomplished prior to the development of renal dysplasia and early enough in gestation to allow for lung development. The accurate prenatal measurement of renal function is still being examined, and prospective studies are needed to determine the benefit, if any, of these therapeutic approaches. Furthermore, individual skill in performing fetal surgery is limited by the relatively infrequent occurrence of these lesions and the limited number of centers with sufficient experience with the technique.

Oligohydramnios may also be observed during labor in patients with rupture of the membranes or those who are post-term. Repetitive umbilical cord compression during labor, as demonstrated by the presence of variable decelerations, is more common in the presence of oligohydramnios and may compromise umbilical blood flow with dire consequences. Efforts to increase amniotic fluid volume during labor and prevent umbilical cord compression have been reported (Miyazaki et al., 1985; Wenstrom and Parsons, 1989; Nagoette et al., 1985). These studies demonstrate that large-volume saline amnioinfusions result in improved fetal heart rate patterns and fetal outcomes, and a decrease in cesarean section rate.

Maternal intravascular fluid status appears to be closely tied to that of the fetus. Several instances of oligohydramnios in association with maternal intravascular volume depletion have been noted (Goodlin et al., 1983). Intravenous hydration of such individuals results in resolution of the oligohydramnios. In a prospective study of patients with decreased AFI, a significant, measurable increase has been observed with overnight oral hydration (Kilpatrick et al., 1991). These studies would suggest that the state of maternal hydration should be considered when investigating causes of oligohydramnios, since such abnormalities may be treatable.

POLYHYDRAMNIOS

Prior to the availability of ultrasound examination, polyhydramnios was diagnosed on the basis of an abnormal increase in uterine size for gestation and the inability to palpate fetal parts. More quantitatively, polyhydramnios was defined as an amniotic fluid volume greater than 2000 ml. Based upon these criteria, the incidence of polyhydramnios diagnosed clinically was 0.4 per cent (Queenan and Gadow, 1970). With the use of ultrasound, however, the diagnosis of polyhydramnios is now made in approximately 1 per cent of pregnancies (Hill et al., 1987). Early ultrasound

definitions were subjective and divided into such categories as mild, moderate, and severe. Early attempts to quantify utilized a single vertical amniotic fluid pocket in excess of 8 cm. Currently, the diagnosis is most accurately based upon the four-quadrant AFI, and polyhydramnios may be defined as an AFI greater than the 95th percentile for gestational age (see Fig. 40–2). This definition has been found to be superior to either the descriptive definition or the 8-cm rule (Carlson et al., 1990).

It has long been recognized that polyhydramnios is associated with increases in maternal morbidity as well as perinatal morbidity and mortality (Queenan and Gadow, 1970). Mild increases in amniotic fluid are not usually of clinical significance. Smith et al. (1992) defined mild polyhydramnios as an AFI of 24.1 to 39.9 cm and observed a frequency of 8.2 per cent of 1177 patients late in gestation. None of the pregnancies were complicated by the usual entities associated with excessive amniotic fluid, although there was a significantly greater number of infants with birth weights >4000 gm. Outcome of those pregnancies was comparable to those with a normal AFI. In another study (Hill et al., 1987), an etiology was found in only 16 per cent of patients with mild polyhydramnios. Conversely, when sharply increased volumes of amniotic fluid were observed, defined as a single vertical pocket >16 cm, 21 of the 23 patients had readily apparent causes.

Earlier studies, prior to *in utero* diagnosis by ultrasound, suggested that the cause of polyhydramnios was idiopathic in one-third of all cases (Queenan and Gadow, 1970). More recent data suggest that no cause will be found in two-thirds of patients. The various conditions associated with polyhydramnios are summarized in Table 40–1. More recently, an increased incidence of aneuploidy (3.2 per cent) has been observed in patients with idiopathic polyhydramnios, and chromosome analysis should be considered (Brady et al., 1992).

Maternal diabetes mellitus has long been a known maternal cause of polyhydramnios, and the volume of amniotic fluid is correlated with glycemic control (Cousins, 1987). The presence of polyhydramnios associated with diabetes seems to raise the risk of perinatal morbidity and mortality, but usually is the result of inadequate glycemic control or malformations (Des et al., 1990). Fetal anomalies such as esophageal atresia and other upper gastrointestinal tract obstructive malformations are the most common type of fetal

TABLE 40–1. Maternal and Fetal Conditions Associated with Polyhydramnios

Idiopathic	66.0%
Fetal anomalies	12.7%
Insulin-dependent diabetes	7.8%
Gestational diabetes	6.9%
Multiple gestation	4.9%
Other disorders	1.0%

Adapted from Hill LM et al.: Polyhydramnios: Ultrasonically detected prevalence and neonatal outcome. Obstet Gynecol **69**:21, 1987. Reprinted with permission from the American College of Obstetricians and Gynecologists.

anomalies associated with polyhydramnios (Hill et al., 1987). The presumed mechanism for polyhydramnios with gastrointestinal obstruction is the inability of swallowed amniotic fluid to reach the small bowel and be absorbed. However, even with complete gastrointestinal blockage, polyhydramnios is not universally observed. Esophageal atresia is associated with polyhydramnios in only 10 per cent of cases (Romero et al., 1988), whereas more distal upper intestinal obstruction, such as duodenal and jejunal atresia, is associated with polyhydramnios in 50 per cent of cases (Lloyd and Clatworthy, 1958). The reason for the low frequency with esophageal atresia is that the majority of such malformations have tracheoesophageal fistula with connections from the mouth to the stomach (Bovicelli et al., 1983), thus permitting passage of amniotic and lung fluid. Why one-half of cases of duodenal atresia do not lead to polyhydramnios is unclear, although it may be related to amniotic fluid absorption through an intramembranous pathway (see Chapter 5).

Congenital diaphragmatic hernia may result in a decrease in fetal swallowing and polyhydramnios due to abnormal location of the abdominal viscera, whereby they enter the fetal chest and compress the esophagus. Similarly, other malformations in the fetal chest, such as cystic adenomatous malformation or extrapulmonary sequestration, may interfere with fetal swallowing. Anencephaly is also associated with polyhydramnios, and in rare cases, certain muscular dystrophies may inhibit fetal swallowing (Dunn and Dierker, 1973).

The twin-to-twin transfusion syndrome frequently results in polyhydramnios in the second trimester. In monozygotic twinning, one twin develops polyhydramnios and occasionally hydrops fetalis, while the other twin is growth-retarded and becomes volume-depleted with oligohydramnios. This disorder develops in those monozygotic twins with large arteriovenous anastomoses connecting their placentas (Benirschke and Kaurman, 1990). One twin with a dominant circulation (donor) pumps blood via a placental vessel into the circulation of the other twin (recipient). The recipient twin is at risk for cardiac failure and hydrops fetalis. The oligohydramniotic donor twin is at risk for umbilical cord occlusion, renal failure, and pulmonary hypoplasia. If the diagnosis of twin transfusion syndrome is made prior to 24 weeks of gestation, the perinatal mortality approaches 100 per cent (Bebbington and Wittmann, 1989; Weir et al., 1979). Premature labor is a significant complication of polyhydramnios in the multiple or single gestation and a significant contributor to perinatal morbidity and mortality (Hill et al., 1987; Barkin et al., 1987).

Several modalities, including pharmacologic and mechanical, have been utilized in cases of twin transfusion syndrome diagnosed prior to viability. Inasmuch as the underlying pathology in this syndrome is vascular communication with the monozygotic placentas, De Lia et al. (1990) have attempted to ablate the placental vascular connections with fetoscopically directed laser coagulation. In three cases diagnosed prior to 23 weeks gestation, the perinatal survival rate was 66 per cent. This modality treats the underlying cause of the syndrome but requires highly specialized technology and experience and can only be utilized with posteriorly located placentas. Another promising treatment modality in the twin transfusion syndrome is repetitive, large-volume amniotic fluid reduction utilizing amniocentesis. Sufficient amniotic fluid is removed to reduce the AFI into the normal range (under 25 cm). Frequently, volumes of 4 to 6 liters are required to return the AFI to this upper limit of normal range. The procedure is repeated every one to three weeks as needed until the fetuses have achieved pulmonary maturity or require delivery for other indications. Elliott et al. (1991) have performed amnioreductions on 17 patients and reported a perinatal survival rate of 79 per cent. The mean gestation at the start of amnioreductions was 21.5 weeks, and pregnancy was prolonged to a mean of 33.5 weeks. More recently, a perinatal survival rate of 37 per cent in 19 cases of twin transfusion syndrome treated with massive amnioreductions has been reported (Saunders et al., 1992). In both reports, the survival rate is better than that for historical controls.

Another approach involves the pharmacologic manipulation of fetal urine flow. Fetal urine volumes of 1200 ml enter the amniotic cavity daily (Rabinowitz et al., 1989). Fetal renal blood flow is maintained under normal conditions by prostaglandins (Matson et al., 1981). Cyclooxygenase inhibitors such as indomethacin have been found to decrease fetal renal blood flow and urine flow in animal models (Robillard and Nakamura, 1988). In humans, indomethacin has been used to decrease fetal urine output and decrease amniotic fluid volume (Moise et al., 1988). In many cases, premature labor is associated with polyhydramnios, and indomethacin therapy may be utilized to treat both polyhydramnios and premature labor. Indomethacin has other striking effects on the fetal cardiovascular system such as constriction of the ductus arteriosus. Severe narrowing of the ductus and/or pulmonary hypertension may be more than a theoretical risk. The benefits of indomethacin must be weighed against its significant effects on the fetal vascular system before it is prescribed. Because most of the adverse fetal outcomes associated with indomethacin treatment occur after 33 weeks of gestation, indomethacin should be restricted to fetuses below that gestational age (Gilbert, 1990).

REFERENCES

Barkin SZ, Pretorius DH, Beckett MK, Manchester DK, Nelson TR, Manco-Johnson ML: Severe polyhydramnios: Incidence of anomalies. AJR **148**:155, 1987.

Barss VA, Benacerraf BR, Frigoletto FD: Second trimester oligohydramnios, a predictor of poor fetal outcome. Obstet Gynecol **64**:608, 1984.

Bebbington MW, Wittmann BK: Fetal transfusion syndrome: Antenatal factors predicting outcome. Am J Obstet Gynecol **160**:913, 1989.

Benirschke K, Kaurman P (eds): Pathology of the Human Placenta. New York, Springer-Verlag, 1990, pp 690–702.

Bottoms SF, Welch RA, Zador IE, Sokol RJ: Limitations of using maximum vertical pocket and other sonographic evaluation of amniotic fluid volume to predict fetal growth: technical or physiologic? Am J Obstet Gynecol **155**:154, 1986.

Bovicelli L, Rizzo N, Orsini LF, Pilu G: Prenatal diagnosis and management of fetal gastrointestinal abnormalities. Semin Perinatol **7**:109, 1983.

Brady K, Polzin WJ, Kopelman JN, Read JA: Risk of chromosomal abnormalities in patients with idiopathic polyhydramnios. Obstet Gynecol 79:234, 1992.

Carlson DE, Platt LD, Medearis AL, Horenstein J: Quantifiable polyhydramnios: Diagnosis and management. Obstet Gynecol 75:989, 1990.

Chamberlain PF, Manning FA, Morrison I, Harman CR, Lange IR: Ultrasound evaluation of amniotic fluid volume. I. The relationship of marginal and decreased amniotic fluid volumes to perinatal outcome. Am J Obstet Gynecol 150:245, 1984.

Cousins L: Pregnancy complications among diabetic women: review 1965–1985. Obstet Gynecol Survey 42:140, 1987.

Crombleholme TM, Harrison MR, Golbus MS, et al: Fetal intervention in obstructive uropathy: prognostic indicators and efficacy of intervention. Am J Obstet Gynecol 162:1239, 1990.

De Lia JE, Cruikshank DP, Keye WR: Fetoscopic neodymium:yag laser occlusion of placental vessels in severe twin-twin transfusion syndrome. Obstet Gynecol 75:1046, 1990.

Desmedt EJ, Henry OA, Beischer NA: Polyhydramnios and associated maternal and fetal complications in singleton pregnancies. Br J Obstet Gynaecol 97(12):1115, 1990.

Dunn LJ, Dierker LJ: Recurrent hydramnios in association with myotonia dystrophica. Obstet Gynecol 42:104, 1973.

Elliott JP, Urig MA, Clewell WH: Aggressive therapeutic amniocentesis for treatment of twin-twin transfusion syndrome. Obstet Gynecol 77:537, 1991.

Gilbert WM: Maternal, fetal and neonatal physiology in pregnancy. Curr Opin Obstet Gynecol 2:4, 1990.

Goodlin RC, Anderson JC, Gallagher TF: Relationship between amniotic fluid volume and maternal plasma volume expansion. Am J Obstet Gynecol 146:505, 1983.

Hill LM, Breckle R, Thomas ML, Fries JK: Polyhydramnios: ultrasonically detected prevalence and neonatal outcome. Obstet Gynecol 69:21, 1987.

Jacoby HE, Charles D: Clinical conditions associated with hydramnios. Am J Obstet Gynecol 94:910, 1966.

Kilpatrick SJ, Safford K, Pomeroy T, Hoedt L, Scheerer L, Laros RK: Maternal hydration affects amniotic fluid index (AFI). Am J Obstet Gynecol 164:361, 1991.

Kirshon B: Fetal urine output in hydramnios. Obstet Gynecol 73:240, 1989.

Kurjak A, Kirkinen P, Latin V, Ivankovic D: Ultrasonic assessment of fetal kidney function in normal and complicated pregnancies. Am J Obstet Gynecol 141:266, 1981.

Leveno KJ, Quirk JG, Cunningham FG, Nelson SD, Santos-Ramos R, Toofanian A, DePalma RT: Prolonged pregnancy. I. Observations concerning the causes of fetal distress. Am J Obstet Gynecol 150:465, 1984.

Lloyd JR, Clatworthy HW: Hydramnios as aid to the early diagnosis of congenital obstruction of the alimentary tract: a study of the maternal and fetal factors. Pediatrics 23:903, 1958.

Manning FA, Platt LD, Sipos L: Antepartum fetal evolution: Development of a fetal biophysical profile. Am J Obstet Gynecol 136:787, 1980.

Matson JR, Stokes JB, Robillard JE: Effects of inhibition of prostaglandin synthesis of fetal renal function. Kidney Int 20:621, 1981.

Mercer LJ, Brown LG: Fetal outcome with oligohydramnios in the second trimester. Obstet Gynecol 67:840, 1986.

Miyazaki FS, Miyazaki BA: False reactive nonstress tests in postterm pregnancies. Am J Obstet Gynecol 140:269, 1981.

Miyazaki FS, Neverez F: Saline amnioinfusion for relief of repetitive variable decelerations: A prospective randomized study. Am J Obstet Gynecol 153:301, 1985.

Moise KJ, Huhta JC, Sharif DS, et al: Indomethacin in the treatment of premature labor. N Engl J Med 319:327, 1988.

Moore TR, Cayle JE: The amniotic fluid index in normal human pregnancy. Am J Obstet Gynecol 162:1168, 1990.

Moore TR, Longo J, Leopold G, Gosink B, Cassola G: The reliability and predictive value of an amniotic fluid scoring system in severe second trimester oligohydramnios. Obstet Gynecol 73:739, 1989.

Nagoette FS, Freeman RK, Garite TJ, Dorchester W: Prophylactic intrapartum amnioinfusion in patients with preterm rupture of membranes. Am J Obstet Gynecol 153:557, 1985.

Peeters LLH, Sheldon RE, Jones MD, Makowski EL, Meschia G: Blood flow to fetal organs as a function of arterial oxygen content. Am J Obstet Gynecol 135:637, 1979.

Phelan JP, Ohn MO, Smith CV, Rutherford SE, Anderson E: Amniotic fluid index measurements during pregnancy. J Reprod Med 32:603, 1987.

Queenan JT, Gadow EC: Polyhydramnios: Chronic versus acute. Am J Obstet Gynecol 108(3):349, 1970.

Rabinowitz R, Peters MT, Vyas S, Campbell S, Nicolaides KH: Measurement of fetal urine production in normal pregnancy by real-time ultrasonography. Am J Obstet Gynecol 161:1264, 1989.

Robillard JE, Nakamura KT: Hormonal regulation of renal function during development. Biol Neonate 53:201, 1988.

Romero R, Pilu G, Jeanty P, Ghidini A, Hobbins JC (eds): Prenatal Diagnosis of Congenital Anomalies. Norwalk, CT, Appleton and Lange, 1988, pp 234–236.

Rutherford SE, Phelan JP, Smith CV, Jacobs N: The four quadrant assessment of amniotic fluid volume: an adjunct to antepartum fetal heart rate testing. Obstet Gynecol 70:353, 1987.

Saunders NJ, Snijders RJM, Nicolaides KH: Therapeutic amniocentesis in twin-twin transfusion syndrome appearing in the second trimester of pregnancy. Am J Obstet Gynecol 166:820, 1992.

Schneider AS, Mennuti MT, Zackal EH: High cesarean section rate in trisomy 18 births: A potential indication for late prenatal diagnosis. Am J Obstet Gynecol 140:367, 1981.

Smith CV, Plambeck RD, Rayburn WF, Albaugh KJ: Relation of mild idiopathic polyhydramnios to perinatal outcome. Obstet Gynecol 79:387, 1992.

Wenstrom KD, Parsons MT: The prevention of meconium aspiration in labor using amnioinfusion. Obstet Gynecol 73:647, 1989.

Wier PE, Raten G, Beischer N: Acute polyhydramnios—a complication of monozygous twin pregnancy. Br J Obstet Gynaecol 86:849, 1979.

CHAPTER

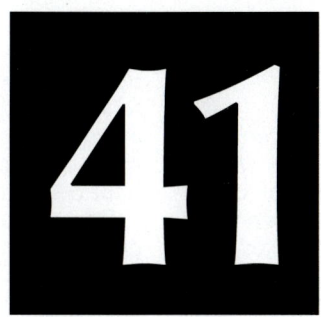

PREMATURE RUPTURE OF THE MEMBRANES

THOMAS J. GARITE, M.D.

Premature rupture of the fetal membranes (PROM), or amniorrhexis, is one of the most common and controversial problems facing the obstetric clinician. The fetal membranes and the amniotic fluid that they encase have functions that are critical for normal fetal protection, growth, and development. The fluid environment allows full fetal movement, enhancing normal muscle development and growth. Fetal swallowing and urination are integral to normal fetal fluid balance and to the development of the gastrointestinal and urinary systems. The amniotic fluid provides a column of fluid within the fetal tracheal-bronchial tree which, during normal fetal inspiratory and expiratory movements, allows for development of the fetal lungs. The amniotic fluid also protects the fetus from traumatic injury and, by allowing the umbilical cord to float freely, protects it from compression during fetal movement or uterine contractions.

Besides encasing the amniotic fluid, the membranes also serve as an important barrier separating the sterile fetus and the amniotic fluid from a bacteria-laden vaginal canal and preventing prolapse of any intra-amniotic contents through the cervix, which often dilates somewhat prior to the onset of labor. Finally, the membranes also function as a repository for substrates for many critical biochemical processes, including storage of phosphoglycerolipids, which release the precursors for prostaglandins. Thus, any disruption in the integrity of the amniotic cavity might potentially interrupt or interfere with any or all of these important functions.

DEFINITION AND INCIDENCE

Premature rupture of membranes (PROM) is defined as rupture of the chorioamniotic membranes prior to the onset of labor. The definition is independent of gestational age, and PROM prior to term is correctly termed *preterm PROM.* The interval between PROM and the onset of labor is referred to as the *latency period.* Although some authors impose an arbitrary latency period for the definition of premature rupture of membranes, varying from 1 to 12 hours, the majority define PROM simply as rupture of the membranes

prior to the onset of contractions. Traditionally, pediatricians are concerned with the duration of ROM, especially in the term gestation—hence the term *prolonged ROM,* usually referring to ROM for more than 24 hours. The reported incidence of PROM varies between 3 and 18.5 per cent (Gunn et al., 1970). This wide variation is attributed to differences in definition (with or without a latency period) and by variation in the incidence of PROM in differing populations. Approximately 8 to 10 per cent of patients at term will present with ROM prior to the onset of labor. Preterm PROM accounts for one-fourth of all cases of PROM and is responsible for about 30 per cent of all premature deliveries (Kaltreider and Kohl, 1980). The contribution of preterm PROM to premature delivery is greater in populations of lower socioeconomic status and those with higher rates of sexually transmitted diseases.

ETIOLOGY

Normal fetal membranes are extremely strong early in pregnancy, to the extent that they withstand rupture from nearly all acute nonpenetrating forces (Parry-Jones and Priya, 1976; Artal et al., 1976). As term approaches, the fetal membranes are subjected to forces that cause them to become progressively weakened (Parry-Jones and Priya, 1976; Artal et al., 1976; Lavery et al., 1982; Skinner et al., 1981; Lavery and Miller, 1979). The combination of stretching of the membranes with uterine growth and the frequent strain caused by normal uterine contractions and fetal movements may contribute to the weakening of this membrane. In addition, significant biochemical changes occur in the membranes near term, including a substantial decrease in the collagen content. Thus, at term PROM may be a physiologic variant rather than a pathologic event. Since membranes are so strong in the preterm gestation, it is likely that either a pathologic intrinsic weakness or extrinsic factors are responsible for preterm PROM. Studies examining membranes from patients with preterm PROM do not show a difference in membrane strength except near the site of rupture (Artal et al., 1976). This local

625

difference suggests an exogenous source of weakening.

Recent evidence would suggest, at least in a substantial number of cases, that local infection ascending from the vagina is responsible for membrane weakening and rupture in a substantial number of cases (Lonky and Hayashi, 1988). It has been shown that patients in early gestation who are carriers of one or more sexually transmitted organisms (e.g., Gonococcus, group B Streptococcus, Chlamydia, Trichomonas, and *Gardnerella vaginalis*) have substantially increased incidences of PROM (Edwards et al., 1978; Regan et al., 1981; Martin et al., 1982; Minkoff et al., 1984). Although data on some of these organisms are inconsistent, the majority of studies show increased risks of preterm PROM in patients who are carriers of group B Streptococcus, Gonococcus, and *Gardnerella vaginalis*. Histologic chorioamnionitis is much more prevalent with preterm than with term PROM (Naeye, 1979). Studies evaluating amniotic fluid and fetal cord blood immunoglobulins suggest that many cases of preterm PROM are infected prior to membrane rupture (Cederqvist et al., 1979). Patients with preterm PROM are much more likely than their term counterparts to have clinical chorioamnionitis and endometritis (Garite and Freeman, 1982; Daikoku et al., 1982), even when corrected for differences in other clinical variables such as duration of membrane rupture and number of pelvic examinations. Recent studies have shown that bacteria, which attach to fetal membranes, elaborate substances such as proteases, which cause membrane weakening and likely membrane rupture (McGregor et al., 1986). Thus, a great body of evidence suggests that in many cases bacteria ascending from the vagina are responsible for membrane weakening and subsequent rupture. It is not clear, however, why some patients who harbor similar organisms do not have preterm PROM or preterm labor. Therefore, it is obvious that some, as yet undefined, host factor or environmental cofactor must be involved.

Occasionally, other etiologies can be identified. Premature PROM is more commonly seen in the setting of polyhydramnios or incompetent cervix, or following such procedures as cervical cerclage or amniocentesis. However, most cases do not have a definable etiology.

Few epidemiologic factors are consistently associated with an increased risk of PROM (Kaltreider and Kohl, 1980; Naeye, 1982). Smoking has been incriminated in some studies. Multiple gestation, abruptio placentae, previous preterm PROM, and previous cervical operations or lacerations are usually shown to correlate with increased risk of PROM. No relationship has been shown between PROM and maternal age, parity, maternal weight or weight gain, trauma, or meconium.

COMPLICATIONS

PROM may lead to a number of complications, and the risk of these complications varies significantly with gestational age. The lack of agreement over the relative contribution of each of these complications to perinatal morbidity and mortality is responsible for much of the controversy that exists over management. Complications associated with PROM include maternal and fetal/neonatal infections, premature labor and delivery, hypoxia and asphyxia secondary to umbilical cord compression, increased cesarean section rates, and fetal deformation.

PREMATURE LABOR. Once membranes rupture, the onset of labor usually follows within a relatively short time. The duration of the latency period varies inversely with gestational age. At term, labor follows PROM within 24 hours in 90 per cent of cases (Gunn et al., 1970). When PROM occurs between 28 and 34 weeks, 50 per cent of patients are in labor within 24 hours and 80 to 90 per cent within one week (Mead, 1980; Garite et al., 1981). Prior to 26 weeks, approximately half the patients begin labor within one week (Taylor and Garite, 1984). Obviously, at term, labor is a desirable sequel to PROM, and only when labor does not spontaneously begin within a short time is there any need for concern. When preterm PROM occurs, subsequent delivery and the resultant complications of prematurity are the most common causes of perinatal mortality and morbidity with this diagnosis. In addition to being associated with the onset of labor, PROM also has an influence on the duration and course of labor. Generally there is a moderate shortening of the first stage but no effect on the duration of the second stage of labor with rupture of membranes, as opposed to labor with intact membranes (Schwarz et al., 1974). It is not clear whether dystocia occurs more frequently in patients with PROM when spontaneous labor ensues; however, among patients with PROM, most studies show a higher rate of cesarean section for failure to progress in labor that has been induced than with spontaneous labor following PROM (Duff et al., 1984).

INFECTION. Both mother and fetus are subjected to increased risk of infection when membranes rupture prior to the onset of labor. Maternal infection is termed *chorioamnionitis*. Fetal infection may occur as septicemia, pneumonia, urinary tract infection, or local infections such as omphalitis or conjunctivitis. Generally, maternal chorioamnionitis precedes such fetal infections; however, serious fetal sepsis may occur before the mother demonstrates clinically evident chorioamnionitis. This is explained by preclinical infection, which occurs when the amniotic sac becomes colonized with virulent bacteria, but before there are clinically evident signs of maternal infection. To clarify this apparent discrepancy, recent authors have used the term *intra-amniotic infection* to include both preclinical and clinical chorioamnionitis (Yoder et al., 1983; Gibbs et al., 1982). The incidence of chorioamnionitis, in association with PROM, varies according to population type. For all pregnancies the incidence is 0.5 to 1 per cent. In prolonged rupture of membranes, it has been reported to occur in 3 to 15 per cent. Chorioamnionitis appears to be more common in preterm PROM, with reported frequencies of 15 to 25 per cent (Garite and Freeman, 1982; Gibbs et al., 1982; Ledger, 1976). The impact of PROM and chorioamnionitis on fetal/neonatal infection also varies with populations and gestational age. The incidence of neonatal sepsis at term is about 1 in 500 babies; with prolonged rupture of membranes, this is increased severalfold; and with chorioamnionitis, the incidence rises to 3 to 5 per cent (Yoder et al., 1983). With preterm PROM perinatal infections are much more common than at term. Major neonatal infections occur in about 5 per cent of all cases of preterm PROM and in 15 to 20 per cent of those with chorioamnionitis developing prior to term (Garite and Freeman, 1982; Ledger, 1976; Gibbs et al., 1980). The preterm baby is much more likely to die of infectious complications than is its term counterpart.

It is conventional teaching that the incidence of infection following PROM increases as the duration of the latency period increases. The proposed explanation is that with increasing duration of ROM, the likelihood of ascending infection from vaginal bacteria increases. However, detailed analysis of this problem (Figs. 41–1 and 41–2) reveals that this is probably true only in the term gestation. In preterm PROM, the incidences of both chorioamnionitis and perinatal infections are not changed with increasing duration of ROM (Johnson et al., 1981). This is probably explained by the fact that many preterm patients are already infected at the time of membrane rupture. Recent findings also suggest that in most cases increased infection rates with prolonged rupture of membranes may correlate more closely with the interval between digital cervical examinations than with the interval between rupture of membranes and the onset of infection (Lewis et al., 1991; Adoni et al., 1990).

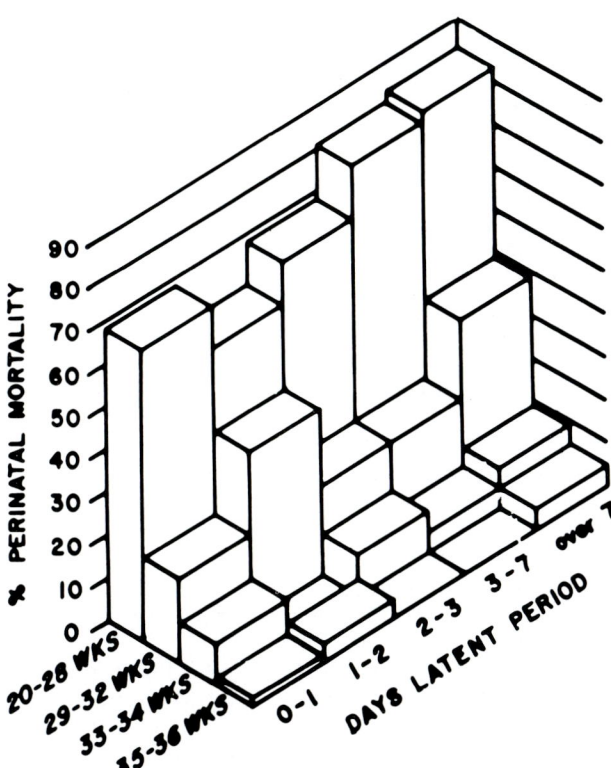

FIGURE 41–2. Perinatal mortality by duration of latent period for preterm deliveries. Within each gestational age group, no significant differences were noted for the various latent period lengths. (From Johnson et al: Premature rupture of the membranes and prolonged latency. Obstet Gynecol **57**:547, 1981.)

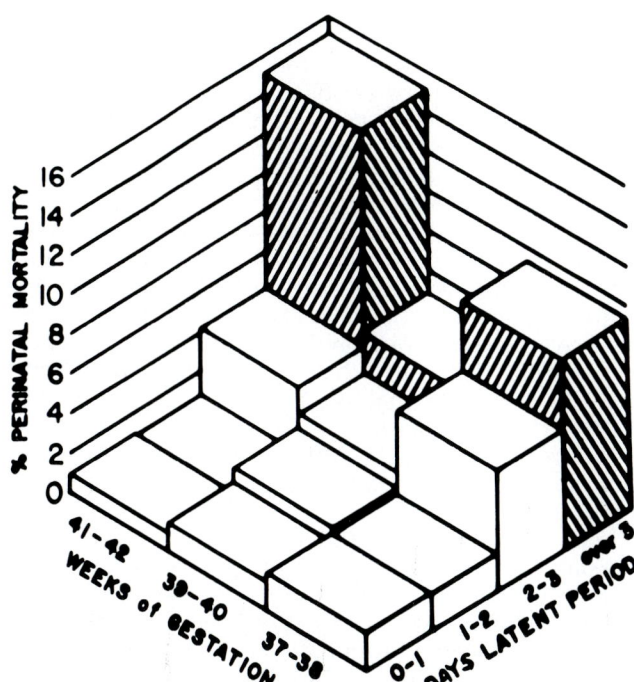

FIGURE 41–1. Perinatal mortality by duration of latent period for term infants. The cross-hatching indicates that the observed perinatal mortality is significantly higher than that noted among infants of the same gestational age with latent periods under one day. (From Johnson et al: Premature rupture of the membranes and prolonged latency. Obstet Gynecol **57**:547, 1981.)

With preterm PROM, the relative contributions of prematurity and perinatal infections to perinatal mortality are responsible for much of the controversy that exists regarding management of patients with this diagnosis. Table 41–1 compares a number of studies that describe the causes of perinatal mortality in specific study populations (Daikoku et al., 1982; Garite et al., 1981; Kappy et al., 1979; Stedman et al., 1981; Varner and Galask, 1981; Schreiber and Benedetti, 1980; Wilson et al., 1982; Barrett and Boehm, 1982; Morales, 1987). In most cases, perinatal mortality consequent to preterm PROM arises from complications of prematurity such as respiratory distress syndrome (RDS), intraventricular hemorrhage (IVH), and necrotizing enterocolitis (NEC). However, combining all gestational ages into one category for the purpose of this analysis may lead to oversimplified conclusions. For example, in the 26-week gestation the relative contribution of prematurity to the risks of perinatal morbidity and mortality far outweigh any risks from infection, and thus all efforts at prolonging gestation to decrease the complications of prematurity would seem warranted. However, in a fetus at 34 weeks gestation, at which point perinatal mortality is not substantially different from that for the fetus at term and complications of morbidity are minor, the contribution of infection becomes much more important. Studies by Garite and Freeman (1982) and by Morales

TABLE 41–1. Perinatal Outcome with Expectant Management of Preterm Labor

STUDY	NO. OF PATIENTS	PND	CAUSE OF DEATH		
			RDS/PREMATURITY	INFECTION	OTHER
Kappy et al.	45	10	4	1	5
Garite et al.	80	5	3	0	2
Stedman et al.	55	3	2	1	0
Varner and Galask	115	4	3	1	0
Daikoku et al.	203	28	8	4	16
Schreiber and Benedetti	90	12	4	1	7
Wilson et al.	143	22	10	4	8
Barrett and Boehm	53	7	5	1	1
Totals	784	91	39 (43%)	13 (14%)	39 (43%)

PND = perinatal deaths; RDS = respiratory distress syndrome.

et al. (1987) have shown that the risks of serious neonatal infections and of respiratory distress syndrome increase several-fold with chorioamnionitis in the preterm pregnancy. In addition, long-term neurologic complications are increased in fetuses delivered subsequent to the onset of maternal infection (Hardt et al., 1985).

HYPOXIA AND ASPHYXIA. It is well known that umbilical cord prolapse occurs more frequently when ROM occurs prior to the onset of labor (incidence about 1.5 per cent) as the presenting fetal part is less likely to occupy the pelvis (Gunn et al., 1970). The combination of PROM and malpresentation increases the frequency of this complication.

Recently, it has also become apparent that umbilical cord compression, even without prolapse, is more common with PROM secondary to oligohydramnios (Rutherford et al., 1987; Gabbe et al., 1976). This may occur prior to labor or during labor. In preterm patients in labor following PROM, Moberg and Garite reported a high incidence of fetal distress, mostly from cord compression, in 8.5 per cent of patients with PROM as compared to only 1.5 per cent of those in premature labor with intact membranes (Moberg et al., 1984). Series of expectantly managed patients with preterm PROM frequently report increased incidences of stillbirth, unexplained by infection, of up to 3 per cent (Johnson et al., 1981; Wilson et al., 1982; Miller et al., 1978). Studies of antepartum testing in patients with preterm PROM suggest a high incidence of antepartum fetal distress requiring intervention for fetal heart rate (FHR) patterns consistent with umbilical cord compression occurring even prior to the onset of labor (Moberg and Garite, 1987). Vintzileos et al. have shown a good correlation between the severity of oligohydramnios and the frequency of severe variable decelerations (Vintzileos et al., 1985b).

FETAL DEFORMATION SYNDROME. The final naturally occurring major complication that may result from PROM is the fetal deformation syndrome. As in fetuses with *Potter's syndrome*, PROM occurring very early in gestation can lead to growth retardation, compression malformations of the fetal face and limbs, and most importantly pulmonary hypoplasia. Prolonged and early oligohydramnios seems to be the cause of all of these problems. Bain et al. described 16 such cases in which there was a maternal history of PROM of 3 to 19 weeks duration (Bain et al., 1964).

The frequency of this syndrome is not clearly defined. A review of retrospectively accumulated case series in patients with PROM prior to 26 weeks reveals a combined frequency of 3.5 per cent (Taylor and Garite, 1984; Moretti and Sibai, 1988; Bengtson and Van-Marter, 1989; Major and Kitzmiller, 1990); however, it is likely that some cases of sublethal pulmonary hypoplasia may go unrecognized.

EVALUATION OF THE PATIENT WITH PROM

Management of the patient with PROM depends on a number of variables. Therefore, the initial evaluation of the patient who presents with a history suspicious for PROM must result in a basic data base which includes confirming the diagnosis, determining gestational age, evaluating for the presence of maternal and/or fetal infection, establishing the onset of labor, and ruling out fetal distress. Only when all of these factors are known, in addition to a complete review of the patient's obstetrical and past medical history, can decisions be made regarding management.

DIAGNOSIS OF PROM. Obviously, making the correct diagnosis of PROM is essential. A patient's history, consisting of a large gush of clear fluid from the vagina followed by persistent leakage, is correct in 90 per cent of cases (Friedman and McElin, 1969). Other explanations for such a history include urinary leakage, excessive vaginal discharge, or rarely bloody show. A watery vaginal discharge is also a common presenting symptom in patients with premature cervical dilation (incompetent cervix), even in the absence of ROM.

The diagnosis of premature rupture of membranes is established by aseptic speculum vaginal examination. Effort should be made in the process of examining the patient to avoid introduction of infection. Digital intracervical examination of the patient who is not in labor, and when immediate induction is not planned, should be avoided altogether; such examinations add little needed information and probably increase the risk of complications from infection (Wagner et al., 1989). Several recent studies have shown that patients with PROM who have digital intracervical infection have shorter latency periods and increased risks of neonatal sepsis (Lewis et al., 1991; Adoni et al., 1990; Wagner et al., 1989; Schutte et al., 1983). Confirmation of the diagnosis by speculum examination includes the identification of a pool of fluid in the posterior fornix (pooling). Prolonged rupture of membranes may result in loss of most of the fluid, and occasionally vaginal mucosa appears only moist. In such cases, either the Valsalva maneuver or pressure on the uterine fundus during speculum examination allows visualization of leakage from the endocervical canal. The next test for confirmation of amniorrhexis is the use of Nitrazine, a pH-sensitive paper strip, which changes color from yellow-green to dark blue at a pH above 6.0 to 6.5. The pH of the vagina in pregnancy is usually 4.5 to 6.0, and amniotic fluid has a pH of 7.1 to 7.3. Hence testing for this alkaline pH usually confirms the presence of amniotic fluid. Nitrazine may become falsely positive from contamination with blood, semen, or alkaline antiseptics (Friedman and McElin, 1969). Vaginal infections may raise the pH of the vagina. Occasionally alkaline urine may cause a false-positive result. If pooling and Nitrazine are not both positive, a swab of the posterior vaginal fornix should be taken, smeared on a slide, allowed to dry, and examined under a microscope for the presence of a typical *ferning* appearance (Fig. 41–3) (Kovacs, 1962). Although a swab inadvertently taken from the endocervical canal may cause a false-positive picture of ferning, the ferns seen from cervical mucus are not the typical lush and elaborate pattern seen with amniotic fluid. Finally, oligohydramnios seen on ultrasonography is usually confirmatory. When the diagnosis remains unclear, as with concomitant bleeding and oligohydramnios, an alternative invasive method may be applied whereby amniocentesis is done and a dye, such as Evans Blue or fluorescein, is injected; the cervix can then be visualized for leakage of dye (Atlay and Sutherst, 1970; Smith, 1976).

At the time of speculum examination, other information is also obtained. The cervix should be visualized to ascertain that no fetal extremity or umbilical cord prolapses through the os. An impression of cervical dilation and effacement can be ascertained

with a moderate degree of reliability. Cultures of the cervix and vagina can be taken for Gonococcus, group B Streptococcus, and Chlamydia. Culturing for other organisms adds little clinically useful information. In certain premature gestations, a sample of amniotic fluid from the posterior fornix can be aspirated and submitted for maturity testing; the presence of phosphatidylglycerol is the most reliable indicator of maturity (Stedman et al., 1981).

ESTABLISHING GESTATIONAL AGE FROM FETAL MATURITY. Menstrual dating, prenatal examinations, and previous ultrasonograms should all be reviewed to carefully establish gestational age, as the most critical factor in determining management of the patient with PROM is fetal age. If any doubt exists, ultrasonography should be performed. In patients with PROM or oligohydramnios from any cause, compression may cause alteration in measurements of biparietal diameter or abdominal circumference (O'Keeffe et al., 1985). Careful biometric evaluation of all routinely measured fetal parameters should be compared to eliminate this potential cause of error. Since cervical examination usually is to be avoided in patients with PROM and not in labor, ultrasonography also is useful in confirming the presentation of the fetus.

RULE OUT CHORIOAMNIONITIS. All patients with premature rupture of membranes, regardless of gestational age and regardless of uterine activity, must be evaluated carefully for signs of infection. The reader is referred to Chapter 42 for a detailed discussion of the diagnosis and management of chorioamnionitis. However, patients with preterm PROM should be evaluated for signs including fever, leukocytosis, maternal and fetal tachycardia, uterine tenderness, and/or malodorous vaginal discharge. In early or less severe cases, any or all of these signs may be missing. The diagnosis of chorioamnionitis, to be based on clinical signs and symptoms alone, must include a fever (temperature ≥ 100.4° F) in the setting of ruptured membranes and in the absence of any other explanation for the elevated temperature. Cervicovaginal cultures for group B Streptococcus, Chlamydia, and Gonococcus are done principally for the purpose of screening the uninfected patients and providing prophylactic antibiotics to prevent perinatal transmission. Since antibiotics will be used in patients with chorioamnionitis regardless and one cannot be assured that the organism isolated from the vagina is actually the organism causing the intra-amniotic infection, a more general cervicovaginal culture is of little value. Other laboratory tests also have limited utility. Maternal WBC count and C-reactive protein may indicate impending infection, but are relatively nonspecific, are elevated in patients in early labor, and must be interpreted along with all other clinical parameters (Ohlsson and Wong, 1990).

In cases of suspected chorioamnionitis, where the diagnosis cannot be clinically confirmed, amniocentesis may be of value and can be performed in the vast majority of patients with premature rupture of membranes. A further discussion of amniocentesis for the purpose of screening for occult intra-amniotic infection will follow in this chapter, but for the purposes of ruling out infection in the patient with subtle but

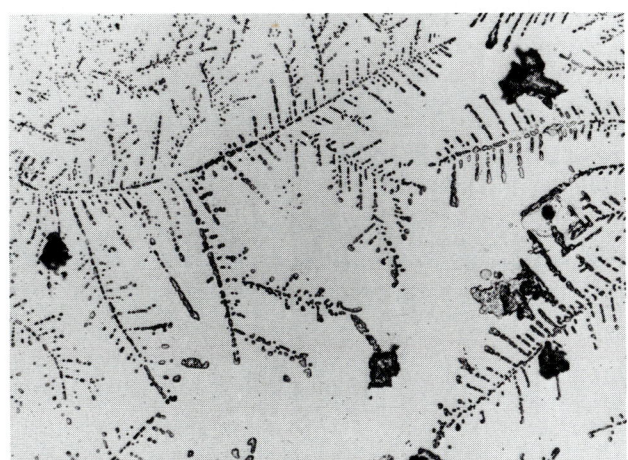

FIGURE 41–3. Typical "ferning" appearance. As seen with a swab from the posterior vaginal fornix, smeared on a slide and allowed to dry, from a patient with PROM.

inconclusive signs, this is a place where amniocentesis may have its greatest value and where the majority of experts might agree on its applicability. Amniotic fluid from patients with chorioamnionitis should have evidence of bacteria on Gram stain and, by the time evidence of infection is clinically present, should also have some white blood cells on Gram stain.

RULE OUT LABOR. The patient who is having regular and painful uterine contractions in the presence of ROM generally is found to be in active labor. However, since digital examinations are generally to be avoided until one is certain of labor, preliminary speculum examination may be used to determine whether cervical dilation is present. Patients who have premature rupture of membranes often experience contractions that stop spontaneously. External electronic fetal monitors may be applied to determine the presence and frequency of contractions and to allow early diagnosis of labor in most cases. In the very early preterm gestation, uterine activity may be difficult to detect on external monitors, and frequently variable decelerations of the FHR will be the first sign of labor (Moberg and Garite, 1987).

RULE OUT FETAL DISTRESS. As previously noted, PROM increases the risk of umbilical cord prolapse and cord compression from oligohydramnios. Continuous fetal heart rate monitoring should be included in the initial evaluations of all patients with this diagnosis if the fetus is of a viable gestational age (i.e., at least 25 weeks). Besides variable decelerations, late decelerations may reveal a coexistent abruption or uteroplacental pathology, and loss of fetal heart rate accelerations (loss of reactivity) and/or fetal tachycardia may suggest fetal sepsis.

CONTROVERSIES IN THE MANAGEMENT OF PROM

Despite the fact that there has been a great deal of investigation reported, including many prospective randomized trials, regarding the management of patients with PROM at varying gestational ages, this topic remains one of the most controversial and enigmatic clinical problems that the obstetrician must face. In a survey of Maternal Fetal Medicine specialists by Capeless and Mead (1987), it was evident that many important issues such as the use of corticosteroids, tocolytic therapy, amniocentesis, and several other diagnostic and therapeutic modalities could not be agreed upon with any degree approaching a consen-

sus. In many areas, however, information is more clear and agreement on management does exist. A patient with a history suggestive of premature rupture of membranes should be brought to the hospital immediately and evaluated to confirm or rule out the diagnosis of PROM. Those in whom the diagnosis is confirmed should be hospitalized and, in most cases, remain in the hospital until delivery. An exception would be the patient with PROM in whom the gestational age is below that of likely neonatal viability; in these patients, fetal status is not an immediate issue and outpatient expectant management may be appropriate. In some patients, leakage stops, and reaccumulation of normal amniotic fluid is noted on ultrasonography (about 11 per cent) (Johnston et al., 1990); their prognosis seems to be similar to that of patients who have never had rupture of membranes, and they can be safely discharged from the hospital once resealing of the membranes is confirmed (Johnston et al., 1990).

Patients with advanced active labor, clinical chorioamnionitis, and irreversible fetal distress obviously all need to be delivered. Otherwise management is dependent principally on gestational age. However, in the patient with PROM who is not in labor, and without evidence of infection or fetal distress, especially in premature gestational ages, there remains a great deal of controversy regarding management.

TOCOLYSIS. Since premature labor is an expected sequela of PROM and prematurity is the leading cause of perinatal morbidity and mortality in such cases, the appeal of agents to prevent or stop premature labor is obvious. It is clear from all studies of tocolytic therapy, regardless of the agent used, that patients with intact membranes are more likely to have labor successfully stopped than those whose membranes are ruptured. Over the past 5 years several prospective randomized controlled trials of tocolytic agents in patients with preterm PROM have been conducted (Table 41–2) (Christensen et al., 1980; Garite et al., 1987; Weiner et al., 1988). While one of these three studies shows prolongation of pregnancy of up to 24 hours in patients with tocolytic therapy (Christensen et al., 1980), the other two showed no difference, and none of these showed any prolongation of pregnancy beyond that point or any difference in any index of perinatal mortality or morbidity measured. Two randomized trials of prophylactic oral tocolytics also failed to show pregnancy prolongation (Levy and Warsof, 1985; Dunlop et al., 1986). In the past some have been concerned about increasing the risk of infection by attempts to prolong pregnancy in patients with PROM; however,

TABLE 41–2. Studies Evaluating Tocolytics to Prolong Pregnancy with Preterm PROM

AUTHOR	N		DELIVERY >24°	DELIVERY >48°	DELIVERY >7cd.	RDS	MORTALITY
Christiansen et al.	30	Rx	14/14	7/14	3/14	2/14	1/14
		Control	10/16*	7/16	1/16	1/16	0/16
Garite et al.	79	Rx	35/39	30/39	12/39	20/39	6/39
		Control	36/40	30/40	13/40	23/40	2/40
Weiner et al.	75	Rx	31/33	29/33	Not stated	15/33	5/33
		Control	39/42	32/42	Not stated	22/40	3/40

*p <.05, All others not significant.

TABLE 41–3. Effect of Corticosteroids on RDS in Preterm PROM (Randomized Controlled Studies Only)

AUTHOR	NUMBER OF PTS STEROIDS	NUMBER OF PTS CONTROL	EFFECT ON RDS
Block	43	26	No difference
Taeusch	17	24	*No difference
Papageorgiou	17	19	Decreased
Young	38	37	Decreased
Garite	80	80	*No difference
Collaborative	153	135	No difference
Iams	38	35	*No difference
Nelson	22	46	*No difference
Simpson	112	105	*More RDS in steroid group
Morales	121	124	Decreased

*Studies also suggesting an increased incidence of maternal and/or neonatal infection in the steroid group.

TABLE 41–4. Combined Frequency of Organisms Cultured From Amniotic Fluid Obtained by Amniocentesis in Patients with Preterm PROM (7 Studies)

Group B Streptococcus	20%
Gardnerella vaginalis	17%
Peptostreptococcus/Peptococcus	11%
Fusobacteria	10%
Bacteroides fragilis	9%
Other streptococci	9%
Bacteroides species	5%

none of these studies showed any difference. Of course, one would not expect a difference in studies that did not show any prolongation of pregnancy.

CORTICOSTEROIDS. In 1972 Liggins and Howie (1972) first demonstrated that when betamethasone was given to mothers threatening to deliver prematurely, the incidence and severity of RDS in their premature neonates were substantially reduced. Many subsequent randomized trials have uniformly confirmed the benefit. Since premature rupture of membranes is an obvious prelude to premature delivery, this seems an ideal circumstance for the application of corticosteroids. Some studies in the past have shown some acceleration of fetal lung maturity from rupture of membranes alone after 24 to 48 hours. Therefore, one could not necessarily apply the data showing benefit of corticosteroids in patients with preterm labor to the situation of preterm PROM. In fact, there are now a large number of prospective randomized controlled trials of corticosteroids with preterm PROM, and the majority of these trials, unlike the unanimity with preterm labor, have not shown a reduction in the rate or severity of RDS in treated patients (Table 41–3) (Garite et al., 1981; Block et al., 1977; Taeusch et al., 1979; Papageorgiou et al., 1979; Young et al., 1980; Collaborative Group on Antenatal Steroid Therapy, 1981; Iams et al., 1985; Nelson et al., 1985; Simpson and Harbert, 1985; Morales et al., 1986). Five of these ten studies have also shown an increase in the risk of maternal and/or neonatal infections in the patients randomized to the corticosteroid group. A recent meta-analysis, combining the data of all of these trials, suggests a minimal reduction in the incidence of RDS with the use of corticosteroids and confirms a statistically small increased risk of infection (Ohlsson, 1989). However, it would seem that the small benefit gained in the reduction of the incidence of RDS, in light of the increased risk of infection, would not appear to justify the use of corticosteroids in such patients.

PROPHYLACTIC ANTIBIOTICS. The use of prophylactic antibiotics in patients with preterm PROM is theoretically appealing from two standpoints: (1) maternal and perinatal risks of infection would be reduced; and

(2) the interval between PROM and delivery might be prolonged (since occult infection is a probable cause of preterm PROM and preterm labor). The first large prospective trial was undertaken in the 1960s and showed no benefit from prophylactic antibiotics (Lebherz et al., 1980). Unfortunately, these authors had little to choose from in the way of broad-spectrum antibiotics, and the drug used, tetracycline, has poor amniotic fluid penetration and probably a poor spectrum of activity for the organisms involved. Table 41–4 illustrates the most commonly identified organisms from amniotic fluid obtained by amniocentesis in patients with preterm PROM (Garite et al., 1979; Miller et al., 1980; Cotton et al., 1984; Zlatnick et al., 1984; Broekhuizen et al., 1985; Gonik and Cotton, 1985; Romero et al., 1988). The predominance of anaerobes and group B Streptococcus indicates a need for antibiotics effective against both types of organism. A number of recent randomized controlled trials of prophylactic antibiotics in patients with preterm PROM are showing some promise. Most of these studies (Table 41–5) show a prolongation of latency period by an average of 5 to 7 days, and some also show a reduction in the incidence of maternal amnionitis and/ or neonatal sepsis (Amon et al., 1988; Morales et al., 1989; Johnston et al., 1990; McGregor and French, 1989; Christmas et al., 1990). Clearly there is no uniformity in antibiotics chosen or in duration of therapy. Many questions remain to be answered including whether or not consistent results will be shown in further studies, whether or not these studies apply to all populations, what is the best antibiotic including route and duration of therapy, and whether or not we can be selective, reserving therapy for a specific group of patients at higher risk.

As discussed in detail in Chapter 42, it is always

TABLE 41–5. Antibiotic Prophylaxis in PROM

AUTHORS	N	ANTIBIOTIC	OUTCOME
Amon et al.	82	Ampicillin IV/PO	PR LAT/<NN INF
Morales et al.	165	Ampicillin IV	<IAI/<NN INF
Johnston et al.		Mezlocin Ampicillin IV/PO	PR LAT/<NN INF/ <IAI
McGregor et al.	54	Erythromycin	PR LAT
Christmas et al.	56	Ampicillin Gentamicin Clindamycin	PR LAT

PR LAT = prolonged latency; NN INF = neonatal infection; IAI = intra-amniotic infection (chorioamnionitis).

necessary to use prophylactic antibiotics for group B Streptococcus infection in patients with preterm ROM or prolonged ROM at term if the patient is a known carrier or if there has been insufficient time to obtain culture results for the presence or absence of this organism. The purpose of this therapy is obviously to prevent perinatal transmission of this devastating organism to the newborn, and many trials now show that intrapartum treatment is effective in significantly reducing the risk of this complication (Regan et al., 1981; Boyer et al., 1983).

RULING OUT OCCULT INTRA-AMNIOTIC INFECTION. There exists a significant controversy over the issue of identifying occult intra-amniotic infection. Clearly, once chorioamnionitis occurs, the incidence of neonatal morbidity and mortality is significantly aggravated (Garite and Freeman, 1982). It would seem logical, therefore, that a method to detect occult or early intra-amniotic infection and to treat this subgroup of patients selectively, with either delivery or antibiotics or with both, would have the potential for improving the outcome in this group. Thus the controversy surrounds two questions: (1) What is the best way to identify such early/occult infection? (2) Is there indeed any benefit in detecting occult intra-amniotic infection before it becomes clinically apparent?

Table 41–6 lists the many reported tests for detecting occult intra-amniotic infection. Clinical signs and symptoms are often nonspecific. Maternal laboratory tests, including white blood cell count and erythrocyte sedimentation rate are particularly nonspecific unless counts are unusually high (Ohlsson and Wong, 1990).

A great deal of debate has surrounded the issue of C-reactive protein. This nonspecific maternal serum marker has been reported to be elevated in patients who are destined to develop intra-amniotic infection prior to delivery. However, results of a large number of studies evaluating this question have been conflicting, with the majority of studies showing inadequate sensitivity and specificity to act on this marker alone (Ohlsson and Wong, 1990).

Amniocentesis, with the Gram stain and subsequent culture, was one of the first described attempts at specifically addressing the problem of intra-amniotic infection (Garite et al., 1979). Many other methods of analyzing the amniotic fluid have subsequently been described. According to a careful analysis of all the available methods for analyzing amniotic fluid by Romero et al., the Gram stain on spun or unspun amniotic fluid and the amniotic fluid glucose determination (with positive values of less than 15 mg/dl) are probably the best combination of methods for amniotic fluid analysis to detect occult infection (Romero, 1991). The Gram stain generally reveals the presence of bacteria that have a high specificity for subsequent development of chorioamnionitis. Patients who have a positive Gram stain but do not develop chorioamnionitis generally deliver within a short time, and thus have not had sufficient opportunity to mount an inflammatory response and systemic reaction that would result in a clinical syndrome of chorioamnionitis. However, the sensitivity of the Gram stain is somewhat low, especially when colony counts are low. Colony counts of approximately 10^5 or greater are generally necessary to effect a positive Gram stain. Similarly, amniotic fluid glucose, when low, has a relatively high specificity but fairly poor sensitivity.

Much attention has been given to the use of various fetal biophysical parameters to detect signs of infection. Vintzileos first introduced the concept of the biophysical profile for detecting occult intra-amniotic and/or fetal infection (Vintzileos et al., 1985a). His initial results showed a high degree of sensitivity and specificity for detecting either or both types of infection. In analyzing the various parameters of the biophysical profile that may detect infection, there is some debate over whether the loss of reactivity or loss of fetal breathing movements provides the better single marker (Vintzileos et al., 1986). In a review of 14 patients from the initial study of Vintzileos (1985) (Table 41–7), one can see that when the fetal heart rate was reactive (3 cases), the remainder of the biophysical profile was normal. In all cases in which the biophysical profile score was low, the FHR was nonreactive. Therefore, based on these data and other studies looking specifically at fetal heart rate as a predictor of infection, it appears that the evaluation of FHR reactivity is a good screening tool for fetal infection, and if heart rate accelerations are absent, the more complete biophysical profile can be used as a back-up test. In all series evaluating these biophysical parameters, testing was done on a daily basis, and it appears that this frequency is necessary to provide adequate fetal evaluation. Not all analyses of the use of biophysical profile for the evaluation of infection have been as supportive of its value as those of Vintzileos (Miller et al., 1990).

Further analysis of the literature evaluating the biophysical profile for detecting infection reveals that this modality detects fetal infection much more accurately than it detects maternal infection—the loss of reactivity, fetal movement, tone, and breathing being similar to the nonspecific signs seen with sepsis in the newborn nursery. The simple presence of bacteria in the amniotic fluid may or may not lead to such fetal depression, although there is some speculation that release of prostaglandins associated with bacterial in-

TABLE 41–6. Reported Tests for the Preclinical Diagnosis of Intra-Amniotic Infection

CLINICAL TESTS
C-reactive protein
WBC
Sedimentation rate
AMNIOTIC FLUID TESTS
Culture
Gram stain
Gas liquid chromatography
Lemulus lysate
Fibronectin
Glucose
Leukocyte esterase
Cytokines
BIOPHYSICAL
Biophysical profile
Amniotic fluid volume
Nonstress test

TABLE 41–7.   Analysis of Biophysical Profile of 16 Infected Cases (Group 1)

CASE NO.	NST	FBM	FM	FT	AF	PL	TOTAL SCORE	DIAGNOSIS
1	2	0	2	2	2	2	10	Amnionitis
2	0	0	2	1	1	2	6	Amnionitis
3	0	0	2	2	1	2	7	Possible neonatal sepsis
4	0	0	2	2	0	2	6	Possible neonatal sepsis
5	0	0	2	2	0	2	6	Possible neonatal sepsis
6	0	0	2	2	1	2	7	Amnionitis—possible neonatal sepsis
7	1	0	0	1	2	2	6	Amnionitis—possible neonatal sepsis
8	0	0	2	2	0	2	6	Amnionitis—possible neonatal sepsis
9	0	0	0	1	0	1	2	Amnionitis—possible neonatal sepsis
10	0	0	1	2	1	2	6	Neonatal sepsis
11	1	0	2	0	2	0	5	Neonatal sepsis
12	0	0	0	0	0	2	2	Neonatal sepsis
13	0	0	0	2	0	2	4	Amnionitis—neonatal sepsis
14	0	0	1	1	0	2	4	Amnionitis—neonatal sepsis
15	0	0	0	2	0	1	3	Amnionitis—neonatal sepsis
16	0	0	0	1	0	2	3	Amnionitis—neonatal sepsis

NST = Nonstress test; FBM = fetal breathing movements; FM = fetal movements; FT = fetal tone; AF = amniotic fluid; PL = placental grading.
From Vintzileos AM et al: The fetal biophysical profile in patients with premature rupture of the membranes: An early predictor of fetal infection. Obstet Gynecol **152**:510, 1985.

vasion has an impact on such biophysical parameters as fetal breathing (Vintzileos et al., 1986).

Based on this information, it would appear that some initial form of careful maternal and fetal assessment on admission, followed by daily evaluation, is necessary to detect early infection. Since fetal infection sometimes may occur in the absence of maternal infection, the use of some fetal evaluation technique is also important. After the initial clinical evaluation on admission, a daily nonstress test and/or a daily biophysical profile would be appropriate adjuncts to the daily clinical examination. The utility of amniocentesis remains controversial, but should be used at least for cases in which clinical suspicion of infection exists but cannot be confirmed and/or in selected gestational age groups in which the risk of infection may become more significant than the risk of prematurity (e.g., greater than 32 weeks).

FETAL MATURITY TESTING. Another important debate regarding the management of PROM involves the question whether fetal lung maturity testing should be incorporated into the management algorithm. The protocol involves taking patients of selected gestational ages in which some reasonable likelihood of fetal lung maturity exists (e.g., ≥ 32 weeks) and selectively managing these patients based on lung maturity. In an initial description of this protocol (1982), I reported that amniotic fluid was successfully obtained in 50 per cent of patients with preterm PROM, and approximately one-half had LS ratios consistent with fetal lung maturity. Sixty-three such patients were delivered with two cases of mild RDS, one case of fetal pneumonia resulting in neonatal death, and no other major complications of prematurity in mature patients. Subsequently, Stedman et al. (1981) tested amniotic fluid—obtained from the posterior vaginal fornix—for the presence or absence of phosphatidylglycerol (PG) and reported similar results. Since amniotic fluid obtained from the vagina may be contaminated by substances present there, the PG test theoretically is the only fetal maturity test

available that is totally unaffected by contamination. However, a significant number of fetuses will have lung maturity in the absence of PG, and PG generally indicates maturity a week or more later than other tests, such as the LS ratio. Therefore, it is advisable to use the PG obtained from the vaginal pool as an initial screening test and to follow with amniocentesis if PG is absent.

One randomized study has subjected such a management scheme to careful scrutiny. Spinnato and coworkers (1987) studied 46 patients, all of whom had fetal lung maturity as documented by amniotic fluid tests. These patients were categorized according to either delivery or expectant management. Patients who were delivered immediately had a lower overall incidence of chorioamnionitis than those managed expectantly. Although there was no difference in the incidence of neonatal sepsis or other newborn complications, the sample size was not large enough to sufficiently test this question. One would infer, however, that if maternal infection rates are higher in the expectantly managed group, the rate of neonatal complications is likely to increase.

MANAGEMENT OF THE PATIENT WITH PROM

As previously stated, the management of patients with PROM remains one of the most controversial problems in obstetrics. All patients who present with symptoms suggestive of PROM should be brought to the hospital and evaluated. Those who are not in advanced active labor should have a speculum examination performed to confirm the diagnosis and to evaluate the status of the cervix. Patients who are in advanced active labor obviously are delivered regardless of gestational age, and cesarean section is performed for the usual obstetric indications. Patients who are found to have clinical chorioamnionitis need to be treated with antibiotics and delivered regardless of gestational age. Although there are a few cases in the obstetric literature in which patients with chorioamnionitis in very early gestational ages were treated with antibiotics and not delivered (Monif, 1983), there are many more cases in which serious maternal infectious complications developed as a result of such management (Webb, 1967). Labor should be induced in patients without other indications for cesarean section and a reasonable trial of labor allowed, as chorioamnionitis in and of itself is not an indication for cesarean section regardless of gestational age. In cases of irreversible fetal distress, usually associated with variable decelerations of heart rate in the face of premature rupture of the membranes, delivery also is indicated. The management of patients who do not exhibit advanced labor, clinical infection, or fetal distress is based primarily on their gestational age on admission.

Management of PROM at Term

At 36 weeks and beyond, the goal of management of PROM is delivery. Patients in active labor should be allowed to progress, and management is the same as for any other term patient. Most of the remaining patients will go into labor within 24 hours following PROM. However, since the risk of neonatal infection increases as the duration of membrane rupture becomes prolonged, many clinicians have aggressively managed term patients by inducing labor with oxytocin shortly after PROM in an effort to shorten the interval between rupture and delivery. However, recent studies have shown that such an aggressive approach with oxytocin induction only serves to increase the cesarean section rate, usually for failed induction or failure to progress in labor, and is not effective in lowering the infection rate (Duff et al., 1984; Kappy et al., 1979). Quite to the contrary, since cesarean section rates are increased with induction, these patients have higher rates of postpartum endometritis. Duff and co-workers (Duff et al., 1984), in a randomized trial of patients managed expectantly versus those aggressively induced with oxytocin, found a cesarean section rate three times higher in those induced and no difference in the incidence of chorioamnionitis or neonatal sepsis. However, not all studies have confirmed this finding (Wagner et al., 1989). In addition, a much larger sample size would be needed to assess the impact of such management on neonatal infection.

More recently a third option has been described utilizing prostaglandin E_2 for preinduction cervical ripening. A randomized trial by Ray and Garite (1992) compared three management schemes: (1) immediate oxytocin induction, (2) placebo prostaglandin (expectant management), and (3) prostaglandin using 3-mg vaginal suppositories, two doses, six hours apart, followed by induction for those patients not in labor. The shortest intervals between admission and delivery were found in the oxytocin and prostaglandin groups. The lowest cesarean section rates were found in the prostaglandin and expectant management groups, and the lowest rate of overall infection was seen in the prostaglandin group. Other nonrandomized studies have described such a protocol with similarly encouraging results (Magos et al., 1983).

Management of Preterm PROM

As previously stated, the major risks to the baby following preterm PROM are related to complications of prematurity. Therefore, management is aimed at prolonging gestation for the patient who is not in labor, not infected, and not experiencing fetal distress. However, based on the previously described controversies and the individual clinician's interpretation of these data, several possible alternative management schemes can be developed.

The most commonly accepted management scheme for the patient at less than 36 weeks with PROM, but with a viable fetus, is expectant management in the hospital, which basically consists of careful observation for signs of infection, labor, or fetal distress in an effort to gain time for fetal growth and maturation. On admission the diagnosis is confirmed by speculum examination. Patients are initially evaluated by prolonged monitoring of fetal heart rate and uterine contractions (i.e., for 12 to 24 hours). For patients who go into labor, develop infection, or develop fetal distress, delivery is warranted; the other patients may be transferred to a regular hospital room for observation, which includes daily clinical evaluation, frequent nonstress tests, and/or biophysical profile evaluation. Patients in early labor are transferred immediately to the labor and delivery suite for careful fetal evaluation and supervision of labor. Although most of these patients commit themselves to delivery by going into labor, some do reach term and the timing of delivery must be decided. When the patient reaches 36 or 37 weeks, delivery is indicated; documented fetal lung maturity may permit a somewhat earlier delivery.

Another management scheme involves the use of selective expectant management. In this algorithm patients are evaluated on admission for fetal lung maturity and delivered if this maturity can be documented. It is reasonable to assume that lung maturity is unlikely at less than 31 weeks gestation, and this group of patients can be managed expectantly. At 32 weeks or more, examination of vaginal pool fluid for phosphatidylglycerol by means of the rapid slide agglutination test will give an answer in a short time. In those negative for PG, amniocentesis can be considered, and if any test of amniotic fluid documents fetal lung maturity, labor can be induced. Fluid obtained at amniocentesis should undergo the Gram stain examination and glucose level determination. The discovery of occult infection is an indication for delivery and antibiotic treatment in these cases. The immature fetal lung and absence of occult infection are indications for expectant management, as already described.

Finally, many clinicians interpret the available data on tocolysis and corticosteroids somewhat differently. Their patients are subjected to aggressive tocolysis with beta-sympathomimetics or magnesium sulfate and given corticosteroids in an effort to accelerate fetal lung maturity. After 48 hours of such therapy, the patient can either be delivered or expectantly managed; both protocols have been described in the literature (Garite et al., 1981; Simpson and Harbert, 1985). Although prolonged tocolytic therapy has not been supported in clinical trials, many elect to continue this therapy with oral tocolytics in an effort to prolong gestation.

One of the main arguments for keeping these patients in the hospital is that once labor begins there is a very high incidence of fetal distress, especially from umbilical cord compression. As Westgren has described (Westgren et al., 1983), fetal distress in the very preterm gestation can be quite different from that in the term gestation. These fetuses progress from mild to severe variable decelerations more rapidly, fetal heart rate variability is lost more rapidly, and there is better correlation between such abnormal heart rate patterns and depressed Apgar scores, umbilical cord acidosis, and neonatal complications (Fig. 41–4). Therefore, it is necessary to promptly evaluate fetal well-being once the patient goes into labor and to quickly deliver the infant should fetal distress develop.

Another important issue is the use of *amnioinfusion* for the prevention of fetal distress. Since the incidence of fetal distress in association with preterm PROM is so high and since this fetal distress is caused most often by umbilical cord compression, this group of patients is ideally suited to amnioinfusion. Nageotte and co-workers (1985) randomly assigned patients with preterm PROM who were in active labor to either prophylactic amnioinfusion or none. Patients given prophylactic amnioinfusion had a lower rate and severity of variable decelerations, higher Apgar scores and cord pH values, and a lower incidence of fetal

distress requiring cesarean section. The advantage of prophylactic amnioinfusion over waiting for abnormal heart rate patterns and then instituting amnioinfusion in these patients is that once fetal distress develops in the very preterm gestation there is insufficient time for the amnioinfusion to work before operative intervention is necessary.

Previable/Preterm PROM. PROM that occurs very early in pregnancy (e.g., less than 25 weeks) presents a special set of problems, as previously described. In these patients there is a relatively low probability (25 to 40 per cent) that a viable gestational age will be achieved and that the patient will deliver a surviving infant. There are real maternal risks (e.g., infection, abruption) associated with the process of waiting. A review of available retrospective series (Taylor and Garite, 1984; Moretti and Sibai, 1988; Bengtson and VanMarter, 1989; Major and Kitzmiller, 1990) (Table 41–8) reveals substantial maternal morbidity and a rather dismal outlook for the fetus, including a high rate of serious neurologic morbidity, in those that are managed expectantly. Not only are maternal chorioamnionitis rates much higher than at later preterm gestational ages (39 per cent), but other serious maternal complications (e.g., need for blood transfusions, serious maternal sepsis) and even death from sepsis have been described in these series.

There is increasing interest in the issue of the *fetal deformation syndrome* in patients with very early and prolonged rupture of membranes. This syndrome, as previously described, includes growth retardation, compression deformities, and pulmonary hypoplasia. The most serious complication, pulmonary hypoplasia, occurs relatively infrequently, but obviously has the most devastating impact. Many efforts have been

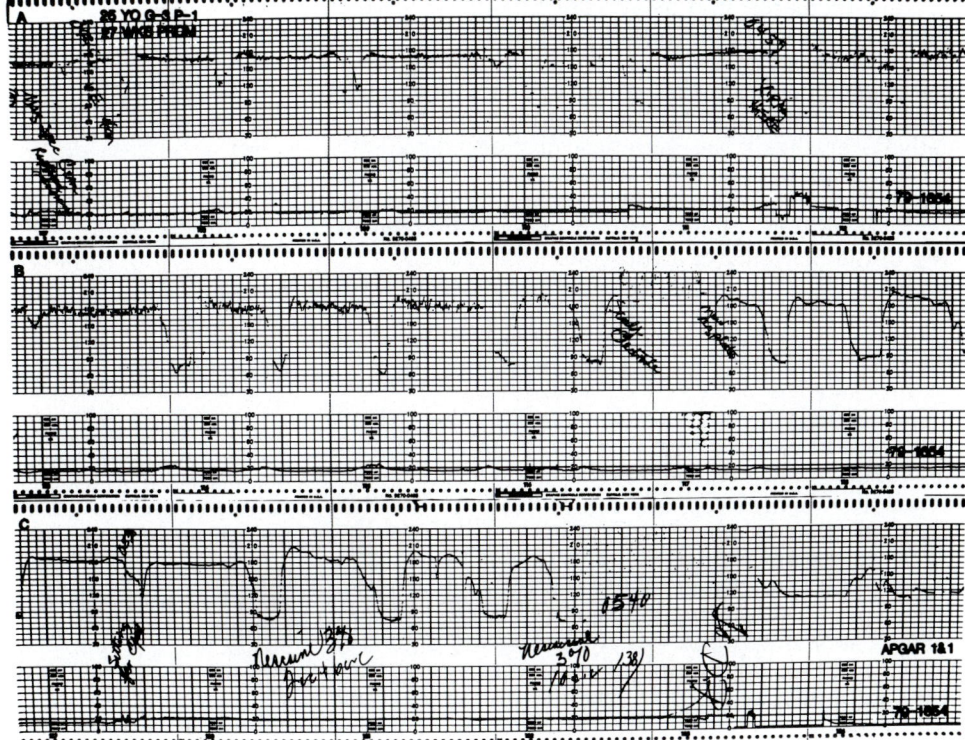

FIGURE 41–4. Rapid progression in depth and duration of variable decelerations in a patient with preterm PROM and oligohydramnios. This is characteristic of the very premature fetus.

TABLE 41–8. Outcome with PROM in Previable Gestations (All Studies <26 weeks)

STUDY	N MOTHER	CHORIOAMNIONITIS	N BABY	NEWBORN SURVIVORS	NORMAL NEUROLOGIC DEVELOPMENT
Taylor and Garite	53	13 (25%)	60	13 (22%)	38%
Major and Kitzmiller	70	30 (43%)	71	46 (65%)	31%
Moretti and Sibai	118	46 (39%)	124	40 (32%)	33%
Bengston and Van Marter	59	27 (46%)	63	32 (51%)	16%
Overall	300	116 (39%)	318	131 (41%)	30%

made to detect pulmonary hypoplasia by means of various sonographic parameters. Measurements used to assess this problem include fetal chest circumference, which can be compared with normograms for gestational age, and various ratios such as fetal chest circumference to abdominal circumference or fetal chest circumference to cardiac circumference. Unfortunately, all of these parameters have shown limited sensitivity and specificity and are far too unreliable for clinical use in making any management decision (Vintzileos et al., 1989).

Management of these patients consists of initial evaluation and, if labor or clinical infection is present, delivery. For the remainder of these patients, there are essentially two options: expectant management and termination. It is crucial, with such a high maternal risk and poor prognosis for good fetal outcome, that the patient be involved in this decision process. In many cases, the patient is admitted to the hospital before she is presented with these options so that, should she elect to terminate her pregnancy, this can be carried out immediately. If the patient chooses expectant management, this can be carried out at home since there is little that can be done for the fetus. The mother is discharged and instructed to maintain bed rest, avoid intercourse, check her temperature regularly, and await contractions. Once the patient reaches a viable gestational age (e.g., 25 to 26 weeks), she can be admitted to the hospital for daily fetal evaluation and prompt intervention should labor occur. For patients who elect termination, several methods are available: high-dose oxytocin or 20-mg prostaglandin suppositories every 4 hours are reasonable options. The diagnosis of incompetent cervix as a cause of PROM in such patients should be considered in the planning of a subsequent pregnancy.

RISK OF RECURRENCE

Very little data has existed regarding the risk of recurrence in patients with preterm PROM. Asrat and co-workers (1991) recently evaluated this issue and looked at subsequent pregnancy outcome in patients who had been managed with preterm PROM in the index pregnancy. Thirty-two per cent of these patients had recurrent preterm PROM at an average of 2 weeks later in the subsequent pregnancy. Therefore, these patients should be counseled regarding the high risk of recurrence of this complication; unfortunately very little can be said at this point about what can be done to prevent it.

SUMMARY

The management of the patient with PROM is a common and perplexing problem faced frequently by the clinician. Despite many efforts, little progress has been made obstetrically toward reducing complications of this problem, especially from prematurity. Primary goals of management of PROM include making the diagnosis promptly without increasing the risk of infection in the process and evaluating the patient for signs of infection, fetal distress, and impending labor. Since prematurity accounts for the majority of perinatal mortality and morbidity with PROM, management designed to minimize complications of prematurity is appropriate. However, complications from infection and asphyxia do occur, and efforts to avoid and minimize these problems are necessary.

REFERENCES

Adoni A, Chetrit AB, Zacut D, et al: Prolongation of the latent period in patients with premature rupture of the membrane by avoiding digital vaginal examination. Int J Gynecol Obstet 32:19, 1990.

Amon E, Lewis SV, Sibai B, et al: Antibiotic prophylaxis in preterm PROM: a prospective randomized study. Am J Obstet Gynecol 159:539, 1988.

Artal JP, Sokol RJ, Neuman M, et al: The mechanical properties of prematurely and non-prematurely ruptured membranes. Am J Obstet Gynecol 125:655, 1976.

Asrat T, Lewis DF, Garite TJ, et al: Rate of recurrence of preterm PROM in consecutive pregnancies. Am J Obstet Gynecol 165:1111, 1991.

Atlay RD, Sutherst JR: Premature rupture of the fetal membranes confirmed by intra-amniotic injection of dye (Evans blue T-1824). Am J Obstet Gynecol 108:993, 1970.

Bain AD, Smith II, Gould IK: Newborn after prolonged leakage of liquor amnii. Br Med J 2:598, 1964.

Barrett JM, Boehm FH: Comparison of aggressive and conservative management of premature rupture of fetal membranes. Am J Obstet Gynecol 144:12, 1982.

Bengtson JM, Van Marter LJ: Pregnancy outcome after premature rupture of the membranes at or before 26 weeks gestation. Obstet Gynecol 73:921, 1989.

Block MF, Kling OR, Crosby WM: Antenatal glucocorticoid therapy for the prevention of respiratory distress syndrome in the premature infant. Obstet Gynecol 50:186, 1977.

Boyer KM, Gadzala CA, Kelly PD, et al: Selective intrapartum chemoprophylaxis of neonatal group B streptococcal early onset disease: II. Predictive value of prenatal cultures. J Infect Dis 148:802, 1983.

Broekhuizen FF, Gilman M, Hamilton PR: Amniocentesis for Gram stain and culture in preterm premature rupture of the membranes. Obstet Gynecol 66:316, 1985.

Capeless EL, Mead PB: Management of preterm premature rupture of membranes: Lack of a national consensus. Am J Obstet Gynecol 157:11, 1987.

Cederqvist LL, Zervoudakis IA, Ewool LC, Litwin SD: The relationship between prematurely ruptured membranes and fetal immunoglobulin production. Am J Obstet Gynecol **134**:784, 1979.

Christensen KK, Ingemarsson I, Leideman T, et al: Effect of ritodrine on labor after premature rupture of membranes. Obstet Gynecol **55**:187, 1980.

Christmas JT, Cox SM, Gilstrap LC, et al: Expectant management of preterm ruptured membranes: effect of antimicrobial therapy on interval to delivery. (Abstract #15.) Presented at the Tenth Annual Meeting of the Society of Perinatal Obstetricians. Houston, Texas, 1990.

Collaborative Group on Antenatal Steroid Therapy: Effect of antenatal dexamethasone administration on the prevention of respiratory distress syndrome. Am J Obstet Gynecol **141**:276, 1981.

Cotton DB, Hill LM, Strassner HT, et al: Use of amniocentesis in preterm gestation with ruptured membranes. Obstet Gynecol **63**:38, 1984.

Daikoku NH, Kaltreider F, Khozami VA, et al: Premature rupture of membranes and spontaneous preterm labor: Maternal endometritis risks. Obstet Gynecol **59**:13, 1982.

Duff P, Huff RW, Gibbs RS: Management of PROM and unfavorable cervix in term pregnancy. Obstet Gynecol **63**:697, 1984.

Dunlop PDM, Crowley PA, Lamont RF, Hawkins DF: Preterm ruptured membranes, no contractions. J Obstet Gynecol **7**:92, 1986.

Edwards LE, Barrada MI, Haaman AA, et al: Gonorrhea in pregnancy. Am J Obstet Gynecol **132**:637, 1978.

Friedman ML, McElin TW: Diagnosis of ruptured fetal membranes: Clinical study and review of the literature. Am J Obstet Gynecol **104**:544, 1969.

Gabbe SG, Ettinger BB, Freeman RK, et al: Umbilical cord compression associated with amniotomy: Laboratory observations. Am J Obstet Gynecol **126**:353, 1976.

Garite TJ, Freeman RK, Linzey EM, et al: The use of amniocentesis in patients with premature rupture of membranes. Obstet Gynecol **54**:226, 1979.

Garite TJ, Freeman RK: Chorioamnionitis in the preterm gestation. Obstet Gynecol **54**:539, 1982.

Garite TJ: What's the best care in preterm PROM? Contemp Obstet Gynecol **19**:178, 1982.

Garite TJ, Keegan KA, Freeman RK, et al: A randomized trial of ritodrine tocolysis vs. expectant management in patients with preterm PROM at 25 to 30 weeks. Am J Obstet Gynecol **157**:388, 1987.

Garite TJ, Freeman RK, Linzey EM, et al: Prospective randomized study of corticosteroids in the management of premature rupture of the membranes and the premature gestation. Am J Obstet Gynecol **141**:508, 1981.

Gibbs RS, Blanco JD, St. Clair PJ, et al: Quantitative bacteriology of amniotic fluid from patients with clinical intra-amniotic infection at term. J Infect Dis **145**:1, 1982.

Gibbs RS, Castillo MS, Rodgers PJ: Management of acute chorioamnionitis. Am J Obstet Gynecol **136**:709, 1980.

Gonik B, Cotton DB: The use of amniocentesis in preterm premature rupture of membranes. Am J Perinatol **2**:21, 1985.

Gunn GC, Mishell DR, Morton DG: Premature rupture of the fetal membranes. A review. Am J Obstet Gynecol **106**:469, 1970.

Hardt NS, Kostenbauder M, Ogborn M, et al: Influence of chorioamnionitis on long-term prognosis in low birth weight infants. Obstet Gynecol **65**:5, 1985.

Iams JD, Talbert ML, Barrows H, et al: Management of preterm prematurely ruptured membranes: a prospective randomized comparison of observation versus use of steroids and timed delivery. Am J Obstet Gynecol **151**:32, 1985.

Johnson JWC, Daikoku NH, Niebyl JR, et al: Premature rupture of the membranes and prolonged latency. Obstet Gynecol **57**:547, 1981.

Johnston JWC, Egerman RS, Moorhead J: Cases with ruptured membranes that "reseal." Am J Obstet Gynecol **163**:1024, 1990.

Johnston MM, Sanchez-Ramos L, Vaughn AJ, et al: Antibiotic therapy in preterm PROM: a randomized prospective double blind trial. Am J Obstet Gynecol **163**:743, 1990.

Kaltreider DF, Kohl S: Epidemiology of preterm delivery. Clin Obstet Gynecol **23**:17, 1980.

Kappy KA, Cetrulo CL, Knuppel RE, et al: Premature rupture of the membranes: A conservative approach. Am J Obstet Gynecol **134**:655, 1979.

Kovacs D: Crystallization test for the diagnosis of ruptured membranes. Am J Obstet Gynecol **83**:1257, 1962.

Lavery JP, Miller CE: Deformation and creep in the human chorioamniotic sac. Am J Obstet Gynecol **134**:366, 1979.

Lavery JP, Miller CE, Knight RD: The effect of labor on the rheologic response of chorioamniotic membranes. Obstet Gynecol **60**:87, 1982.

Lebherz TB, Hellman LP, Madding R, et al: Double blind study of premature rupture of the membranes. N Engl J Med **303**:769, 1980.

Ledger WJ: Amnionitis, endometritis and premature rupture of membranes. *In* Current Concepts. Kalamazoo MI, The Upjohn Co., 1976.

Levy DL, Warsof SL: Oral ritodrine and preterm premature rupture of membranes. Obstet Gynecol **66**:621, 1985.

Lewis DF, Major CA, Towers CV, et al: Effects of digital vaginal exams on latency period in preterm premature rupture of membranes. (SPO Abstract 495.) Am J Obstet Gynecol **164**(2):381, 1991.

Liggins GC, Howie RN: A controlled trial of antepartum glucocorticoid treatment for the prevention of RDS in premature infants. Pediatr **50**:515, 1972.

Lonky NM, Hayashi RH: A proposed mechanism for premature rupture of membrane. Obstet Gynecol Surv **43**(1):22, 1988.

Magos AL, Nobem MCB, Wong Ten Yuen A, Rodeck CH: Controlled study comparing vaginal prostaglandin E$_2$ pessaries with intravenous oxytocin for the stimulation of labour after spontaneous rupture of the membranes. Br J Obstet Gynaecol **90**:726, 1983.

Major CA, Kitzmiller JL: Perinatal survival with expectant management of midtrimester rupture of membranes. Am J Obstet Gynecol **163**:838, 1990.

Martin DH, Koutsky L, Eschenbach DA, et al: Prematurity and perinatal mortality in pregnancies complicated by maternal *Chlamydia trachomatis* infections. JAMA **247**:1585, 1982.

McGregor JA, Lawellin D, Franco-Buff A, et al: Protease production by microorganisms associated with reproductive tract infection. Am J Obstet Gynecol **154**:109, 1986.

McGregor JA, French JI: Double blind, randomized, placebo controlled, prospective evaluation of the efficacy of short course erythromycin in prolonging gestation among women with preterm rupture of membranes. (Abstract #371.) Presented at the Ninth Annual Meeting of the Society of Perinatal Obstetricians. New Orleans, LA, 1989.

Mead PB: Management of the patient with premature rupture of the membranes. Clin Perinatol **7**:243, 1980.

Miller JM Jr, Kho MS, Brown HL, Gabert HA: Clinical chorioamnionitis is not predicted by an ultrasonic biophysical profile in patients with premature rupture of membranes. Obstet Gynecol **76**(6)1051: 1990.

Miller JM, Pupkin MJ, Crenshaw C: Premature labor and premature rupture of the membranes. Am J Obstet Gynecol **132**:1, 1978.

Miller JM, Hill GB, Welt S, et al: Bacterial colonization of amniotic fluid in the presence of ruptured membranes. Am J Obstet Gynecol **137**:451, 1980.

Minkoff H, Grunebaum AN, Schwarz RH, et al: Risk factors for prematurity and premature rupture of membranes: a prospective study of vaginal flora in pregnancy. Am J Obstet Gynecol **150**:965, 1984.

Moberg LJ, Garite TJ, Freeman RK: Fetal heart rate patterns and fetal distress in patients with preterm premature rupture of membranes. Obstet Gynecol **64**:60, 1984.

Moberg LJ, Garite TJ: Antepartum fetal heart rate testing in preterm PROM. Presented at the Seventh Annual Meeting of the Society of Perinatal Obstetricians. Lake Buena Vista, FL, February, 1987.

Monif GRG: Recurrent chorioamnionitis and maternal septicemia. A case of successful *in utero* therapy. Am J Obstet Gynecol **146**:334, 1983.

Morales WF, Diebel ND, Lazar AJ, et al: The effect of antenatal dexamethasone on the prevention of respiratory distress syndrome in preterm gestations with premature rupture of membranes. Am J Obstet Gynecol **154**:591, 1986.

Morales W, Angel J, O'Brien W, et al: Use of ampicillin and corticosteroids in PROM: a randomized study. Obstet Gynecol **73**:721, 1989.

Morales WJ: The effect of chorioamnionitis on developmental outcome of preterm infants at one year. Obstet Gynecol **70**:183, 1987.

Moretti M, Sibai BM: Maternal and perinatal outcome of expectant management of premature rupture of membranes in the midtrimester. Am J Obstet Gynecol **159**:390, 1988.

Naeye RL: Factors that predispose to premature rupture of the fetal membranes. Obstet Gynecol **69**:93, 1982.

Naeye RL: Coitus and associated amniotic fluid infections. N Engl J Med **22**:1198, 1979.

Nageotte MP, Freeman RK, Garite TJ, et al: Prophylactic intrapartum amnioinfusion in patients with preterm premature rupture of membranes. Am J Obstet Gynecol **153**:557, 1985.

Nelson LH, Meis PJ, Hatjis CG, et al: Premature rupture of membranes: a prospective, randomized evaluation of steroids, latent phase and expectant management. Obstet Gynecol **66**:55, 1985.

O'Keeffe DF, Garite TJ, Elliott JP, et al: The accuracy of estimated gestational age based on ultrasound measurement of the biparietal diameter in preterm premature rupture of the membranes. Am J Obstet Gynecol **151**:309, 1985.

Ohlsson A, Wong E: An analysis of antenatal tests to detect infection in preterm PROM. Am J Obstet **162**:809, 1990.

Ohlsson A: Treatments of preterm premature rupture of membranes: A meta-analysis. Am J Obstet Gynecol **160**:890, 1989.

Papageorgiou AN, Desgranges MF, Masson M, et al: The antenatal use of betamethasone in the prevention of respiratory distress syndrome: A controlled double-blind study. Pediatrics **63**:73, 1979.

Parry-Jones E, Priya S: A study of elasticity and tension of fetal membranes and of the relation of the area of the gestational sac to the area of the uterine cavity. Br J Obstet Gynaecol **83**:205, 1976.

Ray DR, Garite TJ: Prostaglandin E$_2$ for induction of labor in patients with PROM at term. Am J Obstet Gynecol **166**:836, 1992.

Regan TA, Chao S, James LS: Premature rupture of membrane, preterm delivery and group B streptococcal colonization of mothers. Am J Obstet Gynecol **141**:184, 1981.

Romero R: Infectious etiology of preterm labor. Presented at the World Symposium of Perinatal Medicine. San Francisco, Oct 31, 1991.

Romero R, Emamian M, Quintero R, et al: The value and limitations of the Gram stain examination in the diagnosis of intra-amniotic infection. Am J Obstet Gynecol **159**:114, 1988.

Rutherford SE, Phelan JP, Smith CV, Jacobs N: The four-quadrant assessment of amniotic fluid volume: An adjunct to antepartum fetal heart rate testing. Obstet Gynecol **70**:353, 1987.

Schreiber J, Benedetti T: Conservative management of preterm premature rupture of the fetal membranes in a low socioeconomic population. Am J Obstet Gynecol **136**:92, 1980.

Schutte MF, Treffers PE, Kloosterman GI, et al: Management of premature rupture of membranes: A risk of vaginal examination to the infant. Am J Obstet Gynecol **146**(4):395, 1983.

Schwarz R, Belizan JM, Nieto F, et al: Third progress report on the Latin American Collaborative Study on the effects of late rupture of membranes on labor and the neonate. *In* Gluck L (ed): Modern Perinatal Medicine. Chicago, Year Book, 1974.

Simpson GL, Harbert GM: Use of betamethasone in management of preterm gestation with premature rupture of membranes. Obstet Gynecol **66**:168, 1985.

Skinner SJM, Campos GA, Higgins GC: Collagen content of human

amniotic membranes: Effect of gestational length and premature rupture. Obstet Gynecol **57**:487, 1981.

Smith RP: A technic for the detection of rupture of the membranes. Obstet Gynecol **48**:172, 1976.

Spinnato JA, Shaver DC, Bray E, et al: Preterm premature rupture of the membranes with fetal pulmonary maturity present: A prospective study. Obstet Gynecol **69**:196, 1987.

Stedman CM, Crawford S, Staten E, et al: Management of preterm premature rupture of membranes: Assessing amniotic fluid in the vagina for phosphatidyl glycerol. Am J Obstet Gynecol **140**:34, 1981.

Taeusch HW, Frigoletto F, Kitzmiller J, et al: Risk of respiratory distress syndrome after prenatal dexamethasone treatment. Pediatrics **63**:64, 1979.

Taylor J, Garite TJ: Premature rupture of membranes before fetal viability. Obstet Gynecol **64**:615, 1984.

Varner MW, Galask RP: Conservative management of premature rupture of the membranes. Am J Obstet Gynecol **140**:39, 1981.

Vintzileos AM, Campbell WA, Nochimson DJ, et al: The fetal biophysical profile in patients with premature rupture of the membranes: An early predictor of fetal infection. Obstet Gynecol **152**:510, 1985a.

Vintzileos AM, Campbell WA, Rodis JF, et al: Comparison of six different ultrasonographic methods of predicting lethal fetal pulmonary hypoplasia. Am J Obstet Gynecol **161**:606, 1989.

Vintzileos AM, Campbell WA, Nochimson DJ, Weinbaum PJ: Fetal breathing as a predictor of infection in premature rupture of the membranes. Obstet Gynecol **67**:813, 1986.

Vintzileos AM, Campbell WA, Nochimson DJ, Weinbaum PJ: Degree of oligohydramnios and pregnancy outcome in patients with premature rupture of the membranes. Obstet Gynecol **66**:162, 1985b.

Wagner MV, Chin VP, Peters CJ, et al: A comparison of early and delayed induction of labor with spontaneous rupture of membranes at term. Obstet Gynecol **74**(1):93, 1989.

Webb GA: Maternal death associated with premature rupture of the membranes: An analysis of 54 cases. Am J Obstet Gynecol **98**:594, 1967.

Weiner CP, Renk K, Klugman M: The therapeutic efficacy and cost effectiveness of aggressive tocolysis for premature labor associated with PROM. Am J Obstet Gynecol **159**:216, 1988.

Westgren LM, Holmquist P, Svenningsen NW, et al: Intrapartum fetal monitoring in preterm deliveries: Prospective study. Obstet Gynecol **90**:726, 1983.

Wilson JC, Levy DC, Wilds PL: Premature rupture of membranes prior to term: Consequences of non-intervention. Obstet Gynecol **60**:601, 1982.

Yoder PR, Gibbs RS, Blanco JD, et al: A prospective, controlled study of maternal and perinatal outcome after intra-amniotic infection at term. Am J Obstet Gynecol **145**:695, 1983.

Young BK, Klein SA, Katz M, et al: Intravenous dexamethasone for prevention of neonatal respiratory distress: A prospective controlled study. Am J Obstet Gynecol **138**:203, 1980.

Zlatnick FJ, Cruikshank DP, Petzold CR, Galask RP: Amniocentesis in the identification of inapparent infection in preterm patients with premature rupture of the membranes. J Reprod Med **29**:656, 1984.

MATERNAL AND FETAL INFECTIONS

CHAPTER

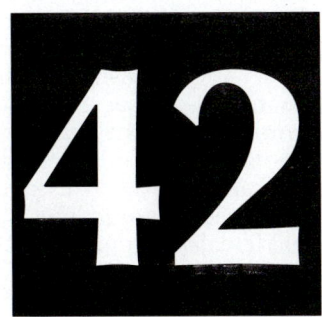

CLINICAL DISORDERS

RONALD S. GIBBS, M.D., AND RICHARD L. SWEET, M.D.

Within the last 25 years, infection and immunology have become central issues in the study of the pregnant woman and her fetus. In practice, clinical infectious disease problems are both common and potentially severe. They involve a wide range of organisms: group A and B streptococci, *Listeria monocytogenes, Escherichia coli*, the anaerobes, human immunodeficiency virus (HIV), herpes virus, rubella virus, cytomegaloviruses, mycoplasma, chlamydia, treponemes, and *Toxoplasma gondii*. They span a range of diseases and situations: premature rupture of the membranes, endometritis and consequent sepsis, pyelonephritis, pneumonia, and venereal diseases. They also lead to a variety of effects: abortion, malformation, congenital diseases, growth restriction, stillbirth, prematurity, sepsis, and shock. Of major importance is the link between immunology and infection on the one hand and two fundamental issues on the other: (1) the very existence of the fetus in the mother and (2) the pathogenesis of premature birth.

Interest and concern have arisen over the effect of human parvovirus and Lyme disease during pregnancy. In addition, new information is presented on hepatitis C (formerly non-A non-B transfusion-associated hepatitis), group B streptococcal infection, and herpes simplex.

BACTERIAL INFECTIONS

Urinary Tract Infections

Urinary tract infections are the most common medical complications of pregnancy. They may be either asymptomatic (asymptomatic bacteriuria of pregnancy) or symptomatic (cystitis, acute pyelonephritis).

Urinary tract infections are more common in females than in males. It has been suggested that this predominance is due to (1) a shorter urethra in the female, (2) continuous contamination of the external third of the urethra by pathogenic bacteria from the vagina and rectum, (3) the high probability that females do not empty their bladders as completely as males, and (4) movement of the bacteria into the female bladder during sexual intercourse.

Epidemiology

Obstetricians have long recognized the frequency and the seriousness of symptomatic urinary tract infections in pregnancy. Beginning in the mid-1950s, Kass demonstrated that significant bacteriuria can occur in the absence of symptoms or signs of urinary tract infections (Kass, 1960a, 1960b, 1973b; Kass and Zinner, 1969, 1973a). He established quantitative bacteriology as the indispensable laboratory aid for the diagnosis, follow-up, and confirmation of cure of urinary tract infection. Kass demonstrated that urinary bacterial counts on midstream voided urine specimens distinguished between contamination and infection with a high degree of accuracy. From these studies evolved the commonly accepted definition of asymptomatic bacteriuria: the presence of 10^5 or more colonies of a bacterial organism per milliliter of urine on two consecutive clean, midstream voided specimens in the absence of signs or symptoms of urinary tract infection. Persistent asymptomatic bacteriuria was identified in 6 per cent of pregnant patients. Acute pyelonephritis developed in 40 per cent of patients with the disorder who received a placebo; when bacteriuria was eliminated, pyelonephritis did not occur. Kass and Zinner also noted that rates of neonatal death and prematurity rates were two to three times greater in bacteriuric women receiving placebo than in nonbacteriuric women or bacteriuric women whose infection was eliminated by antibiotics. Kass concluded that detection of maternal bacteriuria would identify patients at risk for pyelonephritis and premature delivery, and he maintained that pyelonephritis in pregnancy could be prevented by detection and treatment of bacteriuria in early pregnancy. Moreover, Kass estimated that 10 per cent of premature births would be prevented by such a program.

It has long been recognized that symptomatic urinary tract infection is more frequently encountered in pregnant women. This suggests that some factors present during gestation allow bacteria to replicate in the urine and ascend to the upper urinary tract. Several findings support this view. The normal female urinary tract undergoes dramatic physiologic and anatomic changes during pregnancy, as discussed in Chapter 50. Briefly, a decrease in ureteric muscle tone and activity results in a lower rate of passage of urine throughout the urinary collecting system. The upper ureters and renal pelvices become dilated, resulting in a physiologic hydronephrosis of pregnancy. These changes are caused by the effects of progesterone on muscle tone and peristalsis and, more important, by mechanical obstruction by the enlarging uterus. Vesicle changes also occur in pregnancy; these include decreased tone, increased capacity, and incomplete emptying, all of which predispose to vesicoureteric reflux. Hypotonia of the vesicle musculature, vesicoureteric reflux, and dilatation of the uterers and renal pelvices result in static columns of urine in the ureters, which facilitate the ascending migration of bacteria to the upper urinary tract after bladder infection is established. The hypokinetic collecting system reduces urine flow, and urinary stasis occurs, predisposing to infection.

It is also possible that alterations in the physical and chemical properties of urine during pregnancy exacerbate bacteriuria, further predisposing to ascending infection. Because of the increased excretion of bicarbonate, urinary pH rises, encouraging bacterial growth. Glycosuria, which is common in pregnancy, may favor an increase in the rate of bacterial multiplication. The increased urinary excretion of estrogens may also be a factor in the pathogenesis of symptomatic urinary tract infection during pregnancy. It has been demonstrated in animal experiments that estrogen can enhance the growth of strains of *Escherichia coli* that cause pyelonephritis and predispose to renal infection. In addition, the renal medulla is particularly susceptible to infection because its hypertonic environment inhibits leukocyte migration, phagocytosis, and complement activity. The cumulative effect of these physiologic factors is an increased risk that infection in the bladder may ascend to the kidneys.

Pathogenic characteristics of microorganisms such as *E. coli* are major determinants of urinary tract infection. These include: (1) pili (adherence); (2) K antigen (antiphagocytic); (3) hemolysin (cytotoxic); and (4) antimicrobial resistance. Host susceptibility factors include: (1) anatomic or functional abnormalities of the urinary tract; (2) uroepithelial and vaginal epithelial cells with increased attachment of uropathogenic *E. coli*; and (3) nonsecretor status, which uncovers receptors for *E. coli* in uroepithelial and vaginal cells. In addition, an association has been reported between diaphragm plus spermicide use and urinary tract infections (Fihn et al., 1985). The spermicide alters the vaginal flora and promotes *E. coli* vaginal colonization.

It has been shown that most cases of asymptomatic bacteriuria of pregnancy are detected at initial prenatal visits and that relatively few pregnant women acquire bacteriuria after the initial visit. There is no evidence that bacteriuria is acquired between the time of conception and the first antenatal visit. In fact, there is good evidence that in many instances the bacteriuria antedates the pregnancy. The prevalence of asymptomatic bacteriuria in schoolgirls is approximately 1 per cent. There is a considerable increase in the rate of asymptomatic bacteriuria once a woman begins sexual activity. The prevalence of bacteriuria rises to 3.5 per cent in females 15 to 19 years old and increases thereafter at a rate of about 1 per cent for each decade of life. Several studies have shown that nonpregnant women have an incidence of asymptomatic bacteriuria comparable to that found in pregnant women in the same locale. It appears that most women in whom bacteriuria is first discovered during pregnancy have acquired asymptomatic bacteriuria earlier in life, the incidence of infection having increased as a result of sexual activity. Although pregnancy per se does not cause any major increase in incidence of bacteriuria, it does predispose to the development of acute pyelonephritis in bacteriuric patients.

Asymptomatic Bacteriuria

As a result of Kass's initial observations, considerable interest has focused on asymptomatic bacteriuria in pregnant women. It is generally accepted that untreated asymptomatic bacteriuria during pregnancy often leads to acute pyelonephritis. For this reason, it is clear that the presence of bacteriuria must be viewed with concern. Other claims, however, such as that asymptomatic bacteriuria predisposes the patient to anemia, preeclampsia, and chronic renal disease, are controversial and unproven. Even more controversial is the association of bacteriuria with prematurity and low birth weight. The prevalence of asymptomatic bacteriuria in pregnant women ranges from 2 to 11 per cent, a majority of investigations reporting 4 to 7 per cent. An increased prevalence of bacteriuria in females has been associated with the presence of sickle cell trait, lower socioeconomic status, reduced availability of medical care, and increased parity. *Escherichia coli* has been the predominant pathogen isolated in each study of asymptomatic bacteriuria and is cultured in 60 to 90 per cent of cases. The next most common organisms are *Proteus mirabilis*, *Klebsiella pneumoniae*, and the enterococci. Group B beta-hemolytic streptococci and *Staphylococcus saprophyticus* are also potential pathogens in the urinary tract during pregnancy.

BACTERIURIA AND PYELONEPHRITIS. Acute pyelonephritis, one of the most common medical complications of pregnancy, is a serious threat to maternal and fetal well-being. An association between acute pyelonephritis in pregnancy and premature delivery was recognized in the preantibiotic era, with prematurity rates of 20 to 50 per cent being reported. Studies made after the advent of antibiotics have confirmed this association between acute pyelonephritis and an increased risk of premature delivery. Endotoxin produced by gram-negative bacteria results in the release of cytokines such as tumor necrosis factor and interleukin-2, which can initiate the prostaglandin cascade and subsequent myometrial activity.

A significant factor in understanding the pathogenesis of pyelonephritis was the concept of quantitative urine culture, which made it possible to determine whether infection of the urinary tract was present without symptoms or signs. Early studies identified the presence of asymptomatic bacteriuria as the most significant factor associated with the development of acute pyelonephritis of pregnancy. As mentioned, Kass (1960b) noted that 20 to 40 per cent of pregnant women with asymptomatic bacteriuria who were receiving a placebo subsequently developed pyelonephritis. When the bacteriuria was treated and eliminated with antimicrobials, however, pyelonephritis did not occur. Subsequent studies have confirmed that pregnant women with untreated asymptomatic bacteriuria are at high risk (13.5 to 65 per cent) of developing acute pyelonephritis during pregnancy. Detection and treatment of asymptomatic bacteriuria significantly reduces the risk of developing pyelonephritis. Initially, it was believed that pyelonephritis, with its attendant maternal and fetal morbidity and mortality rates, could be completely prevented by detecting and treating bacteriuria early in pregnancy. However, subsequent studies have shown that a small proportion of women without bacteriuria at the first antenatal visit do develop pyelonephritis. The explanation for this phenomenon is that approximately 1 per cent of pregnant women who do not have asymptomatic bacteriuria at the first antenatal visit acquire it later in pregnancy. In pregnant women whose bacteriuria is treated, the reported incidence of pyelonephritis ranges from zero to 5.3 per cent, with an average of 2.9 per cent. In addition, pyelonephritis may develop in women with asymptomatic bacteriuria prior to their initial prenatal visit and thus before screening attempts. Detection and eradication by treatment of bacteriuria early in pregnancy should prevent pyelonephritis in at least 70 to 80 per cent of cases. The prevention rate could be improved if screening for bacteriuria were performed routinely several times throughout pregnancy.

Various techniques have been used to localize urinary infections. Direct methods include ureteric catheterization for culture and renal biopsy. Indirect measures include measurements of maximum urinary concentrating ability, serum antibodies against infecting organisms, antibody-coated bacteria in urinary sediment, pattern of response to therapy, and beta-glucuronidase excretion in urine, and bladder washout techniques. The results of these investigations suggest that renal involvement is already present in many pregnant women with bacteriuria, despite the absence of clinical evidence. On the basis of these attempts to localize the site of asymptomatic urinary tract infection, it has been suggested that 25 to 50 per cent of pregnant women with asymptomatic bacteriuria have renal tissue involvement and silent pyelonephritis. It is this subgroup that is at high risk for symptomatic pyelonephritis during pregnancy.

BACTERIURIA AND HYPERTENSION. An increased incidence of hypertensive disease of pregnancy has been alleged to exist in pregnant women with asymptomatic bacteriuria, although this issue is controversial. Some investigations have confirmed the association, but most studies have failed to document any relationship between bacteriuria and hypertension (Whalley, 1967; Whalley et al., 1965).

BACTERIURIA AND CHRONIC RENAL DISEASE. Although urinary tract infections are related to renal disease, the factors that determine their frequency in the etiology of chronic renal disease have not been defined. It has been estimated that 10 to 15 per cent of bacteriuric pregnant women are destined to have evidence of chronic pyelonephritis 10 to 12 years following delivery (Zinner and Kass, 1971). Renal failure ultimately develops in one of every 3000 pregnant women with bacteriuria. Because persistent bacteriuria, abnormal renal function, and radiologic evidence of chronic pyelonephritis are found so commonly in follow-up studies of patients with asymptomatic bacteriuria of pregnancy, long-term follow-up of women having bacteriuria is essential. Follow-up should include periodic urine cultures, treatment if bacteriuria persists or recurs, and intravenous pyelograms to detect urinary tract abnormalities that may be correctable. Such close surveillance and management may impede or prevent progression to end-stage renal disease.

BACTERIURIA AND LOW BIRTH WEIGHT. That acute pyelonephritis during pregnancy is associated with a significantly increased rate of prematurity is well documented. In contrast, the relationship of asymptomatic bacteriuria to premature delivery, babies who are small for gestational age, and fetal mortality remains controversial. Kass (1973b) initially reported that there is an association between asymptomatic bacteriuria and prematurity and that eradication of bacteriuria with antimicrobial therapy significantly reduces the rate of preterm delivery. He proposed that early detection and treatment of bacteriuria would prevent prematurity in 10 to 20 per cent of cases. It should be pointed out that the diagnosis of "prematurity" in the initial study was based entirely on a birth weight of 2500 gm or less. Subsequently, numerous studies have demonstrated conflicting results regarding bacteriuria and prematurity. Kincaid-Smith and Bullen (1965) first suggested the hypothesis that underlying renal disease was the major cause for the excessive risk of prematurity or low birth weight among bacteriuric pregnant women. The varying definitions for prematurity used in the literature have contributed to the confusion, although the majority of authors base their definitions on birth weight of less than 2500 gm. A possible mechanism for initiating premature labor in such cases could be the release of prostaglandins as a result of decidual necrosis. Studies have shown that certain bacteria, including the gram-negative facultatives such as *E. coli* commonly found in urinary tract infections, can produce the precursors for prostaglandin such as phospholipase A_2 (Bejar et al., 1981).

Bacteriuria is only one of many factors that may influence the onset of premature labor. Because the incidences of both pregnancy bacteriuria and prematurity increase with decreasing socioeconomic status, any relationship between bacteriuria and gestational length and birth weight may be complex and difficult to establish. The design of the majority of studies can be criticized because they involve small numbers of subjects. In an attempt to resolve this controversy, Romero and colleagues utilized the technique of meta-analysis to assess the relationship between ASB and preterm delivery and/or low birth weight (Romero et al., 1989). Although only five of the 17 studies included in the analysis demonstrated a statistically significant increase in low-birth-weight infants among patients with bacteriuria, meta-analysis confirmed a statistically significant increased risk for low-birth-weight infants among bacteriuric women. Similarly, meta-analysis demonstrated a significant association between bacteriuria and preterm delivery, although only two of four accepted studies demonstrated a statistically significant risk. Finally, this meta-analysis confirmed a statistically significant reduction in low birth weight among bacteriurics treated in eight placebo-controlled treatment trials. Thus it appears that maternal ASB is a risk factor for preterm delivery and low birth weight, and this risk can be reduced by screening and treatment of ASB in pregnant women (Mittendorf et al., 1992).

Treatment of Bacteriuria. Detection and treatment of asymptomatic bacteriuria gives the obstetrician an opportunity to prevent a significant medical complication of pregnancy. Screening at the original antenatal visit, appropriate treatment, and eradication of bacteriuria lead to the prevention of antenatal acute pyelonephritis in 70 to 80 per cent of cases. Such a reduction, with its attendant decline in risk to mother and fetus, is itself sufficient justification for such a screening program. In addition, as discussed above, screening and treatment of ASB may also significantly reduce the risk for preterm delivery and low-birth-weight infants.

Treatment should be designed to maintain sterile urine throughout pregnancy, with the shortest possible course of antimicrobial agents in order to minimize the toxic effects of these drugs in mother and fetus. Most antibacterial agents are excreted by glomerular filtration, and, as a result, therapeutic concentrations are readily achieved in the urine. In fact, the concentration of these drugs in the urine greatly exceeds that required for the treatment of most urinary tract infections. Even those drugs that do not reach therapeutic concentrations in serum, such as nitrofurantoin, are present in significant concentrations in urine. Investigations indicate that short courses of treatment (1 to 3 weeks) with sulfonamides, ampicillin, or nitrofurantoin are as effective as continuous therapy and eliminate the bacteriuria in 70 to 90 per cent of patients. No single agent seems better than any other. At present, it is generally accepted that short courses of treatment are preferable because the duration of initial therapy does not affect the recurrence rate, a short course minimizes the adverse drug effects in mother and fetus, emergence of resistant bacteria is discouraged, and costs are kept to a minimum.

When asymptomatic bacteriuria is detected, treatment generally consists of a 10-day course of a short-acting sulfonamide, nitrofurantoin, oral cephalosporin, or ampicillin. *E. coli* has been the offending organism in the vast majority of bacteriuric patients, and most strains of *E. coli* that are not hospital-acquired are sensitive to the urinary drug levels obtained with sulfisoxazole. In the last trimester, ampicillin is the drug of choice because sulfa compounds compete with bilirubin for albumin-binding titer and may theoretically produce hyperbilirubinemia in the newborn.

When short courses of therapy are prescribed for asymptomatic bacteriuria during pregnancy, continuous surveillance for recurrent bacteriuria by repeated urine cultures is essential. Persistent asymptomatic bacteriuria is frequently, although by no means invariably, associated with evidence on excretory urography of some abnormality. Persistent asymptomatic bacteriuria may necessitate continuous antimicrobial therapy for the duration of pregnancy. A single daily dose of nitrofurantoin, 100 mg, preferably after the evening meal, is recommended. Alternatively, short-acting sulfonamide preparations may be prescribed.

It is our policy to treat patients with recurrent asymptomatic bacteriuria with antimicrobials on the basis of the microorganism's sensitivities for the remainder of the pregnancy and 2 weeks postpartum. The duration of therapy for urinary tract infections remains a subject of considerable debate. Although 7 to 14 days still constitute the usual and approved duration, recent studies suggest that this long period is probably not suitable for all infections. An increasing number of reports have confirmed that an uncomplicated urinary tract infection can be treated as well with 4 days or even 1 day of therapy, especially if the bacteria are not antibody-coated. Conversely, if the bacteria are antibody-coated, suggesting renal involvement, prolonged therapy is recommended. However, single-dose therapy for urinary tract infections is substantially less effective in pregnant women than in nonpregnant women. Harris et al. (1982) reported failure rates with single-dose therapy for asymptomatic bacteriuria in pregnancy of 29 per cent, 45 per cent, 27 per cent and 25 per cent for ampicillin 2 gm, cephalexin 2 gm, nitrofurantoin 100 mg, and sulfisoxazole 2 gm respectively. Thus, we favor continued use of the standard 10-day course for treatment of asymptomatic bacteriuria in pregnancy.

Cystitis in Pregnancy

Acute cystitis is a syndrome characterized by urinary urgency and frequency, dysuria, and suprapubic discomfort in the absence of systemic symptoms such as fever and tenderness at the costovertebral angle. Gross hematuria may be present; the urine culture is invariably positive for bacterial growth, with more than 100,000 colonies/ml. Stamm and co-workers (1982) have suggested that a urine culture positive for bacterial growth with more than 100 colonies/ml, in combination with symptoms of dysuria and frequency, is sufficient to confirm the diagnosis of cystitis.

Harris and Gilstrap (1974) reported a recurrence rate of 1.3 per cent for cystitis during pregnancy. Although the increase in diagnosis and treatment of asymptomatic bacteriuria has resulted in a decreasing incidence of pyelonephritis at their institution, the incidence of acute cystitis has remained constant. On initial urine cultures, 64 per cent of the cystitis patients had negative cultures, in contrast to the patients with asymptomatic bacteriuria and acute pyelonephritis, only a minority of whom had negative initial screening cultures. Harris and Gilstrap (1974) noted that the recurrence pattern in patients with acute cystitis was also different from that in patients with either bacteriuria or acute pyelonephritis. Disease recurred in 75 per cent of patients with acute pyelonephritis who were not given suppressive antimicrobial therapy; only 17 per cent of patients with acute cystitis subsequently had positive cultures.

Once cystitis is suspected, either a catheterized specimen or a clean-catch midstream specimen should be obtained prior to the institution of antibiotic therapy, for urinalysis and culture and sensitivity tests. Because of the symptomatology of acute cystitis and the danger of upward extension of the infection to the kidney, it is not possible to await the results of culture. The constellation of symtoms and demonstration by urinalysis of white cells and bacteria should be sufficient grounds for beginning therapy. Pregnant women with acute cystitis should receive immediate therapy with nitrofurantoin, sulfisoxazole, or ampicillin. The organisms most commonly isolated in acute cystitis are *E. coli*, other gram-negative facultative organisms, and group B streptococci, all of which are equally sensitive to the three agents recommended. The duration of therapy in cystitis also remains a subject of considerable debate; the usual recommendation is 7 to 14 days. Although recent observations in nonpregnant women suggest that a shorter course may be effective in the absence of upper urinary tract disease during pregnancy, we prefer the standard 10-day course. Follow-up urine cultures should be performed in order to determine the effectiveness of therapy.

Acute Pyelonephritis in Pregnancy

The most common serious urinary tract complication that occurs during pregnancy is acute pyelonephritis. The overall incidence is reported to be 1 to 2.5 per cent of all obstetric patients. Symptoms and signs of pyelonephritis include shaking chills, fever, flank pain, nausea and vomiting, urinary frequency and urgency, dysuria, and costovertebral angle tenderness; laboratory tests reveal pyuria and bacteriuria. The pregnant woman with pyelonephritis generally has clear-cut signs and symptoms that allow one to easily make the diagnosis; most have chills and documented fever and complain of back pain (85 per cent). A significant number (40 per cent) have symptoms of lower urinary tract infection, e.g., dysuria and frequency. Fever is universal, and the diagnosis should be only tentative in its absence.

Not only is pyelonephritis a serious risk for preterm labor and delivery, but it also poses a serious threat to maternal well-being. Affected patients should be hospitalized for vigorous treatment with intravenous fluids and antimicrobial agents and close monitoring of renal function. Nausea, vomiting, anorexia, and pyrexia frequently result in severe dehydration. Cunningham and co-workers (1987) reported that acute pyelonephritis of pregnancy may be complicated by adult respiratory distress syndrome (ARDS). A recent report by Towers et al. identified the following as risk factors for pulmonary injury in antepartum pyelonephritis: (1) maternal heart rate ≥ 110 per minute; (2) use of a tocolytic agent; (3) use of ampicillin alone; (4) temperature $\geq 103°F$ in first 24 hours; and (5) fluid overload $>3L$ (Towers et al., 1991). Moreover, approximately 20 per cent of affected women have transient renal dysfunction as documented by decreased creatinine clearance (Gilstrap et al., 1981). This latter complication is especially important when the antimicrobial agent used is nephrotoxic or is eliminated by the kidney. For this reason aminoglycosides should be used with caution. Also associated with pyelonephritis are hematologic (thrombocytopenia) and hemodynamic (endotoxinemia, septic shock) dysfunction. Important management points include hydration and lowering of the elevated temperature, monitoring of the renal function with meticulous attention to intake and output, and close observation for the shock that occurs in gram-negative infections. Approximately 10 per cent will be shown to have bacteremia if appropriate blood cultures are taken.

As stated above, administration of aminoglycosides requires particular caution and is not recommended for pregnant patients with pyelonephritis unless the identified microorganism is resistant to, or the patient has had an allergic reaction to, other antimicrobials. The one exception is the patient who appears septic, with possibility of septic shock. In these patients, aminoglycosides should be utilized to cover the more resistant organisms and provide bactericidal activity. The choice of antimicrobials is empiric. The most common isolates are *E. coli*, organisms of the Klebsiella-Enterobacter group, and Proteus species. Dunlow and Duff studied 121 pregnant women with pyelonephritis and noted that the most frequent pathogens were *E. coli* (80 per cent), *Klebsiella pneumoniae* (7.4 per cent), *S. aureus* (6 per cent), and *Proteus mirabilis* (2 per cent) (Dunlow and Duff, 1990). In the past, therapy with ampicillin, 1 to 2 gm intravenously every 6 hours, was sufficient. Clinicians should be aware that in many hospitals even community-acquired *E. coli* may be resistant to ampicillin. In the study by Dunlow and Duff, 26 per cent of their uropathogens were ampicillin-resistant, whereas only 4 per cent were resistant to first-generation cephalosporins (e.g., cephalothin, cefazolin). Thus use of cephalosporins has replaced ampicillin as the choice for single-agent therapy for acute pyelonephritis in pregnancy. In cases of clinical sepsis, the combination of either ampicillin or a cephalosporin with an aminoglycoside, such as gentamicin or tobramycin, is usually indicated. The dosage recommended for aminoglycosides is 3 to 5 mg/kg/24 hours in three divided doses. Serum levels in pregnant women receiving aminoglycosides may be monitored selectively to ensure adequate dosage and prevent toxicity. Alternatively, a third-generation cephalosporin such as ceftriaxone, cefotaxime, or ceftizoxime may be used in such patients. With intravenous antimicrobial therapy, 85 per cent of patients become afebrile within 48 hours and 97 per cent within 4 days. If resolution does not occur and the fever continues, the possibilities of resistant organisms and obstructive uropathy must be considered. A change of antibiotics, on the basis of microorganism sensitivities found on urine culture, may be necessary.

Angel and co-workers (1990) recently suggested that oral outpatient antimicrobial therapy was an acceptable alternative to inpatient parenteral therapy. However, 13 (14 per cent) of the 90 patients had bacteremia, and no clinical finding at presentation was predictive of bacteremia. If the bacteremic patients are included in the analysis, oral therapy was successful in only 71 per cent of cases, which is unacceptable with pyelonephritis and its associated risk for preterm labor and delivery and septic shock. Thus we recommend hospitalization, close monitoring of mother and fetus, and parenteral treatment of acute pyelonephritis in pregnancy.

The incidence of recurrence of acute pyelonephritis during the same gestation is reported to be between 10 and 18 per cent. In a retrospective analysis, Harris and Gilstrap (1974) reported that patients with acute pyelonephritis who did not receive suppressive antimicrobial therapy for the remainder of gestation had a 60 per cent rate of recurrence that required rehospitalization. Incidence of recurrence and rehospitalization in patients who received suppressive antimicrobial therapy for the duration of the gestation was 2.7 per cent. Suppression is accomplished with 100 mg nitrofurantoin each night at bedtime. Alternatively, short-acting sulfonamides or ampicillin may be given in similarly low dosage. An acceptable alternative to suppressive therapy is the continued examination every 2 weeks of urine cultures for bacteriuria with prompt treatment if it is found.

Intra-Amniotic Infection

Bacterial infection of the amniotic cavity is an important cause of perinatal mortality and maternal morbidity. A number of terms have been used, including *clinical chorioamnionitis, amnionitis, intrapartum infection, amniotic fluid infection,* and *intra-amniotic infection* (IAI). The last designation is used here to distinguish this clinical syndrome from asymptomatic bacterial colonization of amniotic fluid and from histologic inflammation of the placenta. Clinically evident IAI occurs in 0.5 to 10 per cent of pregnancies (Gibbs and Duff, 1991).

PATHOGENESIS. With the onset of labor or with rupture of membranes, bacteria from the lower genital tract commonly ascend into the amniotic cavity. This is the most common pathway for development of IAI. Occasional cases of IAI in the absence of membrane rupture or labor support a presumed hematogenous or transplacental route of infection. Fulminant IAI with intact membranes may be caused by *Listeria monocytogenes.* Maternal sepsis with this aerobic gram-positive rod often appears as a maternal flu-like illness and may result in fetal demise. In an outbreak caused by contaminated Mexican-style cheese, several maternal deaths occurred. Less commonly, IAI may develop as a consequence of obstetric procedures such as cervical cerclage, diagnostic amniocentesis, intrauterine transfusion, and percutaneous umbilical blood sampling. The absolute risk is small with all of these procedures—IAI may develop in 2 to 8 per cent of patients after cerclage, 0 to 1 per cent after amniocentesis, and up to 5 per cent after intrauterine transfusion.

MICROBIOLOGY. As with many other pelvic infections, IAI is often polymicrobial in origin. In a controlled study, Gibbs and colleagues (1982) collected amniotic fluid from patients with clinical IAI. Characteristics of these cultures are shown in Table 42–1. In the amniotic fluid of patients with IAI, the most common organisms were *Bacteroides* species, 25 per cent; group B streptococci, 12 per cent; other aerobic streptococci, 13 per cent; *Escherichia coli,* 10 per cent; and other aerobic gram-negative rods, 10 per cent.

A role for genital mycoplasmas has been suggested by case reports isolating them in amniotic fluid of clinically infected patients and by a controlled study reporting that 35 per cent of fluid specimens from patients with IAI yielded *M. hominis,* whereas only 8 per cent of matched control fluids had *M. hominis* (P <0.001) (Blanco et al., 1983). Present evidence suggests a small, if any, role for *Chlamydia trachomatis* in amniotic fluid infections. This organism is rarely isolated from amniotic cells in cases of IAI, and no significant antibody changes to *C. trachomatis* have been noted in sera of women with IAI. Pregnant women with cervical *C. trachomatis* infections have not been found to have higher rates of intrapartum fever (Sweet et al., 1987).

DIAGNOSIS. The diagnosis of intra-amniotic infection requires a high index of suspicion. Usual laboratory indicators of infection, such as positive stains for organisms or leukocytes and positive cultures, are found much more frequently than in clinically evident infection. Diagnosis is usually based upon maternal fever, maternal or fetal tachycardia, uterine tenderness, foul odor of the amniotic fluid, and leukocytosis.

TABLE 42–1. Characteristics of Amniotic Fluid from Patients with Intra-amniotic Infection and from Controls

	PATIENTS WITH INFECTION	MATCHED CONTROLS
Number studied	52	52
Mean number of isolates	2.2	1.2
Number with anaerobes	29	13
Number with 10^2 cfu/ml	42	16
Number with no bacterial growth	3	13
Number with high-virulence isolates	42	12
Number with low-virulence isolates	7	27

In patients with fever, two sets of blood cultures should be drawn; however, studies have found that bacteremia occurs in only 10 per cent. Because peripheral blood leukocytosis occurs commonly in normal labor, this result is not always indicative of infection.

Direct examination of the amniotic fluid may provide important diagnostic information. We have found that samples can be collected by aspiration through an intrauterine pressure catheter in 50 per cent of cases. Positive amniotic fluid Gram stains for bacteria or leukocytes occur significantly more often in cases of IAI than in matched controls (Gibbs et al., 1982). In patients with suspected amnionitis, presence of leukocyte esterase in the amniotic fluid has shown excellent sensitivity and specificity in one study. Low amniotic fluid glucose levels (variously defined as <5 to 25 mg/dl) have been a good predictor of a positive amniotic fluid culture, but a poorer predictor of clinical IAI. Maternal fever is recognized as a high-risk factor for neonatal sepsis. However, immediately after birth, making the diagnosis of neonatal septicemia is difficult. The neonate's response to infection is impaired, and his reaction is often nonspecific.

MANAGEMENT. In broad principle, investigators agree that in this situation delivery of the fetus is necessary for treatment with antibiotics; however, specific points of management are unresolved.

Regarding the timing of delivery, in recent studies excellent maternal-neonatal outcome has been reported without use of arbitrary time limits. Cesarean delivery was performed for standard obstetric indications and not for IAI alone. The mean time from diagnosis of IAI to delivery was between 3 and 5 hours. No critical interval from diagnosis of amnionitis to delivery could be identified. The preferred route of delivery is also unclear. Cesarean section rates are higher among patients with IAI, running two to three times greater than in the general population. Some investigators advocate the extraperitoneal procedure. Although this approach avoids contamination of the abdominal cavity, it is more difficult to execute than the transperitoneal approach. Inadvertent entry into the peritoneum or bladder may also occur, and the teaching of this technique has declined to the extent that most practitioners are not familiar with it. Yonekura and colleagues (1983) compared 26 extraperitoneal (Norton technique) sections with 65 transperitoneal, low-cervical cesarean sections in patients with clinical amnionitis. There were no significant differences in wound infections (11.5 per cent in extraperitoneal versus 14 per cent in transperitoneal sections), postpartum hospital stay (5.31 ± 1.35 days versus 4.81 ± 1.95 days, respectively), or Apgar scores (11 per cent less than 7 at 5 minutes in both groups). There were no cases of septic pelvic thrombophlebitis or pelvic abscess. Thus, there was no advantage to extraperitoneal section.

Also, fundamental questions have been raised regarding antibiotic administration. Many authors begin treatment immediately in the belief that they are limiting maternal sepsis and initiating therapy to the fetus. Others defer antibiotic use until after delivery to avoid masking sepsis of the newborn. Three recent comparative studies have demonstrated a significant

advantage of intrapartum over immediate postpartum antibiotic treatment (Table 42–2). In a randomized trial Sperling and co-workers (1987) reported a lower incidence of neonatal sepsis when antibiotic treatment was begun intrapartum than when treatment was begun immediately postpartum. In a randomized trial, Gibbs and colleagues used ampicillin (2 mg IV every 6 hours) plus gentamicin (1.5 mg/kg every 8 hours), initiating treatment either intrapartum or immediately postpartum. In addition, clindamycin was used after cord clamping if cesarean delivery was performed because of the high failure rate of ampicillin and gentamicin alone. Maternal outcome was improved and confirmed neonatal sepsis was decreased by intrapartum treatment (Gibbs et al., 1988). Other initial regimens employing cefoxitin alone or ampicillin plus a new cephalosporin may be equally effective, but no comparative trials have been performed.

Pharmacokinetic studies in early pregnancy show that ampicillin concentrations in maternal and fetal sera are comparable 120 minutes after administration. Benzylpenicillin (penicillin G) levels in fetal serum are one-third the maternal levels 120 minutes after administration. For this reason, ampicillin may be preferable to penicillin G in the treatment of IAI. In late pregnancy, gentamicin also crosses the placenta rapidly; however, peak fetal levels may be low, especially since maternal levels are often subtherapeutic. An initial gentamicin dose of at least 1.5 to 2.0 mg/kg is indicated. As an alternative, use of a newer penicillin or cephalosporin with excellent aerobic gram-negative activity might be suggested. However, there is no reported experience with these antibiotics in IAI. For ampicillin and aminoglycosides, levels in AF are usually below fetal serum levels, and peak AF concentrations may be attained only after 2 to 6 hours.

OUTCOME. Since 1979, reports have provided systematically collected data on the outcome for mothers and neonates in pregnancies complicated by intraamniotic infection. These studies have generally shown a vastly improved perinatal outcome compared with older studies. In retrospective studies, maternal outcome was excellent, with no deaths, few cases of septic shock, and rare pelvic abscesses. The cesarean delivery rate was increased in all studies, usually because of dystocia. Nearly all abdominal deliveries were by the transperitoneal approach. Hysterectomy was reserved for cases involving additional problems such as hemorrhage.

Perinatal mortality is increased in cases of IAI, but little of the excess mortality can be attributed to infection per se. Among term infants born after IAI, perinatal mortality is less than 1 per cent.

TABLE 42–2. Neonatal Sepsis is Decreased by Intrapartum Antibiotic Treatment in Cases of IAI

	NEONATAL SEPSIS RATE		
STUDY	INTRAPARTUM TREATMENT	P	NEONATAL TREATMENT
Sperling, 1987 (n = 257)	2.8%	.001	19.6%
Gilstrap, 1988 (n = 273)	1.5%	.06	5.7%
Gibbs, 1988 (n = 45)	0	.03	21%

Yoder and colleagues (1983) provided a prospective, case-controlled study of 67 patients with microbiologically confirmed intra-amniotic infection at term. There was only one perinatal death (unrelated to infection). Cerebrospinal fluid cultures were negative in all 49 infants sampled, and there was no clinical evidence of meningitis. Chest radiographs were interpreted as "possible" pneumonia in 20 per cent and as unequivocal pneumonia in only 4 per cent. Neonatal bacteremia was documented in 8 per cent. There was no significant difference in the frequency of low Apgar scores between the IAI and control groups.

Preterm neonates have a higher frequency of complications if they are delivered of mothers with IAI. Garite and Freeman (1982) noted that the perinatal death rate was significantly higher in 47 preterm neonates with IAI than in 204 neonates with similar birth weights. The group with IAI also had a significantly higher number (13 per cent as opposed to 3 per cent, P <.05) with respiratory distress syndrome (RDS) and total infection. Similar results were reported by Morales in a larger study (1987). In a retrospective case-controlled study, Ferguson and co-workers (1985) reported on perinatal outcome after chorioamnionitis. The next liveborn infant matched for birth weight within 100 gm and gestational age within 2 weeks served as the control for each case. Seventy per cent of newborns weighed less than 2500 gm. In 116 matched pairs, the authors found more deaths (20 per cent versus 11 per cent), more sepsis (6 per cent versus 2 per cent), and more asphyxia (27 per cent versus 16 per cent) in the chorioamnionitis group. None of these differences was statistically significant. However, it is possible that these are true differences and that this study may contain a beta error. Hardt and colleagues (1985), in their follow-up of preterm infants (<2000 gm) born after chorioamnionitis, found a significantly lower mental development index (Bayley scale) compared with preterm controls.

Patients with IAI are more likely to have cesarean delivery. Although some physicians may hurry to perform abdominal delivery because of concern for the infant, women with IAI (or with high-virulence bacteria in the amniotic fluid) often have uterine dysfunction, a poorer response to oxytocin, and abnormal cervical dilatation even when uterine activity is adequate. It is likely that these abnormal labor characteristics are the reason for the apparently excessive cesarean section rate. Thus, intra-amniotic infection has a significant adverse effect upon the mother and neonate, but vigorous antibiotic therapy and reasonably prompt delivery result in an excellent prognosis, especially for the mother and the term neonate. When the combination of prematurity and amnionitis occurs, serious sequelae are more likely for the neonate.

Postpartum Infection

Epidemiology

Many studies have reported the incidence of "standard puerperal morbidity," which is defined by the United States Joint Committee on Maternal Welfare as "a temperature of 100.4° (38.0°C), the temperature to occur in any two of the first 10 days postpartum, exclusive of the first 24 hours, and to be taken by mouth by a standard technique at least four times daily." Yet the full criteria of the original definition can no longer be applied because of early patient discharge practices. In addition, many infected patients respond to antibiotics so quickly that they do not meet the temperature criteria for standard disease. Also, in some institutions, antibiotics have been administered so commonly that this practice might be responsible for a deceptively low morbidity rate.

Low-grade fever occurs commonly in the postpartum period and often resolves spontaneously. When fever is caused by infection, the genital tract is the most common source in most reports, but the urinary tract may also be involved. Less common sources of bacterial infection are the breasts and lungs.

At present, the rate of postpartum infection rarely exceeds 3 per cent after vaginal delivery, but is 5 to 10 times higher after cesarean section. Although the absolute risk of death from postpartum infection is extremely low, infection continues to account for about 15 per cent of maternal deaths in the United States.

Risk Factors

Risk factors for puerperal infection are traditionally considered to be as follows (Gibbs, 1980):

CESAREAN SECTION. For both frequency and severity of pelvic infection, cesarean section has emerged in the last few decades as the major predisposing clinical factor. This observation is of particular importance because of increasing cesarean section rates. Compared with patients delivered vaginally, those delivered by cesarean section have a five- to 30-fold increase in risk of puerperal infection. Published accounts of post-cesarean section infection reveal that endometritis occurs in 12 to 51 per cent. Although endometritis usually is a mild infection responding within a few days to antibiotic therapy, serious infectious complications may result. Bacteremia develops in 8 to 20 per cent, and other serious complications—abscess, evisceration, presumed septic pelvic thrombophlebitis—occur in 1 to 2 per cent of indigent patients with endometritis after cesarean section.

Studies have attempted to correlate postoperative infection with results of culture of the amniotic fluid obtained at cesarean section. Simply qualitative cultures have not been satisfactory, inasmuch as positive cultures per se may be obtained in many patients who do not develop infection. Conversely, some patients with sterile amniotic fluid subsequently develop puerperal infection. Better correlations have been obtained when quantitative cultures were obtained and high-virulence organisms were distinguished from low-virulence organisms.

LABOR AND RUPTURE OF THE MEMBRANES. Numerous studies have documented maternal and perinatal problems accompanying either prolonged or premature rupture of membranes. In recent years, reports have emphasized the major influence of rupture and labor on infection following cesarean section.

SOCIOECONOMIC STATUS. Most reports indicate that

indigent patients regardless of race have higher puerperal infection rates than do middle-class patients, especially in the presence of other major risk factors such as premature rupture and cesarean section. Possible explanations may indicate differences in flora, hygiene, nutrition, and amniotic fluid bacterial inhibition. Indigent patients may also have more examinations during labor and longer labor.

VAGINAL EXAMINATION. Two decades ago, clinical studies demonstrated that vaginal examination in labor carried no greater infection risk than did rectal examination. Whether the number of vaginal examinations is a separate risk factor is difficult to determine because it is usually a co-variable of the duration of labor. Using a multivariant analysis, Gibbs and coworkers (1978) found that the number of examinations was a definite risk factor for puerperal infection following cesarean section.

INTERNAL FETAL MONITORING. A fundamental principle of infectious disease prevention is that foreign bodies increase the risk of bacterial infection. Prominent examples are urinary bladder and intravenous catheters. Among gynecologic patients, users of intrauterine devices are at increased risk for pelvic inflammatory disease. It is thus not surprising that the use of internal fetal monitoring has been accompanied by concerns about increased intrauterine infection. Because physicians often use internal fetal monitoring in patients with difficult labor, it is difficult to separate the role of this procedure from other major determinants, notably cesarean section, premature rupture, and labor. Most studies conclude, however, that fetal monitoring plays little or no role (Gibbs et al., 1978).

OTHER RISK FACTORS. It is reasonable to expect that major cervical and vaginal *trauma* will increase the likelihood of infection by providing a weakened host and a favorable environment for bacterial growth; yet only a small percentage of infected women sustain major trauma at delivery. The association of *anemia* with puerperal infection has been well recognized, but a cause-and-effect relationship has not been established; perhaps anemia is merely a marker for poor nutrition or lower socioeconomic status. Among patients undergoing cesarean section, *obesity* has not been a consistent risk factor for genital tract infection, although obesity is a major risk factor for wound infection in general.

Recently, Newton and colleagues (1990) looked at clinical and microbiologic risk factors for endometritis in 607 asymptomatic women in labor, 100 of whom subsequently developed postpartum endometritis. Multivariate analysis using stepwise logistic regression identified cesarean section as the dominant overall predictive factor with a relative risk of 12.8. In patients undergoing cesarean section, prophylactic antibiotics played an important protective role (relative risk 0.54; $p<0.0002$), whereas highly virulent bacteria or *Mycoplasma hominis* in the amniotic fluid increased the risk of infection (relative risk 1.4; $p<0.01$). In patients undergoing vaginal delivery, organisms associated with bacterial vaginosis (i.e., anaerobes, *G. vaginalis* or *M. hominis*) were important for the development of endometritis (relative risk 14.2; $p<0.001$), as were aerobic gram-negative rods in the amniotic fluid (relative risk 4.2; $p<0.01$). Although clinical variables such as duration of labor, duration of rupture of membranes, and internal fetal monitoring were significantly associated with endometritis on univariate analysis, these clinical risk factors were not significant on multivariate analysis. It was concluded that clinical variables actually may be facilitators rather than predictors of endometritis.

Microbiology of Puerperal Infection

In most cases, endomyometritis appears to be a polymicrobial infection, involving organisms that have ascended from the lower genital tract. Because of contamination of "uterine" or "endometrial" samples with lower genital tract bacteria, many studies of the bacteriology of puerperal endometritis must be interpreted cautiously. In attempts to avoid contamination, others have used transfundal needle aspirations, culdocentesis, or double- or triple-lumen catheters. Although these techniques seem to have theoretic advantages, none has provided a satisfactory solution. The transabdominal, transfundal approach to the uterus is fraught with technical difficulties and possible complications (at least after cesarean section). Culdocentesis yields scanty material that may be contaminated with vaginal bacteria. Multiple-lumen catheters offer probable advantages, but may require detailed quantitative techniques to distinguish infected from uninfected patients (Watts et al., 1990).

Further information regarding the bacteriology of endomyometritis can be obtained from amniotic fluid specimens collected at cesarean birth from patients who develop postpartum infection (Newton, 1990). Combining this information with that from uterine samples of patients with postpartum infection, one may obtain the best bacteriologic information about puerperal endometritis. Aerobic isolates are present in about 70 per cent of cultures, and anaerobic isolates in about 80 per cent. The mean number of isolates is approximately two to three, with a range of one to eight or more. Common isolates from genital specimens of patients with endometritis are summarized in Table 42–3. *Neisseria gonorrhoeae* may be isolated, but usually in mixed culture; it does not have a major role. Other species such as *Gardnerella vaginalis* (formerly *H. vaginalis*), *Haemophilus influenzae*, *Streptococcus pneumoniae*, and *Listeria monocytogenes* have been reported as rare causes of endometritis.

In addition to those organisms, a number of others are commonly isolated from genital specimens of both infected and uninfected patients. These are generally organisms of very low virulence (often called "nonpathogens") such as lactobacilli, diphtheroids, *Staphylococcus epidermidis*, and propionibacteria.

Mycoplasma hominis and *Ureaplasma urealyticum* are also regularly found in genital specimens when special techniques are used. (Ureaplasma was formerly called T-mycoplasma.) Both mycoplasma and ureaplasma are distinctly different from bacteria because they have no cell walls. Ureaplasma and *M. hominis* are found in the vagina of a large percentage of women registering at prenatal clinics. Both organisms on occasion have been isolated from the blood of women with postpar-

TABLE 42–3. **Bacterial Isolates in Endometritis**

ORGANISM	FREQUENCY OF ISOLATION (%)	ANTIMICROBIALS OF CHOICE	COMMENTS
GRAM-POSITIVE AEROBES			
Group A streptococci (S. pyogenes)	1–2	Penicillin; erythromycin; cephalosporins	Typically, there is early onset and high fever. May cause epidemics.
Group B streptococci (S. agalacitae)	2–14	Same as for group A	Typical infection same as with group A. Does not cause maternal epidemics. Major cause of neonatal sepsis.
Group D enterococci (S. faecalis)	2–18	Penicillin plus aminoglycoside; ampicillin	Generally of low virulence. Resistant to penicillin alone, cephalosporins, aminoglycosides alone, and clindamycin. Common cause of endocarditis.
Viridans streptococci	10–15	Penicillin, erythromycin, cephalosporins	Low virulence, may be skin contaminant in blood cultures. Common cause of endocarditis.
Staphylococcus aureus	5	Penicillinase-resistant penicillin (oxacillin); cephalosporins; clindamycin	Uncommon but virulent isolate. Vancomycin may be needed in methicillin-resistant species.
GRAM-NEGATIVE AEROBES			
Escherichia coli	5–40	Gentamicin; but most are sensitive to cephalosporins and newer penicillins	Common isolate in bacteremic patients. May cause septic shock.
Klebsiella spp.	5–10	As for E. coli	
Proteus mirabilis	2–5	Usually susceptible to ampicillin	
Enterobacter spp.	1–2	Gentamicin; most are susceptible to cefamandole; usually resistant to ampicillin and older cephalosporins.	
Morganella morganii	1–2	As for Enterobacter spp.	Formerly was classified as Proteus morganii
Pseudomonas spp.	1	Gentamicin; carbenicillin, piperacillin, mezlocillin, cefoperazone, cefotaxime	Infrequent but highly resistant opportunist. Usually found in patients with previous antibiotic therapy.
Gardnerella vaginalis	25–38	Ampicillin	Requires selective media for proper isolation.
GRAM-POSITIVE ANAEROBES			
Peptostreptococci and peptococci (anaerobic staphylococci)	20–90	Penicillin; clindamycin; chloramphenicol; metronidazole; cefoxitin; erythromycin; cephalosporin	One of the most common isolates.
Clostridium perfringens	3–7	As for peptostreptococci	
Other Clostridium spp.	3–5	As for peptostreptococci	
GRAM-NEGATIVE ANAEROBES			
Bacteroides fragilis group	3–20	Clindamycin; chloramphenicol; metronidazole; cefoxitin	Commonly found in pelvic abscesses and presumably with septic pelvic thrombophlebitis. Includes B. fragilis, B. distansonis, B. thetaiotomicron, B. vulgatus, and B. ovatus.
Bacteroides bivius	10–25	Half are susceptible to penicillin; others may be treated like B. fragilis, and are also susceptible to most of the newer cephalosporins and penicillins	Newly recognized but common species.
Bacteroides melaninogenicus	5–20	As for B. bivius	
Fusobacterium spp.	5–20	As for peptostreptococci	
Genital mycoplasmas U. urealyticum	50–100	Erythromycin, tetracycline, quindones	Despite frequency of isolation, their role is unclear. Good response without specific antibiotic therapy.
M. hominis	20–35	Clindamycin, tetracycline, quinolones	
C. trachomatis	3	Erythromycin, clindamycin, tetracycline	

tum fever. The antibiotic of choice for these agents is tetracycline. Clindamycin or lincomycin may also be used to treat *M. hominis,* and erythomycin to treat ureaplasma. Penicillins, cephalosporins, and aminoglycosides are ineffective.

Chlamydia trachomatis, an obligate intracellular bacterium, is responsible for a number of genital infections (see later in this chapter). *C. trachomatis* is found in 5 to 10 per cent of cervical cultures from asymptomatic pregnant women and may be a cause of late postpartum infection, especially after vaginal delivery. Special culture technique employing McCoy cells is required for identification. The antibiotic of choice is tetracycline, with alternatives being erythromycin and sulfonamides.

Diagnosis and Treatment

The diagnosis of endomyometritis is usually based on symptoms of fever, malaise, abdominal pain, and purulent, foul lochia. However, not all patients manifest the complete picture. Indeed, many patients with group A or group B streptococcal bacteremia have no localizing signs at the onset of fever. In most cases, presenting signs and symptoms commonly develop within the first 2 to 7 days after delivery.

Appropriate laboratory procedures include a complete blood count, venous blood cultures, and a uterine tissue culture. Gram stain of the genital culture may be helpful when hemolytic streptococci, clostridia, or other anaerobes are suspected.

With general supportive therapy and appropriate antibiotics, most patients improve within a few days. Well-controlled, large-scale treatment studies are few and are restricted to use of the newer, more potent antimicrobials. Yet, among patients with endomyometritis after vaginal delivery, the rate of response is very high, even to therapy without good anaerobic activity (e.g., penicillin plus gentamicin). Reasonable regimens for treatment of cases of mild endometritis after vaginal delivery include cefoxitin, a broad-spectrum penicillin, a newer cephalosporin, a penicillin-beta lactamase inhibitor combination, or clindamycin-gentamicin. Other regimens may be equally effective. Causes of persistent fever include abscesses, septic pelvic thrombophlebitis, infection of another site, and noninfectious causes such as a drug reaction.

Among patients with endomyometritis after cesarean section, the response to antibiotics is less dramatic. Prospective studies have demonstrated the cure rate to be approximately 70 to 85 per cent for therapy with penicillin plus aminoglycoside. In about half the failures, the causes can be identified; they include a resistant organism, wound infection, pelvic hematoma or abscess, and presumed septic pelvic thrombophlebitis. As with infection after vaginal delivery, the cause of persistent fever may be infection in another site or a noninfectious source.

When initial therapy consists of clindamycin plus gentamicin, the response rate of endomyometritis after cesarean section is higher, and the rate of major infectious complications is reduced (DiZerega et al., 1979).

The combination of gentamicin and clindamycin is

not without its problems, however; in some recent trials, failure rates as high as 20 to 25 per cent were reported, which are considerably higher than the 0 to 14 per cent failure rates reported in the early 1980s. The decrease in response rate may be the result of the emerging importance of enterococci; the isolation of enterococci in endometrial cultures has been associated with an increased failure rate of the clindamycin-gentamicin combination. Furthermore, the use of both clindamycin and an aminoglycoside may be accompanied by potentially serious side effects. Diarrhea develops in 2 to 6 per cent of patients who are being treated with IV clindamycin. Pseudomembranous colitis, although rare in obstetric patients, also may occur, and although such patients are at low risk for aminoglycoside toxicity, nephrotoxicity and ototoxicity are possible. Moreover, pharmacokinetic studies indicate that serum aminoglycoside levels are likely to be below therapeutic levels when standard dosing regimens are used. Accordingly, the proper use of aminoglycosides may require determination of peak and trough levels in some patients. Routine determination of aminoglycoside levels is expensive, however, and may be unnecessary in most patients who are being treated with aminoglycosides for postpartum endometritis. Because most patients are at low risk and respond promptly to standard dosing regimens, the determination of aminoglycoside levels is necessary only in the following cases: in patients who are bacteremic or who do not respond to therapy; in those who are on prolonged therapy (i.e., >5 to 7 days); in obese patients (weight >30 per cent of ideal weight); and in patients who are renally compromised (although use of alternative antibiotics in this group would be preferable). The administration of two drugs may be more timeconsuming and more expensive than administration of a single antibiotic.

During the past decade, a number of new antibiotics were developed that may serve as alternatives to the clindamycin-gentamicin combination. Aztreonam (Azactam), the first monobactam, provides excellent coverage against aerobic gram-negative rods, including those that are resistant to many other antibiotics. It is a relatively safe drug and thus is an alternative to aminoglycosides in patients who are at risk for aminoglycoside toxicity. When used in combination with clindamycin, aztreonam has produced excellent results. In studies of endometritis following cesarean section, aztreonam, 2 gm IV every 8 hours, plus clindamycin, 600 mg every 6 hours, has compared favorably with gentamicin plus clindamycin. Overall, the clinical cure rate was excellent in both groups (91.4 per cent in the aztreonam group and 88.6 per cent in the gentamicin group). No patient experienced nephrotoxicity.

Although relatively little has been reported concerning its efficacy, metronidazole has also been used (in place of clindamycin) in combination with aminoglycosides for the treatment of postpartum endometritis and other pelvic infection. Although metronidazole has a somewhat broader *in vitro* spectrum against anaerobes, clindamycin has performed extremely well in eradicating anaerobic infection and affords the additional advantage of activity against important gram-positive aerobes such as group B streptococci and *Staphylococcus aureus*.

Extended-spectrum cephalosporin-like antibiotics, which were introduced in the mid-1970s, provide a higher degree of safety, favorable pharmacokinetics, and broad activity against obstetric and gynecologic pathogens. One of the first developed of these agents was cefoxitin, which possesses high activity against most organisms encountered in obstetric and gynecologic infection. When used alone, this well-studied antibiotic resulted in a cure rate greater than 90 per cent in most cases. Because of its relatively short half-life, cefoxitin must be administered at least every 6 hours.

A number of related antibiotics with broader activity and a longer half-life than cefoxitin have since been introduced. Some of these compounds, such as cefotetan, provide the advantage of 8- to 12-hour dosing. Even though many of these drugs have broader activity than cefoxitin, the overall response rates are similar. The potential benefits in using these drugs include the longer dosing interval and the lower direct and indirect administration costs.

Although the newer cephalosporins are well tolerated, the infrequent adverse side effects include allergic reactions, transient elevations in liver function test results, and, with some cephalosporins, bleeding disorders. These bleeding disorders have been associated with the presence of the methylthiotetrazole side chain on moxalactam, cefoperazone, and cefotetan. Although concerns about the safety of moxalactam have led to its infrequent use in obstetric and gynecologic infection, bleeding secondary to this agent rarely occurs (0.1 per cent). On the other hand, concerns about bleeding have not been an impediment to the use of cefotetan.

Like the extended-spectrum cephalosporins, the extended-spectrum penicillins (ureidopenicillins) offer increased activity against many of the organisms that cause pelvic infection. These compounds are active against enterococci but not against some aerobic gram-negative rods and some strains of *S. aureus*. The reported cure rate was approximately 75 to 91 per cent, which was comparable to cure rates achieved with cefoxitin or clindamycin plus gentamicin. Side effects of piperacillin occur infrequently and are generally mild; the most common ones are thrombophlebitis (1 to 2 per cent) and allergic reactions. Large doses of piperacillin (e.g., 4 gm every 6 hours) have been used in clinical trials with a correspondingly high cost.

Another therapeutic option involves combination of a penicillin with a β-lactamase inhibitor. Available parenteral combinations include ticarcillin plus clavulanic acid (Timentin) and ampicillin plus sulbactam (Unasyn). Another combination, ampicillin plus clavulanic acid (Augmentin), is available in oral form. These combinations provide a much broader spectrum of activity than the older penicillins alone and are extremely effective against pathogens responsible for obstetric and gynecologic infection. High cure rates have been observed, making these compounds (along with the broader-spectrum cephalosporins and penicillins) single-agent alternatives to the clindamycin-aminoglycoside combination.

Imipenem is the first member of the carbapenem group of antibiotics. Imipenem plus cilastatin (Primaxin) is active against most gram-positive cocci and gram-negative species, including *Pseudomonas* and many other resistant aerobic gram-negative rods. It appears to be as active as metronidazole and clindamycin against anaerobes *in vitro*. Resistant organisms include most methicillin-resistant *S. aureus*, coagulase-negative staphylococci, mycoplasmas, and chlamydia. Enterococci are sensitive *in vitro*, but the imipenem-cilastatin compound has not been proved effective against them in experimental infections. This compound should not be used in conjunction with other β-lactam antibiotics because the effects may be antagonistic. Despite its extremely broad *in vitro* spectrum of activity, the imipenem-cilastatin compound is not substantially more efficacious than other single-agent drugs. Allergic reactions, which occur in 2 to 3 per cent of patients, are the most common adverse effects; no bleeding disorders or renal impairment has been noted. Because of its extremely broad spectrum of activity, most authorities feel that imipenem should not be used in the initial treatment of patients with postpartum endometritis.

When selecting an agent for initial treatment of a patient with postpartum endometritis, the clinician has many alternatives from which to choose. Since it is next to impossible for the individual physician to gain firsthand experience with each of these drugs, it appears wise to select a limited number on the basis of spectrum of activity, clinical performance, side effects, and cost.

In a patient who responds promptly to parenteral antibiotics, therapy should be continued approximately 36 to 48 hours after the patient has become asymptomatic. Intravenous antibiotics may be discontinued and the patient discharged without oral antibiotics, except in cases of bacteremia, particularly if *S. aureus* is involved. Oral antibiotics may add to side effects as well as cost and do not decrease the already low likelihood of late-developing infection (Dismoor et al., 1991).

In a patient with a persistent infection despite appropriate antibiotic therapy, physical examination may reveal a wound infection or a pelvic mass. Radiographic studies, including ultrasonography, computerized tomography, and magnetic resonance imaging, are often helpful in identifying pelvic masses or deep-seated wound infection. In patients who are stable and not seriously ill, an appropriate change in antibiotics (e.g., adding ampicillin to clindamycin plus gentamicin) is effective in about 80 per cent of cases. Subcutaneous masses in the incision should be drained, and retained products of conception should be removed by curettage. Many patients with a hematoma or cellulitis will respond to continued antibiotic therapy. However, in a patient who appears to be acutely ill or who does not respond to antibiotics, drainage is essential. In selected patients, percutaneous drainage of cystic masses may be curative. However, when there is no response to percutaneous drainage or if sepsis is apparent, laparotomy will be necessary. Septic pelvic thrombophlebitis was first recognized more than 35 years ago in autopsies of patients dying of puerperal sepsis. More recently, it has been described as "obscure" or "enigmatic" fever persisting despite long-term therapy with multiple antibiotics.

Patients characteristically appear nontoxic, having either no pain or mild, poorly localized discomfort despite wide swings in temperature. Abdominal and pelvic findings are minimal and vague. Frank septic pulmonary emboli are rare complications. In most cases, the diagnosis has been presumptive and has been based on rapid defervescence (within 48 to 72 hours) after initiation of heparin therapy. In some cases, however, the response to heparin is clouded by the concomitant response to a change of antibiotic. In some reports, the incidence of septic pelvic thrombophlebitis has been zero to 2 per cent of infected patients. Before heparin therapy became popular, laparotomy and ligation of the inferior vena cava and ovarian vessels was recommended, but surgical intervention is now rarely necessary. Blood cultures may be helpful; positive culture results have been reported in approximately 25 per cent of cases. Organisms include aerobic and anaerobic streptococci, *S. aureus*, *E. coli*, and Bacteroides. (Because of the difficulties in diagnosing specific thrombophlebitis clinically, we frequently employ a CT scan, as it may detect an occult abscess or even depict the thrombus.) The required duration of anticoagulant therapy (heparin either alone or followed by coumadin) is not entirely clear, but 10 days of full anticoagulation with heparin has been widely used. It is possible that shorter periods of anticoagulation, such as 7 days, are also adequate.

A thorough discussion of septic shock is beyond the scope of this review (see Chapter 51), but a few points deserve emphasis. First, the most likely causative organism is *E. coli*, although other gram-negative aerobes as well as Clostridium and Bacteroides should be considered. Appropriate antibiotic coverage must therefore be directed at all likely pelvic organisms. Second, although the reported incidence of death from septic shock is about 65 per cent in large series, many of the patients who die have underlying debilitating diseases. In obstetric patients, the overall mortality rate would appear to be much lower. Third, vigorous supportive therapy (including, in some cases, Swan-Ganz catheter measurements) is necessary until the definitive therapy can take effect. Finally, one must consider the need for surgical treatment. If conservative treatment fails to bring about a response, surgery is indicated. Unlike shock accompanying septic abortion, septic shock with term delivery usually involves infection extending beyond the uterine cavity. Therefore, curettage may be performed first, but unless large amounts of necrotic placental tissue are unexpectedly recovered, an abdominal hysterectomy and often bilateral salpingo-oophorectomy with drainage will be the procedure of choice.

Prophylactic Antibiotics

For the past 20 years, interest in the perioperative and prophylactic use of antibiotics for cesarean section has been stimulated by a number of events, including the high rate of postoperative infections, the recent increase in the rate of cesarean section, and the success of infection prophylaxis in vaginal hysterectomy. In over 30 well-designed controlled studies, perioperative antibiotics have been noted to significantly decrease post-cesarean section infectious morbidity (Sweet and Gibbs, 1990). With rare exception, these regimens have resulted in a reduction of infection rates by more than 50 per cent owing mainly to decreases in uterine and wound infections. Several studies have compared one antibiotic to another for prophylaxis and found no significant differences. It should be noted that when cefoxitin was compared to cefazolin in nonelective sections, there was no difference in genital infection rate or hospital stay (Stiver et al., 1983).

Regimens for prophylaxis begun after cord clamping are as effective as those begun preoperatively and may avoid otherwise unneeded "septic work-ups" of the neonate. For several antibiotics, single-dose prophylaxis has been found to be just as effective as three doses (Sweet and Gibbs, 1990). Still, 10 to 20 per cent of patients receiving prophylactic antibiotics have febrile disease, primarily of uterine origin. Furthermore, the administration of perioperative antibiotics in cesarean section may be complicated by other clinical considerations; among these are significant alterations in the flora of patients receiving prophylactic antibiotics and developing pelvic infection. Documentation of a shift in the flora toward organisms such as enterococci, Bacteroides, Enterobacter, and Pseudomonas raises the concern about the emergence of resistant bacteria with the widespread use of antibiotics. In rare instances, there are deaths from anaphylaxis or antibiotic-associated colitis after the administration of prophylactic antibiotics.

Antibiotic prophylaxis in cesarean section should be limited to patients at high risk for infectious disease. Only a short perioperative course of antibiotics should be administered, commencing after cord clamping and continuing for one or two postoperative doses at 6-hour intervals. Potent or potentially toxic antibiotics, such as clindamycin, chloramphenicol, and aminoglycosides, which are required for the treatment of severe infections, should not be used for prophylaxis. Studies have demonstrated that first-generation cephalosporin (cephazolin) is as effective as second- or third-generation cephalosporin (cefoxitin, moxalactam) (Stiver et al., 1983). Patients who develop fever or other signs of infection after prophylaxis need careful evaluation, cultures to rule out resistant organisms, and appropriate therapeutic antibiotics.

Mastitis

No definitive data are available regarding incidence, but mastitis appears infrequently after delivery. Both an epidemic form and an endemic form of puerperal mastitis may occur. *Epidemic* puerperal mastitis has occurred among hospitalized women in conjunction with staphylococcal nursery epidemics. This form of the disease has been described mainly as a mammary adenitis, involving principally the lactiferous glands and ducts. *Endemic* puerperal mastitis occurs sporadically among nonhospitalized nursing women. It usually presents as a lobular, V-shaped cellulitis of the periglandular connective tissue, often with a fissure, crack, or irritation on the nipple. In recent reports, endemic mastitis has been the main form encountered.

In cases of epidemic mastitis, *Staphylococcus aureus* is usually cultured. In endemic mastitis, *S. aureus* is also a common pathogen, in either pure or mixed culture, but other common organisms include group A and B streptococci. *Haemophilus influenzae* and *Haemophilus parainfluenzae* have been reported as well, and in up to 50 per cent of cases only normal skin flora are cultured from breast milk.

Sporadic mastitis most often begins between the second or third week and several months after delivery. Fever commonly higher than 102°F, malaise, and localized breast signs are the usual presenting problems. In untreated patients, breast abscess is a common complication. Stasis of milk due to weaning is often suggested as a precipitating event in mastitis, but in fact, only a minority of women (perhaps 20 per cent) with mastitis have recently stopped nursing. Culture of expressed breast milk is appropriate, although in only a few cases will findings influence management.

Quantitative cultures and leukocyte counts of breast milk may be helpful. Women without breast symptoms have leukocyte counts less than 10^6/ml of milk and bacterial counts of more than 10^3/ml. Thomsen and colleagues (1983) divided women with breast symptoms into three groups: those with milk stasis, those with noninfectious breast inflammation, and those with breast infection. In the stasis group, leukocyte and bacterial counts were similar to those of asymptomatic women. Symptoms resolved spontaneously in an average of 2 days. In the second group, leukocyte counts were more than 10^6/ml, but cultures were similar to those of asymptomatic women. Symptoms lasted an average of 5 days. In the third group, leukocyte counts were more than 10^6/ml and colony counts were more than 10^3/ml; breast abscess developed in 11 per cent of this group.

With early antibiotic treatment, endemic mastitis usually resolves within 24 to 48 hours, and abscess formation is unusual. In one series of 71 cases, abscess developed in only eight (11.5 per cent); in six of these, treatment was not instituted for more than 24 hours. On the basis of the organisms involved and the well-known resistance of even community-acquired staphylococci to penicillin, the choice of initial antibiotic therapy would seem to be a penicillinase-resistant penicillin (such as dicloxacillin) or a cephalosporin. However, empiric treatments with penicillin V, erythromycin, and sulfonamides have all resulted in prompt responses even in the presence of *in vitro* drug resistance. In most cases of mastitis, antibiotics should be given orally because there is no need for hospitalization (Deveraux, 1970; Niebyl et al., 1978).

In addition to antibiotic therapy, adjunctive measures such as ice packs, breast support, and analgesics have been suggested. In most cases, the mother may continue to nurse from both breasts. If the infected breast is too sore, she may pump this breast gently. Regular drainage of the infected breast may be important in preventing abscess. Infants do not seem to suffer any adverse effects from sucking an infected breast unless an abscess has developed. In the unusual case in which an abscess develops, incision and drainage should be done promptly.

Wound Infection After Cesarean Section

Abdominal wound infection following cesarean section is a frequent occurrence, complicating the care in approximately 5 per cent of patients undergoing primary cesarean section. Prospective studies have suggested an increased incidence of wound infection if membranes have been ruptured for longer than 6 hours before delivery. The definition of wound infection, as adopted by the National Academy of Sciences–National Research Council (1964), is a follows: "A wound is defined as infected if pus discharges, and possibly infected if it develops the signs of inflammation or a serous discharge. Possibly infected wounds are inspected daily until pus discharges (infected) or they resolve (not infected)." By this definition, a *clean* wound is one in which the gastrointestinal, respiratory, or genitourinary tract is not entered, no inflammation is encountered, and no break in aseptic technique occurs. One large prospective study has reported that of 36,383 clean wounds, only 624 (1.7 per cent) became infected (Cruse and Foord, 1973). Wounds from elective repeat cesarean section are included in this group. A *clean-contaminated* wound is one in which the gastrointestinal or respiratory tract is entered without significant spillage; included in this category are procedures involving entry into the vagina or the uninfected biliary tract. Cesarean section in the presence of ruptured membranes also falls into this category. An expected infection rate of 10 per cent is generally quoted in these cases. A *contaminated* wound is one in which acute inflammation (without pus formation) is encountered, there is a major break in aseptic technique, or gross spillage from the gastrointestinal tract occurs. Incision into infected biliary or urinary tracts is also included in this category. A cesarean section performed in the presence of chorioamnionitis falls into the category of a contaminated wound. The expected infection rate in contaminated wounds is about 20 per cent. Finally, a *dirty* wound is one that occurs in the presence of pus or a perforated viscus. Traumatic wounds are included here. The definition implies the presence of organisms in ordinarily sterile tissue prior to the operation. A 30 per cent infection rate is considered a reasonable estimate for dirty wounds.

The two major factors that determine whether a wound will become infected are the dose of bacterial contamination and the resistance of the patient. Bacterial contamination is either endogenous (from the patient's own microbial flora) or exogenous (from the environment). The influence of endogenous contamination is readily documented by the progressive increase of the infection rate from 1 to 2 per cent in clean wounds, to 10 per cent in clean-contaminated wounds, to 20 per cent in contaminated wounds, and to 30 per cent in dirty wounds. In general, the source of endogenous bacteria in post-cesarean section abdominal wound infections is the flora of the vagina and cervix. With labor, rupture of membranes, and delivery, the microorganisms from the lower genital tract gain access to the amniotic fluid. At the time of cesarean section, the uterine and abdominal wounds are exposed to the amniotic fluid containing these organisms. The most prevalent bacteria in the lower genital tract include facultative (aerobic) organisms such as lactobacilli, nonhemolytic streptococci, group B beta-hemolytic streptococci, *Staphylococcus epidermidis*, *Escherichia coli*, Proteus species, and Klebsiella species, and anaerobic bacteria such as Peptococcus, Peptostreptococcus, *Bacteroides fragilis*, *Bacteriodes bivius*, and other Bacteroides species. Clostridial organisms have also been noted as part of the normal lower genital tract flora. Because the normal flora is composed of aerobic and anaerobic bacteria, endogenous infections are often of the mixed aerobic and anaerobic, or polymicrobic, type. It requires a relatively large number of bacteria to produce an infection, 10^5 bacteria per milliliter or gram being the crucial inoculum. The presence of a foreign body such as suture material reduces the required inoculum by a factor of 10,000.

Exogenous contamination is the key factor in the clean wound infection rate. Surveillance studies have identified factors that adversely affect this rate. Razor-shaving the operative site, the use of the electrosurgical knife, use of Penrose drains (especially if brought out through the skin incision), and prolonged preoperative hospitalization significantly increase the wound infection rate. Night-time or emergency surgery (e.g., for fetal distress) is associated with a three- to fourfold increase in wound infection rate. Similarly, the rate increases with increasing duration of the surgical procedure. In modern operating rooms, exogenous contamination is less important than the endogenous source of organisms from the patient's vagina or cervix. However, if general host resistance or local resistance is reduced, a smaller inoculum of bacteria can gain a foothold, and exogenous contamination may become a significant cause of wound infection.

The patient's general resistance is an important detriment to infection. Increases in wound infection rate are associated with advancing age, diabetes, malnutrition, obesity, corticosteroid therapy, and immunosuppressive states. The condition of the wound is important in determining local resistance and is to a large extent a reflection of surgical technique. Gentle tissue handling, complete hemostasis, debridement of devitalized tissue, adequate blood supply, obliteration of dead space, and closing of the wound without tension are commonly recognized principles of good surgical technique. The presence of hematomas or foreign bodies in the wound predisposes to the development of infection. Hemoglobin interferes with leukocyte migration and phagocytosis. An inadequate blood supply leads to a lower oxygen tension and acidosis in the wound, with a resultant inability of macrophages to kill bacteria.

EARLY-ONSET WOUND INFECTION. Early-onset wound infection occurs within the first 48 hours after operation. The first signs are elevated temperature and an alteration in appearance of the abdominal wall or the wound; this alteration may be a spreading cellulitis or discoloration of the skin in association with an advancing margin of active infection. Early wound infection is usually caused by a single bacterial pathogen, most commonly group A beta-hemolytic streptococci or *Clostridium perfringens*. A Gram stain of material aspirated from the active margin of infection is diagnostic. Gram-positive rods are strongly suggestive of clostridia, and gram-positive cocci indicate the probable presence of group A beta-hemolytic streptococci. Infection due to group A streptococci should be suspected if the patient develops a diffuse cellulitis or systemic illness or both. In clostridial infection, cellulitis of the skin and subcutaneous tissue is associated with a watery discharge. This is followed by the characteristic bronze appearance of the skin and crepitation in the vicinity of the wound.

The treatment of early wound infection consists of antibiotic therapy and excision of necrotic tissue. Penicillin is the antibiotic of choice for both clostridia and group A streptococci; alternatives include ampicillin, cephalosporins, cefoxitin, erythromycin, and chloramphenicol. Extensive debridement and excision of necrotic tissue may be required. It is crucial to remove all nonviable tissue. Failure to treat aggressively an early-onset wound infection exposes the patient to the risk of necrotizing fasciitis, bacteremia, and disseminated intravascular coagulation.

A rare but potentially lethal condition is toxic shock syndrome (TSS) associated with *Staphylococcus aureus* wound infection. Patients with this condition have the classic findings of TSS: (1) hypotension or syncope, (2) erythematous rash, (3) vomiting and/or diarrhea, and (4) involvement of at least three major organ systems. Management of TSS requires early diagnosis, massive volume replacement, use of necessary life support systems, and antistaphylococcal antibiotic therapy.

LATE-ONSET WOUND INFECTION. Late-onset wound infections occur at about 6 to 8 days postoperatively. They manifest as fever and a swollen, erythematous, draining wound. Following a clean operation, such as an elective repeat cesarean section with intact membranes and no labor, *S. aureus* is the usual pathogen. In clean-contaminated cases in which membranes have been ruptured and labor has occurred, the pathogens are the endogenous bacteria from the vagina and cervix (i.e., mixed aerobes and anaerobes), and multiple bacteria are the rule.

The diagnosis is made clinically with the presence of purulent drainage. The basic treatment for late-onset wound infection is incision and drainage. Antibiotics are not generally required unless there is extensive coexistent cellulitis. Once the wound has been opened and drained and nonviable tissue has been excised, the patient should rapidly become afebrile, usually within 12 hours. If response does not occur within this time, broad-spectrum antibiotic therapy aimed at mixed aerobic and anaerobic bacteria should be instituted, and the possibility of a more extensive infection process such as *necrotizing fasciitis* must be considered. The diagnosis of this latter serious complication is based on the presence of edema and

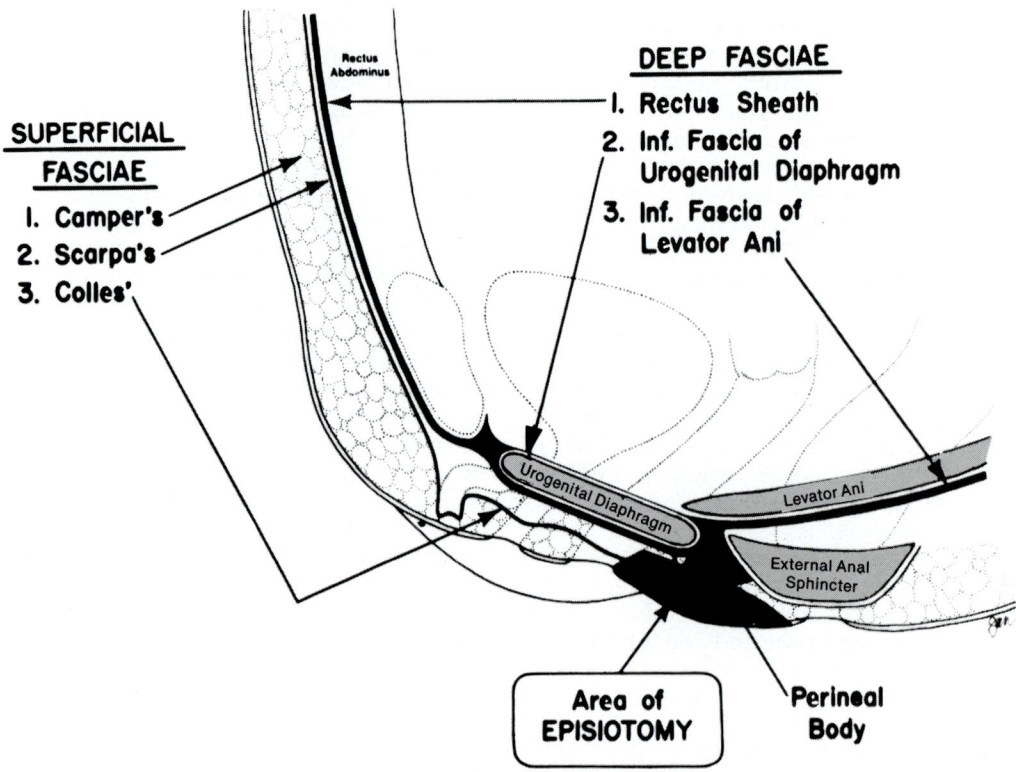

FIGURE 42–1. Paramedian sagittal section of the fascial layers of the perineum. (From Shy KK, Eschenbach DA: Fatal perineal cellulitis from an episiotomy site. Obstet Gynecol **54**:292, 1979. Reprinted with permission of the American College of Obstetricians and Gynecologists.)

necrosis with partial liquefaction of the fascia adjacent to the wound site and the presence of thrombosed microvasculature in the tissue. Necrotizing fasciitis is a polymicrobic infection; its bacterial isolates include such anaerobes as peptostreptococci, peptococci, and *Bacteroides fragilis,* as well as such facultative bacteria as *E. coli,* Klebsiella species, Proteus species, and *S. aureus.*

Although necrotizing fasciitis is a rare clinical entity after cesarean section, the necessity for early recognition, extensive surgical debridement, aerobic and anaerobic cultures, and antimicrobial therapy is well-documented. Treatment must be aggressive and must include extensive drainage and debridement and administration of appropriate antibiotics, as indicated by the Gram stain and cultures, in high dosage as adjunctive therapy. In view of the mixed (aerobic-anaerobic) nature of these infections, appropriate antimicrobial regimens include (1) clindamycin with aminoglycoside, (2) metronidazole with aminoglycoside, (3) cefoxitin, (4) one of the third-generation cephalosporins, imipenem, or (5) one of the extended-action penicillins such as piperacillin or mezlocillin.

Episiotomy Infection and Other Pelvic Infections

Although episiotomy with repair is performed in most vaginal deliveries, infection is an infrequent complication of this operation. However, recent papers have drawn attention to occasional lethal consequences. Shy and Eschenbach (1979) classified episiotomy infections according to the extent of the structures involved (Fig. 42–1).

SIMPLE EPISIOTOMY INFECTION. This form is a localized infection involving only the skin and subcutaneous tissue (including Camper's fascia of the perineum) adjacent to the episiotomy. Signs are local edema and erythema with exudate; more extensive findings should raise the suspicion of a deeper infection. Treatment consists of opening, exploration, and debridement of the perineal wound. Drainage alone is usually adequate, but appropriate antibiotics would be indicated if there is marked superficial cellulitis or isolation of group A streptococci. The episiotomy incision should not be resutured at this time. Most wounds will heal by granulation. Those involving the sphincter muscle or rectal mucosa may be repaired when the field is free of infection.

SUPERFICIAL FASCIAL NECROSIS. This type of episiotomy infection is a variant of necrotizing fasciitis. Both layers of the superficial perineal fascia (i.e., Camper's and Colles' fasciae) become necrotic, and infection spreads along the fascial planes to the abdominal wall, thigh, or buttock. Typically, the deep perineal fascia (i.e., inferior fascia of the urogenital diaphragm) is not involved. Skin findings are variable, but initially include edema and erythema without clear borders. Later, there is progressive, brawny edema of the skin. The skin becomes blue or brown, and bullae or frank gangrene may occur. As the infection progresses, there may be loss of sensation or hyperesthesia.

Associated findings include marked hemoconcentrations, although often after fluid replacement the patient is anemic. Hypocalcemia may also develop owing to saponification of fatty acids. Traditionally, this infection has been associated with group A streptococci, but anaerobic bacteria also play an important role.

In order for therapy to be effective, appropriate antibiotics must be combined with adequate debridement. Indications for surgical exploration include: extension beyond the labia, unilateral edema, signs of systemic toxicity or deterioration, and failure of the infection to resolve within 24 to 48 hours. At surgery, necrotizing fasciitis may be recognized by separation of the skin from the deep fascia, absence of bleeding along incision lines, and a serosanguineous discharge. Dissection should be wide enough to remove all necrotic tissue.

MYONECROSIS. This infection involves the muscle beneath the deep fascia. It is often the result of a myotoxin elaborated by *Clostridium perfringens*, but may occasionally result from an extension of necrotizing fasciitis. Onset may be early and is typically accompanied by severe pain. Treatment for this form is also extensive debridement and high-dose antibiotics, including penicillin when clostridia are suspected.

Not all puerperal vulvar edema signifies serious perineal infection. Indeed, in most cases, vulvar edema results from less serious causes such as hematoma, prolonged bearing down in labor, generalized edema from toxemia, allergic reactions, and trauma without serious infection. In these instances, however, the edema is usually bilateral, does not extend to the buttock and abdominal wall, and is not accompanied by signs of systemic toxicity.

Group B Streptoccal Infection

The hemolytic streptococci cause a variety of infectious syndromes and are significant causes of perinatal morbidity and mortality. Lancefield, in 1933, used serologic techniques to subdivide beta-hemolytic streptococci into specific groups, designated A, B, C, D, and E. Only groups A, B, and D are commonly involved in human disease.

Group A beta-hemolytic streptococcus (*Streptococcus pyogenes*) has long been recognized as a major pathogen in perinatal sepsis. Prior to the introduction of penicillin, this organism was the major cause of puerperal sepsis and was responsible for 75 per cent of maternal mortality due to infection.

The group B streptococci (GBS) are serologically classified into five serotypes on the basis of antigenic structure. They were virtually ignored as human pathogens until 1964, when their role in perinatal infections first became apparent. Subsequently, an increasing number of neonatal infections with GBS have been reported. Recent reports document the growing concern with neonatal sepsis and/or meningitis due to these organisms. Baker (1977) has estimated that 12,000 to 15,000 newborns per year have GBS infection and that the mortality rate is 50 per cent

in this group. Moreover, it has been pointed out that neurologic sequelae are present in 50 per cent of those with meningeal involvement.

Recently, group B streptococci have been reported to cause 1 to 5 per cent of urinary tract infections in pregnancy. In addition, a characteristic early onset of puerperal endomyometritis has been associated with these organisms.

EPIDEMIOLOGY. Asymptomatic vaginal colonization with group B streptococci occurs in 5 to 30 per cent of pregnant women. The reported prevalence of vaginal colonization in gravid women varies according to geographic locale, age, gravidity, duration of gestation, and location and number of sites cultured. The carrier rates seem to be highest for women less than 20 years old and Caucasian. The highest isolation rates are reported from the introitus and the lowest from the cervix. In addition, the choice of culture medium is a crucial determinant of the prevalence of group B streptococci. The highest yield occurs when a selective medium such as Todd-Hewitt broth with sheep blood, nalidixic acid, and gentamicin is used. When selective media are used, genital tract yield for GBS may be increased 50 per cent.

The risk of a baby's being colonized with group B streptococci increases if the mother is colonized. The transmission rate from mother to baby at birth approximates 75 per cent (Silver et al., 1990). Sixteen to 45 per cent of nursery personnel are carriers of GBS infection, and nosocomial acquisition in newborns is common. There is an association between heavy growth of GBS in the maternal genital tract and the development of group B streptococcal sepsis in neonates. Yet, an important portion of neonates with GBS sepsis (perhaps 25 per cent) are born to women with light colonization. Thus, focusing solely on heavily colonized women in preventive approaches is inadequate.

The documented colonization rate for GBS has been far higher than the attack rate in terms of neonatal infection. If 20 per cent is the average proportion of GBS-positive mothers, and the concordance rate is 75 per cent, approximately 15 per cent of all infants are colonized with group B streptococci at birth. This far exceeds the attack rate for these organisms, which is reported to be from 0.6 to 4 per 1000 live births. Various studies have attempted to identify which risk factors exist for colonization and infection. Their results suggest that risk factors such as prematurity, low birth weight, maternal fever, and premature membrane rupture for longer than 12 to 18 hours are extremely valuable in predicting infants at risk for GBS sepsis (Boyer and Gotoff, 1986). However, the full-term appropriate-for-gestational-age infant born after a normal pregnancy and delivery is not immune to such infection. GBS infection among prematures is more serious than in term infants. The chance that an infected premature baby will die of group B streptococcal sepsis is at least twice that for the term infant.

CLINICAL MANIFESTATIONS IN THE NEONATE. Two clinically distinct neonatal GBS infections have been identified (Baker, 1977).

Early-onset infection appears within the first week of life, and usually within 48 hours. It is characterized by rapid clinical deterioration and a high mortality rate. The majority of symptomatic newborns are of low birth weight. In the most fulminant form, early-onset GBS infection manifests as septic shock accompanied by respiratory distress leading to death within several hours despite appropriate antibiotic therapy. The mortality rate ranges from 50 to 70 per cent. In less severe disease, the clinical findings are similar to those seen in respiratory distress syndrome. Although pulmonary disease predominates in early-onset disease, meningitis may be present in about 30 per cent of cases.

Late-onset infection with group B streptococci occurs more insidiously, usually after the first week of life. In the majority of infants, meningitis is the predominant clinical manifestation. Although the mortality rate in late-onset group B streptococcal infection is lower (15 to 30 per cent), up to 50 per cent of babies with meningitis subsequently demonstrate neurologic sequelae. Late-onset disease may result in localized infections involving middle ears, sinuses, conjunctiva, breasts, lungs, bones, joints, and skin. Meningitis appears to be related to the serotype of GBS. More than 80 per cent of early-onset GBS infections with meningitis present are due to type III organisms, and in late-onset disease, 95 per cent of meningitis is attributable to this subtype.

Although early-onset disease had been associated with transmission from the mother's genital tract either prior to labor or during parturition, such a route of transmission is thought to obtain less commonly in late-onset disease. Nosocomial transmission of GBS can occur in the nursery from colonized nursing staff or from other infants.

CLINICAL MANIFESTATIONS IN THE MOTHER. Several recent studies have identified the group B streptococcus as a major cause of puerperal infection. Features of GBS puerperal infection are the development of a high fever within 12 hours of delivery, tachycardia, abdominal distention, and endomyometritis or endomyoparametritis. Some patients have no localizing signs early in the course of the infection. The incidence of bacteremia is approximately 35 per cent. Patients undergoing cesarean section seem particularly at risk for GBS puerperal sepsis.

DIAGNOSIS. Maternal asymptomatic genitourinary or gastrointestinal colonization with GBS can be diagnosed only by culture, preferably using a selective medium. The symptoms of maternal genitourinary tract infection may include fever, chills, uterine tenderness, dysuria, urgency, and pyuria. Because none of these is specific for group B streptococci, the diagnosis must be confirmed by isolation of the organism from culture.

The great majority of colonized neonates are asymptomatic, and diagnosis requires culture and isolation. None of the clinical manifestations of neonatal infection is sufficient for diagnosis in the absence of a positive culture. The diagnosis should be suspected when the clinical manifestations occur in association with a Gram stain of amniotic fluid or gastric aspirate that reveals a predominance of gram-positive cocci.

TREATMENT AND PREVENTION. Penicillin remains the drug of choice for symptomatic group B strepto-

coccal infection in mother or neonate if the infecting organism has been identified. The combination of penicillin with an aminoglycoside may also kill the GBS faster. In most instances, however, treatment must be initiated prior to the availability of culture results. In these instances, a broad-spectrum approach for empirically treating the mother with chorioamnionitis or puerperal sepsis and the neonate with sepsis is required. Ampicillin is frequently used in such situations and provides adequate treatment for group B streptococcal infection.

Because of the severity of early- and late-onset GBS neonatal infection, major efforts have been directed to prophylactic administration of antibiotics to gravid women whose genital tracts are colonized with GBS. Strategies may be classified as antepartum, intrapartum, neonatal, and immunologic. Antepartum strategies to reduce maternal carrier rates have generally been unsuccessful. Hall and colleagues (1976) noted that administration of ampicillin to gravid women with cervical colonization of GBS resulted in a significant decrease in colonization rate within 3 weeks of therapy, but the treated women were often recolonized by the time of parturition. In addition, the infants of the treated mothers were colonized at the same rate as the control infants. Merenstein and co-workers (1980) evaluated the efficacy of an oral penicillin regimen at 38 weeks of gestation. They observed a significant reduction in maternal and infant colonization with GBS in the treatment group (mothers and sexual partners treated). However, this approach is not applicable to the preterm pregnancy, in which the risk for neonatal mortality is greater. Gardner and associates (1979) demonstrated that oral penicillin treatment of couples in the early third trimester of pregnancy was not an effective means of reducing maternal colonization at the time of delivery and reported no difference in colonization rates at delivery between treated and control groups.

Attempts to prevent neonatal GBS infection are complicated by several factors. First, venereal transmission of the organism allows for reinfection. Second, it is difficult to eradicate GBS from the rectum because of the beta-lactamase enzymes that inactivate penicillin and ampicillin and are produced by the Enterobacteriaceae. Third, the high ratio of maternal and neonatal colonization rate to infection rate requires that 100 women (and their sexual partners) must be treated for each possible case of GBS infection. Such widespread use of penicillins and ampicillin imposes a significant risk for allergic reactions to these drugs.

Intrapartum strategies have been most attractive to date. Three variations have been suggested. First, Minkoff and Mead (1986) suggested culturing for GBS in women with risk factors (premature labor, PROM >12 to 18 hours) and treating in the presence of positive culture *or* treating presumptuously if delivery was likely before the culture status was known. Second, others have favored rapid diagnostic techniques to identify colonized women at high risk during labor. These techniques have included the Gram stain, latex agglutinates, enzyme-linked immunosorbent assay (ELISA), and a rapid (5-hr) culture (Morales and Lim, 1987). Some of these "rapid tests" have performed poorly, especially the Gram stain (Carey et al., 1990) and latex agglutinates (Isada and Grossman, 1987). Others, such as rapid culture and ELISA, have been reported to have better predictive values. Yet, even these latter two tests are insensitive in detecting women with light colonization and are therefore unreliable tests in the clinical setting. Third, following the report by Boyer and Gotoff that administration of IV ampicillin intrapartum to women with preterm labor or preterm rupture of membranes (interval longer than 12 to 18 hours) led to a significant decrease in neonatal sepsis from GBS (1986), there has been recent support by some for universal screening for GBS at approximately 26 weeks and selective administration of intrapartum ampicillin when risk factors are present (Gibbs et al., 1992). The American Academy of Pediatrics recently supported universal screening (1992) whereas the American College of Obstetricians and Gynecologists Technical Bulletin noted that there were insufficient data upon which to recommend universal screening (ACOG, 1992). At the University of Colorado, we are currently applying this approach to determine its efficacy in a clinical setting.

Neonatal strategies to prevent neonatal GBS infection have focused on the reports of decreases in neonatal early-onset disease when penicillin is given at birth. In a prospective study of over 18,000 infants, reported by Siegel and co-workers (1978), single IM injections of aqueous penicillin were given within 60 minutes of delivery to more than 9,000 infants. The control group received topical tetracycline for the prevention of gonococcal ophthalmia. The incidence of GBS colonization and early-onset GBS disease fell significantly in penicillin-treated infants. Similarly, Lloyd and associates (1979) have demonstrated that penicillin prophylaxis in neonates weighing less than 2,500 grams reduces the colonization and the attack rates of group B streptococci. No increase in the mortality rate from other infections was noted. Yet, other data (Boyer and Gotoff, 1986) has shown that up to 40 per cent of neonates who develop GBS sepsis are already bacteremic at birth, suggesting that this approach of single dose penicillin may be "too little and too late."

The immunologic approach is appealing, but there currently is no safe immunogenic and effective vaccine. Moreover, such a vaccine would need to be polyvalent to cover all serotypes involved in early-onset sepsis, and some data suggest that pre-existing type-specific antibodies may not be protective of neonatal sepsis (Silver et al., 1990).

For women who have previously delivered an affected neonate, intrapartum prophylaxis in subsequent pregnancies has been suggested regardless of culture status and regardless of pressure of risk factors, but data to support this approach are lacking. Currently there is much debate, and no approach is foolproof.

Listeriosis

Listeriosis is an infection caused by *Listeria monocytogenes*, a motile non-spore-forming gram-positive rod.

Patients who are immunocompromised and pregnant women and their newborns are particularly susceptible to infection with *L. monocytogenes*. Of concern to the obstetrician is the association between maternal listeria infection and preterm labor and fetal infection. High perinatal morbidity and mortality rates have been reported for listeria infection in pregnancy (Charles, 1990; Bortolussi and Seeliger, 1990; Gellin and Broome, 1989; McLauchlin, 1990).

As is the case with group B streptococcal infection, neonatal listeriosis has been divided into two serologically and clinically distinct types. Early-onset disease takes the form of a diffuse sepsis with multi-organ involvement including the lungs, the liver, and the central nervous system. Early-onset listeriosis is associated with a high stillbirth rate and a high neonatal mortality rate and appears to occur more frequently in low-birth-weight infants.

Late-onset listeriosis presents as meningitis, usually in the term infant born to mothers with uneventful perinatal courses. Neurologic sequelae such as hydrocephaly and/or mental retardation are common with late-onset disease. In addition, a mortality rate approaching 40 per cent is reported.

Although Charles (1990) has suggested that an ascending route of infection from cervical colonization with *L. monocytogenes* (even across intact membranes) plays a role in the pathogenesis of neonatal infection, the more important and common route of infection proceeds from maternal infection to placental infection and then to fetal septicemia and multi-organ involvement in the fetus.

Human listeriosis presents in both an epidemic and sporadic form. The epidemic form has clearly been associated with contamination of food and food products. A recent example includes clusters of maternal infection due to contaminated dairy products (Linnan et al., 1988). In Los Angeles, from January 1 through August 15, 1985, 142 cases of human listeriosis were reported in association with ingestion of cheese contaminated by *L. monocytogenes*. Two-thirds of these infections occurred in pregnant women or their offspring, and 30 of the 48 deaths in this epidemic occurred in fetuses or neonates. In a recent report from Finland, a mortality rate of 30 per cent was noted among the neonates infected with *L. monocytogenes*. Among the six pregnant women with listeria, five had fetal complications: three spontaneous abortions and two preterm deliveries. Interestingly, all healthy nonimmunocompromised nonpregnant patients survived their listeria infection. This again demonstrates that listeria is prone to adversely affect immunocompromised adults and fetuses or neonates with immature immune systems.

Many pregnant women with listeriosis remain asymptomatic. When symptomatic they present with a flu-like syndrome that is characterized by fever, chills, malaise, myalgia, back pain, and upper respiratory complaints. Maternal infection tends to be mild and not associated with significant maternal morbidity. On occasion, diffuse sepsis may occur. Unfortunately, no specific clinical manifestations have been demonstrated that help to distinguish listeriosis from other infections that may occur during pregnancy.

Because of the high mortality rate associated with both early- and late-onset neonatal listeria infection, it is crucial that the obstetrician maintain a high index of suspicion that any febrile illness in pregnancy may be due to *L. monocytogenes*. In such patients, cervical and blood cultures should be obtained for *Listeria monocytogenes* as soon as possible. Because colonies of *L. monocytogenes* may be mistaken on the Gram stain for diphtheroids and thus ignored, it is important to inform the microbiologist that listeria is a concern. In febrile pregnant women, a Gram stain revealing gram-positive pleomorphic rods with rounded ends is highly suggestive of, and should be presumed to be, *L. monocytogenes*.

Penicillin G and ampicillin are effective *in vivo* against *L. monocytogenes*. Current opinion holds that optimum therapy includes a combination of ampicillin plus an aminoglycocide. Maternal treatment consists of ampicillin (1 to 2 gm IV every 4 to 6 hours) and gentamicin (2 mg per kg IV every 8 hours). For the newborn, the ampicillin dosage is 200 to 300 mg/kg/day administered in four to six divided doses. The duration of treatment is generally one week. A recent report has suggested that, with documentation via amniocentesis of intrauterine listeria infection, antibiotic treatment without immediate delivery may be successful and result in a normal healthy fetus (Kalstone, 1991).

Lyme Disease

Since Lyme disease was first described in 1977 it has emerged as an important infection. Between 1982 and 1988, the Centers for Disease Control reported nearly 13,500 cases of Lyme disease in the United States (CDC, 1989). From 1982 through 1987, the number of cases increased approximately five-fold, and in 1988 reported cases doubled. Lyme disease is currently the most commonly reported vector-borne disease in the United States and accounts for 50 per cent of vector-borne infections reported to the Centers for Disease Control.

Lyme disease, a tick-borne infection caused by the spirochete *Borrelia burgdorferi*, is a multi-system illness characterized by a distinct lesion, erythema chronicum migrans (ECM), which is often followed by neurologic, cardiac, and/or arthritic manifestations (Steere et al., 1977a, 1977b; Steere, 1989). The Lyme disease spirochete is transmitted by Ixodes ticks. The most common vector is the deer tick, *Ixodes dammini*, whose distribution coincides with endemic areas of the disease in the Northeastern United States. The white-footed mouse is host for the larval and nymph stage of the disease. White-tail deer are the preferred hosts for *I. dammini's* adult stage. In the Western United States, *I. pacificus*, the black-legged deer tick, is responsible for transmission of the disease.

As noted by Steere (1989), Lyme disease generally occurs in stages characterized by differing clinical manifestations. The initial manifestation is erythema migrans, which is followed several weeks or months later by meningitis or Bell's palsy and subsequently followed months or years later by arthritis. Asbrink

and Hoomark (1988) suggested a classification, based on the system used in syphilis, whereby Lyme disease is divided into early and late infection. Early infection consists of stage I (localized erythema migrans), followed within days or weeks by stage II (disseminated infection), and within weeks or months by intermittent symptoms. Late infection or stage III (persistent infection) begins generally a year or more after the onset of disease.

Following transmission of the *B. burgdorferi*, approximately 60 to 80 per cent of individuals develop erythema migrans. This lesion begins as a small erythematous papular macule, which is then followed by a gradual centrifugal expansion over three to four weeks. The initial skin lesion is often accompanied by systemic symptoms including fever, flu-like symptoms with migratory arthralgias, myalgias, headaches, and regional lymphadenopathy (Steere, 1989). Even without treatment, erythema migrans usually fades within three to four weeks. Disseminated infection is often associated with characteristic symptoms involving skin, nervous system, or musculoskeletal system. Nearly half the patients will develop secondarily annular skin lesions that resemble the primary erythema migrans lesions. These are usually smaller and migrate less. Patients commonly develop severe headaches and mild stiffness of the neck, which occur in short attacks. Interestingly, a recent report utilizing a polymerase chain reaction assay for *Borrelia*-specific DNA has demonstrated the presence of *B. burgdorferi* in the central nervous system during acute disseminated infection (Luft et al., 1992). The musculoskeletal pain associated with Lyme disease is migratory in nature, lasting only hours or days in any given location. During the disseminated stage, patients frequently have severe malaise and fatigue. As the infection begins to localize, approximately 15 to 20 per cent of patients develop frank neurologic involvement. The classic triad of neurologic Lyme disease includes meningitis, cranial nerve palsies, and peripheral radiculopathies. The predominant symptoms of Lyme meningitis are severe headaches and mild neck stiffness, which fluctuate for several weeks. Nearly half the cases of meningitis have an associated mild encephalitis that leads to loss of concentration, emotional lability, lethargy, sleep disturbances, or focal cerebral dysfunction. The most commonly affected cranial nerve is the seventh nerve, leading to Bell's palsy. One-third of the patients with Bell's palsy have bilateral involvement. Peripheral radiculopathies are characterized by severe neuritic pain, dysesthesias, focal weakness, and areflexia. Within several weeks from the onset of disease, 5 to 10 per cent of patients have cardiac involvement. Fluctuating degrees of atrioventricular block are the most common abnormalities; this ranges from first-degree to complete heart block. The duration of cardiac abnormalities is usually very brief, lasting from three days to six weeks. Approximately six months after the onset of disease, about 60 per cent of the patients in the United States begin to have brief attacks of asymmetric, oligoarticular arthritis, primarily in the large joints, especially the knee. Stage III or late infection is characterized by episodes of arthritis, often lasting longer during the second and third year of the illness, a chronic arthritis. In addition, several late syndromes of the central nervous system have now been described. These include progressive encephalomyelitis (Ackerman et al., 1988), subacute encephalitis, and a syndrome suggestive of dementia.

Experience with Lyme disease during pregnancy is rather limited (Smith et al., 1991). Concern has arisen because spirochetes such as *Treponema pallidum* cross the placenta and produce adverse effects on the fetus and/or neonate. In 1985, the first case of transplacental transmission of *B. burgdorferi* was documented by identification of the spirochete in multiple organs of an infant who died of congenital heart disease shortly after birth (Schlesinger et al., 1985). Subsequently, Weber et al. (1988) isolated the organism from the brain and liver of an infant who died within the first 24 hours of life. Both of these infants were born to mothers who had erythema migrans in the first trimester. Three cases of stillbirth with recovery of *B. burgdorferi* from multiple organs subsequently were reported in the literature (MacDonald, 1986, 1987; Markowitz et al., 1986). The Centers for Disease Control have evaluated the effect of Lyme disease during pregnancy on two occasions. In a retrospective study, they identified five adverse outcomes in fetuses born to 19 women with Lyme disease (Markowitz et al., 1986). Among the adverse outcomes noted were prematurity, cortical blindness, fetal demise, and syndactyly and rash in the neonate. However, they could not prove a teratogenetic pattern, nor could they show a reduction in fetal morbidity if the mothers had been appropriately treated for Lyme disease. In a prospective study, they evaluated 17 women with documented first-trimester Lyme infection (Ciesielski et al., 1987). Only two of these pregnancies were abnormal, and one of these ended in a spontaneous abortion at 13 weeks. In the second, the infant had syndactyly. In a survey of cord blood sera from 421 infants born in an area endemic for *B. burgdorferi*, Williams et al. (1988) demonstrated no relationship between congenital malformation and the presence of antibody to Lyme disease. In a recent European study, 0.85 per cent of cord bloods obtained from over 1400 pregnancies demonstrated elevated titers to *B. burgdorferi* (Nadel et al., 1989). Of these, only one patient had had clinical disease during her pregnancy, and her infant was noted to have a ventricular septal defect without other anomalies. In the remaining 11 infants with elevated IgG cord titers, six had an abnormal neonatal course: two with hyperbilirubinemia, one with macrocephaly, one with intrauterine growth restriction, and one with supraventricular extrasystoles. However, at an average follow-up of nine months, all these latter six infants were normal. Thus, any relationship between positive IgG titers and abnormalities in the fetus or neonate are inconclusive.

The diagnosis of Lyme disease is hindered by the various manifestations of the disease. The culture or direct visualization of *B. burgdorferi* from patients' specimens is difficult, and thus serology is currently the only practical laboratory diagnosis available. An indirect fluorescent antibody (IFA) and an enzyme-linked immunosorbent assay (ELISA) are the most commonly used tests for the diagnosis of Lyme dis-

ease. In general, the ELISA is the preferred method because of its greater sensitivity and specificity. It is important to recognize that false-positive serologic testing can be seen with other spirochetal diseases, such as infectious mononucleosis, autoimmune disorders, and Rocky Mountain spotted fever. Thus, an indirect screening test for syphilis should be done on all positives to rule out syphilis. False-negative serologic testing may be seen early in the disease, that is, during the first two weeks when infection is localized to the skin or, if antibiotics have been given, before an immune response can be mounted. Because laboratory diagnosis is uncertain a case definition has been developed to aid in the recognition of Lyme disease: (1) the occurrence of erythema migrans no more than 30 days following exposure in an endemic area (i.e., where vector ticks are known to exist), or (2) the involvement of at least one of the three commonly affected organ systems, producing neurologic, cardiovascular, or arthritic symptoms and either a positive serology or isolation of *B. burgdorferi*, or (3) erythema migrans or positive serology without a history of exposure.

Treatment of Lyme disease is most successful when given early. Treatment regimens are listed in Table 42–4. Doxycycline, tetracycline, and amoxicillin have been used with demonstrated good efficacy in the treatment of early disease. Although tetracycline is an effective agent for eradicating *B. burgdorferi*, it is contraindicated in pregnancy. Based on the recent report by Luft et al. demonstrating the presence of *B. burgdorferi* DNA in the CSF during acute disseminated infection, ceftriaxone may become the preferred agent for the treatment of early as well as late disease. The advantages of ceftriaxone are its penetrance into the

TABLE 42–4. Treatment of Lyme Disease in Adults*

DISEASE MANIFESTATION	REGIMEN
Erythema migrans	Tetracycline 250 mg orally qid for 10–30 days†
	Doxycycline 100 mg orally bid for 10–30 days†
	Amoxicillin 500 mg orally qid for 10–30 days‡
Neurologic abnormalities	
Meningitis	Ceftriaxone 2 gm intravenously daily for 14 days
	Penicillin G 20,000,000 U IV daily for 14 days
Isolated cranial nerve palsy	Oral regimens as for Erythema migrans
Cardiac abnormalities	Ceftriaxone 2 g IV daily for 14 days
	Penicillin G 20,000,000 U IV daily for 14 days
Arthritis	Doxycycline 100 mg orally bid for 30 days
	Amoxicillin (plus probenecid) 500 mg orally qid for 30 days
	Ceftriaxone 2 g IV daily for 14 days
	Penicillin G 20,000,000 U IV daily for 14 days

*Modified from Steere AG: Lyme disease. N Engl J Med **321**:586, 1989.
†Tetracyclines should not be used in pregnancy.
‡Penicillin-allergic patients in pregnancy: Erythromycin 250 mg orally qid for 10–30 days.

central nervous system and the fact that it can be given once daily, thereby facilitating compliance with the antibiotic regimen.

VIRAL INFECTIONS

Rubella

The rubella virus produces a mild illness with fever, postauricular or suboccipital lymphadenopathy, arthralgia, and a transient erythematous rash. Although its teratogenic potential was first recognized 40 years ago, most current problems are related to diagnosis of maternal rubella and the consequences of vaccination.

Wild rubella virus is spread by droplets or direct contact with infected persons or articles contaminated with nasopharyngeal secretions. It is primarily a mild disease in children, with peak incidence between 5 and 9 years of age. Only on rare occasions have serious sequelae such as central nervous system involvement and thrombocytopenia developed. By reproductive age, about 75 to 85 per cent of the population has had rubella, about half of whom experienced subclinical infections. Once wild virus infection occurs, even if subclinical, immunity is lifelong.

Before vaccination was available, rubella occurred in cycles of 6 to 9 years, with the last major epidemic in 1964. The primary concern to the obstetrician is maternal infection during early pregnancy, when primary rubella may lead to involvement of the embryo or fetus. Overall, the risk of congenital rubella syndrome is about 20 per cent for primary maternal infection in the first trimester of pregnancy. The risk ranges from 50 per cent in the first month to 10 per cent in the third month. Cataracts, patent ductus arteriosus, and deafness are the most common abnormalities (Mann et al., 1981; Cooper et al., 1969).

DIAGNOSIS. The clinical diagnosis of rubella is often difficult because it resembles a number of other exanthemas. Rubella virus can be isolated from the bloodstream and throat 7 to 10 days after exposure. Shedding of virus from the throat continues for about a week. The rash, which typically starts in the face, generally develops 16 to 18 days after exposure. Rubella infection stimulates a variety of antibody responses, as follows.

Hemagglutinating Inhibition Antibody (HIA). This IgG class antibody has been the most commonly used for screening. After wild virus infection, HIA titers usually remain positive for life. From 5 to 15 per cent of normal women with remote rubella infection have stable HIA titers less than 1:256. A titer of more than 1:8 is conclusive evidence of immunity. Recently there has been controversy as to the interpretation of a titer equal to 1:8. In such cases, the test should be repeated. If a titer equal to 1:8 is again obtained, it most probably indicates long-lasting immunity. On the other hand, if the second titer shows a fourfold rise, the patient has acute rubella infection. Because of variations between laboratories and day-to-day variations within one laboratory, it is essential that paired serum samples be tested on the same day in the same laboratory.

Complement Fixation Test. Also an IgG class anti-

body, complement is one that appears later than HIA and may be useful in some diagnostic situations, as in those patients with high HIA titer or those first seen 1 to 5 weeks after exposure.

ELISA. Many laboratories now use the enzyme-linked immunosorbent assay (ELISA). With this technique, antibody serum is detected by an antihuman globulin conjugated to an enzyme (often alkaline phosphatase). The amount of enzyme conjugate is proportional to the amount of serum antibody; the amount of enzyme is determined colorimetrically and read in absorbance units at a given wavelength. The absorbance is influenced by the incubation times and reagent concentrations in addition to the amount of serum antibody. The advantages of ELISA are rapidity, sensitivity, and economy. Usually an absorbance reading is selected as a breakpoint to correlate with the reference HIA breakpoint of 1:8. Values below this breakpoint are then reported as seronegative (or rubella susceptible), whereas values above the cutoff are seropositive (or rubella-immune). For individuals with suspected acute rubella, quantitative techniques need to be used.

Rubella-Specific IgM. As shown in Figure 42–2, IgM antibodies appear early and last for only a few weeks. This test may be helpful in some diagnostic situations, but is available in few laboratories. Although the presence of rubella-specific IgM is indicative of recent primary rubella infection, its absence does not necessarily exclude infection because in some patients IgM may disappear in less than 4 to 5 weeks.

Other Responses. Other serologic responses are detectable by radioimmunoassay neutralization. At present, these are not useful in clinical situations.

MANAGEMENT. In women with confirmed rubella infection in pregnancy, management principally consists of counseling in regard to risks and types of congenital anomalies. Culture of amniotic fluid does not reliably distinguish reliably the infected fetus from the uninfected one in a pregnancy at risk. By use of percutaneous umbilical blood sampling at mid-pregnancy, rubella-specific IgM has been detected in fetal blood in a small number of patients (Daffos et al., 1984). This information may be used to counsel pa-

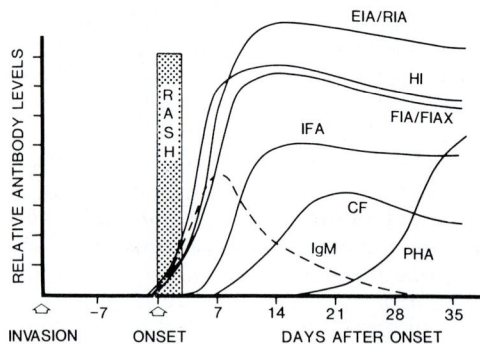

FIGURE 42–2. Schema of immune response in acute rubella infection, as measured by various tests. EIA/RIA = Enzyme immunoassay; HI = Hemagglutination inhibition; IFA, FIA, FIAX = Immunofluorescence; CF = Complement fixation; PHA = Passive hemagglutination. (From Hermann KL: Available rubella serologic tests. Rev Infect Dis 7:S109, 1985.)

tients, but there are serious limitations including (1) risk of this diagnostic procedure, (2) high possibility of absence of clinical congenital rubella syndrome even with IgM in fetal blood, and (3) affected fetuses without IgM detected.

Future techniques, including polymerase chain reaction combined with fetal blood sampling, may offer additional diagnostic possibilities.

Use of immune globulin (IG) after exposure has been recommended by some authors. However, the Advisory Committee to the Centers for Disease Control (1981) notes that IG given after exposure prevents neither infection nor viremia, although it may alter symptoms. Furthermore, infants with congenital rubella have been born to women who received IG shortly after exposure. Thus, IG is not recommended for routine use as postexposure prophylaxis.

PREVENTION. Since January 1979, the rubella vaccine used in the United States has been the RA 27/3, which replaced the HPV–77 vaccine. All rubella vaccines contain live, attenuated virus. RA 27/3 is administered subcutaneously. After vaccination, approximately 95 per cent of susceptible individuals develop HI antibodies, which provide long-term, possibly lifelong protection. Among adults who do not show a positive HI titer after vaccination, nearly all have detectable antibody when a more sensitive test is used. Any detectable rubella antibody or a history of rubella vaccination is presumptive evidence of immunity.

Vaccinated individuals may shed the attenuated virus from the nasopharynx for a few weeks, but there is no evidence that the vaccine virus can be transmitted. Consequently, there appears to be no risk to susceptible pregnant women who have contact with recently vaccinated children or adults. Susceptible women of reproductive age are candidates for immunization, and it is recommended that pregnancy be avoided for 90 days after vaccination. The immediate postpartum period is often suggested as an excellent time for immunization. Vaccinated women may breast-feed without fear of adverse effects on the newborn.

Despite recommendations, many rubella-susceptible pregnant women have received rubella vaccine within 3 months of the time of conception. As of December 1983, 214 of these women who delivered living infants had been reported to the Centers for Disease Control (Bart et al., 1985). After vaccination with the HPV–77 preparation, the virus has been isolated from the products of conception in about 20 per cent of the cases. With the RA 27/3 vaccine, this virus is isolated less frequently (1 of 32, 3 per cent). Even though the virus may be isolated in the products of conception, none of the 214 infants had any anomalies consistent with the congenital rubella syndrome. The maximum theoretical risk for congenital rubella syndrome is 1.7 per cent. Although four infants born to susceptible women had subclinical infection, all were normal (Bart et al., 1985).

Side effects of the vaccine include arthralgias, but true arthritis occurs in less than 1 per cent. In susceptible adult women, joint symptoms are more common and tend to be more severe than in children. Other complaints such as pain and paresthesias have been

rare. Contraindications to vaccination include febrile illnesses, immunosuppression, and pregnancy. Precautions are necessary in the rare individual with neomycin allergy.

Cytomegalovirus

Cytomegalic inclusion disease is due to infection with cytomegalovirus (CMV), a DNA virus of the herpesvirus group. Although the characteristic large cells with prominent intranuclear inclusion bodies seen in this disease have been recognized since the early 20th century, the virus was not isolated until 1956. Initially, cytomegalovirus was considered to be rare, and only the classic clinically severe form of the disease was appreciated. Subsequent studies utilizing isolation of the virus have identified the frequent presence of "silent" CMV infection, in which no clinical manifestations are present. Weller, in 1971, first described the scope and impact of congenital CMV infection (Weller, 1971). The virus is now recognized as the most common cause of intrauterine infection, and congenital infection has been reported to occur in 0.5 to 2.5 per cent of all babies delivered. It has been suggested that 5 to 10 per cent of congenitally infected children will have neurologic sequelae. Severe symptomatic cytomegalic inclusion disease occurs in from one in 10,000 to one in 20,000 newborns.

Asymptomatic infection cannot be considered innocuous. The persistent and progressive nature of this inapparent congenital infection results in CNS disorder and neurologic sequelae, which represent the major impact of cytomegalovirus infection.

The teratogenic potential of cytomegalovirus is unsettled. Although the virus can cause a reduction in the absolute number of cells in various organs, it is not known whether this reduction is due to a direct effect on the cells or whether it is secondary to endothelial and vascular damage. Malformations such as cataracts and congenital heart lesions are seldom seen with cytomegalovirus infections. Their effects appear to be secondary to cytotoxic actions.

Approximately 50 per cent of females in the United States and Europe are susceptible to cytomegalovirus by the time they reach reproductive age, and the highest rate of seroconversion occurs between the ages of 15 and 35. As a result, the possibility that cytomegalovirus disease will coincide with pregnancy is extremely high. Past exposure to CMV relates to sociocultural and to sexual behavior. Chandler and coworkers (1985) have demonstrated that seropositivity correlated with lower socioeconomic status, multigravidity, older age, a first pregnancy when younger than 15 years of age, and a greater total number of sex partners. Absence of these risk factors identifies those women who are most susceptible to primary CMV infection during pregnancy. Thus, nearly 50 per cent of higher-income women are susceptible to acute CMV infection while only 15 per cent of low-income women are. It is estimated that approximately 2 per cent of susceptible pregnant women acquire primary CMV infection during pregnancy in the United States. Although this viral infection is widespread, it produces serious illness only in fetuses, immunodeficient individuals, and patients receiving immunosuppressive therapy.

Cytomegalovirus has developed a remarkably successful form of parasitism in human populations. It is persistently excreted and thus is communicable for long periods. Infants infected congenitally excrete cytomegalovirus for an average of 4 years. Those acquiring CMV at the time of birth excrete it for 2 years. Many seropositive young adults shed cytomegalovirus intermittently. Recurrent excretion of the virus in asymptomatic persons may be due to several possible mechanisms. Following primary infection, a lowgrade chronic infection might be established in which viral excretion periodically reaches detectable levels. Reinfection could occur in immune persons owing to antigenic and genetic disparity among cytomegalovirus strains. Also, like herpes simplex virus, cytomegalovirus may become latent during primary infection and be reactivated in later life by various stimuli.

Asymptomatic infection with excretion is common during pregnancy. CMV can be cultured (cervix and urine) in 2 to 28 per cent of pregnant women. The incidence of cytomegalovirus infection is highest in low-income, young, primiparous, less educated, unmarried women. Longitudinal studies have demonstrated that the average incidence of cervical excretion of the virus in pregnancy increases from 2.6 per cent (range 0 to 7.1) in the first trimester to 7.6 per cent (range 2 to 28 per cent) near term. These asymptomatic infections occur mainly in seropositive women and reflect recurrent CMV infection. Pregnancy itself may either increase a woman's susceptibility to cytomegalovirus infection or reactivate latent infection.

Congenital CMV infection is generally the result of transplacental transmission of CMV, which causes *in-vitro* infection (Demmler, 1991). Between 0.5 and 2.5 per cent of the neonatal population is infected by vertical transmission from mother to fetus during pregnancy. These neonates excrete CMV (urine) at birth. An additional 3 to 5 per cent of liveborn infants acquire cytomegalovirus peripartum, presumably as a result of exposure to infected cervical secretions, infected breast milk, or infected transfused blood. These infants have perinatal CMV infection in which the initial urine culture is negative, but subsequent excretion of CMV is demonstrated several weeks to months after delivery. Thirty to 50 per cent of neonates whose mothers have genital CMV infection at the time of birth will acquire the virus.

The infections transmitted *in utero* are the major concern, especially in relation to infant development. Congenital infections may occur following either primary or recurrent maternal infection. The occurrence of a demonstrably high rate (3.4 to 6 per cent) of congenital infection in infants born to previously immune mothers suggests that recurrent maternal infection is an important cause of intrauterine transmission of cytomegalovirus. The birth of one congenitally infected infant does not preclude the possibility of a subsequent baby's becoming infected *in utero*. However, it is clear that primary cytomegalovirus infection acquired during pregnancy is significantly more dangerous to the fetus than recurrent CMV and associated

in utero transmission. Recently Fowler and colleagues (1992) have demonstrated that only infants with primary infection had symptomatic CMV infection at birth (18 per cent). Infants in the primary infection group had a 25 per cent incidence of one or more sequelae as compared to 8 per cent with the recurrent infection group. Mental impairment was demonstrated in 13 per cent of the infants whose mothers had primary infection during pregnancy, but in none of those whose mothers had recurrent CMV infection. Sensorineural hearing loss was found in 15 per cent of infants born to mothers with primary CMV infection during pregnancy, but in only 5 per cent of those born to women with recurrent infection. Most importantly, bilateral hearing loss was identified only in the children born to primarily infected mothers (8 per cent) (Fowler et al., 1992).

Approximately 10 per cent of neonates born with congenital CMV are symptomatic at birth (Demmler, 1991). These infants often have prematurity, low birth weight, microcephaly, chorioretinitis, hepatosplenomegaly, jaundice, and thrombocytopenic purpura. The long-term prognosis for symptomatic CMV-infected neonates is poor. Approximately 90 per cent will develop some type of significant neurologic sequelae (Pass et al., 1980). Survivors of the symptomatic CMV infection develop a classic tetrad of microcephaly, intracranial calcification, severe mental retardation and chorioretinitis. The sequelae in the survivors with symptomatic CMV include hearing loss, mental retardation, psychomotor development delay, chorioretinitis, seizures, and learning disabilities. Stagno et al. (1982) have demonstrated that adverse outcome with congenital CMV infection is most likely to occur with primary CMV acquired during pregnancy, especially that acquired at less than 20 weeks of gestation. In that time frame there is a 30 to 40 per cent risk of intrauterine transmission.

Ninety per cent of neonates with *in utero* acquired CMV infection are asymptomatic. Five to 15 per cent of these asymptomatic congenitally infected neonates will still develop late sequelae (Hanshaw, 1971; Stagno et al., 1983). These infants have sensorineural hearing loss, subnormal intelligence, and behavior problems.

Approximately 10 per cent of seropositive women in the United States excrete cytomeglovirus from the genital tract at the time of delivery. It is estimated that 50 per cent of infants born to such women acquire CMV during the process of labor and delivery. In addition, approximately 30 per cent of infants nursed by seropositive mothers contract CMV via breast milk transmission. Unlike the situation with *in utero* transmission of CMV, perinatal transmission either intrapartum or postpartum does not have serious implications for the future development of the infant except in the case of extremely low-birth-weight infants (<1200 gm).

There are multiple potential sources of perinatal infection with cytomegalovirus. Transplacental transmission from mother to fetus has been confirmed. In addition, *in utero* infection may possibly be due to ascending infection across intact membranes from an infected cervix. The common presence of the virus in the cervix and birth canal is an obvious source of acquired neonatal infection, as with herpes simplex virus. Cytomegalovirus has also been isolated in breast milk. Another potential source of infection is sibling contact.

The timing of infection during pregnancy is another major determinant of outcome. Monif and colleagues (1972) have shown that the more severely affected infants are those who acquire CMV infection in the first or second trimester of pregnancy. Those born after third-trimester maternal infection were normal at birth, but had cord serum cytomegalovirus IgM antibodies, suggesting "silent" congenital infection. Stern and Tucker (1973) have shown that 50 per cent of infants whose mothers developed a primary infection during pregnancy were excreting virus after delivery. None of the infants of the eight women in their study who had reactivation of infection during pregnancy were excreting virus after delivery. Stagno et al. (1986) similarly noted that primary maternal CMV during the first 20 weeks gestation was significantly more likely to result in infants with sequelae than when infection occurred during the third trimester. Thus, it appears that primary infection is more important than reactivation of latent infection in pregnancy, and primary infection during the first two trimesters presents a greater risk for fetal involvement than infection occurring in the third trimester. However, most women who excrete virus during pregnancy do so as a result of recurrent infection (Stagno and Whitley, 1985). Thus intrauterine CMV infection more often follows recurrent maternal infection than primary infection. On the other hand, primary maternal infection is more often associated with severe clinically apparent congenital CMV.

The prognosis is poor for babies who have clinically apparent disease at birth. CNS and perceptual disabilities usually result in severe mental retardation. The major sites for this chronic disease are the brain and perceptual organs, with resultant seizures, spastic diplegia, optic atrophy, blindness, and sensorineural deafness. Recently, interest has shifted from obviously diseased infants to prognosis of the 90 to 95 per cent of congenitally infected neonates who appear normal at birth. These children do not develop normally, and significant neurologic sequelae may become apparent with time (Reynolds et al., 1974; Hanshaw, 1971; Hanshaw et al., 1976). Long-term longitudinal follow-up studies have documented progressive sensorineural hearing loss and apparently subtle brain damage resulting in lowered IQ and school-associated behavioral problems, which develop over several years following delivery of infants with subclinical cytomegalovirus infection. The prevalence of this viral infection suggests that CMV may be a leading cause of deafness, a major contributor to school-related learning disabilities, and a significant public health problem.

CLINICAL MANIFESTATIONS. Almost all maternal infections, primary and recurrent, are asymptomatic. Occasionally, cytomegalovirus infection manifests as a heterophile-negative mononucleosis syndrome with leukocytosis, relative or absolute lymphocytosis, abnormal liver function readings, abrupt onset of spiking temperature, and constitutional symptoms such as malaise, myalgias, and chills. The mildness of the pharyngitis, minimal lymphadenopathy, and absence of hepatosplenomegaly and jaundice help to differentiate this disease from the infectious mononucleosis syndrome.

The spectrum of disease caused by cytomegalovirus in the fetus and neonate is very broad. Of the congenitally infected infants, 90 to 95 per cent are completely asymptomatic at birth. Clinically apparent disease ranges from isolated organ involvement to the classic multi-organ system disease. In the severely infected neonate, the clinical features include hepatosplenomegaly, jaundice, thrombocytopenic, purpura, microcephaly, deafness, chorioretinitis, optic atrophy, and cerebral calcifications. The cerebral calcifications are characteristically periventricular in the subependymal region. A characteristic tetrad of findings has been described in the infants who have survived fulminant, clinically apparent infection; these are mental retardation, chorioretinitis, cerebral calcifications, and microcephaly.

DIAGNOSIS. Because maternal infection is almost always asymptomatic, the diagnosis is rarely suspected or confirmed in pregnancy. Even when clinical disease occurs, it is generally mild and cytomegalovirus is usually overlooked as a diagnostic possibility.

Several antibody tests are available. The complement fixation (CF) method is no longer preferred because of considerable cross reactivity with other herpesviruses. Indirect hemagglutination (IHA), ELISA, fluorescent antibody (FA), and neutralization tests are available for epidemiologic studies. Because approximately 50 per cent of adults have antibody, a single positive test result does not necessarily indicate recent or current infection. The use of paired specimens, an initial follow-up, and the demonstration of seroconversion (presence of a significant rise in titer) are the best means of documenting a primary infection. If infection has occurred within the previous 4 to 8 months, IgM-specific antibody can be detected in the serum.

The best way to establish the presence of cytomegalovirus infection is by isolating the virus. Isolation does not differentiate primary infection from recurrent. On the other hand, diagnosis of asymptomatic recurrent infection is dependent on viral isolation from the urine or cervix, because no change in antibody levels occurs in normal hosts with recurrent infection. Two to 6 weeks may be required for cytopathic effects of the virus to be seen in tissue culture of cervical swabs or urine samples.

A major concern has been the risk of CMV acquisition by hospital personnel working in areas such as newborn nurseries in which a high rate of CMV infection can be expected. Fortunately, studies in Sweden and the United States have shown that such personnel, including nurses, do not have higher rates of seroconversion than do people working in other patient care areas or with the general population (Balfour and Balfour, 1986).

Most newborns infected with cytomegalovirus are asymptomatic. The few clinically apparent infections are similar in presentation to other congenital infections such as toxoplasmosis, rubella, syphilis, and herpes; the characteristic periventricular calcifications may be helpful in clinically differentiating congenital cytomegalovirus infection. Laboratory confirmation is necessary, however. Although serology can be used as an aid in diagnosis of congenital cytomegalovirus infection, virus isolation is more sensitive and direct. In newborns, as in adults, newer methods such as indirect hemagglutination test, ELISA, and fluorescent antibody test have replaced the complement fixation test.

The great majority of neonates with congenital cytomegalovirus have antibody to the virus when tested with the newer, more sensitive and specific methods. Approximately 80 per cent of congenitally infected infants have IgM-specific antibody in their sera during the first few months of life. This test is rather sophisticated and available in only a few medical research laboratories. Virus isolation is the best method available for documenting newborn infection with cytomegalovirus. Specimens can be taken from the urine, nasopharynx, conjunctiva, or spinal fluid.

The general consensus holds that routine antepartum screening for CMV infection is not indicated. This belief was based on the realization that while approximately 2 per cent of susceptible pregnant women acquire primary CMV during pregnancy, the overwhelming majority are asymptomatic. Thus maternal screening would require a cumbersome (logistically and economically) practice of testing at the initial prenatal visit for anti-CMV IgG and retesting seronegatives at subsequent visits to document seroconversion or to identify anti-CMV IgM antibody in symptomatic women. Further compounding the problem, in the past, has been the lack of effective drug therapy to treat maternal and/or fetal CMV infection or reliable practical methods to determine the presence of fetal infection. However, as effective therapies are introduced and an effective CMV vaccine becomes available, the question of routine screening should be reassessed. For the present, the best alternative for prevention of congenital CMV may be that recommended by Yow and Demmler (1992). They proposed that all women have their CMV-antibody status determined, and those who are CMV-seronegative (i.e., susceptible to primary infection) should be counseled. Seronegative pregnant women should practice careful hygiene and minimize contact with toddlers' urine and saliva.

Recently, significant strides have been made in the prenatal diagnosis of congenital CMV infection (Hohlfield, 1991). Direct fetal sampling by fetoscopy (Lange et al., 1982) and cordocentesis (Hogge et al., 1988) have detected elevated levels of anti-CMV IgM. More recent studies have demonstrated that amniocentesis with culturing of the amniotic fluid may be the optimum method for detection of *in utero* CMV infection (Weiner and Grose, 1990; Hogge et al., 1988; Lamy et al., 1992; Lynch et al., 1991). Grose and Weiner (1990) recommended that amniotic fluid culture for CMV should be obtained in pregnant women with documented primary CMV or when ultrasonography demonstrates IUGR, hydrops, or ascites and CNS abnormalities.

TREATMENT. No effective therapy for maternal CMV infection is approved and clinically available. In moth-ers with the infectious mononucleosis—like syndrome, treatment is symptomatic.

No satisfactory therapy is currently available for the treatment of congenital infection. Attempts have been made to use antiviral agents, such as adenosine arabinoside (ara-A), and cytosine arabinoside (ara-C), for neonates with severe clinical infection. These drugs are toxic, and although they temporarily suppress the excretion of the virus, shedding resumes when the drugs are stopped. Their toxicity precludes treatment of the much more common asymptomatic CMV infection. Recent good results with ganciclovir to treat serious CMV infections (retinitis and esophagitis) in AIDS patients (Collaborative DHPG Treatment Study Group, 1986) and as a prophylactic agent to prevent CMV disease after organ transplantation (Merigan et al., 1992), has led to the hope that ganciclovir will be effective in the management of neonatal symptomatic CMV.

The clinician is faced with a dilemma when dealing with maternal cytomegalovirus infection. The majority of maternal infections are undiagnosable, and serologic status is not predictive of the possibility of fetal infection. Thus, counseling patients about the disease is practically impossible. In those instances in which a primary infection is documented during the first 20 weeks of gestation, after manifesting as a heterophile-negative mononucleosis syndrome, a therapeutic termination of pregnancy should be considered. Counseling a mother who has already given birth to an infected infant is also difficult. In such a situation the incidence of recurrence is unknown. However, it is clear that subsequent congenital infections are associated with a much better prognosis than the initial episode.

The development of a cytomegalovirus vaccine has been suggested as a means of preventing congenital infection with its associated morbidity and mortality (Elek and Stern, 1974). However, the facts that the virus persists in the host even in the presence of high levels of specific antibody and that existing maternal antibody does not invariably protect against congenital infection suggest that such an approach is unlikely to be successful. Other methods of prevention and control are probably required.

Varicella (Chickenpox) and Herpes Zoster

The varicella zoster virus, a member of the herpesvirus family, is a DNA virus. Varicella is the acute primary disease commonly known as chickenpox. Herpes zoster is the recurrent form of infection.

This common childhood disease is usually marked by typical skin lesions, which progress from macules and papules to vesicles and pustules. A highly contagious disorder, varicella is acquired by most persons in the United States prior to reproductive age and is generally self-limited. In adults who contract the disease, constitutional and pulmonary symptoms may be more severe. The special problems for the obstetrician include a possible increase in severity of the disease in the pregnant woman and the effects on the fetus and newborn.

Varicella is an unusual infection in adults and probably occurs with no greater frequency in pregnant women. Varicella pneumonia also is probably no more common in pregnant women than in nonpregnant adults, but there is some evidence that it is more fulminant in pregnancy. A literature review in 1965 reported mortality in 41 per cent of pregnant women with varicella pneumonia compared to 11 per cent in nonpregnant women (Harris and Rhoades, 1965). However, more recent reports suggest that the mortality rate for varicella pneumonia in pregnancy ranges from 0 to 25 per cent, which is similar to that seen in nonpregnant women (Smego and Asperilla, 1991; Paryani and Arvin, 1986). However, most pregnant patients with varicella do not develop pulmonary signs. Although a detailed discussion of varicella pneumonia is not appropriate here, a few points are worth emphasizing. Pulmonary symptoms begin on the second to sixth day after appearance of the rash, usually consisting of a mild nonproductive cough. If the disease is more severe, there may also be pleuritic chest pain, hemoptysis, dyspnea, and frank cyanosis. Physical examination reveals fever, rales, and wheezes. The pregnant patient should be warned to contact her physician immediately if even mild pulmonary symptoms develop. Hospitalization with full respiratory support should then be made available. Although primary varicella zoster (chickenpox) is associated with significant morbidity during pregnancy, morbidity is rare with recurrent herpes-zoster.

Smego and Asperilla reported on their use of acyclovir for the management of severe varicella (e.g., pneumonia) during pregnancy (Smego and Asperilla, 1991). They reviewed 21 cases, of which 12 required intubation and mechanical ventilation. The mortality rate was 14 per cent—all in the third trimester. No adverse drug effects were noted. The dosage recommended for acyclovir is 10 to 15 mg/kg three times daily for 7 days.

Congenital anomalies due to varicella in early pregnancy were not recognized until the mid–1970s (Brozin et al., 1979; Balducci et al., 1992). It is now appreciated that maternal varicella infection in the first 4 months of pregnancy rarely will produce a congenital varicella syndrome, which consists of cutaneous scars, limb hypoplasia, rudimentary digits, and occasionally eye and central nervous system abnormalities including cerebral cortical atrophy and mental retardation (Siegel, 1973).

Paryani and Arvin (1986) reported that while varicella during pregnancy was associated with maternal morbidity and evidence of fetal infection, herpes zoster was not. These investigators prospectively studied 43 pregnancies complicated by varicella and 14 by herpes zoster. Nine of 43 pregnant women with varicella had associated complications including pneumonia, death, and premature delivery. According to clinical or immunologic criteria, eight of 33 infants had evidence of intrauterine varicella infection. The congenital varicella syndrome occurred in one of 11 infants of women with first-trimester varicella. Higa and co-workers (1987) hypothesized that congenital malformations related to the varicella zoster virus (VZV) may not be caused by varicella of the fetus, but rather

can be ascribed to sequelae of herpes zoster infection *in utero*. In particular, recurrent zoster infection would explain the cutaneous and limb abnormalities whereas acute varicella is responsible for the central nervous system/neurologic lesions. The risk for congenital varicella among infants whose mothers develop varicella in the first trimester ranges from 0 to 9 per cent with a cumulative rate of 3 per cent (Table 42–5).

Although the risk of the congenital varicella syndrome is small, some authorities have recommended administration of varicella zoster immune globulin (VZIG) to susceptible pregnant women who have not previously had varicella as soon as possible, but within 96 hours of exposure, in the hope of protecting the fetus during the viremia. However, this treatment is expensive, and no trials have been conducted to establish the benefit of this approach. Treatment with VZIG is safe and does decrease maternal clinical manifestations. Pregnant women exposed to varicella should be questioned as to a history of chickenpox. Only those who do not know or say no should be screened for antibody evidence of previous varicella. From this group only susceptible women (i.e., having no antibodies against varicella zoster) should receive VZIG.

A number of serologic assays detect antibodies to VZV. These techniques include complement fixation, immune adherence hemagglutination (IAHA), fluorescent antibody against membrane antigen (FAMA), and ELISA. Complement fixation is insensitive compared with FAMA or ELISA. Because ELISA is more readily available, it has become the method of choice for measuring antibodies to VZV.

Acquisition of maternal antibody usually protects the fetus. However, if an infant is born after the maternal viremia but before the mother has developed an antibody response, the fetus is at high risk for life-threatening neonatal varicella infection. It has been determined that infants at risk are those whose mothers contract varicella within 5 days before or after delivery. Congenital varicella infection has been reported in 17 per cent of term infants born to mothers who have varicella within 4 to 5 days of delivery, and the case fatality rate is 31 per cent (four of 13) (DeNicola and Hanshaw, 1979). Varicella zoster immune globulin can prevent or moderate clinical varicella in susceptible individuals if given shortly after exposure. VZIG can be obtained from regional offices of the American Red Cross. Infants born to mothers who develop varicella between 5 days before and 2 days after delivery should receive at least 125 U of VZIG.

TABLE 42–5. Risk of Symptomatic Intrauterine Varicella-Zoster Infection After First-Trimester Maternal Varicella

STUDY	NO. INFANTS EXPOSED	NO. INFANTS WITH CONGENITAL VARICELLA
Siegal	27	2 (7.4%)
Paryani & Arvin, 1986	11	1 (9%)
Enders	23	0
Balducci	35	0
TOTAL	96	3 (3%)

In England, no deaths attributable to varicella occurred among 91 VZIG-treated seronegative infants whose mothers had acute varicella up to 2 weeks after delivery (Miller et al., 1989). Interestingly, two-thirds of the infants had evidence of varicella infection, and one-half of those infected had symptomatic disease. Thus, while VZIG may ameliorate the infection it does not universally prevent varicella in the neonate.

Herpes Simplex

In the past few years, important new information has become available regarding perinatal herpes, and this has improved our understanding of its pathogenesis and changed treatment recommendations.

Herpes simplex virus may infect the adult, the newborn, or, on rare occasion, the fetus. In the adult, typical lesions are vesicular or ulcerative, involving only the skin and mucous membranes. More widespread infection involving the central nervous system is an extremely unusual adult complication, most often developing in those with debilitating disease. On the other hand, because of an incompletely developed immune system, the newborn is subject to systemic, frequently lethal, disease.

In adults, the virus commonly causes infection of the oral cavity, skin, and lower genital tract. In the past, herpes simplex virus type 1 was said to be responsible for infection of the mouth and of the skin above the waist, and type 2 virus for infection of the genitalia and of the skin below the waist. Approximately 90 per cent of cases still follow the pattern, but either type may cause infection at either site.

In surveys of adult females, herpesvirus has been isolated from the genitalia of 0.02 to 1 per cent. Among pregnant women, one survey found positive cultures in 0.6 per cent of asymptomatic women. The disease does not appear to be more severe or more protracted in pregnancy. A recent serologic survey with a reliable antibody test for HSV–2 revealed a 32 per cent seroprevalence in a cohort of private patients in California (Kulhanjian et al., 1992).

Clinically, there are three herpetic syndromes in adults. *First-episode primary genital herpes* is the clinical presentation in a patient without antibodies to either HSV–1 or HSV–2. Its clinical manifestations include severe local symptoms, with lesions lasting two to three weeks, regional adenopathy, constitutional symptoms, and, in a small percentage, viral meningitis. It should be noted that as many as two-thirds of women with HSV–2 antibodies have acquired the infection asymptomatically (Kulhanjian et al., 1992). This recent observation represents a major change from previous concepts. *First-episode nonprimary infection* is the initial clinical episode in a patient with antibodies to type 1 or type 2. It is similar in presentation to recurrent episodes. Recurrent genital herpes infections are much milder and shorter, with viral shedding lasting an average of only three to five days.

When primary genital herpes occurs in pregnancy, there is a high risk of fetal and neonatal involvement, especially with infection in the third trimester (Brown et al., 1987). Brown and co-workers found that serious prenatal morbidity occurred in 6 of 15 infants born to women with primary infections in pregnancy and in four of five with primary infection in the third trimester. In addition, asymptomatic viral shedding was more common later in pregnancy.

Transplacental infection of the fetus resulting in congenital infection is a rare sequel to maternal infection, presumably arising from primary infections with viremia. Only a few such documented cases have been reported (Hutto et al., 1987).

When episodes recur in pregnancy, there appears to be no increase in abortion or low-birth-weight infants (Kulhanjian et al., 1992). When nonprimary first episodes occur in pregnancy, the course is similar to that of recurrent infections (Brown et al., 1987).

The major perinatal problem is neonatal herpes infection. Exact estimates of its frequency are subject to error because up to 50 per cent of infants with culture-proven fatal disease may not show typical lesions on the skin or mucous membranes. In addition, viral laboratories have not been widely available, and recent treatment recommendations have probably decreased the incidence of neonatal disease.

Neonatal herpes is acquired perinatally from an infected lower maternal genital tract, most commonly during vaginal delivery. Other cases have occurred in newborns delivered by cesarean section. If primary genital herpes is present in the mother at the time of delivery, the risk of neonatal herpes infection in the infant delivered through the vagina may be as high as 40 per cent. However, the risk is lower among women with recurrent clinically evident infection. In these women, the risk is probably less than 5 per cent. Recent data from Stanford University indicate that the risk to infants born vaginally in women with *asymptomatic recurrent* infection was zero of 34, with 95 per cent confidence limits of zero to 8 per cent (Prober et al., 1987). However, asymptomatically infected patients can give birth to seriously infected neonates. In a referral nursery, 70 per cent of mothers of infected infants had asymptomatic infections. Among infants with disseminated herpes, the risk of death or serious sequelae is about 50 per cent. Thus, maternal antibodies do not offer complete protection to the neonate (Nahmias et al., 1971; Amstey and Monif, 1974).

Diagnosis. The clinical diagnosis of genital herpes is based on typical, painful crops of vesicles and ulcers in various stages of progression. With primary infection, there is apt to be regional lymphadenopathy, fever, and other more marked constitutional symptoms. Primary genital herpes usually lasts 2 to 3 weeks. Clinically detectable recurrences are variable, but about 50 per cent of patients have recurrent disease within 6 months. Recurrences are more mild, with fewer lesions, fewer constitutional symptoms, and a shorter course (usually 10 to 14 days).

One-third of women with genital herpes do not have typical lesions. Thus, for screening procedures, cytologic and culture techniques have been used. Although herpes infection may be suggested by rather typical changes seen in Papanicolaou smears (intranuclear inclusion bodies and multinucleated giant cells), the 20 to 25 per cent rate of false-negative results is too high for this to be used with diagnostic accuracy.

The "gold standard" diagnostic test to rule out the presence of herpesvirus infection is the viral culture, but even the culture has a recognized false-negative rate. For clinical use, it is fortunate that this virus grows rapidly, with most positive cultures being identifiable at 48 to 72 hours. Rapid diagnostic tests are currently available, including a monoclonal antibody and an ELISA. As with rapid techniques for other genital infections, these methods have their best performance in high-prevalence populations. Recent data suggest that they may be reliable in patients with vesicular or ulcerative genital lesions (compared to culture), but the culture remains the diagnostic technique of choice.

Neonatal herpes infection may be limited to the skin or may be systemic with or without cutaneous involvement. Typically, clinical disease begins at the end of the first week of life. Because the findings depend on the organ system involved, the presentation may include skin lesions, cough, cyanosis, tachypnea, dyspnea, jaundice, seizures, and disseminated intravascular coagulation. In infants at risk for, or suspected of having, neonatal herpes, the only reliable diagnostic test is the viral culture.

A few infants have been described with congenital (transplacental) herpes infection. Congenital infection has been manifested by typical cutaneous lesions apparent within 24 to 48 hours of life; fetal infection presumably occurs a few days before birth. In other cases, there have been less specific clinical signs (microcephaly and spasticity), but serologic evidence of infection is present. Transplacental infection presumably results from maternal viremia, which occurs only with primary maternal infection (Hutto et al., 1987).

In the individual patient, commercially available serologic techniques have little utility. Cross-reactivity of antibodies to serotypes 1 and 2 preclude differentiation. One use of these commercial tests is to rule out previous genital herpes in a patient with an unconfirmed or equivocal history by demonstrating absence of antibodies to both HSV–1 and HSV-2. A reliable antibody test to distinguish type 2 from type 1 is available as a research tool. It uses type-specific antibody to type 2 glycoprotein G (Kulhanjian et al., 1992).

TREATMENT. In the last few years, treatment of genital herpes and management of genital herpes in pregnancy have been markedly revised. During clinically evident episodes, treatment consists of supportive measures such as analgesics, hygiene, and good topical anesthetics. Secondary infections such as *Monilia* should also be treated. Many women find that frequent bathing, followed by thorough drying of the affected area with a hair dryer, provides temporary relief.

Acyclovir, an antiviral agent with excellent activity against herpes infection, is a specific inhibitor in viral thymidine kinase. It is available in topical, oral, and intravenous preparations. In nonpregnant individuals, all of the forms have been of value in decreasing the duration of symptoms and of viral shedding in primary genital infection. In immunocompetent individuals, the oral form is also effective in shortening some recurrences significantly (200 mg PO 5 times a day for 5 days) and in suppressing frequent recurrences (200 mg PO 2 to 3 times a day for 6 months). In regard to the use of acyclovir in pregnancy, the benefits must be weighed against the potential risks in each case. Several hundred pregnant women with severe genital herpes infection have received acyclovir without any increase in birth defects to date (Andrews et al., 1992). However, use in pregnancy is not recommended for mild cases; neither is prophylactic use currently recommended. Concerns regarding prophylactic use are (1) whether acyclovir suppresses asymptomatic shedding as well as symptomatic recurrences and (2) whether acyclovir may have unusual kinetics in the fetus that could lead to concentration in such organs as the fetal liver and could cause toxicity. The latter concern is entirely theoretical.

Because of the severity of neonatal herpes infection and the lack of satisfactory therapy, the only current means of preventing neonatal infection is to avoid contact between the fetus and the infected maternal lower genital tract by performing cesarean section. Accordingly, recommendations are for use of cesarean section when typical herpes lesions are present at the time of labor, regardless of duration since membrane rupture (ACOG, 1988; Gibbs et al., 1988).

Major changes have also developed in management of pregnant women with a history of recurrent genital herpes. Until recently, the standard practice has been as follows: Patients with a history of genital herpes should be screened for recurrent herpes of the genital tract at term. In general, weekly cultures should be initiated at 35 or 36 weeks. If premature delivery is anticipated, screening should be started earlier. If the last two cultures taken prior to birth have been negative and there are no new lesions, it is safe to assume that there is no active infection in the maternal genital tract.

If cultures taken in late pregnancy are positive, the patient should be instructed to contact the obstetrician immediately when labor begins or the membranes rupture. When labor seems likely in a patient with active herpes at term, a planned cesarean delivery is appropriate. However, it was not considered necessary to perform cesarean section in all patients with active herpes in late pregnancy because of the possibility that the infection might clear before the onset of labor. Management can be individualized by the use of repeated cultures. Previous recommendations included use of amniocentesis to exclude transplacental herpes prior to performing a cesarean section in a mother with genital herpes. However, the risk of transplacental infection is low (probably lower than the risk of amniocentesis), and the amniotic fluid tests may not correlate with findings in the newborn.

This policy was widely criticized on the basis of four arguments. First, it appeared to overestimate the risk of neonatal sepsis after vaginal delivery of an asymptomatically infected mother. Second, because the duration of viral shedding in an asymptomatic episode is short (3 to 5 days), by the time the culture result was read it would no longer reflect the culture status in the patient. Third, with weekly cultures, most episodes of asymptomatic shedding would be missed. Fourth, the cost of screening programs was high, estimated by one group to be $1.8 million to prevent cases of neonatal sepsis (Binkin et al., 1984).

In 1986, Arvin and colleagues reported herpes simplex virus cultures in a series of 515 pregnant women with recurrent herpes infection. Seventeen had positive antepartum cultures, but none was positive at delivery. Of 354 asymptomatic mothers, five (1.4 per cent) had positive results at delivery, but none had positive antepartum cultures. The likelihood of asymptomatic shedding at delivery was 1.3 per cent. Later, the same group reported a series of 34 neonates born vaginally of women with asymptomatic infection. None became infected, leading to a maximum theoretical risk of 8 per cent (Prober et al., 1987).

We believe these data are convincing and recommend the following plan of management. First, the obstetrician should assume the responsibility of eliciting a history of genital herpes. Second, if the diagnosis of genital herpes has not previously been confirmed by culture, culture should be performed during an active episode. Third, serial cultures in *asymptomatic women* beginning at 34 to 36 weeks, as previously recommended in patients with a history of herpes infection, can be abandoned. Fourth, herpesvirus cultures can be used, however, to document absence of the virus after a clinically evident episode in late pregnancy. Fifth, the patient should be told to come to the hospital early in labor or immediately if she has premature rupture of the membranes. Also, she should be informed of the low risk of asymptomatic infection at delivery (1 per cent) and the low risk of neonatal infection after delivery through an asymptomatically infected genital tract. Sixth, when the patient arrives in labor with membrane rupture, a careful pelvic examination should be performed. If no lesions are present, the delivery can be managed normally. If lesions are observed, cesarean section to prevent neonatal herpes is indicated. Seventh, viral culturing of asymptomatic women with a history of HSV infection has been suggested by some, and culturing of the infants has been suggested by others (ACOG, 1988; Gibbs et al., 1988).

In the nursery, infection control measures for the infant of an infected mother include isolation of the newborn, gown and glove precautions, and double bagging of contaminated disposable materials. The newborn may be brought to the mother provided she performs supervised thorough handwashing, is seated in a chair, and is wearing a clean gown (Kilbrick, 1980).

Newborns of mothers with nongenital herpes do not require any special precautions during labor and delivery. However, after the mother has contact, the newborn is considered suspect for herpes and is handled as just described.

Suspected infants should be cultured for herpesvirus and observed closely by examination. If the parents are reliable, it is not necessary to delay the infant's discharge. Rather, the parents may be informed of signs and symptoms of possible neonatal infection and then contacted regularly by telephone. Kilbrick (1980) recommends that the clinically infected mother be permitted to handle her infant with the precautions just cited. The baby must be brought to her; the mother should not enter the nursery. It is not known whether breast-feeding by a woman with active genital herpes poses any clear risk to the newborn.

Because the woman with nongenital herpes at delivery may also infect her newborn, many of the precautions advised for control of genital herpes are recommended. These include the use of private room, gown and glove precautions, and proper disposal of linen and dressings. In addition, topical applications of agents (such as ethyl ether, povidone-iodine, or benzoin) to hasten crusting of the lesions are recommended. After the lesions have become encrusted, the mother may handle and feed her infant provided precautions used for women with genital herpes are followed. Owing to limited information, several clinical problems exist. For example, there is no consensus regarding management of patients with third-trimester primary herpes. The pregnancy should be monitored for premature birth, fetal status, and growth abnormalities, but there is no scientifically based plan regarding use of antiviral therapy or the method of delivery.

Hepatitis

Acute viral hepatitis is a systemic infection predominantly affecting the liver. A variety of distinct viral agents are now recognized as causing viral hepatitis (Table 42–6). Laboratory diagnosis can be established by testing immunologic responses to these viral agents (Table 42–6). In the past, the term non-A non-B hepatitis was used to describe cases of hepatitis in which hepatitis A (HAV) and hepatitis B (HBV) had been excluded by serologic testing. Recently, two

TABLE 42–6. Nomenclature of Hepatitis Viruses

HEPATITIS VIRUS TYPE	ROUTE OF TRANSMISSION	INCUBATION PERIOD (whs)	CONFIRMATORY TEST	CHRONIC DISEASE
A	Fecal-oral	2–7	Anti-HA IgM	0
B	Parenteral Sexual Peripartum	7–15	HBsAg, HB core antigen, anti-HBc antibody	10%
C	Parenteral Sexual	4–8	Anti-HCV antibody, PRC for viral RNA	50%
D	Parenteral Sexual	4–20	Anti-HDV antibody	5–70%
E	Fecal-oral	2–8	Immune electron microscopy of viral particles in feces, ELISA, anti-HEV antibody	0

TABLE 42–7. Nomenclature of Hepatitis B Antigens and Antibodies

HEPATITIS TYPE	ANTIGEN	ANTIBODY
B	Hepatitis B surface antigen (HBsAg)	Anti-HBs
	Hepatitis B core antigen (HBcAg)	Anti-HBc
	Hepatitis B e antigen (HBeAg)	Anti-HBe

distinct viruses have been identified that cause the majority of non-A non-B hepatitis. These are hepatitis C virus (HCV), which is the major cause of post-transfusion hepatitis, and hepatitis E virus (HEV), which is responsible for the enterically transmitted form. Delta agent (hepatitis D), another cause of hepatitis, requires HBV to replicate. The delta agent is capable of transforming asymptomatic or mild chronic HBV infection into severe, progressive chronic active hepatitis and cirrhosis. It also accelerates the course of chronic active hepatitis. Other viral agents causing hepatitis include cytomegalovirus, Epstein-Barr virus, varicella zoster, coxsackie B, herpes simplex, and rubella viruses. Because the major impact of hepatitis on the fetus and neonate relates to hepatitis B, the emphasis of this discussion will be on the epidemiology, mode of transmission, and clinical aspects of hepatitis B (also see Chapter 58).

Maternal infection during pregnancy with the hepatitis B virus is increasingly recognized as a threat to the fetus and neonate. In addition, clinically apparent icteric hepatitis is now recognized as only a part of the disease spectrum, and "silent" infections may result in chronic and progressive damage.

The nomenclature of HBV antigens and antibodies is summarized in Table 42—7. HBV is a DNA virus 42 mm in diameter. The outer protein coat is the "surface antigen" (HBsAg); this is produced in excess by the liver and appears in the serum. The central core of the virus contains DNA, DNA polymerase, and the "core antigen," HBcAg. This antigen is found only in infected liver cells and not in serum. A third HBV antigen is the "e antigen," HBeAg, which is related to the virus core but is found in serum. Each of these antigens has a corresponding antibody: anti-HBs, anti-HBc, and anti-HBe, respectively.

The e antigen appears early in almost all patients during the acute phase of hepatitis B infection and may persist in patients in whom the infection progresses to chronic active hepatitis. Most important, several significant prognostic and epidemiologic observations have been made with the e system. Persistent carriers of HBsAg who have e antigen-positive blood have a greater chance of developing chronic active hepatitis. Second, it has been demonstrated that HBsAg-positive blood that lacks e antigen but contains anti-e antibody does not cause post-transfusion hepatitis, whereas e antigen-positive blood carries a significant risk for post-transfusion hepatitis B. The third finding relates to pregnancy and transmission of hepatitis B from mother to offspring. Mothers with e antigen-positive blood uniformly transmit HBsAg to their children, whereas those with HBsAg-positive, e antigen-negative blood appear to be less likely to transmit HBsAg to their offspring. Thus, it seems

likely that the presence of e antigen identifies the group that is highly infectious and at greater risk of transmitting hepatitis B virus.

HA virus is a 27-nm RNA virus and may be classified as an enterovirus. Following an incubation period of 15 to 49 days, HAV commonly produces acute hepatitis, which is usually a mild, self-limited disease without chronic sequelae. Death occurs in less than 1 per cent of hospitalized cases. No chronic carrier state exists for HAV. The presence of IgM anti-HA in the serum suggests current or recent infection. The presence of IgG anti-HA indicates that infection has occurred in the past and confers immunity to hepatitis A. Mild and clinically unrecognized infections with HA virus commonly occur in childhood and account for the high incidence of IgG anti-HA in adult populations, a finding reflected in the adequate antibodies present in normal immune serum globulin. HAV is transmitted predominantly by the fecal-oral route. There is no evidence that the course of HAV is altered by pregnancy, nor any suggestion of specific fetal effects or perinatal transmission.

Following the identification of hepatitis C virus (HCV) and development of serologic testing for anti-HCV antibody (Kuo et al., 1989; Chou et al., 1989) it was recognized that HCV is the major etiologic agent of transfusion-associated hepatitis (formerly non-A non-B hepatitis). HCV is a single-stranded RNA virus. The predominant route of transmission is parenteral, but sexual transmission also appears possible (Lynch-Salamon and Coombs, 1992). Among blood donors the seroprevalence of anti-HCV antibody has ranged from 0.5 to 1.4 per cent (Esteban et al., 1989; Stevens et al., 1990; Dawson et al., 1991). Acute HCV is responsible for 5 per cent of all reported cases of hepatitis, and approximately 50 per cent of cases progress to chronic liver disease. To date, identified risk factors for HCV are intravenous drug use, previous blood transfusion, and multiple sexual partners. Previous studies on non-A non-B hepatitis suggested that vertical transmission (based on elevated transaminases) occurred in two-thirds of infants born to mothers with acute disease in the third trimester and that one-third of infected infants developed chronic liver disease. Several serologic studies have suggested that perinatal transmission of HCV can occur (Reesink et al., 1990; Giovannini et al., 1990). Thaler et al. (1991), utilizing the polymerase chain reaction, demonstrated the presence of HCV RNA in six of seven infants whose mothers had circulating HCV RNA. The implication of this finding is unclear as only two infants demonstrated moderate elevation of transaminases. Whether perinatal HCV infection initiates a silent disease process or chronic carrier state that is associated with chronic liver disease or hepatocellular carcinoma remains to be clarified.

The enterically transmitted agent associated with non-A non-B hepatitis has been named hepatitis E virus (HEV). HEV disease occurs in epidemic and sporadic forms, and most outbreaks are associated with fecal contamination of drinking water. The disease occurs predominantly in Asia, Africa, the Middle East, and Central America. Recent outbreaks have been reported in Mexico. The incubation period of

HEV ranges from 2 to 8 weeks. The attack rate is highest among young adults aged 15 to 39. Unlike HAV, hepatitis E can be a severe disease. In epidemics of hepatitis E the case fatality rate is 1 to 2 per cent, with the most severe form occurring in pregnant women during the third trimester and having a case fatality rate of 10 to 20 per cent (Gust and Purcell, 1987). Until recently, diagnosis of hepatitis E has been based on exclusion of HBV and HAV and detection by immune electron microscopy of virus-like particles in fecal specimens. An ELISA that detects anti-HEV, IgM, and IgG antibodies has recently been developed (Goldsmith et al., 1992).

Hepatitis delta virus (HDV) is an incomplete, defective RNA virus that cannot survive on its own. HDV requires the presence of a DNA virus, specifically HBV, for replication and expression (Houfnagle, 1989). Because of this requirement, HDV infection occurs when there is simultaneous acute HDV and HBV infection or when an acute HDV infection is superimposed on chronic HBV infection (HBsAg carrier). HDV contributes to the development of severe fulminant hepatitis B infection. In addition, HDV accelerates the course of chronic HBV infection to cause chronic active hepatitis and cirrhosis. Although only available in research laboratories, both HDV antigen and anti-HDV antibody can be identified. No direct effect on pregnancy or the fetus has been demonstrated.

The comparative clinical and epidemiologic features of types A and B are shown in Table 42–8. It has become clear that distinction between hepatitis A and B cannot be made solely on epidemiologic and clinical grounds. Detection of serum HBsAg has become the important tool for distinguishing between the two. HBsAg is present in approximately one per 1000 adults in the United States and Europe. However, it is present in 2 to 25 per cent of adults in tropical areas and Southeast Asia.

Epidemiologic studies have demonstrated an increasing incidence of hepatitis B in the general population and in hospitalized patients with acute hepatitis. Hepatitis B often causes a more severe infection than hepatitis A. HBV infection is transmitted predominantly by sexual contact, parenteral exposures, and transmission from mother to newborn during the birth process. World-wide vertical transmission of HBV is the major source of hepatitis B infection. HBsAg has been identified in urine, feces, seminal fluid, saliva, intestinal fluid, and gastric juice. Asymptomatic persistence of HBsAg, without abnormalities of liver function, is the most common form of hepatitis B virus infection. Asymptomatic carriers of hepatitis B are estimated to number about 1 million in the United States, and 200 million people world-wide are believed to serve as an epidemiologic reservoir for hepatitis B infection. Approximately 10 per cent of acute HBV infections result in persistent infection characterized by the presence of HBsAg. This group is at risk to develop chronic hepatitis, cirrhosis and hepatocellular carcinoma. As many as 25 per cent of HBV carriers eventually die of cirrhosis or hepatocellular carcinoma. During the childbearing years, 70 per cent of women in the United States are susceptible to hepatitis B. Approximately two cases of overt hepatitis and one chronic carrier of hepatitis B are encountered per 1000 pregnant women in the general United States population. This risk for infection varies greatly depending on occupation, socioeconomic status, drug abuse, and geographic factors.

The incidence of HBV in pregnancy is similar to that in the general population, and the course of the disease is not altered during pregnancy. No increase in fetal wastage or in risk for congenital anomalies has been noted with HBV. With acute severe HBV infection in the third trimester, a possible increased risk for preterm labor and delivery exists. However, the major concern in pregnancy is vertical transmission to the neonate.

Neonatal Infection. Investigations have demonstrated several important epidemiologic and clinical aspects of hepatitis B infection in the neonate

Table 42–8.   Clinical and Epidemiologic Features of Acute Viral Hepatitis

FEATURES	HEPATITIS A	HEPATITIS B
Epidemiologic		
Onset	Acute	Acute and insidious
Age group	Children and adults	All ages
Season	Fall and winter	All year
Parenteral transmission	Rare	Common
Nonparenteral transmission	Common	Common
Incubation period	15–45 days	45–160 days
Clinical		
Prodrome	Common	Common
Severity	Mild	Mild to severe
Prognosis	Benign	More severe in older patients
Chronic disease	No	Occasionally
Prophylaxis with conventional gamma globulin (immune serum globulin)	Partial protection	Low rate of protection unless recent lot with low levels of anti-HBs is used
Hepatitis B immune globulin		Probably protective
Abnormal SGOT	Transient, 1–3 weeks	Usually more prolonged, 1–8 months
Immunity	Previous infection protects	Previous infection protects

(Schweitzer, 1973; Isenberg, 1977). Approximately 80 to 90 per cent of newborns of mothers who develop acute HBV in the third trimester or within 1 month of delivery will be HBsg-positive within 6 months. Biochemical and histologic abnormalities often are present, but they are usually mild. Persistence of HBsAg has been associated with chronic hepatitis and cirrhosis. The mode of transmission is considered to be oral contamination of the neonate by maternal blood and/or feces during delivery. When maternal hepatitis occurs in early pregnancy, HBsAg is detected much less often in the neonate. The frequency of transmission is also relatively low when the mother is an asymptomatic carrier of HBsAg. However, asymptomatic women who are HBeAg-positive transmit HBV to their newborn in 90 per cent of cases. The risk for asymptomatic HBeAg-negative mothers is 10 to 30 per cent and for the asymptomatic anti-HBe-positive group, the transmission rate is zero to 10 per cent.

MORTALITY RATE. In a well-nourished normal population, the mortality rate from hepatitis is low and no greater in pregnant than in nonpregnant individuals (Adams, 1965). In populations in which malnutrition is a problem, the mortality rate is much higher, but is still similar in pregnant and nonpregnant women. The incidence of spontaneous abortion during the first trimester in patients with acute viral hepatitis has been reported to be increased. Similarly, when viral hepatitis occurs during the third trimester, there is a reported increased incidence of preterm labor. However, the incidence of spontaneous abortion and that of preterm delivery are probably no higher with hepatitis than with other febrile illnesses. Although transplacental passage of hepatitis virus has been established, teratogenic damage has never been demonstrated for type B or A.

DIAGNOSIS. In the neonate, the most frequent presentation of hepatitis B infection is asymptomatic chronic hepatitis with histologic evidence of unresolved hepatitis (Isenberg, 1977; Schweitzer, 1973). Clinical illness is relatively uncommon with congenital hepatitis infection. About 10 per cent of newborns with asymptomatic disease become icteric at 3 to 4 months of age.

Specific diagnosis of hepatitis depends on laboratory confirmation. Hepatitis B surface antigen is the primary diagnostic tool for differentiating hepatitis A from hepatitis B. HBsAg is present in the blood 30 to 50 days after exposure and 7 to 21 days before the onset of jaundice. The antigen may disappear with the onset of jaundice or may persist for many weeks. One per cent of patients in the United States are chronic HBsAG carriers. The SGPT levels rise about 50 days after exposure and are increased at the time jaundice appears. The elevated SGPT levels persist for 30 to 60 days.

Hepatitis Be antigen appears early in the disease and persists for days to weeks, in some cases indefinitely. When HBeAg is present the patient is likely to be infectious. When HBe antibody is present, the patient is much less likely to be infectious. Infected newborns can be diagnosed by the demonstrated presence of HBeAg in the blood. These infants have mild to moderate elevations of the serum transaminase levels. Liver biopsy of infected children may show unresolved hepatitis.

TREATMENT AND PREVENTION. Most pregnancies complicated by acute viral hepatitis can be managed on an outpatient basis. No specific treatment exists for hepatitis. Increased bed rest and a high-protein, low-fat diet are recommended. Indications for hospitalization in patients with viral hepatitis include severe anemia, diabetes, intractable nausea and vomiting, a prolonged prothrombin time, low serum albumin level, and a serum bilirubin level greater than 15 mg/100 ml.

Pregnant women and children with household or other short-duration exposure to hepatitis A infection should be given immune-specific globulin in a dosage of 0.02 to 0.05 ml/kg to modify the disease. For prolonged exposure, the dosage should be 0.06 to 0.14 ml/kg.

The risk of acquiring hepatitis B is greatest for those exposed to hepatitis patients or blood containing HBsAg and especially HBeAg; examples include household contact, hospital exposures, and inoculation with contaminated needles. Women with definite exposure to HBV should be given hepatitis B immune globulin (HBIG), 0.05 to 0.07 ml/kg as soon as possible within 7 days of exposure. For those without serologic evidence of previous immunity, a course of HBV vaccination should be started.

Children born to women who have hepatitis B during pregnancy and who are HBsAg-positive should be given HBIG, a single dose of 0.13 ml/kg within 12 hours of delivery. In addition, hepatitis B vaccine should be given within 12 hours of birth and repeated at 1 month and 6 months of life. In order to accomplish this, HBsAg-positive pregnant women must be identified through the screening of prenatal patients. Women at high risk include (1) those of Asian, Pacific basin, or Native Alaskan descent; (2) those who are Haitian, sub-Saharan African, Eastern European, Middle Eastern, Caribbean, or Central or South American born; (3) illicit drug users; and (4) those with acute or chronic liver disease. In the past, only prenatal patients deemed to be at high risk were screened for HBsAg, and the neonates of HBsAg carriers were immunized. Currently the CDC and ACOG recommend universal screening of all prenatal patients for HBsAg. The rationale for this approach is that approximately 50 per cent of HBsAg-positive pregnant women are not identified by selective screening of high-risk categories (Summers et al., 1987; Kumar et al., 1987) and that routine screening of pregnant women and immunization of neonates is cost effective, resulting in savings of over $100 million annually (Arvello and Washington, 1989). Neonates born to HBsAg-positive mothers should receive HBIG, 0.5 ml IM at birth, followed by Recombivax HB, 5 μg IM shortly after birth and at 1 month and 6 months of life. This approach prevents infection in up to 95 per cent of infants born to positive mothers.

Human Parvovirus Infection

The human parvoviruses are a family of DNA viruses of which human parvovirus B19 is the only known human pathogen (Anderson, 1987; Thurn, 1988). Human parvovirus was first identified in 1975. The virus has a predilection for the hematopoietic system and has been shown to be cytotoxic for erythroid progenitor cells. The most common manifestation of human parvovirus B19 is erythema infectiosum (fifth disease). Parvovirus has also been implicated in aplastic crisis in patients with chronic hemolytic anemia.

Human parvovirus B19 is world-wide in distribution and is most common in young children 5 to 14 years of age. The most common manifestation in children is erythema infectiosum, which has a winter and spring seasonality. In children, the disease tends to be clinically mild and presents with a low-grade prodromal fever that precedes the development of a highly characteristic—an erythematous, warm "slap-cheek" facial rash. Thereafter a morbilliform rash appears on the extremities. Among adults, the disease usually presents with fever, adenopathy, arthralgias, and mild arthritis, particularly of the hands, wrists, and knees. Rash is not usually present in adults.

The diagnosis is generally made on clinical grounds, especially in children. Antibody tests for parvovirus B19 have become available. An ELISA method is currently recommended for IgG- and IgM-specific antibodies to human parvovirus B19. In the United States, 50 to 75 per cent of women in the reproductive age group are immune and demonstrate antibodies against human parvovirus B19. The organism is a highly infectious agent and 60 to 80 per cent of susceptible household contacts will become infected when exposed to childhood disease. Among seronegative school teachers who are at risk during epidemics, 20 to 30 per cent will develop the disease (Gillespie et al., 1990). Finally, the risk to the fetus has received tremendous attention over the last decade since initial reports suggested that during pregnancy human parvovirus B19 may result in fetal hydrops and stillbirth (Anand et al., 1987; CDC, 1989; Rodis et al., 1988; Woernele et al., 1987). The pathogenesis of this disease revolves around the predilection of human parvovirus B19 for human erythroid progenitor cells. With intrauterine transmission to the fetus, the fetus is at risk for developing aplastic anemia secondary to this predilection. The rapidly expanding red blood cell volume, a shorter half-life of red blood cells in the fetus and an immature system make the fetus peculiarly susceptible to the effects of B19 parvovirus.

Although early reports suggested a high rate of transmission to the fetus and a significant morbidity and mortality to the fetus with human parvovirus infection, more recent work has demonstrated that maternal infection produces no adverse effect on the fetus in the majority of cases. Early small case studies suggested a high rate of transmission to the fetus. Woernle et al. (1987) reported that four of 12 pregnant women at risk for B19 were IgM-positive. In this group, one of the four fetuses was a stillbirth due to hydrops.

Other previous reports had described 22 pregnant women with serologic evidence of B19 infection in whom nine fetal deaths occurred. Rodis et al. (1988) reviewed 37 reported cases of women exposed and infected during pregnancy. In this retrospective study, they reported that 14 (38 per cent) of the pregnancies had adverse outcomes including spontaneous abortion, intrauterine fetal death, and congenital anomalies. Eleven of the 37 fetuses had intrauterine fetal hydrops. Similarly, Schwartz et al. (1988), in another retrospective study, reported that 10 of 39 (26 per cent) susceptible pregnancies developed fetal hydrops; seven of these infants died *in-utero* and three who had received intrauterine transfusions survived. However, more recent prospective studies have cast doubt on this high rate of fetal transmission. In England, the Public Health Laboratory Service Working Party on Fifth Disease reported, in a large series of 190 pregnancies, a fetal death rate of 16 per cent; however, only six of the 14 fetuses tested were DNA-positive for human parvovirus B19. These authors reported a fetal loss rate of 1 out of 14 (7 per cent) at more than 20 weeks gestation and a 17 per cent loss at less than 20 weeks, which is similar to the rate in the general population (Public Health Laboratory, 1990). In a prospective study undertaken during a 1988 epidemic of erythema infectiosum in Connecticut, Rodis and colleagues reported that among 39 pregnant women with evidence of recent infection during pregnancy, 37 (95 per cent) delivered healthy newborns and only two (5 per cent) had spontaneous abortions of which only one was related to human parvovirus B19 (Rodis et al., 1990). No infants developed fetal hydrops in this series. In a large prospective study that screened 3526 pregnant women, the Centers for Disease Control (1989) concluded that while the risk for fetal death was increased especially in the first 20 weeks gestation, this did not reach statistical significance. They noted no increase in preterm delivery; birth weights were similar to the B19 infected and controls; and no increase in birth defects occurred among the infants affected with B19.

Women exposed to erythema infectiosum during pregnancy should be screened serologically for IgG and IgM antibodies against parvovirus. The presence of IgG antibody denotes immunity against the disease, and these patients can be reassured. Those who are IgG-negative and IgM-negative are susceptible to infection and should be cautioned to reduce their risk of exposure, especially if they are schoolteachers or work in day care centers during epidemics of fifth disease. The group that are IgG-negative and IgM-positive and in whom acute parvovirus infection is thus confirmed, should be closely evaluated and monitored for the development of intrauterine fetal hydrops. For women with a documented infection, maternal serum alpha-fetoprotein (MSAFP) (Bernstein et al., 1989; Carrington et al., 1987) and diagnostic ultrasonography are utilized to detect the development of hydrops. In general, MSAFP will be elevated prior to the onset of hydrops as demonstrated by sonography. Serial MSAFPs are obtained. If the MSAFP becomes elevated, serial sonograms are then obtained. Hydrops usually occurs 4 to 6 weeks after infection. Once intrauterine evidence for hydrops develops, two alternatives are available. Until recently, intrauterine blood transfusion, usually via PUBS, has been proposed for the treatment of the hydropic fetus with B19 parvovirus-induced anemia and has been reported to be successful (Naides and Weiner, 1989; Peters and Nikolaides, 1990; Sahakian et al., 1991; Soothill, 1990). However, several recent studies have noted cases of fetal hydrops associated with acute parvovirus infection that resolved spontaneously over a course of 4 to 6 weeks without intrauterine transfusion (Humphrey et al., 1991). Thus, the role of intrauterine blood transfusion to prevent intrauterine stillbirth due to hydrops secondary to aplastic anemia remains unclear. It is possible that the younger fetus (at less than 20 to 22 weeks gestation) is at risk and requires intrauterine transfusion, whereas the older fetus, in the latter part of the second trimester with a more functional immune system, may be better able to tolerate the insult from the parvovirus infection.

Recently, Torok et al. (1992) reported on the use of polymerase chain reaction (PCR) to antenatally diagnose *in utero* fetal infection with human parvovirus B19.

Influenza

The predominant feature of influenza during pregnancy is the increased likelihood that life-threatening pneumonia will occur as a complication. Reports from the epidemics of 1889 and 1918, as well as from 1957, all indicate that pregnant women were disproportionately represented in groups dying of influenza. It is not clear whether pregnant women are more likely to develop influenza or whether they are more likely to develop influenza pneumonia. It appears, however, that if influenza pneumonia develops in pregnancy, it is more severe. Death of a pregnant woman with influenza may result from secondary bacterial infection (such as with *S. aureus, S. pneumoniae,* or Klebsiella species) and also from primary influenza pneumonia without bacterial superinfection.

Accordingly, in years of epidemics, it is generally considered advisable to vaccinate pregnant women (Larsen, 1982). Flu vaccines are as immunogenic in pregnant women as in other adults, and no unusual complications have been encountered. The vaccines are killed virus preparations.

The effect of influenza on rates of abortion, prematurity, and congenital anomalies is difficult to determine because the evidence is contradictory. In part, confusion may arise from variations of the virus itself from epidemic to epidemic and from the lack of well-controlled studies.

On the whole, the vast majority of women who have influenza in pregnancy have normal outcomes, and there seems to be little influence on the incidences of congenital anomalies, intrauterine growth, prematurity, and stillbirth (Finland, 1973).

Rubeola

Measles is the most communicable of the childhood exanthems. The virus is spread chiefly by droplets expectorated by an infected person and gains access to susceptible people via the nose, oropharynx, and conjunctival mucosa. The incubation time is 10 to 14 days. Measles is most communicable during the prodrome and catarrhal stage.

Prior to the availability of live measles vaccines, epidemics of measles occurred at intervals of 2 to 3 years in the United States. The use of attenuated measles vaccine since 1963 has resulted in significant changes in the epidemiology of this disease.

Measles occurs less commonly during pregnancy than chickenpox or mumps. Prior to the introduction of the measles vaccine, there were 0.4 to 0.6 cases of measles per 10,000 pregnancies. This figure has probably dropped even lower since the measles vaccine was introduced.

The prodrome of fever and malaise begins 10 to 11 days after exposure and is followed within 24 hours by coryza, sneezing, conjunctivitis, and cough. During the next several days the catarrhal phase is exacerbated, with a marked conjunctivitis and photophobia. Koplik's spots appear on the lateral buccal mucosa at the end of the prodrome; they are tiny, granular, slightly raised white lesions surrounded by halos of erythema. The maculopapular rash appears 12 to 14 days after exposure. It begins on the head and neck, usually behind the auricles, and subsequently spreads to the trunk, the upper extremities, and finally the lower extremities.

Complications of measles most commonly involve the respiratory tract. Otitis media and croup are frequent occurrences, but bacterial pneumonia is the complication most commonly associated with mortality. Encephalitis, less common but serious and causing coma and gross cerebral dysfunction, is estimated to occur with a frequency of one per 1000 cases. The incidence is probably higher if drowsiness, irritability, and transient electroencephalographic changes are accepted as evidence of encephalitis. Death occurs in about 11 per cent of encephalitis cases. Other complications of measles include thrombocytopenic purpura, myocarditis, and subacute sclerosing panencephalitis.

MATERNAL EFFECTS OF MEASLES. It is unclear whether pregnant women with measles are at greater risk for serious complications and death than nonpregnant adults. Several studies of large measles epidemics have reported an increased mortality rate among pregnant women. The deaths were usually related to pneumonia. More recent studies in the United States and Australia have noted that measles in pregnant women is only rarely associated with pneumonia or other complications.

FETAL AND NEONATAL EFFECTS OF MEASLES. The consensus among reports in the literature is that there is an increased rate of prematurity in pregnancies complicated by measles, especially when the disease occurs late in gestation. There is no clear evidence that maternal measles is associated with an increased risk of spontaneous abortion. The teratogenic potential of gestational measles for the fetus has not been proved or refuted because of the rarity of measles in pregnancy. No particular constellation of abnormalities has been found among the sporadic instances of congenital defects that have been reported in association with maternal measles. In general, if there is any increased risk of malformations following measles, it is small (Siegal and Fuerst, 1966).

Measles that is clinically apparent at birth or in the first 10 days of life is considered transplacental (congenital) in origin, whereas measles occurring 14 days or more after birth has been acquired postnatally. Postnatally acquired measles usually has a mild course. The spectrum of illness in congenital measles varies from a mild illness, in which the rash is transient and Koplik's spots may be absent, to rapidly fatal disease. In reported cases of congenital measles the mortality rate is 32 per cent. Approximately the same case fatality rate (30 to 33 per cent) was observed whether the rash was present at birth or appeared subsequently. It appears that premature infants with congenital measles have a significantly increased death rate (56 per cent) over that in term infants (20 per cent). Insufficient data are available to evaluate whether transplacentally acquired antibodies to measles virus may diminish the case fatality rate in congenital measles, when the mother's rash occurs more than 48 hours before delivery.

TREATMENT. The treatment of uncomplicated measles is symptomatic. When otitis media or pneumonia develops, appropriate antibiotic therapy should be instituted on the basis of the Gram stain and culture results. Passive immunization is recommended for the prevention of measles in susceptible, exposed pregnant women, neonates, and their contacts in the delivery room or nursery. Immune serum globulin (ISG), in a dose of 0.25 ml/kg administered as soon as possible after exposure, may prevent or at least modify the infection. Children born to women who have measles in the last week of pregnancy or the first week postpartum should be given ISG as soon as possible, in a dose of 0.25 ml/kg.

In the adult, it is recommended that passive prophylaxis be followed in 8 or more weeks by administration of live measles vaccine except during pregnancy, when live attenuated viral vaccines are contraindicated. Also, it is recommended that vaccination in infants be given after the age of 12 months because the induction of immunity and the production of antibodies may be suppressed by residual transplacentally acquired antibodies if the vaccine is given earlier.

Mumps

Mumps, which is an acute generalized nonexanthematous infection with a predilection for the parotid and salivary glands, also may affect the brain, pancreas, and gonads. The mumps virus is a member of the paramyxovirus family and is thus an RNA virus. The mumps virus is transmitted by saliva and droplet contamination and has been recovered from saliva and respiratory secretions from 7 days prior to the onset of parotitis until 9 days afterward. The usual incubation period is 14 to 18 days.

Mumps is primarily a disease of childhood, and only 10 per cent of cases occur in patients over 15 years of age. Many adults are immune as a result of clinical or subclinical infection. However, even among susceptible subjects exposed to household members, the attack rate is low. Mumps occurs more commonly in pregnant women than measles or chickenpox. The incidence in prospective studies has been variously reported as ranging from 0.8 to ten cases per 10,000 pregnancies.

The prodrome of mumps consists of fever, malaise, myalgia, and anorexia. Parotitis occurs within 24 hours and is characterized by a swollen and tender parotid gland. The orifice of Stensen's duct is usually red and swollen. In most cases parotitis is bilateral. The submaxillary glands are involved less often, and almost never without parotid gland involvement. The sublingual glands are rarely affected. Although mumps is generally a self-limited and complication-free disease, it can be a significant cause of morbidity. Orchitis occurs in about 20 per cent of postpubertal males and is the most common manifestation other than parotitis in this group. Oophoritis is far less common and, unlike orchitis, does not lead to sterility. The most common neurologic complication of mumps, especially in males, is aseptic meningitis, the course of which is almost always benign and self-limited. In rare instances, cranial nerve involvement has led to permanent sequelae, the most common of which is sensorineural deafness. In addition, mumps may cause pancreatitis, mastitis, thyroiditis, myocarditis, nephritis, and arthritis.

Mumps in pregnant women is generally benign and is not more severe than in nonpregnant patients. Aseptic meningitis in pregnant patients is neither more common nor more severe. Mortality in association with mumps is extremely rare in both pregnant and nonpregnant patients.

Retrospective studies have suggested that mumps during the first trimester of pregnancy is associated with a twofold increase in the incidence of spontaneous abortion. No significant association between maternal mumps infection and prematurity, intrauterine growth retardation, or perinatal mortality has been demonstrated (Monif, 1974).

The role of mumps virus in congenital disease remains controversial (Gershon, 1990). Despite animal studies in which mumps virus induced congenital malformations, definitive evidence of a teratogenic potential for mumps virus in humans has not been reported. Siegal (1973) has noted that the rate of congenital malformation in infants born to women who had mumps during pregnancy (two of 117) was essentially the same rate as in infants born to uninfected mothers (two of 123). The predominant concern has been the postulated association between maternal mumps infection and the development of subsequent congenital cardiac abnormalities, specifically endocardial fibroelastosis (EFE) (St. Geme et al., 1966). At present the issue remains unresolved.

The treatment of mumps is symptomatic in pregnant as well as in nonpregnant patients. Analgesics, bed rest, and application of cold or heat to the parotids are useful. Maternal mumps is not an indication for termination of pregnancy. The Jeryl Lynn live-attenuated mumps vaccine has been effective in preventing primary mumps. Ninety-five per cent of vaccinated susceptible subjects develop antibodies without clinically adverse reactions. The duration of protection afforded by immunization is not known.

Attenuated virus particles have been recovered from placental tissue in susceptible women vaccinated during pregnancy (Monif, 1976). Immunization with the mumps live virus vaccine in pregnancy is contraindicated on the theoretical grounds that the developing fetus might be harmed. Although the risk to the fetus seems negligible, the innocuous nature of mumps in pregnancy suggests that vaccination is unwarranted.

Echoviruses

The echoviruses are classified as enteroviruses along with polio and coxsackieviruses. Echoviruses are responsible for a variety of illnesses, including respiratory disease, rash, gastroenteritis, conjunctivitis, aseptic meningitis, and pericarditis.

Many neonatally acquired infections caused by a good number of the echoviruses have been reported. The clinical findings associated with neonatal echovirus infection include fever with splenomegaly and lymphadenopathy, macular rashes, diarrhea and vomiting, pneumonitis, otitis media, jaundice, coryza with cough, and septic meningitis.

Echovirus infection in pregnancy has not been associated with abortions, premature delivery, stillbirths, or congenital malformations. However, it has been demonstrated that congenital echovirus infection can produce severe disease and damage in the neonate. Echovirus 14 has been reported to be the cause of a febrile illness that developed at 3 days of life and progressed to cyanotic episodes, hypothermia, hepatomegaly, bradycardia, and purpura, and to death at 7 days of life (Hughes et al., 1972). Echovirus 19 has been reported to be the cause of hepatic necrosis and massive hemorrhage in three infants (Philip and Larsen, 1973). Thus, it appears that echoviruses 14 and 19 can result in perinatal infection and produce severe, even fatal multi-organ disease with thrombocytopenia.

Most infections are acquired in the immediate perinatal period, with 63 per cent of cases occurring between the third and fifth days of life (Modlin, 1986). Nearly 70 per cent of the affected mothers have an acute illness within 1 week of delivery. Of the 61 reported cases of neonatal echovirus infection, 43 (70 per cent) were due to echovirus 11.

No treatment or vaccine is available for echovirus infections.

Coxsackieviruses

Coxsackieviruses are RNA viruses of the enterovirus group. These are divided into group A coxsackieviruses (23 types) and group B coxsackieviruses (6 types). Group A coxsackieviruses do not cause significant perinatal illness, except in rare cases.

Group B coxsackieviruses can cause pleurodynia, meningoencephalitis, and myocarditis. Hepatitis, the hemolyticuremic syndrome, and pneumonia are infrequent but severe manifestations of group B coxsackievirus infection. Transplacental transmission of group B coxsackievirus has been demonstrated, but the magnitude of risk to the fetus has not been defined. The great majority of maternal group B coxsackievirus infections result in no demonstrable adverse effects on the fetus. Myocarditis seems to be a particularly prominent manifestation of group B coxsackievirus infection in the neonate (Van Creveld and deJager, 1956; Verlinde et al., 1956). Infection with coxsackievirus B-4 in the first trimester has been associated with urogenital malformations such as hypospadias, epispadias, and cryptorchidism (Brown and Karunas, 1972). B-3 virus has been recovered from the spinal cord of a stillborn infant.

Diagnosis of coxsackievirus infection is based on virus isolation from throat or rectum and serologic evidence of increasing antibody titer during the convalescent period. Hemagglutination inhibition (HI) or complement fixation (CF) tests may be performed.

No treatment or vaccination is available for the coxsackieviruses.

SEXUALLY TRANSMITTED DISEASES
Syphilis

Syphilis is a chronic infectious process due to the spirochete *Treponema pallidum*. It has been recognized for several centuries that primary, secondary, and early latent syphilis in pregnant women caused infection of the fetus, with resultant congenital abnormalities and active disease at birth. Because of this significant morbidity, great emphasis has been placed on routine screening of all pregnant women for syphilis. Acquisition is generally through sexual contact and is followed by an average incubation time of 3 weeks (range, 10 to 90 days).

EPIDEMIOLOGY. With the introduction of penicillin, the total number of cases of syphilis in the United States progressively decreased from the 1940s until 1957. In 1958 the trend reversed, and the number of reported cases of primary and secondary syphilis (the best indicator of incidence trends) began steadily increasing. The incidence of primary and secondary syphilis in the United States reached a peak of 14.6 cases per 100,000 population in 1982, in large part due to increases among homosexual and bisexual men. A decrease of syphilis was again noted due in large part to a decrease among homosexual males with the advent of the AIDS epidemic. Over the past 5 years, an increased incidence of primary and secondary syphilis has been seen in the United States (Rolfs and Nakoshima, 1990). Coincident with this increase has been a dramatic increase in reported cases of congenital syphilis (Ricci et al., 1989; CDC, 1988). From a low of 108 cases of congenital syphilis in 1978, there were 350 cases reported in 1986 and nearly 3000 cases in 1990. Nearly 80 per cent of congenital syphilis cases occur in Texas, Florida, California, and New York City. Nearly 90 per cent of congenital syphilis cases were among Blacks or Hispanics, and one-half occurred when mothers received no prenatal care. Reasons for this dramatic upsurge include exchange of drugs (e.g., "crack" cocaine) for sex, decreased funding for syphilis control, treatment of penicillinase-producing *Neisseria gonorrhoeae* with spectinomycin, which does not treat incubating syphilis, and the use of revised reporting guidelines for congenital syphilis, which were introduced in 1989. Thus, in the 1990s syphilis is increasingly a disease of young, unmarried, low socioeconomic status individuals of color.

CLINICAL MANIFESTATIONS. After exposure, there is an incubation period ranging from 10 to 90 days (average 21 days) before the primary lesion appears. The chancre is a painless, ulcerated lesion with a raised border and an indurated base. Painless inguinal lymphadenopathy is frequently present. Although chancres on the external genitalia are easily recognized, more commonly the lesion is on the cervix or in the vagina and therefore not detected. Without treatment, the primary chancre spontaneously disappears in 2 to 6 weeks. Following this, the patient enters the secondary or bacteremic stage of syphilis. The clinical manifestations of secondary syphilis include a generalized maculopapular rash involving the palms and soles, mucous patches, condyloma latum, and generalized lymphadenopathy. These findings spontaneously clear within 2 to 6 weeks and the latent stage of syphilis ensues, in which there is no apparent clinical disease. In about 25 per cent of patients, the early latent phase (duration of less than 4 years) may be associated with an exacerbation of secondary syphilis in which the mucocutaneous lesions are infectious. The late latent stage is not infectious by sexual transmission, but the spirochete may still be transmitted transplacentally to the fetus. If treatment for primary, secondary, or latent syphilis is not provided, one-third of patients develop tertiary syphilis, with involvement of the cardiovascular, central nervous, or musculoskeletal system and/or involvement of various organ systems by gummas (late benign tertiary syphilis).

In the past, syphilis was thought to invade the fetus via transplacental infection only after 16 weeks gestation, because it was believed that spirochetes were unable to penetrate Langhan's layer of the placenta. However, research has documented that *T. pallidum* can be transferred across the placenta and infect the fetus as early as 6 weeks gestation (Harter and Benirschke, 1976). Clinical manifestations are not apparent until after 16 weeks gestation, when the fetus develops immunocompetence. Thus, the risk to the fetus is present throughout pregnancy, and the degree of risk is related to the quantity of spirochetes in the maternal blood stream. Women with primary or secondary syphilis are more likely to transmit infection to their offspring than are those with latent disease. Specifically, maternal primary syphilis and secondary syphilis are associated with a 50 per cent probability of congenital syphilis and a 50 per cent rate of perinatal death; maternal early latent syphilis with a 40 per cent risk of congenital syphilis and a 20 per cent mortality rate, and maternal late syphilis with a 10 per cent risk of congenital syphilis (Fiumara and Lessel, 1970). Experience at the University of Miami in the late 1980s confirmed that currently untreated syphilis is associated with significant and frequent adverse effects on pregnancy (Ricci et al., 1989). Among 56 cases of congenital syphilis, 19 (35 per cent) were stillbirths and the perinatal mortality was 464/1000 live births. Preterm labor/delivery was significantly more com-

mon, and infants with congenital syphilis had significantly lower birth weights and 21 per cent were intrauterine growth-retarded. In addition, the manifestations of congenital syphilis are usually less severe in association with long-standing maternal disease than with early syphilis (duration of less than 1 year).

The clinical spectrum in fetal infection includes stillbirth, neonatal death, clinically apparent congenital syphilis during the early months of life (early congenital syphilis), and development of the classic stigmata of late congenital syphilis. Congenital syphilis is a systemic illness. Prematurity and stillbirths are common in mothers with early syphilis. At present, however, pregnant women diagnosed as having syphilis are usually asymptomatic, are in the latent stage, and have had the disease for more than 1 year. Consequently, most infants with early congenital syphilis are asymptomatic at birth and do not develop evidence of active disease for 10 days to 2 weeks. Chancres do not occur unless the disease is acquired at the time of passage through the birth canal. The characteristic manifestations of early congenital syphilis include a maculopapular rash that may progress to desquamation or vesicular and bullae formation, snuffles (a flu-like syndrome associated with a nasal discharge), mucous patches in the oropharyngeal cavity, hepatosplenomegaly, jaundice, lymphadenopathy, pseudoparalysis due to osteochondritis, chorioretinitis, and iritis. Both cutaneous and mucous lesions contain spirochetes that can be seen on darkfield microscope examination of specimens.

If early congenital syphilis is untreated or incompletely treated, the classic manifestations of late congenital syphilis will appear. These include Hutchinson's teeth, mulberry molars, interstitial keratitis, eighth-nerve deafness, saddle nose, rhagades, saber shins, and cardiovascular stigmata (Ingall and Norins, 1976).

DIAGNOSIS. The most specific method for diagnosing syphilis is demonstration of *T. pallidum* on darkfield microscope examination of fresh specimens from the lesions of infected individuals. However, the woman who is diagnosed as having syphilis while pregnant is usually asymptomatic. The diagnosis may be strongly suspected if she has a history of sexual contact with a person(s) known to have syphilis, and is most often based on serologic testing. The serologic tests are classified into two types: nonspecific tests for reagin-type antibodies and specific antitreponemal antibody tests. Nonspecific antibody tests for syphilis include the VDRL test and the rapid plasma reagin (RPR) test. These are used for screening. All pregnant women should be screened at the initial prenatal visit with one of these nontreponemal tests. High-risk patients should be rescreened at 32 to 34 weeks gestation. In areas with high rates of congenital syphilis, rescreening at admission in labor has been recommended. Treponema-specific tests are employed for confirming the diagnosis of syphilis in patients who have reactive VDRL or RPR results. These tests include the *T. pallidum* immobilization (TPI) test, the fluorescent treponemal antibody absorption (FTA-ABS) test, and the micro-hemagglutination test for *T. pallidum* (MHA-TP) (Jaffe, 1975).

It is important to recognize that when the syphilitic chancre first appears, results of both the nonspecific antibody tests (VDRL and RPR) and the treponema-specific tests (FTA-ABS and MHA-TP) may be nonreactive. Therefore, lesion(s) of syphilitic chancre(s) should be sampled for examination under darkfield microscope. The presence of spirochetes on this examination is the sine qua non for the diagnosis of primary syphilis. During the next several weeks, after the chancre appears, these serum test results become positive; by 4 weeks, 100 per cent of patients with primary syphilis have positive nonspecific and specific treponemal serum test results. The FTA-ABS test result is positive slightly earlier than the VDRL test result. Both serum tests will show positive results during the secondary and latent stages of syphilis.

The pregnant woman with a positive nontreponemal test result should promptly be given a quantitative nontreponemal test (usually the VDRL) and a confirmatory treponemal test such as the FTA-ABS. False-positive reactions can occur with all of these tests but are uncommon with the specific treponemal tests. The false-positive results in nontreponemal tests are most often only weak or borderline reactions. In pregnancy, it is best to consider all FTA-ABS or MHA-TP test results to be truly positive in order to maximize treatment of the fetus at risk (Jones and Harris, 1979). A major problem with the diagnosis of syphilis in pregnancy is failure to properly carry out appropriate serologic testing. The RPR is a semi-automated modification of the VDRL and is associated with the prozone phenomenon in which an undiluted specimen leads to a false-negative result. Thus it is important to remember that a negative RPR on an undiluted specimen does not rule out syphilis.

Controversy has arisen over whether all pregnant women who are asymptomatic but have positive serologic diagnoses of syphilis should have a spinal tap for the detection of asymptomatic neurosyphilis. Although the CNS is involved in half the patients with early syphilis (Chesney and Kemp, 1924; Stokes, 1934; Lukehard et al., 1988), less than 10 per cent of untreated syphilis progresses to symptomatic late neurosyphilis (Clark and Danboldt, 1955). Spinal tap ensures proper treatment of neurosyphilis. If a spinal tap is not performed, the patient should be treated as if asymptomatic neurosyphilis were present, which requires a series of penicillin injections. The WHO has recommended that CSF examination be performed if any risk factors for progression to neurosyphilis are present. These include neurologic signs or symptoms, treatment failure, serum nontreponemal titer $\geq 1:32$, other evidence of active syphilis, therapy with a drug other than penicillin, and HIV infection (WHO, 1986).

The diagnosis of reinfection or persistence of active syphilis can be made in patients previously known to have syphilis by following the titer of the quantitative VDRL. With successful therapy the VDRL titer should decrease and become negligible within 6 to 12 months in early syphilis and 12 to 18 months in late syphilis of more than 1 year's duration. A rising titer would indicate a need for further diagnostic measures such as a spinal tap and appropriate treatment.

Congenital syphilis is easily diagnosed in the clinically apparent case in which a jaundiced, hydropic baby with florid disease and a large, edematous placenta are delivered and laboratory studies confirm the presence of the disease. However, the vast majority of infected newborns are asymptomatic at birth, but the cord blood gives a positive nonspecific test result for syphilis. The problem lies in attempting to determine whether this represents merely IgG antibody passively transferred from the mother or IgM antibody indicative of a fetal infection. The FTA-ABS test also detects an IgG antibody that crosses the placenta. An IgM FTA-ABS test has been developed; however, there are problems related to separating the IgM from the IgG, and the test is performed only in specialized laboratories. If an infant's seropositivity is due to passive transfer of maternal IgG antibodies, a progressive decrease in the VDRL titer occurs and the titer becomes negative within 3 months of delivery. Any infant with a positive VDRL result but no clinical evidence of syphilis should be given serial monthly quantitative VDRL tests for at least 9 months. A rising titer indicates active disease and the need for therapy. Infected infants may be asymptomatic and the serum VDRL result may be normal if maternal infection occurred late in pregnancy. Several new laboratory tests have been introduced to facilitate the diagnosis of congenital syphilis. These include: (1) IgMb$_\gamma$, western blot for 47KD protein, (2) polymerase chain reaction, and (3) rabbit infectivity test (RIT).

Recently, the CDC implemented a new case definition for congenital syphilis reporting (Table 42–9). This new case definition includes infants born to women with untreated syphilis and stillbirths. Thus it should provide a truer picture of the epidemiology of congenital syphilis (Zenker, 1991). Use of this new case definition has dramatically contributed to the increase in reported cases of congenital syphilis (Cohen et al., 1990).

TREATMENT. All pregnant women who have (1) a history of sexual contact with a person with documented syphilis, (2) darkfield microscope confirmation of the presence of spirochetes, or (3) serologic evidence of syphilis via a specific treponemal test should be treated. In addition, those in whom the diagnosis cannot be ruled out with certainty or those who have been previously treated but now show evidence of

---

TABLE 42–9. Congenital Syphilis Case Definition

A. *Confirmed case*

Infant in whom *Treponema pallidum* is identified by darkfield microscopy, fluorescent antibody, or other specific stains in specimens from lesions, placenta, umbilical cord, or autopsy material.

B. *Presumptive case*

1. Any infant whose mother had untreated or inadequately treated syphilis at delivery, regardless of signs or symptoms in the infant; or
2. Any infant or child who has a reactive treponemal test for syphilis and any one of the following:
   a. evidence of congenital syphilis on physical examination
   b. evidence of congenital syphilis on long-bone x-ray
   c. reactive cerebrospinal fluid VDRL
   d. elevated CSF cell count or protein (without other cause)
   e. reactive test for FTA-ABS-195-IgM antibody

reinfection, such as darkfield microscope confirmation or a fourfold rise in titer on a quantitative nontreponemal test, should receive appropriate treatment.

Penicillin is the most effective treatment available for syphilis. The secondary drugs are tetracycline and erythromycin. Tetracycline should not be used in pregnancy; penicillin is the only proven therapy that has been widely used for patients with neurosyphilis, congenital syphilis, or syphilis during pregnancy (CDC, 1989). Because the efficacy of erythromycin treatment of syphilis in pregnancy is inadequate, it no longer is recommended as an alternative for pregnant women with syphilis. Recent recommendations have advocated the role of skin testing to confirm penicillin allergy and penicillin desensitization (Wendel et al., 1985; CDC, 1989). This can be accomplished by an oral desensitization regimen (CDC, 1989) or by an intravenous approach (Ziaya et al., 1986). The treatment schedules for syphilis recommended by the United States Public Health Service are presented in Table 42–10.

Central nervous system syphilis may occur at any stage of syphilis. The need for cerebrospinal fluid (CSF) examination in the evaluation of patients without clinical signs of neurosyphilis remains controversial. CSF examination should be performed in patients with clinical symptoms or signs suggestive of neurosyphilis. The CDC suggest that this examination is also desirable for patients with syphilis of longer than 1 year's duration to exclude asymptomatic neurosyphilis. The CDC recommendation for neurosyphilis is aqueous crystalline penicillin G, 2 to 4 million units every 4 hours IV for 10 to 14 days. An alternative regimen (if outpatient compliance can be ensured) is aqueous procaine penicillin G, 2.4 million units IM daily plus probenecid 500 mg orally four times daily, both for 10 to 14 days. Both regimens can be followed

by benzathine penicillin G, 2.4 million units IM weekly for three doses. Neurosyphilis patients with a history of allergy to penicillin should have their allergy confirmed and should be hospitalized for penicillin desensitization and treatment.

Therapy should be monitored with monthly quantitative VDRL titers during pregnancy and then at 3, 6, 9, and 12 months after therapy for early syphilis. Patients with syphilis of more than 1 year's duration should also have titers measured at 18 and 24 months after therapy. Those who show a fourfold rise should be retreated.

Congenital syphilis is unusual if the mother received adequate treatment with penicillin during pregnancy. Infants should be treated if maternal treatment was inadequate, unknown, or with drugs other than penicillin, or if adequate follow-up of the infant is not possible. Any child suspected of having congenital syphilis should have a spinal tap prior to treatment. If the spinal fluid is normal, a single intramuscular injection of benzathine penicillin G, 50,000 U/kg, should be given. If the spinal fluid is abnormal or is not examined, the infant should receive aqueous crystalline penicillin G, 100,000 to 150,000 units/kg daily (50,000 U/kg IV every 8 to 12 hrs) or 50,000 units kg of procaine penicillin IM daily for 10 to 14 days.

Gonorrhea

Gonorrhea is the most commonly reported communicable disease. It is estimated that approximately 3 million cases occur annually in the United States. Infection with *Neisseria gonorrhoeae* in pregnancy is a major concern. Gonococcal ophthalmia neonatorum has long been recognized as a major consequence of maternal infection. Over the past several decades, an association has been recognized between maternal gonococcal infection and disseminated gonococcal infection, amniotic infection syndrome, and perinatal complications such as premature ruptured membranes, chorioamnionitis, prematurity, intrauterine growth retardation, neonatal sepsis, and postpartum endometritis.

EPIDEMIOLOGY. *N. gonorrhoeae* infects both males and females; the primary site of involvement is the genitourinary tract. Female infection is often asymptomatic, and the primary site of involvement is the endocervical canal. Recently it has been recognized that approximately 20 per cent of women with endocervical gonorrhea are symptomatic. Most commonly they have vaginal discharge, dysuria, and abnormal uterine bleeding.

The incidence of gonorrhea in pregnancy has been reported to range from 0.5 to 7 per cent. This frequency depends on the socioeconomic status of the population and the number of sites cultured. Risk factors for the acquisition of *N. gonorrhoeae* infection include young age, numerous sex partners, use of nonbarrier contraceptive methods, and risk-taking behavior patterns. Similar to the situation with syphilis, concern has arisen over "crack" cocaine abuse and a resurgence of gonorrhea.

Transmission of gonorrhea is almost entirely by

TABLE 42–10. **Centers for Disease Control Recommended Treatment Schedule for Syphilis**

DURATION OF DISEASE	RECOMMENDED TREATMENT
Early syphilis (primary, secondary, or latent syphilis of less than 1 year's duration)	Benzathine penicillin G, 2.4 million U, IM in one dose *or* If patient is allergic to penicillin (nonpregnant), Doxycycline 100 mg orally 2 times a day for 2 weeks *or* Tetracycline 500 mg orally 4 times a day for 2 weeks
Syphilis of more than 1 year's duration (latent disease, cardiovascular involvement, or late benign neurosyphilis). For treatment of neurosyphilis, see text	Benzathine penicillin G, 7.2 million U total, given IM at 2.4 million U weekly for 3 consecutive weeks *or* If patient is allergic to penicillin (nonpregnant), Doxycycline 100 mg orally 2 times daily for 4 weeks *or* Tetracycline 500 mg orally 4 times a day for 4 weeks.

Adapted from Centers for Disease Control. MMWR 38(8S), 1989.

sexual contact. The risk of transmission from an infected male to an exposed female is 80 to 90 per cent. There is a short incubation time of 3 to 5 days.

CLINICAL MANIFESTATIONS. Gonococcal infections in pregnant patients are most commonly asymptomatic. When symptoms develop, they usually include vaginal discharge and dysuria. On examination, endocervicitis may be present with erythema and a mucopurulent discharge.

Disseminated gonococcal infection (DGI) is the most common clinical presentation of gonorrhea in pregnancy. Pregnant women, especially during the second and third trimesters, appear to be at an increased risk for DGI. Disseminated gonococcal infection has two stages. The early bacteremic stage is characterized by chills, fever, and typical skin lesions. The dermatitis is characterized by a variety of skin lesions of gonococcal emboli. These lesions appear initially as small vesicles, which become pustules and develop a hemorrhagic base. The center becomes necrotic. These lesions occur on any body region, but are most frequently present on the volar aspects of the arms, hands, and fingers. These skin lesions fade without residual scarring. Blood cultures are positive for *N. gonorrhoeae* in half the patients in whom culture is done during the bacteremic stage. Bacterial endocarditis occasionally ensues. Joint symptoms are frequently present during this stage, as well as in the second, septic arthritis phase (Holmes et al., 1971). This second stage or septic arthritis stage is characterized by a purulent synovial effusion. The knees, ankles, and wrists are most commonly involved. Blood cultures during this stage are usually sterile. Gonococci may be isolated from the septic joints during the second stage.

NEONATAL GONOCOCCAL OPHTHALMIA. Gonococcal ophthalmia neonatorum has been recognized since 1881. Prior to the introduction by Crede of silver nitrate prophylaxis, ophthalmia neonatorum occurred in approximately 10 per cent of infants born in the United States. Introduction of routine prophylaxis resulted in a rapid reduction in this rate. However, the resurgence of gonorrhea in the 1960s and 1970s led to a reappearance of neonatal gonococcal conjunctivitis, the most common clinical manifestation of *N. gonorrhoeae* infection in the newborn.

Most newborns who have gonorrhea acquire it during passage through an infected cervical canal. Gonococcal ophthalmia usually is manifested within 4 days after birth, but incubation periods up to 21 days have been reported. A frank purulent conjunctivitis occurs, usually affecting both eyes. Untreated gonococcal ophthalmia can rapidly progress to corneal ulceration, resulting in corneal scarring and blindness.

GONOCOCCAL INFECTION IN PREGNANCY AND THE NEONATE. In recent years, postabortion gonococcal endometritis and salpingitis have been recognized with increasing frequency after pregnancy termination. Patients undergoing therapeutic abortion who have untreated endocervical gonorrhea are at increased risk for developing postabortion endometritis.

The effects of gonorrheal infection on both mother and fetus have not been fully appreciated until recently. The amniotic infection syndrome is an additional manifestation of gonococcal infection in pregnancy. This entity manifests as placental, fetal membrane, and umbilical cord inflammation that occurs after premature membrane rupture and is associated with infected oral and gastric aspirate, leukocytosis, neonatal infection, and maternal fever. This syndrome is characterized by premature rupture of membranes, premature delivery, and a high rate of infant morbidity (Handsfield et al., 1973).

Studies have identified an association between untreated maternal endocervical gonorrhea and perinatal complications, including an increased incidence of premature rupture of membranes, preterm delivery, chorioamnionitis, neonatal sepsis, and maternal postpartum sepsis. Sarrel and Pruett (1968) noted a high rate of spontaneous abortion and PROM among patients with untreated gonococcal infection. Handsfield and co-workers (1973) reported that 67 per cent of women with positive GC cultures at delivery were preterm. Similarly, Amstey and Steadman (1976) and Edwards et al. (1978) demonstrated that patients from whom *N. gonorrhoeae* was recovered were significantly more likely to have PROM and preterm delivery. In addition, a higher incidence of intrauterine growth restriction has been observed in infants of women with gonococcal infection during pregnancy (Edwards et al., 1978).

DIAGNOSIS. The majority of patients with gonorrhea in pregnancy are asymptomatic. Thus, the diagnosis of these infections depends on sampling potentially infected sites. Ideally, a specimen should be obtained for culture of *N. gonorrhoeae* from every woman during her initial prenatal visit. In patients at high risk for gonorrheal infection, cultures should be repeated in the third trimester. In settings where routine screening of pregnant women for GC is not performed, high-risk patients should be screened. These include (1) partners of men with GC or urethritis, (2) patients known to have other STDs, (3) patients with multiple sexual partners, (4) young unmarried inner city women, (5) IV drug users, and (6) women with symptoms and/or signs of lower genital tract infection. The major site of primary infection in pregnant women is in the endocervix. The anal canal, urethra, and pharyngeal cavity are important sites to consider as well. Unfortunately, microscopic examination of a Gram-stained specimen from the infected site produces a diagnosis in only 60 per cent of affected women, compared with 95 per cent of men. In women, the diagnosis requires isolation of the organism by culture. Clinical isolation is best performed by use of a selective medium for *N. gonorrhoeae*, such as Thayer-Martin. Following inoculation, the medium should be placed in a carbon dioxide incubator or candle jar to provide an adequate concentration of carbon dioxide. Transgrow medium, a modification of the Thayer-Martin medium, is available to clinicians in a bottle sealed under carbon dioxide tension.

The diagnosis of a *N. gonorrhoeae* infection is made by identification of the organism with a typical growth on selective media, a positive oxidase reaction, and observation of a gram-negative diplococcal organism on a Gram stain of the isolated colonies. *N. gonorrhoeae* forms oxidase-positive colonies which are differentiated from other strains of Neisseria by use of the fermentation reaction. Fermentation reactions take advantage of the ability of the gonococcus to ferment glucose, but not sucrose or maltose.

For optimal yield of *N. gonorrhoeae*, either two consecutive endocervical specimens or a combination of an endocervical specimen and an anal specimen should be obtained. A single endocervical swab will miss approximately 10 per cent of gonococcal infections. Gonococcal pharyngitis is more frequently encountered in females. Although these cases often present with clinical symptoms similar to those of other types of pharyngitis, the disease may be asymptomatic. In patients with sore throat or with history of oral-genital contact, cultures should be obtained from the tonsillar area and from the pharynx behind the uvula. While culture remains the "gold standard," a variety of diagnostic tests for *N. gonorrhoeae* are being evaluated, including antigen detection methods, DNA probe, and serologic assays.

TREATMENT. The treatment for pregnant women with gonococcal infection is similar to that for nonpregnant women, with the exception that tetracycline should not be used for concomitant chlamydial infection. Both asymptomatic and symptomatic infections should be treated. The treatment of gonococcal infection in the United States has been influenced by two factors. First, there has been increasing prevalence and spread of infections due to antibiotic-resistant *N. gonorroeae* such as (1) penicillinase-producing *N. gonorrhoeae* (PPNG), (2) tetracycline-resistant *N. gonorrhoeae* (TRNG), and (3) chromosomally mediated resistant *N. gonorrhoeae* (CMRNG) to multiple antibiotics. Currently over 10 per cent of gonorrheal isolates in the United States are resistant to penicillin (Cates and Hinman, 1991). In a recent investigation at public clinics for sexually transmitted diseases in Seattle, Brooklyn, Baltimore, and Denver, 39 per cent of 303 gonococcal isolates demonstrated one or more types of antimicrobial resistance (Handsfield et al., 1991). Second, there is a high frequency of coexisting chlamydial infection in women infected with *N. gonorrhoeae* (20 to 50 per cent). The current recommendations for the treatment of gonorrheal infections by the CDC are listed in Table 42–11. These were revised in 1989. Ceftriaxone in a single IM dose of 250 mg is an effective and safe agent for the treatment of uncomplicated *N. gonorrhoeae* infection of all anatomic sites (Moran and Zenilman, 1990). Alternatives include single-dose oral regimens of ciprofloxacin, norfloxocin (the latter two quinolones should not be used in pregnancy) and cefuroxime axetil or single-dose intramuscular regimens of spectinomycin, ceftizoxime, and cefotaxime. Handsfield and colleagues (1991) noted that a single dose of cefixime (400 or 800 mg) given orally was as effective as ceftriaxone, 250 mg IM, for the treatment of uncomplicated anogenital gonorrhea.

All patients treated for gonorrhea should receive concomitant therapy for *Chlamydia trachomatis* because 20 to 50 per cent of women with gonorrhea are also infected with Chlamydia. In pregnancy erythromycin is the drug of choice for *C. trachomatis*. In pregnant women allergic to beta-lactam agents, spectinomycin, 2.0 gm IM, is recommended. Quinolone agents (cip-

TABLE 42–11. Centers for Disease Control Recommended Treatment Schedule for Gonorrhea in Pregnancy

Uncomplicated Urethral, Endocervical or Rectal Infections
Recommended Regimen
Ceftriaxone 250 mg IM once
plus
Doxycycline* 100 mg orally 2 times a day for 7 days
Alternate Regimens†
Spectinomycin 2 g IM
Ciprofloxocin‡ 500 mg orally once
Norfloxacin‡ 800 mg orally once
Cefuroxime axetil 1 g orally once with probenecid 1 g
Cefotaxime 1 g IM once
Ceftizoxime 500 mg IM once

Pharyngeal Gonococcal Infection
Ceftriaxone 250 mg IM once
Alternative: Ciprofloxocin 500 mg orally as a single dose

Disseminated Gonococcal Infection (DGI)
Ceftriaxone 1 mg IM or IV every 24 hours
or
Ceftizoxime 1 g IV every 8 hours
or
Cefotaxime 1 mg IV every 8 hours
Reliable patients with uncomplicated DGI may be discharged 24–28 hours after symptoms resolve and may complete therapy for a total of 1 week with oral regimen of:
Cefuroxime axetil 500 mg 2 times a day
or
Amoxicillin 500 mg with clavulanic acid (Augmentin) 3 times a day
or
Ciprofloxocin 500 mg 2 times a day (if not pregnant)

*Doxycycline should not be used in pregnancy; erythromycin base or stearate 500 mg orally 4 times a day for 7 days or erythromycin ethylsuccinate 800 mg orally 4 times a day for 7 days may be substituted.

†All these regimens followed by doxycycline 100 mg orally twice daily for 7 days.

‡Quinolones, such as ciprofloxacin and norfloxacin, are contraindicated during pregnancy.

rofloxocin, norfloxacin) should not be used during pregnancy.

With ceftriaxone treatment, follow-up cultures to document eradication of GC are no longer recommended. Rather reculturing in two to three months to identify reinfection is suggested. If other antimicrobial agents are used for the treatment of *N. gonorrhoeae*, follow-up assessment is suggested. Follow-up cultures should be obtained from the infected site(s) 3 to 7 days after completion of treatment. In women, follow-up cultures must be obtained from the anal canal as well as the endocervix; failure to culture the anal canal will result in missing 50 per cent of resistant *N. gonorrhoeae* strains.

Treatment of disseminated gonococcal infection depends on the severity of the disease and the clinical response. Basically, the same antibiotics are used as for uncomplicated gonorrhea, but the dosages are different. Outpatient therapy of DGI is appropriate after initial response occurs with in-hospital parenteral therapy (see Table 42–11). Hospitalization is indicated for the patient who is unreliable or has uncertain diagnosis, purulent joint effusions, or other complications such as endocarditis or meningitis. Whether pregnant patients with DGI should be hospitalized for bed rest and close observation for the occurrence of preterm labor or intrauterine infection has not been established. Until further information is available, hospitalization seems appropriate. Concomitant erythromycin therapy for *C. trachomatis* is indicated.

Although treatment with topical penicillin alone has been advocated for gonococcal ophthalmia neonatorum and is considered effective, the possibility of concomitant infection at other sites argues against the use of local therapy alone. The treatment of choice is parenteral penicillin G combined with local irrigation of the eyes with a saline solution of aqueous penicillin G (10,000 U/ml).

PREVENTION. The increasing frequency of asymptomatic gonorrheal infection in women makes screening for *N. gonorrhoeae* during the antepartum period an important aspect of prevention of the perinatal morbidity associated with this organism. Instillation of a prophylactic agent into the eyes of all newborn infants is recommended by the CDC to prevent gonococcal ophthalmia neonatorum. The recommended regimens include erythromycin (0.5 per cent) ophthalmic ointment, tetracycline (1 per cent) ophthalmic ointment or silver nitrate (1 per cent) aqueous solution.

Most important to any prevention effort is the treatment of sexual contacts. Even those without symptoms must be treated if the circle of infection is to be broken.

Condylomata Acuminata

Condylomata acuminata, often called genital warts, are very common. The disease is sexually transmitted and the etiologic agent has been identified as a type of human papillomavirus (HPV). More than 60 types have been identified, of which 20 affect the epithelium of the genital tract. HPV infection may result in either clinically apparent grossly visible disease or subclinical disease requiring magnification and/or acetic acid for visualization. The majority of the clinically apparent lesions are the classic condyloma accuminatum. In addition, HPV may remain present in a latent form within cells. Application of polymerase chain reaction to amplify and detect the DNA or HPV revealed that approximately 40 per cent of sexually active women carry HPV in their genital tract. HPV types 6 and 11 have been considered to be "low oncogenic risk" viruses and are frequently associated with condyloma accuminatum but not cervical intraepithelial 3 (CIN 3) or invasive cancers. On the other hand, types 16, 18, and 33 are considered "high oncogenic risk" and are often detected in CIN 2, CIN 3 and invasive cancers. This simplistic approach has been questioned as it was recognized that a large number of healthy women with normal Pap smears harbored so called "high risk" HPV types (Roman and Fife, 1989; Singer and Jenkins, 1991).

Condylomata acuminata affect the young, predominantly, with highest prevalence among the 16- to 25-year age group, which is also the age group with the highest rate of pregnancy. Condylomata acuminata grow more rapidly during pregnancy and may involve the cervix, vagina, or vulva so extensively that vaginal delivery is precluded. The reason for the increase in size and number of lesions is not known, but has been postulated to be the decrease in cell-mediated immunity that occurs during pregnancy.

These lesions occur in the urogenital and anorectal areas, which offer a warm, moist environment for viral replication. The risk of acquiring the virus by sexual contact with an infected partner is very high. An infection rate of approximately 65 per cent has been documented, and the incubation period ranges from 3 weeks to 8 months, with an average of 2.8 months.

Condylomata acuminata are pedunculated lesions varying in size from a pinhead to large masses covering the entire vulva. Most warts are so characteristic in appearance that the diagnosis is obvious on physical examination alone. If lesions are atypical-looking and isolated, a biopsy should be obtained to rule out carcinoma in situ.

Management of these lesions in pregnancy presents difficult problems. The application of podophyllin resin, the usual treatment of condylomata acuminata in nonpregnant patients, is contraindicated in pregnancy because absorption of the resin may be harmful to both mother and fetus. This drug has strong antimitotic activity and may be teratogenic. It causes local vascular spasm, ischemia, and necrosis of tissue (Chamberlain et al., 1972). During pregnancy, the lesions are profuse and vascular, predisposing to systemic absorption of podophyllin. Fetal death and maternal neuropathy have been reported to occur with use of the agent in gravid women. An alternate chemical agent used for treatment of condylomata acuminata is 50 per cent trichloroacetic acid, which is also applied weekly. Unlike podophyllum, it does not require washing off; however, it may result in intense burning that lasts 5 to 30 minutes. The best approach to treatment during pregnancy may be the excision of the lesions by cautery or the use of cryosurgery. Care must be taken to prevent extensive scarring or sloughing of tissue. The CO_2 laser is an effective method for managing condylomata acuminata and may be used with local anesthesia. Cure rates greater than 90 per cent have been reported with laser. In addition, laser offers the advantage of less destruction to surrounding normal tissue. However, it is expensive and requires local anesthesia. Interferon has been successfully used to treat nonpregnant patients with recurrent condylomata. Both intralesional and parenteral injections have been used. Thus far, interferon has been limited to research studies and has not been studied in pregnancy for efficacy or safety.

Respiratory papillomatosis (laryngeal papilloma) is a rare disease for which an association with maternal condylomata acuminata has been suggested (Cook et al., 1973). Laryngeal papillomas can be particularly troublesome because they may produce respiratory distress secondary to obstruction and because recurrence following treatment is common. The papillomaviruses recovered from the genital tract and from respiratory papillomatosis are identical; deoxyribonucleic acid sequences of human papillomavirus types 6 and 11 have been recovered from almost all laryngeal papilloma tissues. Potential routes of vertical transmission of HPV include transplacental and intrapartum in the birth canal or during the neonatal period. The route of transmission is unknown at present.

The risk for transmission of the virus from maternal condylomata acuminata to the neonate has not been established. Because genital papillomavirus infection is so common and respiratory papillomatosis is rare, Shah et al. (1986) suggested that the risk of intrapartum transmission is low. These investigators estimated that the risk may be in the order of one case of juvenile respiratory papillomatosis per several hundred to one thousand children born to papillomavirus-infected mothers. Such a low risk requires further definition of risk factors and prospective studies of vertical transmission before cesarean delivery can be advocated to decrease the incidence of juvenile laryngeal papilloma. Currently, the CDC notes that cesarean section for prevention of transmission of HPV infection to the newborn is not indicated (CDC, 1989). Moreover, Shah et al. (1986) reported a case of juvenile respiratory papillomatosis that developed at age 7 months in an infant delivered by elective repeat cesarean section before rupture of the membranes. Recently, it has been reported that HPV is present in maternal blood and can be transmitted transplacentally to the fetus.

Chlamydial Infection

Chlamydial infections of the genital tract and their consequences such as impaired fertility and perinatal complications have received considerable attention. *Chlamydia trachomatis* has long been known as the causative agent of trachoma, a disease that is hyperendemic in many developing countries and is considered to be the leading preventable cause of blindness in the world. However, *C. trachomatis* is now recognized as a major pathogen in industrialized communities, where the predominant mode of spread is sexual. As is true for other sexually transmitted organisms, chlamydial infections have reached epidemic levels. *C. trachomatis* is the most common STD organism in the United States, and it is currently estimated that over 4 million chlamydial infections occur annually in this country. Recently a human strain of *C. psittaci* known as *C. pneumoniae* (formerly the TWAR strain) has been demonstrated to be a common respiratory tract pathogen.

C. trachomatis causes significant diseases in both men and women. In addition, recent investigations have documented the consequences to infants of perinatal exposure to the organism. Although inclusion conjunctivitis of the newborn was studied for 60 years, it was not until recently that we began to appreciate the importance of extraocular chlamydial infections in infants (Beem and Saxon, 1977). It is now clear that inclusion conjunctivitis of the newborn is not a rarity, but probably the most common form of conjunctivitis seen in the first month of life, and that chlamydia is one of the common causes of pneumonia in the first 6 months of life.

The chlamydiae are a genus of obligate intracellular bacteria separated into their own order, Chlamydiales, on the basis of a unique growth cycle that distinguishes them from all other microorganisms. This cycle involves infection of the susceptible host cell by a chlamydia-specific phagocytic process, so that these organisms are preferentially ingested. After attachment and ingestion, the chlamydiae remain in a phagosome throughout the growth cycle, but surface antigens of chlamydiae appear to inhibit phagolysosomal fusion. These two virulence factors, enhanced ingestion and inhibition of phagolysosomal fusion, attest to an exquisitely adapted parasitism. Once in the cell, the chlamydial elementary body, which is the infectious particle, changes to a metabolically active replicating form called the reticulate body, which synthesizes its own macromolecules and divides by binary fission. The chlamydiae are energy parasites that do not synthesize their own ATP; thus, energy-rich compounds must be supplied to them by the host cell. By the end of the growth cycle (approximately 48 hours), most reticulate bodies have reorganized into elementary bodies, which are released as the result of mechanical disruption of host cell to initiate new infectious cycles.

Although chlamydiae do not stain with the Gram stain, in many respects they are similar to bacteria; they contain DNA and RNA, are susceptible to certain antibiotics, have a rigid cell wall similar in structure and content to that of a gram-negative bacteria, and multiply by binary fission. However, they differ from bacteria but are similar to viruses in that they are obligate intracellular parasites and may be regarded as bacteria that have adapted to an intracelluar environment. Thus, they need viable cells for multiplication and survival.

The characteristics of the two species that make up the genus Chlamydia are presented in Table 42–12. *Chlamydia psittaci* is the causative agent of psittacosis, a common pathogen in avian species and lower mammals. The *C. pneumoniae* strain of *Chlamydia psittaci* is a human pathogen. *Chlamydia trachomatis* seems to be a specifically human pathogen (except for a few strains of rodent origin).

Although all chlamydiae share a common genus-specific antigen, *C. trachomatis* may be further differentiated on a serologic basis. There are currently 15 recognized serotypes. Three of these serotypes (L1, L2, L3) represent the agents causing lymphogranuloma venereum (LGV). The other serotypes of *C. trachomatis* represent the agents causing endemic blinding trachoma (A, B, Ba, and C) and the sexually transmitted *C. trachomatis* strains (D through K), which cause inclusion conjunctivitis, newborn pneumonia, urethritis, cervicitis, endometritis, pelvic inflammatory disease, and the acute urethral syndrome.

Epidemiology and Transmission. *C. trachomatis* has long been recognized as the causative agent of trachoma, a chronic conjunctivitis affecting hundreds of millions of people in developing countries and resulting in millions of cases of blindness. However, the child-to-child and intrafamilial infection patterns that predominate in endemic areas have not been proved to cause disease in newborns. The recent studies that focus on the role of *C. trachomatis* in diseases of individuals living in industrialized countries have documented that the major method of transmission of chlamydial infections in these popu-

TABLE 42–12.   Chlamydiae: Taxonomy and Association with Human Disease

ORGANISM	RESPONSE TO SULFON- AMIDE	INCLUSIONS STAIN WITH IODINE	ORIGIN(S)	SEROTYPE(S)	DISEASE(S)
Chlamydia psittaci	Resistant	No	Common pathogen in birds and lower mammals	Many	Psittacosis
Chlamydia pneumoniae			Respiratory tract infections in humans		
Chlamydia trachomatis	Sensitive	Yes	Mostly of human origin	A, B, Ba, C	Hyperendemic blinding trachoma
				D, E, F. G. H. I. J. K.	Inclusion conjunctivitis, nongonococcal urethritis, cervicitis, salpingitis, proctitis, epididymitis, pneumonia of newborn
				L^1, L^2, L^3	Lymphogranuloma venereum

lations is sexual. These chlamydial infections, like other sexually transmitted diseases, have reached epidemic levels. *C. trachomatis* is probably the most common sexually transmitted pathogen in Western industrialized society. Chlamydia causes between one-third and one-half of cases of nongonococcal urethritis in men. Epididymitis is an important complication of chlamydial infection of the male urethra, and chlamydia is the major cause of epididymitis in men under the age of 35. Rectal and pharyngeal infections occur in both sexes.

In the female, a number of clinical conditions can be attributed to chlamydia, among them mucopurulent cervicitis, acute urethral syndrome, urethritis, and salpingitis. Unfortunately, many chlamydial infections of the cervix are clinically inapparent. Thus, asymptomatic and clinically inapparent infections occur in both men and women. They are usually discovered during routine screening procedures or as a result of contact tracing from symptomatic patients. Approximately one-third to one-half of women with chlamydia cervicitis will have signs and symptoms.

Brunham and co-workers (1984) have proposed that mucopurulent cervicitis, which often is chlamydia, is the female equivalent of nongonococcal urethritis in men. Paavonen et al. (1982) described the characteristics associated with mucopurulent endocervicitis and ascribed the majority of such infections to *C. trachomatis*.

As seen in Table 42–13, the prevalence rate of *C. trachomatis* infection among pregnant women can vary broadly with a reported range of 2 to 37 per cent. The general consensus is that the national average in the United States for chlamydial infection of the cervix is 5 per cent in sexually active women. However, high-risk populations can be readily identified. A number of studies have shown that the same populations at high risk for other sexually transmitted infections are at highest risk for chlamydial infections. Among pregnant women risk factors for chlamydial infection include: (1) unmarried; (2) age <20 years old; (3) presence of other STDs; (4) partners with nongonococcal urethritis; (5) presence of mucopurulent endocervicitis; (6) sterile pyuria (acute urethral syndrome); (7) resi-

dent of socially disadvantaged community; and (8) late or no prenatal care. Detection rates as high as 25 to 30 per cent have been reported in screening and prospective studies of such populations.

The infant born to a woman with a chlamydial infection of the cervix is at a 60 to 70 per cent risk of acquiring the infection during passage through the birth canal. Approximately 25 to 50 per cent of exposed infants develop conjunctivitis in the first 2 weeks of life, and 10 to 20 per cent develop pneumonia within 3 to 4 months. *In utero* transmission is not known to occur. Infants born by cesarean section are not at risk of acquiring chlamydial infection, unless the membranes have ruptured prematurely.

In the past, retrospective chart surveys had indicated that *C. trachomatis* was an uncommon form of conjunctivitis, with an incidence of one to four cases per 1000 live births. These estimates, which relied on severe cases of conjunctivitis that were brought to the attention of ophthalmologists, grossly underestimated

TABLE 42–13.   Prevalence of *C. trachomatis* Cervical Infection in Pregnant Women

STUDY	LOCATION	NO. OF WOMEN CULTURE-POSITIVE/ NO. TESTED (%)
Chandler et al., 1977	Seattle	18/142 (13)
Hammerschlag et al., 1979	Boston	6/322 (2)
Frommell et al., 1979	Denver	30/340 (9)
Hammerschlag et al., 1979	Seattle	67/572 (12)
Mardh et al., 1980	Lund	23/273 (9)
Heggie et al., 1981	Cleveland	240/1327 (18)
Harrison et al., 1983	Tucson	73/1046 (7)
Thompson et al., 1982	Atlanta	71/433 (16)
Harrison et al., 1983	Gallup, N.M.	48/200 (24)
Khurana et al., 1985	Manila	61/363 (17)
Ismail et al., 1985	Chicago	44/201 (21)
Fitz-Simmons et al., 1986	Philadelphia	22/221 (15)
Schachter et al., 1986b	San Francisco	262 (7)
Gravett et al., 1986	Seattle	47/534 (9)
Ryan et al., 1990	Memphis	2424/11,544 (21)

the true incidence of inclusion conjunctivitis and the significant risk for vertical transmission of maternal chlamydial infection to the newborn. More recently, prospective studies have shown that in fact this is a most common form of conjunctivitis in infants. Prospective studies aimed at determining the true incidence of vertical transmission of chlamydial infections have demonstrated that roughly 20 to 50 per cent of newborns delivered vaginally to mothers with cervical chlamydial infection will develop conjunctivitis (Table 42–14). In addition, these prospective investigations have revealed that 11 to 20 per cent of infants delivered through a cervix infected with *C. trachomatis* develop chlamydial pneumonia. Studies of serial admission for pneumonia in infants less than 6 months old have documented that *C. trachomatis* could be implicated in 10 to 50 per cent of cases. Thus, chlamydial infection is responsible for a major portion of pneumonias in this age group. Based on serologic assessment of infants born to mothers with untreated cervical chlamydial infection, some 50 to 80 per cent of exposed infants develop serologic evidence of chlamydia infection.

CLINICAL SPECTRUM OF PERINATAL INFECTION

Conjunctivitis. Acute conjunctivitis of the newborn (inclusion conjunctivitis of the newborn, inclusion blennorrhea) was initially described in the first decade of this century. It was recognized that the agent that caused inclusion conjunctivitis of the newborn was also present in the genital tract of the mother; intracytoplasmic inclusion bodies similar to those produced by trachoma were seen in scrapings from the conjunctiva of infants with conjunctivitis and in those from the cervices of their mothers. It is now recognized as the most common conjunctivitis in the first month of life.

The disease often starts with a watery eye discharge that rapidly and progressively becomes purulent. The eyelids are usually markedly swollen. The conjunctivae become reddened and somewhat thickened throughout. The mucopurulent conjunctivitis generally develops more than 5 days after birth. Thus, it is rarely diagnosed accurately because the infant will have left the hospital when the disease develops.

Recent prospective studies have shown that 20 to 50 per cent of infants exposed at birth will develop inclusion conjunctivitis. It is estimated that there are approximately 75,000 cases of inclusion conjunctivitis of the newborn in the United States each year.

In severe cases, diagnosis is readily made by demonstrating the typical inclusion bodies by Giesma staining of conjunctival scrapings. Chlamydiae are also readily cultured from the eye. Serologic diagnosis is not helpful because of the presence of maternally transmitted chlamydial IgG antibody and because of the uncertain appearance of IgM in this disease. Chlamydial infections are unaffected by silver nitrate prophylaxis, and so it seems reasonable to recommend a regimen active against both chlamydia and gonococci for neonatal eye prophylaxis. A preliminary trial of prophylactic erythromycin ointment has been shown to prevent the development of inclusion conjunctivitis of the newborn. Currently the CDC suggests the use of either erythromycin (0.5 per cent) ophthalmic ointment or tetracycline (1 per cent) ophthalmic ointment (CDC, 1989).

Pneumonia. Until 1975, it was assumed that chlamydial infection in the infant was restricted to the conjunctiva. Beem and Saxon (1977) published a series of retrospective and prospective cases of chlamydial pneumonia in young infants. This report was followed by studies from other centers, and the clinical entity of chlamydial pneumonia became well defined. During the years since the first recognition, it has become clear that this disease is very common indeed, probably one of the three most common pneumonias seen in infancy. Many reported series have helped to delineate its clinical features.

The vast majority of infants manifest the disease between the 4th and 11th weeks of life; virtually all are symptomatic before the eighth week. Initially, they have respiratory symptoms. Usually such a patient is afebrile or has only a low-grade fever. The upper respiratory tract symptoms are those of congestion and obstruction of the nasal passages without significant discharge. The finding of abnormal, bulging eardrums is common, occurring in more than half the cases described. The history or presence of conjunctivitis can be elicited in half the cases. Lower respiratory tract symptoms consist of tachypnea and a very prominent "staccato" cough. Some infants have apneic periods, and on occasion the infection is severe enough to warrant intubation. Crepitant inspiratory rales are commonly heard; on the other hand, expiratory wheezes are uncommon. The cough, which often interferes with sleeping and feeding, may be disturbing to the infant and the parents. For the same reason, food intake drops and the patient fails to gain weight.

The radiographic findings are those of hyperexpansion of the lungs, with bilateral symmetrical interstitial infiltrates. The effects of hyperexpansion on the diaphragm may render the liver and spleen easily palpable.

Laboratory findings include a normal white blood cell count and an increase in eosinophils. Blood gas analysis usually indicates a mild or moderate degree

TABLE 42–14. Prospective Studies of Perinatal Chlamydial Infection

STUDY	RATE OF PERINATAL INFECTION (%)		C. TRACHOMATIS % RECOVERED
	CONJUNCTIVITIS	PNEUMONIA	
Chandler et al., 1977	50	Not studied	—
Frommell et al., 1979	44	11	44
Schachter et al., 1979	35	20	70
Hammerschlag et al., 1979	33	16	69
Mardh et al., 1980	23	Not studied	23
Heggie et al., 1981	21	3	28
Alexander and Harrison, 1983	50	Not studied	Not studied
Grossman et al., 1982	18	18	34
Ismail et al., 1985	31	14	44

of hypoxia. Levels of serum immune globulins, both the IgG and IgM varieties, are generally elevated.

Adverse Pregnancy Outcome. Much more controversial is the question whether maternal cervical *C. trachomatis* infection is associated with adverse pregnancy outcome. Some studies have demonstrated an association of cervical chlamydial infection with preterm PROM, preterm labor and delivery, low birth weight, increased perinatal mortality, and/or late-onset postpartum endometritis. Other equally carefully designed studies have failed to demonstrate such an association. Martin et al. (1982) were the first to demonstrate that chlamydia-infected prenatal patients screened prior to 19 weeks gestation had a significantly shorter mean duration of pregnancy (35.9 versus 39.4 weeks), a significantly higher rate of birth weight less than 2500 gm (28 versus 8 per cent), and a ten-fold increase in neonatal death (33 versus 3.4 per cent). Subsequent studies by Heggie et al. (1981), Thompson et al. (1982), Harrison et al. (1983), Hardy et al. (1984), Berman et al. (1987), Ismail et al. (1985), and McGregor et al. (1990) failed to confirm such associations. However, Harrison and co-workers (1983) demonstrated that while cervical infection with *C. trachomatis* did not increase the risk of low birth weight, abortion, stillbirth, prematurity, or PROM, the subgroup of IgM-seropositive chlamydia-infected women had significantly more low-birth-weight infants and a significantly increased incidence of PROM. They postulated that IgM seropositively reflected recent chlamydial acquisition and that such patients were at high risk for adverse pregnancy outcome.

Although Sweet and co-workers (1987) noted that cervical chlamydia infection was not associated with low-birth-weight infants, preterm labor, preterm delivery, PROM, or increased perinatal mortality, they demonstrated, as did Harrison et al. (1983), that the subgroup of chlamydia-infected women who were IgM seropositive had an increased risk for preterm delivery and PROM. However, when controlled for the presence of other sexually transmitted agents (GBS, *M. hominis,* and *U. urealyticum*), this relationship was no longer significant. On the other hand, in a smaller study, Gravett et al. (1986) reported that cervical infection with *C. trachomatis* was associated with preterm labor and low birth weight. Interestingly, preterm delivery was not associated with cervical infection by chlamydia. Serologic results for chlamydial antibody were not assessed in Gravett's study. Martius and co-workers reported (again on the population in Seattle) an increased association between chlamydia and preterm birth (OR 5.4; 95 per cent CI 1.3 to 23.04), which remained significant after adjusting for the presence of bacterial vaginosis (1988). Alger et al. noted that preterm PROM occurred significantly more often among chlamydia-positive women (1988), and Polk et al., in a large prospective study of chlamydial cervical infection during pregnancy, demonstrated that *C. trachomatis* was significantly associated with preterm birth (OR 1.6; 90 per cent CI 1.01 to 2.5) and IUGR (OR 2.4; 90 per cent CI 1.32 to 4.18) (Johns Hopkins Study Group, 1989). While the latter study adjusted for multiple risk factors for preterm delivery they used a 90 per cent confidence level to determine

significance rather than the more common level of 95 per cent. On the other hand in a multi-institutional large collaborative investigation sponsored by the National Institutes of Health, no association between *C. trachomatis* and preterm labor, preterm delivery, preterm PROM or low birth weight has been demonstrated (Personal Communication, Eschenbach DA). A final assessment of the role of *C. trachomatis* in causing adverse pregnancy outcome must await further large-scale prospective studies.

In an additional attempt to address the role of *C. trachomatis* in adverse pregnancy outcome, treatment studies of chlamydial infection in pregnant women have been undertaken. Ryan et al., in a high-prevalence population (21 per cent positive), reported that untreated chlamydia-infected pregnant women had significant increases in occurrences of PROM and low birth weight and decreased perinatal survival compared to treated women or those not infected with chlamydia (1990). Similarly, Cohen and co-workers reported that treatment of chlamydial infection resulted in decreased rates for preterm delivery, PROM, preterm labor, and fetal growth restriction (1990). However, this study compared women successfully treated to those who did not comply with or respond to treatment; it was not a randomized, prospective study and the study of Ryan et al. was a retrospective comparison of two different time periods.

Wager and co-workers (1980) suggested that antepartum cervical chlamydial infection was associated with late-onset postpartum endometritis following vaginal delivery. This relationship could not be confirmed by Thompson et al. (1982), Harrison et al. (1983), Blanco et al. (1985), Berman et al. (1987), Sweet et al. (1987), and McGregor (1990). Studies by Ismail et al. (1985) and Hoyme et al. (1986) have demonstrated that cervical chlamydial infection was associated with a significantly increased risk for postpartum endometritis.

DIAGNOSIS. Schachter and Dawson (1977) have suggested that the principle of diagnosing chlamydial infections is essentially the same as for any other microbial infection. The agent may be demonstrated by cytologic examination of clinical specimens, by serologic demonstration of rising antibody titers to chlamydial antigens, by isolation from culture of the patient's tissues, or with antigen detection methods such as fluorescein-conjugated monoclonal antibody smears or enzyme immunoassay (Amortegui and Meyer, 1985). Cytologic identification of chlamydial infection was the only available diagnostic tool prior to 1957. Direct staining of epithelial cell scrapings with Giemsa or iodine identified the characteristic inclusion bodies of *C. trachomatis*. While it is simple and inexpensive, standard cytology has little practical use as a diagnostic tool in genital tract infection. When compared with culture or antigen detection methods, Papanicolaou smear has poor sensitivity and specificity. On the other hand, cytology is a useful diagnostic tool in detecting newborn inclusion conjunctivitis.

Tissue culture has been the standard diagnostic test for chlamydial detection. However, it requires a cell culture system (most commonly cyclohexamide-treated McCoy cells, is time consuming (up to 7 days may be required), is relatively expensive, and is not widely available to clinicians. The need for a more readily available and rapid diagnostic test for chlamydia has led to the development of direct antigenic detection of fixed genital smears. There are currently two such methods clinically available: (1) fluorescein-conjugated monoclonal antibody staining of a direct smear and (2) enzyme immunoassay. Both of these antigen-detection methods have been demonstrated to be highly sensitive and specific. However, in a low-prevalence population (i.e., ≤5 per cent chlamydia infection), the positive predictive value drops to about 50 per cent; this means that there will be false-positive results. Of these two methods, the monoclonal antibody system has the advantage of rapid processing time and has a built-in quality control for assessing the adequacy of a clinical specimen (i.e., presence of epithelial cells). The advantages of antigen detection methods are that they are less costly than culture, do not require cold chain storage, are more rapid, and are more widely available to clinicians. In a recent review of antigen detection methods, Stamm (1987) reported that the direct immunofluorescence method had an overall sensitivity (89 per cent), specificity (98 per cent), and positive predictive value (90 per cent) in a high-prevalence population. In a moderate-prevalence population he noted sensitivity to be 79 per cent, specificity, 98 per cent, and positive predictive value, 79 per cent. For enzyme immunoassay, the results for high-prevalence population were sensitivity, 90 per cent; specificity, 97 per cent; and positive predictive value, 86 per cent; and for the moderate-prevalence group 89 per cent, 97 per cent, and 73 per cent, respectively. However, reported experience with those tests in low-prevalence populations is lacking, especially for screening purposes in asymptomatic women. In-situ DNA hybridization and polymerase chain reaction (PCR) (Holland et al., 1990) technology have been tried on a limited basis to date, but appear to offer exciting potential as future diagnostic tools in the clinical setting. Moncada et al. reported that the use of a cytobrush to obtain an endocervical specimen significantly improves the sensitivity of culture, direct fluorescence smear, and Chlamydiazyme (Moncada et al., 1989).

The question of which pregnant women should be screened for *C. trachomatis* is controversial. Ideally, all sexually active women should be screened, especially during pregnancy. Practically, at least young, sexually active females attending family planning clinics, prenatal clinics, and abortion clinics should be screened.

Serologic diagnosis has not been useful as a diagnostic test for the routine clinical determination of genital chlamydial infection. On the other hand, chlamydia serology is a helpful epidemiologic tool in large populations and can identify patients who have had previous chlamydial infection. The microimmunofluorescence test is the most commonly used serologic test for detecting IgG and/or IgM antibodies against *C. trachomatis*.

TREATMENT. It has been generally accepted that inclusion conjunctivitis responds to topically applied ophthalmic ointments or drops containing tetracycline, erythromycin, or sulfonamides. The ointment or drops are applied four times a day for 2 weeks. Many infections, however, are slow to clear with this regimen. Outright failures of treatment occur, possibly explained by the difficulty parents have getting the ointment or drops into their baby's eyes. Because failure rates greater than 50 per cent have been reported, and secondarily because the infection usually extends beyond the anatomic reach of ointments, we currently recommend a 2-week course of oral therapy with erythromycin, a dose of 40 mg/kg per day, in divided doses. Systemic therapy for conjunctivitis appears to eradicate the nasopharyngeal carriage of chlamydia and thus to prevent pneumonia as well. There is convincing evidence that this treatment of pneumonia with erythromycin both shortens significantly the clinical course of illness and decreases the duration of nasopharyngeal shedding of *C. trachomatis*. Sulfisoxazole, 150 mg/kg per day in divided doses, has been equally effective in controlled trials. Beyond the specific antimicrobial therapy, the infants require standard supportive measures, attention to nutrition and to fluid and electrolyte balance, and chest physical therapy; oxygen and ventilatory therapy are required in a minority of cases.

Pregnant women who have proven infection with *C. trachomatis* should receive treatment. Many authorities recommend routine screening of all prenatal patients with culture or antigen detection methods for *C. trachomatis*. This screening should occur at the initial prenatal visit, and in high-risk patients repeat screening for acquisition of chlamydia should be undertaken in the third trimester. If chlamydia diagnostic tests are not performed, the CDC recommend that treatment be given to women with mucopurulent endocervicitis, proven gonococcal infection, or sex partners who have nongonococcal urethritis or epididymitis. In pregnancy the recommended treatment for chlamydial infection is erythromycin base, 500 mg by mouth four times daily for 7 days, or erythromycin ethylsuccinate, 800 mg by mouth four times daily for 7 days. For women who cannot tolerate these high-dose regimens, one-half the daily dose four times daily should be given for at least 14 days. Schachter and co-workers (1986a) have demonstrated that erythromycin treatment at 36 to 37 weeks gestation will eradicate maternal cervical chlamydial infection and prevent vertical transmission of *C. trachomatis* to neonates in 90 per cent of cases in which the mother had cervical chlamydial infection. However, there was a 5 per cent drug failure rate, and an additional 5 per cent of patients stopped the erythromycin because of GI upset. Recently, Crombleholme et al. (1990) reported that treatment of pregnant women with amoxicillin, 500 mg 3 times daily for 7 days, was well tolerated, that it eradicated cervical chlamydial infection, and that it prevented vertical transmission of chlamydia to the neonates. Amoxicillin therapy resulted in eradication of cervical chlamydia in 70 (98.6 per cent of) infected women, and 44 (95.6 per cent of) infants had negative cultures and serologic studies for *C. trachomatis*. Not only did this compare favorably with the erythromycin group, but only 2 per cent of the amoxicillin group stopped therapy compared to 13 per cent in the erythromycin group.

Sex partners of patients with *C. trachomatis* infection should be treated. They should receive doxycycline, 100 mg orally 2 times daily for 7 days, or tetracycline, 500 mg orally 4 times a day for 7 days (CDC, 1989). The alternative regimens in nonpregnant patients include erythromycin and ofloxocin, 300 mg twice a day for 7 days (Hooten et al., 1992).

OTHER INFECTIONS
Mycoplasma Infection

The mycoplasmas are a unique group of microorganisms that commonly inhabit the mucosal surfaces of the respiratory and genital tracts. To date, many antigenically distinct species that are infectious in humans have been characterized. These can be divided into respiratory mycoplasmas, mainly *Mycoplasma pneumoniae*, the agent responsible for atypical pneumonia; and the genital mycoplasmas. The most common of these are *M. hominis* and *Ureaplasma urealyticum* (formerly T-mycoplasmas or T strains). Recently, a new species, *M. genitalium*, has been identified and implicated in pelvic inflammatory disease.

Phylogenetically, mycoplasmas fall between bacteria and viruses. All mycoplasmas have these characteristics in common: (1) absence of cell walls, (2) growth in cell-free media, (3) dependence on the availability of sterols for adequate growth (except for Acholeplasmas), (4) inhibition of growth by specific antibody, (5) susceptibility to antimicrobial agents that inhibit protein synthesis, and (6) resistance to agents that affect synthesis of cell walls. They differ from bacteria because they have no cell walls, but rather a nonrigid triple-layered membrane enclosing each cell. Mycoplasmas are the smallest known free-living organisms. The mycoplasmas differ from viruses in that they contain both DNA and RNA and can grow in cell-free media. Viruses are distinguished by the facts that they contain either RNA or DNA and their replication depends on the host cell's metabolic activities.

The major pathogenic genital tract mycoplasmas are distinguished by differences in colonial morphology, metabolic characteristics, and susceptibility to antibiotics (Table 42–15). *M. hominis* is recognizable as forming a "fried-egg" colony. The organism converts

arginine or ornithine with the liberation of ammonia; this reaction has an easily recognized color change when an appropriate pH indicator is incorporated into a broth medium containing arginine. *U. urealyticum* is a microaerophilic organism characterized by small colony size and the ability to hydrolyze urea. Urea is an essential substrate for growth and is converted to ammonia. This reaction can be detected by addition of a pH indicator to the broth or agar medium containing urea.

Epidemiology. Infants become colonized with genital mycoplasmas during the birth process. Presumably the organisms are acquired from a contaminated cervix or vagina, because infants delivered by cesarean section are less frequently colonized with mycoplasmas than those delivered vaginally. Approximately one-third of newborn females have vaginal colonization with *U. urealyticum*, and a smaller percentage harbor *M. hominis*. Mycoplasmas are less frequently recovered from the genital tracts of infant males. Sequential studies have shown a progressive decrease in colonization during the first year of life.

Genital mycoplasmas are uncommon in prepubertal girls. After puberty, colonization with genital mycoplasmas occurs primarily through sexual contact. The organism recovery rate increases dramatically with the onset of sexual intercourse. A wide range in the recovery rate has been reported for *U. urealyticum*, from 40 to 95 per cent, and for *M. hominis*, from 15 to 72 per cent among sexually active women. McCormack and associates (1972) have shown that the colonization rate of genital mycoplasmas is related to the number of sexual partners. Ureaplasma was recovered from only 6 per cent of women without history of sexual contact, from 37.5 per cent of women with one sexual partner, from 55 per cent of women with two sexual partners, and from 75 per cent of women with three or more sexual partners. In this study, recovery of *M. hominis* was less prevalent but followed a similar pattern.

Genital mycoplasmas are commonly isolated from gravid women at approximately the same rate as from nonpregnant women with the same degree of sexual activity. Braun and colleagues (1971) reported that pregnant women had 79 and 48 per cent isolation rates for *U. urealyticum* and *M. hominis*, respectively; both organisms were recovered in 41 per cent of the study group. Genital mycoplasmas have been recovered more frequently from women of lower socioeconomic classes than from private patients and from Black women than from Caucasian women. It is apparent that both *M. hominis* and *U. urealyticum* can be isolated frequently from the female genital tract. Investigations of the role of these organisms in human disease must take into account their high rate of presence in the genital tract.

Spontaneous Abortion and Stillbirth. Investigators have reported the isolation of genital mycoplasmas from the chorion, amnion, and decidua in spontaneous abortions. However, a causal relationship has not been established. The major unresolved issue is whether contamination occurs when the products of conception pass through the cervix and vagina. Stray-Pederson and associates (1978) isolated ureaplasmas

Table 42–15. Characteristics of Genital Tract Mycoplasms

CHARACTERISTIC	UREAPLASMA UREALYTICUM	MYCOPLASMA HOMINIS
Colony morphology	Small, granular	Large, "fried egg"
Colony size	20 to 30 μ	200 to 300 μ
Metabolic substrate	Urea	Arginine
Antibiotic susceptibility		
Tetracycline	+	+
Erythromycin	+	−
Lincomycin	−	+
Clindamycin	−	+
Penicillin	−	−
Cephalosporins	−	−
Aerobic growth	−	+

more often from the endometrium in women who had repeated spontaneous abortions (28 per cent) than from the endometrial cavity in a control group (7 per cent). The results of these studies suggest that there is an association between spontaneous abortion and maternal or fetal infection or both by genital mycoplasmas. It is not clear whether the association is real; however, it is difficult to evaluate the comparability of the study groups, and the role of other microorganisms was not investigated.

The mycoplasmas isolated from abortuses and still-births cannot be explained completely by contamination; these organisms have been isolated from the lungs, brain, heart, and viscera. However, none of these observations provides an answer to the question whether abortion occurs because mycoplasmas invade the fetus and cause its death or because the fetus dies from another cause, with subsequent invasion of necrotic tissue by the mycoplasmas (Taylor-Robinson and McCormack, 1980).

Mycoplasmas are sensitive to antibiotics. Fetal loss, if caused by these organisms, could be prevented by appropriate antimicrobial therapy. Kundsin and coworkers (1967) have reported successful pregnancies after antibiotic therapy in women who were colonized by ureaplasmas and had a history of frequent spontaneous abortions. Stray-Pederson and associates (1978) used doxycycline to treat women who had had repeated spontaneous abortions, many of whom subsequently had normal pregnancies. These findings have led to the concept that subclinical mycoplasma infection is an important cause of spontaneous abortion, especially repeated abortions. However, these studies have not assessed other microorganisms (especially *C. trachomatis* and anaerobes). Most significantly, the effectiveness of antibiotics in preventing spontaneous abortion remains controversial because all the antibiotic trials have been uncontrolled.

In summary, the evidence linking the genital mycoplasmas to spontaneous abortion and stillbirth is mainly anecdotal. Establishment of a causal relationship will require large-scale investigations that assess other potential pathogens and include placebo-controlled trials of antibiotics in patients who have had repeated spontaneous abortions.

Histologic Chorioamnionitis, Intra-Amniotic Infection, and Neonatal Infection. Shurin and colleagues (1975) isolated *U. urealyticum* twice as frequently from neonates whose mothers had histologically severe chorioamnionitis as from newborns whose mothers had less severe or no disease. The histologic chorioamnionitis could be due to any of the other microorganisms that could gain entry to the amniotic cavity at the same time. The data of Shurin and colleagues are significant because they accounted for duration of membrane rupture and still noted a statistically significant association between chorioamnionitis and ureaplasmal infection.

As noted earlier in this chapter, *M. hominis* is found significantly more often in the amniotic fluid of women with intra-amniotic infection than in matched control women, and there is a significant association between symptomatic IAI and a rise in maternal antibodies to *M. hominis*. *U. urealyticum* is found equally in both groups (Blanco, 1983; Gibbs, 1986).

The genital mycoplasmas acquired by the infant during labor generally have not been associated with serious neonatal infection.

Low Birth Weight. Klein and associates (1969), in the first systematic study of the effects of mycoplasma on infants, reported that 22 per cent of infants weighing less than 2500 gm were colonized with *M. hominis* or *U. urealyticum*, a rate significantly higher than the 12 per cent colonization rate among infants weighing more than 2500 gm. The colonized infants had a statistically lower mean birth weight (2605 gm) than those who were not colonized (2952 gm). However, in a recent, multicenter study, antepartum cultures for *U. urealyticum* in 4934 women were found not to correlate with low-birth-weight infants, preterm labor, or preterm birth after adjustment for sociodemographic factors (Carey et al., 1991). This large, powerful study concludes that antepartum culture for ureaplasma to predict pregnancy outcome on a routine basis is not justified.

Postpartum Infection. Like other organisms of the lower genital tract microflora, mycoplasmas can be recovered transiently in the blood stream shortly after delivery. However, genital mycoplasmas are seldom recovered from the blood of postpartum women who are not febrile, whereas they are commonly found in the blood of febrile postpartum women (Lamey et al., 1982). Both genital mycoplasms are isolated commonly in the endometrium of women with endometritis (see Watts, 1990, under Postpartum Infection).

The frequency with which endometritis due to *M. hominis* occurs without blood stream invasion and the percentage of endometritis cases caused by *M. hominis* are not clear. Studies suggest that *M. hominis* is a common cause of postpartum infection (McCormack et al., 1973), but there is an excellent response of endometritis to antibiotics such as cefoxitin and broad spectrum penicillins, therapies without notable activity against the mycoplasms.

Diagnosis. The diagnosis of mycoplasma infection is based on isolation of the organism from a site of infection and demonstration of a rise in antibody titer. For optimal isolation of mycoplasmas, specimens should be inoculated immediately into medium, kept at 4°C, and transported to the laboratory as soon as possible. The basic medium is a beef-heart infusion broth, available commercially as pleuropneumonia-like organism broth, supplemented with fresh yeast extract and horse serum. Antibacterials are added to inhibit bacterial growth.

Various procedures, including ELISA and metabolic inhibition, have been used to detect serologic response to the genital mycoplasmas.

Treatment. The penicillins, the cephalosporins, and vancomycin are ineffective. The antimicrobial agents that inhibit protein synthesis, including the aminoglycosides, tetracyclines, chloramphenicol, lincomycins, and erythromycin, are active against most mycoplasmas. Tetracyclines are effective against both *M. hominis* and *U. urealyticum*. *M. hominis* is sensitive to lincomycin but resistant to erythromycin. Ureaplasmas, on the other hand, are sensitive to erythromycin but not to lincomycin. In addition, *M. hominis* is highly sensitive and ureaplasmas are moderately sensitive to clindamycin.

On the basis of Kass's early controlled antibiotic trials with tetracycline in bacteriuric women, it has been suggested that antimicrobial treatment of the microorganisms such as the mycoplasmas in the lower genital tract would decrease the risk of premature delivery. Kass and co-workers (1981) reported that erythromycin given in the third trimester significantly reduced the risk of premature, low-birth-weight infants in a group of 245 low-income pregnant women at the Boston City Hospital who were found at the initial antenatal visit to have *Mycoplasma* infections. These investigators used a double-blind protocol in which patients received placebo or erythromycin, 1 gm per day for 6 weeks. They reported that the excess prematurity rate associated with mycoplasma infection accounted for half the noted birth weight differences in their study. However, it should be noted that the antibiotic therapy may have acted on other infectious agents as well. In 1991, Eschenbach and co-workers repeated a large, powerful treatment trial attempting to resolve the role of ureaplasma in preterm birth and excluding patients (in this part of their work) with *C. trachomatis*. In this multicenter, double-blind, randomized trial, pregnant women with *U. urealyticum* were treated with erythromycin base or placebo during the third trimester. Erythromycin did not eliminate *U. urealyticum* from the lower genital tract, and there was no association between erythromycin treatment and improved pregnancy outcome.

Treatment should be restricted to clinical situations in which mycoplasmas have been isolated from a body fluid or a focus of infection and appear to be significantly related to the disease process. Thus, erythromycin treatment of pregnant patients for the purpose of resolving repeated abortions, unexplained infertility, and poor late pregnancy outcome should be limited to formal research situations.

Candidiasis (Monilial Vaginitis)

Candida albicans is a saprophytic yeast that exists as part of the endogenous flora of the vagina. The organism is present in the vagina of approximately 25 per cent of sexually active women. It may become an opportunistic pathogen, especially when host defense mechanisms are compromised. Systemic candidiasis is a rare event in gravid patients, occurring only when disease entities with significant debilitation, such as sepsis and malignancy, are present. Candidal vulvovaginitis is a much more common infection. *C. albicans* is the second most common cause (after bacterial vaginosis) of vaginitis. Other yeasts, such as *C. glabrata*, account for approximately 5 to 15 per cent of yeast vaginitis.

Fifteen per cent of pregnant women develop symptomatic candidal vulvovaginitis. It is thought that the hormonal environment of pregnancy, in which high levels of estrogen produce an increased concentration of vaginal glycogen, accounts for the frequency of symptomatic infection in gravid patients. In addition, suppression of cell-mediated immunity in pregnancy may decrease the ability to limit fungal proliferation.

The clinical manifestations in pregnancy are similar to those in the nonpregnant state; they include pruritus and burning, dysuria, dyspareunia, excoriations with secondary infection, and pruritus ani. The vaginal discharge is frequently thick, white, and curd-like.

A presumptive diagnosis of candidiasis is best made by microscopic examination of vaginal secretions for hyphae and yeast forms. The diagnosis can be aided by using 10 per cent potassium hydroxide to facilitate identification of fungus. Since patients with yeast vulvovagnitis may have negative KOH smears, the diagnosis may be confirmed by cultures. Sabouraud's or Nickerson's medium is most commonly employed, but almost any standard microbiologic transport medium is adequate for *C. albicans*.

Yeast vulvovaginitis has not been associated with preterm birth, preterm labor, LBW, or premature rupture of the membranes.

The clinical manifestations of congenital candidiasis range from superficial skin infections to systemic disease with hemorrhage and necrosis of the heart, lungs, kidneys, and other organs. The most common route of infection is by direct contact during delivery through an infected vagina, and oropharyngeal candidiasis of the neonate (thrush) is the most common problem.

Nystatin had previously been used for candidal vulvovaginitis. Tropical drugs for therapy of candidiasis—such as miconazole, clotrimazole, terconazole, and butaconazole—have the advantages of somewhat greater efficacy and a shorter course of therapy. Although data on use of these drugs in the first trimester are not extensive, use especially of miconazole and clotrimazole (the older of these preparations) later in pregnancy has not been accompanied by adverse effects on the fetus.

Bacterial Vaginosis

This condition formerly has been called nonspecific "vaginitis," "*Gardnerella vaginalis* vaginitis," and "*Haemophilus vaginalis* vaginitis" (Pheifer et al., 1978). Bacterial vaginosis seems a preferable term in view of recent progress regarding pathophysiology. The condition is marked by a major shift in vaginal flora from the normal predominance of lactobacilli to a predominance of anaerobes, which are increased 100-fold compared with normal secretions (Spiegel et al., 1980). *Gardnerella vaginalis* is present in 95 per cent of the cases, but is also found to be present in 30 to 40 per cent of normal women when selective media are used. *M. hominis* in vaginal secretions is significantly increased in cases of bacterial vaginosis.

Clinically, the primary symptoms are discharge and odor. Itching is not prominent usually. The odor is characteristically amine-like or fishy and may be accentuated after coitus (due to the alkaline pH of semen). On examination, the discharge is milky or creamy and is most often white to yellow. It has an elevated pH (≥ 4.7), and the amine odor may be detected directly or accentuated by the addition of 10 per cent KOH. A wet mount reveals an increase in numbers and kinds of bacteria, a reduction in numbers of lactobacilli, typically few leukocytes, and true "clue" cells, squamous epithelial cells so heavily stippled with bacteria that the borders are obscured.

A Gram stain of vaginal secretions makes the shift in bacteria and "clue" cells easier to observe.

Bacterial vaginosis is the most common type of infectious vaginitis. In Seattle, approximately 15 per cent of pregnant women had evidence of it, but most were asymptomatic.

Recent evidence has associated bacterial vaginosis with several pregnancy complications: an increase in premature birth (Gravett et al., 1986a, 1986b; Martius et al., 1988), intra-amniotic infection (Silver et al., 1989), endometritis (Newton et al., 1990), and histologic choriamniionitis (Hillier et al., 1988). Yet, treatment of asymptomatic pregnant patients with bacterial vaginosis for the purpose of reducing these complications has not been evaluated.

In nonpregnant women, the most consistent cure rates (90 per cent) have been achieved with metronidazole (e.g., 500 mg twice a day for 5 to 7 days). Lower cure rates (60 to 80 per cent) are observed with 2.0-gm single-dose metronidazole. Treatment with oral tetracycline or ampicillin and amoxicillin has modest cure rates (60 per cent). Some investigators have expressed concern regarding use of metronidazole in the pregnant woman, especially in the first trimester (Robbie and Sweet, 1983). Clindamycin has been shown to be effective orally (300 mg twice a day for 7 days) in treating nonpregnant patients, and oral clindamycin appears safe in pregnancy. Vaginal clindamycin creams (2 per cent) also have been effective in nonpregnant women. The vaginal dose is only 140 mg daily, with very little being absorbed. Accordingly, 2 per cent clindamycin vaginal cream offers an alternative treatment in pregnancy. Although commercial preparations are not available as of this writing, they are expected soon. In the meantime, preparations can be made easily in the pharmacy.

Toxoplasmosis

A widely distributed illness, toxoplasmosis is caused by *Toxoplasma gondii,* an intracellular parasite found in many mammalian species. The cat is the only definitive host. The parasite exists as a trophozoite, a cyst, or an oocyst. Trophozoites are the invasive forms, and the cysts are the latent forms. The oocysts are found only in cats. Human infection may be acquired by consuming cysts in uncooked or undercooked meat or infected animals (especially mutton and lamb) or by contact with oocysts from the feces of an infected cat. The oocysts may be spread to humans or food by hand or by insects and then ingested. Cats acquire toxoplasmosis by eating infected mice and other animals. Oocysts in cat feces do not become infective for 4 to 5 days. Once infected by oocysts or cysts, a pregnant woman may experience a parasitemia during which fetal involvement may occur. Later, *T. gondii* cysts appear in maternal tissues, especially striated muscle and brain, where they persist indefinitely.

Among pregnant women, serologic evidence of past infection with toxoplasmas is common. In one study, in London and New York (Stray-Pederson and Lor-

entzen-Styr, 1977), the prevalence of dye-test antibodies was 22 and 32 per cent respectively; in Paris, the prevalence was 87 per cent (Desmonts, 1974).

Seroconversion during pregnancy occurred in approximately two per 1000 pregnant women in New York. In Oslo, the rate of seroconversion was three to five per 1000 young women per year, while in Paris the rate of seroconversion in young married women was higher (10 per 1000 per year). Note that the latter rates are expressed as cases per year, not in pregnant women (Desmonts and Couvreur, 1974a).

With primary toxoplasmosis during pregnancy, there is approximately a one-third chance of fetal infection (Desmonts and Couvreur, 1974b). One-third of those fetuses infected have clinically detectable illness, and two-thirds have subclinical disease. Furthermore, the *rate* of fetal infection is higher when maternal infection occurs in the third trimester than when it occurs in the first trimester (65 versus 17 per cent). However, the *severity* of fetal infection is greater when maternal infection occurs in the first trimester. Five infants of 30 women with first-trimester toxoplasmosis had clinical disease (4 severe, 1 mild; rate 17 per cent), and two infants of 39 women with third-trimester toxoplasmosis had clinical disease (both mild; rate 5 per cent). As a rule, congenital infection does not affect more than one pregnancy in a particular mother. The role of toxoplasmosis in chronic abortions remains unresolved after 20 years of study (Desmonts, 1974; Desmonts and Couvreur, 1974a, 1976b).

Diagnosis. Subclinical disease is the rule with toxoplasmosis. When apparent clinically, the disease may manifest as a syndrome of fever, fatigue, sore throat, and maculopapular rash accompanied by nontender lymphadenopathy (most commonly cervical) and occasionally hepatosplenomegaly. Examination of the peripheral blood shows lymphocytosis on an occasional atypical lymphocyte. When clinically evident, this disease is often thought to be "flu" or infectious mononucleosis. An occasional adult may have mainly ocular symptoms, including haziness of vision, pain, and photophobia. In these cases, ophthalmologic examination shows clusters of yellow-white patches in the optic fundus, representative of a focal necrotizing retinochoroiditis. In healthy adults, clinical toxoplasmosis is mild and self-limited, but in immunosuppressed individuals it may lead to serious pulmonary or central nervous system involvement (Feldman, 1968; Krogstad et al., 1972).

As noted, most infants with congenital toxoplasmosis have only serologic abnormalities. Of those with clinical disease, few have the full triad of intracerebral calcifications, chorioretinitis, and hydrocephaly commonly suggested in the past. Rather, common findings in symptomatic infants are: chorioretinitis (80 per cent), abnormal spinal fluid (69 per cent), anemia (64 per cent), splenomegaly (56 per cent), jaundice (54 per cent), fever (51 per cent), lymphadenopathy (43 per cent), convulsions (34 per cent), and vomiting (32 per cent). Thus, there is a wide spectrum of disease. In addition, acute primary toxoplasmosis in pregnancy has been associated with abortion, prematurity, and growth retardation (Alford et al., 1974; Stray-Pederson and Lorentzen-Styr, 1977).

Usually, serologic techniques are used to confirm toxoplasmosis. IgG antibodies are detected by the indirect fluorescent antibody test, Sabin-Feldman dye test, indirect hemagglutination inhibition test, and complement fixation test. Acute infection is diagnosed by a serial two-tube (i.e., fourfold) rise in titer of any of these tests, but as with rubella, the specimens should be tested in parallel. Titers resulting from acute infection nearly always rise to more than 1:1000 with the indirect fluorescent antibody test and the dye tests. These antibodies peak within 1 to 2 months of the onset of infection, and low titers persist for years.

IgM antibodies may be detected by an indirect fluorescent antibody technique. They appear within a week and usually last for a matter of months.

For pregnant patients with possible exposure, Krick and Remington (1978) advise use of IgM indirect fluorescent antibody test when the IgG test (conventional indirect fluorescent antibody test or dye test) is positive at any titer. The combination of a negative IgM reading with an IgG titer higher than 1:1000 suggests remote infection. Conventional (IgG) and IgM indirect fluorescent antibody tests are available from the CDC through state laboratories.

In 1988, prenatal diagnosis was assessed in 746 pregnancies at risk for congenital toxoplasmosis (Daffos et al., 1988). Diagnosis of fetal infection was based upon: culture of fetal blood, obtained by cordocentesis; culture of amniotic fluid; presence of IgM to *T. gondii* in fetal blood; nonspecific markers of infection in fetal blood (such as platelet count, WBC, total Igm, eosinophilia, and hepatic enzymes); and ultrasonographic findings. Of 42 fetuses ultimately diagnosed with infection, 39 (93 per cent) were detected *in utero*. Most pregnancies (24 of 39) were terminated, but of the remaining 15, 13 fetuses remained clinically well. The other two had chorioretinitis. All mothers were treated with spiromycin; pyrimethamine and sulfonamide were added to the maternal regimen when fetal infection was diagnosed.

PREVENTION. To prevent toxoplasmosis in pregnancy, most authorities advise: (1) avoiding undercooked meat, (2) handwashing after handling a cat, especially before eating, (3) having someone else change a cat's litter box daily, (4) not permitting indoor cats to go outside, where they may attack an infected mouse, (5) not allowing stray cats in the house, and (6) not feeding raw meat to cats. We do not recommend routine toxoplasmosis screening of pregnant women in the United States.

TREATMENT. Among women with confirmed first-trimester toxoplasmosis, the physician should offer counseling regarding the risk of serious congenital infection (probably 15 per cent) and the possibility of pregnancy termination.

In the United States, the only effective medical therapy is a combination of sulfadiazine (or triple sulfonamide) with pyrimethamine. Because of the marrow toxicity of this combination, folinic acid or baking yeast should be given as well. Spiramycin has been used extensively in Europe, but it is not available in the United States. European studies show that treatment of primary toxoplasmosis in pregnancy decreases, but does not eliminate, the risk of congenital infection in the fetus. However, in the United States, there has been no agreement on treatment in pregnancy to control fetal infection. Some conclude that the pregnant woman should not be treated except in the rare instance of serious disease. Others avoid pyrimethamine but use sulfadiazine in the woman with first-trimester toxoplasmosis who does not choose abortion.

All authorities agree that symptomatic infants with congenital toxoplasmosis should be treated with sulfadiazine, pyrimethamine, and folinic acid supplementation. Dosage regimens are available in a number of the listed references. In the infant with asymptomatic toxoplasmosis at birth, late central nervous system sequelae are possible. Thus, some physicians treat all newborns with toxoplasmosis, and others suggest treatment only for newborns proven to have toxoplasmosis by abnormal cerebrospinal fluid examination.

Trichomoniasis

Trichomonas vaginalis is a common cause of vaginitis, often characterized by intense pruritus, bad odor, and dysuria. Physical examination typically shows a malodorous, yellow-green, frothy discharge, but variations of the gross appearance occur in approximately 50 per cent of cases. The diagnosis may be confirmed by a microscopic examination of a smear of the discharge diluted with saline. The examination reveals many leukocytes and bacteria; trichomonads are recognized by their size (slightly larger than leukocytes) and active flagellae. Cultures for trichomonas may be more sensitive than the smear.

T. vaginalis vaginitis occurs in from less than 10 to as many as 50 per cent of pregnant women, depending on sexual activity and socioeconomic status. Consequently, it has been difficult to establish whether this vaginal infection is truly increased in pregnant women.

The relationship between *T. vaginalis* infection and pregnancy complications remains controversial. One report noted no association between this parasite and low birth weight (Mason and McLure Brown, 1980), and another noted that treatment was not accompanied by an increase in birth weight or gestational age, in a placebo controlled trial (Ross and Middlekoop, 1983). On the other side, in an adolescent clinic, *T. vaginalis* was associated with nearly a threefold increase in low birth weight (18 per cent with infection versus 6.7 per cent without infection, p = .06) (Hardy et al., 1984). Premature rupture of membranes at term has also been associated with positive cultures for *T. vaginalis* (27.5 per cent with versus 12.8 per cent without, p <.03) (Minkoff et al., 1984). Finally, in the large NIH infection and prematurity study, *T. vaginalis* infection at mid-pregnancy was significantly associated with LBW and PROM even after adjustment for confounding factors and other microbes (Cotch et al., 1990).

Standard treatment of trichomoniasis consists of oral metronidazole, either as 250 mg three times daily for 7 to 10 days or as a single 2.0-gm dose. Topical agents are often unsuccessful in relieving symptoms or in eradicating this protozoon. Because of concerns of possible teratogenicity, it is prudent to avoid metronidazole in the first trimester. Later in pregnancy, topical agents may achieve some relief. If symptoms persist, however, use of oral metronidazole in late pregnancy is recommended.

ANTIBIOTICS IN PREGNANCY

Bacterial infections play a prominent role in the morbidity and mortality statistics of obstetric services. As a result, antibiotics are among the drugs most frequently administered during the perinatal period. The clinician is currently confronted with an almost bewildering array of antibiotics available for use. Thus, appropriate use of antibiotics in pregnancy requires a working knowledge of activity, kinetics, toxicity, and cost. In this part of the chapter, we provide an overview of use in pregnancy. More detailed, recent works are available (Sweet and Gibbs, 1990; Kucers and Bennett, 1987).

Antibiotics exert inhibitory effects on bacteria by interfering with their metabolic activities or the function of their structural components. This requires the administration of effective inhibitory concentrations of the agent without the attainment of toxic levels. A bacterium is considered sensitive to an antimicrobial agent if it is inhibited by concentrations of the antibiotic that can be obtained without harm to the host. Ideally, the effect of antibiotics should be directed against bacteria without being toxic to the host. This search for selective antimicrobial toxicity has been the impetus for the development of antibiotics that affect the characteristics and physiologic attributes of bacteria that differ from those of human cells.

Antimicrobial agents may interfere with bacterial metabolism, with the synthesis or integrity of bacterial structural components such as cell wall and plasma membrane, or with biosynthesis of proteins and nucleic acids. In general, the metabolic activities of bacteria are similar to those of mammalian cells. In some cases, however, bacteria synthesize compounds that animal cells must obtain as preformed molecules. Folic acid is an example of such a compound. Thus, the inhibition of folate biosynthesis affects bacterial cells selectively. Bacteria require a cell wall to protect them from osmotic damage and provide a characteristic shape. Because such a cell wall is not present in mammalian cells, it is a selective target for antibiotic action. The cell membrane, which lies inside the cell wall, represents another site for antibiotic action. The bacterial plasma membrane has essentially the same structure as the cell membrane of mammalian cells. As a result, antibiotics that are active against bacterial cell membrane are usually quite toxic to the human host. Bacterial protein synthesis occurs on 70-S ribosomes within the cell. Mammalian ribosomes (except in mitochondria) are 80-S entities, and this difference may account for some selective toxicity of antibiotics that inhibit protein synthesis. Nucleic acid synthesis by bacteria also offers possibilities for antibiotic action.

Mechanisms of Antibiotic Action

Antibiotics are classified as bactericidal or bacteriostatic on the basis of their mode of action. Bactericidal drugs produce a change in the bacterial cell that is incompatible with survival, such as disruption of the cell wall structure or disorganization of the cell membrane. Drugs are considered bacteriostatic if they inhibit certain metabolic events and thus cause suspension of bacterial growth. This blockade of metabolic activity is not immediately lethal, and if the antibiotic is removed from the environment, bacterial growth may resume. The multitude of sites in bacteria where antibiotics can exert their action are summarized in Table 42–16, and a review of their mechanisms of action has been published (Moellering, 1979).

The antimicrobials that inhibit microbial metabolism are among the oldest antibacterial agents. This group includes the sulfonamides, trimethoprim, para-aminosalicylic acid (PAS), and isoniazid. These agents are usually bacteriostatic. Most bacteria cannot incorporate preformed folic acid, but must synthesize their own from para-aminobenzoic acid.

Inhibition of cell wall synthesis leads to the produc-

TABLE 42–16. Classification of Antibiotics by Mechanism of Action

MECHANISM OF ACTION	ANTIBIOTICS
Inhibit the synthesis of essential metabolites	Sulfonamides
	Trimethoprim
	Para-aminosalicylic acid (PAS)
	Isoniazid (INH)
Inhibit cell wall synthesis	Penicillins
	Cephalosporins
	Cephamycins
	Carbapenems
	Vancomycin
	Bacitracin
	Cycloserine
	Ristocetin
Inhibit β-lactamase plus inhibit cell wall synthesis	Amoxicillin plus clavulanic acid
	Ampicillin plus sulbactam
	Ticarcillin plus clavulanic acid
Affect the cell membrane	Polymyxin B
	Colistin
	Amphotericin B
	Nystatin
Inhibit protein synthesis Bactericidal	Streptomycin
	Neomycin
	Kanamycin
	Gentamicin
	Tobramycin
	Amikacin
	Netilmicin
Bacteriostatic	Erythromycin
	Lincomycin
	Clindamycin
	Chloramphenicol
	Tetracylines
	Spectinomycin
Interfere with the synthesis of nucleic acid	Rifampin
	Actinomycin D
	Quinolones

tion of wall-deficient forms (protoplasts) that lyse in an osmotically unprotected environment. Thus, agents that inhibit cell wall structure unique to bacteria are generally nontoxic to host cells. Surrounding the bacterial cell is a macromolecular matrix of peptidoglycan, or short strands of peptides cross-linked to a polysaccharide polymer. In gram-positive organisms, this matrix is covalently bound to teichoic acid or teichoglucuronic acid, whereas in gram-negative organisms, it is bound to the outer membrane. As shown in Figure 42–3, the cell wall of gram-negative organisms contains (from the inside out) the inner membrane, the peptidoglycan layer, the periplasmic space, and the outer membrane. The penicillins and cephalosporins act as inhibitors of transpeptidase and prevent the final step in cell wall synthesis. The cephamycins also act by inhibiting cell wall synthesis. Penicillin-binding proteins, which bind beta-lactam antibiotics and are critical in the action of these antibiotics, project into the periplasmic space. When beta-lactamase enzymes are present, they are located in the periplasmic space. If present in large enough amounts, these enzymes can inactivate the beta-lactam antibiotic (Eschenbach, 1987). In the last few years, novel combination antibiotics consisting of a penicillin plus a beta-lactamase inhibitor have been introduced widely into clinical practice.

The polymyxins (polymyxin B and colistin), the polyenes (nystatin and amphotericin B), nalidixic acid, and novobiocin act at the level of the cell membrane. Mammalian cells also contain binding sites for the polymyxins on their cell membranes, and so these agents are relatively toxic. Nystatin and amphotericin B cause disruption of the cell membrane by binding to sterols in the membrane. Bacterial cells do not have sterols and are thus resistant to these drugs. These agents are effective against fungi, but because mammalian cells also contain sterols, nystatin and amphotericin B are toxic in parenteral form in humans. Nalidixic acid and novobiocin disrupt the integrity of the plasma membrane and affect synthesis of membrane-bound DNA.

The aminoglycosidic aminocyclitols (aminoglycosides) bind to the 30-S subunit of the ribosome and inhibit protein synthesis. Unlike other groups of an-

tibiotics that inhibit protein synthesis and are bacteriostatic, the aminoglycoside group is bactericidal. It is believed that aminoglycosides produce cell death by means of their irreversible binding to the ribosome. The aminoglycoside group includes streptomycin, kanamycin, gentamicin, tobramycin, neomycin, and amikacin. These agents display ototoxicity and nephrotoxicity.

Many additional antibiotics are capable of binding to the ribosomes and inhibiting protein synthesis. However, bacteria can survive for a time with the proteins that are already present when the synthesis of new proteins is blocked. Thus, these agents are not immediately lethal to the bacteria, are bound reversibly, and are thus bacteriostatic. Erythromycin, lincomycin, clindamycin, and chroramphenicol all bind to the 50-S subunit of the ribosome. Although protein synthesis is inhibited, no irreversible damage to the cell occurs. If these bacteriostatic agents are removed, the bacteria resume normal protein synthesis and growth. The tetracyclines bind to the 30-S subunit of the ribosome and block the attachment of transfer RNA to the 50-S subunit. As a result, protein synthesis is inhibited. Spectinomycin is an aminocyclitol antibiotic that binds to the 30-S subunit of the ribosome (like the aminoglycosides); however, this agent inhibits protein synthesis and is therefore bacteriostatic.

Two antibiotics of clinical significance affect nucleic acid synthesis, rifampin and actinomycin D. However, actinomycin D binds to DNA and is toxic to mammalian cells. Its use is thus limited to antineoplastic therapy. Rifampin displays selective toxicity for bacteria and is a useful antibiotic; it indirectly inhibits protein synthesis and is therefore bacteriostatic.

Antibiotic Therapy

The treatment of bacterial infections during the perinatal period must take into account the unique circumstances of pregnancy and the puerperium in order to prevent toxicity and to achieve maximum therapeutic effect. As discussed later in this chapter, the physiologic changes that accompany pregnancy alter the pharmacokinetics of the antibiotics and enhance some of their toxic effects. In addition, the use of antibiotics in pregnancy is complicated by their teratogenic potential. All antibiotics cross the placenta and reach the fetus, and thus have the potential for toxicity in the intrauterine environment (Charles, 1979).

Antibiotics that carry a risk of toxicity for the mother, fetus, and neonate are listed in Table 42–17. These drugs should be avoided in pregnancy whenever possible.

PENICILLINS. The penicillins—penicillin G, ampicillin, and amoxicillin—have been widely used during pregnancy. There are no known or suspected teratogenic effects associated with their use. Plasma levels of ampicillin are significantly lower in pregnant than in nonpregnant women. Ampicillin administration results in a decreased urinary estriol excretion as a consequence of reduction in intestinal flora. The primary indications for penicillin therapy are infections

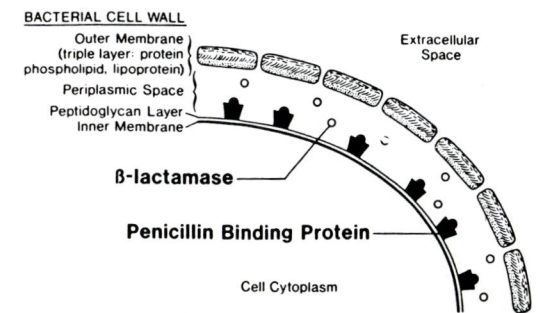

FIGURE 42–3. Schematic representation of gram-negative bacterial cell envelope. (From Eschenbach DA: A review of the role of β-lactamase-producing bacteria in obstetric-gynecologic infections. Reprinted with permission from the American College of Obstetricians and Gynecologists. Am J Obstet Gynecol **156**:495, 1987.)

TABLE 42–17. Perinatal Toxicity of Maternal Antibiotics

ANTIMICROBIAL AGENT(S)	MATERNAL TOXIC EFFECTS	FETAL TOXIC EFFECTS	NEONATAL TOXIC EFFECTS (VIA BREAST MILK)
Sulfonamides	Similar to those in nonpregnant woman	Displacement of bilirubin; low level kernicterus	Same as in fetus
Tetracycline	Fatty liver degeneration, which may be fatal; pancreatitis; renal damage	Discoloration of deciduous teeth; enamel hypoplasia; possible inhibition of bone growth	Same as in fetus
Chloramphenicol	Similar to those in nonpregnant woman (i.e., aplastic anemia)	Theoretical risk of gray syndrome	Gray syndrome in preterm babies
Streptomycin	Similar to those in nonpregnant woman	Eighth nerve damage; deafness	—
Nitrofurantoin	Similar to those in nonpregnant woman	Hemolytic anemia in fetus with G6PD deficiency	Similar to those in fetus
Trimethoprim-sulfamethoxazole	Similar to those in nonpregnant woman	Possible teratogenic effects	—

with aerobic streptococci (except enterococci), pneumococcus, nonpenicillinase-producing *Neisseria gonorrhoeae,* nonpenicillinase staphylococci, and anaerobes other than resistant strains of *Bacteroides,* such as *B. fragilis* and *B. bivius.* Ampicillin has the same indications as penicillin and provides better coverage against enterococci and gram-negative facultative bacteria. During the past decade, however, the resistance of the gram-negative facultative bacteria to ampicillin has been steadily increasing.

A variety of new, expanded-spectrum penicillins have become available clinically. Carbenicillin and ticarcillin were the first to be introduced; subsequently piperacillin and mezlocillin became available. These agents tend to be similar to ampicillin, with an enhanced spectrum of activity (in large doses) against *Pseudomonas aeruginosa* and the beta-lactamase–producing gram-negative anaerobic rods such as *Bacteroides fragilis, B. bivius,* and *B. disiens.* As a result, these agents have been used as a single therapy for mixed aerobic-anaerobic pelvic infections.

Recently, agents that include a compound that blocks the activity of beta-lactamase enzymes have been introduced. Beta-lactamase–producing bacteria are isolated commonly from genital sites and blood of women with postpartum infection (Eschenbach, 1987). Clavulanic acid and sulbactam are examples of such compounds. Clavulanic acid has been combined with amoxicillin or ticarcillin to become Augmentin and Timentin, respectively. Sulbactam has been used in combination with ampicillin or cefoperazone. The use of these enzyme blockers has expanded the spectrum of activity of older agents such as ampicillin to include most gram-negative facultative bacteria (but not *Pseudomonas*), most anaerobes *(S. aureus),* and penicillinase-producing *N. gonorrhoeae.* The use of these antibiotics in obstetric-gynecologic infections has been evaluated in the last few years. Cure rates are high, generally equivalent to other single-agent therapy (e.g., cefoxitin) or clindamycin-gentamicin. Adverse effects are infrequent, and resistant organisms have been relatively uncommon.

Last, a new category of penicillin-type agents has been described. These are known as monobactams, and aztreonam is the first to become available. Az-

treonam is a beta-lactam antimicrobial that is active against gram-negative aerobes, but has no activity against gram-positive aerobes or anaerobic bacteria. It has few adverse effects and favorable kinetics, characteristic of other beta-lactam antibiotics. Current studies have demonstrated that aztreonam is equal in efficacy to aminoglycosides in combination with clindamycin for the treatment of mixed aerobic-anaerobic infections. However, its cost is high compared to the direct cost of gentamicin.

CEPHALOSPORINS AND CEPHAMYCINS. These agents are beta-lactam antibiotics, similar to penicillins. There are no known or suspected teratogenic effects associated with the use of the cephalosporins or cephamycins. First-generation cephalosporins such as cephalothin and cefazolin are the primary agents for *Klebsiella* urinary tract infections. They were commonly used as secondary agents against streptococcus, staphylococcus, E. coli, and anaerobes other than *B. fragilis.* These agents were not effective against enterococci, *Pseudomonas, B. fragilis,* or *B. bivius.* Their most common use during pregnancy was for the treatment of pyelonephritis. In addition, the oral first-generation cephalosporin, cephalexin, was commonly used for urinary tract infections.

The second-generation cephalosporins, cefamandole and cefoxitin, exhibit activity against gram-positive aerobic bacteria, with the exception of the enterococcus. Cefamandole and cefoxitin (the cephamycin antibiotics) are resistant to the action of the beta-lactamase enzymes produced by the Enterobacteriaceae and thus provide enhanced activity against these organisms. In addition, cefoxitin is effective against *B. fragilis* and *B. bivius,* the anaerobes resistant to the first-generation agents. Cefoxitin has been widely used for well over a decade and has a good record of clinical success, with few side effects.

Recently, introduction of the third-generation cephalosporins has expanded the available armamentarium against bacterial microorganisms. The third-generation agents currently available include cefotaxime, moxalactam, cefoperazone, ceftizoxime, ceftazidime, imipenem, and cefotetan. These agents are stable against many beta-lactamase enzymes and thus have enhanced activity against most gram-negative facultative bacteria such as *E. coli, Klebsiella, Proteus,* and *Enterobacter.* In general these agents are not consistently active against *Pseudomonas aeruginosa.* The third-generation cephalosporins have relatively good activity against gram-positive aerobes except *S. aureus.* In addition, many of these agents have good to excellent activity against anaerobic bacteria, including *B. fragilis, B. bivius,* and *B. disiens.* This is especially true for imipenem, moxalactam, and cefotetan. The coverage of ceftazidime against *B. fragilis* remains controversial. Of all of these newer agents, cefotetan has been evaluated more thoroughly in pelvic infections. Clinically it is similar in spectrum to cefoxitin and is commonly used as an alternative. With a longer half-life than cefoxitin, cefotetan can be given less frequently (e.g., every 8 or 12 hours) than cefoxitin (every 6 hours).

TETRACYCLINES. Tetracyclines are not recommended for use in pregnancy. They cross the placenta rapidly and are bound to the developing fetal bone and teeth. They may cause tooth discoloration and enamel hypoplasia. Administration of tetracycline between mid-gestation and the first 6 months of life affects the deciduous (baby) teeth. Tetracycline given intravenously in large doses can produce toxic effects in the mother, including acute fatty necrosis of the liver, pancreatitis, and renal damage. The liver damage appears to be dose-related and may be fatal.

AMINOGLYCOSIDES. Serum gentamicin and kanamycin levels are consistently lower in pregnant than in nonpregnant women. Because the maternal levels are low, the levels in the fetus are usually below the therapeutic range. Eighth-nerve damage has been reported among children whose mothers received long-term streptomycin therapy for tuberculosis during pregnancy. To date, similar effects have not been noted for kanamycin, gentamicin, tobramycin, or amikacin. However, because of concern about the ototoxic potential of these agents, they should be avoided during pregnancy unless required for the treatment of gram-negative facultative bacteria that are resistant to less toxic agents such as ampicillin and the cephalosporins. If an aminoglycoside is required, blood levels should be monitored closely and renal function should be checked frequently.

CHLORAMPHENICOL. Chloramphenicol is poorly detoxified by preterm infants, with resulting high serum levels of this drug. On occasion, gray syndrome, characterized by pallid cyanosis, abdominal distention, vascular collapse, and death, has occurred. Because of the risk of gray syndrome, it has been generally recommended that chloramphenicol not be used during the third trimester of pregnancy. However, it is important to recognize that there are no case reports of gray syndrome in neonates whose mothers received chloramphenicol during pregnancy. All cases have occurred in preterm infants who received chloramphenicol after birth. With the availability and capacity to measure serum chloramphenicol levels, gray syndrome should never occur.

ERYTHROMYCIN. Erythromycin is often administered to pregnant women who have chlamydia or as a replacement for penicillin in patients allergic to penicillin. Although previously an alternative for treatment of syphilis in penicillin-allergic patients, erythromycin is no longer recommended for the treatment of syphilis. Unfortunately, very low levels are achieved in the fetal circulation with the therapeutic doses given to the mother. Maternal serum levels and therefore tissue levels of erythromycin are unpredictable. Erythromycin estolate has been associated with severe hepatotoxicity in pregnancy; this form of erythromycin is contraindicated for pregnant women, and only erythromycin base or ethylsuccinate should be used in pregnancy.

CLINDAMYCIN. Over the past decade, clindamycin has become the mainstay of treatment for resistant anaerobic infections due to organisms such as *B. fragilis* and *B. bivius.* It has been commonly used in postpartum infections but uncommonly during pregnancy. The drug does rapidly cross the placenta and achieves adequate therapeutic levels in the fetus. No teratogenic effects have been reported. The major concern with this agent is the maternal development of pseudomembranous colitis due to a resistant strain of clostridia, *C. difficile;* this occurrence, however, is no more common in pregnancy than in the nonpregnant state. Recently, it has been demonstrated that clindamycin in large doses is effective against *C. trachomatis.* When used, orally (300 mg PO twice daily for seven days) or topically (2 per cent cream, 7 ml every hour for seven days), clindamycin is effective in curing bacterial vaginosis.

SULFONAMIDES. The sulfonamides cause no known damage to the fetus, but their administration during pregnancy may affect the neonate adversely. Sulfonamides compete with bilirubin for binding sites, raise the level of free bilirubin in the serum, and increase the risk of kernicterus in the neonate. Thus, these drugs (especially the long-acting forms) should not be administered to women in the late third trimester of pregnancy. Whether they can be used safely in women who are breast-feeding is unclear. A major indication for these agents during pregnancy is the treatment of asymptomatic bacteriuria or cystitis.

NITROFURANTOIN. Nitrofurantoin may cause hemolysis, anemia, and hyperbilirubinemia in a glucose-G-dehydrogenase–deficient infant born to a mother receiving the drug. Other than the potential for hemolytic anemia in susceptible fetuses, there have been no teratogenic effects reported for this drug. It is commonly used for prophylaxis of urinary tract infections in both pregnant and nonpregnant women.

METRONIDAZOLE. Recent studies have shown that metronidazole is carcinogenic in rodents and mutagenic in bacteria. Whether these findings are applicable to humans is not known. The general consensus is that there is no increase in the incidence of congenital anomalies among infants born to mothers who received metronidazole during pregnancy. It is recommended, however, that this agent not be given during the first trimester. Whether or not to administer the drug during the remainder of pregnancy remains an unsolved dilemma, and generally its use should be limited to those diseases for which it is the only available drug, such as severe trichomoniasis and other parasitic infections.

TRIMETHOPRIM-SULFAMETHOXAZOLE. In animal

studies, trimethoprim has been shown to induce birth defects. Thus there is a theoretical teratogenic risk in humans. Studies with the utilization of trimethoprim-sulfamethoxazole in human pregnancy have not demonstrated an increased occurrence of congenital malformations. Because of the theoretical teratogenic risk, however, the use of trimethoprim-sulfamethoxazole is generally contraindicated in pregnancy. One possible exception would be in the treatment of toxoplasmosis.

ISONIAZID. Isoniazid is a potentially hepatotoxic drug that may have an increased toxicity during pregnancy. If a pregnant woman is exposed to tuberculosis or has a conversion of the skin reaction but does not have active tuberculosis, she needs no prophylactic isoniazid until after pregnancy. The greatest risk of developing active tuberculosis occurs during the puerperium, and this is when isoniazid should be utilized as a prophylactic measure. If she does have active tuberculosis, however, isoniazid therapy during pregnancy is acceptable.

QUINOLONES. Nalidixic acid (Negram) has been widely used in nonpregnant patients for the treatment of urinary tract infection. However, it inhibits nucleic acid formation and is not used in pregnancy. Newer quinolones recently have undergone extensive clinical trials and several are currently available. These are norfloxocin, ciprofloxocin, and ofloxocin. The quinolones in general have excellent coverage against aerobic gram-negative bacteria including *Pseudomonas aeruginosa, N. gonorrhoeae,* and genital tract mycoplasmas. Against gram-positive aerobic bacteria and *C. trachomatis,* the activity of quinolones is less predictable and varies by agent. Anaerobic coverage of the currently available quinolones is poor. Ofloxocin provides better activity against *C. trachomatis* than ciprofloxocin, while norfloxocin has weak antichlamydial activity. It is used primarily for the treatment of urinary tract infection, including *Pseudomonas aeruginosa.* At present these agents are not being used in pregnancy.

Pharmacokinetics

Antimicrobials may be used during pregnancy to treat a coincidental maternal infection such as pneumonia or pyelonephritis, a maternal-fetal infection such as syphilis or intra-amniotic infection, or a predominantly fetal infection such as some cases of toxoplasmosis.

The physiologic changes that occur in pregnancy may have important influences on serum concentrations of antibiotics. The relevant changes include:

1. A marked increase in the volume of distribution (vascular and interstitial fluid volumes and the fetal compartment).
2. A marked increase in cardiac output.
3. A large increase in renal blood flow and glomerular filtration.
4. A decrease in plasma protein concentrations by about 1 gm/100 ml.

In addition, technical and ethical problems may make the determination of antibiotic levels more complex in pregnant women than in nonpregnant women.

Current data regarding serum antibiotic levels in pregnancy are subject to much criticism. First, in many of the studies, patients were given a single dose of drug, and only one maternal sample was obtained, often in relation to delivery. Consequently, the samples represent a different time in each pregnancy with each patient being represented by only one point. Second, the vaginal or cesarean delivery may itself influence drug levels. In only rare studies have healthy pregnant patients been available for comparison. Third, in nearly all studies, levels in pregnant women have been compared with levels measured in nonpregnant women from different populations and in different laboratories. Only rarely has the pregnant subject been her own control; in these studies, levels were determined before and a few weeks after delivery. Fourth, there may be important differences of serum level in early and late gestation; few investigations have reported serum levels in the same woman at varying stages of gestation.

Despite these limitations, lower serum or plasma levels are suspected for a number of antibiotics. For ampicillin, serum levels have been documented to be lower in pregnancy. Overall, the decrease in levels ranges from 10 to 50 per cent. Decreases in serum ampicillin concentrations have been observed after oral and intravenous administration. The reason for the lower levels of antibiotics in pregnant women may be more rapid excretion, a large volume of distribution, or perhaps sequestration of the drug in the fetal compartment.

The therapeutic implication of these findings is not altogether clear, as peak blood levels even in pregnancy are usually many times greater than minimal inhibitory or minimal bactericidal concentrations. Furthermore, in pregnant women given standard doses, there have been few documented cases of antibiotic failure due solely to subtherapeutic levels. Accordingly, it would seem wise to proceed as follows: For agents with wide margins of safety, such as ampicillin and the cephalosporins, use dosages in the upper ranges. For agents with narrower margins of safety, such as the aminoglycosides, use standard doses (on a mg/kg basis). Then, if therapy appears inadequate, consider determining antibiotic serum levels. This subject has been reviewed (Philipson, 1979).

Distribution of Antibiotics

Distribution of drugs into various body fluids depends on the mechanism, which may be either active or passive. The passive mechanism (i.e., mainly diffusion), which is probably more important for antibiotic transfer, is influenced by the concentration gradient, molecular weight, capacity for protein binding, and ionization of the drug. In general, rapid transfer is favored by large concentration gradients, small molecular weight, and low protein-binding activity. The effect of ionization is more complex; only unionized, non–protein-bound drug engages in diffusion across membranes. If all other factors were equivalent, drugs that are weak bases would have a higher concentration in a more acid medium, and drugs that are weak acids would have a higher concentration in a more alkaline medium.

Placental Transfer of Antibiotics

Available clinical experiments of placental transmission have shown that all antibiotics pass into the fetal circulation. Many of the criticisms of studies on antibiotic levels in pregnant women apply even more so to data on placental transmission. Of special importance is the relative inaccessibility of the fetal circulation and, to lesser extent, of the amniotic fluid. Consequently, much of the information comes from "single-dose, single-determination" studies. This is an important limitation because levels of antibiotics in the fetal compartment should increase after repeated, regular maternal administration. An additional point to consider is the likelihood of marked differences in transmission at different gestational ages. Thus, data obtained from mid-trimester pregnancies may not be directly applicable to term pregnancies. This entire topic has been comprehensively reviewed (Charles, 1979).

Although there is wide variation, placental transfer of many antibiotics, including ampicillin, cephalothin, clindamycin, carbenicillin, and the aminoglycosides, follows a general pattern. After an *intravenous* injection, maternal levels achieve peak concentration within 15 minutes and then fall exponentially. Peak umbilical blood concentrations are also achieved rapidly (within 30 to 60 minutes) and also fall exponentially. The ratio of infant to maternal peak serum levels for the above antibiotics ranges from 0.3 to 0.9. Levels in amniotic fluid when drugs are given at term are usually not detectable for a few hours and then gradually increase. The amniotic fluid level of an antibiotic depends to a large extent on the excretion of the agent in fetal urine. Thus, obtaining therapeutic levels of the agent in the amniotic fluid requires a live fetus. This may explain the difficulty in treating chorioamnionitis after fetal demise. For some antibiotics, including erythromycin and dicloxacillin, placental transmission is more limited; the ratio of infant to maternal peak serum levels for these agents is 0.1.

Antibiotic Excretion in Breast Milk

Excretion of antibiotics in breast milk is governed by the same principles that regulate placental transmission. In addition to the influence of concentration gradient, molecular weight, and protein binding, differences in pH between breast milk and serum may be especially important. The pH of breast milk ranges from 6.4 to 7.6. Because the pH of milk is usually lower than that of plasma, antibiotics that are weak bases tend to have higher concentrations in the milk. Conversely, antibiotics that are weak acids tend to have higher concentrations in serum. In addition to the concentration of an antibiotic in breast milk, it may be necessary to consider the amount of milk consumed by the newborn (i.e., concentration × volume consumed).

Breast milk concentration of some antibiotics ranges from 50 to 100 per cent of serum concentration. These antibiotics include erythromycin, lincomycin, tetracycline, sulfonamides, chloramphenicol, and isoniazid. Breast milk concentrations of more commonly used antibiotics such as penicillin G and oxacillin are smaller percentages of maternal serum concentrations (generally, 2 to 20 per cent). Of the aminoglycosides, data are available for the oldest, streptomycin, which is excreted in small amounts in breast milk for some time after IM administration to the mother. The subject of excretion of drugs in breast milk has been reviewed (Knowles, 1965), and the reader is referred to Chapter 10 for a complete summary of drugs secreted into breast milk.

REFERENCES

Bacterial Infections

Urinary Tract Infection and Pyelonephritis

Angel JL, O'Brien WF, Finan MA, et al: Acute pyelonephritis in pregnancy: A prospective study of oral versus intravenous antibiotic therapy. Obstet Gynecol **76**:28, 1990.

Bejar R, Curbelo V, Davis C, Gluck L: Premature labor. II. Bacterial sources of phospholipase. Obstet Gynecol **57**:479, 1981.

Cunningham FG, Lucas MJ, Hankins GDV: Pulmonory injury complicating antepartum pyelonephritis. Am J Obstet Gynecol **156**:797, 1987.

Fihn SD, Latham RH, Roberts P, Running K, Stamm WE: Association between diaphgram use and urinary tract infection. JAMA **253**:240, 1985.

Dunlow DP, Duff P: Prevalence of antibiotic-resistant uropathogens in obstetric patients with acute pyelonephritis. Obstet Gynecol **76**:241, 1990.

Gilstrap LC, Cunningham FG, Whalley PJ: Acute pyelonephritis in pregnancy: An anterospective study. Obstet Gynecol **57**:409, 1981.

Harris RE, Gilstrap LC: Prevention of recurrent pyelonephritis during pregnancy. Obstet Gynecol **44**:637, 1974.

Harris RE, Gilstrap LC, Pretty A: Single-dose antimicrobial therapy for asymptomatic bacteriuria during pregnancy. Obstet Gynecol **59**:546, 1982.

Kass EH: Bacteriuria and pyelonephritis of pregnancy. Arch Intern Med **205**:194, 1960a.

Kass EH: The role of asymptomatic bacteriuria in the pathogenesis of pyelonephritis. *In* Quinn EL, Kass EH (eds): Biology of Pyelonephritis. Boston, Little, Brown, 1960b.

Kass EH, Zinner SH: Bacteriuria and renal disease. J Infect Dis **120**:27, 1969.

Kass EH, Zinner SH: Bacteriuria and pyelonephritis in pregnancy. *In* Charles D, Finland M (eds): Obstetric and Perinatal Infections. Philadelphia, Lea & Febiger, 1973a.

Kass EH: Pregnancy, pyelonephritis and prematurity. Clin Obstet Gynecol **13**:239, 1973b.

Kincaid-Smith P, Bullen M: Bacteriuria in pregnancy. Lancet **1**:395, 1965.

Mittendorf R, Williams MA, Kass EH: Prevention of preterm delivery and low birth weight associated with asymptomatic bacteriuria. Clin Infect Dis **14**:927, 1992.

Romero R, Oyarzum E, Mazur M, et al.: Meta-analysis of the relationship between asymptomatic bacteriuria and preterm delivery/low birth weight. Obstet Gynecol **73**:576, 1989.

Stamm WE, Counts GW, Running KR, et al: Diagnosis of coliform infection in acutely dysuric women. N Engl J Med **307**:463, 1982.

Towers CV, Kaminskas CM, Garite TJ, et al.: Pulmonary injury associated with antepartum pyelonephritis: Can patients at risk be identified? Am J Obstet Gynecol **164**:974, 1991.

Whalley P, Martin F, Peters P: Significance of symptomatic bacteriuria detected during pregnancy. JAMA **193**:879, 1965.

Whalley P: Bacteriuria of pregnancy. Am J Obstet Gynecol **97**:723, 1967.

Zinner SH, Kass EH: Long-term (10–14 years) follow-up of bacteriuria of pregnancy. N Engl J Med **285**:820, 1971.

Intra-Amniotic Infection

Blanco JD, Gibbs RS, Malherbe H, et al: A controlled study of genital mycoplasmas in amniotic fluid from patients with intra-amniotic infection. J Infect Dis **147**:650, 1983.

Ferguson MG, Rhodes PG, Morrison JC, Pucket CM: Clinical amniotic fluid infection and its effect on the neonate. Am J Obstet Gynecol **151**:1058, 1985.

Garite TJ, Freeman RK: Chorioamnionitis in the preterm gestation. Obstet Gynecol **59**:539, 1982.

Gibbs RS, Blanco JD, St. Clair PJ, Castaneda YS: Quantitative bacteriology of amniotic fluid from patients with clinical intra-amniotic infection at term. J Infect Dis **145**:1, 1982.

Gibbs RS, Dinsmoor MJ, Newton ER, Ramamurthy RS: A randomized trial of intrapartum vs. immediately postpartum treatment of intra-amniotic infection. Obstet Gynecol **72**:823, 1988.

Gibbs RS, Duff P: Progress in pathogenesis and management of clinical intra-amniotic infection. Am J Obstet Gynecol **164**:1317, 1991.

Hardt NS, Kostenbauder M, Ogburn M, et al: Influence of chorioamnionitis on long-term prognosis in low birth weight infants. Obstet Gynecol **65**:5, 1985.

Morales WJ: The effect of chorioamnionitis and developmental outcome of preterm infants at one year. Obstet Gynecol **70**:183, 1987.

Sperling RS, Ramamurthyr S, and Gibbs RS: A comparison of intrapartum versus immediate postpartum treatment of intra-amniotic infection. Obstet Gynecol **70**:861, 1987.

Sweet RC, Landers DV, Walker C, Schachter J: *Chlamydia trachomatis* infection and pregnancy outcome. Am J Obstet Gynecol **156**:9829, 1987.

Yoder RP, Gibbs RS, Blanco JD, et al.: A prospective controlled study of maternal and perinatal outcome after intra-amniotic infection at term. Am J Obstet Gynecol **145**:695, 1983.

Yonekura ML, Wallace R, Eglinton WR: Amnionitis—optimal operative management: Extraperitoneal cesarean section vs. low cervical transperitoneal cesarean section. Presented at Third Annual Meeting, Society of Perinatal Obstetricians, Abstract 24A, San Antonio, 1983.

Postpartum Infection

DiZerega G, Yonekura L, Roy S, et al: A comparison of clindamycin/gentamicin and penicillin/gentamicin in the treatment of post-cesarean section endomyometritis. Am J Obstet Gynecol **134**:238, 1979.

Dismoor MJ, Newton ER, Gibbs RS: A randomized, double-blinded, placebo-controlled trial of oral antibiotics following intravenous antibiotic therapy for postpartum endometritis. Obstet Gynecol **77**:60, 1991.

Gibbs RS, Jones PM, Wilder CJY: Internal fetal monitoring and maternal infection following cesarean section. A prospective study. Obstet Gynecol **52**:193, 1978.

Gibbs RS: Clinical risk factors for puerperal infection. Obstet Gynecol **55**:1785, 1980.

Newton ER, Prihoda T, Gibbs RS: Clinical and microbiological analysis of risk factors for puerperal endometritis. Obstet Gynecol **75**:402, 1990.

Stiver HG, Forward KR, Livingstone RA, et al: Multicenter comparison of cefoxitin vs. cefazolin for prevention of infectious morbidity after non-elective cesarean section. Am J Obstet Gynecol **145**:158, 1983.

Sweet RC, Gibbs RS: Infectious diseases of the female genital tract. Baltimore, Williams and Wilkins, 1990, pp 356, 460.

Watts DH, Eschenbach DA, Denny GE: Early postpartum endometritis: The role of bacteria, genital mycoplasmas, and *C. trachomatis*. Obstet Gynecol **75**:52, 1990.

Mastitis

Deveraux WP: Acute puerperal mastitis. Am J Obstet Gynecol **108**:78, 1970.

Niebyl JR, Spence MR, Parmley TH: Sporadic (nonepidemic) puerperal mastitis. J Reprod Med **20**:97, 1978.

Thomsen AC, Hansen KB, Moeller BR: Leukocyte counts and microbiologic cultivation in the diagnosis of puerperal mastitis. Am J Obstet Gynecol **146**:938, 1983.

Wound Infection After Cesarean Section

Cruse PJE, Foord R: A five-year prospective study of 23,649 surgical wounds. Arch Surg **107**:206, 1973.

National Academy of Sciences–National Research Council, Division of Medical Sciences, Ad Hoc Committee on Trauma: Postoperative wound infections: The influence of ultraviolet irradiation of the operative room and of various other factors. Ann Surg **160**(Suppl 2):1, 1964.

Episiotomy Infection and Other Pelvic Infections

Shy KK, Eschenbach DA: Fatal perineal cellulitis from an episiotomy site. Obstet Gynecol **54**:292, 1979.

Group B Streptococcal Infection

ACOG Technical Bulletin: Group B Streptococcal Infections in Pregnancy 1992; No. 170, The American College of Obstetricians and Gynecologists.

Baker CJ: Summary of the workshop on perinatal infections due to group B streptococcus. J Infect Dis **136**:137, 1977.

Boyer KM, Gotoff SP: Prevention of early-onset neonatal group B streptococcal disease with selective intrapartum chemoprophylaxis. N Engl J Med **314**:1665, 1986.

Committee on Infectious Diseases and Committee on Fetus and Newborn: Guidelines for Prevention of GBS Infection by Chemoprophylaxis. Pediatrics **90**:775, 1992.

Carey JC, Klebanoff MA, Regan JA, et al: Evaluation of the Gram stain as a screening tool for maternal carriage of group B beta-hemolytic streptococci. Obstet Gynecol **76**:693, 1990.

Gardner SW, Yow MD, Leeds LJ, et al: Failure of penicillin to eradicate group B streptococcal colonization in the pregnant woman. Am J Obstet Gynecol **135**:1062, 1979.

Gibbs RS, Hall RT, Yow MW, McCrochan GH, Nelson JD: Consensus: perinatal prophylaxis for group B streptococcal infection. Pediatr Infect Dis J **11**:179, 1992.

Hall RE, Barnes W, Krishnan L, et al: Antibiotic treatment of parturient women colonized with group B streptococci. Am J Obstet Gynecol **124**:630, 1976.

Isada N, Grossman JH: A rapid screening test for the diagnosis of endocervical group B streptococci in pregnancy. Obstet Gynecol **70**:139, 1987.

Lloyd DJ, Belgaumkar TK, Scott KE, et al: Prevention of group B beta hemolytic streptococcal septicemia in low-birth-weight neonates by penicillin administered within two hours of birth. Lancet i:713, 1979.

Merenstein GB, Todd WA, Brown G, et al: Group B beta hemolytic streptococcus: Randomized controlled treatment at term. Obstet Gynecol **55**:315, 1980.

Minkoff H, Mead P: An obstetric approach to the prevention of early-onset group B beta-hemolytic streptococcal sepsis. Am J Obstet Gynecol **154**:973, 1986.

Morales WJ, Lim D: Reduction of group B streptococcal maternal and neonatal infections in preterm pregnancies with PROM throughout rapid identification test. Am J Obstet Gynecol **157**:13, 1987.

Siegel JD, McCracken GH, Thrielkeld N, et al: Single-dose penicillin prophylaxis against neonatal group B streptococcal infections. N Engl J Med **45**:685, 1978.

Silver HM, Gibbs RS, Gray BM, et al.: Risk factors for perinatal group B streptococcal disease after amniotic fluid colonization. Am J Obstet Gynecol **163**:19, 1990.

Listeriosis

Charles D: *Infections in Obstetrics and Gynecology*. Philadelphia, WB Saunders, 1990, pp 192–197.

Bartolussi R, Seeliger HPR: Listeriosis. *In* Remington JS, Klein JO (eds): Infectious Diseases of the Fetus and Newborn Infant. Philadelphia, WB Saunders, 1990, p 812.

Gellin BG, Broome CV: Listeriosis. JAMA **261**:1313, 1989.

Kalstone C: Successful antepartum treatment of listeriosis. Am J Obstet Gynecol **164**:57, 1991.

Linnan MJ, Mascola L, Dong LX, et al: Epidemic listeriosis associated with Mexican-style cheese. N Engl J Med **319**:823, 1988.

McLauchlin J: Human listeriosis in Britain. 1967–85. A summary of 722 cases. I. Listeriosis during pregnancy and in the newborn. Epidemiol Infect **104**:181, 1990.

Lyme Disease

Ackerman R, Rehse-Kuppen B, Gallmer E, Schmidt R: Chronic neurologic manifestations of erythema migrans borreliosis. Ann NY Acad Sci **539**:16, 1988.

Asbrink E, Hovmark A: Early and late cutaneous manifestations of *Ixodes*-borne borreliosis (erythema migrans borreliosis, Lyme borelliosis). Ann NY Acad Sci **539**:4, 1988.

Centers for Disease Control: Lyme Disease—United States, 1987 and 1988. MMWR **38**:668, 1989.

Ciesielski CA, Russell H, Johnson S, et al: Prospective study of pregnancy outcome in women with Lyme disease. (Abstract) Twenty-Seventh Interscience Conference Antimicrobial Agents Chemotherapy, 1987.

Luft BJ, Steinman CR, Neimark HC, et al: Invasion of the central nervous system by *Borrelia burgdorferi* in acute disseminated infection. JAMA **267**:1364, 1992.

MacDonald A: Human fetal borreliosis, toxemia of pregnancy, and fetal death. Zentralbl Bakteriol [A] **263**:189, 1986.

MacDonald AB, Benach JL, Burgdorfer W: Stillbirth following Lyme disease. NY J Med **8**:615, 1987.

Markowitz LE, Steere AC, Benach JL, et al: Lyme disease during pregnancy. JAMA **255**:3394, 1986.

Nadel D, Hunziker VA, Bucher HV, et al: Infants born to mothers with antibodies against *Borrelia burgdorferi* at delivery. Eur J Pediatr **148**:426, 1989.

Schlesinger PA, Duray PH, Burke BA, et al: Maternal-Fetal transmission of the Lyme disease spirochete, *Borrelia burgdorferi*. Ann Intern Med **103**:67, 1985.

Smith LG Jr., Pearlman M, Smith LG, Faro S: Lyme disease: a review with emphasis on the pregnant woman. Obstet Gynecol Surv **46**:125, 1991.

Steere AC, Malawista SE, Snydman DR, et al: Lyme arthritis in children and adults in three Connecticut communities. Arthritis Rheum **20**:7, 1977a.

Steere AC, Malawista SE, Hardin JA, et al: Erythema chronicum migrans and Lyme arthritis: the enlarging clinical spectrum. Am Intern Med **86**:685, 1977b.

Steere AC: Lyme disease. N Engl J Med **321**:586, 1989.

Weber K, Bratzke HJ, Neubert U, et al: *Borrelia burgdorferi* in a newborn despite oral penicillin for Lyme borreliosis during pregnancy. Pediatr Infect Dis J **7**:286, 1988.

Williams CL, Benach JL, Curran AS, et al: Lyme disease during pregnancy: a cord blood serosurvey. Ann NY Acad Sci **539**:504, 1988.

Viral Infections

Rubella

Bart SW, Steller HC, Preblud SR: Fetal risk associated with rubella vaccine: An update. Rev Infect Dis **7**:595, 1985.

Centers for Disease Control. Rubella prevention. MMWR **30**(37), 1981.

Cooper LZ, Ziring PR, Ockerse AB, et al: Rubella: Clinical manifestations and management. Am J Dis Child **118**:18, 1969.

Daffos F, Grangeot-Keros L, Leban P, et al: Prenatal diagnosis of congenital rubella. Lancet **2**:1, 1984.

Hermann KL: Available rubella serologic tests. Rev Infect Dis **7**:S109, 1985.

Mann JM, Preblud SR, Hoffman RE, et al: Assessing risks of rubella infection. JAMA **245**:1647, 1981.

Cytomegalovirus

Balfour CL, Balfour HH: Cytomegalovirus is not an occupational risk for nurses in renal transplant and neonatal units. JAMA **256**:1909, 1986.

Chandler SH, Alexander ER, Holmes HR: Epidemiology of cytomegalovirus infection in a heterogeneous population of pregnant women. J Infect Dis **152**:249, 1985.

Collaborative DHPG Treatment Study Group: Treatment of serious cytomegalovirus infection with 9-(1–3-dihydroxypropoxymethyl) quanine in patients with AIDS and other deficiencies. N Engl J Med **314**:801, 1986.

Demmler GJ: Summary of a workshop on surveillance for congenital cytomegalovirus disease. Rev Infect Dis **13**:315, 1991.

Elek SD, Stern H: Development of a vaccine against mental retar-

dation caused by cytomegalovirus infection *in utero*. Lancet **1**:1, 1974.

Fowler KS, Stagno S, Pass RF, et al: The outcome of congenital cytomegalovirus infection in relation to maternal antibody status. N Engl J Med **326**:663, 1992.

Grose C, Weiner CP: Prenatal diagnosis of congenital cytomegalovirus infection: Two decades later. Am J Obstet Gynecol **163**:447, 1990.

Hanshaw JB: Congenital cytomegalovirus infection: A 15-year prospective study. J Infect Dis **123**:555, 1971.

Hanshaw JB, Scheiner AP, Moxley AW, et al: School failure and deafness after "silent" congenital cytomegalovirus. N Engl J Med **295**:468, 1976.

Hogge WH, Thiagarajah S, Brerbridge AN, Harbert GM: Fetal evaluation by percutaneous blood sampling. Am J Obstet Gynecol **158**:132, 1988.

Hohlfeld P, Vial Y, Maillard-Brigno C, et al: Cytomegalovirus fetal infection: Prenatal diagnosis. Obstet Gynecol **78**:615, 1991.

Lamy ME, Mulongo KN, Gadicseux JF, et al: Prenatal diagnosis of fetal cytomegalovirus infection. Am J Obstet Gynecol **166**:91, 1992.

Lange I, Rodeck CM, Morgan-Capner P: Prenatal serological diagnosis of intrauterine cytomegalovirus infection. Br Med J **284**:1673, 1982.

Lynch L, Daffos F, Emmanuel D, et al: Prenatal diagnosis of fetal cytomegalovirus infection. Am J Obstet Gynecol **165**:714, 1991.

Merigan TC, Renlund DG, Keay S, et al: A controlled trial of ganciclovir to prevent cytomegalovirus disease after heart transplantation. N Engl J Med **326**:1182, 1992.

Monif GRG, Egan EA, Held B, et al: The correlation of maternal cytomegalovirus infection during varying stages in gestation and neonatal involvement. J Pediatr **80**:17, 1972.

Pass RF, Stagno S, Meyer GJ, et al: Outcome of symptomatic congenital CMV infection: results of long-term longitudinal follow-up. Pediatrics **66**:758, 1980.

Reynolds DW, Stagno S, Stubbs KG, et al: Inapparent congenital cytomegalovirus infection with elevated cord IgM levels: Causal relation with auditory and mental deficiency. N Engl J Med **290**:291, 1974.

Stagno S, Pass RF, Dworsky ME, et al: Congenital cytomegalovirus infection: relation to auditory and mental deficiency. N Engl J Med **290**:291, 1974.

Stagno S, Pass RF, Dworsky ME, et al: Congenital cytomegalovirus infection. The relative importance of primary and recurrent maternal infection. N Engl J Med **306**:945, 1982.

Stagno S, Pass RF, Dworsky ME, Alford CA: Congenital and perinatal cytomegalovirus infection. Semin Perinatol **7**:302, 1983.

Stagno S, Whitley RJ: Herpesvirus infections of pregnancy. Part I: Cytomegalovirus and Epstein-Barr virus infection. N Engl J Med **313**:1270, 1985.

Stagno S, Pass RF, Cloud G, et al: Primary cytomegalovirus infection in pregnancy: Incidence, transmission to fetus, and clinical outcome. JAMA **256**:1904–8, 1986.

Stern J, Tucker SM: Prospective study of cytomegalovirus infection in pregnancy. Br Med J **2**:268, 1973.

Weiner CP, Grose C: Prenatal diagnosis of congenital cytomegalovirus infection by virus isolation from amniotic fluid. Am J Obstet Gynecol **163**:1253, 1990.

Weller TH: The cytomegaloviruses: ubiquitous agents with protein clinical manifestations. N Engl J Med **285**:203, 267, 1971.

Yow MD, Demmler GJ: Congenital cytomegalovirus disease: 20 years is long enough. N Engl J Med **326**:702, 1992.

Varicella and Herpes Zoster

Balducci J, Rodis JF, Rosengren S, et al: Pregnancy outcome following first-trimester varicella infection. Obstet Gynecol **79**:5, 1992.

Brozin SA, Simkovich JW, Johnson WT: Herpes zoster during pregnancy. Obstet Gynecol **53**:175, 1979.

DeNicola LK, Hanshaw JB: Congenital and neonatal varicella (Editorial). J Pediatr **94**:175, 1979.

Harris RE, Rhoades ER: Varicella pneumonia complicating pregnancy: Report of a case and review of the literature. Obstet Gynecol **25**:734, 1965.

Higa K, Don K, Manabe H: Varicella-zoster virus infections during pregnancy: Hypothesis concerning the mechanisms of congenital malformations. Obstet Gynecol **69**:214, 1987.

Miller E, Cradock-Watson JE, Ridehalgh MK: Outcome in newborn babies given anti-varicella zoster immune globulin after perinatal maternal infection with varicella zoster virus. Lancet **2**:301, 1989.

Paryani SG, Arvin AM: Intrauterine infection with varicella-zoster virus after maternal varicella. N Engl J Med **314**:1542, 1986.

Siegal M: Congenital malformations following chickenpox, measles, mumps, and hepatitis: Results of a chart study. JAMA **226**:1521, 1973.

Smego RA, Asperilla MO: Use of acyclovir for varicella pneumonia during pregnancy. Obstet Gynecol **78**:1112, 1991.

Herpes Simplex

American College Obstetricians and Gynecologists: Perinatal herpes simplex infections. Tech Bull 122. Washington, DC, ACOG, 1988.

Amstey MS, Monif GRG: Herpes virus in pregnancy. Obstet Gynecol **44**:394, 1974.

Andrews EB, Yankaskas BC, Cordero J: Fetal acyclovir in pregnancy Registry: Six years' experience. Obstet Gynecol **79**:7, 1992.

Arvin AM, Hensleigh PA, Prober CG, et al: Failure of antepartum maternal cultures to predict the infant's risk of exposure to herpes simplex virus at delivery. N Engl J Med **315**:796, 1986.

Binkin NJ, Koplan JP, Cates W Jr: Preventing neonatal herpes: The value of weekly viral cultures in pregnant women with recurrent genital herpes. JAMA **251**:2816, 1984.

Brown AZ, Vantuer LA, Benedetti J, et al: Effects on infants of a first episode of genital herpes in pregnancy. N Engl J Med **317**:1246, 1987.

Gibbs RS, Amstey MS, Sweet RS, et al: Management of genital herpes infection in pregnancy. Obstet Gynecol **71**:779, 1988.

Hutto C, Arvin A, Jacobs R, et al: Intrauterine herpes simplex virus infections. Pediatrics **110**:97, 1987.

Kibrick S: Herpes simplex infection at term. What to do with mother, newborn and nursery personnel. JAMA **253**:157, 1980.

Kulhanjian JA, Soroush V, Au DS, et al: Identification of women at unsuspected risk of primary infection with herpes simplex virus type 2 during pregnancy. N Engl J Med **326**:916, 1992.

Nahmias A, Josey WE, Naib ZM, et al.: Perinatal risk associated with maternal genital herpes simplex infection. Am J Obstet Gynecol **110**:825, 1971.

Prober CG, Sullender WM, Yasukawa LL, et al: Low risk of herpes simplex virus infections in neonates exposed to the virus at the time of vaginal delivery to mothers with recurrent genital herpes simplex virus infections. N Engl J Med **316**:240, 1987.

Hepatitis

Adams RMH, Combes B: Hepatitis during pregnancy. JAMA **192**:95, 1965.

Arvelo JA, Washington AE: Cost effectiveness of prenatal screening and immunization for hepatitis B virus. JAMA **259**:365, 1989.

Chou GL, Kuo G, Weiner AJ, et al: Isolation of a cDNA clone derived from a blood-bourne non-A, non-B viral hepatitis genome. Science **244**:359, 1989.

Dawson GJ, Leseniewski RR, Steward KM, et al: Detection of antibodies to hepatitis C in U.S. blood donors. J Clin Microbial **29**:551, 1991.

Esteban JI, Esteban R, Viladominu L, et al: Hepatitis C virus antibodies among high risk groups in Spain. Lancet **ii**:294, 1989.

Giovannini M, Tagger A, Ribero ML, et al: Maternal-infant transmission of hepatitis C virus and HIV infections: A possible interaction. Lancet **i**:1166, 1990.

Goldsmith R, Yarbough PO, Reyes GR, et al: Enzyme-linked immuno-absorbent assay for diagnosis of acute sporadic hepatitis E in Egyptian children. Lancet **339**:328, 1992.

Gust ID, Purcell RH: Report of a workshop: Waterborne non-A, non-B hepatitis. J Infant Dis **156**:630, 1987.

Houfnagle JH: Type D (delta) hepatitis. JAMA **261**:1321, 1989.

Isenberg J: The infant and hepatitis B virus infections. Adv Pediatr **24**:455, 1977.

Kumar ML, Dawson NV, McCullough HJ, et al: Should all pregnant women be screened for hepatitis B? Ann Intern Med **107**:273, 1987.

Kuo G, Choo GL, Alter JH, et al: An assay for circulating antibodies to a major etiologic virus of human non-A, non-B hepatitis. Science **244**:362, 1989.

Lynch-Salamon DI, Coombs CA: Hepatitis C in obstetrics and gynecology. Obstet Gynecol **79**:621, 1992.

Reesink HW, Wong VCW, Ip HMH, et al: Mother-to-infant transmission and hepatitis C virus. Lancet **1**:1216, 1990

Schweitzer I: Viral hepatitis B in neonates and infants. Am J Med **55**:762, 1973.

Stevens CE, Taylor PE, Pindych J, et al: Epidemiology of hepatitis C virus: A preliminary study in volunteer blood donors. JAMA **263**:49, 1990.

Summers PR, Biswas MK, Pastoret JG, et al: The pregnant hepatitis B carrier: Evidence favoring comprehensive antepartum screening. Obstet Gynecol **69**:701, 1987.

Thaler MM, Park CK, Landers DV, et al: Vertical transmission of hepatitis C virus. Lancet **338**:17, 1991.

Human Parvovirus

Anand A, Gray ES, Brown T, et al: Human parvovirus infection in pregnancy and hydrops fetalis. N Engl J Med **316**:183, 1987.

Anderson LJ: Role of parvovirus B19 in human disease: Pediatr Infec Dis **6**:911, 1987.

Bernstein IM, Capeless EL: Elevated maternal serum alphafetoprotein and hydrops fetalis in association with fetal parvovirus B19 infection. Obstet Gynecol **74**:456, 1989.

Carrington D, Gilmore DH, Whittle MJ, et al: Maternal serum alphafetoprotein: A marker of fetal aplastic crisis during intrauterine human parvovirus infection. Lancet **1**:433, 1987.

Centers for Disease Control: Risks associated with human parvovirus B19 infection. MMWR **38**:81, 1989.

Gillespie SM, Cartler ML, Asch S, et al: Occupational risk of human parvovirus B19 infection for school and day-care personnel during an outbreak of erythema infectiosum. JAMA **263**:2061, 1990.

Humphrey W, Magoon M, O'Shaughnessy R: Severe nonimmune hydrops secondary to parvovirus B19 infection: Spontaneous reversal *in utero* and survival of a term infant. Obstet Gynecol **78**:900, 1991.

Naides SJ, Weiner CP: Antenatal diagnosis and palliative treatment of non-immune hydrops fetalis secondary to fetal parvovirus B19 infection. Prenat Diagn **9**:105, 1989.

Peters MT, Nikolaides KH: Cordocentesis for the diagnosis and treatment of human fetal parvovirus infection. Obstet Gynecol **75**:501, 1990.

Public Health Laboratory Service Working Party on Fifth Disease: Prospective study of human parvovirus (B19) infection during pregnancy. Br Med J **300**:1166, 1990.

Rodis JF, Hovick TJ, Quinn DL, et al: Human parvovirus infection in pregnancy. Obstet Gynecol **72**:733, 1988.

Rodis JF, Quinn DL, Gary W, et al: Management and outcomes of pregnancies complicated by human B19 parvovirus infection: A prospective study. Am J Obstet Gynecol **163**:1168, 1990.

Sahakian V, Weiner CP, Naides SJ, et al: Intrauterine transfusion treatment of nonimmune hydrops fetalis secondary to human parvovirus B19 infection. Am J Obstet Gynecol **164**:1090, 1991.

Schwartz TF, Roggendorf M, Hottentrager B, et al: Human parvovirus B19 infection in pregnancy. Lancet **2**:566, 1988.

Soothill P: Intrauterine blood transfusion for non-immune hydrops fetalis due to parvovirus B19 infection. (Letter) Lancet **2**:121, 1990.

Torok TJ, Wang AY, Gary GW, et al: Prenatal diagnosis of intrauterine infection with parvovirus B19 by the polymerase chain reaction technique. Clin Infect Dis **14**:149, 1992.

Thurn J: Human parvovirus B19: Historical and clinical review. Rev Infect Dis **10**:1005, 1988.

Woernle CH, Anderson LJ, Tattersall P, Davison JM: Human parvovirus B19 infection during pregnancy. J Infect Dis **156**:17, 1987.

Influenza

Finland M: Influenza complicating pregnancy. *In* Charles D, Finland M (eds): Obstetric and Perinatal Infections. Philadelphia, Lea & Febiger, 1973.

Larsen JW: Influenza and pregnancy. Clin Obstet Gynecol **25**:599, 1982.

Rubeola

Siegal M, Fuerst HT: Low birth weight and maternal virus disease: A prospective study of rubella, measles, mumps, chicken pox and hepatitis. JAMA **197**:680, 1966.

Mumps

Monif GRG: Maternal mumps infection during gestation: Observations in the progeny. Am J Obstet Gynecol **119**:549, 1974.

Gershon A: Chickenpox, Measles and Mumps. Chapter 11. In Remington JS, Leein JD (eds): Infectious Diseases of the Fetus and Newborn Infant. Philadelphia, WB Saunders Co., 1990.

Monif GRG: Transplacental mumps infection. Am J Obstet Gynecol **125**:875, 1976.

Siegal M: Congenital malformations following chickenpox, measles, mumps, and hepatitis: Results of a chart study. JAMA **226**:1521, 1973.

St Geme JW Jr, Noren GR, Adams P: Proposed embryopathic relationship between mumps virus and primary endocardial fibroelastosis. N Engl J Med **275**:339, 1966.

Echoviruses

Hughes JR, Wilfert CM, Moore M, et al: Echovirus 14 infection associated with fatal neonatal hepatic necrosis. Am J Dis Child **123**:61, 1972.

Modlin JF: Perinatal echovirus infection: Insights from a literature review of 61 cases of serious infection and 16 outbreaks in nurseries. Rev Infect Dis **8**:918, 1986.

Philip AGS, Larsen EJ: Overwhelming neonatal infection with echo 19 virus. J Pediatr **82**:391, 1973.

Coxsackievirus

Brown G, Karunas R: Relationship of congenital anomalies and maternal infection with selected enteroviruses. Am J Epidemiol **95**:207, 1972.

Van Creveld S, deJager H: Myocarditis in newborns caused by coxsackievirus: Clinical and pathological data. Ann Pediatr **187**:100, 1956.

Verlinde J, von Tongeren H, Kret A: Myocarditis in newborns due to group B coxsackievirus: Virus studies. Ann Pediatr **187**:113, 1956.

Sexually Transmitted Diseases

Amstey MS, Steadman KT: Symptomatic gonorrhea and pregnancy. J Am Vener Dis Assoc **3**:14, 1976.

Cates W, Jr, Hinman AR: Sexually transmitted diseases in the 1990s. N Engl J Med **325**:1368, 1991.

Centers for Disease Control: Syphilis and congenital syphilis—United States, 1985–1988. MMWR **37**:486, 1988.

Centers for Disease Control: 1989 Sexually transmitted diseases treatment guidelines. MMWR **38**(Suppl 81), September 1, 1989.

Chamberlain MJ, Reynolds AL, Yeoman WB: Toxic effects of podophyllin: Application in pregnancy. Br Med J **3**:391, 1972.

Chesney AM, Kemp JE: Incidence of Spirochaeta pallida in cerebrospinal fluid during early state of syphilis. JAMA **83**:1725, 1924.

Clark EG, Danboldt N: The Oslo study of the natural history of untreated syphilis. An epidemiologic investigation based on a restudy of the Boeck-Bruusguotd Material: A review and appraisal. J Chronic Dis **2**:311, 1955.

Cohen DH, Boyd D, Pabhudes I, Mascola I: The effects of case definition, maternal screenings, and reporting criteria on rates of congenital syphilis. Am J Public Health **80**:316, 1990.

Cook TA, Cohn AM, Brunchwig JP, et al: Wart viruses and laryngeal papillomas. Lancet **i**:782, 1973.

Edwards LE, Barrada MI, Hamann AA, Hakanson EY: Gonorrhea in pregnancy. Am J Obstet Gynecol **132**:637, 1978.

Fiumara NJ, Lessel S: Manifestations of late congenital syphilis. Arch Dermatol **102**:78, 1970.

Handsfield HH, Hodson A, Holmes KK: Neonatal gonococcal infection. I. Orogastric contamination with Neisseria gonorrhoeae. JAMA **225**:697, 1973.

Handsfield HH, McCormack WM, Hook EW, III, et al: A comparison of single-dose cefixime with ceftriaxone as treatment for uncomplicated gonorrhea. N Engl J Med **325**:337, 1991.

Harter CA, Benirschke K: Fetal syphilis in the first trimester. Am J Obstet Gynecol **124**:705, 1976.

Holmes KK, Counts LW, Beaty HN: Disseminated gonococcal infection. Ann Intern Med **74**:979, 1971.

Ingall D, Norins L: Syphilis. In Remington JS, Klein JO (eds): Infectious Diseases of the Fetus and Newborn Infant. Philadelphia, WB Saunders, 1976.

Jaffe HW: The laboratory diagnosis of syphilis. New concepts. Ann Intern Med **83**:846, 1975.

Jones JE, Harris RE: Diagnostic evaluation of syphilis during pregnancy. Obstet Gynecol **54**:611, 1979.

Lukehard SA, Hook EW III, Baker-Zander SA, et al: Invasion of the central nervous system by Treponema pallidum: Implications for diagnosis and treatment. Ann Intern Med **109**:855, 1988.

Moran JS, Zenilman JM: Therapy for gonococcal infections: Options in 1989. Rev Infect Dis **12**:633, 1990.

Ricci JM, Fojaco RM, O'Sullivan MJ: Congenital syphilis. The University of Miami/Jackson Memorial Medical Center Experience, 1986–88. Obstet Gynecol **74**:687, 1989.

Rolfs RT, Nakoshima AK: Epidemiology of primary and secondary syphilis in the United States, 1981 through 1989. JAMA **264**:1432, 1990.

Roman A, Fife KH: Human papillomaviruses: Are we ready to type? Clin Microbiol Rev **2**:166, 1989.

Sarrel PM, Pruett KA: Symptomatic gonorrhea during pregnancy. Obstet Gynecol **32**:670, 1968.

Shah K, Ashima H, Polk BF, et al: Rarity of cesarean delivery in cases of juvenile-onset respiratory papillomatosis. Obstet Gynecol **68**:795, 1986.

Singer A, Jenkins D: Viruses and cervical cancer. Br Med J **302**:251, 1991.

Stokes JH (ed): Modern Clinical Syphilology. 2nd ed. Philadelphia, WB Saunders, 1934.

Wendel GD, Stark BJ, Jamison RB, et al: Penicillin allergy and desensitization in serious maternal/fetal infections. N Engl J Med **312**:1229, 1985.

WHO Expert Committee on Veneral Diseases and Treponematoses. Sixth Report. Technical report series No. 736. World Health Organization, 1986.

Zenker P: New case definition for congenital syphilis reporting. Sex Transm Dis **18**:44, 1991.

Ziaya RP, Hankins GDV, Gilstrap LC, Haley AB: Intravenous penicillin desensitization and treatment during pregnancy. JAMA **256**:2561, 1986.

Chlamydial Infection

Alexander ER, Harrison HR: Role of Chlamydia trachomatis in perinatal infections. Rev Infect Dis **5**:713, 1983.

Alger LS, Lovchik JC, Hebel JR, et al: The association of Chlamydial trachomatis, Neisseria gonorrhoeae, and group B streptococci with preterm rupture of the membranes and pregnancy outcome. Am J Obstet Gynecol **159**:397, 1988.

Amortegui AJ, Meyer MP: Enzyme immunoassay for detection of Chlamydia trachomatis from the cervix. Obstet Gynecol **65**:523, 1985.

Beem MO, Saxon EM: Respiratory tract colonization and a distinctive pneumonia syndrome in infants infected with Chlamydia trachomatis. N Engl J Med **296**:306, 1977.

Berman SM, Harrison HR, Boyce WT, et al: Low birth weight, prematurity and postpartum endometritis: Association with prenatal cervical Mycoplasma hominis and Chlamydia trachomatis infection. JAMA **257**:1189, 1987.

Blanco JD, Diaz KC, Lipscomb KA, et al: Chlamydia trachomatis isolation in patients with endometritis after cesarean section. Am J Obstet Gynecol **152**:278, 1985.

Brunham RC, Paavonen J, Stevens CE, et al: Mucopurulent cervicitis: The ignored counterpart in women of urethritis in men. N Engl J Med **311**:1, 1984.

Chandler JW, Alexander ER, Pheiffer TH, et al: Ophthalmia neonatorum associated with maternal chlamydial infections. Trans Am Acad Ophthalmol Otolaryngol **83**:302, 1977.

Cohen I, Veille C, Calkins BM, et al: Improved pregnancy outcome following successful treatment of chlamydial infection. JAMA **263**:3160, 1990.

Crombleholme WR, Schachter J, Grossman M, Landers DV, Sweet RL: Amoxicillin therapy for Chlamydia trachomatis in pregnancy. Obstet Gynecol **75**:752, 1990.

Fitz-Simmons J, Callahan C, Shanahan B, Jungkind D: Chlamydial infections in pregnancy. J Reprod Med **31**:19, 1986.

Frommell GT, Rothenberg R, Wang S-P, et al: Chlamydial infection of mothers and their infants. J Pediatr **95**:28, 1979.

Gravett MG, Nelson HP, DeRouen T, et al: Independent associations of bacterial vaginosis and *Chlamydia trachomatis* infection with adverse pregnancy outcome. JAMA **256**:1899, 1986.

Grossman M, Schachter J, Sweet RL, et al: Prospective studies of chlamydia in newborns. *In* Mardh P-A, Holmes KK, Oriel JD, Piot P, Schachter J (eds): Chlamydial Infections. Fernstrom Foundation Series. Amsterdam, Elsevier, 1982, Vol 2, pp 213–216.

Hammerschlag MR, Anderka M, Semine DZ, et al: Prospective study of maternal and infantile infection with *Chlamydia trachomatis*. Pediatrics **64**:142, 1979.

Hardy PH, Hardy JB, Nell EE, et al: Prevalence of six sexually transmitted disease agents among pregnant inner-city adolescents and pregnancy outcome. Lancet ii:333, 1984.

Harrison HR, Alexander ER, Weinstein L, et al: Cervical *Chlamydia trachomatis* and mycoplasmal infections in pregnancy. JAMA **250**:1721, 1983.

Heggie AD, Lumiaco CG, Stuart LA, Gyues MT: *Chlamydia trachomatis* infection in mothers and infants. Am J Dis Child **135**:507, 1981.

Holland SM, Gaydos CA, Quinn TC: Detection and differentiation of *Chlamydia trachomatis, Chlamydia psittaci,* and *Chlamydia pneumoniae* by DNA amplification. J Infect Dis **162**:984, 1990.

Hooton TM, Batteiger BE, Judson FN, et al: Ofloxacin versus doxycycline for treatment of cervical infection with *Chlamydia trachomatis*. Antimicrob Agents Chemother **36**:1144, 1992.

Hoyme UB, Kiviat N, Eschenbach DA: Microbiology and treatment of late postpartum endometritis. Obstet Gynecol **68**:226, 1986.

Ismail MA, Chandler AE, Beem MO, Moawad AH: Chlamydial colonization of the cervix in pregnant adolescents. J Reprod Med **30**:549, 1985.

Johns Hopkins Study Group for Cervicitis and Adverse Pregnancy Outcome: Association of *Chlamydia trachomatis* and *Mycoplasma hominis* with intrauterine growth retardation and preterm delivery. Am J Epidemiol **129**:1247, 1989.

Khurana CM, Deddish PA, delMundo F: Prevalence of *Chlamydia trachomatis* in the pregnant cervix. Obstet Gynecol **66**:241, 1985.

Mardh P-A, Helin I, Bobeck S, et al: Colonization of pregnant and puerperal women and neonates with *Chlamydia trachomatis*. Br J Vener Dis **56**:96, 1980.

Martin DH, Koutsky L, Eschenbach DA, et al: Prematurity and perinatal mortality in pregnancies complicated by maternal *Chlamydia trachomatis* infections. JAMA **247**:1585, 1982.

Martius J, Krohn M, Hillier S, et al: Relationship of vaginal lactobacillus species, cervical *Chlamydia trachomatis* and bacterial vaginosis to preterm birth. Obstet Gynecol **71**:89, 1988.

McGregor JH, French JL, Richter R, et al: Antenatal microbiologic and maternal risk factors associated with prematurity. Am J Obstet Gynecol **163**:1465, 1990.

Moncada J, Schachter J, Shipp M, et al: Cytobrush in collection of cervical specimens for detection of *Chlamydia trachomatis*. J Clin Microbiol **27**:1863, 1989.

Paavonen J, Brunham R, Kiviat N, et al: Cervicitis: etiologic, clinical and histopathologic findings. *In* Mardh P-A, Holmes KK, Oriel JD, Piot P, Schachter J (eds): Chlamydial Infections. Amsterdam, Elsevier-Biomedical Press, 1982, pp 141–145.

Ryan GM, Abdella TN, McNeeley SG, et al: *Chlamydia trachomatis* infection in pregnancy and effect of treatment on outcome. Am J Obstet Gynecol **162**:34, 1990.

Schachter J, Dawson CR: Comparative efficiency of various diagnostic methods for chlamydial infection. *In* Holmes KK, Hobson D (eds): Nongonococcal Urethritis and Related Conditions. Washington DC, American Society for Microbiology, 1977.

Schachter J, Holt J, Goodner E, et al: Prospective study of chlamydial infection in neonates. Lancet **2**:377, 1979.

Schachter J, Sweet RL, Grossman M, et al: Experience with the routine use of erythromycin for chlamydial infections in pregnancy. N Engl J Med **314**:276, 1986a.

Schachter J, Grossman M, Sweet RL, et al: Prospective study of perinatal transmission of *Chlamydia trachomatis*. JAMA **255**:3374, 1986b.

Stamm WE: Diagnosis of *Chlamydia trachomatis* genitourinary infections. Ann Intern Med **108**:710, 1987.

Sweet RL, Landers DV, Walker C, Schachter J: *Chlamydia trachomatis* infection and pregnancy outcome. Am J Obstet Gynecol **156**:824, 1987.

Thompson S, Lopez B, Wong K-H, et al: A prospective study of Chlamydia and Mycoplasma infections during pregnancy: Relation to pregnancy outcome and maternal morbidity. *In* March P-A, Holmes KK, Oriel JD, et al (eds): Chlamydial Infections. Vol 2. Fernstrom Foundation Series. New York, Elsevier-North Holland Inc, 1982, pp 155–158.

Wager GP, Martin DH, Koutsky L, et al: Puerperal infectious morbidity: Relationship to route of delivery and to antepartum *Chlamydia trachomatis* infection. Am J Obstet Gynecol **138**:1028, 1980.

Other Infections

Mycoplasma Infection

Braun P, Lee Y-H, Klein JO, et al: Birth weight and genital mycoplasmas in pregnancy. N Engl J Med **284**:167, 1971.

Carey JC, Blackwelder WC, Nugent RP, Matteson MA, et al: Antepartum cultures for *U. urealyticum* are not useful in predicting pregnancy outcome. Am J Obstet Gynecol **164**:728, 1991.

Eschenbach DA, Nugent RP, Ra AV, et al: A randomized placebo-controlled trial of erythromycin for the treatment of *U. urealyticum* to prevent premature delivery. Am J Obstet Gynecol **164**:734, 1991.

Gibbs RS, Cassel GH, Davis JK, et al: Further studies on genital mycoplasmas in intra-amniotic infection: blood cultures and serologic response. Am J Obstet Gynecol **154**:717, 1986.

Kass EH, McCormack WM, Lin, JS, et al: Genital mycoplasmas as a cause of excess premature delivery. Trans Assoc Am Physicians **94**:261, 1981.

Klein JO, Buckland D, Finland M: Colonization of newborn infants by mycoplasmas. N Engl J Med **280**:1025, 1969.

Kundsin RB, Driscoll SG, Ming PL: Strains of mycoplasma associated with human reproductive failure. Science **157**:1573, 1967.

Lamey JR, Eschenbach DA, Mitchell SH, et al: Isolation of mycoplasmas and bacteria from the blood of postpartum women. Am J Obstet Gynecol **143**:104, 1982.

McCormack WM, Almeida PC, Bailey PE, et al: Sexual activity and vaginal colonization with genital mycoplasmas. JAMA **221**:1375, 1972.

McCormack WM, Lee Y-H, Lin JS, Rankin JS: Genital mycoplasmas in postpartum fever. J Infect Dis **127**:193, 1973.

Shurin PA, Alpert S, Rosner B, et al: Chorioamnionitis and colonization of the newborn infant with genital mycoplasmas. N Engl J Med **293**:5, 1975.

Stray-Pederson B, Erg J, Reikuan TM: Uterine T-mycoplasma colonization in reproductive failure. Am J Obstet Gynecol **130**:307, 1978.

Taylor-Robinson D, McCormack WM: The genital mycoplasmas. N Engl J Med **302**:1003, 1980.

Bacterial Vaginosis

Gravett MG, Hummel D, Eschenbach DA, et al: Preterm labor associated with subclinical amniotic fluid infection and with bacterial vaginosis. Obstet Gynecol **67**:229, 1986a.

Gravett MG, Preston-Nelson HP, DeRouen T, et al: Independent associations of bacterial vaginosis and *Chlamydia trachomatis* infection with adverse pregnancy outcome. JAMA **256**:1899, 1986.

Hillier SL, Martius J, Kohn M, Kinat N, et al: A case-control study of chorioamnionic infection and histology chorioamnionitis in prematurity. N Engl J Med **319**:972, 1988.

Martius J, Krohn MA, Hillier SL, et al: Relationships of vaginal *Lactobacillus* species, cervical *Chlamydia trachomatis*, and bacterial vaginosis to preterm birth. Obstet Gynecol **71**:89, 1988.

Newton ER, Prihoda TJ, Gibbs RS: A clinical and microbiologic analysis of risk factors for puerperal endometritis. Obstet Gynecol **75**:402, 1990.

Pheifer TA, Forsyth PS, Durfee MA, et al: Nonspecific vaginitis: Role of *Haemophilus vaginalis* and treatment with metronidazole. N Engl J Med **298**:1429, 1978.

Robbie MO, Sweet RL: Metronidazole use in obstetrics and gynecology: A review. Am J Obstet Gynecol **145**:865, 1983.

Silver HM, Sperling RS, St Clair PJ, Gibbs RS: Evidence relating bacterial vaginosis to intraamniotic infection. Am J Obstet Gynecol **161**:808, 1989.

Spiegel CA, Amsel R, Eschenbach D, et al: Anaerobic bacteria in nonspecific vaginitis. N Engl J Med **303**:601, 1980.

Toxoplasmosis

Alford CA, Stagno S, Reynolds DW: Congenital toxoplasmosis: Clinical laboratory and therapeutic considerations. Bull NY Acad Med **50**:164, 1974.

Daffos F, Forestier F, Capella-Pavlovsky M, et al: Prenatal management of 746 pregnancies at risk for congenital toxoplasmosis. N Engl J Med **318**:271, 1988.

Desmonts G: Congenital toxoplasmosis. N Engl J Med **291**:366, 1974.

Desmonts G, Couvreur J: Congenital toxoplasmosis: A prospective study of 378 pregnancies. N Engl J Med **290**:1110, 1974a.

Desmonts G, Couvreur J: Toxoplasmosis in pregnancy and its transmission to the fetus. Bull NY Acad Med **50**:146, 1974b.

Feldman HA: Toxoplasmosis. N Engl J Med **279**:1370, 1968.

Krick JA, Remington JS: Toxoplasmosis in the adult—an overview. N Engl J Med **298**:550, 1978.

Krogstad DJ, Juranek DD, Walls KW: Toxoplasmosis. Ann Intern Med **77**:773, 1972.

Stray-Pedersen B, Lorentzen-Styr A: Uterine toxoplasma infections and repeated abortion. Am J Obstet Gynecol **128**:716, 1977.

Trichomoniasis

Cotch MF, et al: Personal communication. Interscience Conference on Antimicrobial Agents and Chemotherapy (ICAAC), 1990.

Hardy PH, Nell EE, Spence MR, et al: Prevalence of six sexually transmitted disease agents among pregnant inner-city adolescents and pregnancy outcome. Lancet **2**:333, 1984.

Mason PR, McLure Brown I: Trichomonas in pregnancy. (Letter) Lancet **2**:1025, 1980.

Minkoff H, Grunebaum AN, Schwarz RH, et al: Risk factors for prematurity and premature rupture of membranes: A prospective study of the vaginal flora in pregnancy. Am J Obstet Gynecol **150**:965, 1984.

Ross SM, Middelkoop AV: Trichomonas infection in pregnancy—does it affect pregancy outcome? South Med J **63**:566, 1983.

Antibiotics in Pregnancy

Charles D: Placental transmission of antibiotics. Obstet Gynecol Annu **8**:19, 1979.

Eschenbach DA: A review of the role of β-lactamase-producing bacteria in obstetric-gynecologic infections. Am J Obstet Gynecol **156**:495, 1987.

Knowles JA: Excretion of drugs in milk: a review. J Pediatr **66**:1068, 1965.

Kucers A, Bennett N McK: The Use of Antibiotics. 4th ed. Philadelphia, JB Lippincott Co, 1987.

Moellering RC Jr: Mechanism of action of antimicrobial agents. Clin Obstet Gynecol **22**:277, 1979.

Philipson A: Pharmacokinetics of antibiotics in pregnancy and labor. Clin Pharmacokinet **4**:297, 1979.

Sweet RC, Gibbs RS: Antimicrobial agents. *In* Sweet RL, Gibbs RS (eds): Infectious Diseases of the Female Genital Tract. 2nd ed. Baltimore, Williams & Wilkins, 1990.

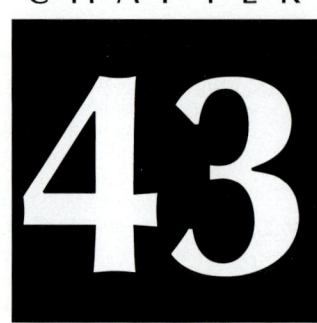

C H A P T E R

43

HUMAN IMMUNODEFICIENCY VIRUS

HOWARD L. MINKOFF, M.D.

At the current time, close to 6000 pregnancies in the United States are complicated by human immunodeficiency virus (HIV) infections. Public health agencies and professional organizations have stressed the important role obstetricians play in identifying and caring for seropositive women. The recent advent of therapeutic trials designed to interrupt perinatal HIV transmission further highlight the critical role of obstetricians in confronting this epidemic. In order to appropriately carry out their role in the overall health care of women, the obstetrician must be cognizant of the virology, pathophysiology, natural history, and standards of clinical management of pregnant women infected with HIV.

EPIDEMIOLOGY

Approximately one million United States citizens are infected with HIV (at least 80,000 women of childbearing age) and more than 100,000 have died. As of July 1991, 18,648 cases of AIDS in women have been reported, with approximately 5000 cases reported in 1991. Half the affected women were Black, a quarter were White and a fifth Hispanic (Centers for Disease Control, 1991a). The rate of new infections is increasing more rapidly among women than among men, and women comprise over 11 per cent of those infected in the United States. In other parts of the world, women comprise almost half of the infected population. AIDS is now the fifth leading cause of death among women of reproductive age in the United States. World-wide it is estimated that by the end of the decade, ten million children will have lost their mothers to AIDS.

In the United States, women's acquisition of HIV is primarily related to sexual exposure and intravenous drug use. The Centers for Disease Control (CDC) estimate that 51 per cent of women acquired their infection through the sharing of needles (Centers for Disease Control, 1991b). This may overstate the contribution of intravenous drug use since the CDC utilizes a hierarchal approach to risk assignment. Thus, for example, if a woman has multiple sexual partners and acknowledges using intravenous drugs one time

she will be categorized as an intravenous drug user. Approximately one-third of infected women acquire their infection heterosexually. However, it should be emphasized that the sexual partners of these women are more often than not intravenous drug users.

More than 80 per cent of cases of pediatric AIDS are secondary to vertical transmission of HIV from mother to fetus (Centers for Disease Control, 1992b). HIV infection is now among the ten leading causes of death among children aged one to four (Centers for Disease Control, 1991c). As of 1990, estimates of the number of children with HIV infection in the United States ranged from 5000 to 10,000 (Hardy, 1991). Based upon national newborn heel stick surveys of HIV prevalence, it is estimated that approximately 6000 children are born to HIV-infected women annually, which would result in 1800 newly infected children per year (Gwinn et al., 1991).

The World Health Organization (WHO) estimates 30 per cent excess infant and child mortality in major United States, Western European, and sub-Saharan African cities where AIDS has become the leading cause of death for women aged 20 to 40 years (Chin, 1990).

VIROLOGY AND PATHOGENESIS

HIV is one of five known human retroviruses. These organisms are single-stranded RNA-enveloped viruses that have the ability to become incorporated into cellular DNA. HIV-1, which used to be called human T cell lymphotrophic virus III (HTLV-III), has a diameter of about 100 nm. The principal core proteins are p18 and p24; the major surface proteins are gp120 and gp41. Recently, much interest has focused on gp120 as a predictor of infectivity and an important focus for vaccine research. The other retroviruses, all of which are significantly less common than HTLV-III, are HTLV-I which causes adult T cell leukemia/lymphoma and tropical spastic paraparesis, HTLV-II which causes hairy cell leukemia, HTLV-IV (also called HIV-2) which causes AIDS, and HTLV-V which causes cutaneous T cell lymphoma/leukemia.

For replication, the virus attaches at the CD4 receptor of the target cell and enters. Cells that have a high density of CD4 on their surface include lymphocytes, monocytes, and neural cells. Some researchers have also identified CD4 on Hofbauer cells. Through the use of a reverse transcriptase, the virus produces a double-stranded DNA that becomes circular and enters the nucleus (Sever, 1989). Subsequently the cell may become stimulated, and the DNA codes for the production of viral RNA and hence viral protein.

Several weeks after acquiring HIV, many individuals will have an acute seroconversion syndrome similar in clinical appearance to an acute episode of mononucleosis. Antibody to HIV generally appears within a few months after infection but in rare instances delays of over a year have been reported. Antigen is detected for a brief period before the appearance of antibody, and some evidence suggests that individuals are particularly infectious during periods of antigenemia. The estimated latent period from infection to AIDS is almost 11 years. Once an individual develops symptoms, the circulating viral load increases markedly as, presumably, does an individual's infectivity.

The principal mechanism whereby HIV leads to immunodeficiency is via its effect on helper (CD4) lymphocytes. These cells play a key role in organizing the body's immune responses. As these cells become progressively depleted, the host becomes susceptible to an expanding array of opportunistic infections. *The presence of a defining opportunistic infection or a CD4 count less than 200 mm³ confirms the diagnosis of AIDS. Once that diagnosis is made, the prognosis is poor.* Although most individuals do not develop opportunistic infections with CD4 counts over 100 mm³, cell counts drop at more rapid rates over time and most individuals with AIDS do not survive two years.

AIDS IN PREGNANCY

Prenatal HIV Testing

Tests for detection of the antibody to HIV were first available for clinical use in the United States in 1985. The two methods that are licensed for use are (1) enzyme-linked immunosorbent assay (ELISA) for initial screening and, (2) Western blot for confirmation. These tests all use antigens derived from disrupted whole virus. The published sensitivity and specificity of the combined tests are about 99 per cent.

Serum samples are first tested and confirmed by the ELISA technique, which depends upon a colorimetric change mediated by an antigen-antibody reaction. The Western Blot test is performed if the ELISA is repeatedly positive. The Western Blot identifies antibodies against specific portions of the virus. The Western Blot is considered positive if the patient has antibody to multiple virus-specific bands—p24, p31, and either gp41 or gp160. If fewer bands are identified, the test is called indeterminate. A small number (15 to 20 per cent) of tests from low-risk patients will be indeterminate and remain so even if repeated over many months. Individuals recently infected may also have indeterminate results, but repeat tests in six months will usually reveal a positive Western Blot. The pa-

tient's final results are considered positive only if *both* the ELISA and the Western Blot are positive.

Counseling

Pretest counseling should be provided to all patients, regardless of their decision to be tested. Such counseling provides an opportunity to educate patients about behaviors that may put them at risk for HIV infection or any other sexually transmitted disease (STD) and to discuss risk-reduction practices. This information can be imparted through clinician-patient discussion, the use of written educational materials or videotapes, or some combination of these methods. The particular mix will depend upon the clinical setting and the prevalence of HIV in the community. Patients should be counseled about HIV and offered the antibody test as early in their pregnancy as possible. Pretest counseling and patients' decisions about testing should be documented in the medical record.

Informational content of pretest counseling should include the following: (1) spectrum of HIV disease and relationship to AIDS, (2) modes of HIV transmission, (3) what the HIV antibody test is and the implications of a negative or positive result, (4) the importance of knowing one's HIV status with regard to pregnancy and perinatal transmission, and (5) risk-reduction behaviors, both sexual and drug-related.

The CDC guidelines for persons who should be offered HIV testing include, as previously outlined, all women of childbearing age who are at risk for HIV infection. Risk assessment depends upon the woman's willingness to self-identify risk factors that may be seen as socially unacceptable or stigmatizing, such as intravenous drug use, prostitution, or history of sex with a drug user. Because many women may not be willing to self-identify such risk behaviors before HIV testing, they should not be required to acknowledge these behaviors as a prerequisite to testing (Landesman et al., 1987). Consequently, it may be prudent in areas of low prevalence to offer all pregnant women the HIV test and in high prevalence areas to routinely recommend that all women take the test.

The post-test session should cover the implications of the patient's positive HIV antibody test result, a brief review of HIV infection and how it is transmitted (and not transmitted), discussion of "safer sex" and "safer needle use" if appropriate, and the implications of HIV infection during pregnancy. The patient should be informed that the chance of having a child who is infected may be 14 to 50 per cent, but that at this time there is no means of predicting whether she will transmit the infection.

Generally, people react to this news in much the same way they have reacted to other stressful news in the past. It is important to allow women enough time during the counseling session to work through some of their initial reactions.

Studies of seropositive womens' pregnancy decisions have shown that women frequently do not choose to terminate the pregnancy and that decisions about abortion are independent of serostatus (Sunderland et al., 1992; Selwyn et al., 1989). A 14 to 50 per cent chance of delivering an infected child may not be a sufficiently compelling reason for a woman to choose abortion. Childbearing and rearing may be of paramount importance; religious and ethical values may preclude abortion.

INTERACTION OF HIV DISEASE AND PREGNANCY

Most recent reports dealing with the relationship of HIV disease to pregnancy outcomes have not found significant effects. In one study, follow-up of 31 asymptomatic seropositive pregnant women and their infants showed that the prevalence of premature delivery, fetal growth retardation, and early neonatal disease was comparable to that of pregnant seronegative drug addicts (Semperini et al., 1987). Others have compared 50 asymptomatic seropositive and 64 seronegative controls throughout their pregnancy and, except for an increased incidence of spontaneous abortion in the seropositive group attributed to the small sample size, found no differences in pregnancy outcome (Johnstone et al., 1988). However, they did note that the incidence of prematurity and LBW infants in both groups of intravenous drug users was about twice that recorded in the general population. Minkoff et al. (1990) studied both drug using and non-drug using HIV infected pregnant women and matched controls in New York City and were unable to demonstrate any differences in birth weight, gestational age, or other outcome parameters.

In order to understand the effect of pregnancy on the course of HIV disease it is essential for the clinician to understand both the normal immune response to foreign antigens and the effect of pregnancy on that response (see also Chapter 6). The main host responses are mediated by two groups of lymphocytes, the "T" or thymus-derived and the "B" or bursa-derived lymphocytes. "T" helper cells are activated by specific foreign antigens, and they in turn stimulate "B" cells to produce immunoglobulins (humeral response). The B cell response initially involves the production of specific IgM antibody and subsequently the production and predominance of IgG antibody. The T lymphocytes have a multitude of functions beyond helping B cells in antibody production. These functions include retaining immunologic memory, suppressing antibody production, identifying antigen, producing delayed hypersensitivity reaction, and lysing specific antigen-bearing target cells (cell-mediated immune response) (Claman, 1987). The different types of T cells can be recognized by their reaction with different monoclonal antibodies and are assigned according to different "cluster designations" (CD). For example, the T helper cells and the cells responsible for the delayed hypersensitivity reaction are designated as CD4 because they react to the OKT4 antigen, and the cytotoxic (suppressor) T cells belong to the CD8 cluster.

The T4 lymphocyte is involved in the initiation of both humeral and cell-mediated immune responses. In the presence of a soluble antigen the T4 cells enlarge, divide to form clones, and produce a variety of soluble protein mediators called lymphokines. Further growth of T cells and B cells then occurs, and the B cells produce antibody. The cytotoxic T cells, which have the ability to directly lyse the target cell, are also activated. Activated T cells can also stimulate bone marrow precursors of granulocytes, macrophages, eosinophiles, and mast cells.

The HIV has a predilection for T4 cells (helper/inducer) as well as macrophages and neural cells. As a result, a reduction in the T4 population occurs, and in the presence of a normal T8 population (suppressor), a reversal of the T4/T8 ratio occurs (Ho et al., 1987; Spickett et al., 1988; Kalish et al., 1985; Bowen et al., 1985). Concomitant with a decrease in proliferation of T4 cells, impairment of lymphokine production occurs, and defective cytotoxic activity by natural killer cells is observed. B cell abnormalities, which have been observed, include poor antibody response to new antigens and inappropriate polyclonal activation with resultant elevated level of serum immunoglobulins, circulating immune complexes, and various autoimmune phenomena (Bowen et al., 1985). These multiple defects in the immune response render the host susceptible to the array of opportunistic infections seen in patients with AIDS.

Pregnancy may also influence immune function. The obstetric literature supports the hypothesis that a pregnant patient is more susceptible to various viral, bacterial, and fungal infections and is more likely to die from these infections than her nonpregnant counterpart. Higher than normal isolation and infection rates have been reported among pregnant patients for other viral infections such as herpes, CMV, and poliomyelitis (Weinberg, 1984). Additionally, the severity of infections such as malaria, Toxoplasma, and listeriosis is greatly increased during pregnancy. Ascertainment bias, however, limits the reliability of much of these data.

Although a slight decrease in total immunoglobulins has been reported during pregnancy and somewhat reduced complement levels have been observed in the first trimester, these changes cannot account for the major decrease seen in immune response (Gall, 1977). Because the response to the majority of the infectious disorders noted above is cell mediated, it is thought that pregnancy may be associated with a decrease in cell-mediated immunity. However, the demonstrated ability of pregnant women to mount a satisfactory response to intradermal skin antigens and their ability to reject skin grafts suggest that only certain selective functions of cell-mediated immunity are depressed during pregnancy. The main focus of interest has been on the role of lymphocytes in the depression of cell-mediated immunity.

It is not entirely clear in what manner T cell function is compromised in pregnancy. Sridama et al. (1982) showed that there was a significant decrease in the relative and absolute number of helper T lymphocytes (CD4) throughout pregnancy and that normalization of these cells occurred during the third and fifth month postpartum. No change in the ratio of other T cells was observed. Bailey et al. (1985) also observed a decrease in T helper cells in pregnancy, but assumed that patients had adequate T helper cell function as determined by *in vitro* immunoglobulin synthesis assay. They did not observe increased B suppressor activity and believed that a decrease in T helper cells was responsible for the immunodeficiency of pregnancy. A small but significant reduction in whole circulating lymphocytes and the T helper subsets has been reported, but no change in the T suppressor and cytotoxic cells (CD8) has been found (Vanderberken et al., 1982).

In contrast, a progressive increase in the total number of T cells during the first two trimesters of pregnancy has been observed, and a decrease noted only in the third trimester (Fiddes et al., 1986). They also reported an increase in the T8 cells which led to a significantly decreased T4/T8 ratio.

Although the cited evidence is conflicting, most investigators agree that there is a decrease in cell-mediated immunity during pregnancy, which is probably mediated through an altered T helper cell: T suppressor cell. Other factors contributing to the immunosuppression of pregnancy may be increased levels of total steroids and other pregnancy-specific plasma proteins and hormones such as HCG, alpha-fetal protein, and pregnancy-associated alpha 2-glycoprotein (Weinberg, 1984).

As noted above, the multiple defects in the immune response seen in AIDS patients renders them susceptible to a variety of opportunistic infections. Since pregnancy may also be associated with a significant depression of cell-mediated immunity, concern has been expressed that pregnancy could have an adverse effect on the natural history of HIV disease by enhancing the relative immuno-incompetence. The initial reports of AIDS in pregnancy seemed to confirm this impression. The first five reported women with AIDS in pregnancy, all with opportunistic infection, died (Minkoff et al., 1986; Wetli et al., 1983; Jensen et al., 1984). As suggested by the authors, however, the poor outcome in pregnant women at that time may have represented reporting bias, delay in diagnosis and treatment, or an actual worsening of the infection in pregnancy. In one report on the follow-up of 34 HIV-positive mothers over a mean of 27.8 ± 21.6 months, it was found that 15 of the women had developed AIDS or ARC (Nossal, 1987). This was higher than the expected progression of the disease in nonpregnant patients and suggested that perhaps pregnancy was responsible for the acceleration of their illness. However, a definitive conclusion could not be drawn from that report since the mothers were identified through the birth of a child who developed AIDS and thus may be representative of a cohort with advanced immunocompromise. Recently, several controlled studies have been reported in which HIV-positive mothers have been prospectively evaluated. Schaeffer et al. (1988) followed 32 HIV-positive women and 40 HIV-negative women during pregnancy and for six months following delivery, and observed no clinical progression of illness during pregnancy among seropositive women. However, 9 per cent of patients developed signs of clinical deterioration during postpartum observation. The authors believed that pregnancy had only a minor effect on the course of HIV disease. Bigger et al. (1988) showed that the direction of immunologic changes seen in HIV-positive mothers were the same as that in HIV-negative control pregnancies except that drops in CD4 counts were 10 to 20 per cent greater among seropositive women.

Other investigators have failed to show any evidence of progression of disease during pregnancy (Nanda and Minkoff, 1989). In a follow-up of 88 postpartum patients, MacCallum et al. (1988) were unable to demonstrate any adverse effect of pregnancy on the course of HIV disease. Similarly, in a study of 23 pregnant patients followed for two years following delivery, compared to matched seropositive nonpregnant controls, no significant differences were observed in the number of opportunistic infections between the two groups (Berrebi et al., 1988).

At present, a significant influence of pregnancy on the course of HIV disease has not been documented. The available evidence suggests that pregnancy may exert only a minor influence on the progression of disease. More prospective, long-term studies are needed before the impact of pregnancy on the disease will be clearly delineated.

TRANSMISSION OF HIV

In 1981, soon after AIDS was initially described in adults, the first pediatric AIDS case was reported, presumably acquired via infected blood products. Shortly thereafter, many other HIV infections of infants and children were reported world-wide. In review of all pediatric AIDS cases reported as of 1984, Thomas et al. (1984) summarized the evidence supporting perinatal transmission by showing that 30 of 35 babies appeared to have acquired the infection from a parent who was from a risk group. In the other five the infection was probably acquired from transfusions of infected blood.

Earlier, it had been suggested that all babies born to HIV-positive mothers be delivered by cesarean section, thus avoiding the possibility of vertical peripartum transmission of the virus during passage through an infected birth canal (Chiodo et al., 1986). Although this recommendation is supported by reports of isolation of HIV or its antibody from cervical-vaginal secretions (Wofsy et al., 1986; Vogt et al., 1986; Archibald et al., 1987) and cervical tissue itself (Pomerantz et al., 1988), the frequency of viral isolation and quantity of virus isolated has been low. There is, at present, no direct evidence that AIDS can be acquired by the infant during its passage through the birth canal. On the contrary, there is clear evidence that cesarean section does not prevent infection in the child (Cowen et al., 1984; Scott et al., 1984; Lapointe et al., 1985; Minkoff et al., 1987).

The timing of perinatal transmission has been difficult to determine. Lapointe et al. (1985) described the case of a 28-week-old fetus delivered from a terminally ill AIDS patient by cesarean section and in whom viral antigen was detected in the thymus. Since this infant was born by cesarean section and had been immediately separated from the mother, the infant apparently had already acquired the infection by 28 weeks. Reports of isolation of HIV in fetuses during the mid-trimester provide further evidence of intrauterine infection and information about the timing of transplacental passage. HIV has been directly isolated from the placenta (Hill et al., 1987) at 34 weeks and from the amniotic fluid (Mundey et al., 1987) and fetuses as early as 15 weeks gestation (Spreacher et al., 1986). The possibility of contamination during the delivery process cannot be ruled out in many of these cases.

More recently, evidence has accumulated suggesting that late transmission, including peripartum, plays an important role in neonatal infection. That evidence includes the seroconversion of infants in the neonatal period (Ehrnst et al., 1991) and the finding that among twins discordant for HIV infection in 18 of 22 reported cases, twin A was that infected twin (Goedert et al., 1991). The latter finding is compatible with the hypothesis that exposure of the presenting twin to virally contaminated vaginal secretions could pose a risk of HIV acquisition.

The efficiency with which vertical transmission occurs also has not been completely elucidated. Several factors appear to modify the risk of transmission. Maternal viremia, lower CD4 counts, clinical illness, recent seroconversion, and p24 antigenemia are all factors associated with enhanced perinatal transmission.

Based on current epidemiologic evidence, it appears that the risk of prenatal transmission of infection transplacentally is between 14 and 50 per cent. Giaquinto et al. (1988) followed 71 babies from the first weeks of life through three years of age and reported that the risk of transmission of HIV was approximately 30 per cent. Similar results have been reported by other investigators (Minkoff et al., 1987; Terrangana et al., 1988). Higher transmission rates have been reported by other investigators (Ciraru-Vigneron et al., 1988; Scott et al., 1985; Ryder et al., 1988). These studies are flawed by short follow-up and variation in the HIV test utilized. The largest study to date is that from the European collaborative group (1991), which reported the lowest overall transmission rate, approximately 14 per cent.

At present there is no doubt that the transplacental route of infection is the major route of infection among infants, accounting for 75 to 80 per cent of all pediatric AIDS cases. Approximately 14 per cent of HIV-infected infants acquired their infection through blood transfusion. Given the current practice of donor screening, this percentage is likely to drop.

Transmission via Breast Milk

Although perinatal acquisition of HIV seems to be the major route of pediatric infection, there are scattered reports of infection acquired by ingestion of infected breast milk (Friedland et al., 1986; Zeigler et al., 1984; Lepage et al., 1987; Van de Perre et al., 1991). In most of these reports the mothers were infected postnatally by blood transfusions from donors who subsequently went on to develop HIV disease. Although pre-transfusion serostatus was generally undocumented, no other source of maternal infection was suspected and no other family members were

known to be infected. These pediatric infections, along with reports of the isolation of free virus from the breast milk of healthy carriers of HIV, make it probable that HIV infection can be acquired by breast-feeding.

However, there is doubt about the efficiency of transmission of HIV through infected breast milk. Zeigler et al. (1988) reported that among breast-fed children, breast milk was a source of infection only when breast-feeding occurred around the time that seroconversion was documented. Among mothers who were HIV antibody-positive, the incidence of infection in their children was the same whether or not they were breast-fed. It is possible that maternal infectivity is maximal at the time of initial acquisition of infection when a viral antigenemia occurs. Since it remains probable that breast-feeding can be a source of transmission of HIV, Centers for Disease Control has recommended that mothers known to have HIV disease avoid breast-feeding. Unfortunately, while these recommendations may make sense in countries where safe alternatives to breast-feeding are readily available, they are not appropriate in areas where breast-feeding is the only realistic source of nutrients.

MANAGEMENT OF PREGNANCIES COMPLICATED BY HIV INFECTION

The guiding principle in the care of HIV-infected pregnant women is to adhere rigorously to standards of care for all other HIV-infected individuals. Infected women should receive Pneumovax, influenza, and hepatitis vaccines, and should be screened for tuberculosis and sexually transmitted diseases.

Perhaps of most importance is the monitoring of immune status with CD4 counts. This should be performed every trimester since some studies have shown rapid changes in count during pregnancy. If the count stays over 500 mm³, the obstetrician can anticipate an unremarkable course. If the count drops under 500 mm³, consideration should be given to the use of azidothymidine (AZT) to delay the onset of clinical illness. If the count drops below 200 mm³, *Pneumocystis carinii* pneumonia (PCP) prophylaxis should be instituted. The specific details of management of the myriad infections to which these women are prone is beyond the scope of this chapter.

PREVENTING PERINATAL TRANSMISSION

Several avenues of investigation are being pursued in an attempt to develop an effective strategy for the prevention of perinatal transmission of HIV. The first clinical trial to assess the benefits of one of these approaches is a trial of AZT in pregnancy. It is hoped that AZT, through its inhibiting effect on reverse transcriptase, will prevent the incorporation of maternal virus into fetal cells. The study is currently ongoing with the outcome still uncertain.

Soluble CD4 linked to IgG is an alternative regimen that is also being tested. It is hypothesized that the soluble CD4 will act as a "false" receptor for the virus, thereby preventing the linkage between the virus and

CD4 on fetal cells. Phase I trials of this agent are underway.

Other approaches will be tested shortly. One will be a trial of HIV immunoglobulin, obtained from asymptomatic HIV-infected individuals, who do not have P24 antigenemia but have high titer antibody against several portions of the virus. One potential problem with this approach is the relatively scarce supply of HIVIG and the relatively large numbers of women in whom it would be required if it proves efficacious in the prevention of perinatal transmission. Phase I vaccine trials are also set to begin, in an attempt to augment an individual's own immune response. Until a clear-cut treatment or vaccine is identified, prevention will be based upon patient education and alteration of behaviors placing individuals at high risk for the disease.

REFERENCES

Archibald DW, Witt DJ, Craven DE, et al: Antibodies to HIV in cervical secretions from women at risk for AIDS. (Letter) J Infect Dis **156**:240, 1987.

Bailey K, Herrod HG, Younger R, et al: Functional aspects of T lymphocytes subsets in pregnancy. Obstet Gynecol **66**(2):211, 1985.

Berrebi A, Puel J, Grandjean H, Herne F, Pontonnier G: The influence of pregnancy on the evolution of HIV infection. Fourth International Conference on AIDS, 1988, Stockholm. Abst. No. 4041.

Bigger RJ, Pahwa S, Landesman S, et al: Helper and suppressor lymphocyte changes in HIV-infected mothers and their infants. Fourth International Conference on AIDS. 1988, Stockholm. Abst. No. 4031.

Bowen DL, Lane HC, Fauci AS: Immunopathogenesis of the acquired immunodeficiency syndrome. Ann Intern Med **103**:704, 1985.

Centers for Disease Control: Update: Acquired immunodeficiency syndrome—United States, 1981–1990. MMWR **40**:357, 1991a.

Centers for Disease Control: HIV/AIDS surveillance report. Atlanta, GA. July, p 9, 1991b.

Centers for Disease Control: MMWR **39**:28, 1991c.

Chin J: Current and future dimensions of the HIV/AIDS pandemic in women and children. Lancet **336**:221, 1990.

Chiodo F, Ricchi E, Costigliola P, et al: Vertical transmission of HTLV111. Lancet **1**:739, 1986.

Ciraru-Vigneron N, Nguyen TL, Bercau G. et al: Prospective study for HIV infection among high risk pregnant women. Fourth International Conference on AIDS, 1988, Stockholm. Abst. No. 4629.

Claman HN: The biology of the immune response. JAMA **258**:2834, 1987.

Cowen MJ, Hellmar G, Chudwin D, et al: Maternal transmission of acquired immune deficiency syndrome. Pediatrics **73**(3):382, 1984.

Ehrnst A, Linocren S, Dictor M, et al: HIV in pregnant women and their offspring: evidence for late transmission. Lancet **338**:203, 1991.

European Collaborative Study: Children born to women with HIV-1 infection. Natural History and risk of transmission. Lancet **337**:25, 1991.

Fiddes TM, O'Rielly DB, Cetrulo CL, et al: Phenotypic and functional evaluation of suppressor cells in normal pregnancy and in chronic aborters. Cell Immunol **97**:407, 1986.

Friedland GH, Saltzman BR, Rogers MF, et al: Lack of transmission of HTLV111/LAV infection to household contacts of patients with AIDS or ARC with oral candidiasis. N Engl J Med **314**(6):3444, 1986.

Gall SA: Maternal immune system during human gestation. Semin Perinatol **1**:119, 1977.

Giaquinto C, DeRossi, A, Elia RD, et al: Natural history of pediatric HIV infection. Fourth International Conference on AIDS, 1988, Stockholm. Abst. No. 7227.

Goedert JJ, Duliege AM, Amos CI, et al: High risk of HIV infection for first-born twins. Lancet **338**:1171, 1991.

Gwinn N, Pappaioanou M, George JR, et al: Prevalence of HIV infection in childbearing women in the United States. JAMA **265**:1704, 1991.

Hardy LM (ed): HIV screening of pregnant women and newborns. *In* Institute of Medicine Report. Washington, DC, National Academy Press, 1991.

Hill WC, Bolton V, Carlson JR: Isolation of acquired immunodeficiency syndrome virus from the placenta. Am J Obstet Gynecol **157**:10, 1987.

Ho DD, Pomerantz RJ, Kaplan JC: Pathogenesis of infections with human immunodeficiency virus. N Engl J Med **317**:278, 1987.

Jensen LP, O'Sullivan MJ, Gomez-del-rio M, et al: Acquired immune deficiency syndrome in pregnancy. Am J Obstet Gynecol **148**:1145, 1984.

Johnstone FD, McCallum L, Brettle R, et al: Does HIV infection affect the outcome of pregnancy. Br Med J **296**:467, 1988.

Kalish RS, Schlossman SF: The T4 lymphocyte in AIDS. N Engl J Med **313**:112, 1985.

Landesman S, Minkoff HL, Holman S, et al: Sero survey of human immunodeficiency virus infection in parturients. JAMA **258**:2701, 1987.

Lapointe N, Michaud J, Pekovik D, et al: Transplacental transmission of HTLV III virus. N Engl J Med **312**:1325, 1985.

Lepage P, Van de Perre P, Careel M, et al: Postnatal transmission of HIV mother to child. Lancet **2**:400, 1987.

MacCallum LR, France AJ, Jones ME, et al: The effects of pregnancy on the progression of HIV disease. Fourth International Conference on AIDS, 1988, Stockholm. Abst. No. 4032.

Minkoff H, DeRegt, RH, Landesman S, et al: Pneumocystis carinii pneumonia associated with acquired immunodeficiency syndrome in pregnancy: A report of three maternal deaths. Obstet Gynecol **67**(2):284, 1986.

Minkoff HL, Henderson C, Mendez H, et al: Pregnancy outcomes among women infected with HIV and matched controls. Am J Obstet Gynecol **163**:1598, 1990.

Minkoff H, Nanda D, Menez R, et al: Pregnancies resulting in infants with acquired immunodeficiency syndrome or AIDS related complex. Obstet Gynecol **69**:285, 1987.

Minkoff H, Nanda D, Menez R, et al: Pregnancies resulting in infants with acquired immunodeficiency syndrome or AIDS related complex: Follow-up of mothers, children and subsequently born siblings. Obstet Gynecol **69**:288, 1987.

Mundey DC, Schinazi RF, Gerber AR, et al: HIV isolated from amniotic fluid. Lancet **2**:459, 1987.

Nanda D, Minkoff HL: HIV in pregnancy—transmission and immune effects. Clin Obstet Gynecol **32**:456, 1989.

Nossal GJV: Current Concepts: Immunology: The basic components of the immune system. N Engl J Med **316**:1320, 1987.

Pomerantz RJ, De la Monte SM, Dongan SP, et al: HIV infection of the uterine cervix. Ann Intern Med **108**:321, 1988.

Ryder RW, Nsa W, Behets F, et al: Perinatal HIV transmission in two African hospitals: One year follow-up. Fourth International Conference on AIDS, 1988, Stockholm. Abst. No. 4128.

Schaefer A, Grosch-Woerner, Friedman I, et al: The effect of pregnancy on the natural course of HIV disease. Fourth International Conference on AIDS, 1988, Stockholm. Abst. No. 4039.

Scott GB, Burke BE, Letterman JG, et al: Acquired immune deficiency syndrome in infants. N Engl J Med **310**:76, 1984.

Scott GB, Fischl MA, Klimas N, et al: Mothers of infants with acquired immune deficiency syndrome. JAMA **253**:363, 1985.

Selwyn DA, Carter RJ, Shoenbaum EE, et al: Knowledge of HIV antibody status and decisions to continue or terminate pregnancy among intravenous drug users. JAMA **261**:2567, 1989.

Semperini AE, Sucetich A, Parti GL, et al: HIV infection and AIDS in newborn babies of mothers positive for HIV antibody. Prev Med **294**:610, 1987.

Sever JL: HIV Biology and immunology. Clin Obstet Gynecol **32**:423, 1989.

Spickett GP, Dalgleish AG: Cellular immunology of HIV infection. Clin Exp Immunol **71**:1, 1988.

Spreacher S, Soumenkoff G, Puissant F, Degueldre M: Vertical transmission of HIV in 15 week fetus. Lancet **2**:288, 1986.

Sridama V, Pacini F, Yang SL, et al: Decreased level of helper T cells: a possible cause of immunodeficiency in pregnancy. N Engl J Med **307**:352, 1982.

Sunderland A, Minkoff HL, Handte J, et al: The influence of serostatus on women's reproductive decisions. Obstet Gynecol **79**:1027, 1992.

Terrangana A, De Maria, Sampietro F, et al: Perinatal HIV infection: Evaluation of the risk for the mother and child. Fourth International Conference on AIDS, 1988, Stockholm. Abst. No. 4028.

Thomas P, Jaffe H, Spira TJ, et al: Unexplained immune deficiency in children—a surveillance report. JAMA **252**:639, 1984.

Van de Perre P, Simonon A, Msellati P, et al: Postnatal transmission of HIV type 1 from mother to infant. N Engl J Med **325**:593, 1991.

Vanderberken Y, Vheghe MP, Velespesse G, et al: Characterization of immunoregulatory T cells during pregnancy by monoclonal antibodies. Clin Exp Immunol **48**:118, 1982.

Vogt MW, Witt DJ, Craven DE: Isolation of HTLV 111/LAV from cervical secretions of women at risk for AIDS. Lancet **1**:525, 1986.

Weinberg ED: Pregnancy-associated depression of cell-mediated immunity. Rev Infect Dis **6**(6):814, 1984.

Wetli CV, Roldan EO, Fujaco RM: Listeriosis as a cause of maternal death: An obstetric complication of acquired immune deficiency syndrome. Am J Obstet Gynecol **147**:7, 1983.

Wofsy CB, Cohen JB, Haven LB, et al: Isolation of AIDS-associated retrovirus from vaginal and cervical secretions from women with antibody for the virus. Lancet **1**:527, 1986.

Zeigler JB, Stewart GJ, Penney R, et al: Breast-feeding and transmission of HIV from mother to infant. Fourth Annual International AIDS Conference, 1988, Stockholm. Abst. No. 5100.

Zeigler JB, Cooper DA, Johnson RO, et al: Postnatal transmission of AIDS-associated retrovirus from mother to infant. Lancet **1**:896, 1984.

MATERNAL BLOOD GROUP IMMUNIZATION

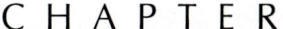

C H A P T E R

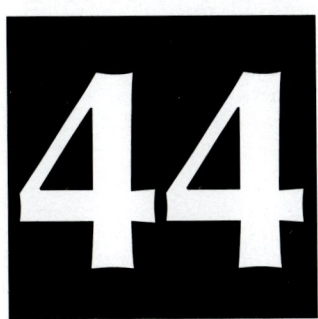

HEMOLYTIC DISEASE
(ERYTHROBLASTOSIS FETALIS)

JOHN M. BOWMAN, M.D.

HISTORICAL ASPECTS

Hemolytic disease of the fetus and newborn (HDN) was reported as early as 1609, when a midwife, writing in the French press, reported the birth of twins. The first-born was grossly edematous (hydrops fetalis) and died promptly. The second-born became severely jaundiced (icterus gravis) and died a few days later.

The cause of HDN, and indeed the fact that hydrops and icterus gravis were related, was unknown until late in the first half of the present century. Diamond et al. (1932) showed that hydrops fetalis, icterus gravis, and anemia of the newborn were simply different aspects of the same disease (a hemolytic process) and that circulating erythroblasts (erythroblastosis) were found in all three. Darrow (1938) postulated the passage of anti-fetal hemoglobin from mother into fetus as a cause of hemolysis. Her maternal-fetal antibody passage theory was correct; her specific antigen (fetal hemoglobin) and her antibody were incorrect.

The correct antibody was discovered in 1940 by Landsteiner and Weiner, who found that rabbits and guinea pigs injected with rhesus monkey red cells produced rhesus monkey red cell antisera. When the rhesus monkey red cell antisera were mixed with blood samples from a group of Caucasians, agglutination occurred in 85 per cent of the samples (rhesus- or Rh-positive) but did not occur in 15 per cent (rhesus- or Rh-negative). This experiment, a landmark in medicine, is the basis of modern immunohematology. Although the rhesus monkey antigen (LW) is not quite the same as the human red cell Rh antigen, this difference in no way reduces the importance of Land-

steiner and Wiener's experiment. It was only following their work that reasonably safe blood transfusion became possible and the etiology and pathogenesis of hemolytic disease of the fetus and newborn were unraveled.

Soon thereafter, it was shown that most transfusion reactions were caused by giving Rh-positive blood to Rh-negative patients (Wiener and Peters, 1940). Subsequently, Levine and colleagues (1941) demonstrated that the development of Rh antibodies in the Rh-negative woman was the usual cause of hemolytic disease of the fetus and newborn.

In the 40 plus years since the work of Landsteiner and Wiener, the complexities of the Rh blood group system have been elucidated and many other blood group systems have been discovered. Very sensitive methods of screening for blood group antibodies have been developed, culminating in the ability to quantitate (in micrograms) the amount of antibody in maternal serum. The pathogeneses of maternal blood group immunization and of hemolytic disease of the fetus and newborn have been defined accurately. Methods of assessing severity of hemolytic disease *in utero* and of managing mother, fetus, and newborn have been developed. Since 1967 a method of preventing Rh immunization has been developed and put into practice.

THE Rh BLOOD GROUP SYSTEM

Although other blood group systems may on occasion cause immunization and hemolytic disease (atypical immunization), which are discussed later in this chapter, the Rh blood group system is the most common and most important. The Rh system is a complex one made up of a family of inherited antigens. Controversy surrounds the nomenclature and the basic genetics of the system. The theory proposed by Wiener and Wexler (1958) of a single locus occupied by a pair of complex agglutinogens may be the most accurate and the numbering system of Rosenfield and colleagues (1962) the most logical. However, the nomenclature and theories of inheritance put forth by Fisher and by Race (1948) are simple and work well in practice.

Fisher's Theory

The Rh antigens are grouped in three pairs: Dd, Cc, and Ee. The presence of D determines that the individual is Rh-positive. Because d, the reciprocal of D, has never been found (no antiserum with anti-d specificity exists), it is the absence of D (not the presence of d) that determines that a person is Rh(D)-negative. It is the production of anti-D in Rh(D)-negative women that causes hemolytic disease in Rh(D)-positive fetuses.

According to the Fisher-Race hypothesis, the antigens are inherited in two sets of three, one set being contributed by each parent. Some sets are more common than others (Table 44–1). CDe(R¹), c(d)e(r), and cDE(R²) are the most common. cDe(R⁰), C(d)e(r'), and c(d)E(r''), are not rare. CDE(Rᶻ) and C(d)E(rʸ) are very uncommon in Caucasians but are not rare in North American Indians and Orientals, respectively.

About 45 per cent of Rh-positive individuals are homozygous for D, having inherited D-containing sets of antigens from both parents; the other 55 per cent are heterozygous, having inherited a D-containing set from one parent and a non-D-containing set from the other parent. The zygosity for D of the Rh-positive husband of an Rh-negative woman is of great importance. If he is homozygous, all of his children will be Rh-positive (Fig. 44–1A); if he is heterozygous, in each pregnancy the chances that the fetus will be Rh-positive or Rh-negative are equal (Fig. 44–1B). Only Rh-positive fetuses will cause Rh immunization, and only Rh-positive fetuses will be affected by the Rh antibody produced.

TABLE 44–1.   Rh Gene Frequencies in a Caucasian Canadian Population of 2000 Unrelated Adults

GENE COMPLEX	FREQUENCY (%)
CDe (R¹)	41
c(d)e (r)	39
cDE (R²)	16
cDe (R⁰)	2.2
C(d)e (r')	1.1
c(d)E (r'')	0.6
CDE (Rᶻ)	0.08
C(d)E (rʸ)	0.00

From Lewis M, Kaita H, Chown B: The inheritance of the Rh blood groups: Frequencies in 1000 unrelated Caucasian families consisting of 2000 parents and 2806 children. Vox Sang 20:502, 1971.

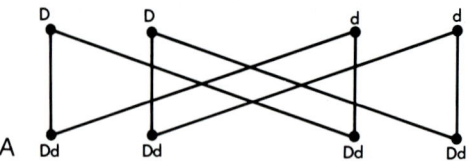

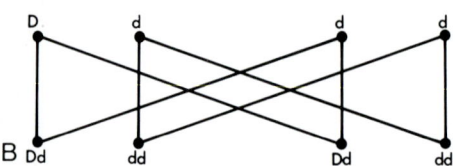

FIGURE 44–1. Rh genotypes of D-positive husband and D-negative wife matings. Husband's gametes are shown on the left, wife's gametes on the right. *A,* With a homozygous D-positive husband and D-negative wife mating, all children will be Rh(D)-positive. *B,* With a heterozygous D-positive husband the probability that a child will be D-positive is 50 per cent; that is, on the average, 50 per cent of children will be D-negative. (From Bowman JM, Friesen RF: Rh-isoimmunization. *In* Goodwin JW, Godden JO, Chance G [eds]: Perinatal Medicine. Copyright © 1976. Reprinted by permission of Williams & Wilkins Company.)

Because anti-d has never been found, the zygosity for D of an Rh-positive husband can be determined for certain only if he fathers two babies who have inherited different sets of Rh-antigens from him. Certain combinations of antigens are more common than others, and so the determination of the presence or absence of C, E, c, and e will indicate the most likely Rh zygosity of the husband (Table 44–2).

The Rh blood group system is much more complex than the five antigens described. Forty other antibodies have been described that delineate other Rh antigens. Cʷ, an allele for C, is not rare. Dᵘ, replacing D, is also not uncommon. On rare occasions, a Dᵘ-positive mother carrying a D-positive fetus may be stimulated to form anti-D, which has on one occasion caused hydrops fetalis (Lacey et al., 1983). Even more rarely, an Rh-negative mother carrying a Dᵘ-positive fetus may become Rh-immunized. Dᵘ positivity is more common in Blacks. Six subgroups of these partial Rh-positive (Dᵘ-positive) individuals have been described (Tippett and Sanger, 1962).

Rh Blood Group Distribution

The absence of the D antigen (Rh negativity) appears to be a Caucasian trait. In most Caucasian countries, the incidence of Rh negativity is 15 to 16 per cent. In Finland it is only 10 to 12 per cent. The Basque population of France and Spain has an incidence of 30 to 35 per cent. Mongoloid races initially were entirely Rh-positive. About 1 to 2 per cent of North American Indians and Inuit are Rh-negative (owing to the presence of Caucasian genes). The incidence in Indo-Eurasians is about 2 per cent, and in Blacks 4 to 8 per

TABLE 44–2. Zygosity for Rh(D) of D-Positive Husband (D-Negative Wife)

ANTIGENS PRESENT IN HUSBAND	A MOST LIKELY Rh GENOTYPE	B LESS LIKELY Rh GENOTYPE(S)	C LEAST LIKELY Rh GENOTYPE
1. CDe	CDe • CDe(R^1R^1)* Homozygous	CDe • Cde(R^1r') Heterozygous	
2. CDce	CDe • cde(R^1r) Heterozygous	CDe • cDe(R^1R^0) Homozygous	Cde • cDe($r'R^0$) Heterozygous
3. CDEce	CDe • cDE(R^1R^2) Homozygous	Cde • cDE($r'R^2$) / CDe • cdE(R^1r'') / CDE • cde(R^2r) Heterozygous	CDE • cDe(R^2R^0) Homozygous
4. DEc	cDE • cDE(R^2R^2)* Homozygous	cDE • cdE(R^2r'') Heterozygous	
5. DEce	cDE • cde(R^2r) Heterozygous	cDE • cDe(R^2R^0) Homozygous	cdE • cDe($r''R^0$) Heterozygous
6. Dce	cDe • cde(R^0r) Heterozygous	cDe • cDe(R^0R^0) Heterozygous	

*Genotypes 1A and 4A can never be proven because the baby will be only one paternal genotype (CDe in 1A and cDE in 4A). The remainder of the husband's possible genotypes can be proven only if he produces children of two different genotypes.
From Bowman, JM: Hemolytic disease of the newborn. In Conn HF, Conn RB Jr (eds): Current Diagnosis 6. Philadelphia, WB Saunders Company, 1980.

cent (about 8 per cent in American Blacks, considerably less in African Blacks).

It is very likely that several thousand years ago Rh negativity was confined to one specific Caucasian group, the modern-day Basques, and that initially all other races were entirely Rh-positive. The present-day incidence of Rh negativity in non-Caucasians is related to the intermingling of Caucasian genes, which is more common in Blacks and North American Indians than in the Japanese and Chinese.

Rh Antigenic Structure

The Rh(D) antigen (approximate molecular weight, 30,000) is associated with the membrane skeleton of the red cell (Gahmberg and Karhi, 1984). It appears to be a proteolipid (Brown et al., 1983). Unlike the ABO antigens, which are ubiquitous, the Rh antigens appear to be confined to the red cell membrane. They are an essential component of the membrane. The rare individuals who lack Rh antigens (Rh-null) have defective red cell membranes and mild-to-moderate hemolytic anemia. There is recent, albeit disputed, evidence that the Rh(D) antigen may be present in human trophoblast (Goto et al., 1980).

THE PATHOGENESIS OF MATERNAL BLOOD GROUP IMMUNIZATION

Blood Transfusion

Prior to the discovery of the Rh blood group system, incompatible blood transfusion was a frequent cause of Rh immunization. It is still the most common cause of atypical (non-D) blood group immunization, because transfused red cells are compatible only for ABO and D in the Rh system. About 1 to 2 per cent of individuals develop atypical blood group antibodies following transfusion. Although many of the antibodies are of little clinical significance, anti-c, Kell, and, to a lesser extent, E, C, and Fyᵃ are quite capable of causing hemolytic disease of the fetus and newborn. Atypical immunization is discussed later in this chapter.

Fetal-Maternal Transplacental Hemorrhage (TPH)

With the interdiction of transfusion of Rh-positive blood into Rh-negative individuals, the incidence of Rh immunization diminished, but only to a limited extent. A significant number of Rh-negative parous women who had never been transfused showed evidence of Rh immunization. Wiener's theory (1948) that transplacental hemorrhage of fetal Rh-positive red cells into the circulation of the Rh-negative mother was the cause of Rh immunization was later confirmed (Chown, 1954). Following the delivery of a very anemic Rh-positive baby, an Rh-negative primipara was found to have 5 per cent Rh-positive fetal red cells in her circulation. She developed a powerful Rh antibody response within 20 days of delivery.

The acid elution test developed by Kleihauer and associates (1957) is a very accurate, sensitive method of differentiating fetal red cells from adult red cells (Fig. 44–2). It has been of great value in determining the incidence and size of fetal transplacental hemorrhage at different gestations, at delivery, and following various obstetric procedures and complications. Unfortunately, it does not lend itself readily to routine laboratory use.

Seventy-five per cent of gravidas have evidence of TPH during pregnancy or immediately after delivery (Bowman et al., 1986). In 60 per cent of such cases, the amount of fetal blood in the maternal circulation is less than 0.1 ml. Less than 1 per cent of such women have more than 5 ml, and less than 0.25 per cent have more than 30 ml of fetal blood in the circulation. Certain obstetric complications and procedures carry

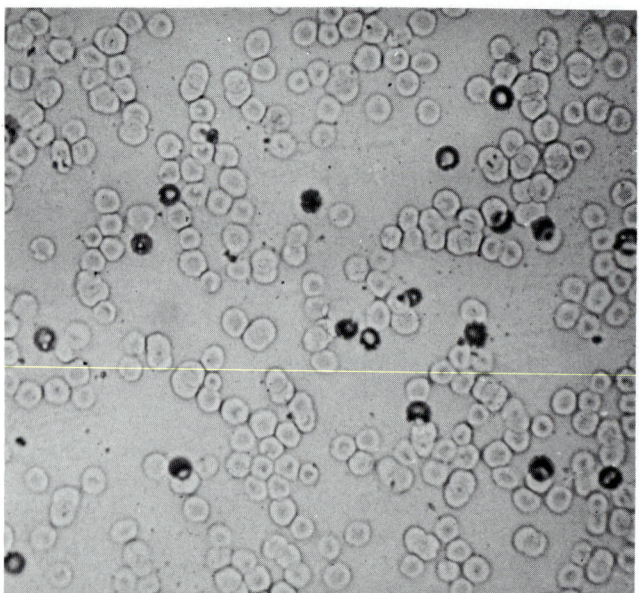

FIGURE 44–2. Acid elution technique of Kleihauer. Fetal red blood cells stain with eosin (appear dark). Adult red blood cells do not stain (appear as ghosts). This maternal blood smear contained 11.2 per cent fetal red blood cells, representing a transplacental hemorrhage of about 450 ml of blood. (From Bowman JM: Hemolytic disease of the newborn. *In* Conn HF, Conn RB [eds]: Current Diagnosis 5. Philadelphia, WB Saunders Company, 1977.)

a risk of more severe TPH: antepartum hemorrhage, toxemia of pregnancy, cesarean section, manual removal of the placenta, and external version.

The incidence and size of transplacental hemorrhage increases as pregnancy advances. There is less than 0.1 ml in 5 to 15 per cent of women by the second month of pregnancy. In the third trimester, 45 per cent of women have evidence of TPH, and in some the volume of fetal blood may be large (Bowman et al., 1986).

Amniocentesis is also a hazard. Peddle (1968) reported that, prior to placental localization, TPH occurred following 46 of 410 amniocenteses (11.2 per cent). In one-half of those tested, there was a prompt increase in antibody titer. Placental localization by ultrasound scanning reduces the risk of TPH due to amniocentesis to 2.5 per cent (Bowman and Pollock, 1985).

Following spontaneous abortion, there is a 5 per cent incidence of transplacental hemorrhage. Contrary to the weak expression of the A and B antigens on the fetal red cell, the Rh(D) antigen is well developed by 30 days gestation. TPH after abortion is usually but not always small. After therapeutic abortion the incidence may be as high as 20 to 25 per cent, and the amount may exceed 0.2 ml of fetal blood in 4 per cent of cases.

The Rh Immune Response

THE PRIMARY RESPONSE. The primary Rh immune response is characteristically slow in development, perhaps owing to the pregnant woman's depressed immune responsiveness and the slow destruction of the Rh-positive fetal red cells in her circulation (1 to 1.5 per cent per day). In experimental exposure of Rh-negative male volunteers to Rh-positive red cells, about 8 to 9 weeks elapse before the primary Rh immune response can be detected. Indeed, it may not appear for 6 months.

The usual primary response is weak and may be mostly IgM. IgM anti-D, which has a molecular weight of 900,000, cannot traverse the placenta and therefore cannot produce fetal red cell hemolysis. However, the majority of Rh-immunized women quickly convert to production of IgG anti-D (molecular weight 160,000), which crosses the placenta and causes fetal red cell hemolysis.

THE SECONDARY RESPONSE. Following the primary Rh immune response, a second exposure to Rh-positive red cells produces a different response. The dose may be small. There is usually a rapid increase in the strength of the Rh antibody (the secondary immune response), which is predominantly IgG. Further exposure may produce even higher anti-D levels. Long periods between exposures to Rh-positive red cells are frequently associated with marked rises in antibody titer and an increased avidity, or binding constant, of the Rh antibody for the antigen. If the antibody has a greater avidity (i.e., a higher binding constant), more of it will bind to Rh antigen on the red cell membrane. An Rh antibody with greater avidity will produce more severe hemolytic disease than an Rh antibody of the same titer but lower avidity.

ANTIBODY DETECTION AND MEASUREMENT

Saline Methods

Rh-positive red cells suspended in isotonic saline are agglutinated only by IgM anti-D. IgG anti-D cannot bridge the gap between two red cells suspended in saline. Although it will coat Rh-positive red cells suspended in saline, it will not agglutinate them. Therefore, a maternal serum containing only IgG anti-D will not agglutinate Rh-positive red cells suspended in saline. In the early 1940s, when saline-suspended red cell antibody screening techniques were the only ones in use, there was great confusion, because many

Rh-negative women giving birth to sick erythroblastotic babies had no demonstrable Rh antibodies in their sera.

Colloid Methods

Wiener (1945) was the first to observe that Rh antibodies (IgG) that produce no agglutination of Rh-positive, saline-suspended red cells promptly agglutinated the same red cells if they were suspended in a more viscous medium such as albumin. The viscous media have higher dielectric constants, which reduce the negative electrical potential of the red cell membrane, causing the red cells to lie more closely together. IgG anti-D is then able to bridge the gaps between the red cells and cause agglutination. Bovine serum albumin is the most frequently used colloid medium (Lewis and Chown, 1957).

Because IgM anti-D also agglutinates Rh-positive red cells suspended in albumin, if saline and albumin titers of about the same level are present, the albumin titer may not be an accurate reflection of the amount of IgG anti-D present. Mixing the serum that contains saline and albumin agglutinating anti-D with dithiothreitol causes disruption of IgM but not of IgG sulfhydryl bonds and destruction of IgM. Subsequent remeasurement of the serum anti-D titer in albumin allows a determination of the true IgG anti-D level.

Indirect Antiglobulin Titer (IDAT)

When human serum (or specific human globulin) is injected into other animal species (rabbits, guinea pigs, or goats), the animals, recognizing the serum as foreign, produce antihuman globulin known as Coombs serum (Coombs et al., 1945).

Rh-positive red cells are incubated with the serum being tested for the presence of anti-D. If anti-D is present in the serum, the antigen will adhere to the Rh-positive red cell membrane. The red cells are then washed three or four times with isotonic saline to remove nonadherent human protein and are then suspended in the antihuman globulin (Coombs) serum. If the red cells are coated with anti-D, they will be agglutinated by the antihuman globulin serum—constituting a positive indirect antiglobulin (Coombs) test result. The reciprocal of the highest dilution of maternal serum that produces agglutination is the indirect antiglobulin titer (IDAT).

IDAT is a more sensitive screening and titration technique than the colloid method. Titers of antibody in the same serum are usually one to three dilutions higher than albumin titers. The relation between the two titers will, however, vary greatly from laboratory to laboratory.

Enzyme Methods

Incubation of red cells with enzymes such as papain, trypsin, and bromelin reduces the electrical potential of the red cell membranes. Red cells treated with enzymes lie closer together when suspended in saline and are agglutinated by IgG anti-D. Enzyme screening methods are the most sensitive manual techniques available for detecting Rh immunization (Lewis et al., 1958).

Automated Analysis

AutoAnalyzer (AA) methods have been developed to detect and measure Rh and other antibodies. The techniques in most common use are the bromelin method (Rosenfield and Haber, 1965) and the low-ionic polybrene method (Lalezari, 1967), and modifications thereof. AutoAnalyzer techniques are the most sensitive automated methods for the detection of Rh antibody. An Rh antibody detected only by automated analysis and not by any manual method must be viewed with caution. In 85 per cent of instances of maternal serum Rh antibody detection by AA only and unconfirmed by other methods, the mother may not be truly Rh-immunized. The AA bromelin method has been modified to allow accurate quantitation of the amount of anti-D in serum (Moore, 1969).

INCIDENCE OF Rh IMMUNIZATION

Amount of Antigen Necessary to Produce Rh Immunization

Relatively small amounts of Rh-positive blood may produce Rh immunization; six of 13 volunteers were immunized by a single injection of 10 ml in one experiment. In other studies, two-thirds of the subjects were Rh-immunized by five injections of 3.5 ml; four out of five by one injection of 0.5 ml of Rh-positive red cells (Woodrow, 1970); and five of 16 by repeated injections of 0.1 ml of red cells (Zipursky and Israels, 1967). The incidence of Rh immunization is dose-dependent; 15 per cent became immunized after 1 ml, 33 per cent after 40 ml, and 65 to 70 per cent after 250 ml of Rh-positive red cells. The secondary immune response is provoked by very small amounts of Rh-positive blood (0.1 to 0.5 ml of red cells).

Periodic Kleihauer fetal cell examinations during pregnancy and at the time of delivery help in determining the risk of Rh immunization in relation to the presence and size of fetal-maternal transplacental hemorrhage (TPH). If the volume of hemorrhage is always less than 0.1 ml, the incidence of Rh immunization demonstrable within 6 months of delivery is 3 per cent; if the volume is greater than 0.1 ml the incidence is 14 per cent (Zipursky and Israels, 1967). If the volume is greater than 0.4 ml the risk is 22 per cent (Woodrow, 1970). Because TPH is usually less than 0.1 ml, however, most affected women are immunized to Rh factor as a result of very small or nondemonstrable amounts of transplacental hemorrhage.

Incidence

The risk that Rh immunization will appear within 6 months of delivery of the first Rh-positive, ABO-compatible baby is 8 to 9 per cent. This is not the entire story, however. Nevanlinna (1953) noted that another group of women, about the same number as those overtly immunized 6 months after delivery, had no detectable Rh-antibodies 6 months after delivery but, by mounting a secondary immune response in the next Rh-positive pregnancy, demonstrated that they also had been immunized as a result of the previous Rh-positive pregnancy. He called this phenomenon "sensibilization," that is, a primary immune response inadequate to produce detectable Rh antibodies but sufficient to produce a prompt secondary immune response in a subsequent Rh-positive pregnancy. Therefore, the total overall risk that Rh immunization will develop as a result of the first ABO-compatible, Rh-positive pregnancy is about 16 per cent. A woman not immunized by a first such pregnancy may be at about the same risk in a second one. As parity increases, however, the number of women able to respond to the Rh antigen decreases owing to prior Rh immunization, leaving a relatively greater number of nonresponders. Thus, with each subsequent ABO-compatible, Rh-positive pregnancy, the risk of Rh immunization in the remaining Rh-negative unimmunized women decreases. Nevertheless, by the time an Rh-negative woman has undergone five Rh-positive, ABO-compatible pregnancies, there is a greater than 50 per cent likelihood that she will have become Rh-immunized. In the pre-prevention era, between 0.5 and 1.0 per cent of *all* pregnant women were Rh-immunized.

The ABO Status of the Fetus and Mother

ABO incompatibility between the Rh-positive fetus and its Rh-negative mother confers partial protection against Rh immunization. In one study, whereas 35 per cent of marriages were ABO-incompatible (husband A or B, wife O; husband B, wife A, and so forth), only 20 per cent of Rh-immunized women had ABO-incompatible husbands. Since about half of ABO-incompatible husbands will be heterozygous for A or B, a considerable number of instances of Rh immunization in ABO-incompatible matings are due to ABO-

compatible, Rh-positive pregnancies. The risk of Rh immunization after an ABO-incompatible, Rh-positive pregnancy is 1.5 to 2 per cent (Woodrow, 1970).

ABO incompatibility confers partial protection, probably because of the rapid intravascular hemolysis of the ABO-incompatible red cells and sequestration of the Rh-positive red cell stroma in the liver, where there are fewer potential antibody-forming lymphocytes than in the spleen.

Rh Immunization During Pregnancy

A significant number of Rh-negative, unimmunized pregnant women become Rh-immunized during pregnancy after 28 weeks gestation or within 3 days after delivery; the number was 1.6 per cent (57 of 3528) of those at risk in one series (Table 44–3). (Bowman et al., 1978). This group (1.6 per cent) represents 12 per cent of all the Rh-negative women who will become Rh-immunized as a result of an Rh-positive pregnancy. Such an observation has significant implications as far as Rh immunization prevention is concerned and is discussed in more detail in the prevention section of the chapter.

Rh Immunization After Abortion

Since fetal red cells have been discovered in the maternal circulation as early as the 10th to 12th week of gestation and following abortion, the woman who has a spontaneous abortion is at risk of becoming Rh-immunized. There is some argument about the degree of risk, estimates varying from 1.1 to 4.3 per cent; it is probably about 2 per cent. The risk is 4 to 5 per cent after therapeutic abortion at 20 weeks gestation. Women immunized as a result of the small transplacental hemorrhage that occurs at the time of abortion are "good responders," and they very frequently have severely affected babies in subsequent pregnancies. The risk of Rh immunization after abortion at 6 to 8 weeks is quite low, becoming more significant by the 10th to the 12th week.

TABLE 44–3.   Rates of Rh Immunization Either During Pregnancy or Within 3 Days of Delivery*

Rh-NEGATIVE MOTHERS	Rh-POSITIVE, ABO-COMPATIBLE PREGNANCIES		Rh-POSITIVE, ABO-INCOMPATIBLE PREGNANCIES		TOTAL	
	No. PATIENTS	No. IMMUNIZED (%)	No. PATIENTS	No. IMMUNIZED (%)	No. PATIENTS	No. IMMUNIZED (%)
Primigravidas	2257	44 (1.9)	511	1 (0.2)	2768	45 (1.6)
Multigravidas	602	14 (2.3)	163	3 (1.8)	765	17 (2.2)
All	2859	58 (2.0)	674	4 (0.6)	3533	62 (1.8)

*Manitoba, March 1, 1967, to December 15, 1974.
Modified from Bowman JM, Chown B, Lewis M, et al: Rh-immunization during pregnancy: Antenatal prophylaxis. Can Med Assoc J **118**:623, 1978.

PATHOGENESIS OF HEMOLYTIC DISEASE OF THE FETUS AND NEWBORN (HDN)

Blood production begins in the human embryo as early as the third week of gestation. Rh antigen has been demonstrated in the red cell membrane by the sixth week. By the eighth to the tenth week, erythropoiesis is present in the liver and spleen. Normally by the sixth month it shifts to the bone marrow and by the time of delivery is confined to the marrow. Under conditions of blood loss or hemolysis (fetal anemia), extramedullary erythropoiesis may persist and may become extreme.

The basic pathogenesis of HDN is the destruction of Rh-positive fetal red cells by maternal Rh antibody (IgG anti-D). Red cell destruction produces fetal anemia, which stimulates greater production and higher concentrations of fetal erythropoietin. When the ability of bone marrow red cell production to keep up with red cell destruction is exceeded, extramedullary sites, primarily the liver and spleen but also the kidney, adrenal, and intestinal mucosa, are stimulated to produce red cells as well. Hepatosplenomegaly is very characteristic of HDN (Fig. 44–3).

When extramedullary erythropoiesis is present, control of erythroid maturation is poor. Many nucleated red cell elements, from mature normoblasts to very immature erythroblasts, appear in the fetal circulation (Fig. 44–4). The synonym for the disease, *erythroblastosis fetalis*, is derived from this common finding.

Mechanisms of Red Cell Destruction

COMPLEMENT-MEDIATED HEMOLYSIS. Antibodies that fix complement, such as anti-A and anti-B, cause severe red cell damage. The fixation of antibody, complement, and antigen on the red cell surface produces large defects in the membrane. Intravascular hemolysis occurs, and there is hemoglobinemia and hemoglobinuria. Red cell agglutinates and red cell debris are predominantly picked up by the liver, where they are engulfed by the reticuloendothelial cells in the hepatic microcirculation.

NON-COMPLEMENT-MEDIATED HEMOLYSIS. The mechanism of red cell destruction by anti-D (either IgG or IgM) is quite different. Although there has recently been an argument as to whether Rh antibody fixes complement or not, the general belief is that it does not. Whether it does or not, the action of Rh antibody on the red cell is more subtle than, but in the end as destructive as, that of anti-A and anti-B.

Anti-D attaches itself to the Rh antigen in the red cell membrane, and chemotaxis (i.e., attraction of phagocytes to the red cells) is increased. The coated red cells adhere to the macrophages, forming rosettes. Adherence and rosette formation occur particularly in the spleen, where the slower circulation and increase in hematocrit bring coated red cells and macrophages closer together. Electron-microscopic examination has shown that the macrophage pseudopods attach themselves to the antibody-coated red cell, puckering and invaginating the red cell membrane (Lobuglio et al., 1967). A portion of the membrane fragments, breaks

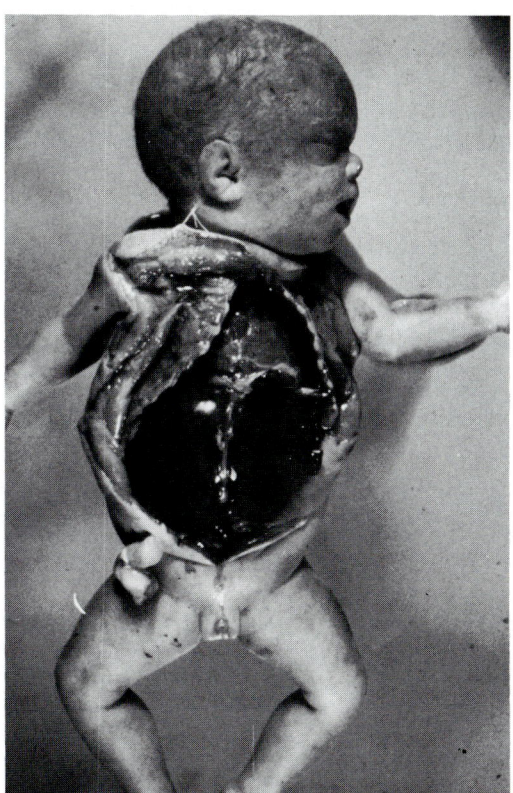

FIGURE 44–3. Hydropic neonate who died a few minutes after birth. Note extreme enlargement of the liver and moderate enlargement of the spleen. (From Bowman JM: Blood-group incompatibilities. *In* Iffy L, Kaminetzky HA [eds]: Principles and Practice of Obstetrics and Perinatology. Copyright © 1981. Reprinted by permission of John Wiley & Sons, Inc.)

away from the red cell and is engulfed. The defect seals, and the macrophage may lose contact with the erythrocyte. Loss of membrane substance produces sphering of the red cell, which is then more rigid and less deformable, with greater osmotic fragility and susceptibility to lysis. Although phagocytosis of entire antibody-coated red cells does occur, it probably does not play a major role in Rh hemolysis.

Severity of Rh Hemolytic Disease

The degrees of severity of hemolytic disease of the fetus and newborn are summarized in Table 44–4.

Mild (No Treatment Required)

Severity of hemolytic disease is determined by the amount of maternal IgG anti-D (titer), its binding constant (avidity for the Rh antigen), and the ability of the affected fetus to respond to hemolysis by erythropoiesis without the development of severe hepatocellular damage, portal obstruction, and hydrops fetalis.

One-half of affected babies do not require treatment. They are only mildly anemic at birth (cord blood hemoglobin concentration greater than 12 to 13 gm/100

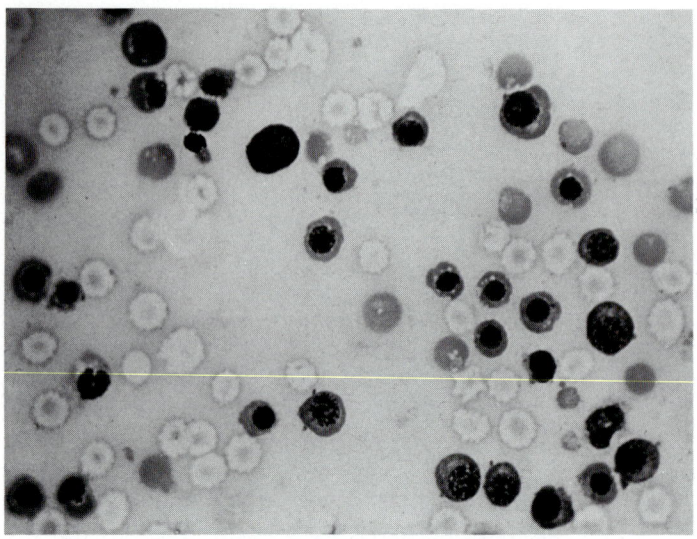

FIGURE 44–4. Cord blood of a baby with severe Rh erythroblastosis fetalis who required multiple fetal transfusions and exchange transfusions. Smear treated by Kleihauer technique and Wright's stain. Note adult donor ghost red cells, dark fetal red cells, and early fetal erythroid series from erythroblasts to normoblasts. (From Bowman JM: Blood-group incompatibilities. *In* Iffy L, Kaminetzky HA [eds]: Principles and Practice of Obstetrics and Perinatology. Copyright © 1981. Reprinted by permission of John Wiley & Sons, Inc.)

ml) and are not dangerously hyperbilirubinemic (cord serum bilirubin levels less than 3.0 to 3.5 mg/100 ml). At the same time, their red cells are coated with anti-D, yielding a positive direct antiglobulin (Coombs) test result. A positive cord blood direct Coombs test result is diagnostic of hemolytic (other than ABO) disease of the fetus and newborn.

In this group of affected babies hemoglobin levels do not drop below 11 to 12 gm/100 ml; nor do serum indirect bilirubin levels exceed 20 mg/100 ml (15 to 18 mg/100 ml in the premature infant) in the neonatal period. In the postneonatal period hemoglobin levels do not drop below 7 to 8 gm/100 ml. No treatment is required. Such infants survive and develop normally, as they did 50 years ago prior to the discovery of the Rh system, when no treatment was available.

Moderate (Without Treatment, Icterus Gravis and Kernicterus Occur)

Intermediate disease is present in 25 to 30 per cent of affected infants. Erythropoiesis is sufficient to maintain an adequate fetal hemoglobin level, but not so great that hepatic dysfunction and circulatory obstruction develop. The fetus is born in good condition at or near term. As long as the fetus is *in utero*, the products of blood destruction are transferred across

the placenta and metabolized by the mother. After birth, the infant has to rely on his own resources to metabolize the products of hemolysis.

Following hemolysis, globin is split from the hemoglobin and released, leaving the pigment heme. Heme is converted to "indirect" bilirubin, which is neurotoxic. With increased hemolysis, there is increased production of indirect bilirubin. The ability of the newborn to metabolize indirect bilirubin is limited because his liver is deficient in both the transport protein Y and the microsomal enzyme glucuronyl transferase. These substances are responsible for intracellular binding of indirect bilirubin, its transport into the cytoplasm of the liver cell, and its conjugation into water-soluble, nontoxic bilirubin diglucuronide ("direct" bilirubin); direct bilirubin is in turn excreted into the biliary canaliculi, down the bile ducts, and into the small bowel.

Water-insoluble indirect bilirubin is lipid-soluble and can circulate only in plasma bound to a protein carrier albumin. When the bilirubin-binding capacity of albumin is exceeded, unbound "free" indirect bilirubin appears. It cannot remain in plasma—a watery medium—and so it diffuses into tissues of high lipid content. Neurones have a high membrane lipid content. "Free" indirect bilirubin passes into the neurone, interferes with mitochondrial function, and produces swelling and ballooning of the mitochondria with neurone cell death. Because of the accumulation of bilirubin within them, the dead neurones appear yellow at postmortem (kernicterus).

Babies who develop kernicterus (bilirubin encephalopathy) become deeply jaundiced. On the third to fifth day they develop signs of cerebral dysfunction, such as lethargy and hypertonicity. They lie in a position of opisthotonos, with the neck extended and the knees, wrists, and elbows flexed (Fig. 44–5). They suck poorly, grasp and Moro reflexes disappear, and they may have convulsions. Finally, they become apneic and die.

About 10 per cent of babies with signs and symptoms of kernicterus do not die. Jaundice fades and hypertonicity is reduced. Initially they may appear to

TABLE 44–4. Classification of Severity of Rh Hemolytic Disease

DEGREE OF SEVERITY	DESCRIPTION	INCIDENCE (%)
Mild	Indirect bilirubin does not exceed 16–20 mg/100 ml. No anemia. No treatment needed.	45–50
Moderate	Fetal hydrops does not develop. Moderate anemia. Severe jaundice with risk of kernicterus unless treated after birth.	25–30
Severe	Fetal hydrops develops *in utero*:	20–25
	before 34 weeks	10–12
	after 34 weeks	10–12

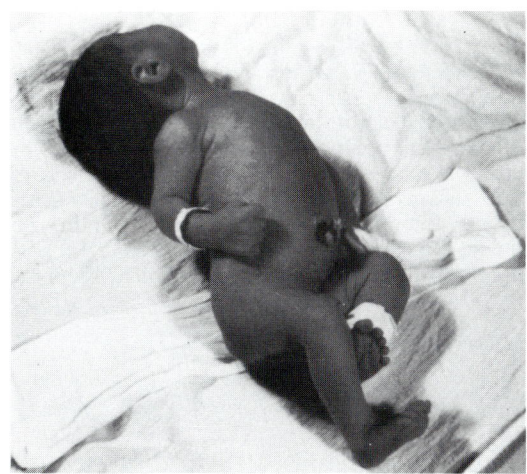

FIGURE 44–5. Infant with kernicterus; note spasticity and opisthotonos. (From Bowman JM: Rh-Isoimmunization 1977. Mod Med Can Vol. 32, 1977.)

be normal. As they become older they show signs of severe neural damage. Most are profoundly deaf. Cerebral palsy of the spastic choreoathetoid type is present. Some children are severely intellectually retarded; others are not but have difficulty learning and functioning because of the deafness.

Severe (Without Treatment, Hydrops Fetalis Occurs)

Despite calling into action all of their red cell production resources, the remaining 20 to 25 per cent of affected fetuses become progressively more anemic. Ascites with generalized edema (anasarca), hydrops fetalis, occurs (Fig. 44–6). One-half of these unfortunate fetuses become hydropic between 18 and 34 weeks gestation, the other half between 34 and 40 weeks.

The original belief that hydrops was due to fetal heart failure is no longer tenable. Although heart failure does develop if the hydropic infant lives long enough (Fig. 44–7), the majority of hydropic infants are not hypervolemic or in heart failure at birth (Phibbs et al., 1974). Hepatic enlargement and hepatocellular damage are more likely causes of hydrops fetalis (James, 1970).

With severe hemolysis and progressively greater extramedullary erythropoiesis, the hepatic cords and hepatic circulation are distorted by the islets of erythropoiesis. Portal and umbilical venous obstruction with portal hypertension occurs. The placenta becomes edematous, and cytotrophoblast persists. Placental perfusion diminishes. Ascites develops. Further distortion of hepatic cords by islets of erythropoiesis interferes with hepatocellular circulation and cell function. Albumin production drops, hypoalbuminemia develops, and generalized edema (anasarca) occurs. Pleural and pericardial effusions appear. In the most extreme cases, compression hypoplasia of the lungs makes oxygenation after birth impossible.

The hepatic damage theory of the pathogenesis of hydrops fetalis explains the inconsistent relationship of hydrops to the degree of anemia in the fetus. Although most hydropic fetuses are severely anemic, some have hemoglobin levels well above 7 gm/100 ml; other fetuses are not hydropic even though they have much lower hemoglobin levels (in one instance, 2.5 gm/100 ml).

MONITORING THE PREGNANT WOMAN AND FETUS AT RISK

Antenatal Blood Testing

Unless antenatal blood group and antibody screening tests are carried out, the physician will not know which patients are Rh-negative and at risk of Rh immunization and which are already Rh-immunized or atypically immunized and have conceptuses at risk of hemolytic disease. A blood sample must be taken from every woman at her first antenatal visit for Rh blood grouping and antibody screening. This policy should be universal and should be carried out no matter what the parity or what screening tests were reported to show in previous pregnancies. Mistyping

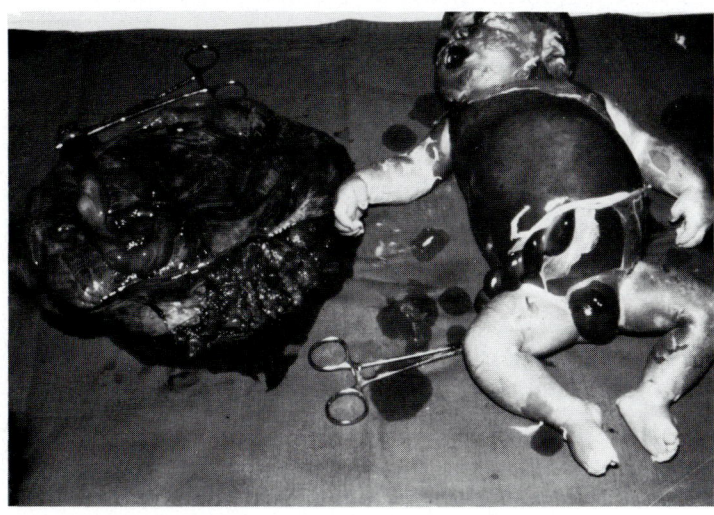

FIGURE 44–6. Stillborn fetus with hydrops fetalis; note the edema and markedly enlarged placenta. (From Bowman JM: Rh-Isoimmunization 1977. Mod Med Can Vol. 32, 1977.)

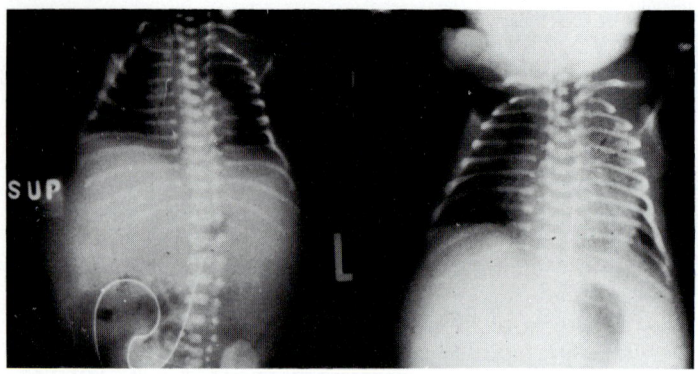

FIGURE 44–7. X-ray of a hydropic newborn at birth and 6 hours later after exchange transfusion. Note the small heart at the time of birth and the very marked increase in heart size and evidence of pulmonary congestion denoting heart failure 6 hours later. The fetus has extreme ascites. (From Bowman JM: Blood-group incompatibilities. *In* Iffy L, Kaminetzky HA [eds]: Principles and Practice of Obstetrics and Perinatology. Copyright © 1981. Reprinted by permission of John Wiley & Sons, Inc.)

of the Rh-negative woman may have occurred in a previous pregnancy. An Rh-positive woman may have atypical blood group antibodies, particularly if she has received transfusions in the past. Some atypical blood group antibodies are capable of producing hemolytic disease every bit as severe as that produced by Rh antibodies.

The Pregnant Woman Without Blood Group Antibodies

The Rh-positive woman who has no demonstrable atypical blood group antibodies early in pregnancy is not likely to develop dangerous atypical immunization as her pregnancy progresses. Because no preventive measures are possible, there is nothing to be gained by frequent retesting of the Rh-positive woman. A second blood sample should be sent from an Rh-positive woman at 27 to 28 weeks gestation to confirm that she is Rh-positive and that she has not developed atypical blood group antibodies.

If the pregnant woman is Rh-negative, her ABO group and the Rh status and ABO group of her husband should be determined. If he is Rh-negative the conceptus should be Rh-negative and the mother should not be at risk of Rh immunization. Because extramarital pregnancies are not unknown, she should be rescreened at 32 to 36 weeks gestation, and the Rh status of the infant should be determined using cord blood obtained at delivery.

If the father is Rh-positive, his ABO group and Rh phenotype should be determined. Depending on his Rh phenotype, the likelihood of his zygosity for D can be determined (see Table 44–2). If he is heterozygous, there is a 50 per cent chance that the conceptus is Rh-negative and the overall risk of Rh immunization is halved. When the mother's blood is group O and her husband's is A, B, or AB, there is a 66⅔ per cent chance that the conceptus is ABO-incompatible, reducing the risk of Rh immunization from 16 to about 1.5 per cent if the fetus is Rh-positive. When the ABO group and Rh phenotype of the father are known, the risk of Rh immunization can be calculated (Table 44–5).

The pregnant Rh-negative woman whose husband is Rh-positive must have further antibody screening tests as her pregnancy progresses. Minimum recommendation is a second test at 18 to 20 weeks gestation followed by monthly tests thereafter. If an Rh antibody appears during pregnancy (as either a primary or a secondary immune response), it rarely does so before 20 weeks gestation.

Meticulous management of the Rh-negative unimmunized woman during labor is most important. If the fetus is Rh-positive, both cesarean section and manual removal of the placenta increase the risk and volume of fetal-maternal transplacental hemorrhage and the risk of Rh immunization. Amniocentesis, carried out for genetic purposes in early pregnancy or for the determination of pulmonary maturity in later pregnancy, also carries a risk of TPH, thereby increasing the hazards of Rh immunization. The risk of TPH in these circumstances can be greatly reduced, but not removed altogether, by real-time ultrasonographic placental localization and direction of the amniocentesis needle.

After delivery, cord and maternal blood samples must be obtained and tested. Cord blood is analyzed for ABO group and Rh type and is subjected to direct antiglobulin (Coombs) testing. Maternal blood is again tested for the presence of Rh antibody and, if a test is available, for maternal-fetal transplacental hemorrhage. Most instances of Rh immunization occur following small or undetectable TPH. However, testing will identify the rare woman (0.23 per cent) into whom

TABLE 44–5. Approximate Risk of Rh Immunization

HUSBAND	BABY	RISK (%)
D-negative	D-negative	0
D-positive homozygous, ABO-compatible		16
D-positive homozygous, ABO incompatible	ABO unknown	7
	D-positive, ABO incompatible	2
D-positive heterozygous, ABO-compatible	Rh unknown	8
D-positive heterozygous, ABO-incompatible	ABO and Rh unknown	3.5

Modified from Bowman JM: Hemolytic disease of the newborn. *In* Conn HF, Conn RB Jr (eds): Current Diagnosis 6. Philadelphia, WB Saunders Company, 1980.

more than 30 ml of fetal blood (15 ml of fetal red blood cells) have passed and who therefore may not be protected by one standard prophylactic dose of Rh immune globulin.

The Immunized Rh-Negative Pregnant Woman

The physician caring for the immunized Rh-negative woman must be able to predict whether the fetus will be affected severely, moderately, minimally, or not at all by the mother's Rh antibody. If the fetus will be severely affected, the physician must know at what stage of gestation hydrops is likely to occur. This information is important because management measures that carry some risk are available to increase the likelihood of survival of the severely affected fetus. Only fetuses doomed to become hydropic before 34 weeks gestation should be subjected to intrauterine fetal transfusions. Only these and fetuses who will become hydropic between 34 weeks and term should be subjected to premature delivery. The latest point in gestation that is compatible with intact survival must be selected for initial fetal transfusion or for premature delivery.

Predicting Severity of Rh Hemolytic Disease

There are six main predictive parameters: (1) history of prior hemolytic disease, (2) maternal antibody titers, (3) cell-mediated maternal antibody functional assays, (4) amniotic fluid spectrophotometric measurements, (5) fetal real time ultrasonographic assessment, and (6) fetal percutaneous umbilical blood sampling. Each is considered in turn.

History of Fetus or Infant with Rh Disease

There are two usual patterns of severity of Rh hemolytic disease. Disease may remain at the same degree of severity from baby to baby or may become progressively worse with each succeeding pregnancy. Occasionally, disease may become less severe. If a pattern of mild disease is established in two or three pregnancies, it tends to remain the same. Occasionally, however, hydrops may affect the fetus of a woman whose previous three or four babies were only mildly affected.

The other pattern, disease that progresses from mild to severe with or without an intervening moderately affected fetus, is just as common. For the woman with one hydropic birth, the likelihood that hydrops fetalis will develop in the next Rh-positive pregnancy is 90 per cent, not 100 per cent.

Medical and obstetric history is of no value in a first sensitized pregnancy, in which the risk of hydrops is 8 to 10 per cent. Obstetric history is also of no help when hydrops fetalis has occurred previously and the husband is heterozygous for D. History of hydrops fetalis does not indicate when during the pregnancy the next affected fetus will become hydropic. Generally, but not invariably, hydrops develops in a later fetus at the same time or earlier in gestation.

Maternal Rh Antibody Measurement

When Rh antibody titrations are carried out in the same laboratory by experienced technologists using the same methods and the same test cells, they are of some value in predicting severity of Rh hemolytic disease. Since factors such as the Rh antibody binding constant, the amount of Rh antigen in the red cell membrane, and the ability of the fetus to maintain an adequate circulating red cell hemoglobin level without compromising hepatic function and umbilical portal venous circulation will vary, the Rh antibody measurement determines only whether the fetus is at risk. It cannot predict severity of Rh disease accurately enough that treatment may be undertaken solely on its basis.

Methods of Rh antibody titration vary from laboratory to laboratory. Therefore, the maternal Rh antibody titer at which there is a significant risk of hydrops fetalis must be decided for each laboratory. In our laboratory, an albumin Rh antibody titer below 1:16, in the absence of a history of fetal hydrops or a neonate requiring exchange transfusion, will not be associated with hydrops and stillbirth before term. A titer of 1:16 carries a 10 per cent risk; of 1:32 a 25 per cent risk; of 1:64 a 50 per cent risk; and of 1:128 a 75 per cent risk. At no antibody titer is the risk 100 per cent.

Indirect antiglobulin titers (IDAT) are preferred by many laboratories. They are more sensitive and are usually one to three dilutions higher than albumin titers. Therefore, the critical IDAT at which the fetus is at risk may be on the order of 1:32 to 1:128. As mentioned, the lowest IDAT at which the fetus is at risk must be determined individually for each laboratory.

Because the Rh antibody titer is the basis for identifying the pregnant woman and her fetus who are at risk and require further investigation, regular Rh antibody measurements must be carried out during pregnancy in an Rh-negative woman. The initial measurement should be made at the first prenatal visit, a subsequent one at 16 to 18 weeks gestation, one at 22 weeks gestation, and every 2 weeks thereafter.

Rh antibody titer and maternal history are insufficient to allow proper management of the Rh-negative mother and her affected fetus. In one major hospital, in a consecutive series of 426 Rh-immunized gravidas seen between 1954 and 1961, there were 67 perinatal deaths and 54 infants who survived because delivery was induced before term, some as early as 32 weeks gestation (Bowman and Pollock, 1965). In only 62 per cent of these 121 most severely affected fetuses was severity of disease predicted accurately. If greater accuracy of prediction had been possible, half of the perinatal deaths might have been prevented by treatment measures available at that time.

Cell-Mediated Maternal Antibody Functional Assays

Because of the relatively poor correlation between blood group antibody titrations and severity of hemolytic disease, various functional assays have been developed, which reflect the binding constant or avidity of the antibody for the antigen on the red cell membrane and therefore its ability to produce severe hemolytic disease. These assays include the monocyte monolayer assay (MMA) (Zupanska et al., 1989; Nance et al., 1989); antibody-dependent cellular cytotoxicity (ADCC), using lymphocytes (Urbaniak et al., 1984); using monocytes (Engelfriet et al., 1986); and monocyte chemiluminescence assay (Hadley et al., 1988).

P. L. Mollison et al. (1991), testing sera from mothers delivering babies with varying degrees of hemolytic disease, revealed correct results as follows: ADCC (monocytes), 60 per cent; ADCC (lymphocytes), 57 per cent; chemiluminescence, 51 per cent; rosetting and phagocytosis with peripheral monocytes, 41 per cent; with U937 cells or cultured macrophages, 32 per cent. The assays appeared to be more helpful in predicting mild or minimal disease, than in predicting very severe disease. Obviously, since all of these assays measure the potential lethality of the maternal antibody, they are quite incapable of differentiating the unaffected antigen-negative fetus from the affected antigen-positive fetus.

A recent report casts doubt upon the ability of the monocyte-macrophage (MMA) assay to predict severity of hemolytic disease of the newborn (Brown et al., 1991). In sera from 41 pregnant women with potentially dangerous blood group antibodies who delivered affected babies, there was no correlation between the hematocrit of a fetal blood sample obtained at cordocentesis and the MMA.

Therefore, although these functional tests may be helpful in more accurately determining the fetus at risk and therefore, in some pregnancies, precluding the need for invasive measures such as amniocentesis and fetal blood sampling, they in no way replace such invaluable perinatal management aids in ultimately differentiating the fetus who requires treatment *in utero* from the fetus who does not.

Amniotic Fluid Optical Density Measurement

Obstetricians have noted for years that, in the presence of a severely erythroblastotic fetus, the amniotic fluid is stained yellow. The yellow pigment is bilirubin, which can be quantitated most accurately by spectrophotometric measurements of the optical density between 420 and 460 nm, the wavelength absorbed by bilirubin.

Amniotic fluid is primarily a fetal product. The fetus swallows it and voids into it. The most likely source of the bilirubin is fetal tracheal and pulmonary secretions, which are quite yellow in babies with severe hemolytic disease.

In 1961, Liley described a method of amniotic fluid spectrophotometric measurement that allows comparison of measurements from different laboratories. Amniotic fluid protected from light, which destroys bilirubin, is centrifuged and filtered. Optical density (OD) readings are made in a good quality spectrophotometer over the 700-nm to 350-nm wavelength range. The readings are plotted on semilogarithmic graph paper, using wavelength as the linear horizontal coordinate and optical density as the vertical logarithmic coordinate (Fig. 44–8). The plotted dots are joined. The deviation from linearity of the optical density reading at 450 nm (the Δ OD 450 reading) is directly related to the severity of hemolytic disease. A second rise at 405 nm, if the fluid is not contaminated with blood, is due to the presence of heme pigment, in itself an indicator of severe hemolysis. To measure the deviation from linearity (Δ OD 450), the readings at 550 nm and 365 nm are connected on the graph. The measurement from where the connecting line intersects 450 nm to the actual reading at 450 nm gives the Δ OD 450.

The 450-nm deviation must then be replotted using gestation as the linear coordinate (Figs. 44–8 and 44–

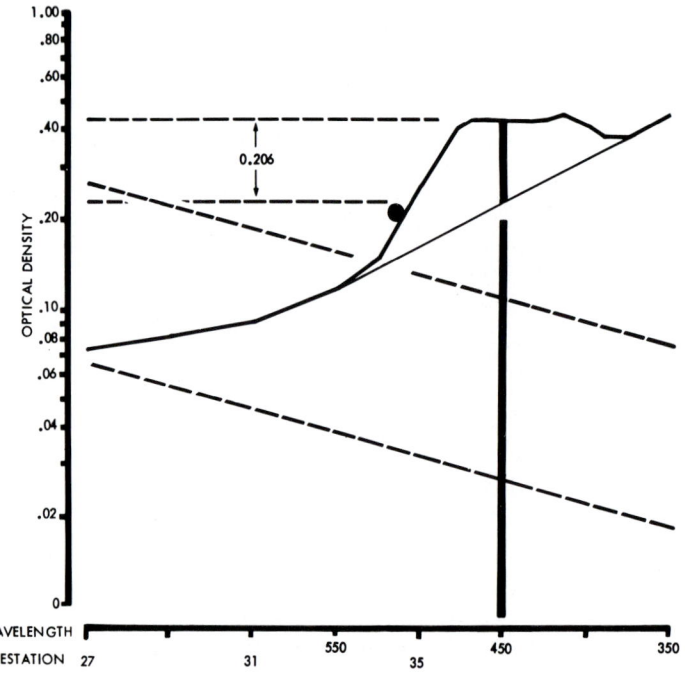

FIGURE 44–8. Amniotic fluid spectrophotometric reading (Liley method) is 0.206 in this example. The value falls into zone 3, indicating impending fetal death. This first affected infant was delivered at 35 weeks gestation with a cord hemoglobin level of 4.0 gm/100 ml and a cord bilirubin level of 8.0 mg/100 ml and required five exchange transfusions in order to survive.

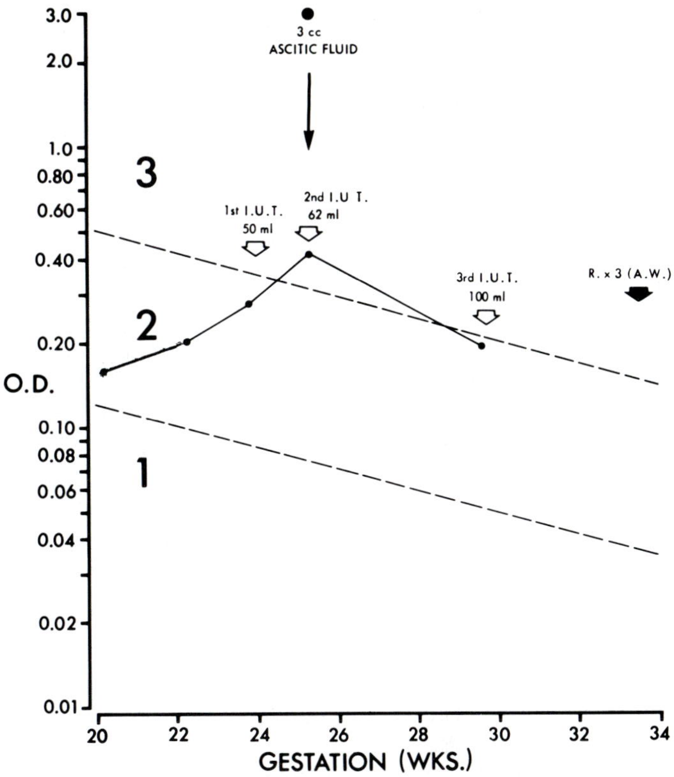

FIGURE 44–9. Serial spectromographic readings (Liley method) in a gravida with a history of two hydropic fetal deaths at 38 and 32 weeks gestation. First IUT was given when reading was at the 80 per cent level in zone 2 at 24 weeks gestation. The fetus required three transfusions and was delivered at 33½ weeks gestation. Only donor red cells were found in the neonatal circulation. Birth weight 2000 gm; cord hemoglobin 12.5 gm/100 ml; cord bilirubin 4.5 mg/100 ml. The neonate required three exchange transfusions in order to survive.

9). Replotting is required because the unaffected fetus produces bilirubin early in gestation. These levels in normal fetuses peak at about 23 to 25 weeks gestation. Liley (1961) in his original study examined fluids from 101 Rh-immunized pregnancies, all after 28 weeks gestation. From his evaluation of the degree of hemolytic disease after birth he was able to divide the spectrophotometric graph into three zones (see Figs. 44–8 and 44–9). Readings in zone 3 (the upper zone) indicate severe hemolytic disease, hydrops, and fetal death probably within 7 to 10 days. Readings in zone 1 (the lowest zone) indicate mild or no hemolytic disease, but a 10 per cent probability that neonatal exchange transfusion will be necessary. Readings in zone 2 (the middle zone) indicate intermediate disease, becoming increasingly severe as the Δ OD 450 readings approached the zone 3 boundary.

The zone boundaries slope, indicating that the amount of bilirubin present in amniotic fluid diminishes as pregnancy progresses. This is certainly true after 25 weeks gestation, when the same Δ OD 450 readings seen in later gestation are indicative of more severe hemolytic disease. Between 18 weeks and 25 weeks gestation, Nicolaides et al. (1986) noted little if any relationship between amniotic fluid Δ OD 450 readings and fetal circulating hemoglobin concentrations. Because of this observation, they recommend direct fetal blood sampling without amniotic fluid spectrophotometric measurements for assessment of severity of hemolytic disease before 26 weeks gestation. A single Δ OD 450 reading in the second trimester of pregnancy may be of little value in predicting severity of hemolytic disease unless it is extremely high ($\geq$0.400), and even then, if noted before 24 weeks gestation, it must be interpreted with caution.

The overall amniotic fluid accuracy of prediction of severity of hemolytic disease is 95 per cent (Table 44–6), but such accuracy can only be achieved with serial Δ OD 450 measurements, the final reading being after 26 to 27 weeks gestation. As noted, Δ OD 450 readings may be relatively inaccurate in early to middle second trimester. In the second trimester the zone boundaries are poorly delineated. We have observed, as have Nicolaides et al. (1986), that Δ OD 450 readings in normal unaffected pregnancies peak at 23 to 25 weeks gestation, rendering the true zone boundaries parabolic. Thus we have recently modified the Liley zone boundaries, declining them downward before 24 weeks gestation at the same angle as the angle of inclination after 24 weeks gestation (Fig. 44–10) (Bowman et al., 1992a). Because fetal blood sampling (described later), followed if necessary by intravascular fetal transfusions, is the most accurate means of determining the presence and severity of hemolytic disease and the preferred treatment *in utero*, we recom-

**TABLE 44–6. Accuracy of Amniotic Fluid
Δ OD 450 Spectrophotometry (Liley Method)***

ZONE OF LAST SAMPLE	NUMBER OF WOMEN	RATE OF INACCURATE PREDICTIONS (%)	RATE OF LIFE-THREATENING INACCURACY (%)
1	253	2.4	1.2
2	530	8.9	3.6
3	314	1.6	0.6
Total	1097	5.3	2.2

*3177 samples examined between December 15, 1961, and July 3, 1981.

LILEY AMNIOTIC FLUID ZONE BOUNDARIES
Modified Before 24 Weeks Gestation

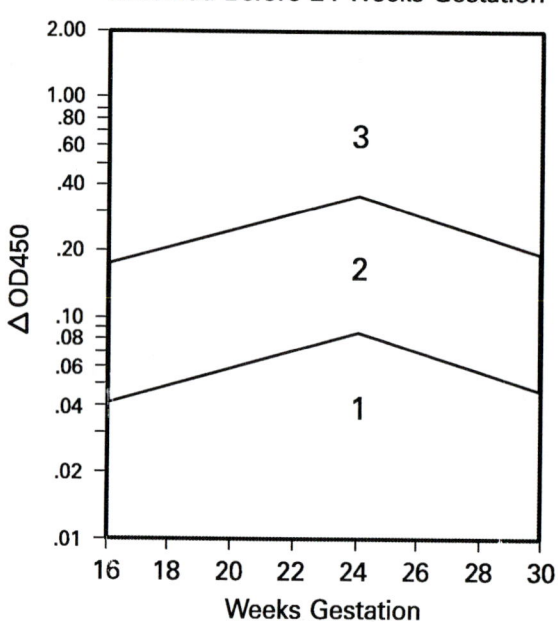

FIGURE 44–10. Modification of Liley Δ OD 450 reading zone boundaries before 24 weeks gestation. Zone boundary angle of declination before 24 weeks gestation is the same as the zone boundary angle of inclination after 24 weeks gestation. (From Bowman JM: Rhesus haemolytic disease. *In* Wald NJ [ed]: Antenatal and Neonatal Screening. 2nd ed. Oxford, Oxford University Press, 1992. By permission of the Oxford University Press.)

mend fetal blood sampling if a single or final Δ OD 450 reading is at the 65 per cent level of zone 2 modified before 24 weeks gestation.

Because of the high risk of fetomaternal transplacental hemorrhage that accompanies fetal blood sampling (at least 50 per cent), we do not recommend abandonment of amniocentesis, which carries a 2 to 2.5 per cent risk of fetal TPH. Serial amniotic fluid Δ OD 450 measurements still have a place in the management of alloimmune hemolytic disease. Nevertheless, recognizing that serial Δ OD 450 measurements before 24 weeks gestation may not be completely accurate, we also recommend proceeding to fetal blood sampling if the antibody titers are high, if there is a prior history of severe hemolytic disease, and if amniotic fluid Δ OD 450 readings are either equivocal (middle of modified zone 2) or unobtainable because of an anterior placenta.

Amniocentesis

Technique of Amniocentesis. Because of the risk of transplacental hemorrhage and of more hemolytic disease if the placenta is traumatized, amniocentesis should be preceded by ultrasound localization of the placental site. Indeed, if the placenta is anteriorly situated, amniocentesis should be carried out under real-time ultrasonographic guidance. If the placenta cannot be avoided, amniocentesis should not be carried out. Fetal blood sampling then is the preferred procedure.

The procedure should be carried out using aseptic technique. A clotted blood sample should be obtained immediately before and 5 minutes after amniocentesis. The site for insertion of the needle is selected on the basis of physical examination and real-time ultrasonographic determination of placental site, fetal position,

and the presence of a suitable pool of amniotic fluid. The site is prepared with a suitable antiseptic, draped, and infiltrated with a local anesthetic. A 20- or 22-gauge lumbar puncture needle is introduced through the abdominal and uterine walls to the depth at which ultrasonography has indicated the presence of amniotic fluid. The stylette is removed, and 10 to 15 ml of fluid are aspirated gently. If fluid is not obtained, the needle is withdrawn slightly and is cautiously inserted more deeply. Rotation of the needle may help the flow of fluid. Amniotic fluid normally is slightly turbid, becoming more so with gestational age. It will also have a varying degree of yellow pigmentation. The amniotic fluid, protected from light, is sent for spectrophotometric measurement and, in a pregnancy beyond 32 weeks, for the determination of fetal pulmonary maturity. The maternal blood samples are sent for fetal cell screening and for antibody titer measurement.

Hazards. Maternal hazards in amniocentesis are minimal. If the procedure is properly carried out the risk of infection is negligible. There have been rare reported instances of precipitation of labor and abruptio placentae following amniocentesis.

Fetal hazards are not great but they should not be minimized. Direct needle trauma has been reported (Rehder and Weitzel, 1978). The major risk has already been described—placental trauma followed by TPH, rising antibody titers, and resulting increased severity of hemolytic disease. Fetal exsanguination has been reported but is very rare.

Sources of Error. Other materials in the amniotic fluid or fetal conditions can distort the amniotic fluid findings and cause serious errors. Maternal or fetal blood produces sharp 580-, 540-, and 415-nm peaks, which obscure the 450-nm peak and make the reading valueless (Fig. 44–11). Smaller amounts of blood will

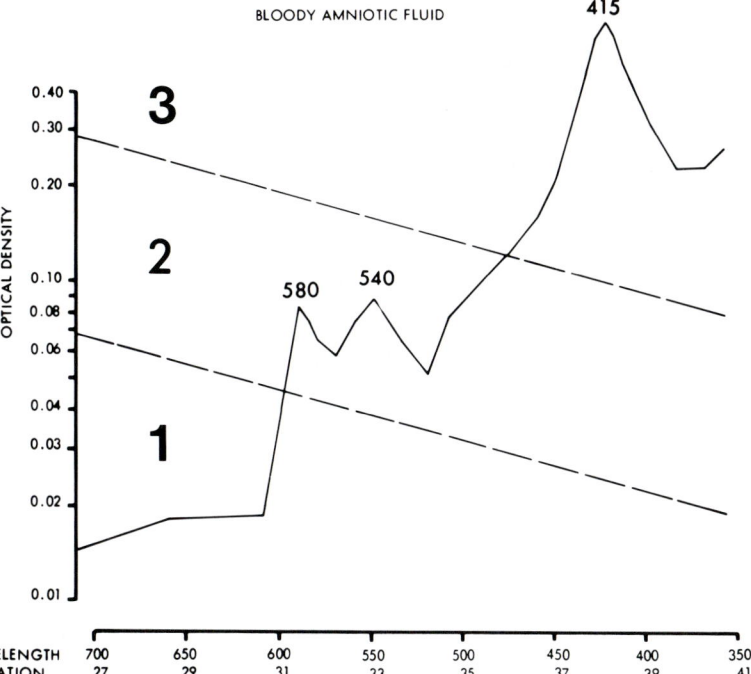

FIGURE 44–11. Spectrophotometric curve (Liley method) of amniotic fluid grossly contaminated with blood. Note sharp peaks at 580, 540, and 415 nm, which obscure the 450-nm rise. (From Bowman JM: Hemolytic disease of the newborn. *In* Conn HF, Conn RB [eds]: Current Diagnosis 5. Philadelphia, WB Saunders Company, 1977.)

not mask the peak, but small amounts of plasma (particularly fetal plasma) will increase the Δ OD 450 reading, with consequent misinterpretation of severity of hemolytic disease. Methemalbumin produces a 405-nm pigment peak, which may depress the Δ OD 450 reading but in itself is usually an indicator of severe hemolytic disease. Meconium in amniotic fluid produces a marked distortion. Inadvertent exposure of amniotic fluid to light (particularly fluorescent light) decolorizes bilirubin and produces an incorrectly low Δ OD 450 value.

Maternal urine may occasionally be aspirated, as may fetal ascitic fluid. Urine produces no 450-nm peak. Ascitic fluid is clear, bright yellow, and more viscous than amniotic fluid. Unless contaminated by blood (as after intrauterine fetal transfusion), ascitic fluid can be differentiated from amniotic fluid by visual examination. Its absorption peak is very much higher (dilution may be necessary).

Certain congenital anomalies of the fetus such as anencephaly and obstructive lesions of the upper gastrointestinal tract (tracheoesophageal fistula, duodenal atresia) produce both hydramnios and marked rises in Δ OD 450 readings, which may be very misleading if the mother is also Rh-immunized.

INDICATIONS FOR AND TIMING OF AMNIOCENTESIS. Because amniocentesis does carry some risk to the fetus, it should be carried out only when history and/or antibody titer indicated that the fetus is at risk of hydrops and death. In 50 per cent of instances of Rh-immunization, amniocentesis can be avoided. If an earlier pregnancy has ended in stillbirth or has produced an infant requiring exchange transfusion, amniocentesis should be carried out at 16 to 18 weeks gestation, irrespective of the antibody titer. In the absence of such a history, amniocentesis should be carried out only if an antibody titer indicates a risk of hydrops and fetal death (1:16 in albumin or higher, in

our laboratory). If the critical titer is present before 20 weeks gestation, the initial amniocentesis is carried out at 16 to 18 weeks. If the critical titer is reached after 20 weeks gestation, amniocentesis is carried out as promptly as possible (i.e., within 3 to 5 days). Amniotic fluid examinations should be repeated at intervals of 5 to 28 days depending on the Δ OD 450 reading from the immediately preceding amniotic fluid sample.

Perinatal Ultrasonography

The development of modern ultrasound linear-array B-scan ultrasound imaging techniques in the mid- to late 1970s has markedly improved management in many areas of maternal blood group immunization. This is particularly so in predicting severity of fetal hemolytic disease.

Because ultrasound techniques are noninvasive, without ionizing radiation, they can be used frequently (even daily) in a serial fashion to determine severity of disease and to monitor improvement or deterioration in relation to time and to treatment measures carried out. Ultrasonography gives an accurate determination of hepatic and placental size (Fig. 44–12). It allows the prompt and accurate diagnosis of hydrops fetalis and, to some extent, the degree of severity of the hydropic state, in that it can show the presence and amount of fetal ascites and edema (Fig. 44–13) and whether the fetus is moribund and not breathing or moving. However, ultrasonography does not give as accurate a prediction of impending hydrops as do serial amniotic fluid Δ OD 450 readings.

When hydrops has occurred, serial ultrasonographic assessments are invaluable in determining (1) whether there is reduction or progression of fetal hydrops after IUT (by showing changes in amounts of ascites and edema); and (2) whether there is improvement or

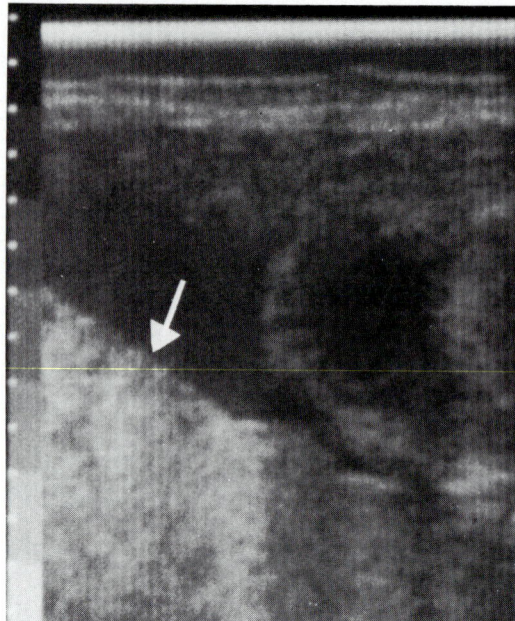

FIGURE 44–12. Ultrasound examination of fetus with hydrops fetalis. Placenta is enormously thickened and edematous *(white arrow)*. Fetal abdomen grossly distended with ascitic fluid appears to the right of the arrow.

deterioration in fetal condition (by showing changes in fetal heart rate or rhythm or fetal tone, movement, or respiration).

Percutaneous Umbilical Fetal Blood Sampling (PUBS)

With the development of sophisticated ultrasound equipment and the availability of perinatologists skilled in its use, percutaneous fetal umbilical blood sampling became available in the mid-1980s. This procedure allows measurements of all blood parameters that can be measured after birth (hemoglobin, hematocrit, blood groups, direct antiglobulin testing, serum bilirubin levels, platelet and leucocyte counts, serum protein levels, erythropoietin levels, and fetal blood gases). Fetal blood sampling is the most accurate means of determining the degree of severity of fetal hemolytic disease, in the absence of hydrops.

In the presence of a history of prior hydrops and a husband heterozygous for the antigen to which the mother is alloimmunized, fetal blood sampling will settle the question of whether the fetus is antigen-positive and affected or antigen-negative and unaffected.

The procedure is relatively benign, carrying with it a traumatic fetal mortality rate of a fraction of 1 per cent (Daffos et al., 1985). Since, as described earlier, it does carry with it a great likelihood of fetomaternal hemorrhage, it should be reserved for situations in which serial amniotic fluid Δ OD 450 readings are equivocal or rise into the upper 65 per cent of modified zone 2 or when an anterior placenta cannot be avoided at amniocentesis and maternal pregnancy history and/or maternal antibody titers place the fetus at risk.

Fetal blood sampling may be possible as early as 18 weeks gestation; it usually is feasible by 20 to 21 weeks gestation.

The preferred sampling site is from the umbilical vessel (preferably the vein) at its insertion into the placenta. For this reason, the procedure is technically easier if the placenta is implanted upon the anterior uterine wall. The technique of fetal blood sampling will be described with the technique of intravascular fetal transfusion (IVT).

TREATMENT OF THE Rh-IMMUNIZED MOTHER AND FETUS

In a Pregnancy Without Risk of Hydrops Fetalis

In the 50 per cent of pregnancies in which history and antibody titers are such that amniocentesis has not been required and in the remaining pregnancies in which serial amniotic fluid Δ OD 450 readings have remained below the middle of zone 2, or fetal blood sampling has revealed normal hemoglobin and hematocrit parameters (≥130 gm/1, ≥0.40 respectively), immunized mothers should be allowed to deliver spontaneously. If the expected date of delivery is certain, labor might be induced and delivery effected at 38½ to 39 weeks. A low zone 2 or zone 1 reading in a woman with a history of severe hemolytic disease of the newborn and/or with a high antibody titer and a husband heterozygous for D indicates that the fetus is Rh-negative and unaffected. The mother should be allowed to deliver spontaneously. If readings rise into the 50 to 70 per cent area of zone 2 by 35 to 37 weeks gestation, delivery should be carried out at 36½ to 38

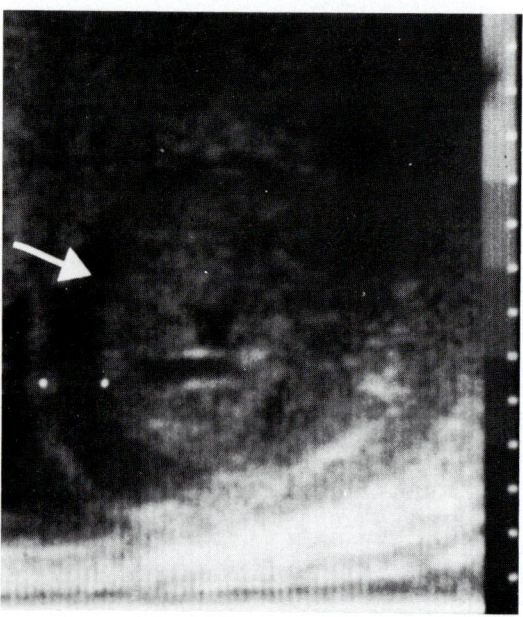

FIGURE 44–13. Ultrasound examination of fetus with hydrops fetalis. Fetal abdomen encloses a large volume of ascitic fluid (under *white arrow*) and a large liver with a dilated ductus venosus.

weeks, as long as there is evidence of fetal pulmonary maturity. Under no circumstances should the pregnancy be allowed to go past 39½ to 40 weeks. The fetus will not be hydropic, but after delivery the infant will probably have a significant degree of hemolytic disease and will require prompt treatment. Such a baby benefits from delivery 2 to 3 weeks before term. If there is any doubt about the gestation of the fetus, amniotic fluid phospholipid analysis should be carried out first to determine whether the fetal lungs are mature.

In a Pregnancy With Risk of Hydrops

Half of the 20 to 25 per cent of fetuses destined to become hydropic will become so after 34 weeks gestation (see Table 44-4). If the Δ OD 450 reading rises into the upper 80 per cent of zone 2 or an initial measurement taken after 34 weeks is in zone 3, prompt delivery should be carried out, provided there is evidence of fetal pulmonary maturity. If there is no evidence of pulmonary maturity, fetal blood sampling with intravascular fetal transfusion at ≥34 weeks gestation is recommended. If fetal venous access is not possible, corticosteroids should be administered followed by delivery 48 hours later.

Intrauterine Fetal Transfusion (IUT)

If delivery is carried out too early in gestation, the neonatal mortality rate from prematurity becomes prohibitive. Before 1963, delivery was performed at 32 weeks gestation because no other treatment was available, and the 25 per cent neonatal death rate was acceptable. Because 8 per cent of affected fetuses are hydropic by 32 weeks, in 1963, 8 per cent was the optimal perinatal death rate from hemolytic disease. Liley (1963) altered the prognosis for these most severely affected fetuses when he reported the use of intrauterine transfusion (IUT) in their management.

The original intrauterine fetal transfusion method introduced by Liley was the technique of placing blood in the peritoneal cavity of the fetus (intraperitoneal fetal transfusion). Fetal blood sampling and direct intravascular transfusion of Rh-negative blood through a needle introduced via a fetoscope was first reported by Rodeck et al. in 1981, followed by direct intravascular transfusions via a needle introduced under ultrasound guidance by Bang et al. in 1982. Direct intravascular transfusion (IVT) represents a major advance in the management of severe Rh immunization. It is now the preferred method of fetal transfusion.

BLOOD FOR IUT. If the ABO blood group of the fetus is unknown, group O red cells—tightly packed (hemoglobin 270 to 290 gm/l, hematocrit 0.85 to 0.90), less than four days old, and negative for the antigen to which the mother is immunized—are used for IUT. If fetal blood sampling has been carried out and the fetal ABO status is known and there is no fetal maternal ABO incompatibility, red cells of the same ABO type as the fetus may be transfused.

Because we have no instance of graft-versus-host disease (GVHD) developing in any of the 313 surviving infants who have had fetal transfusions in Winnipeg with no gamma irradiated red cells, some transfused as early as 18½ to 20 weeks gestation, we believe that the risk of GVHD following IUT with nonirradiated blood in otherwise normal fetuses is minimal. However, because there are isolated reports of GVHD occurring after IUT (Parkman et al., 1974) and since gamma irradiation does not appear to affect the function or shorten the life span of donor red cells, we recommend that blood for IUT be irradiated, if time permits.

SELECTION OF PATIENTS FOR IUT. Because IUT carries distinct risks for the fetus, only fetuses at risk of developing hydrops before 34 weeks gestation are candidates for such treatment.

Prior to the ultrasound and fetal blood sampling era, selection of fetuses for IPT was made on the basis of amniotic fluid Δ OD 450 readings; preferably serial readings falling into the upper 80 to 85 per cent level of zone 2 before 30 weeks gestation, into zone 3 after 30 weeks gestation, or a single reading well into zone 3 at any gestation.

In the present ultrasound and fetal blood sampling era, IUT (IVT) are carried out based upon fetal blood parameters, (hemoglobin less than 100 to 110 gm/l, hematocrit less than 0.30). Fetal blood sampling is carried out on the basis of amniotic fluid, prior history, and antibody titer criteria already outlined.

Ultrasonographic evidence of hydrops is an absolute indication for IUT (nearly always IVT). If the fetus is moribund (i.e., not breathing), immediate IVT should be undertaken. In this situation, in which any delay is likely to be fatal, group O, unmatched, nonirradiated, packed red cells, missing the antigen to which the mother is immunized, are used, the crossmatch being carried out at the same time as the transfusion is being given. Subsequent transfusions are carried out with group O, crossmatched, compatible, irradiated red cells.

The number of candidates for IUT is decreasing as the number of immunized Rh-negative women declines because of the success of Rh prophylaxis. IUT technique, either IPT or IVT, appears simple, but it is not. Complete management of the immunized mother and her baby before and after birth requires not only an experienced obstetrician but also neonatal, ultrasound, radiology, and laboratory personnel and services of the highest order. The procedure should be carried out only in a tertiary level perinatal center. A team approach is essential.

As a minimum, each center in which fetal transfusions are performed should deal with four or five fetuses annually on whom 12 to 16 transfusions are carried out. To reach this volume of patients, the IUT team must have all transfusion candidate referrals from a population base of two million (25,000 to 30,000 deliveries per year). Only under such circumstances will the team's expertise in IUT and overall management of the severely affected fetus and infant with hemolytic disease be maintained.

Intraperitoneal Fetal Transfusions (IPT)

Although intraperitoneal fetal transfusion (IPT) has, to a great extent, been supplanted by intravascular fetal transfusion (IVT), occasionally IVT may be technically impossible. For that reason, the ability to carry out IPT must be maintained.

Red cells injected into the peritoneal cavity are absorbed intact into the circulation via subdiaphragmatic lymphatic lacunae and the right lymphatic duct. About 10 to 13 per cent of the injected red cells are absorbed each 24 hours, absorption being complete within 8 to 10 days. Although absorption of red cells in the presence of ascites is more variable, in some instances it is quite adequate (Lewis et al., 1973). If the fetus is hydropic, moribund, and not breathing, absorption of red cells from the peritoneal cavity into the circulation will not occur (Menticoglou et al., 1987).

The volume of packed red cells injected intraperitoneally is limited by the size of the peritoneal cavity. If intraperitoneal pressure exceeds umbilical venous pressure, umbilical venous blood flow stops and the fetus will die (Crosby et al., 1970). If the following IPT formula is used, intraperitoneal pressure should not exceed umbilical venous pressure; IPT volume = (weeks gestation − 20) × 10 ml.

Calculation of residual donor hemoglobin concentration in the fetus after IPT allows appropriate spacing of IPT and selection of gestation of delivery. Residual donor hemoglobin concentrations can be calculated using the formula:

$$\text{Hemoglobin concentration in gm/100 ml} = \frac{0.85}{125} \times \frac{a}{b} \times \frac{120-c}{120}$$

where 0.85 is the fraction of the transfused red cells in the fetoplacental circulation; 125 is the fetoplacental blood volume in ml/kg estimated fetal body weight; a is the amount of donor red cell hemoglobin transfused; b is the estimated fetal body weight; c is the interval in days from the time of transfusion to the time of donor hemoglobin estimation; and 120 days is the life span of donor red cells. IPT is repeated when the donor hemoglobin level is estimated to have dropped to the 10 gm/100 ml level. Because the donor hemoglobin level cannot be raised to 10 gm/100 ml with one IPT, a second IPT is given 9 to 10 days after the first IPT. Subsequent IPT intervals are about 4 weeks, delivery being planned for 34 to 35 weeks gestation.

Technique of IPT

Although there have been many modifications of Liley's initial IPT technique, our IUT team uses Liley's original catheter method (Bowman et al., 1969), modified by the use of real-time ultrasonography as an aid to the proper placement of the needle and catheter into the fetal peritoneal cavity.

The mother is heavily sedated but not anesthetized. Rigorous asepsis is observed. Under real-time scan guidance, the obstetrician inserts a Tuohy 16-gauge, 17-cm needle into the peritoneal cavity of the fetus. Usually the tip of the needle can be seen indenting the fetal abdomen and then entering it. A shortened epidural catheter with the side holes removed is then threaded down the needle (Fig. 44–14). The needle is withdrawn over the catheter to lie on the maternal abdomen. Whereas prior x-ray studies have been obviated by ultrasonography, determination of the proper position of the catheter tip (free in the peritoneal cavity) must be determined. Injection of shaken saline with dissolved air, the aerated saline, noted by ultrasonography to rise to the top of the peritoneal cavity, may be reasonable evidence that the catheter tip is free in the peritoneal cavity. However, we have made errors with its use (Harman et al., 1989), as have others (Watts et al., 1988). For this reason, it is essential to confirm beyond any doubt that the catheter tip (or needle tip if a catheter is not used) is free in the peritoneal cavity, and this is done by injection of radiopaque contrast medium and a subsequent x-ray (Fig. 44–15).

If the catheter tip is in an organ or embedded

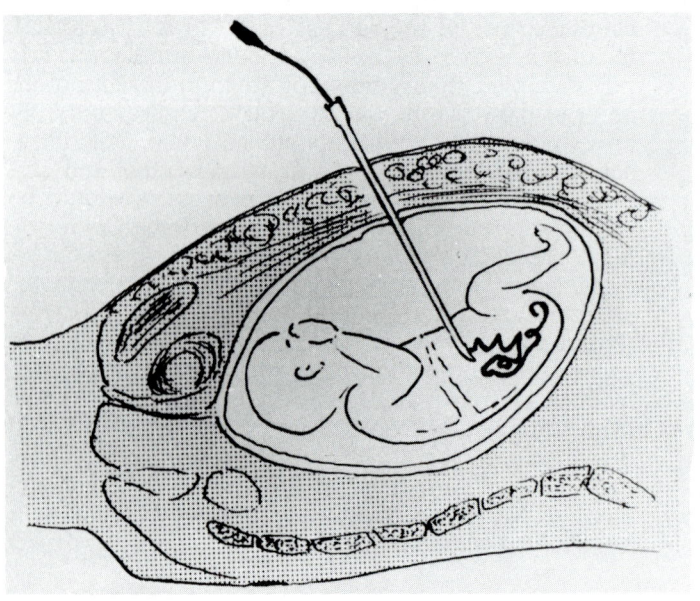

FIGURE 44–14. IPT diagram. The Tuohy needle has been inserted across the maternal abdominal wall and uterine wall into the fetal peritoneal cavity, and the epidural catheter has been threaded into the peritoneal cavity of the fetus. The safest position for the fetus at IPT is not with his abdomen anterior (as shown in this diagram), because the umbilical fetal vessels then lie in the center of the target area. (From Bowman JM: Blood-group incompatibilities. *In* Iffy L, Kaminetzky HA [eds]: Principles and Practice of Obstetrics and Perinatology. Copyright © 1981. Reprinted by permission of John Wiley & Sons, Inc.)

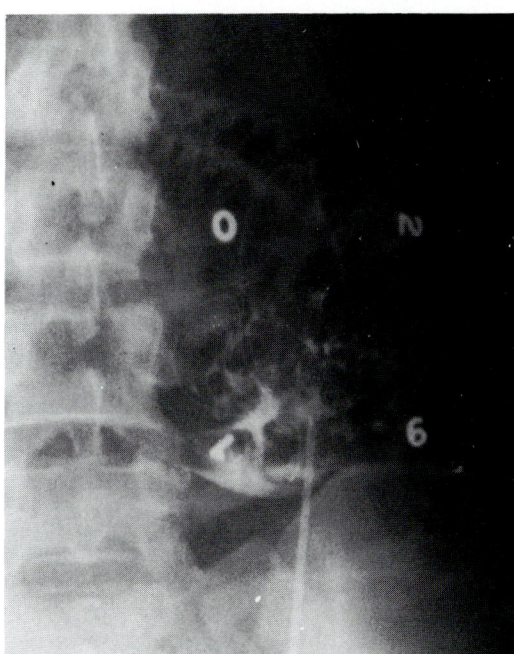

FIGURE 44–15. Successful catheterization of the fetal peritoneal cavity as shown by radiopaque contrast agent in the fetal peritoneal cavity outlining negative shadows of small bowel.

retroperitoneally, injected red cells will not be absorbed and they also may cause lethal trauma.

When the catheter tip has been demonstrated to be free in the peritoneal cavity (Fig. 44–15), the transfusion is carried out in 10-ml aliquots, injection of each 10 ml taking 3 to 5 minutes. The fetal heart rate is monitored by ultrasonography at the end of each infusion and continuously during infusion of the last 10 to 15 ml. The volume of red cells administered is determined according to the formula already discussed. If the fetus is in good condition with an intact autonomic nervous system, the heart rate increases to 160 to 190 beats per minute during the procedure. Bradycardia early in the procedure is uncommon but ominous, usually indicating the probability of fetal death. Fetal bradycardia toward the end of the procedure, a rare occurrence, is an indication for immediate termination of the transfusion because intraperitoneal pressure may be approaching umbilical venous pressure.

When the transfusion has been completed, the catheter is slowly withdrawn during continuous fetal heart rate monitoring. Profound bradycardia of vagal origin may occur. Further catheter removal should be delayed until the bradycardia disappears. The fetal heart rate is monitored periodically after the transfusion.

IPT is contraindicated if the placenta is anterior and must be traversed. It is also contraindicated if the fetus is hydropic. Only if IVT is impossible, in these circumstances, should IPT be considered. If the hydropic fetus is moribund and not breathing, IPT is absolutely contraindicated since red cell absorption will not occur. In this situation, if IVT is impossible, intracardiac transfusion is the only feasible procedure.

Technique for a Hydropic Fetus

When hydrops is present, if IPT, for any reason, must be carried out, an attempt should be made to aspirate some of the fluid through the needle before the catheter is threaded. A volume of ascitic fluid 20 to 30 ml in excess of the planned volume of red cells to be transfused should be aspirated, if possible. The catheter is then inserted and contrast agent is injected. When ascites is present, the dye diffuses into the fluid, and no small bowel half-moons or other landmarks are seen on radiographs (Fig. 44–16). If the x-ray shows marked residual ascites after the catheter is inserted, an attempt should be made to remove more fluid, up to a total of 150 ml. No effort should be made to empty the peritoneal cavity completely. If more ascitic fluid is aspirated than the planned volume of red cells to be infused, the total volume of the transfusion should be increased 20 to 30 per cent.

Direct Intravascular Fetal Transfusion (IVT)

In the mid-1960s attempts were made at direct intravascular exchange transfusions by hysterotomy, either through a fetal blood vessel (Adamsons et al., 1965; Asensio et al., 1966) or via a placental vessel (Seelen et al., 1966). These attempts were abandoned because of the very high associated perinatal mortality, mainly due to precipitation of preterm delivery. In

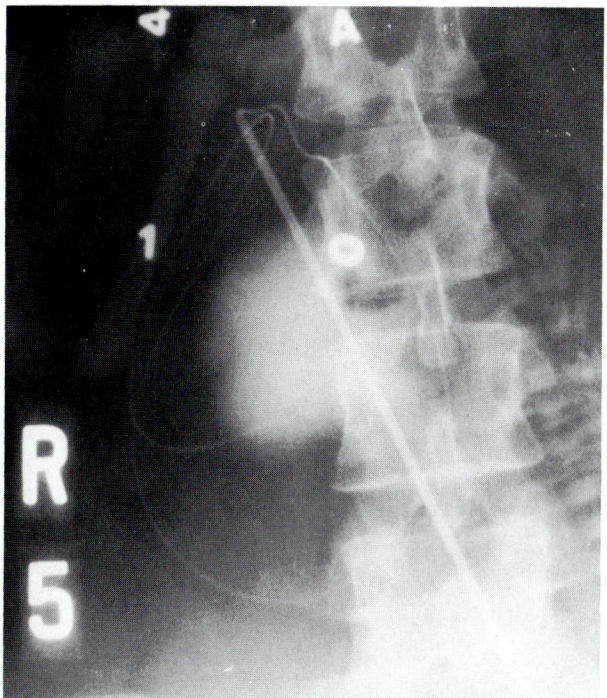

FIGURE 44–16. Hydrops fetalis at IPT. Note gross ascites at first IPT (31½ weeks gestation); ascites was more severe at second IPT given 4 days later (not shown). Severe residual hydrops at emergency cesarean section (33½ weeks gestation). At birth, cord hemoglobin was 6.2 gm/100 ml (99 per cent of donor origin), cord bilirubin 5.4 mg/100 ml. Neonate required five exchange transfusions, respiratory care for 4 days, and intensive nursery care for 3 weeks in order to survive.

1981, Rodeck et al. reported a method of fetal blood sampling and direct intravascular fetal transfusion through a needle introduced via a fetoscope. With this transfusion method they achieved an overall perinatal salvage rate of 72 per cent (Rodeck et al., 1984). However, transfusion via the fetoscopic route requires special equipment and skills available in few tertiary level centers. With the report of successful fetal blood sampling, wherein 606 fetal blood samplings were carried out in 562 pregnancies between 17 weeks and 38 weeks gestation, via a needle tip directed by ultrasonography into the umbilical vein or artery at its insertion into the placenta (Daffos et al., 1985), fetoscopy could be dispensed with and the needle introduced for fetal blood sampling and direct IVT under ultrasonographic guidance alone.

Technique of Fetal Blood Sampling and Direct Intravascular Fetal Transfusion (IVT)

Some investigators have introduced the needle tip for IVT under sonographic guidance into the fetal hepatic portion of the umbilical vein (Bang et al., 1982; de Crespigny et al., 1985). Others have directed the tip of the needle into the umbilical vein (or artery) at its insertion into the placenta (Berkowitz et al., 1986; Seeds and Bowes, 1986). Some advocate paralyzing the fetus immediately prior to transfusion by the intramuscular (or intravenous) injection of pancuronium (de Crespigny et al., 1985). Our group prefers the technique of needle tip insertion into the placental end of the umbilical blood vessel. Paralysis is necessary when fetal limbs or body overlie the placental cord insertion site or when fetal activity is such that the needle tip may be dislodged. The needle is a 22- or 20-gauge spinal needle, 8 cm to 12 cm in length, depending upon the distance of the target (the umbilical blood vessel) from the maternal abdominal wall.

When it has been decided from amniotic fluid and ultrasonographic assessment that fetal blood sampling and direct IVT are required, the mother is heavily premedicated with morphine, scopolamine, and diazepam and transferred to the fetal assessment and therapy unit. A highly skilled, experienced perinatal ultrasonographer is an essential component of the IVT group. Great care and considerable time are spent in identifying the target blood vessel (Fig. 44–17A, B).

After careful aseptic preparation of the maternal abdomen, the obstetrician drapes the maternal abdomen, infiltrates the skin with local anesthetic, and inserts a 22- or 20-gauge spinal needle tip through the maternal skin immediately over the target site selected previously by ultrasound. The ultrasound transducer, enclosed in sterile plastic, with ultrasound transmission gel between plastic and transducer and sterile oil external to the plastic on the maternal abdomen is applied to the maternal abdomen immediately adjacent to the needle insertion site. The transducer is positioned in a plane decided on by the ultrasonographer and venipuncturist, which allows simultaneous ultrasound identification of the blood vessel target site and the needle tip. The needle is guided toward the blood vessel with appropriate ultrasound-directed corrections in needle direction, to keep the tip on target.

In most instances, the needle tip can be identified as it penetrates to the appropriate depth of the target blood vessel. Because the needle tip is being advanced in a three-dimensional plane using ultrasound, which is two-dimensional, one cannot be certain that the needle tip has been correctly inserted into the lumen of the vein. When the tip is at the proper depth, the needle stylette is withdrawn and aspiration is attempted using a lightly heparinized 1-ml tuberculin syringe. If nothing is obtained or if amniotic fluid is aspirated, withdrawal (but not removal) of the needle tip and reinsertion under ultrasound guidance are carried out. If a free-flowing blood sample is aspirated, the tip of the needle is probably properly positioned in the fetal blood vessel lumen. At initial fetal blood sampling and IVT, this may be confirmed by determining that the blood is fetal by alkaline denaturation screening or blood gas analysis. (Time will not allow Kleihauer acid elution confirmation.) After the first IVT, the amount of donor blood present in the fetal circulation obscures any alkaline denaturation test to confirm its fetal origin.

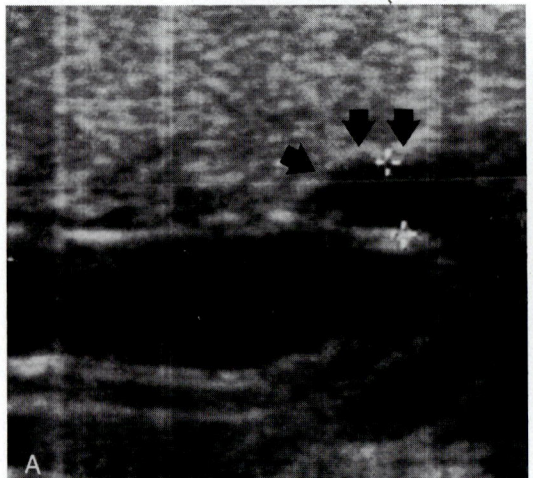 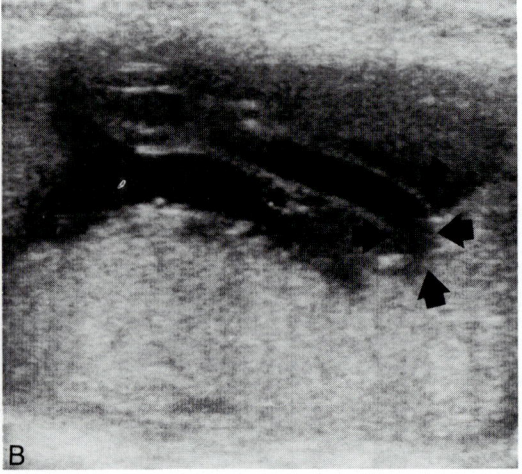

FIGURE 44–17. *A, B,* Real-time scan ultrasound view of insertion of the umbilical vein into the placenta *(arrows); A,* anterior placenta; *B,* posterior placenta. The lumen of the umbilical vein is sonar lucent.

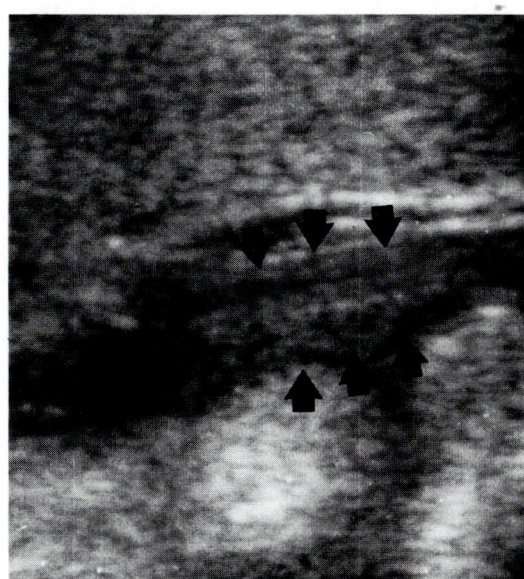

FIGURE 44–18. Donor red cell infusion into the umbilical vein *(arrows)*. In this static picture, the blood is sonar opaque. At the time of infusion, dynamic real-time ultrasound demonstrates the streaming of blood (turbulence) through the vein (between the *arrows*).

Confirmation that the needle tip is properly placed is easily and accurately done at the beginning of injection of the donor packed red cells. If the needle tip is in the vein, streaming ultrasound turbulence is seen as the blood passes down the vein (Fig. 44–18). Conversely, if the needle tip is in the artery, the turbulence of the transfused blood may be seen moving in the opposite direction onto the surface of the placenta. If turbulence can be seen in the amniotic fluid, the needle tip is in the amniotic cavity. If no turbulence can be seen, the needle tip may be dislodged and embedded in the umbilical cord. In this situation, injection should not be carried out, since life-threatening umbilical vein compression may occur. Only if streaming of blood in the vessel can be seen should infusion be continued. While the venipuncturist holds the needle hub and the blood transfusion tubing connector firmly and the ultrasonographer watches the blood flow turbulence in the fetal blood vessel, the transfusionist (the third member of the team) transfuses compatible packed red cells in 10-ml aliquots over one to two minutes until the desired transfusion volume is attained. The usual volume transfused is 50 ml/kg estimated fetal body weight (less if the fetus is hydropic, becomes bradycardiac, or has evidence of marked ventricular dilatation). The fetus tolerates such large transfusion volumes because its circulation is connected to the low-pressure placental vascular bed.

Because there are only 2 or 3 millimeters of needle tip within the fetal blood vessel, which may be as little as 2 to 3 millimeters in diameter, the tip is in great danger of early dislodgement. For this reason, infusion of packed red cells is carried out as rapidly as possible. Red cell infusion rates of 10 ml per 1 to 2 minutes are tolerated quite well. When the volume infused has been reached, the needle is cleared with 0.5 ml of normal saline. A 1-ml post-transfusion blood sample is withdrawn, again into a heparinized tuberculin syringe. The first pretransfusion blood sample is blood grouped and direct Coombs tested. All blood samples, both pre- and post-transfusion, are tested for hemoglobin, hematocrit, bilirubin, Kleihauer fetal adult red cell ratios, plasma protein, and blood gases.

The average increase in circulating donor hemoglobin concentration achieved with each IVT ranges from 5.0 to 10.0 gm/100ml. The usual procedure is to carry out IVT at 2- to 3-day intervals until the final post-IVT hemoglobin concentration is ≥18 gm/100 ml and hematocrit ≥50 per cent. The average donor circulating red cell attrition rate is about 0.4 gm/100 ml per day. Further transfusions are carried out when it is calculated that the donor hemoglobin concentration will have fallen into the 8.0 to 9.0 gm/100 ml range (14 to 28 days). The final transfusion is given at 32 to 36 weeks gestation, with delivery planned at 35½ to 37½ weeks gestation. Because direct IVT volumes by necessity are smaller than IPT volumes, more IVTs will be necessary to bring the fetus to delivery at a reasonable maturity. Whereas rarely if ever are more than four IPTs required to bring a fetus from 21 weeks to 34 weeks gestation, seven or eight IVTs may be required to obtain the same results.

IVT of the Hydropic Fetus

IVT is now the only procedure that should be considered if a fetus is hydropic. It is the only hope for fetal survival if the fetus is moribund and not breathing (Harman et al., 1988a; Menticoglou et al., 1987), because in this situation red cells in the peritoneal cavity are not absorbed. The severely hydropic fetus may be thrombocytopenic and hemorrhage after IVT (Harman et al., 1988b). Platelet concentrates should be available for fetal IVT if necessary.

If venous or arterial access at placental or fetal vessel insertion is impossible and the fetus is moribund and not breathing, cardiac puncture and intracardiac transfusion may be the only possible procedure. Our group has reserved cardiac puncture and transfusion as a last resort when vessel puncture is not possible or fetal hypotension with impaired umbilical blood flow is present. Under ultrasound direction, a 20-gauge spinal needle is introduced into a cardiac chamber, preferably the left or right ventricle, and packed red cells, 30 ml per estimated kilogram of nonhydropic fetal weight, are transfused. Three hydropic fetuses have been "rescued" with intracardiac transfusion; one died despite intracardiac transfusion; in five others the procedure failed. Westgren et al. (1988) report survival of four of six fetuses in whom 25 intracardiac transfusions were carried out because vascular access was not possible.

IUT Hazards

The maternal and fetal risks of IPT and IVT are summarized in Table 44–7.

Maternal infection is avoidable with proper attention to aseptic technique. Some authors recommend the prophylactic use of broad-spectrum antibiotics from 12 hours before to 48 hours after the procedure.

TABLE 44–7. Hazards of IUT

IUT
Maternal
    Infection
    Maternal tissue trauma
IPT
Fetal
    Overtransfusion
    Exsanguination
    Cardiac tamponade
    Infection
    Precipitation of labor
    Graft-versus-host disease
    Radiation damage
    Transient susceptibility to infection
IVT
Fetomaternal
    Fetomaternal TPH
Fetal
    Overtransfusion
    Exsanguination
    Umbilical vein compression
    Cerebral damage
    Graft-versus-host disease

Serious illness may occur if the needle or catheter lodges in maternal tissue. For example, if radiopaque dye is injected into a maternal uterine venous sinus, there is a risk of amniotic fluid embolism. Abruptio placentae, fetal death, maternal shock, and disseminated intravascular coagulation may also occur (Barnes et al., 1965).

SPECIFIC IPT HAZARDS. IPT is also hazardous to the fetus. The risk of overtransfusion has already been described. The other immediate risk is fetal vascular trauma—for example, needle perforation of an artery, major vein, or heart, with death from hemorrhage or cardiac tamponade. The risk of vascular trauma may be reduced by introducing the needle into the peritoneal cavity under direct ultrasonographic guidance, avoiding the placenta when possible, and taking care not to insert the needle too deeply.

Precipitation of labor after IPT is a real risk, occurring in 20 per cent of cases in the Winnipeg Rh Laboratory experience. Fortunately, this does not often occur before 32 weeks gestation. Seventy per cent of babies born following precipitation of labor by IPT in Winnipeg have survived.

GVHD due to donor lymphocyte grafting has been reported (Parkman et al., 1974). Although GVHD following IUT is extremely rare, gamma irradiation of donor red cells to be used for IUT is recommended.

X-ray exposure of the fetus during IPT is significant, up to 3.5 to 4.0 rads (Peddle and Campbell, 1968). Replacing most x-rays now with ultrasonographic examination materially reduces radiation exposure. There are no reports of radiation damage to fetal transfusion survivors. Full knowledge of the radiation hazards of IPT will have to await examination of the next generation. One example of leukemia in a fetal transfusion survivor has been reported (Turner et al., 1974), but this is probably no more than the expected incidence of this disease in a pediatric population.

Transient susceptibility to infection in the first few months of life is a real risk. Acute gram-negative sepsis has occurred, as have acute viral infections of adeno-viral and syncytioviral origin (Bowman, 1978). This hazard appears to be transient, disappearing before the infant is 12 months of age.

SPECIFIC IVT HAZARDS. IVT is surprisingly benign. The risk of exsanguination is low because of the much smaller size of the IVT needle (22- or 20-gauge compared to the 16-gauge IPT needle). Exsanguination almost occurred in one of the IVTs carried out in Winnipeg. On occasion, fetal bleeding into the amniotic fluid does occur owing to inadvertent transfixion of the vessel with the IVT needle. Also, following removal of the needle tip after IVT, bleeding from the vessel usually occurs. In most cases the bleeding is transient, stopping very quickly.

One hazard, which appears to be universal, is that passage of the IVT needle through an anterior placenta into an umbilical vessel is associated with significant fetomaternal TPH and a likelihood of sharply increasing Rh antibody titers. However, this risk simply has to be accepted. It does not further affect the fetus being transfused, since that fetus is already at maximal risk. It has implications as far as the welfare of future fetuses is concerned.

Overtransfusion at IVT is also a hazard but is unlikely to occur with transfusion volumes of 50 ml/kg nonhydropic fetal weight. There has been at least one IVT death caused by overtransfusion. Overtransfusion with consequent hyperviscosity may also cause fetal cerebral damage (Dildy et al., 1991).

The major hazard, which can lead to fetal demise, is the inadvertent injection of blood into the umbilical cord around the umbilical vein, with compression of the vein and compromise of placental fetal umbilical vein blood flow. In one case the fetus had sudden profound bradycardia and was severely asphyxiated at emergency cesarean delivery. Fortunately, the infant survived and is doing well. It is axiomatic that no blood should be injected at IVT unless it can be seen by ultrasound to be streaming into an umbilical blood vessel.

Survival After Fetal Transfusion

There is no doubt that IUT saves lives and represents a major advance in the treatment of maternal blood group alloimmunization. In Winnipeg, prior to the IVT era, 353 alloimmunized women had 863 IPTs carried out. The overall IPT survival rate was 63 per cent (221 fetuses).

In the ultrasound era, 77 fetuses had 204 IPT and 13 fetuses, whose survival was due to IVT not IPT, had a further 18 IPT. These 13 fetuses, plus 98 others, had a total of 451 IVT. The comparative survival rates for IPT and IVT are set out in Table 44–8. As can be seen, survival rates with IVT are significantly better than with IPT (Harman et al., 1990), 86 per cent versus 76 per cent overall; 94 per cent versus 86 per cent for nonhydropic fetuses; 70 per cent versus 60 per cent for hydropic fetuses; 65 per cent (11 of 17) versus 0 (0 of 8) for moribund, nonbreathing, hydropic fetuses. The IVT hydropic survival rates were depressed by failure to refer a known hydropic fetus for 12 days and failure to refer a known hydropic set of twins for 8 days. Many tertiary perinatal centers report similar IVT survival rates.

Table 44-8. Intrauterine Fetal Transfusions (Winnipeg—Ultrasound ERA)

	IPT 204 (July 1980 to October 1986)		IVT 451 (May 1986 to March 1992)	
	Total	Alive (%)	Total	Alive (%)
Fetuses	75	57 (76)	111	96 (86)
Nonhydrops	45	39 (87)	70	66 (94)
Hydrops	30	18 (60)	41	30 (70)
Nonmoribund	22	18 (82)	24	19 (79)
Moribund	8	0 (0)	17	11 (65)

The Pros and Cons of IPT versus IVT

There can be no doubt that IVT, if feasible, is the procedure of choice. What is gratifying is the much lower overall risk with IVT versus IPT (0.8 per cent versus 3.5 per cent per procedure). This is even more dramatically illustrated when the placenta is anterior (0 risk for IVT versus 7 per cent for IPT).

Although the risk of IVT is materially less, this low risk can only be achieved when the obstetrician-ultrasonographer and his or her obstetrician/venipuncturist colleagues have great skill and experience with the procedure. Otherwise there are hazards that will increase the risk of IVT: overtransfusion with cardiac failure; exsanguination (a problem, particularly if the fetus is hydropic and thrombocytopenic and the cord insertion is posterior); and inadvertent injection of blood into the cord around the vein that produces a cord hematoma, compressing and interfering with umbilical blood flow. This third hazard is a real one and has caused fetal deaths. It can be prevented only by an alert and experienced obstetric ultrasonographer.

Despite the great advantages of IVT, there are two situations in which IPT may still be required. Therefore, the skill in carrying out IPT must be maintained. One is the rare situation, early in pregnancy, before 20 to 21 weeks gestation, when the cord vessels may be too small for a successful venipuncture. The other is the more common situation later in pregnancy when (after 30 weeks gestation), after several successful IVTs, increasing fetal size totally obscures a posterior cord vessel insertion, making venipuncture impossible.

Development in Fetal Transfusion Survivors

Physical and intellectual development in most fetal transfusion survivors is normal. Because prematurity may be marked (as early as 29 weeks), however, and residual severity of disease may be great, some problems may be anticipated. In the Winnipeg Rh Laboratory, of 101 children tested at 18 months or later, 87 appeared completely normal, 10 had minor developmental delay—probably transient and due to prematurity—and four were definitely abnormal. One had a normal IQ but spastic hemiparesis; two had IQs of 75 and 85; and the fourth, in whom fetal hydrops had been reversed, had cerebral agenesis that was probably unrelated to the hydrops.

DELIVERY OF THE FETUS WITH HEMOLYTIC DISEASE

Timing and Location

When history, antibody titers, and amniotic fluid Δ OD 450 readings indicate the presence of a mildly affected or unaffected fetus, delivery should be allowed to occur spontaneously. Delivery may take place in a regional perinatal center or a well-equipped community hospital, provided that the necessary personnel and facilities are available to monitor cord and infant blood parameters and to carry out exchange transfusions if necessary. Facilities for fetal heart rate monitoring should be available if labor is being induced.

The severely affected infant with hemolytic disease, who often has undergone fetal transfusions and requires early delivery, needs antenatal and postnatal facilities of the highest order. Such a baby should be delivered in a tertiary-level perinatal center where personnel and resources are available to manage a very sick, premature, possibly hydropic neonate.

If the placenta is not anterior and if serial Δ OD 450 readings indicate the need for intervention at 33 to 34 weeks gestation (IUT or delivery), amniotic fluid should be examined for pulmonary maturity (lecithin-sphingomyelin ratio greater than 2:1 or presence of phosphatidyl glycerol and/or stable foam in amniotic fluid). If the lungs are mature, delivery should be carried out. If they are not mature, fetal transfusion then and again possibly in 10 days with delivery at 35½ to 37 weeks is a recommended alternative. If the placenta is anterior, delivery may be carried out at 34 to 35 weeks or a direct IVT should be performed. No fetus who has undergone intrauterine transfusion should remain undelivered after 38 weeks provided gestational age is accurate.

Mode of Delivery

Once delivery is elected, the method must be decided on. The pros and cons of elective cesarean section versus trial of induction with cesarean section only if the fetus shows signs of distress have been debated. If for any reason delivery must take place prior to 32 weeks gestation, or if the fetus is in a breech position, cesarean section, preferably using epidural anesthesia, is the recommended method. In other circumstances, a trial of labor induction with vaginal delivery is appropriate, and is successful in 80 per cent of cases. Careful fetal heart rate monitoring is mandatory. If labor has not begun within 24 hours of rupture of the membranes, cesarean section should be performed.

The fetal heart rate should be monitored continuously, initially by external tocodynamometry, and subsequently by fetal scalp electrode with simultaneous recording of uterine contractions. If fetal heart rate parameters indicate distress, scalp blood pH should be determined. If fetal heart rate readings and pH demonstrate fetal distress and if immediate vaginal delivery is impossible, the baby should be delivered by prompt cesarean section. Sinusoidal heart rate patterns have been reported in anemic fetuses (Verma et al., 1980).

Every effort should be made to ensure adequate oxygenation and optimal fetal condition during labor and delivery. After delivery, the cord should be clamped promptly, and 10 to 15 ml of heparinized blood should be obtained. Immediate gentle, thorough suction of the baby's oropharynx and nasopharynx is carried out, and the infant is then promptly given into the care of an expert neonatologist. Management of these commonly very ill, premature erythroblastotic infants may tax the resources of the most highly developed tertiary-level neonatal intensive care unit.

SUPPRESSION OF Rh IMMUNIZATION

Since the mid-1940s, attempts have been made to suppress the strength of already developed maternal Rh immunization. The benefit of Rh-positive red cell stroma touted by Bierme and associates (1979) has been refuted by Gold and colleagues (1983). The value of administration of promethazine hydrochloride put forward by Gusdon and co-workers (1976) has not been confirmed by others, including ourselves. Similarly, administration of Rh immune globulin (RhIG), of great value in Rh prevention, has been shown to be quite ineffective in suppressing Rh immunization, no matter how weak, once Rh immunization has begun (Bowman and Pollock, 1984).

The two suppressive modalities of some benefit in reducing maternal antibody levels are intensive plasma exchange (Graham-Pole et al., 1977; Robinson and Tovey, 1980) and administration of intravenous immune serum globulin (IGIV) (Berlin et al., 1985; Margulies et al., 1991). With intensive plasma exchange (10 to 20 liters weekly), maternal alloantibody can be reduced as much as 75 per cent. However, after 6 to 8 weeks, even with continued plasma exchange, antibody levels tend to rebound. Venous access often becomes a problem, with the need for placement of arteriovenous shunts. The plasma removed must be replaced, at least partially, with blood fractions (albumin and IGIV) in order to reduce antibody feedback rebound and to keep maternal serum albumin and IgG at adequate levels (>3gm/dl and >300 mg/dl, respectively). Plasma exchange is tedious, costly, and uncomfortable. It is not without minor risk to the mother, including bacterial sepsis, particularly

if arteriovenous shunts have to be placed. The only expectation with the use of intensive plasma exchange is that fetal treatment measures may be delayed until the fetus is greater than 22 to 24 weeks gestation.

The institution of plasma exchange should never preclude or delay the use of definitive investigative procedures such as amniocentesis or fetal blood sampling. Plasma exchange should be reserved for the mother who has a husband homozygous for the antigen to which she is immunized and who has a prior history of hydrops, at or before 24 to 26 weeks gestation. In this situation, intensive plasma exchange should be begun at 10 to 12 weeks gestation when transfer of maternal IgG is beginning, with initial amniocentesis at 18 weeks gestation and/or fetal blood sampling at 19 to 22 weeks gestation.

There have been reports of the benefits of high-dose IGIV administration in severely alloimmunized pregnant women, (Berlin et al., 1985; Margulies et al., 1991). With doses of 2 gm/kg maternal body weight, circulating maternal alloantibody levels can be reduced by as much as 50 per cent, primarily as a result of the negative feedback produced by total circulating maternal IgG levels of 2.5 to 3 gm/dl, readily achieved by a dose of 2 gm/kg body weight. Further benefits of IGIV therapy may be due to interference with transfer of maternal antibody across the placenta by trophoblastic FC receptor saturation and, similarly, reduction of IgG-coated fetal red cell hemolysis by fetal reticuloendothelial FC receptor saturation with the injected IGIV.

If IGIV therapy is considered, it should be used only in the same situation as intensive plasma exchange, again beginning at 10 to 12 weeks gestation. The recommended dose is 400 mg/kg maternal body weight daily for 5 days, repeated at 3-week intervals, depending upon amniotic fluid and/or fetal blood sampling assessment of fetal disease and the need for definitive fetal therapy. This form of therapy can no longer be considered experimental and has been shown to be of transient benefit, again delaying the need for fetal blood sampling and fetal transfusions until 22 to 24 weeks gestation.

PREVENTION OF Rh IMMUNIZATION

Whereas attempts to suppress Rh immunization have been of questionable value, there can be no doubt that the development of a means of preventing Rh immunization altogether represents a major advance in the management of the pregnant Rh-negative woman. Von Dungern (1900) proved the axiom that formed the basis for Rh prophylaxis 65 years later. He injected a group of rabbits with red cells from an ox. The rabbits obligingly produced ox red cell antibodies. When he injected a second group of rabbits with red cells from the same ox and then gave them sera from the first group of rabbits (containing ox red cell antibodies), the second group of rabbits did not develop ox red cell antibodies. He proved that active immunization to an antigen is prevented by the presence of passive antibody to the antigen. It has been known for many years that the immune response of infants in the first 2 or 3 months of life to diphtheria and tetanus toxoid is poor because of the presence of transplacentally acquired maternal diphtheria and tetanus antitoxin. Suppression of the immune response in these infants is dose-related and can be overcome to some extent if large doses of toxoid are administered.

Trials of Prevention

More than 60 years after Von Dungern's report, the information he provided was first put to use almost simultaneously in New York (Freda et al., 1964) and Liverpool (Clarke et al., 1963) and shortly thereafter in Winnipeg (Zipursky et al., 1967). Initially, experiments were carried out by giving Rh-negative male volunteers Rh-positive red cells coated with Rh antibody (Stern et al., 1961). When Rh immunization did not occur, the volunteers were given Rh-positive red cells followed by Rh antibody in the form of high-titer plasma or Rh immune globulin (RhIG or anti-D IgG). In every experiment, Rh immunization was prevented by administration of Rh antibody.

Clinical trials were then undertaken whereby Rh-negative, unimmunized women were given RhIG intramuscularly following delivery of an Rh-positive baby. All such Rh prevention trials were highly successful in preventing Rh immunization when RhIG was given within 72 hours postpartum (Table 44–9) (Chown et al., 1969).

Rh immune globulin has been licensed since 1968 in North America, where one standard prophylactic dose is about 300 μg, given intramuscularly. Smaller doses, 100 to 125 μg, are standard in Europe and Australia and are just about as effective.

It is almost certain that RhIG always prevents Rh immunization from developing, with two provisos: the agent must be administered before Rh immunization has begun, and it must be given in adequate dosage. The exact mechanism by which Rh antibody given passively prevents Rh immunization is unknown. IgM probably does not, as was once thought, enhance Rh immunization, but it has little if any preventive effect.

Initial Recommendations for Rh Prophylaxis

The clinical protocols in successful Rh prophylaxis trials were based on injection of RhIG within 72 hours after delivery, the interval needed in some instances for cord blood findings to be assessed. Initial recommendations after licensure were the same, i.e., that every Rh-negative woman without evidence of Rh immunization was to be given one prophylactic dose of RhIG intramuscularly within 72 hours after delivering an Rh-positive baby. Because the protection conferred on the fetus by ABO incompatibility is only partial, women delivering Rh-positive babies, irrespective of their ABO status, were to be afforded protection.

Since there are rare but undoubted instances of Rh immunization occurring after delivery, but before 72 hours after delivery (Bowman et al., 1978), the present recommendation is to give RhIG as soon after delivery as cord blood findings indicate the baby to be Rh-positive and the mother to be at risk. If for any reason cord blood findings are not known 72 hours after delivery, the mother should be given RhIG with the understanding that in about one-third of such cases the baby will subsequently be shown to be Rh-negative and the mother not to be at risk. It is preferable to treat a woman unnecessarily than to fail to treat a woman who then becomes Rh-sensitized. Conversely, if a woman at risk is inadvertently not given RhIG within 72 hours after delivery, prophylaxis should not be withheld but should be given, at least up to 14 days after delivery. (In the Winnipeg Rh Laboratory, the recommendation is to give treatment up to 21 to 28 days after delivery.) Experimentally, it has been shown that some protection is afforded after RhIG is given 13 days after exposure to Rh-positive red cells (Samson and Mollison, 1975). It should, however, be understood that if prophylaxis after delivery is delayed it may not be effective.

Remaining Problems in Rh Immunization Prophylaxis

Rh disease prevention programs have been in place for 25 years. They have been very successful, but they

TABLE 44–9. Western Canadian Rh Immunization Prevention Trial (March 1, 1967, to January 31, 1968)

TREATMENT AND PARITY	NUMBER OF PATIENTS IN TRIAL*	PATIENTS Rh-IMMUNIZED 6–9 MONTHS LATER	
		NUMBER	**%**
RhIG, 145–435 μg, given within 72 hours postpartum			
Primiparas	481	0	0
Multiparas	735	0	0
Total	1216	0	0
No treatment			
Primiparas	203	18	8.9
Multiparas	297	18	6.1
Total	500	36	7.2

*Only Rh-negative women who had just produced ABO-compatible, Rh-positive babies were entered in the trial.
Adapted from Chown B, Duff AM, James J, et al: Prevention of primary Rh immunization. First report of the Western Canadian Trial. Can Med Assoc J **100**:1021, 1969.

have not yet eradicated Rh immunization. Some of the problems that remain to be solved are as follows (Table 44–10).

REACTIONS TO Rh IMMUNE GLOBULIN. In most countries, RhIG is prepared by the cold ethanol process developed by Cohn in 1940. RhIG prepared by this method has been highly effective and has had a very low reaction rate. It does have modest amounts of IgA and IgM and traces of other plasma proteins, however. Some previously treated women develop transient skin rashes and pain and swelling at the injection site after a subsequent injection. Severe anaphylaxis has been reported on at least one occasion (Rivat et al., 1970). Because it is anticomplementary, RhIG prepared by the Cohn method cannot be given intravenously. The yield of anti-D in RhIG prepared by this method is only 40 to 50 per cent of that in the starting plasma.

Hoppe and colleagues (1973) have produced RhIG by an ion exchange column method using DEAE Sephadex. The method has been adapted for use in North America, and an ion exchange–prepared RhIG is now licensed for use in Canada (Bowman et al., 1980). The RhIG that results is very pure, with a low total protein content and no demonstrable contaminating IgA or IgM. It has a very low anticomplementary activity and can be given safely intravenously. The efficiency of yield is 85 per cent. RhIG given intravenously is twice as effective, microgram for microgram, as RhIG given intramuscularly. Therefore, a postdelivery dose of 120 μg IV is as protective as 250 to 300 μg IM. Clinical trials and subsequent service programs have shown ion exchange–prepared RhIG to be at least as successful in preventing Rh immunization as the cold ethanol–prepared agent. Its advantages are greater purity and therefore less likelihood of reaction; less discomfort; greater economy because column preparation is less expensive, efficiency of yield is greater, and a lower dose is used. Ion exchange–prepared RhIG has two minor disadvantages. First, because of its great purity, its total protein content is so low that it is unstable in solution and must be prepared in a lyophilized form, which requires reconstitution with 0.9 per cent sterile saline before injection. Second, although it can be given intramuscularly, the higher efficiency is present only when it is given intravenously, a minor inconvenience for the administrator.

FAILURE TO GIVE TREATMENT AFTER DELIVERY. The

TABLE 44–10. Remaining Problems in Prevention of Rh Immunization

Allergic reactions to RhIG
Failure to give treatment after delivery of Rh-positive baby
Failure to give treatment after abortion
Failure to give treatment after amniocentesis
Failure of RhIG to confer protection (because of massive transplacental hemorrhage or inadvertent Rh-positive transfusion)
Occurrence of Rh immunization late in pregnancy or soon after delivery, before prophylaxis is given
Occurrence of Rh immunization during infancy ("grandmother theory")
Very weak Rh antibody in an Rh-negative woman

---

occasional Rh-negative woman is still left unprotected after delivery of an Rh-positive baby. A blood sample should be taken and tested from every pregnant woman at the beginning of each pregnancy. If she is Rh-negative she should be retested regularly. Cord blood must be examined to determine the Rh status of the baby and therefore the need for Rh prophylaxis. If the baby is Rh-positive and is ABO-incompatible with the mother, and the baby's cord blood red cells are weakly direct antiglobulin (Coombs)–positive, RhIG should not be withheld from the mother. The baby has ABO erythroblastosis, which confers only partial protection against Rh immunization (residual 1.5 to 2 per cent risk).

There are several reasons for the failure to give postdelivery Rh prophylaxis. The mother may not have sought prenatal care. The physician may have neglected to have prenatal blood samples tested. The hospital obstetric unit may not have sent postdelivery cord and maternal blood samples to the laboratory for blood grouping and antibody screening. It is essential that the physician giving obstetric care know who his or her Rh-negative pregnant patients are. If they are unimmunized, the physician must make sure that they are given Rh prophylaxis after they deliver Rh-positive babies.

FAILURE TO GIVE TREATMENT AFTER ABORTION. The Rh-negative woman who has an abortion, either spontaneous or therapeutic, is at a 2 to 4 per cent risk of becoming Rh-sensitized. Because hospitalization may be very brief and there is less time for blood grouping studies, her Rh status, particularly at the time of spontaneous abortion, may not be known. The physician managing the woman who aborts must know her Rh status and, if she is Rh-negative, must ensure that she is given RhIG. Failure to protect the Rh-negative teenager undergoing therapeutic abortion may have tragic consequences, i.e., a severely affected hydropic fetus in the next pregnancy. Because transplacental hemorrhage after spontaneous abortion is usually small, smaller doses of RhIG (50 μg), if available, will be protective. If an Rh-negative woman has an antepartum hemorrhage (threatened abortion), she should be given 300 μg of RhIG, and this dose should be repeated every 12 weeks if her pregnancy continues.

FAILURE TO GIVE TREATMENT AFTER AMNIOCENTESIS AND CHORIONIC VILLUS SAMPLING. When the placenta is implanted on the anterior uterine wall, there is a very considerable risk that it will be traversed at amniocentesis, with a consequent transplacental hemorrhage (Peddle, 1968). In the unimmunized Rh-negative woman undergoing amniocentesis in early pregnancy for genetic investigation or in late pregnancy for determination of fetal pulmonary maturity, the resulting transplacental hemorrhage will place her at risk of Rh immunization. Placental localization reduces the risk of TPH to 2.5 per cent (Bowman and Pollock, 1985), but does not remove it completely. For this reason, all Rh-negative, unimmunized women undergoing amniocentesis at any stage of gestation should be given RhIG prophylaxis. Because the RhIG given must exert its protective effect over several weeks, the dose of RhIG given at the time of amniocentesis should be 300 μg. Despite the concerns of some investigators, RhIG given at the time of amniocentesis will not harm the conceptus, as evidenced by the several thousand normal infants born after antenatal Rh prophylaxis. Similarly, chorionic villus sampling carries a significant risk of TPH and requires similar protection. Again the RhIG dose should be repeated every 12 weeks until delivery.

FAILURE OF RhIG TO CONFER PROTECTION

After Massive TPH. The protection afforded by RhIG is dose-dependent. Pollack and associates (1971a) showed experimentally that one prophylactic dose (300 μg) will prevent Rh sensitization to an exposure of as much as 30 ml of Rh-positive blood (12 to 15 ml of Rh-positive red cells). With greater exposure, there is only partial protection. The immunization rate following exposure to 30 to 450 ml of blood and administration of 300 μg of Cohn-prepared RhIG is about 30 per cent (Pollack et al., 1971b). Since only 0.24 per cent of gravidas (as calculated in one series) are exposed to TPH in excess of 30 ml of blood, the Rh immunization rate due to failure to diagnose massive TPH and the consequent routine administration of only 300 μg of anti-D is 0.07 per cent. Although TPH screening at delivery is recommended, failure to diagnose and treat massive TPH is a rare cause of failure of Rh prophylaxis.

Massive transplacental hemorrhage may occur during the latter part of pregnancy but is more common at the time of delivery. If it is diagnosed after delivery of an Rh-positive infant, the following dosage of RhIG is recommended: one vial (300 μg) if the TPH is 25 ml of blood or less; two vials (600 μg) if TPH is between 25 and 50 ml; three vials (900 μg) if TPH is between 50 and 75 ml, and so on. Up to 4 vials (1200 μg) may be given intramuscularly every 12 hours until the total required dose has been given.

On the rare occasion when massive TPH is diagnosed during pregnancy (almost always in the third trimester), three factors must be considered, the risk of Rh immunization, the risk of fetal exsanguination, and the risk that RhIG administered maternally may cross the placenta and destroy the red cells of the Rh-positive fetus.

If massive TPH is found and the fetus is likely to be Rh-positive, 600 μg of RhIG may be given without hazard to the Rh-positive fetus. Larger doses may be safe, but there is no evidence that they are. If the amount of hemorrhage is greater than 50 ml of blood, there is a risk of fetal exsanguination and maternal Rh immunization. If the fetal red cells clear completely and passive anti-D is present after injection of RhIG, Rh immunization of the mother and exsanguination of the fetus is unlikely. If fetal red cells persist or if the original TPH is greater than 100 ml, there is a great risk of maternal Rh immunization and fetal exsanguination. In such cases the fetus should be delivered promptly as long as there is evidence of pulmonary maturity. Immediately after delivery, the infant should be examined for evidence of fetal hemorrhage and shock and transfused if necessary; if the infant is Rh-positive, more RhIG should be given to the mother according to the size of TPH as already discussed.

If the husband is most likely heterozygous for D, the fetus may be either Rh-negative, with the only risk being to the fetus, or Rh-positive, with the three risks previously listed. In this situation, one or two vials of RhIG should be given to the mother depending on the size of the TPH (less or more than 25 ml of blood). If there is no change in the amount of fetal blood circulating in the mother 48 to 72 hours after injection and if passive anti-D is present, the fetus is probably Rh-negative. The pregnancy should be allowed to continue provided (1) the TPH is less than 100 ml of blood, (2) the TPH is not increasing, and (3) fetal assessment reveals an uncompromised fetus. If partial or complete clearing of fetal red cells occurs, the fetus is most likely Rh-positive, and the risk of fetal exsanguination is very high. Management of the mother and newborn as described in the previous paragraph is mandatory.

After Inadvertent Rh-Positive Transfusion. When an Rh-negative woman is inadvertently transfused with large volumes of Rh-positive blood—greater than two units (900 ml)—caution should be used when attempting to prevent Rh immunization because of the risk of severe anemia. The total dose of RhIG should be calculated and given (1200 μg every 12 hours for the Cohn preparation IM, 300 μg every 8 hours for the ion exchange preparation IV), until the total required dose has been administered. If the inadvertent transfusion of Rh-positive blood exceeds two units (900 ml), no attempt should be made to prevent Rh immunization if the patient is past her childbearing years. If Rh prevention is required, a 1.5 blood volume exchange transfusion using cross-matched, ABO-compatible, Rh-negative blood should be carried out. The exchange transfusion will remove 75 per cent of the circulating Rh-positive red cells and provide an adequate number of additional Rh-negative red cells to prevent post–RhIG anemia. The total dose of RhIG necessary is 25 per cent of the volume of Rh-positive blood transfused. It should be administered at the doses and intervals previously listed. Differential agglutination and passive anti-D measurements should be carried out 72 to 96 hours after the last dose of RhIG has been given to ensure, as far as possible, that the patient is protected.

OCCURRENCE OF Rh IMMUNIZATION LATE IN PREGNANCY OR SOON AFTER DELIVERY. Rh immunization occurring in the latter part of pregnancy or within 3 days after delivery, and therefore too early to be prevented by postdelivery prophylaxis, is an important cause of persisting Rh sensitization (see Table 44-3). In Manitoba, from March 1967 to December 1974, 62 of 3533 (1.8 per cent) Rh-negative women, either primigravidas or multigravidas, who were given Rh prophylaxis after every preceding abortion and Rh-positive delivery were found to be Rh-immunized during the latter part of pregnancy or within 3 days after delivery, five of these prior to 28 weeks gestation (Bowman et al., 1978). Exactly similar findings have been reported from Hamilton, Ontario, Canada, and from Sweden (Zipursky and Blajchman, 1979; Bartsch and Sandberg, 1979; Hermann and Kjellman, 1979). Eklund and Nevalinna (1979) report a lower incidence (0.71 per cent) in Finland; however, the overall incidences of Rh negativity and of Rh immunization are lower in Finland. Although no statistics are available with respect to the incidence of Rh immunization during pregnancy in the United States, it does occur (Scott et al., 1977), and there is no reason to expect the incidence to be any less there than in Canada or Sweden.

Rh immunization during pregnancy constitutes 12 to 13 per cent of all instances of Rh immunization if no prophylaxis of any sort is given. In the Manitoba experience, it has been the single most important cause of persisting Rh immunization, accounting for 69 (41 per cent) of the 167 Rh-immunized pregnancies encountered in the 3-year period ending October 31, 1976.

A clinical trial of Rh prophylaxis in which 300 μg of Cohn-prepared RhIG were given at 28 and 34 weeks gestation was very successful, reducing the incidence of Rh immunization during pregnancy from 1.8 to 0.1 per cent (Bowman et al., 1978).

An antenatal Rh prophylaxis service program in which one dose of 300 μg of Cohn-prepared RhIG or one dose of 300 μg of ion exchange–prepared RhIG was given, was equally successful (Table 44–11) (Bowman and Pollock, 1978; Bowman et al., 1980). Antenatal Rh prophylaxis at 28 weeks gestation is now highly recommended and is the accepted standard of Rh prophylactic care in North America.

Administration of RhIG to the mother during pregnancy carries no risk to her fetus. If doses are given at 28 weeks and again at 34 weeks, 35 per cent of babies will have Coombs-positive cord red cells but will show no signs of anemia or hyperbilirubinemia. If one injection is given at 28 weeks gestation, no babies will have cord red cells that are Coombs-positive.

OCCURRENCE OF Rh IMMUNIZATION DURING INFANCY ("GRANDMOTHER THEORY"). It has been theorized that transplacental passage of Rh-positive maternal red cells into the fetus at the time of delivery may produce Rh immunization in infancy (the so-called Grandmother Theory) (Taylor, 1967). Sixty per cent of mothers of Rh-negative babies are Rh-positive. Early studies using cord blood purporting to show a high incidence of maternal-fetal transplacental hemorrhage were refuted by Cohen and Zuelzer (1965). The true

incidence is less than 2 per cent and the volume is usually very small, equivalent to 0.005 ml of a fetal-maternal bleed. There is one report of a massive bidirectional maternal-fetal–fetal-maternal TPH with fetal polycythemia, heart failure, and hydrops (Bowman et al., 1984). The reports of astoundingly high incidences of Rh immunization in infancy—11 per cent (Bowen and Renfield, 1976) and 22.2 per cent (Carapella-de Luca et al., 1978)—have not been substantiated (Bernard et al., 1977).

If maternal-fetal TPH and neonatal Rh sensitization were the reason that Rh immunization appears in a first Rh-positive pregnancy, using the above figures we would expect the incidence of such immunization to be between 6.6 and 13.3 per cent, rather than the 1.8 per cent noted in Manitoba (Bowman et al., 1978). Antenatal Rh prophylaxis should not have been successful in these already sensitized women. In actual fact, the incidence was reduced to 0.1 per cent. Rh immunization of an Rh-negative neonate must be very rare; it is less than 0.1 per cent of Rh-negative babies born of Rh-positive mothers. Prophylactic treatment of Rh-negative infants delivered of Rh-positive mothers is not indicated.

VERY WEAK Rh ANTIBODY IN AN Rh-NEGATIVE WOMAN. The occasional Rh-negative woman will be found to have a very weak Rh antibody, detectable only by AutoAnalyzer (AA) or by AA and manual enzyme technique. In one series studied in Manitoba, 87 per cent (206 of 236) of Rh-negative women with only AA-detectable Rh antibody showed no progression of Rh immunization despite delivering Rh-positive babies. Women with such weak anti-D only may not be truly Rh-immunized, and they should be given the benefit of prophylaxis.

The woman who has an anti-D demonstrable by AA and manual enzyme technique but not by indirect antiglobulin (Coombs) methods is in a quite different position. Attempts to prevent progression of Rh immunization in these women by administration of RhIG at 6-week intervals until delivery have been unsuccessful; 21 of 36 women treated in this manner went on to fully developed Rh immunization and gave birth to babies with hemolytic disease (Bowman and Pollock, 1984). Rh prophylaxis of women in whom anti-D is detectable by manual enzyme methods is not recommended. If the manual enzyme technique shows an extremely weak or equivocal antibody response, however, Rh prophylaxis is advised, with the clear understanding that it may not be effective.

Current Recommendations for Prevention of Rh Disease

1. Every Rh-negative, unimmunized woman who delivers an Rh-positive baby should be given one prophylactic dose of RhIG as soon after delivery as possible, irrespective of the ABO status of her baby.

2. Every Rh-negative, unimmunized woman who aborts should be given at least 50 μg of RhIG unless the father of the conceptus is known to be Rh-negative. If antepartum hemorrhage (threatened abortion) occurs, 300 mcg of RhIG should be given and repeated every 12 weeks if the pregnancy continues.

TABLE 44–11.   Results of Antepartum Rh Prophylaxis, Manitoba, December 1, 1968 to May 31, 1981

Total number of Rh-negative women given antepartum prophylaxis	9423
Number who delivered Rh-positive babies	6517
Women in whom Rh immunization was expected at delivery	104
Those in whom Rh immunization was observed	4*
Women who were reexamined 6 months after delivery	4148
Those in whom Rh immunization was expected	56
Those in whom Rh immunization was observed	2†
Antepartum prophylaxis protection rate	94%

*3 were multigravidas not treated antepartum in a previous pregnancy.
†Both were primigravidas with Rh-positive mothers.

3. Every Rh-negative, unimmunized woman undergoing amniocentesis or chorionic villus sampling should be given one prophylactic dose of RhIG unless the father of the conceptus is known to be Rh-negative. The dose should be repeated every 12 weeks until delivery.

4. One prophylactic dose of RhIG (300 μg) should be given to the Rh-negative, unimmunized pregnant woman at 28 weeks gestation unless the father of the conceptus is known to be Rh-negative. If delivery has not occurred within 12½ weeks of the injection, a second dose should be given antenatally, but it need not be repeated postpartum unless the interval between the second injection and delivery is greater than 3 weeks.

5. If massive transplacental hemorrhage of Rh-positive fetal red cells into an Rh-negative, unimmunized woman is diagnosed after delivery, one prophylactic dose of RhIG should be given for every 25 ml of fetal blood or fraction thereof in the maternal circulation. If massive TPH is diagnosed before delivery, the same management is advised, except that if the TPH exceeds 50 ml, prompt delivery of the infant should be carried out as soon as pulmonary maturity permits; if anemic, the infant should be treated, and further Rh prophylaxis of the mother should be undertaken.

6. One vial of RhIG should be given following delivery of an Rh-positive baby to the Rh-negative woman in whom Rh antibody is detectable only by AA method. Administration of RhIG to the Rh-negative woman in whom Rh antibody is demonstrable by a manual enzyme method as well will be ineffective but should be carried out if there is any doubt about the validity or specificity of the enzyme reactions.

Non-Rh(D) Blood Group Immunization

With the decrease in prevalence of Rh immunization that has occurred owing to Rh prevention programs, non-Rh(D) blood group immunization is becoming a relatively more common and more important cause of hemolytic disease of the fetus and newborn. ABO hemolytic disease and non-Rh(D) non-ABO hemolytic disease will both be considered.

ABO HEMOLYTIC DISEASE. ABO hemolytic disease is quite different from Rh hemolytic disease and other non-Rh(D) hemolytic disease. It should be managed differently. Anti-A and anti-B, which bind complement in adults, produce violent life-threatening intravascular hemolysis after transfusion of ABO-incompatible blood. ABO hemolytic disease is much milder than Rh, c, Kell, and some other forms of "atypical" hemolytic disease. Although kernicterus may develop if the baby with ABO hemolytic disease is left untreated, hydrops rarely, if ever, occurs and anemia at birth is rarely more than moderate.

There are extremely rare reports of severe hemolytic disease, even on occasion hydrops fetalis, due to ABO erythroblastosis (Miller and Petrie, 1963; Cox et al., 1991; Gilja and Shah, 1988). However, in 35 years experience, encompassing in excess of 600,000 deliveries, 120,000 of which were ABO-incompatible, I have never seen a proven instance of severe anemia (≤9.0 gm/100 ml) or hydrops due to ABO erythroblastosis.

Several reasons can be listed for the paradoxical mildness of ABO hemolytic disease. First, there are a smaller number of A and B antigenic sites on the fetal red cell membrane. Second, anti-A and anti-B are mostly IgM, which does not traverse the placenta. Also, anti-A and anti-B do not bind complement on the fetal red cell membrane (Brouwers et al., 1988). Third, the small amounts of IgG anti-A and anti-B that do cross the placenta have myriad antigenic sites other than red cells—other tissues and secretions—to which they may bind. Only a very small proportion of the minor amount of anti-A or anti-B that crosses the placenta adheres to antigen on the red cell membrane. Because there is very little antibody on the red cell, the cord blood direct antiglobulin test in ABO hemolytic disease is only weakly positive and may be negative, unless a sensitive test is used. Not infrequently, capillary blood taken when the infant is 2 or 3 days old yields a negative result no matter how sensitive the test used.

ABO hemolytic disease, which commonly occurs in the first pregnancy, is not a problem for the obstetrician because there is minimal if any risk of hydrops fetalis or severe anemia at birth. Amniocentesis and early delivery are not indicated. Anti-A and anti-B titers are of little value in predicting the likelihood of clinical ABO hemolytic disease before delivery.

In about 25 to 30 per cent of ABO-incompatible babies, cord blood red cells are weakly direct antiglobulin (Coombs)–positive at delivery. Only a small fraction of these infants develop clinical evidence of hemolytic disease (early and severe jaundice). In one hospital from 1954 to 1965, of 9000 ABO-incompatible babies delivered, 2500 had weakly direct antiglobulin-positive red cells and only 41 (less than 2 per cent) required exchange transfusion (Bowman, 1977). Management of ABO erythroblastosis is a pediatric problem involving the appropriate management of hyperbilirubinemia and the prevention of kernicterus.

NON-Rh(D) NON-ABO HEMOLYTIC DISEASE. Non-D non-ABO alloimmunization is frequently produced by a blood transfusion, since so-called compatible blood transfusions are only ABO and D compatible. Transfused red cells have many antigens that are missing in the recipient. Following blood transfusion, 1 to 2 per cent of recipients develop "atypical" blood group antibodies. Many are weak, mostly IgM, and do not produce hemolytic disease, for example anti-Le[a], anti-Le[b], and anti-P. Some, such as anti-M, anti-N, and anti-S, rarely produce clinical problems. Others are quite capable of producing hemolytic disease as severe as anti-D.

Mollison et al. (1987) list the following "atypical" alloantibodies as having been reported to cause hemolytic disease: (1) within the Rh system: anti-c, -C, -C[w], -C[x], -e, -E, -E[w], -ce, -Ce[s], -Rh32, -Go[a], -Be[a], -Evans, -LW; (2) outside the Rh system: anti-K, -k, -K[u], Kp[a], -Kp[b], -Js[a], -Js[b], -Fy[a], -Fy[3], -Jk[a], -Jk[b], -M, -N, -S, -s, -U, -Vw, -Far, -M[v], -Mit, -Mt[a], -Mur, -Hil, -Hut, -En[a], -PP₁p[k], -Lu[a], -Lu[b], -Lu[9], -Di[a], -Di[b], -Yt[a], -Yt[b], -Do[a], -Co[a], -Wr[a]; (3) antibodies to low-incidence antigens: anti-Bi, -By, -Fr[a], -Good, -Rd, -Re[a], -Zd; and (4) antibodies to high-incidence antigens: anti-At[a], -Jr[a], -Lan, -Ge. They state that of all the multitude of antibodies implicated in producing HDN, those reported to produce moderate to severe hemolytic dis-

TABLE 44–12.   Severity of Hemolytic Disease: Manitoba—26 Years (November 1, 1962 to October 31, 1988), Except for Anti-D (November 1, 1975 to October 31, 1988)

ALLOANTIBODY SPECIFICITY	NO. OF PATIENTS	AFFECTED (%)	% NO TREATMENT REQUIRED	% PHOTOTHERAPY AND/OR EXCHANGE TRANSFUSION REQUIRED	% SB HYDROPIC OR HgB <60 gm/l
D (13 yrs)	420	201 (48)	49	32	19
E	350	108 (31)	88	12	—
c, cE	183	119 (65)	62	29	9*
C, Ce, C^w	108	34 (32)	79	21	—
Kell	337	8 (2.4)	75	25	—
Kp^a	6	2 (33)	50	50	—
k	1	1 (100)		100	—
Fy^a	23	5 (22)	80	20	—
S	14	8 (57)	75	25	—

SB = stillborn.
*Anti-c, other than D, was the only cause of hydrops in Manitoba patients in the 26 year period.
From Bowman JM: Treatment options for the fetus with alloimmune hemolytic disease. Transf Med Rev **4**:191, 1990.

ease are all of those in the Rh blood group system plus anti-K, -Jk^a, -Js^a, -Js^b, -Ku, -Fy^a, -M, -N, -s, -U, -PP$_1$P^k, -Di^b, -Lan, -LW, -Far, -Good, -Wr^a, -Zd.

This list appears intimidating, but attention must be paid to the frequency with which such antibodies occur and the frequency with which they cause significant hemolytic disease of the newborn. The numbers of patients referred to Winnipeg with non-Rh(D) alloimmunization for assessment for fetal transfusion have increased from two in the 10-year period ending December 31, 1973 to 19 in the 10-year period ending October 31, 1988. The non-D alloantibodies observed in pregnant Manitoban women during the 26-year period ending October 31, 1988 are listed in Tables 44–12 and 44–13. Although anti-E and anti-Kell were the most common (350 and 337 respectively), only 13 of the 108 affected infants (cord red cells direct antiglobulin-positive) due to anti-E and only two of the eight affected infants due to anti-Kell required exchange transfusion and/or phototherapy. None of them was severely affected. Anti-c, when present, was more likely to cause hemolytic disease (65 per cent

versus 31 per cent and 2.4 per cent for anti-E and anti-Kell), and in those affected it was more likely to cause disease requiring exchange transfusion and/or phototherapy (29 per cent versus 12 per cent and 25 per cent for anti-E and Kell). Anti-c was the only non-D alloantibody in the 26-year period that caused disease so severe that it ended in hydropic stillbirth, fetuses requiring intrauterine transfusions, or infants born with cord hemoglobin levels less than 60gm/l (6 gm/dl).

In a more recent study of Kell alloimmunization in Manitoban women encompassing the years 1944 to 1992, 23 infants born of Kell alloimmunized mothers were Kell-positive and affected with hemolytic disease. Thirteen of the 23 were so mildly affected that they required no treatment. Five were moderately affected and required either exchange transfusion or phototherapy. Five were severely affected (four born before 1955); three were hydropic and died; one, left untreated in a rural hospital, developed kernicterus and died, one severely hydropic at 21 weeks gestation survived following eight intrauterine transfusions.

Anti-C, -Ce, -C^w, -Kp^a, -k, -Fy^a, and -S (Table 44–12) on rare occasions caused hemolytic disease severe enough to require treatment after birth, but in no instance was disease so severe that hydrops developed or that fetal transfusions were required. Other blood group antibodies in these pregnant Manitoban patients (Table 44–13) produced either no clinical disease or mild clinical disease that did not require treatment.

The experience of the Rh Laboratory in Winnipeg over the past 29 years with 27 pregnant non-D alloimmunized women referred from outside of Manitoba, a highly selected group with very severely affected fetuses, drawn from a much greater population base, is somewhat different (Table 44–14). In these referred women there were examples of the following antibodies: Kell (13), c (8), k (1), Jk^a, Fy^a, CC^w, cE, and E (one each), which produced hemolytic disease so severe that intrauterine treatment was required. There are rare instances of other alloantibodies, usually benign, causing severe hemolytic disease, e.g., anti-Kp^b (Dacus and Spinnato, 1984) and anti-M (MacPherson et al., 1961).

TABLE 44–13.   Antibodies Associated With No Treatment Required or No Clinical Disease—Manitoba (November 1, 1962 to October 31, 1988)

NOT AFFECTED	
Lu^a	15
Lu^b	1
P	25
Le^a (Le^b)	88
Wr^a	18
Multiple/rare	11
Nonspecific or high incidence	11
AFFECTED BUT NO TREATMENT REQUIRED	
Fy^b	1 of 3
Jk^a	4 of 7
Jk^b	1 of 2
s	1 of 2
M	2 of 82
LW	1 of 2
Auto	3 of 27

From Bowman JM: Treatment options for the fetus with alloimmune hemolytic disease. Transf Med Rev **4**:191, 1990.

TABLE 44–14. Twenty-seven Non-anti-D Out of Province Referrals to Rh Laboratory (November 1, 1962 to October 31, 1991)

ALLOANTIBODY SPECIFICITY	NO. OF PATIENTS	ANTIGEN NEGATIVE	HYDROPS IN PREGNANCY	HYDROPIC DEATHS	IUT TRAUMATIC DEATHS
Kell	13	1	10	4*	0
c	8	0	1	0	3*
cE	1	0	0	0	0
Fy^a	1	0	0	0	0
Jk^a	1	0	1	0	0
CC^w	1	0	0†	0	0
k	1	0	0††	0	0
E	1	0	0†	0	1

*Three Kell and 1 c death not treated in Winnipeg.
†Prior hydropic death.
††Hgb 60 gm/l.

As noted, anti-c, anti-Kell, and to a lesser extent, anti-E are capable of producing hemolytic disease quite as severe as that produced by anti-D. Anti-Kell is uncommon because it is usually caused by blood transfusion; 91 per cent of husbands of Kell-sensitized women are themselves Kell-negative, and only 0.2 per cent are homozygous for Kell. Anti-c is quite different since 80 per cent of husbands will be c-positive and 40 per cent will be homozygous for c. Hydrops fetalis from anti-c is not uncommon. Anti-E is of intermediate danger, followed by anti-C, anti-e, anti-Ce, and anti-cE. Although we have seen severe hemolytic disease due to E, C and Ce (Bowman et al., 1992b), these

antibodies are usually of low titer and rarely produce severe hemolytic disease.

Pregnant women immunized against any blood groups listed as of common or uncommon risk in Table 44–15, or against any antigen for which the effect on the conceptus of such immunization is not known, should be managed as if they were Rh-negative and Rh-immunized. Antibody measurements should be made at the same intervals and amniocentesis and/or fetal blood sampling should be carried out on the basis of the same history and antibody titer measurements.

A recent report has questioned the validity of amniotic fluid Δ OD 450 measurements in the assessment of severity of anti-Kell erythroblastosis (Caine and Mueller-Heubach, 1986). These investigators report more serious Kell erythroblastosis at lower Δ OD 450 values than usually observed in Rh erythroblastosis.

It has not been my experience that Δ OD 450 readings were low relative to the degree of Kell disease (Bowman et al., 1992a). I believe that amniotic fluid Δ OD 450 measurements in Kell alloimmunization have the same degree of accuracy (or inaccuracy) as in other forms of alloimmunization, since they reflect the degree of fetal hemolysis, irrespective of the antibody causing hemolysis. Interpretation of severity of erythroblastosis in early second trimester, before 24 to 25 weeks gestation, must take into account both amniotic fluid measurements, using the modified zone boundaries described, and careful ultrasonographic assessment parameters. Fetal blood sampling, IUT, and early delivery should be undertaken according to the same history, titer, and amniotic fluid indications as for Rh(D) immunization.

TABLE 44–15. Incidence of Association of HDN With Atypical Maternal Blood Group Antibodies

FREQUENCY OF HDN	ANTIBODY
Common	c
	Kell
	E
Uncommon	e
	C^w
	C
	Ce
	Kp^a
	Kp^b
	cE
	k
	s
	Wr^a
	Fy^a
Very rare	S
	U
	M
	Fy^b
	N
	Do^a
	Co^a
	Di^a
	Di^b
	Lu^a
	Yt^a
	Jk^a
	Jk^b
No occurrence	Le^a
	Le^b
	P

REFERENCES

Adamsons K Jr, Freda VJ, James LS, et al: Prenatal treatment of erythroblastosis fetalis following hysterotomy. Pediatrics 35:848, 1965.
Asensio SH, Figueroa-Longo JG, Pelegrina A: Intrauterine exchange transfusion. Am J Obstet Gynecol 95:1129, 1966.
Bang J, Bock JE, Trolle D: Ultra-sound guided fetal intravenous transfusion for severe rhesus haemolytic disease. Br Med J 284:373, 1982.
Barnes PH, McInnis AC, Friesen RF, et al: Maternal mishap following fetal transfusion. Can Med Assoc J 92:1277, 1965.
Bartsch F, Sandberg L: Incidence of anti-D at delivery in previously

non-immunized Rh-negative mothers with Rh-positive babies. *Presented at* McMaster Conference on Prevention of Rh Immunization, 28–30 September, 1977. Vox Sang 36:50, 1979.

Berkowitz RL, Chitkara U, Goldberg JD, et al: Intrauterine intravascular transfusions for severe red blood cell isoimmunization: Ultrasound-guided percutaneous approach. Am J Obstet Gynecol 155:574, 1986.

Berlin G, Selbing A, Ryden G: Rhesus haemolytic disease treated with high-dose intravenous immunoglobulin. Lancet 1:1153, 1985.

Bernard B, Presley M, Caudillo G, et al: Maternal fetal hemorrhage: Incidence and sensitization (abstract). Pediatr Res 11:467, 1977.

Biermé SJ, Blanc M, Abbal M, et al: Oral Rh treatment for severely immunized mothers. Lancet 1:604, 1979.

Bowen FW, Renfield M: The detection of anti D in Rh (D) negative infants born of Rh (D)-positive mothers. Pediatr Res 10:213, 1976.

Bowman JM: Neonatal management. *In* Queenan JT (ed): Modern Management of the Rh problem. 2nd ed. Hagerstown, Md, Harper & Row, 1977.

Bowman JM: Management of Rh-isoimmunization. Obstet Gynecol 52:1, 1978.

Bowman JM, Chown B, Lewis M, et al: Rh-immunization during pregnancy: Antenatal prophylaxis. Can Med Assoc J 118:623, 1978.

Bowman JM, Friesen RF, Bowman WD, et al: Fetal transfusion in severe Rh isoimmunization. JAMA 207:1101, 1969.

Bowman JM, Friesen AD, Pollock JM, Taylor WE: WinRho: Rh immune globulin prepared by ion exchange for intravenous use. Can Med Assoc J 123:1121, 1980.

Bowman JM, Lewis M, deSa DJ: Hydrops fetalis caused by massive maternofetal transplacental hemorrhage. J Pediatr 104:769, 1984.

Bowman JM, Pollock JM: Amniotic fluid spectrophotometry and early delivery in the management of erythroblastosis fetalis. Pediatrics 35:815, 1965.

Bowman JM, Pollock JM: Antenatal Rh prophylaxis: 28 week gestation service program. Can Med Assoc J 118:627, 1978.

Bowman JM, Pollock JM: Reversal of Rh alloimmunization. Fact or Fancy? Vox Sang 47:209, 1984.

Bowman JM, Pollock JM: Transplacental fetal hemorrhage after amniocentesis. Obstet Gynecol 66:749, 1985.

Bowman JM, Pollock JM, Manning FA, et al: Maternal Kell blood group alloimmunization. Obstet Gynecol 79:239, 1992a.

Bowman JM, Pollock JM, Manning FA, et al: Severe anti-C hemolytic disease of the newborn. Am J Obstet Gynecol 160:1239, 1992b.

Bowman JM, Pollock JM, Penston LE: Fetomaternal transplacental hemorrhage during pregnancy and after delivery. Vox Sang 51:117, 1986.

Brouwers HAA, Overbeeke MAM, Huiskes E, et al: Complement is not activated in ABO haemolytic disease of the newborn. Br J Haematol 68:363, 1988.

Brown PJ, Evans JP, Sinor LT, et al: The Rhesus D antigen. A dicyclohexylcarbodiimide-binding proteolipid. Am J Pathol 110:127, 1983.

Brown SJ, Perkins JT, Sosler SD, et al: The monocyte monolayer assay does not predict severity of hemolytic disease of the newborn. Transfusion 31(S193):53S, 1991.

Caine ME, Mueller-Heubach E: Kell sensitization in pregnancy. Am J Obstet Gynecol 154:85, 1986.

Carapella-de Luca E, Casadei AM, Pascone R, et al: Maternofetal transfusion during delivery and sensitization of the newborn against Rhesus D-antigen. Vox Sang, 34:241, 1978.

Chown B: Anemia from bleeding of the fetus into the mother's circulation. Lancet 1:1213, 1954.

Chown B, Duff AM, James J, et al: Prevention of primary Rh immunization: First report of the Western Canadian Trial. Can Med Assoc J 100:1021, 1969.

Clarke CA, Donohoe WTA, McConnell RB, et al: Further experimental studies in the prevention of Rh-haemolytic disease. Br Med J 1:979, 1963.

Cohen F, Zuelzer WW: The transplacental passage of maternal erythrocytes into the fetus. Am J Obstet Gynecol 93:566, 1965.

Coombs RRA, Mourant AE, Race RR: A new test for the detection of weak and "incomplete" Rh agglutinins. Br J Exp Pathol 26:255, 1945.

Cox MT, Sheils L, Masel D, et al: Fetal hydrops due to anti-B. Transfusion 31(S98):29S, 1991.

Crosby WM, Brobmann GF, Chang ACK: Intrauterine transfusion and fetal death: Relationship of intraperitoneal pressure to umbilical vein flow. Am J Obstet Gynecol 108:135, 1970.

Dacus JV, Spinnato JA: Severe erythroblastosis secondary to anti-Kp[b] sensitization. Am J Obstet Gynecol 150:888, 1984.

Daffos F, Capella-Pavlovsky M, Forestier F: Fetal blood sampling during pregnancy with use of a needle guided by ultrasound: A study of 606 consecutive cases. Am J Obstet Gynecol 153:655, 1985.

Darrow RR: Icterus gravis (erythroblastosis neonatorum, examination of etiologic considerations). Arch Pathol 25:378, 1938.

De Crespigny LC, Robinson HP, Quinn M, et al: Ultrasound-guided fetal blood transfusion for severe rhesus isoimmunization. Obstet Gynecol 66:529, 1985.

Diamond LK, Blackfan KD, Baty JM: Erythroblastosis fetalis and its association with universal edema of the fetus, icterus gravis neonatorum and anemia of the newborn. J Pediatr 1:269, 1932.

Dildy GA III, Smith LG, Moise KJ Jr, et al: Porencephalic cyst, a complication of fetal intravascular transfusion. Am J Obstet Gynecol 165:76, 1991.

Eklund J, Nevanlinna HR: Rh antibody appearance during pregnancy in Finland. *Presented at* McMaster Conference on Prevention of Rh Immunization, 28–30 September, 1977. Vox Sang 36:50, 1979.

Engelfriet CP, Brouwers HAA, Huiskes E, et al: Prognostic value of the ADCC with monocytes and maternal antibodies for haemolytic disease of the newborn. (Abstract) Book of Abstracts XXIst Congr ISH and XIXth Cong ISBT, Sydney, 1986, p. 162.

Freda VJ, Gorman JG, Pollack W: Successful prevention of experimental Rh sensitization in man with an anti-Rh gamma-2-globulin antibody preparation: A preliminary report. Transfusion 4:26, 1964.

Gahmberg CG, Karhi KK: Association of Rh₀(D) polypeptides with the membrane skeleton in Rh₀(D)-positive human red cells. J Immunol 133:334, 1984.

Gilja BK, Shah VP: Hydrops fetalis due to ABO incompatibility. Clin Pediatr 27:210, 1988.

Gold WR Jr, Queenan JT, Woody J, et al: Oral desensitization in Rh disease. Am J Obstet Gynecol 146:980, 1983.

Goto S, Nishi H, Tomoda A: Blood group Rh-D factor in human trophoblast determined by immunofluorescent method. Am J Obstet Gynecol 137:707, 1980.

Graham-Pole J, Barr W, Willoughby MLN: Continuous flow plasmapheresis in management of severe Rhesus disease. Br Med J 1:1185, 1977.

Gusdon JP Jr, Caudle MR, Herbst GA, et al: Phagocytosis and erythroblastosis: I. Modification of the neonatal response by promethazine hydrochloride. Am J Obstet Gynecol 125:224, 1976.

Hadley AG, Kumpel BM, Merry AH: The chemiluminescence response of human monocytes to red cells sensitized with monoclonal anti-Rh(D) antibodies. Clin Lab Haematol 10:377, 1988.

Harman CR, Bowman JM, Manning FA, et al: Intrauterine transfusion. Intraperitoneal versus intravascular approach: A case control comparison. Am J Obstet Gynecol 162:1053, 1990.

Harman CR, Bowman JM, Menticoglou SM, et al: Profound fetal thrombocytopenia in Rhesus disease: serious hazard at intravascular transfusion. Lancet 2:741, 1988b.

Harman CR, Manning FA, Bowman JM, et al: Use of intravascular transfusion to treat hydrops fetalis in a moribund fetus. Can Med Assn J 138:827, 1988a.

Harman CR, Menticoglou SM, Bowman JM, et al: Current technique of intraperitoneal transfusion: Do not throw away the renografin. Fetal Therapy 4:78, 1989.

Hermann M, Kjellman H: Rh prophylaxis with immune globulin anti-D administered during pregnancy and after delivery. *Presented at* McMaster Conference on Prevention of Rh Immunization, 28–30 September, 1977. Vox Sang 36:50, 1979.

Hoppe HH, Mester T, Hennig W, et al: Prevention of Rh-immunization: Modified production of IgG anti-Rh for intravenous application by ion exchange chromatography (IEC). Vox Sang 25:308, 1973.

James LS: Shock in the newborn in relation to hydrops. *In* Robertson JG, Dambrosio F (eds): International Symposium on the Management of the Rh problem. Annali Obstet Ginec Special Number 1970.

Kleihauer E, Braun H, Betke K: Demonstration von Fetalem Hae-moglobin in den Erythrozyten eines Blutausstriches. Klin Wochenschr 35:637, 1957.

Lacey PA, Caskey CR, Werner DJ, et al: Fatal hemolytic disease of the newborn due to anti-D in an Rh positive D^u variant mother. Transfusion 23:91, 1983.

Lalezari P: A polybrene method for the detection of red cell antibodies. Fed Proc 26:756, 1967.

Landsteiner K, Weiner AS: An agglutinable factor in human blood recognized by immune sera for Rhesus blood. Proc Soc Exp Biol Med 43:223, 1940.

Levine P, Katzin EM, Burnham L: Isoimmunization in pregnancy: Its possible bearing on the etiology of erythroblastosis fetalis. JAMA 116:825, 1941.

Lewis M, Chown B: A short albumin method for the determination of isohemagglutinins, particularly incomplete Rh antibodies. J Lab Clin Med 50:494, 1957.

Lewis M, Kaita H, Chown B: Kell typing in the capillary tube. J Lab Clin Med 52:163, 1958.

Lewis M, Bowman JM, Pollock JM, et al: Absorption of red cells from the peritoneal cavity of an hydropic twin. Transfusion 13:37, 1973.

Liley AW: Liquor amnii analysis in management of pregnancy complicated by rhesus immunization. Am J Obstet Gynecol 82:1359, 1961.

Liley AW: Intrauterine transfusion of fetus in hemolytic disease. Br Med J 2:1107, 1963.

Lobuglio AF, Cotran RS, Jandl JH: Red cells coated with immunoglobulin G: Binding and sphering by mononuclear cells in man. Science 158:1582, 1967.

MacPherson CR, Christiansen MJ, Newton WA, et al: Anti-M antibody as a cause of intrauterine death. Am J Clin Pathol 35:31, 1961.

Margulies M, Voto LS, Mathet E, et al: High-dose intravenous IgG for the treatment of severe Rhesus alloimmunization. Vox Sang 61:181, 1991.

Menticoglou SM, Harman CR, Manning FA, et al: Intraperitoneal transfusion: Paralysis inhibits red cell absorption. Fetal Therapy 2:154, 1987.

Miller DF, Petrie SJ: Fatal erythroblastosis due to ABO incompatibility: report of a case. Obstet Gynecol 22:773, 1963.

Mollison PL, Engelfriet CP, Contreras M: Haemolytic Disease of the Newborn. In Mollison PL (ed): Blood Transfusion in Clinical Medicine. 8th ed. Oxford, Blackwell Scientific Publications. 1987, p 639.

Mollison PL (Collaborative study): Results of tests with different cellular bioassays in relation to severity of Rh(D) haemolytic disease. Report from nine collaborating Laboratories. Vox Sang 60:225, 1991.

Moore BPL: Automation in the blood transfusion laboratory: I. Antibody detection and quantitation in the Technicon AutoAnalyzer. Can Med Assoc J 100:381, 1969.

Nance SJ, Nelson JM, Horenstein J, et al: Monocyte monolayer assay: an efficient noninvasive technique for predicting the severity of hemolytic disease of the newborn. Am J Clin Pathol 92:89, 1989.

Nevanlinna HR: Factors affecting maternal Rh immunization. Ann Med Exp Biol (Fenn Suppl 2)31:1, 1953.

Nicolaides KH, Rodeck CH, Mibashan MD, et al: Have Liley charts outlived their usefulness? Am J Obstet Gynecol 155:90, 1986.

Parkman R, Mosier D, Umansky I, et al: Graft versus host disease after intrauterine and exchange transfusions for hemolytic disease of the newborn. N Engl J Med 290:359, 1974.

Peddle LJ: Increase of antibody titer following amniocentesis. Am J Obstet Gynecol 100:567, 1968.

Peddle LJ, Campbell EM: Radiation to the fetus in intrauterine transfusion. Am J Obstet Gynecol 100:366, 1968.

Phibbs RH, Johnson P, Tooley WH: Cardio-respiratory status of erythroblastotic infants: II. Blood volume, hematocrit and serum albumin concentration in relation to hydrops fetalis. Pediatrics 53:13, 1974.

Pollack W, Ascari WQ, Kochesky RJ, et al: Studies on Rh prophylaxis: I. Relationship between doses of anti-Rh and size of antigenic stimulus. Transfusion 11:333, 1971a.

Pollack W, Ascari WQ, Crispin JF, et al: Studies on Rh prophylaxis:

II. Rh immune prophylaxis after transfusions with Rh-positive blood. Transfusion 11:340, 1971b.

Race RR: The Rh genotype and Fisher's theory. Blood 3(Special Issue No. 2):27, 1948.

Render H, Weitzel H: Intrauterine amputations after amniocentesis. Lancet i:832, 1978.

Rivat L, Rivat C, Parent M, et al: Accident survenu après injection de gamma-globulines anti-Rh dú à la présence d'anti-corps anti-γA. Presse Med 7:2072, 1970.

Robinson EAE, Tovey LAD: Intensive plasma exchange in the management of severe Rh disease. Br J Haemat 45:621, 1980.

Rodeck CH, Holman CA, Karnicki J, et al: Direct intravascular fetal blood transfusion by fetoscopy in severe rhesus isoimmunisation. Lancet 1:652, 1981.

Rodeck CH, Nicolaides KH, Warsof SL, et al: The management of severe rhesus isoimmunization by fetoscopic intravascular transfusions. Am J Obstet Gynecol 150:769, 1984.

Rosenfield RE, Allen FH, Swisher SN, et al: A review of Rh serology and presentation of a new terminology. Transfusion 2:287, 1962.

Rosenfield RE, Haber GV: Detection and measurement of homologous human hemagglutinins. Presented at Automation in Analytical Chemistry–Technicon Symposia, 1965.

Samson D, Mollison PL: Effect on primary Rh-immunization of delayed administration of anti-Rh. Immunology 28:349, 1975.

Scott JR, Beer AE, Guy LR, et al: Pathogenesis of Rh immunization in primigravidas. Fetomaternal versus maternofetal bleeding. Obstet Gynecol 49:9, 1977.

Seeds JW, Bowes WA: Ultrasound-guided intravascular transfusion in severe rhesus immunization. Am J Obstet Gynecol 154:1105, 1986.

Seelen J, Van Kessel H, Eskes T, et al: A new method of exchange transfusion in utero: Cannulation of vessels on the fetal side of the human placenta. Am J Obstet Gynecol 95:872, 1966.

Stern K, Goodman HS, Berger M: Experimental isoimmunization to hemoantigens in man. J Immunol 87:189, 1961.

Taylor JF: Sensitization of Rh-negative daughters by their Rh-positive mothers. N Engl J Med 276:547, 1967.

Tippett P, Sanger R: Observations on subdivisions of the Rh antigen D. Vox Sang 7:9, 1962.

Turner JH, Hutchinson DL, Petricciani JC: Chimerism following fetal transfusion: Report of leucocyte hybridization and infant with acute lymphocytic leukaemia. Scan J Haematol 10:358, 1974.

Urbaniak SJ, Greiss MA, Crawford RJ, et al: Prediction of the outcome of Rhesus haemolytic disease of the newborn: additional information using an ADCC assay. Vox Sang 46:323, 1984.

Verma U, Tejani N, Weiss R, et al: Sinusoidal fetal heart rate patterns in severe Rh disease. Obstet Gynecol 55:666, 1980.

Von Dungern F: Beitrage zur Immunitatslehr. Munch Med Wochenschr 47:677, 1900.

Watts DH, Luthy DA, Benedetti TJ et al: Intraperitoneal transfusion under direct ultrasound guidance. Obstet Gynecol 71:84, 1988.

Westgren M, Selbing A, Strangenberg M: Fetal intracardiac transfusions in patients with severe isoimmunization. Br Med J 1:855, 1988.

Wiener AS, Peters HR: Hemolytic reactions following transfusions of blood of the homologous group, with three cases in which the same agglutinogen was responsible. Ann Intern Med 13:2306, 1940.

Wiener AS: Conglutination test for Rh sensitization. J Lab Clin Med 30:662, 1945.

Wiener AS: Diagnosis and treatment of anemia of the newborn caused by occult placental hemorrhage. Am J Obstet Gynecol 56:717, 1948.

Wiener AS, Wexler IB: Heredity of the Blood Groups. New York, Grune & Stratton, 1958.

Woodrow JC: Rh immunization and its prevention. Series Hematologia Vol III. Copenhagen, Munksgaard, 1970.

Zipursky A, Israels LG: The pathogenesis and prevention of Rh immunization. Can Med Assoc J 97:1245, 1967.

Zipursky A, Blajchman M: The Hamilton Rh prevention studies. Presented at McMaster Conference on Prevention of Rh Immunization, 28–30 September, 1977. Vox Sang 36:50, 1979.

Zupanska B, Brojer E, Richards Y, et al: Serological and immunological characteristics of maternal anti-Rh(D) antibodies in predicting the severity of haemolytic disease of the newborn. Vox Sang 56:247, 1989.

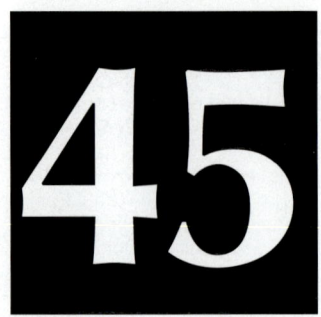

NONIMMUNE HYDROPS

ISABELLE WILKINS, M.D.

Hydrops fetalis is the term used to describe generalized edema in the neonate. This edema is accompanied by collections of fluid in serous spaces. In the past, most cases of hydrops fetalis were due to severe erythroblastosis from Rh alloimmunization. Potter (1943) first described nonimmune hydrops fetalis in a group of infants without erythroblastosis and whose mothers were Rh positive.

Since first described, 50 years ago, nonimmune hydrops (NIH) has become more common than hydrops from alloimmunization. Santolaya et al. (1992) recently reported a series of 76 hydropic fetuses of which 87 per cent were nonimmune. Warsof et al. (1986) reported a 9:1 ratio of nonimmune to immune cases in 1986. Graves and Baskett (1984) examined all babies born at their institution with hydrops and reported that 76 per cent were nonimmune.

The incidence of NIH at delivery in published accounts is approximately 1 in 1500 to 1 in 3800 (Im et al., 1984; Hutchison et al., 1982; Graves and Baskett, 1984). However, in a recent review from an ultrasonography referral center, it was present in 1 in 150 sonographic examinations (Santolaya et al., 1992).

Nonimmune hydrops is a heterogeneous disorder with a large number of possible causes and associations. Overall the prognosis is poor; a 50 to 98 per cent perinatal mortality rate is typical (Im et al., 1984; Watson and Campbell, 1986; Castillo et al., 1986). As treatment and prognosis of this disorder are dependent on etiology or underlying fetal condition, elucidation of etiology is of primary importance, but may be difficult. Although Holzgreve et al., in 1984, reported that they were able to define an etiology in 84 per cent of cases, more commonly this can be done in only 50 to 70 per cent of cases despite multiple investigations (Watson and Campbell, 1986; Castillo et al., 1986; Hutchison et al., 1982; Warsof et al., 1986). As these statistics reflect postnatal and postmortem studies, the elucidation of etiology may be even more unsuccessful before delivery.

PRESENTING SIGNS AND SYMPTOMS

Although NIH is a clinical diagnosis made in the neonate, the diagnosis may be made antenatally on obstetrical sonographic examination. The success rate in making this diagnosis is essentially 100 per cent. The indication for ultrasonography (US) varies in different series. Watson and Campbell, in 1986, found that 63 per cent of cases of nonimmune hydrops were discovered on routine ultrasonography whereas another 30 per cent of patients were referred for this study because of suspected hydramnios. Graves and Baskett (1984) found that NIH was less commonly found on routine ultrasonography than on ultrasonography ordered for a specific indication. The most common indications in their population were hydramnios, large for dates, fetal tachycardia, and maternal pregnancy-induced hypertension. Other frequently cited indications for US evaluation have included decreased fetal movement and antenatal hemorrhage (Warsof et al., 1986).

Maternal complications of pregnancy are increased in NIH. Hydramnios, pregnancy-induced hypertension, severe anemia, postpartum hemorrhage, preterm labor, birth trauma, gestational diabetes, and retained placentas or difficult delivery of the placenta are all frequently mentioned in large series (Hutchison et al., 1982; Macafee et al., 1970; Castillo et al., 1986; Graves and Baskett, 1984).

ULTRASONOGRAPHY

Ultrasonography is essential to the diagnosis of NIH, and criteria for its definition in the fetus are based exclusively on US parameters. The fluid that accumulates may include ascites, pleural effusions, pericardial effusions, and skin edema. Several definitions of fetal NIH have been proposed based on the quantity and distribution of excess fetal water. Variations in these definitions have made direct comparison between published series inexact. Mahoney et al. (1984) defined hydrops as generalized skin edema with or without an associated serous effusion. Although others have also used this definition (Brown, 1986), NIH is more commonly defined as edema with one effusion or more or with effusions in at least two spaces, that is, two of the following must be present:

ascites, pleural effusion, pericardial effusion, and skin edema (Romero et al., 1988; Platt and DeVore, 1982).

The degree or severity of hydrops is generally subjective. Hutchison et al. (1982) described a score based on total number of serous space effusions. As the only requirement for the definition of NIH was edema, it was possible to have a score of 0 with no serous involvement. This score was not predictive of outcome in this series as the overall perinatal mortality was close to 100 per cent. Saltzman et al. (1989) described a different scoring system in which each effusion was quantified. With this system they were able to predict which cases were likely to be due to fetal anemia and which were from other causes. Although they included isoimmunized pregnancies in their series, other forms of anemia followed the same general pattern.

Fluid in one of these spaces may be an early finding in a fetus destined to become hydropic and certainly warrants careful attention. At the very least, a careful search for fluid in other serous sites is warranted. Those fetuses should undergo follow-up over time to ensure that hydrops is not developing.

FETAL FLUID ACCUMULATION

Ascites is seen sonographically as an echolucent rim of varying size in the fetal abdomen (Fig. 45–1). A small rim of ascites may be hard to distinguish from a similarly located area of echo dropout commonly seen in normal fetuses (Platt and DeVore, 1982). One possible distinguishing feature is that a true rim of fluid should be visible all the way around the abdomen in transverse viewing plane. Longitudinally, the edge of the liver, bladder, or diaphragm may be outlined. When ascites is more marked, the entire liver is outlined and the bowel is compressed (Fig. 45–2). In

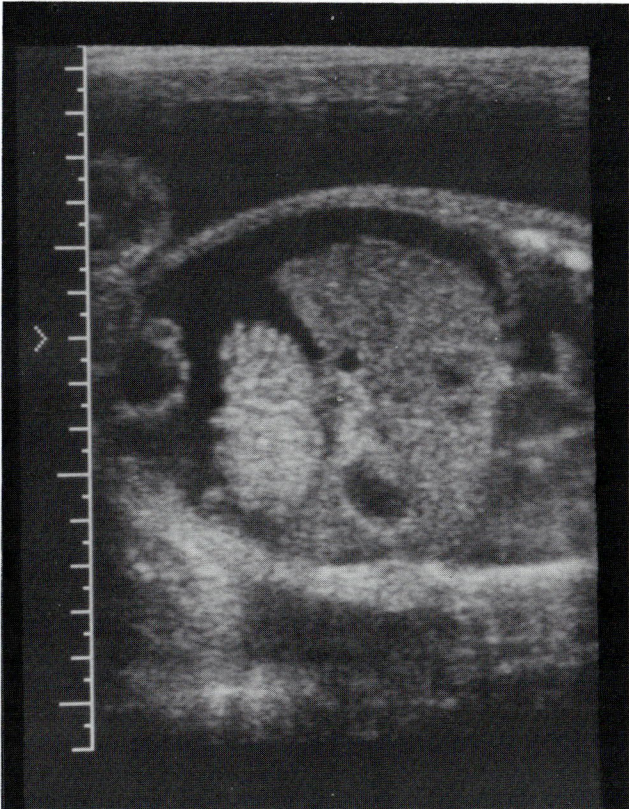

FIGURE 45–2. Longitudinal image of the fetal abdomen with ascitic fluid outlining the liver and compressing bowel.

these more extreme cases the diagnosis is relatively easy. When trying to distinguish early ascites from a normal rim of echolucency, another useful sign is small amounts of fluid surrounding loops of bowel (Fig. 45–3). This was first described by Benacerraf and Frigoletto (1985) and mimics the radiographic signs of free peritoneal air on abdominal x-ray.

Pleural effusions may be unilateral or bilateral. Although they may present as small rims of fluid outlining the pleural space and diaphragm, more commonly they are large and are seen compressing the lung (Figs. 45–4 and 45–5). It is uncommon for a unilateral effusion to shift the mediastinum. In such a case, an extrinsic fluid-filled mass, such as a diaphragmatic hernia, or other space-occupying lesion is likely to be present. Pulmonary hypoplasia is a frequent cause of death in neonates with NIH, and the size of pleural effusions may help to predict this (Castillo et al., 1987).

Pericardial effusions are smaller in total volume and are therefore more difficult to see than ascites or pleural effusions (Fig. 45–6). M-mode examination of the heart can also be useful to illustrate pericardial fluid (Fig. 45–7).

Some authors (Platt and DeVore, 1982) have proposed that pericardial effusions are indicative of cardiac decompensation and that this is the earliest sign of hydrops in fetuses with cardiac lesions. In a group of patients with mixed etiologies, Carlson et al. (1990) found that the biventricular dimension, an indicator of overall cardiac size as measured on M-mode, was highly predictive of survival.

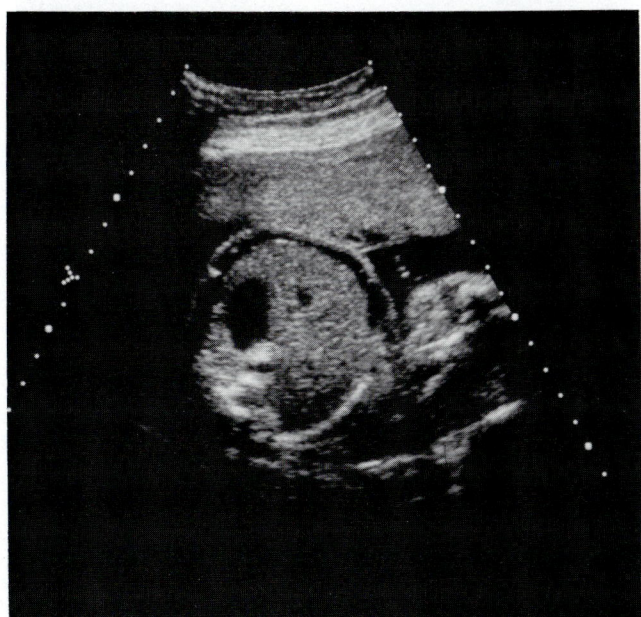

FIGURE 45–1. Transverse image of the abdomen at the level of the fetal stomach. A small rim of ascites is seen within the abdominal wall.

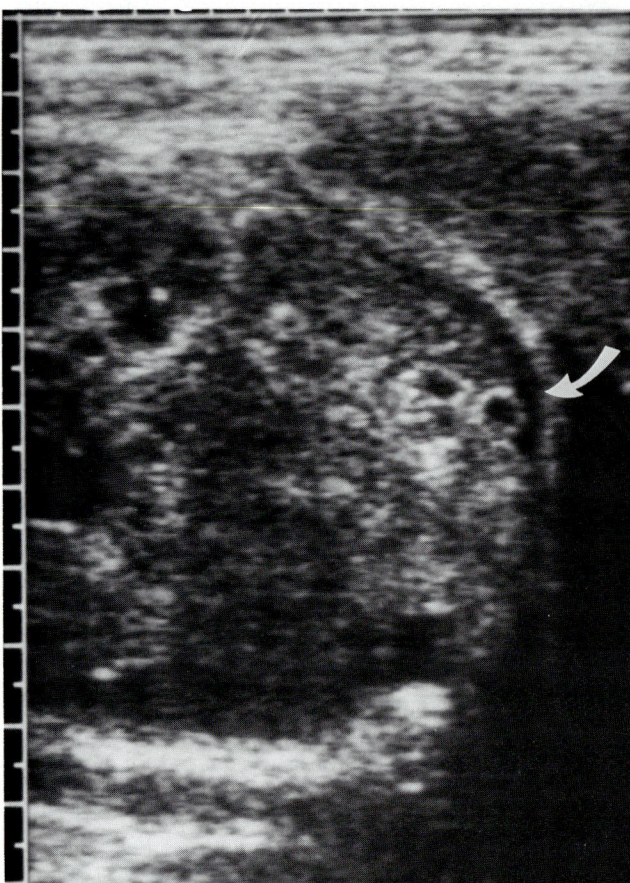

FIGURE 45–3. Fetal abdomen with a small rim of ascites and loops of bowel separated by fluid *(arrow)*.

Skin edema is usually a generalized process, although it is easiest to see with US over the chest wall or scalp, where soft tissue is typically thin and any thickness can be appreciated. The usual definition of edema is greater than 5 millimeters of subcutaneous tissue. This may be misleading if the fetus has redundant skin folds or is macrosomic.

Placental thickening is frequently considered a sign of hydrops as well. Abnormal thickening is usually defined as greater than 6 centimeters (Romero et al., 1988; Chitkara et al., 1988). Others have used a cutoff of 4 centimeters (Hoddick et al., 1985; Fleischer et al., 1981). With hydramnios, the placenta may appear compressed and instead be quite thin. In cases in which therapeutic amniocenteses are performed because of severe hydramnios, the placenta may "thicken" by the end of the procedure, and this occurrence implies that hydrostatic pressure was responsible for the thinned appearance (Elliott et al., 1991).

Hydramnios is present in 40 to 75 per cent of cases of NIH according to various authors. The definition of hydramnios is different in many of these series, but when present it is often severe and therefore present by any quantifying technique (see Chapter 40). In some cases of fetal hydrops, oligohydramnios is present, and this is believed by many authors to be an ominous or late finding. Although oligohydramnios

in general is associated with poor pregnancy outcome, its prognosis in nonimmune hydrops depends on the underlying cause rather than simply on this sonographic feature.

CAUSES OF NONIMMUNE HYDROPS

One of the greatest challenges in the management of a fetus with nonimmune hydrops is ascertaining the etiology of the disorder. Unfortunately, causes are numerous and new associations are continually appearing in the literature. The causes may be divided into several broad categories, which are helpful in organizing an approach to this often frustrating problem (Table 45–1). Many of the conditions listed in Table 45–1 are placed into a category somewhat arbitrarily. For example, many anatomic cardiac lesions have a chromosomal basis. Similarly, viral syndromes that lead to nonimmune hydrops may be associated with fetal anemia, with fetal malformation complexes, or with myocarditis. It is also obvious from Table 45–1 that some of these syndromes are extremely rare, whereas others are more common. In addition, many of these conditions represent congenital anomalies, whereas others are acquired defects. Classifying these

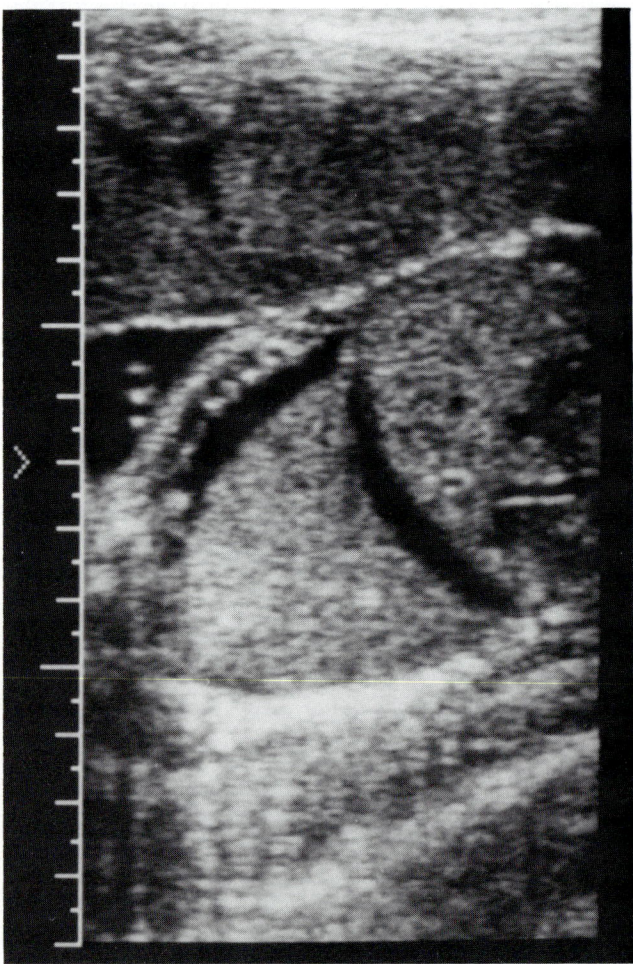

FIGURE 45–4. Small pleural effusion.

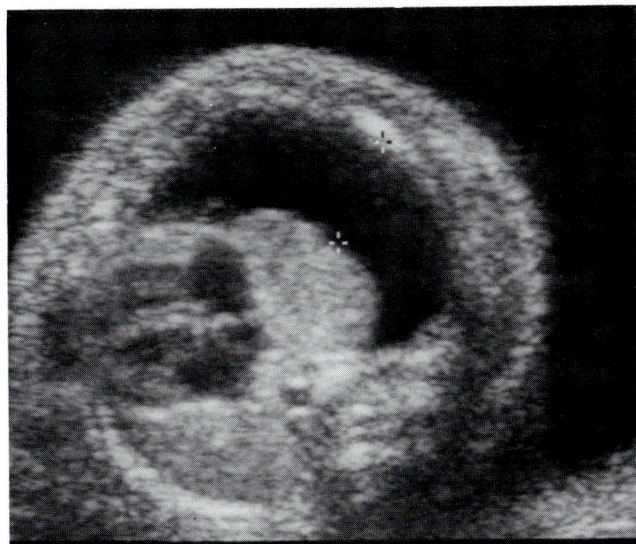

FIGURE 45–5. Large pleural effusion with compressed lung. Also note skin edema overlying ribs.

conditions in a different fashion may be helpful when considering particular problems such as management, recurrence risks, or possible fetal therapy.

It should be noted that Table 45–1 is not a list of etiologies, but rather of conditions associated with nonimmune hydrops. There are only a few cases in which the pathophysiology of nonimmune hydrops is well worked out. Furthermore, it is clear that not all cases have the same pathophysiologic mechanism. A review by Machin (1989) tries to elucidate some of these mechanisms. As he points out, hydrops is generally a common end stage for a variety of diseases reached by several pathways. He proposes five basic

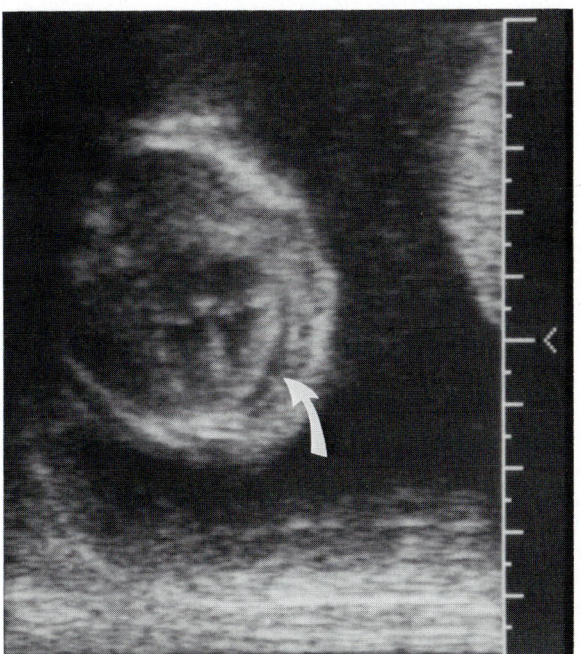

FIGURE 45–6. Four-chamber view of the fetal heart with a pericardial effusion present *(arrow).*

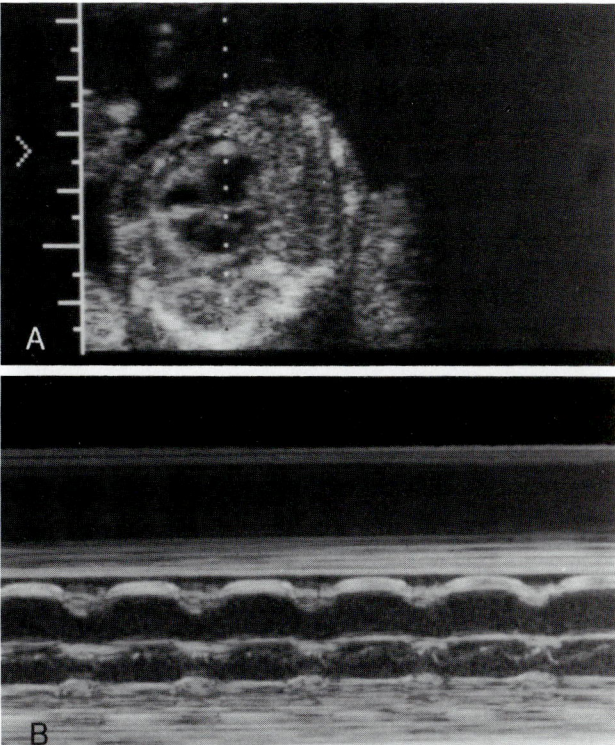

FIGURE 45–7. *A,* Fetal pericardial effusion is seen by 2-D imaging. *B,* The M-mode cursor placed through the suspected effusion is seen more clearly.

disease processes that lead to hydrops, including cardiovascular failure, chromosomal abnormalities, thoracic compression, twinning, and fetal anemia, and believes that each of these has a common pathway for the development of hydrops. Furthermore, he believes that most causes can be classified into one of these large groups in order to explain its pathophysiology.

Cardiovascular Causes of Hydrops

Fetal cardiac abnormalities are among the most common causes of hydrops in most series.

Congenital heart disease is a common problem with an incidence of 8 to 9 per 1000 liveborns. Malformations of the cardiovascular system have varying degrees of complexity and seriousness, but it is not always clear why some of these fetuses develop hydrops, whereas others are born in a well-compensated condition (McFadden and Taylor, 1989). There are no forms of congenital heart disease that reliably lead to hydrops, although one would expect that more minor abnormalities are less likely to cause the ultimate decompensation of the fetus. Overall, a structural malformation of the heart with associated fetal hydrops carries an extremely poor prognosis, with a mortality approaching 100 per cent (Crawford et al., 1988; Allan et al., 1986). The diagnosis of structural heart disease is made by means of US and may be accomplished on a targeted US examination or require referral for more sophisticated fetal echocardiography. In general, regardless of the presence of hydrops,

TABLE 45–1. Conditions Associated with Nonimmune Hydrops

Cardiovascular	Malformation	Hematologic	Alpha-thalassemia
	Left heart hypoplasia		Fetomaternal transfusion
	A-V canal defect		Parvovirus B19 infection
	Right heart hypoplasia		*In utero* hemorrhage
	Closure of foramen ovale		G6PD-deficiency
	Single ventricle		Red cell enzyme deficiencies
	Transposition of the great vessels	Thoracic	Congenital cystic adenomatoid
	VSD		malformation of lung
	ASD		Diaphragmatic hernia
	Tetralogy of Fallot		Intrathoracic mass
	Ebstein's anomaly		Pulmonary sequestration
	Premature closure of ductus		Chylothorax
	Truncus arteriosus		Airway obstruction
	Tachyarrhythmia		Pulmonary lymphangiectasia
	Atrial flutter		Pulmonary neoplasia
	Paroxysmal atrial tachycardia		Bronchogenic cyst
	Wolff-Parkinson-White	Infections	CMV
	Supraventricular tachycardia		Toxoplasmosis
	Bradyarrhythmia		Parvovirus B19 (Fifth disease)
	Other arrhythmia		Syphilis
	High-output failure		Herpes
	Neuroblastoma		Rubella
	Sacrococcygeal teratoma	Malformation	Congenital lymphedema, e.g., Noonan
	Large fetal angioma	sequences and	syndrome
	Placental chorioangioma	genetic	Arthrogryposis
	Umbilical cord hemangioma	syndromes	Multiple pterygia
	Cardiac rhabdomyoma		Neu-Laxova syndrome
	Other cardiac neoplasia		Pena-Shokeir syndrome
	Cardiomyopathy		Myotonic dystrophy
Chromosomal	45,X		Saldino-Noonan syndrome
	Trisomy 21	Metabolic	Gaucher disease
	Trisomy 18		GM$_1$ gangliosidosis
	Trisomy 13		Sialidosis
	18q+		MPS IVa
	13q−	Urinary	Urethral stenosis or atresia
	45,X/46,XX		Posterior urethral valves
	Triploidy		Congenital nephrosis (Finnish type)
	Other		Prune belly syndrome
Chondrodysplasias	Thanatophoric dwarfism	Gastrointestinal	Midgut volvulus
	Short rib polydactyly		Malrotation of the intestines
	Hypophosphatasia		Duplication of the intestinal tract
	Osteogenesis imperfecta		Meconium peritonitis
	Achondrogenesis		Hepatic fibrosis
Twin pregnancy	Twin-twin transfusion syndrome		Cholestasis
	Acardiac twin		Biliary atresia
			Hepatic vascular malformations

cases of cardiac malformation that are diagnosed prenatally have a poor outcome. Crawford et al. (1988) found only a 17 per cent survival in such fetuses. Copel et al. (1988) suggested that 30 per cent of fetuses with prenatally diagnosed structural congenital heart disease have an abnormal karyotype. Thus it is their recommendation that chromosomes be obtained whenever this diagnosis is made. Because of the poor prognosis associated with hydrops in association with an abnormal karyotype, these fetuses generally are not considered candidates for *in utero* fetal therapy or for active intervention with early delivery and vigorous resuscitation.

Cardiac arrhythmias are also an important cause of hydrops, but the prognosis is entirely different from that for structural heart disease. Tachyarrhythmias associated with hydrops generally have a better prognosis than most other causes of nonimmune hydrops (Cameron et al., 1988; Romero et al., 1988). Arrhythmias may be of several types, including tachyarrhyth-

mias, bradyarrhythmia, as well as dysrhythmias. The diagnosis and management of these disorders is discussed more fully in Chapter 21, and therefore it will not be considered in any detail here. If an arrhythmia is associated with underlying structural heart disease, the prognosis is as poor as for heart disease without arrhythmia, as described above (Shenker et al., 1987).

Premature closure of the foramen ovale is generally idiopathic and can occur at any time during gestation. Generally, this diagnosis is only made once hydrops has occurred, and prognosis is therefore poor. Diagnosis can be made by careful US examination of the fetal heart, with Doppler studies and color Doppler as useful adjuncts to imaging. The etiology of premature closure of the foramen ovale is unknown, and if the disorder presents in a fetus with hydrops, prognosis is poor.

Premature closure or narrowing of the ductus arteriosus also has been associated with fetal hydrops (Harlass et al., 1989). In some of these cases the patient was receiving indomethacin for the arrest of preterm labor (Mogilner et al., 1982). Moise et al. (1988) described narrowing of the ductus in response to maternal indomethacin ingestion, but have found this to be measurable and reversible. Vanhaesebrouck et al. (1988) described NIH with neonatal ileal perforation in fetuses exposed to indomethacin for the arrest of preterm labor.

A variety of miscellaneous cardiac abnormalities may lead to hydrops. Neoplasias such as rhabdomyomas may be present with hydrops. In such cases, a family history of tuberous sclerosis should be sought, as this autosomal dominant disorder may present in this fashion (Ostor and Fortune, 1978).

Cardiac failure from myocarditis is responsible for at least some cases of hydrops in fetuses who have congenital infections (Naides and Weiner, 1989). Such cases have been documented in fetal parvovirus B19, cytomegalovirus (CMV), and much more rarely in toxoplasmosis. These are discussed below under infectious causes of hydrops.

Several noncardiac lesions can lead to high-output cardiac failure, a presumed mechanism of hydrops. Sacrococcygeal teratomas are large vascular tumors that act as an arteriovenous shunt and may be associated with hydrops on this basis (Langer et al., 1989; Mostoufi-Zadeh et al., 1985). Langer et al. (1989) reported the open surgical excision of fetal sacrococcygeal teratomas. They were able to demonstrate increased aortic flow, presumably due to shunting within the tumor, which decreased after excision of the tumor. This controversial approach is justified, according to the authors, by the high rate of complications in certain of these tumors. However, as the majority of these tumors are well tolerated by the fetus and do not lead to hydrops (Gross et al., 1987), and as the authors were unsuccessful in preventing an extremely preterm delivery due to maternal and fetal complications (Langer et al., 1989), this approach is still highly experimental.

Other causes of presumed high-output failure associated with fetal hydrops include fetal adrenal neuroblastomas, of which there have been multiple cases reported. These rare tumors presumably lead to heart failure on the basis of high catecholamine release, much as they would in a child with the same lesion. Other angiomas may lead to hydrops and have been described in the placenta as chorioangiomas (Hutchison et al., 1982; Maidman et al., 1980), in the cord (Seifer et al., 1985), and in the fetus in the angioosteohypertrophy syndrome (Mor et al., 1988).

Chromosomal Abnormalities

Chromosomal abnormalities are fairly common in cases of fetal hydrops, and there may be several mechanisms by which they cause hydrops (Machin, 1989). One large group of chromosomally abnormal fetuses with hydrops have cystic hygromas (Holzgreve et al., 1984). Cystic hygromas are among the most common causes of hydrops, particularly among fetuses diagnosed prior to 20 weeks (Santolaya et al., 1992). The most common chromosomal abnormality among these fetuses is 45,X or Turner's syndrome. On the other hand, fetuses with this phenotype may also have trisomy 21 or a normal karyotype (Cullen et al., 1990). Among fetuses with a 45,X karyotype, there are two common structural abnormalities that could lead to the development of hydrops. Certainly one is cystic hygroma, but these fetuses also frequently have a tubular coarctation of the aorta. There is some controversy about which of these is the more important mechanism for causing NIH (Machin, 1989). With the advent of high-resolution first-trimester transvaginal ultrasonography, it is possible to see small cystic hygromas early in gestation. Cullen et al. (1990) reported 30 cases of cystic hygroma in the first trimester. Hydrops was not predictive of poor outcome if chromosomes were normal. This is in marked contrast to the finding of cystic hygroma and hydrops in the second trimester, which is generally considered lethal.

Other chromosomal abnormalities have been described in fetuses with hydrops as well. The most common, as expected, are trisomy 21, trisomy 18, trisomy 13, and triploidy. Sex chromosome abnormalities that result in Turner's syndrome, such as 45,X/46,XX, are also described, as are a large number of more unusual autosomal rearrangements. Structural cardiac lesions are common in aneuploid fetuses and may be associated with hydrops. If no structural cardiac lesion is found, the pathophysiology for the development of hydrops in this situation is not known, but certainly the prognosis is poor, and important information can be given to the parents about recurrence risk and diagnosis in future pregnancies. The overall rate of chromosome abnormality in hydropic fetuses varies widely between 7 and 34 per cent (Landrum et al., 1986; Holzgreve et al., 1984; Santolaya et al., 1992). Obtaining a fetal karyotype is thus an essential part of the work-up of any hydropic fetus.

Thoracic Abnormalities

Increases in intrathoracic pressure may lead to the development of hydrops by obstructing venous return and altering cardiovascular hemodynamics. Most of these conditions involve space-occupying lesions of the thorax.

Cystic adenomatoid malformation of the lung has several different subtypes, depending on the size and distribution of the cysts. In most cases, if pulmonary hypoplasia is not life threatening, this lesion is amenable to surgery in the neonate. However, these fetuses may become hydropic. This diagnosis requires US to examine lung tissue for the presence of cystic structures.

Most of the cases described in detail in the literature have presented with a single large cyst and a shift of the mediastinum. In several cases, continuous drainage of such a solitary cyst via pleuroamniotic shunt placement has been successful (Clark et al., 1987; Blott et al., 1988). In another reported case, extensive microscopic disease in the affected lung apparently accounted for failed therapy with multiple needle aspirations despite resolution of fetal hydrops (Chao and Monoson, 1990).

Harrison et al. (1990a) have performed open fetal surgery for congenital cystic adenomatoid malformation in order to prevent the development of pulmonary hypoplasia and/or fetal hydrops in cases in which cysts are microscopic or otherwise not amenable to shunt placement.

Other types of masses or lesions in the chest may be associated with hydrops as well. These include diaphragmatic hernias, hamartomas or other neoplasms of the lung or chest, pulmonary extralobar sequestration syndrome, and various bronchogenic cysts. Diaphragmatic hernia is the most common of these lesions, but it is unusual for these fetuses to develop hydrops. Once again, *in utero* therapy has been proposed. Benacerraf and Frigoletto (1986) described a fetus that underwent a single thoracentesis to remove ascitic fluid that had entered the chest with subsequent resolution of hydrops. However, the infant died of respiratory complications. Harrison et al. (1990b) have proposed open surgery for this condition in order to prevent pulmonary hypoplasia, although this approach is controversial (Wenstrom et al., 1991).

Unilateral hydrothorax may present as a space-occupying lesion in the chest and is frequently associated with hydrops. When it is bilateral, it may be indistinguishable from other causes of NIH since one of the features of hydrops is pleural effusion. In these cases, the effusions are the primary event and the hydrops a secondary problem. Many authors have considered unilateral or bilateral fetal hydrothorax as analogous to neonatal chylothorax (Booth et al., 1987; Roberts et al., 1986). As there are no chylomicrons in the fetus, this is not known with certainty and in most cases after birth no particular surgery on the presumably abnormal lymphatic system is performed (Rodeck et al., 1988). Overall, these fetuses have a relatively poor prognosis as pulmonary hypoplasia is frequently present (Beischer et al., 1971; Castillo et al., 1987). In the neonate, isolated pleural effusion without hydrops has a much more favorable prognosis with a 15 per cent mortality (Chernick and Reed, 1970).

When the diagnosis of unilateral or bilateral hydrothorax is considered, many authors recommend a diagnostic fetal thoracentesis. The fluid that is obtained contains predominantly lymphocytes in cases of isolated hydrothorax, although Eddleman et al. (1991) recently reported two cases in which this test was misleading. In one of their cases, a single thoracentesis and drainage of the space was satisfactory in that no effusion reaccumulated. However, in most cases reported, serial thoracenteses have been performed as rapid reaccumulation of fluid occurred. This has led some authors to propose placement of a pleuroamniotic shunt for continual drainage of this space. The results of such therapy have been mixed, but in some cases successes have been reported (Rodeck et al., 1988; Booth et al., 1987).

Since it is difficult to predict pulmonary hypoplasia *in utero*, it is also difficult to carefully select appropriate candidates for invasive procedures. In Rodeck's series, the failures occurred at later gestational ages than the successes, and these late cases presumably had pre-existing pulmonary hypoplasia. Various authors have attempted to measure chest size to predict pulmonary hypoplasia. Nimrod et al. (1988) believe that this technique is useful in patients with ruptured membranes, but is not predictive in the presence of pleural effusions.

The rate of aneuploidy in association with fetal hydrothorax or isolated pleural effusion is high. Rodeck et al. (1988) placed shunts prior to the availability of a fetal karyotype, and one of eight fetuses had Down syndrome. Petrikovsky et al. (1991) reported three consecutive cases of pleural effusion, all of which involved aneuploid fetuses.

Twins

When one of a set of twins presents with fetal hydrops, there are special considerations in the differential diagnosis. If it is known that the twins are not monozygotic, then the cause is likely to be unrelated to the twin pregnancy, and the diagnostic approach to the hydropic twin should be similar to that for any other hydropic fetus. In the case of monozygotic twins, the hydrops is probably related to abnormal vessels in the placenta resulting in a twin-to-twin transfusion syndrome. Twin-to-twin transfusion syndrome and other abnormal aspects of twins are discussed in Chapter 38.

In the situation of a twin-to-twin transfusion syndrome, the hydropic fetus may be the donor or the recipient (Macafee et al., 1970). In the classic situation, the donor twin is growth-restricted and has oligohydramnios. The recipient twin is plethoric, has hydramnios, and may be hydropic (Blickstein, 1990; Brown et al., 1989). Presumably this sequence of events results from cardiac overload and congestive heart failure. On the other hand, it is also possible for the donor twin to be hydropic, and in this case the pathophysiology is likely to be related to chronic anemia (Holzgreve et al. 1985).

Twin-to-twin transfusion syndrome carries a poor prognosis, particularly when it is found early in gestation or when hydrops is present (Shah and Chaffin, 1989; Gonsoulin et al., 1990). Various aggressive therapies have recently been proposed including serial amniocenteses and *in utero* laser ablation of communicating placental vessels (Elliott et al., 1991; De Lia et al., 1990). In addition, there have been several reports of attempted selective feticide of one twin. Although selective feticide has been used in situations in which twins are discordant for a variety of genetic or structural defects, success has been poor in the situation of twin-to-twin transfusion (Chitkara et al., 1989). Golbus et al. (1988) reported a high incidence of death in the other twin within a short time from the procedure, presumably because of the vascular anastomoses between them. In addition, it is known that when one monozygotic twin dies *in utero*, the other twin is at risk for a variety of cerebral ischemic events (Carlson and Towers, 1989; D'Alton et al., 1984). This has led others to attempt selective delivery of one twin (Urig et al., 1988; Wittmann et al., 1986). At this time, the best treatment for this situation is unclear, but a poor prognosis exists when hydrops is present (Bebbington and Wittmann, 1989).

Fetal Anemia

Anemia is a well-known cause of fetal hydrops, and the model used to elucidate the pathophysiology of this condition is alloimmunization. Because immune hydrops has been extensively studied, this is the best understood mechanism for the development of non-immune hydrops as well.

One of the most common causes of hydrops in patients from Asia or the Eastern Mediterranean is alpha-thalassemia (Nakayama et al., 1986). This recessive disorder causes formation of abnormal tetramers of the beta chain of hemoglobin, which are not capable of carrying oxygen. Thus, there is massive tissue hypoxia. Fetuses are commonly hydropic as early as 20 weeks gestation. As long-term survival with homozygous alpha-thalassemia is extremely rare, there is no current recommendation for treatment of these fetuses. On the other hand, the proper diagnosis is important for counseling and prenatal diagnosis in future pregnancies.

Fetomaternal hemorrhage is a relatively common occurrence and, in rare instances, may be massive enough to cause fetal hydrops (Owen et al., 1989). In most cases the etiology for the fetomaternal hemorrhage or transfusion is unknown. This diagnosis can easily be made by examination of peripheral maternal blood for the presence of fetal cells with a Kleihauer-Betke stain. It is also possible to detect a fetomaternal bleed by an abnormally elevated maternal serum alpha-fetoprotein. Although this may be a self limited process, if a fetus is hydropic, many have advocated more aggressive management as the fetus is certainly at risk for demise. There have now been several case reports of fetuses who have undergone serial transfusions with resolution of hydrops and an ultimately good outcome (Cardwell, 1988; Thorp et al., 1992; Rouse and Weiner, 1990).

Fetal hemorrhage with subsequent anemia and hydrops formation has also been reported. Most commonly this has been associated with an intracranial hemorrhage, and in the absence of a history of trauma, a fetal coagulation deficiency such as alloimmune thrombocytopenia should be suspected (Bose, 1978; Daffos et al., 1984).

G-6-PD deficiency is a common X-linked enzyme deficiency in African-Americans and people of Mediterranean heritage. Female carriers are usually asymptomatic. This disorder is characterized by hemolytic crises, usually in response to various stimuli including sulfa drugs, aspirin, and fava beans. There are two reports of affected male fetuses presenting with anemia and hydrops after maternal ingestion of these substances (Perkins, 1971; Mentzer and Collier, 1975).

A number of inherited erythrocyte enzyme deficiencies may cause fetal anemia and, in rare cases, fetal hydrops (Ravindranath et al., 1987; Matthay and Mentzer, 1981). Examples include glucose phosphate isomerase deficiency and pyruvate kinase deficiency. These commonly lead to chronic hemolytic anemia, but rarely to severe anemia, in fetal life.

Congenital leukemia may cause anemia and hydrops, and demonstration of leukemic infiltration of myocardium has also been reported (Gray et al., 1986).

Transmission of maternal antibodies to erythroid precursors in a mother who had acquired red cell aplasia has been reported. Transfusions to the fetus reversed the hydrops and resulted in a healthy liveborn with a normal outcome (Oie et al., 1984).

Infection

There is a great deal of literature concerning congenital infection as a cause of nonimmune hydrops. Many different viruses, bacteria, and parasites cause congenital infection, but the fetal effects are variable, and no infection predictably results in hydrops fetalis. In addition, although it has long been felt that the common mechanism for the development of hydrops in these fetuses is anemia, it may also involve myocarditis, hepatitis, or other pathways that have yet to be elucidated.

Congenital syphilis is a well-known cause of fetal hydrops. The diagnosis can be made by obtaining a positive serologic test in the mother. In addition, dark-field examination of amniotic fluid may be helpful (Wendel, 1988). A hydropic fetus with syphilis has a poor prognosis compared with milder cases of congenital syphilis. The treatment remains the same, which is to treat the infection in the mother.

Cytomegalovirus (CMV) is the most common perinatally acquired infection (Demmler, 1991). Although the attack rate is high and vertical transmission to the fetus is high, a much smaller percentage of fetuses are symptomatic. Findings at birth in severe cases may include microcephaly, chorioretinitis, and intracerebral calcifications. These fetuses are frequently growth restricted and also may be hydropic (Demmler, 1991). Maternal infection is ideally demonstrated by documenting seroconversion. Rising titers of CMV IgG antibody may also be used. Primary infection causes prolonged viral shedding, and a positive maternal urine culture also may be helpful. Blood obtained from the fetus can be sent for CMV specific IgM if the fetus is past 20 weeks and is capable of producing IgM. Fetal IgG levels are unhelpful, as they may merely reflect transplacental passage of maternal IgG. Recently, a number of case reports and small series have demonstrated that a simple culture for CMV from amniotic fluid is the most reliable predictor of CMV infection in the fetus (Fadel and Ruedrich, 1988). Lynch et al. (1991) have shown that cultures from blood and serology are less reliable, but advocate their use as amniotic fluid culture is not always positive. At present there is no *in utero* treatment for fetal cytomegalovirus infection.

The most common manifestation of infection with parvovirus B19 is Fifth disease or erythema infectiosum. This common disease may be acquired by a pregnant woman from an affected child. It causes a characteristic rash, flu-like symptoms, and arthralgias that may be mild. Fetal infections clearly occur, but the transmission rate is not established.

A large study in England and Wales (Public Health Laboratory Service Working Party on Fifth Disease, 1990) demonstrated a 33 per cent transplacental infection rate with 9 per cent fetal loss in infected pregnancies. Most fetal losses occurred in the second trimester, and there was only one case of fetal hydrops. The Centers for Disease Control (CDC) published data in the Morbidity and Mortality Weekly Report (MMWR) in 1989 from an ongoing study. They found that among 95 recently infected women, two had fetal losses including one case of hydrops. By contrast, Rodis et al. (1988) found fetal hydrops in three of four women who acquired this infection during pregnancy.

The diagnosis of human parvovirus infection in a hydropic fetus is difficult and requires the isolation of virus from fetal blood, parvovirus specific IgM in fetal serum, or the demonstration of virus in fetal tissues (Samuels and Ludmir, 1990; Weiner et al., 1992). Viral particles may be detected through electron microscopy or DNA in situ hybridization studies (MMWR, 1989; Naides and Weiner, 1989). Fetal serology may be negative in some cases of known fetal infection with hydrops (Peters and Nicolaides, 1990; Carrington et al., 1987; Anderson et al., 1988). A characteristic though nonspecific finding in hydropic fetuses with this infection is an elevated maternal serum alpha-fetoprotein (Anand et al., 1987). Data from Carrington et al. (1987) and from Bernstein and Capeless (1989) suggest that a very elevated MSAFP is a useful marker as it may herald the onset of hydrops in an affected pregnancy. The usual mechanism for the development of hydrops in parvovirus infections is presumably anemia from an aplastic crisis. Fetuses undergoing percutaneous umbilical blood sampling who have parvovirus are severely anemic (Rodis et al., 1988; Carrington et al., 1987). However, virus has been shown to invade myocardium as well, and myocarditis may also account for hydropic changes, particularly in less anemic fetuses (Porter et al., 1988; Naides and Weiner, 1989).

As this virus is not known to be associated with congenital malformations or long-term sequelae, aggressive *in utero* supportive therapy has been attempted. Transfusions of packed cells to the fetus have resulted in some good outcomes (Peters and Nicolaides, 1990; Soothill, 1990; Sahakian et al., 1991).

The transient nature of this infection in the absence of fetal demise has led many investigators to speculate that it may be a causative agent in cases of ascites or hydrops that spontaneously resolve *in utero* (Peters and Nicolaides, 1990; Morey et al., 1991). In addition, it may be more common than previously believed and account for a substantial portion of so-called idiopathic cases of nonimmune hydrops (Porter et al., 1988; Samuels and Ludmir, 1990).

A number of other infectious agents have been related to hydrops in at least a few cases (Spahr et al., 1980; Zornes et al., 1988; Gembruch et al., 1987; Bain et al., 1956; Robb et al., 1986). These include toxoplasmosis, herpes simplex, rubella, and Listeria. In some cases, there is suspicion of an infectious process, but no causative organism can be identified (Zimmer et al., 1986). It is possible that certain influenza viruses, Coxsackie virus, or enteroviruses are also capable of producing fetal hydrops, either in a transient fashion or with subsequent fetal death. An interesting report by Robertson et al. (1985) describes a case in which multiple cultures were negative. Nonetheless, the fe-

tus had continuing evidence of hepatitis for several weeks after delivery with an eventual good outcome.

Metabolic Disease

A variety of genetic metabolic diseases, particularly lysosomal storage diseases, can cause hydrops in the fetus (Gillan et al., 1984). Gaucher's disease, GM_1 gangliosidosis, Salla disease, sialidosis, mucopolysaccharidosis type VII and type IV, Tay-Sachs disease, and others can all present in this manner (Beck et al., 1984; Abu-Dalu et al., 1982). Gaucher's disease is the most common of these disorders and has been reported the most frequently, but the presentation with hydrops is rare (Ginsburg and Groll, 1973). These conditions can recur in subsequent pregnancies, as they are typically inherited in an autosomal recessive fashion. Establishing the correct diagnosis is therefore extremely important. This may be accomplished by analysis of oligosaccharides in fetal or neonatal urine, enzyme analysis and carrier testing in the parents, and histologic examination of appropriate fetal tissues (Gillan et al., 1984). Unfortunately, most of these studies will be performed after fetal or neonatal death as the prognosis is poor.

Other Malformations

A variety of chondrodysplasias may present with fetal hydrops. Pretorius et al. (1986) found all such cases associated with fatal dwarfing syndromes. In these cases, the chest is compressed and the neonates die of respiratory insufficiency. The most common skeletal dysplasias described with fetal hydrops are short-rib polydactyly syndrome, thanatophoric dysplasia, and achondrogenesis. The diagnosis of a skeletal dysplasia is fairly easy to make by US by measurement of the extremities relative to the head size and abdominal size, but it may be difficult to classify the type of chondrodysplasia in a fetus by US alone. After birth, x-ray studies as well as examination of other phenotypic features of the neonate elucidate the specific type of chondrodysplasia. As many of the lethal types are inherited in a recessive fashion, there is a high recurrence rate.

A number of genetic syndromes have also been associated with fetal hydrops. These include congenital myotonic dystrophy, arthrogryposis, multiple fetal pterygia, Neu-Laxova syndrome, and Pena-Shokeir type I (Jauniaux et al., 1990; Afifi et al., 1992; Holzgreve et al., 1984).

Urinary tract malformations have been described in conjunction with hydrops in numerous reports; however, close examination in many of these cases is often unconvincing. On the other hand, urinary ascites is common in any form of urinary tract obstruction. This is generally self-limited and rarely progresses to hydrops.

A number of intra-abdominal processes related to the gastrointestinal tract commonly present with ascites, but in rare cases may be associated with hydrops. These include meconium peritonitis, small bowel volvulus, and various intestinal atresias.

Other Causes

Diabetes is frequently cited as a cause of nonimmune hydrops, and several large series have a few cases in which pre-existing maternal diabetes is the only etiology (Poeschmann et al., 1991). It is not clear whether these fetuses were structurally normal. Others have found no association between maternal diabetes and NIH (Macafee, 1970). The above list of causes is certainly not complete. There are numerous case reports of other syndromes or malformations that have been associated with fetal hydrops. In some of these cases the association may not be causative or may be unproven, but in others it is more convincing. The literature is constantly being updated, not only with series, but with such case reports, and this discussion is therefore not exhaustive.

EXPERIMENTAL MANAGEMENT OF IDIOPATHIC CASES

A number of management strategies have been attempted in cases of NIH of unknown etiology. Shimokawa et al. (1988) injected albumin into the peritoneal cavity of a hydropic fetus on two occasions, and there was subsequent resolution of hydrops. This group subsequently published a series of 21 cases treated with a combination of red cell transfusions and serial albumin injections. Improvements were found only in fetuses without pleural effusions, but the survival rate in this group was 5 out of 7 (72 per cent) (Maeda et al., 1988).

Lingman et al. (1989) attempted direct intravascular albumin transfusion on five occasions in a fetus later found to have a lysosomal storage disease. Doppler studies and blood counts before and after the procedures indicated effective plasma expansion and peripheral vasodilatation.

Goldberg and associates (1986) placed a peritoneal-amniotic shunt in a case of NIH of unknown etiology in the second trimester with massive ascites. Although the ascites resolved, other features of hydrops developed, and the fetus ultimately died.

DIAGNOSTIC APPROACH TO THE HYDROPIC FETUS

The work-up of a patient with the diagnosis of fetal hydrops should be directed at possible causes. Since the diagnosis is confirmed with ultrasonography, this is frequently the first test performed. During a careful US examination, the known causes of nonimmune hydrops should be kept in mind. Many of the fetal conditions, congenital anomalies, and malformation sequences that are known causes of hydrops will be found or eliminated on the initial US examination. Twins, cardiac arrhythmias, and hydrothorax are all examples of obvious US diagnosis. If the examination is unsatisfactory, it should be repeated later to delineate the fetal anatomy as well as possible. Although the underlying diagnosis is far more predictive of outcome than any other US parameters, the initial US examination can be used to assess the severity of the hydrops and to initiate antenatal testing, if appropriate, depending on gestational age. Assessment of the severity of the hydrops is particularly important if the fetus is observed for some length of time or if fetal therapy is initiated. US parameters can be longitudinally followed to predict fetal decompensation or fetal response to *in utero* therapy.

A history should be taken with particular attention to any family history of genetic diseases or congenital anomaly, consanguinity, ethnic background, and recent maternal infections or exposures. Once again, careful scrutiny of the causes of hydrops outlined above will give direction to the types of questions that should be asked of the mother and family.

The initial testing of the mother should include the elimination of immune causes of hydrops with blood typing and the indirect Coombs test. A screen for hemoglobinopathies, a Kleihauer-Betke test to look for fetal blood cells in the maternal circulation, and TORCH titers are also useful at this time. Some of these tests may not be immediately available, but blood should be drawn and sent to the laboratory.

In addition to careful US, fetal echocardiography may be helpful if it is available. A fetal karyotype should be obtained in most cases. How this is accomplished will depend on gestational age and US findings. Before 18 weeks, a karyotype can be obtained by culture of amniotic fluid or chorionic villi. Amniotic fluid should be sent for viral cultures as well. After 18 to 20 weeks gestation, it is usually preferable to perform a fetal blood sampling for karyotype (Hogge et al., 1988; Hsieh et al., 1987). Karyotype from blood is typically available in as little as 72 hours, whereas amniocyte culture and analysis may take over two weeks. This rapidly obtained information will frequently help with management decisions. Furthermore, fetal blood can be used to obtain other information such as a complete blood count and platelet count to rule out fetal anemia or thrombocytopenia. Fetal serum may be frozen or may be sent for other studies such as total IgM or viral specific IgM or IgG if certain infections are highly suspected. Although Delta OD450 levels are increased in many cases of nonimmune hydrops (Appelman et al., 1988), this is not clinically useful information, and therefore the study is not generally indicated. Amniotic fluid should be obtained for viral culture and lung maturity studies when appropriate. A frozen sample of amniotic fluid may be useful for future viral DNA hybridization studies or oligosaccharide analysis.

Because some tests will not be available promptly, numerous tests may need to be ordered before initial results are available. It is important to establish a connection with cooperative laboratory facilities and, when these are not available locally, with reference laboratories to which specimens can be sent.

MANAGEMENT

Management issues are difficult to generalize, as they depend on the prognosis, gestational age, and presenting signs and symptoms. Before fetal viability, parents should be presented the prognosis and given the option of terminating the pregnancy. If the underlying etiology is amenable to fetal therapy, this should be frankly discussed with the family, but overall they should be warned that the possibility of diagnostic error always exists and that the overall prognosis in this condition is still grim.

Unfortunately, many cases of NIH present in the third trimester. If the patient presents in preterm labor or if symptomatic hydramnios exists, difficult decisions need to be made about whether to give the patient tocolytic medications or to allow labor to continue. In many cases, patients have presented in labor and tocolysis has been initiated before the diagnosis of hydrops is made. We would recommend continuing the tocolysis while the fetal work-up is being pursued. If a potentially reversible cause of hydrops is found, every attempt should be made to prolong the pregnancy to maximize fetal survival and initiate *in utero* resuscitation. On the other hand, if a fetal diagnosis with a poor prognosis seems fairly certain, a frank discussion with the family may lead to the discontinuation of tocolytic medication. Patients who present with signs of maternal compromise such as preeclampsia or antenatal hemorrhage should be managed without regard to fetal outcome as it is so poor. Management decisions are particularly difficult in idiopathic cases because the prognosis is uncertain. Even though the overall prognosis is poor in idiopathic cases, every attempt should be made to prolong the pregnancy to 32 or 34 weeks gestation unless there are signs of fetal or maternal decompensation. If significant or symptomatic hydramnios is present, it may be treated with therapeutic amniocenteses, indomethacin, or, more conservatively, with bed rest and conventional tocolytic therapy. Treatment of hydramnios is further discussed in Chapter 40.

Fetal decompensation may be difficult to measure, but the usual biophysical parameters are nonetheless useful. If the fetus has had a reactive heart rate tracing that becomes abnormal, this should be interpreted as a sign of acute decompensation. Similarly, oligohydramnios, a decrease in fetal movement, and poor fetal tone are all ominous signs. Unless there is evidence that hydrops is resolving or that treatment has otherwise been effective, there does not seem to be any reason to prolong a pregnancy past 34 weeks gestation or the attainment of a mature lung profile.

RECURRENCE RISKS

After the delivery of a fetus with nonimmune hydrops, investigation should continue in the nursery if necessary to elucidate its cause. If the fetus is stillborn or dies in the early neonatal period, every attempt should be made to obtain a postmortem examination directed at finding the underlying etiology for the problem. Without this information, counseling the patient and her family about future pregnancies is frustrating. Overall, recurrent hydrops fetalis is unusual, and for most families the prognosis is good for a future normal pregnancy. However, there are numerous case reports of couples who have had recurrent pregnancies with hydropic fetuses (Cumming, 1979; Etches and Lemons, 1979; Schwartz et al., 1981). One must therefore be wary of reassuring families with idiopathic hydrops that the problem is not going to recur, and future pregnancies should be carefully monitored.

DELIVERY CONSIDERATIONS

Delivery of a hydropic fetus should be accomplished with an experienced pediatric team prepared to deal with a sick neonate. Some authors have recommended the liberal use of cesarean section to avoid asphyxia and birth trauma, although no objective data support this (Spahr et al., 1980). Pre-delivery thoracentesis or paracentesis has also been advocated in order to aid immediate postnatal resuscitation or, in the case of a large fetal abdominal girth, to facilitate vaginal delivery (deCrespigny et al., 1980; Holzgreve et al., 1985; Romero et al., 1988).

Immediate problems of the neonate are likely to center on respiratory support and fluid management. Virtually all hydropic neonates require mechanical ventilation, and edema may make intubation difficult (Carlton et al., 1989).

Postnatal drainage of pleural or peritoneal fluid in order to maintain oxygenation may be required. Some authors reserve these procedures for extreme cases whereas others propose a more liberal use of fluid drainage (Davis, 1982; Ringer and Stark, 1989; Carlton, 1989). Fluid restriction, careful management of electrolytes, judicious use of albumin and diuretics, correction of anemia, and continual assessment of intravascular volume are all important issues in the first few days of life.

CONCLUSION

Although there have been many advances in our understanding of the causes of fetal nonimmune hydrops, it remains a difficult clinical problem. Many conditions have been associated with fetal hydrops, but few shed light on the pathophysiology of the development of hydrops. Once the diagnosis of nonimmune hydrops is established, a careful search for causative fetal pathology should be undertaken. The results of such a search may not be available when difficult management decisions need to be made. Recent advances in fetal therapy have increased the number of potentially treatable fetal conditions. However, the overall rates of morbidity to mother and fetus and mortality to the fetus are high.

REFERENCES

Abu-Dalu KI, Tamary H, Livni N, et al: GM$_1$ gangliosidosis presenting as neonatal ascites. J Pediatr **100**:940, 1982.

Afifi AM, Bhatia AR, Eyal F: Hydrops fetalis associated with congenital myotonic dystrophy. Am J Obstet Gynecol **166**:929, 1992.

Allan LD, Crawford DC, Sheridan R, et al: Aetiology of non-immune hydrops: the value of echocardiography. Br J Obstet Gynaecol **93**:223, 1986.

Anand A, Gray ES, Brown T, et al: Human parvovirus infection in pregnancy and hydrops fetalis. N Engl J Med **316**:183, 1987.

Anderson MJ, Khousam MN, Maxwell DJ, et al: Human parvovirus B19 and hydrops fetalis. Lancet **1**:535, 1988.

Appelman Z, Blumberg BD, Golabi M, et al: Nonimmune hydrops fetalis may be associated with an elevated Delta OD$_{450}$ in the amniotic fluid. Obstet Gynecol **71**:1005, 1988.

Bain AD, Bowie JH, Flint WF, et al: Congenital toxoplasmosis disease stimulating haemolytic disease of the newborn. J Obstet Gynecol **63**:826, 1956.

Bebbington MW, Wittmann BK: Fetal transfusion syndrome: Antenatal factors predicting outcome. Am J Obstet Gynecol **160**:913, 1989.

Beck M, Bender SW, Reiter HL, et al: Neuraminidase deficiency presenting as non-immune hydrops fetalis. Eur J Pediatr **143**:135, 1984.

Beischer NA, Fortune DW, Macafee J, et al: Nonimmunologic hydrops fetalis and congenital abnormalities. Obstet Gynecol **38**:86, 1971.

Benacerraf BR, Frigoletto FD, Jr.: Sonographic sign for the detection of early fetal ascites in the management of severe isoimmune disease without intrauterine transfusion. Am J Obstet Gynecol **152**:1039, 1985.

Benacerraf BR, Frigoletto FD Jr: In utero treatment of a fetus with diaphragmatic hernia complicated by hydrops. Am J Obstet Gynecol **155**:817, 1986.

Bernstein IM, Capeless EL: Elevated maternal serum alpha-fetoprotein and hydrops fetalis in association with fetal parvovirus B-19 infection. Obstet Gynecol **74**:456, 1989.

Blickstein I: The twin-twin transfusion syndrome. Obstet Gynecol **76**:714, 1990.

Blott M, Nicolaides KH, Greenough A: Pleuroamniotic shunting for decompression of fetal pleural effusions. Obstet Gynecol **71**:798, 1988.

Booth P, Nicolaides KH, Greenough A, et al: Pleuro-amniotic shunting for fetal chylothorax. Early Human Development **15**:365, 1987.

Bose C: Hydrops fetalis and in utero intracranial hemorrhage. J Pediatr **93**:1023, 1978.

Brown B St J: The ultrasonographic features of nonimmune hydrops fetalis: a study of 30 successive patients. J Can Assoc Radiol **37**:164, 1986.

Brown DL, Benson CB, Driscoll SG, et al: Twin-twin transfusion syndrome: sonographic findings. Radiology **170**:61, 1989.

Cameron A, Nicholson S, Nimrod C, et al: Evaluation of fetal cardiac dysrhythmias with two-dimensional, M-mode, and pulsed Doppler ultrasonography. Am J Obstet Gynecol **158**:286, 1988.

Cardwell MS: Successful treatment of hydrops fetalis caused by fetomaternal hemorrhage: a case report. Am J Obstet Gynecol **158**:131, 1988.

Carlson DE, Platt LD, Medearis AL, et al: Prognostic indicators of the resolution of nonimmune hydrops fetalis and survival of the fetus. Am J Obstet Gynecol **163**:1785, 1990.

Carlson NJ, Towers CV: Multiple gestation complicated by the death of one fetus. Obstet Gynecol **73**:685, 1989.

Carlton DP, McGillivray BC, Schreiber MD: Nonimmune hydrops fetalis: a multidisciplinary approach. Clin Perinatol **16**:839, 1989.

Carrington D, Whittle MJ, Gibson AAM, et al: Maternal serum alpha-fetoprotein—a marker of fetal aplastic crisis during intrauterine human parvovirus infection. Lancet **1**:433, 1987.

Castillo RA, Devoe LD, Hadi HA, et al: Nonimmune hydrops fetalis: Clinical experience and factors related to a poor outcome. Am J Obstet Gynecol **155**:812, 1986.

Castillo RA, Devoe LD, Falls G, et al: Pleural effusions and pulmonary hypoplasia. Am J Obstet Gynecol **157**:1252, 1987.

Chao A, Monoson RF: Neonatal death despite fetal therapy for cystic adenomatoid malformation: a case report. J Reprod Med **35**:655, 1990.

Chernick V, Reed MH: Pneumothorax and chylothorax in the neonatal period. J Pediatr **76**:624, 1970.

Chitkara U, Berkowitz RL, Wilkins IA, et al: Selective second-trimester termination of the anomalous fetus in twin pregnancies. Obstet Gynecol **73**:690, 1989.

Chitkara U, Wilkins I, Lynch L, et al: The role of sonography in assessing severity of fetal anemia in Rh- and Kell-isoimmunized pregnancies. Obstet Gynecol **71**:393, 1988.

Clark SL, Vitale DJ, Minton SD, et al: Successful fetal therapy for cystic adenomatoid malformation associated with second-trimester hydrops. Am J Obstet Gynecol **157**:294, 1987.

Copel JA, Cullen M, Green JJ, et al: The frequency of aneuploidy in prenatally diagnosed congenital heart disease: An indication for fetal karyotyping. Am J Obstet Gynecol **158**:409, 1988.

Crawford DC, Sunder KC, Allan LD: Prenatal detection of congenital heart disease: Factors affecting obstetric management and survival. Am J Obstet Gynecol **159**:352, 1988.

Cullen MT, Gabrielli S, Green JJ, et al: Diagnosis and significance of cystic hygroma in the first trimester. Prenat Diagn **10**:643, 1990.

Cumming DC: Recurrent nonimmune hydrops fetalis. Obstet Gynecol **54**:124, 1979.

Daffos F, Forestier F, Muller JY, et al: Prenatal treatment of alloimmune thrombocytopenia. Lancet **2**:632, 1984.

Davis CL: Diagnosis and management of nonimmune hydrops. J Reprod Med **27**:594, 1982.

D'Alton ME, Newton ER, Cetrulo CL: Intrauterine fetal demise in multiple gestation. Acta Genet Med Gemellol **33**:43, 1984.

deCrespigny LC, Robinson HP, McBain JC: Fetal abdominal paracentesis in the management of gross fetal ascites. Aust NZ J Obstet Gynaec **20**:228, 1980.

De Lia JE, Cruikshank DP, Keye WR: Fetoscopic neodymium: YAG laser occlusion of placental vessels in severe twin-twin transfusion syndrome. Obstet Gynecol **75**:1046, 1990.

Demmler GJ: Summary of a workshop on surveillance for congenital cytomegalovirus disease. Rev Infect Dis **13**:315, 1991.

Eddleman KA, Levine AB, Chitkara U, et al: Reliability of pleural fluid lymphocyte counts in the antenatal diagnosis of congenital chylothorax. Obstet Gynecol **78**:530, 1991.

Elliott JP, Urig MA, Clewell WH: Aggressive therapeutic amniocentesis for treatment of twin-twin transfusion syndrome. Obstet Gynecol **77**:537, 1991.

Etches PC, Lemons JA: Nonimmune hydrops fetalis: report of 22 cases including three siblings. Pediatrics **64**:326, 1979.

Fadel HE, Ruedrich DA: Intrauterine resolution of nonimmune hydrops associated with cytomegalovirus infection. Obstet Gynecol **71**:1003, 1988.

Fleischer AC, Killam AP, Boehm FH, et al: Hydrops fetalis: Sonographic evaluation and clinical implications. Radiology **141**:163, 1981.

Gembruch U, Niesen M, Hansmann M, et al: Listeriosis: A cause of non-immune hydrops fetalis. Prenat Diagn **7**:277, 1987.

Gillan JE, Lowden JA, Gaskin K, et al: Congenital ascites as a presenting sign of lysosomal storage disease. J Pediatr **104**:225, 1984.

Ginsburg SJ, Groll M: Hydrops fetalis due to infantile Gaucher's disease. J Pediatr **82**:1046, 1973.

Golbus MS, Cunningham N, Goldberg JD, et al: Selective termination of multiple gestations. Am J Med Genet **31**:339, 1988.

Goldberg JD, Mitty H, Dische MR, et al: Prenatal shunting of fetal ascites in nonimmune hydrops fetalis. Am J Perinatol **3**:92, 1986.

Gonsoulin W, Moise KJ, Kirshon B, et al: Outcome of twin-twin transfusion diagnosed before 28 weeks of gestation. Obstet Gynecol **75**:214, 1990.

Graves GR, Baskett TF: Nonimmune hydrops fetalis: Antenatal diagnosis and management. Am J Obstet Gynecol **148**:563, 1984.

Gray ES, Balch NJ, Kohler H, et al: Congenital leukaemia: an unusual cause of stillbirth. Arch Dis Child **61**:1001, 1986.

Gross SJ, Benzie RJ, Sermer M, et al: Prenatal diagnosis and management. Am J Obstet Gynecol **156**:393, 1987.

Harlass FE, Duff P, Brady K, et al: Hydrops fetalis and premature closure of the ductus arteriosus: A review. Obstet Gynecol Surv **44**:541, 1989.

Harrison MR, Adzick NS, Jennings RW, et al: Antenatal intervention for congenital cystic adenomatoid malformation. Lancet **336**:965, 1990a.

Harrison MR, Adzick NS, Longaker MT, et al: Successful repair in utero of a fetal diaphragmatic hernia after removal of herniated viscera from the left thorax. N Engl J Med **322**:1582, 1990b.

Hoddick WK, Mahony BS, Callen PW, et al: Placental thickness. J Ultrasound Med **4**:479, 1985.

Hogge WA, Thiagarajah S, Brenbridge AN, et al: Fetal evaluation by percutaneous blood sampling. Am J Obstet Gynecol **158**:132, 1988.

Holzgreve W, Curry CJ, Golbus MS, et al: Investigation of nonimmune hydrops fetalis. Am J Obstet Gynecol **150**:805, 1984.

Holzgreve W, Holzgreve B, Curry CJR: Nonimmune hydrops fetalis: Diagnosis and management. Semin Perinatol **9**:52, 1985.

Hsieh FJ, Chang FM, Tsang-Ming K, et al: Percutaneous ultrasound-guided fetal blood sampling in the management of nonimmune hydrops fetalis. Am J Obstet Gynecol **157**:44, 1987.

Hutchison AA, Drew JH, Yu VYH, et al: Nonimmunologic hydrops fetalis: A review of 61 cases. Obstet Gynecol **59**:347, 1982.

Im SS, Rizos N, Joutsi P, et al: Nonimmunologic hydrops fetalis. Am J Obstet Gynecol **148**:566, 1984.

Jauniaux E, Van Maldergem L, De Munter C, et al: Nonimmune hydrops fetalis associated with genetic abnormalities. Obstet Gynecol **75**:568, 1990.

Landrum BG, Johnson DE, Ferrara B, et al: Hydrops fetalis and chromosomal trisomies. Am J Obstet Gynecol **154**:1114, 1986.

Langer JC, Harrison MR, Schmidt KG, et al: Fetal hydrops and death from sacrococcygeal teratoma: Rationale for fetal surgery. Am J Obstet Gynecol **160**:1145, 1989.

Lingman G, Stangenberg M, Legarth J, et al: Albumin transfusion in non-immune fetal hydrops: Doppler ultrasound evaluation of the acute effects on blood circulation in the fetal aorta and the umbilical arteries. Fetal Ther **4**:120, 1989.

Lynch L, Daffos F, Emanuel D, et al: Prenatal diagnosis of fetal cytomegalovirus infection. Am J Obstet Gynecol **165**:714, 1991.

Macafee CAJ, Fortune DW, Beischer NA: Non-immunological hydrops fetalis. J Obstet Gynaecol Br Commonw **77**:226, 1970.

Machin GA: Hydrops revisited: Literature review of 1,414 cases published in the 1980s. Am J Med Gen **34**:366, 1989.

Maeda H, Shimokawa H, Nakano H, et al: Effects of intrauterine treatment on nonimmunologic hydrops fetalis. Fetal Ther **3**:198, 1988.

Mahoney BS, Filly RA, Callen PW, et al: Severe nonimmune hydrops fetalis: sonographic evaluation. Radiology **151**:757, 1984.

Maidman JE, Yeager C, Anderson V, et al: Prenatal diagnosis and management of nonimmunologic hydrops fetalis. Obstet Gynecol **56**:571, 1980.

McFadden DE, Taylor GP: Cardiac abnormalities and nonimmune hydrops fetalis: A coincidental, not causal relationship. Pediatr Path **9**:11, 1989.

Matthay KK, Mentzer WC: Erythrocyte enzymopathies in the newborn. Clin Haematol **10**:31, 1981.

Mentzer WC, Collier E: Hydrops fetalis associated with erythrocyte G-6-PD deficiency and maternal ingestion of fava beans and ascorbic acid. J Pediatr **86**:565, 1975.

Mogilner BM, Ashkenazy M, Borenstein R, et al: Hydrops fetalis caused by maternal indomethacin treatment. Acta Obstet Gynecol Scand **61**:183, 1982.

Moise KJ, Huhta JC, Sharif DS, et al: Indomethacin in the treatment of premature labor: effects on the fetal ductus arteriosus. N Engl J Med **319**:327, 1988.

Mor A, Schreyer P, Wainraub Z, et al: Nonimmune hydrops fetalis associated with angioosteohypertrophy (Klippel-Trenaunay) syndrome. Am J Obstet Gynecol **159**:1185, 1988.

Morbidity and Mortality Weekly Report, **38**:81, 1989.

Morey AL, Nicolini U, Welch CR, et al: Parvovirus B19 infection and transient fetal hydrops. Lancet **337**:496, 1991.

Mostoufi-Zadeh M, Weiss LM, Driscoll SH: Nonimmune hydrops fetalis: A challenge in perinatal pathology. Hum Pathol **16**:785, 1985.

Naides SJ, Weiner CP: Antenatal diagnosis and palliative treatment of non-immune hydrops fetalis secondary to fetal parvovirus B19 infection. Prenat Diag **9**:105, 1989.

Nakayama R, Yamada D, Steinmiller V, et al: Hydrops fetalis secondary to Bart hemoglobinopathy. Obstet Gynecol **67**:176, 1986.

Nimrod C, Nicholson S, Davies D, et al: Pulmonary hypoplasia testing in clinical obstetrics. Am J Obstet Gynecol **158**:277, 1988.

Oie BK, Hertel J, Seip M, et al: Hydrops foetalis in 3 infants of a mother with acquired chronic pure red cell aplasia: Transitory red cell aplasia in 1 of the infants. Scand J Haematol **33**:466, 1984.

Ostor A, Fortune DW: Tuberous sclerosis initially seen as hydrops fetalis. Arch Pathol Lab Med **102**:34, 1978.

Owen J, Stedman CM, Tucker TL: Comparison of predelivery versus postdelivery Kleihauer-Betke stains in cases of fetal death. Am J Obstet Gynecol **161**:663, 1989.

Perkins RP: Hydrops fetalis and stillbirth in a male glucose-6-phosphate dehydrogenase-deficient fetus possibly due to maternal ingestion of sulfisoxazole. Am J Obstet Gynecol **3**:379, 1971.

Peters MT, Nicolaides KH: Cordocentesis for the diagnosis and treatment of human fetal parvovirus infection. Obstet Gynecol **75**:501, 1990.

Petrikovsky BM, Shmoys SM, Baker DA, et al: Pleural effusion in aneuploidy. Perinatology **8**:214, 1991.

Platt LD, DeVore GR: In utero diagnosis of hydrops fetalis: Ultrasound methods. Clin Perinatol **9**:627, 1982.

Poeschmann RP, Verheijen RHM, Van Dongen WJ: Differential diagnosis and causes of nonimmunological hydrops fetalis: A review. Obstet Gynecol Surv **46**:223, 1991.

Porter JH, Quantril AM, Fleming KA: B19 parvovirus infection of myocardial cells. Lancet **1**:535, 1988.

Potter EL: Universal edema of the fetus unassociated with erythroblastosis. Am J Obstet Gynecol **46**:130, 1943.

Pretorius DH, Rumack CM, Manco-Johnson ML, et al: Specific skeletal dysplasias in utero: sonographic diagnosis. Radiology **159**:237, 1986.

Public Health Laboratory Service Working Party on Fifth Disease: Prospective study of human parvovirus (B19) infection in pregnancy. Br Med J **300**:1166, 1990.

Ravindranath Y, Paglia DE, Warrier I, et al: Glucose phosphate isomerase deficiency as a cause of hydrops fetalis. N Engl J Med **316**:258, 1987.

Ringer SA, Stark AR: Management of neonatal emergencies in the delivery room. Clin Perinatol **16**:23, 1989.

Robb JA, Benirschke K, Mannino F, et al: Intrauterine latent herpes simplex virus infection: Latent neonatal infection. Hum Pathol **17**:1210, 1986.

Roberts AB, Clarson RM, Pattison NS, et al: Fetal hydrothorax in the second trimester of pregnancy: Successful intrauterine treatment at 24 weeks' gestation. Fetal Ther **1**:203, 1986.

Robertson L, Ott A, Mack L, et al: Sonographically documented disappearance of nonimmune hydrops fetalis associated with maternal hypertension. West J Med **143**:382, 1985.

Rodeck CH, Fisk NM, Fraser DI, et al: Long-term in utero drainage of fetal hydrothorax. N Engl J Med **319**:1135, 1988.

Rodis JF, Hovick TJ, Quinn DL, et al: Human parvovirus infection in pregnancy. Obstet Gynecol **72**:733, 1988.

Romero R, Pilu G, Jeanty P, et al: Other anomalies: nonimmune hydrops fetalis. In Romero R, Pilu G, Jeanty P, et al (eds): Prenatal Diagnosis of Congenital Anomalies. Norwalk, Appleton and Lange, 1988, pp 403–431.

Rouse D, Weiner C: Ongoing fetomaternal hemorrhage treated by serial fetal intravascular transfusions. Obstet Gynecol **76**:974, 1990.

Sahakian V, Weiner CP, Naides SJ, et al: Intrauterine transfusion treatment of nonimmune hydrops fetalis secondary to human parvovirus B19 infection. Am J Obstet Gynecol **164**:1090, 1991.

Saltzman DH, Frigoletto FD, Harlow BL, et al: Sonographic evaluation of hydrops fetalis. Obstet Gynecol **74**:106, 1989.

Samuels P, Ludmir J: Nonimmune hydrops fetalis: A heterogeneous disorder and therapeutic challenge. Sem Roentgenol **25**:353, 1990.

Santolaya J, Alley D, Jaffe R, et al: Antenatal classification of hydrops fetalis. Obstet Gynecol **79**:256, 1992.

Schwartz SH, Viseskul C, Laxova R, et al: Idiopathic hydrops fetalis report of 4 patients including 2 affected sibs. Am J Med Gen **8**:59, 1981.

Seifer DB, Ferguson JE, Behrens CM, et al: Nonimmune hydrops fetalis in association with hemangioma of the umbilical cord. Obstet Gynecol **66**:283, 1985.

Shah DM, Chaffin D: Perinatal outcome in very preterm births with twin-twin transfusion syndrome. Am J Obstet Gynecol **161**:1111, 1989.

Shenker L, Reed KL, Anderson CF, et al: Congenital heart block and cardiac anomalies in the absence of maternal connective tissue disease. Am J Obstet Gynecol **157**:248, 1987.

Shimokawa H, Hara K, Fukuda A, et al: Idiopathic hydrops fetalis successfully treated in utero. Obstet Gynecol **71**:984, 1988.

Soothill P: Intrauterine blood transfusion for non-immune hydrops fetalis due to parvovirus B19 infection. Lancet **336**:121, 1990.

Spahr RC, Botti JJ, MacDonald HM, et al: Nonimmunologic hydrops fetalis: A review of 19 cases. Gynaecol Obstet **18**:303, 1980.

Thorp JA, Cohen GR, Yeast JD, et al: Nonimmune hydrops caused by massive fetomaternal hemorrhage and treated by intravascular transfusion. Perinatology **9**:22, 1992.

Urig MA, Simpson GF, Elliott JP, et al: Twin-twin transfusion syndrome: The surgical removal of one twin as a treatment option. Fetal Ther **3**:185, 1988.

Vanhaesebrouck P, Thiery M, Leroy JG, et al: Oligohydramnios, renal insufficiency, and ileal perforation in preterm infants after intrauterine exposure to indomethacin. J Pediatr **113**:738, 1988.

Warsof SL, Nicolaides KH, Rodeck C: Immune and non-immune hydrops. Clin Obstet Gynecol **29**:533, 1986.

Watson J, Campbell S: Antenatal evaluation and management in nonimmune hydrops fetalis. Obstet Gynecol **67**:589, 1986.

Weiner CP, Naides SJ, Pringle K: Fetal survival after human parvovirus B19 infection: Spectrum of intrauterine response in a twin gestation. Am J Perinatol **9**:66, 1992.

Wendel GD: Gestational and congenital syphilis. Clin Perinatol **15**:287, 1988.

Wenstrom KD, Weiner CP, Hanson JW: A five-year statewide experience with congenital diaphragmatic hernia. Am J Obstet Gynecol **165**:838, 1991.

Wittmann BK, Farquharson DF, Thomas WDS, et al: The role of feticide in the management of severe twin transfusion syndrome. Am J Obstet Gynecol **155**:1023, 1986.

Zimmer EZ, Gutterman E, Blazer S: Recurrent nonimmune hydrops. J Reprod Med **31**:193, 1986.

Zornes SL, Anderson PG, Lott RL: Congenital toxoplasmosis in an infant with hydrops fetalis. Southern Med J **81**:391, 1988.

MATERNAL DISORDERS

CHAPTER

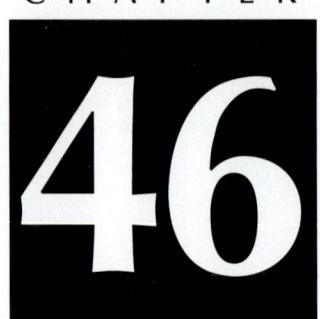

46

CARDIOVASCULAR AND RENAL ADAPTATION TO PREGNANCY

MANJU MONGA, M.D. and ROBERT K. CREASY, M.D.

There are profound changes in the cardiovascular and renal systems during pregnancy. These remarkable adaptations, which occur as a result of the maternal-fetal interaction, begin early after conception and continue as gestation advances, yet in the main are almost totally reversible after pregnancy is complete.

Physiologic adaptations of the cardiovascular system, which include changes in anatomy, blood volume, cardiac output, and systemic vascular resistance, result in cardiac enlargement, sinus tachycardia, cardiac murmurs, and peripheral edema. While these are normal in pregnancy, they are signs of cardiovascular dysfunction in the nonpregnant patient. Similarly, anatomic and functional changes in the renal system, such as dilatation of the collecting systems, could lead one to a misdiagnosis of urinary tract disease.

Preexisting disease, such as cardiac myopathy or chronic renal disease, can be exacerbated by the pregnant state, can adversely affect fetal status leading to low-birth-weight infants, or can lead to the superimposition of preeclampsia. Drug therapy of problems such as seizure disorders may need modification owing to plasma volume changes. Such laboratory values as serum creatinine concentrations that may be normal in the nonpregnant are distinctly abnormal in the pregnant patient.

These physiologic adaptations are usually well tolerated by the pregnant patient, but they must be understood so that the normal can be distinguished from the abnormal. Also, they must be recognized so that the pathophysiology of potentially hazardous disease processes that may occur during a gestation may be recognized.

CARDIOVASCULAR SYSTEM

Blood Volume

Plasma volume increases progressively from 6 to 8 weeks gestation and reaches a maximal volume of 4700 to 5200 ml at 32 weeks, an increase of 45 per cent (1200 to 1600 ml) above nonpregnant values (Pritchard, 1965a; Lund and Donovan, 1967). This increment is greater in multiple gestations and is also correlated with fetal weight (Rovinsky and Jaffin, 1965; Duffus et al., 1971). The mechanism for this plasma volume expansion is unclear but may be related to estrogen stimulation of the renin-angiotensin-aldosterone system, which stimulates sodium and water retention. As maternal hypervolemia is present in cases of hydatidiform mole, it is unlikely that the presence of a fetus per se is necessary for this to occur (Pritchard, 1965b).

Red blood cell mass increases by 250 to 450 ml by term, an increment of 20 to 30 per cent from prepregnancy values. This rise, which is even greater in women receiving exogenous iron supplementation, reflects increased production of red blood cells rather than prolongation of red cell life (Pritchard, 1965a). Placental chorionic somatomammotropin, progesterone, and perhaps prolactin are responsible for this increase in erythropoiesis (Jepson, 1968), which consequently increases the maternal demand for iron by 500 mg during pregnancy. This is in addition to the 300 mg of iron transferred from maternal stores to the fetus and the 200 mg required to compensate for normal daily losses over this time. Erythrocyte 2,3-diphosphoglycerate concentration increases in pregnancy, thus lowering the affinity of maternal hemoglobin for oxygen. This facilitates the dissociation of oxygen from hemoglobin, which enhances oxygen transfer to the fetus (Bille-Brahe and Rorth, 1979).

The forementioned changes result in an increase in circulating blood volume by approximately 45 per cent. This may protect the pregnant woman from hemodynamic instability following antepartum or, more commonly, postpartum blood loss. Since plasma volume increases disproportionately to red blood cell mass, there is a physiologic hemodilution effect resulting in a mild decrease in maternal hematocrit, which is maximal in the middle of the third trimester. This may also have a protective function by decreasing blood viscosity to counter the predisposition to thromboembolic events in pregnancy (Koller, 1982). (See Chapters 48 and 53 for changes in other blood constituents during pregnancy.)

Anatomic Changes

Histologic and echocardiographic studies indicate that ventricular wall muscle mass and end-diastolic volume increase in pregnancy without an associated increase in end-systolic volume or end-diastolic pressures (Lard-Meeter et al., 1979; Rubler et al., 1977). Although the increase in ventricular mass does not continue after the first trimester (Thompson et al., 1986), the increment in end-diastolic volume occurs in the second and early third trimesters (Rubler et al., 1977). As cardiac compliance thus increases (resulting in a physiologically dilated heart), without a concomitant reduction in ejection fraction, it would appear that myocardial contractility must also increase. This is supported by studies of systolic time intervals in pregnancy (Rubler et al., 1972; Burg et al., 1974). Finally, a general softening of collagen occurs in the entire vascular system, associated with hypertrophy of the smooth muscle components (Marazita, 1946). This results in increased compliance of the vascular system.

Cardiac Output

Cardiac output, the product of heart rate and stroke volume, is a measure of the functional capacity of the heart. Cardiac output may be calculated by use of invasive heart catheterization with dye- or thermodilution or by noninvasive methods such as impedance cardiography and echocardiography. Although limited data have been obtained from normal pregnant women by means of invasive methods (Bader et al., 1955; Walters et al., 1966; Clark et al., 1989), M-mode echocardiography (Mashini et al., 1987) and Doppler studies (Easterling et al., 1990a) recently have been used successfully to delineate the alterations in cardiac output during pregnancy. In contrast, thoracic electrical bioimpedance has had poor correlation with thermodilution techniques in pregnancy (Easterling et al., 1989).

Cardiac output increases by 30 to 50 per cent during pregnancy (Bader et al., 1955; Walters et al., 1966; Clark et al., 1989), with 50 per cent of this increase occurring by 8 weeks gestation (Capeless and Clapp, 1989). There is a continued rise, at a slower rate, until the third trimester of pregnancy. Controversy exists as to whether the reported mild decrease in the expanded cardiac output that occurs toward term reflects the supine position in which these women were studied rather than a true decline. Studies performed in the left lateral recumbent position appear to have confirmed a small decline in cardiac output at term (Ueland et al., 1969a; Easterling et al., 1990b).

The documented increase in maternal cardiac output is due to an increase in both stroke volume and heart rate. Stroke volume is primarily responsible for the early increase in cardiac output (Capeless and Clapp, 1989; Robson et al., 1989), probably reflecting the increase in ventricular muscle mass and end-diastolic volume. Stroke volume declines toward term (Ueland et al., 1969), whereas maternal heart rate, which rises from 5 weeks gestation to a maximal increment of 15 to 20 bpm by 32 weeks, is maintained (Ueland et al., 1969; Robson et al., 1989) (Fig. 46–1). Therefore, in the late third trimester, the relatively mild maternal tachycardia is primarily responsible for maintaining cardiac output.

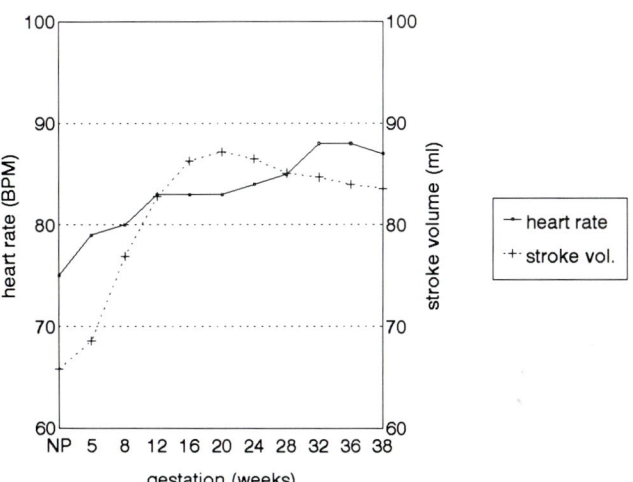

FIGURE 46–1. Alteration in stroke volume and heart rate during pregnancy. Stroke volume increases maximally during the first half of gestation. There is a slight decrease in stroke volume toward term. The mild increase in heart rate begins early in gestation and continues until term. (Adapted with permission from Robson SC, Hunter S, Boys RJ, et al: Serial study of factors influencing changes in cardiac output during human pregnancy. Am J Physiol **256**:H1060, 1989.)

Maternal posture significantly affects cardiac output. Turning from the left lateral recumbent to the supine position at term can result in a drop in cardiac output by as much as 25 to 30 per cent (Ueland et al., 1969). This is due to caval compression by the gravid uterus, which diminishes venous return from the lower extremities, thus decreasing stroke volume and cardiac output. Although most women do not become hypotensive with this maneuver, up to 8 per cent of women will demonstrate the supine hypotensive syndrome, which is manifested by a sudden drop in blood pressure, bradycardia, and syncope (Holmes, 1960). This may be due to inadequacy of the paravertebral collateral blood supply in these women.

There is selective regional distribution of this physiologic increase in cardiac output. Uterine blood flow increases tenfold to between 500 and 800 ml/min (Gant and Worley, 1989). This represents a shift from 2 per cent of total cardiac output in the nonpregnant state to 17 per cent at term. Renal blood flow increases significantly (by 50 per cent) during pregnancy (Chesley and Sloan, 1964), as does perfusion of the breasts and skin (Katz and Sokal, 1980). There does not appear to be any major alteration in blood flow to the brain or liver.

Blood Pressure

Arterial blood pressure decreases in pregnancy beginning as early as the seventh week (Capeless and Clapp, 1989). This early drop probably represents the inability of increased cardiac output to compensate for the fall in peripheral vascular resistance. When measured in the sitting or standing positions, systolic blood pressure remains relatively stable throughout pregnancy, whereas diastolic blood pressure decreases by a maximum of 10 mm at 28 weeks and then increases toward nonpregnant levels by term (Wilson et al., 1980). In contrast, when measured in the left lateral recumbent position, both systolic and diastolic blood pressures decrease to a level 5 to 10 mm Hg and 10 to 15 mm Hg respectively below nonpregnant values. This nadir occurs at 24 to 32 weeks gestation and is followed by a rise toward nonpregnant values at term (Wilson et al., 1980) (Fig. 46–2). As diastolic pressures fall to a greater extent than systolic pressures, there is a slight increase in pulse pressure in the early third trimester. As arterial blood pressures are approximately 10 mm Hg higher in the standing or sitting positions than in the lateral or supine positions, consistency in position during successive blood pressure measurements is essential for the accurate documentation of a trend during pregnancy.

Finally, confusion has arisen with regard to the definition of diastolic blood pressure in pregnancy. Measurement of Korotkoff phase 4 (the point of muffling) results in mean diastolic pressures 13 mm Hg higher than measurement of Korotkoff phase 5 (the point of disappearance) (Wickman et al., 1984). Intraarterial measurements of diastolic pressures may be 15 mm Hg lower than manual determinations (Koller, 1982), whereas they may be significantly higher than automated cuff diastolic measurements (Kirshon et al.,

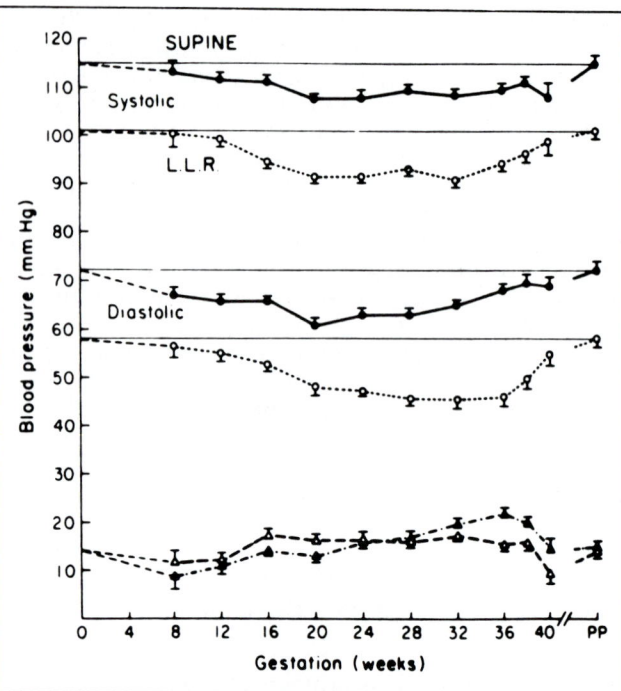

FIGURE 46–2. Sequential changes in blood pressures throughout pregnancy with subjects in supine and left lateral recumbent positions. The change in systolic (*open triangles*) and diastolic (*closed triangles*) blood pressures produced by movement from the left lateral recumbent to the supine position is illustrated in bottom part of figure. (Reproduced with permission from Wilson M, Morganti AD, Zervondakis I, et al: Blood pressure, the renin-aldosterone system, and sex steroids throughout normal pregnancy. Am J Med **68**:97, 1980.)

1987). For these reasons it is also important to be consistent in the method by which blood pressure is recorded throughout pregnancy and to ascertain the definition of diastolic blood pressure when reviewing studies of arterial blood pressure in pregnant women.

Systemic Vascular Resistance

Systemic vascular resistance (SVR) is calculated by the following equation:

$$\frac{[\text{mean arterial pressure } - \text{ central venous pressure}] \times 80 \text{ dynes-sec cm}^2}{\text{cardiac output}}$$

SVR decreases during pregnancy as a result of the vasodilatory effect of progesterone and prostaglandins and perhaps the arteriovenous fistula—like function of the low-resistance uteroplacental circulation (Greiss and Anderson, 1970; Gerber et al., 1981). The fall in SVR reaches a nadir at 14 to 24 weeks gestation and then rises progressively toward term (Bader et al., 1955).

Venous Vascular Bed

Venous compliance increases progressively during pregnancy; this results in a decrease in flow velocity, and subsequent stasis (Fawer et al., 1978). This increase in venous capacitance may be due to the relaxant effect of progesterone on the smooth muscle of the blood vessels or to altered elastic properties of the venous wall. As a result of this decrease in venous vascular resistance, pregnant women are more sensitive to autonomic blockade, which results in further venous pooling, decreased venous return, and a fall in cardiac output manifested as a sudden drop in arterial blood pressure (Assali and Brinkman, 1972). This may be seen in response to conduction anesthesia and ganglionic blockade. Forearm venous pressure increases throughout normal pregnancy by 40 to 50 per cent above nonpregnant values. Calf venous pressures are always higher than that of the forearm, and this difference becomes more exaggerated as gestation advances, owing in part to the enlarging uterus (Barwin and Roddie, 1976; McLennan, 1943) (Fig. 46–3).

Antepartum Hemodynamics

Clark et al. (1989) studied the effect of pregnancy on central hemodynamics by placing Swan-Ganz catheters and arterial lines in 10 normal primiparous women at 35 to 38 weeks gestation and again at 11 to 13 weeks postpartum (Table 46–1). Late pregnancy was characterized by significant elevations in heart rate, stroke volume, and cardiac output in concert with significant decreases in systemic and pulmonary vascular resistance and serum colloid osmotic pressure. There was no significant alteration in pulmonary capillary wedge pressure, central venous pressure, or mean arterial blood pressure. Clark et al. (1989) suggested that pulmonary capillary wedge pressure does not increase, despite significant increases in blood

TABLE 46–1. Hemodynamic Profiles for Nonpregnant and Pregnant Patients in Third Trimester

	NONPREGNANT	PREGNANT	CHANGE
Cardiac output (liters/min)	4.3 ± 0.9	6.2 ± 1.0	+43%
Heart rate (beats/min)	71 ± 10	83 ± 10	+17%
SVR (dyne-cm-sec^{-5})	1530 ± 520	1210 ± 266	−21%
PVR (dyne-cm-sec^5)	119 ± 47	78 ± 22	−34%
CVP (mm Hg)	3.7 ± 2.6	3.6 ± 2.5	NS
COP (mm Hg)	20.8 ± 1.0	18.0 ± 1.5	−14%
PCWP (mm Hg)	6.3 ± 2.1	7.5 ± 1.8	NS
COP-PCWP (mm Hg)	14.5 ± 2.5	10.5 ± 2.7	−28%

Nonpregnant = 11–13 weeks postpartum; pregnant = 36–38 weeks gestation; SVR = systemic vascular resistance; PVR = pulmonary vascular resistance; CVP = central venous pressure; COP = colloid osmotic pressure; PCWP = pulmonary capillary wedge pressure; COP-PCWP = gradient between COP and PCWP. (Adapted with permission from Clark SL, Cotton DB, Lee W, et al: Central hemodynamic assessment of normal term pregnancy. Am J Obstet Gynecol **161**:1439, 1989.)

volume and stroke volume, because of ventricular dilatation and the fall in pulmonary vascular resistance. They noted, however, that pregnant women were still at higher risk for developing pulmonary edema due to the significantly decreased gradient between colloid osmotic pressure and pulmonary capillary wedge pressure (gradient of 10.5 ± 2.7 mm Hg) compared with the nonpregnant state (gradient of 14.5 ± 2.5 mm Hg).

Circulation time demonstrates a slight but progressive decline during pregnancy, reaching a minimal value of 10.2 seconds in the third trimester (Manchester and Loube, 1946). These findings have been interpreted to mean that blood flow velocity increases slightly in pregnancy.

Arterial Blood Gases

As discussed in Chapter 52, maternal tidal volume increases by 40 per cent in pregnancy, and this increase results in maternal hyperventilation and hypocapnia (Awe et al., 1979). There is a decrease in partial pressure of carbon dioxide (P_{CO_2}) from a normal pregnancy level of 39 mm Hg to approximately 28 to 31 mm Hg. This is partially compensated by increased renal secretion of hydrogen ions, with a resultant serum bicarbonate level of 18 to 22 mEq/liter. A mild respiratory alkalosis is therefore normal in pregnancy, with an arterial pH of 7.44 compared to 7.40 in the nonpregnant state. There is also a narrowing of the difference between arterial and central venous oxygen saturation in pregnancy (Guzman and Caplan, 1970). This implies that the increase in cardiac output is more than adequate to compensate for the increased metabolic demands of pregnancy.

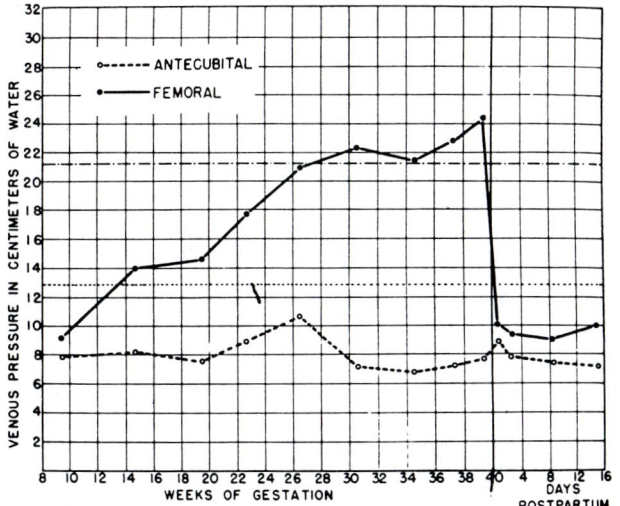

FIGURE 46–3. Alterations in antecubital and femoral venous pressures throughout normal pregnancy and the immediate puerperium. The lower straight dotted line represents the upper limit of normal for antecubital venous pressure, and the upper broken line the upper limit of normal for femoral venous pressure. (Reproduced with permission from McLennan CE: Antecubital and femoral venous pressures in normal and toxemic pregnancies. Am J Obstet Gynecol **45**:568, 1943.)

Symptoms and Signs of Normal Pregnancy

Pregnant women report dyspnea with increased frequency as gestation advances (15 per cent in the first trimester compared with 75 per cent by the third) (Milne et al., 1978). The mechanism for this is unclear, but may relate to the exaggerated ventilatory response (perhaps progesterone-mediated) in response to the increased metabolic demand. Easy fatiguability and decreased exercise tolerance are also commonly reported, although mild-to-moderate exercise is well tolerated under normal circumstances (Kulpa et al., 1987; Wolfe et al., 1989). Increased lower extremity venous pressure, due to compression by the gravid uterus and associated lower colloid osmotic pressure, is commonly manifested as dependent edema—most often found in the distal lower extremities at term.

Cutforth and MacDonald (1966) have clearly documented the alterations in heart sounds and murmurs in pregnancy by phonocardiographic study of 50 normal primigravid women. These changes are summarized in Figure 46–4. Briefly, the first heart sound increases in loudness and is more widely split (30 to 45 msec as compared to 15 msec in the nonpregnant state). This exaggerated splitting of the first heart sound, found in approximately 90 per cent of women, is due to early closure of the mitral valve as demonstrated by the shortened interval between the Q wave of the electrocardiogram and the first heart sound. There is no significant change in the second heart sound until 30 weeks gestation, when there may be persistent splitting that does not vary with respiration. A loud third heart sound is heard in up to 90 per cent of pregnant women, whereas less than 5 per cent will have an audible fourth heart sound. Systolic murmurs develop in more than 95 per cent of pregnant women. These are heard best along the left sternal border and are most often either aortic or pulmonary in origin. Doppler echocardiography has demonstrated an increased incidence of functional tricuspid regurgitation during pregnancy which may also lead to a systolic precordial murmur (Limacher et al., 1985). Although most of these changes in heart sounds are first audible between 12 and 20 weeks gestation and regress by one week postpartum, nearly 20 per cent will have a persistent systolic murmur beyond the fourth postpartum week (Cutforth and MacDonald, 1966).

Systolic murmurs louder than grade 2/4 and diastolic murmurs of any intensity are considered abnormal during pregnancy. However, 14 per cent of women may have a continuous, often bilateral, murmur heard maximally in the second intercostal space which is of mammary vessel origin (Cutforth and MacDonald, 1966).

Uterine growth results in upward displacement of the diaphragm, which is associated with superior, lateral, and anterior displacement of the heart within the thorax. This leads to lateral displacement of the point of maximal impulse. It may also suggest the presence of cardiomegaly on chest radiographs, an appearance further enhanced by straightening of the left heart border and prominence of the pulmonary outflow tracts. However, the cardiothoracic ratio is only slightly increased, if at all, in normal pregnancy (Turner, 1975).

Intrapartum Hemodynamic Changes

Labor results in significant alterations in the cardiovascular measurements discussed above. The first stage of labor is associated with a 15.3 per cent rise in cardiac output, primarily due to a 22 per cent increase in stroke volume (Ueland and Hansen, 1969). The second stage of labor is associated with an even greater increase in cardiac output (49 per cent). Laboring in the left lateral decubitus position or caudal anesthesia decreases the magnitude of this increment. The increase in cardiac output is not completely abolished by relief of pain, however, as during labor each contraction results in the transfer of 300 to 500 ml of blood from the uterus to the general circulation (Adams and Alexander, 1958; Hendricks and Quilligan, 1958). For these reasons, women who have cardiovascular compromise may experience decompensation with labor, especially during the second stage.

Postpartum Hemodynamic Changes

Pregnant women with cardiac disease are perhaps at greatest risk for pulmonary edema in the immediate postpartum period. The immediate puerperium is associated with an 80 per cent increase in cardiac output after vaginal delivery with local anesthesia compared to 60 per cent with caudal anesthesia (Ueland and Metcalfe, 1975). This immediate increase in cardiac output is due to release of venocaval obstruction by the gravid uterus, autotransfusion of uteroplacental blood, and rapid mobilization of extravascular fluid. All of these result in increased venous return to the heart and increased stroke volume. Cesarean section

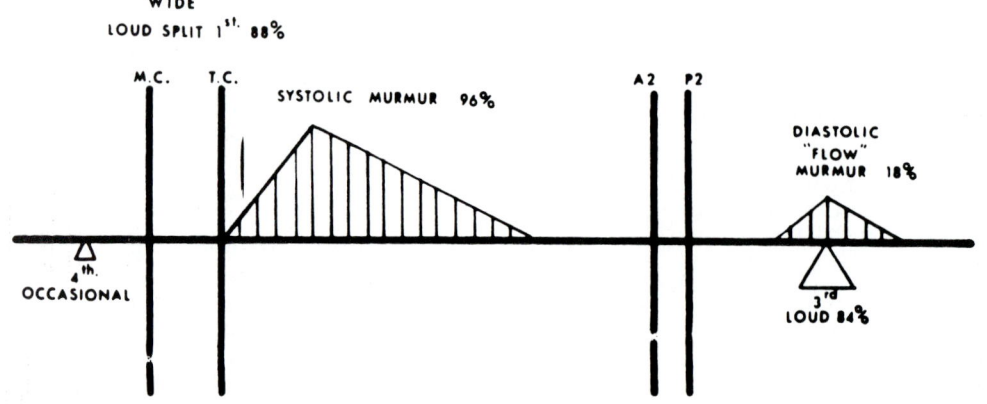

FIGURE 46–4. Summarization of the findings on auscultation of the heart in pregnancy. M.C., mitral closure; T.C., tricuspid closure. AZ and PZ, aortic and pulmonary elements of the second sound. (Reproduced with permission from Cutforth R, MacDonald CB: Heart sounds and murmurs in pregnancy. Am Heart J **71**:741, 1966.)

does not cause as dramatic a shift in hemodynamics, although there is still a 25 per cent increase in cardiac output using the most controlled form of analgesia (epidural anesthesia without epinephrine) (Ueland et al., 1968).

Vaginal delivery is associated with a blood loss of approximately 500 ml as opposed to 1000 ml at cesarean section (Ueland, 1976). The pregnant woman is protected from this blood loss in part by the expansion of blood volume associated with pregnancy. In fact, there may be a slight rise in hematocrit several days after an uncomplicated vaginal delivery owing to the normal postpartum diuresis (Ueland, 1976).

Cardiovascular measurements such as stroke volume, end-diastolic volume, and systemic vascular resistance, as measured by M-mode echocardiography, do not completely return to pre-pregnancy values by 12 weeks postpartum (Capeless and Clapp, 1991). Therefore, the early postpartum period may not accurately reflect the nonpregnant state in studies of pregnancy-related hemodynamic changes.

KIDNEYS AND LOWER URINARY TRACT

The marked hemodynamic and hormonal changes of normal pregnancy are associated with striking alterations in renal physiology involving structure, dynamics, tubular function, and volume homeostasis.

Structure and Dynamics

Renal size and weight increase during pregnancy owing to an increase in renal vascular and interstitial volume. Kidney length increases by approximately 1 cm (Bailey and Rolleston, 1971), and renal volume, as determined by computerized nephrosonography, increases by approximately 30 per cent (Christensen et al., 1989).

More dramatic, however, is dilatation of the urinary collecting system, which occurs in over 80 per cent of gravidas by mid-gestation (Rasmussen and Nielse, 1988). Calyceal and ureteral dilatation are more common on the right side (three-fourths) than the left (one-third) (Schulman and Herlinger, 1975), and the degree of calyceal dilatation is more pronounced on the right than on the left (15 mm versus 5 mm) (Fried et al., 1983). Ureteral dilatation is rarely present beyond the level of the pelvic brim, and sonographic visualization demonstrates tapering of the ureters as they cross the common iliac artery (MacNeily et al., 1991). Therefore, it has been suggested that obstruction or compression of the ureters by the enlarging uterus and ovarian vein plexus is the primary etiology for the physiologic hydronephrosis and hydroureter of pregnancy. This is supported by the prominence of these changes on the right side, which may be due to dextrorotation of the pregnant uterus, the location of the right ovarian vein that crosses the ureter, and the protective "cushion" effect of the sigmoid colon on the left side. Although progesterone may play a concomitant role in ureteral smooth muscle relaxation,

there is no consensus on the influence of hormones on these anatomic alterations (Marchant, 1972).

The dilatation of the urinary collecting system has several important clinical consequences, including an increase in ascending urinary tract infection perhaps related to urinary stasis, difficulty in interpreting radiologic examinations of the urinary tract, and interference with evaluation of glomerular and tubular function as these tests require high urine flow rates. Renal volume returns to normal within the first week of delivery (Christensen et al., 1989), but hydronephrosis and hydroureter may persist for as long as 3 to 4 months postpartum (Fried et al., 1983). This should be considered when radiologic or renal function studies on postpartum women are being interpreted.

Ureteral peristaltic activity in pregnant women does not differ from that in nonpregnant women. However, ureteral tone progressively increases, possibly owing to mechanical obstruction, and then returns to normal shortly after delivery (Sala and Rubi, 1967). Controversy exists with regard to changes in urinary bladder pressures and capacity. In one study, urinary bladder pressure doubled between the first and third trimesters of pregnancy, implying a decrease in bladder capacity (Iosif et al., 1980). Previous studies had demonstrated a relatively hypotonic bladder, with decreased pressure and increased capacity near term (Youssef, 1956). Urethral length and intraurethral closure pressure in pregnancy have also been determined by means of urodynamic studies and have been found to increase by 20 per cent (Iosif et al., 1980). The latter may counter the increase in bladder pressure in an attempt to reduce stress incontinence, which is increased in pregnancy.

Renal Function

Renal plasma flow (RPF), as estimated by para-aminohippurate clearance, increases by 60 to 80 per cent over nonpregnant values by the middle of the second trimester, and then falls to 50 per cent above prepregnancy values in the third trimester (Dunlop, 1981). RPF, like cardiac output, measures significantly higher when the patient is in the left lateral recumbent position than when she is sitting, standing, or supine. This reflects maximal venous return in the left lateral position (Davison and Dunlop, 1984; Equimokhai et al., 1981).

Glomerular filtration rate (GFR) is estimated by determination of either inulin or creatinine clearance. The former is more accurate, as inulin is cleared solely by the glomerulus whereas creatinine is also secreted by the tubules. Creatinine clearance measurements are therefore usually higher than actual GFR; however, both methods of GFR determination have good clinical correlation in the normal range. Creatinine clearance is calculated by dividing the total amount of urinary creatinine (in mg) by the duration of collection (in minutes). This value is then divided by the creatinine concentration in serum (in mg per ml). This yields a creatinine clearance in ml/min.

GFR begins to increase by as early as 6 weeks

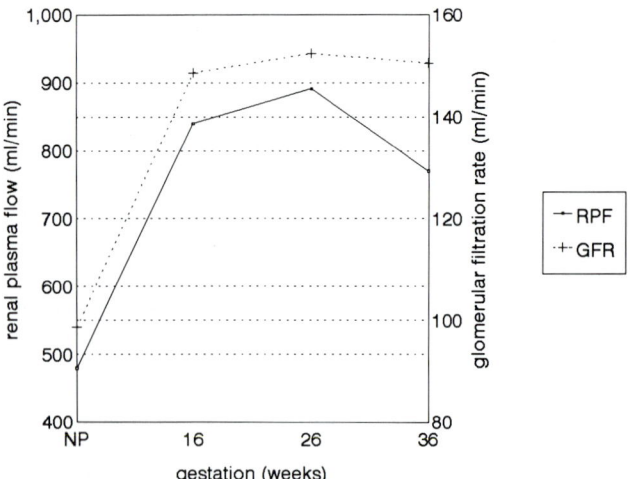

FIGURE 46–5. Patterns of change in renal plasma flow (RPF) (as estimated by PAH clearance) and glomerular filtration rate (GFR) (as estimated by inulin clearance). Initially, the rise in RPF is greater than the rise in GFR, and therefore the filtration fraction (GFR/RPF) falls. Since RPF decreases toward term, whereas GFR remains stable, filtration fraction returns to prepregnancy values of 20 per cent. (Adapted with permission from Dunlop W: Serial changes in renal hemodynamics during normal human pregnancy. Br J Obstet Gynaecol **88**:1, 1981.)

gestation, with a peak of 50 per cent over nonpregnant values by the end of the first trimester (Davison and Dunlop, 1984). Although there are little data on the measurement of GFR after 36 weeks gestation, GFR does not appear to decrease at term. Creatinine clearance is therefore moderately increased in pregnancy (110 to 150 ml/min). This rate has a circadian variation of 80 to 125 per cent, with maximal creatinine excretion between 1400 and 2200 hours and lowest excretion rates between 0200 and 1000 hours (Kalousek et al., 1969).

The mechanisms behind the changes in renal hemodynamics are unclear, although study of pregnant rats would suggest that GFR rises secondary to vasodilatation of pre- and postglomerular resistance vessels without any alteration in glomerular capillary pressure (Baylis, 1987).

As the increment in renal plasma flow is initially greater than the rise in glomerular filtration rate, the filtration fraction (GFR/RPF) decreases until the third trimester of pregnancy, when a fall in renal plasma flow results in the return of the filtration fraction to prepregnancy values of 1/5 (Davison and Dunlop, 1984). This alteration in filtration fraction parallels the change in mean arterial pressure described in the previous section of this chapter, and is inversely related to the changes in RPF. The relationship between modifications in glomerular filtration rate and renal plasma flow in pregnancy is depicted in Figure 46–5.

Filtration capacity, which is estimated by the maximal GFR in response to a vasodilator stimulus, appears to be intact in pregnancy, as documented by studies of amino acid administration in rats (Baylis, 1987) and protein loading in pregnant women (Ronco et al.,

1988). As the resting GFR rises during pregnancy, the functional renal reserve (the difference between the filtration capacity and the resting GFR) decreases. One can therefore assess renal function in pregnant patients with early renal disease by determining filtration capacity but not functional renal reserve (Ronco et al., 1988).

The pregnancy-associated rise in GFR (which occurs without any concomitant increase in production of urea or creatinine) results in decreased serum creatinine and urea concentrations in pregnancy (Davison and Dunlop, 1980). Serum creatinine falls from prepregnancy values of 0.83 mg/100 ml to 0.73, 0.58, and 0.5 mg/100 ml in successive trimesters. Blood urea nitrogen decreases from 12.0 mg/dl in the nonpregnant state to 11, 9, and 10 mg/dl in the first, second, and third trimesters, respectively.

Renal Tubular Function

SODIUM. Several factors promote sodium *excretion* in pregnancy. Perhaps foremost of these is an increase in the filtered load of sodium from approximately 20,000 mEq per day to 30,000 mEq per day as a result of the 50 per cent rise in GFR. Hormones that favor sodium excretion include: progesterone, a competitive inhibitor of aldosterone (Barron and Lindheimer, 1984); vasodilatory prostaglandins (Davison and Dunlop, 1984); and atrial natriuretic factor, although increased pregnancy-related production of atrial natriuretic factor has not been universally demonstrated (Marlettini et al., 1991; Bond et al., 1989). Despite these forces, there is a cumulative *retention* of approximately 950 mg of sodium during pregnancy. This is distributed between the maternal intravascular and interstitial compartments, the fetus, and the placenta (Hytten and Leitch, 1971). The net reabsorption of sodium is one of the most remarkable adaptations of renal tubular function to pregnancy.

Factors that promote this sodium *reabsorption* include the increased production and secretion of aldosterone, deoxycorticosterone, and estrogen (Barron and Lindheimer, 1984) (Fig. 46–6). These hormones may be regulated in part by the rise in plasma progesterone

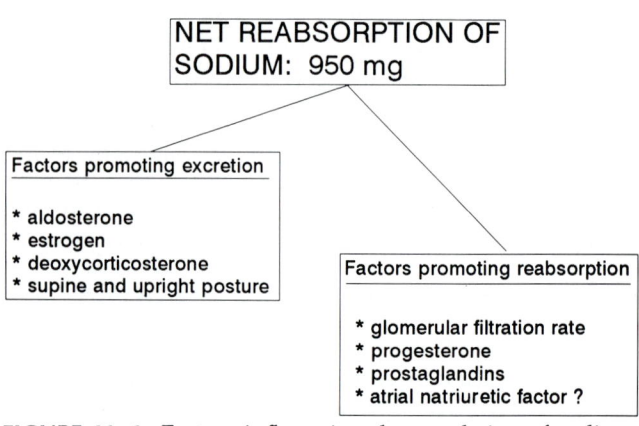

FIGURE 46–6. Factors influencing the regulation of sodium excretion in pregnancy.

and vasodilatory prostaglandins but also appear to be mediated by stimulation of the renin-angiotensin system. Sodium retention is also favored by postural changes in pregnancy; the supine and upright positions are associated with a marked decrease in sodium excretion (Chesley and Sloan, 1964).

POTASSIUM. While the pregnancy-associated increase in plasma aldosterone would favor potassium excretion, a net *retention* of 300 to 350 mEq of potassium actually occurs. Increased kaliuresis may be prevented by the influence of progesterone on renal potassium excretion (Lindheimer et al., 1987). Since potassium reabsorption from the distal tubule and Henle's loop decreases with pregnancy, it has been deduced that a significant increase in proximal tubular reabsorption occurs (Garland and Green, 1982).

CALCIUM. Urinary calcium excretion increases as a result of increased calcium clearance (Roelofsen et al., 1988). This is balanced by increased absorption of calcium from the small intestine, and therefore serum ionic (unbound) calcium levels remain stable. Total calcium levels fall in pregnancy owing to a decrease in plasma albumin.

GLUCOSE. Glucose excretion increases in pregnant women by ten- to 100-fold over nonpregnant values of 100 mg/day (Davison and Hytten, 1975). This glycosuria, which occurs despite increased plasma insulin and decreased plasma glucose levels, was originally thought to be due to the inability of the renal tubules to reabsorb the increased filtered glucose load (Welsh and Sims, 1960). Studies in the rat contradict this, as the proximal tubule demonstrates an increased absorptive capacity greater than that required to handle the increase in filtered glucose load (Bishop and Green, 1981). Rather, glycosuria occurs due to impaired reabsorption by the collecting tubule and Henle's loop of the 5 per cent of the filtered glucose that normally escapes proximal convoluted tubular reabsorption (Bishop and Green, 1981). The clinical significance of this is that glycosuria cannot be accurately used to monitor pregnant women with diabetes mellitus. Also, increased glycosuria may predispose these patients to develop urinary tract infections.

URIC ACID. Plasma uric acid levels decrease by 25 per cent as early as 8 weeks gestation, reaching a nadir or 2.0 to 3.0 mg/dl at 24 weeks gestation and then increase toward nonpregnant levels at term (Lind et al., 1984). This may be due to an alteration in the fractional clearance of uric acid (uric acid clearance/GFR) with a net decrease in renal tubular uric acid reabsorption (Dunlop and Davison, 1977). Conditions that lead to volume contraction, such as preeclampsia, may be associated with decreased uric acid clearance and increased plasma levels.

AMINO ACIDS. The fractional excretion of alanine, glycine, histidine, serine, and threonine increases in pregnancy (Hytten and Cheyne, 1972). Cystine, leucine, lysine, phenylalanine, taurine, and tyrosine excretion increases early in pregnancy but then decreases in the second half of gestation. The excretion of arginine, asparagine, glutamic acid, isoleucine, methionine, and ornithine does not change. The mechanism of this selective amino aciduria is unknown. It is unclear whether renal excretion of albumin decreases

(Misiani et al., 1991) or remains stable (Wright et al., 1987) in normal pregnancy. Urinary protein excretion does not normally exceed 300 mg.

VOLUME HOMEOSTASIS. Body weight increases by an average of as much as 30 to 35 pounds in pregnancy (Abrams and Laros, 1986). Two-thirds of this may be accounted for by an increase in total body water, with 6 to 7 liters gained in the extracellular space and approximately 2 liters gained in the intracellular space. Plasma volume expansion, as outlined earlier in this chapter, accounts for 25 per cent of the increase in extracellular water, with the rest of the increment appearing as interstitial fluid (Hytten, 1981).

As water is retained, plasma sodium and urea levels fall slightly, from 140.3 ± 1.7 mM/liter to 136.6 ± 1.5 mM/liter and from 4.9 ± 0.9 to 2.9 ± 0.5 mM/liter, respectively (Davison et al., 1981). Plasma osmolality decreases to a value 10 mOsm/kg less than nonpregnant women (289 ± 2.1 mOsm/kg to 280.9 ± 2.1 mOsm/kg). Since water deprivation in pregnant women leads to an appropriate increase in vasopressin and urine osmolality, and water loading results in a proportional decrease, it would appear that the osmoregulation system is functioning normally but is "reset" at a lower threshold, (Davison et al., 1984; Davison et al., 1988). Further evidence to support this conclusion is that the osmotic threshold for thirst is decreased by 10 mOsm/kg in pregnancy (Lindheimer et al., 1989). The mechanism for this readjustment of the osmoregulatory system is unclear but may involve placental secretion of human chorionic gonadotropin (Davison et al., 1988).

All components of the renin-angiotensin-aldosterone system increase in the first trimester of pregnancy (Wilson et al., 1980). Renin-substrate production by the liver is stimulated by estrogens and results in elevated renal production of renin, which peaks at 32 weeks gestation. Renin stimulates increased conversion of angiotensinogen to angiotensins I and II. The pregnant woman develops resistance to angiotensin II infusion. It is unknown whether this is a result of a change in the number of available receptors or in the receptor response. Increased sensitivity to angiotensin II infusion in the second trimester has been associated with the subsequent development of preeclampsia (Gant et al., 1974).

REFERENCES

Abrams BF, Laros RK Jr: Prepregnancy weight, weight gain, and birth weight. Am J Obstet Gynecol **154**:503, 1986.

Adams JQ, Alexander AM: Alterations in cardiovascular physiology during labor. Obstet Gynecol **12**:542, 1958.

Assali NS, Brinkman CR III: Disorders of maternal circulatory and respiratory adjustments. *In* Assali NS (ed): Pathophysiology of Gestational Disorders. Vol I: Maternal Disorders. New York, Academic Press, 1972.

Awe RJ, Nicotra MB, Newsom TD, et al: Arterial oxygenation and alveolar-arterial gradients in term pregnancy. Obstet Gynecol **53**:182, 1979.

Bader RA, Bader MG, Rose DJ, et al: Hemodynamics at rest and during exercise in normal pregnancy as studied by cardiac catheterization. J Clin Invest **34**:1524, 1955.

Bailey RR, Rolleston GLI: Kidney length and ureteric dilatation in the puerperium. J Obstet Gynaecol Br Commonw **78**:55, 1971.

Barron WM, Lindheimer MD: Renal sodium and water handling in pregnancy. Obstet Gynecol Annu 13:35, 1984.

Barwin BN, Roddie IC: Venous distensibility during pregnancy determined by graded venous congestion. Am J Obstet 125:921, 1976.

Baylis C: The determinants of renal hemodynamics in pregnancy. Am J Kid Dis 9:260, 1987.

Bille-Brahe NE, Rorth M: Red cell 2,3,-diphosphoglycerate in pregnancy. Acta Obstet Gynecol Scand 58:19, 1979.

Bishop JHV, Green R: Effects of pregnancy on glucose reabsorption by the proximal convoluted tubule in the rat. J Physiol 319:271, 1981.

Bond AL, August P, Druzin ML, et al: Atrial natriuretic factor in normal and hypertensive pregnancy. Am J Obstet Gynecol 160:1112, 1989.

Burg J, Dodek A, Kloster F, et al: Alterations of systolic time intervals during pregnancy. Circulation 49:560, 1974.

Capeless EL, Clapp JF: Cardiovascular changes in early phase of pregnancy. Am J Obstet Gynecol 161:1449, 1989.

Capeless EL, Clapp JF: When do cardiovascular parameters return to their preconception values? Am J Obstet Gynecol 165:883, 1991.

Chesley LC, Sloan DM: The effect of posture on renal function in late pregnancy. Am J Obstet Gynecol 89:754, 1964.

Christensen T, Klebe JG, Bertelsen V, et al: Changes in renal volume during normal pregnancy. Acta Obstet Gynecol Scand 68:541, 1989.

Clark SL, Cotton DB, Lee W, et al: Central hemodynamic assessment of normal term pregnancy. Am J Obstet Gynecol 161:1439, 1989.

Cutforth R, MacDonald CB. Heart sounds during normal pregnancy. Am Heart J 71:741, 1966.

Davison JM, Dunlop W: Renal hemodynamics and tubular function in normal human pregnancy. Kidney Int 18:152, 1980.

Davison JM, Dunlop W: Changes in renal hemodynamics and tubular function induced by normal human pregnancy. Semin Nephrol 4:198, 1984.

Davison JM, Gilmore EA, Durr J, et al: Altered osmotic thresholds for vasopressin secretion and thirst in human pregnancy. Am J Physiol 246:F105, 1984.

Davison JM, Hytten FE: The effect of pregnancy on the renal handling of glucose. J Obstet Gynaecol Br Commonw 82:374, 1975.

Davison, JM, Shiells EA, Philips PR, et al: Serial evaluation of vasopressin and thirst in human pregnancy. Role of human chorionic gonadotropin on the osmoregulatory changes of gestation. J Clin Invest 81:798, 1988.

Davison JM, Vallotton MB, Lindheimer MD: Plasma osmolality and urinary concentration and dilution during and after pregnancy. Br J Obstet Gynaecol 88:472, 1981.

Duffus GM, MacGillivaray I, Dennis KJ. The relationship between baby weight and changes in maternal weight, total body water, plasma volume, electrolytes, and proteins and urinary oestriol excretion. J Obstet Gynaec Br Commonw 78:97, 1971.

Dunlop W: Serial changes in renal hemodynamics during normal human pregnancy. Br J Obstet Gynaecol 88:1, 1981.

Dunlop W, Davison JM: The effect of normal pregnancy upon the renal handling of uric acid. Br J Obstet Gynaecol 84:13, 1977.

Easterling TR, Benedetti TJ, Carlson KL, et al: Measurement of cardiac output in pregnancy by thermodilution and impedance techniques. Br J Obstet Gynaecol 96:67, 1989.

Easterling TR, Carlson KL, Schmucker BC, et al: Measurement of cardiac output in pregnancy by doppler technique. Am J Perinatol 7:220, 1990a.

Easterling TR, Benedetti TJ, Schmucker BC, et al: Maternal hemodynamics in normal and preeclamptic pregnancies: A longitudinal study. Obstet Gynecol 76:1061, 1990b.

Equimokhai M, Davison JM, Philips PR, et al: Non-postural serial changes in renal function during the third trimester of normal human pregnancy. Br J Obstet Gynaecol 88:465, 1981.

Fawer R, Dettling A, Weihs D, et al.: Effect of the menstrual cycle, oral contraception and pregnancy on forearm blood flow, venous distensibility and clotting factors. Eur J Clin Pharm 13:251, 1978.

Fried A, Woodring JH, Thompson TJ: Hydronephrosis of pregnancy. J Ultrasound Med 2:255, 1983.

Gant NF, Chand S, Worley RJ, et al: A clinical test useful for predicting the development of acute hypertension in pregnancy. Am J Obstet Gynecol 120:1, 1974.

Gant NF, Worley RJ: Measurement of uteroplacental blood flow in the human. In Rosenfeld CR (ed): The Uterine Circulation. Ithaca, Perinatology Press, 1989, pp 53–73.

Garland HO, Green R: Micropuncture study of changes in glomerular filtration and ion and water handling in the rat kidney during pregnancy. J Physiol 329:389, 1982.

Gerber JG, Payne HA, Murphy RC, et al: Prostacyclin produced by the pregnant uterus in the dog may act as a circulating vasodepressor substance. J Clin Invest 67:632, 1981.

Greiss FC, Anderson SG: Effect of ovarian hormones on the uterine vascular bed. Am J Obstet Gynecol 107:829, 1970.

Guzman C, Caplan R: Cardiorespiratory response to exercise during pregnancy. Am J Obstet Gynecol 108:600, 1970.

Hendricks CH, Quilligan EJ: Cardiac output during labor. Am J Obstet Gynecol 76:969, 1958.

Holmes F: Incidence of the supine hypotensive syndrome in late pregnancy. J Obstet Gynecol Br Emp 67:254, 1960.

Hytten FE: Weight gain in pregnancy. In Hytten F, Chamberlain G (eds): Clinical Physiology in Obstetrics. Oxford, Blackwell Scientific Publications, 1981.

Hytten FE, Cheyne GA: The aminoaciduria of pregnancy. J Obstet Gynaecol Br Commonw 79:424, 1972.

Hytten FE, Leitch I: The Physiology of Human Pregnancy. 2nd ed. Oxford, Blackwell Scientific Publications, 1971.

Iosif S, Ingemarsson I, Ulmsten U: Urodynamics studies in normal pregnancy and in puerperium Am J Obstet Gynecol 137:696, 1980.

Jepson JH: Endocrine control of maternal and fetal erythropoiesis. Can Med Assoc J 98:884, 1968.

Kalousek G, Hlavecek C, Nedoss B, et al: Circadian rhythms of creatinine and electrolyte excretion in healthy pregnant women. Am J Obstet Gynecol 103:856, 1969.

Katz M, Sokal MM: Skin perfusion in pregnancy. Am J Obstet Gynecol 137:30, 1980.

Kirshon B, Lee W, Cotton DB, et al: Indirect blood pressure monitoring in the obstetric patient. Obstet Gynecol 70:799, 1987.

Koller O: The clinical significance of hemodilution during pregnancy. Obstet Gynecol Surv 37:649, 1982.

Kulpa PJ, White BM, Visscher R: Aerobic exercise in pregnancy. Am J Obstet Gynecol 156:1395, 1987.

Lard-Meeter K, van de Ley G, Bom T, et al: Cardiocirculatory adjustments during pregnancy: An echocardiographic study. Clin Cardiol 49:560, 1979.

Limacher MC, Ware JA, O'Meara ME, et al: Tricuspid regurgitation during pregnancy: Two dimensional and pulsed Doppler echocardiographic observations. Am J Cardiol 55:1059, 1985.

Lind T, Godfrey KA, Otun H: Changes in serum uric acid concentration during normal pregnancy. Br J Obstet Gynaecol 91:128, 1984.

Lindheimer MD, Barron WM, Davison JM: Osmoregulation of thirst and vasopressin release in pregnancy. Am J Physiol 257:F59, 1989.

Lindheimer MD, Richardson DA, Ehrlich EN, et al: Potassium homeostasis in pregnancy. J Reprod Med 32:517, 1987.

Lund CJ, Donovan JC: Blood volume during pregnancy. Am J Obstet Gynecol 98:393, 1967.

MacNeily AE, Goldenberg SL, Allen GJJ, et al: Sonographic visualization of the ureter in pregnancy. J Urol 146:298, 1991.

Manchester B, Loube SD: The velocity of blood flow in normal pregnant women. Am Heart J 32:215, 1946.

Marazita AJD: The action of hormones on varicose veins in pregnancy. Med Rec 159:422, 1946.

Marchant DJ: Effects of pregnancy and progestational agents on the urinary tract. Am J Obstet Gynecol 112:487, 1972.

Marlettini MG, Cassani A, Boschi S et al: Plasma concentrations of atrial natriuretic factor in normal pregnancy and early puerperium. Clin Exp Hypertens A 13:1305, 1991.

Mashini IS, Albazzaz SJ, Fadel HE, et al: Serial noninvasive evaluation of cardiovascular hemodynamics during pregnancy. Am J Obstet Gynecol 156:1208, 1987.

McLennan CE: Antecubital and femoral venous pressure in normal and toxemic pregnancy. Am J Obstet Gynecol 45:568, 1943.

Milne JA, Howie AD, Pack AL: Dyspnoea during normal pregnancy. Br J Obstet Gynaecol 85:260, 1978.

Misiani R, Marchesi D, Tiraboschi G, et al: Urinary albumin excretion in normal pregnancy and pregnancy-induced hypertension. Nephron 59:416, 1991.

Pritchard JA: Changes in the blood volume during pregnancy and delivery. Anethesiology **26**:393, 1965a.

Pritchard JA: Blood volume changes in pregnancy and the puerperium. IV. Anemia associated with hydatidiform mole. Am J Obstet Gynecol **91**:621, 1965b.

Rasmussen PE, Nielse FR: Hydroephrosis during pregnancy: A literature survey. Eur J Obstet Gynaecol Reprod Biol **27**:249, 1988.

Robson SC, Hunter S, Boys RJ, et al: Serial study of factors influencing changes in cardiac output during human pregnancy. Am J Physiol **256**:H1060, 1989.

Roelofsen JMT, Berkel GM, Uttendorfsky OT, et al: Urinary excretion rates of calcium and magnesium in normal and complicated pregnancies. Eur J Obstet Gynaecol Reprod Biol **27**:227, 1988.

Ronco C, Brendolan A, Bragantini L, et al: Renal functional reserve in pregnancy. Nephrol Dial Transplant **2**:157, 1988.

Rovinsky JJ, Jaffin H: Cardiovascular hemodynamics in pregnancy. I. Blood and plasma volumes in multiple pregnancy. Am J Obstet Gynecol **93**:1, 1965.

Rubler S, Damani P, Pinto E: Cardiac size and performance during pregnancy estimated with echocardiography. Am J Cardiol **49**:534, 1977.

Rubler S, Hammer N, Schneebaum R: Systolic time intervals in pregnancy and the postpartum period. Am Heart J **86**:182, 1972.

Sala NL, Rubi RA: Ureteral function in pregnant women. II. Ureteral contractibility during normal pregnancy. Am J Obstet Gynecol **99**:228, 1967.

Schulman A, Herlinger H: Urinary tract dilatation in pregnancy. Br J Radiol **48**:638, 1975.

Thompson JA, Hayes PM, Sagar KB, et al: Echocardiographic left ventricular mass to differentiate chronic hypertension from preeclampsia during pregnancy. Am J Obstet Gynecol **155**:994, 1986.

Turner AF: The chest radiograph during pregnancy. Clin Obstet Gynecol **18**:65, 1975.

Ueland K: Maternal cardiovascular dynamics. VII. Intrapartum blood volume changes. Am J Obstet Gynecol **126**:671, 1976.

Ueland K, Akamatsu TJ, Eng M, et al: Maternal cardiovascular hemodynamics. I. Cesarean section under subarachnoid block anesthesia. Am J Obstet Gynecol **100**:42, 1968.

Ueland K, Hansen JM: Maternal cardiovascular hemodynamics. III. Labor and delivery under local and caudal anesthesia. Am J Obstet Gynecol **103**:8, 1969.

Ueland K, Metcalfe J: Circulatory changes in pregnancy. Clin Obstet Gynecol **18**:41, 1975.

Ueland K, Novy M, Peterson E, et al: Maternal cardiovascular dynamics. IV. The influence of gestational age on the maternal cardiovascular response to posture and exercise. Am J Obstet Gynecol **104**:856, 1969.

Walters WAW, MacGregor WG, Hills M: Cardiac output at rest during pregnancy and the puerperium. Clin Sci **30**:1, 1966.

Welsh GW, Sims EAH: The mechanisms of renal glucosuria in pregnancy. Diabetes **9**:363, 1960.

Wickman K, Ryden G, Wickman G: The influence of different positions and Korotkoff sounds on the blood pressure measurements in pregnancy. Acta Obstet Gynaecol Scand **118**(Suppl):25, 1984.

Wilson M, Morganti AA, Zervoudakis J, et al: Blood pressure, the renin-aldosterone system and sex steroids throughout normal pregnancy. Am J Med **68**:97, 1980.

Wolfe LA, Hall P, Webb KA: Prescription of aerobic exercise during pregnancy. Sports Med **8**:273, 1989.

Wright A, Steeke P, Bennet JR, et al: The urinary excretion of albumin in normal pregnancy. Br J Obstet Gynaecol **94**:408, 1987.

Youssef AF: Cystometric studies in gynecology and obstetrics. Obstet Gynecol **8**:181, 1956.

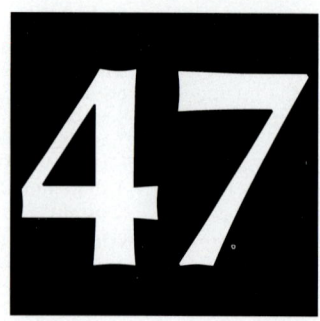

C H A P T E R

47

CARDIAC DISEASES
···························

RALPH SHABETAI, M.D.

DIAGNOSIS OF HEART DISEASE IN PREGNANCY

The significant hemodynamic changes that accompany pregnancy make the diagnosis of certain forms of cardiovascular disease difficult. Pregnant women frequently complain of dyspnea, orthopnea, easy fatigability, dizzy spell, and even syncope. On physical examination, dependent edema, rales in the lower lung fields, visible neck veins, and cardiomegaly are commonly found. Systolic murmurs occur in more than 95 per cent of pregnant women, and internal mammary flow murmurs and venous hums are common. Certain findings, however, indicate heart disease in pregnancy and should increase the suspicion that there is a significant cardiovascular abnormality. The symptoms include severe dyspnea, syncope with exertion, hemoptysis, paroxysmal nocturnal dyspnea, and chest pain related to exertion. Signs of heart disease are cyanosis, clubbing, diastolic murmurs, cardiac arrhythmias, and loud, harsh systolic murmurs.

Once the clinical diagnosis of heart disease is made, confirmatory diagnostic tests should be initiated. It is important that the changes of normal pregnancy be recognized so that the findings are not misinterpreted. For example, nonspecific S-T segment and T wave abnormalities and shifts in the electrical axis can occur on electrocardiogram (ECG) (Boyle and Lloyd-Jones, 1966; Oram and Holt, 1961; Schwartz and Schamroth, 1979). Pregnancy also produces changes in the echocardiogram, including alterations in cardiac dimensions as well as performance. The left ventricular internal dimension is increased, the ejection fraction and stroke volume are concomitantly larger, and the cardiac output is increased (Rubler et al., 1977). Radiographic diagnostic procedures should be avoided during pregnancy unless the procedure is deemed essential for the health and safety of the mother. Similarly, radionuclide procedures to determine intracardiac shunts and left ventricular function should, if possible, be reserved for the nonpregnant patient.

PRECONCEPTION COUNSELING

If the woman plans to become pregnant but knows that she has heart disease, she and her medical atten-

dants must be fully aware of several fundamental principles. The cardiovascular system undergoes specific adaptations to meet the increased demands of the mother and fetus during pregnancy. The most important of these are increases in blood volume, cardiac output, and heart rate. These adaptations exacerbate the symptoms, clinical signs, and laboratory evidence of heart disease or heart failure and may necessitate significant escalation in treatment. On the other hand, although pregnancy in cases of severe heart disease or failure may be extremely uncomfortable and even dangerous, no permanent damage to the heart ensues.

Cardiac risk varies among specific forms of heart disease and with its severity. When counseling a woman and the potential father of her child before pregnancy, the discussion should encompass a description, comprehensible to lay individuals, of the nature of the heart disease. The risk, which may vary from negligible to prohibitive, should be spelled out as clearly as the information available permits. Based on this, the patient may be advised either that the contemplated pregnancy is safe, will be uncomfortable and will necessitate treatment, carries a significantly increased risk, or would be extremely dangerous and should not be undertaken.

In the case of a cardiac condition that can be cured or virtually cured, the patient should be strongly advised to undergo the necessary treatment before pregnancy and allow several months to a year to elapse before becoming pregnant. Examples in this category include the secundum type of atrial septal defect, patent ductus arteriosus, and some cases of coarctation. In other cases, the heart condition can be ameliorated but not cured; examples include mitral stenosis and regurgitation, aortic stenosis, tetralogy of Fallot, ventricular septal defect with moderate pulmonary hypertension, pulmonary stenosis, and a variety of other congenital malformations and acquired heart diseases. Again, it is imperative that the palliative procedure be carried out *before* pregnancy is undertaken and that a year or so elapse before the woman becomes pregnant. Flexibility in clinical judgment, however, is mandatory. A woman with mild to moderately severe valvular disease of the heart may in the future require a prosthetic valve. In such a case,

768

the patient should be advised to have her family before the necessity for valve replacement arises with its associated anticoagulant risk (Born et al., 1992).

As previously noted, some cardiac disorders are so serious in nature that the physiologic changes of a superimposed pregnancy pose prohibitive risks to the mother and carry such a high maternal mortality risk that pregnancy is contraindicated. In such circumstances, patients must be strongly cautioned against becoming pregnant, and if presenting for the first time when already pregnant, termination of the pregnancy is recommended. The most serious of the cardiac disorders are those involving pulmonary hypertension, particularly associated with a right-to-left shunt in cardiac blood flow (Eisenmenger's syndrome). Low cardiac output states and entities in which there is an increased risk of aortic dissection (Marfan's syndrome) also represent an extraordinarily high risk of maternal mortality. These high-risk maternal cardiovascular disorders are listed in Table 47–1.

In some women with specific dangerous cardiovascular diseases, such as cardiomyopathy, primary pulmonary hypertension, Eisenmenger's syndrome, and Marfan's syndrome, pregnancy is contraindicated due to the substantial risk of maternal death. Should patients with these disorders already present pregnant, they should be strongly urged to consider termination. A carefully planned dilation and curettage prior to 13 weeks gestation would place these women at minimal risk. Termination of pregnancy beyond this stage increases the risk to the mother inasmuch as many of the cardiovascular alterations occurring in pregnancy have taken place. The use of prostaglandins E_2 and $F_2\alpha$ and their analogues is successful in evacuating the uterus during the second trimester, but all these agents have significant cardiovascular side effects and should be used with caution. In experienced hands, and with knowledgeable anesthetic consultation, dilation and evacuation performed up to 22 weeks gestation may be an appropriate alternative.

Infective endocarditis often causes rapid and serious deterioration of the cardiac status, posing a major threat to the life and health of the mother and therefore of the fetus as well. Scrupulous attention to prophylaxis against endocarditis is critical during pregnancy. Pregnant women must pay meticulous attention to their dental health; if they have cardiac lesions susceptible to infectious endocarditis, neglect of antibacterial prophylaxis may have dire consequences.

The prospective parents will want to know not only about the risk to the health and life of the future mother but also about the fetal risks. One of the most important questions is whether the mother's heart disease is hereditary and, if so, what is the risk that the infant will be born with the same defect. A detailed family cardiac history must be obtained before pregnancy even if the prospective mother is free from heart disease, although it is especially critical when she is not.

There is a strong familial tendency in certain congenital malformations such as patent ductus arteriosus (Burman, 1961) and atrial septal defect (Johansson and Sievers, 1967). Some of the cardiomyopathies, especially hypertrophic, may be inherited in a Mendelian

manner (Bjarnason et al., 1982). Familial dilated cardiomyopathy has also been described (Mestroni et al., 1990). Mothers with congenital heart disease may also have children with unrelated congenital malformations (Corone et al., 1983).

Mothers with advanced heart disease, especially those with low cardiac output or severe hypoxia, experience a greatly increased incidence of spontaneous abortion, stillbirths, and small or deformed children (Cannell and Vernon, 1963). Furthermore, today's prospective mother wants to know about the risks to her fetus of drugs that must be given to treat heart disease and that other treatments such as electrical cardioversion are safe. Echocardiography poses no threat to the fetus, but radiation incurred with radionuclide angiography, cardiac catheterization with contrast angiography, and computed tomography may pose a potential hazard to the fetus. When these studies are required, they should be performed before the woman becomes pregnant and should be repeated thereafter only when mandated for the safety of the mother and then with pelvic shielding.

Infection of the mother with the virus of German measles (rubella) is associated with a high risk of congenital malformation of the heart of the fetus. If the woman has not had German measles as a child and has never been inoculated against it and her antibody titer confirms the absence of immunity, she should be inoculated some months before becoming pregnant.

Every pregnant woman known or suspected to have heart disease should, at a minimum, be evaluated once by a cardiologist who understands the cardiovascular adaptations to pregnancy. The cardiologist will prescribe necessary diagnostic studies and treatment and, of equal importance, will not allow unnecessary ones. The effects of heart disease can often be ameliorated by correcting anemia, chronic infection, anxiety, thyroid dysfunction, hypertension and arrhythmia, to mention a few of the more obvious disorders.

CARDIOVASCULAR ADAPTATIONS TO PREGNANCY

It is worthwhile to reconsider and emphasize some of the most important cardiovascular changes that occur during pregnancy, inasmuch as they may significantly alter the course of cardiac disease or may themselves be influenced by a specific disorder.

Blood volume and cardiac output increase during pregnancy (Sullivan and Ramanathan, 1985). The uterus hypertrophies, endometrial vascularization is greatly increased, and the placenta becomes a highly vascular structure that functions to some extent as an arteriovenous shunt. In addition, generalized arteriolar dilation develops, mediated most probably by estrogen. These mechanisms combine to lower systemic vascular resistance. Investigators disagree about the extent and rate of blood volume expansion (Ueland et al., 1973), but an increase of 50 per cent is thought to occur commonly. The blood volume thus increases

TABLE 47–1. High-Risk Maternal Cardiovascular Disorders

DISORDER	MATERNAL MORTALITY RATE* (%)
Aortic valve disease	10–20
Coarctation of the aorta	5
Eisenmenger's syndrome	30–70
Marfan's syndrome	25–50 (estimated)
Mitral stenosis with atrial fibrillation	14–17
Peripartal cardiomyopathy	15–60
Primary pulmonary hypertension	50
Tetralogy of Fallot	12

*These figures, compiled from 18 references, represent different study periods and disorders of varying severity; therefore they must be regarded as approximations.

Modified from Ueland K: Cardiovascular disease complicating pregnancy. Clin Obstet Gynecol **21:**429, 1978.

steadily during the first trimester and is increased by almost 50 per cent by the 30th week, remaining more or less constant thereafter (Elkayam and Gleicher, 1990). It is commonly stated that plasma volume increases more than the red blood cell mass, accounting for a "physiologic" anemia that is common in pregnancy (Hytten and Thompson, 1968). However, some authorities believe that if iron intake is appropriately increased, anemia is not a normal manifestation of pregnancy. In any case, iron treatment corrects the anemia which, if untreated, may be significant (hematocrit as low as 33 and hemoglobin 11 gm/dl).

Several mechanisms are responsible for increasing blood volume in pregnancy. They include the steroid hormones of pregnancy, elevated plasma renin activity, and hyperaldosteronism. Human placental lactogen and variations in atrial natriuretic factor and other peptides may also play significant roles in governing changes of blood volume in pregnancy. Hypervolemia also occurs with trophoblastic disease, indicating that a fetus is not essential for its development.

Cardiac output rises during the first few weeks of pregnancy and is 30 to 45 per cent above the nonpregnant level by the 20th week, remaining there until term (Sullivan and Ramanathan, 1985). In late pregnancy, the enlarged uterus partially impedes venous return via the inferior vena cava, accounting for lower cardiac output measured when the patient is supine (Ueland and Hansen, 1969). The drop in cardiac output in the 38th to 40th week of pregnancy is much less pronounced when the patient is not supine. This is one reason why some obstetricians prefer to manage labor with the patient in the Sims's (left decubitus) position. The increase in cardiac output in the first trimester begins rapidly and peaks around the 20th to 26th week. Early in pregnancy the dominant factor is elevated stroke volume, but later increased heart rate predominates (Metcalfe and Ueland, 1974).

Echocardiographic studies indicate an increased velocity of fiber shortening and an enhanced ejection fraction (Perloff, 1988). These changes do not necessarily indicate increased myocardial contractility but may simply be the result of decreased peripheral vascular resistance and increased preload. In any case, stroke volume is increased and cardiac output is fur-

ther augmented by the 10 to 15 per cent increase in cardiac rate that characterizes normal pregnancy (Katz et al., 1978).

Demands on the cardiovascular system increase significantly during labor and delivery. Pain increases sympathetic tone, and uterine contractions induce wide swings in the systemic venous return.

When a chest radiograph is obtained in the pregnant woman, the cardiac silhouette often appears slightly enlarged owing to the combined effects of volume overload and elevation of the diaphragm. Echocardiography shows slight dilation and a degree of hyperactivity of the ventricular walls. Routine echocardiographic studies have demonstrated that a small silent pericardial effusion is quite common (Haiat and Halphen, 1984).

Electrocardiogram

The mean QRS may shift to the left (Carruth et al., 1981) as a result of the elevated diaphragm. In later pregnancy the axis may shift to the right when the fetus descends into the pelvis. Minor ST (Boyle and Lloyd-Jones, 1966) and T wave changes may be observed, usually in lead 3, and sometimes aVF as well. T inversions may, less commonly, appear transiently in the left precordial leads. Small Q waves may occasionally accompany T wave inversion in leads 3 and aVF. These changes are seldom of sufficient magnitude to raise the question of ischemic heart disease, which in any case is uncommon in pregnancy, especially when the mother is young and free from symptoms. Extrasystoles and paraventricular tachycardia are more common during pregnancy.

GENERAL GUIDELINES TO MANAGEMENT

During treatment of all patients with heart disease in pregnancy, priority must be given to maternal health, but all possible therapeutic measures should also be taken to protect the developing fetus. The aspects of management are outlined in Table 47–2.

Because pregnancy increases the demands on the heart, physical exertion frequently must be restricted, especially if it makes the patient symptomatic. Some women with certain forms of cardiac disease, such as significant mitral stenosis and cardiomyopathy, toler-

TABLE 47–2. Cardiac Disease in Pregnancy: Aspects of Management

Activity restriction
Diet modification
Team approach for medical care
Infection control:
  Immunizations
  Prophylaxis against bacterial endocarditis
  Prophylaxis against rheumatic fever
Interruption of pregnancy
Counseling
Contraception or sterilization
Cardiovascular surgery
Cardiovascular drugs

ate pregnancy poorly and are intolerant to physical exertion. They may require strict bed rest for the duration of the pregnancy and particularly during the last trimester. It is important to maintain cardiac demand within the limits of cardiac capacity in all pregnant women with heart disease. There is limited means to increase capacity, and so therapy most frequently is directed at limiting the demands placed on the heart. Limiting physical activity is therefore the cornerstone of this approach to therapy.

Cardiovascular Drugs

Some of the drugs commonly used in the management of patients with cardiovascular disease have potential harmful effects on the developing embryo and fetus. Although analyzing the data in the literature is difficult because of the interaction of numerous variables, there are some drugs that have the potential of being harmful during pregnancy. There is little question that oral anticoagulants are potential teratogens when administered in the first trimester of pregnancy (see also Chapter 12). The "warfarin embryopathy syndrome," consisting of nasal hypoplasia, optic atrophy, digital abnormalities, and mental impairment, may occur in as many as 15 to 25 per cent of cases (Stevenson et al., 1980; Hall et al., 1980). The fetal risks continue beyond the first trimester because the use of these drugs increases the possibility of fetal bleeding as well as maternal intrauterine bleeding. This may represent a significant practical problem in dealing with patients with prosthetic heart valves (Born et al., 1992). In general, heparin offers a safer alternative for both mother and fetus.

Beta-adrenergic blocking agents which are used for the treatment of hypertension and tachyarrhythmia, have been associated with neonatal respiratory depression, sustained bradycardia, and hypoglycemia when administered late in pregnancy or just prior to delivery.

The thiazide diuretics are another group of drugs that have the potential of producing harmful effects on the fetus, especially when used initially in the third trimester of pregnancy or for extended periods. Severe neonatal electrolyte imbalance, jaundice, thrombocytopenia, liver damage, and even death have been reported, although rarely, in association with the use of thiazide diuretics.

Recently, there have been numerous reports of fetal and neonatal renal complications following the use of angiotensin-converting enzyme inhibitors (ACE) during pregnancy (Rosa et al., 1989; Scott and Purohit, 1989). These complications would suggest a profound and deleterious effect on fetal renal function leading to decreased renal function and oligohydramnios, as well as neonatal renal failure. It is currently recommended that the ACE inhibitors are absolutely contraindicated during pregnancy.

The indications and possible adverse effects of commonly prescribed cardioactive drugs during pregnancy are summarized in Table 47–3.

Team Approach to Medical Care

Medical care for pregnant women with heart disease is best provided through the cooperative efforts of a cardiologist familiar with the hemodynamic changes of pregnancy and an obstetrician. Frequent visits to both specialists along with open consultations will provide the patient with consistent advice and reassurance and circumvent the worry and anxiety created by confusing and conflicting information. In addition, the anesthesiologist needs to be consulted during the antepartum period in order to outline the anticipated approach to intrapartum management, a time of maximum risk for the majority of these women.

CONGENITAL HEART DISEASE

A number of simple congenital malformations are compatible with a normal or nearly normal pregnancy. Congenital malformations previously associated with high maternal morbidity and mortality and fetal wastage now frequently end with a satisfactory outcome because of palliative or corrective surgery. The problems associated with most forms of congenital cardiac malformation differ from the congestive heart failure that may supervene in patients with acquired heart disease. Management is correspondingly different. For example, extreme caution in fluid administration is not needed in simple left-to-right shunt and may be frankly dangerous in cyanotic congenital heart disease.

Left-to-Right Shunt

Atrial Septal Defect

Atrial septal defect may be first discovered in women of childbearing age because symptoms are often absent and the physical findings are not blatant. Other causes of left-to-right shunt such as patent ductus arteriosus and ventricular septal defect may still be present at this age, but more often have been discovered and treated in infancy or childhood. Physicians should be alert to the possibility of uncorrected defects in women who have immigrated from an undeveloped country.

Surgical closure of secundum atrial septal defect is straightforward and safe and usually is curative. The operation should therefore be carried out before pregnancy. However, if the patient is unwilling to undergo cardiac surgery, she can be advised that the lesion is unlikely to complicate pregnancy, labor, or delivery (Perloff, 1988; Neilson et al., 1970). In a recent review (Metcalfe et al., 1986), the authors reported one maternal death in 219 pregnancies in 113 women with atrial septal defect. Peripheral vasodilation, if anything, reduces the left-to-right shunt (Metcalfe and Ueland, 1974). Atrial septal defect in young women is not associated with heart failure; therefore digitalis, diuretics, and extreme limitation of intravenous infusion are not warranted. A small percentage of patients with atrial septal defect have atrial flutter, which usually is paroxysmal. This arrhythmia can be man-

AGENT: MATERNAL	INDICATION	ADVERSE EFFECTS: FETAL (FDA PREGNANCY CATEGORY)	ADVERSE EFFECTS: MATERNAL
Digitalis (digoxin, digitoxin):	Heart failure arrhythmia, especially atrial fibrillation	Fetal toxicity and neonatal death have been reported with overdosage Animal studies have not demonstrated teratogenic effects (category C)	Arrhythmias, conduction disturbances, anorexia, nausea, vomiting
Newer inotropic drugs: IV milrinone IV amrinone	Not FDA approved Acute heart failure, cardiogenic shock Approved for intravenous use Do not prescribe for pregnant women	Animal studies conflicting (category C)	Gastrointestinal symptoms, headache, reversible thrombocytopenia, hypotension
Diuretics: Loop diuretics (furosemide, bumetanide)	Heart failure, hypertension, constrictive pericarditis	Growth retardation No adequate well-controlled studies (category C)	Electrolyte disturbances (hyponatremia, hypokalemia), hypotension, increased creatine and urea nitrogen levels
Thiazides (hydrochlorothiazide)	Hypertension	Neonatal jaundice, thrombocytopenia, hemolytic anemia, hypoglycemia (category C)	Same as loop diuretics but less potent
Metolazone	Hypertension, heart failure	(category B)	
Potassium sparing			Same as loop diuretics but more potent
Spironolactone	Excessive edema, hypokalemia	Chronic administration in rats has shown it to be a tumorigen Feminization occurs in male rat fetuses (category C)	Gastrointestinal disturbance, amenorrhea, hirsutism, deepening of voice, hyperkalemia
Triamterene	Excessive edema, hypokalemia	No adequate well-conducted studies done on pregnant women (category B)	Gastrointestinal disturbance, hyperkalemia
Vasodilators (directly acting): Hydralazine, Isosorbide	Heart failure, hypertension, pulmonary hypertension, angina	Teratogenic in animals, thrombocytopenia, leukopenia reported in newborns (category C)	Hypotension, nausea, diarrhea, headache, systemic lupus erythematosus
Vasodilators (ACE inhibitors): Captopril Enalapril	Heart failure, hypertension contraindicated in pregnancy	Renal failure in fetus and neonate	May worsen renal function, cough, hypotension, hyperkalemia, angioedema (1% to 2%)
Vasodilators (alpha-antagonist): Prazosin Terazosin Doxazosin	Hypertension	No well-controlled studies (category C) (category C) (category B)	First dose syncope, nasal congestion, headache, drowsiness
Beta-adrenergic antagonists: Propranolol Metropolol	Angina, hypertrophic cardiomyopathy, hypertension, mitral valve prolapse, arrhythmia	During delivery: bradycardia, hypotension, oliguria, hypoglycemia (category C)	Uterine contraction, bradycardia, hypotension, bronchospasm
Calcium-channel blockers: Diltiazem, Nifedipine, Verapamil	Angina, hypertension, arrhythmia (verapamil)	Teratogenicity in small animals No controlled human studies (category C)	Constipation (verapamil), bradycardia, conduction disturbances, negative inotrope, hypotension
Antiarrhythmics: Quinidine	Arrhythmia	Neonatal thrombocytopenia reported (category C)	Thrombocytopenia, cinchonism, gastrointestinal, life-threatening arrhythmia
Procainamide	Arrhythmia	Quinidine preferred due to more experience	Gastrointestinal disturbance, SLE
Disopyramide Lidocaine Mexilitine Propafenone	Arrhythmia Arrhythmia Arrhythmia Arrhythmia	(category C) (category C) (category B) (category C)	Arrhythmia Anticholinergic Epilepsy, drowsiness, confusion Gastrointestinal disturbance, tremor, lightheadedness, arrhythmia
Flecainide	Arrhythmia	Embryotoxic in animals (category C)	

TABLE 47–3. Indications and Possible Adverse Effects on Mother and Fetus of
Commonly Prescribed Cardioactive Drugs Continued

AGENT: MATERNAL	INDICATION	ADVERSE EFFECTS: FETAL (FDA PREGNANCY CATEGORY)	ADVERSE EFFECTS: MATERNAL
Moricizine	Arrhythmia	Teratogenic in rabbits (category C)	Gastrointestinal disturbance, dizziness, AV block, arrhythmia
Amiodarone	Arrhythmia	(category B)	Gastrointestinal disturbance, dizziness, headache, arrhythmia
		Growth retardation in rats (category C)	Dizziness, nausea, arrhythmia Pulmonary fibrosis, thyroid abnormalities, photosensitivity
Anticoagulants: Coumadin	Valve disease, prosthetic valves, hypercoagulable states, atrial fibrillation, intracardiac thrombus	Fetal hemorrhage, prematurity, stillbirth, congenital malformations (category X)	Hemorrhage
Heparin	Same as Coumadin		Hemorrhage Loss of bone density
Corticosteroids	Myocarditis, recurrent pericarditis, immunosuppression for cardiac transplant recipients	Cleft palate (category C) in laboratory animals; not in humans	Multiple fluid and electrolyte disturbances, osteoporosis, peptic ulcer, mental disturbance
Cyclosporine	Cardiac transplant recipients, myocarditis?	Embryotoxic in animals (category C)	Impaired immunity, hypertension, renal disease, hirsutism, tremor

Category B: Animal studies have not demonstrated a risk to the fetus, but there are no adequate studies in pregnant women.
Category C: Animal studies have shown no adverse effect on the fetus, but there are no adequate studies in humans; benefits may be acceptable despite potential risks.
Category X: Studies demonstrate fetal risk or abnormalities. Risks outweigh potential benefits.
Adapted from FDA Pregnancy Categories, February, 1991.

aged along conventional lines. The prospective mother should be informed that surgical closure of the defect does not prevent arrhythmia.

The patient often has no cardiac symptoms other than those common in normal pregnant women. The murmur is inconspicuous, being a pulmonary ejection systolic murmur and therefore not unlike the physiological murmur of pregnancy. However, the second heart sound is split in expiration as well as inspiration, a distinctly abnormal finding. The ECG shows incomplete right bundle branch block and, in the case of the much more common secundum defect, right axis deviation. In the less common primum defect, marked left axis deviation accompanies incomplete right bundle branch block. The chest x-ray shows cardiac enlargement, involving the right atrium and right ventricle, prominent pulmonary artery segment, and plethoric lung fields. Echocardiography establishes or confirms the diagnosis, obviating cardiac catheterization in many cases.

When atrial flutter recurs frequently and especially when the heart rate is difficult to control, catheter ablation is successful in restoring normal sinus rhythm without the need for antiarrhythmic drugs. Generally this procedure should not be done until after delivery because of the extensive radiation exposure that is needed. In rare instances, labor may be associated with a paradoxical systemic embolus due to preferential flow from the inferior vena cava to the left atrium (Somerville et al., 1973).

In the rare event that the patient is over 35 years old, it is likely that atrial fibrillation will have become the established rhythm and that right heart failure will be incipient or present. A number of women past this

age who have atrial septal defect may have pulmonary hypertension and pulmonary vascular disease. Pregnancy is ill advised if any of these late sequelae of atrial defect are present. If the patient insists upon going through with the pregnancy, prolonged bed rest will be required, and vigorous treatment of heart failure as it develops will be needed. The maternal risk will be increased, and there will be significant fetal wastage.

Infectious endocarditis rarely if ever complicates a simple atrial septal defect; therefore, prophylaxis during labor is not warranted.

Ventricular Septal Defect

The clinical spectrum of ventricular septal defect may range from so mild that it does not affect pregnancy or outcome, to posing a high risk for maternal or fetal death. Small defects in the muscular ventricular septum frequently close spontaneously during childhood. However, these defects occasionally persist, allowing a small left-to-right shunt manifest by a loud pansystolic murmur along the left sternal border accompanied by a coarse thrill. The chest radiograph is normal save for prominence of the main pulmonary artery, and the electrocardiogram likewise is normal. These findings constitute the maladie de Roger. Prophylaxis against infectious endocarditis is indicated; otherwise, this lesion has no effect on pregnancy or labor.

When the defect is in the membranous septum, the left-to-right shunt is larger than in maladie de Roger, and spontaneous closure is rare. In the absence of significant pulmonary vascular disease, the same pansystolic murmur and thrill that characterize maladie de Roger are found. In addition, there is frequently a short mid-diastolic rumbling murmur owing to increased flow through the mitral valve. Because the shunt is larger, it is usually manifest by overcirculation in the lung fields seen on the chest radiograph, which also shows prominence of the pulmonary artery and cardiac enlargement.

The classic electrocardiogram is that of biventricular hypertrophy. In such cases, flow through the pulmonary vascular bed is usually at least twice the systemic cardiac output; such pulmonary hypertension as is found results mainly from the increased cardiac output. Pulmonary vascular resistance is not elevated.

Patients with relatively large uncomplicated left-to-right shunts through a ventricular septal defect tolerate pregnancy well and, in this respect, are comparable to patients with atrial septal defect, except in the latter, infectious endocarditis does not occur. On the other hand, patients with uncomplicated left-to-right shunt through a ventricular septal defect are less prone to arrhythmia than patients with atrial septal defect.

Here it is appropriate to detour from clinical description to pathophysiology. Pulmonary vascular resistance is calculated as the pressure-drop across the pulmonary vascular bed divided by the flow through it, i.e.:

$$R_{clinical\ units} = \frac{PAMP - PWMP\ mm\ Hg}{Q_{pulmonary}\ l/min}$$

where R equals pulmonary vascular resistance, PAMP and PWMP mean pulmonary arterial and wedge (or capillary) pressure, and $Q_{pulmonary}$ equals total pulmonary flow, i.e., cardiac output plus left-to-right shunt. Sometimes resistance is given in dyne/cm • sec^{-5}. The clinical unit has the merit of simplicity and is derived from clinical units of pressure and flow. The more fundamental but less friendly unit can be obtained by multiplying clinical units by 80. Normal vascular resistance is 0.5 to 1.5 units. When a clinician is faced with a pregnant woman with pulmonary hypertension, the key to how safe she will be during pregnancy lies in the pulmonary vascular resistance. High flow per se can be the mechanism for pulmonary hypertension without resistance being dangerously elevated. This mechanism can be appreciated by rewriting the resistance equation to read

$$P = Q \times R$$

where P and Q are pressure drop and flow across the pulmonary vascular bed. A patient at one extreme may have a large shunt with pulmonary flow at 20 l/min and pulmonary vascular resistance at 3 units, yielding a mean pulmonary artery pressure of 55 mm Hg, assuming a normal pulmonary wedge pressure of 5 mm Hg. At the other extreme, a patient with pulmonary vascular disease may have a pulmonary blood flow of 7 l/min and a pulmonary vascular resistance of 7 units, yielding a pulmonary arterial mean pressure of 44 mm Hg (49 minus 5). The higher the pulmonary vascular resistance, the greater the maternal risk. The risk is prohibitive when the pulmonary vascular resistance reaches the systemic level. In borderline cases, e.g., those with pulmonary vascular

resistance between 5 and 8 units, a pulmonary arteriolar vasodilating agent is sometimes administered to determine whether the increased pulmonary vascular resistance is due to excessive arteriolar tone and thus is reversible, or to irreversible damage to the vessels.

Mild increase in pulmonary vascular resistance is in the range of 3 to 4 units, moderate 5 to 7 units, and severe above 8 units, sometimes up to 15 or 20 units. The significance of these numbers can be appreciated by comparison with systemic vascular resistance, which is usually around 15 units.

Ventricular septal defect may be associated with considerable increase in pulmonary vascular resistance, reflecting occlusive disease of the small pulmonary arteries and pulmonary arterioles. This development, if it is to occur, usually does so in early childhood and, unless corrected, leads to the Eisenmenger situation, which is discussed later. However, a small number of adults may survive with ventricular septal defect and pulmonary vascular resistance that is significantly elevated but falls short of the Eisenmenger syndrome. Such patients are at high risk for maternal death during pregnancy or labor, and there is a high risk of fetal impairment or wastage (Neilson et al., 1971). The patient should be told that, in the first trimester, therapeutic abortion would be the safest and wisest option and that later pregnancy would be hazardous and require intensive care. Physical exercise would be strictly curtailed, and prolonged bed rest enforced. The combination of decreased physical activity, pulmonary hypertension, and pulmonary vascular disease would constitute sound reasons for instituting anticoagulation.

Some authorities would strongly advise delivery prematurely by means of cesarean section and urge sterilization at the same operation. These dangers must be thoroughly understood by women in this category who insist on continuing pregnancy.

Patent Ductus Arteriosus

The loud continuous or machinery murmur of typical patent ductus arteriosus with a large left-to-right shunt and no pulmonary vascular disease is so striking that the lesion is almost invariably detected in infancy or childhood; the ductus is therefore usually divided at that time. Occasionally, however, women of childbearing age or pregnant women from underprivileged communities may present with a patent ductus. If the left-to-right shunt is large, the circulation is hyperdynamic with a wide arterial pulse pressure, low arterial diastolic pressure, hyperactive precordium, and warm skin, perhaps with capillary pulsation. The heart may be somewhat enlarged to clinical and radiologic examination, but the electrocardiogram is usually normal. The signs of hyperdynamic circulation due to the ductus are exaggerated by pregnancy.

The murmur of patent ductus arteriosus is systolo-diastolic and thus commonly referred to as a continuous murmur, although sometimes the murmur, while it significantly overlaps the second heart sound, stops short of end diastole. The murmur, because of its characteristics, is also referred to as a machinery murmur. It is maximal in the left infraclavicular region and peaks around the second heart sound. It must be distinguished from the venous hum, which is loudest in the neck, although usually still audible in the infraclavicular area. Venous hum is common in pregnant women (Hardison, 1968). It changes dramatically with changes in the position of the head. Critical examination should easily distinguish venous hum from continuous murmurs.

Division of the ductus should be accomplished before pregnancy is undertaken. If the patient does become pregnant, uncomplicated left-to-right shunt through a patent ductus arteriosus can be managed safely, much as those due to atrial or ventricular septal defect. Endocarditis is a risk in patients with patent ductus arteriosus, another reason for preconception surgical closure of the duct. A lesion forms on the endothelium of the pulmonary artery where the arterial jet strikes and may become the site for infective endocarditis. Embolic complications of infectious endocarditis secondary to patent ductus arteriosus thus usually take the form of infected pulmonary emboli. The patient becomes febrile, has respiratory symptoms, and has a chest radiogram showing multiple opacities and infiltrates.

The leading cause of Eisenmenger's syndrome is a large ventricular septal defect. However, a large patent ductus arteriosus in susceptible individuals also may increase pulmonary vascular resistance, sometimes to the extent of Eisenmenger pathophysiology. As with ventricular septal defect, individuals with patent ductus arteriosus may sustain severe increases in pulmonary vascular resistance with the corresponding pulmonary hypertension and right ventricular hypertrophy, yet fall short of Eisenmenger physiology. The maternal risk during pregnancy is high, being similar to that encountered in ventricular septal defect with equivalent pathophysiology, and treatment is the same (see above). When the pulmonary pressure rises, aortopulmonary shunt decreases, with the result that the murmur becomes progressively quieter and shorter until it finally disappears.

The woman with uncomplicated patent ductus arteriosus tolerates pregnancy well. If pulmonary hypertension supervenes, the risk to the mother becomes significant. If indeed pulmonary hypertension is suspected and documented, termination of pregnancy is strongly recommended. If the pregnancy is uncomplicated, medical management is indicated for other left-to-right shunt disorders (atrial septal and ventricular septal defect).

Eisenmenger's Syndrome

The Eisenmenger syndrome is characterized by a congenital communication between the systemic and pulmonary circulations and increased pulmonary vascular resistance, either to systemic level, so that there is no shunt across the defect, or with pulmonary vascular resistance exceeding systemic, allowing right-to-left shunt. The most common underlying defect is a large interventricular septal defect. The next most common cause of Eisenmenger pathophysiology is a large patent ductus arteriosus. It is less common for

Eisenmenger pathophysiology to develop secondary to atrial septal defect (Craig and Selzer, 1968). Occasionally this type of pathophysiology develops in other less common defects. By the time the syndrome is fully developed, it is often difficult or impossible clinically to diagnose the underlying defect. For the purpose of this discussion, the ventricular septal defect serves as a good model (Fig. 47–1). The cause of cyanosis in this condition compared with that in tetralogy of Fallot can be appreciated by comparing Figure 47–1 with Figure 47–4.

Eisenmenger pathophysiology develops only when the defect is large and is not restrictive, i.e., obligates equal systolic pressure in the two ventricles. It is more common in girls and develops at a young age. When

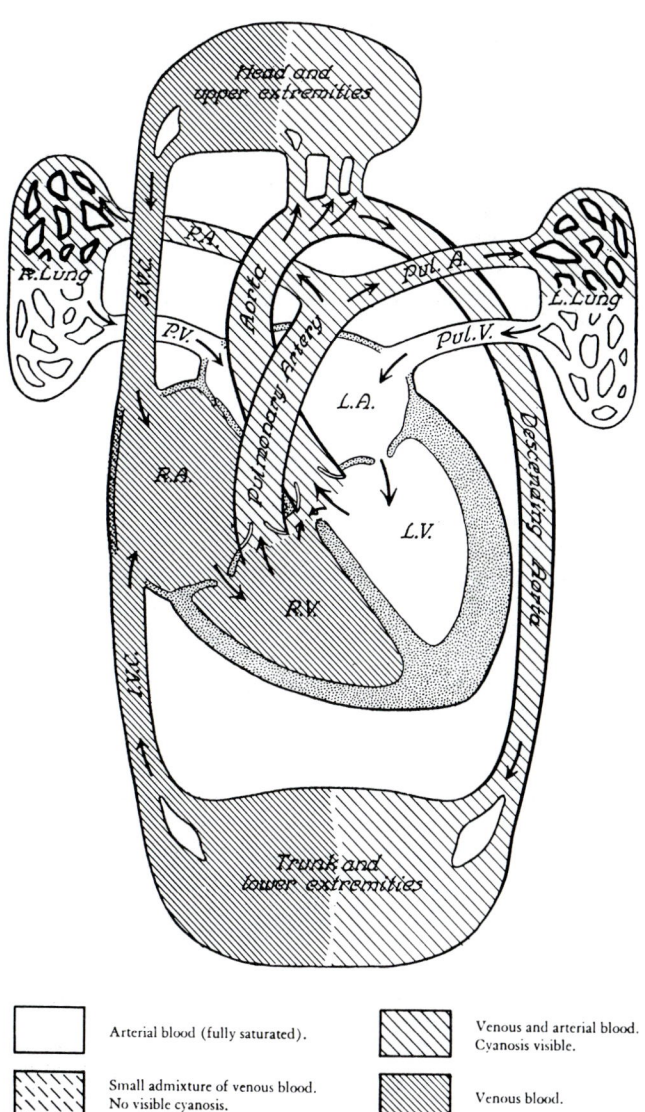

☐	Arterial blood (fully saturated).	▨	Venous and arterial blood. Cyanosis visible.
▨	Small admixture of venous blood. No visible cyanosis.	▨	Venous blood.

FIGURE 47–1. Eisenmenger complex. In comparison with Figure 47–4, note the absence of pulmonary stenosis. Here the cause of right-to-left shunt across the ventricular septal defect is increased pulmonary vascular resistance arising in the small pulmonary arteries and arterioles. (From Taussig HB: Congenital Malformation of the Heart. Cambridge, Harvard University Press, 1960.)

increased pulmonary vascular resistance is detected in a child with a large ventricular septal defect, operative closure must be done as soon as possible to prevent the development of Eisenmenger pathophysiology because, once this has appeared, pulmonary hypertension is irreversible and the defect is inoperable.

The major clues that Eisenmenger pathophysiology is developing or has developed are diminution and final disappearance of evidence of a left-to-right shunt and the appearance of progressive pulmonary hypertension. The pansystolic murmur of ventricular septal defect or the continuous murmur of patent ductus arteriosus is replaced by a short ejection systolic murmur. The lungs are no longer hyperemic but show large central pulmonary arteries and small peripheral arteries characteristic of severe pulmonary hypertension. Because the shunt has disappeared, the radiographic cardiothoracic ratio returns to normal, but the main pulmonary segment is prominent. There is usually a striking right ventricular heave, a loud and palpable pulmonary valve closure sound, and commonly an ejection sound. When concentric ventricular hypertrophy gives way to dilatation and right heart failure, evidence of tricuspid regurgitation appears. Until then, the mean venous pressure is normal, but the amplitude of the *a* wave may be increased, reflecting decreased right ventricular diastolic compliance. When pulmonary vascular resistance is significantly higher than systemic, right-to-left shunt causes cyanosis, clubbing of the fingers and toes, and increased hematocrit. Attempts at surgical correction usually result in the death of the patient (Wood, 1958). Many patients die from right heart failure, pulmonary hypertension, or pulmonary hemorrhage (Haroutunian and Neill, 1972).

The would-be mother must be informed that to become pregnant would be taking a 50 per cent risk of dying (Gleicher et al., 1979) and, even if she survives, the probable outcome for the fetus is likely to be unsatisfactory: fetal mortality exceeds 50 per cent in cyanotic women with Eisenmenger syndrome (Young and Mark, 1971). Sudden death may occur at any time, but labor, delivery, and the early puerperium seem to be the most dangerous periods (Pitts et al., 1977; Spinnato et al., 1981). Any significant fall in venous return, regardless of etiology, impairs the ability of the right heart to pump blood through the high, fixed pulmonary vascular resistance. Therefore, management during pregnancy centers on the maintenance of pulmonary blood flow. If the patient insists on maintaining the pregnancy, limitation of physical activity is essential, as is the use of pressure-graded elastic support hose, low-flow home oxygen, and monthly monitoring of platelet counts. A planned term delivery with central hemodynamic monitoring seems most appropriate, with continued close monitoring postpartum in an intensive care unit until hemodynamic stability is achieved.

OBSTRUCTIVE LESIONS

Some congenital cardiac malformations are characterized by obstruction in the lesser or greater circula-

tion. The more frequent examples include pulmonary stenosis, aortic stenosis, and coarctation of the aorta. The hypoplastic left heart syndrome seldom allows survival to the childbearing age, but when it does, there has usually been a major palliative procedure, such as construction of a ventriculo-aortic-conduit with a prosthetic valve, which would constitute a strong contraindication to pregnancy.

Aortic Stenosis

Bicuspid aortic valve is one of the more common congenital malformations. It leads in later life to calcific aortic stenosis. It may occur as an isolated defect or in combination with other anomalies such as coarctation. This development occurs more commonly in males and usually develops late in life. In the childbearing time of life, while the bicuspid aortic valve may be either stenotic or regurgitant, the lesions are usually not severe. Congenital aortic stenosis, on the other hand, can be a very tight lesion and cause severe left ventricular hypertrophy that strictly limits the ability of the heart to respond to increased demands with appropriately augmented cardiac output. The syndrome is very like adult aortic stenosis except that it is severe at a young age. The pulses are of slow upstroke and diminished amplitude. Unlike adults with acquired aortic stenosis, children with congenital aortic stenosis have an abnormally loud aortic valve closure sound. Left ventricular ejection is prolonged so that the aortic valve closure sound may occur after the pulmonary valve closure sound, resulting in paradoxical splitting of the second heart sound; that is, splitting of the second heart sound is heard in expiration instead of inspiration. There frequently is a loud ejection sound followed by an ejection systolic murmur. The duration of the murmur and the time of its peak intensity increase with increasing severity of aortic stenosis.

The electrocardiogram shows severe left ventricular hypertrophy, and this is confirmed by the echocardiogram. The chest radiograph is characterized by post-stenotic dilatation of the aorta. In the childbearing age, the valve is usually not calcified. Patients may complain of dyspnea, chest pain, and syncope but, in spite of extreme aortic stenosis, may be asymptomatic. The lesion can be recognized and its severity assessed by Doppler echocardiography.

Critical aortic stenosis is usually treated by aortic valve replacement but occasionally by aortic valve repair. If aortic stenosis is severe and especially when it is symptomatic, the woman should be advised against becoming pregnant because the mortality is around 17 per cent (Arias and Pineda, 1978). She should be advised that, if it becomes necessary to replace the aortic valve, pregnancy and labor would be difficult and dangerous owing to the need for anticoagulant treatment. If aortic stenosis is moderately severe, she should be advised to undergo pregnancy before the aortic valve is replaced. Labor can be managed in such cases without a high maternal or fetal risk (Neilson et al., 1970). Strict limits on physical exertion and prolonged periods of bed rest may be required. Left ventricular failure may appear and necessitate the use of diuretics and digitalis; prophylaxis against bacterial endocarditis at delivery is recommended. Vasodilators, helpful in heart failure of other etiology, are dangerous in aortic stenosis because the impeded left ventricle may not be able to fill the dilated peripheral vascular bed. It is important to remember that the lowered systemic vascular resistance of pregnancy adversely affects aortic stenosis. The obstructed left ventricle is limited in its ability to fill the dilated peripheral bed, a situation that can lead to syncope or more serious manifestations of limited, relatively fixed cardiac output.

Pulmonary Stenosis

The murmur of pulmonary stenosis is loud and long and often accompanied by a thrill. The lesion is therefore usually detected in early childhood and should have been corrected before the childbearing age. Expectant mothers who have not had adequate health supervision in childhood may have pulmonary stenosis hitherto unrecognized and certainly untreated.

The diagnosis is suggested by a long, harsh systolic murmur over the pulmonary area sometimes preceded by an ejection sound. The venous pressure is normal, but there are striking *a* waves in the jugular venous pulse. The pulmonary valve closure sound is usually too soft to hear when pulmonary stenosis is severe. Severe pulmonary stenosis causes massive concentric right ventricular hypertrophy manifested by a left parasternal heave and by tall R waves and deeply inverted T waves in the right precordial leads of the electrocardiogram. Tall pointed P waves are also present, marking right atrial hypertrophy. Right ventricular enlargement and poststenotic dilatation of the main pulmonary artery are seen on the chest radiograph, which also shows paucity of peripheral pulmonary vasculature. Doppler echocardiography confirms right ventricular hypertrophy and abnormally rapid velocity of blood flow in the pulmonary artery, and it allows calculation of the right ventricular pressure as well as the systolic pressure gradient across the valve. These pressures can also be measured directly in the hemodynamics laboratory (Fig. 47–2).

Mild or moderate pulmonary stenosis is well tolerated so that neither pregnancy nor labor poses a significant threat. Prophylaxis against infective endocarditis is necessary. More severe pulmonary stenosis requires treatment. However, unlike aortic stenosis, it does not require valve replacement but is treated by balloon valvotomy in the hemodynamics laboratory (Stanger et al., 1990). Surgical pulmonary valvotomy is seldom done for simple pulmonary valve stenosis, its place having been usurped by the less invasive catheter procedure. Ideally this should be carried out before pregnancy is undertaken, but if the woman becomes pregnant, the operation can still be safely performed although at considerable risk to the fetus. Extreme pulmonary stenosis, e.g., with right ventricular systolic pressure above 150 mm Hg, is a contraindication to pregnancy until the lesion has been adequately treated.

Severe Pulmonary Hypertension

Pulmonary arterial pressure and pulmonary vascular resistance may achieve systemic levels in idiopathic

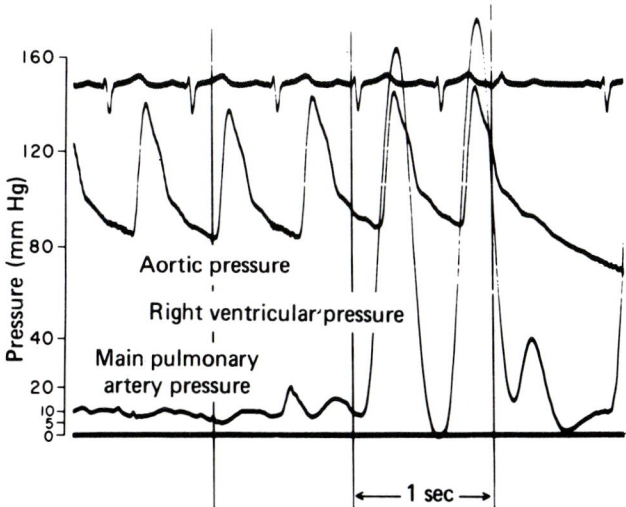

FIGURE 47–2. Pressure tracings in severe pulmonary stenosis. Pulmonary pressure is extremely low and appears damped. Right ventricular pressure is suprasystemic. (Reproduced by permission from Shabetai R, Adolph, RJ: Principles of cardiac catheterization. *In* Fowler NO (ed): Cardiac Diagnosis and Treatment. Hagerstown, Harper & Row, 1980, pp 106–183.)

pulmonary hypertension. This is a disorder associated with poor prognosis even without the additional burden of pregnancy. Severe but somewhat less than systemic pulmonary hypertension and vascular resistance may occur in chronic pulmonary embolism. In both conditions, pregnancy is extremely hazardous (50 per cent mortality) (McCaffrey and Dunn, 1964), and so the patient must be advised in the strongest possible terms to avoid pregnancy or to terminate pregnancy before the end of the first trimester. Although the expectant mother is at risk of death at any time during the pregnancy, the risk peaks during labor and in the first puerperal week. This grim outlook for primary pulmonary hypertension does not differ from that for the Eisenmenger syndrome.

The major physiologic difficulty in pulmonary hypertension is that of maintaining adequate pulmonary blood flow to provide adequate oxygenation. Anything that decreases venous return, such as vasodilatation on the systemic side of the circulation from epidural anesthesia or pooling of blood in the lower extremities from vena caval compression, will decrease preload to the right ventricle and pulmonary blood flow. Because of the precarious physiologic balance, patients should be delivered with intensive care monitoring, including a Swan-Ganz catheter, with provisions for skilled obstetric anesthesia care (Nelson et al., 1983). Anesthetic considerations for this entity are discussed later in this book.

Right-to-Left Shunt Without Pulmonary Hypertension (Tetralogy of Fallot)

The congenital cyanotic heart diseases discussed so far have been those associated with a communication between the pulmonary and systemic circulations and pulmonary vascular resistance sufficiently high to drive the shunt from right to left. Cyanosis characterizes another group of congenital malformations also characterized by a defect between the right and left sides of the heart, but in which obstruction to flow through the right heart is caused by right ventricular outflow obstruction (Fig. 47–3). Examples include the tetralogy of Fallot and tricuspid atresia. Tetralogy of Fallot will be used to illustrate this class of congenital malformation of the heart because it is by far the most common form of cyanotic congenital heart disease encountered in pregnancy. It should also be emphasized that the hereditary risk of this combination of anomalies if one parent has congenital heart disease has been reported to be between 2 and 13 per cent (Whittemore et al., 1982; Morris and Menashe, 1985; Nora et al., 1981). The malformation comprises a large defect high in the ventricular septum, pulmonary stenosis, which may be at the valve itself but more commonly is in the infundibulum of the right ventricle, overriding of the aorta so that the aortic orifice sits astride the ventricular septal defect and looks at least in part directly into the right ventricle, and right ventricular hypertrophy (Fig. 47–4).

There is a wide spectrum of clinical presentations, depending upon the relative cross-sectional areas of the ventricular septal defect through which the right-to-left shunt flows and the narrowing of the pulmonary outflow tract obstructing flow to the lungs and diverting it through the defect. In the typical case, right and left ventricular systolic pressures are equal, but the pulmonary artery pressure is exceedingly low (see Fig. 47–3). A loud, long systolic murmur is audible along the left sternal border. The murmur is caused by an abnormal flow pattern through the obstructed right ventricular outflow tract. The right-to-left shunt through the ventricular septum does not generate a murmur that is audible at the precordium. The pulmonary valve closure sound is usually inaudible. The patients are usually cyanosed, often profoundly so, and often have significant clubbing of the fingers and toes. The electrocardiogram shows severe right ventricular hypertrophy. The chest radiograph is characterized by a normal-sized heart and a concavity in the region where the pulmonary artery should be (Fig. 47–5). As in all malformations of this general type,

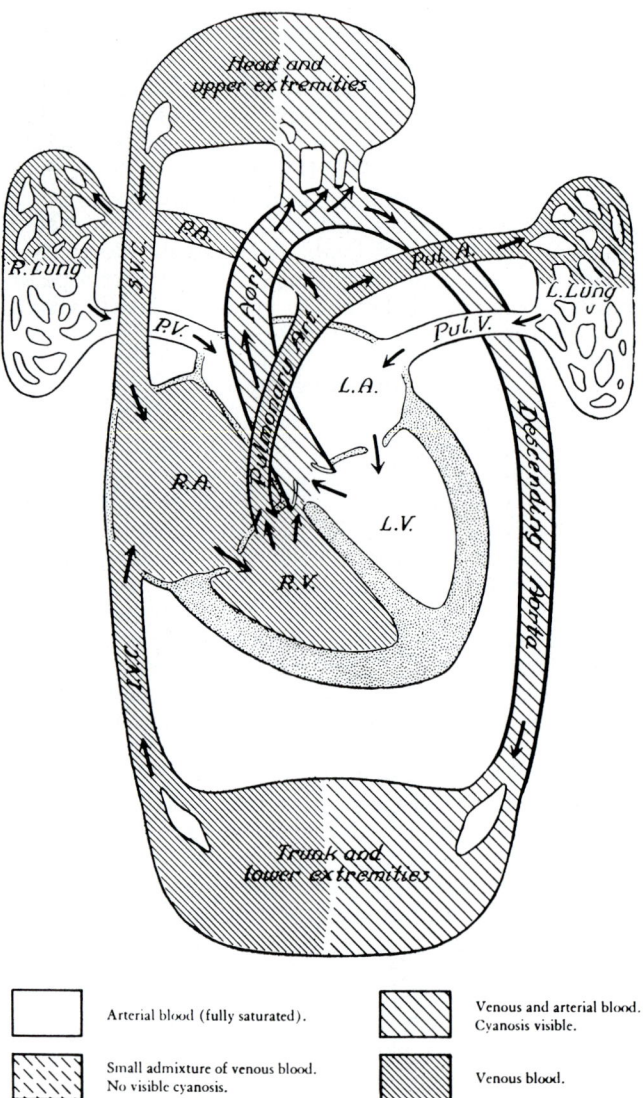

□	Arterial blood (fully saturated).	▨	Venous and arterial blood. Cyanosis visible.
▨	Small admixture of venous blood. No visible cyanosis.	▨	Venous blood.

FIGURE 47–4. In the tetralogy of Fallot, cyanosis is present because blood shunts from left to right through the ventricular septal defect because its flow to the lungs is impeded by pulmonary stenosis. (Taussig HB: Congenital Malformation of the Heart. Cambridge, Harvard University Press, Cambridge, 1960.)

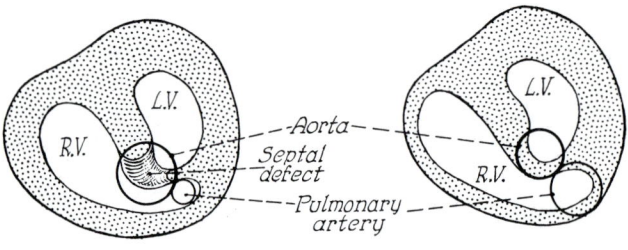

FIGURE 47–3. Tetralogy of Fallot. The anatomic pathology (*left*) compared with normal (*right*). Note the ventricular septal defect, the aorta (which overrides the defect), the pulmonary stenosis, and right ventricular hypertrophy. (Taussig HB: Congenital Malformation of the Heart. Cambridge, Harvard University Press, 1960.)

the lung fields are oligemic, showing small vessels throughout.

The vast majority of adults born with the tetralogy of Fallot and lesions with similar pathophysiology will have undergone prior surgical treatment before reaching young adulthood. They have had the ventricular septal defect closed and the pulmonary stenosis relieved, constituting virtual total repair, rendering them potentially safe candidates for pregnancy, delivery, and motherhood. The operation, however, is not curative. The pulmonary artery sometimes needs to be patched because it is hypoplastic. Significant arrhythmia and conduction defects may occur years after an apparently successful operation.

The cyanotic patient with tetralogy of Fallot has special problems during pregnancy. The reduced systemic vascular resistance of pregnancy causes more

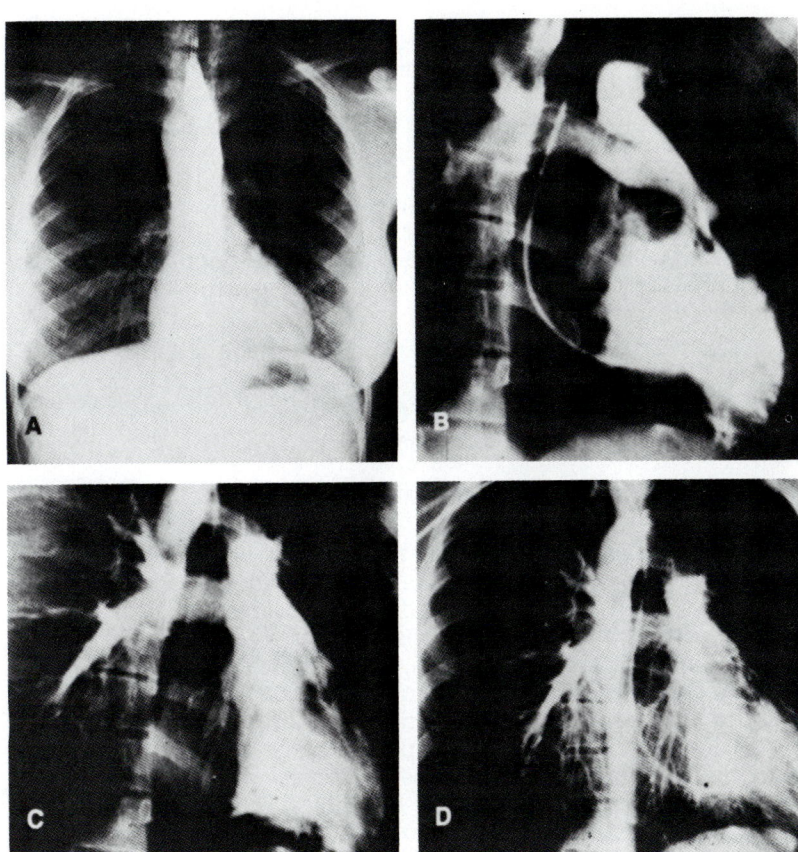

FIGURE 47–5. Tetralogy of Fallot. *A*, Chest radiograph; note concavity in the area of the pulmonary artery, oligemic lungs, and right aortic arch. *B*, Right ventriculogram; note narrow right ventricular outflow tract. *C*, Further clarification of the pulmonary arteries; the left ventricle is slightly opacified via the ventricular septal defect. *D*, The associated right-sided aortic arch is now visible. (Reproduced by permission from Shabetai R, Adolph RJ: Principles of cardiac catheterization. *In* Fowler NO (ed): Cardiac Diagnosis and Treatment. Hagerstown, Harper & Row, 1980, pp 106–183.)

blood to shunt right to left and proportionately less to flow to the pulmonary circulation. Hypoxia is intensified in this way and can lead to syncope or death. Maintenance of venous return is crucial. The most dangerous times for these women are late pregnancy and the early puerperium. Venous return is impeded by the large gravid uterus near term, and following delivery there is pooling of blood in the large dilated veins of the legs. Pressure-graded elastic support hose are recommended. Antibiotic prophylaxis should be used in these susceptible patients at delivery. Blood loss during labor may compromise venous return, and blood volume must be promptly and adequately restored. Anesthetic considerations during delivery are discussed in detail in a later chapter.

Because of the combined high maternal risk and the high incidence of fetal loss, it should again be emphasized that pregnancy is discouraged in women with uncorrected tetralogy of Fallot. If there is a history of repeated syncopal episodes, if the hematocrit exceeds 60 per cent, or if the right ventricular pressure is in excess of 120 mm Hg, the prognosis is particularly bleak. In the event that a young woman with untreated tetralogy of Fallot should request prepregnancy counseling, she should be advised to undergo surgical correction prior to pregnancy. Pregnancy does not represent an increased risk in patients whose lesions have been totally corrected.

Coarctation of the Aorta

The malformation is a congenital narrowing at the isthmus of the aorta where the ligamentum arteriosum and the left subclavian artery insert. It may be simple or complex and is either an isolated malformation or associated with patency of the ductus and other malformations, notably aortic stenosis or aortic regurgitation secondary to a bicuspid aortic valve. It may also be found in association with the Turner XO syndrome. The lesion should be detected and treated surgically or by balloon dilatation in childhood, but may be present in women who are, or want to become, pregnant. The typical features are upper extremity hypertension but lower extremity hypotension, visible and palpable collateral arteries in the scapular area, a late systolic murmur usually well heard or maximal over the interscapular region, femoral pulses that lag behind the carotid pulses and are usually of diminished amplitude, and notching of the inferior rib borders seen on the chest radiogram and due to erosion by the collaterals that bridge the coarctation. Electrocardiographic evidence of severe left ventricular hypertrophy strongly suggests associated aortic stenosis. Surgical resection, graft, or bypass reduces the upper extremity hypertension, but blood pressure does not always return to normal, and hypertension may recur in later life. Whenever possible, the operation should be performed before pregnancy because otherwise maternal mortality is 3 per cent (Deal and Wooley, 1973). Coarctation is associated with congenital berry aneurysm of the circle of Willis. The patients are at risk for dissecting hematoma of the aorta and infectious endocarditis involving an abnormal aortic valve, not the native or postoperative coarctation; these risks increase during pregnancy (Barash et al.,

1975; Deal and Wooley, 1973). Paroxysmal hypertension during the second stage of labor may cause rupture of a berry aneurysm with catastrophic cerebral hemorrhage, but this event fortunately is uncommon. Operation does not require cardiopulmonary bypass and can be carried out with safety for the mother and with less fetal risk than accompanies open heart surgery. If delivery must be undertaken in cases of unoperated coarctation, blood pressure can be titrated with alpha-adrenergic stimulating and blocking agents delivered by intravenous drip.

OTHER CONGENITAL CARDIAC MALFORMATIONS

Ebstein's Anomaly

Ebstein's anomaly is a malformation of the tricuspid valve in which the leaflets are displaced from their normal location. The result is that a considerable volume of the right ventricle behaves hemodynamically as an enlarged right atrium, but electrically as ventricular myocardium. The tricuspid valve may be significantly incompetent or stenotic, depending upon the location of the anomalously placed cusps of the valve. In some cases, the malformation causes impediment to right ventricular outflow. The clinical features are easily recognized by a cardiologist, and the echocardiogram is characteristic and reliable. This anomaly is frequently associated with anomalous atrioventricular conduction pathways so that the Wolff-Parkinson-White syndrome may be found in patients with Ebstein's anomaly. The patients frequently have an atrial-septal defect with right-to-left shunting. Supraventricular tachycardia is common also in patients who do not have the Wolff-Parkinson-White syndrome. The most favored treatment is reconstruction of the tricuspid valve, for which satisfactory techniques have now been developed. The operation should be performed before pregnancy is undertaken. The surgical repair usually interrupts any anomalous atrioventricular conduction pathways, eliminating pre-excitation and the risk of supraventricular tachycardia during pregnancy and delivery.

Congenital Atrioventricular Block

Congenital atrioventricular block differs somewhat from the heart block of adults. The ventricular pacemaker is usually higher, and therefore the QRS complex is normal or only slightly widened and the ventricular rate is more rapid than in acquired atrioventricular block. It has been discovered that, although these patients appear to do very well during childhood and young adulthood, the lesion is associated with an unexpectedly high mortality. Therefore, treatment with a pacemaker is indicated in many of the cases. The pacemaker used should be atrioventricular and rate-responsive so that the patient may enjoy normal cardiovascular dynamics at rest and exercise. Patients who are untreated or have received a pacemaker are at slight or no increased risk during pregnancy.

A number of other malformations may be present in women of childbearing age. These include other left-to-right or right-to-left shunts, transposition of the great vessels, truncus arteriosus, single ventricle, double outlet ventricle, and a variety of obstructive lesions. The malformations may be multiple and complex. Survival to adulthood depends upon at least partial correction, which may have been furnished by surgical operation or be part of the malformation. For example, in transposition the aorta arises from the right ventricle and the pulmonary artery from the left. Prolonged survival requires a route for admixture which may be a naturally occurring defect of the atrial septum or be surgically created. An appropriate stenosis may protect the lung from flooding or pulmonary hypertension. Some of these women with beautifully but delicately balanced lesions bear children, but usually this is not wise. Further discussion of this topic is beyond the scope of this chapter, save to state that the women should be evaluated and followed by a pediatric cardiologist and an obstetrician with special knowledge and experience in managing women with congenital heart disease.

RHEUMATIC HEART DISEASE

Rheumatic Fever

Rheumatic fever seldom occurs for the first time in young adults; usually when it occurs, it has been preceded by an episode in childhood. Rheumatic fever is now distinctly uncommon in the United States, Western Europe, and Great Britain, but is still highly prevalent in less economically developed countries. Many young women emigrate to the Western world and constitute a large proportion of the patients. Women with a prior history of rheumatic fever should take daily penicillin or, if allergic, its equivalent before and throughout pregnancy to prevent a recurrence. Acute rheumatic fever or acute streptococcal infection mandates a full bactericidal dose for 10 days. Acute rheumatic heart disease manifested by pericarditis, symptoms of heart failure, cardiac murmurs, and enlargement of the heart necessitates prompt suppression with prednisone and bed rest.

Rheumatic Heart Disease

In the United States, acute rheumatic fever with carditis has been uncommon for many years, and chronic rheumatic heart disease is becoming uncommon among the native childbearing population, although cases may still be found among the poor. Control of rheumatic fever has largely shifted the burden of mitral stenosis from teenagers to women in the third and fourth decades of life. The characteristic lesion is mitral stenosis, and the next most common is mitral stenosis with aortic regurgitation. The mitral valve lesion may be mixed stenosis and incompetence, and the valve may calcify. Pure mitral regurgitation is almost always nonrheumatic except in young people with acute carditis. Likewise, aortic valve disease without mitral involvement is seldom rheumatic. Tricuspid regurgitation is a late secondary manifestation secondary to pulmonary hypertension and right ventricular enlargement.

Mitral Stenosis

The principal features are enlargement of the left atrium and right ventricle, a diastolic murmur at the cardiac apex and pulmonary hypertension. Inflow to the left ventricle is impeded by the narrowed valve and can be accomplished only by an increased head of pressure in the left atrium (Fig. 47–6). The faster the heart rate, the less is the time for ventricular filling. Left atrial pressure therefore is further elevated by tachycardia. Atrial fibrillation eventually supervenes, causing a fall in cardiac output and escalation of left atrial hypertension, especially if the ventricular rate cannot easily be controlled. Atrial fibrillation substantially increases the probability of thrombus in the left atrial appendage and the threat of an embolic stroke.

Pregnancy drastically stresses the circulation in women with severe mitral stenosis. The increased blood volume, heart rate, and cardiac output raise left atrial pressure to a level that causes severe pulmonary congestion, which may be manifested by progressive exertional dyspnea or orthopnea and progress to paroxysmal nocturnal dyspnea and pulmonary edema. Women who have not been receiving antenatal care often report initially with intractable pulmonary edema. Longstanding cases develop severe right heart failure. Infective endocarditis, pulmonary embolism, and massive hemoptysis may also occur. The maternal risk for death is maximal in the third trimester and in the puerperium (Szekely et al., 1973).

Significant Mitral Stenosis Without Heart Failure

These women should be advised to undergo mitral valvotomy and postpone pregnancy until after full recovery from the operation. If they fail to follow this advice and become pregnant, one reasonable course for some individuals in the first trimester is therapeutic abortion, followed by mitral valve operation and subsequent pregnancy planning. If this is not acceptable, the patient can be advised to remain under frequent close supervision by the cardiologist and obstetrician, accept long periods of rest and prohibition of strenuous activity, salt restriction, and diuretic treatment. When this type of regimen is followed closely and is expertly supervised, maternal mortality is low (Szekely et al., 1973). Atrial fibrillation would signal the need

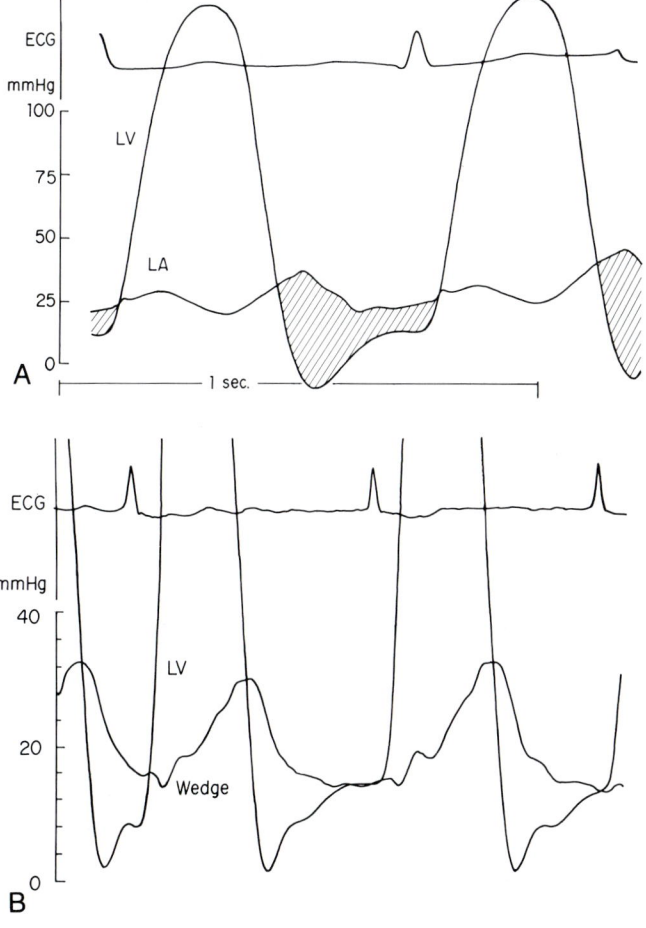

FIGURE 47–6. Hemodynamics of mitral valve disease. *A*, Mitral stenosis. Note the diastolic pressure gradient *(shaded)* between left atrium and left ventricle that persists to end diastole. *B*, Mitral regurgitation. Note the large systolic pressure wave of the pulmonary wedge pressure tracing and that the diastolic pressure gradient is limited to early diastole.

for digitalis, a beta-adrenergic blocking agent, or a calcium channel blocking agent to maintain a normal heart rate. More than one of these drugs may be needed to achieve the desired result without side effects.

Atrial fibrillation with significant mitral stenosis requires anticoagulant treatment. The problems with this (Hall et al., 1980) and the possible role of Coumadin during the second trimester have been mentioned at the beginning of this chapter. In a recent review (Born et al., 1992), it was reported that acute perivalvular thrombosis occurred on three occasions, two of them fatal, during 35 pregnancies in women with mechanical valve replacement receiving anticoagulant. Spontaneous abortion developed in seven of the patients. Prematurity and low birth weight were common, and there were three neonatal deaths. If it is deemed that the valve can be treated by valvotomy and will not require replacement, the operation can be carried out safely for the mother, but the fetus may be lost (Snaith and Szekely, 1967). If it is thought that valve replacement will be needed, the operation should be postponed until after delivery, if at all possible.

Depending on her course, the woman may have to spend many weeks in bed and should be admitted to the hospital well in advance of labor. The supine posture should be avoided as much as possible and delivery in the Sims position is desirable. The lithotomy position with the patient on her back and her feet elevated in stirrups is an invitation to pulmonary edema. The crisis of pulmonary edema may appear in spite of this management. Sedation to drop the heart rate and promote cardiac filling and output and diuretic treatment must then be followed by prompt abdominal delivery if the fetus is viable.

Balloon valvuloplasty is a nonsurgical means to dilate mitral stenosis (Kaplan et al., 1987; McKay et al., 1987a). Fluoroscopy is required to guide the balloon into the mitral orifice, but when the procedure can be put off until after the first trimester, mitral balloon angioplasty may well become the procedure of choice when it is essential to increase the mitral valve orifice (Lefevre et al., 1991).

If a patient is known to have mitral stenosis and right heart failure with severe pulmonary congestion, pregnancy should be avoided. The risk of maternal mortality is high.

MITRAL VALVE PROLAPSE

A degree of prolapse of the mitral valve was considered so prevalent in the general population (Devereux et al., 1976), and particularly among young women, that authorities differed as to whether mitral prolapse should be considered a normal variant or abnormal. More exacting echocardiographic criteria yield more realistic and lower estimates of the prevalence (Wann et al., 1983), which still remains high (Perloff et al., 1986). Mitral prolapse occurs because portions of the mitral valve apparatus are too large for the heart and therefore the leaflets balloon into the left atrium during systole. The leaflets may remain coapted, in which

case prolapse is an isolated phenomenon, or separate causing a variable degree of mitral regurgitation. More severe prolapse may be caused by myxomatous degeneration of the leaflets or redundant chordae. These abnormalities of connective tissue may be isolated to the mitral valve or be a part of Marfan's syndrome. Mitral (and sometimes tricuspid) valve prolapse may be associated with congenital malformations, notably atrial septal defect.

Mitral regurgitation may be absent, intermittent, or permanent and may be of any degree of severity. Severe mitral regurgitation greatly enlarges the left atrium (Fig. 47–7) and ventricle and eventually leads to left ventricular failure and pulmonary hypertension, the latter less severe than with mitral stenosis.

In a minority of cases, mitral prolapse is associated with severe dysfunction of the autonomic nervous system (Perloff et al., 1986), manifested in the main by excessive lability of the heart rate and blood pressure, usually postural hypotension. Dysautonomia (Coghlan et al., 1979) is increased during pregnancy. Less well understood is the association with anxiety and panic attacks, which may be partly related to

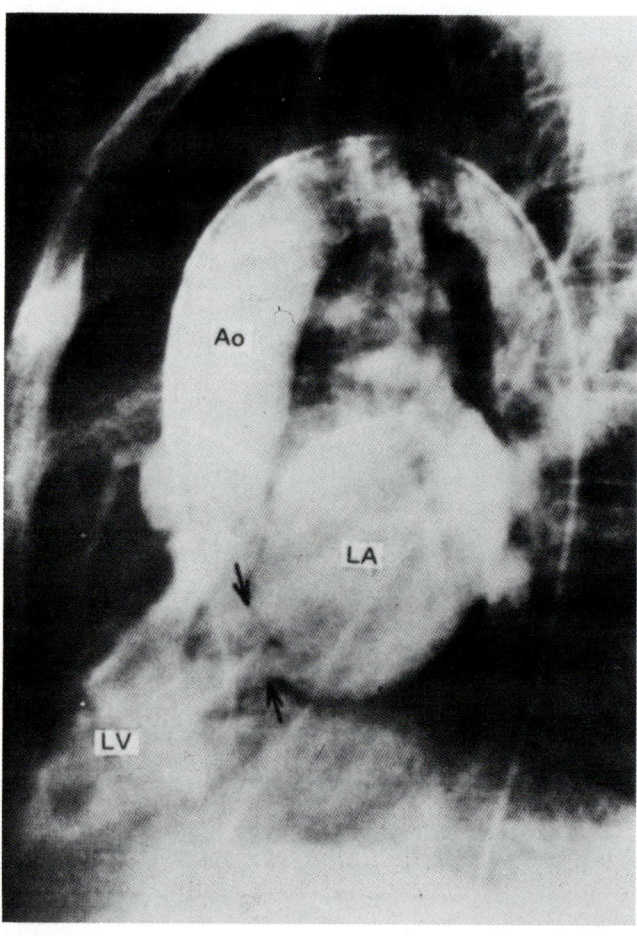

FIGURE 47–7. Mitral regurgitation. Contrast was injected into the left ventricle. Note massive opacification of the enlarged left atrium. (Reproduced by permission from Shabetai R, Adolph RJ: Principles of cardiac catheterization. *In* Fowler NO (ed): Cardiac Diagnosis and Treatment. Hagerstown, Harper & Row, 1980, pp 106–183.)

abnormal catecholamine metabolism and altered function of the sympathetic nervous system. Psychological abnormalities also are more frequent than in the general population (Hartman et al., 1982).

A number of women complain of chest pain, which partly meets the criteria for angina pectoris. Although these women have a normal coronary arteriogram, T-wave inversions, especially in leads 2, 3, and aVF, are found in a small proportion, and the treadmill exercise test may induce ST-segment depression indistinguishable from ischemia (Butman et al., 1982).

Ventricular extrasystoles, supraventricular extrasystoles, and atrial fibrillation may be considerably more frequent and more symptomatic than in the general population of women of childbearing age. In an exceedingly small minority, ventricular tachycardia or fibrillation occurs and, in a small subset of these, has resulted in sudden death. This outcome is so rare (Devereux et al., 1976) that, when counseling, it need not be mentioned and must not be emphasized unless there is convincing evidence that the particular individual is clearly at risk. Stroke is an unusual but definite complication (Sandok and Giuliani, 1982) and is thought to be due to platelet occlusion or embolism, not left atrial thrombus, except when mitral regurgitation is severe. In this connection platelet function is abnormal in some patients with mitral valve prolapse.

Diagnosis

In the majority of cases, the diagnosis is made by the physician providing preconception counseling and antenatal care. Alternatively, the woman may inform the physician that she has prolapse and, because often it is familial (Shell et al., 1969), that other family members have it too. The prepregnancy examination will reveal a systolic click occurring between the first and second heart sounds. The click may or may not be followed by a mid or late systolic murmur. The click and murmur vary with the patient's posture and from time to time.

Simple Mitral Prolapse

In the vast majority, no other abnormality will be found on clinical examination or, with the exception of echocardiography which images the prolapse, on laboratory investigation. In such cases, the patient should be told that pregnancy, labor, and delivery will be safe and unaffected by the prolapse, but the physician should keep a watchful eye on the patient's blood pressure, especially when she is standing, and on her heart rate and rhythm, especially after exercise. Opinion is divided on the need for prophylaxis against infectious endocarditis when the only manifestation of mitral valve prolapse is the systolic click (Clemens et al., 1982). I do not recommend it. When a systolic murmur is present, however, it is evidence of mitral regurgitation and signals the need for such prophylaxis.

Mitral Valve Prolapse With Significant Regurgitation

Patients in this category will be far fewer in number. The murmur is louder, longer, and more consistent and may become pansystolic. Clinical and laboratory evidence of enlargement of the left atrium and ventricle increases with increasing severity and duration of regurgitation. Volume overload of the heart is well tolerated for many years, the enlarged left ventricle maintaining full compensation. However, the inevitable eventual onset of deterioration of left ventricular function is subtle, because resistance to regurgitant flow to the pulmonary venous bed is far less than resistance to flow through the systemic arterioles. This safety valve, or low impedance leak, preserves the pumping function of the left ventricle, even after myocardial damage has occurred as a consequence of the longstanding volume overload (Eckberg et al., 1973). Even modest impairment of left ventricular function, especially when progressive, indicates that pregnancy may well precipitate heart failure and cannot be lightly undertaken. More obvious left ventricular dysfunction—for example, ejection fraction below 35 per cent—indicates that the woman should be strongly advised to avoid pregnancy. She should then be referred for complete cardiologic evaluation (Ross, 1981). In some cases, the valve would then be *repaired*; it seldom needs to be replaced. Thereafter, if the result is good and ventricular function significantly improved, pregnancy may be undertaken, and a successful outcome can be predicted.

Symptomatic Mitral Prolapse

Chest pain, palpitation, tachycardia, dysrhythmia, anxiety, and panic attacks are best managed by blockade of the beta-adrenergic receptors with an agent such as propranolol. When symptoms are unusually pronounced, treatment should be preceded by tests of thyroid function and measurements of plasma catecholamine concentration. The gravid uterus and vasodilation may add to postural hypotension. The woman should therefore be informed that during pregnancy she may experience light-headedness, dizziness, or fainting during prolonged standing. Pronounced arrhythmia that is not ameliorated by beta-receptor blockade requires conventional antiarrhythmic management. The woman should be told of the strong tendency for prolapse to occur in other family members but that the condition is not sufficiently serious for her to consider avoiding pregnancy because of the possibility of prolapse in the offspring (Shell et al., 1969).

Mitral Regurgitation Not Caused By Prolapse

In younger women, the etiology is often rheumatic or congenital. In older women, mitral regurgitation is more often a manifestation of hypertension, ischemia, or idiopathic myocardial disease. Infectious endocarditis can cause severe mitral regurgitation.

Most of the information in the section on mitral regurgitation in prolapse applies here too. In older women the valve is more likely to be calcified; fewer of the valves are amenable to repair and must be replaced. The problems posed by prosthetic valves in pregnant women have been discussed in preceding paragraphs. The hemodynamics are illustrated in Figure 47–6 and the angiography in Figure 47–7.

In patients with far-advanced left ventricular dysfunction or failure who have severe mitral regurgitation, it can be difficult to determine which is the cause and which the result. However, in either case the patient with a greatly enlarged grossly hypokinetic ventricle must be advised against becoming pregnant. Most of the pregnancy would be spent in bed, the course would be punctuated by episodes of uncompensated congestive heart failure, any of which could prove fatal or require therapeutic abortion, and the risk to the fetus would exceed 50 per cent.

Patients with mild or moderate mitral regurgitation can be managed safely by means of a conservative regimen of reduced physical activity, salt restriction, and low doses of diuretic. Low-dose digoxin is helpful, especially when atrial fibrillation supervenes.

Severe or moderate mitral regurgitation is an indication to repair or replace the valve when symptoms and early evidence of declining ventricular function appear. Clearly surgical treatment is best undertaken before pregnancy. If the woman is already pregnant, every effort should be made to carry the pregnancy to term using strict medical measures. This course is particularly important when clinical, radiologic, and echocardiographic criteria suggest that the valve is irreparable and would need to be replaced.

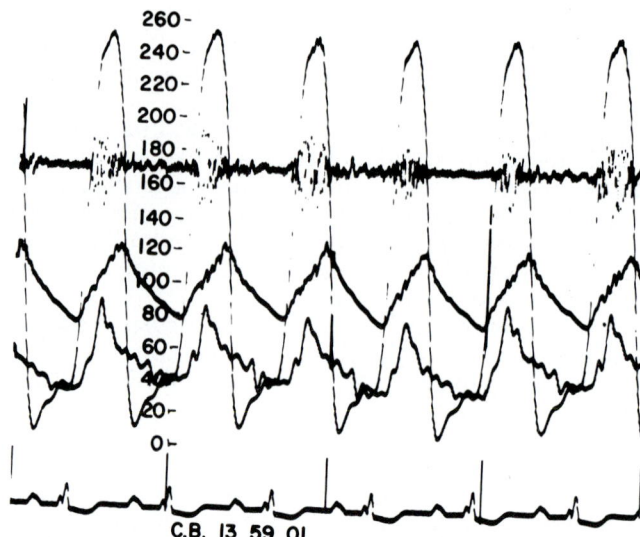

FIGURE 47–8. Hemodynamic data in aortic stenosis. Left ventricular pressure is 250/40 mm Hg (normal 120/10 mm Hg). Aortic systolic pressure is 130 mm Hg lower than left ventricular and shows a slow upstroke and vibrations representing the systolic thrill. The record above the aortic pressure tracing is a phonocardiogram showing the systolic murmur. Also shown is the pulmonary wedge pressure (lowest pressure tracing) which is elevated to equal the left ventricular diastolic pressure. The bottom tracing is the ECG. (Reproduced by permission from Shabetai R, Adolph RJ: Principles of cardiac catheterization. *In* Fowler NO (ed): Cardiac Diagnosis and Treatment. Hagerstown, Harper & Row, 1980. pp 106–183.)

AORTIC VALVE DISEASE

Aortic Stenosis

The etiology of aortic stenosis commonly is degeneration, often of a congenitally bicuspid valve. The problem may be encountered in women a decade or more older than those with rheumatic or congenital aortic valve disease. Frequently the valve is calcified. Critical aortic stenosis leads to severe left ventricular hypertrophy and eventually to left ventricular failure. Even before the advent of overt heart failure, syncope or even sudden death may occur.

The characteristic findings include an ejection systolic murmur—harsher, louder and peaking later than the normal ejection murmur of pregnancy. It is usually loudest at the second right interspace. When aortic stenosis is severe, the pulse shows slow upstroke, and left ventricular hypertrophy is evident on the electrocardiogram. The echocardiogram is a more sensitive and more specific marker of left ventricular hypertrophy. Doppler echocardiographic measurement of the blood flow velocity through the aortic valve permits reliable estimation of the systolic pressure drop across the valve and thus the severity of aortic stenosis. The aortic valve area can be calculated from the Doppler echocardiography imaging. The hemodynamics are illustrated in Figure 47–8.

The left ventricle does not dilate until the ventricle fails. A dilated ventricle in aortic stenosis is an omi-

nous sign calling for rapid intervention to relieve the obstruction to the left ventricular outflow tract. If this is achieved during late pregnancy by balloon valvuloplasty, valve replacement will almost certainly have to be done soon after delivery. When dilated heart failure is severe, the wisest option is to deliver the fetus abdominally and replace the aortic valve.

Heart failure (past or present), syncope, and an episode of cardiac arrest are absolute contraindications to pregnancy in women with uncorrected critical aortic stenosis (Arias and Pineda, 1978). Following valve replacement, a woman who desperately wants a baby and who is prepared to deal with the maternal and fetal risks posed by anticoagulants may, with close supervision, be brought to term with a relatively low maternal risk. Severe cardiac symptoms in pregnant women secondary to tight aortic stenosis can be relieved by aortic balloon valvuloplasty (McKay et al., 1987b), although proper preconception counseling should have spared them this predicament.

Aortic Regurgitation

The etiology is commonly rheumatic fever, in which case mitral stenosis often coexists. Disease of the ascending aorta, e.g., Marfan's syndrome, may cause severe aortic regurgitation. Infectious endocarditis is another important cause. Aortic regurgitation imposes a volume load and as such is usually well tolerated in pregnancy and labor (Sullivan and Ramanathan, 1985).

The diagnosis is usually based on the typical high-pitched blowing diastolic murmur and can be quantified by Doppler echocardiography. Pregnancy itself and the lesion both contribute to hypervolemia and peripheral vasodilatation. A prolonged course without decompensation is characteristic of chronic aortic regurgitation, but once heart failure appears, the course may be rapidly downhill. Traditionally no major action is taken until symptoms of heart failure, notably exertional dyspnea, make their appearance or evidence of left ventricular dysfunction can be detected by pulmonary congestion or abnormal laboratory tests. These include a falling ejection fraction and increasing ventricular echocardiographic dimensions, particularly at end systole. These are the usual indications for aortic valve replacement or, occasionally, repair. Repair of aortic regurgitation is much less often successful than in mitral regurgitation. In the case of women contemplating pregnancy, the need for aortic valve replacement constitutes the grounds on which the medical advisor must recommend against pregnancy and make the woman fully understand the consequences of choosing otherwise. Increased *diastolic* volume of the left ventricle is a consequence of its overload and does not necessarily constitute evidence of heart failure. When left ventricular dysfunction and heart failure are absent, carefully supervised pregnancy is in order, and the woman should be encouraged to complete her family before heart failure and the need to consider valve replacement arise.

In many cases, the cause of aortic regurgitation will not be clarified. Special care must be taken to rule out aortic aneurysm or dissection, especially when associated with Marfan's syndrome, since these conditions may give rise to aortic rupture and constitute strong reasons to advise against the patient's becoming pregnant.

Prophylaxis against infectious endocarditis is mandated in any valvular disease of the heart.

CARDIOMYOPATHY

Cardiomyopathy is an idiopathic disorder of myocardium. Thus, the diagnosis cannot be established in the presence of other causes of myocardial dysfunction such as hypertension or coronary or valve disease.

Dilated Cardiomyopathy

The cardiac chambers are dilated and in consequence, although hypertrophied, are not thick-walled. Ventricular wall tension is increased, and systolic pump function declines. Consequently, cardiac output falls, and filling pressures increase; both these changes cause progressive dyspnea, edema, and fatigue. Serious ventricular arrhythmia develops in the majority. The 5-year prognosis for survival is less than 50 per cent, and during that time heart failure becomes less and less responsive to treatment (Clemens et al., 1982). In a few cases, however, improvement or even return to normal has been noted, but at the time of initial contact, there are no markers enabling the physician

to predict this outcome. Some of the patients who recover may have had unrecognized myocarditis that did not progress to cardiomyopathy.

Dilated cardiomyopathy is thought to be the outcome of an autoimmune response to a myocardial injury, most commonly viral myocarditis. The exact role of alcohol is unclear, but it is at least a major aggravating factor in some cases.

Patients may have symptoms and signs of heart failure for which no cause can be found on clinical and laboratory examination. Weight is increased, the jugular venous pressure is elevated, and the heart is enlarged. A third heart sound gallop is often present, frequently accompanied by the murmurs of mitral and tricuspid regurgitation, which develop as a consequence of cardiac dilatation. The electrocardiogram is usually grossly abnormal, often showing left ventricular hypertrophy or left bundle branch block. Ventricular function tests disclose enlargement and hypocontractility of the ventricles. The patients are subject to mural thrombus in the cardiac chambers and thus to the risk of stroke or pulmonary embolism.

Established dilated cardiomyopathy, even when heart failure is compensated, is a contraindication to pregnancy.

Peripartal Cardiomyopathy

Peripartal cardiomyopathy is dilated cardiomyopathy, arising for the first time in the puerperium or, less commonly, in the last trimester of pregnancy (O'Connell et al., 1986). Whether the peripartal or postpartum state somehow constitutes the original myocardial insult or is an aggravating factor in individuals susceptible to cardiomyopathy for other reasons is not known (Cunningham et al., 1986). Tragically, this devastating disease may affect previously healthy young women.

Perhaps 50 per cent of women with peripartal cardiomyopathy go on to have dilated cardiomyopathy, indistinguishable from idiopathic. The rest show remarkable recovery (Van der Leeuw-Harmsen et al., 1985). Women who recover from peripartal cardiomyopathy must be informed that cardiomyopathy may recur with a subsequent pregnancy. It has been believed for some time that this risk is 50 per cent (Cole et al., 1987). However, a recent report of four women who had peripartal cardiomyopathy with a prior pregnancy, but whose hearts remained normal clinically and by echocardiography in a subsequent pregnancy, indicates that the risk may be less (St. John Sutton et al., 1991). Nevertheless, the women should be counseled against another pregnancy. The clinical and prognostic features of dilated cardiomyopathy overlap those of heart failure of other etiology. These are discussed in a subsequent section of this chapter.

Dilated cardiomyopathy is not ordinarily familial (Shabetai and Shine, 1973), but inherited cases are occasionally observed (Mestroni et al., 1990). The prospective mother can be advised that the risk that her baby will develop dilated cardiomyopathy is small.

In a young woman with severe dilated cardiomyopathy, manifested by greatly impaired ventricular function and drastically reduced exercise capacity, cardiac transplantation should be considered. Eventually such women can have children with reasonable safety (Kossoy et al., 1988; Key et al., 1989).

Acquired Immune Deficiency Syndrome (AIDS)

Myocarditis or cardiomyopathy is frequently discovered when patients with AIDS are examined postmortem (Bestetti, 1989; Lewis, 1989). Symptomatic myocardial disease, while considerably less common, is observed with increasing frequency. If patients with AIDS are screened for cardiac involvement, for example, by echocardiography, cardiac or pericardial involvement is found in almost 75 per cent of the cases (Raffanti et al., 1988). Myocarditis is usually caused by opportunistic infection, but in some cases hybridization studies have proved direct AIDS infection. Dilated cardiomyopathy ranges from clinically silent ventricular dysfunction to severe uncompensated heart failure. Rarely, even Kaposi's sarcoma has been detected in the heart or pericardium. Pericardial effusion, usually occult unless specifically sought out, is one of the more common cardiac manifestations. Malignant lymphoma has been reported involving the myocardium and endocardium.

Cardiac failure ranks low on the list of problems faced by the physician managing pregnancy complicated by AIDS. Nevertheless, physicians need to be on guard lest the patient develop severe dilated cardiomyopathy, myocarditis, or cardiac tamponade, and the family must be prepared for a child with congenital AIDS.

CORONARY ARTERY DISEASE

Premenopausal women enjoy substantial protection against coronary atherosclerosis (Sullivan and Ramanathan, 1985). Ischemic heart disease therefore is rarely relevant to obstetric practice. However, coronary artery disease may be found in women of childbearing age when other risk factors overwhelm the natural protection they should normally enjoy. Lupus erythematosus, especially when treated with steroidal agents, may precipitate premature coronary artery disease (Meller et al., 1975). Coronary atherosclerosis appears in a significant proportion of patients who have received a cardiac transplant (Johnson et al., 1991) and may be found in familial lipid disorders. In the latter instance, the exact nature of the lipid disorder must be defined by detailed analysis of the patient's lipid chemistry and lipoproteins to enable the physician to provide an accurate forecast of the risk that the baby would inherit the lipid disorder and premature coronary artery disease. A risk factor unique to this population is the use of oral contraceptive agents (Ratnoff and Kaufman, 1982).

Angina pectoris on moderate effort may require treatment with nitrates, calcium-channel blocking drugs, or beta-adrenergic blocking drugs, but otherwise should have no effect whatever on pregnancy, labor, or delivery. Likewise, if a woman had in the past sustained a myocardial infarction but had recovered without heart failure, significant left ventricular dysfunction, or unstable angina pectoris, she too can be advised that her pregnancy and labor should not differ significantly from those in women without heart disease.

The major indications that pregnancy and labor would pose a significant threat of morbidity and mortality to women with ischemic heart disease are heart failure (see later section of this chapter), significant enlargement and dysfunction of the left ventricle, and ischemia at rest or provoked by slight effort.

Severe ischemia may be diagnosed when angina occurs at rest or with mild exertion. This unstable angina frequently, but not necessarily, follows a period of classic stable angina pectoris. Unstable angina is a reliable symptom of severe extensive myocardial ischemia and thus is a clear warning of the imminence of major ischemic events such as acute myocardial infarction or a fatal ventricular arrhythmia. Clearly, starting a pregnancy under these circumstances would be unwise.

In some women with advanced heart disease the clinical picture is less dramatic, but a treadmill exercise test demonstrates that profound and dangerous ischemia can be precipitated by minimal exertion. Thus, if the treadmill test provokes more than 3 mm of ST-segment depression at a low level of exercise, and particularly if this abnormal response is accompanied by either angina pectoris or a fall in blood pressure, the woman is at high risk for a serious and possibly fatal myocardial ischemic event and must not undertake pregnancy unless the myocardium can be revascularized.

Patients with unstable angina or severe ischemia must be referred to a cardiology center where the acute problem can be stabilized and the patient can be assessed for revascularization of the myocardium by coronary bypass graft operation or transluminal coronary angioplasty. If the outcome is satisfactory, the patient may then bear children.

Myocardial Infarction

A remote myocardial infarction followed by recovery without angina, major left ventricular dysfunction, or heart failure should not influence pregnancy or labor. Patients should wait a year after infarction before undertaking pregnancy. In many cases coronary arteriography should be done first, so that if critical coronary stenoses are found, myocardial revascularization can be done. Severe left ventricular damage and heart failure are relative contraindications to pregnancy and, when far advanced, absolute contraindications.

Patients with ischemic heart disease may experience episodic myocardial ischemia without having angina. Patients should therefore undergo objective tests such as treadmill exercise tolerance or myocardial perfusion imaging at rest and after peak exercise. Similarly, myocardial infarction may lead to severe depression of left ventricular function, which may or may not be accompanied by evidence of heart failure. Left ventricular function testing by echocardiography or determination of the left ventricular ejection fraction should be carried out, preferably before pregnancy or, failing that, shortly thereafter.

For remote myocardial infarction without evidence of ischemia, heart failure, or severe left ventricular dysfunction, simple electrocardiographic monitoring suffices during labor. In other cases, central venous pressure, pulmonary arterial and pulmonary wedged pressure, and cardiac output should be monitored via a Swan-Ganz catheter together with intra-arterial blood pressure. Cardiac function can also be monitored via transesophageal echocardiography.

Monitoring should be continued until after the completion of labor because, with birth, maternal preload abruptly increases, after which substantial loss of blood accompanies delivery of the placenta. With good care, most women who survive a myocardial infarction during pregnancy can be safely delivered (Husaini, 1971).

HEART FAILURE

Chronic heart failure is a syndrome that develops when the heart cannot meet the metabolic requirements of the normally active individual. It may be defined as ventricular dysfunction causing dyspnea, fatigue, and sometimes arrhythmia.

Primary Myocardial Causes

The primary fault may lie in the myocardium. Examples include myocarditis, the various cardiomyopathies, ischemic heart disease, other specific myocardial disorders such as amyloidosis, and metabolic abnormalities (e.g., myxedema).

Secondary Myocardial Causes

The myocardial response to chronic pressure overload is concentric hypertrophy with increased thickness of the ventricular walls; the response to chronic volume overload is dilatation (eccentric hypertrophy). Eventually contractile power is diminished, decreasing the pump function of the heart. Causes include valve disease, systemic and pulmonary hypertension, and congenital malformations. The clinical manifestations are due in part to the abnormal loading conditions and in part to the damaged myocardium.

Manifestations

The principal manifestations are caused by increased left and right ventricular diastolic pressure, which engenders pulmonary and systemic congestion and reduced cardiac output in severe cases at rest or in less severe cases during exercise. The combined effects of inadequate cardiac output and congestion are dyspnea, fatigue, and edema. In the later stages of heart failure these changes lead to progressive dysfunction of vital organs, principally the liver and kidneys. The prognosis of severe uncorrectable heart failure is less than 50 per cent survival after 5 years.

The critical clinical features that enable physicians to diagnose and follow the course of heart failure are body weight, jugular venous pressure, the third heart sound, the cardiac size, radiologic evidence of pulmonary congestion, lung crepitation, and peripheral edema—in most cases in that order.

Heart failure greatly limits physical activity and requires continuous, usually escalating, treatment with diuretics, positive inotropic agents, vasodilators, salt restriction, and frequently antiarrhythmic agents. Pregnancy imposes a powerful, often intolerable, additional load on the failing heart. Once it has been established that no remediable cause for heart failure exists, it is clear that pregnancy is contraindicated.

Symptoms

The chief symptoms are dyspnea and fatigue. These symptoms are exaggerated by pregnancy, which often induces—in addition—edema, orthopnea, nocturnal dyspnea, and pulmonary edema. Five-year survival is less than 50 per cent (Foster et al., 1981), and the course is apt to be progressively downhill. For all these reasons, such women should be advised in the strongest possible terms against becoming pregnant.

Episodes of cardiac decompensation that do not respond to adjustment of orally administered medicine will necessitate admission to an intensive care unit where the effects of treatment, including heavy sedation, on cardiac output, pulmonary arterial pressure, systemic venous pressure, and pulmonary wedge pressure can be monitored along with the maternal and fetal electrocardiograms. When the hemodynamic parameters and clinical condition indicate continuing deterioration in spite of maximal treatment with diuretics, oxygen, vasodilators, and positive inotropic agents, emergency abdominal delivery may be necessary.

Treatment

Patients who have major clinical manifestations of chronic heart failure secondary to a myocardial disorder have sustained irreversible damage to a large proportion of the ventricular myocardium. Cardiac reserve in such individuals is necessarily greatly restricted and often is inadequate to bear the additional hemodynamic burdens of pregnancy. Usually, in order to remain clinically compensated, such patients must practice significant restriction of sodium intake and receive a variety of drugs typically including a loop diuretic, digitalis, and a vasodilator. Additionally, most patients in this category take potassium supplements, and some receive antiarrhythmic agents as well.

Left Ventricular Dysfunction

There is a remarkable lack of correlation between symptoms of heart failure and objective evidence of left ventricular dysfunction (Engler et al., 1982). Patients with chronic heart disease, for example, following myocardial infarction, may have a considerably enlarged and extremely hypokinetic ventricle and yet be relatively free from symptoms. For this reason any woman who has sustained myocardial damage should have left ventricular function assessed by a radionuclide ventriculogram, an echocardiogram, or in some instances both before deciding on pregnancy. A left ventricular ejection fraction in the range of 20 per cent calls for advice basically the same as that given to patients with overt heart failure, since pregnancy may be the event that transforms the clinical picture from that of compensated left ventricular dysfunction to overt congestive heart failure. Moderately impaired left ventricular systolic function, for instance, as documented by a left ventricular ejection fraction in the range of 40 per cent, is compatible with safe pregnancy and delivery, provided the patient remains under meticulous care from a cardiologist and obstetrician and is prepared to follow a strict regimen throughout pregnancy.

Cardiac Transplantation

Some fortunate women with advanced heart failure may become successful recipients of a cardiac transplant. Successful pregnancy and delivery in patients with cardiac transplantation have been reported (Kossoy et al., 1988; Key et al., 1989). However, they represent complex management problems due to the immunosuppressive drug regimen, and the frequent endomyocardial biopsies that must be done under fluoroscopy, and the uncertain long-term prognosis. Nevertheless, it is likely that more women will be desirous of pregnancy following heart and perhaps heart-lung transplantation.

DISTURBANCES OF CARDIAC RHYTHM

Supraventricular and ventricular extrasystoles are universal and require no treatment. Preconception counseling is simplified by a clear appreciation of several general principles. Arrhythmia that occurs in the absence of organic heart disease is almost always benign and is therefore not an indication for pharmacologic treatment, unless the woman finds palpitation intolerable. Reassuring her of the benign nature of this symptom is often all that is required. It has not been proven that drug treatment of unsustained asymptomatic arrhythmia can prevent death, even when organic heart disease is present. Therefore, the need for pharmacologic treatment is disputed. On the other hand, sustained symptomatic arrhythmia is life-threatening and must be treated pharmacologically, by implantation of an intracardiac defibrillating-pacing device, or by ablation of a pathway that permits abnormal re-entrant tachycardia. Ablation is performed via radio-frequency energy delivered by an electrode catheter located at the site to be ablated, which is identified by intracardiac mapping. This procedure has largely replaced surgical excision.

Pregnancy and labor should be normal and safe except in the group with sustained arrhythmia, with its attendant risk of cardiac arrest and need for vigorous treatment. Pharmacologic treatment for serious arrhythmia is apt to be with newly introduced agents such as amiodarone, for which there is at best limited knowledge of potentially unfavorable effects on the fetus. Pregnancy should be postponed until the arrhythmia has been eliminated or at least controlled, preferably by nonpharmacological means. If antiarrhythmic drugs must be employed, they should, whenever possible, be those that have been used for several decades, allowing prediction of the fetal risk.

High-grade atrioventricular conduction disturbance, especially when symptomatic, is treated by artificial pacing, which should not influence pregnancy, labor, or the fetus. Electrical cardioversion or defibrillation of the mother's heart does not disturb or damage the fetal heart (Schroeder and Harrison, 1971).

It is clearly desirable to evaluate disturbances of cardiac rhythm and conduction before pregnancy, proceeding when indicated to full electrophysiologic testing. This algorithm avoids administering antiarrhythmic agents potentially toxic to the fetus and protects from the radiation associated with electrophysiologic investigation.

MARFAN'S SYNDROME

This variably expressed syndrome is inherited as an autosomal dominant trait. Life expectancy is reduced by half in those who exhibit the classic syndrome (Murdoch et al., 1972). The basic defect is one of connective tissue, and connective tissue weakness in the aorta causes the dangerous complications (Pyeritz and McKusick, 1979).

The symptoms and signs of the syndrome include dyspnea and chest pain, an aortic diastolic murmur, and a mid-systolic click. The best diagnostic test and apparently the most critical for determining the outcome of pregnancy is the echocardiogram. More than 90 per cent of patients have evidence of mitral valve prolapse, whereas 60 per cent have echocardiographic evidence of aortic root dilatation (Brown et al., 1975). Pregnancy is particularly dangerous for patients with this syndrome, because there appears to be a higher risk of aortic rupture and dissection, especially in those women with demonstrable dilatation of the aortic root. It has been stated that women with an aortic diameter exceeding 40 mm are at greatest risk of death during pregnancy and that others may undertake pregnancy relatively safely (Pyeritz, 1981). However, if the woman exhibits all of the manifestation of Marfan's syndrome, it would be prudent to avoid becoming pregnant altogether.

Deficiency of elastic tissue is the cause of myxomatous degeneration of the aortic and mitral valves and cystic medial necrosis of the aorta (Fig. 47–9). This abnormality translates to large aneurysms of the aortic

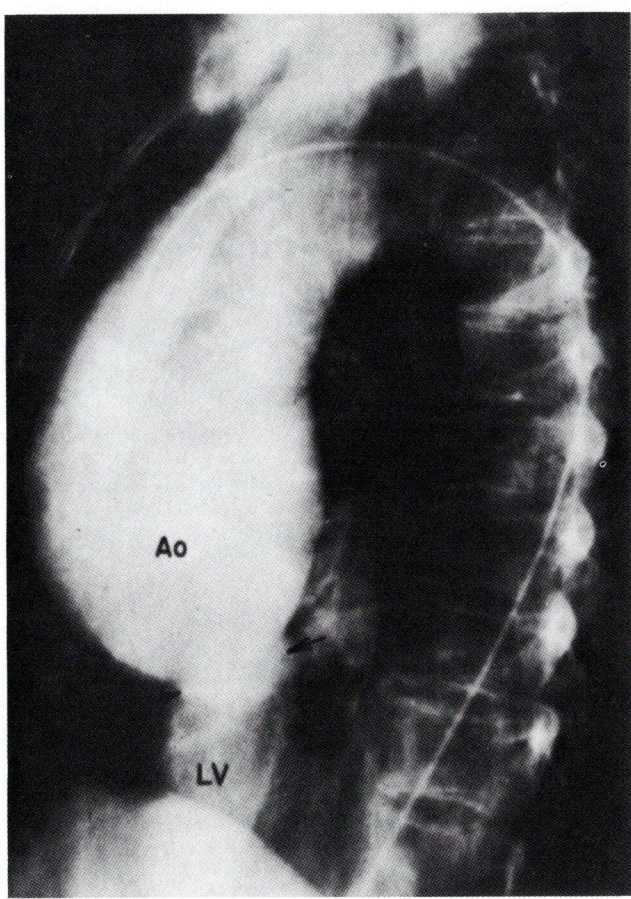

FIGURE 47–9. Aortogram showing an aneurysm of the ascending aorta (Ao) with regurgitation of contrast through an incompetent aortic valve into the left ventricle (LV). (Reproduced by permission from Shabetai R, Adolph RJ: Principles of cardiac catheterization. *In* Fowler NO (ed): Cardiac Diagnosis and Treatment. Hagerstown, Harper & Row, 1980, pp 106–183.)

root, multiple aneurysms elsewhere along the course of the aorta and great vessels, and severe aortic and mitral regurgitation with resulting heart failure. Surgical treatment usually provides only temporary relief of acute cardiovascular problems because of the universal nature of the elastic tissue disease. Nevertheless, surgery is indicated for rapidly expanding aneurysm or when evidence of leaking or dissection is present. The vascular tissues do not hold sutures well, a factor that increases surgical mortality and morbidity. Pregnancy is poorly tolerated under these conditions, and labor may precipitate rupture of an aneurysm or heart failure.

It should be reemphasized that pregnancy in patients with Marfan's syndrome carries a high risk, and that risk is markedly increased with aortic root dilatation. Should the patient elect to continue the pregnancy, therapy is directed at markedly limiting physical activity, preventing hypertensive complications, and decreasing the pulsatile forces on the aortic wall with the use of a beta-blocker. The long-acting cardioselective β_1 blocker atenolol may be the drug of choice during pregnancy. As previously noted, any symptoms of aortic dissection require prompt evaluation.

PREGNANCY IN PATIENTS WITH ARTIFICIAL HEART VALVES

Management of the pregnant patient with a mechanical valve replacement may be extremely complex, owing primarily to maternal and fetal complications of the anticoagulants. As mentioned previously, Born et al. (1992) reported valvular thrombosis in three of 35 pregnant women with two fatalities. Among a group of 64 pregnancies in 40 women, fetal loss was 53 per cent (25/47) in those women treated with coumarin, and two fetal malformations consistent with the "warfarin embryopathy" were observed (Ayhan et al., 1991).

However, other recent reports would suggest a more favorable outcome. Sareli et al. (1989) prospectively followed 50 pregnancies in 49 patients, all of whom received warfarin during the first and second trimesters. Of these pregnancies, 41 went beyond 28 weeks, and in 23 women, warfarin was replaced with heparin at 36 weeks gestation. There were no thromboembolic complications. Fetal birth weight was low primarily due to prematurity. There were seven stillbirths (14 per cent) and two neonatal deaths associated with intracranial hemorrhage. Two of the neonates (4 per cent) demonstrated evidence of warfarin embryopathy.

Treatment with heparin, which does not cross the placenta, is far safer for the fetus in a patient with valve prostheses desiring pregnancy (Ginsberg et al., 1989). Finally, although the long-term outlook for patients with porcine xenografts is guarded, it is likely that they are safer in pregnancy. Prophylactic antibiotics are mandatory during dental and surgical procedures and at delivery because the mortality rate from prosthetic valve endocarditis exceeds 40 per cent. The patient developing endocarditis with a prosthetic valve requires aggressive antibiotic therapy, and if this is unsuccessful, the prosthesis must be replaced.

The patient with a tissue valve replacement has the same risk of bacterial endocarditis, but appears to be less susceptible to thrombosis and thromboembolic events. For this reason, the young woman contemplating pregnancy should receive a tissue valve replacement even though it must be realized that eventual reoperation will be required. Non-anticoagulated individuals with aortic valve tissue prostheses have a 1 to 3 per cent incidence of systemic emboli yearly, and those with mitral valve tissue protheses, an incidence of 3 to 5 per cent (Kloster, 1979). These rates are considerably lower than those encountered with mechanical prostheses.

IDIOPATHIC HYPERTROPHIC SUBAORTIC STENOSIS (IHSS)

Inherited as an autosomal dominant trait with variable penetrants, IHSS is being recognized with increasing frequency. The echocardiographic findings are diagnostic and include marked thickening of the ventricular septum and abnormal systolic movement of the mitral valve. Because of the dynamic characteristics of hypertrophic obstructive cardiomyopathy, one would not expect pregnancy to be well tolerated. The normal fall in peripheral vascular resistance accompanying pregnancy tends to increase outflow tract obstruction. In addition, vena caval obstruction in late pregnancy and blood loss at delivery, both of which may result in hypotension, could have a similar deleterious effect. Outflow tract obstruction may also be aggravated by the increases in circulating catecholamine levels frequently encountered during labor and delivery. Exacerbation of symptoms has been reported during pregnancy in women with obstructive cardiomyopathy.

Treatment is aimed at avoiding hypovolemia and maintaining venous return, as well as diminishing the force of myocardiac contraction by avoiding anxiety, excitement and strenuous activity. Prompt volume replacement and vasopressor therapy should be given along with the use of beta-adrenergic blockers. More recently, calcium-channel blockers such as nifedipine and verapamil have been shown, in a few patients, to be effective in reducing symptoms through improved hemodynamic function (Lorell et al., 1982).

CARDIAC SURGERY DURING PREGNANCY

Clearly, any patient requiring cardiac surgery should have her procedure performed prior to becoming pregnant. Nevertheless, the rare patient will require surgery during pregnancy, and although there does not appear to be an increase in maternal mortality risk, there is substantial risk to the fetus due to the nonpulsatile blood flow and hypotension associated with cardiopulmonary bypass (CPB). CPB has been successfully undertaken during pregnancy, but with substantial risk. The reader is referred to a recent report of ten cases of pregnant women with cardiac disorders requiring surgical intervention, and to an extensive review of the physiologic considerations and of the literature (Strickland et al., 1991).

REFERENCES

Arias F, Pineda J: Aortic stenosis in pregnancy. J Reprod Med **20**:229, 1978.

Ayhan A, Yapar EG, Yuce K, et al: Pregnancy and its complications after cardiac valve replacement. Int J Gynecol Obstet **35**:117, 1991.

Barash PG, Hobbins JC, Hook R, et al: Management of coarctation of the aorta during pregnancy. J Thorac Cardiovasc Surg **69**:781, 1975.

Bestetti RB: Cardiac involvement in the acquired immune deficiency syndrome. Int J Cardiol **22**:143, 1989.

Bjarnason I, Jonsson S, Hardarson T: Mode of inheritance of hypertrophic cardiomyopathy in Iceland. Br Heart J **47**:122, 1982.

Born D, Martinez EE, Almeid PAM, et al: Pregnancy in patients with prosthetic heart valves: The effects of anticoagulation on mother, fetus and neonate. Am Heart J **124**:413, 1992.

Boyle DM, Lloyd-Jones RL. The electrocardiographic ST segment in pregnancy. J Obstet Gynaec (Br Comm) **73**:986, 1966.

Brown OR, DeMots H, Kloster FE, et al: Aortic root dilatation and mitral valve prolapse in Marfan's syndrome: An echocardiographic study. Circulation **52**:651, 1975.

Burman D: Familial patent ductus arteriosus. Br Heart J **23**:603, 1961.

Butman S, Chandraratna PA, Milne N, et al: Stress myocardial

imaging in patients with mitral valve prolapse: Evidence of a perfusion abnormality. Cathet Cardiovasc Diagn **8**:243, 1982.

Cannell DE, Vernon CP: Congenital heart disease and pregnancy. Am J Obstet Gynecol **85**:744, 1963.

Carruth JE, Mivis SB, Brogan DR, et al: The electrocardiogram in normal pregnancy. Am Heart J **102**:1075, 1981.

Clemens JD, Horwitz RI, Jaffe CC, et al: Controlled evaluation of the risk of bacterial endocarditis in persons with mitral valve prolapse. N Engl J Med **307**:776, 1982.

Coghlan HC, Phares P, Cowley M, et al: Dysautonomia in mitral valve prolapse. Am J Med **67**:236, 1979.

Cole P, Cook F, Plappert T: Longitudinal changes in left ventricular architecture and function in peripartum cardiomyopathy. Am J Cardiol **60**:811, 1987.

Corone P, Bonaiti C, Feingold J, et al: Familial congenital heart disease: How are the various types related? Am J Cardiol **51**:942, 1983.

Craig RJ, Selzer A: Natural history and prognosis of atrial septal defect. Circulation **37**:805, 1968.

Cunningham FG, Pritchard JA, Hankins GD, et al: Peripartum heart failure: Idiopathic cardiomyopathy or compounding cardiovascular events? Obstet Gynecol **67**:157, 1986.

Deal K, Wooley CF: Coarctation of the aorta and pregnancy. Ann Intern Med **78**:706, 1973.

Devereux RB, Perloff JK, Reichek N, et al: Mitral valve prolapse. Circulation **54**:3, 1976.

Eckberg DL, Gault JH, Bouchard RL, et al: Mechanics of left ventricular contraction in chronic severe mitral regurgitation. Circulation **47**:1252, 1973.

Elkayam U, Gleicher N: Hemodynamics and cardiac function during normal pregnancy and the puerperium. In Elkayam U, Gleicher N (eds): Cardiac Problems in Pregnancy. New York, Alan B. Liss, 1990.

Engler R, Ray R, Higgins CB, et al: Clinical assessment and follow-up of functional capacity in patients with chronic congestive cardiomyopathy. Am J Cardiol **49**:1832, 1982.

Foster V, Gersh BJ, Giuliani ER, et al: The natural history of idiopathic dilated cardiomyopathy. Am J Cardiol **47**:525, 1981.

Ginsberg JS, Hirsh J, Turner DC: Risks to the fetus of anticoagulant therapy during pregnancy. Thromb Haemost **61(2)**:197, 1989.

Gleicher N, Midwall J, Hochberger D, et al: Eisenmenger's syndrome and pregnancy. Obstet Gynecol Surv **34**:721, 1979.

Haiat R, Halphen C: Silent pericardial effusion in late pregnancy: A new entity. Cardiovasc Intervent Radiol **7**:267, 1984.

Hall JG, Pauli RM, Wilson KM: Maternal and fetal sequelae of anticoagulation during pregnancy. Am J Med **68**:122, 1980.

Hardison JE: Cervical venous hum: A clue to the diagnosis of intracranial arteriovenous malformations. N Engl J Med **278**:587, 1968.

Haroutunian LM, Neill CA: Pulmonary complications of congenital heart disease: hemoptysis. Am Heart J **84**:540, 1972.

Hartman N, Kramer R, Brown T, et al: Panic disorder in patients with mitral valve prolapse. Am J Psychiatry **139**:669, 1982.

Husaini MH: Myocardial infarction during pregnancy. Postgrad Med J **47**:600, 1971.

Hytten FE, Thompson AM: Maternal physiologic adjustments. In Assali NS (ed): Biology of Gestation. New York, Academic Press, 1968.

Johansson BW, Sievers J: Inheritance of atrial septal defect. Lancet **i**:1224, 1967.

Johnson, DE, Alderman EL, Schroeder JS, et al: Transplant coronary artery disease. Histopathologic correlation with angiographic morphology. J Am Coll Cardiol **17**:449, 1991.

Kaplan JD, Isner JM, Karas RH, et al: In vitro analysis of mechanisms of balloon valvuloplasty of stenotic mitral valves. Am J Cardiol **59**:318, 1987.

Katz R, Karliner JS, Resnik R: Effects of a natural volume overload state (pregnancy) on left ventricular performance in normal human subjects. Circulation **58**:434, 1978.

Key TC, Dittrich H, Reisner L, Resnik R. Successful pregnancy following cardiac transplantation. Am J Obstet Gynecol **160**:367, 1989.

Kloster FE: Complications of artificial heart valves. JAMA **241**:2201, 1979.

Kossoy LR, Herbert CM, Wentz AC: Management of heart transplant recipients: guidelines for the obstetrician-gynecologist. Am J Obstet Gynecol 159:490, 1988.

Lefevre T, Bonan R, Serra A, et al: Percutaneous mitral valvuloplasty in surgical high risk patients. J Am Coll Cardiol 17:348, 1991.

Lewis W: AIDS: Cardiac findings from 115 autopsies. Prog Cardiovasc Dis 32:207, 1989.

Lorell BH, Paulus WJ, Grossman W, et al: Modification of abnormal left ventricular diastolic properties by nifedipine in patients with hypertrophic cardiomyopathy. Circulation 65:499, 1982.

McCaffrey RM, Dunn LJ: Primary pulmonary hypertension in pregnancy. Obstet Gynecol Surv 19:567, 1964.

McKay RG, Lock JE, Safian RD, et al: Balloon dilation of mitral stenosis in adult patients: Postmortem and percutaneous mitral valvuloplasty studies. J Am Coll Cardiol 9:723, 1987a.

McKay RG, Safian RD, Lock JE, et al: Assessment of left ventricular and aortic valve function after aortic balloon valvuloplasty in adult patients with critical aortic stenosis. Circulation 75:192, 1987b.

Meller J, Conde CA, Deppisch LM, et al: Myocardial infarction due to coronary atherosclerosis in three young adults with systemic lupus erythematosus. Am J Cardiol 35:309, 1975.

Mestroni L, Miani D, Di Lenarda A, et al: Clinical and pathologic study of familial dilated cardiomyopathy. Am J Cardiol 65:1449, 1990.

Metcalfe J, McAnulty JH, Ueland K: Cardiac Disease and Pregnancy: Physiology and Management. Boston, Little Brown, 1986, p 223.

Metcalfe J, Ueland K: Maternal cardiovascular adjustments to pregnancy. Prog Cardiovasc Dis 16:363, 1974.

Morris CD, Menashe VD: Recurrence of congenital heart disease in offspring of parents with surgical correction. Clin Res 33:68A, 1985.

Murdoch JL, Walker BA, Halpern BL, et al: Life expectancy and causes of death in the Marfan syndrome. N Engl J Med 286:804, 1972.

Neilson G, Galea EG, Blunt A: Congenital heart disease and pregnancy. Med J Aust 1:1086, 1970.

Neilson G, Galea EG, Blunt A: Eisenmenger's syndrome and pregnancy. Med J Aust 1:431, 1971.

Nelson DM, Main E, Crafford W: Peripartum heart failure due to primary pulmonary hypertension. Obstet Gynecol 62:58s, 1983.

Nora JJ, Nora AH, Wexler P: Hereditary and environmental aspects as they affect the fetus and newborn. Clin Obstet Gynecol 24:851, 1981.

O'Connell JB, Costanzo-Nordin MR, Subramanian R, et al: Peripartum cardiomyopathy: Clinical, hemodynamic, histologic and prognostic characteristics. J Am Coll Cardiol 8:52, 1986.

Oram S, Holt M: Innocent depression of the S-T segment and flattening of the T-wave during pregnancy. J Obstet Gynaecol (Br Cwlth) 68:765, 1961.

Perloff JK: Pregnancy and cardiovascular disease. In Braunwald E (ed): A Textbook of Cardiovascular Disease, 3rd ed. Philadelphia, WB Saunders Company, 1988.

Perloff JK, Child JS, Edwards JE: New guidelines for the clinical diagnosis of mitral valve prolapse. Am J Cardiol 57:1124, 1986.

Pitts JA, Crosby WM, Basta LL: Eisenmenger's syndrome in pregnancy: Does heparin prophylaxis improve the maternal mortality rate? Am Heart J 93:321, 1977.

Pyeritz RE: Maternal and fetal complications of pregnancy in Marfan syndrome. Am J Med 71:784, 1981.

Pyeritz RE, McKusick VA: The Marfan syndrome: Diagnosis and management. N Engl J Med 300:772, 1979.

Raffanti SP, Chiaramida AJ, Sen P, et al: Assessment of cardiac function in patients with the acquired immunodeficiency syndrome. Chest 93:592, 1988.

Ratnoff OD, Kaufman R: Arterial thrombosis in oral contraceptive users. Arch Int Med 142:447, 1982.

Rosa FW, Bosco LA, Graham CF, et al: Neonatal anuria with maternal angiotensin-converting enzyme inhibition. Obstet Gynecol 74:371, 1989.

Ross J, Jr: Left ventricular function and the timing of surgical treatment in valvular heart disease. Ann Intern Med 94:498, 1981.

Rubler S, Damani PM, Pinto ER: Cardiac size and performance during pregnancy estimated with echocardiography. Am J Cardiol 40:534, 1977.

Sandok BA, Giuliani ER: Cerebral ischemic events in patients with mitral valve prolapse. Stroke 13:448, 1982.

Sareli P, England MJ, Berk MR: Maternal and fetal sequelae of anticoagulation during pregnancy in patients with mechanical heart valve prostheses. Am J Cardiol 63:1462, 1989.

Schroeder JS, Harrison DC: Repeated cardioversion during pregnancy: Treatment of refractory paroxysmal atrial tachycardia during 3 successive pregnancies. Am J Cardiol 27:445, 1971.

Schwartz DB, Schamroth L: The effect of pregnancy on the frontal plane QRS axis. J Electrocardiog 12:279, 1979.

Scott AA, Purohit DM: Neonatal renal failure: A complication of maternal antihypertensive therapy. Am J Obstet Gynecol 160:1223, 1989.

Shabetai R, Shine I: Heritable and familial aspects of myocardial diseases. In Fowler ND (ed): Myocardial Diseases. New York, Grune & Stratton, 1973.

Shell WE, Walton JA, Clifford ME, et al: The familial occurrence of the syndrome of mid-late systolic click and late systolic murmur. Circulation 39:327, 1969.

Snaith L, Szekely P: Cardiovascular surgery in relation to pregnancy. In Marcus SL, Marcus CC (eds): Advances in Obstetrics and Gynecology. Baltimore, Williams & Wilkins, 1967, p 220.

Somerville J, Khaliq SU, Brewer AC, et al: Clinical pathologic conference. Atrial septal defect with paradoxical embolism. Am Heart J 86:822, 1973.

Spinnato JA, Kraynack BJ, Cooper MW: Eisenmenger's syndrome in pregnancy: Epidural anesthesia for elective cesarean section. N Engl J Med 304:1215, 1981.

St. John Sutton M, Cole P, Plappert M: Effects of subsequent pregnancy on left ventricular function in peripartal cardiomyopathy. Am Heart J 121:1776, 1991.

Stanger P, Cassidy SC, Girod DA, et al: Balloon pulmonary valvuloplasty. Results of the valvuloplasty and angioplasty register. Am J Cardiol 65:775, 1990.

Stevenson RE, Burton M, Ferlanto GJ, Taylor HA: Hazards of oral anticoagulant during pregnancy. JAMA 243:1549, 1980.

Strickland RA, Oliver WC Jr, Chantigian RC et al: Anesthesia, cardiopulmonary bypass, and the pregnant patient. Mayo Clin Proc 66:411, 1991.

Sullivan JM, Ramanathan KB: Management of medical problems in pregnancy—severe cardiac disease. N Engl J Med 313:304, 1985.

Szekely P, Turner R, Snaith L: Pregnancy and the changing pattern of rheumatic heart disease. Br Heart J 35:1293, 1973.

Ueland K, Hansen JM: Maternal cardiovascular dynamics: II. Posture and uterine contractions. Am J Obstet Gynecol 103:1, 1969.

Ueland K, Novy MJ, Metcalfe J: Cardiorespiratory responses to pregnancy and exercise in normal women and patients with heart disease. Am J Obstet Gynecol 115:4, 1973.

Van der Leeuw-Harmsen L, de Graaff J, Chappin JJ: Peripartal cardiomyopathy. Eur J Obstet Gynaecol Reprod Biol 19:59, 1985.

Wann LS, Grove JR, Hess TR, et al: Prevalence of mitral prolapse by two dimensional echocardiography in healthy young women. Br Heart J 49:334, 1983.

Whittemore R, Hobbins JC, Engle MA: Pregnancy and its outcome in women with and without surgical treatment of congenital heart disease. Am J Cardiol 50:641, 1982.

Wood P: The Eisenmenger syndrome or pulmonary hypertension with reversed central shunt. Br Med J 701:755, 1958.

Young D, Mark H: Fate of the patient with the Eisenmenger syndrome. Am J Cardiol 28:658, 1971.

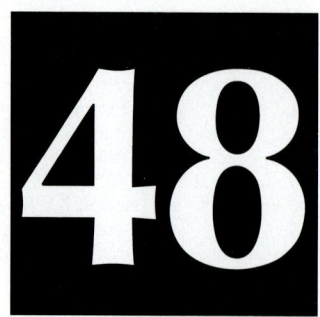

THROMBOEMBOLIC DISEASE

RUSSELL K. LAROS, Jr., M.D.

Thromboembolic disease is the leading nonobstetric cause of postpartum death. As management of sepsis and eclampsia has improved, pulmonary embolism has made a relatively greater impact and in some series is second only to trauma as a cause of maternal mortality (Sachs et al., 1987). Fortunately, it is also a disease in which early recognition and proper treatment can dramatically improve the outcome. The pregnant patient is unique in that she is actually two patients; consequently, the usual diagnostic and therapeutic maneuvers must be modified so as not to affect the fetus adversely.

INCIDENCE AND PATHOPHYSIOLOGY

Incidence

Although thrombophlebitis is serious because of its potentially fatal consequences, it is fortunately quite rare in young women. The reported incidence varies between 0.018 and 0.29 per cent during gestation and between 0.1 and 1 per cent postpartum (Wessler, 1976a). Puerperal patients outnumber antepartum patients by approximately three to one. The difficulty of making an accurate diagnosis accounts for the wide variation in incidence noted by these reports. Although thrombophlebitis can be seen at any stage of gestation, it appears to increase in frequency as pregnancy advances. After delivery, deep venous thrombosis (DVT) is most frequently seen on the second postpartum day. DVT appears in 55 per cent of patients within the first 3 days, but may occur as late as 4 weeks after delivery (Aaro and Juergens, 1971).

The incidence of pulmonary embolism depends on whether or not DVT is adequately treated. Untreated, as many as 24 per cent of patients with antenatal DVT will have pulmonary embolism, with a mortality rate of approximately 15 per cent (Wessler, 1976a). If patients are treated with anticoagulants, embolization will occur in only 4.5 per cent, and the mortality rate is less than 1 per cent (Villasanta, 1965). The importance of proper treatment with anticoagulation is clear.

Pathophysiology

Over a century ago, Virchow described a triad of factors that play an essential role in the initiation of intravascular coagulation: injury to the vessel wall, stasis, and changes in local clotting factors. During pregnancy, thrombosis may occur without any known abnormality of the endothelium. However, vein distensibility increases during the first trimester (McCausland et al., 1961), and by the third trimester the velocity of venous flow in the lower extremities is reduced by half, in part because the gravid uterus provides a mechanical impediment to venous return (Wright et al., 1950). This tendency toward stasis is augmented if the patient requires periods of prolonged bed rest as in preeclampsia, threatened abortion, or premature labor.

Todd and associates (1965) have shown that fibrinogen, factor VIII, and other vitamin K-dependent clotting factors are increased during pregnancy. There is evidence of decreased fibrinolytic activity with reduced levels of available circulating plasminogen activator as well (Nilsson and Kullander, 1967). It is interesting that although pregnancy would appear to be a "hypercoagulable state," the increased risk of thromboembolism seems to be confined primarily to the postpartum period. The risk is enhanced by cesarean section (a ninefold increase over vaginal delivery), instrument delivery, advanced maternal age, increased parity, and suppression of lactation by estrogens. Other risk factors reported include varicosities, trauma or infection, obesity, blood type other than type O, congestive heart failure, dehydration, shock, disseminated cancer, dysproteinemia, polycythemia vera, and anemia (especially sickle cell) (Rickles and Edwards, 1983). Additionally, a history of a prior thrombolic event in the absence of a predisposing cause or a family history of thromboembolism suggests the possibility of a defect in the physiologic antithrombotic mechanisms. Congenital defects in antithrombin III, protein C, protein S, and plasminogen, as well as the presence of lupus anticoagulant, all predispose to thromboembolic events (Taberino et al., 1991; Mueh et al., 1980).

Overall, the risk during pregnancy and postpartum

is 5.5 times greater than that for nonpregnant controls (Hathaway and Bonnar, 1987). With the availability of effective contraceptives, more women are delaying childbearing, and a concomitant increase in the incidence of pulmonary emboli can be expected because of the increase in maternal age.

DIAGNOSIS

It is as important to diagnose thromboembolism as it is difficult. Anticoagulation, although an invaluable therapeutic tool, is not without hazard. Therefore, the physician should be certain of this diagnosis before committing a patient to a lengthy course of treatment.

Deep Venous Thrombosis

The signs and symptoms most commonly used to diagnose deep venous thrombosis are listed in Table 48–1. Leg swelling is a measured difference between leg circumferences of greater than 2 cm. A positive Homans sign is pain in the calf when the great toe is passively dorsiflexed. Unfortunately, many of the complaints listed occur as normal physiologic changes of pregnancy. Haeger (1969) found that not only are none of these symptoms or signs specific, but that their presence in limbs with and without thrombosis occurs with approximately equal frequency. Forty-five per cent of patients thought to have clinically certain DVT had an entirely normal venous system by venography. Conversely, venograms done on patients with pulmonary emboli may demonstrate clots in a totally asymptomatic limb (Cranley et al., 1976). In only 10 per cent of patients is the diagnosis of DVT made before the occurrence of fatal pulmonary embolism (Coon, 1976). It appears that the more symptomatic the thrombus, the more tightly adherent it is to the vessel wall.

Septic pelvic thrombophlebitis may be even more difficult to diagnose, and the only signs may be chills and a hectic febrile course (Duff and Gibbs, 1983). Pelvic examination is frequently unrevealing, and the diagnosis is usually made on the basis of failure to respond to a 48- to 72-hour regimen of adequate antibiotic therapy (including coverage of anaerobes).

DOPPLER ULTRASOUND. Doppler ultrasound has become the diagnostic study of choice in cases of suspected proximal vein occlusion (Cronan, 1991). A 5-mHz transducer is placed over the vein. Venous flow produces a characteristic low-pitched sound that is abolished by venous occlusion. Concomitant evaluation of venous anatomy, flow, augmentation (in-

TABLE 48–1.   Signs and Symptoms of Deep Venous Thrombosis

Muscle pain
Palpable deep linear cord
Tenderness
Swelling
Homans sign
Dilated superficial veins

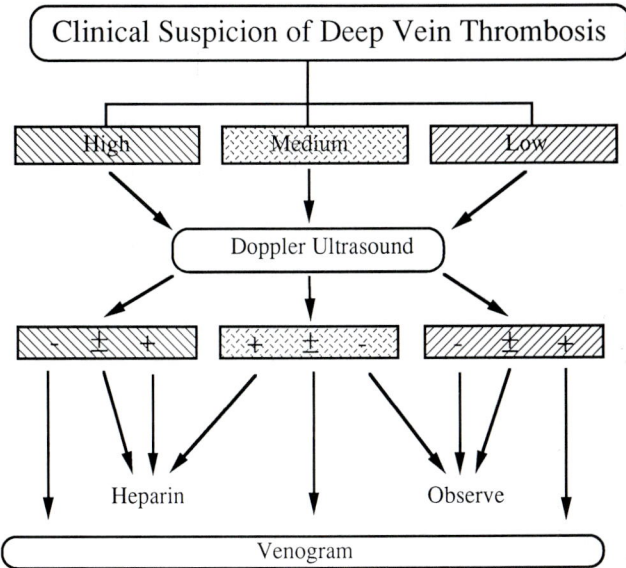

FIGURE 48–1. Diagnostic algorithm for suspected deep vein thrombosis in pregnancy.

creased flow with muscular activity in the calf), and compression (elimination of residual lumen by firm pressure with the transducer probe using one hand) yield a correct diagnosis with a high degree of sensitivity and specificity when compared with venography (Lensing et al., 1989). Although studies in pregnant women are still limited in number, the accuracy appears to be excellent (Greer et al., 1990). The algorithm that the author uses to evaluate pregnant women suspected of having a DVT is shown in Figure 48–1.

VENOGRAPHY. For years venography has been the reference standard against which all other methods are compared. Although it is the most specific, it has limitations—it is invasive, expensive, and difficult to interpret unless all of the deep veins are filled adequately. It cannot be used to demonstrate the pelvic venous plexus. The procedure cannot be repeated frequently, and the contrast material may cause chemical phlebitis. Venography has not been used frequently during pregnancy because of possible hazards to the fetus. However, it may be the only definitive study available, and the fetus can be protected by shielding of the maternal abdomen (Bonnar, 1979).

ISOTOPE SCANNING. ^{125}I fibrinogen uptake scanning is useful in evaluating the lower extremities below mid-thigh. Unfortunately, it loses sensitivity in the upper thigh and pelvis because of the increased background radioactivity levels in the femoral artery and bladder (Gallus, 1975). This is a significant deficiency, since the majority of serious pulmonary emboli are thought to originate from deep veins in the iliofemoral region. This method should rarely be used during pregnancy, because free isotopic iodine crosses the placenta and concentrates in the fetal thyroid.

IMPEDANCE PLETHYSMOGRAPHY. This technique utilizes temporary occlusion of venous return by inflation of a thigh cuff. The occlusion causes an increase in the venous volume of the calf. Release of the cuff results in a rapid decrease in volume as the blood drains proximally. If venous obstruction is present, the rate of outflow is diminished. These changes in blood volume can be detected by measuring electrical resistance in the calf (Toy and Schrier, 1978). Clarke-Pearson and Jelovsek (1981) have documented the reliability of this technique in the gynecologic patient and suggest that it may also be a sensitive and specific test during pregnancy. However, only a few cases of documented DVT during pregnancy have been studied with this technique, and its ultimate place in the diagnostic armamentarium remains unclear.

Ginsberg and colleagues (1989) present data showing that the combination of Doppler ultrasound and photoplethysmography are more reliable than either study alone in predicting the presence or absence of proximal DVT. Unfortunately, pregnant patients were not included in their series.

BLOOD TESTS FOR THROMBOSIS. Hirsh (1981) has summarized several tests that reflect the formation of intravascular fibrin. They are invariably positive when thrombosis has occurred. Unfortunately, they are also positive in the presence of hematomas or inflammatory exudates containing fibrin. The assay for fibrinopeptide A and the fibrin degradation product, D-dimer, are the most sensitive. The finding of a normal level of either of these essentially rules out DVT.

Pulmonary Embolism

Clinical Signs and Symptoms

Although small emboli may go unrecognized by the patient, the hallmark of pulmonary embolism is dyspnea. The major sign is tachypnea. Table 48–2 shows the signs and symptoms most frequently encountered (Sasahara et al., 1983). Small emboli become lodged more peripherally and may produce infarction accompanied by pleural signs, including cough, hemoptysis, pleuritic chest pain with splinting, and a friction rub. However, with many emboli, infarction and its associated symptoms are absent. Leg discomfort and shortness of breath may be the result of uterine enlargement in the third trimester, but may also indicate multiple small emboli. Also, multiple small emboli can mimic a major embolus. Massive pulmonary embolism, defined for clinical purposes as occlusion of at least 50 per cent of the pulmonary arterial circulation, may cause symptoms suggesting a myocardial infarction, including hypotension and occasionally syncope or convulsions.

Tachycardia or a few atelectatic rales may be the only finding on physical examination. However, massive emboli may produce right-sided heart failure with jugular venous distention, an enlarged liver, a left parasternal heave, and fixed splitting of the second heart sound. Cardiac auscultation during normal pregnancy may reveal a variety of "functional" murmurs or an increase in the pulmonic second heart sound; thus these findings are valuable only if they are clearly new.

Laboratory Studies

ELECTROCARDIOGRAM. The EKG is abnormal in 90 per cent of patients; however, tachycardia alone is the most common abnormality. Nonspecific T-wave inversion is found in 40 per cent, and the classic right axis shift with strain pattern ($S_1Q_3T_3$) is found in those patients with extensive embolization.

ARTERIAL PO$_2$. An arterial partial pressure of oxygen (PaO$_2$) of greater than 80 mm Hg with the patient breathing room air makes pulmonary embolism unlikely. In one study, 11.5 per cent of patients with proven pulmonary embolism had a PaO$_2$ of between 80 and 90 mm Hg (Sasahara et al., 1983). Although a PaO$_2$ of 90 mm Hg makes the diagnosis of pulmonary embolism unlikely, if the signs and symptoms persist, additional studies are needed to better define the diagnosis.

LUNG SCANNING AND PULMONARY ARTERIOGRAPHY. Because pulmonary embolism is a diagnosis of such consequence, if it cannot be excluded on the basis of a normal PaO$_2$, a lung scan should be done. The agent of choice is microspheres of macroaggregates labeled with technetium (^{99m}Tc), which has a half-life of 6 hours. Because a 1-millicurie dose given to the mother yields a fetal dose of only about 2 millirads, a perfusion scan is a safe procedure during pregnancy. The radiation doses yielded by the radionuclides commonly used are listed in Table 48–3. The likelihood of a pulmonary embolus depends on the nature of the scan abnormality observed. The specificity of the lung scan is significantly improved if coupled with a ventilation study. This is especially true if the perfusion defects are not typical of embolization or if they are accompanied by chest film abnormalities suggesting consolidation (Hull et al., 1983).

A prospective study of more that 900 patients with acute pulmonary embolism (The PIOPED Investigators, 1990) showed that nearly all patients with an embolus had an abnormal V/Q scan (high, intermediate or low probability). Unfortunately, so did most patients without emboli (sensitivity, 98 per cent; specificity, 10 per cent). The sensitivity of the V/Q scan was 41 per cent for high probability scans, 82 per cent for intermediate- or high-probability scans, and 98 per cent for low-, intermediate-, or high-probability scans. The specificities were 97 per cent, 52 per cent and 10 per cent respectively. The diagnostic algorithm that we currently use is outlined in Figure 48–2 and combines several diagnostic studies including pulmonary arteriography. Pulmonary angiography is indicated if surgical intervention is contemplated. In attempting

TABLE 48–2. Signs and Symptoms of Pulmonary Embolism

Tachypnea	89*
Dyspnea	81
Pleuritic pain	72
Apprehension	59
Cough	54
Tachycardia	43
Hemoptysis	34
Temperature (>37° C)	34

*Percentage of patients with proven pulmonary embolism having these findings.

From Sasahara AA, Sharma GVRK, Barsamian EM, et al: Pulmonary thromboembolism. JAMA **249**:2945, 1983. Copyright 1988, the American Medical Association.

TABLE 48–3. Radiation Doses Produced by Various Radionuclides Used in Lung Scanning

RADIONUCLIDE	HALF-LIFE	USUAL DOSE (mC)	WHOLE BODY RADIATION DOSE (mRads)
^{99m}Tc	6.0 h	3	2
^{133}Xe	5.3 d	10–20	4
^{127}Xe	36.4 d	5–10	1
^{125}I	8.1 d	0.3	300
^{127}I	60.2 d	0.1–0.3	10

to assess anticoagulation failures requiring caval interruption, it is the only method capable of reliably distinguishing between recurrent embolism and fragmentation and distal migration of the original clot.

OTHER LABORATORY STUDIES. Laboratory examinations are typically unrevealing, although the white count, serum LDH, bilirubin, and erythrocyte sedimentation rate may each be elevated. As already discussed, fibrin split products are always present; however, they can be found in uncomplicated pregnancy and in most postoperative patients. Their absence, however, essentially excludes the possibility of embolism (Hirsh, 1981). When a family history of

repeated thromboembolism is encountered, the levels of antithrombin III, protein C, and protein S should be studied (Mackie et al., 1978; Griffin et al., 1981; Comp and Esmon, 1984).

MANAGEMENT

Anticoagulation therapy, which will be discussed later, is the mainstay of therapy for deep thrombophlebitis with or without pulmonary embolism. However, for both entities there are a number of additional modalities useful in achieving symptomatic relief.

Deep Venous Thrombosis

Bed rest with elevation of the involved extremity is valuable initially as it promotes venous return and decreases edema. The Trendelenburg position, obtained by elevating the foot of the bed approximately 8 inches, is preferable to using pillows, which, because they flex the hip, may impede femoral flow. The patient may be supplied with a foot board and instructed in the performance of hourly flexion and extension exercises of both lower extremities. However, as soon as symptoms permit, the patient should be encouraged to ambulate, since bed rest itself may enhance venous stasis. There is no evidence that bed rest will prevent embolus detachment. Sitting with legs dependent is contraindicated. Application of moist heat to involved areas can be beneficial. Although moist heat is more effective than dry heat, it is useless unless hot packs are replaced as frequently as they cool. Analgesic drugs may be required, but those that affect platelet function (e.g., aspirin) must be avoided while anticoagulants are being used. Anti-inflammatory drugs, although useful agents, are generally contraindicated during pregnancy.

When correctly designed, elastic stockings increase the velocity of venous flow. The pressure gradient should decrease from ankle to thigh without a constricting garter at the top. Certain brands designed for ambulatory patients may be overly compressive in the recumbent position. Elastic bandages, once in vogue, are best avoided since they are easily wrapped incorrectly with the greatest pressure ending up at the top and thus impeding venous return.

Pulmonary Embolism

If an embolic source can be traced to the lower extremities, the aforementioned measures can be employed. In addition, specific treatment of the embolus is required. Oxygen therapy is particularly important during pregnancy, because even if the mother survives, the fetus may die or be damaged secondary to maternal hypoxia. The maternal PaO_2 should be maintained above 70 mm Hg. Positive pressure administration may be required if pulmonary edema is present. Meperidine or morphine may be used for pain and apprehension. Bed rest is indicated for at least 5 to 7 days, allowing time for the initial organization of the

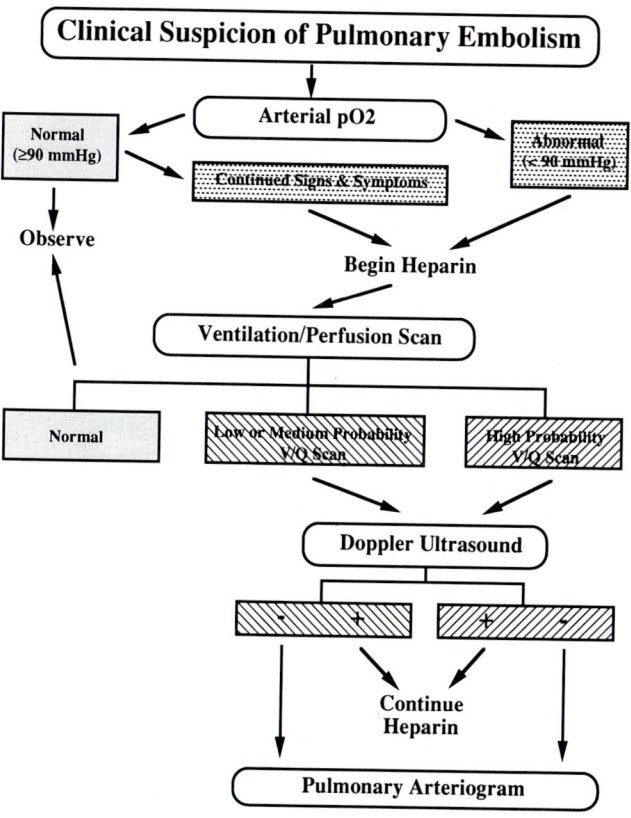

FIGURE 48–2. Diagnostic algorithm for suspected pulmonary embolism in pregnancy. (Adapted from Hull RD, et al: Pulmonary angiography, ventilation lung scanning, and venography for clinically suspected pulmonary embolism with abnormal perfusion lung scan. Ann Intern Med **98**:891, 1983.)

clot. Straining at stool is best avoided, and stool softeners may prove helpful.

A vasoactive amine such as isoproterenol or dopamine is indicated for treatment of shock. The objective is to increase the mean arterial pressure and the flow through the pulmonary vasculature. Isoproterenol (mix 1 mg in 500 ml of normal saline yielding 2µg/ ml) is given at 2 to 8 µg/minute and dopamine (200 mg in 500 ml of normal saline yielding 400 µg/ml) is started at 200 µg/min. Administration of both fluids and vasoactive amines should be monitored via a Swan-Ganz catheter measuring pulmonary artery and wedge pressure (see Chapter 51). Aminophylline and digoxin may also be useful. Aminophylline decreases reflex bronchospasm and has a diuretic action that is particularly useful if pulmonary edema is present. Digoxin can be administered if heart failure is present but is rarely of benefit. Aminophylline (250 mg in 500 ml of normal saline yielding 500 µg/ml) is infused rapidly over 20 minutes to give a dose of 4 to 5 mg/kg of body weight. The infusion is then slowed to 12 to 15 µg/kg/ min. The dosage is adjusted to achieve a serum concentration of 10 to 20 mg/ml. Antibiotics are not indicated unless a septic embolus is suspected.

Anticoagulation

Currently, three major types of therapeutic agents are available for treating thrombosis. Each is directed at a different portion of the coagulation process. They consist of: (1) agents that interfere with platelet adhesion and aggregation, (2) agents that interfere with fibrin formation, and (3) agents that facilitate clot lysis.

Although there is general agreement that proximal DVT should be treated by anticoagulation, the need for treatment of thrombosis below the level of the popliteal fossa remains in dispute. Because approximately 20 per cent of lower leg DVTs will extend proximally and heparin can prevent this spread, many believe that treatment is required (Bentley et al., 1980). In essence, one must balance the risks of anticoagulation with the benefits of prevention of proximal extension. Agents that interfere with fibrin formation are by far the most important in treating thromboembolism, and in the United States they are heparin and the coumarin derivatives. Heparin is the preferred agent in the initial treatment of thromboembolism, but for long-term management in the nonpregnant state,

conversion to a coumarin derivative is usually ideal. For reasons to be discussed later, I believe that heparin should be the preferred drug throughout pregnancy.

Heparin

Heparin is a naturally occurring mucopolysaccharide organic base found within mast cells of most mammals. In plasma it combines with an alpha-globulin known as antithrombin III to become a potent inhibitor of thrombin (thus preventing conversion of fibrinogen to fibrin) and to increase the circulating level of activated factor X (Xa) inhibitor (Rosenberg, 1987). Heparin has only a minimal antiplatelet effect, and does not stimulate fibrinolysis or directly lyse thrombi (Wessler and Gitel, 1979). Commercial preparations of heparin are heterogeneous with molecular weights from 3000 to 30,000 (mean 15,000). Because of its large size and negative charge, it does not cross the placenta or appear in breast milk; both features are advantageous when anticoagulation is required during pregnancy or lactation. If necessary, heparin effects can be reversed rapidly by administering protamine sulfate in a dose of 1 mg/100 U of administered heparin. (When constant infusion methods are used, twice the amount necessary to neutralize the hourly dose should be sufficient.) No more than 50 mg should be given over any 10-minute period, since protamine itself can cause bleeding. Heparin is used primarily to prevent either initiation or propagation of venous thromboembolism. Three different dosage ranges are commonly used, as outlined in Table 48–4.

MEDIUM-DOSE THERAPY. Several studies have provided clear evidence that monitoring the dosage of heparin affects the recurrence rate of thrombotic events (Hirsh, 1991a). Lack of adequate anticoagulation increases the risk of recurrent DVT 11- to 15-fold. Although presumed, it is less clear that monitoring affects hemorrhagic complications. A variety of clotting studies is available for monitoring circulating heparin levels. After reviewing the literature on control of heparin therapy, Estes (1970) and Godal (1974) both agree that partial thromboplastin times (PTT), including activated partial thromboplastin time (aPTT) and whole blood partial thromboplastin time (wBPTT), are more sensitive and accurate tests than is the Lee-White clotting time (LWCT). Although a number of investigators have favored the aPTT, there is evidence that aPTTs greater than 70 seconds are poorly repro-

TABLE 48–4. Heparin Regimens

DOSAGE (USP units/24 h)	ROUTE	CLINICAL INDICATIONS
Medium: 20,000–60,000	Continuous intravenous or intermittent subcutaneous	Active thromboembolism; disseminated intravascular coagulation
High: 60,000–100,000	Continuous intravenous	Massive pulmonary embolism
Low: 10,000–15,000	Intermittent subcutaneous or continuous intravenous	Elective pelvic surgery; disseminated intravascular coagulation
Adjusted minidose: 10,000–20,000	Intermittent subcutaneous	Long-term anticoagulation
Minidose: 10,000	Intermittent subcutaneous	Prophylaxis

ducible and hence unreliable when higher degrees of anticoagulation are assessed. The thrombin clotting time (TCT) seems also to satisfy the requirements for accuracy and ease of performance, and is the method preferred by some (Penner, 1974).

Optimal anticoagulation is usually obtained with a circulating heparin level of 0.2 to 0.4 U per ml by protamine titration (aPTT, 1.5 to 2.5 × control). Spontaneous hemorrhage will frequently occur if the concentration exceeds 0.6 U/ml for periods of time greater than 12 hours (Salzman et al., 1975). The circulating level is a balance between input of new drug, rapid metabolism, and excretion either directly by the kidneys or indirectly by diffusion into extravascular spaces to be metabolized slowly. The half-life of heparin is 30 to 90 minutes and is dose dependent. A stable circulating level is most easily achieved by administration of a loading dose followed by a continuous intravenous infusion. Because normal individuals vary widely in their responses to a given dose, the rate of infusion should be varied to achieve an aPTT within the therapeutic range regardless of the amount of heparin this requires. Table 48–5 gives a schema for continuous intravenous infusion for DVT. A mixture of 30 units of heparin in 500 ml dextrose 5 percent in water yields a concentration of 60 U per ml and is started at 1250 or 1300 U per hour (21 or 22 ml per hour). An aPTT is obtained every 6 hours until stable and the infusion adjusted upward if the aPTT is <60 seconds and down if >85 seconds.

The clinical impression that there is an increased requirement for heparin during pregnancy has been confirmed in the laboratory (Whitfield et al., 1983). This relative resistance during pregnancy is in part caused by an increased volume of distribution, a decrease in plasma albumin concentration, and a significant increase in factors VII, VIII, IX, X, and fibrinogen. Ineffective orally, heparin is well absorbed after subcutaneous administration. The intramuscular route should not be used because of the high incidence of hematoma formation at the injection site. While a steady circulating level can most easily be obtained by continuous intravenous administration, either the intermittent intravenous route or the subcutaneous route can be used. However, intermittent administration produces peaks and valleys in the circulating heparin activity that lead to seven times as many major bleeding complications as with continuous infusion (Hill and Pearson, 1971). When an intermittent subcutaneous regimen is chosen, a starting dose of 17,500 U every 12 hours is used and the dose adjusted to achieve an aPTT of 1.5 to 2.5 × control at 6 hours. Once a stable dose is obtained, monitoring can be decreased to daily, then weekly or less frequently.

TABLE 48–5. Anticoagulation with Medium-Dose Heparin

Loading dose	5000 U intravenously by rapid administration
Continuous infusion	Hourly rate to achieve 30,000 to 35,000 U/24 hours; adjust rate to achieve aPTT 1.5 to 2.5 × control
Long-term anticoagulation	17,500 U every 12 hours; adjust dose to achieve aPTT 1.5 to 2.5 × control at 6 hours

Before therapy is begun, a baseline hematocrit, platelet count, prothrombin time (PT), and aPTT or TCT should be obtained. Heparin should be avoided if the platelet count is less than 50,000 (50 × 10⁹/l) or if platelet function is inadequate.

Continuous intravenous heparin should be maintained for 7 to 14 days for active thromboembolic disease, or until symptoms have resolved and there is no evidence of recurrence. At this point the patient may be switched to subcutaneous heparin or oral coumarin for long-term management. Long-term heparinization is accomplished with the adjusted minidose regimen described below. The patient is instructed in self-administration, using the 20,000 or 40,000 U/ml preparation of heparin, a tuberculin syringe, and a 25-gauge 5/8-inch needle to inject deep into the subcutaneous fat of the anterior abdominal wall. To reduce local hematoma formation, ice is applied to the site for several minutes prior to injection, and the site should be chosen on a rotating daily basis. Intramuscular injections are forbidden, and the patient must be cautioned against the use of aspirin. There are ample data supporting the practicality, safety, and efficacy of chronic heparin therapy in ambulatory pregnant and nonpregnant patients (Spearing et al., 1978; Howell et al., 1983; Hellgren and Nygard, 1982; Stillman et al., 1977; Hirsh and Hull, 1986). Indications for anticoagulant therapy beyond the acute episode include recurrence, pulmonary embolization, and pregnancy. In my practice, an acute first episode of DVT is usually treated for 6 to 12 weeks. If a PE has occurred, treatment is extended for 6 to 12 months. If the DVT has occurred during pregnancy, minidose prophylaxis is continued through labor and delivery and for 2 to 3 weeks postpartum. Similarly, therapy should be extended for patients with iliofemoral venous thrombosis and recurrent venous thrombosis, and this should include either therapeutic or prophylactic doses during labor, delivery, and the early puerperium.

HIGH-DOSE THERAPY. In patients with massive pulmonary embolism, a large dose of heparin should be used during the first 24 hours of treatment. The initial loading dose should be 10,000 to 15,000 units followed by an hourly dose sufficient to yield a total dose of 60,000 units during the first 24 hours (Sasahara et al., 1983). Although there are no guidelines from clinical trials, it has been suggested that high doses are beneficial by relieving vasospasm. Additionally, there is evidence that a patient's heparin requirement is related to the extent of thrombosis (White et al., 1979). The high dosage should be reduced to the medium dose range after 12 to 24 hours of treatment.

LOW-DOSE THERAPY. In recent years the prophylactic use of heparin in minidoses to prevent thromboembolism has received a considerable amount of attention. The rationale for using small doses centers on the concept that a critical concentration of factor Xa (activated factor X) is required for thrombus formation. Factor Xa is the major component of the complex that activates prothrombin and lies at the point at which both intrinsic and extrinsic pathways converge to form the final common pathway of the clotting cascade. Heparin markedly enhances the action of the major plasma inhibitor of Xa, antithrombin III. It takes much less heparin to inhibit factor Xa than to prevent clotting once thrombin has been formed.

Standard regimens employ only 5000 U subcutaneously every 8 or 12 hours. This dose is insufficient to do more than minimally prolong the aPTT; consequently, there is no need to monitor dosage and no increase in hemorrhagic complications or intraoperative transfusion requirements. The only adverse effect reported is a slight increase in the number of wound hematomas. Multiple studies confirm that low-dose heparin prophylaxis in patients undergoing abdominothoracic surgery markedly decreases the incidence of DVT (Hirsh and Hull, 1986; White et al., 1979; Gallus et al., 1973; Nicolaides et al., 1972; Wessler, 1976b). More important, there is proof from a multicenter trial that the incidence of fatal pulmonary emboli is reduced as well (Kakkar et al., 1975).

Following baseline hematologic studies, the prophylactic regimen I prefer is 5000 U subcutaneously every 12 hours. If possible, the patient should not receive antiplatelet-aggregating agents (dipyridamole, clofibrate, acetylsalicylic acid) for 5 days prior to surgery, as low-dose heparin potentiates the aspirin-induced prolongation of the bleeding time observed in certain individuals (Gurewich et al., 1978). When these agents are avoided, there is no apparent increase in operative blood loss or postoperative hematoma formation (Gurewich et al., 1978; Ballard et al., 1973; Gjonnaess and Abildgaard, 1976). When the minidose regimen is used for peripartum prophylaxis, the first dose is given when the patient is admitted in labor. If epidural anesthesia is planned, the catheter should be placed 10 to 12 hours after a dose of heparin and after an aPTT in the normal range has been obtained. The next dose is withheld until the catheter is removed.

Adjusted Minidose Therapy. An alternative low-dose method is the adjusted minidose technique (Hull et al., 1982). In this regimen heparin is given every 12 hours in a dose adjusted to prolong the mid-interval aPTT to 1.5 times control. After initial adjustment, the subcutaneous dose of heparin is fixed and no additional coagulation monitors are performed. This method has been shown to be as effective as therapeutic doses of warfarin in the prevention of recurrent thromboembolism (Hull et al., 1982; Leyvraz et al., 1983).

If a woman has had one pregnancy complicated by a pulmonary embolus, a strong argument can be made for the necessity of prophylaxis during subsequent pregnancies. In one study, two of every 20 patients with pregnancy-related pulmonary emboli had a history of this complication (Baskin et al., 1972).

It is my belief that prophylactic doses of heparin should be used at the time of labor and delivery under the following circumstances: (1) previous pulmonary emboli, (2) previous thrombophlebitis, and (3) in patients at high risk for phlebitis, i.e., individuals with severe varicosities undergoing surgery.

The safety of minidose heparin during pregnancy has been amply documented. While it seems reasonable to extend the efficacy data from nonpregnant to pregnant subjects, there really are as yet no studies documenting efficacy during pregnancy. When con-

duction anesthesia is anticipated for delivery, the regimen is changed so that the first dose is given in early labor. The epidural catheter is placed when appropriate, after an aPTT in the normal range is obtained. Again, the second dose of heparin is not given until after the catheter is removed.

Low-Molecular-Weight Heparin. In recent years there has been a great deal of interest in low-molecular-weight heparin (Hirsh and Levine, 1992). Low-molecular-weight heparins (LMWHs) consist of a portion of the various sized molecules that make up standard heparin. Those molecules having fewer than 18 saccharide moieties (MW <5400) are unable to bind antithrombin III (ATIII) and thrombin simultaneously. Thus they are able to catalyze the inhibition of factor Xa by ATIII, but not the accelerated inactivation of thrombin by ATIII. This property should allow LMWHs to produce less microvascular bleeding while retaining an equivalent antithrombotic effect with standard heparin. Additionally, LMWHs have a longer plasma half-life, and their anticoagulant response to weight-adjusted doses is less variable. While these compounds hold significant promise including outpatient treatment of acute DVTs, there are still many questions to be answered including their safety in pregnancy, and no LMWH is available in the United States for other than experimental use.

Side Effects. The major risk of heparin therapy is hemorrhage. Recent reports show an incidence of approximately 4 per cent in properly monitored nonsurgical patients receiving heparin via the intravenous route (Basu et al., 1972). Heparin also causes osteoporosis when administered in doses greater than 15,000 U per day for more than 6 months (Griffith et al., 1965). This usually is not a problem during pregnancy, because patients rarely require antepartum therapy for periods this long. However, this complication has been reported by de Swiet et al. (1983) and warrants concern. A prospective study by Dahlman and colleagues (1990) found radiologic evidence of osteoporosis in 17 per cent of 25 pregnant women on full-dose heparin. The effect can be blunted by administration of calcium carbonate (1.5 gm daily). Other rare effects of heparin include hypotension, alopecia, allergic reactions, pain at the injection site, and thrombocytopenia. Thrombocytopenia, apparently an immune phenomenon, is characterized by a decline in platelets between the third and eighth days following initiation of therapy, reaching its nadir in 2 or 3 days, with recovery usually following within 5 days of discontinuing heparin (Babcock et al., 1976; Wahl et al., 1978). In most patients the platelet count will return to normal even if heparin is continued (Johnson et al., 1984). A prospective study of 120 nonpregnant patients treated with porcine heparin revealed only a 3 per cent incidence of thrombocytopenia (Power et al., 1979). In two of the four patients who did develop thrombocytopenia, a cause other than heparin was found for the fall in platelet count. Heparin is contraindicated in threatened abortion or if suspicion of significant risk of intracranial hemorrhage exists (e.g., in the eclamptic patient or the patient with severe hypertension). Hemoptysis from pulmonary infarction is not a contraindication.

Coumarin Agents

Of the various coumarin derivatives available, sodium warfarin is the most widely used in managing thromboembolic disease. Its therapeutic efficacy lies in its ability to inhibit the actions of vitamin K. Vitamin K functions in the liver as a cofactor in the synthesis of four essential clotting factors: factor VII, factor IX, factor X, and prothrombin (Hirsh, 1991b).

As a small molecule loosely bound to albumin, warfarin easily crosses the placenta and is excreted in breast milk (Wessler and Gitel, 1984). For these reasons, its use during pregnancy can be extremely hazardous. If administered during the first trimester (especially the fourth through eighth weeks), a syndrome that phenotypically resembles the Conradi-Hunermann type of chondrodysplasia punctata may result (Shaul and Hall, 1977). These children are born with multiple congenital anomalies including nasal cartilage hypoplasia, stippling of bones, slight intrauterine growth retardation, and brachydactyly. Recent reports indicate that warfarin may cause birth defects even if first administered in the second and third trimesters. Three children with microcephaly, bifrontal narrowing, mental retardation, and ophthalmologic abnormalities are known (Stevenson et al., 1980). It is postulated that the first-trimester anomalies may be secondary to either a direct teratogenic effect, use of warfarin, or a vitamin K deficiency effect, whereas the second- and third-trimester defects could result from fetal hemorrhage. The primary problem of warfarin administration during the last two trimesters has been fetal and placental hemorrhage resulting in fetal demise. In a collected series of 214 patients, there were 25 fetal deaths or a fetal mortality rate of 11.7 per cent (Laros, 1975). However, the great majority of such events appear to be secondary to the trauma of delivery itself (Bloomfield, 1970). In a prospective study of 23 women with heart valve prostheses who conceived 40 times, the fetal wastage exceeded 80 per cent (Lutz et al., 1978).

Although most investigators believe that coumarin therapy is contraindicated during pregnancy, Hall and associates (1980) state that two-thirds of pregnancies exposed to coumarin derivatives yielded normal infants and that heparin was not a clearly superior alternative. I disagree with their conclusions and think that coumarin derivatives should be used during pregnancy only in patients who are unable to master self-administration or who exhibit allergic reactions. In this case heparin should be used for the acute episode and until 14 weeks of gestation, at which point warfarin is substituted. Warfarin should be stopped and heparin substituted well in advance of labor. The patient should be fully informed of the potential risks of using coumarin (and all other vitamin K antagonists) during pregnancy.

Evidence suggests that the antithrombotic effect of warfarin is largely related to reduction in circulating levels of factors IX and X, whereas untoward bleeding seems more closely related to the level of factor VII. Large loading doses tend to greatly depress factor VII (which has a half-life of only 6 hours) and produce bleeding. Thus, a good therapeutic dosage schedule aims at a smooth reduction in circulating levels of all of these factors. The usual anticoagulating dose of warfarin is 10 to 15 mg daily until a therapeutic prolongation of the prothrombin time is achieved. An appropriate International Normalized Ratio (INR) for either prevention or treatment of DVT or for an in situ tissue cardiac valve is 2.0 to 3.0. If a mechanical cardiac valve is present, the dose should be adjusted to achieve an INR of 3.0 to 4.5. The INR should be used rather than simply the prothrombin time because it corrects for variations in the potency of the thromboplastins used by different laboratories. Thereafter, a maintenance dose of 3 to 20 mg daily is utilized. Initially the prothrombin time is monitored daily for 5 to 7 days, then twice weekly for one to two weeks and then weekly for several months, depending on the stability of the response. During the first 5 to 7 days of warfarin therapy, heparin is continued. Since heparin can prolong the prothrombin time by 2 to 4 seconds, the prothrombin time should be at least 2.5 times the control value by the time heparin is discontinued. Alternatively, heparin can be withdrawn in gradual decrements.

It is important to remember that a number of drugs affect the activity of the coumarin derivatives (Koch-Weser and Sellers, 1971). Agents increasing the activity of warfarin include salicylates, phenothiazines, phenylbutazone, and antibiotics, while ethyl alcohol and barbiturates decrease its activity. Fever, diarrhea, and change in intake of leafy green vegetables also have an effect.

As already mentioned, warfarin is discontinued and heparin therapy resumed well in advance of labor. The average half-life for disappearance of the drug is 44 hours (Wessler and Gitel, 1984). It is not known exactly how long it takes for the effects of oral anticoagulation on the fetus to wear off, but it is thought to be somewhere between 3 and 14 days (Pridmore et al., 1975). If spontaneous labor should occur while the patient is still taking warfarin, its effects can be reversed by administering vitamin K and fresh-frozen plasma. A single dose of 5 mg of vitamin K3, given orally or subcutaneously, begins to normalize the prothrombin time within 6 hours. Higher doses (e.g., 25 to 50 mg) normalize the prothrombin time slightly more rapidly, but also render the patient refractory to reanticoagulation for a period of 10 days to 2 weeks. Because there is some experimental and clinical evidence that vitamin K crosses the placenta, its administration may enhance the rate of return of fetal clotting factors as well (Hirsh et al., 1972). Immediately after delivery the infant is given 1 mg of vitamin K intramuscularly. If the newborn shows signs of bleeding or is less than 35 weeks of gestation or if it was a difficult instrument delivery, fresh-frozen plasma, 5 ml per kg, may be required as well.

Many surgeons and cardiologists are concerned that there is no large body of literature documenting that heparin is as effective as warfarin at preventing thromboses on prosthetic heart valves. Several case reports of heparin failure have heightened their concerns. An alternative proposed by Lee and associates is a switch to adjusted-dose heparin as soon as pregnancy is confirmed. The heparin is continued throughout the first trimester and reinstituted 3 weeks prior to term. Warfarin is used throughout the second and most of the third trimester (Lee et al., 1986).

Because the relative risks of these alternative approaches are unknown, the author believes that patients already taking coumarin agents and desiring to conceive (e.g., patients with prosthetic heart valves) should be switched to heparin prior to conception. Patients who inadvertently receive oral agents during the first trimester (for longer than the first 14 to 21 days after conception) must be advised of the risks involved and given the option of terminating the pregnancy.

Intrapartum, Intraoperative, and Postpartum Anticoagulation

Selected patients—those with recent pulmonary embolization, those with recent iliofemoral thrombosis, and those with heart valve prostheses—should be continued on medium-dose heparin during delivery or surgery. When hospitalized these patients are converted to a regimen of continuous intravenous heparin. The dose should be adjusted to achieve a circulating heparin level of 0.1 to 0.2 U/ml (aPTT 1.5 to 2.0 × control) during labor and delivery. Continuing this regimen does not increase the incidence of postpartum hemorrhage in a normal delivery. However, there is a slight increase in the incidence of episiotomy hematoma, and it may contribute to blood loss in patients with uterine atonia or retained placenta (Pridmore et al., 1975). Conduction anesthesia is contraindicated in these patients.

Full doses of heparin should be reinstituted 6 hours after delivery or surgery to re-attain a circulating level of 0.2 to 0.4 U/ml. Warfarin may be started (if the patient is not nursing) as soon as the patient resumes oral intake. Heparin is then discontinued 5 to 7 days later, as described above. Oral agents should be continued for 3 to 6 months postpartum, depending on the seriousness of the condition. Clotting factors tend to return to normal approximately 8 weeks after delivery (Lee et al., 1986).

Warfarin may be monitored successfully on an outpatient basis, as described by Davis et al. (1977). In 263 patients followed over a 5-year period by means of serial hematocrits, prothrombin times, and urinalyses, major bleeding episodes developed in only 4 per cent and minor bleeding in another 4 per cent.

A study of 68 patients with deep venous thrombosis indicated that the administration of therapeutic doses of warfarin was superior to long-term administration of minidose heparin at preventing new episodes of thromboembolism (Hull et al., 1979). However, as already discussed, adjusted-dose heparin has been shown to be equivalent to warfarin at preventing recurrent DVT and is associated with a lower risk of bleeding.

Controversy exists as to the safety of allowing women taking warfarin to nurse. There are two studies of warfarin suggesting that it does not pose a major risk to breast-fed infants (Orme et al., 1977; de Swiet and Lewis, 1977). However, other vitamin K antagonists do appear in the breast milk in large quantities

and can lead to hemorrhagic complications (Illingworth and Finch, 1959; Bramel and Hunter, 1950). Estrogen suppression of lactation is contraindicated because of a 10-fold increase in venous thrombosis in mothers over the age of 25 (Daniel et al., 1967).

Alternative Therapy

Fibrinolytic Agents

Fibrinolytic agents have the potential of providing a more rapid return to the normal physiologic state and of diminishing long-term disability. They should be considered an adjunct rather than a substitute for anticoagulant therapy. The challenge for the clinician is proper selection of the patient who will benefit from fibrinolytic therapy and will not have a major hemorrhagic complication. Two first-generation fibrinolytic agents, streptokinase (SK) and urokinase (UK), have undergone extensive clinical trials and are now available for clinical use. Both agents act to increase plasmin formation and thus the rate of clot lysis (Porter and Goodnight, 1977). In acute DVT, SK produces total clot lysis in 30 to 50 per cent of patients. Both SK and UK produce rapid resolution of pulmonary emboli, evident on angiography, as noted by improvement in pulmonary hemodynamics (Urokinase Pulmonary Embolism Trial, 1970; 1974). There are only a few case reports of use during pregnancy and thus conclusions as to safety must be withheld (Ludwig, 1973; Delclos and Davilla, 1986). Because of severe postpartum hemorrhage from the placental site, these agents should not be used for the first 10 postpartum days. Urokinase should not be used in patients who are anticoagulated, and SK must be used with extreme caution, as the combination greatly enhances the risk of overanticoagulation and bleeding.

A group of second- and third-generation fibrinolytic agents is also undergoing clinical investigation. The second-generation agents include recombinant tissue plasminogen activator, acylated plasminogen, streptokinase activator complex, and single-chain urokinase. The third-generation agents are polyethylene glycol–derived, antibody-directed, tailor-made recombinant forms, and hybrid complexes. The thrust of development of these newer agents is to make them more fibrin-specific.

Antiplatelet Agents

These drugs may play a role in arterial thromboembolism, but there is no definitive evidence that they are effective in the treatment or prophylaxis of venous thromboembolism (Genton et al., 1975). Dextran, the most widely used of these agents, must be administered intravenously, yet it is less effective than low-dose subcutaneous heparin for prophylaxis (Macintyre et al., 1974).

Surgical Intervention

Surgery is reserved for those patients for whom anticoagulants are contraindicated or have failed after an adequate course. Lower extremity thrombectomy is justified only if the patient is threatened by impending gangrene resulting from phlegmasia cerulea dolens (Lee et al., 1986). It does not reduce subsequent chronic venous insufficiency because the majority of vessels so treated do not remain patent on long-term follow-up.

Indications for vena caval interruption or insertion of an intracaval device are (1) recurrent pulmonary emboli despite adequate anticoagulation, (2) pulmonary embolization or iliofemoral thrombosis in a patient with an absolute contraindication to anticoagulation, (3) development of hemorrhagic complications of anticoagulation, and (4) following embolectomy (Kempczinski, 1986; Hux et al., 1986). Inferior vena caval ligation, plication, clipping, or insertion of an umbrella is not indicated unless recurrent life-threatening embolization persists despite adequate anticoagulation. A minor recurrence is observed in approximately 10 per cent of patients during the first few days of heparin therapy and should not be considered a failure of therapy. Bilateral ligation of the femoral veins is not fully protective because of the frequent involvement during pregnancy of the pelvic and gluteal veins, which drain into the iliacs above the inguinal ligament. If a pelvic source of embolism is suspected, the left ovarian vein may also require ligation.

Pulmonary embolectomy may be lifesaving, but should be considered only in those patients with angiographically demonstrated massive embolization to the main pulmonary artery with persistent inadequate cardiac output refractory to appropriate measures. In such situations the maternal outcome is of primary concern. Evans et al. (1968) described a patient who underwent interruption of the inferior vena cava, pulmonary angiography, peripheral venography, laparotomy, and thoracotomy on cardiopulmonary bypass with subsequent delivery of a normal baby.

SPECIAL PROBLEMS

Ovarian Hemorrhage During Anticoagulant Therapy

Intraperitoneal hemorrhage secondary to rupture of an ovarian cyst has been reported as a rare complication of anticoagulant therapy. Twenty-nine laparotomies were performed on 25 nonpregnant patients because of hemoperitoneum secondary to ruptured ovarian cysts (Waxman and Baird, 1978; Peters et al., 1979). The patients were receiving a coumarin derivative in 21 instances. This distribution of cases undoubtedly reflects the greater usage of coumarin agents for long-term therapy rather than a therapeutic advantage of heparin. Seventeen of the 21 patients for whom a pathologic diagnosis was given had a ruptured corpus luteum. The clinical presentation of acute onset of lower abdominal pain followed by distention should suggest the diagnosis of a ruptured cyst in any menstruating woman receiving anticoagulant therapy. Culdocentesis is useful in confirming the impression

of intraperitoneal hemorrhage. Although ovarian conservation is warranted, bilateral oophorectomy should be considered in situations in which the patient has a lifelong indication for anticoagulation.

Septic Pelvic Thrombophlebitis

Septic thrombophlebitis is a serious complication of pyogenic pelvic infections. Findings on pelvic examination often are not diagnostic, and recognition depends on a high index of suspicion in postpartum, postabortal, and postoperative patients who develop a spiking fever that persists despite adequate antibiotic therapy (Duff and Gibbs, 1983; Ledger and Peterson, 1970; Cohen et al., 1983). When a presumptive diagnosis of septic thrombophlebitis is made, the patient is begun on a medium-dose heparin regimen. If the diagnosis is correct, the fever should decrease within 12 to 36 hours. Thus heparin is both a diagnostic and a therapeutic tool. In the absence of a significant temperature response, a reassessment of the cause of the fever is indicated.

While there is general agreement as to initiation of therapy, there are no data dealing with how long to continue therapy. It has been my practice to treat these patients the same as those with acute, uncomplicated deep venous thrombosis. Thus, a medium-dose heparin regimen is started, and the patient is then converted to a coumarin agent, which is continued for a total course of anticoagulation of 3 to 6 weeks.

Ovarian Vein Thrombosis

Puerperal ovarian vein thrombosis is a difficult diagnosis to make. The diagnosis was made by laparotomy in 80 per cent of cases (Munsick and Gillanders, 1981). Fever, pain, and a lateral pelvic mass are present in 50 per cent of patients. In my experience and that of others, computed tomography has been helpful in making the diagnosis without operation in some cases (Angel and Knuppel, 1984; Dunnihoo et al., 1991).

REFERENCES

Aaro LA, Juergens JL: Thrombophlebitis associated with pregnancy. Am J Obstet Gynecol **109**:1128, 1971.

Angel JL, Knuppel RA: Computed tomography in diagnosis of puerperal ovarian vein thrombosis. Obstet Gynecol **63**:61, 1984.

Babcock RB, Dumper CM, Scharkman WB: Heparin-induced immune thrombocytopenia. N Engl J Med **295**:237, 1976.

Ballard RM, Bradley-Watson PJ, Johnstone FD, et al: Low doses of subcutaneous heparin in the prevention of deep vein thrombosis after gynaecologic surgery. J Obstet Gynaecol Br Cwlth **80**:469, 1973.

Baskin HF, Murray JM, Harris RE: Low-dose heparin for prevention of thromboembolic disease in pregnancy. Am J Obstet Gynecol **129**:590, 1972.

Basu D, Gallus A, Hirsach J et al: A prospective study of the value of monitoring heparin treatment with the activated partial thromboplastin time. N Engl J Med **287**:324, 1972.

Bentley PG, Kakar VV, Scully MF, et al: An objective study of alternative methods of heparin administration. Thromb Res **18**:177, 1980.

Bloomfield DK: Fetal deaths and malformations associated with the use of coumarin derivatives in pregnancy. Am J Obstet Gynecol **107**:883, 1970.

Bonnar J: Venous thromboembolism. *In* Recent Advances in Obstetrics and Gynecology. London, Churchill Livingstone, 1979.

Bramel CE, Hunter RE: Effect of dicumarol on the nursing infant. Am J Obstet Gynecol **59**:1153, 1950.

Clarke-Pearson DL, Jelovsek FR: Alterations of occlusive cuff impedance plethysmography results in the obstetric patient. Surgery **89**:594, 1981.

Cohen MB, Pernoll ML, Gevirtz CM, et al: Septic pelvic thrombophlebitis: An update. Obstet Gynecol **62**:83, 1983.

Comp PC, Esmon CT: Recurrent venous thromboembolism in patients with partial deficiency of protein S. N Engl J Med **311**:1525, 1984.

Coon WW: The spectrum of pulmonary embolism: Twenty years later. Arch Surg **111**:398, 1976.

Cranley JJ, Canos AJ, Sull WJ: The diagnosis of deep venous thrombosis—fallibility of clinical symptoms and signs. Arch Surg **111**:34, 1976.

Cronan JJ: Contemporary nevous imaging. Cardiovasc Intervent Radiol **14**:87, 1991.

Dahlman T, Lindvall N, Hellgren M. Osteopenia in pregnancy during long-term heparin treatment: A radiologic study postpartum. Br J Obstet Gynaecol **97**:221, 1990.

Daniel DG, Campbell H, Turnbull AC: Puerperal thromboembolism and suppression of lactation. Lancet **2**:287, 1967.

Davis FB, Estruch MT, Samson-Corvera EB, et al: Management of anticoagulation in outpatients. Arch Intern Med **137**:197, 1977.

Delclos GL, Davilla F: Thrombolytic therapy for pulmonary embolism in pregnancy. Am J Obstet Gynecol **155**:375, 1986.

De Swiet M, Lewis PJ: Excretion of anticoagulants in breast milk. N Engl J Med **297**:1471, 1977.

De Swiet M, Ward PD, Fidler J, et al: Prolonged heparin therapy in pregnancy causes bone demineralization. Br J Obstet Gynaecol **90**:1129, 1983.

Duff P, Gibbs RS: Pelvic vein thrombophlebitis: Diagnostic dilemma and therapeutic challenge. Obstet Gynecol Surv **38**:365, 1983.

Dunnihoo DR, Gallaspy JW, Wise RB et al.: Postpartum ovarian vein thrombophlebitis: A review. Obstet Gynecol Surv **46**:415, 1991.

Estes JW: Kinetics of the anticoagulant effect of heparin. JAMA **212**:1492, 1970.

Evans GL, Dalen JE, Dexter L: Pulmonary embolism during pregnancy. JAMA **206**:320, 1968.

Ginsberg JS, Hirsh J, Rainbow AJ, et al: Risk to the fetus of radiologic procedure used in the diagnosis of maternal venous thromboembolic disease. Thromb Haemost **61**:189, 1989.

Gallus AS: ^{123}I-Fibrinogen leg scanning. *In* Fratantoni J, Wessler S (ed): Prophylactic Therapy of Deep Vein Thrombosis and Pulmonary Embolism. Bethesda, National Institutes of Health, 1975, p. 83.

Gallus AS, Hirsh J, Tuttle RJ, et al: Small subcutaneous doses of heparin in prevention of venous thrombosis. N Engl J Med **288**:545, 1973.

Genton E, Gent M, Hersh J, et al: Platelet-inhibiting drugs in the prevention of clinical thrombotic disease. N Engl J Med **293**:1296, 1975.

Gjonnaess H, Abildgaard V: Bleeding in gynecologic surgery: Influence of lowdose heparin. Int J Gynaecol Obstet **14**:9, 1976.

Godal HC: Heparin assay methods for the control of in vivo heparin effects. Thromb Diath Haemorrh **33**:77, 1974.

Greer IA, Barry J, Mackon N, et al.: Diagnosis of deep venous thrombosis in pregnancy: A new role for diagnostic ultrasound. Br J Obstet Gynaecol **97**:53, 1990.

Griffin JH, Evatt B, Zimmerman TS, et al: Deficiencies in protein C in congenital thrombotic disease. J Clin Invest **68**:1370, 1981.

Griffith GC, Nichols G, Asher JD, et al: Heparin osteoporosis. JAMA **193**:185, 1965.

Gurewich V, Nunn T, Kuriakos TTX, et al: Hemostatic effects of uniform, low-dose subcutaneous heparin in surgical patients. Arch Intern Med **138**:41, 1978.

Haeger K: Problems of acute deep venous thrombosis. Angiology **20**:219, 1969.

Hall JG, Pauli RM, Wilson KM: Maternal and fetal sequelae of anticoagulation during pregnancy. Am J Med **68**:122, 1980.

Hathaway WE, Bonnar J: Thrombotic disorders in pregnancy and the newborn. *In* Hemostatic disorders of the pregnant woman and newborn infant. New York, Elsevier Scientific Publishing Company, Inc., 1987.

Hellgren M, Nygard EB: Long-term therapy with subcutaneous heparin during pregnancy. Gynecol Obstet Invest **13**:76, 1982.

Hill WC, Pearson JW: Outpatient intravenous heparin therapy for antepartum iliofemoral thrombophlebitis. Obstet Gynecol **37**:785, 1971.

Hirsh J: Blood tests for the diagnosis of venous and arterial thrombosis. Blood **57**:1, 1981.

Hirsh J: Heparin. N Engl J Med **324**:1565, 1991a.

Hirsh J: Oral anticoagulant Drugs. N Engl J Med **324**:1865, 1991b.

Hirsh J, Hull R: Treatment of venous thromboembolism. Chest **89**:426s, 1986.

Hirsh J, Cade JF, Gallus AS: Anticoagulants in pregnancy: A review of indications and complications. Am Heart J **83**:301, 1972.

Hirsh J, Levine MN: Low molecular weight heparin. Blood **79**:1, 1992.

Howell R, Fidler J, Litsky E, et al: The risk of antenatal subcutaneous heparin prophylaxis: A controlled trial. Br J Obstet Gynaecol **90**:1124, 1983.

Hull R, Delmore T, Carter C, et al: Adjusted subcutaneous heparin versus warfarin sodium in the long-term treatment of venous thrombosis. N Engl J Med **306**:189, 1982.

Hull R, Delmore T, Genton E, et al: Warfarin sodium versus low-dose heparin in the long-term treatment of venous thrombosis. N Engl J Med **301**:855, 1979.

Hull RD, Hirsh J, Carter CJ, et al: Pulmonary angiography, ventilation lung scanning, and venography for clinically suspected pulmonary embolism with abnormal perfusion lung scan. Ann Intern Med **98**:891, 1983.

Hux CH, Wapner RJ, Chayen B, et al: Use of the Greenfield filter for thromboembolic disease in pregnancy. Am J Obstet Gynecol **155**:734, 1986.

Illingworth RS, Finch E: Ethyl biscoumacetate in human milk. J Obstet Gynaecol Br Cwlth **66**:487, 1959.

Johnson RA, Lazarus KH, Henry DH: Heparin-induced thrombocytopenia. Am J Hematol **17**:349, 1984.

Kakkar VV, Corrigan TP, Fossard DP: Prevention of fatal postoperative pulmonary embolism by low doses of heparin: An international multicentre trial. Lancet **2**:45, 1975.

Kempczinski RF: Surgical prophylaxis of pulmonary embolism. Chest **89**:384s, 1986.

Koch-Weser J, Sellers EM: Drug interactions with coumarin anticoagulants. N Engl J Med **285**:547, 1971.

Laros RK Jr: Anticoagulants: Indications and use. Contemp Obstet Gynecol **5**:67, 1975.

Ledger WJ, Peterson EP: The use of heparin in the management of pelvic thrombophlebitis. Surg Gynecol Obstet **131**:1115, 1970.

Lee PK, Wang RYC, Chow JSF, et al: Combined use of warfarin and adjusted subcutaneous heparin during pregnancy in patients with artificial heart valve. J Am Coll Cardiol **8**:221, 1986.

Lensing AWA, Prandoni P, Brandjes D, et al.: Detection of deep-vein thrombosis by real-time B-mode ultrasonography. N Engl J Med **320**:342, 1989.

Leyvraz PF, Richard J, Bachmann F, et al: Adjusted versus fixed-dose subcutaneous heparin in the prevention of deep-vein thrombosis after total hip replacement. N Engl J Med **309**:954, 1983.

Ludwig H: Results of streptokinase therapy in deep vein thrombosis during pregnancy. Postgrad Med J **8**:65, 1973.

Lutz DJ, Noller KL, Spittell JA, et al: Pregnancy and its complications following cardiac valve prostheses. Am J Obstet Gynecol **131**:460, 1978.

Macintyre IMC, Vasilescu C, Jones DRB, et al: Heparin versus dextran in the prevention of deep-vein thrombosis: A multi-unit controlled trial. Lancet **ii**:118, 1974.

Mackie M, Bennett B, Ogston D, et al: Familial thrombosis: Inherited deficiency of antithrombin III. Br Med J **1**:136, 1978.

McCausland AM, Hyman C, Winsor T, et al: Venous distensibility during pregnancy. Am J Obstet Gynecol **81**:472, 1961.

Mueh JR, Herbst KD, Rapaport SI: Thrombosis in patients with lupus anticoagulant. Ann Intern Med **92**:156, 1980.

Munsick RA, Gillanders LA: A review of the syndrome of puerperal ovarian vein thrombophlebitis. Obstet Gynecol Surv **36**:57, 1981.

Nicolaides AN, Desai S, Douglas JN, et al: Small doses of subcutaneous sodium heparin in preventing deep venous thrombosis after major surgery. Lancet 2:890, 1972.

Nilsson I, Kullander S: Coagulation and fibrinolytic studies during pregnancy. Acta Obstet Gynecol Scand 46:273, 1967.

Orme MLE, de Swiet M, Serlin MJ, et al: May mothers given warfarin breastfeed their infants? Br Med J 1:1564, 1977.

Penner JA: Experience with a thrombin clotting time assay for measuring heparin activity. Am J Clin Pathol 61:645, 1974.

Peters WA, Thiagarajah S, Thornton WN: Ovarian hemorrhage in patients receiving anticoagulant therapy. J Reprod Med 22:82, 1979.

PIOPED Investigators: Value of the ventilation/perfusion scan in acute pulmonary embolism. JAMA 263:2753, 1990.

Porter JM, Goodnight SH: The clinical use of fibrinolytic agents. Am J Surg 134:217, 1977.

Power PJ, Cuthbert D, Hirsh J: Thrombocytopenia found uncommonly during heparin therapy. JAMA 241:2396, 1979.

Pridmore BR, Murray KH, McAllen PM: The management of anticoagulant therapy during and after pregnancy. Br J Obstet Gynaecol 82:740, 1975.

Rickles FR, Edwards RL: Activation of blood coagulation in cancer. Blood 62:14, 1983.

Rosenberg RD: The heparin-antithrombin system: A natural anticoagulant mechanism. *In* Colman RW, Hirsh J, Marder VJ Salzman EW (eds): Hemostasis and Thrombosis: Basic Principles and Clinical Practice, 2nd ed. Philadelphia, J. B. Lippincott, 1987.

Sachs BP, Brown DAJ, Driscoll SG, et al: Maternal mortality in Massachusetts. N Engl J Med 316:667, 1987.

Salzman E, Deykin D, Shapiro R, et al: Management of heparin therapy: Controlled prospective trial. N Engl J Med 292:1046, 1975.

Sasahara AA, Sharma GVRK, Barsamian EM, et al: Pulmonary thromboembolism. JAMA 249:2945, 1983.

Shaul WL, Hall JG: Multiple congenital anomalies associated with oral anticoagulants. Am J Obstet Gynecol 127:191, 1977.

Spearing G, Fraser J, Turner G, et al: Long-term self-administered subcutaneous heparin in pregnancy. Br Med J 1:1457, 1978.

Stevenson RE, Burton OM, Ferlauto GJ, et al: Hazards of oral anticoagulants during pregnancy. JAMA 243:1549, 1980.

Stillman RM, Chapa L, Stark ML, et al: A 10-year study of heparin therapy for thrombophlebitis in ambulatory patients. Surg Gynecol Obstet 145:193, 1977.

Taberino MD, Tomas JF, Alberca I, et al: Incidence and clinical characteristics of hereditary disorders associated with venous thrombosis. Am J Hematol 36:249, 1991.

Todd ME, Thompson JH, Bowie EJW, et al: Changes in blood coagulation during pregnancy. Mayo Clin Proc 40:370, 1965.

Toy PTCY, Schrier SL: Occlusive impedance plethysmography. West J Med 129:89, 1978.

Urokinase Pulmonary Embolism Trial Study Group: Urokinase pulmonary embolism trial: Phase 1. JAMA 214:2163, 1970.

Urokinase Pulmonary Embolism Trial Study Group: Urokinase pulmonary embolism trial: Phase 2. JAMA 229:1606, 1974.

Villasanta U: Thromboembolic disease in pregnancy. Am J Obstet Gynecol 93:142, 1965.

Wahl TO, Lipschitz DA, Stechschulte DJ: Thrombocytopenia associated with antiheparin antibody. JAMA 240:2560, 1978.

Waxman M, Baird GJ: Corpus luteum hemorrhage: Cause of abdominal pain in patients receiving anticoagulant therapy. JAMA 239:2270, 1978.

Wessler S: Medical management of venous thrombosis. Ann Rev Med 27:313, 1976a.

Wessler S: Heparin as an antithrombotic agent—-Low-dose prophylaxis. JAMA 236:389, 1976b.

Wessler S, Gitel SN: Heparin: New concepts relevant to clinical use. Blood 53:525, 1979.

Wessler S, Gitel SN: Warfarin. N Engl J Med 311:645, 1984.

White TM, Bernene JL, Marino AM: Continuous heparin infusion requirements. JAMA 241:2717, 1979.

Whitfield LR, Lele AS, Levy G: Effect of pregnancy on the relationship between concentration and anticoagulant action of heparin. Clin Pharmacol Therap 34:23, 1983.

Wright HP, Osborn SB, Edmonds DG: Changes in the rate of flow of venous blood in the leg during pregnancy, measured with radioactive sodium. Surg Gynecol Obstet 90:481, 1950.

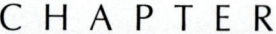
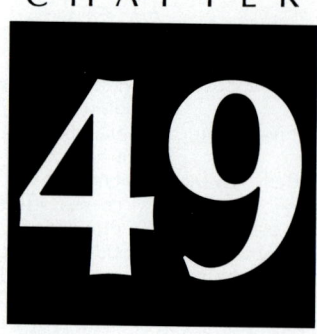
PREGNANCY-RELATED HYPERTENSION

JAMES M. ROBERTS, M.D.

CLASSIFICATION AND DEFINITIONS

The hypertensive disorders of pregnancy challenge the medical and obstetric skills of the health care team. Decisions as to the possible use and appropriate choice of pharmacologic agents require not only an understanding of the pathophysiology of the hypertensive disorders and a recognition of the pharmacokinetic changes occurring during pregnancy, but also an appreciation of the possible fetal effects of such therapeutic agents. Obstetric management demands meticulous maternal observation and use of tests of fetal-placental function and fetal maturity in order to weigh maternal risks and the risks to the infant of intrauterine versus extrauterine existence.

Recent information has provided new insights into the pathophysiology of the hypertensive disorders of pregnancy and has suggested methods of evaluating and treating the patient with these disorders.

The management of elevated blood pressure and the impact of the disorder on the mother and her fetus depend on whether hypertension antedated the pregnancy or appeared as the marker of a specific pregnancy-related vasospastic condition. An attempt to distinguish between the two has led to several systems of nomenclature and classification. The hypertensive disorders of pregnancy were for many years called *toxemias of pregnancy*, a term that originally even included hyperemesis gravidarum and acute yellow atrophy of the liver. This term reflected the opinion that these disorders had, as a common etiology, circulating toxins. Failure to identify these toxins did not lead to a revision of this terminology, signifying the continuing confusion that has plagued the taxonomy of these disorders. This archaic terminology, which neither describes the disorders nor clarifies their etiology, has rightly been abandoned.

One of the difficulties in interpreting studies of the hypertensive disorders of pregnancy is the inconsistency of terminology (Rippman, 1969). Several systems of nomenclature are in use around the world. The system prepared by the Committee on Terminology of the American College of Obstetricians and Gynecologists (Hughes, 1972), and recommended by the NIH working group on hypertension in pregnancy

(Working Group on High Blood Pressure in Pregnancy, 1990), although as imperfect as all such systems, has the advantage of clarity and is available in published form to investigators throughout the world. This classification is as follows:

Chronic hypertension
Preeclampsia-eclampsia
Preeclampsia superimposed upon chronic hypertension
Transient hypertension
Unclassified

The various classifications are explained in the following discussion.

Chronic Hypertension

Chronic hypertension is defined as hypertension that is present and observable prior to pregnancy or is diagnosed before the 20th week of gestation. The Committee has defined *hypertension* as a blood pressure greater than 140/90 mm Hg. Hypertension diagnosed for the first time during pregnancy that persists beyond the 42nd day postpartum is also classified as chronic hypertension.

Preeclampsia-Eclampsia

The diagnosis of preeclampsia is determined by increased blood pressure accompanied by proteinuria, edema, or both. Blood pressure must increase by at least 30 mm Hg systolic or 15 mm Hg diastolic relative to blood pressure prior to 20 weeks gestation. If prior blood pressure is not known, readings of 140/90 after 20 weeks gestation are considered sufficiently elevated for diagnosis of preeclampsia. This elevation must be present at two measurements taken 6 hours apart.

Page and Christianson (1976) advocated the use of mean arterial pressure during pregnancy. Mean pressures are determined by the following relationship:

$$\text{Mean arterial pressure} = \frac{\text{Systolic BP} + (2 <\times> \text{Diastolic BP})}{3}$$

which can be simplified for clinical use to:

$$\text{Mean arterial pressure} = \text{Diastolic pressure} + (1/3 <\times> \text{pulse pressure})$$

The use of mean arterial pressure eliminates confusion regarding the significance of diastolic or systolic hypertension. For example, if one regards a mean arterial pressure of 105 as defining risk, this level may be associated with diastolic "hypertension" (125/95) or systolic "hypertension" (155/80). In addition, mean blood pressures are much easier to deal with statistically. The obvious disadvantage is that obstetricians are not familiar with the use of mean pressures. The Committee defines either an increase in mean arterial pressure of 20 mm Hg or, if a prior blood pressure is not known, a mean arterial pressure of 105 mm Hg as indicative of hypertension.

Proteinuria is defined as the excretion of 0.1 gm/liter of protein in a random specimen or 0.3 gm/liter in a 24-hour specimen. Interestingly, the Committee did not define the minimum amount of protein excreted in 24 hours that can be considered diagnostic. On the basis of usual urinary output, the minimum would be about 0.3 gm/day. Edema is diagnosed as clinically evident swelling, but fluid retention may also be manifest as a rapid increase of weight without evident swelling.

Preeclampsia has mild and severe forms. Severe preeclampsia is diagnosed when the following criteria are present:

1. Blood pressure of 160 mm Hg or more systolic, or 110 mm Hg or more diastolic, recorded on at least two occasions at least 6 hours apart, with the patient at bed rest.
2. Proteinuria of 5 gm or more in 24 hours (3- or 4-plus on qualitative examination).
3. Oliguria (500 ml or less in 24 hours).
4. Cerebral or visual disturbances.
5. Epigastric pain.
6. Pulmonary edema or cyanosis.

Eclampsia is the occurrence of seizures in a preeclamptic patient that cannot be attributed to other causes.

Preeclampsia Superimposed Upon Chronic Hypertension

There is ample evidence that preeclampsia may occur in women already hypertensive and that the prognosis for mother and fetus is much worse than with either condition alone. The Committee on Terminology recommends that the diagnosis be made on the basis of increases of blood pressure (30 mm Hg systolic and 15 mm Hg diastolic, or 20 mm Hg mean arterial pressure) together with the appearance of proteinuria or generalized edema.

Transient Hypertension

Transient hypertension is the development of elevated blood pressure during pregnancy or in the first 24 hours postpartum without other signs of preeclampsia or pre-existing hypertension.

Unclassified Hypertension

Information about these disorders is insufficient for classification. This category should be used for a minority of patients with hypertensive disorders of pregnancy.

Problems with Classification

The degree of blood pressure elevation that constitutes gestational hypertension is controversial. Because average blood pressure in women in their teens to 20s is 120/60 mm Hg, the standard definition of hypertension—blood pressure greater than 140/90 mm Hg—is judged by some investigators to be too high (Vartran, 1966). There is evidence that the rate of perinatal mortality is increased in women with blood pressures even lower than 140/90 (Page and Christianson, 1976).

There are also problems inherent in the use of blood pressures measured in the first trimester to diagnose chronic hypertension or to define basal blood pressure for the diagnosis of preeclampsia. Blood pressure usually decreases early in pregnancy, reaching its nadir at about the stage of pregnancy at which women usually present for obstetric care (Fig. 49–1). The decrease averages 7 mm Hg for diastolic and systolic readings. In some women, obviously, blood pressure decreases more than 7 mm Hg, and in others, the

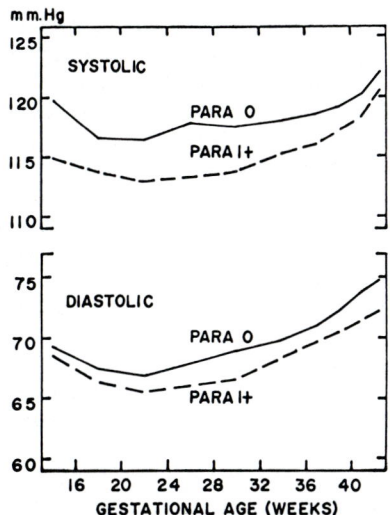

FIGURE 49–1. Mean blood pressure by gestational age in 6000 white women 25 to 34 years of age who delivered single term infants. (From Christianson R, Page EW: Studies on blood pressure during pregnancy. Influence of parity and age. Am J Obstet Gynecol **125**:509, 1976. Copyright 1976 by American College of Obstetricians and Gynecologists.)

early decline and subsequent return of blood pressure to prepregnant levels in late gestation will be sufficient to diagnose preeclampsia. There is evidence that women who are hypertensive prior to pregnancy actually have a greater decrease in blood pressure in early pregnancy than do normotensive women (Chesley and Annitto, 1947) and thus are even more likely to be erroneously diagnosed as preeclamptic according to blood pressure criteria. Also, the diagnosis of chronic hypertension based on the failure of blood pressure to return to normal by 42 days postpartum can be in error. In a long-range prospective study by Chesley (1956), many women who remained hypertensive 6 weeks postpartum were normotensive at long-term follow-up.

Even the triad of proteinuria, edema, and hypertension are nonspecific signs, and their presence in pregnancy could be due to conditions other than preeclampsia. Edema is a physiologic finding that is present in many normal pregnant women. The diagnosis of superimposed preeclampsia is especially difficult. Women fulfilling diagnostic criteria for superimposed preeclampsia may, indeed, have preeclampsia, but in some of these women the origin of signs may instead be renal disease, either causing the hypertension or secondary to it, that may coincidentally worsen during pregnancy. Conversely, many women who actually develop preeclampsia may not have the condition diagnosed. This is a special problem in women receiving antihypertensive therapy, in whom early stages of preeclampsia without proteinuria may be masked by therapeutic lowering of blood pressure. Superimposed preeclampsia is especially difficult to diagnose in the hypertensive woman with proteinuria at the onset of pregnancy. To aid in diagnosis, investigators have suggested the use of increasing serum uric acid (Redman et al., 1976a) and reduced concentrations of antithrombin 3 (Weiner and Brandt, 1982) as indicators of preeclampsia.

Renal biopsy specimens from women clinically diagnosed as having preeclampsia (blood pressure increase and proteinuria) demonstrate these diagnostic difficulties (Table 49–1) (McCartney, 1964). Of 62 women diagnosed as preeclamptic in their first pregnancy, 70 per cent had a glomerular lesion believed to be characteristic of preeclampsia. However, 24 per cent had evidence of chronic renal disease that was not suspected previously. Renal biopsies of multiparous women with a clinical diagnosis of superimposed preeclampsia demonstrate the difficulty of diagnosing this condition. Of 152 subjects, only 3 per cent had

the characteristic glomerular lesion, but 43 per cent had evidence of pre-existing renal or vascular disease.

Preeclampsia has a clinical spectrum ranging from mild to severe forms and then potentially to eclampsia. Affected patients do not "catch" eclampsia but progress through this spectrum. In most cases progression will be slow and the disorder may never proceed beyond mild preeclampsia. In others, the disease may progress more rapidly, changing from mild to severe over days to weeks. In the most serious cases, progression may be fulminant, with mild preeclampsia evolving to severe preeclampsia or eclampsia over hours to days. In a series of eclamptic women analyzed by Chesley (1978), 25 per cent had evidence of only mild preeclampsia in the days preceding convulsions. Thus, for clinical management, we must accept the fact that we are overdiagnosing the condition, because as will be discussed later, a major goal in managing preeclampsia is the prevention of eclampsia, primarily through timing of delivery. It is also evident, however, that studies of preeclampsia will be confounded by inclusion of women diagnosed as preeclamptic who actually have another cardiovascular or renal disorder. Still another problem is that some women with pregnancy-specific pathophysiologic changes identical to those present in preeclampsia will not have the specific signs of preeclampsia sufficient to satisfy the ACOG definition (Goodlin, 1986). These women are nonetheless at increased risk, as are their infants (Weinstein, 1982, Martin et al., 1991) and should be managed as is the more typical preeclamptic patient.

PREECLAMPSIA-ECLAMPSIA

In spite of the difficulty of making a clinical diagnosis of preeclampsia, there is no question that a disorder exists unique to pregnancy and characterized by poor perfusion of many vital organs, including the fetal-placental unit, and completely reversible with the termination of pregnancy. Pathologic, pathophysiologic, and prognostic findings clearly indicate that this condition, which we will call preeclampsia,* is not merely an unmasking of preexisting, underlying hy-

....

*It is tempting to use a new "label" to define this vasospastic condition in pregnancy. However, because there are already too many labels and because the diagnosis of this pregnancy-related condition can be made only retrospectively, i.e., when physiologic functions including blood pressure return to normal after pregnancy, we will use *preeclampsia*, realizing its limitations.

TABLE 49–1. Renal Biopsy Findings in Patients with Clinical Diagnosis of Preeclampsia

BIOPSY FINDINGS	PRIMIGRAVIDAS (N = 62)	MULTIGRAVIDAS (N = 152)
Glomeruloendotheliosis	70%	14% (with or without nephrosclerosis)
Normal histologic appearance	5%	53%
Chronic renal disease (chronic GTN, chronic pyelonephritis)	25%	21%
Arteriolar nephrosclerosis	0	12%

Modified from McCartney CP: Pathological anatomy of acute hypertension of pregnancy. Circulation **30**(Suppl II):37, 1964, by permission of the American Heart Association, Inc.

pertension. Although this fact has been well documented for many years, problems still arise owing to approaches in the management of preeclampsia that are based solely on principles useful in managing hypertension in nonpregnant individuals. The successful management of preeclampsia requires an understanding of the pathophysiologic changes in this condition and the recognition that the signs of preeclampsia—increased blood pressure, proteinuria, and edema—are only signs and not causal abnormalities. The etiology of preeclampsia-eclampsia is not completely understood; however, as Zuspan (1978) has pointed out, we can manage the condition very successfully using the information we do have about its pathophysiology, prognosis, and natural history.

Clinical Presentation

The "Typical" Preeclamptic Patient

Preeclampsia occurs in about 7 per cent of pregnancies not terminating in first-trimester abortions. It would be useful to be able to identify the women at greatest risk. In preeclampsia, as with all diseases, there are no truly "typical" patients. Epidemiologic findings do indicate, however, that certain characteristics are more common in women who develop preeclampsia. The most important is nulliparity. Preeclampsia is primarily a disease of the first pregnancy. At least two-thirds of cases occur in women during the first pregnancy not terminating in a first-trimester loss.

Preeclampsia is thought to be more common in women of lower socioeconomic status. In his study of pregnant women in Aberdeen, Scotland, nearly all of whom were delivered in hospitals, Nelson (1955) found no relationship of preeclampsia-eclampsia to socioeconomic status. In similar studies in Finland (Vara et al., 1965) and Jerusalem (Davies, 1970), no relationship was established between this factor and the incidence of preeclampsia. It remains the current clinical impression of most individuals caring for pregnant women in the United States that preeclampsia is a disease of lower-income women. This impression may be accurate, but it is undoubtedly confounded by the relationship of preeclampsia to age, race, and parity. Eclampsia, on the other hand, is clearly a disease of women of lower socioeconomic status (Nelson, 1955; Vara et al., 1965; Davies, 1970). Eclampsia is preventable by careful obstetric observation and delivery for severe preeclampsia. Therefore, the lack of availability and utilization of good-quality obstetric care to indigent women is undoubtedly a major factor in the increased incidence of eclampsia. It is interesting to note that in past years the clinical impression was that preeclampsia-eclampsia was a disease of women of higher socioeconomic status (Chesley, 1978).

There is a relationship between the extremes of childbearing age and the incidence of eclampsia and preeclampsia. Because most pregnancies, particularly most first pregnancies, occur in young women, most cases of preeclampsia-eclampsia occur in this age group. However, studies of entire populations in Ab-

erdeen, Jerusalem, and Finland do not indicate an increased incidence of preeclampsia in young women if parity is considered. In all of these studies a higher incidence of preeclampsia was found in older women that was not dependent on parity. The information from the Collaborative Study in the United States (Vollman, 1970) does suggest a higher incidence of preeclampsia in younger women, although Davies (1971) has pointed out the deficiencies in this study. It is possible that the incidence of preeclampsia may be greater in young women in the United States but not in other parts of the world; however, even if this is true, increased incidence of the youngest age groups in the Collaborative Study is not nearly as great as that of older patients.

The relationship of preeclampsia and eclampsia to race is equally difficult to evaluate. Data from both the United States Collaborative Study and the Jerusalem study indicate a relationship to race (Vollman, 1970; Davies, 1970). The Jerusalem study revealed the strong correlation of race and age during pregnancy. In the Collaborative Study the incidence of preeclampsia was higher in blacks, in whom hypertension is generally more common. This finding raises the question whether the incidence of preeclampsia is truly race-related or whether the finding is an example of the difficulty in differentiating preeclampsia from unrecognized pre-existing chronic hypertension. Chesley has stated that there is no difference in incidence of preeclampsia between blacks and Caucasians (unpublished observation cited by Davies, 1971).

A characteristic of preeclampsia-eclampsia that is frequently overlooked is the tendency of the condition to occur in daughters and sisters of women with a history of preeclampsia. In Aberdeen, the incidence of proteinuric preeclampsia was found to be four times higher in sisters of women who had preeclampsia in their first pregnancy than in sisters of women who did not (Adams and Finlayson, 1961). In a recent study of the same population the incidence of preeclampsia was 15 per cent in mothers, but only 4 per cent in mothers-in-law, of preeclamptic women (Sutherland et al., 1981). Chesley and Cooper (1986) evaluated preeclampsia in the first pregnancy of sisters, daughters, granddaughters, and daughters-in-law of women who had been eclamptic. The incidence of preeclampsia in sisters was 37 per cent, in daughters 26 per cent, in granddaughters 16 per cent, but in daughters-in-law only 6 per cent. These observed incidences fit closely with inheritance of preeclampsia through a single maternal gene with the frequency of the putative gene being 0.25. Such a genetic predisposition is supported by HLA typing of mothers and fetuses (Kilpatrick et al., 1990; Johnson et al., 1990). Although these data are conflicting, they do suggest that in a given population, certain HLA types are more common in the mother and the fetus from preeclamptic pregnancies.

Certain medical disorders also predispose to preeclampsia. Diabetes is frequently complicated by preeclampsia, with the incidence stated to be as high as 50 per cent of diabetic pregnancies (Chesley, 1978). Preeclampsia is also more common in women with hypertension antedating pregnancy. In several studies

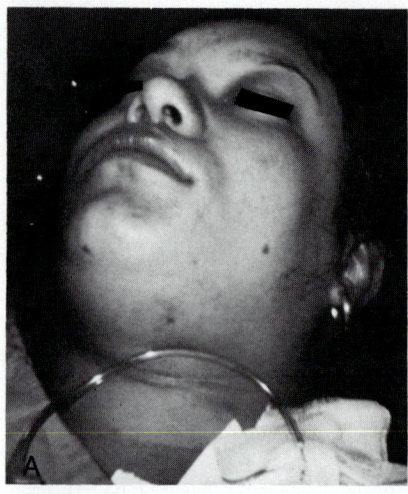
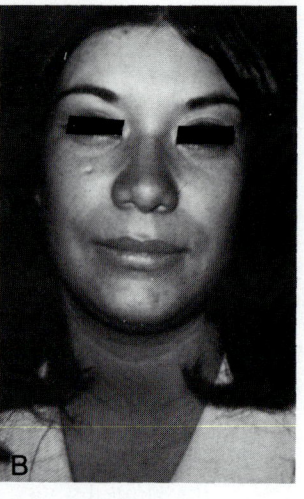

FIGURE 49–2. Facial edema in severe preeclampsia. Markedly edematous facies of this severely preeclamptic woman (*A*) is especially evident when compared with her appearance 6 weeks postpartum (*B*).

the reported incidence is approximately 20 per cent (Roberts and Perloff, 1977).

Certain conditions of pregnancy also increase the risk of preeclampsia. The incidence is approximately 30 per cent in women with twin pregnancies and is increased regardless of parity. In a study by Bulfin and Lawler (1957) the incidence was 70 per cent in primiparas and 20 per cent in multiparas. Preeclampsia is also present in 70 per cent of women with large, rapidly growing hydatidiform moles and occurs earlier than usual in gestation (Page, 1939). In fact, in cases of preeclampsia occurring before 24 weeks, hydatidiform mole should be suspected and sought. An interesting variant of preeclampsia occurs with fetal hydrops, although not with erythroblastosis uncomplicated by hydrops; the incidence is high (approximately 50 per cent), and preeclampsia is not confined to hydrops secondary to isoimmunization, occurring in one series in nine of 11 infants with hydrops of nonimmune etiology (Scott, 1958). This condition may present early in pregnancy and with severe signs and symptoms of preeclampsia. Proteinuria is massive, and blood pressure elevation and edema are marked. In spite of this severity, eclampsia is a rare complication. Preeclampsia is also reported to be more common in pregnancies complicated by polyhydramnios; however, if the association of polyhydramnios with diabetes and multiple pregnancies is accounted for, the relationship is not present (Jeffcoate and Scott, 1959).

Signs of Preeclampsia

The diagnostic signs of preeclampsia usually antedate symptoms. The usual sequence of the appearance of the signs is edema, followed by increased blood pressure and proteinuria; however, any order of appearance may occur (Chesley, 1978).

Edema

Fluid retention can be manifested as a rapid gain in weight prior to demonstrable edema. A gain of 5 lb in one week is cited as a warning sign of preeclampsia. However, rapid weight gain can occur in pregnancy without preeclampsia, and in one group of women who became eclamptic, only 10 per cent manifested this rapid weight gain (Chesley, 1978). Edema in preeclampsia is believed to be related in part to sodium retention and is thus not limited to dependent edema. Edema of the hands and face is more likely to be associated with sodium retention and is therefore a more reliable indicator of preeclampsia than is dependent edema, which may be due to primarily hydrostatic mechanisms. However, sodium retention caused by altered glomerular tubular balance due to postural decreases in glomerular filtration is common in normal pregnancy. Edema of the hands and face occurs in 10 to 15 per cent of women whose blood pressure remains normal throughout pregnancy (Thomson et al., 1967). Edema may be massive, especially in severe preeclampsia, rendering the patient virtually unrecognizable (Fig. 49–2). With such patients it is important to remember that substantial hypoalbuminuria may complicate preeclampsia and contribute to the edema. Therefore, edema is an early and common sign of preeclampsia but is not diagnostic.

Blood Pressure Change

Increased blood pressure is required for the diagnosis of preeclampsia. As discussed previously, however, the changes in blood pressure associated with normal pregnancy may lead to misdiagnosis. In clinical practice the possible impact of preeclampsia on mother and fetus warrants such overdiagnosis. From a pathophysiologic viewpoint, of primary importance is poor tissue perfusion secondary to vasospasm, which is revealed more clearly by blood pressure changes than by absolute blood pressure levels. However, even the relative increase of blood pressure does not always correlate well with decreased tissue perfusion and subsequent damage. Eclampsia and maternal or fetal death can occur in the patient with only modest blood pressure elevation. In two series, 20 per cent of women with eclampsia never had a systolic blood pressure exceeding 140 mm Hg (Chesley, 1978; Dieckman, 1952).

Proteinuria

Among the diagnostic signs of preeclampsia, proteinuria accompanied by hypertension is the most reliable indicator of fetal jeopardy. In two studies of preeclampsia, the perinatal mortality rate tripled in women with proteinuria (MacGillivray, 1958), and the amount of proteinuria correlated with increased perinatal mortality rate and the number of growth-restricted infants (Tervila et al., 1973). If only eclampsia is considered—thus excluding cases of chronic hypertension misdiagnosed as preeclampsia—the relationship of proteinuria to perinatal mortality is even more striking. In the series reported by Nelson (1955) from Aberdeen, there were 15 neonatal deaths in 52 proteinuric women and no neonatal deaths in 17 women who became eclamptic but did not have proteinuria. In spite of the specificity and fetal prognostic significance of proteinuria, however, we must emphasize that eclampsia can occur without proteinuria. In one series of 298 eclamptic patients, 41 per cent did not have proteinuria (Naidoo and Moodley, 1980), and in a series of eclamptic patients reviewed by Chesley (1978), 26 of 199 had either trace (16) or no (10) proteinuria prior to seizures.

Retinal Changes

Important and consistent signs in preeclamptic patients are retinal vascular changes on funduscopic examination. Localized or generalized changes occur in retinal arterioles in at least 50 per cent of women with preeclampsia. These retinal vascular changes are the clinical sign that best correlates with renal biopsy changes of preeclampsia (Pollak and Nettles, 1960). Localized retinal vascular narrowing is visualized as segmental spasm, and the generalized narrowing is indicated by a decrease in the ratio of arteriolar:venous diameter from the usual 3:5 to 1:2 or even 1:3. It may occur in all vessels or, in early stages, in single vessels (Jaffe and Shatz, 1986). Preeclampsia does not cause chronic arteriolar changes; thus the presence of arteriolar sclerosis detected by increased light reflex, copper wiring, or arteriovenous nickling indicates pre-existing vascular disease. Finnerty (1956) described a characteristic "retinal sheen" in preeclamptic patients. In my experience, this finding is present in many young patients, pregnant and nonpregnant, male and female, and has not been a useful sign.

Hyper-reflexia

Hyper-reflexia is a sign given a great deal of clinical attention. Deep tendon reflexes are increased in many women prior to seizures. However, seizures can occur in the absence of hyper-reflexia (Sibai et al., 1981), and many young subjects are consistently hyper-reflexic without being preeclamptic. Changes, or lack of changes, in deep tendon reflexes are not part of the diagnosis of preeclampsia.

Other Signs

Other signs that occur in preeclampsia less commonly are indicators of involvement of specific organs of the preeclamptic process. Thus, patients with marked edema may have ascites and hydrothorax, and those in congestive heart failure have the usual signs—increased neck vein distention, gallop rhythm, and pulmonary rales. Hepatic capsular distention, manifested by hepatic enlargement and tenderness, is particularly ominous, as is disseminated intravascular coagulation sufficient to result in petechiae or generalized bruising and bleeding.

Symptoms of Preeclampsia

It is important to remember that the majority of women with early preeclampsia are asymptomatic. This lack of symptoms is, in fact, an important part of the rationale for frequent obstetric visits in late gestation. In most cases, increased blood pressure, increasing edema, and proteinuria antedate overt symptoms.

The multitude of symptoms that can occur secondary to preeclampsia—especially preeclampsia of increasing severity—are listed in Table 49–2. Because preeclampsia is a disease of poor perfusion to essentially all tissues, the occurrence of symptoms related to many organ systems is not surprising. Tightness of hands and feet and paresthesias secondary to medial or ulnar nerve compression occur because of fluid retention. Although these are of concern to the patient, who may be quite uncomfortable, they are not of prognostic significance. However, certain symptoms are indicators of the severity of the disease. Symptoms of hepatic capsular distention are particularly ominous. These include epigastric pain, "stomach upset," and pain penetrating to the back. Headache and mental confusion indicate poor cerebral perfusion and may be precursors of convulsions. Visual symptoms ranging from scotomata to blindness indicate retinal arterial spasm and edema. In evaluation of the patient with preeclampsia, these signs of poor perfusion are as important indicators of the severity of the disease as the easily quantifiable signs. Other symptoms may also be present secondary to the complications of preeclampsia, such as congestive heart failure and abruptio placentae.

TABLE 49–2. Signs and Symptoms of Preeclampsia-Eclampsia

Cerebral	Headache
	Dizziness
	Tinnitus
	Drowsiness
	Change in respiratory rate
	Tachycardia
	Fever
Visual	Diplopia
	Scotomata
	Blurred vision
	Amaurosis
Gastrointestinal	Nausea
	Vomiting
	Epigastric pain
	Hematemesis
Renal	Oliguria
	Anuria
	Hematuria
	Hemoglobinuria

Laboratory Findings

Proteinuria is, by strict definition, not a sign of preeclampsia-eclampsia. It is a laboratory finding. Because it is a diagnostic feature of the disorder, however, proteinuria has already been discussed. Major changes revealed by laboratory studies occur in severe preeclampsia and eclampsia. In mild preeclampsia, changes in most of these indicators may be minimal or absent.

Renal Function Studies

SERUM URIC ACID CONCENTRATION AND URATE CLEARANCE. The most sensitive indicator of preeclampsia available to clinicians, serum uric acid concentration, has been largely ignored by obstetricians in the United States in recent years. Studies from England and Australia have demonstrated that a decrease in uric acid clearance precedes a measurable decrease in glomerular filtration rate (Gallery and Györy, 1979b). Also, serum uric acid levels were actually a better predictor of perinatal outcome than blood pressure (Redman et al., 1976a). Table 49–3 shows normal uric acid levels during gestation and levels associated with preeclampsia.

SERUM CREATININE CONCENTRATION AND CREATININE CLEARANCE. Creatinine clearance is decreased in the majority of patients with severe preeclampsia, but may be normal in patients with milder forms of the disease. Serum creatinine determinations, if obtained serially, may reflect this decrease in clearance but, unless very elevated, are not helpful because of the wide range of normal single values. The serum creatinine varies as a geometric function of creatinine clearance. Thus, an increase from 0.6 to 1.2 mg/100 ml indicates a halving of creatinine clearance. Interpretation of more subtle variations of serum creatinine concentration depends on the ability to differentiate between small changes in creatinine due to functional changes and those due to variations in laboratory technique. Thus, smaller changes in glomerular filtration are best determined by measurements of creatinine clearance.

BLOOD UREA NITROGEN AND UREA CLEARANCE. Changes in urea clearance and blood urea nitrogen mirror the changes in creatinine clearance. The same caution as with creatinine serum concentrations is necessary, as well as the understanding that blood urea concentration (BUN) also is influenced by protein intake and liver function. BUN will sometimes increase in hospitalized patients in spite of unchanging serum creatinine concentrations, probably owing to an improved diet.

URINARY SEDIMENT. Pollak and Nettles (1960) reported urinary sediment changes in cases of severe preeclampsia. Unfortunately there was no control group, and there is evidence of increased urinary excretion of formed elements in normal pregnancy (Elden and Cooney, 1935). Urinary sediment analysis is probably not a useful aid to differential diagnosis except in individuals with urinary changes pathognomonic of other renal diseases who have clinical signs of mild preeclampsia.

Hematologic Changes

In severe preeclampsia, reduction in plasma volume may be indicated by a rapid increase in hematocrit over values obtained in the preceding week. Hematocrit decreases postpartum or with volume expansion (Dieckman, 1952). In mild preeclampsia, the hematocrit is not usually elevated.

Liver Function Tests

The results of laboratory tests of liver function have been extensively reviewed by Chesley (1978). In reviewing published results of bilirubin, alkaline phosphatase, SGOT and SGPT determinations, and several older tests of liver function in preeclampsia, he concluded that none of these tests is useful prognostically or as a gauge of severity of the disease. However, the association of microangiopathic anemia and elevated SGOT and SGPT has an especially ominous prognosis for mother and baby (Weinstein, 1982; Martin et al., 1991). These findings usually correlate with severity of disease and, when associated with hepatic enlargement, are an ominous sign of impending hepatic rupture. In other cases, however, abnormalities of liver function, coagulation changes, and hemolysis may be present in women who do not show blood pressure and renal changes of preeclampsia (HELLP syndrome) (Weinstein, 1982). This condition has the same implications for maternal and fetal morbidity as the more classic presentation, and its recognition demands a high index of suspicion by the clinician.

TABLE 49–3. Plasma Urate Concentrations in Normotensive and Hypertensive Pregnant Women*

WEEKS GESTATION	NORMOTENSIVES				HYPERTENSIVES			
	MMOL/LITER			MG/100 ML	MMOL/LITER			MG/100 ML
24–28	.18	(20%)		3.02	.24	(20%)		4.03
29–32	.18	(35%)		3.02	.28	(25%)		4.7
33–36	.20	(30%)		3.36	.30	(20%)		5.04
37–40	.26	(20%)		4.4	.31	(23%)		5.28
41–42	.25	(24%)		4.2	.32	(12%)		5.38

*Numbers in parentheses are standard deviation as percentage of the mean values shown. Values for hypertensive and normotensive women are statistically different at all gestational ages (p<.05).

Modified from Shuster E, Weppelman B: Plasma urate measurements and fetal outcome in preeclampsia. Gynecol Obstet Invest **12**:162, 1981.

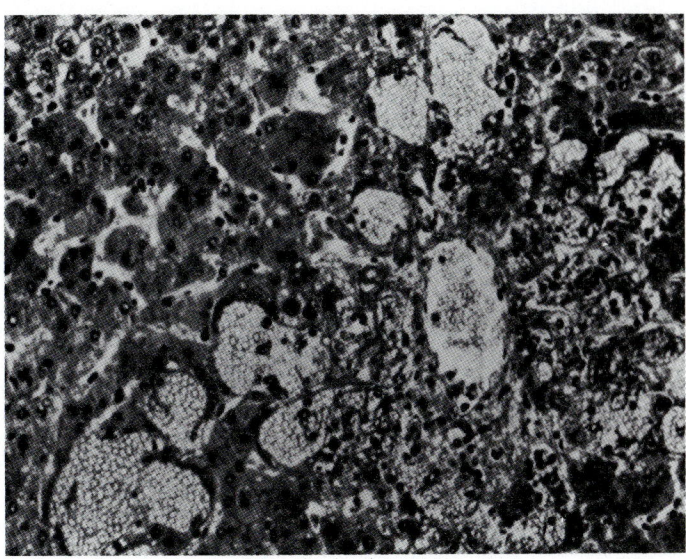

FIGURE 49–3. Hemorrhagic hepatic lesions in eclampsia. Hemorrhage into periportal area with crescentic compression of liver cells. (From Sheehan HL, Lynch JB: Pathology of Toxemia in Pregnancy. London, Churchill Livingstone, 1973.)

Coagulation Factors

In approximately 20 per cent of patients with severe preeclampsia, the usual laboratory evidence of consumption of procoagulants is present (Pritchard et al., 1976). The average platelet count in the patient with mild preeclampsia does not differ from the platelet count in normal pregnant women (Galton et al., 1971); however, careful platelet counts performed sequentially in individual patients may reveal decreased platelets in many patients (Redman et al., 1978). Highly sensitive indicators of activation of the clotting system, reduced serum concentrations of antithrombin III (Weiner and Brandt, 1985) and a decrease in the ratio of factor VIII bioactivity to factor VIII antigen (Redman et al., 1977a), and subtle indicators of platelet dysfunction including alteration of turnover (Inglis et al., 1982) and content (Douglas et al., 1982) are present in even mild preeclampsia and may, in fact, antedate clinically evident disease.

Pathologic Changes

The pathologic changes found in organs of women dying of eclampsia and in biopsy specimens from women with preeclampsia provide strong evidence that preeclampsia is not merely an unmasking of essential hypertension or a variant of malignant hypertension. These findings also indicate that the elevation of blood pressure is probably not of primary pathogenetic importance.

Brain

Cerebral edema was once thought to be a common finding in women dying with eclampsia. Sheenan and Lynch (1973), on the basis of postmortem examinations performed within 2 to 3 hours of death, concluded that the findings previously reported were primarily postmortem changes, and that cerebral edema was actually a rare complication. Recent studies using computer-assisted tomography have once again raised the possibility that cerebral edema is an important pathophysiologic event in some patients with preeclampsia (Naheedy et al., 1985).

Liver

Gross lesions of the liver are visible in about 60 per cent of women dying of eclampsia, and one-third of the remaining livers are microscopically abnormal. Many early investigators thought that the hepatic changes were pathognomonic of eclampsia (Schmorl, 1901). Similar changes, however, have been described in women dying of abruptio placentae (Sheehan, 1950). The most extensive description of the hepatic changes has been provided by Sheehan and Lynch (1973). They describe two types of lesions, which they consider temporally and etiologically distinct. Initially, the hepatic changes are most consistent with hemorrhage into the hepatic cellular columns, with dislocation and deformation of the hepatocytes in their stromal sleeves (Fig. 49–3). These changes are interpreted as hemorrhage secondary to vasodilatation of arterioles. Later, signs of hepatic infarction are present. These changes range from small to large areas of infarction beginning near the sinusoids, but eventually extending into the area adjacent to portal vessels (Fig. 49–4). These changes are believed to be secondary to intense vasospasm. Hemorrhagic changes are present in 66 per cent and necrotic changes in 40 per cent of eclamptic women and in about half as many preeclamptic women. Several authors have described hyalinization and thrombosis of hepatic vessels and have cited this finding as evidence of disseminated intravascular coagulation, although it may be a later stage of the hemorrhagic phenomenon.

Kidney

Pathologic changes in the kidney of preeclamptic and eclamptic women are clearly different from the morphologic changes seen in other hypertensive or renal disorders. Glomerular, tubular, and arteriolar

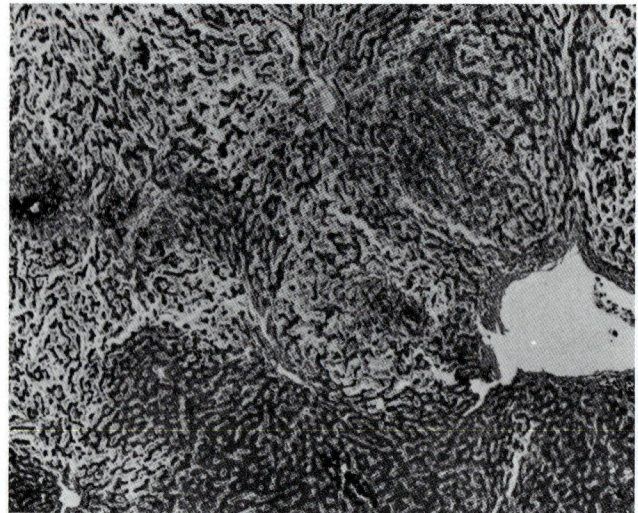

FIGURE 49–4. Hepatic infarction in eclampsia. (From Sheehan HL, Lynch JB: Pathology of Toxemia in Pregnancy. London, Churchill Livingstone, 1973.)

changes have been described. Of these, the most characteristic and consistent is the glomerular lesion, which is in fact considered by some investigators to be pathognomonic of preeclampsia-eclampsia. Identical changes are present, however, in kidneys of women who have placental abruption without evident preeclampsia (Thomson et al., 1972).

GLOMERULAR CHANGES. A number of characteristic changes are seen by light microscopy in glomeruli of preeclamptic women (Pollak and Nettles, 1960). There is a slight decrease in glomerular size, and the glomerular tuft protrudes into the proximal tubule. The diameter of the glomerular capillary lumen is decreased and contains few blood cells. The endothelial-mesangial cells, which are indistinguishable on light microscopy, are larger owing to an increase in cytoplasmic volume and may contain lipoid droplets (Fig. 49–5).

Electron microscopic examination of glomeruli provides a more precise picture (Fig. 49–6). From both examinations it is evident that the primary pathologic change occurs in endothelial cells. These cells, which line the glomerular capillaries, are increased greatly in size and may occlude the capillary lumen; their cytoplasm contains electron-dense material (Spargo et al., 1959). The basement membrane bordering the epithelial cell may be slightly thickened and also contains electron-dense material. The epithelial cell podocytes are not altered. On the basis of these pathologic findings, the lesion has been termed glomerular capillary endotheliosis.

Faith and Trump (1966) believe that the endothelial changes are secondary to phagocytosis of blood-borne materials by these cells, the nature of this material being a matter of controversy. It was originally reported on the basis of immunofluorescent staining studies that immune globulins were not present, but that the material had the antigenic characteristics of fibrinogen (Vassali et al., 1963). In more recent studies using more specific anti-immunoglobulin, IgG, IgM,

and complement have been demonstrated (Petruccho et al., 1974). Fibrin is also found in the glomeruli. Petruccho and colleagues (1974) have suggested that fibrin is present secondary to an immunologic reaction. Other investigators have not consistently found immunoglobulins or fibrin-like material in renal biopsy specimens (Spargo et al., 1976). It is possible that differences can be accounted for by methodology. Kincaid-Smith and co-workers, using fixing techniques designed to maintain antigenicity of the deposits, demonstrated deposition of fibrinogen, IgA, IgG, IgM, complement, and albumin (Kincaid-Smith, 1991).

The glomerular lesion, although not pathognomonic, is highly characteristic of preeclampsia. The more likely the diagnosis of preeclampsia, the more common the glomerular lesion. Thus, characteristic glomerular changes are present in 70 per cent of primiparas but in only 14 per cent of multiparas diagnosed as preeclamptic (McCartney, 1964). In addition, as the clinical condition worsens, the magnitude of the glomerular lesion also increases. The glomerular lesions are reversible after delivery and are not present in repeat biopsy specimens obtained 5 to 10 weeks later (Pollak and Nettles, 1960).

The glomerular changes described correlate more consistently with proteinuria than with hypertension, suggesting that the proteins identified immunohistochemically might simply be trapped in the glomerulus. These staining patterns, however, are not characteristic of findings in other renal disorders in which proteinuria is present.

NONGLOMERULAR CHANGES. Pathologic changes in renal tubules are less consistently or less frequently described than those in glomeruli. Changes described by several investigators include dilatation of proximal tubules with thinning of the epithelium (Sheehan and Lynch, 1973), tubular necrosis (Pollak and Nettles, 1960), enlargement of the juxtaglomerular apparatus (Altchek et al., 1968), and hyaline deposition in renal

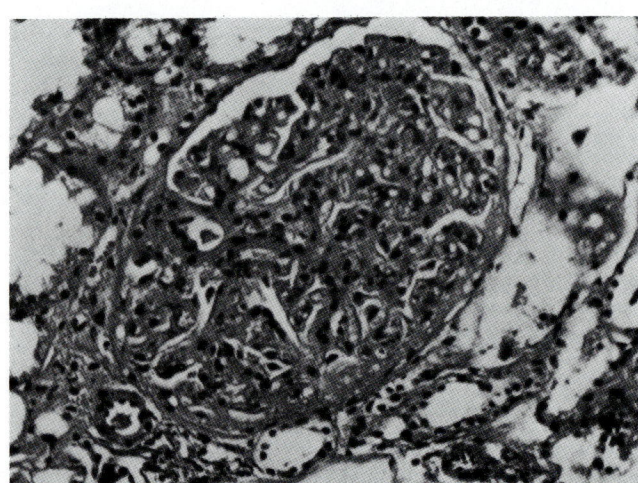

FIGURE 49–5. Glomerular changes in preeclampsia light microscopy. The enlarged glomerulus completely fills Bowman's capsule. Diffuse edema of the glomerular wall is indicated by the vacuolated appearance. The visible capillary loops are extremely narrow, and there are virtually no red blood cells in the capillary tuft.

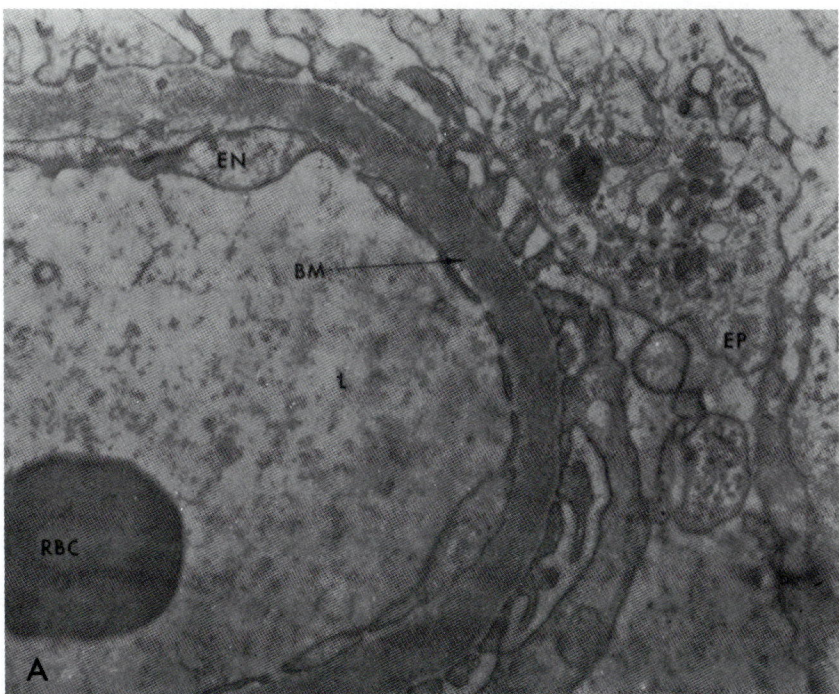

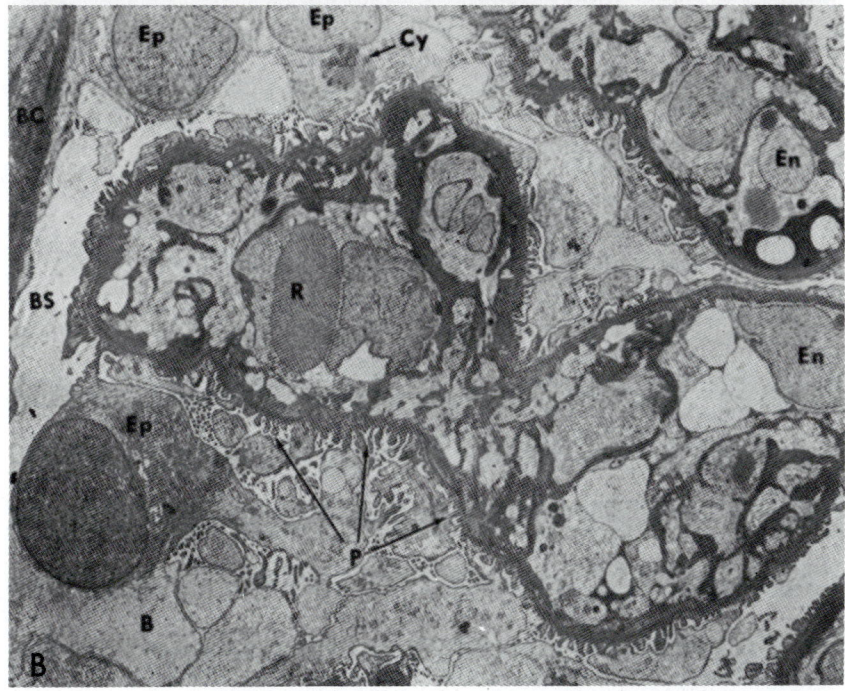

FIGURE 49–6. Electron photomicrographs of renal glomeruli. *A,* Normal anatomy. EN = capillary endothelial cells that line the glomeruli; L = the capillary lumen containing red blood cell (RBC); BM = basement membrane; Ep = renal epithelial cells. *B,* Biopsy specimen from a preeclamptic woman. Endothelial cells (En) are markedly enlarged, obstructing the capillary lumen, and contain electron-dense inclusions. The basement membrane is slightly thickened with inclusions, but the epithelial foot processes (P) are normal. R = red blood cell; P = podocytes; BS = Bowman's space; Cy = cytoplasmic inclusions. (From McCartney CP: Pathological anatomy of acute hypertension of pregnancy. Circulation **30**(Suppl II):37, 1964, by permission of the American Heart Association, Inc.)

tubules (Sheehan and Lynch, 1973). Fat deposition in women with prolonged heavy proteinuria has been reported by Sheehan and Lynch (1973). Altchek and co-workers (1968) described necrosis of the loop of Henle, a change that correlates with the degree of hyperuricemia and is also present in biopsy specimens from people with gout. It is possible that several of the other tubular changes described are also secondary to the glomerular pathophysiology.

Thickening of renal arterioles is also present in some patients with preeclampsia. It is more common in women with a known history of hypertension, and

unlike the glomerular lesion, it does not regress postpartum (Pollak and Nettles, 1960), suggesting that the arteriolar change is due to coincident disease rather than to preeclampsia.

Vascular Changes in the Placental Site

The characteristic changes in the decidual vessels supplying the placental site in normal pregnancy are described in Figure 49–7. In normal pregnancy the spiral arteries (Fig. 49–8) increase greatly in diameter (Ramsey and Harris, 1966). Morphologically, the en-

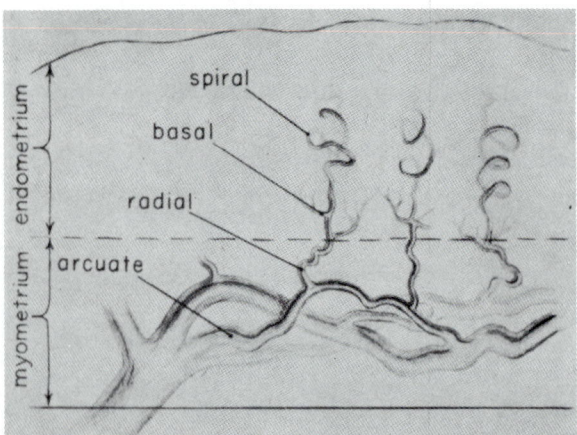

FIGURE 49–7. Schematic representation of uterine arteries. (From Okkels H, Engle ET: Studies of the finer structure of the uterine vessels of the Macacus monkey. Acta Pathol Microbiol Scand **15**:150, 1938.)

dothelium is replaced by trophoblast, and the internal elastic lamina and smooth muscle of the media are replaced by both trophoblast and an amorphous matrix containing fibrin (Brosens et al., 1972) (Fig. 49–8). These changes occur originally in the decidual portion of the spiral arteries, but extend into the myometrium as pregnancy advances and may even involve the distal portion of the uterine radial artery. The basal arteries are not affected. These morphologic changes are considered to be a vascular reaction to trophoblast that results in increased perfusion of the placental site.

In placental site vessels of women with preeclampsia, the normal physiologic changes do not occur or are limited to the decidual portion of the vessels; myometrial segments of spiral arteries in myometrium retain the nonpregnant component of intima and smooth muscle, and the diameter of these arteries is about 40 per cent that of vessels in normal pregnancy (Khong et al., 1986). In addition, some spiral arterioles in decidua and myometrium and some basal and radial arterioles are affected by a change termed acute atherosis (Zeek and Assali, 1950) (Fig. 49–9). The affected vessels are necrotic, and the usual components of the vessel wall are replaced by amorphous material and "foam cells." This lesion is best seen in basal arteries, because these arteries do not undergo the normal changes of pregnancy. It is also present in decidual and myometrial spiral arteries and may progress to vessel obliteration. The obliterated vessels correspond to areas of placental infarction. Although some believe that this change occurs only in preeclampsia, others hold that it is present in placental site vessels in pregnancies with fetal growth restriction and without clinical evidence of preeclampsia. Similar changes occur in decidual vessels of some diabetic women (Kitzmiller et al., 1981).

Investigators have reported changes characteristic of preeclampsia in the decidual vessels of approximately 14 per cent of primiparous women and a lower percentage of multiparous women at the time of first-trimester abortion (Nadji and Sommers, 1973; Lichtig

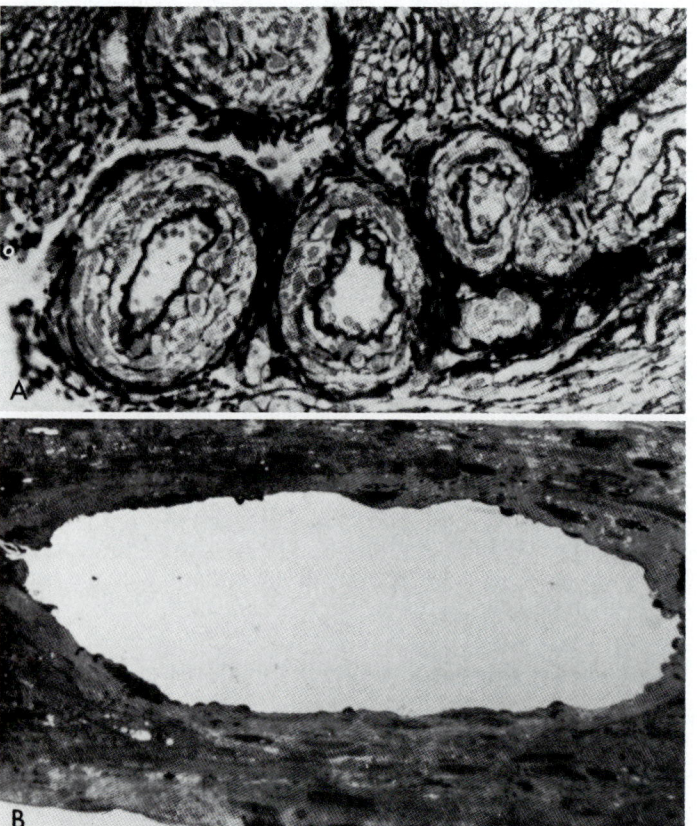

FIGURE 49–8. Spiral arterial changes in normal pregnancy. *A*, Section of spiral arterioles at the junction of endometrium and myometrium in a nonpregnant individual; note inner elastic lamina and smooth muscle. *B*, Section of spiral arteriole in the same scale and from the same location during pregnancy; note markedly increased diameter and absence of inner elastic lamina and smooth muscle. (From Sheppard BL, Bonnar J: Uteroplacental arteries and hypertensive pregnancy. *In* Bonnar J, MacGillivray I, Symonds G (eds): Pregnancy Hypertension. Baltimore, University Park Press, 1980.)

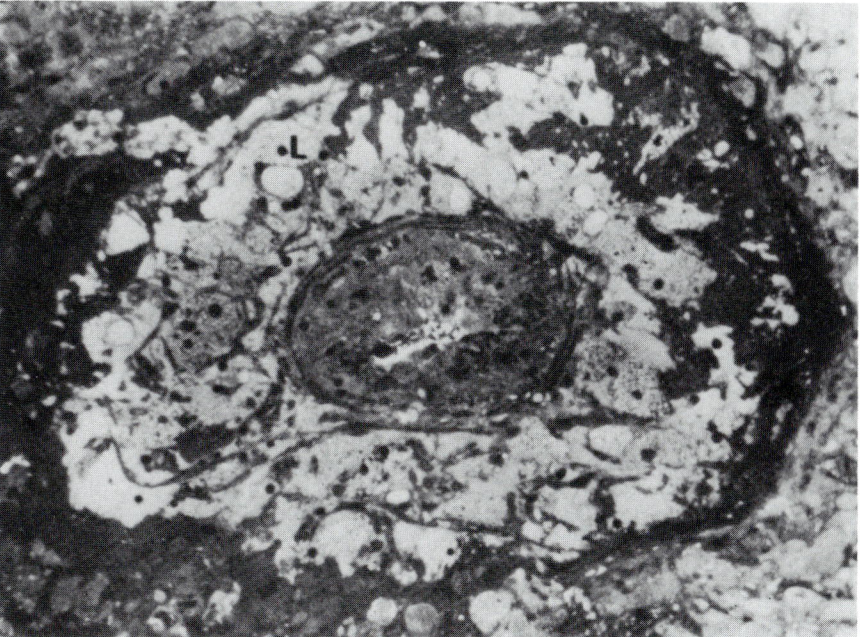

FIGURE 49–9. Atherosis: Numerous lipid-laden cells (*L*) and fibrin deposition (*F*) are present in the media of this occluded decidual vessel. (From Sheppard BL, Bonnar J: Uteroplacental arteries and hypertensive pregnancy. *In* Bonnar J, MacGillivray I, Symonds G (eds): Pregnancy Hypertension. Baltimore, University Park Press, 1980.)

et al., 1985). This finding indicates that preeclampsia may be a disorder of placentation and that characteristic pathologic changes preceded the clinical presentation of this disorder. The etiology of the decidual vascular lesions is not known. The appearance of these vessels is somewhat similar to that of vessels in transplanted kidneys that have undergone rejection. This suggestion of an immunologic etiology is supported by the finding of Kitzmiller and Benirschke (1973), who demonstrated components of complement (C3) in decidual vessels with the lesion.

Placental Pathologic Changes

Ultrastructural examination of placentas from preeclamptics provides details about the pathologic changes. The syncytiotrophoblast is abnormal, containing areas of cell death and degeneration. Viable-appearing syncytiotrophoblast is also abnormal, with decreased density of microvilli, dilated endoplasmic reticulum, and evidence of decreased pinocytotic and secretory activity. The cells of the villous cytotrophoblast cells are increased in number and have higher mitotic activity. The basement membrane of the trophoblast is irregularly thickened, with fine fibrillary inclusions (Jones and Fox, 1980).

The etiology of these anatomic changes is speculative. Similar syncytiotrophoblastic changes are present in placental segments maintained under hypoxic conditions *in vitro* (Fox, 1970). The cytotrophoblastic alterations are also consistent with hypoxia. The cytotrophoblast comprises the stem cells of the trophoblast and responds to damage by proliferation. Although most of the findings are consistent with hypoxia secondary to poor perfusion being the cause of placental change, there is at least one finding suggesting that other factors may be involved. Even though the cytotrophoblastic cells in most instances proliferate, there are also areas in which cytotrophoblast, resistant to

hypoxia *in vitro*, is seen to be degenerating adjacent to normal syncytiotrophoblast, which is very susceptible to hypoxia. This evidence suggests either the absence of a factor other than oxygen that is required more by cytotrophoblast than by syncytiotrophoblast or the presence of factors specifically toxic to cytotrophoblast.

Pathologic Changes in Other Organs

Subendocardial hemorrhages are present in over one-half of women who die of eclampsia. These are located primarily on the left side of the intraventricular septum. Hemorrhage rarely extends into myocardial tissue (Sheehan and Lynch, 1973). In character and location, these hemorrhages are identical to those found in patients dying of hypovolemic shock.

Histologic changes in adrenal tissue obtained inadvertently at percutaneous renal biopsy reveal areas of necrosis and hemorrhage. This observation is in keeping with the changes in adrenals of women dying of eclampsia that were described by Sheehan and Lynch (1973), who noted ischemic cortical changes in approximately one-half of cases.

Summary

Structural changes associated with preeclampsia-eclampsia lead to two important conclusions. First, preeclampsia is not merely an alternate form of malignant hypertension. The renal changes in preeclamptic and eclamptic women and the structural changes in other organs of women dying of eclampsia are quite different from the alterations caused by malignant hypertension. Second, the pathologic findings indicate that the pathogenetic factor of primary importance is not blood pressure elevation, but rather poor tissue perfusion. The histologic data support the clinical impression that the poor perfusion is secondary to profound vasospasm, which also increases total peripheral resistance and blood pressure.

Pathophysiologic Changes

As emphasized in the discussion of signs and symptoms, preeclampsia can cause changes in virtually all organ systems. Several organ systems are consistently and characteristically involved. They are discussed in detail, as they have been extensively studied and provide insight into the pathophysiologic changes in all organ systems.

Cardiovascular Changes

Blood pressure is the product of cardiac output (CO) and total peripheral resistance (TPR). Cardiac output is increased by up to 50 per cent in normal pregnancy, yet blood pressure does not usually increase. As mentioned previously, blood pressure is, in fact, lower during the first half of pregnancy than in the postpartum period, when cardiac output subsides toward nonpregnant levels (see Fig. 49–1). Thus, during normal pregnancy TPR decreases. Although there is some controversy about the status of cardiac output in women with severe preeclampsia (Easterling et al., 1990), the majority of studies of untreated preeclamptic women indicate that cardiac output is normal or slightly reduced (Wallenburg, 1988). Therefore, increased TPR must account for the increase in blood pressure.

There is considerable direct evidence that arteriolar narrowing occurs in preeclampsia. Changes in the caliber of retinal arterioles correlate with the clinical severity of the disorder and with renal biopsy diagnosis of preeclampsia (Pollak and Nettles, 1960). Similar findings are present in vessels of the nail bed and conjunctiva. Measurements of forearm blood flow indicate higher resistance in preeclamptic than in normal pregnant women (Spetz, 1965; Duncan et al., 1968). It is unlikely that this effect is determined by the autonomic nervous system. Although normal pregnant women are exquisitely sensitive to interruption of autonomic neurotransmission by ganglionic blockade and high spinal anesthesia, preeclamptic women are actually less sensitive (Assali and Prystowsky, 1950), suggesting that the arteriolar constriction of preeclampsia is not maintained by the autonomic nervous system and implicating humoral factors.

Assays of concentrations of recognized endogenous vasoconstrictors are limited to determinations of catecholamines and angiotensin II. Results of early studies of urinary catecholamine excretion were inconsistent and difficult to interpret, probably owing to the effect on catecholamine excretion of the renal function changes known to occur in preeclampsia. The limited studies of circulating plasma catecholamines are not subject to the same criticism, because endogenous catecholamines are rapidly metabolized (half-life 30 sec), and renal excretion is a minimal component of catecholamine degradation. Although some studies have found slightly elevated concentrations of circulating catecholamines (Oian et al., 1985), the results in

several studies are quite inconsistent (Poland and Lucas, 1980; Sammour et al., 1980).

Angiotensin II is a potent vasoconstrictor. Nevertheless, serum concentrations of angiotensin II are increased during normal pregnancy. Circulating levels in preeclamptic women, however, have been reported to be increased (Symonds et al., 1976), decreased (Weir et al., 1971), or unchanged (Gordon et al., 1973).

Endothelin-1, a vasoconstrictor produced by endothelial cells, is increased in the blood of preeclamptic women (Taylor et al., 1990). However, concentrations present in these women are much lower than those necessary to stimulate vascular smooth muscle contraction *in vitro*. Whether these circulating concentrations reflect endothelial production sufficient to stimulate vasoconstriction at the site of production, or whether low concentrations of endothelin may potentiate contractile responses to other agonists in preeclampsia will remain speculative until the availability of specific endothelin antagonists.

As indicated by the older term *toxemia*, early investigators suspected that preeclampsia was caused by circulating humors. Several investigators have reported finding pressor substances in blood, decidual extracts, placental extracts, and amniotic fluid of preeclamptic patients, but the results of their studies have been inconsistent and unreproducible. The explanation for the pressor effects was, in some studies, normal endogenous pressors, and in others, faulty methodology and failure to recognize the immunologic difference between the source of the extract and the animals tested. In other experiments, no defect is obvious. At present, probably appropriately, the hypothesis that arteriolar constriction of preeclampsia is caused by new circulating pressors has largely been abandoned (Chesley, 1978).

An alternative explanation for vasospasm in preeclampsia is greater response to normal concentrations of endogenous pressors. Preeclamptic women have higher sensitivity to all endogenous pressors thus far tested. They are exquisitely sensitive to vasopressin (Dieckman and Michel, 1937; Chesley and Valenti, 1958a). Vasopressin can elicit marked blood pressure elevation, seizures, and oliguria in some patients (Dieckman and Michel, 1937). Sensitivity to epinephrine (Zuspan et al., 1964) and norepinephrine (Talledo et al., 1968) is also increased (Fig. 49–10). The most striking difference is seen in the sensitivity of the preeclamptic woman to angiotensin II. Normal pregnant women are less sensitive to angiotensin II than nonpregnant women, requiring approximately two-and-a-half times as much angiotensin to raise their blood pressure a similar increment (Schwarz and Retzke, 1971). Preeclamptic women are much more sensitive to angiotensin II than normal pregnant and nonpregnant women (Talledo et al., 1968), having a striking difference in dose response (Fig. 49–11).

Angiotensin II sensitivity increases many weeks before the development of elevated blood pressure (Fig. 49–12) (Gant et al., 1973). Although resistance to angiotensin II does not decrease to nonpregnant levels until 32 weeks gestation, as early as 14 weeks there are significant differences in sensitivity between women who later become hypertensive and those who remain normotensive.

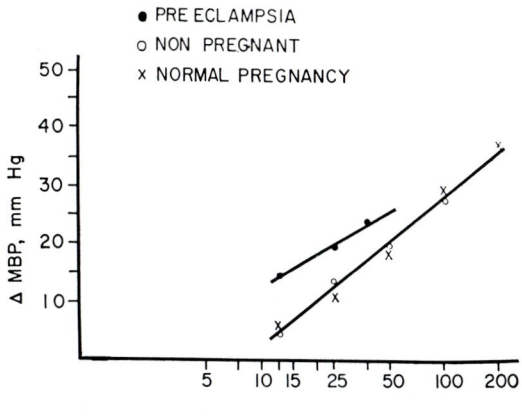

FIGURE 49-10. Mean dose-response lines to norepineph-rine. (From Talledo OE, Chesley LC, Zuspan FP: Renin-angiotensin system in normal and toxemic pregnancies. III: Differential sensitivity to angiotensin II and norepinephrine in toxemia of pregnancy. Am J Obstet Gynecol **100**:218, 1968.)

The decreased sensitivity of normal pregnant women to angiotensin II and the lower TPR in normal pregnancy suggest that arteriolar narrowing in pre-eclamptic women may be the result of decreased vasodilator substances, either circulating or local, rather than of increased circulating pressors. However, this attractive hypothesis is not consistent with the unchanged sensitivities to norepinephrine, epinephrine, and vasopressin in normal pregnancy (Talledo et al., 1968; Zuspan et al., 1964; Dieckman and Michel, 1937).

Coagulation Changes

The syndrome of disseminated intravascular coagulation (DIC) occurs in preeclampsia and has been suggested as a primary pathogenetic factor (McKay, 1972) (also see Chapter 53). The activation of the coagulation system is manifested as the intravascular

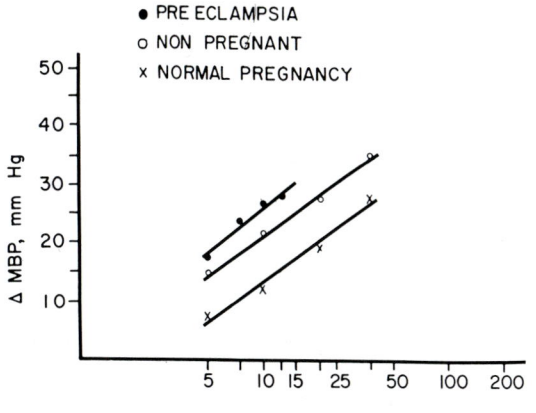

FIGURE 49-11. Mean dose-response lines to angiotensin. (From Talledo OE, Chesley LC, Zuspan FP: Renin-angiotensin system in normal and toxemic pregnancies. III: Differential sensitivity to angiotensin II and norepinephrine in toxemia of pregnancy. Am J Obstet Gynecol **100**:218, 1968.)

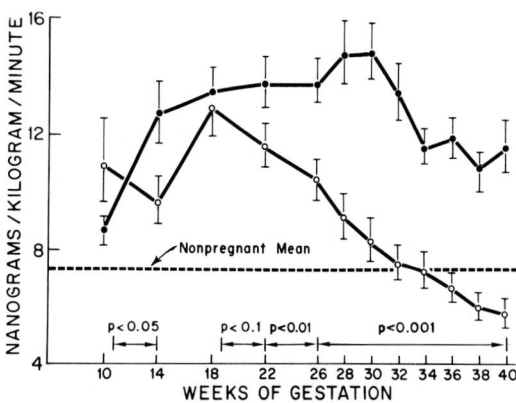

FIGURE 49-12. Angiotensin sensitivity throughout pregnancy: Comparison of the dose of angiotensin II necessary to increase diastolic blood pressure 20 mm Hg in women who developed elevated blood pressure in late pregnancy (o) and those who remained normotensive (•) demonstrates that a significantly lower dose was required in the former group as early as 10 to 14 weeks of gestation. (From Gant NF, Daley GL, Chand S, et al: A study of angiotensin II pressor response throughout primigravid pregnancy. Reproduced from the Journal of Clinical Investigation, 1973, Vol 49, pp 82–86, by copyright permission of the American Society for Clinical Investigation.)

disappearance of procoagulants, the intravascular appearance of degradation products of fibrin, and end-organ damage secondary to the formation of micro-thrombi (Bell, 1980). In the most advanced form of DIC, procoagulants—especially fibrinogen and platelets—decrease to a degree sufficient to produce spontaneous hemorrhage. In milder forms, only highly sensitive indicators of clotting system activation are present. Decreasing platelet concentrations is such a sign, but is usually evident in early cases only if platelet count has been followed serially. An elevated level of fibrin degradation products is a sensitive indicator of intravascular coagulation. This and other sensitive indicators of intravascular coagulation such as increased platelet turnover (Inglis et al., 1982), reduced platelet content (Douglas et al., 1982), increased platelet content in plasma (Socol et al., 1985), reduced levels of antithrombin III (Weiner and Brandt, 1985), and a reduced ratio of factor VIII activity to factor VIII antigen (Denson, 1977) are frequently present when concentrations of procoagulants remain normal.

Abnormalities of blood coagulation sufficient clinically to diagnose disseminated intravascular coagulation are present in approximately 10 per cent of patients with severe preeclampsia or eclampsia (Roberts and May, 1976). Levels of procoagulants are normal in the majority of patients with preeclampsia, suggesting that coagulation changes are secondary, rather than primary, pathogenetic factors (Pritchard et al., 1976). Results of highly sensitive assays of coagulation activation suggest, however, that abnormalities of the coagulation system are present in many patients with mild-to-moderate preeclampsia. Fibrin degradation products in plasma are reported to be a common occurrence in mild-to-moderate preeclampsia by some authors (Beller et al., 1979; McKillop et al., 1976;

Henderson et al., 1970), but not by others (Gordon et al., 1976). The differing results probably reflect different assay specificities and sensitivities. Redman and co-workers (1978) performed serial platelet counts in women at risk for preeclampsia and found a decrease in platelets coinciding with the appearance of clinical signs of the disease. Similarly, subtle signs of platelet dysfunction (Inglis et al., 1982; Douglas et al., 1982; Socol et al., 1985) and reduced antithrombin III (Weiner and Brandt, 1985) and reduction in the ratio of factor VIII bioactivity to factor VIII antigen (Redman et al., 1977a) are present in mild preeclampsia and may precede its clinical signs. Whether even the early appearance of coagulation changes indicates that activation of the clotting system is a primary pathogenetic factor has not been established because another early sign of preeclampsia, increased serum uric acid, may precede any measurable change in coagulation (Redman et al., 1978).

The etiology of the change in coagulation factors is a matter of controversy. Vascular damage secondary to vasospasm may initiate DIC (Pritchard et al., 1976). Although this phenomenon probably has a role in intensifying the activation of the clotting system in severe preeclampsia, its effect is less likely in the early changes preceding the occurrence of vasospasm sufficient to elevate blood pressure. It is also possible that vascular changes in the implantation site that appear to antedate blood pressure elevation may be pathogenetically important. Whether coagulation changes measured in preeclamptic patients are true DIC or a localized consumption of procoagulants in the intervillous space is not clear. Microthrombi and the presence of fibrin antigen have been demonstrated in liver, placenta, and kidney by some investigators (Arias and Muncilla-Jimenez, 1976; Matter and Faulk, 1980; Vassali et al., 1963), but not by others (Sheehan and Lynch, 1973). The early coagulation changes—factor VIII activity-antigen ratios and platelet count—correlate better with fetal outcome as measured by mortality and growth restriction rates than with clinical severity of preeclampsia. Identical coagulation changes are present in normotensive women with growth-restricted fetuses (Whigham et al., 1980). These findings suggest that localized coagulation in the intervillous space may be of major importance. Consistent with this theory is the finding of an increased concentration of fibrin antigen in the placentas of preeclamptics (Matter and Faulk, 1980).

Endothelial Cell Changes

ENDOTHELIAL INJURY. An increasing body of information indicates endothelial injury as a pathophysiologic component of preeclampsia (Roberts et al., 1989). As cited, alterations of glomerular endothelial cells are a consistent feature of preeclampsia. Endothelium from the umbilical arteries of infants of preeclamptic women also demonstrates profound cell disruption, with increased intracellular inclusions, vacuolization, and disruption of intercellular integrity (Dadak et al., 1984). In addition, cellular fibronectin (Lockwood and Peters, 1990; Taylor et al., 1991a), growth factors (Taylor et al., 1990), and factor VIII antigen, peptides

released from injured endothelial cells, are increased in preeclamptic women prior to the appearance of clinical disease (Redman et al., 1977a).

Serum from preeclamptic women alters endothelial cell function when applied to these cells *in vitro*. The release of cellular fibronectin (Taylor et al., 1991b), expression of PDGF B chain (Taylor et al., 1991c), uptake of triglycerides (Lorentzen et al., 1991), and release of ^{51}chromate from cells preloaded with this isotope (Rodgers et al., 1988) are all increased by serum obtained from preeclamptic women prior to delivery compared to effects of serum from the same women postpartum or from normal pregnant women. Although the identity of the factor causing this alteration in function is not established, an attractive hypothesis is that many of these changes could be secondary to oxidative stress and the generation of lipid peroxides (Hubel et al., 1989). Lipid peroxide concentrations are increased in the blood of preeclamptic women (Hubel et al., 1989) in association with reduced antioxidant activity, but not in normal pregnant women (Davidge et al., 1992).

It is now evident that endothelium is a complex tissue with many important functions. Two of these, prevention of coagulation and modulation of vascular tone, have special relevance to preeclampsia. Intact vascular endothelium is resistant to thrombus formation (Rodgers et al., 1983). With vascular injury, endothelial cells can initiate coagulation either by the intrinsic pathway (contact activation) (Wiggins et al., 1980) or by the extrinsic pathway (tissue factor) (Maynard et al., 1987). Platelet adhesion can also occur after injury with exposure of subendothelial components, such as collagen (Baumgartner and Hardenschild, 1977) and microfibrils.

Endothelium also profoundly influences the response of vascular smooth muscle to vasoactive agents. The response to some agents (Furchgott, 1983) can change from dilator to constrictor with the removal of endothelium (one of the changes present in the umbilical vessels of infants of preeclamptic women). Prostacyclin, a very potent vasodilator, is produced by endothelium. Studies show that vessels from preeclamptic women and the umbilical vessels of their neonates generate less prostacyclin than similar vessels from normal pregnant women (Remuzzi et al., 1980; Bussolino et al., 1980; Dadak et al., 1982). A role for prostacyclin in affecting vascular sensitivity is especially relevant to preeclampsia. If potent inhibitors preventing the synthesis of all prostaglandins (including prostacyclin) are administered to pregnant women, the usual resistance to the vasoconstrictor effect of angiotensin II is abolished (Everett et al., 1978). Conversely, if aspirin is used as an inhibitor of prostaglandin synthesis in a manner determined to specifically reduce contractile prostanoids (thromboxane A_2) much more than prostacyclin, the increased angiotensin II sensitivity of preeclamptic women is reduced (Sanchez-Ramos et al., 1987). Nitric oxide (NO, previously known as endothelium-releasing factor (EDRF)), is another bioactive material produced by normal endothelium (Moncada et al., 1991). Its release is stimulated by several hormones and neurotransmitters as well as by hydrodynamic shear stress. NO is quite labile and acts synergistically with prostacyclin as a local vasodilator and inhibitor of platelet aggregation. Production of NO is reduced with endothelial cell injury. Although no information is currently available on production of nitric oxide by endothelial cells of preeclamptic women, production by umbilical vessels of infants of preeclamptic women is reduced (Pinto et al., 1991).

The information currently available indicates that endothelial cell damage can alter both vascular responses and intravascular coagulation in a manner consistent with the pathophysiologic abnormalities present in preeclampsia. Thus, evidence is accumulating that endothelial injury may play a central role in the pathogenesis of preeclampsia.

Renal Function Changes

Renal function changes are consistent and characteristic in women with preeclampsia-eclampsia. Glomerular function changes, manifested by decreased glomerular filtration rate (GFR) and proteinuria, are common findings. Tubular handling of certain substances is abnormal, although other materials apparently are handled normally. Changes in components of the renin-angiotensin system are probably different from those seen in normal pregnancy. Sodium excretion is decreased, resulting in fluid retention and edema.

Glomerular Functional Changes

GLOMERULAR FILTRATION RATE (GFR). Decreased glomerular filtration frequently, but not inevitably, complicates preeclampsia. The decreased GFR is explained only partially by decreased renal plasma flow (RPF), and thus the filtration fraction, GFR/RPF, is decreased (Chesley, 1978). It is possible that the change in the filtration fraction is due to intrarenal redistribution of blood flow, which unfortunately is difficult to test (Hollenberg et al., 1968). A more obvious explanation is that the change is due to glomeruloendotheliosis, in which the occlusion of glomerular capillaries by swollen endothelial cells probably renders many glomeruli nonfunctional.

PROTEIN "LEAKAGE." The pathogenesis of proteinuria in preeclampsia involves primarily glomerular changes. The normal absence of protein from urine is due both to a relative impermeability of glomeruli to large protein molecules and to the tubular reabsorption of smaller proteins that cross the glomeruli. As glomerular damage occurs, permeability to proteins increases. As damage increases, so does the size of the protein molecule that can cross the glomerular membrane. This increase in permeability results in a decrease in selectivity; that is, with minimal glomerular damage or tubular dysfunction, only small protein molecules are excreted, but with greater damage, both large and small proteins are present in urine. In preeclampsia selectivity is low, indicating increased permeability and glomerular damage (Katz and Berlyne, 1974). It is a familiar clinical observation, however, that proteinuria increases and decreases in preeclamptic women. The pattern was quantitated by

Chesley (1938), who found that there was a great variability from hour to hour in the ratio of creatinine to protein in urine of women with preeclampsia that was not present in the urine of individuals with other diseases causing proteinuria. Because structural glomerular changes are obviously constant, proteinuria in preeclamptic women must depend in part on a varying functional cause, for example a variation in the intensity of the renal vascular spasm. That vascular spasm can cause proteinuria has been demonstrated by measuring urinary excretion of protein in individuals subjected to the cold pressor test. Immersing a patient's hand in ice water for 60 seconds increases blood pressure more than 16 mm Hg systolic and diastolic, and an increase in protein excretion almost invariably also occurs (Chesley et al., 1939).

Renal Tubular Functional Changes

URIC ACID CLEARANCE. Three separate processes are involved in the renal excretion of urate. Urate is completely filtered at the glomerulus. It is not bound to plasma proteins under physiologic conditions (Farrell et al., 1974), and glomerular urate concentration is equal to renal arterial plasma concentration. Urate is both secreted and reabsorbed by renal tubules. Most urate (98 per cent) is reabsorbed, and excreted urate is about 80 per cent accounted for by urate secretion. Both of these processes occur predominantly in the proximal tubule. Reabsorption occurs to a greater extent than secretion, and so urate clearance is about 10 per cent of creatinine clearance (Emmerson, 1974).

Abnormalities of uric acid clearance have long been recognized as a consistent phenomenon in preeclampsia (Stander and Cadden, 1934) and have been regarded as a function of decreased glomerular filtration (Schaffer et al., 1943). Several studies have demonstrated the discrepancy between uric acid clearance and both inulin clearance and creatinine clearance (Seitchik, 1953; Hayashi, 1956). Serial studies also reveal that decreased uric acid clearance precedes decreases in GFR (Gallery and Györy, 1979a).

The etiology of the tubular change that results in decreased uric acid clearance is attributed to the lactic acidosis believed to be present in preeclamptic patients (Handler, 1960). Lactic acid infusion will decrease uric acid clearance (Yu et al., 1957), but the clearance of uric acid is frequently decreased in preeclamptic women who have normal acid-base balance and normal lactate levels (Fadel et al., 1976). Urate clearance is also decreased by hypovolemia, presumably as a result of nonspecific stimulation of proximal tubular reabsorption (Suki et al., 1967). Plasma volume depletion is coincident with urate clearance changes (Gallery et al., 1980b), suggesting that volume change may account for the abnormality in urate clearance. However, there is a poor correlation between the degree of volume depletion and the decrease in urate clearance (Gallery et al., 1980b).

Angiotensin II infusion decreases urate clearance even in the presence of normal blood volume (Ferris and Gordon, 1968). The increase in angiotensin II sensitivity seen in preeclampsia might account for the change in renal function. Local effects of angiotensin

II might also be important, because this substance can be produced locally (Sokabe, 1974), unassociated with increased circulating angiotensin II. Furthermore, although circulating lactate concentration cannot explain changes in uric acid excretion, local changes in lactate could be involved. Lactate concentration is greater in the renal medulla than in the renal cortex, presumably owing to greater anaerobic metabolism (Dell and Winters, 1967). The gradient of increasing lactate from cortex to medulla is matched by an increasing gradient of uric acid (Cannon et al., 1970). Renal ischemia increases renal medullary lactic acid and could thus explain changes in urate clearance without associated changes in circulating lactic acid levels.

In summary, uric acid clearance changes earlier in preeclamptic pregnancy than does GFR, suggesting a tubular rather than a glomerular functional explanation. Furthermore, although the exact mechanism for the urate clearance change is not established, the common feature in the suggested mechanisms is decreased renal perfusion, although increased production by poorly perfused tissue cannot be excluded (Parks and Granger, 1986).

URINARY CONCENTRATING CAPACITY. Although there are some problems with studies of increased urinary osmolality in response to water restriction during pregnancy, several investigations have concluded that tubular concentrating capacity is unchanged in normal pregnancy (Kaitz, 1961). Assali and co-workers (1953) suggested that urinary concentrating ability is decreased in hypertensive women. The limitations of these studies include the failure to account for parallel changes in concentrating capacity and GFR (Steele et al., 1969) and the use of specific gravity—an unreliable estimate of osmolality—as the measure of concentration (Chesley, 1978).

In one study evaluating the response to Pitressin administration, normal pregnant women were found to have decreased capacity to concentrate urine (measured as osmolar concentration and corrected for GFR); this decrease was similar to that seen in pregnant women who either were or were destined to become hypertensive (Gallery and Györy, 1979b). Differences between these findings and those of other studies suggesting that tubular concentrating capacity is normal in normal pregnancy probably reflect the failure in other studies to correct for the increased GFR of normal pregnancy, which concomitantly increases concentrating capacity (Steele et al., 1969).

PSP EXCRETION. There are few studies that directly assay tubular function. Phenolsulfonphthalein (PSP) is secreted by proximal tubular cells, and its excretion can be used as a sensitive indicator of proximal tubular function (Gallery and Györy, 1979a). This technique has a number of potential limitations. PSP excretion is altered independent of tubular secretory capacity with increased (Ochwadt and Pitts, 1956) or decreased (Heidland and Reidl, 1968) renal plasma flow, or reduced GFR (Healy et al., 1964), and with increased urinary dead space (an especially pertinent problem in pregnancy). However, when these factors are carefully controlled, reduced PSP excretion indicating abnormal proximal tubular function precedes both changes in GFR and clinically evident disease (Gallery and Györy, 1979a).

Renin-Angiotensin-Aldosterone System

The renin-angiotensin-aldosterone system is an important factor in pressure and volume regulation in normal pregnancy (Ehrlich and Lindheimer, 1972). The components of the renin-angiotensin-aldosterone system in normal pregnancy (Fig. 49–13) have been extensively examined. The components of the system as evaluated by different assays are presented in Table 49–4.

Dramatic changes occur in the renin-angiotensin system during pregnancy (Bay and Ferris, 1979). There are increases in renin substrate, plasma renin activity (PRA) (Weir et al., 1971), plasma renin concentration (PRC), angiotensin II concentration (Gordon et al., 1973; Weir et al., 1971), and aldosterone (Bay and Ferris, 1979). The theory that abnormalities of the renin-angiotensin system may be causal factors in preeclampsia is suggested by (1) the potent vasoconstrictor effect of angiotensin II, (2) the effect of angiotensin II on aldosterone secretion and consequent sodium retention, and (3) the finding that large doses of the substance can cause proteinuria (Langford and Pickering, 1965). This etiologic possibility is further supported by the observation that myometrium and chorion have the capacity to synthesize renin, which is stimulated in experimental animals by uterine ischemia (Ferris et al., 1972).

Most but not all studies agree that renin substrate remains elevated in preeclampsia (Tapia et al., 1972; Weir et al., 1971). There are reports that PRA is increased (Symonds et al., 1976), decreased, and unchanged (Skinner et al., 1972). The same is true of PRC, angiotensin II, and aldosterone concentration. These differences are probably methodologic in origin. PRA and PRC are influenced by posture and sodium intake, and in some studies, hospitalized patients at bed rest have been compared with ambulatory normotensive patients. In many studies, sodium intake has not been controlled. Pregnant women have a high concentration of "pro-renin," which is activated by acid hydrolysis (Skinner et al., 1972); this determination was used in the past by several investigators to inactivate renin substrate in the assay of PRC. Also, pregnant women have a component of renin that is activated by low temperatures (Rowe et al., 1979), and the laboratory practice of storing many samples on ice for different lengths of time prior to assay undoubtedly has affected results.

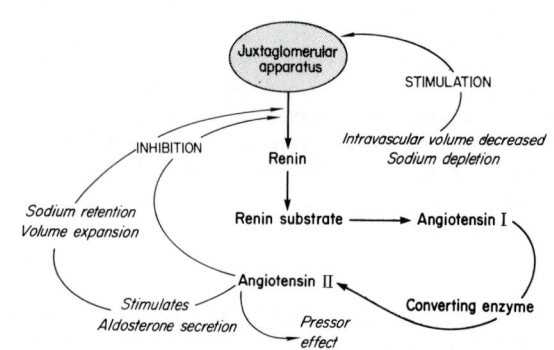

FIGURE 49–13. Schematic representation of the renin-angiotensin system.

TABLE 49–4. Evaluation of Renin-Angiotensin System

TEST	METHOD*	RESULTS DETERMINED BY ENDOGENOUS CONCENTRATIONS OF
Plasma renin activity (PRA)	Incubate plasma and angiotensinase inhibitors	Renin, renin substrate, activators, inhibitors
Plasma renin substrate (PRS)	Incubate plasma, angiotensinase inhibitors, and excess exogenous renin	Renin substrate, activators, inhibitors
Plasma renin concentration (PRC)	Incubate plasma, angiotensinase inhibitors, and excess exogenous substrate	Renin, activators, inhibitors

*All tests use generated angiotensin I or II as the end point.

In a prospective study of chronically hypertensive women in whom posture was controlled and blood collected to avoid cryoactivation, PRA was lower in women in whom superimposed preeclampsia developed (diagnostic blood pressure increase and proteinuria) than in chronic hypertensive women without superimposed preeclampsia or normal pregnant women. Interestingly, values were similar in early pregnancy in all groups and decreased slightly prior to increased blood pressure (August et al., 1990).

In contrast, there is a very strong correlation between diastolic pressure and angiotensin II concentration at all levels of blood pressure in primiparas but not in multiparas (Symonds et al., 1976). Interestingly, there is an inverse relationship between PRA and angiotensin II levels, suggesting that angiotensin II suppresses renin production and, by extrapolation, that PRA is inversely related to diastolic blood pressure.

Attempts to test the role of the renin-angiotensin system by using angiotensin II antagonists or by converting enzyme inhibitors have not, as yet, clarified this point. Administration of the angiotensin antagonist (1-Sar 8 Ile angiotensin II) to pregnant hypertensive women increases blood pressure (Saruta et al., 1981), and because this antagonist is a partial agonist, the increase in blood pressure may perhaps reflect the increased angiotensin sensitivity of hypertensive pregnant women. The administration of either the angiotensin antagonist saralasin (Pipkin et al., 1980) or the converting enzyme inhibitor SQ 20,881 (Sullivan et al., 1978) in the postpartum period has not had significant effects on blood pressure in a mixed group of hypertensive women.

Studies of the renin-angiotensin system in pregnancy are inconclusive. It is clear that no simple relationship exists between components of the renin-angiotensin system and preeclampsia. However, the significance of even unchanged PRA, PRC, and angiotensin II level on blood pressure and sodium excretion in this group of women, who are apparently volume-constricted and exquisitely sensitive to angiotensin II, requires and deserves elucidation.

Atrial Natriuretic Factor

Atrial natriuretic factor (ANF) is a peptide produced primarily in response to atrial stretch with hypervolemia, which regulates intravascular volume by several mechanisms. Among other functions, ANF increases sodium excretion and the egress of fluid from the intravascular compartment. Although the reduced plasma volume of preeclampsia predicts reduced ANF concentration, the concentration is increased (Bond et al., 1989), and this increase precedes clinical disease (Malee et al., 1992). The stimulus for this increase is unclear; however the paradoxical finding of increased circulating ANF and reduced renin concentration with reduced plasma volume in preeclamptic women raises the possibility that this reduced plasma volume is actually increased relative to the constricted vascular compartment.

Changes in Sodium Excretion

Sodium retention has long been considered an integral part of the pathophysiology of preeclampsia. Eclamptic and severely preeclamptic women have very little chloride and sodium in their urine (Zangmeister, 1903). After delivery, however, chloride excretion increases dramatically. Infusion of hypertonic saline into preeclamptic women results in excretion of the infused sodium at about one-half the rate seen in normal pregnant women (Chesley et al., 1958b). Similar results are obtained in women with a renal biopsy diagnosis of glomeruloendotheliosis (Sarles et al., 1968). The majority of studies of exchangeable sodium have indicated an increase in total body sodium in preeclamptic patients (Dieckman et al., 1957; Chesley, 1966).

The etiology of sodium retention in preeclamptic women is difficult to determine, owing to the enormous number of factors that influence sodium excretion in normal pregnancy and, in part, to the many demonstrated anomalies of renal function in preeclampsia that may cause sodium retention (Table 49–5). Any or all of the demonstrated changes in plasma volume, angiotensin sensitivity, and renal function may act on several of the factors listed in Table 49–5 to cause sodium retention. Several investigators have considered the increased sodium retention to be a primary factor inciting the pathogenetic changes in preeclampsia. Although this possibility cannot be definitely excluded on the basis of sequential studies currently available, it is not likely for several reasons: First, angiotensin sensitivity precedes obvious fluid retention by months. Second, sequential studies of thiocyanate space, which is proportional to sodium space, have not indicated that an increase in this space is a valuable predictor of preeclampsia (Chesley and

TABLE 49–5. Factors Affecting Sodium Balance in Normal Pregnancy

Factors affecting glomerular filtration	Blood pressure in critical areas of the kidney
	Relative tonus of afferent and efferent glomerular arterioles
	Plasma oncotic pressure
	Intrarenal redistribution of blood flow
	CNS effects
Factors affecting tubular reabsorption	Aldosterone
	Progesterone (an aldosterone antagonist)
	Renal vascular resistance
	Perfusional pressure in peritubular capillaries
	Oncotic pressure in peritubular capillaries
	Nonreabsorbable anions in the filtrate
	Velocity of flow in tubules
	The reabsorptive capacity of tubules
	Estrogens (stimulate sodium reabsorption, possibly indirectly, through effects on vascular permeability)
	Plasma sodium concentration
	Hematocrit (viscosity effects)
	Changes of plasma volume
	Angiotensin
	Sympathetic nervous system
	Possibly a natriuretic hormone ("third factor")

From Chesley LC: Hypertensive Disorders in Pregnancy. New York, Appleton-Century-Crofts, 1978. Reprinted by permission.

Chesley, 1943). Third, attempts to prevent preeclampsia by restricting dietary sodium or by increasing sodium excretion with diuretics have had no salutary effect on the occurrence of preeclampsia (Weseley and Douglas, 1962; Flowers et al., 1962; Kraus et al., 1966).

Summary

Renal function changes in preeclampsia are consistent and characteristic. Recent investigations indicate that changes in tubular function precede the more widely appreciated changes in glomerular function. At present it appears that these functional changes return completely to normal weeks to months after the termination of pregnancy. Prospective sequential studies of renal function indicate that at least some of these changes antedate the clinical diagnosis of preeclampsia. They do not consistently antedate other sensitive indicators of preeclampsia such as changes in coagulation and plasma volume and are thus unlikely to be causal abnormalities. Although the etiology of these renal functional changes has not been precisely elucidated, they could all be explained by abnormalities of renal perfusion, either general or regional.

Immunologic Changes

Observed changes in components of the immune system and epidemiologic observations have suggested that immunologic changes have a pathogenetic role, and that perhaps fetal-maternal immunologic interactions are etiologically important, in the development of preeclampsia. The predominance of preeclampsia in first pregnancies and the protective effect even of miscarriage suggest a beneficial effect of maternal exposure to fetal antigen. The protective effect of previous pregnancy may be lost if the father is not the same man (Need, 1975). In addition, the exposure to the paternal components of fetal antigen through increased sexual activity preceding the first pregnancy also reduces the risk of preeclampsia (Marti and Herrman, 1977). The pathologic changes in decidual vessels at the placental site are very similar to the vascular changes of acute immunologic rejection (Kitzmiller and Benirschke, 1973).

Several immunologic mechanisms have been suggested (Redman, 1980; Scott and Beer, 1976). Preeclampsia may be an immune complex disease. There is an efflux of fetal antigen into the maternal circulation during pregnancy. If the maternal antibody response is adequate, the complexes are cleared by the reticuloendothelial system and no damage occurs. If the antibody response or clearance mechanisms are inadequate, the pathologic immune complexes thus formed would cause vasculitis, glomerular damage, and activation of the coagulation system. The postulated inadequacy of response might be due to an inadequate maternal antibody response, such as might, for example, occur in first pregnancies. The maternal antibody system could also be overwhelmed by an excess of fetal antigen, a condition compatible with the increased incidence of preeclampsia associated with increased amounts of trophoblastic tissue, as seen with twins, hydatidiform mole, and hydropic placenta. The data supporting this concept are few. The possibility that inadequate maternal antibody response may play a role in preeclampsia-eclampsia is indicated by HLA typing, which demonstrates an increased concordance of the major histocompatibility antigens in maternal-paternal pairs that result in preeclamptic pregnancies (Redman, 1980). The fact that preeclampsia is less common in consanguineous marriages, however, is incompatible with this concept (Stevenson, 1971). Actual measurements of immune complexes are inconsistent, because of widely differing methodologies, and although some studies have not demonstrated circulating immune complexes in preeclamptic pregnancy (Knox et al., 1978), other studies do indicate the presence of these complexes (Stirrat et al., 1978). Changes consistent with deposition of immune complex in the arterioles of the kidney (Petruccho et al., 1974), liver (Arias and Muncilla-Jimenez, 1976), and the uteroplacental bed (Kitzmiller and Benirschke, 1973) are described by some researchers. The evidence for increased consumption of complement, which would be predicted if preeclampsia were an immune complex disease, is also equivocal (Kitzmiller et al., 1973).

Another hypothesis of immunologic etiology is that the vascular changes in the spiral arterioles of the placental implantation site in preeclampsia are a consequence of an allograft rejection between mother and fetus, the question being who is rejecting whom (Redman, 1980)? Should the spiral arteries lined with trophoblast be thought of as fetal vessels, with the fetus rejecting the mother, or as maternal vessels, with the mother rejecting the fetus? If preeclampsia is a rejection of the fetus by the mother, the epidemiologic evidence of the protective effect of previous exposure to antigen would indicate that the preeclamptic mother has a deficit of blocking antibodies or of suppressor cell function. The recent recognition of a unique HLA antigen, HLA-G, on trophoblast (Kavats et al., 1990) raises other possible causes for rejection of the fetus. HLA-G is a class 1 antigen present almost exclusively on cytotrophoblast. Thus far, there has been no heterogeneity noted in the HLA-G antigen. Therefore, unlike classic HLA antigens, which exhibit numerous epitopes, fetal HLA-G in trophoblast is likely to be identical in most (all) fetuses and that of the fetus would be the same as that expressed by the mother during her fetal life. Since an immune cell found in maternal decidua in high numbers, the natural killer cell, is postulated to destroy cells not bearing HLA antigens, a reduced level of HLA-G could render the fetus a target for these cells. Also, unusual epitopes of HLA-G (thus far not recognized) could also activate maternal immune defenses.

The alternative postulate, that the fetus rejects the mother, requires that the preeclamptic woman is deficient in the capacity to destroy fetal immune cells. These alternative hypotheses—one requiring active intervention and the other passive intervention by the maternal immune system—should give disparate results in *in vitro* testing of maternal immune function. The experimental evidence currently available is not consistent enough to confirm or to contradict either hypothesis.

The hypothesis of an immunologic cause of preeclampsia is consistent with much we know about the disorder. The increased delineation of the changes in the immunologic activity in preeclampsia may well provide insight into the etiology of both preeclampsia and normal fetal-maternal compatibility during pregnancy. On the basis of available data, the relationship of the immune system to preeclampsia is speculative at present.

Prognosis for Mother and Infant in Preeclampsia

Perinatal Mortality Rate

The perinatal mortality rate is higher for infants of preeclamptic women (Plouin et al., 1986). Causes of perinatal death are placental insufficiency and abruptio placentae (Naeye and Friedman, 1979), which cause intrauterine death prior to or during labor, and prematurity. As one would expect, the mortality rate is higher in infants of women with more severe forms of the disorder. At any level of disease severity, the perinatal mortality rate is greatest in women with preeclampsia superimposed upon preexisting vascular disease (Lopez-Llera and Horta, 1972).

Growth restriction is more common in infants of preeclamptic women. As with perinatal mortality, intrauterine growth restriction is more common in infants of women with superimposed preeclampsia (Lopez-Llera and Horta, 1972). The dramatic decrease in perinatal mortality rate among infants of preeclamptic women in recent years results from more appropriate

medical and obstetric management (specifically, avoiding the use of profound maternal, and hence neonatal, sedation) and from the ability to assess fetal well-being in the antepartum and intrapartum periods. The primary impact on perinatal mortality rate, however, comes from improvements in neonatal care. It is important to remember that although neonatal survival rates have improved dramatically, delivery before 34 weeks gestation continues to be associated with an increased risk of long-range neurologic disability. The best obstetric management demands a decision for delivery that balances the risks of maternal and fetal mortality and long-range morbidity.

Maternal Mortality and Morbidity

Mortality

Maternal death in association with preeclampsia is due predominantly to complications of abruptio placentae, hepatic rupture, and most significant, eclampsia. The mortality rate of eclamptic women has been most dramatically affected by reduction of iatrogenic complications due to overmedication and overzealous approaches to vaginal delivery. In several series reported from the late 19th century, during which immediate delivery was the practice, the mortality rate of eclamptic women was 20 to 30 per cent. The advent of expectant management with profound maternal sedation with narcotics and hypnotics in the early 20th century was associated with a 10 to 15 per cent mortality rate. In the 1920s and 1930s the change to magnesium as the exclusive agent resulted in maternal mortality of 5 per cent. Although magnesium undoubtedly had a salutary effect, perhaps more important to the improvement was the decreased use of sedatives, because the protocols for magnesium administration in some series would have minimally increased serum magnesium concentration (Chesley, 1978).

The combination of timely delivery and use of magnesium sulfate and hydralazine as sole pharmacologic agents has been associated with a maternal mortality rate of virtually zero (Pritchard and Pritchard, 1975; Sibai et al., 1981), owing to an appreciation of the profound pathophysiologic abnormalities of preeclampsia and to careful cardiopulmonary monitoring. It is important to realize, however, that the largest improvement in survival can be attributed not to what was done, but rather to what was not done.

Later Consequences

Women with the clinical diagnosis of preeclampsia during one pregnancy have an increased chance of developing hypertension in subsequent pregnancies and fixed hypertension in later life. This is not surprising, because this diagnostic group includes women with pre-existing renal or cardiovascular disease. However, two questions important for clinical management must be answered. First, is the risk of recurrence of preeclampsia in subsequent pregnancies high enough and would the recurrence be severe enough to influence the decision for future pregnancies? Second, is there evidence that a hypertensive pregnancy adversely affects the long-range health of the mother? More specifically, does pregnancy accelerate the progression of underlying hypertensive or renal vascular disease, and does preeclampsia in women with normal cardiovascular and renal function cause damage leading to an increased incidence of cardiovascular morbidity, including hypertension, in later years?

RECURRENCE IN SUBSEQUENT PREGNANCIES. The recurrence of preeclampsia in a subsequent pregnancy is influenced by the certainty of the clinical diagnosis in the first pregnancy. Of 225 women with hypertension during pregnancy chosen for study without regard to parity, 70 per cent experienced recurrence in their next pregnancy (Berman, 1930). In a study of primiparas with severe preeclampsia, the recurrence rate was 45 per cent (Sibai et al., 1986). Because the diagnosis in both of these studies was based solely on clinical findings, these groups undoubtedly included patients with unrecognized preexisting blood pressure elevation or underlying renal or cardiovascular disease. Chesley (1980), in an attempt to minimize confusion of prognosis by conditions other than preeclampsia, has followed 270 women with eclampsia for more than 40 years, only two of whom have been lost to follow-up. Twenty women with eclampsia as multiparas had recurrent hypertension in 50 per cent of subsequent pregnancies. In 187 women who had eclampsia in their first pregnancy, only 33 per cent had some hypertensive disorder in any subsequent pregnancy. In the majority of women the condition was not severe in subsequent pregnancies, but 5 per cent did have recurrence of eclampsia. Thus, the woman with a clinical diagnosis of preeclampsia is at increased risk of a hypertensive disorder in subsequent pregnancies. The chances of recurrence decrease as the likelihood of true preeclampsia increases. If the condition does recur, it will usually not be worse, and if preeclampsia truly arose *de novo*, it will probably be less severe in subsequent pregnancies. There are, however, some women who are normotensive between pregnancies but have recurrent preeclampsia. The risk of such recurrence is increased when preeclampsia occurs in the late second or early third trimester (Sibai et al., 1991). The recurrence of severe preeclampsia or eclampsia in one pregnancy predicts its likely recurrence in subsequent pregnancies.

FUTURE HYPERTENSION AND CARDIOVASCULAR MORBIDITY. Several observations indicate that it is extremely unlikely that hypertensive disorders during pregnancy accelerate the progression of preexisting—perhaps unrecognized—hypertension, or cause cardiovascular morbidity or hypertension in normal women. Women eclamptic in the first pregnancy with subsequent hypertensive pregnancies have a greater incidence and earlier age of appearance of hypertension. However, when taken as a group, women eclamptic in first pregnancy have the same incidence of hypertension as an appropriate control group of unselected women. Interestingly, women normotensive in all pregnancies have a lower rate of hypertension than an unselected population of groups of women never pregnant (Chesley, 1980). The findings suggest that pregnancy, with or without eclampsia,

does not accelerate hypertension, but rather that it unmasks hypertension in women who either were not recognized as hypertensive in early pregnancy or are destined to become hypertensive in later life.

Many investigators have correlated preeclampsia with an increased risk of hypertension in later life. Some investigators use this correlation as evidence that residual damage from the preeclamptic process predisposes women to cardiovascular morbidity and mortality (Schreier et al., 1955; Epstein, 1964). There are serious flaws in many of these studies. All are compromised by the uncertainty of the clinical diagnosis of preeclampsia. In some, inappropriate control groups have been used, i.e., not corrected for age and race. Also, as noted earlier, the use of women normotensive in all pregnancies as controls is inappropriate. In all of these studies, as the likelihood that the clinical diagnosis was preeclampsia increased, the incidence of hypertension in later life decreased.

If women with preeclampsia in their first pregnancy are followed, the incidence of hypertension in later life is seen to be lower than in women with preeclampsia as multiparas. In women with proteinuria, the incidence of hypertension in later life is one-half that in women diagnosed with preeclampsia but without proteinuria (Berman, 1930). In a 15- to 20-year follow-up of women with preeclampsia in their first pregnancy, the incidence of diastolic blood pressures greater than 90 mm Hg was 60 per cent in women who had not had proteinuria, 40 per cent in those who had, and 35 per cent in women who were never pregnant (Adams et al., 1961). The definitive information about the long-range impact of preeclampsia-eclampsia comes from the masterful study by Chesley and associates (1976). In women with eclampsia in their first pregnancy who were followed for more than 40 years, there was no excess rate of hypertension (Fig. 49–14) and no increase in cardiovascular mortality or in death rate in general. The follow-up results for women with eclampsia as multiparas supports the concept that preeclampsia rarely arises *de novo* in multiparous women. The incidence of hypertension is greater in these women, as are rates of death from all causes and, specifically, cardiovascular death. The dramatic difference between the prognostic implications of eclampsia for primiparous and multiparous women is indicated in a survey of survival rates (Fig. 49–15). On the basis of this information, it would seem reasonable to conclude that preeclampsia does not cause permanent damage or predispose to chronic hypertension. The increased incidence of hypertension in later life for women with preeclampsia indicates either misdiagnosis or the unmasking of potential to develop hypertension regardless of the pregnancy.

An alternative explanation also deserves careful scrutiny. The duration of preeclampsia in pregnancy may dictate outcome. It is possible that mildly preeclamptic women are less likely to be expeditiously delivered than if they were severely preeclamptic or eclamptic. These women therefore are preeclamptic for a longer time and hence could have a higher chance of hypertension in later life (Epstein, 1964; Schreier et al., 1955). Examination of pathophysiologic changes

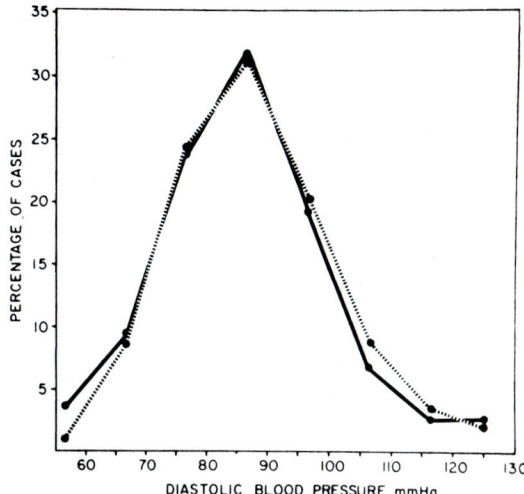

FIGURE 49–14. Distribution of diastolic blood pressures at 20 + -year follow-up of women eclamptic in their first pregnancy (*solid line*) compared with women from an appropriate control group (*broken line*). (From Chesley LC, Annitto JE, Cosgrove RA: Long-term follow-up study of eclamptic women: Fifth periodic report. Am J Obstet Gynecol **101**:886, 1968.)

in preeclampsia, however, indicates that they are present long before symptoms in all patients, whether mildly preeclamptic or eclamptic, and that the clinical stigmata of preeclampsia are present long before those of eclampsia. Also, if one uses the renal biopsy finding of glomeruloendotheliosis to increase the accuracy of the diagnosis of preeclampsia, incidences of hypertension are similar. In 53 women with this renal change, the incidence of hypertension was no higher than expected at follow-up, an average of 6 years after the hypertensive pregnancy (Fisher et al., 1981).

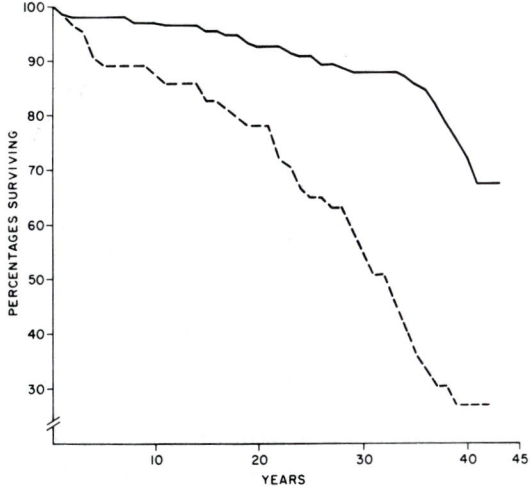

FIGURE 49–15. Survivals of women with eclampsia in the first pregnancy (*solid line*) and those with eclampsia in a later pregnancy (*broken line*). Survival of women with first-pregnancy eclampsia was not different from that of a control group. (From Chesley LC, Annitto JE, Cosgrove RA: The remote prognosis of eclamptic women: Sixth periodic report. Am J Obstet Gynecol **124**:446, 1976.)

Plan of Management for Preeclampsia

General Considerations

Philosophy of Management

On the basis of the pathologic and pathophysiologic changes and the prognosis of preeclampsia, it is possible to formulate a philosophy of management, as follows.

1. Delivery is always appropriate therapy for the mother but may not be so for the fetus. Because we do not yet understand the etiology of preeclampsia, attempts to prevent it by conventional medical approaches have been understandably unsuccessful. In terms of maternal health, the goal of therapy is to prevent eclampsia. Preeclampsia is the precursor of eclampsia, and so careful antepartum observation can identify the woman at risk. Preeclampsia is completely reversible and begins to abate with delivery. Thus, if only maternal well-being were considered, delivery of all preeclamptic women regardless of severity of process or stage of gestation would be appropriate. When the fetus is taken into consideration, however, delivery of infants of mildly preeclamptic women that are immature but have no signs of fetal distress is not sensible. There are two important corollaries of this statement: First, any therapy for preeclampsia other than delivery must have as its successful end point the reduction of perinatal mortality and morbidity. Second, the cornerstone of obstetric management of preeclampsia is based on a decision as to whether the infant is more likely to survive *in utero* or in the nursery.

2. The signs and symptoms of preeclampsia are not of pathogenetic importance. The pathologic and pathophysiologic changes of preeclampsia indicate that poor perfusion, most probably secondary to vasospasm, is the major factor leading to the derangement of maternal physiologic function and to increased perinatal mortality and morbidity rates. This same abnormality also causes increased total peripheral resistance with subsequent elevation of blood pressure and decreased renal perfusion leading to sodium retention and edema. The proteinuria of preeclampsia is at least partially explained by vasospasm and also by reversible glomerular damage due to phagocytosis of abnormal circulating proteins by glomerulocapillary endothelial cells.

Attempts to treat preeclampsia by natriuresis or by the lowering of blood pressure do not alleviate the important pathophysiologic changes. In fact, natriuresis may be counterproductive and may adversely affect fetal outcome because plasma volume is already reduced in preeclamptic women.

3. The pathogenetic changes of preeclampsia are present long before clinical criteria leading to the diagnosis are manifest. Recent studies indicate that changes in vascular reactivity, plasma volume, and renal function antedate, in some cases by months, the increases in blood pressure, protein excretion, and sodium retention. These findings suggest that irreversible changes affecting fetal well-being may be present prior to the clinical diagnosis. This possibility probably explains why dietary, pharmacologic, and postural therapy instituted after the recognition of clinical disease have not been successful when avoidance of perinatal morbidity and mortality is taken as the end point. If there is a rationale for modes of therapy other than delivery, it would be to palliate the maternal condition in order to allow fetal maturation. However, even this rationale is controversial.

Indications for Delivery

FETAL INDICATIONS. The major consideration in decisions for delivery should usually be fetal well-being, for the reasons already cited. Thus, if the maternal condition is stable, delivery is indicated by signs of abnormal fetal function. If fetal growth and well-being remain normal, pregnancy should proceed to spontaneous labor. If the maternal condition is rapidly deteriorating, however, delivery is indicated for fetal well-being. With maternal deterioration, a reflection of increasingly poor perfusion of brain, kidney, and liver, uteroplacental blood flow is also likely to be compromised. In addition, the predictive value of all tests of fetal well-being is invalidated by rapid changes in maternal, and hence fetal, condition.

MATERNAL INDICATIONS. Although fetal considerations usually dictate the timing of delivery, there are important exceptions. In the rare case in which a choice is made to palliate maternal signs and symptoms in order to allow fetal growth or maturation, such efforts must be abandoned if the maternal condition worsens. Also, a potentially lethal complication of preeclampsia, hepatic rupture, cannot be prevented by any mode of therapy other than delivery. It has a mortality rate of 65 per cent. Thus, the woman with hepatic capsular distention manifested by hepatomegaly, liver tenderness, and abnormal liver function values should be delivered regardless of fetal well-being or maturity.

Route of Delivery

Vaginal delivery is preferable to cesarean delivery for preeclamptic women. It is desirable, if possible, to avoid the added stress of surgery because of multiple physiologic abnormalities. Palliation for several hours should not increase maternal risk if performed appropriately. In addition, several investigators have demonstrated that with postural manipulations and fluid infusion for volume expansion, many fetuses, even those with positive contraction stress test results, can tolerate labor. Induction should be carried out aggressively and expeditiously once the decision for delivery is made. In gestation remote from term and complicated by severe preeclampsia, consideration may be given to glucocorticoid treatment to accelerate fetal lung maturation. Although there is evidence that glucocorticoids may be used safely in preeclamptic women (Ricke et al., 1980), fetal or maternal indications for delivery frequently contraindicate 24 to 36 hours of delay to allow such drugs to be effective. The aggressive approach to induction indicates that amniotomy be performed as soon as possible and a clear end point be formulated at the initiation of therapy. The cervical condition is generally predictive of the

likelihood of successful induction. Many authors point out, however, that in individual preeclamptic women the success of induction may be greater than would be predicted by the cervical examination (Zuspan et al., 1968). A trial of induction is warranted regardless of cervical condition. Obviously, if vaginal delivery cannot be effected within the predetermined time frame, cesarean delivery should be performed.

Cesarean delivery should be reserved for the usual obstetric indications, with the following exceptions. Because the probability of fetal compromise in preeclampsia is high, it is mandatory in all vaginal deliveries that the fetus be adequately monitored. Internal monitoring is preferable in order to allow determination of beat-to-beat variability; however, external monitoring, if technically good, is adequate until internal monitoring is feasible. Periodic changes or inadequate long-range variability requires assessment by internal fetal heart rate monitoring. Cesarean delivery is indicated if internal monitoring is not possible. Magnesium sulfate may decrease beat-to-beat variability (Stallworth et al., 1981), but especially if normal variability was never evident, it should be proven by fetal scalp blood sampling that decreased variability is not secondary to asphyxia. The woman with marked hepatic capsular distention should undergo cesarean delivery if vaginal delivery is not imminent. Even several extra hours may be life-threatening, and none of the palliative therapies prevents liver rupture.

Regional anesthesia offers its usual advantages for vaginal and cesarean delivery, but does carry the possibility of extensive sympatholysis with consequent decreased cardiac output, hypotension, and impairment of already compromised uteroplacental perfusion. This problem can be avoided by meticulous attention to anesthetic technique and volume expansion. Regional anesthesia is not a rational means to lower blood pressure because it does so at the expense of cardiac output. Likewise, although analgesia with narcotics is not contraindicated and should be used when necessary, there is abundant evidence that attempting to manage or prevent eclampsia with profound maternal sedation is dangerous and ineffective.

Monitoring of Mother and Fetus

MATERNAL MONITORING. There are two goals for antepartum monitoring of the mother. The first is the early recognition of the condition, because infants of mothers with even mild preeclampsia are at increased risk, and the second is to gauge the rate of progression of the condition, both to prevent eclampsia by delivery and to determine whether fetal well-being can be safely monitored by the usual intermittent observations. Ideally, identification of early changes would allow intervention prior to the advent of clinical symptoms. Hemodynamic, volume, and biochemical changes appear to antedate the diagnostic clinical signs of preeclampsia. In the past, lability of blood pressure, which is a feature of preeclampsia, was suggested as a predictor. However, neither stimulation of sympathetic response by the cold pressor test (Chesley and Valenti, 1958a) nor second-trimester blood pressure "spikes" (Browne, 1933) were found to be specific enough as predictors. More recently, higher early second-trimester blood pressures were measured in groups of women destined to have diagnostic blood pressure increases in later pregnancy (Gallery et al., 1977). The overlap of blood pressure levels between these women and women who remained normotensive, however, was too large to regard this value as a useful predictor for individual women. Brachial artery blood pressure that is higher in the supine than in the lateral position is believed by some investigators to predict the development of sustained blood pressure increases in late pregnancy. Extensive studies of this phenomenon do not support the earlier enthusiastic reports (Kuntz, 1980). Recently, Sobel and co-workers (1980) found that both men and nonpregnant women had higher right arm blood pressure in the supine position than in the left lateral position, the difference being related to the distance of the brachial artery above the heart. However, the increased blood pressure response to angiotensin II (Gant et al., 1973; Oney and Kaulhausen, 1982; Nakamura et al., 1986) in women destined to have elevated blood pressure in late pregnancy appears to be an accurate predictor, but the test is neither simple nor safe enough for extensive clinical use. Changes in renal function, serum urate, and PSP clearance (Gallery and Györy, 1979a) precede clinical signs of preeclampsia. Also, it appears that decreased plasma volume (Arias, 1975) and subtle coagulation changes are also predictors (Redman et al., 1977a). The usefulness of these values as clinical predictors in patient management remains to be confirmed.

At present, clinical management is dictated by the overt clinical signs of preeclampsia. Unfortunately, proteinuria—the most valid clinical indicator of preeclampsia—is often a late change, sometimes even preceded by seizures, and so it is not a useful sign for early recognition. Although rapid weight increase and hand and face edema indicate the fluid and sodium retention characteristic of preeclampsia, they are neither universally present nor uniquely characteristic of preeclampsia. These signs are, at most, a reason for closer observation of blood pressure and monitoring of urinary protein. Early recognition of preeclampsia is based primarily on diagnostic blood pressure increases in the late second and early third trimesters in relation to early pregnancy. Using blood pressure changes without evidence of proteinuria as an indicator does, undoubtedly, result in the diagnosis of preeclampsia in some normal women as well as in some with underlying renal or vascular disease. Because the goal of early diagnosis is to identify patients requiring more careful observation, however, overdiagnosis is preferable to underdiagnosis.

Once the blood pressure changes diagnostic of preeclampsia appear, an office examination within 24 hours is mandatory, or with selected patients, blood pressure and urinary protein must be checked at home. These measures are directed at determining the rapidity of progression of the condition in order to ensure that it is not following a fulminant course. Frequency of subsequent observations is determined by these initial observations and the ensuing clinical progression. If the condition appears stable, weekly observations may be appropriate. If it appears to be accelerating, more frequent observations, perhaps in hospital, are required. The initial appearance of proteinuria is an especially important sign of progression and dictates frequent observation, which is best accomplished in hospital.

If an increasing rate of deterioration is noted, as determined by laboratory findings, symptoms, and clinical signs, the decision to continue the pregnancy is determined day by day. Important clinical signs are blood pressure, urinary output, and fluid retention as evidenced by daily weight increase. Laboratory studies are performed at intervals of no more than 48 hours. These include examination for possible activation of the coagulation system as determined by platelet count and fibrin split products, evaluation of renal function as measured by urinary protein excretion and serum creatinine and urate levels, and determination of hepatic dysfunction as evidenced by increasing SGOT and SGPT. In addition, subjective evidence of central nervous system involvement, such as headache, disorientation, and visual symptoms, and the presence of hepatic distention as indicated by abdominal pain and liver tenderness are equally important indicators of worsening preeclampsia.

FETAL OBSERVATION. Tests to assess fetal well-being provide information for determining whether the infant is safer in the uterus or delivered. Since the perinatal mortality rate is higher for infants of women with even mild preeclampsia, it is mandatory to begin monitoring the fetal condition in any woman with the clinical diagnosis of preeclampsia. If the maternal condition is stable, weekly monitoring of the fetus appears to be adequate. The etiology of fetal demise is apparently placental insufficiency. Thus, biophysical assessment of the fetal oxygenation by observations of periodic changes in fetal heart rate and activity and contraction stress testing are direct and accurate indicators of fetal condition (Freeman, 1975). Unfortunately, no test of fetal well-being is predictive when maternal condition is rapidly deteriorating. The management of the fetus with intrauterine growth restriction, a common complication of preeclampsia, is discussed in Chapter 36. Assessment of amniotic fluid for determination of lung maturity aids in the decision to deliver the fetus with severe intrauterine growth retardation. Jeopardy of fetal well-being rather than lung maturity is the fetal criterion for determining delivery in a pregnancy with preeclampsia that is remote from term.

Prophylaxis for Preeclampsia

Since the recognition of the preeclamptic syndrome, numerous approaches have been used to attempt prevention of preeclampsia. These strategies, which include dietary restriction and supplementation and sodium restriction and supplementation, among other restrictions, have been unsuccessful (Chesley 1978). More recently, several studies of women at high risk for preeclampsia indicate a beneficial effect of low-dose (60 to 80 mg/day) aspirin prophylaxis to prevent preeclampsia and intrauterine growth restriction (Imperiale and Petrulis, 1991). The rationale for this therapy is to prevent generation of the vasoconstrictor/platelet aggregation stimulator by activated platelets while sparing the synthesis of the vasodilator/platelet aggregation inhibitor by endothelial cells. Measurement of these prostanoids confirms this effect in most women using this therapy (Spitz et al., 1988).

In these small groups of patients, therapy was not associated with adverse fetal outcome at short-term follow-up. It is tempting, but unwise, to extrapolate these findings to low-risk women. The potential adverse effects of aspirin militate against this form of prophylaxis until risk/benefit ratio is established in low-risk women. Aspirin as a prostaglandin synthesis inhibitor would be expected to effect recognized prostaglandin-mediated responses in the fetus such as maintenance of ductal patency and glomerular filtration. Perhaps of more concern are the unrecognized effects of prostaglandins on fetal homeostasis. Large studies of low-risk women are currently in progress, and until the results of these studies are completed, therapy should be reserved for women with risk similar to those in the subsets of high-risk patients studied, that is, groups with a predicted incidence of 20 to 40 per cent.

In all of these studies reported, therapy was instituted before clinically evident disease. Aspirin therapy is not effective for the woman with overt preeclampsia (Toppozada et al., 1991).

Antepartum Management in Preeclampsia

There is little evidence that therapeutic efforts alter the underlying pathophysiology of preeclampsia. Therapeutic intervention for clinically evident preeclampsia is palliative. At best, it may slow the progression of the condition, but it is more likely to merely allow continuation of the pregnancy. Bed rest is a usual and reasonable recommendation for the woman with mild preeclampsia, although its efficacy is not clearly established (Mathews, 1977). Prophylactic hospitalization with increased bed rest may reduce the incidence of preeclampsia for women at high risk, as identified by increased angiotensin sensitivity (Hauth et al., 1976). It is unclear, however, which of the several behavioral modifications involved in hospital residence is important. Anecdotal reports of clinical improvement with bed rest must be tempered by the recognition of the unpredictable course of preeclampsia. Strict sodium restriction or diuretic therapy has no role in the prevention or therapy of preeclampsia. In women with marked sodium retention as manifested by significant edema, modest sodium restriction may not alter the course of the disease but may reduce discomfort. Diuretics should not be given because these patients already have decreased plasma volume and further volume depletion could adversely affect the fetus. Attempts to modify the progression of the disease by volume expansion are not conclusive and require more complete evaluation before they can be considered part of routine antepartum management (Goodlin et al., 1978).

Prolonged expectant antepartum management of women with severe preeclampsia is not practiced in most centers. With improvements in neonatal care, many investigators regard delivery of women with severe preeclampsia beyond 30 weeks gestation to be in the best interests of not only the mother but also the fetus. Acute antihypertensive therapy is not used because it masks one important clinical sign of disease progression and blood pressure control does not improve fetal well-being. Diastolic pressure of 110 mm Hg and higher, which puts the mother at increased risk of cerebrovascular accident, is an indication for delivery with control of blood pressure. When gestational age is critical (between 25 and 30 weeks), one might consider control of maternal blood pressure along with meticulous observation of maternal and fetal condition. Delivery is then indicated by worsening maternal symptoms, laboratory evidence of end organ dysfunction, or deterioration of fetal condition. Whether this plan of action can effect a decrease in perinatal morbidity and mortality rates after 30 weeks gestation is not clear. The use of this approach with even very immature fetuses may only replace a nonviable neonate with an extremely premature one, with the attendant risks of long-range neurologic disability. Such an approach should therefore be attempted only in centers equipped to provide meticulous maternal observation and daily assessment of fetal and maternal condition.

Intrapartum Management in Preeclampsia

The intrapartum management of women with preeclampsia tests the obstetric and medical skills of the health care team. The severely preeclamptic or eclamptic woman is acutely ill, with functional derangements of many organ systems. An appreciation of this situation and the availability of methods of accurate maternal monitoring have reduced mortality rates from 5 per cent in earlier series to 1 per cent or less in recent series. Failure to recognize and appropriately manage this grave condition probably accounts for most deaths. Also, even mildly preeclamptic women may experience an acceleration of the process during labor. Delivery terminates the preeclamptic process, and it is tempting to effect immediate delivery, frequently by cesarean section. However, physiologic abnormalities are not immediately corrected by delivery, and adding surgical stress to the abnormal physiologic state is not desirable. It is possible to partially correct many of these abnormalities, and it is imperative to attempt to do so prior to imposing surgical stress. If the fetus can be monitored, several hours of palliation with vaginal delivery are preferable to the added maternal stress of operative delivery.

Baseline information should be obtained to determine renal function, coagulation status, and liver function. Determination of serum protein concentration indicates the choice of appropriate fluid administration. Some investigators advocate the use of intensive cardiovascular monitoring, preferably with Swan-Ganz catheters or with central venous pressure catheters in all severely preeclamptic and eclamptic women (Chapter 51). Such a practice is certainly indicated in oliguric patients whose urinary output does not improve with a modest fluid challenge. The major problems to be managed are those of high blood pressure, intravascular volume, and convulsions. Less commonly, disseminated intravascular coagulation and myocardial dysfunction will require treatment.

Anticonvulsants

PROPHYLAXIS. The majority of seizures occur during the intrapartum and postpartum periods, suggesting that these are the periods in which the preeclamptic process is most likely to accelerate. In many centers outside the United States, anticonvulsant prophylaxis is not used routinely, but rather is reserved for the woman who seems clinically to be at risk for seizures. It is not known whether the risk for seizures is less in these centers than in those in the United States. However, a recent review of eclamptic patients from a major United States center indicates the hazards of this approach (Sibai et al., 1981). None of the clinical signs and symptoms considered to be prognostic of seizures was absolutely reliable. Seventeen per cent of women who had seizures did not have headache, 80 per cent did not have epigastric pain, and 20 per cent had normal deep tendon reflexes (Table 49–6). The lack of absolute correlation with proteinuria is consistent with the observations by Chesley and Chesley (1943) 50 years ago that 24 per cent of patients do not have proteinuria prior to seizure.

The prophylactic use of anticonvulsant therapy, which is the approach strongly recommended by most United States investigators, will protect most women at risk for seizures only if therapy is elected for all women with a blood pressure elevation diagnostic of preeclampsia, whether or not there are other signs and symptoms, including proteinuria. Because this approach will certainly include many women at no risk for seizure, the first requirement for anticonvulsant prophylaxis is that the agent and its dosage must be extremely safe for the mother. The other obvious requirement is safety for the infant, not only as a fetus but also when, as a neonate with appreciable blood levels of the drug, it begins the complex adaptation to extrauterine life.

In the past, a staggering array of drugs and combinations of drugs have been used as therapeutic and prophylactic agents for convulsions (Studd, 1977). Zuspan (1978) and Pritchard and Pritchard (1975), among others, have demonstrated the value of simplifying therapy by reducing the number of agents administered. Both reports advocate the use of magnesium sulfate for anticonvulsant prophylaxis, which is clearly the drug of choice for United States obstetricians. Other anticonvulsant agents, primarily benzodiazepine derivatives, are used in other parts of the world. Investigators worldwide agree with the principle of simplifying therapy by avoiding polypharmaceutical regimens (Studd, 1977).

CHLORMETHIAZOLE AND BENZODIAZEPINES. The use of large doses of diazepam was advocated by some British investigators as an effective means of terminating eclamptic seizures and preventing their recurrence (Studd, 1977). It is now evident that diazepam in these dosages results in hypotonia, hypothermia, and respiratory depression in a high proportion of neonates (Cree et al., 1973). These effects may last for several days owing to the pharmacokinetics of benzodiazepine in the neonate. Lorazepam, a long-acting benzodiazepine derivative, has even more severe fetal effects (Whitelaw et al., 1981). In spite of these findings, benzodiazepines continue to be the major anticonvulsants used in many centers outside the United States. The effects of these agents on the neonate would appear to contraindicate their use as prophylactic agents. Chlormethiazole (clomethiazole) has also been advocated for prophylactic use in preeclamptic women (Duffus et al., 1969). In one series in which this drug was used in combination with diazoxide, however, 13 of 21 infants were severely depressed (hypotonia, hypoventilation) for 24 to 36 hours after birth (Johnson, 1976).

MAGNESIUM SULFATE. Magnesium sulfate offers considerable advantages over the preceding agents for prophylaxis in preeclamptic women. Its pharmacokinetic processes during pregnancy are well established, as are its efficacy and safety for mother and fetus.

Pharmacokinetics, Mechanism of Action, and Maternal Side Effects. The volume of distribution of magnesium is greater than that of sucrose, indicating that the distribution of this ion goes beyond extracellular fluid, also entering bones and cells (Chesley, 1979). Magnesium circulates largely unbound to protein and is almost exclusively excreted in urine. It is reabsorbed in the proximal tubule by a process limited by transport maximum (T_{max}), and its excretion increases as filtered load increases above the transport maximum (Massey, 1977). In patients with normal renal function, the half-time for excretion is about 4 hours (Chesley, 1979). Because excretion depends on delivery of a filtered load of magnesium that exceeds the T_{max}, the half-time of excretion is prolonged in women with decreased glomerular filtration rate. The clinically significant results of elevated serum magnesium are related primarily to its membrane effects. Magnesium slows or blocks neuromuscular and cardiac conducting system transmission, decreases smooth muscle contractility, and depresses central nervous system irritability. The results include a desired anticonvulsant effect and undesirable effects such as decreased uterine and myocardial contractility, depressed respirations, and interference with cardiac conduction. These effects occur at different serum magnesium concentrations (Table 49–7). Doses of magnesium sulfate sufficient for anticonvulsant therapy cause little change in blood pressure. Because the depression of deep ten-

TABLE 49–6. Frequency of Symptoms Preceding Eclampsia

SYMPTOM	PATIENTS IN WHOM PRESENT (%)
Headache	83
Hyper-reflexia	80
Proteinuria	80
Edema	60
Clonus	46
Visual signs	45
Epigastric pain	20

Adapted from Sibai BM, Lipshitz J, Anderson GD, Dilts PV Jr: Reassessment of intravenous MgSO₄ therapy in preeclampsia-eclampsia. Obstet Gynecol 57:199, 1981.

TABLE 49–7. Effects Associated with Various Serum Magnesium Levels

EFFECT	SERUM LEVEL (mEq/liter)
Anticonvulsant prophylaxis	4–6
EKG changes	5–10
Loss of deep tendon reflexes	10
Respiratory paralysis	15
General anesthesia	15
Cardiac arrest	>25

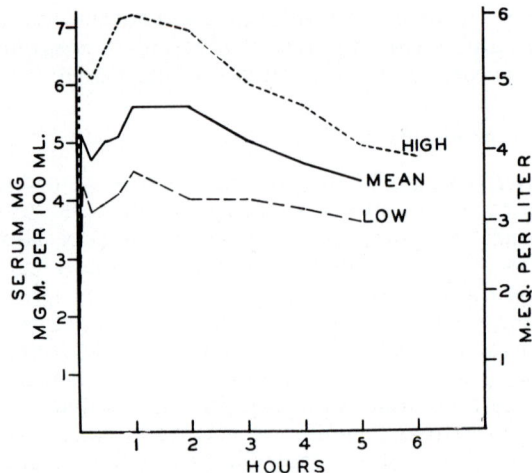

FIGURE 49–16. Serum magnesium concentrations resulting from the concurrent administration of 3 gm magnesium sulfate IV and 10 gm IM. (From Chesley C, Tepper I: Plasma levels of magnesium attained in magnesium sulfate therapy for preeclampsia and eclampsia. Surg Clin North Am **37**:353, 1957.)

don reflexes occurs at serum concentrations lower than those associated with adverse cardiac and respiratory effects, the presence of deep tendon reflexes indicates that serum magnesium concentration is not dangerously high. If deep tendon reflexes are lost, serum magnesium concentration may be greater than 10 mEq/liter. However, any attempt to control magnesium therapy by eliminating deep tendon reflexes is irrational and dangerous, as is the assumption that brisk deep tendon reflexes signify inadequate magnesium dosage.

Dosage. Two regimens of magnesium administration have been used extensively. Pritchard and Pritchard (1975) reported use of a combination of intramuscular and intravenous magnesium ($MgSO_4 \cdot 7H_2O$), with impressive results (Table 49–8). Two to 4 gm are given intravenously over 2 to 4 minutes, and 10 gm are concomitantly administered intramuscularly. The intravenous dosage results in immediate elevation of serum magnesium, which falls rapidly. As serum magnesium from intravenous injection decreases, the absorption of intramuscular magnesium results in a relatively consistent serum concentration. The range of magnesium concentration attained in patients with differing renal functions and body sizes is indicated in Figure 49–16. Serum magnesium levels after initial administration are determined by volume of distribution and not by renal function (Chesley, 1979). The initial dose can be safely administered without knowledge of renal function. It is recommended that 5 gm of $MgSO_4 \cdot 7H_2O$ be readministered intramuscularly every 4 hours. The serum concentration of magnesium after subsequent doses is influenced by renal function, and if the patient is not excreting more than 40 ml/hr

of urine, the dosage must be reduced as determined by serum magnesium levels. Prior to the administration of subsequent doses, deep tendon reflexes must be present and the respiratory rate must be normal.

Because intramuscular administration of large volumes of $MgSO_4 \cdot 7H_2O$ is painful, many investigators advocate the use of a continuous intravenous infusion, in which 2 to 4 gm of $MgSO_4 \cdot 7H_2O$ are given over 5 minutes, followed by controlled continuous infusion of 1.0 gm/hr. Magnesium is administered by continuous infusion because intermittent bolus infusions result in only transient elevations of magnesium level. To ensure consistent infusion and to avoid inadvertent administration of large doses of magnesium, mechanically controlled infusion is mandatory. The rate of infusion is modified for patients with compromised renal function, in whom magnesium levels should be measured. If overdosage, especially with apnea, does occur, calcium gluconate, 10 ml of a 10 per cent solution, injected intravenously over 3 minutes, is an effective antidote.

Both of these approaches have been clinically tested for more than 30 years and are effective and extremely safe for the mother (Table 49–9). It should be emphasized that the "therapeutic concentrations" of magnesium have been empirically determined and are the levels attained with dosages found to be usually effective. No study has yet compared magnesium concen-

TABLE 49–8. Results of Standardized Treatment of Preeclampsia Using Magnesium Sulfate*

Fetuses dead when eclampsia diagnosed	7
Fetuses alive when eclampsia diagnosed	115
Intrapartum death	1†
Live births	114
Neonatal deaths	4‡
Survivors	100
Total fetuses	122

*Includes only fetuses weighing 1000 gm or more at birth, at Parkland Memorial Hospital, 1955 to 1975.
†Weighed 1200 gm.
‡All weighed less than 1800 gm. All 100 fetuses weighing 1800 gm (4 lbs) or more and alive when eclampsia was diagnosed survived.
Modified from Pritchard JA, Pritchard SA: Standardized treatment of 154 consecutive cases of eclampsia. Am J Obstet Gynecol **123**:543, 1975.

TABLE 49–9. Safety and Efficacy of Intravenous $MgSO_4$ Therapy

Treated	1870
Seizures	11 (.6%)
Seizure morbidity	1 (.05%)
Treatment morbidity	0

Adapted from Sibai BM, Lipshitz J, Anderson GD, Dilts PV Jr: Reassessment of intravenous $MgSO_4$ therapy in preeclampsia-eclampsia. Obstet Gynecol **57**:199, 1981.

trations in patients either successfully or unsuccessfully treated with $MgSO_4 \cdot 7H_2O$. Also, magnesium is not a perfect anticonvulsant, and some women have convulsions even with high serum concentrations (Chesley and Tepper, 1957). Attempts to modify this modality, which has been found effective and safe even though liberally administered to many women who do not need the therapy, must be made with caution. There is now extensive experience with the intravenous administration of magnesium at doses up to 2 gm per hour, which appears safe for the patient with normal renal function. However, doses larger than this require that deep tendon reflexes be followed carefully and that serum magnesium concentrations be monitored at least every 2 hours until a steady state has been reached.

Fetal and Neonatal Effects of Magnesium Sulfate. A major advantage of magnesium sulfate therapy is that at effective anticonvulsant doses it is very safe for the fetus and neonate (see Table 49–8). Neonatal serum magnesium concentrations are nearly identical to those of the mother (Pritchard, 1955). Although amniotic fluid magnesium concentrations increase with prolonged infusion owing to fetal renal excretion of the substance, fetal serum magnesium levels do not increase, and there is no evidence of cumulative effects of prolonged magnesium administration on the neonate. In a study of 118 infants of mothers treated with magnesium sulfate, the average serum magnesium concentration was 3.7 mEq/liter and there was no correlation of magnesium level with Apgar scores (Pritchard and Stone, 1967).

PHENYTOIN. Phenytoin is an effective anticonvulsant with pharmacologic effects that would not be predicted to adversely affect the fetus *in utero* or the physiologic events necessary for perinatal adaptation. In several small studies there were no obvious adverse fetal or maternal effects (Crowther, 1990; Appleton et al., 1991). Several authors have championed the use of phenytoin as a prophylactic and therapeutic agent for preeclampsia/eclampsia. There are no controlled trials sufficiently large to judge the relative efficacy of phenytoin and magnesium sulfate. In the comparisons that are available, it is surprising that phenytoin is not evidently more efficacious than magnesium (Crowther, 1990). The incidence of repeated seizures in women receiving phenytoin at dosage sufficient to achieve therapeutic blood levels is 16 to 20 per cent (Tuffnell et al, 1989; Crowther, 1990), which is quite similar to the results with magnesium sulfate in other studies (Pritchard and Pritchard, 1975; Sibai et al., 1981). In addition, although phenytoin should be a safer agent than magnesium, it does have potential severe adverse effects which are magnified by the fact that obstetric personnel are not familiar with its use. At present it would seem prudent to continue to consider magnesium sulfate the first choice as a prophylactic agent. However, phenytoin is likely to be equally effective, and in settings in which magnesium would be best avoided (e.g., markedly compromised renal function, myasthenia gravis), phenytoin is a reasonable alternative.

ANTICONVULSANT THERAPY. If treatment with magnesium has not been given, 4 gm can be safely administered intravenously and intramuscular or intravenous $MgSO_4$ begun as described previously to maintain serum magnesium levels. If the patient is already receiving magnesium, it is safer to terminate seizures with another anticonvulsant agent, such as Valium, 5 mg, or a short-acting barbiturate such as pentobarbital, 125 mg given intravenously. Once seizures are terminated, serum magnesium concentration can be determined and the rate of magnesium infusion can be adjusted accordingly. Because most seizures terminate spontaneously in 1 to 2 minutes, the most important measures for any seizure, which should be taken before pharmacologic therapy is initiated, are prevention of injury and protection of the airway to prevent aspiration.

Antihypertensive Therapy

Antihypertensive agents are not routinely administered to preeclamptic women. There is no evidence that the acute administration of these agents has beneficial fetal effects. The suggestion that lowering blood pressure reduces the risk of seizures has not been tested. Therapy is reserved for women in whom blood pressure is elevated to a degree that might be associated with intracranial bleeding. Treatment is recommended for women with diastolic blood pressure persistently greater than 105 mm Hg. The goal of blood pressure control is not to attain normal blood pressure, but merely to reduce blood pressure to a level that will provide a margin of maternal safety (95 to 100 mm Hg) without compromising adequate uterine perfusion. It is important to remember that these patients have elevated blood pressure with reduced plasma volume and that too-aggressive treatment will lower maternal cardiac output and uterine perfusion and may result in iatrogenic fetal distress. A number of agents available for rapidly lowering blood pressure are listed in Table 49–10; not listed in this table are potent diuretic agents that lower blood pressure rapidly by depleting plasma volume, because the use of these agents in the plasma volume–depleted patient would result in reduced maternal cardiac output and uterine perfusion.

HYDRALAZINE. The agent most widely used to lower blood pressure in severe preeclampsia is hydralazine. A direct vasodilator, it offers two major advantages. Vasodilation with hydralazine results in a reflex increase in cardiac output, which in animal studies leads to the first advantage—increased uterine blood flow. A more important advantage is that the increase in cardiac output blunts the hypotensive effect and makes it difficult to overdose the patient. The important side effects of hydralazine are headache and epigastric pain, which may be confused with worsening preeclampsia. The pharmacokinetics of hydralazine are outlined in Table 49–10. The onset of action is 10 to 20 minutes, and peak action occurs 20 minutes after administration, even when the agent is given intravenously. The duration of action is 3 to 8 hours. On the basis of these facts, the use of continuous intravenous infusions of hydralazine is not sensible, because minute-to-minute control cannot be attained. An alternative approach is to administer the

TABLE 49–10. **Drugs for Treatment of Hypertensive Emergencies**

DRUG	TIME COURSE OF ACTION			IM	DOSAGE IV	INTERVAL BETWEEN DOSES	MECHANISM OF ACTION
	ONSET	MAXIMUM	DURATION				
Hydralazine	10–20 min	20–40 min	3–8 hr	10–50 mg	5–25 mg	3–6 hr	Direct dilatation of arterioles
Trimethaphan camsylate	1–2 min	2–5 min	10 min	—	IV solution, 2 gm/liter; IV infusion rate, 1–5 mg/min		Ganglionic blockade
Sodium nitroprusside	½–2 min	1–2 min	3–5 min	—	IV solution, 0.01 gm/liter; IV infusion rate, 0.2 to 0.8 mg/min		Direct dilatation of arterioles and veins
Labetalol	1–2 min	10 min	6–16 hrs	—	20–50 mg	3–6 hr	Alpha- and beta-adrenergic blocker
Nifedipine	5–10 min	10–20 min	4–8 hrs	—	10 mg orally	4–8 hr	Calcium-channel blocker

drug as a bolus infusion, repeated at 20-minute intervals until the desired control is attained and then repeated as necessary. A test dose of 1.0 mg is given over 1 minute and blood pressure is determined to avoid idiosyncratic hypotensive effects. Four milligrams are then infused over 2 to 4 minutes. After 20 minutes the blood pressure is determined; the dose is repeated if there was no effect, or a lower dose is given if a suboptimal effect was obtained. If diastolic blood pressure is between 90 and 100 mm Hg, therapy is not repeated until diastolic blood pressure increases to 105 mm Hg.

OTHER DRUGS. Rarely, hydralazine will not effectively lower blood pressure to the desired level. If blood pressure control is not adequate after the administration of 20 mg of hydralazine, other hypotensive agents must be used. The calcium entry blocker nifedipine has also been used in doses of 10 mg orally after 30 minutes to rapidly lower blood pressure. It is quite effective and well tolerated (Greer et al., 1989). Some concerns have been raised about synergistic effects of nifedipine and magnesium sulfate (Waisman et al., 1988) although this has not been my experience. The mixed alpha- and beta-adrenergic antagonist, labetalol, is also useful for acutely lowering blood pressure. It is given intravenously as a bolus infusion beginning with 20 mg followed by doses of 10 to 50 mg repeated every 10 minutes as needed for blood pressure control (Mabie et al., 1987). The major reservation with the use of labetalol is that, unlike the vasodilators hydralazine and nifedipine, it does not reduce afterload. Thus, labetalol has theoretical disadvantages in managing cardiac failure associated with the hypertension of preeclampsia. Although alphamethyldopa is a safe and well-tested drug, its delayed onset of action (4 to 6 hours), even when administered intravenously, limits its usefulness for hypertensive emergencies. Clonidine, also a centrally acting vasodilator, reduces blood pressure more rapidly. A dose of 150 μg given in 10 ml of saline over 5 minutes reduces blood pressure within 20 to 30 minutes. Experience with its use in preeclampsia is not extensive, however. Trimethaphan, a ganglion-blocking agent,

effectively reduces blood pressure, but primarily through a reduction of cardiac output via decreased venous return, and thus reduces uteroplacental perfusion. Sodium nitroprusside is a potent, short-acting, direct vasodilator that allows excellent moment-to-moment blood pressure control. In experimental animals there are reports of elevated concentrations of serum cyanide, sometimes to toxic levels, in the fetus (Naulty et al., 1981). Diazoxide is a thiazide analog that has no diuretic effect, but is an extremely potent antihypertensive agent, acting as a direct vasodilator. It is rarely used because of effects on maternal and fetal carbohydrate metabolism and its profound and slowly reversible effect on blood pressure.

On the basis of side effects and experience, the drug of first choice when hydralazine is ineffective is nifedipine or labetalol.

Management of Oliguria

In preeclamptic women, oliguria may be of prerenal or renal origin. Even though there is agreement that plasma volume is decreased in preeclamptic patients, the use of fluids is controversial. Excessive fluid infusion may lead to congestive heart failure and perhaps cerebral edema (Benedetti and Quilligan, 1980); nevertheless, oliguria may be corrected in many patients by fluid infusion.

In order to avoid complications, hypotonic fluids should not be used, because they would worsen dilutional decreases in serum osmolality that may occur with (1) oliguria from renal causes, (2) elevated ADH secondary to stress, or (3) oxytocin treatment. Fluids must be administered with the consideration that oliguria may be of renal origin and that the patient is at risk for fluid overloading. Since acute renal failure resulting in permanent renal damage is extremely rare in pregnancy while pulmonary edema is an almost monthly event on many obstetrical services, oliguria should be defined conservatively, 20 to 30 ml/hr for two hours. If there are no clinical signs or history of congestive heart failure, 1000 ml of isotonic crystalloid can safely be infused in 1 hour. If urine output increases, fluid infusion is maintained as 100 ml/hr of isotonic crystalloids. If the oliguria does not resolve, further fluid infusion should be guided by central venous or, preferably, pulmonary wedge pressures (Chapter 51). In addition, relatively small amounts of intrapartum and postpartum blood loss may result in profound hypovolemia and shock in those patients having already compromised blood volumes. A large peripheral line should be in place at all times in case rapid replacement of blood volume is needed.

Management of Less Common Problems

DISSEMINATED INTRAVASCULAR COAGULATION. Evidence of disseminated intravascular coagulation (DIC) is an important indicator of severity and progression of preeclampsia. DIC will be measurable by the usual clinical tests in 20 per cent of severely preeclamptic and eclamptic women, and will be sufficient to cause coagulation problems in less than 10 per cent. The definitive therapy of DIC is the removal of the inciting factor. In preeclampsia, whether the etiology of the coagulation disorder is endothelial cell damage, release of thromboplastic materials, vasospasm with attendant microangiopathic changes, or local consumption of procoagulants in the choriodecidual space, the inciting factor is clearly pregnancy-related, and definitive therapy is termination of the pregnancy. The long-range follow-up of women with preeclampsia indicates that all organ system functions return to normal. Thus, it is unlikely that occlusion of the microvasculature by thrombi in mild forms of DIC causes permanent damage. Evidence of early disseminated intravascular coagulation is not by itself an absolute indication for immediate delivery. With rapidly deteriorating renal or hepatic function or DIC complicated by spontaneous hemorrhage, however, delivery should be expeditious.

The experience with heparin anticoagulation, either to maintain pregnancies in women with symptomatic DIC or as a prophylactic measure to prevent DIC, indicates that these approaches are not effective (Howie et al., 1975). The question of the use of heparin during labor in women in whom DIC necessitates delivery has not been extensively studied. The experiences already cited, however, indicate that it is unlikely that the benefits outweigh the risks.

If procoagulants decrease to a level associated with spontaneous hemorrhage, appropriate procoagulant therapy should be given prior to delivery, whether the anticipated mode of delivery is vaginal or cesarean (see Chapter 53). The choice of mode of delivery is based on other considerations and is not influenced by the presence or absence of DIC. It is important to remember that with a decrease in procoagulants, vaginal delivery does not necessarily prevent hemorrhage, which may be apparent or may manifest less obviously as vulvar or vaginal hematomas.

PULMONARY EDEMA. Pulmonary edema occurs in a small number of women with preeclampsia. In past years this complication was associated with high maternal mortality rates. The pathogenesis of pulmonary edema is frequently iatrogenic fluid overload, but may be cardiogenic or involve transudation of fluid into alveolae. The noncardiogenic variety is secondary either to decreased colloid oncotic pressure or to a pulmonary vascular leakage and may occur antepartum, intrapartum, or postpartum. Delayed onset of pulmonary edema requires special awareness because the edema usually occurs during postpartum diuresis, when most concerns about the complications of preeclampsia are lessening. The management of pulmonary edema requires intensive monitoring, with the capability to assess pulmonary and cardiac function accurately and perform mechanical ventilation as needed (see Chapter 51). With accurate assessment of cardiopulmonary function and aggressive treatment, the mortality due to pulmonary edema in preeclampsia has been greatly reduced (Cotton and Benedetti, 1980).

Postpartum Management in Preeclampsia

Delivery does not immediately reverse the pathophysiologic changes of preeclampsia, and it is necessary to continue palliative therapy for variable lengths of time. However, some of the constraints on therapy are eliminated by delivery of the fetus. Approximately one-third of convulsions occur in the postpartum period, most within 24 hours and virtually all within 48 hours, although there are rare exceptions. Extending the rationale that it is better to treat prophylactically all women at risk for seizures even though we treat many who do not require therapy, most physicians advocate continuing anticonvulsant therapy for 24 hours postpartum. For simplicity, magnesium sulfate therapy is usually continued, although since there is no need to consider fetal effects, any safe anticonvulsant regimen is reasonable at this time. Anticonvulsant efficacy rather than sedation is the goal, however, and barbiturate anticonvulsants in usual therapeutic doses will require days to achieve effective levels. Likewise, diphenylhydantoin must be administered intravenously in large doses to achieve therapeutic levels within hours, with the attendant dangers of cardiac arrhythmia. Serum magnesium concentrations decrease with increased urinary output, and with puerperal diuresis it is extremely unlikely that serum magnesium concentration is therapeutic at usual doses. In spite of this drawback, with either the intravenous or intramuscular dosage regimen usually used, convulsions rarely occur in the postpartum period, suggesting that rapid diuresis indicates resolution of the preeclamptic process and that therapy may no longer be required. On the basis of these considerations, it appears reasonable to discontinue magnesium sulfate therapy when diuresis occurs before 24 hours postpartum. Some authors recommend continuing magnesium sulfate administration for longer than 24 hours in selected patients, but it is difficult to decide on what basis this selection can be made (see Table 49–6).

Hypertension may take considerably longer than 24 to 48 hours to resolve. Women who are hypertensive 6 weeks postpartum may be normotensive at long-term follow-up (Chesley et al., 1976). The indications for therapy are similar to those for the antepartum period. The patient with diastolic blood pressure greater than 105 mm Hg postpartum should be treated, and the fetus no longer influences therapeutic choices. If rapid blood pressure control is necessary, sodium nitroprusside is more effective and better tolerated than hydralazine. Also, diuretics and conventional oral antihypertensive agents can be started to achieve smooth control. The woman who remains hypertensive, with greater than 100 mm Hg diastolic blood pressure, should be sent home with continued antihypertensive therapy. Lesser elevations require no therapy. The choice of drugs is based on the usual step method of antihypertensive therapy. It is important that the patient sent home on therapy be warned of symptoms of hypotension and that she be seen at weekly intervals because in some patients the need for therapy diminishes rapidly.

Follow-up in Preeclampsia

Although it is evident from the studies cited that preeclampsia does not cause higher cardiovascular risk or hypertension in later life, the correlation between a clinical diagnosis of preeclampsia and hypertension in later life is also well proven. Because the early recognition and treatment of significant blood pressure elevation reduces morbidity, all women with a clinical diagnosis of preeclampsia deserve long-range follow-up. Decisions for evaluation and treatment should be deferred until 12 weeks postpartum because some women who are hypertensive at 6 weeks are normotensive years later. The woman who is normotensive at 12 weeks should be advised of her slightly increased risk for hypertension and should be counseled to have her blood pressure checked at least yearly.

CHRONIC HYPERTENSION

The differentiation of the pregnant woman with chronic hypertension from the preeclamptic is difficult but important. Even more important is the difficult discrimination between the exacerbation of preexisting hypertension and the onset of superimposed preeclampsia. The rate of progression and the effect on mother and baby of these conditions are quite different in the two diseases. Management of the woman with hypertension in early pregnancy requires early recognition of blood pressure elevation, baseline testing to aid in the later diagnosis of superimposed preeclampsia, and meticulous maternal and fetal observation. If a decision is made to use antihypertensive therapy, antihypertensive drugs must be chosen on the basis of considerations specific to pregnancy.

Effects of Chronic Hypertension on the Mother

Blood pressure elevation during pregnancy without the superimposition of preeclampsia has the same impact as blood pressure increases in any other 10-month period. That is, if diastolic blood pressure exceeds 105 mm Hg, it is possible that morbid events may occur over even this short time, whereas at pressures of 95 to 100 mm Hg diastolic, morbidity is

extremely unlikely. This is not the case with superimposed preeclampsia, which occurs in 20 per cent of hypertensive women, compared with a 7 per cent incidence of preeclampsia in women previously normotensive. In addition, maternal morbidity and mortality rates are greater in superimposed preeclampsia than in preeclampsia arising *de novo*. Blood pressure elevation is also greater, increasing the possibility of intracranial bleeding. Whereas two-thirds of cases of eclampsia occur in first pregnancies, two-thirds of maternal deaths occur in pregnancies other than the first pregnancy, in which underlying hypertension is a common disposing factor (Neutra and Neff, 1975).

Effects of Chronic Hypertension on the Fetus

The perinatal mortality rate is higher in infants of hypertensive women, increasing along with rising maternal blood pressure (Tervila et al., 1973). Prior to the advent of antihypertensive therapy, a woman with a systolic pressure of 200 mm Hg or a diastolic pressure of 120 mm Hg had only a 50 per cent chance of bearing a living infant. The perinatal mortality rate is strikingly higher in hypertensive women with proteinuria, indicating the impact of superimposed preeclampsia on the fetus. The perinatal mortality rate for infants of women with superimposed preeclampsia is greater than for infants of women in whom the condition arises *de novo* (Lin et al., 1982). There are two explanations for this difference. First, the decidual vessels of women with even mild pre-existing hypertension demonstrate vascular changes very similar to the changes in renal arterioles that occur in women with long-standing hypertension (Robertson et al., 1967). Decreased uteroplacental perfusion secondary to this change is probably at least additive and perhaps synergistic with the decidual vascular changes of preeclampsia. The decidual vascular changes also probably explain the higher incidence of abruptio placentae in women with superimposed preeclampsia. In addition, preeclampsia appears earlier in pregnancies of hypertensive women than of normotensive women. Intrauterine growth restriction is also common in infants of hypertensive women and increases in frequency and severity with increasing maternal blood pressure (Tervila et al., 1973).

Some investigators argue that hypertension without preeclampsia has no adverse effect on the fetus (Redman, 1980; Sibai et al., 1983a). Although this opinion is controversial, clinical management is not influenced by the argument. In view of the difficulty of diagnosing superimposed preeclampsia, the infants of all hypertensive women should be considered at increased risk and monitored accordingly.

Efficacy of Antihypertensive Therapy in the Reduction of Maternal and Fetal Morbidity and Mortality

Antihypertensive therapy reduces maternal mortality as effectively during pregnancy as at any other time. Reduction of markedly elevated blood pressure (diastolic pressure greater than 100 mm Hg) will reduce the risk of morbid events over even 10 months, whereas the impact of such reduction on the minimal morbidity associated with less elevated pressures is unlikely.

A major benefit of antihypertensive therapy to mother and fetus would be the reduction of the incidence of superimposed preeclampsia. Unfortunately, such a reduction has not been evident in large studies of antihypertensive therapy administered during pregnancy. On the basis of findings that pathologic and pathophysiologic changes are present as early as 14 weeks gestation, it is possible that, in these studies, in which patients were identified and treated as late in gestation as 28 weeks, therapy was begun too late to be effective. In reports of series of women in whom therapy was begun early in pregnancy, it has been suggested that antihypertensive therapy prevented or delayed the appearance of superimposed preeclampsia (Arias and Zamora, 1979).

The ability of antihypertensive therapy to reduce rates of perinatal mortality and morbidity is controversial. Agreement as to the effect of antihypertensive agents on uterine perfusion in experimental animals is lacking (Ladner et al., 1970; Brinkman and Assali, 1976). In all clinical studies, however, antihypertensive therapy has not increased perinatal mortality rates (Roberts and Perloff, 1977; Naden and Redman, 1985). Thus, if therapy is indicated for maternal considerations (diastolic pressure greater than 100 mm Hg), it is safe for the fetus if the choice of drug is appropriate (Kincaid-Smith et al., 1966).

Controlled studies have shown lower perinatal mortality rates for infants of mildly hypertensive women given antihypertensive agents (Table 49–11). There was, however, an excess of second-trimester losses in the control group (a complication not usually ascribed to hypertension) in the studies reported by Redman and co-workers (1976b) and Leather and colleagues (1968). This first group has proposed that the reduction of perinatal mortality with alpha-methyldopa therapy might be the result of some other, nonhypertensive effect of the drug. If cases of premature labor and incompetent cervix are excluded, however, there does appear to be a relationship between hypertension and second-trimester losses (Silverstone et al., 1980). In a more recent well-designed and controlled study (Sibai et al., 1990), no difference in perinatal mortality, or perinatal morbidity as indicated by growth restric-

tion, or low Apgar scores, was seen in a group of women untreated or treated with alpha-methyldopa or labetalol. Thus the impact of antihypertensive therapy in mild hypertension to improve fetal outcome remains unproven and controversial.

Summary

Antihypertensive therapy can be used safely when indicated by maternal condition. Therapy reduces the maternal risks of markedly elevated pressures. It is controversial whether therapy can delay or prevent preeclampsia if begun early in pregnancy or reduce rates of perinatal mortality and morbidity. The decision to use antihypertensive therapy is based on these considerations. If therapy is chosen for fetal indications, then it should be used in all women with *persistent* diastolic blood pressure elevation to more than 90 mm Hg in early pregnancy. Attempts should be made to document that blood pressure is persistently elevated—perhaps with home blood pressure determinations—as early in pregnancy as possible. The vascular changes in decidual vessels in cases of hypertension described by Robertson and associates (1967), as well as the presence of demonstrable physiologic changes in preeclamptic women in early pregnancy, argue for early initiation of therapy. There is no evidence that antihypertensive therapy begun after 30 weeks has any beneficial fetal effect.

If one concludes that antihypertensive therapy does not reduce perinatal mortality and morbidity rates, such therapy is reserved for women with diastolic pressure greater than 100 mm Hg. In addition, women using hypertensive therapy when they become pregnant, regardless of pretreatment blood pressure, would best be served by continuation of therapy. There is no evidence that antihypertensive therapy presents a risk to the fetus, and it is very possible that discontinuation of therapy may adversely affect long-range compliance with drug therapy, clearly increasing the risk to the mother.

Choice of Antihypertensive Agents

The presence of a fetus requires special considerations in the choice of antihypertensive agents. Of great concern is the possible teratogenic effect of such drugs. None of the currently available antihypertensive agents has been associated with morphologic teratogenic effects. Because development obviously does not end with gross organ development, however, the ultimate test of drug safety depends on long-range follow-up. At present, information from careful long-range follow-up is available only for alpha-methyldopa. Children of mothers treated with this agent during pregnancy showed no signs of neurologic or somatic abnormalities in a 7½-year follow-up (Ounsted, 1983).

It is important to remember that maternal drug therapy also "treats" the fetus. In animal studies, maternal treatment with propranolol reduces fetal as well as maternal cardiac output (Oakes et al., 1976). Because of the potential pharmacokinetic differences

TABLE 49–11. Fetal Outcome with Maternal Antihypertensive Therapy

STUDY		PREGNANCIES	TOTAL FETAL DEATHS	TRIMESTER FETAL DEATHS
Redman et al.	Control	125	9	5
(1976b)	Treated	127	1	1
Leather et al.	Control	24	5	2
(1986)	Treated	23	0	0
Sibai et al.	Control	90	1	1
(1990)	Treated	174	2	1

TABLE 49–12. Antihypertensive Agents in Pregnancy

AGENT	MECHANISM OF ACTION	CARDIAC OUTPUT	RENAL BLOOD FLOW	SIDE EFFECTS	
				MATERNAL	NEONATAL
Thiazide	*Initial*: decreased plasma volume and cardiac output	Decreased	Decreased	Electrolyte depletion, serum uric acid increase, thrombocytopenia, hemorrhagic pancreatitis	Thrombocytopenia
	Later: decreased TPR	Unchanged	Unchanged or increased		
Methyldopa	False neurotransmission, CNS effect	Unchanged	Unchanged	Lethargy, fever, hepatitis, hemolytic anemia, positive Coombs' test result	
Hydralazine	Direct peripheral vasodilation	Increased	Unchanged or increased	Flushing, headache, tachycardia, palpitations, lupus syndrome	
Prazosin	Direct vasodilator and cardiac effects	Increased or unchanged	Unchanged	Hypotension with first dose; little information on use in pregnancy	
Clonidine	CNS effects	Unchanged or increased	Unchanged	Rebound hypertension; little information on use in pregnancy	
Propranolol	Beta-adrenergic blockade	Decreased	Decreased	Increased uterine tone with possible decrease in placental perfusion	Depressed respiration
Labetalol	Alpha- and beta-adrenergic blockade	Unchanged	Unchanged	Tremulousness, flushing, headache	See Propranolol
Reserpine	Depletion of norepinephrine from sympathetic nerve endings	Unchanged	Unchanged	Nasal stuffiness, depression, increased sensitivity to seizures	Nasal congestion, increased respiratory tract secretions, cyanosis, anorexia
Enalapril	Angiotensin converting enzyme inhibitor	Unchanged	Unchanged	Hyperkalemia, dry cough	Neonatal anuria
Nifedipine	Calcium channel blocker	Unchanged	Unchanged	Orthostatic hypotension, headache, tachycardia	None demonstrated in humans

between mother and fetus, appropriate dosage for the mother may be excessive for the fetus (Rane and Tomson, 1980). Also, drug effects of minimal importance to mother and fetus may be of great importance to the infant as a neonate. For example, nasal congestion as a complication of reserpine therapy is annoying to the mother and of no importance to the fetus, but is potentially lethal to the neonate, an obligate nose-breather.

Another important consideration is the effect of drugs upon uterine blood flow. This issue is especially pertinent with antihypertensive drugs, which lower blood pressure by reducing either cardiac output or total peripheral resistance, with consequent changes in blood flow distribution. Making a rational drug choice requires avoiding agents that reduce uterine and hence uteroplacental blood flow. Agents that reduce cardiac output are best avoided because they almost inevitably reduce uterine blood flow. Antihypertensive drugs that lower blood pressure through effects on total peripheral resistance could increase, decrease, or not change uterine perfusion, depending on the pattern of blood flow redistribution. Unfortunately, there is little reliable information on the effects of antihypertensive drugs on human uterine blood

flow. Data on potential effects of these drugs are based on studies of pregnant animals in which it was assumed that humans and sheep respond identically or in which blood flow to the kidney, an exquisitely autoregulated organ that usually receives 10 per cent of cardiac output, was compared with blood flow to the uterus, an organ whose perfusion increases 500-fold over several months. Within these limitations, Table 49–12 outlines the available information about antihypertensive agents currently used in pregnancy.

A few drugs require special comment. The use during pregnancy of the two common classes of drugs for antihypertensive therapy, diuretics and beta-adrenergic blockers, is especially controversial. The indiscriminate use of diuretic agents during pregnancy has been appropriately condemned. In an epidemiologic assessment of 8000 pregnancies, a small but significant increase in perinatal mortality rate was demonstrated in women receiving continued or intermittent diuretic therapy for nonmedical indications, especially when the drug was begun late in pregnancy (Christianson and Page, 1976). Also, lack of expansion of intravascular volume during pregnancy has adverse prognostic significance (Arias, 1975; Soffronoff et al., 1977). In women taking diuretics from early pregnancy, plasma volume does not expand as much as in normal pregnancy (Sibai et al., 1983b, 1984). Because of this, several investigators recommend that diuretics not be used during pregnancy (Redman, 1980; Feitelson and Lindheimer, 1972). In the United States, however, diuretics are frequently used for antihypertensive therapy in nonpregnant patients, and their efficacy, safety, and infrequency of side effects are extensively documented (Jandhyala et al., 1974). The combination of diuretics with other antihypertensive drugs allows the use of lower doses of the other agents by preventing sodium retention. Also in spite of the theoretic concerns, when continuous diuretic therapy is begun before 24 to 30 weeks gestation there is no evidence of increased perinatal mortality rate or decreased neonatal weight (Kraus et al., 1966; Flowers et al., 1962). However, diuretic therapy should never be instituted if there is any evidence of reduced uteroplacental perfusion, as is the case with intrauterine growth restriction or preeclampsia. Another problem with diuretic therapy is the resultant increase in uric acid that renders serum uric acid determinations invalid for determination of superimposed preeclampsia.

Beta-adrenergic antagonists are the initial antihypertensive agents for nonpregnant patients in many settings. These agents reduce blood pressure by reducing cardiac output and perhaps by interfering with renin release. They are especially valuable adjuncts to hydralazine therapy, increasing the efficacy of this vasodilator by reducing the reflex increase in cardiac output. In spite of earlier concerns (Reed et al., 1974; Gladstone et al., 1975), while a review of the use of beta antagonists during pregnancy (Rubin, 1981) found no increase in perinatal mortality or growth restriction, a recent trial by the same group (Butters et al., 1989) indicated that infants of mothers receiving the beta antagonist, atenolol, weighed 500 gm less than infants of control mothers.

It is important to remember that not all beta-adrenergic antagonists are identical. Some of these agents are beta-1-adrenergic subtype-specific (e.g., metoprolol and atenolol) and as such should have less effect on beta$_2$-receptors in myometrium. In addition, variations in lipid solubility of these drugs results in different effects on the central nervous system and probably on placental transfer. Also, some of the beta-adrenergic antagonists, such as oxprenolol, actually have beta-agonist effects as well. Labetalol, in addition to its beta-adrenergic antagonist effects, is an alpha-adrenergic antagonist. The decision, both theoretical and empiric, about the safety and efficacy of these drugs requires evaluation of the pharmacologic characteristics of each drug rather than consideration of them as a class.

Hydralazine would appear to be an ideal antihypertensive drug for pregnant women. However, side effects such as headache and palpitations due to reflex increase in cardiac output usually prevent its use in effective dosages. Alpha-methyldopa, the drug used in the largest study and the only drug whose safety for infants has been demonstrated in long-range follow-up, is the benchmark of antihypertensive therapy. It frequently causes drowsiness, however, especially when used in the large doses necessary when diuretics

are not used concomitantly, occasionally to a degree that is incapacitating, particularly for ambulatory patients (Redman et al., 1977b). In the original examination of infants whose mothers received alpha-methyldopa, there was a small but statistically significant decrease in head circumference, although this effect was not found in follow-up studies (Ounsted, 1983).

Several newer antihypertensive drugs are available that might offer theoretic advantages for use in pregnancy. The widespread use of these newer drugs during pregnancy, however, requires clinical testing of efficacy and immediate and long-range safety.

One agent that is widely used in nonpregnant patients is the angiotensin converting enzymes (ACE) inhibitor, enalapril. Animal studies with another ACE inhibitor, captopril, suggested caution in the use of this drug in pregnancy. There was unexplained fetal death when pregnant ewes and rabbit does were treated (Pipkin et al., 1982). These concerns have been borne out by clinical experience. Although there are no reports of fetal death, a number of infants have been born with neonatal renal dysfunction which, in some cases, has been permanent (Rosa et al., 1989). However, there are no reports of teratogenesis (Working Group on High Blood Pressure in Pregnancy, 1990), these findings being limited to infants of mothers who received these drugs in late pregnancy. Thus the drug should be discontinued during pregnancy. However, the woman becoming pregnant while receiving enalapril can be reassured that permanent damage to the fetus is unlikely if the drug was taken only in early pregnancy.

Recommendations

On the basis of the preceding information, a plan for the pharmacologic management of hypertension in pregnancy can be advanced. The use of ganglionic blockers—rare in the 1990s—should be discontinued because of the extreme sensitivity of pregnant women to these agents and the potential fetal risk of meconium ileus. ACE inhibitors should also be discontinued. No other drugs are absolutely contraindicated. The drug regimens suggested in the following paragraphs are preferred because of currently available information regarding efficacy, side effects, and long-term follow-up. If a woman has established excellent blood pressure control, however, especially after unsuccessful trials of other agents, she should continue the successful regimen upon becoming pregnant. This is especially pertinent to beta-adrenergic antagonist use. Women receiving propranolol should switch if possible to a less lipid-soluble and perhaps more selective beta-adrenergic antagonist of equivalent efficacy. The use of diuretic therapy is associated with few acute adverse effects and potentiates other drug effects. Although the use of diuretics from early pregnancy appears safe (Kraus et al., 1966; Weseley and Douglas, 1962; Flowers, 1962), theoretic concerns raised by the effects of these agents upon plasma volume militate against their use as initial therapy. Diuretics are also contraindicated for women with evidence of decreased uterine perfusion manifested as intrauterine growth restriction or preeclampsia. Furthermore, there is no evidence that after 30 weeks of gestation diuretics do not adversely affect survival or growth. Another major consideration in the use of diuretics is the fact that they render uric acid determination invalid as an indicator of superimposed preeclampsia.

Aldomet is the drug of choice for the initiation of antihypertensive therapy in pregnancy. The initial dosage is 250 mg at night and then 250 mg twice daily, increasing to a maximum of 1 gm twice daily. If side effects prevent the use of maximal doses or if 2 gm daily does not sufficiently control blood pressure, another agent should be added (not substituted). The use of small doses of diuretic will usually dramatically increase the efficacy of Aldomet. If the pregnancy is less than 30 weeks, available information indicates the safety of these drugs, in spite of theoretic concerns. The initial dose should be 25 mg of hydrochlorothiazide equivalent, increasing at 2- to 4-day intervals to 50 mg/day. In view of the vagaries of electrolyte balance during pregnancy, it is prudent to supplement dietary potassium and, more important, to avoid stringent sodium restriction.

If this addition does not achieve adequate blood pressure control or if diuretics are contraindicated, prazosin, or nifedipine, or hydralazine may be added. Although there has been most experience with hydralazine during pregnancy, the side effects with other agents are usually much less. If hydralazine is chosen, dosage is begun at 10 mg daily, increasing to a maximum of 100 mg twice daily. Prazosin can be initiated at 1 mg a day increasing to 10 mg twice daily. The woman should take the first dose at bedtime and be warned of the orthostatic hypotension that may accompany the first dose of prazosin. Nifedipine can be started at 10 mg twice a day increasing to 90 mg day. If doses of 30 mg or greater are necessary, 30-mg long-acting tablets can be substituted for multiple daily dosing. When used in this supplemental manner, these drugs usually are successful at low dosages.

Alternatively, alpha-methyldopa can be discontinued and single-agent therapy with nifedipine, prazosin, or labetalol initiated. Of the three, there is most experience with labetalol in pregnancy (Sibai et al., 1990). It is begun at 100 mg twice a day and the dosage increased incrementally to a maximum of 2400 mg/day. Prazosin and nifedipine dosing is as described as adjuncts above.

Obstetric Management in Chronic Hypertension

Obstetric management of the woman with chronic hypertension comprises (1) early recognition of superimposed preeclampsia, (2) monitoring of fetal well-being, and (3) ruling-out of pheochromocytoma. Early in pregnancy, studies of renal function (creatinine clearance and 24-hour protein excretion) and serum urate determination should be performed. These studies serve as a baseline to aid in the diagnosis of superimposed preeclampsia later in pregnancy. These baseline studies are especially helpful in determining whether increased blood pressure in later pregnancy is due to exaggeration of the usual blood pressure changes of pregnancy or to the superimposition of

preeclampsia. Because preeclampsia occurs earlier in pregnancy in hypertensive women, these patients should be seen every other week beginning at 26 weeks gestation and weekly beginning at 30 weeks.

Ultrasonographic evaluation of the fetus between 18 and 24 weeks gestation allows accurate dating and also provides a baseline to determine incremental growth in suspicion of growth retardation.

The majority of hypertensive pregnant women have essential hypertension. Thorough evaluation for most secondary forms of hypertension is best reserved for the postpartum period because of the obfuscation of many of these forms by physiologic changes of pregnancy as well as the risks of diagnostic procedures to mother and fetus. Pheochromocytoma is a potentially lethal complication, especially during the intrapartum period. This condition can be simply, accurately, and inexpensively diagnosed in many individuals with fixed hypertension by determination of serum or urinary catecholamine concentration. Hypertensive women in whom this parameter has not been measured in the past should undergo this determination in early pregnancy. Coarctation of the aorta, a rare cause of hypertension in women of reproductive age, can be readily diagnosed by determination of a lag between radial and femoral pulses, which should be sought as part of the physical examination of hypertensive patients.

Because of the controversy about effects of hypertension uncomplicated by preeclampsia on perinatal mortality, and since the origin of the increased mortality of this condition is placental insufficiency, extensive fetal surveillance should be reserved for infants with evidence of growth restriction or whose mothers are preeclamptic.

REFERENCES

Adams EM, Cantab MA, Aberd MD, MacGillivary I: Long-term effect of pre-eclampsia on blood pressure. Lancet 2:1373, 1961.

Adams EM, Finlayson A: Familial aspects of preeclampsia and hypertension in pregnancy. Lancet 2:1357, 1961.

Altchek A, Allbright NL, Sommers C: The renal pathology of toxemia of pregnancy. Obstet Gynecol 31:595, 1968.

Appleton MP, Kuehl TJ, Raebel MA, Adams HR, Knight AB, Gold WR: Magnesium sulfate versus phenytoin for seizure prophylaxis in pregnancy-induced hypertension. Am J Obstet Gynecol 165:907, 1991.

Arias F: Expansion of intravascular volume and fetal outcome in patients with chronic hypertension and pregnancy. Am J Obstet Gynecol 123:610, 1975.

Arias F, Muncilla-Jiminez R: Hepatic fibrinogen deposits in preeclampsia. N Engl J Med 295:578, 1976.

Arias F, Zamora J: Antihypertensive treatment and pregnancy outcome in patients with mild chronic hypertension. Obstet Gynecol 53:489, 1979.

Assali NS, Kaplan SA, Fomon SJ, Douglass RA Jr: Renal function studies in toxemia of pregnancy. Excretion of solutes and renal hemodynamics during osmotic diuresis in hydropenia. J Clin Invest 32:44, 1953.

Assali NS, Prystowsky H: Studies on autonomic blockade. I. Comparison between the effects of tetraethylammonium chloride (TEAC) and high selective spinal anesthesia on blood pressure of normal and toxemic pregnancy. J Clin Invest 29:1354, 1950.

August P, Lenz T, Ales KL, et al: Longitudinal study of the renin-angiotensin-aldosterone system in hypertensive pregnant women:

Deviations related to the development of superimposed pre-eclampsia. Am J Obstet Gynecol 63:1612, 1990.

Baumgartner HR, Hardenschild C: Adhesion of platelets to subendothelium. Ann NY Acad Sci 201:22, 1977.

Bay WH, Ferris TF: Factors controlling plasma renin and aldosterone during pregnancy. Hypertension 1:410, 1979.

Bell WR: Disseminated intravascular coagulation. Johns Hopkins Med J 146:289, 1980.

Beller FK, Ebert CH, Dame WR: High molecular fibrin derivatives in preeclamptic and eclamptic patients. Europ J Obstet Gynec Reprod Biol 9:105, 1979.

Benedetti TJ, Quilligan EJ: Cerebral edema in severe pregnancy-induced hypertension. Am J Obstet Gynecol 137:861, 1980.

Berman S: Observations in the toxemic clinic, Boston Lying-In Hospital, 1923–1930. Obstet Gynecol 203:361, 1930.

Bond AL, August P, Druzin ML, et al: Atrial natriuretic factor in normal and hypertensive pregnancy. Am J Obstet and Gynecol 160:1112, 1989.

Brinkman CR, Assali NS: Uteroplacental hemodynamic response to antihypertensive drugs in hypertensive pregnant sheep. In Ludheimer GD, Katz AI, Zuspan FP (eds): Hypertension in Pregnancy. New York, John Wiley & Sons, 1976.

Brosens IA, Robertson WB, Dixon HG: The role of the spiral arteries in the pathogenesis of preeclampsia. Obstet Gynecol Annu 1:171, 1972.

Browne FJ: The early signs of preeclampsia toxaemia, with special reference to the order of their appearance, and their interrelation. J Obstet Gynaecol Br Emp 40:1160, 1933.

Bulfin MJ, Lawler PE: Problems associated with toxemia in twin pregnancies. Am J Obstet Gynecol 73:37, 1957.

Bussolino F, Benedetto C, Massobrio M, Camussi G: Maternal vascular prostacyclin activity in pre-eclampsia. (Letter) Lancet ii:702, 1980.

Butters L, Kennedy S, Rubin P: Atenolol and fetal weight in chronic hypertension during pregnancy. (Abstract) Clin Exp Hypertens [A]BA:468, 1989.

Cannon PJ, Svahn DS, DeMartini FE: The influence of hypertonic saline infusion upon the fractional reabsorption of urate and other ions in normal and hypertensive man. Circulation 41:97, 1970.

Chesley LC: Renal function tests in the differentiation of Bright's disease from so-called specific toxemia of pregnancy. Surg Gynecol Obstet 67:481, 1938.

Chesley LC, Markowitz I, Wetchler BB: Proteinuria following momentary vascular constriction. J Clin Invest 18:51, 1939.

Chesley LC, Chesley ER: An analysis of some factors associated with the development of preeclampsia. Am J Obstet Gynecol 45:748, 1943.

Chesley LC, Annitto JE: Pregnancy in the patient with hypertensive disease. Am J Obstet Gynecol 53:372, 1947.

Chesley LC, Tepper I: Plasma levels of magnesium attained in magnesium sulfate therapy for preeclampsia and eclampsia. Surg Clin North Am 37:353, 1957.

Chesley LC, Valenti C: The evaluation of tests to differentiate preeclampsia from hypertensive disease. Am J Obstet Gynecol 75:1165, 1958a.

Chesley LC, Valenti C, Rein H: The excretion of sodium loads by nonpregnant and pregnant normal, hypertensive and preeclamptic women. Metabolism 7:575, 1958b.

Chesley LC: Sodium retention and preeclampsia. Am J Obstet Gynecol 95:127, 1966.

Chesley LC, Annitto JE, Cosgrove RA: Long-term follow-up study of eclamptic women: Fifth periodic report. Am J Obstet Gynecol 101:886, 1968.

Chesley LC, Annitto JE, Cosgrove RA: The remote prognosis of eclamptic women: Sixth periodic report. Am J Obstet Gynecol 124:446, 1976.

Chesley LC: Hypertensive Disorders in Pregnancy. New York, Appleton-Century-Crofts, 1978.

Chesley LC: Parenteral magnesium sulfate and the distribution, plasma levels, and excretion of magnesium. Am J Obstet Gynecol 133:1, 1979.

Chesley LC: Hypertension in pregnancy: Definitions, familial factor, and remote prognosis. Kidney Intl 18:234, 1980.

Chesley LC, Cooper DW: Genetics of hypertension in pregnancy: Possible single-gene control of pre-eclampsia and eclampsia in

the descendants of eclamptic women. Br J Obstet Gynaecol 93:898, 1986.

Christianson RE: Studies on blood pressure during pregnancy. 1. Influence of parity and age. Am J Obstet Gynecol 125:509, 1976.

Christianson R, Page EW: Diuretic drugs and pregnancy. Obstet Gynecol 48:647, 1976.

Cotton DB, Benedetti TJ: Use of the Swan-Ganz catheter in obstetrics and gynecology. Obstet Gynecol 56:641, 1980.

Cree JE, Meyer J, Hailey DM: Diazepam in labour: Its metabolism and effect on the clinical condition and thermogenesis of the newborn. Br Med J 4:251, 1973.

Crowther C: Magnesium sulfate versus diazepam in the management of eclampsia: A randomized controlled trial. Br J Obstet Gynaecol 97:110, 1990.

Dadak C, Kefalides A, Sinzinger H, Weber G: Reduced umbilical artery prostacyclin formation in complicated pregnancies. Am J Obstet Gynecol 144:792, 1982.

Dadak C, Olrich W, Sinzinger H: Morphological changes in the umbilical arteries of babies born to pre-eclamptic mothers: An ultrastructural study. Placenta 5:419, 1984.

Davidge ST, Hubel CA, Brayden RD, Capeless EC, McLaughlin MK: Sera antioxidant activity in uncomplicated and preeclamptic pregnancies. Obstet Gynecol 79(6):897, 1992.

Davies AG: Geographical Epidemiology of the Toxemias of Pregnancy. Springfield, IL, Charles C Thomas, 1971.

Davies AM, Czaczkes JW, Sadovsky E, et al: Toxemia of pregnancy in Jerusalem. I. Epidemiological studies of a total community. Isr J Med Sci 6:253, 1970.

Dell RB, Winters RW: Lactate gradients in the kidney of the dog. Am J Physiol 213:301, 1967.

Denson KWE: The ratio of factor VIII-related antigen and factor VIII biological activity as an index of hypercoagulability and intravascular clotting. Thromb Res 10:107, 1977.

Dieckman WJ: The Toxemias of Pregnancy. 2nd ed. St Louis, CV Mosby, 1952.

Dieckman WJ, Michel HL: Vascular-renal effects of posterior pituitary extracts in pregnant women. Am J Obstet Gynecol 33:131, 1937.

Dieckman WJ, Pottinger RE: Total exchangeable sodium and space in normal and preeclamptic patients determined with sodium[22]. Am J Obstet Gynecol 74:816, 1957.

Douglas JT, Shah M, Lowe GDO, et al: Plasma fibrinopeptide and beta-thromboglobulin in pre-eclampsia and pregnancy hypertension. Thromb Haemost 47:54, 1982.

Duffus GM, Tunstall ME, Condie RG, MacGillivray I: Chlormethiazole in the prevention of eclampsia and the reduction of perinatal mortality. J Obstet Gynaec Br Cwlth 76:645, 1969.

Duncan SLB, Ginsburg J, Bernard AG: Arteriolar distensibility in hypertensive pregnancy. Am J Obstet Gynecol 100:222, 1968.

Easterling TR, Benedetti TJ, Schmucker BC, Millard SP: Maternal hemodynamics in normal and preeclampsia pregnancies: A longitudinal study. Obstet Gynecol 76:1061, 1990.

Ehrlich EN, Lindheimer MD: Sodium metabolism, aldosterone and the hypertensive disorders of pregnancy. (Editorial) J Reprod Med 8:106, 1972.

Elden CA, Cooney JW: The Addis sediment count and blood urea clearance test in normal pregnant women. J Clin Invest 14:889, 1935.

Emmerson BT: Effect of drugs on the renal handling of urate. In Edwards DK (ed): Drugs and the Kidney. (Progr Biochem Pharmacol Vol 9) Basel, S Karger, 1974.

Epstein FH: Late vascular effects of toxemia of pregnancy. N Engl J Med 271:391, 1964.

Everett RB, Worley RJ, McDonald PC, et al: Effect of prostaglandin synthetase inhibitors on pressor response to angiotensin II in human pregnancy. J Clin Endocrinol Metab 46:1007, 1978.

Fadel HE, Northrop G, Misenheimer HR: Hyperuricemia in pre-eclampsia. A reappraisal. Am J Obstet Gynecol 125:640, 1976.

Faith GC, Trump BF: The glomerular capillary wall in human kidney disease: Acute glomerulonephritis, systemic lupus erythematosus, and preeclampsia-eclampsia. Lab Invest 15:1682, 1966.

Farrell PC: Protein binding of urate ions in vitro and in vivo. In Edwards DK (ed): Drugs and the Kidney. (Progr Biochem Pharmacol Vol 9) Basel, S Karger, 1974.

Feitelson PJ, Lindheimer MD: Management of hypertensive gravidas. J Reprod Med 8:111, 1972.

Ferris TF, Gordon P: Effect of angiotensin and norepinephrine upon urate clearance in man. Am J Med **44**:359, 1968.

Ferris TF, Stein JH, Kauffman J: Uterine blood flow and uterine renin secretion. J Clin Invest **51**:2827, 1972.

Finnerty FA: Toxemia of pregnancy as seen by an internist. An analysis of 1,081 patients. Ann Intern Med **44**:358, 1956.

Fisher KA, Luger A, Spargo BH, Lindheimer MD: Hypertension in pregnancy: Clinical-pathological correlations and remote prognosis. Medicine **60**:267, 1981.

Flowers CE, Grizzle JE, Easterling WE, Bonner OB: Chlorothiazide as a prophylaxis against toxemia of pregnancy. A double-blind study. Am J Obstet Gynecol **84**:919, 1962.

Fox H: Effect of hypoxia on trophoblast in organ culture. Am J Obstet Gynecol **107**:1058, 1970.

Freeman RK: The use of the oxytocin challenge test for antepartum clinical evaluation of uteroplacental respiratory function. Am J Obstet Gynecol **121**:481, 1975.

Furchgott RF: Role of endothelium in the response of vascular smooth muscle. Circ Res **53**:558, 1983.

Gallery EDM, Györy AZ: Glomerular and proximal renal tubular function in pregnancy-associated hypertension: A prospective study. Eur J Obstet Gynec Reprod Biol **9**:3, 1979a.

Gallery EDM, Györy AZ: Urinary concentration, white blood cell excretion, acid excretion, and acid-base status in normal pregnancy: alterations in pregnancy-associated hypertension. Am J Obstet Gynecol **135**:27, 1979b.

Gallery EDM, Hunyor SN, Ross M, Györy AZ: Predicting the development of pregnancy-associated hypertension: The place of standardised blood-pressure measurement. Lancet **1**:1273, 1977.

Gallery EDM, Saunders DM, Boyce ES, Györy AZ: Relation between plasma volume and uric acid in the development of hypertension in pregnancy. In Bonnar MA, MacGillivray I, Symonds MS (eds): Pregnancy Hypertension. Baltimore, University Park Press, 1980b.

Galton M, Merritt K, Veller FK: Coagulation studies on the peripheral circulation of patients with toxemia of pregnancy: A study for the evaluation of disseminated intravascular coagulation in toxemia. J Reprod Med **6**:78, 1971.

Gant NF, Daley GL, Chand S, et al: A study of angiotensin II pressor response throughout primigravid pregnancy. J Clin Invest **52**:2682, 1973.

Gladstone GR, Hordof A, Gersony WM: Propranolol administration during pregnancy: Effects on the fetus. J Pediatr **86**:962, 1975.

Goodlin RC: Expanded toxemia syndrome or gestosis. Am J Obstet Gynecol **154**:1227, 1986.

Goodlin RC, Cotton DB, Haesslein HC: Severe edema-proteinuria-hypertension gestosis. Am J Obstet Gynecol **132**:595, 1978.

Gordon RD, Symonds EM, Wilmhurst EG, Pawsey CGK: Plasma renin activity, plasma angiotensin and plasma and urinary electrolytes in normal and toxaemic pregnancy, including a prospective study. Clin Sci Molec Med **45**:115, 1973.

Gordon YB, Ratky SM, Baker LRI, et al: Circulating levels of fibrin/fibrinogen degradation fragment E measured by radioimmunoassay in preeclampsia. Br J Obstet Gynaecol **83**:287, 1976.

Greer IA, Walker JJ, Bjornsson S, Calder AA: Second line therapy with nifedipine in severe pregnancy induced hypertension. Clin Exper Hyperten **B8**:277, 1989.

Handler JS: The role of lactic acid in the reduced excretion of uric acid in toxemia of pregnancy. J Clin Invest **39**:1526, 1960.

Hauth JC, Cunningham FG, Whalley PJ: Management of pregnancy-induced hypertension in the nullipara. Am J Obstet Gynecol **48**:253, 1976.

Hayashi T: Uric acid and endogenous creatinine clearance studies in normal pregnancy and toxemias of pregnancy. Am J Obstet Gynecol **71**:859, 1956.

Healy JK, Edwards KDG, Whyte HM: Simple tests of renal function using creatinine, phenolsulfonphthalein and pitressin. J Clin Pathol **17**:557, 1964.

Heidland A, Reidl E: Klinisch-experimentelle Untersuchung uber den renalen Phenolsulfonphthalein-Transport. Arch Klin Med **214**:163, 1968.

Henderson AH, Pugsley DJ, Thomas DP: Fibrin degradation products in preeclamptic toxaemia and eclampsia. Br Med J **3**:545, 1970.

Hollenberg NK, Epstein M, Rosen SM, et al: Acute oliguric renal failure in man: Evidence for preferential renal cortical ischemia. Medicine **47**:455, 1968.

Howie PW, Prentice CRM, Forbes CD: Failure of heparin therapy to affect the clinical course of severe preeclampsia. Br J Obstet Gynecol **82**:711, 1975.

Hubel CA, Roberts JM, Taylor RN, et al: Lipid peroxidation in pregnancy: New perspectives on preeclampsia. Am J Obstet Gynecol **16**(4):1025, 1989.

Hughes EC (ed): Obstetric-Gynecologic Terminology. Philadelphia, FA Davis, 1972.

Imperiale TF, Petrulis AS: A meta-analysis of low-dose aspirin for the prevention of pregnancy-induced hypertensive disease. JAMA **266**:261, 1991.

Inglis TCM, Stuart J, George AJ, Davies AJ: Haemostatic and rheological changes in normal pregnancy and pre-eclampsia. Br J Haematol **50**:461, 1982.

Jaffe G, Schatz H: Ocular manifestations of preeclampsia. Am J Ophthalmol **103**:309, 1986.

Jandhyala BS, Clarke DE, Buckley JP: Effects of prolonged administration of certain antihypertensive agents. J Pharm Sci **63**:1497, 1974.

Jeffcoate TNA, Scott JS: Some observations on the placental factor in pregnancy toxemia. Am J Obstet Gynecol **77**:475, 1959.

Johnson N, Moodley J, Hammond MG: HLA status of the fetus born to African women with eclampsia. Clin Exper Hyper in Preg **B9**(3):311, 1990.

Johnson RA: Adverse neonatal reaction to maternal administration of intraveous chlormethiazole and diazoxide. Br Med J **601S**:943, 1976.

Jones CJP, Fox H: An ultrastructural and ultrahistochemical study of the human placenta in maternal preeclampsia. Placenta **1**:61, 1980.

Kaitz AL: Urinary concentrating ability in pregnant women with asymptomatic bacteriuria. J Clin Invest **40**:1331, 1961.

Katz M, Berlyne GM: Differential renal protein clearance in toxaemia of pregnancy. Nephron **13**:212, 1974.

Kavats S, Main EK, Librach C, et al: Class I antigen, HLA-G, expressed in human trophoblasts. Sci **248**:220–223, 1990.

Khong, TY, De Wolf F, Robertson WB, Brosens I: Inadequate maternal vascular response to placentation in pregnancies complicated by pre-eclampsia and by small-for-gestational age infants. Br J Obstet Gynaecol **93**:1049, 1986.

Kilpatrick DC, Gibson G, Livingston J, Liston WA: Preeclampsia is associated with HLA-DR4 sharing between mother and fetus. Tissue Antigens **35**:178–181, 1990.

Kincaid-Smith P: The renal lesion of preeclampsia revisited. Am J Kidney Dis **144**:148, 1991.

Kincaid-Smith P, Bullen M, Mills J: Prolonged use of methyldopa in severe hypertension in pregnancy. Br Med J **1**:274, 1966.

Kitzmiller JL, Benirschke K: Immunofluorescent study of placental bed vessels in pre-eclampsia. Am J Obstet Gynecol **115**:248, 1973.

Kitzmiller JL, Stoneburner L, Yelenosky PF, Lucas WE: Serum complement in normal pregnancy and pre-eclampsia. Am J Obstet Gynecol **117**:312, 1973.

Kitzmiller JL, Watt N, Driscoll SG: Decidual arteriopathy in hypertension and diabetes in pregnancy: Immunofluorescent studies. Am J Obstet Gynecol **141**:773, 1981.

Knox GE, Stagno S, Volanakis JE, Huddleston JF: A search for antigen-antibody complexes in pre-eclampsia: Further evidence against immunologic pathogenesis. Am J Obstet Gynecol **132**:87, 1978.

Kraus GW, Marchese JR, Yen SSC: Prophylactic use of hydrochlorothiazide in pregnancy. JAMA **198**:1150, 1966.

Kuntz WD: Supine pressor (roll-over) test: An evaluation. Am J Obstet Gynecol **137**:764, 1980.

Ladner CN, Weston PV, Brinkman CR, Assali NS: Effects of hydralazine on uteroplacental and fetal circulations. Am J Obstet Gynecol **108**:375, 1970.

Langford HG, Pickering GW: The action of synthetic angiotensin on renal function in the unanesthetized rabbit. J Physiol (London) **177**:161, 1965.

Leather HM, Humphreys DM, Baker P, Chadd MA: A controlled trial of hypotensive agents in hypertension in pregnancy. Lancet **2**:488, 1968.

Lichtig C, Deutsch M, Brandes J: Immunofluorescent studies of endometrial arteries in the first trimester of pregnancy. Am J Clin Pathol **83**:633, 1985.

Lin CC, Lindheimer MD, River P, Moawad AH: Fetal outcome in hypertensive disorders of pregnancy. Am J Obstet Gynecol **142**:255, 1982.

Lockwood CJ, Peters JH: Increased plasma levels of ED1+ cellular fibronectin precede the clinical signs of preeclampsia. Am J Obstet Gynecol **162**:358, 1990.

Lopez-Llera M, Horta JLH: Perinatal mortality in eclampsia. J Reprod Med **8**:281, 1972.

Lorentzen B, Endresen MJ, Haug THE, Henriksen T: Sera from preeclamptic women increase the content of triglycerides and reduce the release of prostacyclin in cultured endothelial cells. Thromb Res **363**:372, 1991.

Mabie WC, Gonzalez AR, Sibai BM, Amon E: A comparative trial of labetalol and hydralazine in the acute management of severe hypertension complicating pregnancy. Obstet Gynecol **170**:328, 1987.

MacGillivray I: Some observations on the incidence of preeclampsia. J Obstet Gynaecol **65**:536, 1958.

Malee MP, Malee KM, Azuma SD, et al: Increases in plasma atrial natriuretic peptide concentration antedate clinical evidence of preeclampsia. J Clin Endocrinol Metab **74**:1095, 1992.

Marti JJ, Herrman U: Immunogestosis. A new concept of "essential" EPH gestosis, with special consideration of the primagravid patient. Am J Obstet Gynecol **128**:489, 1977.

Martin JN, Blake PG, Pery KG, et al: The natural history of HELLP syndrome: Patterns of disease progression and regression. Am J Obstet Gynecol **164**:1500, 1991.

Massey SG: Pharmacology of magnesium. Ann Rev Pharmacol Toxicol **17**:67, 1977.

Mathews DD: A randomized controlled trial of bed rest and sedation or normal activity and non-sedation in the management of non-albuminuric hypertension in late pregnancy. Br J Obstet Gynaecol **84**:108, 1977.

Matter L, Faulk WP: Fibrinogen degradation products and factor VIII consumption in normal pregnancy and preeclampsia: Role of the placenta. In Bonnar MA, MacGillivray I, Symonds MS (eds). Pregnancy Hypertension. Baltimore, University Park Press, 1980.

Maynard JR, Dreyer BE, Stemerman MB, Pitlick FA: Tissue factor coagulant activity of cultured human endothelial and smooth muscle cells and fibroblasts. Blood **50**:387, 1987.

McCartney CP: Pathological anatomy of acute hypertension of pregnancy. Circulation **30**(Suppl II):37, 1964.

McKay DG: Hematologic evidence of disseminated intravascular coagulation in eclampsia. Obstet Gynecol Surv **27**:399, 1972.

McKillop C, Howie PW, Forbes CD, Prentice CRM: Soluble fibrinogen/fibrin complexes in preeclampsia. Lancet **1**:56, 1976.

Moncada S, Palmer RMJ, Higgs EA: Nitric oxide: Physiology, pathophysiology, and pharmacology. Pharmacol Rev **43**:109, 1991.

Naden RP, Redman CWG: Antihypertensive drugs in pregnancy. Clin Perinatol **12**:521, 1985.

Nadji P, Sommers SC: Lesions of toxemia in first trimester pregnancies. Am J Clin Pathol **59**:344, 1973.

Naeye RL, Friedman EA: Causes of perinatal death associated with gestational hypertension and proteinuria. Am J Obstet Gynecol **133**:8, 1979.

Naheedy MH, Biller J, Schiffer M, et al: Toxemia of pregnancy: Cerebral findings. J Comput Assist Tomogr **9**:497, 1985.

Naidoo DV, Moodley J: A survey of hypertension in pregnancy at the King Edward VIII Hospital, Durban. S Afr Med J **58**:556, 1980.

Nakamura T, Ito M, Matsui K, et al: Significance of angiotensin sensitivity test for prediction of pregnancy-induced hypertension. Obstet Gynecol **67**:388, 1986.

Naulty J, Cefalo RC, Lewis PE: Fetal toxicity of nitroprusside in the pregnant ewe. Am J Obstet Gynecol **139**:708, 1981.

Need JA: Pre-eclampsia in pregnancies by different fathers: Immunological studies. Br Med J **1**:548, 1975.

Nelson TR: A clinical study of preeclampsia, Parts I and II. J Obstet Gynaecol Br Emp **62**:48, 1955.

Neutra R, Neff R: Fetal death in eclampsia: II. The effect of nontherapeutic factors. Br J Obstet Gynaecol **82**:390, 1975.

Oakes GK, Walker AM, Ehrenkranz RA, Chez RA: Effect of propranolol infusion on the umbilical and uterine circulations of pregnant sheep. Am J Obstet Gynecol **126**:1038, 1976.

Ochwadt B, Pitts RF: Disparity between phenol red and Diodrast clearances in the dog. Am J Physiol **187**:318, 1956.

Oian P, Kjeldsen SE, Eide I, Norman N: Adrenaline and preeclampsia. Acta Med Scand (Suppl) **693**:29, 1985.

Okkels, H, Engle ET: Studies of the fever structure of the uterine vessels of the Macacus monkey. Acta Pathol Microbiol Scand **15**:150, 1938.

Oney T, Kaulhausen H: The value of the angiotensin sensitivity test in the early diagnosis of hypertensive disorders in pregnancy. Am J Obstet Gynecol **142**:17, 1982.

Ounsted M, Cockburn J, Moar VA, Redman CWG: Maternal hypertension with superimposed preeclampsia: Effects on child development at 7½ years. Br J Obstet Gynaecol **90**:644, 1983.

Page EW: The relation between hydatid moles, relative ischemia of the gravid uterus, and placental origin of eclampsia. Am J Obstet Gynecol **37**:291, 1939.

Page EW, Christianson R: The impact of mean arterial blood pressure in the middle trimester upon the outcome of pregnancy. Am J Obstet Gynecol **125**:740, 1976.

Parks DA, Granger DN: Xanthine oxidase: Biochemistry, distribution and physiology. Acta Physiol Scand (Suppl) **584**:87, 1986.

Petruccho OM, Thomson NM, Lawrence JR, Weldon MW: Immunofluorescein studies in renal biopsies in preeclampsia. Br Med J **1**:473, 1974.

Pinto A, Sorrentino R, Sorrentino P, et al: Endothelial-derived relaxing factor released by endothelial cells of human umbilical vessels and its impairment in pregnancy-induced hypertension. Am J Obstet Gynecol **164**:507, 1991.

Pipkin FB, Oats JJ, Symonds EM: The effect of a specific AII antagonist (saralasin) on blood pressure in the immediate puerperium. In Bonnar MA, MacGillivray I, Symonds MS (eds): Pregnancy Hypertension. Baltimore, University Park Press, 1980.

Pipkin FB, Symonds EM, Turner SR: The effect of captopril (SQ 14,225) upon mother and fetus in the chronically cannulated ewe and in the pregnant rabbit. J Physiol **323**:415, 1982.

Plouin PF, Chatellier G, Breart G, et al: Frequency and perinatal consequences of hypertensive disease of pregnancy. Adv Nephrol **57**:69, 1986.

Poland ML, Lucas CP: Plasma epinephrine and norepinephrine in normotensive and pregnancy-induced hypertensive pregnancies. In Bonnar MA, MacGillivray I, Symonds MS (eds): Pregnancy Hypertension. Baltimore, University Park Press, 1980.

Pollak VE, Nettles JB: The kidney in toxemia of pregnancy: A clinical and pathologic study based on renal biopsies. Medicine **39**:469, 1960.

Pritchard JA: The use of the magnesium ion in the management of eclamptogenic toxemias. Surgery **100**:131, 1955.

Pritchard JA, Cunningham FG, Mason RA: Coagulation changes in eclampsia: Their frequency and pathogenesis. Am J Obstet Gynecol **124**:855, 1976.

Pritchard JA, Pritchard SA: Standardized treatment of 154 consecutive cases of eclampsia. Am J Obstet Gynecol **123**:543, 1975.

Pritchard JA, Stone SR: Clinical and laboratory observations on eclampsia. Am J Obstet Gynecol **99**:754, 1967.

Ramsey EM, Harris HWS: Comparison of uteroplacental vasculature and circulation in the rhesus monkey and man. Contributions to Embryology. No. 261. Carnegie Institution of Washington **38**:59, 1966.

Rane A, Tomson G: Prenatal and neonatal drug metabolism in man. Eur J Clin Pharmacol **18**:9, 1980.

Redman CWG, Beilin LJ, Bonnar J, Wilkinson RH: Plasma urate measurements in predicting fetal death in hypertensive pregnancy. Lancet **i**:1370, 1976a.

Redman CWG, Beilin LJ, Bonnar J, Ounsted MK: Fetal outcome in trial of antihypertensive treatment in pregnancy. Lancet **2**:753, 1976b.

Redman CWG, Denson KWE, Beilin LJ, et al: Factor-VIII consumption in preeclampsia. Lancet **2**:1249, 1977a.

Redman CWG, Beilin LJ, Bonnar J: Treatment of hypertension in pregnancy with methyldopa: Blood pressure control and side effects. Br J Obstet Gynaecol **84**:419, 1977b.

Redman CWG, Bonnar J, Beilin L: Early platelet consumption in preeclampsia. Br Med J **1**:467, 1978.

Redman CWG: Treatment of hypertension in pregnancy. Kidney Int **18**:267, 1980.

Reed RL, Cheney CB, Fearon RE, et al: Propranolol therapy throughout pregnancy: A case report. Anes Analg Curr Res **53**:214, 1974.

Remuzzi G, Marchesi D, Zoja C, et al: Reduced umbilical and placental vascular prostacyclin in severe preeclampsia. Prostaglandins 20:105, 1980.

Ricke PS, Elliott JP, Freeman RK: Use of corticosteroids in pregnancy-induced hypertension. Obstet Gynecol 55:206, 1980.

Rippman ET: Pra-eklampsie oder Schwangerschaftsspatgestose? Gynaecologia 167:478, 1969.

Roberts JM, May WJ: Consumptive coagulopathy in severe preeclampsia. Obstet Gynecol 48:163, 1976.

Roberts JM, Perloff DL: Hypertension and the obstetrician-gynecologist. Am J Obstet Gynecol 127:316, 1977.

Roberts JM, Taylor RN, Musci TJ, et al: Preeclampsia: An endothelial cell disorder. Am J Obstet Gynecol 161(5):1200, 1989.

Robertson WB, Brosens I, Dixon HG: The pathological response of the vessels of the placental bed to hypertensive pregnancy. J Pathol Bacteriol 93:581, 1967.

Rodgers GM, Greenberg CS, Shuman MA: Characterization of the effects of cultured vascular cells on the activation of blood coagulation. Blood 61:1155, 1983.

Rodgers GM, Taylor RN, Roberts JM: Preeclampsia is associated with a serum factor cytotoxic to human endothelial cells. Am J Obstet Gynecol 159:908, 1988.

Rosa FW, Bosco LA, Graham CF, et al: Neonatal anuria with maternal angiotensin-converting enzyme inhibition. Obstet Gynecol 74:371, 1989.

Rowe J, Gallery EDM, Györy AZ: Cryoactivation of renin in plasma from pregnant and nonpregnant subjects, and its control. Clin Chem 25:11, 1979.

Rubin PC: Beta-blockers in pregnancy. N Engl J Med 305:1323, 1981.

Sammour MB, Ammar AR, Tash F, Sawaud S: Plasma catecholamines during labor in normal and preeclamptic pregnancies. In Bonnar J, MacGillivray I, Symonds G (eds): Pregnancy Hypertension. Baltimore, University Park Press, 1980.

Sanchez-Ramos L, O'Sullivan MJ, Carrido-Calderon J: Effects of low-dose aspirin on angiotensin II pressor response in human pregnancy. Am J Obstet Gynecol 156:193, 1987.

Sarles HE, Hill SS, LeBlanc AL, et al: Sodium excretion patterns during and following intravenous sodium chloride loads in normal and hypertensive pregnancies. Am J Obstet Gynecol 102:1, 1968.

Saruta T, Nakamura R, Nagahama S, et al: Effects of angiotensin II analog on blood pressure, renin and aldosterone in women on oral contraceptives and toxemia. Gynecol Obstet Invest 12:11, 1981.

Schaffer NK, Dill LV, Cadden JF: Uric acid clearance in normal pregnancy and preeclampsia. J Clin Invest 22:201, 1943.

Schmorl G: Zur pathologischen Anatomie Untersuchung uber Puerperal-Eklampsie. Verhandl Dtsch Gesellsch Gyneakol 9:303, 1901.

Schreier PC, Adams JQ, Turner HB, Smith MJ: Toxemia of pregnancy as an etiological factor in hypertensive vascular disease. JAMA 159:105, 1955.

Schwarz R, Retzke U: Cardiovascular response to infusion of angiotensin II in pregnant women. Obstet Gynecol 38:714, 1971.

Scott JR, Beer AA: Immunologic aspects of pre-eclampsia. Am J Obstet Gynecol 125:418, 1976.

Scott JS: Pregnancy toxaemia associated with hydrops foetalis, hydatidiform mole and hydramnios. J Obstet Gynaecol Br Emp 65:689, 1958.

Seitchik J: Renal tubular reabsorption of uric acid. I. Normal pregnancy and abnormal pregnancy. Am J Obstet Gynecol 65:981, 1953.

Sheehan HL: Pathologic lesions in the hypertensive toxaemias of pregnancy. In Hammond J, Browne FJ, Wolstenholm GEW (eds): Toxaemias of Pregnancy, Human and Veterinary. Philadelphia, Blakiston, 1950.

Sheehan HL, Lynch JB: Pathology of Toxemia in Pregnancy. London, Churchill Livingstone, 1973.

Sheppard BL, Bonnar J: Uteroplacental arteries and hypertensive pregnancy. In Bonnar J, MacGillivray I, Symonds G. (eds): Pregnancy Hypertension. Baltimore, University Park, 1980.

Shuster E, Weppelman B: Plasma urate measurements and fetal outcome in preeclampsia. Gynecol Obstet Invest 12:162, 1981.

Sibai BM, Abdella TLN, Anderson GD: Pregnancy outcome in 211 patients with mild chronic hypertension. Obstet Gynecol 61:571, 1983a.

Sibai BM, Abdella TN, Anderson GD, Dilts PV: Plasma volume findings in pregnant women with mild hypertension: Therapeutic considerations. Am J Obstet Gynecol 15:539, 1983b.

Sibai BM, El-Nazer A, Gonzales-Ruiz A: Severe preeclampsia-eclampsia in young primigravid women: Subsequent pregnancy outcome and remote prognosis. Am J Obstet Gynecol 155:1011, 1986.

Sibai BM, Grossman RA, Grossman HG: Effects of diuretics on plasma volume in pregnancies with long-term hypertension. Am J Obstet Gynecol 150:831, 1984.

Sibai BM, Lipshitz J, Anderson GD, Dilts PV Jr: Reassessment of intravenous MgSO4 therapy in preeclampsia-eclampsia. Obstet Gynecol 57:199, 1981.

Sibai BM, Mabie WC, Shamsa F, Villar MA, Anderson GD: A comparison of no medication versus methyldopa or labetalol in chronic hypertension during pregnancy. Am J Obstet Gynecol 162:960, 1990.

Sibai BM, Mercer B, Sarinoglu C: Severe preeclampsia in the second trimester: Recurrent risk and long-term prognosis. Am J Obstet Gynecol 165:1408, 1991.

Silverstone A, Trudinger BJ, Lewis PJ, Bulpitt CJ: Maternal hypertension and intrauterine fetal death in midpregnancy. Br J Obstet Gynaecol 87:457, 1980.

Skinner SL, Lumbers ER, Symonds EM: Analysis of changes in the renin-angiotensin system during pregnancy. Clin Sci 42:479, 1972.

Sobel B, Laurent D, Ganguly S, et al: Hydrostatic mechanism in the roll-over test. Obstet Gynecol 55:285, 1980.

Socol ML, Weiner CP, Louis G, et al: Platelet activation in preeclampsia. Am J Obstet Gynecol 151:494, 1985.

Soffronoff EC, Kaufmann BM, Connaughton JF: Intravascular volume determinations and fetal outcome in hypertensive diseases of pregnancy. Am J Obstet Gynecol 127:4, 1977.

Sokabe H: Phylogeny of the renal effects of angiotensin. Kidney Int 6:263, 1974.

Spargo BH, Lichtig C, Luger AM, et al: The renal lesion in preeclampsia: Examination by light-, electron- and immunofluorescence-microscopy. In Lindheimer MD, Katz AI, Zuspan FP (eds): Hypertension in Pregnancy. New York, John Wiley & Sons, 1976.

Spargo BH, McCartney CP, Winemiller R: Glomerular capillary endotheliosis in toxemia of pregnancy. AMA Arch Pathol 68:593, 1959.

Spetz S: Peripheral circulation in pregnancy complicated by toxaemia. Acta Obstet Gynecol Scand 44:243, 1965.

Spitz B, Magness RR, Cox SM, et al: Low-dose aspirin. Am J Obstet Gynecol 159:1035, 1988.

Stallworth JC, Yeh SY, Petrie RH: The effect of magnesium sulfate on fetal heart rate variability and uterine activity. Am J Obstet Gynecol 140:702, 1981.

Stander HJ, Cadden JF: Blood chemistry in preeclampsia and eclampsia. Am J Obstet Gynecol 28:856, 1934.

Steele TW, Györy AZ, Edwards KDG: Renal function in analgesic nephropathy. Br Med J 2:231, 1969.

Stevenson AC, Davison BCC, Say B, et al: Contribution of fetal/maternal incompatibility to aetiology of preeclamptic toxaemia. Lancet 2:1286, 1971.

Stirrat GM, Redman CWG, Levinsky RJ: Circulating immune complexes in pre-eclampsia. Br Med J 1:1450, 1978.

Studd J: Pre-eclampsia. Br J Hosp Med 18:52, 1977.

Suki WN, Hull AR, Rector FC Jr, et al: Mechanism of the effect of thiazide diuretics on calcium and uric acid. J Clin Invest 46:1121, 1967.

Sullivan JM, Palmer EI, Schoeneberger AA, et al: SQ 20,811: Effect on eclamptic-preeclamptic women with postpartum hypertension. Am J Obstet Gynecol 131:707, 1978.

Sutherland A, Cooper DW, Howie PW, et al: The incidence of severe preeclampsia amongst mothers and mothers-in-law of preeclamptics and controls. Br J Obstet Gynaecol 88:785, 1981.

Symonds EM, Pipkin FB, Craven DJ: Changes in the renin-angiotensin system in normotensive and hypertensive women during pregnancy and parturition. Isr J Med Sci 12:495, 1976.

Talledo OE, Chesley LC, Zuspan FP: Renin-angiotensin system in normal and toxemic pregnancies. III. Differential sensitivity to angiotensin II and norepinephrine in toxemia of pregnancy. Am J Obstet Gynecol 100:218, 1968.

Tapia HR, Johnson CE, Strong CG: Renin-angiotensin system in normal and in hypertensive disease of pregnancy. Lancet **2**:847, 1972.

Taylor RN, Heilbron DC, Roberts JM: Growth factor activity in the blood of women in whom preeclampsia develops is elevated from early pregnancy. Am J Obstet Gynecol **163**(6):1839, 1990a.

Taylor RN, Varma M, Teng NNH, Roberts JM: Women with preeclampsia have higher plasma endothelin levels than women with normal pregnancies. J Clin Endocrinol Metab **71**(6):1675, 1990b.

Taylor RN, Casal DC, Jones LA, et al: Selective effects of preeclamptic sera on human endothelial cell procoagulant protein expression. Am J Obstet Gynecol **165**:1705, 1991b.

Taylor RN, Crombleholme WR, Friedman SA, et al: High plasma cellular fibronectin levels correlate with biochemical and clinical features of preeclampsia but cannot be attributed to hypertension alone. Am J Obstet Gynecol **165**:895, 1991a.

Taylor RN, Musci TJ, Rodgers GM, Roberts JM: Prepartum preeclamptic sera stimulate platelet-derived growth factor mRNA and protein production by cultured human endothelial cells. Am J Reprod Immunol **25**:105, 1991c.

Tervila L, Goecke C, Timonen S: Estimation of gestosis of pregnancy (EPH-gestosis). Acta Obstet Gynecol Scand **52**:235, 1973.

Thomson AM, Hytten FE, Billewicz WZ: The epidemiology of oedema during pregnancy. J Obstet Gynaecol Br Cwlth **74**:1, 1967.

Thomson D, Paterson WG, Smart GE, et al: The renal lesions of toxemia and abruptio placentae studies by light and electron microscopy. J Obstet Gynaecol Br Cwlth **79**:311, 1972.

Toppozada M, Darwish EA, Osman YF, Abd-Rabbo MS: Low dose acetyl salicylic acid in severe preeclampsia. Int J Gynecol Obstet **35**:311, 1991.

Tuffnell D, O'Donovan P, Lilford RJ, et al: Phenytoin in preeclampsia. Lancet **1**:274, 1989.

Vara P, Timonen S, Lokki O: Toxaemia of late pregnancy: A statistical study. Acta Obstet Gynecol Scand **44**(Suppl):3, 1965.

Vartran CK: Hypertension in pregnancy: A new look. Proc R Soc Med **59**:841, 1966.

Vassali P, Morris RH, McCluskey RI: The pathogenic role of fibrin deposition in the glomerular lesions of toxemia of pregnancy. J Exper Med **118**:467, 1963.

Vollman RF: Rates of toxemia by age and parity. *In* Die Spat gestose (E and H-Gestose). Basel, Schwabe, 1970.

Waisman GD, Mayorga LM, Camera MI, et al: Magnesium plus nifedipine: Potentiation of hypotensive effect in preeclampsia? Am J Obstet Gynecol **159**:308, 1988.

Wallenburg HCS: Hemodynamics in hypertensive pregnancy. *In* Rubin PC (ed): *Hypertension in Pregnancy*. (Handbook of Hypertension, vol 10). Amsterdam, Elsevier, p 66, 1988.

Weiner CP, Brandt J: Plasma antithrombin III activity: An aid in the diagnosis of preeclampsia-eclampsia. Am J Obstet Gynecol **142**:275, 1982.

Weinstein L: Syndrome of hemolysis, elevated liver enzymes, and low platelet count: A severe consequence of hypertension in pregnancy. Am J Obstet Gynecol **142**:159, 1982.

Weir RJ, Paintin DB, Brown JJ, et al: A serial study in pregnancy of the plasma concentrations of renin, corticosteroids, electrolytes and proteins; and of haematocrit and plasma volume. J Obstet Gynecol Br Cwlth **78**:590, 1971.

Weseley AC, Douglas GW: Continuous use of chlorothiazide for prevention of toxemias of pregnancy. Obstet Gynecol **19**:355, 1962.

Whigham KAE, Howie PW, Shah MM, Prentice CRM: Factor VIII related antigen/coagulant activity ratio as a predictor of fetal growth retardation: A comparison with hormone and uric acid measurements. Br J Obstet Gynaecol **87**:797, 1980.

Whitelaw AGL, Cummings AJ, McFadyen IR: Effect of maternal lorazepam on the neonate. Br Med J **282**:1106, 1981.

Wiggins RC, Loskutoff DJ, Cochrane CG, et al: Activation of rabbit Hageman factor by homogenates of cultured rabbit endothelial cells. J Clin Invest **65**:197, 1980.

Working Group on High Blood Pressure in Pregnancy (Gifford RW, August P, Chesley LC, et al): National High Blood Pressure Education Program Working Group Report on High Blood Pressure in Pregnancy. Am J Obstet Gynecol **163**:1691, 1990.

Yu TF, Sirota JH, Berger L, et al: Effect of sodium lactate infusion on urate clearance in man. Proc Soc Exp Biol (NY) **96**:809, 1957.

Zangmeister W: Untersuchungen uber die Blutbeschaffenheit und die Harnsekretion bei Eklampsie. Z Geburtschilfe Gynaekol **50**:385, 1903.

Zeek PM, Assali NS: Vascular changes in the decidua associated with eclamptogenic toxemia. Am J Clin Pathol **20**:1099, 1950.

Zuspan FP: Problems encountered in the treatment of pregnancy-induced hypertension. Am J Obstet Gynecol **131**:591, 1978.

Zuspan FP, Nelson GH, Ahlquist RP: Epinephrine infusions in normal and toxemic pregnancy. I. Nonesterified fatty acids and cardiovascular alterations. Am J Obstet Gynecol **90**:88, 1964.

Zuspan FP, Talledo E, Rhodes K: Factors affecting delivery in eclampsia. Am J Obstet Gynecol **100**:672, 1968.

CHAPTER

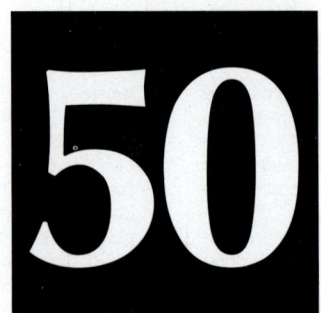

RENAL DISORDERS

·······················

JOHN M. DAVISON, M.D., and MARSHALL D. LINDHEIMER, M.D.

Among the various physiologic alterations that occur in normal pregnancy, few are as striking as those affecting the urinary tract. These changes and various diagnostic pitfalls for the unwary clinician have already been discussed in Chapter 46. There is no doubt that improvements in our knowledge of background physiology, in prenatal care generally, in technology for fetal surveillance, and in neonatal intensive care have meant better care for women with renal problems and their newborns. With this in mind, this chapter focuses on urinary tract infection, chronic renal disease, pregnancy in dialysis patients, gestation in renal allograft patients, and acute renal failure that occurs during pregnancy.

INFECTION OF THE URINARY TRACT

Definitions and Pathogenesis

Urinalysis during pregnancy is especially likely to be hampered by contamination at the time of collection with bacteria from urethra, vagina, or perineum. This problem can be overcome by suprapubic aspiration of bladder urine, but the rather inconvenient procedure is distasteful to many patients and obstetricians. Another approach is to obtain a fresh mid-stream urine specimen collected by a clean-catch technique. In the latter instance, nurse-supervised multiple vulvar washings give reproducible cultures more than 95 per cent of the time. With the suprapubic technique, all growth is significant, whereas with mid-stream urine specimens, true bacteriuria is traditionally defined as the presence of more than 100,000 bacteria per milliliter of urine of the same species in two consecutive mid-stream specimens. One should be aware, however, that lower colony counts may still represent active infection (Stamm et al., 1982). A number of presumptive tests based on changes in chemical indicators exist, but these are not reliable enough for clinical practice.

Asymptomatic or covert bacteriuria designates true bacteriuria in the absence of symptoms or signs of acute urinary infection. When there is symptomatic urinary tract infection (UTI), two clinical syndromes

are recognized: lower UTI or cystitis and upper UTI or acute pyelonephritis. It must be remembered, though, that pregnant women often complain of, or will admit to, frequency of micturition, dysuria, urgency, and nocturia, singly or in combination, and such symptoms are not in themselves diagnostic of UTI (Editorial, 1985).

It is probable that bacteria originate from the large bowel and colonize the urinary tract transperineally. By far the most common infecting organism is *Escherichia coli*, which is responsible for 75 to 90 per cent of bacteriuria during pregnancy. The pathogenic virulence of this organism, which is not the most plentiful in feces, appears to involve a number of factors, including resistance to vaginal acidity, rapid division in urine, adhesions (characterized as fimbriae) allowing adherence to uroepithelial cells, and production of chemicals that decrease ureteric peristalsis and inhibit phagocytosis (McFadyen, 1986). Other organisms frequently responsible for UTI include Klebsiella, Proteus, coagulase-negative staphylococci, and Pseudomonas.

The stasis associated with ureteropelvic dilatation and/or partial ureteric obstruction (see Chapter 46), increased nutrient content of the urine, and the presence of potential pathogens are characteristic of most pregnant women, and yet only a small minority develop bacteriuria. Susceptible women may differ immunologically from those who resist infection: they are less likely to express antibody to the O antigen of *E. coli* on the vaginal epithelium and may display less effective leukocyte activity against the organism.

Finally, it should be noted that urinary sediments may be misleading in pregnancy. Although urine replete with white blood cells, casts, and bacteria is informative, cultures have been positive when fewer than five white blood cells were present in the sediment.

Asymptomatic Bacteriuria

Covert bacteriuria is a heterogeneous entity. Several methods have been used to try to differentiate between upper and lower urinary tract bacteriuria—renal biopsy, urethral catheterization, bladder washout tests, urinary concentration tests, and serum antibody tests. The first two methods are too invasive for clinical practice and the remainder are insufficiently precise to confidently localize infection. The utility of another predictor of the presence and site of a UTI, the determination of antibody-coated bacteria in the urine, also remains controversial (McNeeley et al., 1987).

The reservoir of young women with covert bacteriuria acquired during childhood is about 5 per cent, but only 1.2 per cent are infected at any one time. The incidence increases after puberty and is approximately equal in both the pregnant and nonpregnant populations (2 to 10 per cent). One antenatal study (Stenqvist et al., 1989), in which 99 per cent of women took part in at least one screening, indicates that the risk of onset of bacteriuria was highest between the 9th and 17th gestational weeks. The 16th week was the optimal time for a single screening for bacteriuria calculated as the numbers of bacteria-free gestational weeks gained by treatment.

During pregnancy, 40 per cent of the infected group, if untreated, develop acute symptomatic UTI. Thus, treating patients with covert bacteriuria should prevent approximately 70 per cent of all potential cases of symptomatic UTI infection in pregnancy. However, about 1.5 per cent of those with initial negative cultures develop acute infections, and this accounts for the remaining 30 to 40 per cent of all cases of acute UTI in pregnancy.

Asymptomatic bacteriuria has been alleged to be associated with several complications of pregnancy, notably low birth weight, fetal loss, preeclampsia, and maternal anemia. Several of these apparent correlations may have resulted from inaccuracies in matching cases and controls, and none appears to be supported by more recent studies (Davison et al., 1984; Martinell et al., 1990). However, when evidence of previous damage is present, there may be a greater propensity to hypertension (McGladderry et al., 1992).

Not all untreated bacteriuric women will develop symptoms of acute UTI during pregnancy; by the same token, those who are found to have sterile urine when screened antenatally will contribute substantially to the pool of symptomatic women. It has therefore been argued that screening programs are not cost effective (Lawson and Miller, 1973; Campbell-Brown et al., 1987). Furthermore, it has been suggested that as a predictor of symptomatic urinary infection, the presence of bacteriuria has a specificity of 89 per cent but a sensitivity of only 33 per cent and a false-positive rate of almost 90 per cent (Chang and Hall, 1982). However, the patients referred to by those making this claim were screened by means of a single urine test only, and their results showed an unusually high prevalence (11.8 per cent) of bacteriuria. Interestingly, it has been suggested that women who have a history of previous UTI as well as current bacteriuria are 10 times more likely to develop symptoms during pregnancy than women without either feature. Furthermore, women with renal scarring and persistent reflux are more likely to develop acute pyelonephritis (Martinell et al., 1990).

Management in Pregnancy

Most obstetricians treat asymptomatic bacteriuria despite the screening controversy (Campbell-Brown et al., 1987; Andriole and Patterson, 1991). We favor this approach, noting the need for further carefully conducted research. The agent chosen must not only be effective against the organism identified, but also be acceptable for use during pregnancy. The Physicians' Desk Reference now lists pregnancy risk factors for all medications. Antibiotics in categories A and B may be used throughout gestation; C should be relegated to beyond the teratogenic period, whereas categories D and X should not be prescribed for pregnant women.

Ampicillin and the cephalosporins are commonly prescribed, but it should be remembered that short-acting sulfonamides may be equally effective. Sulfonamides should be avoided during the last few weeks of pregnancy, however, because they competitively inhibit the binding of bilirubin to albumin and may increase the risk of neonatal hyperbilirubinemia. Nitrofurantoin, with its common side effect of nausea, may not be readily tolerated in pregnancy. Furthermore, it should be avoided during late pregnancy because of the risk of hemolysis due to deficiency of erythrocyte phosphate dehydrogenase in the newborn. The tetracyclines are contraindicated during pregnancy because of problems of dental staining in the child.

A 2-week course of therapy is usually adequate. Recurrent infection is common, however, affecting some 30 per cent of bacteriuric women; after two courses of treatment about 15 per cent will continue to have positive urinary cultures. Recurrence may be caused by relapse, when the same organism is found within 6 weeks of the initial infection, or by reinfection, when a different organism is detected more than 6 weeks after treatment. About 25 per cent of pregnant women will have a recurrence and need a second course of treatment, but only about 40 per cent will have the covert bacteriuria cleared. Persistent infections may merit continuous treatment to the time of delivery.

Long-Term Prognosis

In the longer term, there is little evidence that treatment during pregnancy affects the subsequent prevalence of bacteriuria (Brumfitt, 1981) or that persistent bacteriuria in women with a normal urinary tract contributes to the development of chronic renal disease. Some 20 per cent of bacteriuric women have some abnormality of the urinary tract (Powers, 1991), but in most cases the abnormality is minor and not clearly related to the disease. Postpartum evaluation such as intravenous urography or renal ultrasound is probably therefore best reserved for bacteriuric women with a history of acute symptomatic infections before or during pregnancy, those in whom bacteriuria is difficult to eradicate, and those in whom there is a postpartum recurrence of disease (Andriole and Patterson, 1991).

Acute Cystitis

This occurs in about 1 per cent of pregnant women, of whom 60 per cent have a negative initial screening.

The symptoms are often difficult to distinguish from those due to pregnancy itself. Features indicating a true infection include hematuria, dysuria, and suprapubic discomfort, as well as a positive urine culture. The bacteriology is the same as in women with covert bacteriuria. Similar treatment is recommended with the aims of abolishing symptoms and preventing occurrence of acute pyelonephritis.

Acute Pyelonephritis

This is the most common urinary tract complication of pregnancy, occurring in approximatley 2 per cent of all pregnancies (Cunningham, 1987; Andriole and Patterson, 1991). Its presentation in pregnant women is similar to that in nonpregnant women, with fever, flank pain, nausea, and vomiting with or without frequency, urgency, and dysuria. Physical examination usually confirms the presence of pyrexia and flank tenderness on the affected side. Causative organisms are similar to those in the general population, with P-fimbriated *E. coli* representing approximately 75 per cent. At least 25 per cent of patients experience a transient decrease in glomerular filtration rate and a rise in blood creatinine. Ultrasonographic examination of the renal tract in gravidas with pyelonephritis has revealed significantly increased pelvicalyceal dilatation compared to normal physiologic dilatation of pregnancy, but as treatment did not produce a consistent decrease, their anomaly may antedate the acute infection (Twickler et al., 1991).

Acute pyelonephritis may or may not play a role in the etiology of hypertension and intrauterine deaths, but upper tract infections certainly may mimic and/or precipitate premature labor. Bacteremia occurs in approximately 10 to 20 per cent of all cases. Pregnant women are more vulnerable to endotoxins (lipopolysaccharide) than are the nonpregnant, which is one reason they tolerate acute pyelonephritis poorly. Some even develop septic shock (on occasion in association with instrumentation of the infected urinary tract), adult respiratory distress syndrome (Cunningham et al., 1987; Pruett and Faro, 1987), and/or anemia, all probably due to lipopolysaccharide-induced cell membrane damage (Cox et al., 1991).

Management in Pregnancy

Treatment of acute pyelonephritis requires early hospitalization and adequate intravenous hydration. After appropriate cultures are obtained, treatment with broad-spectrum intravenous antibiotics should be started. Antibiotic therapy should be adjusted to organism sensitivities when known. Most patients treated appropriately respond clinically within 48 hours. Lack of clinical improvement by 72 hours suggests inadequate or improper antibiotic use, an underlying anatomic urinary tract problem (e.g., obstruction by stone), and a need to reconsider the diagnosis. The overall recurrence rate is estimated at approximately 20 per cent. After resolution of an episode of acute pyelonephritis, the patient should be treated for at least 3 weeks and then should be followed with frequent urine cultures. Continuous antimicrobial suppression with close follow-up until term may be used in the noncompliant patient or in instances when an underlying urinary tract abnormality is present or suspected, if assessment of this can be safely postponed until the puerperium. It should not be forgotten that there is an association between UTI and sudden unexpected postperinatal death (Carpenter et al., 1983).

Differential Diagnosis

HEMATURIA DURING PREGNANCY. Spontaneous gross or microscopic hematuria can have a variety of causes (Danielli et al., 1987). If associated with congenital anomalies, UTI can be difficult to eradicate and may predispose to hematuria. Rupture of small veins around the dilated renal pelvis may also cause bleeding. Rarely, hematuria may be secondary to complications such as acute glomerulonephritis, calculi, neoplasm, hemangiomas, calculi, and fungal diseases (Klein et al., 1987). Endometriosis, inflammatory bowel lesions, leukoplakia, and granulomas may involve the urinary tract and also produce hematuria. A bleeding ureteral stump after a nephrectomy (for either benign or malignant disease) should be ruled out.

Investigation of hematuria may be deferred until after delivery, but the clinician should decide whether or not it takes absolute priority. In any event, ultrasonic techniques should be utilized, and magnetic resonance is quite safe for diagnostic use during pregnancy. In the absence of any demonstrable cause, hematuria can be classified as idiopathic, and recurrences are unlikely in the current or subsequent pregnancy.

ACUTE HYDRONEPHROSIS AND HYDROURETER. There is a broad spectrum of the so-called overdistention syndrome (Meyers et al., 1985). This is not to be confused with the massive ureteral and renal pelvic dilatation (and slight reduction in cortical width) that can occasionally occur in normal pregnancy without ill effect (Brown, 1990). With the overdistention syndrome there are definite symptoms; some women have transient mild flank pain whereas others have recurrent episodes of severe flank or lower abdominal pain radiating to the groin. There are also functional abnormalities characterized by small increments in serum creatinine levels, but urinalysis contains few or no red cells and repeat mid-stream specimens are sterile.

The variations in symptoms with changes in posture and position are hallmarks of this condition. Diagnosis can be confirmed using limited excretory urography or sonar scanning. Positioning of the patient in lateral recumbency or the knee-chest position often gives relief. If this fails, ureteral catheterization or sonographically guided percutaneous nephrostomy may be necessary, so that surgery is delayed until the postpartum period (Van Sonnenberg et al., 1992).

NONTRAUMATIC RUPTURE OF THE URINARY TRACT. The intrusion of unremitting pain and hematuria upon the course of pyelonephritis or the overdistention syndrome suggests rupture of the urinary tract. Furthermore, this complication can masquerade as other obstetric and surgical abdominal catastrophes, including appendicitis, pelvic abscess, cholecystitis, stone disease (see later), and abruptio placentae. Prompt recognition may prevent extension or expansion or both of a small tear and urine leak, treatable by postural or tube drainage. Rupture of the renal parenchyma, with hemorrhagic shock, formation of a flank mass, or dissection of urinary tract contents intraperitoneally, compels prompt surgical intervention, usually with nephrectomy.

CHRONIC RENAL DISEASE

The majority view is that, with the exception of certain specific disease entities such as systemic lupus erythematosus (SLE), renal polyarteritis nodosa, and scleroderma, obstetric outcome is usually successful, provided renal function is at most moderately compromised and hypertension is absent or minimal. Furthermore, pregnancy does not adversely affect the natural history of the renal disease (Katz et al., 1980). There are also four entities about which controversy exists: IgA nephropathy, membranoproliferative glomerulonephritis, focal glomerular sclerosis, and reflux nephropathy; some investigators believe that gestation affects the course of these disorders adversely (reviewed by Abe 1991a,b; Imbasciati and Ponticelli, 1991; Jungers et al., 1991).

Renal Function and Obstetric Considerations

Normal Pregnancy and Renal Assessment

Glomerular filtration rate (GFR), measured as 24-hour creatinine clearance, increases shortly after conception. Serum levels of creatinine and urea nitrogen (SUN), which average 0.8 mg/100 ml and 13 mg/100 ml, respectively, in nonpregnant women, decrease to mean values of 0.6 mg/100 ml and 9 mg/100 ml in pregnant women. Near term, a 15 to 20 per cent decrement in GFR occurs, which affects serum creatinine minimally.

Values of creatinine of 0.9 mg/100 ml and SUN of 14 mg/100 ml, which are acceptable in nonpregnant subjects, are suspect in pregnancy. However, caution is necessary when one is assessing renal function by serum creatinine levels alone. This is because creatinine is both filtered and secreted by the kidney, the ratio of creatinine/inulin clearance normally falling between 1.1 and 1.2. As renal disease progresses, a greater portion of urinary creatinine is formed due to secretion (clearance ratios rising to 1.4 to 1.6 when serum creatinine is 1.4). Therefore, the glomerular filtration may be overestimated by 50 per cent.

Although serum creatinine—its reciprocal or its logarithm—often is used to estimate or even calculate GFR (in relation to age, height, and weight), this approach should not be used in pregnancy, because body weight or size does not reflect kidney size.

Ideally, evaluation of renal function in pregnancy should be based on the clearance of creatinine rather than its serum concentration. Creatinine levels may increase by up to 0.15 mg/100 ml shortly after ingestion of cooked meat (because cooking converts preformed creatine into creatinine) and the timing of the blood sample during a clearance period must take into account meals and their content.

Renal Dysfunction and Preconception Counseling

Initiating and sustaining pregnancy are basically related to the degree of functional impairment. Fertility is diminished as renal function falls. When preconception serum creatinine and SUN exceed 3 mg/100 ml and 30 mg/100 ml, respectively, normal pregnancy is unusual, but successes have been documented in women with moderate-to-severe disease, including some treated with dialysis (Davison, 1991).

Ideally, pregnancy is probably best restricted to women whose preconception serum creatinine levels are less than 2 mg/100 ml and diastolic blood pressure is 90 mm Hg or less. If hypertension requiring more than one drug for control is also present, prognosis becomes substantially poorer. Some physicians extend this limit to 2.5 mg/100 ml, and others believe it should be no higher than 1.5 mg/100 ml. We tend to favor the lower number. Whatever level is utilized, one should recognize that degrees of impairment not causing symptoms or disrupting homeostasis in nonpregnant individuals certainly can jeopardize pregnancy.

The question has to be asked, "Is pregnancy advisable?" If a woman with chronic renal disease wishes to have a family, the sooner she starts the better. In some of these patients, renal function continues to decline with time. Women are not always counseled prior to conception. A patient with suspected or known renal disease may present already pregnant, and then the question is whether to continue the pregnancy.

Renal Dysfunction and Impact of Pregnancy

Because of the different obstetric and remote prognoses in women with different degrees of renal insufficiency, the impact of pregnancy should be considered by categories of functional renal status before conception (Tables 50–1 to 50–3).

PRESERVED OR MILDLY IMPAIRED RENAL FUNCTION AND MINIMAL HYPERTENSION. Women with chronic renal disease, but normal or only mildly decreased renal function at conception, usually have a successful obstetric outcome, and pregnancy does not appear to adversely affect the course of their disease (Katz et

TABLE 50–1. Categories of Pre-pregnancy Functional Renal Status

CATEGORY	SERUM CREATININE mg/100 ml
Preserved/mildly impaired renal function	< 1.4
Moderate renal insufficiency	> 1.4 to < 2.5
Severe renal insufficiency	> 2.5

TABLE 50–2. **Pregnancy and Renal Disease: Functional Renal Status and Prospects**

PROSPECTS	CATEGORY (See Table 50–1)		
	MILD	**MODERATE**	**SEVERE**
Pregnancy	25%	47%	86%
Successful obstetric outcome	96% (85)	90% (59)	47% (8)
Long-term sequelae	<3% (9)	25% (71)	53% (92)

Estimates are based on 1862 women/2799 pregnancies (1973–1992) and do not include collagen diseases.

Numbers in parentheses refer to prospects (%) when complication(s) develop before 28 weeks gestation.

al., 1980; Katz and Lindheimer, 1985; Barcelo et al., 1986; Abe, 1991 a,b; Imbasciati and Ponticelli, 1991). Although this holds true for most patients, there are exceptions. Most authors strongly advise against pregnancy in women with scleroderma and periarteritis nodosa. Others suggest that this statement be tempered somewhat in cases involving lupus nephropathy, membranoproliferative glomerulonephritis, and perhaps IgA and reflux nephropathies, which appear more sensitive to intercurrent pregnancy.

Most of these patients show increments in GFR, but less than those of normal pregnant women. Increased proteinuria is common, occurring in 50 per cent of pregnancies (although this is unusual in women with chronic pyelonephritis), and it can be massive (often exceeding 3 gm in 24 hours), with nephrotic edema. Two recent retrospective studies emphasize several important issues: Abe (1991a) analyzed 240 pregnancies in 166 women and Jungers et al. (1991) 254 in 148 women, all with biopsy proven disease. Perinatal outcome was jeopardized by the presence of uncontrolled hypertension, nephrotic range proteinuria in early gestation, and/or glomerular filtration rate ≤70 ml/min prior to conception or in the initial trimester, whatever the type of renal disease.

Hypertension, renal functional abnormalities, and proteinuria are considerably lessened in prevalence, as well as in their severity, between pregnancies and during long-term follow-up. When renal failure does supervene, it usually reflects the inexorable course of a particular renal disease.

MODERATE RENAL INSUFFICIENCY. Prognosis is more guarded when renal function is moderately impaired before pregnancy (serum creatinine 1.4 to 2.5 mg/100 ml). It is difficult to draw firm conclusions about pregnancy in these women, chiefly because the

number of cases reported is still small. In one series, a high incidence of renal morbidity occurred early in pregnancy; nearly half (five of 11) developed serious deterioration of renal function culminating in terminal renal failure several months postpartum (Kincaid-Smith et al., 1980). Due to this experience and the fact that apparent deterioration also was seen in an occasional patient with stable renal function, Kincaid-Smith and co-workers have adopted a rather pessimistic approach to pregnancy in women with both mild and moderate renal disease.

Another study of the influence of pregnancy (Bear, 1978) revealed no immediate loss of renal function in 29 patients whose creatinine levels were less than 1.5 mg/100 ml. In contrast, four of eight patients with initial creatinine levels above 1.6 mg/100 ml experienced significant further increases during pregnancy, which was complicated in virtually every case. Four patients in this group progressed to end-stage renal failure within 18 months of delivery. It is now recognized that uncontrolled hypertension is an extremely important factor in overall deterioration (Imbasciati et al., 1986; Hou et al., 1985; Cunningham et al., 1990; Jungers et al., 1991).

Our customary recommendation has been that pregnancy is best avoided in women who have lost 50 per cent of their kidney function. More recent studies, however, have reopened the question. Hou and her colleagues (1985) recorded a successful obstetric outcome in 92 per cent of the pregnancies in 22 women with creatinine levels of 1.7 to 2.7 mg/100 ml whose pregnancies were allowed to go beyond the second trimester. Cunningham et al. (1990) had successful obstetric outcome in 85 per cent of pregnancies in 26 women. However, many of the patients in both series had escalating and occasionally severe hypertension. Furthermore, GFR did not increase at all in pregnancy in half the women and in 25 per cent there was an accelerated decline in renal function. Because of these two complications, especially the former, we usually try to dissuade most women with moderate renal insufficiency from conceiving.

SEVERE RENAL INSUFFICIENCY. Most women in this category (serum creatinine ≥ 2.5 mg/100 ml) are amenorrheic or anovulatory or both. The likelihood of conception, let alone of having a normal pregnancy and delivery, is low; however, it is not impossible (Cunningham et al., 1990), as some patients have been led to believe. Moreover, the risk of severe maternal complications is greater than the probability of a successful obstetric outcome.

TABLE 50–3. **Renal Disease and Pregnancy: Improvements in Perinatal Mortality Over 4 Decades**

RENAL DISEASE	PREGNANCY OUTCOME	1950s	1960s	1970s	1980s	1990s
Mild	Preterm delivery	8%	10%	19%	25%	25%
	Perinatal mortality	18%	15%	7%	<5%	<3%
Moderate	Preterm delivery	15%	21%	40%	52%	57%
	Perinatal mortality	58%	45%	23%	10%	10%
Severe	Preterm delivery	100%	100%	100%	100%	100%
	Perinatal mortality	100%	91%	58%	53%	51%

Estimates are based on 2952 women/4011 pregnancies (1954–1992) and do not include cases of SLE.

It must be admitted, however, that there are reports of women with severe chronic renal failure having successful pregnancies managed without dialysis (Grunebaum and Minkoff, 1987), and in one gravida the serum creatinine was 8 mg/100 ml at the time of spontaneous delivery (Vogt et al., 1989). There are also reported cases in which dialysis has been instituted prophylactically during pregnancy to increase the chances of successful outcome (Redrow et al., 1988; Jakobi et al., 1992). Nevertheless, we believe that these women should not take additional health risks. The aim should be to preserve what little renal function remains and/or to achieve renal rehabilitation via dialysis and transplantation, after which the question of pregnancy can be considered if appropriate.

Antenatal Strategy and Decision-Making

Patients should be seen at 2-week intervals until 32 weeks gestation—after this, assessment should be weekly. Routine serial antenatal observations should be supplemented with (1) assessment of renal function by 24-hour creatinine clearance and protein excretion on approximately a monthly basis, (2) careful monitoring of blood pressure for early detection of hypertension and then assessment of its severity, (3) early detection of superimposed preeclampsia (after midtrimester), (4) biophysical assessment of fetal size, development, and well-being, and (5) early detection of asymptomatic bacteriuria or confirmation of UTI.

RENAL FUNCTION. If renal function deteriorates, reversible causes should be sought, such as UTI, subtle dehydration, or electrolyte imbalance, occasionally precipitated by inadvertent diuretic therapy. Near term, a 15 to 20 per cent decrement in function, which affects serum creatinine minimally, is permissible. Failure to detect a reversible cause of a significant decrement is reason to end the pregnancy by elective delivery. When proteinuria occurs and persists but blood pressure is normal and renal function is preserved, the pregnancy can be allowed to continue.

BLOOD PRESSURE. Most of the specific risks of hypertension appear to be mediated through superimposed preeclampsia. There is still controversy about the incidence of preeclampsia in those women with preexisting renal disease. The diagnosis cannot be made with certainty on clinical grounds alone because hypertension and proteinuria may be manifestations of the underlying renal disease (Lindheimer and Katz, 1992). Treatment of hypertension in pregnancy is considered in Chapter 49.

High blood pressure in the presence of an underlying kidney disorder is treated more aggressively than are other hypertensive complications of pregnancy. This is because such actions preserve function longer.

It should be borne in mind that in pregnancy renal artery stenosis may present as chronic hypertension or as recurrent isolated preeclampsia (Heybourne et al., 1991). Renal angiography is the most sensitive and specific diagnostic technique and concomitant therapeutic percutaneous transluminal angioplasty may be undertaken (Easterling et al., 1991).

FETAL SURVEILLANCE AND TIMING OF DELIVERY. Serial assessment of fetal well-being is essential because renal disease can be associated with intrauterine growth restriction, and when complications do arise, the judicious moment for intervention is influenced by fetal status (Thacker and Berkelman, 1986). Current technology should minimize the risk of intrauterine fetal death as well as neonatal morbidity and mortality. Regardless of gestational age, most babies weighing 1500 gm or more are better off in a special-care nursery than in a hostile intrauterine environment. Deliberate preterm delivery may be necessary if renal function deteriorates substantially or for the usual maternal and fetal causes such as uncontrollable hypertension and signs adduced by monitoring of fetal jeopardy.

Problems Associated with Specific Renal Disease

An in-depth review by Imbasciati and Ponticelli (1991) describes outcomes in over 1000 patients with a variety of specific disorders, usually documented by kidney biopsy (Tables 50–4 to 50–6). (Therapeutic abortions were excluded from calculation of pregnancy success rates.)

Acute and Chronic Glomerulonephritis

The acute disease is a rare complication of pregnancy, and it can be mistaken for preeclampsia. With

TABLE 50–4. Fetal and Maternal Outcome of Pregnancies in Women with Primary Glomerulonephritis

HISTOLOGY	PREGNANCIES/ PATIENTS	SPONTANEOUS ABORTION	PERINATAL LOSS	PRETERM DELIVERY	RENAL FUNCTION DECREASE		BLOOD PRESSURE INCREASE	
					REVERSIBLE	PROGRESSIVE	REVERSIBLE	PERMANENT
Focal glomerulosclerosis	85/61	2/58 (3%)	19/81 (23%)	25/79 (32%)	11/84 (13%)	4/84 (5%)	27/84 (32%)	8/84 (10%)
Membranous nephropathy	110/70	11/95 (12%)	4/92 (4%)	28/79 (35%)	3/97 (3%)	2/97 (2%)	21/97 (22%)	3/97 (3%)
Membranoproliferative	165/98	23/138 (17%)	11/133 (85)	25/134 (19%)	9/164 (6%)	5/164 (3%)	31/164 (20%)	20/164 (12%)
IgA nephritis	268/166	12/229 (5%)	36/246 (15%)	43/208 (21%)	28/230 (12%)	5/230 (2%)	58/230 (25%)	27/230 (12%)
Mesangial proliferative	278/163	14/275 (5%)	32/261 (12%)	19/223 (9%)	14/243 (2%)	7/243 (3%)	88/243 (36%)	16/243 (7%)
All types	906/558	62/795 (8%)	102/813 (13%)	140/723 (19%)	65/818 (8%)	23/818 (3%)	225/818 (27%)	74/818 (9%)

From Imbasciati E, Ponticelli C: Pregnancy and renal disease: Predictions for fetal and maternal outcome. Am J Nephrol **11**:353, 1991. With permission. See journal article for details of the 6 reports surveyed in this Table.

TABLE 50–5. Outcome of Pregnancy in Women with Diabetic Nephropathy, Polycystic Kidney Disease, Reflux Nephropathy

NEPHROPATHY	PREGNANCIES/ PATIENTS	PERINATAL LOSS	PRETERM DELIVERY	RENAL FUNCTION DECREASE	BLOOD PRESSURE INCREASE	PROGRESSIVE COURSE AFTER DELIVERY
Diabetic nephropathy	97/94	5/88 (6%)	32/88 (36%)	31/97 (32%)	56/97 (58%)	10/77 (13%)
Polycystic disease	464/242	11/378 (3%)	23/228 (10%)	3/276 (3%)	38/276 (14%)	1/276 (0.3%)
Reflux nephropathy	137/53	8/119 (7%)	18/119 (15%)	1/137 (0.7%)	15/137 (11%)	3/137 (3%)

From Imbasciati E, Ponticelli C: Pregnancy and renal disease: Predictions for fetal and maternal outcome. Am J Nephrol 2:353, 1991. With permission. See journal article for details of the 6 reports surveyed in this table.

chronic glomerulonephritis, one view warns of aggravation because of the hypercoagulable state accompanying pregnancy, with patients more prone to superimposed preeclampsia or hypertensive crises earlier in pregnancy. The consensus, however, is that if renal function is stable and hypertension is absent, most pregnancies are successful.

In a recent review of 906 pregnancies in 558 women, Imbasciati and Ponticelli (1991) endorse the above generalizations. In addition, several specific issues were highlighted.

1. Complications developed more frequently in women who already had some dysfunction and/or hypertension in early gestation.

2. De novo hypertension or worsening of preexisting hypertension occurred in 25 per cent of pregnancies, but usually reverted post-delivery, suggesting superimposed preeclampsia, a diagnosis that is not easy in this group of patients.

3. In 10 per cent of pregnancies hypertension persisted after delivery, especially in focal and segmental glomerulosclerosis, membranoprolifrative glomerulonephritis, and IgA nephropathy.

4. Higher rates of fetal loss observed in these particular women can be accounted for by the greater prevalence of severe hypertension and renal insufficiency.

5. Primary glomerulonephritis should also be considered per se as a contraindication to pregnancy.

Other smaller series have concentrated on particular glomerular lesions. For example, Abe (1991b) examined the impact of IgA nephropathy and pregnancy on each other in 168 pregnancies in 118 women. Always the message emerges that (1) pregnancy is well tolerated without effect on the course of the disease if blood pressure is normal and GFR >70 ml/min before conception and (2) with hypertension the rate of live births is low if it exists before pregnancy and/or is not well controlled during gestation.

Hereditary nephritis, an uncommon disorder, may first become manifested or exacerbated during pregnancy, but most gestations succeed. Of interest is a variant of hereditary nephritis, involving disordered platelet morphology and function. In these cases, pregnancy has been successful but at times complicated by bleeding problems, especially at delivery.

Chronic Pyelonephritis (Tubulointerstitial Disease)

Tubulointerstitial disease in pregnancy may be either infectious or noninfectious. The prognosis in pregnancy is similar to that for patients with glomerular disease, in that outcome is best in patients with adequate renal function and normal blood pressure. Compared with the nonpregnant state, frequency of symptomatic infections is greater in pregnant women, but these patients have a more benign antenatal course than do women with glomerular disease.

Reflux Nephropathy

This term is used to describe renal morphologic and functional changes that relate to past (and usually present) vesicoureteric reflux, often complicated by recurrent infection. Reflux nephropathy is frequently associated with hypertension and moderate or severe renal dysfunction, features that, as discussed earlier, adversely affect pregnancy outcome (Jungers et al., 1987). Specific obstetric concerns in affected patients include severe fetal intrauterine growth retardation and the risk of sudden rapid worsening of hypertension and renal function with accelerated progression to renal failure. Currently there is disagreement about the natural history of reflux nephropathy in gestation. We agree with Jungers et al. (1987) that women with preserved function and no hypertension do as well as patients with other diseases.

Urolithiasis

The prevalence of urolithiasis in pregnancy is 0.03 to 0.35 per cent (Coe et al., 1978). Renal and ureteric calculi are common causes of nonuterine abdominal pain severe enough to necessitate hospital admission during pregnancy. Most are calcium oxalate, the more benign type, but occasionally the more malicious struvite stones (e.g., staghorn) are seen. Uric acid and cystine are much more infrequent.

Management should be conservative initially, with adequate hydration, appropriate antibiotic therapy, and pain relief with systemic analgesics. The use of

TABLE 50–6. SLE and Pregnancy

LITERATURE	PREGNANCIES	SPONTANEOUS ABORTIONS, %	PERINATAL LOSS, %	FETAL LOSS, %
1952–1970	587	20	9	29
1971–1980	184	20	5	25
1981–1988	224	13	13	26

From Imbasciati E, Ponticelli C: Pregnancy and renal disease: Predictors for fetal and maternal outcome. Am J Nephrol 11:353, 1991. With permission. (See journal article for details of the 6 reports surveyed in this table.)

continuous segmental (T11 to L2) epidural block has been advocated, as in nonpregnant patients with ureteric colic, and may even favorably influence spontaneous passage of the stone(s). With good pain relief, the patient micturates without difficulty, moves without assistance, and is less at risk from thromboembolic problems than if drowsy, nauseated, and bedridden with pain.

When there are complications that might need surgical intervention, pregnancy should not be a deterrent to intravenous pyelography (IVP), even though the clinician may be reluctant to consider radiologic investigation. Specific clinical criteria should be met before a limited IVP is done: (1) microscopic hematuria, (2) recurrent urinary tract symptoms, and (3) sterile urine culture when pyelonephritis is suspected; the presence of two of these indicates a diagnosis of calculi in 60 per cent of women (Miller and Kakkis, 1982).

Alternative management in which x-rays are avoided during pregnancy has recently been proposed. This involves the cystoscopic placement of an internal ureteral tube, or stent, between bladder and kidney, under local anesthesia (Loughlin and Bailey, 1986). The stent retains its position because it has a pigtail or J-like curve at each end (double-J) and can be changed every 8 weeks to prevent encrustation. Early empiric use for presumed stone obstruction in pregnant women with flank pain is recommended, especially when hydration, analgesia, and antibiotics do not resolve pain and/or fever. When the pregnancy is over, the usual x-ray films can be obtained and standard management resumed.

Sonographically guided percutaneous nephrostomy is another effective and safe method of treating gravidas with ureteric colic or symptomatic obstructive hydronephrosis (Van Sonnenberg et al., 1992). The procedure is rapid, requires minimal anesthesia, and is perhaps a preferable alternative to retrograde stenting or more invasive surgery.

In patients with cystinuria, assiduous maintenance of high fluid intake is the mainstay of management. Although D-penicillamine appears relatively safe, it should be used only for severe cases, when urinary cystine excretion is known to be very high (Gregory and Mansell, 1983).

Polycystic Renal Disease

This entity may remain undetected during pregnancy, but careful questioning for a history of familial problems and the use of ultrasonography may lead to earlier detection. Patients do well when functional impairment is minimal and hypertension absent, as is often the case in childbearing years. They do, however, have an increased incidence of hypertension late in pregnancy and a higher perinatal mortality compared with that in pregnancies of sisters unaffected by this autosomal dominant disease.

Women with advanced renal failure are best advised against pregnancy although use of prophylactic dialysis has been advocated, despite lack of controlled studies, for just this type patient (Alcalay et al., 1992). If one or the other prospective parent has evidence of polycystic renal disease, the couple may seek genetic counseling. There will be a 50 per cent chance of transmitting the disease to the offspring. DNA probe techniques are now being developed so that antenatal diagnosis is possible by chorionic villus sampling, allowing women to undergo selective termination of pregnancy (Reeders et al., 1986).

Diabetic Nephropathy

Since many patients have been diabetic since childhood, they probably already have microscopic changes in the kidneys (Hayslett and Reece, 1987). During pregnancy, diabetic women have an increased prevalence of covert bacteriuria (and may be more susceptible to symptomatic urinary tract infection), peripheral edema, and preeclampsia (Cousins, 1987).

The consensus is that most women with diabetic nephropathy demonstrate normal GFR increments (and perhaps significant proteinuria), and pregnancy does not accelerate renal deterioration (Reece et al., 1988 and 1990; Combs and Kitzmiller, 1991). There is, however, a report of diabetic women with moderate renal dysfunction (serum creatinine >1.4 mg/100 ml) whose renal function permanently deteriorated in pregnancy in comparison to the changes before and afterward—GFR declines of 1.8 ml/min per month in pregnancy and 1.4 ml/min per month postpartum until the start of dialysis (Biesenbach et al., 1992). Such changes occurred despite good metabolic control and might have been related to hypertension, which often accelerates in the third trimester, regardless of intensified treatment (McCance et al., 1992). It should be noted, however, that there were no controls for this study. The condition of nongravid diabetics with creatinine levels >1.4 mg per cent too often progresses rapidly to renal failure.

Hypertension should be treated more intensively in diabetics (Parving et al., 1987). As with other renal disorders during pregnancy, we believe that more aggressive antihypertensive therapy is a reasonable objective. Of course, some of the agents used before conception may be contraindicated during gestation (Lancet Editorial, 1989).

Systemic Lupus Erythematosus (SLE)

This relatively common disease has a predilection for childbearing age, and coincidence with pregnancy poses complex clinical problems due to the profound disturbance of the immunologic system and multiple-organ involvement in SLE and the complicated immunology of pregnancy itself (Mor-Yosef et al., 1984). Transient improvements, no change, and a tendency to relapse have all been reported (see Chapter 59).

Decisions regarding the status of the disease and the importance of having a baby to the patient and her partner should be made on an individual basis. The majority of pregnancies succeed, especially when the maternal disease has been in complete clinical remission for 6 months prior to conception, even if there were marked pathologic changes in the original renal biopsy and heavy proteinuria in the early stages of the disease (Hayslett and Lynn, 1980; Jungers et al., 1982; Hayslett, 1992). Continued signs of disease activity or increasing renal dysfunction reduce the likelihood of an uncomplicated pregnancy and the clinical course thereafter.

The effects of gestation on SLE activity and on the course of lupus nephritis have long been debated. Taking into account both extrarenal manifestations and renal changes at least 50 per cent of women show some change in clinical status—often called "lupus flare" (Petri et al., 1991). Admittedly, increments in proteinuria and/or blood pressure could be due to preeclampsia, but from recent reviews of the literature (Imbasciati and Ponticelli, 1991; Nicklin, 1991), it appears that as many as 19 per cent (progressive in 8 per cent) and 42 per cent experience decrements in GFR and hypertension, respectively. The figures become worse if renal insufficiency (serum creatinine >1.4 mg/dl) antedates the pregnancy.

Lupus nephropathy may sometimes become manifest during pregnancy and, when accompanied by hypertension and renal dysfunction, may be mistaken for preeclampsia. Some patients have a definite tendency to relapse, occasionally severely in the puerperium; therefore, some clinicians prescribe or increase steroids at this time (Leikin et al., 1986). Rarely, a particularly severe postpartum syndrome may develop consisting of pleural effusion, pulmonary infiltration, fever, EKG abnormalities, and even cardiomyopathy, with extensive IgG, IgM, IgA, and C3 deposition in the myocardium (Kochenour et al., 1987).

The above views, especially that of a "stormy puerperium," are disputed (Lockshin et al., 1984; Hayslett and Lynn, 1980). In fact, many now observe postpartum patients and do not institute or increase steroid therapy unless signs of increased disease activity are noted.

SLE sera may contain a bewildering array of autoantibodies (lupus serum factor) against nucleic acids, nucleoproteins, cell surface antigens and phospholipids. Antiphospholipid antibodies (APA) exert a complicated effect on the coagulation system. This led to the rather enigmatic definition of a lupus (LE) anticoagulant, found in 5 to 10 per cent of patients with SLE. This is discussed in detail in Chapter 31. Because treatment with heparin and aspirin may lead to successful pregnancies, it is important to screen for LE anticoagulant in women with SLE and perhaps also those with a history of recurrent intrauterine death or thrombotic episodes in order to identify this particular cohort.

An increased incidence of congenital cardiac anomalies occurring in the offspring of women with SLE, and particularly in patients with anti-Ro (SS-A) antibodies, is discussed in Chapter 59.

Periarteritis Nodosa

In contrast to lupus nephropathy, the outcome of pregnancy in women with renal involvement due to periarteritis nodosa is very poor, largely because of the associated hypertension, frequently malignant. Many cases noted in the literature have involved maternal demise. It should be noted, however, that this dismal prognosis is based primarily on selected

anecdotal reports, and a few successful pregnancies have been reported. Still, until more data are available (perhaps through a registry), we continue to advise early therapeutic termination in the best interests of the mother.

Systemic Sclerosis

Scleroderma is a term that includes a heterogeneous group of limited and systemic conditions causing hardening of the skin. Systemic sclerosis implies involvement of both skin and other sites, particularly certain internal organs. Renal involvement is thought to occur in about 60 per cent of these patients, usually within 3 to 4 years of diagnosis. The presentation may take one of three forms: sudden onset of malignant hypertension, rapidly progressive renal failure, or slowly increasing azotemia (Magmon and Fejgin, 1989).

The combination of systemic sclerosis and pregnancy is unusual because the disease occurs most often in the fourth and fifth decades, and affected patients are usually infertile. When it has its onset in pregnancy, there is a greater tendency for deterioration. Patients with scleroderma and no evidence of renal involvement prior to conception have developed severe kidney disease in gestation. There are also instances in which pregnancy has been uneventful and successful, but marked reactivation occurred unexpectedly in the puerperium. Most maternal deaths involve rapidly progressive scleroderma with severe pulmonary complications, infections, hypertension, and/or renal failure.

The extent of systemic involvement is probably more important than the duration of the disease, and limited mild disease carries a better prognosis. Sclerosis usually spares the abdominal wall skin, but there is one report of hydronephrosis, presumed secondary to thickened skin and decreased abdominal wall compliance, in a twin pregnancy complicated by polyhydramnios (Moore et al., 1985).

Wegener's Granulomatosis

There is a paucity of information on the outcome of pregnancy in women with granulomatosis. Proteinuria (± hypertension) is common from early in pregnancy (Fields et al., 1991) and reports to date have described both complicated and uneventful pregnancies (Murty et al., 1991). Experience with Cytoxan in pregnancy is limited, and the risks to embryo and fetus must be weighed in relation to the course of the disease if such therapy were to be withheld from the mother.

Previous Urinary Tract Surgery

Permanent urinary diversion is still used in the management of patients with congenital lower urinary tract defects, but its use has declined for neurogenic bladder since the introduction of self-catheterization. The most common complication of pregnancy is urinary infection. Premature labor occurs in 20 per cent; the use of prophylactic antibiotics throughout pregnancy may reduce its incidence. Decline in renal function may occur, invariably related to infection or intermittent obstruction or both. With an ileal conduit, elevation and compression by the expanding uterus can cause outflow obstruction, whereas with a ureterosigmoid anastomosis, actual ureteral obstruction may occur (Barrett and Peters, 1983). The changes usually reverse after delivery.

The mode of delivery is dictated by obstetric factors. Abnormal presentation accounts for a cesarean section rate of 25 per cent. Vaginal delivery is safe, but because the continence of a ureterosigmoid anastomosis depends on an intact anal sphincter, this must be protected with a mediolateral episiotomy.

During the last 10 years, urinary tract reconstruction by means of augmentation cystoplasty, with or without artificial genitourinary sphincter, has become more commonplace. Deterioration of renal function as well as urinary tract obstruction and/or infection can occur at any time in pregnancy (Hill et al., 1990). Delivery by cesarean section is recommended for these gravidas because of the potential for disruption of the continence mechanism.

Solitary Kidney

Some patients have either a congenital absence of one kidney or marked unilateral renal hypoplasia. Most, however, have had a previous nephrectomy because of pyelonephritis (with abscess or hydronephrosis), unilateral tuberculosis, congenital abnormalities, or a tumor. It is important to know the indication for and the time elapsed since the nephrectomy (Klein, 1984). In patients with an infectious and/or a structural renal problem, sequential prepregnancy investigation is needed to detect any persistent infection.

It makes no difference whether the right or left kidney remains, as long as it is located in the normal anatomic position. If function is normal and stable, women with this problem seem to tolerate pregnancy well despite the superimposition of GFR increments on already hyperfiltering nephrons. Single kidneys are most often associated with the rare instances of acute renal failure due to obstruction during pregnancy (Lindheimer et al., 1993).

Ectopic kidneys (usually pelvic) are more vulnerable to infection and are associated with decreased fetal salvage, probably because of associated malformations of the urogenital tract. If infection occurs in a solitary kidney during pregnancy and does not quickly respond to antibiotics, termination may have to be considered for preservation of renal function.

Nephrotic Syndrome

The most common cause of nephrotic syndrome in late pregnancy is preeclampsia, which has a poorer fetal prognosis than preeclampsia with less heavy proteinuria (Fisher et al., 1981). Other causes include proliferative or membranoproliferative glomerulonephritis, lipid nephrosis, lupus nephropathy, hereditary nephritis, diabetic nephropathy, renal vein thrombosis, and amyloidosis. Some of these do not respond to, and may even be seriously aggravated by, steroids; this emphasizes the importance of a tissue diagnosis before steroid therapy is begun (Uribe et al., 1991).

If renal function is adequate and hypertension is absent, there should be few complications during pregnancy. However, several of the physiologic changes occurring during pregnancy may mimic aggravation or exacerbation of the disease. For example, increments in renal hemodynamics as well as increases in renal vein pressure may enhance protein excretion. Serum albumin levels usually decrease by 0.5 to 1.0 gm/100 ml during normal pregnancy, and further decreases due to nephrotic syndrome may enhance the tendency toward fluid retention. Because of decreased intravascular volume, diuretics could compromise uteroplacental perfusion or aggravate the increased tendency to thrombotic episodes.

Nephropathy Associated with Human Immunodeficiency Virus

Over the past decade there have been increasing reports of a nephrotic syndrome and severe renal impairment in patients infected with the human immunodeficiency virus (HIV). This entity may be seen in HIV seropositive patients, patients with acquired immunodeficiency syndrome (AIDS), or patients with AIDS-related complex. The condition is characterized by severe proteinuria and rapid progression to end-stage renal disease (Carbone et al., 1989). The distinctive features seen on histologic evaluation of renal biopsy are glomerulosclerosis, visceral epithelial cell hypertrophy, tubular microcysts, and tubular degenerative changes (Bourgoigne and Pardo, 1991). The incidence of this HIV-associated nephropathy appears to be increasing, particularly in the black population and in cases of intravenous drug abuse (Frassetto et al., 1991). Although there have not been any cases of this nephropathy reported in pregnant women, with the rising incidence of AIDS in women this form of renal disease should be considered in HIV infected patients presenting with severe proteinuria.

Precis

The problems associated with the specific disorders discussed in this section are summarized in Table 50-7. In general our conclusions are: Preserved renal function and the absence of hypertension prior to conception predict successful fetal outcome and few maternal complications regardless of the nature of the disorder. Exceptions include several collagen disorders associated anecdotally with serious maternal problems. There is some controversy between authorities regarding four specific diseases (Table 50-7), and we are with the optimists. Finally, we reiterate that these conclusions are based on poorly controlled retrospective data, underscoring the need for registries and for prospectively acquired data.

Remote Prognosis

Pregnancy does not adversely affect the natural history of the renal lesion if kidney dysfunction is minimal and hypertension is absent at conception, with the exception of certain collagen disorders; how-

TABLE 50–7. Chronic Renal Disease and Pregnancy

RENAL DISEASE	EFFECTS
Chronic pyelonephritis (infectious tubulointerstitial disease)	Bacteriuria in pregnancy and may lead to exacerbation.
Chronic glomerulonephritis and focal glomerular sclerosis (FGS)	Increased incidence of high blood pressure late in gestation but usually no adverse effect if renal function preserved and hypertension absent prior to gestation. Some disagree, believing coagulation changes in pregnancy exacerbate disease, especially IgA nephropathy, membranoproliferative glomerulonephritis, and FGS.
Systemic lupus erythematosus	Controversial; prognosis most favorable if disease in remission 6 or more months prior to conception. Some authorities increase steroid dosage in immediate postpartum period.
Periarteritis nodosa	Fetal prognosis is poor. Associated with maternal deaths. Therapeutic abortion should be considered.
Scleroderma	If onset during prenancy, there can be rapid overall deterioration. Reactivation of quiescent scleroderma can occur during pregnancy and postpartum.
Diabetic nephropathy	No adverse effect on the renal lesion. Increased frequency of infections, edema, and/or preeclampsia.
Polycystic disease	Functional impairment and hypertension usually minimal in childbearing years.
Reflux nephropathy	Controversial; some cite risks of sudden escalating hypertension and worsening of renal function. Others say results are satisfactory when preconception function only mildly affected and hypertension absent.
Urolithiasis	Ureteral dilatation and stasis do not seem to affect natural history, but infections can be more frequent. Stents have been successfully placed and sonographically controlled ureterostomy performed during gestation.
Previous urologic surgery	Depending on original reason for surgery, there may be other malformations of the urogenital tract. Urinary tract infection common during pregnancy, and renal function may undergo reversible decrease. No significant obstructive problem, but cesarean section might be necessary for abnormal presentation and/or to avoid disruption of the continence mechanism if artificial sphincters or neourethras are present.
After nephrectomy, solitary and pelvic kidney(s)	Pregnancy well tolerated. Might be associated with other malformations of the urogenital tract. Dystocia rarely occurs with a pelvic kidney.

ever, there is still debate concerning IgA and reflux nephropathies (Lindheimer and Katz, 1992; Becker et al., 1986). An important factor in remote prognosis is the sclerotic effect that hyperfiltration might already have had in the residual (intact) glomeruli of kidneys of patients with renal insufficiency. Theoretically, further progressive loss of renal function could ensue in pregnancy, but it is encouraging that this is not the case in animals when pregnancy is superimposed on experimental glomerulonephritis (Baylis, 1987; Baylis et al., 1989).

The superimposition of pregnancy hyperfiltration on the compensatory changes already present in a single kidney could lessen the life span of the kidney. The crux of this hypothesis is the implication that increases in glomerular pressure and/or glomerular plasma flow cause sclerosis within the glomerulus and that in pregnancy further physiologic hyperfiltration augments the damage. In health, it seems unlikely that there are long-term renal sequelae (Baylis and Rennke, 1985). Clearly, more human and animal research is needed because patients with renal disease can have unpredicted, accelerated, and irreversible renal decline in pregnancy or immediately afterward, and the mechanisms are unknown (Baylis, 1987).

HEMODIALYSIS PATIENTS AND PREGNANCY

It has been several decades since the first description of conception and successful delivery in a patient on chronic hemodialysis, and since then further case reports and registry data have been published. Any optimism must be tempered by the thought that clinicians are reluctant to publish failures or disasters, and consequently the true incidence of unsuccessful pregnancies in women on dialysis cannot be determined. The high surgical abortion rate in these patients indicates that those who become pregnant do so accidentally, probably because they are unaware that pregnancy is a possibility.

Counseling and Early Pregnancy Assessment

In spite of irregular or absent menstruation and impaired infertility, women on dialysis should use contraception if they wish to avoid pregnancy. The introduction of recombinant human erythropoeitin (rHuEpo) to the treatment of women with renal failure appears to be associated in some cases with return of normal menses (and ovulation), probably because of correction of hyperprolactinemia and/or improved overall health (Schaefer et al., 1989).

There are substantial arguments against pregnancy, not least of which are the risks to the patient herself and the fact that even when therapeutic termination of pregnancy are excluded, there is at best only a 20 to 40 per cent likelihood of successful outcome (Nageotte and Grundy, 1988; Kobayashi et al., 1981; Hou, 1987; Davison, 1991; Souqiyyeh et al., 1992).

Early diagnosis of pregnancy is difficult. A missed period will usually be ignored. The mistake the clinician may make is failure to consider the possibility of pregnancy. Urine pregnancy tests are unreliable, and early diagnosis and estimation of gestational age are best accomplished by sonar technology.

Antenatal Strategy and Decision-Making

For a successful outcome, scrupulous attention must be paid to blood pressure control, fluid balance, increased hours of dialysis, and provision of good nutrition (Cohen et al., 1988; Redrow et al., 1988; Yasin and Beydoun, 1988; Durant, 1989; Barri et al., 1991; Elliott et al., 1991).

Dialysis Policy

Some patients show increments in GFR despite the fact that the level of renal function is too poor to sustain life without hemodialysis whereas other women remain completely anuric (Amoah and Arab, 1991). Women with some residual renal function and satisfactory daily urine volumes, in whom dialytic control is easier, are more likely to become pregnant (Hou, 1987).

The planning of dialysis strategy should have seven aims: (1) Maintain SUN <80 mg/100 ml; some would argue lower (e.g., <50 mg/100 ml). Intrauterine death is more likely if levels are much in excess of 80 mg/100 ml, but success has been achieved despite levels of 100 mg/100 ml for many weeks. (2) Avoid hypotension during dialysis, which could be damaging to the fetus. In late pregnancy the gravid uterus and the supine posture may aggravate this by decreasing venous return. (3) Ensure good control of blood pressure. (4) Ensure minimal fluctuations in fluid balance and limit volume changes. (5) Scrutinize carefully for preterm labor, as dialysis and uterine contractions are associated. (6) Watch calcium levels closely and avoid hypercalcemia. (7) Limit interdialysis weight gain to about 1 kg until late pregnancy. Also after midpregnancy, the classic 0.5 kg/week weight gain should be taken into account when considering dry weight. This should mean a 50 per cent increase in hours and frequency of dialysis. Frequent dialysis renders dietary management and control of weight gain much easier.

In a recent report from Saudi Arabia (Souqiyyeh et al., 1992) of 27 pregnancies in 22 women only 10 went beyond 28 weeks gestation and 8 of these were successful. Comparing the pregnancies that ended before 28 weeks with those that went beyond, the authors found no significant differences in blood pressure, hemoglobin, creatinine levels, type of dialysate, past obstetric history, or duration on hemodialysis, but dialysis hours were significantly longer in the successful group.

Anemia

Patients with severe renal insufficiency are usually anemic. This anemia is usually aggravated further in pregnancy; therefore, blood transfusion may be needed, especially before delivery. Caution is necessary because transfusion may exacerbate hypertension and impair the ability to control circulatory overload, even with extra dialysis. Fluctuations in blood volume can be minimized if packed red cells are transfused during dialysis.

Recently rHuEpo has been used in pregnancy with-out ill effect (Barri et al., 1991; McGregor et al., 1991). In particular, the theoretical risks of hypertension and thrombotic complications have not been encountered so far. No adverse effects have been noted in neonates in whom normal hematologic indices and erythropoietin concentrations for gestational age suggest that rHuEpo does not have significant transplacental effects.

Unnecessary blood sampling should be avoided in the face of anemia and lack of venipuncture sites. The protocol for various tests usually performed in a particular unit should be followed strictly, with no more blood removed per venipuncture than is absolutely necessary.

Hypertension

Affected patients have abnormal lipid profiles and possibly accelerated atherogenesis, and so it is difficult to predict the cardiovascular capacity to tolerate pregnancy. Diabetic women on dialysis who have become pregnant are those in whom cardiovascular problems are most evident. In these and other women with renal disease, a normotensive state at conception is reassuring. Unfortunately, blood pressure tends to be labile and hypertension is a common problem, although it may be possible to help control it by dialysis.

Nutrition

Despite more frequent dialysis, relatively free dietary intake should be discouraged. A daily oral intake of 70 gm protein, 1500 mg calcium, 50 mM potassium, and 80 mM sodium is advised, with supplements of dialyzable vitamins. Vitamin D supplements can be difficult to judge in patients who have had parathyroidectomy. In addition, the placenta produces hydroxyvitamin D, one reason why oral supplementation may have to be curtailed. All this poses risks for fetal nutrition, plus the fact that the exact impact of the uremic environment is difficult to assess. The use of parenteral nutrition supplementation in pregnancy in these gravidas has been advocated (Brookhyser, 1989).

Fetal Surveillance and Timing of Delivery

What has been said with regard to chronic renal disease applies here as well. Cesarean section should be necessary only for purely obstetric reasons. It could be argued, however, that elective cesarean section in all cases would minimize potential problems during labor. In fact, preterm labor is generally the rule and may commence during hemodialysis. The role of cesarean section in this situation needs to be carefully considered.

Peritoneal Dialysis Patients and Pregnancy

Since 1976 chronic ambulatory peritoneal dialysis (CAPD) and chronic cycling peritoneal dialysis (CCPD) have been utilized more frequently in the management of patients with all forms of renal insufficiency. Several features of peritoneal dialysis (PD) make it an attractive approach for the management of renal failure in pregnancy: (1) maintenance of a more stable environment for the fetus in terms of fluid and electrolyte concentrations, (2) avoidance of episodes of abrupt hypotension—a frequent occurrence during hemodialysis which can cause fetal distress, (3) continuous allowance for extracellular fluid volume control so that blood pressure control is augmented, (4) refraining from systemic heparin use, (5) achievement of better maternal nutrition by allowing less restricted diet, (6) better blood sugar control in patients with diabetes mellitus via intraperitoneal insulin, and (7) theoretically permitting safe use of intraperitoneal magnesium, facilitating prevention and treatment of premature labor and possibly preeclampsia.

Young women can be treated with this approach, and a number of successful pregnancies have been reported (Kioko et al., 1983; Hou, 1987; Redrow et al., 1988; Elliott et al., 1991). Although anticoagulation and some of the fluid balance and volume problems of hemodialysis are avoided in these women, they nevertheless face the problems of placental abruption, premature labor, sudden intrauterine death, and hypertension. It should be remembered that peritonitis, which can be a severe complication of continuous ambulatory peritoneal dialysis, accounts for the majority of therapy failures. Superimposed on a pregnancy, this can present a confusing diagnostic picture and then a whole series of treatment problems.

It has been argued that if dialysis is to be used in pregnancy, CAPD is the method of choice, and if a woman is already on hemodialysis, a change should be considered (Redrow et al., 1988). We, however, prefer that women continue on the mode of dialysis in place at conception.

RENAL TRANSPLANT PATIENTS AND PREGNANCY

After transplantation, renal and endocrine functions return rapidly, and normal sexual activity can ensue. About 1 in 50 women of childbearing age with a functioning renal transplant becomes pregnant. Of the conceptions, 40 per cent do not go beyond the initial trimester because of spontaneous or therapeutic abortion. Over 90 per cent of pregnancies that do continue past the first trimester end successfully (Davison, 1991; Rizzoni et al., 1992).

Transplants have been performed with the surgeons unaware that the recipient was in early pregnancy. Obstetric success in such cases does not negate the importance of contraception counseling for all renal failure patients and the exclusion of pregnancy prior to transplantation.

Counseling and Early Pregnancy Assessment

A woman should be counseled from the time the various treatments for renal failure and the potential for optimal rehabilitation are discussed. Information regarding potential reproductive capacity must be included. Even after transplantation, stress will still be a major factor in everyday life, which will always have a "baseline of uncertainty." Couples who want a child

should be encouraged to discuss all the implications, including the harsh realities of maternal prospects of survival.

Preconception Guidelines. Individual centers have their own specific guidelines (Ehrich et al., 1991; Lindheimer and Katz, 1992). In most, a wait of 18 months to 2 years post-transplant is advised. This has turned out to be good advice because, by then, the patient will have recovered from the major surgery and any sequelae, graft function will have stabilized, and immunosuppression will be at maintenance levels. Also, if function is well maintained at 24 months, there is a high probability of allograft survival at 5 years.

A suitable set of guidelines is given here, but the criteria are only relative: (1) good general health for about 2 years since transplantation, (2) stature compatible with good obstetric outcome, (3) no or minimal proteinuria, (4) absence of hypertension, (5) no evidence of graft rejection, (6) absence of pelvicalyceal distention on a recent intravenous urogram, (7) stable renal function with plasma creatinine of 2 mg/100 ml or less (preferably less than 1.5 mg/100 ml), and (8) drug therapy reduced to maintenance levels: prednisone, 15 mg/day or less, and azathioprine, 2 mg/kg body weight/day or less. Safe doses of cyclosporin A have not yet been established because of limited clinical experience (Flechner et al., 1985; Cockburn et al., 1989), but 5 mg/kg body weight per day or less is quoted anecdotally.

Ectopic Pregnancy. Ectopic pregnancy occurs in at least 0.5 per cent of all conceptions. The diagnosis can be difficult because irregular bleeding and amenorrhea accompany deteriorating renal function or even an intrauterine pregnancy. Patients may be at higher risk of ectopic pregnancy because of pelvic adhesions due to previous urologic surgery, peritoneal dialysis, pelvic inflammatory disease, or overzealous use of intrauterine contraceptive devices. The main clinical problem is that symptoms secondary to genuine pelvic pathology are erroneously attributed to the transplant.

Antenatal Strategy and Decision-Making

Patients must be monitored as high-risk cases. Management requires attention to serial assessment of renal function, diagnosis and treatment of rejection, blood pressure control, early diagnosis or prevention of anemia, treatment of any infection, and meticulous assessment of fetal well-being.

Antenatal visits should be every 2 weeks up to 32 weeks and weekly thereafter. Monthly, the following tests should be undertaken: full blood count, including platelets; urea nitrogen, creatinine, electrolytes, and urate levels; 24-hour creatinine clearance and protein excretion; and mid-stream urine specimens for microscopy and culture.

Liver function tests, plasma protein, and calcium and phosphate levels should be checked at 6-week intervals. Tests for cytomegaloviruria and herpes hominis virus should be done during each trimester if the initial screening is negative. Although immunosuppressive therapy is usually maintained at pre-pregnancy levels, adjustments may be needed if there are decreases in the maternal white cell and platelet counts. Hematinics should be prescribed if the various hematologic indices show deficiency (Davison et al., 1985).

ALLOGRAFT FUNCTION. Serial data on renal function are needed to supplement routine antenatal observations, which are summarized above. The anatomic changes (Absy et al., 1987) and the increased and then sustained GFR characteristic of early pregnancy are evident, even though the allograft is ectopic, denervated, potentially damaged by previous ischemia, and immunologically different from both recipient and fetus. The better the pre-pregnancy GFR, the greater the increment in pregnancy. Transient reductions in GFR can occur during the third trimester and usually do not represent a deteriorating situation with permanent impairment. In 15 per cent of patients, significant renal functional impairment develops during pregnancy and may persist following delivery. However, as a gradual decline in function is common in nonpregnant patients, it is difficult to delineate a specific effect of pregnancy. Of interest is a renal transplant patient tolerating five term pregnancies and one spontaneous abortion without any long-term kidney function deterioration (Scott and Branch, 1986).

Subclinical chronic rejection with declining renal function may occur following an episode of acute rejection or if immunosuppression becomes suboptimal. Increases in proteinuria, often to abnormal levels, occur near term in 40 per cent of patients; this regresses postpartum and, in the absence of hypertension, is not significant. Whether or not cyclosporin A is more nephrotoxic in pregnancy, compared to the blunting of augmentation in GFR in the nonpregnant patient, is not known. Consequently, advice to switch to standard immunosuppressive regimens in pregnant women is based purely on clinical anecdote, and evaluations are urgently needed in pregnancy.

ALLOGRAFT REJECTION. Serious rejection episodes occur in 9 per cent of pregnant women. While this incidence of rejection is no greater than that expected for nonpregnant transplant patients, it is unusual because it has been assumed that the privileged immunologic state of pregnancy would benefit the transplant. Also, it occasionally occurs during pregnancy in women who have had years of stable function before conception. Rejection also can occur in the puerperium and may be caused by return to a normal immune state (despite immunosuppresion) or possibly a rebound effect from the altered immunoresponsiveness of pregnancy.

Chronic rejection may be a problem in all recipients, having a progressive subclinical course. Whether a pregnancy influences the course of subclinical chronic rejection is unknown. No factors consistently predict which patients will develop rejection during pregnancy. Some have hypothesized a nonimmune contribution to chronic graft failure owing to the damaging effect of hyperfiltration through remnant nephrons, perhaps even exacerbated during pregnancy (Feehally et al., 1986). From the clinical viewpoint, several points are important. Because rejection is difficult to diagnose, when any of the clinical hallmarks is present (such as fever, oliguria, deteriorating renal function,

renal enlargement, and tenderness), the diagnosis should be considered. Although ultrasonography may prove helpful, without renal biopsy, rejection cannot be distinguished from acute pyelonephritis, recurrent glomerulopathy, possibly severe preeclampsia, and even cyclosporin A nephrotoxicity. Renal biopsy is indicated before aggressive antirejection therapy is begun.

IMMUNOSUPPRESSION. Immunosuppressive therapy is usually maintained at pre-pregnancy levels, but adjustments may be needed if the maternal leukocyte or platelet count decreases. When white blood cell counts are maintained within physiologic limits for pregnancy, the neonate usually is born with a normal blood count (Davison et al., 1985). Azathioprine liver toxicity has been noted occasionally during pregnancy and responds to dose reduction.

The most sensitive method of monitoring azathioprine dosage and bioavailability is the measurement of red blood cell (RBC) 6-thioguanine nucleotides (6-TGN), metabolites of both azathioprine and 6-mercaptopurine whose formation of 6-TGN is catalyzed by RBC thiopurine methyltransferase (TPMT) (Lennard et al., 1987). Low TPMT activity may be a risk factor for the development of thiopurine toxicity because there are wide individual variations in RBC 6-TGN among patients receiving identical azathioprine dosage (Lennard et al., 1987). One in 300 patients lacks TPMT activity on a genetic basis. Identification of such patients could be important, especially in pregnancy, if side effects are to be avoided.

At present there are only limited reports of (noncomplicated) pregnancies in patients taking cyclosporin A (Flechner et al., 1985; Derfler et al., 1988; Pickrell et al., 1988; Haugen et al., 1991). More recently a registry has been started by Vincent Armenti, M.D., who can be contacted at Thomas Jefferson University, Philadelphia, PA. Numerous adverse effects are attributed to this drug in nonpregnant transplant recipients, including renal toxicity, hepatic dysfunction, tremor, convulsions, diabetogenic effects, hemolytic uremic syndrome, and neoplasia (Meyers, 1986; Al-Khader et al., 1988). In pregnancy, some of the maternal adaptation that normally occurs could theoretically be blunted or abolished by cyclosporin A—especially plasma volume expansion and renal hemodynamic augmentation. Further assessments are needed.

HYPERTENSION AND PREECLAMPSIA. The appearance of hypertension in the third trimester, its relationship to deteriorating renal function, and the possibility of chronic underlying pathology and preeclampsia are diagnostic problems. Hypertension, particularly before 28 weeks gestation, is associated with adverse perinatal outcome (Sturgiss and Davison, 1991), which may be due to covert cardiovascular changes that accompany or are aggravated by chronic hypertension. Preeclampsia is diagnosed clinically in about 30 per cent of pregnancies. When eclampsia supervenes, its development may be rapid.

INFECTIONS. Patients should be carefully monitored for all types of infection throughout pregnancy. Prophylactic antibiotics must be given before any surgical procedure, however trivial.

DIABETES MELLITUS. As the results of renal transplantation have improved in those women whose renal failure was caused by juvenile onset diabetes mellitus, pregnancies are now being reported in these women. Pregnancy complications occur with at least twice the frequency seen in the nondiabetic patient, and this may be due to the presence of generalized cardiovascular pathology (Ogburn et al., 1986; Endler et al., 1987). A few successful pregnancies have been reported after confirmed pancreas-kidney allograft (Calne et al., 1988; Tyden et al., 1989), and in one woman the pancreatic graft was unexpectedly lost in acute rejection immediately after delivery, having functioned normally for 3 years prior to the pregnancy.

FETAL SURVEILLANCE AND TIMING OF DELIVERY. The points given for chronic renal disease are equally applicable. Preterm delivery is common (45 to 60 per cent) because of intervention for obstetric reasons and the common occurrence of premature labor or premature rupture of membranes. Premature labor frequently is associated with poor renal function, but in some it has been postulated that long-term steroid therapy may weaken connective tissues and contribute to the increased incidence of premature rupture of membranes.

Vaginal delivery should be the aim, and usually there is no mechanical injury to the transplant. Unless there are specific obstetric problems, spontaneous onset of labor can be awaited.

MANAGEMENT DURING LABOR. Careful monitoring of maternal fluid balance, cardiovascular status, and temperature is essential; aseptic technique is important for every procedure. Surgical induction of labor (by amniotomy) and episiotomy warrant antibiotic coverage. Pain relief is conducted as for healthy women. Augmentation of steroids is necessary to cover delivery.

ROLE OF CESAREAN SECTION. The kidney does not usually obstruct the birth canal. Cesarean section is necessary for the usual obstetric reasons. Several factors are important when deciding on the delivery route. Transplant patients may have pelvic osteodystrophy related to their previous renal failure (and dialysis) or prolonged steroid therapy, particularly before puberty. Antenatal diagnosis of these problems is important and permits the planning of elective cesarean delivery. If there is a question of disproportion or kidney compression, simultaneous intravenous pyelography and x-ray pelvimetry could be performed (with limitation of the IVP to one to three films) at 36 weeks gestation. When a cesarean section is performed, a lower segment approach is usually feasible. However, previous urologic surgery and/or peritonitis may make this difficult.

Pediatric Management

IMMEDIATE PROBLEMS. Over 50 per cent of liveborns have no neonatal problems. Preterm delivery is common (45 to 60 per cent), small-for-dates infants are delivered in at least 20 per cent of cases, and occasionally the two factors coexist. Although management is the same as in neonates of other mothers, some specific problems exist (Table 50–8). Adrenocortical

insufficiency due to the maternal steroid therapy potentially increases the risk of overwhelming neonatal infection.

BREAST-FEEDING. There are substantial benefits to breast-feeding. It could be argued that because the baby has been exposed to azathioprine and its metabolites in pregnancy, breast-feeding should be allowed. However, little is known about the quantities of azathioprine and its metabolites in breast milk and whether or not the levels are biologically trivial or substantial. Even less is known about cyclosporin A in breast milk except that levels are usually greater than those in a simultaneously taken blood sample. Until the many uncertainties are resolved, breast-feeding should not be encouraged.

LONG-TERM ASSESSMENT. Azathioprine can cause abnormalities in the chromosomes of leukocytes, which may take almost 2 years to disappear spontaneously. In tissues not yet studied, however, these anomalies may not be as temporary. The sequelae could be eventual development of malignant tumors in affected offspring or abnormalities in the reproductive performance in the next generation. There are some worrying animal data. For instance, fertility problems affect the female offspring of mice that have received low doses of 6-mercaptopurine, the major metabolite of azathioprine (equivalent to 3 mg/kg). These offspring subsequently proved to be sterile or, if they conceived, had smaller litters and more dead fetuses than did unexposed dams (Reimers and Sluss, 1978). Thus, exposure *in utero* may not affect otherwise normal females until they attempt childbearing. Finally, the long-term sequelae of *in utero* exposure to cyclosporin A are not known.

Maternal Follow-up After Pregnancy

The ultimate measure of transplant success is the long-term survival of the patient and the graft. As it is only 30 years since this procedure became widely employed in the management of end-stage renal failure, there are few long-term data from sufficiently large series from which to draw conclusions. Furthermore, it must be emphasized that the long-term results for renal transplants relate to a period when many aspects of management would be unacceptable by present-day standards. Average survival figures of large numbers of patients worldwide indicate that 70

TABLE 50–8. Neonatal Problems in Offspring of Renal Transplant Patients

Preterm delivery/small for gestational age
Respiratory distress syndrome
Depressed hematopoiesis
Lymphoid/thymic hypoplasia
Adrenocortical insufficiency
Septicemia
CMV infection
Hepatitis B surface antigen carrier state
Congenital abnormalities
Immunologic problems
    Reduced lymphocyte PHA-reactivity
    Reduced T lymphocyte
    Reduced immunoglobulin levels
    Chromosome aberrations in leukocytes

to 80 per cent of recipients of kidneys from related living donors are alive 5 years after transplantation. With cadaver kidneys, the figure is 40 to 50 per cent (Briggs and Junor, 1992). If renal function was normal 2 years after transplant, survival increased to about 80 per cent. This is why women are counseled to wait about 2 years before attempting conception.

A major concern is that the mother may or may not survive or remain well enough to rear the child she bears. Pregnancy does occasionally and sometimes unpredictably cause irreversible declines in renal function. However, the consensus at present is that pregnancy has no effect on graft function or survival (Sturgiss and Davison, 1992).

It has been calculated that 10 per cent of these mothers will be dead within 7 years of pregnancy and 50 per cent dead within 15 years (Crespigny and d'Apice, 1986). Nevertheless, many women will choose parenthood in an effort to re-establish a normal life and possibly in defiance of the sometimes-negative attitudes of the medical establishment. More long-term studies are needed to assess this area, especially with the advent of new immunosuppressive drugs, so that counseling can be enhanced and can be based on recorded experience rather than clinical anecdote.

CONTRACEPTION. It is unwise to offer the option of sterilization at the time of transplantation; this decision should not take place at this time. Oral contraceptives cause or aggravate hypertension or thromboembolism and can produce subtle changes in the immune system, but this does not necessarily contraindicate their use. Careful surveillance is important.

An intrauterine contraceptive device (IUD) may aggravate menstrual problems, which in turn may obscure signs and symptoms of abnormalities of early gestation, such as threatened abortion and ectopic pregnancy. The increased risk of pelvic infection associated with the IUD in an immunosuppressed patient makes this method worrisome. Indeed, as insertion or replacement of an IUD is associated with bacteremia of vaginal origin in at least 13 per cent, antibiotic coverage is essential at this time (Murray et al., 1987). The efficacy of the IUD may be reduced by immunosuppressive and anti-inflammatory agents, possibly because of modification of the leukocyte response. Careful counseling and follow-up are essential.

GYNECOLOGIC PROBLEMS. There is a danger that symptoms secondary to genuine pelvic pathology may be erroneously attributed to the transplant because of its location near the pelvis. Transplant patients might be at slightly higher risk of ectopic pregnancy because of pelvic adhesions resulting from previous urologic surgery, pelvic inflammatory disease, or the overzealous use of IUDs. Diagnosis can be overlooked because irregular bleeding and amenorrhea may be associated with deteriorating renal function as well as intrauterine pregnancy.

Transplant recipients receiving immunosuppressive therapy have a malignancy rate estimated to be 100 times greater than normal (Penn, 1990), and the female genital tract is no exception (Caterson et al., 1984; Halpert et al., 1986). This association is probably related to factors such as loss of immune surveillance,

chronic immunosuppression allowing tumor proliferation, and/or prolonged antigenic stimulation of the reticuloendothelial system. Therefore, regular gynecologic assessment is essential. Management should be on conventional lines, with the outcome unlikely to be influenced by stopping or reducing immunosuppression.

ACUTE RENAL FAILURE PARTICULAR TO PREGNANCY

Acute renal failure severe enough to require dialysis occurs in less than 1:20,000 gestations (Lindheimer et al., 1993), although complications with transient decrements in GFR of a mild to moderate degree probably occur in 1:8000 deliveries (Krane, 1988). This section emphasizes specific problems in obstetric practice (Table 50–9) and focuses on avoidance of diagnostic errors (Hirsch et al., 1992) that can further compound this serious obstetric emergency. Usually, acute renal failure occurs in women with previously healthy kidneys, but it can complicate the course of patients with preexisting renal disease (Hayslett, 1985; Lindheimer et al., 1993; Turney et al., 1989). Table 50–10 suggests an approach to patients with sudden decrements in urinary volumes, focusing on tests to differentiate acute tubular necrosis from pre-renal failure. Before anuria or oliguria is ascribed to acute renal failure, obstruction to renal outflow must be excluded. Hydronephrosis leading to acute renal failure in late pregnancy can be due to obstruction from an enlarging uterus (with or

TABLE 50–9.   Obstetric Acute Renal Failure

Volume contraction/ hypotension	Antepartum hemorrhage due to placenta praevia
	Postpartum hemorrhage: from uterus or extensive soft tissue trauma
	Abortion
	Hyperemesis gravidarum
	Adrenocortical failure; usually failure to augment steroids to cover delivery in patient on long-term therapy
Volume contraction/hypotension and coagulopathy	Antepartum hemorrhage due to abruptio placentae
	Preeclampsia/eclampsia
	Amniotic fluid embolism
	Incompatible blood transfusion
	Drug reaction(s)
	Acute fatty liver of pregnancy
	Hemolytic uremic syndrome
Volume contraction/ hypotension, coagulopathy, and infection	Septic abortion
	Chorioamnionitis
	Pyelonephritis
	Puerperal sepsis
Urinary tract obstruction	Polyhydramnios
	Damage to ureters: during cesarean section and repair of cervical/vaginal lacerations
	Pelvic hematoma
	Broad ligament hematoma
	Calculus or clot in ureters primarily of single kidney

TABLE 50–10. Differential Diagnosis of Oliguria

	PRERENAL FAILURE	ACUTE TUBULAR NECROSIS
History	Vomiting, diarrhea, other causes of dehydration	Dehydration, ischemic insult, ingestion of nephrotoxin; no specific history in 50% of cases
Physical examination	Decreased blood pressure, increased pulse rate, poor skin turgor	May have signs of dehydration, but physical examination often normal
Urinalysis	Concentrated urine; few formed elements on sediment, but many hyaline cases	Isosthenuria; sediment contains renal tubular cells and pigmented casts, but may be normal
Urinary sodium	<20 mEq/L; most <10 mEq/L	≥25, usually >60 mEq/L
Urine-plasma (U/P) ratios	High	Low
Osmolality	Often ≥1.5	<1.1
Urea	≥20	≤3
Creatinine	>40	<15
Fractional sodium excretion ($U/P_{Na}/U/P_{creatinine}$)	<1%	>1%
Renal failure index ($U/P_{Na}/U/P_{creatinine}$)	<1	>1
	<1	>1

From Lindheimer MD, Davison JM: Renal disorders. *In* Barron WM, Lindheimer MD (eds): Medical Disorders During Pregnancy. St. Louis, Mosby-Year Book, 1991. With permission.

without polyhydramnios), a situation that resolves immediately after amniotomy (Brandes and Fritsche, 1991); if delivery is not appropriate, ultrasound-guided percutaneous nephrostomy is safe and reliable (Van Sonnenberg et al., 1992). Furthermore, the urinary tract may be unwittingly damaged when surgery is performed for obstetric emergencies such as postpartum hemorrhage, which can themselves be the cause of acute renal failure.

Septic Abortion

There are many reasons why acute renal failure is associated with septic abortion. Dehydration and hypotension can lead to considerable renal ischemia. Soap and Lysol, common abortifacients, may have specific nephrotoxic effects. However, the marked hemolysis caused by some bacteria and chemical abortifacients is sufficient to provoke the renal shutdown. Most pregnancy sepsis is due to gram-negative bacteria, and clostridia are responsible for only 0.5 per cent of cases in which patients develop shock. It is the latter bacterium that is responsible for one of the most devastating syndromes complicating gestation.

Presentation can be quite dramatic, with an abrupt rise in temperature (to 40°C), often associated with myalgias, vomiting, and diarrhea, the latter occasionally bloody. Once symptoms begin, hypotension, tachypnea, and progression to frank shock occur rapidly. The patient is usually jaundiced with the bronze-like color characteristic of the association of jaundice with cutaneous vasodilation, cyanosis, and pallor. Despite the presence of fever, the extremities are often cold and display purplish areas that may be precursors of small patches of necrosis on the toes, fingers, and nose. Generalized muscular pains, often most intense in the thorax and abdomen, may lead to confusion with intra-abdominal inflammatory processes; this is especially true when a history of provoked abortion is denied or not sought, since heavy vaginal bleeding is often not a prominent feature (see Chapter 51).

Acute Renal Failure and Preeclampsia

Preeclampsia is accompanied by a characteristic renal lesion in which the glomeruli enlarge and become ischemic due to swelling of the intracapillary cells—glomerular endotheliosis and mesangiosis. Most preeclamptic patients experience moderate decreases in GFR, but occasionally this decrease is accompanied by acute renal failure. The kidney failure is usually due to acute tubular necrosis, but acute cortical necrosis may also occur. It is possible that acute tubular necrosis is the obligatory outcome of glomerular cell swelling that can lead to complete obliteration of the capillary lumen (see Chapter 49). This might be aggravated by inappropriate drug therapy, abruptio placentae, and/or hemorrhage in the antenatal and peripartum periods (Brown et al., 1990). If the renal failure is related solely to preeclampsia without chronic hypertension, renal disease or both before pregnancy, then long-term normal renal function is evident in about 80 per cent of cases. Underlying chronic problems reduce this to 20 per cent, with the rest needing long-term dialysis (Sibai et al., 1990). Treatment should follow the standard approach (see below), although recently more specific therapies for this group of patients have been tested, such as prostacyclin infusion (Fox et al., 1991).

Acute Renal Failure and Pyelonephritis

In the absence of complicating features such as obstruction, calculi, papillary necrosis, and analgesic nephropathy, it is extremely rare for acute pyelonephritis to cause acute renal failure in nonpregnant subjects, but this association appears to be more frequent in pregnant women. It is known that acute pyelonephritis in pregnancy is accompanied by marked decrements in GFR, in contrast to test results in nonpregnant patients (Thompson et al., 1986). It has been suggested that the vasculature in pregnancy may be more sensitive to the vasoactive effect of bacterial endotoxins.

Acute Fatty Liver of Pregnancy

Acute fatty liver of pregnancy, also called obstetric pseudoacute yellow atrophy, is a rare complication of late pregnancy or the early postpartum period, occurring in approximately 1 in 13,000 deliveries (see Chapter 49). It is characterized by jaundice, severe hepatic dysfunction, including coma, and varying degrees of renal failure. It may also be associated with hypertension and with coagulation and platelet abnormalities that lead to diagnostic confusion with preeclampsia. In the past tetracyclines were associated with this condition. In addition, reversible urea cycle enzyme deficiencies (ornithine transcarbamylase and carbamoyl phosphate synthetase) resembling those seen in Reye's syndrome have been described.

Idiopathic Postpartum Renal Failure

Idiopathic postpartum renal failure is also called postpartum malignant nephrosclerosis, irreversible postpartum renal failure, and postpartum hemolytic uremic syndrome (HUS). It is a rare and frequently fatal syndrome, characterized by the onset of renal failure 3 to 10 weeks into the puerperium (Hayslett, 1985; Li et al., 1988) after the patient has had an uneventful pregnancy and delivery. The patient develops marked azotemia and severe hypertension, frequently associated with microangiopathic hemolytic anemia and platelet aggregation with formation of microthrombi in the terminal portions of the renal vasculature (see also Chapter 49).

There is uncertainty concerning the management of this condition, as many patients succumb despite treatment with dialysis, plasmapheresis, exchange transfusion, immunosuppression, heparin, streptokinase, dipyridamole, aspirin, or corticosteroids alone or combined. Others have survived but required dialysis and/or transplantation. One theory of the etiology implicates lack of prostacyclin, a powerful vasodilator and potent endogenous inhibitor of platelet aggregation, which may be counteracted by exchange transfusion or even plasma infusion alone. Prolonged prostacyclin infusions have been tried with the aim of restoring the deficiency, thus controlling the hypertension and reversing the platelet consumption, but such therapy remains to be proved effective. It has been argued that disseminated intravascular coagulation (DIC) is significant (with placental thromboplastin being released during labor) and that antithrombin III (AT-III) may have a protective effect. Again such claims are anecdotal.

Cortical Necrosis in Pregnancy

Renal cortical necrosis is an extremely rare complication that at one time seemed to be more common in pregnant than in nonpregnant populations, but most recently its incidence during gestation has decreased to below 1:80,000 (Lindheimer et al., 1993). This pathologic entity is characterized by tissue death throughout the cortex with sparing of the medullary portions.

Acute cortical necrosis may develop in patients with DIC or overwhelming septicemia, but most cases present in the third trimester or the puerperium. Multigravidas beyond the age of 30 are more likely to develop cortical necrosis. The condition tends to be associated with specific obstetric complications, mainly placental abruption, unrecognized long-standing intrauterine death, and occasionally preeclampsia (Pertuiset and Grünfeld, 1987).

Although cortical necrosis may involve the entire renal cortex, resulting in irreversible renal failure, it is the "patchy" variety that occurs more often in pregnancy. This is characterized by an initial episode of severe oliguria, which lasts much longer than in uncomplicated acute tubular necrosis, followed by a variable return of function and stable period of moderate renal insufficiency. Years later, for reasons still obscure, renal function may decrease again, often leading to end-stage renal failure.

Miscellaneous Causes

Acute renal failure can occur during pregnancy in a variety of situations similar to those causing sudden renal dysfunction in nonpregnant patients. These situations include primary renal diseases (i.e., acute nephritis, sarcoidosis, lymphoma, and Goodpasture syndrome); those related to systemic illnesses such as endocarditis; the ingestion of nephrotoxins; incompatible transfusions; and those in which there is structural infiltration of the kidneys secondary to an extrarenal disease (Warren et al., 1988; Maikranz and Katz, 1991; Sheil et al., 1991; Yankowitz et al., 1992). Finally, the literature suggests that some pregnant women with underlying renal disease but well-preserved GFR are prone to develop acute tubular necrosis, especially when pregnancy is complicated by superimposed preeclampsia or another cause of increased blood pressure (Katz et al., 1980).

MANAGEMENT

Treatment of sudden renal failure resembles that in nonpregnant populations and aims at retarding the appearance of uremic symptomatology, acid-base and electrolyte disturbances, and volume problems (i.e., overhydration when the patient is oliguric and dehydration during the polyuric phase) (Lindheimer et al., 1993; Krane, 1988). One must also be aware of the propensity of patients with acute renal failure to develop infection, a complication that can be serious in pregnant women. Many of the aforementioned problems will respond to judicious conservative management, but if such an approach is unsuccessful, dialysis will be necessary.

Dialysis in patients with acute renal failure is prescribed "prophylactically," that is, prior to the appearance of electrolyte and/or acidemia, or uremic symptoms. Such "prophylactic" dialysis appears even more necessary in prepartum patients with an immature fetus and in whom temporization is desired. Problems during dialysis peculiar to pregnancy were discussed in detail earlier.

Peritoneal dialysis is effective and safe as long as the catheter is inserted high in the abdomen under direct vision through a small incision. In fact, as discussed earlier, chronic ambulatory peritoneal dialysis may become the preferred dialysis approach in the prepartum woman because it minimizes rapid metabolic perturbations. Volume shifts during hemodialysis should be minimized to avoid impairment of uteroplacental blood flow.

Controlled anticoagulation with heparin (preferably including monitoring to verify that activated clotting time is maintained between 150 and 180 sec) is desirable during hemodialysis. Observation for vaginal bleeding is also important.

As discussed previously, premature contractions or the onset of labor frequently occurs during or immediately after dialysis. Therefore, when possible, early delivery (as dictated by fetal maturity) should be undertaken. Blood losses should be replaced quickly to the point of overtransfusing slightly, because in the pregnant patient uterine bleeding may be concealed and thus underestimated.

When delivery is imminent, nursery personnel should be advised that the neonate is subject to rapid dehydration. This is due to increased levels of urea and other solutes within the fetal circulation that precipitate an osmotic diuresis shortly after birth.

SUMMARY

Changes in the urinary tract during normal pregnancy are so marked that norms in the nonpregnant cannot be used for obstetric management. Awareness of all alterations is essential if kidney problems in pregnancy are to be suspected or detected and then handled correctly.

Most women with mild and moderate renal disease tolerate pregnancy well and have a successful obstetric outcome without adverse effect on the natural history of the underlying renal lesion. Crucial determinants are renal functional status at conception, the presence or absence of hypertension, and the type of renal disease. There is disagreement regarding pregnancy outcome in the presence of focal glomerular sclerosis, IgA and reflux nephropathies, mesangio-proliferative glomerulonephritis, while patients with certain collagen disorders (especially periarteritis nodosa and scleroderma) do poorly. In general, prognosis is good if renal dysfunction is minimal and hypertension is absent.

Pregnancy in women on dialysis can be excessively complicated. Increased frequency and duration of dialysis are needed. There is high fetal wastage at all stages of pregnancy.

In the absence of severe maternal problems, the hazards of pregnancy in renal transplant patients are minimal, and successful obstetric outcome is the rule.

Acute obstetric renal failure can occur in women with previously healthy kidneys. Pathology peculiar to pregnancy must always be considered.

REFERENCES

Abe S: An overview of pregnancy in women with underlying renal disease. Am J Kidney Dis **17**:112, 1991a.

Abe S: Pregnancy in IgA nephropathy. Kidney Int **40**:1098, 1991b.

Absy M, Metreweli C, Mathews C, et al: Changes in transplanted kidney volume measured by ultrasound. Br J Radiol **60**:525, 1987.

Alcalay M, Blau A, Barkai G, et al: Successful pregnancy in a patient with polycystic disease and advanced renal failure: the use of prophylactic dialysis. Am J Kidney Dis **19**:382, 1992.

Al-Khader A, Absy M, Al-Hasani MK, et al: Successful pregnancy in renal transplant recipients treated with cyclosporine. Transplantation **45**:987, 1988.

Amoah E, Arab H: Pregnancy in a hemodialysis patient with no residual renal function. Am J Kidney Dis **17**:585, 1991.

Andriole VT, Patterson TF: Epidemiology, natural history and management of urinary tract infection in pregnancy. Med Clin North Am **75**:359, 1991.

Barcelo P, Lopez-Lillo J, Del Rio G: Successful pregnancy in primary glomerular disease. Kidney Int **30**:914, 1986.

Barrett RJ, Peters WA: Pregnancy following urinary diversion. Obstet Gynecol **62**:582, 1983.

Barri YM, Al-Furayh O, Qunibi WY, et al: Pregnancy in women on regular hemodialysis. Dial Transpl **20**:652, 1991.

Baylis C: Glomerular filtration and volume regulation in gravid animal models. Clin Obstet Gynaecol (Bailliere) **1**:789, 1987.

Baylis C, Reese K, Wilson CB: Glomerular effects of pregnancy in a model of glomerulonephritis in the rat. Am J Kidney Dis **14**:452, 1989.

Baylis C, Rennke HG: Renal hemodynamics and glomerular morphology in repetitively pregnant aging rats. Kidney Int **28**:140, 1985.

Bear RA: Pregnancy in patients with chronic renal disease. Can Med Assoc J **48**:13, 1978.

Becker GJ, Ihle BO, Fairley KF, et al: Effect of pregnancy on moderate renal failure in reflux nephropathy. Br Med J **294**:796, 1986.

Biesenbach G, Stoger H, Zaztgarnik J: Influence of pregnancy on progression of diabetic nephropathy and subsequent requirement of renal replacement therapy in female type 1 diabetic patients with impaired renal function. Nephrol Dial Transpl **7**:105, 1992.

Bourgoigne JJ, Pardo V: The nephropathology in human immunodeficiency virus (HIV-1) infection. Kidney Int **35**:S19, 1991.

Brandes JC, Fritsche C: Obstructive acute renal failure by a gravid uterus: a case report and review. Am J Kidney Dis **18**:398, 1991.

Briggs JD, Junor BJR: Long-term complications and results in the transplant patient. In Cameron JS, Davison AM, Grunfeld JP, Kerr DNS, Ritz E (eds): Oxford Textbook of Nephrology. New York, Oxford University Press, 1992, pp 1570–1594.

Brookhyser J: The use of parenteral nutrition supplementation in pregnancy complicated end-stage renal disease. J Am Diet Assoc **89**:93, 1989.

Brown MA: Urinary tract dilation in pregnancy. Am J Obstet Gynecol **164**:641, 1991.

Brown MA, Child RP, O'Connor M, et al: Pregnancy-induced hypertension and renal failure: clinical importance of diuretics, plasma volume and vasospasm. Aust NZ J Obstet Gynaecol **30**:230, 1990.

Brumfitt W: The significance of symptomatic infection in pregnancy. Contrib Nephrol **25**:23, 1981.

Calne RY, Brons EGM, Williams PF, et al: Successful pregnancy after panatopic segmental pancreas and kidney transplantation. Brit Med J **298**:1709, 1988.

Campbell-Brown M, McFadyen IR, Seal DV, et al: Is screening for bacteriuria in pregnancy worthwhile? Br Med J **294**:1579, 1987.

Carbone L, D'Agati V, Cheng JT, et al: Course and prognosis of human immunodeficiency virus-associated nephropathy. Am J Med. **87**:389, 1989.

Carpenter RG, Gardner A, Jepson M, et al: Prevention of unexpected infant death. Lancet **1**:723, 1983.

Caterson RJ, Furber J, Murray J, et al: Carcinoma of the vulva in the two young renal allograft recipients. Transplant Proc **16**:559, 1984.

Chang PK, Hall MH: Antenatal prediction of urinary tract infection in pregnancy. Br J Obstet Gynaecol **89**:8, 1982.

Cockburn I, Krupp P, Monka C: Present experience of Sandimmun in pregnancy. Transpl Proc **21**:3730, 1989.

Coe FL, Parks JH, Lindheimer MD: Nephrolithiasis during pregnancy. N Engl J Med **298**:324, 1978.

Cohen D, Frenkel Y, Maschiach S, et al: Dialysis during pregnancy in advanced chronic renal failure patients: outcome and progression. Clin Nephrol **29**:144, 1988.

Combs GA, Kitzmiller JL: Diabetic nephropathy and pregnancy. Clin Obstet Gynecol **34**:505, 1991.

Cousins L: Pregnancy complications among diabetic women: Review, 1965—1985. Obstet Gynecol Surv **42**:140, 1987.

Cox SM, Shelburne P, Mason RA, et al: Mechanisms of hemolysis and anemia associated with acute antepartum pyelonephritis. Am J Obstet Gynecol **164**:587, 1991.

Crespigny PCD, d'Apice AJF: Parenthood after renal transplantation. Aust NZ J Med **16**:245, 1986.

Cunningham FG: Urinary tract infections complicating pregnancy. Clin Obstet Gynaecol (Bailliere) **1**:891, 1987.

Cunningham FG, Cox SM, Harstad TW, et al: Chronic renal disease and pregnancy outcome. Am J Obstet Gynecol **163**:453, 1990.

Cunningham FG, Lucas MJ, Hawkins GDV: Pulmonary injury complicating antepartum pyelonephritis. Am J Obstet Gynecol **156**:797, 1987.

Danielli L, Korchazak D, Beyar H, et al: Recurrent hematuria during multiple pregnancies. Obstet Gynecol **69**:446, 1987.

Davison JM: Dialysis, transplantation and pregnancy. Am J Kidney Dis **27**:127, 1991.

Davison JM, Dellagrammatikas H, Parkin JM: Maternal azathioprine therapy and depressed haemopoiesis in the babies of renal allograft recipients. Br J Obstet Gynaecol **92**:233, 1985.

Davison JM, Sprott MS, Selkon JB: The effect of covert bacteriuria in schoolgirls on renal function at 18 years and during pregnancy. Lancet **2**:651, 1984.

Derfler K, Schaller A, Herd CH, et al: Successful outcome of a complicated pregnancy in a renal transplant recipient taking cyclosporine A. Clin Nephrol **29**:96, 1988.

Durant AQ: Treatment guidelines in a pregnant hemodialysis patient. Dial Transpl **18**:86, 1989.

Easterling TR, Brateng D, Goldman ML, et al: Renal vascular hypertension during pregnancy. Obstet Gynecol **78**:921, 1991.

Editorial: Urinary tract infection during pregnancy. Lancet **2**:190, 1985.

Ehrich JHH, Rizzoni G, Brunner FP, et al: Combined report on regular dialysis and transplantation of children in Europe, 1989. Nephrol Dial Transpl **6**:37, 1991.

Elliott JP, O'Keefe DF, Schon DA, et al: Dialysis in pregnancy: A critical review. Obstet Gynecol Surv **46**:319, 1991.

Endler M, Derfler K, Schaller A, et al: Schwangerschaft und Geburt nach Nierentransplantation unter Cyclosporin A. Fallb Literat Gesurt Fran **47**:660, 1987.

Feehally J, Bennett SE, Harris KPG: Is chronic renal transplant rejection a nonimmunological phenomenon? Lancet **2**:486, 1986.

Fields CL, Ossorio MA, Roy TM, et al: Wegener's granulomatosis complicated by pregnancy. A case report. J Reprod Med **36**:463, 1991.

Fisher K, Luger A, Spargo BH, et al: Hypertension in pregnancy: Clinical-pathological correlations and remote prognosis. Medicine **60**:267, 1981.

Flechner SM, Katz AR, Rogers AJ, et al: The presence of cyclosporine in body tissues and fluids during pregnancy. Am J Kidney Dis **5**:60, 1985.

Fox JG, Sutcliffe NP, Walker JJ, et al: Postpartum eclampsia and acute renal failure: treatment with prostaglandin. Case report. Br J Obstet Gynaecol **98**:400, 1991.

Frassetto L, Schoenfeld PY, Humphreys MH: Increasing incidence of human immuno-deficiency virus-associated nephropathy at San Franciso Hospital. Am J Kidney Dis **18**:655, 1991.

Gregory MC, Mansell MA: Pregnancy and cystinuria. Lancet **2**:1158, 1983.

Grunebaum AN, Minkoff H: Twin gestation and perinatal follow-up in a woman with severe chronic renal failure managed without dialysis. A case report. J Reprod Med **32**:463, 1987.

Halpert R, Fruchter RG, Sedlis A, et al: Human papillomavirus and lower genital neoplasia in renal transplant patients. Obstet Gynecol **68**:251, 1986.

Haugen G, Fauchald P, Sodal G, et al: Pregnancy outcome in renal allograft recipients: influence of cyclosporin A. Eur J Obstet Gynecol Reprod Biol **39**:25, 1991.

Hayslett JP: Postpartum renal failure. N Engl J Med **312**:1556, 1985.

Hayslett JP: The effect of systemic lupus erythematosus on pregnancy and pregnancy outcome. Am J Reprod Immunol **28**:199, 1992.

Hayslett JP, Lynn RI: Effect of pregnancy in patients with lupus nephropathy. Kidney Int **18**:207, 1980.

Hayslett JP, Reece EA: Managing diabetic patients with nephropathy and other vascular complications. Clin Obstet Gynaecol (Bailliere) **1**:939, 1987.

Heybourne KD, Schultz MF, Goodlin RC, et al: Renal artery stenosis during pregnancy. A review. Obstet Gynecol Surv **46**:509, 1991.

Hill DE, Chantigian PM, Kramer SA, et al: Pregnancy after augmentation cystoplasty. Surg Gynecol Obstet **170**:485, 1990.

Hirsch DJ, Jindal KK, Trillo AA: An unusual case of renal failure after pregnancy. Am J Kidney Dis **19**:86, 1992.

Hou S: Peritoneal and hemodialysis in pregnancy. Clin Obstet Gynaecol (Bailliere) **1**:1009, 1987.

Hou SH, Grossman SD, Madias NE: Pregnancy in women with renal disease and moderate renal insufficiency. Am J Med **78**:185, 1985.

Imbasciati E, Pardi G, Capetta P, et al: Pregnancy in women with chronic renal failure. Am J Nephrol **11**:193, 1986.

Imbasciati E, Ponticelli C: Pregnancy and renal disease: Predictors for fetal and maternal outcome. Am J Nephrol **2**:353, 1991.

Jakobi P, Ohel G, Szylman P, et al: Continuous ambulatory dialysis as the primary approach in the management of severe renal insufficiency in pregnancy. Obstet Gynecol **79**:808, 1992.

Jungers P, Dougados M, Pelissies C, et al: Lupus nephropathy and pregnancy. Arch Int Med **142**:771, 1982.

Jungers P, Houillier P, Forget D: Reflux nephropathy and pregnancy. Clin Obstet Gynaecol (Bailliere) **1**:955, 1987.

Jungers P, Houillier P, Forget D, et al: Specific controversies concerning the natural history of renal disease in pregnancy. Am J Kidney Dis **17**:116, 1991.

Katz AI, Davison JM, Hayslett JP, et al: Pregnancy in women with kidney disease. Kidney Int **28**:192, 1980.

Katz AI, Lindheimer MD: Does pregnancy aggravate primary glomerular disease? Am J Kidney Dis **6**:261, 1985.

Kincaid-Smith P, Whitworth JA, Fairley KF: Mesangial IgA nephropathy in pregnancy. Clin Exp Hypertens **2**:821, 1980.

Kioko M, Shaw KM, Clarke AD, et al: Successful pregnancy in a diabetic patient treated with chronic ambulatory peritoneal dialysis. Diabetes Care **6**:298, 1983.

Klein EA: Urologic problems of pregnancy. Obstet Gynecol Surv **39**:605, 1984.

Klein VR, Laifer S, Timoll EA: Renal cell carcinoma in pregnancy. Obstet Gynecol **69**:531, 1987.

Kobayashi H, Matsumoto Y, Otsubo O, et al: Successful pregnancy in a patient undergoing chronic hemodialysis. Obstet Gynecol **57**:382, 1981.

Kochenour NK, Branch DW, Rote NS, et al: A new postpartum syndrome associated with antiphospholipid antibodies. Obstet Gynecol **69**:460, 1987.

Krane NK: Acute renal failure in pregnancy. Arch Intern Med **148**:2327, 1988.

Lancet Editorial: Are ACE inhibitors safe in pregnancy? Lancet **2**:482, 1989.

Lawson DH, Miller AWF: Screening for bacteriuria in pregnancy: A critical reappraisal. Arch Intern Med **132**:904, 1973.

Leikin JB, Arof HM, Pearlman LM: Acute lupus pneumonitis in the postpartum period: A case history and review of the literature. Obstet Gynecol **68**:295, 1986.

Lennard L, van Loon JA, Lilleyan JS, et al: Thiopurine pharmacogenetics in leukemia: Correlation of erythrocyte thiopurine methyl-transferase activity and 6-thioguanine nucleotide concentrations. Clin Pharmacol Ther **41**:18, 1987.

Li PK, Lai FM, Tam JS, et al: Acute renal failure due to postpartum haemolytic uraemic syndrome. Aust NZ J Obstet Gynaecol **28**:228, 1988.

Lindheimer MD, Davison JM: Renal disorders. *In* Barron WM, Lindheimer MD (eds): Medical Disorders During Pregnancy. St. Louis, Mosby-Year Book, 1991.

Lindheimer MD, Katz AI: Renal physiology disease in pregnancy. *In* Seldin DW, Giebisch G: The Kidney: Physiology and Pathophysiology, 2nd ed. New York, Raven Press, 1992a.

Lindheimer MD, Katz AI: Pregnancy in the renal transplant patient. Am J Kidney Dis **19**:173, 1992.

Lindheimer MD, Katz AL, Ganeval D, et al: Acute renal failure in pregnancy. *In* Brenner BM, Lazarus JM (eds): Acute Renal Failure, 3rd ed. New York, Churchill Livingstone, 1993.

Lockshin MD, Reinitz E, Druzin NL, et al: Lupus pregnancy: Case-control prospective study demonstrating absence of lupus exacerbation during or after pregnancy. Am J Med **77**:893, 1984.

Loughlin KR, Bailey RB: Internal ureteral stents for conservative management of ureteral calculi during pregnancy. N Engl J Med **315**:1647, 1986.

Magmon R, Fejgin M: Scleroderma in pregnancy. Obstet Gynecol Surv **44**:530, 1989.

Maikranz P, Katz AI: Acute renal failure in pregnancy. Obstet Gynecol Clin North Am **18**:333, 1991.

Martinell J, Jodal U, Lidiu-Janson G: Pregnancies in women with and without renal scarring after urinary infections in childhood. Br Med J **300**:840, 1990.

McCance S, Lowe SA, Rubin PC: The pharmacological management of hypertension in pregnancy. J Hypertens **10**:201, 1992.

McGladdery SL, Aparicio S, Verrier-Jones K: Outcome of pregnancy in an Oxford-Cardiff cohort of women with previous bacteriuria. Q J Med **83**:533, 1992.

McGregor E, Stewart G, Junor BJR: Successful use of recombinant human erythropoietin in pregnancy. Nephrol Dial Transpl **6**:292, 1991.

McFadyen IR: Urinary tract infection in pregnancy. *In* Andréucci VE (ed): The Kidney. Boston, Martinus Nijhoff, 1986.

McNeeley SG, Baselski VS, Ryan GM: An evaluation of two rapid bacteriuria screening procedures. Obstet Gynecol **69**:550, 1987.

Meyers BD: Cyclosporine nephrotoxicity. Kidney Int **30**:964, 1986.

Meyers SJ, Lee RV, Munschauer RW: Dilatation and nontraumatic rupture of the urinary tract during pregnancy. A review. Obstet Gynecol **66**:809, 1985.

Miller DR, Kakkis J: Prognosis, management and outcome of obstructive renal disease in pregnancy. J Reprod Med **27**:199, 1982.

Moore M, Saffran JE, Barof HSB, et al: Systemic sclerosis and pregnancy complicated by obstructive uropathy. Am J Obstet Gynecol **153**:893, 1985.

Mor-Yosef S, Navot D, Rabinowitz R, et al: Collagen disease in pregnancy. Obstet Gynecol Surv **39**:67, 1984.

Murray S, Hickey J, Houang E: Significant bacteremia associated with replacement of intrauterine contraceptive device. Am J Obstet Gynecol **156**:698, 1987.

Murty GE, Davison JM, Cameron DS: Wegener's granulomatosis complicating pregnancy: first report of a case with a tracheostomy. J Obstet Gynecol **10**:399, 1991.

Nageotte MP, Grundy HO: Pregnancy outcome in women requiring chronic hemodialysis. Obstet Gynecol **72**:456, 1988.

Nicklin JL: Systemic lupus erythematosus and pregnancy at the Royal Women's Hospital, Brisbane 1979–1989. Aust NZ J Obstet Gynaecol **31**:128, 1991.

Ogburn PL, Kitzmiller JL, Hare JW, et al: Pregnancy following renal transplantation in Class T diabetes mellitus. JAMA **255**:911, 1986.

Parving H-H, Andersen AR, Smidt UM, et al: Effect of antihypertensive treatment on kidney function in diabetic nephropathy. Br Med J **294**:1443, 1987.

Penn I: Cancers complicating organ transplantation. N Engl J Med **323**:1767, 1990.

Pertuiset N, Grünfeld J-P: Acute renal failure in pregnancy. Clin Obstet Gynaecol (Bailliere) **1**:873, 1987.

Petri M, Howard D, Repke J: Frequency of lupus flare in pregnancy: The Hopkins Lupus Pregnancy Center Experience. Arthritis Rheum **34**:1538, 1991.

Pickrell MD, Sawers R, Michael J: Pregnancy after renal transplantation: severe intrauterine growth retardation during treatment with cyclosporin A. Br Med J **296**:825, 1988.

Powers RD: New directions in the diagnosis and therapy of urinary tract infections. Am J Obstet Gynecol **164**:1387, 1991.

Pruett K, Faro S: Pyelonephritis associated with respiratory distress. Obstet Gynecol **69**:444, 1987.

Redrow M, Cherem L, Elliott J: Dialysis in the management of pregnant patients with renal insufficiency. Medicine **67**:199, 1988.

Reece EA, Coustan DR, Hayslett JP, Holford T, Couleham J, Occoner TZ, Hobbins JC: Diabetic nephropathy. Pregnancy performance and fetal outcome. Am J Obstet Gynecol **159**:56, 1988.

Reece EA, Winn HN, Hayslett JP et al: Does pregnancy alter the rate of progression of diabetic nephropathy? Am J Perinatol **7**:193, 1990.

Reeders ST, Brenning MH, Corney G, et al: Two genetic markers closely linked to adult polycystic kidney disease on chromosome 16. Br Med J **292**:851, 1986.

Reimers TJ, Sluss PM: 6-Mercaptopurine treatment of pregnant mice: Effects on second and third generations. Science **202**:65, 1978.

Rizzoni G, Ehrich JHH, Broyen M, et al: Successful pregnancies in women on renal replacement therapy: Report from EDTA Registry. Nephrol Dial Transpl **7**:1, 1992.

Schaefer RM, Kokot F, Wernze H: Improved sexual function in hemodialysis patients on recombinant erythropoietin: a possible role for prolactin. Clin Nephrol **31**:1, 1989.

Scott JR, Branch DW: The effect of repeated pregnancies on renal allograft function. Transplantation **42**:695, 1986.

Shiel O, Redman CWG, Pugh C: Renal failure in pregnancy due to primary renal lymphoma. Case Report. Br J Obstet Gynaecol **98**:216, 1991.

Sibai BM, Villar MA, Mabie BC: Acute renal failure in hypertensive disorders of pregnancy. Pregnancy outcome and remote prognosis in 31 consecutive cases. Am J Obstet Gynecol **162**:777, 1990.

Souqiyyeh MZ, Huraib SO, Mohd Saleh A, et al: Pregnancy in chronic hemodialysis patients in the Kingdom of Saudi Arabia. Am J Kidney Dis **19**:235, 1992.

Stamm WE, Counts GW, Running KR, et al: Diagnosis of coliform infection in acutely dysuric women. N Engl J Med **307**:463, 1982.

Stenqvist K, Dahlen-Nilsson I, Lidin-Janson G, et al: Bacteriuria in pregnancy. Frequency and risk of acquisition. Am J Epidemiol **129**:372, 1989.

Sturgiss SN, Davison JM: Perinatal outcome in renal allograft recipients: prognostic significance of hypertension and renal function before and during pregnancy. Obstet Gynecol **78**:573, 1991.

Sturgiss SN, Davison JM: Effect of pregnancy on longterm function of renal allografts. Am J Kidney Dis **19**:167, 1992.

Thacker SB, Berkelman RL: Assessing the diagnostic accuracy and efficacy of selected antepartum fetal surveillance techniques. Obstet Gynecol Surv **41**:121, 1986.

Thompson C, Verami R, Evanoff G, et al: Suppurative bacterial pyelonephritis as a cause of acute renal failure. Am J Kidney Dis **8**:271, 1986.

Turney JH, Ellis CM, Parsons FM: Obstetric acute renal failure—1956–1987. Br J Obstet Gynaecol **96**:679, 1989.

Twickler D, Little BB, Satin AJ, et al: Renal pelvicalyceal dilatation in antepartum pyelonephritis: ultrasonographic findings. Am J Obstet Gynecol **165**:1115, 1991.

Tyden G, Brattstrom C, Bjorkman U, et al: Pregnancy after combined pancreas-kidney transplantation. Diabetes **38**:43, 1989.

Uribe LG, Thakur VD, Krane NK: Steroid-responsive nephrotic syndrome with renal insufficiency in the first trimester of pregnancy. Am J Obstet Gynecol **164**:568, 1991.

Van Sonnenberg E, Casola G, Talner LB, et al: Symptomatic renal obstruction or urosepsis during pregnancy: treatment by sonographically guided percutaneous nephrostomy. Am J Roentgenol **158**:91, 1992.

Vogt K, Kensch G, Baumann U, et al: Successful pregnancy in advanced renal failure without dialysis. Paediatr Nephrol **3**:189, 1989.

Warren GV, Sprague SM, Corwin HL: Sarcoidosis presenting as acute renal failure during pregnancy. Am J Kidney Dis **12**:161, 1988.

Yankowitz J, Kuller JA, Thomas RL: Pregnancy complicated by Goodpasture syndrome. Obstet Gynecol **79**:806, 1992.

Yasin SY, Beydoun SN: Hemodialysis in pregnancy. Obstet Gynecol Surv **43**:655, 1988.

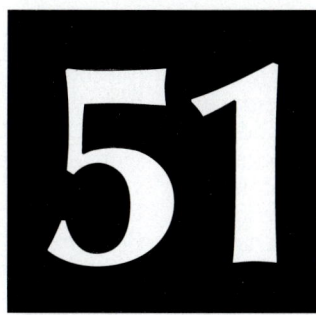

INTENSIVE CARE MONITORING OF THE CRITICALLY ILL PREGNANT PATIENT

BERNARD GONIK, M.D.

As our specialty continues to develop, we become more aware of the need for a better understanding of critical care medicine as it applies to obstetrics (Mabie and Sibai, 1990). This issue is not based on the fact that maternal mortality is increasing in the United States or Europe, because demographic statistics demonstrate continuing declines in maternal mortality. Neither does this approach advocate the exclusion of other traditional health care providers in the area of critical care medicine. However, it does point out that the gravid patient who becomes critically ill is best served by individuals who appreciate both maternal and fetal physiology, in addition to those needs associated with the acute medical or surgical pathologic condition at hand. This chapter addresses basic critical care monitoring in obstetrics and specifically discusses conditions in which more intensive care management of the pregnant patient may be indicated.

MATERNAL MORTALITY

Maternal mortality is defined as the number of maternal deaths per 100,000 live births. This vital statistic is periodically surveyed by various local, state, and national agencies. Because these maternal mortality committees frequently utilize death certificates as their only data base, some have suggested that these numbers underestimate this mortality rate by as much as 20 to 50 per cent (Kaunitz et al., 1985). Variations in the definition of "maternal" death, medicolegal concerns, and physicians untrained in the proper completion of death certificates further confuse these investigations. To address these concerns, Shanklin and associates (1991) have recently attempted to more strictly define the various classifications of maternal mortality. Until these newer guidelines are universally adopted, the following general conclusions regarding maternal mortality from recent analyses are presented below (Kaunitz et al., 1985; Gabel, 1987; Centers for Disease Control, 1985; Atrash et al., 1990).

As can be seen in Figure 51–1, mortality rates have steadily declined in the United States over the last two decades (Atrash et al., 1990). Although this is true for all races, wide discrepancies still exist between the white and nonwhite populations. These differences have been attributed mainly to socioeconomic factors limiting adequacy of health care for minority groups.

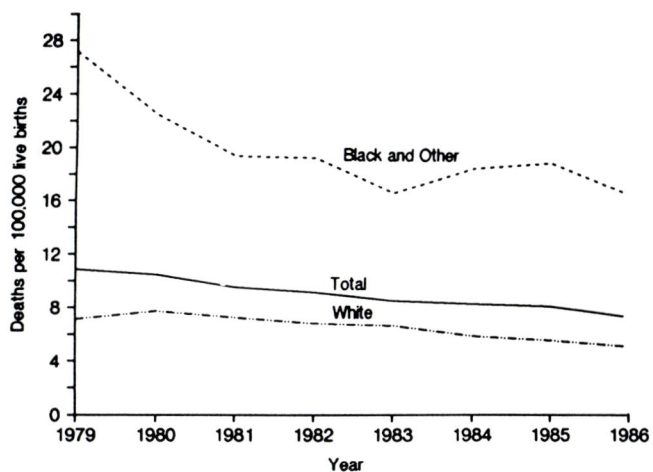

FIGURE 51–1. Maternal mortality rates in the United States, 1979–1986. (From Atrash HK, Koonin LM, Lawson HW, et al: Maternal mortality in the United States, 1979–1986. Obstet Gynecol **76**:1055, 1990.)

Geographic differences also appear to exist in maternal mortality. Rates are highest in the South and lowest in the Western states. Here again, racial differences within each region of the country appear to be the factor influencing these discrepancies. The current overall maternal mortality rate for the United States is 9.1/100,000 (5.1/100,000 whites, 16.6/100,000 nonwhites).

Advanced maternal age is a recognized risk factor for death. This appears to be due to the increased age-associated incidence of chronic illness such as hypertension, diabetes, and obesity rather than age alone. In addition, advancing age is usually accompanied by increasing parity, which is associated with an increased incidence of abruptio placentae, placenta previa, and uterine rupture.

Variables related to health care delivery systems, such as hospital size, have also been correlated with maternal mortality. Both very large delivery services and very small obstetric units have higher maternal death rates as compared with medium-sized institutions. The underlying reasons for these discrepancies in mortality rates are distinctly different. For larger hospitals, patients tend to come from higher-risk groups, i.e., blacks, tertiary care referrals, and so on. As for smaller hospitals, less sophisticated blood banking facilities and limited intensive care technology make them less able to handle acute life-threatening conditions.

Table 51–1 outlines the causes of maternal death in the United States over a 4-year period, excluding those associated with abortive outcomes (Kaunitz et al., 1985). As can be seen, the most commonly identified causes of death were embolism, hypertensive disease, obstetric hemorrhage, and infection. This report differs from previous reports because of the preeminence of embolic disease. Other recent investigations have substantiated the prominence of embolic disease as a cause of maternal mortality (Centers for Disease Control, 1985; Gabel, 1987). Two factors have been suggested for this change. First, embolism tends to be less easily recognized and less successfully treated by current intensive care methodologies than the other causes of maternal death. Second, embolic disease may be overreported because of its more nebulous diagnosis.

CRITICAL CARE FACILITIES ON AN OBSTETRIC UNIT

Recent advances in critical care medical knowledge and instrumentation have influenced many directors of obstetric services to develop full cardiovascular hemodynamic monitoring capabilities within their labor and delivery suites or in nearby special care units. As these special facilities are located on the obstetric ward, one is able to provide for intensive fetal surveillance in addition to maternal care equivalent to that of most medical or surgical intensive care units. Precise information regarding which patients would most benefit from admission to these units and the cost effectiveness of such facilities has yet to be established. It is important to point out that in recent literature this issue has been confused by failure to make appropriate distinctions between clinical and research necessities.

The overall dimensions of a room designated for this purpose need to be large for several reasons. These include the need for a variety of large pieces of monitoring equipment along with the expectation that many members of the management team will be in the room at any given time. In addition, it is necessary that capabilities be available within the room or nearby for emergency cesarean section. If a vaginal delivery is anticipated, this should be performed within the intensive care room itself to minimize the need for switching monitors or transporting the critically ill patient.

The basic monitoring equipment should preferably include a 4- or 8-channel hemodynamics unit, oscilloscope, pressure transducers, electrocardiograph module, a cardiac output computer, and a pulse oximeter. Although direct oscilloscopic or digital display readings are usually adequate, a hard-copy chart recorder may be desirable for evaluating complex pressure tracings or for times when a patient's respiratory efforts add too much variation to the displayed values. The fetal surveillance equipment should include capabilities for both external and internal heart rate monitoring along with pressure transducer tracings. A hand-held or desk top computer can be programmed to calculate extrapolated hemodynamic variables. A pH/blood gas analyzer, co-oximeter, and oncometer are also preferred in order to complete the hemodynamic requirements of the unit. Most often, these latter pieces of equipment do not need to be individually purchased if the institution has an established stat laboratory facility.

The most important component to the successful operation of a critical care unit is adequate health care provider training. Nursing supervisory staff should designate individuals from each work shift interested in working in these units. Training should include critical care patient management, Swan-Ganz data interpretation, and equipment maintenance. Frequently, this requires periodic assignments to the surgical or medical intensive care units of the hospital. Refresher courses to maintain these skills should also be planned at regular intervals, depending on the amount of utilization of the facility.

INVASIVE HEMODYNAMIC MONITORING

Indications for Pulmonary Artery Catheterization

Current indications for the use of invasive pulmonary artery catheterization in obstetrics are based on

TABLE 51–1. **Causes of Maternal Mortality**

Embolism	24%
Hypertensive disease	20%
Obstetric hemorrhage	16%
Sepsis	10%
Cerebrovascular accident	5%
Anesthesia-related	5%
Other or unspecified	20%

Modified from Kaunitz AM, Hughes JM, Grimes DA: Causes of maternal mortality in the United States. Obstet Gynecol 65:605, 1985. Reprinted with permission from the American College of Obstetricians and Gynecologists.

individual experiences and empiric thinking. Controlled trials evaluating this new technology in the management of the critically ill pregnant woman have yet to be carried out. These comparisons may never be made because of the limited clinical exposure to these types of patients in obstetrics and the fact that too many confounding variables exist to make meaningful comparisons possible. Robin (1985) has pointed out that invasive monitoring should be used in the clinical setting only when the data obtained will specifically influence acute management; too often this tenet is not followed. The following are some of the suggested indications for invasive monitoring of the obstetric patient: (1) hypovolemic shock that is unresponsive to initial volume resuscitation attempts; (2) septic shock when vasopressor therapy may be needed; (3) pregnancy-induced hypertension complicated by oliguria; (4) need for rapid intravenous antihypertensive therapy; (5) adult respiratory distress syndrome (ARDS) requiring intubation; (6) cardiac disease, class 3 or 4, in labor or requiring surgery; (7) amniotic fluid embolism; (8) isolated pulmonary hypertension in labor or during surgery; and (9) pulmonary edema, from any etiology, that is unresponsive to initial therapy (ACOG Technical Bulletin, 1988).

Central venous pressure (CVP) monitoring should not be considered equivalent to pulmonary artery catheter monitoring. Recent data evaluating the relationship between serial CVP measurements and pulmonary capillary wedge pressure (PCWP) readings in severe pregnancy-induced hypertension are shown in Figure 51–2 (Cotton et al., 1985a). Although statistically a linear relationship was noted, there was large variation between patients for a given CVP measurement. For instance, a CVP reading of 8 mm Hg could be associated with a PCWP of between 8 and 21 mm

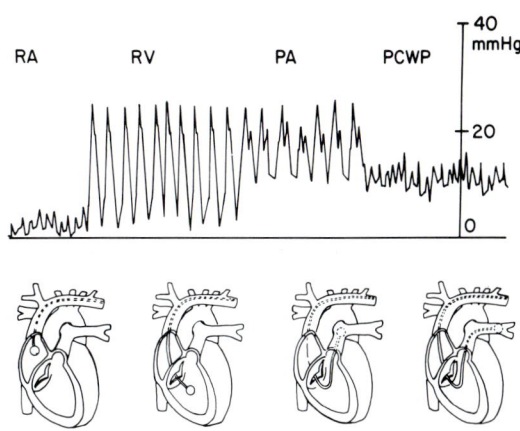

FIGURE 51–3. Pressure wave-forms in relation to pulmonary artery catheter position. (From Hankins GDC: Principles of invasive hemodynamic monitoring. *In* Cotton DB, Clark SL (eds): Clinics in Perinatology. Philadelphia, WB Saunders Company, 1986.)

Hg. Thus, from a clinical perspective, CVP measurement would not appear to be as satisfactory a measure of left atrial filling pressure as PCWP. Whether this holds true for pregnant women with critically ill disease states other than pregnancy-induced hypertension remains unknown. From a pathophysiologic perspective, CVP remains an important consideration in the development of lung edema because it inversely influences pulmonary lymph drainage.

Pulmonary Artery Catheterization

DESCRIPTION AND INSERTION TECHNIQUE. In 1970 Swan and associates first described the use of a balloon-tipped pulmonary artery catheter that allowed for invasive serial hemodynamic measurements. The original instrument has undergone numerous modifications and improvements. It is now commercially available through several suppliers in the United States and abroad. The Swan-Ganz catheter, a No. 7 French polyvinylchloride multilumen device, is capable of directly measuring right atrial pressure (CVP), pulmonary artery pressure (PA), and PCWP. Cardiac output (CO) can be intermittently measured by thermodilution, and mixed venous oxygen saturation can be continuously measured by reflection spectrophotometry.

By percutaneous insertion, the catheter is directed into place via the internal or external jugular, subclavian, basilic, or femoral vein. Some of the more peripheral access sites make catheter positioning more difficult but may be preferred when a coagulopathy is present. Characteristic oscilloscopic pressure wave-forms (Fig. 51–3) are utilized to establish the catheter's location when it is advanced. Simultaneous continuous EKG monitoring is needed to identify catheter-related arrhythmias. These arrhythmias tend to be transient and generally do not require intervention except for withdrawal of the catheter. Inflation of the balloon assists in positioning of the catheter because the device is carried through the heart's chambers by

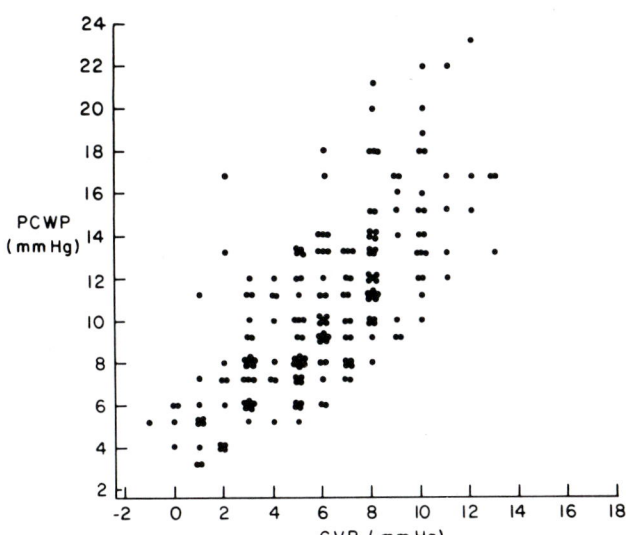

FIGURE 51–2. Relationship of central venous pressure (CVP) to pulmonary capillary wedge pressure (PCWP) in severe pregnancy-induced hypertension. (From Cotton DB, Gonik B, Dorman K, et al: Cardiovascular alterations in severe pregnancy-induced hypertension: Relationship of central venous pressure to pulmonary capillary wedge pressure. Am J Obstet Gynecol **151**:762, 1985.)

established venous and cardiac flow patterns. Once the inflated balloon reaches the pulmonary artery, a dampened tracing (PCWP) usually indicates that the balloon is situated in the proper "wedged" position. When it is deflated, return of an identifiable pulmonary artery systolic and diastolic pressure tracing should occur. Periodic manipulation of the catheter may be needed to maintain accurate readings and to avoid permanent wedging of the catheter. A portable chest x-ray can be utilized to verify the catheter's approximate location.

COMPLICATIONS OF PULMONARY ARTERY CATHETERS. Recognized complications associated with insertion and maintenance of a pulmonary artery catheter are listed in Table 51–2. The initial complications seem to be most closely correlated with the technical skills and experience of the clinician. Many of the later complications can be minimized by having available ancillary health care personnel familiar with the catheter and its functioning.

As indicated earlier, cardiac arrhythmias are most often transient in nature, although fatal ventricular fibrillation has been reported. Their overall incidence during insertion has been reported to be between 15 and 50 per cent (Swan et al., 1970; Sprung et al., 1982). The occurrence of a significant arrhythmia is more common when underlying cardiac disease is present or when metabolic disturbances are left uncorrected. Additional specific risk factors include hypocalcemia, hypokalemia, hypoxemia, and acidosis. With these latter two factors, some have noted a greater than 80 per cent risk for ventricular tachyarrhythmias (Sprung et al., 1982). One should therefore have available lidocaine hydrochloride in case bolus administration is needed, when attempting catheter placement. In addition, appropriate resuscitation equipment should be at hand for acute cardiopulmonary complications should they occur.

Pulmonary infarction may occur as a result of direct catheter tip occlusion of a pulmonary artery tributary or from thrombus dislodgement and embolization around the catheter. It is typically diagnosed by radiographic findings of a wedge-shaped infiltrate distal to the catheter tip. Although originally thought to occur in 35 per cent of catheter placements, it is a much less common event today, with a suggested incidence of 1.3 to 7.2 per cent (Boyd et al., 1983). This probably relates to an overall better understanding of invasive monitoring techniques and the routine use of a continuous heparin flush.

Sepsis from continuous catheter usage occurs approximately 2 to 8 per cent of the time (Boyd et al., 1983). One must distinguish between true infection and catheter tip contamination (or colonization), which can occur in up to 35 per cent of catheter insertions. These two entities are distinguished by clinical evidence of septicemia with the same blood- and catheter-identified organisms, in the first case, and organism-positive catheter cultures only for the latter case. Risk factors for sepsis include underlying infection, prolonged catheter usage (more than 3 days), and nonsterile repositioning of the catheter after initial placement. This latter event has been minimized by the recent introduction of a sterile/clean catheter sheath system that allows for catheter advancement under more aseptic conditions.

The other potential complications of using a pulmonary artery catheter listed in Table 51–2 occur infrequently. Pneumothorax risks (incidence 1 to 6 per cent) can be minimized by using an alternate site for insertion rather than the subclavian approach. Catheter knotting can be avoided during placement if the operator remains aware of the centimeter markings on the advancing catheter. As a general rule, the right ventricle is almost always reached when the catheter has been inserted 25 to 30 cm from the jugular vein site. Few patients require more than 50 cm of catheter to reach the pulmonary artery. Inflated catheter balloons should be checked prior to insertion to reduce the risk of air leakage and balloon rupture. In addition, overinflation of the balloon with air (greater than 1.5 ml) should be avoided. Pulmonary artery rupture—generally a fatal complication—is uncommon (0.2 per cent incidence); the major risk factor is existing pulmonary artery hypertension and distal migration of the catheter. Valvular damage can occur from chronic catheter irritation or during insertion when the catheter balloon is not deflated prior to retrograde movement.

HEMODYNAMIC VARIABLES. Utilizing a pulmonary artery catheter, the following hemodynamic variables can be *directly measured* in the patient: heart rate (HR) (beats per minute), CVP (mm Hg), pulmonary artery systolic and diastolic pressures (PAS, PAD) (mm Hg), PCWP (mm Hg), and CO (liters per minute). By use of a sphygmomanometer or by peripheral artery catheterization, direct measurements of systemic arterial pressures can also be obtained. Mean pressure values for both the arterial and pulmonary circulations can be calculated by the following formula:

$$\text{Mean arterial pressure (MAP)} = \frac{\text{Systolic pressure} + 2\,(\text{Diastolic pressure})}{3}$$

Listed below are other *calculated* hemodynamic variables, along with their respective formulas:

$$\text{Stroke volume (SV)} = \frac{\text{CO}}{\text{HR}} \text{ (ml/beat)}$$

$$\text{Systemic vascular resistance (SVR)} = \frac{\text{MAP} - \text{CVP}}{\text{CO}} \times 80 \text{ (dyne} \times \text{sec} \times \text{cm}^{-5})$$

TABLE 51–2. Potential Pulmonary Artery Catheter Complications

At Insertion	After Placement
Pneumothorax	Pulmonary infarction
Thrombosis	Pulmonary artery rupture
Arterial puncture	Infection
Air embolization	Balloon rupture
Catheter knotting	Endocardial/valvular
Cardiac arrhythmias (transient, sustained)	damage

Pulmonary vascular resistance (PVR) =
$$\frac{PAP - PCWP}{CO} \times 80 \text{ (dyne} \times \text{sec} \times \text{cm}^{-5})$$

Left ventricular stroke work (LVSW) =
$$SV \times MAP \times 0.0144 \text{ (gm} \times M/M^2)$$

Many times these hemodynamic parameters are expressed in an "indexed" fashion (i.e., cardiac index). In order to do this, the original nonindexed cardiac output value must be divided by body surface area (BSA). Since standard BSA calculations have never been established specifically for pregnancy, this traditional way of expressing hemodynamic data is somewhat controversial in obstetrics. Those who argue for its use point out that indexing allows direct comparison of hemodynamic parameters for pregnant women of different sizes, a critical issue when interpreting these values.

Presented in Table 51–3 are mean hemodynamic measurements for pregnant and nonpregnant patients. These are paired data from 10 healthy subjects, taken between 36 and 38 weeks gestation and between 11 and 13 weeks postpartum (Clark et al., 1989). Using the noninvasive technique of M-mode echocardiography, Capeless and Clapp (1989) demonstrated that many of these physiologic alterations in hemodynamics begin in the early phases of pregnancy. Clark and associates (1991) demonstrated that position changes late in pregnancy significantly influenced central hemodynamic stability. The standing position resulted in a 50 per cent increase in pulse, a 21 per cent fall in left ventricular stroke work index (LVSWI), and a 54 per cent rise in peripheral vascular resistance (PVR). It is interesting that the pregnant state, when compared with the nonpregnant state, seemed to result in a *buffering* of orthostatic-related hemodynamic changes. The authors speculated that the increased intravascular volume during pregnancy accounted for this stabilizing effect.

TABLE 51–3.   Normal Central Hemodynamic Parameters in Healthy Nonpregnant and Pregnant Patients

	NONPREGNANT	PREGNANT
Cardiac output (l/min)	4.3 ± 0.9	6.2 ± 1.0
Heart rate (beats/min)	71 ± 10	83 ± 10
Systemic vascular resistance (dyne × cm × sec⁻⁵)	1530 ± 520	1210 ± 266
Pulmonary vascular resistance (dyne × cm × sec⁻⁵)	119 ± 47	78 ± 22
Colloid oncotic pressure (mm Hg)	20.8 ± 1.0	18.0 ± 1.5
Colloid oncotic pressure— pulmonary capillary wedge pressure (mm Hg)	14.5 ± 2.5	10.5 ± 2.7
Mean arterial pressure (mm Hg)	86.4 ± 7.5	90.3 ± 5.8
Pulmonary capillary wedge pressure (mm Hg)	6.3 ± 2.1	7.5 ± 1.8
Central venous pressure (mm Hg)	3.7 ± 2.6	3.6 ± 2.5
Left ventricular stroke work index (gm × m × m⁻²)	41 ± 8	48 ± 6

From Clark SL, Cotton DB, Lee W, et al: Central hemodynamic assessment of normal term pregnancy. Am J Obstet Gynecol **161**:1439 1989.

Hemodynamic Considerations for Specific Conditions

This section deals specifically with hemodynamic considerations for various pathologic conditions in the pregnant woman. A complete discussion of these conditions can be found in various other chapters of this text.

MITRAL VALVE STENOSIS. The principal hemodynamic problem associated with severe mitral valve stenosis in pregnancy relates to an obstruction in left ventricular filling. The resultant fixed cardiac output limits the parturient's ability to tolerate large fluctuations in intravascular volume. During the intrapartum and postpartum periods, shunted blood returning to the heart may easily overload the cardiovascular system. The immediate clinical implication is the development of pulmonary congestion and edema. Other factors, such as increases in heart rate, can also limit ventricle diastolic filling and therefore can precipitate pulmonary edema more easily in patients with this condition. Management goals center on the prophylactic maintenance of a relatively nonoverloaded or slightly constricted (for pregnancy) intravascular volume in anticipation of fluid shifts known to occur during the peripartum period. Adequate analgesia and anesthesia during labor and delivery also reduce excessive cardiac demands associated with pain and anxiety.

The other important hemodynamic consideration in the patient with mitral valve stenosis relates to the potential for misinterpretation of the invasive monitoring data. Because of the stenotic mitral valve, PCWP readings do not accurately reflect left ventricular diastolic pressure. In some instances, very high PCWP values are recorded (and are needed to maintain an adequate cardiac output). Overt pulmonary edema is usually not associated with these high readings. Therefore, during attempts at maintaining a relatively "constricted" intravascular volume, cardiac output should be concomitantly monitored and maintained. For each individual patient, optimal PCWP and cardiac output values should be determined (i.e., those values that maintain blood pressure and tissue perfusion).

AORTIC STENOSIS. The major problem encountered with aortic stenosis centers on the patient's potential inability to maintain cardiac output. Factors that cause a reduction in blood flow to the heart can trigger sudden decreases in cardiac output and death. Hypotension from conduction anesthesia, positioning changes, and acute blood loss are particularly hazardous to the laboring woman. Unlike mitral stenosis, aortic valve stenosis requires that attempts be made to maintain the patient in a relatively hypervolemic state. Spinal or conduction anesthesia would appear to be relatively contraindicated because of their associated risks for hypotension.

PULMONARY HYPERTENSION. Maternal mortality rates for patients with pulmonary hypertension have been reported to be as high as 50 to 80 per cent. The underlying problem in this condition is obstruction to right ventricular outflow caused by a fixed and elevated pulmonary vascular resistance. When systemic vascular resistance is reduced, there is a tendency for right-to-left shunting of deoxygenated blood with resultant hypoxemia. In addition, reductions in blood return to the heart can decrease right ventricular pressure so that the pulmonary vasculature is hypoperfused. The resultant hypoxemia has been associated with sudden death. Intrapartum management requires maintenance of a relatively "hypervolemic" state, with any interventions that would lead to significant preload reduction specifically avoided.

AMNIOTIC FLUID EMBOLISM. Confusion exists about the hemodynamic events associated with amniotic fluid embolization. In part, this relates to discrepancies between experimental animal data and a limited amount of anecdotal human observations. In an attempt to reconcile these differences, Clark et al. (1985a) have postulated that a biphasic hemodynamic response pattern exists. First, an initial transient period of intense pulmonary vasospasm leads to acute right heart failure and hypoxemia. This initial event may explain the 50 per cent occurrence of maternal deaths during the acute episode. Subsequently, however, the predominant feature is one of left ventricular heart failure with only mild to moderate elevations in pulmonary artery pressure. Characteristically, in this phase is seen an elevated PCWP and a reduction in LVSW.

Treatment should be directed toward the latter hemodynamic response, with optimization of cardiac output using crystalloid fluids to replenish intravascular volume depletion and vasopressor therapy for acute hypotension and congestive heart failure. Previous therapeutic recommendations aimed at selective reductions in pulmonary artery vasospasm would not appear to be helpful unless this finding is specifically identified by hemodynamic monitoring. Recent reports have demonstrated the recovery of squamous epithelial cells from the pulmonary artery in a variety of conditions *not* associated with amniotic fluid embolism, including septic shock, pregnancy-induced hypertension, and severe cardiac disease (Clark et al., 1986). Therefore, this finding may not be pathognomonic for amniotic fluid embolism, and other differential diagnoses need to be considered.

PREGNANCY-INDUCED HYPERTENSION. Thus far, most of the clinical hemodynamic monitoring studies in obstetrics have taken place in patients with pregnancy-induced hypertension. From a purely clinical perspective, clear indications for this invasive technology have not been established. Arguments for its use center on reports demonstrating a broad and variable spectrum of hemodynamic findings in this group of patients. For those identified to be relatively hypovolemic, optimizing intravascular volume status should improve uteroplacental perfusion, reduce systemic vascular resistance, and blunt hypotensive complications associated with conduction anesthesia and antihypertensive therapy. Oliguria (particularly if unresponsive to fluid therapy) and pulmonary edema, both recognized complications of severe pregnancy-induced hypertension, can also be better defined and managed with invasive monitoring.

Vasospasm is a central feature of pregnancy-induced hypertension. Empirically, one would assume that an elevated systemic vascular resistance is a constant finding with this disease state. Interestingly, Phelan and Yurth (1982) examined several clinical reports in the literature in which systemic vascular resistance data were available and found a wide range of values with an apparent inverse relationship to cardiac output. These observations were unfortunately marred by several critical factors. Many of the study patients were pretreated with a variety of antihypertensive agents, magnesium sulfate, and intravenous fluids before catheter insertion. These treatments have been shown to influence the hemodynamic status of preeclamptic patients (Hankins et al., 1984; Cotton et al., 1984, 1985b). Interestingly, Visser and Wallenburg (1991) have recently presented preliminary hemodynamic data in 51 untreated preeclamptic patients that resuggest a uniform picture of an elevated systemic vascular resistance. In all likelihood, pregnancy-induced hypertension represents an overall vasoconstrictive condition that is frequently influenced by underlying disease processes such as chronic hypertension, duration and severity of illness, and various therapeutic modalities.

Unlike systemic vascular resistance, relatively uniform agreement exists regarding cardiac function in pregnancy-induced hypertension. Utilizing ventricular function curves (Fig. 51–4) that correlate PCWP (preload) with LVSWI (myocardial contractility), investi-

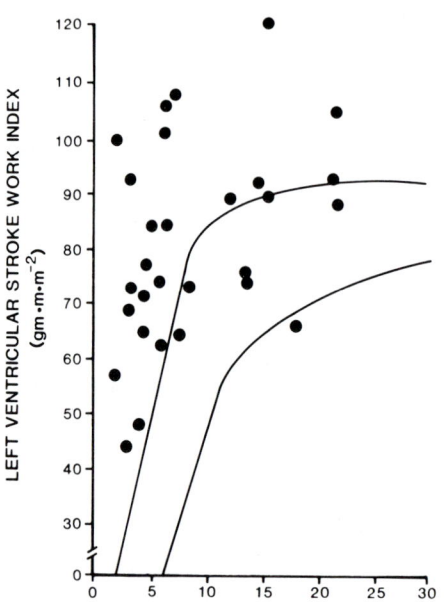

FIGURE 51–4. Ventricular function in pregnancy-induced hypertensive patients. (Combined data from Benedetti TJ, Cotton DB, Read JC, et al: Hemodynamic observations in severe pre-eclampsia with a flow-directed pulmonary artery catheter. Am J Obstet Gynecol 136:465, 1980; Hankins GDV, Wendel GP, Cunningham FG, et al: Longitudinal evaluation of hemodynamic changes in eclampsia. Am J Obstet Gynecol 15:506, 1984; Phelan JP, Yurth DA: Severe preeclampsia. I. Peripartum hemodynamic observations. Am J Obstet Gynecol 144:17, 1982; Rafferty TD, Berkowitz RL: Hemodyamics in patients with severe toxemia during labor and delivery. Am J Obstet Gynecol 138:263, 1980.)

gators have found that most preeclamptic and eclamp-tic patients fall into a relatively hyperdynamic range (Benedetti et al., 1980; Hankins et al., 1984). The values shown in Figure 51–4 are superimposed on ventricular function graphs derived from nonpregnant subjects. Therefore, the preeclamptic patient probably has at least a normal, and probably a somewhat hyperdy-namic, functioning heart for pregnancy. As suggested earlier, this cardiac function, as estimated by cardiac output, appears to be inversely related to peripheral vascular resistance.

Recently, some investigators have recommended that patients with pregnancy-induced hypertension be classified by different hemodynamic subsets so that management protocols can be tailored to individual patient needs. Clark et al. (1988) first reported the use of this approach for dealing with the oliguric pre-eclamptic patient. He noted that these patients either had low PCWP values (hypovolemic) and were se-verely vasoconstricted (elevated SVR) or were volume replete with normal to elevated vascular resistances. A third group had markedly elevated PCWP and SVR readings with depressed cardiac function. Manage-ment for these groups of oliguric patients would be varied. In the first subset, patients respond favorably to volume expansion therapy. Conversely, the next two groups of patients are best managed with vaso-dilators and aggressive afterload reduction therapy.

Another important clinical issue in the oliguric pa-tient with pregnancy-induced hypertension relates to the use of standard urinary diagnostic indices (UDI) such as urine-to-plasma ratios of osmolality, urea nitrogen, and creatinine or fractional excretion of so-dium. Although these urinary parameters are rou-tinely used in nonobstetric patients to differentiate prerenal and renal etiologies of oliguria, they have proved to be unreliable in the preeclamptic patient (Lee et al., 1987). In preeclampsia complicated by oliguria, urinary diagnostic indices have been shown to suggest a prerenal picture in spite of a true func-tional intravascular volume, which is normal by inva-sive pressure measurement determinations. From a physiologic standpoint, it is postulated that the kidney misinterprets local renal artery vasospasm to indicate a volume-depleted state.

BETA-ADRENERGIC AGONIST TOCOLYTIC THERAPY. There has been an increasing awareness of major cardiovascular side effects associated with the use of beta-adrenergic agonist tocolysis for preterm labor (Katz et al., 1981; Robertson et al., 1981). The most significant side effect, by virtue of its frequency and severity, is pulmonary edema. Very limited hemody-namic data are currently available that help clarify the etiology of this untoward complication. Presented in Table 51–4 are available data examining hemodynamic changes associated with beta-adrenergic agonist ther-apy. Of note is the fact that these findings are rela-tively uniform across different experimental animal species and in human subjects. In particular, the consistent rise seen in PCWP over time may be a crucial finding when extrapolating a cardiogenic cause for pulmonary edema. This PCWP rise occurs in spite of marked elevations in cardiac output. Therefore, the fluid retention known to occur with beta-adrenergic

TABLE 51–4.   A Comparison of Species Differences in Hemodynamic Responses to Beta-adrenergic Agonist Therapy*

	BABOON†	SHEEP‡	HUMAN§
HR	↑	↑ (50%)	↑ (18%)
MAP	↑	Slight ↓	Slight ↓
PAP	NC	↑	↑ (72%)
PCWP	↑ (282%)	↑	↑ (57%)
CO	↑ (60%)	↑ (40%)	↑ (50%)
SVR	↓ (35%)	↓ (70%)	—
PVR	NC	↓ (15%)	↓ (15%)

*Data expressed as increased (↑), decreased (↓), or no change (NC). When available, maximal percentage change (%) from control or baseline measurements given.

†From Hankins GD, Hauth JC, Kuehl TJ, et al: Ritodrine hydrochloride infusion in pregnant baboons. II. Sodium and water compartment alterations. Am J Obstet Gynecol 147:254, 1983.

‡From Kleinman G, Nuwayhid B, Rudelstorfer R, et al: Circulatory and renal effects of β-adrenergic-receptor stimulation in pregnant sheep. Am J Obstet Gynecol 149:865, 1984.

§From Wolff F, Carstens V, Behrenbeck D, et al: The effect of fenoterol and betamethasone on pulmonary circulation—results of intensive monitoring of pregnant women using cardiac catheter for prevention of pulmonary edema. In Jung H, Lamberti G (eds): Betamimetic Drugs in Obstetrics and Perinatology. New York, Thieme-Stratton, Inc., 1982.

agonist therapy may be a dominant factor leading to fluid overload in a hyperdynamic functioning cardio-vascular system (Hankins et al., 1983). Anecdotal clinical experiences with fluid restriction during intra-venous tocolytic therapy support these conclusions, in that apparent reductions in the incidence of pul-monary edema have been noted.

One cannot, however, ignore two other factors as they relate to pulmonary edema and beta-adrenergic agonist therapy. Myocardial ischemia has been re-ported in association with beta-agonist therapy. Al-though the underlying etiology is unknown, it has usually been attributed to high output demands on the heart. The possibility of a direct catecholamine-induced cardiac muscle necrosis suggested by *in vitro* work (Haft, 1974) has not been supported to date by *in vivo* data (Zebe et al., 1982).

The second factor that needs to be addressed relates to the fact that some preterm labor patients who develop pulmonary edema during betamimetic ther-apy have been shown to have normal or low PCWP readings, supporting a noncardiogenic etiology. Be-nedetti (1986) has suggested that incipient or overt infection may induce transient injury to pulmonary capillary beds leading to increased permeability and edema. This mechanism of pulmonary injury has recently been supported by studies of pyelonephritis and associated pulmonary disease in pregnancy (Cun-ningham et al., 1987).

SEPTIC SHOCK. Septic shock represents a generic term describing vascular collapse associated with an infectious process. Although septic shock has been well described in the nonobstetric literature, only anecdotal reports are available for obstetric patients. A paucity of clinical data is as yet available regarding hemodynamic parameters in this same critically ill obstetric population. Lee and colleagues (1988) have studied the hemodynamic profiles of ten obstetric patients, at various gestational ages, identified to have

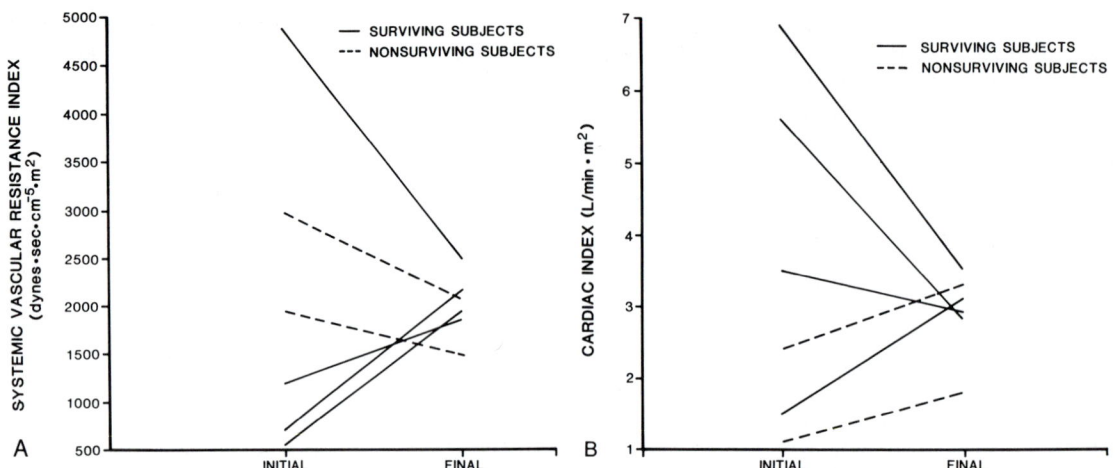

FIGURE 51–5. *A,* Serial measurements of systemic vascular resistance index for pregnant women in septic shock. Initial measurements taken at time of pulmonary artery insertion. Final measurements taken just before catheter removal (n = 4) or immediately prior to profound alterations associated with rapid decompensation and death (n = 2). *B,* Serial measurements of cardiac index for gravidas in septic shock. (From Gonik B, et al: Septic shock in obstetrics: Clinical perspective and hemodynamic observations. (Abstract) Infectious Disease Society for Obstetrics and Gynecology, 1987.)

septic shock and requiring invasive monitoring. Prolonged rupture of membranes with the subsequent development of chorioamnionitis or postpartum endometritis were risk factors that commonly preceded the diagnosis of septic shock in these patients. Figure 51–5 schematically describes the wide range of hemodynamic alteration seen in a subset of six of these patients, studied serially (Gonik et al., 1987). With successful therapy, SVR and CO are shown to be restored to more intermediate and normal ranges. Additionally, consistent improvements in cardiac function (Fig. 51–6) are demonstrated for those subjects who survived. Although preliminary, these findings suggest that, depending on duration and severity, septic shock in the pregnant woman can involve a

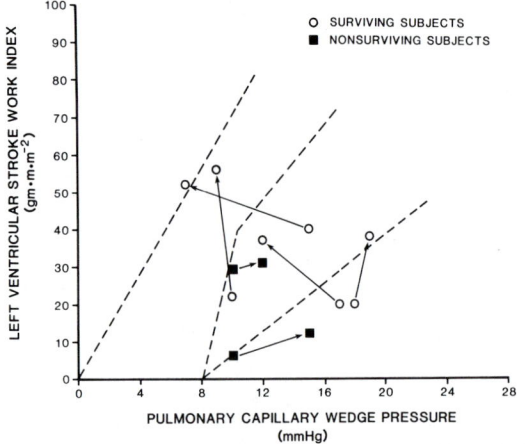

FIGURE 51–6. Effects of fluid and vasopressor therapy on ventricular function in gravidas with septic shock. (From Gonik B, Lee W, Giebel R, et al: Septic shock in obstetrics: Clinical perspectives and hemodynamic observations. (Abstract) Infectious Disease Society for Obstetrics and Gynecology, 1987.)

wide variety of hemodynamic alterations. Patients may benefit from pharmacologic interventions in which these marked initial differences in cardiovascular hemodynamics are specifically taken into account. With the use of a bedside-generated cardiac function curve, one should be able to serially monitor patient status and predict outcome.

MYOCARDIAL INFARCTION. Although considered a rare condition associated with pregnancy, with national trends reporting delayed childbearing and with the increasing use of illicit substances, myocardial infarction may become a more frequently observed pregnancy complication. Hankins et al. (1985), in reviewing the 68 cases presented in the world literature, noted that the majority of maternal deaths occurred at the time of the initial infarction. Additionally, the risk was greatest if this event occurred late in pregnancy. For those who survived the initial infarction, delivery within two weeks was associated with reinfarction during labor and an increased mortality rate. The authors speculated that the increasing cardiovascular demands late in pregnancy and during labor seriously compromised women with ischemic heart disease. From a hemodynamic standpoint, efforts should be made to (1) limit myocardial oxygen consumption by bed rest, sedation, and pain relief during labor; (2) avoid, if possible, delivery too soon after the acute infarction; and (3) recognize and treat any associated congestive heart failure. Oxytocin, in dilute concentrations, is not specifically contraindicated during labor. Nitrate therapy for angina has been used in a very limited fashion during pregnancy without apparent adverse fetal effects.

NONINVASIVE HEMODYNAMIC AND VENTILATORY MONITORING

The noninvasive evaluation of cardiovascular hemodynamics in the pregnant woman has recently been explored. Utilizing M-mode echocardiography in combination with electrocardiography and phonocardiography, Mashini and associates (1987) have demonstrated the ability to measure or calculate heart rate, stroke volume (as a function of left ventricular dimensional changes during systole and diastole), CO, PVR, and PCWP. Although some of these noninvasively extrapolated hemodynamic parameters have been closely correlated to concomitant invasive determinations in the nonpregnant subject (Abdulla et al., 1980; Askenazi et al., 1981), minimal data are available in the pregnant woman to validate this new technology. Recently, Easterling et al. (1987) reported on the use of Doppler ultrasonography to measure CO in both healthy pregnant women and those with pregnancy-induced hypertension. As a part of their study, 12 patients underwent concomitant pulmonary artery catheterization with thermodilutionally determined measurements of CO. In this pilot study, the noninvasive Doppler technique accurately estimated CO with a high degree of correlation. This same group (Easterling et al., 1990) have recently reported on a longitudinal study of preeclamptic women, demonstrating a long-standing elevation in CO, which precedes other hemodynamic alterations. Additional work is needed with these tools to provide new insights into the natural history of both physiologic and pathologic cardiovascular alterations in pregnancy.

Since its introduction into clinical medicine in the early 1980s, the pulse oximeter has gained widespread acceptance in the critical care area. As a noninvasive alternative to arterial blood gas sampling, the pulse oximeter is capable of providing rapid and continuous determinations of maternal blood oxygen saturation. The instrument consists of a sensor, a miniature computer, and a connecting cable. The sensor can be attached to any pulsatile tissue bed (e.g., fingertip). It transmits rapidly alternating beams of red and infrared light through the tissue bed to a photoelectric cell. The oxygen saturation is calculated by means of an algorithm based on the differential absorption of the two colors of light, during pulsation of arterial blood through the tissue. Previous studies have shown that the pulse oximeter accurately reflects oxygenation status in both healthy and decompensated subjects (Yelderman and New, 1983). Studies in pregnancy have shown this noninvasive device to be useful in the early detection of amniotic fluid embolization (Quance, 1988), and to describe the effects of labor and delivery (Deckardt et al., 1987) and conduction anesthesia on oxygen saturation during cesarean section (Brose and Cohen, 1989).

COLLOID OSMOTIC PRESSURE

Definitions and Determinations

Colloid osmotic pressure (COP) describes the ability of the intravascular (or interstitial) space to retain fluid by the presence of large molecules that, by virtue of their inability to traverse the semipermeable endothelial membrane, set up an "osmotic" gradient. Al-

though it is discussed separately in this section, one should recognize this as artificial in that COP is intimately associated with hydrostatic pressure (PCWP) as originally defined by Starling (1896):

$$Q = K (P_c - P_i) - k (\pi_c - \pi_i)$$

where Q = fluid flux; K = filtration coefficient; P = hydrostatic pressure in the capillary vascular bed (P_c) and the interstitium (P_i); k reflection coefficient, and π = the osmotic pressure in the plasma (π_c) and the interstitium (π_i). Thus PCWP is a clinical determinant of P_c and COP a clinical measure of π_c in the equation. Albumin and globulin are the major components in plasma that influence COP. This close relationship to plasma proteins (TP) is sometimes used to indirectly calculate COP by the equation

$$COP = 2.1 (TP) + 0.16 (TP)^2 + 0.009 (TP)^3$$

More often, COP can be directly measured by use of an oncometer. This device is in essence a two-chambered instrument divided by a semipermeable membrane. Prepared clinical specimens can be directly injected into the first chamber, establishing an osmotic gradient that draws isotonic fluid from the second chamber. This net flux is electronically calculated and digitally displayed.

Predicting Pulmonary Edema: The COP to PCWP Gradient

In the presence of a normal COP, PCWP readings around 18 mm Hg are usually associated with early evidence of pulmonary congestion. Between 20 and 25 mm Hg, congestion becomes more overt, and beyond 25 mm Hg, frank pulmonary edema occurs. On the basis of Starling's equation and clinical experience (Stein et al., 1974), we can say that pulmonary edema will occur at lower PCWP readings if COP is reduced. Rackow et al. (1977) have suggested that a COP to PCWP gradient of less than 4 mm Hg substantially increases the risk of pulmonary edema in critically ill nonpregnant patients. These same observations have been reported in the obstetric population as well (Benedetti et al., 1985; Cotton et al., 1985a). One should recognize this as a simplified approach to the understanding of pulmonary edema. Other critical factors such as alterations in pulmonary capillary permeability or changes in interstitial fluid components (via changes in lymph flow) can equally influence the development of pulmonary edema. The utility of the COP to PCWP gradient concept centers on the fact that these are the only clinically measurable forces in the Starling relationship.

COP in Obstetrics

Mean ($\pm$ SD) COP values of 25.4 $\pm$ 2.3 mm Hg have been reported for nonpregnant ambulatory adults. Prolonged supine positioning reduces this value slightly due to redistribution of compartmental fluids. Several investigators have studied COP alterations in pregnancy with consistent findings of a steady decline until approximately 36 weeks gestation (Wu et al., 1983). Mean values at term are reported to be 22.4 ± 0.5 mm Hg.

With delivery, a more substantial decrease in COP has been noted. In addition to fluid redistribution, other intrapartum factors such as acute blood loss and aggressive intravenous crystalloid administration have been suggested as causes for this decline (Gonik and Cotton, 1984; Cotton et al., 1984). Postpartum values of 15.4 ± 2.1 mm Hg have been reported (Cotton et al., 1984). Interestingly, no differences are seen between patients undergoing vaginal delivery and those delivered by cesarean section. These COP reductions are also noted to be independent of type of anesthesia utilized. Follow-up studies demonstrate that nadir values are reached by 6 hours postpartum (Fig. 51–7) (Gonik et al., 1985b). Fluid restriction, under these same circumstances, has been shown to significantly moderate these reductions in COP, suggesting that overzealous intravenous hydration is an important component to these observed puerperal COP declines (Gonik and Cotton, 1984). Although none of the aforementioned studies reported clinical findings consistent with pulmonary edema in these otherwise healthy parturients, others have shown frequent incipient evidence of pulmonary interstitial fluid leakage during the postpartum period (Hughson et al., 1982).

Under certain pathologic conditions in obstetrics, COP changes should be more carefully evaluated. Pulmonary edema is a recognized complication of pregnancy-induced hypertension and of tocolytic therapy in preterm labor patients, both conditions occasionally being associated with fluid retention in the pregnant woman. In addition, traditional peripartum management strategies for these conditions have been shown to cause marked reductions in COP (Benedetti and Carlson, 1979; Gonik et al., 1985b).

Benedetti and Carlson (1979) have reported mean COP values of 17.9 ± 0.7 mm Hg and 13.7 ± 0.5 mm

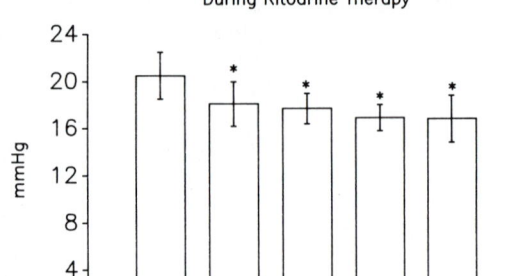

FIGURE 51–8. Colloid osmotic pressure changes during ritodrine therapy in preterm labor subjects (n = 9). (From Gonik B, Creasy RK, Chambers SL: Colloid osmotic pressure alterations with ritodrine hydrochloride therapy. (Abstract) Eighth Annual Midwestern Conference in Perinatal Research, 1985.)

Hg during the antepartum and postpartum periods, respectively, in patients with pregnancy-induced hypertension. The potential significance of these observations in COP can best be appreciated by examining PCWP alterations during this same time period. It has been reported that in patients with severe preeclampsia, from delivery and continuing into the postpartum period, PCWP measurements may rise to levels as high as 23 mm Hg (Rafferty and Berkowitz, 1980). These acute hemodynamic changes in the patient with pregnancy-induced hypertension can result in a narrowing of the previously described critical PCWP–COP gradient; therefore, they increase the potential for pulmonary edema.

Again, minimal data are currently available for COP fluctuations during tocolytic therapy. Our group has prospectively studied nine preterm labor patients undergoing parenteral ritodrine hydrochloride tocolysis, serially measuring COP changes (Gonik et al., 1985a). In this study, maintenance intravenous and oral fluids were restricted to less than 2500 ml/24 hr. Over the ensuing 24-hour study period, mean COP levels progressively fell to a low of 16.8 ± 2.0 mm Hg (Fig. 51–8). This represented an overall 18 per cent decline from baseline values. The etiology for this drop in COP is most likely related to alterations in renal sodium and water retention known to occur potentially with this class of tocolytic agents (Hankins et al., 1983).

Use of COP Determinations

The appropriate clinical use of COP determinations in obstetrics is as yet unclear. From the previous discussions, significant alterations do occur under certain clinical conditions and management protocols may benefit from this additional perspective. Controlled studies to demonstrate the clinical value and role in obstetric patients of COP measurement are

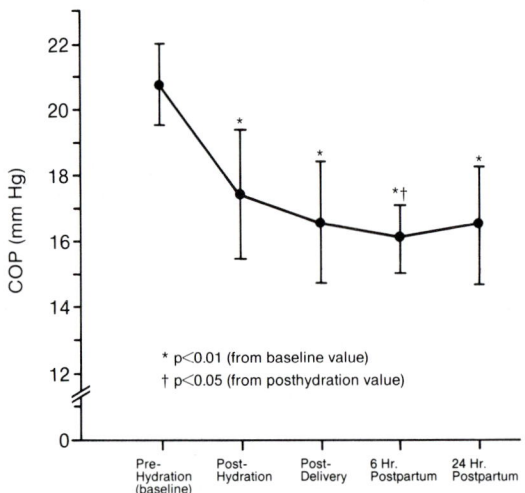

FIGURE 51–7. Serial colloid osmotic pressure (COP) determinations during the peripartum period. (From Gonik B, Cotton DB, Spillman T, et al: Peripartum colloid osmotic changes: Effects of controlled fluid management. Am J Obstet Gynecol 151:812, 1985.)

currently lacking. Empirically, the following clinical circumstances may benefit from COP monitoring:

1. In conjunction with peripartum invasive hemodynamic monitoring of the severely preeclamptic patient. Here, serial assessments of the COP to PCWP gradient may reduce risks for pulmonary edema, because PCWP can be clinically altered by pre- or afterload reduction. Whether one should administer colloid fluids in an attempt to improve COP status is controversial. Although COP can be artificially increased with the use of these colloid solutions (i.e., albumin, hetastarch), arguments against their use are based on the transient nature of these improvements and the inability to predict subsequent capillary "leakage," thus potentially prolonging interstitial fluid accumulation.

2. During intravenous beta-adrenergic agonist tocolytic therapy, in particular under circumstances when it is anticipated that baseline COP values are low (i.e., multiple gestation or after previous unknown amounts of intravenous hydration). On occasion, betamimetic tocolysis has been empirically decreased or discontinued on the basis of an extremely low (<12 mm Hg) COP alone. The other possibility might be to utilize invasive hemodynamic monitoring in those preterm labor patients with initial low COP values (<15 mm Hg) when use of aggressive tocolytic therapy is unavoidable. Under these unusual circumstances, pulmonary artery catheterization data would be available to calculate COP to PCWP relationships and to confirm an adequate, yet not overexpanded, intravascular volume status.

SHOCK IN OBSTETRICS

Pathogenesis of Shock

The term "shock" represents a morbid condition in which the patient's functional intravascular blood volume is below that of the capacity of the body's vascular bed. This pathologic state results in a lowering of blood pressure and decreased tissue perfusion. If left untreated, resulting cellular acidosis and hypoxia lead to end-organ tissue dysfunction and death.

Types of shock include hypovolemic and hemorrhagic shock, which are conditions associated with acute blood volume loss; cardiogenic shock, related to pump failure; and neurogenic shock, caused by a loss of sympathetic control of resistance vessels. When the inciting cause stems from an infectious focus, the term *septic shock* is usually applied. With septic shock, a combination of both hypovolemic and cardiogenic shock frequently coexists. Since hemorrhagic shock and septic shock make up the overwhelming majority of cases identified in the obstetric patient, the remainder of this section will deal with these two entities. However, with the increasing use of conduction anesthesia, neurogenic shock may become a more prominent iatrogenic cause in the future. Likewise, the rare development of severe myocardial ischemia reported to occur with beta-adrenergic agonist tocolytics may result in cardiogenic shock, related to myocardial dysfunction.

The central issue in shock relates to a deficiency in effective tissue perfusion. This is thought to occur as a direct result of physiologic homeostatic responses in the patient, leading to prolonged generalized vasoconstriction. In the case of experimentally induced hemorrhagic shock in the dog preparation, both amount of blood loss and time elapse until replacement begins critically influence the degree of vasoconstriction, via alpha-adrenergically mediated mechanisms (Lillehei et al., 1964). Until approximately 15 to 20 per cent of total blood volume is lost, localized nonessential areas of vasoconstriction along with HR increases can maintain effective perfusion pressure. In pregnancy, this is particularly interesting since this would suggest that the patient's normally expanded blood volume will allow for a much larger absolute blood loss before clinical evidence of shock (hypotension) appears. Beyond this amount, generalized intense vasoconstriction involving both essential and nonessential organ systems develops in response to hypotension.

As indicated earlier, rapid intervention in the experimental animal also influences the overall vasoconstrictive sympathoadrenal response. Hemorrhagic shock, and its subsequent vasoconstriction, is best reversed if retransfusion occurs within 2 hours (Lillehei et al., 1964). Beyond 4 hours, even with adequate retransfusion, irreversible sympathetic-induced cellular changes led to animal demise 80 per cent of the time.

In septic shock, a more complex series of events leads to the aforementioned vasoconstrictive responses. With gram-negative sepsis, endotoxin appears to be the critical factor mediating the initial pathophysiologic derangements of shock (Sugerman et al., 1981). Endotoxin is a complex lipopolysaccharide present in the cell wall of aerobic gram-negative bacteria, which is released when the organism is destroyed. For gram-positive sepsis, similar events are thought to be initiated by the release of a variety of exotoxins produced within the organism (Kwann and Weil, 1969). Most of our current knowledge of septic shock is based upon studies using endotoxin-induced septic shock models.

Endotoxin-induced activation of the complement cascade leads to leukocyte migration and release of a variety of vasoactive substances such as histamine, serotonin, and bradykinin (Fearon et al., 1975). These, in turn, increase capillary permeability, induce endothelial damage, and promote vasodilatation. Phagocytosis and killing of the bacteria by leukocytes potentiate two further events: an increased release of endotoxin and generalized, systemic exposure to intracellular toxins such as superoxide free radials, lysosomes, and hydrogen peroxide. These local vasodilatory events then induce intact reflex sympathetic responses to produce profound vasoconstriction, as discussed earlier.

At a cellular level, intense vasoconstriction further worsens local capillary leakage and intravascular fluid loss. In addition, resultant reductions in tissue perfusion potentiate cellular hypoxia and acidosis. Individual cells become metabolically inadequate, losing their ability to utilize available oxygen supplies. The end result of this pathologic sequence leads to a loss of cellular control of capillary vessel responsiveness, marked reductions in peripheral resistance, and extensive capillary pooling of blood. As the number of dilated capillary beds increases, an increasing disparity between effective intravascular volume and intravascular space develops. Tissue perfusion continues to deteriorate, as does venous return to the heart. This latter event again reduces CO. In addition, some have suggested that a circulating substance, myocardial depressant factor (MDF), is released from ischemic tissue which further attenuates cardiac function (Lefer et al., 1967). Endogenous opiates, endorphins, are also released and are believed to cause a profound reduction in blood pressure (Holaday and Faden, 1978). The overall end-stage clinical complex is usually termed "secondary shock" and is considered irreversible regardless of intervention strategy.

Septic Shock

INCIDENCE IN OBSTETRICS. Although both lower and upper genital tract infections are commonly identified on an obstetric service, septic shock in the obstetric patient tends to be an uncommon event. When an obstetric patient has clinical evidence of local sepsis, the incidence of bacteremia appears to be low (approximately 8 to 10 per cent) (Blanco et al., 1981; Ledger et al., 1975; Bryan et al., 1984). More striking is the fact that obstetric patients with bacteremia rarely develop overt septic shock. Ledger and associates (1975) identified only a 4 per cent rate of shock in parturients with bacteremia. This value is in agreement with other investigators, who have reported a 0 to 12 per cent incidence of septic shock in bacteremic obstetric and gynecologic subjects (Blanco et al., 1981; Ledger et al., 1975; Bryan et al., 1984; Chow and Guze, 1974). Table 51–5 lists the types of bacterial infections, by incidence, specifically identified in the obstetric patient associated with the development of septic shock. Of those listed, the use of prophylactic antimicrobial agents has dramatically reduced the incidence of postcesarean section endometritis; septic abortion has also become a less common event since the legalization of elective pregnancy termination.

MORTALITY ASSOCIATED WITH SEPTIC SHOCK. The mortality rate in medical and surgical specialty fields is extremely high in the face of septic shock, but tends to be low in obstetrics. The incidence of death from sepsis is estimated at 0 to 3 per cent in obstetric patients as compared with 10 to 81 per cent in nonobstetric patients (Blanco et al., 1981; Ledger et al., 1975; Cavanagh et al., 1982; Wernstein et al., 1983). Suggested reasons for these improved outcomes include: (1) younger age group, (2) transient nature of the bacteremia, (3) type of organisms involved, (4) primary site of infection (pelvis) more amenable to both surgical and medical intervention, and (5) lack of other underlying disease that could negatively influence the prognosis for recovery. This last factor is supported by investigators who have demonstrated increased mortality when patients had significant underlying diseases in addition to their sepsis (Freid and Vosti, 1968). Regardless of these optimistic perspectives, sepsis still constitutes a major source of obstetric maternal deaths because mortality in the gravida from all causes is so uncommon (Gibbs and Locke, 1976).

ENDOTOXIN-INDUCED SEPTIC SHOCK AND PREGNANCY. In the experimental animal model utilizing endotoxin-induced septic shock, pregnant animals have a much more pronounced metabolic acidosis in response to fixed doses of lipopolysaccharide than do nonpregnant controls, with earlier cardiovascular collapse (Beller et al., 1985). These findings are in agreement with other investigators who have demonstrated an increased susceptibility to the harmful effects of endotoxin during pregnancy in several animal species at term (Morishima et al., 1978; Bech-Jansen et al., 1972; O'Brian et al., 1985). It is interesting to note that the fetus and newborn are much more resistant to the direct deleterious effects of endotoxin in the experimental setting. Bech-Jansen and associates (1972) have demonstrated that the fetus and the immediate neonate are capable of tolerating doses ten times greater than those proving to be lethal in the adult pregnant sheep. They hypothesized that these altered effects related to the immature status of the vasoactive response in the fetus (and newborn). Conversely, Morishima et al. (1978) demonstrated profound asphyxia and rapid deterioration in the fetus when the pregnant baboon is administered endotoxin. These effects are thought to be mediated by maternal factors such as hypotension and increased myometrial activity, both of which contribute to a reduction in placental perfusion.

CLINICAL MANIFESTATIONS OF SEPTIC SHOCK. In the early phase of septic shock, bacteremia is typically heralded by a shaking chill, sudden rise in temperature, tachycardia, and warm extremities. Although the patient may appear "infected," the diagnosis of septic shock may be somewhat deceptive until blood pressure readings are ascertained. In addition, patients may initially present with nonspecific complaints such as nausea, vomiting, and at times profuse diarrhea. Abrupt alterations in behavior may also herald the onset of septic shock; this symptom has been attributed to reductions in cerebral blood flow. Tachypnea and shortness of breath may be present, with minimal physical examination findings. This may represent a direct effect of endotoxin on the respiratory center or may immediately precede the development of ARDS.

Laboratory findings are variable during the early stages of septic shock. The white blood cell count may,

TABLE 51–5. **Incidence of Different Bacterial Infections in the Obstetric Patient**

	INCIDENCE (%)
Postpartum endometritis	
Following cesarean section	15–87
Following vaginal delivery	1–4
Urinary tract infections (lower tract)	1–4
Pyelonephritis	1–2
Septic abortion	1–2
Chorioamnionitis	0.5–1
Necrotizing fasciitis (postoperative)	<1
Toxic shock syndrome	<1

TABLE 51–6. Initial Laboratory and Radiographic Studies in Patients with Suspected Septic Shock

CBC with differential and platelet count
Coagulation profile (PT, PTT, FSP, fibrinogen, thrombin time)
Arterial blood gases
Electrolytes, creatinine, BUN, glucose
Colloid osmotic pressure
Urinalysis and culture
Blood cultures, Gram stain
Cultures of suspected infectious foci (aerobic and anaerobic)
Chest x-ray
Abdominal series and pelvic x-ray if suspected source of infection
Special radiographic studies if needed to help localize infectious focus (e.g., ultrasound, CT scan)

at first, be ironically depressed; soon afterward a marked leukocytosis is usually evident. Although there is a transient increase in blood glucose levels secondary to catecholamine release and tissue underutilization, hypoglycemia may later prevail as a reduction in gluconeogenesis occurs from hepatic dysfunction. Early evidence of disseminated intravascular coagulation (DIC) may be represented by decreased platelet count, decreased fibrinogen, elevated fibrin split products, and an elevation in thrombin time. Initial arterial blood gases may show a transient respiratory alkalosis. These parameters later reflect an increasing metabolic acidosis as tissue hypoxia and lactic acid levels increase. Presented in Table 51–6 is a list of laboratory studies that may be helpful in initial diagnosis.

As the septic process continues, generalized vasoconstriction leads to more typical findings of shock, which include cold extremities, oliguria, and peripheral cyanosis. Profound metabolic acidosis, electrolyte imbalances, and generalized DIC should now be anticipated. Terminally, CO will be markedly depressed and a generalized peripheral vasodilatation picture is reflected by a low systemic vascular resistance. Multiple end-organ failures usually become evident before coma and death.

MANAGEMENT OF SEPTIC SHOCK. Initial intervention modalities in the septic shock patient should be directed at the following goals: (1) improvement in functional circulating intravascular volume, (2) establishment and maintenance of an adequate airway to facilitate management of respiratory failure, (3) initiation of diagnostic evaluations to determine septic focus, and (4) use of empiric antimicrobial therapy to eradicate most likely pathogens. If the patient is pregnant, regardless of gestational age, priorities should be focused toward maternal concerns even in the face of the suggested deleterious effects of septic shock on the fetus. Since the fetus appears to be compromised mainly from maternal cardiovascular decompensation, improvements in the maternal status should also have a positive effect on the fetus. Furthermore, attempts at delivery in this tenuous situation may lead to increased risks of fetal distress and the need for more aggressive obstetric management. In a mother who is already partially decompensated, these iatrogenic insults can precipitate adverse results. This, of course, is presuming that the fetal compartment is not the

source of sepsis, in which case appropriate therapy would mandate removal of the infected focus.

Fluid Management. The mainstay of immediate management of septic shock centers on volume expansion to correct for either an absolute or a relative hypovolemia (Rackow and Astiz, 1991; Packman and Rackow, 1983; Hawkins, 1980). Correction of this pathologic event is almost always needed in these patients and correlates closely with improvement in CO, oxygen delivery, and survival (Weil and Nishijima, 1978). At times, considerable quantities of fluid are needed to maintain effective tissue perfusion because of profound vasodilatation, increased capillary permeability, and extravasation of fluid into extravascular spaces. The best practical means of monitoring this crucial component of therapy is the use of a flow-direct pulmonary artery catheter, i.e., Swan-Ganz catheter (Swan et al., 1970).

One method of monitoring the "fluid challenge" administered to the patient has been suggested by Shubin et al. (1977), who recommended administering 5 to 20 ml/min of intravenous fluid over 10 minutes. If the PCWP increases by more than 7 mm Hg (from the starting value), the next fluid bolus should be withheld. However, if after this 10-minute test period the PCWP does not exceed 3 mm Hg, a repeat challenge should be administered. The optimal range for the PCWP is 10 to 12 mm Hg. An elevated PCWP may reflect an overexpanded intravascular space or a reduction in left ventricular function or both. Calculation of the LVSWI and construction of a ventricular function curve can help one to differentiate between these possibilities (Shoemaker et al., 1983). Pre- and afterload reduction therapy or inotropic support—separately or in combination—can then be instituted as indicated.

Inotropic Support. At times, fluid resuscitation proves inadequate in restoring optimal cardiovascular function. Under these circumstances, the use of vasopressor agents is indicated. The most widely used initial agent in this regard is dopamine hydrochloride, a drug with dose-dependent alpha- and beta-adrenergic effects (Goldberg, 1974). In lower doses (<10 μg/kg/min), the predominant effect increases myocardial contractility and CO without increasing myocardial oxygen consumption. In addition, a selective increase in mesenteric and renal blood flow occurs. As the dosage is increased, alpha effects predominate, with marked vasoconstriction leading to further reductions in peripheral tissue perfusion. Dopamine is administered as a continuous infusion starting at 2 to 5 μg/kg/min and titrated according to clinical and hemodynamic responses. Interestingly, Rolbin et al. (1979) have demonstrated that dopamine decreases uterine blood flow in the hypotensive pregnant sheep. Therefore, dopamine may actually compromise the fetal status while improving the maternal condition. This adds support to the need for external fetal monitoring in the gestationally viable fetus during initial maternal resuscitation attempts. Listed in Table 51–7 are other commonly used vasopressor agents, along with their recommended dosages and hemodynamic effects.

Adult Respiratory Distress Syndrome (ARDS). Special mention should be made of ARDS because this

TABLE 51–7. **Inotropic Drugs for Management of Shock**

AGENT	DOSE	HEMODYNAMIC EFFECT
Dopamine		
Low dose	<10 µg/kg/min	↑ CO, vasodilation of renal arteries
High dose	10–20 µg/kg/min	↑ CO, ↑ SVR
Dobutamine	2.5–15 µg/kg/min	↑ CO, ↓ SVR or ↑ SVR
Phenylephrine	40–180 µg/min	↑ SVR
Norepinephrine	2–12 µg/min	↑ CO, ↑ SVR
Isoproterenol	0.5–5 µg/min	↓ CO, ↑ SVR

complication is common in septic shock. The diagnosis is made on the basis of progressive hypoxemia, a normal PCWP, diffuse infiltrates on chest x-ray, and decreased pulmonary compliance (Sugerman et al., 1981). These findings are consistent with a pathophysiologic state in which an increase in capillary permeability leads to extensive extravasation of fluid into the pulmonary interstitium. The cornerstone of therapy involves intubation and ventilatory support to maintain adequate gas exchange at nontoxic levels of FiO_2. Positive end-expiratory pressure (PEEP) is often necessary to accomplish this goal, and serial monitoring of arterial blood gases is essential. It is necessary to remember that even in the face of overt pulmonary capillary leakage, intravenous hydration must be continued as outlined earlier to promote the desired increase in systemic perfusion. In addition, when interpreting hemodynamic values, one must take into account the fact that PEEP may artificially increase PCWP measurements. Therefore, momentary discontinuation of PEEP support may be needed to record PCWP readings accurately.

Evaluation of Sepsis and Antimicrobial Therapy. In concert with attempts at restoring normal cardiovascular function, one must initiate a careful investigation into the underlying etiology of the sepsis. Because the course of septic shock can be short and fulminant, this must be carried out without delay so that empiric antimicrobial therapy can be started. Microbiologic specimens from blood, sputum, urine, wound, and any other site of suspected infection should be collected. Even though mixed flora are usually identified in transvaginal cultures, a careful sampling of the endometrial cavity should be carried out if this is the suspected source of infection (Duff et al., 1983). In patients thought to have chorioamnionitis, transabdominal amniocentesis or cultures taken from a freeflowing internal pressure transducer catheter are useful (Gibbs, 1982).

Since empiric therapy in the obstetric patient should include coverage for a wide variety of both aerobic and anaerobic bacteria, I prefer to use a combination of aqueous penicillin (5,000,000 units/6 hours), an aminoglycoside (80 to 120 mg/8 hours), and clindamycin (600 mg/6 hours). If *Staphylococcus aureus* is a suspected pathogen, a semisynthetic penicillin should be substituted for aqueous penicillin. In patients who have received previous cephalosporin prophylaxis or therapy, empiric coverage for enterococcus may be warranted. Enterococcus is not uncommonly identified as part of the vaginal flora in the infected parturient, although its pathogenicity is still somewhat controversial. Other alternative antimicrobial treatment regimens are available, including the use of single-agent therapy with some of the newer advanced-generation antibiotics. However, the clinician must be familiar with the administration, potential pitfalls, and toxic effects of these drugs.

Few, if any, antimicrobial agents are absolutely contraindicated in the critically ill obstetric patient. Tetracycline has been demonstrated to cause growth and color abnormalities in developing bone and teeth and therefore should be avoided during the period of fetal organogenesis in pregnancy. Aminoglycosides have been associated with fetal, as well as maternal, nephrotoxicity and ototoxicity, although this is rarely used as an argument for withholding this class of agents in the critically ill pregnant patient. If aminoglycosides are used, however, careful monitoring of peak (6 to 10 mg/ml) and trough (<2 µg/ml) levels is indicated.

A new class of antimicrobial agents, the quinolones, have been shown to have excellent gram-negative coverage. However, this group of agents should not be used in pregnancy because of reported cartilage formation abnormalities seen in experimental animals.

Surgical Approach to Septic Shock. Most clinicians would agree that in a life-threatening condition such as septic shock, extirpation of infected tissues may be needed, even in the face of a compromised or debilitated host, to ensure survival. In patients with septic abortion, surgical attempts at evacuating the uterus should begin promptly after antibiotics have been initiated and after initial attempts have been made to stabilize the patient's condition. Septic shock in association with chorioamnionitis and a gestationally viable fetus is best treated by expeditious evacuation of the uterus; this can be accomplished by the vaginal route if maternal hemodynamic parameters are stable. If this is not the case, the ethical decision of performing a cesarean section is perhaps weighted toward this more aggressive surgical approach given the increased chance of survival of the fetus and the uncertain risks to the mother if the nidus for infection is not removed rapidly. Antibiotic therapy should be initiated prior to delivery. The protective effect to the fetus of intrapartum antibiotic therapy for maternal sepsis has never been carefully evaluated. However, Bray and associates (1966) demonstrated measurable levels of ampicillin in amniotic fluid and fetal blood when that drug was administered intravenously to the mother.

In the postpartum patient, hysterectomy may be needed if microabscess formation is identified within the myometrial tissues or if there is clinical evidence of deterioration in the patient's condition with appropriate antibiotic therapy. When the diagnosis of septic pelvic thrombophlebitis is entertained, treatment with heparin in combination with broad-spectrum antibiotics is appropriate. If this proves unsuccessful, again a surgical approach with ligation of the involved vessels is the treatment of choice (Collins, 1970).

Controversial Therapeutic Modalities. A variety of adjuvant therapeutic modalities have also been suggested in the treatment of septic shock. Corticosteroids can theoretically exert a beneficial effect in the septic shock patient by stabilization of cellular membranes, inhibition of inflammatory responses, and improvements in myocardial performance. However, given the difficulty in evaluating this isolated variable in the clinical arena, numerous conflicting reports exist (Sprung et al., 1984). Current recommendations limit the use of systemic steroids in septic shock patients to those who have demonstrable diminished adrenal reserve.

Investigators have used prostaglandin synthetase inhibitors with some success in blunting the prostaglandin-related pathophysiologic responses of sepsis in experimental animals (Cefalo et al., 1980; Makabalie et al., 1983; Rao et al., 1981; O'Brian et al., 1981). Antilipopolysaccharide immunoglobulin has also been used in preliminary clinical trials to reduce both morbidity and mortality in the obstetric and gynecologic septic shock patient (Lachman et al., 1984). In a much larger clinical trial involving nonobstetric subjects, adjunctive therapy with a human monoclonal antibody against endotoxin similarly reduced mortality in those with gram-negative sepsis (Ziegler et al., 1991). Studies have suggested that beta-endorphin, an opiate-like substance produced in the central nervous system, may have a deleterious effect on the outcome of septic shock (Holaday and Faden, 1978). Several anecdotal reports now exist suggesting that narcotic antagonists such as naloxone can reverse these effects. This finding is particularly interesting in regard to the obstetric patient, in whom beta-endorphin levels are known to progressively increase throughout gestation (Genazzani et al., 1981).

Additional Supportive Measures in Septic Shock. Additional measures that require the attention of the clinician include management of electrolyte imbalances, correction of metabolic acidosis, stabilization of coagulation defects, and monitoring of renal function. Patients in septic shock may have either hypokalemia (secondary to losses from the alimentary canal) or hyperkalemia (secondary to acute cation shifts). Lactic acidosis from anaerobic metabolism should be monitored by serial arterial blood gases and serum lactate levels. Normal saline infusions with 1 to 2 ampules of sodium bicarbonate can be periodically administered to help correct these alterations. Serum glucose levels may be elevated, normal, or depressed.

Laboratory coagulation abnormalities tend to reflect a generalized picture similar to that of DIC. Unless the patient has clinical evidence of bleeding or requires surgical intervention, aggressive attempts at correcting these defects (see Chapters 39 and 53) should not be undertaken because spontaneous improvement will occur when the overall clinical picture improves.

Renal function is best monitored by an indwelling catheter and with serial creatinine and blood urea nitrogen determinations. Although acute tubular necrosis most often presents with oliguria, occasionally a high output picture can be seen. Regardless, tests of tubular function will demonstrate increased fractional excretion of sodium and an impaired concentrating ability. In addition, serum creatinine determinations should be monitored when the course of acute tubular necrosis is being followed. Provided that irreversible damage has not occurred, correction of the hemodynamic and perfusion deficits should result in restoration of renal function.

Hemorrhagic Shock

INCIDENCE AND ETIOLOGY. Obstetric hemorrhage continues to be one of the leading causes of maternal mortality. Excluding pregnancies associated with abortive outcomes, postpartum hemorrhage accounts for over 50 per cent of these hemorrhagic deaths (Kaunitz et al., 1985). Although lack of adequate blood banking facilities does contribute to some of these maternal deaths, most are due to lack of anticipation of excessive bleeding or gross underestimation of blood loss. The diagnosis and management of the various causes of intrapartum and postpartum hemorrhage have been already discussed in Chapter 39. Presented in Table 51–8 are some of the more common peripartum etiologies, along with their approximate incidences. As can be appreciated from this table, most often evidence of hemorrhage is obvious. Concealed types of hemorrhage, however, such as those that occur with pelvic fracture or with abruptio placentae, can also result in unrecognized, extremely large blood losses and hemodynamic instability. Although the causes of obstetric hemorrhage (arbitrarily defined as an estimated blood loss of more than 500 ml) and their incidences have been frequently reported, there is a lack of information on the actual incidence of obstetric hemorrhagic shock.

CLINICAL STAGING OF HEMORRHAGE. Traditional signs of hypovolemic shock in the nonpregnant subject will not become evident until approximately 15 to 20 per cent of total blood volume is lost. Table 51–9 outlines the clinical manifestations of hemorrhagic shock, depending on severity. It should be noted that although shock is most often clinically identified by the finding of hypotension in a previously normotensive individual, this is too simplistic an approach. Most of the significant aberrations of shock relate to inadequate tissue oxygenation and perfusion. Therefore a broader observational base including an evalu-

TABLE 51–8. Etiologies of Obstetric Hemorrhage

	INCIDENCE PER DELIVERY
Late Pregnancy	
Abruptio placentae	1:120
Placenta previa	1:200
Toxemia-associated	1:20
Delivery and postpartum	
Cesarean section	1:6
Obstetric lacerations	1:8
Uterine atony	1:20
Retained placenta	1:160
Uterine inversion	1:2300
Placenta accreta	1:7000

Modified from American College of Obstetricians and Gynecologists: Hemorrhagic Shock. ACOG technical bulletin 82. Washington, D.C., ACOG, 1984, p. 1.

Obstetric hemorrhage is usually defined as an acute blood loss in excess of 500 ml.

Table 51–9. Clinical Staging of Hemorrhagic Shock by Volume of Blood Loss

SEVERITY OF SHOCK	FINDINGS	% BLOOD LOSS
None	None	Up to 15–20
Mild	Tachycardia (<100 beats/min)	20–25
	Mild hypotension	
	Peripheral vasoconstriction	
Moderate	Tachycardia (100–120 beats/min)	25–35
	Hypotension (80–100 mm Hg)	
	Restlessness	
	Oliguria	
Severe	Tachycardia (>120 beats/min)	>35
	Hypotension (<60 mm Hg)	
	Altered consciousness	
	Anuria	

ation of mental status, respiratory rate, peripheral perfusion, and urinary output is indicated.

MANAGEMENT OF HEMORRHAGIC SHOCK. The two basic goals in the management of hemorrhagic shock are restoration of blood volume and oxygen-carrying capacity and definitive treatment of the underlying disorder causing hemorrhage. Ideally, stabilization of the patient should take priority before definitive therapy is begun. This is frequently impractical because of the degree of obstetric hemorrhage encountered. A minimum of laboratory diagnostics is needed prior to initial resuscitation attempts. These include a sample of blood for type and cross-matching and hematocrit, and a red-topped tube to evaluate the patient's gross blood clotting capabilities. This latter bedside diagnostic evaluation is a modification of the Lee-White whole blood clotting time test, which crudely estimates clot formation and platelet retraction. Although an established protocol is not available detailing the methodology for this test, by convention a tube of blood is collected and observed for clot formation, which should occur within 6 to 8 minutes.

Volume Replacement Therapy. In the case of hemorrhagic shock, the best agent for intravascular volume replacement is blood. Unfortunately, acute management frequently must be initiated prior to the availability of type-specific or cross-matched or type O negative blood. Large-gauge intravenous access lines should be secured and rapid crystalloid (approximately 2 to 3 ml per 1 ml estimated blood loss) or colloid fluid boluses should be administered. As suggested for septic shock, a useful means of evaluating fluid replacement therapy is based on PCWP responses to intermittent fluid challenges. It should be anticipated that if crystalloids are used, two to three times the volume will be needed as would be with colloid solutions (Rackow and Weil, 1983). Colloids in the form of 5 per cent albumin or 67 per cent hetastarch have been recommended by some investigators (Rackow and Weil, 1983). Fresh-frozen plasma should not be used for volume replacement alone (NIH Consensus Conference, 1985). This relates to its excessive costs, its greater need in other more critical conditions such as for specific blood factor deficiencies, and the low but recognized risk of infectious disease transmission.

Blood Component Therapy. Various blood components available for clinical use along with suggested indications are given in Table 51–10 (see also Chapters 39 and 53). If hemorrhage is massive, fresh whole blood is preferable but usually not readily available. Packed red blood cells can be exchanged for whole blood with the recognition that additional components such as fresh frozen plasma may be needed concomitantly for dilutional coagulopathies. In this regard, there is no evidence that prophylactically administered fresh frozen plasma in the massively transfused patient is of any benefit. Therefore, transfusion protocols should not arbitrarily include this component after every four to six units of packed red cells (NIH Consensus Conference, 1985). As indicated in Table 51–10, fresh-frozen plasma should be reserved for identifiable coagulation defects or the need for specific blood factor replacement. Similarly, platelet packs should not be utilized for thrombocytopenia that is otherwise asymptomatic. The two exceptions to this statement are when the patient is scheduled for surgery with a preoperative platelet count of less than 50,000 or at any time the platelet count is less than 20,000. In the first case, hemostasis is more easily achieved intraoperatively when a more adequate number of platelets are available. Since the life span of these previously frozen platelets is limited, transfusion should be given within 6 to 12 hours of the planned surgery. In the latter case, spontaneous pulmonary hemorrhage has been reported when platelet counts are below 20,000.

Transfusion reactions can be grouped into two categories: "minor" reactions, in which case the blood being administered may be continued depending upon circumstances, and "major" reactions, which mandate immediate discontinuation of the transfusion. Within the first category are included allergic reactions and low-grade febrile responses. Allergic reactions occur in approximately 4 per cent of all recipients of whole blood or packed red blood cells. This is caused by passive transfer of donor antigens to a sensitive recipient. Symptoms may include fever, chills, urticaria, and hives. Low-grade febrile reactions (2 per cent incidence) are caused by leukocyte or platelet agglutinins present in the donor blood. The usual approach to these two minor reactions includes continuation of the transfusion, diphenhydramine 50 mg by parenteral administration, and antipyretics.

Table 51–10. Indications for Blood Component Replacement Therapy

BLOOD COMPONENT	INDICATION FOR USE
Whole blood	Active bleeding and > 25% blood volume loss or active bleeding and > 4 units RBC used
Red blood cells (RBC)	Hypovolemia and decreased oxygen-carrying capacity or > 15% blood volume loss or hematocrit < 24%
Platelets	< 20,000 or surgery and < 50,000
Fresh-frozen plasma (FFP)	Coagulation deficiencies with PTT > 60, PT > 16, or specific factor deficiency
Cryoprecipitate	Hemophilia A, von Willebrand's disease, decreased fibrinogen, or factor XIII deficiency

Severe reactions are less common, with acute hemolysis from administration of grossly incompatable blood occurring in 0.03 per cent of blood transfusions and bacteremia (usually due to cold-growing organisms) in less than 0.01 per cent of transfusions. These more serious reactions can be seen within the first few moments after the transfusion has been initiated or may be delayed for several hours to days. Symptoms can include acute decompensation with shock, DIC, fever, and renal failure. Delayed responses may be suspected only when jaundice develops distant from the transfusion period. Treatment involves discontinuation of the transfusion and supportive care. A blood sample from the recipient and the transfusion bag should be immediately sent to the laboratory for repeat cross-matching.

One is frequently asked about the risks of hepatitis and acquired immunodeficiency syndrome (AIDS) with blood transfusion. The incidence of nonicteric and icteric hepatitis after multiple transfusions ranges between 3 and 10 per cent (NIH Consensus Conference, 1985). Post-transfusion hepatitis can be caused by a variety of blood-borne viral entities including hepatitis B, hepatitis C, hepatitis D, and cytomegalovirus. Cases of "non-A/non-B hepatitis" not attributable to the above pathogens also exist. Most occurrences are self-limited, although a small percentage of cases progress to chronic or fulminant hepatitis. Specific risks for hepatitis B are estimated in Table 51–11. As indicated, the incidence of hepatitis B transmission varies according to the blood component utilized. The reason for these differences relates to the fact that some blood components are "pooled" from a large number of donor sources, increasing the risk of hepatitis contamination.

Previous surveys have suggested that approximately 1 per cent of the reported cases of AIDS are transfusion-associated (Curran et al., 1984). In 1985, 0.04 per cent of blood donations were positive for the human immunodeficiency virus (HIV) antibody by Western blot assay (Centers for Disease Control, 1987). The prevalence of blood donor–positive antibody testing for HIV varies considerably among different communities (range 0.011 to 0.11 per cent) (Schorr et al., 1985). Because of the variable pattern of viral antigenemia and the uncertain latency period before antibody production, HIV transmission in screened blood products can still occur. It is currently estimated that the risk of HIV transmission through blood transfusion is 1 in 153,000 per unit transfused (Cumming et al., 1989).

It is expected that transfusion-related transmission rates for both hepatitis and HIV will continue to decline. Factors associated with this expectation include the more judicious use of blood components, the further availability of genetically engineered products (e.g., factor VIII), and the development of better and more specific diagnostic screening tools for viral antigen (e.g., HIV p24), surrogate markers (e.g., transaminases), and new viruses (e.g., hepatitis C and D).

Additional Measures. Certain basic resuscitation maneuvers should be instituted concomitantly with blood volume replacement therapy. Blood loss not only reduces circulating volume but also significantly impairs the body's oxygen-carrying capabilities. Therefore, supplemental oxygen should always be administered by face mask. In addition, simple methods of autotransfusion such as elevating the lower extremities and use of the Trendelenburg position can increase perfusion to more vital organs until blood volume replacement is accomplished. A more sophisticated means of autotransfusion involves the use of antishock trousers (Gunning, 1983). This device, popularized in wartime applications, has two beneficial features. One is the ability to redistribute approximately 500 to 1000 ml of blood from the lower extremities to the central vasculature. The other is the ability to induce external pressure tamponade of actively bleeding pelvic and intra-abdominal structures. Actual experience with this unit is limited in obstetrics (Sandberg and Pelligra, 1983). In all likelihood, its primary use will be in those situations in which inadequate hospital facilities mandate patient transfer or when emergency medical personnel on a "scene" are unable to control hemorrhage locally. There are no data on use of antishock trousers during pregnancy because of the presumed deleterious effects on uteroplacental perfusion.

Specific guidelines should be followed in the use of antishock trousers. The device typically has three separate inflatable compartments. After each lower extremity compartment is inflated individually, the abdominal compartment should be inflated. Starting pressures should be in the 5 mm Hg range, increasing in increments of 5 mm Hg until the desired effect is achieved. The average pressure needed to control hemorrhage ranges between 20 and 25 mm Hg. The antishock trousers can be left inflated for up to 12 hours. When the chambers are decompressed, deflation should take place over at least 30 minutes, with chamber pressures decreased by 5 mm Hg increments. Complications of antishock trousers usually occur at higher pressures and include peripheral metabolic acidosis and impairment of renal function.

Definitive Therapy for Hemorrhagic Shock. The approach to definitive therapy of hemorrhagic shock must take into account individual circumstances. In the case of immediate postpartum hemorrhage, conventional methods to control bleeding such as uterine massage or direct compression are the first lines of treatment. One useful maneuver is to manually elevate the uterine fundus above the symphysis pubis for easier continual uterine massage. Confirmation that

TABLE 51–11. Incidence of Hepatitis B Transmission by Blood Component Type

COMPONENT	% RISK OF HEPATITIS
Whole blood	0.2–0.7
Packed RBC	<0.1
Serum albumin	0
Platelet packs	0.1–0.2
Fresh-frozen plasma	0.1–0.2
Cryoprecipitate	0.1–0.2
Factor VIII or IX concentrate	10–20

Modified from Baker RJ: Blood component therapy and transfusion reactions. *In* Condon RE, Nyhus LM (eds): Manual of Surgical Therapeutics. 6th ed. Boston, Little Brown, 1982.

TABLE 51–12.   **Pharmacologic Agents Useful for Controlling Uterine Atony**

AGENT	DOSE	ROUTE
Oxytocin	10–20 units	IV drip,* IM, intramyometrial (multiple sites)
Methylergonovine	0.2 mg	IM
Prostaglandin $F_{2\alpha}$	1 mg	Intramyometrial
Prostaglandin 15 methyl	0.25 mg	IM, intramyometrial (multiple sites)

*IV bolus administration of oxytocin can result in premature ventricular contractions and hypotension.

the uterine cavity is adequately clean of residual placental fragments should be undertaken without hesitation. Pharmacologic agents useful in controlling hemorrhage from an atonic uterus are listed in Table 51–12. Oleen and Mariano (1990) have reported a 95 per cent success rate in the use of these agents for the control of refractory atonic postpartum hemorrhage. Checking for a bleeding diathesis (as a cause or result of hemorrhage) should also be done.

At times a surgical approach to severe hemorrhage is needed. Careful examination of the lower genital tract following delivery can disclose significant vaginal or cervical lacerations requiring repair. For uterine hemorrhage that is unresponsive to medical management, several approaches have been advocated. Ligation of the ascending branches of the uterine arteries is perhaps the easiest of procedures to perform from a technical perspective. O'Leary (1980) reported significant success using this technique in more than 100 patients with postcesarean hemorrhage. The uterine arteries are usually identified anteriorly near the vesicouterine peritoneal reflection. A suture ligature with No. 0 chromic suture is passed through the broad ligament, around the uterine artery, and then into 2 to 3 cm of adjacent myometrium (Fig. 51–9). Another approach is to displace the uterus anteriorly out of the pelvis in order to visualize the uterine vessels coursing through the broad ligament from the posterior view. The individual vessels should not be divided. Recanalization is reported to occur, and subsequent pregnancies are apparently unaffected by this procedure

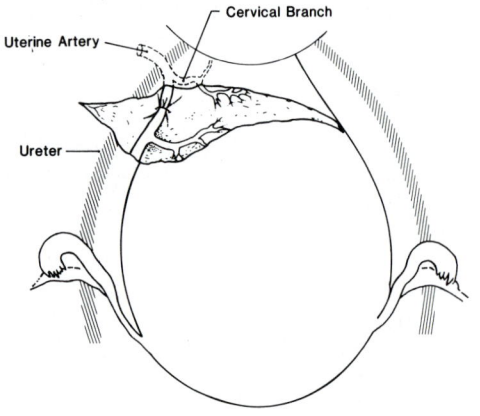

FIGURE 51–9. Uterine artery ligation technique (anterior approach) for postpartum obstetric hemorrhage.

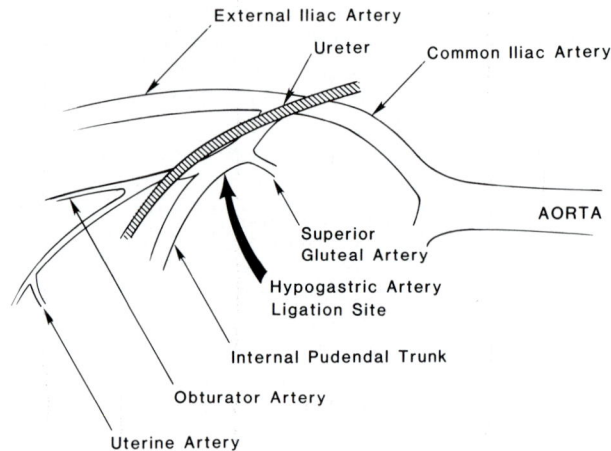

FIGURE 51–10. Localization of the hypogastric artery along the right pelvic sidewall.

(O'Leary, 1980). As an additional measure, if necessary, some investigators have suggested that an additional suture be placed beneath the ovarian ligament at its junction with the uterus (Clark et al., 1985b). This ligature should further reduce blood flow to the uterus by occluding ovarian artery anastomoses.

Hypogastric artery ligation is a procedure that is technically more difficult to perform. The success of this procedure depends on an overall decrease in pulse pressure to the uterus and is best accomplished by a bilateral approach. Access to the retroperitoneal space is obtained by division of the round ligament and gentle dissection of the loose areolar tissue along the pelvic side wall (Fig. 51–10). The ureter should always be identified beneath the medial margins of the peritoneum and retracted away. A right-angle clamp is placed below and lateral to the hypogastric artery approximately 2 to 3 cm distal to the bifurcation of the common iliac artery. Care must be taken to avoid injury to the hypogastric vein, which lies posterior and medial to the artery. Although some have suggested that ligation should take place below the posterior division of the hypogastric artery (superior gluteal artery) to prevent gluteal muscle ischemia, this area frequently cannot be easily identified. Two zero silk ties should be placed around the vessel and doubly ligated (see Fig. 51–10). The artery should not be surgically divided.

Clark et al. (1985b) have reviewed the effectiveness of hypogastric artery ligation for control of obstetric hemorrhage. This procedure was found to be effective in controlling bleeding in only 42 per cent of the cases studied. The remainder of patients required subsequent hysterectomy to control hemorrhage. Additionally, there was an increased incidence of complications, including cardiac arrest and ureteral injury, in those patients requiring hysterectomy for intractable bleeding after attempted hypogastric artery ligation. Clark and colleagues concluded that this procedure should be reserved for hemodynamically stable patients of low parity in whom future childbearing potential is of concern.

The incidence of emergency hysterectomy for ob-

TABLE 51–13. Obstetric Hemorrhage Indications for Emergency Hysterectomy

Uterine atony	43%
Placenta accreta	30%
Uterine rupture	13%
Incision extension	10%
Fibroid uterus	3%

Modified from Clark SL, Sze-Ya Y, Phelan JP: Emergency hysterectomy for obstetric hemorrhage. Obstet Gynecol **64**:376, 1984.

stetric hemorrhage ranges between 0.02 and 0.7 per cent (Clark et al., 1984). This procedure is more commonly needed following cesarean section than vaginal delivery. Uterine atony is the most common indication cited in more recent reports (Clark et al., 1984; Plauche et al., 1981). Other indications for emergency hysterectomy in a large obstetric population are listed in Table 51–13 (Clark et al., 1984). In this study, the estimated blood loss averaged 3575 ml, substantially more than the 1400 ml reported by Pritchard (1965) in elective hysterectomy cases. Much of this difference was attributed to intraoperative attempts at conservative management prior to proceeding with hysterectomy. Other complications encountered during emergency hysterectomy following delivery are summarized in Table 51–14. The choice between total and subtotal hysterectomy should be based on patient stability and availability of blood components. However, if hysterectomy is being performed for placenta accreta occurring in the lower uterine segment, adequate hemostasis may not be achieved with a subtotal procedure. Under these circumstances, the source of bleeding may be the cervical branch of the uterine artery.

Pelvic Artery Embolization. Within the field of radiology, arteriography has become a well-accepted and refined tool for both diagnostic and therapeutic purposes. Internal iliac artery embolization utilizing this new technology has already proved effective in the management of pelvic hemorrhage due to malignancy and trauma. It is therefore surprising that only a few isolated cases have been reported in the obstetric population with regard to arteriographic control of postpartum hemorrhage (Pais et al., 1980; Rosenthal and Colapinto, 1985; Chin et al., 1989). In a small series of ten patients, reported by Gilbert et al. (1992), the angiographically directed embolization procedure was 100 per cent successful in controlling hemorrhage. Gelfoam or another type of particulate material has been used for embolization, as have a variety of pharmacologic vasoconstrictive agents, with varying success. Precise catheter placement and manipulation require fluoroscopic imaging with optimal resolution. The femoral artery is usually chosen as the access route to the pelvic vessels. After diagnostic arteriography is used to demonstrate dye extravasation, the involved artery is selectively catheterized and the embolic material is injected. Placement of the material into the target vessel can be fluoroscopically monitored. The contralateral hypogastric artery should be examined arteriographically as well after the successful embolization to make certain that no other sites of hemorrhage exist. Pelvic arteriography and embolization can often be completed within 2 hours from the start of the procedure. Reported complications include excess ischemia or tissue necrosis and contrast media–associated nephrotoxicity. It should be recognized that failure of this approach does not preclude a subsequent surgical attempt at hemorrhage control. Conversely, once hypogastric artery ligation is performed, successful arteriographic embolization is much more difficult to achieve.

Other Approaches. Several recent reports have surfaced, reintroducing the use of uterine (Irani and Penkar, 1990) and vaginal (Hallak et al., 1991; Robie et al., 1990) pressure packs to control life-threatening postpartum hemorrhage. In these reports, other more conventional approaches were first exhausted prior to proceeding to this technique. In each case, the pack was removed vaginally approximately 24 to 48 hours later, with good hemostasis noted. No rebleeding was reported in these selected cases, and no pack-related morbidity was identified. Use of this technique allowed for the stabilization of the patient and reversal of any consumptive coagulopathy that was severely hampering attempts at obtaining hemostasis.

TRAUMA IN PREGNANCY

Epidemiology

Trauma continues to be a leading cause of death in women of childbearing age (ACOG Technical Bulletin, 1991a). For the pregnant woman, accidental injury has been estimated to occur in 6 to 7 per cent of all pregnancies (Peckham and King, 1963). According to one report from a large regional medical center, three to four women per 1000 giving birth sustained injuries sufficiently severe to require hospitalization (Lavin and Polsky, 1983). With regard to types of trauma, motor vehicle accidents are the leading cause of severe maternal trauma and death (Bremer and Cassata, 1986). This is followed by violent assaults and suicide. Current estimates suggest that these figures will continue to rise in the future because of the trend for women to remain actively employed during pregnancy, an increase in jobs for women which are considered more hazardous, and the trend toward a more violent society.

TABLE 51–14. Complications of Emergency Hysterectomy for Obstetric Hemorrhage

Blood transfusion	96%
Febrile morbidity	50%
Wound infection	12%
Coagulopathy	6%
Uretheral injury	4%
Cardiac arrest	4%
Septic pelvic thrombophlebitis	3%
Maternal death	1%

Modified from Clark SL, Sze-Ya Y, Phelan JP: Emergency hysterectomy for obstetric hemorrhage. Obstet Gynecol **64**:376, 1984. Reprinted with permission from the American College of Obstetricians and Gynecologists.

Influence of Physiologic Alterations in Pregnancy on Trauma

Pregnancy is accompanied by a variety of physiologic and anatomic alterations. Many of these changes can specifically influence both patterns of injuries and host responses (Pearlman et al., 1990a). Near term, the pregnant patient has been shown to have a 35 to 40 per cent increase in total blood volume. Since clinical signs of shock tend to present as a function of percentage of total blood loss, the pregnant patient will have an increased absolute amount of blood loss, as compared with her nonpregnant counterpart, for the same clinically determined degree of shock (see section on Hemorrhagic Shock). It should therefore be anticipated that a large volume of blood and fluid will be needed during urgent resuscitation attempts. Additionally, the pregnant patient at term will at times be able to temporarily maintain hemodynamic stability in the face of acute volume depletion only at the expense of the fetal status. Reflex vasoconstrictive responses can significantly decrease uteroplacental perfusion, thereby insidiously compromising the fetal compartment.

Several other hemodynamic alterations in pregnancy could potentially confuse the picture of shock. For example, although CO is increased by 40 per cent near term, supine positioning can significantly decrease blood return to the heart, leading to overt hypotension and loss of consciousness. Simple maneuvers such as lateral displacement of the uterus will dramatically improve this event. Pulse rate increases by approximately 15 per cent and maternal blood pressure falls in the mid-trimester; both these findings may signal early signs of shock in the nonpregnant subject but are physiologic in pregnancy.

From an anatomic viewpoint, the genitourinary tract is the most significantly affected organ system in pregnancy, as it pertains to trauma. The uterus, which in early pregnancy is a pelvic organ well protected by bony structures, becomes a prominent abdominal organ beyond 12 weeks gestation. This results in an overall increase in risk of injury to the uterus and fetus as pregnancy advances. A parallel increase in blood supply to the uterus adds the additional risk of significant hemorrhage in the event of injury to this organ. Similarly, the urinary bladder is more prone to injury due to its proximity to the enlarging uterus. The ureters and renal pelvis are actually somewhat protected by the uterus later in pregnancy. However, the radiologist who is unfamiliar with these principles may misinterpret normal physiologic dilatation of these structures as abnormal.

The enlarging uterus also has profound influences on the gastrointestinal tract; the bowel is pushed into the upper abdominal cavity late in pregnancy. It is not surprising, therefore, that upper abdominal trauma frequently involves injury to both the small and large bowel. For this same reason, most investigators would agree that paracentesis or peritoneal lavage is more risky in pregnancy and is of limited value. Others, however, have advocated this diagnostic procedure in pregnancy, utilizing a modified approach (Rothenberger et al., 1977; Stuart et al., 1980).

Lastly, due to decreased GI motility and gastric emptying, traumatized pregnant patients requiring general anesthesia are subject to a much higher risk of aspiration during intubation.

Several hematologic factors regarding the pregnant patient should be kept in mind. First, pregnancy represents a hypercoagulable state that may increase risks of thrombosis after injury. Since DIC is a common component of severe trauma, one should recall that the normal fibrinogen level in pregnancy ranges between 350 and 400 mg per cent. Values ranging from 80 to 180 mg per cent may be normal in the nonpregnant patient but could indicate early DIC in pregnancy. Careful screening for sepsis is also a routine part of the management of the traumatized patient. Pregnancy frequently has an associated mild leukocytosis, probably caused by demargination of peripheral leukocytes in the circulation. Therefore, the diagnosis of sepsis should not be made on the basis of a moderately elevated white blood cell count alone.

Effects of Trauma on the Fetus

As suggested earlier, during the first trimester the developing fetus is well protected from external forces by the bony pelvis, the fluid-filled amniotic sac, and soft tissues surrounding the pelvis. In a review of 240 noncatastrophic trauma cases in early pregnancy, no differences were apparent between the traumatized subjects and pregnant controls in terms of pregnancy losses (Fort and Harlin, 1970). There are some uncommon, but recognized, traumatic causes for fetal loss in the first trimester. Direct causes include severe pelvic fractures and penetrating injuries to the lower abdomen and lower genital tract. Potential indirect etiologies for early pregnancy loss include generalized sepsis, maternal shock, and iatrogenic causes such as excessive radiation exposure.

Later in pregnancy, the fetal compartment extends beyond the protective pelvis, becoming more vulnerable to injury. Penetrating trauma can result in membrane rupture or direct fetal injury. Blunt trauma can induce inertial types of fetal injury, including skull fracture and intracranial hemorrhage. Disruption of uteroplacental exchange by premature separation of the placenta has also been reported. Nonfatal injuries to the fetus may heal *in utero* and potentially lead to later recognized sequelae such as neurologic deficits. Because these are recognized remote from the traumatic event, a cause-and-effect relationship is difficult to establish. With regard to fetal death, studies have shown that this event is most often the result of maternal death. In circumstances in which there is fetal death with maternal survival, placental abruption has been implicated as the most frequent cause. With traumatic rupture of the uterus, fetal mortality approaches 100 per cent.

Blunt Abdominal Trauma

The protuberant abdomen of a pregnant patient is a common target site for injury. Most instances of mild to moderate blunt trauma to the abdomen are well tolerated by the fetus and mother; however, more severe blunt trauma has adverse consequences in pregnancy. It would appear that automobile-associated trauma is the most common cause of severe blunt injury in the pregnant patient (Bremer and Cassata, 1986). Maternal deaths occurring as a direct result of motor vehicle accidents are primarily attributed to head trauma and intra-abdominal hemorrhage. In support of this finding, Rothenberger et al. (1978) reviewed 103 cases of blunt trauma and noted that hemorrhagic shock was a consistent feature of all maternal deaths. Pathophysiologically, an acute deceleration phenomenon is thought to occur, which would lead to the shearing of intracranial and intra-abdominal blood vessels. A similar proposal has been suggested by Crosby (1986) regarding uteroplacental vasculature injuries leading to abruptio placentae.

The safety of seat belt use in pregnancy has been questioned. Crosby's experimental work on pregnant baboons in automobile accidents (1986) demonstrated profound alterations in intrauterine pressure following collisions equivalent to a decelerative force of 20 gm (35 miles per hour, head-on collision). Use of seat belt restraints significantly improved both maternal and fetal outcomes. Current recommendations are that pregnant women wear three-point restraint seat belts during automobile travel (ACOG, 1991b). Care should be taken to place the lower portion of the seat belt across the lap and not over the dome of the uterus.

Pelvic fracture is also a commonly reported injury in the bluntly traumatized pregnant woman. Several significant points should be remembered regarding this type of injury. First, pelvic fracture is often associated with extensive hidden blood losses due to the rich vasculature of the pelvic structures during pregnancy. Additionally, pelvic fracture has been associated with a 10 to 15 per cent incidence of lower urinary tract injury. Lastly, the decision to allow vaginal delivery following pelvic fracture should be based on timing and stability of the fracture. Well-healed fractures do not specifically prohibit vaginal delivery unless clear anatomic compromise, suggestive of cephalopelvic disproportion, is demonstrated by clinical and radiologic studies.

Penetrating Abdominal Trauma

Penetrating injuries to the abdomen in pregnancy are less frequently encountered than blunt trauma. As in the nonpregnant subject, patient prognosis depends on the type of instrument used to create the injury and the number of organs injured. It is of interest that the mortality in these patients is thought to be lower (0 to 9 per cent) than in nonpregnant counterparts because the uterus acts as a shield for vital abdominal structures during penetrating trauma. Buchsbaum (1968) reported only a 19 per cent incidence of injury to intra-abdominal organs, other than the uterus, following gunshot wounds to the abdomen in pregnancy. Unfortunately, the fetus fares less well, with a reported injury rate of 59 to 80 per cent and a perinatal mortality rate of 41 to 71 per cent.

Management of Trauma in Pregnancy

The acute management of trauma in pregnancy differs little from that in the nonpregnant state. As suggested previously, stabilization of the mother's condition is the most critical issue and will result in improved maternal and fetal survival. Critical care management as well as fluid and blood replacement therapy have already been discussed. Several salient features involving the care of the traumatized pregnant woman are still worthy of comment. During acute resuscitative attempts, prolonged supine positioning should be avoided. Placement of a wedge along the right side of the patient to achieve lateral displacement of the uterus should be routine. One should anticipate the need for large fluid requirements for the patient in shock, as suggested earlier. If dopamine or other vasoactive agents are used for hemodynamic stability, it should be recognized that uteroplacental vasoconstriction may lead to fetal compromise.

With regard to the fetus, an attempt at establishing an accurate gestational age should be undertaken as soon as possible. In the gestationally viable fetus, constant external monitoring is recommended. Since abruptio placentae is a common sequela of trauma to the abdomen, one should monitor for classic features of this complication. This would include marking the top of the uterine fundus and serially measuring for evidence of change. Pepperell et al. (1977) reported that only six of 16 cases of placental abruption severe enough to cause fetal death involved vaginal bleeding.

There are no clear rules related to the management of the gravid uterus if laparotomy is needed following abdominal trauma. Under no circumstances should the enlarged uterus be allowed to compromise the surgical exploration. Conversely, laparotomy is not an automatic indication for hysterotomy. If the uterus has not been significantly injured and the fetus is dead, vaginal delivery following exploratory surgery is an appropriate approach. Management of the live fetus under these same circumstances should be handled in a much more individualized fashion. If uterine injury has occurred and the fetus had reached a viable gestational age, delivery during the laporatomy procedure is probably indicated. Similarly, if it is expected that the maternal condition may continue to deteriorate, more aggressive fetal intervention would seem warranted.

Few diagnostic studies or therapeutic modalities utilized in the care of traumatized patients are absolutely contraindicated during pregnancy. Real-time ultrasonography for assessment of the fetus and Betke-Kleihauer stain analysis to evaluate for fetal-maternal hemorrhage are certainly recommended procedures. Radiographic studies should be carefully selected, in particular during the first trimester, and pelvic and abdominal shielding should be used whenever possible. As mentioned earlier, the use of paracentesis or peritoneal lavage in pregnancy remains controversial. Indications for diagnostic lavage include unexplained abdominal signs or symptoms, altered sensorium, unexplained shock, major thoracic injury, and multiple major orthopedic injuries. If these are utilized, Rothenberger et al. (1977) have recommended surgical

TABLE 51–15. Interpretation of Diagnostic Peritoneal Lavage Findings Following Blunt Trauma

Positive*
  Grossly bloody lavage fluid
  RBC count > 100,000/mm³
  WBC count > 175/dl
  Amylase > 175/dl
  Lavage fluid identified in Foley catheter
Indeterminate†
  RBC count > 50.000 but < 100,000/mm³
  WBC count > 100 but < 500/mm³
  Amylase > 75 but < 175/dl
Negative
  RBC count < 50,000/mm³
  WBC count < 100/mm³
  Amylase < 75/dl

(Modified from Rothenberger DA, Quattlesbaum FW, Zabel J, et al: Diagnostic peritoneal lavage for blunt trauma in pregnant women. Am J Obstet Gynecol 129:479, 1977.) Peritoneal lavage performed with 1 liter Ringer's lactated solution.
*Positive lavage (any one criterion) suggests need for surgical exploration.
† Recommendations are to repeat lavage.

opening of the peritoneum and insertion of a peritoneal dialysis catheter in the direction of the pelvis. Interpretations of peritoneal lavage findings are summarized in Table 51–15.

Choice of antibiotic(s) for the infected patient should be modified according to known teratogenic factors and pharmacokinetic alterations that occur in pregnancy (see Septic Shock). Tetanus toxoid prophylaxis should be used for the same indications as in the nonpregnant patient. RhoGAM administration may be needed in the case of the traumatized Rh-negative woman, based on the laboratory detection of a feto-maternal hemorrhage. Under these circumstances when RhoGAM is administered, the blood bank should be aware of this therapy so that confusion during subsequent blood typing does not occur.

Duration of fetal monitoring after blunt trauma remains controversial. Although earlier reviews empirically suggested continuous fetal monitoring for longer than 24 hours, recent studies (Goodwin and Breen, 1990; Pearlman et al., 1990b) support a shorter observation interval—*provided* that the patient does not have significant uterine activity or tenderness, vaginal bleeding, a worrisome fetal HR monitor pattern, or a positive Betke-Kleihauer stain. Although these positive clinical findings do not necessarily mandate immediate delivery, they may signify abruptio placenta.

PERIMORTEM CESAREAN SECTION

Perimortem cesarean section represents a new and somewhat empiric approach to the care of a gestationally viable fetus when immediate maternal survival is in question. *Postmortem* delivery has been previously recognized to have limited success in terms of fetal survival. Katz et al. (1986) recently reviewed these data and raised several crucial issues that need to be readdressed in modern obstetrics. In particular, they noted that the causes of maternal mortality have shifted from more chronic forms of illness to acute

situations such as anesthetic complications, embolic disease, and cerebrovascular accidents. Under these circumstances, it is anticipated that more often the mother can be saved with aggressive intervention. In addition, it is less likely that the fetus has been chronically compromised prior to the acute events that lead to the maternal cardiopulmonary arrest.

The benefit of earlier attempts at delivery of the fetus have been argued from the perspectives of *both* the mother and the fetus. Successful cardiopulmonary resuscitation (CPR) depends on maintaining an adequate cardiac output by chest compression. In the best of circumstances, CPR can generate 30 per cent of the normal cardiac output. Supine positioning in pregnancy near term further reduces blood return to the heart due to vena caval occlusion (Lee et al., 1986). Anecdotal case reports have suggested more successful outcomes with CPR with emptying of the uterus (DePace et al., 1982; Marx, 1982). From the infant's perspective, survival seems to be dependent on the timing of the operation. Few cases of surviving healthy infants have been reported for those delivered beyond 10 minutes after CPR was initiated. Clinical experience and laboratory experimentation suggest that an intact fetus can usually be delivered if total asphyxia is limited to 4 to 6 minutes (Katz et al., 1986; Windle, 1968).

On the basis of these perspectives, some authorities have suggested that appropriate management during a perimortem event include the following principles: (1) Attempts at delivery of the gestationally viable fetus should be begun within 4 minutes after maternal cardiac arrest. (2) CPR should be continued during and after the procedure in cases in which the potential for maternal survival exists. (3) Time should not be wasted preparing a sterile field. (4) Because there have been isolated reports of infant survival well beyond the 4- to 6-minute time limit, attempts at delivery usually should be undertaken at any time after maternal death if signs of fetal life are present. It is important to point out that no current data are available to document whether this approach actually improves maternal or fetal outcome. Comprehensive assessment of this approach will need to be carried out in future analyses, and at present, each case must be individualized. Three additional points need to be emphasized: (1) It should be recognized that cesarean delivery is associated with significant blood loss and this may further compromise maternal stability unless blood volume is replaced. (2) Cesarean section should not be performed in an unstable patient because of anticipated cardiac arrest. Under these tenuous circumstances, this iatrogenic insult will precipitate a poorer outcome. (3) If a patient undergoes successful CPR before an attempt is made to deliver the infant, this operative procedure should not be performed because successful *in utero* resuscitation is likely.

BURNS IN PREGNANCY
Epidemiology and Definitions

Each year approximately 75,000 people in the United States require hospitalization for significant burn in-

TABLE 51–16. Estimating Area of Burn Wound Injury

ANATOMIC AREA	PERCENTAGE OF BODY SURFACE AREA
Head	9
Upper extremity (each)	9
Lower extremity (each)	18
Anterior trunk	18
Posterior trunk	18
Neck	1

juries (Smith et al., 1983). Current estimates suggest that 4 to 7 per cent of the reproductive age women in this group are pregnant (Smith et al., 1983; Matthews, 1982a). Limited data demonstrate that pregnancy does not increase the incidence or change the etiology of burn injuries, when these women are compared with nonpregnant women. The approach to management of the burn victim depends on two basic issues: depth of the burn and size of the area involved. Partial-thickness burns are those in which sufficient numbers of epithelial cells allow for spontaneous re-epithelialization after injury. These were previously classified as first- and second-degree burns. Full-thickness burns, formerly called third-degree burns, are those in which total destruction of the skin does not allow for regeneration of the epithelial surface.

"Minor" burns are usually defined as partial-thickness injuries covering less than 10 per cent of the total body surface. "Major" burns are partial- or full-thickness injuries covering more than 10 per cent. These major burns can be further subclassified as moderate (10 to 19 per cent), severe (20 to 39 per cent), and critical (≥40 per cent). The term major can also be used in less extensive injuries if the host is significantly debilitated or when accompanying injuries are significant enough to be life-threatening. Table 51–16 demonstrates one method of rapidly determining the percentage of total body surface burned. This represents estimates for the nonpregnant patient; a similar chart has not been established for the pregnant patient.

Effect on Pregnancy

Severe burns are morbid events with significant short- and long-term consequences. Pregnancy (or gestational age) does not appear to have any direct influence on maternal prognosis following burn injury. As should be anticipated, maternal survival is most dependent on the severity of the burn itself (Table 51–17). Similarly, a favorable fetal outcome is primarily determined by maternal survival. However, one investigator has advocated prompt delivery of the second- and third-trimester fetus, in the mother's interest, if the burn exceeds 50 per cent of the BSA (Matthews, 1982a). Matthews analyzed only a limited number of cases during pregnancy, in a retrospective fashion, and compared these results with previously published data in nonpregnant patients. Although this recommendation has been propagated through the literature (Rayburn et al., 1984), as of this writing it would appear that the existing data are insufficient to firmly support this management approach.

Management of Burns in Pregnancy

As with most critical conditions in pregnancy, the management of a severe burn differs little from that in the nonpregnant patient. A detailed description of burn wound management is beyond the scope of this chapter. Basically, management in pregnancy can be divided into three components. Management in the acute phase centers on providing fluid and electrolyte therapy, establishing hemodynamic and ventilatory stability, and, when a fetus is involved who has reached a viable gestational age, evaluating fetal well-being. With regard to this latter issue, stillbirth or preterm delivery usually occurs within the first few days after injury and is most often associated with instability of the mother's condition. If fetal compromise can be minimized during this acute phase, prognosis is much improved.

Frequently, the question of tocolytic therapy is raised during this acute management period because of the common occurrence of preterm labor. Burns are uniformly associated with elevated prostaglandin levels. No ideal approach to therapy has been established. Clearly, burn patients are at high risk for beta-agonist tocolytic complications due to their high output state, extensive fluid requirements, and capillary permeability problems. Magnesium sulfate therapy may also be dangerous in this setting because of the known vasodilatory effects of this drug and the already existing electrolyte disturbances related to the burn injury. This leaves few therapeutic alternatives. In the near-term fetus, perhaps the best approach is expectant management. Gestational age cutoffs for this nonintervention approach should be based on each individual institution's perinatal mortality statistics. In the very preterm infant, there may be success in delaying delivery with indomethacin therapy for 48 to 72 hours. After this point, if the patient's condition becomes stable, tocolytic therapy can be altered to more traditional agents or discontinued completely.

During the convalescent recovery period, careful monitoring for sepsis is critical. As burn areas demarcate healthy from devitalized tissues, serial débridements are necessary, as are grafting procedures. Topical agents such as silver sulfadiazine are typically used to dress the burn wounds; these are not specifically contraindicated in pregnancy. Early ambulation is especially important in the pregnant patient to reduce risks of thromboembolic disease. Route of delivery should be based on obstetric considerations.

Only a limited amount of information is currently available concerning remote consequences of severe burn injuries. By most reports, after severe abdominal

TABLE 51–17. Crude Mortality Rates Following Maternal Burn Injuries

PERCENTAGE OF BODY SURFACE INJURED	MATERNAL MORTALITY	PERINATAL MORTALITY
< 40%	3%	22%
50%	25%	53%
> 80%	100%	100%

burns, the abdominal wall is able to expand sufficiently in subsequent pregnancies to allow for normal uterine enlargement and fetal growth (Matthews, 1982b; Rai and Jackson, 1975). Daw and Mohandas (1983), however, followed 11 pregnant patients with scarring from previous severe burns, noting frequent complaints of itching and painful abdominal tightness with advancing gestation. In 6 of 11 patients, delivery was prematurely induced because of these complaints. Others have described surgical decompression procedures during pregnancy for abdominal scarring (Haeseker and Green, 1981).

REFERENCES

Abdulla AM, Kavouras T, Rivas F, et al: Determination of mean pulmonary capillary pressure by a noninvasive technique. JAMA **243**:1539, 1980.

ACOG Technical Bulletin: Automobile passenger restraints for children and pregnant women **151**:1, 1991b.

ACOG Technical Bulletin: Trauma during pregnancy **161**:1, 1991a.

ACOG Technical Bulletin: Invasive hemodynamic monitoring in obstetrics and gynecology. **121**:1, 1988.

Askenazi J, Koenigsberg DI, Ziegler JA, et al: Echocardiographic estimates of pulmonary artery wedge pressure. N Engl J Med **305**:1566, 1981.

Atrash HK, Koonin LM, Lawson HW, Franks AL, Smith JC: Maternal mortality in the United States, 1979–1986. Obstet Gynecol **76**:1055, 1990.

Baker RJ: Blood component therapy and transfusion reaction. *In* Condon RE, Nyhus LM (eds): Manual of Surgical Therapeutics. 6th ed. Boston, Little Brown, 1985.

Bech-Jansen P, Brinkman CR, Johnson GH, et al: Circulatory shock in pregnant sheep. Am J Obstet Gynecol **112**:1084, 1972.

Beller FK, Schmidt EH, Holzfreve W, et al: Septicemia during pregnancy: A study in different species of experimental animals. Am J Obstet Gynecol **151**:967, 1985.

Benedetti TJ: Life-threatening complications of betamimetic therapy for preterm labor inhibition. Clin Perinatol **13**:843, 1986.

Benedetti TJ, Carlson RW: Studies of colloid osmotic pressure in pregnancy-induced hypertension. Am J Obstet Gynecol **135**:308, 1979.

Benedetti TJ, Cotton DB, Read JC, et al: Hemodynamic observations in severe preeclampsia with a flow-directed pulmonary artery catheter. Am J Obstet Gynecol **136**:465, 1980.

Benedetti TJ, Kates R, Williams V: Hemodynamic observations of severe preeclampsia complicated by pulmonary edema. Am J Obstet Gynecol **152**:330, 1985.

Blanco JD, Gibbs RS, Castaneda YS: Bacteremia in obstetrics: Clinical course. Obstet Gynecol **58**:621, 1981.

Boyd KD, Thomas SJ, Gold J, et al: A prospective study of complications of pulmonary artery catheterizations in 500 consecutive patients. Chest **84**:245, 1983.

Bray RE, Boe RW, Johnson WL: Transfer of ampicillin into fetus and amniotic fluid from maternal plasma in late pregnancy. Am J Obstet Gynecol **96**:938, 1966.

Bremer C, Cassata L: Trauma in pregnancy. Nurs Clin North Am **21**:705, 1986.

Brose WG, Cohen SE: Oxyhemoglobin saturation following cesarean section in patients receiving epidural morphine, PCA, or IM meperidine analgesia. Anesthesiology **70**:948, 1989.

Bryan CD, Reynolds KL, Moore EE: Bacteremia in obstetrics and gynecology. Obstet Gynecol **64**:155, 1984.

Buchsbaum HJ: Accidental injury complicating pregnancy. Am J Obstet Gynecol **102**:752, 1968.

Capeless EL, Clapp JF: Cardiovascular change in early phase of pregnancy. Am J Obstet Gynecol **161**:1449, 1989.

Cavanagh D, Knuppel RA, Shepherd JH, et al: Septic shock and the obstetrician/gynecologist. South Med J **75**:809, 1982.

Cefalo RC, Lewis PE, O'Brian WF, et al: The role of prostaglandins

in endotoxemia: Comparisons in response in the nonpregnant, maternal, and fetal models. Am J Obstet Gynecol **137**:53, 1980.

Centers for Disease Control: Maternal mortality: Pilot surveillance in seven states. MMWR **34**:709, 1985.

Centers for Disease Control: Epidemiologic notes and reports: Human immunodeficiency virus infection in transfusion recipients and their family members. March, 1987.

Chin HG, Scott DR, Resnik R, et al: Angiographic embolization of intractable puerperal hematomas. Am J Obstet Gynecol **160**:434, 1989.

Chow AW, Guze LB: Bacteroidaceae bacteremia: Clinical experience with 112 patients. Medicine **53**:93, 1974.

Clark SL, Cotton DB, Lee W, et al: Central hemodynamic assessment of normal term pregnancy. Am J Obstet Gynecol **161**:1439, 1989.

Clark SL, Cotton DB, Pivarnik JM, et al: Position change and central hemodynamic profile during normal third-trimester pregnancy and postpartum. Am J Obstet Gynecol **164**:883, 1991.

Clark SL, Greenspoon J, Aldahl D, et al.: Severe preeclampsia with persistent oliguria: Management of hemodynamic subsets. Am J Obstet Gynecol **159**:604, 1988.

Clark SL, Montz FJ, Phelan JP: Hemodynamic alterations associated with amniotic fluid embolism: A reappraisal. Am J Obstet Gynecol **15**:617, 1985a.

Clark SL, Pavova Z, Horenstein J, et al: Squamous cells in the maternal pulmonary circulation. Am J Obstet Gynecol **154**:104, 1986.

Clark SL, Phelan JP, Sze-Ya Y, et al: Hypogastric artery ligation for obstetric hemorrhage. Obstet Gynecol **66**:353, 1985b.

Clark SL, Sze-Ya Y, Phelan JP: Emergency hysterectomy for obstetric hemorrhage. Obstet Gynecol **64**:376, 1984.

Collins CG: Suppurative pelvic thrombophlebitis. Am J Obstet Gynecol **108**:681, 1970.

Cotton DB, Gonik B, Dorman K, et al: Cardiovascular alterations in severe pregnancy-induced hypertension: Relationship of central venous pressure to pulmonary capillary wedge pressure. Am J Obstet Gynecol **151**:762, 1985a.

Cotton DB, Gonik B, Dorman KF: Cardiovascular alterations in severe pregnancy-induced hypertension: Acute effects of intravenous hydralazine bolus. Surg Gynecol Obstet **16**:240, 1985b.

Cotton DB, Gonik B, Spillman T, et al: Intrapartum to postpartum changes in colloid osmotic pressure. Am J Obstet Gynecol **149**:174, 1984.

Crosby W: Trauma in the pregnant patient. Conn Med **50**:251, 1986.

Cumming PD, Wallace EL, Schorr JB, et al: Exposure of patients to human immunodeficiency virus through the transfusion of blood components that test antibody-negative. N Engl J Med **321**:941, 1989.

Cunningham FG, Lucas MJ, Hankins GDV: Pulmonary injury complicating antepartum pyelonephritis. Am J Obstet Gynecol **156**:797, 1987.

Curran JW, Lawrence DN, Jaffe H, et al: Acquired immunodeficiency syndrome (AIDS) associated with transfusions. N Engl J Med **310**:69, 1984.

Daw E, Mohandas I: Pregnancy in patients after severe abdominal burns. Br J Obstet Gynaecol **90**:69, 1983.

Deckardt R, Fembacher PM, Schneider KTM, et al: Maternal arterial oxygen saturation during labor and delivery: Pain-dependent alterations and effects in the newborn. Obstet Gynecol **70**:21, 1987.

DePace NL, Betesh SS, Kotter MN: "Postmortem" cesarean section with recovery of both mother and offspring. JAMA **248**:971, 1982.

Duff P, Gibbs RS, Blanco JD, et al: Endometrial culture techniques in puerperal patients. Obstet Gynecol **61**:217, 1983.

Easterling TR, Benedetti TJ, Schmucker BC, et al: Maternal hemodynamics in normal and preeclamptic pregnancies: A longitudinal study. Obstet Gynecol **76**:1061, 1990.

Easterling TR, Watts DH, Schmucker BC, et al: Measurement of cardiac output during pregnancy: Validation of doppler technique and clinical observations in preeclampsia. Obstet Gynecol **69**:845, 1987.

Fearon DT, Ruddy S, Schur PH, et al: Activation of the properdin pathway of complement in patients with gram-negative bacteremia. N Engl J Med **292**:937, 1975.

Fort AT, Harlin RS: Pregnancy outcome after noncatastrophic maternal trauma during pregnancy. Obstet Gynecol **35**:912, 1970.

Freid MA, Vosti KL: The importance of underlying disease in patients with gram-negative bacteremia. Arch Intern Med **121**:418, 1968.

Gabel HD: Maternal mortality in South Carolina from 1970 to 1984: An analysis. Obstet Gynecol **69**:307, 1987.

Genazzani AR, Facchinetti F, Parrini D: β-Lipotrophin and β-endorphin plasma levels during pregnancy. Clin Endocrinol **14**:409, 1981.

Gibbs CE, Locke WE: Maternal deaths in Texas, 1969 to 1973. Am J Obstet Gynecol **126**:687, 1976.

Gibbs RS: Quantitative bacteriology of amniotic fluid. J Infect Dis **145**:1, 1982.

Gilbert WM, Moore TR, Resnik R, et al: Angiographic embolization in the management of hemorrhagic complications of pregnancy. Am J Obstet Gynecol **166**:493, 1992.

Goldberg LI: Dopamine—clinical uses of an endogenous catecholamine. N Engl J Med **291**:707, 1974.

Gonik B, Creasy RK, Chambers SL: Colloid osmotic pressure alterations with ritodrine hydrochloride therapy. (Abstract) Eighth Annual Midwestern Conference on Perinatal Research, 1985a.

Gonik B, Cotton DB: Peripartum colloid osmotic pressure changes: Influence of intravenous hydration. Am J Obstet Gynecol **150**:99, 1984.

Gonik B, Cotton DB, Spillman T, et al: Peripartum colloid osmotic changes: Effects of controlled fluid management. Am J Obstet Gynecol **151**:812, 1985b.

Gonik B, Lee W, Giebel R, et al: Septic shock in obstetrics: Clinical perspectives and hemodynamic observations. (Abstract) Infectious Disease Society for Obstetrics and Gynecology, 1987.

Goodwin TM, Breen MT: Pregnancy outcome and fetomaternal hemorrhage after noncatastrophic trauma. Am J Obstet Gynecol **162**:665, 1990.

Gunning JE: For controlling intractable hemorrhage: The gravity suit. Contemp Gynecol Obstet **22**:23, 1983.

Haeseker B, Green MF: A complication in pregnancy due to severe burns in childhood. Br J Plast Surg **34**:102, 1981.

Haft JI: Cardiovascular injury induced by sympathetic catecholamines. Prog Cardiovasc Dis **17**:73, 1974.

Hallak M, Dildy GA, Hurley TJ, et al: Transvaginal pressure pack for life threatening pelvic hemorrhage secondary to placenta accreta. Obstet Gynecol **78**:938, 1991.

Hankins GD, Hauth JC, Kuehl TJ, et al: Ritodrine hydrochloride infusion in pregnant baboons. II. Sodium and water compartment alterations. Am J Obstet Gynecol **147**:254, 1983.

Hankins GD, Wendel GD Jr, Cunningham FG, et al: Longitudinal evaluation of hemodynamic changes in eclampsia. Am J Obstet Gynecol **150**:506, 1984.

Hankins GD, Wendel GD Jr, Leveno KJ, et al: Myocardial infarction during pregnancy: A review. Obstet Gynecol **65**:139, 1985.

Hawkins DF: Management and treatment of obstetric bacteremia shock. J Clin Pathol **33**:895, 1980.

Holaday JW, Faden AI: Naloxone reversal of endotoxin hypotension suggests role of endorphins in shock. Nature **275**:450, 1978.

Hughson WG, Friedman PJ, Feigin DS, et al: Postpartum pleural effusion: A common radiologic finding. Ann Intern Med **97**:856, 1982.

Irani SA, Penkar SJ: Packing of uterus at cesarean section for refactory postpartum haemorrhage: Revival of a time tested technique. J Obstet Gynecol India **40**:72, 1990.

Katz M, Robertson PA, Creasy RK: Cardiovascular complications associated with terbutaline treatment for preterm labor. Am J Obstet Gynecol **139**:605, 1981.

Katz VL, Dotters DJ, Droegemueller W: Perimortem cesarean delivery. Obstet Gynecol **68**:571, 1986.

Kaunitz AM, Hughes JM, Grimes DA: Causes of maternal mortality in the United States. Obstet Gynecol **65**:605, 1985.

Kleinman G, Nuwayhid B, Rudelstorfer R, et al: Circulatory and renal effects of β-adrenergic-receptor stimulation in pregnant sheep. Am J Obstet Gynecol **149**:865, 1984.

Kwann HM, Weil MH: Differences in the mechanism of shock caused by bacterial infections. Surg Gynecol Obstet **1**:37, 1969.

Lachman E, Pitsoe SB, Gaffin SL: Anti-lipopolysaccharide immunotherapy in management of septic shock of obstetric and gynaecologic origin. Lancet **1**:981, 1984.

Lavin JP, Polsky SS: Abdominal trauma during pregnancy. Clin Perinatol **10**:423, 1983.

Ledger WJ, Norman M, Gee C, et al: Bacteremia on an obstetric-gynecologic service. Am J Obstet Gynecol **121**:205, 1975.

Lee RV, Rodgers BD, White LM, et al: Cardiopulmonary resuscitation of pregnant women. Am J Med **81**:311, 1986.

Lee W, Clark SL, Cotton DB, et al: Septic shock during pregnancy. Am J Obstet Gynecol **159**:410, 1988.

Lee W, Gonik B, Cotton DB: Urinary diagnostic indices in pre-eclampsia-associated oliguria: Correlation with invasive hemodynamic monitoring. Am J Obstet Gynecol **156**:100, 1987.

Lefer AM, Cowgill R, Marshall FF, et al: Characterization of a myocardial depressant factor present in hemorrhagic shock. Am J Physiol **213**:492, 1967.

Lillehei RC, Longerbeam JK, Bloch JH, et al: The nature of irreversible shock: Experimental and clinical observations. Ann Surg **160**:682, 1964.

Mabie WC, Sibai BM: Treatment in an obstetric intensive care unit. Am J Obstet Gynecol **162**:1, 1990.

Makabali GL, Mandal AK, Morris JA: An assessment of the participatory role of prostaglandins and serotonin in the pathophysiology of endotoxic shock. Am J Obstet Gynecol **145**:439, 1983.

Marx GF: Cardiopulmonary resuscitation of late-pregnant women. (Letter) Anesthesiology **56**:156, 1982.

Mashini IS, Albazzaz SJ, Fadel HE, et al: Serial noninvasive evaluation of cardiovascular hemodynamics during pregnancy. Am J Obstet Gynecol **156**:1208, 1987.

Matthews RN: Obstetric implications of burns in pregnancy. Br J Obstet Gynecol **89**:603, 1982a.

Matthews RN: Old burns and pregnancy. Br J Obstet Gynaecol **89**:610, 1982b.

Morishima HO, Niemann WH, James LS: Effects of endotoxin on the pregnant baboon and fetus. Am J Obstet Gynecol **131**:899, 1978.

NIH Consensus Conference: Fresh frozen plasma. JAMA **253**:551, 1985.

O'Brian WF, Cefalo RC, Lewis PE, et al: The role of prostaglandins in endotoxemia and comparisons in response in the nonpregnant, maternal, and fetal models. Am J Obstet Gynecol **139**:535, 1981.

O'Brian WF, Golden SM, Davis SE, et al: Endotoxemia in the neonatal lamb. Am J Obstet Gynecol **151**:671, 1985.

O'Leary JA: Pregnancy following uterine artery ligation. Obstet Gynecol **55**:112, 1980.

Oleen MA, Mariano JP: Controlling refractory atonic postpartum hemorrhage with Hamabate sterile solution. Am J Obstet Gynecol **162**:205, 1990.

Packman MI, Rackow EC: Optimum left heart filling pressure during fluid resuscitation of patients with hypovolemic and septic shock. Crit Care Med **11**:165, 1983.

Pais SO, Glickman M, Schwartz P, et al: Embolization of pelvic arteries for control of postpartum hemorrhage. Obstet Gynecol **55**:754, 1980.

Pearlman MD, Tintinalli JE, Lorenz RP: Blunt trauma in pregnancy. N Engl J Med **323**:1609, 1990a.

Pearlman MD, Tintinalli JE, Lorenz RP: A prospective controlled study of outcome after trauma during pregnancy. Am J Obstet Gynecol **162**:1502, 1990b.

Peckham CH, King RW: A study of intercurrent conditions observed during pregnancy. Am J Obstet Gynecol **87**:609, 1963.

Pepperell RJ, Rubinstein E, MacIssac IA: Motor-car accidents during pregnancy. Med J Aust **1**:203, 1977.

Phelan JP, Yurth DA: Severe preeclampsia. I. Peripartum hemodynamic observations. Am J Obstet Gynecol **144**:17, 1982.

Plauche WC, Gruich FG, Bourgeois MO: Hysterectomy at the time of cesarean section: Analysis of 108 cases. Obstet Gynecol **58**:459, 1981.

Pritchard J: Changes in blood volume during pregnancy and delivery. Anesthesiology **26**:393, 1965.

Quance D: Amniotic fluid embolism: Detection by pulse oximetry. Anesthesiology **68**:951, 1988.

Rackow EC, Astiz ME: Pathophysiology and treatment of septic shock. JAMA **266**:548, 1991.

Rackow EC, Fein IA, Leppo J: Colloid osmotic pressure as a prognostic indicator of pulmonary edema and mortality in the critically ill. Chest **72**:709, 1977.

Rackow EC, Weil MH: Recent trends in diagnosis and management of septic shock. Curr Surg **40**:181, 1983.

Rafferty TD, Berkowitz RL: Hemodynamics in patients with severe toxemia during labor and delivery. Am J Obstet Gynecol **138**:263, 1980.

Rai YS, Jackson DM: Childbearing in relation to the scarred abdominal wall from burns. Burns **1**:167, 1975.

Rao PS, Cavanagh D, Gaston LW: Endotoxic shock in the primate: Effects of aspirin and dipyridamole administration. Am J Obstet Gynecol **140**:914, 1981.

Rayburn W, Smith B, Feller I, et al: Major burns during pregnancy: Effects on fetal well-being. Obstet Gynecol **63**:392, 1984.

Robertson PA, Herron M, Katz M, et al: Maternal morbidity associated with isoxsuprine and terbutaline tocolysis. Eur J Obstet Gynecol Reprod Biol **11**:317, 1981.

Robie GF, Morgan MA, Payne GC, et al: Logothetopulos pac for the management of uncontrollable postpartum hemorrhage. Am J Perinatol **7**:327, 1990.

Robin ED: The cult of the Swan-Ganz catheter. Ann Intern Med **103**:445, 1985.

Rolbin SH, Levinson G, Shnider DM, et al: Dopamine treatment of spinal hypotension decreases uterine blood flow in the pregnant ewe. Anesthesiology **51**:36, 1979.

Rosenthal DM, Colapinto R: Angiographic arterial embolization in the management of postoperative vaginal hemorrhage. Am J Obstet Gynecol **151**:227, 1985.

Rothenberger D, Quattlebaum FW, Perry JF, et al: Blunt maternal trauma: A review of 103 cases. J Trauma **18**:173, 1978.

Rothenberger DA, Quattlebaum FW, Zabel J, et al: Diagnostic peritoneal lavage for blunt trauma in pregnant women. Am J Obstet Gynecol **129**:479, 1977.

Sandberg EC, Pelligra R: The medical antigravity suit for management of surgically uncontrollable bleeding associated with abdominal pregnancy. Am J Obstet Gynecol **146**:519, 1983.

Schorr JB, Berkowitz A, Cumming PD, et al: Prevalence of HTLV-III antibody in American blood donors. N Engl J Med **313**:384, 1985.

Shanklin DR, Sommers SC, Brown DAJ, et al: The pathology of maternal mortality. Am J Obstet Gynecol **165**:1127, 1991.

Shoemaker WC, Appel PL, Bland R, et al: Clinical trial of an algorithm for outcome prediction in acute circulatory failure. Crit Care Med **11**:165, 1983.

Shubin H, Weil MH, Carlson RW: Bacterial shock. Am Heart J **94**:112, 1977.

Smith BK, Rayburn WF, Feller I: Burns and pregnancy. Clin Perinatol **10**:383, 1983.

Sprung CL, Caralis PV, Marcial EH, et al: The effects of high-dose corticosteroids in patients with septic shock. N Engl J Med **311**:1137, 1984.

Sprung CL, Pozen RG, Rozanski JJ, et al: Advanced ventricular arrhythmias during bedside pulmonary artery catheterization. Am J Med **72**:203, 1982.

Starling EH: On the absorption of fluids from the connective tissue spaces. J Physiol **19**:312, 1896.

Stein L, Bernard J, Cavanilles J, et al: Pulmonary edema during fluid infusion in the absence of heart failure. JAMA **229**:65, 1974.

Stuart GC, Harding PG, Davies EM: Blunt abdominal trauma in pregnancy. Can Med Assoc J **122**:901, 1980.

Sugerman HJ, Peyton JWR, Greenfield LJ: Gram-negative sepsis. *In* Thal A (ed): Current Problems in Surgery. Chicago, Year Book Medical Publishers, Inc., 1981.

Swan HJ, Ganz W, Forrester J, et al: Catheterization of the heart in man with use of a flow-directed balloon-tipped catheter. N Engl J Med **283**:447, 1970.

Visser W, Wallenburg HCS: Central hemodynamic observations in untreated preeclamptic patients. Hypertension **17**:1072, 1991.

Weil MH, Nishijima H: Cardiac output in bacterial shock. Am J Med **64**:920, 1978.

Wernstein MP, Murphy JR, Retter LB, et al: The clinical significance of positive blood cultures: A comparative analysis of 500 episodes of bacteremia and fungemia in adults. Rev Infect Dis **5**:54, 1983.

Windle WF: Brain damage at birth. JAMA **206**:1967, 1968.

Wolff F, Carstens V, Behrenbeck D, et al: The effect of fenoterol and betamethasone on pulmonary circulation—results of intensive monitoring of pregnant women using cardiac catheter for prevention of pulmonary edema. *In* Jung H, Lamberti G (eds): Betamimetic Drugs in Obstetrics and Perinatology. New York, Thieme-Stratton, Inc., 1982.

Wu PYK, Udani V, Chan L, et al: Colloid osmotic pressure: Variations in normal pregnancy. J Perinatol **11**:193, 1983.

Yelderman M, New W: Evaluation of pulse oximetry. Anesthesiology **59**:349, 1983.

Zebe H, Roth V, Lorenz U, et al: Investigations into the effect on myocardial function of chronic intravenous tocolysis using noninvasive test methods. *In* Jung H, Lamberti G (eds): Betamimetic Drugs in Obstetrics and Perinatology. New York, Thieme-Stratton, Inc., 1982.

Ziegler EJ, Fisher CJ, Sprung CL, et al: Treatment of gram-negative bacteremia and septic shock with HA-1A human monoclonal antibody against endotoxin. N Engl J Med **324**:429, 1991.

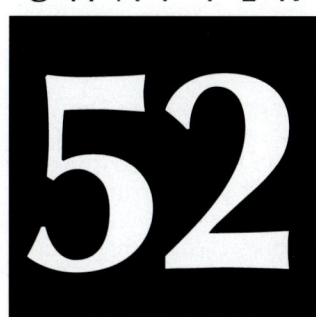

C H A P T E R

52

PULMONARY DISORDERS

....

MICHAEL DE SWIET, M.D.

This chapter considers first the biological adaptation of the maternal respiratory system to the presence and needs of pregnancy and then the interrelationships of various specific respiratory disorders and pregnancy. The changes in pulmonary physiology occurring in pregnancy are well documented, but pulmonary diseases in pregnancy are not as well understood, perhaps because although there is a considerable increase in ventilation in pregnancy, respiratory failure is rare (Gaensler et al., 1953). The most common problem in the management of respiratory disease in pregnancy is currently the effect of medications on the developing fetus.

PHYSIOLOGIC ADAPTATION TO PREGNANCY

Consumption and Partial Pressure of Oxygen, P-50

During pregnancy, oxygen (O_2) consumption rises by 32 to 58 ml/min (Alaily and Carrol, 1978; Gazioglu et al., 1970; Ueland et al., 1973), and the maximum oxygen consumption "at rest" varies between 249 and 331 ml/min (Knuttgen and Emerson, 1974; Emerson et al., 1972; Pernoll et al., 1975). Assuming that the basal metabolic rate of the fetus is the same as that of its mother (O_2 consumption 3.65 ml/kg/min), its oxygen consumption at term would be about 12 ml/min. The placenta can consume approximately 4 ml/min; the increased work associated with higher cardiac output and ventilation accounts for approximately 7 and 2 ml/min, respectively, and the kidneys need about 7 ml/min more to deal with extratubular reabsorption of sodium. A further 5 ml/min can be accounted for by the extra tissue of breasts and uterus (de Swiet, 1991). Thus, we can identify a total of 37 ml/min of the extra oxygen consumption associated with pregnancy, which corresponds nicely with the observed increase of 32 to 58 ml/min. Any remaining extra oxygen consumption could be explained by the extra work of absorption from the gastrointestinal tract and by the growth of maternal tissues and the fetus.

This increase in oxygen consumption is achieved with little change in the partial pressure of oxygen in arterial vessels (PaO_2). It has been reported that there is a small increase in PaO_2, from 85 mm Hg at 10 weeks gestation to 92 mm Hg at term (Lucius et al., 1970); however, a PaO_2 of 85 mm Hg is abnormally low, even by nonpregnant standards, and others have reported PaO_2 values from about 107 mm Hg in early pregnancy to about 103 mm Hg at term (Anderson et al., 1969; Templeton and Kelman, 1976; Eng et al., 1975). It is likely that changes in posture account for some of these discrepancies, owing to a combination of alterations in maternal hemodynamics (see Chapter 46) and changes in functional residual capacity and closing volumes (to be discussed).

Because of the shape of the hemoglobin dissociation curve, small changes in PaO_2 have little effect on oxygen content at normal atmospheric pressures. However, at high altitudes (4200 m), where the PaO_2 in men is 48 mm Hg, women at term have a PaO_2 of 61 mm Hg (Sobrevilla et al., 1971); this figure represents a very real increase in oxygen content of 5 to 10 per cent (Comroe, 1974). Similar differences have been found at altitude between pregnant and nonpregnant women (Hellegers et al., 1959). In addition, P–50, a measure of affinity of hemoglobin for oxygen, is progressively increased from 26 mm Hg in the nonpregnant state to 30 mm Hg at term (Kambam et al., 1983). This represents a decrease in affinity induced by pregnancy and would allow easier unloading of oxygen from maternal blood to fetal blood in the placenta. Mild acute hypoxia of travel in modern pressurized aircraft (maternal $PaO_2 \approx 65$ mm Hg) has no effect on fetal heart rate, and therefore presumably on fetal well being (Huch et al., 1986).

The increase in oxygen consumption is associated with a corresponding increase in carbon dioxide output. Since the respiratory quotient increases from 0.76 before pregnancy to 0.83 in late pregnancy, the increase in CO_2 production is proportionately greater than the increase in oxygen uptake (Knuttgen and Emerson, 1974; Emerson et al., 1972). This effect is likely to be due to an increase in the proportion of carbohydrates to fat metabolized during pregnancy.

Lung Volumes

Oxygen consumption rises during pregnancy, the PaO_2 does not alter, and the arteriovenous oxygen difference decreases (Bader et al., 1955), and so there must be an increase in ventilation (granted that pulmonary gas transfer is a limiting factor). The increase in resting ventilation of 40 per cent is impressive, exceeding that in oxygen consumption (about 20 per cent), so that women "hyperventilate" in pregnancy. Ventilation is increased by the rise in tidal volume from about 500 ml to 700 ml in each breath (Fig. 52–1) (Cugell et al., 1953; Lehmann and Fabel, 1973a; Prowse and Gaensler, 1965). There is no change in respiratory rate (Knuttgen and Emerson, 1974; Lehmann and Fabel, 1973a; Pernoll et al., 1975), so that minute ventilation rises from about 7.5 to 10.5 liters/min. In studies in which changes in ventilation are measured serially from early pregnancy, ventilation is seen to increase in the first trimester and to remain at that level, not to increase further, as pregnancy progresses (Milne et al., 1977c). Although the physiologic dead space is increased by about 60 ml in pregnancy (Pernoll et al., 1975), perhaps owing to dilation of the small airways, an increase in tidal volume is clearly a more efficient way of increasing alveolar ventilation than a proportionately equal increase in respiratory rate.

Alveolar ventilation is further increased by the reduction during pregnancy of the residual volume by about 20 per cent (Cugell et al., 1953), from about 1200 ml to 1000 ml (Lehmann and Fabel, 1973b; Gazioglu et al., 1970; Milne, 1979) (see Fig. 52–2). A reduction in alveolar volume reduces the amount by which the tidal volume is diluted at each breath and thus increases the effective alveolar ventilation.

The increase in alveolar ventilation and the decrease in residual volume lead to a reduction in the "pulmonary mixing index," the percentage of nitrogen remaining in the lungs after 7 minutes of breathing pure oxygen (Cugell et al., 1953). An increase in venous admixture may be the reason that arterial

oxygen saturation has been reported to decrease from 95 per cent at the end of pregnancy to 89 per cent at the end of the second stage of labor (Esteban-Altirriba, 1960). However, labor is really not a steady state, and so it is difficult to obtain reliable arterial blood samples during its progress. The vital capacity, the maximum volume of gas that can be expired after a maximum inspiration, probably does not change in pregnancy (Cugell et al., 1953; Heidenreich et al., 1971; Lehmann and Fabel, 1973b; Sims et al., 1976; Alaily and Carrol, 1978; Milne, 1979).

Partial Pressure of Carbon Dioxide

The increase in ventilation of 40 per cent, compared with the increase in oxygen consumption of 20 per cent, causes a considerable increase in ventilatory equivalent (the minute volume divided by oxygen consumption), which rises from 3.2 to 4.0 liters/min/100 ml oxygen consumed. Therefore, the partial pressure of arterial carbon dioxide ($PaCO_2$) falls in pregnancy, from nonpregnant levels of between 35 and 40 mm Hg to about 30 mm Hg (Eng et al., 1975; Lucius et al., 1970; Kelman and Templeton, 1975). The $PaCO_2$ falls early in pregnancy in parallel with the change in ventilation, although there may be a further progressive fall in $PaCO_2$ (Lucius et al., 1970; Boutourline-Young and Boutourline-Young, 1956). The fall in $PaCO_2$ is even greater at altitudes where the mother is hyperventilating further in an attempt to maintain the PaO_2 as high as possible (Hellegers et al., 1959; Sobrevilla et al., 1971).

The fall in $PaCO_2$ is matched by an equivalent fall in plasma bicarbonate concentration, and all the evidence suggests that arterial pH is not altered from the normal nonpregnant level of about 7.4.

The Stimulus to Hyperventilation

The increase in ventilation and associated fall in $PaCO_2$ that occur in pregnancy are due to progesterone. This effect was first shown by Döring and Loeschcke (1947), who found that estrogen also stimulates respiration and that progesterone and estrogen are synergistic in action. Not all "progestational" compounds stimulate respiration; for example, anhydrohydroxyprogesterone, 1,2-dihydroprogesterone, and 19-norethinyltestosterone are ineffective (Tyler, 1960). Wilbrand and colleagues (1959) showed that progesterone lowers the CO_2 threshold of the respiratory center. In addition, during pregnancy, the sensitivity of the respiratory center increases (Lyons and Antonio, 1959) so that an increase in $PaCO_2$ of 1 mm Hg increases ventilation by 6 liters/min in pregnancy, compared with 1.5 liters/min in the nonpregnant state (Prowse and Gaensler, 1965; Pernoll et al., 1975, Eng et al., 1975). It is also possible that progesterone acts as a primary stimulant to the respiratory center independently of any change in CO_2 sensitivity or threshold (Skatrud et al., 1978).

Progesterone not only stimulates ventilation but also probably increases levels of carbonic anhydrase B in

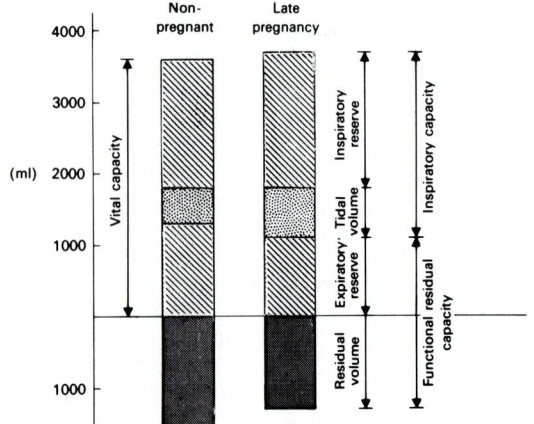

FIGURE 52–1. Subdivisions of lung volume and their alterations in pregnancy. (From de Swiet M: The respiratory system. *In* Hytten F, Chamberlain G (eds): Clinical Physiology in Obstetrics. Oxford, Blackwell Scientific, 1991.)

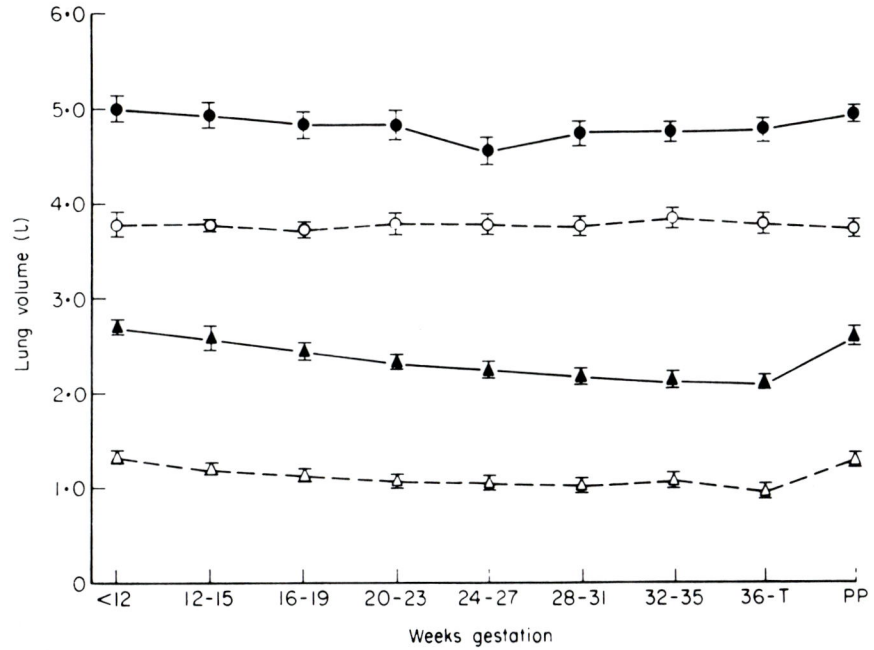

FIGURE 52–2. Serial values of static lung volume during normal pregnancy and postpartum (PP). (Values are mean ± SEM.) *Solid circles* = total lung capacity; *open circles* = vital capacity; *solid triangles* = functional residual capacity; *open triangles* = residual volume. (From Milne J: The respiratory response to pregnancy. Postgrad Med J **55**:318, 1979.)

the red cell (Paciorek and Spencer, 1980). Schenker and associates (1972) showed that carbonic anhydrase levels increase in pregnant patients and in patients taking oral contraceptives. A close relationship has been shown to exist between the levels of carbonic anhydrase and plasma progesterone in pregnancy, in the menstrual cycle, and during oral contraception (Milne et al., 1977a). An increase in carbonic anhydrase level facilitates carbon dioxide transfer and also tends to decrease $PaCO_2$ independently of any change in ventilation.

The respiratory-stimulant effect of progesterone has been used in the treatment of respiratory failure and emphysema (Cullen et al., 1959; Lyons and Huang, 1968; Sutton et al., 1975).

A similar but smaller increase in ventilation is observed during the luteal phase of the menstrual cycle (England and Farhi, 1976; Milne et al., 1977b) and in patients taking some oral contraceptives (Milne, 1979).

Anatomic Changes

The findings of no change in vital capacity and a reduction in residual volume are in keeping with the observed changes in the configuration of the chest during pregnancy. Radiologic studies made early in pregnancy have shown that the subcostal angle increases from 68 to 103 degrees before there is any mechanical pressure from the enlarging uterus (Thomson and Cohen, 1938). The level of the diaphragm rises by about 4 cm and the transverse diameter of the chest increases by 2 cm (Klaften and Palugyay, 1926, 1927; Möbius, 1961). These changes account for the

decrease in residual volume because the lungs would be relatively compressed during forced expiration. However, the excursion of the diaphragm in respiration is about 1.5 cm farther in pregnancy than in the nonpregnant state (Möbius, 1961; McGinty, 1938).

The effect of pregnancy on pulmonary mechanics has been compared to the effect of a pneumoperitoneum; in both situations the residual lung volume is decreased but ventilation remains unimpaired.

Airways Resistance

Large Airways

The work done in breathing may be partitioned into work done in overcoming airways resistance where the resistance of large airways (greater than 2 mm in diameter) is more important than small airways function (Macklem and Mead, 1967) and work done in expanding the lungs and chest wall (lung compliance). The simplest clinical measures of this work are those of forced expiratory volume in one second (FEV_1) and peak expiratory flow rate. These are indirect measurements that depend on both airways resistance and lung compliance (FEV_1 and peak flow do not change in pregnancy) (Rubin et al., 1956; Cugell et al., 1953; Sims et al., 1976; Gazioglu et al., 1970; Knuttgen and Emerson, 1974; Milne, 1979). By means of whole-body plethysmography, it is possible to measure airways conductance independently of lung compliance. Airways conductance does not change in pregnancy (Milne et al., 1977c), nor, as might be expected, does lung compliance (Gee et al., 1967).

The lack of change in airways resistance during

pregnancy is likely to be the sum of several factors acting in opposite directions. Prostaglandin $F_{2\alpha}$ is a bronchoconstrictor, whereas prostaglandins E_1 and E_2 are bronchodilators (Hyman et al., 1978); the levels of both series of prostaglandins increase in pregnancy, although prostaglandin E levels do so only at the end of pregnancy (Whalen et al., 1978). Progesterone causes bronchodilation, possibly by increasing beta-adrenergic activity (Raz et al., 1973). In opposition are the bronchoconstrictor effects of a reduced residual volume (Briscoe and Dubois, 1958) and a reduction in $PaCO_2$ (Newhouse et al., 1964).

Small Airways

Bevan and colleagues (1974) found an increased closing volume in pregnancy, with closure beginning during normal tidal volume in half their subjects. This would suggest that the caliber of small airways less than 2 mm in diameter decreases in pregnancy to the point where some airways close during quiet respiration. This finding was confirmed by Garrard and associates (1978); however, these authors note that the subjects had difficulty in complying with the measurement of vital capacity, and many of Bevan's subjects had hypertension. Those with hypertension had the greatest increase in closing volume (Farebrother and McHardy, 1974). Since pregnancy hypertension is associated with abnormal pulmonary blood flow (Littler et al., 1973), the increase in closing volume may have been a feature of hypertensive rather than normotensive pregnancy. Others (Craig and Toole, 1975; Baldwin et al., 1977; Russell and Chambers, 1981) have found no change in the point of airways closure during normal pregnancy. If some airways do close during tidal volume, impairment of ventilation-perfusion ratio and a decreased efficiency of pulmonary gas exchange would result.

Gas Transfer

Gas transfer (pulmonary diffusing capacity) is a measure of the ease with which carbon monoxide and therefore oxygen are transported across the pulmonary membrane (Ogilvie et al., 1957). Although early studies showed no change in transfer factor during pregnancy (Bedell and Adams, 1962; Krumholtz et al., 1964), Lehmann and Fabel (1973b) and Milne and colleagues (1977b) have shown more recently that there is a marked decrease in transfer factor early in pregnancy (Fig. 52–3). The mucopolysaccharides of the alveolar capillary wall might be affected by estrogen (Pecora et al., 1963), but correlation between the decrease in transfer factor level and estrogen status is lacking (Milne et al., 1977a). Interestingly, the transfer factor level may remain significantly reduced for up to 12 months after delivery (Milne et al., 1977b). A reduction in transfer factor would be one effect acting against the increase in ventilation to improve the efficiency of gas exchange in pregnancy.

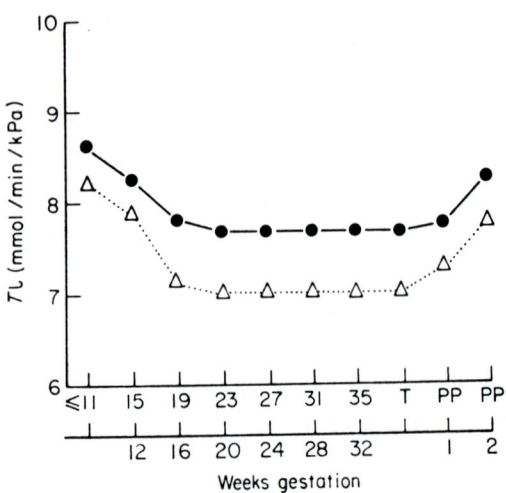

FIGURE 52–3. Change in pulmonary transfer factor during normal pregnancy and postpartum *(PP). Closed circles =* corrected for Hb alveolar volume; *open triangles =* observed values. (From Milne J: The respiratory response to pregnancy. Postgrad Med J **55**:318, 1979.)

Dyspnea in Pregnancy

The degree to which patients are aware of the profound changes in ventilation in the form of breathlessness varies enormously between patients and in the same patient in different pregnancies. Approximately 50 per cent of women are aware of breathlessness before 20 weeks gestation, and the maximum incidence of breathlessness at rest occurs between 28 and 31 weeks gestation (Milne et al., 1978). The symptom of breathlessness cannot be correlated with any single parameter of respiratory function in pregnancy (Cugell et al., 1953). This is not surprising, however, since it has been suggested (Wassermann, 1981) that dyspnea occurs when the ratio of ventilatory requirement to ventilatory capacity increases (Wassermann, 1981). Ventilatory requirement depends on CO_2 production, the fraction of the breath required to ventilate the functional dead space, and the level at which $PaCO_2$ is being regulated. The ventilatory capacity is affected by airways resistance and maximum alveolar ventilation. The variability of these determinants of the ratio of ventilatory requirements to ventilatory capacity between patients and throughout pregnancy could well account for the variability in individual patients' awareness of dyspnea.

Although breathlessness may be a feature of normal pregnancy, it is a worrisome symptom for the clinician because it can also be caused by pulmonary embolism or diffuse lung conditions such as pulmonary lymphangioleiomyomatosis (see below), which may worsen during pregnancy. In the absence of other symptoms of cardiorespiratory disease, normal findings on examination and a chest x-ray should be sufficient to exclude pathology in many cases. Another useful test is to measure oxygen saturation transcutaneously at rest and on exercise. The normal saturation is greater than 95 per cent, and it should not fall on moderate exercise. The equipment to do this should be available in anesthetic departments for monitoring during general anesthesia. Additional tests that may be necessary are measurement of arterial blood gases and transfer factor.

Exercise

The interactions between pregnancy and exercise are of particular relevance in view of the current interest in physical fitness. However, the capacity for exercise in pregnancy has not been fully tested (Lotgering et al., 1984). This is because weight-bearing exercise such as treadmill walking or step testing is heavily influenced by the change in weight associated with pregnancy. Sitting exercise (bicycle ergometry) should be less affected (Edwards et al., 1981). Also, the capacity for maximum exercise depends on many other variables such as motivation, which may themselves be altered by pregnancy. The question of interest is whether in pregnancy exercise costs more or is performed less efficiently. Artal et al. (1986) found on treadmill testing in late pregnancy that women could not increase oxygen consumption as much as in the nonpregnant state, that the ventilatory equivalent increased with higher grades of exercise, and that ventilation was less efficient at extreme exercise. Nevertheless, short-term exercise does not appear to affect the normal fetus, at least as measured in terms of fetal cardiac function assessed by M-mode echocardiography (Sørensen et al., 1986). Prolonged exercise (lasting more than 20 minutes) does increase fetal heart rate, although the mechanism is unknown (Clapp, 1985). Changes in uterine blood flow induced by maternal exercise may be compensated for by hemoconcentration (increasing oxygen capacity) and increased oxygen extraction by the placenta (Lotgering et al., 1984). Certainly moderate exercise is to be recommended in previously fit pregnant women (Huch and Erkkola, 1990) and is associated with a better pregnancy outcome than that in nonexercising controls (Hall and Kaufmann, 1987).

DISORDERS OF THE RESPIRATORY SYSTEM IN PREGNANCY

Pregnancy puts much less stress on the respiratory system than on the cardiovascular system. During pregnancy the minute ventilation increases by about 40 per cent and oxygen consumption by about 15 per cent. During exercise in nonpregnant patients, however, minute ventilation may increase by 1000 per cent (Comroe et al., 1962). Cardiac output also rises by approximately 40 per cent in pregnancy, but the maximum cardiac output achieved during exercise in nonpregnant patients is probably no greater than 300 per cent. Thus, although cardiac output and minute ventilation both increase by approximately 40 per cent in pregnancy, the increase in cardiac output represents a far greater proportion of the maximum of which the body is capable than does the increase in ventilation. For this reason, the clinical status of a patient with respiratory disease is much less likely to deteriorate in pregnancy than that of a patient with cardiac disease.

Bronchial Asthma

Asthma is a relatively common medical problem, affecting approximately 3 per cent of women of reproductive age (Littlejohn et al., 1989), and the prevalence may well be increasing (Burnley et al., 1990). It is also an extremely variable condition, its severity depending on the season of the year, which influences the patient's exposure to allergens such as pollen; on the presence of respiratory infections, which also depends on the season of the year in some countries; and on the patient's emotional state. If enough patients are studied to allow for these influences, pregnancy appears to have no consistent effect on asthma. A review of more than 1000 pregnant asthmatics reported in nine different publications revealed that 48 per cent of patients show no change, 29 per cent show improvement, and 23 per cent show deterioration (Gluck and Gluck, 1976). In serial measurement of FEV_1 in patients with asthma in pregnancy, Sims and colleagues (1976) were unable to discern any consistent changes during pregnancy or between pregnancy and the nonpregnant state. More recently Juniper et al (1989) followed airways responsiveness and treatment requirements (among other variables) in 16 patients from before conception and showed that both improved significantly during pregnancy. One reason that asthma in pregnant patients sometimes improves in pregnancy may be the elevation in serum cortisol. Although much of the increase in total cortisol level is in the protein-bound, non–metabolically active fraction, this does not account for the whole increase. The free cortisol index, which adjusts the cortisol level for an increase in binding protein, doubles in the last trimester of pregnancy over the value in the nonpregnant state (Nolten and Rueckert, 1981). For other series and general reviews, see Stablein and Lockey (1984), Greenberger (1985), White et al. (1989), and Spector (1983).

Schatz and colleagues (1975) found no excess risk to fetuses of 70 patients receiving corticosteroids for asthma, apart from a slightly higher rate of prematurity, which was also noted by Bahna and Bjerkedal (1972). Sims and colleagues (1976) found no extra risk to the fetus if the mother suffered from asthma in pregnancy, although there was a tendency toward growth retardation, particularly among fetuses of mothers taking oral steroids. These patients were more severely affected by asthma and may have been intermittently hypoxic. Although the results of one study suggested that the perinatal mortality is doubled in asthmatic patients (Gordon et al., 1970), this effect was largely confined to a socioeconomically deprived population. By contrast, Apter et al. (1989) found no excess fetal morbidity in 21 adolescent patients with asthma even though these patients required aggressive treatment with multiple hospital admissions. In view of these reports, it seems reasonable to conclude that there may be a slight increased risk to the fetus of the mother with asthma, but this effect is small and should not be exaggerated when one is counseling the individual patient.

The management of patients with asthma in pregnancy depends on a consideration of the likely fetal effects of the drugs used. Beta-sympathomimetic agents, such as albuterol (salbutamol in the UK) and terbutaline, are widely used and are given by inhalation rather than orally. Because of concern that beta$_2$-agonists, particularly fenoterol (Spitzer et al., 1992) may be responsible for the increasing mortality from asthma (Burrows and Liebowitz, 1992) the trend is to use inhaled glucocorticoids (see below) for first-line maintenance therapy and to reserve beta$_2$-agonists for break-through symptoms (Haahtela et al., 1991). The long-acting inhaled beta$_2$-agonist salmeterol is likely to prove effective and popular (Fitzpatrick et al., 1990). Because very little inhaled salmeterol enters the blood, it is unlikely that the fetus will be affected. However, at present there are insufficient data to recommend the use of salmeterol in pregnancy. The dose of beta$_2$-agonists is limited in pregnancy as in the nonpregnant state by tachycardia and tremor. They are also widely used to relax the pregnant uterus, particularly in cases of preterm labor (Lewis et al., 1980). The side effects of particular concern in obstetric practice are pulmonary edema and hyperglycemia with acidosis (Philips et al., 1980). Pulmonary edema has occurred when high doses of these drugs have been used for premature labor, particularly with intravenous administration (see Chapter 33). This is unlikely to be a problem in the treatment of asthma because lower doses are used and the drugs are normally not given intravenously.

Hyperglycemia could be a problem in patients who also have impaired glucose tolerance, because maintenance of the normal blood glucose is so important in the treatment of diabetes in pregnancy. Asthma and diabetes rarely coexist in pregnancy, and the hyperglycemia associated with beta-sympathomimetic drug therapy is amenable to treatment with diet or insulin. The use of beta-sympathomimetic agents for asthma might be expected to delay the onset of normal labor, but there are no data supporting this possibility.

Aminophylline has been widely used in pregnancy with no reported side effects. Disodium cromoglycate also appears to be safe for both mother and fetus (Weinstein et al., 1979). Anticholinergic drugs such as atropine have also been given for asthma (Van Arsdel and Paul, 1977). Fetal tachycardia is the only likely side effect.

Chest infection should be treated vigorously in pregnancy as in the nonpregnant state. Of the commonly used broad-spectrum antibiotics, tetracycline should be avoided because it can cause permanent staining of the infant's teeth and abnormalities of bone formation. Iodine-containing cough mixtures should not be used because the iodine may block thyroxine synthesis in the fetus, causing hypothyroidism or goiter (Carswell et al., 1970; Galina et al., 1962).

There is considerable controversy concerning the use of steroids for asthma in pregnancy. Inhaled steroids (e.g., beclomethasone) represent a considerable advance in treatment of asthma and have been widely used with success in pregnancy (Morrow

Brown and Storey, 1975). Little of the drug enters the blood (Harris, 1975); therefore, there is little potential for harm to the fetus. Furthermore, current opinion favors the use of inhaled corticosteroids rather than inhaled sympathomimetics (see above). Oral corticosteroids have been reported to cause cleft palate in fetal rabbits, but so far this risk does not appear to apply in humans. Clinical studies have not shown any excess fetal risk to be associated with maternal steroid therapy (Schatz et al., 1975; Snyder and Snyder, 1978).

In theory, the pituitary-adrenal axis of the fetus may be suppressed by maternal steroid therapy, rendering the neonate liable to collapse (Warrell and Taylor, 1968). In practice this does not happen. However, it is usual to give the mother additional steroid therapy to cover the stress of labor if she has taken oral steroid therapy for more than 2 weeks within the previous year. Hydrocortisone, 100 mg IM every 6 hours during labor, is more than adequate.

Patients may be reassured that it is surprisingly uncommon to have asthma "attacks" during labor. The reasons are not clear; perhaps there is a genuine increase in adrenal secretion of cortisol. If prostaglandins are used in labor for ripening of the cervix or induction of labor (or earlier for termination of pregnancy), prostaglandin E$_2$, which is a bronchodilator, should be given rather than prostaglandin F$_{2\alpha}$, which has bronchoconstrictor actions and has caused status asthmaticus in susceptible patients (Fishburne et al., 1972a, 1972b; Smith, 1973; Hyman et al., 1978).

Acute severe asthma remains a dangerous condition (MacDonald et al., 1976), and the risk may be especially high in pregnancy (Gordon et al., 1970). It is particularly easy for both patients and clinicians to underestimate the seriousness of acute severe asthma (MacDonald et al., 1976). Respiratory function may deteriorate before the patient is aware of it. Peak flow monitoring at home allows the patient to increase treatment (usually with inhaled or oral glucocorticoids) before her symptoms deteriorate. The treatment of acute severe asthma should be given in the hospital in consultation with a respiratory specialist as soon as possible (Hernandez et al., 1980). If intensive therapy fails to improve the condition of the patient with acute severe asthma, termination of pregnancy may be life-saving (Gelber et al., 1984).

Conclusion. Pregnancy rarely puts any extra burden on the woman with asthma, although it is possible that the patient with very severe asthma requiring large doses of oral prednisone might not be able to sustain the extra ventilation required to increase basal oxygen consumption by 20 per cent. Such women are rare, certainly less than 1 per cent of all patients with asthma. Similarly, the fetus is likely to be affected by growth retardation only in severe asthma and then not necessarily so. The major problems lie in realizing that the majority of drugs used in the treatment of asthma do not harm the fetus, maintaining the treatment of a potentially life-threatening illness despite pregnancy, and underestimating the severity of acute severe asthma.

Cystic Fibrosis

Cystic fibrosis (CF) is the most common semilethal genetic disorder in Caucasians, having a gene frequency of one in 20 (Cystic Fibrosis Foundation, 1976). Since heterozygotes are asymptomatic, homozygous patients who suffer from the condition are relatively common. The incidence is about one in 2500 live births (British Paediatric Association Working Party on Cystic Fibrosis, 1988). Recently the mortality rate has improved remarkably, and many more women are surviving to become pregnant. More than 70 per cent of children whose disease is identified in the first year of life now survive beyond 12 years (Mearns, 1974), and better than 30 per cent live longer than 30 years (Matthews and Drotar, 1984). The possibility of heart and lung transplantation may make a big difference in the future (Scott et al., 1988). In 1989 it was estimated that there were 1500 cystics past the age of 15 years in the United Kingdom (Hodson, 1989), of whom about 500 would have been female. The decrease in mortality rate has come from improved prophylactic bronchial toilet and widespread use of antibiotics rather than any single therapeutic advance. In addition, pancreatic enzymes can now be added to a high-protein, low-starch, low-fat diet.

Because of the large number of cystic fibrosis mutations that have been identified (more than 150), only 80 per cent of all heterozygotes can be identified (Wald, 1991). However, first-trimester prenatal diagnosis is possible on genetic material prepared from chorionic villi using linked DNA probes in about two-thirds of couples having one affected child. The expected false-negative and false-positive rates of this procedure are 2 and 6 per cent, respectively (Farrall et al., 1986). Biochemical analysis of amniotic fluid is not sufficiently accurate at present to detect or exclude the affected fetus. The patient should also be aware that her child will be heterozygous for cystic fibrosis, even if it is not homozygous. This, in turn, is likely to increase the future genetic load in the community.

A survey of 119 medical centers in North America revealed 129 pregnant CF patients delivered before 1975 (Cystic Fibrosis Foundation, 1976). Although 19 per cent of patients had therapeutic abortions, the incidence of spontaneous abortion (5 per cent) was not elevated. However, both the perinatal mortality rate (11 per cent) and the maternal mortality rate (12 per cent within 6 months of delivery) were considerably higher than in the general population. Although the maternal mortality rate was alarming, it was no greater than has been reported for patients with cystic fibrosis who are not pregnant (Warwick et al., 1975).

Pregnant patients with cystic fibrosis show a decrease in residual volume, like normal women in pregnancy, but they are unable to maintain vital capacity. Although they increase oxygen uptake, they do not show the "hyperventilation" normally associated with pregnancy (Novy et al., 1967).

Because most physicians have experience with relatively few cases, there is a wide diversity of clinical opinion regarding the advisability of pregnancy in patients with cystic fibrosis. Several indices have been suggested as a guide to the success of pregnancy, based on the presence or absence of emphysema, cor pulmonale, and such abnormalities in respiratory function as vital capacity less than 50 per cent predicted (Schwachman and Kulczyki, 1958; Taussig et al., 1973; Larsen, 1972). A patient with vital capacity of less than 50 per cent predicted may, however, have a normal pregnancy. Since cystic fibrosis patients die because of uncontrollable, recurrent chest infection and cor pulmonale, which is in turn related to hypoxemia, it is suggested that these be the parameters considered when counseling patients about pregnancy. If there is any doubt about the presence of hypoxemia, arterial blood gases should be measured. It would appear that an arterial PO_2 of less than 60 mm Hg in a patient free from infection is associated with an NIH score of less than 50, which is the score at which pulmonary hypertension is present (Di Sant'Agnese and Davis, 1979; Siassi et al., 1971). Pulmonary hypertension has a particularly poor outcome in pregnancy as has been documented for primary pulmonary hypertension, in which the mortality rate is 53 per cent (McCaffrey and Dunn, 1964) and for Eisenmenger's syndrome, in which the mortality rate is 31 per cent (Morgan Jones, 1965). Presumably, the pulmonary vasculature cannot dilate sufficiently to accommodate the increased cardiac output of pregnancy. Further arterial desaturation occurs, leading to a declining spiral of myocardial hypoxia, a decrease in cardiac output, and an increase in hypoxemia. If there is any doubt about the presence of pulmonary hypertension, pulmonary artery pressures should be measured. If the pulmonary artery systolic pressure is less than 35 mm Hg, the patient does not have cor pulmonale; this is much more reliable evidence than inference from clinical signs, chest radiographs, or electrocardiography.

Obstetricians should be aware that patients with cystic fibrosis may also have liver disease (Psacharopoulos et al., 1981). However, the reported incidence of cirrhosis varies between 0.5 per cent (Crozier, 1974) and 90 per cent (Isenberg and L'Heureuse, 1976). Cirrhosis has not yet been reported to be a problem in pregnancy.

Apart from a high level of medical and obstetric care, no special measures need be taken in the antenatal period for patients with cystic fibrosis. Because of the ototoxic and renal side effects of the aminoglycosides, these antibiotics should be avoided if possible in pregnancy, and the penicillins should be used instead. It is reassuring, however, that there were no congenital abnormalities in the 129 pregnancies reviewed by Cohen and associates (1980), in 26 of which the mothers received aminoglycosides during pregnancy.

During labor, particular attention should be given to fluid and electrolyte balance. Patients with cystic fibrosis lose large quantities of sodium in sweat and may easily become hypovolemic. However, they are also very intolerant of overhydration if there is any degree of cor pulmonale. Oxygen may be freely administered. Because of the risk of postanesthetic atelectasis, inhalation anesthesia is better avoided in favor of epidural or caudal anesthesia.

The baby of a woman with cystic fibrosis should be breast-fed only after the sodium content of her milk has been estimated. It may be as high as 280 mmol/liter (Whitelaw and Butterfield, 1977).

Chronic Bronchitis, Emphysema, and Bronchiectasis

Since these conditions are rarely important in women of childbearing age, there is little information about their effects on pregnancy. Chest infection and airways obstruction should be managed as in the patient with asthma. The success of pregnancy in any of these disorders would be limited only by the presence of pulmonary hypertension and hypoxemia, as discussed in the previous section on cystic fibrosis.

Kyphoscoliosis

I have successfully managed patients with kyphoscoliosis who have vital capacities of less than 1 liter. As in cystic fibrosis, the limiting factors are hypoxemia and pulmonary hypertension rather than the results of particular respiratory function tests. In one case of kyphoscoliosis, severe chronic maternal hypoxia (PaO_2 5.9 kpA) has caused fetal brain damage (Barrett et al., 1991). These patients are more likely to require cesarean section because of associated abnormalities of the bony pelvis. Notwithstanding the spinal deformities, epidural anesthesia is preferable to general anesthesia.

Tuberculosis

Pulmonary tuberculosis is now a rare complication of pregnancy in developed countries. Before antituberculous drugs were available, the results of pregnancy for both mother and fetus were poor, and there was a particular tendency for the maternal condition to deteriorate in the puerperium (Cohen et al., 1952; Hedvall, 1953; Barnes, 1974). More recently, de March (1975) was unable to detect any deleterious effect of pregnancy in a comparison of 100 tuberculosis patients who had been pregnant and 108 tuberculosis patients who had not been pregnant. Tuberculosis rarely affects the fetus by transplacental passage (Kapllan et al., 1980). Infection may occur when the fetus swallows infected amniotic fluid or it may be blood-borne via the umbilical vein. If the diagnosis is made early, for which a high index of clinical suspicion is necessary, the outlook for the neonate is good. The mother may have tuberculosis infection of any severity from subclinical to miliary tuberculosis (Snider, 1984).

The problem in managing a pregnant patient with tuberculosis is not the potential maternal respiratory impairment but the possible fetal effects of the chemotherapeutic agents. This subject has been extensively reviewed by Snider and co-workers (1980). The drugs for which there is considerable information are ethambutol, isoniazid, streptomycin, and rifampicin. In addition, it is believed that ethionamide is teratogenic (Potworoska et al., 1966). However, before starting chemotherapy for tuberculosis, the obstetrician or internist or both may consult a chest physician, because with the general decline of tuberculosis in the community, chest physicians are the only specialists sufficiently experienced in the treatment regimens used.

Ethambutol has replaced para-aminosalicylic acid (PAS) as a principal antituberculous drug because it is easier for patients to take, although ethambutol has in turn been replaced by pyrazinamide in nonpregnant patients (see below). Although ethambutol may cause retrobulbar neuritis in adults (Citron, 1969), there is no evidence from abortion specimens or neonatal examination that maternal ethambutol affects the fetus (Lewit et al., 1974; Brobowitz, 1974). In 655 pregnancies treated with ethambutol, only 14 infants or fetuses were found to have abnormalities and none had optic nerve abnormality (Snider et al., 1980). This drug must therefore be considered safe in pregnancy.

The safety of isoniazid has also been established. Only 16 abnormal fetuses have been reported in a total of 1480 pregnancies in which isoniazid was given (Snider et al., 1980). This abnormality rate is lower than that of the normal hospital population. Four of the five abnormal fetuses in a series of 125 patients treated with isoniazid had CNS abnormalities (Monnet et al., 1967). Isoniazid is known to cause peripheral neuritis, which also is a potential problem with its use during pregnancy. The reported high incidence of CNS abnormalities was seen only in one group of patients, however, all of whom had also received ethionamide. Because of the possible higher requirement of pyridoxine in pregnancy, all patients taking isoniazid in pregnancy should also take pyridoxine 50 mg/day (Atkins, 1982) to reduce the risk of peripheral neuritis (Brummer, 1972).

There is real concern about the use of streptomycin and rifampicin during pregnancy. At one time streptomycin was considered to be relatively innocuous in pregnancy, on the basis of a study by Conway and Birt (1965); however, eight children in this study had abnormal caloric test results and/or abnormal audiograms. It has since been shown that the incidence of eighth nerve damage in infants of mothers treated with streptomycin during pregnancy is approximately 15 per cent (Snider et al., 1980). Variable and severe fetal malformations have also been seen in 14 of 442 patients treated with rifampin (Snider et al., 1980; Steen and Stainton-Ellis, 1977). There is one curious report of a nearly 5-fold increase in the risk of deep vein thrombosis in patients treated with rifampicin for tuberculosis but this study was not performed in pregnant patients (White 1989). Pyrazinamide is increasingly used in antituberculous regimens because it rapidly renders the sputum negative for acid-fast bacilli and because 6-month rather than 9-month treatment periods are effective (Cole, 1985). However, as of this writing there is inadequate information concerning the safety of pyrazinamide in the first trimester; therefore, it should not be used until after 14 weeks gestation.

The patient presenting with tuberculosis in the first trimester of pregnancy should be treated with isoniazid and ethambutol unless the disease is widespread or the patient's condition is deteriorating. After organogenesis is complete at 16 weeks gestation, it should be safe to use rifampicin and pyrazinamide if necessary.

After birth, babies should only be isolated from their mothers if the mothers are still smear positive. Since modern antituberculosis regimens render the sputum sterile within 2 weeks and markedly reduce the number of organisms within 24 hours, this should not occur frequently. The neonate should be treated with prophylactic isoniazid for 3 months. After this period, BCG vaccination is given in the United Kingdom but not in the United States (Lancet, 1990). It is not clear whether neonatal BCG vaccination adds any further protection to isoniazid prophylaxis. It is not without risks, such as skin ulceration, osteitis, and occasionally disseminated disease, particularly if the mother has an immunodeficiency state. As isoniazid therapy does not affect the immunogenicity of BCG vaccine, there is no longer any rationale for the use of isoniazid-resistant BCG neonatal vaccination (Lancet, 1990).

Sarcoidosis

Pulmonary sarcoid is a rare complication of pregnancy affecting at most 0.05 per cent of all pregnancies. In addition, fewer than five cases have been reported in which there was marked impairment in respiratory function (Grossman and Littner, 1976; Reisfield et al., 1969). Only one maternal death has been reported, in a patient who also had preeclampsia (Given and DiBenedetto, 1963). If sarcoidosis changes during pregnancy it usually improves, perhaps owing to the increase in free cortisol as well as the total cortisol level. There is, however, a tendency for the condition to relapse in the puerperium (Weinberger et al., 1980; O'Leary, 1962; Fried, 1964; Scadding, 1961). Nevertheless, such a relapse is unlikely to be serious and should not be a contraindication to pregnancy except in the rare woman with severe disease.

No special management is necessary for sarcoidosis in pregnancy. Angiotensin-converting enzyme levels have been reported to fall (Cugini et al., 1989) or to remain unchanged in normal pregnancy (Erskine et al., 1985). In addition, they showed diurnal variation (Cugini et al., 1989). Also the level of the enzyme has been reported to vary markedly in a patient with sarcoid in pregnancy independent of apparent disease activity. Thus, converting enzyme levels may no longer be useful in monitoring patients with sarcoid who become pregnant (Erskine et al., 1985). If disease is severe, systemic steroids should not be withheld. The condition is not transmitted to the fetus (Barnes, 1974). Because women often take extra vitamins in pregnancy, the sarcoidosis patient should be particularly warned not to take extra vitamin D, to which she may be very sensitive (James, 1970).

Wegener's Granulomatosis

This is a rare form of systemic vasculitis in which necrotizing granulomatosis lesions affect the upper respiratory tract (particularly the nose, causing perforation of the septum) and the lungs; the kidneys are affected by glomerulonephritis. It causes nasal symptoms, hemoptysis, general malaise, and renal failure. Untreated, it is rapidly fatal. The condition is now being diagnosed more frequently during (Talbot et al.,

1984; Murty et al., 1990) or before (Cooper et al., 1970) pregnancy as less severe cases are recognized and treated with prednisone and cyclophosphamide. The latter drug, an alkylating agent, is potentially teratogenic; at least three case reports have documented various abnormalities in the infant following first-trimester use (Toledo et al., 1971; Coates, 1970; Greenberg and Tanaka, 1964). Therefore, patients who conceive while taking cyclophosphamide should be offered termination and patients who have Wegener's granulomatosis should wait until the disease is in remission so that cyclophosphamide can be stopped before pregnancy. As of this writing, it is unknown whether the course of Wegener's granulomatosis is affected by pregnancy.

Pulmonary Lymphangioleiomyomatosis

This is a very rare condition, but it has attracted much interest and is of particular relevance since it occurs in young women during their childbearing years (Corrin et al., 1975, Silverstein et al., 1974, Taylor 1990). Pulmonary lymphangioleiomyomatosis is characterized by proliferation of smooth muscle in pulmonary mediastinal and retroperitoneal lymphatics, in pulmonary vessels and in the smaller airways (Corrin et al., 1975). Patients present with breathlessness or with symptoms from pneumothorax or chylothorax.

Chest radiologic examination may be normal initially or show interstitial thickening, pneumothorax, or pleural effusion (Silverstein et al., 1974). High-resolution CT scanning may be necessary to show the typical small cystic changes. Lung function tests show air flow obstruction and characteristically low gas transfer factor; the latter, it should be noted, is decreased in pregnancy (see under Gas Transfer). The differential diagnosis of pulmonary infiltration includes eosinophilic granuloma, sarcoidosis, and idiopathic pulmonary fibrosis. Diagnosis is usually confirmed by lung biopsy, which can be performed safely in pregnancy.

Early reports (Corrin et al., 1975) suggested that most patients died within 10 years of diagnosis. More recent studies, possibly in patients diagnosed earlier in the course of disease, are more optimistic. Taylor et al., (1990) found that 78 per cent of patients were alive 8 years after diagnosis. The evidence that estrogen (Shen et al., 1991) and pregnancy (Hughes and Hodder, 1987; Murata et al., 1989) cause the condition to deteriorate is anecdotal. Nevertheless, in the desire to give some form of active treatment for an otherwise fatal condition, patients have been offered oophorectomy with or without additional progesterone and tamoxifen therapies (Taylor et al., 1990). Lung transplantation has been performed for some patients (Raffin et al., 1991).

Pre-pregnancy counseling and decisions about termination of pregnancy can be based only on a frank discussion of the uncertainty about the natural history of this fascinating condition.

Adult Respiratory Distress Syndrome

Adult respiratory distress syndrome (ARDS) is the final result of several different types of obstetric complications, such as inhalation of gastric contents during anesthesia, disseminated intravascular coagulation (DIC) in preeclampsia, eclampsia, abruptio placentae, dead fetus syndrome, and amniotic fluid embolism. It also occurs in hypovolemic shock from postpartum hemorrhage with or without sepsis (Andersen et al., 1980), in metastatic cancer, and in hydatidiform mole (Orr et al., 1980).

Adult respiratory distress syndrome in association with pyelonephritis in pregnancy seems a particular problem in the United States (Towers et al., 1991; Ridgway et al., 1991; Cunningham et al., 1987). Particular risk factors for the development of adult respiratory distress syndrome in a patient with pyelonephritis include maternal heart rate greater than 110 per minute, pyrexia greater than 39.4°C in patients with gestational age greater than 20 weeks, and the use of tocolytic agents.

In a group of 14 obstetric cases with adult respiratory distress syndrome, 12 were caused by strictly obstetric factors such as preeclampsia or hemorrhage. The mortality was 43 per cent (Smith et al., 1990).

The apparent frequency of pregnancy as an underlying cause of adult respiratory distress in women may relate to the physiologic changes caused by pregnancy. Alternatively, it may be that secondary causes, such as anesthesia, shock from hemorrhage, and DIC are more likely to occur in pregnancy than in the nonpregnant state.

The clinical picture of ARDS consists of severe hypoxemia despite a high inspired oxygen concentration (Ashbaugh et al., 1967) with diffuse infiltrates seen on the chest radiograph, although radiologic signs may take 24 hours to develop. The primary problem is assumed to be in the lung, where compliance and permeability are reduced owing to extravasation of liquid, rather than in the heart. It is important, however, to exclude primary cardiac abnormality by demonstrating a normal wedge pressure by means of a Swan-Ganz catheter. The Swan-Ganz will also be of great assistance for management because it will permit measurements to be made of pulmonary artery pressure and cardiac output. Peripheral edema, elevated jugular pressure, and cardiomegaly are unusual findings in ARDS and suggest cardiac rather than pulmonary disease.

The available therapeutic options are correction of the underlying cause, artificial ventilation, and administration of vasoactive drugs, inotropes, and steroids. In addition, manipulation of the circulating blood volume is helpful. Correction of the underlying cause is usually limited to reversal of DIC with fresh-frozen plasma and treatment of overt infection. Ventilation, preferably with an inspired oxygen concentration of less than 60 per cent, and maintenance of an end-expiratory pressure of 5 to 35 cm H_2O are suggested, with the goal to achieve arterial PO_2 greater than 60 mm Hg (Andersen et al., 1980). The use of positive pressure at the end of expiration is believed to force extravasated water back into the circulation and to reverse atelectasis.

Fluid balance is crucial in adult respiratory distress syndrome. If the patient is hypovolemic, cardiac output and perfusion will decrease; hence infusion of albumin or blood is often helpful. If the patient is hypervolemic, extravasation of fluid and preload will increase, and oxygenation and cardiac output will decrease. Diuretic therapy will then be necessary. The indication for and effect of manipulating blood volume can be determined by repeated measurement of pulmonary artery wedge pressure and cardiac output via the Swan-Ganz catheter. Corticosteroids may reverse excess capillary permeability (Wilson, 1972), but they may also increase susceptibility to infection (Blaisdell and Schlobohm, 1973), and a recent study suggests that they do not affect outcome (Bernard et al., 1987).

Despite these measures, the mortality rate in adult respiratory distress syndrome is 50 to 60 per cent (Shanies, 1977). It is hoped, although not proven, that early aggressive treatment can reduce this death rate (Andersen et al., 1980).

Anesthetic Considerations

A survey of the 265 maternal deaths occurring in the United Kingdom between 1985 and 1987 indicated that only one of the deaths was due to inhalation of stomach contents (Department of Health and Social Security, 1991). Much of modern obstetric practice involves prevention of the complication of gastric aspiration. It is common to proscribe oral intake during labor, but the stomach continues to secrete fluid, although in reduced quantities. Also, gastric emptying from meals taken before the onset of labor is reduced. On the assumption that it is the acid component of gastric contents that is harmful, patients in labor are often given up to 30 ml of antacid (magnesium trisilicate mixture) to keep the pH higher than 3.5 (Cohen, 1979). The confidential maternal mortality series (Department, 1979), however, indicates that the number of deaths from aspiration from 1973 to 1975, when antacid administration was widespread, was no less than the number occurring from 1970 to 1972, before antacids were generally used (Scott, 1978). Furthermore, Bond et al. (1979) have described pulmonary aspiration syndrome after inhalation of stomach contents of pH 6.4 in a patient who had been given regular antacid therapy with magnesium and aluminum hydroxide. This would suggest that the hydrogen ion concentration is not the only determinant of the pulmonary aspiration syndrome. Either the antacid itself or other constituents of the gastric fluid must contribute. For these reasons large-scale studies are still necessary to compare cimetidine therapy, which decreases acid secretion, metoclopramide therapy, which increases gastric emptying (Howard and Sharp, 1973), and conventional antacid therapy.

In the laboring patient with respiratory impairment, general anesthesia should be avoided because of the slight risk of intrapartum hypoxia due to deteriorating ventilation-perfusion imbalance, and the greater risk of postoperative atelectasis. Epidural, caudal, or spinal anesthesia may, obviously, be used instead.

Summary

The respiratory system adapts easily to pregnancy, having the ability to increase ventilation much more than is needed. Because of this reserve in ventilatory capacity, and because most chronic respiratory conditions affect older patients, respiratory failure is rare in pregnancy. Respiratory failure may become more common as more patients with cystic fibrosis become pregnant, but the usual cause is some catastrophe such as amniotic fluid embolus or inhalation of gastric contents. Most management problems in the pregnant patient with respiratory disease concern the effect of drugs on the fetus rather than the effect of pregnancy on maternal respiratory status.

REFERENCES

Alaily AB, Carrol KB: Pulmonary ventilation in pregnancy. Br J Obstet Gynaecol 85:518, 1978.

Andersen HF, Lynch JP, Johnson TRB: Adult respiratory distress syndrome in obstetrics and gynecology. Obstet Gynecol 55:291, 1980.

Anderson GJ, James GB, Mathers NP, et al: The maternal oxygen tension and acid base status during pregnancy. Am J Obstet Gynecol 100:1, 1969.

Apter AJ, Greenberger PA, Patterson R: Outcomes of pregnancy in adolescents with severe asthma. Arch Intern Med 149:2571, 1989.

Artal R, Wiswell R, Romem Y, Dorey F: Pulmonary responses to exercise in pregnancy. Am J Obstet Gynecol 154:378, 1986.

Ashbaugh DG, Bigelow DB, Petty TL: Acute respiratory distress in adults. Lancet 2:319, 1967.

Atkins NA: Maternal plasma concentrations of pyridoxal phosphate during pregnancy: Adequacy of Vitamin B6 supplementation during isoniazid therapy. Am Rev Resp Dis 126:714, 1982.

Bader RA, Bader ME, Rose DJ, Braunwald E: Haemodynamics at rest and during exercise in normal pregnancy as studied by cardiac catheterization. J Clin Invest 34:1524, 1955.

Bahna SL, Bjerkedal T: The course and outcome of pregnancy in women with bronchial asthma. Acta Allergol 27:397, 1972.

Baldwin GR, Moorthi DS, Whelton JA, MacDoneal KF: New lung functions and pregnancy. Am J Obstet Gynecol 127:235, 1977.

Barnes CG: Medical Disorders in Obstetric Practice. Oxford, Blackwell Scientific Publications, 1974.

Barrett JFR, Dear PRF, Lilford RJ: Brain damage as a result of chronic intrauterine hypoxia in a baby born of a severely kyphoscoliotic mother. J Obstet Gynaecol 11:260–261, 1991.

Bedell GN, Adams RS: Pulmonary diffusing capacity during rest and exercise. A study of normal persons and persons with atrial septal defect, pregnancy and pulmonary disease. J Clin Invest 41:1908, 1962.

Bernard GR, Luce JM, Sprung CL, et al: High-dose corticosteroids in patients with adult respiratory distress syndrome. N Engl J Med 317:1565–1570, 1987.

Bevan DR, Holdcroft A, Loh L, et al: Closing volume and pregnancy. Br Med J 1:13, 1974.

Blaisdell FW, Schlobohm RM: The respiratory distress syndrome: A review. Surgery 74:251, 1973.

Bond VK, Stoetling RK, Gupta CD: Pulmonary aspiration syndrome after inhalation of gastric fluid containing antacids. Anesthesiology 51:452, 1979.

Boutourline-Young H, Boutourline-Young E: Alveolar carbon dioxide levels in pregnant, parturient and lactating subjects. J Obstet Gynaecol Br Emp 63:509, 1956.

Briscoe WA, Dubois AB: The relationship between airway resistance, airway conductance and lung volume in subjects of different age and body size. J Clin Invest 37:1279, 1958.

British Paediatric Association Working Party on Cystic Fibrosis: Cystic fibrosis in the United Kingdom. Br Med J 297:1599–1602, 1988.

Brobowitz ID: Ethambutol in pregnancy. Chest 66:20, 1974.

Brummer DL: Letter to the editor. Am Rev Resp Dis 106:785, 1972.

Burnley PG, Chinn S, Rowa RJ: Has the prevalence of asthma increased in children? Evidence from the national study of health and growth. Br Med J 300:1306, 1990.

Burrows B, Lebowitz MD: The β_2-agonist dilema. N Engl J Med 8:36, 1992.

Carswell F, Kerr MM, Hutchinson JH: Congenital goitre and hypothyroidism produced by maternal ingestion of iodides. Lancet 1:1241, 1970.

Citron KM: Ethambutol: A review with special reference to ocular toxicity. Tubercle, March Supplement, pp. 32–36, 1969.

Clapp JF: Fetal heart rate response to running in midpregnancy and late pregnancy. Am J Obstet Gynecol 153:251, 1985.

Coates A: Cyclophosphamide in pregnancy. Aust NZJ Obstet Gynaecol 10:33, 1970.

Cohen JD, Patton EA, Badger TL: The tuberculous mother. Am Rev Tuberc 65:1, 1952.

Cohen LF, Di Sant'Agnese PA, Friedlander J: Cystic fibrosis and pregnancy. A national survey. Lancet ii:842, 1980.

Cohen SE: Aspiration syndromes in pregnancy. Anesthesiology 41:375, 1979.

Cole RB: Modern management of pulmonary tuberculosis. Prescribers Journal 25:110, 1985.

Comroe JH: Physiology of Respiration. 2nd ed. Chicago, Year Book Medical Publishers, Inc, 1974.

Comroe JJ, Forster RE, Dubois AB, et al: The Lung: Clinical Physiology and Pulmonary Function Tests. Chicago, Year Book Medical Publishers, Inc, 1962.

Conway N, Birt BD: Streptomycin in pregnancy: Effect on fetal ear. Br Med J 2:260, 1965.

Cooper K, Stafford J, Turner Warwick M: Wegener's granuloma complicating pregnancy. Br J Obstet Gynaecol 77:1028, 1970.

Corrin B, Liebow AA, Friedman PJ: Pulmonary lymphangiomyomatosis. Am J Pathol 79:374, 1975.

Craig DR, Toole MA: Airway closure in pregnancy. Can Anaesth Soc J 22:665, 1975.

Crozier MD: Cystic fibrosis—a not-so-fatal disease. Pediatr Clin North Am 21:935, 1974.

Cugell DW, Frank NR, Gaensler EA, Badger TL: Pulmonary function in pregnancy. Serial observations in normal women. Am Rev Tuberc 67:568, 1953.

Cugini P, Letizia C, Di Palma L, Caserta D, Moscarini M, Scavo D: Circadian variation in serum angiotensin converting enzyme activity in normal and hypertensive pregnancy. J Obstet Gynaecol 10:124, 1989.

Cullen JH, Brum VC, Reid TWH: The respiratory effects of progesterone in severe pulmonary emphysema. Am J Med 27:551, 1959.

Cunningham FG, Lucas MJ, Hankins GDV. Pulmonary injury complicating antepartum pyelonephritis. Am J Obstet Gynecol 156:797, 1987.

Cystic Fibrosis Foundation: 1974 Report on Survival of Patients with Cystic Fibrosis. Rockville, Maryland, Cystic Fibrosis Foundation, 1976.

de March AP: Tuberculosis and pregnancy: Five- to ten-year review of 215 patients in their fertile age. Chest 68:800, 1975.

Department of Health and Social Security: Report on Confidential Enquiries into Maternal Deaths in England and Wales, 1973–1975. London, Her Majesty's Stationery Office, 1979.

Department of Health and Social Security: Report on Confidential Enquiries into Maternal Deaths in England and Wales, 1979–1981. London, HMSO, 1986.

Department of Health and Social Security: Report on Confidential Enquiries into Maternal Deaths in England and Wales. London, Her Majesty's Stationery Office, 1991.

de Swiet M: The respiratory system. In Hytten F, Chamberlain G (eds): Clinical Physiology in Obstetrics. 2nd ed. Oxford, Blackwell Scientific Publications, 1991.

Di Sant'Agnese PA, Davis PB: Cystic fibrosis in adults. Am J Med 66:121, 1979.

Döring GK, Loeschcke HH: Atmung und Sauer—Basengleichgewicht in de Schwangershaft. Pflugers Arch 249:437, 1947.

Edwards MJ, Metcalfe J, Dunham MJ, Paul MS: Accelerated respiratory response to moderate exercise in late pregnancy. Respir Physiol 45:229, 1981.

Emerson K, Saxena BN, Poindexter EL: Colonic effect of normal pregnancy. Obstet Gynecol 40:786, 1972.

Eng M, Butler J, Bonich JJ: Respiratory function in pregnant obese women. Am J Obstet Gynecol 123:241, 1975.

England SJ, Fahri LE: Fluctuations in alveolar CO_2 and in base excess during the menstrual cycle. Respir Physiol 26:157, 1976.

Erskine KJ, Taylor KS, Agnew RAL: Serial estimation of serum angiotensin converting enzyme activity during and after pregnancy in a woman with sarcoidosis. Br Med J 290:269, 1985.

Esteban-Altirriba J: A comparative study of oxygen saturation of the peripheral arterial blood during pregnancy, labour and post partum period. Gynecologica 150:33, 1960.

Farebrother MJB, McHardy GJR: Closing volume and pregnancy. Br Med J 1:454, 1974.

Farrall M, Law H, Rodeck CH, et al: First-trimester prenatal diagnosis of cystic fibrosis with linked DNA probus. Lancet 1:1402, 1986.

Fishburne JI Jr, Brenner WE, Braaksma JT, Hendricks CH: Bronchospasm complicating intravenous prostaglandin F$_{2\alpha}$ for therapeutic abortion. Obstet Gynecol 39:892, 1972a.

Fishburne JI Jr, Brenner WE, Braaksma JT, et al: Cardiovascular and respiratory responses to intravenous infusion of prostaglandin F$_2$ in the pregnant woman. Am J Obstet Gynecol 114:765, 1972b.

Fitzpatrick MF, Mackay T, Driver H, Douglas NJ: Salmeterol in nocturnal asthma: a double blind, placebo-controlled trial of a long acting inhales β$_2$-agonist. Br Med J 301:1365, 1990.

Fried KH: Sarcoidosis and pregnancy. Acta Med Scand 176(Suppl 425):218, 1964.

Gaensler EA, Patton WE, Verstraeten JM, et al: Pulmonary functions in pregnancy. III. Serial observations in patients with pulmonary insufficiency. Am Rev Tuberc 67:779, 1953.

Galina MP, Avnet NL, Einhorn A: Iodides during pregnancy: Apparent cause of fetal death. N Engl J Med 267:1124, 1962.

Garrard CG, Littler WAW, Redman CWL: Closing volume during normal pregnancy. Thorax 33:484, 1978.

Gazioglu K, Kaltreider NL, Rosen M, Yu PN: Pulmonary function during pregnancy in normal women and in patients with cardiopulmonary disease. Thorax 25:445, 1970.

Gee JBL, Packer BS, Millen JE, Robin ED: Pulmonary medicines during pregnancy. J Clin Invest 46:945, 1967.

Gelber M, Sidi Y, Gassner S, et al: Uncontrollable life-threatening status asthmaticus—an indicator for termination of pregnancy by cesarean section. Respiration 46:320, 1984.

Given FR, DiBenedetto RL: Sarcoidoses and pregnancy. Obstet Gynecol 22:355, 1963.

Gluck JC, Gluck PA: The effects of pregnancy on asthma. A prospective study. Ann Allergy 37:164, 1976.

Gordon M, Niswander KR, Berendes H, Kantor AG: Fetal morbidity following potentially anoxigenic obstetric conditions. VII. Bronchial asthma. Am J Obstet Gynecol 106:421, 1970.

Greenberg LM, Tanaka KR: Congenital anomalies probably induced by cyclophosphamide. JAMA 188:423, 1964.

Greenberger PA: Pregnancy and asthma. Chest 87:855, 1985.

Grossman JH II, Littner MD: Severe sarcoidosis in pregnancy. Obstet Gynecol 50(Suppl):81, 1976.

Haahtela T, Jarvinen M, Kava T, Kiviranta K, Koskinen S, Lehtonen K, Nikander K, Persson T, Reinikainen K, Selroos O, Sovijärvi A, Stenius-Aarniala B, Svahn T, Tammivaara R, Laitinen L: Comparison of a β$_2$-agonist, terbutaline, with an inhaled corticosteroid, budesonide, in newly detected asthma. N Engl J Med 325:388, 1991.

Hall DC, Kaufmann DA: Effects of aerobic and strength conditioning on pregnancy outcomes. Am J Obstet Gynecol 157:1199, 1987.

Harris DM: Some properties of beclomethasone dipropionate and related steroids in man. Postgrad Med J 51(Suppl 4):20, 1975.

Hedvall E: Pregnancy and tuberculosis. Acta Med Scand 147(Suppl 286):1, 1953.

Heidenreich J, Kafarnik D, Westenburger U, Beck L: Statische und Dynamische Ventilationgrössen in der Schwangerschaft und im Wochenbett. Archiv für Gynakologie 210:208, 1971.

Hellegers A, Metcalfe J, Huckabee W, et al: The alveolar Pco$_2$ and Po$_2$ in pregnant and non-pregnant women at altitude. Clin Invest 38:1010, 1959.

Hernandez E, Angel CS, Johnson JWC: Asthma in pregnancy: Current concepts. Obstet Gynecol 55:739, 1980.

Hodson M: Managing adults with cystic fibrosis. Br Med J 298:471, 1989.

Howard FA, Sharp DS: Effect of metoclopramide on gastric emptying during labour. Br Med J 1:446, 1973.

Huch R, Baumann H, Fallenstein F, Schneider KTM, Holdener F, Huch A: Physiologic changes in pregnant women and their fetuses during jet air travel. Am J Obstet Gynecol 154:996, 1986.

Huch R, Erkkola R: Pregnancy and exercise—exercise and pregnancy. A short review. Br J Obstet Gynecol 97:208, 1990.

Hughes G. Hodder RV: Pulmonary lymphangiomyomatosis complicating pregnancy. A case report. 32:553, 1987.

Hyman AL, Spannhake EW, Kadowitz QJ: Prostaglandins and the lung: State of the art. Am Rev Respir Dis 117:111, 1978.

Isenberg JN, L'Heureuse DR: Clinical observation on the biliary system in cystic fibrosis. Am J Gastroenterol 65:134, 1976.

James DG: Sarcoidosis. Disease-A-Month, February 1970, p. 1.

Juniper EF, Daniel EE, Roberts RS, Line PA, Hargreave FE, Newhouse MT: Improvement of airway responsiveness and asthma severity during pregnancy. Am Rev Respir Dis 140:924, 1989.

Kambam JR, Mandte RE, Brown WR, Smith BE: Effect of pregnancy on oxygen dissociation. Anesthesiology 59:A395, 1983.

Kapllan C, Benirschke K, Tarzy B: Placental tuberculosis in early and late pregnancy. Am J Obstet Gynecol 137:858, 1980.

Kelman GR, Templeton A: Maternal blood gases during human pregnancy. Physiology 244:66, 1975.

Klaften E, Palugyay J: Zr Physiologie der Atmung in der Schwangerschaft. Arch Gynkol 129:414, 1926.

Klaften E, Palugyay J: Verleichende Untersuchungen über Lage und Ausdehnung von Herz und Lunge in der Schwangerschaft und im Wochenbett. Arch Gynäkol 131:347, 1927.

Knuttgen HG, Emerson K: Physiological response to pregnancy at rest and during exercise. J Appl Physiol 36:549, 1974.

Krumholz RA, Echt CR, Ross JC: Pulmonary diffusing capacity, capillary blood volume, lung volumes and mechanics of ventilation in early and late pregnancy. J Clin Med 63:648, 1964.

Lancet Editorial. Perinatal prophylaxis of tuberculosis. Lancet 336:1479, 1990.

Larsen JW: Cystic fibrosis and pregnancy. Obstet Gynecol 39:880, 1972.

Lehmann V, Fabel H: Lungenfunktionsuntersuchungen an Schwangeren. I: Lungenvolumina. Z Geburtshilfe Perinatol 177:387, 1973a.

Lehmann V, Fabel H: Lungenfunktionsuntersuchungen an Schwangeren. II. Ventilation, Atemmechanik und Diffusionkapazitt. Z Geburtshilfe Perinatol 177:397, 1973b.

Leontic EA: Respiratory disease in pregnancy. Med Clin North Am 61:111, 1977.

Lewis PJ, de Swiet M, Boyland P, Bulpitt CJ: How obstetricians in the United Kingdom manage preterm labour. Br J Obstet Gynaecol 87:574, 1980.

Lewit T, Nebel L, Terracina S, Karman S: Ethambutol in pregnancy: Observations on embryogenesis. Chest 66:25, 1974.

Littlejohn PI, Ebrahim S, Anderson R. Prevalence and diagnosis of chronic respiratory symptoms in adults. Br Med J 289:1556, 1989.

Littler WA, Redman CWG, Bonnar J, et al: Reduced pulmonary arterial compliance in hypertensive pregnancy. Lancet i:1274, 1973.

Lotgering FK, Gilbert RD, Longo L: The interactions of exercise and pregnancy: A review. Am J Obstet Gynecol 149:560, 1984.

Lucius H, Gahlenbeck H, Kleine HO, et al: Respiratory functions, buffer system and electrolyte concentrations of blood during human pregnancy. Respir Physiol 9:311, 1970.

Lyons HA, Antonio R: The sensitivity of the respiratory centre in pregnancy and after the administration of progesterone. Trans Assoc Am Physicians 72:173, 1959.

Lyons HA, Huang CT: Therapeutic use of progesterone in alveolar hypoventilation associated with obesity. Am J Med 44:881, 1968.

McCaffrey RM, Dunn LJ: Primary pulmonary hypertension and pregnancy. Obstet Gynecol Surv 19:567, 1964.

MacDonald JB, MacDonald ET, Seaton A, Williams DA: Asthma deaths in Cardiff 1963–1974: 53 deaths in hospital. Br Med J 2:721, 1976.

McGinty AP: The comparative effect of pregnancy and phrenic nerve interruption on the diaphragm and their relation to pulmonary tuberculosis. Am J Obstet Gynecol 35:237, 1938.

Macklem PT, Mead J: Resistance of central and peripheral airways measured by a retrograde catheter. J Appl Physiol 22:395, 1967.

Matthews LW, Drotar D: Cystic fibrosis—a challenging long-term chronic disease. Pediatr Clin North Am 31:133, 1984.

Mearns MR: Cystic fibrosis. Br J Hosp Med 12:497, 1974.

Milne JA, Pack AI, Coutts JRT: Gas exchange and acid-base status during the normal human menstrual cycle and in subjects taking oral contraceptives (proceedings). J Endocrinol 75:17P, 1977a.

Milne JA, Pack AI, Coutts JRT: Maternal gas exchange and acid-base status during normal pregnancy. Scott Med J 22:108, 1977b.

Milne JA, Mills RJ, Howie AD, Pack AI: Large airways functions during normal pregnancy. Br J Obstet Gynaecol 84:448, 1977c.

Milne JA, Howie AD, Pack AI: Dyspnoea during normal pregnancy. Br J Obstet Gynaecol 84:448, 1978.

Milne JA: The respiratory response to pregnancy. Postgrad Med J 55:318, 1979.

Möbius WV: Abrung und Schwangerschaft. Mnchener Med Woschr 103:1389, 1961.

Monnet P, Kalb JC, Pujol M: De l'influence nocive de l'isoniazide fur le produit de conception. Rev Lyon Med 218:431, 1967.

Morgan Jones A: Eisenmenger syndrome in pregnancy. Br Med J 1:1627, 1965.

Morrow Brown H, Storey G: Treatment of allergy of the respiratory tract with beclomethasone dipropionate steroid aerosol. Postgrad Med J 51(Suppl 4):59, 1975.

Murata A, Takeda Y, Usuki J, et al: A case of pulmonary lymphangiomyomatosis induced by pregnancy. Nippon Kyobu Shikkan Gakkai Zasshi 27:1106, 1989.

Murty GE, Davison JM, Cameron DS: Wegener's granulomatosis complicating pregnancy. Br J Obstet Gynaecol 10:399–400, 1990.

Newhouse MT, Becklaile MR, Macklem PT, McGregor M: Effect of alterations in endtidal CO_2 on flow resistance. J Appl Physiol 19:745, 1964.

Nolten WE, Rueckert PA: Elevated free cortisol index in pregnancy: Possible regulating mechanisms. Am J Obstet Gynecol 139:492, 1981.

Novy MJ, Tyler JM, Schwachman H, et al: Cystic fibrosis and pregnancy. Obstet Gynaecol 30:530, 1967.

Ogilvie CM, Forster RE, Blakemore WS, Morton JW: A standardized breath holding technique for the clinical measurement of the diffusing capacity of the lung for carbon monoxide. J Clin Invest 36:1, 1957.

O'Leary JA: Ten year study of sarcoidosis and pregnancy. Am J Obstet Gynecol 84:462, 1962.

Orr JW, Austin JM, Hatch KD, et al: Acute pulmonary edema associated with molar pregnancy: A high-risk factor for development of persistent trophoblastic disease. Am J Obstet Gynecol 136:412, 1980.

Paciorek J, Spencer N: An association between plasma progesterone and erythrocyte carbonic anhydrase I concentration in women. Clin Sci 58:161, 1980.

Pecora LJ, Putnam LR, Baum GL: Effects of intravenous estrogens on pulmonary diffusing capacity. Am J Med Sci 246:48, 1963.

Pernoll ML, Metcalfe J, Kovach PA, et al: Ventilation during rest and exercise in pregnancy and postpartum. Respir Physiol 25:295, 1975.

Philips PJ, Vendig AE, Jones PL, et al: Metabolic and cardiovascular side effects of the β-adrenoceptor agonists salbutamol and rimiterol. Br J Clin Pharmacol 9:483, 1980.

Potworoska M, Sianozeka E, Szufladowicz R: Ethionamide treatment and pregnancy. Pol Med J 5:1152, 1966.

Prowse CM, Gaensler EAL: Respiratory and acid base changes during pregnancy. Anaesthesiology 26:31, 1965.

Psacharopoulos HT, Howard ER, Portmann B, et al: Hepatic complications of cystic fibrosis. Lancet 2:78, 1981.

Raffin TA, Taylor JR, Ryu J, Colby TV: Treatment of lymphangiomyomatosis. N Engl J Med 325:63, 1991.

Raz S, Ziegler M, Caine M: The effect of progesterone on the adrenergic receptors of the urethra. Br J Urol 45:131, 1973.

Reisfield DR, Yahia C, Laurenz GA: Pregnancy and cardiorespiratory failure in Boeck's sarcoid. Surg Gynecol Obstet 109:412, 1969.

Ridgway LE, Martin RW, Hess LW, et al: Acute gestational pyelonephritis: The impact of colloid osmotic pressure plasma fibronectin, and arterial oxygen saturation. Am J Perinatol 8:222, 1991.

Rubin A, Russo N, Goucher D: The effect of pregnancy upon pulmonary function in normal women. Am J Obstet Gynecol 72:963, 1956.

Russell IF, Chambers WA: Closing volume in normal pregnancy. Br J Anaesth 53:1043, 1981.

Scadding JG: Prognosis of intrathoracic sarcoidosis in England: A review of 136 cases after five years' observation. Br Med J 2:1165, 1961.

Schatz M, Patterson R, Zietz S: Corticosteroid therapy for the pregnant asthmatic patient. JAMA 233:804, 1975.

Schenker JG, Ben-Yoseph Y, Shapira E: Erythrocyte carbonic anhydrase B levels during pregnancy and use of oral contraceptives. Obstet Gynaecol 39:237, 1972.

Schwachman H, Kulczyki LL: Long-term study of one hundred and five patients with cystic fibrosis. Am J Dis Child 96:6, 1958.

Scott DB: Mendelson's syndrome. (Editorial) Br J Anaesth 50:81, 1978.

Scott J, Higenbottam T, Hutter J, Hodson M, Steward S, Penketh A, Wallwork J: Heart-lung transplantation for cystic fibrosis. Lancet i:192, 1988.

Shanies HM: Noncardiogenic pulmonary edema. Med Clin North Am 61:1319, 1977.

Shen A, Iseman MD, Waldron JA, King TE: Exacerbation of pulmonary lymphangiomyomatosis by exogenous estrogens. Chest 5:782, 1991.

Siassi B, Moss AJ, Dooley RR: Clinical recognition of cor pulmonale in cystic fibrosis. J Pediatr 78:794, 1971.

Silverstein EF, Ellis K, Wolff M, Jaretzki A: Pulmonary lymphangiomyomatosis. Am J Roentgenol Rad Ther Nucl Med 120:833, 1974.

Sims CD, Chamberlain GVP, de Swiet M: Lung function tests in bronchial asthma during and after pregnancy. Br J Obstet Gynecol 88:434, 1976.

Skatrud JB, Dempsey JA, Kaiser DG: Ventilatory response to medroxy-progesterone acetate in normal subjects: Time course and mechanism. J Appl Physiol 44:939, 1978.

Smith APL: The effects of intravenous infusion of graded doses of prostaglandins $F_{2\alpha}$ and E_2 on lung resistance in patients undergoing termination of pregnancy. Clin Science 44:17, 1973.

Smith JL, Thomas F, Orme JF, Clemmer TP: Adult respiratory distress syndrome during pregnancy and immediately postpartum. West J Med 153:508, 1990.

Snider DE, Layde PM, Johnson MW, Lyle HA: Treatment of tuberculosis during pregnancy. Am Rev Respir Dis 122:65, 1980.

Snider DE: Pregnancy and tuberculosis. Chest 86:105, 1984.

Snyder RD, Snyder DL: Corticosteroids for asthma during pregnancy. Ann Allergy 41:340, 1978.

Sobrevilla LA, Cassinelli MT, Carcelen A, Malaga JW: Human fetal and maternal oxygen tension and acid-base status during delivery at high altitude. Am J Obstet Gynecol 111:111, 1971.

Sørensen KE, Børlum K: Fetal heart function in response to short-term maternal exercise. Br J Obstet Gynaecol 93:310, 1986.

Spector SL: The treatment of the asthmatic mother during pregnancy and lactation. Ann Allergy 51:173, 1983.

Spitzer WO, Suissa S, Ernst P, Horwitz RI, Habbick B, Cockcroft D, Boivin J, McNutt M, Buist AS, Rebuck AS: The use of β₂-agonists and the risk of death and near death from asthma. N Engl J Med 323:1254, 1992.

Stablein JF, Lockey RF: Managing asthma during pregnancy. Compre Ther 10:45, 1984.

Steen JSM, Stainton-Ellis DM: Rifampicin in pregnancy. Lancet 2:604, 1977.

Sutton FD, Zwillich CW, Creagh CE, et al: Progesterone for outpatient treatment of Pickwickian syndrome. Ann Intern Med 83:476, 1975.

Talbot SF, Main DM, Levinson AI: Wegener's granulomatosis: First report of a case with onset during pregnancy. Arthritis Rheum 27:109, 1984.

Taussig LM, Kattwinkel J, Friedwald WT, di Sant'Agnese PA: A new prognostic score and clinical evaluation system for cystic fibrosis. J Pediatr 82:380, 1973.

Taylor RJ, Ryu J, Colby TV, Raffin TA: Lymphangiomyomatosis—Clinical Course in 32 patients. N Engl J Med 323:1254–1260, 1990.

Templeton AA, Kelman GR: Maternal blood-gases, (PaO_2–PaO_2) physiological shunt and VD/VT in normal pregnancy. Br J Anaesth 48:1001, 1976.

Thomson KJ, Cohen ME: Studies on the circulation in normal pregnancy. II. Vital capacity observations in normal pregnant women. Surg Gynecol Obstet 66:591, 1938.

Toledo TM, Harper RC, Moser RM: Fetal effects during cyclophosphamide and radiation therapy. Ann Intern Med 74:87, 1971.

Towers GV, Kaminskas CM, Carite TJ, et al: Pulmonary injury associated with antepartum pyelonephritis: Can patients at risk be identified? Am J Obstet Gynecol 164:974, 1991.

Tyler JM: The effect of progesterone on the respiration of patients with emphysema and hypercapnia. J Clin Invest 39:34, 1960.

Ueland K, Novy MJ, Metcalfe J: Cardiorespiratory responses to pregnancy and exercise in normal women and patients with heart disease. Am J Obstet Gynecol **115**:4, 1973.

Van Arsdel PP Jr, Paul GH: Drug therapy in the management of asthma. Ann Intern Med **87**:68, 1977.

Wald NJ: Couple screening for cystic fibrosis. Lancet **338**:1318–1319, 1991.

Warrell DW, Taylor R: Outcome for the fetus of mother receiving prednisolone during pregnancy. Lancet **i**:117, 1968.

Warwick WJ, Progue RE, Gerber HM, Nesbitt CJ: Survival patterns in cystic fibrosis. J Chronic Dis **28**:609, 1975.

Wassermann K: Physiology of gas exchange and exertional dyspnoea. Clin Sci **61**:7, 1981.

Weinberger WE, Weiss ST, Cohen WR, et al: Pregnancy and the lung. Am Rev Respir Dis **121**:559, 1980.

Weinstein AM, Dubin BD, Podleski WK, et al: Asthma and pregnancy. JAMA **214**:1161, 1979.

Whalen JB, Clancey CJ, Farley DB, Van Orden DE: Plasma prostaglandins in pregnancy. Obstet Gynecol **51**:52, 1978.

White NW: Venous thrombosis and rifampicin. Lancet **ii**:434, 1989.

Whitlaw A, Butterfield A: High breast milk sodium in cystic fibrosis. Lancet **ii**:1288, 1977.

Wilbrand U, Porath CH, Matthaes P, Jaster R: Der einfluss der Ovarialsteroide auf die Funktion des Atemzentrums. Arch Gynkol **191**:507, 1959.

Wilson JW: Treatment or prevention of pulmonary cellular damage with pharmacological doses of corticosteroids. Surg Gynecol Obstet **134**:675, 1972.

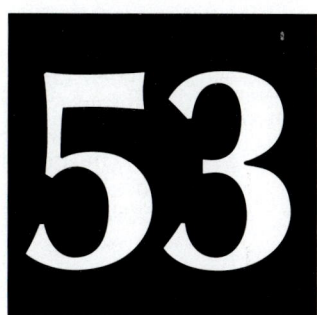

MATERNAL HEMATOLOGIC DISORDERS

RUSSELL K. LAROS, JR., M.D.

ABNORMALITIES OF THE RED AND WHITE BLOOD CELLS

Anemia

Definition

Anemia is usually defined as "hemoglobin (Hgb) value below the lower limits of normal not explained by the state of hydration." The normal hemoglobin level for the adult female is 14.0 ± 2.0 gm/dl (Laros, 1986; Thorup, 1987). The above definition has physiologic validity in that it is the amount of Hgb per unit volume of blood that determines the oxygen-carrying capacity of blood. Based on the aforementioned normal value, 20 to 60 per cent of prenatal patients will be found to be anemic at some time during their pregnancy. Some centers have chosen to use slightly lower Hgb values (11.0 or 10.5 gm/dl) to define anemia during pregnancy. Although this practice will decrease the number of gravidas found to be anemic, it does so by calling some mildly anemic patients normal and thus delaying additional hematologic evaluation. Such a decision is practical and appropriate as long as the practitioner remembers to obtain a follow-up hemogram to be sure that there is not a progression of the anemia.

Clinical Presentation

Symptoms due to anemia are those of tissue hypoxia, of the cardiovascular system's attempts to compensate for the anemia, and/or symptoms due to an underlying disease. Tissue hypoxia produces fatigue, lightheadedness, weakness, and exertional dyspnea. Cardiovascular compensation leads to a hyperdynamic circulation with the attendant symptoms of palpitations and tachycardia. Clinical situations commonly associated with anemia include multiple pregnancy, trophoblastic disease, chronic renal disease, arthritis, chronic liver disease, and chronic infection. However, in obstetric patients anemia is most commonly discovered because a complete blood count (CBC) is obtained as part of routine laboratory evaluation either at the initial prenatal visit or at repeat screening at 28 to 32 weeks gestation.

Additional history of value is the use of "tonics," a family history of anemia or splenectomy, a history of gastrointestinal bleeding and melena, genitourinary bleeding, and exposure to oxidant drugs in individuals at risk for glucose-6-phosphate dehydrogenase (G6PD) deficiency.

Utilization of the Complete Blood Count (CBC)

Anemia is not a diagnosis but rather a sign, as is fever or edema. The key issue in the evaluation of anemia is to define the mechanism or disease process. Although a mild anemia during pregnancy caused by iron deficiency is of little consequence to either the mother or the fetus, a similarly mild anemia caused by carcinoma of the colon has grave implications. One must also keep in mind the genetic implications of many anemias such as the hemoglobinopathies or hereditary spherocytosis.

Table 53–1 presents a classification of anemia based on the pathophysiologic mechanism involved. Although a mechanistic classification of anemia provides an exhaustive catalog of diagnoses, it does not lend itself to a systematic investigation of an individual patient (Horowitz and Laros, 1979). Rather, one wants to know: (1) Is the patient anemic? (2) What is the morphology of the anemia? (3) What is the reticulocyte count? Developing the answers to these questions allows one to make a first approximation of a specific diagnosis and answer the following questions: (1)What is the mechanism of the anemia? (2) Is there an underlying disease? (3) What is appropriate treatment?

The CBC and the reticulocyte count provide the answers to the first three questions and really represent the hematologist's "critical biopsy." These data allow a morphologic classification of the anemia and indicate whether the marrow is hyper- or hypoproliferative. Table 53–2 presents normal values for women. The Hgb is determined by converting the pigment to cyanmethemoglobin and quantitating the amount spectrophotometrically. The remainder of the values are obtained by flow cytometry with an electronic cell counter. Based on the size of the RBCs, anemia can be classified as microcytic, normocytic, or macrocytic. The appearance of the RBCs may also

TABLE 53—1. Anemia Classified by Pathophysiologic Mechanism

I. Dilutional (Expansion of the Plasma Volume)
  A. Pregnancy
  B. Hyperglobulinemia
  C. Massive splenomegaly
II. Decreased Red Blood Cell Production
  A. Bone marrow failure
    1. Decreased building blocks or stimulation
      a. Iron, protein
      b. Chronic infection, chronic renal disease
    2. Decreased erythron
      a. Hypoplasia (hereditary, drugs, radiation, toxins)
      b. Marrow replacement (tumor, fibrosis, infection)
  B. Ineffective production
    1. Megaloblastic (B_{12} and folate deficiency, myelodysplasia, erythroleukemia)
    2. Normoblastic (refractory anemia, thalassemia)
III. Increased Red Cell Loss
  A. Acute hemorrhage
  B. Hemolysis
    1. Intrinsic RBC disorders
      a. Hereditary
        (1) Hemoglobinopathies
        (2) RBC enzyme deficiency
        (3) Membrane defects
        (4) Porphyrias
      b. Acquired
        (1) Paroxysmal nocturnal hemoglobinuria
        (2) Lead poisoning
    2. Extrinsic RBC disorders
      a. Immune
      b. Mechanical
      c. Infection
      d. Chemical agents
      e. Burns
      f. Hypersplenism
      g. Liver disease

provide a clue to the mechanism of the anemia. For example, hypochromic microcytic cells associated with a low reticulocyte count suggest iron deficiency, thalassemia trait, sideroblastic anemia, or lead poisoning. Oval macrocytes combined with a low reticulocyte count and hypersegmented polymorphonuclear leukocytes suggest megaloblastic anemia (B_{12} or folate deficiency). Oval microcytes and an elevated reticulocyte count are characteristic of hereditary spherocyto-

sis. Various poikilocytes such as sickle cells, acanthrocytes, target cells, and schistocytes suggest sickle cell disease, acanthrocytosis, hemoglobin C disease, and mechanical RBC destruction, respectively.

The peripheral blood smear also allows evaluation of the white cells (WBCs). In most cases of leukemia, abnormal granulocytes or lymphocytes appear. The presence of nucleated RBCs in association with marked poikilocytosis suggests erythroleukemia, myeloid metaplasia, or marrow infiltration with solid tumor or granulomatous infection.

Additional Laboratory Studies

Although the CBC is an excellent first step in the approximate diagnosis of anemia, additional studies are usually necessary to confirm the diagnosis. Table 53–3 lists laboratory studies frequently used in the evaluation of an anemic patient. Serum Hgb and serum haptoglobin levels are useful in defining intravascular hemolysis. When a low or absent serum haptoglobin is associated with an elevated serum Hgb, the presence of intravascular hemolysis is established. Further studies are necessary to rule in or out specific causes of intravascular hemolysis, such as severe autoimmune hemolytic anemia (direct Coombs' test), paroxysmal nocturnal hemoglobinuria (osmotic fragility) and hemoglobinopathies such as sickle cell disease

TABLE 53–2. Normal Values for Red Blood Cells

Erythroid values	
Hemoglobin (Hgb)	12–16 gm/dl
Hematocrit (Hct)	36–41 ml/dl
Red cell count (RBC)	$4.0–5.2 \times 10^{12}/l$
Erythroid indices	
Mean corpuscular volume (MCV)	80–100 fl
Mean corpuscular hemoglobin concentration (MCHC)	31–36 gm/dl
Red cell morphology	
Anisocytosis	Variation in cell size
Poikilocytosis	Variation in cell shape
Polychromatophilia	Amount of "blueness"
Hypochromia	Amount of central pallor
Platelet estimate	5–10 platelets per oil immersion field
Reticulocyte count	$48–152 \times 10^9/l$
White blood cell count	$5–14 \times 10^9/l$

TABLE 53–3. Laboratory Studies Useful in Evaluation of Anemia

STUDY	NORMAL VALUE
Serum hemoglobin	<1.0 mg/dl
Serum haptoglobin	30–200 mg/dl
Total bilirubin	0.1–1.2 mg/dl
Direct Coombs' test	Negative
G6PD	
Electrophoresis	B+
	(A+, A−, B−, 150 others are abnormal)
Quantitative study	4–8 U/gm of Hgb
Hemoglobin electrophoresis	>98% A
	<3.5% A_2
	<2% F
RBC enzymes	Multiple types; pyruvate kinase most common
Osmotic fragility	Preincubation: 0.40–0.46% NaCl
	Postincubation: 0.48–0.60% NaCl
Serum ferritin	>10 µg/l
Free erythrocyte protoporphyrin (FEP)	<3.0 µg/gm
Plasma iron	40–175 µg/dl
Plasma total iron binding capacity	216–400 µg/dl
Transferrin saturation	16–60%
Stool guaiac	Negative
Folate level	
Serum	6–12 µg/l
RBC	165–760 ng/l
Serum B_{12}	190–950 ng/l
Anti-intrinsic factor antibody (AIF)	Negative
Bone marrow	Normal distribution of erythroid and myeloid precursors

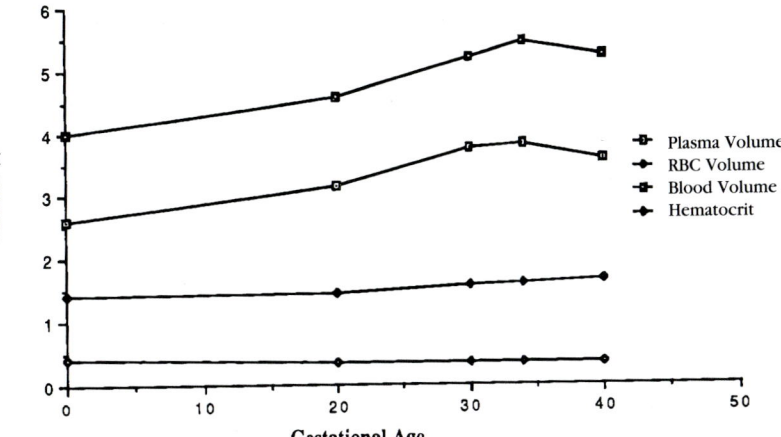

FIGURE 53–1. Hematologic changes during pregnancy. (Redrawn from Peck and Arias: Hematologic changes associated with pregnancy. Clin Obstet **22**:785, 1979.)

and thalassemia major (hemoglobin electrophoresis). The total bilirubin is elevated modestly in hemolytic anemia (rarely >4 mg/dl). The increase is due predominantly to an increase in the indirect fraction. However, significant hemolysis can occur without an elevation in the bilirubin. Thus the bilirubin level is helpful only when elevated. The direct Coombs' test uses antihuman globulin to detect globulins attached to the surface of RBCs. A positive test indicates an immune cause for a hemolytic anemia. In such cases it is important to search for underlying causes for autoimmunity such as connective tissue disease, lymphoma, carcinoma, and sarcoidosis. The diagnosis and management of G6PD and of the various hemoglobinopathies will be discussed later in this chapter.

The free erythrocyte protoporphyrin (FEP) (Schifman et al., 1987), plasma iron, plasma total iron binding capacity (Ho et al., 1987), and serum ferritin level (Foulkes and Goldie, 1982; Puolakka et al., 1980) are useful in establishing a diagnosis of iron deficiency. Iron is transported in the plasma bound to transferrin. In the iron-deficient state the plasma iron decreases, the iron binding capacity increases, and the per cent saturation decreases. In contrast, with chronic infection, both the plasma iron and the iron binding capacity are decreased and the per cent saturation remains normal. Serum ferritin correlates closely with body iron stores, and in the iron-deficient state the serum ferritin level is <20 μg/liter. Both the plasma iron and serum ferritin levels are increased following the ingestion of iron (Seligman et al., 1983; Taylor et al., 1982). Thus iron therapy must be discontinued for 24 to 48 hours before these studies are carried out. In iron deficiency the FEP increases approximately fivefold. It is still debatable which of the aforementioned studies is the most sensitive and specific for making the diagnosis of iron deficiency. Whenever a diagnosis of iron deficiency anemia is made, it is essential to rule out gastrointestinal bleeding as the cause for the iron deficit. This is accomplished by testing the stool for the presence of occult blood with guaiac or some other equally sensitive reagent.

Serum folate, RBC folate, and serum B_{12} levels are useful in defining the cause of macrocytic anemia. Because the RBC folate more accurately reflects the body's folate stores, many laboratories no longer offer the serum folate determination. The presence of serum intrinsic factor antibodies is specific for pernicious anemia. However, since they are absent in approximately 40 per cent of cases, the absence of these antibodies does not rule out a diagnosis of pernicious anemia.

Examination of the bone marrow by aspiration and/or biopsy can add much useful information. In addition to providing a ratio of myeloid to erythroid (M:E) production (normally approximately 3:1), it provides a measure of iron stores, allows a differential count of myeloid and erythroid precursors, provides evidence of infiltration with neoplasm, and allows histologic and bacteriologic confirmation of infection.

Normal Hematologic Events Associated with Pregnancy

Blood Volume Changes

During pregnancy there is normally a 36 per cent increase in the blood volume, the maximum being reached at 34 weeks gestation (Peck and Arias, 1979). The plasma volume increases 47 per cent and the RBC mass only 17 per cent. The latter reaches its maximum at term. As shown in Figure 53–1, there is relative hemodilution throughout pregnancy, and this reaches its maximum at 28 to 34 weeks. While this dilutional effect will lower the Hgb, Hct, and RBC count, it causes no change in the mean corpuscular volume (MCV) or in the mean corpuscular hemoglobin concentration (MCHC). Thus, serial evaluation of these two indices is useful in differentiating dilutional anemia from progressive iron deficiency anemia during pregnancy. In the former, the indices do not change; while in the latter, they decrease progressively.

Iron Kinetics

The classic study by Scott and Pritchard (1967) shows that iron stores in healthy women are marginal at best. They evaluated iron stores found in the bone marrow of healthy, white, college students who had never been pregnant and had never donated blood. Approximately two-thirds had minimal iron stores. In another study, Pritchard and colleagues (1969) demonstrated that almost 50 per cent of healthy primagravidas had minimal iron stores in their marrow during the first trimester of pregnancy.

The major reason for poor iron stores is thought to be menstrual loss. Monsen's data indicate that the usual menstrual loss is 25 to 30 ml whole blood (1967). This is equivalent to 12 to 15 mg elemental iron since each milliliter of blood contains 0.5 mg of iron. To meet the iron loss for menses alone, a woman requires that 1.5 to 2.0 mg elemental iron be absorbed from her diet each day. Because only 10 per cent of dietary iron is usually absorbed and the average diet contains only 6 mg per 1000 kilocalories, a woman's iron balance is precarious at best.

Pregnancy presents substantial demands on iron balance above and beyond what is saved by 9 months of amenorrhea (Pritchard et al., 1969). Table 53–4 lists the iron requirements for pregnancy. If there is insufficient iron available to meet the demands of pregnancy, iron-deficient erythropoiesis will result. Fenton and colleagues (1977) used the serum ferritin level to evaluate iron stores in pregnant women and found significantly higher ferritin levels in those receiving iron supplementation than in those who were not.

Thus most young women enter their first pregnancy with marginal iron stores. Pregnancy places a large demand on iron balance which cannot be met with the usual diet. In the absence of supplementation, iron deficiency develops. The usual sequence of events with iron deficiency is an absence of iron in the marrow followed by the development of abnormal plasma iron studies (transferrin, ferritin, or free red cell protoporphyrin). The RBCs first become microcytic, then hypochromic. Finally, anemia develops.

Folate

Folic acid is a water-soluble vitamin that is generally widely available in the diet. Dietary folates are in fact a family of compounds and generally appear as polyglutamates. In humans the only source of folate is the diet, and absorption is primarily in the proximal jejunum. Before folate can be absorbed it must be reduced to the monoglutamate form (Herbert et al., 1975). Pancreatic conjugases within the intestine are responsible for this process. The activity of conjugase is decreased by anticonvulsants, oral contraceptives, alcohol, and sulfa drugs (Shojania and Hornady,

1973). Thus, in addition to an absolute diminution in the dietary intake, the combination of increased need (as in multiple pregnancy and hemolytic anemia) and decreased absorption can lead to folate deficiency (Iyengar, 1975; Johan and Magnus, 1981; Pritchard et al., 1970).

During pregnancy there is a significant increase over the nonpregnant state requirement of 50 μg/day to 800 to 1000 μg/day (Kitay, 1969; Pritchard et al., 1969). When folate depletion occurs, the usual sequence of events is a decreased serum folate, hypersegmentation of polymorphonuclear leukocytes, a decrease in RBC folate, the appearance of ovalocytes in the blood, development of an abnormal marrow, and finally anemia (Herbert et al., 1975).

Women who have had a pregnancy resulting in a fetus with a neural tube defect should be advised to take additional folic acid before and during the early part of their next pregnancy. A dose of 4 mg per day of folic acid should be started at least 4 weeks before conception and continued through the first 3 months of pregnancy (CDC, 1991).

Vitamin B₁₂

Vitamin B_{12} is also abundantly available in the diet bound to animal protein. Absorption requires hydrochloric acid and pepsin to free the cobalamin molecule from protein. Intrinsic factor is also essential for absorption. Once absorbed, transport occurs by binding to transcobalamin II. Most of the vitamin B_{12} is stored in the liver, and most humans have a 2- to 3-year store available (Ho et al., 1987).

Morphologic Classification of Anemia

As already discussed, a CBC allows placement of a given case of anemia into one of three major groups based on size and hemoglobin content of the RBCs. The classification is augmented by the reticulocyte count, which adds information about the bone marrow's activity.

Microcytic Anemia

This group of anemias is characterized by abnormal Hgb synthesis with normal RBC production. A logical progression of diagnostic steps requires first that iron deficiency anemia be ruled out. If it is present, it is essential to consider whether or not chronic blood loss from the gastrointestinal or genitourinary tract is a factor in the etiology. When a microcytic anemia is not due to iron deficiency, one must then seek other causes such as hemoglobinopathy, chronic infection, or the various sideroblastic anemias. For this purpose, the following tests are indicated: plasma iron (PI) and iron binding capacity (TPIBC), FEP, hemoglobin electrophoresis, DNA probing for a-genes, and bone marrow examination. Anemia of chronic disorders is associated with a decreased PI and TPIBC and/or an elevated FEP. If the PI and TPIBC are normal or increased and/or the FEP is normal, one usually is dealing with thalassemia or a sideroblastic anemia.

TABLE 53–4.   Iron Requirements for Pregnancy

REQUIRED FOR	AVERAGE (mg)	RANGE (mg)
External iron loss	170	150–200
Expansion of RBC mass	450	200–600
Fetal iron	270	200–370
Iron in placenta and cord	90	30–170
Blood loss at delivery	150	90–310
Total requirement	980	580–1340
Requirement less RBC expansion	840	440–1050

Hemoglobin electrophoresis and DNA probes are used to define the thalassemias, and ring sideroblasts are present in the bone marrow of individuals with hereditary or acquired sideroblastic anemia.

Normocytic Anemia

Evaluation of normocytic anemia is the most difficult owing to the diverse nature of this group. The reticulocyte count varies depending on whether RBC production is increased, normal, or decreased. If erythropoiesis is increased, one must then differentiate between hemorrhage and an increased rate of destruction. The blood smear may reveal a type of RBC that is virtually diagnostic. Fragmented cells are seen in microangiopathic hemolysis (the HELLP syndrome of preeclampsia/eclampsia and thrombotic thrombocytopenic purpura) and in association with prosthetic heart valves. Other types of poikilocytes identified include sickle cells, target cells, stomatocytes, ovalocytes, spherocytes, elliptocytes, and acanthocytes.

The Coombs' test will differentiate immune from nonimmune causes of hemolysis. Immune hemolysis is related to alloantibodies, drug-induced antibodies, and autoantibodies. Nonimmune causes of hemolysis include various hemoglobinopathies, hereditary disorders of the RBC membrane (spherocytosis and elliptocytosis), hereditary deficiency of a RBC enzyme, and the porphyrias. Acquired, nonimmune hemolysis is due to either paroxysmal nocturnal hemoglobinuria or lead poisoning. Bone marrow examination is essential for the evaluation of patients with hypoproliferative anemias with normal iron studies. If erythropoiesis is megaloblastic, folate or B_{12} deficiency are likely causes. If sideroblastic, both acquired and hereditary forms of sideroblastic anemia must be considered. Finally, if erythropoiesis is normoblastic, etiologies fall into two major categories. The first group shows M:E ratios of >4:1 and includes aplasia, infiltration, effects of chronic diseases, and endocrine disorders such as hypothyroidism and hypopituitarism. In the second group, there is ineffective erythropoiesis, usually associated with an M:E ratio of <2:1.

Macrocytic Anemia

Macrocytic anemia is associated with either (1) an increased rate of RBC production and release of less than fully mature RBCs or (2) disorders of impaired DNA synthesis. Early use of a bone marrow examination is helpful in pointing the investigation in the correct direction. When maturation is megaloblastic, serum B_{12} and RBC folate levels will allow a diagnosis of B_{12} or folate deficiency. When folate deficiency is diagnosed, the various causes of decreased deconjugation of the polyglutamate and malabsorption must be considered. If anti-intrinsic factor antibodies are present, a diagnosis of pernicious anemia (PA) is assured. If absent, a Schilling test is required to differentiate between PA and a small bowel malabsorption syndrome.

Anemia and Perinatal Morbidity and Mortality

The Effects of Anemia

Although it has been traditionally taught that significant maternal anemia is associated with suboptimal fetal outcome, data supporting this concept are scarce. Several studies carried out in developing countries have compared fetal outcome in groups of women with hemoglobins above or below 6 to 7 gm/dl. Although these studies show improved reproductive function in women with higher hemoglobin levels, they do not control for protein malnutrition and chronic parasitic infestation.

Maternal anemia has been reported in association with placental gigantism (>900 gm) (Beischer et al., 1968a) and with low plasma estriol values (Beischer et al., 1968b). The study of Sagen et al. showed an inverse relation among placental weight, fetal weight, and maternal Hct (1984). These data are interpreted as evidence of chronic hypoxia. Studies in sheep show that fetal oxygen consumption is maintained until the maternal Hct is reduced by >50 per cent (Paulone et al., 1987). Furthermore, there are several anecdotal reports in which fetal distress noted in a fetal heart rate tracing was completely relieved by correction of maternal anemia. Thus, while profound maternal anemia can have adverse effects on the fetus, the margin of safety appears to be large.

The Effects of Specific Nutritional Defects

Fortunately, the fetal compartment preferentially obtains iron (Galbraith et al., 1980; Okuyama et al., 1985), folate, and B_{12} (Johan and Magnus, 1981) from and at the expense of the mother. In the study of Fenton et al. (1977), the cord blood ferritin levels of infants whose mothers were iron deficient were reduced below that of infants whose mothers were not iron deficient. However, the infants whose ferritins were low were not anemic and had normal iron kinetics, and their serum ferritin values were not in the iron-deficient range. In a study of newborns of women with severe folate deficiency, Pritchard and colleagues (1969) found normal neonatal levels of folate.

Genetic Implications

It is important to remember that many of the hemolytic anemias are inherited as either autosomal dominant or recessive traits. Thus, once the correct diagnosis has been made, the genetic implications should be thoroughly discussed with the patient and her partner. When appropriate, the discussion should include antenatal diagnosis.

Specific Anemias

Space does not allow a detailed discussion of the diagnosis and treatment of literally hundreds of different anemias. Instead, we have presented a scheme of diagnostic studies useful in evaluating any anemia and will limit discussion of specific anemias to only a few commonly seen during the course of pregnancy.

Iron Deficiency Anemia

Iron deficiency is among the most common causes of anemia in pregnant women. We have already discussed the demands placed on iron metabolism by both menstruation and pregnancy. Clinical symptoms include easy fatigue, lethargy, and headache. Pica involving clay, dirt, ice, or starch is a classic manifestation of iron deficiency. Clinical findings include pallor, glossitis, and cheilitis. Koilonychia has been associated with iron deficiency anemia but is a rare finding. The laboratory characteristics of iron deficiency anemia are a microcytic, hypochromic anemia with evidence of depleted iron stores. The plasma iron is low, the total iron binding capacity is high, the serum ferritin is low, and/or the FEP is elevated. If a bone marrow examination is done, stainable iron is markedly depleted or absent.

The specific treatment is oral iron, most commonly ferrous sulfate, 320 mg three times daily. Other iron preparations are more expensive and do not offer any advantage over ferrous sulfate if equal amounts of elemental iron are given. Reticulocytosis should be observed after 7 to 10 days of therapy, and the Hgb can rise by as much as one gram per week in severely anemic individuals. Absorption from the gastrointestinal tract can be enhanced by administration of 500 mg of ascorbic acid with each dose of iron. Gastrointestinal symptoms associated with iron therapy include nausea, vomiting, abdominal cramps, diarrhea, and constipation. These symptoms relate to the dose of elemental iron ingested, and if troublesome, the dose of iron should be reduced. Ferrous sulfate syrup is an effective way of tailoring the dose to the patient's tolerance. Once the anemia has resolved, the patient should continue to receive iron therapy for an additional 6 months in order to replace iron stores. Parenteral administration of iron dextran is rarely indicated and should be reserved for patients with a malabsorption syndrome or patients who absolutely will not take oral iron and who are significantly anemic (Hgb <8.5 gm/dl) (Hamstra et al., 1980). We prefer to administer the total calculated dose by the intravenous route. Because severe anaphylaxis can occur, a test dose should be administered first. In the absence of any reaction, the full dose can be administered at a maximum rate of 1 ml per minute. The required dose of iron dextran to correct anemia and replenish stores can be calculated as below.

Megaloblastic Anemia

Megaloblastic anemia is the second most common nutritional anemia seen during pregnancy. Most com-

monly folate deficiency is the etiology, but a deficiency in vitamin B_{12} also must be considered. Patients with folate deficiency present with the typical symptoms of anemia plus roughness of the skin and glossitis. The CBC reveals a macrocytic, normochromic (or normocytic, normochromic) anemia with hypersegmentation of the polymorphonuclear leukocytes. The reticulocyte count is normal or low, and the WBC and platelet count are frequently decreased. Bone marrow examination usually is not necessary for diagnosis, but if done, it shows megaloblastic erythropoiesis. The RBC folate is decreased to <165 μg/dl (serum folate <6 μg/l), and the vitamin B_{12} level is normal.

Treatment consists of the administration of oral folic acid in a dose of 1 mg three times daily. Parenteral folic acid may be indicated in individuals with malabsorption. A reticulocyte response should be seen in 48 to 72 hours, and the platelet count will normalize within a few days. The neutrophils will normalize after 1 to 2 weeks.

In addition to anemia, individuals with B_{12} deficiency may also manifest neurologic defects relating to damage to the posterior columns of the spinal cord. It is critical that individuals with B_{12} deficiency not be treated with folic acid alone. Such treatment may well improve the anemia but will have absolutely no salutary effect on the neuropathy and in fact may make it worse. As with folate deficiency, vitamin B_{12} deficiency is associated with either dietary deficiency or an increased requirement or both. Except in strict vegetarians who avoid all animal products, dietary deficiency is rare. The most common causes are inadequate production of intrinsic factor (PA), inadequate production of intrinsic factor after gastrectomy, or the presence of a malabsorption syndrome. The morphologic features of B_{12} deficiency are similar to those of folate deficiency. In this instance the serum B_{12} level is low and the folate normal. Because ineffective erythropoiesis is a prominent feature, evidence of low-grade hemolysis may be present (increased bilirubin and decreased haptoglobin) The Schilling test and measurement of anti-intrinsic factor antibodies are useful. Because the Schilling test requires ingestion of a radionuclide, its performance is not advised during pregnancy.

Treatment consists of 1000 μg of vitamin B_{12} administered parenterally weekly for 6 weeks followed by monthly administration for life in cases of PA. Again a prompt reticulocyte response is anticipated after 3 to 5 days of therapy.

Hereditary Spherocytosis and Elliptocytosis

Spherocytosis is the most common form of inherited hemolytic anemia. The inheritance is as an autosomal dominant trait with variable penetrance. The exact

$$\text{Iron dextran (ml)} = (14 - \text{patient's Hgb}) \times (\text{wt in kg}) \times (0.0476) + \frac{\text{wt in kg}}{5} \text{ [maximum 14]}$$

defect in the RBC leading to the anemia is unknown, but is most likely a structural defect in the cell wall. The classic characteristic is an increased RBC osmotic fragility. The prevalence of the gene is 2.2×10^{-4}, which should account for over 650 pregnancies annually in women with spherocytosis. A hemolytic crisis can be precipitated by many conditions such as infection, trauma, or pregnancy itself (Moore et al., 1976). A relationship between increased hemolysis and increased maternal blood volume and splenic blood flow has been suggested. An alternative suggestion is an increased osmotic fragility during the third trimester of pregnancy (Magid et al., 1982).

The diagnosis is suspected on the basis of family history and findings in the CBC and reticulocyte count that suggest a hyperproliferative anemia. Confirmation is obtained with the osmotic fragility test. Prenatal care of women with hereditary spherocytosis who have not had a splenectomy requires vigilance for hemolytic crisis and folate supplementation to ensure adequate marrow function (Maberry et al., 1992). A hemolytic crisis can be treated conservatively with replacement transfusions or with splenectomy. Splenectomy is mechanically difficult to accomplish during the third trimester of pregnancy unless preceded by cesarean section. In the absence of severe, untreated anemia, spherocytosis does not contribute to perinatal morbidity or mortality.

Hereditary elliptocytosis, also inherited as an autosomal dominant trait, is a milder hemolytic state also caused by a structural defect in the RBC wall. The signs and symptoms are similar to those of spherocytosis but not so severe. Most cases diagnosed during pregnancy have been successfully treated with supportive therapy alone (Breckenridge and Riggs, 1968).

Autoimmune Hemolytic Anemia

There are two major types of antibodies responsible for autoimmune hemolytic anemia (AIHA), warm-reactive and cold-reactive. Most warm-reactive antibodies are of the IgG class and are directed against some component of the Rh system on the surface of the red cell. In contrast, most cold-reactive antibodies are IgM and usually are specific for anti-I or anti-i. AIHA with warm-reactive antibodies is frequently seen in association with various hematologic malignancies (chronic lymphocytic leukemia, lymphoma), lupus erythematosus, viral infections, and drug ingestion. Penicillin, stibophen, and alpha-methyldopa all have been reported to cause AIHA. Cold-reacting antibodies can be seen in association with mycoplasma infections, infectious mononucleosis, and lymphoreticular neoplasms. Unfortunately, in a large number of cases no specific inciting event can be identified (Sacks et al., 1981). Diagnosis is suspected when a hyperproliferative, macrocytic anemia is identified. The stained smear of the peripheral blood often reveals microcytes, polychromatophilia, poikilocytosis, and the presence of normoblasts. Leukocytosis is frequently seen and is a result of marrow hyperactivity. The critical study to confirm the diagnosis is a positive direct Coombs' test.

Treatment of AIHA is directed toward both the hemolytic process and the underlying disease. Blood transfusion, corticosteroid therapy, immunosuppression and splenectomy are the most frequently used measures. In cases with warm-reactive antibodies, corticosteroid should be tried initially because approximately 80 per cent of patients will respond dramatically. Splenectomy is an effective form of treatment in approximately 60 per cent of patients with warm-reactive antibodies. If the patient is refractory to both corticosteroid therapy and splenectomy, a trial of immunosuppression is warranted. The treatment of cold-reactive antibodies depends on the severity of the hemolytic process. In patients with mild anemia, avoidance of cold temperatures is all that is required. Corticosteroid therapy and splenectomy usually are not effective if the majority of RBC breakdown occurs intravascularly. In patients with severe anemia, a trial of immunosuppression or plasmapheresis should be considered.

Enzymopathies: G6PD Deficiency and Others

More than 20 different hereditary red cell enzyme defects have been described, most with an associated hemolytic anemia. Of these, only G6PD deficiency occurs with more than occasional frequency. The genetic locus controlling G6PD synthesis is on the X chromosome, and males with an abnormal gene may suffer hemolysis, especially if exposed to oxidant drugs that stress the pentose phosphate pathway of the erythrocyte; female heterozygotes are generally clinically unaffected by similar exposure. The G6PD activity of the red cells of heterozygous females is usually intermediate between that of hemizygous males and that of normal subjects. Some female carriers, however, have normal G6PD activity while others have activity that falls within the range in affected males. It has been proposed that this is consistent with the Lyon hypothesis: one of the two X chromosomes of every female cell is randomly inactivated in early embryonic life and continues to be inactive throughout all cell divisions (Beutler, 1991). Thus a few heterozygous women will be severely deficient, but most will have enough G6PD activity to withstand added stress on this critical metabolic pathway in erythrocytes.

The ethnic groups in which variants of the deficiency occur with greatest frequency are blacks, Mediterranean peoples, Sephardic and Oriental Jews, and selected Asian populations. Twelve per cent of black males in the United States are reported to be deficient. Most affected individuals are hematologically normal unless exposed to certain drugs, chemicals, metabolic disturbances, or infections that precipitate an acute hemolytic episode. Most affected US blacks carry a variant with these properties. Their hemolytic episodes are relatively mild. Greeks, Sardinians, and Sephardic Jews are more likely to carry G6PD Mediterranean, in which hemolysis is characteristically more severe, and favism (hemolysis induced by ingestion of fava beans) occurs. G6PD-deficient American blacks have not been reported to experience favism.

It is relatively unusual for a pregnant woman to experience severe difficulty because of G6PD deficiency. However, Silverstein and associates (1974) reported a Hct of less than 30 per cent in 62 per cent of 180 G6PD-deficient women. Prudence would argue against exposure of a known carrier to precipitants of hemolysis. Sulfonamides, sulfones, some antimalarials, nitrofurans, naphthalene, probenecid, para-aminosalicylic acid-isoniazid, and nalidixic acid are among the medications and commonly occurring environmental chemicals known to precipitate red cell destruction.

One report has suggested an increased incidence of low-birth-weight infants born to G6PD-deficient mothers, but no correction for the effects of anemia or urinary tract infection was made (Perkins, 1976). Affected male infants born of carrier females have a higher incidence of neonatal hyperbilirubinemia—sometimes severe—than normal infants, and careful observation of those at risk is strongly advised. The incidence of severe jaundice in deficient newborn males is approximately 5 per cent, rising to 50 per cent if there is a history of a prior icteric sibling. Occasionally hemolysis has also been reported in breast-fed infants whose mothers have eaten fava beans or have been exposed to an oxidant. The neonatal manifestations of G6PD deficiency and other enzymopathies have been reviewed by Matthay and Mentzer (1981).

If a hemolytic episode should occur during pregnancy because of G6PD deficiency in a female heterozygote (or the very rare homozygote), management should include prompt discontinuation of any medication or other agent that may be responsible, treatment of any intercurrent illness, and, if clinically indicated, transfusion support. In patients with the variant common in US blacks, the G6PD activity of young red cells is, even in the male hemizygote, much higher than in cells that have circulated for weeks and months. Old cells may be totally devoid of activity. Hence the hemolytic episode recognized early is generally relatively mild and can be limited to the oldest population of circulating red cells if the inciting agent is eliminated.

Aplastic and Hypoplastic Anemia

Aplastic anemia is characterized by a reduction in the number of circulating RBCs, neutrophils, and platelets, and by the presence of a hypocellular bone marrow. Three mechanisms have been postulated to explain the development of aplastic anemia: (1) insufficient stem cells either because of an intrinsic defect or a reduction in number after exposure to some noxious agent; (2) the presence of some suppressor substance that inhibits the maturation of the myeloid precursors; and (3) the development of autoimmune reaction that causes death of the stem cells. Such agents as benzene, ionizing radiation, nitrogen mustard, antimetabolites, antimitotic agents, certain antibiotics, and toxic chemicals predictably lead to marrow aplasia. In another category are agents such as chloramphenicol, anticonvulsants, analgesics, and gold salts, which induce aplasia only in an occasional patient. Finally, there are literally hundreds of agents of various types that have been implicated in several cases as causes of aplastic anemia. Unfortunately, in about half the cases, careful search does not reveal any causative agent.

In 1953, Holly described eight patients with hypoplastic anemia diagnosed during pregnancy that remitted spontaneously after delivery. The bone marrow was described as hypocellular with an increase in megakaryocytes. To date, approximately 80 cases have been reported (Fleming, 1973; Snyder et al., 1991). However, these cases present a spectrum of clinical and bone marrow findings that make it difficult to substantiate that a hypoplastic anemia specifically related to pregnancy does in fact exist. Support for such a hypothesis is found only in those cases in which recovery occurred after delivery, an entirely normal marrow is documented between pregnancies, and relapse occurs with a subsequent pregnancy. Patients with aplastic anemia seek medical attention because of symptoms relating to profound anemia, bleeding, or infection. The CBC reveals pancytopenia with a hypoproliferative reticulocyte count. Examination of the bone marrow reveals hypoplasia with normoblastic erythropoiesis. Severe aplastic anemia is fatal for more than 50 per cent of affected patients (Lynch et al., 1975). Bone marrow transplantation is now the treatment of choice, and long-term survival of 50 to 70 per cent can be expected. Several survivors have had successful pregnancies following transplantation (Deeg et al., 1983; Schmidt et al., 1987; Doney et al., 1985). During pregnancy, supportive therapy remains the major objective. In recent years, with modern supportive therapy, the maternal mortality rate has been only 15 per cent and more than 90 per cent of patients survive in remission.

Treatment consists of maintenance of Hbg levels by periodic transfusion, prevention and treatment of infection, stimulation of hematopoiesis with androgens, splenectomy, therapeutic abortion and premature delivery, intravenous gamma globulin and marrow transplantation (McGuire et al., 1987). Androgen therapy can be effective at stimulating erythropoiesis. However, androgens are contraindicated during pregnancy unless the fetus is demonstrated to be male. Agents commonly used include fluoxymesterone (0.25 mg/kg per day), oxymetholone (3 to 5 mg/kg per day), nandrolone decanoate (3 to 4 mg/kg weekly), or testosterone ethanate (1 to 3 mg/kg per week). Adrenocorticosteroids have also been widely used with some benefit. Unfortunately, the remission rate with steroids is only 12 per cent. Bone marrow transplantation is now the treatment of choice for patients with severe aplastic anemia. Another therapy that shows promise is administration of anti-human thymocyte globulin. Unfortunately, neither of these modalities can be used safely during pregnancy.

Because of the anecdotal reports of complete remission following pregnancy termination, it is tempting to consider therapeutic abortion. However, thorough examination of the available literature indicates that abortion or premature termination of pregnancy is not associated with a more favorable outcome. The only reason to terminate pregnancy prematurely is the inability to support the patient satisfactorily with transfusion alone and thus the need to proceed to either marrow transplantation or antithymocyte globulin therapy.

Paroxysmal nocturnal hemoglobinuria (PNH) hemolysis occurs due to an unexplained structural defect in the RBC. There are distinct cohorts of long-lived and short-lived cells. The inherent defect makes the RBCs unusually susceptible to lysis by complement. PNH usually begins insidiously; there is no familial tendency. Considerable variability exists in severity of the disease, and the classic presentation of hemoglobinuria is seen in only 25 per cent of patients. Exacerbations of the hemolytic process are precipitated by infection, menstruation, transfusion, surgery, and ingestion of iron. The most serious complications are marrow aplasia, thrombosis, and infection. Thrombosis accounts for 50 per cent of deaths and is of particular concern during pregnancy. Although anemia is the most prominent hematologic feature of PNH, leukopenia and thrombocytopenia also occur frequently. The diagnosis of PNH is based on a series of special tests that demonstrate the sensitivity of the patient's RBCs to complement.

The ideal treatment for PNH is replacement of the abnormal stem cell with cells capable of producing the normal cellular components. This has been accomplished by bone marrow transplantation. The major therapeutic modalities during pregnancy are iron therapy, androgen treatment if the fetus is male, corticosteroids, and transfusions (Frakes et al., 1976; Hurd et al., 1982; Solal-Celigny et al., 1988). Iron can be administered orally to replace the considerable amount lost in the urine. Unfortunately, in significantly iron-deficient patients, such treatment may lead to a burst of erythropoiesis with delivery of a cohort of cells susceptible to the lytic action of complement. If a hemolytic episode follows iron therapy, it should be treated with either suppression of erythropoiesis by transfusion or suppression of hemolysis with corticosteroids. Prednisone in a dose of 1 mg/kg per day is an effective regimen.

When acute hemolytic episodes occur, treatment is aimed at diminishing hemolysis and preventing complications. Because patients with PNH have frequent episodes of venous thrombosis, this must be watched for carefully. In cases of acute deep venous thromboses, anticoagulation should be begun. Care must be taken in the use of heparin as hemolytic episodes clearly can be related to its use. During pregnancy, heparin is the anticoagulant of choice; however, during the puerperium or nonpregnant state, warfarin is preferred. Only a few pregnancies have been reported in women with PNH, and both spontaneous abortion and thrombotic events appear to be increased in frequency.

Hemoglobinopathies

Our understanding of the molecular genetics of the hemoglobinopathies and the ability to make specific diagnoses have evolved rapidly over the past three decades (Bunn and Forget, 1986; Weatherall and Clegg,. 1981; Steinberg and Adams, 1982). The hemoglobinopathies can be broadly divided into two general types. In the thalassemia syndromes, normal hemoglobin is synthesized at an abnormally slow rate.

In contrast, the structural hemoglobinopathies occur because of a specific change in the amino acid content of hemoglobin. These structural changes may have either no effect or profound effects on the function of hemoglobin, including instability of the molecule, reduced solubility, methemoglobinemia, and increased or decreased oxygen affinity.

Thalassemia Syndromes

The thalassemia syndromes are named and classified by the type of chain that is inadequately produced. The two most common are α- and β-thalassemia, both of which affect the synthesis of hemoglobin A. Reduced synthesis of γ or δ chains and combinations in which two or more globin chains are affected are relatively rare. In each instance, the thalassemia is a quantitative disorder of globin synthesis.

α-Thalassemia

In α-thalassemia, one or more structural genes are physically absent from the genome. The various α-thalassemia genotypes are summarized in Figure 53–2. In blacks, the most common two-gene deletion state consists of one gene missing on each chromosome. However, in Asians most commonly both genes are missing from the same chromosome. In the homozygous stage, all four genes are deleted and no chains are produced. Thus the fetus is unable to synthesize normal hemoglobin F or any adult hemoglobins. This deficiency results in high-output cardiac failure, hydrops fetalis, and stillbirth (Higgs et al., 1989).

The most severe form of α-thalassemia compatible with extrauterine life is hemoglobin H disease, which results from deletion of three α genes. In these patients, abnormally high quantities of both hemoglobin H (β_4) and hemoglobin Barts (γ_4) accumulate. Because hemoglobin H precipitates within the red cell, the cell is removed by the reticuloendothelial system, leading to a moderately severe hemolytic anemia.

In α-thalassemia minor (α-thalassemia 1) two genes are deleted, leading to a mild, hypochromic, microcytic anemia that must be differentiated from iron deficiency. A single gene deletion (α-thalassemia 2) is clinically undetectable and is called the "silent carrier" state. Thus, the α-thalassemia trait presents in the adult as mild, hypochromic, microcytic anemia. Diagnosis is presumptive by exclusion of iron deficiency and β-thalassemia. Although α-thalassemia trait does not present a hazard to the adult, it does have serious genetic implications when a mating of two individuals with the trait occurs. Under these circumstances, a specific diagnosis must be made using restriction endonuclease techniques or a DNA probe before undertaking antenatal diagnosis (Miller, 1982; Kan et al., 1976).

β-Thalassemia

In β-thalassemia no gene deletions have been demonstrated. The best evidence to date suggests that underproduction of beta globulin chains is caused by a quantitative reduction in messenger RNA leading to

GENOTYPE

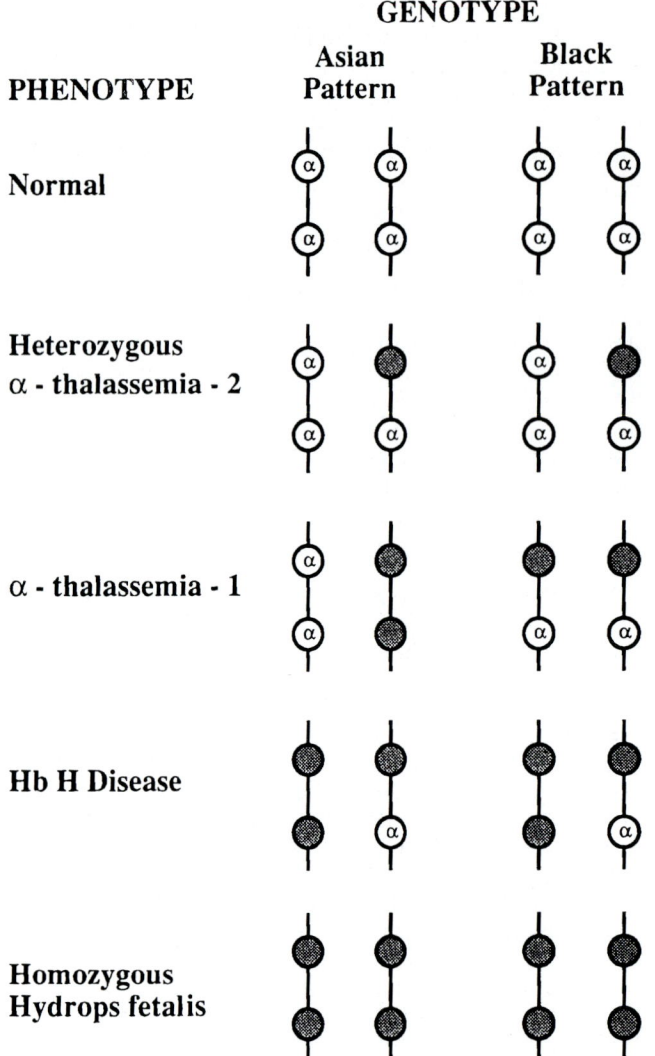

FIGURE 53–2. Genotypes of the various α-thalassemia syndromes.

eral smear resembling iron deficiency. Hemoglobin electrophoresis characteristically shows an elevation of hemoglobin A_2. β-Thalassemia trait does not impair fertility, and the incidence of prematurity, low-birth-weight infants, and infants of abnormal size for gestational age are identical to those in normal women (Alger et al., 1979; Fleming and Lynch, 1967). The clinical characteristics and hematologic findings of the various thalassemias are summarized in Table 53–5.

Again, the mating of two individuals who are heterozygous for β-thalassemia is an indication for antenatal diagnosis. A detailed program of prenatal identification and antenatal diagnosis has been described by Alger and associates (1979).

Structural Hemoglobinopathies

To date several hundred variants of α, β, γ, and δ chains have been identified. Most differ from normal chains by only one amino acid. The nomenclature and frequency of the most common hemoglobinopathies in American blacks are depicted in Table 53–6 (Motulsky, 1973). Diagnosis of a specific hemoglobinopathy requires identification of the abnormal hemoglobin by means of hemoglobin electrophoresis.

Sickle Cell Trait

Women with sickle cell trait do well during pregnancy and labor, but caution must be observed in the use of anesthesia, to ensure good oxygenation. Because there is a twofold increase in the rate of urinary tract infection, prenatal patients should be screened for asymptomatic bacteriuria (Whalley et al., 1963; Blattner et al., 1977; Whalley et al., 1964). These patients may become iron deficient, and supplementation during pregnancy is indicated.

Sickle Cell Anemia

Patients with sickle cell anemia (SCA) suffer from lifelong complications in part caused by the markedly shortened life span of their red blood cells. Most observers believe that the pre-pregnancy course of a women is a good index of how she will fare during pregnancy. Although series reported before 1979 indicated a high perinatal mortality and incidence of infants weighing less than 2500 gm (Horger, 1972; Pritchard et al., 1973), recent series showed generally good fetal outcomes (Morrison and Wiser, 1976; Cunningham et al., 1983).

Virtually all of the signs and symptoms of SCA are secondary to hemolysis, vaso-occlusive disease, or an increased susceptibility to infection (Table 53–7). Clinical manifestations may affect growth and development, with growth restriction and skeletal changes secondary to expansion of the marrow cavity. Painful crises may occur in the long bones, abdomen, chest, or back. The cardiovascular manifestations are those of a hyperdynamic circulation, and pulmonary signs may be secondary to either infection or vaso-occlusion. In addition to painful vaso-occlusive episodes, patients may exhibit hepatomegaly, signs and symptoms of hepatitis, cholecystitis, and painful splenic infarcts.

a decreased rate of transcription. In the homozygous β-thalassemia condition, α chain production is unimpeded, and these highly unstable chains accumulate and eventually precipitate. Markedly ineffective erythropoiesis and severe hemolysis result in a condition known as thalassemia major or Cooley's anemia. The fetus is protected from severe disease by α chain production. However, this protection disappears rapidly after birth, with the affected infant becoming anemic by 3 to 6 months of age. The infant has splenomegaly and requires blood transfusions every 3 to 4 weeks. Death generally occurs by the third decade of life and is usually secondary to myocardial hemochromatosis. Those female infants surviving until puberty are usually amenorrheic with severely impaired fertility (Kazazian and Boehm, 1988; Fosburg and Nathan, 1990).

β-thalassemia minor results in a variable degree of illness depending on the rate of β chain production. The characteristic findings include a relatively high RBC, moderate to marked microcytosis, and a periph-

TABLE 53–5. Hematologic and Clinical Aspects of the Thalassemia Syndromes

| CONDITION | HEMOGLOBIN (Hb) PATTERN* | | | | CLINICAL SEVERITY |
	HB LEVEL	HB A$_2$	HB F	OTHER HB	
Homozygotes					
α-thalassemia	↓↓↓↓	0	0	80% Hb Barts, remainder Hb H and Hb Portland Some Hb A	Hydrops fetalis
β$^+$-thalassemia	↓↓↓	variable	↑↑	Some Hb A	Moderately severe Cooley's anemia
β^0-thalassemia	↓↓↓↓	variable	↑↑↑	No Hb A	Severe Cooley's anemia
δβ^0-thalassemia	↓↓	0	100%	No Hb A	Thalassemia intermedia
Heterozygotes					
α-thalassemia silent carrier	N	N	N	1–2% Hb Barts in cord blood at birth	N
α-thalassemia trait	↓	N	N	5% Hb Barts in cord blood at birth	Very mild
Hb H disease	↓↓	N	N	4–30% Hb H in adults; 25% Hb Barts in cord blood	Thalassemia intermedia
β$^+$-thalassemia	↓ to ↓↓	↑	↑	None	Mild
β^0-thalassemia	↓ to ↓↓	↓	↑↑↑	None	Mild

* ↑ = increased; ↓ = decrease. Number of arrows indicates relative intensity; N = normal.

Genitourinary signs include hyposthenuria, hematuria, and pyelonephritis.

Treatment for patients with SCA has been largely symptomatic, with the major objective being to end a painful crisis and combat infection. Urinary tract and pulmonary infections should be promptly diagnosed and vigorously treated with appropriate antibiotics. During the third trimester, fetal surveillance with either non-stress or stress tests should be carried out regularly. Transfusion therapy has been used widely for years in the treatment of symptomatic patients with SCA. More recently, partial exchange transfusions and/or prophylactic transfusions have been advocated (Cunningham et al., 1979; Francis and Johnson, 1991). The transfusion protocol utilized at the our institution is outlined in Table 53–8. The objective of the partial exchange transfusion is to achieve a hematocrit of >35 per cent and a hemoglobin A level of >40 per cent. Exchange transfusion is repeated when the hematocrit falls to less than 25 per cent or the hemoglobin A level to less than 20 per cent, or when crisis or labor occurs.

A prospective, randomized study of 72 patients with SCA showed no significant difference in perinatal outcome between women treated with prophylactic transfusion and those transfused only if their hemoglobin fell below 6 gm/dl or hematocrit below 18 per cent (Koshy et al., 1988). Sixty-six patients with sickle cell–hemoglobin C disease and 23 with sickle cell–β-

thalassemia were only transfused for hematologic reasons and experienced similar perinatal outcomes. Prophylactic transfusion significantly reduced the incidence of painful crises and other sickle cell disease–related complications. However, the benefits attained must be balanced against a 25 per cent incidence of

TABLE 53–7. Clinical Manifestations of Sickle Cell Anemia

I. Growth and Development
  A. Retarded growth
  B. Skeletal changes
  C. Decreased life span
II. Sickle Cell Crisis
  A. Painful vaso-occlusive episode: bones, abdomen, chest, and back.
III. Cardiovascular manifestations of hyperdynamic circulation
  A. Cardiomegaly
  B. Systolic murmurs
  C. Failure
IV. Pulmonary Signs
  A. Infection—pneumococcal, mycoplasma, hemophilus, salmonella
  B. Vascular occlusion
V. Abdominal Involvement
  A. Painful vaso-occlusive episodes
  B. Hepatomegaly
  C. Hepatitis
  D. Cholecystitis
  E. Splenic infarction
VI. Bone and Joint Changes
  A. Bone marrow infarction
  B. Osteomyelitis—salmonella
  C. Arthritis
VII. Genitourinary Signs
  A. Hyposthenuria
  B. Hematuria
  C. Pyelonephritis
VIII. Neurologic Manifestations
  A. Vascular occlusion
  B. Convulsions
  C. Hemorrhage
  D. Visual disturbances
IX. Ocular Manifestations
  A. Conjunctival vessel changes
  B. Vitreous hemorrhage

TABLE 53–6. Nomenclature and Frequency of the Most Common Hemoglobinopathies in Adult US Blacks

HEMOGLOBINOPATHY	ABBREVIATED NAME	FREQUENCY
Sickle cell trait	Hb SA	1:122
Sickle cell anemia	Hb SS	1:708
Sickle cell–hemoglobin C disease	Hb SC	1:757
Hemoglobin C disease	Hb CC	1:4790
Hemoglobin C trait	Hb CA	1:41
Hemoglobin S–β-thalassemia	Hb S–β-thal	1:1672
Hemoglobin S–high F	Hb S-HPFH	1:3412

TABLE 53–8. Protocol for Partial Exchange Transfusion

I. Begin: at 24–28 weeks of gestation
II. Baseline laboratory studies
   A. Hb, Hct, WBC, reticulocyte count
   B. Hb electrophoresis
III. Type and crossmatch blood: 4 units of fresh, buffy coat–poor, Hb S–free, washed, packed RBCs
IV. Exchange
   A. In morning
     1. Infuse 500 ml crystalloid over 1–2 h
     2. Remove 500 ml by phlebotomy over same time period
     3. Infuse 2 units of packed RBCs over 1–2 h
   B. In afternoon: Repeat morning procedure
V. Repeat laboratory evaluation following morning
   A. Hb, Hct
   B. Hb electrophoresis
VI. Additional exchange (2–4 units) if
   A. Hct <35%
   or
   B. Hb A level <40%

Hb = hemoglobin; Hct = hematocrit; WBC = white blood cell count; RBC = red blood cell.

alloimmunization and 20 per cent delayed transfusion reaction.

During labor and delivery, care must be taken to be sure that the patient is well oxygenated and well hydrated. Anesthesia-related hypovolemia and/or hypoxia is contraindicated. In an untransfused patient regional anesthesia should be administered with great caution (Maduska et al., 1975; Finer et al., 1988). Careful fetal monitoring should be carried out throughout labor. However, if an exchange transfusion protocol has been utilized and the hemoglobin A level is >40 per cent, painful crises are distinctly unusual (Morrison et al., 1978).

Hemoglobin SC Disease

Women who are doubly heterozygous for both the hemoglobin S and the hemoglobin C genes are said to have hemoglobin SC disease (Hgb SCD). Hemoglobin electrophoresis reveals approximately 60 per cent hemoglobin C and 40 per cent hemoglobin S. Patients with Hgb SCD generally have a normal habitus, a healthy childhood, and a normal life span. If a systematic screening program has not been utilized, many women are first diagnosed during the latter part of pregnancy when a complication occurs. At the beginning of pregnancy, most women are mildly anemic and splenomegaly is present. Examination of a peripheral blood smear will show numerous target cells. Hemoglobin electrophoresis will ensure the correct diagnosis (Laros, 1967; Maberry et al., 1990).

During pregnancy, 40 to 60 per cent of patients with Hb SCD will behave as if they had SCA. In contrast to patients with SCA, they frequently experience rapid and severe anemic crises due to splenic sequestration. Also, they have a greater tendency to experience bone marrow necrosis with the release of fat-forming marrow emboli. The clinical manifestations of Hb SCD are otherwise similar to SCA but milder. The general management of symptomatic patients with Hb SCD is identical to that for patients with SCA. Although

several authors have reported good results with vigorous transfusion protocols for all patients with Hb SCD, I have reserved exchange transfusion for those patients who are symptomatic or whose hematocrit is <25 per cent. Considerations for the management of labor are the same as with SCA.

Hemoglobin S–β-thalassemia

In this condition the patient is heterozygous for the sickle cell and the β-thalassemia gene. In addition to decreased β chain production, there is a variably increased production of hemoglobin F and hemoglobin A_2. Because of this variable production rate, hemoglobin electrophoresis reveals a spectrum of hemoglobin concentrations. Hemoglobin S may account for 70 to 95 per cent of the hemoglobin present, with hemoglobin F rarely exceeding 20 per cent (Laros and Kalstone, 1971). Because of the thalassemia influence, hemoglobin S concentration exceeds hemoglobin A concentration. This is in sharp contrast to patients with sickle cell trait, in whom hemoglobin A levels exceed the concentration of hemoglobin S.

The diagnosis is made in an anemic patient by demonstrating increased hemoglobin A_2 and hemoglobin F levels in association with a level of hemoglobin S exceeding that of hemoglobin A. The peripheral smear reveals hypochromia and microcytosis with anisocytosis, poikilocytosis, basophilic stippling, and target cells. The clinical manifestations of this disorder parallel those of SCA but are generally milder. Painful crises may occur; however, these patients have a normal body habitus and frequently enjoy an uncompromised life span. I believe that the role of exchange transfusion should be similar to that in patients with Hb SCD; that is, exchange transfusion is reserved for the woman who experiences painful crises or whose anemia leads to a hematocrit of <25 per cent.

Hemoglobin C Trait and Disease

Hemoglobin C trait is an asymptomatic trait without reproductive consequences. Target cells are found in the peripheral smear, but anemia is not present. Hemoglobin C disease is the homozygous state and is a mild disorder usually discovered during a medical evaluation. Mild hemolytic anemia with a hematocrit in the range of 25 to 35 per cent is characteristic. The red blood cells show microspherocytes and characteristic targeting. There is no increased morbidity or mortality associated with pregnancy, and no specific therapy is indicated.

Hemoglobin E Disease

The recent resettlement of persons of Southeast Asian extraction has resulted in an increase in the number with hemoglobin E trait and disease. The clinical and laboratory manifestations of the various hemoglobin E syndromes are outlined in Table 53–9 (Wong and Ali, 1982; Ferguson and O'Reilly, 1985). Most individuals have a mild, microcytic anemia that is of no clinical significance and requires no treatment. Those peoples homozygous for hemoglobin E have a

TABLE 53-9. Various Genotypes of Hemoglobin E and Their Phenotypic Expression

| GENOTYPE | DEGREE OF ANEMIA* | MCV† | ELECTROPHORESIS (%) | | | | PHENOTYPE EXPRESSION |
			A + A₂	E	F	S	
A/E	0	↓	68	30	<2	0	None
E/E	0 to +	↓↓	<4	94	<2	0	None
E/α-thal	+ to + +	↓	50	15	35	0	None
S/E	+ +	↓	0	40	0	60	None
E/β⁺-thal	+ +	↓↓	10	60	30	0	Splenomegaly
E/β⁰-thal	+ + +	↓↓	0	60	40	0	Splenomegaly

*Number of + symbols indicates relative severity.
†MCV = mean corpuscular volume; number of arrows indicates relative amount of decrease.

greater degree of microcytosis and are frequently anemic. Target cells are prominent. As with hemoglobin C trait and disease, no specific therapy is required and reproductive outcome is normal.

Anemias Associated with Systemic Disease

The normal bone marrow has the capacity to increase its red cell production six- to eightfold in response to anemia. This compensatory mechanism, responsible also for the increase in red cell mass in normal pregnancy, is triggered by tissue hypoxia and mediated by erythropoietin. The response may be absent or blunted in some circumstances, most commonly in chronic disorders. Chronic infections, rheumatoid arthritis, and other inflammatory states are characterized by a mild normocytic, normochromic (or sometimes hypochromic, microcytic) anemia with low serum iron concentration, low transferrin level, inappropriately low reticulocyte count and generous but poorly utilized stores of reticuloendothelial iron. Although the bone marrow is normally cellular, it fails to respond appropriately to the mildly accelerated red cell destruction typical of chronic inflammation. Studies thus far have failed to establish conclusively whether or not the defect in erythropoiesis can be attributed to inadequate erythropoietin secretion. In the absence of pregnancy, the hemoglobin is, in these chronic states, frequently 9 to 10 gm/100 ml and the hematocrit about 30 per cent. The hydremia of pregnancy may lower these values somewhat.

A similar but frequently more complicated anemia accompanies renal failure. Here, more often perhaps than in chronic inflammatory states, blood loss and hemolysis are contributory factors, and the serum iron and transferrin changes noted previously are less regular. In many of these situations, diminished erythropoietin is important in the pathogenesis.

Renal failure and chronic inflammation are rare in pregnancy, so that management of the associated anemias is seldom a clinical problem in obstetric patients. Occasionally, however, it is the anemia that calls attention to the underlying disease. These anemias do not respond to hematinics or steroid hormones (unless the adrenal steroids play some role in controlling the underlying disease, as in rheumatoid arthritis or lupus). Erythropoietin is useful in treating patients with chronic renal disease and can often obviate repeated RBC transfusion (Erslev, 1991)

Neutropenia and Agranulocytosis

White Blood Cells

Pregnancy is associated with an increase in the neutrophilia count beginning during the second month. The total WBC increases because of this increase in neutrophils. The neutrophilia begins in the first trimester and reaches a plateau in the second or third trimester, when total counts usually range between 9 and 15 × 10⁹ cells per liter. Kuvin and Brecher (1962) reported that 20 per cent of their group of 88 normal pregnant women had total counts greater than 10.0 × 10⁹ cells per liter. One-quarter of those with these higher counts had occasional myelocytes and metamyelocytes on peripheral blood smears. A similar proportion of those with total counts less than 10.0 × 10⁹ cells per liter also had these immature forms in their peripheral blood. The authors concluded that this left shift is a common occurrence in normal pregnancy. If the normal pregnant woman should develop any complicating illness usually associated with a polymorphonuclear leukocytosis (i.e, a bacterial infection), a substantial rise in white count can be seen. In the absence of complications, the total WBC falls to within the normal range for nonpregnant women by the sixth postpartum day.

Döhle bodies, blue-staining cytoplasmic inclusions seen in granulocytes stained with Romanovsky dyes (Wright's stain, Giemsa stain) and initially identified in individuals with bacteremia, are found on nearly all peripheral smears from pregnant women. By means of electron microscopy they have been identified as aggregates of rough endoplasmic reticulum. Minor increases in eosinophils have been reported during pregnancy, and basophils decrease slightly. No systematic changes in monocytes have been observed. The absolute lymphocyte count is not changed by pregnancy, nor are the relative numbers of T and B cells. However, cell-mediated immunity is depressed. The mechanisms responsible are poorly understood; however, the process is certainly in part directed by the physiologic hormonal changes accompanying normal pregnancy.

Neutropenia

Isolated neutropenia is uncommon in pregnant women. It has become standard practice among physicians experienced in the chemotherapy of leukemias and other neoplastic diseases to regard 1×10^9 per liter as a "safe" number, sufficient to cope with most infections against which neutrophils would provide defense. While translation of this lower limit of acceptability into other clinical situations has not been established, a count above 1×10^9 per liter is probably "safe" in most situations. As most cases of neutropenia among pregnant women are caused by drugs or other environmental agents, the importance of recognizing a low WBC is to alert the physician to the possible presence of a dangerous drug or chemical or a complicating disorder. Neutropenia may occasionally herald the appearance of lupus erythematosus, acute leukemia, neoplasia involving the marrow, or other serious intercurrent disease. Megaloblastic anemia is often accompanied by neutropenia. When an isolated low WBC is observed, a careful history of medication and other exposure should be taken. Clues suggesting systemic disorders should be sought, and if these efforts are unrewarding, the bone marrow should be examined.

Management is supportive. Complicating illness should be treated and potentially myelosuppressive substances should be excluded from the patient's medications and environment. A partial list of drugs reported to cause neutropenia is given in Table 53–10. Deficiencies should be corrected, and supportive care, with prompt evaluation and treatment of infection, should be instituted. White blood cell transfusions have been of limited value.

Hematologic Neoplasia and Pregnancy

Advances in the past 25 years in the management of some leukemias, Hodgkin's disease, and the non-Hodgkin's lymphomas have substantially improved

TABLE 53–10. Some Common Agents Occasionally Reported to Cause Neutropenia

Analgesics and anti-inflammatory agents
  Aminopyrine
  Phenylbutazone
Anticonvulsants
  Diphenylhydantoin sodium
  Trimethyloxazolidine
Tranquilizers
  Phenothiazines
  Meprobamate
  Haloperidol
Antimicrobials
  Chloramphenicol
  Metronidazole
  Isonicotinic acid hydrazide
  Sulfonamides
Diuretics
Oral hypoglycemics
Antithyroid drugs
  Propylthiouracil
  Methimazole
Miscellaneous
  Penicillamine
  Cimetidine
  Quinine
  Gold salts

the prognosis for most patients with these malignancies. The former high mortality rates and poor reproductive potential for children and young adults with hematologic neoplastic disease no longer apply in all cases, and an increasing number of these patients now achieve complete, durable remissions and even cure. This improved prognosis has raised new questions concerning both the possibility and the outcome of pregnancy.

Acute Leukemia

The classification of the acute leukemias by cell type has become increasingly important in evaluation of studies designed to identify therapeutic regimens most likely to succeed in a given case. Identification of cell surface markers, histochemical staining, and careful study of the neoplastic cells in peripheral blood and bone marrow stained by conventional methods have allowed more precise classification and subclassification, and these carry reasonably accurate therapeutic and prognostic implications. For purposes of this discussion, the terms acute lymphoblastic leukemia (ALL) and acute nonlymphoblastic leukemia (ANLL) are used.

ALL, the most common acute leukemia of childhood, is the disorder in which prolonged remissions and even cures have most often been achieved. In general, the probability of a favorable outcome of therapy usually is inversely related to age, young children being more likely to do well. The disorder occurs occasionally in young adults with a less favorable prognosis. ANLL may occur at any age but is rare in childhood. Its many variants are the common acute leukemias of adults, and whereas hematologic remissions are being achieved in an increasing proportion of cases, ultimate relapse and resistance to further therapy remains the rule. Newer techniques, including bone marrow transplantation, show some promise for improving the survival in these cases, but these therapeutic modalities continue to have many biologic and practical limitations.

Prepubertal girls who are successfully treated for ALL with chemotherapy and irradiation usually experience normal sexual development (Siris et al., 1976). Catanzarite and Ferguson (1984) were able to identify ten mothers cured of childhood ALL who bore a total of 13 children, all carried to term and all apparently normal at birth. Dara and co-workers (1981) have reported a successful outcome in a pregnancy that began while the mother was receiving 6-mercaptopurine and methotrexate maintenance therapy for ALL in remission. Relapse occurred in the fourth month, but additional chemotherapy induced a second hematologic remission. The infant appeared normal at birth and had normal growth and development during the first 6 months. Pregnancy in women with ANLL is a rare event, and ANLL complicating an established pregnancy is equally uncommon. In a published review in 1977, Lilleyman and associates determined that if ANLL is diagnosed during the first half of pregnancy, a live healthy baby will be produced in fewer than half the cases. Abortion, stillbirth, or maternal death undelivered accounted for the fetal wastage. In only one of the 32 cases included in the report was a fetal abnormality (trisomy C) identified, although nearly two-thirds of the mothers received cytotoxic drugs.

Careful analysis of the reported cases of acute leukemia in pregnancy strongly suggests that the course of the leukemia is not directly influenced by the pregnancy. Some women (and their physicians), however, may be reluctant to expose the fetus to possibly teratogenic or mutagenic drugs. There is no question that acute leukemia untreated or in relapse exerts a potentially devastating effect on both the pregnancy and the mother. The natural history of both ALL and ANLL managed without cytotoxic drugs is one of death from bleeding and/or infection in, at best, a few months. Measures to avoid conception are strongly advocated for young women with acute leukemia requiring chemotherapy, and a solid case for interruption of pregnancy in this same group of patients can be made. However, this advice is not acceptable to all patients.

The frequency and the severity of the teratogenic effects of the drugs employed in the treatment of acute leukemia is not known with certainty because the collected series are small (Pizzuto et al., 1980) and single cases are uncommon (Schafer, 1981; Plows, 1982; Sanz and Rafecas, 1982). The occurrence of leukemia in a newborn delivered from a leukemic mother is exceedingly rare, however. Even less is known about the late effects of antileukemic therapy on the surviving offspring of women exposed to these agents during pregnancy. More information is available about the children of individuals themselves treated in childhood for a variety of neoplasms (Li et al., 1979). In 286 completed pregnancies in which one or the other parent had been treated for childhood cancer, there was no excess of congenital anomalies in comparison with published figures for the general population. Additional information is recorded about the obstetric experience of women treated with chemotherapy for trophoblastic neoplasms (Walden and Bagshawe, 1979). In those successfully treated there was no increase in the rate of abnormal pregnancies or fetal abnormalities.

It is therefore evident that some pregnant women who develop acute leukemia and some women with leukemia who become pregnant can be delivered of live healthy infants. Chemotherapy is not invariably teratogenic, but the precise risk of a congenital abnormality is not known. The risk of fetal abnormality may be greater if treatment is started in the early weeks of pregnancy rather than in the latter half, but this hazard must be balanced against the real threat inherent in untreated leukemia. The patient should be encouraged to make her decision in the light of all the available information, including that about her own life expectancy. Management will often be difficult, and the skills of experienced obstetricians and specialists in hematologic neoplasia will be taxed to their utmost. Not only will their technical skills be required, but they must be prepared to provide understanding support and the best-informed advice in an area of uncertainty to a patient and her family burdened with problems that are emotionally charged to an unusual degree.

Chronic Leukemia

Chronic myelogenous leukemia (CML), also sometimes called chronic granulocytic leukemia, occurs most often in those over 40 but occurs occasionally in women in the reproductive years. In most cases significant elevation of the white cell count (in the absence of infection), with a marked left shift including variable numbers of myelocytes and myeloblasts, calls attention to the possibility of a blood dyscrasia. In early cases anemia is usually absent or mild and the platelet count is often increased. About 75 per cent of the patients have splenomegaly. Many patients are treated with busulfan, an agent often responsible for amenorrhea and ovarian failure; on this account pregnancy in a patient with established and treated CML is very rare. However, a number of women have been discovered to have CML after pregnancy has begun. As the life-threatening complications so common in acute leukemia (hemorrhage secondary to thrombocytopenia and infection) are rarely encountered in the early months in patients with CML, the pregnancy can usually be carried to term without the use of chemotherapy or other modalities except, in some cases, transfusion for significant anemia. In this way the risks to the fetus of potentially mutagenic or teratogenic interventions can be avoided. Splenomegaly can be a problem of clinical importance. A large spleen may be uncomfortable, may be the site of recurrent infarction with perisplenitis, or may compete for space in an abdomen already attempting to accommodate an enlarging uterus. Richards and Spiers (1975), employing localized radiation therapy, have reported successful reduction in spleen size with no obstetric or detectable fetal complications.

The overall average duration of survival from time of diagnosis in CML is between 3 and 4 years. Young women frequently experience a more prolonged survival. Although cures are virtually nonexistent, most patients treated with oral agents enjoy a prolonged clinical remission. Ultimately, the disease becomes refractory to therapy or assumes an accelerated phase that resembles acute leukemia morphologically but is generally resistant to treatment. Successful marrow transplantation for chronic phase CML has been increasingly reported, but the good outcomes have usually been limited to those transplants done in young patients whose donors were HLA-identical siblings (Champlin et al., 1988). The other forms of chronic leukemia occur so infrequently in patients under 50 years of age that they are not discussed here.

Hodgkin's Disease

Several factors have conspired to make Hodgkin's disease a hematologic neoplasm of increasing importance in obstetric practice: (1) it is a disease with a peculiar predilection for young adults of both sexes; (2) long-term cures in selected cases following adequate and appropriate radiation therapy are well known; and (3) at present, more commonly than for any other tumor (except childhood acute leukemia), durable remissions and cures occur in patients with advanced (extensive) disease treated with both combination chemotherapy and high-dose radiation. An increasing number of young women who have been treated successfully for Hodgkin's disease wish to and do become pregnant. In addition, the management decisions (by both patient and physician) necessary when the disorder first manifests during pregnancy have become increasingly complex. Data are being accumulated that can assist physicians as they advise both groups of patients about the effect of Hodgkin's disease and its treatment on fertility, pregnancy, and the fetus. It is now well established that pregnancy per se does not affect Hodgkin's disease, although it must be conceded that treatment plans may have to be modified if the fetus is to be protected.

Young women who have been successfully treated for Hodgkin's disease with total lymphoid irradiation, combination chemotherapy, or combined radiation and chemotherapy frequently experience amenorrhea (Horning et al., 1981; Schilsky et al., 1981). Absence of menses may occur even in radiation treated patients in whom mid-line oophoropexy had been done in an attempt to provide increased protection for the ovaries during radiation therapy. For some, the amenorrhea is temporary. Persistent amenorrhea occurs more often in those receiving combination therapy (radiation and cytotoxic drugs) and in those who are 25 years or older at the initiation of treatment. In a series reported by Horning and colleagues (1981), pregnancy occurred after treatment for Hodgkin's disease in 28 women. Twenty of these resulted in 21 normal live births, including a set of twins; there were two premature infants, one low-birth-weight infant, and five elective therapeutic abortions. Schilsky and associates (1981) reported a total of 15 pregnancies in 27 treated women; two elective abortions were carried out, but the remaining 13 pregnancies were uneventful and the infants appeared normal. Holmes and Holmes (1978) have reported an excess of unfavorable outcomes in pregnancies among women given combination therapy. The treatment programs employed in their study, which covered patients treated between 1944 and 1975, were variable and can probably not be fairly compared with the more recently reported series. One can conclude, therefore, that women successfully treated with irradiation alone, combination chemotherapy alone, or irradiation and chemotherapy may suffer premature ovarian failure, but this occurrence is not universal, and successful pregnancies without obvious neonatal malformations can occur. Some of the late effects of intensive radiation and chemotherapy, especially the appearance of second neoplasms in some individuals cured of Hodgkin's disease, are well-recognized risks of modern treatment with curative intent. Only careful follow-up of Hodgkin's patients and their progeny will provide meaningful and more precise information concerning the frequency of these late complications. It is too early to offer a sound opinion concerning the possibility that delayed complications or toxic effects may appear in the offspring.

The special problems surrounding pregnancy and Hodgkin's disease are focused on the limitations pregnancy imposes on both evaluation of extent of disease (staging) and treatment. It is well established that the chances for successful treatment and cure are greatly enhanced if the full extent of disease can be determined and therapy can be planned to eradicate present or suspected tumor. Optimal staging often includes numerous radiographic and scanning procedures and possibly even exploratory laparotomy and splenectomy, procedures that are generally contraindicated in pregnancy. Similarly, exposure of the fetus to potentially mutagenic and teratogenic drugs or to therapeutic radiation, especially in the first trimester, is undesirable. Most experienced authorities recommend interruption of pregnancy if Hodgkin's disease is discovered early or if the patient has been treated with radiation or cytotoxic drugs during the first trimester. If the diagnosis is made in later pregnancy, or relapse of previously known disease occurs at that time, thorough staging evaluations and treatment can sometimes be deferred until after delivery, especially if early delivery is feasible. Carefully planned supradiaphragmatic radiation has occasionally been necessary during pregnancy, and rare patients with progressive, symptomatic disease have been given systemic chemotherapy during late pregnancy without apparent untoward effects on the neonate (Thomas and Peckham, 1976; Jacobs et al., 1981). Management of the patient with Hodgkin's disease during pregnancy must be individually tailored. Young women about to be treated for the disease should undergo tests for pregnancy before therapy is initiated. Effective measures to avoid conception should be stressed as treatment is undertaken. If pregnancy occurs, interruption should be recommended during the first trimester. The management of the patient with Hodgkin's disease who wishes to continue a pregnancy or who has suffered relapse during pregnancy will require the advice of physicians experienced in the use of modern radiation and chemotherapeutic modalities and familiar with the behavior of the many subtypes of this neoplasm.

Non-Hodgkin's Lymphoma

The non-Hodgkin's lymphomas, the collective term currently employed for malignant disorders primarily affecting lymphoid tissues excluding Hodgkin's disease and the lymphoid leukemias, are extremely rare in pregnancy. Falkson and co-workers (1980), in a review of the literature, found 13 cases to which they added one of their own. Of the 14 women, only two were successfully treated during pregnancy; in both, combination chemotherapy was used and apparently normal infants were delivered.

ABNORMALITIES OF COAGULATION

The Coagulation Mechanism

The initial coagulation mechanism for thrombus formation *in vivo* is adhesion of platelets to the injured vessel walls (Shattil and Bennett, 1981). Exposed subendothelium of the injured tissue initiates adhesion, which is promptly followed by a change in shape of the platelet:

(1) Injury + platelets $\xrightarrow[\text{aggregation}]{\text{adhesion}}$ platelet factors + ADP

Both the platelet membrane and release of the contents of δ-, α-, and γ-granules are involved in platelet adhesion and aggregation as well as the initiation of the plasma phase of coagulation. The adenosine diphosphate (ADP) released from platelets attracts more platelets to the area, resulting in *platelet aggregation*. The aggregation phenomenon tends to perpetuate itself, because newly attracted platelets in turn release ADP and attract additional platelets. Increasingly large amounts of platelet factors become available for initiation of the plasma phase of coagulation.

Table 53–11 presents some of the properties of the coagulation factors (Colman et al., 1987). With the exceptions of fibrinogen, prothrombin, and calcium, the coagulation factors are trace proteins. Factor III is not listed in the table and is, in fact, the tissue factor thromboplastin. The preferred descriptive name and several common synonyms for the coagulation factors are as follows: V, proaccelerin or labile factor; VII, proconvertin or serum prothrombin conversion accelerator; VIII, antihemophilic factor or antihemophilic globulin; IX, plasma thromboplastin component or Christmas factor; X, Stuart factor or Prower factor; XI, plasma thromboplastin antecedent; XII, Hageman factor or glass or contact factor; and XIII, fibrin-stabilizing factor.

The third column in the table indicates the site of biosynthesis for each factor. It is noteworthy that prothrombin, factor VII, factor IX, and factor X are dependent on vitamin K for their synthesis and, thus, are the factors depleted when a patient is receiving a vitamin K antagonist such as sodium warfarin. The biologic half-life is also listed for each factor and can be used to estimate roughly the frequency of replacement therapy needed during an acute bleeding problem.

The remainder of the coagulation process can be broadly divided into three phases: the extrinsic pathway, intrinsic pathway, and common pathway. The pathway of function for each of the plasma factors is also noted in Table 53–11. The remainder of the coagulation scheme can be summarized by the following six schematized formulas:

(2) Tissue thromboplastin + VII $\xrightarrow[\text{Ca}^{++}]{\text{Ca}^{++}}$ extrinsic activator

(3) XII + XI + IX + PF3 + VIII $\longrightarrow$ intrinsic activator

(4) X + V + PF3 + Ca^{++} $\xrightarrow[\text{intrinsic activator}]{\text{extrinsic activator}}$ common activator

(5) Prothrombin $\xrightarrow[\text{Ca}^{++}]{\text{common activator}}$ thrombin

(6) Fibrinogen $\xrightarrow{\text{thrombin}}$ fibrin polymer

(7) Fibrin polymer + VIII $\xrightarrow{\text{Ca}^{++}}$ stabilized fibrin

The basic feature of coagulation is the conversion of circulating fibrinogen into a stabilized fibrin clot; it occurs in two steps. First, fibrinogen is enzymatically converted to fibrin monomer by the action of thrombin, and the fibrin monomeric units polymerize (formula 6). Next, the resulting fibrin clot is strengthened and further rendered insoluble by the action of factor XIII (formula 7).

In order for fibrinogen to be converted to fibrin, thrombin must be generated from its precursor prothrombin. This reaction is catalyzed by a complex, common activator which consists of the activated form of factor X, factor V, calcium, and platelet factors (formula 5). The production of the common activator

---

TABLE 53–11. Some Properties of Coagulation Factors

FACTOR	BIOCHEMISTRY	SITE OF BIOSYNTHESIS	BIOLOGIC HALF-LIFE (h)	FUNCTION
Fibrinogen (I)	Glycoprotein; MW* 340,000; 3 globular subunits	Liver	72–120	Common pathway; fibrin precursor
Prothrombin (II)	Monomeric glycoprotein; MW 69,000	Liver; vitamin K†	67–106	Common pathway; proenzyme precursor of thrombin
Calcium (IV)	Ionic calcium	—		Extrinsic, intrinsic, and common pathways
Factor V	Multimeric; MW 200,000–400,000	Liver	12–36	Common pathway
Factor VII	Monomeric glycoprotein; MW 63,000	Liver; vitamin K	4–6	Extrinsic pathway; proenzyme
Factor VIII	Multimeric glycoprotein; MW 330,000; circulates bound to multimeric von Willebrand factor	Probably by liver	10–14	Intrinsic pathway
Factor IX	Monomeric glycoprotein; MW 62,000	Liver; vitamin K	24	Intrinsic pathway; coenzyme
Factor X	Two-chain glycoprotein; MW 59,000	Liver; vitamin K	24–60	Common pathway; proenzyme
Factor XI	Two-chain glycoprotein; MW 200,000	Liver	48–84	Intrinsic pathway; proenzyme
Factor XII	Monomeric glycoprotein; MW 80,000	Unknown	52–60	Intrinsic pathway; proenzyme
Factor XIII	Multimeric glycoprotein; MW 320,000; 4 subunits	Liver; megakaryocytes	72–168	Common pathway; proenzyme; transglutaminase
von Willebrand	Series of macromolecules; MW 1–15 × 10⁶	Endothelial cells and megakaryocytes	12–36	Intrinsic pathway; forms a stable complex with factor VIII

*MW = molecular weight.
†Vitamin K required for synthesis.

TABLE 53–12. Screening Coagulation Tests

STUDY	MEASURES	NORMAL VALUES
Bleeding time	Platelets and vascular integrity	1–5 min (Ivy)
Platelet count	Number of platelets	140–440 × 10^3/mm³
Partial thromboplastin time	II, V, VIII, IX, X, XI	24–36 sec
Prothrombin time	II, V, VII, X	11–12 sec
Thrombin time	I, II, circulating split products, heparin	16–20 sec
Plasma fibrinogen	II (fibrinogen)	175–433 mg/dl
Fibrin D-dimer	Fibrin degradation	<0.05 μg/ml

can occur as a result of two different pathways, the intrinsic and extrinsic (formula 4). The intrinsic is so named because all its components are present in the circulating plasma (formula 3). This pathway is probably triggered by both endothelial damage and platelet factors. The extrinsic pathway is so named because it is triggered by tissue thromboplastin (formula 2). Finally, the fibrinolytic system must be briefly considered. Fibrinolysis is the major physiologic means by which fibrin is disposed of after its hemostatic function has been fulfilled. The mechanism of fibrinolysis is schematically summarized by formulas 8 and 9:

$$(8) \quad \text{Plasminogen} \xrightarrow{\text{activators}} \text{plasmin}$$

$$\begin{array}{l}\text{Fibrin}\\\text{Fibrinogen}\\(9) \quad \text{Complement} \xrightarrow{\text{plasmin}} \text{degradation products}\\\text{Factor VIII}\end{array}$$

Plasminogen is a beta-globulin with a molecular mass of 81,000 daltons. It circulates in the plasma in concentrations of 10 to 20 mg/dl. It is activated by a heterogeneous group of substances termed "plasminogen activators" (formula 8). Activators reside within the lysozyme of most cells, and urokinase and streptokinase are examples of specifically identified activators. The activated form of plasminogen, plasmin, is a proteolytic enzyme with a wide spectrum of activity. It cleaves arginyl-lysine bonds in a large variety of substrates, including fibrinogen, fibrin, factor VIII, and various components of complement (formula 9). It has a very short life in plasma owing to its inactivation by humoral antiplasmins.

There are also a number of plasma proteases that function as inhibitors of coagulation and fibrinolysis. They serve to control both the speed and extent of coagulation and fibrinolysis. The major inhibitor of the extrinsic phase is C1 inhibitor, which inactivates factor VII$_a$ and kallikrein. The major inhibitor of the intrinsic phase is antithrombin III, which inhibits factor IX$_a$, factor X$_a$, and thrombin. Other inhibitors are α_1-antitripsin, α_2-macroglobulin, and α_2-antiplasmin. Protein C is also a potent inhibitor of coagulation. Activated protein C (with its cofactor, protein S) reacts with factors V and VIII to destroy their coagulation property.

Laboratory Methods for Study of Blood Coagulation

There is no single test that is suitable as an overall laboratory screening study of hemostasis and blood

coagulation. Commonly, the combination of bleeding time, platelet count, activated partial thromboplastin time (aPTT), prothrombin time (PT), and thrombin time (TT) is used as a screening battery. Table 53–12 indicates which factors are measured by each study and indicates the normal value for the study in question. A large number of additional studies define specific abnormalities of platelet function or allow measurements of a specific plasma clotting factor. The Rumpel-Leede test, platelet adhesiveness, platelet aggregation, whole blood prothrombin activation rate, and clot retraction are all examples of studies that further define abnormalities of platelet function.

Precise levels of each circulating plasma factor can be defined by either the thromboplastin generation test or cross-correction studies with normal plasma and plasma known to be deficient in the factor being assayed. A specific assay for factor XIII is also available. Several accurate methods are now available for the quantitative assay of plasma fibrinogen. Normal values range from 175 to 430 mg/dl and are abnormal in acquired hypofibrinogenemia secondary to disseminated intravascular coagulation and in the hereditary afibrinogenemias and dysfibrinogenemias.

Studies used in the evaluation of fibrinolysis include the euglobulin clot lysis time and the demonstration of fibrin-fibrinogen degradation products by a variety of techniques. The D-dimer study is specific for identifying fibrinolysis in contrast to fibrinogenolysis. It is important to remember that the screening coagulation studies do not provide a specific etiologic diagnosis. Such a diagnosis is important because only then is it possible to optimally treat excessive bleeding should it occur during surgery. Furthermore, the presence of an adequate coagulation screen in a patient suspected of having a coagulation abnormality does not diminish the necessity of pursuing a specific diagnosis and making available specific therapy should it be needed.

Several extensive reviews indicate that the utility of the bleeding time has not been enhanced by standardization of the method, that there is no clinically useful correlation between the bleeding time and platelet count in thrombocytopenic individuals, and that no evidence exists that the bleeding time is a predictor of the risk of either spontaneous or surgically induced hemorrhage (Rodgers and Levin, 1990; Lind, 1991).

Diagnosis and Treatment of Specific Coagulation Disorders

Acquired disorders are far more common than congenital, and those seen most frequently include idiopathic thrombocytopenic purpura (ITP), disseminated intravascular coagulation (DIC), liver disease, and anticoagulant therapy. The congenital disorders seen most frequently are von Willebrand's disease and factor XI deficiency.

Platelet Disorders

Thrombocytopenia is the most common platelet disorder and is due to either diminished production or increased destruction of platelets. The severity of bleeding in thrombocytopenia is roughly proportional to the degree to which the platelet count has been lowered. A specific diagnosis is obviously essential for the proper total management of a patient with thrombocytopenia. However, when hemorrhage is due to thrombocytopenia, platelet transfusions are frequently of value (Cash, 1972). The success of platelet transfusion therapy is dependent on the functional integrity of the transfused platelets, the underlying cause of the platelet defect in the recipient, and the presence and level of antiplatelet antibodies. Platelet transfusions are available both as platelet-rich plasma and as platelet concentrates. When platelet concentrates are used, a relatively large number of platelets remain in the bag and can be harvested by adding a small amount of normal saline solution after evacuation of each bag to resuspend platelets remaining in the bag. One can expect an increase in platelet count of 5 to 10 $\times$ 10^9 per liter per unit of platelets transfused. The exact incremental rise and the length of platelet survival are dependent on both the underlying disease process and the freshness of the platelets.

The complications of platelet transfusion are less common and less serious than those accompanying transfusion of whole blood. They include bacterial contamination, infectious hepatitis, febrile transfusion reaction, and post-transfusion purpura.

IDIOPATHIC THROMBOCYTOPENIC PURPURA. Also called isoimmune thrombocytopenic purpura, ITP is an autoimmune disorder in which platelet destruction is caused by an antiplatelet antibody that results in the destruction of platelets by the reticuloendothelial system. The antibody is usually of the IgG class and is directed against a platelet-associated antigen. Although the spleen is usually the major site of antibody production, bone marrow cells are also able to synthesize antiplatelet IgG.

Most patients with ITP have increased levels of platelet-associated IgG (PA-IgG), and an inverse relationship exists between the PA-IgG level and the platelet count. Another group of patients have activated complement C3, causing elevated levels of both C3 and PA-IgG. A third group of patients, constituting 10 to 30 per cent of cases of ITP, has normal levels of PA-IgG but elevated levels of PA-C3.

Both direct and indirect techniques are available for measuring antiplatelet antibodies (Cines et al., 1982). In the direct technique the patient's platelets are incubated with ^{125}I-labeled anti-IgG, and the platelet-associated radioactivity is measured after washing. This test is equivalent to the direct Coombs' test for detecting RBC antigen-antibody complexes. In the indirect test, normal platelets are incubated with the patient's plasma and washed, and then the radioactivity is measured as in the direct technique. This study is analogous to the indirect Coombs' test. Samuels and associates (1990) have reported a correlation between the level of indirect antibody and the fetal platelet count.

The diagnosis of ITP is made according to established criteria that include a normal blood count, except for thrombocytopenia, a normal bone marrow, with adequate or increased megalokaryocytes, a blood smear showing an increased percentage of large platelets, normal coagulation studies, increased levels of platelet-associated IgG, and no other obvious cause of thrombocytopenia.

Management of ITP during pregnancy requires concern for both mother and fetus (Laros and Kagan, 1984; Cook et al., 1991). The goal of treatment for patients with ITP is remission, not cure. Thus therapy is stepwise: corticosteroids, then splenectomy, and, following that, consideration of immunosuppressive therapy or plasmapheresis. Each step is determined by the severity of the clinical situation. The management of ITP in pregnancy requires special consideration because the human placenta is known to have receptors for the F_c portion of the IgG molecule. IgG and antibodies are actively transferred from the mother to the fetus and cause neonatal thrombocytopenia in 50 to 70 per cent of neonates.

Most obstetricians and hematologists would agree that the overall management of pregnant women with this disorder should be similar to that of a nonpregnant patient. Initially one should employ corticosteroids such as prednisone in a dose of 0.5 to 1 mg/kg. If a response to corticosteroids has not been achieved, splenectomy is indicated and should be carried out if at all possible during the middle trimester. Corticosteroids have been used for the last 30 years and owe their efficacy to both an immunosuppressive effect and a slowing of the rate of platelet destruction by the reticuloendothelial system. By themselves, corticosteroids produce a transient remission in 75 per cent of cases in adults, but a sustained remission in only 14 to 33 per cent of cases. More recently immunosuppression with high-dose serum immune globulin has been found to be useful and now is often used during pregnancy before resorting to splenectomy. Other agents include danazol, cyclophosphamide, azathioprine, vincristine, and vinblastine. Danazol is relatively contraindicated if the patient is carrying a male fetus, and the various chemotherapeutic agents are used only as a last resort (Brunskill, 1992).

The major controversial issue in the management of ITP has been the mode of delivery. Because of the theoretic risks of intracranial hemorrhage to thrombocytopenic fetuses, many investigators have advocated cesarean section for all women with ITP. A review summarizes data on 165 cases (Kagan and Laros, 1983). Of the 134 infants delivered vaginally, 50 (37 per cent) either had or developed platelet counts below 100 $\times$ 10^9 per liter and 28 (21 per cent) had counts below 30 $\times$ 10^9 per liter. Only one infant was described as having intracerebral bleeding and this was not fatal. By contrast, of the 31 infants delivered by cesarean section, 17 (55 per cent) had platelet counts below 100×10^9 per liter and 9 (29 per cent) below 30×10^9 per liter. There were three serious hemorrhages, one of which was intracranial hemorrhage at 3 days of age. These data do not support the premise that delivery by cesarean section is beneficial for thrombocytopenic infants of women with ITP. A more recent report describing 31 pregnancies from 25 women with immune thrombocytopenic purpura managed at a single institution also concluded that the route of delivery may not affect the incidence of intracranial hemorrhage in infants with thrombocytopenia (Cook et al., 1991).

In an attempt to define those fetuses really at risk, Scott and associates (Scott et al., 1980) have suggested the use of fetal platelet counts obtained by fetal scalp blood sampling in early labor. They have documented the reliability of the technique and suggest cesarean section only for those infants with platelet counts proven to be below 30×10^9 per liter. An alternative technique is percutaneous umbilical cord blood sampling performed at 38 weeks gestation (Moise et al., 1988; Scioscia et al., 1988). Similarly, Samuels and associates (1990) and Kelton and associates (1982) have studied the value of platelet-associated IgG in predicting the significantly thrombocytopenic infant. Unfortunately, the antibody studies do not allow the prospective detection of those infants with marked thrombocytopenia. Because there is no evidence substantiating that cesarean section offers benefits to a thrombocytopenic infant, I believe that the decision on route of delivery should be based on obstetric indications alone.

Three recent reports concern the use of epidural catheters in 14 patients with platelet counts $<100 \times 10^9$ per liter without any neurologic sequelae (Waldman et al., 1987; Rolbin et al., 1988; Rasmus et al., 1989). Hew-Wing and associates (1989) conclude that "the current belief, that epidural anesthesia is contraindicated in patients whose platelet counts are below 100×10^9 per liter, has no supporting data."

NEONATAL ALLOIMMUNE THROMBOCYTOPENIA. This is a disorder of the fetus, not of the mother. It is the platelet analog of Rh disease of the newborn; the mother mounts an immune response to platelet antigens present in the fetus, and the antibody crosses the placenta and attacks fetal platelets. Although fetomaternal incompatibility with ABO, HLA class I, and platelet-specific antigens on the platelet surface is possible, most cases of NATP are the result of antibodies directed against the platelet-specific antigens Zw (Pl^A), Pl^E, Bak, Yuk, Br, and DUZO. The frequency of NATP is only one to two per 10,000 births, and it is virtually never anticipated until a mother has an affected infant (Taaning and Skibsted, 1990). In more than 50 per cent of the cases, NATP occurs in a first pregnancy and the recurrence risk is over 80 per cent (Muller, 1988). Unfortunately, prepartum serum studies do not predict the severity, but in subsequent affected children the disorder will be as severe as or more severe than the index case. The major threat to the fetus is from intracranial hemorrhage, which can occur before, during, or after labor and delivery.

Diagnosis is made by demonstrating maternal-paternal platelet antigen incompatibility, the presence of antiplatelet antibody in the maternal serum, and platelet-bound antibody on the platelets of the fetus or newborn. Fetal antigen type and platelet count can be obtained by percutaneous umbilical blood sampling (PUBS) as early as 20 weeks gestation. If significant thrombocytopenia exists, transfusion with irradiated maternal platelets (Daffos et al., 1984) and/or high-dose intravenous immune globulin (Bussel et al., 1988) can be started (see Chapter 24). After birth, either platelet or exchange transfusion with maternal blood is effective treatment (McIntosh et al., 1973). The fetal platelet count should be sampled by PUBS before either vaginal or cesarean delivery. Sia and associates (1985) have reported two cases of intracranial hemorrhage despite delivery by cesarean section.

TRANSFUSION-INDUCED THROMBOCYTOPENIA. Thrombocytopenia may be induced by blood transfusion by one of two mechanisms. The first is simply dilutional and may occur in any patient who rapidly receives large volumes of red cells or stored whole blood (6 units or more) for replacement in a major hemorrhage. Addition of platelet concentrates to the replacement fluids is the treatment of choice, if correction must be made promptly. Megakaryocytic hyperplasia and the appearance of newly produced endogenous platelets will follow the acute thrombocytopenia if the marrow reacts normally. A second rare type of transfusion-related thrombocytopenia may occur in women who were previously sensitized by transfusion or pregnancy to naturally occurring platelet antigens. After this sensitization, they demonstrate abrupt onset of severe thrombocytopenia and purpura about 10 days after receiving subsequent transfusion of even a single unit of red cells, whole blood, or plasma. Exchange transfusion has been dramatically effective treatment in two reported cases (Shulman et al., 1961; Cimo and Aster, 1972).

FUNCTIONAL PLATELET DEFECTS. Such defects are far less common than quantitative disorders. Primary hemostasis is normally accomplished by the interaction of vasoconstriction, endothelial cell reaction to injury, and a series of biochemical events involving platelets that promote adhesion and aggregation, with the formation of the initial hemostatic platelet plug. Normal platelets also contribute significantly to the initiation of blood coagulation and thus the formation of fibrin, and are necessary for clot retraction. Platelet prostaglandin cyclooxygenase plays a key role in the generation of the intermediate cyclic endoperoxides, which are converted into the active thromboxanes and prostaglandins important in the initiation and modulation of the platelet release reaction, the process by which a variety of biologically active substances stored in platelet granules and dense bodies are extruded from the platelet to participate in the ongoing hemostatic and coagulation process.

Bleeding may occur because of acquired or congenital abnormalities of platelet function. Except for the platelet defect seen in von Willebrand's disease, the recognized hereditary disorders are rare and beyond the scope of this text; Weiss (1980) has recently provided a comprehensive review. On the other hand, acquired platelet dysfunction is a common occurrence because it can be produced by a great many biologically active compounds and may accompany a wide variety of disorders. Such disorders, which include uremia, myeloproliferative syndromes, and cyanotic congenital heart disease, are themselves unusual in pregnancy, but drug-induced platelet abnormalities may be responsible for mild bleeding manifestations in many pregnant women and may create more serious problems in those whose hemostatic and clotting mechanisms are already compromised by thrombocytopenia, the use of anticoagulants, or the presence of some other coagulation defect.

Of the drugs in common use that have a significant effect on platelet function, aspirin is the most important because of its ubiquity and duration of effect. Aspirin inhibits the platelet release reaction by acetylating platelet cyclooxygenase; this effect persists in the platelet for the duration of its life span and results in prolongation of the bleeding time and deficient platelet aggregation in the presence of collagen. Patients taking aspirin may note increased bruisability and minor bleeding symptoms, manifestations that persist for several days following a single dose. Ordinarily these symptoms are inconsequential, but during pregnancy and especially at term, hemorrhagic complications can be of more than trivial importance. Normal pregnant women given usual doses of aspirin within 10 days of delivery have been shown to have increased intrapartum or postpartum blood loss, and their infants sustained a higher incidence of hemostatic abnormalities than did control maternal-neonatal pairs (Stuart et al., 1982). Low doses of aspirin (60 to 80 mg) in preliminary studies to prevent preeclampsia have not appeared to cause hemostatic problems, and large studies of this issue are currently under way.

Most other nonsteroidal anti-inflammatory agents inhibit prostaglandin synthesis and have been shown to affect platelet function. In general, they are less powerful and shorter-acting antagonists than aspirin, but they should be avoided in pregnancy except for extraordinary indications. Acetaminophen is a safe antipyretic from the standpoint of platelet function; the choice of an analgesic that is safe in pregnancy must be made on an individual basis.

Several antimicrobials have been shown to impair platelet aggregation and the release reaction. In general these effects have been of no clinical significance, but carbenicillin has been reported to be responsible for serious hemorrhage. Numerous other classes of drugs, when tested, have demonstrated at least *in vitro* effects on platelet activity. One of importance because it is commonly included in over-the-counter cough and cold remedies is glyceryl guaiacolate. Pregnant women should be warned to avoid preparations containing this compound.

The diagnostic hallmark of platelet dysfunction is a significantly prolonged template bleeding time. Devices for performing the Ivy bleeding time test by the template technique are readily available commercially and provide reasonably reproducible results in the hands of experienced operators. Prolonged bleeding times may be seen in thrombocytopenic states (platelet counts less than 100×10^9 per liter) and most cases of von Willebrand's disease. The differential diagnosis among these three entities is generally readily accomplished.

Drug-induced disorders of platelet function are best managed prophylactically: medications influencing platelet activity should be used with great care in pregnancy and only for compelling reasons. If, however, they are employed and serious bleeding ensues, platelet transfusion will generally be beneficial in controlling the hemorrhage.

Acquired and Congenital Plasma Factor Disorders

VON WILLEBRAND'S DISEASE. This inherited autosomal dominant trait is characterized by abnormal bleeding of varying severity. The pathophysiologic basis for the disease is a marked decrease or absence of both clottable and antigenic factor VIII. Criteria for laboratory diagnosis are as yet not completely satisfactory, but include slight-to-moderate reduction in the aPTT, a clottable factor VIII level 15 to 30 per cent of normal, a prolonged bleeding time, abnormal platelet adhesiveness, a lack of ristocetin-induced platelet aggregation, and a factor VIII coagulant activity to factor VIII antigen ratio of 1 (Veltkamp and van Tilburg, 1974; Weiss et al., 1973). The factor VIII level should be checked periodically during the antenatal course and pretreatment reserved for patients with levels <25 per cent of normal. DDAVP (l-deamino-8-D-argenine-vasopressin) should be used instead of cryoprecipitate for cases known to be responsive (type I and some IIa). Treatment is begun when the patient presents in labor. The dose is 0.3 μg/kg of DDAVP given over 30 minutes with the total dose not greater than 25 μg. Treatment is repeated every 12 hours with infusions being progressively less effective.

The specific treatment for serious hemorrhagic manifestations in patients with von Willebrand's disease (vWD) who are not responsive to DDAVP is cryoprecipitate or fresh frozen plasma. Serious bleeding (and thus treatment) is rare if the factor VIII level is >25 per cent of normal and/or the bleeding time is <15 minutes. If cesarean section is required for obstetrical reasons, treatment is indicated if the level is <40 per cent. Cryoprecipitate, given in a dose 24 to 36 U/kg (0.24 to 0.39 bags/kg) is followed by one-half the dose every 12 hours for 3 to 8 days. If possible, treatment should be started 24 hours preoperatively to allow new factor VIII synthesis in addition to the elevation obtained from the therapeutic material. When unanticipated acute bleeding is encountered or immediate cesarean section planned, the initial therapeutic dose should be increased by approximately 50 per cent and a second dose should be given approximately 12 hours later (Shulman, 1967). Levels should be checked daily after vaginal delivery or cesarean section and therapy given if the level falls below 25 per cent or bleeding occurs (Noller et al., 1973; Krishanamurth and Miotti, 1977; Lipton et al., 1982; Cohen and Goldiner, 1989). The various glycine-precipitated antihemophilic factors available for treatment of classic hemophilia should not be used in vWD. Although they are effective at raising factor VIII levels, they do not correct the bleeding time, the ristocetin platelet aggregation defect, or, in fact, the clinical bleeding.

LIVER DISEASE. Virtually every hemostatic function

may be impaired in liver disease. Deficiencies of prothrombin and of factors VII, IX, and X generally result from decreased synthesis by the damaged liver. Factor V and fibrinogen are also synthesized by the liver; however, their levels are usually not so severely depressed. The diversity of the coagulation abnormality will be reflected in the laboratory studies by abnormalities in the aPTT, PT, and fibrinogen levels and by abnormal fibrinolysis.

Treatment consists of both vitamin K administration and procoagulant replacement therapy. Vitamin K can be administered as vitamin K_1 in a dose of 50 mg intramuscularly; it will produce improvement in approximately 30 per cent of patients with liver disease. Replacement therapy is accomplished with fresh frozen plasma in a dose of 10 to 20 ml/kg (Spector and Corn, 1967).

FACTOR XI DEFICIENCY. Also called plasma thromboplastin antecedent deficiency, this hereditary disorder is transmitted as an incompletely recessive autosomal trait manifested either as a major defect in homozygous individuals with factor XI levels below 20 per cent or as a minor defect in heterozygous individuals with levels ranging from 30 to 65 per cent of normal (Leiba et al., 1965). However, severity of bleeding does not always correlate with the level of factor XI (Rimon et al., 1976; Purcell and Nossel, 1970). The aPTT is usually prolonged in individuals with factor XI deficiency, and the specific diagnosis is confirmed when the factor XI level is shown to be below 65 per cent of normal.

Despite the fact that factor XI normally decreases during pregnancy (Phillips et al., 1973), most gravidas do not encounter bleeding problems. In one series, nine women went through 17 pregnancies without a major hemorrhage (Rapaport et al., 1961). Therapy is based on maintaining the factor XI level above 40 per cent for minor procedures (including delivery) and above 50 per cent for major procedures. Treatment consists of a loading dose of fresh frozen plasma of 10 ml/kg followed by a maintenance dose of 5 mg/kg/day.

HEMOPHILIA A (FACTOR VIII DEFICIENCY) AND HEMOPHILIA B (FACTOR IX DEFICIENCY). These disorders are transmitted as sex-linked recessive traits. Therefore, severe genetically determined disease is unlikely to occur in pregnant women. The heterozygous carrier of factor VIII or IX deficiency is usually free of bleeding manifestations. Occasionally, carriers whose normal X chromosome has been inactivated in early fetal life may have unusually low levels of factor VIII or IX (Lusher and McMillan, 1978). They may be troubled with menorrhagia (usually responsive to oral contraceptives) and even hemarthroses, but pregnancy and delivery usually have been free of serious hemorrhage. Successful treatment for bleeding in the factor VIII—deficient woman has been accomplished with the administration of cryoprecipitate or factor VIII concentrate. Factor IX—deficient individuals have received fresh frozen plasma or factor IX concentrate for bleeding or surgery.

Sons born to hemophilia A or B carriers have a 50 per cent chance of being affected with the disease. Carrier detection in hemophilia A, employing the techniques of procoagulant and antigenic assay for factor VIII, is reliable even during pregnancy. Intrauterine detection of hemophilia is being accomplished in a few special laboratories (Alter, 1984; Weatherall, 1985; White and Shoemaker, 1989), either using a specific DNA probe or taking advantage of restriction-fragment length polymorphism linked to the factor VIII gene. Affected sons born to carriers have remarkably little bleeding during vaginal delivery, but there are anecdotal reports of massive cephalohematomas in such infants subjected to fetal scalp monitoring during labor. The presence or absence of the disease in newborn males can generally be established by simultaneous assays of maternal and cord blood. Factors VIII and IX do not cross the placenta.

Most female carriers for hemophilia B have no clinical manifestations; however, carriers with levels as low as 10 per cent have been reported (Lusher and McMillan, 1978). Women with low levels are at risk for intrapartum and postpartum bleeding and should be given factor IX concentrate if their factor IX level is less than 25 per cent at term (Rust et al., 1975). The appropriate dose of factor IX is 50 U/kg, which usually calculates to 2500 to 3000 U as an initial dose followed by 1500 units every 12 to 24 hours. The half-life of factor IX varies in individual patients, and the dosage schedule should be modified based on analysis of each patient's factor IX level after transfusion.

Carrier detection for factor IX relies on coagulation assay for factor IX, and carriers have a broad overlap with the normal range. Prenatal diagnosis of fetuses at risk is difficult. Direct fetal blood sampling may be contaminated by factor IX activity in amniotic fluid, and most families do not have revealing polymorphism (Miller and Hoyer, 1986).

FACTOR XIII DEFICIENCY. Probably transmitted as an autosomal recessive trait, factor XIII deficiency is extremely rare. It is included in this discussion primarily because two manifestations of the disorder are especially pertinent to any consideration of hematologic problems in obstetrics: (1) persistent, even fatal bleeding from the umbilical stump has been reported as a common event in infants affected by the disorder, and (2) affected women experience a very high incidence of spontaneous abortion (Kitchens and Newcomb, 1979; Lorand et al., 1980). Other clinical manifestations include intracranial bleeding after trivial trauma (an incidence of 30 per cent is reported in some series, much higher than that observed in most coagulation defects) and defective wound healing. The diagnosis is established by demonstrated dissolution of the clot in 5 M urea; results of all other commonly employed coagulation tests are normal.

Successful results of replacement therapy with fresh and stored plasma, whole blood, and cryoprecipitate have all been reported. Levels adequate for normal hemostasis are low, and transfusion of small amounts of normal plasma given infrequently has served as adequate therapy or prophylaxis. One reported pregnant woman was treated with 300 ml of plasma every 10 days during pregnancy and had a successful outcome (Fisher et al., 1966).

ANTIBODIES TO FACTOR VIII. These antibodies produce a rare but often dramatic hemorrhagic disease.

The onset is usually in the postpartum period, but occasionally it may be as long as a year after parturition. The disorder is caused by the spontaneous development of an inhibitor to factor VIII. The pathogenesis of the disorder is unknown. The inhibitor is an immunoglobulin, usually an IgG but occasionally an IgM. Polyclonal inhibitors have been described. The clinical manifestations mimic those seen in hemophilia A, with soft tissue bleeding and even hemarthroses after minimal trauma. A prolonged partial thromboplastin time that is not corrected by addition of normal plasma after incubation of the mixture is characteristic. All other screening coagulation studies are normal, but the level of factor VIII is low when specific assays are carried out. The natural history of the illness is one of gradual disappearance of the inhibitor over time.

The clinical course in patients with spontaneously occurring factor VIII inhibitors can often be modified by the use of prednisone. The infant of an affected mother is rarely affected, and subsequent pregnancies, when they have occurred, have usually not been marred by recurrence of the inhibitor (Coller et al., 1981).

DISSEMINATED INTRAVASCULAR COAGULATION. This disorder is really a syndrome produced as part of an underlying disease that in some way leads to initiation of the clotting mechanisms (Laros, 1986). In the area of obstetrics and gynecology, DIC is seen in association with placental abruption (Colman et al., 1987), the dead fetus syndrome (Sutton et al., 1971), amniotic fluid embolism (Phillips et al., 1964), gram-negative sepsis (Phillips and Davidson, 1972), saline abortions (Phillips et al., 1967), and severe preeclampsia-eclampsia (Laros and Penner, 1976; Davidson and Phillips, 1972; Pritchard et al., 1976).

The first result of DIC is a disturbance of the coagulation mechanism. This results from the consumption of plasma factors and from the production of anticoagulants by the fibrinolytic system. The coagulation factors consumed are platelets, fibrinogen, prothrombin, factor V, and factor VIII. The body has a limited capacity to produce circulating plasma factors and platelets necessary for clot formation. When the available plasma factors are consumed by intravascular coagulation, the circulating blood becomes deficient in clotting factors. Without sufficient clotting factors, a severe bleeding diathesis may result. Activation of the fibrinolytic system produces fibrin degradation products (FDPs). These split products serve to further interfere with the coagulation mechanism. The pathophysiology of DIC is summarized in Figure 53–3.

The second major result of DIC is the presence of small clots in the microcirculation. These clots can cause plugging of small vessels and ischemia of various organs. DIC occurs when the coagulation mechanism is inappropriately triggered by any of several underlying disease processes that have in common the ability to disrupt the normal coagulation mechanism.

Disease entities associated with DIC fall into three major groups based on the mechanisms by which the primary disease initiates intravascular clotting. The underlying mechanism in the first group is the intra-

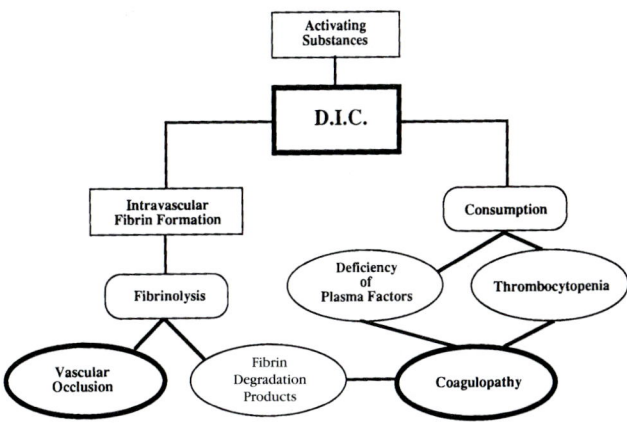

FIGURE 53–3. Pathophysiology of disseminated intravascular coagulation.

vascular infusion of thromboplastic substances, tissue thromboplastins that activate the extrinsic coagulation system. Placental abruption and the dead fetus syndrome fall into this category. They differ in that with abruption consumption is rapid and fulminant; with the dead fetus syndrome, the consumption is very slow, occurring over a period of days.

The second group of pathologic conditions causing DIC includes those conditions associated with endothelial damage. Both the extrinsic and the intrinsic coagulation systems are activated by endothelial damage. Eclampsia/preeclampsia is thought to fall into this category. Several prospective studies have documented subclinical changes in the coagulation system of patients with eclampsia/preeclampsia. However, the specific changes noted and the frequency of the changes have varied widely (Pritchard et al., 1976; Kitzmiller et al., 1974; Kelton et al., 1985; O'Brien et al., 1986; Socol et al., 1985; Stubbs et al., 1984; Weenink et al., 1984; Weiner and Brandt, 1982).

Although Weinstein (1985) first coined the term HELLP (*h*emolysis, *e*levated *l*iver enzymes, *l*ow *p*latelets), the syndrome had been known for years. Weinstein described nausea and vomiting, epigastric pain and right upper quadrant tenderness in over 80 per cent of cases. Liver enzymes (SGOT and SGPT) were elevated and platelets decreased in all patients. Proteinuria, fragmented RBCs, hyperbilirubinemia, elevated creatinine, and abnormal PT, aPTT, and fibrinogen were described in 100, 96, 86, 62, 53, and 4 per cent of cases respectively. Table 53–13 compares findings in the various syndromes having in common thrombocytopenia and RBC fragmentation.

The third group of diseases associated with DIC encompasses nonspecific or indirect effects of certain diseases. This group includes amniotic fluid embolism, gram-negative sepsis, and saline abortions.

In DIC, the signs and symptoms are basically those of the underlying disease. The clinical presentation may be hemorrhagic, thrombotic, or both. With acute presentation, hemorrhagic problems predominate and vice versa. Hemorrhagic presentations of DIC involving the skin or mucous membranes include ecchymoses, petechiae, epistaxis, gingival bleeding, hematuria, gastrointestinal bleeding, and venipuncture

TABLE 53–13. Comparison of Syndromes Associated with
Thrombocytopenia and Red Cell Fragmentation

FINDINGS*	DISEASE			
	PE/E	DIC	HUS	TTP
Neurologic findings	±	±	±	+
Fever	−	±	±	+
Hypertension	+	±	+	±
Renal dysfunction	+	±	+	±
Thrombocytopenia	±	+	+	+
Hemolytic anemia	±	±	+	+
Elevated FDPs	±	+	±	±
Low fibrinogen	±	+	−	−

*(+) usually present; (±) variably present; (−) absent; PE/E = preeclampsia/eclampsia; DIC = disseminated intravascular coagulation; HUS = hemolytic uremic syndrome; TTP = thrombotic thrombocytopenic purpura.

oozing. Intracranial or intracerebral bleeding are also hemorrhagic manifestations that may occur. Thrombotic presentations of DIC may be neurologic—as seen in multifocal lesions, delirium, and coma—or dermatologic, with focal ischemia and superficial gangrene. Renal examples of thrombotic presentation are cortical necrosis and uremia. Acute ulceration with bleeding is an example of a gastrointestinal thrombotic presentation. Infarcts and emboli represent pulmonary vascular obstruction, whereas phlebitis and peripheral gangrene are results of thrombotic effects within peripheral veins and arteries.

The laboratory diagnosis of full-blown DIC can be relatively easy. All the routine screening tests of coagulation yield grossly abnormal results. The platelet count is almost always decreased or falls progressively, the fibrinogen is low, and circulating FDPs are increased. The PT and aPTT may be normal, prolonged or shortened. The shortening occurs early in the progression of the syndrome when excess amounts of activated factor V and X are in circulation, but before much consumption of these factors has occurred and before the level of FDPs with their antithrombin properties has increased, leading to prolongation of the PT and aPTT. Indirect evidence of an obstructed microcirculation can be found by examining a peripheral blood smear. As normal red cells are forced through the obstructed capillary beds, they tend to fragment. Bizarre cell forms called schistocytes and helmet cells are formed and can be readily identified. If the rate of red cell destruction is brisk, the patient may show evidence of intravascular hemolysis by the appearance of an elevated plasma hemoglobin level and hemoglobinuria.

The most important step in treating DIC is recognition and treatment of the underlying disease process. Bleeding poses the greatest threat to the patient with DIC, and administration of procoagulants is essential. Platelets are administered as platelet concentrates with one unit raising the count 5 to 10 × 10⁹/liter. The clotting factors may be replaced with fresh frozen plasma. Factor VIII and fibrinogen may be replaced with cryoprecipitate. Appropriate doses are 10 to 20 ml/kg of fresh, frozen plasma or 0.1 to 0.2 bags/kg.

Heparin is rarely required in the treatment of DIC,

but should be considered when there is evidence of progressive renal dysfunction, gangrene of the digits, or other special circumstances. Heparin is administered in a dose of 500 to 1000 units per hour intravenously following a loading dose of 5000 units. Laboratory control of heparin therapy may be difficult; however, unless the fibrinogen level is very low, an adequate endpoint can usually be obtained and consists of an increased TT or aPTT to approximately one and one-half times the control value. Platelet transfusions are particularly important if heparin is to be administered in the face of significant thrombocytopenia (<30 × 10⁹ per liter).

Fortunately, in obstetric practice those diseases associated with DIC are usually cured by delivery. Therefore, specific treatment for the coagulopathy produced by the DIC is also limited in scope. After delivery, the DIC will ameliorate and the coagulation abnormalities return to normal. Because of the liver's immense capacity for protein synthesis, the plasma factors will return to normal within 24 hours of cessation of DIC. The return of the platelet count to normal will be slow (5 to 7 days) because of the time required for generation, maturation, and release by the bone marrow.

THROMBOTIC THROMBOCYTOPENIC PURPURA. This acute and occasionally chronic or recurrent disorder is characterized by a pentad of clinical and laboratory manifestations: hemolytic anemia, thrombocytopenia, neurologic symptoms, renal abnormalities, and fever. It occurs in either sex and at any age but is most common in women in their 20s and 30s. Numerous variants have been described (acute, chronic, familial), and in some instances the clinical manifestations have appeared in association with other conditions (including neoplasia, connective tissue disorders, infection, pregnancy, and the puerperium), but many cases remain idiopathic. Bukowski's comprehensive review (1982) summarizes the available clinical and pathologic data as well as the results of the several therapies proposed over the past three decades.

The clinical diagnosis of acute idiopathic thrombotic thrombocytopenic purpura (TTP) is usually reasonably straightforward. Presenting symptoms include some or all of the following: abnormal bleeding (usually into skin and from mucous membranes; vaginal bleeding is common), jaundice, neurologic symptoms (including cranial nerve palsies, headache, alterations of consciousness, paresis, organic brain syndromes, syncope, seizures, visual disturbance) that typically fluctuate in severity and may be transient, and fever. A variety of other complaints have been reported less commonly. Noteworthy physical findings are pallor, jaundice, purpura, and neurologic abnormalities; splenic enlargement is unusual. The peripheral blood is characteristic: moderate-to-severe anemia with numerous fragmented erythrocytes, polychromatophilia (indicating a brisk reticulocytosis), and numerous nucleated red blood cells are found together with a moderate polymorphonuclear leukocytosis and moderate-to-severe thrombocytopenia. The bone marrow shows intense normoblastic erythroid hyperplasia and an adequate-to-increased number of megakaryocytes. This hematologic appearance has been termed microangiopathic hemolysis, in reference to the fragmentation of red cells within the microcirculation. The indirect serum bilirubin and the LDH levels are elevated, and hematuria is commonly found. Elevations of BUN and creatinine, sometimes not found at first presentation, usually develop but seldom go beyond 100 mg/dl and 3 mg/dl, respectively. The Coombs' antiglobulin reaction is almost invariably negative. The natural history of the disease is nearly always one of progressive deterioration, and survival beyond 3 months from onset is unusual unless therapy is successful.

At presentation, diagnostic considerations often include lupus erythematosus, Evans' syndrome, and sepsis (particularly *Clostridium perfringens* endometritis in young women with vaginal bleeding) with DIC, but these conditions can usually be promptly excluded on clinical, immunologic, and bacteriologic grounds. Hemolytic uremic syndrome (HUS) presents a more difficult problem in differential diagnosis because microangiopathic hemolysis, thrombocytopenia, and renal failure are the hallmarks of this condition. Features that help to distinguish the two disorders clinically are as follows: (1) history of a viral or bacterial gastrointestinal illness, especially with diarrhea, is common in HUS but rare in TTP; (2) early, severe renal failure with oliguria, anuria, and hypertension are typical of HUS, but less common, less severe and later in appearance in TTP; (3) HUS is predominantly a disease of childhood, although bona fide cases have been reported in adults of all ages, as well as during pregnancy and the postpartum period (Segonds et al., 1979; Lazebnik et al., 1985); (4) bleeding and thrombocytopenia are generally more severe in TTP; and (5) neurologic manifestations (except for alterations of consciousness and even seizures consistent with profound renal failure and hypertensive encephalopathy) are unusual in HUS. None of these differential points can be considered absolute, but taken together they are helpful in making the distinction between the two conditions. The differential diagnosis has been considered of some importance because of the differences in prognosis, although postpartum HUS carries a much higher mortality rate than the HUS of childhood. Whether better supportive care and plasmapheresis, plasma infusion, and antiplatelet agents individually or in combination will modify the outcome of postpartum HUS in an increasing number of patients remains to be seen.

Further compounding the diagnostic difficulties when microangiopathic hemolysis is recognized in pregnancy and the postpartum period is the observation that some women with severe toxemia or eclampsia are noted to have fragmentation hemolytic anemia, thrombocytopenia, and renal failure. In 1978, Schwartz and Brenner reviewed the reported cases of TTP in pregnancy and concluded that in most instances the diagnosis of TTP was in error, and that treatment for eclampsia should take precedence over that for TTP unless there is positive evidence that TTP either preceded pregnancy or occurred without evidence of toxemia. This review cites several eclamptics with microangiopathy who were successfully managed with the measures directed toward control of eclampsia; whereas treatments directed at control of TTP (with heparin, antiplatelet agents, dextrose, steroids, dialysis, and splenectomy in various combinations) in many cases had disastrous results. In this retrospective review, plasmapheresis or plasma infusions are not mentioned as treatment for TTP, and there is limited experience with such therapy in pregnant or postpartum women suspected of having TTP. Neame (1980) reports briefly the apparently successful use of plasma exchange in a single patient in whom the TTP syndrome, which was previously noted but in remission for 7 years, recurred after delivery. Weiner (1987) cites several patients satisfying his criteria for TTP in pregnancy whose cases were successfully managed with plasma manipulations.

Current opinion about treatment of TTP in the absence of pregnancy leans toward plasma exchange or plasma infusions. It is proposed that the patient's plasma contains some substance favoring platelet aggregation or lacks some material that protects endothelial cells from platelet adhesion. Certainly, recent uncontrolled therapeutic trials of each of these modalities, usually with added antiplatelet agents, have yielded more survivors than have been reported as historical controls. It is reasonable to consider the employment of these measures in a pregnant or postpartum woman in whom the diagnosis of eclampsia can be excluded. Whether such measures, in addition to the usual modalities employed for the management of eclampsia, should be considered in those patients in whom information about the time sequence of proteinuria, hypertension, hemolysis, thrombocytopenia, seizures, and renal failure is unavailable cannot at present be stated with certainty.

HEMOLYTIC UREMIC SYNDROME. This disorder shares many of the clinical and laboratory features of TTP. However, it occurs primarily in children and produces a paucity of neurologic symptoms and a far greater degree of renal dysfunction. In nonpregnant adults it is now often treated with plasma exchange, because the more benign course seen in young children and successfully treated with careful supportive measures (sometimes including dialysis) is less commonly observed in older patients. Uncontrolled reports suggest that plasma exchange is often the key to beginning improvement in renal function and hematologic status. With the present state of our knowledge, acceptance of these reports makes diagnostic certainty between TTP and HUS less important. It is not known whether plasma exchange influences the course of HUS in postpartum patients.

LUPUS ANTICOAGULANT. First described more than 30 years ago in two patients who had established systemic lupus erythematosus and a hemorrhagic diathesis caused by a circulating inhibitor, lupus anticoagulants (or lupus inhibitors) are immunoglobulins that interfere with phospholipid dependent coagulation tests but do not inhibit the activity of specific coagulation factors (Shapiro and Thiagarajan, 1982). The overall incidence of the abnormality in patients with lupus is 34 per cent, and most patients with lupus anticoagulant (LAC) do not have lupus (Love and Santoro, 1990). Furthermore, although patients with LAC have abnormal coagulation tests, they rarely have significant bleeding.

A related group of patients are those with anticardiolipin antibodies (ACA). Although these antibodies do not produce abnormalities in phospholipid-dependent coagulation studies, they are associated with a similar clinical syndrome and are found in 44 per cent of lupus patients (Love and Santoro, 1990).

The clinical syndrome associated with both LAC and ACA includes recurrent venous and/or arterial thrombosis, thrombocytopenia, recurrent abortion, recurrent fetal loss, and early-onset preeclampsia (Kalunian et al., 1988; Harris et al., 1986; Petri et al., 1987; Branch et al., 1989). Extensive placental infarction has been found in some of these cases of fetal loss, and it is suggested that the peripheral thromboses and placental infarction share pathogenic mechanisms related to the lupus inhibitor (De Wolf et al., 1982). The pathophysiology and treatment of both LAC and ANA are discussed in greater detail in Chapter 31.

Laboratory findings characteristic of the presence of the lupus inhibitor include a prolonged aPTT or Russell Viper time not corrected by the addition of an equal volume of normal plasma (Thiagarajan et al., 1986).

Patients who have experienced either arterial or venous thromboembolism are usually treated with anticoagulants for life. Full anticoagulating doses of warfarin are used when the woman is not pregnant and heparin is used during pregnancy (Rosove et al., 1990). If the aPTT is not prolonged, heparin is administered subcutaneously every 12 hours in a dose sufficient to prolong the aPTT to 1½ to 2 times control at 6 hours. When the aPTT is prolonged, a dose is chosen that prolongs the aPTT to 2 to 2½ times control at 6 hours without prolonging the PT by more than 2 seconds. The role of low-dose aspirin and heparin therapy in patient with recurrent pregnancy loss is also discussed in Chapter 31.

REFERENCES

Alger LS, Golbus MS, Laros RK Jr: Thalassemia and pregnancy. Am J Obstet Gynecol 134:662, 1979.

Alter BP: Advances in prenatal diagnosis of hematologic disease. Blood 64:329, 1984.

Beischer NA, Holsman M, Kitchen WH: Relation of various forms of anemia to placental weight. Am J Obstet Gynecol 101:801, 1968a.

Beischer NA, Townsend L, Holsman M, et al.: Urinary estriol excretion in pregnancy anemia. Am J Obstet Gynecol 102:819, 1968b.

Beutler E: Glucose-6-phosphate dehydrogenase deficiency. N Engl J Med 324:169, 1991.

Blattner P, Dar H, Nitowski HM: Pregnancy outcome in women with sickle cell trait. JAMA 238:1392, 1977.

Branch DW, Andres R, Digre KB, et al.: The association of antiphospholipid antibodies with severe preeclampsia. Obstet Gynecol 73:541, 1989.

Breckenridge RL, Riggs JA: Hereditary elliptocytosis with hemolytic anemia complicating pregnancy. Am J Obstet Gynecol 101:861, 1968.

Brunskill PJ: The effects of fetal exposure to danazol. Br J Obstet Gynaecol 99:212, 1992

Bukowski RM: Thrombotic thrombocytopenic purpura: A review. Prog Hemost Thromb 6:287, 1982.

Bunn HF, Forget BJ: Human Hemoglobins. Philadelphia, W.B. Saunders Company, 1986.

Bussel JB, Berkowitz RJ, McFarland JG, et al.: Antenatal treatment of neonatal alloimmune thrombocytopenia. N Engl J Med 319:1374, 1988.

Cash JD: Platelet transfusion therapy. Clin Hematol 1:395, 1972.

Catanzarite VA, Ferguson JE II: Acute leukemia and pregnancy: A review of management and outcome, 1972–1982. Obstet Gynecol Surv 39:663, 1984.

CDC: Use of folic acid for prevention of spina bifida and other neural tube defects—1983–1991. MMWR 40:513, 1991.

Champlin RE, Goldman JM, Gale RP: Bone marrow transplantation in chronic myelogenous leukemia. Semin Hematol 25:74, 1988.

Cimo PL, Aster RH: Post-transfusion purpura: Successful treatment with exchange transfusion. N Engl J Med 287:290, 1972.

Cines D, Dussk B, Tomaski A, et al.: Immune thrombocytopenic purpura and pregnancy. N Engl J Med 306:106, 1982.

Cohen S, Goldiner PL: Epidural analgesia for labor and delivery in a patient with von Willebrand's disease. Regional Anesth 14:95, 1989.

Coller BS, Hultin MB, Hoyer LW, et al.: Normal pregnancy in a patient with a prior postpartum factor VIII inhibitor: With observations on pathogenesis and prognosis. Blood 58:619, 1981.

Colman RW, Hirsh J, Marder VJ, Salzman EW: Hemostasis and Thrombosis. Philadelphia, J. B. Lippincott Company, 1987.

Cook RL, Miller RC, Katz VL, Cefalo RC: Immune thrombocytopenic purpura in pregnancy: A reappraisal of management. Obstet Gynecol 78:578, 1991.

Cunningham FG, Pritchard JA, Mason RA: Pregnancy and sickle cell hemoglobinopathies. Obstet Gynecol 62:419, 1983.

Cunningham FG, Pritchard JA, Mason RA, Chase G: Prophylactic transfusion of normal red blood cells during pregnancy complicated by sickle cell hemoglobinopathies. Am J Obstet Gynecol 135:994, 1979.

Daffos F, Forestier F, Muller JY, et al.: Prenatal treatment of alloimmune thrombocytopenia. Lancet 2:632, 1984.

Dara P, Slater LM, Armentrout SA: Successful pregnancy during chemotherapy for acute leukemia. Cancer 47:845, 1981.

Davidson EC, Phillips LL: Coagulation studies in the hypertensive toxemias of pregnancy. Am J Obstet Gynecol 113:905, 1972.

Deeg HJ, Kennedy MS, Sanders JR, et al.: Successful pregnancy after marrow transplantation for severe aplastic anemia and immunosuppression with cyclosporine. JAMA 250:647, 1983.

De Wolf F, Carreras LO, Moermman P, et al.: Decidual vasculopathy and extensive placental infarction in a patient with repeated thromboembolic accidents, recurrent fetal loss, and a lupus anticoagulant. Am J Obstet Gynecol 142:829, 1982.

Doney K, Storb R, Buckner CD, et al.: Marrow transplantation for treatment of pregnancy-associated aplastic anemia. Exp Hematol 13:1080, 1985.

Erslev AJ: Erythropoietin. N Engl J Med 324:1339, 1991.

Falkson HC, Simson IW, Falkson G: Non-Hodgkin's lymphoma in pregnancy. Cancer 45:1679, 1980.

Fenton V, Cavill J, Fisher J: Iron stores in pregnancy. Br J Haematol 37:145, 1977.

Ferguson JE, O'Reilly RA: Hemoglobin E and pregnancy. Obstet Gynecol 66:136, 1985.

Finer P, Blair J, Rowe P: Epidural analgesia in the management of labor pain and sickle cell crisis. A case report. Anesthesiology 68:799, 1988.

Fisher S, Rikover M, Naor S: Factor XIII deficiency with severe hemorrhagic diathesis. Blood 28:34, 1966.

Fleming AF: Hypoplastic anaemia in pregnancy. Clin Haematol 2:477, 1973.

Fleming AF, Lynch W: Beta-thalassemia minor during pregnancy with particular reference to iron status. J Obstet Gynaecol Br Comm 76:451, 1967.

Fosburg MT, Nathan DG: Treatment of Cooley's anemia. Blood 76:435, 1990.

Foulkes J, Goldie DJ: The use of ferritin to assess the need for iron supplements in pregnancy. J Obstet Gynecol 3:11, 1982.

Frakes JT, Burmeister RE, Giliberti JJ: Pregnancy in a patient with paroxysmal nocturnal hemoglobinuria. Obstet Gynecol 47(s):22, 1976.

Francis RB, Johnson CS: Vascular occlusion in sickle cell disease: Current concepts and unanswered questions. Blood 77:1405, 1991.

Galbraith GMP, Galbraith RM, Temple A, et al.: Demonstration of transferrin receptors on human placental trophoblast. Blood 55:240, 1980.

Hamstra RD, Block MH, Schocket AL: Intravenous iron dextran. JAMA 233:1726, 1980.

Harris EN, Chan JKH, Asherson RA, et al.: Thrombosis, recurrent fetal loss, and thrombocytopenia. Arch Intern Med 146:2153, 1986.

Herbert V, Colman N, Spivack M: Folic acid deficiency in the United States: Folate assays in a prenatal clinic. Am J Obstet Gynecol 123:175, 1975.

Hew-Wing R, Rolbin SH, Hew E, Amato D: Epidural anesthesia and thrombocytopenia. Anaesthesia 44:775, 1989.

Higgs DR, Vickers MA, Wilkie AOM, et al.: A review of the molecular genetics of the human a-globin gene cluster. Blood 73:1081, 1989.

Ho CH, Yuan CC, Yeh SH: Serum ferritin, folate and cobalamin levels and their correlation with anemia in normal full-term pregnant women. Eur J Obstet Gynecol Reprod Biol 26:7, 1987.

Holly RG: Hypoplastic anemia in pregnancy. Obstet Gynecol 1:533, 1953.

Holmes GE, Holmes FF: Pregnancy outcome of patients treated for Hodgkin's disease. A controlled study. Cancer 41:1317, 1978.

Horger E: Sickle cell and sickle cell-Hgb C disease during pregnancy. Obstet Gynecol 39:873, 1972.

Horning SJ, Hopp RT, Kaplan HS, Rosenberg SA: Female reproductive potential after treatment for Hodgkin's disease. N Engl J Med 304:1377, 1981.

Horowitz JJ, Laros RK Jr: Anemia and pregnancy: A review of the pathophysiology, diagnosis and treatment. J C E Obstet Gynecol 1:9, 1979.

Hurd WW, Miodovnik M, Stys SJ: Pregnancy associated with paroxysmal nocturnal hemoglobinuria. Obstet Gynecol 60:742, 1982.

Iyengar L: Folic acid absorption in pregnancy. Br J Obstet Gynaecol 82:20, 1975.

Jacobs C, Donaldson SH, Rosenberg SA, Kaplan HS: Management of the pregnant patient with Hodgkin's disease. Ann Intern Med 95:669, 1981.

Johan E, Magnus EM: Plasma and red blood cell folate during normal pregnancy. Acta Obstet Gynecol Scand 60:247, 1981.

Kagan R, Laros RK Jr: Immune thrombocytopenia. Clin Obstet Gynecol 26:537, 1983.

Kalunian KC, Peter JB, Middlekauff HR, et al.: Clinical significance of a single test for anti-cardiolipin antibodies in patients with systemic lupus erythematosus. Am J Med 85:602, 1988.

Kan YW, Golbus MS, Dozy AM: Prenatal diagnosis of alpha-thalassemia. N Engl J Med 295:1165, 1976.

Kazazian HH, Boehm CD: Molecular basis and prenatal diagnosis of β-thalassemia. Blood 72:1107 1988.

Kelton JG, Hunter DJS, Neame PB: A platelet function defect in preeclampsia. Obstet Gynecol 65:107, 1985.

Kelton JG, Inwood MJ, Barr RM, et al.: The prenatal prediction of thrombocytopenia in infants of mothers with clinically diagnosed immune thrombocytopenia. Am J Obstet Gynecol 144:449, 1982.

Kitay DZ: Folic acid deficiency in pregnancy. Am J Obstet Gynecol 104:1067, 1969.

Kitchens CS, Newcomb TF: Factor XIII. Medicine (Balt) 58:413, 1979.

Kitzmiller JL, Lang JE, Yelenosky PF, et al.: Hematologic assays in preeclampsia. Am J Obstet Gynecol 118:362, 1974.

Koshy M, Burd L, Wallace D, et al.: Prophylactic red-cell transfusion in pregnant patients with sickle cell disease. N Engl J Med 319:1447, 1988.

Krishanamurth M, Miotti AB: Von Willebrand's disease and pregnancy. Obstet Gynecol 49:244, 1977.

Kuvin SF, Brecher G: Differential neutrophil counts in pregnancy. N Engl J Med 266:877, 1962.

Laros RK Jr: Sickle cell hemoglobin C disease in pregnancy. Pa Med 70:73, 1967.

Laros RK Jr (ed): Blood Disorders in Pregnancy. Philadelphia, Lea & Febiger, 1986.

Laros RK Jr, Kagan R: Route of delivery for patients with immune thrombocytopenic purpura. Am J Obstet Gynecol 148:901, 1984.

Laros RK Jr, Kalstone C: Sickle cell beta-thalassemia and pregnancy. Obstet Gynecol 37:67, 1971.

Laros RK Jr, Penner JA: Pathophysiology of disseminated intravascular coagulation in saline-induced abortion. Obstet Gynecol 48:353, 1976.

Lazebnik N, Jaffa AJ, Peyeser R: Hemolytic-uremic syndrome in

pregnancy. Review of the literature and report of a case. Obstet Gynecol Surv 40:618, 1985.

Leiba H, Ramot B, Many A: Heredity and coagulation studies in ten families with factor XI deficiency. Br J Haematol 11:654, 1965.

Li FP, Fine W, Jaffe N, et al.: Offspring of patients treated for cancer in childhood. JNCI 62:1193, 1979.

Lilleyman JS, Hill AS, Anderton KJ: Consequences of acute myelogenous leukemia in early pregnancy. Cancer 40:1300, 1977.

Lind SE: The bleeding time does not predict surgical bleeding. Blood 77:2547, 1991.

Lipton RA, Ayromlooi J, Coller BS: Severe von Willebrand's disease during labor and delivery. JAMA 248:1355, 1982.

Lorand L, Losowsky MS, Miloszewski KJM: Human factor XIII: Fibrin-stabilizing factor. Prog Hemost Thromb 5:245, 1980.

Love PE, Santoro SA: Antiphospholipid antibodies: Anticardiolipin and the lupus anticoagulant in systemic lupus erythematosus (SLE) and in non-SLE disorders. Prevalence and clinical significance. Ann Intern Med 112:9, 1990.

Lusher JM, McMillan CW: Severe factor VIII and factor IX deficiency in females. Am J Med 65:637, 1978.

Lynch RE, Williams DM, Reading JC, et al.: The prognosis in aplastic anemia. Blood 45:517, 1975.

Maberry MC, Mason RA, Cunningham FG, Pritchard JA: Pregnancy complicated by hemoglobin CC and C-β-thalassemia disease. Obstet Gynecol 76:324, 1990.

Maberry MC, Mason RA, Cunningham FG, Pritchard JA: Pregnancy complicated by hereditary spherocytosis. Obstet Gynecol 79:735, 1992.

Maduska AL, Guinee WS, Heaton AJ, et al.: Sickling dynamics of red blood cells and other physiologic studies during anesthesia. Anesth Analg 54:361, 1975.

Magid MS, Perkins M, Gottfried EL: Increased erythrocyte osmotic fragility in pregnancy. Am J Obstet Gynecol 144:910, 1982.

Matthay KK, Mentzer WC: Erythrocyte enzymes in the newborn. Clin Haematol 10:31, 1981.

McGuire WA, Yang HH, Bruno E, et al.: Treatment of antibody-mediated pure red-cell aplasia with high-dose intravenous gammaglobulin. N Eng J Med 317:1004, 1987.

McIntosh S, O'Brien RT, Schwartz AD, et al.: Neonatal isoimmune purpura: Response to platelet infusions. J Pediatr 82:1020, 1973.

Miller JM: Alpha thalassemia minor in pregnancy. J Reprod Med 27:207, 1982.

Miller CH, Hoyer LW: Prenatal diagnosis of two sporadic cases of hemophilia. N Engl J Med 314:584, 1986.

Moise KL Jr, Carpenter RJ Jr, Cotton DB, et al.: Percutaneous umbilical cord blood sampling in the evaluation of fetal platelet counts in pregnant patients with autoimmune thrombocytopenic purpura. Obstet Gynecol 72:346, 1988.

Monsen ER, Kuhn JH, Finch CA: Iron status of menstruating females. Am J Clin Nutr 20:842, 1967.

Moore A, Sherman MM, Strongin MJ: Hereditary spherocytosis with hemolytic crisis during pregnancy. Obstet Gynecol 47(s):19, 1976.

Morrison JC, Whybrew WD, Bucovary ET: Use of partial exchange transfusion preoperatively in patients with sickle cell hemoglobinopathies. Am J Obstet Gynecol 132:59, 1978.

Morrison JC, Wiser WL: The use of prophylactic partial exchange transfusion in pregnancies associated with sickle cell hemoglobinopathies. Obstet Gynecol 48:510, 1976.

Motulsky AG: Frequency of sickling disorders in U.S. Blacks. N Engl J Med 288:31, 1973.

Muller JY: Alloimmune thrombocytopenia in the newborn. Curr Stud Hematol: Blood Transf 55:94, 1988.

Neame PB: Immunologic and other factors in thrombotic thrombocytopenic purpura (TTP). Semin Thromb Hemostas 6:416, 1980.

Noller KL, Bowie EJW, Kempers RD, Owen CA Jr: Von Willebrand's disease in pregnancy. Obstet Gynecol 41:865, 1973.

O'Brien WF, Saba HI, Knuppel RA, et al.: Alterations in platelet concentration and aggregation in normal pregnancy and preeclampsia. Am J Obstet Gynecol 155:486, 1986.

Okuyama T, Tawada T, Furuya H, et al.: The role of transferrin and ferritin in the fetal-maternal-placental unit. Am J Obstet Gynecol 152:344, 1985.

Paulone ME, Edelstone DI, Shedd A: Effects of maternal anemia on uteroplacental and fetal oxidative metabolism in sheep. Am J Obstet Gynecol 156:230, 1987.

Peck TM, Arias F: Hematologic changes associated with pregnancy. Clin Obstet 22:785, 1979.

Perkins RP: The significance of glucose-6-phosphate dehydrogenase deficiency in pregnancy. Am J Obstet Gynecol 125:215, 1976.

Petri M, Golbus M, Anderson R, et al.: Antinuclear antibody, lupus anticoagulant, and anticardiolipin antibody in women with idiopathic habitual abortion. A controlled, prospective study. Arthritis-Rheum 30:601, 1987.

Phillips LL, Davidson EC: Procoagulant properties of amniotic fluid. Am J Obstet Gynecol 113:911, 1972.

Phillips LL, Rosano L, Skrodelis V: Changes in factor XI levels during pregnancy. Am J Obstet Gynecol 116:1114, 1973.

Phillips LL, Skrodelis V, Kers TA: Hypofibrinogenemia and intrauterine fetal death. Am J Obstet Gynecol 89:903, 1964.

Phillips LL, Skrodelis V, Quigley HJ: Intravascular coagulation in septic abortion. Obstet Gynecol 30:350, 1967.

Plows CW: Acute myelomonocytic leukemia in pregnancy. Report of a case. Am J Obstet Gynecol 143:41, 1982.

Pizzuto J, Aviles A, Noriega L, et al.: Treatment of acute leukemia during pregnancy: Presentation of nine cases. Cancer Treat Rep 64:679, 1980.

Pritchard JA, Cunningham FG, Mason RA: Coagulation changes in eclampsia. Am J Obstet Gynecol 124:855, 1976.

Pritchard JA, Scott DE, Whalley PJ, Cunningham FG, Mason RA: The effects of maternal sickle cell hemoglobinopathies and sickle cell trait on reproductive performance. Am J Obstet Gynecol 117:662, 1973.

Pritchard JA, Whalley PJ, Scott DE: The influence of maternal folate and iron deficiency on intrauterine life. Am J Obstet Gynecol 104:388, 1969.

Pritchard JA, Whalley PJ, Scott DE: Infants of mothers with megaloblastic anemia due to folate deficiency. JAMA 211:1982, 1970.

Puolakka A, Janne O, Pararinen A, et al.: Serum ferritin in the diagnosis of anemia during pregnancy. Acta Obstet Gynecol Scand 95(Suppl):57, 1980.

Purcell G, Nossel HL: Factor XI (PTA) deficiency. Obstet Gynecol 35:69, 1970.

Rapaport SI, Proctor RR, Patch MJ, Yettra M: The mode of inheritance of PTA disease. Blood 18:149, 1961.

Rasmus KT, Rottman RL, Kotelko DM, et al.: Unrecognized thrombocytopenia in parturients: A retrospective review. Obstet Gynecol 71:943, 1989.

Richards HGH, Spiers ASD: Chronic granulocytic leukemia in pregnancy. Br J Radiol 48:261, 1975.

Rimon A, Schiffman S, Feinstein D, Rapaport SI: Factor XI activity and factor XI antigen in homozygous and heterozygous factor XI deficiency. Blood 48:165, 1976.

Rodgers RPC, Levin J: A critical reappraisal of the bleeding time. Semin Thromb Hemostas 16:1, 1990.

Rolbin SH, Abbott D, Musclow E, et al.: Epidural anesthesia in pregnant patients with low platelet counts. Obstet Gynecol 71:918, 1988.

Rosove MH, Tabsh K, Wasserstrum N, et al.: Heparin therapy for women with lupus anticoagulant or anticardiolipin antibodies. Obstet Gynecol 75:630, 1990.

Rust LA, Goodnight SH, Freeman RK, Johnson CS: Pregnancy and delivery of a woman with hemophilia B. Obstet Gynecol 46:483, 1975.

Sacks DA, Platt L, Johnson CS: Autoimmune hemolytic anemia during pregnancy. Am J Obstet Gynecol 140:942, 1981.

Sagen N, Nilsen ST, Kim HC, et al.: Maternal hemoglobin concentration is closely related to birth weight in normal pregnancies. Acta Obstet Gynecol 63:245, 1984.

Samuels P, Bussel JB, Braitman LE, et al.: Estimation of the risk of thrombocytopenia in the offspring of pregnant women with presumed immune thrombocytopenic purpura. N Engl J Med 323:229, 1990.

Sanz MA, Rafecas FJ: Successful pregnancy during chemotherapy for acute promyelocytic leukemia. N Engl J Med 306:939, 1982.

Schafer AI: Teratogenic effects of antileukemia chemotherapy. Arch Intern Med 141:514, 1981.

Schifman RB, Thomasson JE, Evers JM: Red blood cell zinc protoporphyrin testing in iron-deficiency anemia in pregnancy. Am J Obstet Gynecol 157:304, 1987.

Schilsky R, Sherins R, Hubbard S, et al.: Long term follow-up of ovarian function in women treated with MOPP chemotherapy for Hodgkin's disease. Am J Med 71:552, 1981.

Schmidt H, Ehninger G, Dopfer R, et al.: Pregnancy after bone marrow transplantation for severe aplastic anemia. Bone Marrow Transpl 2:329, 1987.

Schwartz ML, Brenner WE: The obfuscation of eclampsia by thrombotic thrombocytopenic purpura. Am J Obstet Gynecol 131:18, 1978.

Scioscia AL, Grannum PAT, Copel JA, Hobbins JC: The use of percutaneous umbilical blood sampling in immune thrombocytopenic purpura. Am J Obstet Gynecol 159:1066, 1988

Scott DE, Pritchard JA: Iron deficiency in healthy young college women. JAMA 199:147, 1967.

Scott JR, Cruikshank DP, Kochenour NK, et al.: Fetal platelet counts in the obstetric management of immunologic thrombocytopenic purpura. Am J Obstet Gynecol 136:495, 1980.

Segonds A, Louradour N, Suc JM, Orfila C: Postpartum hemolytic uremic syndrome: A study of three cases with a review of the literature. Clin Nephrol 12:229, 1979.

Seligman PA, Caskey JH, Frazier JI, et al.: Measurements of iron absorption from prenatal multivitamin-mineral supplements. Obstet Gynecol 61:356,1983.

Shapiro SS, Thiagarajan P: Lupus anticoagulants. Prog Hemost Thromb 6:263, 1982.

Shattil SJ, Bennett JS: Platelets and their membranes in hemostasis: Physiology and pathophysiology. Ann Intern Med 94:108, 1981.

Shojania AM, Hornady GJ: Oral contraceptives and folate absorption. J Lab Clin Med 82:869, 1973.

Shulman NR: The physiologic basis for therapy of classic hemophilia and related disorders. Ann Intern Med 67:856, 1967.

Shulman NR, Aster RH, Leitner A, Hiller MC: Immunoreactions involving platelets. V. Posttransfusion purpura due to a complement-fixing antibody against a genetically-controlled platelet antigen: A proposed mechanism for thrombocytopenia and its relevance in autoimmunity. J Clin Invest 40:1597, 1961.

Sia CG, Amigo NC, Harper RG, et al.: Failure of cesarean section to prevent intracranial hemorrhage in siblings with isoimmune neonatal thrombocytopenia. Am J Obstet Gynecol 153:79, 1985.

Silverstein E, Roadman C, Byers, RH, et al.: Hematologic problems in pregnancy. III. Glucose-6-phosphate dehydrogenase deficiency. J Reprod Med 12:153, 1974.

Siris ES, Leventhal BG, Vaitukaitis JL: Effects of childhood leukemia and chemotherapy on puberty and reproductive function in girls. N Engl J Med 294:1143, 1976.

Snyder TE, Lee LP, Lynch S: Pregnancy-associated hypoplastic anemia: A review. Obstet Gynecol Surv 46:264, 1991.

Socol ML, Weiner CP, Louis G, et al.: Platelet activation in preeclampsia. Am J Obstet Gynecol 151:494, 1985.

Solal-Celigny P, Tertian G, Fernandez H, et al.: Pregnancy and paroxysmal nocturnal hemoglobinuria. Arch Intern Med 148:593, 1988.

Spector I, Corn M: Laboratory tests of hemostasis: The relation to hemorrhage in liver disease. Arch Intern Med 119:577, 1967.

Steinberg MH, Adams JG: Thalassemia: Recent insights into molecular mechanisms. Am J Hematol 12:81, 1982.

Stuart MJ, Gross SJ, Elred H, Graeber JE: Effects of acetylsalicylic acid ingestion on maternal and neonatal hemostasis. N Engl J Med 307:909, 1982.

Stubbs TM, Lazarchick J, Horger EO: Plasma fibronectin levels in preeclampsia: A possible biochemical marker for vascular endothelial damage. Am J Obstet Gynecol 150:885, 1984.

Sutton DMC, Hauser R, Kulaping S, Bachmann F: Intravascular coagulation in abruptio placentae. Am J Obstet Gynecol 109:604, 1971.

Taaning E, Skibsted L: The frequency of platelet alloantibodies in pregnant women and the occurrence and management of neonatal alloimmune thrombocytopenic purpura. Obstet Gynecol Surv 45:521, 1990.

Taylor DJ, Mallen C, McDougall N, et al.: Effect of iron supplement on serum ferritin levels during and after pregnancy. Br J Obstet Gynaecol 89:1011, 1982.

Thiagarajan P, Pengo V, Shapiro SS: The use of the dilute Russell Viper Venom Time for the diagnosis of lupus anticoagulant. Blood 68:869, 1986.

Thomas PRM, Peckham MJ: The investigation and management of Hodgkin's disease in the pregnant patient. Cancer 38:1443, 1976.

Thorup OA (ed.): Fundamentals of Clinical Hematology. Philadelphia, W.B. Saunders Company, 1987.

Veltkamp JJ, van Tilburg NH: Autosomal haemophilia. Br J Haematol **26**:141, 1974.

Walden PAM, Bagshawe KD: Pregnancies after chemotherapy for gestational trophoblastic tumours. Lancet **2**:1241, 1979.

Waldman SD, Feldstein GS, Waldman HJ, et al.: Caudal administration of morphine sulfate in anticoagulated and thrombocytopenic patients. Anesth Analg **66**:267, 1987.

Weatherall DJ: The New Genetics and Clinical Practice. Oxford/New York: Oxford University Press, 1985.

Weatherall DJ, Clegg JB: The Thalassemia Syndromes. 2nd ed. Oxford, Blackwell Scientific, 1981.

Weenink GH, Treffers PE, Vijn P, et al.: Antithrombin III levels in preeclampsia correlate with maternal and fetal morbidity. Am J Obstet Gynecol **148**:1092, 1984.

Weiner CP: Thrombotic microangiopathy in pregnancy. Semin Hematol **24**:119, 1987.

Weiner CP, Brandt J: Plasma antithrombin III: An aid in the diagnosis of preeclampsia-eclampsia. Am J Obstet Gynecol **142**:275, 1982.

Weinstein L: Preeclampsia/eclampsia with hemolysis, elevated liver enzymes, and thrombocytopenia. Obstet Gynecol **66**:657, 1985.

Weiss HJ: Congenital disorders of platelet function. Semin Hematol **17**:228, 1980.

Weiss HJ, Hoyer LW, Rickles FR, et al.: Quantitative assay of a plasma factor deficient in von Willebrand's disease that is necessary for platelet aggregation. J Clin Invest **52**:2708, 1973.

Whalley PJ, Martin FG, Pritchard JA: Sickle cell trait and urinary tract infections during pregnancy. JAMA **189**:903, 1964.

Whalley PJ, Pritchard JA, Richards JR: Sickle cell trait and pregnancy. JAMA **186**:1132, 1963.

White GC, Shoemaker CB: Factor VIII gene and hemophilia A. Blood **73**:1, 1989.

Wong SC, Ali MAM: Hemoglobin E disease. Am J Hematol **13**:15, 1982.

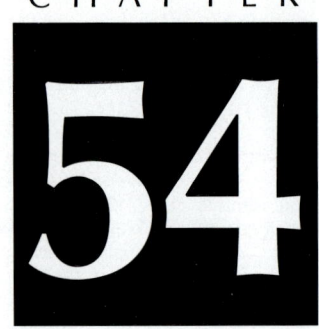

DIABETES IN PREGNANCY

THOMAS R. MOORE, M.D.

THE SPECTRUM OF DIABETES IN PREGNANCY

One in every 200 pregnancies occurs in a woman with insulin-requiring diabetes. A recent report from a statewide diabetes registry estimated that 60 per cent of pregnant women with pre-existing diabetes have the insulin-dependent, ketosis-prone form of disorder (IDDM, type I) and 40 per cent have the non–insulin-dependent form (NIDDM, type II) (Cousins, 1991).

Pregnancies in women with poorly managed insulin-deficient diabetes may be complicated by diabetic ketoacidosis, deterioration in visual acuity and renal function, marked elevation in blood pressure, severe preeclampsia, and multisystem organ failure. Hydramnios and preterm labor are common. The fetus is at increased risk for congenital anomalies, growth restriction, stillbirth, and postnatal metabolic instability.

The social and economic cost of inadequately treated type I diabetic pregnancies is enormous (Elixhauser et al., 1992). The cost of corrective surgery for a single infant with a diabetes-associated cardiac malformation such as ventricular septal defect or transposition of the great vessels averages $154,000 per survivor (Watson et al., 1986). The cost of maternal hospital admission for diabetic ketoacidosis averages approximately $5000 (Faich et al., 1983).

On the other hand, programs that foster early and comprehensive care of diabetic pregnancy reduce not only morbidity but overall health care expenditures. A recent study of the California Diabetes and Pregnancy Program demonstrated that early prenatal care reduced hospital days by 25 per cent and hospital costs by 30 per cent. For each dollar spent in the program, over $5 were saved, when compared to diabetic patients delivered outside the program (Scheffler et al., 1992).

Approximately an equal number of pregnancies are complicated by pre-existing adult-onset diabetes. Although many women with the nonketotic type of diabetes are asymptomatic, they are at substantial risk for significant maternal ophthalmologic, cardiovascular, renal, and obstetric complications. The fetus/neonate in these pregnancies is plagued by excessive growth, increased risk of stillbirth, shoulder dystocia, birth injury, and long-term obesity.

Transitory glucose intolerance (gestational diabetes, GDM) confined to pregnancy occurs in 1 to 4 per cent of all pregnancies, and this rate is much higher in some populations, notably in those of Hispanic descent and in older age groups (Hollingsworth et al., 1991). Although gestational diabetes is associated with relatively minor maternal risks during pregnancy, serious fetal and neonatal sequelae occur in the offspring in as many as half the cases.

Today, even with optimal management, diabetic pregnancy is accompanied by higher overall morbidity and mortality risks for both mother and infant. Comprehensive maternal, fetal, and infant care to optimize outcomes in diabetic pregnancy is labor-intensive. When contemporary outcomes are compared to those of even a decade ago, remarkable strides have been made in "normalizing" the course of diabetic pregnancy. These achievements, and the unmet challenges of the future, are best appreciated against the background of a historical perspective (Gabbe, 1992).

A HISTORY OF DIABETIC PREGNANCY

Until the late nineteenth century, pregnancy among diabetic women was virtually unknown, owing to the severe effects of unchecked hyperglycemia and functional starvation associated with insulin deficiency. The first review of diabetic pregnancy (Duncan, 1882) reported the course of 22 pregnancies in 15 women aged 21 to 38 years. Only 10 children survived, and only six of the patients were alive one year after delivery. In Williams' 1909 review of 66 cases, maternal mortality was 50 per cent and perinatal survival was 59 per cent. Joslin (1916) reported seven pregnant women with severe insulin-dependent diabetes, five of whom died of diabetic complications. Later descriptions of diabetic pregnancies by Craigin and Ryder (1916), DeLee (1920), and Williams (1925) reported an overall 30 per cent incidence of abortion and premature labor, stillbirth in over half, infant death in one-in-seven.

The discovery of insulin in 1922 by Banting and Best began a remarkable period in which the health of diabetics vastly improved. With insulin injections, women formerly condemned to a life of starvation, inanition, recurrent coma, and early death began to live longer, experience improved fertility, and hope for improvement in pregnancy outcome. Priscilla White's pioneering contribution to improving pregnancy outcomes at Boston's Joslin Clinic in this period cannot be overestimated. In 1932, she had reported the use of insulin treatment in three pregnant women. By 1939, she had reviewed 245 such pregnancies, noting that the incidence of maternal diabetic ketoacidosis (DKA) had fallen dramatically and the frequency of antepartum fetal death was half that recorded in the pre-insulin period. However, macrosomia and perinatal death remained persistent problems.

The next three decades brought the recognition that pregnancy outcome and metabolic control were closely linked (Peel, 1972). Closer maternal surveillance and the use of extended-action insulins permitted more "physiologic" blood sugar control during pregnancy (Karlsson and Kjellmer, 1972). Maternal death became a rarity. In the 1960s, the advent of the neonatal intensive care unit and pediatricians specialized in the care of high-risk newborns improved infant survival. Perinatal mortality fell from 35 per cent to 10 per cent during this period.

The formal development of the subspecialties of perinatology and neonatology in the 1970s led to a more concerted approach to diabetic pregnancy care in which obstetrician, dietician, and neonatologist collaborated in management. The impact of delivery timing on neonatal respiratory distress was recognized, and the relationship of glycemic control to congenital anomalies was defined. The sequential application of fetal heart rate testing, ultrasonographic biophysical profiling, fetal movement counting, and Doppler umbilical velocimetry contributed to such a marked improvement in antepartum fetal death rates that perinatal mortality in recent reports has approached that observed in nondiabetic women (Lassman-Vague and Thiers, 1990; Johnstone et al., 1990). Better techniques of insulin delivery and blood glucose monitoring have raised the future prospect of essentially "normal" metabolic control even in women with long-standing diabetes and vascular disease (Gabbe, 1981).

Nevertheless, major problems with both fetal and maternal management persist. While stillbirth rates have fallen dramatically, expensive biophysical testing and disturbingly high rates of preterm birth and cesarean section have been the cost. Congenital fetal anomalies, many of them life-threatening and debilitating, remain three to four times more frequent in diabetic than in nondiabetic pregnancies. Macrosomia and birth injury occur ten times more frequently in diabetic fetuses.

As for maternal management, metabolic control relies on periodic sampling of blood sugar and responsive injection of one or more insulin preparations, just as it did when White began her studies in the 1930s. Our understanding of the interrelation of diet, activity, stress, glucose level, and fetal well-being continue to be rudimentary. The ideal diet prescription for the pregnant diabetic woman remains elusive, and the role of exercise in metabolic control is poorly defined. Finally, on a practical level, in spite of a wealth of data linking birth defects and poor maternal metabolic status during embryogenesis, only a minority of women with preexisting diabetes achieve excellent glycemic control prior to pregnancy. This not only predisposes to an excess of congenital fetal structural anomalies and macrosomia, but may precipitate maternal retinal deterioration and degrade metabolic control throughout the remainder of the pregnancy. Progress in diabetes research in the next decades must address these important challenges.

RECENT DEVELOPMENTS IN THE UNDERSTANDING OF THE PATHOGENESIS OF DIABETES

Genetics of Diabetes

The predilection for clustering of glucose intolerance in families has been recognized for decades. However, it is only recently that the genetic determinants of this susceptibility have been relatively clearly defined (Reece et al., 1991). Diabetes mellitus is a chronic autoimmune disorder that occurs in genetically susceptible individuals. However, it is now clear that IDDM and NIDDM arise from separate genetic loci (Cudworth and Woodrow, 1975). NIDDM is possibly inherited as an incompletely penetrating autosomal dominant trait, while the major histocompatibility haplotypes within the HLA complex (on the short arm of chromosome 6) strongly influence susceptibility to IDDM. The region associated with IDDM lies within the D region (class II) of the HLA gene, with over 90 per cent of patients with IDDM possessing the HLA subtypes DR3 or DR4. Among asymptomatic patients who have both the DR3 and DR4 alleles, the risk of developing IDDM is 15 times higher than if only one allele is inherited (Thompson, 1984). The absolute risk for IDDM in Caucasians is 1 in 42 for the highest-risk HLA phenotype (DR3/DR4 heterozygote) (Rotter et al., 1983; MacLaren and Henson, 1986), whereas those with DR2 and DR5 have a risk of 1:2500.

The pathophysiology and characteristics of IDDM differ in DR3 and DR4 individuals, as shown in Table 54–1 (Rotter and Rimoin, 1987). Diabetic patients with the DR3 phenotype possess an inherited propensity for autoimmune disease in general, as evidenced by the higher frequency of autoimmune thyroiditis, Addison's disease, and autoimmune gastritis. In contrast, DR4 individuals have a heightened antibody response to both endogenous (even before clinical disease is apparent) and exogenous insulin and increased risk of proliferative retinopathy. Differences in these IDDM subgroups are important because they affect the course of pregnancy.

However, other genes in the D region of the HLA complex may be equally important. Analysis of DNA sequences from diabetics indicates that alleles in the DQ complex enhance susceptibility to IDDM conferred by HLA-D4 genes. Sequence analysis of the HLA-DQ3

TABLE 54–1. **Heterogeneity within IDDM: DR3 Compared with DR4**

CHARACTERISTIC	DR3	DR4
Production of insulin antibodies	Low or absent	High response
Islet cell antibodies	Persistent	Disappear shortly after diagnosis
Antipancreatic cell-mediated immunity	Increased	Not increased
Thyroid and other autoimmune endocrine diseases	Frequent	Less frequent
Onset	Any age	Young age
Seasonal variation in onset	None	Yes
Residual β-cell function, short-term after diagnosis	High	Low
Can present as NIDDM	Yes	No
Association with proliferative retinopathy	Not increased	Increased
Gene preferentially transmitted by mothers	Yes	No
Gene preferentially transmitted by fathers	Yes	Yes

From Rotter JI, Rimoin DL: The genetics of diabetes. Hosp Pract **22**:5 May 1987, p. 86.

gene product has demonstrated that a single amino acid difference at position 57 influences both disease susceptibility and resistance (Todd et al., 1987, 1988). Patients who are homozygous-negative for aspartic acid at position 57 are at highest risk.

Tillil and Köbberling (1987) reported the age-corrected empirical genetic risk estimates for first-degree relatives of DM probands. They calculated the lifetime recurrence risk to age 80 to be 6.6 ± 1.1 per cent for siblings and 4.9 ± 1.7 per cent for children. Regardless of age at onset, offspring of male probands always have a higher risk than offspring of female probands. Among all probands, fathers were significantly more often affected with IDDM (about twice) than mothers (4.1 ± 0.9 versus 1.7 ± 0.6 per cent, respectively). The risk for further siblings of the proband was significantly increased when there was an IDDM parent (25.2 ± 10.3 versus 5.8 ± 1.0 per cent for the remaining probands).

Monozygotic twin studies indicate that genetic factors account for only 50 to 70 per cent of IDDM (Rotter and Landaw, 1984). Thus the factors contributing to the phenotypic manifestation of genetically susceptible genotypes is complex, possibly involving the interaction susceptibility genes, cytokine production (Nerup et al., 1987), and environmental factors. Reece et al. (1991) have proposed a six-stage model to describe the events linking the DR3 and DR4 genotype to clinical expression of IDDM (Table 54–2).

In its final form, IDDM results from complete destruction of the pancreatic islet cells by the patient's own cellular immune mechanisms. Current theories postulate a genetically determined defect in recognition/protection of self-antigens on the islet cells, coincident environmental factors such as viral infections

stress and rapid skeletal growth (Jenson et al., 1980), and activation of T lymphocytes and macrophages with subsequent progressive destruction of insulin production capability (Palmer et al., 1983; Doberson et al., 1980; Srikanta et al., 1985). In the future, more detailed delineation of the mechanisms by which cell-mediated immune destruction of pancreatic tissue will be necessary if the hope of preventing or arresting this process in susceptible individuals is to be realized.

Insulin Resistance

Non–insulin-dependent diabetes mellitus (NIDDM, type II) is the most common form of diabetes (90 per cent of patients). Obesity and age greater than 40 are common risk factors. The contemporary trend to delaying pregnancy into the mid- to late thirties has increased the number of women with NIDDM who become pregnant. There are no proven genetic markers for NIDDM, but strong genetic associations are clearer than in IDDM as evidenced by the almost 100 per cent concordance rates among monozygotic twins (Pyke, 1979). Genetic heterogeneity is also apparent in NIDDM, and an autosomal dominant form of transmission has been described in some families (Fajans, 1982). No HLA association or polymorphic sequences in DNA near the insulin gene have been established.

In contrast to IDDM, in which insulin deficiency underlies the clinical syndrome, NIDDM patients have normal or increased insulin secretion (Perley and Kipnis, 1966). In some type II diabetic patients, insulin secretion in response to a glucose load is delayed, but all patients demonstrate decreased tissue sensitivity to a given plasma level of insulin, resulting in inadequate glucose disposal from the blood stream and subsequent hyperglycemia (Ginsberg et al., 1975).

TABLE 54–2. **A Model of IDDM Pathogenesis**

STAGE	EVENT	EXAMPLES
1	Genetic susceptibility	HLA-DR3/DR4, HLA-DQ3
2	Triggering factors	Stress, rapid skeletal growth, viral infections
3	Active autoimmunity	Anti-islet cell and anti-insulin antibodies
4	Progressive blunting of glucose-induced insulin secretion	Subclinical phase detectable in relatives of IDDM
5	Overt diabetes—early phase	"Easily controlled" IDDM
6	Overt diabetes—complete beta cell destruction	"Brittle" IDDM

Adapted from Reece et al: Insulin-dependent diabetes mellitus and immunogenetics: maternal and fetal considerations. Obstet Gynecol Surv **46**:225, © by Williams & Wilkins, 1991.

The mechanism of tissue resistance to the effects of insulin in NIDDM has been the subject of intense investigation (Kolterman et al., 1981; Olefsky et al., 1982; Revers et al., 1984). Reduced or defective cellular insulin receptors have been hypothesized but refuted by the finding that in type II diabetics both receptor number and binding kinetics are normal. Rather, the defect in glucose handling appears to occur after binding of insulin to the receptor (post-receptor defect) (Puavilai et al., 1982). Ciaraldi et al. (1991) studied insulin kinetics and glucose disposal in adipocytes of NIDDM patients. Basal and maximally insulin-stimulated rates of 3-O-methylglucose transport in adipocytes from NIDDM subjects were 50 per cent lower than the values in cells from normal subjects. They concluded that adipocytes from NIDDM subjects display defects in the kinetics of insulin action, slower activation and accelerated deactivation of glucose transport, that mirror the defects observed in vivo.

The thesis that insulin resistance results from a defective insulin action after receptor binding was further explored by Brillon and colleagues (1989) in an investigation of tyrosine kinase activity in the insulin receptors of adult nonpregnant subjects with NIDDM. Tyrosine kinase activity was identified in 43 ± 8 per cent of the receptors in normal subjects compared to only 14 ± 6 per cent of NIDDM receptors ($P < .05$), suggesting that human adipocytes contain two distinct receptor populations, both of which bind insulin but only one of which is capable of insulin-stimulated tyrosine phosphorylation. In nondiabetic subjects, 40 to 50 per cent of the receptors that bind insulin are capable of insulin-stimulated tyrosine autophosphorylation, whereas the proportion of "ineffective" receptors is markedly increased in NIDDM.

NORMAL PREGNANCY AND INSULIN RESISTANCE. It appears that an insulin-resistant state similar to NIDDM may be characteristic of normal pregnancy. Catalano et al. (1991) documented the changes in insulin release and insulin resistance in nonobese pregnant women before pregnancy and throughout gestation by using a euglycemic, hyperinsulinemic clamp technique. The first and second phases of the insulin secretory response to glucose challenge were significantly elevated during normal pregnancy and peripheral insulin sensitivity decreased by 56 per cent ($p = 0.0003$) as pregnancy progressed. In contrast to NIDDM, however, insulin receptor tyrosine kinase activity appears to be intact during pregnancy (Camps et al., 1990). Placental steroid (estrogens, progestins) and peptide hormones (human chorionic somatomammotropin) have been implicated in the mechanism of insulin resistance in normal pregnancy, as the degree of resistance parallels the maternal plasma level of these substances.

GESTATIONAL DIABETES. It is now clear that gestational diabetes mellitus (GDM) arises from a pathophysiology distinct from the abnormalities of type I and type II diabetes. Botta et al. (1988) demonstrated that the pancreatic insulin secretory pattern of gestational diabetic women was delayed and blunted compared to that of normals. They also noted that impaired peripheral glucose utilization characteristic of GDM was associated with increased peripheral resistance similar to that observed in NIDDM. Kuhl (1991) reported both quantitative and qualitative differences in insulin secretion between pregnant women with normal glucose tolerance and women with GDM. Insulin responses to oral glucose and protein-rich meals were lower in women with GDM than in normals, despite significantly higher mean plasma glucose concentrations in the women with GDM. Furthermore, peak plasma insulin concentrations occurred later in women with GDM than in pregnant control subjects.

MATERNAL METABOLIC ADJUSTMENTS DURING NORMAL AND DIABETIC PREGNANCY

In normal women, pregnancy is accompanied by remarkable changes in metabolic homeostasis to favor fetal growth, maturation, and survival. To achieve a proper metabolic milieu for a constantly feeding fetus and an intermittently feeding mother, a well-integrated metabolic shift must occur. Fetal nutritional needs take precedence over maternal, demanding a continuous supply of fuel. In the first few weeks of pregnancy, maternal carbohydrate metabolism is affected by a rise in maternal estrogen and progesterone levels, which stimulates pancreatic β-cell hyperplasia and insulin excretion. At the same time, tissue glycogen storage and peripheral glucose utilization increase while hepatic glucose production and maternal fasting plasma glucose levels decrease. Thus, normal pregnancy results in relative hypoglycemia, increased turnover of plasma lipids, hypoaminoacidemia, and marked sensitivity to food deprivation.

GLUCOSE METABOLISM IN NORMAL PREGNANCY. Pregnancy in normal women is characterized by hyperinsulinemia and progressive insulin resistance (Yen, 1978). Yet as pregnancy progresses, maternal levels of glucose actually decrease, with a shift toward increased mobilization of free fatty acids and ketones. Figure 54–1 (Cousins et al., 1980) demonstrates the change in glucose profiles in response to feeding around the clock in normal pregnant women in the second and third trimesters, with postpartum values as the nonpregnant control. The mean values for fasting blood sugar decline by approximately 11 mg/dl compared to postpartum control as the patient enters the third trimester. During the nonfeeding nighttime hours, plasma glucose level falls progressively as the fetus continues to consume nutrients. Post–mean peak blood sugar values are relatively unchanged from the nonpregnant and rarely exceed 140 mg/dl at one hour, and 120 mg/dl two hours postprandially.

Pancreatic islet cells hypertrophy, and owing to peripheral tissue insensitivity, glucose-stimulated insulin secretion increases. Although glucose excursions in normal women are relatively small after meals (30 to 35 mg/dl), there is a marked increase in insulin response, with mean 24-hour plasma values about one-third higher than those of nonpregnant women (Cousins et al., 1980; Phelps et al., 1981; Hollingsworth, 1985).

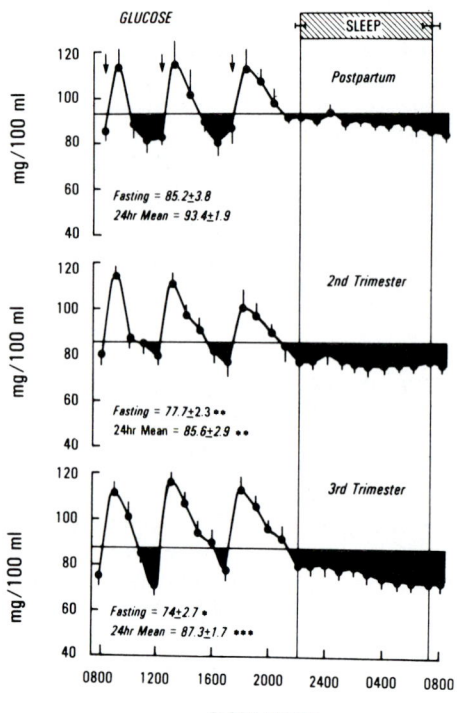

FIGURE 54–1. Profile of blood glucose over 24 hours in the second and third trimesters of pregnancy, with postpartum observations used as a control. Error bars = SE. (From Cousins et al: The 24-hour excursion and diurnal rhythm of glucose, insulin and C peptide in normal pregnancy. Am J Obstet Gynecol **136**:483, 1980.)

During the latter half of pregnancy (Table 54–3), pancreatic reserve is further stressed by the insulin-blunting effects of rising levels of placental human chorionic somatomammotropin (hCS) and prolactin, and maternal cortisol and glucagon. Freinkel and colleagues described these combined effects as "accelerated starvation" during the fasting state and "facilitated anabolism" after feeding (Freinkel, 1964).

INTEGRATION OF NUTRIENTS BY THE MATERNAL-PLACENTAL-FETAL UNIT. Figure 54–2 depicts the central role played by the placenta in the delivery and regulation of maternal fuels to the fetus. Glucose is transported across the placenta by carrier-mediated diffusion in direct proportion to blood glucose levels up to a saturable maximum. Placental amino acid uptake is regulated by intracellular amino acid concentrations. Concentrations of most amino acids are higher in the fetal circulation and are maintained against a concentration gradient within the placenta. There is negligible

transport of acidic amino acids (glutamate, aspartate), with fetal requirements met by fetal synthesis (Shambaugh, 1986).

FREE FATTY ACIDS (FFA). These readily cross the placenta in amounts exceeding those necessary to fulfill lipid storage requirements. Although the placentas of all species investigated appear to be virtually impermeable to esterified lipids, FFA derived from maternal triglyceride (TG) have been shown to cross the placenta in rabbits and humans (Elphick et al., 1978; Thomas et al., 1984; Knopp et al., 1986). There is considerable storage of triglyceride within the placenta and hydrolysis of very low-density lipoprotein (VLDL) (guinea pig). FFA transported to the fetus are rapidly taken up and esterified by the fetal liver and released into the circulation as VLDL.

INSULIN. The role of insulin in placental regulation of metabolic fuels has not been established. Insulin does not ordinarily cross the placenta, although immunologically facilitated transport into the fetal circulation has been documented (Menon et al., 1990). A large polypeptide, insulin binds to placental microvilli where it is normally degraded. Steel and associates (1977) have suggested that the abundance of placental insulin receptors might play a role in regulation of glucose uptake, glycogen metabolism, or lipolysis, because these processes are physiologic effects of the hormone in other tissues.

Although the placenta has a critical role in the transfer of nutrients from mother to fetus, it also serves as a modulator of maternal metabolic fuels by synthesizing hormones and steroids that are lipolytic and antagonistic to insulin. Human chorionic somatomammotropin stimulates the secretion of maternal insulin, which in turn may regulate the availability of glucose to the fetus (Kalkhoff et al., 1978). In the latter half of gestation hCS stimulates lipolysis, which ensures adequate transfer of glucose and amino acids for the period of accelerated fetal growth.

AMINO ACIDS. The transfer of maternal amino acids to the fetus via the placenta results in maternal hypoaminoacidemia, particularly involving alanine, which is a key precursor for gluconeogenesis in the maternal liver. Freinkel and Metzger (1979) and Phelps and associates (1981) have reported distinct alterations in plasma levels of individual amino acids in women with even very mild gestational diabetes. Postprandial increments in plasma levels of the branched-chain amino acid isoleucine seem to persist longer after meals. Because amino acids cross the placenta readily and may independently stimulate fetal islet cell insulin release (Milner, 1979), higher maternal postprandial levels of some amino acids could have important

TABLE 54–3. Carbohydrate Metabolism in Late Pregnancy (20 to 40 weeks)

HORMONAL CHANGE	EFFECT	METABOLIC CHANGE
↑ hCS	"Diabetogenic" ↓ Glucose tolerance	Facilitated anabolism during feeding *and*
↑ Prolactin	Insulin resistance	Accelerated starvation during fasting ↓
↑ Bound and free cortisol	↓ Hepatic glycogen stores ↑ Hepatic glucose production	Ensures glucose and amino acids to fetus

PLACENTAL TRANSFER OF MATERNAL NUTRIENTS

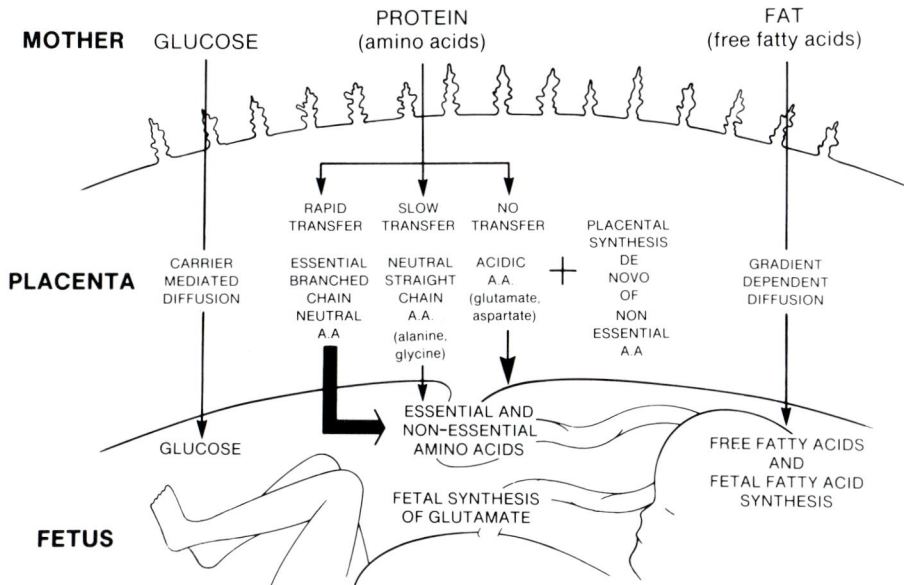

FIGURE 54–2. The transport of maternal fuels to the placental and fetal compartments. The placenta serves as a modulator for the total parenteral alimentation of the fetus. (From Hollingsworth DR: Alterations of maternal metabolism in normal and diabetic pregnancies in insulin-dependent, non–insulin-dependent, and gestational diabetes. Am J Obstet Gynecol **146**:417, 1983.)

implications for in utero hyperinsulinemia and fetal growth.

LIPIDS. During normal pregnancy all aspects of lipid metabolism are modified. The changes reflect anabolic fat storage early in pregnancy and maternal adipose tissue catabolism as pregnancy approaches term, when fetal utilization of glucose and amino acids accelerates (McDonald-Gibson et al., 1975). In early pregnancy, insulin plays a leading role in transport of glucose into fat cells and in increased synthesis of fat; lipolysis is inhibited and fat cell hypertrophy occurs. Late in pregnancy, high concentrations of placental hCS oppose the action of insulin and stimulate lipolysis.

The most striking lipid change during pregnancy is the increase in plasma TG. During the last trimester of human pregnancy, hypertriglyceridemia results primarily from an increase of VLDL (Warth et al., 1975). Concentrations of cholesterol and phospholipid also increase during normal pregnancy. Figure 54–3 depicts

differences in total plasma TG and cholesterol levels at 3 months postpartum (control) and in the second and third trimesters in normal women.

Lipid abnormalities are common in diabetes and vary in individual patients because of the heterogeneity of carbohydrate intolerance. Hyperlipidemia results from the interaction of the diabetic syndrome, the genetic background of the patient, and the environment (Goldberg, 1982). Pregnancy is associated with progressive, hormone-related, increments in plasma levels of cholesterol (CHOL), phospholipids, and TG. It therefore evokes a metabolic stress that exaggerates the heterogeneous characteristics of diabetic women, who may already have lipid abnormalities associated with insulin deficiency, insulin resistance, obesity, or abnormal genetic factors in addition to varying degrees of hyperglycemia.

Recently, investigators in the Diabetes In Early Pregnancy study (DIEP) (Peterson et al., 1992) reported that pregnant women with IDDM actually have lower

FIGURE 54–3. Fasting levels of total plasma cholesterol and triglyceride (±SD) in normal-weight women in the second trimester, third trimester, and 3 months postpartum. (From Hollingsworth DR: Alterations of maternal metabolism in normal and diabetic pregnancies in insulin-dependent, non–insulin-dependent, and gestational diabetes. Am J Obstet Gynecol **146**:417, 1983.)

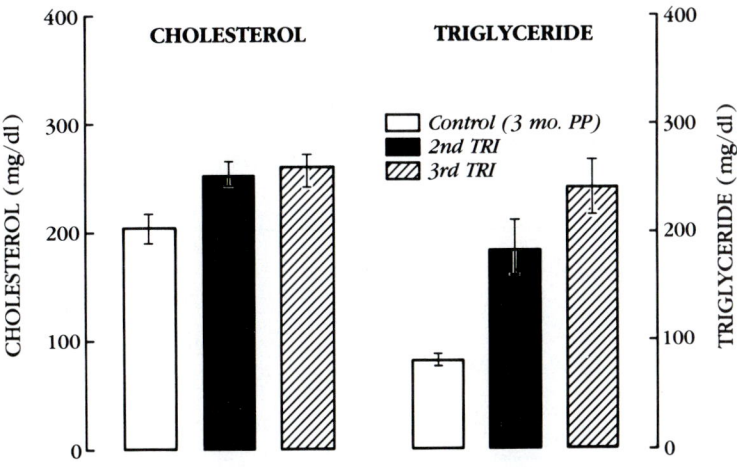

Table 54-4.   White's Classification of Diabetes in Pregnancy

WHITE'S CLASS	AGE AT ONSET (YEARS OLD)	DURATION (YEARS)	COMPLICATIONS
A	Any	Any	Diagnosed prior to pregnancy; no vascular disease
B	≥20 or	<10	No vascular disease
C	10–19 or	10–19	No vascular disease
D	<10 or	≥20	Background retinopathy only or hypertension
E			Calcification of pelvic arteries (no longer used)
F			Nephropathy (>500 mg/day proteinuria)
H			Arteriosclerotic heart disease
R			Proliferative retinopathy or vitreous hemorrhage
T			After renal transplantation

Adapted from Hare and White: Gestational diabetes and the White classification. Diabetes Care 3:394, 1980. Copyright © 1980 by American Diabetes Association, Inc.)

CLASSIFICATION OF DIABETES IN PREGNANCY

Because diabetes mellitus is not a single disease but a genetically and clinically heterogeneous group of disorders that have in common carbohydrate intolerance (Fajans et al., 1982; Rotter and Rimoin, 1987), it is important to define and classify the specific metabolic syndrome as accurately as possible. This specificity has particular relevance during pregnancy, when the metabolic adjustments of gestation are superimposed upon a variety of forms of carbohydrate intolerance that require highly individualized management programs.

In earlier descriptions of diabetic pregnancies, physicians have relied on the classification of White (1974). This nomenclature was based primarily on historical factors: age at onset, duration of disorder, and complications. Because of this, patients were often reclassified during the course of pregnancy, which caused inconsistencies that hampered the assessment of clinical data. Table 54-4 summarizes the White Classification of diabetes in pregnancy.

A classification of glucose intolerance in pregnancy derived from the pathophysiology of hyperglycemia was developed by the National Diabetes Data Group

(NDDG) of the National Institutes of Health (1979) (Table 54-5). This nomenclature is a useful guide, although it is already clear that considerable heterogeneity exists within each major type of diabetes. Use of this classification scheme is recommended since it differentiates the various types of glucose intolerance encountered in pregnancy by underlying pathophysiology. In addition, the complications of pregnancy and the course, treatment, and outcome of both maternal and fetal complications are vastly different in women with the four major types of hyperglycemia. The clinical features that differentiate type I and type II diabetes are listed in Table 54-6.

OVERT DIABETES IN PREGNANCY: IDDM AND NIDDM

Maternal Complications

Women with diabetes prior to pregnancy are at risk for a number of obstetric and medical complications. However, the relative risk of these problems can be graded against the duration and severity of disease (Table 54-7).

Diabetic Retinopathy

Diabetic retinopathy is the leading cause of blindness in women between the ages of 24 and 64 years (Elman et al., 1990). Some form of retinopathy is present in virtually 100 per cent of women with type I diabetes for 25 years or more, of which approximately 1 in 5 is legally blind (Klein et al., 1984).

The terminology and clinical features of the various stages of diabetic retinopathy are presented in Table

Table 54-5.   Classification of Glucose Intolerance in Pregnancy

NOMENCLATURE	OLD NAMES	CLINICAL FEATURES
Type I Insulin-dependent diabetes mellitus (IDDM)	Juvenile-onset diabetes	Ketosis-prone, insulin-deficient
Type II Non—insulin-dependent diabetes (NIDDM)	Adult-onset diabetes	Ketosis-resistant, insulin-resistant; obesity, family history, and age are common factors
Type III Gestational diabetes (GDM)	Gestational diabetes	Occurs only during pregnancy; established by glucose tolerance testing; obesity and age are common risk factors
Type IV Secondary diabetes	Glucose intolerance	Secondary to other medical conditions, e.g., cystic fibrosis, Cushing's syndrome, acromegaly

TABLE 54–6.   Differentiating Features of Type I and Type II Diabetes*

CLINICAL FEATURES	IDDM (TYPE I)	NIDDM (TYPE II)
Obesity at onset	Uncommon	Common; often of central or masculine type
Metabolic ketoacidosis	Prone to ketosis	Ketosis less likely
Age at onset	Predominantly young (< 30 yr)	Predominantly older (> 30 yr)
Seasonal trend	Fall and winter	None
Insulin levels	Low to absent	Variable
Appearance of symptoms	Acute or subacute	Variable, usually slow
Inflammatory cells in islets	Present initially	Absent
Treatment	Insulin is required for life	Diet control or oral hypoglycemics may be sufficient, although insulin may be required to control hyperglycemia
Family history of diabetes	Uncommon, but increased prevalence of IDDM	Common with increased prevalence of NIDDM
Twin studies	20% to 50% concordance in monozygotic twins	Close to 100% concordance in monozygotic twins
Association with other autoimmune endocrine diseases and antibodies	Yes	No
Islet cell antibodies	Yes	No
HLA associations	Yes	No
Further subtypes	DR3, DR4 associated	MODY, mutant insulins

MODY = maturity-onset diabetes of the young.
*Both types may present initially during pregnancy as gestational carbohydrate intolerance.

54–8. The earliest stage, "background" retinopathy, is present in 98 per cent of patients who have had diabetes for 15 years or more (Klein, 1987). This lesion is characterized by outpouching of blood vessels and extravasation of plasma into the layers of the retina. Later, small, localized hemorrhages and exudates are seen. As the process advances into the frankly proliferative stage, ischemic lesions ("cotton-wool" infarcts) become common. Finally, neovascularization of the retina proceeds, stimulated by retinal ischemia. The abnormal vasculature invades the inner membrane of the retina and may extend into the vitreous humor. Not only do capillary rupture and hemorrhage obstruct the vitreous, but, as healing occurs, contraction of the vitreous and detachment of the retina may follow. Significant visual disability is evident in patients with preproliferative or proliferative retinopathy.

Since the prevalence of diabetic retinopathy is high in patients with long-standing diabetes, and progression to significant visual disability is frequent, the effect of pregnancy on this process is of critical importance.

EFFECT OF DIABETES SEVERITY AND DURATION. Sinclair et al. (1984) have observed that the severity of

diabetes and its duration are of greater prognostic significance than the occurrence of pregnancy. Evidence for this view includes the minimal risk of retinopathy reported in women with gestational diabetes or those with diabetes diagnosed within 5 years of pregnancy. Horvat et al. (1980) conducted a 12-year prospective study comparing 172 women with clinical diabetes and 107 women with latent diabetes. In the diabetic group, background retinopathy was documented in 40 (23 per cent). Eleven women had prepregnancy proliferative retinopathy, and an additional four progressed to the proliferative stage during pregnancy. These individuals had an average duration of diabetes of 21 years in contrast to 13.5 years for women with background retinopathy. No progression of retinal disease was noted in the group with "latent diabetes."

Moloney and Drury (1982) subjected 53 pregnant women with IDDM to follow-up by retinal photography every 6 weeks and for 6 months postpartum. Thirty-three (62 per cent) had retinopathy at first

TABLE 54–7.   Maternal Morbidity Associated with Diabetic Pregnancy by White's Classification

COMPLICATION	GDM	B,C	D,F,R	TOTAL
Preeclampsia	10%	8%	16%	12%
Chronic hypertension	10%	8%	17%	10%
All hypertension	15%	15%	31%	18%
Ketoacidosis	8%	7%	9%	
Hydramnios	5%		18%	18%
Preterm labor	8%	5%	10%	
Cesarean section	12%	44%	57%	—

Adapted from Cousins: Pregnancy complications among diabetic women: Review. Obstet Gynecol Surv **42**:140, © by Williams & Wilkins, 1987.

TABLE 54–8.   Classification and Clinical Features of Diabetic Retinopathy

LESION	CLINICAL FEATURES
Background retinopathy	Retinal microaneurysms, dot or blot hemorrhages, hard exudates
Preproliferative retinopathy	Ischemic lesions: "cotton-wool spots," venous beading, and duplications
Proliferative retinopathy	Neovascularization: may extend into vitreous, lead to hemorrhage, clot retraction, vitreous "scarring," retinal detachment

Adapted from Elman et al: Diabetic retinopathy in pregnancy: a review. Obstet Gynecol **75**:119, 1990. Reprinted with permission from the American College of Obstetricians and Gynecologists.

examination and eight others (15 per cent) developed it as pregnancy advanced. A moderate increase in microaneurysms and hemorrhages was observed in 56.6 per cent, and appearance of soft exudates in 28 per cent. Four women had neovascularization, which further deteriorated with advancing pregnancy. However, by 6 months after delivery, all of the background changes had returned to control levels. Those with neovascularization showed some regression. Most importantly, progression of retinopathy was related to duration of disease. Pregnancy had no visible effect in the retina of patients who had diabetes for less than 2 years.

Serup (1986) conducted a prospective study of the influence of pregnancy on diabetic retinopathy in 145 women. Of those enrolled in the study, about half with retinopathy experienced deterioration during pregnancy, but all had partial regression following delivery. This study demonstrated that patients with White's class B or C diabetes do not have significant risk of developing persistent retinopathy during pregnancy, and class D patients, with a 50 per cent risk of progression during pregnancy, can expect regression of those changes postpartum.

EFFECT OF RAPID GLYCEMIC CONTROL. Several studies have suggested that rapid induction of glycemic control in early pregnancy stimulates retinal vascular proliferation (Laatikainen et al., 1987; Kroc, 1988). Phelps et al. (1986) observed a highly significant correlation between worsening retinopathy, the degree of hyperglycemia at entry into prenatal care, and the magnitude of improvement in glycemic control. However, the majority of the lesions evolving during induction of glycemic control in this study were relatively minor.

OPHTHALMOLOGIC MANAGEMENT OF THE PREGNANT DIABETIC. These findings place the obstetrician and ophthalmologist in opposing positions: optimal obstetric management requires rapid and strict glycemic control, yet such aggressive metabolic management may threaten the patient's vision. This further underlines the importance of preconception glycemic control to avoid worsening of retinopathy during pregnancy. Because duration of diabetes is also important, pregnancies should be planned, if possible, within 10 years of the diagnosis of IDDM. Achievement of good diabetic control well in advance of conception (6 to 12 months) helps to minimize or prevent retinopathy.

For those in poor metabolic control at onset of pregnancy, it is preferable to begin rigorous glucose regulation as early as possible in favor of reduced risk of fetal maldevelopment, even though the patient's ophthalmologic status may require intensive surveillance and therapy. An examination by a retinal specialist early in pregnancy is imperative. Prompt laser therapy for preexisting proliferative disease is indicated (see below). Patients with minimal disease should be reexamined at least once each trimester and 3 and 6 months postpartum. Those with significant retinal disease may require monthly follow-up.

MANAGEMENT OF PROLIFERATIVE RETINOPATHY AND VITREOUS HEMORRHAGE. Laser photocoagulation of severe proliferative retinopathy can reduce the rate of progression to blindness by 50 per cent (Diabetic

Retinopathy Study Research Group, 1982). Several studies indicate that photocoagulation of retinal lesions before conception may be more protective than performance of the procedure during pregnancy (Dibble et al., 1982; Gerke and Meyer-Schwiekerath, 1982). Pregnant women with severe disc neovascularization or with marked progression should have photocoagulation therapy as soon as the diagnosis is confirmed.

Management of the patient with significant recent or old vitreous hemorrhage is controversial. Theoretically, the cardiovascular transients associated with labor and, particularly, bearing-down efforts during delivery may increase the risk of retinal detachment. However, the corresponding ophthalmologic risk associated with cesarean section complicated by hemorrhage or hypotension has not been quantified. Currently, presence of vitreous hemorrhage is not, of itself, indication for operative delivery. Consideration can be given to limiting the second stage through vacuum or forceps assistance.

Similarly, the role of pregnancy termination in patients with advanced retinopathy is unclear. At present, there is no evidence that ultimate visual outcome is improved substantially by interrupting the pregnancy. Abortion decisions in women with progressive proliferative retinopathy should be based upon personal considerations by the patient and her partner. The most recent information available as well as a sympathetic factual explanation and discussion help to facilitate these decisions.

Diabetic Nephropathy

Microvascular renal lesions in IDDM are a serious and life-threatening complication. Late microangiopathic renal complications represent the most important causes of death and disability in IDDM (Pontiroli et al., 1986). Nephropathy accounts for about 30 per cent of deaths in patients with onset of diabetes before age 31 (Deckert et al., 1986). The pathogenesis of this problem has not been established, and the relative roles of genetic susceptibility, control of hyperglycemia, and hypertension have not been delineated. Additional complications such as repeated urinary tract infections, excessive glycogen deposition, and papillary necrosis all hasten deterioration of renal function. For diabetic women, assessment of potential effects of childbearing on renal function is an important issue.

The kidney is normal at the outset of IDDM, but within 1.5 to 2.5 years, thickening of glomerular basement membrane can be appreciated. By 5 years, there is expansion of the glomerular mesangium (diffuse diabetic glomerulosclerosis), which becomes the dominant pathologic process (Mauer et al., 1986). A minority of patients progress to the most marked expression of mesangial expansion, the Kimmelstiel-Wilson syndrome. All individuals with marked mesangial expansion have more than 400 mg of urinary protein excretion in 24 hours.

The peak incidence of nephropathy occurs after about 16 years of diabetes; approximately 40 to 45 per cent of patients with IDDM develop overt diabetic nephropathy and die at an earlier age than those without this complication. Why almost half those with IDDM escape this problem is a mystery; their mortality rate differs little from that of the background population. Microscopic proteinuria is defined as >0.5 gm protein per 24 hours or >300 mg albumin per 24 hours. Onset of this process indicates incipient diabetic nephropathy and increased risk for later development of clinical nephropathy (Mogensen and Christiansen, 1984; Kupin et al., 1987; Cohen et al., 1987). Figure 54–4 shows the relationship of clinical nephropathy to duration of IDDM.

The relationship of diabetic control to progression of nephropathy has not been established, but two Scandinavian reports suggest a relationship. In Denmark, Feldt-Rasmussen et al. (1986a, 1986b) reported the effect of 2 years of strict metabolic control on progression of incipient nephropathy in 36 patients with Albustix-negative urine and IDDM randomly assigned to conventional treatment or insulin pump therapy for 2 years. None of the patients managed on the insulin pump progressed to clinical nephropathy, whereas five in the conventional treatment did. In a Norwegian study (Dahl-Jorgensen, 1986), near-normal glucose levels for 2 years did not have an effect on microalbuminuria. After 4 years, a reduction in urinary albumin secretion was demonstrated in the intensively treated groups. In a subgroup of patients with urine albumin excretion in excess of 200 mg per 24 hours, 12 of 15 patients on multiple injections of insulin or the insulin pump improved their excretion rates.

COURSE OF NEPHROPATHY IN TYPE I DIABETIC PREGNANCY. In general, the physiologic changes associated with normal pregnancy increase renal blood flow and glomerular filtration by 30 to 50 per cent. Most type I diabetic women with preexisting nephropathy also experience an improvement in renal function, especially during the second trimester (Jovanovic and Jovanovic, 1984). During the third trimester, when mean arterial pressure and peripheral vascular resistance rise, diabetic women with microvascular disease may have marked diminution of renal function associated with an increase in pre-existing hypertension or the onset of pregnancy-induced hypertension (PIH).

Frank renal failure may follow (Dicker et al., 1986), but is extremely rare with meticulous medical surveillance.

Elevated maternal blood pressure and a rapid decrease in creatinine clearance are among the most common precipitating events leading to preterm delivery. Although the timing and severity of the decline in renal function in mid- to late pregnancy are difficult to predict, Hayslett and Reece (1987) suggest that if patients with the most severe forms of nephropathy are excluded (poorly controlled first-trimester hypertension despite medical therapy, serum creatinine greater than 1.5 mg/dl, proteinuria more than 3 gm/24 hr in the first trimester), both maternal and fetal outcomes are good (Main et al., 1984). In a study of renal function for 4 years before and 4 years after pregnancy in 11 patients with diabetic nephropathy, Reece et al. (1990b) showed that the gradual rise in serum creatinine over that period was unaffected by the intervening pregnancy. These findings confirm the earlier reports by Lindheimer and Katz (1977) and by Early and Gottschalk (1979).

Some physicians have strongly discouraged pregnancy in women with diabetic renal disease, especially if there is impairment of renal function or hypertension (Grenfell, 1986). Currently, however, specialists accustomed to managing diabetic pregnancy regard informed reproductive decisions as the responsibility of the patient and her partner. With well-coordinated multidisciplinary care, pregnancy outcomes in these patients are acceptable and often excellent. Counseling regarding the risks and potential complications of pregnancy in the patient with diabetic renal disease should be complete, honest, and sensitive to individual circumstances. These considerations are pertinent also for women who are receiving peritoneal dialysis or hemodialysis or those who have had a kidney transplant.

RENAL DIALYSIS IN PREGNANT WOMEN WITH TYPE I DIABETES. Neither chronic hemodialysis nor chronic peritoneal dialysis corrects uremia. Instead, these modes of therapy limit uremia to a level that allows a tolerable degree of health and rehabilitation (Ward,

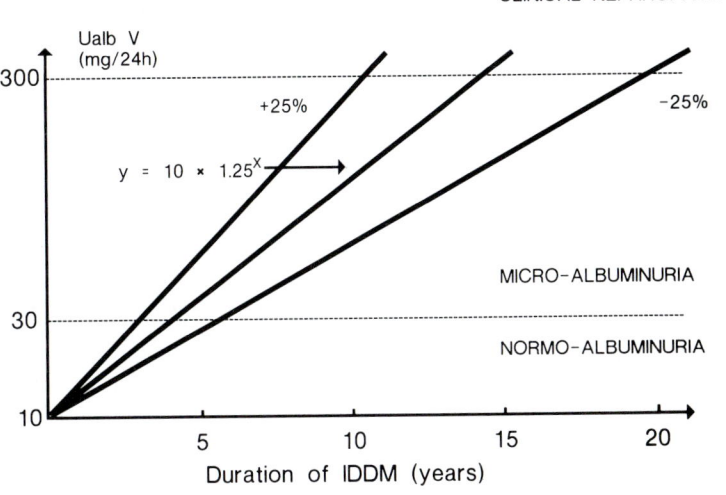

FIGURE 54–4. Development of proteinuria and clinical nephropathy in IDDM. There is a gradual increase in the excretion of urinary albumin over time in IDDM with microalbuminuria. (From Deckert T, Feldt-Rasmussen B, Borch-Johnsen K, et al: Clinical assessment and prognosis of complications of diabetes. Transplant Proc **18:**1636, 1968.)

1988). Although women receiving maintenance dialysis for end-stage renal failure are usually amenorrheic or at least anovulatory, several have conceived and at least 50 have borne healthy children (Wing et al., 1980).

Nevertheless, the prognosis for successful gestation in diabetic patients with end-stage renal disease is poor. Fetal loss is common in the second-trimester, and third-trimester intrauterine or neonatal death is frequent. About 60 per cent of births are premature, often requiring early delivery because of maternal or fetal complications, or resulting from premature labor, which often begins during hemodialysis (Johnson et al., 1979). Of the 20 or 25 per cent of pregnancies ending in live births, 40 per cent of babies are below the tenth percentile.

A major practical problem with hemodialysis involves judiciously adjusting maternal vascular volume. Dialysis teams are accustomed to "taking off fluid" at each session. However, the pregnant patient requires a progressive increase in vascular volume to at least 20 to 30 per cent above nonpregnant values from 8 to 30 weeks gestation. This volume augmentation appears to be necessary to maintain uteroplacental perfusion. Pregnancies in which vascular volume increases do not occur have a high incidence of fetal growth restriction and stillbirth. Difficulties with vascular underfill (hypotension, poor fetal growth, asphyxia) and overfill (and hypertension) are common in pregnant hemodialysis patients and often difficult to rectify.

The poor prognosis associated with hemodialysis, together with other considerations, has prompted increased interest in continuous ambulatory peritoneal dialysis (CAPD). Several successful pregnancies have been reported (Galler et al., 1983; Davison, 1987). Although fluid and chemical balance is constant and heparinization is not necessary, intrauterine deaths, abruption, prematurity, hypertension, and fetal distress still occur. At present, the best strategy for most diabetic women on dialysis desiring pregnancy is to obtain a kidney transplant.

RENAL TRANSPLANTATION. Patients with successful kidney transplants are relieved of their uremia and usually regain near–normal fertility. After transplant, delay in pregnancy of at least 2 years is recommended to avoid the problems of graft rejection and infection, which are more common in this period. Criteria of allograft stability sufficient to allow pregnancy (Marushak et al., 1986; Davison, 1987) include stable function (serum creatinine less than 2 mg/dl), no proteinuria, no significant hypertension, no evidence of allograft rejection, no evidence of hydronephrosis, and modest doses of immunosuppressives (prednisone <15 mg/day and <2 mg/kg/day of azathioprine).

Results of pregnancy in renal transplant recipients have been extensively documented. Davison (1987) reviewed data from 1569 pregnancies in 1009 women. Therapeutic abortions were performed in 22 per cent (for unwanted pregnancy, uncertain maternal prognosis, or maternal medical problems); 16 per cent aborted spontaneously (the same incidence as in normal women). Of the 60 per cent of pregnancies that extended beyond the first trimester, 92 per cent resulted in a viable infant. Preeclampsia occurred in 30 per cent, preterm delivery in about 50 per cent, and intrauterine growth restriction in 20 per cent. Patients with the worst renal function had the poorest pregnancy outcomes.

Graft survival and renal function are not compromised by pregnancy. Renal allograft rejection episodes occur in about 9 per cent of pregnancies, which is similar to the rate in nonpregnant patients. However, there may be difficulty distinguishing acute rejection from preeclampsia. Magnetic resonance imaging or renal biopsy may be helpful in diagnosing rejection. The reader is referred to Chapter 50 for a more detailed review of renal transplantation and pregnancy.

Cardiovascular Complications

Cardiovascular complications experienced by diabetic pregnant women include chronic hypertension, PIH, and, rarely, atherosclerotic heart disease. In composite studies of all types of diabetic pregnancies, the incidence of hypertensive disorders during pregnancy varies from 15 to 30 per cent (Gabbe et al., 1977a, 1977b; Kitzmiller et al., 1978; Tevaarwerk et al., 1981).

CHRONIC HYPERTENSION AND PREECLAMPSIA. Chronic hypertension (defined as blood pressure at or above 140/90 mm Hg before the 20th week of gestation) complicates approximately one in ten diabetic pregnancies overall, and 17 per cent of diabetics with preexisting renal or retinal vascular disease (Cousins, 1987). The perinatal problems encountered with chronic hypertension include intrauterine growth restriction and increased risk of maternal stroke, superimposed preeclampsia and abruptio placentae. In type I diabetes, the prevalence of chronic hypertension increases with duration of diabetes and is closely associated with nephropathy (Peiris and Gustafson, 1986). As noted in Table 54–7, White's class A and B diabetics have a risk profile similar to that of nondiabetic patients. However, women with evidence of renal or retinal vasculopathy (classes D, F, R) have a 50 per cent risk of hypertensive complications over the rate observed in normals.

A recent study by the DIEP group suggests that type I diabetics have higher mean blood pressures throughout pregnancy than normal controls (Peterson et al., 1992) (Fig. 54–5). This raises the question of the proper definition of hypertension during pregnancy in these patients. Whether the overall higher pressures represent subclinical vasculopathy or a hypertensive response to elevated insulin levels is unclear. Pregnant women with type II diabetes have a higher prevalence of hypertension, hyperlipidemia, and decreased levels of high-density lipoprotein cholesterol. Lipid abnormalities are also common in type I women in poor control and during episodes of diabetic ketoacidosis. All diabetic women should be screened before conception for hypertension and abnormal fasting plasma lipid concentrations so that appropriate treatment can be advised if necessary.

Underlying chronic hypertension should be suspected when the patient's systolic blood pressure exceeds 130 mm Hg or diastolic exceeds 80 mm Hg before the third trimester. The diagnosis is strength-

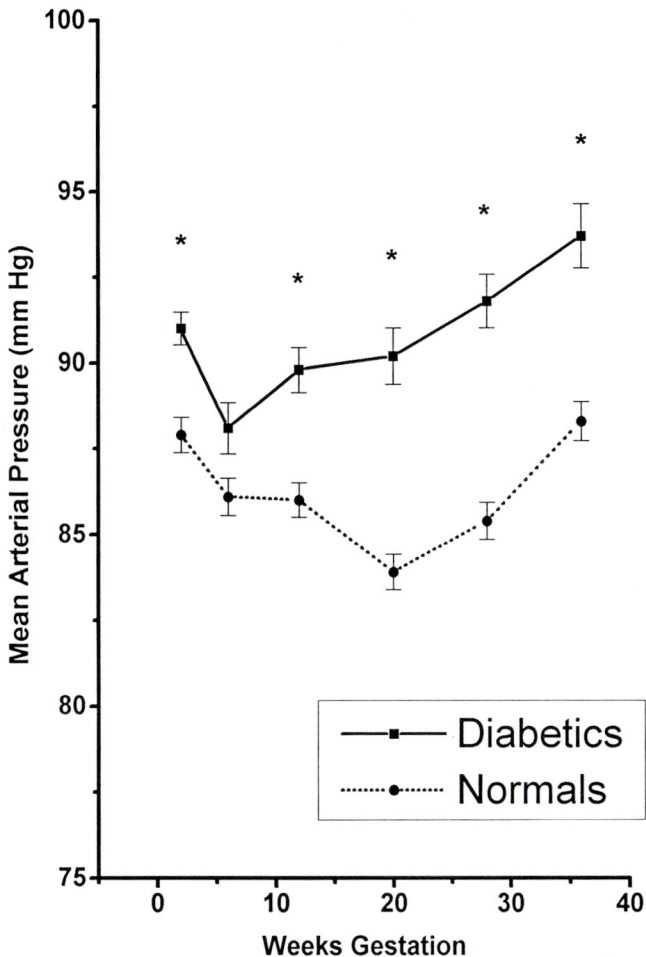

FIGURE 54–5. Mean arterial pressure in normals and diabetic patients during gestation. (Adapted from Peterson CM et al: The Diabetes in Early Pregnancy Study: Changes in cholesterol, triglycerides, body weight, and blood pressure. Am J Obstet Gynecol **166**:513, 1992.)

ened by finding (1) a failure of mean blood pressure to decline normally in the late second trimester and/or (2) elevation in blood urea nitrogen (BUN) above 10 mg/dl and/or (3) serum creatinine greater than 1.0 mg/dl and/or (4) creatinine clearance less than 100 ml/min. As blood pressure normally rises in the third trimester, differentiating isolated increased vascular resistance from preeclampsia can be difficult. Renal function assessments in each trimester are recommended in diabetics with overt vascular disease, and in those who have had diabetes for more than 10 years. Significant proteinuria, plasma uric acid levels >6.0 mg/dl, or evidence of the HELLP syndrome should prompt a work-up for preeclampsia.

Preeclampsia occurs in approximately 12 per cent of insulin-requiring diabetics, as compared to 8 per cent in the nondiabetic population (Moore et al., 1985). Diamond et al. (1985) observed PIH in 19 per cent of diabetics, noting that risk of preeclampsia was related to maternal age and duration of preexisting diabetes. Fetal deaths were increased in the diabetics with PIH in that series. In the chronically hypertensive diabetic

patient, preeclampsia may be difficult to distinguish from near-term blood pressure elevations. The onset is typically insidious and not confidently recognized until severe.

HEART DISEASE. Coronary heart disease is rarely encountered in pregnant women with type I or type II diabetes. Airaksinen and colleagues (1986) studied cardiac function in pregnant normal and type I women, comparing left ventricular function during gestation and postpartum by means of serial echocardiography. Diabetic women had less than the normal increase in left ventricular size and stroke volume. In addition, heart rate increases were lower, which resulted in a smaller increment in cardiac output. These investigators concluded that the normal hemodynamic adjustments to pregnancy are impaired in type I diabetic women. They speculated that preclinical cardiomyopathy and autonomic neuropathy may be involved in the observed alterations.

Altered maternal cardiac function and decreased uteroplacental blood flow may be of clinical importance when other factors such as anemia or placental vasculopathy compromise fetal oxygen supply (Nylund et al., 1982). Physical exertion may also induce left ventricular dysfunction (Hilsted et al., 1982). Because most diabetic pregnant women do not have overt cardiovascular symptoms or physical findings, pathology which may become significant during intrapartum stress may be overlooked. Women with microvascular disease or autonomic complications should be evaluated carefully and advised about physical activity during gestation.

Although uncommon, atherosclerotic heart disease (White's class H) may afflict diabetic patients in the reproductive years. Patients with this complication are typically older (mean age 34 years) and have other evidence of diabetic vascular involvement (White's class D or R) (Silfen et al., 1980). Pregnancy outcome is dismal for the diabetic with cardiac involvement, with 75 per cent maternal mortality and 29 per cent perinatal loss. Recognition of cardiac compromise in the pregnant diabetic may be difficult because of the decrease in exercise tolerance which occurs in normal pregnancy. Compromised cardiac function in patients who are restricted to bed rest for hypertension or poor fetal growth may also be difficult to detect. Thus it is prudent to obtain a detailed cardiovascular history on all diabetic patients and to consider electrocardiography and more extensive cardiology evaluation in type I diabetic patients over the age of 30. With intensive monitoring, successful pregnancy is possible albeit hazardous for women with significant cardiac disease (Reece et al., 1986).

Diabetic Ketoacidosis

Pregnant women with type I diabetes are at increased risk for diabetic ketoacidosis (DKA). Emesis and the use of beta-sympathomimetic drugs were the most common precipitating factors in a study by Rodgers and Rodgers (1991). Patient noncompliance and physician management errors were considered etiologic in 24 per cent and contributory in 16 per cent. Severe DKA is life-threatening to mother and fetus.

TABLE 54–9.   Treatment Protocol for Diabetic Ketoacidosis*

	INITIAL PHASE	RECOVERY PHASE
Insulin	10–20 U insulin IV bolus plus 5–10 U/h IV (infusion), IM, or SC. IV route should be used in any hypotensive patient† Increase hourly dose if serum glucose does not fall despite adequate fluid therapy	As acidosis is reversed, decrease to 5–10 U/q 2–4 hr When patient is eating, begin long-acting insulin
Fluids	0.9% NaCl at 1000 ml/hr Replace sodium deficit in 4–6 hours (average 500 mEq)	When BP is stable, urine output brisk, and serum glucose falling, decrease to 0.45% NaCl at 250–500 ml/hr When serum glucose <250 mg/100 ml, add 5% glucose to IV fluids Replace H$_2$O deficit over 12–24 hr (average 5–10 liters)
Potassium	If serum K$^+$ high, begin KCl at 20 mEq/hr after urine output is established If serum K$^+$ low or normal, begin KCl at 20 mEq/hr immediately; reduce rate by 50% if patient is oliguric Monitor EKG; measure serum K$^+$ q 2–4 hr	Adjust dose of KCl according to serum K$^+$ measurements Continue oral KCl replacement for 1 week to correct total deficit
Bicarbonate	If pH <7.0, give as needed to raise pH to 7.0 If pH 7.0–7.2, ± small amounts (not >88 mEq) If pH >7.2, give no bicarbonate	Give no bicarbonate
Phosphorus	If patient not oliguric, potassium phosphate may be given at 10 mEq/hr (decrease dosage of KCl accordingly) Measure serum phosphorus and calcium frequently	Give no phosphorus
General measures	If patient is comatose, establish nasogastric tube and bladder catheter Identify and treat any precipitating illness Consider low-dosage heparin	Remove catheter as soon as possible Continue to observe for signs of precipitating or complicating illness

*Note: These are general guidelines. Because there may be wide variation in individual patient needs, there is no substitute for careful monitoring of each patient, particularly in the initial phase of therapy.

†In pregnant women, constant IV insulin infusion with an IVAC is preferable.

Adapted from Porte D Jr, Halter JB: The endocrine pancreas and diabetes mellitus. *In* Williams RH (ed): Textbook of Endocrinology. 6th ed. Philadelphia, WB Saunders Company, 1981.

Prompt treatment is essential, because fetal well-being is in jeopardy until maternal metabolic homeostasis is reestablished. High levels of plasma glucose and ketones are readily transported to the fetus, who may be unable to secrete sufficient quantities of insulin to prevent DKA *in utero*.

The pathogenesis of diabetic ketoacidosis derives from a deficiency in insulin, which initiates a chain of events leading to increased hepatic glucose production and decreased or absent tissue disposal of glucose with resulting hyperglycemia. The subsequent osmotic diuresis results in loss of water and electrolytes, hyperosmolality, and volume depletion. The release of stress hormones (catecholamines, glucagon, growth hormone, and cortisol) further impairs insulin action and contributes to insulin resistance. This combination of events leads to decreased tissue uptake and increased hepatic production of ketones and ketonemia.

Early in the illness an elevation of plasma glucose and an increase in plasma ketones (acetoacetic and β-hydroxybutyric acids) occurs. If hyperglycemia is not corrected, marked diuresis, dehydration, and hyperosmolality follow. In pregnant women with mild illness, the early stages of ketoacidosis respond quickly to appropriate treatment of the initiating cause, additional doses of regular insulin, and adjustment of food and fluid intake.

Pregnant women with advanced diabetic ketoacidosis present with typical findings, including hyperventilation, normal or obtunded mental state (depending on severity of the acidosis), dehydration,

hypotension, and a fruity odor to the breath. Abdominal pain and vomiting may be prominent symptoms. The diagnosis of DKA is confirmed by the presence of hyperglycemia (glucose more than 300 mg/dl) and ketonemia demonstrated by a positive nitroprusside reaction in undiluted plasma. This procedure is unsatisfactory for quantifying ketonemia, however, and a specific ketone titer should be obtained from the laboratory.

Table 54–9 contains a protocol for treatment of DKA. When DKA occurs after 28 weeks gestation, the fetal heart rate should be closely monitored. If fetal distress is documented, correction of the maternal metabolic disorder should be the first priority, rather than resorting to emergency delivery. Conservative measures (hydration, maintenance of blood pressure) and correction of ketoacidosis are usually effective in improving fetal biophysical status (Hughes, 1987).

Obstetric Complications

HYDRAMNIOS. Poor diabetic control is associated with increased amniotic fluid volume. The frequency in pregnancy varies from 1 to 2 per cent in normal subjects to 18 per cent among diabetics. The pathophysiology of hydramnios in diabetic pregnancy has not been well elucidated, but current theories center on four principal mechanisms: excessive fetal urination (Miller, 1946), decreased or absent fetal swallowing (Chung and Myrianthopoulos, 1975), abnormal amniotic/maternal osmotic balance, and congenital anomalies, especially those of the central nervous system, thorax, and gastrointestinal tract (Alexander et al., 1982).

Ultrasonographic studies of human fetal urination have shown an increase in fetal urinary production rates of some fetuses of diabetic mothers (Wladimiroff et al., 1981; Kurjak et al., 1981). The concept that amniotic fluid in diabetic pregnancy has increased osmolality associated with elevated glucose levels is also attractive. Nevertheless, data supporting this theory are lacking, other than the observation that hydramnios tends to occur in diabetic pregnancies with poor metabolic control (Sivit et al., 1987). Congenital anomalies can contribute to excessive amniotic fluid through obstruction of fetal swallowing or in conjunction with fetal hydrops. Esophageal atresia or obstruction by a thoracic mass can prevent fetal swallowing. Thoracic masses including diaphragmatic hernia, pulmonary sequestrations and cystic adenomatoid malformations have been associated with this disorder.

The clinical definition of hydramnios varies, including >2000 ml amniotic fluid recorded at delivery and various measures of amniotic fluid pocket depths as observed on ultrasonography (Chamberlain et al., 1984; Moore and Cayle, 1990). In practice, polyhydramnios is usually diagnosed when any single vertical pocket of amniotic fluid is deeper than 8 cm (equivalent to the 97th percentile) or when the sum of four pockets from each quadrant of the uterus (Amniotic Fluid Index) exceeds approximately 250 mm (95th percentile). Ideally, the sonographic measurements of amniotic fluid volume should be referenced against the appropriate gestational age norms (Moore and Cayle, 1990).

Diagnosing hydramnios is important because of its association with fetal anomalies and preterm labor (Leucht et al., 1986). A rapid increase in fundal height should prompt a thorough ultrasonographic examination by a skilled examiner. Esophageal atresia should be ruled out by careful evaluation of the fetal stomach, as should gastroschisis and omphalocele. Finally, fetal hydrops and hydramnios may occur in conjunction with fetal cardiac anomalies, which are observed more frequently in diabetic patients (Rowland et al., 1973).

Management of the patient with hydramnios is summarized in Table 54–10. Once significant fetal structural defects have been excluded, the clinician should focus on prevention of premature labor. Enhanced patient awareness of contractions and the

TABLE 54–10. Work-Up and Management of Hydramnios in the Diabetic Patient

1. Measure amniotic fluid volume using the four-quadrant technique.
2. *Rule Out:*
   Esophageal atresia
   Omphalocele and gastroschisis
   Fetal cardiac anomaly and hydrops
   Anencephaly and spina bifida
3. Evaluate and improve maternal glycemic control
4. Educate patient about signs of preterm labor
5. Schedule frequent office visits to detect early cervical change

signs and subtle sensations of preterm labor is essential. The patient should be seen weekly for cervical examination. Hospital admission and tocolysis should be considered in patients with advanced cervical dilation.

PRETERM LABOR. Preterm labor, defined as contractions resulting in cervical change prior to fetal maturity, can occur in diabetic patients as late as 38 to 39 weeks, given the late onset of fetal pulmonary maturity. Mimouni et al. (1987) reported a rate of 31.1 per cent preterm labor among well-controlled diabetics, compared to a 20 per cent rate in nondiabetics at their institution.

The onset of premature labor in diabetic women is not linked to metabolic control, suggesting that vigilance for premature contractions is indicated in all diabetic pregnancies. Certain historical factors should be noted in assessing increased risk for preterm labor: twins, prior premature delivery, uterine anatomic abnormalities such as large myoma or bicornuate uterus, history of diethylstilbestrol (DES) exposure, and prior cervical surgery (e.g., cone biopsy). Patients with these risk factors should have intensive surveillance from 20 weeks onward, including education regarding signs and symptoms of preterm labor and frequent cervical examinations. With more than four uterine contractions per hour, the risk of premature delivery is increased (Katz et al., 1986).

Once preterm labor is diagnosed, the risk of premature birth should be assessed. Contraindications to tocolysis should be reviewed and excluded prior to initiation of labor suppression. Careful review of obstetric dates should precede further intervention. If fetal lung maturity is suspected (gestational age >34 weeks), amniocentesis for phospholipid profile, Gram stain, and culture should be performed while initial tocolysis efforts are under way. Because neonatal transition is frequently difficult for the premature infant of a diabetic mother, every effort should be made to suppress labor if fetal lung maturity cannot be ascertained.

Choice of tocolytic agent depends on the practitioner's experience, the difficulty encountered in suppressing contractions and the degree of prematurity involved. However, many of the pharmacologic agents conventionally used to manage preterm labor significantly affect the diabetic patient's metabolic control. Available agents include β-mimetic agents such as ritodrine and terbutaline (Merkatz et al., 1980), indomethacin (Niebyl et al., 1980), and magnesium sulfate (Miller et al., 1982), and calcium channel blockers. At present, the only FDA-approved agent for inhibition of preterm labor is the β-mimetic agent ritodrine. Although highly controversial, this medication has been shown to be effective in prevention of preterm delivery in both nondiabetic (King et al., 1985) and diabetic subjects (Miodovnik et al., 1985a).

Merkatz et al. (1980) demonstrated the efficacy of beta-mimetic agents in inhibition of contractions associated with preterm labor. However, the side effects of these agents on maternal glucose and mineral metabolism (hyperglycemia, hyperinsulinemia, and acidosis) make their use undesirable in diabetic pregnancy. In the study by Miodovnik et al., most patients were significantly hyperglycemic during tocolysis (mean blood glucose 200 mg/dl) and required high-dose insulin infusions (up to 3.5 U/hr) to maintain even modest levels of control. For these reasons, most experts avoid the use of mimetics in diabetic women. If ritodrine is used for tocolysis, it should be mixed in a non–glucose-containing solution (0.45 per cent NaCl) and infused with a separate continuous insulin infusion (0.5 to 1.5 U/hr) to maintain glucose levels in the 80 to 100 mg/dl range (Barrett et al., 1980).

Magnesium sulfate offers the advantage of equivalent efficacy to β-adrenergic agents without hyperglycemic side effects (Elliott, 1984). Indeed, when beta-mimetics and magnesium sulfate were compared, the cardiovascular side effects were so markedly greater with the adrenergic agents (38 per cent versus 2 per cent) that the increased rate of failed therapy with these medications (42 per cent versus 30 per cent) was attributable primarily to side effects (Beall et al., 1985). Hollander (1987) reported an 88 per cent success rate with magnesium sulfate versus 79 per cent with ritodrine in a study of nondiabetic pregnancies. Magnesium sulfate was better tolerated because of fewer cardiovascular adverse effects. Consequently, this drug is considered to be the first choice for tocolysis.

For the patient who continues progressive cervical dilatation despite therapeutic magnesium levels, a second agent or, less frequently, switching medications may be considered. Both prostaglandin inhibitors (indomethacin) and calcium channel blockers (nifedipine) have been helpful in weaning the difficult to manage patient from therapeutic levels of magnesium to less toxic doses (Niebyl et al., 1980; Ferguson et al., 1990). Courses of indomethacin, limited to a 48-hour duration, have been demonstrated safe for the fetus. Because of concern regarding constriction of the ductus arteriosus during therapy (Mari et al., 1989), gestations later than 33 weeks and fetuses with marginal oxygenation, IUGR, or cardiac anomalies should be excluded from this second-line therapy.

ANTENATAL CORTICOSTEROIDS. During treatment of preterm labor, many specialists add corticosteroids to hasten fetal lung maturation. Use of high-dose steroids reduces the risk of newborn respiratory distress syndrome (RDS) by 30 to 50 per cent (Liggins and Howie, 1972). However, before corticosteroids are administered, the following should be considered: (1) The hyperglycemic effects of dexamethasone or betamethasone will persist for 48 to 72 hours. Diabetic patients will require increased doses of insulin and intensive glucose monitoring during this phase. (2) The beneficial effect of steroids is not observed if the fetus is delivered in less than 24 hours or more than 7 days after treatment. (3) Steroid administration to a woman whose fetus has already gained pulmonary maturity will expose the diabetic patient unnecessarily to alterations in metabolic status (DKA) that may actually endanger the fetus. Therefore, the management strategy for the diabetic preterm labor patient should include assessment of gestational age, amniocentesis to determine the relative maturity of the pulmonary system if gestational age is beyond 34 weeks, aggressive tocolysis if the fetus is immature, and intensive fetal and maternal monitoring during labor suppression regardless of agent used.

Fetal Complications

ABORTION. The possibility that the rate of abortion is increased in diabetic women has been debated extensively. A recent review of the available literature by Kalter (1987) concluded that the aggregate spontaneous abortion rate of 12.7 per cent among 8041 diabetic pregnancies was not significantly different from the rate observed among nondiabetic women.

Mills et al. (1988) performed a careful study of 386 insulin-dependent women and 432 control subjects. The early pregnancy losses among diabetic (16.1 per cent) and control women (16.2 per cent) were not different. After adjustment for known risk factors, the rate was still not higher among diabetic patients. However, the patients in this study primarily had excellent metabolic control. Among those who had poorer control, they noted an increase in the risk of miscarriage of 3.1 per cent for each standard deviation above the normal range in the first-trimester glycosylated hemoglobin. Among those who miscarried, there was a correlation between risk of abortion and fasting glucose levels (p<.01), but an even stronger correlation with postprandial blood sugars (p<.001).

Since fetuses with structural malformations are found more frequently in abortion material than in term pregnancies, an elevation in the early pregnancy loss rate, particularly in patients with poor metabolic control, is at least theoretically likely (Pedersen and Mantoni, 1983). In support of this view, a retrospective study by Sutherland and Pritchard (1986) of 164 diabetic pregnancies managed during a period of relatively relaxed glycemic control demonstrated a spontaneous abortion rate of almost double the expected rate. Key et al. (1987) reported increased pregnancy loss only in patients with elevated glycohemoglobin concentrations.

Wright et al. (1983) documented a markedly increased spontaneous abortion rate among women with diabetes in poor control. The glycosylated hemoglobin levels were significantly higher in those who aborted than in those who delivered successfully (12.8 per cent versus 11.2 per cent). Miodovnik et al. (1984) studied spontaneous abortion in diabetic pregnancy prospectively and found an increasing rate among patients with more advanced classes of diabetes (rates for C, D, and F were 25, 44, and 22 per cent, respectively). The same group compared diabetic patients with preconceptional control with postconceptional registrants and noted that poorer glycemic control in the late-care group was associated with a threefold increase in spontaneous abortion (Rosenn et al., 1991). Dicker et al. (1988) confirmed these observations.

It therefore appears that diabetic women with excellent glycemic control have a risk of miscarriage equivalent to that of the nondiabetic patient (Miodovnik et al., 1985b). These facts can be used to effectively counsel the diabetic patient preconceptionally and to urge her to maintain excellent control prior to the onset of her pregnancy. On the other hand, patients in early pregnancy who have suboptimal glycohemoglobin values can be reassured that the overall elevation and risk of miscarriage is modest. For patients whose glycohemoglobin is 2 or 3 standard deviations above the norm, intense early pregnancy surveillance is indicated. Documenting the normal appearance of the yolk sac, appropriate progression of the crown-rump length, and pulsations of the fetal heart may help to identify the patient at risk for embryonic demise.

CONGENITAL ANOMALIES. In infants of diabetic mothers (IDM), congenital malformations occur about two to three times as often as in those of nondiabetic women (Mills, 1982; Reece and Hobbins, 1986). They represent the most common cause of death in newborn IDM (approximately 40 per cent) (Fig. 54–6).

Kucera (1971), in a summary of world literature, found a malformation rate of 4.8 per cent in IDM. A control group from World Health Organization (WHO) data showed a rate of 1.65 per cent. In the U.S. Collaborative Perinatal Project (CPP), involving 48,437 infants from 14 geographic areas examined throughout the first year of life, Caucasian IDM had a major malformation rate of 17.7 per cent compared with 8.3 per cent in infants of nondiabetics. In Blacks the findings were 17.3 per cent versus 8.5 per cent (Chung and Myrianthopoulos, 1975).

There is, however, no increase in birth defects in progeny of diabetic fathers, babies born to prediabetic women, or those who develop gestational diabetes during the latter half of pregnancy, suggesting that the periconceptional metabolic milieu is a critical factor in diabetic teratogenesis. Miller and co-workers (1981), in a study of 116 IDM, reported 15 with major anom-

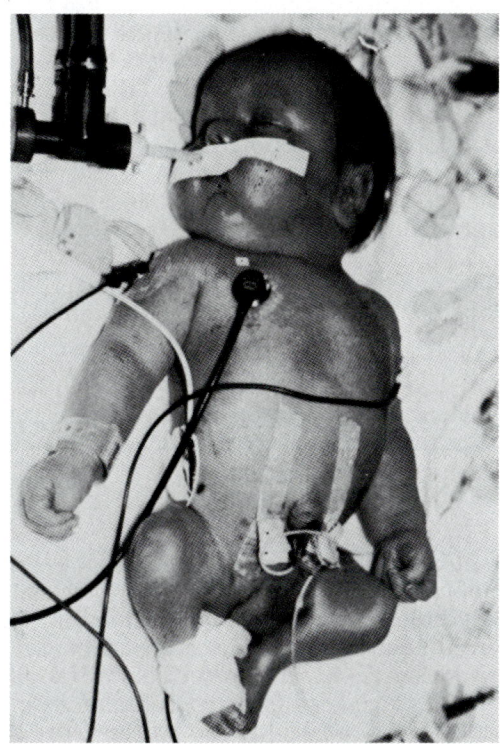

FIGURE 54–6. Newborn infant with caudal regression syndrome, flexion contractures, and hypoplasia of the lower extremities. The mother had type I diabetes and an HbA_1c concentration of 13.5 per cent when first seen for prenatal care at 12 weeks gestation.

alies that were correlated with elevated concentrations of HbA_1. Ylinen and associates (1984) also reported a higher risk of minor and major malformations in infants of diabetic mothers with elevated HbA_1 concentrations. A recent multicenter study in France reported the outcomes of 483 pregnancies complicated by diabetes. They noted that HbA_1c levels in the 13 pregnancies with congenital malformations were significantly higher than those with normally formed fetuses (Gestation and Diabetes in France Study Group, 1991).

Lucas et al. (1989) reported experience with 105 diabetic patients in which the overall malformation rate was 13.3 per cent. However, the risk of delivering a malformed infant was closely linked to glycohemoglobin level in early pregnancy: No malformations when HbA_1 <7.1, 14 per cent with HbA_1 7.2 to 9.1, 23 per cent with HbA_1 9.2 to 11.1, and 25 per cent when HbA_1 was >11.2 (p<.05). This graded risk suggests that periconceptional glycemic control produces a dose-response effect. The studies of Leslie et al. (1978), Fuhrmann et al. (1983), Molsted-Pedersen and Pedersen (1985), and Kitzmiller et al. (1991) provide additional support to this notion.

The observations, however, do not confirm the relationship of hyperglycemia to malformations. Other events such as ketonemia, wide variations in blood glucose levels with episodes of hypoglycemia, altered lipid and amino acid fluxes, and genetic susceptibility may also be critical factors. In mammalian embryos, hypoglycemia and nutritional abnormalities are also important causes of malformations (Duraiswami, 1959; Kalter and Warkany, 1959; Smithberg and Runner, 1963; Freinkel, 1984; Seller, 1987).

Pedersen's hypothesis (1977), that maternal hyperglycemia stimulates premature fetal pancreatic maturation and hypertrophy, which in turn leads to hyperanabolism and macrosomia, was expanded by Freinkel (1980) to include the concept that the altered fuel mixture in early diabetic pregnancy (hyperglycemia, abnormal amino acid and lipid milieu) adversely influences fetal organogenesis (fuel-mediated teratogenesis). Evidence for this theory is abundantly available from animal and in vitro studies. Rodent embryos subjected to high concentrations of glucose in culture display growth restriction and increased structural malformations (Cockroft and Coppolla, 1977; Sadler, 1980). Ketones (β-hydroxybutyrate) promote malformations in rat embryos independently (Horton and Sadler, 1983) and in concert with hyperglycemia (Lewis et al., 1983). In a study of embryonic fuel mixture in the diabetic rat model, Styrud and Eriksson (1991) correlated embryonic malformations with maternal serum concentrations of glucose, triglycerides, a number of amino acids, creatinine, urea, and IGF-1.

The precise mechanism by which hyperglycemia disturbs embryonic organ development has not been delineated; reduced arachidonic acid and myo-inositol levels, and accumulation of sorbitol and trace metals in the conceptus, have been suggested (Eriksson et al., 1991). A plausible pathophysiologic mechanism of diabetic teratogenesis centers on the abnormal production of oxygen free radicals. This theory states that hyperglycemia produces increased electron transport in the mitochondria, which in turn generates oxygen free radicals (Morriss and New, 1979). These highly chemically reactive agents enhance peroxidation of native lipid compounds, leading to the formation of hydroperoxides. Hydroperoxides are recognized inhibitors of prostacyclin, which possibly alter the balance of thromboxane and prostacyclin in the growing conceptus (Warso and Lands, 1983). In support of this theory, addition of prostaglandin inhibitors to the culture medium in one recent study prevented glucose-induced embryopathy (Pinter et al., 1986).

The most common congenital defects and their time of occurrence in IDM are shown in Table 54–11. These data were obtained from the Metropolitan Atlanta Congenital Defects Program, a prospective study of 4929 infants with major malformations (Becerra et al., 1990). The risk estimates are adjusted for the effect of maternal age, drug intake, and race. The majority of lesions involve the central nervous system and the cardiovascular system, although other series have reported an excess of genitourinary and limb defects as well (Cousins, 1991). The *caudal regression syndrome* (see Fig. 54–6), a severe congenital malformation consisting of agenesis of the sacrum and lumbar spine and hypoplasia of the lower extremities, is almost never seen except in IDM (Mills et al., 1979). Although the relative risk of caudal regression syndrome is 10 to 15 times higher than the relative risk of cardiac anomalies, cardiovascular malformations constitute a much more significant clinical problem because congenital heart disease occurs in 1 in 40 infants while only one in 350 will have caudal regression.

The syndrome of diabetic embryopathy may also include abnormal postnatal neurologic development secondary to severe maternal ketosis or hypoglycemia. The long-term effects of maternal hyperglycemia and an abnormal supply of all classes of nutrients to the fetus are unknown (Eriksson et al., 1984).

TABLE 54–11. Congenital Malformations in Infants of Insulin-Dependent Diabetic Mothers

ANOMALY	RISK RATIO (95% CI)	PERCENT RISK (Risk/100 Cases)	GESTATIONAL AGE AT OCCURRENCE (Menstrual Weeks)
All cardiac anomalies	18 (3.9,83)	8.5%	7–10
VSD	20.2 (3.8,108)		
Transposition of great vessels	27.2 (3.5,209)		
All CNS anomalies	15.5 (3.3,74)	5.3%	5–7
Anencephaly	13.1 (1,178)		
Spina bifida	19.8 (2.6,153)		
All congenital anomalies	7.9 (1.9,34)	18.4%	

Adapted from Becerra et al: Diabetes mellitus during pregnancy and the risks for specific birth defects: A population based case-control study. Pediatrics 85:1, 1990.

Fetal Growth Disturbances

MACROSOMIA. Macrosomia, defined variously as birth weight above the 90th percentile for gestational age or birth weight greater than 4000 grams, occurs in 15 to 45 per cent of diabetic pregnancies (Lavin et al., 1983; Gyves et al., 1977; Coustan et al., 1980; Cousins, 1991). Excessive size contributes to increased risk of intrapartum injury (shoulder dystocia, brachial plexus and facial nerve injuries, and asphyxia). Macrosomia is also a major factor in the increased rate of cesarean delivery among diabetic women. The incidence of macrosomia in the California Diabetes and Pregnancy Program is indicated in Table 54–12 (California Department of Health Services, 1991). The risk of macrosomia is fairly constant across all classes of diabetes, suggesting that the effect of first trimester metabolic abnormalities has less effect on fetal growth than events occurring in the third trimester.

The pathophysiology of excessive fetal growth is complex and reflects the end result of delivery of an abnormal nutrient mixture to the fetoplacental unit. As already noted, Pedersen's (1952) hypothesis that maternal hyperglycemia stimulates fetal hyperinsulinemia, which in turn mediates accelerated fuel utilization and growth, established a potential link between maternal metabolic control and fetal growth. The features of the diabetic growth disturbance include abnormal adipose deposition and distribution, visceral organ hypertrophy and hyperplasia, and acceleration of skeletal growth (Ogata et al., 1980). Freinkel and Metzger (1979) further suggested that abnormal fetal growth was related to altered levels of lipids, amino acids, and ketones entering the uterine circulation.

A corollary to the "Pedersen Hypothesis" would suggest that strict control of maternal glucose levels should reduce the incidence of fetal macrosomia. However, the data to support this concept are conflicting. Willman (1986) analyzed 205 diabetic pregnancies and found an increased risk of fetal macrosomia only in patients whose mean glucose levels exceeded 130 mg/dl (65 per cent versus 27 per cent, P<.01). Jovanovic and Jovanovic (1984) reported a small series of patients with advanced diabetic vascular complications whose HbA$_1$c levels were normal throughout pregnancy. All infants were of normal weight except two patients with the highest maternal glycohemoglobin levels (7.3 per cent). Newborn weights in those patients were above the 90th percentile.

On the other hand, Coustan et al. (1980) reported that the risk of macrosomia (11 per cent) in strictly controlled diabetic pregnancies did not correlate with mean maternal glucose values. Other investigators have similarly failed to demonstrate a relationship between good glycemic control and normalization of birth weights in some infants (Knight et al., 1983; Dandona et al., 1984). Moore et al. (1987) failed to alter a macrosomic fetal growth profile in an insulin-resistant, obese, type II diabetic whose fetus was at the 90th percentile at 28 weeks. Continuous, subcutaneous insulin infusion normalized the mean blood glucose from over 200 to less than 100 mg/dl at 28 weeks, but fetal growth velocity and macrosomia actually accelerated.

TABLE 54–12. Incidence of Growth Abnormalities in Diabetic Pregnancy by White's Classification

	GESTATIONAL	CLASS A,B,C	CLASS D,F,R	TOTAL
Macrosomic (> 90th Percentile)	22%	31%	22%	24%
Small for Dates (< 10th Percentile)	4%	5%	5%	4%

Adapted from California Department of Health Services, Maternal and Child Health Branch: Status Report of the Sweet Success California Diabetes and Pregnancy Program 1986–1989. March 31, 1991.

However, recent data from the DIEP project suggest that maternal metabolic control is indeed highly predictive of macrosomia (Jovanovic-Peterson et al., 1991). In this study of diabetic women who received meticulous care in early pregnancy, the correlation with fasting glucose levels was not significant, but second- and third-trimester postprandial levels were strongly predictive of both birth weight and the overall percentage of macrosomic infants (P = 0.009). With postprandial glucose values averaging 120 mg/dl, approximately 20 per cent of infants were macrosomic; a 30 per cent rise in postprandial levels to 160 mg/dl resulted in a predicted percentage of macrosomia of 35 per cent. The implications of these data for clinical management of diabetic patients are enormous. The DIEP study suggests that while control of fasting glucose levels is important, limiting the magnitude of post-feeding glucose excursions is critical.

Other recent data indicate that maternal insulin levels, in addition to glucose, may influence fetal growth. In a study of insulin levels in umbilical cord sera of newborns delivered of diabetic women taking either animal or human insulin, Menon et al. (1990) demonstrated a significant correlation between the maternal and cord-serum concentrations of anti-insulin antibody and the concentration of animal insulin in the baby. Detection of significant levels of maternally administered animal insulin in the fetal blood suggests that the animal insulin was transferred across the placenta as an insulin-antibody complex. Macrosomic infants in this study had animal insulin levels in the umbilical cord blood almost three times higher than that observed in infants of normal weight. These data suggest that, under certain circumstances, insulin can be transferred transplacentally and retain its biological activity. High maternal anti-insulin antibody titers appear to favor this process.

Alteration in growth parameters of the fetus in diabetic pregnancy may extend into childhood. Silverman et al. (1991) reported follow-up of offspring of 205 women with diabetes from birth through age 8 years. During pregnancy these women maintained good to fair glycemic control (mean fasting glucose = 105 ± 21 mg/dl in insulin-requiring patients, = 91 ± 13 in gestational diabetics). However half the infants weighed >90th percentile for gestational age at birth. After delivery, all infants were followed with yearly evaluations of height and weight. Childhood growth was evaluated by comparing weight and height to population norms. An index of obesity, the symmetry index (SI), was calculated by dividing relative weight (observed weight/median weight for age) by relative height. The weight curve demonstrated that at 12 months of age, both the controls and diabetic offspring had equivalent body mass. However, at age 8 years,

approximately half weighed more than the heaviest 10 per cent of the nondiabetic children. The symmetry index was 30 per cent higher in diabetic offspring than in the controls by age 8 years. Interestingly, SI at birth did not correlate with SI at 8 years. Rather the maternal prepregnant body weight and amniotic fluid insulin values were most predictive.

In summary, fetal macrosomia occurs in almost one-third of diabetic pregnancies regardless of class. Abnormal fetal fat stores lead to difficult labor, dystocia, and birth injury as well as postnatal metabolic transition. The abnormal body fat distribution at birth may destine some of these infants to life-long obesity. Abnormal fetal growth in diabetic pregnancy appears to occur with any elevation in maternal glucose levels, however modest. Detection of macrosomia is therefore a major goal of diabetic pregnancy management.

INTRAUTERINE GROWTH RESTRICTION (IUGR). Although the weights of diabetic infants are generally skewed into the upper range, IUGR occurs with concerning frequency in diabetics with underlying vascular disease. Additional factors in diabetic pregnancy which increase the risk of IUGR include the higher incidence of structural anomalies and maternal hypertension. Typically the IUGR infant exhibits loss of truncal adipose stores, oligohydramnios, uteroplacental insufficiency, hypoxia, poor tolerance of labor, fetal distress, and intrauterine or neonatal death (Battaglia and Lubchenko, 1967).

Intrinsic IUGR is typically associated with chromosomal abnormalities, severe intrauterine infection, teratogenic insults, and genetic factors. In the case of diabetic pregnancy, intrinsic IUGR is most frequently associated with severe congenital anomalies and chromosomal defects. Extrinsic IUGR in diabetic pregnancy results from nutrient limitation associated with maternal hypertension and advanced diabetic vasculopathy. On ultrasonography, extrinsic growth restriction is characterized by slowing abdominal growth and plateau or cessation in weight gain. If allowed to progress unchecked, extrinsic IUGR leads to oligohydramnios, hypoxia, asphyxia, or fetal death. In diabetic pregnancy, asymmetrical IUGR is most commonly observed in patients with vasculopathy (retinal, renal, chronic hypertension). This association suggests that a uteroplacental vasculopathy may restrict fetal growth in these patients.

Asphyxia and Perinatal Mortality

Outcome of the diabetic gestation has improved markedly since the discovery of insulin (1922) and intensive obstetrical and infant care. Perinatal mortality in diabetic pregnancy has decreased 30-fold in this period. The present perinatal mortality rate of 2 per cent and lower (Fig. 54–7) since the 1970s has been associated with the development of regional perinatal centers and neonatal intensive care nurseries. In geographic areas where a regionalized perinatal team approach to high-risk pregnancies is not available, infant mortality rates are higher. The declining rate of iatrogenic respiratory distress syndrome has also contributed, with better timing of deliveries on the basis of amniotic fluid lipid profiles.

The currently reported perinatal mortality rates among diabetic women remain approximately twice those observed in the nondiabetic population (Rust et al., 1987; California Department of Health Services, 1991) (Table 54–13). Unexplained intrauterine demise, congenital malformations, and respiratory distress syndrome account for most perinatal deaths in contemporary diabetic pregnancy. In the past decade, fewer intrauterine deaths have been reported, probably reflecting more careful monitoring of these pregnancies. Nevertheless, intrapartum asphyxia and fetal demise remain a persistent problem.

Identification of the individual fetus at risk is difficult. Although the association of fetal death and poor maternal glycemic control has been recognized for decades, only recently has a plausible pathophysiology been elucidated. Several investigators have suggested that fetal hyperglycemia and hyperinsulinemia

TABLE 54–13.   Perinatal Mortality Rates in Diabetic Pregnancy

	GESTATIONAL	OVERT	NORMALS*
Fetal mortality	4.7	10.4	5.7
Neonatal mortality	3.3	12.2	4.7
Perinatal mortality	8.0	22.6	10.4

Mortality Rates = Deaths/1000 births
*Normal = California Data 1986, Birth weight, sex, and race corrected.

in the poorly controlled diabetic patient leads to progressive fetal hypoxemia, acidosis, and eventually death.

HYPERGLYCEMIA, HYPERINSULINEMIA, AND HYPOXIA. Miodovnik et al. (1982) infused betahydroxybutyrate into the hind-limb vein of the chronically prepared sheep fetus and demonstrated that fetal oxygenation was significantly reduced during periods of hyperketonemia. Phillips and co-workers (1985) experimentally induced hyperglycemia in the fetal sheep and noted that fetal oxygenation fell progressively during the period of elevated glucose levels. In several experiments, the induced hypoxemia was severe enough to precipitate fetal demise. In another study, Miodovnik et al. (1989), using alloxan-induced diabetic pregnant sheep, found that maternal hyperglycemia caused fetal hyperinsulinemia (more than twofold increase), fetal hypoxemia (37 per cent fall), and stillbirth.

In human pregnancy, pathologic changes in the fetal heart rate (decreased variability, late decelerations) have been recorded during periods of poor maternal glycemic control (Teramo et al., 1983; Kariniemi et al., 1983; Hughes, 1987). Bradley et al. (1991) performed umbilical cord sampling in 28 diabetic pregnancies and found significantly elevated fetal lactate levels and acidemia in the third trimester. Oxygen and carbon dioxide tensions were normal. These investigators did not correlate the elevated lactic acid levels with maternal glucose level, however. Edelberg et al. (1987) studied the effect of maternal hyperglycemia on fetal biophysical status associated with maternal glucose infusion. Using ultrasound to monitor fetal activity during hyperglycemia, they documented that fetal movements decreased significantly when maternal plasma glucose levels were raised to 120 mg/dl.

Other studies have linked reduced short-term variability of the fetal heart rate tracing to periods of maternal hyperglycemia (Kariniemi et al., 1983). Furthermore, studies utilizing Doppler waveform analysis of fetal umbilical blood flow have documented increased placental vascular resistance when maternal glucose levels were elevated (Bracero et al., 1986).

These findings strongly indicate that oxygen delivery to the fetus is adversely affected by maternal glucose control. The pathophysiology of this phenomenon may involve constriction of placental vasculature in response to fetal hyperglycemia or hyperinsulinemia but more likely is related to augmented fetal glucose metabolism and coincident increase in oxygen utilization in excess of supply.

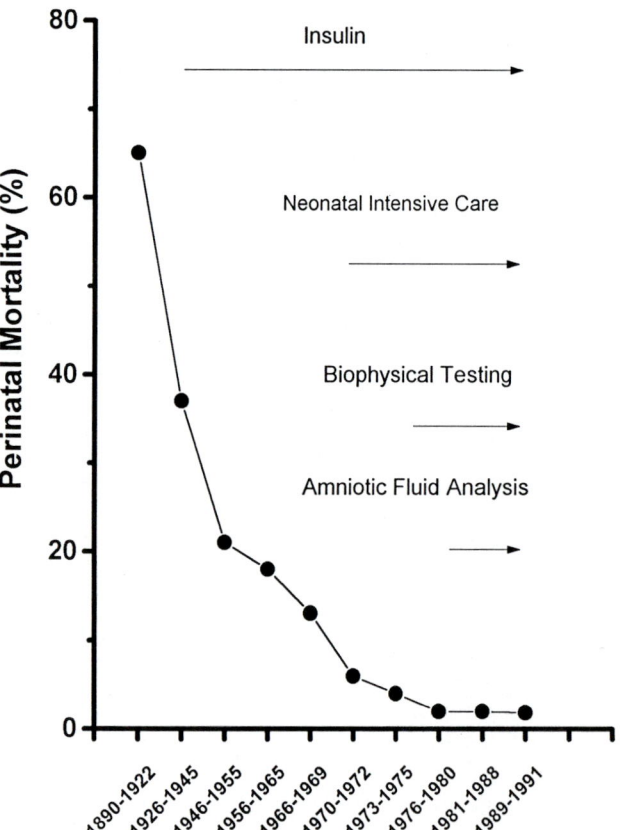

FIGURE 54–7. Perinatal mortality rate in diabetic pregnancy from 1890 to 1981. Plotted from numerical reports of Cragin and Ryder (1916), DeLee (1920), Williams (1925), Pedersen (1977), Gabbe (1978), Jorge et al (1981), French Diabetes Study Group (1991).

NEONATAL COMPLICATIONS

The postnatal course of infants of diabetic pregnancy continues to be more complicated than that experienced by offspring of normal women. Table 54–14 shows the incidence of neonatal morbidity among 2112 IDM followed in the California Diabetes and Pregnancy Program from 1986 to 1989. The reader is also referred to Chapter 63.

Prematurity and Respiratory Distress Syndrome

PRETERM BIRTH. Premature delivery of IDM remains a persistent problem even with meticulous control of maternal plasma glucose levels. Diabetic women have a higher incidence of maternal complications that require early timing of delivery (PIH, declining renal function, and uteroplacental insufficiency). Lavin (1981) reported a 19 per cent preterm delivery rate despite moderately good maternal control, and Coustan (1980) delivered 40 per cent of diabetic women before 38 weeks gestation in a group managed with "tight" glycemic regulation.

NEONATAL RESPIRATORY DISTRESS SYNDROME (RDS). Until recently, RDS was the most common and most serious disease in IDM. In the 1970s, improved prenatal maternal management for diabetes and new techniques in obstetrics for timing and mode of delivery resulted in a dramatic decline in its incidence from 31 to 3 per cent (Frantz and Epstein, 1979).

Nevertheless, neonatal pulmonary function of the IDM is suboptimal compared to infants of nondiabetic women matched for gestational age (Kjos et al., 1990). This may be due to inadequate alveolar surfactant production or abnormal pulmonary maturation and function. Kulovich and Gluck (1979) reported abnormal timing of phospholipid production in diabetic pregnancy, as indicated by a delay in the appearance of phosphatidylglycerol in the amniotic fluid. In their study, maturational delay occurred only in gestational diabetes (White's class A patients); other diabetic women had normal or accelerated maturation of pulmonary phospholipid profiles.

Some investigators have disagreed with the above findings. Ferroni et al. (1984), Tyden et al. (1984), and Landon et al. (1987) reported that fetal lung maturity occurred later in pregnancies with poor glycemic control (mean plasma glucose level >110 mg/dl) regardless of class of diabetes when these infants were stratified

by maternal plasma glucose levels. These observations agree with similar findings by Cunningham et al. (1978) and by Ylinen (1987). The biochemical mechanism of delayed surfactant production remains uncertain, but Bourbon et al. (1986) proposed that elevated maternal plasma levels of myo-inositol observed in diabetic women may inhibit or delay the production of phosphatidylglycerol in the fetus.

It is possible that poor neonatal respiratory performance in the IDM may have a histologic basis instead of, or in addition to, a biochemical etiology. Studies of fetal lung ion transport in the diabetic rat by Pinter et al. (1991) demonstrated decreased fluid clearance and lack of thinning of the lung's connective tissue compared to controls. Bhavnani et al. (1988) reported higher lung glycogen levels and reduced pulmonary compliance in offspring of diabetic rabbits compared to controls. In humans, Kjos et al. (1990) noted "respiratory distress" in 18 of 526 infants delivered of diabetic gestations (3.4 per cent). However, surfactant-deficient airway disease accounted for less than one-third of cases, with transient tachypnea, hypertrophic cardiomyopathy, and pneumonia responsible for the majority.

Thus, the near-term infant of a poorly controlled diabetic mother is more likely to have neonatal respiratory distress syndrome than the baby of a nondiabetic mother at the same gestational age. This unfortunate circumstance further compounds the diabetic infant's metabolic and cardiovascular difficulties after birth. The observations of Kulovich et al. (1979) indicate that the nondiabetic fetus achieves pulmonary maturity at a mean gestational age of 34 to 35 weeks. By 37 weeks, more than 99 per cent of normal newborn infants have mature lung profiles as assessed by phospholipid assays. In a diabetic pregnancy, however, it is unwise to assume that the risk of respiratory distress has passed until after 38.5 gestational weeks have been completed. Any delivery contemplated before 38.5 weeks for other than the most urgent fetal and maternal indications should be preceded by documentation of pulmonary maturity by amniocentesis.

Postnatal Hematologic and Metabolic Disturbances

POLYCYTHEMIA AND HYPERVISCOSITY. Polycythemia (central venous hemoglobin concentration >20 gm/dl or hematocrit >65 per cent) is not uncommon in IDM

TABLE 54–14. **Perinatal Morbidity in Diabetic Pregnancy**

MORBIDITY	GESTATIONAL DIABETES	TYPE I DIABETES	TYPE II DIABETES
Hyperbilirubinemia	29%	55%	44%
Hypoglycemia	9%	29%	24%
Respiratory distress	3%	8%	4%
Transient tachypnea	2%	3%	4%
Hypocalcemia	1%	4%	1%
Cardiomyopathy	1%	2%	1%
Polycythemia	1%	3%	3%

Adapted from California Department of Health Services, Maternal and Child Health Branch: Status Report of the Sweet Success California Diabetes and Pregnancy Program 1986–1989. March 31, 1991.

and apparently is related to glycemic control. The pathogenesis of increased erythropoiesis in IDM was investigated by Widness et al. (1990). These investigators documented a strong correlation between maternal antepartum glucose control and elevated fetal hematocrit and erythropoietin levels. They concluded that hyperglycemia is a powerful stimulus to fetal erythropoietin production, probably mediated by decreased fetal oxygen tension. Untreated, neonatal polycythemia may promote vascular sludging, ischemia, and infarction of vital tissues, including the kidneys and central nervous system.

Neonatal Hypoglycemia. The hyperinsulinemic fetus of a diabetic mother is at increased risk for low plasma glucose levels after birth. This complication is usually much milder and less common in the infant whose insulin-dependent diabetic mother is well controlled throughout the entire pregnancy and euglycemic during labor and delivery. Unrecognized postnatal hypoglycemia may lead to neonatal seizures, coma, and brain damage. Thus it is imperative that the nursery receiving the IDM have a protocol for frequent monitoring of the infant's blood sugars until metabolic stability is assured.

Meticulous antepartum and intrapartum maternal glucose control combined with early neonatal feeding in the first hours of life reduces the necessity for intravenous glucose infusions. The use of bolus infusions of hypertonic glucose excessively stimulates the hypertrophied pancreatic β cells and tends to perpetuate a hyperinsulinemia–hypoglycemia cycle. Oh (1979) recommends an intravenous glucose infusion administered at the rate of 6 mg/kg/min utilizing a constant-infusion pump as standard treatment for neonatal hypoglycemia. In a few infants, hypoglycemia may persist beyond 24 to 28 hours. In these instances, the use of glucocorticoids is recommended.

Neonatal Hypocalcemia. Low levels of serum calcium (less than 7 mg/dl) have been reported in up to 50 per cent of IDM during the first 3 days of life. Tsang and co-workers (1979) have studied this problem extensively. They have reported normal levels of parathyroid hormone in cord blood of IDM, indicating normal fetal parathyroid function. Decreased parathyroid function in such infants was associated with decreased serum calcium levels and increased serum phosphorus values. These changes in infants of insulin-dependent diabetics did not evoke an increase in serum parathyroid hormone. The resulting functional hypoparathyroidism was judged to be related to (1) prematurity, (2) birth asphyxia, or (3) suppressed parathyroid function secondary to hypercalcemia in utero. A fourth possibility, hypersecretion of calcitonin, has also been suggested, but serum calcitonin levels in IDM are not different from those in normal term infants (Cruikshank et al., 1980).

Neonatal Hypomagnesemia. Tsang and co-workers (1976) followed 56 diabetic mothers and their infants prospectively from birth and noted that 38 per cent of the infants had a serum magnesium level of less than 1.5 mg/dl on at least one occasion during the first 3 days of life. Decreased levels of serum magnesium were related to low maternal age and gravidity, severity of maternal diabetes, and prematurity. Neuromuscular irritability in infants was not correlated with decreased serum magnesium alone or with decreased ionized or total calcium. In IDM, decreased serum magnesium levels were associated with decreased maternal serum magnesium, decreased ionized and total calcium, increased serum phosphorus, and decreased parathyroid function. Later studies from this group (Shaul et al., 1987) have confirmed that magnesium plays an important role in neonatal calcium metabolism. Parathyroid hormone (PTH) and calcium responses to magnesium sulfate infusions were found to be inversely related to neonatal serum magnesium concentrations. Magnesium infusions, however, did not affect serum calcitonin concentrations.

Hyperbilirubinemia. The risk of hyperbilirubinemia is higher in IDM than in normal infants (Taylor et al., 1963; Peevy et al., 1980) and represents one of the most common postnatal problems. There are multiple causes of hyperbilirubinemia in IDM, but prematurity and polycythemia are the primary contributing factors. Increased destruction of red blood cells contributes to the risk of jaundice and kernicterus. Treatment of this complication is usually by phototherapy, but exchange transfusions may be necessary if bilirubin levels are markedly elevated.

Hypertrophic and Congestive Cardiomyopathy. In some macrosomic, plethoric infants of poorly controlled diabetic mothers, a thickened myocardium and significant asymmetric septal hypertrophy (ASH) has been described (Gutgesell et al., 1976; Schwartz et al., 1986). The prevalence of clinical and subclinical ASH in IDM has been estimated to be 30 per cent at birth, with resolution by 1 year of age (Mace et al., 1979). As noted in the report by Kjos et al. (1990), cardiac dysfunction associated with this entity often leads to respiratory distress, which may be mistaken for hyaline membrane disease.

IDM who manifest cardiomegaly and signs of congestive heart failure may have either congestive or hypertrophic cardiomyopathy. This condition is often asymptomatic and unrecognized. Echocardiograms show a hypercontractile, thickened myocardium, often with septal hypertrophy disproportionate to the ventricular free walls. The ventricular chambers are often smaller than normal, and there may be anterior systolic motion of the mitral valve producing left ventricular outflow-tract obstruction.

The pathogenesis of hypertrophic cardiomyopathy in IDM is unclear, although it is recognized to be associated with poor maternal metabolic control. There is evidence that the fetal myocardium is particularly sensitive to insulin during gestation, and Susa et al. (1979) reported a 100 per cent increase in cardiac mass in fetal hyperinsulinemic rhesus monkeys. The myocardium is known to be richly endowed with insulin receptors (Steven and Whitsett, 1979).

Cooper et al. (1992) performed serial echocardiography on the fetuses of 61 pregnant diabetic women and correlated the findings with indices of glycemic control. Although there was a persistent antenatal trend toward excessive ventricular septal thickness in the fetuses with postnatally diagnosed ASH (n = 19, 46 per cent), this became statistically significant only

TABLE 54–15. Preconceptional Evaluation of the Diabetic Patient

PROCEDURE	TESTS	RECOMMENDATIONS
Medical history, family history, review of symptoms	Selected patients: fasting and postprandial C-peptide determinations to clarify type of diabetes	Avoid pregnancy until HbA₁c is in the normal, nonpregnant range
Physical examination Positive findings:		
Hypertension	EKG, cardiac, renal evaluation	Antihypertensive medications
Retinopathy	Retinal evaluation	Ophthalmology consultation
Goiter	T4, TSH, antibodies	
Neuropathy		Vascular, podiatric evaluation
Obesity		Exercise, weight loss
Proteinuria	24-hour urine for protein, creatinine	Nephrology consultation if renal function abnormal
Diabetes assessment Glycemic control	HbA₁c Home glucose monitoring Stable glycemic profile	
Nutrition		Dietitian consultation
Occupational and family life assessment		Help prepare patient for life-style commitments necessary for tight glycemic control

after 31 weeks. When the ASH newborns were compared to normals, birth weights (4009 gm versus 3457 gm, P<.01) and maternal glycosylated hemoglobin levels (6.7 per cent versus 5.7 per cent) were higher in the infants with cardiomyopathy. This study demonstrates the association of fetal septal hypertrophy and poor maternal glycemic control.

IDM may also have congestive cardiomyopathy without hypertrophy. On echocardiogram the myocardium is overstretched and poorly contractile. This condition is often rapidly reversible with correction of neonatal hypoglycemia, hypocalcemia, and polycythemia; it responds to digoxin or diuretics or both. In contrast, treatment of hypertrophic cardiomyopathy with an inotropic or diuretic agent tends to decrease further the size of the ventricular chambers and leads to obstruction of blood flow. Echocardiographic examination of IDM with enlarged hearts is recommended to detect and treat clinically silent cardiomyopathy.

PREGNANCY MANAGEMENT OF OVERT DIABETICS

Preconceptional Care

Preconceptional counseling and a detailed medical risk assessment is recommended for all women with overt diabetes and those with a history of gestational diabetes during a previous pregnancy. Ideally, this information should be provided to the patient at numerous intervals during her life, beginning in puberty. The role of the pediatrician, adolescent specialist, internist, and endocrinologist in providing this ongoing counseling cannot be overstated. Significant impact on the maternal and neonatal complications of diabetic pregnancy will not be realized until meticulous preconceptional metabolic control is achieved in all women contemplating pregnancy.

More realistically, preconceptional counseling is frequently provided by the obstetrician or perinatologist.

The important elements to be considered in preconceptional counseling of the diabetic patient are listed in Table 54–15. Preconceptional counseling should, optimally, be accompanied by a thorough medical evaluation. Key aspects of the medical evaluation of at-risk patients is outlined in Table 54–16. Ultimately, preconceptional medical evaluation and risk assessment should be directed into a comprehensive program of metabolic control. The major goals of a prepregnancy metabolic program include: (1) establishing personal habits that permit frequent and regular monitoring of capillary glucose level, (2) adopting an insulin dosing regimen that results in smooth interprandial glucose profile (fasting glucose 80 to 100 mg/dl, 2-hour postprandial glucose <120 mg/dl, no reactions between meals or at night), (3) bringing HbA₁c level into the normal range for nondiabetics, and (4) developing family, financial, and personal resources to assist patient should pregnancy complications require lost time from job and/or bed rest.

TABLE 54–16. Preconceptional Counseling of Diabetic Women

TOPIC	KEY POINTS
Maternal medical risks	Individualized counseling. Consider patient's retinal, cardiovascular, renal status; use current statistics regarding impact of maternal medical status on pregnancy outcome
Fetal and neonatal risks	Congenital anomalies and glycemic control; prematurity, macrosomia, birth injury; neonatal metabolic abnormalities; use current statistics
Obstetric complications	Exacerbation of hypertension; risk of preeclampsia, premature labor; need for bed rest, cesarean section
Family and social supports	Spousal or significant other's level of involvement and support; personal resources to facilitate meticulous glycemic control, accommodate bed rest if necessary
Economic considerations	Insurance coverage and limitations; ability to interrupt occupation, accommodate job absence

Pregnancy Care

Team Management

Since management of diabetic pregnancy is complex and time consuming, and has profound short- and long-term implications for mother and infant, many perinatal clinics have adopted a team approach (Table 54–17). Optimal care of the diabetic patient requires the intense and steadfast commitment of the patient herself. Involvement of her spouse or a significant other is not essential but is associated with improved outcome.

The remainder of the diabetes management team consists of a perinatologist, who has the primary responsibility for prenatal and obstetric decisions, including timing of delivery, amniocentesis, fetal monitoring, and management of labor and delivery; a medical diabetologist, who assists in metabolic management of the patient and advises on decisions concerning insulin administration and problems with hyperglycemia, hypoglycemia, and ketosis; a dietician, who works closely with the physicians to monitor the patient's nutrition, dietary compliance, and appropriate weight gain during pregnancy; and a nurse clinician, who has a critical role in patient education, coordination of medical care, and collection of appropriate laboratory samples for monitoring control. A social worker's assistance is frequently needed to help with stress management, resolution of financial problems and coordination of job and career interruptions necessitated by the patient's intensive prenatal care regimen. Although it is possible to provide integrated "team care" between the offices of the internist and the obstetrician, many centers find that centralizing the resources in a "diabetic center" helps to promote optimal patient compliance and minimizes oversights and errors in management.

Fetal Surveillance

Fetal surveillance in diabetic pregnancy begins, ideally, in the preconceptual phase and continues throughout the pregnancy, utilizing an array of techniques to detect the fetus in jeopardy. A recommended sequence in fetal evaluation during diabetic pregnancy is presented in Table 54–18.

DETECTION OF CONGENITAL MALFORMATIONS. Preconceptional counseling and metabolic control have the effect of preventing the occurrence of congenital malformations, thus saving countless hours of anguish and the considerable economic consequences of an IDDM born with significant handicaps. In an Israeli study (1986), 75 patients managed preconceptionally

TABLE 54–17. The Diabetic Pregnancy Care Team

The patient
The patient's spouse/significant other
Obstetrician or perinatologist
Endocrinologist or internist
Diabetes nurse educator
Dietitian
Social worker

TABLE 54–18. Fetal Surveillance in Type I and II Diabetic Pregnancies

TIME		TEST
Preconception		Maternal glycemic control
8–10	Weeks	Sonographic crown-rump measurement
16	Weeks	Maternal serum alpha-fetoprotein level
20–22	Weeks	High-resolution sonography, fetal cardiac echography in women in suboptimal diabetic control (abnormal HbA$_{1c}$) at first prenatal visit
24	Weeks	Baseline sonographic growth assessment of the fetus
28	Weeks	Daily fetal movement counting by the mother
32	Weeks	Repeat sonography for fetal growth
34	Weeks	Biophysical testing: 2 × weekly NST or Weekly CST or Weekly biophysical profile
36	Weeks	Estimation of fetal weight by sonography
37–38.5	Weeks	Amniocentesis and delivery for patients in poor control (persistent daily hyperglycemia)
38.5–40	Weeks	Delivery without amniocentesis for patients in good control who have excellent dating criteria*

*See text for description.
Abbreviations: NST = non-stress test; CST = contraction stress test.

were compared to 31 women whose tight glycemic control began after pregnancy registration. First trimester glycohemoglobin levels were lower in the preconceptional patients (7.4 versus 10.4 per cent), as was the occurrence rate of fetal malformations (0 versus 9.6 per cent). These results are echoed by the reports of Fuhrmann et al. (1983), Lucas et al. (1983), and Hod et al. (1991).

Once the pregnancy is ongoing, early detection of fetal anomalies is of paramount importance, particularly if maternal glycemic control has been suboptimal. A secondary goal is to provide the anxious diabetic gravida with reassuring information about the structural integrity of her baby while, should a major anomaly be discovered, permitting her the opportunity to choose appropriate therapeutic options in management, pre- and postnatally. Since the risk of discovering a fetal anomaly in diabetic pregnancy is clearly related to the level of early glycemic control (Pinter et al., 1986), all type I and type II diabetic women should undergo careful fetal screening for anomalies.

Precise documentation of obstetric dates facilitates management later in pregnancy when issues of fetal maturity may become prominent. Measurement of the fetal crown-rump length at 9 to 12 weeks provides highly accurate gestational dating (±3 days). The possibility of early detection of the anomalous embryo during this early dating sonogram was suggested by Pedersen et al. (1986). This group noted a delay in progression of the crown-rump length sonographically among fetuses later noted to be structurally abnormal. Although other investigators have not confirmed this finding (Cousins et al., 1988), careful ultrasonographic scrutiny of the embryo at 9 to 12 weeks not only establishes obstetric dates, but will occasionally disclose a fetus with anencephaly or cystic hygroma.

Neural Tube Defects. In the second trimester, maternal serum alpha-fetoprotein screening (MSAFP) should be performed. Since the frequency of neural tube defects is increased more than ten times in diabetic pregnancy (Milunsky et al., 1982), MSAFP screening at 16 ± 2 weeks is an important diagnostic maneuver for all type I and type II diabetics. A normal MSAFP result lowers the risk of undetected spina bifida by a factor of 100.

At approximately 18 weeks, after the MSAFP screening result is available, level II sonography with targeted imaging of the fetal anatomy should be conducted. This examination should include detailed images of the cranium and its contents, the spinal axis, heart (chambers and outflow tracts), abdominal contents, kidneys, bladder, genitalia, umbilical cord insertion, and limb morphology. The study should be performed with highest resolution equipment available by a knowledgeable sonologist. If, because of fetal position or maternal obesity, views are considered suboptimal by the sonographer, a repeat examination prior to 24 weeks must be scheduled.

Cardiac Anomalies. Cardiac anomalies are increased fourfold in diabetic pregnancy and represent a defect with potentially major impact on the fetus. However, the precise level of glycohemoglobin which marks the threshold of increased risk of fetal cardiac anomalies is as yet undefined. Since the risk of fetal malformations increases with any elevation in maternal glycemic control, detailed views of the fetal heart should be obtained in all patients with first-trimester glycohemoglobin above the normal range. If a qualified fetal echocardiologist is available, fetal echocardiography should be offered to all diabetic patients whose glycohemoglobin was above normal at registration. If such expertise is not available, a normal four-chamber view of the heart during the level II examination will rule out over 90 per cent of significant cardiac malformations. In a study of 43 type I diabetic pregnancies, Gomez et al. (1988) confirmed the efficacy of second-trimester screening ultrasonography (100 per cent specificity, 67 per cent sensitivity) for cardiac lesions.

Detection of Macrosomia. The dynamics of fetal growth in diabetic pregnancy have only recently become clear. Until the early third trimester, differentiation of diabetic from nondiabetic fetuses by ultrasonography is extremely difficult. However, from 24 weeks onward, the path of growth followed by the abdominal circumference in particular begins to deviate from normal. Ogata et al. (1980) demonstrated that growth of the abdominal circumference differentiates the growth of a diabetic fetus from normals. This difference was reliably detectable by 30 weeks gestation (Fig. 54–8).

Reece et al. (1990a) prospectively studied fetal growth in 45 insulin-dependent diabetics utilizing ultrasonographic measurements of the fetal head. They found that the fetus of the diabetic mother exhibits head growth velocities similar to those of normals, even when advanced degrees of maternal vascular disease were present. Landon et al. (1989a, 1989b) also conducted serial ultrasonographic examinations to characterize the dynamics of fetal growth. Head and femur length growth did not differ statistically from

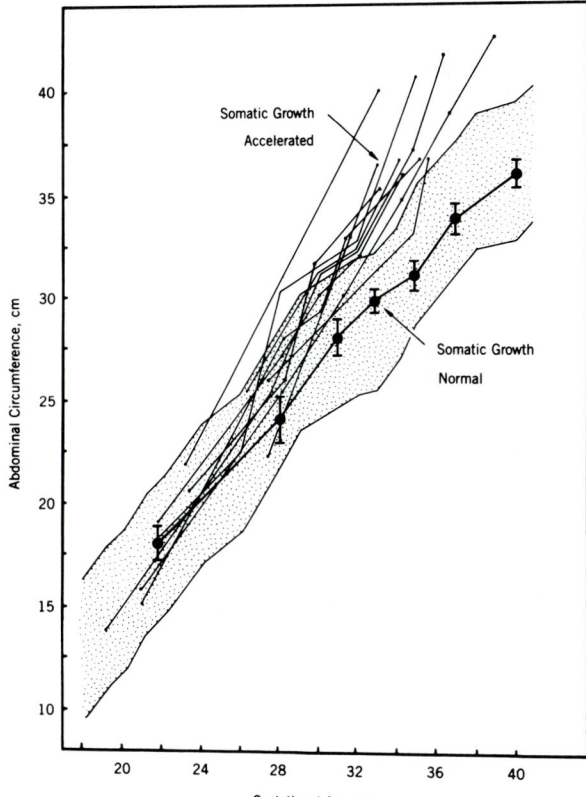

FIGURE 54–8. Serial measurements of the fetal abdominal circumference during diabetic pregnancy. The 95 per cent confidence band for nondiabetic pregnancy is also shown. (From Ogata et al: Serial ultrasonography to assess evolving fetal macrosomia. Studies in 23 pregnant diabetic women. JAMA **243**:2405, 1980. Copyright 1980, The American Medical Association.)

normals. Abdominal circumference growth diverged from normals beginning at 32 weeks (abdominal circumference growth in diabetics = 1.36 cm/wk versus 0.901 cm/wk in normals, P <.001). Using a cutoff value of a growth velocity of 1.2 cm/wk from 32 to 39 weeks, these investigators were able to identify macrosomic infants with 84 per cent sensitivity and 85 per cent specificity.

A good deal of effort has been expended in identifying a regression formula that will accurately predict the weight of the diabetic fetus from sonographic parameters. A number of polynomial formulas utilizing a combination of head, abdominal, and limb measurements have been proposed (Shepherd et al., 1982). Unfortunately, small errors in individual measurements of the head, abdomen, and femur are multiplied together in such formulas. Perhaps this is why no single formula has proved to be adequate in identifying the macrosomic fetus (Tamura et al., 1985). Benson and colleagues (1987) studied 160 fetuses of diabetic pregnancies using a variety of sonographic formulas to predict fetal weight before delivery. Although 77 per cent of fetuses sonographically predicted to weigh over 4000 gm were indeed macrosomic at birth (false-positive rate of 23 per cent), over half of the total macrosomic group were incorrectly predicted to be of normal weight.

Tamura et al. (1985) noted that the most widely used formulas for calculation of fetal weight using sonographic measurements underestimate actual weight by 300 to 1000 grams. In a later study (Tamura et al., 1986), a combination of sonographic fetal weight estimation and abdominal circumference above the 90th percentiles was used to define potential macrosomia. This study predicted macrosomia correctly in 72 per cent. Only 8% of normal-weight infants were incorrectly predicted to be macrosomic. Typical accuracy in estimation of fetal weight near-term is ± 15 per cent.

While precise prediction of fetal weight is not possible at present, serial trending of ultrasonographic parameters offers an estimate of overall weight percentile. The growth percentile can be estimated from two or three third-trimester examinations. Use of three sets of measurements compensates for inaccuracies in individual observations. When assessing the likelihood of whether a fetus is macrosomic, all of the measurements should be taken into account. Particular attention should be paid to the percentiles of the abdominal circumference and calculated weight. If both are consistently above the 90th percentile, the likelihood of macrosomia is high.

In the case where a decision about fetal macrosomia must be based upon a single measurement, several investigators have proposed the use of biometric ratios. Bracero et al. (1985) has investigated the use of the fetal abdominal diameter/femur length ratio to define potential macrosomia. This technique produced an 83 per cent positive predictive value for macrosomia with a sensitivity of 79 per cent when the ratio exceeded 1.385. However, four of 23 (17 per cent) of the babies identified as macrosomic were in fact of normal weight. Similarly disappointing results were reported by Landon et al. (1987), who reported a correct diagnosis of only 37 per cent of macrosomic fetuses.

Hadlock et al. (1982) suggested the use of the femur length to abdominal circumference ratio (FLAC), because it is relatively constant at 22 per cent ± 2 per cent throughout the latter half of pregnancy. Unfortunately, this measure is not sufficiently sensitive or specific for clinical management except in the most extreme cases. Elliott et al. (1982) proposed a macrosomia index, calculated by subtracting the biparietal diameter from chest diameter. In cases where the macrosomia index was 1.4 cm or greater, shoulder dystocia was encountered in 25 per cent of patients. This macrosomia index has not been widely applied, possibly because ultrasonographic measurement of the chest diameter is difficult and subject to a high degree of variation. As of this writing, therefore, fetal weight estimations by sonographic measurements or calculations of ratios of fetal dimension are not accurate enough to be used independently to diagnose macrosomia. Nevertheless, these techniques are useful as indicators of macrosomia. If estimated fetal weight exceeds 4500 gm, and if the fetal abdominal circumference is above the 90th percentile, cesarean delivery is the preferred mode of delivery. In pregnancies with estimated fetal weights between 4000 and 4300 gm with a diabetic morphologic profile (abdominal circumference > head circumference), vaginal delivery

should be approached with caution (Landon et al., 1990).

PREVENTION OF FETAL ASPHYXIA AND DEATH. Antenatal fetal heart rate testing remains the cornerstone of fetal surveillance in the third trimester. However, the choice of test and selection of testing interval remain highly controversial. Although the majority of perinatal centers use the non-stress test (NST) as the primary biophysical test, a multicenter comparison of NST and contraction stress test (CST) documented a significantly lower risk of antepartum death with the CST (7.8 versus 1.1/1000 births, P<.05) (Freeman et al., 1982).

Examining the effectiveness of the NST in diabetic pregnancy, Keegan noted that the NST failed to predict two perinatal deaths in 342 pregnancies when the test was performed weekly (Keegan and Paul, 1980). A subsequent report (Golde et al., 1984), administering the NST *twice weekly*, documented no perinatal losses in 107 cases. Olofsson et al. (1986a, 1986b), compared the NST and CST retrospectively in 99 diabetic pregnancies. This study documented no differences in the predictive value of a reassuring test performed weekly but found the CST to be superior in that there were fewer falsely pathologic tests that precipitated unwarranted intervention. On the basis of these data, the NST should be performed twice weekly if used in diabetic pregnancy. Available information indicates that the CST and biophysical profile can be performed weekly without excessive fetal risk. Testing should be performed from 32 to 34 weeks onward unless fetal growth restriction, significant maternal hypertension, or oligohydramnios dictates that these tests begin sooner.

Despite an abundance of data to suggest that antepartum fetal heart rate monitoring is adequate in diabetic pregnancy, many authorities believe that some form of daily testing, such as fetal movement assessment, is a valuable adjunct (Landon and Gabbe, 1985). A review of the diagnostic accuracy of various antepartum surveillance techniques by Thacker and Berkelman (1986) reported that fetal movement counting had the highest sensitivity and specificity for predicting fetal death. The "count-to-ten" method used has been shown to decrease perinatal mortality in a moderate-risk population (Moore and Piacquadio, 1989) and has become a standard of care at most large centers. Fetal movement counting should begin at 28 weeks. Figure 54–9 shows a "kick count card" for recording fetal movements.

Many centers now utilize umbilical arterial Doppler velocimetry as an adjunct to fetal testing. Umbilical Doppler sonography detects the velocity wave-form of the blood circulating from the fetal heart to the placenta. Increased Doppler up-shift during cardiac systole and reduced flow velocity in diastole are indicative of increased placental resistance. Absence of diastolic flow or reversed diastolic flow is associated with fetal distress and in utero demise. Fetuses at risk for these phenomena include severe fetal growth restriction and gravidas with marked hypertension or autoimmune disease (e.g., lupus erythematosus, anticardiolipin antibodies).

Landon et al. (1989a) used umbilical systolic/diastolic

FETAL MOVEMENT RECORD

Name:_____

Due Date:_____

Start Date	Number of weeks pregnant

INSTRUCTIONS

1. Count the baby's movements **EVERY NIGHT**.

2. A movement may be a kick, swish or roll. Do not count hiccups or small flutters.

3. You can start counting any time in the evening when the baby is active. BUT: COUNT EVERY NIGHT.

4. Count baby's movements while lying down, preferably on your left side.

5. Mark down the **time** you feel the baby move for the first time.

6. Mark down the **time** you feel the 10th fetal movement.

7. You should feel at least 10 fetal movements within one hour. Call Labor and Delivery **immediately** if

   a) you do not feel 10 movements within 1 hour.

   b) it takes longer and longer for your baby to move 10 times.

   c) you have not felt the baby move all day.

DO NOT WAIT UNTIL TOMORROW.

Date	Time First Movement Felt	Time 10th Movement Felt	Total Time
EXAMPLE 11/4/91	6:50 p.m.	7:28 p.m.	38 minutes

FIGURE 54–9. A Fetal Movement card. The patient is instructed to note the time at which she begins monitoring fetal movements, then to note the time at which the tenth movement is felt. If she has not recorded 10 movements in one hour, she is to call her physician.

(SD) ratios together with traditional biophysical testing in 35 diabetics. The SD ratio did not correlate with glycohemoglobin level or mean blood glucose level. However, the mean SD ratios were higher in patients with vascular disease. Among IUGR infants in the series, 80 per cent were identified by an elevated SD ratio. In three cases, the ratio became abnormal before sonographic documentation of IUGR was made. Ishimatsu et al. (1991) studied Doppler wave-forms in the umbilical circulation of 16 diabetic patients. They found no correlation with overall maternal glucose level, but observed abnormal Doppler results in two cases with glucose levels >300 mg/dl. These normalized when glycemic control was restored. Johnstone et al. (1992) studied umbilical flow velocity wave-forms in 128 diabetics and 170 controls in the third trimester. No relationship between Doppler studies and maternal glycemic control was observed, and umbilical resistances in diabetics were similar to those of controls. High umbilical resistance was associated with IUGR in nine cases. As of this writing, Doppler studies complement rather than substitute for effective traditional antepartum testing measures, and routine antenatal testing of diabetic pregnancy with Doppler velocimetry is not recommended. Selective use of umbilical Doppler studies in pregnancies at high risk for IUGR may be helpful in identifying the fetus as risk for demise.

Maternal Surveillance

Many women with type I diabetes become pregnant after a prolonged period of poor control having interrupted their medical care when they ceased being pediatric patients and failed to select a new family physician or internist in their young adult years. Such patients may have neglected their metabolic control, developed background or more severe retinopathy, or experienced asymptomatic hypertension. To achieve successful pregnancy outcome, intensive glycemic control and meticulous organ system monitoring are essential. Although meticulous management of diabetic women during pregnancy requires careful planning, frequent visits, and liberal use of consultation, the strategy is simple: achieve and maintain maternal euglycemia, avoid or promptly detect cardiovascular, renal, ophthalmologic, and renal complications, and judiciously select the timing and route of delivery.

CARDIOVASCULAR AND RENAL MONITORING. Specific recommendations for preconception and early postconception renal care were described earlier. It should be noted that women with creatinine clearance of less than 80 ml per minute or a 24-hour urinary protein loss of more than 500 mg per day are at higher risk for poor pregnancy outcome. Assessment of renal function (creatinine clearance and total urinary protein excretion) should be performed each trimester and more often if blood pressure elevations occur. In women with normal blood pressures and diabetes of less than 8 years duration, a single baseline renal evaluation may be sufficient. Renal function tests should be repeated promptly if an unexplained decline in insulin requirement occurs since this may reflect decreased renal insulin clearance or placental failure.

Close monitoring of the diabetic patient's cardiovascular status and early detection of PIH are essential to optimize pregnancy outcome. The effect of hormonal changes during pregnancy on peripheral vascular resistance typically improves blood pressure in the second trimester. In the third trimester, when peripheral resistance and mean arterial pressures rise by 10 to 50 per cent over first-trimester values, differentiation of PIH from chronic hypertension can be extremely difficult.

Management of the hypertensive diabetic patient requires a combination of bed rest and, when indicated, antihypertensive medications. The goal of therapy is to limit maternal blood pressure elevation to minimize the risk of stroke and abruptio placentae while maintaining adequate uterine perfusion to sustain fetal growth. However, the precise level of hypertension that should prompt the initiation of medical management has not been defined. Indeed, Sibai et al. (1983) have shown that pharmacotherapy in nondiabetics with mild-to-moderate hypertension does not improve perinatal outcome. Nevertheless, antihypertensive medications are commonly prescribed when systolic pressures consistently exceed 150 to 160 mm Hg or diastolics are persistently above 100 mm Hg.

Selection of antihypertensive agents should be individualized. Most experts utilize methyldopa as the first-line drug. It is common practice to adjust the dose of antihypertensive agents to keep the patient's diastolic pressure in the low 90s and systolic pressure under 160 mm Hg. This theoretically maintains adequate uterine perfusion pressure yet minimizes the risk of hypertensive complications such as intracerebral hemorrhage, renal compromise, and abruptio placentae although conclusive data supporting this approach are lacking. Having the patient obtain multiple blood pressures at home between office visits is helpful in ensuring that blood pressure control is based on accurate data.

When a single agent is ineffective in controlling hypertension, a beta-blocker such as propranolol or atenolol may be added (Oloffson et al., 1986a, 1986b). Hydralazine or a calcium-channel blocker is a reasonable second choice. Certain antihypertensive agents are relatively contraindicated during pregnancy. Diuretics, either thiazides or furosemide, reduce circulating blood volume and may compromise uterine blood flow and fetal growth (Gant et al., 1975). Angiotensin-converting enzyme (ACE) inhibitors (e.g., captopril and enalapril), used with increasing frequency in the nonpregnant hypertensive patient, have been linked to poor fetal growth, severe fetal anuria, and death in the newborn (Brent and Beckman, 1991). These medications should be avoided in the second and third trimesters. Patients who require the addition of a third antihypertensive agent should be monitored closely since these patients frequently experience poor fetal growth and early onset of preeclampsia. The therapeutic goal of antihypertensive therapy should be to keep blood pressure in the 140/90 mm Hg range.

The use of antihypertensive medications does not alter the severity or timing of onset of superimposed PIH. Clues that worsening PIH is responsible for late-pregnancy hypertension include: (1) an abrupt drop in creatinine clearance, (2) an increase in serum uric acid above 7.0 mg/dl, (3) the appearance of marked nondependent edema, and (4) falling platelet counts (<150,000/mm^3). Bed rest should be instituted promptly when a diabetic patient develops PIH before 36 weeks gestation. When the signs of mild PIH appear near term, amniocentesis for fetal lung maturity and induction of labor should be considered.

Glycemic Control and Glucose Monitoring. The goals of metabolic management in diabetic pregnancy are to: (1) prevent diabetic ketoacidosis, (2) prevent episodes of symptomatic or asymptomatic hypoglycemia (plasma glucose <60 mg/100 ml (3.33 mM/liter), (3) achieve a normal HbA$_1$c concentration (<6.5 per cent), (4) maintain fasting glucose levels <100 mg/100 ml (5.5 mM/liter), (5) keep 1-hour postprandial glucose levels below 140 mg/100 ml (7.7 mM/liter) and 2-hour postprandial plasma glucose levels <120 mg/dl. These goals can be achieved easily in type II, GDM, and many type I patients. The task is much more difficult in type I women with zero levels of C peptide, hypoglycemia unawareness, and lack of counter-regulatory responses to abnormally low blood sugar levels. Jovanovic and associates (1980) demonstrated the feasibility of maintaining normal glucose profiles in 10 type I pregnant diabetic women in a program that emphasized dietary education, three subcutaneous injections of insulin a day, and home monitoring of plasma glucose levels by the patients. They reported an excellent outcome in all the women and their infants.

The role of hospitalization in management of diabetic pregnancies has changed in the past two decades. Confinement of the patient for 2 to 4 weeks before delivery (chiefly to permit the performance of daily urinary estriol measurements) is no longer considered necessary or desirable. The studies of Golde et al. (1984) indicate that ideal patients who maintain good outpatient glycemic control need not be hospitalized before delivery. In early pregnancy, many diabetes and pregnancy services routinely hospitalize patients briefly for intensive metabolic, renal, ophthalmologic, and obstetric assessment and to establish tight glycemic control. Jovanovic et al. (1981) maintained their patients on an outpatient basis except for a brief admission at 24 weeks to assess control. Recently, many specialists have found that the activity and dietary environment of the hospital is so dissimilar from the patient's own that little is gained by this practice at relatively large economic cost. Intensive outpatient care, on the other hand, with frequent telephone contact supplemented by once- or twice-weekly clinic visits, may be more efficient since dietary and insulin adjustments are made in a more realistic environment. Regardless of the techniques used, there is no substitute for frequent and personal contact with the patient, especially during the first trimester.

Dietary Therapy. Dietary therapy has been used more intensively for treatment of diabetes than for any other disease in medical history. Extreme approaches have varied from total starvation to emphasis on a particular class of foods such as fats or carbohydrates. For both nonpregnant and pregnant diabetic patients, nutritionists and physicians are still struggling to find the best way to regulate the quantity and quality of food intake.

Pregnancy Weight Gain. The controversy over ideal weight gain in pregnancy is decades old. During the 1940s and 1950s, limitation of weight gain to 10 kg or less was highly recommended. More recently, as data have shown that maternal weight-for-height influences pregnancy outcome independent of weight gain, more liberal guidelines, with more individualization have been the rule (Kleinman, 1990). Additionally, adolescent women and women of African-American descent benefit by increased weight gains when compared to Caucasian women of the same body mass. Table 54–19 outlines the current recommendations for total pregnancy weight gain stratified by weight-for-height categories. In general, these guidelines are applicable to the wide spectrum of lean and obese patients with diabetes during pregnancy.

Dietary Content. Arky and colleagues (1982) examined current dietary recommendations for individuals with diabetes. They noted that the nutrition committees of the American Diabetes Association (1979), British Diabetic Association (1980), and Canadian Diabetes Association (1980) have all called attention to the disadvantages of "traditional" low-carbohydrate diabetic diets which, inevitably, overemphasize dietary fat. All three organizations recommend lowering of fat content and the inclusion of complex carbohydrates and carbohydrate sources associated with fiber as the major proportion of carbohydrate calories. The dietary composition now recommended contains 50 to 60 per cent carbohydrate, 12 to 20 per cent protein, less than 10 per cent saturated fatty acids, and up to 10 per cent polyunsaturated fatty acids, with the remainder of ingested fat derived from monounsaturated forms.

Manipulation of the type of carbohydrate in the diet can provide additional benefits in glycemic control. Crapo et al. (1981) compared the blood glucose excursions induced by the ingestion of 50 gm of carbohydrate from dextrose, rice, potato, corn, and bread. They observed that the highest glucose response occurred with dextrose and potato, with much lower peaks after intake of corn and rice. This has led Jenkins et al. (1981) to propose that foods be classified by a "glycemic index" related to their tendency to induce hyperglycemia. In general, foods with a low glycemic index are associated with a more gradual release of glucose into the circulation from the gut. Although data are conflicting, complex carbohydrate (rather than simple sugars) and foods with higher soluble fiber content have this profile (Ney et al., 1982).

The Committee on Dietary Allowances, Food and Nutrition Board (1990) advises an additional food intake for pregnancy of 300 calories per day above basal requirements (38 kcal/kg or 2000 to 2400 kcal), up to 10 gm additional protein per day, and 30 mg of elemental supplemental iron. This committee does not recommend routine dietary supplementation of other vitamins and minerals if a balanced diet is maintained. The typically prescribed prenatal vitamin provides additional amounts of all vitamins and minerals including 250 mg of calcium and 800 μg more of folacin.

TABLE 54–19. Recommended Total Weight Gain Ranges for Pregnant Women by Pre-pregnancy Body Mass Index

BODY MASS INDEX*	RECOMMENDED TOTAL WEIGHT GAIN	
	lb	**kg**
Low (BMI <19.8)	28–40	12.5–18
Normal (BMI 19.8–26)	25–35	11.5–16
High (BMI 26–29)	15–25	7–11.5
Very high (BMI >29)	≥15	≥6

*BMI = weight-for-height = kg/cm^2

Adapted from National Academy of Sciences, Subcommittee on Nutritional Status and Weight Gain During Pregnancy, Subcommittee on Dietary Intake and Nutrient Supplements During Pregnancy and Lactation, Food and Nutrition Board, Institute of Medicine: Nutrition During Pregnancy. Part I. Weight Gain. Washington DC, National Academy Press, 1990.

DIETARY COUNSELING OF PREGNANT WOMEN WITH TYPE I DIABETES. In counseling type I diabetic women, one must consider several variables. These include the stage of pregnancy when the patient is first seen, lifestyle, cultural food preferences, timing of meals, level of physical activity, and energy needs for gestation.

During the first trimester, food intake may drop appreciably with symptoms of nausea or vomiting and decreased physical activity. These patients commonly present with episodes of hypoglycemia and ketonuria. Dietary advice and insulin readjustment should be coordinated to maintain reasonable control of plasma glucose levels. In the second trimester, increased energy and physical activity, coupled with renewed appetite, usually require additional calories and insulin. As fetal glucose needs rise, the tendency to nocturnal and between-meal hypoglycemia increases, requiring close attention to timing and content of meals.

Early in pregnancy, a detailed dietary history should be obtained. A diet is prescribed to ensure sufficient calories and frequency of food intake to prevent ketosis. Foods in the diet plan should be ethnically appropriate. Timing of meals has a significant effect on glycemic control during pregnancy. For type I patients who continue to experience insulin activity for up to 4 to 6 hours after a dose of regular insulin, prolonged periods without food intake increase the risk of hypoglycemic episodes. In these patients, a consistent program of three meals plus snacks at mid-morning, mid-afternoon, and bedtime provides ideal intervals between food intakes. Because nocturnal hypoglycemia is often a severe and common problem in type I pregnant patients, emphasis is placed on the bedtime snack, which should contain a minimum of 25 gm of complex carbohydrate. Inclusion of a small amount of dietary protein or fat at this time helps to prolong release from the gut. Since the course of pregnancy represents a dynamic state, the dietary prescription is continually adjusted according to the patient's weight gain, insulin requirement, and pattern of exercise. Weekly medical and dietary evaluations help to ensure optimal control.

DIETARY CONSIDERATIONS FOR WOMEN WITH TYPE II DIABETES. Many obese type II diabetics have non–insulin-dependent diabetes before pregnancy, but are unaware of significantly impaired glucose tolerance. Because their diabetes may be asymptomatic, they often seek medical attention late in gestation, after macrosomia and polyhydramnios have occurred. These individuals present special problems, because exaggerated insulin resistance during pregnancy makes control of plasma glucose levels more difficult. Their dietary habits, which may have contributed to their glucose intolerance, may be difficult to modify. Practitioners may be timid in prescribing adequate doses of insulin to overcome endogenous resistance, resulting in unnecessary delay until glycemic control is achieved.

Calorie Reduction and Ketosis. Are the weight gain recommendations (10 kg) for women of normal body habitus reasonable for obese patients? Pitkin (1977), Mintz et al. (1978), and Schulman and associates (1979) believe that caloric restriction of obese pregnant women is contraindicated and that pregnancy is not a time for weight reduction. However, excessive weight gain in obese patients may result in increased perinatal mortality (Naeye, 1979) (Fig. 54–10). Other studies have shown an increase in preterm birth among obese women with weight gains above 15 kg (Kleinman, 1990). Thus it is tempting to recommend calorie restriction in obese pregnant women, particularly those with NIDDM. The controversy is further complicated by the risk of inducing ketosis.

Churchill and associates (1969) and Stehbens and colleagues (1977) reported that ketonuria during pregnancy is associated with impairment of neuropsychological development of offspring. This report has resulted in admonitions to avoid caloric reduction in any pregnant woman. However, Coetzee and associates (1980) have raised serious questions about the experimental protocols and methodology of the Churchill study. The evidence for ketonuria was obtained from many different hospitals by having a nurse check a single urine sample for ketones on the day of delivery. No measurements or correlations were made of urinary ketones, serum ketones, plasma glucose levels, or complications during pregnancy, labor, delivery, and the neonatal period.

Coetzee and associates (1980) reported their findings in 18 pregnant women with diabetes on a 1000-calorie diet, 17 nonobese diabetic pregnant patients on a 1400- to 1800-calorie diet, and 35 normal pregnant women on a free diet (1600 kcal/day). They found morning ketonuria, as measured by reagent strips, in 19 per cent of women with insulin-independent diabetes on the 1000-calorie diet, 14 per cent of diabetics on the 1400- to 1800-calorie diet, and 7 per cent of normal pregnant women on the free diet. The reagent strip test result was never positive in blood samples, even

when it was 2+ in urine samples. Serum acetoacetate levels in all subjects were always below 1 mM/liter. These levels are considered nontoxic. It is of interest that despite the restrictive 1000-calorie diet in obese diabetic patients, mean infant birth weight was 3463 gm for the women with ketonuria and 3389 gm for the women without ketonuria. This was in contrast to birth weights of 2908 to 3109 gm for normal women on a 1,600-calorie diet. There were no untoward neonatal events in infants of ketonuric mothers.

The nutritional prescription for normal and diabetic pregnancies must take into account both maternal and fetal needs. Hytten (1979) has observed that the fetus may be much less vulnerable to the vagaries of maternal diet than previously thought. During the first half of pregnancy, maternal fat stores increase with eating to appetite. In these circumstances the usual weight gain of 12.5 kg is in excess of the total increment attributed to the products of conception, growth of uterus and breasts, and expansion of blood and other body fluids. The difference includes the addition of 3.5 kg of body fat resulting from the change in energy balance. The control of energy balance during gestation is not well understood, but it is known to include the influence of larger appetite, less physical activity, and a decrease in the plasma levels of glucose and most nutrients (except lipids). The changes in nutrient levels may favor placental transfer to the fetus.

Although poor nutrition is associated with suboptimal reproductive performance, under most circumstances the effect is marginal and can be demonstrated only in studies of large population groups. The long-term consequences of maternal calorie restriction on fetal growth are not clear. In the extreme food deprivation (700 calories daily) associated with famine in Holland in 1944 to 1945, the average birth weight in pregnancies subjected to third-trimester starvation decreased by only 300 to 400 gm compared to prefamine births. Stein and co-workers (1975) reported that the infants born to starving Dutch women during that period appear to have suffered no permanent effect on subsequent growth and intellectual development. In general, the fetus who is deprived because the mother does not eat enough is not particularly stunted but merely lean, and the 300-gm deficit that distinguishes it from the fetus of a well-fed or supplemented mother may be largely the luxury of a subcutaneous fat store.

In the final analysis, all nutritionists and diabetologists agree that severe maternal ketosis, as reflected by ketonemia, that affects maternal acid-base balance is unfavorable for mother and fetus. The unanswered question is: Are the large infants of significantly obese women on diets exceeding 2000 kcal/day at more or less risk for perinatal and long-term problems than infants of mothers on restricted caloric intake who have occasional ketonuria (without significant ketonemia) during pregnancy?

GLUCOSE MONITORING. *Glycosylated Hemoglobin and Fructosamine.* Measurements of glycosylated hemoglobin have proved to be a useful index of long-term (4 to 6 weeks) glycemic control during diabetic pregnancy. HbA$_1$c is a normal minor hemoglobin that has glucose linked to the N-terminal end of the beta

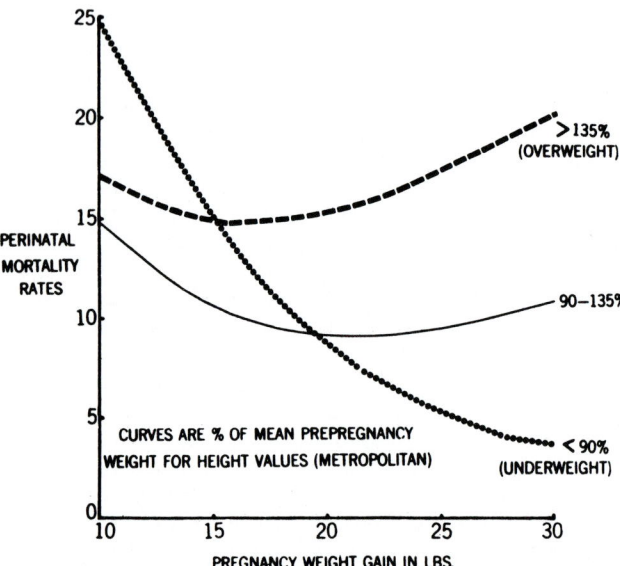

FIGURE 54–10. A plot of perinatal mortality (per 100 births) and pregnancy weight gain. Curves are referenced to per cent of ideal body weight, Metropolitan Life Insurance Co. (From Naeye: Weight gain and the outcome of pregnancy. Am J Obstet Gynecol **135**:3, 1979.)

TABLE 54–20. Timing of Home Capillary Glucose Monitoring

CAPILLARY GLUCOSE ASSESSMENT	ADVANTAGE	DISADVANTAGE
Pre-Meal	Permits prospective adjustment of food intake, supplementation of pre-meal insulin	Pre-meal or fasting glucose levels correlate poorly with fetal morbidity; significant postprandial hyperglycemia may go undetected
Post-Meal	Permits supplementation of insulin to reduce postprandial glucose overshoots; improved postprandial control correlates with improved fetal/neonatal outcome	Results are obtained after food intake
Bedtime	Permits adjustment of calories at bedtime snack, adjustment of bedtime insulin	
3–4 AM	Permits detection of nocturnal hypoglycemia	Interrupts sleep; may increase stress

chain. Glycosylation of hemoglobin occurs nonenzymatically throughout the life span of the red blood cell. HbA$_1$c levels correlate closely with the mean circulatory glucose levels to which the erythrocyte is exposed during its 120-day life span. HbA$_1$c levels provide information about glucose control when erythrocyte survival time is normal and are not as accurate or useful in sickle cell anemia or other disorders with shortened RBC life span. HbA$_1$c concentrations vary with different methods and in various laboratories. During pregnancy, excellent diabetic control implies a normal HbA$_1$c value for the laboratory method employed. Several reports have shown that HbA$_1$c concentrations are of little value in the diagnosis of NIDDM among patients with abnormal glucose tolerance in pregnancy (Santiago et al., 1978; Saibene et al., 1978; Miller et al., 1979).

Fructosamine, another glycosylated plasma protein, has been used in the nondiabetic patient to assess medium-to-short-term glycemic control. However, Doery et al. (1990) found this test to be of little value in metabolic management of diabetic pregnancy. On the other hand, Pasi et al. (1989) demonstrated a positive correlation between maternal serum fructosamine levels and the incidence of macrosomia. Suhonen et al. (1989) compared HbA$_1$c, glycosylated hemoglobin and fructosamine to the 24-hour glycemic profile in pregnant patients. HbA$_1$c was more accurate.

Clinical use of glycosylated hemoglobin levels during diabetic pregnancy provides both a confirmation of the patient's reported capillary glucose levels and a numeric index of the patient's overall compliance. Although assessing HbA$_1$c levels every 4 to 6 weeks during pregnancy rarely alters management significantly, it provides the patient with a "score" by which she can rate the success of her hourly efforts to keep blood sugars within a narrow band.

Home Glucose Monitoring (HGM). The advent of chemical test strips which reflect capillary glucose concentration has revolutionized the management of diabetes. The availability of portable meters to read these reagent strips and store the glucose values with date and time of sampling has brought further convenience and accuracy to the management of diabetic pregnancy. It should now be considered the standard of care to monitor multiple capillary glucose samples daily in all diabetic pregnancies.

The discipline of measuring and recording blood glucose levels before and after meals may have the effect of improving glycemic control. Goldberg et al. (1986) compared the outcomes of gestational diabetic pregnancies managed by weekly clinic glucose measurement with the outcomes of home glucose monitoring and noted that the incidence of macrosomia and mean birth weights were less in the HGM group.

Caution must be exercised, however, in the interpretation of HGM results. Clinical problems include (1) missing values or questionable records, (2) improper technique, (3) meter malfunction or poor calibration, (4) failure to monitor glucose values during hypoglycemic episodes or illnesses, and (5) misinterpretation of high blood glucose values following inapparent hypoglycemic episodes or many hours following exercise. Errors of interpretation are most common in type I patients. Insulin doses should never be selected or changed on the basis of numbers without a careful patient history and review of dietary and exercise practices. These problems are accentuated if one confidently relies upon the printout of built-in memory meters without putting the results in perspective by assessing the patient's history, lifestyle, and emotional status and the presence or absence of minor or major infections.

The frequency and timing of HGM should be individualized (Table 54–20). A typical schedule involves blood sugar checks on rising in the morning, 1 or 2 hours after breakfast, before and after lunch, before dinner, and before bedtime. An additional blood sugar check in the 3 AM to 4 AM time frame is helpful in guiding insulin therapy both at bedtime and before breakfast.

INSULIN THERAPY. No insulin delivery method now available approaches the precise secretion of the hormone from the human pancreas. The therapeutic goal of exogenous insulin therapy during pregnancy is to achieve diurnal glucose excursions similar to those of nondiabetic pregnant women. As shown in Figure 54–1, normal pregnant women maintain their postprandial blood sugar excursions within a relatively narrow range. As pregnancy progresses, the fasting and between-meal blood sugar levels drop progressively lower, owing to the continual uptake of glucose from the maternal circulation by the growing fetus. This phenomenon is accentuated during the night while the patient sleeps. Any insulin regimen for pregnant women must be designed to avoid excessive unopposed insulin action during the fasting state.

However, the goal of "physiologic" glycemic control

in pregnancy will not be met by simply avoiding hypoglycemia. The data summarized above regarding fetal macrosomia and postnatal morbidity emphasize the key role of excessive postprandial glucose excursions. Thus close attention must be paid to both pre- and postprandial glycemic profiles.

Choice of Insulin. Patients may enter pregnancy accustomed to the use of a wide variety of insulin types and schedules. At present, the human insulin preparations manufactured by recombinant DNA methodology, semisynthetic human insulin derived from porcine insulin, and highly purified monocomponent porcine insulin are favored over the older beef or pork insulins to reduce the formation of anti-insulin antibodies. Short-acting soluble insulin (regular), medium-acting isophane (NPH), and zinc suspensions (Lente) are the main types of insulin in use during diabetic pregnancies. These insulins are used singly or in combination regimens two to four times each day. Some diabetic patients may begin pregnancy using a long-acting insulin (Ultralente) because of the convenience of once-daily dosing. The practitioner should be familiar with the pharmacodynamics of each of the insulin types in use in order to optimize glycemic control and minimize hypoglycemic episodes. Long- and intermediate-acting insulins, in particular, may peak in activity during fasting periods (e.g., sleep) and must be carefully timed.

Insulin Pharmacokinetics. Subcutaneous insulin regimens are based on the assumption that insulin absorption and availability are predictable and reproducible. However, many factors influence insulin absorption and availability. Variation in insulin absorption from day to day in a single individual is 25 per cent and between patients is up to 50 per cent (Binder et al., 1984). There are regional differences in insulin absorption, attributable to variations in blood flow. Absorption is fastest from the abdomen, followed by the arm, buttocks, and thigh. The variation is sufficiently great that Skyler (1986) recommends that random rotation of injection sites should be avoided. He advises that any given injection—e.g., prebreakfast—should be administered in the same region to decrease day-to-day variability.

The generally accepted understanding of the pharmacokinetics of subcutaneous regular insulin has implied a rapid onset of insulin action in less than 1 hour, a peak effect in 2 to 4 hours, and a total duration of 6 to 8 hours. However, in studies of type I diabetic patients reported by Gardner et al. (1986) the onset of insulin action was at 1.2 ± 0.1 ($\pm$ SEM) hours, the peak effect at 5.7 ± 0.3 hours, and the duration of action 16.2 ± 1.2 hours. Bressler and Galloway (1971) and Bhaskar et al. (1980) reported similar delays. These findings are of particular importance for women who may take regular insulin to suppress between-meal or nocturnal hyperglycemia, since hypoglycemia 4 to 6 hours later may ensue.

Insulin type and dosing frequency should be individualized. Use of regular insulin prior to each major meal helps to limit postprandial hyperglycemia. To provide basal insulin levels between feedings, a longer-acting preparation is necessary. Ultralente has the advantage of a single injection in the morning, but typically leads to uncontrollable hypoglycemia during the hours of sleep. For this reason, most experts utilize an injection of NPH or Lente insulin in the morning and another later in the day. Typical dose ratios are two-thirds of total insulin in the morning, consisting of two-thirds intermediate-acting and one-third regular insulin.

Adequate doses of morning NPH or Lente insulin will regularly cause hypoglycemia in late morning unless a snack is taken. Additional intermediate-acting insulin is needed to cover basal insulin needs during sleep. However, if this dose is given prior to the evening meal, the peak of action (8 hours later) occurs at approximately 2 to 3 AM. Delaying the evening dose of NPH or Lente until bedtime will move the peak in action to 4 to 6 AM, a time when increasing insulin action is needed.

Continuous Subcutaneous Insulin Infusion (CSII) During Pregnancy. Achieving optimal glycemic control with multiple subcutaneous injections (MSI) requires meticulous blood sugar monitoring and multiple dosing. Recently, more type I diabetic women have been using the continuous subcutaneous insulin infusion (CSII) pump and wish to continue with this method during pregnancy because of convenience and the opportunity to achieve enhanced control. Several investigators have reported successful outcomes with use of CSII in pregnancy (Potter et al., 1981; Rudolf et al., 1981; Cohen et al., 1982; Hertz et al., 1984). Caruso (1987) compared CSII with intensive MSI in 12 pregnant patients. Poorly controlled patients on MSI achieved excellent control with CSII. Patients with good control with MSI experienced a reduction in the variation of glucose excursions and a reduction in the total daily insulin requirement. Jennings et al. (1991) compared glycemic control in type II diabetics with CSII and conventional therapy. Those with CSII had lower HbA$_1$c levels and better overall control. Haakens et al. (1990) performed a similar comparison in type I diabetic patients and reported not only improved glycemic control but patient preference for the control and convenience of CSII.

Nevertheless, Mecklenburg et al. (1984) reported that while diabetes control improved significantly with insulin pump therapy, 42 per cent of patients experienced at least one major complication, such as diabetic ketoacidosis (DKA), infection, or hypoglycemic coma. Significantly, episodes of DKA increased markedly after institution of pump therapy when compared with the patients' own control period of MSI.

Problems with pump malfunction, precipitation of insulin inside the pump mechanism, and abscess formation at the infusion site are now less common. CSII clearly offers the prospect of significantly smoother metabolic control for some women, particularly for those who are highly motivated and meticulous. Successful diabetic pregnancy management with CSII requires a motivated and knowledgeable patient, a diabetologist or perinatologist experienced with pump therapy, and prompt availability of emergency counseling and assistance on a 24-hour basis (Carta et al., 1986).

From a practical viewpoint, use of programmable insulin infusion rates allows tailoring of the insulin administration profile to the patient's individual metabolic and lifestyle rhythms. A typical regimen is shown in Table 54–21. The enhanced ability for the patient to check her blood sugar and administer extra insulin outside of the home is of great value in improving the smoothness of glycemic control.

Hypoglycemia. Because of absent pancreatic reserve, the risk of significant hypoglycemia is much higher in women with type I diabetes. Blood glucose levels less than 50 mg/dl are usually accompanied by autonomic symptoms and/or mental confusion in most patients. The range of symptoms is variable, and each patient tends to have a characteristic pattern. The earliest symptom may be a sensation of circumoral numbness followed by tremulousness, tremor, increased sweating, tachycardia, a feeling of intense hunger, or headache. In some individuals, the only premonitory sensation is a feeling of fatigue.

The most common cause of hypoglycemia is overinsulinization by a zealous patient and/or her physician in the attempt to achieve perfect control. Wilson (1983) reviewed the biochemical effects and clinical repercussions of excessive insulin therapy. Low blood glucose levels often occur (particularly in type I patients) during excessive or unplanned exercise when appropriate dietary adjustments have not been made in advance. Mild episodes are easily controlled by a snack consisting of milk and crackers or orange juice. Pregnant diabetic women should be advised to carry a thermos of milk and crackers with them at all times. Ingestion of sucrose and unrefined sugars is not recommended for treatment because this results in very high levels of plasma glucose that disturb glycemic control for many hours and sometimes an entire day or longer. Spouses or other housemates should be trained in managing hypoglycemic episodes.

Exercise. Exercise is generally recommended for pregnant women, but the advice is usually nonspecific. It is noteworthy that little evidence exists to support the popular notion that regular exercise will improve the outcome of pregnancy. Those studies that have been done reveal no change in the length or quality of labor and no reduction in the number of maternal or fetal complications (Berkowitz et al., 1983). There is some evidence that increased occupational activity and heavy endurance exercise shorten the length of gestation and result in lower infant weights (ACOG, 1985).

Since ancient times, exercise has been recommended as an important adjunct in the treatment of diabetes. However, data documenting the beneficial or deleterious effects of exercise in diabetic pregnancy are few. Reviews of the available data regarding the metabolic and cardiovascular effects of exercise in normal and diabetic pregnancies have been published (Artal and Wiswell, 1986; Hollingsworth and Moore, 1987). Evidence to support the benefit of an exercise program in pregnant diabetic individuals is limited, but Jovanovic-Peterson and colleagues (1991a) recently reported a series of investigations pertinent to these issues. In one study (Durak et al., 1990b), the effects of various exercise machines on uterine activity were studied. They found that exercise stimulated significant uterine activity when the bicycle (50 per cent), rowing ergometer (10 per cent), or treadmill (40 per cent) was used, whereas no increase in contractions was observed when the recumbent bicycle or arm ergometer was utilized. In another study, they reported the results of an upper body aerobic exercise program for women with GDM, with patients divided into diet-only and diet-exercise groups. After six weeks, they demonstrated significant improvement in mean fasting and postprandial blood sugars in the exercising group, as well as lower HbA$_1$c levels (p<.01). At least four weeks of physical training were necessary to observe a statistically significant difference. A study by Hollingsworth and Moore (1987), utilizing walking exercise, in 13 IDDM women, demonstrated a reduction in plasma lipids but no significant effect on glycemic control.

For type I diabetic women who are in good physical condition and metabolic control it seems reasonable to continue exercise along the lines recommended by the American College of Obstetricians and Gynecologists (1985). They should, of course, be aware of the special precautions suggested to avoid hyper- and hypoglycemia, and exercise should not be prescribed for those with antecedent hypertension, pregnancy-induced hypertension, evidence of macro- or microvascular disease, autonomic dysfunction, or lack of normal counter-regulatory mechanisms to counteract hypoglycemia. Durak et al. (1990a) have suggested that exercise specialists be employed to tailor the exercise prescription to the patient's own risk profile.

Pregnant women with type II and gestational diabetes appear to have the most to gain and least to risk from a moderate exercise program, yet many of these patients are obese and ill-disposed to exercise regularly or vigorously. Whether metabolic control is more easily achieved and maintained without risk when exercise is added to treatment with diet and insulin remains to be firmly established. As discussed earlier, regular physical exercise may improve insulin resistance and, in some GDM and NIDDM patients, render insulin therapy unnecessary. In any case, all pregnant women with established or gestationally provoked diabetes who engage in exercise programs should do so only with the close supervision of their physician.

TABLE 54–21. A Typical Administration Profile Using Continuous Subcutaneous Insulin Infusion Pump

TIME	BASAL RATE*	BOLUS	COMMENT
4 AM	1.3 U/hr		Higher basal rate opposes the "dawn effect" of rising serum glucose from 4–6 AM
7 AM		8 U	Pre-breakfast bolus
10 AM	1.0 U/hr		Lower basal rate to match increased physical activity, decreased insulin needs
12 Noon		4 U	Pre-lunch bolus
6 PM		4 U	Pre-dinner bolus
10 PM	0.6 U/hr		Lower basal rate for sleep

*Regular insulin.

Timing and Mode of Delivery

Prevention of Birth Injury. Shoulder dystocia is defined as difficulty in delivery of the fetal body after expulsion of the fetal head. This obstetric emergency occurs in .3 to .5 per cent of vaginal deliveries among normal pregnant women. Under the influence of hyperinsulinemia of diabetic pregnancy, fetal shoulder and abdominal widths can become massive and extremely difficult to deliver vaginally. Although 48 per cent of shoulder dystocia occurs in infants of average birth weight (2500 to 4000 grams) (Acker et al., 1986), the incidence of shoulder dystocia rises tenfold to 3 per cent among infants weighing 4000 grams or more. Among diabetic women with infants of more than 4000 grams, 16 per cent sustained shoulder dystocia in a recent series.

The clinical features signaling increased risk of shoulder dystocia include (1) protracted active phase labor, (2) prolonged second stage (pushing for more than two hours), and (3) the use of mid-forceps. An attempt by Sandmire et al. (1988) to predict shoulder dystocia on the basis of risk factors concluded that the majority of cases of shoulder dystocia occur without recognizable antecedent warning signs. Gross et al. (1987) found that birth weight, prolonged deceleration phase, and length of second stage contributed to the risk of shoulder dystocia, but that only 16 per cent of the cases of shoulder dystocia with trauma could be predicted by this multifactorial model.

In spite of these data, IDM are more likely to experience shoulder dystocia than normal fetuses of the same weight. Acker et al. (1986) documented a three-fold increase in the risk of shoulder dystocia (31 per cent) in diabetic neonates weighing more than 4000 grams as opposed to nondiabetic macrosomic infants. These investigators recommended cesarean section for all diabetic patients whose estimated fetal weight is greater than 4000 grams. Landon et al. (1990) surveyed maternal-fetal medicine specialists and found that over half of these practitioners recommend cesarean delivery when estimated fetal weight is over 4500 grams, but only one-third opted for cesarean section when the weight estimation was 4000 to 4500 grams.

On the basis of available evidence, the decision to perform cesarean section for the indication of macrosomia should be individualized. Most importantly, application of forceps after protracted active phase or prolonged second stage should be considered with great caution.

Delivery Timing. Determining delivery timing is a critical issue in diabetic pregnancy to minimize both maternal and neonatal morbidity and mortality. Delaying delivery until term is likely to maximize cervical ripeness and improve the chances of vaginal delivery, yet the risks of fetal macrosomia and unexpected fetal death increase as the due date approaches. Although it was common practice to perform amniocentesis and deliver diabetic women at 37 weeks gestation in the past, recent data indicate that with meticulous antepartum fetal assessment practices, delivery can frequently be delayed until nearly 40 weeks without increasing maternal morbidity, fetal demise, neonatal mortality, or neonatal morbidity.

Drury et al. (1983) allowed diabetes patients at the National Maternity Hospital of Dublin to wait until obstetric indications for delivery were present or spontaneous labor occurred. The cesarean section rate was 20 per cent. Murphy and colleagues (1984) compared earlier management techniques (delivery at 37 weeks) to a policy of expectant management. Average fetal age at delivery increased from 37.5 weeks to 39.4 weeks, with 14 per cent spontaneous labor in the early group and 38 per cent in the expectantly managed group. Perinatal mortality was not affected. Indications for delivery are summarized in Table 54–22. Delivery before 38.5 weeks gestation without documented fetal lung maturity should be performed only for compelling maternal or fetal reasons. After 38.5 weeks, the obstetrician can await spontaneous labor if the fetus is not macrosomic and biophysical testing is reassuring. After 40 plus weeks, the benefits of continued conservative management are likely to be less than the danger of fetal compromise. Induction of labor before 42 weeks in diabetic pregnancy, regardless of the readiness of the cervix, is prudent.

Fetal pulmonary maturity is an important prerequisite to labor induction, planned cesarean section, or termination of tocolysis. Documenting a lecithin/sphingomyelin (L/S) ratio >2.0 is insufficient reassurance in diabetic pregnancy. Phosphatidylglycerol must be present in at least a 3 per cent concentration to ensure relatively normal respiratory function after birth (Dudley and Black, 1985). For deliveries planned at or beyond 38.5 weeks, amniocentesis should be performed for confirmation of fetal maturity unless obstetric dates are absolutely certain (Table 54–23).

Delivery Route. Given the aforementioned considerations, choice of vaginal delivery or cesarean must be based on limited scientific data. The patients past history (of macrosomia, shoulder dystocia), present estimation of fetal weight (macrosomia or IUGR), fetal adipose profile (abdomen larger than head), and clinical pelvimetry should all be considered. Cervical ripening with prostaglandins may be helpful in improving inducibility and have no effect on glycemic control.

Most large series of diabetic pregnancies report a cesarean section rate of 30 to 50 per cent (California Department of Health Services, 1991). The ideal means by which this rate can be lowered is by early and strict glycemic control in pregnancy. Conducting long labor inductions in patients with a large fetus and marginal

Table 54–22. Indications for Delivery in Diabetic Pregnancy

Fetal	Nonreactive, positive CST
	Reactive postive CST, mature fetus
	Sonographic evidence of fetal growth arrest
	Decline in fetal growth rate with decreased amniotic fluid
	40–41 weeks gestation
Maternal	Severe preeclampsia
	Mild preeclampsia, mature fetus
	Markedly falling renal function (creatinine clearance < 40 ml/min)
Obstetric	Preterm labor with failure of tocolysis
	Mature fetus, inducible cervix

TABLE 54–23. Confirmation of Fetal Maturity Before Induction of Labor or Planned Cesarean Delivery in Diabetic Pregnancy

1. Phosphatidylglycerol > 3 per cent in amniotic fluid collected from vaginal pool or by amniocentesis
2. Completion of 38.5 weeks gestation
3. Normal last menstrual period
4. First pelvic examination before 12 weeks confirms dates
5. Sonogram before 24 weeks confirms dates
6. Documentation of more than 18 weeks of unamplified (fetoscope) fetal heart tones

pelvis may increase, rather than lower, morbidity and costs.

INTRAPARTUM GLYCEMIC CONTROL. Maintenance of intrapartum metabolic homeostasis is essential to avoid fetal hypoxemia. Unfortunately, strict maternal euglycemia during labor and delivery does not lessen the likelihood of hypoglycemia in infants with macrosomia and long-established islet cell hypertrophy. Several investigators have advocated the use of a combined insulin and glucose infusion to maintain maternal euglycemia during labor. Although initial reports suggested that this technique reduced the risk of neonatal hypoglycemia (Yeast et al., 1978), subsequent studies indicate that the primary benefit of continuous infusion is smooth maternal glycemic control (Caplan et al., 1982).

Golde and co-workers (1982) found that during use of continuous glucose and insulin infusions in labor for type I diabetic patients, almost half required no insulin after labor was established. Moreover, the incidence of neonatal hypoglycemia in infants of patients who received only glucose was similar to patients who received the combined therapy (17.6 per cent versus 12.5 per cent). Jovanovic and Peterson (1983) studied the maternal response to continuous insulin infusion in labor and found glucose requirements (2.55 mg/kg/min) unchanged over the course of labor and delivery, but insulin requirements dropped to zero during active phase labor. A protocol for administration of a continuous insulin infusion in labor, based on these data, is outlined in Table 54–24.

POSTPARTUM MANAGEMENT. Following delivery, an immediate decrease in insulin requirement occurs, probably related to the abrupt loss of the placenta and the associated rapid disappearance of the steroid and peptide hormones it produced. Type II patients typically require little or no insulin for 1 to 3 days following delivery, whereas type I patients require small doses of regular insulin determined on the basis of regular measurements of plasma glucose levels. Once the patient returns to relatively normal feeding, plasma glucose levels can be assessed before meals, at bedtime, and at 3:00 AM. Regular insulin is administered in 2- to 10-unit doses when plasma glucose levels exceed 150 mg/100 ml. By the third or fourth day postpartum, the type I patient can be shifted to about two-thirds of her pre-pregnancy dosage divided into two or three daily injections. The insulin requirement varies appreciably from one patient to another and must be carefully adjusted for each individual. Postpartum complications such as infections increase the insulin requirement.

Hospital discharge usually coincides with an increased requirement for insulin and the onset of lactation. All diabetic patients should continue home blood glucose monitoring and have careful supervision of diabetic control. Women who breast-feed frequently find that episodes of hypoglycemia are common 30 to 45 minutes after nursing. These can be prevented if the patient drinks a glass of milk or the equivalent before or during each breast-feeding session.

At home, most patients become more casual about their diabetic control with the added responsibility of a new baby and more irregular eating and sleeping patterns. Rigg et al. (1980) reported that women 6 to 12 weeks postpartum were markedly underinsulinized and in poorer control than at any time during pregnancy. The diabetes-pregnancy team that manages the patient during gestation should arrange *before delivery* for the supervision of the patient's diabetes by a diabetologist or diabetes center immediately following hospital discharge. This approach minimizes periods of poor glycemic control that are so frequent in new diabetic mothers.

GESTATIONAL DIABETES

The term *gestational diabetes* is used to describe carbohydrate intolerance that occurs (or is first recognized) during pregnancy. The incidence of gestational diabetes is 10 times higher than that of overt diabetes (Roversi et al., 1980), with clustering among certain ethnic groups. Hollingsworth et al. (1991) demon-

TABLE 54–24. Intrapartum Maternal Glycemic Control

1. *Insulin Infusion Method*
   a. Withhold AM insulin injection.
   b. Begin and continue glucose infusion (5% dextrose in water) at 100 ml/hr throughout labor.
   c. Begin infusion of regular insulin at 0.5 U/hr.
   d. Begin oxytocin as needed.
   e. Monitor maternal glucose levels hourly using capillary reflectance meter at bedside and/or laboratory determinations.
   f. Adjust insulin infusion.

Plasma/Capillary Glucose (mg/100 ml)	Infusion Rate (Units/hour)
< 80	Insulin Off
80–100	0.5*
101–140	1.0
141–180	1.5
181–220	2.0*
>220	2.5*

2. *Intermittent Subcutaneous Injection Method*
   a. Give one-half the usual insulin dose in A.M.
   b. Begin and continue glucose infusion (5% dextrose in water) at 100 ml/hr throughout labor.
   c. Begin oxytocin as needed.
   d. Monitor maternal glucose levels hourly using capillary reflectance meter at bedside and/or laboratory determinations.
   e. Administer regular insulin in small (2–5 units) doses to maintain glucose 80–120 mg/100 ml.

*Bolus 2–5 units IV when rate increased.

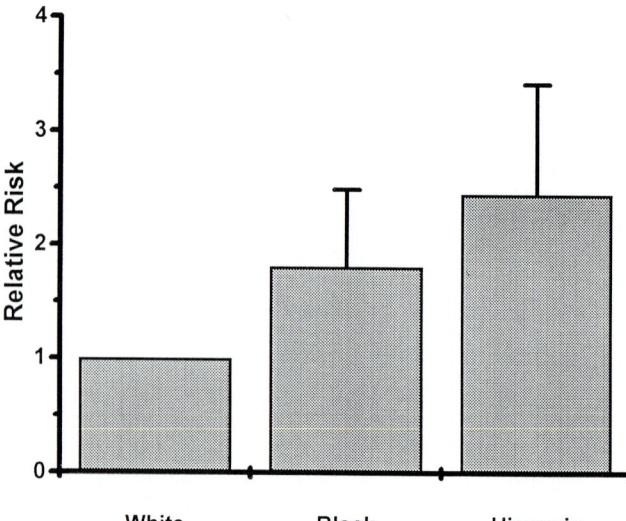

FIGURE 54–11. Relative risk of gestational diabetes. Adjusted for maternal age and pre-pregnant body weight. Error bars denote the 95 per cent confidence interval, compared to white race. (Adapted from Dooley et al: The influence of demographic and phenotypic heterogeneity on the prevalence of gestational diabetes mellitus. Int J Gynecol Obstet 35:13, 1991.)

Table 54—25. Prevalence of Neonatal Complications in GDM Pregnancy (Per Cent)

COMPLICATION	GESTATIONAL DIABETES N = 878	NORMALS N = 380
Macrosomia	17.9 **	5.6
Hyperbilirubinemia	16.5 **	8.2
Polycythemia	13.3 **	4.9
Hypocalcemia	5.5	2.7
Hypoglycemia	5.1	0.9
Hyaline membrane disease	1.3	1.4

**P <.05
Adapted from Hod et al: Prevalence of congenital anomalies and neonatal complications in the offspring of diabetic mothers in Israel. Isr J Med Sci 27:498, 1991.

strated a 4.5 per cent incidence among Hispanic patients in California, compared to 1.5 per cent in Caucasians. Dooley et al. (1991) studied women in the Midwest and found an overall prevalence of GDM of 3.5 per cent, with a significantly increased relative risk among Black, Hispanic, and Asian women (Fig. 54–11). Advanced maternal age and obesity are also strong cofactors in the risk for developing glucose intolerance during pregnancy (Coustan et al., 1989).

Although the maternal morbidity associated with gestational diabetic pregnancy is less severe and less frequent than that experienced by type I patients, there is no less risk of fetal macrosomia, birth trauma, neonatal hypoglycemia, or morbidity (Table 54–25). Prospective studies have demonstrated that women with GDM have a higher than normal perinatal mortality rate (O'Sullivan et al., 1974) and morbidity rate (O'Sullivan et al., 1973; Gabbe et al., 1977a). There is, however, no increased risk of congenital malformations (Cousins, 1991).

Do these considerations justify administering a glucose tolerance test to every pregnant woman, and is the procedure cost effective? If so, which tests are the most practical and valuable?

Screening and Diagnostic Measures. The Landon survey (1990) indicated that 90 per cent of perinatologists screen all pregnant women at 24 to 28 weeks, but only 75 per cent of board-certified obstetricians do so. The remainder screen only women with "risk factors" for GDM (Table 54–26). However, O'Sullivan and colleagues (1973) found the incidence of GDM to be no higher in a group of patients with risk factors than in the whole of their antenatal population. Lavin and co-workers (1981) conducted screening tests in 2077 pregnant women. The number of cases of GDM detected was similar in women who had clinical risk factors (1.5 per cent) and those who did not (1.4

per cent). However, since only 25 per cent of pregnant women have recognizable risk factors for GDM, restricting screening to the "risk" population would have overlooked approximately 75 per cent of patients with gestational glucose intolerance. These studies are persuasive arguments for evaluation of glucose tolerance in all pregnant women.

A continuing controversy revolves around the laboratory procedures used to screen patients for GDM. A screening test should be diagnostically accurate, cost effective, and acceptable to the patient. Two major diagnostic protocols are advocated at present: a single 75-gm 2-hour test (World Health Organization, 1980) and the two-step system recommended by the National Diabetes Data Group (1979) involving a 50-gm 1-hour challenge and 100-gm 3-hour oral glucose tolerance test for those with an abnormal glucose response challenge. The WHO testing scheme has the advantages of a single set of criteria for the diagnosis of adult diabetes during or outside of pregnancy and widespread use throughout the world. A disadvantage of the WHO criteria is that three times as many patients are identified as having impairment of glucose tolerance during pregnancy as when the NDDG methods are used. In epidemiologic studies, WHO criteria are most often used for diagnosis of diabetes in both pregnant and nonpregnant subjects. Until the differences in the criteria for diagnosis and methods for measurement of glucose values can be reconciled, accurate information will be unavailable on the inci-

Table 54—26. Risk Factors for Gestational Diabetes

Patients with any of these factors should be screened for GDM at the first prenatal visit:
1. Maternal age >25 years
2. Previous macrosomic infant
3. Previous unexplained fetal demise
4. Previous pregnancy with GDM
5. Strong immediate family history of NIDDM or GDM
6. Obesity (>90 kg)
7. Fasting glucose >140 mg/dl (7.8 mM) or random glucose >200 mg/dl (11.1 mM)

TABLE 54–27. WHO Diagnostic Criteria for Diabetes Mellitus (Venous Plasma Glucose)

DIAGNOSIS	FASTING	2 HOUR
Normal	<140 mg/dl (<7.8 mM)	<200 mg/dl (<11.1 mM)
Impaired glucose tolerance	<140 mg/dl (<7.8 mM)	>140 mg/dl and 200 mg/dl (≥7.8 and <11 mM)
Diabetes	≥140 mg/dl (>7.8 mM)	≥140 mg/dl (>11.1 mM)

Note: For diagnosis of NIDDM after pregnancy, the NDDG requires a 1-hour value >200 mg/dl in addition to abnormal fasting and 2-hour values.

TABLE 54–28. Diagnostic Criteria for Gestational Diabetes (100-Gram 3-Hour Glucose Tolerance Test)

Test prerequisites
1. 1-hour 50-gram glucose challenge result ≥140 mg/dl
2. Overnight fast of 8–14 hours
3. Unrestricted diet and activity for 3 days including ≥150 gm carbohydrate
4. Seated, not smoking during test

Diagnosis of gestational diabetes: two or more values must be met or exceeded

	Venous Plasma
Fasting	105 mg/dl
1 hour	190 mg/dl
2 hour	165 mg/dl
3 hour	145 mg/dl

From Metzger B and the Organizing Committee: Diabetes **40** (Suppl 2):197–201, 1991. Copyright © 1991 by the American Diabetes Association, Inc.

dence and management of pregnancy-evoked hyperglycemia and maternal and fetal outcome in these patients. Table 54–27 shows the WHO criteria for the diagnosis of diabetes mellitus.

The Third International Workshop-Conference on Gestational Diabetes Mellitus (1991) has recommended continued use of the two-stage screening/diagnosis system first proposed by O'Sullivan and Mahan (1964). A 50-gm oral glucose challenge test is the preferred screening test because it takes less time and is better tolerated than the more specific 3-hour oral glucose tolerance test. The patient need not be fasting. Indeed, Coustan et al. (1986) have shown that tests performed in fasting subjects are more likely to be falsely elevated than tests conducted shortly after a meal. Of patients screened with the 50-gram glucose challenge, approximately 3 to 5 per cent will have a value above 140 mg/dl. Patients with a 1-hour plasma glucose value of >140 mg/100 ml should undergo a 3-hour 100-gm oral GTT.

The risk of GDM is directly related to the result of the 1-hour glucose challenge. Dooley et al. (1991) calculated the probability of GDM at various levels of glucose response (Fig. 54–12). These data show that, among non-Caucasian women, the risk of GDM with a 1-hour glucose value >200 mg/dl is >90 per cent. For Caucasians, approximately two-thirds will have GDM. For this reason, Coustan and Lewis (1978) have recommended that no further testing be ordered for those with 1-hour challenge responses above 200 mg/dl. Dooley et al. argue that most patients, especially Caucasians, should have definitive testing (100-

gram 3-hour GTT) before the diagnosis of GDM is made. Many clinicians omit the 3-hour GTT in these patients.

GLUCOSE TOLERANCE TESTING. In the United States, the current recommendations for detection of abnormal glucose tolerance during pregnancy are those published as the Proceedings of the Third International Workshop-Conference on Gestational Diabetes (1991). Measurements of glycosylated hemoglobin have not been shown to be sensitive diagnostic indicators for gestational diabetes.

The normal values for the 3-hour GTT are shown in Table 54–28. Abnormal glucose tolerance is defined as two or more venous blood glucose values more than two standard deviations above the mean. The workshop attendees did not think that capillary blood measurements using glucose oxidase–impregnated strips were accurate enough for diagnostic purposes. Nevertheless, because many clinics utilize these strips, the equivalent values using the Accu-chek bG II (Biodynamics, a Boehringer Mannheim Co., Indianapolis, IN) meter to determine capillary glucose values are shown (Weiner, 1987).

Management of Gestational Diabetes

DIET THERAPY. Treatment recommendations during pregnancy vary for patients with gestational diabetes (Table 54–29). Dietary modification with elimination

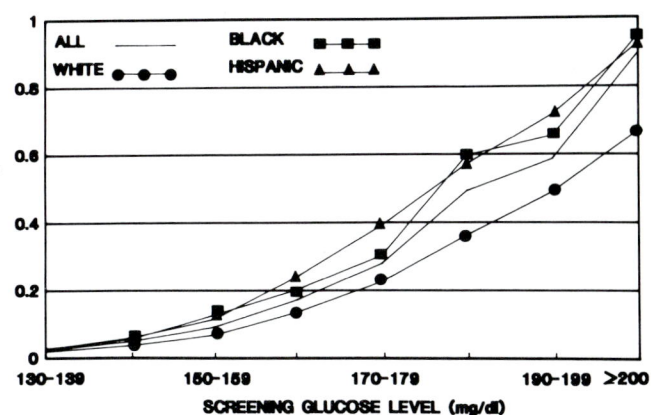

FIGURE 54–12. The risk of gestational diabetes at various levels of glucose response (mg/dl) one hour after a 50-gram glucose load. (From Dooley et al: The influence of demographic and phenotypic heterogeneity on the prevalence of gestational diabetes mellitus. Int J Gynecol Obstet **35**:13, 1991.)

of concentrated sweets and prevention of excessive weight gain constitute the usual and conservative approach. Diets for individual patients are devised from the dietary history, with attention focused on total calories and their distribution during the 24-hour day. The dietary history is useful in screening food intake for excessive sucrose; for example, unsweetened fruit juices and carbonated beverages (unless specified otherwise) have high sugar content. In GDM, dietary therapy alone as an initial approach to maintain plasma glucose in the range of 70 to 120 mg/dl is successful in approximately 90 per cent of patients. Insulin therapy is added when hyperglycemia is not controlled by a modified diet.

In women with GDM, many clinicians obtain a single HbA₁c level at first diagnosis. In patients with mildly elevated plasma glucose levels and normal concentrations of HbA₁c, dietary modifications alone and a modest increase in exercise are often sufficient to normalize plasma glucose levels. Conversely, patients with significantly elevated HbA₁c levels are more likely to have preexisting NIDDM, which was serendipitously discovered during pregnancy.

GLUCOSE MONITORING. The frequency and methods of glucose monitoring in GDM vary widely, even among experts in the field. Although weekly testing of fasting or postprandial glucose in the office or clinic was a standard for GDM patients in the past, abundant evidence now supports the efficacy of home self-glucose monitoring in improving glycemic control and reducing perinatal morbidity (Goldberg et al., 1986). Ideally, all patients with GDM should be lent a reflectance meter and taught the techniques of capillary glucose monitoring. The optimal range of glucose levels in GDM is the same as for IDDM and NIDDM (fasting <100 mg/dl, postprandial <140 mg/dl at 1 hour, <120 mg/dl at 2 hours). Patients who exceed these values consistently should be considered candidates for insulin therapy.

INSULIN THERAPY. The use of insulin in gestational diabetes remains controversial. Gyves and co-workers (1980) treated GDM primarily by dietary management. Insulin was prescribed for patients in whom the 2-hour postprandial blood glucose level exceeded 120 mg/100 ml (15 per cent of patients). These and other studies have shown that therapeutic interventions in GDM reduce perinatal mortality rate to within the range of the general population but may not prevent

macrosomia (Gabbe et al., 1977a; Gabbe, 1980; Hoet, 1980). This may be because GDM is often diagnosed after macrosomia is already apparent. There are no reports in the literature of reversible macrosomia or even a reduction in fetal growth velocity in response to treatment with diet or insulin.

Landon's survey of perinatologists (1990) indicates that most utilize the criteria of persistent abnormal fasting blood sugar or elevated postprandial levels (>120 mg/dl) as an indication for initiation of insulin. However, the persistent demonstration of 15 to 45 per cent macrosomia rates even in "well-controlled" GDM pregnancy has led some investigators to consider routine prophylactic insulin therapy in all GDM patients. Coustan and Lewis (1978) randomized 72 patients with gestational diabetes to treatment with insulin (20 U NPH and 10 U regular) plus diabetic diet, diet alone, or neither. They found that only 7 per cent of patients treated with diet and insulin had infants weighing more than 8.5 lb. This was in contrast to 36.4 per cent of mothers who received only dietary therapy and 50 per cent of untreated mothers who had large infants. O'Sullivan (1975) has also shown that treatment of gestational diabetes with insulin normalizes infant birth weight, in contrast to the outcome of babies whose mothers were treated with diet alone.

The insulin regimen should be devised to minimize postprandial glycemic overshoots since most patients have relatively normal pre-meal blood sugar levels. Use of long- or intermediate-acting insulin does not provide this type of control. For this reason, many clinicians utilize doses of regular insulin prior to each major meal, and add NPH at bedtime for the occasional patient with abnormal morning fasting glucose levels.

The first step in devising an individualized insulin regimen is to develop a 24-hour blood sugar profile on the patient's accustomed diet and activity in her home or workplace. If insulin is begun while the patient is hospitalized, the insulin prescription will have to be extensively revised after the patient is discharged. Capillary glucose levels should be obtained pre- and postprandially and at bedtime for several days prior to starting insulin.

Next, the postprandial capillary blood sugars should be reviewed and regular insulin given prior to all major meals when blood sugars are persistently >120 mg/dl (6.6 mM). Because of the relatively increased insulin resistance in the morning, a typical starting regimen is 8 units regular human insulin prior to breakfast and 6 units prior to lunch and dinner. Finally, if the AM fasting glucose levels are above 105 mg/dl (5.83 mM), NPH or Lente insulin should be administered at bedtime. A starting dose of 2 U is typical. Patients who are obese will require substantially higher doses of insulin than lean patients.

An alternative to this regime is a combination of NPH and regular insulin in the AM, with NPH added at bedtime if fasting glucose levels are elevated. While this method has the advantage of only 1 or 2 insulin injections daily, it does not focus on controlling the postprandial glucose responses to feeding, which are presently believed to be the principal mediator of macrosomia (Jovanovic-Peterson et al., 1991b).

TABLE 54–29. Treatment of the Woman with Gestational Carbohydrate Intolerance (GCI)

1. Dietary modification:
   a. Eliminate concentrated sweets (American Diabetes Association, 1979).
   b. Monitor caloric intake to prevent excessive weight gain (more than 25 lb).
2. Insulin administration: none or small doses of regular insulin before meals.*
3. Delivery at term.

*The use of insulin in mild GCI varies in different clinics. When 2-hour postprandial glucose values exceed 120 mg/100 ml, insulin administration is usually indicated.

After insulin is begun, telephone contact with the patient daily, then twice weekly in addition to clinic visits, is crucial to ensure compliance. This practice allows a rapid increase in the insulin regimen with a goal of achieving euglycemia within 10 days.

MONITORING FETAL WELL-BEING. The optimal regimen for fetal heart rate surveillance in gestational diabetes is controversial. Although previous studies by Gabbe et al. (1977a) indicate that the stillbirth rate for gestational diabetic patients is similar to that for nondiabetic patients up to 40 weeks, most diabetes and pregnancy centers now employ antepartum fetal heart rate surveillance for gestational diabetics prior to 40 weeks. There is unanimous agreement that gestational diabetics should undergo non-stress testing twice weekly, or contraction stress testing once weekly, beginning at the expected date of confinement (EDC).

The data summarized earlier regarding the influence of hyperglycemia on fetal oxygenation suggests that fetal risk roughly parallels maternal glycemic control. The timing and intensity of antepartum surveillance should therefore be gauged against maternal metabolic state. Gestational diabetics requiring insulin should generally undergo the same testing regimen as type I and type II diabetics. A typical protocol involves fetal movement counting beginning at 28 weeks and non-stress tests on a weekly basis from 36 to 40 weeks.

INTRAPARTUM AND POSTPARTUM MANAGEMENT OF GDM. Intrapartum management of women with gestational diabetes is only a little different from that of normoglycemic pregnant women. Glucose-containing intravenous solutions should be avoided or minimized. The possibility of fetal macrosomia and shoulder dystocia should be considered. Ultrasonographic screening for estimated fetal weight and abdominal circumference can provide clues. A gestational diabetic woman with a suspected macrosomic infant should not be subjected to mid-pelvic delivery after a prolonged second stage of labor if the risk of significant fetal injury is to be avoided.

In the postpartum period, fasting and 2-hour after-breakfast glucose levels should be checked with a meter each day until discharge because it may not be clear until postpartum testing at a later date whether the patient has gestational diabetes or preexisting NIDDM.

GDM patients should be tested for persistent diabetes at the 6-week postpartum visit using the 75-gram 2-hour oral glucose tolerance test. The patient is then reclassified by NDDG or WHO criteria as: (1) normal, (2) impaired glucose tolerance, or (3) diabetes. Diabetic women should be referred to a diabetologist. Women who have normal or mildly impaired glucose tolerance should be informed of the significant risks of developing subsequent NIDDM.

RISK OF OVERT DIABETES FOLLOWING A GDM PREGNANCY. A follow-up study of women who exceeded the O'Sullivan and Mahan criteria in their 1964 study showed that 29 per cent became diabetic. The more abnormal the oral GTT result during pregnancy, the higher the risk of later diabetes. Women whose glucose value exceeded the mean by three standard deviations had a 60 per cent chance of becoming

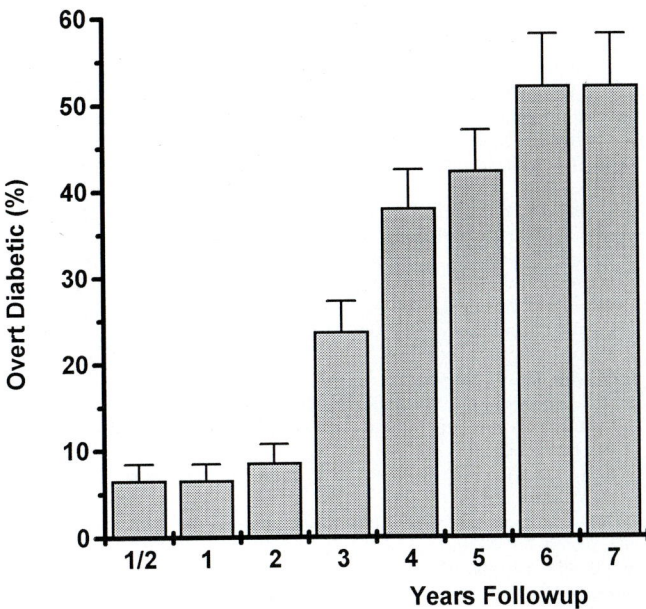

FIGURE 54–13. The incidence of overt diabetes following a pregnancy complicated by gestational diabetes. Error bars represent the standard error of the mean. (Adapted from O'Sullivan: Diabetes mellitus after GDM. Diabetes **40**:131, 1991. Copyright © 1991 by American Diabetes Association, Inc.)

diabetic in the 8-year follow-up period. The results of a more recent follow-up study reported by O'Sullivan (1991) are shown in Figure 54–13. Taking all patients with gestational diabetes as a whole, the risk of overt NIDDM within the next 5 years is approximately 50 per cent.

SUMMARY AND FUTURE DIRECTIONS

In summary, glucose intolerance during pregnancy poses significant risks for both mother and fetus. Consistently successful pregnancy outcomes require meticulous supervision of the pregnancy by a skilled and knowledgeable practitioner. The patient and her family must be motivated to dedicate virtually every minute of the gestational period to maximizing both the fetal and maternal metabolic milieu. With these principles in mind, the clinician should be able to promise most pregnant women with glucose intolerance an infant with intellectual and physical potential that differ little from those of an infant of a normal mother.

Future progress must be made in assisting women with overt, pre-pregnancy diabetes to achieve glycemic control sufficient to reduce the excess of congenital anomalies. Better understanding of fetal and maternal fuels should permit better dietary therapy and help to prevent the present 30 per cent rate of macrosomia in "diet controlled" gestational diabetics. Finally, progress in pancreatic transplantation and the immunology of diabetes may soon permit women with IDDM to regain normal insulin function and, in those with late-onset diabetes, correction of the inborn prediliction to glucose intolerance.

REFERENCES

Acker DB, Sachs BP, Friedman EA: Risk factors for shoulder dystocia in the average weight infant. Obstet Gynecol 67:614, 1986.

Airaksinen KEJ, Ikaheimo MJ, Salmela PI, et al: Impaired cardiac adjustment to pregnancy in Type I diabetes. Diabetes Care 9:376, 1986.

Alexander ES, Spitz HB, Clark RA. Sonography of polyhydramnios. Am J Roentgenol 138:343, 1982.

American College of Obstetricians and Gynecologists (ACOG): Technical Bulletin, Exercise during pregnancy and the postnatal period. Washington, DC, ACOG, 1985.

American Diabetes Association: Principles of nutrition and dietary recommendations for individuals with diabetes mellitus: 1979. Diabetes 28:1027, 1979.

Arky R, Wylie-Rose J, El-Beheri B: Examination of current dietary recommendations for individuals with diabetes mellitus. Diabetes Care 5:59, 1982.

Artal R, Wiswell RA: Exercise in pregnancy. Baltimore, Williams and Wilkins, 1986.

Banting FG, Best CH: The internal secretion of the pancreas. J Lab Clin Med 7:251, 1922.

Barrett AH, Stubbs SM, Mander AM: Management of premature labor in diabetic pregnancy. Diabetologia 18:365, 1980.

Battaglia FC, Lubchenco LO: A practical classification of newborn infants by weight and gestational age. J Pediatr 71:159, 1967.

Beall MH, Edgar BW, Paul RH: A comparison of ritodrine, terbutaline and magnesium sulfate for the suppression of preterm labor. Am J Obstet Gynecol 153:854, 1985.

Becerra JE, Khoury MJ, Cordero JF, et al: Diabetes mellitus during pregnancy and the risks for specific birth defects: a population based case-control study. Pediatrics 85:1, 1990.

Benson CB, Doubilet PM, Saltzman DH: Sonographic determination of fetal weights in diabetic pregnancies. Am J Obstet Gynecol 156:441, 1987.

Berkowitz GS, Kelsey JL, Holford TR, et al: Physical activity and the risk of spontaneous preterm delivery. J Reprod Med 28:581, 1983.

Bhaskar R, Chou MCY, Field JB: Time-reaction characteristics of regular and NPH insulin in insulin-treated diabetics. Diabetes 50:475, 1980.

Bhavnani BR, Enhorning G, Ekelund L, et al: Maternal diabetes and its effect on biochemical and functional development of rabbit fetal lung. Biochem Cell Biol 66:396, 1988.

Binder C, Lauritzer T, Faber O, et al: Insulin pharmacokinetics. Diabetes Care 7:188, 1984.

Botta M, Sinagra D, Donatelli M, et al: Evaluation of B-cell secretion and peripheral insulin resistance during pregnancy and after delivery in gestational diabetes mellitus with obesity. Acta Diabetol Lat 25:81, 1988.

Bourbon JR, Doucet E, Rieutort M, et al: Role of myo-inositol in impairment of fetal lung phosphatidylglycerol biosynthesis in the diabetic pregnancy: Physiological consequences of a phosphatidylglycerol deficient surfactant in the newborn rat. Exp Lung Res 11:195, 1986.

Bracero L, Schulman H, Fleischer A, et al: Umbilical artery velocimetry in diabetes and pregnancy. Obstet Gynecol 68:654, 1986.

Bracero LA, Baxi LV, Rey HR, et al: Use of ultrasound in antenatal diagnosis of large-for-gestational-age infants in diabetic gravid patients. Am J Obstet Gynecol 152:43, 1985.

Bradley RJ, Brudenell JM, Nicolaides KH: Fetal acidosis and hyperlacticaemia diagnosed by cordocentesis in pregnancies complicated by maternal diabetes mellitus. Diabet Med 8:464, 1991.

Brent RL, Beckman DA: Angiotensin-converting enzyme inhibitors, an embryopathic class of drugs with unique properties: Information for clinical teratology counsellors. Teratology 43:543, 1991.

Bressler R, Galloway JA: Insulin treatment of diabetes mellitus. Med Clin North Am 55:861, 1971.

Brillon DJ, Freidenberg GR, Henry RR, Olefsky JM: Mechanism of ineffective insulin-receptor kinase activity in NIDDM. Evidence for two receptor populations. Diabetes 38:397, 1989.

California Department of Health Services, Maternal and Child Health Branch. Status Report of the Sweet Success California Diabetes and Pregnancy Program 1986—1989. March 31, 1991.

Camps M, Guma A, Testar X, et al: Insulin resistance of skeletal muscle during pregnancy is not a consequence of intrinsic modifications of insulin receptor binding or kinase activities. Endocrinology. 127:2561, 1990.

Canadian Diabetes Association: Guidelines for the nutritional management of diabetes mellitus: 1980. J Can Dietet Assoc 42:110, 1981.

Caplan RH, Pagliara AS, Beguin EA, et al: Constant intravenous insulin infusion during labor and delivery in diabetes mellitus. Diabetes Care 5:6, 1982.

Carta Q, Meriggi E, Trossarelli GF, et al: Continuous subcutaneous insulin infusion versus intensive conventional insulin therapy in Type I and Type II diabetic pregnancy. Diabetes Metab 12:121, 1986.

Caruso A, Lanzone A, Bianchi V, et al: Continuous subcutaneous insulin infusion (CSII) in pregnant diabetic patients. Prenat Diagn 7:41, 1987.

Catalano PM, Tyzbir ED, Roman MM, et al: Longitudinal changes in insulin release and insulin resistance in nonobese pregnant women. Am J Obstet Gynecol 165:1667, 1991.

Chamberlain PF, Manning FA, Morrison I, et al: Ultrasound evaluation of amniotic fluid volume. II. The relationship of increased amniotic fluid volume to perinatal outcome. Am J Obstet Gynecol 150:250, 1984.

Chung CS, Myrianthopoulos NC: Factors affecting risks of congenital malformations. II. Effect of maternal diabetes. Birth Defects Series. Vol. XI, No. 10, 1975.

Churchill JA, Berendes HW, Nemore J: Neuropsychological deficits in children of diabetic mothers. Am J Obstet Gynecol 105:257, 1969.

Ciaraldi TP, Molina JM, Olefsky JM. Insulin action kinetics in adipocytes from obese and noninsulin-dependent diabetes mellitus subjects: identification of multiple cellular defects in glucose transport. J Clin Endocrinol Metab 72:876, 1991.

Cockroft DL, Coppolla PT. Teratogenic effects of excess glucose on head-fold rat embryos in culture. Teratology 16:141, 1977.

Coetzee EJ, Jackson WPU, Berman PA: Ketonuria in pregnancy—with special reference to calorie-restricted food intake in obese diabetics. Diabetes 29:177, 1980.

Cohen AW, Liston RM, Mennuti MT, et al: Glycemic control in pregnant diabetic women using a continuous subcutaneous insulin infusion pump. J Reprod Med 27:651, 1982.

Cohen D, Dodds R, Viberti G: Effect of protein restriction in insulin-dependent diabetics at risk of nephropathy. Br Med J 294:795, 1987.

Committee on Dietary Allowances, Food and Nutrition Board: Recommended Dietary Allowances. 9th ed. Washington DC, National Academy of Sciences, 1990.

Cooper MJ, Enderlein MA, Tarnoff H, et al: Asymmetric septal hypertrophy in infants of diabetic mothers: fetal echocardiography and the impact of maternal diabetic control. Am J Dis Child 146:226, 1992.

Cousins L: Pregnancy complications among diabetic women: Review. Obstet Gynecol Surv 42:140, 1987.

Cousins L: The California Diabetes and Pregnancy Programme: a statewide collaborative programme for the pre-conception and prenatal care of diabetic women. Balliere's Clin Obstet Gynecol 5:443, 1991.

Cousins L, Key TC, Schorzman L, et al: Ultrasonographic assessment of early fetal growth in insulin treated diabetic pregnancies. Am J Obstet Gynecol 159:1186, 1988.

Cousins L, Rigg L, Hollingsworth D, et al: The 24-hour excursion and diurnal rhythm of glucose, insulin and C peptide in normal pregnancy. Am J Obstet Gynecol 136:483, 1980.

Coustan DR, Berkowitz RL, Hobbins JC: Tight metabolic control of overt diabetes in pregnancy. Am J Med 68:845,1980.

Coustan DR, Lewis SB: Insulin therapy for gestational diabetes. Obstet Gynecol 51:306, 1978.

Coustan DR, Nelson C, Carpenter MW, et al: Maternal age and screening for gestational diabetes: a population-based study. Obstet Gynecol 73:557, 1989.

Coustan DR, Widness JA, Carpenter MW, et al: Should the 50 gram one-hour screening test for gestational diabetes be administered in the fasting or the fed state? Am J Obstet Gynecol 154:1031, 1986.

Craigin EB, Ryder GH: Obstetrics. A Practical Textbook for Students and Practitioners. Philadelphia, Lea & Febiger, 1916.

Crapo PA, Insel J, Sperling M, et al: Comparison of serum glucose, insulin and glucagon responses to different types of complex carbohydrate in non-insulin-dependent diabetic patients. Am J Clin Nutr 34:184, 1981.

Cruikshank DP, Pitkin RM, Reynolds WA, et al: Altered maternal calcium homeostasis in diabetic pregnancy. J Clin Endocrinol Metab 50:264, 1980.

Cudworth AG, Woodrow JC: HLA system and diabetes mellitus. Diabetes 24:245, 1975.

Cunningham MD, Desai NS, Thompson SA, et al: Amniotic fluid phosphatidylglycerol in diabetic pregnancy. Am J Obstet Gynecol 131:712, 1978.

Dahl-Jorgensen K: Near-normoglycemia and late diabetic complications. The Oslo Study. Acta Endocrinol 115(Suppl):1, 1986.

Dandona P, Besterman HS, Freedman DB, et al: Macrosomia despite well-controlled diabetic pregnancy. Letter Lancet i:737, 1984.

Davison JM: Renal transplantation in pregnancy. Am J Kidney Dis 9:374, 1987.

Deckert T, Feldt-Rasmussen B, Borch-Johnsen K, et al: Clinical assessment and prognosis of complications of diabetes. Transplant Proc 18:1636, 1986.

DeLee JB: The Principles and Practice of Obstetrics. 3rd ed. Philadelphia, WB Saunders Company, 1920.

Diabetic Retinopathy Study Research Group: Photocoagulation treatment of proliferate diabetic retinopathy. Clinical application of diabetic retinopathy study (DRS) findings. Report No. 8. Ophthalmology 88:583, 1982.

Diamond MP, Shah DM, Hester RA, et al: Complication of insulin-dependent diabetic pregnancies by pre-eclampsia and/or chronic hypertension: analysis of outcome. Am J Perinatol 2:263, 1985.

Dibble CM, Kochenour NK, Worley RJ, et al: Effect of pregnancy on diabetic retinopathy. Obstet Gynecol 59:699, 1982.

Dicker D, Feldberg D, Peleg D, et al: Pregnancy complicated by diabetic nephropathy. J Perinat Med 14:299, 1986.

Dicker D, Feldberg D, Samuel N, et al: Spontaneous abortion in patients with insulin dependent diabetes mellitus: the effect of preconceptional diabetic control. Am J Obstet Gynecol 158:1161, 1988.

Doberson MJ, Scharff JE, Ginsberg-Fellner F, et al: Cytotoxic auto-antibodies to beta cells in the serum of patients with insulin-dependent diabetes mellitus. N Engl J Med 303:1493, 1980.

Doery JCG, Healy D, Bishop S, et al: Fructosamine in gestational diabetes. Am J Obstet Gynecol 162:1635, 1990.

Dooley SL, Metzger BE, Cho N, et al: The influence of demographic and phenotypic heterogeneity on the prevalence of gestational diabetes mellitus. Int J Gynecol Obstet 35:13, 1991.

Drury MI, Stronge JM, Foley ME, et al: Pregnancy in the diabetic patient. Obstet Gynecol 62:279, 1983.

Dudley DK, Black DM: Reliability of lecithin/sphingomyelin ratios in diabetic pregnancy. Obstet Gynecol 66:521, 1985.

Duncan JM: On puerperal diabetes. Trans Obstet Soc Lond 24:256, 1882.

Duraiswami P: Insulin-induced skeletal anomalies in developing chickens. Br Med J 2:384, 1959.

Durak EP, Jovanovic-Peterson L, Peterson CM: Physical and glycemic responses of women with gestational diabetes to a moderately intense exercise program. Diabetes Educ 16:309, 1990a.

Durak EP, Jovanovic-Peterson L, Peterson CM: Comparative evaluation of uterine response to exercise on five aerobic machines. Am J Obstet Gynecol 162:754, 1990b.

Early LE, Gottschalk CW: Circulatory, metabolic and toxic effects on the kidney. In Early LW, Gottschalk CW (eds): Strauss and Welt's Diseases of the Kidney. 3rd ed. Boston, Little, Brown, 1979.

Edelberg ST, Dierker LR, Kalhan S, et al: Decreased fetal movements with sustained maternal hyperglycemia using the glucose clamp technique. Am J Obstet Gynecol 156:1101, 1987.

Elixhauser A, Weschler JM, Kitzmiller JL, et al: Financial implications of implementing standards of care for diabetes and pregnancy. Diabetes Care 15:22, 1992.

Elliott JP, Garite TJ, Freeman RK, et al: Ultrasonographic prediction of fetal macrosomia in diabetic patients. Obstet Gynecol 60:159, 1982.

Elliott JP: Magnesium sulfate as a tocolytic agent. Am J Obstet Gynecol 147:277, 1984.

Elman KD, Welch RA, Frank RN, et al: Diabetic retinopathy in pregnancy: a review. Obstet Gynecol 75:119, 1990.

Elphick MC, Filshie GM, Hull D: The passage of fat emulsion across the human placenta. Br J Obstet Gynaecol 85:610, 1978.

Eriksson UJ, Borg LAH, Forsberg H, et al: Diabetic embryopathy: studies with animal and in vitro models. Diabetes 40(Suppl):94, 1991.

Eriksson UJ, Lewis NJ, Freinkel N: Growth retardation during organogenesis in embryos of experimentally diabetic rats. Diabetes 33:281, 1984.

Faich GA, Fishbein HA, Ellis SE: Epidemiology of diabetic acidosis, a population-based study. Am J Epidemiol 117:551, 1983.

Fajans SS: Heterogeneity between various families with non–insulin-dependent diabetes of the MODY type. In Kobberling J, Tattersall R (ed): The Genetics of Diabetes Mellitus. Proceedings of The Serono Symposia. Vol 47. London, Academic Press, 1982.

Feldt-Rasmussen B, Mathiesen ER, Deckert T: Effect of two years of strict metabolic control on progression of incipient nephropathy in insulin-dependent diabetes. Lancet ii:1300, 1986b.

Feldt-Rasmussen B, Mathiesen ER, Hegedus L, et al: Kidney function during 12 months of strict metabolic control in insulin-dependent diabetic patients with incipient nephropathy. N Engl J Med 314:665, 1986a.

Ferguson JE, Dyson DC, Schutz T, et al: A comparison of tocolysis using nifedipine or ritodrine: analysis of efficacy and maternal, fetal and neonatal outcome. Am J Obstet Gynecol 163:105, 1990.

Ferroni KM, Gross TL, Sokol RJ, et al: What affects fetal pulmonary maturation during diabetic pregnancy? Am J Obstet Gynecol 150:270, 1984.

Frantz ID III, Epstein MF: Fetal lung development in pregnancies complicated by diabetes. In Merkatz IR, Adam PAJ (eds): The Diabetic Pregnancy: A Perinatal Perspective. New York, Grune & Stratton, 1979.

Freeman RK, Anderson G, Dorchester W: A prospective multi-institutional study of antepartum fetal heart rate monitoring. I. Risk of perinatal mortality and morbidity according to antepartum fetal heart rate results. Am J Obstet Gynecol 143:771, 1982.

Freinkel N: Effects of the conceptus on maternal metabolism during pregnancy. In Leibel BS, Wrenshall GA (eds): On the Nature and Treatment of Diabetes. Amsterdam, Excerpta Medica, 1964.

Freinkel N: Banting Lecture 1980: Of pregnancy and progeny. Diabetes 29:1023, 1980.

Freinkel N, Lewis NJ, Akazawa S: The honeybee syndrome—implications of the teratogenicity of mannose in rat-embryo culture. N Engl J Med 310:223, 1984.

Freinkel N, Metzger BE: Pregnancy as a tissue culture experience: The critical implications of maternal metabolism for fetal development. In Pregnancy Metabolism, Diabetes and the Fetus. CIBA Foundation Symposium 63 (new series). Amsterdam, Excerpta Medica, 1979.

Fuhrmann K, Reiher H, Semmler K, et al: Prevention of congenital malformations in infants of insulin-dependent diabetic mothers. Diabetes Care 6:219, 1983.

Gabbe SG: Effects of identifying a high-risk population. Diabetes Care 3:486, 1980.

Gabbe SG: Diabetes mellitus in pregnancy: Have all the problems been solved? Am J Med 70:613, 1981.

Gabbe SG: A story of two miracles: the impact of the discovery of insulin on pregnancy in women with diabetes mellitus. Obstet Gynecol 79:295, 1992.

Gabbe SG, Mestman JH, Freeman RK, et al: Management and outcome of diabetes mellitus. Am J Obstet Gynecol 127:465, 1977a.

Gabbe SG, Mestman JH, Freeman RK, et al: Management and outcome of diabetes mellitus, classes B to R. Am J Obstet Gynecol 129:723m 1977b.

Galler M, Spinowitz B, Charytan C, et al: Reproductive function in dialysis patients: CAPD vs hemodialysis. Perit Dial Bull 3:30S, 1983.

Galloway JA, Spradlin CT, Nelson RL, et al: Insulin concentration and blood glucose responses after injections of regular insulin and various insulin mixtures. Diabetes Care 4:366, 1981.

Gant NF, Madden JD, Siiteri PK, et al: The metabolic clearance rate of dehydroisoandrosterone sulfate. III. The effect of thiazide diuretics in normal and future pre-eclamptic pregnancies. Am J Obstet Gynecol **123**:159, 1975.

Gardner DF, Wilson HK, Podet EJ, et al: Prolonged action of regular insulin in diabetic patients: Lack of relationship to circulating insulin antibodies. J Clin Endocrinol Metab **62**:621, 1986.

Gerke E, Meyer-Schwiekerath G: Proliferative diabetische retinopathie und schwangerschaft. Klin Mbl Augenkeilkd **181**:170, 1982.

Gestation and Diabetes in France Study Group: Multicenter survey of diabetic pregnancy in France. Diabetes Care **14**:994, 1991.

Ginsberg H, Kimmerling G, Olefsky JM, et al: Demonstration of insulin resistance in untreated adult onset diabetic subjects with fasting hyperglycemia. J Clin Invest **55**:454, 1975.

Goldberg RB: Lipid disorders in diabetes. Diabetes Care **4**:561, 1982.

Goldberg JD, Franklin B, Lasser D, et al: Gestational diabetes: impact of home glucose monitoring on neonatal birth weight. Am J Obstet Gynecol **154**:546, 1986.

Golde SH, Good-Anderson B, Nontoro M, et al: Insulin requirements during labor: A reappraisal. Am J Obstet Gynecol **144**:556, 1982.

Golde SH, Montoro M, Good-Anderson B, et al: The role of NST, fetal biophysical profile and CST in the outpatient management of insulin-requiring diabetic pregnancies. Am J Obstet Gynecol **148**:269, 1984.

Gomez KJ, Dowdy K, Allen G, et al: Evaluation of ultrasound diagnosis of fetal anomalies in women with pregestational diabetes: University of Florida experience. Am J Obstet Gynecol **159**:584, 1988.

Grenfell A, Brudenell JM, Doddridge MC, et al: Pregnancy in diabetic women who have proteinuria. Quart J Med (New series 59) **228**:379, 1986.

Gross SJ, Shime J, Farine D: Shoulder dystocia: predictors and outcome. A five year review. Am J Obstet Gynecol **156**:334, 1987.

Gutgesell HP, Mullins CE, Gillette PC, et al: Transient hypertrophic subaortic stenosis in infants of diabetic mothers. J Pediatr **89**:120, 1976.

Gyves MT, Rodman HM, Littlke AB, et al: A modern approach to management of pregnant diabetics: A two-year analysis of perinatal outcomes. Am J Obstet Gynecol **128**:606, 1977.

Gyves MT, Schulman PK, Merkatz IR: Results of individualized intervention of gestational diabetes. Diabetes Care **3**:495, 1980.

Haakens K, Hanssen KF, Dahl-Jorgensen K, et al: Continuous subcutaneous insulin infusion (CSII), multiple injections (MI) and conventional insulin therapy (CT) in self-selecting insulin-dependent diabetic patients. J Intern Med **228**:457, 1990.

Hadlock FP, Deter RL, Harrist RB, et al: A date independent predictor of intrauterine growth retardation: femur length/abdominal circumference ratio. Am J Roentgenol **141**:979, 1982.

Hare JW and White P: Gestational diabetes and the White classification. Diabetes Care **3**:394, 1980.

Hayslett JP, Reece EA: Effect of diabetic nephropathy on pregnancy. Am J Kidney Dis **9**:344, 1987.

Hertz RH, King KC, Kalhan SC: Management of third-trimester diabetic pregnancies with use of continuous subcutaneous insulin infusion therapy: Pilot study. Am J Obstet Gynecol **149**:256, 1984.

Hilsted J, Galbo H, Christensen NJ, et al: Hemodynamic changes during graded exercise in patients with diabetic autonomic neuropathy. Diabetologia **22**:318, 1982.

Hod M, Merlob P, Friedman S, et al: Prevalence of congenital anomalies and neonatal complications in the offspring of diabetic mothers in Israel. Isr J Med Sci **27**:498, 1991.

Hoet JJ: Effect of intervention in gestational diabetes. Diabetes Care **3**:497, 1980.

Hollander DI, Nagey D'A, Pupkin MJ: Magnesium sulfate and ritodrine hydrochloride: A randomized comparison. Am J Obstet Gynecol **156**:631, 1987.

Hollingsworth DR: Maternal metabolism in normal pregnancy and pregnancy complicated by diabetes mellitus. Clin Obstet Gynecol **28**:457, 1985.

Hollingsworth DR, Moore TR: Postparandial walking exercise in pregnant insulin-dependent Type I diabetic women. Reduction of plasma lipid levels but absence of a significant effect on glycemic control. Am J Obstet Gynecol **157**:1359, 1987.

Hollingsworth DR, Vaucher Y, Yamamoto TR: Diabetes in pregnancy in Mexican Americans. Diabetes Care. **14**:695, 1991.

Horton WE Jr, Sadler TW: Effects of maternal diabetes on early embryogenesis: alterations in morphogenesis produced by the ketone body, B-hydroxybutyrate. Diabetes **32**:610, 1983.

Horvat M, Maclean H, Goldberg L, et al: Diabetic retinopathy in pregnancy: A 12-year prospective survey. Br J Ophthalmol **64**:398, 1980.

Hughes AB: Fetal heart rate changes during diabetic ketosis. Acta Obstet Gynecol Scand **66**:71, 1987.

Hytten FE: Nutrition in pregnancy. Postgrad Med J **55**:295, 1979.

Ishimatsu J, Yoshimura O, Manabe A, et al: Umbilical artery blood flow velocity waveforms in pregnancy complicated by diabetes mellitus. Arch Gynecol Obstet **248**:123, 1991.

Jenkins DJA, Wolever TMS, Taylor RH, et al:. Glycemic index of foods: a physiological basis for carbohydrate exchange. Am J Clin Nutr **34**:362, 1981.

Jennings AM, Lewis KS, Murdoch S, et al: Randomized trial comparing continuous subcutaneous insulin infusion and conventional insulin therapy in type II diabetic patients poorly controlled with sulfonylureas. Diabetes Care **14**:73, 1991.

Jenson AB, Rosenberg HS, Notkins AL: Pancreatic islet cell damage in children with fatal viral infections. Lancet **2**:354, 1980.

Johnson TR, Korenz RP, Menon KMJ, et al: Successful outcome of a pregnancy requiring dialysis. J Reprod Med **22**:217, 1979.

Johnstone FD, Nasrat AA, Prescott RJ: The effect of established and gestational diabetes on pregnancy outcome. Br J Obstet Gynecol **97**:1009, 1990.

Johnstone FD, Steel JM, Haddad NG, et al: Doppler umbilical artery flow velocity waveforms in diabetic pregnancy. Br J Obstet Gynecol **99**:135, 1992.

Jorge CS, Artal R, Paul RH, et al: Antepartum fetal surveillance in diabetic patients. Am J Obstet Gynecol **141**:641, 1981.

Joslin EP: The Treatment of Diabetes Mellitus; With Observations Upon the Disease Based Upon One Thousand Cases. Philadelphia, Lea & Febiger, 1916.

Jovanovic L, Druzin M, Peterson CM: Effect of euglycemia on the outcome of pregnancy in insulin-dependent diabetic women as compared with normal control subjects. Am J Med **71**:921, 1981.

Jovanovic R, Jovanovic L: Obstetric management when normoglycemia is maintained in diabetic pregnant women with vascular compromise. Am J Obstet Gynecol **149**:617, 1984.

Jovanovic L, Peterson CM: Insulin and glucose requirements during the first stage of labor in insulin-dependent diabetic women. Am J Med **74**:607, 1983.

Jovanovic L, Peterson CM, Saxena BB, et al: Feasibility of maintaining normal glucose profiles in insulin-dependent pregnant diabetic women. Am J Med **68**:105, 1980.

Jovanovic-Peterson L, Peterson CM: Is exercise safe or useful for gestational diabetic women? Diabetes **40**:179, 1991a.

Jovanovic-Peterson L, Peterson CM, Reed GF, et al: Maternal postprandial glucose levels and infant birth weight: the Diabetes in Early Pregnancy Study. The National Institute of Child Health and Human Development—Diabetes in Early Pregnancy Study. Am J Obstet Gynecol **164**:103, 1991b.

Kalkhoff RK, Kissebah AH, Kim H-K: Carbohydrate and lipid metabolism during normal pregnancy: Relationship to gestational hormone action. Semin Perinatol **2**:291, 1978.

Kalter H: Diabetes and spontaneous abortion: A historical review. Am J Obstet Gynecol **156**:1243, 1987.

Kalter H, Warkany J: Experimental production of congenital malformations in mammals by metabolic procedure. Physiol Rev **39**:69, 1959.

Kariniemi V, Forss M, Siegberg R, et al: Reduced short term variability of fetal heart rate in association with maternal hyperglycemia during pregnancy in insulin dependent diabetic women. Am J Obstet Gynecol **147**:793, 1983.

Karlson K, Kjellmer I: The outcome of diabetic pregnancies in relation to the mother's blood sugar level. Am J Obstet Gynecol **112**:213, 1972.

Katz M, Newman RB, Gill PJ: Assessment of uterine activity in ambulatory patients at high risk of preterm labor and delivery. Am J Obstet Gynecol **154**:44, 1986.

Keegan KA, Paul RH: Antepartum fetal heart rate testing. IV. The nonstress test as a primary approach. Am J Obstet Gynecol **136**:75, 1980.

Key TC, Giuffrida R, Moore TR: Predictive value of early pregnancy glycohemoglobin in the insulin-treated diabetic patient. Am J Obstet Gynecol **156**:1096, 1987.

King JF, Keirse JNC, Grant A, et al: Tocolysis—The case for and against. *In* Beard RW, Sharp F (eds): Preterm Labour And Its Consequences. London, Royal College of Obstetricians and Gynaecologists, 1985, p. 199.

Kitzmiller JL, Cloherty JP, Younger MD, et al: Diabetic pregnancy and perinatal morbidity. Am J Obstet Gynecol **131**:560, 1978.

Kitzmiller JL, Gavin LA, Gin GD, et al: Preconception care of diabetes. Glycemic control prevents congenital anomalies. JAMA **265**:731, 1991.

Kjos SL, Walther FJ, Montoro M, et al: Prevalence and etiology of respiratory distress in infants of diabetic mothers: predictive value of fetal lung maturation tests. Am J Obstet Gynecol **163**:898, 1990.

Klein R: The epidemiology of diabetic retinopathy: findings from the Wisconsin Epidemiologic Study of Diabetic Retinopathy. Int Ophthalmol Clin **27**:230, 1987.

Klein R, Klein BE, Moss SE, et al: The Wisconsin epidemiologic study of diabetic retinopathy. II. Prevalence and risk of diabetic retinopathy when age at diagnosis is less than 30 years. Arch Ophthalmol **102**:520, 1984.

Kleinman JC: Maternal weight gain during pregnancy: determinants and consequences. NCHS Working Paper Series No. 33. National Center for Health Statistics, Public Health Service, U.S. Department of Health and Human Services, Hyattsville, MD, 1990.

Knight G, Worth RC, Ward JD: Macrosomy despite a well-controlled diabetic pregnancy. Lancet **2**:1431, 1983.

Knopp RH, Warth MR, Charles D, et al: Lipoprotein metabolism in pregnancy, fat transport to the fetus and the effects of diabetes. Biol Neonate **50**:297, 1986.

Kolterman OG, Gray RS, Griffin J, et al: Receptor and post receptor defects contribute to the insulin resistance in non-insulin-resistant diabetes mellitus. J Clin Invest **68**:957, 1981.

Kroc Collaborative Study Group. Diabetic retinopathy after two years of intensified insulin treatment; followup of the Kroc Collaborative Study. JAMA **260**:37, 1988.

Kucera V: Rate and type of congenital anomalies among offspring of diabetic women. J Reprod Med **7**:61, 1971.

Kuhl C: Insulin secretion and insulin resistance in pregnancy and GDM. Implications for diagnosis and management. Diabetes **40**:18, 1991.

Kulovich MV, Gluck L: The lung profile. II. Complicated pregnancy. Am J Obstet Gynecol 136:64, 1979.

Kulovich MV, Hallman MB, Gluck L: The lung profile. I. Normal pregnancy. Am J Obstet Gynecol **135**:57, 1979.

Kupin WL, Cortes P, Dumler F, et al: Effect on renal function of change from high to moderate protein intake in Type I diabetic patients. Diabetes **36**:73, 1987.

Kurjak A, Kirkinen P, Latin V, et al: Ultrasonographic assessment of fetal kidney function in normal and complicated pregnancies. Am J Obstet Gynecol **141**:266, 1981.

Laatikainen L, Teramo K, Hieta-Heikurainen, et al: A controlled study of the influence of continuous subcutaneous insulin infusion treatment on diabetic retinopathy during pregnancy. Acta Med Scand **221**:367, 1987.

Landon MB, Gabbe SG: Glucose monitoring and insulin administration in the pregnant diabetic patient. Clin Obstet Gynecol **28**:496, 1985.

Landon MB, Gabbe SG, Bruner JP, et al: Doppler umbilical artery velocimetry in pregnancy complicated by insulin-dependent diabetes mellitus. Obstet Gynecol **73**:961, 1989a.

Landon MB, Gabbe SG, Piana R, et al: Neonatal morbidity in pregnancy complicated by diabetes mellitus: Predictive value of maternal glycemic profiles. Am J Obstet Gynecol **156**:1089, 1987.

Landon MB, Gabbe SG, Sachs L: Management of diabetes mellitus and pregnancy: a survey of obstetricians and maternal-fetal specialists. Obstet Gynecol. **75**:635, 1990.

Landon MB, Mintz MC, Gabbe SG: Sonographic evaluation of fetal abdominal growth: predictor of the large for gestational age infant in pregnancies complicated by diabetes mellitus. Am J Obstet Gynecol **160**:115, 1989b.

Lassman-Vague V, Thiers D: Maternal and fetal prognosis during pregnancy in diabetic women. Diabete Metab **16**:149, 1990.

Lavin JP, Barden TP, Miodovnik M: Clinical experience with a screening program for gestational diabetes. Am J Gynecol **141**:491, 1981.

Lavin JP, Lovelace DR, Miodovnik M, et al: Clinical experience with

one hundred seven diabetic pregnancies. Am J Obstet Gynecol **147**:742, 1983.

Leslie RDG, Pyke DA, John PN, et al: Hemoglobin A1c in diabetic pregnancy. Lancet **ii**:958, 1978.

Leucht W, Rabe D, Hendrik HJ, et al: Sonographic evaluation of the amount of amniotic fluid. I. Polyhydramnios—significance for the course of pregnancy and labor. Geburtshilfe Frauenheilkd **46**:157, 1986.

Lewis NJ, Akazawa S, Freinkel N: Teratogenesis from beta hydroxybutyrate during organogenesis in rat embryo organ culture and enhancement by subteratogenic glucose. (Abstract) Diabetes **32**(Suppl):11a, 1983.

Liggins GC, Howie RN: A controlled trial of antepartum glucocorticoid treatment for the prevention of the respiratory distress syndrome in premature infants. Pediatrics **50**:515, 1972.

Lindheimer MD, Katz AI: Kidney disease. *In* Lindheimer MD, Katz AI (eds): Kidney Function and Disease in Pregnancy. Philadelphia, Lea & Febiger, 1977.

Lucas MJ, Leveno KJ, Williams ML, et al: Early pregnancy glycosylated hemoglobin, severity of diabetes, and fetal malformations. Am J Obstet Gynecol **161**:426, 1989.

Mace S, Hirschfeld SS, Riggs T, et al: Echocardiographic abnormalities in infants of diabetic mothers. J Pediatr **95**:1013, 1979.

MacLaren NK, Henson V: The genetics of insulin-dependent diabetes. Growth, Genetics and Hormones **2**:1, 1986.

Main EK, Main DM, Gabbe SG: Factors predicting perinatal outcome in pregnancies complicated by diabetic nephropathy (Class F). Diabetes **33**:(Suppl 1):201, 1984.

Mari G, Moise KJ Jr, Deter RL, et al: Doppler assessment of the pulsatility of the middle cerebral artery during constriction of the fetal ductus arteriosus after indomethacin therapy. Am J Obstet Gynecol **161**:1528, 1989.

Marushak A, Weber T, Bock J, et al: Pregnancy following kidney transplantation. Acta Obstet Gynecol Scand **65**:557, 1986.

Mauer SM, Ellis EN, Bilous RW, et al: The pathology of diabetic nephropathy. Transplant Proc **18**:1629, 1986.

McDonald-Gibson RG, Young M, Hytten FE: Changes in plasma, nonesterified fatty acids and serum glycerol in pregnancy. Br J Obstet Gynaecol **82**:460, 1975.

Mecklenburg RS, Benson EA, Benson JW Jr, et al: Acute complications associated with insulin infusion pump therapy: Report of experience with 161 patients. JAMA **252**:3265, 1984.

Menon RK, Cohen RM, Sperling MA, et al: Transplacental passage of insulin in pregnant women with insulin-dependent diabetes mellitus. Its role in fetal macrosomia. N Engl J Med **323**:309, 1990.

Merkatz IR, Peter JB, Barden TP: Ritodrine hydrochloride. A betamimetic agent for use in preterm labor. II: Evidence of efficacy. Obstet Gynecol **56**:7, 1980.

Metzger BE, and the Organizing Committee. Summary and recommendations of the third international workshop—Conference on gestational diabetes mellitus. Diabetes **40**:197, 1991.

Miller E, Hare JW, Cloherty JP, et al: Elevated maternal HbA1c in early pregnancy and major congenital anomalies in infants of diabetic mothers. N Engl J Med **304**:1331, 1981.

Miller HC: The effect of diabetic and prediabetic pregnancies on the fetus and newborn infant. J Pediatr **29**:455, 1946.

Miller JM, Crenshaw C Jr, Welts I: Hemoglobin A1c in normal and diabetic pregnancy. JAMA **242**:2785, 1979.

Miller JM, Keane MWD, Horger EO III: A comparison of magnesium sulfate and terbutaline for the arrest of premature labor. J Reprod Med **27**:348, 1982.

Mills JL: Malformations in infants of diabetic mothers. Teratology **25**:385, 1982.

Mills JL, Baker L, Goldman AS: Malformations in infants of diabetic mothers occur before the seventh gestational week. Diabetes **28**:292, 1979.

Mills JL, Simpson JL, Driscoll SG, et al. Incidence of spontaneous abortion among normal women and insulin-dependent diabetic women whose pregnancies were identified within 21 days of conception. N Engl J Med **319**:1617, 1988.

Milner RGG: Amino acids and beta cell growth in structure and function. *In* Merkatz IR, Adam PAJ (eds): The Diabetic Pregnancy: A Perinatal Perspective. New York, Grune & Stratton, 1979.

Milunsky A, Alpert E, Kitzmiller JL, et al: Prenatal diagnosis of neural tube defects. VIII. The importance of serum alpha fetoprotein screening in diabetic pregnant women. Am J Obstet Gynecol 142:1030, 1982.

Mimouni F, Miodovnik M, Tsang RC, et al: Decreased maternal serum magnesium concentration and adverse fetal outcome in insulin dependent diabetic women. Obstet Gynecol 70:85, 1987.

Mintz DH, Skyler JS, Chez RA: Diabetes mellitus and pregnancy. Diabetes Care 1:49, 1978.

Miodovnik M, Lavin JP, Harrington DJ, et al: Cardiovascular and biochemical effects of infusion of beta hydroxybutyrate into the fetal lamb. Am J Obstet Gynecol 144:594, 1982.

Miodovnik M, Lavin JP, Knowles HC, et al: Spontaneous abortion among insulin-dependent diabetic women. Am J Obstet Gynecol. 150:372, 1984.

Miodovnik M, Mimouni F, Berk M, et al: Alloxan-induced diabetes mellitus in the pregnant ewe: metabolic and cardiovascular effects on the mother and her fetus. Am J Obstet Gynecol 160:1239, 1989.

Miodovnik M, Peros N, Holroyde JC, et al: Treatment of premature labor in insulin dependent diabetic women. Obstet Gynecol 65:621, 1985a.

Miodovnik M, Skillman C, Holroyde JC, et al: Elevated maternal glycohemoglobin in early pregnancy and spontaneous abortion among insulin-dependent diabetic women. Am J Obstet Gynecol 153:439, 1985b.

Mogensen CE, Christiansen CK: Predicting diabetic nephropathy in insulin-dependent patients. N Engl J Med 311:89, 1984.

Moloney JBM, Drury MI: The effect of pregnancy on the natural course of diabetic retinopathy. Am J Ophthalmol 93:745, 1982.

Molsted-Pedersen L, Pedersen JF: Congenital malformations in diabetic pregnancies. Clinical viewpoints. Acta Paediatr Scand 320(Suppl):79, 1985.

Moore TR, Cayle JE: The amniotic fluid index in normal human pregnancy. Am J Obstet Gynecol 162:1168, 1990.

Moore TR, Hollingsworth DR, Kolterman O, et al: Continuous subcutaneous insulin infusion in an obese insulin-resistant pregnant woman with Type II diabetes: Accelerated fetal growth and neonatal complications. Obstet Gynecol 70:480, 1987.

Moore TR, Key TC, Reisner LS, et al: Evaluation of the use of continuous lumbar epidural anesthesia for hypertensive pregnant women in labor. Am J Obstet Gynecol 152:85, 1985.

Moore TR, Piacquadio K: A prospective assessment of fetal movement screening to reduce fetal mortality. Am J Obstet Gynecol 160:1075, 1989.

Morriss GM, New DAT: Effect of oxygen concentration on mortphogenesis of cranial neural folds and neural crest in cultured rat embryos. J Embryol Exp Morphol 54:17, 1979.

Murphy J, Peters P, Morris TM, et al: Conservative management of pregnancy in diabetic women. Br Med J 288:1203, 1984.

Naeye RL: Weight gain and the outcome of pregnancy. Am J Obstet Gynecol 135:3, 1979.

National Academy Of Sciences, Subcommittee on Nutritional Status and Weight Gain During Pregnancy, Subcommittee on Dietary Intake and Nutrient Supplements During Pregnancy, Committee on Nutritional Status During Pregnancy and Lactation, Food and Nutrition Board, Institute of Medicine: Nutrition During Pregnancy. Part I, Weight Gain. Washington DC, National Academy Press, 1990.

National Diabetes Data Group: Classification and diagnosis of diabetes mellitus and other categories of glucose intolerance. Diabetes 28:1039, 1979.

Nerup J, Mandrup-Poulsen T, Molvig J: The HLA-IDDM association: Implications for etiology and pathogenesis of IDDM. Diabet Metab Rev 3:779, 1987.

Ney D, Hollingsworth DR, Cousins L: Decreased insulin requirement and improved control of diabetes in pregnant women given a high-carbohydrate, high-fiber, low-fat diet. Diabetes Care 5:529, 1982.

Niebyl JR, Blake DA, White RD, et al: The inhibition of premature labor with indomethacin. Am J Obstet Gynecol 136:114, 1980.

Nutrition Sub-Committee of the British Diabetic Association's Medical Advisory Committee: Dietary Recommendations for Diabetics for the 1980's. London, British Diabetic Association, 1982.

Nylund L, Lunell N-O, Lewander R, et al: Uteroplacental blood flow in diabetic pregnancy: Measurements with indium113m and a computer-linked gamma camera. Am J Obstet Gynecol 144:298, 1982.

O'Sullivan JB: Prospective study of gestational diabetes and its treatment. In Sutherland HW, Stowers JM (eds): Carbohydrate Metabolism in Pregnancy and the Newborn. Edinburgh, Churchill Livingstone, 1975.

O'Sullivan JB: Diabetes mellitus after GDM. Diabetes 40:131, 1991.

O'Sullivan JB, Mahan CM: Criteria for the oral glucose tolerance test in pregnancy. Diabetes 13:278, 1964.

O'Sullivan JB, Mahan CM, Charles D: Screening criteria for high-risk gestational diabetic patients. Am J Obstet Gynecol 116:895, 1973.

O'Sullivan JB, Mahan CM, Charles D, et al: Medical treatment of gestational diabetic. Obstet Gynecol 43:817, 1974.

Ogata ES, Sabbagha R, Metzger BE, et al: Serial ultrasonography to assess evolving fetal macrosomia. Studies in 23 pregnant diabetic women. JAMA 243:2405, 1980.

Oh W: Neonatal care and long-term outcome of infants of diabetic mothers. In Meskatz IR, Adam PAJ (eds): The Diabetic Pregnancy: A Perinatal Perspective. New York, Grune & Stratton, 1979.

Olefsky JM, Kolterman OG, Scarlett JA, et al: Insulin action and resistance in obesity and non-insulin dependent Type II diabetes mellitus. Am J Physiol 243:E15, 1982.

Olofsson P, Sjoberg NO, Solum T: Fetal surveillance in diabetic pregnancy. I. Predictive value of the nonstress test. Acta Obstet Gynecol Scand 65:241, 1986a.

Olofsson P, Sjoberg NO, Solum T: Fetal surveillance in diabetic pregnancy. II. The nonstress test versus the oxytocin challenge test. Acta Obstet Gynecol Scand 65:357, 1986b.

Palmer JP, Asplin CM, Clemons P, et al: Insulin antibodies in insulin-dependent diabetics before insulin treatment. Science 222:1337, 1983.

Pasi KJ, Toop MJ, Cockrill BL, et al: Serum fructosamine in diabetic pregnany. Diabete Metab. 15:151, 1989.

Pedersen J: Diabetes and pregnancy. Blood Sugar of Newborn Infants. Copenhagen, Danish Science, 1952.

Pedersen J: Hyperglycemia-Hyperinsulinism Theory and Birth Weight in the Pregnant Diabetic and Her Newborn. 2nd ed. Baltimore, Williams & Wilkins, 1977.

Pedersen JF, Mantoni M: The prognostic significance of fetal size in early diabetic (and normal?) pregnancy and in threatened abortion. Ultrasound Med Biol 6(Suppl 2):573, 1983.

Pedersen JF, Molsted Pedersen L, Lebech PE: Is the early growth delay in the diabetic pregnancy accompanied by a delay in placental development? Acta Obstet Gynecol Scand 65:675, 1986.

Peel J: A historical review of diabetes and pregnancy. J Obstet Gynecol Br Cwlth 79:385, 1972.

Peevy KJ, Landaw SA, Gross SJ: Hyperbilirubinemia in infants of diabetic mothers. Pediatrics 66:417, 1980.

Peiris AN, Gustafson AB: Review. Current therapeutic concepts in diabetic hypertension. Diabetes Care 9:409, 1986.

Perley M, Kipnis DM: Plasma insulin responses to glucose and tolbutamide of normal weight and obese diabetic and nondiabetic subjects. Diabetes 15:867, 1966.

Peterson CM, Jovanovic-Peterson L, Mills JL, et al: The Diabetes in Early Pregnancy Study: Changes in cholesterol, triglycerides, body weight, and blood pressure. The National Institute of Child Health and Human Development—The Diabetes in Early Pregnancy Study. Am J Obstet Gynecol 166:513, 1992.

Phelps RL, Metzger BE, Freinkel N: Carbohydrate metabolism in pregnancy, XVIII: Diurnal profiles of plasma glucose, insulin, free fatty acids, triglycerides, cholesterol and individual amino acids in late normal pregnancy. Am J Obstet Gynecol 140:730, 1981.

Phelps RL, Sakol P, Metzger BE, et al: Changes in diabetic retinopathy during pregnancy. Correlations with regulation of hyperglycemia. Arch Ophthalmol 104:1806, 1986.

Phillips AF, Rosenkrantz TS, Raye J: Consequences of perturbations of fetal fuels in ovine pregnancy. Diabetes 34(Suppl 2):32, 1985.

Pinter E, Peyman JA, Snow K, et al: Effects of maternal diabetes on fetal rat lung ion transport. Contribution of alveolar and bronchiolar epithelial cells to Na+,K(+) ATPase expression. J Clin Invest 87:821, 1991.

Pinter E, Reece EA, Leranth CS, et al: Yolk sac failure in embryopathy due to hyperglycemia. Ultrastructural analysis of yolk sac differentiation associated with embryopathy in rat conceptuses under hyperglycemic conditions. Teratology 33:73, 1986.

Pinter E, Reece EA, Leranth CZ, et al: Arachidonic acid prevents hyperglycemia-associated yolk sac damage and embryopathy. Am J Obstet Gynecol **155**:691, 1986.

Pitkin RM: Nutritional influences during pregnancy. Med Clin North Am **1**:3, 1977.

Pontiroli AE, Calderara A, Bonisolli L, et al: Genetic and metabolic risk factors for the development of microangiopathic complications of type I diabetes mellitus (DM). Transplant Proc **18**:1806, 1986.

Potter JM, Reckless JPD, Cullen DR: The effect of continuous subcutaneous insulin infusion and conventional insulin regimens on 24-hour variations of blood glucose and intermediary metabolism in the third trimester of diabetic pregnancy. Diabetologia **21**:534, 1981.

Proceedings of the Third International Workshop-Conference on Gestational Diabetes Mellitus. November 8–10, 1990, Chicago, IL. Diabetes **40**:1–201, 1991.

Puavilai G, Drobny EC, Domont LA, et al: Insulin receptors and insulin resistance in human pregnancy: Evidence for a post receptor defect in insulin action. J Clin Endocrinol Metab **54**:247, 1982.

Pyke DA: Diabetes: The genetic connections. Diabetologia **17**:333, 1979.

Reece EA, Egan JFX, Coustan DR, et al: Coronary artery disease in diabetic pregnancies. Am J Obstet Gynecol **154**:150, 1986.

Reece EA, Hagay Z, Hobbins JC. Insulin-dependent diabetes mellitus and immunogenetics: maternal and fetal considerations. Obset Gynecol Surv **46**:255, 1991.

Reece EA, Hobbins JC: Diabetic embryopathy: Pathogenesis, prenatal diagnosis and prevention. Obstet Gynecol Surv **41**:325, 1986.

Reece EA, Winn HN, Smikle C, et al: Sonographic assessment of growth of the fetal head in diabetic pregnancies compared with normal gestations. Am J Perinatol **7**:18, 1990a.

Reece EA, Winn HN, Hayslett JP, et al: Does pregnancy alter the rate of progression of diabetic nephropathy? Am J Perinatol **7**:193, 1990b.

Revers RR, Fink RI, Griffin J, et al: Influence of hyperglycemia on insulin's in vivo effects in Type II diabetes. J Clin Invest **73**:664, 1984.

Rigg L, Cousins L, Hollingsworth DR, et al: Effects of exogenous insulin on excursions and diurnal rhythm of plasma glucose in pregnant diabetic patients with and without residual β-cell function. Am J Obstet Gynecol **136**:537, 1980.

Rodgers BD, Rodgers DE: Clinical variables associated with diabetic ketoacidosis during pregnancy. J Reprod Med **36**:797, 1991.

Rosenn B, Miodovnik M, Combs CA, et al: Pre-conception management of insulin-dependent diabetes: improvement of pregnancy outcome. Obstet Gynecol **77**:846, 1991.

Rotter JI, Anderson CE, Rubin R, et al: HLA genotypic study of insulin-dependent diabetes. The excess of DR3/DR4 heterozygotes allows rejection of the recessive hypothesis. Diabetes **32**:169, 1983.

Rotter JI, Landaw EM: Measuring the genetic contribution of a single locus to multilocus disease. Clin Genet **26**:529, 1984.

Rotter JI, Rimoin DL: The genetics of diabetes. Hosp Pract **22**:79, 1987.

Roversi GD, Gargiulo M, Nicolini U, et al: Maximal tolerated insulin therapy in gestational diabetes. Diabetes Care **3**:489, 1980.

Rowland TW, Hubbell JP, Nadas AS: Congenital heart disease in infants of diabetic mothers. J Pediatr **83**:815, 1973.

Rudolf MCJ, Coustan DR, Sherwin RS, et al: Efficacy of the insulin pump in the home treatment of pregnant diabetics. Diabetes **30**:891, 1981.

Rust FP, Rust KJ, Williams RL: 1980-1984 Maternal and Child Health Data Base, Descriptive Narrative. California Department of Health Services, 1987.

Sadler TW: Effects of maternal diabetes on early embryogenesis. II. Hyperglycemia-induced exencephaly. Teratogenesis **21**:349, 1980.

Saibene V, Brembilla L, Bertoletti A, et al: Combined OGTT and glycosylated hemoglobin detection for carbohydrate intolerance diagnosis. Diabetologia **15**:267, 1978.

Sandmire HF, OHalloin TJ: Shoulder dystocia: its incidence and associated risk factors. Int J Gynaecol Obstet **26**:65, 1988.

Santiago JV, Davis JE, Fisher F: Hemoglobin A1c levels in a diabetes detection program. J Clin Endocrinol Metab **47**:578, 1978.

Scheffler RM, Feuchtbaum LB, Phibbs CS: Prevention: the cost-effectiveness of the California Diabetes and Pregnancy Program. Am J Public Health **82**:168, 1992.

Schulman PK, Gyves MT, Merkatz IR: Role of nutrition in the management of the pregnant diabetic patient. *In* Merkatz IR, Adam PAJ (eds): The Diabetic Pregnancy: A Perinatal Perspective. New York, Grune & Stratton, 1979.

Schwartz JB, Warburton D, Gordon LS: Neonatal cardiology case book. J Perinatol **6**:350, 1986.

Seller MJ: Nutritionally induced congenital defects. Proc Nutr Soc **46**:227, 1987.

Serup L: Influence of pregnancy on diabetic retinopathy. Acta Endocrinol **112**(Suppl 277):122, 1986.

Shambaugh GE III: Carbohydrate, fat and amino acid metabolism in the pregnant woman and fetus. *In* Falkner F, Tanner JM (eds): Human Growth, A Comprehensive Treatise. 2nd ed, Vol. 1. Development Biology and Prenatal Growth. New York, Plenum Press, 1986.

Shaul PW, Mimouni F, Tsang R, et al: The role of magnesium in neonatal calcium homeostasis: Effects of magnesium infusion on calciotropic hormones and calcium. Pediatr Res **22**:319, 1987.

Shepherd MJ, Richards VA, Berkowitz RL, et al: An evaluation of two equations for predicting fetal weight by ultrasound. Am J Obstet Gynecol **142**:47, 1982.

Sibai BM, Abdella TN, Anderson GD: Pregnancy outcome in 211 patients with mild chronic hypertension. Obstet Gynecol **61**:571, 1983.

Silfen SL, Wapner RJ, Gabbe SG: Maternal outcome in Class II diabetes mellitus. Obstet Gynecol **55**:749, 1980.

Silverman BL, Rizzo T, Green OC, et al: Long-term prospective evaluation of offspring of diabetic mothers. Diabetes **40**(Suppl 2):121, 1991.

Sinclair SH, Nesler C, Foxman B, et al: Macular edema and pregnancy in insulin-dependent diabetes. Am J Ophthalmol **97**:154, 1984.

Sivit CJ, Hill MC, Larsen JW, Lande IM: Second-trimester polyhydramnios: evaluation with US. Radiology **165**:467, 1987.

Skyler JS: Lesions from studies of insulin pharmacokinetics. Diabetes Care **9**:666, 1986.

Smithberg M, Runner MN: Teratogenic effects of hypoglycemic treatments in inbred strains of mice. Am J Anat **113**:479, 1963.

Srikanta S, Ganda OP, Rabizadeh A, et al: First-degree relatives of patients with type I diabetes: Islet-cell antibodies and abnormal insulin secretion. N Engl J Med **313**:461, 1985.

Steel RB, Mosley JD, Smith CH: Insulin and placenta: Degradation and stabilization, binding to microvillous membrane receptors, and amino acid uptake. Am J Obstet Gynecol **135**:408, 1977.

Stehbens JA, Baker GL, Kitchell M: Outcome at ages 1, 3 and 5 years of children born to diabetic women. Am J Obstet Gynecol **127**:408, 1977.

Stein Z, Susser M, Saenger G, et al: Famine and Human Development: The Dutch Hunger Winter of 1944–45. New York, Oxford University Press, 1975.

Steven J, Whitsett JA: Insulin binding to neonatal human, guinea pig and rat myocardial membranes. Pediatr Res **13**:482, 1979.

Styrud J, Eriksson UJ: In vitro effects of glucose and growth factors on limb bud and mandibular arch chondrocytes maintained at various serum conditions. Teratology **44**:65, 1991.

Suhonen L, Stenman UH, Koivisto V, et al: Correlation of HbA1C, glycated serum proteins and albumin, and fructosamine with the 24 h glucose profile of insulin dependent pregnant diabetics. Clin Chem **35**:922, 1989.

Susa JB, McCormick KL, Widness JA, et al: Chronic hyperinsulinemia in the fetal rhesus monkey. Effects of fetal growth and composition. Diabetes **25**:1058, 1979.

Sutherland HW, Pritchard CW: Increased incidence of spontaneous abortion in pregnancies complicated by maternal diabetes mellitus. Am J Obstet Gynecol **155**:135, 1986.

Tamura RK, Sabbagha RE, Dooley SL, et al: Real-time ultrasound estimations of weight in fetuses of diabetic gravid women. Am J Obstet Gynecol **153**:57, 1985.

Tamura RK, Sabbagha RE, Depp R, et al: Diabetic macrosomia: accuracy of third trimester ultrasound. Obstet Gynecol **67**:828, 1986.

Taylor PM, Wolfson JH, Bright NH, et al: Hyperbilirubinemia in infants of diabetic mothers. Biol Neonate **5**:289, 1963.

Teramo K, Ammala P, Ylinen K, et al: Pathologic fetal heart rate associated with poor metabolic control in diabetic pregnancies. Obstet Gynecol **61**:559, 1983.

Tevaarwerk GJM, Harding PGR, Milne KJ, et al: Pregnancy in diabetic women: Outcome with a program aimed at normoglycemia before meals. Can Med Assoc J **125**:435, 1981.

Thacker SB, Berkelman RL: Assessing the diagnostic accuracy and efficacy of selected antepartum fetal surveillance techniques. Obstet Gynecol Surv **41**:121, 1986.

Thomas CR, Lowy C, St Hillaire RJ, et al: Studies on the placental hydrolysis and transfer of lipids to the fetal guinea pig. In Miller RK, Thiede HA (eds): Fetal Nutrition, Metabolism and Immunology. The Role of the Placenta. New York, Plenum Press, 1984.

Thompson G: HLA-DR antigens and susceptibility to insulin-dependent diabetes mellitus. Am J Hum Genet **36**:1309, 1984.

Tillil H, Köbberling J: Age-corrected empirical genetic risk estimates for first-degree relatives of IDDM patients. Diabetes **36**:93, 1987.

Todd JA, Bell JI, McDevitt HO: HLA-DQ gene contributes to susceptibility and resistance to insulin-dependent diabetes mellitus. Nature **329**:599, 1987.

Todd JA, Bell JI, McDevitt HO: A molecular basis for genetic susceptibility to insulin-dependent diabetes mellitus. Trends Genet **4**:129, 1988.

Tsang RC, Brown DR, Steicher JJ: Diabetes and calcium: Calcium disturbances in infants of diabetic mothers. In Merkatz IR, Adam PAJ (eds): The Diabetic Pregnancy: A Perinatal Perspective. New York, Grune & Stratton, 1979.

Tsang RC, Strub R, Brown DR, et al: Hypomagnesemia in infants of diabetic mothers: Perinatal studies. J Pediatr **89**:115, 1976.

Tyden O, Berne C, Erikkson UJ, et al: Fetal maturation in strictly controlled diabetic pregnancy. Diabetes Res **1**:1314, 1984.

Ward DM: Hypertension, renal diseases and kidney transplantation. In Hollingsworth DR, Resnik R (eds): Medical Counseling Before Pregnancy. New York, Churchill Livingstone, 1988.

Warso MA, Lands WEM: Lipid peroxidation in relation to prostacyclin and thromboxane physiology and pathophysiology. Br Med Bull **39**:277, 1983.

Warth MR, Arky RA, Knopp RH: Lipid metabolism in pregnancy. III. Altered lipid composition in intermediate, very low, low, and high-density lipoprotein fractions. J Clin Endocrinol Metab **41**:649, 1975.

Watson DC, Bradley LM, Medgley FM, et al: Costs and results of cardiac operations in infants less than four months old: Are they worthwhile? J Thorac Cardiovasc Surg **91**:667, 1986.

Weiner CP, Faustich MW, Burns J, et al: Diagnosis of gestational diabetes by capillary blood samples and a portable reflectance meter: Derivation of threshold values and prospective validation. Am J Obstet Gynecol **156**:1085, 1987.

White P: Diabetes in childhood and Adolescence. Philadelphia, Lea & Febiger, 1932, pp 224–225.

White P: Diabetes mellitus in pregnancy. Clin Perinatol **1**:331, 1974.

White P, Titus RS, Joslin EP: Prediction and prevention of late pregnancy accidents in diabetes. Am J Med Sci **198**:482, 1939.

Widness JA, Teramo KA, Clemons GK, et al: Direct relationship of antepartum glucose control and fetal erythropoietin in human type 1 (insulin dependent) diabetic pregnancy. Diabetologia **33**:378, 1990.

Williams JW: The clinical significance of glycosuria in pregnant women. Am J Med Sci **137**:1, 1909.

Williams JW: Obstetrics. A Textbook for the Use of Students and Practitioners. New York, D. Appleton, 1925.

Willman SP, Leveno KJ, Guzick DS, et al: Glucose threshold for macrosomia in pregnancy complicated by diabetes. Am J Obstet Gynecol **154**:470, 1986.

Wilson DE: Review. Excessive insulin therapy: Biochemical effects and clinical repercussions. Current concepts of counter-regulation in type I diabetes. Ann Intern Med **98**:219, 1983.

Wing AJ, Brunner FP, Brynger H, et al: Successful pregnancies in women treated by dialysis and kidney transplantation. Br J Obstet Gynecol **87**:839, 1980.

Wladimiroff JW, Barentsen R, Wallenburg HCS, et al: Fetal urine produciton in a case of diabetes associated with polyhydramnios. Obstet Gynecol **46**:100, 1975.

World Health Organization. WHO Expert Committee on Diabetes Mellitus: Second Report. (Tech. Rep. Ser. 646) Geneva, World Health Organization, 1980.

Wright AD, Nicholson HO, Pollock A, et al: Spontaneous abortion and diabetes mellitus. Postgrad Med J. **59**:295, 1983.

Yeast JD, Porreco RP, Ginsberg HN: The use of continuous insulin infusion for the peripartum management of pregnant diabetic women. Am J Obstet Gynecol **131**:861, 1978.

Yen SSC: Metabolic homeostasis during pregnancy. In Yen SSC, Jaffe RF (eds): Reproductive Endocrinology. Philadelphia, WB Saunders Company, 1978.

Ylinen K: High maternal levels of hemoglobin A1c associated with delayed fetal lung maturation in insulin-dependent diabetic pregnancies. Acta Obstet Gynecol Scand **66**:263, 1987.

Ylinen K, Aula P, Stenman U-H, et al: Risks of minor and major malformations in diabetics with high haemoglobin A1c values in early pregnancy. Br Med J **289**:345, 1984.

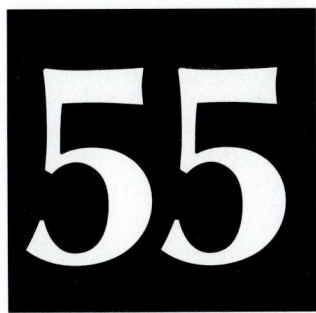

CHAPTER

55

THYROID DISEASE AND PREGNANCY

·····················

B. LYNN SEELY, M.D., and GERARD N. BURROW, M.D.

Thyroid disease is common in women during their reproductive years. Abnormal thyroid function can significantly affect a woman's ability to become pregnant, the course of an established pregnancy, the health of the fetus, and the condition of both the mother and the neonate in the postpartum period. Pregnancy also significantly alters the course of autoimmune disease in general and thyroid disease in particular. Knowledge of normal thyroid hormone physiology and how pregnancy affects thyroid function is essential for the accurate diagnosis and management of thyroid disease during pregnancy and the postpartum period.

In this chapter we will describe normal thyroid function before discussing the impact of pregnancy on normal thyroid hormone economy. We will then proceed with a description of hypo- and hyperthyroid states occurring in pregnancy and a discussion of their management. Finally, the varying facets of postpartum thyroiditis will be covered. Throughout this chapter, the underlying message will be that appropriate management of thyroid disease in pregnancy requires frequent evaluation of both mother and fetus to achieve adequate treatment of the mother without under- or overtreating the fetus.

MATERNAL-FETAL THYROID PHYSIOLOGY

Normal Thyroid Physiology

The normal adult thyroid gland weighs about 15 to 25 gm and consists of two lobes connected by an isthmus. Each thyroid lobe is divided into lobules consisting of 20 to 40 follicles. There are approximately three million follicles in an adult thyroid, and each follicle consists of a ring of follicular cells surrounding large amounts of colloid (Fig. 55–1). The thyroid gland is responsible for synthesizing and secreting thyroid hormones, L-thyroxine (T_4) and L-triiodothyronine (T_3). The concentration of circulating free thyroid hormone is closely regulated by the hypothalamic-pituitary-thyroid axis. Free thyroid hormone enters the cell where T_4 is converted to T_3. T_3 then controls metabo-

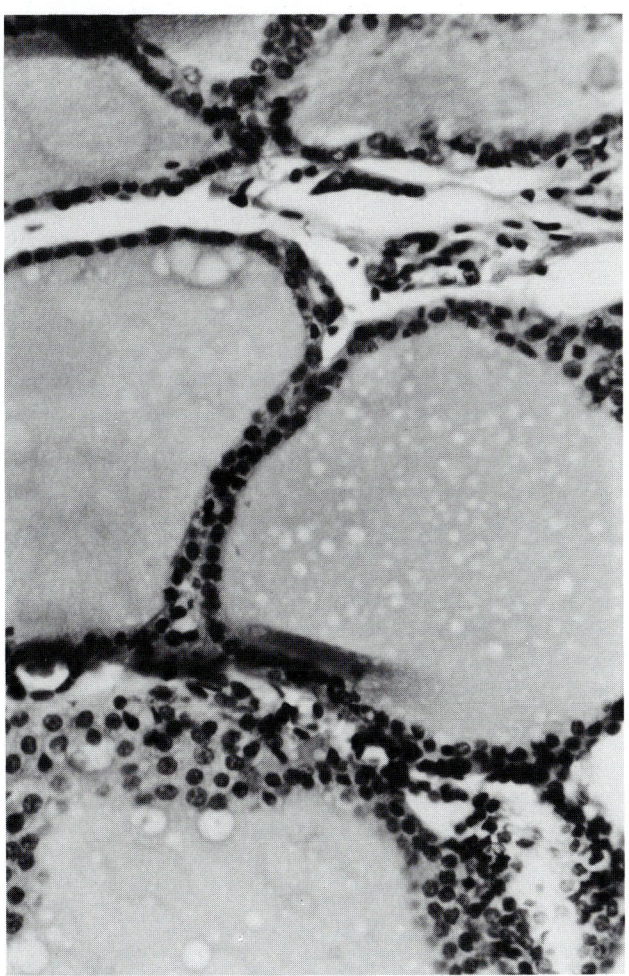

FIGURE 55–1. An individual thyroid follicle filled with colloid and surrounded by thyroid follicular cells.

lism largely by regulating gene expression and protein synthesis (Oppenheimer, 1985).

The synthesis of hormone by the thyroid gland requires iodine. T_4 has four iodine atoms per molecule and T_3 has three iodine atoms per molecule. In a nonpregnant woman, approximately 80 to 100 μg of iodine must be taken up by the gland daily to maintain a steady state with the iodine being secreted from the gland in the form of T_3 and T_4. Dietary iodine is reduced to iodide and is absorbed in the small intestine. Eighty per cent of circulating iodide is cleared by the kidney and 20 per cent is cleared by the thyroid. Movement of iodide from blood into thyroid cells is an active process known as trapping. Energy is required to move iodide into the thyroid gland because the concentration of iodide is 30-fold higher in the cell than in the blood. Iodide transport is under the control of TSH and is the rate-limiting step in thyroid-hormone biosynthesis.

After transport into the gland, iodide undergoes organification, a process involving the conversion of iodide back to iodine, binding to tyrosyl residues, and subsequent synthesis of iodothyronines catalyzed by the enzyme peroxidase. Thionamide drugs inhibit peroxidase activity as they compete with iodine for the enzyme. Congenital deficiency of peroxidase results in cretinism (Lever et al., 1983; Cooper, 1984).

Iodine is stored in the thyroid gland as thyroglobulin, a prohormone with a molecular weight of 660,000 containing six molecules of T_3 and T_4 and iodotyrosines (monoiodotyrosines and diiodotyrosines). Thyroglobulin is stored in the colloid of the thyroid follicles. With TSH stimulation, the prothyroid hormone is brought back into the thyroid cell and is digested by proteases to cause the secretion of T_4 and T_3 (DeGroot and Niepomnizcze, 1977).

Thyroid-stimulating hormone (TSH, thyrotropin) is responsible for stimulating the transport of iodide into the gland, iodide organification, thyroglobulin synthesis, and ultimately, thyroglobulin digestion and secretion of T_4 and T_3. TSH signals these actions by binding to specific receptors on the thyroid plasma membrane and activating adenylate cyclase, the enzyme catalyzing the formation of cyclic adenosine monophosphate (cAMP). The thyroid hormone receptor belongs to the superfamily that contains steroid hormone receptors and is, in fact, the cellular counterpart of the viral oncogene v-erb-A (Weinberger et al., 1986; Sap et al., 1986).

Approximately 90 μg of T_4 and 30 μg of T_3 are secreted by the thyroid each day. T_4 and T_3 both circulate predominantly bound to serum proteins. T_4 is more highly protein bound and has a half-life of about one week. Because of this long half-life, five to six weeks are necessary before a change in the dose of levothyroxine therapy is reflected in steady-state serum T_4 values. The daily turnover of T_4 is only 10

per cent. T_3 has a significantly larger free fraction than that of T_4 (0.3 per cent versus 0.03 per cent) and has a half-life of one day with a daily turnover of 75 per cent. The T_4- and T_3-binding proteins are synthesized by the liver. Thyroxine-binding globulin (TBG) accounts for 75 per cent of T_4 binding, while 15 per cent is bound to thyroxine-binding prealbumin (TBPA) and 10 per cent is bound to albumin. It is the free, unbound hormone that gains access to the cell and is the active compound (Oppenheimer, 1968, 1979).

All the T_4 in the body is secreted by the thyroid gland, but only about 20 per cent of T_3 comes directly from the thyroid. In most human tissues, particularly the liver and the kidney, T_4 is metabolized to T_3 by deiodination. T_3 then diffuses across the cell membrane and cytoplasm to enter the nucleus, where it binds to nuclear receptors and signals its cellular responses (Dillmann, 1985; Oppenheimer, 1985). T_3 has a 10-times greater affinity for the nuclear receptor than does T_4, a fact that probably accounts for the greater biological activity of T_3. Tissues such as liver and kidney, which are sensitive to thyroid hormone, have a high number of nuclear binding sites, whereas tissues that are relatively resistant to thyroid hormone have few T_3 nuclear receptors. In the rare syndrome of thyroid hormone resistance, circulating free hormone levels are high, but nuclear T_3 receptors are abnormal (Cooper et al., 1982).

The 5′-deiodination of T_4 to form T_3 involves removal of an iodine from the outer ring of T_4 (Schimmel and Utiger, 1977). Removal of an iodine from the inner ring of T_4 rather than the outer ring results in the formation of reverse T_3 (rT_3) (Fig. 55–2). Reverse T_3 (3,3′,5′-triiodothyronine) has no metabolic activity and is, in essence, a mechanism for inactivation of T_4. In health, approximately 35 per cent of T_4 is converted to T_3 and 40 per cent to rT_3. This balance is shifted dramatically in favor of rT_3 production during starvation, severe illness, or other catabolic states. Reverse T_3 levels are also elevated in fetal life, but fall to normal levels after birth (Wartofsky and Burman, 1982).

The production of T_4 and T_3 by the thyroid is controlled by TSH. TSH, which accelerates all steps of thyroid hormone biosynthesis, is synthesized in the anterior pituitary gland and is a glycoprotein composed of an alpha and a beta subunit. The alpha subunit of TSH is identical to the alpha subunits of human chorionic gonadotropin (hCG) and luteinizing hormone (LH). There is also significant homology in the beta subunits of these hormones, which may have

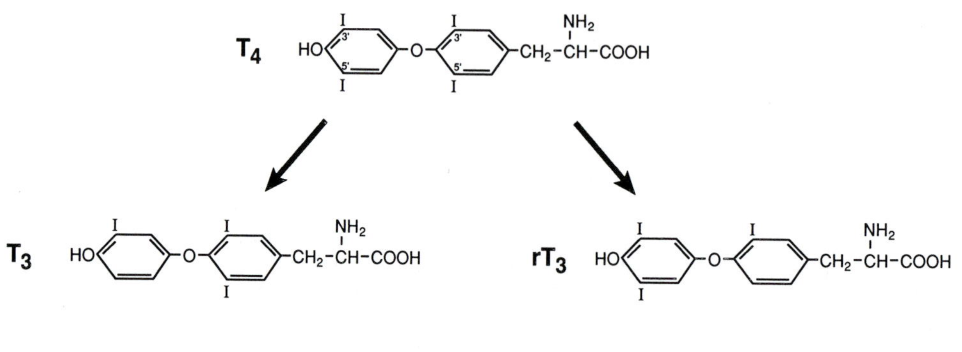

FIGURE 55–2. Removal of an iodine by 5′-monodeiodination from the outer ring of T_4 results in formation of metabolically active T_3. Removal of an iodine from the inner ring results in formation of the metabolically inactive rT_3.

been derived from the same ancestral gene (Saxena and Rathnam, 1983). TSH is regulated by circulating levels of free T_3 and T_4. Elevated levels of T_3 and T_4 provide negative feedback to the pituitary and result in suppression of TSH. Suppression of TSH occurs by interaction of T_3 with the nuclear receptor of the thyrotroph. T_4 mediates TSH suppression by rapid monodeiodination to T_3 (Silva and Larsen, 1977).

Thyrotropin-releasing hormone (TRH) is a tripeptide that is secreted by the hypothalamus and stimulates TSH release. This was the first hypothalamic hormone to be synthesized and injected into humans. TRH binds to thyrotroph receptors and stimulates secretion of TSH. This hypothalamic TRH does not reach the systemic circulation, and so serum TRH levels are not helpful in evaluating thyroid pathophysiology (Gershengorn, 1982).

Although circulating levels of free thyroid hormone and TRH stimulation are the major regulators of free thyroid hormone levels, somatostatin, dopamine, estrogens, and catecholamines also play a role. For example, dopamine and dopamine agonists such as bromocriptine suppress the TSH response to TRH, whereas dopamine antagonists such as metoclopramide increase serum TSH values (Scanlon et al., 1979).

Maternal Thyroid Physiology

The healthy pregnant woman is considered to be euthyroid, although remarkable perturbations can take place in her thyroid function values. The role of maternal thyroid hormones in fetal growth and development remains controversial, but much new information has been gained. In this section, we will review what is known about changes in maternal thyroid physiology during pregnancy and the development of the fetal hypothalamic-pituitary-thyroid axis.

Goiter and Iodine Deficiency

An ancient Roman poet eloquently described the practice of diagnosing pregnancy by measuring the swelling in the neck of a recently married young woman (Medvei, 1982). Egyptians similarly documented pregnancy when a reed tied around a young woman's neck broke from the strain of progressive swelling (Becks and Burrow, 1991). Mild thyroid enlargement does occur as a result of glandular hyperplasia and increased vascularity (Stoffer et al., 1957), but frank goiter developing during pregnancy signifies iodine deficiency or, in regions of high iodine intake, other thyroid disease.

The use of radioiodine is absolutely contraindicated in the pregnant woman. However, early studies using [132]I, an isotope with a half-life of 2.3 hours, demonstrated a threefold enhancement of the thyroid clearance of iodine in pregnant women (Abdoul-Khair et al., 1964). Similar studies in 25 pregnant women also revealed a marked increase in radioactive iodine thyroid uptake during pregnancy as compared with nonpregnant and postpartum control values (Halnan, 1958).

Increased maternal renal iodine clearance during pregnancy may result in iodine deficiency in areas of borderline iodine intake. The mean renal clearance of iodine almost doubles during pregnancy and remains enhanced until delivery. This is probably secondary to the normal rise in cardiac output, stroke volume, and heart rate coupled with the decreased systemic vascular resistance regularly observed in pregnant women. There is a resultant increase in renal blood flow and a rise in glomerular filtration rate by as much as 50 per cent (Ferris, 1988). If the iodide concentration in urine samples is greater than 5 µg/dl or an excretion rate of iodine greater than 100 µg/24 hr is documented, it can be assumed that the patient's iodine intake is adequate (Beckers, 1991). The World Health Organization recommends a daily iodine intake of at least 150 µg for pregnant women to prevent iodine deficiency (Delange, 1988).

In the United States, the increased need for iodine is inconsequential as the average iodine intake is substantially above that required. In a study of pregnant American adolescents, only 6 per cent had a goiter compared to 5 per cent in a nonpregnant control group. Of the goiters in the pregnant group, 50 per cent were nontoxic, 28 per cent were of autoimmune etiology, and 22 per cent were associated with subacute thyroiditis (Long et al., 1985). In another United States study, 49 pregnant and 49 nonpregnant controls were examined by several blinded observers, and no increase in goiter during pregnancy was reported (Levy et al., 1980). Ultrasound studies from areas replete in iodine have confirmed these findings (Nelson et al., 1987; Brander and Kivisaari, 1989).

In Scotland and Ireland, areas of known iodine deficiency, 70 per cent of a group of pregnant women developed a visible or palpable goiter (Crooks et al., 1967). A more recent study of pregnant women in Belgium, an area of marginal iodine intake, revealed that 9 per cent had a goiter (thyroid volume >23 ml by ultrasonography) at delivery, whereas 73 per cent had a measurable increase in thyroid volume during pregnancy, with an average increase of 20 per cent. There was no direct correlation between urinary iodine excretion and thyroid volume, but thyroid volume was negatively correlated with serum TSH concentrations during pregnancy (Glinoer et al., 1991).

Thus, a goiter is not a normal finding in pregnancy and requires further evaluation, that is, a search for iodine deficiency in areas of marginal iodine intake or a search for other thyroid diseases in areas of excessive iodine intake. Etiologies of goiter other than iodine deficiency include: Graves' disease, Hashimoto's thyroiditis, excessive iodine intake, lymphocytic thyroiditis, thyroid cancer, lymphoma, and therapy with lithium or thioamides.

Thyroxine-Binding Globulin, T_4 and T_3

One of the most notable changes in maternal thyroid physiology during pregnancy is an increase in TBG in response to elevated estrogen levels. Hyperestrogenemia is believed to cause the sialylation of TBG, thus decreasing clearance by the liver (Ain et al., 1987; Ain and Refetoff, 1988; Ain et al., 1988). This rise in TBG is associated with a concomitant increase in total T_4

and T$_3$. In many situations of TBG elevation, such as in women taking oral contraceptives, the total T$_4$ and T$_3$ levels rise in conjunction with the TBG levels, free hormone concentrations are unchanged, and the women remain euthyroid. Free hormone levels during pregnancy consistently remain within the normal range (Yamamoto et al., 1979), but recent data indicate that the rise in serum T$_4$ and T$_3$ concentrations may not be as great during pregnancy as the rise in TBG, and the result is relative hypothyroxinemia (Glinoer et al., 1991). This study was done in Belgium, which is an area of marginal iodine intake.

Glinoer et al. studied a cohort of 606 pregnant women. Free T$_4$ levels fell from 17.9 pM/liter in the first trimester to 13.4 pM/liter in the third trimester (normal range = 10 to 26 pM/liter). A similar fall was seen in the free T$_3$ levels, although again the hormone values did not decrease out of the normal range. This same trend for normal to mildly elevated free T$_3$ and free T$_4$ values early in pregnancy and low-normal or just subnormal levels in the third trimester have been reported by several investigators using a variety of free hormone assays (Harada et al., 1979; Yamamoto et al., 1979; Guillaume et al., 1985; Price et al., 1989). There was a concomitant rise in the serum TSH levels (Glinoer et al., 1991).

While TBG levels increase, TBPA and albumin levels fall during pregnancy. Interestingly, free T$_3$ measurements correlate with T$_4$-TBPA and T$_4$-albumin concentrations, not with free T$_4$ concentrations. Thyroglobulin levels also rise during pregnancy, but return to normal by the sixth postpartum week (Rasmussen et al., 1989). In summary, pregnancy results in a rise in maternal TBG associated with a concomitant rise in total T$_3$ and T$_4$ levels. The free hormone concentrations actually do not fall below the normal range, but decrease by about 30 per cent in late pregnancy compared to free T$_4$ values in early pregnancy.

Human Chorionic Gonadotropin and Thyroid-Stimulating Hormone

The elevation of hCG seen during pregnancy has an interesting impact on maternal thyroid hormone regulation. Because of structural similarity, hCG has a TSH-like activity and can stimulate thyroid hormone production in normal pregnancy (Yoshikawa et al., 1989; Kimura et al., 1990). The placental syncytiotrophoblast secretes hCG early in pregnancy to support the corpus luteum through the 10th week of pregnancy. The hCG levels rise to a peak of 50,000 to 100,000 mIU/ml, then fall to a plateau of 10,000 to 20,000 mIU/ml at 20 weeks. Early in pregnancy there appears to be an indirect correlation between peak hCG levels and TSH levels. As the hCG levels rise, TSH is decreased and there is a linear relationship between hCG and free T$_4$ concentrations (Kasagi et al., 1989; Kennedy and Darne, 1991). In the second and third trimesters, there is a plateau or gradual increase in the mean serum TSH concentrations (Glinoer et al., 1991; Ballabio et al., 1991; Thorpe-Beeston et al., 1991b). Profound rises in hCG seen with gestational trophoblastic disease can result in clinical hyperthyroidism.

It has been calculated from *in vitro* data that 25,000 IU/L hCG is roughly equivalent to 1.0 mU/L TSH (Kennedy et al., 1990). The rising levels of hCG could therefore affect thyroid hormone production early in pregnancy. However, free T$_4$ levels in the thyrotoxic range are unusual. It is widely held that hCG is responsible for the high free hormone levels observed in the first trimester of pregnancy, but data from the third trimester of pregnancy have been less convincing. Pregnancy serum stimulates iodide uptake in FRTL-5 cells, a rat thyroid cell line, in good correlation with hCG levels in the first trimester (Kennedy et al., 1990). However, recent evidence demonstrates a poor correlation between thyroid-stimulating activity and hCG and TSH levels late in pregnancy or after termination (Kennedy et al., 1992). Further studies are necessary to explain this discrepancy.

Thyrotropin-Releasing Hormone

Women scheduled to undergo therapeutic abortion have been given TRH, 400 μg, intravenously to further characterize the hypothalamic-pituitary-thyroid axis during pregnancy. Overall, there was minimal difference in the TRH response between pregnant and nonpregnant women. In first-trimester pregnancies, however, the TSH response was blunted as compared to second trimester pregnancies, but it was not flat as is seen in hyperthyroidism. The free T$_4$ levels were higher in the first trimester than in the second, and these data were interpreted to show normal negative feedback inhibition at the pituitary (Guillaume et al., 1985). The augmented second-trimester response has also been observed in women taking oral contraceptives and is believed to be secondary to increased estrogen levels (Burrow et al., 1975).

TRH testing is generally not recommended as TRH does cross the placenta and may interfere with the fetal pituitary-thyroid axis (Thorpe-Beeston et al., 1991a; Moya et al., 1991). Other side effects of TRH include urinary urgency, mild nausea, light-headedness, a sensation of facial flushing, and a peculiar taste sensation. A significant transient rise in both systolic and diastolic blood pressures is not uncommon. Sensitive third-generation TSH assays provide comparable information without the risk and have, for the most part, rendered TRH testing unnecessary.

Placental-Fetal Thyroid Physiology

Placental Transfer of Thyroid Hormone

Many questions still remain about just how maternal thyroid hormones affect fetal development. Early studies suggested that fetal growth is largely independent of maternal thyroid hormones and that placental transport of thyroid hormone in humans is minimal (Fisher and Klein, 1981; Fisher and Polk, 1989). When thyroxine therapy was given to term pregnant women at doses of 500 to 8000 μg/day, elevated levels of butanol-extractable iodine were found only in the neonates of mothers treated with 8000 μg/day, and then only 2.8 per cent of the 8000-μg dose was transferred over a

16-hr diffusion period. The increase was dramatically less than that found in the butanol-extractable iodine levels in maternal serum. Similarly, the administration of 300 μg/day of T_3 for several weeks to pregnant women produced only a modest increase in mean cord serum free T_3 levels at delivery (Fisher et al., 1964). Chronically treating pregnant women on propylthiouracil with up to 500 μg of T_4 per day does not prevent the development of fetal goiter, again demonstrating the poor placental transfer of thyroid hormone (Fisher et al., 1977).

Some believe the maternal rise in T_4 and the concomitant rise in TBG may provide a protective role in the early neural development of the fetus (Elkins, 1985). Any thyroid hormone required by the fetus prior to 10 to 12 weeks of gestation must be supplied by maternal thyroid hormones. The existence of thyroid hormone receptors and the measurement of thyroid hormone in fetal tissues before fetal serum T_4 levels increase imply that placental transfer of hormones occurs (Bernal and Pekonen, 1984). Nonetheless, the development and initiation of function by the fetal thyroid gland appears to be unrelated to maternal thyroid function. The fetus, however, is known to be completely dependent upon the mother for its supply of iodine (Fisher and Polk, 1989).

In rats, substantial evidence exists documenting the transfer of maternal thyroid hormones to the fetus (Morreale de Escobar et al., 1987, 1988, 1989, 1990). Maternal hypothyroidism in rats results in fetal hypothyroxinemia early in gestation when the fetal thyroid has not yet completed development. Once the human fetal thyroid gland becomes functional, during the 10th to 12th week of gestation, the gland can compensate for the maternal deficiencies, except in settings of fetal thyroid compromise such as iodine deficiency.

Recent studies in humans suggest that transfer of T_4 and T_3 can occur across the placenta in late pregnancy or at term. Vulsma et al. showed that 40 infants with congenital hypothyroidism (25 with a total organification defect and 15 with thyroid agenesis) had significant serum levels of T_4 at birth (35 to 70 μM/liter), although the levels were subnormal (normal range 80 to 170 μM/liter). Maternal thyroxine levels were normal (Vulsma et al., 1989).

Thorpe-Beeston has published a series of thyroid hormone values from 62 fetuses from 17 to 37 weeks of gestation. The serum samples were obtained by cordocentesis. In this study, fetal serum concentrations of TSH, total and free T_4, total and free T_3, and TBG increased progressively throughout gestation, and there were no significant associations between the values in maternal and fetal serum (Thorpe-Beeston et al., 1991b).

Placental Transfer of Drugs Affecting Thyroid Function

The placenta can further impact the fetal hypothalamic-pituitary-thyroid development by readily transferring several agents affecting thyroid function. These include iodide, thioamides, beta-adrenergic receptor blockers, somatostatin, exogenous TRH (maternal

TRH serum levels are low and are unlikely to affect the fetus), and dopamine agonists and antagonists (Burrow et al., 1977; Delange, 1991). TSH and other glycoproteins do not cross the placenta in significant amounts, but the thyroid-stimulating immunoglobulins (TSI) found in Graves' disease cross the placenta easily (Roti et al., 1983).

The transfer of exogenous TRH by the placenta has been extensively studied because of potential therapeutic benefits. Following TRH administration to women at term, cord serum TSH was substantially elevated in response to TRH, a response that was followed by a rise in serum T_3 and T_4 (Roti et al., 1981). Antenatal thyroid hormone given by intraamniotic injection has been shown to stimulate the synthesis of surfactant in premature neonates. Recent trials have been performed using glucocorticoids and TRH administration to stimulate T_4 release and prevent the respiratory distress syndrome in newborns (Smith, 1984). Morales et al. have demonstrated that TRH therapy improves the lecithin/sphingomyelin ratio, decreases time on the ventilator, and decreases the frequency of bronchopulmonary dysplasia, a major complication of the respiratory distress syndrome (Morales et al., 1989).

Development of Fetal Thyroid Function

Thyroid hormone plays a significant role in mammalian development, stimulating growth and development of the central nervous system as well as the development of adequate thermogenesis. Study of the development of fetal thyroid function in man has revealed that TRH can be detected in the fetal hypothalamus and TSH in the pituitary by the 12th week of gestation, the time when the fetal thyroid can begin to concentrate iodine. Pituitary and serum TSH are measurable by 8 to 10 weeks of gestation, and they rise gradually prior to delivery. Serum total T_4 levels in the fetus rise between the 10th and 30th weeks of gestation, paralleled by a rise in serum TBG (Fisher and Polk, 1989, Thorpe-Beeston et al., 1991b).

This unusual positive correlation between fetal free T_4 and TSH levels indicates insensitivity to T_4 and greater sensitivity to T_3 by the pituitary as there is no negative feedback inhibition by the rising T_4 levels, or there is an enhanced stimulus of TRH from the hypothalamus (Thorpe-Beeston et al., 1991b) (Fig. 55–3). This positive correlation of TSH and free T_4 was also reported by Ballabio, although the study ended at 31 weeks of gestation (Ballabio, 1989). Previously a fall in TSH had been reported in the 30th week of gestation in conjunction with a rise in free T_4 and it was believed that this indicated the fetal hypothalamic-pituitary-thyroid axis was fully functional (Fisher et al., 1977).

Free T_3 levels are substantially lower than adult levels throughout gestation, labor, and delivery (Fig. 55–3). Immediately after birth, there is a surge of TRH and TSH followed by a significant rise in T_3 and a more moderate rise in T_4 (Fisher and Klein, 1981). The elevation in T_3 results partially from increased thyroidal secretion and partially from increased peripheral conversion of T_4 to T_3 (Fisher and Polk, 1989). Enhanced T_4 to T_3 conversion in brown adipose tissue

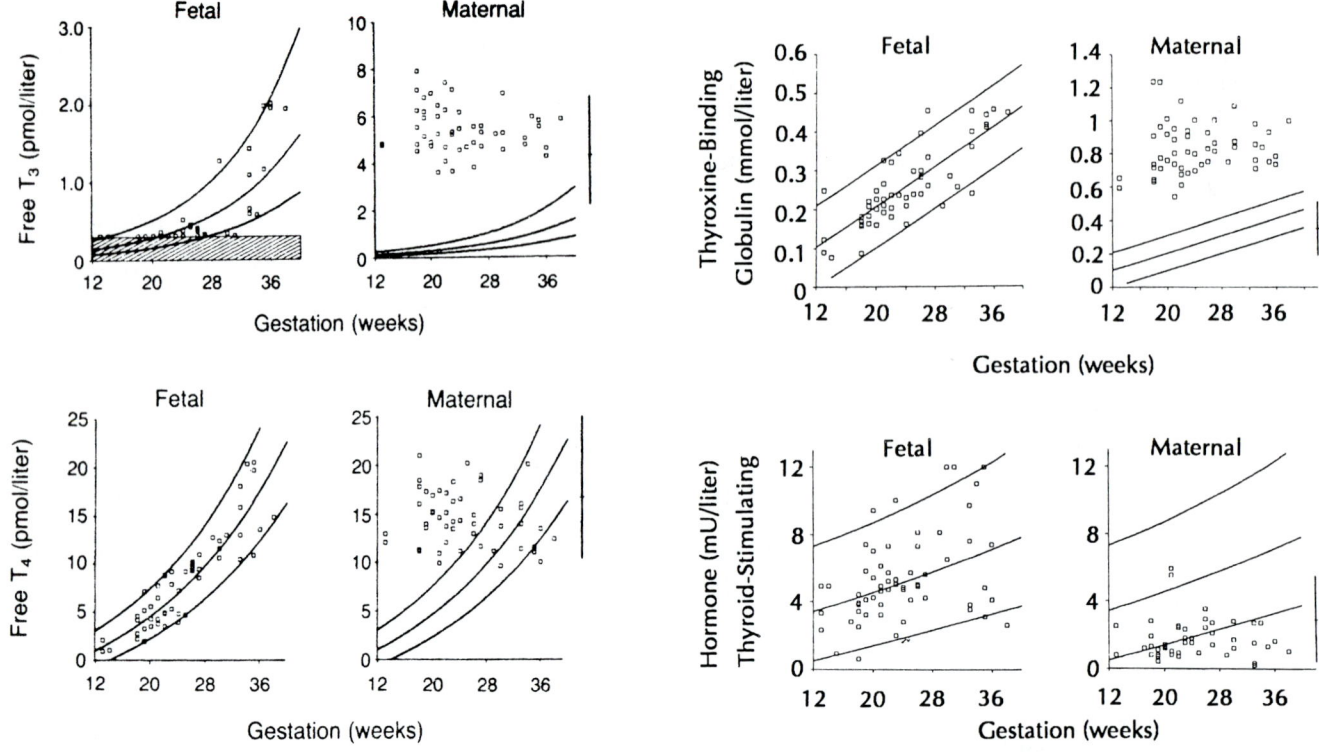

FIGURE 55–3. Individual fetal and maternal free T_3, free T_4, thyroxine-binding globulin, and TSH concentrations plotted as a function of length of gestation. The curved lines are the mean and the 5th and 95th percentile values. The vertical lines to the right are the normal ranges in nonpregnant adults (Reprinted by permission from Thorpe-Beeston JG, Nicolaides KH, Felton CV, et al: Maturation of the secretion of thyroid hormone and thyroid-stimulating hormone in the fetus. N Engl J Med **324**:532, 1991.)

may improve the neonate's thermogenic response (Polk, 1988).

The rise in the TSH level at birth abates to normal adult levels within a few days as a result of negative feedback inhibition by T_4 and T_3 at the pituitary and the hypothalamus, and the neonatal T_4 and T_3 levels then fall to normal adult levels in four to six weeks (Fisher and Polk, 1989). The impetus for this transient hyperthyroxinemia is not known, but it may be triggered by neonatal cooling, and it may be a requisite for the successful adaptation of thermogenesis and the cardiovascular system to extrauterine life (Fisher et al., 1977; Polk, 1988; Dussault, 1991).

Although the fetal total and free T_3 levels are very low through labor and delivery, levels of rT_3 are present in high concentrations after 28 weeks in the serum, the amniotic fluid, and the cord serum (Fisher and Klein, 1981). The same enzyme that controls the extrathyroidal conversion of T_4 to T_3 is responsible for the degradation of rT_3. Low activity of this enzyme, an α ring 5'-deiodinase, in the fetus could result in both the low serum T_3 levels and the elevated rT_3 levels, thus contributing to the placental barrier to maternal thyroid hormones (Kaplan, 1983; Roti et al., 1983). In premature neonates, low free T_4 levels, normal TSH levels, and a normal TSH response to TRH are seen. The T_4 levels are inversely proportional to gestational age. These babies classically have a transient 4- to 20-week course of immature hypothalamic hypothyroidism, but their growth and development

are normal (Fisher and Klein, 1981). Treatment with thyroxine is not recommended, as the abnormality resolves with time and is of no apparent clinical consequence (Fisher and Foley, 1989; Dussault, 1991).

Levels of TSH, T_4, T_3, and rT_3 are measurable in the amniotic fluid and appear to correlate with fetal rather than maternal serum taken at the same gestational age (Morley et al., 1979). The fetus may be able to absorb thyroid hormones from the amniotic fluid. A fetus at risk of ^{131}I-induced hypothyroidism was treated with injections of levothyroxine into the amniotic fluid, and the neonate was born euthyroid (Lightner et al., 1977). Intra-amniotic injections of 200 to 500 μg of T_4 were also used to successfully treat a case of fetal goiter and hypothyroidism (Davidson et al., 1991).

Pregnancy, the Immune System, and Thyroid Disease

Marked perturbations in the maternal-placental-fetal immune systems also occur during pregnancy, changes that allow the fetus, with its complete set of paternal antigens, to survive. These changes profoundly impact the courses of autoimmune thyroid disease and other autoimmune diseases including systemic lupus erythematosus, myasthenia gravis, and idiopathic thrombocytopenia. It is well known, for example, that the severity of Graves' disease is ameliorated during pregnancy, particularly in the second and third trimesters. Two to three months postpartum, there is a resurgence in disease activity. Levels of thyroid-stimulating immunoglobulins fall during pregnancy, then rebound in the postpartum period. The precise immunologic mechanism(s) for these observations are incompletely defined.

The immune tolerance that develops during pregnancy is primarily maternal-placental tolerance rather than maternal-fetal tolerance. It is the trophoblastic cell, and later the placenta, that interacts with the maternal immune system (Colbern and Main, 1991). Many hypotheses have arisen to explain this tolerance including the placenta as an anatomic barrier, weakly expressed fetal antigens, and suppression of the maternal immune response (Medawar, 1953). The reader is referred to Chapter 6 for a detailed review of pregnancy immunology.

Studies in animals and in man have shown that fetal T cells can suppress proliferation of maternal lymphocytes, presumably by elaboration of a soluble factor such as transforming growth factor-β (Froelich, 1980; Clark et al., 1986). Many *in vitro* studies of cellular immunity in pregnant women have demonstrated diminished lymphocyte responses to mixed lymphocyte cultures and to soluble antigens. A significant decrease in the relative and absolute numbers of helper T lymphocytes was also found in the peripheral blood of normal pregnant women. The helper T lymphocyte numbers subsequently returned to normal during the third to fifth postpartum months. There is no change during pregnancy in the absolute number of B cells (Sridama et al., 1982). Further work showed that the percentage and absolute number of helper T lymphocytes also fell significantly during pregnancy in patients with Graves' disease, while there was no significant change in the suppressor T lymphocytes from pre-pregnancy levels. The levels of helper T lymphocytes returned to normal in the postpartum period (Bizzarro et al., 1987).

There is increasing evidence to suggest that a significant amount of immune modulation occurring during pregnancy is happening at the maternal-placental interface by such mechanisms as nonexpression of classic class I major histocompatibility complex (MHC) or class II MHC antigens at the syncytiotrophoblast cell surface, a coating of sialomucin on the trophoblast "hiding" surface antigens from recognition, and the expression of HLA-G (a nonclassic class I antigen) by the extravillous cytotrophoblasts (Colbern and Main, 1991). Much remains to be learned about the immu-

nology of autoimmune thyroid disease during pregnancy.

LABORATORY EVALUATION OF THYROID FUNCTION IN PREGNANCY

TSH and Free T$_4$

In interpreting the thyroid function laboratory values of a pregnant woman, one must keep in mind the stage of her pregnancy to avoid misdiagnosis of borderline values (Table 55–1). A third-generation TSH determination and a free T$_4$ concentration are the best tests to evaluate the thyroid function of a pregnant woman. Total T$_4$ and T$_3$ levels are generally not of value. They are consistently elevated because of the decreased clearance of TBG stimulated by the hyperestrogenemic state (Ain et al., 1987).

Free T$_3$ and T$_4$ levels are frequently in the high normal range early in pregnancy, perhaps because of the stimulatory effects of hCG. The free hormone levels then fall by approximately 30 per cent over the course of a normal pregnancy, but they usually do not decrease below the lower limit of the normal range (Glinoer et al., 1991). TSH may be low early in pregnancy in conjunction with the rise in free T$_3$ and T$_4$ levels, again presumably from the TSH-like activity of the peak levels of hCG seen in the first trimester of pregnancy.

The second- and third-generation TSH determinations are helpful indicators of thyroid function in pregnant women because of the improved sensitivity for low values. It is now possible to reliably differentiate those with hyperthyroidism and suppressed TSH values from those who are euthyroid with low normal TSH values. The old TSH assays, or so-called first-generation assays, were done by radioimmunoassay (RIA) and generally were insensitive below the lower limit of the normal range. Cross reactivity with the gonadotropins and hCG, hormones sharing a common alpha subunit, was also a significant disadvantage. In 1984, a number of immunoradiometric assays (IRMA) utilizing monoclonal antibodies were introduced and proved to have a much greater sensitivity at lower TSH concentrations than the standard radioimmunoassay and are now known as second-generation assays. Most recently, an immunochemiluminometric

TABLE 55–1.   Biochemical Parameters of Thyroid Function During Gestation

	TRIMESTER		
	First	Second	Third
Total T$_4$ (3.9–11.6 μg/dl)	10.7 +/− 0.2	11.5 +/− 0.2*	11.5 +/− 0.2†
Total T$_3$ (90.9–208 ng/dl)	205 +/− 2.0	231 +/− 3.0*	233 +/− 2.0†
Molar T$_3$/T$_4$ (10–23 × 10^3)	23.1 +/− 0.3	24.3 +/− 0.3‡	24.8 +/− 0.3†
Thyroxine-binding globulin (11–21 mg/liter)	21.2 +/− 0.3	28.5 +/− 0.4*	31.5 +/− 0.3*
TBG saturation (28–60%)	39.3 +/− 0.6	30.9 +/− 0.4*	27.9 +/− 0.3*
Free T$_4$ (0.8–2.0 ng/dl)	1.4 +/− 0.02	1.1 +/− 0.01*	1.0 +/− 0.01*
Free T$_3$ (190–710 pg/dl)	330 +/− 0.06	270 +/− 0.06*	250 +/− 0.06*
TSH (0.2–4.0 mU/liter)	0.75 +/− 0.04	1.1 +/− 0.04*	1.29 +/− 0.04*
hCG (IU/liter × 10^3)	38.5 +/− 1.5	16.4 +/− 0.9*	13.0 +/− 1.5†

*P<.001; †P = NS; ‡P<.005

(ICMA) TSH assay has become clinically available. This is a sandwich assay using an immobilized monoclonal TSH antibody and an affinity-purified goat anti-TSH antibody with a chemiluminescent molecule. This assay has a tenfold greater sensitivity over the second-generation immunoradiometric assays (Spencer et al., 1990) (Table 55–2).

The free thyroid hormone determination complements the TSH concentration and circumvents the prior difficulty in interpretation of total T_4 values caused by changes in TBG (Table 55–3) (Surks et al., 1990). Even in the rare instance of congenital absence of TBG, the free T_4 hormone level is normal despite very low total T_4 levels. Total thyroxine concentrations have previously been ascertained by measuring the serum protein-bound iodine or the butanol-extractable iodine. These assays have been replaced by radioimmunoassays. The active or free form of the hormone can be precisely determined by equilibrium dialysis.

In this technically difficult procedure, ^{125}I-T_4 is incubated with a diluted serum sample in a system allowing the free hormone to diffuse across a permeable membrane. Protein-bound hormone cannot escape the dialysis tubing. The dialyzable T_4 is determined directly, and the total T_4 is measured by radioimmunoassay. The free T_4 value is calculated by multiplying the dialyzable T_4 value by the total T_4 value. This highly accurate but tedious method is generally used only for research purposes. Two-step radioimmunoassay kits are commercially available and are now widely used. When these tests are performed carefully, they can provide results comparable to equilibrium dialysis measurements (Sturgess et al., 1987).

If free hormone determinations are not available, the T_3 resin uptake can be measured, although this test is rarely performed anymore. It provides an inverse correlation with thyroid hormone—binding capacity. In a normal pregnancy, the T_3 resin uptake should be low. If it is normal or elevated in the presence of an elevated total T_4, hyperthyroidism is likely (Burrow et al., 1975). The product of the total T_4 and the T_3 resin uptake levels, commonly referred to as the free thyroxine index, is low or normal in a euthyroid pregnancy. Total T_4 levels in excess of 15 mg/dl and total T_3 levels greater than 250 ng/dl are rarely seen in a normal pregnancy (Burrow, 1985; Glinoer et al., 1990).

In hypothyroidism, the free T_4 will be subnormal and the TSH will be elevated. In hyperthyroidism, the TSH will be suppressed in the setting of a free T_4 level

TABLE 55–2. Three Generations of TSH Assays

	FUNCTIONAL SENSITIVITY LIMIT*
First-generation	
Radioimmunoassay (RIA)	0.5–1.0 mU/liter
Second-generation	
Immunoradiometric assay (IRMA)	0.1–0.2 mU/liter
Third-generation	
Immunochemiluminescent assay (ICMA)	0.01–0.02 mU/liter

*Technical advancements have improved tenfold the functional sensitivity limit of each generation of TSH assay.

TABLE 55–3. Factors That Influence Thyroxine-Binding Globulin

INCREASE	DECREASE
Oral contraceptives	Testosterone
Pregnancy	Corticosteroids
Estrogens	Severe illness
Hepatitis	Cirrhosis
Acute intermittent porphyria	Nephrotic syndrome
Inherited	Inherited

above the normal range. If the free T_4 is normal in the setting of a suppressed TSH, a free T_3 level should be obtained to rule out the unusual case of isolated T_3 elevation or "T_3 toxicosis." If the TSH is elevated concurrently with an elevated free T_4, the TSH level is inappropriate, and a diagnosis of secondary hyperthyroidism should be entertained.

Resistance to thyroid hormone is a rare diagnosis and may present as an increased free T_4 concentration and an inappropriately elevated TSH. Resistance to thyroid hormone is a descriptive term encompassing a number of different defects, but in certain patients the pituitary is resistant to thyroid hormone, either alone or in conjunction with other peripheral tissues. Patients with thyroid hormone resistance have normal alpha subunit concentrations, whereas those with a TSH-secreting pituitary tumor often have elevated serum alpha subunit levels (Weintraub, 1981).

TSH Receptor Antibodies

Determination of TSH receptor antibodies can help one to identify the etiology of hyper- or hypothyroidism. Antibodies to the TSH receptor were first described in Graves' disease as thyroid stimulators. Since then, numerous abbreviations have been introduced to describe thyroid antibodies with different binding and functional characteristics. To measure the biological activity of anti–TSH receptor antibodies, a measure of cAMP in FRTL-5, a rat thyroid cell line, is most commonly used. This assay can differentiate thyroid-stimulating antibodies (frequently referred to as TSAb) from blocking antibodies (TSBAb). In a radioreceptor assay that does not assess antibody function, anti–TSH receptor antibodies inhibit binding of labeled TSH to the TSH receptor, and these antibodies are called TSH-binding inhibitory immunoglobulins (TBII) (Amino, 1988) (Table 55–4).

Antithyroid Antibodies

The two most commonly determined antithyroid antibodies are those to thyroglobulin and to microsomes. The thyroid microsomal antigen has been found to be thyroid peroxidase, and antimicrosomal antibodies are sometimes referred to as antithyroid peroxidase antibodies (Mariotti, 1989). The presence of antimicrosomal antibodies is almost invariably associated with thyroid autoimmune disease. Pregnant women with positive titers of these antibodies have

TABLE 55–4.   Antibodies to the TSH Receptor*

Bioassay	
Stimulating activity	
Increase of cAMP	Thyroid-stimulating antibody (TSAb)
Blocking activity	
Inhibition of TSH-induced cAMP increase	Thyroid stimulation blocking antibody (TSBAb)
Binding Assay	
Radioreceptor assay	
Inhibition of ^{125}I-TSH-binding to TSH receptor	TSH-binding inhibitory immunoglobulin (TBII)
	Thyroid-stimulating immunoglobulin (TSI)
	Thyroid receptor antibodies (TRAb)

*The nomenclature for TSH-receptor antibodies is based upon either functional (bioassay) characteristics or binding characteristics.

an increased risk of postpartum thyroiditis (Scherbaum, 1987).

Drugs and Thyroid Function

Multiple drugs can affect the interpretation of thyroid function tests. Estrogens increase total T_4 and T_3 levels, as exemplified by pregnancy and oral contraceptive use. Iodine, lithium, and sulfonylureas all inhibit thyroid function. Propranolol, amiodarone, and ipodate can block the conversion from T_4 to T_3 and stimulate release of TSH from the pituitary. These patients will have an increased serum T_4 concentration, a normal or low T_3 concentration, and an elevated TSH level. Glucocorticoids inhibit conversion of T_4 to T_3, but decrease release of TSH from the pituitary. Dopamine, dopamine agonists, and somatostatin can decrease the TSH concentration, whereas cimetidine and dopamine antagonists will raise the serum TSH concentration. Phenytoin can result in a decline in total T_4 levels by 20 to 30 per cent because it inhibits the binding of thyroid hormone to binding proteins but also increases thyroxine clearance. TSH levels are not elevated and patients usually remain euthyroid (Table 55–5).

Nonthyroidal Illness and Thyroid Function

Assessing the thyroid function of severely ill patients can be difficult. The clinical diagnosis can be virtually impossible, making the biochemical diagnosis of paramount importance. Patients with nonthyroidal illness commonly present with a low serum free T_3 concentration because the conversion of T_3 to T_4 is shifted in favor of increased conversion to rT_3. Reverse T_3 levels are substantially elevated because of this increased conversion, as well as from an impairment in metabolic clearance. In this "euthyroid sick syndrome," the TSH concentration may be low, normal, or elevated, but is generally not elevated greater the 20 μU/ml (Wartofsky and Burman, 1982).

In the setting of a mildly elevated TSH, an elevated serum rT_3 level may be useful in differentiating non-

thyroidal illness from the low levels of rT_3 routinely seen in hypothyroidism (Oppenheimer, 1979). The serum T_4 concentration may be low, normal, or high. The more severe the illness, the lower the total T_4 values are. The total T_4 concentration in severe nonthyroidal illness has been used as a prognostic indicator because a high correlation has been demonstrated between a low serum T_4 concentration and a fatal outcome (Brent and Hershman, 1986). Despite the low T_4 and T_3 states, this does not represent true hypothyroidism and should not be treated with supplemental levothyroxine. It may, in fact, represent an adaptation to stress (Wartofsky and Burman, 1982).

THYROID DYSFUNCTION AND INFERTILITY

Hypothyroidism

Maintaining normal thyroid hormone levels is of particular importance in the reproductive years for those who desire pregnancy because both hypo- and hyperthyroidism can affect fertility. In hypothyroidism, libido is decreased in both sexes. Excessive menstrual bleeding is common in hypothyroid women and fertility decreases. The mechanism is unclear, but the metabolism of sex hormones is altered and sex hormone–binding proteins are decreased (Goldsmith et al., 1952). Mild hypothyroidism is associated with mild hyperprolactinemia and may be responsible for a luteal-phase defect resulting in infertility for some (Del Pozo et al., 1979; Bohnet et al., 1981).

Severe hypothyroidism is more commonly associated with infertility. Injections of TRH cause a release of prolactin, and the consistently elevated TRH levels

TABLE 55–5.   Drug Effects on Thyroid Hormone Tests

1. Inhibit thyroid function
    Iodine
    Lithium
    Sulfonylureas
2. Inhibit T_4 to T_3 conversion
    Glucocorticoids
    Ipodate
    Propranolol
    Amiodarone
    Propylthiouracil
3. Increase TSH
    Iodine
    Lithium
    Dopamine antagonists
    Cimetidine
4. Decrease TSH
    Glucocorticoids
    Dopamine agonists
    Somatostatin
5. Inhibit T_4 and T_3 binding to transport proteins
    Phenytoin
    Sulfonylureas
    Diazepam
    Furosemide
    Salicylates
6. Inhibit GI absorption of thyroid hormone
    Cholestyramine
    Cholestipol

seen in primary hypothyroidism can also elevate serum prolactin levels. Amenorrhea, anovulation, and in rare cases, galactorrhea are all seen in hypothyroidism (Honbo et al., 1978; Thomas and Reid, 1987; Johnson and McGregor, 1990). Because LH levels are also elevated, it has been hypothesized that diminished dopamine secretion in hypothyroidism might result in loss of inhibitory influences on the gonadotropes and lactotropes, partially explaining the elevated prolactin and LH levels (Thomas and Reid, 1987) (Fig. 55–4).

In severe hypothyroidism, the pituitary enlarges from thyrotrophic hyperplasia. The combination of an enlarged pituitary and elevated prolactin levels has led to some unnecessary interventions for a presumed prolactinoma (Khalil et al., 1984). In one case report, ovarian hyperstimulation and multiple giant follicular cysts were described in association with primary hypothyroidism (Rotmensch and Scommegna, 1989).

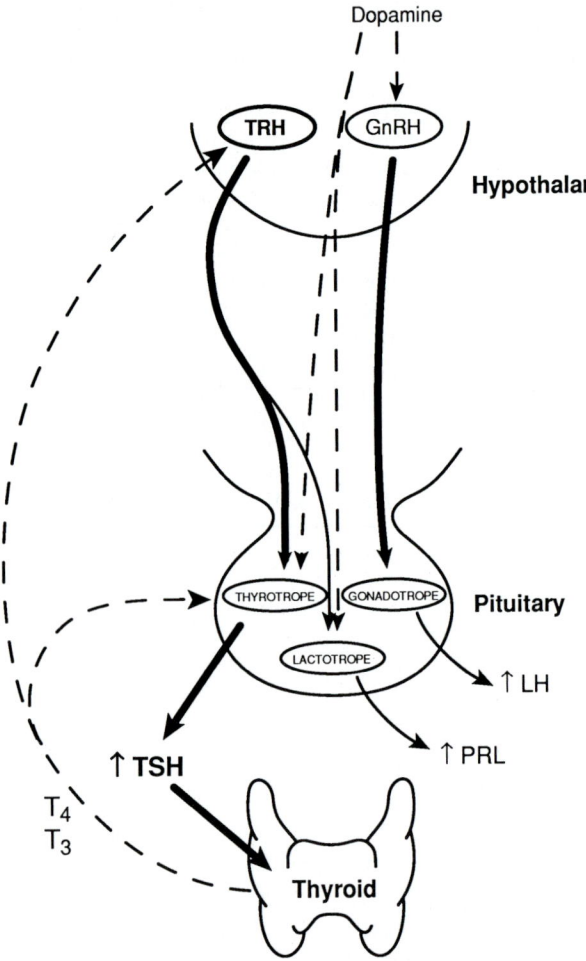

FIGURE 55–4. Primary hypothyroidism results in enhanced production of TRH. TRH stimulates release of TSH and prolactin from the pituitary. A fall in dopaminergic inhibition in the hypothalamus may also stimulate TSH and prolactin production, as well as increase gonadotropin levels. Solid lines represent stimulation; dotted lines represent inhibition. (Adapted from Thomas and Reid: Thyroid disease and reproduction dysfunction. Obstet Gynecol **70**:789, 1987. Reprinted with permission from the American College of Obstetricians and Gynecologists.)

These disorders resulting from hypothyroidism and affecting fertility are all correctable with appropriate thyroxine therapy (Montoro et al., 1981).

Rates of recurrent spontaneous abortions in a prospective study were reported to be higher in hypothyroid than in euthyroid pregnant women (Jones and Man, 1969). Early replacement with thyroxine improves fetal outcome in the setting of hypothyroidism (Greenman, 1962; Winikoff and Malinek, 1975). Because evidence exists suggesting an association between autoimmune thyroid disease and recurrent spontaneous abortion, thyroid antibodies should be obtained in women with recurrent spontaneous abortion (Beer, 1986). However, there is no documented benefit from treating euthyroid women with recurrent spontaneous abortions with L-thyroxine.

Women with insulin-dependent diabetes have a relatively high incidence of hypothyroidism and should be routinely screened with a free T_4 and a TSH serum level prior to attempting conception (Bech et al., 1991b). Gerhard et al. further recommend that TRH stimulation testing should routinely be part of the evaluation of infertile women in order to detect and treat subclinical thyroid dysfunction. In a series of 185 infertile women without clinical signs of thyroid dysfunction, they reported that women with high stimulated TSH values, low T_4 levels, and positive antimicrosomal antibodies had lower spontaneous pregnancy rates than women without these findings. An association was found between positive antimicrosomal antibody levels and spontaneous early abortion (Gerhard et al., 1991). The third-generation TSH determination should supplant the TRH test to diagnose subclinical hypothyroidism.

Hyperthyroidism

Although mild hyperthyroidism does not appear to have a major impact on fertility (Becks and Burrow, 1991), severe thyrotoxicosis is rarely seen in early pregnancy, implying a negative effect upon fertility. Menstrual irregularity and amenorrhea occur commonly in those with thyrotoxicosis, but it is important to note that many women with mild-to-moderate thyrotoxicosis remain ovulatory (Goldsmith et al., 1952). The evaluation of amenorrhea in the thyrotoxic patient should always begin with a pregnancy test.

The infertility caused by severe hyperthyroidism is not well understood. It probably results from alteration by thyrotoxicosis of any combination of a number of factors involved in conception. Weight loss can be substantial, and the patient's overall nutritional, psychological, and emotional status frequently are affected (Rogers, 1958). Women with hyperthyroidism have multiple modifications in their sex hormone levels, which have unknown effects on fertility. For example, serum estrogen levels are two to three times higher than in euthyroid women throughout the menstrual cycle, but the levels of sex hormone–binding globulin are also elevated (Ruder et al., 1971; Tulchinsky and Chopra, 1973; Akande, 1974).

Estrogen action is enhanced as sex hormone–binding globulin levels rise. Relatively more testosterone binds to the sex hormone–binding globulin than does estrogen, because testosterone has a higher affinity for the binding protein. The clearance rate of testosterone is also decreased in hyperthyroid women, and plasma levels of both testosterone and androstenedione are elevated; these elevations may contribute to the increased estrogen levels seen in these patients (Southern et al., 1974).

Interestingly, mean LH levels are also increased in both the follicular and the luteal phases of the menstrual cycles of hyperthyroid patients. The high LH levels in the follicular and luteal phases in the setting of elevated estrogen levels implies a change in the pituitary set point. The tonically elevated gonadotropins are believed to result in a diminished or absent mid-cycle LH surge in many patients, indicating a further abnormality in hypothalamic-pituitary function, which exacerbates infertility (Akande and Hockaday, 1972; Tanaka et al., 1981).

HYPERTHYROIDISM AND PREGNANCY

Signs and Symptoms

Hyperthyroidism occurs in two of every 1000 pregnant women. This common disease of pregnancy may go undiagnosed because the clinical presentation of thyrotoxicosis is difficult to distinguish from the apparent "hypermetabolic" state of pregnancy, particularly in the second and third trimesters. The basal metabolic rate rises between 15 and 20 per cent during the fourth to eighth months of a normal pregnancy. An elevated basal metabolic rate was the best method of documenting hyperthyroidism in nonpregnant individuals prior to the advent of biochemical parameters.

Many of the classic signs of hyperthyroidism—including heat intolerance, diaphoresis, warm skin, fatigue, anxiety, emotional lability, tremulousness, tachycardia, and a wide pulse pressure—are also seen during a normal pregnancy. Helpful differentiating signs seen in thyrotoxicosis, but rarely in a normal pregnancy, are weight loss, onycholysis, and a heart rate faster than 100 beats/min that does not decrease with the Valsalva maneuver (Burrow, 1978; Burrow, 1985; Seely and Burrow, 1991). Thyromegaly and infiltrative ophthalmopathy frequently accompany the thyrotoxicosis of Graves' disease, but their presence in a pregnant woman does not necessarily reflect active disease.

Vomiting may be a presenting sign of either hyperthyroidism or pregnancy (Rosenthal et al., 1976). Other clinical signs and symptoms that may be seen in association with thyrotoxicosis include diarrhea, proximal myopathy, and lymphadenopathy. In a study of 60 pregnant women with thyrotoxicosis, 12 per cent developed congestive heart failure. These women also had associated complications such as preeclampsia, infection, or anemia and probably represented particularly severe cases of thyrotoxicosis.

Biochemical confirmation of a presumed diagnosis of hyperthyroidism is mandatory. An elevated serum free T_4 and a suppressed TSH are diagnostic of hyperthyroidism. TSH values <0.05 μU/ml are diagnostic of hyperthyroidism in the absence of pituitary disease. Occasionally, the TSH concentration is suppressed, but the free T_4 is normal. A free T_3 determination may reveal "T_3 toxicosis" or an isolated elevation of T_3, but is not ordinarily required. A normochromic normocytic anemia, mild neutropenia, elevated liver function tests (alkaline phosphatase, transaminases, and bilirubin), mild hypercalcemia, and hypomagnesemia are other laboratory abnormalities that have been reported in association with thyrotoxicosis, particularly Graves' disease.

The initial screening for a pregnant woman with possible hyperthyroidism includes only tests for free T_4 and TSH. A test for free T_3 is added when the diagnosis remains unclear. Pregnant women and their unborn children generally tolerate mild-to-moderate hyperthyroidism well, and so it is reasonable to wait 3 to 4 weeks to repeat the laboratory determinations in borderline cases. Once thyrotoxicosis has been confirmed, a complete blood count, liver profile, and serum calcium, albumin, and magnesium determinations should follow. Thyroid-stimulating antibody probably should be measured in the third trimester of all pregnant women with active thyroid disease or a history of autoimmune thyroid disease, because, as will be discussed later, the level can be helpful in predicting neonatal thyrotoxicosis (Zakarija and McKenzie, 1983; Mortimer et al., 1990).

Differential Diagnosis

Graves' Disease

The term *hyperthyroidism* describes a set of clinical and biochemical features, but the etiology of the hyperthyroidism must still be determined (Table 55–6). Ninety to 95 per cent of pregnant women with hyperthyroidism will have Graves' disease, an etiology that can be diagnosed with confidence in the presence of a goiter and ophthalmopathy. The goiter is nontender, diffusely enlarged, firm, and homogeneous and frequently exhibits a bruit. Distinguishing features of Graves' ophthalmopathy include retraction of the upper eyelids, widened palpebral fissures, lid lag on downward gaze, and infrequent blinking (Werner, 1977). Infiltrative dermopathy—including pretibial myxedema and acropachy (clubbing)—is also occasionally present. An elevated thyroid-stimulating immunoglobulin level confirms the diagnosis. Radioactive uptake scans to demonstrate an increased

TABLE 55–6. Etiology of Thyrotoxicosis in Pregnancy

1. Graves' disease
2. Toxic multinodular goiter
3. Toxic adenoma
4. Hyperemesis gravidarum
5. Gestational trophoblastic neoplasia
6. Pituitary hypersecretion of TSH
7. Metastatic follicular cell carcinoma
8. Exogenous T_4 or T_3
9. De Quervain's thyroiditis
10. Silent lymphocytic thyroiditis
11. Struma ovarii

thyroidal uptake are contraindicated during pregnancy.

Graves' disease is an autoimmune disease mediated by antibodies that recognize the TSH receptor, attach to the receptor, and activate the thyroid follicular cell (Smith et al., 1988). Most commonly these TSH-receptor antibodies are stimulatory, but some have been reported to inhibit TSH action. The basic immunologic defect that incites this disease is unknown, but it is particularly common in young women, affecting 3 per cent of all women of reproductive age (Varner, 1991).

The same vaguely defined mechanisms that suppress the maternal immune response and prevent the rejection of the fetus similarly ameliorate the course of Graves' disease. The thyrotoxicosis may worsen in the first trimester from the stimulatory effects of the rising hCG levels, but as the pregnancy progresses, the thyroid-stimulating immunoglobulins fall and the signs and symptoms of the disease abate (Salvi and How, 1987). Women commonly are able to taper their antithyroid medication as pregnancy continues, but the disease frequently resurges in the postpartum period as the maternal immune system suppression disappears (Jansson et al., 1988; Salvi and How, 1987).

Gestational Trophoblastic Disease

Human chorionic gonadotropin has TSH-like stimulatory activity, as has been previously discussed. Gestational trophoblastic disease such as hydatidiform mole and choriocarcinoma can be associated with hCG levels more than 1000 times normal and can cause hyperthyroidism. The potency and composition of tumor hCG differs from that of pregnancy hCG and the increased thyrotrophic potency of some tumor hCG appears to be related to particular variant forms (Mann et al., 1986; Kennedy and Darne, 1991). Approximately half the women with gestational trophoblastic disease will have biochemical evidence of hyperthyroidism.

A diagnosis of gestational trophoblastic neoplasm must be considered in all pregnant women with hyperthyroidism. The clinical signs are usually mild, but weight loss and fatigue are common. The thyroid is usually small; goiter is rare. The treatment of choice is removal of molar tissue and/or chemotherapy. Treatment with antithyroid drugs and beta blockers is appropriate when necessary to control symptoms of hyperthyroidism (Morgan, 1990).

Hyperemesis Gravidarum

Thyrotoxicosis can present as hyperemesis gravidarum, probably mediated by hCG (Jeffcoate and Bain, 1982; Goodwin et al., 1992) (Fig. 55–5). Affected patients rarely have signs of hyperthyroidism other than nausea and vomiting, and the thyroid gland is not enlarged. Thyroid antibody levels are not elevated. Fifty to 70 per cent of patients with hyperemesis gravidarum have elevated free T_4 and free T_3 levels in the first trimester, values that return to normal as the hyperemesis remits and the pregnancy progresses (Becks and Burrow, 1991).

In a recent prospective study, Goodwin et al. eval-

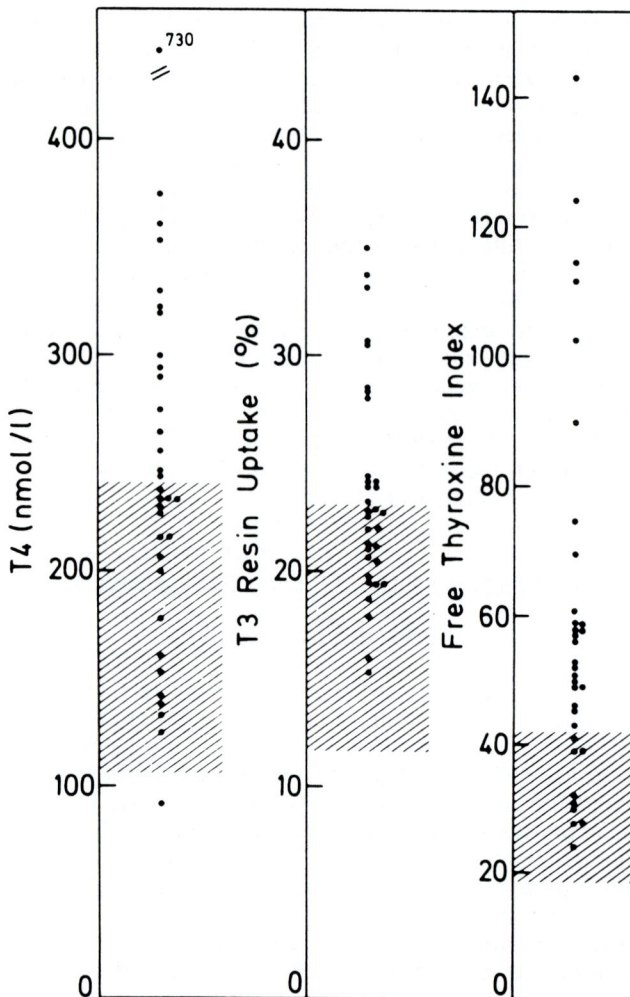

FIGURE 55–5. Thyroid function values in a series of patients with hyperemesis gravidarum. Hatched area represents normal values. (From Jeffcoate and Bain: Recurrent pregnancy-induced thyrotoxicosis presenting as hyperemesis gravidarum. Br J Obstet Gynaecol **92**:413, 1982.)

uated the biochemical parameters of 57 patients with hyperemesis gravidarum without history or evidence of thyroid disease and those of matched controls. Sixty per cent of patients with hyperemesis had suppressed TSH values at presentation. Serum levels of hCG correlated negatively with TSH and positively with free T_4 over the whole population. These authors concluded that hCG plays an important role in the causation of hyperemesis gravidarum (Goodwin et al., 1991).

Treatment of hyperemesis gravidarum is controversial. The vomiting is not always controlled by normalization of thyroid hormone levels with antithyroid drugs. Since no parenteral forms of thioamide drugs are available, therapy can be difficult in the hyperemetic patient. Methimazole suppositories are often successful, and it is reasonable to consider this therapy for symptomatic women past 20 weeks gestation with documented hyperthyroxinemia.

The use of erythrocyte zinc levels has been recommended to differentiate Graves' thyrotoxicosis from that of hyperemesis gravidarum. Erythrocyte zinc levels, an assay for thyroid hormone analogous to assay of glycosylated hemoglobin for hyperglycemia, are low in patients with hyperthyroidism. Hyperthyroxinemia inhibits the synthesis of erythrocyte carbonic anhydrase, a zinc metalloenzyme. At the time of diagnosis, women with hyperemesis gravidarum have normal erythrocyte zinc levels, which can be differentiated from the low levels found in women with the pre-existing thyrotoxicosis of Graves' disease (Chin et al., 1990).

Morning sickness may also be related to thyroid hormone excess, although no conclusive data exist. Some studies show no difference in thyroid hormone levels between those with vomiting and those without (Evans et al., 1986). Other studies report a direct correlation between hCG levels and the degree of nausea and vomiting (Mori et al., 1988). In separate studies, hCG levels have been shown to correspond directly with free T_4 levels and indirectly with TSH levels (Burrow, 1985).

Other Causes

If Graves' disease and hCG-mediated thyrotoxicosis are eliminated as possible diagnoses, other less common etiologies must be considered. Thyrotoxicosis factitia, the surreptitious ingestion of exogenous thyroid hormone, does occur. Thyroglobulin is normally secreted with T_3 and T_4. Thyroglobulin levels should be elevated if the thyroid gland is hyperfunctioning, whereas they will be suppressed with intake of exogenous thyroid hormone (Mariotti et al., 1982).

Thyrotoxicosis secondary to a toxic multinodular goiter generally occurs in those with large glands. The lumpy-bumpy, heterogeneous glands are palpable, and the diagnosis is readily made on the basis of clinical and biochemical findings. Radioactive iodine scanning is contraindicated in pregnancy. Occasionally, hyperthyroidism may be precipitated in women with nodular goiters by exogenous iodide administration, a phenomenon known as jodbasedow. Some patients will have Plummer's disease or a solitary autonomous toxic nodule. The diagnosis is again based on clinical findings. Antithyroid drugs should be used in both conditions until more definitive therapy (radioactive iodine or thyroidectomy) can be safely undertaken.

Rare causes of hyperthyroidism in pregnancy include struma ovarii, a mature ovarian teratoma containing thyroid tissue, advanced metastatic follicular thyroid carcinoma, and secondary hyperthyroidism (pituitary hypersecretion of TSH). A transient thyrotoxicosis may rarely be seen with de Quervain's or acute painful thyroiditis and silent lymphocytic thyroiditis. Antithyroid agents are not indicated in thyrotoxicosis from thyroiditis because the hyperthyroidism results from destruction of the gland and release of stored hormone rather than from increased thyroid hormone synthesis and secretion as in Graves' disease. Treatment should be aimed at controlling symptoms only. Mild cases should receive no therapy. Aspirin or nonsteroidal anti-inflammatory agents may be used for pain relief in acute painful thyroiditis, and beta blockers may be used briefly if necessary to control severe adrenergic symptoms.

Treatment of Hyperthyroidism

Hyperthyroidism is best treated prior to conception because the outcome for early treatment before pregnancy is better than that for treatment administered during pregnancy (Davis et al., 1989). Untreated or inadequately treated hyperthyroid women deliver babies with a higher incidence of minor fetal anomalies (Momotani et al., 1984) and have more complications during pregnancy and delivery. Thyrotoxicosis in pregnancy should be treated, except for the mildest cases.

The value of early and aggressive treatment has been underscored by a retrospective study of 60 thyrotoxic pregnant women. Preterm delivery, perinatal mortality, and maternal heart failure were significantly increased in women who remained thyrotoxic despite treatment and in those never treated. Thyroid hormone status at delivery correlated directly with pregnancy outcome (Davis et al., 1989).

Thionamide Therapy

The goal of therapy is to gain control of the thyrotoxicosis while avoiding any fetal or neonatal transient hypothyroidism (Momotani et al., 1986). The maternal thyroxine level should be maintained in the high normal or slightly elevated range characteristic of pregnancy. The thionamide drugs are used most commonly for treatment of thyrotoxicosis during pregnancy. Propylthiouracil (PTU) is prescribed more frequently in the United States; carbimazole, a drug metabolized to methimazole, is predominantly used in Europe. The thionamides inhibit the iodination of thyroglobulin and thyroglobulin synthesis by competing with iodine for the enzyme peroxidase. PTU, but not methimazole, inhibits the conversion from T_4 to T_3.

PTU is usually started at a dose of 100 to 150 mg every 8 hours, but doses should be increased as necessary to gain control of the thyrotoxicosis. Some patients may require doses of 600 to 900 mg per day. The risk of uncontrolled maternal thyrotoxicosis is greater than that of high-dose thionamide therapy (Davis et al., 1989). Because the drug inhibits thyroid hormone synthesis, response is not seen until hormone stored in the thyroid colloid is depleted. Most patients begin to show clinical improvement at the end of the first week. Once the patient is rendered euthyroid, free T_4, free T_3, and TSH levels should be measured monthly and the dose of thionamides tapered as the pregnancy progresses to achieve euthyroidism at the lowest possible dose of thionamide (Cheron et al., 1981).

Maternal side effects of the thionamide drugs do not occur with great frequency. One to 5 per cent of patients develop pruritus, skin rash, drug fever, a metallic taste, nausea, bronchospasm, oral ulcerations, hepatitis, or a lupus-like syndrome. An alternative thionamide can be used when these symptoms develop, although cross-sensitivity develops in 50 per cent of patients.

Agranulocytosis is the most serious side effect of therapy, but it develops in only 0.1 per cent of patients and is more likely to occur in those older than 40 and those on very high doses (Cooper et al., 1983). A baseline white blood cell count should be ordered in all patients at the onset of therapy and in all patients who develop a fever while on therapy. Some recommend routine white blood cell count monitoring throughout therapy (Tajiri et al., 1990). Agranulocytosis, to be distinguished from a mild transient leukopenia, is a contraindication to further thionamide therapy. The blood count gradually improves over days to weeks.

Antithyroid agents do not seem to be highly teratogenic. In the mid-1980s, methimazole fell into disfavor because of reports of fetal aplasia cutis, a reversible scalp defect. A European study of neonates of mothers with Graves' disease showed a rate of fetal anomaly of less than 1 per cent that was indistinguishable from euthyroid untreated controls and revealed no correlation between the rate of malformations and the dose of methimazole (Mujtaba and Burrow, 1975). In fact, recent studies indicate that untreated hyperthyroidism results in a higher rate of congenital anomalies than does treatment with antithyroid drugs (Davis et al., 1989; Messer et al., 1990). All thionamides cross the placenta and are excreted into breast milk. PTU crosses the placenta four times less than methimazole and into breast milk ten times less than methimazole, because it is more highly protein bound and has poorer solubility than methimazole (Cooper, 1984; Cooper, 1987).

Because thionamides cross the placenta with ease, there is concern that *in utero* hypothyroidism caused by drug therapy may impair neurologic development. Currently, there are no data to document this (Burrow et al., 1968; Burrow, 1978; Cheron et al., 1981). However, it is imperative to avoid overtreating the mother and to monitor the fetus closely. Thionamide levels that result in a euthyroid state in the mother may be excessive for the fetus. The fetus should be evaluated ultrasonographically for signs of hypothyroidism such as goiter, bradycardia, and intrauterine growth retardation. In worrisome cases, cordocentesis may prove helpful; reference ranges have recently been reported (Thorpe-Beeston et al., 1991b).

Some have recommended combined thionamide-levothyroxine therapy to ensure that adequate thyroid hormone is available to the fetus while the mother is kept euthyroid with thionamide therapy. No benefit from this approach has been demonstrated, and a possible increase in congenital anomalies was reported in those on combined therapy (Ramsay et al., 1983). However, a recent study, has suggested that the addition of thyroxine decreases the recurrence rate by suppressing TSH stimulation of Graves' disease (Hashizume et al., 1991).

When thyrotoxicosis is severe, additional antithyroid agents may be needed temporarily to gain control of the symptoms. This is particularly necessary when labor and delivery, cesarean section, infection, or eclampsia threatens to precipitate thyroid storm. Beta blockers and iodide can be used safely for brief courses of therapy, but glucocorticoids have not been shown to be safe in pregnancy and should be avoided.

Beta Blockers

Beta blockers are particularly useful for rapid control of the adrenergic symptoms of thyrotoxicosis. These drugs do not alter the synthesis or secretion of hormone, and thus only mask the underlying disease. Propranolol, 20 to 40 mg two or three times a day, or atenolol, 50 to 100 mg a day, will keep the maternal heart rate at 80 to 90 beats/min. Prolonged therapy can result in the fetal side effects of intrauterine growth retardation, diminution of the placenta, fetal bradycardia, hypoglycemia, and a subnormal response to hypoxemic stress (Gladstone et al., 1975; Habib and McCarthy, 1977). The successful use of esmolol, an ultrashort-acting cardioselective intravenous beta blocker, in a thyrotoxic pregnant woman unresponsive to high doses of propranolol has been reported in a patient requiring emergency surgery (Isley et al., 1990).

Iodides

Iodides are often used in combination with thioureas and beta blockers in cases of severe thyrotoxicosis or incipient thyroid storm. Therapy is generally instituted after the thionamide drug has been initiated. Iodides will decrease serum T_4 and T_3 by 30 to 50 per cent in 10 days by acutely inhibiting the release of stored thyroid hormone. Sodium ipodate, a radiographic contrast agent, has the added benefit of inhibiting the extrathyroidal conversion of T_4 to T_3. Although it is used commonly in hyperthyroidism, there are no data documenting the safety of this drug in pregnancy. Potassium iodide (SSKI), 5 to 10 drops twice a day, is recommended.

Iodide therapy is an important adjunctive therapy in severe cases of hyperthyroidism, but it should only be used for a short-term course lasting not longer than two weeks. Iodine readily crosses the placenta, and the fetus is particularly sensitive to the inhibitory effects of excessive iodine. Goiter will occur with prolonged therapy. Inconspicuous use of iodides must also be avoided. Exposure can occur from betadine vaginal suppositories, betadine-containing cleansing solutions applied topically, and, in asthmatic women, iodide-containing bronchodilator products. The use of amiodarone, a drug high in iodide content, should be avoided during pregnancy except in cases of life-threatening, drug-resistant arrhythmias because fetal hypothyroidism, goiter, and low birth weights have been reported (Widerhorn et al., 1991). Iodides are also to be avoided during lactation, as they are readily transferred into breast milk.

[131]Iodine thyroid ablation is contraindicated during pregnancy because the radioactive iodine readily crosses the placenta and is concentrated in the fetal thyroid gland after 10 to 12 weeks of gestation. In the unfortunate case in which the ^{131}I is inadvertently given to a pregnant woman, treatment should be instituted immediately with SSKI to limit recycling.

Therapy also should include a thionamide to block organification and thus reduce radiation exposure to the fetal thyroid by a factor of 100 and the fetal whole-body by a factor of 10. Treatment must be given within the first 7 to 10 days after exposure to be of any benefit.

Surgery

Thyroidectomy may be advised in cases of thyrotoxicosis with severe complications from or poor compliance with medical therapy. Surgery is usually recommended during the second trimester following two weeks of preoperative preparation with iodine to decrease the vascularity of the gland and thionamides and beta blockers for biochemical and symptomatic control. Subtotal thyroidectomy may also be performed in the first or third trimesters if necessary (Burrow, 1985). The risks of thyroidectomy include an anesthetic complication, hypoparathyroidism, and recurrent laryngeal nerve paralysis.

Fetal and Neonatal Thyrotoxicosis

Fetal Thyrotoxicosis

Careful fetal monitoring is recommended during a thyrotoxic pregnancy so that hypo- or hyperthyroidism in the fetus might be avoided. Thyroid-stimulating immunoglobulins readily cross the placenta and can activate the fetal thyroid gland. This is a rare complication, occurring in only 1 per cent of babies born to women with a history of Graves' disease or Hashimoto's thyroiditis, but it may have serious consequences if not recognized.

The level of thyroid-stimulating immunoglobulins should be measured in the third trimester in all pregnant women with either active or quiescent Graves' disease. High levels, more than five times normal, are seen more commonly in the mothers of babies with neonatal hyperthyroidism. It should be stressed that thyroid-stimulating antibodies can only be measured in a functional assay. It is well recognized that TSH-receptor antibodies are heterogeneous and can have stimulating or blocking activity resulting in fetal hyper- or hypothyroidism (Matsuura et al., 1980; Isekei et al., 1983; Clavel et al., 1990). Neonatal syndromes have been described for the transplacental passage of both stimulating and blocking antibodies (Zakarija et al., 1986). The activity of the mother's disease does not correlate with fetal or neonatal disease (Mortimer et al., 1990; Clavel et al., 1990). In those pregnancies considered to be at high risk, the fetus should be closely monitored.

Fetal thyrotoxicosis is suggested by a heart rate greater than 160 beats/min, growth retardation, advanced bone age, and craniosynostosis, all of which can be detected by ultrasonography (Becks and Burrow, 1991). The fetal thyroid becomes susceptible to maternal stimulating immunoglobulins between 20 and 24 weeks gestation. Occasionally, thyrotoxicosis results in fetal death with characteristic pathologic findings including pulmonary hypertension, viscero-

megaly, generalized adenopathy, decreased subcutaneous fat, and thyromegaly (Page et al., 1988). *In utero*, most cases are probably treated unknowingly by placental transfer of thionamide therapy. Difficulty arises in the rare event that the mother is euthyroid, but the fetus is hyperthyroid (Houck et al., 1988). Combination therapy to treat the fetus and levothyroxine therapy to keep the mother euthyroid are reasonable (Porreco and Bloch, 1990). Cordocentesis may be used to confirm the diagnosis and monitor therapy.

Neonatal Thyrotoxicosis

In many cases neonatal thyrotoxicosis is not evident at birth when the mother has been treated with thioamides. Thionamide levels fall in the neonate, and irritability, tachycardia, poor feeding, and failure to gain weight are noted 5 to 10 days after delivery. Usually the disease is self-limited over 1 to 3 months. As the circulating maternal immunoglobulins fall with a half-life of 8 to 20 days, the disease wanes (Fig. 55–6). In severe disease, goiter with resultant respiratory distress, exophthalmos, tachycardia, diarrhea, failure to thrive, heart failure, hyperthermia, jaundice, and thrombocytopenia may be present.

If the diagnosis is missed, the mortality rate can be as high as 25 per cent (Delange, 1991). A careful physical examination seeking signs of thyroid dysfunction should be done immediately after delivery. Cord blood serum free T_4, TSH, and thyroid-stimulating immunoglobulins should be measured promptly because they will describe the *in utero* environment. These hormone values should be repeated on the second day of life as the maternal antithyroid drug effects will have fallen.

Treatment of neonatal thyrotoxicosis is similar to that used in an adult. Thionamides, beta blockers, and iodine are used most commonly. Ipodate is the iodine of choice as it also blocks the deiodinase converting T_4 to T_3. Digitalis, glucocorticoids, and sedatives may all be helpful in severe cases. The ultimate effect of thyrotoxicosis on psychomotor, emotional, and behavioral consequences remains unresolved.

HYPOTHYROIDISM AND PREGNANCY

Signs and Symptoms

Hypothyroidism occurs in pregnant women in the United States with a frequency of about 6 per 1000 (Niswander and Gordon, 1972). Yet, like hyperthyroidism, this relatively common condition is difficult to diagnose in the pregnant patient. Making a diagnosis is crucial to the outcome of the pregnancy. Women with hypothyroidism have a higher incidence of preeclampsia, placental abruption, and low-birth-weight and stillborn infants, outcomes that can be improved with early levothyroxine therapy (Davis et al., 1988).

The symptoms of hypothyroidism in the adult are insidious without definable onset, and they are often masked by the hypermetabolism of the pregnant state.

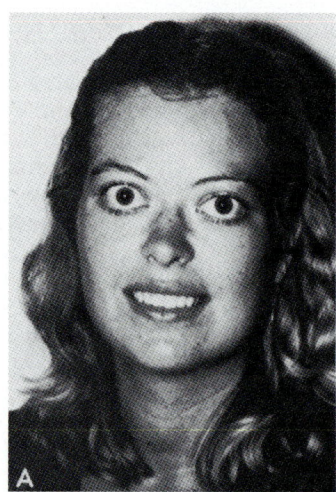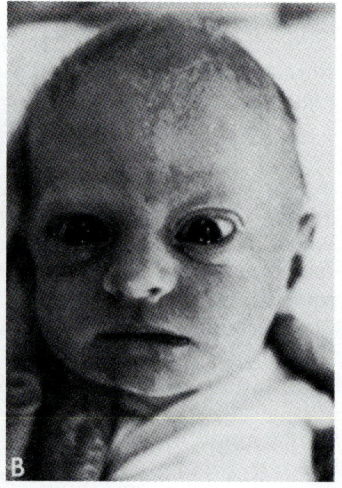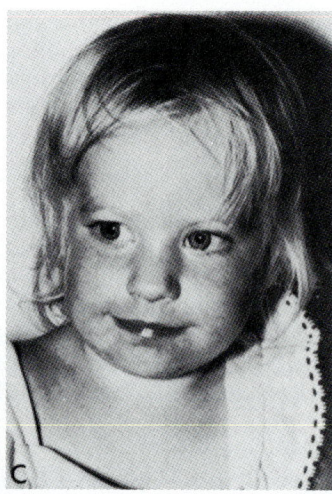

FIGURE 55–6. *A,* Hypothyroid 21-year-old mother who developed Graves' disease at age 7 and was treated by subtotal thyroidectomy. She was given maintenance therapy with Synthroid, 0.15 mg, throughout pregnancy. *B,* Her daughter was born at term with severe Graves' disease, goiter, and exophthalmos that persisted for 6 months. *C,* Child was normal at age 20 months.

All pregnant women should be carefully questioned about any personal or family history of thyroid disease or treatment directed at the thyroid gland, particularly of external radiation to the head and neck. Past or present therapy with lithium and the use of iodine-containing products or prescriptions should be ascertained.

Typically, patients present complaining of modest weight gain or inability to lose weight with dieting; morbid obesity does not result from hypothyroidism. A decrease in exercise capacity, general lethargy, and intolerance of cold are usually present. Muscle cramps are common, but muscle weakness is infrequent. Constipation, a hoarse voice, hair loss, brittle nails, and dry skin are also often reported.

The classic cases of hypothyroidism can be diagnosed with confidence from the physical examination; subtle cases must await laboratory confirmation. The thyroid gland may be enlarged, but it may also be nonpalpable. A scar at the neck signals prior thyroidectomy. The heart rate is generally slowed and hypothermia may be present. Carpal tunnel syndrome results from nerve compression by myxedematous infiltration (Rao et al., 1980), and delay in the relaxation phase of the deep tendon reflexes is seen commonly in hypothyroidism but may also occur in pregnancy. In severe cases—often called myxedema—somnolence, slow speech, poor concentration, cerebellar ataxia, ascites, ileus, pleural and pericardial effusions, and nonpitting edema of the hands, face, and ankles have all been reported, but are rarely seen today as the diagnosis is usually made earlier in the disease course. Gestational hypertension is more common in women with hypothyroidism (Leung et al., 1992).

The best biochemical tests for diagnosing hypothyroidism are a serum sensitive TSH level and a free T_4 level. In primary hypothyroidism, the TSH will be elevated and the free T_4 will be low. If the TSH is elevated and the free T_4 is normal, the patient may have subclinical hypothyroidism. An elevation of TSH is the most sensitive indication of early hypothyroidism. This condition of subclinical hypothyroidism is particularly prevalent in pregnant women and is frequently associated with thyroid autoantibodies. The impact of this condition on fetal brain development is unknown (Klein et al., 1991).

In secondary or pituitary hypothyroidism, the TSH will be normal or low in the setting of a low free T_4. TRH testing is no longer necessary for the diagnosis of hypothyroidism and free T_3 levels are of no benefit for this purpose. Antithyroid antibodies are helpful in making the diagnosis of Hashimoto's thyroiditis and in predicting the occurrence of neonatal hypothyroidism and postpartum thyroiditis (Dussault and Rousseau, 1987; Orgiazzi et al., 1991).

Other laboratory abnormalities seen in hypothyroidism include a modestly elevated creatine phosphokinase, serum oxaloacetic transaminase, lactate dehydrogenase, serum cholesterol, and serum carotene. Anemia occurs commonly. In the reproductive years of hypothyroid women, an iron deficiency anemia results from the menorrhagia. Ten per cent of patients with hypothyroidism have pernicious anemia, but neither B_{12} nor folate deficiencies explain the macrocytic anemia seen in approximately one-third of patients with hypothyroidism and anemia (Tudhope and Wilson, 1960; Klein and Levely, 1984). Most commonly, hypothyroidism is associated with a mild normochromic, normocytic anemia. Some patients also exhibit an acquired coagulation defect that is reversible with levothyroxine therapy and reminiscent of the abnormalities seen in von Willebrand's disease (Klein and Levely, 1984). Prolactin levels can be elevated with chronic elevation of TSH.

Patients with insulin-dependent diabetes mellitus should be watched closely for the development of hypothyroidism during pregnancy. Subclinical hypothyroidism can become overt because of marked proteinuria. In a study of 51 pregnant women with type

I diabetes, 26 developed elevated TSH levels or antimicrosomal antibodies or both. All had normal T_4 levels before conception. Importantly, replacement therapy with thyroxine resulted in increased insulin requirements (Jovanovic-Peterson and Peterson, 1988). Bech et al. confirmed the high incidence of antithyroid antibodies in pregnant women with insulin-dependent diabetes mellitus but not the increased rate of hypothyroidism (Bech et al., 1991b).

Differential Diagnosis

Hashimoto's Thyroiditis

Hashimoto's thyroiditis, an autoimmune disorder, is the most common cause of hypothyroidism during pregnancy in the United States. Also referred to as *chronic lymphocytic thyroiditis* and *autoimmune thyroiditis*, it may occur in 8 to 10 per cent of women of reproductive age. The disease is characterized by the presence of antimicrosomal and antithyroglobulin antibodies. Hashimoto's disease occurs in patients who have a predilection for other autoimmune disorders including Addison's disease, diabetes mellitus, pernicious anemia, and myasthenia gravis.

Hashimoto's thyroiditis often presents with a goiter. The goiter is usually firm, diffusely enlarged, and bosselated, although occasionally it can be multinodular. It is most often painless. When thyroid atrophy rather than goiter formation occurs and the antibody titers are negative, the disease is labeled idiopathic hypothyroidism, although this disease is likely to be a variant of Hashimoto's thyroiditis. Seventy-five to 80 per cent of patients with Hashimoto's thyroiditis are euthyroid, but overt and subclinical hypothyroidism are seen with relative frequency. Although Hashimoto's thyroiditis is characterized by infiltration of the gland with plasma cells and lymphocytes, biopsy is seldom necessary to make the diagnosis.

The diagnosis can usually be confirmed with elevated antimicrosomal and antithyroglobulin antibody titers. Seronegative Hashimoto's thyroiditis has been reported (Baker et al., 1988), but this may reflect the sensitivity of the assay. Elevated titers of antithyroglobulin antibodies are found in 50 to 70 per cent of patients with Hashimoto's thyroiditis. Antimicrosomal antibodies are found in almost all patients with Hashimoto's thyroiditis (Weetman and McGregor, 1984).

Autoimmune thyroid disease appears to represent a spectrum ranging from Graves' thyrotoxicosis caused by antibodies stimulating the TSH receptor to the thyroid destruction by antithyroid antibodies seen in Hashimoto's thyroiditis. Patients with Graves' disease can occasionally develop hypothyroidism from a switch from TSH-receptor–stimulating antibodies to TSH-receptor–blocking antibodies (Shigemasa et al., 1990), and Graves' disease and Hashimoto's thyroiditis can present together in a condition referred to as "hashitoxicosis." As in Graves' disease, pregnancy has a beneficial effect on the course of Hashimoto's thyroiditis, with a relapse frequently seen after delivery (Salvi and How, 1987). Hashimoto goiters decline in size coincident with the fall in thyroid microsomal and thyroglobulin antibodies during pregnancy (Amino et al., 1978).

Post-therapy Hypothyroidism

The prior treatment of Graves' disease with radioactive iodine or thyroidectomy results in hypothyroidism and is the second leading cause of hypothyroidism during pregnancy. Ten to 20 per cent of patients who receive radioactive iodine will be rendered hypothyroid within the first 6 months of therapy. Two to 4 per cent more will become hypothyroid each year thereafter (Werner, 1977), a phenomenon some believe is due to the development of TSH-receptor–blocking antibodies (Konishi et al., 1985; Miyauchi et al., 1988).

Suppurative and Subacute Thyroiditis

Hypothyroidism may develop from other forms of thyroiditis including suppurative thyroiditis and subacute thyroiditis. Postpartum thyroiditis will be discussed later. Suppurative thyroiditis is not difficult to diagnose as these patients complain of severe pain and swelling in the neck and are febrile. The infection, which usually occurs in terminally ill patients, may result either from bacteria, such as *Staphylococcus aureus* or *Streptococcus hemolyticus*, or from fungus, such as *Aspergillus fumigatus*.

Subacute thyroiditis is believed to be of viral origin and is generally self-limited. Patients experience a painful, firm goiter and a clinical course typically consisting of an early hyperthyroid phase from leakage of thyroid hormone from damaged follicles, a euthyroid phase, and then, in about 20 per cent of patients, a transient hypothyroid phase. The duration of illness is from 6 weeks to 6 months (Fig. 55–7).

Immunologic factors appear to play a substantial role in the subset of patients who develop hypothyroidism. Tamai has studied a group of 68 nonpregnant patients with subacute thyroiditis with negative thyroid autoantibodies. Those patients who developed hypothyroidism had a significantly higher incidence of development of TSH-blocking antibodies, as well as thyroid-stimulating immunoglobulins. These data

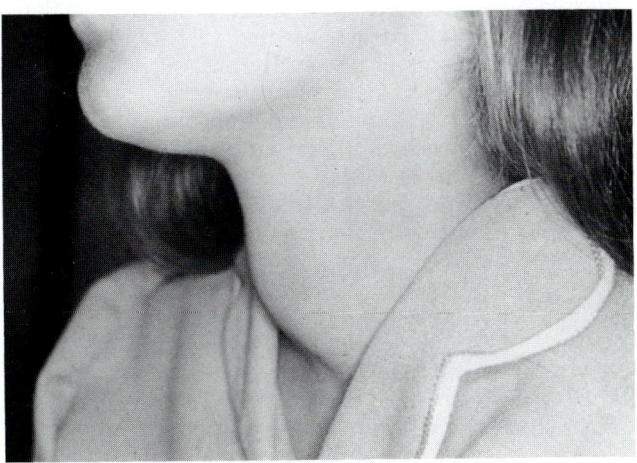

FIGURE 55–7. A young woman who developed a viral illness and an enlarged, tender thyroid gland.

suggest that the initial thyroid damage causes release of antigens which cause the immunologic abnormalities (Tamai, 1991).

Drugs

Thionamide therapy, iodides, and lithium, drugs commonly implicated in hypothyroidism, are all well known to inhibit the synthesis and/or secretion of thyroid hormones. Infiltration of the thyroid gland with lymphoma, metastatic carcinoma, sarcoidosis, or amyloidosis can cause hypothyroidism but rarely present during pregnancy.

Lymphocytic Hypophysitis

Hypothalamic-pituitary disorders do occur, but are rare. Recently, however, attention has centered on lymphocytic hypophysitis, an uncommon disease that may go unrecognized. First described in 1962 in an autopsy series, this is a disorder in which the pituitary gland is infiltrated with mononuclear cells, predominantly lymphocytes. Almost all patients with this disorder are women, and many are postpartum at the time of diagnosis. An association with postpartum thyroiditis has been reported (Amino, 1988).

Six reported cases of lymphocytic hypophysitis have been diagnosed during pregnancy. The disease frequently presents as a pituitary mass or as pituitary dysfunction during pregnancy or in the postpartum period. Many patients previously described with Sheehan's syndrome may, in fact, have had lymphocytic hypophysitis. Treatment consists of hormone replacement and possibly a course of steroids. Recovery of pituitary function may occur (Bitton et al., 1991).

Iodine Deficiency

Iodine deficiency is a common cause of hypothyroidism in many parts of the world, although it is exceedingly rare in the United States. The hypothalamic-pituitary axis responds to iodine deficiency with a hypersecretion of TSH that is probably responsible for the formation of goiters and nodules. The goiter frequently increases in size during pregnancy, and multiple pregnancies result in much larger goiters than those seen in nulliparous women (Fig. 55–8). Many women may be clinically euthyroid, but show biochemical hypothyroidism upon careful testing. The treatment is iodine supplementation, most practically by adding potassium iodide to salt. Intramuscular injection of iodized poppyseed oil, which releases iodide slowly and requires treatment once every 3 to 5 years, is used in some areas of the world.

Treatment of Hypothyroidism

Hypothyroxinemia is to be avoided during pregnancy because of its potential impact on pregnancy outcome as well as on neonatal and childhood development. As soon as the diagnosis is made, full-dose replacement with 0.1 to 0.15 mg per day of levothyroxine should be initiated. The dose should be in-

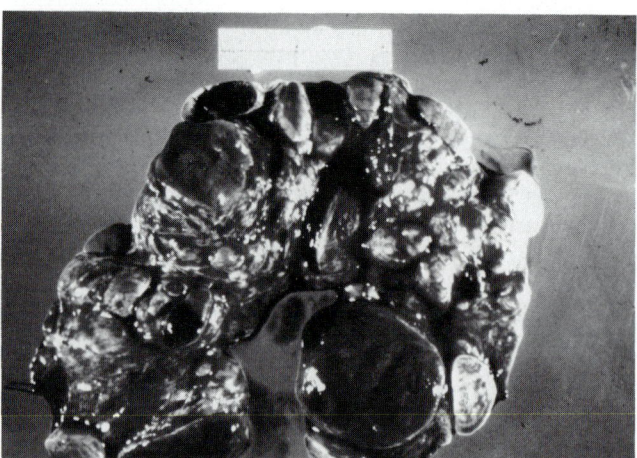

FIGURE 55–8. Surgical specimen from a multiparous woman with iodine deficiency and a multinodular goiter.

creased every 4 weeks until the TSH is returned to the low normal range. Women on thyroid hormone replacement prior to conception should continue this therapy. Some women may require an increase in their dosage as the pregnancy progresses.

In a study of 12 pregnant women with primary hypothyroidism, nine required a higher levothyroxine dose, with a mean dosage increase of 45 per cent. This rise in requirement occurred in the first trimester and persisted throughout pregnancy (Mandel et al., 1990). Tamaki et al. reported that pregnant women with autoimmune hypothyroidism are likely to have a decrease in their thyroid replacement requirements, whereas those with hypothyroidism as a result of thyroidectomy have increased requirements (Tamaki et al., 1990).

Fetal and Neonatal Hypothyroidism

The danger of hypothyroidism during pregnancy is heavily underscored by the condition of cretinism resulting from maternal, fetal, and neonatal thyroid hormone deficiency in iodine-deficient regions (Fig. 55–9). Severe cretinism is characterized by marked mental retardation, deaf mutism, spasticity, strabismus, and abnormal sexual maturation. Congenital hypothyroidism occurs with an incidence of approximately 10 per cent in severely iodine-deficient areas (Hetzel, 1987). In addition to possibly resulting in poor neurologic development in the fetus, maternal hypothyroidism during pregnancy is associated with a twofold increase in stillbirths (Niswander and Gordon, 1972) and increased rates of perinatal mortality and congenital anomalies (Davis et al., 1988).

Severe neurologic deficits can also be seen in children with congenital deficiency of thyroid hormone unrelated to iodine deficiency. These children appear well and normal at birth, but if not diagnosed and treated by three months of age, they have remarkably poor progression in their neurologic development. In the United States, screening of all neonates for thyroid hormone deficiency is recommended by the American Academy of Pediatrics and, in some states, is man-

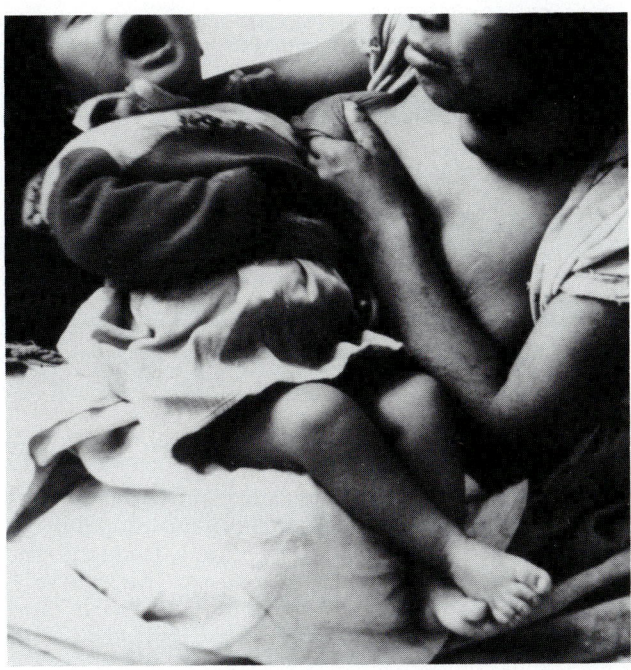

FIGURE 55–9. A woman with a multinodular goiter from iodine deficiency breast-feeding her infant.

datory. With early replacement therapy, the growth and neurologic development of these children are essentially normal (Fisher and Polk, 1989).

Causes of primary hypothyroidism in the newborn also include thyroid dysgenesis and the inborn errors of thyroid function such as thyroid peroxidase deficiency. Some believe thyroid dysgenesis results from maternal blocking antibodies that are transferred to the fetus and prevent thyroid growth and development or block fetal thyroid stimulation by TSH (Dussault and Rousseau, 1987; Bogner et al., 1989). Congenital pituitary and hypothalamic hypothyroidism are extremely rare (Table 55–7).

It is known that thyroid hormone deficiency can profoundly affect neurologic development, but controversy remains over the stages of development in which this dependency upon thyroid hormone exists, the duration and the severity of thyroid hormone deficiency necessary to impair neurologic development, and whether or not normal maternal thyroid function can fully protect a fetus with congenital hypothyroidism. Whether or not transient maternal hypothyroxinemia can result in a drop in the mean intelligence quotient (IQ) of the offspring remains to be determined (Burrow et al., 1978; Morreale de Escobar et al., 1987).

TABLE 55–7. Etiology and Incidence of Congenital Hypothyroidism

Primary hypothyroidism
    Thyroid dysgenesis (1 in 4000)
    Inborn errors of thyroid function (1 in 30,000)
    Drug-induced (1 in 10,000)
    Endemic hypothyroidism (1 in 7)
Secondary and tertiary hypothyroidism (1 in 60,000)

The neonatal screening programs diagnose most cases of congenital hypothyroidism. Abnormal clinical findings often do not exist. Occasionally, evidence of respiratory and feeding difficulty, abdominal distention, icterus, dry skin, postmaturity, a large posterior fontanelle, macroglossia, an umbilical hernia, and hypothermia allow the diagnosis to be made on clinical grounds. Cretinism, extremely rare in the United States, may resemble Down's syndrome.

A longitudinal study of 85 children in Quebec tested at the age of 7, and 25 children again tested at the age of 12, has demonstrated that the initial biochemical status of neonates with congenital hypothyroidism at birth determines their intellectual outcome based on Wechsler Intelligence Scales for Children, Revised. As a group, the patients had results within the normal range of the test. The children with severe hypothyroidism at birth, however, clearly had lower scores than those with more moderate hypothyroidism. Furthermore, the severely affected children scored significantly lower than their siblings, whereas there was no significant difference in test results between those who were moderately affected with hypothyroidism at birth and their normal siblings (Glorieux, 1991) (Table 55–8). Studies from Australia, Norway, and Britain also indicate that children with low thyroxine levels at birth have lower mean IQs than matched controls (Richards et al., 1989; Heyerdahl et al., 1991).

Treatment with levothyroxine, 10 to 15 μg/kg per day or 50 μg daily, is initiated as soon as the diagnosis of hypothyroidism is made, even though it is recognized that 10 per cent of cases will be transient, particularly in cases of prematurity, iodine deficiency or excess, or blocking antibody-mediated disease, or in those cases related to drug therapy (Fisher and Foley, 1989). In a recent study from Japan, 23 neonates of mothers with autoimmune thyroiditis during pregnancy were described (Matsuura and Konishi, 1990). All babies had transient neonatal hypothyroidism from maternal TSH-binding inhibitory antibodies. Babies born to mothers who were severely hypothyroid during pregnancy because of poor compliance had a mean IQ of only 66. In contrast, the children of mothers who were treated appropriately and remained euthyroid throughout the pregnancy had normal intelligence with a mean IQ of 104. Most other variables were comparable between the two groups of infants including the levels of antibody, TSH, and T_4 at birth; the therapy provided at birth; and the duration of therapy. This study reinforces the prevalent belief that maternal thyroid hormone status *in utero* affects fetal, neonatal, and childhood neurointellectual development (Delange, 1991).

The placental transfer of blocking antibodies is rare and thus does not warrant screening with anti–TSH receptor antibody assays in every pregnant woman with autoimmune thyroiditis. When a neonate of a mother with autoimmune thyroiditis is diagnosed with hypothyroidism, however, antibody titers should be measured. An elevated titer in the neonate implies that the hypothyroidism is likely to be transient, and discontinuation of therapy can be attempted after several months (Delange, 1991). In women with idiopathic hypothyroidism, also known as atrophic hy-

Table 55–8. WISCR Results at the Age of 7 Years*

SEVERE HYPOTHYROIDISM		SIBLINGS n = 12 PAIRS	
	mean SD	mean SD	
Global IQ	86 +/− 13	103 +/− 13	P<.01
Verbal IQ	83 +/− 11	98 +/− 12	P<.01
Performance IQ	93 +/− 14	109 +/− 16	P<.03
MODERATE HYPOTHYROIDISM		SIBLINGS n = 30 PAIRS	
	mean SD	mean SD	
Global IQ	102 +/− 12	104 +/− 8	N.S.
Verbal IQ	97 +/− 12	100 +/− 10	N.S.
Performance IQ	108 +/− 12	109 +/− 8	N.S.

*Results of Wechsler Intelligence Scales for Children, Revised (WISC-R) comparing children 7 years of age born with either severe or moderate hypothyroidism with their normal siblings.

From Glorieux: Developmental outcome of children with congenital hypothyroidism: long-term assessment. *In* Beckers C, Reinwein D (eds): The Thyroid and Pregnancy. New York, Wiley, 1992.

pothyroidism, anti–TSH receptor assays are predictive of neonatal hypothyroidism and should be measured during the third trimester of pregnancy (Tamaki et al., 1989; Orgiazzi et al., 1991).

Fetuses at high risk for the development of hypothyroidism have been born euthyroid after treatment by intra-amniotic injections of levothyroxine (Lightner et al., 1977), but therapy for *in utero* hypothyroidism is unquestionably difficult. Treatment of the mother with oral levothyroxine is not particularly helpful, because to deliver significant amounts of hormone to the fetus, the mother must be made markedly hyperthyroid (Fisher et al., 1964).

Because we do not know the neurologic effects of transient *in utero* hypothyroidism and because it is difficult to treat, it is imperative to carefully monitor the mother and the fetus in high-risk cases. For example, mothers on thionamide therapy or levothyroxine replacement therapy should be seen at least monthly once a euthyroid state has been achieved. The fetus should undergo ultrasonography in search of goiter, bradycardia, and intrauterine growth retardation. As cordocentesis becomes a more routine and accepted procedure, prenatal diagnosis and treatment may become more satisfactory (Davidson et al., 1991).

THYROID NODULES, MALIGNANT TUMORS, AND NONTOXIC GOITER AND PREGNANCY

The finding of a solitary nodule during pregnancy requires fine-needle aspiration to investigate the possibility of malignancy. Free T$_4$ and TSH levels should be obtained to rule out the possibility of a toxic nodule or an unusual presentation of Hashimoto's thyroiditis. Radioisotope scanning is contraindicated during pregnancy. Ultrasonography may or may not be helpful.

Thyroid carcinoma rarely presents during pregnancy. Previous studies have reported that pregnancy does not affect the prognosis of thyroid cancer (Rosvoll and Winship, 1965; Hill et al., 1966). More recent reports suggest that there may be a small impact on the progression of thyroid cancer (Fukuda et al., 1991). In the rare case of thyroid carcinoma diagnosed during pregnancy, surgery is recommended. [131]Iodine-ablation therapy should be postponed until after delivery.

The great majority of thyroid cancers in young women are of well-differentiated papillary, mixed papillary-follicular, or follicular histology. Cure is frequent, and even in the case of residual disease, the course is generally indolent. When including the much more aggressive anaplastic and medullary thyroid carcinomas, the overall mortality may reach 10 per cent.

A nontoxic goiter may enlarge during pregnancy. Existing data do not point to the appropriate treatment for iodine-replete pregnant women who had a nontoxic goiter prior to conception. Some authors recommend treatment with levothyroxine to prevent further enlargement (Koutras, 1991).

POSTPARTUM THYROIDITIS

Signs and Symptoms

Abnormalities in thyroid function are frequent following pregnancy, occurring in 4 to 7 per cent, or one in every 20, postpartum women (Gerstein, 1990). This condition often goes undiagnosed because symptoms occur after the standard 6-week postpartum follow-up appointment and the symptoms are often attributed by the patient and her family to the added stress of the newborn. The first report of thyroid dysfunction

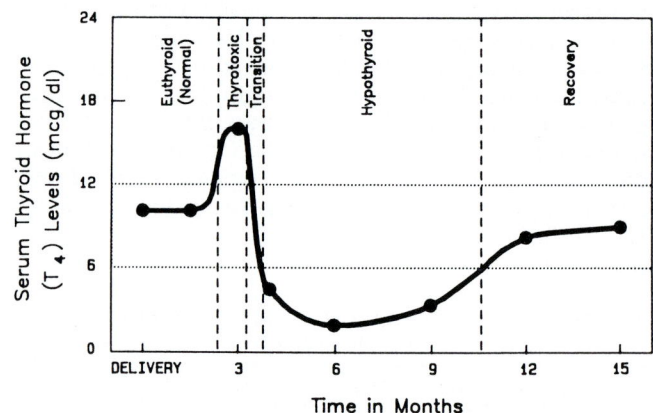

FIGURE 55–10. Thyroid function during postpartum thyroiditis. (From Smallridge et al: Postpartum thyroiditis. The Bridge 3:3, 1988. Newsletter of the Thyroid Foundation of America, Inc.)

following pregnancy appeared in 1874 (Gull, 1874), but it was not until more than 100 years later that the link to autoimmune thyroid disease was described (Amino et al., 1976).

The hallmark of postpartum thyroiditis, or silent thyroiditis as it is sometimes called, is its transient nature (Jansson et al., 1988). Careful study has delineated a typical clinical course for this disease (Fig. 55–10). Initially, 75 per cent of women will experience a thyrotoxic phase beginning about 2 to 3 months postpartum. Symptoms of fatigue, weight loss, palpitations, and dizziness experienced in the thyrotoxic phase are accepted by many new mothers as a natural part of a normal postpartum course. The following hypothyroid phase, seen about 4 to 8 months postpartum, is usually more clinically evident with complaints primarily of fatigue and weight gain. Dry skin, constipation, and cold intolerance are not common. Goiter, which appears in 50 per cent of the patients, may be noted at this time, and some women experience depression. Most patients return to the euthyroid state after 3 to 5 months, although 10 to 30 per cent develop permanent hypothyroidism. Although there is marked variability in presentations between patients, recurrence in a single patient with a similar course and intensity usually occurs after subsequent pregnancies (Amino et al., 1982; Jansson et al., 1984; Tachi et al., 1988).

The association of postpartum depression and psychosis with postpartum thyroiditis has yet to be confirmed. Postpartum depression has an incidence of 10 to 15 per cent and usually develops in the third postnatal week, although the diagnosis often is not made until the fourth or fifth month postpartum. It is a self-limited disease, and two-thirds of the patients recover by the end of the first year (Watson et al., 1984). This depression follows a time course not unlike that of postpartum thyroiditis.

Hamilton has successfully treated more than 200 women with postpartum depression with thyroid hormone, and depressive symptoms have been well documented to occur with an increased frequency in women with postpartum hypothyroidism (Hayslip et al., 1988). A recent study of 95 women with positive antithyroid peroxidase antibodies and 150 antibody-negative women were observed by follow-up for 9 months postpartum. The group with positive antithyroid peroxidase antibodies developed significantly more depressive symptomatology than the control group (Lazarus et al., 1991). Although suggestive, the relationship between postnatal depression and thyroid dysfunction remains speculative.

Psychosis can occur with thyrotoxicosis (Spratt et al., 1982), but Jansson (1984) has reported normal thyroid hormone values in women with postpartum psychosis, and Stewart et al. found antimicrosomal antibodies present in only 5 per cent of women with psychosis. These patients did have an elevated free T_4 index and a lower TSH than controls, but the values remained within normal limits (Stewart et al., 1988). Although the association between psychiatric disturbance and postnatal thyroid dysfunction remains ill defined, any woman with depression or other psychiatric symptoms in the year after delivery should be carefully examined and evaluated with a TSH and a free T_4.

Etiology, Screening, and Diagnosis

Postpartum thyroiditis is characterized histologically as a destructive, lymphocytic thyroiditis, and thyroid antimicrosomal antibodies can be detected in most women with this condition (Jansson et al., 1984). Antithyroid antibody levels decrease as pregnancy progresses, but there is a postpartum resurgence reaching a peak at about six months, coinciding with the peak incidence of postpartum hypothyroidism. As antibody titers fall, the hypothyroidism resolves (Figs. 55–10 and 55–11).

Postpartum thyroiditis is thus an autoimmune disease, and as with many other autoimmune diseases, the pathogenesis is not clearly understood. DeGroot has hypothesized that multiple factors interact to supply the backdrop for the development of this disease. Inheritance plays a role as those with histocompatibility antigen DR-5 have a six-fold greater risk of developing postpartum thyroiditis (Weetman and McGregor, 1984). Evidence of both humoral and cellular immune dysfunction exists because antimicrosomal antibody titers are elevated in the postpartum period, as is the ratio of helper to T suppressor cells (Sridama et al., 1982). Environment may also be an active factor as geographic differences exist in the incidence of this disease (Jansson et al., 1988).

The level of antimicrosomal antibody in the first trimester of pregnancy may be used to predict the development of postpartum thyroiditis in those at risk. Hemagglutination titers of 1:6400 or higher routinely predict postpartum thyroiditis, while those less than 1:100 virtually exclude it (Jansson et al., 1984). First-trimester screening with antimicrosomal antibodies is advisable for any woman with a personal or family history of thyroid disease. If the titer is positive, the patient should be followed throughout pregnancy and the postpartum period, carefully monitoring the TSH and free T_4 concentrations (Ramsay, 1986). Measuring antimicrosomal antibodies on the second postpartum

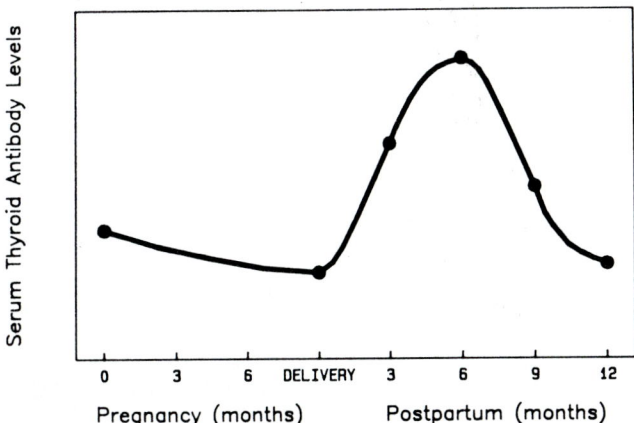

FIGURE 55–11. Thyroid antibody levels during and after pregnancy. (From Smallridge et al: Postpartum thyroiditis. The Bridge 3:3, 1988. Newsletter of the Thyroid Foundation of America, Inc.)

day is also predictive of the development of postpartum thyroiditis and may be more cost effective than evaluating all symptomatic women with thyroid hormone tests (Hayslip et al., 1988).

The diagnosis of postpartum thyroiditis is made by abnormal free T_4 and TSH values in the postpartum period coupled with a positive titer of antimicrosomal antibodies. Although rarely necessary, confirmation can be obtained by documenting a low uptake on radioactive iodine thyroid scanning. [123]Iodine should be used because of its shorter half-life, and breast-feeding should be interrupted for at least 5 days after the test.

Treatment

Treatment of postpartum thyroiditis is based on symptoms and usually is not necessary. If symptoms of hypothyroidism become prominent, replacement therapy with levothyroxine should be initiated. Therapy should be withdrawn gradually one year postpartum to determine whether the condition is permanent. Those who develop marked symptoms early in the postpartum period without goiter are more likely to have permanent hypothyroidism (Jansson et al., 1988).

Symptoms of thyrotoxicosis can be temporarily treated with beta blockers if necessary. A depressed radioiodine thyroid uptake differentiates postpartum thyroiditis from Graves' disease. Those with Graves' disease usually do not have antimicrosomal antibody titers and often develop the thyrotoxicosis later than 3 to 4 months after delivery. Thionamide therapy is not indicated for treatment of postpartum thyrotoxicosis because the thyroid hormone excess results from release of stored hormone by the damaged gland, rather than from increased synthesis and secretion.

All women who have experienced postpartum thyroiditis should be followed closely as they are at high risk (10 to 25 per cent) for a recurrence after subsequent pregnancies, as well as for the development of permanent hypothyroidism (Walfish and Chan, 1985; Tachi et al., 1988; Roti et al., 1991). Other autoimmune conditions such as Addison's disease or premature ovarian failure syndrome may develop.

REFERENCES

Abdoul-Khair SA, Crooks J, Turnbull AC, et al: The physiological changes in thyroid function during pregnancy. Clin Sci 27:195, 1964.

Ain KB, Mori Y, Refetoff S: Reduced clearance rate of thyroxine-binding globulin (TBG) with increased sialylation: A mechanism for estrogen-induced elevation of serum TBG concentration. J Clin Endocrinol Metab 65:689, 1987.

Ain KB, Refetoff S: Relationship of oligosaccharide modification to the cause of serum thyroxine-binding globulin excess. J Clin Endocrinol Metab 66:1037, 1988.

Ain KB, Refetoff S, Sarne DH, et al: Effect of estrogen on the synthesis and secretion of thyroxine-binding globulin by a human hepatoma cell line, HEP G2. Molec Endocrinol 2:313, 1988.

Akande EO: The effect of oestrogen on plasma levels of luteinizing hormone in euthyroid and thyrotoxic postmenopausal women. Br J Obstet Gynecol 81:795, 1974.

Akande EO, Hockaday TDR: Plasma luteinizing hormone levels in women with thyrotoxicosis. J Endocrinol 53:173, 1972.

Amino N: Autoimmunity and hypothyroidism. Baillieres Clin Endocrinol Metab 2:591, 1988.

Amino N, Kuro R, Tanizawa O, et al: Changes of serum antithyroid antibodies during and after pregnancy in autoimmune thyroid diseases. Clin Exp Immunol 31:30, 1978.

Amino N, Miyai K, Onishi T, et al: Transient hypothyroidism after delivery in autoimmune thyroiditis. J Clin Endocrinol Metab 42:296, 1976.

Amino N, Mori H, Iwatani Y, et al: High prevalence of transient postpartum thyrotoxicosis and hypothyroidism. N Engl J Med 306:849, 1982.

Baker JR Jr, Saunders NB, Wartofsky L, et al: Seronegative Hashimoto's thyroiditis with thyroid autoantibody production localized to the thyroid. Ann Intern Med 108:26, 1988.

Ballabio M, Nicoline U, Jowett T, Ruiz de Elvira MC, Ekins RP, Rodeck CH: Maturation of thyroid function in normal human foetuses. Clin Endocrinol 31:565, 1989.

Ballabio M, Poshyachinda M, Ekins RP: Pregnancy-induced changes in thyroid function: Role of human chorionic gonadotropin as putative regulator of maternal thyroid. J Clin Endocrinol Metab 73:824, 1991.

Bech K, Hertel, Rasmussen NG, et al: Effect of maternal thyroid autoantibodies and post-partum thyroiditis on the fetus and neonate. Acta Endocrinol (Copenh) 125:146, 1991a.

Bech K, Hoier-Madsen, Feldt-Rasmussen U, et al: Thyroid function and autoimmune manifestations in insulin-dependent diabetes mellitus during and after pregnancy. Acta Endocrinol (Copenh) 124:534, 1991b.

Beckers C: Iodine economy in and around pregnancy. In Beckers C, Reinwein D (eds): The Thyroid and Pregnancy. New York, Wiley, 1992.

Becks GP, Burrow G: Thyroid disease and pregnancy. Med Clin North Am 75:121, 1991.

Beer AE: New horizons in the diagnosis, evaluation and therapy of recurrent spontaneous abortion. Clin Obstet Gynaecol 13:115, 1986.

Bernal J, Pekonen F: Ontogenesis of nuclear 3,5,3' triiodothyronine receptors in human fetal brain. Endocrinology 114:677, 1984.

Bitton RN, Slavin M, Decker RE, et al: The course of lymphocytic hypophysitis. Surg Neurol 36:40, 1991.

Bizzarro A, Fontano A, De Bellis A, et al: T-lymphocyte subsets in pregnant women with Graves' disease. Acta Endocrinol (Copenh) 114:218, 1987.

Bogner U, Gruters A, Sigle B, et al: Cytotoxic antibodies in congenital hypothyroidism. J Clin Endocrinol Metab 68:671, 1989.

Bohnet HG, Fiedler K, Leidenberger FA: Subclinical hypothyroidism and infertility. Lancet 2:1278, 1981.

Brander A, Kivisaari L: Ultrasonography of the thyroid during pregnancy. J Clin Ultrasound 17:403, 1989.

Brent GA, Hershman JM: Thyroxine therapy in patients with severe nonthyroidal illnesses and low serum thyroxine concentration. J Clin Endocrinol Metab 63:1, 1986.

Burrow GN: Hyperthyroidism during pregnancy. N Engl J Med 298:150, 1978.

Burrow GN: The management of thyrotoxicosis in pregnancy. N Engl J Med 313:562, 1985.

Burrow GN: The thyroid gland and reproduction. In Yen SSC, Jaffe R: Reproductive Endocrinology, 3rd ed. W.B. Saunders, 1991, p 292.

Burrow GN, Bartsocas L, Klatskin EH, et al: Children exposed in utero to propylthiouracil: Subsequent intellectual and physical development. Am J Dis Child 116:161, 1968.

Burrow GN, Klatskin EH, Genel M: Intellectual development in children whose mothers received propylthiouracil in pregnancy. Yale J Biol Med 51:151, 1978.

Burrow GN, May PB, Spaulding SW, Donabedian RK: TRH and dopamine interactions affecting pituitary hormone secretion. J Clin Endocrinol Metab 45:65, 1977.

Burrow GN, Polackwich R, Donabedian R: Perinatal Thyroid Physiology and Disease. New York, Raven Press, 1975, p 1.

Cheron RG, Kaplan MM, Larsen PR, et al: Neonatal thyroid function after propylthiouracil therapy for maternal Graves' disease. N Engl J Med 304:525, 1981.

Chin RKH, Lao TT, Swaminathan R, et al: A longitudinal study of changes in erythrocyte zinc concentration in hyperemesis gravidarum. Gynecol Obstet Invest 29:22, 1990.

Clark DA, Slapsys R, Chaput A, et al: Immunoregulatory molecules of trophoblast and decidual suppressor cell origin at the maternofetal interface. Am J Reprod Immunol Microbiol 10:100, 1986.

Clavel S, Madec AM, Bornet H, et al: Anti TSH-receptor antibodies in pregnant patients with autoimmune thyroid disorder. Br J Obstet Gynaecol 97:1003, 1990.

Colbern GT, Main EK: Immunology of the maternal-placental interface in normal pregnancy. Semin Perinatol 15:196, 1991.

Cooper DS: Antithyroid drugs. N Engl J Med 311:1353, 1984.

Cooper DS: Antithyroid drugs: To breastfeed or not to breastfeed. Am J Obstet Gynecol 157:234, 1987.

Cooper DS, Goldminz D, Levin AA, et al: Agranulocytosis associated with antithyroid drugs. Ann Intern Med 98:26, 1983.

Cooper DS, Ladenson PW, Nisula BC, et al: Familial thyroid hormone resistance. Metabolism 31:504, 1982.

Crooks J, Tulloch MI, Turnbull AC, et al: Comparative incidence of goiter in pregnancy in Iceland and Scotland. Lancet 2:625, 1967.

Davidson KM, Richards DS, Schatz DA, et al: Successful in utero treatment of fetal goiter and hypothyroidism. N Engl J Med 324:543, 1991.

Davis LE, Leveno KJ, Cunningham FG: Hypothyroidism complicating pregnancy. Obstet Gynecol 72:108, 1988.

Davis LE, Lucas MJ, Hankins GDV, et al: Thyrotoxicosis complicating pregnancy. Am J Obstet Gynecol 160:63, 1989.

DeGroot LJ, Niepomnizcze H: Biosynthesis of thyroid hormone: Basic and clinical aspects. Metabolism 26:665, 1977.

Delange F: Neonatal hypothyroidism: recent developments. Baillieres Clin Endocrinol Metab 2:637, 1988.

Delange F: Effect of maternal thyroid function during pregnancy on fetal development. In Beckers C, Reinwein D (eds): The Thyroid and Pregnancy. New York, Wiley, 1992.

Del Pozo E, Wyss H, Tolis G, et al: Prolactin and deficient luteal function. Obstet Gynecol 53:282, 1979.

Dillmann WH: Mechanism of action of thyroid hormones. Med Clin North Am 69:849, 1985.

Dussault JH: Development of thyroid function. In Beckers C, Reinwein D (eds): The Thyroid and Pregnancy. Schattauer, 1991, pp 3–6.

Dussault JH, Rousseau F: Immunologically-mediated hypothyroidism. Endocrinol Metab Clin North Am 16:417, 1987.

Elkins R: Roles of serum thyroxine binding proteins and maternal thyroid hormones in fetal development. Lancet i:1129, 1985.

Evans AJ, Li TC, Selby C, et al: Morning sickness and thyroid function. Br J Obstet Gynecol 93:520, 1986.

Ferris TF: Renal disease. In Burrow GN, Ferris TF (eds): Medical Complications During Pregnancy. Philadelphia, WB Saunders Co., 1988.

Fisher DA, Dussault JH, Sack J, et al: Ontogenesis of hypothalamic-pituitary-thyroid function and metabolism in man, sheep and rat. Recent Progr Horm Res 3:59, 1977.

Fisher DA, Foley BL: Early treatment of congenital hypothyroidism. Pediatrics 83:785, 1989.

Fisher DA, Klein AH: Thyroid development and disorders of thyroid function in the newborn. N Engl J Med 304:702, 1981.

Fisher DA, Lehman H, Lackey C: Placental transport of thyroxine. J Clin Endocrinol Metab 24:393, 1964.

Fisher DA, Polk DH: Development of the thyroid. Baillieres Clin Endocrinol Metab 3:627, 1989.

Froelich CJ: Pregnancy, a temporary fetal graft of suppressor cells in autoimmune disease? Am J Med 69:329, 1980.

Fukuda K, Hachisuga T, Sugimori H, et al: Papillary carcinoma of the thyroid occurring during pregnancy. Acta Cytologica 35:725, 1991.

Gerhard I, Becker T, Eggert-Kruse W, et al: Thyroid and ovarian function in infertile women. Hum Reprod 6:338, 1991.

Gershengorn MC: Thyrotropin releasing hormone. Mol Cell Biochem 45:163, 1982.

Gerstein HC: How common is postpartum thyroiditis? Arch Intern Med 150:1397, 1990.

Gladstone GR, Hordof A, Gersony WM: Propranolol administration during pregnancy: effects on the fetus. J Pediatr 86:962, 1975.

Glinoer D, De Nayer P, Bourdoux P, et al: Regulation of maternal thyroid during pregnancy. J Clin Endocrinol Metab 71:276, 1990.

Glinoer D, Soto MF, Bourdoux P, et al: Pregnancy in patients with mild thyroid abnormalities: Maternal and neonatal repercussions. J Clin Endocrinol Metab 73:421, 1991.

Glorieux J: Developmental outcome of children with congenital hypothyroidism: long-term assessment. In Beckers C, Reinwein D (eds): The Thyroid and Pregnancy. New York, Wiley, 1992.

Goldsmith RE, Sturgis SH, Lerman J, et al: The menstrual pattern in thyroid disease. J Clin Endocrinol Metab 12:846, 1952.

Goodwin TM, Montoro M, Mestman JH, et al: The role of chorionic gonadotropin in transient hyperthyroidism of hyperemesis gravidarum. Trans Assoc Am Physicians CIV:233, 1991.

Goodwin TM, Montoro M, Mestman JH: The role of chorionic gonadotropin in transient hyperthyroidism of hyperemesis gravidarum. J Clin Endocrinol Metab 75:1333, 1992.

Greenman GW, Gabrielson MO, Howard-Flanders J, Wessel MA: Thyroid dysfunction in pregnancy. Fetal loss and follow-up evaluation of surviving infants. N Engl J Med 267:426, 1962.

Guillaume J, Schussler GC, Goldman J: Components of the total serum thyroid hormone concentrations during pregnancy: High free thyroxine and blunted thyrotropin (TSH) response to TSH-releasing hormone in the first trimester. J Clin Endocrinol Metab 60:678, 1985.

Gull WW: On a cretinoid state supervening in adult life in women. Trans Clin Soc London 7:180, 1874.

Habib A, McCarthy JS: Effects on the neonate of propranolol administered during pregnancy. J Pediatr 91:808, 1977.

Halnan KE: The radioiodine uptake of the human thyroid in pregnancy. Clin Sci 17:281, 1958.

Harada A, Hershman JM, Reed AW, et al: Comparison of thyroid stimulators and thyroid hormone concentration in the sera of pregnant women. J Clin Endocrinol Metab 48:793, 1979.

Hashizume K, Ichikawa K, Sakurai A, et al: Administration of thyroxine in treated Graves' disease. N Engl J Med 4:324(14):947, 1991.

Hayslip CC, Fein HG, O'Donnell VM, et al: The value of serum antimicrosomal antibody testing in screening for symptomatic postpartum thyroid dysfunction. Am J Obstet Gynecol 159:203, 1988.

Hetzel BS: Progression in the prevention and control of iodine deficiency disorders. Lancet ii:266, 1987.

Heyerdahl S, Kase BF, Lie SO: Intellectual development in children with congenital hypothyroidism in relation to recommended thyroxine treatment. J Pediatr 118:850, 1991.

Hill CS, Clark RL, Wolf M: The effect of subsequent pregnancy on patients with thyroid carcinoma. Surg Gynecol Obstet 122:1219, 1966.

Honbo KS, Van Herle AJ, Kellett KA: Serum prolactin levels in untreated primary hypothyroidism. Am J Med 64:782, 1978.

Houck JA, Davis RE, Sharma HM: Thyroid-stimulating immunoglobulin as a cause of recurrent intrauterine fetal death. Obstet Gynecol 71:1018, 1988.

Iseki M, Shimizi YM, Oikawa T, et al: Sequential serum measurements of thyrotropin binding inhibition immunoglobulin G in transient familial neonatal hypothyroidism. J Clin Endocrinol Metab 57:384, 1983.

Isley WL, Dahl S, Gibbs H: Use of esmolol in managing a thyrotoxic patient needing emergency surgery. Am J Med 89:122, 1990.

Jansson R, Bernander S, Karlsson A, et al: Autoimmune thyroid dysfunction in the postpartum period. J Clin Endocrinol Metab 58:681, 1984.

Jansson R, Dahlberg PA, Karlsson F: Postpartum thyroiditis. Baillieres Clin Endocrinol Metab 2:619, 1988.

Jeffcoate WJ, Bain C: Recurrent pregnancy-induced thyrotoxicosis presenting as hyperemesis gravidarum: Case report Br J Obstet Gynaecol 92:413, 1982.

Johnson MR, McGregor AM: Endocrine disease and pregnancy. Baillieres Clin Endocrinol Metab 4:313, 1990.

Jones WS, Man EB: Thyroid Function in human pregnancy. VI. Premature deliveries and reproduction failure of pregnant women with low butanol extractable iodines. Am J Obstet Gynecol 104:909, 1969.

Jovanovic-Peterson L, Peterson CM: De novo clinical hypothyroidism in pregnancies complicated by type I diabetes, subclinical hypothyroidism and proteinuria. Am J Obstet Gynecol 159:442, 1988.

Kaplan NM: Metabolism of thyroid hormones. In Dussault JH, Walker P (eds): Congenital Hypothyroidism. New York, Marcel Dekker, 1983, pp 11–35.

Kasagi K, Hidaka A, Hatabu H, et al: Stimulation of cAMP production in FRTL-5 thyroid cells by crude immunoglobulin fractions of serum from pregnant women. Clin Endocrinol **31**:267, 1989.

Kennedy RL, Darne J: The role of hCG in regulation of the thyroid gland in normal and abnormal pregnancy. Obstet Gynecol **78**:298, 1991.

Kennedy RL, Darne J, Cohn M, et al: Human chorionic gonadotropin may not be responsible for thyroid-stimulating activity in normal pregnancy serum. J Clin Endocrinol Metab **74**:260, 1992.

Kennedy RL, Darne J, Griffiths H, et al: Thyroid-stimulatory effects of human chorionic gonadotropin in early pregnancy. In vivo and in vitro studies. Horm Res **33**:117, 1990.

Khalil A, Kovacs K, Sima AAF, et al: Pituitary thyrotroph hyperplasia mimicking prolactin-secreting adenoma. J Endocrinol Invest **7**:399, 1984.

Kimura M, Amino N, Tamaki H, et al: Physiologic thyroid activation in normal early pregnancy is induced by circulating hCG. Obstet Gynecol **75**:775, 1990.

Klein I, Levely GS: Unusual manifestations of hypothyroidism. Arch Intern Med **144**:123, 1984.

Klein RZ, Haddow JE, Faix JD, et al: Prevalence of thyroid deficiency in pregnant women. Clin Endocrinol **35**:41, 1991.

Konishi J, Iida Y, Kasagi K, et al: Primary myxedema with thyrotrophin-binding inhibitor immunoglobulins: clinical and laboratory findings in 15 patients. Ann Intern Med **103**:26, 1985.

Koutras DA: Prevention and treatment of nontoxic goiter during pregnancy. In Beckers C, Reinwein D (eds): The Thyroid and Pregnancy. New York, Wiley, 1992.

Lazarus JH, Othman S, Harris B, et al: Postpartum thyroiditis and psychiatric aspects. In Beckers C, Reinwein D (eds): The Thyroid and Pregnancy. New York, Wiley, 1992.

Leung AS, Millar LK, Koonings PP, et al: Perinatal outcome in hypothyroid patients. Obstet and Gynecol **81**:349, 1993.

Lever EG, Medeiros-Neto GA, DeGroot LJ: Inherited disorders of thyroid metabolism. Endocrinol Rev **4**:213, 1983.

Levy RP, Newman DM, Rejali LS, et al: The myth of goiter in pregnancy. Am J Obstet Gynecol **137**:701, 1980.

Lightner ES, Fisher DA, Giles H, et al: Intra-amniotic injections of thyroxine (T_4) to a human fetus. Am J Obstet Gynecol **127**:487, 1977.

Long TJ, Felice ME, Hollingsworth DR: Goiter in pregnant teenagers. Am J Obstet Gynecol **152**:670, 1985.

Mandel SJ, Larsen PR, Seely EW, et al: Increased need for thyroxine during pregnancy in women with primary hypothyroidism. N Engl J Med **323**:91, 1990.

Mann K, Schneider N, Hoermann R: Thyrotropic activity of acidic isoelectric variants of human chorionic gonadotropin from trophoblastic tumors. Endocrinology **118**:1558, 1986.

Mariotti S, Martino E, Cupini C: Low serum thyroglobulin as a clue to the diagnosis of thyrotoxicosis factitia. N Engl J Med **307**:410, 1982.

Mariotti S, Chiovato L, Vitti P, et al: Recent advances in the understanding of humoral and cellular mechanisms implicated in thyroid autoimmune disorders. Clin Immunol Immunopath **50**:573, 1989.

Matsuura N, Konishi J: Transient hypothyroidism in infants born to mothers with chronic thyroiditis. A nationwide study of 23 cases. Endocrinol Jpn **37**:369, 1990.

Matsuura N, Yamada Y, Nohara Y, et al: Familial neonatal transient hypothyroidism due to maternal TSH-binding inhibitor immunoglobulins. N Engl J Med **103**:738, 1980.

Medawar PB: Some immunological and endocrinological problems raised by the evolution of viviparity in vertebrates. Symp Soc Exp Biol **7**:320, 1953.

Medvei VC: A History of Endocrinology. Boston, MTP Press, 1982, pp 57–58.

Messer PM, Hauffa BP, Olbricht T, et al: Antithyroid drug treatment of Graves' disease in pregnancy: Long-term effects on somatic growth, intellectual development and thyroid function of the offspring. Acta Endocrinol (Copenh) **123**:311, 1990.

Miyauchi A, Amino N, Tamaki H, et al: Coexistence of thyroid-stimulating and thyroid-blocking antibodies in a patient with Graves' disease who had transient hypothyroidism. Am J Med **85**:418, 1988.

Momotani N, Ito K, Hamada N, et al: Maternal hyperthyroidism and congenital malformation in the offspring. Clin Endocrinol **20**:695, 1984.

Momotani N, Noh J, Oyanagi H, et al: Antithyroid drug therapy for Graves' disease during pregnancy. N Engl J Med **315**:24, 1986.

Montoro M, Collea JV, Frasier SD, et al: Successful outcome of pregnancy in women with hypothyroidism. Ann Intern Med **94**:31, 1981.

Morales WJ, O'Brien WF, Angel JL, et al: Fetal lung maturation: the combined use of corticosteroids and thyrotropin-releasing hormone. Obstet Gynecol **73**:111, 1989.

Morgan LS: Hormonally active gynecologic tumors. Semin Surg Oncol **6**:83, 1990.

Mori M, Amino N, Tamaki H, et al: Morning sickness and thyroid function in normal pregnancy. Obstet Gynecol **72**:355, 1988.

Morley JE, Bashore RA, Reed A, et al: Thyrotropin-releasing hormone and thyroid hormones in amniotic fluid. Am J Obstet Gynecol **134**:581, 1979.

Morreale de Escobar G, Calvo R, Obregon MJ, et al: Contribution of maternal thyroxine to fetal thyroxine pools in normal rats near term. Endocrinology **126**:2765, 1990.

Morreale de Escobar G, Obregon MJ, Escobar del Rey F: Fetal and maternal thyroid hormones. Horm Res **26**:12, 1987.

Morreale de Escobar G, Obregon MJ, Ruiz de Ona C, et al: Transfer of thyroxine from the mother to the rat fetus near term: effects on brain 3,5,3'-triiodothyronine deficiency. Endocrinology **122**:1521, 1988.

Morreale de Escobar G, Obregon MJ, Ruiz de Ona C, et al: Comparison of maternal to fetal transfer of 3,5,3'-triiodothyronine versus thyroxine in rats, as assessed from 3,5,3'-triiodothyronine levels in fetal tissues. Acta Endocrinol (Copenh) **120**:20, 1989.

Mortimer RH, Tyack SA, Galligan JP, et al: Graves' disease in pregnancy: TSH receptor binding inhibiting immunoglobulins and maternal and neonatal thyroid function. Clin Endocrinol **32**:141, 1990.

Moya F, Mena P, Foradori A, et al: Effect of maternal administration of thyrotropin releasing hormone on the preterm fetal pituitary-thyroid axis. J Pediatr **119**:966, 1991.

Mujtaba Q, Burrow GN: Treatment of hyperthyroidism in pregnancy with PTU and methimazole. Obstet Gynecol **46**:282, 1975.

Nelson M, Wickus GG, Caplan RH, et al: Thyroid gland size in pregnancy. J Reprod Med **32**:888, 1987.

Niswander KR, Gordon M (eds): The collaborative perinatal study of the National Institute of Neurological Disease and Stroke: the women and their pregnancies. US Department of Health, Education and Welfare, 1972, pp 246–249.

Oppenheimer JH: Role of plasma proteins in the binding, distribution and metabolism of the thyroid hormones. N Engl J Med **278**:1153, 1968.

Oppenheimer JH: Thyroid hormone action at the cellular level. Science **203**:971, 1979.

Oppenheimer JH: Thyroid hormone action at the nuclear level. Ann Intern Med **102**:374, 1985.

Orgiazzi J, Rodien P, Morel Y, et al: Thyroid autoimmune disorders and pregnancy. In Beckers C, Reinwein D (eds): The Thyroid and Pregnancy. New York, Wiley, 1992.

Page DV, Brady K, Mitchell J, et al: The pathology of intrauterine thyrotoxicosis: two case reports. Obstet Gynecol **72**:479, 1988.

Polk DH: Thyroid hormone effects on neonatal thermogenesis. Semin Perinatol **12**:151, 1988.

Porreco RP, Bloch CA: Fetal blood sampling in the management of intrauterine thyrotoxicosis. Obstet Gynecol **76**:509, 1990.

Price A, Griffiths H, Morris BW: A longitudinal study of thyroid function in pregnancy. Clin Chem **35**:275, 1989.

Ramsay I: Postpartum thyroiditis—an underdiagnosed disease. Br J Obstet Gynaecol **93**:1121, 1986.

Ramsay I, Kaur S, Krassas G: Thyrotoxicosis in pregnancy: Results of treatment by antithyroid drugs combined with T_4. Clin Endocrinol **18**:73, 1983.

Rao SN, Katiyar BC, Nair KRP, et al: Neuromuscular status in hypothyroidism. Acta Neurol Scand **61**:167, 1980.

Rasmussen NG, Hornnes PJ, Hegedus L, et al: Serum thyroglobulin during the menstrual cycle, during pregnancy, and postpartum. Acta Endocrinol (Copenh) **121**:168, 1989.

Richards A, Coakley J, Francis I, et al: Results at follow-up at 5 years in a group of hypothyroid Australian children detected by newborn screening. *In* Delange F, Fisher DA (eds): Research in Congenital Hypothyroidism. New York, Plenum, 1989, pp 3111.

Rogers J: Menstruation and systemic disease. N Engl J Med **259**:676, 1958.

Rosenthal FD, Jones C, Lewis SI: Thyrotoxic vomiting. Br Med J **2**:209, 1976.

Rosvoll RN, Winship T: Thyroid carcinoma and pregnancy. Surg Gynecol Obstet **121**:1039, 1965.

Roti E, Gnudi A, Braverman LE: The placental transport, synthesis and metabolism of hormones and drugs which affect thyroid function. Endocrinol Rev **4**:131, 1983.

Roti E, Gnudi A, Braverman LE, et al: Human cord blood concentrations of thyrotropin, thyroglobulin and iodothyronines after maternal administration of thyrotropin-releasing hormone. J Clin Endocrinol Metab **53**:813, 1981.

Roti E, Minelli R, Gardini E, et al: Impaired intrathyroidal iodine organification and iodine-induced hypothyroidism in euthyroid women with a previous episode of postpartum thyroiditis. J Clin Endocrinol Metab **73**:958, 1991.

Rotmensch S, Scommegna A: Spontaneous ovarian hyperstimulation syndrome associated with hypothyroidism. Am J Obstet Gynecol **160**:1220, 1989.

Ruder H, P Corvol, Mahoudeau JA, et al: Effects of induced hyperthyroidism on steroid metabolism in man. J Clin Endocrinol Metab **33**:382, 1971.

Salvi M, How J: Pregnancy and autoimmune thyroid disease. Endocrinol Metab Clin North Am **16**:431, 1987.

Sap J, Munoz A, Damm K, et al: The c-erb-A protein is a high-affinity receptor for thyroid hormone. Nature **324**:635, 1986.

Saxena BB, Rathnam P: Human chorionic gonadotropin in early pregnancy. Curr Top Exp Endocrinol **4**:97, 1983.

Scanlon MF, Weightman DR, Shale DJ, et al: Dopamine is a physiological regulator of thyrotrophin (TSH) secretion in normal man. Clin Endocrinol **10**:7, 1979.

Scherbaum WA: On the clinical importance of thyroid microsomal and thyroglobulin antibody determination. Acta Endocrinol (Copenh) **281**(Suppl):325, 1987.

Schimmel M, Utiger RD: Thyroidal and peripheral production of thyroid hormones. Ann Intern Med **87**:760, 1977.

Seely BL, Burrow GN: Thyrotoxicosis in pregnancy. The Endocrinologist **6**:409, 1991.

Shigemasa C, Mitani Y, Taniguchi S, et al: Development of postpartum spontaneously resolving transient Graves' hyperthyroidism followed immediately by transient hypothyroidism. J Intern Med **228**:23, 1990.

Silva JE, Larsen PR: Pituitary nuclear 3,5,3'-triiodothyronine and thyrotropin secretion: an explanation for the effect of thyroxine. Science **198**:617, 1977.

Smallridge RC, Fein HG, Hayslip CC: Postpartum thyroiditis. The Bridge **3**:3, 1988.

Smith BR, Mclachlan SM, Furmaniak J: Autoantibodies to the thyrotropin receptor. Endocrinol Rev **9**:106, 1988.

Smith BT. Pulmonary surfactant during fetal development and neonatal adaptation: hormonal control. *In* Robertson B, Van Golder LMG, Batenburg JJ (eds): Pulmonary Surfactant. New York, Elsevier Science, 1984, pp 357–382.

Southern AL, Olivio J, Gordon GG, et al: The conversion of androgens to estrogens in hyperthyroidism. J Clin Endocrinol Metab **38**:207, 1974.

Spencer CA, LoPresti JS, Patel A, et al: Applications of a new chemiluminometric thyrotropin assay to subnormal measurement. J Clin Endocrinol Metab **70**:453, 1990.

Spratt DI, Pont A, Miller MB, et al: Hyperthyroxinemia in patients with acute psychiatric disorders. Am J Med **73**:41, 1982.

Sridama V, Pacini F, Yang SL, et al: Decreased levels of helper T cells. N Engl J Med **307**:352, 1982.

Stewart DE, Addison AM, Robinson GE, et al: Thyroid function in psychosis following childbirth. Am J Psychiatry **145**:1579, 1988.

Stoffer RP, Koencke IA, Chesky VE, et al: The thyroid in pregnancy. Am J Obstet Gynecol **74**:300, 1957.

Sturgess ML, Weeks I, Evans PI, et al: An immunochemiluminometric assay for serum free thyroxine. Clin Endocrinol **27**:383, 1987.

Surks MI, Chopra IJ, Mariash CN, et al: American Thyroid Association guidelines for use of laboratory tests in thyroid disorders. JAMA **263**:1529, 1990.

Tachi J, Amino N, Tamaki H, et al: Longterm follow-up and HLA associations in patients with postpartum hypothyroidism. J Clin Endocrinol Metab **66**:480, 1988.

Tajiri J, Noguchi S, Murakami T, et al: Antithyroid drug-induced agranulocytosis. Arch Intern Med **150**:621, 1990.

Tamai H: TSH-blocking antibodies during the hypothyroid phase of subacute thyroiditis. J Clin Endocrinol Metab **73**:245, 1991.

Tamaki H, Amino N, Aozasa M, et al: Effective method for prediction of transient hypothyroidism in neonates born to mothers with chronic thyroiditis. Am J Perinatol **6**:296, 1989.

Tamaki H, Amino N, Takeoka K, et al: Thyroxine requirement during pregnancy for replacement therapy of hypothyroidism. Obstet Gynecol **76**:230, 1990.

Tanaka T, Tamai H, Kuma K, et al: Gonadotropin response to luteinizing hormone releasing hormone in hyperthyroid patients with menstrual disturbances. Metabolism **30**:323, 1981.

Thomas R, Reid RL: Thyroid disease and reproductive dysfunction. Obstet Gynecol **70**:789, 1987.

Thorpe-Beeston JG, Nicolaides KH, Snijders RJM, et al: Fetal thyroid-stimulating hormone response to maternal administration of thyrotropin-releasing hormone. Am J Obstet Gynecol **164**:1244, 1991a.

Thorpe-Beeston JG, Nicolaides KH, Felton CV, et al: Maturation of the secretion of thyroid hormone and thyroid-stimulating hormone in the fetus. N Engl J Med **324**:532, 1991b.

Tudhope GR, Wilson GM: An anemia in hypothyroidism. Q J Med **29**:513, 1960.

Tulchinsky D, Chopra IJ: Competitive ligand-binding assay for measurement of sex hormone-binding globulin (SHBG). J Clin Endocrinol Metab **37**:873, 1973.

Varner MW: Autoimmune disorders and pregnancy. Semin Perinatol **15**:238, 1991.

Vulsma T, Gons MH, De Vijlder JJM: Maternal-fetal transfer of thyroxine in congenital hypothyroidism due to a total organification defect or thyroid agenesis. N Engl J Med **321**:13, 1989.

Walfish PG, Chan JYC: Postpartum hyperthyroidism. Clin Endocrinol Metab **14**:417, 1985.

Wartofsky L, Burman KD: Alterations in thyroid function in patients with systemic illness: the "euthyroid sick syndrome." Endocrinol Rev **3**:164, 1982.

Watson JP, Elliot SA, Rugg AJ, et al: Psychiatric disorder in pregnancy and the first postnatal year. Br J Psychiatry **144**:453, 1984.

Weetman AP, McGregor AM: Autoimmune thyroid disease; developments in our understanding. Endocrinol Rev **5**:309, 1984.

Weinberger C, Thompson CC, Ong ES, et al: The c-erb-A gene encodes a thyroid hormone receptor. Nature **324**:641, 1986.

Weintraub BD: Inappropriate secretion of thyroid-stimulating hormone. Ann Intern Med **95**:339, 1981.

Werner SC: Modification of the classification of eye changes of Graves' disease: recommendation of the Ad Hoc committee of the American Thyroid Association. J Clin Endocrinol Metab **44**:203, 1977.

Widerhorn J, Bhandari AK, Bughi S, et al: Fetal and neonatal adverse effects profile of amiodarone treatment during pregnancy. Am Heart J **122**:1162, 1991.

Winikoff D, Malinek M: The predictive value of thyroid "test profile" in habitual abortion. Br J Obstet Gynaecol **82**:760, 1975.

Yamamoto T, Amino N, Tanizawa O, et al: Longitudinal study of serum thyroid hormones, chorionic gonadotropin and thyrotrophin during and after normal pregnancy. Clin Endocrinol **10**:459, 1979.

Yoshikawa N, Nishikawa M, Horimoto M, et al: Thyroid-stimulating activity in sera of normal pregnant women. J Clin Endocrinol Metab **69**:891, 1989.

Zakarija M, McKenzie JM: Pregnancy-associated changes in the thyroid-stimulating antibody to Graves' disease and the relationship to neonatal hyperthyroidism. J Clin Endocrinol Metab **57**:1036, 1983.

Zakarija M, McKenzie JM, Hoffman WH: Prediction and therapy of intrauterine and late-onset neonatal hyperthyroidism. J Clin Endocrinol Metab **62**:368, 1986.

CHAPTER

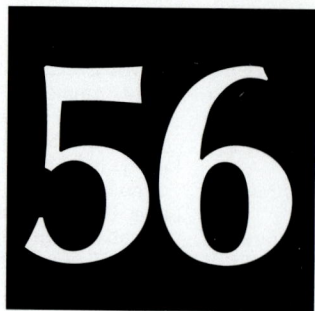

OTHER ENDOCRINE DISORDERS OF PREGNANCY

SHAHLA NADER, M.D.

The staggering advancements in endocrinology over the last few decades have permitted precise descriptions and scientific delineation of derangements of normal physiology. In tandem, technologic and pharmaceutical advances have followed that allow correction and management of prevailing problems with a precision that is lacking in many other fields of medicine. When pregnancy is superimposed upon abnormal endocrine function in the mother, there may be adverse consequences for the mother and/or the fetus, sometimes disastrous. This, combined with the knowledge that accurate diagnostic and therapeutic measures are often available, places a substantial burden on the obstetrician caring for the pregnant patient. The aim of this chapter is to summarize the normal maternal endocrine adaptation to pregnancy and to outline maternal disorders, some of which are almost specific to pregnancy.

HYPOTHALAMUS AND PITUITARY

The sella turcica of the sphenoid bone, lined by dura mater, is occupied by the pituitary gland. The dura covering the roof, called the diaphragm sella, is perforated centrally by the pituitary stalk. Directly above this diaphragm, and anterior to the stalk, lies the optic chiasm. The gland consists of two lobes, anterior (adenohypophysis) and posterior (neurohypophysis), the former accounting for five-sixths of the volume of the gland. The pituitary stalk not only comprises the direct neural connections between the hypothalamic nuclei and the posterior lobe, but also is the vascular link between the hypothalamus and the anterior lobe, thus enabling hypothalamic neurohumoral secretions to influence the activity of the anterior lobe cells. Paired superior hypophyseal arteries, arising from the internal carotids, anastomose around the upper part of the stalk. These terminate within elongated coiled capillary loops into which the hypothalamic hormones are discharged. The capillary bed drains into portal veins that empty into sinusoids

of the anterior lobe (Fig. 56–1). Paired inferior hypophyseal arteries supply the posterior lobe. The venous drainage of both lobes is into the cavernous sinuses.

Figure 56–2 is a diagrammatic representation of the

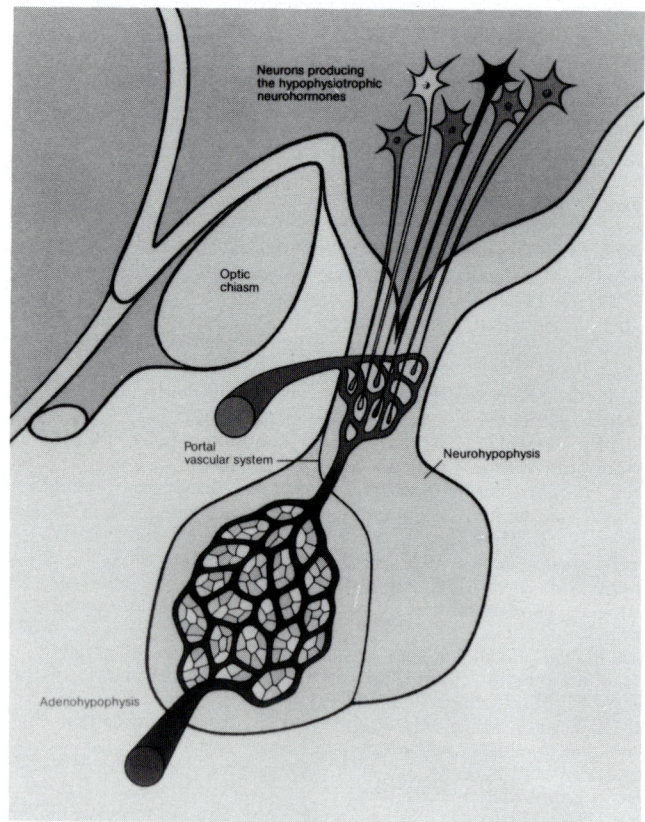

FIGURE 56–1. Schematic illustration of the hypothalamus, pituitary, and neurohumoral mechanism controlling the anterior pituitary. Halasz B: Introduction to Neuroendocrinology. *In* Fluckiger E, Muller EE, Thorner MO: Basic and Clinical Aspects of Neuroscience: The Dopaminergic System. Berlin, Heidelberg, Springer-Verlag, 1985, pp. 1–9. Courtesy of Sandoz, East Hanover, NJ.

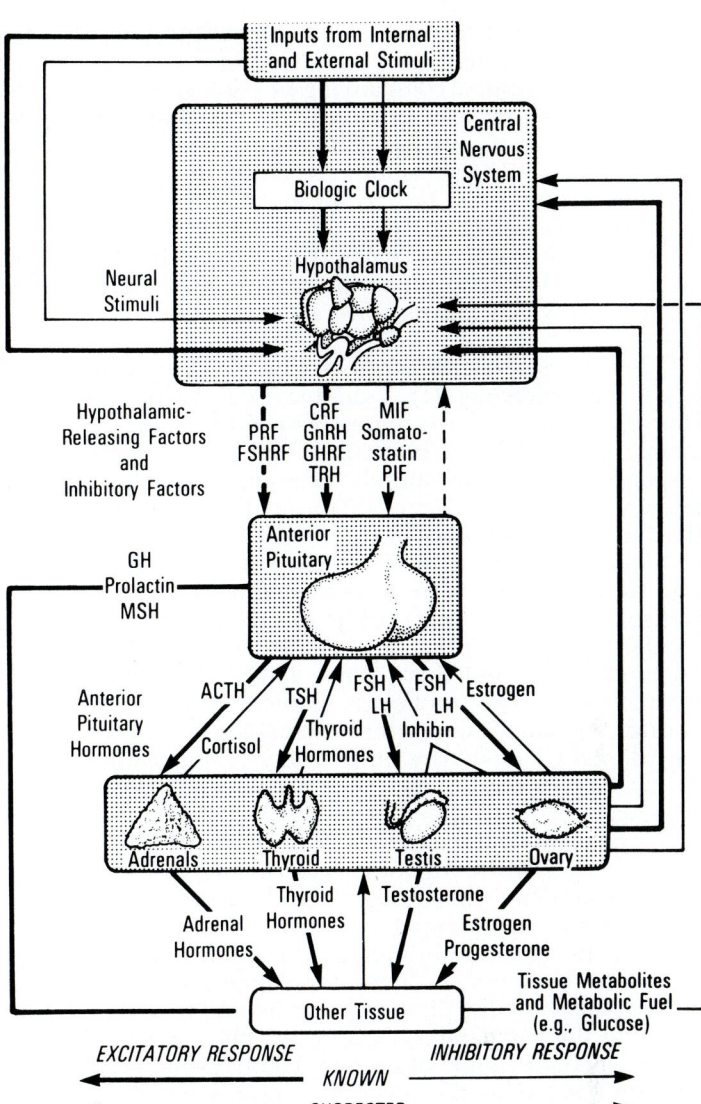

FIGURE 56–2. Schematic drawing of the relationships and feedback mechanism of the neuroendocrine system. The components include the central nervous system, hypothalamus, anterior pituitary, and target glands and tissues. *Heavy lines* indicate hormone secretion, *thin lines* indicate inhibitory effect, and *dotted lines* indicate suspected pathways. CRF = corticotropin-releasing factor; GnRH = gonadotropin-releasing hormone; GHRF = growth hormone–releasing factor; TRH = thyrotropin-releasing factor; MIF = melanocyte-stimulating hormone–inhibiting factor; PIF = prolactin-inhibiting factor; GH = growth hormone; MSH = melanocyte-stimulating hormone; ACTH = adrenocorticoptropin; TSH = thyroid-stimulating hormone; FSH = follicle-stimulating hormone; LH = luteinizing hormone. (Reprinted with permission from Frohman LA: Neurotransmitters as regulators of endocrine function. *In* Krieger DR, Hughes JC (eds): Neuroendocrinology. A Hospital Practice Book. Sunderland, Mass., Sinauer Associates, 1980. Illustration by Nancy Kou Gahan and Albert Miller.)

inter-relationships and feedback mechanisms of higher brain centers, hypothalamus, pituitary, and target endocrine glands in normal nonpregnant women (Frohman, 1980). The adenohypophysis produces gonadotropins (luteinizing hormone [LH], follicle-stimulating hormone [FSH]), growth hormone, thyrotropin (TSH), prolactin, and corticotropin (ACTH) and its related peptide β-lipotropin, from which melanocyte-stimulating hormone β-MSH is derived. Since 1947, when the concept that the control of the anterior pituitary is exerted through a neurohumoral mechanism was formulated, several peptides have been isolated from the hypothalamus that indeed function in this capacity. Thus, thyrotropin-releasing hormone (TRH) causes release of TSH (and also of prolactin); growth hormone–releasing hormone (GHRH) releases growth hormone; gonadotropin-releasing hormone (GnRH) allows release of LH and FSH; and corticotropin-releasing factor (CRF) releases ACTH. In addition, substances with an inhibitory rather than stimulatory influence have been identified: somatostatin inhibits the release of growth hormone (and many other hormones), and dopamine inhibits the release of prolactin. This inhibition of the lactotroph is clinically important; disturbances of the stalk or vascular dissociation of the hypothalamus from the anterior pituitary results in deficiency of all anterior pituitary hormones with the exception of prolactin. Thus, the lactotroph is normally under predominantly inhibitory control.

Physiologic Changes During Pregnancy

During pregnancy, the anterior lobe may double or triple in size due to hyperplasia and to hypertrophy of lactotrophs. This is evident at one month and continues throughout gestation. At delivery, involution of pregnancy cells occurs for a period of several months but seems to be retarded by lactation (Scheithauer et al., 1990). Magnetic resonance imaging studies of normal primigravid patients have confirmed progressively increasing pituitary volumes during gestation (Gonzalez et al., 1988): at the end of pregnancy there is an overall increase in pituitary gland size of 136 per cent as compared with control nulliparous subjects. The major accompanying physiologic change is a progressive increase in serum prolactin concentrations (Tyson et al., 1972), with approximately a tenfold increase during gestation (Fig. 56–3). Its role is in the preparation of the breasts for initiation and maintenance of lactation. Despite this dramatic increase, the lactotroph maintains its ability to respond to TRH, its releasing hormone (in contradistinction to prolactinomas, in which this response is usually blunted or absent).

Other physiologic changes during pregnancy include the following: (1) a decline in gonadotropin concentrations with a progressively diminishing response to GnRH; (2) blunting of growth hormone response to its normal stimuli: for example, insulin or arginine; (3) an increase in CRF during the second and third trimester, probably of placental origin; (4) a two- to fourfold increase in ACTH concentrations, occurring despite a rise in both bound and free plasma cortisol, suggesting that factors beside cortisol may regulate its release or that an alternate source of ACTH exists (Itskovitz and Rosenwaks, 1989). The diurnal variation of cortisol, although blunted, is preserved during pregnancy (for further discussion see section on Adrenal Glands). Thyrotropin, decreasing slightly in the first trimester, is otherwise essentially unchanged.

The posterior pituitary is a storage terminal for the neurohypophyseal hormones, oxytocin and vasopressin. Produced by the supraoptic and paraventricular hypothalamic nuclei, along with their respective binding proteins or neurophysins, they are transported as neurosecretory granules along the supraoptico-hypophyseal tract to the pituitary, and hence find their way into the circulation. Vasopressin plays a central role in osmolarity and volume regulation. Osmoreceptors are located in the anterior hypothalamus, and

vasopressin release increases when plasma osmolality rises (Fig. 56–4). Early in pregnancy, plasma osmolality decreases to values 5 to 10 mOsm/kg below the normal mean of 285 mOsm/kg in nonpregnant women (Davison et al., 1983). However, plasma levels of vasopressin and its response to water loading and dehydration are normal in pregnancy, indicating a resetting of the threshold, that is, vasopressin is secreted at a lower plasma osmolality (Fig. 56–4). Similarly, the plasma osmolality at which thirst is experienced is lowered in the pregnant state. Along with these changes, the metabolic clearance of vasopressin increases markedly between gestational week 10 and mid-pregnancy. This is paralleled by the appearance and increase of circulating vasopressinase (Lindheimer et al., 1991).

Oxytocin is involved in the process of parturition (Dawood and Khan-Dawood, 1990) and in suckling. Although the role of oxytocin in the initiation of labor is unclear, there is significant preterm increase in plasma concentrations of oxytocin. During nursing, nipple stimulation initiates a neurogenic reflex which is transmitted to the hypothalamus, thus triggering oxytocin release from the posterior pituitary. Oxytocin then induces contraction of the myoepithelial cells and mammary duct smooth muscle, resulting in milk ejection.

Fetal Hypothalamic and Pituitary Development

Figure 56–5 shows the gradual development of the structural and functional aspects of the neuroendocrine system in the fetus. By 10 to 13 weeks gestation, fetal pituitary and hypothalamic tissues can respond *in vitro* to stimulatory or inhibitory stimuli. By midgestation, the fetal hypothalamic-pituitary axis is a functional and autonomous unit subject to feedback control mechanisms. The posterior lobe of the fetal pituitary serves as a storage depot for neuropeptides.

Disorders of the Hypothalamus

Disorders of the hypothalamus may be congenital (Lawrence-Moon-Bardet-Biedl syndrome) or acquired inflammatory (meningitis, encephalitis), space-occupying (tumors, cysts), vascular or degenerative. In many of these conditions, reproduction is impossible or undesirable. In the autosomal recessive Lawrence-Moon-Bardet-Biedl syndrome of polydactyly, obesity, retinitis pigmentosa, and mental retardation, 45 to 53 per cent of affected females are hypogonadal, but several pregnancies have been reported in such patients (Green et al., 1989). Craniopharyngiomas are derived from vestigial remnants of Rathke's pouch or craniopharyngeal anlage. Manifestations may include headaches, visual disturbances, and hypothalamic dysfunction including diabetes insipidus. There are two case reports of craniopharyngiomas, previously undiagnosed, that have presented with diabetes insipidus in pregnancy (Hiett and Barton, 1990). In one of these the patient also had visual field disturbances and symptoms of raised intracranial pressure. Surgery

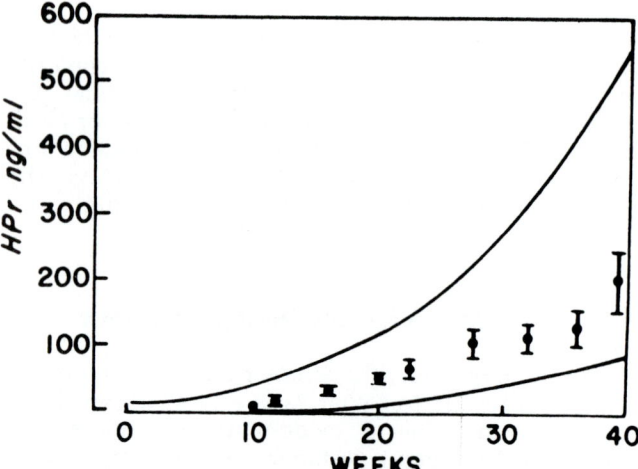

FIGURE 56–3. Basal serum prolactin (HPr) levels throughout normal gestation. The points represent the mean ± SEM; the solid lines represent the range of prolactin levels found in pregnancy. (From Tyson JE, Hwang P, Guyden H, et al: Studies of prolactin secretion in human pregnancy. Am J Obstet Gynecol **113**:14, 1972.)

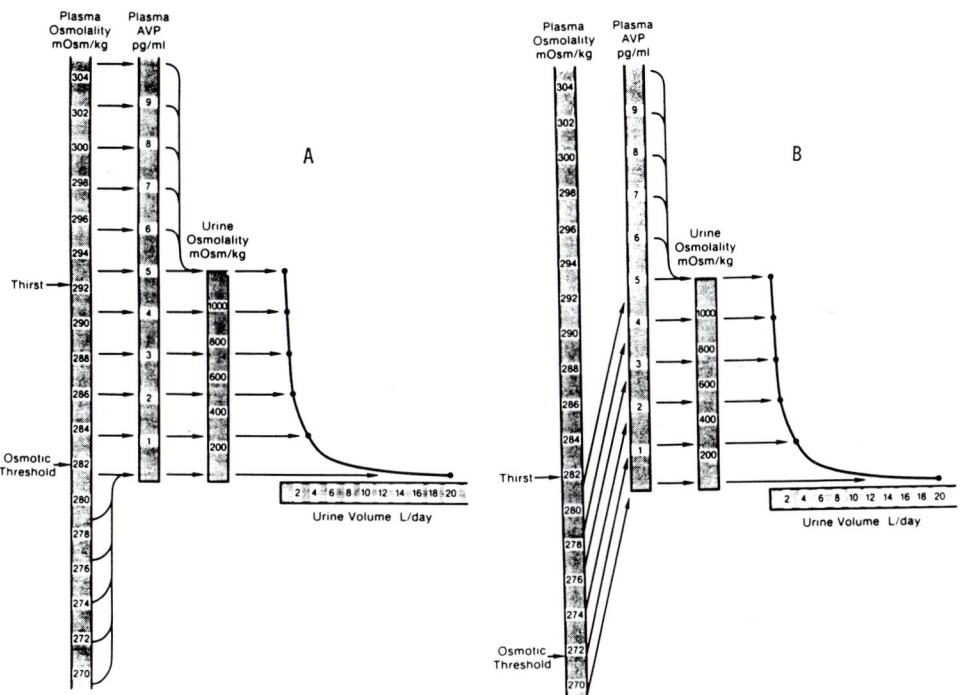

FIGURE 56–4. *A,* An idealized schematic of normal physiologic relationships showing the direct relationship between plasma osmolality and plasma vasopressin and the direct relationship between plasma vasopressin and urine osmolality. The osmotic threshold is illustrated as a floor for plasma osmolality below which the plasma osmolality will not normally fall becasue of excretion of a high volume of dilute urine. Thirst is illustrated as a physiologic ceiling for plasma osmolality because above this level thirst will be sensed and water imbibed to avoid further elevation of plasma osmolality. *B,* Idealized schematic of the reset osmostat (as occurs in pregnancy). Note that for the patient to function normally around a lower osmolality, it is necessary that both thirst and the osmotic threshold be lowered and maintain their relative relationship one to the other. Urine osmolality and urine volume follow appropriately for the level of vasopressin in plasma. The subjects will experience extreme thrist if the osmolality is raised into the normal range. (From Robinson AG: Disorders of antidiuretic hormone secretion. Clin Endocrinol Metab **14**:55, 1985.)

was performed three days postpartum after delivery at 34 weeks gestation because of deteriorating visual acuity.

Disorders of the Pituitary: Anterior Lobe

Most commonly, tumors, and less commonly, vascular mishaps and inflammatory changes may afflict the anterior lobe. In their evaluation, consideration has to be given to both anatomic derangements and the effects of excess or deficient hormones that may accompany these disorders. Given the additional physiologic changes in pregnancy outlined above, the combination of pregnancy and pituitary disorders poses a challenge to the obstetrician and endocrinologist in their endeavor for a safe outcome for both mother and child.

Pituitary Tumors

Pituitary tumors may be classified into hormonally functioning and functionless lesions. Examples of the former include growth hormone–producing tumors resulting in acromegaly, ACTH-producing tumors giv-

ing rise to Cushing's disease, and prolactinomas. Prolactinoma is by far the most common pituitary tumor encountered in pregnancy. Less commonly, hormonally functionless pituitary tumors may occur (although some of these may produce subunits of pituitary hormones, they are hormonally functionless clinically). As these are relatively asymptomatic in their early stages, they tend to be larger at the time of diagnosis. If diagnosed, the patient should be appropriately treated surgically before becoming pregnant.

Prolactinoma

The advent of prolactin radioimmunoassay in the early 1970s permitted the correct diagnosis of prolactinomas to be made in many patients previously thought to have functionless pituitary tumors. Because of the negative impact of excess prolactin on the hypothalamic-pituitary-gonadal axis, the majority of these women, who were also in their childbearing years, presented with amenorrhea and consequently infertility. Parallel with the development of the prolactin assay and improved radiologic techniques for diagnosing these tumors came the development and refinement of trans-sphenoidal microsurgical tech-

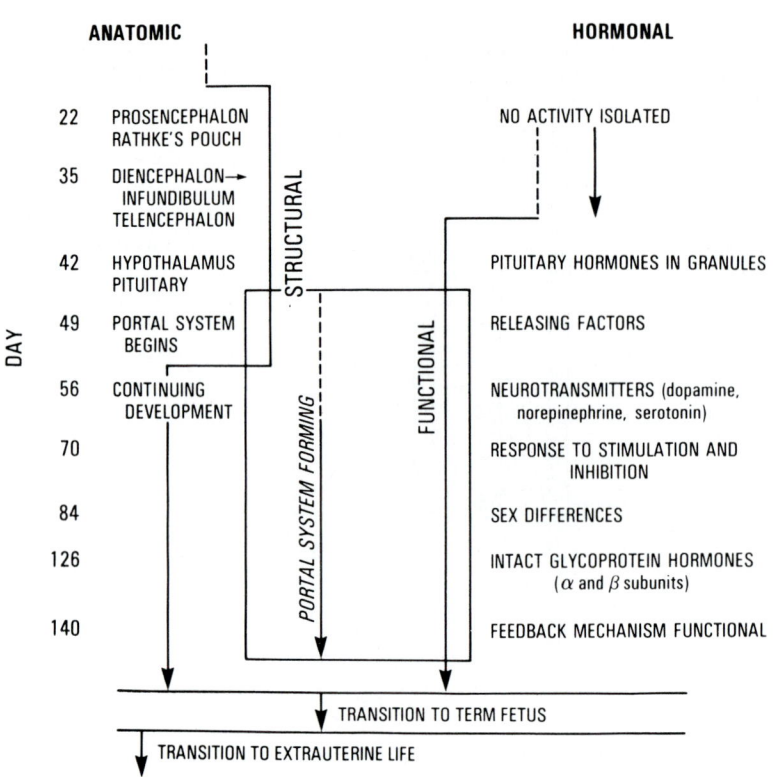

FIGURE 56–5. The structural and functional development of neuroendocrine tissue in the human fetus. (From Decherney A, Naftolin F: Hypothalamic and pituitary development in the fetus. Clin Obstet Gynecol **23**:749, 1980.)

niques and a powerful new drug, bromocriptine mesylate, which is capable of suppressing elevated prolactin concentrations to normal. Numerous pregnancies resulted from restoring normal gonadal function in these women, and over the last decade information concerning these pregnancies has been consolidated. Given the physiologic changes that occur in the pituitary in a normal pregnancy, namely enlargement of the gland and hyperplasia of the lactotrophs with a tenfold increase in serum prolactin, concerns about women with prolactinomas becoming pregnant were very reasonable.

EFFECT OF PROLACTINOMA AND ITS TREATMENT ON PREGNANCY AND THE FETUS: SAFETY OF BROMOCRIPTINE IN PREGNANCY. Bromocriptine mesylate is an ergot derivative with potent dopamine receptor agonist activity. Administered orally, it is a potent inhibitor of prolactin secretion, the effects lasting usually only for the duration of treatment. Numerous accounts of the use and safety of bromocriptine in pregnancy are available, but they are best summed up by Krupp and Monka (1987) from the Drug Monitoring Center, Clinical Research, Sandoz, Basel, Switzerland. They collected data from 2587 pregnancies in 2437 women treated with bromocriptine during some stage of gestation. The results showed that its use was not associated with an increased risk of spontaneous abortion, multiple pregnancy, or the occurrence of congenital malformation in their progeny. In addition, they followed 546 children postnatally up to 9 years and found no adverse effect on postnatal development. In the majority of women treated, bromocriptine was discontinued upon confirmation of pregnancy. These results are important insofar as investigations indicate that

bromocriptine crosses the placental barrier and can be found in dose-related concentrations in fetal blood and in the amniotic fluid (del Pozo and Krupp, 1984).

EFFECTS OF PREGNANCY ON THE PROLACTINOMA. Prolactinomas are subclassified, according to their size, into microadenomas (<10 mm in size: see Fig. 56–6) and macroadenomas (≥10 mm in size). In a review of the subject with data collected and combined from many studies, Albrecht and Betz (1986) noted the following: of 352 pregnant patients with untreated microadenomas, eight (2.3 per cent) developed visual disturbances, 17 (4.8 per cent) developed headaches, and 2 (0.6 per cent) had diabetes insipidus; the corresponding figures for 144 pregnant women with macroadenomas were visual disturbances in 22 (15.3 per cent), headaches in 22 (15.3 per cent), and diabetes insipidus in two (1.4 per cent). In the same review, outcome of 318 pregnancies in patients with micro- and macroadenomas treated (surgery, radiation therapy, or both) prior to pregnancy were analyzed. There were visual disturbances in ten (3.1 per cent), headaches in 12 (3.8 per cent), and diabetes insipidus in one (0.3 per cent). Symptoms related to a pregnancy-induced increase in the size of a pituitary tumor may begin as early as the first trimester, with a mean time for the onset of visual symptoms at 14 weeks gestation (Magyar and Marshall, 1978); headaches usually precede visual changes. The time from beginning of pregnancy to onset of symptoms in 91 pregnancies in women with previously untreated tumors is shown in Figure 56–7.

Based on these data, patients with prolactinomas planning pregnancy can be counseled, and definitive treatment of macroadenomas before pregnancy is cur-

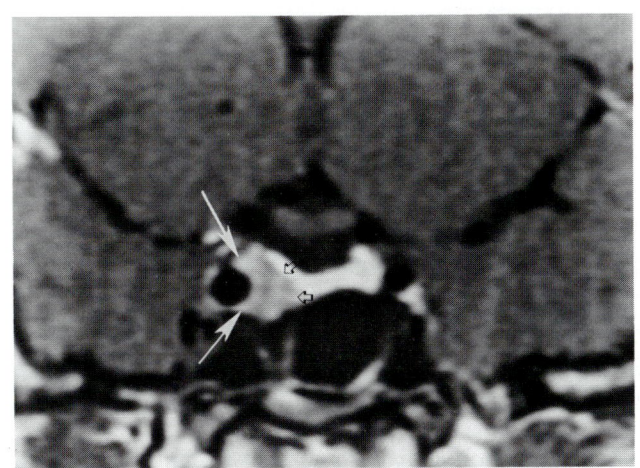

FIGURE 56–6. Prolactinoma in a 26-year-old woman. Coronal magnetic resonance image (SE 600/25) after injection of gadolinium-DTPA reveals a 9 × 8 mm solid mass *(black open arrows)* of intermediate signal intensity, involving the R side of the pituitary gland. The mass is abutting the dura *(white solid arrows)*, which is surrounding the R internal carotid artery. The gadolinium-DTPA has increased the signal intensity of normal pituitary tissue, enhancing the contrast between normal and adenomatous areas.

rently recommended, especially if associated with destruction of the sella turcica or with suprasellar extension. Recommendations for management of patients with prolactinomas are outlined in Tables 56–1 and 56–2. Despite prior surgical intervention, complications still may occur during pregnancy (Belchetz et al., 1986). Monthly measurement of serum prolactin is not necessary. Prolactin concentrations measured in a group of patients with surgically untreated microadenomas were found to be elevated early in gestation but did not increase further with advancing gestation (Divers and Yen, 1983), in contrast to normal pregnant controls (Fig. 56–8).

MANAGEMENT OF PROLACTINOMA COMPLICATIONS DURING PREGNANCY. Before the bromocriptine era and in the early stages of its use, the management of tumor complications in pregnancy was difficult and included surgery, radiotherapy, and/or early delivery. Fortuitously, it was soon observed that bromocriptine may, in addition to its prolactin-lowering effects, shrink the volume of pituitary tumors, including large macroadenomas causing visual field defects. Given the lack of known adverse effects of bromocriptine use in pregnancy, and the predicament of a pregnant patient with symptomatic tumor enlargement, bromocriptine has been successfully used in the treatment of such complications and is the treatment of choice (Molitch, 1985). It should be administered with food and the dose adjusted according to symptoms (e.g., 2.5 to 5 mg, two or three times daily). Glucocorticoids may also be given to expedite recovery of visual defects. Surgery is recommended only if there is no response to bromocriptine.

As indicated previously, the majority of patients with microadenomas have uncomplicated pregnancies, whereas a disturbing number of patients with untreated macroadenomas have symptomatic tumor

enlargement. Given the tumor-shrinking properties of bromocriptine, it is not surprising that the continuous use of bromocriptine in pregnancy has been advocated and indeed carried out in patients with macroadenomas (Ruiz-Velasco and Tolis, 1984). However, until the safety of such therapy on the developing fetus is more fully established, such therapy cannot be recommended at present except in special circumstances. Although the rates of abortion and perinatal mortality do not differ in women with pituitary tumors that are untreated or treated before or during pregnancy, there is a significant increase in prematurity in those treated (surgery and/or radiotherapy) during pregnancy as compared with those not requiring such treatment or those treated *prior* to pregnancy (Magyar and Marshall, 1978). Pituitary apoplexy, itself a rare event, has also been reported in a patient with a macroadenoma in early pregnancy (O'Donovan et al., 1986).

BREAST-FEEDING AND POSTPARTUM CARE. There is no reason to avoid breast-feeding when a patient wishes to nurse her child. In a small study of 14 women with microadenomas who breast-fed 6 to 14 months, serum prolactin was not significantly higher than before pregnancy (Zarate et al., 1979). In another, the increase in prolactin associated with suckling was absent in women with pathologic hyperprolactinemia. For those wishing to inhibit lactation, bromocriptine is the treatment of choice, a dose of approximately 2.5 mg three times daily with food usually being appropriate. Estrogen should not be used to inhibit lactation, as expansion of the tumor can occur. Ophthalmologic

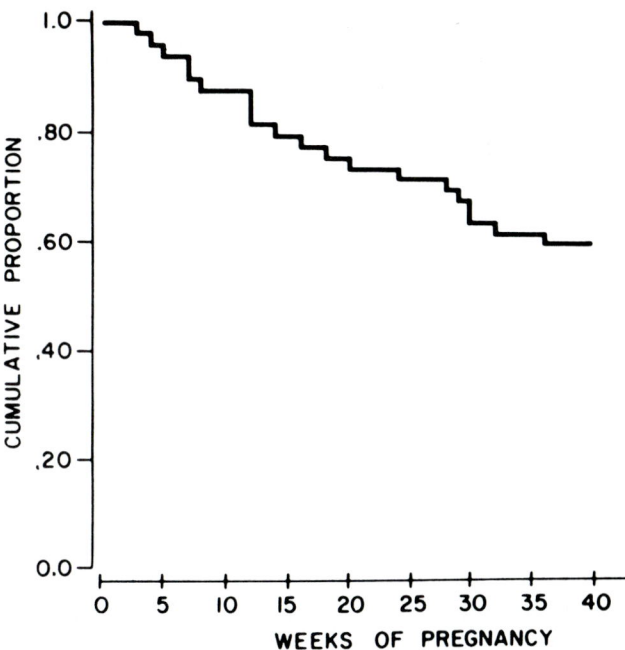

FIGURE 56–7. Time from beginning of pregnancy to onset of symptoms (i.e., headache or visual disturbances) in 91 pregnancies in women with previously untreated pituitary tumors. Sixty-one per cent failed to develop either headache or visual disturbance during pregnancy. Occurrence of symptoms is fairly evenly distributed throughout pregnancy. (From Magyar DM, Marshall JR: Pituitary tumors and pregnancy. Am J Obstet Gynecol **132**:739, 1978.)

TABLE 56–1.   Recommendations for Treatment of Patients with Prolactinomas Who Desire Pregnancy

Treatment	Microadenomas	Macroadenomas
Primary	Bromocriptine	Transsphenoidal surgery followed by bromocriptine
Alternative	Transsphenoidal surgery followed by bromocriptine (if necessary)	(i) Radiotherapy plus bromocriptine (ii) Continuous bromocriptine (see text)

and radiologic evaluation and determination of serum prolactin concentrations are in order 6 to 8 weeks after delivery. In most instances, the sella returns to its original size and prolactin decreases to previous levels. Further pregnancies are not contraindicated in patients with prolactinomas.

Acromegaly

Acromegaly is the result of excessive growth hormone secretion in adults, this usually being associated with acidophilic or chromophobic pituitary adenomas. Women with acromegaly slowly develop coarse facial features, prognathism, and spade-like hands and feet. When clinical evidence exists, a glucose tolerance test is performed; lack of suppression of growth hormone below 5 ng/ml during this test is in keeping with a diagnosis of acromegaly. Because the biologic effect of growth hormone is mediated through somatomedin C, elevation of serum concentration of this growth factor not only is considered a useful confirmatory test but also has been used to monitor the progression of the disease. However, in the context of pregnancy, somatomedin C concentrations should be interpreted with caution as they may be elevated (Furlanetto et al., 1978).

Menstrual irregularity or amenorrhea is an extremely frequent finding in acromegalic women. Nonetheless, pregnancy may occur in women with acromegaly and may be accompanied by tumor expansion necessitating hypophysectomy. Despite other soft tissue changes, no major changes occur in the genital tract that would complicate delivery. Definitive treatment before conception is the treatment of choice in acromegalics desiring children.

The observation that L-dopa causes a paradoxical decrease in growth hormone in acromegaly led to the use of dopaminergic agonists in the treatment of acromegaly. In two reported cases, pregnancy occurred in acromegalics during bromocriptine therapy, and with continuation of treatment during pregnancy, tumor expansion was not observed (Luboshitzky et al., 1980).

Should acromegaly be diagnosed in a pregnant patient, management will depend on the activity of the disease, the tumor size, and the stage of pregnancy. Active disease during pregnancy may respond to bromocriptine until fetal lung maturation is documented. If signs and symptoms related to suprasellar extension do not abate with bromocriptine, transsphenoidal surgery may be necessary. In a case reported by Yap et al. (1990), acromegaly was diagnosed in the second trimester. Bromocriptine corrected visual field defects and suppressed prolactin secretion but did not reduce fasting growth hormone levels. It was suggested that suppression of physiologic lactotroph hyperplasia by bromocriptine may permit noninvasive management of the pituitary adenoma in pregnancy. The maternal-fetal transfer of growth hormone has been said to be negligible, and apart from the effect of glucose intolerance, the fetus is not thought to be affected by acromegaly.

Cushing's Syndrome

Cortisol secretion is controlled by the hypothalamic-pituitary axis (see above and section on Adrenal Glands, which follows). Cushing's syndrome is a state of hypercortisolism and may arise from excess ACTH produced by the pituitary or an ectopic ACTH source such as a tumor, both of which may lead to bilateral adrenal hyperplasia. In addition, an adrenal lesion (adenoma or carcinoma) may itself be the direct source of excess cortisol. Pregnancy is uncommon in patients with this syndrome because of its association with a high incidence of menstrual disturbances and anovu-

TABLE 56–2.   Management of Patients Harboring Prolactinomas During Gestation

	MICROADENOMAS	MACROADENOMAS
Asymptomatic patient	STOP bromocriptine Routine obstetric care with evaluation for symptoms of tumor expansion Check visual fields each trimester	STOP bromocriptiine Monthly evaluation for symptoms of tumor expansion Check visual fields each month
Symptomatic patient	Check visual fields Measure serum prolactin concentration Magnetic resonance imaging of pituitary gland Initiate bromocriptine ± dexamethasone for visual complications Transsphenoidal surgery if unresponsive to bromocriptine	

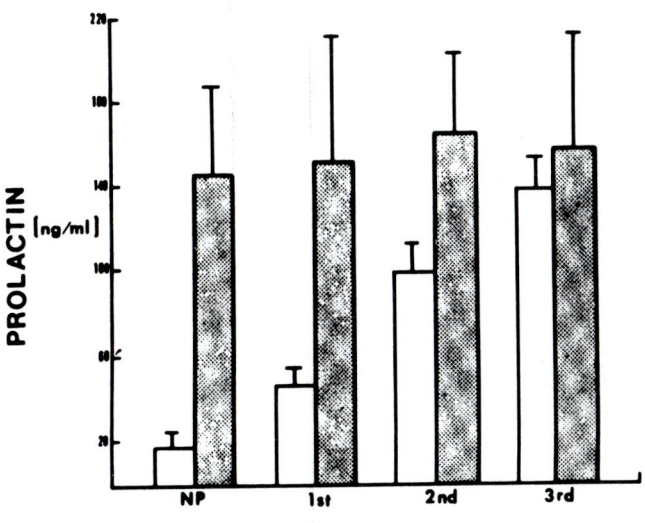

FIGURE 56–8. Maternal serum prolactin concentration (mean ± SEM) in microadenoma patients (*shaded bars,* n = 237) and controls (*open bars,* n = 215) while nonpregnant (NP) and during each trimester of pregnancy. (From Divers WA, Yen SSC: Prolactin producing microadenomas in pregnancy. Obstet Gynecol **62**:425, 1983. Reprinted with permission of the American College of Obstetricians and Gynecologists.)

lation. Pituitary-dependent Cushing's (also called Cushing's disease), gives rise to bilateral adrenal hyperplasia and a state of hypercortisolism. Although the most common etiology in nonpregnant patients, pituitary-dependent Cushing's is relatively less commonly associated with pregnancy, hyperfunctioning adrenal tumors being relatively more common in pregnant patients with this syndrome. A possible explanation for this discrepancy may be a greater degree of ovulatory disturbance in patients with pituitary-dependent Cushing's (Buescher et al., 1992).

In a recent series of 67 pregnancies (in 58 patients), incorporating 63 pregnancies from the world literature and four new cases (Aaron et al., 1990), there were 23 patients with adrenal adenoma (40 per cent), six patients with adrenal cortical carcinoma (10 per cent), and one case of ectopic ACTH syndrome resulting from an ACTH-secreting pheochromocytoma (2 per cent). In four the etiology was not determined (7 per cent), and in the remaining 24 (41 per cent) bilateral adrenal hyperplasia was found, suggestive of pituitary-dependent Cushing's. However, since the placenta may elaborate both CRF-like and ACTH-like compounds, these could conceivably lead to adrenal stimulation. This phenomenon would also explain apparent exacerbation of Cushing's in pregnancy with amelioration or remission after pregnancy (Pickard et al., 1990; Buescher et al., 1992).

DIAGNOSIS. The diagnosis of Cushing's syndrome in pregnancy may be rendered more difficult because weight gain, hypertension, striae, edema, and pigmentation may occur in normal pregnancy. More specific signs such as thinning of the skin, spontaneous bruising, and muscle weakness should be

sought. Furthermore, the laboratory diagnosis is complicated by the changes in adrenal function that occur during normal pregnancy, namely an elevation of plasma cortisol and diminished diurnal variation. It should be noted that urinary free cortisol excretion (<100 μg/24 hours in the nonpregnant state) is elevated during normal pregnancy (averaging 127 μg/24 hours in the third trimester, with values ranging from 68 to 252 μg/24 hours). Bearing these changes in mind, and while it is still useful as a test of Cushing's syndrome, a low-dose dexamethasone suppression test (2 mg/day), preferably for 8 days (rather than the customary 2 days) is the more appropriate test for diagnosis, and failure of suppression is in keeping with Cushing's syndrome. However, even dexamethasone suppressibility of plasma cortisol, as judged by standard criteria (<6 μg/ml), may be impaired (as is also seen in patients receiving estrogen therapy), and to be more certain, both plasma cortisol and 24-hour urinary steroids (free cortisol, 17 ketogenic and 17 ketosteroids) should be measured during dexamethasone suppression tests in pregnancy. To distinguish pituitary-dependent Cushing's from hyperfunctioning adrenal tumors, a high-dose dexamethasone suppression test is recommended (8 mg/day for at least 2 days). Significant (≥50 per cent) suppression of plasma cortisol is the rule in pituitary-dependent Cushing's, and failure of suppression to high-dose dexamethasone, along with low or undetectable ACTH concentrations, would strongly suggest an adrenal source. The pituitary (and also the adrenal) may be evaluated during pregnancy by means of magnetic resonance imaging (Schultz et al., 1984; Gonzalez et al., 1988).

MATERNAL-FETAL COMPLICATIONS. Although congenital malformations are not seen more frequently than in normal pregnancy (Pickard et al., 1990), maternal and fetal complications may occur. In the series of Aaron et al. (1990), premature birth occurred in 35 of 57 cases (61 per cent) and was associated with morbidity and mortality. There were seven spontaneous abortions (pregnancies terminating before 20 weeks gestation) and six stillbirths. Intrauterine growth restriction is prevalent, occurring in approximately one-third of reported cases (Buescher et al., 1992). Possible etiologies include hypertension and cortisol excess itself. Neonatal adrenal insufficiency has also been reported and is presumably due to suppression of the fetal hypothalamic-pituitary-adrenal axis from transplacental transport of excess maternal cortisol (see Fig. 56–5). Maternal complications include hypertension (87 per cent), abnormal carbohydrate metabolism (61 per cent), congestive heart failure, decreased wound healing, and maternal death in three of the 67 cases (Aaron et al., 1990).

THERAPY. Given the poor fetal outcome, therapy aimed at controlling the hypercortisolism has been attempted. The following recommendations for treatment have been suggested and would seem reasonable (Van der Spuy and Jacobs, 1984). In the first trimester, pituitary surgery for pituitary-dependent Cushing's and adrenal surgery for those of adrenal origin (especially to rule out carcinoma) should be performed. In the third trimester, early delivery of the fetus—

preferably vaginally—may be attempted. Metyrapone therapy (to block cortisol secretion) may reduce hypercortisolism until fetal maturity is attained. In the second trimester, treatment should be individualized, the alternatives being definitive surgery versus medical therapy aimed at ameliorating hypercortisolism. The risk of treatment with metyrapone and aminoglutethimide, which also blocks cortisol secretion, is uncertain since transplacental passage occurs and fetal adrenal steroid synthesis may be affected (Gormley et al., 1982).

NELSON'S SYNDROME. When a patient with pituitary-dependent Cushing's has bilateral adrenalectomy as definitive treatment for hypercortisolism and the pituitary lesion is not adequately addressed, a syndrome of hyperpigmentation along with an expanding intrasellar ACTH-producing tumor may result and is called *Nelson's syndrome*. The association of this syndrome and pregnancy is rare. In a series involving ten cases, five required postpartum treatment of their pituitary tumors, four had observation only, and one required surgical treatment during the pregnancy, with successful outcome for both mother and child (Surrey and Chang, 1985).

Hypopituitarism

Diminished or decreased production of anterior pituitary hormones results in inadequate activity of target organs such as thyroid, adrenal, and gonads. The deficiency may be partial, affecting trophic hormones in varying degrees, or it may be complete, resulting in panhypopituitarism. The role of the obstetrician-gynecologist in this context is twofold: (1) to be alert to and aware of the possibility of two disease processes that may affect the pregnant patient, namely Sheehan's syndrome and lymphocytic hypophysitis, and (2) to recognize and treat hypopituitarism in a pregnant patient, thus avoiding undesirable consequences.

Sheehan's Syndrome

In 1937, Sheehan drew attention to the relationship between postpartum hemorrhage and anterior pituitary necrosis. Because the syndrome is distinctly uncommon with other conditions associated with shock and vascular collapse, it is assumed that the hyperplastic gland in pregnancy is more vulnerable to an inadequate blood supply. In a retrospective survey by Hall (1962), pregnant patients admitted for hemorrhagic collapse were subsequently traced and evaluated for hypopituitarism, the incidence being approximately 3.6 per cent. There is said to be no direct correlation between the severity of the hemorrhage and the occurrence of Sheehan's syndrome, but the major part of the pituitary must be destroyed before symptoms become evident (Hall, 1962).

In a series of 25 cases (Drury and Keelan, 1966), half the patients had permanent amenorrhea, the remainder having rare and scanty menses. Only one had normal menstruation, and in most lactation was poor or absent. There was a surprisingly long interval between the obstetric event and diagnosis (more than 10 years) in over half the cases.

Although pregnancy in hypopituitary patients is rare, failure to establish the diagnosis and institute proper therapy may have lethal consequences for both mother and fetus. In a review by Grimes and Brooks (1980), pregnancies among patients with Sheehan's syndrome were reviewed. There were 87 per cent live births, 13 per cent abortions, and no stillbirth or maternal death in 15 pregnancies in patients receiving hormonal therapy. In sharp contrast, in 24 pregnancies among 11 women, in whom hormone replacement was not provided, there were 58 per cent live births, 42 per cent abortions, a stillbirth, and three maternal deaths.

In nonpregnant patients suspected of having Sheehan's syndrome, the diagnosis and the extent of pituitary damage can be determined by tests of target organ function (e.g., thyroid function tests, cortisol concentration) as well as tests of pituitary reserve (Lufkin et al., 1983). An ongoing pregnancy does not constitute evidence against the diagnosis of Sheehan's syndrome, and it should be considered in all patients with a past history of postpartum hemorrhage, especially if symptomatic. The finding of a low serum thyroxine and low TSH is in keeping with secondary hypothyroidism, and low cortisol concentrations (compared with those of normal pregnant women) with failure of cortisol and ACTH to increase during times of stress would be in keeping with diminished ACTH reserve.

Treatment of pituitary insufficiency during pregnancy does not present special problems. Oral L-thyroxine (0.1 to 0.2 mg/day) and cortisol (20 mg AM, 10 mg PM) or prednisone (5 mg AM, 2.5 mg PM) are administered. There is no need for mineralocorticoids. As in the nonpregnant state, glucocorticoid requirements may increase during episodes of intercurrent illness. During labor a good state of hydration should be maintained and parenteral glucocorticoids administered. This is most easily achieved by the intravenous infusion of hydrocortisone (cortisol). The dose may be adjusted as appropriate for the patient's state, ranging from 25 mg to 75 mg every 6 hours. Following delivery, parenteral glucocorticoids should be continued, in the smaller doses, for a few days along with intravenous fluids.

Pituitary Necrosis

Spontaneous pituitary necrosis and hypopituitarism may occur in pregnant diabetic patients, possibly related to diabetic vascular changes and the general susceptibility of the anterior pituitary to ischemia in pregnancy. It is manifested by severe, midline headaches and vomiting, during the third trimester, followed by a decrease in insulin requirements. In three of eight patients reported, the condition was associated with fetal death followed by maternal death (Dorfman et al., 1979), hence the need for early recognition and prompt management.

Lymphocytic Hypophysitis

In 1962, Goudie and Pinkerton described the case of a 22-year-old woman who died of circulatory collapse 8 hours after appendectomy. She was 14 months postpartum following a normal pregnancy and delivery but had developed secondary amenorrhea postpartum. Autopsy revealed lymphocytic infiltration of the pituitary and also of the thyroid, and the authors postulated an autoimmune mechanism to explain both.

In a review of the literature (English language) since then, a total of 44 pathologically documented cases have been found, 43 of which were in women (Cosman et al., 1989; Feigenbaum et al., 1991; Stelmach and O'Day, 1991; Bitton et al., 1991). In addition, a number of cases have been reported that fit the description just given, but for which pathologic confirmation is not available because surgery was not performed (Nader and Orlander, 1990). In 32 of the 43 women with pathologically documented lymphocytic hypophysitis, the disease occurred in relation to pregnancy. The features of these 32 patients are outlined in Table 56–3. In 13, the symptoms were noted postpartum; in the other 19, symptoms occurred during the pregnancy and included headache, lethargy, weight loss, and in one case collapse and death in labor. Twenty-two of the cases had varying degrees of hypopituitarism, and 18 had visual disturbances. Eight cases had inappropriate hyperprolactinemia and/or galactorrhea; pituitary stalk disturbance with relative lack of the prolactin inhibitory factor, dopamine, has been suggested as the mechanism likely to explain this phenomenon. In seven the diagnosis was made at autopsy; in the remaining 25, pituitary surgery was performed for suspected tumor.

Seven of the women had evidence of an autoimmune disease. Given this association, antipituitary antibodies have been sought and found in both pregnancy-related and unrelated cases (Nader and Orlander, 1990). The close temporal association of this disease with pregnancy is most intriguing. Flare-up of autoimmune disease processes in the postpartum period has been well documented, but given the relative immunologic tolerance during pregnancy, the occurrence of lymphocytic hypophysitis during a pregnancy is less well explained. Exacerbation of the disease postpartum, even when it initially presents in pregnancy, has also been described (Meichner et al., 1987). The association of this disease with pregnancy is also highlighted in an immunohistochemical study performed on pituitary material obtained at autopsy in 69 women who were pregnant or postpartum; among these, five cases of mild lymphocytic hypophysitis were found (Scheithauer et al., 1990). In four of these five, the patients died at 38 to 41 weeks gestation.

The importance of this condition is that it is a potentially life-threatening but treatable disease affecting young women during or after pregnancy. Thus the diagnosis should be considered in women of reproductive age presenting with signs and symptoms of anterior pituitary hormone deficiencies, isolated or in combination, antepartum or postpartum (especially in the absence of significant bleeding during labor). It should also be considered in pregnant or postpartum women with visual symptoms and changes. In the absence of a threat to vision, such patients should be treated medically with hormone replacement and their progress observed. Magnetic resonance imaging should be used to delineate and follow the anatomic defects. It is also noteworthy that the use of steroids has been associated with amelioration of visual symptoms (Stelmach and O'Day, 1991; Bitton et al., 1991), and the sellar mass has been shown to regress spontaneously. In another reported case (Bitton et al., 1991), partial hypopituitarism resolved postpartum in a biopsy-diagnosed case of lymphocytic hypophysitis. Finally, in a case reported by Brandes and Cerletty (1989) in which the data strongly supported a presumptive diagnosis of lymphocytic hypophysitis, and despite persistent partial hypopituitarism, the patient's menses resumed, she became pregnant and had an uncomplicated pregnancy while on thyroid and cortisol replacement.

Disorders of the Pituitary: Posterior Lobe

Diabetes Insipidus

Vasopressin and oxytocin, produced in the supraoptic and paraventricular nuclei of the hypothalamus, are released into the posterior lobe and hence into the circulation. No disease process has yet been described with oxytocin deficiency or excess. However, lack of vasopressin results in diabetes insipidus, and this may occur as a primary or idiopathic disorder (approximately 30 per cent of cases) or be acquired secondary to a variety of pathologic lesions including cranial injuries (16 per cent), infections, sellar and suprasellar tumors (25 per cent), and vascular lesions. The main symptoms are polyuria, polydipsia, and low urinary specific gravity. The diagnosis is made by water deprivation. During this test, increasing serum osmolality, in the face of low urine osmolality, is diagnostic of diabetes insipidus; a return toward normal after vasopressin administration confirms vasopressin deficiency.

EFFECT OF DIABETES INSIPIDUS ON PREGNANCY. Hendrichs (1954), in a comprehensive review, concluded that the prior existence of diabetes insipidus in a woman did not appear to alter her fertility, the course

TABLE 56–3. **Characteristics of 32 Women with Pregnancy-Related and Pathologically Documented Lymphocytic Hypophysitis**

Age	Mean 28 years
	Range 18–38 years
History of onset	19 during gestation
	13 postpartum
Hypopituitary*	22 cases
Visual disturbance*	18 cases
Hyperprolactinemia/galactorrhea	8 cases
Associated disorders	
Thyroiditis	4
Thyroiditis and adrenalitis	1
Pernicious anemia	1
Positive smooth muscle antibody	1
Diagnosis	
Autopsy	7
Biopsy (tumor suspected)	25

*Not documented in one of the cases.

of pregnancy, the effectiveness of labor, or lactation. Since oxytocin is also produced in the same hypothalamic nuclei, diabetes insipidus is of particular interest in the pregnant woman because of the possible relationship of decreased oxytocin with decreased uterine contractions during labor. Despite one report of uterine atony (Maranon, 1947), it would appear that labor is normal in most patients with diabetes insipidus.

Effect of Pregnancy on Diabetes Insipidus. The effect of pregnancy on established diabetes insipidus is variable. In a review of the subject, Hime and Richardson (1978) found that 58 per cent deteriorated, 20 per cent improved, and 15 per cent remained the same. The metabolic clearance of vasopressin markedly increases between gestational week 10 and midpregnancy and is associated with parallel increases in circulating vasopressinase. Placental inactivation of vasopressin with the production of large quantities of vasopressinase by the placenta may contribute to this increase in clearance rate (Lindheimer et al., 1991). Interestingly, in a few patients in whom preeclampsia had developed, the diabetes insipidus improved. The decreased contribution of the placenta to destruction of vasopressin is thought to explain this improvement (Campbell, 1980).

Transient Diabetes Insipidus of Pregnancy. A number of authors have described transient states of diabetes insipidus in relation to pregnancy (Krege et al., 1989; Iwasaki et al., 1991). The patients described have been cases of both central and nephrogenic diabetes insipidus, and some have involved unmasking of mild defects in vasopressin production (central) or action (nephrogenic). Increased destruction of normal, or previously subnormal (subclinical) concentrations of vasopressin could account for the transient appearance of diabetes insipidus in pregnancy (Robinson and Amico, 1991). For example, in patients with previously compensated nephrogenic diabetes insipidus (with secondarily increased vasopressin concentrations), the increased disposal of vasopressin could lead to decompensation and thus unmasking of nephrogenic diabetes insipidus, as could, also, a change in the renal sensitivity to vasopressin (Iwasaki et al., 1991). In addition, lowering of the osmotic threshold for thirst which occurs in pregnancy (see Fig. 56–4) would cause polydipsia and hence unacceptable polyuria in a patient with previously compensated (mild dehydration, mild thirst, and acceptable urine volume) nephrogenic diabetes insipidus (Robinson and Amico, 1991).

The occurrence of transient diabetes insipidus postpartum has also been reported (Nakamura et al., 1991). It is more difficult to explain as the high vasopressinase concentrations of pregnancy are rapidly reduced to undetectable levels within a few days of delivery (Robinson and Amico, 1991). Prostaglandin-related decreased renal sensitivity to vasopressin has been proposed (Nakamura et al., 1991).

Treatment. The current treatment of choice for central diabetes insipidus is L-deamino-8-d-arginine vasopressin (DDAVP) or desmopressin acetate, a synthetic analog of vasopressin, administered intranasally. Because of lack of information, DDAVP has not been recommended in pregnancy, but the drug has been used successfully in pregnant women (Sack et al., 1980). Dosages range from 1.0 to 2.5 μg given once or twice daily. In a study by Burrow et al. (1981), the drug was administered and DDAVP concentrations measured as vasopressin by radioimmunoassay in maternal serum and breast milk. Whereas maternal serum concentrations rose about sevenfold, breast milk concentrations showed little change. This suggested that, given the low levels of DDAVP in milk, these mothers might also breast-feed. It is also noteworthy that DDAVP has little pressor or uterotonic action and is not affected by vasopressinase.

ADRENAL GLANDS

Disorders of the Adrenal Cortex

The adrenal cortex plays an important and essential metabolic role in the human. Adrenal steroidogenesis leads to the production of three types of steroids. Mineralocorticoids are produced by the zona glomerulosa, glucocorticoids primarily in the zona fasciculata, and sex steroids in the zona reticularis. Figure 56–9 depicts the biosynthetic pathways diagrammatically.

Control of Adrenocortical Hormones

Aldosterone is primarily under the control of the renin-angiotensin system, although ACTH and hyperkalemia also have a stimulatory role. Renin, which is secreted by the juxtaglomerular apparatus of the kidney, converts angiotensinogen, an a_2-globulin produced by the liver, to angiotensin I, which is itself converted to angiotensin II. Angiotensin II, in addition to its pressor action, stimulates aldosterone secretion. In turn, while an increase in angiotensin II suppresses renin production, volume and sodium depletion stimulate its release.

Cortisol secretion is controlled by the hypothalamic-pituitary axis. Corticotropin-releasing factor (CRF) is secreted by the paraventricular nucleus of the hypothalamus. It is a $1\text{-}41\text{-}NH_2$ polypeptide which binds to the corticotroph membrane, activating the adenyl cyclase system. ACTH is a 1-39 polypeptide derived from a much larger precursor, proopiomelanocortin (POMC). This precursor is processed mainly into ACTH. There is a diurnal rhythm of cortisol secretion, the main secretory phase occurring during the late hours of sleep and early morning. There are long- and short-loop negative feedbacks operating. In the long loop the adrenal inhibits the anterior pituitary through the plasma cortisol by inhibiting ACTH release and also by inhibition of the genome responsible for POMC synthesis. In the short loop, ACTH regulates its own secretion by inhibition of CRF release.

While control of adrenal androgens is not understood, ACTH has a stimulatory effect. The major androgens are androstenedione, dehydroepiandrosterone, and its sulfate. Androstenedione is converted peripherally to testosterone as well as to estrone and estradiol.

FIGURE 56–9. Adrenal steroidogenic pathways of mineralocorticoid, glucocorticoid, and androgen synthesis. Major pathways are indicated by *thick arrows*, minor ones by *thin arrows*. Extra-adrenal conversion of sex steroids is denoted by *double arrows*. The *numbers* indicate enzymatic steps as follows: (1) 20α-hydroxylase, 22-hydroxylase, 20-22-desmolase; (2) 17α-hydroxylase; (3) 3β-hydroxysteroid dehydrogenase, 5-4 isomerase; (4) 21-hydroxylase; (5) 11β-hydroxylase; (6) C17-20-lyase; (7a) 18-hydroxylase; (7b) 18-dehydrogenase; (8) 17β hydroxysteroid dehydrogenase; (9) aromatase; (10) sulfatase.

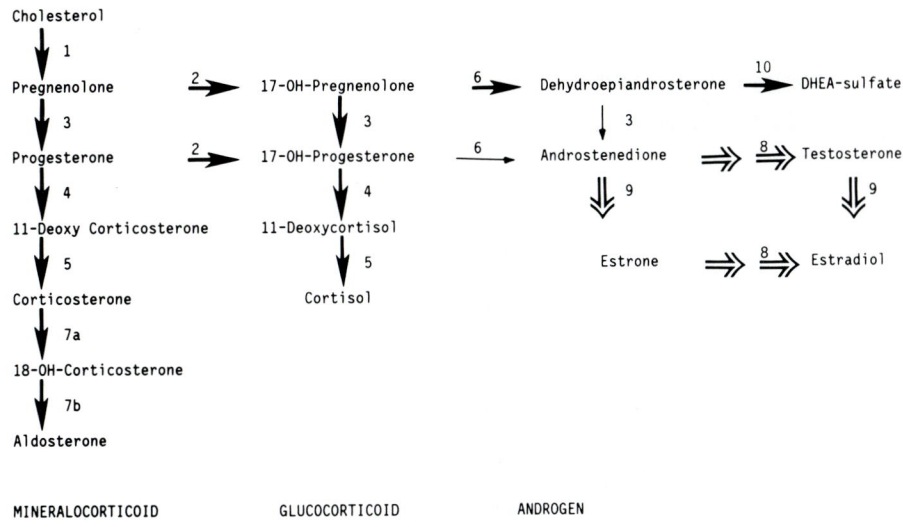

Physiologic Changes During Pregnancy

Plasma CRF increases progressively during the second and third trimester, peaking at delivery. The placenta is the likely source (Sasaki et al., 1984). ACTH concentrations also increase during pregnancy and may be of placental origin (Rees et al., 1975); the diurnal variation of both cortisol and ACTH, while blunted, is maintained. Corticosteroid-binding globulin concentrations increase threefold during pregnancy, resulting in an increase in the total plasma cortisol and a fall in its metabolic clearance. However, the unbound fraction also increases, and this is reflected by a rise in urinary free cortisol. These changes are depicted in Figure 56–10. The 9 AM plasma cortisol ranges between 25 and 46 μg/100 ml and the urinary free cortisol excretion between 68 and 252 μg/24 hr in the third trimester.

Renin activity increases early, peaking at 12 weeks gestation, with a decline in the third trimester (Wilson et al., 1980), the decline probably being related to the rise in angiotensin II that occurs at this time. Thus plasma aldosterone concentrations reach values five to eight times that of the nonpregnant state by the third trimester. Total testosterone increases in pregnancy due to an increase in sex hormone–binding globulin with a reduction in the per cent unbound; although the amount of free testosterone is low normal in the first 28 weeks, it increases thereafter, values often exceeding the normal range for nonpregnant women. Mean levels of androstenedione also increase in the latter part of pregnancy, while dehydroepiandrosterone sulfate concentrations fall due to a major rise in the metabolic clearance rate.

Fetal Adrenal Development

The fetal adrenal can synthesize cortisol *in vitro* by 8 weeks gestation. *In vivo*, placental 5-pregnenolone and 4-progesterone are utilized to synthesize steroids (Peterson, 1977). Two adrenal cortical zones can be identified in the fetus. The inner, or fetal zone, which

represents about 80 per cent of the cortex *in utero*, involutes in the first few months of extrauterine life. The outer zone becomes the adult adrenal cortex.

Disorders of the Adrenal Cortex During Pregnancy

Disrupted reproductive function commonly accompanies significant genetic or acquired abnormalities of adrenal cortical function, thus these are usually diagnosed prior to conception. In patients with already recognized adrenal disorders, replacement hormone therapy is continued throughout gestation, and the patient monitored, bearing in mind the pregnancy associated changes in normal values.

Primary Adrenocortical Insufficiency (Addison's Disease)

Atrophy of the adrenals on an autoimmune basis is the most common cause of adrenal failure, accounting for 75 per cent of the cases. Other causes include hemorrhage, associated usually with sepsis and burns, infections (viral, fungal, or tuberculous), and infiltrative disorders including metastases, lymphoma, and amyloidosis. With the availability of hormone replacement, pregnancy is no longer contraindicated.

DIAGNOSIS DURING PREGNANCY. The diagnosis of Addison's disease in pregnancy is uncommon and may relate to fetal contribution to maternal steroids. The symptoms include weakness, lassitude, nausea with or without vomiting, pigmentation, weight loss, anorexia, and abdominal pain. Some of these symptoms are also commonly noted in normal pregnant women. Thus, the index of suspicion should be raised when a thin pregnant woman complains of prolonged nausea and vomiting, weakness, postural hypotension, and personality changes. A history of polyendocrine autoimmune disorders, type I diabetes, adrenogenital syndrome, tuberculosis, and acquired immune deficiency syndrome places the pregnant

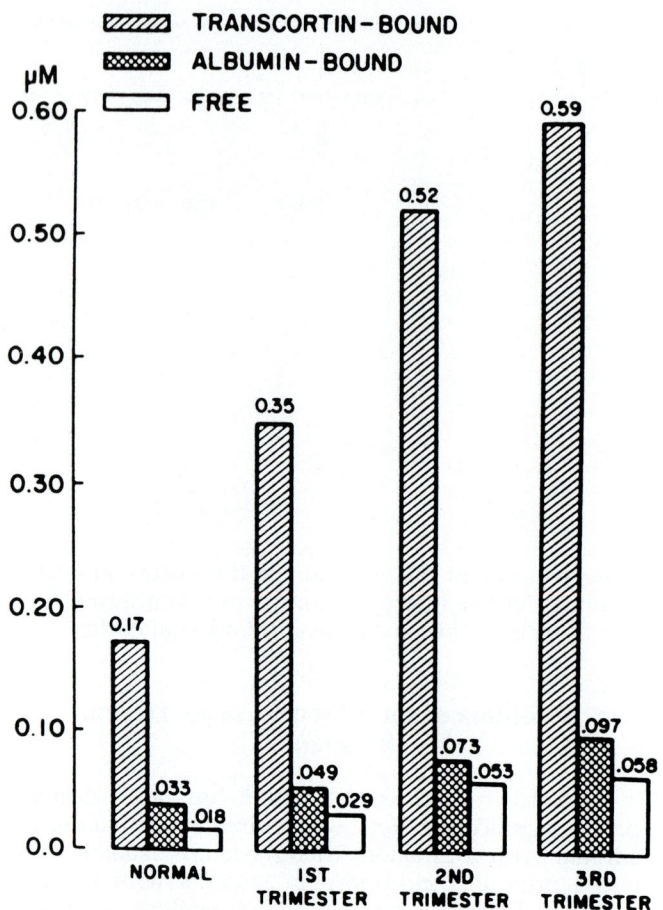

μM CORTISOL

FIGURE 56–10. Absolute distribution of bound and free cortisol in μM/liter pregnancy plasma. (From Rosenthal HE, Slaunkwhite WR, Sandberg AA: Transcortin: A corticosteroid-binding protein of plasma X cortisol and progesterone interplay and unbound levels of these steroids in pregnancy. J Clin Endocrinol Metab 29:352, 1969. © The Endocrine Society.)

woman at increased risk for adrenocortical insufficiency.

The signs and symptoms and laboratory tests are outlined in Table 56–4. In acutely ill patients, replacement therapy must be initiated immediately and the diagnosis confirmed retrospectively by obtaining a pretreatment serum or plasma sample for electrolytes, cortisol, and ACTH. In patients whose illness is less severe, a rapid ACTH stimulation test using synthetic ACTH may be performed; 250 μg is administered IV and blood samples obtained at baseline, 30 and 60 minutes. While a cortisol level exceeding 18 μg per cent and an increment exceeding 7 μg per cent is considered normal in the nonpregnant state, the mean increments have been reported as 18, 23, and 26 μg per cent in the first, second, and third trimester of pregnancy, respectively (Nolten et al., 1978).

TREATMENT. Replacement regimens are similar to those used in nonpregnant women. This is usually accomplished by hydrocortisone (cortisol) 20 mg in the morning and 10 mg in the evening along with 9α-fludrocortisone, 0.05 to 0.1 mg daily. The dose of 9α-fludrocortisone is increased if postural hypotension or hyperkalemia persists and is decreased if hypertension or hypokalemia occur. The dose of cortisol should be doubled or tripled in any situation associated with stress, including systemic illness, trauma, or surgery.

Breast-feeding has been discouraged because of the potential hazard of corticosteroids passing into the maternal milk, but some investigators disagree (Albert et al., 1989).

ACUTE ADRENAL INSUFFICIENCY DURING PREGNANCY, LABOR, DELIVERY, OR THE PUERPERIUM. Addi-

TABLE 56–4.   **Diagnosis of Primary Adrenal Insufficiency During Pregnancy**

Signs and Symptoms
  Nausea with or without vomiting, anorexia
  Systolic BP <100 mm Hg with postural fall
  Increased pigmentation
  Abdominal pain
  Personality changes
  Weakness, fatigue
  Muscle and joint pain
  Salt craving
Laboratory Findings
  Decreased sodium
  Increased potassium, BUN, creatinine
  Hypoglycemia
  Plasma cortisol below normal pregnancy level
  Urinary-free cortisol: 24-hour excretion below normal pregnancy level
  Increased plasma ACTH
  Abnormal cortisol response to rapid ACTH stimulation test

sonian crisis is a rare but life-threatening event in pregnant women (Seaward et al., 1989). The onset may be confused with an abdominal surgical emergency because of the prominence of abdominal pain, nausea, vomiting, and shock. After necessary blood samples are obtained for electrolytes, cortisol, and ACTH determinations, intravenous therapy should be started immediately with 100 mg hydrocortisone sodium succinate along with an infusion of normal saline and 5 per cent glucose. During the first 24 hours, 300 to 400 mg intravenous hydrocortisone sodium succinate should be given continuously, and this may conveniently be added to the replacement fluids administered. Recovery occurs quickly, and by 24 hours the patient may be able to return to oral feedings and replacement doses of oral hydrocortisone and 9α-fludrocortisone. If not, hydrocortisone may be continued intravenously, usually in diminished dosage. An effort should be made to determine the cause of the adrenal crisis, and the patient should have careful post-pregnancy supervision. Patients with mild deficiency are especially at risk during labor, delivery, and the immediate postpartum period (Albert et al., 1989).

EFFECT OF MATERNAL ADDISON'S DISEASE ON THE NEWBORN. Infants born to mothers with Addison's disease usually do not have any recognizable defects. Fetal growth may, however, be suboptimal with lower-than-normal birth weights, especially if the diagnosis is made late in pregnancy or during the postpartum period (Drucker et al., 1984). Maternal antibodies to the adrenal cortex do cross the placenta but do not significantly affect neonatal adrenal function.

Cushing's Syndrome

Cushing's syndrome results from an excess of glucocorticoids and is rare during pregnancy. For a full discussion of this syndrome, the reader is referred to the sections on Hypothalamic and Pituitary Disorders earlier in this chapter and to a recent review (Buescher et al., 1992).

Primary Hyperaldosteronism

The autonomous secretion of aldosterone in this syndrome may be due to an adrenal adenoma, bilateral hyperplasia, or—rarely—an adrenocortical carcinoma. In pregnancy the clinical picture of hyperaldosteronism is similar to that of the nonpregnant patient with hypertension, hypokalemia, and often kaliuresis and elevated serum bicarbonate (Lotgering et al., 1986). The electrolyte disturbances and hypertension may be first apparent in the peripartum period, coinciding with the removal of the protective antialdosterone effect of progesterone. All but one (Neerhof et al., 1991) of the pregnancy-related cases of hyperaldosteronism have harbored adenomas.

DIAGNOSIS. After standardizing for dietary sodium (100 to 150 mEq daily) and posture (recumbent) and the replacement of plasma potassium, renin activity and aldosterone concentrations are measured. The renin activity is lower and the aldosterone concentration higher than those found in normal pregnancy

(Lotgering et al., 1986). Suppression of the aldosterone axis may also be attempted with salt loading (200 to 300 mEq per day for 3 to 5 days), the hallmark of primary hyperaldosteronism being lack of suppression of serum aldosterone concentration.

TREATMENT. Medical treatment with standard antihypertensive drugs along with potassium supplements should be provided. Surgery in the second trimester may be required if medical treatment fails. Spironolactone is contraindicated in pregnancy, especially in the first trimester, because of its possible feminizing effects. In the first case report of a pregnant patient with hyperaldosteronism associated with bilateral hyperplasia reported by Neerhof et al. (1991), enalapril maleate, an angiotensin-converting enzyme inhibitor, successfully lowered blood pressures in a patient unresponsive to other medications. The safety of this type of medication in pregnancy remains to be established; there are some reports of potential adverse effects (Kreft-Jais et al., 1988), including fetal skull ossification defects, preterm birth, low birth weight, and oligohydramnios.

Congenital Adrenal Hyperplasia

In the congenital adrenal hyperplasias (CAH), there are inherited enzymatic defects of adrenal steroidogenesis. The most severe and life-threatening disorders occur early in the biosynthetic cascade and are usually fatal or incompatible with successful reproduction. Deficiency of 21-hydroxylase is the most common defect (see Fig. 56–7), accounting for 90 to 95 per cent of cases with an incidence of about 1 in 14,000, although in some areas, for example Alaska, it is more frequent (Pang et al., 1988). The second most common form is 11-hydroxylase deficiency.

Genetics

All CAHs are autosomal-recessive disorders. Thus the parents of an affected child have at least one haplotype for the defect, giving each subsequent offspring a 25 per cent chance of having the condition and a 50 per cent chance of being a carrier. An affected individual will produce 100 per cent carriers if her partner is nonaffected; if her partner is a carrier, 50 per cent of the offspring will be affected and the other 50 per cent carriers. Siblings or spouses who want to know if they are heterozygotes for 21-hydroxylase deficiency can be tested by measuring adrenal steroids, notably 17-hydroxyprogesterone, before and after ACTH stimulation (White et al., 1987a).

21-Hydroxylase Deficiency

This deficiency arises due to genetic mutations at a site linked to the HLA histocompatibility complex on the short arm of the sixth chromosome. The variation in severity of the deficiency can be accounted for by allelic variation at the gene locus (White and New, 1992). The enzyme block results in inadequate synthesis of 11-deoxycortisol and cortisol; the resulting excess ACTH stimulates adrenal precursors, notably 17-hydroxyprogesterone. Consequent to shunting of these excess precursors, excess androgens result, leading to masculinization of genitalia of the female fetus and excess masculinization of the male infant. If the defect is severe, mineralocorticoid deficiency is also seen with salt wasting. Diagnosis is made by the finding of excess basal 17-hydroxyprogesterone concentrations; in milder forms, ACTH stimulation is necessary and shows an excessive rise in 17-hydroxyprogesterone. Physiologic replacement doses of glucocorticoids (usually cortisol) are used as therapy, dosage being based upon surface area. Concentrations of 4-androstenedione, testosterone, and 17-hydroxyprogesterone are used to monitor adequacy of suppression. Fludrocortisone is indicated in salt-losing forms. Virilized females may require surgical reconstruction of the genitalia to provide for a normal appearance, intercourse, and pregnancy.

MATERNAL AND FETAL CONSIDERATIONS. While poor control of CAH results in irregular or absent menses, well-controlled patients may achieve pregnancy, although not so often as one might predict, possibly owing to intervals of excess androgen exposure postnatally. Usually the same dose of cortisol can be continued through gestation, with additional amounts given during labor, delivery, and the immediate postpartum period. Cesarean section rates are higher because of abnormal maternal external genitalia or a small bony pelvis from premature closure of the epiphyses (Mori and Miyakawa, 1970). Most children of CAH mothers are normal, although women receiving suboptimal doses of replacement therapy will have elevated circulating androgens, which may cross the placenta and virilize the fetus. Conversely, excessive glucocorticoid therapy of the CAH mother may result in suppression of fetal adrenals with resulting transient adrenocortical insufficiency of the neonate.

PRENATAL DIAGNOSIS AND TREATMENT. Prenatal diagnosis of 21-hydroxylase deficiency is possible for offspring of known heterozygotes. Elevated levels of amniotic fluid 17-hydroxyprogesterone provide the diagnosis (White et al., 1987b). In addition, HLA typing of amniotic cells may provide confirmation. However, these tests are usually done after masculinization of the affected females has already begun. An alternative test, namely chorionic villus sampling, using DNA probes for HLA genes in comparison with parental chromosomes will allow earlier diagnosis (Mornet et al., 1986). Prenatal treatment of the mother with high-dose glucocorticoids has been shown to be effective in preventing virilization of the affected female fetus; the glucocorticoid crosses the placenta and suppresses ACTH secretion from the fetal pituitary (White et al., 1987b). The present-day approach is to treat all such mothers with glucocorticoids. Chorionic villus sampling is then performed. If the fetus is male, maternal treatment is discontinued; if female, the treatment is continued until the DNA/HLA test results are available. The glucocorticoids are discontinued only if the female fetus is considered unaffected.

11-Hydroxylase Deficiency

This enzyme defect, which is not HLA-linked, results in blocked production of cortisol and aldosterone

with resulting excess precursors, 11-deoxycortisol and deoxycorticosterone (White et al., 1987b). A shunt toward excess androgens occurs, and the presentation is that of androgen excess and hypertension. Diagnosis is based upon elevated 11-deoxycortisol and deoxycorticosterone concentrations either basally or following ACTH stimulation. Heterozygotes have no demonstrable biochemical abnormality even with ACTH stimulation. Treatment is with glucocorticoid replacement. Prenatal diagnosis is made by measuring amniotic fluid 11-deoxycortisol concentrations (Rosler et al., 1979), and prenatal treatment of the mother with dexamethasone, as in 21-hydroxylase deficiency, should be possible.

Other CAH Enzyme Deficiencies

There are a few other rare forms of CAH (see Fig. 56–9). In 17-hydroxylase deficiency the sex steroid pathway is blocked both in the adrenal cortex and gonad, resulting in a hypogonadal state and primary amenorrhea. Deficiency of 3β-hydroxysteroid dehydrogenase, if severe, will present as lack of pubertal development. Milder forms present pubertally with hyperandrogenism (Rosenfeld et al., 1980).

Long-Term Therapy with Pharmacologic Doses of Steroids

The occurrence of congenital anomalies, in particular cleft palate, in animal experiments raised concern about pregnant women receiving glucocorticoids during pregnancy. However, in a review involving 260 pregnancies in which glucocorticoids had been administered to women in pharmacologic doses, there were only two infants with cleft palate (Bongiovanni and McPadden, 1960). Both mothers had received steroids in large doses early in pregnancy. Since closure of the palatal process occurs by the 12th week, it is possible that the anomaly was related to the medication. Other, smaller studies have been negative (Snyder and Snyder, 1978). It is also important to remember that the hypothalamic-pituitary-adrenal axis is suppressed with long-term supraphysiologic doses of glucocorticoids, and abrupt withdrawal should be avoided, as it may precipitate maternal adrenocortical insufficiency. Glucocorticoids are excreted in breast milk and have the potential to cause growth restriction in the neonate. In addition, neonatal adrenal insufficiency, while rare, may occur in infants born to mothers being treated with exogenous glucocorticoids (Bongiovanni and McPadden, 1960).

Disorders of the Adrenal Medulla During Pregnancy

Pheochromocytoma

Pheochromocytomas are tumors of chromaffin cells. These cells predominantly cluster in the adrenal medulla, and 90 per cent of pheochromocytomas are found in this location. Extra-adrenal tumors range in site from the carotid body to the pelvic floor. They

TABLE 56–5. Changes in Maternal and Fetal Mortalities in Over 200 Pregnancies Complicated by Pheochromocytoma, Spanning Several Decades

TIME OF DIAGNOSIS	MATERNAL MORTALITY			FETAL MORTALITY		
	BEFORE 1969	**1969–1979**	**1980–1987**	**BEFORE 1969**	**1969–1979**	**1980–1987**
During pregnancy	18%	4%	0%	50%	42%	15%
Postpartum	58%	50%	17%	56%	56%	35%

occur either sporadically or as part of the familial multiple endocrine neoplasia, type 2 syndrome. Approximately 12 per cent are malignant, although the percentage is higher in those occurring in extra-adrenal sites.

SYMPTOMS. Pheochromocytoma is a rare but potentially lethal cause of hypertension in pregnancy. Its possibility should be considered in women with intermittent, labile hypertension or paroxysmal symptoms such as anxiety, diaphoresis, headache, and palpitations. Other symptoms include chest or abdominal pain, unusual reactions to drugs affecting catecholamine release and actions, visual disturbances, convulsions, and collapse. Symptoms tend to be similar in pregnant and nonpregnant women. The occurrence of symptoms during pregnancy only, with recurrence in subsequent pregnancies, has also been described. Increased vascularity of the tumor in pregnancy as well as the mechanical effect of an enlarging uterus may explain this phenomenon. In many cases, severe symptoms develop in the peri- and postpartum periods.

LABORATORY DIAGNOSIS. Laboratory diagnosis involves biochemical demonstration of elevated vanillylmandelic acid, catecholamines, and metanephrines in the 24-hour urine specimen. Plasma catecholamines can also be determined. Values in pregnant women are similar to those of nonpregnant subjects. As methyldopa interferes with catecholamine measurements, it should be discontinued prior to testing. If necessary, the tumor may be localized during pregnancy by means of ultrasonography (Griffin et al., 1984) or magnetic resonance imaging (Glazer et al., 1986).

TREATMENT. Treatment of pheochromocytoma in pregnancy is somewhat controversial. Most agree that when the diagnosis is made in the second half of pregnancy, alpha-adrenergic blockade with phenoxybenzamine is the treatment of choice; it is given orally, starting with 10 mg twice daily, gradually increasing by 10 to 20 mg daily until hypertension is controlled. When fetal maturity is achieved, cesarean section should be performed, with simultaneous or subsequent excision of the tumor (Fudge et al., 1980; Harper et al., 1989) during adrenergic blockade. In tumors diagnosed before the 24th week, surgery during pregnancy has been advocated (Harper et al., 1989) to avoid fetal wastage. However, a number of such cases have been successfully managed during pregnancy with alpha and beta blockade with good fetal outcome (Lyons and Colmorgen, 1988; Oliver et al., 1990). The arguments against medical therapy are the unknown effects of alpha- and beta-blockade on the fetus in the long term, the teratogenic potential of phenoxybenzamine, and the risk of a malignant lesion. Beta-blockade alone should not be used without prior alpha-blockade, as unopposed alpha-adrenergic activity may lead to generalized vasoconstriction and a steep rise in blood pressure. Anesthetic management of pheochromocytoma resection during pregnancy requires special consideration (Mitchell et al., 1987).

PROGNOSIS. It is a life-threatening disease, both for the mother and the fetus, although with better management and the availability of α and β-adrenergic blockade, the prospects for both have improved. Table 56–5 reflects the changes in maternal and fetal mortalities over the last few decades and also indicates the better prognosis when the diagnosis is made during pregnancy (Schenker and Granat, 1982; Harper et al., 1989). Fetal growth restriction may occur secondary to reduced uteroplacental perfusion, and fetal death may occur during acute hypertensive crises.

Four cases of malignant pheochromocytomas in pregnancy were reviewed by Ellison et al. (1988), and another by Devoe et al. (1986); alpha-methyl paratyrosine, a dopamine synthesis inhibitor, was used in the latter case. Six cases of pregnancy with pheochromocytoma as part of multiple endocrine neoplasia, type 2, have also been reported (Harper et al., 1989).

HIRSUTISM AND VIRILIZATION IN PREGNANCY

This subject was recently reviewed by McClamrock and Adashi (1992). Women and their female fetuses are protected from the increased concentrations of androgens by the enhanced binding to sex hormone–binding globulin, competition by progestins either for binding to the androgen receptor or for disposition of androgens to more biologically potent compounds, and also by placental aromatization of androgens. Nevertheless, maternal hirsutism and virilization may occur in pregnancy, nearly always secondary to ovarian disease (or iatrogenic insult). In addition, the female fetus may be affected by elevated circulating maternal androgens. Differentiation of the female external genitalia occurs between the 7th and 12th week of gestation, and exposure to excess androgens may result in partial or complete labial fusion and cliteromegaly. Cliteromegaly may still occur after the 12th week. The approach to maternal hirsutism and virilization in pregnancy is outlined in Table 56–6.

The two major causes of gestational hyperandrogenism are luteomas and hyperreactio luteinalis (gestational ovarian theca-lutein-cysts). Luteomas are benign, solid tumors of the ovary; they are often multinodular and bilateral, and usually yellow/tan in color. Regardless of their virilizing effect, luteomas

Table 56–6.   Approach to Maternal Hirsutism and Virilization in Pregnancy

HISTORY	
Acute onset in pregnancy: Investigate as indicated below. Androgenic drug exposure: Stop drug.	
PHYSICAL EXAM/OVARIAN ULTRASOUND	POSSIBLE VIRILIZATION OF FEMALE FETUS
Bilateral cystic: Theca lutein cysts R/O high hCG states	No
Bilateral solid: Luteoma very likely	Yes
Unilateral solid: Surgery to R/O malignancy	Yes
No ovarian mass: Investigate adrenal glands	Yes

have been associated with elevated circulating maternal androgens. Not all luteomas cause maternal virilization (overall incidence of virilization 35 per cent); this may depend upon the amount of androgen secreted, the end-organ sensitivity, and the degree of aromatization by the placenta to nonandrogenic steroids. Approximately 80 per cent of female infants born to mothers with virilizing luteomas are virilized, usually exhibiting cliteromegaly. Although luteomas are considered intrapartum lesions that regress postpartum, this concept has recently been challenged and may account for recurrence of virilization in subsequent pregnancies (Shortle et al., 1987). In contrast to hyperreactio luteinalis, luteomas occur more frequently in black multiparas, and are not associated with toxemia, erythroblastosis, or multiple gestation.

Hyperreactio luteinalis is characterized by ovarian enlargement with multiple large-follicle cysts and/or corpora lutea with marked edema of the stroma. It is generally bilateral, affecting white primigravidas, and is often associated with conditions resulting in increased human chorionic gonadotropin (hCG) such as molar pregnancies and multiple gestation. Maternal hirsutism or virilization has been documented in approximately 30 per cent of reported cases. There are no reported cases of fetal masculinization, even if the mother is virilized. It has been suggested that the condition may represent an excessive ovarian sensitivity to hCG. The lack of fetal virilization in this condition is intriguing and has been attributed to androgen aromatization in the placenta. As with luteomas, recurrence of hyperreactio luteinalis in consecutive pregnancies has been reported (Bachman et al., 1974).

Other ovarian lesions that may cause maternal virilization include Sertoli-Leydig cell tumors (arrhenoblastomas), Krukenberg tumors, Brenner tumors, lipoid cell tumors, dermoid cysts, and mucinous and serous cystadenocarcinomas. The majority of Sertoli-Leydig cell tumors coexisting with pregnancy are associated with maternal virilization, and virilization of the female fetus may occur. The malignancy rate for these tumors is high (44 per cent), with substantial maternal (31 per cent) and perinatal (50 per cent) mortality rates. Krukenberg tumors, which are gastrointestinal tumors metastatic to the ovary, are often bilateral and have caused maternal and fetal virilization in all reported cases.

Adrenal tumors, including adrenocortical carci-

noma, may cause maternal and fetal virilization (Miyata et al., 1989). Finally, masculinization of the female fetus has been associated with the gestational administration of progestins and androgens and may be unaccompanied by maternal virilization.

PARATHYROID GLANDS AND CALCIUM METABOLISM

Maternal and Fetal Physiology and Lactation

Serum calcium is tightly regulated and maintained within normal limits by parathyroid hormone (PTH) and vitamin D. Vitamin D can be synthesized in the skin under the influence of ultraviolet irradiation or may be absorbed from dietary sources via the gastrointestinal tract. Vitamin D is 25-hydroxylated in the liver and then 1-hydroxylated in the kidney. The physiologically active form of vitamin D is $1,25(OH)_2$ D, which is responsible for increasing intestinal absorption of calcium and also bone resorption. The parathyroid glands, which produce PTH, are stimulated by hypocalcemia and suppressed by high concentrations of calcium, magnesium, and $1,25(OH)_2$ D, and also by hypomagnesemia. Parathyroid hormone influences calcium metabolism, not only by directly resorbing bone, but also by stimulating $1,25(OH)_2$ D formation. There are three major forms of circulating calcium, namely ionized, protein-bound, and chelated fractions. The ionized fraction is physiologically active and homeostatically regulated.

Although the mechanisms responsible for placental transport of calcium are poorly understood, large amounts of calcium and phosphorus are transferred against a concentration gradient from the mother to the fetus (Pitkin, 1985), the net fetal accumulation of calcium being 25 to 30 gm by term (mostly in the third trimester). Maternal calcium absorption, mediated through increases in PTH and $1,25(OH)_2$ D synthesis, rises during pregnancy to meet these demands. Depending on calcium intake, the net effect of pregnancy on the maternal skeleton could be positive or negative; under normal conditions there is little influence on bone mineral content. Paralleling a decline in serum albumen, total serum calcium concentrations decline during gestation (Fig. 56–11), with little change in ionized calcium (Pitkin et al., 1979).

In response to placental calcium transfer as well as an expanding extracellular volume and increased urinary calcium loss, maternal PTH concentrations rise during pregnancy (Fig. 56–12). Serum 25(OH)D concentrations remain essentially unchanged, while $1,25(OH)_2$ D levels also rise during pregnancy, peaking at term (Steinchen et al., 1980); there may be a placental contribution to the latter. There are no consistent changes in calcitonin concentrations in pregnancy.

Fetal parathyroid tissue has been identified by 6 weeks gestation, and skeletal mineralization is apparent by the eighth week. Total and ionized calcium concentrations are elevated in the fetus at term and decrease to normal in the newborn period. PTH levels are low in the fetus and increase after birth (Pitkin,

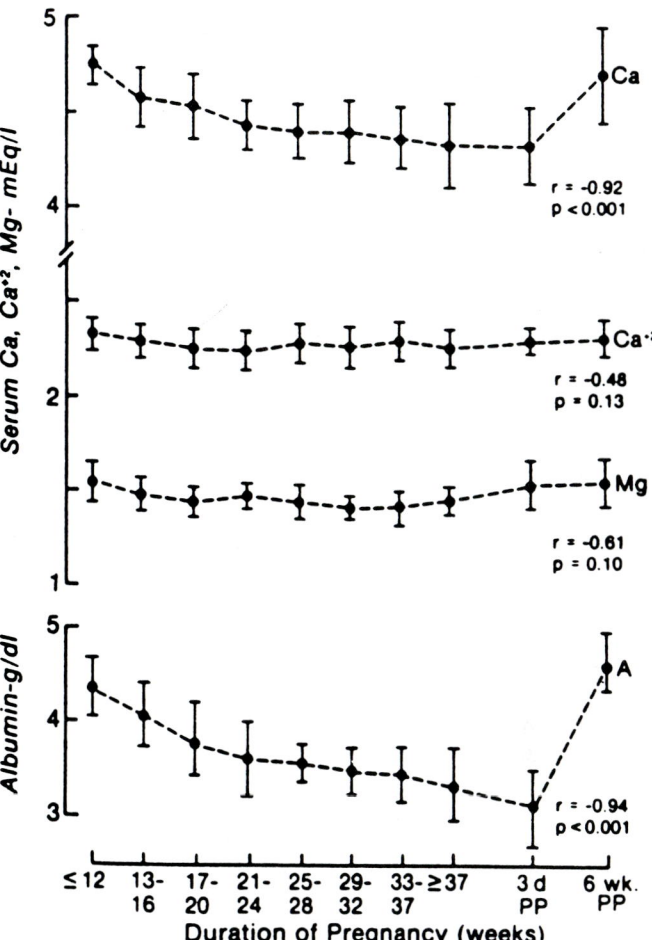

FIGURE 56–11. Mean (± SD) levels of calcium (Ca), ionized calcium (Ca⁺²), magnesium (Mg), and albumin during pregnancy and the puerperium. (From Pitkin RM, Reynolds WA, Williams GA, et al: Calcium metabolism in normal pregnancy: A longitudinal study. Am J Obstet Gynecol **133**:781, 1979.)

1985). Calcitonin is elevated in the fetus. These events are summarized in Table 56–7. During lactation the average daily loss of calcium in human milk is 220 to 340 mg. There is a small drop in serum calcium, accompanied by a rise in PTH and 1,25(OH)₂ D concentrations.

Disorders of the Parathyroid Glands

Primary Hyperparathyroidism and Hypercalcemia

As in nonpregnant women, the histopathology of hyperparathyroidism in pregnant women involves a single adenoma in the vast majority, although hyperplasia and carcinoma have also been reported (Kristofferson et al., 1985; Gelister et al., 1989). While many are asymptomatic, clinical features of the associated hypercalcemia are summarized in Table 56–8. In the 102 pregnancies (in 73 women) reported by Kristofferson et al. (1985), the clinical history was known in 45. Abdominal symptoms, including nausea, vomiting, pain, and renal colic, were the most frequent, followed by muscular weakness, mental symptoms, and polyuria; 20 per cent were asymptomatic. The diagnosis of hyperparathyroidism during pregnancy is suggested by hypercalcemia. The fall in total serum calcium

during pregnancy may mask the diagnosis (or be associated with a postpartum flare-up), and ionized serum calcium should be measured in patients suspected of having primary hyperparathyroidism. The diagnosis is then confirmed by finding inappropriately elevated PTH concentrations as well as an increase in urinary nephrogenic cyclic adenosine monophosphate levels (cAMP). The differential diagnosis of hypercalcemia includes malignant disease, granulomatous disease, thyrotoxicosis, hypervitaminosis D or A, and immobilization as well as familial hypocalciuric hypercalcemia, which is an autosomal dominant, inherited form of mild, benign hyperparathyroidism associated with low urinary calcium excretion.

During pregnancy, there is a degree of protection in the mother against hypercalcemia provided by calcium transport across the placenta, this being greatest in the third trimester. Loss of this protection with delivery may cause acute postpartum maternal hypercalcemia. In many patients the diagnosis is made postpartum following the occurrence of neonatal tetany. Ten of 15 cases of hyperparathyroidism reported recently by Gelister et al. (1989) presented in this way, the others presenting with hyperemesis, hypertension, and a jaw fracture in a patient who turned out to have a parathyroid carcinoma.

COMPLICATIONS. Complications of hyperparathyroidism affect both mother and infant. Maternal com-

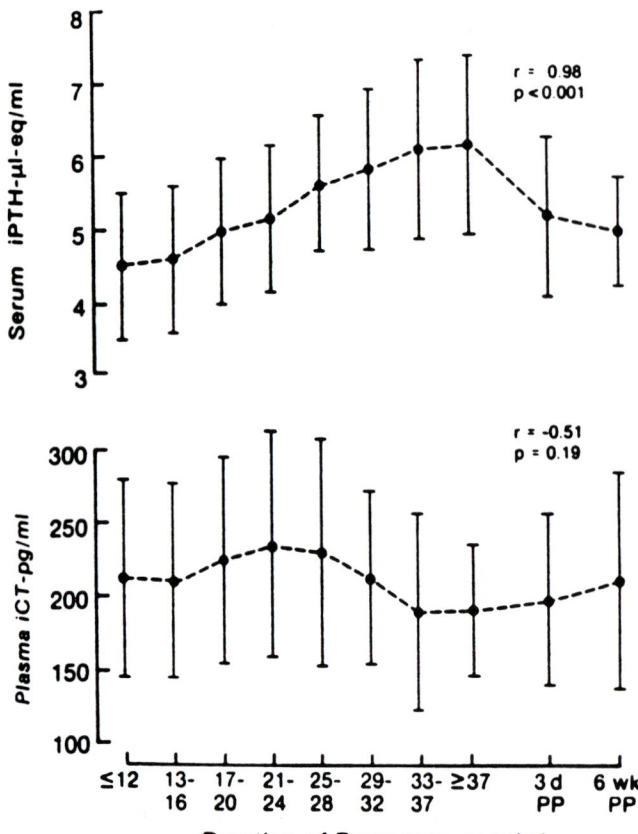

FIGURE 56–12. Mean (± SD) levels of immunoreactive parathyroid hormone (iPTH) and immunoreactive calcitionin (iCT) during pregnancy and the puerperium. (From Pitkin RM, Reynolds WA, Williams GA, et al: Calcium metabolism in normal pregnancy: A longitudinal study. Am J Obstet Gynecol **133**:781, 1979.)

plications include hyperemesis, weakness, renal calculi, pancreatitis, and psychiatric problems. The overall maternal mortality remains low (one out of 73 in the collected series of Kristofferson et al., 1985). However, fetal morbidity and mortality are significant. In the 102 pregnancies, involving 73 women, reviewed by Kristofferson et al. (1985), there were 53 (52 per cent) normal children, 24 (23.5 per cent) cases of neonatal tetany, 10 (9.8 per cent) stillbirths, and a few cases of prematurity and neonatal death. In the series of Gelister et al. (1989), 10 of 15 presented with

TABLE 56–7. Minerals and Hormones Involved in Calcium Homeostasis

MINERAL/ HORMONE	MOTHER	FETUS	NEWBORN
Total calcium	Low	High	Falls†
Ionized calcium*	Low normal	High	Falls
Magnesium*	Low normal	High normal	Falls
Phosphorus*	Low	High	Rises†
PTH	High	Low	Rises
Calcitonin	Normal	High	Falls
25(OH)D*	Variable	Variable	Variable
1,25(OH)₂D	High	Low	Rises

*Placental transfer
†Toward nonpregnant adult values

TABLE 56–8. Maternal Features of Hypercalcemia

Urinary system:	nephrolithiasis
	nephrocalcinosis
	polyuria
Neuromuscular:	weakness
Gastrointestinal:	peptic ulcer disease
	constipation
	anorexia
	nausea/vomiting
Cardiovascular:	hypertension
	arrhythmias
Skeletal:	osteitis fibrosa cystica
	osteopenia and fractures
Neuropsychiatric:	depression
	psychosis
	obtundation
	coma
Miscellaneous:	thirst
	pruritus

neonatal hypocalcemia and there was one stillbirth. Although neonatal hypocalcemia with tetany is usually a transient phenomenon related to suppression of fetal parathyroid glands resulting from maternal-fetal hypercalcemia, it may be more prolonged in less mature infants or infants with birth asphyxia.

TREATMENT. For hyperparathyroidism presenting during pregnancy, standard practice favors surgical treatment. In the collected series of Kristoffersen et al. (1985), there were 79 pregnancies among 50 women who did not undergo surgery; there were complications in 41 of the pregnancies (52 per cent), and neonatal tetany occurred in 21 (26.6 per cent). This was contrasted with the more favorable outcome in 23 pregnancies involving 23 women who had surgical treatment during pregnancy; five had complications (22 per cent) and there were three cases of neonatal tetany (13 per cent). Surgery should be performed in the second trimester, when fetal organs are developed and the uterus less likely to undergo labor (Nudelman et al., 1984). Conservative treatment of mild asymptomatic patients has also been suggested (Lowe et al., 1983).

The treatment of life-threatening hypercalcemia may be problematic and may require hydration, furosemide, phosphates, and even hemodialysis (Monturo et al., 1980; Kleinman et al., 1991). This is summarized in Table 56–9. Calcitonin inhibits bone resorption; its effects are generally short-lived, and it does not cross the placenta. In life-threatening situations mithramycin (plicamycin) will lower calcium by inhibiting bone resorption. It is an antineoplastic agent and toxic to the fetus. In nonpregnant patients diphosphonates, such as etidronate, given intravenously are also effective in lowering calcium. There are no data on their use in pregnancy.

Hypoparathyroidism

Hypoparathyroidism in pregnancy usually occurs in patients with previous neck surgery, but may be seen in other less common circumstances (Table 56–10). The diagnosis is made by the combination of hypocalcemia, with low PTH, 1,25(OH)₂D, and nephrogenous

TABLE 56–9. **Treatment of Hypercalcemia**

TREATMENT	ADVERSE EFFECTS
General	
Hydration	
Discontinue offending drugs	
Restrict calcium	
Increase renal calcium excretion	
0.9% saline 200–500 ml/hr	Volume overload
Furosemide 20–60 mg IV q2–4h	Volume depletion
	Hypokalemia
Dialysis	
Calcium chelation with phosphates	Extraskeletal
Oral: Neura-phos 500–750 mg	Calcification
q6–8h	
Rectal: Phosphosoda 5 ml q6–8h	
IV: 50 mM phosphate over 8–12	
hours	
Decrease bone resorption	
Calcitonin 4–8 IU/kg IM or Sc	Allergic reaction
every 6–12 hours*	Nausea
Etidronate (diphosphonate)† 7.5	Renal toxicity
mg/kg IV daily in 250 ml	
normal saline	
Mithramycin 25 μg/kg IV‡ every	Low platelets
48–72 hours	Renal toxicity
	Hepatotoxicity

*No reports of congenital defects; does not cross placenta
†No reports on use in pregnancy
‡No reports on use in pregnancy; antineoplastic

cAMP concentrations. Other hypocalcemic states that need to be distinguished from hypoparathyroidism include vitamin D deficiency (high PTH found), excessive chelation (following blood transfusion), pancreatitis, and septic states.

Clinical features include tetany, which may be elicited in latent form using the Chvostek's (tapping of the facial nerve) and Trousseau's tests (the occurrence of tetany within three minutes of the induction of ischemia in the upper extremity). Other symptoms include paresthesia, stridor, muscle cramps, and mental changes including frank psychosis. The electrocardiogram may reveal prolongation of the Q-T interval.

COMPLICATIONS. Neonatal hyperparathyroidism may develop secondary to maternal hypocalcemia. This may cause fetal bone demineralization and growth restriction (Fleischman, 1980). Although this is transient, death from complications of skeletal fractures may occur. Loughhead et al. (1990) reviewed 16 cases of congenital hyperparathyroidism secondary to maternal hypocalcemia; bone features of hyperpara-

TABLE 56–10. **Classification of Hypoparathyroid Disorders**

DEFECT	ETIOLOGY
Absence of PTH or insufficiency	Previous thyroid or parathyroid surgery
	Idiopathic hypoparathyroidism (familial or sporadic)
	Di George's syndrome
	Iron overload (rare)
	Previous irradiation with [131]I (rare)
Absence of and resistance to PTH	Magnesium depletion
PTH resistance	Pseudohypoparathyroidism

thyroidism were documented in 13 cases. Six of the neonates died within the first three months of life. In their conclusion they stated that the presentation was highly variable, ranging from clinically and radiologically silent cases to neonates with severe skeletal disease and bone demineralization.

TREATMENT. The maternal serum calcium level should be maintained within normal limits. Vitamin D (50,000 to 100,000 units/day or more) and calcium salts (1.0 or 1.5 gm elemental calcium per day) are given to maintain normocalcemia. More recently, calcitriol (1,25[OH]$_2$ D), which has a more rapid onset of action, has been used, the usual dose being 0.5 to 1.0 μg/day (Salle et al., 1981). The normal replacement dose of vitamin D in a hypoparathyroid woman may need to be increased, possibly due to increased binding of vitamin D to vitamin D binding protein. In a patient treated with calcitriol, the dose had to be doubled during pregnancy to maintain normocalcemia, similar to the physiologic twofold rise in 1,25(OH)$_2$ D during pregnancy (Sadeghi-Nejad et al., 1980). The aim should be serum calcium concentrations in the 8 to 9 mg/dl range with avoidance of hypercalciuria (>250 mg/24 hr), which may lead to nephrolithiasis. A prompt decrease to prepregnancy doses of vitamin D is necessary postpartum, to avoid hypercalcemia (Caplan and Beguin, 1990). Although lactating women usually require continuation of pregnancy doses of vitamin D, hypercalcemia has been reported (Caplan and Beguin, 1990) and close monitoring would be prudent. One advantage to the use of calcitriol is its shorter half-life.

Acute symptomatic hypocalcemia is a medical emergency and should be treated with intravenous calcium, for example, 10 ml of 10 per cent calcium gluconate over ten minutes followed by an infusion of 0.5 to 2.0 mg/kg/hour of elemental calcium, diluted with dextrose to avoid irritation to veins.

Infants receiving breast milk from mothers consuming large doses of vitamin D should have periodic calcium determinations, as the breast milk will have higher than normal levels of vitamin D (Greer et al., 1984), which may cause hypercalcemia and impaired linear growth in the infant.

REFERENCES

Hypothalamus and Pituitary Disorders

Aaron D, Schwall AM, Sheeler LR: Cushing's syndrome and pregnancy. Am J Obstet Gynecol 162:244, 1990.
Albrecht BH, Betz G: Prolactin-secreting pituitary tumors and pregnancy. In Olefsy JM, Robbins RJ (eds). Contemporary Issues in Endocrinology and Metabolism: Prolactinomas. Vol 2. New York, Churchill Livingstone, 1986, p. 195.
Belchetz PE, Carty A, Clearkin LG: Failure of prophylactic surgery to avert massive pituitary expansion in pregnancy. Clin Endocrinol 25:325, 1986.
Bitton RN, Slavin M, Decker RE, et al: The course of lymphocytic hypophysitis. Surg Neurol 36:40, 1991.
Brandes JC, Cerletty JM: Pregnancy in lymphocytic hypophysitis. Wis Med J 88:29, 1989.
Buescher MA, McClamrock HD, Adashi EY: Cushing syndrome in pregnancy. Obstet Gynecol 79:130, 1992.
Burrow GN, Wassenaar W, Robertson GL, et al: DDAVP treatment

of diabetes insipidus during pregnancy and the postpartum period. Acta Endocrinol **97**:23, 1981.

Campbell JW: Diabetes insipidus and complicated pregnancy. JAMA **243**:1744, 1980.

Cosman F, Post KD, Holub DA, et al: Lymphocytic hypophysitis. Report of 3 cases and review of the literature. Medicine **68**:240, 1989.

Davison JM, Gilmore EA, Durr JS, et al: Altered osmotic thresholds for vasopressin secretion and thirst in human pregnancy. Am J Physiol **246**:105, 1983.

Dawood MY, Khan-Dawood FS: The posterior pituitary pathway. In Droegemveller W, Sciarra J (eds): Gynecology and Obstetrics. Vol. 5. Philadelphia, J.B. Lippincott Co., 1990.

Decherney A, Naftolin F: Hypothalamic and pituitary development in the fetus. Clin Obstet Gynecol **23**:749, 1980.

Del Pozo E, Krupp P: Endocrine effects of dopamine receptor stimulation on the feto-maternal unit. In Krauer B, et al (eds): Drugs and Pregnancy. London, England, Academie, 1984, p. 191.

Divers WA, Yen SSC: Prolactin-producing microadenomas in pregnancy. Obstet Gynecol **62**:425, 1983.

Dorfman SG, Dillaplain RP, Gambrell RD: Antepartum pituitary infarction. Obstet Gynecol **53**(suppl):21S, 1979.

Drury MI, Keelan DM: Sheehan's syndrome. J Obstet Gynaecol Br Commonw **73**:802, 1966.

Feigenbaum S, Martin MC, Wilson CB, et al: Lymphocytic adenohypophysitis: A pituitary mass lesion occurring in pregnancy. Am J Obstet Gynecol **164**:1549, 1991.

Frohman LA: Neurotransmitters as regulators of endocrine function. In Krieger DT, Hughes JC (eds): Neuroendocrinology. Sunderland, Sinauer Associates, Inc., 1980.

Furlanetto RW, Underwood LE, Van Wyk JJ, et al: Serum immunoreactive somatomedin-C is elevated late in pregnancy. J Clin Endocrinol Metab **47**:695, 1978.

Gonzalez JF, Elizondo G, Saldivar D, et al: Pituitary gland growth during normal pregnancy: An in vivo study using magnetic resonance imaging. Am J Med **85**:217, 1988.

Gormley MJJ, Hadden DR, Kennedy TL, et al: Cushing's syndrome in pregnancy—Treatment with metyrapone. Clin Endocrinol **16**:283, 1982.

Goudie RB, Pinkerton PH: Anterior hypophysitis and Hashimoto's disease in a young woman. J Pathol Bacteriol **83**:585, 1962.

Green JS, Parfrey PS, Harnett JD, et al: The cardinal manifestations of Bardet-Biedl syndrome, a form of Lawrence-Moon-Biedl syndrome. N Engl J Med **321**:1002, 1989.

Grimes HG, Brooks MH: Pregnancy in Sheehan's syndrome: Report of a case and review. Obstet Gynecol Surv **35**:481, 1980.

Hall MRP: Incidence of anterior pituitary deficiency following postpartum hemorrhage: Cases reviewed from the Oxfordshire and Buckinghamshire area. Proc Soc Med **55**:468, 1962.

Hendricks CH: The neurohypophysis in pregnancy. Obstet Gynecol Surv **9**:323, 1954.

Hiett AK, Barton JR: Diabetes insipidus associated with craniopharyngioma in pregnancy. Obstet Gynecol **76**:982, 1990.

Hime MC, Richardson JA: Diabetes insipidus and pregnancy: Case report, incidence and review of literature. Obstet Gynecol Surv **33**:375, 1978.

Itskovitz J, Rosenwaks Z: Pituitary disease in pregnancy. In Brody S, Velard K (eds): Endocrine Disorders in Pregnancy. Norwalk, CT, Appleton & Lange, 1989.

Iwasaki Y, Oiso Y, Kondo K, et al: Aggravation of subclinical diabetes insipidus during pregnancy. N Engl J Med **324**:522, 1991.

Krege J, Katz VL, Bowes WA: Transient diabetes insipidus of pregnancy. Obstet Gynecol Surv **44**:789, 1989.

Krupp P, Monka C: Bromocriptine in pregnancy: Safety aspects. Klin Wochenschr **65**:823, 1987.

Lindheimer MD, Barron WM, Davison JM: Osmotic volume control of vasopressin release in pregnancy. Am J Kidney Dis **17**:105, 1991.

Luboshitzky R, Dickstein G, Barzilai D: Bromocriptine induced pregnancy in an acromegalic patient. JAMA **244**:584, 1980.

Lufkin EG, Kao PC, O'Fallon WM, et al: Combined testing of anterior pituitary gland with insulin, thyrotropin-releasing hormone and luteinizing hormone-releasing hormone. Am J Med **75**:471, 1983.

Magyar DM, Marshall JR: Pituitary tumors and pregnancy. Am J Obstet Gynecol **132**:739, 1978.

Maranon G: Diabetes insipidus and uterine atony. Br Med J **2**:769, 1947.

Meichner RH, Riggio S, Manz HJ, et al: Lymphocytic adenohypophysitis causing pituitary mass. Neurology **37**:158, 1987.

Molitch ME: Pregnancy and the hyperprolactinemic woman. N Engl J Med **312**:1364, 1985.

Nader S, Orlander P: Lymphocytic hypophysitis: A case report and review of the literature. Infertility **13**:145, 1990.

Nakamura Y, Takagi H, Sakurai S, et al: Transient diabetes insipidus during and after pregnancy. N Engl J Med **325**:285, 1991.

O'Donovan PA, O'Donovan PJ, Ritchie EH: Apoplexy into a prolactin secreting macroadenoma during early pregnancy with successful outcome. Br J Obstet Gynaecol **93**:389, 1986.

Pickard J, Jochen AL, Sadur CN, Hofeldt FD: Cushing's syndrome in pregnancy. Obstet Gynecol Surv **45**:87, 1990.

Robinson AG: Disorders of antidiuretic hormone secretion. Clin Endocrinol Metab **14**:55, 1985.

Robinson AG, Amico JA: "No−sweet" diabetes of pregnancy. N Engl J Med **324**:556, 1991.

Ruiz-Velasco V, Tolis G: Pregnancy in hyperprolactinemic women. Fertil Steril **41**:793, 1984.

Sack J, Friedman E, Katznelson D, et al: Long-term treatment of diabetes insipidus with a synthetic analog of vasopressin during pregnancy. Isr J Med Sci **16**:406, 1980.

Scheithauer BW, Sano T, Kovacs KT, et al: The pituitary gland in pregnancy: A clinicopathologic and immunohistochemical study of 69 cases. Mayo Clin Proc **65**:461, 1990.

Schultz CL, Haaga JR, Fletcher BD, et al: Magnetic resonance imaging of the adrenal glands: A comparison with computed tomography. AJR **143**:1235, 1984.

Sheehan HL: Post-partum necrosis of the anterior pituitary. J Pathol Bacteriol **45**:189, 1937.

Stelmach M, O'Day J: Rapid change in visual fields associated with suprasellar lymphocytic hypophysitis. J Clin Neuroophthalmol **11**:19, 1991.

Surrey ES, Chang RJ: Nelson's syndrome in pregnancy. Fertil Steril **44**:548, 1985.

Tyson JE, Hwang P, Guyden A et al: Studies of prolactin secretion in human pregnancy. Am J Obstet Gynecol **113**:14, 1972.

Van der Spuy ZM, Jacobs HS. Management of endocrine disorders and pregnancy. Part II. Pituitary, ovarian, and adrenal disease. Postgrad Med J **60**:312, 1984.

Yap AS, Clouston WM, Mortimer RH, Drahe RF: Acromegaly first diagnosed in pregnancy: The role of bromocriptine therapy. Am J Obstet Gynecol **163**:477, 1990.

Zarate A, Canales ES, Alger M: The effect of pregnancy and lactation on pituitary prolactin secreting tumors. Acta Endocrinol **92**:407, 1979.

Adrenal Glands

Albert E, Dalaker K, Jorde R, et al: Addison's disease and pregnancy. Acta Obstet Gynecol Scand **68**:185, 1989.

Bongiovanni AM, McPadden AJ: Steroids during pregnancy and possible fetal consequences. Fertil Steril **11**:181, 1960.

Buescher MA, McClamrock HD, Adashi EY: Cushing syndrome in pregnancy. Obstet Gynecol **79**:130, 1992.

Devoe LD, O'Dell BE, Castillo RA, et al: Metastatic pheochromocytoma in pregnancy and fetal biophysical assessment after maternal administration of α-adrenergic, β-adrenergic, and dopamine antagonists. Obstet Gynecol **68**:155, 1986.

Drucker D, Shumak S, Angel A: Schmidt syndrome presenting with intrauterine growth retardation and postpartum Addisonian crises. Am J Obstet Gynecol **149**:229, 1984.

Ellison GT, Mansberger JA, Mansberger AR: Malignant recurrent pheochromocytoma during pregnancy. Case report and review of the literature. Surgery **103**:484, 1988.

Fudge TL, McKinnon WMP, Greary WL: Current surgical management of pheochromocytoma during pregnancy. Arch Surg **115**:1224, 1980.

Glazer GM, Woolsey EJ, Borrello J, et al: Adrenal tissue characterization using MR imaging. Radiology **158**:73, 1986.

Griffin J, Brooks N, Patricia F, et al: Pheochromocytoma in pregnancy. Diagnosis and collaborative management. South Med J **77**:1325, 1984.

Harper A, Murnaghan GA, Kennedy L, et al: Pheochromocytoma in pregnancy. Five cases and a review of the literature. Br J Obstet Gynecol 96:594, 1989.

Kreft-Jais C, Plovin PF, Tchobrovtsky C, et al: Angiotensin-converting enzyme inhibitors during pregnancy: A survey of 22 patients given captopril and nine given enalapril. Br J Obstet Gynaecol 95:420, 1988.

Lotgering FK, Derhx FMH, Wallenburg HCS: Primary hypoaldosteronism in pregnancy. Am J Obstet Gynecol 155:986, 1986.

Lyons CW, Colmorgen GHC: Medical management of pheochromocytoma in pregnancy. Obstet Gynecol 72:450, 1988.

Mitchell SZ, Freilich JD, Brant D, et al: Anesthetic management of pheochromocytoma resection during pregnancy. Anesth Analg 66:478, 1987.

Mori N, Miyakawa I: Congenital adrenogenital syndrome and successful pregnancy. Obstet Gynecol 35:394, 1970.

Mornet E, Couillin P, Kutten F, et al: Associations between restriction fragment length polymorphisms detected with a probe for human 21-hydroxylase and two clinical forms of 21-hydroxylase deficiency. Hum Genet 74:402, 1986.

Neerhof MG, Shlossman PA, Ludomirsky A, et al: Idiopathic aldosteronism in pregnancy. Obstet Gynecol 78:489, 1991.

Nolten WE, Lindheimer MD, Oparil S, et al: Deoxycorticosterone in normal pregnancy. Am J Obstet Gynecol 132: 414, 1978.

Oliver MD, Brownjohn AM, Vinali PS: Medical management of pheochromocytoma 1-pregnancy. Aust NZ J Obstet Gynaecol 30:268, 1990.

Pang S, Wallace MA, Hofman L, et al: Worldwide experience in newborn screening for classical congenital adrenal hyperplasia due to 21-hydroxylase deficiency. Pediatrics 81:866, 1988.

Peterson RE: Cortisol. In Fuchs F, Klopper A (eds): Endocrinology of Pregnancy. 2nd ed. Hagerstown, Harper & Row, 1977.

Rees LH, Burke CW, Chard T, et al: Possible placental origin of ACTH in normal human pregnancy. Nature 254:620, 1975.

Rosenfeld RL, Rich BL, Wolfsdorf JI, et al: Pubertal presentation of congenital 5-3B-hydroxysteroid dehydrogenase deficiency. J Clin Endocrinol Metab 51:345, 1980.

Rosenthal HE, Slaunwhite WR, Sandberg AA: Transcortin: A corticosteroid binding protein of plasma. X. Cortisol and progesterone interplay and unbound levels of these steroids in pregnancy. J Clin Endocrinol Metab 29:352, 1969.

Rosler A, Leiberman E, Rosenmann A, et al: Prenatal diagnosis of 11 beta hydroxylase deficiency congenital adrenal hyperplasia. J Clin Endocrinol Metab 49:546, 1979.

Sasaki A, Liotta AS, Luckey MM, et al: Immunoreactive corticotropin-releasing factor is present in human maternal plasma during the third trimester of pregnancy. J Clin Endocrinol Metab 59:812, 1984.

Schenker JG, Granat M: Pheochromocytomas and pregnancy—an updated appraisal. Aust NZ J Obstet Gynaecol 22:1, 1982.

Seaward PGR, Guidozzi F, Sonnendecker EWW: Addisonian crisis in pregnancy: Case Report. Br J Obstet Gynaecol 96:1348, 1989.

Snyder RD, Snyder D: Corticosteroids for asthma during pregnancy. Ann Allergy 41:340, 1978.

White PC, New MI: Genetic basis of endocrine disease. 2: Congenital adrenal hyperplasia due to 21-hydroxylase deficiency. J Clin Endocrinol Metab 74:6, 1992.

White PC, New MI, Dupont BO: Congenital adrenal hyperplasia. N Engl J Med 316:1519, 1987a.

White PC, New MI, Dupont BO: Congenital adrenal hyperplasia. N Engl J Med 316:1580, 1987b.

Wilson M, Morganti AA, Zervoudakis I, et al: Blood pressure, the renin-aldosterone system and sex steroids throughout normal pregnancy. Am J Med 68:97, 1980.

Hirsutism and Virilization

Bachman R, Gennser G, Hakfelt B, et al: Steroid studies in a case of ovarian hyperluteinization with virilism in two consecutive pregnancies. Acta Endocrinol 76:747, 1974.

McClamrock HD, Adashi EY: Gestational hyperandrogenism. Fertil Steril 57:257, 1992.

Miyata M, Nishihara M, Tokunaka KS, et al: A maternal functioning adrenocortical adenoma causing fetal female pseudohermaphroditism. J Urol 142:806, 1989.

Shortle BE, Warren MP, Tsin D: Recurrent androgenicity in pregnancy: A case report and literature review. Obstet Gynecol 70:462, 1987.

Parathyroid Disorders and Hypercalcemia

Caplan RH, Beguin EA: Hypercalcemia in a calcitriol-treated hypoparathyroid woman during lactation. Obstet Gynecol 76:485, 1990.

Fleischman AR: Fetal parathyroid gland and calcium homeostasis. Clin Obstet Gynecol 23:791, 1980.

Gelister JSK, Sanderson JD, Chapple CR, et al: Management of hyperparathyroidism in pregnancy. Br J Surg 76:1207, 1989.

Greer FR, Hollis BW, Napoli JL: High concentrations of vitamin D_2 in human milk associated with pharmacologic doses of vitamin D_2. J Pediatr 105:61, 1984.

Kleinman GE, Rodriguez H, Good MC, et al: Hypercalcemic crisis in pregnancy associated with excessive ingestion of calcium carbonate antacid: Successful treatment with hemodialysis. Obstet Gynecol 78:496, 1991.

Kristofferson A, Dahlgren S, Lithner F, et al: Primary hyperparathyroidism and pregnancy. Surgery 97:326, 1985.

Loughead JL, Mughal Z, Mimouni F, et al: Spectrum and natural history of congenital hyperparathyroidism secondary to maternal hypocalcemia. Am J Perinatol 7:350, 1990.

Lowe DK, Orwoll ES, McClung MR, et al: Hyperparathyroidism and pregnancy. Am J Surg 145:611, 1983.

Monturo MN, Collea JV, Mestman JH: Management of hyperparathyroidism in pregnancy with oral phosphate therapy. Obstet Gynecol 55:431, 1980.

Nudelman J, Deutsch A, Sternberg A, et al: The treatment of primary hyperparathyroidism during pregnancy. Br J Surg 71:217, 1984.

Pitkin RM: Calcium metabolism in pregnancy and the perinatal period. A review. Am J Obstet Gynecol 151:99, 1985.

Pitkin RM, Reynolds WA, Williams GA, et al: Calcium metabolism in normal pregnancy: A longitudinal study. Am J Obstet Gynecol 133:781, 1979.

Sadeghi-Nejad A, Wolfsdorf JI, Senior B: Hypoparathyroidism and pregnancy: treatment with calcitriol. JAMA 243:254, 1980.

Salle BL, Berthezene F, Glorieux FH, et al: Hypoparathyroidism during pregnancy: treatment with calcitriol. J Clin Endocrinol Metab 52:810, 1981.

Steinchen JJ, Tsang RC, Grafton TL, et al: Vitamin D homeostasis in the perinatal period: 1,25-dihydroxyvitamin D in maternal, cord and neonatal blood. N Engl J Med 302:315, 1980.

CHAPTER

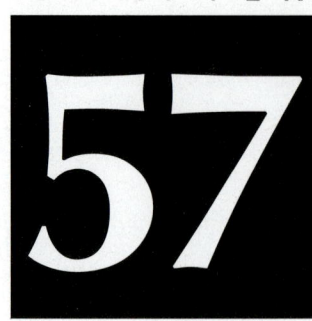

GASTROINTESTINAL DISEASE IN PREGNANCY

LARRY D. SCOTT, M.D.

Gastrointestinal function may be altered during pregnancy with a variety of problems and complaints resulting. Moreover, the unique hormonal and metabolic environment created by pregnancy may alter the course of preexisting gastrointestinal disease with the potential for both favorable and unfavorable effects. Lastly is the possibility for gastrointestinal disease either itself or through its management, specifically pharmacologic agents, to alter the course of pregnancy and affect its outcome. The interrelationships of pregnancy and gastrointestinal function, symptoms, and disease on all these levels are to be the focus of the material presented in this chapter.

GASTROINTESTINAL SYMPTOMS DURING PREGNANCY

Although many complaints and problems are commonly thought to be pregnancy-related, surveys which actually define and quantify gastrointestinal symptoms that might be unique to pregnancy are few in number. In one such study (Table 57–1), 12 symptoms were experienced more frequently by pregnant women during one, two, or all three trimesters than by a group of nonpregnant women from the same population; respondents to a questionnaire regarding a total of 35 digestive symptoms comprised the study population and were largely from a low socioeconomic group attending a university teaching clinic (Scott et al., 1986). Although several of these symptoms (e.g., gastroesophageal reflux) are consistent with long-held concepts, 22 other digestive symptoms were evenly distributed among the four groups and did not appear to be related to pregnancy (Table 57–2). One example, which is contrary to traditional beliefs, was constipation (hard or dry stools, straining at defecation, hemorrhoids); further, a need to use laxatives actually was noted more frequently in the nonpregnant women (see Table 57–1). No firm conclusions can be drawn from one survey, and personal experience may well dictate alternative views; nonetheless, the survey does imply that it is not always possible to state unequivocally which symptoms and conditions are causally related to pregnancy.

Although categorical statements regarding gastrointestinal symptomatology during pregnancy may not be possible, there are some symptoms that have been evaluated in more detail. One of these is heartburn, the cardinal symptom of gastroesophageal reflux. In the study noted above, 48.5 per cent of third-trimester women reported heartburn, a figure similar to the 48 per cent incidence in late pregnancy reported by Nagler and Spiro 30 years ago (Nagler and Spiro, 1962). If one looks at daily occurrence, the frequency of heartburn to this degree was more than twofold that reported by nonpregnant women. The mechanisms that might underlie increased occurrence of gastroesophageal reflux during pregnancy will be discussed below.

Increased appetite, while not specifically a gastrointestinal symptom, nonetheless can reflect gastrointestinal function. Teleologically, this finding is consistent with increased nutritional demands during pregnancy. Influences of sex steroids on appetite have been described, with progesterone thought to be an appetite stimulant (Van Thiel and Schade, 1986).

Nausea and vomiting are clearly pregnancy-related, and again the proposed mechanisms will be discussed below. Other symptoms of gastric origin may also be seen; for example, early satiety is common in third-trimester pregnancy. This may reflect the mechanical effect of an enlarging uterine fundus but also raises questions about gastric emptying, which may be impaired. Reports regarding this possibility are conflicting (Hunt and Murray, 1958; Davison et al., 1970; Schade et al., 1984a). If delayed gastric emptying does occur during pregnancy, it may be, at term, possibly related to drugs given during labor (La Salvia and Steffen, 1950); as such, it does not reflect a pregnancy-related phenomenon.

The issue of constipation is an interesting one; in the survey reported here, it was not, by the definition used, more common during pregnancy. In a study of 1000 Israeli women, half the study population reported no change in bowel frequency during pregnancy with an additional third reporting an increase in bowel frequency (Levy et al., 1971). This is in contrast to statements in several obstetrical textbooks but does

1026

TABLE 57–1. Symptoms Showing Significant Differences in Distribution Among the Study Population (n = 550)*

SYMPTOM	1st TRIMESTER (n = 85)	2nd TRIMESTER (n = 149)	3rd TRIMESTER (n = 225)	NOT PREGNANT (n = 91)
Xerostomia	42.6†	47.5	46.5	37.5
Regurgitation	53.6†	33.5	49.2†	34.0
Heartburn	29.2	29.4	48.5†	27.5
Eructation	31.5†	28.2†	34.0†	13.5
Improved appetite	47.8†	52.1†	52.1†	23.6
Early satiety	43.3	57.0	59.8†	41.3
Epigastric pain	28.7†	20.8	21.9	19.2
Nocturnal pain	21.7	21.0	36.6†	24.0
Nausea	65.8†	59.8†	45.8	35.1
Vomiting	44.2†	32.5	28.4	17.0
Laxative usage	22.7	19.8	21.7	35.9‡
Black stools	13.3	25.4†	34.6†	12.0
Pruritus	31.5†	44.1†	47.6†	28.3

*Data shown are for symptoms with significant differences in distribution of responses among the four groups; numbers reflect per cent of subjects experiencing symptoms regardless of frequency.
†Denotes group within which frequency of occurrence differed significantly from nonpregnant group.
‡Denotes group within which frequency of occurrence differed significantly from each pregnant group.

serve to point out the confusion over what is and what is not pregnancy-related.

In summary, the data reported in Table 57–1, while statistically significant, may not be reproducible in another population. The four groups studied (each trimester plus nonpregnant) were similar demographically and with respect to habits; however, other variables such as medications and co-morbid conditions can certainly affect symptomatology of any kind. That digestive symptoms can be pregnancy-related is not surprising, and in specific individuals, pregnancy may be the key in symptom production. Generalities, however, with the few exceptions just noted, may be difficult if not impossible to make.

ALTERATIONS IN GASTROINTESTINAL FUNCTION (Table 57–3)

The Esophagus

The function of the esophagus is to transport the swallowed bolus from the pharynx to the stomach. At the same time, it must defend itself against reflux of

TABLE 57–2. Symptoms *Not* Showing Significant Differences in Distribution Among the Study Population (n = 550)

Sialorrhea	Antacid usage
Bitter taste	Reduced appetite
Water brash	Postprandial bloating
Solid or liquid dysphagia	Epigastric pain after meals
Odynophagia	
Chest pain	Clay-colored stools
	Dark urine
Oily-appearing stools	Jaundice
Hard or dry stools	Abdominal pain radiating to
Unformed or watery stools	back
Antidiarrheal drug usage	
Straining at defecation	
Flatulence	
Hematochezia	
Hemorrhoids	

gastric or gastroduodenal contents that might injure the esophageal mucosa or be subject to aspiration with subsequent pneumonitis, laryngitis, bronchospasm, or other harmful effects. This function of transport and defense is largely the province of esophageal motility. With swallowing, under normal circumstances sequential peristaltic contractions propel the bolus caudally through a relaxed lower esophageal sphincter, which then regains tone, serving as a barrier against gastroesophageal reflux. Should reflux occur, a primary (swallow-induced) or secondary (distention-induced) peristaltic sequence returns the refluxed contents back to the gastric lumen.

There have been limited observations of esophageal motility in pregnancy. In one series, amplitude and duration of contractions were similar in pregnant and nonpregnant women, although the velocity of spread of wave-forms in the lower third of the esophageal body was decreased by about a third in the former; however, the values for both groups were still within normal limits (Ulmsten and Sundstrom, 1978). Another study of heartburn in pregnancy showed no differences in motility in the body of the esophagus between pregnant and nonpregnant women (Nagler and Spiro, 1961). Although observations have been limited, it is probably safe to conclude that peristaltic motility of the esophageal body is unaltered in pregnancy.

Such is not the case with the lower esophageal sphincter (LES), which is traditionally evaluated by intraluminal measurements of resting pressure. In animal models, as well as in most observations in human pregnancy, resting pressures are lowered (Nagler and Spiro, 1961; Schulze and Christensen, 1977; Van Thiel et al., 1977; Ostick et al., 1976); in a study of early pregnancy, pressures were not affected by pregnancy, but the response of the LES to stimulation by various agonists was reduced (Fisher et al., 1978). Perhaps the most convincing observation was by Van Thiel, who serially measured LES pressure in the same group of women during each trimester of pregnancy and during the postpartum period, showing a stepwise reduction in relation to duration of gestation with

TABLE 57–3. Implications of Alterations in Gastrointestinal Function in Pregnancy

PHYSIOLOGIC ALTERATIONS	CLINICAL IMPLICATIONS
ESOPHAGUS	
Reduction in resting LES* pressure	Gastroesophageal reflux Heartburn
Reduction in responsiveness of LES to pharmacologic and physiologic stimulation	Uncertain risk for erosive esophagitis and stricture formation
Questionable changes in wave-form characteristics and spread	
STOMACH	
Slow gastric emptying with increased residual volume (term)	Gastroesophageal reflux (?) Nausea and vomiting (?) Risk of aspiration with general anesthesia for delivery
Equivocal changes in acid + pepsin secretion	Decreased incidence of duodenal ulcer
SMALL INTESTINE	
Increased transit time	Stasis and bacterial overgrowth
Changes in propulsive motility	Sequestration of bile acids
Reduced contractile responsiveness of intestinal muscle *(in vitro)*	Pseudo-obstruction syndrome
Increased activity of brush border enzymes, gut hypertrophy, and increased villus height	Enhanced efficiency of absorption of some nutrients
Folate malabsorption (?)	Megaloblastic anemia
COLON	
Increased transit time (?)	Constipation and its attendant symptoms
Contractile responsiveness of colonic smooth muscle reduced	Pseudo-obstruction syndrome
Increased sodium and water absorption	

*LES = Lower esophageal sphincter.

recovery following delivery (Van Thiel et al., 1977) (Fig. 57–1). This phenomenon may well be a major variable in the genesis of gastroesophageal reflux and heartburn, to be discussed below.

The explanation for these changes has not been determined with certainty. The theory most often put forward is that reduced LES pressure is due to high circulating levels of progesterone, which has been shown to have an inhibitory effect on gastrointestinal as well as uterine smooth muscle (Kumar, 1962; Bruce and Behsudi, 1980; Ryan and Pellechia, 1982). While this is a plausible theory, the evidence remains circumstantial; at least in one study, the degree of reduction in LES pressure did not correlate with the concentration of progesterone in the peripheral blood (Ostick et al., 1976).

The Stomach

Gastric function is primarily secretory and motor; the former is manifest in the production of hydrogen ion by the parietal cell located in fundic mucosa of the gastric body. The production of acid creates a hostile environment for potentially pathogenic microorganisms while also providing the optimal pH for activation of pepsinogen to pepsin, which has proteolytic function. The presence of acid may also facilitate absorption of certain elements such as ionic iron and ascorbic acid. In practice, however, the importance of this function is limited as patients with achlorhydria do not appear to experience an increased risk from infections and are not jeopardized nutritionally. On the other hand, acid, while serving the physiologic role just discussed, also can serve as a pathogenetic factor in the production of both duodenal ulcer as well as gastroesophageal reflux disease. It is thus reasonable to ask whether acid secretion is altered by pregnancy and, if so, are there physiologic or perhaps pathophysiologic consequences?

Most of the studies of gastric physiology were carried out several years ago in experimental animals and to a lesser extent in small groups of pregnant women. As will be discussed later, it has been observed clinically that ulcer patients experience fewer symptoms during pregnancy, suggesting that acid secretion is reduced. At least two studies addressing acid secretion in pregnancy have concluded that a reduction in both basal acid secretion and stimulated acid secretion in fact does occur during pregnancy (Murray et al., 1957; Hunt and Murray, 1958); however, other studies report no change (Waldum et al., 1980) or even an increase in acid production in the third trimester (Gryboski and Spiro, 1956). Clearly, this issue is unsettled. The implications of changes in acid secretion may be more relevant to ulcer symptoms in patients so affected. For the reasons stated above, it is unlikely that any changes that might occur would have adverse effects on nutrition or susceptibility to infection.

Motor function of the stomach has received more attention in recent publications, although investigations remain somewhat limited because of methodology (e.g., radioisotope scanning), which is precluded in pregnancy. The motor function of the stomach is designed both to receive ingested food or fluids, a process called receptive relaxation, and to prepare the gastric contents for digestion and absorption by grinding solid material into very fine particles prior to intermittently emptying small amounts into the duodenum (Minami and McCallum, 1984). This latter function is carried out by peristaltic contractions in the gastric antrum and the variable size of the pyloric lumen at the gastroduodenal junction. Gastric motility and emptying in pregnancy have been of interest for two reasons. The first of these is the common occurrence of nausea and vomiting, particularly early in pregnancy, and the possibility of altered gastric motor function, regardless of the cause, which might underlie this complaint. The other is the concern expressed by anesthesiologists about gastric contents in a pregnant woman at term undergoing sedation or even general anesthesia without adequate preparation, and the attendant risk for aspiration. A variety of methods have been utilized to examine this question. All have led to the conclusion that there is no influence of pregnancy on gastric emptying (Hunt and Murray, 1958; Schade et al., 1984a; La Salvia and Steffen, 1950; Wyner and Cohen, 1982; Radberg et al., 1989) in

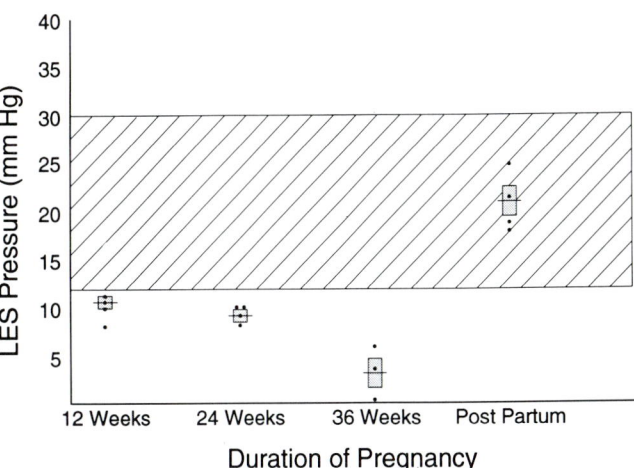

FIGURE 57–1. Lower esophageal sphincter (LES) pressure recorded in 4 volunteer women during pregnancy and in the postpartum period. The *shaded* area shows the range of values for LES pressure in normal nonpregnant women. The *horizontal bars and stippled* areas represent the mean ± SEM for each time period. (From Van Thiel DH, Gavaler J, Joshi SN, et al: Heartburn in pregnancy. Gastroenterology **72:**666, 1977, © by The American College of Gastroenterology.)

first-, second-, and third-trimester women. In some cases, slowing of emptying has been seen at term, but appears to be related to analgesics and sedative agents used during labor (La Salvia and Steffen, 1950; O'Sullivan et al., 1987). In summary, any effects of pregnancy on gastric function, be it secretory or motor, are limited.

Small Intestine

As the site where digestion and absorption of nutrients occur, the function of the small intestine assumes considerable importance during pregnancy because of the unique nutritional demands that occur. Pancreaticobiliary function is also intrinsic to nutrient digestion and absorption and is discussed in Chapter 58.

One way to measure small intestinal function is to look at the movement of intraluminal contents through the duodenum, jejunum, and ileum. Both animal (Datta et al., 1974; Ryan, 1982; Scott and DeFlora, 1983) and human studies (Parry et al., 1970a; Wald et al., 1982; Lawson et al., 1985; Braverman et al., 1988) are in agreement that transit time through the small intestine is prolonged during pregnancy (Fig. 57–2). In one animal study, propulsive motility, as reflected

in the cycling characteristics of the migrating motor complex, was altered (Scott and DeFlora, 1983). However, the observations are sufficiently limited so that it is difficult to conclude in which part of pregnancy this phenomenon is most likely to occur, although in one series, transit time was longest in third-trimester women and returned to normal postpartum (Wald et al., 1982). As transit time, a function of intestinal motility, is prolonged, it could theoretically have both beneficial and negative effects; certainly, prolonged contact of nutrients with the mucosal surface could facilitate absorption. However, mixing of chyme with digestive enzymes and bile salts, also a function of motility, contributes significantly to digestion and absorption as well and is not measured in these studies. On the other hand, delayed transit conceivably could give rise to unpleasant symptoms such as bloating and distention or possibly bacterial overgrowth, which could have an adverse effect on absorption. These absorption questions remain unanswered. Progesterone is again offered as a possible explanation for the prolonged transit time because of its inhibitory effect on gastrointestinal smooth muscle (Wald et al., 1982; Lawson et al., 1985).

Teleologically, it would not be surprising if absorptive function were enhanced during pregnancy, and reference has been made to such a possibility in earlier

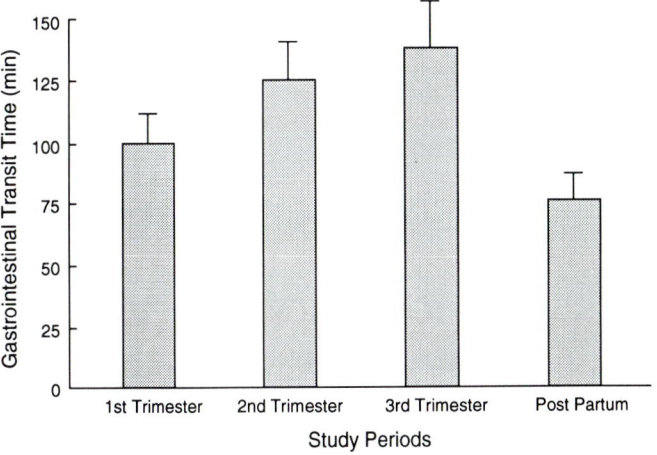

FIGURE 57–2. Oro-cecal gastrointestinal transit time in women in the first (n = 8), second (n = 12), and third (n = 22) trimesters of pregnancy and postpartum (n = 17); data shown are mean values ± SD. Transit time was longest in second- and third-trimester women and was similar in the first-trimester and postpartum women. (Adapted from Lawson et al: Gastrointestinal transit time in human pregnancy, prolongation in the second and third trimesters followed by postpartum normalization. Gastroenterology **89:**996, 1985, © by The American College of Gastroenterology.)

discussions of this issue (Parry et al., 1970a). Vitamin B$_{12}$ absorption, for example, is increased during pregnancy in laboratory animals (Brown et al., 1977), and transport of certain amino acids is increased (Dugas et al., 1970; Butt and Fleshler, 1971); on the other hand, folic acid deficiency may occur (Rothman, 1970). Absorptive efficiency or capacity is difficult to measure, and there are virtually no studies in human pregnancy that answer this question. Animal studies have shown an increase in small intestinal weight during pregnancy, much of which is mucosal (Burdett and Reek, 1979), and morphologically, increase in villus height has been seen (Cripps and Williams, 1975). Activities of some but not all brush border changes are actually more pronounced during lactation and then resolve following weaning (Cripps and Williams, 1975; Elias and Dowling, 1976). Whether these presumed adaptive changes are in response to increased nutrient intake or hormonal factors or both is not clear (Dowling, 1982).

The Colon

Little is known about colonic function in pregnancy. Normally, the proximal colon is a major site of electrolyte and water absorption, concentrating and desiccating the largely fluid material that enters from the ileum. Colonic motility is responsible for periodic transfer of luminal contents from the proximal colon to the distal colon and rectum with subsequent evacuation of stool, which, while still 60 to 85 per cent water in composition, is normally in solid form (Powell, 1991). As has been suggested for other regions of the gastrointestinal tract, it is generally thought that colonic motility is reduced. This has only been measured in animal models of pregnancy. Colonic smooth muscle in pregnant guinea pigs is less responsive to stimulation by agonists (Scott and DeFlora, 1989), and transit time is increased in pregnant rats, although not out of proportion to other circumstances in which sex steroid levels are increased (Ryan and Bhojwani, 1986). In pharmacologic experiments, progesterone does exert an inhibitory effect on colonic smooth muscle, again supporting the hypothesis that this steroid mediates the general inhibition of gut motility during pregnancy (Gill et al., 1985). There is also evidence for increased activity of endogenous opioids during pregnancy, and theoretically this might also inhibit colonic motility (Iwasaki et al., 1991).

In a study in early pregnancy of women scheduled for therapeutic abortion, sodium and water absorption in the proximal colon was increased, possibly on the basis of increased mineralocorticoid activity (Parry et al., 1970b). If these limited observations are valid, it would not be surprising that constipation is often thought to be a problem during pregnancy.

SPECIFIC DISORDERS
Nausea and Vomiting

While obviously not a specific disease, the occurrence of nausea, sometimes accompanied by vomiting,

is so common during pregnancy that it is necessarily included in any discussion of gastrointestinal disorders during pregnancy. In the survey of gastrointestinal symptoms noted earlier, 66 per cent of first-trimester women had some degree of nausea, and 44 per cent complained of vomiting; 18 per cent of the total population surveyed had experienced vomiting more than once daily. The problem is typically more prevalent during the first trimester; other reports cite a frequency of occurrence of up to 70 per cent (Midwinter, 1971; Klebanoff et al., 1985; Jarnfelt-Samsioe et al., 1983; Walker et al., 1985). The term hyperemesis gravidarum is used for the rare patient with vomiting in whom fluid and electrolyte, as well as nutritional, status may be jeopardized as a result of the severity and duration of the problem. This latter condition is unusual and occurs in up to 3.9 per 1000 pregnancies (Van Thiel and Schade, 1986).

The complaint of nausea, sometimes with vomiting, implies a specific disorder of the upper gastrointestinal tract. For example, the nausea and vomiting that sometimes complicate diabetes (gastroparesis diabeticorum) are thought to be due to a primary disturbance of gastric motility in which propulsive activity is reduced or absent (Janssens et al., 1990); a similar phenomenon may be seen following vagotomy or even in the absence of an identifiable underlying disease process (Malagelada, 1982). However, as noted earlier, although gastrointestinal motility may be reduced during pregnancy, studies attempting to document a defect in gastric emptying, as a measure of gastric motility, have generally been unrevealing. A recent report used a technique called *electrogastrography* to measure gastric electrical activity, a correlate of motility, in pregnant women and found abnormalities in patients complaining of nausea (Koch et al., 1990). In this study, surface electrodes placed on the skin of the upper abdomen recorded electrical events in the wall of the stomach, and abnormalities correlated with a higher nausea score as determined subjectively. In a small subgroup who had nausea, the abnormalities subsequently disappeared following delivery. While a study of this type associates disturbed motility with nausea, it does not preclude the possibility that disturbances in gastric function are the result of disturbances elsewhere; in this construct, the stomach may be more the "innocent bystander" than the primary site of the problem.

In fact, this seems to be a more likely possibility. Although nausea and vomiting can be a reflection of an intrinsic abnormality of the stomach, it can also reflect influence by central control mechanisms, sometimes referred to as the vomiting center or, more specifically, the chemoreceptor trigger zone (Ouyang, 1991). This mechanism of nausea is common; examples include adverse reaction to medication (e.g., morphine) or the nausea that accompanies severe pain. It is likely during pregnancy that factor or factors create disturbances in gastroduodenal motility through central effects. Hormonal factors believed to be of possible importance include hCG, thyroxine, and cortisol, as well as the sex steroids estrogen and progesterone; however, there are no clear-cut relationships between circulating levels, increased or decreased, and women with these complaints (Jarnfelt-Samsioe, 1987; Andrews and Whitehead, 1990). Alternatively, it may be that the chemoreceptor trigger zone in some individuals may be more sensitive to otherwise normal levels of a particular hormone or metabolite (Jarnfelt-Samsioe, 1985). Alterations in metabolic function in the liver have also been theorized to play a role in this phenomenon (Andrews and Whitehead, 1990). Regardless of the factors involved, the problem is much more likely to be central than peripheral.

Clinically, management is seldom effective although, fortunately, as noted above, the problem often lessens as the pregnancy progresses. One must be sure that the symptom does not represent the development of other disorders in which nausea may sometimes occur; for example, biliary disease, pancreatitis, and peptic ulcer disease should be considered, although usually there are distinguishing features that assist in differential diagnosis. Symptomatic management with attention to fluid balance is the mainstay of management; small meals with avoidance of potential irritants are often recommended. Pharmacologic agents can be used; however, as with any situation during pregnancy, they should be used judiciously. In the past, pyridoxine has been advocated; although efficacy is not predictable, this agent, vitamin B$_6$, is probably innocuous. Metoclopramide (Reglan) has been used more often in recent years and appears to be safe; placental transfer does occur, but the experience has been favorable, justifying a "B" rating by the United States Food and Drug Administration (FDA) (no evidence of risk in humans); a similar rating has been received by meclizine (Antivert). Phenothiazines (promethazine, prochlorperazine, and others) are also probably safe, although experience to date is less consistently favorable; promethazine, for example, is FDA category "C," in which risk cannot be ruled out (Physicians' Desk Reference, 1992). In severe cases with hyperemesis, more aggressive support may be required to include both fluid and nutritional resuscitation (Levine and Esser, 1988).

Looking at this problem from the other perspective, vomiting per se, despite its prevalence, does not appear to affect pregnancy unfavorably; the potentially important variable is the pharmacologic agent used to treat the problem (Klebanoff and Mills, 1986).

Gastroesophageal Reflux Disease (GERD)

Gastroesophageal reflux disease, if defined as the abnormal reflux of acidic gastric content into the esophagus, is a very common disorder in the general population (Nebel et al., 1976; Talley et al., 1992); the cardinal symptom, heartburn, is one experienced by many people, although only a fraction actually have a problem severe enough to cause them to seek medical attention. Symptoms, however, do not always mean esophagitis as defined by demonstration of mucosal injury and inflammation; in fact, while some patients with heartburn have esophagitis, the majority of patients with these complaints actually have normal esophageal mucosa. There is yet a third group of patients with reflux and esophageal injury, but with

few or no symptoms; these are at highest risk for complications, primarily stricture, because the disease is not recognized until these late problems develop. During pregnancy, conditions may develop that favor the occurrence of gastroesophageal reflux; however, virtually all of these patients fall into the group of symptomatic patients without overt esophagitis, possibly in part because the duration of the problem is limited. Endoscopically determined esophagitis and stricture have been reported during pregnancy, but in this case it was a sequela of protracted vomiting in a patient with hyperemesis gravidarum (Swinhoe et al., 1981). For the most part, therefore, the problem is one of symptoms, often severe, but one in which esophageal injury is unlikely to occur.

The major determinants of reflux are primarily four in number (Dodds et al., 1981). The first and the one most often cited is the strength of the antireflux barrier. Contributing to this barrier is the closure tension, also known as *resting pressure,* of the lower esophageal sphincter, a zone of high pressure associated with specialized circular muscle located anatomically at the gastroesophageal junction. There are also mechanical factors defined by the anatomic configuration of the esophagogastric junction, the diaphragm, and associated supporting structures. The other variables include the potency and volume of refluxed fluid, a function of both acid secretion and gastric emptying; esophageal clearance, a function of propulsive motility in the esophageal body; and tissue resistance, which is poorly understood but probably influenced by nutritional factors and blood flow.

Although a large body of information has been generated regarding these variables in normals and patients with reflux, little is known about them during pregnancy. However, as noted earlier, there is some evidence for reduced lower esophageal sphincter resting pressure during pregnancy, and if true, the barrier against reflux may be jeopardized. Moreover, in addition to the possible changes in the antireflux barrier, the abdominothoracic pressure gradient may be increased by the enlarging uterine fundus and contribute to the tendency for reflux to occur. Observations of esophageal motility are sufficiently limited that no conclusions are possible, although the one report of reduced contractile amplitude and wave-form velocity would imply a possible defect in esophageal clearance of refluxed acid (Ulmsten and Sundstrom, 1978). The information available regarding gastric function, however, would lead one to conclude that alterations here are not likely to play a role in pregnancy-related reflux. What is lacking are observations of intraesophageal pH in ambulatory patients over time, 24 hours or more (Mattox and Richter, 1990; Hewson et al., 1991), and in the absence of this kind of information, conclusions about the magnitude and pathogenesis of the problem remain speculative.

As noted earlier, heartburn of pregnancy occurs in about 50 per cent of third-trimester women. Management of the reflux problem involves some degree of lifestyle modification and, if needed, pharmacologic intervention. Many physicians have a therapeutic nihilistic view of reflux during pregnancy, primarily because it is a limited problem with resolution during the postpartum period. Standard antireflux measures, including head of bed elevation while sleeping, small meals, reduced fat diet, smoking cessation, and others are of some value. On the other hand, attempts to decrease intra-abdominal pressure with, for example, avoidance of tight clothing are of little value during pregnancy. Antacids that neutralize refluxed acid may be useful for symptoms and are generally safe if not taken in excess. Adverse reactions associated with excessive use of antacids include diarrhea and metabolic and electrolyte alterations such as hypercalcemia, hypermagnesemia, hypophosphatemia, and others. However, the mainstay of symptomatic management for severe cases of reflux is inhibition of acid secretion using one of the four available H_2 receptor antagonists. While use of these agents cannot be encouraged in pregnancy, selected patients may benefit. As a group of drugs, they are among the safest available, and their use during pregnancy, while not sanctioned by the FDA, appears to be safe despite transfer of the drug across the placenta (Dicke et al., 1988) (Table 57–4). Cimetidine, ranitidine, and famotidine are all rated category B drugs for use during pregnancy, while nizatidine (Axid) is category C (Physicians' Desk Reference, 1992). Human experience with these agents in pregnancy is largely anecdotal and, for the most part, restricted to cimetidine and ranitidine, the first two H_2 receptor antagonists to be introduced into clinical practice. These two drugs are among the most commonly prescribed agents worldwide. With use in pregnancy, rare complications have been reported, both fetal abnormalities and spontaneous abortions, although their relationship to the drug given was equivocal (Colin-Jones et al., 1985; Koren and Zemlickis, 1991; Cipriani et al., 1983). Although there are case reports of successful use of H_2 antagonists in pregnant patients with both reflux esophagitis and peptic ulcer disease, favorable experience is generally not reported (Armentano et al., 1989; Corrazza et al., 1982). There is an extensive literature on limited use of these drugs in obstetric anesthesia to reduce the risk of acid aspiration pneumonitis (Hodgkinson et al., 1983, Colman et al., 1988; Sacco et al., 1986; Takacs, 1989) with no unfavorable outcomes noted.

Omeprazole (Prilosec), to be discussed later, is also a powerful inhibitor of acid secretion and is indicated in severe cases of reflux esophagitis with mucosal erosion and ulceration. There is no experience in pregnancy, and the clinical picture that might suggest its use is so rare in pregnancy-related reflux disease that it probably will never be used.

Prokinetic agents, such as metoclopramide (Reglan), which have limited use in the management of GERD in general, would predictably be of little benefit during pregnancy. Their major effect is to promote gastric emptying which, as noted earlier, has not been shown unequivocally to be delayed during pregnancy. However, gastric emptying in heartburn of pregnancy has not been specifically studied.

Peptic Ulcer Disease (PUD)

Views are conflicting regarding any significant change in gastric function during pregnancy, be it motor or secretory; hence, based on those observations, one might not expect any alteration in the clinical expression of peptic ulcer disease during pregnancy. In addition, ulcer is more a problem in males than in females. Surprisingly, for several years there has been the general feeling that pregnancy has a salutary effect on the course of ulcer in women who already carry that diagnosis, and new-onset ulcer during pregnancy is rare (Clark, 1953; Spiro et al., 1959; Baird, 1966). In the largest series reported, of 313 pregnancies that took place following the diagnosis of ulcer, 45 per cent had no symptoms, 44 per cent improved, and only 12 per cent experienced no change (Clark, 1953). This is somewhat surprising and to an extent paradoxical if in fact heartburn, which also is an acid-related process, occurs more frequently. Although there may be no change in acid secretion, there has been the suggestion that estrogen via unknown mechanisms may exert a protective effect on gastroduodenal mucosa (Truelove, 1960; Doll et al., 1965) to explain this phenomenon. We think of ulcer disease pathogenetically as a balance between aggressive factors, of which acid is a necessary ingredient, and defensive factors, to which are contributed not only resistance to injury but also accelerated restitution if injury occurs. Thus, in the absence of documented decrease in aggressive factors, a logical explanation for a reduction in occurrence of ulcer is enhanced defense. The recent finding of colonization of the stomach by the bacterium *Helicobacter pylori* in most patients with PUD has not been investigated in pregnancy (Peterson, 1991). If the role of this organism in ulcer pathogenesis is one of impaired defense, its status in pregnancy may be of particular interest.

Despite what appears to be a reduced occurrence of ulcer, complications, primarily perforation, have been reported during pregnancy (Baird, 1966; Paul et al., 1976). As with many conditions that present during pregnancy, symptoms may not be classic and diagnosis may be delayed. Although bleeding as an ulcer complication is more common than perforation in the general population, the reverse may be true in pregnancy. Of one series of 12 pregnant women with upper gastrointestinal bleeding, none was due to peptic ulcer disease (Palmer, 1961), in contrast to a 20 per cent expectancy in the nonpregnant population presenting with this problem (Graham, 1989). Although uncommon, hemorrhage from ulcer is more likely to occur late in pregnancy or in the early postpartum period (Aston et al., 1991).

As in the nonpregnant state, diagnosis of uncomplicated ulcer in pregnancy, while infrequent, should be a clinical one and treatment initiated empirically (Kahn and Greenfield, 1985); obviously, this is easier in the patient with established ulcer disease who develops recurrent dyspepsia, although there may be confusion with heartburn of pregnancy. In the general population, the diagnosis of uncomplicated ulcer can often be made in an otherwise healthy individual based on presenting symptoms; for example, epigastric burning pain, worse on an empty stomach, often awakening the patient in the early morning hours, and relieved with food or antacids is highly suggestive of duodenal ulcer. Empiric therapy in this setting would include a therapeutic dosing regimen of an H_2 receptor antagonist; if the patient responds, 8 weeks of therapy should be completed. If there is a failure of response within 10 to 14 days, a diagnostic study, usually upper gastrointestinal endoscopy, would be indicated. For the patient presenting for the first time during pregnancy, a decidedly unusual event, empiric treatment of suggestive symptoms is certainly appropriate; however, because of concern regarding use of drugs that are placentally transferred, this management—in contrast to that of the nonpregnant patient, might not include H_2 antagonists without first establishing the diagnosis. One would be left with attention to diet with regular meals, avoidance of symptom-producing foods, judicious use of antacids, and avoidance of potentially adverse factors such as smoking, coffee and caffeine-containing foods, alcohol, and aspirin and other nonsteroidal anti-inflammatory drugs. Sucralfate, as a nonabsorbed agent that accelerates healing of ulcer by improving mucosal defense at the ulcer site, is an attractive alternative. Practically speaking, however, the safety profile of many of the H_2 antagonists is so favorable, as already noted, that one need not hesitate to use such agents, although preferably in the patient with documented disease. The use of endoscopy during pregnancy is discussed below.

The newest drug in the therapeutic armamentarium for ulcer disease is omeprazole, which blocks the proton pump (H^+, K^+ = ATPase) located on the apical membrane of the parietal cell in the gastric secretory epithelium. This is the final common pathway in acid secretion, and inhibition of acid secretion at this point markedly reduces acid secretion. This category of antisecretory agents, of which omeprazole is the only commercially available drug at present, represents the most potent agents available. Therapeutically, this translates into healing rates of duodenal ulcer which are faster than the H_2 receptor antagonists; 90 per cent healing rates are seen after 4 weeks of treatment, a rate usually requiring 8 weeks of treatment with H_2 blockers (Maton, 1991). A faster healing rate theoretically may reduce complications. Transplacental transfer of omeprazole probably occurs, albeit in small amounts (Ching et al., 1986), and to date there are no published reports of teratogenicity or maternal-fetal toxicity. Nonetheless, at present, the use of this drug during pregnancy is limited and is a category "C" drug according to the FDA classification (Table 57–4). Given the favorable experience with cimetidine and ranitidine during pregnancy, it is unlikely that omeprazole would be needed in this setting.

Inflammatory Bowel Disease (IBD)

Inflammatory bowel disease is the one gastrointestinal disorder whose relationship with pregnancy generates the most controversy. Several studies examining similar issues often draw conflicting conclusions. Further, there may well be differences between chronic ulcerative colitis and Crohn's disease, the two disorders that comprise IBD, with respect to their impact on pregnancy as well as the impact of pregnancy on the disease.

Ulcerative colitis is primarily a mucosal disease, always involving the rectum and extending proximally in a continuous fashion; the extent of involvement is variable, but in some patients it affects the entire colon. Other regions of the gastrointestinal tract are spared. Symptoms are primarily diarrhea, often with bleeding, and some degree of abdominal pain. Crohn's disease, on the other hand, is a transmural granulomatous inflammatory process that involves the rectum only about 50 per cent of the time. It may involve any region of the gastrointestinal tract, but is most commonly found in the colon and terminal ileum. Although diarrhea and hematochezia may occur, these symptoms are less predictable, particularly in the absence of significant colonic disease, and the diagnosis may be elusive. Abdominal pain is almost always a problem, and nutritional deficiencies occur more often than in ulcerative colitis. Fistulous complications, including rectovaginal fistula, can be particularly troublesome.

In the past, fertility was thought to be jeopardized in patients with IBD of either type (DeDombal et al., 1965); today, that seems to be less likely. In the most often quoted study, women with ulcerative colitis had a fertility rate of 81 per cent with an incidence of involuntary infertility of 7 per cent. If one looked at the number of children per family as an index of fertility, the numbers were similar to those of the general population (Willoughby and Truelove, 1980). Most reviews of this topic also conclude that, at least in ulcerative colitis, fertility rate is unaffected (Singer and Brandt, 1991; Fagan, 1989; Hanan and Kirsner, 1986). The effect of Crohn's disease on fertility is less clear-cut; one might predict that, at least in some patients with small bowel disease with extensive perienteric inflammation—often with fistulous tracts, pelvic inflammation with infertility could easily occur. Again, studies present conflicting results, but the critical variable is probably the degree of disease activity; fertility is highest in women in remission or following surgical resection of active disease (DeDombal et al., 1972; Donaldson, 1985). Much of the controversy surrounding this issue reflects in large part the lack of a consistent definition of infertility. Infertility may result from anatomic causes, but in large population surveys, other variables such as physician advice, impaired sexuality due to psychological as well as physical components of the illness, and even male infertility are not usually considered.

More pertinent questions with respect to pregnancy is the impact of the disease on the course of gestation and its outcome on the one hand, and the effect of pregnancy per se on disease activity on the other. These two questions may also not be mutually exclusive, one conceivably affecting the other. While some studies report an increased risk of preterm birth for women with ulcerative colitis (Baird et al., 1990; Fedarkow et al., 1989), the general consensus is that this disorder does not have an adverse effect on pregnancy outcome as measured by the occurrence of spontaneous abortion, stillbirth, congenital abnormality, or premature delivery (DeDombal et al., 1972; Baiocco and Korelitz, 1984; Mogadam et al., 1981a; Porter and Stirrat, 1986; Nielson et al., 1983). This conclusion should be qualified, however, by noting that most studies report that women with inactive disease have the most favorable course (Willoughby and Truelove, 1980). Should disease activity become severe during pregnancy, a favorable outcome may be less predictable, and certainly the need for surgery for complications such as hemorrhage or toxic megacolon imposes a great risk for fetal survival (Fedarkow et al., 1989; Korelitz, 1985). Similar conclusions may be drawn for women with Crohn's disease. There is probably no adverse effect on outcome, particularly if one looks at individuals with inactive or quiescent disease; again, the emergence of disease activity either at the outset of gestation or during its course increases the risk for an unfavorable outcome (Mogadam et al., 1981a; Nielson et al., 1984; Fedarkow et al., 1989; Khosla et al., 1984). The rate of cesarean section at term does not appear to be affected by an underlying diagnosis of IBD (Porter and Stirrat, 1986; Nielson et al., 1984; Homan and Thorbjarnarson, 1976; Schade et al., 1984b; Crohn et al., 1956).

Having looked at the effect of IBD on the course and outcome of pregnancy, one must also consider the reverse; does pregnancy pose a risk for the patient with IBD? In most patients, the answer is probably no, although the key variable again appears to be the degree of activity of IBD at the time of conception. If activity is quiescent, the odds are favorable that it will remain so for the duration of the pregnancy (Willoughby and Truelove, 1980; Nielson et al., 1983). Relapses do occur but do not seem to be in excess of those occurring in the nonpregnant population (Nielson et al., 1983). Initial presentation of IBD may also occur during pregnancy, possibly more often in ulcerative colitis than in Crohn's disease (Hanan and Kirsner, 1986), and, along with exacerbations of already established IBD, are more likely to occur early in gestation, primarily the first trimester (Korelitz, 1985; Nielson et al., 1983; MacDougall, 1956). The postpartum period at one time was thought to be a particularly high-risk time for exacerbation of previously quiescent IBD or for onset of new disease; this does not now appear to be the case (Willoughby and Truelove, 1980; Khosla et al., 1984; Korelitz, 1982; Mogadam et al., 1981a). The degree of activity at term is probably what would be expected during the postpartum period. The anatomic distribution of Crohn's disease has been speculated to be important, with patients with small bowel disease more likely to do well than those with colitis, but this remains a controversial issue (Fagan, 1989).

Whereas pregnancy may or may not affect IBD or vice versa, it does seem clear that active IBD and pregnancy together, while not a common occurrence, can be problematic from a management as well as an evaluation standpoint. Complaints of diarrhea, particularly with bleeding, and abdominal pain should at least alert one to the possibility of IBD. Constitutional symptoms of fever, anorexia, and anemia may also be seen. Pregnancy per se, particularly in the first trimester, may be accompanied by some of these complaints, and suspicion of underlying IBD would not be as great

as it might be in other clinical situations. As a process involving primarily mucosa and always involving at least the distal colon, if not the more proximal large bowel, ulcerative colitis may be more quickly recognized and diagnosis more easily attained via proctoscopy. Rectal bleeding to some degree is almost always seen, and the change in bowel habit toward diarrhea varies with the extent of colonic involvement. By sparing the rectum in many patients and having the possibility of small as well as large intestinal involvement, the diagnosis of Crohn's disease may be more elusive. As noted above, de novo occurrence of these disorders during pregnancy is not common so that this dilemma is unusual (Singer and Brandt, 1991); in the patient with known disease, one's index of suspicion is necessarily heightened already. The feasibility of various diagnostic modalities, which can certainly come into play with these disorders, will be discussed later.

Pharmacologic management of IBD is a topic that in the past has been controversial; more recent experience as well as published reports suggest the more uniform conclusion that most drugs useful in managing IBD in nonpregnant women are also useful and, more importantly, safe in pregnant women (Singer and Brandt, 1991; Fagan, 1989; Hanan and Kirsner, 1986). Clearly, however, the issue is more complex than that seen with GERD or PUD, for which symptomatic therapy without the use of systemic agents is often the first-line approach. In these patients, drug administration generally has already been initiated, and the decision required is not so much whether to start medication as it is whether to discontinue the drug or alter the dosage. As noted above, disease that is quiescent in women who become pregnant more often than not remains quiescent, but in many cases, particularly with ulcerative colitis, this quiescence or remission is medication-dependent. In the unusual situation in which IBD is initiated during pregnancy, one must be confident in the ability of early use of these agents to control the disease.

Over time the major agents in the management of IBD have been corticosteroids, in particular prednisone, and sulfasalazine (Table 57–4). The latter is a particularly interesting agent in that the active moiety, 5-amino salicylate, works locally within the colonic lumen, but only because its absorption in the small intestine following oral ingestion is largely prevented by its coupling with sulfapyridine. It is the colonic bacteria that break the bond, releasing the salicylate, which exerts an anti-inflammatory effect through inhibition of both the cyclooxygenase and lipoxygenase pathways of arachidonic acid metabolism (Stenson and MacDermott, 1991). Sulfapyridine has no active role in treating IBD, serving only as a vehicle for transport of 5-amino salicylate; it is, however, absorbed in the colon, and is responsible for the orange color of the urine noted by many patients, as well as the adverse reactions, notably headache and hypersensitivity, that can occur during sulfasalazine therapy. Sulfapyridine can also cross the placenta and appears in breast milk in small concentrations, raising concern about the potential to displace unconjugated bilirubin from albumin and cause kernicterus in the breast-fed new-

TABLE 57–4. **Major Gastrointestinal Drugs Used in Pregnancy**

DRUG	POTENTIAL USAGE	FDA CATEGORY*
Metoclopramide	nausea/GERD	B
Cimetidine	GERD/PUD	B
Ranitidine	GERD/PUD	B
Famotidine	GERD/PUD	B
Nizatidine	GERD/PUD	C
Sucralfate	PUD	B
Omeprazole	GERD/PUD	C
Sulfasalazine	IBD	B
Prednisone	IBD	B

GERD = gastroesophageal reflux disease; PUD = peptic ulcer disease; IBD = inflammatory bowel disease.
*B (no evidence of risk in humans); C (risk cannot be ruled out).

born. Outcome studies, however, have shown no increase in neonatal jaundice in women taking sulfasalazine (Willoughby and Truelove, 1980; Baiocco and Korelitz, 1984; Mogadam et al., 1981b; Nielson et al., 1984; Khosla et al., 1984; Nielson et al., 1983). Moreover, the drug is safe during pregnancy, with no evidence of adverse effect on mother or fetus (Willoughby and Truelove, 1980; Mogadam et al., 1981b; Khosla et al., 1984; Nielson, 1983). There should be no hesitation, therefore, regarding the use of sulfasalazine during pregnancy. Folic acid supplements, a mainstay of nutritional management of pregnancy anyway, are of particular importance in pregnant women who are taking this drug, which may inhibit absorption and metabolism of folate, and should be prescribed.

Similar conclusions have been drawn regarding the use of prednisone, which is rapidly metabolized to prednisolone in the maternal liver and does not cross the placenta in significant amounts (Singer and Brandt, 1991). The experience with prednisone is greater than that with sulfasalazine because of its use in other disorders as well as IBD. Comparative studies of women taking and not taking prednisone have failed to show any detrimental effect on either maternal or fetal outcome (DeDombal et al., 1972; Mogadam et al., 1981b; Khosla et al., 1984).

Recently, newer formulations of 5-ASA have been developed which lack the sulfapyridine moiety with a hoped-for reduction in adverse reactions. Olsalazine is the one currently available for prescription in the United States, and there is no published use in pregnancy. Its FDA rating is category "C", however, and in view of the vast and favorable experience with sulfasalazine, this or any similar agents would be considered only if sulfasalazine could not be used because of a prior adverse reaction. Immunosuppressive therapy with azathioprine or 6-mercaptopurine, sometimes used in IBD, has been reported to be safe when used during pregnancy (Miller, 1986; Alstead et al., 1990), but experience is limited. Decisions regarding the use of these agents during pregnancy should be on a case-by-case basis. Likewise, other agents occasionally used, such as metronidazole and more recently novel therapy with methotrexate or cyclosporine, probably would not be needed and should not be used anyway in the absence of well-documented safety (Peppercorn, 1990). Total parenteral nutrition, while not primary therapy for IBD, is nonetheless a potentially useful adjunct in some patients, particularly those with Crohn's disease and associated nutritional deficiencies. While experience is limited, there are increasing numbers of reports of successful use during pregnancy (Amato and Quercia, 1991; Watson et al., 1990; Nutrition Reviews, 1988; Lang et al., 1987).

Other Gastrointestinal Disorders

The above represent the major gastrointestinal problems that may arise during pregnancy and present management difficulties. One other condition often mentioned in discussions of this type is constipation; the lack of precise data regarding this phenomenon has already been alluded to when considering specific symptoms that might be pregnancy-related. The definition of the term varies from person to person; scientifically, fecal water content might be used as an index of constipation. Normal stool weight is 200 gm per day, up to 80 per cent of which is water; a reduction in the water content might therefore be considered constipation. However, patients are not going to use this definition, and there are no studies in which stool weights and water content are measured during pregnancy. Frequency of bowel movements is a more commonly used index. In a general population, "normal" was considered anywhere from three per day to three per week (Connell et al., 1965), and any reduction in the normal pattern for that patient might be considered constipation (Drossman et al., 1982; Everhart et al., 1989). A subjective report of desiccated stools requiring straining for evacuation might be another definition. Although there may be no data supporting the occurrence of constipation as a pregnancy-related problem, the issue is not a crucial one. Constipation is common in the general population, and it is not surprising that it is seen during pregnancy with some regularity. Diagnostic studies as to cause are seldom required, and empiric management is appropriate in most cases. As in the nonpregnant patient, attention to adequate dietary fiber is fundamental to this management along with increasing oral fluid intake. Although inadequate fiber cannot be implicated as a cause of constipation occurring during pregnancy (Anderson, 1986), fiber supplements have been shown to be effective with increasing frequency of bowel movements and production of a softer stool consistency (Anderson and Whichelow, 1985). One source of supplemental fiber is in the form of psyllium preparations, and if necessary, judicious use of an osmotic laxative such as milk of magnesia (magnesium hydroxide), which mobilizes fluid within the gut lumen, may be considered. There has been a favorable experience during pregnancy with senna preparations, and intermittent use is probably safe and effective (Biggs and Vesey, 1980).

There are rare reports of actual development of colonic ileus during pregnancy or the early postpartum period which, in effect, is colonic pseudo-obstruction (Moore et al., 1986; Slemmons and Williams, 1938; Charles and Stronge, 1972). In this condition, in other settings sometimes called Ogilvie's syndrome, the gas-filled colon is acutely dilated in the absence of distal obstruction (Nanni et al., 1982). The patient is often distended and may have obstructive symptoms. Constipation and ileus can be added to the list of conditions that are consistent with the notion that gut motility is reduced during pregnancy. While the gestational metabolic and hormonal environment may predispose to this, ileus may also occur during pregnancy under other circumstances; for example, it is a recognized complication or tocolytic therapy for premature labor using magnesium sulfate (Hill et al., 1985; Dudley et al., 1989). Colonoscopic decompression can be successfully used in selected patients with this disorder and appear to be safe in pregnancy and the postpartum period (Moore et al., 1986) (see Gastrointestinal Endoscopy below).

The occurrence of pancreatitis and biliary disease during pregnancy is discussed in Chapter 58. In addition, the pregnant patient is not protected from other gastrointestinal disorders, and there are case reports dealing with carcinoma of the stomach (Sommerville et al., 1991; Davis and Chen, 1991), carcinoma of the colon (Nesbitt et al., 1985; Shushan et al., 1992; Jaffe et al., 1989), intestinal obstruction (Davis and Bohon 1983), celiac sprue (Ogborn, 1975; Molteni et al., 1990), giardiasis (Kreutner et al., 1981), and amebiasis (Wig et al., 1984) occurring during pregnancy. Undoubtedly, other conditions have been seen as well, and all present unique problems in evaluation and management which must be considered on a case-by-case basis.

DIAGNOSTIC MODALITIES

Imaging Studies

The use of imaging techniques during pregnancy, including barium contrast studies and computed tomography, in the diagnosis and management of gastrointestinal problems is limited, primarily because of the potential adverse effects of ionizing radiation on the fetus (Brent, 1989; American Academy of Pediatrics, 1978). Such studies have undoubtedly been carried out inadvertently in the first trimester of pregnancy, and the impact of such studies is difficult to quantify. Nonetheless, while such exposure may be

harmless in some cases, the risk is significant. Of perhaps equal importance, however, is the fact that the need to perform these studies in any of the disorders discussed above is small due to, depending on the problem, the response to empiric therapy, the self-limited nature of the problem, and the ease and safety of gastrointestinal endoscopy in diagnosing and treating the occasional patient with a difficult clinical dilemma. In contrast to conventional radiographic techniques, ultrasonography appears to pose no risk to mother or fetus during pregnancy; however, its application to the hollow viscus disorders discussed in this chapter is limited. Ultrasound has its major application in pancreatic and hepatobiliary disease.

Gastrointestinal Endoscopy

The major indications for gastrointestinal endoscopy, as outlined by the American Society for Gastrointestinal Endoscopy, are displayed in Table 57–5 (American Society for Gastrointestinal Endoscopy, 1988). These indications would apply to the pregnant mother insofar as timely conduction of the procedure would affect the care of the patient. This would usually be a situation in which empiric management was without benefit or the urgency of the situation warranted prompt intervention. An example of the latter would be upper gastrointestinal hemorrhage. On the other hand, endoscopy, for example, for surveillance for colon cancer in a high risk patient could usually be deferred until after delivery.

Concern regarding the safety of gastrointestinal endoscopy is twofold: the effects of medication given during the procedure, as premedication is often used, and the effects of the manipulation of the endoscope per se, if any. There is very little in the way of published information on either of these issues, particularly the latter, apart from case reports of unusual gastrointestinal problems that occurred during pregnancy; in many of these, gastrointestinal endoscopy was utilized in the care of the patient and note is made that no ill effects occurred (Moore et al., 1986;

TABLE 57–5. Major Indications for Gastrointestinal Endoscopy in a General Population

Esophagogastroduodenoscopy (EGD)
  Persistent upper abdominal distress
  Upper abdominal distress associated with symptoms/signs of serious organic disease
  Dysphagia or odynophagia
  Gastrointestinal bleeding
  Concomitant disease in which the presence of upper gastrointestinal pathology might have impact on management
Colonoscopy
  Gastrointestinal bleeding suggestive of colorectal origin
  Unexplained iron deficiency anemia
  Surveillance of colorectal neoplasia
  Evaluation of suspected or known inflammatory bowel disease
  Clinically significant, unexplained diarrhea

Modified and adapted from American Society for Gastrointestinal Endoscopy: Appropriate use of gastrointestinal endoscopy. Gastrointest Endosc 34(Suppl):15, 1988, © by The American Society for Gastrointestinal Endoscopy.

Sommerville et al., 1991; Davis and Chen, 1991; Hirabayashi et al., 1987). One survey was published in 1986 regarding the safety and efficacy of gastrointestinal endoscopy in the pregnant patient. From a questionnaire circulated to the membership of the American Society for Gastrointestinal Endoscopy, experience with 110 procedures was reported (Rustgi et al., 1986). This was distributed among upper gastrointestinal endoscopy (73), flexible sigmoidoscopy and colonoscopy (26), and rigid proctosigmoidoscopy (11). No complications or ill effects were reported. Over half the patients received premedication—usually meperidine, diazepam, or a combination—without apparent difficulty. Fetal outcome was not specifically looked at in the survey, but note was made of 1 spontaneous abortion at 14 weeks, 4 weeks post-procedure, and 1 premature delivery at 8 months in a patient who had undergone esophagogastroduodenoscopy at 3 weeks. The conclusion of the authors reporting these results was that gastrointestinal endoscopy was safe when performed during pregnancy and, in some cases, may be the procedure of choice given limitations imposed by radiation risks plus accuracy of diagnosis. This has been the experience of the author, although no formal study has been carried out.

The primary indication for upper gastrointestinal endoscopy in 73 patients was nausea with vomiting, some of which was hematemesis (Rustgi et al., 1986). Thirty-two of these procedures were carried out during the first trimester, reflecting the prevalence of this complaint at that point in gestation, and the diagnoses most often made were gastritis and esophagitis. There was the occasional surprise as well, including one patient with adenocarcinoma of the stomach. Virtually all the cases of colorectal endoscopy were done for bleeding, some of which was in patients with IBD.

Although its application is in pancreaticobiliary disease, endoscopic retrograde cholangiopancreatography (ERCP) can also be safely performed during pregnancy if special precautions are taken (Baillie et al., 1990; Hoffman and Cunningham, 1992).

Careful and judicious use of endoscopy can have an important role in the management of selected pregnant patients in whom prompt diagnosis is deemed necessary for successful management.

CONCLUSION

Pregnancy is a unique metabolic and hormonal state with effects on many body systems, not the least of which is the gastrointestinal tract. Many symptoms and complaints result from these changes. Likewise, patients with chronic gastrointestinal disorders may experience changes in symptoms or develop problems for which diagnosis and management can be a challenge. Careful selection of diagnostic and therapeutic options can result in successful outcomes for both mother and fetus.

REFERENCES

Alstead EM, Ritchie JK, Lennard-Jones JE, et al: Safety of azathioprine in pregnancy in inflammatory bowel disease. Gastroenterology 99:443, 1990.

Amato P, Quercia RA: A historical perspective and review of the safety of lipid emulsion in pregnancy. Nutr Clin Pract 6:189, 1991.

American Academy of Pediatrics Committee on Radiology. Radiation of pregnant women. Pediatrics 61:117, 1978.

American Society for Gastrointestinal Endoscopy: Appropriate use of gastrointestinal endoscopy. Gastrointest Endosc 34(Suppl):1S, 1988.

Anderson AS: Dietary factors in the aetiology and treatment of constipation during pregnancy. Br J Obstet Gynaecol 93:245, 1986.

Anderson AS, Whichelow MJ: Constipation during pregnancy: dietary fibre intake and the effect of fibre supplementation. Hum Nutr Appl Nutr 39:202, 1985.

Andrews P, Whitehead S: Pregnancy sickness. NIPS 5:5, 1990.

Armentano G: Bracco PL, DiSilverio C: Ranitidine in the treatment of reflux oesophagitis in pregnancy. Clin Exp Obstet Gynecol 4:130, 1989.

Aston NO, Kalaichandran S, Carr JV: Duodenal ulcer hemorrhage in the puerperium. Can J Surg 34:482, 1991.

Baiocco PJ, Korelitz BI: The influence of inflammatory bowel disease and its treatment on pregnancy and fetal outcome. J Clin Gastroenterol 6:211, 1984.

Baillie J, Carins SR, Putnam WS, et al: Endoscopic management of choledocholithiasis during pregnancy. Surg Gynecol Obstet 171:1, 1990.

Baird DD, Narendranathan M, Sandler RS: Increased risk of preterm birth for women with inflammatory bowel disease. Gastroenterology 99:987, 1990.

Baird RM: Peptic ulcer in pregnancy: Report of a case with perforation. Can Med Assoc J 94:861, 1966.

Biggs JSG, Vesey EJ: Treatment of gastrointestinal disorders of pregnancy. Drugs 19:70, 1980.

Braverman DZ, Herbet D, Goldstein R, et al: Postpartum restoration of pregnancy-induced cholecystoparesis and prolonged intestinal transit time. J Clin Gastroenterol 10:642, 1988.

Brent RL: The effect of embryonic and fetal exposure to x-ray, microwaves, and ultrasound: Counseling the pregnant and non-pregnant patient about these risks. Semin Oncol 16:347, 1989.

Brown J, Robertson J, Gallagher N: Humoral regulation of vitamin B_{12} absorption by pregnant mouse small intestine. Gastroenterology 72:881, 1977.

Bruce LA, Behsudi TM: Differential inhibition of regional gastrointestinal tissue to progesterone in the rat. Life Sci 27:427, 1980.

Burdett K, Reek C: Adaptation of the small intestine during pregnancy and lactation in the rat. Biochem J 184:245, 1979.

Butt J, Fleshler B: Increase in maternal gut amino acid transport in late gestation in the guinea pig. (Abstract) J Lab Clin Med 78:827, 1971.

Charles D, Stronge J: Special problems of the colon and rectum in obstetric practice. Clin Obstet Gynecol 15:522, 1972.

Ching MS, Morgan DJ, Mihaly GW, et al: Placental transfer of omeprazole in maternal and fetal sheep. Dev Pharmacol Ther 9:323, 1986.

Cipriani S, Conti R, Vella G: Ranitidine in pregnancy; three case reports. Clinica Europea 22:1, 1983.

Clark DH: Peptic ulcer in women. Br Med J 1:1254, 1953.

Colin-Jones DG, Langman MJS, Lawson DH, et al: Post-marketing surveillance of the safety of cimetidine: 12-month morbidity report. Quart J Med 54:253, 1985.

Colman RD, Frank M, Loughnan BA, et al: Use of intramuscular ranitidine for the prophylaxis of aspiration pneumonitis in obstetrics. Br J Anaesth 61:720, 1988.

Connell AM, Hilton C, Irvine G, et al: Variation of bowel habit in two population samples. Br Med J 2:1095, 1965.

Corrazza GR, Gasbarrini G, DiNisio O, et al: Cimetidine in peptic ulcer therapy during pregnancy. Clin Trials J 19:91, 1982.

Cripps AW, Williams VJ: The effect of pregnancy and lactation on food intake, gastrointestinal anatomy and the absorptive capacity of the small intestine in the albino rat. Br J Nutr 33:17, 1975.

Crohn BB, Yarnis H, Korelitz BI: Regional ileitis complicating pregnancy. Gastroenterology 31:615, 1956.

Datta S, Hey VM, Pleuvry BJ: Effects of pregnancy and associated hormones in mouse intestine, in vivo and in vitro. Pflugers Arch 346:87, 1974.

Davis JL, Chen MD: Gastric carcinoma presenting as an exacerbation of ulcers during pregnancy. A case report. J Reprod Med 36:450, 1991.

Davis MR, Bohon CJ: Intestinal obstruction in pregnancy. Clin Obstet Gynecol **26**:832, 1983.

Davison JS, Davison MC, Hay DM: Gastric emptying time in late pregnancy and labour. J Obstet Gynaecol Br Commonw **77**:37, 1970.

DeDombal FT, Burton IL, Goligher JC: Crohn's disease and pregnancy. Br Med J **3**:550, 1972.

DeDombal FT, Watts JM, Watkinson G, et al: Ulcerative colitis in pregnancy. Lancet **2**:599, 1965.

Dicke JM, Johnson RF, Henderson GI, et al: A comparative evaluation of the transport of H_2-receptor antagonists by the human and baboon placenta. Am J Med Sci **295**:198, 1988.

Dodds WJ, Hogan WJ, Helm JF, et al: Pathogenesis of reflux esophagitis. Gastroenterology **81**:376, 1981.

Doll R, Hill ID, Hutton CF: The treatment of gastric ulcer with carbenoxalone sodium and estrogens. Gut **6**:10, 1965.

Donaldson RM: Management of medical problems in pregnancy: inflammatory bowel disease. N Engl J Med **312**:1616, 1985.

Dowling RH: Small bowel adaptation and its regulation. Scand J Gastroenterol **17**(Suppl 74):53, 1982.

Drossman DA, Sandler RS, McKee DC, et al: Bowel patterns among subjects not seeking health care. Gastroenterology **83**:529, 1982.

Dudley D, Gagnon D, Varner M: Long-term tocolysis with intravenous magnesium sulfate. Obstet Gynecol **73**:373, 1989.

Dugas MC, Hazlewood RC, Lawrence AL: Influence of pregnancy and/or exercise on intestinal transport of amino acids in rats. Proc Soc Exp Biol Med **135**:127, 1970.

Elias E, Dowling RH: The mechanism for small bowel adaptation in lactating rats. Clin Sci Mol Med **51**:427, 1976.

Everhart JE, Go VLW, Johannes RS, et al: A longitudinal survey of self-reported bowel habits in the United States. Dig Dis Sci **34**:1153, 1989.

Fagan EA: Disorders of the gastrointestinal tract. *In* de Swiet M (ed): Medical Disorders in Obstetric Practice. 2d ed. Oxford, Blackwell Scientific Publications, 1989, pp 521–583.

Fedarkow DM, Persaud D, Nimrod CA: Inflammatory bowel disease: A controlled study of late pregnancy outcome. Am J Obstet Gynecol **160**:98, 1989.

Fisher RS, Roberts GS, Grabowski CJ, et al: Altered lower esophageal sphincter function during early pregnancy. Gastroenterology **74**:1233, 1978.

Gill RC, Bowes KL, Kingma YJ: Effect of progesterone on canine colonic smooth muscle. Gastroenterology **88**:1941, 1985.

Graham DY: Complications of peptic ulcer disease and indications for surgery. *In* Sleisenger MH, Fordtran JS (eds): Gastrointestinal Disease. 4th ed. Philadelphia, W.B. Saunders Co., 1989, pp 925–938.

Gryboski WA, Spiro HM: The effect of pregnancy on gastric secretion. N Engl J Med **255**:1131, 1956.

Hanan IM, Kirsner JB: Inflammatory bowel disease in pregnancy. *In* Rustgi VK, Cooper JN (eds): Gastrointestinal and Hepatic Complications in Pregnancy. New York, John Wiley & Sons, 1986, pp 69–86.

Hewson EG, Sinclair JW, Dalton CB, et al: Twenty-four hour esophageal pH monitoring: the most useful test for evaluating non-cardiac chest pain. Am J Med **90**:576, 1991.

Hill WC, Gill PJ, Katz M: Maternal paralytic ileus as a complication of magnesium sulfate tocolysis. Am J Perinatol **2**:47, 1985.

Hirabayashi M, Veo H, Okudaira Y, et al: Early gastric cancer and a concomitant pregnancy. Am Surg **53**:730, 1987.

Hodgkinson R, Glassenberg R, Joyce TH, III, et al: Comparison of cimetidine with antacid for safety and effectiveness in reducing gastric acidity before elective caesarean section. Anesthesiology **59**:86, 1983.

Hoffman BJ, Cunningham JT: Radiation exposure to the pregnant patient during ERCP. (Abstract) Gastrointest Endosc **38**:253, 1992.

Homan WP, Thorbjarnarson B: Crohn's disease and pregnancy. Arch Surg **111**:545, 1976.

Hunt JN, Murray FA: Gastric function in pregnancy. J Obstet Gynaecol Br Commonw **65**:78, 1958.

Iwasaki H, Collins JG, Saito Y, et al: Naloxone-sensitive, pregnancy-induced changes in behavioral responses to colorectal distension: Pregnancy-induced analgesia to visceral stimulation. Anesthesiology **74**:927, 1991.

Jaffe R, Schwartz I, Freund U, et al: Perforated adenocarcinoma of the colon during pregnancy. Int J Gynaecol Obstet **30**:371, 1989.

Jarnfelt-Samsioe A: Nausea and vomiting in pregnancy: A review. Obstet Gynecol Surv **42**:422, 1987.

Jarnfelt-Samsioe A, Eriksson B, Waldenstrom J: Some new aspects on emesis gravidarum. Relations to clinical data, serum electrolytes, and creatinine. Gynecol Obstet Invest **19**:174, 1985.

Jarnfelt-Samsioe A, Samsioe G, Velinder G: Nausea and vomiting in pregnancy; a contribution to its epidemiology. Gynecol Obstet Invest **16**:221, 1983.

Janssens J, Peeters TL, Vantrappen G, et al: Improvement in gastric emptying in diabetic gastroparesis by erythromycin: Preliminary studies. N Engl J Med **322**:1028, 1990.

Kahn K, Greenfield S (for Health and Public Policy Committee, American College of Physicians): Endoscopy in the evaluation of dyspepsia. Ann Intern Med **102**:266, 1985.

Khosla R, Willoughby CP, Jewell DP: Crohn's disease and pregnancy. Gut **25**:52, 1984.

Klebanoff MA, Koslowe PA, Kaslow R, et al: Epidemiology of vomiting in early pregnancy. Obstet Gynecol **66**:612, 1985.

Klebanoff MA, Mills JL: Is vomiting during pregnancy teratogenic? Br Med J (Clin Res Ed) **292**:724, 1986.

Koch KL, Stern RM, Vasey M, et al: Gastric dysrhythmias and nausea of pregnancy. Dig Dis Sci **35**:961, 1990.

Korelitz BI: Epidemiological and psychosocial aspects of inflammatory bowel disease with observations on children, families, and pregnancy. Am J Gastroenterol **77**:929, 1982.

Korelitz BI: Pregnancy, fertility and inflammatory bowel disease. Am J Gastroenterol **80**:365, 1985.

Koren G, Zemlickis DM: Outcome of pregnancy after first-trimester exposure to H_2 receptor antagonists. Am J Perinatol **8**:37, 1991.

Kreutner AK, Del Bene VE, Amstey MS: Giardiasis in pregnancy. Am J Obstet Gynecol **140**:895, 1981.

Kumar D: In vitro inhibitory effect of progesterone on extrauterine human smooth muscle. Am J Obstet Gynecol **84**:1300, 1962.

Lang CE, Johnson DJ, Sax HC, et al: Total parenteral nutrition in pregnancy: A case report. J Pediatr Perinat Nutr **1**:61, 1987.

La Salvia LA, Steffen EA: Delayed gastric emptying time during labor. Am J Obstet Gynecol **59**:1075, 1950.

Lawson M, Kern F, Jr, Everson GT: Gastrointestinal transit time in human pregnancy, prolongation in the second and third trimesters followed by postpartum normalization. Gastroenterology **89**:996, 1985.

Levine MJ, Esser D: Total parenteral nutrition for the treatment of severe hyperemesis gravidarum: maternal nutritional effects and fetal outcome. Obstet Gynecol **72**:102, 1988.

Levy N, Lemberg E, Sharf M: Bowel habit in pregnancy. Digestion **4**:216, 1971.

MacDougall I: Ulcerative colitis and pregnancy. Lancet **2**:641, 1956.

Malagelada JR: Gastric emptying disorders. Clinical significance and treatment. Drugs **24**:353, 1982.

Maton PN: Omeprazole. N Engl J Med **324**:965, 1991.

Mattox HE, Richter JE: Prolonged ambulatory esophageal pH monitoring in the evaluation of gastroesophageal reflux disease. Am J Med **89**:345, 1990.

Midwinter A: Causes of vomiting in pregnancy. Practitioner **206**:743, 1971.

Miller JP: Inflammatory bowel disease in pregnancy: A review. J R Soc Med **79**:221, 1986.

Minami H, McCallum RW: The physiology and pathophysiology of gastric emptying in humans. Gastroenterology **86**:1592, 1984.

Mogadam M, Korelitz BI, Ahmed SW, et al: The course of inflammatory bowel disease during pregnancy and postpartum. Am J Gastroenterol **75**:265, 1981a.

Mogadam M, Dobbins WD, Korelitz BI, et al: Pregnancy in inflammatory bowel disease: Effect of sulfasalazine and corticosteroids on fetal outcome. Gastroenterology **80**:72, 1981b.

Molteni N, Bardella MT, Bianchi PA: Obstetrical and gynecological problems in women with untreated celiac sprue. J Clin Gastroenterol **12**:37, 1990.

Moore JG, Gladstone NS, Lucas GW, et al: Successful management of post-caesarean section acute pseudo-obstruction of the colon (Ogilivie's syndrome) with colonoscopic decompression. A case report. J Reprod Med **31**:1001, 1986.

Murray FA, Erskine JP, Fielding J: Gastric secretion in pregnancy. J Obstet Gynaecol Br Commonw **64**:373, 1957.

Nagler R, Spiro HM: Heartburn in late pregnancy; manometric studies of esophageal motor function. J Clin Invest **40**:954, 1961.

Nagler R, Spiro HM: Heartburn in pregnancy. Am J Dig Dis **7**:648, 1962.

Nanni G, Garbini A, Luchetti P, et al: Ogilvie's syndrome (acute colonic pseudo-obstruction): Review of the literature (October 1948 to March 1980) and report of four additional cases. Dis Colon Rectum **25**:157, 1982.

Nebel OT, Fornes MF, Castell DO: Symptomatic gastroesophageal reflux: Incidence and precipitating factors. Dig Dis Sci **21**:953, 1976.

Nesbitt JC, Moise KJ, Sawyers JL: Colorectal carcinoma in pregnancy. Arch Surg **120**:636, 1985.

Nielson OH, Andreasson B, Bondesen S, et al: Pregnancy in ulcerative colitis. Scand J Gastroenterol **18**:735, 1983.

Nielson OH, Andreasson B, Bondesen S, et al: Pregnancy in Crohn's disease. Scand J Gastroenterol **19**:724, 1984.

Nutritional Reviews: Maintenance of pregnancy by total parenteral nutrition. Nutr Rev **46**:220, 1988. (No authors cited)

Ogborn ADR: Pregnancy in patients with coeliac disease. Br J Obstet Gynaecol **82**:293, 1975.

Ostick DG, Cowley DJ, Hey VM, et al: A study of gastroesophageal reflux in late pregnancy. In Vantrappen G (ed): Proceedings of the Fifth International Symposium on Gastrointestinal Motility. Herentals, Belgium, Typoff Press, 1976, pp 358–362.

O'Sullivan GM, Sutton AJ, Thompson SA, et al: Noninvasive measurement of gastric emptying in obstetric patients. Anesth Analg **66**:505, 1987.

Ouyang A: Approach to the patient with nausea and vomiting. In Yamada T (ed): Textbook of Gastroenterology. Philadelphia, J.B. Lippincott Co., 1991, pp 647–659.

Palmer ED: Upper gastrointestinal hemorrhage during pregnancy. Am J Med Sci **242**:223, 1961.

Parry E, Shields R, Turnbull AC: Transit time in the small intestine in pregnancy. J Obstet Gynaecol Br Commonw **77**:900, 1970a.

Parry E, Shields R, Turnbull AC: The effect of pregnancy on the colonic absorption of sodium, potassium, and water. J Obstet Gynaecol Br Commonw **77**:616, 1970b.

Paul M, Tew WL, Holliday RL: Perforated peptic ulcer in pregnancy with survival of mother and child: Case report and review of the literature. Can J Surg **19**:427, 1976.

Peppercorn MA: Advances in drug therapy for inflammatory bowel disease. Ann Intern Med **112**:50, 1990.

Peterson WL: Helicobacter pylori and peptic ulcer disease. N Engl J Med **324**:1043, 1991.

Physicians Desk Reference. Montvale, NJ, Medical Economics Co., 1992, p 329.

Porter RJ, Stirrat GM: The effects of inflammatory bowel disease on pregnancy: A case-controlled retrospective analysis. Br J Obstet Gynaecol **93**:1124, 1986.

Powell DW: Approach to the patient with diarrhea. In Yamada T (ed): Textbook of Gastroenterology. Philadelphia, J.B. Lippincott Co., 1991, pp 732–778.

Radberg G, Asztely M, Cautor P, et al: Gastric and gallbladder emptying in relation to the secretion of cholecystokinin after a meal in late pregnancy. Digestion **42**:174, 1989.

Rothman D: Folic acid in pregnancy. Am J Obstet Gynecol **108**:149, 1970.

Rustgi VK, Cooper JN, Colcher H: Endoscopy in the pregnant patient. In Rustgi VK, Cooper JN (eds): Gastrointestinal and Hepatic Complications in Pregnancy. New York, John Wiley & Sons, 1986, pp 104–123.

Ryan JP, Pellechia D: Effect of ovarian hormone pretreatment on gallbladder motility in vitro. Life Sci **31**:1445, 1982.

Ryan JP: Effect of pregnancy on intestinal transit: comparison of results using radioactive and nonradioactive test meals. Life Sci **31**:2635, 1982.

Ryan JP, Bhojwani A: Colonic transit in rats: effect of ovariectomy, sex steroid hormones, and pregnancy. Am J Physiol **251**:G46, 1986.

Sacco T, Corinaldesi R, Miglioli M, et al: The prevention of Mendelson's syndrome. Oral and intravenous administration of ranitidine. Clin Trials J **23**:193, 1986.

Schade RR, Pelekanos MJ, Tauxe WN, et al: Gastric emptying during pregnancy. (Abstract) Gastroenterology **86**:1234, 1984a.

Schade RR, Van Thiel DH, Gavaler JS: Chronic idiopathic ulcerative colitis. Pregnancy and fetal outcome. Dig Dis Sci **29**:614, 1984b.

Schulze K, Christensen J: Lower sphincter of the opossum esophagus in pseudopregnancy. Gastroenterology **73**:1082, 1977.

Scott LD, DeFlora E: Cholinergic responsiveness of intestinal muscle in the pregnant guinea pig. Life Sci **44**:503, 1989.

Scott LD, DeFlora E: Intestinal transit in female rats; effect of pregnancy, estrous cycle and castration. (Abstract) Gastroenterology **84**:1303, 1983.

Scott LD, Lester R, Van Thiel DH, Wald A: Pregnancy-related changes in small intestinal myoelectric activity in the rat. Gastroenterology **84**:301, 1983.

Scott LD, Kozinetz C, Gonik B: Gastrointestinal function in pregnancy. (Abstract) Gastroenterology **90**:1624, 1986.

Shushan A, Stemmer SN, Reubinoff BE, et al: Carcinoma of the colon during pregnancy. Obstet Gynecol Surv **47**:222, 1992.

Singer AJ, Brandt LJ: Pathophysiology of the gastrointestinal tract during pregnancy. Am J Gastroenterol **86**:1695, 1991.

Slemmons JM, Williams NH: Ileus in pregnancy. West J Surg Obstet Gynecol **46**:84, 1938.

Sommerville M, Koonings PP, Curtin JP, et al: Gastrointestinal signal ring carcinoma metastatic to the cervix during pregnancy. J Reprod Med **36**:813, 1991.

Spiro HM, Schwartz RD, Pilot ML: Peptic ulcer in pregnancy. A serial study of gastric secretion during pregnancy. Am J Dig Dis **4**:289, 1959.

Stenson WF, MacDermott RP: Inflammatory bowel disease. In Yamada T (ed): Textbook of Gastroenterology. Philadelphia, J.B. Lippincott Co., 1991, pp 1588–1645.

Swinhoe JR, Cochrane GW, Wishart R: Oesophageal stricture due to reflux oesophagitis of pregnancy. Br J Obstet Gynaecol **88**:1249, 1981.

Takacs G: Usefulness of acid and gastric juice secretion decreasing action of cimetidine in anaesthesia for the prevention of aspiration. Ther Hung **37**:43, 1989.

Talley NJ, Zinsmeister AR, Schleck C, et al: Natural history of gastroesophageal reflux: A population-based study. (Abstract) Gastroenterology **102**:A28, 1992.

Truelove SC: Stilboestrol, phenobarbitone and diet in chronic duodenal ulcer. Br Med J **2**:559, 1960.

Ulmsten V, Sundstrom G: Esophageal manometry in pregnant and non-pregnant women. Am J Obstet Gynecol **132**:260, 1978.

Van Thiel DH, Gavaler J, Joshi SN, et al: Heartburn of pregnancy. Gastroenterology **72**:666, 1977.

Van Thiel DH, Schade RR: Pregnancy: Its physiologic course, nutrient cost, and effects on gastrointestinal function. In Rustgi VK, Cooper JN (eds): Gastrointestinal and Hepatic Complications in Pregnancy. New York, John Wiley & Sons, 1986, pp 1–29.

Wald A, Van Thiel DH, Hoechstetter L, et al: Effect of pregnancy on gastrointestinal transit. Dig Dis Sci **27**:1015, 1982.

Waldum HL, Straume BK, Lundgren R: Serum group I pepsinogens during pregnancy. Scand J Gastroenterol **15**:61, 1980.

Walker AW, Walker BF, Jones J, et al: Nausea and vomiting and dietary cravings and aversions during pregnancy in South African women. Br J Obstet Gynaecol **92**:484, 1985.

Watson LA, Bommarito AA, Marshall JF: Total peripheral parenteral nutrition in pregnancy. J Paren Enteral Nutr **14**:485, 1990.

Wig JD, Bushnurmath SR, Kaushik SP: Complications of amoebiasis in pregnancy and puerperium. Ind J Gastroenterol **3**:37, 1984.

Willoughby CP, Truelove SC: Ulcerative colitis and pregnancy. Gut **21**:469, 1980.

Wyner J, Cohen SE: Gastric volume in early pregnancy. Anesthesiology **57**:209, 1982.

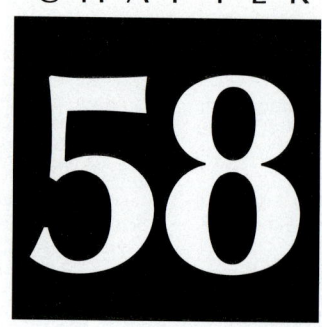

DISEASES OF LIVER, BILIARY SYSTEM, AND PANCREAS

ELIZABETH ANN FAGAN, M.Sc., M.D., MRCP

The lifetime experience of the individual obstetrician, internist, and hepatologist in managing disorders of the liver, pancreas, and biliary system in pregnancy is likely to be limited. General principles of management often are difficult to extrapolate from the literature, and reports tend to select the atypical case with especially severe disease. These limitations can lead to delays in diagnosis and appropriate management. This chapter focuses on practical management issues in: (1) maternal disorders that are unique to pregnancy, and (2) maternal disorders that are coincidental to pregnancy. Primary diseases of the liver remain rare in pregnancy; only 50 cases were recorded in 56,000 pregnancies (less than 0.1 per cent) in one center (Klebanoff et al., 1985). The majority do not adversely affect maternal and fetal well-being. Early identification of the exceptions and careful, interdisciplinary management can improve outcome.

THE LIVER IN NORMAL PREGNANCY

The liver rotates to a more superior and posterior position in the third trimester. Displacement to the right reduces dullness to percussion. A palpable liver usually indicates disease. Liver size and absolute hepatic blood flow (normally 24 to 35 per cent of cardiac output) do not change significantly. Clearance of drugs with high hepatic extraction ratios is unlikely to be altered significantly. Redistribution of the excess circulating volume through the portal veins and vena cava can be seen at endoscopy as engorgement of the esophageal veins in more than 50 per cent of healthy pregnancies. Palmar erythema and spider nevi are common in pregnancy. These no longer are considered diagnostic of chronic liver disease and can be seen in acute liver failure. The histopathology of the liver may show mild fatty change. The correct diagnosis of many chronic liver diseases relies predominantly on characteristic histopathologic features. Reliance on liver serum biochemistry alone to monitor disease activity can be misleading at times. Clinical liver chemistry

tests in normal pregnancy are summarized in Table 58–1.

MATERNAL DISORDERS UNIQUE TO PREGNANCY

Intrahepatic Cholestasis of Pregnancy (IHCP)

Maternal Effects

This is the most common liver disorder unique to pregnancy and second only to viral hepatitis as a cause of jaundice (Rolfes and Ishak, 1986; Schorr-Lesnick et al., 1991). IHCP is prevalent (up to 2 per cent of deliveries) in Chile (Reyes, 1976), Scandinavian and

TABLE 58–1. Clinical Liver Chemistry Tests in Normal Pregnancy

SERUM TESTS	LEVELS IN PREGNANCY
Prothrombin time	
Total bilirubin	
AST/SGOT	No change
ALT/SGPT	
Alkaline phosphatase (liver)	
Gamma-GT	
5-Nucleotidase	
RISES	
Total alkaline phosphatase	Accelerated 3rd trimester*
Globulins alpha and beta	Progressive to term
Lipids	Progressive to term
Fibrinogen	Progressive to term
Ceruloplasmin	
Transferrin	
FALLS	
Albumin	20% first trimester
Globulins: gamma	Minor or unchanged

AST = aspartate aminotransferase; ALT = alanine aminotransferase; Gamma GT = gamma glutamyl transpeptidase.
*Placental and skeletal isoenzymes only.

Mediterranean countries, Canada, Poland, Australia, and China (Berg et al., 1986).

IHCP probably arises from a genetic predisposition and increased sensitivity and altered membrane composition of bile ducts and hepatocytes to estrogens and progestogens. A family history is present in up to half of the patients in association with the histocompatability antigen haplotypes HLA B8 and HLA BW16. This genetic predisposition favors an autosomal dominant trait, and fathers transmit the susceptibility to daughters (Holtzbach et al., 1983). Multiple pregnancies increase the severity of the disease. A central theory has been suggested for the pruritus and increased availability of brain opiate receptors for binding their agonist ligands in cholestasis (Jones and Bergasa, 1990). Seasonal variations in countries of high prevalence suggest some additional environmental factor.

In IHCP, generalized pruritus develops usually after 30 weeks of gestation, becomes progressively severe to term, and is relieved within days following delivery. Nocturnal itching of trunk, palms, and soles can be severe with associated insomnia and fatigue. Anorexia, malaise, epigastric discomfort, steatorrhea, and dark urine are common. Jaundice develops 2 to 4 weeks later and resolves rapidly postpartum, but may recur in up to 45 per cent of subsequent pregnancies (Shaw et al., 1982). This is a mild, predominantly conjugated hyperbilirubinemia (<6 times upper normal) with minor elevations in serum aspartate aminotransferase (AST) and alkaline phosphatase. Any elevation in prothrombin ratio indicates vitamin K deficiency and is rapidly corrected by replacement therapy. Serum levels of cholesterol, triglycerides, and phospholipids are higher in IHCP than in controls. Untypically, pruritus may begin as early as the sixth week, and jaundice may persist for several weeks postpartum.

Any hepatomegaly, splenomegaly, pain, or other abnormal features should alert the physician to exclude other causes of pruritus and jaundice, especially the cholestatic phase of viral hepatitis, biliary obstruction, autoimmune chronic liver diseases, hepatotoxic drugs, and congenital defects of bilirubin metabolism. The risk of formation of gallstones is increased with the enlarged gallbladder volume, reduced bile flow, and rise in serum bile acids. Ultrasonography should be used to exclude cholelithiasis and pancreatic abnormalities. Histologic examination of the liver may be required to diagnose atypical cases. Percutaneous biopsy should be carried out after administration of vitamin K and under ultrasound guidance to avoid the enlarged gallbladder. Liver biopsy is safe in experienced hands within the limitations of normal coagulation. Histopathologic findings are limited to acinar cholestasis.

Cholestyramine up to 20 gm/day and phenobarbitone have been used to treat the pruritus, but results are disappointing (Shaw et al., 1982). Cholestyramine, a nonabsorbable anion-exchange resin, binds bile acids, anionic drugs, and fat-soluble vitamins such as vitamin K and can lead to elevations in the prothrombin ratio. Vitamin K_1 should be administered throughout pregnancy and before delivery, particularly to mothers taking cholestyramine, to reduce the risk of postpartum hemorrhage (Shaw et al., 1982). Results from controlled trials of intravenous S-adenosyl-L-methionine (800 mg daily) have shown variable relief of pruritus with lessening of jaundice. This agent seems to be nontoxic to the fetus.

Fetal Effects

Intrauterine death and stillbirth are well-recognized complications. The improved outcomes reported recently probably reflect milder cases. Serum levels of bile acids and their derivatives rise before other biochemical tests, including serum estriols, and indicate an increased risk of fetal distress, premature labor and meconium staining, and intrauterine death (Berg et al., 1986; Reyes, 1976). The risks of fetal distress and intrauterine death increase as term approaches. Estimations of lung maturity should be performed regularly and provision made to induce labor after the 37th week or for fetal distress. Vitamin K_1 therapy should be administered immediately to the newborn to prevent intracranial bleeding, particularly if the mother has taken cholestyramine.

Preeclampsia, Eclampsia, the HELLP Syndrome, Acute Fatty Liver of Pregnancy, and Liver Rupture and Infarction

Many liver diseases occurring in late pregnancy are associated with hypertension. HELLP syndrome, acute fatty liver, and hepatic rupture and infarction (Krueger et al., 1990; Freund and Arvan, 1990; Schorr-Lesnick et al., 1991) form a spectrum, but their etiology and interrelations remain unclear. The liver is not involved primarily in preeclampsia but becomes the target organ in severe cases. Recent improvements in noninvasive imaging techniques, specialized hematologic tests, and liver histology have led to reappraisal of the involvement of the liver (see also Chapters 48 and 49). Early clinical features of these diseases overlap and are vague such as upper abdominal pain from hepatic tenderness, nausea, and vomiting; overt jaundice is uncommon in mild cases. Elevated levels of serum aspartate aminotransferase (AST, SGOT) are common to many conditions, including those unrelated to pregnancy (Table 58–2) (Goodlin, 1991).

HELLP Syndrome

Patients with hypertension, typically primaparae in the third trimester, may present principally with hepatic dysfunction. The combination of *H*emolytic anemia, *E*levated *L*iver transaminases and a *L*ow *P*latelet count has been defined as the HELLP syndrome (Weinstein, 1982). Occasionally, presentation is as early as the 20th week or as late as the postpartum period. Elevations in levels of unconjugated (indirect) bilirubin and creatinine are common. Hematologic abnormalities include a reduction in hematocrit disproportionate to estimated blood loss, microangiopathic hemolytic anemia with disseminated intravascular coagulation (platelet count below 100×10^9/liter

Table 58–2.   Differential Diagnosis of Hypertension-Related Hepatic Disorders with Elevated Serum Transaminase Levels*

> Acute fatty liver
> Viral hepatitis
> Budd-Chiari syndrome
> Pancreatitis
> Idiopathic thrombocytopenia
> Thrombotic thrombocytopenia
> Hemolytic-uremic syndrome
> Systemic lupus erythematosus
> Cholecystitis
> Biliary colic
> Peptic ulcer
> Pyelonephritis
> Septicemia
> Cocaine abuse
> Dissecting aortic aneurysm
> Other causes of disseminated
>   intravascular coagulation

*Aspartate aminotransferase (AST; SGOT)

[100,000 mm^{-3}]), abnormal erythrocyte forms, elevated levels of fibrin degradation products, and reduced levels of antithrombin III. Liver synthetic function, as measured by prothrombin and partial thromboplastin times, and the fibrinogen levels are frequently normal.

The HELLP syndrome was diagnosed in up to 15 per cent of all patients with preeclampsia and eclampsia in two North American referral centers (Crosby, 1991). Confusion with many conditions (Table 58–2) may delay appropriate management. Most authorities will accept raised levels of aspartate aminotransferase (AST, SGOT) above 50 IU/liter (N<40) and lactate dehydrogenase above 180 IU/liter with a platelet count below 100 × 10^9/liter and hemolysis as criteria for its diagnosis. The AST level usually is below 10 × upper normal limits but occasionally can exceed 1000 IU/liter.

Some milder cases present with epigastric pain, elevated levels of serum AST, and disseminated intravascular coagulation, but with normal or only a mildly raised blood pressure and no proteinuria. Improvements with conservative management may occur before delivery, but the risk of intrauterine growth restriction remains (Aarnoudse et al., 1986).

Deposition of fibrin has been demonstrated in the liver in periportal regions and sinusoids and accompanies the focal parenchymal necrosis, but there is no inflammatory infiltrate. Thrombi can be detected in portal tract capillaries and occasionally in branches of the larger hepatic arteries and even in the portal vein (Rolfes and Ishak, 1986). These features resemble disseminated intravascular coagulation and thrombotic thrombocytopenic purpura. They are unlikely to be primary events. Coagulation abnormalities can occur but are not common, and they can also occur in viral hepatitis, drug-related hepatotoxicities, and acute fatty liver of pregnancy.

The etiology of these related conditions remains unclear. A vascular theory is favored (Rolfes and Ishak, 1986). Segmental vasospasm in the liver results in injury to endothelial cells. Exposure of the subendothelial collagen leads to platelet adherence and aggregation and deposition of fibrin. This injury is reflected in changes in levels of fibronectin and prostaglandins, but measurements of plasma levels are variable. Dilated segments show separation of endothelial cells. The increased intraluminal pressure may result in hemorrhage and rupture of anastomoses between branches of hepatic artery, portal vein, and sinusoids. Other less common but serious complications of severe preeclampsia, eclampsia, and the HELLP syndrome are hepatic rupture and infarction (see below).

Diagnosis of HELLP and related conditions may require specific tests to search for elevations in levels of lactate dehydrogenase (LDH), fibrin degradation products, fibrin D-dimer, plasminogen activator inhibitor, protein C, and anaphylotoxins (C3a, C5a). Levels of antithrombin III often are reduced, whereas the prothrombin ratio is normal or minimally elevated. Unfortunately, many of these values show too much variation for clinical use. Elevation in levels of serum AST and unconjugated (indirect) bilirubin reflect the severity of the hematologic disturbances, but do not correlate with trimester of presentation, clinical severity, and propensity for complications and recovery. Typically, the serum level of AST will recover within 72 hours after delivery, whereas the thrombocytopenia may be protracted.

Acute Fatty Liver of Pregnancy (AFLP)

The first documentation of idiopathic AFLP is attributed to Stander and Cadden (1934), but similar features (acute yellow atrophy) were recognized by Rokitansky (1843) and by Tarnier (1857). Sheehan (1940) separated the idiopathic form from acute liver failure related to infections and toxins.

Idiopathic AFLP remains uncommon; estimates of occurrence being approximately 1 in 10,000 deliveries. (Pockros et al., 1984; Purdie and Walters, 1988). The previous dismal prognosis with maternal and fetal mortalities above 70 per cent has improved to about 25 per cent (Burroughs et al., 1982; Bernuau et al., 1983; Pockros et al., 1984) with improved management and inclusion of milder cases. Common associations include preeclampsia, twin pregnancy (Burroughs et al., 1982), and a male fetus (Kaplan, 1985). Age and race are similar to normal obstetric practice (Rolfes and Ishak, 1985). The association with parity is less clear with the milder cases (Pockros et al., 1984; Rolfes and Ishak, 1985). AFLP has been reported as late as the eleventh gestation.

The more severe cases show rapid deterioration with coma, often related to profound hypoglycemia, acute liver failure, renal failure, metabolic acidosis, bleeding diatheses, and death (Burroughs et al., 1982; Pockros et al., 1984; Kaplan, 1985; Rolfes and Ishak, 1985). Other, more variable, features reported include pruritus, fever, ascites, polydipsia, necrotizing enterocolitis, and pancreatitis.

Laboratory findings in the typical severe case include a marked neutrophil leukocytosis often above 13,000 mm^{-3}, and occasionally above 30,000 mm^{-3} with left shift. Hematologic data overlap with those of the HELLP syndrome. The serum level of uric acid often is disproportionately raised in relation to the impairment in renal function, but this is no longer considered diagnostic. Serum levels of bilirubin may be normal but rise if delivery is delayed. The serum aspartate aminotransferase (AST) typically is between 3 and 10 times above normal limits but may exceed 1000 IU/liter with shock, hepatic ischemia, and profound hypoglycemia (Rolfes and Ishak, 1985). Profound hypoglycemia is common, independent of clinical severity, and contributes significantly to maternal and fetal mortality. The modest elevations in levels of serum AST and the disproportionately high serum alkaline phosphatase and uric acid are also found in other hepatic disorders.

At autopsy severe cases show widespread fatty infiltration and hemorrhages in the gastrointestinal tract, pancreas, kidney, and bone marrow (Rolfes and Ishak, 1985; 1986). At autopsy, the liver is small and yellow with microscopic steatosis. The distribution characteristically is panlobular with sparing of periportal areas. Deposition of fibrinogen is common in the hepatic sinusoids. Other pathologic features include intrahepatic cholestasis with canalicular plugs of bile and an acute cholangiolitis along with extramedullary hemopoiesis and hyperplastic collections of Kupffer cells.

Microvesicular steatosis has also been described in alcoholic hepatitis, hepatotoxicity (due to tetracycline, sodium valproate, and salicylates); Reye's syndrome, vomiting disease of Jamaica, yellow fever, Wolman's disease, and deficiencies of congenital urea cycle enzymes with fatty acid oxidation. Lipid metabolism may be important in AFLP as well as in alcoholism, obesity, diabetes mellitus, and starvation (Rolfes and Ishak, 1986). Free fatty acids can be cytotoxic. More recently, abnormalities in neutral triglycerides and fatty acid oxidation have been implicated (Schoeman et al., 1991).

OVERLAP WITH PREGNANCY-INDUCED HYPERTENSION. Preeclampsia is present in 30 to 100 per cent (Burroughs et al., 1982; Riely et al., 1987) of cases of AFLP. The typical patient with both AFLP and HELLP presents in the third trimester with nonspecific symptoms, abdominal pain, nausea, vomiting, headache, and jaundice. Hematologic disturbances and histologic distinctions in milder cases of AFLP and HELLP overlap with findings in preeclampsia (Burroughs et al., 1982; Pockros et al., 1984; Heilmann et al., 1991). In a detailed study in Japan using oil red O on frozen liver sections, microvesicular fat was detected in all of 41 women presenting with preeclampsia, including some with normal liver function tests (Minakami et al., 1988). Importantly, the fat may be overlooked with only conventional histologic stains. Electron microscopic examination of hepatocytes is sensitive for detecting microvesicular fat. Perinatal mortality rises with the quantity of fat, which also correlates with elevations in serum uric acid levels and, inversely, with the platelet count.

MANAGEMENT PRINCIPLES FOR HELLP AND AFLP. Measurements of liver function and platelet counts should be carried out on all pregnant women with suspected HELLP or AFLP syndromes (Sibai, 1990). Optimal management for abnormal liver function and hypertension involves early discussion and

transferral to a tertiary referral center with intensive care facilities for managing hepatologic, hematologic, and obstetric-related emergencies. General measures include bed rest and strict control and frequent monitoring of arterial blood pressure, blood sugars, coagulation status, and acid-base balance. Hypoglycemia may be profound and should be anticipated.

In AFLP, ultrasonographic studies may show increased reflectivity. Computed tomographic (CT) scanning and magnetic resonance imaging (MRI) may show low attenuation. Overall, these tests have been disappointing. Negative results do not exclude AFLP or related conditions. Liver histology occasionally may help in the timing of delivery in untypical presentations with clinically mild disease and an immature fetus. Percutaneous biopsy often is precluded by abnormal coagulation. Management depends on clinical assessment of disease severity (see Acute Liver Failure, below). Maternal and fetal outcome do not correlate with the AST levels.

Management of patients with HELLP syndrome and AFLP should be interdisciplinary in a setting with full intensive care facilities. Treatment of the hypertension with magnesium sulfate and hydralazine followed by delivery by cesarean section is appropriate for presentations beyond 34 weeks gestation. Milder cases may reach term, and spontaneous vaginal delivery is possible, but close monitoring is essential to anticipate further impairment of liver function. Massive hepatic necrosis and a variety of neurologic and cardiac abnormalities have been reported in several cases. Replacement of clotting factors with fresh frozen plasma and factor concentrates and platelets may be necessary. For cesarean section and vaginal delivery, platelet transfusions should be given for counts below 30 to 50 × 10^9/liter. Plasma exchange (Martin et al., 1990) and antithrombotic agents (Sibai, 1990), including infusions of prostaglandin derivatives and inhibitors of thromboxane synthetase, have shown benefit in some severe cases of HELLP syndrome (Martin et al., 1990).

General anesthesia should be carried out by an anaesthetist experienced in managing hepatic and renal dysfunction. Epidural anaesthesia without adverse effect has been successful despite thrombocytopenia. The catheter should be removed as soon as possible after delivery. The nadir in the platelet count occurs typically 24 to 72 hours postpartum and may precipitate hemorrhage.

Neonatal abnormalities seen with HELLP, such as fetal growth restriction, are less common with severe AFLP. However, widespread fatty infiltration in the offspring has been reported after several months of age (Schoeman et al., 1991). Whether these families represent distinct recessive genetic errors of fatty metabolism, requires further study (see Congenital Disorders of Liver Metabolism, below).

Following delivery, intensive care facilities should be available (see Acute Liver Failure, below). The risk of liver rupture and infarction, hypoglycemia, pancreatitis and pseudocyst formation, and neurologic complications continues postpartum. Liver transplantation for severe AFLP has been successful, and subsequent normal pregnancies have been reported for survivors of HELLP, AFLP, and liver rupture. There are isolated reports of histologically proven recurrent AFLP and of HELLP in a successive pregnancy. A maternal defect in oxidation of long-chain fatty acids was demonstrated in one woman with AFLP occurring in successive pregnancies. Both infants died within the first year, and autopsy revealed widespread fatty infiltration of their livers (Schoeman et al., 1991). Recurrences may be more common than realized. In addition, some multiparous patients presenting with AFLP have documented hypertension in a preceding pregnancy.

Liver Rupture and Infarction

Spontaneous rupture has been reported for one in every 45,000 live births (Smith et al., 1991). In pregnancy, the majority occur with severe preeclampsia and eclampsia (Steven, 1981) and the HELLP syndrome. The pathogenesis remains unclear. Subcapsular hemorrhages in the liver are found at autopsy in 80 per cent of cases of preeclampsia and eclampsia (Margolis and Naidoo, 1974). Vascular malformations, polyarteritis nodosa, mycotic aneurysms, fibromuscular dysplasia, amebic abscess, and tumors account for a minority of cases of liver rupture in pregnancy. Occlusion of the hepatic artery does not lead to widespread infarction because additional blood is supplied from the portal vein. Hepatic infarction more likely results from several factors including gross ischemia and obstruction to sinusoidal blood flow by deposited fibrin and relative hypovolemia. Differential diagnosis and management are the same as for acute liver failure (see below).

Rupture and infarction can occur at any time including in the puerperium. Onset is sudden with upper abdominal pain, nausea, vomiting, and fever. Rapid deterioration in consciousness occurs from hepatic encephalopathy and hypoglycemia. Rupture may be heralded by shock, hypotension, and absent fetal heart sounds. The lower abdomen usually is soft and non-tender. Hemoperitoneum and the subcapsular tear, usually involving the anterior superior aspect of the right lobe, may be discovered at laparotomy for suspected perforated viscus, abruptio placenta, or ruptured uterus. Levels of serum transaminases typically are grossly elevated (>10 times upper normal limits), and the prothrombin ratio is prolonged. Until recently, diagnosis was delayed and maternal mortality exceeded 60 per cent. The triad of preeclampsia, right upper quadrant pain particularly with referral to the shoulder tip, and shock should point to suspect hepatic rupture, and a general surgeon and obstetrician should proceed to the operating theater. Bleeding per vaginam may signify a bleeding diathesis. The left lobe of the liver is involved in 10 per cent of cases, and a subcapsular hematoma can be overlooked at surgery. Bleeding also may occur into the brain, chest, and retroperitoneum.

The prognosis of liver rupture has improved with advances in imaging techniques and increased awareness of HELLP and its complications. Serial scanning for suspected hematoma, hepatic rupture, and infarction is essential. CT and MRI may be necessary if ultrasonography is negative. CT imaging typically re-veals a crescentic or oval lesion of low attenuation without distortion of the hepatic vasculature (absence of mass effect). In hepatic infarction, enhancement after intravenous contrast medium is not seen, unlike that with hemorrhage, infection, and malignancy. Percutaneous diagnostic peritoneal lavage under aseptic technique should be carried out for suspected liver rupture. Combined surgical and obstetric intervention is urgent due to hemodynamic instability. Packing of the rupture with drainage is preferred to radical hepatic resection (Feliciano et al., 1986). Cesarean section should follow hemodynamic stability. Diagnostic hepatic arteriography offers the option of transcatheter embolization in hemodynamically stable patients without hemorrhage into the peritoneal cavity.

Hyperemesis Gravidarum: Effects on Liver

Minor elevations in levels of serum aspartate aminotransferase (AST <4 times upper normal) occur in 15 to 25 per cent of women with hyperemesis gravidarum and reverse rapidly with restoration of fluid balance, improved nutrition, and cessation of vomiting (Larrey et al., 1984; Morali and Braverman, 1990). Synthetic function (the prothrombin time) remains normal except with marked cholestasis and vitamin K deficiency (see Chapter 53). Abnormal liver function tests can occur when severe ketonuria is present. (Morali and Braverman, 1990).

Pathogenetic mechanisms are unclear. Earlier reports included viral hepatitis, drug-related hepatotoxicity, and coincidental thyrotoxicosis. Current hypotheses favor a multifactorial origin for the liver injury, including the adverse effects of starvation and dehydration, high levels of estrogens, and a genetic predisposition (Morali and Braverman, 1990).

VIRAL HEPATITIS

Viral hepatitis remains the most common cause of jaundice in pregnancy. General reviews have been published in the nonpregnant patient (Rothschild et al., 1991; Hollinger et al., 1991). Only those areas relating to maternal and fetal outcome will be considered here. The main hepatotropic agents likely to be seen in pregnancy are listed in Table 58–3. Incubation periods and clinical features overlap. Diagnosis relies on the detection of specific serologic markers of acute or chronic infection. Presentation typically is delayed until the cholestatic phase with pruritus, jaundice, and steatorrhea and may be confused with cholestasis from alcoholic hepatitis, biliary obstruction, intrahepatic cholestasis of pregnancy, drugs, or autoimmune liver diseases (see below), which may present in pregnancy.

Hepatitis A to E

Management principles in pregnancy are the same as for the nonpregnant population. Hepatitis A and B are the most common viruses causing acute hepatitis in pregnancy in North America and Europe. Acute

TABLE 58–3. Serologic Diagnosis of Acute Viral Hepatitis

NOMENCLATURE	ANTIBODIES AND OTHER TESTS
Hepatitis A: HAV	IgM anti-HAV (high-titer)
Hepatitis B: HBV	IgM anti-HBc (high titer)
Hepatitis C: HCV	Core region*, HCV RNA*
Hepatitis D: HDV	IgM/and IgG anti-HDV, HDV antigen
Hepatitis E: HEV	IgM/and IgG antibodies*
Herpes viruses:	IgM antibodies
Epstein-Barr (EBV) ⎫	
Varicella zoster ⎪	
Herpes simplex ⎬	Urine and bone marrow cultures
Cytomegalovirus ⎭	
Exotic viruses	IgM antibodies (panels)
	Cell cultures

*Being evaluated

infection presents more frequently as pregnancy progresses, with a peak onset in the third trimester. In the West there is no increase in severity for hepatitis A to D in pregnancy and no increased risk of spontaneous abortion, stillbirth, intrauterine growth restriction, and congenital abnormalities.

In contrast, data from developing countries show conflicting outcomes and may reflect the preponderance of hepatitis B and hepatitis E (see below), varying standards of medical care, and biased reporting of severe cases. Hepatitis A is uncommon in adults in developing countries. Exposure and immunity are almost universal in childhood. Other adverse factors include extreme malnutrition, enhanced coagulopathy, hormonal changes that might impair cellular immunity, and intercurrent HIV infection.

Hepatitis A

This RNA enterovirus is found worldwide. Spread occurs predominantly by the swallowing of water and food contaminated with sewage (feco-oral route). Illness follows a short incubation period of approximately 4 weeks (range 14 to 50 days). Symptoms often begin abruptly but are nonspecific with a flu-like illness, headache, fatigue, anorexia, nausea, vomiting, and diarrhea. Presentation with cholestasis commonly occurs a few days later with jaundice and pale stools, dark urine, and pruritus. Hepatitis A is self-limiting; chronic hepatitis A has not been recognized in humans. Occasionally, recovery may be delayed beyond six weeks with protracted cholestasis and a biphasic illness. Very rarely, acute liver failure will develop, but there is no special predisposition in pregnancy, unlike that of hepatitis E.

The prevalence of antibodies, indicating past infection and immunity (IgG anti-HAV), relates inversely to standards of sanitation and hygiene. Consequently, hepatitis A occurring in pregnancy is uncommon in Asia, the East, Africa, India, certain Mediterranean countries, and South America. In contrast, in the West, including the United States, hepatitis A is becoming more frequent in adults because herd immunity among children has fallen with improved stan-

dards of hygiene. In these low prevalence areas the infection typically shows seasonal variation. The peaks in the autumn and early winter may indicate virus imported from abroad. In pregnancy, diagnosis (high-titer IgM anti-HAV) is mandatory for reassurance. The presence of IgG anti-HAV confirms immunity for contacts of an infectious person and travellers.

HAV is excreted in large amounts in the stool before onset of symptoms and jaundice. Thereafter, the risk of transmission to others declines. Exposure to HAV is almost universal in promiscuous individuals who engage in oral-anal intercourse. Intravenous drug users are at special risk, presumably from poor standards of hygiene.

Immunoprophylaxis

In 1992, at least one inactivated, whole-virus hepatitis A vaccine has been licensed in Europe for parenteral administration. No information is available for pregnancy, but early data are encouraging on safety and immunogenicity in the nonpregnant population.

Immune globulin (IG) contains antibodies to hepatitis A (and also to hepatitis B; see below). IG has been an effective passive form of immunoprophylaxis for more than 40 years. IG is safe if prepared to standards of the World Health Organization and when administered intramuscularly (MMWR, 1990). A protective efficacy rate of 80 per cent can be achieved short-term following a single dose of 0.02 ml/kg given by deep, intramuscular injection immediately following an exposure. IG can protect against, or attenuate, the illness if given within 2 weeks following exposure.

Pregnant women travelling to high-prevalence areas should be pre-screened for IgG anti-HAV antibodies to prevent unnecessary immunization. There are no specific recommendations for administering IG during pregnancy. Immunoglobulin is recommended prior to travel abroad and also following sexual and other close contacts with an index case and during epidemics. Daycare centers for children, schools, institutions for custodial care, the military, and catering personnel (food handlers) are important sources for transmission. Immediate contacts of an index case should receive immunoprophylaxis.

In view of the increased rate of preterm deliveries to women with viral hepatitis in the third trimester, it would seem prudent to administer IG following close contact with an index case. Shedding of virus in the stool may continue, and isolation of potentially infectious subjects is important in limiting spread in epidemics.

The Neonate

Rarely, the newborn may contract HAV from fecal contamination if maternal incubation coincides with delivery. Neonatal infection should be considered if a mother develops acute hepatitis in the puerperium or has been given IG, which can prolong fecal excretion. Most neonatal infections are mild and followed by recovery and lifelong immunity.

Hepatitis E

Hepatitis E virus (epidemic, waterborne non-A, non-B hepatitis) has been identified in stool. Cloning of the RNA genome has shown some homology to caliciviruses. This agent (like hepatitis A) is transmitted by the feco-oral route and is prevalent in countries with poor sanitation. Surprisingly, attack rates are highest in young adults, suggesting limited immunity. There is a predilection for severe, including fulminant, hepatitis in pregnancy with mortalities as high as 20 per cent.

Hepatitis E is uncommon within the United States. Most cases are in travelers returning from areas of high prevalence such as Mexico, the Indian subcontinent, regions of the former Soviet Union (Commonwealth of Independent States), Nepal, Burma, and Africa. Fragility of the virus has hampered the development of diagnostic tests.

A pregnant woman with suspected hepatitis E should be managed in a center with expertise in maternal and fetal intensive care, hepatology, and infectious diseases (see Acute Liver Failure below). Although secondary spread to contacts is uncommon, contact with feces should be minimized by washing hands thoroughly and by disposing of contaminated clothes and fomites by autoclaving and incineration.

Hepatitis B

The relevance of hepatitis B to maternal-fetal medicine is the high risk of vertical transmission from carrier mother to child, the propensity of the infected newborn to become a chronic carrier, and the potential for eradication by immunization. In the West, the chronic carrier rate is between 1 and 5 per cent of the general population. The pool of infectious carriers in the USA is estimated to be as high as one million (MMWR, 1991a). Transmission generally takes place horizontally from person to person in adolescents and young adults. In the USA more than 300,000 individuals each year become infected. Up to 30,000 of these can be expected to become HBsAg seropositive chronic carriers. Each year, more than 4000 individuals die from HBV-related cirrhosis and 800 from primary liver cancer (Hoofnagle et al., 1987; MMWR, 1991a).

Consecutive surveys from the Center for Disease Control (CDC) (Alter et al., 1990) between 1981 and 1988 showed that the cases of acute hepatitis B attributed to parenteral drug use and heterosexual contact rose by 80 per cent and 38 per cent respectively. The peak prevalence was in those aged 15 to 29 years, compared with less than one per cent for ages below 15 years and 26 per cent for those aged 30 to 44 years. Heterosexual contact was the most significant factor in young females. The impact of hepatitis B virus in children and young adults probably is greatly underestimated. Transmission typically goes unnoticed because of nonspecific symptoms. Delay between virus transmission and manifestation of disease can be many years. Serologic responses remain the cornerstone of diagnosis of acute and chronic HBV infection.

Acute Hepatitis B

Acute infection may be symptomless and anicteric. Any malaise, anorexia, nausea, vomiting, and occasionally rashes and arthralgias cannot be distinguished clinically from hepatitis caused by drugs, alcohol, and autoimmune diseases.

Hepatitis B surface antigen (HBsAg) is detectable in blood 2 to 8 weeks before detection of abnormal serum liver biochemistry and symptoms. Serum HBsAg remains detectable usually until the convalescent phase. Hepatitis B "e" antigen (HBeAg) becomes detectable soon after HBsAg and is closely associated with the inner core (HBcAg) and HBV DNA. A pregnant woman with acute, especially fulminant, hepatitis B may be misdiagnosed as having non-B hepatitis if only serum HBsAg is sought and may be negative due to the "window" phase (see below). Also, additional infection with delta virus can lead to an inhibition of the serologic markers of hepatitis B (see hepatitis D below). Therefore serologic testing for high-titer IgM-anti-HBc is necessary at times for the diagnosis of acute infection.

Clinical recovery is associated with the rapid disappearance of serum HBV DNA followed by clearance of HBeAg and HBsAg antigenemia within 1 to 3 months when IgG anti-core (anti-HBc) and anti-HBe antibodies become detectable. In the "window" phase, defined as the serologic presence of anti-HBc without HBeAg and anti-HBs may persist for 2 to 16 weeks. This ends with detection of anti-HBs which signal recovery, viral clearance, and immunity. Clinical recovery from uncomplicated infection may take several months, and a biphasic illness with elevated serum levels of transaminase and bilirubin is common. At the other end of the spectrum is acute liver failure, associated with a mortality of more than 50 per cent (see below). There is no evidence that the course is especially severe in pregnancy, as is the case with hepatitis E. The frequency of preterm delivery is increased following acute hepatitis B in the third trimester.

The Chronic Carrier

Between 1 and 10 per cent of presumed healthy adults, and over 90 per cent of infected babies, may fail to clear the virus following acute infection. Chronic carriers remain HBsAg seropositive in the absence of IgM anti-HBc for more than 6 months. Serum IgG anti-HBc is detectable in HBsAg-positive carrier mothers and may play an important role in immunomodulation of fetal responses to HBV infection. Factors favoring chronic carriage are incompletely understood, but include infection early in life, symptomless infection, underlying immunosuppression, including that from the human immunodeficiency virus (HIV), and Down's syndrome. The term chronic carrier is somewhat misleading as up to 50 per cent of symptomless carriers have chronic active hepatitis, which predisposes to cirrhosis. Chronic persistent hepatitis can progress silently to chronic active hepatitis and cirrhosis.

Spontaneous seroconversion from HBsAg to anti-

HBs is uncommon in the West. Some HBeAg seropositive chronic carriers seroconvert spontaneously to anti-HBe and this is followed by a reduction in liver inflammation. However, in at least 20 per cent of HBsAg and anti-HBe seropositive Westerners and up to 40 per cent of Orientals, virus replication continues (detectable serum HBV DNA) with progressive liver damage. Furthermore, anti-HBe seropositive carriers have a propensity for delta virus (hepatitis D) superinfection, which aggravates the liver disease. Eventually, about half of the long-term chronic carriers will die from HBV-related liver disease, including chronic active hepatitis, cirrhosis, and its complications. The lifetime risk of a neonatally infected chronic carrier developing primary liver cancer may be 40 per cent (Beasley, 1982).

Mechanisms of Liver Damage

The extent of liver damage relates to the host's immunologic attack. Cytotoxic T cells recognize the core antigen (HBcAg) of the virus together with HLA (histocompatibility) antigens displayed on the membrane of infected hepatocytes. Acute liver failure is associated with an exaggerated immune attack, which destroys the liver to clear the virus. Chronic liver damage is caused by relentless inflammatory activity from continuing virus replication recognized by the presence of HBV DNA and HBeAg in serum.

Maternal Aspects

In prospective studies from Sydney (Britton et al., 1985) and Quebec (Delage et al., 1986), the prevalence of HBsAg positivity among blood donors was below 2 per cent. The Quebec questionnaire was completed by 30,315 pregnant women from nine hospitals between 1982 and 1984. Of the 29 French Canadians who tested positive for HBsAg, 16 (56 per cent) declared one or more risk factors including a past medical history of hepatitis, birth overseas, occupational exposure, blood transfusion, contact with a subject with hepatitis, and living in an institution. Exposure to intravenous recreational drugs was not sought, but was found to be common in the Australian study.

Vertical Transmission

In a study from California (Tong et al., 1981), the risk of transmission from mothers with acute hepatitis B was found to be 0 per cent in the first trimester and 6 per cent in the second trimester, being significantly lower than for the third trimester (67 per cent) and within 5 weeks postpartum (100 per cent). Transmission is most likely with maternal virus replication (HBeAg, HBV DNA, DNA polymerase activity) and occurs regardless of ethnic origin. The high frequency of HBeAg seropositivity among carrier mothers from the Far East and Southeast Asia (Beasley, 1982) results in a very high number (around 95 per cent) of infected neonates. Vertical transmission can occur in up to 25 per cent of HBeAg seronegative carrier mothers and in up to 12 per cent when the mother is anti-HBe positive (MMWR 1990; MMWR 1991c).

Suggested mechanisms for transmission during labor and peripartum have included mixing of maternal with fetal blood, contact with cervicovaginal epithelial cells shown to be positive for HBV DNA, and ingestion of amniotic fluid and breast milk. Transplacental transmission may explain failure to protect some neonates born of HBsAg-positive mothers despite optimum timing of immunoprophylaxis (Stevens et al., 1985; Tang, 1990). Also, avoidance of breast-feeding, delivery by cesarean section, and immediate separation from the infectious mother do not prevent subsequent infection within the first 6 months.

The risk of becoming chronically infected in neonatal life from exposure to an HBsAg-positive mother does not depend upon gestational age, birth weight, or subtype of the virus (Gerety and Schweitzer, 1977). Worldwide, transmission from mother to child around the time of birth accounts for up to 40 per cent of all chronic carriers and more than one million deaths each year from HBV-related liver disease (Kane et al., 1988). Transplacental transmission may be more frequent than recognized previously as HBV DNA was detected in 44 per cent of livers of fetuses from HBsAg-seropositive Chinese mothers (Tang, 1990).

Levels of anti-HBs rise about 3 months after perinatal administration of hepatitis B immune globulin (HBIG) which contains high-titer anti-HBs and anti-HBc. This pattern suggests passive-active immunity from exposure predating passive immunoprophylaxis. Anti-HBc can immunomodulate responses, but other factors must influence the preferential development of chronicity following neonatal infection. Maternal anti-HBc crosses the placenta and immunomodulates fetal responses to the virus, including suppressed expression of viral antigens (HBsAg, HBcAg). Maternal IgG-anti-HBc may block recognition of virus-infected cells by cytotoxic T cells. Early exposure to soluble virus protein may induce a state of immune tolerance to antigen via induction of specific T-suppressor cells which also serve to inhibit the host's cytotoxic attack (Thomas et al., 1986).

Virus replication in the fetus only responds to HBV-associated antigens. HBIG may prevent neonatal infection by protracting the time period of effective levels of inhibitory antibody on virus replication (Alexander and Eddleston, 1986). Maturation of the fetal immune system occurs after the first 2 to 3 months of life, and thereafter the baby can mount the immune response necessary to clear HBV.

Neonatal Outcome

Rapid reduction in titer of HBeAg after birth may predict clearance of virus and seroconversion to anti-HBs. Chronic carriage in the baby is uncommon following acute maternal hepatitis B in the third trimester of pregnancy (Gerety and Schweitzer, 1977). In contrast, over 90 per cent of those born of HBeAg-seropositive, HBV DNA-positive carriers will become chronic carriers. Persistence of HBeAg in the serum of the baby beyond the second month is predictive of chronic carriage.

Neonates of HBsAg-positive carrier mothers without HBeAg and anti-HBe rarely become chronic carriers, but may develop severe, including fulminant, hepatitis (Tong et al., 1984; Beath et al., 1992). Survivors show serologic evidence of clearance of virus and subsequent immunity (anti-HBs) to future infection.

There is no increase in risk of congenital abnormalities for babies born to mothers with HBV infection, even when exposure began in embryo during *in vitro* fertilization (van Os et al., 1991).

Horizontal Transmission

Transmission from person to person is the most common route in the West and plays an important role in Alaska, the American Pacific Islands, and Africa (Greenfield et al., 1986). Importantly, children born to HBsAg-seropositive mothers who seem to escape perinatal infection have up to a 60 per cent chance of becoming infected within 5 years (Margolis et al., 1992). Spread of HBV from an infected neonate to susceptible members of an adopted household can also occur (Nordenfelt and Dahlquist, 1978).

Strategies for Prevention of HBV Infection

Maternal Screening

All pregnant women should be screened for HBsAg to target neonatal immunoprophylaxis. Universal prenatal screening in the USA is estimated to identify 22,000 HBsAg-seropositive women per year. This strategy could prevent 3000 chronic infections per year and is cost-saving (MMWR, 1991c). Guidelines for selective screening of high-risk women extrapolated from the National Center of Health Statistics up to 1988 have shown less than 50 per cent sensitivity. High-risk mothers included first- and second-generation immigrants and refugees from Indochina and Southeast Asia, the Philippines, the Arctic (Eskimos), Haiti and the Dominican Republic, and the American Pacific Islands. Apart from Asian descent, no other risk factor was identified easily from histories (Alter et al., 1990).

Cesarean section does not prevent transmission of HBV from HBsAg-positive mothers. Breast-feeding is not contraindicated (MMWR, 1991c) in the immunized neonate, and lactation is not a contraindication to receiving the hepatitis B vaccine. Isolation and barrier nursing is unnecessary, but direct contact with blood-soaked dressings and pads should be avoided. All attendants should wear protective clothing, cover exposed cuts and abrasions, and handle body fluids with care. Goggles and masks should be worn for anticipated splashes onto ocular and mucosal surfaces (MMWR, 1991b). Five of 12 clusters in which HBV was transmitted from health-care personnel to patients have involved obstetricians and gynecologists performing invasive procedures (MMWR, 1991b). The US Occupational Safety Health Administration (OSHA) directive that all health-care personnel be immunized against hepatitis B was recommended in 1990 (Federal Register, 1989).

Diagnosis of hepatitis B in the mother should prompt screening of all children and intimate household contacts. Seronegativity for HBsAg, anti-HBc,

and anti-HBs will identify susceptible individuals who require vaccination. Testing for HBsAg should be repeated in late pregnancy and postpartum in seronegative mothers considered at risk (MMWR, 1991c). Mothers with suspected acute infection may also need to be screened for high-titer IgM-anti-HBc (Tables 58–3, 58–4).

A high-risk mother who presents in labor with unknown HBV status should be treated by the attending staff as positive for HBV until results are known. Neonatal immunoprophylaxis should be instigated if there is any delay in obtaining serologic results. Babies born to mothers who test positive at the postnatal visit should be screened for HBsAg, anti-HBc, and anti-HBs. Seronegative babies should receive vaccine without delay.

Immunoprophylaxis

Immune Globulin. Hepatitis B immune globulin (HBIG) contains high-titer anti-HBs and anti-HBc and offers good passive protection (0.06 ml/kg, intramuscularly) if given within 36 hours of exposure (MMWR, 1991c). Immune globulin (IG: gammaglobulin) contains moderate titers of anti-HBs (and anti-HAV antibodies) and should be used if HBIG is not available. Intramuscularly administered preparations made to the specifications of the World Health Organization (WHO) do not transmit any blood-borne infections including the human immunodeficiency viruses (HIV) implicated in AIDS (MMWR, 1991c). No specific adverse effects have been reported among many women given HBIG later discovered to be pregnant.

HBIG and IG are expensive, limited in supply, and effective only if given immediately following a definite exposure, and they offer temporary protection. Vaccine should be considered in many because of future risk of exposures to HBV.

Hepatitis B Vaccines. These have been extensively reviewed elsewhere (Hollinger et al., 1991; Alter et al., 1990; Margolis et al., 1992). Safe, efficacious vaccines have been licensed for clinical practice in the USA since 1982. Their safety has been endorsed by the World Health Organization (Deinhardt and Zuckerman, 1985) and the Immunization Practices Advisory Committee (MMWR, 1991c). Recombinant vaccines comprise subunits engineered by means of molecular

Table 58–4.   Serologic Diagnosis of Hepatitis B

STATUS	KEY MARKER	OTHER MARKERS
Acute hepatitis B	IgM anti-HBc (high titer)	HBsAg, HBeAg, HBV DNA
Chronic hepatitis B with high virus replication	HBsAg in the absence of high-titer IgM anti-HBc	HBV DNA, HBeAg
With low virus replication		Anti-HBe and no HBV DNA
With pre-core mutation*		HBeAg seronegative with HBV DNA

*Results in failure of HBeAg production; HBcAg is unaffected (see text).

biology techniques and have superseded the plasma-derived subunit vaccines in the West. Serious adverse reactions are rare. Soreness at the site of injection and a low-grade fever occur in less than 5 per cent of the vaccine recipients. Immunization should be delayed with intercurrent infection to avoid exacerbation of fever.

MATERNAL ASPECTS. Immunization is not offered routinely in pregnancy. However, there are no specific contraindications to the administration of a licensed hepatitis B vaccine and HBIG in maternal medicine. After careful assessment and counseling, vaccine should be offered to women at risk of contracting HBV infection during pregnancy provided there is no specific contraindication such as allergy to the components (MMWR, 1991c). Retrospective evaluation of women given vaccine prior to recognizing pregnancy shows no excess teratogenicity.

Postvaccination immunogenicity testing (anti-HBs levels) is sensible for adults because up to 20 per cent can give suboptimal responses, and this rises with age. Levels of anti-HBs fall exponentially in all vaccine recipients, with an anticipated fall by more than 80 per cent of the test level within 2 years. In the initial responder, anti-HBs levels rise exponentially after challenge indicating immune memory. The duration of protection from HBV infection outlives levels of anti-HBs in the initial responder, but not in the poor responder (Hadler et al., 1986).

The minimum level of anti-HBs antibody that guarantees protection from HBV infection is not known. Intercurrent HIV infection reduces the protective efficacy of HBV vaccination (Carne et al., 1987). The safest policy for poor responders is to assume no protection and to accept HBIG.

COMBINED IMMUNOPROPHYLAXIS FOR NEONATAL HBV INFECTIONS. Immunoprophylaxis should be given to all infants born of HBsAg-positive mothers regardless of maternal ethnic origin and HBeAg/anti-HBe status (Table 58–5). In the USA, the Immunization Practices Advisory Committee has recommended universal immunization of all babies, regardless of maternal HBV status, and of teenagers and young adults among whom intravenous drug use and sexually transmitted diseases are common (MMWR 1991c). Attention should be paid especially to immigrants and refugees from high-prevalence regions such as Alaska, Pacific Islands, Afghanistan, Angola, Bulgaria, Cambodia, Vietnam, Africa, and the Middle and Far East.

TABLE 58–5. Hepatitis B Virus Perinatal Post-exposure Recommendations of the Immunization Practices Advisory Committee

HBIG		VACCINE*	
DOSE	**TIMING**	**DOSE†**	**TIMING**
0.5 ml (250 IU)	within 12 hr	5–10 µg IM	within 12 hr

*First dose given concurrently with HBIG, *but* at different intramuscular sites. Schedules for basic course: 0, 1 and 6 months or 0, 1, 2, and 12 months.
†Dose and schedule depend on manufacturers' recommendations.
Adapted from Morbidity Mortality Weekly Report (MMWR): Update on adult immunization. Recommendations of the Immunization Practices Advisory Committee. MMWR RR12 **40**:33, 1991c.

Combined passive (HBIG) and active (vaccine) immunoprophylaxis offers the best protection of neonates born to mothers with acute and chronic HBV infection (Stevens et al., 1985). These should be administered at different sites as soon as possible after delivery (see Table 58–5). Failing this, the first dose of vaccine is effective up to 7 days later. Testing for HBsAg, anti-HBs, and anti-HBc is recommended at 12 months to assess efficacy. Although maternal anti-HBc may persist beyond 12 months, detection of IgM-anti-HBc indicates recent infection. There is no contraindication to the concurrent administration of other vaccines such as polio, diphtheria, tetanus, or pertussis (MMWR, 1991c).

Immunization Failures. The licensed vaccines are highly immunogenic and efficacious, especially in neonates. Until recently testing for anti-HBs was considered unnecessary in the majority of babies. Data from Senegal (Coursaget et al., 1987) and the United States (Stevens et al., 1985) show that poor responders and nonresponders are not protected from infection. Immunization failures arise from (1) a genetically predetermined response, (2) infection *in utero*, (3) immunosuppression from intercurrent infection, in particular HIV (Carne et al., 1987), (4) other diseases, and (5) the emergence of antibody escape variants of HBV (Carman et al., 1990; Harrison et al., 1992). Normally, anti-HBs antibody neutralizes HBV by binding to the dominant epitopes—the "a" determinant—on HBsAg. Some babies have tested positive for HBsAg beyond six months despite the presence of circulating anti-HBs. A point mutation (glycine substituted for arginine) in the second loop of the "a" determinant abrogated the neutralizing effects of anti-HBs antibody (Carman et al., 1990; Harrison et al., 1992).

Antiviral Therapies. HBV DNA seropositive mothers should be considered for interferon therapy after delivery. Clearance of HBsAg and seroconversion to anti-HBs can be achieved in up to half of women with chronic active hepatitis and recent infection. The disappointing results with neonatally acquired infection (Lok et al., 1986) reflect integration of HBV DNA and impaired cell-mediated host defenses with tolerance (Thomas et al., 1986).

Hepatitis Delta Virus

HBsAg-seropositive individuals are at risk from hepatitis delta virus (HDV) (Negro and Rizzetto, 1991). HDV has been found wherever hepatitis B virus is endemic, is spread by similar routes, and accounts for significant morbidity and mortality in patients with hepatitis B infection. In the USA, 25 to 75 per cent of HBsAg-seropositive intravenous drug users and persons receiving clotting factor concentrates have anti-delta antibodies (MMWR, 1991c). This highly pathogenic RNA-containing virus is very small and relies on hepatitis B for helper functions. Prevention of hepatitis B via immunoprophylaxis will protect against HDV.

HDV can suppress virus replication of HBV leading to transmission in an apparently HBsAg-seronegative person. Serologic testing must include HDVAg, HDV

RNA, anti-HDV, and markers of HBV infection including HBV DNA and IgM anti-HBc.

Simultaneous co-infection with HDV and HBV can cause acute liver failure, especially in intravenous drug abusers and their sexual partners. Horizontal transmission may explain clustering of HDV infection within HBsAg-positive families, especially among anti-HBe-seropositive HBV carriers. Vertical transmission of HDV is much less common than that of HBV and requires high levels of HBV DNA (virus replication) to establish HDV infection. Vertical transmission is unlikely to be a major route of spread compared with hepatitis B because the majority with HDV have sufficient liver disease to impair fertility and preclude pregnancy.

Hepatitis C

This RNA-containing virus is related to the pestiviruses and flaviviruses. HCV is a major cause of parenterally transmitted (post-transfusion non-A, non-B) hepatitis. All blood donors in the USA and Europe have been tested routinely since 1990. HCV, like HBV and HDV, is blood-borne and common among intravenous drug users and persons receiving repeated transfusions. In addition, HCV seems to be a major cause of sporadic (nonparenteral) hepatitis. In the USA the estimated number of new infections annually is between 150,000 and 170,000 (MMWR, 1991a). Chronic hepatitis and cirrhosis commonly follow acute infection. Primary liver cancer has been associated with cirrhosis, especially in countries such as Japan, where the majority of cases are HBsAg-seronegative. Vertical and sexual transmission can occur but are less frequent than for hepatitis B. The FDA has not recommended exclusion of seronegative sexual partners of anti-HCV-seropositive donors from being blood donors. There are no specific recommendations against pregnancy for anti-HCV-seropositive individuals and no special precautions for pregnant women or their babies (MMWR, 1991a).

First-line diagnosis detects antibodies to a panel of recombinant (cDNA) antigens, synthetic peptides (sp) and glycoproteins (gp) representing the more conserved regions of the virus genome. First-generation serologic tests detected antibodies to nonstructural (NS) components of the virus and are unreliable. Second-generation antibody tests (recombinant immunoblot assays: RIBA-2, RIBA-4, and enzyme-linked immunosorbent assays: ELISA) show improved sensitivity and specificity and correlate well with results using the polymerase chain reaction (PCR). Diagnosis of acute hepatitis C can be missed with the antibody tests. Seroconversion to current tests can be delayed many weeks, and discrimination between acute and chronic infection is difficult. The gold standard test is the PCR, but this is labor-intensive, expensive, and difficult to adapt to large-scale routine testing (Fagan, 1991).

Trials of antiviral therapies, especially interferons, are currently under way. Normalization of serum AST levels is easier to achieve with lower doses and more rapid than for chronic HBV infection. Interferons are contraindicated in pregnancy.

Other Hepatitis Viruses

Herpes simplex hepatitis is uncommon but severe, with mortalities exceeding 90 per cent in the third trimester of pregnancy (Taina et al., 1985). Nonspecific features can delay the diagnosis. Jaundice is not invariable, and mucocutaneous stigmata are absent in nearly half the cases. Why the virus can disseminate during pregnancy remains unclear. Antiviral therapy during pregnancy can be successful (Klein et al., 1991) (see Chapter 42). Hepatitis due to varicella zoster is rare, but its occurrence in the fetus has been reported (Da Silva et al., 1990).

Cytomegalovirus (CMV) probably is the most common cause of post-transfusion hepatitis in seronegative neonates and children in the West. In addition, cytomegalovirus commonly accompanies the immunodeficiency virus (HIV). CMV has been isolated from cultures of bile and body fluids. Virus can be detected in liver biopsy specimens by visualizing inclusions and using monoclonal antibodies and cDNA probes (see Chapter 42).

Although transmission of Epstein-Barr virus (EBV) via blood is uncommon, hepatitis has occurred in hemodialysis units. Hepatitis with infectious mononucleosis typically is symptomless except in epidemics. Acute liver failure due to EBV is uncommon but shows some predilection for the pregnant woman.

AIDS AND THE LIVER

Concurrent liver disease is common in late HIV infection and AIDS (see Chapter 43). Liver disease accounted for 4 per cent of deaths in US women aged 15 to 44 years with HIV infection prior to 1987 (Chu et al., 1990). The wide range of histologic changes include viral hepatitis and granulomata from opportunistic infections and drugs. Opportunistic infections, especially cryptosporidium and cytomegalovirus, can cause biliary abnormalities resembling sclerosing cholangitis and extrahepatic duct obstruction. Cryptococcosis, histoplasmosis and, rarely, pneumocystis may cause granulomatous hepatitis. The presenting features are protean, with fever, hepatosplenomegaly, and elevated serum levels of alkaline phosphatase and gamma glutamyl transpeptidase. Differential diagnosis is correspondingly wide and includes all causes of cholestatic jaundice and biliary tract infections. Liver biopsy can provide a valuable source of fresh tissue for culture and fixed material to assist in the diagnosis of many opportunistic infections.

ACUTE LIVER FAILURE

This is a rare and complex medical emergency beyond the scope of successful management in most general hospitals (O'Grady and Williams, 1987; O'Grady et al., 1988).

Fulminant hepatic failure (FHF) is defined as the development of hepatic encephalopathy caused by severe liver dysfunction within 8 weeks of onset of symptoms in a patient with a previously normal liver (Trey and Davidson, 1970). Late-onset hepatic failure (LOHF; subacute hepatic necrosis) defines the development of encephalopathy 8 to 26 weeks after onset of symptoms (Gimson et al., 1986). Early diagnosis is essential. Prognosis without transplantation depends on etiology. Referral should be made to a specialized unit with facilities for grafting before grade III encephalopathy, which is associated with clinical onset of cerebral edema. Travel exacerbates encephalopathy.

Survival is greatest when the interval between onset of encephalopathy and first symptoms and jaundice is less than 8 days, as is typical for hepatitis A and B. This interval often exceeds 7 days in non-A, non-B, non-C hepatitis, especially in LOHF, and correlates with a poor prognosis. Delivery of the mother generally has no specific effect on the course of the liver failure when the etiology is viral hepatitis or drug induced, but leads to improvement if the etiology is acute fatty liver or HELLP syndrome.

In a liver-oriented medical intensive care unit in one center, between 1973 and 1985, survival rates, without grafting, of 233 patients with severe liver failure (grade III-IV encephalopathy) from viral hepatitis were 44.7 per cent for A, 23.3 per cent for B, and 9 per cent for non-A, non-B. Survival for hepatitis A and B without transplantation has improved. The prognosis for non-A, non-B remains very poor without grafting. Early identification of those who require grafting has led to survival rates above 50 per cent.

The major areas of concern for maternal and fetal medicine are (1) the differential diagnosis, which may alter obstetric management, (2) when to refer the patient to a specialized unit, and (3) the timing of delivery.

Maternal Aspects

In the West, sporadic (nonparenteral) non-A, non-B non-C, non-E is the most common presumed viral cause of acute liver failure, but data pertaining to pregnancy are lacking. Viral causes, especially hepatitis E and B, are more prevalent among series reported in Europe and the developing countries. Fulminant hepatitis A and hepatitis B are rare in pregnancy, but isolated reports for hepatitis B have shown survival of mother and child after grafting (Mallia and Nancekivell, 1982; Baker and Cefalo, 1985; Fair et al., 1990; Laifer et al., 1990). Other causes, though rare, include idiosyncratic reactions to drugs, acetaminophen (paracetamol) overdose, carbon tetrachloride, halothane, poisonous mushrooms (*Amanita phalloides),* and herpes viruses.

Etiology is the most important variable for predicting survival without transplantation. Specific serologic tests are necessary because clinical features overlap with other causes of acute liver failure. Tests should include specific IgM class antibodies for hepatitis A (IgM-HAV), hepatitis B (IgM-anti-HBc), hepatitis delta (IgM-anti-delta), and the herpes viruses among others.

Seronegativity for HBsAg is not sufficient to exclude hepatitis B since this antigen is abnormally rapidly cleared in fulminant hepatitis B. Persistent, high-titer HBsAg points to another cause of hepatic failure, especially superinfection of a chronic carrier with other viruses. Multiple viral etiologies also should be considered, especially in intravenous drug users. Tests should be repeated if negative. Hepatitis delta antibodies may be negative in the early phase of fulminant delta and B co-infection, and this is only excluded after repeated testing.

Differential diagnosis in pregnancy includes viral hepatitis, acute fatty liver of pregnancy, severe preeclampsia and toxemia of pregnancy, the HELLP syndrome, and overlapping conditions such as thrombotic thrombocytopenic purpura (TTP) and the hemolytic-uremic syndrome. Severe hyperemesis gravidarum, Budd-Chiari syndrome, alcoholic hepatitis, pancreatitis, septicemias, and infective conditions such as leptospirosis may present with drowsiness, renal impairment, and jaundice. Chronic liver diseases, especially Wilson's disease and autoimmune chronic active hepatitis, and malignant infiltrations of the liver may be clinically indistinguishable.

Clinical features of acute liver failure are not diagnostic. Cutaneous stigmata such as spider nevi and palmar erythema can be seen in acute liver failure, chronic liver disease, and healthy pregnancy. Systolic hypertension may be marked when complicated by cerebral edema. The liver is usually small; a palpable liver in pregnancy may indicate infiltration. Splenomegaly is uncommon but is found in Wilson's disease and some other chronic liver diseases.

Test findings previously believed to be discriminant, such as polymorphonuclear leukocytosis in acute fatty liver and hematologic disturbances in disseminated intravascular coagulation, are common in all patients with acute liver failure because of sepsis, including fungal infection. The presence of hemolytic anemia should prompt consideration of Wilson's disease. Low levels of serum transaminase (AST or ALT) have been reported in acute fatty liver, the toxemias, and the HELLP syndrome, but these can rise above 2000 IU/liter with hepatic ischemia, rupture, and infarction. Relatively low levels of bilirubin and serum transaminase indicate extensive hepatocellular necrosis, lack of regeneration of hepatocytes, and a poor prognosis. Histologic documentation only of massive hepatocyte necrosis is of limited practical use.

Limited data are available regarding pregnant patients with acetaminophen (paracetamol) overdose, but drug levels should be sought in young women of childbearing age. Hepatotoxicity of the fetal liver from metabolites of acetaminophen can lead to impaired coagulation and intraventricular hemorrhage (Kurzel, 1990). *N*-acetylcysteine, given up to 36 hours following the overdose, can prevent the onset of hepatic encephalopathy (O'Grady and Williams, 1987). The very limited information suggests that this antidote is safe in pregnancy (Kurzel, 1990).

General management principles are the same for all patients with acute hepatic failure, regardless of etiology or pregnancy. Assessment includes the potential for recovery and suitability for liver transplantation based on prognostic indicators (Table 58–6). Progression beyond grade III encephalopathy increases the risk of complications, such as the development of cerebral edema. The onset of encephalopathy is variable and may predate jaundice. Early discussion with, and referral to, a specialized center is essential in cases of hepatic encephalopathy (grades II, III, IV), elevated prothrombin ratio (e.g., >2 times normal control), renal impairment, metabolic acidosis (blood pH <7.3), hypotension, hyponatremia, and thrombocytopenia (O'Grady and Williams, 1987). The blood group is important for matching available grafts, and tests should be commenced to exclude Wilson's disease.

The prothrombin time, which is the most sensitive indicator of severity of liver dysfunction and prognosis, should be measured repeatedly. Administration of fresh frozen plasma without overt bleeding does not alter outcome and obscures results of the prothrombin time. Fresh blood and blood products should be available to support any obstetric or surgical intervention and following delivery. Parenteral vitamin K_1 and folic acid should be given routinely. Gastrointestinal bleeding from gastric erosions is decreased by the prophylactic administration of an H_2 antagonist. A nasogastric tube should be put in place and the stomach emptied hourly to prevent aspiration of gastric contents, which is common in the presence of increasing drowsiness and vomiting. Elective endotracheal intubation may be required to protect the airway, particularly prior to any movement—such as that required for travel and surgical procedures including delivery—and before the development of overt cerebral edema. Intubation must be performed by an experienced anesthetist. All sedation should be withdrawn.

Hypoglycemia remains a common cause of fetal and maternal death. Blood glucose levels should be closely monitored and immediate provision made to administer large quantities of glucose (10 to 50 per cent solutions) via a central venous catheter. Early manifestations of cerebral edema include peaks of systolic hypertension and a tachycardia and should be treated by mannitol-induced diuresis (100 ml bolus of 20 per cent solution) and assisted hyperventilation to reduce the blood P_{CO_2} and hence cerebral blood flow. However, mannitol is potentially nephrotoxic and ineffective in renal failure. Ultrafiltration and hemodialysis may be required to remove excess fluid. Levels of

blood urea may be misleadingly low. Renal function is best monitored by serial levels of blood creatinine and creatinine clearance. Detailed microbiologic cultures and analysis should be performed serially on all body fluids including blood, urine, and sputum because infections are common in liver failure. Hemoperfusion techniques using columns of charcoal and albumin-coated resin and plasmapheresis have been superseded by general advances in specialized medical and nursing care in liver-oriented intensive care units (O'Grady et al., 1988).

Health-care personnel should handle patients with care and be provided with protective clothing. Pregnant and nonimmunized (for hepatitis A and B) personnel should not be allowed to nurse such patients, particularly those with suspected hepatitis B and E.

Fetal survival is exceptional. Fetal heart sounds are absent on presentation in the most severe cases, and this absence often relates to profound fetal and maternal hypoglycemia.

The place for agents that inhibit virus replication, such as phosphonoformate trisodium and interferons, seems limited, as indicated by results of small, uncontrolled trials, mostly for hepatitis B. Interferons have been given to three pregnant women with fulminant viral hepatitis, and two of these survived (Levin et al., 1989). Data on controlled trials in fulminant hepatitis are lacking. In fulminant B and D, virus replication is less than in uncomplicated acute infection and may have ceased before presentation. For continuing replication, the extent of liver damage may preclude regeneration.

Corticosteroids are without benefit in controlled trials. The increased risks of microbial infection and known adverse effects on virus replication are sufficient to outweigh any marginal benefits. Insulin-glucagon infusions promoted rapid liver cell regeneration in controlled studies in animal models, but results in humans are conflicting. Prostaglandin E_1 by continuous infusion was associated with improvements and no mortality in acute liver failure from hepatitis B and presumed non-A, non-B hepatitis. Results from larger, controlled studies are awaited.

Liver Transplantation

Grafting during pregnancy has been successful for acute liver failure and Budd-Chiari syndrome. The uniformly poor survival for acute liver failure, excluding hepatitis A and B, has emphasized the place of early liver grafting. Successful maternal and fetal outcomes have been reported for pregnant women grafted for fulminant hepatitis B and acute fatty liver. Subsequent pregnancy in women grafted previously and who were maintained on azathioprine, corticosteroids, and cyclosporin has been reported for acute and chronic liver diseases including Budd-Chiari syndrome and acute liver failure.

Reinfection following transplantation in nonpregnant survivors has been documented for acute liver failure and chronic hepatitis B and D and non-A, non-B with variable clinical outcomes. Data on the efficacy of immunoprophylaxis and antiviral therapies are

TABLE 58–6. Poor Prognostic Indicators in Acute Liver Failure*

ACETAMINOPHEN	OTHER CAUSES
All three:	Any three of these:
Grade III encephalopathy	Etiology, e.g., non-ABC
Prothrombin time >100 sec	Age <10 or >40 yrs
Creatinine >300 μM/l	Prothrombin time >50 sec
	Serum bilirubin >300 μM/l
	Jaundice >7 days before
	encephalopathy
And/or:	Or:
Arterial pH <7.3	Prothrombin >100 sec

*These are for guidance only; other factors must be considered.

sparse. Reinfection seems less likely for hepatitis B and D if HBIG is used.

The menstrual cycle returns to normal soon after successful grafting (Cundy et al., 1990; de Koning and Haagsma, 1990; Brown and Lucey, 1991); continuing amenorrhea may signify early pregnancy. Patients should be offered early advice on contraception. Pregnancy does not increase the risk of graft rejection, but deferral of pregnancy beyond the first year seems sensible because morbidity and mortality are greatest within this time.

Pregnancy in recipients of hepatic allografts is associated with good perinatal outcome, but there is an increased risk of preeclampsia, worsening hypertension, anemia, and preterm delivery. Graft function and survival seem unaffected by pregnancy (Laifer et al., 1990; Scantlebury et al., 1990). Shared management is essential between transplant specialists and perinatologists. Oral contraceptive drugs may enhance hepatotoxicity of cyclosporin (Deray et al., 1987). In addition, these are contraindicated in patients with thrombogenic disorders such as Budd-Chiari syndrome.

CHRONIC LIVER DISEASE, CIRRHOSIS, AND PORTAL HYPERTENSION

In the United States, chronic liver diseases rank within the six major causes of death, disability, and medical expenditure (Mason et al., 1987).

Chronic Persistent and Chronic Active Hepatitis

Chronic persistent hepatitis (CPH) is a histologic description of a chronic inflammatory infiltrate confined to the portal tracts. Chronic active hepatitis (CAH) describes the infiltrate extending beyond the limiting plate into the hepatic lobule and surrounding islands of hepatocytes (piecemeal necrosis). If severe, bridging necrosis occurs toward the central hepatic vein and is associated with progression to cirrhosis. CPH and CAH may result from many insults including chronic viral hepatitis (commonly B and C), autoimmune conditions, Wilson's disease, and drugs such as methyldopa and isoniazid. Although CPH is considered the more benign disease, in some cases it will progress to CAH and cirrhosis. The majority of patients with CAH are young women with autoimmune disease. Features include hypergammaglobulinemia and autoantibodies to smooth muscle, specific proteins (anti-liver specific proteins), and nuclear factor (ANF).

Untreated autoimmune CAH is associated with amenorrhea and infertility, and therefore pregnancy with advanced cirrhosis, regardless of etiology, is uncommon (Cundy et al., 1991). The use of corticosteroids and azathioprine has improved fertility (Steven et al., 1979) and overall prognosis. Liver function is preserved during pregnancy with well-controlled disease activity. Although fetal prematurity, fetal loss, and low birth weight are common, the incidence of congenital malformations is not increased (Steven et

al., 1979). Common obstetric complications include urinary tract infections and toxemia.

Prednisone therapy for autoimmune CAH should be continued in conventional doses (10 to 20 mg/day) and increased with suspected relapse, although this is unusual (Steven et al., 1979). Azathioprine (up to 1.5 mg/kg/day) is also an established therapy for autoimmune CAH with prednisolone (Steven et al., 1979). Uncontrolled disease should prompt reappraisal and exclusion of other conditions such as Wilson's disease. No specific adverse effects on the fetus have been reported except rare pancytopenia (Lawson et al., 1984). Some nonpregnant patients with well-controlled disease can be maintained on azathioprine alone after cautious withdrawal of corticosteroids (Keating et al., 1987). Dual therapy is recommended in pregnancy to minimize the chances of relapse. In chronic viral hepatitis, immunosuppressant drugs are contraindicated in view of the adverse effects on virus replication. Following delivery, the woman who is HBsAg-positive with serologic evidence of virus replication (HBV DNA and HBeAg) should be considered for antiviral therapy. Drug-induced clearance of HBsAg and HBeAg has been documented in up to half the adult females following treatment with interferons. Trials of antiviral therapies are in progress for chronic hepatitis C. Their impact on future risks of developing cirrhosis and primary liver cancer is unknown.

Cirrhosis

Pregnancy in advanced cirrhosis was first reported in 1923 (Scaglione, 1923) but remains uncommon (Cheng, 1977; Britton, 1982; Schreyer et al., 1982; Krol Van Straaten and De Maat, 1984; Teisala and Tuimala, 1985). Information from two series (Cheng, 1977; Britton, 1982) and a collective review of well-documented cases (Schreyer et al., 1982) has helped to clarify the prognosis for mother and fetus. It should also be remembered that transient esophageal varices have been documented on endoscopy in up to 60 per cent of healthy pregnant women (Schreyer et al., 1982).

Effects on the Pregnancy

Fetal loss is high with advanced cirrhosis. In the first trimester, the risk of spontaneous abortion is around 10 per cent (Britton, 1982) and worsens (17 per cent) without portosystemic decompression (Cheng, 1977; Schreyer et al., 1982). In late pregnancy, stillbirth may occur in as many as 25 per cent of cases and neonatal deaths in up to 7 per cent (Schreyer et al., 1982). The prognosis for the fetus was better following portosystemic shunts (median 3 years) prior to delivery. In one series of 30 pregnancies there were 80 per cent live births, 13.7 per cent stillbirths, and one preventable neonatal death (Schreyer et al., 1982).

Effects of Pregnancy on Disease

In a literature survey (Cheng, 1977), 54 per cent of women with documented severe cirrhosis had successful, uneventful term pregnancies. Maternal prognosis depends on the degree of hepatic dysfunction more than the etiologic type. Compensated biliary and postnecrotic cirrhosis carry the best prognosis. Spontaneous improvements in liver function during pregnancy have been reported for primary biliary cirrhosis and Wilson's disease.

Bleeding from esophageal varices remains the most significant complication of cirrhosis in pregnancy (Schalm and van Buuren, 1985). The maximum risk is after the first trimester. This coincides with a progressive increase in circulating blood volume, elevations in portal pressure, and compression of the inferior vena cava by the uterus; a greater proportion of the venous return is diverted through the azygos system. In a review of the literature prior to 1982 (Schreyer et al., 1982), gastrointestinal hemorrhage, from presumed esophageal varices, occurred in 13.3 per cent of cases without previous surgical portal decompression and was associated with high (70 per cent) maternal mortality. No control group was included. However, outcomes for pregnant women who had previously undergone portosystemic shunting (median 3 years) prior to delivery were good; only 1 of 23 pregnancies (21 mothers) resulted in maternal death. Hepatic coma, unrelated to overt bleeding, occurred postpartum. Surgical portal decompression was uneventful in seven mothers during pregnancy. Bleeding occurred on 38 occasions of 160 pregnancies with coexisting esophageal varices (Britton, 1982). Potential postpartum complications include maternal bleeding and death, uterine hemorrhage, hepatic coma, and ascites.

Management

Pregnancy with compensated cirrhosis, in the absence of jaundice and previously impaired liver function, should be allowed to proceed to term. The patient should be encouraged to rest and take vitamin supplements. Protein intake should be limited in advanced cirrhosis and following surgical portal decompression. Maneuvers that increase portal pressure, such as straining and stooping, and alcohol consumption should be avoided. No specific measures to protect the esophagus are of proven benefit in the absence of esophageal reflux (Schalm and van Buuren, 1985). Vaginal delivery is safe in most cases, but a protracted second stage should be avoided and interrupted early by forceps delivery to avoid excessive straining. Forceps-assisted deliveries may account for better fetal outcomes in the shunted groups (26.6 per cent) than in the nonshunted groups (13.0 per cent) (Schreyer et al., 1982).

Delivery should take place in a unit with intensive care facilities and expertise in handling bleeding esophageal varices. Excess blood loss should be anticipated, especially in the puerperium. Vitamin K_1, fresh frozen plasma, and additional coagulation factors and platelets may be required. Sedation should generally be avoided. Anesthetics and diuretics should be used cautiously since these and other factors—including excess blood loss, hypotension, infection, hypoglyce-

mia, and constipation—can precipitate hepatic encephalopathy.

Management of ascites requires restriction of dietary sodium and, in severe cases, fluid restriction. Spironolactone is the mainstay drug therapy in the nonpregnant patient with ascites, but spironolactone, triamterene, frusemide (BAN for furosemide), and bumetanide cross the placenta, and their safety has not been established in prospective trials in pregnancy. The thiazide diuretics can precipitate hepatic coma in pregnant patients with cirrhosis. Frusemide and a metabolite of spironolactone cross into breast milk, and breast-feeding is not recommended. Ascitic fluid should be analyzed for leukocytosis (>250 cells/mm^{-3}), microbial organisms, and an acid pH (<7.35). Peritonitis may be present without fever and peripheral blood leukocytosis. The prognosis with untreated infection is poor and frequently confounded by recurrent gastrointestinal bleeding. Appropriate antimicrobial therapy to cover fecal organisms should be instigated without delay.

Cesarean section should be reserved to save the infant in the presence of rapidly deteriorating maternal liver function, but the prognosis in these circumstances remains poor for both mother and child (Cheng, 1977). Abdominal surgery may be difficult due to the large collateral circulation and adhesions from previous shunt surgery. Local anesthesia, such as an epidural or pudendal block, can be performed safely, but the raised venous pressure and abnormal coagulation increase the risk of bleeding. Elective termination of pregnancy in the first trimester should be considered only for advanced decompensated cirrhosis. A woman presenting in pregnancy with suspected cirrhosis and portal hypertension requires full investigation including upper esophagogastroduodenoscopy and, if necessary, liver biopsy. Both techniques are safe in expert hands, with the usual reservations regarding normal coagulation and ultrasonographic guidance for liver biopsy.

Cirrhosis is the main cause of portal hypertension in the West. Other noncirrhotic causes requiring different medical therapies include schistosomiasis, sarcoidosis, tuberculosis, malignancy, Gaucher's disease (Menton et al., 1990), polycystic liver (Everson, 1990; Gabow et al., 1990), congenital hepatic fibrosis, and acute fatty liver of pregnancy.

Management of bleeding esophageal varices has been simplified with sclerosing agents used to obliterate venous channels. This is equally successful at arresting bleeding in both pregnant and nonpregnant patients (Kochhar et al., 1990). Several controlled trials have shown endoscopic sclerotherapy to be superior to surgical intervention (portosystemic shunting, esophageal transection) for reducing rebleeding episodes in nonpregnant patients who present with bleeding (Schalm and van Buuren, 1985). Portal pressure may also be reduced with beta-blockers or vasoconstrictor agents and a nitrate. Upper endoscopy must be repeated early for each bleeding episode to optimize interventional sclerotherapy and identify other causes. Protection of the airway is essential to prevent aspiration of gastric contents.

Primary Biliary Cirrhosis (PBC)

Primary biliary cirrhosis is a term applied to a wide spectrum of diseases and variable natural history (Nir et al., 1989). The pregnant woman may be symptomless with elevated levels of serum alkaline phosphatase (liver isoenzyme) and gamma glutamyl transpeptidase (GGT). Subsequent diagnosis relies on detection of mitochondrial antibodies in almost all cases and characteristic liver histology in the absence of other biliary diseases. Differential diagnosis includes intrahepatic cholestasis of pregnancy, which resolves in the puerperium, and sclerosing cholangitis, which may be associated with covert inflammatory bowel disease and cholelithiasis.

Maternal and fetal outcomes are variable. Prognosis is better for well-compensated PBC compared with other (nonbiliary) forms of cirrhosis. Drug therapy is nonspecific and aimed at relieving symptoms such as pruritus. Cholestyramine resin binds fat-soluble vitamins (A, D, E, K), and vitamin K_1 supplements should be given, especially before delivery. There are no studies relating to the prognosis of PBC presenting in pregnancy.

Wilson's Disease

Successful pregnancy is uncommon in untreated and advanced disease because of subfertility, amenorrhea, and spontaneous abortions. Wilson's disease should be considered in any young patient with liver disease including acute liver failure. The demonstration of Kayser-Fleischer rings by slit-lamp analysis is useful for diagnosis, but these discolorations can be absent in patients with predominant hepatic disease and present in primary biliary cirrhosis. Detection of symptomless liver disease is common in siblings. Spontaneous improvements in neurologic status and liver function have been recorded in pregnancy and attributed to extraction of copper by the fetus.

In 44 pregnant women who received D-penicillamine or triethylene tetramine dihydrochloride (trientine), good maternal and fetal outcomes were reported (Walshe, 1986). Chelating agents in pregnancy generally are considered safe and should not be discontinued because subsequent relapse rate is high. D-penicillamine can be toxic in doses exceeding 1500 mg/day. The dose for successful cupruresis during pregnancy probably is less than that in the nonpregnant patient and can be cautiously reduced by 25 to 50 per cent should toxic symptoms occur. A full dose should be resumed immediately after delivery. Chelating agents reduce serum levels of iron and zinc and should not be administered simultaneously with oral iron supplements. Pyridoxine (vitamin B_6) should be given as a supplement in a minimum dose of 50 mg/week to counteract the antipyridine effects of D-penicillamine.

D-penicillamine crosses the placenta. Congenital abnormalities described probably are due to copper deficiency. Abnormalities of skin and connective tissue have been described in babies whose mothers took 0.9 to 2.0 gm/day of D-penicillamine during pregnancy. Reversible neonatal cutis laxa followed maternal D-

penicillamine therapy (1.5 gm/day) for Wilson's disease (Linares et al., 1979). Oral zinc has been used in the treatment of Wilson's disease, but there are no data relating to pregnancy.

Liver grafting has been successful in nonpregnant patients with severe hepatic and neurologic dysfunction, but there are no reports of grafting in pregnancy.

Fetal Alcohol Syndrome

For a discussion of this syndrome, see Chapter 13.

Budd-Chiari Syndrome

This syndrome is defined as obstruction of the large hepatic veins producing congestion and necrosis of the centrilobular areas of the liver (Benhamou and Lebrec, 1985). Other, related disorders include thrombosis of the high inferior vena cava, veno-occlusive disease, and peliosis hepatis, conditions that share similarities in clinical presentation, abnormalities in hematologic profiles, and possible etiologies. The first case described by Chiari in 1899 followed childbirth. By 1984, more than 30 cases were reported as presenting during pregnancy or, more commonly, postpartum. The Budd-Chiari syndrome is associated with a hypercoagulable state, but exact mechanisms remain obscure. The increased incidence in pregnancy may relate to the physiologic lowering of concentrations of antithrombin III at delivery. More than 75 per cent of cases of idiopathic Budd-Chiari syndrome occur in females (Van Thiel, 1987). Of 105 patients with Budd-Chiari syndrome, 15 presented between 4 days and 4 weeks postpartum and one during pregnancy (Khuroo and Datta, 1980). There is also an increased incidence of Budd-Chiari syndrome with oral contraceptive therapy (Khuroo and Datta, 1980). In the past, affected females were dissuaded from pregnancy for fear of increased risks of hepatic venous thrombosis. Although activities of clotting factors are altered in pregnancy, no specific abnormality has been found in studies of Budd-Chiari syndrome following pregnancy.

Clinical features include rapid abdominal distention from painless ascites. The liver is enlarged and occasionally tender. The serum liver biochemistry shows an elevation of alkaline phosphatase above that reflecting normal placental function. The serum level of aspartate aminotransferase (AST, ALT) usually is modestly raised. Marked elevations may cause diagnostic confusion with viral hepatitis. Rarely, the clinical presentation is indistinguishable from fulminant hepatic failure (see above). The protein content of the ascitic fluid typically is above 40 gm/liter but can be variable. Diagnosis in pregnancy is best achieved by ultrasonographic Doppler imaging and percutaneous liver biopsy. Percutaneous hepatic venous catheterization is diagnostic should these techniques fail. Liver histology is not specific. Features show centrizonal venous congestion, hemorrhage, hepatocellular necrosis, dilatation of the sinusoids and central veins, and features compatible with outflow block. A search should also be made for causes of abnormal coagulation, such as antithrombin III deficiency and lupus anticoagulant, and hematologic tests should be performed for paroxysmal nocturnal hemoglobinuria and hemolytic anemia. Bone marrow should be examined for abnormalities in erythroid precursors and detection of polycythemia rubra vera.

Fetal outcome is not affected directly, but rather depends on maternal outcome (Steven, 1981), wherein management has been disappointing. The ascites often is resistant to medical therapy. The safety in human pregnancy of many commonly used diuretics—such as spironolactone, amiloride, triamterene, and thiazides—has not been established. Maternal mortality is high following such surgical interventions as portocaval, splenorenal, or mesocaval and meso-atrial shunts, but individual pregnancies have been successful after a mesocaval or cavoatrial shunt (Huguet et al., 1984; Vons et al., 1984). Liver transplantation has been successful, but recurrent thrombosis occurs even with long-term anticoagulant therapy.

INFLAMMATORY BOWEL DISEASE AND THE LIVER

A significant proportion of patients with Crohn's disease and ulcerative colitis have abnormal liver function tests and histologic abnormalities primarily affecting the biliary tract, including sclerosing cholangitis (see Chapter 57). Surgical and autopsy liver specimens show histologic abnormalities in 50 to 95 per cent of cases. The hepatic abnormalities do not seem to correlate with severity of inflammatory bowel disease. Associations with HLA have been described, but pathogenetic mechanisms remain obscure. There are no specific reports relating to pregnancy.

HEPATIC PORPHYRIAS

Acute intermittent porphyria has been reported with variable degrees of hepatic dysfunction and maternal and fetal outcomes (Kanaan et al., 1989; Milo et al., 1989).

HEPATIC ABSCESS

Amebic abscess typically presents in the third trimester and puerperium (Cowan and Houlton, 1978; Mitchell and Teare, 1984) with vague, nonspecific symptoms of abdominal discomfort and intermittent fever and, occasionally, rupture or pulmonary features such as a pleural effusion, chest pain, and elevated right diaphragm. Diagnosis is often mistaken for other abdominal conditions, especially appendicitis. Serologic diagnosis is based on a strongly positive complement fixation test. Serum levels of immunoglobulin may be normal. There is no special predilection for presentation and excess severity in pregnancy. Survival has improved with earlier diagnosis by ultrasonographic techniques and treatment with effective antimicrobial agents such as metronidazole. Ultra-sonographic analysis can differentiate between a pyogenic hepatic abscess and a cyst due to *Echinococcus granulosus* (hydatid cyst). Hydatid disease must be excluded before aspiration because dissemination of daughter scoleces can prove fatal.

CONGENITAL DISORDERS OF LIVER METABOLISM

The congenital hyperbilirubinemias are associated with excess levels of unconjugated (Gilbert's disease) and conjugated (Dubin-Johnson and Rotor syndromes) bilirubins. Presentation with jaundice and dark urine may be precipitated by pregnancy, oral contraceptive drugs, excess alcohol, fasting, exercise, and stress. The maternal and fetal outcomes are good except for isolated reports of severe jaundice and fetal death in the Dubin-Johnson syndrome (Seligsohn and Shani, 1977). Kernicterus is rare. Differential diagnosis includes all causes of jaundice, especially the cholestatic phase of viral hepatitis, intrahepatic cholestasis of pregnancy, and gallstones. Unconjugated bilirubinemia is found in hemolytic disorders and Wilson's disease. Pruritus and elevations in serum alkaline phosphatase and gamma glutamyl transpeptidase do not occur in the Dubin-Johnson syndrome.

Hepatic steatosis has been described in many defects in fatty acid metabolism. Carnitine deficiency may be precipitated in susceptible pregnant individuals due to physiologic alterations of fatty acid oxidation. Whether similar events are implicated in the pathogenesis of acute fatty liver of pregnancy (Schoeman et al., 1991) requires further study.

HEPATIC TUMORS

Benign and Malignant Neoplasms

Hepatic adenomata are vascular, and fatal rupture has been reported in pregnancy. Successful pregnancy has followed partial hepatectomy for removal of multiple adenomata. Some adenomata have areas of focal nodular hyperplasia and carcinoma, casting doubt on their benign classification. Development of primary hepatocellular carcinoma has been linked with low-dose and high-dose estrogens in oral contraceptive drugs (Neuberger et al., 1986), hepatitis B and C infection, and smoking. The clinical findings are similar to those in the nonpregnant population. Typical but not invariable findings are marked elevation in alpha-fetoprotein and cirrhosis. The main differential diagnosis consists of other causes of a rapidly expanding mass including benign hepatic tumors, abscess, and metastases. Tests should include screening for markers of hepatitis B and C and an amebic complement fixation test.

Serum levels of carcinoembryonic antigen (CEA) and beta–human choriogonadotropin (bHCG) may be raised in primary liver cancer, a finding that causes confusion with gestational trophoblastic disease. Primary liver cancer in pregnancy is associated with rapid growth of the tumor and an abysmal prognosis. Cholangiocarcinoma is rare and presents with signs of extrahepatic cholestasis and pruritus. The main differential diagnosis is extrahepatic bile duct obstruction due to cholelithiasis and enlargement of the head of the pancreas.

Polycystic Liver Disease

Differential diagnosis of an enlarged liver in pregnancy is wide but includes polycystic liver disease and congenital hepatic fibrosis. Polycystic liver disease is an autosomal dominant condition found most often in multiparous women with concurrence of renal cysts (Gabow et al., 1990). Several factors—including age, female sex, pregnancy, the degree of renal cystic disease, and the extent of renal functional impairment—may modify the expression of hepatic cystic disease (Everson, 1990). Complications include abdominal pain and infection of the cysts during pregnancy.

THE GALLBLADDER AND BILIARY TRACT

Gallbladder size increases through pregnancy (Bartoli et al., 1984), but effects on gallbladder function remain controversial. A recent study using ultrasonographic techniques showed similar rates of contraction and emptying between pregnant and nonpregnant women (Radberg et al., 1989). However, there is general agreement that residual and fasting volumes are increased in late pregnancy. The mean diameter of the common bile duct has been shown to be greater in pregnant women than in nonpregnant women (Radberg et al., 1990), but this finding is not invariable (Mintz et al., 1985). Altered gallbladder function has been attributed to the relaxant action of progestogens on smooth muscle. However, the progressive rise in serum progestogens after the 11th week does not correlate with earlier gallbladder dysfunction. Estrogens may impair water absorption by the gallbladder by inhibiting the sodium-potassium ATPase pump (Braverman et al., 1980; Mintz et al., 1985).

Cholesterol gallstones are common in the West, especially in women taking oral contraceptive steroids (Bennion and Grundy, 1978; Radberg et al., 1990). The Food and Drug Safety Administration (FDA) requires that risks of gallbladder disease be included with instructions on oral contraceptive steroids. A large case-controlled study was conducted in Australia (Scragg et al., 1984) on the interrelation between oral contraceptive steroids, pregnancy, and gallbladder disease. The risk of developing gallstones rose with parity in young, but not older, women. The risk declined with rising age at first pregnancy. The risk of cholesterol cholelithiasis also rises with obesity, small bowel disorders with malabsorption of bile salts such as Crohn's disease and resections, liver diseases, and diabetes mellitus.

Stone formation requires the hepatic secretion of lithogenic bile. In the nonpregnant female (compared with the male), there is a reduction in total bile acid pool, in particular for chenodeoxycholic acid (CDCA).

The ratio of cholate to CDCA is reduced in contraceptive steroid users, rendering the bile more saturated and lithogenic (Van Thiel, 1987). After the first trimester, there is a progressive decrease in the size of the CDCA, but not cholic acid, pools. As the rate of cholesterol secretion is unchanged, its relative concentration to the diminishing bile acid pool is increased, rendering the bile more lithogenic. Estrogens and progestogens have marked and different effects on metabolism of bile salts, cholesterol, and biliary lipids. Ethinyl estradiol causes an increase in cholesterol content within the liver, but decreases the secretion of bile salts. Progesterone increases the rate of esterification, but not synthesis, of cholesterol and an increase in bile salt–independent bile secretion. The net effect is to increase saturation of the bile with cholesterol.

Cholelithiasis in Pregnancy

Gallbladder disease remains the second most common nonobstetric surgical condition in pregnancy after acute appendicitis (Woodhouse and Haylen, 1985). Acute cholecystitis requiring surgery occurs in approximately 1:1000 deliveries. The presentation and management of acute cholecystitis and biliary obstruction in pregnancy are the same as in the nonpregnant patient. The classic presentation consists of pain in the right upper quadrant, sometimes radiating to the back, and nausea and vomiting. Weight loss, intolerance to fatty food, and fever above 37.5°C are uncommon. The gallbladder usually is not palpable. Differential diagnosis is wide and includes other causes of cholestatic jaundice such as viral hepatitis, alcoholic hepatitis, pyelonephritis, sepsis, and infections such as AIDS. Cirrhosis and intrahepatic cholestasis of pregnancy are associated with cholelithiasis.

General medical management includes bed rest, withdrawal of oral feeding, rehydration with intravenous fluids, and antibiotics. Diagnostic ultrasonographic techniques are safe in pregnancy, but do not determine the state of the papilla or the presence of a biliary stricture, and they may fail to detect coexisting pancreatitis when gas from a small bowel ileus obscures the views. The false-negative rate for imaging of the common bile duct is higher than for the gallbladder. Although radiographic imaging techniques have largely been replaced by pre- and intraoperative ultrasonographic analysis, it may occasionally be necessary to outline the biliary tree by means of a technetium[99] HIDA scan with minimal irradiation to the fetus (Hiatt et al., 1986). Endoscopic retrograde cholangiopancreatography (ERCP) and percutaneous transhepatic cholecystography should be avoided if the fetus cannot be shielded from the significant dose of irradiation required. Fiberoptic endoscopic cannulation for retrieval of stones may be successful in skilled hands.

Cholecystectomy should be considered because recurrent attacks throughout pregnancy are common (Woodhouse and Haylen, 1985). Laparoscopic cholecystectomy may be very difficult because of risks of bleeding and visual limitations imposed by the enlarged uterus. Medical management often is less successful postpartum, and there is an increase in postoperative complications such as deep venous thrombosis. Fetal outcome is optimal following surgery in the second trimester, when there is less risk from spontaneous abortion and when enlargement of the uterus has not displaced the liver significantly.

Coincident pancreatitis is common, especially when there are stones in the common bile duct (Hiatt et al., 1986). Maternal and fetal mortality rise significantly with pancreatitis or pancreatic pseudocyst (Kammerer et al., 1979; Printen and Ott, 1978).

Jaundice in pregnancy due to stones in the common bile duct alone (large duct obstruction) is not common. The patient may present with cholestasis without pain but with features of cholangitis: a high fever, rigors, and polymorphonuclear leukocytosis. Surgical intervention is obligatory to avoid recurrent attacks, cholangitis, pancreatitis, and empyema of the gallbladder. Rarely, biliary obstruction may be due to cholangiocarcinoma or parasites. HIV infection is associated with acalculous cholangitis and large duct dilatation. Management is similar to that in the nonpregnant patient.

Dissolution of cholesterol gallstones with chenodeoxycholic acid, ursocholic acid, and their congeners is contraindicated in pregnancy (Palmer and Heywood, 1974). Bile acids cross the placenta, and chenodeoxycholic acid has been linked to liver toxicity and teratogenicity in animals. Lithotrypsy is contraindicated in pregnancy.

The prevalence of symptomless gallstones detected by ultrasonographic investigation during pregnancy differs from that seen in the nonpregnant matched female population—2.5 per cent (Chesson et al., 1985) versus 11.3 per cent (Williamson and Williamson, 1984). Detection has improved with noninvasive imaging. Symptomless stones are found most often in the obese and multiparous patient, but detection is independent of trimester. Echogenic bile (biliary sludge) was detected ultrasonographically in 36 per cent of serially examined pregnant women (Bartoli et al., 1984). The role of elective surgery remains controversial.

THE PANCREAS

The normal range for serum amylase is wide, and interpretation of changes during healthy pregnancy remains controversial. Amylase is produced by the normal salivary, sweat, and lactating mammary glands, and by the pancreas (Garrison, 1986). Secretion of amylase by the fallopian tube accounts for the high levels found in ruptured ectopic pregnancy. A markedly elevated level of serum amylase remains the cornerstone for diagnosing acute pancreatitis. Elevated levels of amylase in urine and in ascitic and pleural fluids may persist after serum levels return to normal. Diagnosis in pregnancy may be difficult because the serum level and its ratio with creatinine and serum lipases may be misleadingly low in the first trimester or remain normal despite severe acute pancreatitis. Serum triglycerides rise in late pregnancy. High levels

are associated with pancreatitis but can interfere with estimation of amylase. Although renal clearances of amylase and creatinine are elevated in pregnancy, the superiority of using the ratio with creatinine over a single elevated level of serum amylase remains debatable. The serum lipase rises in parallel with serum amylase; however, data on its use in pregnancy are lacking.

Acute Pancreatitis

This is an uncommon cause of abdominal pain in pregnancy and has been reported in 1:1066 to 3800 pregnancies (Jouppila et al., 1974) or 1:1100 to 11,000 live births (Corlett and Mishell, 1972; Wilkinson, 1973). Although no specific predilection for pancreatitis has been associated with pregnancy and the puerperium, gallstones, atony of the biliary tract, bile stasis in the duodenum, and reflux secondary to the actions of progesterone may play some role (Van Thiel, 1987). Elevated serum lipids seen in normal pregnancy could unmask a lipid disorder, in particular those associated with high levels of very-low-density lipoproteins (VLDL) and chylomicrons (e.g., type V hyperlipidemia) and type I hyperlipidemia. There seems to be no relationship with parity and maternal age (Klein, 1986). It has been suggested, but not proved, that the vomiting of toxemia raises abdominal pressure, thereby causing elevation of intrapancreatic pressure, rupture of the ducts, and release of enzymes. Recognized associations in nonpregnant populations are gallstones and biliary tract disease, alcoholism, diuretics, toxemia, and acute fatty liver of pregnancy. Rare associations are corticosteroids, chlorothiazides, primary hyperparathyroidism and parathyroid carcinoma, and viral infections.

The morbidity and mortality from acute pancreatitis remain high but may reflect biased reporting of severe cases. More recent data suggest that maternal mortality is no greater than for the nonpregnant population with acute pancreatitis and that fetal losses are about 10 per cent (Klein, 1986).

Clinical presentation occurs typically in late pregnancy, possibly coinciding with the peak in serum levels of triglyceride, but can occur at any time. Abdominal pain is maximal in the epigastrium, is often constant, and may radiate through to the back. Pain is not invariable. Nausea and vomiting may be confused with hyperemesis gravidarum. Severe hemorrhagic pancreatitis typically is associated with profound shock, hypotension, marked hypovolemia, ecchymoses, pleural effusions, hypoxia due to adult respiratory distress syndrome, milky ascites, and a paralytic ileus. Pancreatitis with gallstones in the common bile duct usually is associated with elevated levels of gamma-glutamyl transpeptidase and alkaline phosphatase beyond that attributed to placental growth. Ultrasonographic analysis may be negative and difficult to perform due to the overlying bowel gas and enlarged uterus. Gallstones may point to underlying pancreatitis.

The differential diagnosis in pregnancy includes all other causes of abdominal pain and nausea and vomiting: acute appendicitis, peptic ulceration, hyperemesis gravidarum, preeclamptic toxemia, and many renal and hepatic disorders and infections (pyelonephritis, perinephric abscess, hepatitis, hepatic abscess, and acute cholecystitis). The differentiation from ruptured ectopic pregnancy and ruptured spleen may be difficult in the presence of bloody ascites. Acute pancreatitis in the puerperium can also pose diagnostic problems leading to a delay in diagnosis and poor maternal outcome.

In most pregnant patients with acute, uncomplicated pancreatitis, the disease settles spontaneously with conservative treatment aimed at resting the gastrointestinal tract and preventing complications. The traditional use of nasogastric suction lacks proven efficacy. Suction may increase comfort but can promote elevations in serum amylase and delay the return of bowel sounds. There are no specific therapies for acute pancreatitis. Uncontrolled trials have found variable benefits for anticholinergic agents, glucagon, corticosteroids, prostaglandins, vasopressin, trypsin inhibitors, and epsilon-aminocaproic acid. The H_2 antagonists inhibit the acid stimulus to pancreatic secretion, but have no demonstrable effect on biliary and pancreatic secretion. Total parenteral nutrition has been successful in malnourished, pregnant alcoholics with acute pancreatitis and when complicated by a pseudocyst and marked hypoalbuminemia, which is associated with intrauterine growth restriction.

Complications are reduced with correction of the marked hypovolemia by means of colloid and crystalloid solutions. Blood volumes are best assessed with Swan-Ganz central pressure monitoring. Other common complications include acid-base imbalance and electrolyte disturbances (especially hypocalcemia and hypomagnesemia), carbohydrate intolerance, renal failure, fat necrosis, hemorrhage including disseminated intravascular coagulation, venous thrombosis, ascites, peritonitis, intestinal damage, jaundice, and hepatic and metabolic encephalopathy. Pulmonary edema, pleural effusions, and respiratory distress syndromes may produce profound hypoxia requiring assisted respiratory support and oxygen therapy.

Early termination of pregnancy is rarely indicated and does not influence maternal outcome. Elective induction of labor in the third trimester remains controversial and offers no guarantee of recovery.

Pancreatic Malignant Tumors

In a 3-year survey from the Center for Disease Control (CDC), 2.8 per cent of cancers in the reproductive age group were due to carcinoma of the pancreas (Donegan, 1983). Isolated cases of adenocarcinoma and insulinoma have been reported in pregnancy and the puerperium. In insulinoma, early recognition of the hypoglycemia, neurologic features, and elevated levels of insulin and C-peptide can lead to early diagnosis, surgery, and successful outcome of pregnancy (Galun et al., 1986). The outcome of malignant tumors of the pancreas is poor.

REFERENCES

Aarnoudse JG, Houthoff HJ, Weits, et al: A syndrome of liver damage and intravascular coagulation in the last trimester of normotensive pregnancy. A clinical and histopathological study. Br J Obstet Gynaecol 93:145, 1986.
Alexander GJ, Eddleston AWLF: Does maternal antibody to core antigen prevent recognition of the transplacental transmission of hepatitis B virus infection? Lancet i:296, 1986.
Alter MJ, Hadler SC, Margolis HS, et al: The changing epidemiology of hepatitis B in the United States. Need for alternative vaccination strategies. JAMA 263:1218, 1990.
Baker VV, Cefalo RC: Fulminant hepatic failure in the third trimester of pregnancy. A case report. J Reprod Med 30:229, 1985.
Bartoli E, Calonaci N, Nenci R: Ultrasonography of the gallbladder in pregnancy. Gastrointest Radiol 9:35, 1984.
Beasley RP: Hepatitis B virus as the etiologic agent in hepatocellular carcinoma-epidemiologic considerations. Hepatology 2(Suppl):21S, 1982.
Beath SV, Boxall EH, Watson RM, et al: Fulminant hepatitis B in infants born to anti-HBe hepatitis B carrier mothers. Br Med J 304:1169, 1992.
Benhamou JP, Lebrec D: Non-cirrhotic intrahepatic portal hypertension in adults. Clin Gastroenterol 14:21, 1985.
Bennion LJ, Grundy SM: Risk factors for the development of cholelithiasis in man (second of two parts). N Engl J Med 299:1221, 1978.
Berg B, Helm G, Petersohn L, et al: Cholestasis of pregnancy. Clinical and laboratory studies. Acta Obstet Gynecol Scand 65:107, 1986.
Bernuau J, Degott C, Nouel O, et al: Non-fatal acute fatty liver of pregnancy. Gut 24:340, 1983.
Braverman D, Johnson ML, Vern F: Effects of pregnancy and contraceptive steroids on gallbladder function. N Engl J Med 302:362, 1980.
Brown KA, Lucey MR: Liver transplantation restores female reproductive endocrine function. Hepatology 13:1255, 1991.
Britton RC: Pregnancy and esophageal varices. Am J Surg 4:421, 1982.
Britton WJ, Parsons C, Gallagher ND, et al: Risk factors associated with hepatitis B infection in antenatal patients. Aust NZ J Med 15:641, 1985.
Burroughs AK, Seong NH, Dojcinar DM, et al: Idiopathic acute fatty liver of pregnancy in 12 patients. Q J Med 204:481, 1982.
Carman WF, Zanetti AR, Karayiannis P, et al: Vaccine-induced escape mutant of hepatitis B virus. Lancet 336:325, 1990.
Carne CA, Weller IVD, Waite J, et al: Impaired responsiveness of homosexual men with HIV antibodies to plasma derived hepatitis B vaccine. Br Med J 294:866, 1987.
Cheng YS: Pregnancy in liver cirrhosis and/or portal hypertension. Am J Obstet Gynecol 128:812, 1977.
Chesson RR, Gallup DG, Gibbs RL, et al: Ultrasonographic diagnosis of asymptomatic cholelithiasis in pregnancy. J Reprod Med 30:920, 1985.
Chu SY, Buehler JW, Berkelman RL: Impact of the human immunodeficiency virus epidemic on mortality in women of reproductive age, United States. JAMA 264:225, 1990.
Corlett RC, Mishell DR: Pancreatitis in pregnancy. Am J Obstet Gynecol 113:281, 1972.
Coursaget P, Yvonnet B, Chotard J, et al: Age and sex-related study of hepatitis B virus chronic carrier state in infants from an endemic area (Senegal). J Med Virol 22:1, 1987.
Cowan DB, Houlton MC: Rupture of an amoebic liver abscess in pregnancy. A case report. S Afr Med J 53:460, 1978.
Crosby ET: Obstetrical anaesthesia for patients with the syndrome of haemolysis, elevated liver enzymes and low platelets. Can J Anaesth 38:227, 1991.
Cundy TF, O'Grady JG, Williams R: Recovery of menstruation and pregnancy after liver transplantation. Gut 31:337, 1990.
Cundy TF, Butler J, Pope RM, et al: Amenorrhoea in women with non-alcoholic chronic liver disease. Gut 32:202, 1991.
Da Silva O, Hammerberg O, Chance GW: Fetal varicella syndrome. Pediatr Infect Dis J 9:854, 1990.
Deinhardt F, Zuckerman AJ: Against hepatitis B: a report on a

WHO meeting on viral hepatitis in Europe. J Med Virol **17**:209, 1985.

de Koning ND, Haagsma EB: Normalization of menstrual pattern after liver transplantation: Consequences for contraception. Digestion **46**:239, 1990.

Delage G, Montplaisir S, Remy-Prince S, et al: Prevalence of hepatitis B virus infection in pregnant women in the Montreal area. Can Med Assoc J **134**:897, 1986.

Deray G, le Hoang P, Cacoub P, et al: Oral contraceptives interaction with cyclosporin. (Letter) Lancet **1**:158, 1987.

Donegan WL: Cancer and pregnancy. Cancer **33**:194, 1983.

Everson GT: Hepatic cysts in autosomal dominant polycystic kidney disease. (Comment) Mayo Clin Proc **65**:933, 1990.

Fagan EA: Testing for hepatitis C. Br Med J **303**:535, 1991.

Fair J, Klein AS, Feng T, et al: Intrapartum orthotopic liver transplantation with successful outcome of pregnancy. Transplantation **50**:534, 1990.

Federal Register. US Department of Labor, Occupational Safety Health Administration: Occupational exposure to bloodborne pathogens: Proposed rule and notice of hearing. Fed Register **54**:23042, 1989.

Feliciano DV, Mattox KL, Jordan GL, et al: Management of 1000 consecutive cases of hepatic trauma (1979–1984). Ann Surg **204**:438, 1986.

Freund G, Arvan DA: Clinical biochemistry of preeclampsia and related liver diseases of pregnancy: a review. Clin Chim Acta **191**:123, 1990.

Gabow PA, Johnson AM, Kaehny WD, et al: Risk factors for the development of hepatic cysts in autosomal dominant polycystic kidney disease. Hepatology **11**:1033, 1990.

Galun E, Ben-Yehuda A, Berlatzki J, et al: Insulinoma complicating pregnancy: a case report and review of the literature. Am J Obstet Gynecol **155**:64, 1986.

Garrison R: Amylase. Emerg Med Clin North Am **4**:315, 1986.

Gerety RJ, Schweitzer IL: Viral hepatitis, type B during pregnancy, the neonatal period and infancy. J Pediatr **90**:368, 1977.

Gimson AES, O'Grady J, Ede RJ, et al: Late-onset hepatic failure: Clinical, serological and histological features. Hepatology **6**:288, 1986.

Goodlin RC: Preeclampsia as the great impostor. Am J Obstet Gynecol **164**:1577, 1991.

Greenfield C, Osidiana V, Karayiannis P, et al: Perinatal transmission of hepatitis B virus in Kenya: Its relation to the presence of serum HBV DNA and anti-HBe in the mother. J Med Virol **19**:135, 1986.

Hadler SC, Francis DP, Maynard JE, et al: Long-term immunogenicity and efficacy of hepatitis B vaccine in homosexual men. N Engl J Med **315**:209, 1986.

Harrison TJ, Zuckerman AJ: Variants of hepatitis B virus. Vox Sang **63**:161, 1992.

Heilmann L, Hojnacki B, Spanuth E: Hemostasis and preeclampsia. (German) Gerburtshilfe Frauenheilkd **51**:223, 1991.

Hiatt JR, Hiatt JC, Williams RA, et al: Biliary disease in pregnancy: strategy for surgical management. Am J Surg **151**:263, 1986.

Hollinger FB, Lemon SM, Margolis HS (eds): Viral Hepatitis and Liver Disease. Proceedings of the 1990 International Symposium, Houston, Texas. Baltimore, Williams & Wilkins, 1991, pp 1–916.

Holtzbach RT, Sivack DA, Braun WE: Familial recurrent intrahepatic cholestasis of pregnancy: A genetic study providing evidence for transmission of a sex-linked dominant trait. Gastroenterology **85**:175, 1983.

Hoofnagle J, Shafritz DA, Popper H: Chronic type B hepatitis and the "healthy" HBsAg carrier state. Hepatology **7**:758, 1987.

Huguet C, Deliere T, Ollivier JM, et al: Budd-Chiari syndrome with thrombosis of the inferior vena cava: long-term patency of mesocaval and cavoatrial prosthetic bypass. Surgery **95**:108, 1984.

Jones EA, Bergasa NU: The pruritus of cholestasis: From bile acids to opiate antagonists. Hepatology **11**:884, 1990.

Jouppila P, Mokka R, Larmi TK: Acute pancreatitis in pregnancy. Surg Gynecol Obstet **139**:879, 1974.

Kammerer WS: Non-obstetric surgery during pregnancy. Med Clin North Am **6**:1157, 1979.

Kanaan C, Veille JC, Lakin M: Pregnancy and acute intermittent porphyria. Obstet Gynecol Surv **44**:244, 1989.

Kane MA, Hadler SC, Margolis HS, et al: Routine prenatal screening for hepatitis B surface antigen. JAMA **259**:408, 1988.

Kaplan MM: Acute fatty liver of pregnancy. N Engl J Med **313**:367, 1985.

Keating JJ, O'Brien CJ, Stellon AJ, et al: Influence of aetiology, clinical and histological features on survival in chronic active hepatitis: An analysis of 204 patients. Q J Med **62**:59, 1987.

Khuroo MS, Datta DV: Budd-Chiari syndrome following pregnancy. Report of 16 cases with roentgenologic, hemodynamic and histologic studies of the hepatic outflow tract. Am J Med **8**:113, 1980.

Klebanoff MA, Koslowe PA, Kaslow R et al: Epidemiology of vomiting in early pregnancy. Obstet Gynecol **66**:612, 1985.

Klein KB: Pancreatitis in pregnancy. In Rustgi VK, Cooper JN (eds): Gastrointestinal and Hepatic Complications in Pregnancy. New York, John Wiley & Sons, 1986, pp 138–161.

Klein NA, Mabie WC, Shaver DC, et al: Herpes simplex hepatitis in pregnancy. Two patients successfully treated with acyclovir. Gastroenterology **100**:239, 1991.

Kochhar R, Goenka MK, Mehta SK. Endoscopic sclerotherapy during pregnancy. Am J Gastroenterol **85**:1132, 1990.

Krol Van Straaten J, De Maat CE: Successful pregnancies in cirrhosis of the liver before and after portacaval anastomosis. Neth J Med **27**:14, 1984.

Krueger KJ, Hoffman BJ, Lee WM: Hepatic infarction associated with eclampsia. Am J Gastroenterol **85**:588, 1990.

Kurzel RB: Can acetaminophen excess result in maternal and fetal toxicity? South Med J **83**:953, 1990.

Laifer SA, Darby MJ, Scantlebury VP, et al: Pregnancy and liver transplantation. Obstet Gynecol **76**:1083, 1990.

Larrey D, Rueff B, Feldmann G, et al: Recurrent jaundice caused by recurrent hyperemesis gravidarum. Gut **25**:1414, 1984.

Lawson DH, Lovatt GE, Gurton CS, et al: Adverse effects of azathioprine. Adverse Drug React Acute Poisoning Rev **3**:161, 1984.

Levin S, Leibowitz E, Torten J, et al: Interferon treatment in acute progressive and fulminant hepatitis. Isr J Med Sci **25**:364, 1989.

Linares A, Zarranz JJ, Rodriguez-Alarson J, et al: Reversible cutis laxa due to maternal D-penicillamine treatment. (Letter) Lancet **2**:43, 1979.

Lok ASF, Lai C-L, Wu PC: Interferon therapy of chronic hepatitis B virus infection in Chinese. J Hepatol **3**(Suppl 2):S209, 1986.

Mallia CP, Nancekivell AF: Fulminant virus hepatitis in late pregnancy. Ann Trop Med Parasitol **76**:143, 1982.

Margolis HS, Alter MJ, Hadler SC: Hepatitis B: Evolving epidemiology and implications for control. Semin Liver Dis **11**:84, 1992.

Margolis K, Naidoo BN: Spontaneous postpartum subcapsular haematoma of the liver. S Afr Med J **48**:1997, 1974.

Martin JN, Files JC, Blake PG, et al: Plasma exchange for preeclampsia-eclampsia with HELLP syndrome. Am J Obstet Gynecol **162**:126, 1990.

Mason JO, Koplan JP, Layde PM: The prevention and control of chronic diseases: reducing unnecessary deaths and disability—a conference report. Public Health Rep **102**:17, 1987.

Menton M, Frauz M, Harzer K, et al: Morbus Gaucher und Schwangerschaft [Gaucher's disease and pregnancy]. Geburtshilfe Frauenheilkd **50**:410, 1990.

Milo R, Neuman M, Klein C, et al: Acute intermittent porphyria in pregnancy. Obstet Gynecol **73**:450, 1989.

Minakami H, Oka N, Sato T, et al: Preeclampsia: A microvesicular fat disease of the liver. Am J Obstet Gynecol **159**:1043, 1988.

Mintz MC, Grumbach K, Arger PH, et al: Sonographic evaluation of bile duct size during pregnancy. Am J Roentgenol **145**:575, 1985.

Mitchell RW, Teare AJ: Amoebic liver abscess in pregnancy. Case report. Br J Obstet Gynaecol **91**:393, 1984.

Morali GA, Braverman DZ: Abnormal liver enzymes and ketonuria in hyperemesis gravidarum. A retrospective review of 80 patients. J Clin Gastroenterol **12**:303, 1990.

Morbidity Mortality Weekly Report (MMWR): Centers for Disease Control: Protection against viral hepatitis. Recommendations of the Immunization Practices Advisory Committee (AICP). MMWR **39**:5, 1990.

Morbidity Mortality Weekly Report (MMWR): Public Health Service Interagency guidelines for screening donors of blood, plasma, organs, tissues, and semen for evidence of hepatitis B and hepatitis C. MMWR RR4 **40**:1, 1991a.

Morbidity Mortality Weekly Report (MMWR): Recommendations

for preventing transmission of human immunodeficiency virus and hepatitis B virus to patients during exposure-prone invasive procedures. MMWR RR8 **40:**1, 1991b.

Morbidity Mortality Weekly Report (MMWR): Update on adult immunization. Recommendations of the Immunization Practices Advisory Committee. MMWR RR12 **40:**33, 1991c.

Negro F, Rizzetto M: Pathobiology of delta virus. *In* Hollinger FB, Lemon SM, Margolis HS (eds): Viral Hepatitis and Liver Disease. Proceedings of the 1990 International Symposium, Houston, Texas. Baltimore, Williams & Wilkins, 1991, pp 477–480.

Neuberger J, Forman D, Doll R, et al: Oral contraceptives and hepatocellular carcinoma. Br Med J **292:**1355, 1986.

Nir A, Sorokin Y, Abramovici H, Theodor E: Pregnancy and primary biliary cirrhosis. Int J Gynaecol Obstet **28:**279, 1989.

Nordenfelt E, Dahlquist E: HBsAg positive adopted children as a cause of intrafamilial spread of hepatitis B. Scand J Infect Dis **10:**161, 1978.

O'Grady J, Williams R: Emergency medicine: Management of acute liver failure. Hosp Update **13:**481, 1987.

O'Grady J, Gimson ASE, O'Brien CJ, et al: Controlled trials of charcoal haemoperfusion and prognostic factors in fulminant hepatic failure. Gastroenterology **94:**1186, 1988.

Palmer AK, Heywood R: Pathological changes in the rhesus fetus associated with oral administration of chenodeoxycholic acid. Toxicology **2:**239, 1974.

Pockros PJ, Peters RI, Reynolds TB: Idiopathic fatty liver of pregnancy: findings in ten cases. Medicine (Baltimore) **63:**1, 1984.

Printen KJ, Ott RA: Cholecystectomy during pregnancy. Am J Surg **44:**432, 1978.

Purdie JM, Walters BN: Acute fatty liver of pregnancy: Clinical features and diagnosis. Aust NZ J Obstet Gynaecol **28:**62, 1988.

Radberg G, Asztely M, Cantor P, et al: Gastric and gallbladder emptying in relation to the secretion of cholecystokinin after a meal in late pregnancy. Digestion **42:**174, 1989.

Radberg G, Friman S, Svanvik J: The influence of pregnancy and contraceptive steroids on the biliary tract and its reference to cholesterol gallstone formation. Scand J Gastroenterol **25:**97, 1990.

Reyes H, Ribalda J, Gonzalez-Ceron M: Idiopathic cholestasis in a large kindred. Gut **17:**709, 1976.

Riely CA, Latham PS, Romero R, et al: Acute fatty liver of pregnancy. A reassessment based on observations in nine patients. Ann Intern Med **106:**703, 1987.

Rolfes DB, Ishak KG: Acute fatty liver of pregnancy: A clinicopathologic study of 35 cases. Hepatology **5:**1149, 1985.

Rolfes DB, Ishak KG: Liver disease in pregnancy. Histopathology **10:**555, 1986.

Rothschild MA, Berk PD, Dienstag JL: Viral hepatitis. Semin Liv Dis **11:**1, 1991.

Scaglione S: Cirrosi di Laennec in gravidanza. Riv Ital di Ginecol **1:**489, 1923.

Scantlebury V, Gordon R, Tzakis A, et al: Childbearing after liver transplantation. Transplantation **49:**317, 1990.

Schalm SW, van Buuren HR: Prevention of recurrent variceal bleeding: non-surgical procedure. Clin Gastroenterol **14:**209, 1985.

Schoeman MN, Batey RG, Wilcken B: Recurrent acute fatty liver of pregnancy associated with a fatty-acid oxidation defect in the offspring. Gastroenterology **100:**544, 1991.

Schorr-Lesnick B, Lebovics E, Dworkin B, et al: Liver diseases unique to pregnancy. Am J Gastroenterol **86:**659, 1991.

Schreyer P, Caspi E, El-Hindi JM, et al: Cirrhosis, pregnancy and delivery: a review. Obstet Gynecol Surv **37:**304, 1982.

Scragg RKR, McMichael AJ, Baghurst PA, et al: Oral contraceptives, pregnancy and endogenous oestrogen in gall stone disease—a case control study. Br Med J **288:**1795, 1984.

Seligsohn U, Shani M: The Dubin-Johnson syndrome and pregnancy. Acta Hepatogastroenterol **24:**167, 1977.

Shaw D, Frohlich J, Wittmann BA, et al: A prospective study of 18 patients with cholestasis of pregnancy. Am J Obstet Gynecol **142:**621, 1982.

Sheehan HL: The pathology of hyperemesis and vomiting of late pregnancy. J Obstet Gynaecol Br Emp **46:**685, 1939.

Sheehan HL: The pathology of acute yellow atrophy and delayed chloroform poisoning. J Obstet Gynaecol Br Emp **47:**49, 1940.

Sibai BM: The HELLP syndrome (Hemolysis, elevated liver enzymes, and low platelets): much ado about nothing? Am J Obstet Gynecol **162:**311, 1990.

Smith LG, Moise KJ, Dildy GA, et al: Spontaneous rupture of the liver during pregnancy: current therapy. Obstet Gynecol **77:**171, 1991.

Stander HJ, Cadden JF: Acute yellow atrophy of the liver in pregnancy. Am J Obstet Gynecol **28:**61, 1934.

Steven MM, Buckley JB, Mackay IR: Pregnancy in chronic active hepatitis. Q J Med **48:**519, 1979.

Steven MM: Pregnancy and liver disease. Gut **22:**592, 1981.

Stevens CE, Toy PT, Tong MJ, et al: Perinatal hepatitis B virus transmission in the United States. Prevention by passive-active immunization. JAMA **253:**1740, 1985.

Taina E, Hanninen P, Gronoos M: Viral infections in pregnancy. Acta Obstet Gynecol Scand **64:**167, 1985.

Tang S: [Chinese] Study on the HBV intrauterine infection and its rate. Chung Hua Liu Hsing Ping Hsueh Tsa Chih **11:**328, 1990.

Tarnier M: Note sur l'etat grasseux due foie dans la fievire puerperale. 1856 Comptes Rendus Seances et Memoires Societe De Biologie **III:**209, 1857.

Teisala K, Tuimala R: Pregnancy and esophageal varices. Ann Chir Gynaecol **197**(Suppl):65, 1985.

Thomas HC, Lever AML, Scully LJ, et al: Approaches to the treatment of hepatitis B virus and delta-related liver disease. Semin Liver Dis **6:**34, 1986.

Tong MJ, Sinatra FR, Thomas DW, et al: Need for immunoprophylaxis in infants born to HBsAg-positive carrier mothers who are HBeAg negative. J Pediatr **105:**945, 1984.

Tong MJ, Thursby M, Rakela J, et al: Studies on the maternal-infant transmission of the viruses which cause acute hepatitis. Gastroenterology **80:**999, 1981.

Trey C, Davidson CS: The management of fulminant hepatic failure. Prog Liver Dis **3:**282, 1970.

van Os HC, Drogendijk HC, Fetter WP, et al: The influence of contamination of culture medium with hepatitis B virus in the outcome of in vitro fertilization pregnancies. Am J Obstet Gynecol **165:**152, 1991.

Van Thiel D: Effects of pregnancy and sex hormones on the liver. Semin Liver Dis **7:**1, 1987.

Vons C, Smadja C, Franco D, et al: Successful pregnancy after Budd-Chiari syndrome. (Letter) Lancet **2:**975, 1984.

Walshe JM: The management of pregnancy in Wilson's disease treated with trientine. Q J Med **58:**81, 1986

Weinstein L: Syndrome of hemolysis, elevated liver enzymes, and low platelet count; a consequence of hypertension in pregnancy. Am J Obstet Gynecol **142:**159, 1982.

Wilkinson EJ: Acute pancreatitis in pregnancy: a review of 98 cases and a report of 8 new cases. Obstet Gynecol Surv **28:**281, 1973.

Williamson SL, Williamson MR: Cholecystosonography in pregnancy. J Ultrasound Med **3:**329, 1984.

Woodhouse DR, Haylen B: Gallbladder disease complicating pregnancy. Aust NZ J Obstet Gynaecol **25:**233, 1985.

CHAPTER

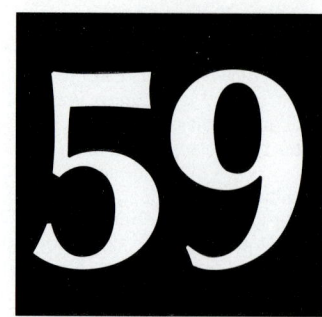

RHEUMATOLOGIC AND CONNECTIVE TISSUE DISORDERS

MICHAEL DE SWIET, M.D.

The common rheumatic disorders, often called the collagen diseases, are chronic inflammatory processes involving primarily the joints and connective tissues, through mechanisms that are still obscure but are clearly autoimmune in nature. These diseases—disseminated lupus erythematosus, rheumatoid arthritis, ankylosing spondylitis, scleroderma, periarteritis nodosa, polymyositis and Sjögren's syndrome—tend to occur with highest frequency in young women.

Problems of management of the rheumatic diseases in pregnancy center on the effects of pregnancy on the disease state and the effects of drug treatment on the fetus. These topics will be covered in this chapter together with some of the effects of the disease state on the fetus. With regard to the last category, the most important feature is the effect of anticardiolipin antibodies and/or lupus anticoagulant (the cardiolipin syndrome) on the outcome of pregnancy. This, together with other features of the cardiolipin syndrome such as thrombosis, is considered in Chapter 31.

SYSTEMIC LUPUS ERYTHEMATOSUS

Systemic lupus erythematosus (SLE), in part due to the associated cardiolipin syndrome (see Chapter 31), is undoubtedly the connective tissue disease that poses the greatest challenge to the obstetrician and internist; indeed it can be one of the greatest problems in fetomaternal medicine.

Most, if not all, manifestations of SLE seem directly related to antigen-antibody complexes in the serum or to autoantibodies reacting to fixed tissue antigens in vessel walls. This may also be an important cause of placental pathology and the reason for much of the fetal wastage in this syndrome.

SLE is a multisystem disease that most frequently affects young women. It is therefore relatively common in pregnancy, and it is certainly the connective tissue disease that has been studied most intensively. The apparent prevalence has increased as more mild forms of the disease are recognized. In 1974, Fessel

found a prevalence of one in 700 women aged 15 to 64 years. In black women the prevalence was one in 245. Minority women have an excess risk five times that of white women.

Clinical Forms

It is unusual to make the diagnosis "de novo" in pregnancy, but dramatic and catastrophic illnesses that were recognized as SLE in the first half of this century are still encountered. However, most patients complain of vague and sometimes severe pain around the joints as well as in the muscles. Lassitude, malaise, and difficulty in coping with small problems at home or at work may suggest a diagnosis of psychoneurosis. Low-grade fever (100° to 101°F), which may come and go, is helpful as a diagnostic sign if present. The characteristic butterfly rash over the nose and cheeks is absent in most patients or is subtle and difficult to distinguish from ordinary sunburn or the increased pigmentation of pregnancy. Pleurisy is a common early feature of lupus, but the pain is rarely severe, and sometimes the history emerges only during direct questioning. Vasospastic Raynaud's phenomenon may be subtle and is particularly unusual in pregnancy. The finding of protein, red cells, and casts in urine will help toward a diagnosis of SLE. Central nervous system (CNS) manifestations are common and often subtle, occurring in about half the patients and consisting mainly of disorders of thought content and of mood. CNS disease may make the patient inattentive, difficult to communicate with, poorly compliant with therapy, or simply vexing to her physician. These CNS manifestations are occasionally heralded by seizures and may be overtly manifested by stroke-like symptoms. Chorea is a rare manifestation of lupus that may be estrogen-induced, i.e., in pregnancy or with the combined oral contraceptive (Donaldson and Espiner, 1971; Lubbe and Walker, 1983).

Laboratory Testing and Diagnosis

In pregnancy, proteinuria and thrombocytopenia can lead to confusion with preeclampsia. The clinical features of preeclampsia—which usually run a much more acute course, remit after delivery, and are not associated with other well-known features of SLE such as arthritis—normally distinguish the two conditions. In preeclampsia, however, proteinuria may occasionally appear early in pregnancy, the process may not be so acute, and in this situation, measurement of antinuclear factor helps to distinguish SLE from other renal conditions and preeclampsia.

The fluorescent antinuclear antibody test (ANA, FANA) is the mainstay of diagnosis. However, with the best technology, about 2 per cent of patients with SLE have negative ANA, presumably because their antibody or antibodies are not detectable with the test substance. Patients develop antibodies to many different chemical moieties within nuclei, as well as to components of cytoplasm and of cell membrane, and these different antigen-antibody reactions may explain the varied manifestations of systemic lupus erythematosus as a single disease or a closely related family of diseases. Commonly tested antibodies, with a brief comment on their clinical relevance, particularly to pregnancy, are listed in Table 59–1.

In addition to tests for specific autoantibodies, the sedimentation rate is usually elevated in lupus and tends to mirror activity of the disease. Unfortunately, the ESR varies considerably in normal pregnancy, and so this is not so helpful for monitoring disease activity in pregnant patients (although values greater than 50 are likely to be abnormal, even in pregnancy). Therefore, in pregnancy, assays for total serum complement C_3 or C_4 help to correlate clinical and laboratory observations of SLE activity (Buyon et al., 1986). High levels of antibodies to double-stranded DNA, as measured in an ELISA assay, often reflect clinical exacerbations.

Course During Pregnancy

As is the case with most illnesses that run a fluctuating course, such as asthma or disseminated sclerosis, it is difficult to document any special effect of pregnancy on SLE. Certainly a simple comparison of the prevalence of autoantibodies in a normal population has shown no difference between pregnancy and the nonpregnant state (Patton et al., 1987). The general consensus is that pregnancy does not affect the long-term prognosis of SLE (Garsenstein et al., 1962), but that pregnancy itself may be associated with more "flare ups," particularly in the puerperium (Fraga et al., 1964; Mund et al., 1963). Since patients are usually observed more closely in pregnancy, this is not surprising. However, in a comparison with the pre-pregnancy period, Garsenstein et al. (1962) found that the exacerbation rate was three times greater in the first half of pregnancy, one and one-half times greater in the second half, and at least six times greater in the puerperium. By contrast, Gimovsky et al. (1984) found more "flares" requiring admission in each trimester of pregnancy than in the first 3 months after delivery.

Kincaid-Smith et al. (1988), in Melbourne, found specific renal biopsy changes in patients with renal "flares" in pregnancy. These were similar to those found in hemolytic-uremic syndrome (HUS) and were also associated with microhemangiopathic hemolytic anemia. Treatment directed toward HUS (aspirin, fresh frozen plasma, plasmapheresis) in pregnancy may be helpful for renal "flares," which may be an endothelial disease.

In summary, pregnancy can cause problems for the mother with lupus, although this is less likely if the disease is under good control at the onset of gestation. So-called "flares" of the disease during pregnancy may not be related to the classic concept of activity reflecting antigen-antibody reactions but may reflect other mechanisms such as preeclampsia. As the fetus is at increased risk (roughly proportionate to disease activity in the mother), management of complications during pregnancy requires careful attention to both mother and fetus and prompt therapeutic decisions based on likely pathogenetic mechanisms. It is interesting that successive pregnancies do not necessarily affect an individual in the same way (Estes and Larson, 1965).

Effect of SLE on Pregnancy

There are three ways in which SLE affects pregnancy and its outcome. First, SLE increases the risks of late pregnancy loss due to hypertension and renal compromise; second, it is an important cause of heart block and other cardiac defects in the newborn. This may be part of a more general neonatal lupus syndrome. Third, SLE increases the risk of abortion in particular as part of the cardiolipin syndrome and therefore in association with venous and sometimes

TABLE 59–1.   Antibody Tests Helpful in Perinatal Assessment of Lupus Erythematosus

ANTIBODY	CLINICAL PERTINENCE
Antinuclear antibody (ANA)	Diagnosis of lupus erythematosus
Antideoxynucleoprotein (Anti-DNA)	Associated with disease activity and nephritis
Anti-Ro (Anti-SSA)	Specific for SLE and Sjögren's; associated with nephritis; highly correlated with neonatal lupus and congenital heart block
Anti-La (Anti-SSB)	Negatively associated with nephritis in anti-Ro positive patients
Anticentromere	90% in CREST variant of scleroderma
Anticardiolipins	Vascular thromboses Multiple abortions/miscarriages Thrombocytopenic purpura
Anti-ribonucleoprotein (n-RNP*)	Mixed connective tissue disease

*A soluble RNP-protein antigen.
From Hollingsworth DR, Resnik R (eds): Medical Counseling Before Pregnancy. New York, Churchill Livingstone, 1988.

arterial thromboembolism. Although technically most of the latter cases, being pregnancy losses before 28 weeks, should be classified as abortions, it is clear that they are quite different from most abortions, which occur at about 12 weeks. The losses in association with SLE may occur at gestations up to and even after 28 weeks. Even if the fetus does not die, it is at risk of developing fetal distress as judged by abnormal fetal heart rate tracings (Lockshin et al., 1985). In addition, there appears to be an extra risk of first-trimester abortion in patients with the cardiolipin syndrome, but the extent of this risk is not well defined.

If the lupus patient does not have hypertension, renal impairment, or the cardiolipin syndrome, her chances of a normal pregnancy are good and may indeed be no worse than those of a normal patient (Loizou et al., 1988).

Hypertension and Renal Impairment

To assess the risks of renal disease in SLE, Houser et al. (1980) studied 18 pregnancies in patients with SLE. Ten occurred in patients with no evidence of renal disease and were uncomplicated. The remaining eight occurred in patients with renal disease. There were four abortions (one elective), three premature deliveries, and only one normal term delivery. It is difficult to be precise as to what level of renal impairment is significant, but a creatinine clearance of less than 65 ml/min/m³ or proteinuria greater than 2.4 gm/24 hours would be ominous. Hayslett and Lynn (1980) noted a 50 per cent fetal loss rate in mothers with a serum creatinine in excess of 132 mM/liter (1.5 mg/dl). The presence of antiplatelet antibodies is an additional risk factor (McCormack et al., 1991).

The Neonatal Lupus Syndrome

This includes hematologic complications, cardiac abnormalities, babies in whom skin lesions are present (Lockshin et al., 1983), and neonates who develop clinical SLE (Hardy et al., 1979). Maternal IgG antibodies have been shown to cross the placenta (Hardy et al., 1979), and it is likely that SLE is one of the conditions—such as rhesus disease, Graves' disease, and myasthenia gravis—in which transplacental passage of antibodies harms the fetus. In SLE, however, the precise antibody or antibodies that affect the fetus have not been identified; also, the fetal outcome cannot be correlated with fetal (or maternal) antibody levels apart from the relationship between congenital heart block and certain maternal antibodies (see below).

The hematologic abnormalities are hemolytic anemia, leukopenia, and thrombocytopenia. Since maternal IgG antibodies do not persist in the neonate, they are usually transient and not a major problem (Nathan and Snapper, 1958).

The cardiac pathology has been well defined by McCue et al. (1977) and by Scott and Esscher (1979). By far the most common abnormality is complete heart block, which may be present and detected antenatally (Altenburger et al., 1977). Although the majority of infants born to mothers with SLE are normal, at least one in three mothers (28 per cent) who deliver babies with isolated congenital heart block has, or will have, a connective tissue disease (Scott and Esscher, 1979).

About 60 per cent of mothers who deliver a child with congenital heart block have antibodies to soluble tissue ribonucleoprotein antigen (anti-Ro and anti-La antibodies). Since the production of anti-Ro and anti-La antibodies is correlated with the presence of HLA antigen DR3, which is more common in patients with Sjögren's syndrome (Hughes, 1984), congenital heart block is even more common in patients with Sjögren's syndrome than in those with lupus (Paredes et al., 1983; Veille et al., 1985). The risk of congenital heart block is far greater in association with anti-Ro than with anti-La. Anti-Ro antibodies are quite common in connective tissue disease, so that the risk of congenital heart block in the presence of anti-Ro is only about 1 in 20, although this increases to 1 in 3 if the mother has already had a child with congenital heart block (Olaf and Gee, 1991).

In one series, anti-Ro and/or anti-La were invariably present in the mothers with SLE who delivered an affected child, and they were also present in some of those asymptomatic women who had a child with congenital heart block (Maddison et al., 1983). There is therefore strong circumstantial evidence to implicate antibodies to soluble tissue ribonucleoprotein in the pathogenesis of congenital heart block. Antibody has been found in the site of the conducting tissue in the heart of a fetus that died with complete heart block. However, since it was both IgG and IgA antibody (Litsey et al., 1985), the IgA antibody, which does not cross the placenta, was presumably derived from the fetus. More recently it has been shown that the mothers and their offspring may also have an IgG antibody that reacts with fetal cardiac tissue (Taylor et al., 1986). This antibody may also be involved in the pathogenesis of congenital heart block, and the presence of this and other autoantibodies may explain why the fetal prognosis is not invariably good even in the absence of well-established markers for fetal death, such as anticardiolipin antibodies. Thus, although the baby usually survives the perinatal period, and often does not require pacing, in a few cases with congenital heart block and without cardiolipin antibodies the fetus dies antenally or during labor (Singsen et al., 1985). Perhaps the antibodies directed against cardiac muscle are causing a fetal cardiomyopathy (McCue et al., 1977). This would certainly be in keeping with the findings of diffuse IgG antibody in all cardiac tissue of a fetus that died in association with high maternal titers of anti-Ro in early pregnancy (Venning et al., 1988) and with the occasional clinical presentation before delivery of nonimmune hydrops. In addition, the syndrome may be associated with endomyocardial fibrosis (Scott and Esscher, 1979), pericarditis (Fox and Hawkins, 1990), or pericardial effusion (Shenker et al., 1987). Of course fetuses may have congenital heart block because of a primary cardiac malformation, frequently an atrioventricular canal defect (Shenker et al., 1987). Under these circumstances there is usually no association with maternal connective tissue disease.

McCuistion and Schoch (1954) first described discoid skin lesions in a neonate whose mother subsequently developed SLE. The lesions are usually on the face or the scalp and are present at birth. They have normally disappeared by one year of life, and only rarely are they associated with other organ involvement (Vonderheid et al., 1976). Some skin lesions have been associated with maternal and fetal antibodies to U1 RNP (nRNP), a protein found in normal human skin cells (Provost et al., 1987).

Management of SLE in Pregnancy

Maternal Considerations

The drugs most frequently used for the treatment of SLE (Buyon et al., 1987) are simple analgesics such as paracetamol and nonsteroidal anti-inflammatory drugs including aspirin. In more severe cases, antimalarial drugs, cortiocosteroids, and cytotoxic agents are used.

Paracetamol has been used widely in pregnancy with no adverse effects in normal therapeutic doses. Aspirin has been extensively studied (Buckfield, 1973; Stuart et al., 1982). Three large prospective studies, including the Perinatal Collaborative Project, of over 14,000 women exposed to aspirin in the USA (Buckfield, 1973) have shown no teratogenic risk. However, aspirin in high dosage and other nonsteroidal anti-inflammatory agents have been associated with neonatal hemorrhage because of their action in inhibiting platelet function (Turner and Collins, 1975; Stuart et al., 1982; Lancet Editorial, 1980). In addition, there is the risk that prostaglandin synthetase inhibitors will cause premature closure of the ductus arteriosus and pulmonary hypertension (Lancet Editorial, 1980). This appears to be more a theoretic than a practical risk (Heymann, 1985). The more widespread use of aspirin to prevent preeclampsia is likely to vindicate at least low-dose aspirin treatment in pregnancy.

So far, only occasional cases of ductus arteriosus—related problems have been reported following maternal indomethacin treatment (Goudie and Dossetor, 1979). Even so, there were no such complications in over 200 infants exposed to indomethacin to treat preterm labor (Dudley and Hardie, 1985; Niebyl and Witter, 1986). Chloroquine may cause choroidoretinitis (Rees and Maibach, 1963) and should be avoided. Prednisone, at least in doses up to 30 mg/day, and hydrocortisone should be considered safe in pregnancy (Schatz et al., 1975; Turner et al., 1980). Although an association between steroid therapy and facial clefts in the fetus has been claimed (Francis and Smellie, 1964), the only data to support this are in rabbits (Fainstall, 1954) (see Chapter 12). Understandably, there is a concern that steroid hormones may cross the placenta, suppressing the fetal hypothalamo-pituitary-adrenal axis. In practice this occurs very rarely, if at all, probably because these steroids, in contrast to dexamethasone and betamethasone, are metabolized by the placenta (Levitz et al., 1978) and therefore do not enter the fetal circulation in significant quantities (Beitins et al., 1972). Patients who have

serious "flares" with renal or CNS involvement may need prednisone 60 mg/day or more for several weeks. Patients who are taking steroids should be regularly checked for gestational diabetes. If a woman has taken regular glucocorticoid therapy for more than one month in the year before delivery, parenteral steroid such as hydrocortisone, 100 mg every 6 hours, should be given to prevent maternal addisonian collapse during labor and delivery.

Azathioprine has been used rather widely in pregnancy, chiefly in patients with renal transplants. There have not been any specific ill effects reported in the fetus (Davison, 1989). The worry concerning azathioprine is that it induces chromosome breaks. These have been observed in peripheral blood leukocytes of neonates exposed to maternal azathioprine therapy. They disappear as the infant grows older. Since the female fetus contains all the ova that the woman will ever shed during ovulation, it is theoretically possible that these ova may be affected and that azathioprine will have impaired the future reproductive capacity of the female fetus (Davison, 1989).

In summary, paracetamol is the best agent to use as an analgesic and an antirheumatic in pregnancy. High-dose salicylate and nonsteroidal anti-inflammatory agents are best avoided in normal therapeutic doses in the last trimester, and if a patient requires extra therapy for this relatively short time, corticosteroids should be used. Because of the risk of dangerous exacerbation of SLE in the puerperium, steroid dosage should only be reduced with great care after delivery. The use of azathioprine should be reserved for cases in which steroid therapy has failed or is contraindicated.

Plasmapheresis has been successfully used in pregnancy for maternal reasons in patients with severe proximal myopathy induced by steroids (Thomson et al., 1985) and with a very bad obstetric history (Frampton et al., 1987). A single successful case raises the possibility that plasmapheresis and steroid therapy may decrease the risk of the development of complete heart block in the fetus of a patient who is anti-Ro—positive (Barclay et al., 1987).

In breast-feeding women, the nonsteroidal anti-inflammatory drugs with short half-lives and rapidly eliminated or inactive metabolites are best, i.e., ibuprofen, flurbiprofen, and diclofenac (Doshi et al., 1980). High-dose salicylate and antimalarial drugs should be avoided for reasons given above. Minute quantities of prednisone are secreted in breast milk, and this drug should therefore be considered safe.

Patients who also have a past history of thromboembolism, arterial or venous, should be treated with subcutaneous heparin, 10,000 units twice daily (Fox et al., 1990), throughout pregnancy in addition to any aspirin and prednisone therapy that might be considered necessary (see Chapter 48). Although this treatment may increase bone loss associated with steroid therapy, I believe it to be necessary in view of the possible dire consequences, particularly of cerebral arterial thrombosis (Farquharson et al., 1985). Patients with lupus anticoagulant and/or cardiolipin antibodies and no history of thromboembolism are treated with low dose aspirin alone (75 mg per day) unless it is judged that they also require steroids for protection of the fetus.

Fetal Considerations

The management of the cardiolipin syndrome is considered in Chapter 31.

Congenital heart block should be diagnosed, before delivery, by means of routine auscultation of the fetal heart and subsequent cardiotocography when bradycardia is discovered. This should be distinguished from sinus bradycardia by a detailed ultrasound examination of the fetal heart (Fox et al., 1990). This will show atrioventricular dissociation confirming heart block and also demonstrate any structural heart disease, which is present in 15 to 20 per cent of cases (Stephensen et al., 1981) and may occur in the absence of maternal connective tissue disease (Shenker et al., 1987). If the fetus has complete heart block (see Chapter 21), it is difficult to assess its general condition *in utero* since accurate assessment usually depends on measurement of fetal heart rate and its variability. Measurement of umbilical blood flow by Doppler ultrasound can be of value, and antenatal fetal blood sampling to measure fetal blood gases (Nicholaides et al., 1986, Soothill et al., 1986) could be of real value. The fetus also can be monitored by repeated fetal blood scalp sampling during labor (Paredes et al., 1983), but understandably many such fetuses are delivered by elective cesarean section.

The management of the occasional fetus that develops hydrops and cardiac failure in association with heart block before viability is a real problem (see Chapter 45). Many of these fetuses may also have an element of cardiomyopathy owing to the presence of anticardiac smooth muscle antibodies. Steroids that cross the placenta, such as dexamethasone or betamethasone, may be helpful (Fox and Hawkins, 1990), but often they are not and the fetus dies.

RHEUMATOID ARTHRITIS

The most common systemic rheumatic disease, rheumatoid arthritis, occurs in young women. Although the exact prevalence of rheumatoid arthritis during the childbearing years is difficult to calculate, the disease probably complicates pregnancy in 1:1000 to 1:2000 cases. The disease is a relatively selective inflammation of synovial (hinged) joints. The association with the tissue antigen HLA-D4 explains the modest familial aggregation of the disease. The pathologic findings of the condition, lymphocytic and monocytic infiltration of the synovia, suggest immune mechanisms. Similarly, rheumatoid arthritis is strongly associated with rheumatoid factor, an autoantibody against gamma globulin and, more characteristically, against macrolin (IgM). Such antibodies are noted in many other chronic inflammatory and infectious diseases, but the titer is higher in rheumatoid arthritis, and the antibody is present in 80 to 90 per cent of patients with typical inflammatory rheumatoid arthritis.

Onset of the disease is usually insidious, with pain and swelling in one or more joints in the upper extremities—classically the wrist joint, the metacarpophalangeal joints, and the proximal finger joints—leading to spindle-shaped deformity. Proximal finger joint swelling is one of the classic features. Within the first weeks or months, the disease tends to settle in the joints symmetrically, with the lower extremities (knees, ankles, toes) becoming involved. Involvement of distal finger joints is rare in rheumatoid arthritis. In the spine, lumbar and dorsal vertebral articulations are almost never involved, but the cervical vertebrae constitute a common site, with neck arthritis a significant cause of disability in rheumatoid arthritis. The hip joints are also involved, but fortunately from the standpoint of pregnancy and the necessity to abduct hips for vaginal delivery, hip disease in the rheumatoid patient is an uncommon and a late synovial joint manifestation. By contrast, involvement of the temperomandibular joints and larynx is quite common in young patients, and this is important because it may cause difficulties with intubation for general anesthesia.

Diagnosis of Rheumatoid Arthritis

Unfortunately, rheumatoid arthritis carries no absolute diagnostic criteria until the disease is far advanced. Rheumatoid factor, usually measured as antiglobulin antibody–agglutinating latex particles coated with IgG (the latex test), should be positive within a year. Titers of 1:160 or higher are strongly supportive of the diagnosis in a patient with compatible history and examination. However, positive titers for rheumatoid factor are found in all sorts of other chronic inflammatory diseases, such as tuberculosis and subacute bacterial endocarditis. Other rheumatic diseases, such as lupus erythematosus, are commonly accompanied by positive tests for rheumatoid factor.

Although rheumatoid arthritis is likely to remain primarily a synovial process, lesions occur elsewhere, although this is uncommon in pregnancy. Typical nonarticular lesions are rheumatoid nodules in the skin, lungs, and heart; pleurisy; pericarditis; and vasculitis similar to that of polyarteritis nodosa.

The finding by Hench (1938) that rheumatoid arthritis improved in 24 of 30 pregnancies, coupled with a belief that cortisol levels were markedly elevated in pregnancy, was so important that it led to the successful use of steroids in patients with rheumatoid arthritis who were not pregnant. These observations have been confirmed by Kaplan and Diamond (1965), and difficulties in the management of rheumatoid arthritis are rare in pregnancy, although exacerbations may occur in the puerperium. The subject has been extensively reviewed by Thurnau (1983). Unger et al. (1983) have correlated the improvement in rheumatoid arthritis with the level of pregnancy-associated α_2-glycoprotein, which has immunosuppressive action. However, pregnancy induces many other changes in the immune system; therefore, there may be other reasons why rheumatoid arthritis improves.

In contrast to SLE, there is no increased risk of abortion in patients with rheumatoid arthritis (Kaplan and Diamond, 1965). As indicated above, there is a small risk of congenital heart block in the newborn.

Management

The most common difficulty involves drug administration. As indicated above, the dangers of steroid therapy have been exaggerated, and paracetamol is a better analgesic for use in pregnancy than aspirin. However, if paracetamol is inadequate, it seems reasonable to use aspirin and other prostaglandin antagonists at least in the first two trimesters. However, there are case reports of convulsions in a breast-fed infant after the mother had taken indomethacin for analgesia (Eeg-Olofsson et al., 1978; Fairhead, 1978), and therefore indomethacin should only be used with caution in women who are breast-feeding.

Gold causes blood dyscrasias, drug rashes, and nephropathy, and the fetus is therefore theoretically at risk from maternal treatment. However, gold is strongly protein-bound, and little appears to cross the placenta (Rocker and Henderson, 1976).

Antimalarial drugs such as chloroquine are also used in the treatment of rheumatoid arthritis. Chloroquine has been reported to cause chromosome damage, but there is no evidence that this results in stable chromosome abnormalities, which might be of genetic or neoplastic significance (Gifford, 1975). A greater worry is that chloroquine may cause retinopathy in the neonate because it is concentrated in the fetal uveal tract (Ullberg et al., 1970). Congenital deafness has also been reported (Hart and Nauton, 1964). Antimalarial drugs should therefore not be used in the treatment of rheumatoid arthritis in pregnancy, particularly since alternative treatments exist. Nevertheless, the risks of their use have probably been exaggerated. Since there is no alternative, women must, and do, take antimalarial drugs for the treatment or prophylaxis of malaria in pregnancy (Lewis et al., 1973); a high incidence of fetal damage associated with malaria has not been reported.

Sulfasalazine is increasingly used as a second-line treatment for rheumatoid arthritis. Its safety in pregnancy has been demonstrated in patients with inflammatory bowel disease (Mogadam et al., 1981).

Immunosuppressive drugs are occasionally used in the treatment of rheumatoid arthritis. Azathioprine is the drug that has been used most frequently, and it appears to be relatively safe, although it does induce chromosome breaks in fetuses exposed to maternal azathioprine therapy (see above, under SLE). Methotrexate is now widely used in nonpregnant patients with rheumatoid arthritis because it is effective and relatively nontoxic, and it does not cause delayed cancer or lymphomas. However, methotrexate should not be used in the first trimester of pregnancy because it is teratogenic. Penicillamine is also used in the treatment of rheumatoid arthritis. There are occasional reports of suspected teratogenesis (Solomon et al., 1977) and neonatal abnormalities of connective tissue (Mjolnerod et al., 1971), which may be irreversible or reversible (Linares et al., 1979). However, there are two series totalling 56 pregnancies in which the only abnormality (which could have occurred by chance) was a small ventricular septal defect in one child (Lyle, 1978; Scheinberg and Sternlieb, 1975). It would therefore seem that penicillamine is reasonably safe in pregnancy.

In summary, if a patient with rheumatoid arthritis requires treatment in pregnancy, she should be given paracetamol. If this does not give adequate relief in the first two trimesters, aspirin or other nonsteroidal anti-inflammatory drugs may be used. If these are inadequate and pregnancy is in the last trimester, corticosteroids should be used notwithstanding concern about joint damage or the risk of long-term complications such as vasculitis. Penicillamine treatment also appears to be safe. Injections of long-acting corticosteroids into involved joints usually provide good symptomatic relief of the injected joint, lasting for several months, and may be used at any time in pregnancy.

ANKYLOSING SPONDYLITIS

Ankylosing spondylitis presents clinically as insidious low back pain and stiffness, which is worse in the morning and improves with moderate physical activity during the day. The spinal involvement usually moves upward from the sacroiliac joints to encompass the entire spine, leaving the spine fused by calcification and the patient bowed forward and stooped. Clinically, this description is seen most commonly in young men (ages 15 to 40); young women have milder disease manifested by back pain (Calin and Fries, 1975). Thus, although the disease seems to occur with about equal frequency in both sexes, the diagnosis is often missed in women, in whom the disease rarely progresses rapidly. Patients with ankylosing spondylitis who become pregnant are not improved by pregnancy (Ostensen and Romberg, 1982), in sharp contrast to the situation in rheumatoid arthritis. The treatment of ankylosing spondylitis is similar to that described above for rheumatoid arthritis.

SCLERODERMA

Scleroderma is a connective tissue disease affecting the skin, gastrointestinal tract (esophagus), kidneys, and lungs. The cause is unknown, and there is no known cure or disease-modifying therapy. There have been five series of 108 patients (Johnson et al., 1964; Leinwold and Dirgee, 1954; Slate and Graham, 1968; Haynes, 1969; Black and Stevens, 1989) and several case reports (Karlen and Cook, 1974; Ballou et al., 1984) and a review (Gopelrud, 1983) describing the interaction of scleroderma and pregnancy. In the localized cutaneous form, the scleroderma process is localized, usually to the hands; it is associated with Raynaud's phenomenon and there is no organ involvement. The prognosis is good in general and in particular in pregnancy. Diffuse cutaneous scleroderma has more widespread cutaneous manifestations and is a more aggressive illness. Raynaud's phenomenon is less common, and the patient may have SCL-70 antibodies. The heart, lungs, and kidneys are often involved. The prognosis in pregnancy is far worse. Since many patients deteriorate, often with hypertensive crises (Black and Stevens, 1989), they have been advised against pregnancy, particularly because they may not be able to look after their children even if they survive pregnancy. However, it is not clear whether pregnancy itself accelerates the inevitable deterioration in these patients.

Captopril has been advocated as treatment for crises in patients with scleroderma (McKenna et al., 1983). It is usually used as an antihypertensive drug but should be avoided in pregnancy because of concern about the fetus in patients taking angiotensin-converting enzyme inhibitors (see Chapter 49).

The fetal outcome in diffuse cutaneous scleroderma is also poor. In a review of 17 pregnancies reported in the literature, Karlen and Cook (1974) documented five perinatal deaths and five instances of premature delivery. These patients often have sclerotic skin and blood vessels, making venipuncture, venous access, and blood pressure measurement difficult. Both regional and general anesthesia are associated with technical problems, particularly the difficulty of endotracheal intubation (Thompson and Conklin, 1983). Such patients should see an anesthesiologist early in their pregnancy so that anesthetic management can be planned rather than guessed at in an emergency.

SJÖGREN'S SYNDROME AND OTHER LESS COMMON CONDITIONS

Sjögren's syndrome is a rare autoimmune disorder that primarily affects the lacrimal and salivary glands, with intense lymphocytic infiltration of these organs and loss of tears and saliva (thus the synonym, keratoconjunctivitis sicca or sicca syndrome). The syndrome is accompanied by the most intense and varied autoantibodies of any disease—antibodies to tissues of several types, rheumatoid factors, and a large family of antinuclear antibodies Ro(SSA) and La(SSB). As in lupus, anti-Ro(SSA) in the idiopathic Sjögren's patient has been associated with congenital heart block in the infant; indeed, congenital heart block is particularly common in patients with Sjögren's syndrome because of the strong association with HLA antigen DR3 and anti-Ro antibody. The sicca syndrome is often seen in patients with clinically evident rheumatoid arthritis or lupus erythematosus.

Mixed connective tissue disease is characterized serologically by antibodies to soluble nuclear antigens such as ribonucleoprotein and by the usual antinuclear antibodies as well. The disease resembles mild lupus with sclerodermatous overlay and has fetal risks similar to those of SLE (Kaufman and Kitridou, 1982).

Other connective tissue diseases that rarely complicate pregnancy are polyarteritis nodosa (Debeukelaer et al., 1973), dermatomyositis (Speira, 1980), and Wegener's granulomatosis (Murty et al., 1990). In all these conditions there is insufficient experience to be confident of the effect of pregnancy. Since some patients have deteriorated in pregnancy, termination has been suggested for cases of polyarteritis nodosa (Nagey et al., 1983), but this may not be justified.

REFERENCES

Altenburger KM, Jedziniak M, Roper WL, Hernandez J: Congenital complete heart block with hydrops fetalis. J Pediatr **91**:618, 1977.

Ballou SP, Morley JJ, Kushner I: Pregnancy and systemic sclerosis. Arthritis Rheum **27**:295, 1984.

Barclay CS, Frency MAH, Ross LD, Sokol RJ: Successful pregnancy following steroid therapy and plasma exchange in a woman with anti-Ro (SS-A) antibodies. Case report. Br J Obstet Gynaecol **94**:369, 1987.

Beitins R, Baynard F, Ances IG, Kowarsk A, Migeon CJ: The transplacental passage of prednisone and prednisolone in pregnancy near term. J Pediatr **81**:936, 1972.

Black CM, Stevens WM: Scleroderma. Rheum Dis Clin North Am **15**:193, 1989.

Buckfield P: Major congenital faults in newborn infants: A pilot study in New Zealand. NZ Med J **78**:159, 1973.

Buyon JP, Cronstein BN, Morris M, et al: Serum complement values (C3 and C4) to differentiate between systemic lupus activity and pre-eclampsia. Am J Med **81**:194, 1986.

Buyon JP, Swersky SH, Fox HE, et al: Intrauterine therapy for presumptive fetal myocarditis with acquired heart block due to systemic lupus erythematosus. Experience in a mother with a predominance of SS-B (La) antibodies. Arthritis Rheum **30**:44, 1987.

Calin A, Fries JF: Striking prevalence of ankylosing spondylitis in "healthy" W27 positive males and females. N Engl J Med **293**:835, 1975.

Davison J: Renal disease. In de Swiet M (ed): Medical Disorders in Obstetric Practice. Oxford, Blackwell Scientific Publications, 1989, p 226.

Debeukelaer MM, Travis LB, Roberts DK: Polyarteritis and pregnancy: Report of a successful outcome. South Med J **66**:613, 1973.

Donaldson LM, Espiner EA: Disseminated lupus erythematosus presenting as chorea gravidarum. Arch Neurol **25**:240, 1971.

Doshi N, Smith B, Klionsky B: Congenital pericarditis due to maternal lupus erythematosus. J Pediatr **96**:699, 1980.

Dudley DKL, Hardie KJ: Fetal and neonatal effects of indomethacin used as a tocolytic agent. Am J Obstet Gynecol **151**:181, 1985.

Eeg-Olofsson O, Malmros I, Elwin C, Steen B: Convulsions in a breast-fed infant after maternal indomethacin. Lancet **2**:215, 1978.

Estes D, Larson DL: Systemic lupus erythematosus and pregnancy. Clin Obstet Gynecol **8**:307, 1965.

Fainstall T: Cortisone-induced congenital cleft palate in rabbits. Endocrinology **55**:520, 1954.

Fairhead FW: Convulsions in a breast-fed infant after maternal administration. Lancet **2**:576, 1978.

Farquharson RG, Compson A, Bloom AL: Lupus anticoagulant: A place for prepregnancy treatment? Lancet **2**:842, 1985.

Fessel WJ: Systemic lupus erythematosus in the community. Incidence, prevalence, outcome and first symptoms; the high prevalence in black women. Arch Intern Med **134**:1027, 1974.

Fox R, Hawkins DF: Fetal-pericardial effusion in association with congenital heart block and maternal systemic lupus erythematosus. Case report. Br J Obstet Gynaecol **97**:638, 1990.

Fox R, Lumb MR, Hawkins DF: Persistent fetal sinus bradycardia associated with maternal anti-Ro antibodies. Case report. Br J Obstet Gynaecol **97**:1151, 1990.

Fraga A, Mintz G, Orozco J, Orozco JH: Sterility and fertility rates, fetal wastage and maternal morbidity in systemic lupus erythematosus. J Rheumatol **1**:293, 1964.

Frampton G, Pameron JA, Thomas M, Jones S, Raftery M: Successful removal of anti-phospholipid antibody during pregnancy using plasma exchange and low-dose prednisolone. Lancet **2**:1023, 1987.

Francis HH, Smellie J: General disease in pregnancy. Br Med J **1**:887, 1964.

Garsenstein M, Pollak VE, Karik RM: Systemic lupus erythematosus and pregnancy. N Engl J Med **267**:165, 1962.

Gifford RH: Rheumatic disease. In Burrow GN, Ferris TF (eds): Medical Complications during Pregnancy. Philadelphia, W.B. Saunders Co., 1975.

Gimovsky ML, Montoro M, Paul RH: Pregnancy outcome in women with SLE. Obstet Gynecol **63**:684, 1984.

Gopelrud CP: Scleroderma. Clin Obstet Gynaecol **26**:587, 1983.

Goudie BM, Dossetor JFB: Effect on the fetus of indomethacin given to suppress labour. Lancet **2**:1185, 1979.

Hardy JD, Solomon S, Banwell GS, Beach R, Wright V, Howard FM: Congenital complete heart block in the newborn associated with maternal systemis lupus erythematosus and other connective tissue disease. Arch Dis Child **54**:7, 1979.

Hart CW, Nauton RF: The ototoxicity of chloroquine phosphate. Arch Otolaryngol 80:407, 1964.

Haynes DM: Medical Complications in Pregnancy. *In* Haynes MM (ed): New York, McGraw-Hill, 1989.

Hayslett JP, Lynn RI: Effect of pregnancy in patients with lupus nephropathy. Kidney Int 18:207, 1980.

Hench AB: The ameliorating effect of pregnancy on chronic atrophic (infectious rheumatoid) arthritis; fibrositis and intermittent hydrothosis. Proc Mayo Clin 13:161, 1938.

Heymann MA: Non-steroidal anti-inflammatory agents. In Drug Therapy During Pregnancy. *In* Eskes TKAB, Finster M (eds): London, Butterworths, 1985, p 85.

Houser MT, Fish AJ, Tagatz GE, Williams PP, Michael AF: Pregnancy and systemic lupus erythematosus. Am J Obstet Gynecol 138:409, 1980.

Hughes GRV: Autoantibodies in lupus and its variants: Experience in 1,000 patients. Br Med J 289:339, 1984.

Johnson TR, Banner EA, Winkelmann RK: Scleroderma and pregnancy. Obstet Gynecol 23:467, 1964.

Kaplan D, Diamond H: Rheumatoid arthritis and pregnancy. Clin Obstet Gynecol 8:286, 1965.

Karlen JG, Cook WA: Renal scleroderma and pregnancy. Obstet Gynecol 44:349, 1974.

Kaufman RL, Kitridou RC: Pregnancy in mixed connective tissue disease: Comparison with systemic lupus erythematosus. J Rheumatol 9:549, 1982.

Kincaid-Smith P, Fairley KF, Kloss M: Lupus anticoagulant associated with renal thrombotic microangiopathy and pregnancy related renal failure. Q J Med 69:795, 1988.

Lancet Editorial: PG-synthetase inhibition in obstetrics and after. Lancet 2:185, 1980.

Leinwald I, Durgee AW: Scleroderma? Ann Intern Med 41:1033, 1954.

Levitz M, Jansen V, Dancis J: The transfer and metabolism of corticosteroid in the perfused human placenta. Am J Obstet Gynecol 132:363, 1978.

Lewis R, Lauersen NH, Birn Baum S: Malaria associated with pregnancy. Obstet Gynecol 42:696, 1973.

Linares A, Zarranz JJ, Rodriguez-Alarcon J, Diaz-Perez JL: Reversible cutis laxa due to maternal d-penicillamine treatment. Lancet 2:43, 1979.

Litsey SE, Noonan JA, O'Connor WM, Cottril CM, Mitchell B: Maternal connective tissue disease and congenital heart block. Demonstration of immunoglobulin in cardiac tissue. N Engl J Med 312:98, 1985.

Lockshin MD, Gibofsky A, Peebles CL, Gigli I, Fotino M, Hurwitz S: Neonatal lupus erythematosus with heart block: family study of a patient with anti-SS-A and SS-B antibodies. Arthritis Rheum 26:210, 1983.

Lockshin MD, Druzin ML, Goei S, Qamar T, Magid MS, Jovanovic L, Ference M: Antibody to cardiolipin as a predictor of fetal distress or death in pregnant patients with systemic lupus erythematosus. N Engl J Med 131:152, 1985.

Loizou S, Byron MA, Englert HJ, David J, Hughes GR, Walport MJ: Association of quantitative anticardiolipin antibody levels with fetal loss and time of loss in systemic lupus erythematosus. Q J Med 68:525, 1988.

Lubbe WF, Walker EB: Chorea gravidarum associated with lupus anticoagulant: Successful outcome of pregnancy with prednisone therapy. Br J Obstet Gynaecol 90:487, 1983.

Lyle WH: Penicillamine in pregnancy. Lancet 1:606, 1978.

Maddison PJ, Skinner RP, Esscher E, Taylor PV, Scott O, Scott JS: Serological studies in congenital heart block. Ann Rheum Dis 42:218, 1983.

McCormack MJ, Adu D, Weaver J, Michael J, Kelley J: Anti-platelet antibodies: A prognostic marker in pregnancies associated with lupus nephritis. Case reports. Br J Obstet Gynaecol 98:324, 1991.

McCue CM, Matakas ME, Tinglesrad JB, Ruddy S: Congenital heart block in newborns of mothers with connective tissue disease. Circulation 56:82, 1977.

McCuistion CH, Schoch EP: Possible discoid lupus erythematosus in a newborn infant: Report of case with subsequent development of acute systemic lupus erythematosus in mother. Arch Dermatol Syphilol 70:782, 1954.

McKenna F, Martin MFR, Bird MA, Wright V: Captopril. Br Med J 287:1299, 1983.

Mjolnerod IK, Rasmussen K, Dommerud SA, Gjeruldsen ST: Congenital connective tissue defect probably due to D-penicillamine treatment in pregnancy. Lancet 1:673, 1971.

Mogadam M, Dobbins WO, et al: Pregnancy in inflammatory bowel disease: Effect of sulphasalazine and corticosteroids on fetal outcome. Gastroenterology 80:72, 1981.

Mund A, Simson J, Rothfield N: Effect of pregnancy on course of systemic lupus erythematosus. JAMA 183:917, 1963.

Murty GE, Davison JM, Cameron DS: Wegener's granulomatosis complicating pregnancy. Br J Obstet Gynaecol 10:399, 1990.

Nagey DA, Fortier KJ, Linder J: Pregnancy complicated by periarteritis nodosa: Induced abortion as an alternative. Am J Obstet Gynecol 147:103, 1983.

Nathan DJ, Snapper I: Simultaneous placental transfer of factors responsible for LE cell formation and thrombocytopenia. Am J Med 25:647, 1958.

Nicolaides KH, Soothill PW, Rodeck CH, Campbell S: Ultrasound-guided sampling of umbilical cord and placental blood to assess fetal well being. Lancet 1:1065, 1986.

Niebyl JR, Witter FR: Neonatal outcome after indomethacin treatment for preterm labour. Am J Obstet Gynecol 155:747, 1986.

Olaf KS, Gee H: Fetal heart block associated with maternal anti-Ro (SS-A) antibody—current management. A review. Br J Obstet Gynaecol 98:751, 1991.

Ostensen M, Romberg O: Ankylosing spondylitis and motherhood. Arthritis Rheum 25:140, 1982.

Paredes RA, Morgan H, Lachelin GCL: Congenital heart block in a fetus associated with maternal Sjorgren's syndrome. Case report. Br J Obstet Gynaecol 90:970, 1983.

Patton PE, Coulam CB, Bergstralh E: The prevalence of autoantibodies in pregnant and nonpregnant women. Am J Obstet Gynecol 157:134, 1987.

Provost TT, Watson R, Gammon WR, Radowsky M, Harley JB, Riechlin M: The neonatal lupus syndrome associated with U RNP (nRNP) antibodies. N Engl J Med 316:1135, 1987.

Rees RB, Maibach HH: Chloroquine: A review of reactions and dermatologic indications. Arch Dermatol 88:96, 1963.

Rocker I, Henderson WJ: Transfer of gold from mother to fetus. Lancet 2:1246, 1976.

Schatz M, Patterson R, Zeitz S: Corticosteroid therapy for the pregnant asthmatic patient. JAMA 233:804, 1975.

Scheinberg IH, Sternlieb I: Pregnancy in penicillamine-treated patients with Wilson's Disease. N Engl J Med 293:1300, 1975.

Scott JS, Esscher E: Congenital heart block and maternal systemic lupus erythematosus. Br Med J 1:1235, 1979.

Shenker L, Reed KL, Anderson CF, Marx GR, Sobonya LE, Graham AR: Congenital heart block and cardiac anomalies in the absence of maternal connective tissue disease. Am J Obstet Gynecol 157:248, 1987.

Singsen BM, Arhter SE, Weinstein MW, Sharp GC: Congenital complete heart block and SS-A antibodies: Obstetric implications. Am J Obstet Gynecol 152:655, 1985.

Slate WG, Graham AR: Scleroderma and pregnancy. Am J Obstet Gynecol 101:335, 1968.

Solomon L, Abrams G, Dinner M, Berman L: Neonatal abnormalities associated with D-Penicillamine treatment during pregnancy. N Engl J Med 296:54, 1977.

Soothill PW, Nicolaides KH, Rodeck CH, Campbell S: The effect of gestational age on blood gas and acid-base values in human pregnancy. Fetal Ther 7:166, 1986.

Speira IE: Connective tissue disease in pregnancy. Mt Sinai J Med 47:438, 1980.

Stephensen O, Cleland WP, Hallidie-Smith K: Congenital heart block and persistent ductus arteriosus associated with maternal systemic lupus erythematosus. Br Heart J 46:104, 1981.

Stuart MJ, Gross SJ, Elrad H, Graeber JE: Effects of acetylsalicylic-acid ingestion on maternal and neonatal hemostasis. N Engl J Med 307:902, 1982.

Taylor PV, Scott JS, Gerlis LM, Essecher E, Scott O: Maternal autoantibodies against fetal cardiac antigens in congenital complete heart block. N Engl J Med 315:667, 1986.

Thompson J, Conklin KA: Anesthetic management of a pregnant patient with scleroderma. Anesthesiology 59:69, 1983.

Thomson BJ, Watson ML, Liston WA, Lambie AT: Phasmapharesis in pregnancy complicated by acute systemic lupus erythematosus. Case report. Br J Obstet Gynaecol 92:523, 1985.

Thurnau GR: Rheumatoid arthritis. Clin Obstet Gynecol **26**:558, 1983.

Turner G, Collins E: Fetal effects of regular salicylate ingestion in pregnancy. Lancet **2**:338, 1975.

Turner ES, Greenberger PA, Patterson R: Management of the pregnant asthmatic patient. Ann Intern Med **6**:905, 1980.

Ullberg S, Lindquist NG, Sjostrand SE: Accumulation of retinotoxic drugs in the foetal eye. Nature **227**:1257, 1970.

Unger A, Kay A, Griffin AJ, Panayi GS: Disease activity and pregnancy associated α 2-glycoprotein in rheumatoid arthritis during pregnancy. Br Med J **286**:750, 1983.

Veille JC, Sunderland C, Bennett RM: Complete heart block in a fetus associated with maternal Sjögren's syndrome. Am J Obstet Gynecol **151**:660, 1985.

Venning MC, Burn DJ, Ward RM, Henry JA, Davison JM: Neonatal lupus syndrome: Optimism justified? Lancet **1**:640, 1988.

Vonderheid EC, Koblenzer PJ, Ming P, Ming J, Burgoon CF: Neonatal lupus erythematosus, report on four cases with a review of literature. Arch Dermatol **112**:698, 1976.

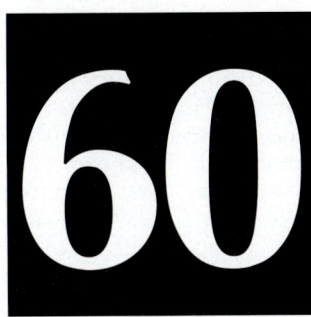
NEUROLOGIC DISORDERS

MICHAEL J. AMINOFF, M.D., FRCP

Women are as liable to neurologic disorders during gestation as at other times, and certain disorders may be aggravated or influenced by pregnancy. Moreover, the investigation and management of many neurologic disorders may be complicated by the pregnancy and by concern for the safety of the developing fetus. This chapter is intended not to provide a detailed account of all aspects of neurologic disease, which is available in a number of standard textbooks dealing with disorders of the nervous system, but rather to provide an account of some of the special problems posed by neurologic disorders during pregnancy and, conversely, by pregnancy in patients with neurologic disorders.

EPILEPSY

Epileptic women should be advised about possible interactions between anticonvulsant drugs and oral contraceptive agents. Whether oral contraceptives affect seizure frequency or blood levels of antiepileptic drugs is unclear, but certain anticonvulsants (phenytoin, phenobarbital, primidone, and carbamazepine) may interfere with the effectiveness of oral contraceptives, leading to unwanted pregnancy (Janz et al., 1989).

Between 0.3 and 0.6 per cent of pregnant women have epilepsy (Niswander and Gordon, 1972; South, 1972; Bjerkedal and Bahna, 1973). Pregnancy may affect the seizure disorder, and the disorder may itself affect the course of the pregnancy and the manner in which it is best managed. Moreover, recurrent seizures and drugs given to the mother in an attempt to control them may affect fetal development.

Effect of Pregnancy on Seizure Disorders

Pregnancy has an unpredictable and variable influence on epilepsy. In 153 pregnancies in one series of 59 patients with epilepsy, seizure frequency increased in 45 per cent, was reduced in 5 per cent, and remained unchanged in the remainder (Knight and Rhind, 1975). When seizure frequency increased, it most commonly did so in the first trimester and usually reverted to the pregestational pattern at the conclusion of the pregnancy, although in a few patients there was a permanent deterioration in seizure control. In general, control in patients with frequent seizures (i.e., more than one per month) before pregnancy was likely to deteriorate during the gestational period, whereas only about 25 per cent of patients with infrequent attacks (i.e., less than one every 9 months) experienced an exacerbation during pregnancies. In a more recent prospective study of 136 pregnancies in 122 epileptic women, seizure frequency increased in 50 pregnancies (37 per cent), often in association with noncompliance with therapeutic regimen (Schmidt et al., 1983). Among several other series published between 1938 and 1985, seizures increased during pregnancy in 23 to 75 per cent of instances (Yerby, 1991).

It is generally not possible to predict the outcome in individual cases, regardless of the maternal age, the outcome of previous pregnancies or any apparent relationship between seizures and the menstrual cycle. None of these provides a guide to the effect that pregnancy will have on the course of epilepsy. Moreover, attacks may occur during pregnancy in patients who have been seizure-free for several years.

Indeed, epilepsy may appear for the first time during or immediately after pregnancy. Less than 25 per cent of women in this latter group will have seizures only in relation to pregnancy and at no other time (i.e., gestational epilepsy) (Montouris et al., 1979). About one-third of patients with true gestational epilepsy experience recurrent seizures during pregnancy, and the remainder have only a single convulsion (Knight and Rhind, 1975). Even in this group of patients, however, the occurrence of seizures in one pregnancy is no guide to the course of subsequent gestations.

The seizures that occur during pregnancy do not differ clinically from those occurring in other circumstances, although in women in whom seizures occur for the first time during pregnancy, the attacks and/or any electroencephalographic (EEG) abnormalities are often focal (Dimsdale, 1959; Knight and Rhind, 1975). Improved compliance with an anticonvulsant drug regimen may sometimes account for the reduction in seizure frequency that occasionally occurs during pregnancy in an epileptic (Suter and Klingman, 1957).

The increase in seizure frequency that occurs in some epileptic patients during pregnancy may relate to the metabolic, hormonal, or hematologic changes of the gestational period, or to fatigue or sleep deprivation. A rapid and excessive gain in weight sometimes occurs prior to an increase in seizure frequency (Suter and Klingman, 1957; Dimsdale, 1959), providing some support for the belief that fluid retention may occasionally be a factor, perhaps by a dilutional effect on anticonvulsant drug concentration. It is also certainly tempting to relate any change in seizure frequency to hormonal factors (Marcus et al., 1966; Timiras, 1969; Backstrom, 1976), because estrogens are epileptogenic in experimental animals and progesterone has both convulsant and anticonvulsant properties.

There is sometimes difficulty in maintaining adequate treatment with anticonvulsant drugs during pregnancy. Phenytoin and phenobarbital requirements increase at this time and decline again in the puerperium, as determined by the relationship between plasma levels and daily dose of each drug (Lander et al., 1977). Similar findings have been noted with other drugs, including carbamazepine, primidone, and ethosuximide (Mygind et al., 1976; Ramsay et al., 1978; Landon and Kirkley, 1979; Niebyl et al., 1979). An increase in dosage is frequently required to maintain plasma levels at pre-pregnancy values.

The reason for such changes in drug requirements is unclear. Among the various possibilities are the dilutional effect of increasing plasma volume and extracellular fluid volume. Poor compliance with anticonvulsant drug regimen, perhaps relating to nausea and vomiting, or to concerns about the effect of medication on the fetus, may also be an important contributory factor, as may decreased plasma protein binding and changes in the absorption and excretion of drugs.

Folic acid therapy may certainly lower the plasma phenytoin level, sometimes to below the therapeutic range, and may thereby precipitate seizures (Baylis et al., 1971; Strauss and Bernstein, 1974). Plasma phenytoin levels can decline, however, even when a pregnant patient is not given folate supplements (Dam et al., 1979). Moreover, the fall in plasma phenytoin level may precede the commencement of folate therapy, and a postpartum increase in plasma phenytoin level may occur despite continued folic acid therapy (Eadie et al., 1977). Folic acid may conceivably influence seizure control in other ways. For example, it is known to have convulsant properties when applied topically to the cerebral cortex in experimental situations (Mauguiere et al., 1975). Other drugs taken concomitantly with an anticonvulsant medication may also lead to reduced plasma levels of the anticonvulsant. Antacids and antihistamines merit particular mention here because it is not uncommon for them to be taken during pregnancy.

The increased metabolic capacity of the maternal liver in pregnancy, and possible fetal and/or placental metabolism of part of the anticonvulsant dose, may also bear on the changes in anticonvulsant drug requirements that occur in epileptic women during pregnancy.

Status epilepticus sometimes complicates pregnancy and may occur without any preceding increase in seizure frequency (Knight and Rhind, 1975), occasionally because of the injudicious discontinuation of anticonvulsant drugs. Fortunately, this is a rare occurrence, but it may lead to a fatal outcome for mother or fetus. The absence of hypertension, proteinuria, and edema help in distinguishing this condition from eclamptic convulsions. As in the nonpregnant patient, it is essential to obtain control of the seizures as rapidly as possible, but the former practice of terminating pregnancy is usually unnecessary now. Status epilepticus is treated by anticonvulsant drug therapy, with the pregnancy being allowed to continue to term. Intravenous diazepam, 10 to 30 mg, usually provides temporary control of the seizures, but other anticonvulsant drugs are generally needed as well if seizures are not to recur. Intravenous phenytoin administration is probably the most satisfactory initial approach, but other drugs, such as phenobarbital, may also be required (Ramsay et al., 1978). The usual loading dose of phenytoin is between 15 and 18 mg/kg, given intravenously at a rate of 50 mg per minute or less. It is of paramount importance to maintain control of the airway and of glucose and electrolyte balance.

Effect of Epilepsy on Pregnancy and Lactation

Only a few studies have attempted to document the effect of epilepsy on pregnancy, and their results are often hard to evaluate because of the limited number of cases reported; the lack of comparative data on nonepileptic women attending the same institutions; differences in the severity of the epilepsy and how it has been treated; differences in age, medical background, and socioeconomic status of the patients reported; and the lack of information concerning such relevant social habits as cigarette smoking and alcohol ingestion.

The incidence of vaginal hemorrhage and of toxemia during 371 gestations in epileptic women was found by Bjerkedal and Bahna (1973) to be almost twice that in an unmatched group of 112,530 control pregnancies. Others, however, have not found any meaningful difference in incidence of toxemia between epileptic and nonepileptic women (Watson and Spellacy, 1971). In a large collaborative study, bleeding occurred during pregnancy in 26 per cent of those with no history of convulsive disorder, in 29.8 per cent of those with such a history, and in 33.7 per cent of those who regularly took phenytoin during early pregnancy (Monson et al., 1973).

Whether preterm labor occurs more commonly in epileptic women, as reported by Bjerkedal and Bahna (1973), is unclear. There is a significantly higher rate of stillbirths in epileptics, but there does not seem to be an increased incidence of low-birth-weight infants (Niswander and Gordon, 1972; Monson et al., 1973; Shapiro et al., 1976). Fetal death can certainly result from maternal seizures (Burnett, 1946), presumably in relation to the accompanying hypoxia and acidosis (Orringer et al., 1977). The effect on placental blood flow of maternal seizures is not established, but changes in fetal heart rate suggestive of hypoxia have been described (Teramo et al., 1979); they may relate to reduced placental blood flow or to metabolic changes in the mother.

An increased incidence of neonatal death has been reported in the offspring of epileptic mothers (Speidel and Meadow, 1972; Bjerkedal and Bahna, 1973). The increase in perinatal mortality may relate to a number of factors, including congenital malformations, iatrogenic neonatal hemorrhage, seizures per se, socioeconomic factors, and preterm delivery.

Anticonvulsant drugs taken by the mother may be present in breast milk, but their concentration is usually insufficient to have any major effect on the infant. The transmission rate of different antiepileptic drugs into breast milk varies with the agent, being about 2 per cent for valproic acid, between 30 and 45 per cent for phenytoin, phenobarbital, and carbamazepine, 60 per cent for primidone, and 90 per cent for ethosuximide (Janz et al., 1989). When obvious sedation develops in an infant and is likely to relate to antiepileptic drugs in breast milk, breast-feeding should be discontinued and the baby observed for signs of drug withdrawal. Breast-feeding need not otherwise be discouraged, at least not for reasons related to its content of anticonvulsant medication.

Effect of Maternal Epilepsy and Anticonvulsant Drugs on the Fetus and Neonate

The epileptic woman who becomes pregnant usually is concerned about the possibility that her unborn child might inherit a similar susceptibility to seizures. The risk of the child having epilepsy depends on the nature of the mother's seizure disorder, being greater in idiopathic than in acquired maternal epilepsy. Precise quantification of the risk is not possible at this time, but it is probably about 2 to 3 per cent. It is curious, however, that although the offspring of women with epilepsy have a significantly higher incidence of epilepsy than the general population, the offspring of affected men do not (Annegers et al., 1976). The cause of this increased risk to the offspring of epileptic mothers is unclear. It may relate to genetic factors, seizures arising during pregnancy, or the metabolic and toxic consequences of seizures or anticonvulsant drugs. In general, pregnancy in epileptic women need not be discouraged on these grounds, but reassurance and support are necessary.

A major problem relating to the management of epileptic patients during pregnancy is the possibility that certain anticonvulsant drugs may induce fetal abnormalities, but controversy still exists regarding the potential teratogenicity of these drugs. In reviewing the available data, one must bear in mind that epilepsy has a relatively low prevalence rate, can occur for a multitude of different reasons, can vary markedly in severity, can be treated by a variety of different drugs either singly or in combination, and can itself be associated with an increased risk of fetal malformations. Moreover, some patients may have a common genetic predisposition to seizures and to fetal malformation. Finally, environmental factors may be important in the genesis of congenital abnormalities, and socioeconomic backgrounds must be matched as far as is possible when comparisons are made of the incidence of malformations in different patient populations.

A number of reports have suggested that anticonvulsant drugs are teratogenic (South, 1972; Speidel and Meadow, 1972; Fedrick, 1973; Lowe, 1973; Monson et al., 1973; Annegers et al., 1974; Janz, 1975). Agreement on this point is lacking, however (Kuenssberg and Knox, 1973; Livingston et al., 1973; Shapiro et al., 1976). The most commonly observed malformations in the offspring of mothers taking anticonvulsant drugs are cleft lip, cleft palate, and congenital heart disease.

In a detailed study by Annegers and colleagues (1974), the incidence of malformations per 1000 live births was 71 for epileptic mothers taking anticonvulsant drugs and 18 for those not taking such medications. The two groups were similar with regard to the types of seizure experienced, but it was not possible to determine whether there were differences between them in seizure frequency during pregnancy or in the familial occurrence of malformations. The incidence of congenital heart disease in this series was 43 per 1000 live births for epileptic mothers receiving anticonvulsant drugs, zero for epileptic mothers not taking such medication, and 5.7 among the general population subserved by the Mayo Clinic. Corresponding figures for cleft lip or palate were 21, zero, and 1.9, respectively. These figures therefore imply an increase in the incidence of such malformations among the children of epileptic women taking anticonvulsant drugs during pregnancy.

Starreveld-Zimmerman and colleagues (1974) have suggested that seizure frequency tends to be higher among epileptic mothers with malformed offspring than among those with normal babies, and the results of studies in Finland and the United States raise the possibility that fetal damage sometimes attributed to phenytoin and other anticonvulsant drugs may be due to the epilepsy itself (Shapiro et al., 1976). The studies confirmed that treated maternal epilepsy is associated with an increased incidence of malformations, especially of cleft anomalies. The malformation rate in children exposed antenatally to phenytoin daily during early pregnancy, however, was similar to that of children born to unexposed epileptic mothers. Moreover, there was no evidence for fetal damage in women taking phenobarbital for indications other than epilepsy.

All of the commonly used antiepileptic drugs are teratogenic to some extent, and malformation rates are higher in the offspring of mothers taking drug combinations (Fedrick, 1973; Lindhout et al., 1984). Although the evidence concerning carbamazepine was unclear until recently, the study of Jones et al. (1989) revealed a relatively high incidence of craniofacial defects, fingernail hypoplasia and developmental delay in children exposed prenatally to this drug. Its use during pregnancy, particularly in combination with other drugs, has also been associated with an increased risk of spina bifida (Rosa, 1991). Valproic acid, however, has an especially high (1 to 2 per cent) rate of neural tube defects (Robert and Guibaud, 1982; Bjerkedal et al., 1982). Trimethadione seems particularly dangerous (German et al., 1970; Speidel and Meadow, 1972; Feldman et al., 1977), having been reported to cause fetal malformations and mental retardation in more than 50 per cent of exposed infants. This drug should therefore be avoided during pregnancy when possible.

Animal studies lend support to the belief that some anticonvulsants are teratogenic (Harbison and Becker, 1969; Elshove, 1969). The mechanism involved is unclear but may relate to folate deficiency or antagonism (Evans et al., 1951; Hibbard and Smithells, 1965), although there appears to be no clear relationship between maternal plasma or serum folate levels and congenital malformations (Scott et al., 1970; Hall, 1972). Other teratogenic mechanisms have been proposed. For example, anticonvulsant therapy has been shown to lead to chromosomal abnormalities in both experimental animals (Roman and Caratzali, 1971) and humans (DeToni et al., 1967; Ayraud et al., 1968; Muniz et al., 1969; Marquez-Monter et al., 1970).

Maternal use of phenytoin during pregnancy has been associated with a specific syndrome, the so-called *fetal hydantoin syndrome*, characterized by prenatal and postnatal growth deficiency, microcephaly, dysmorphic facies, and mental deficiency. It is alleged that some 11 per cent of infants exposed to phenytoin *in utero* have enough clinical features to be classified as having this syndrome, and that almost three times as many more show lesser degrees of impairment of performance and/or morphogenesis (Hanson et al., 1976). Other reports have been unable to confirm the relationship of this syndrome to maternal ingestion of specific anticonvulsants (Shapiro et al., 1976, 1977). The syndrome is not unlike that ascribed to phenobarbital (Seip, 1976) and carbamazepine (Jones et al., 1989), and it resembles the fetal alcohol syndrome. A consistent facial phenotype has also been reported in children exposed to valproic acid or sodium valproate *in utero* (DiLiberti et al., 1984).

Maternal use of barbiturates (60 to 120 mg daily) in late pregnancy may be associated with neonatal withdrawal symptoms beginning a week after birth, including restlessness, constant crying, irritability, tremulousness, difficulty in sleeping, and vasomotor instability, but not seizures (Desmond et al., 1972).

Clinical or subclinical coagulopathy may also occur in the neonate whose mother received anticonvulsants during pregnancy. In a prospective study of neonates born to mothers taking anticonvulsant drugs, seven of 16 infants were found to have a severe coagulopathy, one had a mild defect, and the remainder were normal (Mountain et al., 1970). No evidence of a coagulopathy was found in the mothers. In affected infants, factors II, VII, IX, and X are decreased, and factors V and VIII and fibrinogen are normal. The abnormalities are therefore similar to those produced by vitamin K deficiency. Bleeding in affected infants

tends to occur within 24 hours of birth, rather than on the second or third day as in classic hemorrhagic diseases of the newborn, and at relatively unusual sites such as the pleural and abdominal cavities. Prevalence rates average about 10 per cent, but mortality may exceed 30 per cent (Yerby, 1991). Bleeding may also occur *in utero*, resulting in stillbirth (Speidel and Meadow, 1972). Maternal ingestion of vitamin K_1 during the last month of pregnancy may prevent these hemorrhagic complications in the offspring of treated epileptic mothers (Deblay et al., 1982). Vitamin K_1 administration to the newborn infant will usually reverse the bleeding tendency, but the baby may die despite such therapy (Bleyer and Skinner, 1976). It is therefore recommended that prothrombin and partial thromboplastin times of cord blood be measured at delivery of a child born to a woman receiving anticonvulsant drugs; if the value is abnormally low or if there is clinical evidence of a coagulopathy during the neonatal period, treatment with infusion of fresh-frozen plasma or concentrates of factors II, VII, IX, and X may have to be considered in addition to the routine administration of vitamin K_1.

General Therapeutic Approaches

It is clearly difficult at present to make other than general therapeutic recommendations about pregnancy in the epileptic. If a nonpregnant epileptic woman asks about pregnancy, it is appropriate to indicate that there is a small risk of her having a malformed child because of either the seizure disorder or the drugs used in its treatment. This risk is probably about double that for the nonepileptic (Speidel and Meadow, 1972; Janz, 1975; Smithells, 1976), but is still a very good (i.e., greater than 90 per cent) chance that she will have a normal child. The data currently available concerning the relative safety and therapeutic effectiveness of different anticonvulsant drugs in the management of pregnant epileptic patients are insufficient to guide the physician responsible for the care of such patients. It seems clear, however, that trimethadione should not be used, and valproic acid is probably best avoided. If valproic acid must be used, amniocentesis is advisable to detect any increase in alpha-fetoprotein levels (which is associated with neural tube defects), so that therapeutic abortion can be considered if necessary. Substitution of one anticonvulsant drug for another in epileptic women who are initially seen after the first trimester of pregnancy is best avoided, because major malformation of the fetus has probably occurred already if it is going to occur at all.

The principles of drug management of a seizure disorder in the pregnant woman are the same as in the nonpregnant woman. Anticonvulsant drugs are as necessary to epileptic patients during pregnancy as at other times. A detailed account of the drugs used in the treatment of epilepsy is unnecessary here; the interested reader is referred to standard neurologic textbooks for information in this regard. Several points are, however, worthy of comment. In the first place, a solitary seizure, unrelated to toxemia, should not lead to a diagnosis of epilepsy because there may be no further attacks. Only time will tell whether an individual who has a single seizure is going to have further attacks, thereby justifying a diagnosis of epilepsy and necessitating prophylactic anticonvulsant drug treatment. Although some physicians will start a patient on anticonvulsant medication following one convulsion, others prefer to withhold medication until the patient has had at least two seizures, at least in the nonpregnant state. During pregnancy, however, many physicians elect to initiate anticonvulsant therapy after even a single seizure and arrange for neurologic re-evaluation following delivery. This approach merits emphasis because many patients with so-called gestational epilepsy will have only a single convulsion, and continued treatment in such circumstances may therefore be unnecessary. Simple medical and neurologic investigations are indicated in an adult who has an isolated seizure and is otherwise well with no neurologic signs—hematologic and biochemical screening tests, EEG, and, particularly in the nonpregnant patient, magnetic resonance imaging (MRI) of the head and a chest x-ray. If the findings of such investigations are unremarkable, I discuss the controversial issue of anticonvulsant drug treatment with the patient but generally recommend that treatment be withheld unless a future attack occurs. Pregnant women experiencing two or more seizures clearly merit prophylactic anticonvulsant drug treatment. In those with a progressive history, abnormal neurologic signs, or a focal EEG abnormality, it is also necessary to exclude an underlying structural lesion by means of MRI of the head. The management of such a lesion is considered later in this chapter.

If prophylactic anticonvulsant drug treatment is necessary, it is generally continued until the patient has been seizure-free for at least 4 or 5 years. Treatment is started with a small dose of one of the anticonvulsants shown in Table 60–1, *depending on the type of seizure experienced by the patient and the considerations outlined earlier.* The dose is increased until seizures are controlled, blood concentrations reach the upper end of the optimal therapeutic range, or side effects limit further increments. If seizures continue despite optimal blood levels of the anticonvulsant drug selected, a second drug should be substituted for the first. Patients often respond preferentially to one or another of the various drugs that are available.

Patients must take medication as prescribed, and treatment should be controlled by frequent monitoring of the plasma anticonvulsant drug concentration. Monthly follow-up visits during pregnancy usually permit satisfactory supervision of the patient. In general, the most common reason for the plasma concentration of anticonvulsant medication to be lower than anticipated for the prescribed dose is the patient's poor compliance with her drug regimen, although as indicated earlier, other factors also can be responsible. Compliance can often be improved by encouragement and by explanation of the importance of taking medication regularly. Simplifying the dosage schedule so that medication is taken just once or twice daily may be helpful. As the pregnancy continues, the dose of anticonvulsant drug commonly needs to be increased to maintain plasma concentration at a level previously known to be effective. Indeed, in some instances, the required dose may reach a level that would probably cause toxic side effects in a nonpregnant patient. If anticonvulsant dosage is increased during the pregnancy, reductions will probably be necessary in the puerperium to prevent toxicity, but this change must be based on clinical evaluation and measurement of plasma concentration of the drug, because the period over which drug requirements decline varies considerably.

Folic acid supplements are often prescribed routinely during pregnancy, but it may be more sensible to withhold them from epileptic women experiencing more than about one seizure per month despite regular anticonvulsant drug treatment, unless the supplements are specifically indicated on hematologic grounds. Due to the poorly defined risks of increased obstetric complications among pregnant epileptic women, close supervision of such patients by the obstetrician is mandatory, and delivery in hospital is advised.

After delivery, the infant must be inspected for congenital malformations and given an injection of vitamin K_1 (1 mg/kg intramuscularly). Clotting factors should be studied after about 4 hours, and further

TABLE 60–1.   Drug Treatment of Seizures

TYPE OF SEIZURE	DRUG	USUAL DAILY DOSE* (mg/kg)	TIME TO REACH STEADY STATE (days)	OPTIMAL THERAPEUTIC BLOOD CONCENTRATION	MINIMUM NUMBER OF DAILY DOSES
Generalized tonic-clonic (grand mal) and/or simple or complex partial (focal)	Phenytoin	4–8	5–10	10–20 µg/ml	1
	Carbamazepine	5–25	3–4	4–8 µg/ml	2
	Phenobarbital	2–5	14–21	10–40 µg/ml	1
	Primidone	5–20	4–7	5–15 µg/ml	3
	Valproic acid	10–60	2–4	50–100 µg/ml	3
Absence (petit mal)	Ethosuximide	20–35	5–10	40–100 µg/ml	2
	Valproic acid	10–60	2–4	50–100 µg/ml	3
	Clonazepam	0.05–0.2	?	20–80 ng/ml	2
Myoclonus	Valproic acid	10–60	2–4	50–100 µg/ml	3
	Clonazepam	0.05–0.2	?	20–80 ng/ml	2

From Aminoff MJ: Drug treatment of epilepsy. Compr Ther 7:6, 1981.
*Nonpregnant.

injections of vitamin K_1 should be given if necessary. If hemorrhage occurs, infusions of fresh-frozen plasma or of factors II, VII, IX, and X may also be necessary. Breast-feeding of a healthy infant by an epileptic mother should not be discouraged.

HEADACHE

Headache is a common complaint and may have many causes. Among patients attending headache clinics, symptoms are most frequently attributed to migraine, tension, or depression. Tension headaches are commonly chronic, last all day, are worse in the evening, may have a tight quality to them, may be accompanied by local soreness and concern about lumps or bumps on head, and are often accompanied by poor concentration and nonspecific symptoms such as dizziness. The pain frequently commences, or is most intense, in the neck and the back of the head. If treatment with mild tranquilizers (such as diazepam or chlordiazepoxide) is unsuccessful, a trial of antimigraine preparations may be worthwhile. Depression headaches are somewhat similar but are often worse in the mornings, may be accompanied by other symptoms of depression, and often respond, to a limited extent, to tricyclic antidepressant drugs.

Most patients presenting with headache do not have severe underlying structural disease, but it is important to bear this possibility in mind. About a third of patients with brain tumors present with a primary complaint of headache. The headache in such patients is often an intermittent, dull, nonthrobbing ache that is exacerbated by exercise and may be associated with nausea or vomiting, but these features do not in themselves permit any reliable distinction from migraine. Similarly, the severity of the headache is unhelpful in this regard. Headaches that disturb sleep are, however, more suggestive of an underlying structural lesion, as also are exertional headaches and late-onset paroxysmal headaches. The duration and course of a headache also provide a guide to the underlying cause. A long history of chronic headache without other accompaniments is unlikely to reflect serious disease unless associated with drowsiness, visual disturbances, limb symptoms, seizures, intellectual changes, or other neurologic symptoms. The sudden development of severe headache in a previously well patient is more ominous and may well be due to acute intracranial abnormality such as subarachnoid hemorrhage, to glaucoma, or to another condition requiring specific treatment.

The evaluation of patients with headaches demands a full general and neurologic examination together with an assessment of mental status. It may be necessary to include examination of the teeth, eyes, paranasal sinuses, and urine and various investigative procedures may be indicated depending on the initial clinical impression. If intracranial disease is suspected on the basis of the history or the presence of neurologic signs, the need for a CT scan or MRI of the head, EEG, and examination of the cerebrospinal fluid must be decided on an individual basis. Both cranial arteritis and cervical spondylosis are important causes of headache but would not be expected among patients in the childbearing age group. Post-traumatic headaches generally pose no diagnostic problem because of the relationship to previous injury, and they usually respond to simple analgesics, mild tranquilizers, or antimigraine preparations. Acute sinusitis typically produces a localized throbbing headache accompanied by tenderness; the relationship of symptoms to a respiratory tract infection, and the radiologic findings, permit the diagnosis to be made with confidence, and treatment is directed at the underlying infection.

Migraine

Among women of childbearing age, migraine is an important cause of headache. In classic migraine, episodic headache is preceded by visual, sensory, or motor symptoms, but in other types there may be no premonitory focal symptoms. Headaches may be lateralized or generalized, generally have a gradual onset, and usually last for less than a day, although they may persist for longer. They may be dull or throbbing, are commonly accompanied by nausea, vomiting, and photophobia, and are often also associated with blurring of vision, lightheadedness, and scalp tenderness. Photopsia, fortification spectra, and/or other focal neurologic symptoms may precede or accompany the headache, and consciousness is sometimes impaired or lost (syncopal attacks or seizures).

About 60 per cent of women with migraine link the periodicity of some of their attacks to the menstrual cycle, the headaches occurring usually just before or during menstruation (Lance, 1973). Occasional patients may have headaches that occur only in relationship to the menstrual cycle, although this pattern is much less common. Several studies have failed to show any abnormality of hormonal cycles in women with migraine relating to menstruation (Somerville, 1972a; Epstein et al., 1975); however, migraine headache can be postponed by artificial maintenance of elevated plasma estradiol levels, even though menstruation occurs at the expected time (Somerville, 1972a). The manner in which such hormonal factors provoke migraine remains unclear at present.

Migraine headaches are commonly exacerbated in women using oral contraceptives, but improvement can occur in some patients (Ryan, 1978). Such exacerbation usually becomes apparent within the first few months of oral contraceptive use (Ryan, 1978). Preparations with a relatively higher estrogen content are most likely to influence the headache pattern and are generally not so well tolerated as low-estrogen preparations. Recurrent headache provoked by the use of oral contraceptives may persist despite withdrawal of the offending medications, but whether this is anything more than fortuitous is unclear (Raskin, 1988). Of special concern is evidence suggesting that women with migraine exacerbated by oral contraceptives have an increased risk of cerebral infarction (Collaborative Group, 1975), perhaps due to intimal hyperplasia of arteries supplying the brain (Irey et al., 1978).

Migraine often improves considerably after the first trimester of pregnancy, but it occasionally worsens or occurs for the first time during pregnancy, most commonly during the first 3 months of the gestational period (Somerville, 1972b). Lance (1973) found that relief occurred with pregnancy in 64 per cent of those whose attacks were menstrual and in 48 per cent of those with migraine unrelated to the menstrual cycle. The response of migraine to pregnancy does not correlate with sex of the fetus or with differences in plasma progesterone levels, although it may relate to changes in the pattern of circulating estrogens (Somerville, 1972b). Rotton and co-workers (1959) have suggested that the failure of migraine to improve during pregnancy implies a greater liability to pre-eclampsia, but further clinical studies are necessary to determine whether this is indeed the case.

The treatment of migraine consists of the avoidance of precipitating factors coupled with prophylactic or symptomatic drug treatment, if necessary. In general populations, when simple analgesics do not provide relief, treatment with extracranial vasoconstrictors (e.g., ergotamine or dihydroergotamine), beta-adrenergic blockers (propranolol), serotonin antagonists (e.g., methysergide), tricyclic antidepressants (amitriptyline), or other drugs may be necessary.

In general, treatment of headache during pregnancy should be with simple analgesics whenever possible, but acetaminophen is best used in preference to aspirin because aspirin usage in large doses in late pregnancy may prolong labor and increase the incidence of stillbirth (Niederhoff and Zahrodnik, 1983). A specific effort should be made to avoid ergotamine-containing preparations because of the effect that this drug may have on the gravid uterus. A comparison of the reproductive histories of 777 women with and 182 women without migraine revealed the incidence of miscarriage, stillbirth, and toxemia of pregnancy to be very similar (Wainscott et al., 1978). Also the incidence of congenital malformations among offspring of women with migraine was no greater than in the control group or in the general population, but the drug histories of the patients with migraine were incomplete. Large doses of ergotamine given to experimental animals in early pregnancy cause a number of complications, including fetal death, abortion, cataracts, and various developmental anomalies (Griffith et al., 1978). Ergonovine may induce chromosomal aberrations (Raskin, 1988). Propranolol is also best avoided during pregnancy, because it may mildly impair fetal growth (Schoenfeld et al., 1978) and may lead to beta-adrenergic blockade in the fetus or newborn. Such inhibition of normal beta-adrenergic responsiveness to asphyxia or to other stresses could theoretically increase the harmful effects of the latter (Rosen et al., 1979). Other reported neonatal complications include prematurity, respiratory depression, hypoglycemia, and hyperbilirubinemia (Ueland et al., 1981; Jackson and Fishbein, 1986).

Thus, management of migraine during pregnancy may be difficult. Treatment consists primarily of simple analgesics and—in some instances—sedatives. Beta blockers such as propranolol, which are usually effective and well tolerated, may have to be used for chronic or recurrent headaches despite their potential effects on the neonate. Cyproheptadine (4 to 16 mg daily as tolerated) may also help prophylactically. Dietary and other precipitants of headache should be avoided.

Postnatal Headache

In the order of one-third of women experience headaches in the week after delivery, and most of them have either a past or family history of migraine (Stein, 1981). The headaches, which are usually mild and bifrontal, generally respond well to simple analgesics and are self-limited.

TUMORS

Any type of intracranial tumor can occasionally appear during the gestational period, and accurate diagnosis may then be delayed because symptoms are erroneously ascribed to toxemia of pregnancy. In addition, although the relationship between the tumor and pregnancy is usually fortuitous, pituitary adenomas, meningiomas, neurofibromas, hemangioblastomas, and vascular malformations occasionally exhibit relapses in relation to pregnancy, with symptoms developing or rapidly worsening during gestation, remitting to some extent after delivery, and recurring in a subsequent pregnancy. In this chapter, attention is confined to those aspects of intracranial tumors that relate to pregnancy rather than to a more general account of intracranial neoplasms.

A number of early reports suggested that visual field defects sometimes develop during pregnancy and clear after delivery, owing to physiologic variation in size of the normal pituitary gland. This concept is now largely discounted, and it seems likely that the defects previously described did not have an organic basis (Walsh and Hoyt, 1969). It is important, however, to examine carefully the visual fields of patients complaining of impaired vision during pregnancy, because other causes of visual disturbance must be excluded, such as pituitary adenoma and craniopharyngioma.

Meningiomas in the suprasellar or parasellar region or on the medial sphenoidal wing may also produce symptoms, such as diplopia or unilateral scotoma or ptosis, that relapse and remit in relation to pregnancy over several years (Bickerstaff et al., 1958). Symptoms tend to develop in the last 4 months of gestation and often lead to a mistaken initial diagnosis of multiple sclerosis. Early surgical intervention may help to preserve vision and prevent other neurologic catastrophes.

Symptoms due to acoustic neuroma may begin or may be aggravated in the latter stages of pregnancy (Allen et al., 1974). Such symptoms in different patients include hearing loss, tinnitus, headaches, vertigo, dysequilibrium, facial weakness, and diplopia. Aggravation of symptoms in one pregnancy does not necessarily indicate that exacerbation will occur in subsequent ones.

In one study, six of 12 female patients with cerebellar hemangioblastomas were pregnant at the time of their first symptoms, but in each case at least one normal pregnancy had preceded the onset of symptoms (Robinson, 1965). Two underwent surgery in early pregnancy; one aborted shortly afterward, and the other carried her child to term. The other four patients all went into normal labor and were successfully treated for the tumors later.

How pregnancy may precipitate or exacerbate symptoms due to intracranial tumors is unclear, but the most likely explanation is that pregnancy leads to a slight increase in the size of the tumor, as can be demonstrated angiographically (Michelsen and New, 1969). Tumors with symptoms consistently related to pregnancy are usually so placed that only slight enlargement will lead to significant involvement of important neural structures. Thus, symptoms of spinal meningiomas may be exacerbated by pregnancy (O'Connell, 1962), but convexity meningiomas, which have room for expansion, are unlikely to show any particular relationship of symptoms to pregnancy. Several possibilities have been advanced to account for the manner in which pregnancy might influence tumor size. Suggested mechanisms include accelerated growth rate (Davis et al., 1950), vascular engorgement (King, 1950), and increased fluid content (Weyand et al., 1951); supportive evidence for these proposals is lacking. Nevertheless, there is accumulating evidence for sex steroid–binding sites in a number of human tumors, especially meningiomas (Schipper, 1986).

Patients with intracranial neoplasms may have non-specific symptoms of cerebral dysfunction, with evidence of raised intracranial pressure or with some characteristic combination of symptoms and signs that reflect the location of the lesion. As always, the history and physical findings guide the manner in which such patients are evaluated further. The judicious use of a number of investigative procedures—psychometry, EEG, cerebral evoked potential techniques, audiology, electronystagmography, lumbar puncture—may help to advance the diagnosis without exposing the pregnant patient or developing fetus to any risk. Magnetic resonance imaging or CT scanning of the head (Figs. 60–1 and 60–2) can now provide an enormous amount of additional information noninvasively. When radiologic investigations are necessary, shielding may help to protect the fetus from excessive radiation.

Each patient must be treated on an individual basis, and essential neurosurgical treatment should not be delayed because of the pregnancy. For pituitary adenomas or other benign tumors encountered in the latter half of pregnancy, operations can sometimes be delayed until a more propitious time, provided the patient is carefully followed. However, signs of increased intracranial pressure, visual deterioration, an increasing neurologic deficit, or the clinical features of an infratentorial lesion indicate the need for early or immediate intervention. For patients with pituitary adenomas, however, pharmacologic intervention (for example, with corticosteroids or bromocriptine) may be adequate, and in most instances visual disturbances improve spontaneously after delivery regardless of any pharmacologic measures (Simon, 1988).

In general, pregnancy can be allowed to proceed—at least until the fetus is viable, and often to term—in

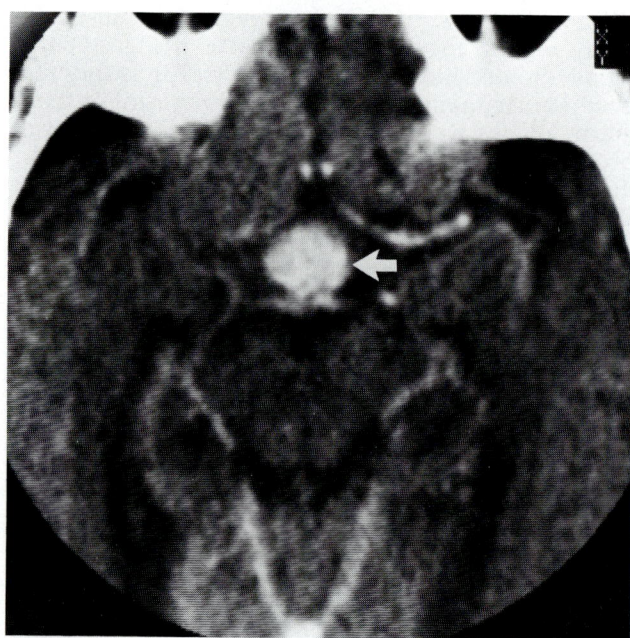

FIGURE 60–1. CT scan of a patient with a pituitary adenoma, showing an enhancing lesion *(arrow)* in the suprasellar cistern. More inferior axial scans showed this lesion to arise from the sella.

patients with intracranial neoplasms, but therapeutic abortion may well be justifiable for some patients with malignant brain tumors. It may also be justifiable if significant symptoms such as uncontrollable seizures occur during pregnancy, particularly when the tumor cannot be removed completely (Kempers and Miller,

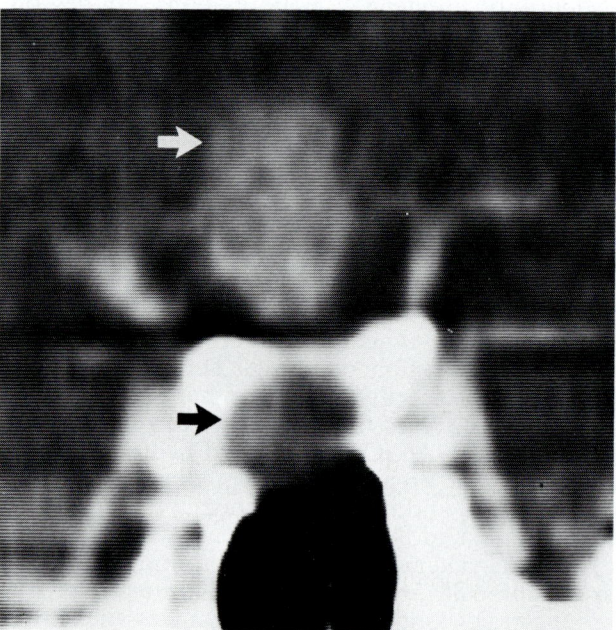

FIGURE 60–2. Coronal reformation of CT scan of same patient as in Figure 60–1. The intrasellar extent *(black arrow)* and suprasellar extent *(white arrow)* of the pituitary adenoma can be seen.

1963). Obstetric management must also be determined on an individual basis. Some investigators have proposed that delivery by cesarean section is safer than spontaneous vaginal delivery in women with cerebral tumors because the vaginal delivery may enhance any increase in intracranial pressure due to the neoplasm (Reeves, 1952). Vaginal delivery with adequate regional anesthesia and judicious shortening of the second stage of labor by use of low forceps (to prevent any increase in intracranial pressure that may be associated with the abdominal pushing efforts of this stage) is usually satisfactory, however.

PSEUDOTUMOR CEREBRI

There is a well-recognized association of benign intracranial hypertension with pregnancy and also with oral contraceptive preparations. When symptoms do develop during pregnancy, they are most likely to occur in the first trimester or the month after delivery, but they may occur at any time during the gestational period. Symptoms consist of headache and visual disturbances due to papilledema, and diplopia due to abducens weakness may also occur. The patient looks well despite the grossly abnormal appearance of the optic disks, and neither EEG nor MRI reveals any evidence of a space-occupying lesion. Although lumbar puncture will show the pressure of the cerebrospinal fluid to be increased, the composition of the fluid is unremarkable. The possibility of intracranial venous sinus thrombosis must be kept in mind when the patient is being evaluated. Although benign intracranial hypertension is self-limiting, remission may not occur till well after delivery, and the disorder sometimes recurs in a subsequent pregnancy. If the condition is left untreated, there is a risk of secondary optic atrophy and subsequent permanent impairment of vision. A number of different therapeutic approaches to lowering intracranial pressure have been reported, including use of high-dose steroids, acetazolamide, furosemide, repeated lumbar punctures, and lumboperitoneal or other shunting procedures. If the response to these measures is unsatisfactory and intracranial pressure remains high enough to endanger vision, optic nerve decompression may require consideration, as also may early delivery of the fetus. There are no specific obstetric complications, and the patient can be expected to give birth to a normal infant.

OCCLUSIVE CEREBROVASCULAR DISEASE

Cerebrovascular disease may develop during an otherwise normal pregnancy, owing to either arterial or venous disease. Pregnancy increases the risk of cerebral infarction to about 13 times the rate expected outside of pregnancy (Wiebers, 1985).

Arterial Occlusive Disease

Arterial disease is not unusual, even in the absence of diabetes or severe hypertension, in women of childbearing potential. Major arterial occlusion accounts for approximately two-thirds of the cases of nonhemorrhagic hemiplegia that develop during pregnancy or the puerperium (Jennett and Cross, 1967). Numerous cases of occlusion of the middle cerebral artery or one of the other major intracranial arteries have been described during pregnancy, occlusion generally occurring in the third trimester or the postpartum period. Such a stroke is usually due to the development of a thrombus on a preexisting atheromatous plaque, but predisposing factors may be anemia, hormonal influences, hypertension, changes in blood coagulation factors during late pregnancy, preeclamptic toxemia with hypertension, and puerperal septicemia. Other causes of stroke in young women include an arteritis, meningovascular syphilis, sickle cell disease, polycythemia and other hematologic disorders, and cardiomyopathy. An embolus secondary to rheumatic or ischemic heart disease, subacute bacterial endocarditis, or a cardiac myxoma may occur, and rare instances of arterial occlusion by paradoxic embolization from a pelvic vein via a patent foramen ovale have also been described (Sauer, 1955). Rarely, fat, air, or amniotic fluid embolism may occur in relation to childbirth.

Transient cerebral ischemic attacks may precede occlusion of one of the major intracranial arteries. The neurologic disorder and the underlying arterial disease must be investigated and treated as in nonpregnant patients. Investigations should include complete blood count, blood smear, sedimentation rate, serum cholesterol and triglyceride levels, prothrombin and partial thromboplastin times, EKG, echocardiography, and radiologic procedures. CT scanning is an important means of excluding intracranial hemorrhage. Angiography enables the major cerebral vessels to be visualized and may permit recognition of degenerative atherosclerotic disease that is remediable by disobliterative surgery (Fig. 60–3). When there is surgically inaccessible disease of the intracranial arteries, the possibility that the obstruction is serving as a source of emboli must be borne in mind, and consideration must therefore be given to treatment with anticoagulants or aspirin. Warfarin is best avoided if possible because it crosses the placenta and increases hemorrhagic complications, and especially during the first trimester because of the risks of teratogenicity and fetal wastage (Wiebers, 1985). Patients requiring anticoagulation during pregnancy are maintained instead on subcutaneously administered heparin, which usually is discontinued when labor begins and resumed about 12 hours after vaginal delivery or 24 hours after cesarean section. With regard to subsequent obstetric management, vaginal delivery, unless specifically contraindicated, is preferable to cesarean section.

Other diseases that may be associated with arterial occlusive disease in pregnancy, such as eclampsia or thrombotic thrombocytopenia purpura, are considered in detail in Chapters 48 and 49.

Intracranial Venous Occlusive Disease

Intracranial venous occlusive disease is an uncommon complication of pregnancy or childbirth. When

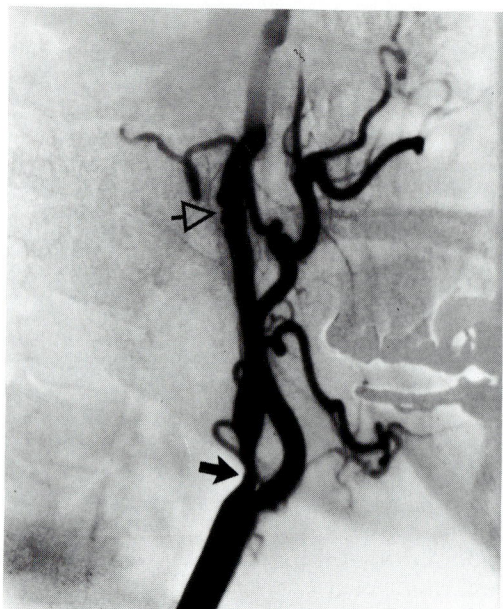

FIGURE 60–3. Common carotid angiogram showing atherosclerotic narrowing of the internal carotid artery *(solid arrow)* at its origin. There is some corrugation of the internal carotid artery more rostrally at the level of C1 and C2, reflecting fibromuscular dysplasia *(open arrow)*.

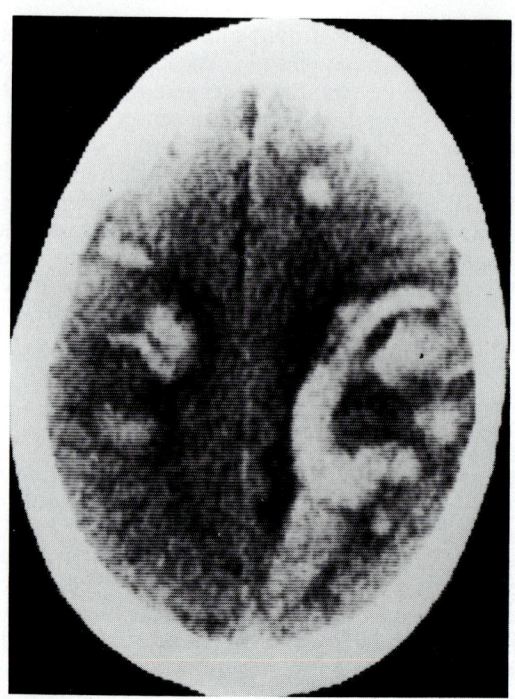

FIGURE 60–4. Patient with superior sagittal sinus thrombosis. CT scan showing curvilinear areas of high density representing cortical venous thromboses and adjacent parenchymal venous infarcts.

the thrombosis occurs in the first trimester of pregnancy, it usually follows some complication such as spontaneous abortion (Symonds, 1940), therapeutic abortion (Lunz, 1926), or stillbirth (Martin, 1941), but it may occur in an otherwise normal pregnancy (Fishman et al., 1957; Stevens and Ammerman, 1959; Eckerling et al., 1963). Intracranial venous thrombosis is more likely to occur in the third trimester or the puerperium (Kendall, 1948; Hyland, 1950) and is sometimes related to preeclampsia (Carroll et al., 1966).

Intracranial venous thrombosis is characterized clinically by headache, paresis, focal or generalized convulsions, drowsiness, and confusion; disturbances of speech, sensation, or vision are not uncommon, and a mild pyrexia may be present. There may be signs of meningeal irritation caused by subarachnoid bleeding secondary to cortical infarction, and fluctuating hypertension is sometimes found (Stevens, 1954; Goldman et al., 1964). Papilledema may be present, particularly if the superior sagittal sinus is involved. The cerebrospinal fluid pressure may be increased, and often the protein or cell content is elevated; occasionally the fluid is frankly blood-stained. The diagnosis may be confirmed by CT scanning and MR angiography, which are also necessary to exclude arterial pathology and vascular malformation (Figs. 60–4 and 60–5).

The symptoms and signs of intracranial venous thrombosis are sometimes ascribed mistakenly to eclampsia, but the absence of previous signs of preeclampsia should help in preventing diagnostic confusion.

The prognosis is not encouraging. In about one-third of cases, intracranial venous thrombosis has a

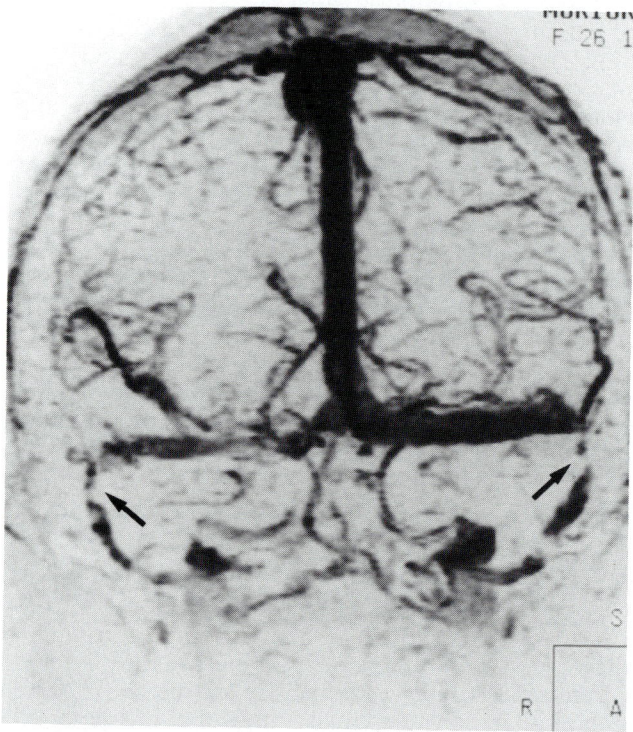

FIGURE 60–5. A 26-year-old woman presented in the middle trimester of pregnancy with headache and had bilateral papilledema. Imaging studies of the brain were normal. This coronal view of her MR venogram (obtained using a two-dimensional time-of-flight technique) shows loss of flow-related enhancement in both transverse sinuses *(arrows)* consistent with thrombus formation.

fatal outcome. Moreover, if patients do survive, thrombosis may recur later in the same pregnancy or the puerperium (Koller et al., 1957; Goldman et al., 1964), or in subsequent pregnancies (Garcin and Pestel, 1949).

The etiologic basis of aseptic intracranial venous thrombosis is uncertain; coagulation abnormalities, changes in the constituents of the peripheral blood, and intimal damage to the dural sinuses (Kendall, 1948) are possible causes. Martin (1941) suggested that retrograde venous embolism from the pelvic veins via their connections with the vertebral venous system may be responsible. Kendall (1948) argued against this hypothesis, however, and Carroll and associates (1966) found that in only seven of 34 cases of autopsy-verified cerebral venous thrombosis was there evidence of thrombosed pelvic or leg veins.

The treatment of intracranial venous thrombosis is controversial. It may include anticonvulsant drugs if seizures have occurred, and antiedema agents such as dexamethasone and mannitol to reduce the intracranial pressure. Anticoagulant drugs have been used in the belief that they may prevent extension of thrombosis, but may provoke hemorrhagic intracranial complications (Gettelfinger and Kokmen, 1977). The risk of intracranial hemorrhage has probably been exaggerated, and a recent study suggests that anticoagulation with dose-adjusted intravenous heparin is effective treatment for venous sinus thrombosis (Einhaupl et al., 1991).

Labor can usually be allowed to commence spontaneously, with forceps assistance of delivery, if the thrombosis has occurred early in pregnancy. If thrombosis occurs shortly before or during labor, however, cesarean section may be necessary.

PITUITARY INFARCTION. Sheehan's syndrome is a well-recognized complication of the peripartum period; it is discussed in detail in Chapter 56.

INTRACRANIAL (SUBARACHNOID) HEMORRHAGE

When intracranial hemorrhage occurs during pregnancy, it is usually, at least in part, into the subarachnoid space. Sudden severe headache, sometimes accompanied by nausea and vomiting, is the main symptom, and examination reveals signs of meningeal irritation that may be accompanied by depressed consciousness, cranial nerve abnormalities, and a neurologic deficit in the limbs.

In one series of 21 patients in whom subarachnoid hemorrhage complicated otherwise normal pregnancies, the underlying source was an aneurysm in 12, an angioma in four, and undetermined in five (Cannell, 1959). In a more recent series of 52 patients the corresponding figures were 21, 19, and 12, respectively (Amias, 1970). Although bleeding may occur at any time during the pregnancy, aneurysms are somewhat more likely to bleed in the latter half of the gestational period.

Cerebral angiomas, which are located supratentorially in at least 70 per cent of patients, may appear at any age. Intracranial or subarachnoid hemorrhage is the most common presentation. The peak age for hemorrhage is between 15 and 20 years, and about 70 per cent of all angiomas that are going to bleed will have done so by the time patients reach the age of 40 (Perret and Nishioka, 1966). The mortality rate from an initial hemorrhage is approximately 10 per cent, and the survivors are more likely to develop further hemorrhage than patients who have never had one. Other patients with intracranial angiomas may present with focal or generalized seizures, headache, focal neurologic deficits, or nonspecific neurologic symptoms. Robinson and colleagues (1974) reported that pregnancy has a deleterious effect on intracranial angiomas, making them more likely to bleed, but their impression has not been substantiated by others (Parkinson and Bachers, 1980; Horton et al., 1990).

Intracranial saccular aneurysms arise from a developmental arterial defect, and with increasing age they become more common sources of hemorrhage than angiomas. They are generally located at sites of vessel branching, occurring with particular frequency in relation to the anterior or posterior communicating arteries. Although such aneurysms sometimes cause focal symptoms that relate to compression of neighboring structures, patients generally present with hemorrhage that occurs without warning, owing to aneurysmal rupture. In addition to the signs of subarachnoid hemorrhage, focal or lateralizing neurologic signs may be present and help to localize the source of bleeding.

In the evaluation of patients presenting with symptoms of intracranial hemorrhage, the first diagnostic study now performed is usually a CT scan of the head, which is a reliable means of detecting recent subarachnoid or intracerebral hemorrhage and may permit the source of bleeding to be localized (Fig. 60–6). In patients with angiomas, nonhomogeneous areas of mixed density with irregular calcifications are typical, and vermiform areas of enhancement are seen after infusion of contrast material. Aneurysms are seen as small round dense areas after infusion of contrast material, and are sometimes evident even without contrast. If the CT findings are normal, the cerebrospinal fluid should be examined, and angiography should be undertaken if the fluid is blood-stained or xanthochromic.

Angiography permits the identity of the lesion to be established with certainty and provides important additional information concerning its anatomic features (Fig. 60–7). Special shielding during this and other radiologic procedures should be provided for pregnant patients. All of the major intracranial vessels should be opacified; feeding vessels to angiomas sometimes arise from the contralateral side, and it is not uncommon for aneurysms to be multiple. Angiography fails to reveal the malformation in the occasional patient with a suspected angioma, possibly because the lesion was small and destroyed itself when it bled ("cryptic malformation"). Nevertheless, if angiography shows neither an angioma nor an aneurysm in a patient presenting with subarachnoid hemorrhage, the study should be repeated after about 14 days, because vascular spasm following a bleed may obscure an aneurysm.

The management of subarachnoid hemorrhage consists of bed rest, with sedation and analgesia as necessary and operative treatment of the underlying lesion if feasible. Surgical treatment is aimed at preventing further hemorrhages, but induction of hypotension during the course of the intracranial operation should be avoided unless it is essential because it may be followed by premature labor or fetal death; hypothermia is well tolerated (Robinson et al., 1974). If the anomalous vessels constituting an angioma are surgically accessible and do not involve a critical vessel or area of the brain, they can often be excised. Such surgery is commonly preceded by embolization of the main vessels feeding the malformation, in an attempt to reduce the size of the latter. A number of other obliterative techniques are being developed (Aminoff, 1983). In the patient with an aneurysm that has bled, there is a much greater risk of further bleeding, especially in the weeks following the initial hemorrhage. Accordingly, operative treatment, if indicated by the angiographic findings and the condition of the patient, should not be delayed because of the pregnancy.

In patients with aneurysms that have been successfully obliterated or that ruptured before the last trimester, pregnancy and delivery can generally be allowed to proceed normally. In patients with incompletely obliterated or unoperated aneurysms that ruptured in the last 2 months of pregnancy, cesarean section is probably advisable at 38 weeks gestation. Some authorities also advocate delivery by elective cesarean section at 38 weeks in patients with arteriovenous malformations and further recommend that concomitant sterilization be considered (Robinson et al., 1974),

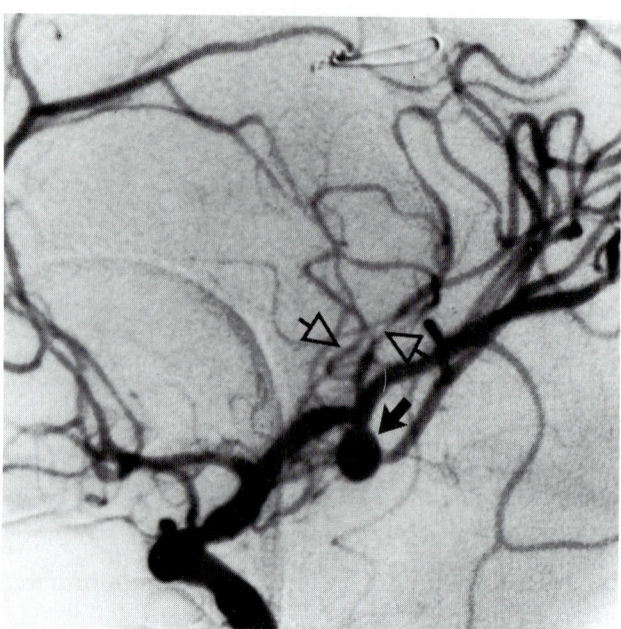

FIGURE 60–7. Carotid angiogram of the same patient as in the previous figure. An aneurysm *(solid arrow)* is shown at the trifurcation of the middle cerebral artery. There is some spasm of vessels in the vicinity of the aneurysm *(open arrows).*

presumably if the malformation itself is inoperable. However, the need for either procedure in this context is unclear, and arguments for them are without adequate foundation. In patients showing a steady deterioration in neurologic status and for whom a fatal outcome seems likely, preparations will have to be made so that the fetus—if viable—can be delivered before it dies from anoxia.

In rare instances, intracranial hemorrhages result from mycotic aneurysms, vasculitides, and various hematologic disorders, or are manifestations of choriocarcinoma. Treatment is of the underlying cause.

VASCULAR ANOMALIES AND THE NERVOUS SYSTEM

The most important vascular anomalies that occur in relation to the nervous system are intracranial aneurysms and cerebral angiomas, which are considered in the preceding discussion of subarachnoid hemorrhage. Several other types of vascular anomalies may, however, become manifested during pregnancy and merit brief discussion.

Intracranial Dural Vascular Anomalies

Certain intracranial dural vascular anomalies may become evident for the first time during pregnancy. They consist of abnormal arteriovenous shunts involving meningeal branches of the carotid and vertebral arteries and the dural veins and sinuses. Although some represent a developmental anomaly, others are acquired in adult life, occasionally following trauma,

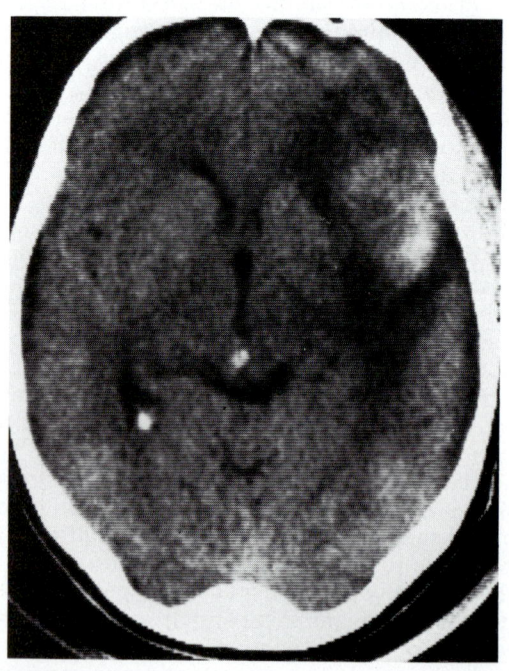

FIGURE 60–6. CT scan showing hemorrhage into the sylvian fissure and adjacent parenchyma, with surrounding edema and/or ischemia. The findings are indicative of subarachnoid and intracerebral hemorrhage, and localize the source of bleeding to the middle cerebral artery.

presumably because of the close anatomic relationship of certain meningeal arteries and veins. A detailed account of these anomalies is provided by Aminoff (1983).

Shunts involving the anterior-inferior group of dural sinuses (cavernous, intercavernous, sphenoparietal, superior and inferior petrosal, and basilar plexus) are characterized clinically by unilateral orbital or head pain, diplopia, a red or protruding eye, and/or tinnitus. The onset of symptoms sometimes follows abortion or relates to the postpartum period (Newton and Hoyt, 1970; Taniguchi et al., 1971), possibly because of rupture of the thin-walled dural arteries during the straining of labor or because of the circulatory changes that occur in pregnancy. On examination, there is usually a mild proptosis, distended conjunctival veins, increased intraocular pressure, a transient sixth nerve palsy, and/or a bruit over the eye. Angiography reveals a low-volume shunt supplied from meningeal branches of the internal and/or external carotid arteries, sometimes from the contralateral side. Drainage may be directly into the cavernous sinus or into a more distant dural sinus or venous structure that communicates with the cavernous sinus. The fistula may close spontaneously, but if it remains patent, embolization of the feeding vessels may help to relieve intolerable symptoms or failing vision.

Arteriovenous shunts to the superior-posterior group of dural sinuses (superior and inferior sagittal, straight, transverse, sigmoid, and occipital) may also occur, with a female predominance among the reported cases. Symptoms and signs may relate to the shunt itself, to subarachnoid hemorrhage, to increased intracranial pressure, or to cerebral ischemia. Tinnitus is the most common complaint, but headache, visual deterioration, subarachnoid hemorrhage, seizures, and various neurologic deficits may also occur. A bruit is often present and may be the sole finding on examination; it is best heard over the mastoid region or behind the ear. Papilledema may be present, and other neurologic signs are sometimes encountered. The arterial supply is commonly from branches of the external carotid artery, tentorial branches of the internal carotid artery, and meningeal branches of the vertebral artery. Ligation or embolization of feeding vessels or a direct surgical approach to the lesion may be helpful in patients with disabling symptoms or a history of hemorrhage.

Dural and Intradural Spinal Angiomas

Spinal angiomas are uncommon but are important to recognize because most are readily treated by surgery. The majority are arteriovenous malformations, and most of these are dural; if intradural, they are commonly extramedullary, are posterior to the cord, and are fed by one or more arteries that either fail to supply the cord or contribute only to the posterior spinal circulation (Aminoff, 1976).

Spinal arteriovenous malformations may lead to spinal subarachnoid hemorrhage but more commonly give rise to a gradual disturbance in function of cord, nerve roots, or both. Spinal subarachnoid hemorrhage

is much more common in patients with a cervical malformation than a more caudal lesion, may sometimes occur from an associated (arterial) aneurysm, and is associated with an overall mortality of at least 15 per cent. It may be the first symptom produced by the lesion. Approximately half of the patients who survive the first hemorrhage have a second, and half of the subsequent survivors have further bleeding episodes unless the underlying malformation is treated. The spinal source of the hemorrhage may not be recognized until the later development of symptoms and signs of cord dysfunction, despite the local occurrence of sudden severe pain at the onset of bleeding, accompanied by signs of meningeal irritation.

Myelopathy or radiculopathy, or both, of gradual or sudden onset, is the more common mode of presentation, and by the time of diagnosis approximately two-thirds of patients complain of leg weakness, sensory symptoms, pain, and a sphincter disturbance. In some patients, symptoms, especially pain, are precipitated or aggravated by exercise and relieved by rest, whereas in other patients they may relate to specific postures, such as sitting or bending forward. Symptoms occasionally relate to pregnancy, the menstrual cycle, nonspecific infective illness, a transient increase in body temperature, or trauma. On examination, signs of an upper or lower motor neuron disturbance—or of a mixed motor deficit—are usually found in the legs; sensory deficits are common and are usually extensive, but occasionally are restricted to a radicular distribution. There may be a coexisting cutaneous angioma that occasionally relates segmentally to the spinal lesion, and a bruit may be audible over the spine on auscultation.

Numerous case reports illustrating the influence of pregnancy on these lesions have been published. In one case encountered personally by me, symptoms occurred during each of three pregnancies, with complete clearing after delivery, and their basis was not recognized until the patient later developed leg weakness and urinary retention that necessitated immediate hospitalization; myelography and spinal angiography then demonstrated an arteriovenous malformation that was treated surgically. The relationship of symptoms to pregnancy in such cases may be based in part on enhancement of preexisting cord ischemia by hemodilution and anemia; moreover, pressure on pelvic and abdominal veins by an enlarged uterus may aggravate symptoms of caudally situated malformations by obstructing venous return to the heart, with a consequent reduction in intramedullary arteriovenous pressure gradient and thus in cord blood flow (Aminoff, 1976).

Diagnosis depends on radiologic investigations, which must not be postponed out of concern for the developing fetus, because any delay in establishing the diagnosis may lead to increased, often irreversible, disability in the mother. Spinal MRI may fail to detect the lesion. At myelography, the characteristic abnormality consists of vermiform defects due to vascular impressions in the column of contrast material, usually without any obstruction in the subarachnoid space. If myelography suggests a vascular malformation, spinal angiography is undertaken to determine the level and extent of the vascular abnormality; the position of the arteriovenous shunt in relation to the cord; the number, origin, and anatomic location of arteries feeding the malformation; and the main supply to the cord in the region of the malformation.

Treatment is indicated in all patients who have progressive symptoms or functional incapacity or have had a hemorrhage. Delay in these cases may lead to irreversible disability or even death. When the angioma is dural or intradural but mainly or completely extramedullary, is posterior to the cord, and is fed by vessels that do not contribute to the anterior spinal circulation, surgical treatment or embolization generally poses no specific problem. Feeding vessels are obliterated, and the fistulous portion of the malformation is removed. Malformations located anterior to or within the cord are more difficult to treat because of their inaccessibility and because they are often supplied by the anterior spinal artery or one of its feeders. Such lesions are often regarded as inoperable, and experience in their treatment remains limited.

INFECTIONS

The central nervous system may be infected by bacterial, viral, fungal, or other organisms through the blood supply, by extension from infected adjacent structures, or by direct inoculation such as may follow trauma. The neural parenchyma may be involved diffusely (as in encephalitis) or focally (as with cerebral abscess), or infection may primarily involve the meninges and parameningeal structures (such as in meningitis or subdural empyema). Although the resulting neurologic disorder may complicate pregnancy or delivery or may necessitate antimicrobial therapy that can harm the developing fetus, the clinical features, diagnosis, and management of such infections during pregnancy are essentially the same as at other times. Accordingly, further discussion is limited to certain infections that either pose some particular problem when they occur during pregnancy or are especially likely to develop in relation to pregnancy.

Poliomyelitis

The development of an effective vaccine has all but eradicated paralytic poliomyelitis in developed countries. Nevertheless, the disorder still occurs in unprotected persons and remains common in many parts of the world. Moreover, patients with residual disability from previous poliomyelitis are still seen fairly regularly in most large medical centers; obstetric management of such patients may be complicated by their neurologic deficits.

Most patients infected with polio virus either are asymptomatic or have only minor, nonspecific respiratory or gastrointestinal symptoms. Nervous system involvement occurs in only a few instances; its clinical manifestations are described in standard neurologic textbooks. Patients with neurologic involvement should be hospitalized, care being taken to provide

for any circulatory or respiratory complications that may develop. Simple analgesics can be provided for relief of pain, and physical therapy may be helpful once muscle weakness has stabilized.

Pregnancy increases the susceptibility of women to clinical poliomyelitis (Weinstein et al., 1951). In one large series of patients admitted with poliomyelitis, 34 per cent of the married women and 26 per cent of all the women of reproductive age were pregnant (Hunter and Millikan, 1954). It is unclear, however, whether pregnant women become more susceptible to the initial viral infection or whether they merely become more susceptible to invasion of the nervous system. Pregnancy may also alter the course of the infection. The course is unaffected in women who develop poliomyelitis early in pregnancy, but an increase in severity or distribution of the muscle weakness may occur if childbirth takes place during the acute phase or shortly thereafter (Weinstein et al., 1951).

In early pregnancy, and especially during the first trimester, spontaneous abortion may occur either in association with a febrile reaction in the acute phase of poliomyelitis, or in relation to apparently mild, nonparalytic attacks of the disease. Abortion or fetal loss may also occur spontaneously in the second or third trimester, but often then with maternal illness of such severity that assisted respiration may be necessary.

Even patients with severe poliomyelitis necessitating respirator assistance can usually be managed supportively, and labor managed similarly to that in normal women, unless there are specific obstetric indications for operative delivery or induction of labor. The uterine muscle is not paralyzed.

Fetal poliomyelitis is exceedingly rare; normal offspring can generally be anticipated, although Schaeffer and colleagues (1954) reported the presence of the virus in both fetus and placenta following spontaneous abortion that occurred 11 days after a clinical attack of poliomyelitis in a 24-year-old woman. Neonatal cases of poliomyelitis are well-recognized (Abramson et al., 1953). If an infant is affected within the first 5 days of life, the disorder is assumed to be secondary to transplacental transmission of the virus. Such neonatal cases are associated with a mortality rate of at least 50 per cent, but subclinical infection with poliovirus may certainly also occur in newborn infants (Shelokov and Habel, 1956).

Tetanus

This worldwide disease is rarely encountered in developed countries where immunization procedures are freely available. *Clostridium tetani* infection via tetanus spores may follow injury, surgical procedures, childbirth, abortion, and injections. If the spores are converted into vegetative gram-positive rods and favorable anaerobic conditions are present, tetanospasmin, a toxin that is responsible for the symptoms of tetanus, is produced.

The incubation period is variable. In generalized tetanus the most common presenting symptom is trismus, and the disorder itself is characterized by frequent spasms of various muscles that can be provoked by minor external stimuli and may occur against a background of continuous tonic muscle contractions. Typically, the trunk is hyperextended, the arms are flexed, and the legs are extended; laryngospasm may lead to respiratory obstruction.

Localized tetanus is more benign. It is characterized by persistent rigidity of muscles close to the site of inoculation with the organism. A splanchnic form is described following abdominal and pelvic operations or uterine trauma, with prominent involvement of the muscles of deglutition and respiration.

The morbidity and mortality rates also vary. Respiratory complications are a leading cause of death, as is the autonomic hyperactivity that sometimes complicates tetanus. Treatment is directed at neutralizing unbound toxin with antitoxin; reducing further toxin production by surgical toilet and antibiotic treatment; controlling tetanic spasms by drugs such as diazepam, chlorpromazine, and barbiturates; assisting respiration mechanically if necessary; and undertaking general supportive measures.

Tetanus may develop as a complication of childbirth or abortion, especially in underdeveloped countries. Adadevoh and Akinla (1970) reported 27 cases of tetanus in relation to pregnancy that were seen at a university teaching hospital in Africa between 1963 and 1967. Twenty-two of the cases were associated with abortion and carried a mortality rate of 50 per cent, and one of the five postpartum cases also ended in death. Even higher mortality rates have been reported in other series of patients with postpartum or postabortion tetanus. In addition to the measures just listed, evacuation of products retained in the uterus may be necessary, and hysterectomy is sometimes required (Speroff, 1966; Reid, 1967).

Tetanus is also a common cause of neonatal death in underdeveloped countries. Infection usually results from a lack of hygiene during delivery, with consequent contamination of the umbilical cord. The clinical manifestations differ from those in older children or adults in that dysphagia and respiratory problems are often more marked, fever is usually higher, and the disease is generally more severe, often fulminating. Most affected infants are 6 to 9 days old when admitted and have a typical history of continuous crying for up to 48 hours, followed by cessation of sucking and then of crying, accompanied by convulsions and often by fever; the overall mortality rate was 73 per cent in a series of 319 cases, most deaths occurring within 48 hours of admission (Athavale and Pai, 1965).

In regions where neonatal tetanus is common, the mortality rate may approach 10 per cent of births. Improvement of delivery practices and obstetric services may prevent the disorder, as may the active immunization of pregnant women. Unfortunately, in most areas with a high incidence of tetanus neonatorum, there are no widely available maternity services, and any prophylactic approach that depends on the early identification of pregnant women is impractical. In one series, however, immunization of women with two or three intramuscular injections of tetanus toxoid resulted in complete absence of neonatal tetanus among the children of subsequent pregnancies for more than 4 years (Newell et al., 1966).

Miscellaneous Maternal Infections

Clinical or subclinical maternal infection may involve the fetus and may affect the developing nervous system, and thus the neonate. The resulting neurologic complications merit brief comment here. Fetal infection may be inconsequential or may result in abortion, stillbirth, growth retardation, congenital disease, or developmental anomalies. Gestational age at the time of infection influences the effects (see Chapter 42 for further details).

Infection with *Listeria monocytogenes* is an important cause of habitual abortion and may also lead to a variety of other manifestations in pregnant women. In neonates, infection may take an early-onset, predominantly septicemic form characterized by prematurity, respiratory distress, heart failure, and increased neonatal mortality, or a late-onset, predominantly meningitic or meningoencephalitic form. Diagnosis depends on the bacteriologic and serologic findings. Treatment consists of appropriate antibiotic therapy, usually with ampicillin.

Maternal rubella, especially when it occurs in the first 2 months of pregnancy, may cause fetal infection and a congenital syndrome characterized by ocular abnormalities, deafness, mental retardation, seizures, focal neurologic deficits, cardiac anomalies, hepatosplenomegaly, and other abnormalities in a variety of combinations. In rare patients with congenital rubella, pyramidal and extrapyramidal signs, seizures, and dementia occur as part of a progressive panencephalitic illness during the second decade of life; high antibody titers to rubella virus occur in blood and cerebrospinal fluid, and the virus may even be isolated from the brain (Townsend et al., 1975; Weil et al., 1975).

In *congenital toxoplasmosis*, seizures and pyramidal defects may result from meningoencephalitis, together with chorioretinitis, obstructive hydrocephalus, and cerebral calcification. There may be respiratory and feeding difficulties. Later mental development may be retarded. For prophylactic purposes, pregnant women should be advised to avoid contact with cat feces and ingestion of raw or undercooked meat.

Fetal infections with *cytomegalovirus* may cause hepatosplenomegaly, jaundice, petechiae, ocular defects, cardiac defects, and other abnormalities. Involvement of the nervous system may lead to cerebral malformation, microcephaly, mental retardation, seizures, obstructive hydrocephalus, cerebral calcification, deafness, or chorioretinitis.

Herpes simplex virus infection in the neonate is characterized primarily by visceral involvement, but the brain may be affected. Seizures, irritability, motor deficits, increased intracranial pressure, and depression of consciousness may all occur, sometimes in the apparent absence of more widespread disease.

Children born to women infected with the *human immunodeficiency virus* (HIV) are at risk of developing acquired immunodeficiency syndrome (AIDS) after an interval ranging from several months to several years. This leads typically to developmental delay and regression due to a progressive encephalopathy. A variety of systemic manifestations may also develop (Shannon and Amman, 1985).

The possibility of *syphilitic infection* must be borne in mind during the evaluation of all pregnant women. Effective treatment of maternal syphilis at an early stage of pregnancy generally prevents fetal involvement, and treatment in later pregnancy affects both mother and fetus. Syphilis may severely affect pregnancy, leading to increased chances of abortion and perinatal mortality and to symptomatic congenital syphilis in many of the surviving infants. Infants may also be infected at birth if they come into contact with an infective lesion. The possibility of congenital infection can be confirmed by various serologic tests. The clinical features of congenital neurosyphilis, which may become apparent after the first few weeks of life or may be delayed for several years, are essentially the same as those of neurosyphilis in adults. Infants with clinical or laboratory evidence of infection require treatment to prevent its occurrence, penicillin being the drug of choice.

METABOLIC DISORDERS

A number of metabolic disorders are considered elsewhere in this chapter, including Wilson's disease, hepatic porphyria, and the Wernicke-Korsakoff syndrome. In this section, attention is confined to two other disorders that are important to recognize for therapeutic purposes.

Vitamin B$_{12}$ Deficiency

Vitamin B$_{12}$ deficiency is a well-known cause of neurologic disease (myelopathy characterized predominantly by pyramidal and posterior column deficits, polyneuropathy, mental changes, optic neuropathy) in adults, in whom it may arise from malabsorption, dietary inadequacy, or other causes. There is often an accompanying megaloblastic anemia, but this may be obscured if folic acid supplements have been taken. Clinical presentation during pregnancy does not differ from that in the nongestational period. Treatment with parenteral vitamin B$_{12}$ prevents further progression and may lead to improvement, at least in part, of the neurologic disorder.

It is not widely recognized that maternal vitamin B$_{12}$ deficiency during pregnancy and the puerperium may lead to a similar deficiency in the fetus and neonate. A reduced content of vitamin B$_{12}$ in maternal milk may then lead to frank deficiency in breast-fed infants. The resulting clinical syndrome among such infants is characterized by megaloblastic anemia, cutaneous pigmentation, apathy, developmental delay or regression, and involuntary movements (Jadhav et al., 1962). The clinical and biochemical abnormalities are rapidly corrected by vitamin supplementation.

Phenylketonuria

An autosomal recessive disorder, phenylketonuria (PKU), is an important cause of mental retardation, which develops in the absence of adequate dietary treatment. Screening programs for neonates with phenylketonuria have permitted the identification and treatment of affected infants to prevent intellectual deterioration, but the optimal duration of treatment remains unclear (for a review, see Scriver and Clow, 1980). It has become apparent that women with PKU have a high rate of spontaneous abortion, and that their nonphenylketonuric (heterozygote) offspring have a high incidence of certain abnormalities. Among the offspring resulting from pregnancies during which the maternal PKU is untreated, there are marked increases in the incidence of mental retardation, microcephaly, and congenital heart disease compared with the normal population, and these increases correlate with maternal blood levels of phenylalanine (Lenke and Levy, 1980).

The cause of these fetal effects of maternal PKU is not entirely clear. Dietary treatment during pregnancy has not proved effective in preventing the fetal effects, but treatment of women known to have PKU may have to be re-initiated before conception—and to be in effect at conception—for maximal benefit in this regard. Even so, a normal child cannot be assured. The mother with undiagnosed PKU poses different problems. Antenatal screening for maternal PKU—or testing for PKU at the first antenatal visit of a woman with a family history of the disease, low intelligence of uncertain etiology, or a history of microcephalic offspring—may well be justifiable (Lancet, 1979).

The newborn offspring of a mother with PKU will be homozygous or heterozygous for the disorder. The homozygotes clearly require a diet low in phenylalanine, but the proper nutritional management of heterozygotes is less clear. The mother, however, should be advised against breast-feeding because her milk will contain a high concentration of phenylalanine (Lancet, 1979).

There is only minimal elevation of blood phenylalanine during pregnancy in mothers who are heterozygous for the disorder, and the incidence of congenital anomalies and brain damage is not excessive in their offspring, save for congenital pyloric stenosis (Scriver and Clow, 1980).

MOVEMENT DISORDERS

Chorea Gravidarum

The term chorea refers to involuntary rapid muscle jerks that occur unpredictably in different parts of the body. When the disorder is florid, choreic limb movements and facial grimacing are unmistakable and distort any concomitant voluntary activity, but in mild cases there may be no more than a persistent restlessness and clumsiness.

Sydenham's chorea is generally regarded as a complication of infection with group A hemolytic streptococci, the underlying pathology possibly being an arteritis. When it occurs during pregnancy, it is referred to as *chorea gravidarum*. This disease occurs most commonly in primigravidas, with symptoms tending to occur in the early part of pregnancy and remitting after delivery. A history of chorea and rheumatic fever is obtained in about two-thirds of patients, and the other third have clinical signs of rheumatic heart disease. Psychological disturbance may occasionally be conspicuous. Willson and Preece (1932) found 20 per cent of women with the disorder to have a recurrence in later pregnancies. Death, due primarily to underlying rheumatic heart disease, is rare (Beresford and Graham, 1950). Symptomatic benefit follows bed rest and sedation, and there is no indication for termination of pregnancy. The prognosis is essentially that of any cardiac complication. No specific obstetric complications are associated with chorea gravidarum, and a normal, healthy infant can generally be anticipated.

Although many cases of chorea gravidarum relate to preceding streptococcal infection, in other instances there is no clinical or laboratory evidence of such an association and clinical impression suggests instead that pregnancy has, in some way, merely exacerbated some preexisting disturbance that then becomes clinically evident. Similarly, chorea is occasionally induced by oral contraceptives in women with preexisting basal ganglia abnormalities due to various causes. The dyskinesia in such cases usually begins within about 3 months of the introduction of contraceptive therapy, evolves subacutely, is often asymmetric or unilateral, and resolves with discontinuation of the offending substance. The pathophysiologic basis of hormonal contraceptive-induced chorea is uncertain, but a vascular mechanism (Lewis and Harrison, 1969), an immunologic mechanism (Gamboa et al., 1971), and a hormone-dependent alteration in central dopaminergic activity (Nausieda et al., 1979) have tentatively been advanced as the underlying causes.

Barber and colleagues (1976) described a young woman with hemichorea that developed with the use of oral contraceptives, later recurred in early pregnancy, and cleared after therapeutic abortion. Subsequent challenge with a combined estrogen/progestogen pill led to recurrence of chorea, but the patient was then successfully managed on progestogen alone without further symptoms, suggesting that the estrogen component was responsible for the dyskinesia. Estrogens may certainly influence catecholamine turnover rates in parts of the brain (Yen, 1977), and this process may therefore be the mechanism by which both chorea gravidarum and contraceptive-induced chorea occur in patients with previous damage, subclinical or evident, to the basal ganglia. Other observations, summarized by Nausieda and co-workers (1979), imply that more complex interaction between estrogenic and progestational hormonal levels is involved.

Chorea developing for the first time during pregnancy must not automatically be regarded as a variant of Sydenham's chorea because it may arise for other reasons. The choreic movements of Huntington's disease occasionally occur for the first time during pregnancy (Bolt, 1968), but the subsequent course of events and the family history will point to the correct diagnosis. Systemic lupus erythematosus may also cause chorea that sometimes commences during pregnancy (Donaldson and Espiner, 1971), and a thorough search for evidence of this disorder should therefore be made in all patients without clear evidence of a rheumatic basis for chorea. Finally, as in nonpregnant patients, chorea may relate to polycythemia vera rubra, thyrotoxicosis, hypocalcemia, Wilson's disease, and treatment with phenytoin or one of the major tranquilizing drugs.

Restless Legs Syndrome

More than 10 per cent of pregnant patients are said to experience unpleasant creeping sensations deep in the legs and occasionally in the arms. Symptoms generally occur when patients are relaxed, especially at night, and induce a need to move about. These symptoms usually develop in the latter half of pregnancy, subsiding soon after delivery (Ekbom, 1970). Similar symptoms may also occur without any relation to pregnancy. No abnormalities are found on neurologic examination. The cause of the disorder is unknown, but symptoms sometimes resolve following correction of any coexisting anemia or iron deficiency. Persistent or intolerable symptoms may respond to treatment with drugs such as diazepam or clonazepam. Other drugs that are sometimes helpful include levodopa, bromocriptine, carbamazepine, propranolol, and baclofen, but these are probably better avoided during pregnancy if possible.

Wilson's Disease

An autosomal recessive disorder, Wilson's disease is characterized by the accumulation of copper in the brain, liver, and other organs. Neurologic and mental symptoms (see Chapter 58) such as intellectual disturbances, abnormal movements of all sorts, dysarthria, dysphagia, and rigidity, are common presenting complaints. Once neurologic signs are present, careful examination of the eyes invariably shows the presence of Kayser-Fleischer rings—brown deposits of copper along the edge of the cornea in Descemet's membrane. Clinical evidence of hepatic involvement may be present, but is not invariable. The diagnosis is suggested by the family history, low serum copper and ceruloplasmin concentrations, and increased 24-hour urinary excretion of copper. Treatment with a low-copper diet and with penicillamine, a chelating agent that promotes copper excretion, may lead to marked improvement of neurologic and hepatic status.

There is a high miscarriage rate in patients with untreated Wilson's disease. Pregnancy generally proceeds normally in patients who have received adequate chelation therapy and carries no particular hazard for mother or fetus. There is no clinical evidence that penicillamine gives rise to fetal connective tissue abnormalities when its use is continued during pregnancy (Scheinberg and Sternlieb, 1975; Walshe, 1977). Nevertheless, it has been suggested that chelating agents may cause fetal abnormalities by inhibiting the synthesis and maturation of collagen (Marsh and Fraser, 1973), and one infant has reportedly been born with a connective tissue abnormality to a woman with cystinuria who was being treated with penicillamine in a dose almost double that generally prescribed in Wilson's disease (Mjolnerod et al., 1971). It may be prudent to reduce the dose of penicillamine to 250 mg daily about 6 weeks before delivery if cesarean section is planned, however, in order to avoid impairment of wound healing (Scheinberg and Sternlieb, 1975).

MULTIPLE SCLEROSIS

Multiple sclerosis is a disorder in which plaques of demyelination develop at different times and in different sites throughout the central nervous system. Its etiology remains uncertain; clinical onset is usually in early adult life. There is considerable variability in the tempo and character of neurologic symptoms and signs. The disorder is classically associated with unpredictable exacerbations during which neurologic deficits develop, followed by remissions during which symptoms and signs may partially or completely resolve. With time, patients become increasingly disabled, although perhaps not for many years after appearance of the initial symptoms. In other patients, the disorder follows a progressive course from its onset.

Several epidemiologic studies have suggested that there is an increased frequency of multiple sclerosis exacerbations in the first 3 to 6 months after childbirth (Millar et al., 1959; Schapira et al., 1966; Korn-Lubetzki et al., 1984; Birk and Rudick, 1986) but that pregnancy itself, or number of pregnancies, has no effect on subsequent neurologic disability (Thompson et al., 1986; Weinshenker et al., 1989). Similarly, multiple sclerosis does not influence the natural course of pregnancy or childbirth (Sweeney, 1953; Kulig and Schaltenbrand, 1956; Poser and Poser, 1983).

The possibility of a familial incidence of multiple sclerosis is widely known, but this pattern is uncommon and tends to involve siblings rather than different generations. It may merely reflect common exposure to some currently unrecognized etiologic agent rather than genetic predisposition to the disorder. With these points in mind, enquiries by a pregnant woman with multiple sclerosis concerning the possibility that her child may later develop the disease should be met with firm reassurance. A patient with multiple sclerosis need not be discouraged from pregnancy unless she is already so disabled by the disorder that she will clearly be incapable of coping with the responsibilities and physical demands of parenthood. Patients with minimal incapacity who are anxious to have a child will usually do so anyway, and need not be discouraged as long as they have some understanding of the nature of their disorder and its unpredictable course. In discussions between such patients and physicians, it seems reasonable to provide optimistic assurance that multiple sclerosis does not shorten life and that significant disability may not occur for many years, if at all.

The management of multiple sclerosis during pregnancy is supportive. The treatment of acute exacerbations generally consists of bed rest and prescription of a brief course of steroids, which may hasten recovery without necessarily influencing its extent. Patients with sphincter disturbances or who are paraplegic may experience increased difficulties during pregnancy. The method of delivery should depend solely on obstetric factors.

OPTIC NEURITIS

Any type of optic neuropathy may develop fortuitously during gestation. Thus, optic neuritis may develop during pregnancy in patients with established multiple sclerosis or in patients who will later develop other manifestations of that disorder. Optic nerve involvement by tumors or vascular malformations may also appear for the first time in the gestational period, as may the optic neuropathy that sometimes complicates vitamin deficiency. Optic nerve involvement may complicate hyperemesis gravidarum, with rapid onset of marked, usually bilateral visual loss; the entity is rare, but if the vomiting is unresponsive to treatment, it may be necessary to terminate pregnancy (Walsh and Hoyt, 1969).

Leber's optic atrophy is a hereditary disorder that usually occurs in early adult life. It commonly has a sex-linked recessive mode of inheritance, so that the male offspring of women carriers of the disorder may be affected, but other modes of inheritance have also been described. The clinical deficit commences abruptly with visual loss and leads ultimately to bilateral central scotoma with optic atrophy. There are no abnormalities to be found in the neonate. Other forms of hereditary optic atrophy have also been described in which the disorder is congenital or develops in infancy or early childhood and may have either a dominant or a recessive mode of transmission (Walsh and Hoyt, 1969). The family pedigree is thus important for diagnostic and counseling purposes in all such instances.

TRAUMATIC PARAPLEGIA

When spinal cord injury resulting in paraplegia occurs during the course of an established pregnancy, it may be followed by spontaneous abortion or stillbirth. If the pregnancy continues, the detailed radiologic investigations that will be needed to determine the nature and extent of the spinal injury may be hazardous to the developing fetus, especially if it is still very immature (see Chapter 12). In such circumstances, however, the interests of the mother are of paramount importance.

Many patients with established paraplegia are eager to experience motherhood, and because they are capable of sexual intercourse, they inquire about the possibility and potential hazards of childbirth. Urinary tract infection, a common complication of paraplegia, can be exacerbated by pregnancy, but this is not a contraindication to pregnancy provided there is no gross impairment of renal function. In the management of paraplegics, it is important to re-educate the paralyzed bladder so that only a minimal amount of residual urine remains after micturition. If this is achieved, difficulty with micturition can usually be postponed to the last stages of pregnancy, when catheterization will often be necessary.

Pregnancy may render a paraplegic more likely to develop pressure sores. Patients and their families should be informed about the cause of these sores and the manner in which prolonged pressure can be avoided (Guttmann, 1963). Anemia lowers the resistance of paraplegics to infection and pressure, and so particular care must be taken to prevent its development during pregnancy.

The uterus itself is able to contract normally in labor despite interruption of its nerve supply. However, patients with complete spinal cord lesions above the tenth thoracic segment will not appreciate the onset of labor or feel any pain during it because afferent fibers from the uterus enter the cord more caudally. Medical attendants will then need to examine the state of the cervix to identify the onset of labor with certainty. Because labor often commences before term in such circumstances, the cervix should be examined at each antenatal visit after the 24th to 26th week of pregnancy; the patient should be hospitalized if the cervix is found to be dilated (Robertson, 1972). Routine hospitalization after the 32nd week should be considered. In patients with cord lesions below the 10th or 11th thoracic segment, uterine contractions produce normal pain sensations. A patient with spasticity resulting from the cord lesion may develop painful flexor spasms and ankle clonus during uterine contractions.

Pregnant women with complete cord lesions above the fifth or sixth thoracic segment, i.e., above the splanchnic outflow, may develop the syndrome of autonomic hyper-reflexia with excessive activity of a viscus. This is characterized by throbbing headache, hypertension, reflex bradycardia, sweating, nasal congestion, and cutaneous vasodilatation and piloerection above the level of the lesion. During labor, these symptoms are most conspicuous with uterine contractions, and they become especially prominent just before delivery. Electrocardiographic monitoring may facilitate recognition of any changes in cardiac rate or rhythm that occur during uterine contractions. Symptoms are due to the sudden release of catecholamines (Garnier and Gertsch, 1964), and treatment has generally been with reserpine (which depletes catecholamines from sympathetic nerve terminals but also can cause potentially dangerous nasal congestion in the nasal-breathing neonate), atropine, clonidine, glyceryl trinitrate, or hexamethonium (a ganglion blocker). This syndrome, if unrecognized, may be mistaken for preeclampsia.

Cesarean section is not indicated by paraplegia per se, but it may be required because of bony deformity of the spine or pelvis; if the patient has a permanent suprapubic cystostomy, a vertical incision rather than a lower-segment transverse incision must be used. Forceps delivery is often required because the muscles responsible for the expulsive efforts of the second stage are paralyzed and because severe hypertension sometimes necessitates shortening the second stage (Robertson, 1963). Absorbable sutures such as catgut are poorly absorbed in paraplegics, and sterile abscesses commonly form around buried catgut, so that nonabsorbable sutures such as nylon are preferred for

repairing an episiotomy (Robertson, 1963). Paraplegic and quadriplegic patients can successfully breast-feed their babies and have a normal letdown (milk ejection) reflex during suckling (Robertson, 1972).

ROOT LESIONS

Prolapsed Intervertebral Disk and Pregnancy

Pregnancy is one etiologic factor in the development of prolapsed lumbar intervertebral disks (O'Connell, 1960). From a review of the case notes of 347 consecutive women with verified disk prolapse, O'Connell (1960) found that low back pain and/or sciatic pain attributable to the prolapse occurred commonly during or immediately after pregnancy. O'Connell (1944) suggested that the postural and mechanical stresses of pregnancy may well be responsible, particularly if hormonal factors render the lumbar intervertebral disks more vulnerable to stress by inducing changes in them analogous to those occurring in the pelvic joints. Other authors have concluded, however, that acute herniation of a lumbar disk during pregnancy is uncommon (King, 1950).

The symptoms and signs of lumbar disk protrusion during pregnancy are similar to those occurring in nonparous women. Radicular and low back pain are usually conspicuous features, and there may be a segmental motor and sensory disturbance in the limbs. When the disk prolapses centrally rather than laterally, symptoms and signs in the legs may be bilateral, and sphincter disturbances occur more commonly.

Lumbar disk protrusion must be distinguished from other causes of leg weakness developing during or soon after pregnancy. Lumbosacral palsy may arise during labor from compressive injury of the plexus, but tenderness and rigidity of the lumbar spine, sciatica, and signs of root tension favor the diagnosis of protruded disk. The distribution of muscular weakness may also be helpful; depending on their location, plexus lesions cause weakness and sensory symptoms in a polyradicular or peripheral nerve distribution in the legs. Moreover, because only the anterior primary rami contribute to the plexus, a proximal radiculopathy can be distinguished from a plexus lesion by electromyographic examination of muscles supplied by the posterior primary rami, namely the paraspinal muscles, involvement of which therefore favors a root lesion.

In patients with lateral protrusion of a lumbar disk, the best treatment is bed rest, together with simple analgesics for symptomatic relief. Imaging studies and surgery can usually be deferred until after childbirth. However, laminectomy and excision of the protruded disk may be necessary during pregnancy, especially if symptoms are bilateral or if there is any disturbance of sphincter function.

Other Lumbosacral Root Lesions

Most disk lesions involve the L5 or S1 roots. Although a disk lesion may occasionally affect the L4 root, involvement of an upper lumbar nerve root raises the distinct possibility of other compressive disease. Moreover, in a patient presenting with an L5 or S1 radiculopathy, there may be a more rostrally situated lesion if no abnormality, such as a protruded disk, is seen in the L4-L5 or L5-S1 region, because the spinal cord ends at the lower border of L1 and the roots then descend intradurally before exiting through their respective intervertebral foramina. In such circumstances the possibility of other compressive lesions must be considered. As with nonpregnant patients, each case is best managed on an individual basis; the reader is referred to standard neurologic textbooks for further details.

PLEXUS LESIONS AND PERIPHERAL MONONEUROPATHIES

Certain peripheral entrapment neuropathies are particularly liable to develop in pregnancy and may lead to troublesome symptoms. Recognition of the basis of such symptoms is important because, with reassurance about their benign nature, most patients can tolerate them until they give birth, when the symptoms generally subside spontaneously. A number of other peripheral nerve or plexus lesions may develop during labor or obstetric surgical procedures as a result of compression or stretch of nerves, especially in anesthetized patients.

Disorders of peripheral nerves may be characterized by slowing or block of conduction along intact axons or by axonal degeneration. The former carries a much more favorable prognosis for recovery than the latter because once axonal degeneration has occurred recovery can take place only by regeneration, a process that may take many months and may never be complete.

Electrophysiologic Evaluation

In the evaluation of patients with suspected nerve lesions, electrophysiologic techniques have been helpful in several ways (Aminoff, 1987). Electromyography can aid in determining whether weakness is neurogenic; if so, the electromyographically demonstrated pattern of affected muscles may indicate the location of the lesion, i.e., whether root, plexus, or individual peripheral nerve has been affected. The electromyographic findings may also indicate whether neurogenic weakness is a consequence of impaired conduction along otherwise intact axons or of axonal degeneration, a distinction which is of prognostic importance.

The motor responses to nerve stimulation provide complementary information. If axonal degeneration results from a focal lesion in a peripheral nerve, the motor responses to electrical stimulation either proximal or distal to the lesion become small or absent about a week after injury, depending on the completeness of the lesion. In contrast, in patients with a conductive disturbance due to an acute focal lesion, the motor responses to stimulation beyond (distal to) the lesion are generally normal, whereas those elicited by more proximal stimulation may be small.

Motor and sensory conduction velocity can be measured in various accessible segments of peripheral nerves, and focal slowing may provide confirmatory evidence of an underlying entrapment or focal neuropathy. Moreover, in patients presenting with a mononeuropathy, nerve conduction studies can be used to exclude the real possibility of an underlying subclinical polyneuropathy.

Lumbosacral Plexus Lesion

The roots of the sciatic nerve may be compressed in the pelvis by the fetal head or obstetric forceps, and the brunt of the resulting motor deficit is then borne by muscles supplied by the common peroneal fibers because of their relationship to the bony pelvis (Sunderland, 1968). This type of injury to the maternal lumbosacral plexus is more likely when a short patient with a small pelvis carries a rather large baby, so that labor is complicated by minor disproportion, or when mid-forceps are used during delivery because of malpresentation. The features of the pelvis that predispose to this complication include a straight sacrum, a flat wide posterior pelvis, posterior displacement of the transverse diameter of the inlet, wide sacroiliac notches, and prominent ischial spines (Whittaker, 1958).

Symptoms are generally unilateral. They usually develop immediately after delivery but may not be noticed until the patient is allowed out of bed. When the common peroneal fibers are involved, the main complaint is of leg weakness, which is sometimes erroneously attributed to a painful episiotomy, and in more severe cases there is footdrop. Numbness and paresthesias may occur over the dorsum of the foot and lateral aspect of the leg, and cutaneous sensation may be impaired in this distribution.

Unless the injury has been severe, the predominant pathologic change is demyelination of the affected fibers, and this is reflected in the electrophysiologic findings. With mild injuries, the prognosis for recovery is excellent, but if wallerian degeneration has occurred, recovery may take many months and may never be complete.

Physical therapy is all that is needed for the treatment of mild cases, but calipers and night casts may be required in more severe instances in order to prevent contracture.

Subsequent pregnancies can be allowed to proceed normally if an easy vaginal delivery is anticipated. Low forceps can be used with caution if necessary, but the use of mid-forceps may be hazardous. If the infant is clearly very large, or if premonitory symptoms suggesting nerve compression occur with attempted engagement of the fetal head in the pelvic brim during the last 4 weeks of pregnancy in a patient with a history of obstetric lumbosacral plexus palsy, it would seem sensible to advise cesarean section.

Acute Familial Brachial Neuritis

Several reports document the rare occurrence of brachial plexus neuropathy on a familial basis. Taylor

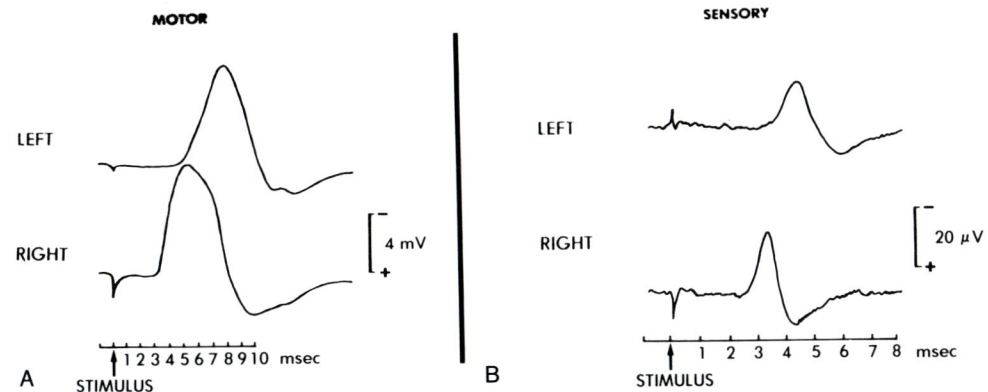

FIGURE 60–8. Nerve conduction studies in a patient with carpal tunnel syndrome. *A,* Responses of the abductor pollicis brevis muscle to surpamaximal electrical stimulation of the median nerves at the wrist. The prolonged latency of the response on the left is evident. *B,* The sensory action potentials recorded over the median nerve at the wrist after electrical stimulation of digital sensory fibers in the index fingers. Those on the left are smaller in amplitude and more prolonged in latency than those on the right. Maximal motor conduction velocity in the forearm segments of the median nerves were normal.

(1960) reported that 24 of 119 members of a family covering five generations had experienced single or multiple attacks of acute brachial neuropathy. This was characterized by pain, weakness, atrophy, and sensory loss that was usually unilateral but occasionally bilateral and from which gradual recovery generally occurred. Both males and females were affected, but among females there was a striking association of attacks with pregnancy or the puerperium, in contrast to the more common idiopathic disorder, which is rarely associated with pregnancy. In some instances of the familial disease there were involvement of lower cranial nerves and isolated mononeuropathies of the other extremities. Ungley (1933) described a similar syndrome in a mother and both of her daughters, and other cases have also been described. Treatment with oral steroids may be helpful in relieving pain but does not seem to affect the rate of recovery.

Carpal Tunnel Syndrome

Compression of the median nerve may occur in the carpal tunnel at the wrist, especially when (1) the normal size of the carpal tunnel is reduced, as by degenerative arthritis, or (2) the volume of its contents is increased, as in inflammatory disorders involving the tendons and connective tissues at the wrist. The carpal tunnel syndrome develops not uncommonly during pregnancy, perhaps because of excessive fluid retention. Pain and paresthesias are early symptoms and frequently occur at night, awakening the patient from sleep. The symptoms usually involve the first three digits and the lateral border of the ring finger, but some patients report that all digits are affected; pain may also occur in the forearm and, occasionally, in the upper arm. With time, weakness of the thenar muscles may develop. On examination, it is often possible to elicit Tinel's sign (percussion of the nerve at the wrist causing paresthesias in its distal distribution), and Phalen's maneuver (flexion at the wrist for more than a minute) sometimes reproduces or en-

hances symptoms. There may be mild weakness and wasting of the abductor pollicis brevis and opponens pollicis muscles, impaired cutaneous sensation in a median nerve distribution in the hand, or both motor and sensory signs.

Electrophysiologic testing usually provides information that suggests or confirms the diagnosis (Fig. 60–8). In the evaluation of patients, it is important to remember that the carpal tunnel syndrome is commonly bilateral even though it may be unilaterally symptomatic, and that an entrapment neuropathy may be the first manifestation of a subclinical polyneuropathy. These possibilities can be excluded by appropriate electrophysiologic studies.

Symptoms developing or worsening during pregnancy usually respond to the nocturnal use of a wrist splint and generally clear within about 3 months of delivery, although they may recur in subsequent pregnancies. The splint is placed on the dorsal surface with the intention of maintaining the wrist in a neutral or slightly flexed position. Some patients are helped by injection of steroids into the carpal tunnel and others by treatment with diuretics. Time must be taken to explain to the patient that her symptoms are benign and will generally subside spontaneously after the pregnancy. With such reassurance, most patients will accept their symptoms without difficulty, but surgical division of the anterior carpal ligament may be necessary if symptoms are intolerable or fail to clear in the weeks following delivery. Surgical treatment may similarly be necessary in a patient with clinical or electrophysiologic evidence of increasing nerve dysfunction despite conservative measures, but can usually be avoided during the pregnancy itself.

Meralgia Paresthetica

The lateral femoral cutaneous nerve, a purely sensory nerve derived from the L2 and L3 roots, is particularly susceptible to compression or stretch injury during pregnancy, especially during the third trimester. Obesity and diabetes mellitus are other predisposing factors. The nerve usually runs under the outer portion of the inguinal ligament to reach the thigh, but the ligament sometimes splits to enclose the nerve. In the latter circumstance, hyperextension of the hip or an increased lumbar lordosis, such as occurs during pregnancy, will lead to compression of the nerve by the posterior fascicle of the ligament (Pearson, 1957; Rhodes, 1957). Entrapment of the nerve at any point along its course may lead to similar symptoms, however, and several anatomic variations, summarized by Sunderland (1968), may predispose the nerve to damage when it is stretched. Pain, paresthesias, and numbness may occur about the outer aspect of the thigh; these symptoms are sometimes relieved by sitting. Symptoms are unilateral in approximately 80 per cent of cases. Little may be found on physical examination, but in severe cases cutaneous sensation is disturbed in the affected area. Symptoms, which are usually mild, subside spontaneously in the puerperium or within a few weeks of delivery. Accordingly, patients should be reassured about the benign nature of the disorder. In a few instances, however, pain has been so severe that labor has had to be induced early. Hydrocortisone injections in the region where the nerve lies medial to the anterior superior iliac spine may relieve persistent symptoms for a time, and nerve decompression by transposition may provide more lasting relief (Keegan and Holyoke, 1962), but is required very rarely.

Traumatic Mononeuropathies

The causes and clinical features of those traumatic mononeuropathies that are likely to develop in relation to obstetric procedures are listed here.

The *obturator nerve* originates within the psoas muscle from the L2, L3, and L4 nerves, emerges from the medial border of psoas, and enters the pelvis immediately in front of the sacroiliac joint. It sweeps round the lateral pelvic wall and then passes through the obturator foramen, dividing into branches that supply the adductor, gracilis, and obturator externus muscles, the skin over part of the medial thigh, and the hip joint. The nerve may be injured during genitourinary operations involving the lithotomy position, owing to angulation as it leaves the obturator foramen (Sunderland, 1968), or by compression between the fetal head (or a pelvic mass) and the bony pelvic wall. An obturator nerve palsy leads to impaired gait because of weakness of the adductor muscles, and to a sensory disturbance involving particularly the medial part of the mid-thigh and lower thigh. Pain may also occur, and it tends to radiate from the groin down the inner side of the thigh.

The *femoral nerve* originates within the psoas muscle from the L2, L3, and L4 nerves and passes beneath the inguinal ligament to enter the thigh. It innervates the iliacus, sartorius, pectineus, and quadriceps femoris muscles, and its cutaneous branches supply anterior and medial portions of the thigh and—through the saphenous nerve—the medial portions of the lower leg. Weakness and, in severe cases, wasting of the quadriceps muscle, sensory impairment over the anteromedial aspect of the thigh and occasionally of the leg to the medial malleolus, and depression or absence of knee jerk are the clinical features of a femoral nerve palsy. Such a palsy can occur as an isolated phenomenon in the patient with diabetes mellitus, a bleeding tendency, or retroperitoneal neoplasm, and it may sometimes arise by angulation and pressure from the inguinal ligament when the thighs are markedly flexed and abducted, as in the lithotomy position in anesthetized patients (Sunderland, 1968).

The *saphenous nerve*, the branch of the femoral nerve that supplies sensation to the medial aspect of the leg below the knee, may itself be damaged by pressure from leg braces when the patient is improperly suspended in the lithotomy position (Slocum et al., 1948; Britt and Gordon, 1964), leading to numbness and paresthesias that are usually fairly short-lived.

Sciatic or *common peroneal nerve palsies* are easy to confuse with a plexus palsy because, as already indicated, their constituent fibers are susceptible to compressive injury in the sacral plexus during labor. Misplaced deep intramuscular injections are probably still the most common cause of sciatic nerve palsy. The sciatic nerve may also be injured by stretch when a patient is positioned in stirrups on the obstetric table. To avoid this injury, the knee and hip joints should be well flexed, and extreme external rotation of the hip should be avoided (Burkhart and Daly, 1966). In patients with a sciatic nerve palsy, the resulting weakness and sensory disturbance depend on whether the entire nerve has been affected or certain fibers are selectively involved. In general, the peroneal fibers of the sciatic nerve are much more likely to be damaged than fibers destined for the tibial nerve. Accordingly, the clinical features of a sciatic nerve lesion may simulate those of a peroneal neuropathy, although electromyographic evidence of involvement of the short head of the biceps femoris muscle favors the former. The common peroneal nerve itself is vulnerable to compression or direct trauma in the region of the head and neck of the fibula and may certainly be injured at this site by pressure from the leg braces of the obstetric table, especially in anesthetized patients. Weakness of dorsiflexion and eversion of the foot is accompanied by numbness or blunted sensation of the anterolateral aspect of the calf and the dorsum of the foot.

Bell's Palsy

Sir Charles Bell first established the motor function of the seventh cranial nerve in the early 19th century. His name soon came to be associated with all forms of facial paralysis, but the designation Bell's palsy is now used for facial paresis of lower motor neuron type when no specific etiologic agent can be found. Most neurologists presume it to be due to an inflammatory reaction involving the facial nerve near the stylomastoid foramen or in the bony facial canal.

Although a possible association with pregnancy was alluded to by Bell himself, it is only recently that such an association has been substantiated. The incidence of Bell's palsy in nonpregnant women of childbearing age is 17.4 per 100,000 per year, whereas the incidence during pregnancy is 45.1 per 100,000 births (Hilsinger et al., 1975). Per year of exposure, the risk to pregnant women is more than three times that to nonpregnant women of similar age, with approximately 85 per cent of cases appearing in the third trimester or immediate puerperium (Hilsinger et al., 1975). No causal relationship with toxemia, hypertension, or primigravidity is proved, although such a relationship with toxemia has been suggested (Pope and Kenan, 1969; Robinson and Pou, 1972).

The clinical features of Bell's palsy are well known. The facial paresis is generally abrupt in onset, although it may worsen over the following day. Pain around the ear may precede or accompany the weakness in about half the cases but usually lasts for only a few days. The face itself feels stiff and pulled to one side. It may be hard to close the eye on the affected side, and ipsilateral epiphora may occur. There may be difficulty with eating and with fine facial movements (as when applying cosmetics, for example). A disturbance of taste, due to involvement of chorda tympani fibers, is common, and hyperacusis, due to involvement of fibers to the stapedius, is occasionally troublesome.

The treatment of Bell's palsy is controversial. Most patients recover without treatment, and only about 10 per cent of all patients are seriously dissatisfied with the final outcome because of permanent disfigurement or other long-term sequelae. Clearly, therefore, treatment is best reserved for patients in whom an unsatisfactory outcome can be predicted soon after onset. It is generally accepted that, to be effective, treatment must commence within the first 5 or 6 days.

The best clinical guide to prognosis at such an early stage is the severity of the palsy. Patients who have clinically complete palsy when first seen are less likely to make a full recovery than those with an incomplete palsy. Other clinical indicators for a poor prognosis for recovery include advancing age, hyperacusis, and the presence of severe initial pain.

The only medical treatment that may influence the outcome of Bell's palsy is with steroids (Taverner et al., 1966, 1967, and 1971; Adour et al., 1972), although rigorously controlled trials have failed to demonstrate any benefit from steroids (May et al., 1976; Wolf et al., 1978). Despite, or because of, the uncertainty about their effectiveness, many physicians routinely prescribe steroids to patients with Bell's palsy who are seen within 5 days of onset. There is no evidence that surgical procedures to decompress the facial nerve are of any benefit.

POLYNEUROPATHIES

There were several early reports of the occasional occurrence of a polyneuropathy during pregnancy, but there does not appear to be any specific "polyneuritis of pregnancy." Any type of polyneuropathy (such as that due to diabetes mellitus) may, in fact, develop during the gestational period, and discussion here is limited to those most likely to become manifest clini-

cally or to pose a management problem during pregnancy.

Nutritional Neuropathies

Nutritional deficiency may well be the most probable cause of peripheral nerve involvement in patients who come from underdeveloped countries or have hyperemesis. Signs of peripheral nerve involvement may be found in patients with hyperemesis gravidarum who have Wernicke's encephalopathy (Campbell and Biggart, 1939; Barnes, 1962). In the limbs, numbness, paresthesias, and dysesthesias are accompanied by cutaneous sensory loss, depressed tendon reflexes, and distal weakness. Retrobulbar neuropathy may also occur, and tachycardia, postural hypotension, exertional dyspnea, and sphincter disturbances are sometimes conspicuous. The polyneuropathy is accompanied by ophthalmoplegia (horizontal and vertical nystagmus, impaired lateral gaze, conjugate gaze palsies), ataxia of gait, and a confusional state. The features of Korsakoff's psychosis, which consists of impaired memory and an inability to acquire new information, sometimes accompanied by confabulation, may also be conjoined. Diagnosis is confirmed by the finding of a marked reduction in blood transketolase activity and a marked thiamine pyrophosphate effect. Treatment is with thiamine, 50 mg being given once intravenously and then intramuscularly for several days until a satisfactory dietary intake is assured.

In other instances, a severe polyneuropathy may develop without an accompanying encephalopathy, presumably in relation to a nutritional deficiency, although the specific factors responsible for the peripheral nerve involvement are not known. Patients may complain of pain, paresthesias, and dysesthesias in the extremities, of limb weakness, or of ataxia, and there may be accompanying cardiac involvement with tachycardia, exertional dyspnea, and heart failure. Treatment consists of a balanced diet and supplements of vitamins, especially those of the B group.

Vitamin B_{12} deficiency may lead to maternal polyneuropathy and other neurologic abnormalities, and can also affect the fetus and neonate.

Acute Idiopathic Polyneuritis (Guillain-Barré Syndrome)

An acute or subacute polyneuropathy that sometimes follows infective illnesses, inoculations, or surgical procedures, but often occurs without any obvious preceding event characterizes acute idiopathic polyneuritis. The disorder may have an immunologic basis, but the precise mechanism is currently unclear. It can pose an especially difficult management problem when it occurs during pregnancy. The main complaint is of weakness that varies widely in severity in different patients, is often more marked proximally than distally, and is often symmetric in distribution. It usually begins in the legs, frequently comes to involve the arms, and often affects one side or both sides of the face. Weakness may progress to total paralysis and may be life-threatening if the muscles of respiration or deglutition are involved. Sensory symptoms are common but are usually less conspicuous than motor symptoms. Autonomic dysfunction may be manifested by tachycardia, cardiac irregularities, hypotension or hypertension, facial flushing, disturbances of sweating, disturbed pulmonary function, and other signs and symptoms. Examination of the cerebrospinal fluid reveals characteristic changes: the protein content is significantly increased but the cell content is normal. Measurement of motor and sensory conduction velocity in the peripheral nerves may reveal marked slowing, but the chronology of this reduction does not necessarily parallel that of the clinical disorder; in some patients the conduction velocity remains normal, presumably because disease is restricted to the nerve roots or proximal segments of the nerves. Most patients eventually make a good recovery, but it may take many months and some patients are left with persisting disability.

There is no convincing evidence that the Guillain-Barré syndrome occurs more commonly during gestation than at other times, and the course of the disorder does not seem to be influenced by pregnancy. Improvement in neurologic status may certainly occur before delivery and is not necessarily delayed until the baby is born. Treatment is symptomatic, attention being directed at the prevention of complications such as respiratory failure and vascular collapse, but plasmapheresis or treatment with intravenous immunoglobulins is helpful in patients with rapidly advancing or severe disease. Severely affected patients are best managed in intensive care units, where respiratory and circulatory function can be monitored and assisted respiration can be started as soon as is necessary.

Approximately 3 per cent of patients with acute idiopathic polyneuritis have one or more relapses, sometimes several years after the initial illness. Such relapses, which are clinically similar to the original illness, occasionally occur in relation to pregnancy (Calderon-Gonzalez et al., 1970; Novak and Johnson, 1973; Jones and Berry, 1981).

Porphyric Neuropathy

In the hepatic forms of porphyria both the central and peripheral nervous systems may be affected. Acute intermittent porphyria, inherited as an autosomal recessive trait, is characterized by increased production and urinary excretion of porphobilinogen and δ-aminolevulinic acid. The Watson-Schwartz test, a useful qualitative test for increased urinary porphobilinogen, is of great value in establishing the diagnosis (Tschudy et al., 1975). Colicky abdominal pain is often the most conspicuous symptom, but the usual neurologic manifestation is a polyneuropathy, predominantly motor but sometimes with pronounced autonomic involvement, that may take weeks or months to regress, depending on its severity. Cerebral manifestations may also occur, often preceding the development of a severe polyneuropathy and similarly clearing after a variable time. Clinical indicators of

disease activity include tachycardia, fever, and a peripheral leukocytosis. In variegate porphyria, cutaneous sensitivity to sunlight is an additional clinical feature.

Attacks may be precipitated by pharmacologic agents such as barbiturates, sulfonamides, and estrogens. Some women have found that relapses are most likely to occur premenstrually; long-term combination oral contraceptives may prevent attacks in these patients (Perlroth et al., 1965). In other patients, oral contraceptives may precipitate exacerbations, and so this form of contraception is probably best avoided in the woman with a blood relative who has a hepatic type of porphyria (Donaldson, 1978). Pregnancy may also lead to an acute exacerbation and may even have a fatal outcome, but in many patients it is tolerated without apparent ill effect. When relapses occur they usually do so in early pregnancy and may lead to spontaneous abortion (Donaldson, 1978). However, exacerbations may occur at any time during pregnancy or postpartum. The implications and uncertain outcome must therefore be explained to patients who are contemplating pregnancy, and close supervision should be provided during the gestational period. Latent cases may be exacerbated by medication used during or after labor, and particular care must therefore be exercised in this regard. In general, if the pregnancy proceeds satisfactorily, a healthy infant can be anticipated.

MYASTHENIA GRAVIS

Variable weakness and fatigability of skeletal muscles, due to defective neuromuscular transmission, are the clinical hallmarks of myasthenia gravis. The disorder has an autoimmune basis. It is characterized by a reduced number of available acetylcholine receptors at the neuromuscular junctions. Myasthenia gravis is more common in females. In some patients the external ocular muscles or levator palpebrae are especially affected, in others the facial and bulbar muscles are selectively involved, and in yet others the limb muscles, especially the proximal ones, are predominantly affected. Weakness may remain localized to a few muscle groups or may become generalized, and it can be life-threatening if the muscles of respiration or deglutition are involved. Patients are particularly sensitive to even small doses of neuromuscular blocking agents such as tubocurarine, but improvement results from treatment with acetylcholinesterase inhibitors. Thymectomy often leads to a remission of symptoms, and myasthenia gravis may be associated with thymoma. Repetitive supramaximal electrical stimulation of motor nerves may lead to an abnormal decline in size of the evoked muscle action potentials; this finding is sometimes of diagnostic help, as is the finding of elevated levels of circulating acetylcholine receptor antibodies and the clinical response to edrophonium or neostigmine. In addition to thymectomy in appropriate cases, treatment may involve the use of anticholinesterases, steroids, and plasmapheresis; the reader is referred to general neurologic textbooks for further details of the standard medical management of this disease.

Exacerbations of myasthenia gravis sometimes occur shortly before the onset of the menstrual period and tend to improve once menstruation has begun (Osserman, 1958). Such an association may disappear following thymectomy (Keynes, 1952).

Myasthenia gravis may first appear during or shortly after pregnancy (Osserman, 1958), but it is difficult to predict the influence that pregnancy will have on an established case. Moreover, the effect of pregnancy may vary on different occasions, so that the outcome in individual cases cannot be predicted on this basis. Viets and associates (1942) reported that relapses are not uncommon in early pregnancy, partial or complete remission often occurring at a later stage. Others hold, however, that a relapse is more likely to occur in the puerperium than during the pregnancy itself (Fraser and Turner, 1963). Osserman (1955) reported that definite remission occurred during pregnancy in approximately one-third of his patients, relapse occurred in another one-third, and the remaining patients showed no change in severity of myasthenia during pregnancy. It may be tempting to terminate a pregnancy because of the severity of myasthenic symptoms—death has been reported in pregnancy complicated by myasthenia gravis (Thomson, 1963)—and because of the difficulties in their treatment, but termination does not necessarily lead to clinical benefit. This disorder must therefore be managed in pregnant patients just as in nonpregnant patients.

Myasthenia gravis has little effect on the pregnancy itself. Moreover, in labor there may be a marked contrast between the strength of uterine contractions in the second stage and the skeletal muscle weakness exhibited by the patient. If the expulsive phase of labor is prolonged, instrumental assistance may help to avoid maternal exhaustion (Fraser and Turner, 1963). Cesarean section should be reserved for patients in whom it is indicated on obstetric grounds. Regional analgesia is preferable to general anesthesia, and use of muscle relaxant drugs is avoided if at all possible. Similarly, the use of magnesium sulfate for eclampsia should be avoided as it may precipitate myasthenic crisis.

Infants born to myasthenic patients should be carefully watched during the week following delivery for signs of neonatal myasthenia. Such signs include a poor cry, respiratory difficulties, weakness in sucking, a weak Moro reflex, and feeble limb movements, and they usually become apparent within the first 72 hours of birth. Symptoms are usually not evident immediately after birth, and this delay has been attributed to protection of the baby by placental transfer of maternal anticholinesterase drugs.

Neonatal myasthenia is a transient disorder that presumably relates to placental transfer of maternal antibody against acetylcholine receptors (Keesey et al., 1977). The disease may occur in the newborn of a myasthenic mother who has undergone thymectomy or who did not take anticholinesterases during pregnancy, and so it cannot be attributed to the maternal thymus gland or the effect of maternal drug treatment. It does not seem to be related to the duration or severity of maternal illness, although disease in mothers of myasthenic newborns is usually generalized rather than localized (Namba et al., 1970). The incidence of neonatal myasthenia among babies born to myasthenic mothers is 10 to 15 per cent (Namba et al., 1970).

The neonatal disorder, which can be treated with anticholinesterase drugs, usually subsides within 6 weeks of delivery, but it may result in death due to aspiration or to respiratory failure. Facilities should thus be available for the immediate resuscitation of affected infants or of those at risk of being affected. Of some interest, in view of the recent development of plasmapheresis as a method of treating adults with myasthenia gravis, is the observation that exchange transfusion for hyperbilirubinemia led to rapid resolution of symptoms in a 2-day-old infant with neonatal myasthenia (Dunn, 1976).

The birth of a child with neonatal myasthenia does not necessarily imply that future children will also have the disorder, although they often do. Namba and colleagues (1970) found that following the birth of affected infants, 11 of the mothers had a second child with the disorder, but five mothers had at least one more child who was unaffected.

The transient neonatal disorder that may occur in the offspring of a myasthenic mother must not be confused with congenital myasthenia gravis. The latter is rare, occurs in children born of healthy mothers, resembles the adult form of the disorder, and is usually permanent.

DISORDERS OF MUSCLE

Myotonic Dystrophy

Myotonic dystrophy is a slowly progressive, dominantly inherited disorder that usually appears in early adult life but may become manifested in childhood. Myotonia is accompanied by weakness of the facial, sternomastoid, and distal limb muscles. There may be a number of associated features, including cataracts, frontal baldness, cardiac and endocrine disturbances, and intellectual changes. During pregnancy, the weakness and myotonia may be aggravated, and the course of the disorder is sometimes accelerated (Davis, 1958; Gardy, 1963; Hopkins and Wray, 1967; Shore and MacLachlan, 1971). When deterioration does occur, it often begins at about the sixth or seventh month of pregnancy.

In the antepartum period, the major reported obstetric complications of myotonic dystrophy include threatened, spontaneous, and habitual abortion (Holland and Hill, 1956; Pruzanski, 1965; Shore and MacLachlan, 1971). Hydramnios, which may also occur, has been attributed to decreased fetal swallowing, as demonstrated radiographically by intra-amniotic injection of radiopaque dye (Dunn and Dierker, 1973), suggesting fetal muscle involvement. Premature onset of labor in patients with myotonic dystrophy has been attributed in some instances to abnormalities of uterine muscle (Shore and MacLachlan, 1971). Labor may also be abnormal in patients with myotonic dystrophy, owing to a failure of the uterus to contract normally (Sciarra and Steer, 1961; Hopkins and Wray, 1967; Shore and MacLachlan, 1971). Thus, the first stage may be prolonged, and retention of the placenta and postpartum hemorrhage may occur. Manual removal of the placenta is sometimes necessary. Skeletal muscle weakness may also lead to poor voluntary assistance in the second stage (Davis, 1958; Gardy, 1963).

Myotonic dystrophy may become manifested in infancy, occurring congenitally among the offspring of mothers who have the disorder, sometimes only very mildly. In such cases, it is often possible to obtain a history of hydramnios or reduced fetal movements during the latter part of pregnancy. Some affected infants die within hours or a few days of birth. The clinical features in affected infants include facial diplegia, hypotonia, neonatal respiratory distress, feeding difficulties, delayed motor development, and mental retardation (Harper, 1979). Myotonia, a cardinal feature of the adult disease, is absent in the congenital form. The neonatal respiratory distress may be due to involvement of the respiratory muscles, pulmonary immaturity, aspiration pneumonia, and impaired neural control of respiration. Talipes is present at birth in about half of all cases and may require surgical correction.

Familial studies have indicated that in almost every case of congenital myotonic dystrophy, transmission has occurred via the mother. Such transmission does not fit with an autosomal dominant pattern of inheritance. Genetic data suggest that the congenital form results from the combination of the gene responsible for the disorder in adults with some additional maternally transmitted factor (Harper, 1979). The nature of this maternal factor is unclear at present. Others have argued that the maternal transmission of the congenital form relates to relative male infertility.

The management of patients requiring anesthesia for obstetric or other reasons merits brief comment. Hook and co-workers (1975) have emphasized that depolarizing muscle relaxant drugs should be avoided because they may cause myotonic spasm, and that nondepolarizing agents, such as tubocurarine, can be used but should be given in reduced dosage to patients receiving quinine for myotonia. Pentothal may lead to marked respiratory depression and is best avoided, as also are other respiratory-depressant drugs, especially if the patient already has impaired respiratory function. Electrocardiographic monitoring will permit the early recognition of any cardiac arrhythmias, to which patients with myotonic dystrophy are prone. For these reasons, regional analgesia is the preferred method of management.

Myotonia Congenita

The dominant form of myotonia congenita (Thomsen's disease) is usually present from birth, although symptoms may not appear until early childhood. Patients complain of muscle stiffness (myotonia) that is enhanced by cold or inactivity and is relieved by exercise; power is full, but the muscles may be diffusely hypertrophied. Pregnancy may aggravate the myotonia, especially in the latter half of the gestational period, with improvement occurring after delivery. Several illustrative case reports have been published (Gardiner, 1901; Hakim and Thomlinson, 1969).

Polymyositis

In polymyositis or dermatomyositis, which can occur at any age, there is weakness and wasting, especially of the proximal musculature, due to inflammatory infiltration of muscles and destruction of muscle fibers. The muscles are often painful and tender. There may be an association with malignancy or with one of the collagen diseases. The erythrocyte sedimentation rate and serum creatine phosphokinase levels are elevated. Histologic examination of a muscle biopsy specimen usually permits the diagnosis to be made with confidence so that treatment with steroids can be instituted. Pregnancy has a variable effect on the muscle weakness, but a high perinatal mortality rate has been reported (Tsai et al., 1973).

PSYCHIATRIC DISORDERS

Pregnancy may occur during the course of established psychiatric illness, and conversely, psychiatric disorders may first develop during or shortly after pregnancy, although there are no specific disorders that relate to this period. In the evaluation of patients with psychiatric disorders, it must be borne in mind that pregnancy can have a number of different psychopathologic implications, depending on the patient's social, cultural, educational, emotional, and medical background. The attitude of a patient to pregnancy, especially with regard to whether it was desired, influences her psychological response, and her capacity to cope with pregnancy depends on her acceptance of it. If the pregnancy was planned, the factors that motivated it are also of some relevance, since the aim may have been to overcome marital disharmony, to keep up with peers, and so on. These aspects clearly govern the response of an individual patient to pregnancy.

Therapeutic abortion is sometimes requested for psychosocial reasons. Termination may be followed by bitter feelings of guilt and remorse, and although they are often short-lived, they sometimes lead to more serious psychiatric complications, especially in the patient with a history of mental illness. Such a patient is also more likely to develop a serious psychiatric disturbance if her request for termination is denied, however, and there is no clear solution to this dilemma. It is sometimes helpful to bear in mind the welfare of the unborn child; a woman who genuinely does not wish for motherhood generally does not make a good mother if her pregnancy is allowed to proceed. Each case must be considered individually, and the motives for rejection of the developing fetus should carefully be sought. Patients with a history of psychiatric disorder merit special consideration. Suicidal threats are difficult to evaluate but always provide cause for particular concern in patients who have previously attempted suicide, who are dependent on drugs or alcohol, or who have made any form of preparation for taking their own lives.

During pregnancy, it is not uncommon for a woman to experience feelings of inadequacy, envy, and even hostility toward herself, the developing fetus, and other family members. Such feelings may lead to symptoms with which the patient can manipulate others to her own advantage, in order to avoid domestic, sexual, or other undesirable obligations. Moreover, fears about the outcome and possible complications of pregnancy and childbirth may color the emotional responses of a patient and evoke various defense reactions. In this regard, education and informed reassurance can do much to reduce distress.

Following delivery a woman may experience a profound but transient sense of anticlimax. She may develop feelings of guilt about her emotional response to the newborn if it is deemed to be inadequate. Often she becomes anxious about her ability to adopt a maternal role. Apathy, irritability, anorexia, malaise, fatigability, moodiness, anxiety, withdrawal, depression, and tearfulness may occur to variable degrees in the postpartum period and may persist for some weeks, and loss of sexual interest may continue for even longer.

Psychotic illness develops infrequently in association with pregnancy, and its occurrence during one pregnancy does not necessarily imply that similar reactions will occur in subsequent pregnancies. The prognosis for recovery is similar to that in nonpregnant patients. About half of the mental illnesses associated with pregnancy or the postpartum period are schizophrenic, about 25 per cent are manic depressive, and 20 per cent are psychoneurotic reactions (Kolb, 1973). The form of any psychosis is predetermined by the background of the patient rather than the pregnancy itself, but symptoms possibly relate, at least in part, to hormonal as well as psychological factors.

The management of psychiatric disorders that either have continued into or have developed during pregnancy is generally the same as for similar disturbances occurring at other times. Hormonal therapy is of no particular benefit. In conjunction with local community services, appropriate steps must be taken to ensure the safety of the child if there are grounds for believing that it is endangered by the nature of the mother's illness. The interested reader is referred to standard textbooks for further details of treatment.

There is natural concern about the effects on the fetus of drugs taken during pregnancy in the treatment of psychiatric disease. Such drugs have often been prescribed for patients who have long-standing mental illness and have become pregnant during the course of the disorder. This issue is addressed in Chapter 12.

REFERENCES

Abramson H, Greenberg M, Magee MC: Poliomyelitis in the newborn infant. J Pediatr **43**:167, 1953.

Adadevoh BK, Akinla O: Postabortal and postpartum tetanus. J Obstet Gynaecol Br Commonw **77**:1019, 1970.

Adour KK, Wingerd J, Bell DN: Prednisone treatment for idiopathic facial paralysis (Bell's palsy). N Eng J Med **287**:1268, 1972.

Allen J, Eldridge R, Koerber T: Acoustic neuroma in the last months of pregnancy. Am J Obstet Gynecol **119**:516, 1974.

Amias AG: Cerebral vascular disease in pregnancy. 1. Haemorrhage. J Obstet Gynaecol Br Commonw **77**:100, 1970.

Aminoff MJ: Spinal Angiomas. Oxford, Blackwell Scientific Publications, 1976.

Aminoff MJ: Angiomas and fistulae involving the nervous system. In Ross Russell RW (ed): Vascular Disease of the Central Nervous System. 2nd ed. Edinburgh, Churchill Livingstone, 1983.

Aminoff MJ: Electromyography in Clinical Practice. 2nd ed. New York, Churchill Livingstone, 1987.

Annegers JF, Elveback LR, Hauser WA, Kurland LT: Do anticonvulsants have a teratogenic effect? Arch Neurol **31**:364, 1974.

Annegers JF, Hauser WA, Elveback LR, et al: Seizure disorders in offspring of parents with a history of seizures—a maternal-paternal difference? Epilepsia **17**:1, 1976.

Athavale VB, Pai PN: Tetanus neonatorum—clinical manifestations. J Pediatr **67**:649, 1965.

Ayraud N, Kermarec J, Martinon J: Effects cytogénétiques des médicaments anticonvulsivants. A propos d'une observation d'anomalies transmises pendant la vie intrautérine. Ann Genet (Paris) **11**:253, 1968.

Backstrom T: Epilepsy in women. Oestrogen and progesterone plasma levels. Experientia **32**:248, 1976.

Barber PV, Arnold AG, Evans G: Recurrent hormone dependent chorea: Effects of oestrogens and progestogens. Clin Endocrinol **5**:291, 1976.

Barnes J: Obstetrical complications in neurological disorders. Proc R Soc Med **55**:575, 1962.

Baylis EM, Crowley JM, Preece JM, et al: Influence of folic acid on blood-phenytoin levels. Lancet **1**:62, 1971.

Beresford OD, Graham AM: Chorea gravidarum. J Obstet Gynaecol Br Emp **57**:617, 1950.

Bickerstaff ER, Small JM, Guest IA: The relapsing course of certain meningiomas in relation to pregnancy and menstruation. J Neurol Neurosurg Psychiatry **21**:89, 1958.

Birk K, Rudick R: Pregnancy and multiple sclerosis. Arch Neurol **43**:719, 1986.

Bjerkedal T, Bahna SL: The occurrence and outcome of pregnancy in women with epilepsy. Acta Obstet Gynecol Scand **52**:245, 1973.

Bjerkedal T, Czeizel A, Goujard J, et al: Valproic acid and spina bifida. Lancet **2**:1096, 1982.

Bleyer WA, Skinner AL: Fatal neonatal hemorrhage after maternal anticonvulsant therapy. JAMA **235**:626, 1976.

Bolt JMW: Abortion and Huntington's chorea. Br Med J **1**:840, 1968.

Britt BA, Gordon RA: Peripheral nerve injuries associated with anaesthesia. Can Anaesth Soc J **11**:514, 1964.

Burkhart FL, Daly JW: Sciatic and peroneal nerve injury: A complication of vaginal operations. Obstet Gynecol **28**:99, 1966.

Burnett CWF: A survey of the relation between epilepsy and pregnancy. J Obstet Gynaecol Br Emp **53**:539, 1946.

Calderon-Gonzalez R, Gonzalez-Cantu N, Rizzi-Hernandez H: Recurrent polyneuropathy with pregnancy and oral contraceptives. N Engl J Med **282**:1307, 1970.

Campbell ACP, Biggart JH: Wernicke's encephalopathy (polioencephalitis haemorrhagica superior): Its alcoholic and nonalcoholic incidence. J Pathol Bacteriol **48**:245, 1939.

Cannell DE: Subarachnoid haemorrhage in pregnancy. Proc R Soc Med **52**:950, 1959.

Carroll JD, Leak D, Lee HA: Cerebral thrombophlebitis in pregnancy and the puerperium. Q J Med **35**:347, 1966.

Collaborative Group for the Study of Stroke in Young Women: Oral contraceptives and stroke in young women. Associated risk factors. JAMA **231**:718, 1975.

Dam M, Christiansen J, Munck O, Mygind KI: Antiepileptic drugs: Metabolism in pregnancy. Clin Pharmacokinet **4**:53, 1979.

Davis HA: Pregnancy in myotonica dystrophia. J Obstet Gynaecol Br Emp **65**:479, 1958.

Davis L, Martin J, Padberg F, Anderson RK: A study of 182 patients with verified astrocytoma, astroblastoma and oligodendroglioma of the brain. J Neurosurg **7**:299, 1950.

Deblay MF, Vert P, Andre M, Marchal F: Transplacental vitamin K prevents haemorrhagic disease of infant of epileptic mothers. Lancet **1**:1247, 1982.

Desmond MM, Schwanecke RP, Wilson GS, et al: Maternal barbiturate utilization and neonatal withdrawal symptomatology. J Pediatr 80:190, 1972.

DeToni E, Vianello MG, Massimo L, Dagna-Bricarelli F: Observazione di cellule tetraploidi ed eteroploidi in culture di sangue di tre Lattanti, figli di madri sottoposte prima e durante la gravidanza a terapia con farmaci anticonvulsivanti. Minerva Pediatr 19:2092, 1967.

DiLiberti JH, Farndon PA, Dennis NR, Curry CJR: The fetal valproate syndrome. Am J Med Genet 19:473, 1984.

Dimsdale H: The epileptic in relation to pregnancy. Br Med J 2:1147, 1959.

Donaldson IM, Espiner EA: Disseminated lupus erythematosus presenting as chorea gravidarum. Arch Neurol 25:240, 1971.

Donaldson JO: Neurology of Pregnancy. Philadelphia, WB Saunders, 1978.

Dunn JM: Neonatal myasthenia. Am J Obstet Gynecol 125:265, 1976.

Dunn LJ, Dierker LJ: Recurrent hydramnios in association with myotonia dystrophica. Obstet Gynecol 42:104, 1973.

Eadie MJ, Lander CM, Tyrer JH: Plasma drug level monitoring in pregnancy. Clin Pharmacokinet 2:427, 1977.

Eckerling B, Goldman JA, Gans B: Intracranial sinus thrombosis, a rare complication of early pregnancy. Report of three cases. Obstet Gynecol 21:368, 1963.

Einhaupl KM, Villringer A, Meister W, et al: Heparin treatment in sinus venous thrombosis. Lancet 338:597, 1991.

Ekbom KA: Restless legs. In Vinken PJ, Bruyn GW (eds): Handbook of Clinical Neurology. Vol 8. Amsterdam, North Holland, 1970.

Elshove J: Cleft palate in the offspring of female mice treated with phenytoin. Lancet 2:1074, 1969.

Epstein MT, Hockaday JM, Hockaday TDR: Migraine and reproductive hormones throughout the menstrual cycle. Lancet 1:543, 1975.

Evans HM, Nelson MM, Asling CW: Multiple congenital abnormalities resulting from acute folic acid deficiency during gestation. Science 114:479, 1951.

Fedrick J: Epilepsy and pregnancy: A report from the Oxford record linkage study. Br Med J 2:442, 1973.

Feldman GL, Weaver DD, Lovrien EW: The fetal trimethadione syndrome. Report of an additional family and further delineation of this syndrome. Am J Dis Child 131:1389, 1977.

Fishman RA, Cowen D, Silbermann M: Intracranial venous thrombosis during the first trimester of pregnancy. Neurology 7:217, 1957.

Fraser D, Turner JWA: Myasthenia gravis and pregnancy. Proc R Soc Med 56:379, 1963.

Gamboa ET, Isaacs G, Harter DH: Chorea associated with oral contraceptive therapy. Arch Neurol 25:112, 1971.

Garcin R, Pestel M: Thrombo-phlébites Cerebrales. Paris, Masson, 1949.

Gardiner CF: A case of myotonia congenita. Arch Pediatr 18:925, 1901.

Gardy HH: Dystrophia myotonica in pregnancy. Obstet Gynecol 21:441, 1963.

Garnier B, Gertsch R: Autonome Hyperreflexie und Katecholaminausscheidung beim Paraplegiker. Schweiz Med Wochenschr 94:124, 1964.

German J, Kowal A, Ehlers KH: Trimethadione and human teratogenesis. Teratology 3:349, 1970.

Gettelfinger DM, Kokmen E: Superior sagittal sinus thrombosis. Arch Neurol 34:2, 1977.

Goldman JA, Eckerling B, Gans B: Intracranial venous sinus thrombosis in pregnancy and puerperium. Report of fifteen cases. J Obstet Gynaecol Br Commonw 71:791, 1964.

Griffith RW, Grauwiler J, Hodel C, et al: Toxicologic considerations. In Berde B, Schild HO (eds): Ergot Alkaloids and Related Compounds. (Handbook of Experimental Pharmacology, Vol 49.) New York, Springer-Verlag, 1978.

Guttmann L: The paraplegic patient in pregnancy and labour. Proc R Soc Med 56:383, 1963.

Hakim CA, Thomlinson J: Myotonia congenita in pregnancy. J Obstet Gynaecol Br Commonw 76:561, 1969.

Hall MH: Folic acid deficiency and congenital malformation. J Obstet Gynaecol Br Commonw 79:159, 1972.

Hanson JW, Myrianthopoulos NC, Harvey MAS, Smith DW: Risks to the offspring of women treated with hydantoin anticonvul-

sants, with emphasis on the fetal hydantoin syndrome. J Pediatr 89:662, 1976.

Harbison RD, Becker BA: Relation of dosage and time of administration of diphenylhydantoin to its teratogenic effect in mice. Teratology 2:305, 1969.

Harper PS: Myotonic Dystrophy. Philadelphia, WB Saunders, 1979.

Hibbard ED, Smithells RW: Folic acid metabolism and human embryopathy. Lancet 1:1254, 1965.

Hilsinger RL, Adour KK, Doty HE: Idiopathic facial paralysis, pregnancy, and the menstrual cycle. Ann Otol Rhinol Laryngol 84:433, 1975.

Holland CM, Hill SR: Myotonia dystrophica: Report of six cases in one family, with an analysis of the metabolic defects. Ann Intern Med 44:738, 1956.

Hook R, Anderson EF, Noto P: Anesthetic management of a parturient with myotonia atrophica. Anesthesiology 43:689, 1975.

Hopkins A, Wray S: The effect of pregnancy on dystrophia myotonica. Neurology 17:166, 1967.

Horton JC, Chambers WA, Lyons SL, et al: Pregnancy and the risk of hemorrhage from cerebral arteriovenous malformations. Neurosurgery 27:867, 1990.

Hunter JS, Millikan CH: Poliomyelitis with pregnancy. Obstet Gynecol 4:147, 1954.

Hyland HH: Intracranial venous thrombosis in the puerperium. JAMA 142:707, 1950.

Irey NS, McAllister HA, Henry JM: Oral contraceptives and stroke in young women: A clinicopathologic correlation. Neurology 28:1216, 1978.

Jackson CD, Fishbein L: A toxicological review of beta-adrenergic blockers. Fundam Appl Toxicol 6:395, 1986.

Jadhav M, Webb JKG, Vaishnava S, Baker SJ: Vitamin-B_{12} deficiency in Indian infants. A clinical syndrome. Lancet 2:903, 1962.

Janz D: The teratogenic risk of antiepileptic drugs. Epilepsia 16:159, 1975.

Janz D, Beck-Mannagetta G, Andermann E, et al: Guidelines for the care of epileptic women of childbearing age. Epilepsia 30:409, 1989.

Jennett WB, Cross JN: Influence of pregnancy and oral contraception on the incidence of strokes in women of childbearing age. Lancet 1:1019, 1967.

Jones KL, Lacro RV, Johnson KA, Adams J: Pattern of malformations in the children of women treated with carbamazepine during pregnancy. N Engl J Med 320:1661, 1989.

Jones MW, Berry K: Chronic relapsing polyneuritis associated with pregnancy. Ann Neurol 9:413, 1981.

Keegan JJ, Holyoke EA: Meralgia paresthetica. An anatomical and surgical study. J Neurosurg 19:341, 1962.

Keesey J, Lindstrom J, Cokely H, Herrmann C: Anti-acetylcholine receptor antibody in neonatal myasthenia gravis. N Engl J Med 296:55, 1977.

Kempers RD, Miller RH: Management of pregnancy associated with brain tumors. Am J Obstet Gynecol 87:858, 1963.

Kendall D: Thrombosis of intracranial veins. Brain 71:386, 1948.

Keynes G: Obstetrics and gynaecology in relation to thyrotoxicosis and myasthenia gravis. J Obstet Gynaecol Br Emp 59:173, 1952.

King AB: Neurologic conditions occurring as complications of pregnancy. Arch Neurol Psychiatry 63:471, 1950.

Knight AH, Rhind EG: Epilepsy and pregnancy: A study of 153 pregnancies in 59 patients. Epilepsia 16:99, 1975.

Kolb LC: Modern Clinical Psychiatry. 8th ed. Philadelphia, WB Saunders, 1973.

Koller T, Stamm H, Hauser GA, Klingler M: Die Zerebralen Venen- und Sinusthrombosen in der Geburtshilfe. Thromb Haemost 1:37, 1957.

Korn-Lubetzki I, Kahana E, Cooper G, Abramsky O: Activity of multiple sclerosis during pregnancy and puerperium. Ann Neurol 16:229, 1984.

Kuenssberg EV, Knox JDE: Teratogenic effect of anticonvulsants. Lancet 1:198, 1973.

Kulig K, Schaltenbrand G: Statistische Untersuchungen zum Problem der Multiplen Sklerose. Dtsch Z Nervenheilk 174:460, 1956.

Lance JW: The Mechanism and Management of Headache. 2nd ed. London, Butterworths, 1973.

Lancet: The growing problems of phenylketonuria. (Editorial) Lancet 1:1381, 1979.

Lander CM, Edwards VE, Eadie MJ, Tyrer JH: Plasma anticonvulsant concentrations during pregnancy. Neurology 27:128, 1977.

Landon MJ, Kirkley M: Metabolism of diphenylhydantoin (phenytoin) during pregnancy. Br J Obstet Gynaecol 86:125, 1979.

Lenke RR, Levy HL: Maternal phenylketonuria and hyperphenylalaninemia: An international survey of the outcome of untreated and treated pregnancies. N Engl J Med 303:1202, 1980.

Lewis PD, Harrison MJG: Involuntary movements in patients taking oral contraceptives. Br Med J 4:404, 1969.

Lindhout D, René JE, Höppener A, Meinardi H: Teratogenicity of antiepileptic drug combinations with special emphasis on epoxidation (of carbamazepine). Epilepsia 25:77, 1984.

Livingston S, Berman W, Pauli LL: Maternal epilepsy and abnormalities of the fetus and newborn. Lancet 2:1265, 1973.

Lowe CR: Congenital malformations among infants born to epileptic women. Lancet 1:9, 1973.

Lunz G: Zbl Gynak 50:2710, 1926. (Cited by Carroll JD, Leak D, Lea HA: Cerebral thrombophlebitis in pregnancy and the puerperium. Q J Med 35:347, 1966.)

Marcus EM, Watson CW, Goldman PL: Effects of steroids on cerebral electrical activity. Arch Neurol 15:521, 1966.

Marquez-Monter H, Ruiz-Fragoso E, Velasco M: Anticonvulsant drugs and chromosomes. Lancet 2:426, 1970.

Marsh L, Fraser FC: Chelating agents and teratogenesis. Lancet 2:846, 1973.

Martin JP: Thrombosis in the superior longitudinal sinus following childbirth. Br Med J 2:537, 1941.

Mauguiere F, Quoex C, Bello S: Epileptogenic properties of folic acid and N⁵ methyltetrahydrofolate in cat. Epilepsia 16:535, 1975.

May M, Wette R, Hardin WB, Sullivan J: The use of steroids in Bell's palsy: A prospective controlled study. Laryngoscope 86:1111, 1976.

Michelsen JJ, New PFJ: Brain tumour and pregnancy. J Neurol Neurosurg Psychiatry 32:305, 1969.

Millar JHD, Allison RS, Cheeseman EA, Merrett JD: Pregnancy as a factor influencing relapse in disseminated sclerosis. Brain 82:417, 1959.

Mjolnerod OK, Rasmussen K, Dommerud SA, Gjeruldsen ST: Congenital connective-tissue defect probably due to D-penicillamine treatment in pregnancy. Lancet 1:673, 1971.

Monson RR, Rosenberg L, Hartz SC, et al: Diphenylhydantoin and selected congenital malformations. N Engl J Med 289:1049, 1973.

Montouris GD, Fenichel GM, McLain LW: The pregnant epileptic. A review and recommendations. Arch Neurol 36:601, 1979.

Mountain KR, Hirsh J, Gallus AS: Neonatal coagulation defect due to anticonvulsant drug treatment in pregnancy. Lancet 1:265, 1970.

Muniz F, Houston E, Schneider R, Nusyowitz M: Chromosomal effects of diphenylhydantoins. Clin Res 17:28, 1969.

Mygind KI, Dam M, Christiansen J: Phenytoin and phenobarbitone plasma clearance during pregnancy. Acta Neurol Scand 54:160, 1976.

Namba T, Brown SB, Grob D: Neonatal myasthenia gravis: Report of two cases and review of the literature. Pediatrics 45:488, 1970.

Nausieda PA, Koller WC, Weiner WJ, Klawans HL: Chorea induced by oral contraceptives. Neurology 29:1605, 1979.

Newell KW, Lehmann AD, Leblanc DR, Osorio NG: The use of toxoid for the prevention of tetanus neonatorum. Final report of a double-blind controlled field trial. Bull WHO 35:863, 1966.

Newton TH, Hoyt WF: Dural arteriovenous shunts in the region of the cavernous sinus. Neuroradiology 1:71, 1970.

Niebyl JR, Blake DA, Freeman JM, Luff RD: Carbamazepine levels in pregnancy and lactation. Obstet Gynecol 53:139, 1979.

Niederhoff H, Zahrodnik H-P: Analgesics during pregnancy. Am J Med 75(Suppl):117, 1983 (Suppl on Antipyretic Analgesic Therapy).

Niswander KR, Gordon M: The Collaborative Perinatal Study of the National Institute of Neurological Diseases and Stroke. The Women and Their Pregnancies. (DHEW Publication No. NIH 73–379) Washington DC, Department of Health, Education and Welfare, 1972.

Novak DJ, Johnson KP: Relapsing idiopathic polyneuritis during pregnancy. Arch Neurol 28:219, 1973.

O'Connell JEA: Maternal obstetrical paralysis. Surg Gynecol Obstet 79:374, 1944.

O'Connell JEA: Lumbar disc protrusions in pregnancy. J Neurol Neurosurg Psychiatry 23:138, 1960.

O'Connell JEA: Neurosurgical problems in pregnancy. Proc R Soc Med 55:577, 1962.

Orringer CE, Eustace JC, Wunsch CD, Gardner LB: Natural history of lactic acidosis after grand mal seizures. N Engl J Med 297:796, 1977.

Osserman KE: Pregnancy in myasthenia gravis and neonatal myasthenia gravis. (Discussion) Am J Med 19:720, 1955.

Osserman KE: Myasthenia Gravis. New York, Grune & Stratton, 1958.

Parkinson D, Bachers G: Arteriovenous malformations. Summary of 100 consecutive supratentorial cases. J Neurosurg 53:285, 1980.

Pearson MG: Meralgia paresthetica with reference to its occurrence in pregnancy. J Obstet Gynaecol Br Emp 64:427, 1957.

Perlroth MG, Marver HS, Tschudy DP: Oral contraceptive agents and the management of acute intermittent porphyria. JAMA 194:1037, 1965.

Perret G, Nishioka H: Report on the cooperative study of intracranial aneurysms and subarachnoid hemorrhage. Section VI. Arteriovenous malformations. J Neurosurg 25:467, 1966.

Pope TH, Kenan PD: Bell's palsy in pregnancy. Arch Otolaryngol 89:830, 1969.

Poser S, Poser W: Multiple sclerosis and gestation. Neurology 33:1422, 1983.

Pruzanski W: Myotonic dystrophy—a multisystem disease. Report of 67 cases and a review of the literature. Psychiatr Neurol 149:302, 1965.

Ramsay RE, Strauss RG, Wilder BJ, Willmore LJ: Status epilepticus in pregnancy: Effect of phenytoin malabsorption on seizure control. Neurology 28:85, 1978.

Raskin NH: Headache. 2nd Ed. New York, Churchill Livingstone, 1988.

Reeves DL: Tumors of the brain complicating pregnancy. West J Surg Obstet Gynecol 60:211, 1952.

Reid DE: Assessment and management of the seriously ill patient following abortion. JAMA 199:805, 1967.

Rhodes P: Meralgia paraesthetica in pregnancy. Lancet 2:831, 1957.

Robert E, Guibaud P: Maternal valproic acid and congenital neural tube defects. Lancet 2:937, 1982.

Robertson DNS: The paraplegic patient in pregnancy and labour. Proc R Soc Med 56:381, 1963.

Robertson DNS: Pregnancy and labour in the paraplegic. Paraplegia 10:209, 1972.

Robinson JL, Hall CS, Sedzimir CB: Arteriovenous malformations, aneurysms, and pregnancy. J Neurosurg 41:63, 1974.

Robinson JR, Pou JW: Bell's palsy. A predisposition of pregnant women. Arch Otolaryngol 95:125, 1972.

Robinson RG: Aspects of the natural history of cerebellar haemangioblastomas. Acta Neurol Scand 41:372, 1965.

Roman IC, Caratzali A: Effects of anticonvulsant drugs on chromosomes. Br Med J 4:234, 1971.

Rosa FW: Spina bifida in infants of women treated with carbamazepine during pregnancy. N Engl J Med 324:674, 1991.

Rosen TS, Lin M, Spector S, Rosen MR: Maternal, fetal, and neonatal effects of chronic propranolol administration in the rat. J Pharmacol Exp Ther 208:118, 1979.

Rotton WN, Sachtleben MR, Friedman EA: Migraine and eclampsia. Obstet Gynecol 14:322, 1959.

Ryan RE: A controlled study of the effect of oral contraceptives on migraine. Headache 17:250, 1978.

Sauer HHA: Paradoxical embolism in pregnancy. Review of the literature and report of a case. J Obstet Gynaecol Br Emp 62:906, 1955.

Schaeffer M, Fox MJ, Li CP: Intrauterine poliomyelitis infection. Report of a case. JAMA 155:248, 1954.

Schapira K, Poskanzer DC, Newell DJ, Miller H: Marriage, pregnancy and multiple sclerosis. Brain 89:419, 1966.

Scheinberg IH, Sternlieb I: Pregnancy in penicillamine-treated patients with Wilson's disease. N Engl J Med 298:1300, 1975.

Schipper HM: Neurology of sex steroids and oral contraceptives. Neurol Clin 4:721, 1986.

Schmidt D, Canger R, Avanzini G, et al: Change of seizure frequency in pregnant epileptic women. J Neurol Neurosurg Psychiatry 46:751, 1983.

Schoenfeld N, Epstein O, Nemesh L, et al: Effects of propranolol during pregnancy and development of rats. 1. Adverse effects during pregnancy. Pediatr Res **12**:747, 1978.

Sciarra JJ, Steer CM: Uterine contractions during labor in myotonic muscular dystrophy. Am J Obstet Gynecol **82**:612, 1961.

Scott DE, Whalley PJ, Pritchard JA: Maternal folate deficiency and pregnancy wastage. II. Fetal malformation. Obstet Gynecol **36**:26, 1970.

Scriver CR, Clow CL: Phenylketonuria: Epitome of human biochemical genetics. N Engl J Med **303**:1336, 1980.

Seip M: Growth retardation, dysmorphic facies and minor malformations following massive exposure to phenobarbitone in utero. Acta Paediatr Scand **65**:617, 1976.

Shannon KM, Amman AJ: Acquired immune deficiency syndrome in childhood. J Pediatr **106**:332, 1985.

Shapiro S, Slone D, Hartz SC, et al: Anticonvulsant and parental epilepsy in the development of birth defects. Lancet **1**:272, 1976.

Shapiro S, Slone D, Hartz SC, et al: Are hydantoins (phenytoins) human teratogens? J Pediatr **90**:673, 1977.

Shelokov A, Habel K: Subclinical poliomyelitis in a newborn infant due to intra-uterine infection. JAMA **160**:465, 1956.

Shore RN, MacLachlan TB: Pregnancy with myotonic dystrophy. Course, complications and management. Obstet Gynecol **38**:448, 1971.

Simon RH: Brain tumors in pregnancy. Semin Neurol **8**:214, 1988.

Slocum HC, O'Neal KC, Allen CR: Neurovascular complications from malposition on the operating table. Surg Gynecol Obstet **86**:729, 1948.

Smithells RW: Environmental teratogens of man. Br Med Bull **32**:27, 1976.

Somerville BW: The role of estradiol withdrawal in the etiology of menstrual migraine. Neurology **22**:355, 1972a.

Somerville BW: A study of migraine in pregnancy. Neurology **22**:824, 1972b.

South J: Teratogenic effect of anticonvulsants. Lancet **2**:1154, 1972.

Speidel BD, Meadow SR: Maternal epilepsy and abnormalities of the fetus and newborn. Lancet **2**:839, 1972.

Speroff L: Bacterial shock in obstetrics and gynecology, with emphasis on the surgical management of septic abortion. Am J Obstet Gynecol **95**:139, 1966.

Starreveld-Zimmerman AAE, van der Kolk WJ, Elshove J, Meinardi H: Teratogenicity of antiepileptic drugs. Clin Neurol Neurosurg **77**:81, 1974.

Stein GS: Headaches in the first postpartum week and their relationship to migraine. Headache **21**:201, 1981.

Stevens H: Puerperal hemiplegia. Neurology **4**:723, 1954.

Stevens H, Ammerman HH: Intracranial venous thrombosis in early pregnancy. Am J Obstet Gynecol **78**:104, 1959.

Strauss RG, Bernstein R: Folic acid and dilantin antagonism in pregnancy. Obstet Gynecol **44**:345, 1974.

Sunderland S: Nerves and Nerve Injuries. Edinburgh, Churchill Livingstone, 1968.

Suter C, Klingman WO: Seizure states and pregnancy. Neurology **7**:105, 1957.

Sweeney WJ: Pregnancy and multiple sclerosis. Am J Obstet Gynecol **66**:124, 1953.

Symonds CP: Cerebral thrombophlebitis. Br Med J **2**:348, 1940.

Taniguchi RM, Goree JA, Odom GL: Spontaneous carotid-cavernous shunts presenting diagnostic problems. J Neurosurg **35**:384, 1971.

Taverner D, Cohen SB, Hutchinson BC: Comparison of corticotrophin and prednisolone in treatment of idiopathic facial paralysis (Bell's palsy). Br Med J **4**:20, 1971.

Taverner D, Fearnley ME, Kemble F, et al: Prevention of denervation in Bell's palsy. Br Med J **1**:391, 1966.

Taverner D, Kemble F, Cohen SB: Prognosis and treatment of idiopathic facial (Bell's) palsy. Br Med J **4**:581, 1967.

Taylor RA: Heredofamilial mononeuritis multiplex with brachial predilection. Brain **83**:113, 1960.

Teramo K, Hiilesmaa V, Bardy A, Saarikoski S: Fetal heart rate during a maternal grand mal epileptic seizure. J Perinat Med **7**:3, 1979.

Thompson DS, Nelson LM, Burns A, et al: The effects of pregnancy in multiple sclerosis: A retrospective study. Neurology **36**:1097, 1986.

Thomson RM: Myasthenia gravis and pregnancy. (Discussion). Proc R Soc Med **56**:381, 1963.

Timiras PS: Role of hormones in the development of seizures. In Jasper HH, Ward AA, Pope A (eds): Basic Mechanisms of the Epilepsies. Boston, Little Brown, 1969.

Townsend JJ, Baringer JR, Wolinsky JS, et al: Progressive rubella panencephalitis. Late onset after congenital rubella. N Engl J Med **292**:990, 1975.

Tsai A, Lindheimer MD, Lamberg SI: Dermatomyositis complicating pregnancy. Obstet Gynecol **41**:570, 1973.

Tschudy DP, Valsamis M, Magnussen CR: Acute intermittent porphyria: Clinical and selected research aspects. Ann Intern Med **83**:851, 1975.

Ueland K, McAnulty JH, Ueland FR, Metcalfe J: Special considerations in the use of cardiovascular drugs. Clin Obstet Gynecol **24**:809, 1981.

Ungley CC: Recurrent polyneuritis in pregnancy and the puerperium affecting three members of a family. J Neurol Psychopathol **14**:15, 1933.

Viets HR, Schwab RS, Brazier MAB: The effect of pregnancy on the course of myasthenia gravis. JAMA **119**:236, 1942.

Wainscott G, Sullivan FM, Volans GN, Wilkinson M: The outcome of pregnancy in women suffering from migraine. Postgrad Med J **54**:98, 1978.

Walsh FB, Hoyt WF: Clinical Neuro-ophthalmology. 3rd ed. Baltimore, Williams & Wilkins Co, 1969.

Walshe JM: Pregnancy in Wilson's disease. Q J Med **46**:73, 1977.

Watson JD, Spellacy WN: Neonatal effects of maternal treatment with the anticonvulsant drug diphenylhydantoin. Obstet Gynecol **37**:881, 1971.

Weil ML, Itabashi HH, Cremer NE, et al: Chronic progressive panencephalitis due to rubella virus simulating subacute sclerosing panencephalitis. N Engl J Med **292**:994, 1975.

Weinshenker BG, Hader W, Carriere W, et al: The influence of pregnancy on disability from multiple sclerosis: a population-based study in Middlesex County, Ontario. Neurology **39**:1438, 1989.

Weinstein L, Aycock WL, Feemster RF: The relation of sex, pregnancy and menstruation to susceptibility in poliomyelitis. N Engl J Med **245**:54, 1951.

Weyand RD, MacCarty CS, Wilson RB: The effect of pregnancy on intracranial meningiomas occurring about the optic chiasm. Surg Clin North Am **31**:1225, 1951.

Whittaker WG: Injuries to the sacral plexus in obstetrics. Can Med Assoc J **79**:622, 1958.

Wiebers DO: Ischemic cerebrovascular complications of pregnancy. Arch Neurol **42**:1106, 1985.

Willson P, Preece AA: Chorea gravidarum. Arch Intern Med **49**:471, 1932.

Wolf SM, Wagner JH, Davidson S, Forsythe A: Treatment of Bell palsy with prednisone: A prospective, randomized study. Neurology **28**:158, 1978.

Yen SSC: Neuroendocrine aspects of the regulation of cyclic gonadotropin release in women. In Martini L, Besser GM (eds): Clinical Neuroendocrinology. New York, Academic Press, 1977.

Yerby MS: Pregnancy and epilepsy. Epilepsia **32**(Suppl 6):S51, 1991.

CHAPTER

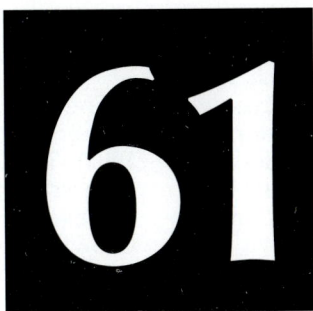

THE SKIN AND PREGNANCY

RONALD P. RAPINI, M.D., and ROBERT E. JORDON, M.D.

The physical and hormonal alterations induced by pregnancy, childbirth, and the puerperium are associated with numerous cutaneous changes. Some of these occur so frequently that they are not considered abnormal and vary only in degree. This chapter will discuss these physiologic changes and will also discuss the pathologic rashes of pregnancy and the effects of pregnancy on preexisting dermatologic diseases.

COMMON SKIN CHANGES INDUCED BY PREGNANCY

Pigmentary Changes

Hyperpigmentation occurs to some degree in at least 90 per cent of pregnant women (Wong and Ellis, 1989). Much of this is presumed to be due to the effects of increased levels of melanocyte-stimulating hormone (MSH) (Ances and Pomerantz, 1974) or estrogen and progesterone (Snell and Bischitz, 1960) on the melanocytes in the epidermis (see Chapter 26 for details of endocrine changes in pregnancy). Altmeyer et al. (1989) showed a significant increase in the levels of alpha-MSH, melatonin, ACTH, and progesterone from the first to the third trimester. Nearly all pregnant women develop mild generalized hyperpigmentation with accentuation in the areolae and genital skin. Hyperpigmentation of the linea alba is referred to as "linea nigra." All of these pigmentary changes generally regress following delivery.

Melasma is diffuse macular hyperpigmentation of the face, usually involving the forehead, cheeks, and bridge of the nose. Although chloasma is often used as a synonym, some authors restrict the term to those cases occurring during pregnancy ("mask of pregnancy"). Melasma occurs in about 70 per cent of pregnant women, but also may be seen in women who are not pregnant, especially those taking oral contraceptives. The hyperpigmentation is usually blotchy and poorly demarcated and is bilaterally symmetrical. In most cases it will resolve postpartum; however, sometimes it may persist for months or years. An increased incidence of thyroid abnormalities has been reported in patients with melasma (Lutfi et

al., 1985), but in many instances this is mild and subclinical. Avoidance of the sun during pregnancy helps to prevent or minimize the formation of melasma. Topical sunscreen lotions or creams with sun protective factor ratings of 15 or greater are helpful. For troublesome hyperpigmentation that persists after delivery, topical hydroquinone bleaching creams are sometimes useful. They must be applied carefully to avoid hypopigmentation, and treatment is frequently prolonged for months. Cosmetics are useful for covering irregular pigmentation. Additional therapeutic options for melasma persisting after pregnancy include topical tretinoin and chemical peels with trichloroacetic acid or phenol.

Pregnancy may induce the appearance of *new melanocytic nevi* or enlargement of preexisting nevi (Foucar et al., 1985). Such lesions should be excised immediately if they show signs suggestive of malignant melanoma (Gormley, 1990). Local anesthetics such as lidocaine are generally regarded as safe. The use of epinephrine in low doses along with lidocaine may help to expedite surgery. Most melanomas exhibit asymmetry, an irregular border, variegated colors (red or white in addition to black or blue), and a diameter greater than 6 mm. The subject of malignant melanoma during pregnancy is addressed in Chapter 62.

Vascular Changes

Pregnancy induces dilation and proliferation of blood vessels. Although this is thought to be largely due to estrogen, the mechanism is not completely understood. *Telangiectasias* occur that resemble those seen with chronic sunlight or radiation exposure. *Spider angiomas* are characterized by a central arteriole with radiating vascular "legs" resembling those of a spider and are most prevalent in sun-exposed areas. In addition to pregnancy, spider angiomas may be seen in liver disease (due to decreased hepatic estrogen catabolism), estrogen therapy, and in normal nonpregnant women. These lesions may regress spontaneously. Persistent lesions are best treated with light electrocoagulation or laser ablation. *Palmar erythema* is seen in many normal pregnant women and also may be associated with liver disease, estrogen therapy, and collagen vascular diseases. These vascular changes require no therapy, usually resolving after delivery.

Pyogenic granuloma is a misnomer for a juicy red nodular, often pedunculated, exuberant proliferation of granulation tissue. These lesions may occur anywhere on the skin but are especially common on the gums, often occurring as a result of gingivitis or trauma. The terms *lobular capillary hemangioma, pregnancy tumor*, and *granuloma gravidarum* are synonyms for pyogenic granuloma (Wong and Ellis, 1989). Therapy consists of surgical excision or electrosurgical destruction; however, this can often be delayed until after delivery, as some lesions will spontaneously regress. Immediate biopsy should be performed if there is any doubt about the clinical diagnosis, because occasional neoplasms such as an amelanotic melanoma may resemble a pyogenic granuloma.

Venous congestion and increased vascular permeability during pregnancy commonly causes edema of the skin and subcutaneous tissue, particularly of the vulva and lower legs. *Severe labial edema* has occasionally been reported during pregnancy (Morris et al., 1990), and sometimes a search for other causes may be warranted. *Varicosities* are common on the legs and around the anus (hemorrhoids). These may regress after delivery, but usually not completely (Wong and Ellis, 1989).

Connective Tissue Changes

The mechanisms by which collagen and other connective tissue elements are influenced during pregnancy are poorly understood. Some changes are thought to be induced by hormones such as estrogen and corticosteroids (Poidevin, 1959).

Striae represent linear tears in dermal collagen and appear as pink or purple atrophic bands over the abdomen, breasts, thighs, buttocks, groin, and axillae. Genetic susceptibility may be involved, since no striae form in pregnant women with Ehlers-Danlos syndrome and some normal women fail to develop them. They are less common in Asians and blacks. The degree of skin distention does not appear to correlate with the development of striae (Poidevin, 1959). Despite numerous anecdotal claims of therapeutic efficacy, no topical therapy prevents or affects the course of striae, which ordinarily become less apparent as the pink or purple color fades postpartum. Topical emollients or antipruritics may be helpful in those patients who experience itching in association with striae. Davey (1972) claims that abdominal striae are less common when the skin is massaged with oil, but this has not been substantiated by others.

Skin tags (acrochordons or *"molluscum fibrosum gravidarum")* are soft papular or pedunculated growths of fibrous and epithelial tissue that commonly occur in obesity as well as in pregnancy. They are usually flesh-colored to brown and most commonly appear on the neck, axillae, or groin. Skin tags persist after delivery and may be easily electrocoagulated or snipped off with scissors.

Hair Cycle and Growth Changes

The hair growth cycle is divided into three phases: anagen, catagen, and telogen (Rook and Dawber, 1982). The duration of the growing phase (anagen) of each scalp hair follicle persists 3 to 4 years, with an average daily growth rate of approximately 0.34 mm. Growth activity is followed by a relatively short transitional (catagen) phase, lasting about 2 weeks, followed by a resting phase (telogen), lasting several weeks. When the next hair cycle starts, newly forming hair causes shedding of the older telogen hairs.

The activity of each of about 100,000 follicles on the human scalp cycles randomly and independently from the activity of neighboring follicles. At any given time, approximately 10 to 15 per cent of hair follicles are in telogen. If the average duration of growth of each follicle is approximately 1000 days (3 years), it can be calculated that about 100 hairs should be shed normally each day, a figure that agrees with observations. Estrogen decreases the rate of hair growth and lengthens the duration of anagen (Hale and Ebling, 1975). In late pregnancy, the proportion of hairs in telogen may be only about 5 to 10 per cent (Lynfield, 1960). Following hormone withdrawal in the postpartum period, the percentage of telogen hairs may rise to 35 or more, resulting in a transient hair loss peaking about 3 to 4 months after parturition (Schiff and Kern, 1963). This suggests that estrogen also slows the entry of anagen hairs into catagen and telogen.

The diffuse hair loss beginning one to five months following delivery has been called *telogen effluvium*. The severity varies greatly, and it takes a total hair loss of 40 to 50 per cent to be noticeable. Telogen effluvium is generally easy to distinguish from other causes of hair loss (Rook and Dawber, 1982), and patients should be reassured that regrowth is likely to occur by 9 months postpartum without any treatment.

Hirsutism of the lower facial or sexual skin areas is uncommon, but may occasionally occur in the second half of pregnancy and may be accompanied by acne. The cause is presumed to relate to the effects of ovarian and placental androgens on the pilosebaceous unit. The possibility of an underlying androgen-secreting tumor of the ovary, of a luteoma, or of a lutein cyst should be considered, although polycystic ovary disease appears to be the most frequent cause (Fayez et al., 1974).

Several different *nail changes* have been reported during pregnancy, but none occur regularly. These include transverse grooving, increased brittleness, softening, or distal onycholysis (Wong and Ellis, 1989).

SKIN CONDITIONS SPECIFIC TO PREGNANCY

Table 61–1 lists the rashes specific to pregnancy. Because of a lack of understanding of the pathogenesis of most of these conditions and the lack of specific diagnostic criteria, the terminology has been confusing (Holmes and Black, 1983). Many of these diseases have been described by different authors using different names for the same conditions (Winton and Lewis,

TABLE 61–1. Rashes of Pregnancy

	ESTIMATED % OF ALL PREGNANCIES	LESION MORPHOLOGY	MOST COMMON LOCATION	IMPORTANT LABORATORY FEATURES	USUAL TRIMESTER OF ONSET	INCREASED FETAL MORTALITY
Pruritus gravidarum	1.5–2.0	Pruritus, no rash	Anywhere	Sometimes increased bile salts	3	Yes (?)
Prurigo gestationis (Besnier)	0.3–2	Excoriated papules	Extremities	None	2	No
Papular dermatitis (Spangler)	0.03	Papules	Trunk, extremities	Decreased estrogen, increased hCG	1, 2, or 3	Yes (?)
Pruritic uriticarial papules and plaques of pregnancy (PUPPP, PEP)	0.5	Papules, plaques, urticaria	Abdomen, thighs	None	3	No
Herpes gestationis (pemphigoid gestationis)	0.01	Papules, vesicles	Anywhere	Direct IF biopsy	2 or 3	Yes (?)
Impetigo herpetiformis	Very rare	Pustules	Intertriginous, trunk	Biopsy subcorneal pustule	1, 2, or 3	Yes
Autoimmune progesterone dermatitis	Only three reported cases	Acneiform, urticarial	Buttocks, extremities	Progesterone intradermal skin test	1	Yes (?)

LFT = Liver function tests; hCG = human chorionic gonadotropin; IF = immunofluorescence.

1982). In general, all tend to be pruritic and usually resolve following delivery. They all may recur in subsequent pregnancies except the polymorphic eruption of pregnancy and prurigo gestationis. Four of the diseases have been claimed to be associated with increased fetal mortality. It is important to keep in mind that pregnant women may also develop other dermatoses besides those specific to pregnancy. For example, contact dermatitis, eczema, superficial fungal infections, folliculitis (Zoberman and Farmer, 1981), erythema multiforme, vasculitis, viral exanthems, scabies, secondary syphilis, and drug eruptions may all occur, and it may be difficult to distinguish these from some of the pregnancy rashes discussed here.

The same general treatment principles apply to all of the specific dermatoses of pregnancy (Sasseville et al., 1981). Few drugs have been proved safe during pregnancy, and the benefit/risk ratio must be considered. Milder disease is treated with topical emollients, cool compresses or baths, and topical steroids. Nearly all topical steroids (such as hydrocortisone and triamcinolone) are classified as FDA Pregnancy Risk Category C, but they are still widely used during pregnancy when the possible benefits outweigh the risks of minimal percutaneous absorption. Many oral antihistamines, including the non-sedating terfenadine and astemizole, are labeled as FDA Pregnancy Risk Category C, since insufficient data are available. Hydroxyzine is contraindicated in early pregnancy. Those oral antihistamines classified as Category B (such as azatadine, chlorpheniramine, cyproheptadine, diphenhydramine, dexchlorpheniramine, or tripelennamine) may be worth trying for those patients with bothersome pruritus (Jurecka and Gebhart, 1989). The favorite appears to be diphenhydramine (Benadryl), even though it produces annoying drowsiness. Use of systemic steroids such as prednisone or prednisolone for patients with severe disease appears to be relatively safe in humans. Although cleft palates have occurred in offspring of pregnant rabbits undergoing such therapy (Sasseville et al., 1981), this relationship has not been demonstrated in humans. Infants of mothers treated with prednisone should be monitored by a pediatrician for evidence of adrenal insufficiency.

Pruritus Gravidarum

Pruritus gravidarum is defined as generalized itching, often associated with some degree of biliary obstruction. Cholestatic itching correlates better with serum bile acid levels than with other biochemical "liver function tests" such as alkaline phosphatase, SGOT, LDH, and bilirubin. Levels of bile salts in the skin correlate better than the serum concentrations (Schoenfield, 1969). The mechanism of biliary obstruction in pregnancy is discussed in Chapter 58.

Pruritus associated with cholestasis occurs in 1.5 to 2.0 per cent of pregnant women, with onset usually in the third trimester; frank clinical jaundice occurs in only 0.02 per cent of pregnancies. The degree of itching is variable but is usually more severe on the extremities than on the trunk. Superficial excoriation may occur. Pruritus limited to the anterior abdominal wall is common and is usually due to skin distention and development of striae rather than cholestasis.

Pruritus usually disappears shortly after delivery but recurs in approximately 50 per cent of subsequent pregnancies. An increased incidence of cholelithiasis has been observed in pregnant women with pruritus and recurrent cholestasis (Furhoff, 1974). Oral contraceptives may precipitate recurrent symptoms in this group. Reported increases in rates of premature delivery and perinatal mortality appear to be restricted to those in whom frank clinical jaundice develops (Friedlander and Osler, 1967). Slightly shortened gestational times, lower birth weights, and increased meconium staining occur in pregnancies without clinical jaundice; their clinical significance awaits further information.

Treatment is symptomatic, and mild cases usually respond to adequate skin lubrication and topical anti-pruritics. Ultraviolet light treatment or judicious sun exposure may also decrease pruritus. In more severe cases, bile-sequestering agents such as cholestyramine, supplemented with fat-soluble vitamins, may be beneficial (Laatikainen, 1978). Oral antihistamines may be of some benefit, as discussed previously.

Prurigo Gestationis

The pathogenesis of this disorder is unknown. The general term prurigo designates an intensely pruritic skin eruption in which excoriation predominates, suggesting a prominent emotional component. Many of these patients have a genetic predisposition toward atopic dermatitis. Prurigo gestationis was first described by Besnier in 1904 and is similar to the early prurigo of pregnancy later described by Nurse in 1968. The lesions consist of excoriated papules or nodules mostly over the extremities, usually beginning in the middle of pregnancy (Fig. 61–1). Although elevated liver function tests have been reported in some cases, this probably represents an overlap of patients with pruritus gravidarum. The eruption usually clears by 3 months after delivery, and the recurrence rate in subsequent pregnancies is low. Treatment depends upon the severity, as discussed earlier.

Papular Dermatitis of Pregnancy

Patients with this rare disease present with pruritic, excoriated, erythematous papules over the trunk and extremities (Michaud et al., 1982). It was separated out as a distinct entity by Spangler et al. (1962) on the basis of the presence of markedly elevated levels of 24-hour urinary human chorionic gonadotropin (hCG) for that stage of pregnancy, decreased levels of plasma and urinary estriol and plasma cortisone, and a short-

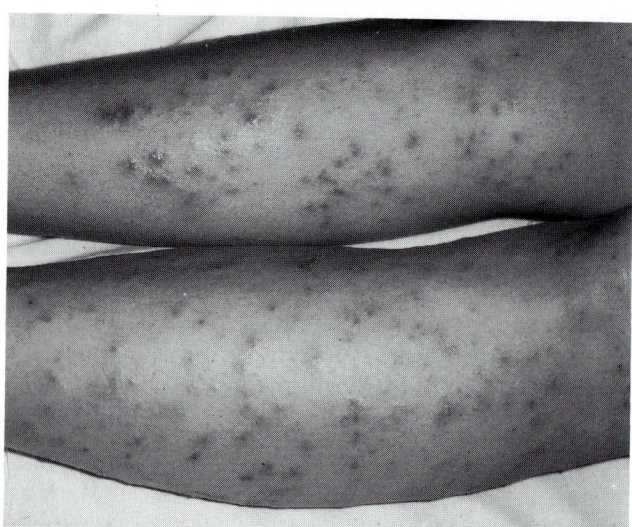

FIGURE 61–1. Prurigo gestationis. The predominant lesions are excoriated papules.

ened plasma cortisone half-life. In addition, the lesions were noted to be more widespread than in the other pregnancy rashes. Whether or not these criteria are sufficient to determine a separate disease is questionable. There have been very few case reports, and some of the reported cases of papular dermatitis have been questionable because appropriate laboratory studies were not done to exclude the other pregnancy rashes discussed here (Pruett and Kim, 1980). Also, hormonal studies have not been performed in detail in most reported cases of other pregnancy dermatoses. Some cases of papular dermatitis of pregnancy might actually represent examples of widespread prurigo gestationis (Black, 1989). Certainly, the clinical lesions themselves are not distinct from other papular eruptions of pregnancy. Histologic findings are nonspecific. The etiology is unknown. It has been suggested that allergic sensitization to an unidentified placental antigen may play a role because patients with this disease develop inflammatory reactions to intradermal injections of placental extracts from other patients with the disease. No such reactions occur with extracts of placentas from normal patients.

As in most of the rashes of pregnancy, the papules usually resolve following delivery, and recurrence during subsequent pregnancies is common. It is often listed as one of the dermatoses of pregnancy in which fetal mortality is increased (30 per cent). However, the actual mortality rate may not be increased because Rh incompatibility probably played a role in some of the reported deaths, and some of the deaths occurred in pregnancies in which the patient was unaffected by the eruption. Also, the authors used no control group, and included patients who aborted in the first trimester, which is common in the normal population. Treatment with systemic steroids has been claimed to decrease the fetal mortality on the basis of small numbers of patients.

Pruritic Urticarial Papules and Plaques of Pregnancy (PUPPP)

PUPPP (Lawley et al., 1979) is a poorly defined disorder characterized by erythematous papules, plaques, and urticarial lesions that usually begins in the third trimester. Vesicles only rarely occur (Schwartz et al., 1981). The rash has also been named *polymorphic eruption of pregnancy (PEP)* by Holmes and Black (1982), and this term is preferred in Europe. It is almost always pruritic, and itching is severe in 80 per cent of patients. The eruption has also been called *toxemic rash of pregnancy* (Bourne, 1962) and *late-onset prurigo of pregnancy* (Nurse, 1968).

The lesions begin on the abdomen in 80 to 90 per cent of cases, often sparing the umbilicus (Fig. 61–2). The striae become involved in 67 per cent of cases, suggesting that abdominal distention may contribute to the inflammation seen in this rash. In many cases, the eruption spreads to the proximal thighs, buttocks, and proximal arms. The face is nearly always spared (Holmes, 1989). Sometimes erythema multiforme–like target lesions are present. The rash usually resolves before or within several weeks after delivery. The

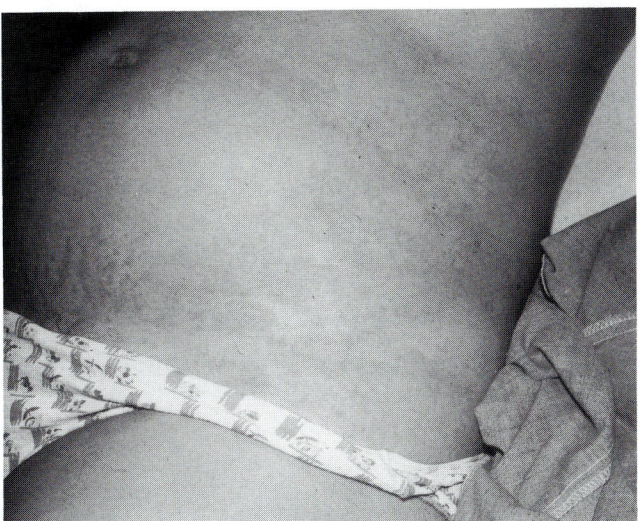

FIGURE 61–2. Polymorphic eruption of pregnancy (pruritic urticarial papules and plaques of pregnancy, PUPPP). Urticarial lesions on the abdomen.

disease is most prevalent in primigravidas. There appears to be an association with increased maternal weight gain, increased newborn birth weight, and an increased twin pregnancy rate of 10 per cent of cases (Cohen et al., 1989). Unlike most of the other rashes of pregnancy, PUPPP does not tend to recur with subsequent pregnancies (Yancey et al., 1984). There is no increase in the fetal mortality rate. Routine skin biopsies show nonspecific changes: there is variable parakeratosis, spongiosis, acanthosis, dermal edema, and a perivascular infiltrate of lymphocytes, histiocytes, and eosinophils (Callen and Hanno, 1981). The etiology is unknown. Hormonal levels appear to be normal (Alcalay et al., 1988). Unlike herpes gestationis, direct immunofluorescence of skin biopsies is negative (Moreno et al., 1985), but in a few cases very weak linear deposition of C3 at the basement membrane zone has been reported (Alcalay et al., 1987). This is probably a nonspecific finding, just like the finding of linear IgM at the dermal/epidermal junction in the absence of other immunoglobulins (Helm and Valenzuela, 1992). Treatment depends upon the severity, as discussed earlier for pregnancy rashes in general.

Herpes Gestationis

Herpes gestationis is a rare, intensely pruritic blistering dermatosis of pregnancy and the immediate postpartum period (Kolodny, 1969; Yancy, 1990). It is not related to infection of herpes virus; the unfortunate name refers to the grouped (herpetiform) nature of the blisters (which are often not really herpetiform at all). The onset usually occurs during the second or third trimester, but cases beginning in the first trimester or the immediate postpartum period have been well documented (Hertz et al., 1976; Lawley et al., 1978). This disorder has been rarely associated with choriocarcinoma of pregnancy and hydatidiform mole

(Tillman, 1950; Dupont, 1974). A high frequency of HLA haplotypes B8 and DR3/DR4 has been reported in patients with herpes gestationis, particularly in those patients whose husbands are DR2 (Shornick et al., 1983).

The clinical presentation is somewhat variable. Erythematous plaques, urticaria-like lesions, vesicles (often in annular configurations), and large tense bullae all may be present (Figs. 61–3 and 61–4). The extent of the disease process and the degree of accompanying pruritus may be mild to severe. Lesions usually begin on the abdomen, often within the umbilicus. Other commonly involved areas include the trunk, buttocks, and extemities. The face and mucous membranes are rarely affected.

An increased mortality of infants born to affected mothers has been estimated to be as high as 30 per cent (Lawley et al., 1978), although this has been disputed by others (Holmes and Black, 1983; Shornick and Black, 1992). A relationship between disease severity (as judged by the need for more vigorous therapy) and fetal complications has also been reported. With systemic steroid treatment of severe cases, there appears to be minimal fetal risk (Holmes and Black, 1983). There is an increase in prematurity and small-for-gestational-age infants (Shornick and Black, 1992). Most infants do not exhibit skin lesions, although transient urticarial and vesicular lesions thought to be due to transplacental antibody transfer have been noted in less than 5 per cent of infants born of affected mothers (Katz et al., 1977; Chorzelski et al., 1976).

Postpartum flares occur in 50 to 75 per cent of patients with herpes gestationis. Exacerbation typically begins within 24 to 48 hours after delivery and may last several weeks or several months. Skin lesions have been reported to persist more than a year in women who do not breast-feed, as compared to those who do breast-feed (average postpartum duration is 1 to 6 months) (Yancey, 1990; Black and Stephens, 1992). Subsequent pregnancies often result in an earlier onset and more severe involvement of herpes gestationis. Flares may also occur with subsequent menses, ovulation, or treatment with estrogen or progesterone. About 20 to 50 per cent of patients who have had herpes gestationis develop recurrent skin lesions when treated with oral contraceptives (Yancey, 1990).

Although not diagnostic, the histopathologic features are characteristic. Blistering lesions are usually subepidermal but sometimes can be intraepidermal as a result of spongiosis. Focal necrosis of basal keratinocytes may be observed. There is a perivascular lymphohistiocytic infiltrate in the dermis with a significant number of eosinophils. Ultrastructurally, the earliest findings appear to be vacuolar degeneration of the endoplasmic reticulum of the basal cells with destruction of their plasma membranes (Hertz et al., 1976). Thus, basal cell degeneration with fluid accumulation in the lamina lucida region of the skin basement membrane zone (BMZ) may be part of the mechanism of blistering in herpes gestationis.

Immunopathologically, herpes gestationis and bullous pemphigoid (an autoimmune disease of the elderly) are strikingly similar. Heavy linear deposits of

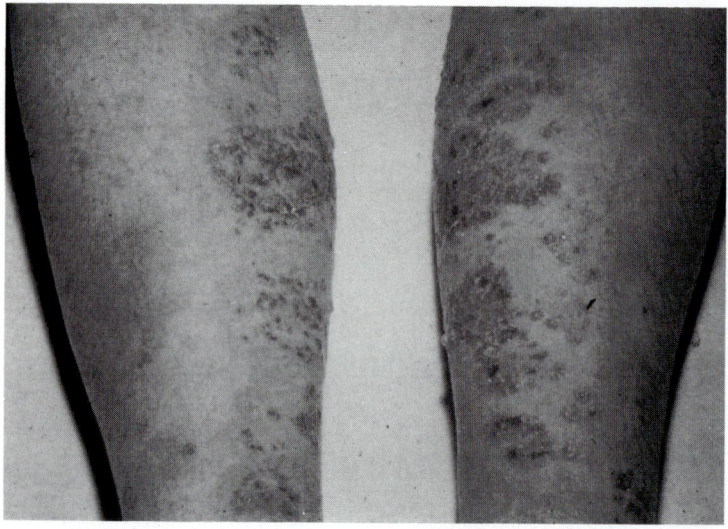

FIGURE 61–3. Herpes gestationis. Vesicular lesions on the arm with a tendency to be annular and grouped (herpetiform).

C3 are present in the BMZ of herpes gestationis perilesional skin (Fig. 61–5), usually in the absence of IgG deposits when tested using direct immunofluorescence (IF) staining methods (Jordon et al., 1976; Katz et al., 1976). Other complement components, in particular properdin and factor B of the alternate pathway, may also be present in lesional tissue. BMZ C3 deposits have also been described in some infants born to affected mothers (Chorzelski et al., 1976). Again, these deposits usually occur in the absence of concomitant immunoglobulin deposition. By immunoelectron microscopy, the C3 deposits are localized to the lamina lucida region of the BMZ as they are in bullous pemphigoid. Because of this relationship to bullous pemphigoid, and because the confusion regarding the name "herpes," a proposal has been made to change the name of herpes gestationis to "pemphigoid gestationis" (Holmes and Black, 1983).

Unlike bullous pemphigoid, however, circulating anti-BMZ IgG are measurable by indirect IF in only 10 to 20 per cent of cases of herpes gestationis (Jordon et al., 1976; Katz et al., 1976). When present, titers are usually low, again in contrast to bullous pemphigoid. In the vast majority of herpes gestationis sera, how-

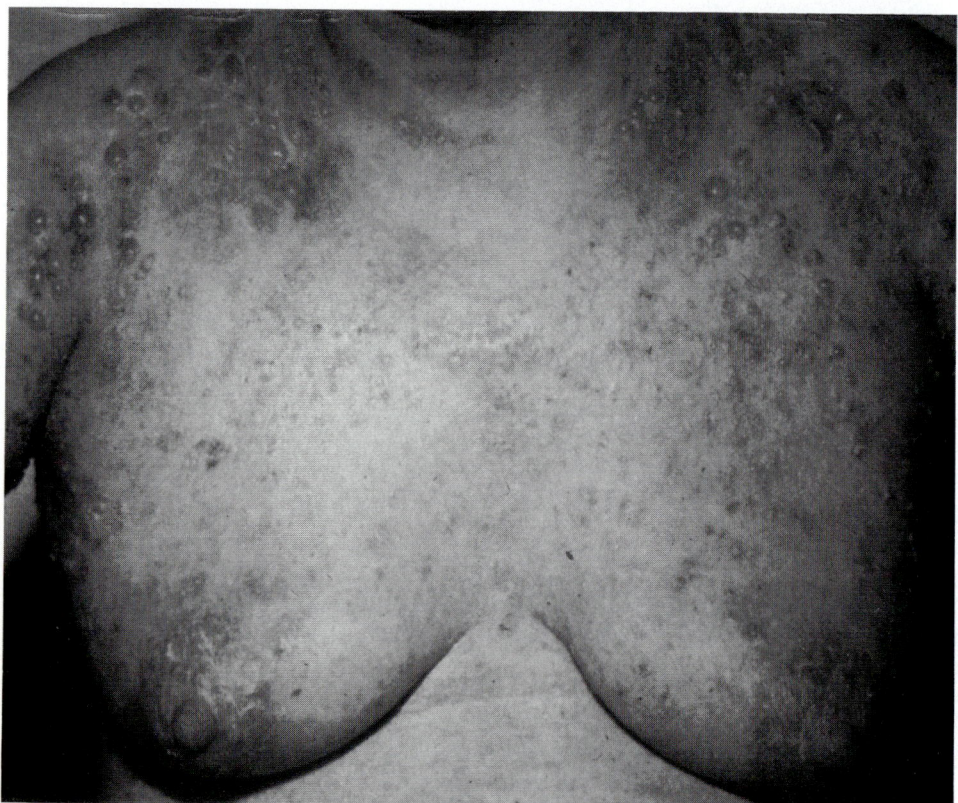

FIGURE 61–4. Herpes gestationis. Bullous lesions on the trunk.

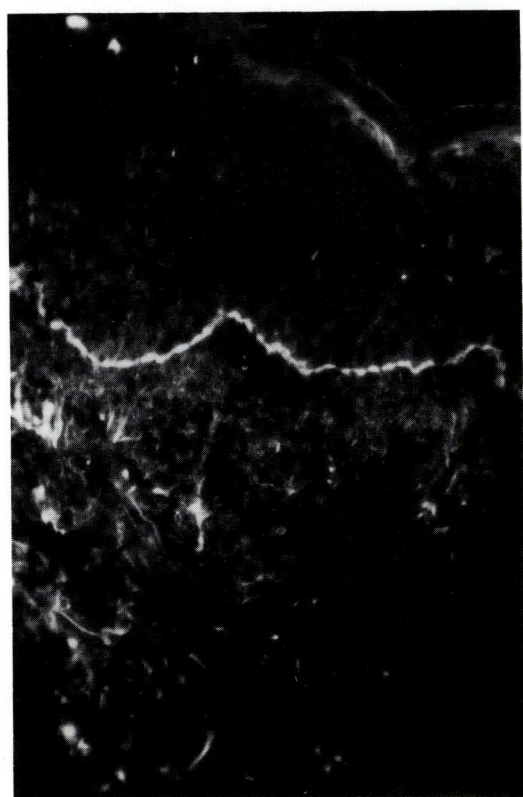

FIGURE 61–5. Herpes gestationis. This skin biopsy taken for direct immunofluorescence demonstrates a linear band of C3 at the basement membrane zone.

ever, a complement-fixing (C3) factor (HG factor) is present that reacts with the BMZ. HG factor is an IgG$_1$ autoantibody to the BMZ, which avidly fixes complement. It is present in such low levels, however, that it often escapes detection by routine methods. HG factor activates complement via the classical pathway in the same fashion as bullous pemphigoid antibodies, but bullous pemphigoid IgG subclasses are more heterogeneous, with IgG$_4$ being predominant over IgG$_1$ (Kelly et al., 1989). By immunoblotting, herpes gestationis autoantibodies react with a 180 kD protein associated with hemidesmosomes of basal keratinocytes (Kelly et al., 1990; Morrison et al., 1988), whereas bullous pemphigoid autoantibodies are reactive with two protein bands, a 240 kD band in addition to the 180 kD band.

Treatment of herpes gestationis should not be designed to suppress the disease process entirely. Instead, therapy should be directed toward suppressing the appearance of new lesions and relieving the intense pruritus (Jordon, 1988). In moderate-to-severe cases, prednisone, 20 to 40 mg/day, is often adequate to suppress new blister formation and relieve symptoms. Once new blister formation has been suppressed, the prednisone dose may be tapered to lower doses or just enough to maintain control and relieve symptoms. At this point, alternate-day therapy might be more appropriate and should be attempted. Immunosuppressive agents such as azathioprine obviously are contraindicated unless used in non-nursing

mothers in the postpartum period. If the disease flares in the immediate postpartum period, treatment with prednisone, 20 to 40 mg/day, should be reinstituted. Higher doses at this time may be instituted if necessary. It is important to remember that systemic steroids will suppress placental estrogen production, making urinary or serum estriol testing worthless as a guide for determining placental function (Winton and Lewis, 1982). Infants of mothers treated with prednisone should be monitored by a pediatrician for evidence of adrenal insufficiency. Other treatment modalities useful for all pregnancy rashes were discussed earlier. Pyridoxine has produced dramatic responses in uncontrolled case reports (Burkhart, 1982).

Impetigo Herpetiformis

First described in 1872 by von Hebra, impetigo herpetiformis represents a severe generalized pustular dermatosis associated with pregnancy. The name is unfortunate, as it is unrelated to either bacterial infection (impetigo) or herpes virus infection. The onset of the disease usually occurs in the third trimester, but well-documented cases have been seen as early as the first trimester (Sasseville et al., 1981). The disease usually subsides between pregnancies but will recur with subsequent pregnancies and usually earlier in the pregnancy (Beveridge et al., 1966). Hypoparathyroidism and hypocalcemia have also been associated with this condition (Sasseville et al., 1981), but the etiology of this disease remains unknown.

Clinically, the disease is characterized by hundreds of translucent white sterile pustules (Fig. 61–6) that arise on irregular erythematous bases or plaques. These lesions extend peripherally while central pustules rupture, owing to their superficial location, leaving denuded surfaces with crusts as seen in some forms of pemphigus. Common areas of involvement include the axillae, inframammary areas, umbilicus, groin, and gluteal crease. Pustular lesions may also occur on the hands and involve the nails with subsequent nail loss or onycholysis. Constitutional symptoms are often present and include fever, chills, nausea, vomiting, and diarrhea with severe dehydration. Delirium, tetany, and convulsions are rare complications usually associated with hypocalcemia. Death may occur, again in association with these complications and septicemia. Because impetigo herpetiformis has been described in nonpregnant individuals, it is now thought to represent a form of generalized pustular psoriasis seen during pregnancy. The clinical presentation and histopathology of both disease entities are identical (Baker and Ryan, 1968; Oosterling et al., 1978).

Histopathologically, impetigo herpetiformis is characterized by subcorneal pustule formation (spongiform pustules of Kogoj) consisting of neutrophils and degenerated keratinocytes. Again, this histopathologic picture is identical to generalized pustular psoriasis. Other laboratory abnormalities include a high sedimentation rate during flares and hypocalcemia usually associated with hypoparathyroidism. Cultures of pus-

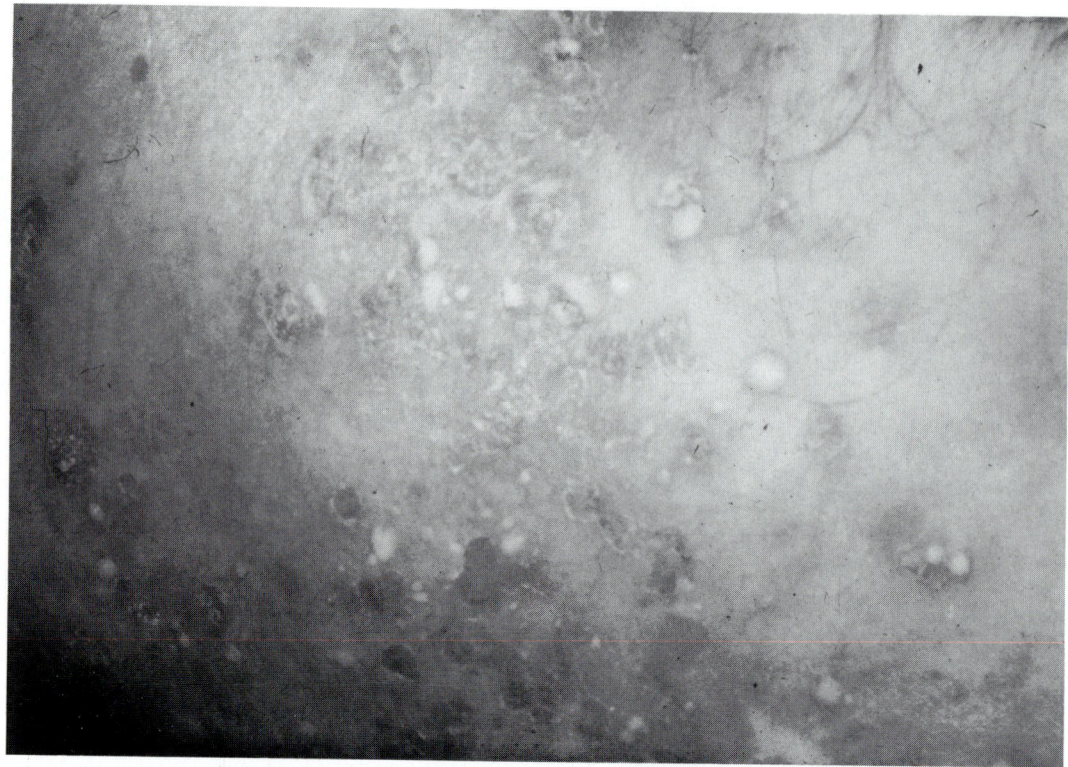

FIGURE 61–6. Impetigo herpetiformis. Sterile pustular lesions.

tular lesions are usually negative unless secondarily infected.

Systemic corticosteroid therapy is the treatment of choice for impetigo herpetiformis. Usually, 20 to 40 mg of prednisone per day is sufficient to control new lesion formation. Systemic antibiotics may help when secondary infection is present. Topical measures, such as wet compresses with or without topical steroid preparations, are also useful, as discussed earlier for all pregnancy rashes. Etretinate (a synthetic vitamin A derivative) and methotrexate, both considered treatment options for generalized pustular psoriasis, are contraindicated during pregnancy. Fetal condition may be assessed as discussed under herpes gestationis.

Autoimmune Progesterone Dermatitis

This dermatosis is a rare, poorly defined urticarial, papular, and pustular eruption thought to be caused by hypersensitivity to progesterone, usually associated with menstruation (Shelley et al., 1964; Jones and Gordon, 1969; Tromovitch and Heggli, 1967). About 24 cases have been reported (Stephens and Black, 1989). Only three cases report onset or worsening of this condition with pregnancy (Stephens and Black, 1989; Bierman, 1973). Two of these cases were associated with spontaneous abortion. In other cases of autoimmune progesterone dermatitis, the rash improved or cleared during pregnancy. There is some controversy whether autoimmune progesterone dermatitis during pregnancy really exists as a specific entity.

This disease has been documented by the use of intradermal or intramuscular test injections of progesterone. Intradermal tests generally produce a local urticarial reaction. Intramuscular challenges have caused exacerbations of the rash, or even angioedema. An indirect basophil degranulation test has also been used to support the concept of autosensitivity to progesterone in this disorder. In this test, the patient's serum is mixed with synthetic progesterone and rabbit basophils (Stephens and Black, 1989). Specific therapy for this condition has not been reported during pregnancy. Nonpregnant patients have responded to estrogens, the antiestrogen tamoxifen, or oophorectomy.

SKIN DISORDERS AFFECTED BY PREGNANCY

The effect of pregnancy on skin diseases is often variable. Table 61–2 lists some skin diseases that improve or become aggravated by pregnancy, although it must be emphasized that the course of a disease in a given patient is not always predictable. Cutaneous infections are covered in Chapter 42, while connective tissue diseases involving the skin are discussed in Chapter 59. Some infectious, autoimmune, or rheumatic diseases tend to worsen during pregnancy.

Acne Vulgaris

Acne is a disease of the pilosebaceous unit. It is partially influenced by androgens such as testosterone

TABLE 61-2.   Effect of Pregnancy on Skin Diseases

IMPROVED BY PREGNANCY (USUALLY)
  Fox-Fordyce disease (Cornbleet, 1952)
  Hidradenitis suppurativa (Cornbleet, 1952)
AGGRAVATED BY PREGNANCY (USUALLY)
  Condylomata acuminata (Lynch, 1985)
  Ehlers-Danlos syndrome (Winton, 1989)
  Erythema multiforme
  Erythema nodosum (Salvatore et al., 1980)
  Herpes simplex (Winton, 1989)
  Lupus erythematosus (Lockshin, 1985)
  Neurofibromatosis (Swapp and Main, 1973)
  Pemphigus (Winton, 1989)
  Pityriasis rosea
  Porphyrias (Winton, 1989)
  Pseudoxanthoma elasticum (Winton, 1989)
  Scleroderma (increased renal disease) (Mor-Yosef et al., 1984)
  Tuberous sclerosis (increased seizures)
UNPREDICTABLE RESPONSE TO PREGNANCY
  Acne
  Acquired immunodeficiency syndrome (Winton, 1989)
  Atopic dermatitis (Kemmett and Tidman, 1991)
  Dermatomyositis (Tsia et al., 1973)
  Malignant melanoma (Winton, 1989)
  Psoriasis

and dehydroepiandrosterone sulfate (DHEA-S), which have been shown to increase sebaceous gland activity (Held et al., 1984). Progesterone does not seem to stimulate sebaceous gland activity except in very large doses. Estrogen reduces sebaceous gland size and activity, but this is probably a function of negative feedback upon androgen production by the ovary.

Acne consists of erythematous papules, pustules, comedones, and cysts on the face, back, and chest. Some cases reported as "pruritic folliculitis of pregnancy" of widespread locations may actually represent hormonally induced acne (Black, 1989). Pregnancy has a variable effect upon acne, probably because there are many other factors involved in its pathogenesis besides the hormonal influences discussed.

Acne may be controlled during pregnancy with topical benzoyl peroxide, salicylic acid, or topical antibiotics such as erythromycin or clindamycin (Jurecka and Gebhart, 1989). Topical and oral sulfonamides should be avoided near term. Topical metronidazole is contraindicated during the first trimester and should be used later in pregnancy only if other alternatives have failed. More severe disease can be treated with oral erythromycin, starting with 1 gm daily (FDA Pregnancy Category B). Tetracycline should be avoided because of its potential adverse effects on fetal dentition. Vitamin A derivatives (retinoids), such as oral isotretinoin, are contraindicated because of teratogenic effects. Topical tretinoin is not contraindicated, but it would probably be best to use a different topical drug during pregnancy.

Atopic Dermatitis

Atopic dermatitis is a skin disease of uncertain origin characterized by intensely pruritic eczematous der-

matitis. Lesions become lichenified when patients are caught in a scratch-itch cycle. There appears to be an inherited irritability of the skin, and many patients have a personal or family history beginning in childhood of eczema, asthma, hayfever, or allergic rhinitis. This disease may worsen (52 per cent) or improve (24 per cent) during pregnancy (Kemmett and Tidman, 1991). Treatment with topical emollients, topical steroids, and oral antihistamines is usually effective. Patients should be instructed to use soap sparingly and should always apply topical emollient lotions or creams after bathing. Exceptional patients may require systemic steroids.

Erythema Nodosum

Erythema nodosum is characterized by tender nodules on the anterior lower legs, usually considered to be a reaction to a drug or an infection somewhere else. Sarcoidosis and inflammatory bowel disease are also frequent etiologies. Erythema nodosum is known to be precipitated by pregnancy as well as oral contraceptives, suggesting an estrogen influence on this disease (Salvatore and Lynch, 1980).

Fox-Fordyce Disease

This is a rare disease often called "apocrine miliaria" because it can be thought of as being similar to the "prickly heat" or "heat rash" involving eccrine glands. Fox-Fordyce disease occurs mainly in women, with onset usually shortly after puberty. Multiple pruritic dome-shaped follicular papules develop in the axillae and anogenital region, areas rich in apocrine glands. The disease usually improves during pregnancy or with oral contraceptive therapy, probably because of an estrogen effect. Apocrine activity appears to be decreased during pregnancy (Cornbleet, 1952), unlike eccrine activity. Response to topical steroids is variable.

Genodermatoses

A long list of inherited severe cutaneous diseases involving the mother or other family members may affect fetal mortality or morbidity. New technologies making it possible to study the molecular, enzymatic, and ultrastructural basis of these conditions are continually evolving. It is impossible to provide up-to-date information on this rapidly changing field in a textbook. More details of prenatal diagnosis are given in Chapter 2. Modalities useful for diagnosing severe fetal skin diseases include chorionic villus sampling, amniocentesis, and fetoscopy with fetal skin biopsy (Sybert et al., 1992). Although ichthyosis and epidermolysis bullosa represent the two most important groups of disorders, prenatal diagnosis has been successful in many other skin diseases (Esterly and Elias, 1983). For ichthyosis and epidermolysis bullosa, fetal skin biopsies have proved to be reliable for the detection of fetal involvement.

There are four major types of ichthyosis, all of which exhibit extensively thickened scaly skin resembling the scales of a fish. A variety of ichthyotic syndromes have been described that involve other abnormalities besides the skin. Ichthyosiform erythroderma is subdivided into dominant and recessive forms, and generalized involvement is usually present at birth. The collodion and harlequin fetuses are severe examples of ichthyosis in which an infant with grotesque deformities, often resulting in death, is born encased in a horny sheet.

The multiple forms of epidermolysis bullosa are characterized by extensive blistering that may contribute to excessive fluid loss or predispose to fatal neonatal infection. The dystrophic and letalis forms of the disease can be distinguished from the less severe simplex form by determining the level of blistering in the skin by electron microscopy or by immunofluorescent staining of basement membrane zone antigens.

REFERENCES

Alcalay J, Ingber A, David M, et al: Pruritic urticarial papules and plaques of pregnancy: A review of 21 cases. J Reprod Med 32:315, 1987.

Alcalay J, Ingber A, Kafri B, et al: Hormonal evaluation and autoimmune background in pruritic urticarial papules and plaques of pregnancy. Am J Obstet Gynecol 158:417, 1988.

Altmeyer P, Bernd A, Holzmann H, et al: Alpha-MSH and pregnancy. Z Hautkr 64:577, 1989.

Ances JG, Pomerantz SH: Serum concentrations of beta-MSH in human pregnancy. Am J Obstet Gynecol 119:1062, 1974.

Baker H, Ryan TJ: Generalized pustular psoriasis. A clinical and epidemiological study of 104 cases. Br J Dermatol 80:771, 1968.

Beveridge GW, Harkness RA, Livingston JRB: Impetigo herpetiformis in two successive pregnancies. Br J Dermatol 78:106, 1966.

Bierman SM: Autoimmune progesterone dermatitis of pregnancy. Arch Dermatol 107:896, 1973.

Black MM: Prurigo of pregnancy, papular dermatitis of pregnancy, and pruritic folliculitis of pregnancy. Semin Dermatol 8:23, 1989.

Black MM, Stephens CJM: The specific dermatoses of pregnancy: The British perspective. Adv Dermatol 7:105, 1992.

Bourne G: Toxaemic rash of pregnancy. J R Soc Med 55:462, 1962.

Burkhart CG: Pyridoxine-responsive herpes gestationis. Arch Dermatol 118:535, 1982.

Callen JP, Hanno R: Pruritic urticarial papules and plaques of pregnancy (PUPPP). J Am Acad Dermatol 5:401, 1981.

Chorzelski TP, Jabloska S, Beutner EH, et al: Herpes gestationis with identical lesions in the newborn. Arch Dermatol 112:1129, 1976.

Cohen LM, Capeless EL, Krusinski PA, Maloney ME: Pruritic urticarial papules and plaques of pregnancy and its relationship to maternal-fetal weight gain and twin pregnancy. Arch Dermatol 125:1534, 1989.

Cornbleet T: Pregnancy and apocrine diseases: Hidradenitis, Fox-Fordyce disease. Arch Dermatol Syph 65:12, 1952.

Davey CMH: Factors associated with the occurrence of striae gravidarum. J Obstet Gynecol Br Commonw 79:1113, 1972.

Dupont C: Herpes gestationis with hydatidiform mole. Trans St John's Hosp Dermatol Soc 60:103, 1974.

Esterly NB, Elias S: Antenatal diagnosis of genodermatoses. J Am Acad Dermatol 8:655, 1983.

Fayez JA, Bunch TR, Miller GL: Virilization in pregnancy associated with polycystic ovary disease. Obstet Gynecol 44:511, 1974.

Foucar E, Bentley TJ, Lanbe DW, et al: A histopathologic evaluation of nevocellular nevi in pregnancy. Arch Dermatol 121:350, 1985.

Friedlander P, Osler M: Icterus and pregnancy. Am J Obstet Gynecol 97:894, 1967.

Furhoff AK: Itching in pregnancy. Acta Med Scand 196:403, 1974.

Gormley DE: Cutaneous surgery and the pregnant patient. J Am Acad Dermatol 23:269, 1990.

Hale PA, Ebling FJ: The effects of epilation and hormones on the activity of rat hair follicles. J Exp Zool 191:49, 1975.

Held BL, Nader S, Rodriguez-Rigan LJ, et al: Acne and hyperandrogenism. J Am Acad Dermatol 10:223, 1984.

Helm TN, Valenzuela R: Continuous dermoepidermal junction IgM detected by direct immunofluorescence: A report of nine cases. J Am Acad Dermatol 26:203, 1992.

Hertz KC, Katz SI, Maize J, et al: Herpes gestationis: A clinical-pathologic study. Arch Dermatol 112:1543, 1976.

Holmes RC, Black MM: The specific dermatoses of pregnancy: A reappraisal with specific emphasis on a proposed simplified clinical classification. Clin Exp Dermatol 7:65, 1982.

Holmes RC, Black MM: The specific dermatoses of pregnancy. J Am Acad Dermatol 8:405, 1983.

Holmes RC: Polymorphic eruption of pregnancy. Semin Dermatol 8:18, 1989.

Jones WN, Gordon VH: Autoimmune progesterone eczema. Arch Dermatol 99:57, 1969.

Jordon RE, Heine KG, Tappeiner G, et al: The immunopathology of herpes gestationis: Immunofluorescence studies and characterization of HG factor. J Clin Invest 57:1426, 1976.

Jordon RE: Herpes Gestationis. In Provost TT, Farmer ER (eds): Current Therapy in Dermatology, 1987–1988. St. Louis, CV Mosby, 1988.

Jurecka W, Gebhart W: Drug prescribing during pregnancy. Semin Dermatol 8:30, 1989.

Katz A, Minta JO, Toole JWP, et al: Immunopathologic study of herpes gestationis in mother and infant. Arch Dermatol 113:1069, 1977.

Katz SI, Hertz KC, Yaoita H: Herpes gestationis. Immunopathology and characterization of the HG factor. J Clin Invest 57:1434, 1976.

Kelly SE, Bhogal BS, Wojnarowska F, et al: Western blot analysis of the antigen in pemphigoid gestationis. Br J Dermatol 122:445, 1990.

Kelly SE, Cerio R, Bhogal BS, Black MM: The distribution of IgG subclasses in pemphigoid gestationis: PG factor is an IgG1 autoantibody. J Invest Dermatol 92:695, 1989.

Kemmett D, Tidman MJ: The influence of the menstrual cycle and pregnancy on atopic dermatitis. Br J Dermatol 125:59, 1991.

Kolodny RC: Herpes gestationis. Am J Obstet Gynecol 104:39, 1969.

Laatikainen M: Effect of cholestyramine and phenobarbital on pruritus and serum bile acid levels in cholestasis of pregnancy. Am J Obstet Gynecol 132:501, 1978.

Lawley TJ, Stingl G, Katz SI: Fetal and maternal risk factors in herpes gestationis. Arch Dermatol 114:552, 1978.

Lawley TJ, Hertz KC, Wade TR, et al: Pruritic urticarial papules and plaques of pregnancy. JAMA 241:1696, 1979.

Lockshin MD: Lupus pregnancy. Clin Rheum Dis 11:611, 1985.

Lutfi RJ, Fridmanis M, Misiunas AL, et al: Association of melasma with thyroid autoimmunity and other thyroidal abnormalities and their relationship to the origin of melasma. J Clin Endocrinol Metab 61:28, 1985.

Lynch PJ: Condyloma acuminata (anogenital warts). Clin Obstet Gynecol 28:142, 1985.

Lynfield YL: Effect of pregnancy on the human hair cycle. J Invest Dermatol 35:323, 1960.

Michaud RM, Jacobson D, Dahl MC: Papular dermatitis of pregnancy. Arch Dermatol 118:1003, 1982.

Moreno A, Noguera J, DeMoranas JM: Polymorphic eruption of pregnancy: Histopathologic study. Acta Dermatol Venereol (Stockh) 65:313, 1985.

Morris LF, Rapini RP, Hebert AA, Katz AR: Massive labial edema in pregnancy. South Med J 83:846, 1990.

Morrison LH, Labib RS, Zone JJ, et al: Herpes gestationis autoantibodies recognize a 180 kD human epidermal antigen. J Clin Invest 81:2023, 1988.

Mor-Yosef S, Navot D, Rabinowitz R, et al: Collagen diseases in pregnancy. Obstet Gynecol Surv 39:67, 1984.

Nurse DS: Prurigo of pregnancy. Australas J Dermatol 9:258, 1968.

Oosterling RJ, Nobrega RE, Duboeuff JA, et al: Impetigo herpetiformis or generalized pustular psoriasis. Arch Dermatol 114:1527, 1978.

Poidevin LOS: Striae gravidarum: Their relationship to adrenal cortical hyperfunction. Lancet ii:436, 1959.

Pruett KA, Kim R: Papular dermatitis of pregnancy. Obstet Gynecol **55**(Suppl):38S, 1980.

Rook A, Dawber R (eds): Diseases of the Hair and Scalp. Oxford, Blackwell Scientific Publications, 1982.

Salvatore MA, Lynch PT: Erythema nodosum, estrogens and pregnancy. Arch Dermatol **116**:557, 1980.

Sasseville D, Wilkinson R, Schnader J: Dermatoses of pregnancy. Int J Dermatol **20**:223, 1981.

Schiff BL, Kern AB: A study of postpartum alopecia. Arch Dermatol **87**:609, 1963.

Schoenfield LJ: The relationship of bile acids to pruritus in hepatobiliary disease. *In* Schiff L, Carey JB, Dietschy J (eds): Bile salt metabolism. Springfield, Charles C Thomas, 1969.

Schwartz RA, Hansen RC, Lynch PJ: Pruritic urticarial papules and plaques of pregnancy. Cutis **27**:425, 1981.

Shelley WB, Purcel R, Stout S: Autoimmune progesterone dermatitis. Cure by oophorectomy. JAMA **190**:35, 1964.

Shornick JK, Stastny P, Gilliam JN: Paternal histocompatibility (HLA) antigen and maternal anti-HLA antibodies in herpes gestationis. J Invest Dermatol **81**:407, 1983.

Shornick JK, Black MM: Fetal risks in herpes gestationis. J Am Acad Dermatol **26**:63, 1992.

Snell RS, Bischitz PG: The effect of large doses of estrogen and estrogen and progesterone on melanin production. J Invest Dermatol **35**:73, 1960.

Spangler AS, Reddy W, Bardawil WA, et al: Papular dermatitis of pregnancy: A new clinical entity? JAMA **181**:577, 1962.

Spangler AS, Emerson K: Estrogen levels and estrogen therapy in papular dermatitis of pregnancy. Am J Obstet Gynecol **110**:534, 1971.

Stephens CJM, Black MM: Perimenstrual eruptions: Autoimmune progesterone dermatitis. Semin Dermatol **8**:26, 1989.

Swapp GH, Main RA: Neurofibromatosis in pregnancy. Br J Dermatol **88**:431, 1973.

Sybert VP, Holbrook KA, Levy M: Prenatal diagnosis of severe dermatologic diseases. Adv Dermatol **7**:179, 1992.

Tillman WG: Herpes gestationis with hydatidiform mole and chorion epithelioma. Br Med J **1**:1471, 1950.

Tromovitch TA, Heggli WF: Autoimmune progesterone urticaria. Calif Med **106**:211, 1967.

Tsia A, Lindheimer MD, Lamberg SI: Dermatomyositis complicating pregnancy. Obstet Gynecol **41**:570, 1973.

Winton GB, Lewis CW: Dermatoses of pregnancy. J Am Acad Dermatol **6**:977, 1982.

Winton GB: Skin diseases aggravated by pregnancy. J Am Acad Dermatol **20**:1, 1989.

Wong RC, Ellis CN: Physiologic skin changes in pregnancy. Semin Dermatol **8**:7, 1989.

Yancey KB: Herpes gestationis. Dermatol Clin **8**:727, 1990.

Yancey KB, Hall RP, Lawley TJ: Pruritic urticarial papules and plaques of pregnancy: Clinical experience in twenty-five patients. J Am Acad Dermatol **10**:473, 1984.

Zoberman E, Farmer ER: Pruritic folliculitis of pregnancy. Arch Dermatol **117**:20, 1981.

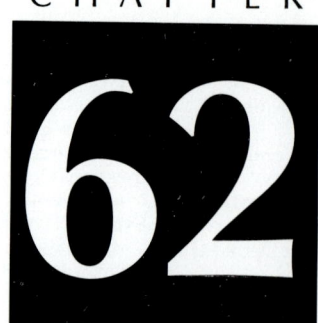

PELVIC MALIGNANCIES, GESTATIONAL TROPHOBLASTIC NEOPLASIA, AND NONPELVIC MALIGNANCIES

MICHAEL L. BERMAN, M.D., and PHILIP J. DiSAIA, M.D.

The frequency of cancer in association with pregnancy is only approximately 1 per 1000 live births; nevertheless, it is difficult to conceive a set of circumstances more stressful for patient and physicians than the discovery of a malignancy in a pregnant woman. Several issues immediately come to mind: (1) Is it necessary to terminate the pregnancy while the fetus is immature? (2) Can the tumor metastasize to the fetus? (3) Will treatment for the malignancy adversely affect the conceptus? (4) Can definitive therapy be deferred safely until the fetus is viable? (5) Does pregnancy adversely affect prognosis for the pregnant patient? Because the coexistence of pregnancy with malignant disease is a relatively rare occurrence, and since pregnancy typically occurs at an earlier age than that associated with most cancer diagnoses, clear therapeutic decisions may not be readily at hand when the diagnosis is made. On the other hand, the increasing trend to delay childbearing to the latter portion of the reproductive years by many women will undoubtedly result in an increased frequency of a cancer diagnosis in older parturients.

In 1963, Barber and Brunschwig reviewed 700 cases of cancer in pregnancy. The most common malignancies in order of frequency were breast cancer, leukemia and lymphomas as a group, melanoma, gynecologic cancer, and bone tumors. The relative frequencies of cancer in pregnancy by site apparently have not changed since that report.

In theory, the hormonal, metabolic, hemodynamic, and immunologic changes that occur during pregnancy impose many possible adverse effects on the malignant state. These theoretic concerns are greatest for tumors arising in tissues and organs that are under hormonal control or that respond to hormonal stimulation. Increased vascularity in the breasts and pelvic organs, enhanced lymphatic drainage of many organs, and the state of immunologic tolerance which characterizes pregnancy might contribute to early dissemination of the malignant process. This indirect and hypothetical reasoning in most instances has not been substantiated and often has led to erroneous conclusions resulting in a recommendation for therapeutic abortion. Although these hypotheses are intellectually stimulating, much of the material that follows suggests that in most instances the validity of such conclusions lacks solid supporting clinical data.

PELVIC MALIGNANCIES IN PREGNANCY

Cervical Cancer

Cervical cancer is the most frequently diagnosed invasive neoplasm in pregnancy, occurring in approximately 1 per 2000 to 2500 pregnancies and comprising approximately 25 per cent of all malignancies in pregnant women. Nearly 3 per cent of all cervical cancers are found during pregnancy, emphasizing the need for careful evaluation of all pregnant women for cervical cancer and its precursor lesions.

As part of every first prenatal visit, the physician should obtain a Papanicolaou smear from both the cervix and endocervical canal. Occult malignancies in the endocervix often are not detected if this area is not evaluated with either a cotton-tipped applicator or an endocervical aspirator. A wire brush sampling device should be avoided in pregnancy because of the small risk of rupturing the fetal membranes. Negative cytology is reassuring in that vaginal bleeding occurring later in pregnancy will not be attributed to cervical cancer, and its treatment will not be complicated by this diagnosis. Although the Papanicolaou smear is a sensitive screening tool, one should not rely upon it to rule out invasive disease in the presence of a suspicious cervical lesion, as up to 30 per cent of invasive cancers can be associated with negative cytology. Thus, office punch biopsy of suspicious lesions should be done even in the presence of a normal Papanicolaou smear. The moderate bleeding that ensues can be controlled adequately with Monsel's solution and silver nitrate.

Although cervical cancer is an uncommon cause of bleeding in pregnancy, a high index of suspicion will avoid unnecessary delays in the diagnosis of the occasional case. Thus, a careful speculum examination of the lower genital tract to rule out the existence of a friable exophytic lesion is essential to evaluate this complaint. Other nonobstetric causes of bleeding such as a cervical polyp and vaginal laceration can also be excluded in this manner.

The methods used for diagnosis and treatment of cervical cancer and its precursors in either pregnant or postpartum patients are the same as those utilized in the nonpregnant patient. Although the Papanicolaou smear is helpful in detecting preclinical disease in the cervix, its accuracy in invasive disease can be compromised by the presence of blood and a marked inflammatory reaction that might obscure the underlying diagnosis. The major diagnostic difficulty lies in the hesitancy to take a biopsy specimen of the cervix of a pregnant patient. Such specimens are unquestionably necessary and, in the absence of a visible lesion, should be carried out with colposcopic visualization.

The general philosophy for diagnosis and treatment of intraepithelial neoplasia of the cervix detected during pregnancy is one of expectant therapy after careful diagnosis. The pregnant patient who has an abnormal Papanicolaou smear should undergo colposcopically directed biopsy of suspicious areas to rule out invasive disease. Depending on the experience of the colposcopist, areas of abnormality that clearly are not invasive, such as those with minimal white epithelium without underlying vascular changes, may be observed without biopsy until the postpartum period.

Patients with intraepithelial neoplasia of the cervix may deliver vaginally with subsequent reassessment performed postpartum. Interestingly, many of these patients do not demonstrate persistent intraepithelial neoplasia when re-evaluated 6 weeks postpartum. Although an explanation for these changes is obscure, it probably results from either spontaneous regression or traumatic loss of the epithelium during the birth process.

When suspicion of invasion exists, based on clinical or cytologic assessment, a carefully directed incisional biopsy of sufficient depth to permit an accurate diagnosis should be carried out. A diagnosis of microinvasion on biopsy must be followed as soon as possible by a cone biopsy to rule out frankly invasive disease (Table 62–1). This is the only absolute indication for conization during pregnancy. Conization will distinguish patients with microinvasion whose pregnancy can proceed to term without appreciable maternal risk from those with frank invasion in whom consideration must be given to early interruption of the pregnancy. "Microinvasion" or "early stromal invasion" of the cervix is defined in our clinic as an invasive cancer that does not penetrate the stroma more than 3 mm below the basement membrane of the surface epithelium, does not manifest vascular or lymphatic invasion, is free of confluent tongues of tumor, and does not extend to the margins of the surgical specimen. By FIGO staging criteria, these lesions must be less

TABLE 62–1. Recommendations for Management of the Pregnant Patient With Abnormal Cytologic Findings

RESULTS OF COLPOSCOPICALLY DIRECTED BIOPSY	MANAGEMENT
CIN* I–III (cytology consistent with CIN)	Deter further diagnostic and therapeutic procedures until 6 weeks postpartum
CIN I–III (cytology consistent with invasive cancer)	Cone biopsy†
Microinvasive tumor	Cone biopsy†
Invasive cancer	Radical hysterectomy or radiotherapy

Adapted from DiSaia PJ, Creasman WT: Clinical Gynecologic Oncology. St. Louis, CV Mosby, 1981.
*Cervical intraepithelial neoplasia.
†Proceed to radical hysterectomy or radiotherapy if invasive cancer is present.

than 7 mm in diameter, as larger lesions are included in the stage IB category and must not be treated expectantly. When these histologic criteria have been met, the patient is advised that pregnancy may continue safely to term. Cesarean section is not necessary for this group of patients, and the route of delivery should be determined by obstetric indications. A recommendation for postpartum hysterectomy is not essential in these patients with "early stromal invasion" if they desire to bear more children.

The performance of a cone biopsy in the pregnant patient is a formidable undertaking with an increased risk of hemorrhage and spontaneous abortion. In reviewing the scientific literature, Hannigan (1990) compiled data that showed a 12 to 13 per cent risk of bleeding complications associated with this procedure. In order to reduce this potentially serious effect, we recommend using six hemostatic sutures evenly distributed around the portio of the cervix close to the vaginal reflection (Fig. 62–1). These sutures will reduce blood flow to the cone bed, evert the squamocolumnar junction, and facilitate performance of a shallow cone biopsy with little interruption of the endocervical ca-

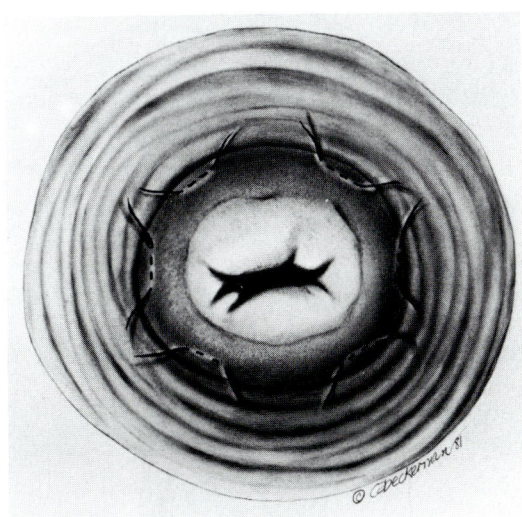

FIGURE 62–1. Location of six hemostatic sutures made in the cervix after cone biopsy.

nal. Fortunately, pregnancy itself causes the squamo-columnar junction to be everted, thereby limiting the need for sampling tissue high in the endocervix. The surgical procedure described for pregnancy might be envisioned as excising a "coin" rather than a cone tissue (Fig. 62–2). The LEEP procedure is especially well adapted to excision of a shallow cone of sufficient breadth and depth to permit treatment decisions while ruling out a more extensive invasive process.

The effect of pregnancy on cervical cancer and the effect of cervical cancer on pregnancy remain controversial. Although many early reports suggested that pregnancy might accelerate the growth of carcinoma of the cervix, more recent studies show that pregnancy has little effect on its growth. In general, cancer patients under the age of 35 tend to have a poorer prognosis than those in whom disease is diagnosed after this age. The difference in 5-year survival percentage between these two age categories is approximately 15 to 20 per cent for each stage of disease, possibly reflecting more aggressive histologic subtypes of cancer in younger patients. Because cervical cancer in pregnancy usually occurs in the younger group of patients, survival status for these women must be compared with that in a group of nonpregnant cervical cancer patients whose age distribution is similar to that of the group of pregnant patients. When such comparisons are made, pregnancy is found to have little adverse effect on the overall survival for this disease. In addition, those patients with DES-associated clear cell carcinoma of the cervix (and vagina) diagnosed during pregnancy have a 5- and 10-year survival rate that is not significantly different from what is reported for nonpregnant women at the time of diagnosis. This reported survival—stage for stage—is approximately equal to that of women with squamous cell cancers.

Confusion concerning the course of this disease in pregnancy has been attended by disagreement concerning optimal therapy. Support can be found for therapeutic approaches that include radiation therapy,

radical surgery, or a combined approach. These controversies are contrasted in two large series, by Waldrop and Palmer (1963) from Roswell Park Memorial Institute and by Bosch and Marcial (1966) from the I. Gonzalez Martinez Oncology Hospital in Puerto Rico. The dissenting opinions are not resolved easily because most reports contain limited numbers of cases from which conclusions can be drawn. As is often true when many therapeutic approaches are advocated for a given disease, in some instances there are clear advantages of one approach over another, and in other situations any of several approaches is satisfactory. The therapeutic modalities and their respective roles are discussed in detail later.

In deciding on the therapy for invasive cervical cancer in pregnancy, the physician must consider both the stage of disease and the duration of pregnancy. The decision often can be influenced by the religious convictions of the patient and family and the desire of the mother for the child. Since pregnancy has not been shown convincingly to have an adverse effect on prognosis, short delays of several weeks in definitive therapy, until the fetus has reached viability, are appropriate. The former beliefs that pregnancy might accelerate tumor growth and that parturition might squeeze viable cells into the vascular system and increase the incidence of metastatic spread have not been substantiated either by hormone receptor data or by clinical observation. Even cervical adenocarcinomas have low or absent sex steroid hormone receptors, supporting the data which show that, except for undifferentiated and small cell cancers, stage for stage, the outcome for the pregnant patient with cervical cancer is approximately that for the young nonpregnant patient.

An outline of recommended treatment for cervical cancer in pregnancy is shown in Table 62–2. For stage I and stage IIA lesions, radical hysterectomy with bilateral pelvic lymphadenectomy is acceptable during any trimester. Ovarian preservation is appropriate and desirable for these patients. Since some also might

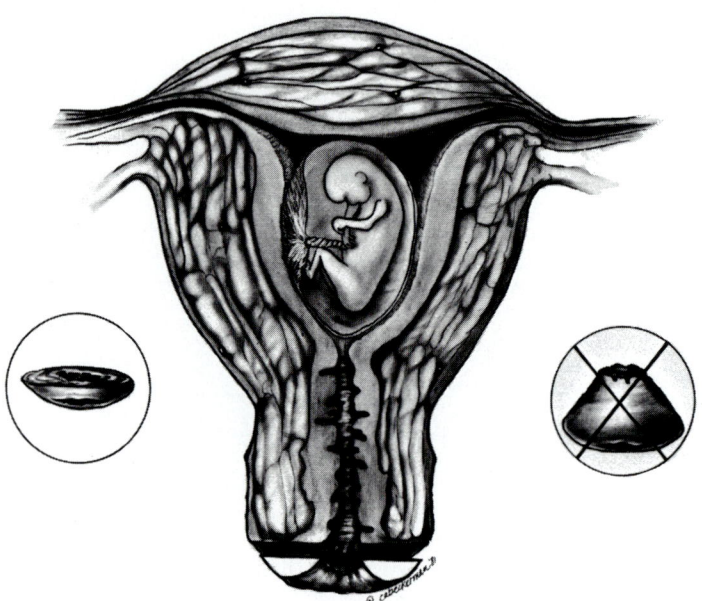

FIGURE 62–2. The shallow "coin biopsy" of the cervix appropriate in pregnancy.

TABLE 62–2. Suggested Therapy for Cervical Cancer in Pregnancy*

LENGTH OF PREGNANCY	STAGE OF CANCER	
	I-IIA	**IIB-IIIB**
Up to 20 weeks	4,500 WP: If spontaneous abortion, 6,000 B If no abortion, modified radical hysterectomy	5,000 WP: If spontaneous abortion, 5,000 B If no spontaneous abortion, Type II radical hysterectomy, no lymphadenectomy
	or Radical hysterectomy with bilateral pelvic lymphadenectomy	*or*
Beyond 20 weeks	Cesarean section when fetus viable followed by 5,000 WP and 5,000 B	Cesarean section when fetus viable followed by 5,000–6,000 WP and 4,000–5,000 B
	or Cesarean radical hysterectomy with bilateral pelvic lymphadenectomy	

*WP = whole-pelvis irradiation, with number indicating rads; B = brachytherapy—vaginal radium in two applications with number indicating mg/hr.
Modified from DiSaia PJ, Creasman WT: Clinical Gynecologic Oncology. St. Louis, CV Mosby, 1981.

require adjuvant radiotherapy following surgery, bilateral ovarian transposition out of the pelvis is recommended to avoid their destruction. The complication rate of radical hysterectomy with bilateral pelvic lymphadenectomy should not exceed that for nonpregnant patients. Although vascular supply to the pelvis is increased, normal tissue planes are very distinct, thereby facilitating easier pelvic dissection.

Generally, patients in the first half of pregnancy are advised to undergo definitive therapy immediately, and thus interruption of the pregnancy usually is advised. Exceptions to this philosophy in patients with "early stromal invasion" have been discussed. Cesarean radical hysterectomy at 34 weeks gestation usually will ensure fetal viability while delaying definitive therapy a maximum of 14 weeks for patients diagnosed during the second half of pregnancy. If studies of fetal lung maturity at this time suggest that respiratory distress syndrome is likely, surgery should be postponed until lung maturity is assured, with repeat tests done on a weekly basis. Such an approach necessitates careful coordination of efforts between the gynecologic oncologist and the perinatologist to ensure the best possible outcome for both mother and fetus. Implicit in this concept is the need for a neonatal intensive care unit for care of the preterm newborn.

Radiation therapy is equally efficacious in patients with early-stage cervical cancer and is the treatment of choice with more advanced stages. In the first 20 weeks of gestation, when the pregnancy is to be disregarded, treatment should begin with whole pelvis irradiation. Spontaneous abortion usually occurs within 5 weeks of therapy if begun in the first trimester and by 7 weeks if begun in the second trimester. Treatment then is completed with intracavitary radium

or cesium applications. If spontaneous abortion does not occur by completion of the external beam therapy, a modified hysterectomy without pelvic lymphadenectomy should be carried out to excise the remaining central neoplasm. This strategy delivers potentially curative doses of radiation in pelvic lymph nodes, followed by surgical resection of the remaining central tumor. This approach is preferable because the gravid uterus is not suitable for intracavitary radium or cesium. Although some clinics prefer an extended extrafascial hysterectomy following 5000 rads of whole-pelvis irradiation in patients with early lesions, we prefer the more extensive modified radical hysterectomy. This approach accomplishes adequate excision of the cervix, accompanying medial parametria, and upper vagina, thereby including all the tissues that would have been effectively irradiated by the pear-shaped isodose distribution of a tandem and ovoid application of brachytherapy. Those who advocate an extrafascial hysterectomy often advise further vaginal vault irradiation following the surgical procedure in order to treat the upper vagina and medial parametria more completely. An alternative approach in the patient who has not aborted is to evacuate the uterus by means of a hysterotomy followed by conventional intracavitary irradiation delivered within 1 to 2 weeks.

Patients who are at least 20 weeks pregnant may delay therapy until fetal viability is reached, unless hemorrhage necessitates earlier intervention. The timing of cesarean delivery is determined by the status of fetal lung maturity as described previously. If a radical hysterectomy with pelvic lymphadenectomy is not performed at the time of cesarean section, whole-pelvis irradiation is begun immediately after the abdominal incision is healed, approximately 10 to 14 days following surgery. Intracavitary radiation can follow completion of treatment to the whole pelvis. The basic radiotherapeutic plan employed for cancer of the cervix in the nonpregnant patient generally can be used for patients in whom only cesarean section has been performed. The Wertheim-type radical hysterectomy at the time of cesarean section, on the other hand, allows the patient to return home with her infant without needing further therapy, permits preservation of ovarian function, and is associated with less frequent sexual dysfunction than following radiotherapy. The most common adverse effect of this approach is bladder dysfunction, which is seen to some degree in the majority of women undergoing radical hysterectomy.

Stages IB and IIA can be treated with either surgery or radiation. The question of which is preferable remains the subject of endless debate. Although Creasman and colleagues (1970) demonstrated the effectiveness of radiation therapy used exclusively or as an important part of the therapy in 108 pregnant patients with cervical cancer, there is a lack of conclusive evidence that either approach offers better survival. The choice of therapy often appears to be determined by either the institutional preference or the expertise of the gynecologic or radiation therapy service. We prefer an approach using radical hysterectomy with bilateral pelvic lymphadenectomy because of the overall result, including ovarian preservation, improved sexual function, and elimination of unnecessary delays for the patient.

As expected, the prognosis for this disease is a function of stage and tumor volume. When primary surgery or a staging laparotomy is done, the survival probability can be refined further based on the status of lymph nodes in the pelvis and along the aorta. The impact of histology on prognosis relates primarily to two small subsets of patients with either small cell, undifferentiated cancers or poorly differentiated adenosquamous cancer, both associated with a dismal outlook. Overall, the 5-year survival in pregnancy is similar to that reported in nonpregnant women.

Ovarian Cancer

Of all malignancies arising in the pelvic region, ovarian cancers are second in frequency to cervical cancer but are exceedingly rare and occur in only 1 in 20,000 to 30,000 pregnancies. The differential diagnosis of ovarian masses during pregnancy is complicated by their location outside the pelvis during the second half of pregnancy, and the difficulty in distinguishing between the consistency of a gravid uterus and an ovarian neoplasm. Despite this diagnostic dilemma, the routine use of ultrasound to assess fetal development and investigate potential fetal anomalies increases the likelihood of finding unexpected ovarian masses. The routine use of ultrasound, however, also creates the clinical dilemma of identifying subclinical masses which rarely prove to be malignant, but which may necessitate some type of intervention.

The finding of an ovarian mass presents challenging problems in diagnosis and management. Eastman and Hellman (1966) reported finding ovarian cysts in one of 81 pregnancies, and Grimes and co-workers (1954) reported a cyst "large enough to be hazardous" in 0.3 per cent of pregnancies. Management of ovarian cysts can be complicated by pelvic impaction, obstructed labor, torsion, hemorrhage into the tumor, rupture of the cyst, infection, and, last but not least, malignancy. Although malignancy is relatively uncommon and the least acute complication in pregnancy, it should always be foremost in the clinician's mind.

Torsion of an ovarian neoplasm is particularly common in pregnancy, with a reported incidence of 10 to 15 per cent. Most torsions occur either when the uterus is growing at a rapid rate between the eighth and 16th weeks of gestation or when the uterus is involuting rapidly during the puerperium. About 60 per cent of the cases occur in the first half of pregnancy and most of the remaining cases in the puerperium. The usual sequence of events is sudden lower abdominal pain, nausea with vomiting, and, in some instances, a shock-like syndrome. The abdomen is often tense and tender, and there may be rebound tenderness with guarding.

Most ovarian enlargements found in pregnancy are follicular or corpus luteum cysts and usually are no more than 5 cm in diameter. Their management in early pregnancy should be expectant, because more than 90 per cent of these functional cysts disappear as pregnancy progresses and are undetectable by the

14th week of gestation. As the uterus begins to rise out of the pelvis and at the end of the first trimester, ovarian enlargement is evaluated best by pelvic and abdominal ultrasound because the ovaries often are not easily palpated. Guidelines for the management of an ovarian mass during pregnancy are similar to those generally recommended in the nonpregnant premenopausal woman. Specifically, if a cyst remains unchanged or increases in size during a 6-week observation period, the patient should undergo abdominal exploration. For solid ovarian masses of any size or cystic enlargement more than 8 cm in diameter, an observation period is not required before surgical intervention because such masses rarely are functional and usually are neoplastic. In the asymptomatic patient with a pelvic mass who is thought to be at low risk for a malignancy on the basis of pelvic examination and ultrasound, operative intervention is best delayed until the second trimester. This cautious approach will minimize the risk of interfering with the pregnancy while permitting spontaneous regression of a mass that would prove to be a functional cyst.

It is especially difficult to distinguish an ovarian tumor in pregnancy from other pelvic structures because of the size and cystic consistency of the gravid uterus. When the tumor is palpable within the pelvis, it must be differentiated from a retroverted pregnant uterus, a pedunculated uterine leiomyoma, carcinoma of the rectosigmoid colon, a pelvic kidney, and a uterine congenital anomaly such as an accessory uterine horn. In the patient with a mass that is suspicious for malignancy, diagnostic studies should involve an ultrasound of the abdomen and pelvis to detect ascites when present and to be certain that the mass is extrauterine in origin. Additional studies can include an intravenous pyelogram to rule out pelvic kidney and possible ureteral obstruction as well as a limited barium enema to be certain that colon cancer is not present. These radiologic studies should be avoided, if possible, during the first trimester of pregnancy in order to prevent the potential mutagenic effects of ionizing radiation to the developing fetus during organogenesis. In the latter half of pregnancy, ovarian tumors are particularly difficult to detect because the adnexa are found in the abdomen beyond the reach of examining fingers in the vaginal area. Abdominal examination, the chief method of diagnosis in the second half of pregnancy, is unreliable even when ascites is present because of the large uterus.

When an ovarian tumor is not detected during the first half of pregnancy, it frequently is not diagnosed until labor or delivery. If the ovarian mass obstructs the birth canal during labor, exploratory laparotomy is indicated for both delivery of the infant and management of the ovarian neoplasm. Allowing a labor to proceed while an ovarian neoplasm obstructs the birth canal can result in rupture of the ovarian mass followed by hemorrhage, peritonitis, tumor dissemination, or shock. Even if an ovarian cyst does not rupture, the trauma of labor can cause hemorrhage into the tumor followed by necrosis and suppuration. On the other hand, Brodsky et al. (1980) reported up to a fivefold increase in second trimester pregnancy loss associated with operative intervention for a pelvic mass. Despite this adverse effect of operative intervention, the authors believe that the benefits of earlier cancer diagnosis and prevention of subsequent complications outweigh the risks of avoiding operative intervention during the second trimester.

Epithelial tumors, which include serous, mucinous, endometroid, and clear cell cancers, account for approximately half of malignant ovarian neoplasms found in pregnancy. The diagnosis is usually fortuitous; the tumor is found at exploratory laparotomy for an adnexal mass or at cesarean section. Characteristically, these tumors are of early stage and low grade; indeed, many epithelial cancers of the ovary are borderline tumors.

Should the surgeon find an ovarian malignancy in pregnancy, the first obligation is to stage the patient's disease properly as outlined in Table 62–3, while providing operative intervention. Treatment should be appropriate for the stage of the disease, regardless of the pregnancy. It is our philosophy to treat stage IA lesions conservatively with a unilateral salpingo-oophorectomy, provided a thorough exploration of the abdominal cavity has been carried out. The exploration should be performed through a mid-line or paramedian incision extending above the umbilicus and should include visualization of the liver and diaphragms, biopsy of the omentum and peritoneum in the pelvis and pericolic areas, careful evaluation of the pelvic and periaortic lymph nodes, and obtaining of peritoneal fluid or washings for cytologic evaluation. We believe that more advanced lesions should not be treated conservatively unless the tumor is of the borderline variety, in which case definitive surgical therapy sometimes can be deferred until fetal viability is achieved. Needless to say, the decision regarding the degree of surgical intervention, which might include hysterectomy while the fetus is still immature, ultimately rests with the patient and her desire to continue the pregnancy.

The pregnant state does not appear to have a direct adverse effect on the prognosis of the patient with an ovarian malignancy, although its continuation can compromise both the initial operation and the initiation of postoperative therapy. Ovarian cancers are not sensitive to either exogenous or endogenous sources of sex steroids; therefore, the prognosis is unaffected by the pregnancy and by subsequent hormonal replacement therapy following removal of the ovaries.

Germ cell tumors are the most common ovarian neoplasms in pregnancy. The malignant tumors include dysgerminoma, embryonal carcinomas, immature teratomas, and endodermal sinus tumors. Sometimes a mixture of these various elements is present within the same malignancy (mixed germ cell tumor). Of the malignant germ cell tumors, dysgerminomas are the most commonly reported. The most common germ cell tumors, however, are mature teratomas, which are almost always benign in this age group. Indeed, they are by far the most common neoplastic cysts found in pregnancy. Attempts should be made to remove them in the early part of the second trimester whenever they are recognized radiographically during the first trimester in order to avoid torsion, rupture, or obstruction of the birth canal during parturition. The uninvolved ovarian tissue usually can be preserved because mature teratomas are well encapsulated and can easily be dissected off the remainder of the ovary.

Malignant germ cell neoplasms usually can be managed with a unilateral salpingo-oophorectomy because they are usually stage IA, and the prognosis for this stage is not improved with more extensive surgery (Fig. 62–3). Adjuvant chemotherapy in this group of highly malignant tumors plays an important role in treating all except the dysgerminoma. Combined chemotherapy has improved survival markedly and can permit preservation of childbearing capacity when the disease is stage I. If the diagnosis is made during the

TABLE 62–3. FIGO Stage Grouping for Primary Carcinoma of the Ovary (1985)

Stage I. Growth limited to the ovaries
IA. Growth limited to one ovary; no ascites. No tumor on the external surface; capsule intact
IB. Growth limited to both ovaries; no ascites. No tumor on the external surfaces; capsules intact
IC*. Tumor either stage IA or IB but with tumor on the surface of one or both ovaries; or with capsule ruptured; or with ascites present containing malignant cells or with positive peritoneal washings

Stage II. Growth involving one or both ovaries with pelvic extension
IIA. Extension and/or metastases to the uterus and/or tubes
IIB. Extension to other pelvic tissues
IIC*. Tumor either stage IIA or IIB but with tumor on the surface of one or both ovaries; or with capsule(s) ruptured; or with ascites present containing malignant cells or with positive peritoneal washings

Stage III. Tumor involving one or both ovaries with peritoneal implants outside the pelvis and/or positive retroperitoneal or inguinal nodes. Superficial liver metastasis equals stage III. Tumor is limited to the true pelvis but with histologically verified malignant extension to small bowel or omentum
IIIA. Tumor grossly limited to the true pelvis with negative nodes but with histologically confirmed microscopic seeding of abdominal peritoneal surfaces
IIIB. Tumor of one or both ovaries with histologically confirmed implants of abdominal peritoneal surfaces, none exceeding 2 cm in diameter; nodes negative
IIIC. Abdominal implants >2 cm in diameter and/or positive retroperitoneal or inguinal nodes

Stage IV. Growth involving one or both ovaries with distant metastasis. If pleural effusion is present there must be positive cytologic test results to allot a case to stage IV; parenchymal liver metastasis equals stage IV

These categories are based on findings at clinical examination and/or surgical exploration. The histologic characteristics are to be considered in the staging, as are results of cytologic testing as far as effusions are concerned. It is desirable that a biopsy be performed on suspicious areas outside the pelvis.
*In order to evaluate the impact on prognosis of the different criteria for allotting cases to Stage IC or IIC, it would be of value to know if rupture of the capsule was (1) spontaneous or (2) iatrogenic and if the source of malignant cells detected was (1) peritoneal washings or (2) ascites.

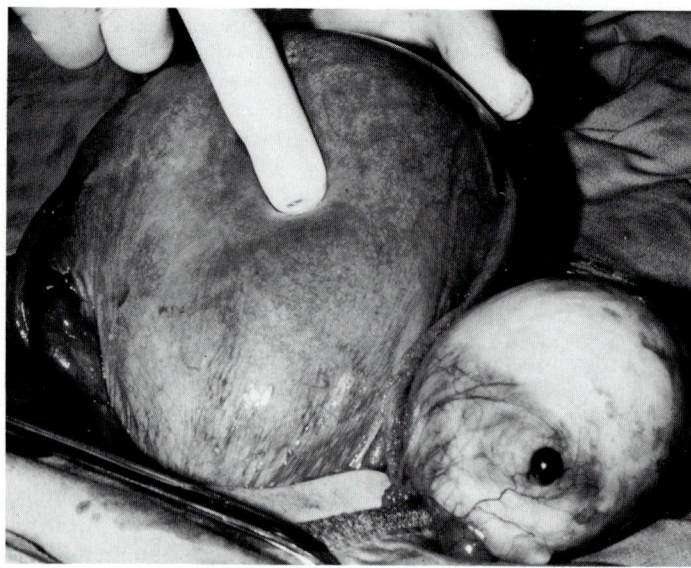

FIGURE 62–3. A unilateral stage II immature teratoma in a patient at 16 weeks gestation.

first or second trimester, the difficult treatment choices include interrupting the pregnancy and initiating chemotherapy immediately postoperatively, preserving the pregnancy and beginning chemotherapy with the fetus in situ, or preserving the pregnancy and delaying chemotherapy until the fetus either is more mature or is delivered. The last of these three choices is least acceptable because these tumors grow rapidly and recur within months when therapy is withheld. Indeed, the high success rate obtained with adjuvant chemotherapy in nonpregnant patients has been recorded utilizing this modality in the immediate postoperative period. The effect of a treatment-free interval of several months prior to the commencement of adjuvant chemotherapy has not been tested adequately. Thus, the patient with a stage IA embryonal carcinoma, endodermal sinus tumor, or immature teratoma early in pregnancy is faced with a dilemma for which incomplete data are available.

Initiation of adjuvant chemotherapy during pregnancy is a subject that is controversial and for which little experience exists. This subject is discussed under Cancer Therapy in Pregnancy, but we must emphasize that all chemotherapeutic agents are theoretically teratogenic. Although retrospective studies have not shown frequent congenital abnormalities in patients treated in the second and third trimesters, many newer agents have not been used frequently in pregnancy.

Therapeutic decisions for patients with more advanced stages of these tumors also are difficult and controversial. Many such patients can be cured with chemotherapy after surgery. As in earlier stages, the uterus and opposite ovary can be preserved if metastatic tumor is not found in these locations. Delay in or withholding of chemotherapy is not warranted, however, and uterine evacuation often is carried out because of fear of potential teratogenic effects.

Because of the uncertain effects of chemotherapy in the second and third trimester of pregnancy and the risk of early recurrence of cancer in the patient for whom adjuvant chemotherapy is delayed for several months, the patient and her family must be counseled carefully concerning the risks versus benefits of all treatment options. The best available data suggest that the fetal risk of antineoplastic agents when administered other than in the first trimester is small, and continuation of the pregnancy probably will not result in congenital malformations. Nevertheless, many patients and their families are unwilling to face the uncertainties associated with a continued pregnancy. Whether or not the pregnancy is interrupted, the initial operation after the first trimester should be followed by prompt initiation of chemotherapy prior to the third trimester for patients even with early-stage malignant germ cell tumors, excluding dysgerminomas.

Ovarian dysgerminomas are unique among the malignant germ cell tumors because of their overall good prognosis in stage I when treated by surgery alone and their exquisite sensitivity to radiation therapy. In this latter regard they behave in a fashion that is identical to seminoma of the testis, which shares the same histologic and biologic features. We believe that these tumors can be managed with a unilateral adnexectomy and continuation of the pregnancy without additional therapy in stage IA. Optimal staging is mandatory and should include a pelvic and periaortic lymphadenectomy on the side of the tumor mass because dysgerminomas metastasize primarily via the lymphatic system to the ipsilateral pelvic and periaortic lymph nodes. Lymphangiography and computerized axial tomography, which are recommended in the evaluation of the nonpregnant patient, are contraindicated when the pregnancy is to be continued. Patients who are not explored adequately at the initial operation should therefore be re-explored before one recommends no further therapy and continuation of the pregnancy. Appropriate diagnostic studies, including lymphangiography and CT scan of the abdomen and pelvis, should be evaluated by CT scan–directed fine-needle aspiration or at re-exploration.

Emergency surgical intervention and obstetric complications are common in patients with dysgerminomas. Karlen and associates (1979) reviewed 27 cases of dysgerminoma associated with pregnancy. Torsion and incarceration were found commonly in this group of patients with rapidly enlarging neoplasms, averaging 25 cm in diameter. Obstetric complications occurred in nearly half the patients and fetal demise in one-fourth of the reviewed cases. Recurrences occurred in 30 per cent of 23 stage IA tumors treated by unilateral oophorectomy, therefore casting doubt on the philosophy of treating these patients conservatively. The extent to which these patients were surgically explored was not known in most cases, however, and therefore accuracy of staging cannot be assessed. This information is crucial to interpret these findings appropriately.

In our experience, lesions confined to one ovary have a 10 per cent recurrence rate. Although most of these recurrences appear in the first 2 years following initial surgery, this group of patients can continue pregnancy safely once appropriate surgical staging has been performed, thereby ruling out extra-ovarian spread of the cancer. Because chemotherapy or radiation therapy is successful in curing over 75 per cent of patients even with metastatic or recurrent dysgerminoma, and because there is a low incidence of recurrence in carefully staged patients with stage IA disease, we favor a conservative approach to these tumors when they are diagnosed during pregnancy.

The role of chemotherapy in the management of patients with advanced-stage ovarian dysgerminoma has been controversial, mainly because radiotherapy has proved so effective in controlling extra-ovarian or recurrent disease. Nevertheless, recent data suggest that multi-agent chemotherapy for these advanced-stage or recurrent dysgerminomas can be curative and is an important new therapeutic tool in management of this disease. The most effective drugs available for this disease include a combination of etoposide with cisplatin and bleomycin.

Rarely, ovarian tumors of stromal cell origin, such as granulosa-theca cell tumors and Sertoli-Leydig cell tumors, are found in pregnancy. It is recommended that these be managed conservatively as in the young nonpregnant patient because these are neoplasms with low malignant potential.

In summary, diagnosing and treating an ovarian tumor in pregnancy is a complex matter for the clinician, the solution of which often is not clear-cut. One must have a high index of suspicion and must endeavor to diagnose early and treat promptly, preferably early in the second trimester of pregnancy. The difficulty arises when both patient and physician resist an abdominal exploration during pregnancy because of the fear of precipitating fetal loss. We believe that the potential danger to the mother exceeds the hypothetical danger to the fetus. Most of the dangers seen with ovarian tumors are those created by acts of omission rather than of commission. The possibility of an ovarian cancer must be kept foremost in the minds of physicians caring for pregnant patients, and any adnexal mass in pregnancy persisting after the 14th week of gestation should be surgically removed.

Other Pelvic Malignancies

Carcinoma of the bladder is seen most frequently after the childbearing years but occasionally is diagnosed in pregnancy. Ninety-five per cent of cases are transitional cell carcinomas, starting in the region of the trigone and spreading by direct extension via lymphatics or, less commonly, by the hematogenous route to regional and distant sites. A metastatic lesion of the lumbar spine or pelvis is common and can be a source of intractable pain. The prognosis is directly related to the extent of disease and grade of tumor. Well-differentiated lesions that are superficial can be managed by local fulguration laser therapy or intravesical chemotherapy, whereas others require partial or total urinary bladder removal with lymphadenectomy for cure. Radiation therapy also has been utilized with curative intent, but a gravid uterus can complicate this situation markedly. The mode of delivery of the fetus must be individualized according to the length of gestation as well as patient and physician preference. Neither cystectomy nor pelvic irradiation is appropriate during pregnancy if the patient wishes to ensure fetal viability. Scattered attempts at surgical extirpation with preservation of the pregnancy have resulted in high rates of fetal wastage.

Sixty per cent of all colorectal cancers are found in the distal colon and rectum, a distribution which is not affected by age or pregnancy status. Fortunately, this is a rare complication in pregnancy, with a reported frequency of 1 in 50,000 to 100,000 pregnancies, because the peak age of incidence is after the usual reproduction period. A delay in diagnosis can occur because rectal bleeding, which often provides the first clue, is commonly ascribed to hemorrhoids, a universal complaint among pregnant women.

The principles of en bloc dissection of the tumor and its lymph nodes and wide margins of tumor-free tissue are necessary during pregnancy and in the nonpregnant state. The gravid uterus often presents technical problems of exposure deep in the pelvis that can necessitate modifying the usual operative approach. At times, hysterotomy or hysterectomy must be done to facilitate exposure, as will be discussed later.

Colorectal cancer found in the first trimester of pregnancy generally should be treated as in nonpregnant patients. Radical surgery at this stage frequently is followed by abortion, and simultaneous hysterotomy should be considered seriously. The fallopian tubes, ovaries, and uterus should be resected if metastases or tumor fixation to these areas is found. Oophorectomy is recommended for all low-lying colonic tumors because of the high incidence of metastatic disease to the ovaries; at times occult metastases are found even in the normal-appearing ovary. Barber and Brunschwig (1968) advocated routine hysterectomy between 10 and 20 weeks of gestation to provide better exposure for adequate margins in resection. The treatment of colorectal cancer during the third trimester remains controversial. Some surgeons believe that with adequate exposure the cancer can be removed without disturbing the uterus and its contents. Others hold that resection should be carried out 2 weeks after cesarean section, at which time the patient has regained her strength and the uterus and pelvic vasculature are less troublesome to the surgeon. As in cancer of the cervix, ovary, and bladder, colon cancer appears to have equivalent prognoses, stage for stage, in pregnant and nonpregnant patients.

Retroperitoneal sarcomas may occur during pregnancy and may present great technical difficulties at surgical removal. Most of the lesions are neurofibrosarcomas or of similar histologic nature, and their course depends greatly on the grade of the neoplasm. Therapy of low-grade sarcomas can be deferred until the postpartum period when resection should be technically much easier, but if such a tumor extends into the pelvis, cesarean delivery is often required. High-grade lesions have a poor prognosis, and therapy must be individualized according to the length of gestation and preference of the patient.

GESTATIONAL TROPHOBLASTIC NEOPLASIA

Gestational trophoblastic neoplasia (GTN) is a clinical diagnosis that includes the histologic diagnoses of hydatidiform mole, invasive mole, and choriocarcinoma. GTN is used for this spectrum of disease because in most instances the histologic diagnosis is unknown when treatment is initiated. Prior to the revolutionary developments in detection and treatment in the 1950s, the prognosis for this group of diseases was quite dismal. In 1956 Li and associates reported the first complete and sustained remissions in patients with metastatic choriocarcinoma after methotrexate therapy. Since that time the treatment has evolved to a point where GTN is the most curable gynecologic malignancy and, indeed, the most curable cancer known to medicine. Several distinct features of these tumors account for the dramatic change in prognosis. First, a sensitive marker, human chorionic gonadotropin (hCG), is secreted by the tumor, and the amount of this hormone measured in serum is directly related to the number of viable tumor cells. Second, these malignancies are exquisitely sensitive to various chemotherapeutic agents. Third, subgroups of affected patients with various high-risk factors have been identified, permitting individualization of treatment. Fourth, the neoplastic cells are highly antigenic and represent a true allograft.

Hydatidiform Mole

Hydatidiform mole occurs in one of every 1200 pregnancies in the United States but much more frequently in other areas of the world. In the Far East and tropics it is reported in one of every 120 pregnancies, and its frequency increased dramatically in the Philippines during World War II, suggesting a relationship to stress and diet. Molar pregnancies occur relatively more frequently at both ends of the reproductive spectrum, with patients at greater risk in the early teens and perimenopausally. There appears to be no difference in parity between patients with molar pregnancy and those with normal pregnancy. Age, parity, and gestational age at the time of diagnosis do not appear to affect the risk of malignant sequelae.

Several clinical presentations including hyperemesis, preeclampsia, uterine size inconsistent with gestational age, and hyperthyroidism often are associated with hydatidiform mole and can suggest the diagnosis. Essentially all patients with hydatidiform mole have amenorrhea and can experience characteristic, often exaggerated signs and symptoms of pregnancy. Vaginal bleeding occurs in most patients, usually during the first trimester, ranging from a dark brown discharge to brisk hemorrhage sometimes requiring blood transfusions. Excessive nausea and vomiting are reported to occur in almost one-third of patients with hydatidiform mole, although Curry and associates (1975) noted only a 14 per cent incidence in 347 patients they studied. Preeclampsia diagnosed in the first trimester of pregnancy is almost pathognomonic of a hydatidiform mole, although only 12 per cent of patients studied by Curry and associates (1975) had this complication. Hyperthyroidism occurs rarely, but when present can precipitate a clinical emergency. As many as 10 per cent of patients manifest laboratory evidence of hyperthyroidism, although less than 1 per cent of the patients studied by Curry and associates (1975) had clinical evidence of this disease. The clinical manifestations of hyperthyroidism disappear once the molar pregnancy is evacuated; thyroid suppression can be indicated in the symptomatic patient, however, with discontinuation of therapy after uterine evacuation. Hyperthyroidism in molar pregnancy results from the production of thyrotropin by molar tissue.

There is often a discrepancy between uterine size and the duration of pregnancy in women with hydatidiform moles. Uterine size is excessive for gestational age in about 50 per cent of patients; however, in approximately one-third of the patients the uterus is smaller than expected. Theca-lutein cysts of the ovary, due to hyperstimulation of the ovaries from excessive hCG production by the molar pregnancy, can be quite large. About 50 per cent of patients with molar pregnancy have palpable theca-lutein cysts. A patient with either a uterus that is large for dates or a theca-lutein cyst appears to have a greater likelihood of malignant sequelae than a patient with normal ovaries and a uterus that is normal or small for dates. More than half the women with both enlarged cystic ovaries and excessive uterine enlargement require therapy for malignant sequelae.

The first evidence to suggest the diagnosis of hydatidiform mole is, in most cases, the spontaneous passage of vesicles from the uterus. Histologically the tissue is characterized by the presence of avascular edematous villi with varying degrees of trophoblastic hyperplasia. Cytogenetic studies have shown these tissues to be diploid, XX with the entire genetic composition to be paternally derived. Several techniques are available to substantiate this diagnosis when pathologic material is not available. An unusually elevated hCG level along with an enlarged uterus and vaginal bleeding strongly suggests the diagnosis of hydatidiform mole; however, a single hCG determination cannot be diagnostic. Occasionally a markedly elevated hCG titer may be seen with a normal single or multiple pregnancy or in a condition such as erythroblastosis fetalis. Conversely, an hCG titer that is appropriate for the computed gestational age can be seen with a mole.

Definitive diagnosis prior to spontaneous passage of vesicles can be made by ultrasonography. Indeed, ultrasonography is specific in differentiating between a normal pregnancy and a hydatidiform mole. In a normal pregnancy a gestational sac is seen early and a fetal pole with cardiac motion is seen at approximately 6 to 7 weeks gestation. In a molar pregnancy, the characteristic ultrasonogram notes multiple echoes, which are formed by the interface between the molar villi and the surrounding tissue in the absence of a gestational sac or fetus. With the new and more refined ultrasound techniques, the diagnosis of a molar pregnancy can be substantiated in almost all cases.

Rarely, a fetus coexists with a mole, thereby confusing the typical ultrasonographic findings. In addition, a partial or "transitional" mole has been described in which a fetus can coexist with hydropic villi having lesser degrees of trophoblastic hyperplasia. Excessive uterine size, toxemia, and hyperthyroidism are rare with this diagnosis, usually thought to be a missed or incomplete abortion on clinical assessment prior to uterine evacuation. Cytogenetic studies show these tissues to be triploid, unlike the "classic" mole, usually with two-thirds of the genetic material derived from the father and one-third from the mother. In some series, 35 per cent of molar pregnancies were partial moles, with approximately one-third of the partial moles demonstrating fetal parts. The clinical implications of this diagnosis have not been defined completely. However, approximately 10 per cent of patients with partial moles will require chemotherapy for nonmetastatic gestational trophoblastic disease. Prompt response to chemotherapy and failure to metastasize have been characteristic of this diagnosis. This clinical entity also can provide a confusing picture on ultrasonography.

Techniques used to evacuate a molar pregnancy in the past have included dilatation and curettage, hysterotomy, hysterectomy, and various chemical and mechanical induction techniques. Before the use of suction curettage, hysterectomy frequently was used for uteri greater than 12 to 14 weeks in size because of the excessive risk of hemorrhage when evacuation was attempted by sharp curettage. Suction curettage now is the method of choice for evacuating a mole, and hysterectomy is limited to older patients who have finished childbearing, in whom the risk of malignant sequelae can be reduced by this means, and to the occasional younger patient with major hemorrhage. Suction curettage can be carried out even when the uterus is the size of that in a term pregnancy. It is recommended that all patients with molar pregnancy who desire to maintain fertility undergo suction curettage with a laparotomy set-up available in case evacuation is not successful. After a moderate amount of tissue has been removed, intravenous oxytocin usually is begun. It is important to avoid uterine stimulation with oxytocin prior to evacuation. Uterine contractions can cause trophoblastic tissue to be engulfed by the large venous sinusoids in the uterus, resulting in embolization of trophoblastic tissue (deportation) to the lungs. When deportation is excessive, severe respiratory embarrassment can occur. A sharp curettage is recommended after suction curettage has been completed and involution has begun.

If a primary hysterectomy is selected for initial therapy, the ovaries can be left undisturbed even when theca-lutein cysts are encountered. These functional cysts regress completely when hCG is no longer present in the serum. Even when hysterectomy is used for therapy, the patient must be followed with serial hCG determinations as if the uterus had not been removed (Table 62–4).

After uterine evacuation, the patient should have serial serum quantitative beta-hCG determinations every 1 to 2 weeks until hCG is undetectable on two consecutive determinations. Two negative readings indicate spontaneous remission and will occur in 80 to 85 per cent of patients. The hCG titer should then be repeated every 1 to 2 months for at least a year. It is imperative that the patient use some type of contraceptive during this interval because a subsequent pregnancy will cause secretion of hCG, suggesting recurrence of GTN. Unless otherwise contraindicated, oral contraceptives should be used, although one report suggests that their administration should be delayed until hCG titer approaches undetectable levels (Bagshawe, 1976). This finding, which suggests that earlier administration of birth control pills can increase the risk of malignant sequelae requiring chemotherapy, has not been confirmed but currently is under investigation by the member institutions of the Gynecologic Oncology Group (NCI). Regular pelvic examinations should be performed at 4-week intervals until the hCG titer is undetectable. Repeat examinations should be performed at 3-month intervals during the first year. After 1 year of negative hCG titers, contraception can be discontinued and further pregnancies may be attempted.

A repeat molar pregnancy will occur in only 1 per cent of subsequent pregnancies; however, this small subset of patients will have a low likelihood of subsequent viable pregnancies. Most patients with a history of molar pregnancy who have desired further childbearing have subsequently had a normal gestation without difficulty, although there might be a slightly increased risk of spontaneous abortion.

TABLE 62–4. Postevacuation/Posthysterectomy Management of Hydatidiform Mole

1. hCG determination (radioimmunoassay) every week until negative two times, then monthly for 1 year.
2. Physical examination including pelvis every 4 weeks until remission; then every 3 months for 1 year.
3. Chest film as a baseline study and again should chemotherapy be required.
4. Chemotherapy started immediately if:
   hCG titer rises or plateaus during follow-up *or* metastases are detected at any time.

Modified from DiSaia PJ, Creasman WT: Clinical Gynecologic Oncology. St. Louis, CV Mosby, 1981.

The hCG titer will plateau or rise during the observation period in up to 25 per cent of patients, indicating persistent GTN. Interestingly, this risk of malignant sequelae varies among different trophoblastic disease centers, with some reporting chemotherapy employed in only 6 to 8 per cent of patients. The variation in part probably reflects different patient populations and variable criteria used among different treatment centers to decide when chemotherapy should be administered. Some authors have suggested starting chemotherapy if hCG titers are still measurable 60 days following uterine evacuation, because at least half such patients will subsequently manifest persistent GTN. Subsequent data indicate that the patient in whom hCG titers are still falling at 60 days can be followed as long as the titer does not plateau or rise and there is no evidence of metastasis. Although most patients who have not demonstrated a normal regression curve characterized by a weekly 50 per cent or greater drop in hCG levels probably will require chemotherapy, in many such patients the hCG titer will become normal spontaneously. Thus, careful continued observation of hCG titers will minimize the number of patients given chemotherapy. There also remains considerable controversy concerning which factors place a patient with a hydatidiform mole at high risk for malignant sequelae; nevertheless, there is good agreement that titers that plateau for 3 consecutive weeks or rise more than 50 per cent over a 2-week interval necessitate evaluation for metastatic disease followed by prompt chemotherapy.

Goldstein and his colleagues (1967, 1970, 1978) have shown that actinomycin D, administered prophylactically at the time of uterine evacuation, can decrease the likelihood of malignant sequelae. This approach has not been accepted widely, however, because the 80 per cent of patients who would have a spontaneous remission will be treated unnecessarily in this fashion and because overall survival remains close to 100 per cent even if treatment is delayed until hCG titers and clinical evaluations suggest persistent disease. For these reasons, prophylactic chemotherapy should no longer be considered appropriate for patients with hydatidiform mole; however, this therapeutic approach may be considered for the occasional patient who is likely to be lost to follow-up.

Data from the era prior to effective chemotherapy for these diseases in which a tissue diagnosis usually was known showed that approximately half the patients with choriocarcinoma had an antecedent molar gestation and the remainder of cases were approximately evenly divided between term gestation and abortion. Because most patients requiring chemotherapy have an invasive mole, which is always preceded by hydatidiform mole, most patients undergoing therapy for GTN will have had a documented molar gestation.

Delays in diagnosis and inappropriate treatment are seen commonly in patients with GTN, especially when the initial manifestation of the malignancy results from sequelae associated with extrauterine disease. These unfortunate events often occur because of errors in interpreting biopsy findings and a low level of suspicion for this disease process by the clinician. Patients with apparent metastatic tumor frequently undergo biopsy procedures and extensive operations when serum hCG determinations by the alert clinician with a high index of suspicion would provide the diagnosis. Metastatic tumors have been resected from the lower genital tract, the gastrointestinal tract, liver, lung, brain, and other sites, and unfortunately, many of these lesions have been reported as "anaplastic tumor," compounding the problem of inappropriate surgery with further delays in diagnosis. It should be apparent that any patient of reproductive age presenting with symptoms of metastatic malignancy should have a quantitative hCG determination to rule out GTN. This approach will obviate biopsy and other surgical evaluations and permit immediate treatment.

The performance of a diagnostic uterine curettage has been a common practice in evaluating patients who might have persistent GTN following evaluation of a molar pregnancy. However, this procedure is unnecessary, rarely is helpful, and occasionally can result in uterine perforation, massive hemorrhage, and the need for a hysterectomy. It is true that if malignant trophoblastic disease is identified pathologically, the diagnosis and need for chemotherapy is confirmed, but GTN is often deep in the myometrium and unobtainable by curettage. Thus the need for chemotherapy is not altered either by the presence or absence of molar tissue or choriocarcinoma on repeat uterine curettage. In many instances, patients with GTN have metastases in the absence of disease within the uterus.

Hammond and associates (1973) have suggested a useful clinical classification for GTN in which it is recognized that tissue diagnoses of chorioadenoma destruens and choriocarcinoma usually are known in patients undergoing treatment for GTN. In this classification, subgroups of patients at high risk for failure of conventional single-agent chemotherapy are identified (Table 62–5). Thus, by identifying GTN as a spectrum of neoplasia and identifying high-risk factors in this disease process, one is able to individualize therapy.

Proper diagnostic evaluation is essential. The workup for a diagnosis of persistent gestational trophoblastic neoplasia should consist of:

History and physical examination
Chest x-ray with CT scan of lungs
Liver and brain scans or CT scans
Liver function tests (LFTs)
Hematologic survey
Pretreatment hCG titer

Initial studies should include computed tomography (CT) of the liver and brain to evaluate for metastases in these sites. We recommend full-lung tomograms or preferably a CT scan of the lungs in addition to the chest x-ray, because the lungs are the most common site of metastases in GTN and occasionally these studies will document metastases in the presence of a normal chest x-ray. Pretreatment blood studies will help to exclude factors that might influence the choice of chemotherapeutic agents. For example, patients with abnormal LFTs should not be treated with methotrexate because of its potential hepatotoxicity. In

TABLE 62–5. Classification of Gestational Trophoblastic Neoplasia

I. Nonmetastatic disease: No evidence of disease outside uterus.
II. Metastatic disease: Any disease outside uterus.
  A. Good-prognosis metastatic disease.
    1. Short duration (last pregnancy <4 months prior).
    2. Low pretreatment hCG titer (<100,000 IU/24 hr urine specimen or <40,000 mIU/ml of serum).
    3. No metastasis to brain or liver.
    4. No prior chemotherapy failure.
  B. Poor-prognosis metastatic disease (any one of the following):
    1. Long duration (last pregnancy >4 months prior).
    2. High pretreatment hCG titer (>100,000 IU/24 hr urine specimen or >40,000 mIU/ml of serum).
    3. Brain or liver metastasis.
    4. Failed prior chemotherapy.

Modified from DiSaia PJ, Creasman WT: Clinical Gynecologic Oncology. St. Louis, CV Mosby, 1981.

TABLE 62–7. Management of Single-Agent Chemotherapy for Gestational Trophoblastic Neoplasia

Agent and dosage as listed in Table 62–6; course repeated every 7 to 10 days, depending on toxicity, until hCG titer is normal.
Contraception begun.
Chemotherapy postponed in presence of:
  Severe oral or gastrointestinal ulceration.
  Febrile course associated with leukopenia.
Chemotherapy repeated when:
  WBC >3,000 cells/mm³.
  Polymorphonuclear leukocyte count >1,500 cells/mm³.
  Platelet count >100,000 cells/mm³.
  BUN, SGOT, SGPT essentially normal.
Chemotherapeutic agent changed if:
  hCG titer rises (twofold or more) or plateaus.
  Evidence of new metastasis appears.
Remission is defined as three consecutive weekly titers with undetectable levels of hCG.

addition, normal renal function is necessary when methotrexate is used, since the drug is cleared by the kidneys. A careful pelvic examination will rule out metastases to the cervix, vagina, and vulva. Once the tests have been obtained, categorization of disease can be made and specific therapy initiated.

Nonmetastatic Trophoblastic Disease

Nonmetastatic trophoblastic disease is the most common diagnosis within the spectrum of GTN and, as expected, has the best prognosis, with 100 per cent of patients expected to achieve complete sustained remission. This designation is applied when the results of evaluation for metastases are negative, implying that disease is limited to the uterus. Patients with nonmetastatic trophoblastic disease are treated with single-agent chemotherapy (Table 62–6). Both methotrexate and actinomycin D have been used successfully as single agents. Recently, the use of higher doses of methotrexate with folinic acid has been advocated over the use of lower doses of methotrexate without folinic acid or actinomycin D because of its lower toxicity and comparable effectiveness. Single-agent therapy should be repeated as soon as possible, allowing 7 to 10 days between courses. Toxicity should be monitored carefully, as noted in Table 62–7, with longer intervals between courses indicated if stomatitis or bone marrow suppression is present when the subsequent course of chemotherapy is due. The therapy should be continued until three negative weekly hCG titers are obtained. Employing the methotrexate with folinic

acid regimen, Berkowitz et al. (1986) reported complete remissions in 90 per cent of 163 patients so treated. The remaining patients achieved complete sustained remissions with the subsequent treatment with actinomycin D or multi-agent chemotherapy regimens. If the hCG titer rises or plateaus after two or more courses of chemotherapy, alternative drugs should be instituted. In general, failure of either actinomycin D or methotrexate warrants switching to the other of these two drugs. The patient with subsequent failure of the second drug can still be treated successfully either with intra-arterial infusion of the drug into the uterus, multiple-agent chemotherapy as described later for metastatic disease with poor prognosis, or hysterectomy. When either hysterectomy or intra-arterial chemotherapy is contemplated, a pelvic arteriogram should be done to verify a resistant focus of tumor within the uterus. Evidence of new metastasis while the patient is being treated is also an indication for changing the chemotherapy. Once the hCG value has returned to normal levels, appropriate follow-up with monthly hCG titers for 1 year is mandatory (Table 62–8). An effective contraceptive must be used during this time. A patient who has remained in remission for 1 year and desires more children should be advised that childbearing may be resumed.

Metastatic Trophoblastic Neoplasia with Good Prognosis

Patients with GTN who have metastases are categorized as having a good prognosis when none of the following is present: (1) brain or liver metastasis, (2) serum beta-hCG titer greater than 40,000 mIU/ml, (3)

TABLE 62–6. Single-Agent Chemotherapy for Gestational Trophoblastic Neoplasia

AGENT	DOSAGE*
Methotrexate	20–25 mg/day IM for 5 days
Actinomycin D	10–12 μg/kg/day IV for 5 days
Methotrexate with	1 mg/kg IM on days 1, 3, 5, and 7
Folinic acid	0.1 mg/kg IM on days 2, 4, 6, and 8

*Intervals of 7 to 10 days between courses, if possible, for all three modalities.

TABLE 62–8. Follow-up Protocol for GTN After Spontaneous or Chemotherapy-Induced Remission

Three consecutive normal weekly hCG assays
hCG titer determinations monthly for 12 months; then every 6 months
Contraception for 1 year

previous chemotherapy, or (4) interval since last pregnancy greater than 4 months. Recent data suggest that an antecedent term pregnancy should exclude a patient with metastatic GTN from the good-prognosis category; however, there is no general agreement about this matter because most such patients also have other clinical features that exclude them from this category. The therapy for good-prognosis metastatic GTN is the same as described for nonmetastatic disease.

Once a normal hCG value has been achieved, one additional course beyond the first negative reading is required. Should resistance to the initial choice of chemotherapy occur, manifested either by rising or plateauing titers or by the development of new metastasis, therapy should be changed as described for patients with nonmetastatic GTN. If resistance to both methotrexate and actinomycin D develops, the patient should be given multiple-agent therapy as described below. The Southeastern Trophoblastic Center reported on 55 patients with good-prognosis metastatic GTN who were treated at their center (Hammond et al., 1980). Thirty-five of 40 patients treated with chemotherapy alone went into complete remission, and the remaining five, all of whom had resistant focus of disease in the uterus despite complete resolution of the metastatic disease, had a hysterectomy after failing drug therapy, with complete remissions in all cases. The other 15 patients had chemotherapy and hysterectomy performed primarily, all of whom had remission. Thus, complete, sustained remission was achieved in all 55 patients with good-prognosis metastatic gestational trophoblastic neoplasia. Many other centers have reported similar results in large numbers of patients, most of whom had presented with lung or pelvic metastases, emphasizing the appropriateness of the term "good-prognosis" GTN.

Metastatic Trophoblastic Neoplasia with Poor Prognosis

The following features indicate a poor prognosis in metastatic trophoblastic neoplasia:

Brain or liver metastases
Serum beta-hCG >40,000 mIU/ml
Unsuccessful prior chemotherapy
Antecedent pregnancy longer than 4 months before diagnosis
Gestational trophoblastic neoplasia after term pregnancy

Patients whose disease has been characterized as having a poor prognosis present the physician and the medical team with a serious challenge. Many of them have been treated previously with chemotherapy and have developed resistance to that treatment while their bone marrow reserves have been depleted. Multiple-agent chemotherapy is recommended in this disease, and a multi-modality approach is essential for many patients. They should be treated in centers where there are teams of physicians with special interest and expertise in this problem. A health care

team of physicians often can include a gynecologic oncologist (who should direct therapy), radiation therapist, neurologist, neurosurgeon, psychiatrist, physiatrist, and others. Essential support personnel include a well-trained team of nurse oncologists and specialists in social service, physical therapy, respiratory therapy, occupational therapy, and speech therapy to deal with some of the many problems patients with this disease can have. Many patients require hospitalization for several months. They develop life-threatening toxicity from therapy and, in some instances, require specialized care, such as total parenteral nutrition, isolation, respirators, and other life support measures during long periods when their host defense mechanisms are depleted and their medical condition requires continuing monitoring and care.

Beginning in 1969 in several centers nationwide, patients with poor-prognosis metastatic GTN were started on multiple-agent chemotherapy for primary treatment because poor-prognosis patients treated initially with single-agent chemotherapy and later with multiple agents rarely were salvaged. A combination of methotrexate, actinomycin D, and cyclophosphamide (MAC) was utilized every 12 to 14 days as permitted by bone marrow toxicity (Table 62–9). Cerebral or hepatic metastases were treated concurrently with 2000 to 3000 cGy in 10 to 15 days to the whole brain or liver. Concurrently, Bagshawe developed a complex seven-drug regimen employed over 8 days per course for treatment of these high-risk patients (Table 62–10). Originally believed to be less toxic than the three-drug regimen already described, it has proved to be difficult to administer; it is no more effective and actually more toxic than the combination of methotrexate, actinomycin D, and chlorambucil. Since 1979, with the recognition of the exceptional clinical activity of etoposide in GTN, Bagshawe's group has employed a five-drug regimen of etoposide, methotrexate, and actinomycin D (EMA) plus vincristine and cyclophosphamide (CO), alternating the two- and three-drug regimens weekly in the treatment of poor-prognosis patients. Available data for this EMA/CO regimen have suggested its superiority over other regimens currently employed for these patients. Bagshawe's group has reported an 84 per cent overall survival rate, including patients in whom prior chemotherapy had failed, and a 94 per cent survival rate in those who had not received any prior chemotherapy (Newlands, 1986).

In treating patients with poor-prognosis GTN, adjunctive modalities including radiation therapy and surgery must be considered at all times. These modalities can include hysterectomy, resection of meta-

TABLE 62–9. Treatment for Poor-Prognosis Gestational Trophoblastic Neoplasia

MODALITY OR AGENT	DOSAGE
Methotrexate	15 mg/day IM for 5 days
Actinomycin D	10–12 μg/kg/day IV for 5 days
Chlorambucil	10 mg/day PO for 5 days
Brain or liver radiation therapy	2,000–3,000 in 10–15 days

TABLE 62–10. Modified Bagshawe Chemotherapy

DAY	HOUR	TREATMENT
1	0600	Hydroxyurea 500 mg PO
	1200	Hydroxyurea 500 mg PO
	1800	Hydroxyurea 500 mg PO
	1900	Actinomycin D 200 μg IV
	2400	Hydroxyurea 500 mg PO
2	0700	Vincristine 1 mg/m² IV
	1900	Methotrexate 100 mg/m² IV
		Methotrexate 200 mg/m² infused over 12 hr
		Actinomycin D 200 μg IV
3	1900	Actinomycin D 200 μg IV
		Cytoxan 500 mg/m² IV
		Folinic acid 14 mg IM
4	0100	Folinic acid 14 mg IM
	0700	Folinic acid 14 mg IM
	1300	Folinic acid 14 mg IM
	1900	Folinic acid 14 mg IM
		Actinomycin D 500 μg IV
5	0100	Folinic acid 14 mg IM
	1900	Actinomycin D 500 μg IV
6	No treatment	
7	No treatment	
8	1900	Cytoxan 500 mg/m² IV
		Adriamycin 30 mg/m² IV

From DiSaia PJ, Creasman WT: Clinical Gynecologic Oncology. St. Louis, CV Mosby, 1981.

static lesions in the lungs or elsewhere, and/or irradiation of nonresectable lesions. As in good-prognosis GTN and nonmetastatic GTN, complete remission is documented only after three consecutive normal weekly hCG titers. Individuals with poor prognosis GTN should have at least four courses of chemotherapy after the first negative hCG titer. Follow-up evaluations after complete remission are the same as for hydatidiform mole and nonmetastatic and good-prognosis metastatic GTN. Those patients with brain and liver metastases have the poorest prognosis: less than a 50 per cent success rate with metastases at either site and a lower remission rate if both are involved.

Most patients with GTN have been cured with chemotherapy and many have desired future childbearing. Major concerns in this regard have included the potential for chemotherapy-induced sterility or congenital malformations in their offspring. Rustin et al. (1984) studied these issues in 445 long-term survivors treated with chemotherapy at the Charing Cross Hospital in London, England. Ninety-seven per cent of women who wished to conceive did so, and 86 per cent achieved at least one live birth. Women who had received combination chemotherapy were found to be less likely to have a live birth than those treated with methotrexate alone. There was no excess of congenital malformations in the offspring of these women as compared with that expected for women of comparable age who had never received chemotherapy.

CANCER THERAPY IN PREGNANCY

Chemotherapy

Most cytotoxic agents useful in treating malignant neoplasms theoretically are both teratogenic and mu-

tagenic in human fetuses when administered early in pregnancy. Their use evokes complex moral and philosophical questions as well as difficult medical decisions. Both mother and fetus are at risk, the mother from the cancer and the fetus from its treatment. The use of cytotoxic drugs can result in abortion, fetal death, malformations, or growth retardation. The long-term effect on the viable infant is unknown but requires careful study. The need for long-term observation has been emphasized dramatically with the recognition of DES-related adenocarcinomas of the vagina and cervix and other congenital effects on reproductive organs which can affect subsequent fertility in young women exposed in utero to this drug during the first trimester of pregnancy, often decades earlier. A similarly devastating long-term effect might be found in the offspring of women treated with chemotherapeutic agents during pregnancy. The theoretic dangers to the fetus must be weighed against the possible detrimental effect of withholding these agents from the mother.

The oncologist treating pregnant women with cytotoxic agents should be aware of the many physiologic changes during pregnancy that can affect drug absorption, distribution, and excretion. The effect of pregnancy on gastrointestinal motility may markedly alter the absorption of agents taken orally. Similarly, the expanded blood volume and total body water have a marked effect on drug distribution, while the increase in renal blood flow accelerates the excretion of agents eliminated by the kidneys. The complex interaction of these various physiologic changes, coupled with the infrequency of cytotoxic drug administration in pregnancy, has precluded well-done pharmacokinetic studies to determine appropriate dosing strategies during pregnancy. In the absence of such data, conventional treatment approaches used in nonpregnant patients are employed when administering these agents during pregnancy.

Most available data suggesting a teratogenic and mutagenic effect of chemotherapeutic agents have been derived from experiments on gravid laboratory animals. Extrapolation of data from these experiments provides the basis for much of the concern about the potential danger to the human fetus. In addition, because all cytotoxic chemotherapeutic agents profoundly affect rapidly growing tissues, and because a high rate of cell division is characteristic of fetal tissues, one would expect a high likelihood of fetal damage from these drugs. There is surprisingly little information in humans, but what does exist suggests a favorable pregnancy outcome in most instances, belying both the findings in laboratory animals and the theoretic concerns.

Unquestionably, the first trimester of pregnancy, in which organogenesis is established, is that period in which the fetus is most vulnerable to anticancer agents. Potential injury can result in either the death of the fetus or induction of abnormalities inadequate to cause fetal demise. During the second and third trimester, organogenesis is completed; however, neuronal growth in the brain continues. In general, adverse effects of these drugs have not been reported when initiated after the first trimester. Nevertheless, the potential adverse effects, especially related to cortical brain function, warrant careful longitudinal investigation of these children.

Several publications that address the reported adverse effects of cytotoxic chemotherapy emphasize the risk of such therapy in the first trimester, but also demonstrate that these effects are not inevitable. Sokal and Lessman (1960) collected 50 reports of pregnant women receiving anticancer chemotherapy. They found eight instances of fetal abnormalities, 16 spontaneous abortions, and seven therapeutic abortions. Although serious congenital anomalies and spontaneous abortions did occur in some patients receiving chemotherapy in the first trimester of pregnancy, such complications were not inevitable. No obvious fetal malformations were observed in the infants of those women who received chemotherapy after the first trimester of pregnancy. Similarly, Nicholson (1968) collected 185 reports of human pregnancies during which anticancer chemotherapy was administered. Of 110 women treated during the first trimester, fetal or infant status was recorded in only 68 cases, in which there were 15 instances of fetal abnormalities. Ten of the 15 women received folic acid antagonists, two had taken busulfan, and one each had been treated with 6-mercaptopurine, chlorambucil, and cyclophosphamide. No malformations were reported in the offspring of 75 women who received chemotherapy during the second and third trimesters of pregnancy, although infant status was recorded in only 73 cases. In a review of this subject by Schapira and Chudley (1984), the incidence of teratogenicity of chemotherapeutic agents given to women during the first trimester of pregnancy was 12.7 per cent, representing a fivefold increase over that of the offspring of noncancer patients. These data are consistent with that from a recent review by Doll et al. (1989), in which first-trimester drug exposure in 139 reported cases resulted in 24 infants with malformations (17 per cent). The frequency of malformations was slightly higher in fetuses exposed to antimetabolites (15 of 77 cases, 19 per cent), including all three reported cases of exposure to methotrexate, as compared with alkylating agents (6 of 44 cases, 14 per cent). Surprisingly, exposure to combinations of cytotoxic agents did not increase the frequency of malformations in the cases reviewed in this report (7 of 45 affected newborns, 16 per cent).

Although the greatest concern about cytotoxic therapy in pregnancy is focused on the first trimester, attention must be given to the effects of drug administration late in the third trimester. While commonly employed agents cross the placenta to the fetus, drug elimination by the fetus is effected through metabolism by the fetal liver, excretion by the fetal kidney, and transplacental passage back to the mother. The role of placental excretion has not been defined, but its absence following delivery, coupled with an underdeveloped ability to metabolize or excrete the drug by the neonate, can lead to leukopenia and subsequent neutropenic sepsis as well as thrombocytopenia and a risk of hemorrhage. Reynoso et al. (1987) estimated that one-third of fetuses exposed to chemotherapy near term will experience pancytopenia based on the

experience of the Toronto Leukemia Study Group. In order to avoid these potential risks, these agents should be withheld, if possible, during the last month of pregnancy. A complete blood count should be done on the newborn, and breast-feeding is contraindicated inasmuch as all of these agents can be secreted in breast milk.

Of the drugs used to treat cancers, the group most commonly associated with teratogenic effects are the folic acid antagonists. The two drugs in this group, aminopterin and methotrexate, almost invariably result in either spontaneous abortion or an abnormal fetus when given in the first trimester of pregnancy. The most frequent effects of exposure to these agents include delayed ossification of the bones of the calvarium (cranial dysostosis), hypertelorism, micrognathia, limb deformities, and cerebral anomalies. Speech and intelligence can be affected severely. Therefore, these drugs should not be administered to a pregnant woman in the first trimester unless she has life-threatening disease for which all other drugs are established to be less than effective. If the antifolic is used, and the mother does not abort spontaneously, therapeutic abortion should be offered. Minimal data on the use of these drugs later in pregnancy indicate that they do not harm the fetus after the first trimester.

Although most other antitumor drugs—including 6-mercaptopurine, azathioprine, 5-fluorouracil, the alkylating agents, vinca alkaloids, and procarbazine—are teratogenic in laboratory animals, there have been few case reports of fetal abnormalities resulting from the use of these agents in the first trimester of human pregnancy. An explanation for this apparent discrepancy is unclear, but the differences might result from variations in placental structure, placental transfer of drugs, and different dosage regimens in the experimental animals and humans. On the other hand, there have been isolated reports of fetal abnormalities with virtually every drug, emphasizing the importance of avoiding their use especially in the first trimester of pregnancy. These findings also emphasize the importance of effective contraception for any woman of childbearing age receiving chemotherapy to prevent pregnancy and potential fetal abnormalities.

The lack of adequate observation of the long-term status of the offspring of patients treated during pregnancy prevents definite conclusions as to the relative safety or danger of anticancer chemotherapy to the viable offspring who appears normal at birth. Long-term observation is necessary in order to establish normality because many defects might not be obvious on inspection and might emerge as impairments of growth, development, learning abilities, reproductive function, carcinogenesis, or even a teratogenic effect, which might be delayed until the next generation.

A major concern to patients of reproductive age who are taking cytotoxic chemotherapeutic agents is the potential effect on subsequent reproductive capacity. Indirect evidence of the possible gonadal effects of these drugs can be found in the studies of reproduction following renal transplantation. Recipients are maintained on immunosuppressive therapy with azathioprine and prednisone, drugs with immunologic effects similar to those of many anticancer agents. The literature concerning the effects of this therapy on reproductive capacity and fetal outcome contains optimistic and pessimistic reports. Women who become pregnant while immunosuppressed appear to deliver healthy babies, barring prematurity and other obstetric problems. In addition, Penn and co-workers (1971) reported 19 men on immunosuppressive therapy who fathered 23 pregnancies that resulted in one spontaneous abortion and 19 live births, including one infant with a meningomyelocele; three pregnancies were not delivered at the time of the report. Most comparable data for women on cytotoxic drug therapy concern those with GTN treated with methotrexate or actinomycin D as reported above and those receiving alkylating agents. Studies of 596 women reported by Rustin et al. (1984) and by Goldstein et al. (1984) show no excess of fetal malformations in the offspring of women treated previously with chemotherapy for GTN. It is unknown whether this favorable experience found for patients treated mainly by methotrexate or actinomycin D will also carry over to those treated successfully with other agents for other types of malignancies seen in younger women, including breast and hematologic malignancies.

The effect of chemotherapy on subsequent fertility has been addressed by Byrne et al. (1987). In their review of a large retrospective cohort study of 2283 childhood and adolescent cancer survivors, they found no decrease in fertility in either sex following chemotherapy that excluded alkylating agents. Therapy with alkylating agents reduced fertility in males by nearly 60 per cent, but did not affect fertility in women. The adverse effect in males results from a loss of spermatogenic function, which relates to dose and duration of therapy. Alkylating agents in general, and especially cyclophosphamide when employed for more than 6 months in women older than 35 years, can also produce amenorrhea and hormonal evidence of ovarian failure. This rarely is seen in younger women or in those treated for shorter durations.

Radiation Therapy

The primary dilemmas of radiation therapy during pregnancy include the effect on the fetus including the risk of abortion, malformations, and impaired reproductive capacity, and the effect on the maternal gonads that might contribute to reproductive difficulties in the future. Thus, the concerns about and potential adverse effects of radiation are identical to those for chemotherapy. Yet unlike those of chemotherapy, these adverse effects occur with alarming and predictable frequency in patients undergoing radiation therapy. The embryo represents the most radiosensitive stage in human life, and radiation injury to the embryo results in marked developmental and structural anomalies. These exaggerated effects result from a combination of factors. First, many cells in the embryo are differentiating and therefore are highly sensitive to ionizing radiation. Second, there is a high rate of mitotic activity in the cells of the embryo, and mitosis is the most radiosensitive period in the cell cycle. Third, if the embryonic cell is genetically altered

or killed during its development, the adult form will either be functionally or structurally altered or will not survive.

The sensitivity to ionizing radiation of different tissues within the human embryo varies markedly. In addition, the adverse effects vary with both the duration of gestation and the dose of radiation. Of the abnormalities attributed to radiation of the embryo, microcephaly and associated central nervous system conditions have been reported most frequently. Other abnormalities most frequently encountered in surviving children include microphthalmus, cataracts, pigmentary degeneration of the retina, and skeletal and genital tract anomalies. Mental retardation and stunted growth are also frequent sequelae. Experimental studies confirm that fetal anomalies consistently result from a dose of 200 to 300 rads delivered during the first trimester of pregnancy. An accurate prediction of incidence of specific anomalies for a given dose of radiation has not been possible.

The adverse effects of radiation on the human gonads include both genetic damage, which can be transmitted from generation to generation, and sterility. Any irradiation of gonadal tissue can result in genetic damage because the photons cause gene mutation or chromosome breakage with subsequent translocation, loss deletion, and abnormal fusion of chromosomal material. These effects are additive and cumulative, and generally the changes are proportional to the total dose. Unfortunately, there is no threshold dose below which genetic damage does not occur, and thus even very small doses of radiation can cause potentially harmful gene mutation. It is estimated that 1 rad produces five mutations for every 1 million genes exposed. Fortunately, most mutants are recessive and many are not harmful. Mutant effects are not seen in the first generation and might not be visible for many generations, until two people with the same mutation mate. Most estimates of genetic damage are empiric, but it is estimated that 25 to 150 rads must be given from birth to the end of reproductive age to double the rate of spontaneous gene mutation. As additional clinical and theoretic data are accumulated, frequent changes are made in what is considered the permissible cumulative body dose of radiation. Current maximal dose recommendations range from 10 to 14 rads during the first 30 years of life. This includes ionizing radiation from both medical and background sources.

The fetus is most sensitive to ionizing radiation between days 11 and 56, but after 56, primary organ systems have developed, and much larger doses of x-rays or gamma rays are necessary to produce serious abnormalities. Therefore, there are three periods of embryogenesis during which similar amounts of radiation can have markedly different radiobiologic effects.

1. *Preimplantation and early implantation (days 0 to 10).* In this phase, radiation produces an all-or-none effect, in that it either destroys the embryo or has no apparent adverse effect.

2. *Organ system formation.* During this period, from days 11 to 56, radiation exposure often causes visceral organ or somatic damage. Microcephaly, anencephaly,

eye damage, growth retardation, spina bifida, and foot damage have been reported with doses of 4 rads or less, quantities consistent with a barium enema or IVP. Cause and effect have not been proved with these lower doses. It is believed, however, that doses as low as 10 rads can result in a measurable increase in fetal anomalies and that doses of 100 rads or more during this crucial phase of fetal development results in anomalies in all surviving children, based on observations in the atomic bomb survivors in Hiroshima and Nagasaki.

3. *After day 56.* After organ system formation is complete, larger doses are required to produce external malformations. At this time the nervous system is especially vulnerable to injury, and doses over 50 rads can produce mental retardation and microcephaly even in the second trimester. These effects have been reported as late as 20 weeks of gestation; however, after this time a surviving child is not likely to exhibit overt abnormalities. Some infants exposed late in pregnancy do exhibit skin erythema, abnormal pigmentation, epilation, or hematologic deficiencies.

Because the developing fetus can be exquisitely sensitive to ionizing radiation and because there is no threshold dose of radiation below which the fetus cannot be harmed, diagnostic radiologic procedures should be avoided during the first and second trimesters of pregnancy. The exposure to the fetus and maternal gonads will vary with the procedure performed and the precautions taken. A chest x-ray will result in an exposure of 300 millirads per plate to the chest and a much lower exposure to the pelvic structures. The pelvic dose can be negligible if the patient wears a lead apron. On the other hand, a barium enema may result in a total dose to the gonads and pelvis, which cannot be shielded during this study, of approximately 6 rads. In a pregnant patient the barium enema is obviously a greater threat because of the greater dosage to the ovaries and developing fetus. Procedures in which multiple x-rays of the pelvis are taken during pregnancy, including a barium enema, IVP, and x-ray pelvimetry, are of special concern because there is evidence to suggest that an exposure of only 3 to 5 rads can result in an increase in benign or malignant tumors in the child after birth. For example, pelvimetry at term has been reported to be associated with an increased risk for childhood leukemia in exposed offspring.

The ovary is sensitive to radiation at higher doses than the testis. This difference is presumably due to the constant cell division that occurs during spermatogenesis, in contrast to the ovary's meiotic activity of only a few cells in each cycle. The dose of radiation to the ovaries required to produce complete and permanent sterility varies with the age at the time of radiotherapy or, more precisely, with the number of oocytes that remain. This range of doses fits nicely with the "target theory" of radiation effect, which postulates that the dose that produces total cell kill in any population is proportional to the total number of cells that must be destroyed.

The threshold values for permanent and temporary sterility have not been defined clearly. In females 40 years of age and older, 600 rads can induce subsequent menopause. Teenage girls treated with 2000 rads fractionated over 5 to 6 weeks have a 95 per cent likelihood of permanent sterility. With conventional doses, any field that includes the ovaries will cause sterility. This is the case with the standard inverted Y field used in the treatment of Hodgkin's disease. In an effort to prevent this effect in young women with this disease who might desire subsequent childbearing, oophoropexy, or surgical movement of the ovaries out of the treatment field, is performed at the time of staging laparotomy. Two locations are used: the ovaries can be displaced either laterally beyond the planned radiation field or medially behind the uterus, where they are shielded during treatment.

NONPELVIC MALIGNANCIES IN PREGNANCY

Melanoma

Malignant melanoma might be one of the few malignancies that pregnancy adversely affects. There are many case reports in which pregnancy has been incriminated in the induction or exacerbation of a melanoma. This concept is supported on theoretic grounds by numerous observations. Melanocyte-stimulating hormone (MSH) of the pituitary increases after the second month of pregnancy, suggesting that pregnancy indirectly stimulates the growth of these tumors. Pregnancy is also associated with increased ACTH production, resulting in heightened intrinsic MSH activity. Thus, increased pigmentation is characteristic of pregnancy, occurring in the nipple, vulva, linea nigra, and, on occasion, preexisting nevi. In addition, estrogens, which are produced in enormous quantities during pregnancy, have been shown to control melanocyte activity in the guinea pig. Despite these anecdotal observations and theoretic concerns, there are no studies that demonstrate a curative benefit of therapeutic abortion, spontaneous delivery, or oophorectomy.

All melanomas masquerade as nevi prior to their diagnosis, indicating a possible role for prophylactic removal in childhood. Unfortunately, there are an average of 15 to 20 nevi per person, and removal of each lesion is hardly practical. Nevertheless, nevi at greatest risk for malignant degeneration, including those on the feet, palms, genitals, and areas of persistent irritation from clothing, should be removed during childhood. Pigmented lesions with irregular borders or surface contour and those that have undergone enlargement or a color change must be excised to rule out the presence of a melanoma. Variations in the color of a lesion should lead the clinician to be suspicious. Shades of red or pink suggest inflammation, while a bluish hue may result from pigmented cells within the dermis, both conditions suggesting a malignant diagnosis. A policy of waiting and watching a suspicious pigmented lesion may be detrimental, since early excision of a melanoma often is lifesaving.

Approximately one-third of women with melanomas are of childbearing age, and they account for 8 per cent of all cancers in pregnancy. Their biologic behavior in pregnancy has been evaluated by many investigators, with conflicting data from different studies. In 1961, White and colleagues reported a study of 71 women with melanomas between 15 and 30 years old, 30 of whom were pregnant. The 5-year survival rate in the pregnant patients was 73 per cent, and that in nonpregnant patients was 53 per cent. The authors concluded that differences in survival were not significant between the two groups. Thus, no deleterious effect of pregnancy on survival of a group with melanoma was demonstrated in this series. George and associates (1960) compared the outcome of 115 cases of melanoma in pregnancy with 330 nonpregnant controls from the same institution. They found that spread to regional nodes appeared to be more rapid in the pregnant patient, but stage for stage, there was no significant difference in the outcomes. These data disagreed with an earlier report from the same institution and directly contradicted an earlier philosophy popularized by Pack and Scharnagel (1951) that melanoma was indeed aggravated by the pregnant state.

The reported low incidence of tumor metastases to products of conception probably is due to a number of factors, including the unexplained resistance of the placenta to invasion of maternal cancer that has been demonstrated in many animal studies. Metastasis of maternal cancer to products of conception is rare despite the sizable number of pregnancies at risk. In a comprehensive review of the subject by Dildy et al. (1989), there were only 53 cases of malignancy metastatic to the products of conception reported between 1866 and 1987, including 12 which metastasized to the fetus. Although melanoma accounts for only 8 per cent of cancers associated with pregnancy, 30 per cent of all tumors metastasizing to the placenta and more than half metastasizing to the fetus are melanomas. In contrast, breast and cervix combined account for more than half the cases in pregnant women; however, only 8 cases have been reported to spread to the products of conception, none of which involve the fetus.

Breast Cancer

Because breast cancer is uncommon in women under the age of 35, it is a rare complication of pregnancy. The incidence rate is approximately one new case per 3500 to 10,000 deliveries. There is a markedly increased incidence of breast cancer in certain families, the overall risk doubling in the woman whose mother or sister has had the disease. Risk factors appear to be cumulative: women with multiple risk factors of early menarche, previous benign breast disease, and nulliparity or initial pregnancy after the age of 34 can have a likelihood of developing breast cancer several times that of women without similar risk factors. For example, the risk in daughters of women who developed bilateral cancer premenopausally is increased ninefold, the greatest risk in these offspring occurring during the premenopausal period. These data have led some investigators to advocate prophylactic subcutaneous mastectomy in women at greatest risk for this disease.

Pregnant patients tend to present with a larger primary tumor and a higher incidence of positive nodes than nonpregnant patients. The prognosis is poorer in pregnancy than in nonpregnant women because regional lymph node metastases frequently are associated with occult distant metastases. Conversely, patients with negative nodes in pregnancy have a prognosis that is similar to that of nonpregnant patients with early-stage disease. The more advanced stage of disease in most pregnant patients has been attributed to multiple factors. First and foremost, the breast engorgement that occurs in pregnancy can delay the diagnosis by obscuring a mass for many months. Second, breast cancer is more difficult to palpate or visualize radiographically in the young premenopausal patient than in the postmenopausal woman in whom normal breast tissue has been replaced largely by fatty tissue. In addition, there is increased vascularity and lymphatic drainage from the breast in pregnancy, which theoretically might assist the metastatic process. Rarely, a pregnant woman will present with metastatic carcinoma in the absence of a known primary lesion. In such instances, breast cancer should be suspected since it is the most common tumor presenting in this fashion during pregnancy.

Obstetricians more than any other physicians have the opportunity to detect breast cancer early in pregnancy through regular examinations and indirectly by educating patients in self-examination. Needle aspiration of masses will distinguish a cyst or galactocele from a solid tumor; if bloody fluid is obtained, it should be examined cytologically, with biopsy indicated to make a definitive diagnosis. Fine-needle aspiration cytology of solid masses has a reported sensitivity and specificity approaching 95 per cent, according to Bottles and Taylor (1985), and therefore can help in the evaluation of suspicious masses in pregnant women. Other investigators report similar specificity but a sensitivity as low as 50 to 66 per cent. Biopsy should be done on masses from which fluid cannot be aspirated and from suspicious masses in which fine-needle aspiration cytology is nondiagnostic. The risk of breast biopsy to mother and fetus is reported to be small. Mammography seldom is useful during pregnancy owing to the great radiographic density of the breast. Even in nonpregnant women under the age of 35 years with a palpable malignant breast mass, mammography will be negative in the majority of instances.

The histopathology of breast cancers found in pregnant women is similar to that reported in matched-age nonpregnant controls. Even inflammatory carcinoma, once thought to occur more frequently in pregnancy, occurs with equal frequency in these two patient populations, approximately 1.5 to 4.0 per cent of cases.

Staging of breast cancer currently conforms to a complicated system recommended jointly by the International Union Against Cancer and the American Joint Committee. The Haagensen clinical staging classification for breast cancer is more useful, however, because it takes into account the bad prognostic indicators in this disease process (Table 62–11).

One to 2 per cent of patients with breast cancer are pregnant when diagnosed, constituting a difficult chal-

TABLE 62–11. Haagensen Clinical Classification for Staging of Breast Carcinoma

Stage A 1. No clinically involved axillary nodes.
        2. No edema or ulceration of skin. Tumor not solidly fixed to chest wall.
Stage B 1. Clinically involved movable axillary nodes less than 2.5 cm in transverse diameter.
        2. No edema or ulceration of skin. Tumor not solidly fixed to chest wall.
Stage C Any one of five grave signs of advanced breast carcinoma.
        1. Edema of skin of limited extent involving less than one-third of the skin over the breast.
        2. Ulceration of skin.
        3. Solid fixation of tumor to chest wall.
        4. Axillary lymph nodes 2.5 cm or more in transverse diameter.
        5. Fixation of axillary nodes to overlying skin or deeper structures of axilla.
Stage D All other patients with more advanced breast carcinoma, including:
        1. A combination of any two or more of the five grave signs listed under Stage C.
        2. Extensive edema of skin (involving more than one-third of the skin over the breast).
        3. Satellite skin nodules.
        4. The inflammatory type of carcinoma.
        5. Clinically involved supraclavicular lymph nodes.
        6. Internal mammary metastases as evidenced by a parasternal tumor.
        7. Edema of the arm.
        8. Distant metastases.

From Haagensen CD, Bodian C, Haagensen DE Jr: Breast Carcinoma; Risk and Detection. Philadelphia, WB Saunders, 1981.

lenge in counseling and treatment. The best evidence indicates that pregnancy does not augment the rate of growth or spread of breast cancer and that abortion does not improve the prognosis. Initial treatment usually is surgical if the pregnancy is allowed to continue and can consist of radical, modified radical, or simple mastectomy, depending on the extent of disease and the histologic type of tumor. Lumpectomy and quadrantectomy rarely are employed because the lesions usually are large with less well-defined clinical margins than in the nonpregnant patient. These operations are tolerated well during pregnancy, and the results of treatment are much the same, stage for stage, as in the nonpregnant state. If a cancer is diagnosed early, is less than 2 cm in diameter, is well-differentiated, and there are no metastases to regional lymph nodes, the chance of survival is the same as in the nonpregnant patient, from 70 to 80 per cent. If, on the other hand, there is involvement of the subareolar region, inflammatory carcinoma, edema or ulceration of the skin, fixation of the tumor to the chest wall, or involvement of high axillary, supraclavicular, or internal mammary lymph nodes, the prognosis is very poor.

Despite the trend toward limited surgery combined with radiotherapy for breast conservation, this approach should not be employed in pregnancy because the dose to the fetus from radiation scatter would be unacceptably high. Even in early pregnancy, when the distance between the breast and uterus is the greatest, radiation scatter within the body to the fetus

might be as low as 10 to 20 rads for the total treatment course. Later in pregnancy, when the fundus approaches the xiphoid process, 100 rads or more might be delivered to the fetus. Even the lower dose is unacceptable in early pregnancy when organogenesis occurs. The woman with an early cancer who insists on breast conservation might be considered for management by tumor excision and axillary node dissection followed by full breast irradiation postpartum.

Optimal treatment of breast cancer during pregnancy is confusing. The confusion is compounded by the lack of controlled studies evaluating survival of comparable patients in different treatment groups. Most studies report small numbers of patients undergoing varying treatment plans in a nonrandomized fashion. Most authorities recommend a radical or modified radical mastectomy for patients with stage I or stage II disease. The extent of surgery in treating advanced breast cancer is currently a subject of extensive debate throughout the world.

The timing of surgery for breast cancer diagnosed late in pregnancy is controversial. Some reports suggest that patients treated postpartum survive better than those treated in the second and third trimesters. This suggests that postponement of therapy for patients near term may be of benefit. However, it is probable that selection bias existed among these retrospective reports. Delays in definitive therapy may have occurred frequently for the patients with the most favorable prognosis, with immediate treatment carried out more frequently in patients with more extensive disease with a less favorable prognosis. If such treatment bias exists, prompt treatment would not be expected to correlate with good results, and treatment after delivery would appear to be better owing to a preponderance of favorable cases in the second group.

The reported overall survival rate for women first diagnosed as having breast cancer during a pregnancy is poor, reflecting the more advanced stage of disease at diagnosis in most of them. Holleb and Farrow (1962) reported a series of 283 patients with carcinoma of the breast in pregnancy; 73 had inoperable disease and 210 received surgery with or without postoperative radiation. Ninety-three per cent of patients with inoperable disease died within 2 years of the diagnosis, including all seven who had undergone interruption of pregnancy. The majority of the remaining 210 patients had radical mastectomy and were given postoperative radiation therapy. Seven of 28 patients whose disease was diagnosed in the first trimester survived for 5 years. One-half of these 28 patients were allowed to deliver normally, and the other half underwent termination of pregnancy. The interruption of pregnancy did not seem to affect survival rate, which was 33 per cent in the group of patients who carried to term but only 17 per cent in those who underwent abortion. For the small subgroups of patients, these survival differences were not significant. Peters and Meakin (1965) reported 70 patients with breast cancer in pregnancy, all of whom were treated with preoperative or postoperative radiotherapy in conjunction with radical mastectomy. The overall survival rate in this series was 32.9 per cent at 5 years and 19.5 per cent at 10 years. Three of 12 patients treated during the first and second trimesters survived 5 years. Only one of the nine patients treated during the third trimester survived 5 years, and she had active disease at the time of the report. The remaining 49 patients who were treated postpartum had a 39 per cent 5-year survival, prompting the authors to suggest that a delay in the treatment of breast carcinoma until after delivery should be considered.

The massive endogenous hormonal production in pregnancy might influence the course of breast cancer adversely. The striking rise in estrogen production during pregnancy has been of sufficient concern that pregnancy termination has been considered by many to be an important therapeutic objective and avoidance of further pregnancies a principle of continuing care. Whether the stimulatory effect of increased estrogen production has an adverse effect on prognosis, or whether the disproportionate rise of estriol, a relatively weak estrogen and possibly an antagonist of estrone and estradiol, confers some measure of protection, is unknown.

Additional hormonal substances secreted in increased quantities in pregnancy that might influence neoplastic growths in the breast include the glucocorticoids and prolactin. Because glucocorticoids can reduce cellular immunity and perhaps promote the implantation and growth of malignant neoplasms, their increased production has grave clinical implications for the patient with breast cancer. Similarly, elevated quantities of prolactin produced by the hypophysis and human placental lactogen by the placenta late in pregnancy and during milk production might affect breast cancer adversely. Prolactin promotes the growth of dimethyleneanthracene-induced mammary tumors in mice. Its role is not established in humans but is a subject of current investigation. Prolactin suppression with either ergot compounds or L-dopa has not been proved to be of therapeutic value; yet the observation that women with bone pain from metastatic breast cancer sometimes obtained relief from prolactin suppression implicates prolactin as a possible promoter of breast cancer in humans.

Although many clinicians believe that localized breast cancer in the first trimester of pregnancy is a valid reason to recommend pregnancy termination, therapeutic abortion has not been found to increase survival, and the presence of a fetus does not compromise proper surgical management. Thus, we do not believe that pregnancy termination is an essential component of effective treatment of early disease despite the theoretic advantage of removing the source of massive estrogen production.

In advanced breast cancer when tumor tissue is estrogen receptor—positive, on the other hand, therapeutic abortion is usually necessary for effective palliation. Surgical castration is the usual step in managing these women with disseminated mammary cancer, and castration would be useless unless accompanied by therapeutic abortion to remove the placental source of hormones. In the first trimester of pregnancy, this can be accomplished by suction curettage of the uterus; later in pregnancy, termination is accomplished by prostaglandin vaginal suppositories, hysterotomy, or hysterectomy. When pregnancy enters the third trimester, the decision for premature delivery depends heavily on the patient's wishes and the urgency for treatment. A short wait until the fetus is viable might not be accompanied by significant progress of the neoplasm. Continued gestation represents no threat to the fetus because the risk that cancer will traverse the placenta and metastasize to the fetus is negligible.

In many instances, hormonal dependence of these tumors cannot be demonstrated. Indeed, Nugent and O'Connell (1985) found that only 30 per cent of breast cancers in pregnancy were estrogen receptor—positive. It is unclear whether this observation reflects true hormone receptor negativity or whether the high levels of circulating estrogen occupy all available estrogen receptor binding sites, resulting in false-negative receptor assays. The relatively infrequent responsiveness to oophorectomy in patients who develop cancers while pregnant suggests that these tumors frequently are receptor-negative. In this situation the pregnant patient with advanced disease might elect to undergo primary cytotoxic chemotherapy without hormonal ablation by abortion plus castration. After the first trimester of pregnancy, the apparent risks of chemotherapy to the fetus are small and pregnancy can be allowed to proceed.

Prophylactic surgical castration in early-stage breast cancer has been advocated to prevent further pregnancy, which might cause recrudescence of the disease through hormonal stimulation, and also to eliminate the ovarian source of estrogen production in the hope of preventing or delaying subsequent recurrence if the tumor was receptor-positive. Neither argument to support this approach is substantiated by published data. Indeed, pregnancy following mastectomy has not been shown to influence the prognosis, and a few reports have even suggested that future pregnancies might be protective. The rationale for eliminating the ovarian source of estrogens in the primary treatment of early disease is based on the observation that castration in the presence of observable recurrence results in partial or complete temporary tumor regression in approximately one-third of cases. This argument is refuted, however, by two large clinical trials conducted in the United States that fail to demonstrate a significant benefit from castration as adjuvant therapy. In one trial, the National Surgical Adjuvant Breast Project, 199 premenopausal breast cancer patients were randomized, with 129 undergoing surgical castration and 70 serving as controls without hormonal ablation (Radvin et al., 1970). After observation for up to 60 months, there was no evidence that those who were castrated derived any benefit from the procedure.

As many as 7 per cent of premenopausal women have one or more pregnancies after mastectomy for breast cancer, 70 per cent of which can be expected within the first 5 years after treatment. How should the physician advise the patient who has had a mastectomy for breast cancer about future pregnancies? Should they be avoided? Should they be terminated if they occur? The recommendations should be influenced by two major considerations: (1) whether pregnancy promotes recurrence of cancer and (2) the probability of having achieved a cure. It is generally observed that women who become pregnant after mastectomy survive surprisingly well, far better than those whose pregnancy coexisted with the primary tumor, and often better than mastectomy patients overall. This phenomenon of a favorable outcome for patients who became pregnant following treatment for breast cancer might be a function of selection, because most women will wait at least 2 years following treatment, during which many tumors destined to recur will do so. In addition, only women with a good prognosis are likely to achieve counsel recommending subsequent pregnancies. Finally, even though hormonal stimulation by a pregnancy might accelerate a recurrence in a patient with cancer, it is probable that, in the pregnant patient whose cancer recurs, the cancer would have recurred eventually even had she not become pregnant. Thus, the issue becomes one of disease-free interval and duration of survival in these patients rather than probability of cure. Although it may be presumptuous to conclude on the basis of retrospective studies that pregnancy protects against recurrence after mastectomy, it is reasonably safe to conclude that it does not increase the risk of recurrence. Consequently, if a pregnancy occurs, there appears to be no justification for recommending its termination in patients without evidence of recurrence. The converse, that early pregnancy in the face of recurrence should be terminated and that an uneventful pregnancy in no way guarantees against subsequent recurrence, is also true. Indeed, there are cases on record in which multiple pregnancies eventually have been followed by recurrence. We usually recommend that women with favorable tumors without regional or distant spread wait at least 3 years before attempting pregnancy. All such patients should undergo extensive evaluation before conception, including bone and liver scans, chest x-rays, and mammography of the opposite breast, and all must be followed closely during pregnancy.

There is no uniform agreement about the role of breast-feeding in the postpartum patient with breast cancer. Because many data implicate a viral etiology for breast cancer in laboratory animals, there is concern that a virus might cause human breast cancer as well. Therefore, the possibility exists that the contralateral breast is contaminated with the etiologic agent, which might even be passed on to the fetus. This theory has never been borne out in fact, but most surgeons recommend artificial feeding in such cases to avoid vascular enrichment in the opposite breast, which also might contain a neoplasm. This approach is especially important if systemic cytotoxic chemotherapy is planned, since antineoplastic agents are detectable in breast milk and might cause neonatal bone marrow suppression. There are, however, no convincing data that nursing affects the prognosis of breast cancer patients adversely.

Chemotherapy has been used after the first trimester to palliate advanced disease. Alkylating agents, 5-fluorouracil, and vincristine are relatively safe and have been utilized while the fetus is still *in utero*. Methotrexate should be avoided, if possible. Chemotherapy should be administered only when the patient is reluctant to have the pregnancy terminated and the disease appears to be progressing at an alarming rate. The possible role for adjuvant chemotherapy is still uncertain; however, recent reports suggest that both single-agent and combination chemotherapy may significantly improve survival in premenopausal patients when used in an adjuvant setting. The National Institutes of Health currently recommends adjuvant systemic chemotherapy for selected patients including premenopausal women with axillary node metastases, a category into which most pregnant breast cancer patients fall. These women are most likely to benefit from either an alkylating agent alone or cyclophosphamide and 5-fluorouracil with either Adriamycin or methotrexate. Ten- and 15-year follow-ups are always necessary in breast cancer because late recurrences occur frequently.

Leukemia

Leukemia rarely complicates pregnancy, occurring in 1 per 100,000 pregnancies. Approximately 90 per cent of newly diagnosed pregnant leukemic patients have acute leukemia, two-thirds of which are acute myelogenous (AML) and one-third are lymphoblastic (ALL). Almost all chronic leukemia patients who are pregnant have chronic myelogenous leukemia (CML) since chronic lymphocytic leukemia is seen primarily in the elderly.

Prior to the era of effective chemotherapy, the median survival of patients with acute leukemias was 2 to 3 months, while that with CML was characteristically several years. With the development of effective multi-agent chemotherapy regimens, 65 to 75 per cent of patients with acute leukemias will achieve complete remissions, and with the increasing use of bone marrow transplantation many can be cured. Thus, while chemotherapy can be withheld safely for many months in pregnant patients with CML, the coexistence of pregnancy with acute leukemia precludes any treatment delay at any stage of gestation. Although therapy for CML is palliative in most instances, delays in therapy do not appear to affect the duration of survival adversely. In fact, there is no evidence that pregnancy alters the natural history or prognosis of any of the types of leukemia.

Lymphoma

Since the average age of women with Hodgkin's lymphoma is between 30 and 35 years, this cancer is seen in pregnancy with relatively greater frequency than other, more prevalent cancers, that occur in an older population. While non-Hodgkin's lymphomas occur approximately a decade later than Hodgkin's disease, lymphomas as a group represent the fourth most frequent cancer associated with pregnancy, seen in approximately one in 5000 deliveries. Symptomatically, these patients typically present with painless adenopathy, fever, night sweats, weight loss, and pruritus. The diagnosis is confirmed by biopsy, usually of an enlarged lymph node, as well as careful staging employing chest x-ray, bone marrow biopsies, bipedal lymphangiography and abdominal imaging with MRI. MRI is preferable to CT because the former does not expose the fetus to ionizing radiation. When a lymphangiogram is done for staging purposes, only a single x-ray 24 hours following injection of dye should provide adequate information to assess the disease status. Findings on careful staging provide important prognostic information and markedly influence treatment decisions.

Treatment choices should be made based on the cell type and extent of disease. In general, low-grade non-Hodgkin's lymphoma should be treated after delivery of the pregnancy near term. In the intermediate- and high-grade non-Hodgkin's lymphomas, treatment should be effected as soon as the diagnosis is certain, since improved cure rates result from early treatment, and delay in treatment may compromise the expected 33 to 70 per cent cure rates associated with early and intensive multi-agent chemotherapy regimens.

Hodgkin's disease, even when advanced, is potentially curable. Thus, unlike intermediate- and high-grade non-Hodgkin's lymphomas, delays in therapy until the second trimester (if diagnosed early in pregnancy) or following delivery (if diagnosed in the third trimester) is an option. Disease confined to a single lymph node group above the diaphragm can be treated with radiotherapy even with the fetus in situ early in pregnancy. Careful shielding of the abdomen and pelvis is mandatory. As the fundal height approaches the diaphragm in the third trimester, localized extra-abdominal radiotherapy late in pregnancy is contraindicated, and therapy should either be withheld until following delivery or should be administered as chemotherapy. Curative chemotherapy regimens include combinations of Mustargen, oncovin, procarbazine, and prednisone (MOPP) and Adriamycin, bleomycin, vinblastine, and dacarbazine (ABVD), both of which can be given after the first trimester with little teratogenic risk to the fetus.

Bone Tumors

Both benign and primary or metastatic malignant bone tumors can be found in pregnant women and can pose problems in diagnosis and treatment. The diagnosis frequently can be suspected from the characteristic radiographic findings in a patient with bony asymmetry or pain. When the diagnosis is uncertain and malignancy is suspected, a biopsy must be done.

Benign bone tumors rarely are a problem in pregnancy; however, two benign tumors that can affect pregnancy and delivery are endochondromas and benign exostosis, both of which can develop at the pelvic brim. These neoplasms may interfere with progression of labor and engagement of the fetal head by causing mechanical obstruction at the pelvic inlet, necessitating cesarean section.

The most common primary malignant tumors seen in the childbearing years are Ewing's sarcoma, osteogenic sarcoma, and osteocystoma. These tumors usually involve the clavicle, sternum, spine, humerus, or femur and are associated with local pain, mass, and disability. Signs and symptoms of myelitis with radiating pain, paresthesias, and weakness can be produced by primary sarcoma of the spine.

Primary bone cancer is aggressive, frequently metastasizing by the hematogenous route at the time of diagnosis. It is treated initially with surgical excision, usually without regard for the pregnancy. In the past, x-ray therapy and chemotherapy were delayed until delivery if the tumor had not metastasized at the time of diagnosis in the pregnant patient. Because pregnancy does not affect the growth of bone cancers and because these tumors do not affect the pregnancy, indications for pregnancy termination did not exist. Unfortunately, survival in the group of patients for whom chemotherapy was delayed was uniformly poor, most patients dying of disseminated cancer within 24 months. Within the past 15 years, the treatment of osteogenic sarcomas has become much more successful, combining adjuvant chemotherapy often with more limited surgery than advocated previously. Aggressive chemotherapy administered soon after amputation or resection is crucial to prevent the development of clinically detectable metastases in patients with these tumors. Therefore, it is appropriate to recommend early termination of pregnancy for patients whose cancer is discovered in the first or early second trimester. If the diagnosis is made later in pregnancy, early delivery of the infant should be effected, and intensive multiple-agent chemotherapy with doxorubicin, methotrexate, and cyclophosphamide should be instituted. Alternatively, because the risk of fetal malformations induced by chemotherapy during the second half of the pregnancy is low, continuation of pregnancy despite administration of a methotrexate-containing multiple-drug regimen can be considered. Because most recurrences from bone malignancy appear within the first 3 years of initial therapy, recommendations for future pregnancies should be deferred until that interval has passed.

In women of childbearing age, the most common malignancies that metastasize to bone are those of breast, cervix, thyroid, and kidney. Metastases occur most frequently in the skull, ribs, spine, and long bones, except for those from the cervix, which can extend directly to involve the pelvis. Patients can present with pain, a pathologic fracture, or paralysis, but some asymptomatic patients are identified by routine chest x-ray during pregnancy. This finding necessitates careful evaluation for a primary site, with definitive therapy dictated by the source of tumor and the duration of pregnancy at the time of diagnosis.

Thyroid Cancer

Both benign diseases and cancers of the thyroid gland occur more commonly in women than in men. Approximately 65 per cent of all patients with carcinoma of the thyroid are women. Although the majority of patients with thyroid carcinoma are in their 50s and 60s, about 15 per cent are below age 30. Some younger patients with thyroid cancer have an antecedent history of thymic radiation during infancy or facial skin radiation in the treatment of adolescent acne.

Thyroid nodules can be present in approximately 1 per cent of women of childbearing age. Since approximately 15 per cent of solitary thyroid nodules are malignant, prompt investigation of these nodules is warranted. Since thyroid scanning in pregnancy is contraindicated, evaluation should consist of measuring serum-free T_4 and T_3, to rule out a benign toxic adenoma, and ultrasonography, to rule out a cystic mass, which is rarely (<2 per cent) malignant. If a solitary solid cold nodule is found, fine-needle aspiration or percutaneous needle biopsy is warranted.

The diagnosis of carcinoma of the thyroid during pregnancy is not an absolute indication to terminate the pregnancy; neither is pregnancy a contraindication to necessary surgery. Most reports suggest that pregnancy does not adversely affect these usually slow-growing tumors. Radioactive iodine therapy must be withheld until after delivery, but only rarely would it be indicated for this disease. The recurrence rate is not influenced by subsequent pregnancies but is related to many other factors. Younger patients with thyroid cancer have been reported to have a better prognosis than older ones. Additional prognostic factors include tumor size and grade, and anaplastic cancers are associated with a dismal outlook.

REFERENCES

Bagshawe KD: Risk and prognostic factors in trophoblastic neoplasia. Cancer 38:1373, 1976.

Barber HRK, Brunschwig A: Carcinoma of the bowel: Radiation and surgical management and pregnancy. Am J Obstet Gynecol 100:926, 1968.

Barber HRK, Brunschwig A: Gynecologic cancer complicating pregnancy. Am J Obstet Gynecol 85:156, 1963.

Berkowitz RS, Goldstein DP, Bernstein MR: Ten years' experience with methotrexate and folinic acid as primary therapy for gestational trophoblastic disease. Gynecol Oncol 23:111, 1986.

Bosch A, Marcial VA: Carcinoma of the uterine cervix associated with pregnancy. Am J Roentgenol 96:92, 1966.

Bottles K, Taylor R: Diagnosis of breast masses in pregnant and lactating women by aspiration cytology. Obstet Gynecol 66:765, 1985.

Brodsky JB, Cohen EN, Brown BW, et al: Surgery during pregnancy and fetal outcome. Am J Obstet Gynecol 138:1165, 1980.

Byrne J, Mulvihill JJ, Myers MH, et al: Effects of treatment on fertility in long-term survivors of childhood or adolescent cancer. N Engl J Med 317:1315, 1987.

Creasman WT, Rutledge F, Fletcher G: Carcinoma of the cervix associated with pregnancy. Obstet Gynecol 36:495, 1970.

Curry SL, Hammond CB, Tyrey L, et al: Hydatidiform mole; diagnosis, management, and long-term follow-up of 347 patients. Obstet Gynecol 45:1, 1975.

Dildy GA, Moise KJ, Carpenter RJ, Klima T: Maternal malignancy metastatic to the products of conception: A review. Obstet Gynecol Surv 44(7):535, 1989.

Doll DC, Ringenberg QS, Yarbro JW: Antineoplastic agents and pregnancy. Semin Oncol 16(5):337, 1989.

Eastman NJ, Hellman LM: Ovarian tumors in pregnancy. In Eastman NJ, Hellman LM (eds): Williams' Obstetrics. 13th ed. New York, Appleton-Century-Crofts, 1966.

George PA, Fortner JG, Pack GT: Melanoma with pregnancy; report of 115 cases. Cancer 13:854, 1960.

Goldstein DP, Reid D: Recent developments in management of molar pregnancy. Clin Obstet Gynecol 10:313, 1967.

Goldstein DP: Five years' experience with the prevention of trophoblastic tumors by the prophylactic use of chemotherapy in patients with molar pregnancy. Clin Obstet Gynecol 13:945, 1970.

Goldstein DP, Saracco P, Osathanondh R, et al: Methotrexate with citrovorum factor rescue for gestational trophoblastic neoplasms. Obstet Gynecol 53:93, 1978.

Goldstein DP, Berkowitz RS, Bernstein MR: Reproductive performance after molar pregnancy and gestational trophoblastic tumors. Clin Obstet Gynecol 27:221, 1984.

Grimes WH, et al: Ovarian cysts in pregnancy. Am J Obstet Gynecol 68:594, 1954.

Hammond CB, Borchert LG, Tyrey L, et al: Treatment of metastatic trophoblastic disease; good and poor prognosis. Am J Obstet Gynecol 115:4, 1973.

Hammond CB, Weed JC Jr, Currie JL: The role of operation in the current therapy of gestational trophoblastic disease. Am J Obstet Gynecol 136:844, 1980.

Hannigan EV: Cervical cancer in pregnancy. Clin Obstet Gynecol 33(4):837, 1990.

Holleb AI, Farrow JH: The relation of carcinoma of the breast and pregnancy in 283 patients. Surg Gynecol Obstet 115:65, 1962.

Karlen JR, Akbari A, Cook WA: Dysgerminoma associated with pregnancy. Obstet Gynecol 53:330, 1979.

Li M, Hertz R, Spencer DB: Effects of methotrexate therapy upon choriocarcinoma and chorioadenoma. Proc Soc Exp Biol Med 93:361, 1956.

Newlands ES, Bagshawe KD, Begent RH, et al: Developments in chemotherapy for medium- and high-risk patients with gestational trophoblastic tumours. Br J Obstet Gynecol 93:63, 1986.

Nicholson HO. Cytotoxic drugs in pregnancy. J Obstet Gynaecol Br Cwlth 75:307, 1968.

Nugent P, O'Connell T: Breast cancer and pregnancy. Arch Surg 120:1221, 1985.

Pack GT, Scharnagel IM: The prognosis for malignant melanoma in the pregnant woman. Cancer 4:324, 1951.

Penn I, Makowski E, Droegemueller W, et al: Parenthood in renal homograft recipients. JAMA 216:1755, 1971.

Peters MV, Meakin JW: The influence of pregnancy in carcinoma of the breast. Prog Clin Cancer 1:471, 1965.

Radvin RG, Lewison EF, Slack NH, et al: The results of a clinical trial concerning the worth of prophylactic oophorectomy for breast cancer. Surg Gynecol Obstet 131:1055, 1970.

Reynoso EE, Shepherd FA, Messner HA, et al: Acute leukemia during pregnancy: The Toronto leukemia study group experience with long-term follow-up of children exposed in utero to chemotherapeutic agents. J Clin Oncol 5(7):1098, 1987.

Rustin GJ, Booth M, Dent J, et al: Pregnancy after cytotoxic chemotherapy for gestational trophoblastic tumours. Br Med J (Clin Res) 14:288, 1984.

Schapira DV, Chudley AE: Successful pregnancy following continuous treatment with combination chemotherapy before contraception and throughout pregnancy. Cancer 54:800, 1984.

Sokal JE, Lessman EM: The effects of cancer chemotherapeutic agents on the human fetus. JAMA 172:1765, 1960.

Waldrop GM, Palmer JP: Carcinoma of the cervix associated with pregnancy. Am J Obstet Gynecol 86:202, 1963.

White LP, Linden G, Breslow L, et al: Studies on melanoma. The effect of pregnancy on survival in human melanoma. JAMA 117:235, 1961.

NEONATAL PROBLEMS

C H A P T E R

IDENTIFICATION AND MANAGEMENT OF HIGH-RISK PROBLEMS IN THE NEONATE

AVROY A. FANAROFF, M.B. (RAND), FRCPE,
RICHARD J. MARTIN, M.D., and
MARTHA J. MILLER, M.D., Ph.D.

RESUSCITATION

During the last decade, increasing obstetric skill in identification of high-risk pregnancies has been paralleled by improved knowledge of the pathophysiology and treatment of prematurity and neonatal asphyxia. When a high-risk delivery is identified, coordination of the referring hospital with a tertiary center that is expert in high-risk obstetric and neonatal care may well reduce attendant morbidity and mortality for both the mother and her child. The current state of the art of perinatal care includes a team composed of perinatologist and/or obstetrician, neonatologist, and skilled nursing staff whose expertise greatly improves preparedness for obstetric emergencies. The cost of such care continues to increase, but this cost is balanced by important improvement in infant outcome. The ability to sustain this momentum in improved perinatal care of both mother and infant rests on continuing research into the transitional physiology of the infant and mother as well as on scrupulous training of all personnel in the most advanced techniques of neonatal resuscitation.

To that end, The Working Group on Pediatric Resuscitation and the National Task Force on Neonatal Resuscitation of the Section on Perinatal Pediatrics of the American Academy of Pediatrics have assembled guidelines for training of health professionals in neonatal resuscitation (Standards, 1992). This curriculum unifies the principles of neonatal resuscitation developed over the last two to three decades of clinical experience in neonatology. The following discussion will review the physiology of normal and abnormal postnatal adaptation as well as the current recommendations for delivery room management.

Pulmonary and Circulatory Adaptations at Birth

Following delivery, a remarkable series of physiologic adaptations take place that allow the infant to make a smooth transition from intrauterine to extrauterine life. After birth, the infant must establish the lungs as the site of gas exchange, and the circulatory pattern that had shunted blood away from the lungs in the fetus must now perfuse the pulmonary vasculature. The first few breaths clear amniotic fluid from the lungs and establish a functional residual capacity (FRC). Clearance of lung fluid is also aided by chest compression as the infant passes through the vaginal canal. Furthermore, expansion of the lungs stimulates surfactant release, which reduces surface tension and stabilizes the infant's FRC. These changes in lung function coincide with the complex circulatory changes that surround delivery. The very act of expansion of the lungs lowers pulmonary vascular resistance and increases pulmonary blood flow. When the cord is clamped, the low-resistance placental circulation is cut off, and the infant's systemic blood pressure rises. These effects combine to decrease right-to-left shunting of blood at the ductus arteriosus and at the foramen ovale. Furthermore, the increase in PaO_2, which occurs as the infant breathes, stimulates closure of the ductus arteriosus over the first few days of life. These important circulatory events reroute right heart blood to the infant's lungs and result in an adult-type circulatory pattern in the healthy newborn by 24 to 48 hours of life.

Initial Steps in Resuscitation

In most instances, resuscitation is not required, and the infant's transition to extrauterine life may be assisted by a few simple steps.

Thermal Management

Immediately after birth, the newborn infant should be placed on a preheated radiant warmer. In order to avoid evaporative heat loss, the infant should be thoroughly dried and the wet blankets promptly removed. These initial steps are important in minimizing heat loss, particularly in premature infants (Fig. 63–1) (Sinclair, 1978). In these patients, heat loss is exaggerated by the infant's lack of subcutaneous fat as well as the increased ratio of surface area to weight. Moreover, the preterm infant is poorly equipped to generate additional heat because of reduced stores of brown fat and glycogen. Hypothermia may precipitate a cascade of dangerous physiologic changes including hypoglycemia, metabolic acidosis, and a reversion to the fetal circulation pattern, with resulting hypoxemia. To avoid these effects, it is recommended that the infant be kept in a neutral thermal environment in which oxygen consumption is minimal. This can be achieved by caring for the newborn on a servocontrolled radiant warmer, with the goal of maintaining a normal rectal temperature of 36.5 to 37.5°C. Placement of a knitted cap on the infant's head in the delivery room is an important additional step, which also decreases evaporative heat loss.

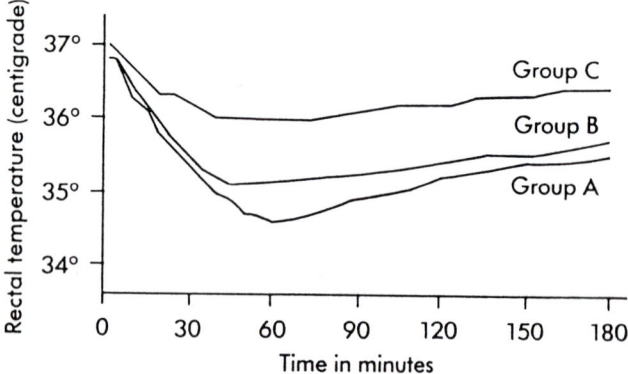

FIGURE 63–1. Mean core temperatures in three groups of infants showing the effect of drying and thermal protection immediately after birth. Group A: open crib, bathed within one hour; Group B: open crib, no bath; Group C: preheated incubator, dried immediately after birth, no bath. (From Miller DL, Oliver TK: Body temperature in the immediate neonatal period: The effect of reducing thermal losses. Am J Obstet Gynecol 94:964, 1966. With permission.)

Respiratory Evaluation

The next step in initial care should be to clear the pharynx and nose of fluid. This can be accomplished easily by using a bulb syringe to suction first the infant's mouth, then the nose. The special management needed for infants with meconium-stained amniotic fluid will be discussed later in this section. During the first minute of life, the caretaker must evaluate the infant's respirations, heart rate, and color. The mildly depressed infant may experience primary apnea at birth. This type of apnea is due to mild depression of the brain stem respiratory control area by hypoxia and/or reflex inhibition and has been found to respond well to tactile stimulation and exposure to oxygen. Thus, if the infant is still apneic after initial drying and suctioning, tactile stimulation may be provided through flicking the soles of the feet or rubbing the infant's back.

Cardiovascular Assessment

The next step in initial stabilization of an infant is evaluation of the heart rate. If the heart rate is above 100 beats/minute and the perfusion is normal, the infant can be considered to be adapting normally to extrauterine life. If the heart rate is below 100 beats/minute, initiation of positive pressure ventilation may be required to provide adequate oxygenation to the heart and brain. In most mildly depressed infants, positive pressure ventilation will promptly restore a heart rate that is above 100 beats per minute.

If the infant is breathing and the heart rate is over 100, the infant's color should be assessed. If peripheral cyanosis is present, supplemental oxygen is not required, but the infant should be evaluated to determine whether core temperature is low and warming is necessary. If central cyanosis is present, free-flow 100 per cent oxygen should be provided by nasal mask, and further evaluation of the cause of the cyanosis should be undertaken.

The Apgar Score

These simple steps, the ABCs of newborn resuscitation, can often be completed before the end of the first minute of life, and are sufficient for the initial delivery room care of the majority of healthy infants. The next step in an infant's evaluation is assessment of the Apgar score at 1 and 5 minutes of life. The Apgar score is a qualitative measure of the infant's success in adapting to the extrauterine environment (Table 63–1). This score consists of two vital signs (respiratory effort and heart rate), color, and two neurologic responses (response to stimulation and general tone). Each of these components is given a score of 0 to 2, with 2 being the best score, and 0 indicating no response. Each component is evaluated at 1 and 5 minutes, and a total score is calculated. When the Apgar score is less than 6 at 5 minutes, it is recommended that a 10- or even 15-minute score be calculated.

Although the Apgar score is useful in the initial steps of evaluation, resuscitation of the infant should

TABLE 63–1. Components of the Apgar Score

SCORE	SCORE 0	1	2
Heart rate	Absent	100 beats/min	100 beats/min
Respiratory effort	Absent	Slow, irregular	Good cry
Color	Cyanotic, pallid	Acrocyanotic	Pink
Muscle tone	Limp	Minimal	Active
Reflex response	Absent	Minimal	Active

not be delayed until the 1-minute Apgar. The initial Apgar scores at 1 and 5 minutes are in fact of limited use in predicting degree of asphyxia or neurologic outcome (Nelson and Ellenberg, 1981). However, the Apgar score assigned at 10 or 15 minutes may indicate the infant's risk of a later neurologic deficit. In premature infants ≤32 weeks gestation or <1500 grams at birth, care must be used in interpretation of a low Apgar score, which can occur in such patients in the absence of asphyxia (Tooley et al., 1977). As of this writing, no testing procedure is available for use within the first weeks of life which can accurately predict the infant's eventual neurologic outcome.

CARE OF THE DEPRESSED NEWBORN INFANT

Antenatal monitoring and anticipatory management of the mother-infant dyad have increasingly been utilized to decrease the possibility of antenatal or perinatal birth asphyxia. Even with our current level of expertise, however, infants may be born who have suffered a degree of hypoxia and/or hypoperfusion *in utero*. For such infants, advanced skill in resuscitation is required, with each step designed to reverse as much as possible the effects of asphyxia.

Hypoxic-ischemic injury *in utero* may lead to a form of severe central depression of respiration which is termed "secondary apnea." An infant with this form of apnea is unresponsive to stimulation, and artificial ventilation with oxygen must be initiated at once if the infant fails to respond to the initial ABCs of resuscitation. Ventilation should be promptly provided through positive pressure ventilation with a bag and mask. When effective, this will rapidly restore oxygenated blood to the brain, and the infant's own respiratory drive will resume. While positive pressure ventilation is being provided to the depressed infant, the heart rate should also be assessed. If the infant has suffered prolonged asphyxia, the heart rate may be depressed, and bag and mask ventilation may restore a normal heart rate over 100 beats per minute, accompanied by an improvement in cardiac output. After stabilization, such infants should be carefully monitored for recurrence of apnea, and oxygen provided until all cyanosis has resolved.

The more profoundly asphyxiated the infant is, the harder it is to establish spontaneous respirations, normal heart rate, and oxygenation. If the infant fails to respond to bag and mask ventilation and the heart rate remains below 80 beats per minute, two further steps in resuscitation must be considered and performed as quickly as possible. If after 15 to 30 seconds of positive-pressure ventilation the infant's heart rate fails to rise, chest compressions should be started at 120 times per minute and continued so as to provide circulatory support and minimize the effects of hypoperfusion. Furthermore, endotracheal intubation should be promptly performed if the infant is not responding to positive-pressure ventilation, or if prolonged positive-pressure ventilation is required to support respiration. Intubating a newborn infant takes practice and skill, and the procedure should be undertaken by individuals specifically trained and experienced in neonatal resuscitation. Even in the moderately depressed infant, restoration of circulation and artificial ventilation will usually dramatically improve color and perfusion before 5 minutes of life, and prolonged cardiorespiratory support may not be necessary.

ADVANCED RESUSCITATION AND THE SPECIFIC PROBLEMS OF THE SEVERELY ASPHYXIATED NEWBORN

The use of medications to support circulation may be required in those rare infants who have a heart rate below 80 despite adequate ventilation and chest compressions for a minimum of 30 seconds, or who have an undetectable heart rate (Table 63–2). Epinephrine, volume expanders, and sodium bicarbonate are the medications for advanced newborn resuscitation which should be available in all delivery rooms.

Two routes are available for administration of such medications to a newborn in an emergency. Epinephrine may be given intratracheally, from which site rapid absorption into the circulation occurs. For administration of volume expanders or bicarbonate, placement of an umbilical venous line provides prompt and convenient access.

Epinephrine is the first drug to be considered during advanced resuscitation. Epinephrine increases the strength and rate of cardiac contractions and may be given at a dose of 0.1 to 0.3 ml/kg (concentration 1:10,000) by the intravenous or intratracheal route, and repeated every 5 minutes if required. Usually within 15 to 30 seconds an improvement in heart rate and perfusion occurs.

The severely depressed infant may present with circulatory shock at birth, owing to such problems as asphyxia, hemorrhage, sepsis, pulmonary insufficiency, or structural heart disease. The antenatal history may give valuable clues allowing anticipation of shock in the infant, e.g., if the mother has abruptio

Table 63–2.   Medications Used During Resuscitation

	CONCENTRATION	DOSAGE	ROUTE
Epinephrine	1:10,000	0.1–0.3 ml/kg	IV or ET
Volume expanders	Whole blood	10 ml/kg	IV
	5% Albumin		
	Normal saline		
	Ringer's lactated solution		
Sodium bicarbonate	0.5 mEq/ml (4.2% solution)	2 mEq/kg IV	IV. Give slowly over at least 2 min; give only if infant being effectively ventilated
Naloxone	0.4 mg/ml or 1.0 mg/ml	0.1 mg/kg	IV, ET, preferred IM, SQ acceptable

placentae, or if severe fetal depression has been diagnosed prior to delivery. Clinical signs of hypovolemia in the infant include pallor, weak pulses, cold extremities, poor capillary refill, poor response to resuscitation, or low blood pressure. In the delivery room, the infant's blood pressure may be measured by the noninvasive Dynamap technique; however, this may underestimate hypotension in low-birth-weight infants. More accurate monitoring of blood pressure can be achieved by an indwelling umbilical arterial catheter. Tachypnea, poor urine output, metabolic acidosis, and central nervous system depression may also accompany the picture of shock.

The management of shock depends on the underlying mechanism of the hypotension. Three mechanisms that may contribute to shock are decreased blood volume (usually due to perinatal blood loss or twin-twin transfusion), decreased cardiac contractility (asphyxia, congenital heart disease), and decreased peripheral vascular resistance (sepsis).

Volume expansion is the first line of treatment of the clinical picture of shock. This is effective for infants with reduced volume due to blood loss as well as septic vasodilated infants with effective reduction of blood volume. The four most commonly used volume expanders are: normal saline, 5 per cent albumin/saline, whole blood (cross-matched with mother), and Ringer's lactated solution. Volume expanders are given intravenously at a dose of 10 ml/kg over 5 to 10 minutes. Care should be taken, however, not to administer excessive fluids to the infant with asphyxia and myocardial dysfunction. In such infants, a combination of fluid administration at the dose indicated above and use of inotropic agents such as dopamine, dobutamine, and isuprel may yield the best outcome. Within minutes of restoration of peripheral circulation, there may be a remarkable and rapid improvement in blood pressure, color, peripheral perfusion, and neurologic state as function is restored to all organ systems.

During prolonged asphyxia, diminished oxygen delivery to the tissues may result in a buildup of lactic acid, with a resultant metabolic acidosis. When ventilation of the asphyxiated infant has been established and metabolic acidosis is documented or strongly suspected on clinical grounds, sodium bicarbonate may be administered intravenously at a dose of 2 mEq/kg of a 0.5 mEq/ml (4.2 per cent) solution. Resolution of the metabolic acidosis will reverse pulmonary vasoconstriction and aid in establishment of normal aerobic metabolism. Bicarbonate should not be administered if ventilation has not been established because this will result in an accumulation of CO_2 in the blood and superimpose a respiratory acidosis on a preexisting metabolic acidosis.

Hypoglycemia may accompany profound asphyxia. The provision of glucose is invaluable for the recovery of all tissues of the asphyxiated infant. Therefore, if asphyxia is suspected, the serum glucose level should be promptly assessed and intravenous glucose infusion provided so as to normalize glucose concentration in the blood.

SPECIAL PROBLEMS OF THE NEWBORN INFANT

Meconium Aspiration

Meconium staining of the amniotic fluid or fetus occurs *in utero* in 8 to 20 per cent of all deliveries and may be indicative of fetal distress, as in infants who are small for gestational age or postmature, those with cord complications, or those in whom other factors are compromising oxygen delivery to or circulation of the infant. Meconium is almost never observed in the amniotic fluid before 34 weeks gestation. The passage of meconium should alert the delivery room team to the possibility of a depressed fetus, and a professional skilled in infant resuscitation should be present in the delivery room.

Meconium in the amniotic fluid may stain the umbilical cord, placenta, and fetus. Normally, the infant exhibits phasic respirations *in utero*, which may increase markedly in depth if asphyxia occurs. Inhaled meconium may penetrate the infant's airways and if the consistency of the meconium is pea soup or particulate, the material may cause obstruction of airways and atelectasis. Occasionally, pulmonary air leaks such as pneumothorax or pneumomediastinum develop after birth, which may severely compromise the infant's cardiorespiratory status.

Management of this problem begins with the obstetrician, who should facilitate clearing of the upper airway by suctioning the pharynx and nares, preferably with wall suction (Carson et al., 1976) after the head has been delivered. Approximately 10 per cent of infants will have residual meconium left in the trachea below the vocal cords. In cases of particulate or thick meconium, endotracheal intubation of the infant by a health professional is recommended to clear the airway of this residual meconium. If the infant has only light meconium and is not depressed at birth, intubation may not be required (Table 63–3).

Drug-Depressed Infants

Meperidine is a narcotic analgesic that may be administered to laboring mothers. If the medication is given intramuscularly within 1½ to 2 hours before delivery, the drug concentration will be at its maximum in the serum of the mother and fetus at the time of birth. Narcotic depression of the infant may appear as apnea and hypotonia. Such an infant is treated with naloxone, 0.01 mg/kg, administered either intramuscularly or intravenously. Typically, the infant's tone and respiratory effort improve dramatically. However, meperidine may create acute drug withdrawal in infants whose mothers are on methadone or are addicted to narcotics, and in such cases, naloxone administration is contraindicated.

Recognizing Congenital Diaphragmatic Hernias

Persistent cyanosis and a scaphoid abdomen in a cyanotic infant who has been intubated should make one suspicious of a diaphragmatic hernia. Congenital diaphragmatic hernia (CDH) results from failure of closure of the posterolateral pleuroperitoneal folds during the eighth to ninth week of gestation, which causes herniation of intestine (90 per cent) and liver (50 per cent) into the thoracic cavity. Most commonly, hernias involve the left hemidiaphragm; in these infants breath sounds are absent over the left lung and the cardiac sounds shift to the right. A right-sided

TABLE 63–3. Prevention of Meconium Aspiration Syndrome

RESOLVED ISSUES
Meconium aspiration may develop in utero
Careful, thorough suctioning of the oropharynx before the first breath is the most important preventive measure
Suctioning via endotracheal tube is indicated for depressed infants before initiation of positive pressure ventilation
UNRESOLVED ISSUES
The role of meconium *thickness* in determining management is undetermined
The ability to recognize evidence for cardiorespiratory depression *immediately* at birth has not been attained
RECOMMENDATIONS
All infants born with meconium-stained fluid should receive endotracheal suctioning if:
Positive pressure ventilation is needed.
Meconium is thick, contains particulate material, or has pea soup consistency.
Oropharyngeal suctioning has not been performed at the perineum.
Antenatal monitoring shows evidence of fetal distress.
Endotracheal suctioning is probably not indicated if meconium is thin, the infant is vigorous at birth, and the oropharynx has been suctioned at delivery.

From Miller MJ et al: Neonatology-Perinatal Medicine. St. Louis, Mosby/Year Book, 1992.

pneumothorax may give similar auscultatory findings but is usually associated with abdominal distention rather than a scaphoid abdomen. When the hernia is on the right side, the diagnosis is more difficult because the clinical signs are not as striking. In general, it is a good practice to obtain a chest x-ray immediately in any infant who fails to respond to cardiopulmonary resuscitation. When a diaphragmatic hernia is diagnosed, a nasogastric tube must be placed to decompress the gastrointestinal tract and prevent cardiac tamponade by the overdistended bowel. Successful management of the infant with CDH depends on early recognition of the defect, stabilization of acid-base components, and adequate ventilation through an endotracheal tube.

Further management may require pulmonary vasodilation (tolazoline), paralysis (pancuronium), and hyperventilation. If the infant survives the first 5 to 7 days and ventilatory insufficiency continues, one should suspect reversal of the shunt, from right-to-left to left-to-right, through a patent ductus arteriosus (PDA). Closure of the PDA at this time may improve survival (Sills et al., 1984).

BIRTH TRAUMA/BIRTH INJURIES

Birth injuries reportedly occur in two to seven per 1000 live births. They are not entirely avoidable and may be noted even after the most skilled and careful obstetric care. The fetus may be injured by antenatal as well as intrapartum interventions in addition to delivery. Amniocentesis, cordocentesis, fetal surgical manipulations, intrauterine transfusions, and even fetal heart rate monitoring via the scalp electrode all present some degree of risk for the fetus. Labor and delivery, however, account for the vast majority of birth injuries. The most vulnerable infants are those who are macrosomic or premature or who have an abnormal presentation. Prolonged labor, dystocia, and cephalopelvic disproportion predispose to injury, as does instrumental intervention with forceps or vacuum extractor. Delivery by cesarean section does not ensure freedom from birth trauma. Furthermore, the neonate may be traumatized during resuscitation.

Cephalohematomas are confined by the sutures, because these represent subperiosteal hemorrhages. There are often associated hairline fractures of the skull, most frequently noted over the parietal bones. A cephalohematoma presents as a fluctuant swelling on the second day of life and, if large enough, may account for anemia and subsequent jaundice. Bilateral cephalohematomas are not uncommon. Cephalohematomas should be differentiated from caput succedaneum, which has overlying bruising and less well-defined margins because the caput is not confined by the suture lines. A caput resolves more rapidly. No therapy is needed for a cephalohematoma, and the fluid should never be aspirated. Blood transfusion may rarely be required.

Facial nerve palsy may result from compression of the facial nerve by forceps or from spontaneous compression against the sacral promontory. The paralyzed side appears smooth and full, with obliteration of the nasolabial fold; the eye remains persistently open and the corner of the mouth droops. With crying, the mouth is drawn to the side that is not paralyzed. If the eye remains open, it is necessary to use a pad and methylcellulose drops to prevent corneal injury. Spontaneous resolution of these lesions usually occurs; however, neurologic evaluation and follow-up may be warranted if the paralysis does not show improvement.

Fractures of the clavicle or long bones may be observed, most notably following shoulder dystocia or a difficult breech delivery. The clavicle is the most frequently fractured bone during labor and delivery. A cracking sound may be audible. The fractures may be asymptomatic or confirmed radiologically after detection of swelling, discoloration, tenderness, or an asymmetric Moro reflex. The affected arm and shoulder are immobilized for 7 to 10 days.

Fractures of the long bones are usually in the midshaft region and are sustained most commonly during manipulation of the arms or legs in a breech delivery. The diagnosis is usually self-evident as a result of the swelling, pain, deformity, shortening, and lack of movement of the affected limb. Treatment is directed at immobilization, with little concern for careful alignment because of the great capacity for remodeling noted in the newborn. Complete union is anticipated within 3 to 4 weeks.

Brachial plexus injuries are classified according to the site of the lesion. The most common is Erb's palsy, which involves the roots of C5 and C6. Klumpke's palsy refers to lesions of the lower brachial plexus C8 to T1. Rarely there is involvement of the whole brachial plexus with a global palsy of the arm. Lesions of C3, C4, and C5 will result in phrenic nerve paralysis, diaphragmatic paralysis, and respiratory compromise. Most cases of brachial palsy follow prolonged labor and difficult deliveries in which traction is exerted on the neck (Allen et al., 1991). However, a significant number (often bilateral and in association with other nerve palsies) occur *in utero* and in the absence of birth trauma. During a breech presentation the plexus is injured as a result of traction on the shoulder when delivery of the head is attempted. In situations with shoulder dystocia, lateral traction on the head and neck away from one of the shoulders may injure the brachial plexus.

Infants with Erb's palsy will hold the arm limply alongside the body with the forearm pronated. There is loss of movement and reflexes of the affected limb including the Moro response. The grasp reflex remains intact. In Klumpke's paralysis the hand is paralyzed, there are no voluntary movements of the wrist, and the grasp reflex is absent. A claw hand may result. X-rays are indicated to exclude fractures of the spine and arm. Treatment is expectant, with splinting to avoid contractures and physiotherapy. Because most injuries are mild, recovery can be anticipated in 3 to 6 months.

RESPIRATORY DISORDERS
Lung Development

The respiratory system plays a critical role in successful early adaptation to extrauterine life. At birth,

interruption of the fetal-placental circulation requires the newborn infant immediately to achieve effective gas exchange. Sufficient prenatal maturation of the respiratory system therefore is an essential aspect of intrauterine development. Differentiation of the lung requires carefully regulated coordination of anatomic, physiologic, and biochemical processes. The ultimate result of these maturational events is for the lung to have adequate surface area, blood supply, and metabolic capability to sustain oxygenation and ventilation during the early neonatal period. Particularly important from a biochemical viewpoint is the capacity for rapid synthesis of surface-active phospholipids, which are necessary in establishing normal lung function after birth.

Fetal lung development is discussed in detail in Chapter 28. For brief review, it is known that in early gestation the epithelial cells of the lung are simple and columnar in type and show few signs of organelle differentiation. During the last 10 to 20 per cent of gestation in most species, certain lining cells of the terminal respiratory units undergo alterations, permitting them to be distinguished as type II pneumonocytes. Although type II pneumonocytes have been identified in the human fetus between 22 and 26 weeks of gestation, these cells become more prominent at 34 to 36 weeks of gestation. The major change allowing these cells to be readily identified is the appearance of osmiophilic lamellar bodies in the cytoplasm. Histochemical and ultrastructural techniques have confirmed the role of the type II pneumonocyte in the synthesis, storage, and secretion of pulmonary surfactant. These studies also have indicated that the osmiophilic lamellar bodies are the intracellular deposits of surfactant. Because of its thin nature and proximity to capillary endothelial cells, the other major cell type (type I pneumonocyte) is ideally suited for the transfer of oxygen and carbon dioxide. Therefore, gas exchange occurs primarily across that portion of the respiratory epithelium composed of type I pneumonocytes.

Through recent advances, pulmonary surfactant is now understood to be an antiatelectasis factor located in the alveolar lining layer, which provides a low and variable surface tension and imparts hysteresis to the air-tissue interface. Surface-active material is, therefore, capable of performing the twofold function of (1) decreasing the pressure required to distend the lung and (2) maintaining alveolar stability over a wide range of local volumes. Once the mature lung has been expanded, the surfactant film lining the alveoli and terminal bronchioles tends to increase surface tension at high lung volumes, promoting emptying, and lowering it at diminished lung volume. Lowering surface tension as the size of terminal air spaces decreases prevents collapse at end expiration. The remaining volume of gas, termed *functional residual capacity*, acts as a reservoir that prevents wide fluctuations in blood oxygen and carbon dioxide levels during respiration. Furthermore, a partially expanded air space requires less effort to reexpand than one that is completely collapsed.

Although many substances are present in pulmonary surfactant, the predominant and functionally essential constituent is saturated phosphatidylcholine, or lecithin (Fig. 63–2). Lung cells and bronchoalveolar fluid are unique in showing high concentrations of saturated phosphatidylcholine and significant amounts of phosphatidylglycerol. The highly saturated nature of lung phosphatidylcholine molecules appears to be essential in relation to the surface tension-lowering capability of the alveolar lining layer. The proteins present in pulmonary surfactant are also unique, and there may be as many as 20 different nonserum proteins associated with surfactant material (King, 1985).

The major emphasis of present research deals with regulatory mechanisms for phosphatidylcholine synthesis and study of pharmacologic agents that accelerate the process of fetal lung development. Various hormones are known to influence the rate of phosphatidylcholine biosynthesis in fetal lung cells. These include corticosteroids, thyroid hormones, estrogens, and theophylline. In addition, labor or oxytocin or both have been shown to stimulate the process of fetal lung development; it is possible that the mechanism for this effect involves endogenous corticoids secreted in increased concentrations as a response to stress. Exogenous maternal corticosteroid administration at least 24 hours prior to delivery appears to decrease the incidence and severity of respiratory distress syndrome (RDS). This is more effective in female infants and prior to 34 weeks gestation but not in very immature infants (Collaborative group, 1981). Other studies indicate that some hormones such as insulin may retard surfactant formation. This might explain the clinical observation that hyperinsulinemic fetuses (principally in gestations complicated by maternal diabetes) often show delayed lung maturation.

Respiratory Distress Syndrome

Clinical Features

Respiratory distress syndrome (RDS) is one of the major causes of mortality and morbidity in newborn babies, although lack of a precise clinical definition necessitates cautious interpretation of statistics regarding incidence, mortality, and outcome. The diagnosis

can usually be established biochemically by documentation of surfactant deficiency in amniotic fluid or in tracheal or gastric aspirate. Approximately 10 to 15 per cent of babies weighing less than 2.5 kg at birth will manifest RDS, although a higher incidence is observed among the lowest-birth-weight groups. The greatest risk factor appears to be gestational age, whereas other risk factors include maternal diabetes and perinatal asphyxia, which may be secondary to placental abruption. The improved outcome in RDS, which can be attributed directly to many therapeutic advances, has raised questions as to whether this disorder is still the major cause of death in low-birth-weight infants. With improved survival there has been a dramatic increase in the sequelae due to the disease process as well as its modes of treatment, such as bronchopulmonary dysplasia, patent ductus arteriosus, and intracranial hemorrhage.

Impaired or delayed surfactant synthesis appears to be key to the pathogenesis of RDS (Fig. 63–3). The resultant decrease in lung compliance leads to alveolar hypoventilation and ventilation-perfusion imbalance. The resultant hypoxemia may cause metabolic acidosis, and both may contribute to pulmonary vasoconstriction. The relative roles of surfactant deficiency and pulmonary hypoperfusion in the overall clinical picture of RDS will vary somewhat with each patient.

Infants with RDS typically are initially seen with a combination of tachypnea, nasal flaring, subcostal and intercostal retractions, cyanosis, and expiratory grunting. Retractions are prominent and are the result of the very compliant rib cage being drawn in on inspiration as the infant generates high intrathoracic pressures to expand the poorly compliant lungs. The typical expiratory grunt is thought to result from partial closure of the glottis during expiration and in this way acts as a means of trapping alveolar air and maintaining lung volume. It should be noted that, although these signs are characteristic for neonatal respiratory distress, they may result from a wide variety of nonpulmonary causes such as hypothermia, hypoglycemia, anemia, polycythemia, or metabolic acidosis. Furthermore, such nonpulmonary conditions may complicate the clinical course of RDS.

A constant feature of RDS is the early onset of clinical signs of the disease, typically within one hour of delivery. Inadequate observation may lead to the impression of a symptom-free period of several hours. The uncomplicated clinical course is characterized by a progressive worsening of symptoms with a peak severity by days 2 to 3 and onset of recovery by 72 hours. When the disease process is severe enough to require assisted ventilation or is complicated by the development of air leaks, significant shunting through a patent ductus arteriosus, or bronchopulmonary dysplasia, the infant's recovery may be delayed for days to months.

The typical roentgenographic features consist of a diffuse reticulogranular pattern in both lung fields with superimposed air bronchograms. These cannot be reliably differentiated from those of neonatal pneumonia, most commonly caused by group B streptococci. This problem has been the major reason for the widespread use of antibiotics in the initial manage-

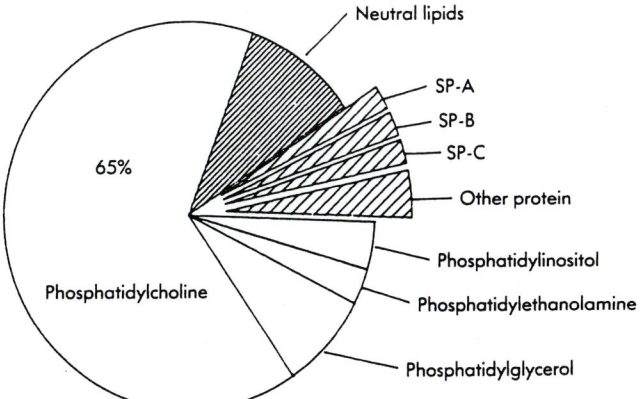

FIGURE 63–2. Composition of surface-active material which constitutes pulmonary surfactant.

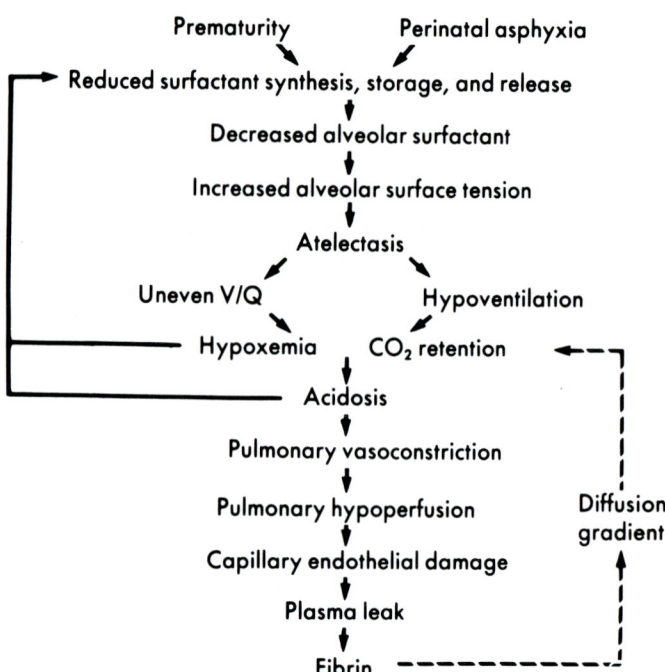

FIGURE 63–3. Pathophysiology of neonatal RDS. (From Martin RJ, Fanaroff AA: The respiratory distress syndrome and its management. *In* Fanaroff A, Martin RJ (eds): Neonatal-Perinatal Medicine. 5th ed. St. Louis, Mosby-Year Book, 1992.)

ment of infants with RDS. The increased use of various means of ventilatory support and the enhanced survival of infants with more severe pulmonary disease have resulted in the more frequent roentgenographic recognition of early signs of bronchopulmonary dysplasia.

Management and Outcome

In an infant with respiratory symptoms, there is a tendency to conclude that underlying pulmonary parenchymal disease is present; however, the differential diagnosis is extensive and includes nonpulmonary problems. Disorders of the major airways, chest wall, central nervous system, cardiovascular system, and musculoskeletal system—together with hematologic and metabolic problems or sepsis—easily may be confused with lung disorders. To avoid serious diagnostic and therapeutic errors, there must be a thorough review of historical information related to pregnancy, delivery, and the neonatal transition. Meticulous observation and careful physical examination of the infant must follow. Analysis of simple laboratory data includes blood gases, hematocrit, blood sugar, and white cell count with differential, together with appropriate radiographic studies. Therapy for RDS comprises the careful application of general supportive measures, administration and regulation of oxygen therapy, specific measures for controlling and/or assisting ventilation, and exogenous surfactant therapy.

Infants with respiratory difficulty require an optimal thermal environment to minimize oxygen consumption and oxygen requirements. The ability to supply an adequate caloric intake to the critically ill infant receiving respiratory assistance has been facilitated by the availability of intravenous hyperalimentation and lipid solutions. The role of nutritional support for these infants cannot be overemphasized. Therefore it

has become commonplace to start administration of hyperalimentation on the second or third day of life, especially for infants weighing less than 1500 gm and receiving mechanical ventilation. An alternative is to begin small-volume gavage feeds of formula or breast milk at this time. Fluid and electrolyte balance must be individualized and closely monitored, since overenthusiastic attention to calories may result in fluid overload, patent ductus arteriosus, and congestive heart failure. The resultant increase in ventilatory support may contribute to development of bronchopulmonary dysplasia (Costarino et al., 1992). Spontaneous diuresis often precedes improvement in lung function and recovery from RDS, suggesting a causal relationship.

Metabolic acidosis is most often encountered when the infant has been depressed at birth and required resuscitation. A subsequent metabolic acidosis out of proportion to the degree of respiratory distress may signify hypoperfusion, sepsis, or an intraventricular hemorrhage. It usually is not necessary to correct a metabolic or respiratory acidosis if the pH is greater than 7.25, whereas a pH of less than 7.20 typically requires intervention. In the case of respiratory acidosis, alkali therapy should be withheld until some form of assisted ventilation has been initiated.

It is customary to maintain a venous hematocrit of at least 40 per cent during the acute phase of RDS to support an adequate oxygen-carrying capacity. Arterial oxygen tension (PaO_2) is maintained between about 50 and 80 mm Hg. Although umbilical arterial catheters still form the basic means of arterial sampling in infants with RDS, the list of catheter-related thrombotic, embolic, and/or ischemic complications is formidable. For infants with mild or resolving respiratory distress, noninvasive measurement of PO_2 and PCO_2 via transcutaneous electrodes is extremely valuable and may make it unnecessary to insert an arterial catheter. Because poor perfusion, hyperoxemia, and advancing postnatal age may make transcutaneous Po_2 ($TcPo_2$) somewhat unreliable as a measure of Pao_2, the technique of continuous noninvasive measurement of oxygen saturation has gained widespread acceptance. As hyperoxic levels of Pao_2 are approached, however, saturation becomes less sensitive, with flattening of the hemoglobin dissociation curve, and large changes in Pao_2 will cause only minor alterations in saturation. Thus, in the absence of arterial sampling, both oxygen saturation and $TcPo_2$ must be interpreted with caution if hyperoxemia is to be avoided (Martin et al., 1986a).

Assisted ventilation has contributed substantially to improving the outcome of infants with respiratory distress. Nonetheless, the complications listed in Table 63–4 are commonly the result of therapeutic interventions. It is important to consider the mechanical characteristics of the respiratory system to understand the physiologic rationale for the blood gas responses that occur after ventilator setting changes. This is especially true in neonates with RDS whose disease is characterized by rapidly changing pulmonary mechanics and in whom high ventilatory frequencies are often employed. Carbon dioxide elimination is a function of alveolar ventilation and is determined by both the pressure gradient between expiration and inspiration and ventilator frequency. Oxygen uptake is not only affected by ventilation, but also largely depends on the matching of perfusion with ventilation. During assisted ventilation, oxygenation is largely determined by the mean airway pressure, which is a measure of the average pressure to which the lungs are exposed during the respiratory cycle. Changes in inspired oxygen concentration also alter alveolar oxygen tension and thus oxygenation (Carlo and Martin, 1986).

New modes of assisted ventilation (including high-frequency jet ventilation and high-frequency oscillation) deliver small volumes of gas at high frequencies and limit the development of high airway pressure. Since high ventilatory pressures and the resultant pulmonary barotrauma and cardiovascular compromise are thought to be major contributory factors to complications associated with assisted ventilation, these new modes of ventilation in neonates have aroused considerable interest. Neither high-frequency jet ventilation nor oscillation has reduced the incidence of bronchopulmonary dysplasia or mortality rate in controlled trials (Carlo et al., 1990; HIFI study group,

TABLE 63–4. Major Complications of Neonatal Assisted Ventilation

Pulmonary air leaks: pneumothorax, pneumomediastinum, pulmonary interstitial emphysema
Endotracheal tube complications: displacement, dislodgment, occlusion, atelectasis after extubation, palatal grooves
Tracheal lesions: erosion, granuloma, subglottic stenosis, necrotizing tracheobronchitis
Infection: pneumonia, septicemia
Chronic lung disease: bronchopulmonary dysplasia
Patent ductus arteriosus
Intracranial hemorrhage
Retinopathy of prematurity

TABLE 63–5. Surfactant Therapy for RDS

KNOWN
Major ingredient: Dipalmitoyl phosphatidylcholine
Administration of fluid suspension requires endotracheal tube
Optimal benefit requires retreatment
Improvement in arterial oxygenation
Decrease in incidence of air leaks
Lower incidence of BPD in infants >1.25 kg
Improved mortality from RDS
UNKNOWN
Optimal preparation: Natural versus synthetic; role of protein
Timing and technique of administration
Duration of retreatment
Effect on BPD rate in infants <1 kg
Metabolism of surfactant preparation
Interaction with endogenous surfactant
Risk of pulmonary hemorrhage
Immunologic effects

1989). Nonetheless high-frequency jet ventilation does appear to benefit infants in whom RDS is complicated by pulmonary interstitial emphysema (Keszler et al., 1991). Finally, preliminary experience with oxygenated perfluorocarbon liquid ventilation suggests that this technique holds promise for supporting pulmonary gas exchange in very immature infants (Wolfson and Shaffer, 1990).

The discovery that surfactant deficiency was key in the pathophysiology of RDS led several early investigators to administer artificial aerosolized phospholipids to infants with RDS. In these studies only limited therapeutic success was encountered. In contrast, animal models in which natural surfactant compounds were used yielded more promising results, and this stimulated development of a mixture of both natural and synthetic surface-active lipids for use in humans. The goal was to achieve alveolar stability with less potential risk for a reaction to foreign protein than would be the case with exclusively natural surfactant. Some of the major resolved and unresolved issues related to exogenous surfactant administration are summarized in Table 63–5 (Martin and Fanaroff, 1992). The major recent focus has been on collaborative multicenter trials in which purely synthetic and mixed natural/synthetic preparations have been employed. The former studies have utilized protein-free synthetic phospholipid products, such as Exosurf, which contain alcohol to act as a spreading agent for dipalmitoyl phosphatidylcholine at the air/fluid alveolar interface (Long et al., 1991). The latter investigations have employed a protein-containing extract of minced calf lung supplemented with dipalmitoyl phosphatidylcholine, tripalmitin, and palmitic acid and marketed as Survanta (Liechty et al., 1991). No direct comparison is as yet available between synthetic and natural preparations in human infants.

All regimens of surfactant therapy appear to decrease the incidence of air leaks and improve oxygenation of ventilated preterm infants (Enhorning et al., 1985; Merritt et al., 1986) (Table 63–6). More strikingly, mortality from RDS, and even overall mortality of ventilated preterm infants, appears to be reduced when multiple-dose surfactant therapy is used for these infants. It is still unclear whether a preventive

TABLE 63–6. **Effect of Surfactant on Complications of RDS and Prematurity**

	SURFACTANT	CONTROL	P VALUE
Number*	157	150	
Pneumothorax	12%	31%	P<.02
P.I.E.	8%	37%	P<.01
P.D.A.	60%	57%	N.S.
B.P.D.	34%	41%	N.S.
Deaths	12%	31%	P<.02

*Hallman et al., 1985; Enhorning et al, 1985; Kwong et al., 1985; Shapiro, Merrit et al., 1986; Gitlin et al., 1987; Raju et al., 1987.

dose administered endotracheally during the first 10 minutes of life has any advantage over waiting until clinical evidence of RDS appears. The incidence of intraventricular hemorrhage and patent ductus arteriosus appears unaltered in most studies. Bronchopulmonary dysplasia is reduced in larger infants weighing at least 1250 gm (Long et al., 1991). Preliminary data have suggested slightly higher pulmonary hemorrhage rates in association with surfactant therapy, and this, together with other as yet unknown factors, will need close observation. The optimal technique for surfactant administration also needs to be intensely scrutinized. The presence of an endotracheal tube appears to be essential for surfactant therapy. Current guidelines call for its administration in divided doses, over the first 48 hours, and body position changes may be utilized to enhance distribution throughout the lung.

Since the genes that code for certain surfactant proteins have been characterized, recombinant DNA technology will make modified human surfactant proteins available. In combination with synthetic phospholipids, this will make a protein-containing artificial surfactant widely available. This assumes that the protein contained in natural surfactant plays an important clinical role in the prevention and management of RDS. Although no adverse immunologic consequences of foreign tissue protein administration have yet been reported in the recipients of natural surfactant therapy, close follow-up of these high-risk survivors of neonatal intensive care is imperative.

The developmental outcome for infants with mild or moderate RDS is probably comparable to that of infants without RDS. Birth weight and gestational age have a much stronger influence on mental and motor developmental scores of preterm infants at 2 years than either the presence or severity of RDS. There is some evidence that late abnormalities of pulmonary function are detectable in the premature survivors of RDS. Nonetheless, in the absence of progression to bronchopulmonary dysplasia in infancy, this has not been a clinical problem in childhood. Bronchopulmonary dysplasia or chronic neonatal lung injury is a consequence of the effects of barotrauma and high inspired oxygen concentration on an immature respiratory system. The risk of later neurodevelopmental handicap is proportional to the duration of supplemental O_2 beyond 28 days of life. Respiratory support, nutritional management, and bronchodilator therapy form the mainstay of management for these infants.

Corticosteroids often facilitate ventilator weaning but are not without potential complications (Bancalari and Gerhardt, 1986; Bancalari, 1992).

Meconium Aspiration and Persistent Fetal Circulation

Although knowledge of the pathophysiologic stimuli in the fetus that govern passage of meconium in response to stress is incomplete, this phenomenon is almost never observed before a gestational age of 34 weeks and is a frequent complication of postmaturity. Many infants with meconium-stained amniotic fluid exhibit no sign of cardiorespiratory depression, although some brief period of asphyxia may well have induced the passage of meconium before delivery. Nonetheless, the presence of meconium in the amniotic fluid necessitates careful supervision of labor and close monitoring of fetal well-being. The key to management of meconium aspiration syndrome (MAS) lies in its prevention.

Several studies have demonstrated clearly that a combined obstetric and pediatric approach can almost entirely eliminate this major neonatal problem. On average, 10 per cent of deliveries will show evidence for meconium staining of amniotic fluid, but the incidence of clinically significant MAS has fallen to around 3 per cent of these deliveries, or 3 per 1000 overall deliveries (Wiswell et al., 1990). In the presence of thick (particulate or pea soup) meconium, or abnormal fetal monitor tracings, the risk for MAS is greatest (Rossi et al., 1989). The cooperative team approach should begin with routine upper airway suctioning by the obstetrician after delivery of the head (Carson et al., 1976). Tracheal suctioning under direct vision is ideally performed before the first breath and always must be completed before the initiation of positive-pressure ventilation when an infant is resuscitated. Controversy remains as to whether all infants with meconium staining of the amniotic fluid should be suctioned, especially when meconium staining is light, the infant is vigorous at birth, and suctioning has been performed at the perineum (Cunningham et al., 1990).

The subsequent management of MAS consists of supportive respiratory therapy. Little can be done to enhance the mechanisms by which meconium is phagocytosed and removed from distal portions of the respiratory tract. Pathophysiologically, the pulmonary problems relate to complete airway obstruction, a ball valve phenomenon created by the presence of meconium within the airways and chemical inflammation. Thus, areas of atelectasis resulting from pneumonia and total small airway obstruction are adjacent to areas of overexpansion from gas trapping in areas with partial obstruction. Air leaks, including pneumomediastinum and pneumothorax, often occur after aspiration of meconium and cellular debris (Fig. 63–4).

The syndrome of persistent fetal circulation (PFC syndrome) can be a major clinical problem in infants with MAS, although the etiology of the accompanying pulmonary hypertension is somewhat controversial. Hypoxic pulmonary arterial vasoconstriction is most likely responsible for the PFC, with right-to-left shunt-

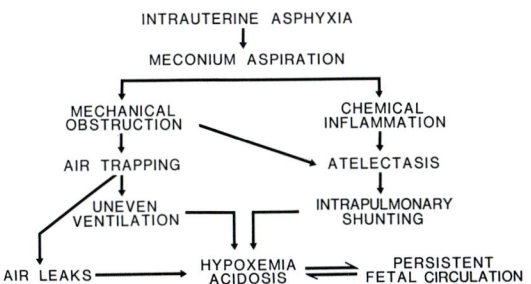

FIGURE 63–4. Pathophysiology of meconium aspiration syndrome. (From Fanaroff A, Martin RJ, Miller MJ: Other pulmonary problems. *In* Fanaroff A, Martin RJ (eds): Neonatal-Perinatal Medicine. 5th ed. St. Louis, Mosby-Year Book, 1992.)

ing at the foramen ovale and ductus arteriosus. Morphometric techniques have been used to study the pulmonary vascular bed in infants with fatal meconium aspiration (Murphy et al., 1984). In almost all cases there was abnormal muscularization of the smallest intra-acinar arteries that must have developed before birth. Thus both prenatal and perinatal maladaptation of the pulmonary circulation may contribute to the development of PFC in infants with MAS.

Apart from complicating birth asphyxia and meconium aspiration, PFC may also be associated with neonatal sepsis, hyperviscosity secondary to polycythemia, or pulmonary hypoplasia of any etiology. It is particularly difficult to differentiate PFC from cyanotic congenital heart disease that is associated with right-to-left shunting. Although PFC and structural heart disease, including total anomalous pulmonary venous return, both cause cyanosis, infants with PFC typically manifest clinical respiratory distress, and their hypoxemia may be relieved by administration of 100 per cent oxygen and hyperventilation to induce respiratory alkalosis. Echocardiographic assessment of infants with PFC is essential to exclude congenital heart disease.

Extracorporeal membrane oxygenation (ECMO) is an innovative technique that is currently being utilized as a means of supporting life during intractible respiratory failure in selected patients with persistent fetal circulation. It may be employed as an alternative to respirator therapy in the hope of decreasing acute and chronic lung damage. Perfusion and gas exchange are maintained by means of prolonged venoarterial or venovenous cardiopulmonary bypass through a membrane lung. This bypass circuit allows the infant's heart and lungs to recover at low ventilator settings and inspired oxygen concentrations. This approach to the management of neonatal respiratory failure has resulted in survival rates exceeding 80 per cent for all diagnostic criteria other than congenital diaphragmatic hernia. Short-term outcome data compare favorably with term infants surviving respiratory failure and PFC with conventional management (Glass et al., 1989).

Other Neonatal Respiratory Disorders

Transient tachypnea is very common and has many overlapping features with respiratory distress caused by surfactant deficiency. The preferred explanation for the clinical features is delayed resorption of fetal lung fluid; therefore, it is seen more commonly after cesarean section in nonasphyxiated term infants or preterm infants who are close to term. The clinical features comprise various combinations of cyanosis, grunting, flaring, retracting, and tachypnea in the first few hours after birth. The chest roentgenogram demonstrates prominent perihilar streaking and fluid in the interlobar fissures. Transient tachypnea of the newborn by definition is self-limiting (up to 72 hours duration) and is characterized by either no oxygen requirement or only a transient one. For these infants, there is no risk of recurrence of residual pulmonary dysfunction.

Neonatal pneumonia may be acquired by the fetus via transplacental passage of organisms, although ascending infection from the genital tract before or during labor appears to be the most common route. Thus, prolonged rupture of membranes in excess of 24 hours is a major predisposing factor. It is possible, however, that bacteria may gain access to the fetus by ascent through intact membranes. Because bacterial contamination of the infant always occurs during vaginal delivery, neonatal pneumonia may well occur in the absence of prolonged rupture of membranes or any maternal symptoms. Major pathogens producing neonatal pneumonia are group B streptococci, *Listeria*, pneumococci, and various gram-negative organisms. The nonspecific clinical signs such as tachypnea, cyanosis, or apnea make a high index of suspicion the key to early diagnosis. Other alerting features include thermal instability, abdominal distention, and jaundice. Latex agglutination assay of body fluids for group B streptococcal polysaccharide antigen allows a specific diagnosis to be made before results of blood and CSF cultures are known. Treatment almost invariably is instituted before the pathogenic organism is identified and its antibiotic sensitivities determined.

Apnea requiring ventilatory support or pharmacologic intervention occurs in at least 50 per cent of surviving infants weighing less than 1500 gm at birth. The incidence of apnea in these babies is inversely correlated with gestational age and may begin by the second day of life in preterm infants without respiratory disease. The peak occurrence of apnea is later in the first week in babies who initially have uncomplicated respiratory distress, often coinciding with resolution of the lung disease.

Neonatal apnea may be associated with a specific precipitating factor or pathophysiologic disorder other than prematurity, many of which are summarized in Figure 63–5. It appears that the respiratory centers responsible for generation of breathing patterns in preterm infants are quite sensitive to a bewildering array of peripheral stimuli that may trigger apnea. Thus apneic episodes are a common response of the infant's respiratory regulatory mechanisms to stimuli that are considerably less potent in an older child or adult.

Apneic episodes generally are defined as periods during which there is cessation of respiration for at least 10 to 15 seconds, frequently complicated by cyanosis, pallor, hypotonia, or bradycardia. Since a fall in heart rate frequently occurs early in the apneic

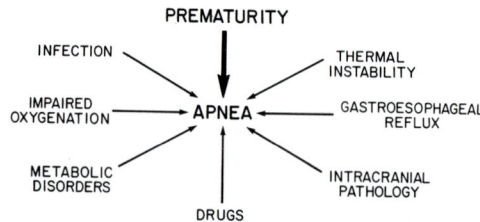

FIGURE 63–5. Some diverse factors that predispose to apnea in preterm infants. (From Martin RJ, Miller MM, Carlo WA: Pathogenesis of apnea in preterm infants. J Pediatr **109**:733, 1986b.)

episode, bradycardia may result primarily from vagal influences on central cardiorespiratory control.

In preterm infants, as in adults, 70 to 80 per cent of apneic episodes may be accompanied by airway obstruction at the level of the pharynx. The most common type of apnea observed in premature infants is mixed apnea, in which a central respiratory pause is preceded or followed by obstructed breaths. Negative pharyngeal pressure generated during inspiration can produce pharyngeal collapse, particularly if upper airway dilator muscle activity is decreased. Diaphragmatic activity may then continue, although no net airflow results. During apnea with an obstructive component, clinical cardiorespiratory monitoring may demonstrate only bradycardia as respiratory movements continue during the period of obstruction.

Clinical judgment will dictate the vigor with which a specific precipitating cause will be pursued. A rational approach to management requires a clear understanding of the difference between a normal respiratory pattern in immature infants and a pathologic event worthy of intervention. Periodic breathing characterized by regularly recurring ventilatory cycles interrupted by short pauses is normal in preterm infants. Although periodic breathing may share common features with the severe apneic episodes that occur in some infants, a common link between periodicity and apneic spells has not been clearly demonstrated. For example, although hypoxemia enhances periodic breathing, infants with apnea (as a group) do not have levels of PaO$_2$ lower than those of comparable infants without apnea.

The first step in evaluating apnea is to rule out treatable causes. When this has been accomplished, the apnea can be considered to be idiopathic. Theophylline therapy has become the mainstay of pharmacologic therapy in apnea of premature infants.

Methylxanthines appear to decrease the frequency of central, mixed, and obstructive episodes. Significant levels of caffeine can be detected in the blood of premature infants receiving only theophylline therapy. It appears that the newborn human infant has the unique ability to methylate theophylline to caffeine. Elimination of these drugs is exceedingly slow in the neonatal period; however, infants are relatively free of toxicity at plasma levels of 5 to 10 µg/ml and 8 to 20 µg/ml for theophylline and caffeine, respectively.

In those infants with persistent apnea on theophylline therapy requiring intervention, nasal continuous positive airway pressure (CPAP) at 2 to 5 cm water

has proved effective. It appears that CPAP exerts its beneficial effect in infants by splinting the upper airway with positive pressure throughout inspiration and expiration rather than by reflex activation of upper airway dilating muscles (Miller et al., 1990).

Developmental anomalies of the respiratory system frequently become apparent during the transition from fetal to neonatal life. Pulmonary hypoplasia may be either unilateral or bilateral. It may be seen as an isolated entity (so-called primary pulmonary hypoplasia) or may be secondary to lesions restricting lung growth. Bilateral pulmonary hypoplasia commonly occurs in association with oligohydramnios caused by either renal disease in the fetus or chronic leakage of amniotic fluid. The presence of pulmonary hypoplasia is well recognized in infants with bilateral renal agenesis, although it has since become apparent that a similar picture of lethal pulmonary hypoplasia is seen in conjunction with bilaterally dysplastic kidneys. Characteristic features include premature birth in the breech position, a typical facial appearance, limb malformations, and severe respiratory insufficiency often complicated by air leaks and invariably resulting in a fatal outcome.

Unilateral pulmonary hypoplasia commonly occurs in infants with diaphragmatic hernia. The clinical course of infants with this type of hypoplasia depends on the degree of herniation and adequacy of surgical repair, in addition to the extent of the pulmonary hypoplasia and accompanying increase in pulmonary vascular resistance.

Less frequently, cystic malformations of the lungs are found at birth, or diagnosed by antenatal ultrasound. These include congenital lobar emphysema, congenital lung cysts, and more diffuse cystic adenomatoid malformation. Infants with chylothorax and congenital pulmonary lymphangiectasia may present with respiratory distress in the newborn period. Both are manifestations of congenitally defective lymphatic structures.

Chronic neonatal lung disease (or bronchopulmonary dysplasia) is a challenging problem in neonatal intensive care (Bancalari and Gerhardt, 1986). The increased incidence of chronic respiratory disease can be directly related to the more aggressive respiratory management and increased survival of small preterm infants. Oxygen toxicity and barotrauma secondary to mechanical ventilation have been most widely implicated in the etiology of chronic lung disease, but immaturity, infection, cor pulmonale, and growth failure all play a role (Fig. 63–6). Weaning from oxygen and assisted ventilation may be a long, slow process, taking many months in extreme cases. The prognosis for these infants has been greatly improved by the institution of steroid therapy (Collaborative Dexamethasone Trial, 1991). In theory, steroid treatment decreases chronic inflammation in the lung, allowing more normal lung growth and remodeling.

GENERAL PROBLEMS
Intrauterine Growth Restriction (IUGR)

Although different rates and patterns of intrauterine growth have been observed for many years, it was

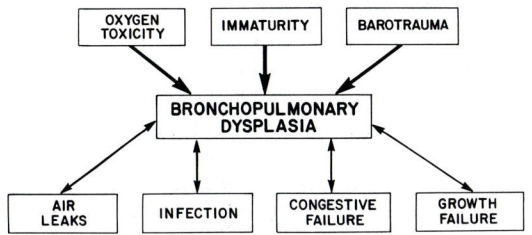

FIGURE 63–6. Pathophysiologic events contributing to neonatal chronic lung disease (bronchopulmonary dysplasia). (From Fox WW, Morray JP, Martin RJ: Chronic neonatal lung disease. *In* Fanaroff A, Martin RJ (eds): Neonatal-Perinatal Medicine. 5th ed. St. Louis, Mosby-Year Book, 1992.)

not until some 40 years ago that the clinical significance of these patterns was recognized. Technologic advances, as outlined throughout this book, have permitted close monitoring of fetal anatomy, growth, well-being, and maturity. Furthermore, the majority of infants with intrauterine growth problems are now identified prior to delivery, permitting better planning of the delivery and preparation for resuscitation of the neonate (see Chapter 36). This represents a quantum leap from a decade ago when less than a third of infants with such problems were anticipated prior to labor and delivery, a time of great stress and danger for the growth-restricted fetus.

Classification of infants, according to tables relating birth weight to gestational age, are utilized to determine whether growth has occurred at a normal, accelerated, or diminished rate *in utero*. As noted in the table from Koops et al. (1982), mortality is determined by birth weight and infants undergrown *in utero* remain at great risk (Fig. 63–7). From a statistical standpoint, only infants born at any gestational age with a birth weight greater than two standard deviations below the mean are truly small for gestational age (SGA). However, because they share common clinical problems, all infants with birth weights below the 10th percentile for gestational age are regarded as SGA.

Furthermore, many infants, particularly those born beyond term, will have birth weights above the 10th percentile but demonstrate evidence of weight loss and should be considered within the spectrum of the growth-restricted infant.

Low birth weight (<2500 gm) accounts for 75 percent of poor perinatal outcomes. Strategies to improve the outcome in these infants have focused on antenatal prevention of conditions associated with low birth weight together with intensive education, extensive intrapartum evaluation and monitoring, and sophisticated and aggressive care of the low-birth-weight fetus and infant. Simple measures in antenatal care, such as elimination of cigarette smoking, improved nutrition, eradication of genitourinary tract infection, and increased awareness of the hazards of preterm birth, have led to lower rates of prematurity in some centers.

There are many conditions resulting in abnormal growth *in utero*. The etiology, as well as the timing, duration, and severity of the insult, will modify the patterns of growth and hence the problems observed in the fetus and newborn. During the first trimester, global insults including perinatal infections (TORCH), ingested teratogens (such as anticonvulsants, alcohol, anticoagulants, and the like), chromosomal abnormalities (trisomy 21, 18, and 13 and Turner's syndrome) and narcotic drug abuse initiate profound failure of growth of the fetus, resulting in a short infant of low birth weight and often reduced head circumference and hence brain capacity. These infants with reduction of all growth parameters are referred to as having symmetric growth retardation.

Later onset of fetal growth failure results from disorders of the fetus or placenta or from maternal problems. Delivery of oxygen and nutrients is impeded by maternal and/or placental factors in what is referred to as *placental insufficiency*. A dramatic effect of oxygen administration enhancing growth and correcting metabolic acidosis in a small group of growth-restricted infants was reported by Nicolaides and co-workers. These factors may become operative at

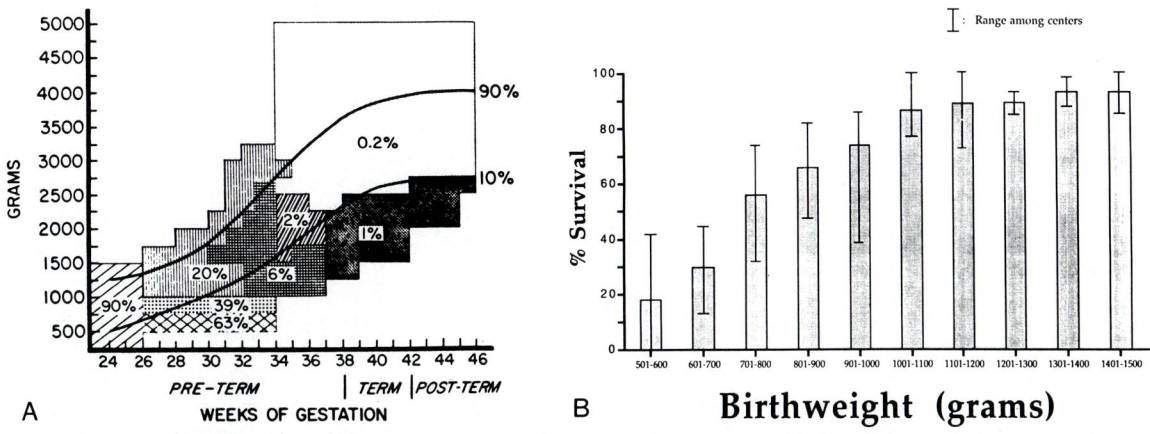

FIGURE 63–7. *A*, Mortality risk according to birth weight–gestational age relationship. Based on 14,413 live births at University of Colorado Health Science Center (1974–1980). (From Koops BL, Morgan LJ, Battaglia FC: Neonatal mortality risk in relation to birth weight and gestational age: Update. J Pediatr **101**:969, 1982.) *B*, Per cent survival by birth weight. (From Hack M, Horbar JD, Malloy MH, et al: Very low birth weight outcomes of the National Institute of Child Health and Human Development Neonatal Network. Pediatrics **87**:587, 1991. Reproduced by permission of Pediatrics.)

variable times during pregnancy, resulting in less predictable effects on fetal growth. Examples of these factors include, among others, maternal hypertension (preeclampsia and essential hypertension), smoking, malnutrition (undernutrition), and varied forms of maternal vascular and renal diseases. They result in asymmetric growth restriction characterized by weight at or below the 10th percentile, with length and head circumference above the 10th percentile. These infants have the potential for normal growth and development yet are extremely vulnerable to perinatal asphyxia, which must be assiduously avoided. Perhaps equally vulnerable and often overlooked are the group of infants, frequently post-term, with birth weight above the 10th percentile but evidence of recent weight loss as indicated by loose folds of skin, the result of loss of subcutaneous tissue.

Recent follow-up data (Hack and Fanaroff, 1984) suggest that intrauterine growth restriction as a consequence of malnutrition secondary to either maternal malnutrition or impaired uteroplacental transfer of nutrients is accompanied by a favorable outcome for the infant. This prompted Warshaw (1985) to question, in a provocative editorial, whether "IUGR resulting from restricted nutrient supply really represents pathology or is it a favorable adaptation of the fetus to maximize the prospects of good outcome? A strong case can be made for the latter." He further emphasizes that decreased fetal size with sparing of brain growth, acceleration of pulmonary maturation, and mild polycythemia—common features in the growth-restricted fetus—initially represents important adaptive strategies that become pathologic when deprivation becomes extreme and fetal distress supervenes. In the typical newborn with nutritionally induced IUGR, body proportions are asymmetric at birth with brain growth and head circumference spared at the expense of both weight and linear growth. It is postulated that redistribution of the blood flow favors brain growth at the expense of the viscera and skeletal muscles.

Another group of infants with disordered intrauterine growth includes those infants in whom specific genetic, inherited metabolic, or chromosome anomalies severely restrict the growth potential. The products of multiple gestation and those with other specific syndromes and congenital malformations may also be SGA. In many infants no cause is identified for their diminished growth. Exposure to tobacco may be significant in this latter group. The variable etiologies and timing of the onset of the insults results in less predictability of growth, with both symmetric and asymmetric patterns observed. Nonetheless, more precise antenatal evaluation of fetal growth is permitting a more rational approach to the perinatal management of these complex problems and has resulted in a significant reduction in the incidence of stillbirths.

In pregnancies with compromised fetal growth, every effort must be made to avoid asphyxia and ensure an atraumatic delivery. The fetus is closely monitored during labor and delivery accomplished surgically if distress supervenes. When fetal compromise is established before labor, elective cesarean section is performed. Personnel skilled and experienced in neonatal resuscitation should be present at the delivery. A depressed infant with low Apgar scores should be anticipated. Resuscitative efforts, designed to clear the airway, establish ventilation, support the circulation, and correct any metabolic acidosis as already detailed, are promptly initiated. The thermal environment should result in minimal oxygen consumption. If the amniotic fluid contains meconium, the airway is first cleared prior to delivery of the body and subsequently the trachea may need to be intubated and aspirated.

Assessment of Gestational Age

Once the initial transfer of extrauterine existence has been accomplished, the first order of business is to establish the birth weight—gestational age relationship.

The clinical course and strategy for management are dependent on early identification of SGA infants. Thus it is essential to classify all infants as soon as possible as small, appropriate, or large for gestational age. Historically, the gestational age is determined from a combination of the mother's dates and antenatal parameters including ultrasonographic examination when available, quickening, and detection of fetal heartbeat. When the antenatal dating is not reliable, the neonatal assessment of gestational age is obtained from a combination of assessment of physical and neurologic characteristics according to the method of Dubowitz (1970). Ballard and colleagues (1979) have produced an abbreviated version (Fig. 63–8) that has become extremely popular and has been statistically validated. The Ballard maturational score has been refined and expanded (Ballard et al., 1991) to be more accurate and include extremely premature infants (Fig. 63–8). This new Ballard score has been validated in 578 neonates following accurately dated pregnancies and found to be a valid, accurate gestational assessment tool for extremely premature infants and remains valid for the entire newborn population. It is recommended that for infants below 26 weeks gestation the assessment should be made before age 12 hours. It is important to plot the weight, length, and head circumference against normal standards and determine first whether growth has been restricted and if so whether there is symmetric or asymmetric growth restriction. The Babson charts (birth to one year) are extremely useful for this (Fig. 63–9). If the infant plots out to be SGA, the etiology of the growth retardation must be sought and a management plan enacted which will anticipate, prevent, and treat those conditions most prominent in these infants and outlined in Table 63–7.

After the infant has been stabilized in the delivery room, a careful physical examination and additional measurements are necessary to confirm that the infant is SGA. For example, the ponderal index, which relates length to weight, is useful in order to further subclassify symmetric or asymmetric growth restriction and identify wasted infants. Physical and laboratory data are utilized to distinguish those infants with congenital malformations or congenital infections from those undergrown as a consequence of placental in-

Neuromuscular Maturity

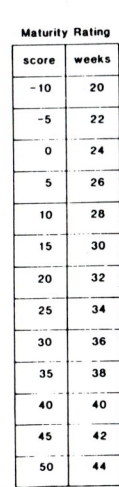

	-1	0	1	2	3	4	5
Posture							
Square Window (wrist)	>90°	90°	60°	45°	30°	0°	
Arm Recoil		180°	140°-180°	110° 140°	90-110°	<90°	
Popliteal Angle	180°	160°	140°	120°	100°	90°	<90°
Scarf Sign							
Heel to Ear							

FIGURE 63–8. New Ballard score, expanded to include extremely premature infants (Ballard JL, Khoury JC, Wedig K, Wang L, Eilers-Walsman BL, et al Univ of Cincinnati; Children's Hosp Research Found; Children's Hosp Med Ctr, Good Samaritan Hosp, Cincinnati. J Pediatr 119:417–423, 1991.)

Physical Maturity

Skin	sticky friable transparent	gelatinous red, translucent	smooth pink, visible veins	superficial peeling &/or rash, few veins	cracking pale areas rare veins	parchment deep cracking no vessels	leathery cracked wrinkled
Lanugo	none	sparse	abundant	thinning	bald areas	mostly bald	
Plantar Surface	heel-toe 40-50mm: -1 <40mm: -2	>50mm no crease	faint red marks	anterior transverse crease only	creases ant. 2/3	creases over entire sole	
Breast	imperceptible	barely perceptible	flat areola no bud	stippled areola 1-2mm bud	raised areola 3-4mm bud	full areola 5-10mm bud	
Eye/Ear	lids fused loosely:-1 tightly:-2	lids open pinna flat stays folded	sl. curved pinna; soft; slow recoil	well-curved pinna; soft but ready recoil	formed &firm instant recoil	thick cartilage ear stiff	
Genitals male	scrotum flat, smooth	scrotum empty faint rugae	testes in upper canal rare rugae	testes descending few rugae	testes down good rugae	testes pendulous deep rugae	
Genitals female	clitoris prominent labia flat	prominent clitoris small labia minora	prominent clitoris enlarging minora	majora & minora equally prominent	majora large minora small	majora cover clitoris & minora	

Maturity Rating

score	weeks
-10	20
-5	22
0	24
5	26
10	28
15	30
20	32
25	34
30	36
35	38
40	40
45	42
50	44

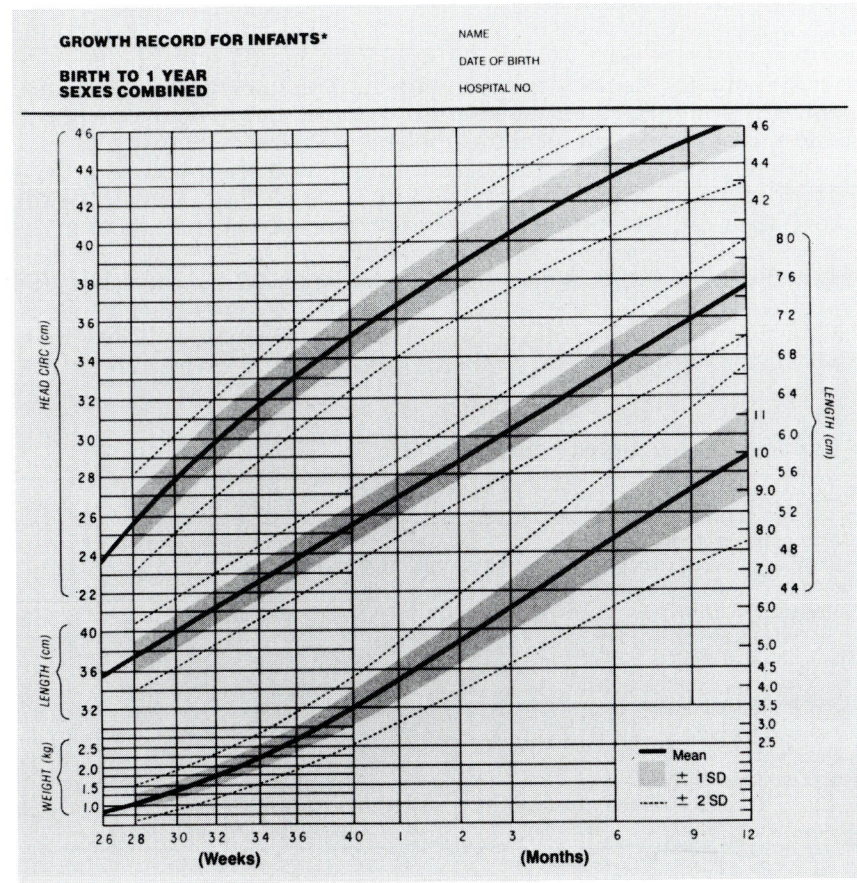

GROWTH RECORD FOR INFANTS*

BIRTH TO 1 YEAR
SEXES COMBINED

NAME

DATE OF BIRTH

HOSPITAL NO.

Mean
± 1 SD
± 2 SD

FIGURE 63–9. Infant growth record. (From Babson SG, Benda GI: Growth graphs for the clinical assessment of infants of varying gestational age. J Pediatr **89**:814, 1976.)

TABLE 63–7.   Comparison of Problems of Small-for-Gestational-Age and Immature Newborn Infants

	IMMATURE AGA	IMMATURE SGA	MATURE SGA (Symmetric)	MATURE SGA (Asymmetric)
Early weight change	5–10% loss, then slow gain	5–10% loss, then slow gain	5–10% loss, then slow gain	≤5% loss, then rapid gain
Congenital infection	+	+ +	+ +	±
Respiratory problems	Hyaline membrane disease	Hyaline membrane disease	Unusual	Aspiration syndrome Pneumomediastinum Pneumothorax
Persistent fetal circulation	+	+	0	+ +
Apneic spells	+ + + +	+ + + +	0	0
Polycythemia	0	0	±	+ +
Hyperbilirubinemia	+ + + +	+ + + +	+	+ +
Hypoglycemia	+	+	+	+ + +
Hypocalcemia	+	+	±	+
Congenital malformation	±	+		±
Intracranial hemorrhage	+ + +	+ + +	±	+
Asphyxia	+ +	+ +	±	+ +
Growth (linear)	Normal	Subnormal (rare catch-up)	Subnormal (rare catch-up)	Normal
Neurobehavioral residua	+ + (most in very-low-birth-weight infant)	+ + +	+ + +	+ (more if asphyxia is severe)

From Klaus MH, Fanaroff AA: Care of the High Risk Neonate. 4th ed. Philadelphia, WB Saunders Company, 1993.

sufficiency. This is critical to determine the prognosis for the infant.

SGA infants have relatively large heads for their wasted trunks and extremities, although approximately 50 per cent of SGA very-low-birth-weight infants will have head circumferences below the third percentile at birth. There is reduced subcutaneous tissue as evidenced by skinfold thickness determinations, and because of a lack of vernix, the skin is often desquamating and stained with meconium. Physical indicators of gestational age including sole creases, breast dimensions, and external appearance of the genitalia may be misleading because of variable effects of malnutrition, and the neurologic examination is usually more reliable and indicative of true gestational age. The neurologic examination may show accelerated maturation as a result of intrauterine stress and is obviously not reliable in infants who have been severely asphyxiated.

Many postmature infants demonstrate evidence of late intrauterine growth restriction. Characteristically their length is on a higher percentile than their birth weight and they have an anxious, alert appearance. The skin is dry, cracked, and wrinkled from loss of subcutaneous tissue; lacks vernix; and is often stained brownish green or yellow. The nails are long and the skull excessively firm. In common with the SGA infants, perinatal complications include asphyxia, meconium aspiration syndrome, and hypoglycemia.

The clinical problems and the underlying physiologic mechanisms resulting in these problems in SGA infants are outlined in Table 63–8. It is worth noting that combinations of problems frequently occur in the same infant. Furthermore, the reserves of these SGA infants may have been depleted by the labor and delivery process. This renders them extremely vulnerable to physiologic deviations that are readily compensated for by their appropriately grown counterparts.

TABLE 63–8.   Perinatal Adaptive Problems

PROBLEM	PATHOGENESIS	PREVENTION
Perinatal asphyxia	↓ Placental reserve (insufficiency) ↓ Cardiac glycogen stores	Antepartum, intrapartum FHR monitoring
Meconium aspiration	Hypoxic/stress phenomenon	Oral-pharyngeal-tracheal suction
Fasting hypoglycemia	↓ Hepatic glycogen ↓ Gluconeogenesis	Early alimentation
Alimented hyperglycemia	"Starvation diabetes"	Avoid excessive carbohydrate loads
Polycythemia-hyperviscosity	Fetal hypoxia. ↑ erythropoietin Placental transfusion	Neonatal partial exchange transfusion
Temperature instability	↓ Adipose tissue ↑ Heat loss	Ensure neutral thermal environment
Pulmonary hemorrhage (rare)	Hypothermia ↓ O₂/DIC	Avoid cold stress, hypoxia
Immunodeficiency	"Malnutrition" effect	Unknown

From Gregory GA: Pediatric Anesthesiology. New York, Churchill Livingstone, 1984.

The most common problems include asphyxia neonatorum, hypoglycemia, polycythemia and hyperviscosity, congenital malformations, and congenital infections. Jones and Robertsen (1986) from Cambridge reviewed the hospital course and outcome of 164 infants less than 5 per cent for gestation-specific birth weight and greater than or equal to 37 weeks gestation. Finding a very low incidence of malformations (4 per cent), congenital infections, and significant complications, they concluded that SGA infants of 37 weeks gestation or more have few neonatal problems and do not require admission to the intensive care unit. They nonetheless still require close observation in well-baby nurseries. Nine infants (5 per cent) did become hypoglycemic, but only one with associated respiratory distress required intravenous glucose.

The long-term prognosis for SGA infants has slowly emerged. In view of the many variables affecting growth and development and the heterogeneous group of infants covered by the definition of SGA, it is not surprising that reports of outcome range from extremely optimistic to depressingly pessimistic. The ultimate picture is dependent upon the etiology of the aberrant growth, including the presence of congenital infections or malformations, timing and duration of the insult, severity of growth retardation, degree of intrauterine or postnatal asphyxia, postnatal course, and above all the socioeconomic status of the family. Recent reports identify and attempt to control for these variables facilitating interpretation of the results.

Very few preterm infants who are SGA at birth catch up in growth during the neonatal period. Superimposed on their intrauterine causes of growth failure are a variety of postnatal problems that further affect their growth. In our experience, 91 per cent of SGA infants will still be less than 2 standard deviations below the norms at 40 weeks corrected age. Varying patterns of growth are observed during the first year of life, with the most rapid catch-up occurring during this period. Some infants who failed to grow during the neonatal period demonstrate an accelerated growth velocity and catch-up; others may demonstrate a normal growth velocity but remain small and never catch up. A few have a decreased growth velocity and frankly "fail to thrive." Growth during infancy is influenced by many factors, including the persistence of perinatal problems such as bronchopulmonary dysplasia, necrotizing enterocolitis, cholestasis, and malabsorption. Additional factors influencing growth include the need for rehospitalization and the presence of caretaking disorders and feeding problems in children with neurologic impairment. SGA infants rarely catch up in weight after the first year, and at 3 years some 50 per cent of SGA infants still have subnormal weight (Fig. 63–10). There is very little evidence in the literature to support the concept that they will catch up later in life. Caretakers must thus make every effort during the first year of life to ensure maximal nutritional support and to utilize nutritional and non-nutritive techniques to optimize caloric utilization.

It is important to follow the growth of the head, as this indicates brain size and correlates well with intellectual development. It is noteworthy that the SGA infant with small head size at birth may still turn out

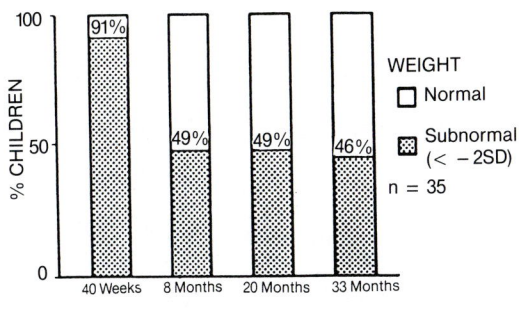

FIGURE 63–10. Catch-up growth in SGA babies. (From Hack M: The outcome of growth failure associated with preterm birth. *In* Merkatz I (ed): Clinical Obstetrics and Gynecology. Philadelphia, Harper & Row, 1984.)

to be developmentally normal. Some 50 per cent of SGA infants will have a small head circumference at birth—catch-up indicates a good outlook. At times it is difficult to distinguish catch-up head growth from hydrocephalus. We use ultrasonography liberally to detect, among other things, congenital or acquired anatomic abnormalities, evidence of bleeding, and ventricular size. CT scans are utilized to clarify suspicious lesions.

The timing, duration, and etiology of the intrauterine growth restriction together with the degree of catch-up growth determines the outcome of both term and preterm growth-restricted infants. The outcome reports of SGA term infants have varied. Normal IQ predominates; however, language delay, behavioral problems, and potential school difficulties despite a normal IQ are emerging as significant problems. As already indicated, early reports on SGA preterm infants were devastating and depressing. Recent reports excluding infants with congenital infections and major malformations have not found significant differences between SGA and AGA preterm infants. This has been attributed to many factors, including earlier recognition, more precise intrauterine monitoring, appropriate delivery with avoidance of asphyxia and trauma, avoidance of hypoglycemia, and improved postnatal nutrition. SGA infants nonetheless do appear to exhibit more minor neurologic abnormalities. Infants at greatest risk for poor neurodevelopmental outcome include those weighing <1 kg at birth, those with asphyxia and seizures in the neonatal period, those with congenital infections and major malformations, and those who do not catch up in any of the growth parameters.

The follow-up of the SGA infant presents a continuing challenge. All infants should be considered at risk, and every effort should be made by the caretakers to ensure that all the available resources at the medical center are used so that these infants can achieve their maximal potential.

Head circumference correlates with brain volume, brain weight, and cellularity during infancy and childhood. It is an excellent predictor of outcome. Those infants with perinatal growth failure as reflected by subnormal head circumference persisting through the first 8 months of life will demonstrate the poorest cognitive function, academic achievement, and behavior at age 8 years (Hack et al., 1991).

Infants of Diabetic Mothers

The metabolic derangements are the major abnormality affecting individuals with diabetes mellitus. Pregnant women with diabetes should be managed by suitably trained individuals and teams who comprehensively monitor mother and fetus throughout pregnancy. Optimal care of women with diabetes must begin prior to conception because it has been demonstrated that careful preconception control of diabetes reduces the incidence of major anomalies. All pregnancies should be screened so that women with gestational diabetes can be identified and appropriately managed.

The pathophysiologic alterations induced by pregnancy in diabetic mothers are discussed in Chapter 54. Many problems may be anticipated in the offspring. The major problems include macrosomia, birth asphyxia, hypoglycemia, cardiorespiratory disorders, and congenital malformations. The improved ability to monitor fetal growth, maturity, and well-being antenatally and during labor has significantly reduced the incidence of stillbirth and severe birth asphyxia, as well as respiratory distress syndrome. Despite tight control of maternal glucose homeostatis, macrosomia remains a significant problem in approximately one-third of diabetic pregnancies. Cesarean section may be indicated for cephalopelvic disproportion; shoulder dystocia is a constant concern for the perinatal team, as this may result in a traumatic delivery with an asphyxiated, depressed infant.

(Procedures for resuscitation have been outlined previously.)

A complete physical examination will determine the presence of malformations and whether birth trauma or injury has occurred. Brachial plexus injury is the most common nerve injury of the newborn. Brachial plexus stretching, the result of traction of the head and neck in a vertex delivery, results in Erb's palsy (C5, C6) characterized by an adducted shoulder and internally rotated arm with the elbow extended, forearm pronated, and wrist flexed. Diaphragmatic paralysis may occur on the same side.

Congenital malformations are observed two to six times more frequently in offspring of diabetes. Whereas any organ system may be involved, anomalies of the cardiovascular system and skeleton predominate. There is an association between maternal HbA_{1c} and malformations, with fewer malformations noted in those pregnancies in which the HbA_{1c} remains in the normal range. There is thus a major thrust to rigid control of maternal blood glucose before conception and during the first trimester to reduce the malformation rate. Animal studies demonstrate that this concept is valid. The rationale of the preconception program for a diabetic woman is to optimize the pregnancy outcome for herself and her offspring. Strict glucose control at this time reduces the frequency of congenital malformations and may also diminish other perinatal complications including intrauterine death,

macrosomia, and neonatal disorders. Although this concept has been well accepted, not all prospective studies have documented a clear reduction in the incidence of malformations (Mills et al., 1988).

Hypoglycemia remains a prevalent problem in the offspring of women with type I and type II diabetes. Because the clinical manifestations of hypoglycemia may be subtle and the neurologic sequelae of sustained hypoglycemia devastating, it is important to screen all infants at risk in order to identify them early and correct hypoglycemia. Screening is accomplished by means of either Dextrostix or Chemstrips. If the screen value is below 25 mg per cent, a quantitative blood sugar specimen is drawn. In term infants hypoglycemia is defined as a blood sugar level below 30 mg/100 ml on two occasions during the first 72 hours of life (20 mg/100 ml in preterm infants). Most clinicians attempt to maintain the blood glucose above 40 mg per cent on the basis of the data from Srinivasan (Fig. 63—11), which reveal that the blood glucose in the normal neonate does not decline below 40 mg per cent after the first 2 hours of life. There is continuing debate with regard to the definition of hypoglycemia. The debate revolves around broad principles including whether the definition is statistical or functional. Because there may be far-reaching consequences of hypoglycemia, it appears wiser to be conservative and maintain the blood glucose above 40 mg per cent.

Hypoglycemia may be manifested dramatically with seizures or more likely has an insidious onset that may be overlooked. A wide range of symptoms have been attributed to hypoglycemia. These include apa-

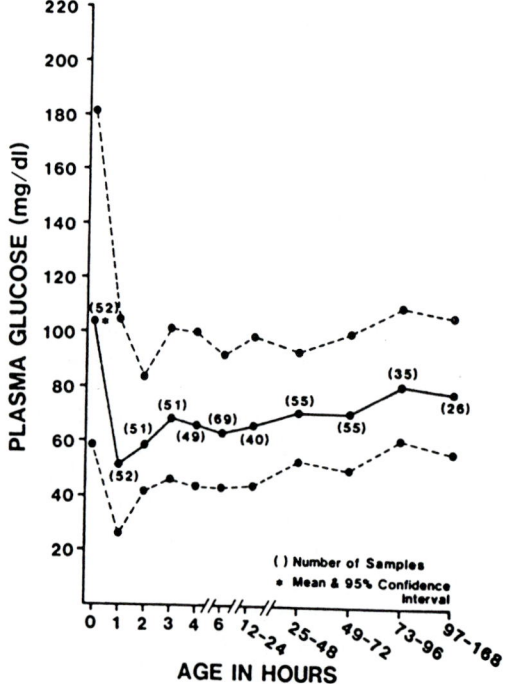

FIGURE 63–11. Predicted plasma glucose values during first week of life in healthy term neonates appropriate for gestational age. (From Srinivasan G, Pildes RS, Cattamanchi G, et al: Plasma glucose values in normal neonates: A new look. J Pediatr **109**:114, 1986.)

thy, poor feeding, apnea, high-pitched or weak cry, hypotonia, and eye rolling. Many of these are non-specific symptoms frequently observed in normoglycemic infants. In all diabetic offspring hypoglycemia should be anticipated and the blood glucose monitored hourly initially and then every 2 to 4 hours until it has stabilized in the normal range. Efforts are made to establish early oral feeds and the environment optimized to minimize energy demands. Intravenous infusions are used liberally, with glucose infused by pump at rates of 4 to 9 mg/kg/min or greater if necessary. If the infant is symptomatic with hypoglycemia, 2 ml/kg of 10 per cent dextrose are infused rapidly followed by an infusion rate of 8 mg/kg/min, increasing with 2 mg/kg/min increments to achieve normoglycemia.

Glucocorticoids are added when the rate of glucose infusion exceeds 14 mg/kg/min. Neurologic sequelae may be noted in 30 to 50 per cent of symptomatic hypoglycemic neonates.

In 1973 Pildes reported that problems of neonatal adaptation could be anticipated in 50 per cent of offspring of insulin-dependent diabetics and 10 to 20 per cent of offspring of gestational diabetics. Since then the enhanced ability to evaluate and monitor fetal maturity and well-being has resulted in a marked reduction in respiratory disorders. Functional and anatomic cardiovascular abnormalities have therefore assumed a more significant role. Technologic advances, including Doppler ultrasonography and two-dimensional echocardiography, permit precise definition of the cardiac problems. The unique cardiomyopathy complicating diabetic pregnancies is only part of the spectrum of heart disease, which includes a fourfold increase in the incidence of congenital heart disease, arrhythmias, persistence of the fetal circulation, disorders of blood pressure, and the effects of asphyxia on myocardial function. The diabetic cardiomyopathy is characterized by cardiomegaly with interventricular septal hypertrophy resulting in functional obstruction akin to the hypertrophic cardiomyopathy observed in adults. The septal hypertrophy can be observed in the fetus and appears to correlate with maternal control as evidenced by HbA_{1c}.

There is a wide spectrum of clinical presentation observed in infants with a cardiomyopathy. Congestive or hypertrophic symptoms may predominate, and cyanosis, mottling, tachypnea, tachycardia, and features of congestive heart failure may be apparent. The heart is enlarged on x-ray and the disorder is confirmed echocardiographically. Treatment is symptomatic with careful management of fluids, correction of polycythemia, maintenance of normoglycemia, as well as close monitoring and correction of electrolyte disorders or hypocalcemia. Although diuretics are used if there is clear evidence of fluid overload, digitalis and inotropic agents are avoided unless poor myocardial contractility is documented. In symptomatic infants with cardiomyopathy, propranolol may be useful.

The disease is self-limited and in general symptoms and clinical features resolve within a few weeks, although the septal and wall hypertrophy may take months to resolve.

Nutrition

Meeting the nutritional and metabolic needs of the increasing number of extremely immature, small, and sick infants who now survive presents a major challenge to the neonatologist. Although the ideal growth rates have yet to be defined, we attempt to achieve intrauterine growth rates. Immaturity of the gastrointestinal tract, together with altered metabolic rates induced by illness, compound the problem. Many infants will fail to thrive during their nursery sojourn, as evidenced by declining growth percentiles. Follow-up data indicate that relatively brief periods of failure to thrive are well tolerated, and provided catch-up growth has been achieved by 8 months corrected age, normal neurodevelopment can be anticipated.

A better understanding of the physiology and development of the gastrointestinal tract is emerging. This should permit a more rational approach to this most important aspect of care. The full-term infant is better equipped to tolerate periods of starvation than the preterm infant, who has extremely low reserves, particularly of fat and glycogen. In all infants every effort is made to avoid even brief periods of starvation, and energy is supplied intravenously commencing on the first day of life. With a combination of intravenous and oral alimentation the immature and diseased gastrointestinal tract is not overburdened, and sufficient calories, fluid, minerals and essential amino acids, fatty acids, and glucose can be administered while maturation or recovery occur. Immaturity, ileus, cardiorespiratory failure, and gastrointestinal or other associated anomalies may all result in an infant too sick to absorb nutrients from the gastrointestinal tract. The provision of 60 calories/kg/day intravenously, provided 10 per cent of these are in the form of protein, will prevent tissue catabolism.

Extrauterine adaptation should be normal before oral alimentation is begun. The technique of feeding is determined by weight, gestational age, and condition of the infant. Oral feeding is commenced only when there is clear-cut evidence of a gag reflex (usually 34 weeks gestation). Whereas formerly infants with arterial catheters receiving assisted ventilation received nothing by mouth, this practice is being reviewed at a number of centers. It appears that even small amounts of food placed in the stomach will accelerate gastrointestinal functional maturation.

Basic problems in feeding the preterm infant include lack of coordination between suck and swallow until 34 weeks gestation, diminished gastric capacity, gastroesophageal reflux (poor sphincter development), diminished gastrointestinal motility, and malabsorption. Alterations in motility and propulsion are accentuated in asphyxiated infants. During the first weeks of life nutritional needs are met primarily with intravenous alimentation, and oral feedings are gradually introduced. In order to ensure adequate growth (15 to 30 grams per day) it is necessary to provide approximately 120 calories/kg/day.

Breast milk or especially modified humanized formula may be used. There has been a hot debate concerning the adequacy of breast milk for the preterm infant. Although the protein, calcium, and iron content, for example, is theoretically inadequate to meet the growth needs of the premature infant, the unique physical and immunologic properties of human milk make it highly desirable. This translates into reducing the incidence of necrotizing enterocolitis (see below). Lucas and Cole (1990) were able to document that preterm infants who received either complete or partial enteral alimentation with breast milk had a reduced rate of necrotizing enterocolitis. The milk may be supplemented or fortified. Formula has been modified to resemble human milk and may be offered as 20 to 24 calories per ounce. Because of low-birthweight infants' limited gastric capacity and delicate fluid balance with a tendency to fluid overload, 24-calorie preparations are popular for them. The nutritional needs of the preterm infant are presented in Table 63–9.

Various feeding strategies have been attempted and there are proponents and opponents of the various regimens. The daily water requirements are dependent upon the thermal environment, maturity, physical environment (i.e., radiant warmers and phototherapy), rate of growth, and intercurrent conditions. Immature infants with high evaporative water losses require large fluid intakes when compared with adults or term infants. Renal immaturity and limited endocrine control further strain the system, diminishing the margins for error. Excess fluid administration has been implicated in the incidence of patent ductus arteriosus, necrotizing enterocolitis, and bronchopulmonary dysplasia. Fluid balance is monitored by closely determining intake/output, body weight, serum and urine osmolarity, urine specific gravity, and urine and serum electrolytes.

Total parenteral nutrition remains an integral part of the feeding program of premature infants and the mainstay of nutritional support for infants with major gastrointestinal anomalies or short bowel following surgical resection. Protein, carbohydrates, fat, electrolytes, trace minerals, vitamins, and water are all provided intravenously. Because of the high complication rate associated with central lines, every effort is made to administer the parenteral nutrition via peripheral veins. This is not always possible, particularly for extremely immature infants and those with short bowel who require prolonged parenteral nutrition. Complications with use of central venous catheters include infections, metabolic derangements, and thromboses (Table 63–10).

Fluid Requirements

In utero the fetus participates in an exchange of water involving the mother, fetus, and the amniotic fluid. Remarkably large volumes of water are exchanged between the mother and the fetus—approximately 3500 ml/hr at term with the net flux being in the maternofetal direction. Ultrasonographic studies reveal that fetal swallowing of amniotic fluid amounts to about 20 ml/hr at term and micturition adds approximately 28 ml/hr at term. Together, swallowing and micturition contribute only about 10 per cent of

TABLE 63–9.   Recommended Dietary Allowances for Infants

	00–0.5 YEARS	0.5–1.0 YEARS	1–3 YEARS
Calories	108 kcal/kg	98 kcal/kg	102 kcal/kg
Protein	2.2 gm/kg	1.6 gm/kg	1.2 g/kg
Vitamins			
A	1250 IU/d	1250 IU/d	1330 IU/d
D	300 IU/d	400 IU/d	400 IU/d
E	3 IU/d	4 IU/d	6 IU/d
K	5 mcg/d	10 mcg/d	15 mcg/d
C	30 mg/d	35 mg/d	40 mg/d
Thiamin	300 mcg/d	400 mcg/d	700 mcg/d
Riboflavin	400 mcg/d	500 mcg/d	800 mcg/d
B_6	300 mcg/d	600 mcg/d	1000 mcg/d
B_{12}	0.3 mcg/d	0.5 mcg/d	1.7 mcg/d
Niacin	5 mg/d	6 mg/d	9 mg/d
Folic acid	25 mcg/d	35 mcg/d	50 mcg/d
Pantothenic acid	2 mg/d*	3 mg/d*	3 mg/d*
Biotin	10 mcg/d*	15 mcg/d*	20 mcg/d*
Minerals			
Magnesium	40 mg/kg	60 mg/kg	80 mg/kg
Iron	6 mg/d	10 mg/d	10 mg/d
Iodine	40 mcg/d	50 mcg/d	70 mcg/d
Zinc	5 mg/d	5 mg/d	10 mg/d
Copper	400–600 mcg/d*	600–700 mcg/d*	700–1000 mcg/d*
Manganese	300–600 mcg/d*	600–1000 mcg/d*	1000–1500 mcg/d*
Chloride	180 mg/d†	300 mg/d†	350–500 mg/d†
Sodium	120 mg/d†	200 mg/d†	225–300 mg/d†
Potassium	500 mg/d†	700 mg/d†	1000–1400 mg/d†
Calcium	400 mg/d	600 mg/d	800 mg/d
Phosphorus	300 mg/d	500 mg/d	800 mg/d

*Safe and adequate ranges.
†Estimated *minimum* requirements for sodium, potassium, and chloride.
From National Research Council: Recommended Dietary Allowances, 10th ed. Report of the Subcommittee on the Tenth Edition of the RDS, Food and Nutrition Board, Commission of Life Sciences, Washington, DC, National Academy Press, 1989.

TABLE 63–10. Complications of Parenteral Nutrition

METABOLIC COMPLICATIONS
Hyper- and hypoglycemia
Hyperammonemia
Prerenal azotemia
Essential fatty acid deficiency
Trace mineral deficiency
Hypertriglyceridemia
Cholestasis
Abnormal liver function
Electrolyte imbalances
Hyper- and hypophosphatemia
Hyper- and hypocalcemia
Hyper- and hypomagnesemia
Hyper- and hypokalemia
Hyperchloremic acidemia
Hypochloremic alkalosis
Metabolic acidosis
MECHANICAL COMPLICATIONS
CATHETER INSERTION
  Pneumothorax
  Hemothorax
  Hydromediastinum
  Subclavian artery injury
  Subclavian hematoma
  Subclavian vein laceration
  Arteriovenous fistula
  Air embolism
  Catheter embolism
  Catheter malposition
  Thoracic duct laceration
  Cardiac perforation and tamponade
  Brachial plexus injury
  Horner's syndrome
  Phrenic nerve paralysis
  Carotid artery injury
CATHETER USE
  Venous thrombosis
    Superior vena cava syndrome
    Pulmonary embolus
  Catheter dislodgement
  Perforation and/or infusion leaks (pericardial,
    pleural, mediastinal)
SEPTIC COMPLICATIONS
CATHETER
  Contamination and infection at catheter site
    due to improper catheter care
  Catheter "seeding" from distant site of
    infection
PARENTERAL NUTRITION SOLUTION
  Improper mixing/handling/administration of
    solutions

the hourly water exchange between the fetus and amniotic fluid. The large fetal renal output is noteworthy; clearly, water conservation is not a priority of the fetal kidney.

The total body water content of the fetus is high and diminishes with advancing gestational age. Total body water accounts for about 90 per cent of fetal weight at 13 weeks, 86 per cent at 26 weeks, and 70 per cent at term. In addition, as maturation proceeds, intracellular water forms a greater percentage of total body water as extracellular water decreases.

Both full-term and preterm infants show appreciable weight loss during the first week of life. This appears to be accounted for by loss of extracellular fluid. *Insensible water loss* is a major source of water loss following delivery. There is an inverse relationship between birth weight, gestational age, and insensible water loss. Hence immature, low-birth-weight infants have the largest losses—in some infants exceeding 100 ml/kg/day. Mechanisms accounting for this excess water loss include the relatively large surface area to body weight, the minimal amount of subcutaneous tissue, and the highly vascularized, permeable, very thin epidermis. Insensible water loss correlates with metabolic rate and hence water losses increase with cold stress, crying, and activity. Metabolic rate increases with advancing postnatal age in all weight groups and gestational ages. The excessive losses in immature, low-birth-weight infants occur independently of their metabolic rates. One investigator noted that evaporative heat losses account for 65 per cent of heat loss in the first week of life and 43 per cent in the second week in healthy preterm infants. Additional factors increasing evaporative water losses up to two- to three-fold include radiant warmers and phototherapy.

Insensible water loss may be reduced by the interposition of a heat shield in an isolette or by the use of double-walled isolettes, thermal blankets, or even Saran wrap when the infants are nursed under a radiant warmer. Topical application of petrolatum will also reduce evaporative water losses, which may significantly influence fluid balance but is not used clinically.

It becomes apparent that water requirements will vary enormously with the weight and gestational age of the infant as well as the environmental conditions. The state of the infant will also be of vital importance in determining fluid management. For example, infants on ventilators will, in general, have no respiratory water losses and may even gain water via the respiratory tract. Fluid management is thus determined by frequent assessment of the infant, taking into account clinical status, vital signs, perfusion, weight, urine output, urine specific gravity and osmolality, hematocrit, BUN, electrolytes, and creatinine levels. Guidelines for fluid management are to commence with 50 to 60 ml/kg/day on the first day and then be adjusted upward thereafter on the basis of the aforementioned determinations and observations. Indications for increasing the daily fluid intake include a failing urine output accompanied by rising specific gravity or osmolality, excessive weight loss (more than 2 to 3 per cent/day), and rising BUN and hematocrit. Increased fluid administration is also necessary in infants with third-space losses, as in peritonitis.

Administration of too little fluid may cause dehydration. Lorentz et al. (1982), however, documented that weight loss up to 15 per cent was tolerated in the first week of life provided that hypoglycemia was prevented. Excess fluid administration (generally greater than 140 ml/kg/day) has been associated with clinical patent ductus arteriosus, pulmonary edema, necrotizing enterocolitis, and bronchopulmonary dysplasia.

In summary, total body water is greater in the less mature infants. All infants lose weight and water during the first week of life. Large insensible water losses should be anticipated in low-birth-weight infants. Daily fluid management is based on clinical observations and measurements together with biochemical monitoring. Excessive fluid administration is possibly more harmful than too little.

Hypocalcemia and Bone Mineralization

Calcium is transferred across the placenta against an uphill maternal-fetal calcium gradient. Fetal levels are about 1 mg/100 ml above maternal levels. Maternal parathormone and 1,25-dihydroxyvitamin D_3 concentrations are elevated during pregnancy, the latter accounting for increased gastrointestinal calcium absorption. In contrast, fetal levels of 1,25-dihydroxyvitamin D_3 are low as a consequence of minimal placental transfer and decreased fetal production. Bone mineralization *in utero* is dependent upon an adequate supply of calcium (130 to 150 mg/kg/day), phosphate, magnesium, and the appropriate balance between parathormone, calcitonin, and vitamin D. From 28 weeks until term as fetal weight triples, the calcium content increases fourfold and bone mineral density increases progressively.

At birth the constant infusion of calcium from the mother stops abruptly and serum calcium starts to fall, stimulating parathormone. 1,25-Dihydroxyvitamin D_3 levels increase to adult levels by 24 hours of life as the neonate prepares to defend the serum calcium and enhance gastrointestinal calcium absorption. However, with a net absorption of only 20 to 25 per cent of the enteral calcium, neither breast milk nor humanized proprietary formulas deliver the same calcium supply to the neonate as that provided the fetus. Consequently, under usual circumstances, bone mineralization in the preterm infant nurtured in the nursery lags behind that achieved *in utero*. Manipulation of the formula to provide additional calcium and phosphate can correct this process.

Despite the physiologic hormonal adaptive process, there is normally a fall in serum calcium in the first 24 to 48 hours before stabilization. Early neonatal hypocalcemia represents an exaggerated physiologic fall in serum calcium during this time and is noted in 30 to 40 per cent of low-birth-weight infants. Other infants at risk include asphyxiated term infants, infants of diabetic mothers, and those with respiratory disorders, sepsis, and hypoglycemia. Serum calcium should be monitored in infants identified at risk and calcium infusions given to symptomatic infants.

Symptoms of hypocalcemia cover a wide spectrum from normal behavior through jitteriness, twitching, and even convulsions. Nonspecific features including vomiting, poor feeding, cyanosis, and high-pitched cry may be observed. Chvostek's sign is unreliable and the diagnosis is confirmed by serum calcium determinations.

Classic neonatal tetany observed on days 5 to 7 of life is associated with hyperphosphatemia. This is secondary to increased phosphate intake. Lactoengineering resulting in better balance between calcium and phosphorus in formulas has made this entity much less common. Hypocalcemia is also seen after exchange transfusions, in neonates with uremia, and as a consequence of chronic diuretic therapy, which may produce hypercalciuria and renal stones.

Treatment of hypocalcemia is to provide 24 to 35 mg/kg/day of calcium. Calcium gluconate (USP), providing 9 mg calcium/ml, and calcium gluceptate injection (Lilly), which contains 18 mg calcium/ml, are most frequently utilized. Infusion is given extremely slowly by pump, as calcium may cause severe bradycardia or even cardiac arrest if administered too rapidly. In acute situations such as an infant who is having seizures, a push of calcium gluconate using a dose up to 3 mg/kg may be used. Heart rate must be closely monitored and only a secure IV line used because calcium is extremely irritating to tissue and has produced extensive tissue necrosis when solutions containing calcium infiltrate the tissues.

Hematologic Problems

Anemia

There are many causes of anemia in the neonatal period. Anemia may result from any of three causes: hemorrhage, hemolysis, and failure of red cell production. The presence of severe anemia at the time of delivery or on the first day of life is usually the result of hemorrhage or hemolysis due to isoimmunization. When the anemia is secondary to acute blood loss at the time of birth, there may be evidence of circulatory insufficiency.

Oski and Naiman (1982) classify hemorrhage leading to anemia at birth or early in the neonatal period broadly into five categories:

1. OBSTETRIC ACCIDENTS AND MALFORMATIONS OF THE PLACENTA AND CORD. This subgroup includes rupture of a normal or abnormal umbilical cord. Rupture of the normal umbilical cord is rare and may result from an unattended precipitous delivery. Severe fetal hemorrhage may accompany placenta previa, abruptio placentae, or accidental incision of the placenta or umbilical cord during cesarean section. Failure of the infant to receive the usual placental transfusion during the section and clamping the cord with the infant above the placenta will aggravate the situation, as fetoplacental hemorrhage will occur. Infants delivered with tight nuchal cords are also at risk for fetoplacental hemorrhage and should be evaluated for signs and symptoms of acute blood loss including pallor, tachycardia, tachypnea or gasping respiration, hypotension, and evidence of poor perfusion with slow capillary refill. The hemoglobin content may initially be normal but, as circulating volume is restored, will drop precipitously. Anemia is defined as a hemoglobin level less than 12 gm/100 ml in the first week of life. The hemoglobin and hematocrit levels both rise 2 to 3 gm/100 ml and 3 to 6 per cent respectively to peak at 3 to 12 hours of age. The capillary values for both hemoglobin and hematocrit are consistently higher than venous or arterial measurements.

It may be extremely difficult to distinguish the infant with hypovolemic shock from the severely asphyxiated newborn; both may be extremely pale with evidence of poor perfusion and circulatory insufficiency. Both conditions may be present in the same patient. Hypotension is noted when circulating volume has been reduced 25 per cent.

When a depressed pale infant is to be treated, the resuscitative plan outlined early in this chapter should be followed. Blood pressure and a venous hematocrit are quickly ascertained. Attempts are made to oxygenate and ventilate the patient, to restore cardiac output and circulating volume, to correct metabolic acidosis, and then to correct the anemia with transfusion. Anemia as a result of obstetric accidents or malformations of the placenta and cord is usually diagnosed from historical information and close inspection of the placenta, cord, and membranes.

2. OCCULT HEMORRHAGE PRIOR TO BIRTH. Although some degree of hemorrhage from the fetus into the maternal circulation occurs during 50 per cent of pregnancies, it has been estimated that in only 1 per cent will the amount of fetal loss exceed 40 ml and cause anemia in the newborn. Massive fetomaternal hemorrhage, defined as more than 150 ml of fetal blood in the maternal circulation, is said to account for 3 per cent of perinatal mortality and occurs in approximately 1:800 deliveries. Some of the causes of fetomaternal hemorrhage include amniocentesis, external version, fundal pressure during the second stage of labor, the use of intravenous oxytocics, trauma, placenta previa, and abruptio placentae (Moya et al., 1987).

The clinical manifestations of fetomaternal hemorrhage depend on the timing and acuity. Chronic bleeding will result in a very pale infant, not necessarily in distress or manifesting any features of shock but with enlargement of the liver and spleen. The blood smear is typically microcytic and hypochromic and there is no evidence of hemolysis. Fetal cells can be demonstrated in the maternal circulation, usually by means of the acid elution technique of Kleihauer and Betke. If fetomaternal hemorrhage of significant proportions has occurred acutely, the clinical features of shock and hypoperfusion as already described will predominate. The red cell morphology is normocytic and normochromic, and no hepatosplenomegaly is present. In contrast to the infants with chronic loss who require only iron supplementation, these latter infants are in dire need of intravenous therapy and whole blood transfusions.

Occult hemorrhage may also be noted with intrauterine twin-to-twin transfusions. The donor twin is pale and usually smaller than the plethoric recipient. Both twins are at risk and need close observation and appropriate intervention.

3. INTERNAL HEMORRHAGE. There are many potential sites for blood loss in the newborn. The detection of anemia during the first days of life should initiate a careful evaluation to determine the source of blood loss. The finding of a large cephalohematoma or extensive swelling of the scalp associated with a subaponeurotic collection of blood is one common site of blood loss. Infants delivered in the breech position may have significant blood loss into the muscles and will manifest bruising but not necessarily swelling. The advent of ultrasound and CT scanning has facilitated the search for intracranial and intraabdominal sites of blood loss.

Adrenal hemorrhage, rupture of the liver, and rupture of the spleen traditionally all accompany difficult and traumatic deliveries of both macrosomic and premature infants and are more likely to be noted with breech presentation. The usual clinical manifestations of shock are accompanied by specific abdominal findings. In some instances adrenal hemorrhage may be confirmed only by the incidental finding of adrenal calcification. Rupture of the liver is usually contained by the capsule, and the infant only decompensates after about 48 hours.

4. IATROGENIC BLOOD LOSS. Iatrogenic blood loss is associated with excess blood withdrawal, bleeding from inadequate clamping of the umbilical cord, bleeding associated with improper management of the umbilical arterial catheters, or excessive bleeding following procedures such as circumcision. It is important to monitor closely the volume of blood withdrawn from sick neonates, to restrict the number of laboratory investigations, and to draw the minimal volume of blood necessary. Strict adherence to protocols regarding care of catheters will diminish the risks of hemorrhage from this source.

Hemolytic Anemias

There are many causes of hemolytic disease in the newborn. The presence of jaundice distinguishes the hemolytic disorders from those characterized by blood loss. Major categories of hemolysis of significance in the neonatal period are:

1. Isoimmunization
2. Congenital defects of the red cell
3. Acquired defects of the red cell

The problem of isoimmunization is dealt with in Chapter 44. Congenital defects of the red cell, which include the enzymatic defects, are characterized by specific morphology of the red cell or the presence of abnormal hemoglobin. Among the causes of acquired defects of the red cell are a variety of bacterial and viral infections and a multitude of drugs and toxins.

In summary, hemorrhage is the most common cause of early anemia. The cause is usually apparent from the history. The initial evaluation requires a complete blood count with smear and reticulocyte count, total and direct bilirubin, blood type and Coombs' test, and Kleihauer-Betke test on maternal blood. TORCH titers, a full coagulation profile, red cell enzymes, and hemoglobin electrophoresis are analyzed as indicated by the history and physical examination.

If significant hemorrhage has occurred and the neonate manifests shock with a reduced blood pressure and metabolic acidosis, arrangements are made for immediate blood transfusion. In the meantime, circulation is supported with expansion of the intravascular volume, and mechanical ventilation optimizes oxygenation.

Polycythemia

Polycythemia is defined by a venous hematocrit above 65 per cent. In appropriately grown newborns the incidence is approximately 4 per cent, rising to 18 to 45 per cent in SGA infants. The high hematocrit is thought to be the result of intrauterine hypoxia stimulating erythropoietin but may also be secondary to a twin-to-twin transfusion. Infants with high hematocrits may have hyperviscosity as well as reduced red cell deformability. They are susceptible to thrombotic complications. Symptoms attributable to polycythemia include respiratory distress, lethargy, jitteriness, edema, and priapism. Polycythemic infants are also more prone to hypoglycemia and jaundice.

The tendency has been to empirically reduce the hematocrit by means of partial exchange transfusion if the hematocrit is greater than 70 per cent or greater than 65 per cent if the infant is symptomatic. Partial isovolemic transfusion most effectively lowers the viscosity if normal saline or 5 per cent albumin is used. The volume necessary to exchange in order to achieve the desired reduction of hematocrit to approximately 55 per cent is calculated as follows:

$$\text{Volume (ml)} = \text{Blood volume} \times \frac{(\text{hct 1} - \text{hct 2})}{\text{hct 1}}$$

where hct 1 = initial hematocrit and hct 2 = desired hematocrit.

Currently, indications for intervention in polycythemic neonates remain largely empirical extrapolations from studies of blood viscosity. Some recent studies indicate that the whole blood viscosity is lower in neonates than adults at every level of hematocrit and that this is the result of a lower plasma viscosity. Intervention is not undertaken lightly. The major risk of partial exchange transfusion is an increased incidence of bowel necrosis and necrotizing enterocolitis.

Murphy and associates (1986) evaluated the cardiac function in infants with polycythemia. M-Mode echocardiograms were performed before and after a partial exchange transfusion and repeated 48 hours later. The polycythemic presumed hyperviscous infants had slower heart rates and findings consistent with elevated pulmonary vascular resistance. Elevated right ventricular pre-ejection–right ventricular ejection time corrected with the partial exchange. An unexplained fractional shortening was noted in the polycythemic infants 48 hours after the exchange.

Jaundice

Hyperbilirubinemia is the most common problem encountered in the full-term neonate. Hyperbilirubinemia is of clinical relevance in the neonate because it has been associated with kernicterus (yellow staining of the basal ganglia and hippocampus). Bilirubin appears to be responsible for the central nervous system damage, although the precise mechanism and predisposing conditions remain under investigation. The interrelationships between total bilirubin, total albumin and bilirubin-binding capacity, the integrity of the blood-brain barrier, and the factors determining the uptake of bilirubin into the cell are all under close scrutiny. Most reports indicate that in term infants, without evidence of hemolysis, kernicterus is unlikely to occur if the serum bilirubin is maintained below 25 mg per cent, although kernicterus has been reported at autopsy in low-birth-weight infants when the serum

bilirubin never exceeded 10 mg per cent. Recent reports suggest that in the absence of sepsis the overall incidence of kernicterus appears to have declined.

Clinical manifestations of kernicterus in the full-term infant include temperature instability, lethargy, poor feeding, high-pitched cry, vomiting, and hypotonia. Subsequently, irritability, opisthotonus, sunsetting appearance of the eyes, and seizures may occur. "Wind-milling" movements of the extremities have been reported. Pulmonary or gastric hemorrhage may occur as a terminal event. Long-term sequelae include the spastic or athetoid form of cerebral palsy, hearing loss (especially high tone), paralysis of upward gaze, and enamel hypoplasia. Many reports suggest, however, that bilirubin encephalopathy may be asymptomatic in the newborn and subsequently produce neurodevelopmental abnormalities. In the preterm infant, fisting, apnea, and increased tone may be the only acute manifestations. The search continues for a methodology of identifying infants at greatest risk to identify if and when encephalopathy is imminent.

Bilirubin is produced from breakdown of hemoglobin, myoglobin cytochromes, and other heme-containing compounds mainly in the liver, spleen, and bone marrow. The indirect bilirubin so formed is water insoluble but fat soluble, hence potentially toxic to the central nervous system. Bilirubin is transported in the blood bound to albumin and accepted into the hepatic cells by a receptor ligandin. Under the influence of the enzyme glucuronyl transferase, the bilirubin is conjugated to form bilirubin diglucuronide, which is water soluble and excreted in the bile. Bilirubin diglucuronide is deconjugated in the gut by glucuronidase, reabsorbed, and recirculated to the liver—the so-called enterohepatic circulation of bilirubin. Prior to delivery, the indirect bilirubin is transported across the placenta.

Jaundice is usually observed in term infants on the third day of life and progresses from the head and neck to the trunk and limbs. It disappears in the reverse direction. The onset of jaundice within the first 36 hours of life, persistence beyond the first week of life, a serum bilirubin exceeding 13 mg per cent, and/or elevation of the direct bilirubin are all indications for investigation of the jaundice. The level of 13 mg per cent has been selected as the upper limit for "physiologic jaundice" from multiple studies. These revealed that the serum bilirubin ranges between 6 and 7 mg per cent between days 2 and 4. Two standard deviations above this is 13 mg per cent. In a sample of 2421 infants admitted to their nursery Maisels and Gifford (1986) noted that the mean serum bilirubin on the second to third day of life was 6.2 ± 3.7 mg per cent. The incidence of infants with bilirubin levels above 12.9 mg per cent was 6.1 per cent—virtually identical to the Caucasian infants in the collaborative study completed in the early 1960s (99 per cent of the Hershey, Pennsylvania, population was Caucasian). This suggests, contrary to some opinion, that the incidence of nonphysiologic jaundice has not decreased with serum bilirubin levels. The boundary between physiologic and pathologic jaundice is not a distinct one. Although the value of 13 mg per cent is a useful guideline, it is noteworthy that this number will often be exceeded in breast-fed and Oriental infants. On the other hand, it would be less commonly reached in black or bottle-fed infants. Thus race and method of feeding are taken into consideration when deciding to investigate jaundice in an infant.

The major causes of jaundice are listed in Table 63–11. Important historical data include the blood types of the parents and the isoimmune status, ethnic origin of parents, maternal drug history, gestation, mode of delivery, past history with regard to jaundiced neonates, stooling pattern, and method of feeding. Jaundice associated with breast-feeding is the most common cause of hyperbilirubinemia in the otherwise healthy full-term infant.

The presence of plethora, bruising, and cephalohematoma should be sought. Hepatosplenomegaly accompanied by pallor, purpura, and rashes may indicate congenital infection or hemolytic disease. The initial evaluation should always include a complete blood count with smear and reticulocyte count, blood type of mother and infant, Coombs' test, total and direct bilirubin level, and urinalysis to rule out infection and galactosemia. If the infant is sick with the jaundice, a blood culture, spinal tap, and chest x-ray are also indicated. If the direct bilirubin exceeds 10 per cent of the total, this is indicative either of biliary obstruction or hepatocellular damage. Therefore, in addition to the aforementioned studies, serum protein and protein electrophoresis, serum transaminases, alpha-1 antitrypsin concentration, hepatitis-associated antigens and titers, TORCH titers, sweat chloride, and clotting profile are indicated (Table 63–12). An abdominal ultrasound may prove extremely productive, as may CT scan of the liver. A liver biopsy may be indicated.

TABLE 63–11.   Causes of Neonatal Hyperbilirubinemia

OVERPRODUCTION	UNDERSECRETION	MIXED
A. Hemolytic disorders 　1. Fetomaternal blood group Incompatibility ABO, Rh, others 　2. Genetic causes of hemolysis 　　a. Hereditary spherocytosis 　　b. Enzyme defects: G6PD, pyruvate kinase, others 　　c. Hemoglobinopathies: α-Thalassemia, β-γ-Thalassemia, others 　3. Drug-induced hemolysis—vitamin K B. Extravascular blood: petechiae, hematoma, pulmonary and cerebral hemorrhage, swallowed blood C. Polycythemia 　1. Chronic fetal hypoxia 　2. Maternal-fetal or fetofetal transfusion 　3. Placental transfusion (cord stripping) D. Exaggerated enterohepatic circulation 　1. Mechanical obstruction 　　a. Atresia and stenosis 　　b. Hirschsprung's disease 　　c. Meconium plug syndrome 　2. Reduced peristalsis 　　a. Fasting or underfeeding 　　b. Drugs (hexamethoniums, atropine) 　　c. Pyloric stenosis	E. Decreased hepatic uptake of bilirubin 　1. Persistent ductus venosus shunt 　2. Cytosol receptor protein (y) blocked by: 　　a. Drugs 　　b. Abnormal human milk inhibitor (? NEFA, ? may belong in D. or F.) F. Decreased bilirubin conjugation 　1. Congenital reduction in glucuronyl transferase activity 　　a. Familial nonhemolytic jaundice (types I and II) 　　b. Gilbert's syndrome* 　2. Enzyme inhibitor 　　a. Drugs and hormones: novobiocin, ? pregnanediol 　　b. Galactosemia (early) 　　c. Lucey-Driscoll syndrome 　　d. Abnormal human milk G. Impaired transport of conjugated bilirubin out of hepatocyte 　1. Congenital transport defect: Dubin-Johnson and Rotor's syndromes 　2. Hepatocellular damage secondary to metabolic disorders 　　a. Galactosemia (late) 　　b. Alpha-1-Antitrypsin deficiency* 　　c. Tyrosinemia 　　d. Hypermethioninemia 　　e. Hereditary fructose intolerance* 　3. Toxic obstruction (IV alimentation) H. Obstruction to bile flow 　1. Biliary atresia 　2. choledochal cyst* 　3. Cystic fibrosis* 　4. Extrinsic obstruction (tumor or band)	I. Prenatal infection 　1. Toxoplasmosis 　2. Rubella 　3. Cytomegalovirus (CMV) 　4. Herpesvirus hominis 　5. Syphilis 　6. Hepatitis 　7. Others J. Postnatal infections (sepsis) K. Multisystems disorders 　1. Prematurity ± RDS 　2. Infants of diabetic mothers 　3. Severe erythroblastosis

*Not seen early in the neonatal period.
From Poland RL, Ostrea EM Jr: Neonatal hyperbilirubinemia. *In* Klaus MH, Fanaroff AA: Care of the High Risk Neonate. 4th ed. Philadelphia, WB Saunders Company, 1993.

TABLE 63–12.   Conjugated Hyperbilirubinemia of Early Infancy

SUGGESTED WORK-UP
1. History and physical examination*
2. CBC and reticulocyte count
3. Coombs' test
4. Urinalysis, including reducing substances
5. Serum bilirubin concentration, total and direct-reacting
6. Total serum protein and protein electrophoresis
7. Serum transaminases
8. Alpha-1-antitrypsin concentration
9. Hepatitis-associated antigen and titers
10. Sweat chloride concentration
11. Serologic titers for rubella, CMV, etc.
12. Clotting factors, platelet count
13. Liver biopsy

*May lead one to order other diagnostic tests not listed.
From Poland RL, Ostrea EM Jr: Neonatal hyperbilirubinemia. In Klaus MH, Fanaroff AA: Care of the High Risk Neonate. 4th ed. Philadelphia, WB Saunders Company, 1993.

Persistent elevation of the indirect bilirubin is seen predominantly with hemolytic disease, hypothyroidism, or breast milk jaundice. The latter has been attributed at various times to hormones in the breast milk, to nonesterified fatty acids in the breast milk that inhibit glucuronyl transferase, and more recently to the presence of β-glucuronidase in human milk, which will enhance the enterohepatic circulation of bilirubin. ABO incompatibility is the most common cause of hemolytic disease in the newborn. A very high anti-A or anti-B antibody titer may be found in the maternal serum; the infant's blood smear reveals abundant spherocytes, and the reticulocyte count may be elevated. Hemolytic disease of the newborn, secondary to Rh compatibility, has become extremely rare with the widespread screening and utilization of Rh immune globulin.

TREATMENT. No treatment should be instituted without an investigation of the cause of the jaundice. It is important to ensure adequate hydration of jaundiced neonates. This has generated considerable controversy because proponents of breast-feeding are convinced that supplementation with formula or water decreases the success of breast-feeding. Evidence is strongly mounting to indicate that a reduced calorie and/or fluid intake is responsible for the early elevated bilirubin levels noted among breast-fed infants. Breast-feeding should not be discontinued during the first days of life. However, if there is prolonged elevation of indirect bilirubin attributed to breast milk, discontinuing breast-feeding for 24 hours will reduce the serum bilirubin.

Phototherapy has been extensively used for the treatment of jaundice. Light reduces bilirubin levels predominantly by photoisomerization and, to a lesser extent, photosensitized oxidation. Essentially during photoisomerization bilirubin is rapidly converted from a relatively insoluble state to water-soluble photoisomers. When bilirubin is exposed to light (Fig. 63–12), native bilirubin is converted to photobilirubin and the structural isomer lumirubin. Lumirubin appears to be the principal route of pigment elimination during phototherapy. Before phototherapy is ordered, the cause of the hyperbilirubinemia should be investigated. Most recent studies on the natural history of jaundice reveal that the early use of phototherapy offers no advantage, and prophylactic phototherapy, even in tiny immature infants, has not proved to be necessary. Guidelines for the use of phototherapy and exchange transfusions are outlined in Table 63–13. It is important to recognize that these are only guidelines. Therapy should always be dictated by the clinical condition and clinical evaluation, not merely by laboratory tests. In bruised, asphyxiated, acidotic, or potentially septic infants more liberal indications for treatment are often utilized. Since the advent of Rh immune globulin, the number of exchange transfusions has diminished markedly.

Infection

Infection remains a significant cause of neonatal morbidity and mortality. The incidence of neonatal septicemia is inversely related to gestational age; 1 in 250 premature infants and 1 in 1500 term infants experience a systemic bacterial infection in the first month of life. Although the spectrum of organisms involved has changed, the overall incidence of infections has decreased little in the last decade. On the positive side, mortality rates have continued to decline as a result of earlier detection and better supportive care, combined with specific antibiotic therapy.

Immune Response

Because the immune system of the newborn is defective in many respects, infants are predisposed to a higher risk of infection. The abnormalities in immune defense mechanisms which have been described include abnormal chemotaxis, phagocytosis and bactericidal activity, abnormal opsonic activity, and defects in the complement pathway. In addition, the infant's host defense mechanisms are not intact at birth, and the IGM and IgG responses to infection are depressed as compared to the adult. The preterm infant is particularly deficient in circulating immunoglobulin because the serum IgG is acquired transplacentally after the 17th week of gestation. Therefore, the infant's IgG level tends to be less than the maternal level and is directly related to gestational age. IgM is, in fact, the principal antibody synthesized by the neonate in response to infection *in utero*.

Environmental Risk Factors

The infant *in utero* is surrounded by sterile amniotic fluid which inhibits the growth of most microorganisms. The infant's protected status may be breached by microorganisms via two routes: by hematogenous spread from the maternal circulation and, more commonly, by ascending infection when normal vaginal flora gain access to the uterine cavity. Colonization and infection of the infant by the latter route are more common following rupture of fetal membranes for more than 24 hours. During vaginal delivery, the infant also may become contaminated by an assort-

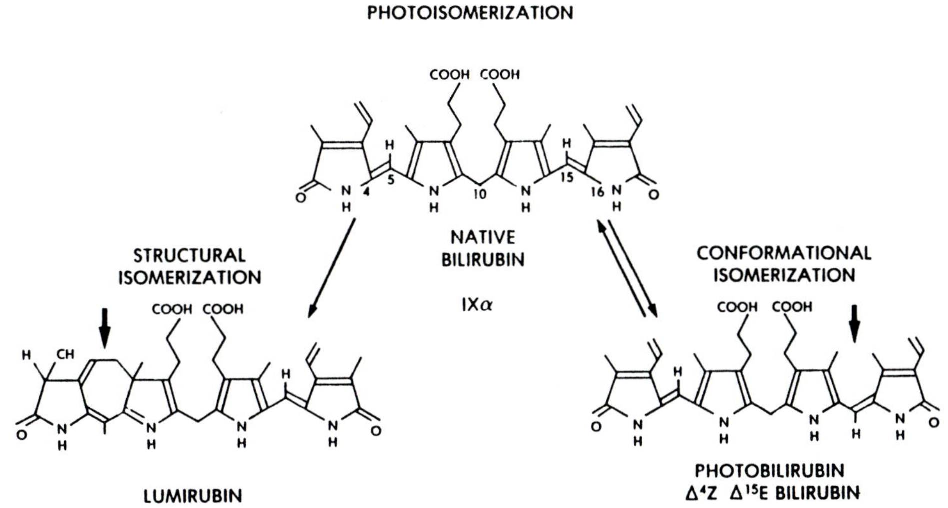

PHOTOISOMERIZATION

FIGURE 63–12. The photoiso-merized conversion of bilirubin IX-α (Z,Z) to water-soluble bili-rubin IX-α (Z,E) and lumirubin. (From Poland RL, Ostrea EM Jr: Neonatal Hyperbilirubinemia. *In* Klaus M, Fanaroff A (ed): Care of the High Risk Neonate. 4th ed. Philadelphia, WB Saunders Company, 1993.)

ment of vaginal flora. Serious infection via this route is more common the heavier the degree of colonization of the infant's skin, e.g., with the group B streptococcal organism.

Evaluation of the Newborn

The signs of sepsis in the newborn are nonspecific and may include poor feeding, apnea, weak suck, lethargy, hypoglycemia, and tachypnea, as well as temperature instability. These signs, when combined with an abnormal CBC (increased total leukocytes,

increased band count) and/or spinal fluid leukocytosis, may warrant initiation of antibiotic therapy prior to definitive isolation of the infecting organism. Ampicillin (100 to 200 mg/kg/day) and gentamicin (5 mg/kg/day) are given intravenously for 7 to 10 days in cases of suspected sepsis to provide broad coverage for the bacteria that commonly produce neonatal infection.

Infections of the Term Newborn

GROUP B STREPTOCOCCUS. The *group B streptococci* are the principal gram-positive organisms responsible

---

TABLE 63–13.   Guidelines for Use of Phototherapy and Exchange Transfusions

☐ Observe

☐ Investigate jaundice

Follow guidelines in the next highest bilirubin level category in the presence of any of the following:

1. Perinatal asphyxia

2. Respiratory distress

3. Metabolic acidosis (pH ≤7.25)

4. Hypothermia (<35C)

5. Low serum protein level (≤5 gm/100 ml)

6. Low birth weight (<1,500 gm)

7. Signs of clinical or CNS deterioration

Serum bilirubin (mg/100 ml)	Birth weight	<24 hr	24–48 hr	49–72 hr	>72 hr
<5	All weights				
5–9	All weights	Phototherapy if hemolysis			
10–14	<2.500 gm	Exchange transfusion if hemolysis*	Phototherapy		
10–14	> 2.500 gm			Investigate if bilirubin is >12 mg/100 ml	
15–19	>2.500 gm	Exchange transfusion*		Consider exchange*	
15–19	<2.500 gm			Phototherapy	
20 and greater	All weights	Exchange transfusion*			

*Use phototherapy after all exchange transfusions.

From Klaus MH, Fanaroff AA: Care of the High Risk Neonate, 4th ed. Philadelphia, WB Saunders Company, 1993.

TABLE 63–14. Sexually Transmitted Diseases That Can Infect the Fetus

ORGANISM	CLINICAL MANIFESTATIONS	PROGNOSIS	TREATMENT
Herpes simplex	Cutaneous vesicles CNS infection, hepatitis, pneumonitis	50–70 mortality; survivors often mentally retarded	Acyclovir
Treponema pallidum	Asymptomatic; skin rash, chorioretinitis, meningitis, periostitis, hepatosplenomegaly	Excellent if treated	Penicillin
N. gonorrhea	Sepsis, ophthalmia neonatorum	Blindness if untreated	Eye prophylaxis Penicillin
Chlamydia vaginalis	Conjunctivitis Late-onset pneumonia	Excellent	Erythromycin
Human Immunodeficiency virus	Asymptomatic, CNS symptoms	Poor; high morbidity under 1 year of age	AZT may delay onset of full clinical disease

for neonatal septicemia and meningitis. This bacterial pathogen may be acquired from the colonized vaginal tract of the mother, with maternal colonization rates varying between 4 and 30 per cent. The attack rate for colonized infants is low, however, less than 1 per cent, possibly due to passive immunization of the newborn by transplacental protective antibody. Early-onset streptococcal infection presents as a multisystem disease, with such symptoms as apnea, respiratory distress, and hypotension. Unless the illness is promptly detected and treated, the infant can rapidly develop a shock-like picture. Fortunately, with early treatment of the septicemic infant, a full recovery is expected. Detection of maternal colonization, coupled with antibiotic therapy to decrease the carrier state, appears to be a promising therapeutic technique for preventing infection of the newborn infant by *group B streptococcus* (Boyer and Gotoff, 1986; Garland and Fliefner, 1991).

SEXUALLY TRANSMITTED DISEASE. Over the last 5 years, sexually transmitted diseases have increased in frequency, with a corresponding increase in the number of congenitally affected infants. These infections may be acquired by either the hematogenous or ascending route, or from the vaginal tract after delivery (see also Chapter 42). Infection may occur early in gestation (e.g., herpes, syphilis) and result in the death of the fetus, or the infant may be born with multisystem involvement attributable to intrauterine infection. Early identification may allow appropriate

treatment and a good prognosis in some but not all of these diseases (Table 63–14). Identification and treatment of the affected mother and her contacts early in gestation hold the greatest promise for eradication of this class of neonatal infection.

CONGENITAL VIRAL INFECTION. Maternal viral infection that occurs during pregnancy may be relatively asymptomatic (see also Chapter 42). Cytomegalovirus infection is most commonly encountered (Table 63–15) (Stagno, 1986). However, in some specific types of infection, the viremia may spread to the newborn, resulting in intrauterine infection with potential long-term sequelae. In many cases, antenatal diagnosis of the infection has not occurred, and the complications of infection are only apparent at delivery (Table 63–16).

TABLE 63–15. Incidence of Congenital and Perinatal Infections in the United States

	CONGENITAL (PER 100 LIVE BIRTHS)	PERINATAL (PER 100 LIVE BIRTHS)
CMV	0.2–2.0	1.5–12
HSV	rare	0.005–0.05
Rubella	very rare	—
Hepatitis B	very rare	0.01–0.03
Varicella	very rare	—
Toxoplasma	0.05–0.01	—
Syphilis	0.01	—
Chlamydia	—	1–7

TABLE 63–16. Diagnostic Aids for Congenital and Perinatal Infections

Cytomegalovirus:	Isolation of virus from urine within 2 weeks of age
Rubella:	Isolation of virus from throat (and stools, conjunctiva, or urine) within 1 month of age. Serial determination of antibody between 3 and 9 months of age
Syphilis:	Darkfield examination of lesions if present. Antibody determination with both reagin (VDRL) and fluorescent antibody (FTA-ABS) test
Toxoplasma:	Isolation of *T. gondii* from placenta, CSF, or blood. Serial determination of IgG antibody (IFA) between 1 and 6 months of age. Determination of IgM antibody in cord serum
Enteroviruses:	Isolation of virus from feces, CSF, throat, nasopharynx
Hepatitis B:	Serial determination of hepatitis B surface antigen (HBsAg), antibody to the surface antigen (Anti HBs), and antibody to the hepatitis B core antigen (Anti HBc)
Herpes Simplex:	Isolation of virus from skin vesicles conjunctiva, throat, CSF, and stools
Varicella:	Isolation of virus from skin lesions
Chlamydia:	Isolation or direct staining of organism from conjunctiva and nasopharynx
Epstein-Barr:	Serial determination of antibodies, culture of cord lymphocytes
AIDS:	Serial determination of antibodies, culture of blood

Modified from Stagno S: Diagnosis of viral infections of the newborn infant. Clin Perinatol **8:**579, 1981.

Modified from Stagno S: Diagnosis of viral infections of the newborn infant. Clin Perinatol **8:**579, 1981.

Treatment at this stage is either incompletely effective or not available.

OPHTHALMIA NEONATORUM. The increased incidence of sexually transmitted diseases in the last four years carries with it a risk for an increase in occurrence of ophthalmia neonatorum caused by *N. gonorrhoeae* and *C. trachomatis*. In developing countries, gonococcus remains a common pathogen responsible for ophthalmia. Prevention of gonococcal ophthalmia is best achieved by recognition and treatment of the infection in the mother prior to delivery, so as to avoid exposure of the neonate. Cultures of the mother for *N. gonorrhoeae* are recommended in both the first and third trimester because 30 per cent of women with gonococcal cervicitis in the first trimester will have a recurrence during the third trimester. Similarly, treatment of the mother with *C. trachomatis* infection will reduce the risk of infection of the infant. All infants now receive eye prophylaxis against these infections immediately after delivery. Erythromycin ointment (0.5 per cent) has emerged as the agent of choice. In addition to being an effective agent against the common pathogens, erythromycin is better tolerated and causes less chemical conjunctivitis than silver nitrate.

Clinical features of conjunctivitis in the infant include purulent discharge, erythema, and swelling of the eyelids, with intense congestion of the conjunctivae. Conjunctival exudates and transudates forming pseudomembranes may often be seen with ophthalmia secondary to Chlamydia, and the palpebral conjunctivae may bleed when touched with a cotton swab. The presence of keratitis suggests serious infection with herpes simplex virus. The onset of clinical symptoms usually occurs on the second day and rarely is seen beyond the 10th day of life; bilateral involvement is common.

Laboratory investigation of the affected infant must include a conjunctival smear, bacterial culture for gonococci or staphylococci, and specific rapid antigen detection tests for Chlamydia. Chlamydial conjunctivitis in young infants is treated with oral erythromycin (50 mg/kg/day) for 14 days. Infants with evidence of gonococcal ophthalmia must be hospitalized. Susceptibility testing of the strain of Gonococcus is recommended because multiple forms of resistance have been reported. Recommended antimicrobial therapy for gonococcal ophthalmia is ceftriaxone, 25 to 50 mg/kg/day intravenously or IM for 7 days. Topical therapy cannot eradicate neonatal ophthalmia due to Gonococcus or Chlamydia.

If the mother and/or her sexual partner are infected with either *N. gonorrhoeae* or *C. trachomatis* at the time of delivery, both should be treated and eye prophylaxis of the infant should be instituted. The infant's eyes should be checked daily during the hospital stay or, with early discharge, the eye condition should be followed closely by the visiting nurse (Laga et al., 1986; Sandstrom, 1986).

Infections of the Premature Infant

The premature infant, as discussed above, has a poorly developed immune system with which to resist infection. In addition, the essential barrier of skin integrity may be breached many times in the hospitalized infant, allowing a portal of entry for microorganisms. These factors predispose the premature baby to several unusual types of infection not seen in the term newborn.

S. EPIDERMIDIS. These organisms are part of the normal human skin flora and, in the adult or term infant, do not cause systemic illness. However, recently it has been recognized that these microorganisms represent an increasing source of morbidity and mortality in the most premature infants. Infected infants often present after the first week of in-hospital life with recurrent apnea, bradycardia, and temperature instability. Both septicemia and meningitis due to *S. epidermidis* have been reported. Parenteral therapy with vancomycin usually results in an effective cure and full recovery.

C. ALBICANS. Colonization of the newborn skin with *C. albicans* is common, and superficial infection presents usually with oral thrush or a diaper dermatitis. However, the premature infant is subject to invasive disease from this yeast-like organism, which may cause both septicemia and meningitis. The portal of entry for infection, as in the case of *S. epidermidis*, may be via indwelling catheters. However, deep spread from contagious surface infection can occur. When promptly recognized through blood, CSF, and urine culture, this infection may be treated successfully with intravenous amphotericin B, although the treatment course may require several weeks of therapy.

NECROTIZING ENTEROCOLITIS. Premature infants are subject to an unusual and potentially fatal disorder of the gastrointestinal tract termed necrotizing enterocolitis. This disorder may present in several different ways, ranging from mild abdominal distention with gastric aspirates to fulminant peritonitis, shock, and disseminated intravascular coagulation (Fig. 63–13). A hallmark feature is the documentation of pneumatosis intestinalis or portal venous gas on abdominal x-ray, both of which may precede intestinal perforation. The injury to the bowel resembles ischemic necrosis, most commonly of the small intestine, although the entire GI tract below the esophagus may be involved. The cause of this disorder is unknown. One hypothesis implicates early feeding of a premature infant in colonization of the bowel with pathogenic organisms which then become invasive (Fig. 63–14). In some series of affected infants, bacteremia with gram-negative or gram-positive organisms has been reported; however, this is not true of all cases. Treatment usually consists of bowel rest, supportive fluid therapy, and broad-spectrum antibiotic coverage (Table 63–17). In some cases, surgical consultation and resection of necrotic bowel may be required. The prognosis for full recovery is best if the segment of the bowel involved is small and surgery is not required.

Cardiovascular Problems

Patent Ductus Arteriosus

Patent ductus arteriosus is a common and potentially serious problem in preterm infants. As a result

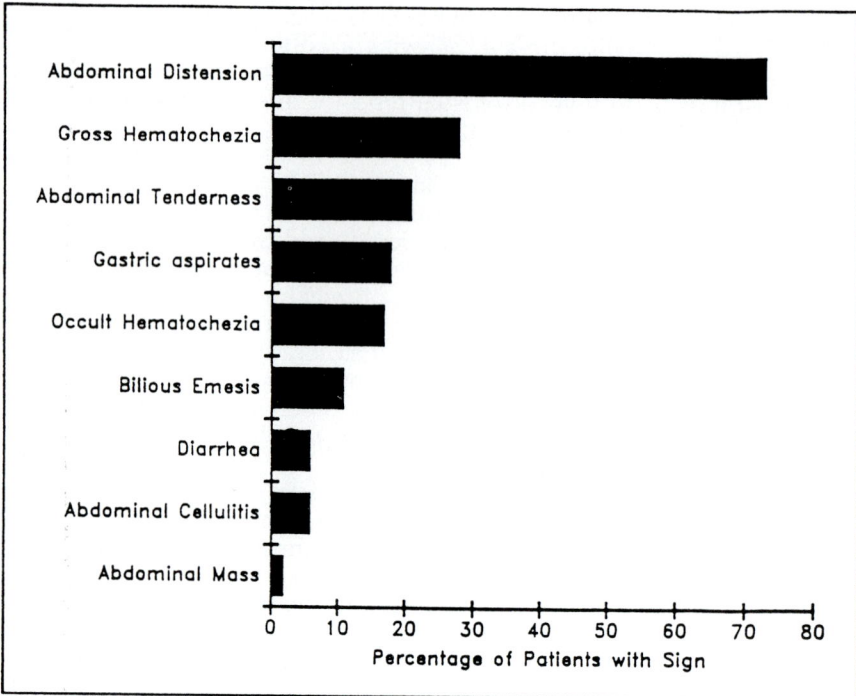

FIGURE 63–13. Presenting clinical features of NEC. (From Walsh MC, Kliegman R: Necrotizing enterocolitis: Treatment based on staging criteria. Pediatr Clin North Am **33**:179, 1986.)

of the postnatal increase in blood oxygen tension, the ductus arteriosus normally constricts shortly after delivery and closes during the first week of life. Prostaglandins are increasingly recognized as the mediators of this phenomenon. The process of ductal closure is delayed in premature infants, and the ductus may remain patent, particularly in infants with respiratory disorders. Paradoxically, in infants with cyanotic congenital heart disease, such as pulmonic atresia in which ductal flow is critical to maintenance of pulmonary blood flow, ductal closure may occur early in life.

Patent ductus arteriosus may result in tachypnea with evidence of congestive heart failure. Apnea may also accompany the onset of clinical symptoms. The peripheral pulses are full and bounding, the precordium is active, and a murmur is present. The characteristic murmur is audible in both systole and diastole; however, in many infants only a systolic murmur is

present, and some infants, depending on pulmonary artery pressure, may have no murmurs at all (Gersony, 1986). The ductus may play a significant role in the pathogenesis of respiratory disorders and may also be responsible for continued dependence on the ventilator. The diagnosis is established echocardiographically. Present technology permits not only delineation of the size of the ductus but also of the degree and direction of flow. In the collaborative study 20 per cent of infants with birth weights below 1750 gm had a hemodynamically significant patent ductus and needed ventilatory support.

The initial approach to management of patent ductus arteriosus is to restrict the fluid intake and commence diuretic therapy. Indomethacin, a prostaglandin synthetase inhibitor, effectively constricts the ductus. The traditional approach is to use indomethacin intravenously (0.2 mg/kg repeated every 12 hours for three doses) in infants who do not respond to 36 to 48 hours of conservative treatment and provided there are no contraindications to its use (Gersony, 1986). Contraindications include poor renal function, thrombocytopenia, a bleeding tendency, and necrotizing enterocolitis. Repeat doses are not necessary if the ductus closes in response to the first dose. Indomethacin is usually successful in about 75 per cent of infants. Treatment failures and infants ineligible for indomethacin may undergo surgical ligation (Strange et al., 1985). Some centers elect to pharmacologically close the ductus before it is symptomatic in premature infants with respiratory disorders.

In situations in which it is imperative to maintain patency of the ductus, prostaglandin E administration has proved to be most efficacious. These include, but are not limited to, cyanotic lesions with reduced pulmonary blood flow, hypoplastic left heart and interrupted aortic arch syndromes, critical aortic stenosis,

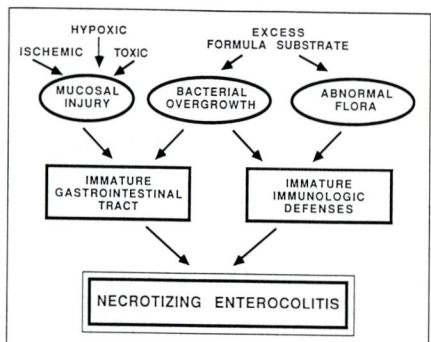

FIGURE 63–14. Pathogenesis of NEC. (From Walsh MC, Kliegman R: Necrotizing enterocolitis: Treatment based on staging criteria. Pediatr Clin North Am **33**:179, 1986.)

TABLE 63–17.   Modified Bell's Staging Criteria for NEC

STAGE	SYSTEMIC SIGNS	INTESTINAL SIGNS	RADIOLOGIC SIGNS	TREATMENT
IA. Suspected NEC	Temperature instability, apnea, bradycardia, lethargy	Elevated pre-gavage residuals, mild abdominal distention, emesis, guaiac-positive stool	Normal or intestinal dilation, mild ileus	NPO, antibiotics ×3d pending culture
IB. Suspected NEC	Same as above	Bright red blood from rectum	Same as above	Same as above
IIA. Definite NEC Mildly ill	Same as above	Same as above, *plus* absent bowel sounds, +/− abdominal tenderness	Intestinal dilation, ileus, pneumatosis intestinalis	NPO, antibiotics ×7–10d if exam is normal in 24–48 hours
IIB. Definite NEC Moderately ill	Same as above, *plus* mild metabolic acidosis, mild thrombocytopenia	Same as above, *plus* absent bowel sounds, definite abdominal tenderness, +/− abdominal cellulitis or right lower quadrant mass	Same as IIA, *plus* portal vein gas, +/− ascites	NPO, antibiotics ×14d NaHCO₃ for acidosis
IIIA. Advanced NEC Severely ill, bowel intact	Same as IIB, *plus* hypotension, bradycardia, severe apnea, combined respiratory and metabolic acidosis, disseminated intravascular coagulation, neutropenia	Same as above, *plus* signs of generalized peritonitis, marked tenderness, and distention of abdomen	Same as IIB, *plus* definite ascites	Same as above, *plus* 200 + ml/kg fluids, inotropic agents, ventilation therapy, paracentesis
IIIB. Advanced NEC Severely ill, bowel perforated	Same as IIIA	Same as IIIA	Same as IIB, *plus* pneumoperitoneum	Same as above, *plus* surgical intervention

From Walsh MC, Kliegman R: Necrotizing enterocolitis: Treatment based on staging criteria. Pediatr Clin North Am **33**:179, 1986.

coarctation of the aorta, and transposition of the great vessels. Prostaglandin E1 and E2 have both been used. Oral and intravenous preparations are both effective, although for critically ill neonates the intravenous route is preferred because absorption is irregular. Manipulation of the ductus has changed the course of the management strategy for some forms of cyanotic congenital heart disease, allowing stabilization of infants for transfer to tertiary units and preoperative stabilization.

Neonatal Hypertension

Systemic arterial hypertension may be detected in 2 per cent of infants admitted to intensive care units (Leder et al., 1986). In defining hypertension in the neonate it is essential to take into consideration birth weight, gestational age, and postnatal age, as well as the clinical history of the infant. In a prospective study of blood pressure during the first month of life, Stork et al. (1984) noted that blood pressure rises acutely during the first 5 days of life and thereafter more gradually. The blood pressure relates to birth weight and remains greater in infants with higher birth weights. No diurnal variation of blood pressure has been found in newborn infants.

Hypertension in the otherwise healthy newborn is usually secondary to renal disease and, in our experience, is most commonly due to renovascular hypertension. Hypertension is also noted in association with raised intracranial pressure; coarctation of the aorta; endocrine disorders including hyperthyroidism, congenital adrenal hyperplasia, or (rarely) pheochromocytoma; and drugs such as phenylephrine, epinephrine, dopamine, and pancuronium. Hypertension may also occur due to intra-aortic thrombosis caused by an indwelling umbilical artery line. Stork et al. found that hypertension occurred with equal frequency when arterial lines were placed in the thoracic or abdominal aorta.

Symptoms associated with hypertension include tachypnea, respiratory distress, mottling of the skin, and even congestive heart failure. Retinopathy may occur soon after onset of hypertension and appears to have features similar to those observed in adults.

Clinical investigation of the infant with hypertension should include ultrasonograms of the kidney and the aorta. The onset of hypertension in a neonate is a significant finding, usually indicative of a potentially life-threatening disorder. Therapy should be directed at control of the hypertension, which commonly responds well to hydralazine therapy. It has been reassuring to note that upon follow-up the hypertension resolves spontaneously in many infants, and there is no evidence of permanent renal impairment.

Neonatal Seizures

Seizures are the most common and distinctive signal of neurologic disturbance in the first month of life (Volpe, 1986). Convulsions have been noted in 1.5 to 3 per 1000 births. However, the true incidence may be obscured by the fact that in many infants the manifestations are extremely subtle and may not be recognized. Newborn infants have less well organized seizure patterns than those observed in adults. Considerable debate surrounds the mechanism and clinical manifestations of neonatal seizures. Technologic developments permitting continuous monitoring of electrical brain activity together with videotape recordings of neonatal activity may result in reclassification of neonatal seizure disorders (Mizrahi and Kellaway, 1984; Mizrahi, 1986).

The etiology of neonatal seizures has been more clearly established as a result of ultrasound, CT scans, and magnetic resonance imaging. Whereas in 1977 the etiology could not be determined in 30 per cent of neonatal seizure disorders, a similar survey in 1986 showed no established etiology in only 2 per cent. It is apparent from Table 63–18 that hypoxic ischemic events are the major cause of neonatal seizures.

Types of Convulsive Patterns

Five patterns of seizure activity are recognized in the newborn (Volpe, 1986). This includes the most common variety designated as *subtle*, wherein sucking, chewing, bicycling, or swimming movements are observed in combination with drooling, apnea, tonic deviation of the eyes, and fluttering of the eyelids. *Multi-focal clonic seizures* are manifested by migratory movements commencing in one or two limbs and moving in a nonorderly fashion to other parts of the body. *Focal seizures* are well-localized and not usually accompanied by unconsciousness. They begin in a single limb and spread to other body parts on the same side. *Tonic seizures* may resemble the decerebrate or decorticate posturing seen in older patients, with tonic extension of all limbs or flexion of upper limbs with extension of the lower limbs. *Myoclonic seizures* are characterized by single or multiple jerks with

flexion of upper or lower limbs. They are rare in the newborn period.

It is important to distinguish seizures from *jitteriness*, which is a stimulus-sensitive series of synchronous movements not accompanied by other signs and which can be terminated with passive flexion. There are no abnormalities of gaze or other eye movements in jittery neonates. The onset, nature, and duration of seizures are all important considerations regarding the prognosis for neonatal seizures. If the seizures are easily controlled and the electroencephalogram returns to normal, the outcome is usually good. Persistence of clinical and electrical seizure activity is ominous.

Anticonvulsant Therapy

It is important to recognize and treat the many metabolic disturbances that may result in neonatal seizures. Included among these are hypoglycemia, hypocalcemia, urea cycle disorders, pyridoxine deficiency, ketotic and non-ketotic hyperglycinemia, and other inborn errors of metabolism. Withdrawal from drugs rarely causes seizures.

Phenobarbital is the mainstay of anticonvulsant therapy. It limits the spread of seizure activity and may elevate the seizure threshold by increasing the activity of the inhibitory neurotransmitters. Phenobarbital is readily absorbed orally, and CSF and brain tissue levels are equal to serum levels. The majority of the phenobarbital is metabolized in the liver; the rest is excreted directly via the kidney.

A loading dose of 20 mg/kg is given intravenously and may be followed with 5 mg/kg every 5 minutes up to a total loading dose of 40 mg/kg in order to control status epilepticus. A maintenance dose of 3 to 4 mg/kg/day is recommended and a serum level of 30 μg/ml is desirable for seizure control (Volpe, 1986). Phenytoin may be used in combination with phenobarbital. It is not absorbed orally, but its activity is similar to that of phenobarbital.

The duration of anticonvulsant therapy is determined by the clinical course. Medication may be discontinued during the first month of life if clinical recovery appears to be complete as evidenced by a normal neurologic examination together with absence of seizures electrically and clinically (Bergman et al., 1983; Goldberg et al., 1986).

Legido et al. (1991) used electroencephalography (EEG) to relate neonatal seizures to the neurologic outcome in 40 infants with seizures of varying cause. The outcome was unfavorable in 70 per cent with the development of epilepsy in 56 per cent, cerebral palsy in 63 per cent, and developmental delay in 67 per cent. The onset of seizures on the first day of life, seizure frequency (more than 2 per hour), and an abnormal EEG background predicted a poor outcome.

Congenital Malformations

As a result of advances in the care of immature low-birth-weight infants, congenital malformations and genetic disorders have assumed an important role as

TABLE 63–18. Etiology of Neonatal Seizures

	1977	1986
Hypoxic ischemic encephalopathy	36%	46%
Intracranial hemorrhage	—	15%
Cerebral infarction	—	6%
Hypoglycemia	4%	5%
Hypocalcemia	12%	0%
Intracranial infection	12%	17%
Developmental defects	5%	8%
Drug withdrawal	0%	0%
Unknown	30%	2%

a cause of morbidity and mortality during the first month of life. Not all malformations will be detected at birth. Thus surveys may underestimate the true incidence. Nonetheless, as noted in a study of 18,155 newborns, Holmes (1976) documented that 2 per cent of newborns have a serious malformation that has surgical or cosmetic importance. Furthermore, the National Foundation of March of Dimes of New York estimates that genetic errors afflict more than 15 million persons in the United States with mental retardation, diabetes, complete or partial blindness, impaired hearing, defects in specific organ systems, and congenital bone, muscle, or joint disease.

There are multiple causes of birth defects or genetic disorders ranging from chromosomal abnormalities, single gene disorders, environmental agents, multifactorial disorders, and many still classified as unknown. It is important that a comprehensive evaluation be offered to the infants and families when birth defects are noted. This includes a careful history noting family pedigree and history of pregnancy, physical and laboratory studies of both the infant and family members if indicated, genetic counseling, and provision of psychosocial support for the family. The type and etiology of major malformations are shown in Table 63—19.

As noted in Chapters 14 and 15, birth defects have been recognized with increasing frequency antenatally. Some of the factors that may raise the index of suspicion, prompting a careful anatomic survey of the fetus, include a positive family history, advanced maternal age, exposure during the pregnancy to teratogens including drugs (anticonvulsants and so on), or the detection antenatally of abnormalities in the volume of amniotic fluid, elevated alpha-fetoprotein,

or fetal growth restriction. After delivery, all infants are carefully examined for birth defects and should be more closely observed and followed if they are undergrown or have abnormal facial features, multiple minor malformations, and a single umbilical artery or single palmar crease. Clinical examination may be complemented by ultrasonographic, radiographic, hematologic, biochemical, and chromosomal studies.

Esophageal Atresia and Tracheoesophageal Fistula

Normal division of the foregut into trachea and esophagus occurs during the fourth week of gestation. Any interruption in embryonic septation will result in esophageal atresia (EA) and tracheoesophageal fistula (TEF). These abnormalities commonly occur together but occasionally appear separately. The most common form of malformation is EA with distal TEF (87 per cent). Isolated esophageal atresia and isolated tracheoesophageal fistula occur 8 and 4 per cent of the time, respectively (Ashcraft and Holder, 1976). The overall incidence is one in 3000 births. The diagnosis should be suspected when there is a history of prematurity (35 per cent) and polyhydramnios. The latter is present in 32 per cent of infants with EA and distal TEF and in 85 per cent of infants with isolated EA.

The presence of excess mucus ("juicy baby") within the first few hours after birth suggests EA with or without TEF. There may be associated respiratory distress marked by tachypnea and cyanosis. Early diagnosis is important to avoid complications of aspiration and chemical pneumonitis. Resistance to a nasogastric tube 9 to 13 cm from the nares suggests EA. A roentgenogram of the chest and abdomen will show the radiopaque catheter lying in a blind esophageal pouch. Associated abnormalities are found in 50 per cent of infants with EA and TEF. Air in the gastrointestinal tract indicates patency of the fistula. Cardiac and vertebral anomalies may be seen as part of the VATER (vertebral, vascular, anal, tracheoesophageal, renal, and radial) association (Smith, 1982).

Early management requires gastrostomy and continuous suction of the blind upper pouch. Definitive surgical repair usually is undertaken later when the infant's condition is stable. Primary repairs depend upon how closely the esophageal ends are juxtaposed. Postoperative complications are the result of leakage of fluid from the esophageal anastomosis and of poor distal esophageal peristalsis. Outlook is good in infants with isolated EA or TEF.

Abdominal Wall Defects

Defects in the abdominal wall may result from obstruction of the omphalomesenteric vessel, resulting in gastroschisis, or from failure of normal embryonic regression of intestine from umbilical stalk into the abdominal coelom during the 10th gestational week, resulting in the development of an omphalocele. Understanding this basic embryology allows the clinician to differentiate these entities (Table 63–20).

Initial treatment should be directed at maintaining body temperature and fluid balance and preventing

TABLE 63–19.   Type and Etiology of Major Malformations in 18,155 Newborns

MALFORMATION		NUMBER
Multifactorial inheritance		128 (0.7%)
Anencephaly-myelomeningocele- encephalocele	25	
Cardiac anomalies	45	
Cleft lip and/or palate	14	
Clubfoot	21	
Congenital hip dislocation	12	
Hypospadias	8	
Omphalocele	2	
Bilateral renal agenesis	1	
Mendelian inheritance		67 (0.4%)
Autosomal dominant disorders (excluding polydactyly)	57	
Autosomal recessive disorders	9	
X-linked recessive disorders	1	
Chromosome abnormalities		27 (0.2%)
Down's syndrome	21	
Trisomy 13	3	
Other	3	
Teratogenic conditions		15 (0.1%)
Infants of diabetic mothers	14	
Effects of warfarin	1	
Unknown		107 (0.6%)
Total number affected		344 (2%)

Reproduced by permission from Kurczynski TW: Congenital malformations. *In* Fanaroff AA, Martin RJ (ed): Neonatal-Perinatal Medicine. 5th ed. St. Louis, Mosby-Year Book, 1992.

TABLE 63–20. Differential Diagnosis: Omphalocele vs. Gastroschisis

	OMPHALOCELE	GASTROSCHISIS
Incidence	1 per 5,000 births	1 per 50,000 births
Location of defect	Central abdomen	Right paraumbilical area
Covering sac	Amnion and peritoneum	Absent
Umbilical ring	Absent	Normal
Herniation of liver	Common	Rare
Associated anomalies	Beckwith syndrome	Intestinal atresia (15%)
	Trisomy 13 or 18	
	Exstrophy of bladder and cloaca	

From Grosfeld JL, Davies L, Weber TR: Congenital abdominal wall defects: Current management and survival. Surg Clin North Am **61**:1037, 1981.

infection. A nasogastric catheter should be placed. Exposed viscera should be covered with warm saline dressings. Frequently, a staged operative closure with the use of a Silastic (silicone) "chimney" is performed. Postoperative complications consist of respiratory embarrassment and pulmonary hypertension, small bowel perforation, and intestinal obstruction. Malrotation of the bowel is present in both conditions.

The mortality rate in infants with gastroschisis can be as high as 60 per cent, but improved survival has been noted with the introduction of total parenteral nutrition (Grosfeld et al., 1981). Outlook for infants with omphalocele relates directly to the presence of associated anomalies.

Neural Tube Defects (Meningomyelocele)

Meningomyelocele results from failure of neural tube closure during the third to fourth week of gestation. The incidence is one to three per 1000 births, 2 to 3 per cent in a second child with one previous affected sibling, and 5 per cent in a third child with two previous affected siblings.

Physical examination demonstrates a thin membrane covering the defect. Leakage of spinal fluid is not uncommon and predisposes the infant to infection. Prognosis for ambulation is determined by identifying the level of sensory and motor function. Hydrocephalus will occur in 60 to 85 per cent of low lumbar and sacral defects and in 96 per cent of high lumbar and thoracic lesions. Outcome is poor with high lumbar or thoracic defects, severe hydrocephalus (less than 1 cm of frontal cerebral mantle), or other brain malformations and/or associated anomalies (Gross et al., 1983). Immediate closure of the defect confers a 90 per cent chance of survival.

Once the defect is closed, a multidisciplinary approach, involving a neurosurgeon, orthopedist, urologist, pediatrician, social worker, physical therapist, and psychologist, is required.

Neonatal Screening for Metabolic Diseases

The American Academy of Pediatrics has recommended metabolic screening of the infant's blood as a preventive public health measure that should be performed on all neonates prior to discharge from the nursery. All states in the US currently screen for the disorders phenylketonuria and congenital hypothy-

roidism. Screening for sickle cell disease has also been recommended by a National Institute of Health Consensus Conference, and many states in addition screen for galactosemia and homocystinuria. These disorders have been selected for early screening because detection and prompt treatment in infancy can prevent mental retardation or severe life-threatening illness.

The most common disorder detected by screening is sickle cell disease, with an incidence as high as 1 in 400 births. Early identification allows prevention of infection in childhood, as well as prompt medical intervention if sickle cell crisis develops. Hypothyroidism occurs in 1 in 5000 deliveries, and may result in permanent mental retardation unless detected and treated with thyroid hormone replacement. Phenylketonuria is a rare defect in phenylalanine metabolism (1 in 14,000 deliveries) in which severe mental retardation may develop if the infant is not provided with a special formula low in phenylalanine. Galactosemia is also a rare metabolic defect (1 in 50,000 births) in which life-threatening toxic effects of elevated blood galactose may occur in the affected infant after feeding. A special galactose-free diet is essential for survival and normal development of these infants. Homocystinuria is a disorder of methionine metabolism, which may result in mental retardation and severe disability unless detected in infancy and treated with dietary management.

Blood specimens for these disorders are obtained from every neonate before the baby is discharged from the nursery. The specimens are forwarded to the responsible laboratory, and results of the tests are returned to the physician ordering them. Infants with abnormal screening tests are then referred for definitive medical evaluation. Earlier discharge of the mother-infant dyad has prompted reorganization of the testing procedure, with home screening when necessary. The positive cost:benefit ratio of newborn metabolic screening continues to justify the personnel and financial commitment to these disorders.

NEURODEVELOPMENTAL OUTCOME

Advances in both perinatal and neonatal care have largely been responsible for improved survival in high-risk neonates. Following the introduction of modern neonatal intensive care in the 1960s, there was a decrease in adverse neurodevelopmental sequelae as compared to the preceding era. During the 1970s and

1980s, there has been a continued decrease in mortality, so that the absolute number of both healthy and neurologically impaired very-low-birth-weight survivors has actually increased (Horwood et al., 1982). It is important to realize, however, that conditions of presumed genetic and prenatal origin account for more children with neurodevelopmental disorders than problems arising out of the perinatal period. Also, because more infants are born full-term, more term children probably have cerebral palsy than preterm infants. Infants who are at risk for later neurodevelopmental problems include those who had severe asphyxia, extensive intraventricular hemorrhage, periventricular leukomalacia, meningitis, or seizures, as well as infants with multisystem congenital malformations and those of very low birth weight.

Comparisons are inevitably made between results of neurodevelopmental follow-up from various tertiary perinatal centers (Hack et al., 1983). Weight-selected samples from different units may not be comparable, however, since outcome is heavily influenced by (1) the socioeconomic status of the parents, (2) the incidence of extreme prematurity, (3) admission policies, and (4) the proportion of inborn patients at any center. Although regional results do reflect a more accurate picture of outcome because they include all infants born in an area, such expensive and time-consuming studies are rarely available.

General Problems

Neonatal intensive care has resulted in an increased morbidity resulting from various medical complications, including chronic neonatal lung disease, increased susceptibility to respiratory infection, sequelae of necrotizing enterocolitis, and cholestatic jaundice. These in turn may contribute to multiple rehospitalizations, poor physical growth, and an increase in postneonatal deaths. Up to 33 per cent of infants with birth weight less than 1.5 kg are rehospitalized during the first year of life and up to 10 per cent during the second and third years (Hack et al., 1983). Children with neurologic sequelae such as cerebral palsy and hydrocephalus have an even higher rate of rehospitalization for such reasons as shunt complications, orthopedic correction of spasticity, and eye surgery.

Intracranial Hemorrhage

Intracerebral hemorrhage occurs in up to 50 per cent of very low-birth-weight infants and is thought to represent a substantial cause of morbidity and mortality in these patients. Bleeding occurs in the subependymal germinal matrix and may extend to the lateral ventricles and brain parenchyma. Potential etiologic factors include capillary fragility, abnormal regulation of cerebral blood flow, air leaks, and blood gas derangements. Follow-up studies demonstrate that only grade IV intraventricular hemorrhages (which demonstrate intraparenchymal extension) have a poor prognosis for neurologic outcome. Grade I (subependymal) and grade II (subependymal plus intraventric-

ular) hemorrhages are not thought to impair the changes for a normal neurodevelopmental prognosis. Grade III hemorrhage is associated with ventricular dilatation; the prognosis will depend, in part, on the extent of the resultant hydrocephalus. Recent studies indicate that leukomalacia or intraparenchymal lesions that demonstrate echodensity on ultrasound may occur independently of intraventricular hemorrhage, are the result of necrosis secondary to ischemia, and carry a poor prognosis for subsequent normal development (Guzzetta et al., 1986; Hanigan et al., 1991).

Growth Delay

Intrauterine and/or neonatal growth retardation occur in up to 50 per cent of very-low-birth-weight infants. The poor neonatal growth is related to inadequate nutrition during the acute phase of neonatal disease and to chronic medical sequelae that result in increased caloric requirements. These include chronic lung disease and malabsorption secondary to necrotizing enterocolitis or cholestatic liver disease. Poor feeding in neurologically impaired children and the lack of an optimal nurturing environment in the nursery may also affect neonatal growth. As these conditions gradually resolve and an optimal home environment is provided, catch-up body growth may occur during the first 2 to 3 years of life.

Growth after discharge is a good measure of physical, neurologic, and environmental well-being. To promote optimal catch-up growth of high-risk infants, neonatal nutrition needs to be maximized and sufficient calories provided during the recovery phase. This is especially important because catch-up of head circumference in both appropriate and small-for-gestational-age children occurs only during the first 6 to 12 months after term.

Neurodevelopmental Disorders

A very high incidence of *transient* neurologic abnormalities occurs in high-risk infants. These include abnormalities of muscle tone such as hypotonia and hypertonia. Some degree of physiologic hypertonia normally exists during the first 3 months, and so it may be difficult to diagnose early spasticity related to cerebral palsy. Children who will develop cerebral palsy have hypotonia initially (poor head control and back support), and spasticity of the extremities develops only later. Spasticity during the first 3 to 4 months is a poor prognostic sign. Persistence of primitive reflexes might also be a sign of early cerebral palsy. Although mild hypertonia or hypotonia persisting at 8 months usually resolves by the second year, it might indicate later subtle neurologic dysfunction (Georgieff et al., 1986).

Major neurologic sequelae can usually be diagnosed during the latter part of the first year of life in up to 10 per cent of high-risk newborns, or even earlier if signs are severe. Major neurologic handicap is usually classified as cerebral palsy (spastic diplegia, spastic quadriplegia, spastic hemiplegia, or paresis), hydro-

Table 63–21. Very-low-birth-weight (<1.5 kg) Infant Outcome: Inborn Infants at Rainbow Babies and Childrens Hospital* 1986–1987 (n = 255)

SURVIVAL/OUTCOME	%
20–month survival	78
20–month outcome	
Neurosensory impairment and/or developmental quotient <80	16
Neurosensory impairment and/or developmental quotient <70	10
Neurodevelopmental outcome	
Normal outcome	84
Major congenital malformation	2
Neurosensory abnormality	7†
Developmental quotient <80	7‡

*Cleveland, Ohio.

†Includes spastic diplegia (4%), severe visual impairment (1.2%), and hypotonia (1.8%).

‡Excluding children with neurosensory abnormality. Ten children had Bayley developmental quotients 70–80 and two had developmental quotients <70.

cephalus (with or without accompanying cerebral palsy or sensory deficits), blindness (usually caused by retrolental fibroplasia), seizures, or deafness (Table 63—21). The intellectual outcome of these children may differ greatly according to the neurologic diagnosis. For example, children with spastic quadriplegia usually have severe mental retardation, whereas children with spastic diplegia or hemiplegia may have intact mental functioning. This is not always measurable until after 2 or 3 years of age.

Most neurologic or physical problems either resolve or become permanent during the first year of life. There is a close relationship between abnormal neurologic findings at one year in very-low-birth-weight infants and school performance at as late as 7 years (Vohr and Garcia Coll, 1985). During the second year the environmental effects of maternal education and social class begin to play a major role on the various cognitive outcome measures. Further problems may emerge, such as subtle motor, visual, and behavioral difficulties. These are best diagnosed and treated in a psychologic and educational rather than a medical follow-up setting.

REFERENCES

Allen R, Sorab J, Gonik B: Risk factors for shoulder dystocia: an engineering study of physician applied forces. Obstet Gyneol **77**:352, 1991.

Ashcraft KW, Holder TM: Esophageal atresia and tracheoesophageal fistula malformations. Surg Clin North Am **56**:299, 1976.

Babson SG, Benda GI: Growth graphs for the clinical assessment of infants of varying gestational age. J Pediatr **89**:814, 1976.

Ballard JL, Novak KK, Driver M: A simplified score for assessment of fetal maturation of newly born infants. J Pediatr **95**:769, 1979.

Ballard JL, Khoury JC, Wedig K, et al: New Ballard score, expanded to include extremely premature infants. J Pediatr **119**:417, 1991.

Ballard RA, Ballard PL, Creasy RK, et al: Respiratory distress in very-low-birth-weight infants after prenatal thyrotropin-releasing hormone and glucocorticoid. Lancet **339**:510, 1992.

Bancalari E, Gerhardt T: Bronchopulmonary dysplasia. Pediatr Clin North Am **33**:1, 1986.

Bancalari E: Neonatal chronic lung disease: *In* Fanaroff AA and

Martin RJ (eds): Neonatal-Perinatal Medicine. 5th ed. St. Louis, CV Mosby, 1992.

Becerra JE, Khoury MJ, Cordero JF, et al: Diabetes mellitus during pregnancy and the risks for specific birth defects: A population-based case-control study. Pediatrics **85**:1, 1989.

Bergman I, Painter MJ, Hirsch RP, et al: Outcome in neonates with convulsions treated in an intensive care unit. Ann Neurol **1**:219, 1983.

Bergsma D (ed): Birth Defects Compendium. 2nd ed. National Foundation, March of Dimes, New York, Alan R. Liss, Inc., 1977.

Black VD, Lubchenco LO, Koops BL et al: Neonatal hyperviscosity: randomized study of effect of partial plasma exchange transfusion in long-term outcome. Pediatrics **75**:1048, 1985.

Bloss RS, Aranda JV, Beardmore HE, et al: Congenital diaphragmatic hernia: Pathophysiology and pharmacologic support. Surgery **89**:518, 1981.

Boucher M, Yonekura ML: Perinatal listeriosis (early onset): Correlation of antenatal manifestations and neonatal outcome. Obstet Gynecol **68**:593, 1986.

Boyer UM, Gotoff SP: Prevention of early-onset neonatal group B streptococcal disease with selective intrapartum chemoprophylaxis. N Engl J Med **314**:1665, 1986.

Brann BS IV, Qualls C, Papile L, et al: Measurement of progressive cerebral ventriculomegaly in infants after grades III and IV intraventricular hemorrhages. J Pediatr **117**:615, 1990.

Brunskill AJ, Rossing MA, Connell FA, et al: Antecedents of macrosomia. Pediatr Perinat Epidemiol **5**:392, 1991.

Carlo WA, Martin RJ: Principles of neonatal assisted ventilation. Pediatr Clin North Am **33**:221, 1986.

Carlo WA, Siner B, Chatburn RL, et al: Early randomized intervention with high-frequency jet ventilation in respiratory distress syndrome. J Pediatr **117**:765, 1990.

Carson BS, Losey RW, Bowes WA Jr, et al: Combined obstetric and pediatric approach to prevent meconium aspiration syndrome. Am J Obstet Gynecol **126**:12, 1976.

Collaborative Group on Antenatal Steroid Therapy: Effect of antenatal dexamethasone administration on the prevention of respiratory distress syndrome. Am J Obstet Gynecol **141**:276, 1981.

Collaborative Dexamethasone Trial Group: Dexamethasone therapy in neonatal chronic lung disease: An international placebo-controlled trial. Pediatrics **88**:421, 1991.

Costarino AT, Gruskay JA, Corcoran L, et al: Sodium restriction versus daily maintenance replacement in very-low-birth-weight premature infants. J Pediatr **120**:99, 1992.

Cunningham AS, Lawson EE, Martin RJ, et al: Tracheal suction and meconium: a proposed standard of care. J Pediatr **116**:153, 1990.

Dubowitz L, Dubowitz V, Goldberg C: Clinical assessment of gestational age in the newborn infant. J Pediatr **77**:1, 1970.

Enhorning G, Shennan A, Possmayer F, et al: Prevention of neonatal respiratory distress syndrome by tracheal installation of surfactant: A randomized clinical trial. Pediatrics **76**:145, 1985.

Ennever FJ, Knox I, Speck WT: Differences in bilirubin isomer composition in infants treated with green and white phototherapy. J Pediatr **109**:119, 1986.

Garland SM, Fliegner JR: Group B streptococcus (GBS) and neonatal infections: the case for intrapartum chemoprophylaxis. Aust NZ J Obstet **31**:119, 1991.

Georgieff MK, Bernbaum JC, Hoffman-Williamson M, Daft A: Abnormal truncal muscle tone as a useful early method for developmental delay in low birth weight infants. Pediatrics **77**:659, 1986.

Gersony WM: Patent ductus arteriosus in the neonate. Pediatr Clin North Am **33**:545, 1986.

Glass P, Miller M, Short B: Mortality for survivors of extracorporeal membrane oxygenation: neurodevelopmental outcome at 1 year of age. Pediatrics **83**:72, 1989.

Goldberg RN, Moscosco P, Bauer GR, et al: Use of barbiturate therapy in severe perinatal asphyxia: A randomized controlled trial. J Pediatr **109**:851, 1986.

Grosfeld JL, Dawes L, Weber TR: Congenital abdominal wall defects: Current management and survival. Surg Clin North Am **61**:1037, 1981.

Gross RH, Cox A, Tatyrek R, et al: Early management and decision making for the treatment of myelomeningocele. Pediatrics **72**:450, 1983.

Guzzetta F, Shackelford GD, Volpe S, Perlman JM, Volpe JJ: Periventricular intraparenchymal echodensities in the premature newborn: Critical determinant of neurologic outcome. Pediatrics **78:**995, 1986.

Hack M, Breslau N, Weissman B, et al: Effect of very low birth weight and subnormal head size on cognitive abilities at school age. N Engl J Med **325:**231, 1991.

Hack M, Caron B, Rivers A, Fanaroff AA: The very-low-birth-weight infant: The broader spectrum of morbidity during infancy and early childhood. J Develop Behavior Pediatr **4:**243, 1983.

Hack M, Fanaroff AA: Changes in the delivery room care of the extremely small infant (<750 gram): Effects on morbidity and outcome. N Engl J Med **314:**660, 1986.

Hack M, Fanaroff AA: Outcome of growth failure associated with preterm birth. Clin Obstet Gynecol **27:**647, 1984.

Hanigan WC, Morgan AM, Anderson RJ, et al: Incidence and neurodevelopmental outcome of periventricular hemorrhage and hydrocephalus in a regional population of very-low-birth-weight infants. Neurosurgery **29:**701, 1991.

HIFI Study Group: High-frequency oscillatory ventilation compared with conventional mechanical ventilation in the treatment of respiratory failure in preterm infants. N Engl J Med **320:**88, 1989.

Holmes LB: Type and etiology of major malformations in 18,155 newborns. N Engl J Med **195:**204, 1976.

Horwood SP, Boyle MH, Torrance GW, Sinclair JC: Mortality and morbidity of 500 to 1,400 gram birth weight infants live-born to residents of a defined geographic region before and after neonatal intensive care. Pediatrics **69:**612, 1982.

Jobe AH: The developmental biology of the lung. *In* Fanaroff AA, Martin RJ (eds) Neonatal-Perinatal Medicine, 5th ed. St. Louis, CV Mosby, 1992.

Jones RAK, Robertsen NRC: Small for dates babies: Are they really a problem? Arch Dis Child **61:**877, 1986.

Jovanovic-Peterson L, Peterson CM, Reed GF, et al: Maternal postprandial glucose levels and infant birth weight: The diabetes in early pregnancy study. J Obstet Gynaecol **164:**103, 1991.

Keszler M, Donn SM, Bucciarelli RL, et al: Multicenter controlled trial comparing high frequency jet ventilation in newborn infants with pulmonary interstitial emphysema. **119:**85, 1991.

King RJ: Composition and metabolism of the apolipo-proteins of pulmonary surfactant. Ann Rev Physiol **47:**775, 1985.

Klein N, Hack M, Gallagher J, Fanaroff AA: Preschool performance of children with normal intelligence who were very low birth weight infants. Pediatrics **75:**531, 1985.

Kliegman RM, Fanaroff AA: Developmental metabolism and nutrition. *In* Gregory GA (ed): Pediatric Anaesthesia. New York, Churchill Livingstone, 1983.

Koops BL, Morgan LJ, Battaglia FC: Neonatal mortality risk in relation to birth weight and gestational age: Update. J Pediatr **101:**969, 1982.

Laga M, Naamara, Brunham RC, et al: Single-dose therapy of gonococcal ophthalmia neonatorum with ceftriaxone. N Engl J Med **315:**1382, 1986.

Leder ME, Kligman RM, Fanaroff AA: Epidemiology and management of severe symptomatic neonatal hypertension. Am J Perinatol **3:**235, 1986.

Legido A, Clancy RR, Berman PH (Children's Hospital of Philadelphia; University of Pennsylvania): Neurologic outcome after electroencephalographically proven neonatal seizures. Pediatrics **88:**583, 1991.

Liechty EA, Donovan E, Purohit D, et al: Reduction of neonatal mortality after multiple doses of bovine surfactant in low birth weight neonates with respiratory distress syndrome. Pediatrics **88:**19, 1991.

Long W, et al: A controlled trial of synthetic surfactant in infants weighing 1250 g or more with respiratory distress syndrome. N Engl J Med **325:**1696, 1991.

Lorentz JM, Kleinman LI, Kotagel UR, Reller MD: Water balance in very low birth weight infants: Relationship to water and sodium intake and effect on outcome. J Pediatr **101:**423, 1982.

Lowe J, Papile L: Neurodevelopmental performance of very-low-birthweight infants with mild periventricular, intraventricular hemorrhage: Outcome at 5 to 6 years of age. Am J Dis Child **144:**1242, 1990.

Lucas A, Cole TJ (MRC Dunn Nutrition Unit, Cambridge, England): Breast milk and neonatal necrotising enterocolitis. Lancet **336:**1519, 1990.

Maisels MJ, Gifford K: Normal serum bilirubin levels in the newborn and the effect of breast-feeding. Pediatrics **78:**837, 1986.

Maisels MJ, Plunkett JW, Roloff DW, Pasick PL, Stiefel GS: Growth and development of preterm infants with respiratory distress syndrome and bronchopulmonary dysplasia. Pediatrics **77:**345, 1986.

Martin RJ, Klaus MH, Fanaroff AA: Respiratory problems. *In* Klaus MH, Fanaroff AA (eds): Care of the High Risk Neonate. 3rd ed. Philadelphia, WB Saunders Company, 1986a.

Martin RJ, Miller MJ, Carlo WA: Pathogenesis of apnea in preterm infants. J Pediatr **109:**733, 1986b.

Martin RJ, Fanaroff AA: The respiratory distress syndrome and its management. *In* Martin RJ, Fanaroff AA (eds): Neonatal-Perinatal Medicine. 5th ed. St. Louis, CV Mosby, 1992.

Merritt TA, Hallman M, Bloom BT, et al: Prophylactic treatment of very premature infants with human surfactant. N Engl J Med **315:**785, 1986.

Miller MJ, DiFiore JM, Strohl KP, Martin RJ. Effect of nasal CPAP on supraglottic and total pulmonary resistance in preterm infants. J Appl Physiol **6:**141, 1990.

Mills JL, Knapp RH, Simpson JL, et al: Lack of relation of increased malformation rates in infants of diabetic mothers to glycemic control during organogenesis. N Engl J Med **318:**671, 1988.

Mizrahi EM: Neonatal electroencephalography: Clinical features of the newborn, techniques of recording, and characteristics of the normal EEG. Am J EEG Technol **26:**81, 1986.

Mizrahi EM, Kellaway P: Seizures of neonates and young infants with and without accompanying EEG epileptiform activity: An EEG/polygraph/video monitoring study. Epilepsia **25:**668, 1984.

Moya ER, Perez A, Reece EA: Severe fetomaternal hemorrhage: A report of 4 cases. J Reprod Med **32:**243, 1987.

Murphy DJ Jr, Reller MD, Meyer RA, Kaplan S: Left ventricular function in normal newborn infants and asymptomatic infants with neonatal polycythemia. Am Heart J **112:**542, 1986.

Murphy JD, Vawter GF, Reid LM: Pulmonary vascular disease in fatal meconium aspiration. J Pediatr **104:**758, 1984.

National Institute of Child Health and Human development: Randomized, controlled trial of phototherapy for neonatal hyperbilirubinemia. Pediatrics **75**(Suppl 2, part 2): 1985.

Nelson KB, Ellenberg JH: Apgar scores as predictors of chronic neurologic sequelae. Pediatrics **68:**36, 1981.

Newman TB, Maisels MJ: Evaluation and treatment of jaundice in the term newborn: A kinder, gentler approach. Pediatrics **89:**809, 1992.

Nicolaides KH, Bradley RJ, Soothill PW, et al: Maternal oxygen therapy for intrauterine growth retardation. Lancet **i:**942, 1987.

Oski FA, Naiman JL: Hematologic problems in the newborn. *In* Problems in Clinical Pediatrics. Philadelphia, WB Saunders Company, 1982.

Pildes R: Infants of diabetic mothers. N Engl J Med **289:**902, 1973.

Pildes RS, Lilien LD: Carbohydrate disorders. *In* Fanaroff AA, Martin RJ (eds): Neonatal-Perinatal Medicine. St. Louis, CV Mosby, 1987.

Rossi EM, Philipson EH, Williams TG, et al: Meconium aspiration syndrome: intrapartum and neonatal attributes. Am J Obstet Gynecol **161:**1106, 1989.

Sandstrom I: Ophthalmia neonatorum with special reference to chlamydia trachomatis: Diagnosis and treatment. Acta Paediatr Scand Suppl 330, 1986.

Sills J, Davis R, Randel R, et al: Left to right patent ductus arteriosus shunting in term infants recovering from persistent pulmonary hypertension. (Abstract) Clin Res 128A, 1984.

Sinclair JC: Temperature Regulation and Energy Metabolism in the Newborn. New York, Grune & Stratton, 1978.

Skalina (Leder) ME, Kliegman RM, Fanaroff AA: Epidemiology and management of severe symptomatic neonatal hypertension. Am J Perinatol **3:**235, 1986.

Smith DW: Recognizable patterns of human malformation. Philadelphia, WB Saunders Company, 1982.

Srinivasan G, Pildes RS, Cattamanchi G, et al: Plasma glucose values in normal neonates. A new look. J Pediatr **109:**114, 1986.

Stagno S, Pass RF, Cloud G, et al: Primary cytomegalovirus infection in pregnancy: Incidence, transmission to fetus and clinical outcome. JAMA **256:**1904, 1986.

Standards for CPR and ECC, Part VII: Neonatal advanced life support. JAMA **268:**2276, 1992.

Stolar C, Dillon P, Reyes C: Selective use of extracorporeal membrane oxygenation in the management of congenital diaphragmatic hernia. J Pediatr Surg **23:**207, 1988.

Stork EK, Carlo WA, Kliegman R, Fanaroff AA: Hypertension redefined for critically ill neonates. Pediatr Res **18:**321A, 1984.

Strange MJ, Myers G, Kirklin JK, et al: Surgical closure of patent ductus arteriosus does not increase the risk of intraventricular hemorrhage in the preterm infant. J Pediatr **107:**602, 1985.

Sweet AY: Classification of the low-birth-weight infant. *In* Klaus MH, Fanaroff AA (ed): Care of the High-Risk Neonate. Philadelphia, WB Saunders Company, 1986.

Tooley WH, Phibbs RH, Sohleuter MA: Intrauterine asphyxia and the Developing Fetal Brain. Chicago, Year Book Medical Publishers, 1977.

Veen S, Ens-Dokkum MH, Schreuder AM, et al: Impairments, disabilities, and handicaps of very preterm and very-low-birth-weight infants at five years of age. Lancet **338:**33, 1991.

Veille JC, Sivakoff M, Fanaroff AA: Ontogeny of diabetic cardiomyopathy. Pediatr Res **21:**389A, 1987.

Victorian Infant Collaborative Study Group: Eight-year outcome in infants with birth weight of 500 to 999 grams: Continuing regional study of 1979 and 1980 births. J Pediatr **118:**761, 1991.

Vohr BR, Garcia Coll CT: Neurodevelopmental and school performance of very low birth weight infants: A seven-year longitudinal study. Pediatrics **76:**345, 1985.

Volpe JJ: Neurology of the Newborn. 2nd ed. Philadelphia, WB Saunders Company, 1986.

Walsh MC, Klugman R: Necrotizing enterocolitis: Treatment based on staging criteria. Pediatr Clin North Am **33:**179, 1986.

Walther FJ, Ramaekers LHJ: Neonatal morbidity of SGA infants in relation to their nutritional status at birth. Acta Paediatr Scand **71:**437, 1982.

Walther F, Siassi B, King J, et al: Cardiac output in infants of insulin-dependent diabetic mothers. J Pediatr **107:**109, 1985.

Warshaw JB: Intrauterine growth retardation: Adaptation or pathology? Commentary. Pediatrics **76:**998, 1985.

Weber HS, Copel JA, Reece EA, et al: Cardiac growth in fetuses with good metabolic control. J Pediatr **118:**103, 1991.

Wiswell TE, Tuggle JM, Turner BS: Meconium aspiration syndrome: Have we made a difference? Pediatrics **85:**715, 1990.

Wolfson MR, Shaffer TH: Liquid ventilation during early development: theory, physiologic processes and application. J Develop Physiol **13:**1, 1990.

ANESTHETIC CONSIDERATIONS

C H A P T E R

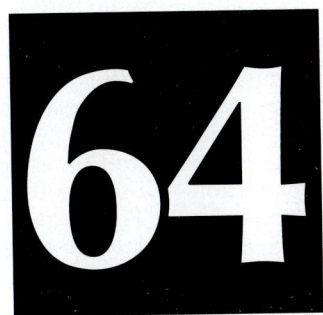

ANESTHETIC CONSIDERATIONS IN THE COMPLICATED OBSTETRIC PATIENT

LAURENCE S. REISNER, M.D., and KATHLEEN P. NICHOLS, M.D.

The physiologic changes that occur during normal pregnancy have striking implications upon the anesthesiologist when selecting the most appropriate and safest anesthetic drugs and techniques. When pregnancy is complicated by a significant medical disorder, the anesthetic considerations are even more challenging. This chapter will review the special concerns posed by the more common and complex medical disorders superimposed on pregnancy, as well as the most prudent technical solutions to the specific problems.

PREECLAMPSIA

The patient with preeclampsia has multiple organ system alterations, which impact on the selection of analgesia and anesthesia for labor and delivery. The patient with mild preeclampsia rarely poses a major anesthetic problem. Consequently, the focus will be upon the patient with severe preeclampsia and eclampsia. Throughout this chapter, there will be numerous references to intensive care monitoring and the use of pulmonary artery occlusion pressure monitoring. The reader is referred to Chapter 51 for a detailed review of this subject.

Intravascular volume depletion is a well-recognized occurrence with severe preeclampsia (Hays et al., 1985). The anesthesiologist is concerned about inducing epidural or spinal anesthesia in the face of a relative hypovolemia because the ensuing sympathetic blockade may lead to precipitous declines in blood pressure, which could seriously impair critical organ

and uteroplacental blood flow. Aggressive preanesthetic fluid replacement is utilized to prevent this undesired effect with reasonably good success. Such replacement often requires the use of central venous pressure or pulmonary artery pressure monitoring (Cotton et al., 1985). Because many patients with preeclampsia have low central filling pressures, they often require large volumes of fluid to bring their pressures into the middle of the normal range. However, this may result in pulmonary edema in the postpartum period, when colloid osmotic pressure reaches its nadir (Benedetti et al., 1985). More judicious fluid management with slow advancement of an epidural block, particularly for those undergoing cesarean section, is proving to be effective at maintaining maternal blood pressure while minimizing the risk of fluid overload.

The choice of fluid—crystalloid or colloid—still remains controversial. Studies have demonstrated the beneficial effects of albumin administration for these patients (Kirshon et al., 1988). Its use is justified in part by the fact that preeclamptic subjects tend to have significant reductions in plasma protein levels and colloid osmotic pressure as a result of protein loss through the kidney. Arguments against its routine use emphasize that the functional changes in membranes that allow edema to occur will also allow protein to leak into the tissues, thus making removal of interstitial fluid more difficult. In order to avoid volume overload, the judicious administration of crystalloid solution up to 2000 ml is guided by central venous or pulmonary artery occlusion pressure monitoring. This is accomplished with simultaneous advancement of the regional block, in effect titrating the effects of one against the other. If the patient has marked edema or low colloid osmotic pressure or has not responded to crystalloid infusion, 25 per cent salt-poor albumin is administered to maintain intravascular volume. The objective is to provide sufficient volume to allow the patient to undergo anesthesia and maintain an adequate urine flow rather than to totally correct an estimated volume deficit.

Vascular reactivity is enhanced in preeclampsia, and the increased sensitivity to vasopressor agents such as angiotensin II and catecholamines is well-documented (Gant et al., 1973; Zuspan, 1977). Systemic vascular resistance may be increased and uteroplacental crucial organ blood flow compromised. The anesthesiologist must consider the possibility that the administration of regional anesthesia and its attendant sympathetic blockade to a patient who is already experiencing volume depletion and vasoconstriction may result in sudden hypotension. However, it has been demonstrated that the initiation of epidural blockade with maintenance of an acceptable maternal blood pressure results in increases in uteroplacental blood flow (Joupilla et al., 1979). An acceptable maternal blood pressure is defined as no more than a 25 per cent reduction in systolic blood pressure.

The vasoreactivity also alerts the anesthesiologist to utilize lower doses of vasopressors to correct maternal hypotension. An arterial catheter may be helpful in monitoring beat-to-beat blood pressure responses in those patients requiring aggressive therapy. Patients who undergo general anesthesia for cesarean section are at risk for developing hypertensive crisis at the time of laryngoscopy and intubation due to the associated increase in sympathetic tone. This can lead to intracranial hemorrhage or pulmonary edema, and measures should be taken to block this response when general anesthesia is required (Fox et al., 1977).

Coagulation system changes are frequently observed in patients with severe preeclampsia. The most common alteration is a decrease in platelet count. This is usually not a concern unless it falls below 100,000/mm³. Many anesthesiologists are reluctant to administer regional anesthesia when the platelet count is at or below this level for fear that an epidural hematoma may occur. A platelet functional defect has also been identified in these patients (Kelton et al., 1985). This results in a prolonged IV bleeding time in spite of a normal platelet count. The absolute limit beyond which it is thought unwise to perform regional anesthesia is arbitrary and variable, although many use a figure between 10 and 12 minutes (normal range 3 to 7 minutes). It should be emphasized that there are no documented reports of an epidural hematoma occurring in association with epidural anesthesia in preeclamptic patients with either lowered platelet counts or a prolonged IV bleeding time. In fact, there is retrospective evidence to suggest that many epidurals have been placed in such patients without incident (Rolbin et al., 1988). Nevertheless, the potential complication is so serious that somewhat arbitrary limits are generally utilized until a true risk is defined. In general, if the bleeding time is less than 12 minutes it is probably safe to utilize regional anesthesia even if the platelet count is below 100,000/mm³. Other tests

of coagulation may be altered if the patient develops disseminated intravascular coagulation, although this is an infrequent occurrence.

Edema is a frequent finding in patients with preeclampsia. Limb edema may make vascular access difficult. Edema in the neck may obscure landmarks for performing internal jugular vein cannulation for central line insertion. The most worrisome edema for the anesthesiologist is that which may occur in the pharynx and larynx. Indeed, difficult or impossible intubation situations have been encountered with severe maternal consequences. General anesthesia for markedly edematous preeclamptic patients is avoided, and when absolutely necessary, preparation for alternate methods of securing the airway must be made. Postextubation airway obstruction due to edema at the level of the glottis is a serious complication and occurs frequently in these patients. Pulmonary edema is another complication of preeclampsia; the majority of these patients have normal cardiac function with imbalances in pulmonary artery pressure and colloid osmotic pressure. The observed reduction of colloid osmotic pressure in normal pregnancy is further decreased in preeclampsia. This is due to the loss of albumin, which is the major contributor to colloid osmotic pressure. Modest elevations in pulmonary artery occlusion pressure from exogenous fluid administration and mobilization of endogenous fluid will alter the gradient between colloid osmotic pressure and pulmonary artery pressure so that transudation of fluid into the interstitium is likely.

Pharmacologic agents are often required to treat the preeclamptic patient. These drugs may interact with anesthetics to produce an undesired effect, and both obstetrician and anesthesiologist should be aware of the pharmacology of the drugs employed, their dosages, and the time of administration. Magnesium sulfate is the most commonly administered agent in the management of preeclampsia. It effectively prevents convulsions and transiently lowers blood pressure. Adverse effects are few when it is administered appropriately, and overdosage is easily treated with intravenous calcium. Magnesium exerts several important effects at the neuromuscular junction. It inhibits the release of acetylcholine from the presynaptic nerve terminal, depresses the post-junctional membrane response, and depresses the response of the underlying myofibrils (Foldes, 1959). These effects are responsible for the muscle weakness and respiratory depression observed with overdosage. Neuromuscular blocking agents are utilized to facilitate endotracheal intubation and to maintain a relaxed surgical field when general anesthesia is provided for cesarean section. Magnesium will potentiate and prolong the action of depolarizing agents (e.g., succinylcholine) as well as nondepolarizing agents (e.g., D-tubocurarine, vecuronium, atracurium, pancuronium) (Ghoneim and Long, 1970). Therefore, lower doses of these drugs will be necessary, and electronic monitoring of the neuromuscular junction is helpful. It is essential that the patient be carefully evaluated at the end of the procedure to ensure that she has regained sufficient muscle function to maintain and protect the airway and to maintain adequate ventilation. Since drugs used to provide anesthesia are anticonvulsant in nature, it is prudent to discontinue magnesium sulfate therapy in the operating room when general anesthesia is used and to reinitiate use after the patient has regained full neuromuscular function.

The anesthetic options for a patient with severe preeclampsia depend on the mode of delivery. Analgesia for the first stage of labor will reduce maternal catecholamine output and perhaps maintain or improve uteroplacental blood flow. Systemic analgesia with narcotics is acceptable, although continuous lumbar epidural analgesia provides the best pain relief with minimal, if any, sedation. The use of segmental epidural analgesia avoids extensive sympathetic blockade. Opioids may be added to the local anesthetic solution to enhance the quality of pain relief without additional sympathetic or motor blockade. If sympathetic blockade must be totally avoided, the use of intrathecal narcotics (e.g., morphine, fentanyl, sufentanil, or meperidine) may be preferable by either single injection or continuous technique. Anesthesia for vaginal delivery may be provided by pudendal nerve block, low spinal anesthesia, or lumbar or caudal epidural anesthesia. Although the choice of anesthetic in the patient who is to undergo cesarean delivery has, in the past, been controversial, it is now well established that the careful use of epidural anesthesia, with meticulous attention to left uterine displacement and fluid management, is associated with good maternal and fetal outcome and is the preferred approach (Moore et al., 1985).

When general anesthesia is required, measures must be taken to avoid the hypertensive response to laryngoscopy and intubation as well as to extubation. Labetalol administered just before induction, in doses up to 1 mg/kg, have proved effective in reducing this response. Alternative or adjunctive drugs such as sodium nitroprusside or nitroglycerin may also be utilized. Sodium nitroprusside, because of its short half-life, provides the advantage of allowing for minute-to-minute blood pressure control. Large doses and long-term administration before delivery have been associated with fetal compromise, presumably because of cyanide toxicity (Naulty et al., 1981).

Since failure to secure the airway is the leading cause of maternal death associated with general anesthesia, alternative means of providing oxygenation and ventilation must be readily available, such as transtracheal jet ventilation. This technique has been demonstrated to adequately oxygenate and ventilate pregnant patients (Benumof and Scheller, 1989). If airway difficulty is anticipated, an awake intubation may be necessary, perhaps aided by a fiberoptic bronchoscope.

Spinal anesthesia is not recommended for cesarean delivery of severe preeclamptic patients due to the rapid onset of profound sympathetic blockade. However, with the use of a continuous catheter, the block may be titrated in a fashion similar to epidural anesthesia. On occasion, some patients technically meet the criteria for severe preeclampsia but do not have evidence of significant volume contraction or vasospasm and may be suitable candidates for spinal anesthesia.

NEUROLOGIC DISORDERS

Multiple Sclerosis

Multiple sclerosis is a disease of young adults that may occur in young pregnant women. Although there have been many attempts to associate anesthesia and surgery with relapses of symptoms, no controlled studies have directly linked any form of anesthesia to exacerbation (Kytta and Rosenberg, 1984). Routine use of anticholinergic agents is not recommended because they may induce an elevation in temperature, known to be associated with exacerbations. There has been a theoretic concern that local anesthetics might be more histotoxic to nervous tissue already damaged by multiple sclerosis. All local anesthetics are neurotoxic in concentrations well above those used clinically. Enhanced neurotoxicity from local anesthetic drugs has not been demonstrated in patients with multiple sclerosis, and epidural analgesia and anesthesia have been successfully used for labor and delivery (Crawford et al., 1981; Bader et al., 1988). The lowest concentration of local anesthetic capable of producing the desired effect should be selected. Epidural and intrathecal narcotics have also been administered without apparent adverse effect.

Paraplegia

The paraplegic patient is able to maintain a far better state of health than in the past, and many do elect to become pregnant. The level and extent of the lesion will determine the patient's response to labor. If the spinal cord lesion is below the tenth thoracic dermatome, the patient will have the sensation of labor. If it is above this level, she will have minimal if any awareness of contractions. Paraplegic parturients tend to have a normal course of labor but a higher percentage of forceps-assisted deliveries because of weakness of the abdominal muscles and consequent impairment of the ability to effectively bear down in the second stage. The major anesthetic issues are the management of analgesia and anesthesia for labor and delivery, the possibility of autonomic hyperreflexia, and hyperkalemia with the administration of succinylcholine.

The phenomenon of *autonomic hyperreflexia* occurs in patients who have their spinal cord lesion at the seventh thoracic dermatome or higher and is characterized by severe hypertension, bradycardia, headache, premature ventricular contractions, flushing, sweating, and pilomotor erection. The hypertension can be severe and, if uncontrolled, may lead to central nervous system hemorrhage, cardiac decompensation, or death. It is triggered by stimulation below the level of the spinal cord lesion. Common initiating events are bladder or rectal distention, rubbing of the skin, genital stimulation, and contraction of any hollow viscus including the uterus. The triggering impulse is conducted to the spinal cord, where a reflex response occurs that cannot be modulated or inhibited by higher centers, owing to the isolation invoked by the cord lesion. This results in an uncontrolled adrenergic discharge with norepinephrine release from the peripheral sympathetic nerve endings (Schonwald et al., 1981). The release of adrenal catecholamines may also be involved. While a large percentage of patients at risk do develop this reflex, some do not. A careful history should reveal those who exhibit such a response. Since preterm labor may be unrecognized by these patients, the sudden onset of paroxysmal hypertension should prompt a search for uterine contractions before considering the diagnosis of pregnancy-induced hypertension.

During labor, adequate blockade of the afferent impulses can be provided by regional anesthesia even if no pain is perceived by the patient. Continuous epidural anesthesia with both local anesthetics and narcotics has been successfully employed to treat autonomic hyperreflexia during labor and delivery (Baraka, 1985). Spinal anesthesia, both single-injection and continuous, has also been utilized to control blood pressure (Lambert et al., 1982). With regional anesthesia it is difficult to determine whether an adequate block is present, since the usual sensory tests are useless below the level of the lesion. The block must therefore be titrated to just above the existing sensory level. Autonomic hyperreflexia may also be controlled by a variety of antihypertensive agents, such as phentolamine and sodium nitroprusside.

Finally, general anesthesia can also effectively inhibit the hyperreflexia response (Wanner et al., 1987). However, if a general anesthetic is required for a complex vaginal delivery or cesarean section, the anesthesiologist will need to determine when the spinal cord injury initially occurred, owing to the fact that there is a significant release of potassium from the denervated muscle following use of succinylcholine for endotracheal intubation, if it is administered 6 months to 1 year after the injury (Gronert and Theye, 1975). The elevation in serum potassium may reach life-threatening levels.

Generally, although a general anesthetic may be utilized safely, an epidural anesthetic is preferred. Regional anesthesia has the advantage of blocking afferent input, thereby avoiding autonomic hyperreflexia. In addition, if the lesion is in the upper thoracic region, the patient will have weak abdominal and thoracic musculature. The use of epidural anesthesia is preferable to spinal anesthesia as the degree of motor impairment is less and profound muscle relaxation is not required. The block can be advanced gradually, thus avoiding sudden hypotension from a rapid extensive sympathetic blockade.

Subarachnoid Hemorrhage

Subarachnoid hemorrhage from an intracranial vascular lesion is an infrequent but extremely serious complication of pregnancy and has been reviewed (Horton et al., 1990; Dias and Sekkar, 1990). It is possible that the stress induced by the increased cardiac output and blood volume, combined with the softening of vascular connective tissue by the hormonal changes of pregnancy, may predispose to such an event. The diagnosis may be obscured initially because nausea and vomiting are common findings

during pregnancy. Treatment is usually surgical if the lesion is an aneurysm because this significantly improves maternal chances of survival. The decision to treat surgically should not be influenced by the pregnancy but rather by the site and type of lesion, the clinical condition of the patient, and the presence or absence of vasospasm. Medical management appears to be as effective as surgical management for arteriovenous malformations during pregnancy. Once a patient has had surgical correction of an aneurysm, there are no special considerations for anesthetic management of labor and delivery.

The anesthetic concerns regarding the patient without surgical correction are focused on two different clinical situations. The first relates to the patient undergoing neurosurgery for a ruptured aneurysm; the second is anesthetic management of labor and delivery for a patient who has not had surgical repair. Anesthesia for the patient having a neurosurgical procedure has the same primary goals as for all patients having surgery during pregnancy, namely, maintaining uteroplacental blood flow and fetal oxygenation and preventing preterm delivery (Leicht, 1990).

The usual neurosurgical anesthetic approach to patients with these types of lesions includes controlled hypotension to reduce the risk of cerebral hemorrhage, hypothermia to reduce cerebral metabolism, hyperventilation to reduce cerebral blood flow and brain size, and diuresis to promote shrinkage of the brain. Controlled hypotension may be induced with a volatile anesthetic, sodium nitroprusside, nitroglycerin, or trimethaphan. Each carries its own potential hazards in addition to reduction in uteroplacental blood flow. It is generally acknowledged that a reduction in systolic blood pressure of 25 to 30 per cent or a mean arterial blood pressure of less than 70 mm Hg will lead to reductions in uteroplacental blood flow. The hypotensive agents also cross the placenta and may induce hypotension in the fetus. Further, nitroprusside is converted to cyanide and cyanide accumulation in the fetus, and toxicity is at least a theoretical risk in the human. If this agent is used, it should be for only a short time and should be discontinued if the required infusion rate exceeds 0.5 mg/kg/hr, maternal metabolic acidosis ensues, or if resistance to the agent is apparent.

Nitroglycerin has yet to be associated with adverse fetal effects. It is metabolized to nitrites, which have experimentally produced methemaglobinemia. However, it is less predictable in its hypotensive effect than is sodium nitroprusside. Trimethaphan often leads to tachyphylaxis and interacts with neuromuscular blocking agents. It is a ganglionic blocker, thus intensifying the effects of some of the nondepolarizing muscle relaxants. Fetal heart rate monitoring should be employed and hypotension limited to the shortest period of time possible. Although it is preferable to avoid or limit the period of hypotension in the pregnant patient, successful neonatal outcome after induced hypotension with careful control has been observed (Donchin et al., 1978; Minielly et al., 1979).

Hypothermia is occasionally used to decrease cerebral metabolic requirements and blood flow. The usual goal is to achieve a temperature of approximately 30°C. This will induce similar temperature changes in the fetus, and fetal bradycardia will occur. The heart rate will increase again with rewarming (Stange and Halldin, 1983). Hyperventilation is commonly utilized during neuroanesthesia, as the decrease in P_{CO_2} reduces cerebral blood flow. The goal is to reach a P_{CO_2} of approximately 20 to 25 mm Hg, and this degree of moderate respiratory alkalosis should not be a problem for the healthy fetus. Fetal heart rate monitoring should alert the anesthesiologist to compromises in fetal oxygenation, and adjustments may be made accordingly.

Diuresis is often accomplished with osmotic agents or loop diuretics to shrink the brain both intra- and postoperatively. These may cause significant negative fluid shifts for the fetus. Obviously, these agents should be used only as necessary and not strictly by protocol for the pregnant patient.

The objectives in managing a patient for labor and delivery who has not undergone surgical repair are to avoid hypertension and to avoid elevations in intracranial pressure. The Valsalva maneuver should be avoided, as the sudden pressure changes at the end of the maneuver may produce a gradient that favors rupture of the lesion. Epidural analgesia and anesthesia can most effectively provide conditions to meet these goals. It may be relatively contraindicated for patients who already have marked increases in intracranial pressure inasmuch as an unintentional dural puncture could lead to herniation of the cerebellum. There is also a theoretical risk of further increasing intracranial pressure from the volume of fluid placed in the epidural space. However, this pressure rise is minimal and transient in the normal parturient when the amount administered is kept relatively small and the rate of injection slow. Other commonly used forms of analgesia may be utilized as long as maternal respiratory depression is avoided. Cesarean section anesthesia is best provided by the continuous epidural technique. Spinal anesthesia may be used if intracranial hypertension does not exist. If general anesthesia is required, the steps outlined previously for preventing the hypertensive response to laryngoscopy and intubation will be necessary.

RESPIRATORY DISORDERS

In order to understand the implications of anesthesia superimposed upon a pregnant woman with respiratory disease, an understanding of the physiologic alterations in the respiratory tract during pregnancy is required. These are reviewed in Chapter 52.

Asthma

Asthma is the most common respiratory problem encountered in the population of childbearing age. The disease is characterized by bronchial constriction, bronchial secretions, and bronchial edema. Therapy commonly includes theophylline preparations, inhaled beta-adrenoceptor agonists, anticholinergics,

corticosteroids, and occasionally cromolyn sodium. Magnesium sulfate has also been found effective at alleviating acute symptoms (Lindeman et al., 1989). The effect of pregnancy on the condition of the asthmatic has been controversial, but it does appear that with proper management and prompt attention to acute episodes, most patients do well (Greenberger, 1990). Maintenance of the patient's medications and hydration are of major importance during labor and delivery.

Analgesia and anesthesia for labor and delivery of the asthmatic patient serve to alleviate anxiety and hyperventilation. Hyperventilation may precipitate an attack and may lead to increased fluid losses and dehydration. Narcotic analgesia administered in a judicious fashion may be utilized, but narcotics are bronchoconstrictors and should be avoided if the patient is actively wheezing or in respiratory distress. Epidural analgesia with local anesthetics, opioids, or both is extremely beneficial as pain may be relieved while avoiding respiratory depression (Younker et al., 1987). If the patient is a severe asthmatic, it is essential to avoid a high and dense level of anesthesia as accessory muscles of respiration may be impaired. A high thoracic level may completely block sympathetic pathways, and the unopposed parasympathetic tone may lead to bronchoconstriction. Either low spinal anesthesia or pudendal block is a reasonable selection for vaginal delivery if epidural analgesia is not utilized.

Regional anesthesia is preferred because the insertion of an endotracheal tube at the light levels of anesthesia traditionally favored for obstetrics frequently results in bronchospasm (Benatar, 1981). Even though pulmonary mechanics are reasonably well maintained under spinal or epidural anesthesia to the fourth thoracic dermatome, the patient should receive an inhaled beta$_2$ agonist prior to the procedure and bring her inhaler with her to the operating room as bronchospasm may occur (McGough and Cohen, 1990). Appropriate attention to hydration and maintenance of blood pressure are required and supplemental oxygen recommended.

General anesthesia for cesarean section in the asthmatic patient poses additional risk, requires careful attention to detail to avoid life-threatening bronchospasm, and should be utilized only if regional anesthesia is contraindicated. Preoperative preparation should include adequate hydration, intravenous aminophylline, treatment with a beta$_2$ agonist inhaler, antacid therapy, and sufficient time for preoxygenation (a minimum of 3 minutes). Then a rapid-sequence induction may be undertaken. The induction agent of choice is ketamine because it is a bronchodilator and does not release histamine (Corssen et al., 1972). Thiopental administered in the commonly used doses for cesarean section produces a plane of anesthesia that is too light to prevent bronchospasm. Larger doses are an alternative to ketamine and may be employed with the small risk that the newborn will be depressed from the anesthetic in the immediate postdelivery period. The patient requiring a general anesthetic for cesarean section with active wheezing may require a slower induction. Anesthesia is induced intravenously, a muscle relaxant administered, cricoid pressure applied and maintained, and the patient ventilated by mask with a volatile anesthetic agent to promote bronchodilation. When a deep plane of anesthesia is reached, the patient is intubated. This technique exposes the patient to a greater risk of regurgitation and aspiration of gastric contents and should be employed only when there are no other reasonable options.

Once anesthesia is induced and the patient successfully intubated, maintenance will include the administration of a volatile agent in a humidified gas mixture because all in current use (halothane, enflurane, isoflurane) produce direct bronchial muscle relaxation (Hirshman et al., 1982). If intraoperative wheezing should occur, a beta$_2$ agonist may be aerosolized via the endotracheal tube. Although their effect is synergistic with the halogenated agents, two potential problems must be considered. First, halothane administration in the presence of therapeutic or higher levels of aminophylline has been associated with serious ventricular arrhythmias and cardiac arrest (Richards et al., 1988). Isoflurane or enflurane are acceptable alternatives. Second, the volatile agents tend to relax uterine musculature at concentrations that are effective as bronchodilators, and the possibility of enhanced uterine bleeding exists. This effect can usually be counteracted by the administration of oxytocin. The use of prostaglandins to control hemorrhage is not recommended as prostaglandin F$_2\alpha$ is a bronchoconstrictor. Once delivered, ventilation with bag and mask oxygen will eliminate the majority of the volatile agent in a few minutes.

Muscle relaxation can be maintained with a succinylcholine infusion or with a nondepolarizing agent. Curare, metocurine, and atracurium are associated with histamine release in large doses, whereas pancuronium and vecuronium are not. When a nondepolarizing agent is used, it usually must be reversed at the end of the procedure with an anticholinesterase such as neostigmine or edrophonium. This group of drugs can produce bronchoconstriction and increased production of secretions. Consequently, a sufficient dose of an anticholinergic such as atropine or glycopyrrolate must be administered prior to their use. The nonpregnant asthmatic patient is usually extubated in a deep plane of anesthesia to avoid the stimulus of the endotracheal tube, but the pregnant patient should be extubated awake because of the risk of vomiting and aspiration. Intravenous lidocaine may prevent coughing and bronchoconstriction upon emergence. Postoperative care should include humidified oxygen, incentive spirometry, and the required pharmacologic agents. Epidural and intrathecal narcotics provide excellent postoperative analgesia with minimal sedation.

Cystic Fibrosis

The meticulous use of pulmonary toilet and aggressive antibiotic therapy has made it possible for many women with cystic fibrosis to survive well into their childbearing years (Canny et al., 1991). The pulmonary complications of patients with cystic fibrosis provide significant anesthetic challenges. Thick, excessive mu-

cus production results in obstruction of the small and medium-sized airways with subsequent bronchitis and bronchiectasis. Pneumothorax, atelectasis, progressive hypoxemia, and cor pulmonale are all commonly seen with the disease.

Therapy consists of postural drainage and chest percussion, often on a daily basis, antibiotics for symptoms of infection, bronchodilators for wheezing, intermittent mucolytic therapy (N-acetylcysteine), vitamins, and pancreatic enzyme replacement. Preoperative evaluation should include pulmonary function studies, cardiac evaluation, and measurement of arterial blood gases. Successful completion of gestation with careful attention to medical management is now well documented (Valenzuela et al., 1988; Canny et al., 1991).

Analgesia during the first stage of labor is optimally provided by continuous lumbar epidural. Management concerns are similar to those of the severe asthmatic patient. The state of hydration needs to be maintained as these patients often lose a great deal of fluid through sweating. Narcotics should be used in very small amounts because they suppress the cough reflex and produce respiratory depression. Nitrous oxide should probably be avoided because of the frequency of pneumothorax from ruptured bullae. Anesthesia for vaginal delivery may be provided with low spinal, epidural, or pudendal nerve block.

Anesthesia for cesarean section also carries with it the same management concerns as for the severe asthmatic, and carefully titrated continuous epidural anesthesia is recommended. Although general anesthesia can be utilized safely for patients with cystic fibrosis, the risk of maternal hypoxemia during induction is greater, and there exists the possibility of pneumothorax during positive pressure ventilation. Anticholinergics (drying agents) and narcotics are usually excluded from the regimen, and gases should be humidified. Patients with very advanced disease may require postoperative mechanical ventilation until they regain their full preoperative capabilities.

MORBID OBESITY

Morbid obesity is defined as an accumulation of adipose tissue that causes the body mass index to increase by 30 per cent or more (BMI = Weight[kg]/Height[m^2]). Substantial change takes place over time in the respiratory system. A restrictive lung disease pattern develops, and pulmonary function testing reveals a decrease in expiratory reserve volume, vital capacity, inspiratory capacity, and total lung capacity. There is decreased compliance and increased work of breathing. There is also a ventilation-perfusion imbalance, leading to hypoxemia, particularly in the supine or Trendelenburg position.

Pregnancy imposes changes in lung volumes similar to those resulting from obesity. While it would be presumed that these effects are additive, this is not the case. A study evaluating 12 obese pregnant women revealed that the usual pulmonary changes of pregnancy occurred, but they were not accentuated by the obesity. Hypoxemia existed but was not worsened by pregnancy (Eng et al., 1975).

Labor should be conducted in the sitting or semi-recumbent position with left uterine displacement. Supplemental oxygen administration and pulse oximeter monitoring are advised. Epidural analgesia is recommended but may be technically difficult to perform. Other forms of analgesia including intrathecal narcotics, intravenous narcotics, and inhalation of nitrous oxide/oxygen are all suitable. The anesthetic for vaginal delivery may be any of the commonly used forms; the patient should remain semi-sitting if at all possible to prevent small airway closure.

Cesarean section anesthesia may be provided by either spinal or epidural routes. Again, technical difficulties may be encountered, and the dosage of drug needs to be reduced because spread in both the subarachnoid and epidural space is enhanced with morbid obesity (Hodgkinson and Husain, 1980). Care must be taken to avoid a significant motor block as this may compromise ventilation and result in hypoxemia. The Trendelenburg position should be avoided because it will shift the weight of the abdominal viscera and the panniculus toward the chest and diaphragm, further compromising respiration.

Technically, a general anesthetic poses several challenges. First, the airway must be secured. Endotracheal intubation can be extremely difficult due to excessive tissue and edema. Exceedingly large breasts can interfere with the insertion of a conventional laryngoscope. A careful assessment of the airway must be made, and if it appears difficult, an awake fiberoptic intubation is recommended. If a rapid sequence induction is attempted and the airway cannot be secured, an alternative means such as transtracheal jet ventilation must be at hand, since hypoxia and acidosis can develop at an extremely rapid rate. After the airway is secured, mechanical ventilation will be required, and the pressures generated will need to be high to move the large body mass. Large tidal volumes will help to prevent airway closure. Extubation should be performed only when the patient is fully awake and has regained her full strength. Postoperative analgesia, preferably by the epidural route, is extremely helpful in allowing for deep breathing exercises to avoid atelectasis and pneumonia.

CARDIAC DISEASE

The pregnant patient with heart disease represents a unique challenge to the anesthesiologist. Determination of the appropriate analgesic and anesthetic modalities requires a thorough understanding of the parturient's pathophysiology as well as pharmacologic therapy and how these interact with anesthetic care.

Over the past two decades, greater awareness of the physiologic burden that pregnancy places upon an already compromised cardiovascular system in this subset of pregnant women has led to more accurate counseling before conception and major advances in treatment. Formerly, rheumatic heart disease was the most common cardiac disorder in pregnancy, with mitral stenosis the single most prevalent resulting

lesion. However, in recent years the improved surgical management of patients with congenital heart disease has increased the survivability of these patients to childbearing age (Spielman, 1986). Also, as more women delay childbearing to later reproductive years, ischemic cardiac disease may be expected to become increasingly prevalent (Roberts and Chestnut, 1987).

General Considerations

Pregnancy normally results in dramatic changes in the cardiovascular system, and these, as well as cardiac disorders in pregnancy, are extensively reviewed in Chapter 47. Four principal changes that present unique problems to the patient with cardiac disease have been well delineated (Clark, 1991) and have special anesthetic implications. First, there is a 50 per cent increase in intravascular volume that generally peaks by the early-to-middle third trimester. This relative volume overload may be poorly tolerated in patients whose cardiac output is limited by myocardial dysfunction from ischemia or intrinsic or valvular lesions.

Second, there is a progressive decrease in systemic vascular resistance (SVR) throughout pregnancy so that mean arterial pressure (MAP) is preserved at normal values despite a 30 to 40 per cent increase in cardiac output (CO). This may be of importance in those patients at risk for right-to-left shunting as well as for patients with some types of valvular disease (e.g., aortic stenosis).

Third, the compromised cardiovascular system is further stressed by the marked fluctuations in cardiac output that are observed during labor. Pain and apprehension may precipitate an increase in cardiac output to as much as 45 to 50 per cent over those levels seen in the late second stage of labor (Ueland and Hansen, 1969a). Further, each uterine contraction serves in effect as an autotransfusion to the central blood volume, resulting in an increase in CO of 10 to 25 per cent (Ueland and Hansen, 1969b). The Valsalva maneuver results in wide swings in both venous and arterial pressures, which have been associated with acute cardiac decompensation. The increases in CO reach a maximum of 80 per cent higher than antepartum levels immediately following delivery secondary to relief of inferior vena cava obstruction and a final autotransfusion of approximately 500 ml from uterine contraction.

The final consideration in these patients is the hypercoagulability associated with pregnancy and the possible need for appropriate anticoagulation, especially in those patients at increased risk for arterial thrombosis and embolization (prosthetic heart valve or chronic atrial fibrillation). Therapeutic anticoagulation will affect the options for anesthetic management, perhaps the location of invasive monitors, and will increase the risk for postpartum hemorrhage.

Optimal anesthetic management requires a thorough assessment of the anatomic and functional capacity of the diseased heart along with an analysis of how the described major physiologic changes are likely to affect the specific limitations imposed by the intrinsic disease. Specifically, in order to determine the most appropriate anesthetic regimen, the anesthesiologist must consider the patient's tolerance to pain during labor or surgery, the impact of uterine contraction–induced autotransfusion, the postpartum changes induced by relief of vena caval obstruction, the potential for postpartum hemorrhage, and the use of uterine oxytocics.

The most basic principles of obstetric anesthesia management must always apply: provisions for maintenance of uteroplacental perfusion by avoidance of aortocaval compression, minimizing sympathetic blockade coupled with intravascular volume maintenance, standard-of-care monitoring of parturient and fetus, and provision for aspiration prophylaxis (Malinow and Ostheimer, 1987).

Analgesia during the first stage of labor is focused on reducing the pain-related rises in catecholamine levels and avoiding aortocaval compression. Intravenous fluid management should be carefully monitored to avoid both a lack of and excess of fluids. Arterial, central venous, and/or pulmonary artery monitoring may be required to optimally manage the patient. While such lines are generally reserved for symptomatic women, patients who have tight aortic stenosis, coarctation of the aorta, aortic aneurysm, right-to-left shunts, or primary pulmonary hypertension may benefit from invasive monitoring even with minimal symptoms. Appropriate analgesia should be supplied during the first stage. All of the available modalities have application for some patients. Continuous lumbar epidural analgesia with local anesthetics, narcotics, or both is frequently optimal. Limited sympathetic blockade may prove helpful with mitral valve lesions because of the effect on both preload and afterload. For a patient whose condition is so compromised that even the modest changes induced by segmental epidural analgesia are worrisome, the use of intrathecal narcotic analgesia by single injection or continuous catheter may be beneficial since all of the hemodynamic alterations of sympathetic blockade are avoided.

Once the patient with significant cardiac disease has entered the second stage of labor, it is prudent to avoid pushing. The Valsalva maneuver results in wide swings in both venous and arterial pressures, which have been associated with acute cardiac decompensation. The lithotomy position may need to be avoided for patients with lesions such as mitral stenosis inasmuch as this causes an acute increase in central blood volume. Analgesia for uterine contractions and anesthesia of the perineum are the objectives for second-stage management. Uterine contractions will spontaneously bring the infant's head to a deliverable position, and delivery may then be assisted by the application of the vacuum extractor or forceps. Again, a regional technique is optimal. Epidural analgesia/anesthesia may be continued. Attention must be paid to extension of the sympathetic blockade. If an epidural is not utilized, a low spinal anesthetic may be appropriate. Pudendal nerve block, while not providing as complete analgesia as the former, may be satisfactorily employed as an adjunct to regional anesthesia, or used alone.

It is generally held that cesarean delivery should be reserved for obstetric indications only and that the presence of heart disease should not influence that decision. The overall stresses of labor and vaginal delivery, as measured by alterations in cardiac output, are approximately the same as with cesarean section. However, there may be occasional circumstances that would lead to the decision to perform an elective cesarean section. The choice of anesthesia depends upon the lesion and its severity. Epidural anesthesia has been shown to provide the least amount of alteration in hemodynamics during cesarean section. However, general anesthesia can be equally as safe when the abrupt changes associated with laryngoscopy and intubation, as well as suction and extubation, are blunted by the appropriate choice of pharmacologic agents and anesthetic technique.

Valvular Heart Disease

Rheumatic fever continues to be the predominant etiology of valvular heart disease in pregnancy. Complications during pregnancy include uni- or biventricular failure, atrial dysrhythmias, systemic or pulmonary embolism, and infective endocarditis, with an overall incidence of complications estimated at 15 per cent of all patients with valvular disease. In general, regurgitant lesions are well tolerated during pregnancy as the increased plasma volume and lowered systemic vascular resistance results in increased cardiac output. By sharp contrast, stenotic valvular disease is poorly tolerated with advancing pregnancy, owing to the inability to increase cardiac output sufficient to accommodate the augmented plasma volume, leading to pulmonary venous congestion and possibly frank pulmonary edema.

Mitral stenosis (MS) may occur as an isolated lesion or in conjunction with right-sided or aortic valvular disease. It accounts for nearly 90 per cent of rheumatic heart disease (RHD) in pregnancy, with 25 per cent of patients first developing symptoms during pregnancy (Sugrue et al., 1981). The principal pathophysiologic derangement is a decrease in mitral valve orifice, resulting in obstruction to left ventricular filling. This hemodynamic aberration leads to a relatively fixed cardiac output. Although initially the left atrium may overcome this obstruction, with disease progression left atrial volume and pressure will ultimately increase and lead to a progressive and chronic rise in pulmonary capillary wedge pressure and pulmonary venous pressure; pulmonary hypertension and right ventricular hypertrophy and failure may ensue. An anatomically moderate lesion may become functionally severe with the marked increase in cardiac output that accompanies normal pregnancy, labor, and delivery.

Anesthetic management is oriented toward the avoidance of tachycardia, as the time required for left ventricular diastolic filling is prolonged. Patients who are asymptomatic at term generally require increased vigilance but should not require invasive monitoring. Patients with marked symptoms are at significant risk in the peripartum period and should receive arterial and pulmonary artery catheter monitoring in the puerperium, continuing through a minimum of 24 hours postpartum (Clark et al., 1985). An increase in central circulating blood volume may occur suddenly in the immediate postpartum period, and tolerance of this intravascular load may be poor, especially for patients with a fixed cardiac output (Ueland, 1988; Ducey and Ellsworth, 1989).

Anesthesia for labor and vaginal delivery may be best accomplished with segmental lumbar epidural anesthesia to avoid changes in monitored hemodynamic parameters. A sudden decrease in systemic vascular resistance (SVR) may be tolerated poorly following the development of reflex tachycardia. Although other analgesic modalities may be employed, segmental epidural analgesia allows for careful titration to the desired result while minimizing undesirable changes. The addition of opioids such as fentanyl to the dilute local anesthetic mixture enhances the quality of analgesia yet does not add to the sympathetic blockade. Opioids alone may be administered by the epidural or intrathecal route for the critically ill patient. Adequate segmental and perineal anesthesia reduces catecholamine-induced increases in heart rate as well as the urge to push, allowing fetal descent to be accomplished by uterine contractions and avoiding the deleterious effects of the Valsalva maneuver during the second stage of labor. When epidural anesthesia has not been utilized, a low spinal anesthetic may be administered to allow for a controlled second stage and delivery. Caudal anesthesia is another reasonable option. Pudendal nerve block will provide adequate, although not ideal, pain relief for some patients.

Anesthetic options for cesarean delivery must take into account the additional potential hazards of marked fluid shifts secondary to anesthetic technique, operative blood loss, and the mobilization of fluid in the postpartum period. Either regional or general anesthesia may be used. Epidural anesthesia is preferred over spinal anesthesia because the former results in slower onset of blockade and thus more controllable hemodynamic alterations. Prophylactic ephedrine and arbitrary intravascular volume loading are best avoided; instead, a careful titration of anesthetic level allows judicious and appropriate intravenous fluid administration, which should be guided by hemodynamic monitoring in the symptomatic patient. These patients may be prone to hypotension with epidural anesthesia, secondary to a combination of venous pooling and prior beta-adrenergic blockade and diuretic therapy (Ziskind et al., 1990). The usual vasopressor choice of ephedrine should be avoided, as it may result in tachycardia. Instead, judicious use of metaraminol or low-dose (20 to 40 μg) phenylephrine will assist in restoration of maternal blood pressure with little or no unwanted effect on uteroplacental perfusion.

General anesthesia may also provide a very stable hemodynamic course if the sympathetic stimulation associated with laryngoscopy and intubation as well as with suction and extubation is minimized. This may be accomplished with anesthetic agents and/or beta-adrenergic blockade. Induction of general anesthesia should be carefully accomplished without drugs that commonly produce tachycardia. Depending on the severity of the disease, the need to blunt the hemo-

dynamic response to endotracheal intubation may necessitate the use of a high-dose narcotic-based technique. This also serves to avoid myocardial depression and the decreases in SVR that may occur with commonly employed short-acting barbiturates. Anesthesia is maintained with narcotics, muscle relaxants, nitrous oxide, and oxygen. Emergence must be carefully controlled to ensure return of protective reflexes and avoidance of tachycardia.

Aortic stenosis (AS) is a rare complication of pregnancy, primarily because the natural history of this lesion occurring secondary to rheumatic heart disease typically requires 3 to 4 decades to yield severity adequate to produce symptoms. However, women with congenitally bicuspid aortic valves and patients with a history of bacterial endocarditis may present in pregnancy with severe AS. Unlike mitral stenosis, symptoms of CHF, angina, and syncope develop relatively late in the course of the disease. The pathophysiology of severe AS entails narrowing of the valve orifice to less than 1 cm², associated with a transvalvular gradient of 50 mm Hg, resulting in significant increases in afterload to left ventricular ejection. The LV appropriately and concentrically hypertrophies and becomes markedly less compliant, although contractility is usually well preserved. The transvalvular gradient increases progressively throughout pregnancy as a result of increasing blood volume and decreasing SVR (Raymond et al., 1987).

Anesthetic management encompasses the goals of avoiding tachycardia, maintaining adequate preload in order that the LV may generate an adequate cardiac output across the stenotic valve, and maintaining hemodynamic parameters within a narrow therapeutic window. Patients with transvalvular gradients greater than 50 mm Hg and patients with symptomatic AS warrant invasive monitoring with arterial and pulmonary artery catheters in the peripartum period (Easterling et al., 1988).

Provision of labor analgesia with segmental epidural anesthesia remains a controversial issue because these patients may not be able to tolerate the decreases in preload and afterload that may attend epidural analgesia and its associated sympathetic blockade (Sugrue et al., 1981). A recent report describes a series of four patients with moderate-to-severe AS who were successfully managed with epidural anesthesia without untoward sequelae; adequate time was allowed to carefully titrate the level of block and initiate appropriate compensatory actions to correct hemodynamic alterations associated with the anesthetic (Easterling et al., 1988). Intrathecal or epidural opioids, whether alone or in combination with an epidural segmental anesthetic, are other appropriate choices. Spinal opioids have no cardiovascular effects. In particular, myocardial contractility is unaltered, preload is preserved, and most importantly, SVR is not diminished by this technique (Forster and Joyce, 1989). Local anesthetics and opioids are believed to act synergistically, allowing for a decrease in concentration of both drugs when used together. Effective analgesia can prevent the tachycardia associated with labor pain.

For cesarean section, either judiciously titrated epidural anesthesia or general endotracheal anesthesia may be utilized. General anesthesia may be accomplished with the same caution that applies for parturients with mitral stenosis; myocardial depression associated with halogenated volatile anesthetics should be avoided.

Mitral valve insufficiency and regurgitation (MR) is the second most prevalent valvular lesion in pregnancy. Chronic left ventricular volume overload and work are usually well tolerated, with symptoms developing relatively late in life after childbearing age, thus most patients with MR tolerate pregnancy well. Complications include an increased risk of atrial fibrillation during pregnancy, bacterial endocarditis requiring antibiotic prophylaxis, systemic embolization, and pulmonary congestion during pregnancy. In one review of maternal deaths associated with rheumatic valvular lesions, no patient died from complications of MR without the presence of coexisting mitral stenosis (Hibbard, 1975). Congenital mitral valve prolapse (MVP) is much more common during pregnancy than MR and may be present in 10 to 17 per cent of pregnancies. It is a well-tolerated and generally benign form of MR, and so therapeutic interventions are rarely necessary (Rayburn and Fontana, 1981; Gianopoulos, 1989).

The pathophysiology of regurgitation through an incompetent mitral valve results in chronic volume overload of the left ventricle and dilatation. If left ventricular compromise is sufficiently long-standing and severe, the increase in plasma volume with pregnancy progression may result in pulmonary venous congestion. By contrast, the decreasing systemic vascular resistance associated with pregnancy may serve to improve forward flow across the aortic valve at the expense of regurgitant flow. Increases in SVR, which occur with labor pain, uterine contractions, or surgical stimulation, may result in a rise in the proportion of regurgitant blood flow, perhaps leading to acute LV failure.

Anesthetic management of labor and delivery can be safely provided via any of the available techniques including segmental lumbar epidural anesthesia. Adequate analgesia and anesthesia will minimize the peripheral vasoconstriction and thus attenuate the increase in LV afterload associated with labor pain and thereby augment the forward flow of blood. Minimal sympathectomy will also serve to decrease SVR and be beneficial in this regard; the caveat here is that venous capacitance will increase, and one must be prepared to augment preload cautiously with IV fluid infusion to maintain LV filling volume.

Asymptomatic patients at term are unlikely to warrant invasive monitoring. Continuous ECG monitoring is a reasonable addition to basic standards of peripartum monitoring. In symptomatic patients, invasive monitoring with arterial and pulmonary arterial catheter should be utilized.

Aortic insufficiency (AI) may be congenital or acquired. If congenital, it is commonly associated with other lesions; if acquired, it may be secondary to rheumatic heart disease or endocarditis in association with aortic root dissection. Symptoms of AI following rheumatic fever usually develop during the fourth or fifth decade of life; thus most women in whom this is the dominant lesion have uneventful pregnancies.

The basic pathophysiology is of chronic volume overloading of the left ventricle resulting in hypertrophy and dilatation associated with increased compliance. Because of hypertrophy, myocardial oxygen requirements are higher than normal, yet perfusion pressure and thus oxygen supply may be decreased by a decrease in diastolic pressure and an increased left ventricular end-diastolic pressure. Anesthetic considerations thus center on minimizing pain and therefore catecholamine-induced increases in SVR; avoiding bradycardia, which serves to increase time for regurgitant flow; and avoiding myocardial depressants, which may exacerbate failure. Since the anesthetic concerns are similar to those for patients with mitral regurgitation, epidural anesthesia for labor and delivery is desirable in order to prevent increases in peripheral vasoconstriction. Epidural anesthesia is also appropriate as a surgical anesthetic, as is general anesthesia with judicious avoidance of direct myocardial depressants. Invasive monitoring is a requirement in any patient presenting with symptoms of congestive heart failure.

Congenital Heart Disease

Congenital cardiac disease is becoming the most common cardiac problem encountered in the pregnant patient (Gianopoulos, 1989). These patients are increasingly likely to survive to childbearing age with the advent of palliative surgery or total correction of their defects. Many can be expected to have an uneventful pregnancy and delivery. The major congenital cardiac diseases can be classified into three distinct functional groups for discussion; left-to-right shunts, right-to-left shunts, and congenital valvular or vascular lesions.

Left-to-Right Shunts

Ventricular septal defect (VSD) occurs in 7 per cent of adults with congenital heart disease. Patients with uncorrected lesions in the absence of pulmonary hypertension will do well during pregnancy. In the small percentage of patients with large VSDs and coexisting pulmonary hypertension, maternal mortality ranges from 7 to 40 per cent. Severe right ventricular failure with shunt reversal (Eisenmenger's syndrome) is the major ensuing complication. During pregnancy, elevation of plasma volume, cardiac output (CO), and heart rate (HR) may increase left-to-right shunt and further worsen the degree of pulmonary hypertension.

The major goals in peripartum management include awareness that marked increases in peripheral vascular resistance and heart rate may be poorly tolerated, with ventricular failure a distinct possibility. Conversely, acute increases in pulmonary vascular resistance and right ventricular compromise may lead to shunt reversal and hypoxia.

Anesthesia for labor and vaginal delivery is optimally achieved with segmental epidural anesthesia utilizing local anesthetics, opioids, or their combination to permit control of painful stimuli, thus minimizing changes in HR and SVR. Anesthesia for cesarean section may be accomplished either with slow titration of an epidural anesthetic to allow time for correction of pressure changes or with a general anesthetic that combines opioid and inhalation technique to depress the adrenergic response to endotracheal intubation and minimize myocardial depression.

Atrial septal defect (ASD) is one of the most common congenital cardiac lesions in women of childbearing age, and pregnancy is generally well tolerated even when pulmonary blood flow is increased. However, the risk of LV failure is increased during pregnancy. Increases in atrial volume result in biatrial enlargement, and thus supraventricular dysrhythmias are likely.

Pregnancy-associated increases in plasma volume and cardiac output serve to accentuate the left-to-right shunt, right ventricular volume work, and pulmonary blood flow, with development of pulmonary hypertension and left and right ventricular failure possible. Peripartum management centers on avoiding vascular resistance changes that may increase the degree of shunt. Increases in SVR or decreases in PVR may not be well tolerated.

Although all of the common methods of providing labor analgesia are useful, lumbar epidural analgesia for labor, vaginal delivery, or cesarean section attenuates the hazards of increased SVR. General anesthesia for cesarean section is also well tolerated provided that increases in SVR are avoided and sinus rhythm maintained.

Patent ductus arteriosis (PDA) accounts for 15 per cent of all CHD, with the majority of patients with a large PDA (> 1 cm) now receiving early surgical intervention. Patients with a small PDA have typically normal pregnancies. However, in those pregnant women with superimposed pulmonary hypertension, maternal mortality may reach 5 to 6 per cent from ventricular failure. The progressive decrease in SVR developing throughout pregnancy can be associated with shunt reversal and peripheral cyanosis.

Anesthetic considerations include avoidance of increases in SVR and hypervolemia. Conversely, acute decreases in SVR may result in reversal of shunt in patients with preexisting pulmonary hypertension and right ventricular compromise. Again, all modalities may be utilized depending on the severity of the disease. Continuous lumbar epidural analgesia for labor and delivery diminishes the increase in SVR associated with pain. Epidural or general anesthesia is appropriate for cesarean section provided increases in SVR associated with endotracheal intubation and surgical stimulation are adequately addressed.

Right-to-Left Shunts

Eisenmenger's syndrome consists of pulmonary hypertension, a right-to-left intracardiac shunt resulting from pulmonary hypertension superimposed on a previously left-to-right shunt, and arterial hypoxemia. Pregnancy is not well tolerated in this condition, with maternal mortality estimated at 30 to 50 per cent. This entity is responsible for approximately 50 per cent of the maternal mortality in parturients with congenital heart disease (Spielman, 1986).

Anesthetic considerations center on avoidance of any decrease in SVR and thus hypotension or myocardial depression. Hypotension from any cause, including conduction block or hemorrhage, can progress to insufficient right ventricular pressures to perfuse the hypertensive pulmonary arterial bed and may result in sudden death.

Analgesia for vaginal delivery may be accomplished with systemic narcotics, intrathecal narcotics, or cautious application of a segmental epidural provided that systemic vascular resistance is maintained. Epidural or intrathecal opioid administration during the first stage of labor would be a useful adjunct, and its sole administration has been recommended as the safest approach (Abboud et al., 1983). If an epidural is employed, epinephrine should be omitted from the test dose as peripheral beta-adrenergic effects may cause a decrease in SVR. A caudal epidural for second-stage analgesia and anesthesia may be preferable to the lumbar route because dense perineal analgesia can be provided without extensive sympathetic blockade. Delivery by cesarean section is most safely accomplished via general anesthesia, although there are reports of regional anesthesia provided for elective cesarean delivery (Spinnato et al., 1981; Hytens and Alexander, 1986).

Regardless of the anesthetic technique employed, the postpartum period is probably the most likely time for life-threatening complications of hypoxemia, cardiac dysrhythmias, and thromboembolic events to occur (Gilman, 1991); the majority of maternal deaths, in fact, occur in the first postpartum week (Cobb et al., 1982). The use of invasive monitoring is highly recommended in management of these patients in the peripartum period; pulmonary artery catheters and serial arterial blood gases may allow early detection of changes in cardiac output, pulmonary artery pressures, and shunt fraction. Serial measurements of CO and especially SVR are useful in this regard. It should be recognized that technical difficulty in passage of a pulmonary artery catheter and obtaining wedge pressures is well documented (Schwalbe et al., 1990; Pollack et al., 1990).

Tetralogy of Fallot comprises 15 per cent of all congenital heart disease and is the most common etiology of right-to-left shunt in women of childbearing age. Particularly poor prognostic signs include a history of syncope, polycythemia (hematocrit greater than 60), decreased arterial oxygen saturation (saturation less than 80 per cent), right ventricular hypertension, and congestive heart failure. Increased right-to-left shunt may accompany pregnancy-induced decreases in SVR. The stress of labor may increase PVR and thus increase the degree of shunt. Most complications occur in the postpartum period when SVR is lowest, thus exacerbating the right-to-left shunting of blood and worsening the degree of arterial hypoxemia.

Anesthetic considerations must focus on minimizing the hemodynamic changes that would exacerbate the degree of shunt. Strict avoidance of decreased SVR and decreased venous return and myocardial depression are of paramount importance. Analgesia for labor and vaginal delivery in these patients is most safely provided by systemic medication, inhalational nitrous oxide analgesia, or pudendal block. Intrathecal opioids may prove optimal in some circumstances. Regional anesthetic techniques should be used with extreme caution as the decrease in SVR may result in increased shunt. Low-dose ketamine may prove a reasonable option for forceps-assisted deliveries. Anesthesia for cesarean section should be provided by a general anesthetic.

Invasive monitoring with arterial and pulmonary artery catheters to evaluate cardiac filling pressures and SVR is warranted in those patients with uncorrected tetralogy or only palliative correction.

Primary pulmonary hypertension predominantly affects women of childbearing age and is associated with a high maternal mortality (> 50 per cent), most deaths occurring during labor and the puerperium (Mangano, 1987; Slomka et al., 1988; Roberts and Keast, 1990). Signs and symptoms depend on severity of the disease and are due to a fixed low cardiac output, the degree of pulmonary hypertension, and the degree of right ventricular compromise. The anesthetic considerations are focused upon evaluating the severity of the disease and its responsiveness to therapy, maintenance of hemodynamic stability, and the appropriate administration of analgesia and anesthesia for labor and delivery.

In the selection of an analgesic and/or anesthetic regimen, the prevention of increases in PVR from underventilation, pharmacologic agents, pulmonary hyperinflation, and stress must be a primary consideration. Furthermore, decreases in right ventricular volume from intravascular volume depletion, venodilation, or aortocaval compression are poorly tolerated. Significant decreases in systemic vascular resistance from sympathetic blockade from regional anesthesia or volatile anesthetic agents may produce severe decompensation as the cardiovascular system may be unable to compensate for the decline in afterload (Slomka et al., 1988). Finally, right ventricular contractility may be marginal, and the addition of negative inotropic anesthetic agents may lead to marked depression in cardiac function. The parturient should be monitored with ECG, pulse oximetry, radial artery catheter, and a pulmonary artery catheter throughout labor and the postpartum period. This will allow early detection of changes in pulmonary vascular resistance (PVR) or right ventricular function and serve as a guide to fluid and pharmacologic therapy.

Labor and vaginal delivery may best be managed by the judicious use of systemic narcotic analgesics and pudendal nerve block. Epidural analgesia with local anesthetics may be provided only if the block is slowly titrated in a limited dermatomal fashion from T10 to L1 to avoid extensive sympathetic blockade. Intrathecal or epidural opioids also provide effective first-stage analgesia. Vaginal delivery can be managed by the addition of a caudal catheter or pudendal block. Regional anesthesia is best avoided for cesarean delivery, and a slow induction with either high-dose narcotics or an inhalation agent is recommended. This is necessary to avoid marked increases in PVR with laryngoscopy. Cricoid pressure must be maintained throughout the induction to prevent the aspiration of gastric contents. Ventilation must be adequate, but pulmonary hyperinflation must be avoided. Uterine stimulants may best be omitted as they can be associated with significant elevations in PVR.

Coronary Artery Disease (CAD)

CAD is uncommon in women of childbearing age, with a reported incidence of 1 in 10,000 pregnancies. In a recent review, it was determined that only 13 per cent of gravidas who had a myocardial infarction (MI) had a known history of CAD; overall maternal mortality was 37 per cent, increasing to 45 per cent if the infarction occurred in the third trimester (Hankins et al., 1989; Burlew, 1985).

The pathophysiology and clinical manifestations are identical to those in the nonpregnant patient. It is important to note that the hemodynamic demands that pregnancy places upon the myocardium represent a stress to the coronary circulation. General management guidelines currently include efforts to reduce the cardiac work load with means such as bed rest, nitrate therapy for preload reduction, and conduction anesthesia during delivery. Cardiac medications such as beta-blockers and nitrates should be continued throughout the pregnancy, labor, delivery, and puerperium. Effort must be directed toward optimizing myocardial oxygen supply; supplemental oxygen should be provided, anemia treated, and respiratory depression secondary to sedation meticulously avoided.

Although reasonable pain relief can be achieved with systemic narcotic analgesia, the early institution of continuous regional anesthesia for labor and delivery is recommended to minimize the pain and stress that could precipitate ischemia and angina (Rosenlund and Marx, 1988). Beneficial effects may also include decreased preload and afterload so that myocardial work is diminished. Marked and sudden decreases in afterload must be avoided as coronary artery perfusion is dependent upon diastolic pressure. Also, significant decreases in SVR can precipitate reflex tachycardia, which may increase cardiac work load sufficiently to produce ischemia. Epidural anesthesia effectively attenuates the progressive rise in CVP and CO that occurs during labor in the unanesthetized parturient. Multiple-lead ECG monitoring should be instituted early in labor so that ischemia can be promptly detected and treated.

When one is establishing epidural blockade, it is recommended that epinephrine be omitted from the test dose to avoid potential tachycardia and that the block be established by administration of slower-onset local anesthetics such as bupivacaine. Additionally, supplementation of a dilute local anesthetic solution with an epidural opioid has been advocated (Hands et al., 1990). It is recommended that fetal descent during the second stage of labor be by force of uterine contraction, with avoidance of the Valsalva maneuver based upon the patient's baseline ejection fraction and analysis of the hemodynamic response to contractions. When epidural analgesia for first-stage labor is not employed, a low spinal anesthetic (saddle block) provides excellent conditions for an assisted delivery with minimal hemodynamic trespass.

Elective cesarean section can be safely performed with a slowly titrated level of epidural anesthesia, allowing judicious intravenous fluid infusion to maintain pulmonary capillary wedge pressure and BP (Aglio and Johnson, 1990). Spinal anesthesia is much less desirable given the rapid onset of sympathetic block with great potential for hypotension and reflex tachycardia. General anesthesia for cesarean section must take into consideration the importance of minimizing the cardiovascular response to the stress of endotracheal intubation and surgery. In the absence of CHF, an inhalation technique is recommended.

Patients with a history of recent MI (especially third trimester) of less than 6 weeks, congestive heart failure, or unstable or crescendo angina warrant invasive monitoring with arterial and pulmonary artery catheters (Frenkel et al., 1991). Monitoring should be continued for a minimum of 24 hours into the postpartum period to monitor for increases in PCWP as intravascular volume increases following delivery and anesthesia subsides.

Asymmetric Septal Hypertrophy (Idiopathic Hypertrophic Subaortic Stenosis)

Asymmetric septal hypertrophy (ASH) or idiopathic hypertrophic subaortic stenosis (IHSS) is a disease without a defined etiology, but at least one-third of the subjects have a familial history and it appears to be an autosomal dominant trait. The primary features of this cardiomyopathy include marked hypertrophy of the left ventricle and interventricular septum and obstruction of the left ventricular outflow tract during systole by the hypertrophied muscle. The anterior leaflet of the mitral valve may be displaced by the hypertrophied muscle and thus contribute to the obstruction in some patients. The disease commonly presents during the second to fourth decades of life. Common symptoms include angina pectoris, dizziness, and exertional dyspnea. Physical findings include signs of left ventricular hypertrophy, a systolic ejection murmur, and a third heart sound. The electrocardiogram will indicate left ventricular hypertrophy and, in many cases, evidence of Wolff-Parkinson-White syndrome and evidence of abnormal Q waves. There is wide variability in both the findings and the symptoms of the disease.

The hemodynamic limitations of ASH are produced as the ventricle contracts. The hypertrophied walls narrow the outflow region during systole. The determinants of the degree of obstruction are the volume of the left ventricle at systole, the force of left ventricular contraction, and the degree of left ventricular distension during systolic contraction. The patient therefore requires a high preload in order to maintain a full left ventricle, a reduced contractile force in order to minimize outflow tract narrowing, and a high systemic vascular resistance to maintain distention of the left ventricle during systole. Therapy is primarily focused upon the administration of beta-adrenergic blocking agents to reduce myocardial contractility and

heart rate. Some patients may receive calcium channel–blocking drugs as well. Patients with ASH do not tolerate hypovolemia, decreased systemic vascular resistance, or increases in myocardial contractility very well. The cardiovascular and hemodynamic changes of pregnancy will have a variable effect on patients with ASH, depending upon both the severity and nature of their disorder. The increase in blood volume associated with pregnancy should yield a beneficial effect as it increases preload. The usually observed increase in heart rate and stroke volume during pregnancy could have a negative effect, and the decrease in systemic vascular resistance, which begins during the second trimester, could also have a negative impact on cardiac performance. While the potential for left ventricular failure and cardiac arrhythmias during pregnancy is real, the outcome of patients with ASH has been reasonably good (Oakley et al., 1979).

The objectives during parturition should be to minimize pain-associated increases in catecholamine levels, to maintain preload by adequate intravenous fluid administration, and to avoid the Valsalva maneuver, which abruptly decreases preload. Invasive monitoring with both an arterial line and a pulmonary artery catheter will yield the information necessary to provide precise management. Recommendations for analgesia during the first stage of labor have been to utilize systemic narcotics, inhaled analgesics, or paracervical block. Regional analgesia has been considered a substantial risk because of the potential for both venodilation (decreased preload) and arterial dilation resulting in decreased systemic vascular resistance (Oakley et al., 1979). This could possibly be avoided, however, if careful incremental titration of continuous lumbar epidural analgesia is carried out. A limited segmental level of analgesia from T10 to L2 will provide adequate analgesia with minimal sympathetic blockade, thus preserving preload. Dilute solutions of local anesthetic with the addition of a narcotic such as fentanyl will provide optimal analgesia (Minnich et al., 1987). Intrathecal narcotics may also be utilized, thereby eliminating the risk of sympathetic blockade but adding the potential side effects of respiratory depression, pruritus, and nausea, all of which are easily treated. Vaginal delivery may be accomplished with pudendal block, carefully extended epidural analgesia, or low spinal anesthesia (saddle block). The saddle block involves the spinal segments from L2 to S5 and thus avoids the majority of sympathetic nerve elements. Regional anesthesia is effective at blocking the uncontrollable urge to bear down. If hypotension necessitating a vasopressor does occur, the use of ephedrine is relatively contraindicated because it causes tachycardia and increased myocardial contractility. Metaraminol or a pure vasoconstricting drug such as phenylephrine (20 to 40 μg) should be employed in the lowest effective doses to minimize its effect on the uterine arteries.

Anesthesia for cesarean delivery offers additional challenges. Left uterine displacement must be maintained and volume requirements carefully assessed in view of the greater blood loss. Invasive monitoring will need to be employed. Regional anesthesia is usually avoided for the aforementioned reasons, and clearly the level of anesthesia required is likely to produce extensive sympathetic blockade with undesirable consequences (Oakley et al., 1979; Loubser et al., 1984). Nonetheless, a carefully titrated epidural anesthetic with ongoing compensation for the induced hemodynamic changes could prove acceptable. General anesthesia is preferred by many, although the ideal technique is yet to be established and experience is limited (Boccio et al., 1986). Although the use of volatile anesthetic agents is advantageous because they reduce myocardial contractility, they also decrease uterine contractility and systemic vascular resistance. Modest doses should have a minimal effect on both. As with the preeclamptic patient, the stimulating effects of laryngoscopy and intubation will need to be pharmacologically blunted. Oxytocin must be administered cautiously as it tends to decrease systemic vascular resistance and result in tachycardia when administered rapidly. The parturient with ASH requires careful attention by means of appropriate monitoring and the immediate availability of the necessary vasopressors, beta-blockers, and intravenous volume expanders.

Marfan's Syndrome

Marfan's syndrome is an autosomal dominant disorder characterized by connective tissue abnormalities of the cardiovascular, skeletal, and ocular systems. The principal cardiovascular involvement in this syndrome is weakness of the aortic media, which can result in progressive aortic dilatation or acute dissection. This dilatation may begin as early as the first year of life and typically occurs first in the coronary sinuses. Profound aortic regurgitation may predate clinical evidence of aortic dissection, and dissection may not be heralded by the classic chest pain with radiation to the back that usually accompanies aortic dissection from other causes. These patients also may suffer coronary artery involvement, pulmonary artery dilatation, redundant chordae tendineae, or an increased incidence of aortic coarctation.

The literature is sparse with respect to anesthetic management options for labor and delivery or cesarean section. In one case report of two patients with Marfan's syndrome and evidence of aortic dissection, epidural anesthesia was successfully provided for cesarean section with invasive monitoring via pulmonary artery catheter and arterial line (Mor-Yosef et al., 1988). In the asymptomatic patient without cardiovascular manifestations and a normal echocardiographic examination, segmental epidural anesthesia for labor and vaginal delivery without invasive hemodynamic monitoring is appropriate and inherently safe provided the severity of associated scoliosis does not preclude the success of this technique. It is apparent that adequate analgesia, as provided by an epidural block, would be distinctly advantageous in decreasing pain and catecholamine output, thus diminishing the stress on the aortic wall. Anesthesia for cesarean delivery may be provided by either regional or general technique.

General anesthesia for cesarean section in the face of cardiovascular complications must be tailored to minimize the hemodynamic response to endotracheal intubation and surgical stimuli. Prophylactic beta-adrenergic blockade and inhalational agents that produce decreased myocardial contractility and slow the force of cardiac ejection have both been advocated (Wells, 1987). Control of blood pressure alone with vasodilators may only serve to increase left ventricular ejection velocity and, unless combined with beta-blockade, may not prevent dissection. There also exists the potential for temporomandibular joint laxity and dislocation upon endotracheal intubation, though difficult intubation has not been reported.

SPINAL ABNORMALITIES

Kyphoscoliosis occurs in approximately 0.4 to 1.0 per cent of the population in the United States and is associated with both obstetric and anesthetic concerns during pregnancy and delivery (Kafer, 1980). Specific obstetric concerns relate to concomitant disease as well as the risk of dystocia in labor. Lesions involving the upper spine are commonly associated with disordered cardiorespiratory function. Natural history of an untreated severe curve is progression of deformity over time, resulting in early death from cardiorespiratory failure.

Anesthetic management for labor and vaginal delivery must be designed to minimize respiratory depression from systemic opioids or respiratory embarrassment from excessive intercostal muscle paralysis during high levels of regional anesthesia in patients with preexisting pulmonary dysfunction (Daley et al., 1990). It is equally important to emphasize the need for adequate analgesia in order to minimize catecholamine-induced increases in cardiac output that can precipitate high-output right-sided heart failure. A closely monitored segmental epidural analgesic technique would serve all of these purposes and avoid systemic opioid-induced respiratory depression.

It is apparent that although an epidural analgesic is optimal for the aforementioned reasons, it may be difficult to achieve in the kyphoscoliotic obstetric patient. Distortion of the spinal column and the epidural space may either prevent proper placement of an epidural catheter or prevent uniform distribution of the local anesthetic solution resulting in incomplete block. Subarachnoid catheter placement and segmental block have been reported for use in labor and vaginal delivery when epidural anesthesia had been unsuccessful (Elam, 1970).

Both continuous epidural and subarachnoid approaches have been utilized to provide surgical anesthesia for cesarean section. Both techniques offer the distinct advantage of slow titration of anesthetic level, which allows time for assessment of adequacy of respiratory function and for compensatory hemodynamic mechanisms to become operative. Another significant factor favoring regional anesthesia is that it provides superior analgesia in the post–cesarean section patient with scoliosis and respiratory impairment. Some investigators have noted attenuation of the decrease in vital capacity following abdominal surgery when epidural anesthesia has been continued post-operatively (Bromage, 1967). Others note that patients undergoing a variety of regional anesthetic and spinal opioid techniques invariably have better pulmonary function than patients receiving systemic opioids (Bromage et al., 1980; Shulman et al., 1984).

General anesthesia for cesarean delivery is indicated in those patients in whom severe scoliosis and cardio-respiratory impairment (cor pulmonale) are apparent at presentation, since they are likely to develop respiratory embarrassment if given a high regional anesthetic block. These patients also warrant invasive monitoring of CVP and serial arterial blood gas measurements.

Previous Spinal Surgery

Previous spinal surgery has been thought by some to represent a relative contraindication to regional anesthesia. Potential problems cited include obliteration of the epidural space from adhesions, which can limit spread of local anesthetics as well as increase the risk of dural puncture. Insertion of an epidural needle in the fused area may be relatively contraindicated or impossible to perform because of the presence of bone graft material and scar tissue, degenerative changes that occur in the spine after fusion, persistent back pain, and the risk of introducing infection in the area of foreign bodies (Daley et al., 1990a). Finally, these patients may express considerable anxiety and reluctance regarding catheter insertion in their backs.

There are a number of complications related to epidural anesthesia for these patients. Generally these include failure to place an epidural catheter, inadequate or patchy anesthesia, and increased risk of dural or vascular puncture. There is an increased risk of failure if the fusion extends to the L5-S1 interspace; significantly higher success rates are noted when the inferior limit of surgery is at L3 (Crosby and Halpern, 1989). Patients with previous spinal surgery should be seen in antepartum consultation by the anesthesiologist and the options for analgesia and anesthesia for labor and delivery discussed in detail (Hubbert, 1985). Epidural anesthesia may be offered, provided that the patient accepts the higher incidence of complications and failure rate. Alterations in dosage with larger than usual doses of local anesthetics required have been described, and with adjustments and vigilance this technique has been successfully used (Daley et al., 1990b).

ACHONDROPLASTIC DWARFISM (AD)

Although AD is a rare complication of pregnancy, these patients may have a number of anatomic and physiologic abnormalities that contribute to problems with the administration of an anesthetic. The airway in achondroplasia typically has narrowed nasal passages and pharyngeal and maxillary hypoplasia. The base of the skull is shortened (because of early fusion of constituent bones) and angulated, yielding limited extension and making endotracheal intubation poten-tially difficult. However, easy-mask general anesthetic ventilation has been described (Mayhew et al., 1986). Kyphoscoliosis is a common associated clinical finding in dwarfs, and so respiratory problems due to decreased functional residual capacity secondary to scoliosis and advancing enlargement of the uterus throughout pregnancy may be encountered (Kalla et al., 1986). Obstructive sleep apnea has become recognized as an insidious cause of morbidity in achondroplasia and is more common than central apnea due to cervicomedullary cord compromise (Reid et al., 1987). Acquired pulmonary hypertension leading to cor pulmonale may occur in achondroplasia, with contributions by restrictive lung disease associated with scoliosis, chronic upper airway obstruction, and sleep apnea.

Abnormalities of the spinal cord may result from severe kyphosis and scoliosis, or from odontoid hypoplasia with cervical instability leading to spinal cord and nerve root compression. The vertebral bodies are abnormally shallow, with underdeveloped vertebral arches yielding narrowing of the subarachnoid and epidural space. Additionally, adults with AD have hypoplastic intervertebral discs that may easily prolapse into a congenitally stenotic canal and produce neural compression. All of the foregoing may make regional anesthesia difficult or impossible to achieve, with unpredictable spread of local anesthetic solutions and increased risk of unintentional dural puncture.

Cesarean section delivery is inevitable in AD because the maternal pelvis is invariably small and contracted, resulting in cephalopelvic disproportion. In this setting, the aforementioned problems must be fully understood by the anesthesiologist in order to facilitate the safe delivery of anesthesia with the further requirements of the full-term parturient—minimizing the risk of maternal aspiration and avoiding fetal depression.

Pregnancy in achondroplasia compounds many of the outlined problems and presents a unique challenge to the obstetrician and anesthesiologist. General endotracheal anesthesia has traditionally been considered the technique of choice in achondroplasia even though there are case reports detailing difficult endotracheal intubation (Walts et al., 1975). In those instances, extension of the neck was difficult or impossible. These patients warrant early discussion of the probability of awake intubation following a thorough examination of the airway and review of any cervical radiographs available.

Technically challenging problems are also associated with regional anesthesia due to the skeletal abnormalities encountered. Epidural anesthesia has been successfully administered (Cohen, 1980; Wardall and Frame, 1990). A relative contraindication to regional anesthesia has been a concern regarding neurologic sequelae being attributed to the anesthetic. Those patients who have received successful epidural anesthesia have not experienced preoperative or postoperative neurologic dysfunction. It is important to note that epidural anesthesia is theoretically preferable to spinal anesthesia as this technique lends itself to titration of the level of block. Less anesthetic agent than usual may be required owing to maternal short stature and kyphoscoliosis. The dangers of intraoperative hypotension and high or total spinal block are greater than with epidural anesthesia.

REFERENCES

Abboud JK, Raya J, Noueihed R, et al: Intrathecal morphine for relief of labor pain in a parturient with severe pulmonary hypertension. Anesthesiology 59:477, 1983.

Aglio LS, Johnson MD: Anesthetic management of myocardial infarction in a parturient. Br J Anaesth 65:258, 1990.

Bader AM, Hunt CO, Datta S, et al: Anesthesia for the pregnant patient with multiple sclerosis. J Clin Anesth 1:21, 1988.

Baraka A: Epidural meperidine for control of autonomic hyperreflexia in a paraplegic parturient. Anesthesiology 62:688, 1985.

Benatar SR: Anaesthesia for the asthmatic. S Afr Med J 59:409, 1981.

Benedetti TJ, Cotton DB, Williams V: Hemodynamic observations in severe preeclampsia complicated by pulmonary edema. Am J Obstet Gynecol 152:330, 1985.

Benumof JL, Scheller MS: The importance of transtracheal jet ventilation in the management of the difficult airway. Anesthesiology 71:769, 1989.

Boccio RV, Chung JH, Harrison DM: Anesthetic management of cesarean section in a patient with idiopathic hypertrophic subaortic stenosis. Anesthesiology 65:663, 1986.

Bromage PR: Extradural analgesia for pain relief. Br J Anaesth 39:721, 1967.

Bromage PR, Comporesi EM, Chestnut D: Epidural narcotics for postoperative analgesia. Anesth Analg 59:474, 1980.

Burlew BS: Managing the pregnant patient with heart disease. Clin Cardiol 13:757, 1990.

Canny GJ, Corey M, Livingstone RA, et al: Pregnancy and cystic fibrosis. Obstet Gynecol 77:850, 1991.

Clark SL: Cardiac disease in pregnancy. Crit Care Obstet 18:237, 1991.

Clark SL, Phelan JP, Greenspoon J, et al: Labor and delivery in the presence of mitral stenosis: Central hemodynamic observations. Am J Obstet Gynecol 152:984, 1985.

Cobb T, Gleicher N, Elkayam V: Congenital heart disease and pregnancy. In Elkayam V, Gleicher N (eds): Cardiac Problems in Pregnancy. New York, Alan R. Liss, 1982, p. 61.

Cohen SE: Anesthesia for cesarean section in achondroplastic dwarfs. Anesthesiology 52:264, 1980.

Corssen G, Gutierrez J, Reves JG, et al: Ketamine in the anesthetic management of asthmatic patients. Anesth Analg 51:588, 1972.

Cotton DB, Gonik B, Dorman K, Harrist R: Cardiovascular alterations in severe pregnancy induced hypertension: Relationship of central venous pressure to pulmonary capillary wedge pressure. Am J Obstet Gynecol 151:762, 1985.

Crawford JS, James FM, Nolte H, et al: Regional analgesia for patients with chronic neurological disease and similar conditions. Anaesthesia 36:821, 1981.

Crosby ET, Halpern SH: Obstetric epidural anaesthesia in patients with Harrington instrumentation. Can J Anaesth 36:693, 1989.

Daley MD, Rolbin SH, Hew EM, et al: Epidural anesthesia for obstetrics after spinal surgery. Reg Anesth 15:280, 1990a.

Daley MD, Rolbin S, Hew E, et al: Continuous epidural anaesthesia for obstetrics after major spinal surgery. Can J Anaesth 37:S112, 1990b.

Dias MS, Sekhar LM: Intracranial hemorrhage from aneurysms and arteriovenous malformations during pregnancy and the puerperium. Neurosurgery 25:855, 1990.

Donchin Y, Amirav B, Sahar A, et al: Sodium nitroprusside for aneurysm surgery in pregnancy. Br J Anaesth 50:849, 1978.

Ducey JP, Ellsworth SM: The hemodynamic effects of severe mitral stenosis and pulmonary hypertension during labor and delivery. Int Care Med 15:192, 1989.

Easterling TR, Chadwick HS, Otto CM, et al: Aortic stenosis in pregnancy. Obstet Gynecol 72:113, 1988.

Elam JO: Catheter subarachnoid block for labor and delivery; A differential segmental technique employing hyperbaric lidocaine. Anesth Analg 49:1007, 1970.

Eng M, Butler J, Bonica JJ: Respiratory function in pregnant obese women. Am J Obstet Gynecol 123:241, 1975.

Foldes FF: Factors which alter the effects of muscle relaxants. Anesthesiology 20:464, 1959.

Forster R, Joyce T: Spinal opioids and the treatment of the obstetric patient with cardiac disease. Clin Perinatol 16:955, 1989.

Fox EJ, Sklar GS, Hiu CH, et al: Complications related to the pressor response to endotracheal intubation. Anesthesiology 47:524, 1977.

Frenkel Y, Etchin A, Barkai G, et al: Myocardial infarction during pregnancy: A case report. Cardiology 78:363, 1991.

Gant NF, Daley GL, Chand S, et al: A study of angiotensin II pressor response throughout primigravid pregnancy. J Clin Invest 52:2682, 1973.

Ghoneim MM, Long IP: Interaction between magnesium and other neuromuscular blocking agents. Anesthesiology 32:23, 1970.

Gianopoulos JG: Cardiac disease in pregnancy. Med Clin North Am 73:639, 1989.

Gilman DH: Caesarean section in undiagnosed Eisenmenger's syndrome: Report of a patient with a fatal outcome. Anaesthesia 46:371, 1991.

Greenberger PA: Asthma during pregnancy. J Asthma 27:341, 1990.

Gronert GA, Theye RA: Pathophysiology of hyperkalemia induced by succinylcholine. Anesthesiology 43:89, 1975.

Hands ME, Johnson MD, Saltzman DH, et al: The cardiac, obstetric, and anesthetic management of pregnancy complicated by acute myocardial infarction. J Clin Anesth 2:258, 1990.

Hankins GD, Wendel GD, Leveno KJ, et al: Myocardial infarction during pregnancy: A review. Obstet Gynecol 65:139, 1985.

Hays PM, Cruikshank DP, Dunn LJ: Plasma volume determination in normal and preeclamptic pregnancies. Am J Obstet Gynecol 151:958, 1985.

Hibbard LT: Maternal mortality due to cardiac disease. Clin Obstet Gynecol 18:27, 1975.

Hirshman CA, Edelstein G, Peetz S, et al: Mechanisms of action of inhalational anesthesia on airways. Anesthesiology 56:107, 1982.

Hodgkinson R, Husain J: Obesity and the cephalad spread of analgesia following epidural administration of bupivacaine for cesarean section. Anesth Analg 59:89, 1980.

Horton JC, Chambers WA, Lyons SL, et al: Pregnancy and the risk of hemorrhage from cerebral arteriovenous malformations. Neurosurgery 27:867, 1990.

Hubbert CH: Epidural anesthesia in patients with spinal fusion. Anesth Analg 64:843, 1985.

Hytens L, Alexander JP: Maternal and neonatal death associated with Eisenmenger's syndrome. Acta Anaesth Belg 37:45, 1986.

Joupilla R, Joupilla P, Hollmen A, Koivala A: Epidural analgesia and placental blood flow during labor in pregnancies complicated by hypertension. Br J Obstet Gynaecol 86:969, 1979.

Kafer ER: Respiratory and cardiovascular function in scoliosis and the principle of anesthetic management. Anesthesiology 52:339, 1990.

Kalla GN, Fening E, Obiaya MO: Anaesthetic management of achondroplasia. Br J Anaesth 58:117, 1986.

Kelton JG, Hunter DJ, Neame PB: A platelet function defect in preeclampsia. Obstet Gynecol 65:107, 1985.

Kirshon B, Moise KJ Jr, Cotton DB, et al: Role of volume expansion in severe preeclampsia. Surg Gynecol Obstet 167:367, 1988.

Kytta J, Rosenberg P: Anaesthesia for patients with multiple sclerosis. Ann Chir Gynaecol 73:299, 1984.

Lambert DH, Deane RS, Mazuzan JE: Anesthesia and the control of blood pressure in patients with spinal cord injury. Anesth Analg 61:344, 1982.

Leicht CH: Anesthesia for the pregnant patient undergoing nonobstetric surgery. Anesth Clin North Am 8:131, 1990.

Lindeman KS, Hirshman CA, Freed AN: Effect of magnesium sulfate on bronchoconstriction in the lung periphery. J Appl Physiol 66:2527, 1989.

Loubser P, Suh K, Cohen S: Adverse effects of spinal anesthesia in a patient with idiopathic hypertrophic subaortic stenosis. Anesthesiology 60:228, 1984.

Malinow AM, Ostheimer GW: Anesthesia for the high-risk parturient. Obstet Gynecol 69:951, 1987.

Mangano DT: Anesthesia for the pregnant cardiac patient. In Shnider SM, Levinson G (eds): Anesthesia for Obstetrics. 2nd ed. Baltimore, Williams & Wilkins, 1987, p 345.

Mayhew JF, Katz J, Miner M, et al: Anaesthesia for the achondroplastic dwarf. Can J Anaesth 33:216, 1986.

McGough EK, Cohen JA: Unexpected bronchospasm during spinal anesthesia. J Clin Anesth 2:35, 1990.

Minielly R, Yupze AA, Drake CG: Subarachnoid hemorrhage secondary to ruptured cerebral aneurysm during pregnancy. Obstet Gynecol 53:64, 1979.

Minnich ME, Quirk JG, Clark RB: Epidural anesthesia for vaginal delivery in a patient with idiopathic hypertrophic subaortic stenosis. Anesthesiology 67:590, 1987.

Moore TR, Key TC, Reisner LS, et al: Evaluation of the use of continuous lumbar epidural anesthesia for hypertensive pregnant women in labor. Am J Obstet Gynecol 152:404, 1985.

Mor-Yosef S, Younis J, Granat M, et al: Marfan's syndrome in pregnancy. Obstet Gynecol Surv 43:382, 1988.

Naulty J, Cefalo RC, Lewis PE: Fetal toxicity of nitroprusside in the pregnant ewe. Am J Obstet Gynecol 139:708, 1981.

Oakley GDG, McGarry K, Limb DG, et al: Management of pregnancy in patient with hypertophic cardiomyopathy. Br Med J 1:1749, 1979.

Pollack KL, Chestnut DH, Wenstrom KD: Anesthetic management of a parturient with Eisenmenger's syndrome. Anesth Analg 70:212, 1990.

Rayburn WF, Fontana ME: Mitral valve prolapse and pregnancy. Am J Obstet Gynecol 141:9., 1981.

Raymond R, Underwood DA, Moodie DS: Cardiovascular problems in pregnancy. Cleveland Clinic J Med 54:95, 1987.

Reid CS, Pyeritz RE, Kopits SE, et al: Cervicomedullary compression in young patients with achondroplasia: Value of comprehensive neurologic and respiratory evaluation. J Pediatr 110:522, 1987.

Richards W, Thompson J, Lewis G, et al: Cardiac arrest associated with halothane anesthesia in a patient receiving theophylline. Ann Allergy 61:83, 1988.

Roberts NV, Keast PJ: Pulmonary hypertension and pregnancy—a lethal combination. Anaesth Intensive Care, 18:366, 1990.

Roberts SL, Chestnut DH: Anesthesia for the obstetric patient with cardiac disease. Clin Obstet Gynecol 30:601, 1987.

Rolbin SH, Abbott D, Musclow E, et al: Epidural anesthesia in pregnant patients with low platelet counts. Obstet Gynecol 71:918, 1988.

Rosenlund RC, Marx GF: Anesthetic management of a parturient with prior myocardial infarction and coronary artery bypass graft. Can J Anaesth 35:515, 1988.

Schonwald G, Fish KJ, Perkash I: Cardiovascular complications during anesthesia in chronic spinal cord injured patients. Anesthesiology 55:550, 1981.

Schwalbe SS, Deshmuk SM, Marx GF: Use of pulmonary artery catheterization in parturients with Eisenmenger's syndrome. Anesth Analg 71:442, 1990.

Shulman M, Sandler AN, Bradley JW, et al: Post-thoracotomy pain and pulmonary function following epidural and systemic morphine. Anesthesiology 61:569, 1984.

Slomka F, Salmeron S, Zetlaoui P, Cohen H, et al: Primary pulmonary hypertension and pregnancy: Anesthetic management for delivery. Anesthesiology 69:959, 1988.

Spielman FJ: Anaesthetic management of the obstetric patient with cardiac disease. Clin Anaesth 4:247, 1986.

Spinnato JA, Kraynack BJ, Cooper MW: Eisenmenger's syndrome in pregnancy: Epidural anesthesia for elective cesarean section. N Engl J Med 304:1215, 1981.

Stange K, Halldin M: Hypothermia in pregnancy. Anesthesiology 58:460, 1983.

Sugrue D, Blake S, MacDonald D: Pregnancy complicated by maternal heart disease at the National Maternity Hospital, Dublin, Ireland: 1969 to 1978. Am J Obstet Gynecol 139:1, 1981.

Ueland K: Intrapartum management of the cardiac patient. Clin Perinatol 8:155, 1988.

Ueland K, Hansen J: Maternal cardiovascular dynamics. II. Posture and uterine contractions. Am J Obstet Gynecol 103:1, 1969a.

Ueland K, Hansen J: Maternal cardiovascular dynamics III. Labor and delivery under local and caudal analgesia. Am J Obstet Gynecol 103:8, 1969b.

Valenzuela GJ, Comunale FL, Davidson BH, et al: Clinical management of patients with cystic fibrosis and pulmonary insufficiency. Am J Obstet Gynecol 159:1181, 1988.

Walts LF, Finerman G, Wyatt GM: Anaesthesia for dwarfs and other patients of pathological small stature. Can J Anaesth 22:703, 1975.

Wanner MB, Rageth CJ, Zach GA: Pregnancy and autonomic hyperreflexia in patients with spinal cord lesions. Paraplegia 25:482, 1987.

Wardall GJ, Frame WT: Extradural anaesthesia for caesarean section in achondroplasia. Br J Anaesth 64:367, 1990.

Wells DG: Anaesthesia and Marfan's syndrome: Case report. Can J Anaesth 34:311, 1987.

Younker D, Clark R, Tessem J, et al: Bupivacaine-fentanyl epidural analgesia for a parturient in status asthmaticus. Can J Anaesth 34:609, 1987.

Ziskind S, Etchin A, Frenkel Y, et al: Epidural anesthesia with the Trendelenburg position for cesarean section with or without a cardiac surgical procedure in patients with severe mitral stenosis: A hemodynamic study. J Cardiothorac Anesth 3:354, 1990.

Zuspan FP: Pregnancy-induced hypertension. I. Role of the sympathetic nervous system and adrenal gland. Acta Obstet Gynecol Scand 56:283, 1977.

INDEX
. . . .

Note: Page numbers in *italics* indicate illustrations;
those followed by t indicate tables.

ISBN 0-7216-6590-X